Success in the Classroom, in Clinicals, and on th

Classroom

- Detailed lecture notes organized by learning outcome
- Suggestions for classroom activities
- Guide to relevant additional resources
- Comprehensive PowerPoint™ presentations integrating lecture, images, animations, and videos
- Classroom Response questions
- Image Gallery
- Video and Animation Gallery
- Online course management systems complete with instructor tools and student activities available in a variety of formats

PEARSON **mynursinglab**

- Saves instructors time by providing quality feedback, ongoing formative assessments and customized remediation for students.
- Provides easy, one-stop access to a wealth of teaching resources, such as test item files, PowerPoint™ slides, and video suggestions.
- A built-in electronic gradebook tracks students' progress on assessment and remediation activities.

Clinical

- Suggestions for Clinical Activities and other clinical resources organized by learning outcome

Real Nursing Simulations Facilitator's Guide: Institutional Edition

- 25 simulation scenarios that span the nursing curriculum
- Consistent format includes learning objectives, case flow, instructions for set up, student debriefing questions and more!
- Companion online course cartridge with student exercises, activities, videos, skill checklists, and reflective questions also available for adoption

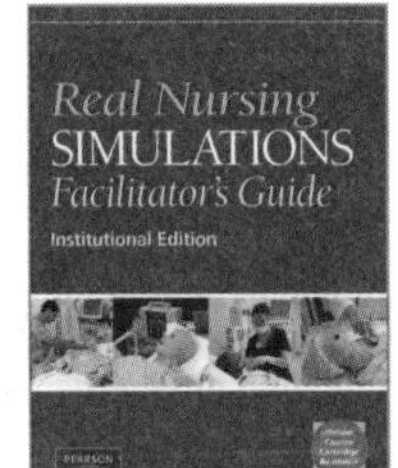

NCLEX-RN®

- Test Item Files with NCLEX®-style questions and complete rationales for correct and incorrect answers mapped to learning outcomes. *available in TestGen, Par Test, and MS Word*

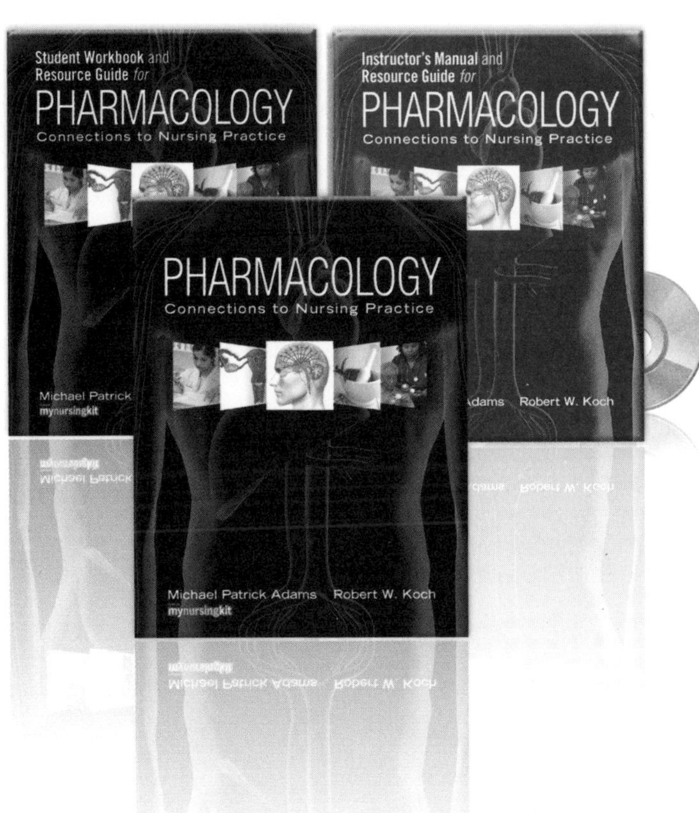

More *information and instructor resources*
visit www.mynursingkit.com

Instructor Resources

Brief Table of Contents

UNIT 1 Fundamental Principles of Pharmacology

CHAPTER 1 Introduction to Pharmacology: Concepts and Connections 2
CHAPTER 2 Drug Regulations 12
CHAPTER 3 Principles of Drug Administration 23
CHAPTER 4 Pharmacokinetics 40
CHAPTER 5 Pharmacodynamics 55
CHAPTER 6 Adverse Drug Effects and Drug Interactions 65
CHAPTER 7 Medication Errors and Risk Reduction 79
CHAPTER 8 Pharmacology of Substance Abuse 92

UNIT 2 Pharmacology and the Nurse–Patient Relationship

CHAPTER 9 Pharmacology and the Nursing Process 114
CHAPTER 10 Pharmacotherapy During Pregnancy and Lactation 122
CHAPTER 11 Pharmacotherapy of the Pediatric Patient 133
CHAPTER 12 Pharmacotherapy of the Geriatric Patient 146
CHAPTER 13 Psychosocial, Gender, and Cultural Influences on Pharmacotherapy 156
CHAPTER 14 Pharmacotherapy in the Community 163
CHAPTER 15 The Role of Complementary and Alternative Therapies in Pharmacotherapy 171

UNIT 3 Pharmacology of the Autonomic Nervous System

CHAPTER 16 Review of Neurotransmitters and the Autonomic Nervous System 184
CHAPTER 17 Cholinergic Agonists 198
CHAPTER 18 Cholinergic Antagonists 212
CHAPTER 19 Adrenergic Agonists 228
CHAPTER 20 Adrenergic Antagonists 245

UNIT 4 Pharmacology of the Central Nervous System

CHAPTER 21 Review of the Central Nervous System 264
CHAPTER 22 Pharmacotherapy of Anxiety and Insomnia 273
CHAPTER 23 Pharmacotherapy of Mood Disorders 297
CHAPTER 24 Pharmacotherapy of Psychoses 325
CHAPTER 25 Pharmacotherapy of Degenerative Diseases of the Central Nervous System 346
CHAPTER 26 Pharmacotherapy of Seizures 370
CHAPTER 27 Pharmacotherapy of Muscle Spasms and Spasticity 396
CHAPTER 28 Central Nervous System Stimulants and Drugs for Attention Deficit/Hyperactivity Disorder 411
CHAPTER 29 Pharmacotherapy of Severe Pain and Migraines 427
CHAPTER 30 Anesthetics and Anesthesia Adjuncts 457

UNIT 5 Pharmacology of the Cardiovascular System

CHAPTER 31 Review of the Cardiovascular System 482
CHAPTER 32 Pharmacotherapy of Hyperlipidemia 495
CHAPTER 33 Calcium Channel Blockers 515
CHAPTER 34 Drugs Affecting the Renin-Angiotensin-Aldosterone System 528
CHAPTER 35 Diuretic Therapy and the Pharmacotherapy of Renal Failure 544
CHAPTER 36 Pharmacotherapy of Hypertension 566
CHAPTER 37 Pharmacotherapy of Angina Pectoris and Myocardial Infarction 587
CHAPTER 38 Pharmacotherapy of Heart Failure 606
CHAPTER 39 Pharmacotherapy of Dysrhythmias 622
CHAPTER 40 Pharmacotherapy of Coagulation Disorders 641
CHAPTER 41 Pharmacotherapy of Hematopoietic Disorders 667
CHAPTER 42 Pharmacotherapy of Fluid Imbalance, Electrolyte, and Acid–Base Disorders 686

UNIT 6 Pharmacology of Body Defenses

CHAPTER 43 Review of Body Defenses and the Immune System 708
CHAPTER 44 Pharmacotherapy of Inflammation and Fevers 716
CHAPTER 45 Immunostimulants and Immunosuppressants 733
CHAPTER 46 Immunizing Agents 754

UNIT 7 Pharmacology of Infectious and Neoplastic Disease

CHAPTER 47 Basic Principles of Anti-Infective Pharmacotherapy 774
CHAPTER 48 Antibiotics Affecting the Bacterial Cell Wall 786
CHAPTER 49 Antibiotics Affecting Bacterial Protein Synthesis 807
CHAPTER 50 Fluoroquinolones and Miscellaneous Antibacterials 825
CHAPTER 51 Sulfonamides and the Pharmacotherapy of Urinary Tract Infections 836
CHAPTER 52 Pharmacotherapy of Mycobacterial Infections 850
CHAPTER 53 Pharmacotherapy of Fungal Infections 868
CHAPTER 54 Pharmacotherapy of Protozoan and Helminthic Infections 885
CHAPTER 55 Pharmacotherapy of Non-HIV Viral Infections 907
CHAPTER 56 Pharmacotherapy of HIV-AIDS 926
CHAPTER 57 Basic Principles of Antineoplastic Therapy 949
CHAPTER 58 Pharmacotherapy of Neoplasia 964

UNIT 8 Pharmacology of the Gastrointestinal System

CHAPTER 59 Review of the Gastrointestinal System 998
CHAPTER 60 Pharmacotherapy of Peptic Ulcer Disease 1006
CHAPTER 61 Pharmacotherapy of Bowel Disorders and Other Gastrointestinal Conditions 1028
CHAPTER 62 Vitamins and Minerals 1051
CHAPTER 63 Enteral and Parenteral Nutrition 1067
CHAPTER 64 Weight Reduction Strategies and the Pharmacotherapy of Obesity 1085

UNIT 9 Pharmacology of the Endocrine System

CHAPTER 65 Review of the Endocrine System 1098
CHAPTER 66 Hypothalamic and Pituitary Drugs 1104
CHAPTER 67 Pharmacotherapy of Diabetes Mellitus 1119
CHAPTER 68 Pharmacotherapy of Thyroid Disorders 1146
CHAPTER 69 Corticosteroids and Drugs Affecting the Adrenal Cortex 1160
CHAPTER 70 Estrogens, Progestins, and Drugs Modifying Uterine Function 1176
CHAPTER 71 Drugs for Modifying Conception 1199
CHAPTER 72 Drugs for Disorders and Conditions of the Male Reproductive System 1218

UNIT 10 Pharmacology of the Respiratory System and Allergy

CHAPTER 73 Pharmacotherapy of Asthma and Other Pulmonary Disorders 1238
CHAPTER 74 Pharmacotherapy of Allergic Rhinitis and the Common Cold 1261

UNIT 11 Miscellaneous Drugs

CHAPTER 75 Pharmacotherapy of Bone and Joint Disorders 1282
CHAPTER 76 Pharmacotherapy of Dermatologic Disorders 1314
CHAPTER 77 Pharmacotherapy of Eye and Ear Disorders 1337
CHAPTER 78 Emergency Preparedness: Bioterrorism and Management of Poisoning 1357

Appendices

A Answers to Critical Thinking Questions, Case Study, and NCLEX-RN® Review 1372
B Top 100 Drugs Ranked by Number of Prescriptions 1437
C Canadian Drugs and Their U.S. Equivalents 1438
D ISMP's List of High-Alert Medications 1441

Glossary 1442
Credits 1460
Index 1461

Your steps to success.

EXPLORE PEARSON mynursingkit™

MyNursingKit is your one stop for online chapter review materials and resources. Prepare for success with additional NCLEX®-style practice questions, interactive assignments and activities, web links, animations and videos, and more!

Register your access code with the instructions below

STEP 1: Register

All you need to get started is a valid email address and the access code below. To register, simply:

1. Go to **www.mynursingkit.com**.
2. Find and click on the appropriate book cover. Cover must match the textbook edition being used for your class.
3. Click "**Students**" under "**First-time users**".
4. Click "**I already have an access code**".
5. Read the License Agreement and Private Policy. If you accept, click "**I Accept**."
6. Leave "**No**" selected under "**Do you have a Pearson account?**"
7. Using a coin scratch off the silver coating below to reveal your access code. Do not use a knife or other sharp object, which can damage the code.
8. Enter your access code in lowercase or uppercase.
9. Follow the on-screen instructions to complete registration.

During registration, you will establish a personal login name and password to use for logging into the Website. You will also be sent a registration confirmation email that contains your login name and password. Be sure to save this email.

Your Access Code is:

Note: If there is no silver foil covering the access code, it may already have been redeemed, and therefore may no longer be valid. In that case, you can purchase access online using a major credit card. To do so, go to www.mynursingkit.com. click "Students" under "First Time Users," find the cover of your textbook, then click "Buy Access," and follow the on-screen instructions.

STEP 2: Log in

1. Go to **www.mynursingkit.com** and click "**Students**" under "**Existing Users**."
2. Enter the login name and password that you created during registration. If unsure of this information, refer to your registration confirmation email.
3. Click "**Login**."

Got technical questions?

Customer Technical Support: To obtain support, please visit us online anytime at http://247pearsoned.custhelp.com where you can search our knowledgebase for common solutions, view product alerts, and review all options for additional assistance.

SYSTEM REQUIREMENTS

For the latest updates on System Requirements, go to www.mynursingkit.com. Click "**Support**" and choose "**System Requirements**". Click on "**Need help**" at bottom of page for site requirements and other frequently asked questions.

Important: Please read the Subscription and End-User License agreement, accessible from the book website's login page, before using the mynursingkit *website. By using the website, you indicate that you have read, understood, and accepted the terms of this agreement.*

PHARMACOLOGY

Connections to Nursing Practice

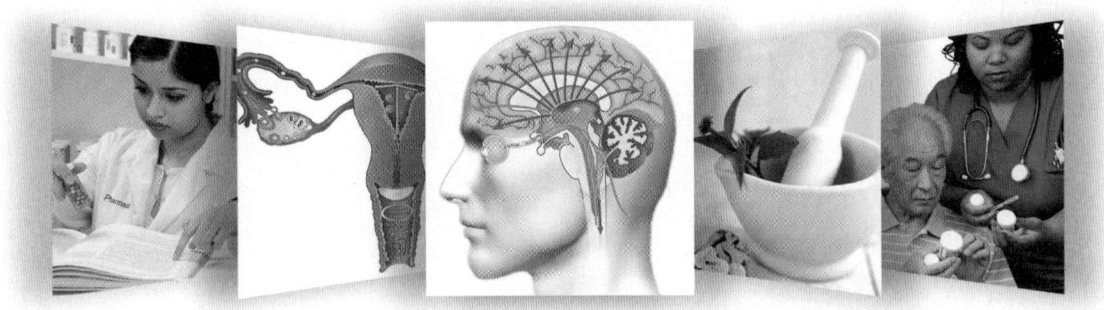

Michael Patrick Adams, PhD

Professor, Biological Sciences
Formerly Dean, Health Occupations
Pasco-Hernando Community College

Robert W. Koch, DNSc, RN

Associate Dean
Loewenberg School of Nursing
University of Memphis

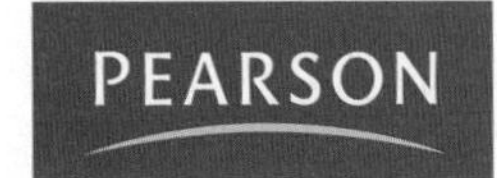

Upper Saddle River, New Jersey

Library of Congress Cataloging-in-Publication Data

Adams, Michael, 1951-

Pharmacology : connections to nursing practice / Michael Patrick Adams, Robert W. Koch.

p. ; cm.

Includes bibliographical references and index.

ISBN-13: 978-0-13-152599-3

ISBN-10: 0-13-152599-9

1. Pharmacology. 2. Nursing. I. Koch, Robert W. II. Title.

[DNLM: 1. Drug Therapy--nursing. 2. Drug Administration Routes. 3. Drug Administration Schedule. 4. Medication Errors--prevention & control. 5. Nursing Records. 6. Pharmacology--Nurses' Instruction. WY 100 A215p 2010]

RM300.A33 2010

615'.1--dc22

2008049030

Publisher: Julie Levin Alexander
Assistant to Publisher: Regina Bruno
Editor-in-Chief: Maura Connor
Assistant to the Editor-in-Chief: Marion Gottlieb
Senior Acquisitions Editor: Kelly Trakalo
Editorial Assistant: Lauren Sweeney
Development Editor: Teri Zak
Media Product Manager: Travis Moses-Westphal
Director of Marketing: Karen Allman
Senior Marketing Manager: Francisco del Castillo
Marketing Specialist: Michael Sirinides
Marketing Assistant: Crystal Gonzalez
Managing Editor, Production: Patrick Walsh
Production Editor: Mary Tindle, S4Carlisle Publishing Services
Production Liaison: Anne Garcia
Media Project Manager: Lorena Cerisano
Art Editor: Patricia Gutierrez
Art Studio: Argosy
Manufacturing Manager: Ilene Sanford
Senior Design Coordinator: Kathryn Foot
Interior Design: Kathryn Foot
Cover Design: Kathryn Foot
Manager, Rights and Permissions: Zina Arabia
Manager, Visual Research: Beth Brenzel
Manager, Cover Visual Research & Permissions: Karen Sanatar
Image Permission Coordinator: Debbie Latronica
Composition: S4Carlisle Publishing Services
Printer/Binder: Quebecor/Versailles
Cover Printer: Lehigh-Phoenix Color/Hagerstown

Pearson Education Ltd., London
Pearson Education Singapore, Pte. Ltd
Pearson Education Canada, Inc., Toronto
Pearson Education—Japan
Pearson Education Australia PTY, Limited
Pearson Education North Asia, Ltd., Hong Kong
Pearson Educación de Mexico, S.A. de C.V.
Pearson Education Malaysia, Pte. Ltd.
Pearson Education Upper Saddle River, New Jersey

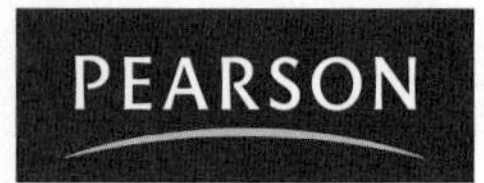

Notice: Care has been taken to confirm the accuracy of information presented in this book. The authors, editors, and the publisher, however, cannot accept any responsibility for errors or omissions or for consequences from application of the information in this book and make no warranty, express or implied, with respect to its contents.

The authors and publisher have exerted every effort to ensure that drug selections and dosages set forth in this text are in accord with current recommendations and practice at time of publication. However, in view of ongoing research, changes in government regulations, and the constant flow of information relating to drug therapy and reactions, the reader is urged to check the package inserts of all drugs for any change in indications or dosage and for added warning and precautions. This is particularly important when the recommended agent is a new and/or infrequently employed drug.

10 9 8 7 6 5 4 3 2
ISBN-13: 978-0-13-152599-3
ISBN-10: 0-13-152599-9

About the Authors

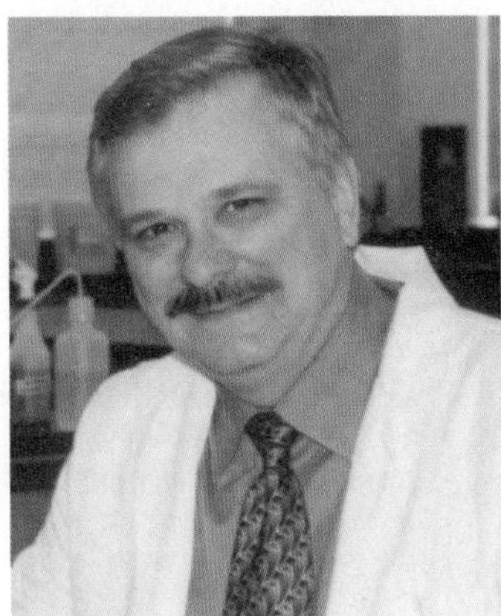

Michael Patrick Adams, PhD, is an accomplished educator, author, and national speaker. The National Institute for Staff and Organizational Development in Austin, Texas, named Dr. Adams a Master Teacher. He has published two other textbooks with Pearson Publishing: *Core Concepts in Pharmacology* and *Pharmacology: A Pathophysiologic Approach.*

Dr. Adams obtained his Master's degree in Pharmacology from Michigan State University and his Doctorate in Education at the University of South Florida. Dr. Adams was on the faculty of Lansing Community College and St. Petersburg College, and was Dean of Health Programs at Pasco-Hernando Community College for 15 years. He is currently Professor of Biological Sciences at Pasco-Hernando Community College.

I dedicate this book to nursing educators, who contribute every day to making the world a better and more caring place.

—MPA

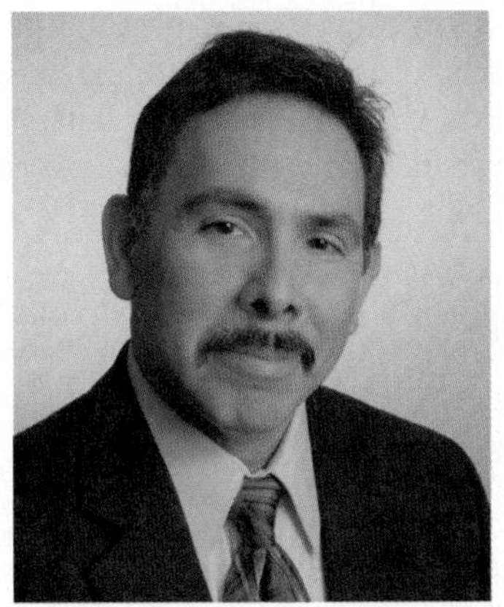

Robert W. Koch, DNS, RN, serves as Associate Dean and director of graduate studies at Loewenberg School of Nursing, University of Memphis. He holds baccalaureate and Master's degrees in nursing from the University of Tennessee Medical Center and a doctorate in nursing administration from Louisiana State University Medical Center in New Orleans. He holds memberships in Sigma Theta Tau International, the National League of Nursing, and the American Organization of Nurse Executives.

Dr. Koch's areas of academic expertise include nursing administration and leadership and nursing education. He has extensive administrative experience in acute care and in academic settings. Dr. Koch is a published author, an accomplished presenter, and a skilled researcher in nursing administration, gerontology, and educational technology. He teaches pharmacology in the undergraduate program.

Lee Iacocca once stated, "The only rock I know that stays steady, the only institution I know that works, is the family." Simply stated, I owe my gratitude to my family for being my rock in supporting me through this publishing process. My wife, Marylane, and daughter, Meredith, understood the sacrifices of my time and my energy that were necessary to bring this book to fruition. Now we can enjoy the pleasure of a work well done. Thanks be to God.

—RWK

Thank You

The authors wish to convey their special thanks to the many nurse contributors and reviewers who provided their unique knowledge and expertise to this project. Their insights, suggestions, eye for detail, and dedication to quality nursing education were evident and enabled us to prepare an accurate, relevant, and useful pharmacology textbook.

Contributors

Textbook Contributors

Diane Benson, RN, EdD
Humboldt State University, Arcata, CA
Chapter 29

Rebecca Boehne, RN, PhD
Linfield College, Portland, OR
Chapter 74

Jacqueline Rosenjack Burchum, APRN, BC
The University of Tennessee Health Science Center, Memphis, TN
Chapter 73

Pamela Evans-Smith, RN, MSN
University of Missouri-Columbia, Columbia, MO
Chapter 57

Geralyn Frandsen, RN, MSN, EdD,
Maryville University, St. Louis, MO
Chapters 26, 27, 28, 30, and 44

Denise Marie McEnroe-Ayers, RN, MSN
Kent State University at Tuscarawas, New Philadelphia, OH
Chapters 67, 72, 75, 76, and 77

Mariann Montgomery, RN, MSN
Kent State University at Tuscarawas, New Philadelphia, OH
Chapters 66, 67, 68, 75, 76, and 77

Kim Alexander Noble, RN, PhD
Temple University, Philadelphia, PA
Chapter 46

G. Elaine Patterson, RNC, MA, FNP-C Ed.D
Ramapo College of New Jersey, Mahwah, N.J.
Chapters 10, 11, 12, 70, and 71

Janice Lynn Reilley, RN, C, MSN, EdD
Widener University, Chester, PA
Chapter 63

Luann G. Richardson, RN, PhD
Duquesne University, Pittsburgh, PA
Chapter 60

Roberta Shea, RN, CCNS, MSN
Indiana University School of Nursing, Bloomington, IN
Chapters 9, 66, 67, and 68

Pat Teasley, RN, MSN, APRN, BC
Central Texas College, Killeen, TX
Chapters 22, 23, 24, 25, 57, and 58

Supplement Contributors

Amanda Barton, DNP, FNP, RN
Hope College, Holland, Michigan
Instructor's Navigation Guide, PowerPoint Slides, Test Item File, MyNursingLab, MyNursingKit

Sharon Burke, RN, MSN, APRN, BCEN
Thomas Jefferson University, Philadelphia, Pennsylvania
Instructor's Navigation Guide, PowerPoint Slides, Test Item File, MyNursingLab, MyNursingKit

Julie Chew, RN, MS
Mohave Community College, Colorado City, Arizona
Instructor's Navigation Guide, PowerPoint Slides, Test Item File, MyNursingLab, MyNursingKit

Lisa Cranwell-Bruce, MS, RN, FNP-C
Georgia State University, Atlanta, Georgia
Instructor's Navigation Guide, PowerPoint Slides, Test Item File, MyNursingLab, MyNursingKit

Debra Dickman, MS, RN, CNE
Blessing-Rieman College of Nursing, Quincy, Illinois
Instructor's Navigation Guide, PowerPoint Slides, Test Item File, MyNursingLab, MyNursingKit

Jennifer Dykstra, MSN, FNP, RN
Hope College, Holland, Michigan
Instructor's Navigation Guide, PowerPoint Slides, Test Item File, MyNursingLab, MyNursingKit

Katherine Gallia, PhD, RN, AOCN
University of North Carolina at Chapel Hill, Chapel Hill, North Carolina
Instructor's Navigation Guide, PowerPoint Slides, Test Item File, MyNursingLab, MyNursingKit

Marge Gingrich, RN, MSN
Harrisburg Area Community College, Harrisburg, Pennsylvania
Instructor's Navigation Guide, PowerPoint Slides, Test Item File, MyNursingLab, MyNursingKit

Jean Graham, MSN, CRNP, CNOR
Faulkner State, Bay Minette, Alabama
Instructor's Navigation Guide, PowerPoint Slides, Test Item File, MyNursingLab, MyNursingKit

Patrick Heyman, PhD, ARNP-BC
Palm Beach Atlantic University, West Palm Beach, Florida
Instructor's Navigation Guide, PowerPoint Slides, Test Item File, MyNursingLab, MyNursingKit

Darcus Kottwitz, BSN, MSN
Fort Scott Community College, Fort Scott, Kansas
Instructor's Navigation Guide, PowerPoint Slides, Test Item File, MyNursingLab, MyNursingKit

Robbie Murphy, RNC, BSN
San Jacinto College, Houston, Texas
Instructor's Navigation Guide, PowerPoint Slides, Test Item File, MyNursingLab, MyNursingKit

Pam Newland PhD, MSN, BSN
Southern Illinois University Edwardsville, Edwardsville, Illinois
Instructor's Navigation Guide, PowerPoint Slides, Test Item File, MyNursingLab, MyNursingKit

Havovi Patel, MS, MBBS
Oakwood University, Huntsville, Alabama
Instructor's Navigation Guide, PowerPoint Slides, Test Item File, MyNursingLab, MyNursingKit

Linda Ruholl, RN, PhD
Lake Land College, Mattoon, Illinois
Instructor's Navigation Guide, PowerPoint Slides, Test Item File, MyNursingLab, MyNursingKit

Jeff Sherer, PharmD, MPH, BCPS, CGP
University of Houston, Houston, Texas
Instructor's Navigation Guide, PowerPoint Slides, Test Item File, MyNursingLab, MyNursingKit

Michelle Skipper, MSN, FNP-BC
East Carolina College of Nursing, Greenville, North Carolina
Instructor's Navigation Guide, PowerPoint Slides, Test Item File, MyNursingLab, MyNursingKit

Sharon Souter, RN, PhD, CNE
University of Mary Hardin-Baylor, Belton, Texas
Instructor's Navigation Guide, PowerPoint Slides, Test Item File, MyNursingLab, MyNursingKit

Claudia Stoffel, BSN, MSN
Kentucky Technical and Community College System, Paducah, Kentucky
Instructor's Navigation Guide, PowerPoint Slides, Test Item File, MyNursingLab, MyNursingKit

Sharon Wallace, MSN, RN, CCRN
South Puget Sound Community College, Olympia, Washington
Instructor's Navigation Guide, PowerPoint Slides, Test Item File, MyNursingLab, MyNursingKit

Julia Ward, PhD, RN
Thomas Jefferson University, Philadelphia, Pennsylvania
Instructor's Navigation Guide, PowerPoint Slides, Test Item File, MyNursingLab, MyNursingKit

Reviewers

Academic Reviewers

Sharon Abbate, EdD, MS, BSN, RN
University of St. Francis-Joliet

Gail Acre, MSN, CRNP
University of Alabama at Birmingham

Judith Azok, MSN, GNP-BC, GCNS, ARNP
University of South Alabama

Cally Baker, MSN
Rogue Community College

Sophia Beydoun, MSN, RN
Henry Ford Community College

Kathryn Blair, PhD, FNP-BC, FAANP
University of Colorado-Colorado Springs

Audrey Bopp, RN, MSN, CNS
University of Northern Colorado

Patricia Brown, PhD, MN, CNE
Kansas Wesleyan University

Amy Bruno, RN, MSN, ANP-C
University of Massachusetts-Dartmouth

Cheryl Buchanan, MSN, RN
University of Akron

Sharon Burke, RN-C, BA, MSN
Thomas Jefferson University

Tammy Chapin, RN, MSN
The University of Wisconsin Oshkosh

Dennis Cheek, RN, PhD, FAHA
Texas Christian University

Kathleen Courtney, RN, CNM, MSN, LCCE, CKC
Case Western Reserve University

Ellen Cram, PhD, RN
University of Iowa

Lisa Cranwell-Bruce, MS, RN, FNP-C, APRN
Georgia State University

Marge Dean, RN, CS, GNP-BC, MSN
West Texas A&M University

Joseph DeRanieri, DM, MSN, RN CPN, BCECR
Thomas Jefferson University

Debra Dickman, MS, RN, CNE
Blessing-Rieman College of Nursing

Joyce Dienger, PhD, RN
University of Cincinnati

Teresa Dobrzykowski, DNS, APRN, BC
Indiana University at South Bend

Tanya Drake, MS, RN
Rockland Community College

Alison Dura, MS, RN
Binghamton University

Jennifer Dykstra, MSN, FNP, RN
Hope College

Nancy Ebersole, RN, PhD
Salem State College

Shawn Elliot, RN, MSN
Adams State College

Margaret Falahee, FNP-BC, MSN, FNP-C
Wayne State University

Barbara Jo Foster, RN, MSN
Copiah-Lincoln Community College

Karen Franklin, PhD
Cumberland University

Cliff Fuhrman, PhD
University of South Carolina

Melissa Geist, APRN, BC, ED.C
Tennessee Technical University

Nancy Goodman, RNC, MSN
Texas A&M University

Susan Growe, RN, MSN, OCN
Nevada State College

Lorrie N. Hegstad, PhD, APRN, BC, ANP, GNP
University of Texas

Patrick Heyman, BSN, MSN, PhD
Palm Beach Atlantic University

Gary Hicks, MS, RN, CNE
Villa Julie College

Linda Howe, PhD, APRN, CNE
Clemson University

Esther Jacobs, PhD, RN
Loyola University

Alice Kindschuh, RN, MSN
Northeast Community College

Shirley King, RN, PhD
Mount Royal School of Nursing

Trudy Klein, MS, RN
Walla Walla University

Julie Ann Koch, MSN, FNP-C
Valparaiso University

Stephen Krau, PhD, RN, CNE, CT
Vanderbilt University

Melissa Lambert, MSN, RN
St. Mary's School of Nursing

Rachelle Lancaster, MSN, RN
University of Wisconsin

Lori Lauver, PhD, MSN, RN
Thomas Jefferson University

Kate Lein, MS, APRN, BC
Michigan State University

Patrick Murphy, PhD
Seattle University

Teak Nelson, MS, RN, NP-C
Truman State University

Lynn Nichols, PhD, RN
St. John Fisher College

Nancy O'Donnell, BSN, MSN, RN
J. Sargeant Reynolds Community College

Allen Orsi, PhD, RN
San Francisco State University

Barbara Phillips, RN, MSN, CNE
Athens Technical College

Karen Piotrowski, RN, MSN
D'Youville College

Susan Pocotte, PhD
University of Toledo

Lori Przymusinski, MSN, RN
Oakland Community College

Linda Ruholl, RN, PhD
Lake Land College

Tracy Saddler, DNP, APRN, ACNP-BC, CEN, CCRN
Union University

Deborah Schiavone, PhD, PMHCNS, BC
Georgetown University

Sharon Schultz, MS, RN
Front Range Community College

Carrie Scotto, PhD, RN, CCRN
University of Akron

Sharon Souter, RN, PhD
Patty Hanks Shelton School of Nursing

Robert Stanton, BS, MBA, Pharm-D, BCTS
Marshall University

Sandy Stewart, RN, BSN, MA
Camosun College School of Nursing

David Taylor, PhD, FCP
East Carolina University

Michelle Taylor-Skipper, MS, FNP-BC
East Carolina University

Victoria Teske, MSN
Minnesota State University

Sharyl Eve Toscano, PhD, APRN, BC
University of Vermont

Peggy Verhoff, RN, MSN
Southern Union State Community College

Laura Waight, MSN, RN
West Texas A&M University

Sharon Wallace, MSN
Thomas Jefferson University

Julia Ward, PhD, RN
Thomas Jefferson University

Sandra Wardell, MSN
Suny Orange

Jacquelyn Warren Smith, FNP, RN
Kirtland Community College

Carolyn White, RN, MSN, CRNP, FNP, PNP, CCRN, JD
University of South Alabama

Diana White, RN, MS
University of Maine

Kristin Windon, MSN, RN, GCNS-BC, CNE
Southside Virginia Community College

Toni Wortham, MSN
Madisonville Community College

Mary Yost, MSN, RN
Drexel University

Nicole Zeller, MSN, RN
Lake Land College

Kathy Zurilla, RNP, MSN
Orange County Community College

Clinical Reviewers

Brenda Baranowski, AND, RN, CMSRN, CHPN, TNCC
Froedtert Hospital

Janice Boundy, RN, PhD
Saint Francis Medical Center

Robin Caldwell, PhD, RN, CLNC
Collin County Community College

Patricia G. Christy, MSN
Capri Wellness Clinic

Damon B. Cottrell, MS, RN, CCNS, CCRN, APRN-BC, CEN
The Washington Hospital Center

Janice Cousino, RN, MSN, CNS, BC
Hartford Hospital

Diane K. Daddario, MSN, APN, BC, RN, CMSRN
Evangelical Community Hospital, Pennsylvania College of Technology

Joyce Foresman-Capuzzi, RN, BSN, CEN, CPN, CCRN, CTRN, EMT
Lankenau Hospital

Karen Groller, MSN, RN, BC, CMSRN
Lehigh Valley Hospital

Melody H. Hale, MSN, APRN, BC
New River Health Association

Linda Howe, PhD, CNS, CNE
Clemson University

Laura Jaroneski, MSN, RN, OCN
Macomb Community College, Baker Community College

Michael J. Kingan, MSN
Washington Hospital Center

Noreen C. Kostelecky, RN, MSN
OSF Saint Francis Medical Center

Angela L. Kouri, RNC, BSN
OSF Saint Francis Medical Center

Marilyn Leshko, RN, CCRN
Lehigh Valley Hospital

Maureen Matthews, MS
OSF Healthcare

Maxine L. Morris, BSN (MSN in progress)
Graduate Nurse Student

Lois A. Pine, MS, RN, ICCE, CLC
University of Wyoming

Maureen Mulhern Prewitt, BA, BSN, RNC, CCE
Women's Health Clinical Research Center

Cristin M. Rassi, APN, CNS, TNS, CNRN
OSF Saint Francis Medical Center

Jana L. Reed, APN-BC, ACNP, CNOR
Associated University Neurosurgeons, SC

Jami Riggenbach-Hays, MSN, CFNP
OSF Saint Francis Medical Center

Carlene A. Schultz, MS, FNP-BC
Roswell Park Cancer Institute

Remedios A. Solarte, MSN, RN, NP
Oakland Community College

Kelly Timbers, MSN, CRNP
Women's Health Center, University of Pennsylvania

Eileen Trigoboff, RN, DNS
Buffalo Psychiatric Center

Drug Table Reviewers

Melissa Devlin, PharmD
excelleRx

Antoine T. Jenskins, PharmD, BCPS
OSF, Staint Francis Medical Center

John T. Johnson, PharmD, CDE
University of Georgia

Paul R. Lockman, PhD
Texas Tech University

Preface

Pharmacology is one of the most challenging and dynamic subjects for professional nurses today. Of all the core nursing subjects, pharmacology is the most dynamic. Each month new drugs are being introduced, and new applications are being developed for existing medications. Medications that were considered the drugs of choice only a decade ago are now rarely or never used. Current knowledge of drug action, interactions, and applicable legislation is mandatory for nurses to provide safe and effective patient care in all health care settings. Pharmacotherapeutics remains a critical and ever changing component of patient care.

The subtitle of this text, *Connections to Nursing Practice*, has guided its development. At a fundamental level, pharmacology is a series of interrelated essential concepts. Some key concepts are borrowed from, or shared with, the natural and applied sciences. Prediction of drug action requires a thorough knowledge of anatomy, physiology, chemistry, and pathology as well as the social sciences of psychology and sociology. This interdisciplinary nature of pharmacology makes the subject difficult to learn but fascinating to study.

The discipline of pharmacology is far more than a collection of isolated facts. To effectively learn this discipline, the student must make connections to nursing practice and, ultimately, connections to patient care. Patients expect to receive effective and safe medication administration from a nurse who is competent in the study of pharmacology. *Pharmacology: Connections to Nursing Practice* identifies key pharmacologic concepts and mechanisms and clearly connects them to current nursing theory and practice for providing optimal patient care.

Pharmacology: Connections to Nursing Practice recognizes that pharmacology is not an academic discipline to be learned for its own sake, but a critical tool to prevent disease and promote healing of illness. This connection to patients, their assessment, diagnoses, and interventions, supports basic nursing practice. Like other core nursing subjects, the focus of pharmacology must be to teach and promote wellness for patients.

STRUCTURE OF THE TEXT

This text is organized according to body systems (units) and diseases (chapters). Unit I, the first eight chapters, identifies fundamental pharmacologic principles that are applied throughout the entire text. Although new drugs are constantly being developed, these eight chapters build the structural framework for understanding the applications of all drugs.

Unit II connects pharmacology, the nurse, and the patient, with an emphasis on positive patient outcomes. These seven chapters recognize the essential role of nurse–patient interactions in providing optimum patient care throughout the life span. The role of complementary and alternative therapies, which are used by many patients, is included in the context of holistic care.

Units III through XI provide the concepts and connections that are necessary to understand the actions and adverse effects of individual drugs on different body systems. Many of the units begin with a chapter that briefly reviews relevant anatomy and physiology, which is a useful feature for the student when studying drug actions. Each chapter clearly identifies the concepts and connections necessary for safe and effective pharmacotherapy. Pharmacology is intimately related to the study of disease processes. The connections between pharmacology and pathophysiology are clearly established for each drug class in every chapter.

A Practical Approach to Learning Pharmacology

UNIT 4 Pharmacology of the Central Nervous System

CHAPTER 21 Review of the Central Nervous System 264
CHAPTER 22 Pharmacotherapy of Anxiety and Insomnia 273
CHAPTER 23 Pharmacotherapy of Mood Disorders 297
CHAPTER 24 Pharmacotherapy of Psychoses 325
CHAPTER 25 Pharmacotherapy of Degenerative Diseases of the Central Nervous System 346
CHAPTER 26 Pharmacotherapy of Seizures 370
CHAPTER 27 Pharmacotherapy of Muscle Spasms and Spasticity 396
CHAPTER 28 Central Nervous System Stimulants and Drugs for Attention Deficit/Hyperactivity Disorder 411
CHAPTER 29 Pharmacotherapy of Severe Pain and Migraines 427
CHAPTER 30 Anesthetics and Anesthesia Adjuncts 457

◄ **Disease and Body System Approach.** The organization by body systems (units) and diseases (chapters) clearly places the drugs in context with how they are used therapeutically. This organization connects pharmacology and pathophysiology to nursing care.

PROTOTYPE DRUG Neostigmine (Prostigmin)

Classification: Therapeutic: Agent for MG

Pharmacologic: Indirect-acting cholinergic agonist, AchE inhibitor

Therapeutic Effects and Uses: Approved in 1939, neostigmine is available by both oral and parenteral routes for the symptomatic treatment of MG. Affecting the neuromuscular synap- neostigmine increases the strength of skeletal muscle- tion and delays fatigue. A major disadvantage of

◄ **Prototype Approach.** The vast number of drugs that the practicing nurse must learn is staggering. To facilitate learning, this text uses a prototype approach in which the most representative medications in each classification are introduced in detail.

► **Drug Tables.** Easy to understand tables provide average dosages for most medications. **Unique** to this text is a listing of the most common and the most serious adverse effects for each drug or drug class. This allows the student to immediately recognize important safety information regarding the drug(s) he or she is administering.

TABLE 17.2 Cholinergic Agonists

Drug	Route and Adult Dose (maximum dose where indicated)	Adverse Effe
Direct Acting (Muscarinic Agonists)		
bethanechol chloride (Duvoid, Urecholine)	PO: 10–50 mg tid or qid (max: 200 mg/day) Subcutaneous: 2.5–5 mg tid or qid (max: 40 mg/day)	*Increased saliv skin, miosis, bl* Orthostatic hy tachycardia, co
carbachol (Miostat, Isopto Carbachol)	Topical: 1–2 drops of 0.75–3% solution tid in lower conjunctival sac every 4–8 h	
cevimeline HCl (Evoxac)	PO: 30 mg tid (max: 90 mg/day)	
pilocarpine (Isopto-Carpine, Ocusert, Salagen)	Topical: 1–2 drops in affected eye tid or qid for chronic glaucoma PO: 5–10 mg tid for xerostomia (max: 10 mg/dose, 30 mg/day)	
Indirect Acting (Anticholinesterase Agents)		
ambenonium (Mytelase)	PO: 2.5–5 mg tid or qid; may increase every 1–2 days to 50–75 mg tid or qid if necessary	*Involuntary co miosis, increas* Bradycardia, h cholinergic cris
donepezil (Aricept)	PO: 5–10 mg (max: 10 mg/day)	
edrophonium (Tensilon)	Edrophonium test for myasthenia gravis IV: Inject 2 mg over 15–30 seconds; if no reaction after 45 seconds, inject additional 8 mg. May repeat test in 30 min IM: Inject 10 mg; if cholinergic reaction occurs, retest after 30 min with 2 mg to rule out false-negative reaction	
galantamine hydrobromide (Razadyne)	PO: 4 mg bid for 4 weeks; may increase by 4 mg bid every 4 weeks to target dose of 12 mg bid as tolerated (max: 24 mg/day)	
neostigmine (Prostigmin)	PO: Start 15 mg every 8 h and increase as necessary IM/IV/subcutaneous: every 2–3 hours (max: 375 mg/day mg/day IM/IV/subcutaneous)	

Connections to Nursing Practice

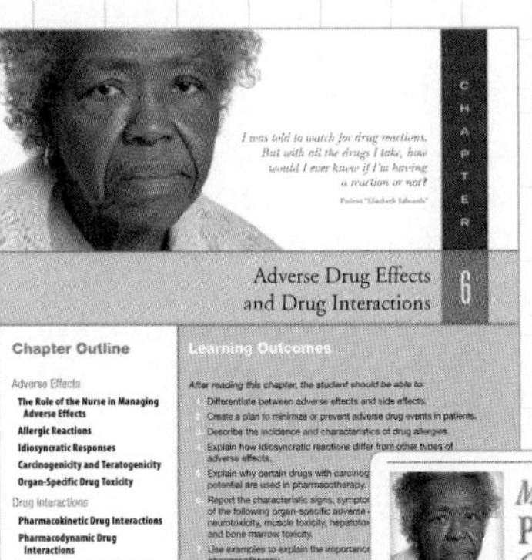

◄ **Making the Patient Connection** is a feature that opens each chapter with a quote and a photo of a patient. This opening scenario is revisited at the end of the chapter.

Making the PATIENT *Connection*

Remember the patient "Elizabeth Edwards" at the beginning of the chapter? Now read the remainder of the case study. Based on the information presented within this chapter, respond to the critical thinking questions that follow.

The more medication an individual takes, the more likely it is that an adverse reaction may occur. For Elizabeth Edwards this is a real possibility because she takes multiple medications for various physical problems. Ms. Edwards is a 77-year-old African American woman with several chronic conditions that require pharmacotherapy, including diabetes, heart failure, arthritis, and depression. She has been wheelchair bound since her stroke 2 years ago and has lost functional ability of her left side.

Unfortunately, she does not have a regular health care provider. Elizabeth obtains all her health care from a clinic operated for lower income individuals. The primary health care providers in the clinic are medical residents and interns who rotate every month as part of their medical training. Therefore, it is unlikely that she will see the same prescriber more than a couple of times. Her medical record is quite extensive and spans her health history for the last 15 years. Because her medical history record is so lengthy, Elizabeth fears that the new doctors will not take the time to read the entire chart before prescribing the newest treatment or therapy.

Critical Thinking Questions

1. Identify ways that you can minimize or prevent adverse drug events in this patient.
2. What existing conditions make Elizabeth more susceptible to a drug reaction?
3. Discuss how drug reactions can affect pharmacokinetics.
4. Differentiate among additive, synergistic, and antagonist drug effects.

Case Study

As the triage nurse in the emergency department, you determine the patient's chief complaint, obtain vital signs, collect past medical history information, and ask about drug and food allergies. While assessing a patient with a suspected ankle fracture, she tells you that she is allergic to codeine because it makes her nauseated and sleepy.

1. What further questions would you ask the patient about drug allergies?
2. Differentiate among adverse effect, side effect, and drug allergy.
3. Is this patient experiencing an idiosyncratic reaction? Explain.

▼ **CONNECTIONS: Treating the Diverse Patient** identify gender and cultural influences that are important modifiers of drug action.

CONNECTIONS **Treating the Diverse Patient**

Enzyme Deficiencies in Ethnic Populations

Pharmacogenetics has identified ethnic populations of people, such as males of Mediterranean and African descent, who are deficient in glucose-6-phosphate dehydrogenase (G6PD), an enzyme that is essential in carbohydrate metabolism. G6PD deficiency is the most common enzyme deficiency with about 400 million people affected worldwide. Caused by mutations in the DNA structure that encode for G6PD, the disorder results in one or more amino acid changes in the enzyme molecule. When certain oxidative drugs are given, such as primaquine, sulfonamides, or nitrofurantoin (Macrobid), an acute hemolysis of red blood cells (RBCs) occurs due to the breaking of chemical bonds in the hemoglobin molecule, with up to 50% of the circulating RBCs being destroyed. Genetic typing does not always predict toxicity. Patients may report a history of severe "allergy" to fava beans, which induce the hemolytic symptoms. The role of the nurse is critical in observing patients carefully for 24 to 72 hours following administration of these medications. Prevention is the best treatment. Fortunately, good alternative choices for these medications are available (Frank, 2005).

CONNECTIONS **Complementary and Alternative Therapies** Lecithin

Description: Lecithin is a mixture of phospholipids that occurs naturally in nervous tissue and is a primary component of pulmonary surfactant. Lecithin contains about 10% to 20% phosphatidylcholine, the agent that is responsible for lecithin's biological effects. When lecithin is taken, the GI tract breaks down the phosphatidylcholine to choline, a B-vitamin. As its name implies, choline is essential to the nervous system as a metabolic precursor of the neurotransmitter acetylcholine. Lecithin protects cells from oxidation. In nature, it is found in high amounts in certain vegetables, such as peanuts, cauliflower, and cabbage, and in fruits, such as oranges. Commercial sources are primarily soybeans and egg yolks.

History and Claims: Lecithin has been used primarily to lower serum cholesterol. More recently, however, lecithin has been claimed to benefit patients with Alzheimer's disease, in whom Ach is deficient in certain regions of the brain. Phosphatidylcholine is also marketed in Germany as a treatment for liver disorders, including protecting the liver from alcohol damage. In addition to its purported role in the nervous system and the liver, choline is widely marketed as a dietary supplement to increase muscle strength and stamina and to promote weight loss.

Standardization: There are several forms of lecithin supplements. Typical supplements contain 20% to 30% phosphatidylcholine. The U.S. Food and Drug Administration (FDA) recommended intake of choline for adults is 550 mg/day for men and 425 mg/day for women. Although quite safe, the most serious adverse effect from high intake of choline is hypotension with possible cholinergic adverse effects (e.g., sweating and diarrhea) and fishy body odor. The upper intake level for adults is 3.5 g/day.

Evidence: The best evidence for lecithin has been from clinical trials showing a hepatoprotective effect in patients suffering from liver damage due to alcohol or viral hepatitis. Clinical trials of lecithin on cholesterol levels have given mixed results and no clear benefit has been established. Research has not demonstrated a clear benefit of treating memory loss or other neurologic disorders with lecithin. Until further research indicates so, patients should not consume more than the recommended FDA intake.

◄ **CONNECTIONS: Complementary and Alternative Therapies** present herbal therapies, dietary supplements, or interventional therapeutic techniques that may be considered as complementary or alternatives to conventional drugs.

CONNECTIONS

Evidence-Based Practice — Controlling Symptoms of Attention Deficit/Hyperactivity Disorder

Clinical Question

What role does pharmacotherapy play in reducing the symptoms of ADHD in children, adolescents, and adults?

Evidence

ADHD is a CNS disorder that is characterized by developmentally inappropriate behavior with inattention. Pharmacotherapy plays an important role in controlling the symptoms of ADHD. The literature supports the premise that compounds that possess dopaminergic and norepinephrine properties are the most effective in treating ADHD. The literature possesses a great deal of research on pharmacologic effects among children and adolescents but research remains limited among the adult population. Stimulant therapy is still considered the first-line treatment for ADHD among the adult population.

Implication

Data support that atomoxetine in adults is useful in treating ADHD. It has also been proven effective in the treatment of ADHD and accompanying anxiety reactions. Tricyclic antidepressants and bupropion have not been studied but appear to be effective in patients who do not respond to stimulant therapy.

Critical Thinking Question

Atomoxetine is useful in treating ADHD in adults. What is the action of this medication? What client education should be provided to the client prescribed this medication?

See Answers to Critical Thinking Questions in Appendix A.

Source: From "Drug Therapy for Adults with Attention Deficit Hyperactivity Disorder," by T. C. Wilens, 2003, *Drugs, 63*(22), pp. 2395–2411.

◄ **CONNECTIONS: Evidence-Based Practice** supply connections to nursing or pharmacology research, which show the short-term and long-term direction of pharmacotherapeutics. A critical thinking question is presented at the end of each feature to challenge the student to connect evidence to practice.

CONNECTIONS: Patient Safety ► present brief patient–nurse scenarios that illustrate potential pitfalls that nurses encounter and can lead to medication errors. This feature enables the student to be alert for similar situations and to deliver medications safely.

CONNECTIONS

Patient Safety

Proper Use of the EpiPen®

The EpiPen® is an autoinjector containing epinephrine that is used to prevent and treat anaphylaxis and severe allergic reactions to insect stings, foods, or drugs. The device is easy to operate, although the word *auto* sometimes gives people a false sense of security. An Australian study in 2007 reported that of 100 hospital-based pediatricians, only 2 were able to demonstrate the correct way to administer the drug using the EpiPen® (Mehr, Robinson, & Tang, 2007). Even after reading instructions, only 40% got most of the steps right. In 37% of cases, epinephrine would not have reached the patient's circulation.

The nurse has a key responsibility in teaching parents and older children the correct use of the EpiPen®. The following is important safety information regarding this device.

- Exert sufficient pressure to activate the EpiPen®.
- Hold the device in place for 5 to 10 seconds.
- The EpiPen® is designed for a single injection; discard after use, preferably in a hospital emergency department or health care provider's office.
- The EpiPen® is not a replacement for proper medical care; seek emergency treatment as soon as possible.
- Check the expiration date often and replace when needed.
- Keep the EpiPen® in a cool, dark place; refrigeration is not recommended.

CONNECTIONS: Lifespan Considerations ► clearly identify geriatric and pediatric impacts on pharmacotherapy that may affect nursing care.

CONNECTIONS

Lifespan Considerations

Cost of Prescription Medications

The elderly population is affected more than any other age group by the high cost of prescription drugs. Americans over age 65 comprise only 13% of the population but account for about 34% of all prescriptions dispensed and 40% of all over-the-counter (OTC) medications. Over 80% of all seniors take at least one prescribed drug each day. The average older person is taking more than four prescription medications at once, plus two OTC medications. Many of these medicines, such as those for hypertension and heart disease, are taken on a permanent basis.

Seniors are less likely than younger people to have insurance that covers the cost of prescription medications. On a fixed an-

CONNECTIONS

To the Community — Myasthenia Gravis—Medications and Nutrition

Although all people need good nutrition for optimal health, persons with chronic disease may have special needs. Persons with myasthenia gravis (MG) may face certain nutritional challenges due to difficulty related to fatigue, chewing, swallowing, and medications.

If possible, meals should be planned for times when the person's strength is best. If the person gets fatigued later in the day, smaller, more frequent feedings may help. Modifications such as the consistency of food or body position at meals can help improve tolerance of meals.

When taking an anticholinergic drug like Mestinon, the person should eat a meal about an hour after taking the medicine. Sometimes these drugs can cause diarrhea or cramping. The person should notify the health care provider and not take OTC medications. Foods with high-fat content, spicy foods, or dairy products can aggravate diarrhea. Coffee, tea, or chocolate can stimulate the intestinal system because they contain caffeine.

Diarrhea can result in loss of body fluid and minerals. Therefore, easy to digest foods that are high in minerals should be added to the person's diet. Foods such as applesauce, ripe bananas, white rice, and baked or broiled chicken or fish may help. Light nutritious soups are good choices as well.

When a person takes corticosteroids such as prednisone for an extended time, bone thinning may result. Taking adequate amounts of calcium and vitamin D is important. Foods to include are milk products, cooked dark green vegetables, salmon, dried beans, and calcium-fortified juices and cereals. Because corticosteroids can cause fluid retention, salt substitutes or spices may be healthy alternatives to table salt. Avoid cured or smoked meats, canned vegetables and soups, salty snacks, and pickled foods.

◄ **CONNECTIONS: To the Community** provide important information that patients will require for effective pharmacotherapy after they leave the hospital or clinical setting. This feature also explores the relationship of lifestyle habits to pharmacology.

Unique to this text, **Connection Checkpoints** ► ask the student to recall past concepts from previous chapters that are related to current study. This reinforces that material learned in previous chapters has direct application to the current chapter.

CONNECTION *Checkpoint* 17.1

From what you learned in Chapter 16, would you expect the cholinergic agonists to have similar or opposite effects to the following: adrenergic agonists, adrenergic antagonists, cholinergic antagonists? See Answer to Connection Checkpoint 17.1 in Appendix A.

Pharm*FACT*

Myasthenia gravis affects females more often than males. The disorder has a peak incidence from age 20 to 30 and again after age 50. In rare cases, pregnancy can trigger the onset of MG. *Source:* Newton & Testa, 2007.

◄ **PharmFacts** connect relevant statistics to the presented material. They add interest to the subject, and place it in perspective with other nursing concepts.

► **Nursing Responsibilities** are provided for each prototype drug in a bulleted list format. These focus on the priorities of safe drug administration with a separate bulleted list emphasizing patient and family education.

Nursing Responsibilities:

- Monitor pulse, respiration, and blood pressu during the initial therapy period of dosage ad the treatment of myasthenia gravis. If below 60 or other established parameter, notify the n

NURSING PROCESS APPLICATION

Patients Receiving Anticholinergic Drug

Assessment

Prior to administration:

- Obtain a complete health history, including drug history, to determine possible drug interactions and allergies.
- Assess the reason for drug administration.
- Assess for heart rate, blood pressure, temperature, and elimination patterns (initially and throughout therapy).

Planning: Patient Goals and Expected

The patient will:

- Exhibit a decrease in symptoms for which the medication is prescribed.

◄ **Nursing Process Applications** concisely connect the nursing process to the major drug class(es) in each drug chapter. Each nursing intervention includes the rationale and associated patient and family teaching.

► **MyNursingKit™** tabs in the margins of the textbook link students to assets found on the MyNursingKit website.

MyNursingKit | Virtual Anesthesia Textbook

Learning Through Visuals and Media

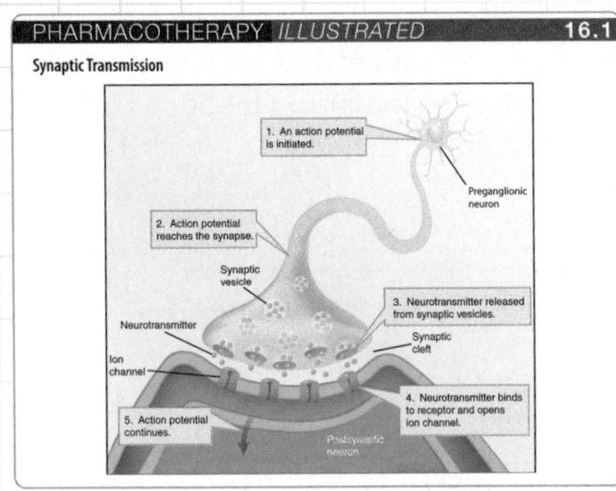

◄ **Pharmacotherapy Illustrated** boxes visually illustrate the mechanism of action of over 20 of the prototype drugs, showing students specifically how drugs counteract the effects of disease.

▲ **Vivid and Colorful Illustrations** help students review the anatomy, physiology, and pathophysiology of a body system to better understand the impact of disease on that system.

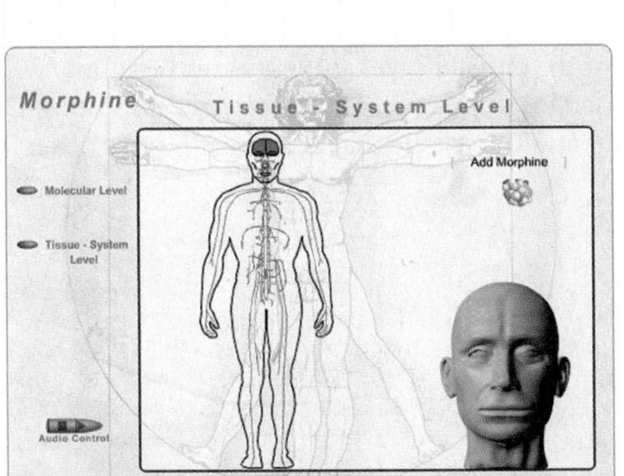

▲ **Mechanism of Action** animated tutorials can be found on the MyNursingKit website that accompanies this textbook. Each animation shows the drug action at the molecular, tissue, organ, and system levels. These interactive animations correlate to the Prototype Drugs and Pharmacotherapy Illustrated boxes.

Mechanism of Action Animations

acetaminophen Ch. 44	doxazosin Ch. 36	lidocaine Ch. 30	reteplase Ch. 40
acyclovir Ch. 55	epinephrine Ch. 19	lisinopril Ch. 34	salmeterol Ch. 73
amiodarone Ch. 39	epoetin alfa Ch. 41	methotrexate Ch. 58	saquinavir Ch. 56
atorvastatin Ch.32	escitalopram Ch. 22	methylphenidate Ch. 28	sildenafil Ch. 72
calcitriol Ch. 75	estradiol Ch. 70	morphine Ch. 29	spironolactone Ch. 35
ciprofloxacin Ch. 50	fluconazole Ch. 53	naproxen Ch. 44	tegaserod Ch. 61
cyclobenzaprine Ch. 27	fluoxetine Ch. 23	nifedipine Ch. 33	valproic acid Ch. 26
cyclophosphamide Ch. 58	furosemide Ch. 35	omeprazole Ch. 60	venlafaxine Ch. 23
diazepam Ch. 26	glipizide Ch. 67	oxycodone Ch. 29	warfarin Ch. 40
digoxin Ch. 38	heparin Ch. 40	penicillin Ch. 48	zidovudine Ch. 56
diphenhydramine Ch. 74	interferon alfa Ch. 45	propranolol Ch. 20	zolpidem Ch. 22
dopamine Ch. 19	levodopa Ch. 25	ranitidine Ch. 60	

Understanding the Chapter

The most chapter review in its class! **Understanding the Chapter** ▸ begins with a **Key Concepts Summary**, which quickly identifies the numbered key concepts from the chapter. An expanded review of key concepts can be found on the MyNursingKit website that accompanies this textbook.

UNDERSTANDING THE CHAPTER

Key Concepts Summary

16.1 The two major subdivisions of the nervous system are the central nervous system and the peripheral nervous system.

16.2 The peripheral nervous system is divided into somatic and autonomic components.

16.3 The autonomic nervous system is divided into two mostly opposing components: the sympathetic and parasympathetic branches.

16.4 Synaptic transmission allows information to be communicated between two nerves or from nerves to muscles or glands.

16.5 Autonomic drugs exert their effects by acting at synapses.

16.6 Acetylcholine is the neurotransmitter released at cholinergic receptors, which may be nicotinic or muscarinic.

16.7 Norepinephrine is the primary neurotransmitter released at adrenergic receptors, which may be alpha or beta.

16.8 The adrenal medulla is a specialized type of sympathetic nervous system tissue that secretes epinephrine and norepinephrine.

16.9 The autonomic nervous system is influenced by higher levels of control in the cerebral cortex and hypothalamus.

16.10 Autonomic drugs are classified by which receptors they stimulate or block.

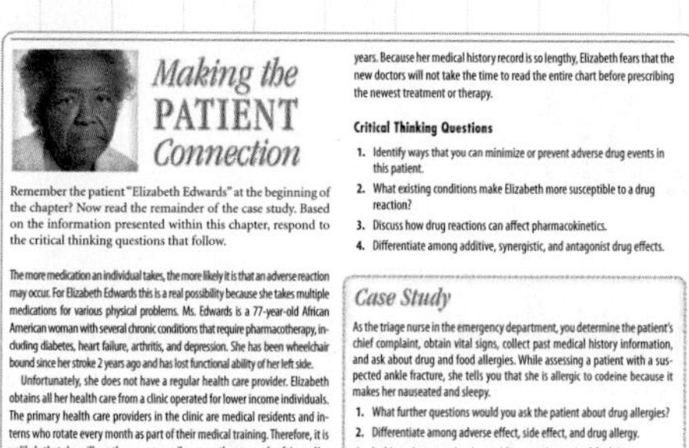

Making the PATIENT Connection

Remember the patient "Elizabeth Edwards" at the beginning of the chapter? Now read the remainder of the case study. Based on the information presented within this chapter, respond to the critical thinking questions that follow.

The more medication an individual takes, the more likely it is that an adverse reaction may occur. For Elizabeth Edwards this is a real possibility because she takes multiple medications for various physical problems. Ms. Edwards is a 77-year-old African American woman with several chronic conditions that require pharmacotherapy, including diabetes, heart failure, arthritis, and depression. She has been wheelchair bound since her stroke 2 years ago and has lost functional ability of her left side.

Unfortunately, she does not have a regular health care provider. Elizabeth obtains all her health care from a clinic operated for lower income individuals. The primary health care providers in the clinic are medical residents and interns who rotate every month as part of their medical training. Therefore, it is unlikely that she will see the same prescriber more than a couple of times. Her medical record is quite extensive and spans her health history for the last 15 years. Because her medical history record is so lengthy, Elizabeth fears that the new doctors will not take the time to read the entire chart before prescribing the newest treatment or therapy.

Critical Thinking Questions

1. Identify ways that you can minimize or prevent adverse drug events in this patient.
2. What existing conditions make Elizabeth more susceptible to a drug reaction?
3. Discuss how drug reactions can affect pharmacokinetics.
4. Differentiate among additive, synergistic, and antagonist drug effects.

Case Study

As the triage nurse in the emergency department, you determine the patient's chief complaint, obtain vital signs, collect past medical history information, and ask about drug and food allergies. While assessing a patient with a suspected ankle fracture, she tells you that she is allergic to codeine because it makes her nauseated and sleepy.

1. What further questions would you ask the patient about drug allergies?
2. Differentiate among adverse effect, side effect, and drug allergy.
3. Is this patient experiencing an idiosyncratic reaction? Explain.

◂ **Making the Patient Connection** reconnects the student to the patient mentioned at the beginning of the chapter. The student learns more about the patient and participates in critical thinking questions about the scenario. This allows application of knowledge obtained in the chapter.

▸ **NCLEX-RN® Review** prepares students for course exams on chapter content and gives exposure to all formats of NCLEX-RN®-style questions. Answers and rationales are provided in Appendix A.

NCLEX-RN® Review

1. Prior to the administration of an antibiotic, the client informs the nurse that 4 years ago the client experienced an allergic reaction. Based on this information what should the nurse do first?
   1. Ask the client to describe the reaction further.
   2. Notify the health care provider on call about the client's statements.
   3. Administer the dose and observe the client for a reaction.
   4. Check the medical administration record for documented allergies.
2. The nurse is researching a new drug prior to administration. The drug handbook states that the adverse effects are "dose related." The nurse is aware that this means that:
4. On physical examination, the nurs like welts covering the client's trur also complains of intense itching a medication. The nurse will suspec adverse effect?
   1. Angioedema
   2. Stevens–Johnson syndrome
   3. Urticaria
   4. Phototoxicity
5. When observing a client for bone nurse would monitor for:
   1. Increased complai lower extr

Case Study

As the triage nurse in the emergency department, you determine the patient's chief complaint, obtain vital signs, collect past medical history information, and ask about drug and food allergies. While assessing a patient with a suspected ankle fracture, she tells you that she is allergic to codeine because it makes her nauseated and sleepy.

1. What further questions would you ask the patient about drug allergies?
2. Differentiate among adverse effect, side effect, and drug allergy.
3. Is this patient experiencing an idiosyncratic reaction? Explain.

◂ A **Case Study** at the end of the chapter gives students another opportunity to apply their knowledge to patient care. Additional case studies can be found on the MyNursingKit website that accompanies this textbook.

Detailed **References** ▸ provide the basis for evidence-based nursing practice and support the currency and accuracy of textbook content.

References

Akamine, D., Filho, M. K., & Peres, C. M. (2007). Drug-nutrient interactions in elderly people. *Current Opinion in Clinical Nutrition and Metabolic Care, 10*(3), 304–310.

Boullata, J. (2005). Natural health product interactions with medication. *Nutrition in Clinical Practice, 20*(1), 33–51.

Boulatta, J., & Armenti, V. T. (2004). *Handbook of drug-nutrient interactions.* Totowa, NJ:

Herr, S. M. (2005). *H handbook* (3rd ed.). C Street Books.

Hu, Z., Yang, X., Ho, P. C. P. W. (2005). Herb- literature review. *Dru*

Lazarou, J., Pomeranz, (1998). Inciden in hosp

PEARSON

EXPLORE mynursingkit™

MyNursingKit is your one stop for online chapter review materials and resources. Prepare for success with additional NCLEX®-style practice questions, interactive assignments and activities, web links, animations and videos, and more!

Register your access code from the front of your book at **www.mynursingkit.com**

Each chapter provides a reminder to visit ◂ **MyNursingKit™** (www.mynursingkit.com) for additional chapter review and resources.

Contents

UNIT 1 Fundamental Principles of Pharmacology

CHAPTER 1 Introduction to Pharmacology: Concepts and Connections 2
Brief History of Pharmacology 3
Pharmacology: The Study of Medicines 4
Characteristics of an Ideal Drug 5
Classification of Drugs 5
Drug Prototypes 6
Naming Drugs 7
Connecting Pharmacology to Clinical Nursing Practice 8

CHAPTER 2 Drug Regulations 12
Patent Medicines 13
Brief History of Drug Legislation 13
Drug Standards 15
The U.S. Food and Drug Administration (FDA) 16
Drug Approval 17
Changes to the Drug Approval Process 18
Prescription and Over-the-Counter Drugs 19
Drug Schedules 20
Canadian Drug Standards 20

CHAPTER 3 Principles of Drug Administration 23
Drug Administration and Patient Adherence 24
Drug Storage and Expiration Dates 25
Prescription Writing 25
Dosing Intervals 26
Measurement of Drug Doses 27
Documenting Drug Administration 28
Routes of Drug Administration 28
Tablets and Capsules 29 • Sublingual and Buccal Drug Administration 31 • Nasogastric and Gastrostomy Drug Administration 31 • Transdermal Delivery System 32 • Ophthalmic Administration 32 • Otic Administration 32 • Intranasal Administration 33 • Vaginal Administration 33 • Rectal Administration 34 • Intradermal and Subcutaneous Administration 35 • Intramuscular Administration 35 • Intravenous Administration 36

CHAPTER 4 Pharmacokinetics 40
Introduction to Pharmacokinetics 41
Primary Processes of Pharmacokinetics 43
Time–Response Relationships 49

CHAPTER 5 Pharmacodynamics 55
Interpatient Variability 56
Therapeutic Index 56
Dose–Response Relationship 57
Potency and Efficacy 58
Receptor Theory 60
Agonists and Antagonists 61
Pharmacogenetics 62

CHAPTER 6 Adverse Drug Effects and Drug Interactions 65
Adverse Effects 66
Drug Interactions 70

CHAPTER 7 Medication Errors and Risk Reduction 79
Medication Errors and Their Impact on Health Care 80
Factors Contributing to Medication Errors 80
Drug Names and Medication Errors 84
Reporting Medication Errors 86
Strategies for Reducing Medication Errors 87

CHAPTER 8 Pharmacology of Substance Abuse 92
Fundamental Concepts of Substance Abuse 93
Legislation of Controlled Substances 94 • Addiction and Dependence 94 • Tolerance 97
Central Nervous System Depressants 97
Sedatives and Related Agents 98 • Opioids 98 • Alcohol (Ethanol) 99
Cannabinoids—Marijuana 102
Hallucinogens 103
LSD and Similar Hallucinogens 103 • Club Drugs and Miscellaneous Hallucinogens 105
Central Nervous System Stimulants 105
Amphetamines and Methylphenidate 105 • Cocaine 106 • Caffeine 107
Nicotine 107
Inhalants 108
Anabolic Steroids 108

UNIT 2 Pharmacology and the Nurse–Patient Relationship

CHAPTER 9 Pharmacology and the Nursing Process 114
Assessment 115
Diagnosis 115
Planning 117
Implementation 118
Evaluation 119

CHAPTER 10 Pharmacotherapy During Pregnancy and Lactation 122
Rationale for Drug Use During Pregnancy and Lactation 123
Pharmacotherapy During Pregnancy 123
Pharmacotherapy During Lactation 127

CHAPTER 11 Pharmacotherapy of the Pediatric Patient 133
Testing and Labeling of Pediatric Drugs 134
Pharmacokinetic Variables in Pediatric Patients 136
Pharmacologic Implications Associated with Growth and Development 137
Medication Safety for Pediatric Patients 139
Determining Pediatric Drug Dosages 140
Adverse Drug Reactions in Children and Promoting Adherence 140

CHAPTER 12 Pharmacotherapy of the Geriatric Patient 146
Polypharmacy 147
Physiological Changes Related to Aging 148
Pharmacokinetic and Pharmacodynamic Changes in the Older Adult 148
Adherence and Drug Misuse Among Older Adults 150
Adverse Drug Reactions in Older Adults 151

CHAPTER 13 Psychosocial, Gender, and Cultural Influences on Pharmacotherapy 156
Holistic Pharmacotherapy 157
Psychosocial Influences 157
Cultural and Ethnic Variables 158
Genetic Influences 159
Gender Influences 160

CHAPTER 14 Pharmacotherapy in the Community 163
Roles of the Nurse in the Community 164
Nurses as Community Resources 167

CHAPTER 15 The Role of Complementary and Alternative Therapies in Pharmacotherapy 171
Types of Complementary and Alternative Therapies 172
History of Herbal Therapies 172
Standardization of Herbal Products 174
Dietary Supplement Regulation 175
Herb–Drug Interactions 177
Specialty Supplements 179

UNIT 3 Pharmacology of the Autonomic Nervous System

CHAPTER 16 Review of Neurotransmitters and the Autonomic Nervous System 184
Basic Structure of the Nervous System 185
Structure and Function of the Autonomic Nervous System 185
Synaptic Transmission 188
Cholinergic Transmission 190
Cholinergic Receptors and Neurotransmitters 190 • Termination of Acetylcholine Action 192
Adrenergic Transmission 192
Alpha-Adrenergic Receptors 192 • Beta-Adrenergic Receptors 193 • Termination of Norepinephrine Action 194
Regulation of Autonomic Functions 195
Classifying Autonomic Drugs 196

CHAPTER 17 Cholinergic Agonists 198
Cholinergic Receptors 199
Muscarinic Agonists 200
PROTOTYPE DRUG: **Bethanechol Chloride (Duvoid, Urecholine)** 203
Drugs Similar to Bethanechol Chloride (Duvoid, Urecholine) 204 • Cholinergic Crisis 205
Pharmacotherapy of Myasthenia Gravis 205
PROTOTYPE DRUG: **Neostigmine (Prostigmin)** 206
Drugs Similar to Neostigmine (Prostigmin) 207
Nursing Process Application Patients Receiving Cholinergic Agonists 207
Nicotinic Agonists 209

CHAPTER 18 Cholinergic Antagonists 212
Classification of Cholinergic Antagonists 213
Muscarinic Antagonists 214
PROTOTYPE DRUG: **Atropine** 216
Drugs Similar to Atropine 217
Nicotinic Antagonists: Ganglionic Blockers 218
PROTOTYPE DRUG: **Mecamylamine (Inversine)** 218
Nicotinic Antagonists: Neuromuscular Blockers 220
PROTOTYPE DRUG: **Succinylcholine (Anectine)** 222
Drugs Similar to Succinylcholine chloride (Anectine) 223
PROTOTYPE DRUG: **Tubocurarine** 223
Drugs Similar to Tubocurarine 224
Nursing Process Application Patients Receiving Anticholinergic Drug Therapy 225

CHAPTER 19 Adrenergic Agonists 228
Actions of Adrenergic Agonists 229
Mechanisms of Action of Adrenergic Agonists 229
Classification of Adrenergic Agonists 230
Nonselective Adrenergic Agonists 231
PROTOTYPE DRUG: **Epinephrine (Adrenalin)** 233
Drugs Similar to Epinephrine (Adrenalin) 235
Alpha-Adrenergic Agonists 236
PROTOTYPE DRUG: **Phenylephrine (Neo-Synephrine)** 236
Drugs Similar to Phenylephrine (Neo-Synephrine) 238
Beta-Adrenergic Agonists 238
PROTOTYPE DRUG: **Isoproterenol (Isuprel)** 239
Drugs Similar to Isoproterenol (Isuprel) 240
Nursing Process Application Patients Receiving Adrenergic Agonists Therapy 241

CHAPTER 20 Adrenergic Antagonists 245
Actions of Adrenergic Antagonists 246
Alpha-Adrenergic Antagonists 246
PROTOTYPE DRUG: **Prazosin (Minipress)** 249
Drugs Similar to Prazosin (Minipress) 250
Beta-Adrenergic Antagonists 251
PROTOTYPE DRUG: **Propranolol (Inderal)** 253
Drugs Similar to Propranolol (Inderal) 254
PROTOTYPE DRUG: **Metoprolol (Lopressor, Toprol)** 256
Drugs Similar to Metoprolol (Lopressor, Toprol) 257
Nursing Process Application Patients Receiving Adrenergic Antagonist Therapy 258

UNIT 4 Pharmacology of the Central Nervous System

CHAPTER 21 Review of the Central Nervous System 264
Scope of Central Nervous System Pharmacology 265
Neurons and Neurotransmission 266
Major Structural Components of the Central Nervous System 267
Functional Systems of the Central Nervous System 269

CHAPTER 22 Pharmacotherapy of Anxiety and Insomnia 273
Anxiety Disorders 274
Sleep Disorders 277
Management of Anxiety and Insomnia 280
Pharmacotherapy of Anxiety and Insomnia 283
PROTOTYPE DRUG: **Lorazepam (Ativan)** 284
Drugs Similar to Lorazepam (Ativan) 285
PROTOTYPE DRUG: **Zolpidem (Ambien, Tovalt)** 287
Drugs Similar to Zolpidem (Ambien, Tovalt) 288
PROTOTYPE DRUG: **Phenobarbital (Luminal)** 291
Drugs Similar to Phenobarbital (Luminal) 292
Nursing Process Application Patients Receiving Therapy for Anxiety or Sleep Disorders 293

CHAPTER 23 Pharmacotherapy of Mood Disorders 297
Types of Mood Disorders 298
Major Depressive Disorder 298
Pathophysiology of Depression 299

Assessment of Depression 300
Nonpharmacologic Therapies for Depression 301
Pharmacotherapy of Depression 303
Tricyclic Antidepressants 303
PROTOTYPE DRUG: Imipramine (Tofranil) 306
Drugs Similar to Imipramine (Tofranil) 307 • Selective Serotonin Reuptake Inhibitors 307
PROTOTYPE DRUG: Fluoxetine (Prozac, Sarafem) 308
Drugs Similar to Fluoxetine (Prozac, Sarafem) 310 • Atypical Antidepressants 311
PROTOTYPE DRUG: Venlafaxine (Effexor) 311
Drugs Similar to Venlafaxine (Effexor) 312 • Monoamine Oxidase Inhibitors 313
PROTOTYPE DRUG: Phenelzine (Nardil) 314
Drugs Similar to Phenelzine (Nardil) 315
Nursing Process Application Patients Receiving Antidepressant Therapy 315
Bipolar Disorder 317
Drugs for Bipolar Disorder 318
PROTOTYPE DRUG: Lithium carbonate (Eskalith, Lithobid) 318
Drugs Similar to Lithium Carbonate (Eskalith, Lithobid) 320
Nursing Process Application Patients Receiving Therapy for Bipolar Disorder 321

CHAPTER 24 Pharmacotherapy of Psychoses 325
Characteristics of Psychoses 326
Symptoms of Schizophrenia 326
Etiology of Schizophrenia 328
Management of Psychoses 328
Antipsychotic Drugs 330
First-Generation Antipsychotics 332
PROTOTYPE DRUG: Chlorpromazine 333
Drugs Similar to Chlorpromazine 334
PROTOTYPE DRUG: Haloperidol (Haldol) 335
Drugs Similar to Haloperidol (Haldol) 336 • Second-Generation (Atypical) Antipsychotics 336
PROTOTYPE DRUG: Risperidone (Risperdal) 336
Drugs Similar to Risperidone (Risperdal) 339
PROTOTYPE DRUG: Aripiprazole (Abilify) 340
Drugs Similar to Aripiprazole (Abilify) 341
Nursing Process Application Patients Receiving Antipsychotic Therapy 342

CHAPTER 25 Pharmacotherapy of Degenerative Diseases of the Central Nervous System 346
Degenerative Diseases of the Central Nervous System 347
Parkinson's Disease 348
Pharmacotherapy of Parkinson's Disease 349
PROTOTYPE DRUG: Levodopa (L-Dopa, Dopar, Larodopa) 350
PROTOTYPE DRUG: Pramipexole (Mirapex) 353
Drugs Similar to Levodopa (L-Dopa, Dopar, Larodopa) and Pramipexole (Mirapex) 354
PROTOTYPE DRUG: Benztropine (Cogentin) 355
Drugs Similar to Benztropine (Cogentin) 356
Nursing Process Application Patients Receiving Therapy for Parkinson's Disease 357
Alzheimer's Disease 358
Pharmacotherapy of Alzheimer's Disease 359
PROTOTYPE DRUG: Donepezil (Aricept) 361
Drugs Similar to Donepezil (Aricept) 362
Nursing Process Application Patients Receiving Therapy for Alzheimer's Disease 363
Multiple Sclerosis 364
Amyotrophic Lateral Sclerosis 366

CHAPTER 26 Pharmacotherapy of Seizures 370
Characteristics of Seizure Disorders 371
Classification of Seizure Disorders 374
Generalized Seizures 374 • Partial Seizures 375
Antiseizure Drugs 379
PROTOTYPE DRUG: Diazepam (Valium) 382
Drugs Similar to Diazepam (Valium) 383
PROTOTYPE DRUG: Phenytoin (Dilantin, Phenytek) 384
Drugs Similar to Phenytoin (Dilantin, Phenytek) 385
PROTOTYPE DRUG: Carbamazepine (Tegretol, Tegretol XR, Carbatrol, others) 386
Drugs Similar to Carbamazepine (Tegretol, Tegretol XR, Carbatrol, Others) 387
PROTOTYPE DRUG: Ethosuximide (Zarontin) 388
Drugs Similar to Ethosuximide (Zarontin) 388
PROTOTYPE DRUG: Gabapentin (Neurontin) 389
PROTOTYPE DRUG: Valproic acid (Depacon, Depakene, Depakote) 390
Other Miscellaneous Drugs 391
Nursing Process Application Patients Receiving Antiepileptic Medications 392

CHAPTER 27 Pharmacotherapy of Muscle Spasms and Spasticity 396
Etiology and Pathophysiology of Muscle Spasms 397
Nonpharmacologic Therapies for Muscle Spasms 397
Pharmacotherapy of Muscle Spasms 398
Centrally Acting Skeletal Muscle Relaxants 398
PROTOTYPE DRUG: Cyclobenzaprine (Amrix, Flexeril) 399
Drugs Similar to Cyclobenzaprine (Amrix, Flexeril) 401
Etiology and Pathophysiology of Muscle Spasticity 402
Nonpharmacologic and Pharmacologic Therapies for Spasticity 403
PROTOTYPE DRUG: Dantrolene sodium (Dantrium) 403
Drugs Similar to Dantrolene Sodium (Dantrium) 406
Skeletal Muscle Relaxants as Surgical Adjuncts 406
Nursing Process Application Patients Receiving Pharmacotherapy for Muscle Spasms and Spasticity 407

CHAPTER 28 Central Nervous System Stimulants and Drugs for Attention Deficit/Hyperactivity Disorder 411
Characteristics of Central Nervous System Stimulants 412
Etiology and Pathophysiology of Attention Deficit/Hyperactivity Disorder 413
Pharmacotherapy of Attention Deficit/Hyperactivity Disorder 414
PROTOTYPE DRUG: Amphetamine sulfate (Racemic amphetamine, Adderall) 415
Drugs Similar to Amphetamine Sulfate (Racemic Amphetamine, Adderall) 417
PROTOTYPE DRUG: Atomoxetine (Strattera) 418
Drugs Similar to Atomoxetine (Strattera) 419

Pharmacotherapy of Narcolepsy 419
PROTOTYPE DRUG: Modafinil (Provigil, Alertec) 420
Drugs Similar to Modafinil (Provigil, Alertec) 421
Methylxanthines 421
PROTOTYPE DRUG: Caffeine 421
Drugs Similar to Caffeine 422
Nursing Process Application Patients Receiving Pharmacotherapy for Attention Deficit/ Hyperactivity Disorder and Narcolepsy 423

CHAPTER 29 Pharmacotherapy of Severe Pain and Migraines 427
General Principles of Pain Management 428
Pharmacotherapy of Acute and Chronic Pain 434
PROTOTYPE DRUG: Morphine sulfate (Astramorph PF, Duramorph RF, Roxanol, others) 437
Drugs Similar to Morphine Sulfate (Astramorph PF, Duramorph RF, Roxanol, Others) 439
Nursing Process Application Patients Receiving Opioid Analgesics 441
PROTOTYPE DRUG: Tramadol (Ultram) 442
Drugs Similar to Tramadol (Ultram) 444
Nursing Process Application Patients Receiving Nonopioid Analgesics 445
Pharmacotherapy with Opioid Antagonists 447
PROTOTYPE DRUG: Naloxone (Narcan) 447
Drugs Similar to Naloxone (Narcan) 448
Pharmacotherapy of Migraines 449
PROTOTYPE DRUG: Sumatriptan (Imitrex) 451
Drugs Similar to Sumatriptan (Imitrex) 452

CHAPTER 30 Anesthetics and Anesthesia Adjuncts 457
Types of Anesthesia 458
Principles of General Anesthesia 458
Intravenous Anesthetic Agents 459
PROTOTYPE DRUG: Thiopental sodium (Pentothal) 459
Drugs Similar to Thiopental Sodium (Pentathol) 461
PROTOTYPE DRUG: Fentanyl (Actiq, Duragesic, Sublimaze) 461
Drugs Similar to Fentanyl (Actiq, Duragesic, Sublimaze) 462
PROTOTYPE DRUG: Midazolam (Versed) 463
Drugs Similar to Midazolam (Versed) 464
PROTOTYPE DRUG: Ketamine (Ketalar) 464
Drugs Similar to Ketamine (Ketalar) 465 • Inhalation General Anesthetic Agents 465
PROTOTYPE DRUG: Nitrous oxide 466
Drugs Similar to Nitrous Oxide 467
PROTOTYPE DRUG: Isoflurane (Forane) 468
Drugs Similar to Isoflurane (Forane) 469
Nursing Process Application Patients Receiving General Anesthesia 470
Local Anesthetics 471
PROTOTYPE DRUG: Procaine (Novocaine) 472
Drugs Similar to Procaine (Novocaine) 474
PROTOTYPE DRUG: Lidocaine (Anestacon, Dilocaine, Xylocaine, others) 474
Drugs Similar to Lidocaine (Anestacon, Dilocaine, Xylocaine, Others) 475
Nursing Process Application Patients Receiving Local Anesthesia 476
Adjuncts to Anesthesia 477

UNIT 5 Pharmacology of the Cardiovascular System

CHAPTER 31 Review of the Cardiovascular System 482
Structure and Function of the Cardiovascular System 483
Functions and Properties of Blood 483
Cardiac Structure and Function 486
Hemodynamics and Blood Pressure 491

CHAPTER 32 Pharmacotherapy of Hyperlipidemia 495
Types of Lipids and Lipoproteins 496
Measurement and Control of Serum Lipids 499
Drugs for Dyslipidemias 501
PROTOTYPE DRUG: Atorvastatin (Lipitor) 504
Drugs Similar to Atorvastatin (Lipitor) 505
PROTOTYPE DRUG: Cholestyramine (Questran) 507
Drugs Similar to Cholestyramine (Questran) 508
PROTOTYPE DRUG: Gemfibrozil (Lopid) 509
Drugs Similar to Gemfibrozil (Lopid) 510 • Cholesterol Absorption Inhibitors 510
Nursing Process Application Patients Receiving Drugs for Hyperlipidemia 511

CHAPTER 33 Calcium Channel Blockers 515
Physiological Role of Calcium Channels in Muscle Contraction 516
Types of Calcium Channels 517
Consequences of Calcium Channel Blockade 518
Classification of Calcium Channel Blockers 518
PROTOTYPE DRUG: Nifedipine (Adalat, Procardia XL) 520
Drugs Similar to Nifedipine (Adalat, Procardia XL) 521
PROTOTYPE DRUG: Verapamil (Calan, Isoptin) 523
Drugs Similar to Verapamil (Calan, Isoptin) 524
Nursing Process Application Patients Receiving Calcium Channel Blocker Therapy 525

CHAPTER 34 Drugs Affecting the Renin-Angiotensin-Aldosterone System 528
Components of the Renin-Angiotensin-Aldosterone System 529
Physiological Effects of the Renin-Angiotensin-Aldosterone System 531
Drugs Affecting the Renin-Angiotensin-Aldosterone System 532
PROTOTYPE DRUG: Lisinopril (Prinivil, Zestril) 534
Drugs Similar to Lisinopril (Prinivil, Zestril) 535
Nursing Process Application Patients Receiving Angiotensin-Converting Enzyme (ACE) Inhibitor Therapy 537
PROTOTYPE DRUG: Losartan (Cozaar) 539
Drugs Similar to Losartan (Cozaar) 540

CHAPTER 35 Diuretic Therapy and the Pharmacotherapy of Renal Failure 544
Review of Renal Physiology 545
Pharmacotherapy in Patients with Renal Failure 546
Diuretic Therapy 548
Loop (High-Ceiling) Diuretics 549
PROTOTYPE DRUG: Furosemide (Lasix) 551
Drugs Similar to Furosemide (Lasix) 553 • Thiazide and Thiazide-Like Diuretics 553
PROTOTYPE DRUG: Hydrochlorothiazide (HydroDIURIL, HCTZ) 553
Drugs Similar to Hydrochlorothiazide (HydroDIURIL, HCTZ) 555 • Potassium-Sparing Diuretics 555

PROTOTYPE DRUG: Spironolactone (Aldactone) 556

Drugs Similar to Spironolactone (Aldactone) 558 • Osmotic Diuretics 558

PROTOTYPE DRUG: Mannitol (Osmitrol) 559

Drugs Similar to Mannitol (Osmitrol) 560 • Carbonic Anhydrase Inhibitors 560

PROTOTYPE DRUG: Acetazolamide (Diamox) 560

Nursing Process Application Patients Receiving Diuretic Therapy 562

Drugs Similar to Acetazolamide (Diamox) 563

CHAPTER 36 Pharmacotherapy of Hypertension 566

Definition and Classification of Hypertension 567

Etiology and Pathogenesis of Hypertension 568

Nonpharmacologic Management of Hypertension 569

Pharmacologic Management of Hypertension 570

Initial Drug of Choice 570 • Adding Drugs to the Antihypertensive Regimen 571 • Promoting Patient Adherence 572 • Antihypertensives in African Americans 573

Drug Classes for Hypertension 573

PROTOTYPE DRUG: Methyldopa (Aldomet) 577

Drugs Similar to Methyldopa (Aldomet) 578

PROTOTYPE DRUG: Hydralazine (Apresoline) 579

Drugs Similar to Hydralazine (Apresoline) 580

Management of Hypertensive Emergency 581

PROTOTYPE DRUG: Nitroprusside sodium (Nipride, Nitropress) 582

Drugs Similar to Nitroprusside Sodium (Nipride, Nitropress) 582

Nursing Process Application Patients Receiving Direct Vasodilators 583

CHAPTER 37 Pharmacotherapy of Angina Pectoris and Myocardial Infarction 587

Pathophysiology of Myocardial Ischemia 588

Myocardial Oxygen Supply 588 • Myocardial Oxygen Demand 588

Etiology of Coronary Artery Disease 588

Pathophysiology of Angina Pectoris 589

Nonpharmacologic Therapy of Coronary Artery Disease 590

Pharmacologic Management of Angina Pectoris 590

Drug Classes for Angina Pectoris 592

PROTOTYPE DRUG: Nitroglycerin (Nitrostat, Nitro-Bid, Nitro-Dur, others) 593

Drugs Similar to Nitroglycerin (Nitrostat, Nitro-Bid, Nitro-Dur, Others) 594

Nursing Process Application Patients Receiving Nitroglycerin 596

PROTOTYPE DRUG: Atenolol (Tenormin) 597

Drugs Similar to Atenolol (Tenormin) 598

Pathophysiology of Myocardial Infarction 598

Pharmacologic Management of Myocardial Infarction 599

Aspirin 600 • ADP Receptor Blockers 600 • Glycoprotein IIb/IIIa Inhibitors 600 • Anticoagulants 600 • Nitrates 602 • Beta-Adrenergic Blockers 602 • Angiotensin-Converting Enzyme Inhibitors 602 • Pain Management 602

CHAPTER 38 Pharmacotherapy of Heart Failure 606

Etiology of Heart Failure 607

Pathophysiology of Heart Failure 607

Ventricular Hypertrophy 608 • Activation of the Sympathetic Nervous System 608 • Increased Plasma Volume and Preload 608 • Natriuretic Peptides and Neurohumoral Factors 609

Pharmacologic Management of Heart Failure 610

Drugs for Heart Failure 610

PROTOTYPE DRUG: Digoxin (Lanoxin, Lanoxicaps) 615

Drugs Similar to Digoxin (Lanoxin, Lanoxicaps) 616

Nursing Process Application Patients Receiving Cardiac Glycosides 617

Beta-Adrenergic Agonists (Sympathomimetics) 618 • Phosphodiesterase III Inhibitors 618

PROTOTYPE DRUG: Milrinone lactate (Primacor) 618

Drugs Similar to Milrinone Lactate (Primacor) 619

CHAPTER 39 Pharmacotherapy of Dysrhythmias 622

Etiology of Dysrhythmias 623

Phases and Measurement of the Cardiac Action Potential 623

Classification of Dysrhythmias 625

General Principles of Dysrhythmia Management 627

Drugs for Dysrhythmias 627

Sodium Channel Blockers: Class I 628

PROTOTYPE DRUG: Procainamide (Procan SR, Pronestyl) 630

Drugs Similar to Procainamide (Procan SR, Pronestyl) 632 • Beta-Adrenergic Antagonists: Class II 633 • Potassium Channel Blockers: Class III 634

PROTOTYPE DRUG: Amiodarone (Cordarone, Pacerone) 634

Drugs Similar to Amiodarone (Cordarone, Pacerone) 635 • Calcium Channel Blockers: Class IV 636 • Miscellaneous Antidysrhythmics 636

Nursing Process Application Patients Receiving Antidysrhythmic Therapies 637

CHAPTER 40 Pharmacotherapy of Coagulation Disorders 641

Disorders of Hemostasis 642

Overview of Coagulation Modifiers 644

Parenteral Anticoagulants 644

PROTOTYPE DRUG: Heparin (Hep-Lock, Monoject) 646

Drugs Similar to Heparin (Hep-Lock, Monoject) 647

PROTOTYPE DRUG: Lepirudin (Refludan) 648

Drugs Similar to Lepirudin (Refludan) 649

Oral Anticoagulants 650

PROTOTYPE DRUG: Warfarin (Coumadin) 650

Drugs Similar to Warfarin (Coumadin) 652

Nursing Process Application Patients Receiving Anticoagulant Therapy 652

Antiplatelet Agents 653

PROTOTYPE DRUG: Clopidogrel (Plavix) 654

Drugs Similar to Clopidogrel (Plavix) 655

PROTOTYPE DRUG: Abciximab (ReoPro) 655

Drugs Similar to Abciximab (ReoPro) 657

Thrombolytics 657

PROTOTYPE DRUG: Alteplase (Activase) 658

Drugs Similar to Alteplase (Activase) 659

Hemostatics 660

Nursing Process Application Patients Receiving Thrombolytic Therapy 660

PROTOTYPE DRUG: Aminocaproic acid (Amicar) 661

Drugs Similar to Aminocaproic Acid (Amicar) 662

Drugs for Hemophilia 662
von Willebrand's Disease 664

CHAPTER 41 Pharmacotherapy of Hematopoietic Disorders 667
The Physiology of Hematopoiesis 668
Hematopoietic Growth Factors 668
PROTOTYPE DRUG: Epoetin alfa (Epogen, Procrit) 669
Drugs Similar to Epoetin Alfa (Epogen, Procrit) 671
Nursing Process Application Patients Receiving Epoetin Alfa 672
PROTOTYPE DRUG: Filgrastim (Neupogen) 673
Drugs Similar to Filgrastim (Neupogen) 674
PROTOTYPE DRUG: Oprelvekin (Neumega) 675
Drugs Similar to Oprelvekin (Neumega) 675
Classification of Anemias 675
Antianemic Agents 677
PROTOTYPE DRUG: Ferrous sulfate (Feosol, Feostat, others) 678
Drugs Similar to Ferrous Sulfate (Feosol, Feostat, Others) 679
Nursing Process Application Patients Receiving Iron Supplementation 681
PROTOTYPE DRUG: Cyanocobalamin (Crystamine, others) 682
Drugs Similar to Cyanocobalamin (Crystamine, Others) 683

CHAPTER 42 Pharmacotherapy of Fluid Imbalance, Electrolyte, and Acid–Base Disorders 686
Fluid Imbalance 687
Fluid Replacement Agents 688
PROTOTYPE DRUG: Normal serum albumin (Albuminar, Plasbumin, others) 690
Drugs Similar to Normal Serum Albumin (Albuminar, Plasbumin, Others) 691
PROTOTYPE DRUG: 5% Dextrose in water (D_5W) 691
Drugs Similar to 5% Dextrose in Water (D_5W) 692
PROTOTYPE DRUG: Dextran 40 (Gentran 40, Hyskon, 10% LMD, Rheomacrodex) 692
Nursing Process Application Patients Receiving Fluid Replacement Therapy 693
Drugs Similar to Dextran 40 (Gentran 40, Hyskon, 10% LMD, Rheomacrodex) 694
Physiology of Electrolytes 694
Pharmacotherapy of Electrolyte Imbalances 695
PROTOTYPE DRUG: Sodium chloride (NaCl) 696
Drugs Similar to Sodium Chloride (NaCl) 697
PROTOTYPE DRUG: Potassium chloride (KCl) 698
Drugs Similar to Potassium Chloride (KCl) 699
PROTOTYPE DRUG: Magnesium sulfate ($MgSO_4$) 700
Drugs Similar to Magnesium Sulfate ($MgSO_4$) 700
Pharmacotherapy of Acid–Base Imbalances 701
PROTOTYPE DRUG: Sodium bicarbonate 702
Drugs Similar to Sodium Bicarbonate 703
PROTOTYPE DRUG: Ammonium chloride 703
Drugs Similar to Ammonium Chloride 704

UNIT 6 Pharmacology of Body Defenses

CHAPTER 43 Review of Body Defenses and the Immune System 708
Organization of the Lymphatic System 709
Nonspecific (Innate) Body Defenses 709
Inflammation 711
Specific (Adaptive) Body Defenses 712
Humoral Immune Response 713 • Cell-Mediated Immune Response 713

CHAPTER 44 Pharmacotherapy of Inflammation and Fever 716
Pathophysiology of Inflammation and Fever 717
Pharmacotherapy of Inflammation 718
Nonsteroidal Anti-Inflammatory Drugs 718
Salicylates 718
PROTOTYPE DRUG: Aspirin (Acetylsalicylic Acid) 721
Drugs Similar to Aspirin (Acetylsalicylic Acid) 723 • Ibuprofen-Like Agents 723
PROTOTYPE DRUG: Ibuprofen (Advil, Motrin, others) 725
Drugs Similar to Ibuprofen (Advil, Motrin, Others) 727 • Cyclooxygenase-2 Inhibitors 727
PROTOTYPE DRUG: Celecoxib (Celebrex) 727
Drugs Similar to Celecoxib (Celebrex) 728
Antipyretic and Analgesic Agent 728
PROTOTYPE DRUG: Acetaminophen (Tylenol) 729
Nursing Process Application Patients Receiving NSAID Therapy 729
Drugs Similar to Acetaminophen (Tylenol) 730

CHAPTER 45 Immunostimulants and Immunosuppressants 733
Immunostimulants 734
PROTOTYPE DRUG: Interferon alfa-2b (Intron A) 735
Drugs Similar to Interferon alfa-2b (Intron A) 736
PROTOTYPE DRUG: Aldesleukin (Proleukin), IL-2 738
Drugs Similar to Aldesleukin (Proleukin), IL-2 739
Immunosuppressants 740
PROTOTYPE DRUG: Cyclosporine (Neoral, Sandimmune) 743
Drugs Similar to Cyclosporine (Neoral, Sandimmune) 744
PROTOTYPE DRUG: Azathioprine (Azasan, Imuran) 745
Drugs Similar to Azathioprine (Azasan, Imuran) 746
PROTOTYPE DRUG: Muromonab-CD3 (Orthoclone, OKT3) 747
Drugs Similar to Muromonab-CD3 (Orthoclone, OKT3) 749
Nursing Process Application Patients Receiving Immunomodulators 750

CHAPTER 46 Immunizing Agents 754
The Discovery of Vaccines 755
Vaccines and the Immune System 755
Types of Vaccines 756
General Principles of Vaccine Administration 757
Active Immunity: Bacterial Immunizations 758
Diphtheria 759 • Pertussis (Whooping Cough) 759 • Tetanus 759 • Pneumococcus 759 • Meningococcus 760
Active Immunity: Viral Immunizations 760
Hepatitis B 761
PROTOTYPE DRUG: Hepatitis B vaccine (Engerix-B, Recombivax HB) 761
Drugs Similar to Hepatitis B Vaccine (Engerix-B, Recombivax HB) 762 • Hepatitis A 762 • Influenza 763 • Rabies 763 • Measles, Mumps, and Rubella 764 Immunization 764 • Polio 764 • Varicella Zoster 765 • Human Papillomavirus 765 • Rotavirus 766
Passive Immunity 767
PROTOTYPE DRUG: Rh_0[D] immune globulin (RhoGAM) 767
Drugs Similar to Rh_0[D] Immune Globulin (RhoGAM) 769
Nursing Process Application Patient Receiving Immunizations 770

UNIT 7 Pharmacology of Infectious and Neoplastic Disease

CHAPTER 47 Basic Principles of Anti-Infective Pharmacotherapy 774
Pathogenicity and Virulence 775
Describing and Classifying Bacteria 776
Classification of Anti-Infectives 776
Mechanisms of Action of Anti-Infectives 776
Inhibition of Cell Wall Synthesis 778 • Inhibition of Protein Synthesis 778 • Disruption of the Plasma Cell Membrane 778 • Inhibition of Nucleic Acid Synthesis 778 • Inhibition of Metabolic Pathways (Antimetabolites) 778 • Other Mechanisms of Action 778
Acquired Resistance 779
Mechanisms of Resistance 779 • Promotion of Resistance 780 • Prevention of Resistant Strains 781
Indications and Selection of Specific Anti-Infectives 782
Host Factors Affecting Anti-Infective Selection 783
Host Defenses 783 • Local Conditions 783 • Allergy History 784 • Other Host Factors 784
Superinfections 784

CHAPTER 48 Antibiotics Affecting the Bacterial Cell Wall 786
Structure of Bacterial Cell Walls 787
Penicillins 788
Natural Penicillins 791
PROTOTYPE DRUG: Penicillin G 791
Drugs Similar to Penicillin G 792 • Broad-Spectrum Penicillins 792
PROTOTYPE DRUG: Ampicillin (Principen) 792
Drugs Similar to Ampicillin (Principen) 793 • Extended-Spectrum (Antipseudomonal) Penicillins 793 • Penicillinase-Resistant (Antistaphylococcal) Penicillins 794
Cephalosporins 795
PROTOTYPE DRUG: Cefazolin Sodium (Ancef, Kefzol) 797
Drugs Similar to Cefazolin Sodium (Ancef, Kefzol) 798
Carbapenems 798
Nursing Process Application Patients Receiving Penicillins or Cephalosporins 799
PROTOTYPE DRUG: Imipenem-cilastatin (Primaxin) 800
Drugs Similar to Imipenem-cilastatin (Primaxin) 801
Miscellaneous Cell Wall Inhibitors 802
PROTOTYPE DRUG: Vancomycin HCl (Vancocin) 802
Drugs Similar to Vancomycin HCl (Vancocin) 803

CHAPTER 49 Antibiotics Affecting Bacterial Protein Synthesis 807
Bacterial Protein Synthesis 808
Tetracyclines 809
PROTOTYPE DRUG: Tetracycline (Sumycin, others) 811
Drugs Similar to Tetracycline (Sumycin, Others) 812
Macrolides 813
PROTOTYPE DRUG: Erythromycin base (E-mycin, others) 814
Drugs Similar to Erythromycin Base (E-mycin, Others) 815
Aminoglycosides 816
PROTOTYPE DRUG: Gentamicin (Garamycin) 817
Drugs Similar to Gentamicin (Garamycin) 818
Nursing Process Application Patients Receiving Tetracyclines, Macrolides, and Aminoglycosides 819
Miscellaneous Inhibitors of Bacterial Protein Synthesis 820

CHAPTER 50 Fluoroquinolones and Miscellaneous Antibacterials 825
Bacterial DNA Replication 826
Inhibition of DNA Replication 826
Fluoroquinolones 827
Adverse Effects 828
PROTOTYPE DRUG: Ciprofloxacin HCl (Cipro) 829
Drugs Similar to Ciprofloxacin HCl (Cipro) 830
Nursing Process Application Patients Receiving Fluoroquinolones 831
Miscellaneous Antibacterials 832

CHAPTER 51 Sulfonamides and the Pharmacotherapy of Urinary Tract Infections 836
Pathophysiology of Urinary Tract Infections 837
Pharmacotherapy of Urinary Tract Infections 837
Acute Uncomplicated Cystitis 838 • Complicated Urinary Tract Infection 838 • Infants and Children 839 • Pregnancy 839 • Older Adults 839 • Recurring Urinary Tract Infections 840
Sulfonamides 840
Adverse Effects 842
PROTOTYPE DRUG: Trimethoprim-sulfamethoxazole (Bactrim, Septra) 842
Drugs Similar to Trimethoprim-Sulfamethoxazole (Bactrim, Septra) 843
Nursing Process Application Patients Receiving Sulfonamides 844
Urinary Antiseptics 845
PROTOTYPE DRUG: Nitrofurantoin (Furadantin) and nitrofurantoin macrocrystals (Macrobid, Macrodantin) 846
Drugs Similar to Nitrofurantoin (Furadantin) and Nitrofurantoin Macrocrystals (Macrobid, Macrodantin) 847

CHAPTER 52 Pharmacotherapy of Mycobacterial Infections 850
Types of Mycobacterial Infections 851
Pathogenesis and Diagnosis of Tuberculosis 851
Pharmacotherapy of Tuberculosis 853
Standard Regimen 856 • HIV-Positive Patients 856 • Pregnant Patients 856 • Chemoprophylaxis Patients 857
PROTOTYPE DRUG: Isoniazid (INH) 857
Drugs Similar to Isoniazid (INH) 859
Drugs for Leprosy 862
PROTOTYPE DRUG: Dapsone (DDS) 862
Drugs Similar to Dapsone (DDS) 863
Drugs for *Mycobacterium Avium* Complex (MAC) Infections 863
Nursing Process Application Patients Receiving Antituberculosis Agents 864

CHAPTER 53 Pharmacotherapy of Fungal Infections 868
Characteristics of Fungi and Fungal Infections 869
Drugs for Systemic Fungal Infections 871
PROTOTYPE DRUG: Amphotericin B deoxycholate (Fungizone) 872
Drugs Similar to Amphotericin B Deoxycholate (Fungizone) 874
Drugs for Both Systemic and Superficial Fungal Infections 875
PROTOTYPE DRUG: Fluconazole (Diflucan) 875
Drugs Similar to Fluconazole (Diflucan) 876
Drugs for Superficial Fungal Infections 877

PROTOTYPE DRUG: Nystatin (Mycostatin, Nystop, others) 880
Drugs Similar to Nystatin (Mycostatin, Nystop, Others) 880
Nursing Process Application Patients Receiving Antifungal Therapy 881

CHAPTER 54 Pharmacotherapy of Protozoan and Helminthic Infections 885
Classification and Pathogenesis of Protozoan Infections 886
Drugs for Malaria 887
PROTOTYPE DRUG: Chloroquine (Aralen) 889
Drugs Similar to Chloroquine (Aralen) 890
Drugs for Nonmalarial Protozoan Infections 890
PROTOTYPE DRUG: Metronidazole (Flagyl) 893
Drugs Similar to Metronidazole (Flagyl) 894
PROTOTYPE DRUG: Pyrimethamine and sulfadiazine (Fansidar) 897
Drugs Similar to Pyrimethamine and Sulfadiazine (Fansidar) 898
Classification and Pathogenesis of Helminthic Infections 898
Nursing Process Application Patients Receiving Pharmacotherapy for a Protozoan Infection 899
Drugs for Helminthic Infections 901
PROTOTYPE DRUG: Mebendazole (Vermox) 902
Drugs Similar to Mebendazole (Vermox) 903
Nursing Process Application Patients Receiving Antihelminthic Agents 904

CHAPTER 55 Pharmacotherapy of Non-HIV Viral Infections 907
Characteristics of Viruses 908
Pharmacotherapy of Non-HIV Viral Infections 910
Agents for Herpesviruses 911
PROTOTYPE DRUG: Acyclovir (Zovirax) 913
Drugs Similar to Acyclovir (Zovirax) 914
Agents for Influenza Viruses 915
PROTOTYPE DRUG: Amantadine (Symmetrel) 916
Drugs Similar to Amantadine (Symmetrel) 917
Agents for Hepatitis Viruses 917
PROTOTYPE DRUG: Lamivudine (Epivir) 921
Drugs Similar to Lamivudine (Epivir) 922
Nursing Process Application Patients Receiving Antiviral Agents for Non-HIV Viral Infections 923

CHAPTER 56 Pharmacotherapy of HIV-AIDS 926
Pathogenesis of HIV Infection 927
General Principles of HIV Pharmacotherapy 929
Classification of Antiretroviral Drugs 932
Antiretroviral Drugs 932
PROTOTYPE DRUG: Zidovudine (Retrovir, AZT) 934
Drugs Similar to Zidovudine (Retrovir, AZT) 935
PROTOTYPE DRUG: Efavirenz (Sustiva) 936
Drugs Similar to Efavirenz (Sustiva) 937
PROTOTYPE DRUG: Lopinavir with ritonavir (Kaletra) 938
Drugs Similar to Lopinavir with Ritonavir (Kaletra) 939
Nursing Process Application Patients Receiving Antiretroviral Agents 941
Prophylaxis of HIV Infections 942
Pharmacotherapy of Opportunistic Infections Associated with HIV-AIDS 944

CHAPTER 57 Basic Principles of Antineoplastic Therapy 949
Characteristics of Cancer 950
Etiology of Cancer 951
Detection and Prevention of Cancer 951
Goals of Chemotherapy 952
Staging and Grading of Cancer 953
The Cell Cycle and Growth Fraction 954
Cell Kill Hypothesis 955
Improving the Success of Chemotherapy 956
Combination Chemotherapy 957 • Dosing Schedules 957 • Route of Administration 957
Toxicity of Antineoplastic Agents 958
Hematologic System 958 • Gastrointestinal Tract 959 • Cardiopulmonary System 959 • Urinary System 959 • Reproductive System 960 • Nervous System 960 • Skin and Soft Tissue 960 • Other Effects 960
Chemotherapeutic Medications and the Nurse 960
Psychological Issues for the Patient Receiving Chemotherapy 961

CHAPTER 58 Pharmacotherapy of Neoplasia 964
Classification of Antineoplastic Agents 965
Nursing Responsibilities for the Patient Undergoing Chemotherapy 965
Nursing Responsibilities 965 • Patient and Family Education 966
Antineoplastic Medications 966
Alkylating Agents 966
PROTOTYPE DRUG: Cyclophosphamide (Cytoxan) 967
Drugs Similar to Cyclophosphamide (Cytoxan) 969
Antimetabolites 972
PROTOTYPE DRUG: Methotrexate (MTX, Rheumatrex, Trexall) 972
Drugs Similar to Methotrexate (MTX, Rheumatrex, Trexall) 974 • Antitumor Antibiotics 976
PROTOTYPE DRUG: Doxorubicin (Adriamycin) 977
Drugs Similar to Doxorubicin (Adriamycin) 978 • Hormones and Hormone Antagonists 979
PROTOTYPE DRUG: Tamoxifen (Nolvadex, Soltamox) 981
Drugs Similar to Tamoxifen (Nolvadex, Soltamox) 982 • Natural Products 984
PROTOTYPE DRUG: Vincristine (Oncovin) 985
Drugs Similar to Vincristine (Oncovin) 986
Nursing Process Application Patients Receiving Cancer Chemotherapy 988
Biologic Response Modifiers and Monoclonal Antibodies 990 • Miscellaneous Antineoplastics 991
Drugs for Reducing Adverse Effects 993
Preparing and Administering Antineoplastics 993

UNIT 8 Pharmacology of the Gastrointestinal System

CHAPTER 59 Review of the Gastrointestinal System 998
Overview of the Digestive System 999
Physiology of the Upper Gastrointestinal Tract 1000
Physiology of the Lower Gastrointestinal Tract 1001
Physiology of the Accessory Organs of Digestion 1001
Regulation of Digestive Processes 1004
Nutrient Categories and Metabolism 1004

CHAPTER 60 Pharmacotherapy of Peptic Ulcer Disease 1006
Physiology of the Upper Gastrointestinal Tract 1007
Etiology and Pathogenesis of Peptic Ulcer Disease 1007

Etiology and Pathogenesis of Gastroesophageal Reflux Disease 1010
Pharmacotherapy of Peptic Ulcer Disease and Gastroesophageal Reflux Disease 1010
Pharmacotherapy with Proton Pump Inhibitors 1013
PROTOTYPE DRUG: **Omeprazole (Prilosec)** 1014
Drugs Similar to Omeprazole (Prilosec) 1015
Pharmacotherapy with H_2-Receptor Antagonists 1016
Nursing Process Application Patients Receiving Proton Pump Inhibitor Therapy 1017
PROTOTYPE DRUG: **Ranitidine (Zantac)** 1018
Drugs Similar to Ranitidine (Zantac) 1019
Pharmacotherapy with Antacids 1019
Nursing Process Application Patients Receiving H_2-Receptor Antagonists 1020
PROTOTYPE DRUG: **Aluminum hydroxide (AlternaGEL, others)** 1021
Drugs Similar to Aluminum hydroxide (AlternaGEL, Others) 1023 • Pharmacotherapy of Helicobacter pylori *Infection 1023 • Miscellaneous Drugs Used for Peptic Ulcer Disease and Gastroesophageal Reflux Disease 1024*

CHAPTER 61 Pharmacotherapy of Bowel Disorders and Other Gastrointestinal Conditions 1028
Pathophysiology of Constipation 1029
Pharmacotherapy with Laxatives 1030
PROTOTYPE DRUG: **Psyllium mucilloid (Metamucil, others)** 1031
Drugs Similar to Psyllium Mucilloid (Metamucil, Others) 1032
Pathophysiology of Diarrhea 1032
Pharmacotherapy of Diarrhea 1033
PROTOTYPE DRUG: **Diphenoxylate with atropine (Lomotil)** 1034
Drugs Similar to Diphenoxylate with Atropine (Lomotil) 1035
Pharmacotherapy of Inflammatory Bowel Disease 1035
Nursing Process Application Patients Receiving Antidiarrheal Therapy 1036
PROTOTYPE DRUG: **Sulfasalazine (Azulfidine)** 1037
Drugs Similar to Sulfasalazine (Azulfidine) 1038
Pharmacotherapy of Irritable Bowel Syndrome 1039
Pathophysiology of Nausea and Vomiting 1040
Pharmacotherapy of Nausea and Vomiting 1041
PROTOTYPE DRUG: **Prochlorperazine (Compazine)** 1044
Drugs Similar to Prochlorperazine (Compazine) 1045
Pharmacotherapy of Pancreatitis 1045
Nursing Process Application Patients Receiving Antiemetic Therapy 1046
PROTOTYPE DRUG: **Pancrelipase (Cotazym, Pancrease, others)** 1047
Drugs Similar to Pancrelipase (Cotazym, Pancrease, Others) 1048

CHAPTER 62 Vitamins and Minerals 1051
Role of Vitamins in Health and Disease 1052
Regulation of Vitamins 1053
Recommended Dietary Allowance 1054
Fat-Soluble Vitamins 1055
Vitamin A (Aquasol A, Del-Vi-A) 1055 • Vitamin D (Ergocalciferol, Calcitriol) 1056 • Vitamin E (Tocopherols) 1057 • Vitamin K (Phytonadione) 1057
Water-Soluble Vitamins 1058
Thiamine (Vitamin B_1 [Thiamine Hydrochloride]) 1058 • Riboflavin (Vitamin B_2) 1059 • Pyridoxine (Vitamin B_6) 1059 • Cyanocobalamin (Vitamin B_{12}) 1060 • Folic Acid (Vitamin B_9) 1060 • Vitamin C (Ascorbic Acid) 1061
Minerals 1061
Nursing Process Application Patients Receiving Vitamin or Mineral Supplementation 1064

CHAPTER 63 Enteral and Parenteral Nutrition 1067
Enteral Nutrition 1068
Methods of Administration 1069 • Enteral Formulations 1069 • Elements of Enteral Nutrition 1070 • Complications of Enteral Therapy 1070 • Drug and Food Interactions 1074
Nursing Process Application Patients Receiving Enteral Nutrition Therapy 1075
Parenteral Nutrition 1076
Components of Total Parenteral Nutrition Solutions 1077 • Monitoring the Patient on Total Parenteral Nutrition 1078 • Complications of Parenteral Therapy 1079 • Drug and Food Interactions 1080
Nursing Process Application Patients Receiving Total Parenteral Nutrition 1081

CHAPTER 64 Weight Reduction Strategies and the Pharmacotherapy of Obesity 1085
Etiology of Obesity 1086
Pathogenesis of Obesity 1086
Measurement of Obesity 1087
Nonpharmacologic Therapies for Obesity 1087
Pharmacotherapy of Obesity 1089
PROTOTYPE DRUG: **Sibutramine (Meridia)** 1090
Drugs Similar to Sibutramine (Meridia) 1091
PROTOTYPE DRUG: **Orlistat (Alli, Xenical)** 1091
Drugs Similar to Orlistat (Alli, Xenical) 1092
Adjuncts to Obesity Therapy 1093
Nursing Process Application Patients Receiving Drugs for Weight Reduction 1093

UNIT 9 Pharmacology of the Endocrine System

CHAPTER 65 Review of the Endocrine System 1098
Overview of the Endocrine System 1099
Hormone Receptors 1099
Negative Feedback Mechanisms 1099
Hormone Pharmacotherapy 1101

CHAPTER 66 Hypothalamic and Pituitary Drugs 1104
Functions of the Hypothalamus 1105
Functions of the Pituitary Gland 1106
Pharmacotherapy of Growth Hormone Disorders 1106
PROTOTYPE DRUG: **Somatropin (Accretropin, Genotropin, Humatrope, Norditropin, Nutropin, Saizen, Serostim, Zorbtive)** 1108
Drugs Similar to Somatropin (Accretropin, Genotropin, Humatrope, Norditropin, Nutropin, Saizen, Serostim, Zorbtive) 1110
PROTOTYPE DRUG: **Octreotide (Sandostatin)** 1111
Drugs Similar to Octreotide (Sandostatin) 1112
Pharmacotherapy of Antidiuretic Hormone Disorders 1112
Nursing Process Application Patients Receiving Growth Hormone Therapy 1113

PROTOTYPE DRUG: **Desmopressin (DDAVP, Stimate) (Antidiuretic hormone)** 1114
Drugs Similar to Desmopressin (DDAVP, Stimate) (Antidiuretic Hormone) 1115
Nursing Process Application Patients Receiving Antidiuretic Hormone Therapy 1116

CHAPTER 67 Pharmacotherapy of Diabetes Mellitus 1119
Physiology of Serum Glucose Control 1120
Pathophysiology of Diabetes Mellitus: Types of Diabetes 1121
Symptoms and Diagnosis of Diabetes 1122
Complications of Diabetes Mellitus 1123
PROTOTYPE DRUG: **Glucagon (GlucaGen)** 1124
Drugs Similar to Glucagon (GlucaGen) 1125
Drug Therapy for Diabetes: Insulin 1126
Insulin Adjunct 1128
PROTOTYPE DRUG: **Human regular insulin (Humulin R, Novolin R)** 1128
Drugs Similar to Human Regular Insulin (Humulin R, Novolin R) 1129
Nursing Process Application Patients Receiving Insulin Therapy 1131
Drug Therapy for Diabetes: Oral Antidiabetic Agents 1132
Sulfonylureas 1132
PROTOTYPE DRUG: **Glyburide (DiaBeta, Glynase, Micronase)** 1134
Drugs Similar to Glyburide (DiaBeta, Glynase, Micronase) 1135
Biguanides 1135
PROTOTYPE DRUG: **Metformin (Glucophage, Glucophage XR, Glumetza)** 1135
Drugs Similar to Metformin (Glucophage, Glucophage XR, Glumetza) 1136 • Meglitinides 1136
PROTOTYPE DRUG: **Repaglinide (Prandin)** 1136
Drugs Similar to Repaglinide (Prandin) 1137 • Thiazolidinediones 1137
PROTOTYPE DRUG: **Rosiglitazone (Avandia)** 1137
Drugs Similar to Rosiglitazone (Avandia) 1138 • Alpha-Glucosidase Inhibitors 1138
PROTOTYPE DRUG: **Acarbose (Precose)** 1138
Drugs Similar to Acarbose (Precose) 1139 • Oral Combination Products 1139
Nursing Process Application Patient Receiving Oral Antidiabetic Therapy 1140
Drug Therapy for Diabetes: Incretin Therapies 1141
PROTOTYPE DRUG: **Sitagliptin (Januvia)** 1141
Drugs Similar to Sitagliptin (Januvia) 1142

CHAPTER 68 Pharmacotherapy of Thyroid Disorders 1146
Physiology of the Thyroid Gland 1147
Diagnosis of Thyroid Disorders 1148
Hypothyroid Disorders 1148
Pharmacotherapy of Hypothyroid Disorders 1150
PROTOTYPE DRUG: **Levothyroxine (Levothroid, Levoxyl, Synthroid, Thyro-Tabs, Unithroid)** 1151
Drugs Similar to Levothyroxine (Levothroid, Levoxyl, Synthroid, Thyro-Tabs, Unithroid) 1152
Hyperthyroid Disorders 1152
Nursing Process Application Patients Receiving Thyroid Hormone Replacement Therapy 1153
Pharmacotherapy of Hyperthyroid Disorders 1154
PROTOTYPE DRUG: **Propylthiouracil (Propyl-Thyracil, PTU)** 1155
Drugs Similar to Propylthiouracil (Propyl-Thyracil, PTU) 1156
Nursing Process Application Patients Receiving Antithyroid Therapy 1157

CHAPTER 69 Corticosteroids and Drugs Affecting the Adrenal Cortex 1160
Physiology of the Adrenal Gland 1161
Overview of Corticosteroid Pharmacotherapy 1163
Adverse Effects of Corticosteroids 1163
Replacement Therapy with Corticosteroids 1165
PROTOTYPE DRUG: **Hydrocortisone (Aeroseb-HC, Alphaderm, others)** 1166
Drugs Similar to Hydrocortisone (Aeroseb-HC, Alphaderm, Others) 1168
Corticosteroids for Nonendocrine Conditions 1168
Mineralocorticoids 1169
PROTOTYPE DRUG: **Fludrocortisone (Florinef)** 1170
Drugs Similar to Fludrocortisone (Florinef) 1171
Antiadrenal Agents 1171
Nursing Process Application Patients Receiving Systemic Corticosteroid Therapy 1172

CHAPTER 70 Estrogens, Progestins, and Drugs Modifying Uterine Function 1176
Hormonal Regulation of Female Reproductive Function 1177
Estrogens 1177
PROTOTYPE DRUG: **Conjugated estrogens (Cenestin, Enjuvia, Premarin)** 1179
Drugs Similar to Conjugated Estrogens (Cenestin, Enjuvia, Premarin) 1181
Progestins 1181
Nursing Process Application Patients Receiving Estrogen Therapy 1182
PROTOTYPE DRUG: **Medroxyprogesterone acetate (Provera)** 1183
Drugs Similar to Medroxyprogesterone Acetate (Provera) 1184
Hormone Replacement Therapy 1184
Nursing Process Application Patients Receiving Progestin Therapy 1185
Uterine Stimulants: Oxytocics 1186
PROTOTYPE DRUG: **Oxytocin (Pitocin)** 1188
Drugs Similar to Oxytocin (Pitocin) 1189
Uterine Relaxants: Tocolytics 1189
Nursing Process Application Patients Receiving Oxytocin (Pitocin) 1190
Pharmacotherapy of Infertility 1191
PROTOTYPE DRUG: **Clomiphene citrate (Clomid, Milophene, Serophene)** 1194
Drugs Similar to Clomiphene Citrate (Clomid, Milophene, Serophene) 1195

CHAPTER 71 Drugs for Modifying Conception 1199
Options and Choices for Birth Control 1200
Combination Oral Contraceptives 1200
PROTOTYPE DRUG: **Estradiol and Norethindrone (Ortho-Novum)** 1204
Drugs Similar to Estradiol and Norethindrone (Ortho-Novum) 1206
Progestin-Only Oral Contraceptives 1206

Adverse Effects of Combined Oral Contraceptives 1206

Nursing Process Application Patients Receiving Oral Contraceptive Therapy 1207

Drugs for Long-Term Contraception and Newer Contraceptive Delivery Methods 1209

Spermicides 1210

PROTOTYPE DRUG: Nonoxynol-9 1211

Drugs Similar to Nonoxynol-9 1212

Emergency Contraception 1212

Drugs for Pharmacologic Abortion 1212

PROTOTYPE DRUG: Mifepristone (RU-486) 1214

Drugs Similar to Mifepristone (RU-486) 1215

CHAPTER 72 Drugs for Disorders and Conditions of the Male Reproductive System 1218

Regulation of Male Reproductive Function 1219

Pharmacotherapy with Androgens 1220

PROTOTYPE DRUG: Testosterone 1221

Drugs Similar to Testosterone 1223

Anabolic Steroids 1223

Nursing Process Application Patients Receiving Androgen Therapy 1224

Etiology of Male Sexual Dysfunction 1225

Pharmacotherapy of Male Infertility 1225

Pharmacotherapy of Erectile Dysfunction 1226

PROTOTYPE DRUG: Sildenafil (Viagra) 1228

Drugs Similar to Sildenafil (Viagra) 1229

Pathophysiology of Benign Prostatic Hyperplasia 1229

Pharmacotherapy of Benign Prostatic Hyperplasia 1231

PROTOTYPE DRUG: Finasteride (Proscar) 1232

Drugs Similar to Finasteride (Proscar) 1233

Nursing Process Application Patients Receiving Therapy with 5-Alpha Reductase Inhibitors 1233

UNIT 10 Pharmacology of the Respiratory System and Allergy

CHAPTER 73 Pharmacotherapy of Asthma and Other Pulmonary Disorders 1238

Physiology of the Lower Respiratory Tract 1239

Pathophysiology of Asthma 1240

Administration of Pulmonary Drugs via Inhalation 1241

Principles of Asthma Pharmacotherapy 1242

PROTOTYPE DRUG: Albuterol (Proventil, Ventolin, VoSpire) 1246

Drugs Similar to Albuterol (Proventil, Ventolin, VoSpire) 1247

PROTOTYPE DRUG: Ipratropium (Atrovent, Combivent) 1248

Drugs Similar to Ipratropium (Atrovent, Combivent) 1249

PROTOTYPE DRUG: Beclomethasone (Beconase AQ, Qvar) 1251

Drugs Similar to Beclomethasone (Beconase AQ, Qvar) 1252

PROTOTYPE DRUG: Cromolyn (Intal) 1252

Drugs Similar to Cromolyn (Intal) 1253

PROTOTYPE DRUG: Zafirlukast (Accolate) 1253

Drugs Similar to Zafirlukast (Accolate) 1254

PROTOTYPE DRUG: Theophylline (Slo-Phyllin, Theochron, Theolair, Uniphyl) 1255

Drugs Similar to Theophylline (Slo-Phyllin, Theochron, Theolair, Uniphyl) 1256

Chronic Obstructive Pulmonary Disease 1256

Nursing Process Application Patients Receiving Therapy for Asthma and Chronic Obstructive Pulmonary Disease 1257

CHAPTER 74 Pharmacotherapy of Allergic Rhinitis and the Common Cold 1261

Physiology of the Upper Respiratory Tract 1262

Pathophysiology of Allergic Rhinitis 1263

Pharmacotherapy of Allergic Rhinitis 1263

PROTOTYPE DRUG: Fexofenadine (Allegra) 1267

Drugs Similar to Fexofenadine (Allegra) 1268

Nursing Process Application Patients Receiving Antihistamine Therapy 1269

PROTOTYPE DRUG: Fluticasone (Flonase) 1270

Drugs Similar to Fluticasone (Flonase) 1271

Decongestants 1271

Nursing Process Application Patients Receiving Intranasal Corticosteroid Therapy 1272

PROTOTYPE DRUG: Pseudoephedrine (Sudafed) 1273

Drugs Similar to Pseudoephedrine (Sudafed) 1274

Drugs for the Common Cold 1274

Antitussives 1275

PROTOTYPE DRUG: Dextromethorphan (Robitussin, Sucrets, others) 1275

Drugs Similar to Dextromethorphan (Robitussin, Sucrets, Others) 1277

Expectorants and Mucolytics 1277

UNIT 11 Miscellaneous Drugs

CHAPTER 75 Pharmacotherapy of Bone and Joint Disorders 1282

Role of Calcium in Body Homeostasis 1283

Regulation of Calcium Balance 1284

Pharmacotherapy of Hypocalcemia 1287

PROTOTYPE DRUG: Calcium salts 1287

Drugs Similar to Calcium Salts 1289

Nursing Process Application Patients Receiving Calcium Supplements 1289

Pathophysiology of Metabolic Bone Disease 1290

Pharmacotherapy of Metabolic Bone Disease 1292

PROTOTYPE DRUG: Calcitriol (Rocaltrol) 1292

Drugs Similar to Calcitriol (Rocaltrol) 1293

PROTOTYPE DRUG: Alendronate (Fosamax) 1296

Drugs Similar to Alendronate (Fosamax) 1297

PROTOTYPE DRUG: Raloxifene (Evista) 1297

Nursing Process Application Patients Receiving Bisphosphonates 1298

Drugs Similar to Raloxifene (Evista) 1299

Pathophysiology and Pharmacotherapy of Joint Disorders 1300

PROTOTYPE DRUG: Hydroxychloroquine (Plaquenil) 1304

Drugs Similar to Hydroxychloroquine (Plaquenil) 1305

Pharmacotherapy of Gout 1306

PROTOTYPE DRUG: Colchicine 1308

Drugs Similar to Colchicine 1309

PROTOTYPE DRUG: Allopurinol (Zyloprim) 1309

Drugs Similar to Allopurinol (Zyloprim) 1310

Nursing Process Application Patients Receiving Antigout Therapy 1311

CHAPTER 76 Pharmacotherapy of Dermatologic Disorders 1314
Anatomy of the Integumentary System 1315
Classification of Skin Disorders 1316
Pharmacotherapy of Skin Infections 1317
Scabicides and Pediculicides 1318
PROTOTYPE DRUG: Permethrin (Acticin, Elimite, Nix) 1319
Drugs Similar to Permethrin (Acticin, Elimite, Nix) 1320
Pharmacotherapy of Acne and Rosacea 1320
Nursing Process Application Patients Receiving Drug Therapy for Lice or Mite Infestation 1321
PROTOTYPE DRUG: Tretinoin (Avita, Retin-A, Trentin-X) 1323
Drugs Similar to Tretinoin (Avita, Retin-A, Trentin-X) 1324
Pharmacotherapy of Dermatitis 1325
Nursing Process Application Patient Receiving Tretinoin (Retin-A) or Isotretinoin (Accutane) 1326
Pharmacotherapy of Psoriasis 1328
Topical Drugs 1328 • Systemic Drugs 1329
Pharmacotherapy of Minor Skin Burns 1331
PROTOTYPE DRUG: Benzocaine (Americaine, Anbesol, others) 1332
Drugs Similar to Benzocaine (Americaine, Anbesol, Others) 1333
Pharmacotherapy of Alopecia 1333

CHAPTER 77 Pharmacotherapy of Eye and Ear Disorders 1337
Anatomy of the Eye 1338
Pathophysiology of Glaucoma 1338
Pharmacotherapy of Glaucoma 1340
PROTOTYPE DRUG: Latanoprost (Xalatan) 1342
Drugs Similar to Latanoprost (Xalatan) 1342
PROTOTYPE DRUG: Timolol (Betimol, Istalol, Timoptic) 1344
Drugs Similar to Timolol (Betimol, Istalol, Timoptic) 1345
Nursing Process Application Patients Receiving Ophthalmic Solutions for Glaucoma 1346
Pharmacotherapy for Eye Examinations 1347
Pharmacotherapy for Other Eye Conditions 1347
Anatomy of the Ear 1349
Pharmacotherapy with Otic Preparations 1350
Nursing Responsibilities for Otic Medications 1352 • Patient and Family Education for Otic Medications 1352
Nursing Process Application Patients Receiving Pharmacotherapy for Otitis Media 1353

CHAPTER 78 Emergency Preparedness: Bioterrorism and Management of Poisoning 1357
Emergency Preparedness, Bioterrorism, and Nursing 1358
Biological Agents 1360
Chemical and Physical Agents 1362
Management of Poisoning 1363
PROTOTYPE DRUG: Activated charcoal (CharcoAid) 1365
Drugs Similar to Activated Charcoal (CharcoAid) 1365
PROTOTYPE DRUG: Edetate calcium disodium (Calcium EDTA) 1366
PROTOTYPE DRUG: Dimercaprol (BAL in Oil) 1367
Nursing Process Application Patients Experiencing Poisoning or Overdose 1368

Appendices
A Answers to Critical Thinking Questions, Case Study, and NCLEX-RN® Review 1372
B Top 100 Drugs Ranked by Number of Prescriptions 1437
C Canadian Drugs and Their U.S. Equivalents 1438
D ISMP's List of High-Alert Medications 1441

Glossary 1442

Credits 1460

Index 1461

UNIT 1

Fundamental Principles of Pharmacology

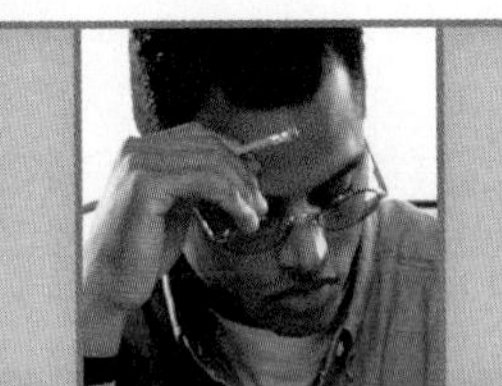
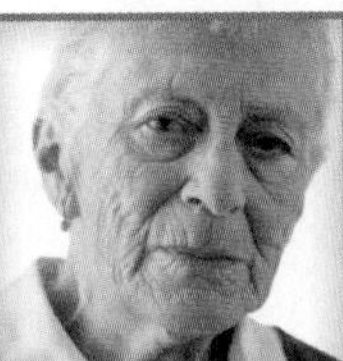
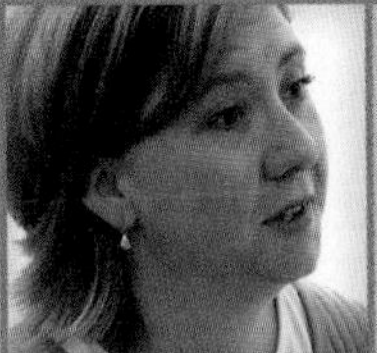
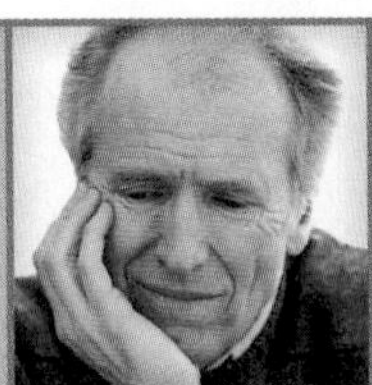

CHAPTER 1 Introduction to Pharmacology: Concepts and Connections

CHAPTER 2 Drug Regulations

CHAPTER 3 Principles of Drug Administration

CHAPTER 4 Pharmacokinetics

CHAPTER 5 Pharmacodynamics

CHAPTER 6 Adverse Drug Effects and Drug Interactions

CHAPTER 7 Medication Errors and Risk Reduction

CHAPTER 8 Pharmacology of Substance Abuse

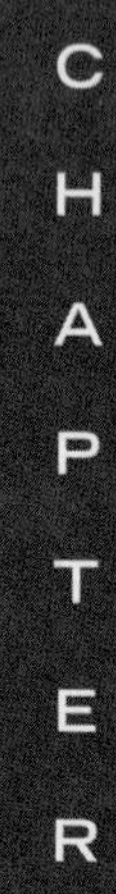

"Wow, I just left my first pharmacology class and my head is swirling. How will I ever remember all this?"

Student "Josh Remming"

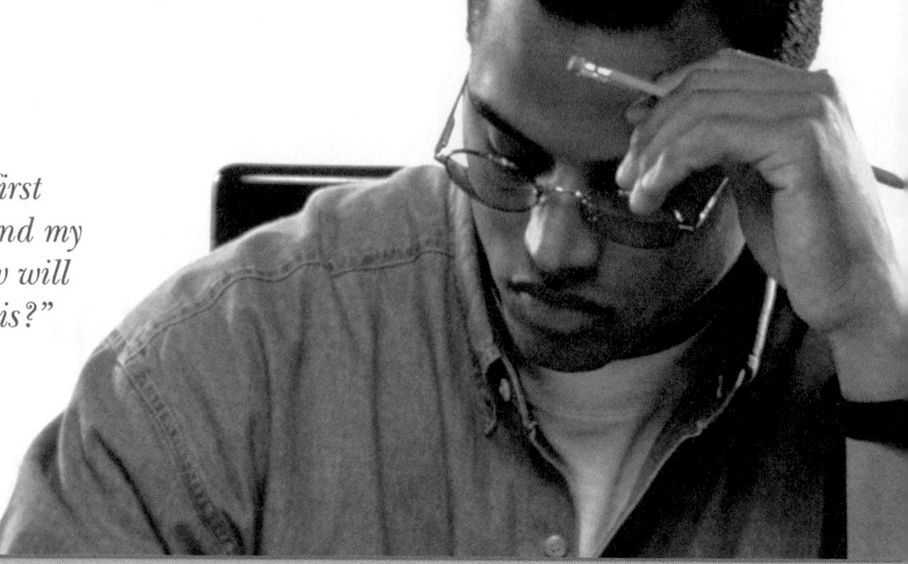

1 Introduction to Pharmacology: Concepts and Connections

Learning Outcomes

After reading this chapter, the student should be able to:

1. Identify key events in the history of pharmacology.
2. Compare and contrast the terms *drug, pharmacology,* and *pharmacotherapy.*
3. Recognize the characteristics of an ideal drug.
4. Explain the importance of pharmacotherapy to clinical nursing practice.
5. Using specific examples, explain the difference between the pharmacologic and therapeutic methods of classifying drugs.
6. Identify the importance of using prototype drugs to study pharmacology.
7. Classify drugs by their chemical, generic, and trade names.
8. Compare the advantages and disadvantages of a pharmaceutical company being granted exclusivity for the development of a new drug.
9. Analyze possible differences between generic drugs and their brand-name equivalents.
10. Assess the responsibilities of the nurse in drug administration.

Chapter Outline

Brief History of Pharmacology

Pharmacology: The Study of Medicines

Characteristics of an Ideal Drug

Classification of Drugs

Drug Prototypes

Naming Drugs

Connecting Pharmacology to Clinical Nursing Practice

Key Terms

bioavailability, 8
chemical names, 7
combination drugs, 7
drug, 4
exclusivity, 7
generic names, 7
indications, 5
pharmacologic classification, 5
pharmacology, 4
pharmacotherapy, 4
prototype drug, 6
therapeutic classification, 5
trade names, 7

More drugs are being administered to consumers than ever before. Over 3 billion prescriptions are dispensed each year in the United States, and the number is rapidly approaching 4 billion. The applications of pharmacology to medicine have evolved over the centuries and the nurse now serves a key role in ensuring the success of pharmacotherapy. The purpose of this chapter is to introduce fundamental concepts of pharmacology and to emphasize the connections between drug therapy and clinical nursing practice.

PharmFACT

According to the National Association of Chain Drug Stores (NACDS), the average cost of a prescription drug has risen from $22.06 in 1990 to $45.79 in 2000 to $64.86 in 2005. This is almost a 200% increase in 15 years. *Source:* NACDS, 2007.

Brief History of Pharmacology

1.1 The practice of applying products to relieve suffering has been recorded throughout history by virtually every culture.

The story of pharmacology is rich and exciting, filled with accidental discoveries and landmark events. Its history likely began when a human first used a plant to relieve symptoms of disease. One of the oldest forms of health care, herbal medicine has been practiced in virtually every culture dating to antiquity. The Babylonians recorded the earliest surviving "prescriptions" on clay tablets in 3000 BC, although magic and the art of reading omens were probably considered as legitimate to healing as the use of drug remedies. At about the same time, the Chinese recorded the *Pen Tsao* (Great Herbal), a 40-volume compendium of plant remedies dating to 2700 BC. The Egyptians followed in 1500 BC by archiving their remedies on a document known as the Eber's papyrus, which contains over 700 magical formulas and remedies. Galen, the famous Greek physician, described over 1,000 healing preparations using plant products before his death in AD 201.

Little is known about pharmacology during the Dark Ages. Although it is likely that herbal medicine continued to be practiced, especially in monasteries and in centers of Arabic culture, few historical events related to drug therapy were recorded. Pharmacology, and indeed medicine, could not advance until the discipline of science was eventually viewed differently than magic and superstition.

The first recorded reference to the word *pharmacology* was found in a text entitled "Pharmacologia sen Manuductio and Materiam Medicum" by Samuel Dale in 1693. Before this date, the study of herbal remedies was called "Materia Medica." Indeed, the term *Materia Medica* likely originated from a Latin term meaning "medical matters" in the Roman Empire that continued into the early 20th century.

Although the exact starting date is obscure, modern pharmacology is thought to have begun in the early 1800s. At that time, chemists were making remarkable progress in separating specific substances from complex mixtures. This enabled chemists to isolate the active agents morphine, colchicine, curare, cocaine, and other early drugs from their natural plant products. Pharmacologists could then study their effects in animals more precisely, using standardized amounts. Some of the early researchers even used themselves as test subjects. Frederich Serturner, who first isolated morphine from opium in 1805, injected himself and three of his friends with a huge dose of 100 mg of his new product. He and his cohorts suffered acute morphine intoxication for several days afterward.

Pharmacology as a distinct discipline was officially recognized when the first Department of Pharmacology was established in Estonia in 1847. John Jacob Abel, who is considered the father of American pharmacology due to his many contributions to the field, founded the first pharmacology department in the United States at the University of Michigan in 1890.

In the 20th century, the pace of change in all areas of medicine became exponential. Pharmacologists no longer needed to rely on the slow, laborious process of isolating active agents from scarce natural products. They could synthesize drugs "from scratch" in the laboratory. Hundreds of new drugs could be synthesized and tested in a relatively short time span. More importantly, it became possible to understand how drugs produced their effects, right down to their molecular mechanism of action.

The current practice of pharmacology is extremely complex and has progressed far beyond its early, primitive history. The nurses and other health professionals who practice it, however, must never forget its early roots: the application of products to relieve human suffering. Whether it is a substance extracted from the Pacific yew tree, one isolated from a fungus, or one created totally in a laboratory, the central purpose of pharmacology is focused on the patient and improving the quality of life.

CONNECTION *Checkpoint* 1.1

Opium, colchicine, and cocaine are drugs obtained from natural products that were used hundreds, and perhaps thousands, of years ago. Are any of these products still used as drugs today? Use a drug guide or encyclopedia to determine the modern names of these drugs and what they are used to treat. See Answer to Connection Checkpoint 1.1 in Appendix A.

Pharmacology: The Study of Medicines

1.2 Pharmacology is the study of medicines.

The word *drug* has already been used numerous times in this text. What exactly is a drug? Is everything a drug, including water, vitamin C, or perhaps a can of cola? What about substances naturally found in the body, such as estrogen or testosterone? Is it even possible to define a drug?

The definition of a drug is indeed difficult but is nevertheless important to the health care profession. There are many definitions, but perhaps the clearest is that a **drug** is any substance that is taken to prevent, cure, or reduce symptoms of a medical condition. Considering the substances listed earlier, which, then, are drugs? Although it may seem vague, the correct answer is, "it depends."

- Water is usually not considered a drug. However, when someone is dehydrated, solutions of water (saline) may be infused into this patient to treat this condition. In this case water, or more specifically saline, is a drug.
- Vitamin C, if ingested as part of an orange or tomato, is food. Food is not a drug. However, someone with a vitamin C deficiency may be administered vitamin C to cure scurvy. For this patient, vitamin C is then considered a drug.
- A can of cola is certainly not listed in any drug guide. However, if a patient with diabetes is experiencing a hypoglycemic reaction, the glucose in a can of soda may raise the patient's blood sugar and prevent a coma; thus the glucose in the cola may be considered a drug in this example.
- Substances normally found in the body are not considered drugs unless they are administered to treat a condition. For example, the hormone estrogen circulating in the blood is not a drug. However, if it is taken as an oral contraceptive to prevent a condition (pregnancy), estrogen is considered a drug.

Once the meaning of drug is understood, the next essential term is *pharmacology.* The word **pharmacology** is derived from two Greek words, *pharmakon,* which means "medicine" or "drug," and *logos,* which means "study." Thus, pharmacology is most simply defined as the study of medicines. **Pharmacotherapy,** or pharmacotherapeutics, is the application of drugs for the purpose of disease prevention and treatment of suffering. Pharmacology is an expansive subject, ranging from understanding how drugs are administered, to where they travel in the body, to the actual responses they produce.

Drugs are a form of medical intervention given to improve a patient's condition or to prevent harm. Pharmacotherapy often begins when the patient experiences signs or symptoms that cause dissatisfaction with current or future health status. A major role of the nurse is to design interventions that meet the desired health goals of the patient. Pharmacotherapy is a critical intervention for many conditions. The rationale for pharmacotherapy is illustrated in Figure 1.1.

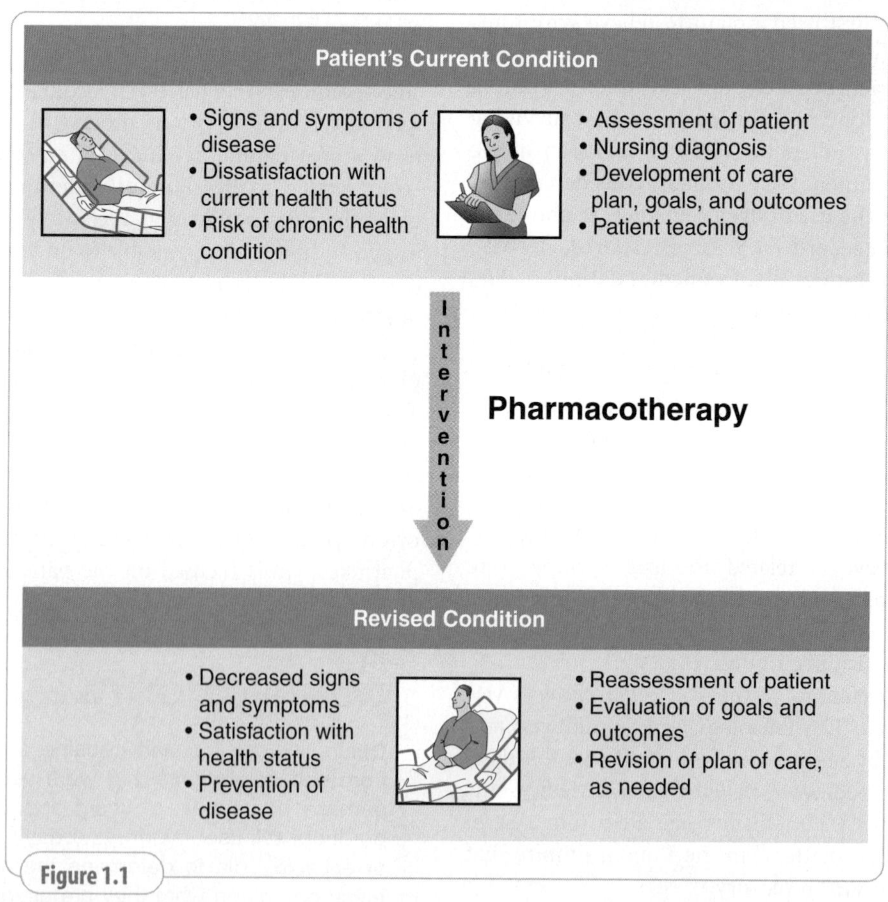

Figure 1.1

Rationale for pharmacotherapy: A partnership between the patient and the health care provider.

Over 11,000 brand-name and generic drugs and combination agents are currently available for pharmacotherapy. Each has its own characteristic set of therapeutic applications, interactions, adverse effects, and mechanism of action. Many drugs are prescribed for more than one disease and most produce multiple effects on the body. Further complicating the study of pharmacology is the fact that drugs may elicit different responses depending on individual patient factors such as age, gender, race, body mass, health status, and genetics. Indeed, learning the applications of existing medications and staying current with new drugs introduced every year are an enormous challenge for the nurse. The task, however, is a critical one for both the patient and the health care provider. If applied properly, drugs can dramatically improve patients' quality of life. If applied improperly, the consequences of drug action can cause permanent disability and even death.

There are important exceptions to the drug definition mentioned earlier. What about crack cocaine, ecstacy, LSD, or the fumes in glues and paint thinners? These are certainly drugs, but they are not taken "to prevent, cure, or reduce symptoms of a medical condition." In fact, they are taken to produce a biologic effect viewed as desirable or pleasurable by the user (see Chapter 8). There are a few exceptions to the drug definition, and these will become apparent as the student studies pharmacology.

Characteristics of an Ideal Drug

1.3 The perfect drug is safe and effective.

As they begin their journey in mastering pharmacology, nurses should start with a notion of the ideal or "perfect drug." Learning the characteristics of an ideal drug gives a basis for comparison to "real drugs." It is always the goal of pharmacotherapy to select the perfect or ideal drug for the patient. Just what is a perfect drug? It is one that:

- Effectively treats, prevents, or cures the patient's condition.
- Produces a rapid, predictable response at relatively low doses.
- Produces no adverse effects or long-term adverse effects.
- Can be taken conveniently, usually by mouth.
- Can be taken infrequently, usually once a day, and for a short length of time.
- Is inexpensive and easily accessible.
- Is quickly eliminated by the body after it produces its beneficial effect.
- Does not interact with other medications or food.

The student should easily recognize that there is no such thing as a perfect drug. Some drugs meet most of the preceding criteria, whereas others meet very few. At the very least, it is expected that all prescription drugs have some degree of effectiveness at treating or preventing a health condition. The conditions for which a drug is approved are its **indications.** Every prescription drug has at least one indication, and most have multiple indications. Some drugs are used for conditions for which they have not been approved; these are called unlabeled or off-label indications.

As a general rule, the more a medicine strays from the "perfect drug" profile, the less commonly it is used. This is because whenever possible, health care providers strive to prescribe the most effective, safest, and most convenient medication for the patient. In the home care setting, drugs that cause annoying adverse effects, have inconvenient dosing schedules, or are expensive are often not taken by patients, potentially worsening their condition and causing failure of treatment outcomes. Of course, some essential drugs do produce serious adverse effects or must be given by invasive routes, such as intravenously. In these cases, the drug is either administered in a clinical setting by a skilled nurse, or the patient receives careful instructions and regular monitoring on an outpatient basis.

Classification of Drugs

1.4 Drugs may be organized by their therapeutic classification or pharmacologic classification.

In the U.S. Food and Drug Administration (FDA) document *Approved Drug Products with Therapeutic Equivalence Evaluations,* informally called the "Orange Book," over 11,000 approved drugs are listed. With the vast number of drugs available, it is essential that methods be used to group similar agents to aid in their study and understanding. The two basic classifications of drugs are therapeutic and pharmacologic. Both categories are widely used in classifying prescription and nonprescription drugs. The key difference is that the **therapeutic classification** describes what is being treated by the drug, whereas the **pharmacologic classification** describes how the drug acts.

CONNECTIONS

Lifespan Considerations

Cost of Prescription Medications

The elderly population is affected more than any other age group by the high cost of prescription drugs. Americans over age 65 comprise only 13% of the population but account for about 34% of all prescriptions dispensed and 40% of all over-the-counter (OTC) medications. Over 80% of all seniors take at least one prescribed drug each day. The average older person is taking more than four prescription medications at once, plus two OTC medications. Many of these medicines, such as those for hypertension and heart disease, are taken on a permanent basis.

Seniors are less likely than younger people to have insurance that covers the cost of prescription medications. On a fixed annual income, many seniors must choose between buying medications and purchasing adequate food or material necessities. The annual drug spending per senior grew from an average of $559 in 1992 to over $1,914 in 2004.

TABLE 1.1 Organizing Drug Information by Therapeutic Classification

Therapeutic Focus: Drugs Affecting Cardiovascular Disease

Therapeutic Usefulness	Therapeutic Classification
Influence blood clotting	Anticoagulants
Lower blood cholesterol	Antihyperlipidemics
Lower blood pressure	Antihypertensives
Restore normal cardiac rhythm	Antidysrhythmics
Treat angina	Antianginals

TABLE 1.2 Organizing Drug Information by Pharmacologic Classification

Focus on How a Drug Works: Pharmacotherapy of Hypertension

Mechanism of Action	Pharmacologic Classification
Lowers plasma volume	Diuretic
Blocks heart calcium channels	Calcium channel blocker
Blocks hormonal activity	Angiotensin-converting enzyme inhibitor
Blocks physiologic reactions to stress	Adrenergic antagonist (or blocker)
Dilates peripheral blood vessels	Vasodilator

Drugs are placed into therapeutic classes based on their usefulness in treating a specific disease. Table 1.1 shows the method of therapeutic classification, using cardiovascular drugs as an example. Many different types of drugs affect cardiovascular function. Some drugs influence blood coagulation, whereas others lower cholesterol levels or prevent the onset of stroke. Drugs may be used to treat hypertension, heart failure, abnormal cardiac rhythm, chest pain, myocardial infarction (MI), or circulatory shock. Thus, drugs that treat cardiovascular disorders may be placed in several therapeutic classes, for example, anticoagulants, antihyperlipidemics, and antihypertensives. The key to therapeutic classification is to simply state what condition is being treated by the particular drug. Other examples of therapeutic classifications include antidepressants, antipsychotics, drugs for erectile dysfunction, and antineoplastics. Notice how the prefix *anti-* often refers to a therapeutic classification.

The pharmacologic classification addresses a drug's mechanism of action or how a drug produces its effect in the body. Table 1.2 illustrates the use of pharmacologic classification, using hypertension as an example. A diuretic treats hypertension by lowering plasma volume. Calcium channel blockers treat this disorder by decreasing the force of cardiac contractions. Other drugs block components of the renin-angiotensin system. Notice that each example describes how hypertension might be controlled. A drug's pharmacologic classification is more specific than its therapeutic classification and requires an understanding of biochemistry and physiology. Pharmacologic classifications may use a drug's chemical name.

Although classifications help to organize drugs, the process is by no means easy or standardized. Most drugs have multiple classifications. For example, the drug epinephrine is classified as a vasoconstrictor, an autonomic nervous system agent, an adrenergic agonist, a sympathomimetic, a bronchodilator, an agent for anaphylaxis, an ocular mydriatic, an antiglaucoma agent, a catecholamine, and a topical hemostatic. It should be noted that this is clearly a mix of therapeutic (e.g., antiglaucoma) and pharmacologic (e.g., catecholamine) classifications. Which one(s) should the student remember? Unfortunately for beginning students of pharmacology, the answer is all of them. The classification chosen primarily depends on the specific clinical use of the drug (What condition of the patient is the nurse treating?). Sometimes it is simply a preference of the attending nurse or health care provider. Although challenging, remembering the different classifications will pay dividends as the student's pharmacology course progresses.

CONNECTION *Checkpoint* 1.2

State whether each of the following classifications for aspirin is therapeutic or pharmacologic: anticoagulant, salicylate, central nervous system agent, analgesic, antipyretic. Use a drug guide, if needed. See Answer to Connection Checkpoint 1.2 in Appendix A.

Drug Prototypes

1.5 A prototype drug is the agent to which all other drugs in a class are compared.

As discussed in Section 1.4 learning thousands of drugs is simplified, at least somewhat, by grouping similar drugs together into broad classifications. Just knowing its therapeutic or pharmacologic classification can reveal important information about a drug. There is an additional strategy that is helpful when learning pharmacology. It is a common and useful practice to select a single drug from a class and compare all other medications in the class to this representative medication. This is called a **prototype drug.** By learning the prototype drug in depth, the actions and adverse effects of other drugs in the same class may be predicted. For example, by learning the actions and effects of penicillin V, students can extend this knowledge to all other drugs in the penicillin class of antibiotics. In this textbook, the drug prototypes are clearly identified, and detailed information regarding their therapeutic effects, mechanism of action, adverse effects, contraindications, precautions, nursing responsibilities, and patient and family education are included.

Selecting a drug to serve as the prototype for a class is not always a simple matter; health care providers and textbooks sometimes disagree. The traditional prototype approach uses the oldest and best understood drug in the class. Sometimes, however, newer drugs are developed in the same class that are more effective, or have a more favorable safety profile. Over time, an older prototype drug may be infrequently prescribed and a different, more clinically useful prototype may be chosen for the class. This textbook uses a practical approach to drug prototypes, selecting a combination of traditional drugs and those most widely used. Regardless of the approach, the student must remember that the prototype is the drug to which all others in a class are compared.

Naming Drugs

1.6 Drugs have chemical, generic, and trade names.

Despite the utility of using drug classes and prototypes when studying pharmacology, it remains a major challenge to learn thousands of drug names. Adding to this difficulty is that most drugs have multiple names. The three basic types of drug names are chemical, generic, and trade names.

Chemical names are assigned using standard nomenclature established by the International Union of Pure and Applied Chemistry (IUPAC). A drug has only one chemical name. This chemical name is sometimes helpful in predicting a drug's physical and chemical properties. Although chemical names convey a clear and concise meaning about the nature of a drug to the chemist, these names are often complicated and difficult to remember or pronounce. For example, it is unlikely that the nurse would remember that the chemical name for alprazolam (Xanax) is 8-chloro-1-methyl-6-phenyl-4H-5-triazo[4,3-a][1,4]-benzodiazepine. In only a few cases, usually when the name is brief and easily remembered, will nurses use chemical names. Examples of easy to remember chemical names of common drugs include lithium carbonate, calcium gluconate, and sodium chloride.

Drugs are sometimes named and classified by a portion of their chemical structure, known as the chemical group name. In the Xanax example, a portion of the chemical name, benzodiazepine, is used as a drug class. Other examples include the fluoroquinolones, aminoglycosides, phenothiazines, and thiazides. Although these names may seem complicated when first encountered, knowledge of chemical group names will become invaluable as the nursing student begins to learn and understand the actions of the drugs in the major drug classes.

The **generic name** of a drug is assigned by the United States Adopted Name Council. With few exceptions, generic names are less complicated and easier to remember than chemical names. Many organizations, including the FDA, the *United States Pharmacopeia,* and the World Health Organization routinely describe a medication by its generic name. Because there is only one generic name for each drug, health care providers often use this name, and students must memorize it.

A drug's **trade name,** sometimes called the proprietary, product, or brand name, is assigned by the pharmaceutical company marketing the drug. The trade name is intentionally selected to be short and easy to remember so that patients will remember it (and ask for it by name). The term *proprietary* suggests ownership. In the United States, the FDA grants the pharmaceutical company exclusive rights to name and market a drug for a certain number of years after it approves a new drug application. During the period of **exclusivity,** competing companies are not allowed to market generic versions of the product. The rationale for exclusivity is that the developing pharmaceutical company needs sufficient time to recoup the millions of dollars in research and development costs involved in designing and testing the new drug. Without the guarantee of exclusivity, there is little incentive to pharmaceutical companies to develop new and unique drugs. When exclusivity expires, competing companies may sell a generic equivalent drug, sometimes using a different name, which the FDA must approve. The typical length of exclusivity for a new drug is 5 years; however, this may be extended by 3 additional years if the drug is determined to have a new indication, can be delivered by a different route, or is made available in a different dosage form. If, for example, the pharmaceutical company completes pediatric studies and determines the dosage and safety of a drug in this population, the FDA adds 6 months of exclusivity. Orphan drugs (see Chapter 2) have 7 years of exclusivity. Pharmaceutical companies can make millions of dollars in sales from exclusivity; thus they usually make great efforts to receive extensions from the FDA. Expiration dates for the exclusivity of specific drugs are listed in the Orange Book.

Trade names are a challenge for students to learn because there may be dozens of product names containing the same drug. In addition, many products contain more than one active ingredient. Drugs with more than one active generic ingredient are called **combination drugs.** This poses a problem in trying to match one generic name with one product name. As an example, refer to Table 1.3 and consider the drug diphenhydramine (generic name), also called Benadryl (one of many trade names). Low doses of diphenhydramine may be purchased OTC. Higher doses require a prescription. If the nurse is looking for diphenhydramine, it may be listed under many trade names such as Benadryl, Nytol QuickCaps, Sominex, and Unisom, formulated alone or in combination with other active ingredients. Acetaminophen and aspirin are additional examples of agents that appear in many combination drugs with

TABLE 1.3 Examples of Generic Drugs Contained in Brand-Name Products

Generic Drugs	Brand Names
aspirin	Acetylsalicylic Acid, Acuprin, Anacin, Aspergum, Bayer, Bufferin, Ecotrin, Empirin, Excedrin, Maprin, Norgesic, Salatin, Salocol, Salsprin, Supac, Talwin, Traphen-10, Vanquish, Verin, ZORprin
diphenhydramine	Allerdryl, Benadryl, Benahist, Bendylate, Caladryl, Compoz, Diahist, Diphenadril, Eldadryl, Fenylhist, Fynex, Hydramine, Hydril, Insomnal, Noradryl, Nordryl, Nytol, Tusstat, Wehdryl
ibuprofen	Advil, Amersol, Apsifen, Brufen, Haltran, Medipren, Midol 200, Motrin, Neuvil, Novoprofen, Pamprin-IB, Rufen, Trendar

dozens of different trade names. To avoid this confusion, generic names should be used when naming the active ingredients in a combination drug. When referring to a drug, it is conventional to write the generic name in lower case first, followed by the trade name in parentheses with the first letter capitalized. Examples include alprazolam (Xanax) and acetaminophen (Tylenol).

1.7 Generic drugs are less expensive than brand-name drugs, but they may differ in bioavailability.

During the years of exclusivity for a new drug, the pharmaceutical company determines the price of the medication. Because there is no competition, the price is generally quite high. Once the exclusive rights end, competing companies market the generic equivalent drug for less money, and consumer savings may be considerable. In some states, pharmacists may routinely substitute a generic drug when the prescription calls for a brand name. In other states, the pharmacist must dispense drugs directly as written by a physician or obtain approval before providing a generic substitute.

PharmFACT

In 2007, the average cost of a generic drug was $34.34. In the same year, the average cost of a trade name drug was $119.51. *Source:* NACDS, 2007.

Pharmaceutical companies marketing brand-name drugs often lobby aggressively against laws that might restrict the routine use of certain brand-name drugs. The lobbyists claim that there are significant differences between a trade name drug and its generic equivalent, and that switching to the generic drug may be harmful for the patient. Consumer advocates on the other hand argue that generic substitutions should always be permitted because of the cost savings to patients.

Are there really significant differences between a brand-name drug and its generic equivalent? The answer is unclear. Despite the fact that the dosages may be identical, drug formulations are not always the same. The two drugs may have different inert ingredients. If in tablet form, the active ingredients may be more tightly compressed in one of the preparations. Liquid drugs may use different solvents such as water or alcohol.

The key to comparing brand-name drugs and their generic equivalents lies in measuring the bioavailability of the two agents. **Bioavailability** is defined by the Federal Food, Drug and Cosmetic Act (see Chapter 2) as the rate and extent to which the active ingredient is absorbed from a drug product and becomes available at the site of drug action to produce its effect. Bioavailability may be affected by many factors, including inert ingredients and tablet compression. Anything that affects the absorption of a drug or its travel to the target cells can certainly affect drug action. Measuring how long a drug takes to exert its effect (onset time) gives pharmacologists a crude measure of bioavailability. If the trade and generic products have the same rate of absorption and have the same onset of therapeutic action, they are said to be bioequivalent.

The importance of bioavailability differences between a trade name drug and its generic equivalent depend on the specific circumstances of pharmacotherapy. For example, if a patient is in circulatory shock and the generic equivalent drug takes 5 minutes longer to produce its effect, that may indeed be significant. However, if a generic medication for arthritis pain relief takes 45 minutes to act, compared to the brand-name drug that takes 40 minutes, it probably does not matter which drug is used, and the inexpensive product should be prescribed to provide cost savings to the consumer. As a general rule, bioavailability is of most concern when using critical care drugs and those with a narrow safety margin. In these cases, the patient should continue taking the brand name drug and *not* switch to a generic equivalent, unless approved by the health care provider. For most other drugs, the generic equivalent may be safely substituted for the trade name drug.

In the age of Internet pharmacies, the issue of exclusive marketing rights has drastically changed. Other countries are not bound to U.S. drug laws, and it is easy for patients to obtain brand-name drugs through the mail at a fraction of the U.S. cost For example, a pharmaceutical company may have exclusivity for selling Cialis in the United States but companies in India and China sell the identical drug through Internet pharmacies and ship it to customers in the United States. In some cases, they even sell the drug to consumers without a prescription. Other countries do not have the same quality control standards as the United States, and the patient may be purchasing a useless or even harmful product. Furthermore, although Internet sites may appear to be based in the United States, they may instead be obtaining their medications from unreliable sources. Nurses must strongly urge their patients not to purchase drugs from overseas pharmacies because there is no assurance that the drugs are safe or effective.

PharmFACT

The way Americans are filling their prescriptions is rapidly changing. While the number of total prescriptions dispensed increased 5% from 2003 to 2005, the number of prescriptions dispensed by mail order pharmacies increased 29% during this 2-year period. *Source:* NACDS, 2005.

Connecting Pharmacology to Clinical Nursing Practice

1.8 Pharmacology is intimately connected to nursing practice and is a key intervention in relieving and preventing human suffering.

The importance of pharmacology to nursing clinical practice cannot be overstated. As nursing students progress toward their chosen specialty, pharmacology is at the core of patient care and is integrated into the nursing process. The connection between pharmacology and clinical nursing practice is emphasized in Chapter 9, but it is integrated throughout this entire textbook. Indeed, pharmacology would not be an important science without its connections to nursing practice.

Whether administering medications or supervising drug use, the nurse is expected to understand the pharmacotherapeutic principles for all medications received by each patient. Given the large number of different drugs and the potential consequences of medication errors, this is indeed an enormous task. A major goal of this textbook is to prepare the nurse for the responsibilities of drug administration. Chapters 2 through 5 of this textbook provide the legal and scientific bases for pharmacotherapeutics. The nurse's responsibilities include knowledge and understanding of the following:

- What drug is ordered
  - Name (generic and trade) and drug classification
  - Intended or proposed use
  - Effects on the body
  - Contraindications
  - Special considerations, such as how age, weight, body fat distribution, and pathophysiologic states affect pharmacotherapeutic response
  - Expected and potential adverse events
- Why the drug has been prescribed for this particular patient
- How the drug is supplied by the pharmacy
- How the drug is to be administered, including dose ranges
- What nursing process considerations related to the drug apply to this patient

A major goal in studying pharmacology is to eliminate medication errors and to limit the number and severity of adverse drug events. Many adverse effects are preventable. Professional nurses can routinely avoid many serious adverse drug effects in their patients by applying their experience and knowledge of pharmacotherapeutics to clinical practice. Some adverse effects, however, are not preventable. It is vital that the nurse be prepared to recognize and respond to potential adverse effects of medications. The nursing management of adverse effects and medication errors are discussed in Chapters 6 and 7, respectively.

Before any drug is administered, the nurse must obtain and process pertinent information regarding the patient's medical history, physical assessment, disease processes, and learning needs and capabilities. Growth and developmental factors must always be considered. It is important to remember that a large number of variables influence a patient's response to drugs throughout the life span. Having a firm understanding of these variables can increase treatment success. Unit 2 of this textbook, Chapters 9 through 15, addresses these aspects of pharmacotherapy.

Despite its essential nature, the study of pharmacology should be viewed in proper perspective. Drugs are just one of many tools available to the nurse for preventing or treating human suffering. Although pharmacology is a key intervention in many cases, nurses must use all the healing sciences in treating their patients. The effectiveness of a drug in treating disease can never substitute for skilled, compassionate nursing care. Too much reliance on drug therapy can diminish the importance of the nurse–patient relationship.

UNDERSTANDING THE CHAPTER

Key Concepts Summary

1.1 The practice of applying products to relieve suffering has been recorded throughout history by virtually every culture.

1.2 Pharmacology is the study of medicines.

1.3 The perfect drug is safe and effective.

1.4 Drugs may be organized by their therapeutic classification or pharmacologic classification.

1.5 A prototype drug is the agent to which all other drugs in a class are compared.

1.6 Drugs have chemical, generic, and trade names.

1.7 Generic drugs are less expensive than brand-name drugs, but they may differ in bioavailability.

1.8 Pharmacology is intimately connected to nursing practice and is a key intervention in relieving and preventing human suffering.

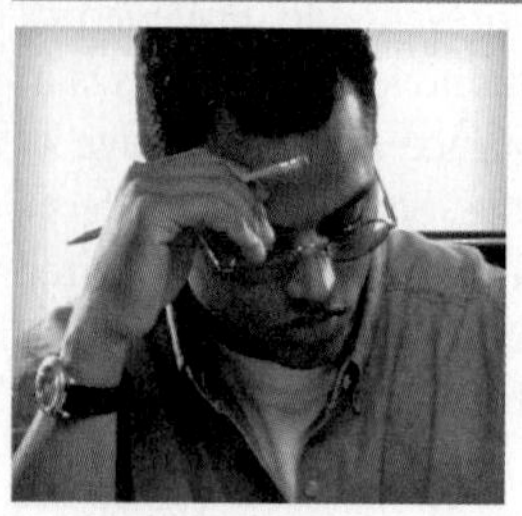

Making the PATIENT Connection

Remember the student "Josh Remming" at the beginning of the chapter? Now read the remainder of the case study. Based on the information presented within this chapter, respond to the critical thinking questions that follow.

Josh Remming, a 23-year-old student, is in his first semester of nursing school. He thought that nursing would provide him with a great career and lots of opportunity. He enjoys helping people and has always been fascinated with health care. However, after the first pharmacology class, Josh is worried because it seems like an overwhelming amount of content to learn in just one semester.

At the end of the class, Josh talks with other students who are concerned and a bit anxious. Much of the conversation centers around lecture content provided by the professor. Following are some of the questions from Josh's classmates. How would you respond?

Critical Thinking Questions

1. What is the difference between therapeutic classification and pharmacologic classification?
2. What classification is a barbiturate? macrolide? birth control pills? laxatives? folic acid antagonist? antianginal agent?
3. What is a prototype drug, and what advantages does a prototype approach to studying pharmacology offer?
4. Why do nurses need to know all this pharmacology?

Case Study

Sarah Hawkins, an elderly woman who lives on a fixed income, is on multiple medications. She says that all her friends are taking the generic form of their medication. While you are visiting her, she asks you, "What do you think of generic medicines? Are they safe? Are they as good? Are they worth it?"

1. How do generic equivalent drugs differ from a proprietary (trade name) drug?
2. What would you recommend that Sarah do about accepting generic drugs?

NCLEX-RN® Review

1 The nurse is using a drug handbook to determine the indications for the drug furosemide (Lasix). The term *indications* is defined as the:

1. Way a drug works on the target organs.
2. Amount of the drug to be administered.
3. Conditions for which a drug is approved.
4. Reason that the drug should not be given.

2 While completing the health history, the nurse asks the client, "What medications do you take regularly?" The nurse would expect the client to use which of the following drug names in providing the answer?

1. Chemical
2. Generic
3. Trade
4. Standard

3 When providing nursing care for the client, the nurse understands that drugs are:

1. One of many tools available to prevent or treat human suffering.
2. The most important part of the therapeutic treatment plan.
3. Primarily the concern of the health care provider and not included in nursing care.
4. Substances that should be relied on for health and wellness.

4 Which of the following client characteristics, if noted in the client's medical record, would the nurse consider important information that may affect the physiological response to various types of drug therapy? Select all that apply.

1. 82-year-old and female
2. Asian and obese
3. Past medical history of kidney disease
4. Mother and sister with diabetes
5. Has no medical insurance

5 When a drug has been absorbed, is available at the site of action, and produces its effect in the client, the nurse knows which process has occurred?

1. Biotransformation
2. Bioavailability
3. Bioengineering
4. Biochemistry

See Answers to Critical Thinking Questions, Case Study, and NCLEX-RN® Review in Appendix A.

References

Arias, D. (2005). Comparison of costs, safety and effectiveness of drugs now online: Consumers Union debuts "best buy drugs." *The Nation's Health, 35*(1), 1–8.

Gandey, A. (2007). Drug costs pushing companies to abandon promising therapies. *Medscape Medical News.* Retrieved March 14, 2008, from http://www.medscape.com/viewarticle/554048

Haas, J. S., Phillips, K. A., Gerstenberger, E. P., & Seger, A. C. (2005). Potential savings from substituting generic drugs for brand-name drugs: Medical expenditure panel survey, 1997–2000. *Annals of Internal Medicine, 142,* 891–897.

Kazmi, S. Z. (2007). Controversies in drug substitution. *Medscape Pharmacists.* Retrieved March 18, 2008, from http://www.medscape.com/viewarticle/563959

National Association of Chain Drug Stores. *Statistical data.* Retrieved October 27, 2008, from http://www.nacds.org

Openshaw, M. (2006). The economics of prescription drug prices, government intervention, and the importation of drugs from Canada. *Nursing Economic$, 23*(6), 307–311.

U.S. Food and Drug Administration (FDA). (2007). *Electronic orange book: Approved drug products with therapeutic equivalence evaluations* (27th ed.). Washington, DC: U.S. Department of Health and Human Services. Retrieved November 2, 2007, from http://www.fda.gov/cder/ob/default.htm

CHAPTER

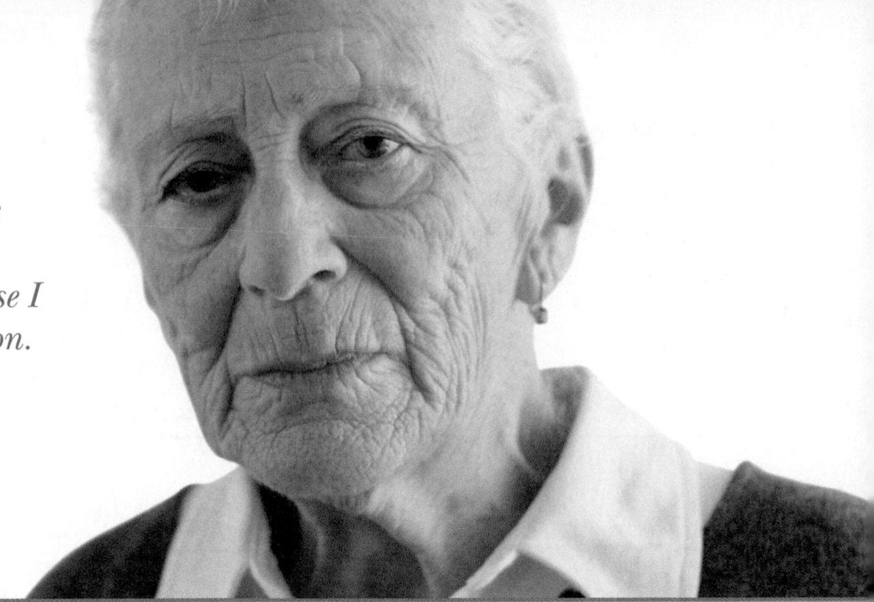

This headache medicine I bought at the grocery store must be safe because I didn't need a prescription.

Patient "Gertrude Stone"

2 Drug Regulations

Learning Outcomes

After reading this chapter, the student should be able to:

1. Explain the role of patent medicines in the history of pharmacology and the legislation of drugs.
2. Outline the key U.S. drug regulations and explain how each has ensured the safety and effectiveness of medications.
3. Describe how the *United States Pharmacopeia-National Formulary* (USP-NF) controls drug purity and standards.
4. Evaluate the role of the U.S. Food and Drug Administration in the drug approval process.
5. Categorize the four stages of new drug approval.
6. Explain the role of a placebo in new drug testing.
7. Discuss how recent changes to the approval process have increased the speed at which new drugs reach consumers.
8. Compare and contrast prescription and over-the-counter drugs.
9. Explain how scheduled drugs are classified and regulated.
10. Describe the Canadian drug approval process and identify similarities to how drugs are approved in the United States.

Chapter Outline

Patent Medicines

Brief History of Drug Legislation

Drug Standards

The U.S. Food and Drug Administration (FDA)

Drug Approval

Changes to the Drug Approval Process

Prescription and Over-the-Counter Drugs

Drug Schedules

Canadian Drug Standards

Key Terms

clinical phase trials, 17
controlled substance, 20
dependence, 20
formulary, 15
Investigational New Drug (IND), 17
New Drug Application (NDA), 18
orphan disease, 14
patent medicines, 13
pharmacopeia, 15
placebo, 18
postmarketing surveillance, 18
preclinical research, 17
scheduled drugs, 20
U.S. Food and Drug Administration (FDA), 16

Laws govern all aspects of the drug approval, labeling, marketing, manufacturing, and distribution process. The purpose of this legislation is to inform the public and to protect it from unsafe and ineffective products. This chapter examines standards and legislation regulating drugs in the United States and Canada.

Patent Medicines

2.1 Early American history saw the rise of patent medicines and the lack of adequate drug regulations.

People have an expectation that the drug they are taking is effective at treating their condition, whether it be asthma, diabetes, or a headache. They expect the label to contain clear and accurate instructions on how the product should be taken. They expect that the drug will be safe if the instructions are correctly followed. Are these reasonable assumptions? In the United States and Canada, the answer is yes. But Americans have not always had this reassurance. Although drugs have been used for thousands of years, it was not until the 20th century that extensive standards and regulations were developed to protect the public from unsafe and ineffective products.

In early America, there were few attempts to regulate drugs. This period saw the rise of **patent medicines.** Although the term *patent* implies a legal right to manufacture or sell a drug, this was not the case. Patent medicines contained a brand name that clearly identified the product, such as William Radam's Microbe Killer, Stanley's Snake Oil, Dr. Kilmer's Swamp Root, or Dr. Moore's Indian Root Pills. Because there were no laws to the contrary, these products claimed to cure just about any symptom or disease. Dr. William's Pink Pills for Pale People, which contained iron oxide and magnesium sulfate, claimed to cure rheumatism, nervous headache, palpitations, grippe, neuralgia, locomotor ataxia, partial paralysis, sallow complexion, and all forms of weakness in men or women. A typical advertisement from this era is shown in Figure 2.1.

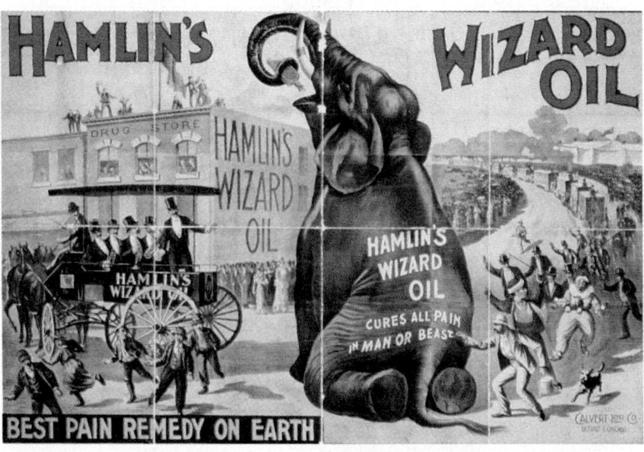

Figure 2.1 Patent medicines contained a name brand that clearly identified the product and claimed to cure just about any symptom or disease.

Source: © Calvert Litho Company/CORBIS. All Rights Reserved.

Patent medicines were often harmless (and ineffective), containing coloring, flavoring, and an aromatic substance that "smelled like medicine." At their worst, some contained hazardous levels of dangerous or addictive substances. In fact, cocaine, heroin, and morphine were freely distributed in patent medicines; some elixirs contained up to 50% morphine, which indeed caused many painful disorders to "disappear." Addictive ingredients were purposely added to guarantee repeat customers for their products. (Note the similarity with nicotine added to tobacco and caffeine added to soft drinks.) In the late 1800s, the familiar Coca-Cola soft drink was a patented beverage that contained an estimated 9 mg of cocaine per serving and was claimed to cure headache, dyspepsia, hysteria, morphine addiction, and impotence. The need for stricter regulation became more apparent in the 1860s as cocaine was synthesized, and the use of opiates as pain killers during the Civil War caused thousands of soldiers to become addicted.

Although the marketing and use of patent medicines may seem humorous and even unbelievable to modern consumers, a few of these products are still available over-the-counter (OTC). Examples of patent medicines that "survived" drug regulations of the 1900s include Smith Brothers Throat Drops, Fletcher's Castoria, Doan's Pills, Vick's VapoRub, and Phillip's Milk of Magnesia. Of course, the ingredients of these products have changed over time so that they conform to modern regulations regarding labeling, safety, and effectiveness.

Brief History of Drug Legislation

2.2 In the 1900s, drug legislation was enacted to make drugs safer and more effective.

Although individual states attempted to regulate drugs, the first national law was the Drug Importation Act, passed in 1848, which attempted to stop the entry of unsafe drugs into the United States. In the early 1900s, the United States began to develop and enforce tougher drug legislation to protect the public. This was, in part, spurred by the tragic deaths of 13 children in St. Louis in 1901 who were given diphtheria antitoxin that was contaminated with tetanus. In 1902, the Biologics Control Act was passed to standardize the quality of sera, antitoxins, and other blood-related products. Passed shortly thereafter, the Pure Food and Drug Act (PFDA) of 1906 was a significant and powerful piece of drug legislation that gave the government authority to control the labeling of medicines. Essentially, this law required that drug labels accurately reflect the contents. Prior to this date, many labels did not contain any indication of the active ingredient within the bottle or its amount.

Unfortunately, the PFDA did not address false therapeutic claims because although the ingredients had to be labeled accurately, a drug could still be marketed for any disease. In 1912, the Sherley Amendment to the PFDA prohibited the sale of drugs labeled with false therapeutic claims that were intended to defraud the consumer. A major weakness, as borne out in subsequent legal battles, was the difficulty in proving that the false claim made by the seller was intentional.

It is surprising that up to this point in American history there was no attempt to legislate the use of addictive drugs. The Harrison Narcotic Act of 1914 was passed to require prescriptions for high doses of narcotic drugs and to mandate that pharmacists and physicians keep narcotic records. Since 1914, hundreds of additional state and federal laws have been passed to regulate drugs with abuse potential, including the landmark Comprehensive Drug Abuse Prevention and Control Act (see Section 2.8). Additional details on the history of the regulation of controlled substances are included in Chapter 8.

Unfortunately there were still two essential components missing from the regulation of drugs in the early 20th century. Although the PFDA and other legislation required that ingredients be listed on the label and prohibited intentional false claims, manufacturers did not have to prove that the drug was effective. Furthermore, product safety did not have to be tested before the drug was marketed. Bringing the issue to the forefront was an incident in 1937 in which an elixir of sulfanilamide containing a poisonous chemical (diethylene glycol) killed 107 persons, mostly children.

In 1938, Congress passed the landmark Food, Drug, and Cosmetic Act (FDCA), which corrected certain loopholes in previous laws. This was the first law preventing the sale of newly developed drugs that had not been thoroughly tested for safety before marketing. Drug labels were required to contain instructions for safe use. The FDCA was also the first attempt at regulating cosmetics and medical devices. Unfortunately, the FDCA did not clearly define "prescription" or specify which drugs required a prescription. Most drugs, including many addictive and harmful substances, were sold by the corner druggist, sometimes legally, other times illegally. In 1951, the Durham-Humphrey Amendment to the FDCA delineated the difference between safer drugs, which may be sold OTC, and more dangerous drugs, which require prescriptions.

In the late 1950s, the drug thalidomide was found to produce severe birth defects in the children of women taking the drug as a sleeping pill and to treat morning sickness during pregnancy. Although the drug was not approved in the United States, it is estimated that over 20,000 Americans received the drug, because it was widely distributed to physicians without FDA approval. As with other drug legislation, it took a tragedy to convince Congress to pass tougher regulations. Passage of the Kefauver-Harris Amendment to the FDCA in 1962 mandated that manufacturers prove their drugs were effective for specific purposes, as well as safe, through the conduct of "adequate and well-controlled" studies. This law was applied retroactively to all drugs introduced since the passage of the FDCA. This amendment also required all significant adverse reactions to be reported to the FDA and that complete information about adverse effects be included in literature distributed to health care providers. For the first time, informed consent was required from patients participating in experimental drug research.

The emphasis on effectiveness continued as the FDA contracted with the National Academy of Sciences and the National Research Council in 1966 to evaluate the effectiveness of 4,000 drugs that were approved between 1938 and 1962 based only on their safety. Approximately 40% of all drugs introduced between 1938 and 1962 were found to be ineffective and were subsequently removed from the market. In 1972, a review of OTC drugs began to examine the safety and effectiveness of these products.

In the 1980s, the public placed considerable political pressure on the FDA to find drugs to treat rare or unusual disorders. Pharmaceutical companies were reluctant to develop drugs for these disorders because there would not be enough sales to recoup their research and development costs. To encourage development of such drugs, the Orphan Drug Act became law in 1983. An **orphan disease** is defined as a serious, though rare, disease that affects less than 200,000 people in the United States. With the passage of this legislation, drug manufacturers are now offered development grants, tax credits for clinical investigation expenses, and 7 years of exclusivity to market an orphan drug. Over 700 medications have been approved as orphan drugs since the passage of this act.

A major focus in the 1990s was to speed the drug approval process, which could be prolonged for many years. The Prescription Drug User Fee Act (PDUFA) of 1992 assessed fees from drug manufacturers to be used specifically for reducing the review time for new drug applications. From 1992 to 2002, the fees collected exceeded a billion dollars and the number of full-time equivalent employees examining new drug applications at the FDA increased from 1,277 to 2,337. The PDUFA was reauthorized in 1997 with the passage of the Food and Drug Administration Modernization Act, which also included provisions to accelerate the review of medical devices, regulate the advertising of unapproved uses of drugs, and regulate health claims for foods.

In reaction to the rising popularity of dietary supplements, Congress passed the Dietary Supplement Health and Education Act of 1994 to control misleading industry claims. Due in part to intense lobbying from the dietary supplement industry, the regulation of these products remains less stringent than prescription or OTC drugs. The regulation of herbal products and dietary supplements is discussed in detail in Chapter 15.

In early 2000, the focus of drug regulation turned to access. Advocacy groups claimed that the high cost of drugs caused unequal access to adequate health care for the poor, the uninsured/underinsured, and the elderly. After lengthy debate, the Medicare Prescription Drug Improvement and Modernization Act of 2003 was passed. This legislation provides for a standard benefit that pays 75% of prescription drug spending up to the first $2,250. Those qualifying for the low-income criteria may have their premiums and cost subsidized by the government. Participants are protected against catastrophic costs at $3,600 per year with most beneficiaries paying a 5% co-pay amount. A brief time line of major events in U.S. drug regulation is shown in Table 2.1.

TABLE 2.1 Historical Time Line of Regulatory Acts, Standards, and Organizations

Year	Regulatory Acts, Standards, and Organizations
1820	Physicians establish the first comprehensive publication of drug standards, the *United States Pharmacopeia* (USP).
1848	The Drug Importation Act requires that all drugs (as defined by the newly established pharmacopeia) entering the United States be inspected and analyzed for "quality, purity, and fitness for medical purposes."
1852	Pharmacists found the American Pharmaceutical Association (APhA). The APhA establishes the *National Formulary* (NF), a standardized publication focusing on pharmaceutical ingredients. The USP continues to catalog all drug-related substances and products.
1862	The Federal Bureau of Chemistry, established under the administration of President Lincoln, eventually becomes the Food and Drug Administration (FDA).
1902	The Biologics Control Act controls the quality of sera and other blood-related products.
1906	The Pure Food and Drug Act prohibits the manufacture and sale of adulterated or misbranded foods, drugs, and medications.
1912	The Sherley Amendment makes medicines safer by prohibiting the sale of drugs labeled with false therapeutic claims.
1914	The Harrison Narcotics Act requires those who dispensed opium, cocaine, and related substances to keep records of the drugs they dispensed and makes it illegal to possess narcotics without a prescription. This act allows physicians to prescribe narcotics only for treatment, not to addicts.
1938	The Food, Drug, and Cosmetic Act is the first law preventing the marketing of drugs not thoroughly tested.
1944	The Public Health Service Act is enacted and covers many health issues, including biologic products and the control of communicable diseases.
1970	The Comprehensive Drug Abuse Prevention and Control Act (also known as the Controlled Substance Act) organizes regulated drugs (including opiates, cocaine, cannabis, stimulants, depressants, and hallucinogens) into five schedules and imposed restrictions and penalties.
1975	The *United States Pharmacopeia* and *National Formulary* become a single standardized publication, the USP-NF.
1986	The Anti-Drug Abuse Act increases sentences and imposes mandatory minimum sentences for those convicted of illegal drug activity based on the type and quantity of drug involved.
1986	The Childhood Vaccine Act authorizes the FDA to acquire information about patients taking vaccines, to recall biologics, and to recommend civil penalties if guidelines regarding biologic use were not followed.
1988	The FDA officially establishes as an agency of the U.S. Department of Health and Human Services.
1992	The Prescription Drug User Fee Act requires that nongeneric drug and biologic manufacturers pay fees to be used for improvements in the drug review process.
1994	The Dietary Supplement Health and Education Act requires clear labeling of dietary supplements and gives the FDA the power to remove supplements that cause a significant public risk.
1997	The FDA Modernization Act reauthorizes the Prescription Drug User Fee Act, representing the largest reform effort of the drug review process since 1938.
2002	The Best Pharmaceuticals for Children Act improves safety and efficacy medicines for children and continues the exclusivity provisions for pediatric drugs as mandated under the Food and Drug Administration Modernization Act of 1997.
2003	The Medicare Prescription Drug Improvement and Modernization Act provides seniors and those with disabilities a prescription drug benefit and better benefits under Medicare.

Drug Standards

2.3 The standardization of drug purity and strength is specified by the *United States Pharmacopeia-National Formulary*.

Until the 1800s, drugs were prepared from plants that were available in the natural environment. The strength and purity of the products varied considerably because they were entirely dependent on the experience (and integrity) of the druggist preparing the product and the quality of the local ingredients. Potency and safety varied from region to region and, indeed, from batch to batch. Consider the simple analogy of baking. If 100 people across the world were asked to bake a loaf of bread, the final products would vary considerably in size, taste, and nutritional value. It is likely that no two loaves would be the same. It is obvious that a standard recipe must be followed. Similarly, to obtain consistency in the preparation and potency of drugs, standards (recipes) are needed.

Among the first standards used by pharmacists was the **formulary,** or list of pharmaceutical products and drug recipes. In the United States, the first comprehensive publication of drug standards, the *United States Pharmacopeia (USP)*, was established in 1820. A **pharmacopeia** is a medical reference summarizing standards of drug purity, strength, and directions for synthesis. From 1852 until 1975, two major compendia maintained drug standards in the United States, the USP and the *National Formulary (NF)*, which were established by the

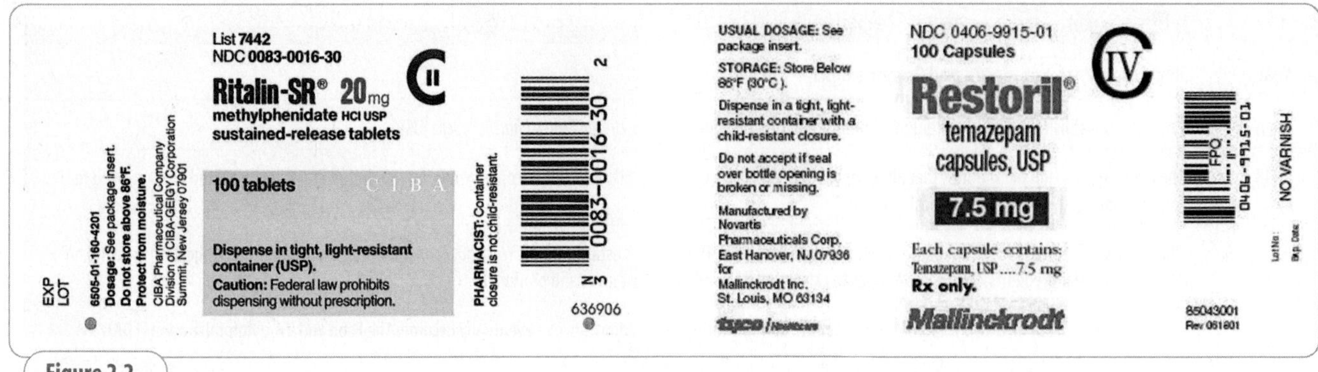

Figure 2.2

Examples of USP labels.

Source: (left) Copyright Novartis Pharmaceuticals Corporation. Reprinted with permission.

American Pharmaceutical Association (APhA). All drug products were covered in the USP, whereas the NF focused on nondrug ingredients. In 1975, the two were merged into a single publication named the *United States Pharmacopeia-National Formulary (USP-NF).* The current document consists of about 2,400 pages and contains 3,777 drug monographs in more than 164 chapters. The USP-NF is published annually, with two supplements being issued throughout the year. Today, the USP label can be found on many medications verifying the purity and exact amounts of ingredients found within the container. Drugs marketed in the United States must conform to USP-NF standards to avoid possible charges of adulteration and misbranding. Sample labels are illustrated in Figure 2.2. The USP also provides a voluntary program for verifying the label accuracy of dietary supplements (see Chapter 15).

The U.S. Food and Drug Administration (FDA)

2.4 The regulatory agency responsible for ensuring that drugs and medical devices are safe and effective is the Food and Drug Administration.

The establishment of a regulatory agency for food and drugs in the United States began with a single chemist appointed by President Lincoln in 1862. The **U.S. Food and Drug Administration (FDA)** was established by the PFDA of 1906 and later expanded to carry out the provisions of the FDCA of 1938. It is one of the oldest drug regulatory agencies in the world. The FDA states its mission as follows:

- Protecting the public health by assuring the safety, efficacy, and security of human and veterinary drugs, biological products, medical devices, the nation's food supply, cosmetics, and products that emit radiation
- Advancing the public health by helping to speed innovations that make medicines and foods more effective, safer, and more affordable
- Helping the public get the accurate, science-based information they need to use medicines and foods to improve their health

With such an important and vast mission, the FDA is organized around six branches, as shown in Figure 2.3. The Center for Drug Evaluation and Research (CDER) states its mission as facilitating the availability of safe, effective drugs; keeping unsafe or ineffective drugs off the market; improving the health of Americans; and providing clear, easily understandable drug information for safe and effective use. All new drugs must be approved by the CDER before they can be marketed. This includes prescription drugs, OTC drugs, and all generic equivalents. After marketing, the CDER is responsible for continued monitoring of safety and may issue additional warnings to health care providers or consumers as additional information becomes available.

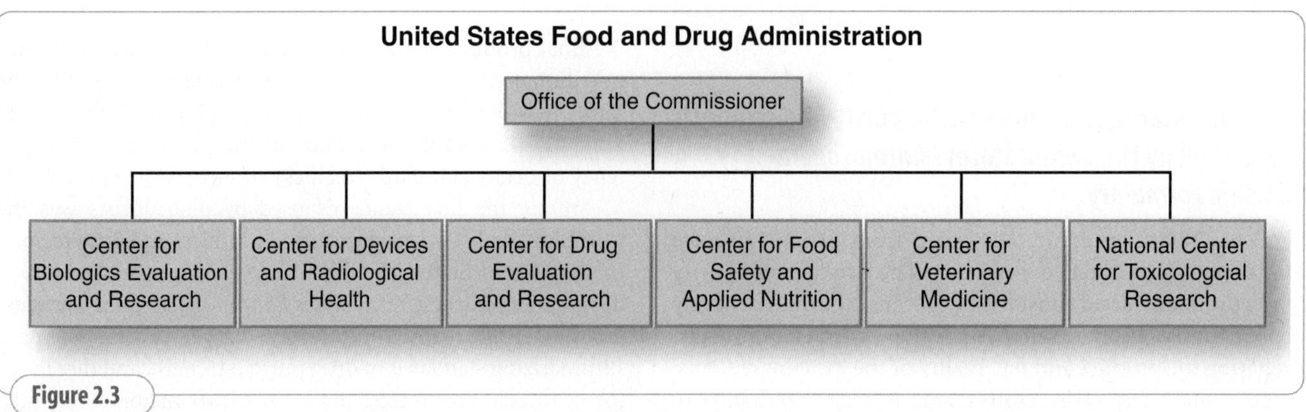

Figure 2.3

Organization of the Food and Drug Administration showing the six centers that regulate human and veterinary drugs, biologic products, medical devices, the nation's food supply, cosmetics, and products that emit radiation.

The Center for Biologics Evaluation and Research (CBER) regulates the use of biologics, including sera, vaccines, and blood products. One historical achievement involving biologics is the 1986 Childhood Vaccine Act. This act authorizes the FDA to acquire information about patients taking vaccines, to recall biologics, and to recommend civil penalties if guidelines regarding biologics are not followed. The mission of the CBER was recently expanded to include the regulation of gene therapy and treatment with human cells or tissue-based products.

The FDA also oversees the administration of herbal products, dietary supplements, and cosmetics through the Center for Food Safety and Applied Nutrition (CFSAN). Although it does not require testing of herbal or dietary supplements prior to marketing, the CFSAN is responsible for taking action against any supplement that is deemed to be unsafe.

The CFSAN also regulates cosmetics, which are legally defined by the FDCA of 1938 as "articles intended to be rubbed, poured, sprinkled, or sprayed on, introduced into, or otherwise applied to the human body . . . for cleansing, beautifying, promoting attractiveness, or altering the appearance." Examples of products considered cosmetics are skin moisturizers, perfumes, lipsticks, fingernail polishes, eye and facial makeup preparations, shampoos, toothpastes, and deodorants. Can a product be both a cosmetic and a drug? In most cases, cosmetics are not drugs; however, it depends on a product's intended use. For example, if a shampoo is marketed to treat a condition such as dandruff, the active ingredient is considered a drug. If a skin cream claims to provide sunscreen protection, it may be considered a drug. Cosmetics do not require approval by the CFSAN prior to marketing, and regulations are much less restrictive compared to drug approval. Manufacturers of cosmetics are generally careful not to promote unwarranted therapeutic claims, such as that a product prevents or treats a condition or disease. This would cause the product to be considered a drug by the FDA, and it would be subject to tighter regulations.

Drug Approval

2.5 The drug approval process established by the Food and Drug Administration ensures that drugs sold in the United States are safe and effective.

Drugs are discovered in any number of ways. Penicillin was discovered purely by accident while the scientist was studying an unrelated topic. Many drugs have been isolated from natural substances, including plants and bacteria. Some drugs are "me too" drugs, whereby the pharmacologist simply took a well-known drug and slightly modified the chemical structure to produce a very similar agent. As molecular biology and genetics have progressed into the modern era, drugs have been purposefully designed to fit into specific receptor sites on enzymes or cells.

Regardless of the path to discovery, all drugs must be approved by the FDA before they can be sold in the United States. The FDA drug review and approval process follows a well-developed and organized plan, summarized in Figure 2.4.

The first stage of drug development is **preclinical research,** which involves extensive laboratory testing by the pharmaceutical company. Scientists perform testing on human and microbial cells cultured in the laboratory. Studies are performed in several species of animals to examine the drug's effectiveness at different doses and to look for adverse effects. The goals of this extensive testing on cultured cells and in animals are to determine drug action and to predict whether the drug will cause harm to humans. Because laboratory tests do not accurately reflect the precise way the human body will respond to the drug, preclinical research results are always inconclusive. Most drugs do not proceed past the preclinical research stage because they are either too toxic or simply not effective. The FDA does not regulate preclinical testing.

If a drug appears promising, the pharmaceutical company submits an **Investigational New Drug (IND)** application to the FDA that contains all the animal and cell testing data. Scientists at the FDA study the data and must be convinced that the drug is safe enough to allow human testing. Approval from the FDA is necessary before the next stage can begin.

Clinical investigation, the second stage of drug testing, takes place in three different stages termed **clinical phase trials.** These clinical trials are the longest part of the drug approval process and occur in sequential stages.

- Phase 1: Testing is conducted on 20 to 80 healthy volunteers for several months to determine proper dosage and to assess for adverse effects. The focus of phase 1 trial is on safety. If unacceptable levels of toxicity are noted, the clinical trials are stopped.
- Phase 2: Several hundred patients with the disease to be treated are given the drug. The primary focus of the phase 2 trial is on effectiveness, although safety data continue to be recorded. In most cases, the effectiveness of the new drug is

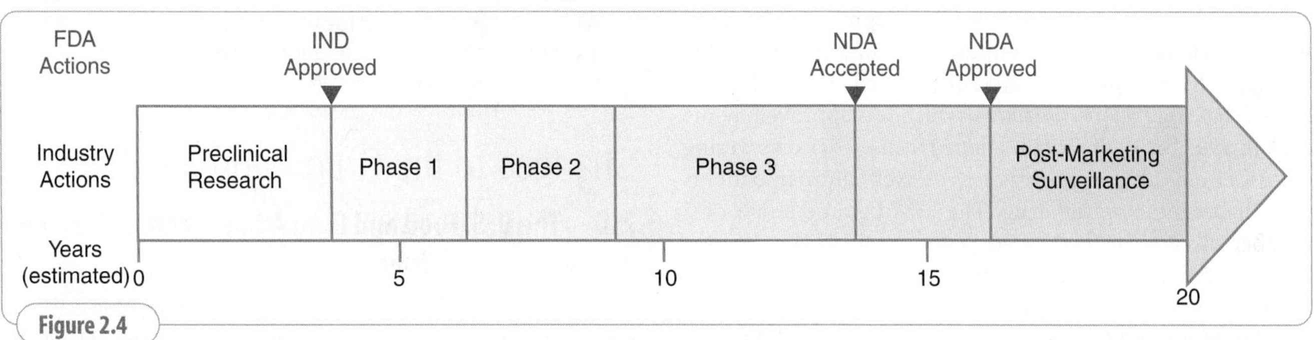

Figure 2.4

Drug development time line.

compared to an inert substance, or **placebo,** which serves as a control "nontreatment" group. In other cases the new drug is compared to a standard drug used for the same condition. For example, a new drug for reducing fever may be compared to acetaminophen (Tylenol). If the new drug is found to have the same (or less) effectiveness and safety profile compared to the standard drug, the pharmaceutical company may stop the clinical trials. This phase may take several years.

- Phase 3: Large numbers of patients with the disease are given the drug to determine patient variability. Potential drug–drug interactions are examined. Patients with chronic conditions such as cardiac, renal, or hepatic impairment are given the drug to determine safety in these important populations. Assessment of effectiveness and safety continues for several years and thousands of patients may be given the new drug during phase 3.

If the drug continues to show promise through the clinical phase trials, a **New Drug Application (NDA)** is submitted to the FDA. The NDA signals that the pharmaceutical company is ready to sell the new drug. During the NDA review, the FDA examines all the preclinical and clinical data to assess whether the proposed new drug is safe and effective. By law, the CDER is obligated to act on at least 90% of the NDAs for standard drugs within 10 months of submission. For priority drugs, the benchmark is 6 months. If the NDA is approved, the manufacturer may begin selling the new drug. If the NDA is rejected, the FDA indicates whether the drug is "approvable" or "not approvable." "Approvable" means that the drug will likely be approved if the pharmaceutical company conducts additional testing or addresses specific issues identified by the FDA. A designation of "not approvable" indicates that the drug has significant barriers to approval. **Postmarketing surveillance,** stage 4 of the drug approval process, begins after the NDA review has been completed. The purpose of stage 4 testing is to survey for harmful drug effects in a larger population. Some adverse effects are very subtle, take longer to appear, and are not identified until a drug is prescribed for large numbers of people. Adverse drug reactions are reported by the manufacturers, health care providers, and patients to the Adverse Event Reporting System (AERS), a computerized database designed to support the FDA's postmarketing surveillance program.

The FDA holds public meetings annually to receive comments from patients, professional organizations, and pharmaceutical companies regarding the effectiveness and safety of new drug therapies. If the FDA discovers a serious problem, it will mandate that a drug be withdrawn from the market. One example of successful postmarketing surveillance is the diabetes drug troglitazone (Rezulin), which was approved by the FDA in 1997. In 1998, Britain banned its use after discovering at least one death and several cases of liver failure in patients with diabetes taking the drug. The FDA became aware of a number of cases in the United States in which Rezulin was linked with liver failure. Consumer advocates also claimed that the drug caused several cases of heart failure. Rezulin was recalled in March 2000 after health professionals asked the FDA to reconsider its therapeutic benefits versus its identified risks. The FDA withdrew 11 prescription drugs from the market from 1997 to 2000.

There are several important limitations to the drug approval process. Historically, drug trials have used Caucasian males as their test population. Because there may be gender and racial differences in how drugs are handled by the body, data obtained during clinical trials may not be representative of the population as a whole. Pharmaceutical companies are now including a more diverse population in their clinical trials. Most drugs have not been tested in children: Pediatric doses and responses are often based on experience rather than research data. Although clinical trials test drugs in pregnant laboratory animals and examine for possible birth defects, these data may not be representative of how drugs affect pregnant women or their fetuses. Finally, adverse effects may occur at such a low level that they are statistically insignificant in clinical trials using a few thousand patients. Several million patients may need to take the drug before these effects can be identified.

Another limitation of the drug approval process relates to off-label uses. When a new drug is tested by a pharmaceutical company it is for a specific indication; FDA approval is based on this indication. After several years of clinical experience, however, health care providers may find that the drug is also useful for indications not approved by the FDA. Once initially approved by the FDA for any indication, health care providers may prescribe the drug for other indications they feel appropriate, despite the fact that the drug was never tested or approved for these additional conditions. How widespread is off-label prescribing? It is estimated that over 20% of prescriptions are for indications not approved by the FDA. The use of off-label drugs is particularly prevalent in treating cancer and in pediatric patients. Although the FDA does not regulate off-label uses of drugs, laws prohibit pharmaceutical companies from advertising or promoting their drugs for off-label uses. It has not been clearly established whether or not off-label prescriptions increase risks to patients.

PharmFACT

It takes about 12 years of research and development before a drug is submitted to the FDA for review.

Source: Drug Information Online.

CONNECTION *Checkpoint* 2.1

In 2003, aprepitant (Emend), an antiemetic, and enfuvirtide (Fuzeon), an antiretroviral, were approved. Which of these is a therapeutic classification? Which is a pharmacologic classification? See Answer to Connection Checkpoint 2.1 in Appendix A.

Changes to the Drug Approval Process

2.6 The U. S. Food and Drug Administration has sped up the process of drug review.

The process of synthesizing a new drug and testing it in cells, experimental animals, and humans takes many years. The NDA can include dozens of volumes of experimental and clinical data that must be examined during the FDA drug review process. Some NDAs contain over 100,000 pages of data. Even after all experiments have been concluded and clinical data have been gathered, the FDA review process can take several years.

Expenses associated with development of a new drug can cost the drug developer millions of dollars. Recent studies estimate the cost of bringing a new drug to market at over $802 million. Pharmaceutical companies are often critical of the regulatory process and are anxious to get the drug marketed to recoup their high research and development expenses. The public is also anxious to receive new medications, particularly for diseases that have a high mortality rate. Although the criticisms of government regulatory agencies are certainly understandable, and sometimes justified, the fundamental priority of the FDA is to ensure the safety of medications. Without an exhaustive review of scientific data, the public could be exposed to dangerous or ineffective drugs.

In the early 1990s, due to pressures from organized consumer groups and various drug manufacturers, government officials began to plan how to speed up the drug review process. Reasons identified for the delay in the FDA drug approval process included outdated guidelines, poor communication, and not enough staff to handle the workload.

In 1992, the PDUFA was passed, requiring drug and biologic manufacturers to provide yearly product user fees. This added income allowed the FDA to hire more employees and to restructure its organization to more efficiently handle the processing of a greater number of drug applications. The result of restructuring was a resounding success. The average NDA review time for new medications approved in 2002 was 12.5 months: less than half the time it took for approval in the early 1990s. Although the approval time has decreased, the actual number of new drugs approved each year has declined from 110 (1996–1999) to 58 (2002–2004), a 47% decline.

As part of the FDA modernization, priority drugs now receive accelerated approval. These are drugs intended to treat serious and life-threatening conditions such as cancer and AIDS, that lack effective treatments. In some cases, the FDA may grant accelerated approval before the drug has completed phase 3 trials. The FDA usually requires the pharmaceutical company to file subsequent reports confirming the effectiveness of the drug.

Pharm*FACT*

For every 5,000 chemicals that enter preclinical testing, only 5 make it to human testing. Of these five potential drugs, only one is finally approved. *Source:* NIH, 2003.

Prescription and Over-the-Counter Drugs

2.7 Over-the-counter drugs are usually safe and effective when used according to label instructions.

The 1951 Durham-Humphrey Amendment to the FDCA clearly established the difference between prescription and OTC drugs. In order to obtain a prescription drug, an order must be given authorizing the patient to receive the medication. Prescription medications are judged by the FDA to be potentially addictive or too harmful for self-administration. In some cases, they are used to treat conditions too complex for self-diagnosis by the consumer or the drug may require a skilled nurse or health care provider to administer.

The advantages of requiring a prescription are numerous. The health care provider has an opportunity to examine the patient and determine a specific diagnosis. The prescriber can maximize therapy by ordering the proper drug for the patient's condition and by controlling the amount and frequency of the drug to be dispensed. In addition, the health care provider has an opportunity to teach the patient proper use of the drug and its expected adverse effects.

In contrast to prescription drugs, OTC drugs do not require an order from a health care provider. In most cases, patients may treat themselves safely if they carefully follow instructions included with the medication. A key point to remember is that no drug is without risk; if patients do not follow the guidelines on the label, serious adverse effects may result.

Patients prefer to take OTC medications for many reasons. OTC drugs may be obtained more easily than prescription drugs. No appointment with a health care provider is required, thus saving time and money. Without the assistance of a health care provider, however, choosing the proper medication for a specific problem can be challenging for a patient. OTC drugs may interact with foods, herbal products, prescription drugs, or other OTC drugs. Patients may not be aware that some OTC medications can impair their ability to function safely. Self-treatment is sometimes ineffective, and the potential for harm may increase if the disease is allowed to progress.

During the past decade, consumer groups have pushed for the reclassification of certain drugs from prescription to OTC in cases whereby a high margin of safety exists with the medicines. For example, prior to 1996, substances that were used to assist in smoking cessation, such as nicotine patches and gum, were available by prescription only but are now available OTC. Other recent switches from prescription to OTC include famotidine (Pepcid AC), cimetidine (Tagamet HB), omeprazole (Prilosec), cetirizine (Zyrtec), and loratadine (Claritin). Over the past 20 years, 700 products have been changed from prescription to OTC. The decision to reclassify a drug may be initiated by the manufacturer or mandated by the FDA during its review process.

Herbal products and dietary supplements are also widely available OTC. Herbal products and dietary supplements are not considered drugs; they are not marketed to treat any disease and they are not subject to the same regulatory process as drugs. Some of these products can, however, cause adverse effects and interact with medications. Nurses should always inquire about their patients' use of herbal products and dietary supplements and caution them that the FDA has not tested these products for effectiveness or safety. In some cases, herbal products are contraindicated. For example,

St. John's wort should not be taken concurrently with antidepressant medications.

PharmFACT

Some OTC drugs are taken in large amounts, sometimes by teens, to get "high." An estimated 12,584 emergency department visits (0.7% of all drug-related emergency department visits) involved pharmaceuticals containing dextromethorphan, a drug found in cold and flu products. *Source:* Drug Abuse Warning Network, 2006.

Drug Schedules

2.8 Drugs with a potential for abuse are categorized into schedules.

Dependence is a powerful physiological or psychological need for a substance. Some drugs are frequently abused or have a high potential for dependence; thus the selling and distribution of these drugs are highly restricted. Drugs that have a significant potential for abuse are placed into five categories called schedules. These **scheduled drugs** are classified and regulated according to their potential for abuse. Concepts of dependence and drug schedules are discussed in detail in Chapter 8.

In the United States, **controlled substances** are drugs whose use is restricted by the Comprehensive Drug Abuse Prevention and Control Act of 1970 and its later revisions. Hospitals and pharmacies must register with the Drug Enforcement Administration (DEA) and use their registration numbers to purchase scheduled drugs. They must maintain complete records of all quantities purchased and sold. Drugs with the highest abuse potential have additional restrictions. For example, providers must use a special order form to obtain Schedule II drugs, and orders must be written and signed by the provider. Telephone orders to a pharmacy are not permitted. Refills for Schedule II drugs are not permitted; patients must visit their doctor first. Health providers convicted of unlawful manufacturing, distributing, and dispensing of controlled substances face severe penalties.

CONNECTION *Checkpoint* 2.2

Once a new drug is approved, it is assigned names. What are the two basic types of drug names and who assigns them? See Answer to Connection Checkpoint 2.2 in Appendix A.

Canadian Drug Standards

2.9 Canadian regulations ensure safe and effective drug use in the provinces and territories.

There are many similarities between how drugs are regulated in Canada and in the United States. In Canada, as in the United States, drug testing and risk assessment are major priorities. The steps in the Canadian drug approval process are shown in Table 2.2.

Health Canada is the federal department working in partnership with provincial and territorial governments. The Health Products and Food Branch (HPFB) of Health Canada is responsible for ensuring that health products and foods approved for sale to Canadians are safe and of high quality. The HPFB regulates the use of therapeutic products through directorates. The Therapeutic Products Directorate (TPD) authorizes marketing of a pharmaceutical drug or medical device, once a manufacturer presents sufficient scientific evidence of the product's safety, efficacy, and quality as required by the Food and Drugs Act and Regulations. The Biologics and Genetic Therapies Directorate (BGTD) regulates biologic drugs (drugs derived from living sources) and radiopharmaceuticals. Products regulated by the BGTD include blood products, vaccines, tissues, organs, and gene therapy products. The Natural Health Products Directorate (NHPD) is the regulating authority for natural health products for sale in Canada.

The Canadian Food and Drugs Act is an important regulatory document specifying that drugs cannot be marketed without a Notice of Compliance (NOC) and Drug Identification Number (DIN) from Health Canada. Foods, drugs, cosmetics, and therapeutic devices must follow established guidelines for approval. Any drug that does not comply with standards established by recognized pharmacopeias and formularies in the United States, Europe, Britain, or France cannot be labeled, packaged, sold, or advertised in Canada.

TABLE 2.2 Steps of Approval for Drugs Marketed Within Canada

Step 1	Preclinical studies or experiments in culture, living tissue, and small animals are performed, followed by extensive clinical trials or testing done on humans.
Step 2	A drug company completes a drug submission to Health Canada. This report details important safety and effectiveness information, including testing data, how the drug product will be produced and packaged, and expected therapeutic benefits and adverse reactions.
Step 3	A committee of drug experts, including medical and drug scientists, reviews the drug submission to identify potential benefits and drug risks.
Step 4	Health Canada reviews information about the drug product and passes on important details to health providers and consumers.
Step 5	Health Canada issues a Notice of Compliance (NOC) and Drug Identification Number (DIN). Both permit the manufacturer to market the drug product.
Step 6	Health Canada monitors the effectiveness of the drug and any concerns after it has been marketed. This is done by regular inspection, notices, newsletters, and feedback from consumers and health care providers.

UNDERSTANDING THE CHAPTER

Key Concepts Summary

2.1 Early American history saw the rise of patent medicines and the lack of adequate drug regulations.

2.2 In the 1900s, drug legislation was enacted to make drugs safer and more effective.

2.3 The standardization of drug purity and strength is specified by the *United States Pharmacopeia-National Formulary.*

2.4 The regulatory agency responsible for ensuring that drugs and medical devices are safe and effective is the Food and Drug Administration.

2.5 The drug approval process established by the Food and Drug Administration ensures that drugs sold in the United States are safe and effective.

2.6 The U.S. Food and Drug Administration has sped up the process of drug review.

2.7 Over-the-counter drugs are usually safe and effective when used according to label instructions.

2.8 Drugs with a potential for abuse are categorized into schedules.

2.9 Canadian regulations ensure safe and effective drug use in the provinces and territories.

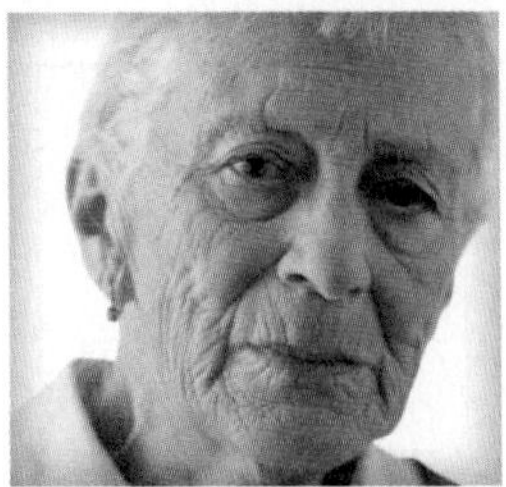

Making the PATIENT *Connection*

Remember the patient "Gertrude Stone" at the beginning of the chapter? Now read the remainder of the case study. Based on the information presented within this chapter, respond to the critical thinking questions that follow.

Gertrude Stone lives alone in the same house she has owned for 46 years. Although she is seldom sick, when she needs to see a health care provider she must ride the public bus system. The trip requires two bus transfers and can be tiring.

Because Gertrude lives only one block from a grocery store, she often self-medicates using over-the-counter (OTC) drugs. She strongly believes in the use of herbs, vitamins, and home remedies.

As a parish nurse, you assist with the health fair at a church where Gertrude is an active member.

Critical Thinking Questions

1. How would you respond to Gertrude about the danger of OTC drugs?
2. What are the advantages and disadvantages of OTC medications?
3. How can Gertrude be certain that OTC medications are safe for her?

Case Study

Your 12-year-old nephew is preparing a report for school about the Food and Drug Administration (FDA) and the drug approval process. You, the nurse in the family, are often called on by family members to answer questions about anything health related. Below are his questions. How would you respond?

1. What is the role of the FDA?
2. What role does the FDA play in regulating herbal and dietary supplements?
3. How quickly can a new drug be approved by the FDA?

NCLEX-RN® Review

1 The nurse knows that governmental drug legislation requires the drug manufacturer to prove that a drug is both safe and:

1. Free of adverse effects and potential reactions.
2. Effective for a specified purpose.
3. Reasonable in cost and easily accessible.
4. Beneficial to various population groups.

2 The drug research participant has been prescribed a placebo as part of an investigative study to examine the effects of a new drug. Which of the following responses would the nurse expect from the client about the drug's response?

1. "Since taking this drug, I now experience a decrease in the symptoms."
2. "Although I am taking the drug, I am not experiencing any type of response."
3. "The symptoms are worsening since I started taking this drug."
4. "I am experiencing additional symptoms since I started taking this drug."

3 When considering various drug therapies, the nurse knows that most drug testing and approval occurs with which of the following populations?

1. Multiple population types and is usually safe for all clients
2. Caucasian males and may not be safe for other populations
3. The elderly, and may be harmful to children and adolescents
4. Animals, which verifies the drug's effectiveness in humans

4 The client requests that a refill prescription of a class II controlled substance be telephoned to the drug store. When responding to the client, the nurse would consider which factor? Refill of class II drugs:

1. Are less costly than the original prescription.
2. Must be listened to by at least two people.
3. Are verified through the local DEA office.
4. Are not permitted under federal law.

5 The nurse knows that drugs that are subject to stricter regulations are those:

1. With a high potential for abuse or dependency.
2. That are most costly and difficult to produce.
3. With adverse effects and high occurrence of drug or food interactions.
4. That have taken years to prove efficiency in the laboratory.

See Answers to Critical Thinking Questions, Case Study, and NCLEX-RN® Review in Appendix A.

References

Berndt, E. R., Gottschalk, A., Philipson, T., & Strobeck, M.W. (2004). *Assessing the impacts of the Prescription Drug User Fee Acts (PDUFA) on the FDA approval process* (NBER Working Paper No. W10822). Retrieved April 10, 2008, from http://ssrn.com/abstract=603642

Dickson, M., & Gagnon, J. P. (2004). Key factors in the rising cost of new drug discovery and development. *Nature Reviews Drug Discovery, 3*(5), 417–429.

DiMasi, J. A., Hansen, R. W., & Grabowski, H. G. (2003). The price of innovation: New estimates of drug development costs. *Journal of Health Economics, 22*(2), 151–185.

Drug Abuse Warning Network. (2006). Emergency department visits involving dextromethorphan. *The New Dawn Report, 32.* Retrieved August 12, 2008, from http://dawninfo.samhsa.gov/files/TNDR10DXMforHTML.pdf

Drug Information Online. Retrieved March 18, 2008, from http://www.drugs.com

Markel, H. (2005). Why America needs a strong FDA. *Journal of the American Medical Association, 294*, 2489–2491.

NIH: Moving research from the bench to the bedside. Hearing before the Subcommittee on Health of the Committee on Energy and Commerce House of Representatives 108th Cong., First Session, July 10, 2003. Retrieved March 18, 2008, from http://energycommerce.house.gov/reparchives/108/Hearings/07102003hearing990/print.htm

Radley, D. C., Finkelstein, S. N., & Stafford, R. S. (2006). Off-label prescribing among office-based physicians. *Archives of Internal Medicine, 166*, 1021–1026.

Roberts, T. G., & Chabner, B. A. (2004). Beyond fast track for drug approvals. *New England Journal of Medicine, 351*, 501–505.

Wood, A. J. (2006). A proposal for radical changes in the drug-approval process. *New England Journal of Medicine, 355*, 618–623.

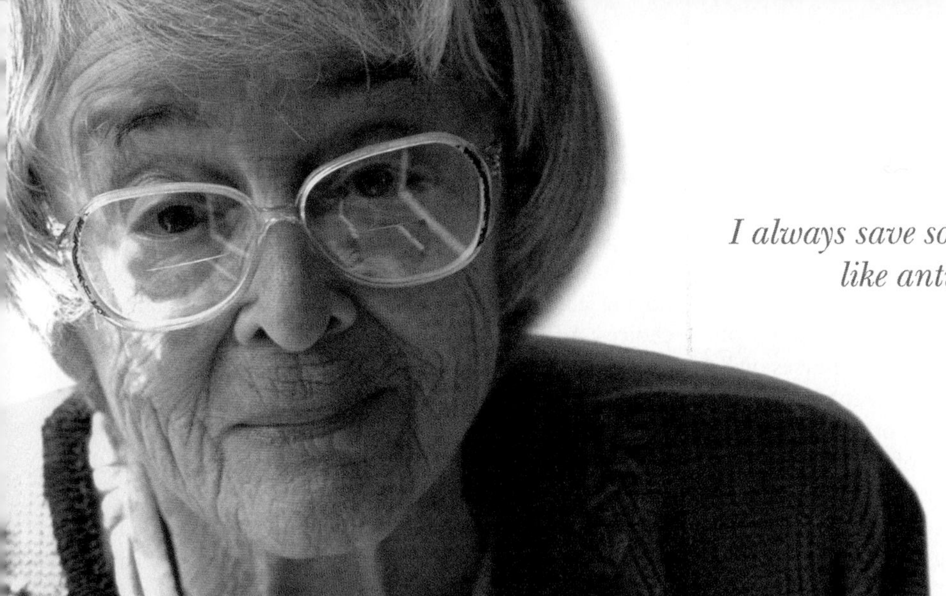

I always save some of my medicines like antibiotics, just in case I need them later.

Patient "Lavenia Deberry"

CHAPTER 3

Principles of Drug Administration

Chapter Outline

Drug Administration and Patient Adherence

Drug Storage and Expiration Dates

Prescription Writing

Dosing Intervals

Measurement of Drug Doses

Documenting Drug Administration

Routes of Drug Administration

Learning Outcomes

After reading this chapter, the student should be able to:

1. Outline a plan for improving patient adherence to the medication regimen.
2. Describe how the storage of drugs can affect their effectiveness.
3. Describe the components of a legal prescription and the abbreviations associated with drug orders.
4. Relate the importance of dosing schedules to successful pharmacotherapeutic outcomes.
5. Compare and contrast the three systems of measurement used in pharmacology.
6. Explain the importance of properly documenting medication administration.
7. Compare and contrast enteral, topical, and parenteral drug administration.

Key Terms

adherence, *24*
apothecary system of measurement, *28*
enteral route, *28*
enteric-coated, *29*
expiration date, *25*
extended release, *29*
household system of measurement, *28*
medication administration record (MAR), *28*
metric system of measurement, *27*
rectal route, *34*
topical route, *31*
transdermal patches, *32*
troches, *29*
vaginal route, *33*

The primary role of the nurse in drug administration is to ensure that medications are taken in a safe manner according to the instructions of the prescriber or as indicated on the label. In the course of drug administration, nurses will collaborate closely with physicians, pharmacists, and other health care providers, and, of course, their patients. The purpose of this chapter is to introduce fundamental principles relating to drug administration that will help nurses to deliver medications safely and effectively.

Drug Administration and Patient Adherence

3.1 Achieving patient adherence with pharmacotherapy is a major challenge for the nurse.

In a hospital setting, the pharmacist, nurse, and physician collaborate to ensure that the patient is receiving the correct drug in the manner designated by the prescriber. In the home setting, the focus shifts to self-administration of medications by the patient. For prescription drugs, health care providers provide the patients with verbal and written instructions on how and when to take the medication. For over-the-counter (OTC) medications, herbal products, and dietary supplements, labels clearly indicate the correct way to take the agent.

Adherence is a major factor affecting pharmacotherapeutic outcomes. As it relates to pharmacotherapy, **adherence** or compliance is defined as taking medications in the manner prescribed by the health care provider. In the case of OTC products, adherence means correctly following the instructions on the label. Patient nonadherence (noncompliance) ranges from not taking the medication at all to taking it at the wrong time or at the wrong dose. Research has confirmed that nonadherence is a major problem in health care, affecting 50% to 75% of patients, and that it is responsible for a significant number of unnecessary hospitalizations and deaths. Studies suggest that about half of all prescriptions never get filled by the patient. Of those that are picked up, about 50% are not taken correctly.

Pharm*FACT*
Patient nonadherence is estimated to cause 125,000 deaths in the United States each year. *Source:* Smith, 2004.

Many factors can influence patient adherence with pharmacotherapy. One of the most common sources of nonadherence is simply forgetting a dose of medication, which occurs frequently when the drug must be taken more than twice daily. Another source of nonadherence is that the drug may be too expensive or not approved by the patient's health insurance plan. Patients often discontinue the use of drugs that have annoying adverse effects or those that impair major lifestyle choices. Adverse effects that often prompt nonadherence are headache, dizziness, nausea, diarrhea, and impotence. About 50% of patients with a chronic disease who must take a drug for a prolonged period have serious problems with adherence that interfere with their ability to obtain optimum clinical benefit (Dunbar-Jacob et al., 2000).

Patients often take medications in an unexpected manner, sometimes "self-adjusting" their doses. Some feel that if one tablet is good, two must be better. Others believe that they will become dependent on the medication if it is taken as prescribed; thus they only take half the necessary dose. Still others simply stop taking the medication when they start feeling better. Patients are usually reluctant to admit or report nonadherence to the nurse for fear of being reprimanded or feeling embarrassed. Because reasons for nonadherence are many and varied, the nurse must be vigilant in questioning patients about taking their medications. When pharmacotherapy fails to produce the expected treatment outcomes, nonadherence should always be considered as a possible explanation.

There are steps that the nurse can take to increase the potential for patient adherence to the therapeutic regimen. All of these steps focus on effective teaching. Before administering a drug, the nursing process should be used to formulate a personalized care plan that will best enable the patient to become an active participant in the treatment (see Chapter 9). This allows the patient to better understand and accept the recommended course of pharmacotherapy based on accurate information that is presented in a manner that addresses individual learning styles in terms that the patient can understand.

In the plan of care, it is important to address essential information that the patient must know regarding the prescribed medications. This includes factors such as the name of the medication, why it has been ordered, expected drug actions, associated adverse effects, and information regarding interactions with other medications, foods, herbal supplements, or alcohol. Patients need to be reminded that they share an active role in ensuring the effectiveness of their medication and their own safety.

For patients receiving outpatient therapy or those being released from a hospital, the nurse must carefully assess the patients' ability to dispense their medications in a safe and effective manner. If the nurse believes that a patient may have difficulty in properly administering the medications, caregivers should be consulted and other arrangements made to ensure that the patient receives the correct drugs using the proper dosing schedule. During follow-up visits, the nurse should reinforce this drug education and assess whether the patient is taking or receiving the drugs correctly. Special considerations related to drug administration to pediatric and geriatric patients are presented in greater detail in Chapters 11 and 12, respectively.

It is imperative to remember that, unless diagnosed as mentally incompetent, a well-informed adult always has the legal option of refusal to take any medication. It is the nurse's re-

CONNECTIONS

Lifespan Considerations Challenges of Pediatric Medication Administration

Administering medication to infants and young children requires special knowledge and techniques. Nurses must have knowledge of growth and developmental patterns and be certain that the prescribed dosages match each child's age and weight.

Children, like adults, want to have choices and control over decisions. Whenever possible, give children a choice of the use of a spoon, cup, dropper, or syringe. Approach children with a matter-of-fact attitude and avoid any dishonesty or threats. Allow time and give medications in a calm environment. Depending on a child's age, oral medications may need to be crushed so that the child can swallow them. Sometimes mixing medications with jelly, honey, flavored syrup, or fruit puree can make their taste more palatable for children. One caution is to avoid mixing medications with needed nutrients or foods such as milk or fruit juice because it may cause some children to dislike these foods in the future.

When children get upset or a medication is distasteful, nausea can be averted by allowing sips of cold carbonated beverages or drinks poured over crushed ice. Offer children crackers or dry cereal before medication administration. Encourage cooperation with praise or a reward system suited to the children's ages and interests.

sponsibility, however, to ensure that the patient has all the necessary information to make an informed decision.

Drug Storage and Expiration Dates

3.2 Drugs should be stored properly and never used past their expiration date.

Drugs, like most chemicals, degrade over time. As they deteriorate, drugs tend to lose their potency and their ability to produce a therapeutic effect. All drugs are packaged with an **expiration date,** which is an approximation as to when the medications will begin to lose their effectiveness. Drugs do not totally lose their effectiveness or become toxic immediately upon expiration. A large study conducted by the U.S. Food and Drug Administration (FDA) regarding expiration dates examined the potency of over 100 prescription and OTC drugs being stored by the military. The results showed that 90% of them were safe and effective even when 15 years past their expiration date.

Although it is likely that drugs retain some effectiveness beyond their expiration date, the nurse should never administer outdated medications. In clinical agencies, nurses and pharmacists rotate their drug stocks so that drugs are less likely to pass their expiration date.

A large number of storage factors can influence drug effectiveness. Some general principles are:

- Temperature. Most drugs should be stored at room temperature because high temperatures encourage faster degradation of the drugs. Some medications require lower temperatures and must be refrigerated or frozen. Drugs should always be administered at room temperature unless otherwise specified by the prescriber.
- Light. Because some chemicals are degraded by exposure to light, medications should be stored in cabinets away from direct light. Light-sensitive drugs are often supplied in amber-colored containers to prevent light entry. Some drugs are so light sensitive that their containers must be covered with foil during an intravenous (IV) infusion.
- Moisture and air. Drugs sometimes interact with atmospheric gases or with water vapor; thus they should be stored with tightly capped lids. Storage in areas with high humidity will enhance deterioration.

Scheduled drugs are stored in narcotics lockers or boxes. Access to these substances is restricted to protect these drugs from theft or misuse. These boxes have special locks and the drugs have additional recording and reporting requirements.

Nurses should become familiar with the specific colors and smells of each medication, because improper storage can sometimes cause changes in the physical characteristics of drugs. A change in color of a liquid drug could indicate contamination or loss of effectiveness. Likewise, for solid drugs, unusual odors, colors, or textures are a cause for concern. Nurses should never administer a drug that appears different from normal without checking with the pharmacist, even if it is within its expiration period. The old adage "when in doubt, throw it out" applies to medicines.

The nurse should teach patients to discard the drugs in their homes that are past their expiration date. Patients tend to keep drugs long past their usefulness, usually in bathroom medicine cabinets. This is an especially dangerous habit in households with small children and is responsible for a large number of accidental poisonings each year. In addition, unused controlled substances are targets for thieves or may be used for intentional overdoses in patients with suicidal ideation. Drugs should always be disposed of properly, as listed in Table 3.1.

Prescription Writing

3.3 Prescriptions must be clearly written and include a heading, a body, and a closing.

An order for a prescription drug follows a standard format, which is designed to ensure that the correct drug is taken by the right patient in the prescribed dose. Each state has specific requirements for what must be included on a legal prescription. Although there are different methods of describing a prescription, all formats must include the following three elements, as shown in Figure 3.1.

- Heading
- Body
- Closing

At the top of a prescription, the heading includes the prescriber's name, address, and phone number. This information is essential, should the pharmacist need to contact the prescriber for questions about the drug order. The patient's name,

TABLE 3.1 Federal Guidelines for Drug Disposal

Take unused, unneeded, or expired prescription drugs out of their original containers and throw them in the trash.	
Mixing prescription drugs with an undesirable substance, such as used coffee grounds or kitty litter, and putting them in impermeable, nondescript containers, such as empty cans or sealable bags, will further ensure that the drugs are not diverted.	
Take advantage of community pharmaceutical take-back programs that allow the public to bring unused drugs to a central location for proper disposal. Some communities have pharmaceutical take-back programs or community solid-waste programs that allow the public to bring unused drugs to a central location for proper disposal. Where these exist, they are a good way to dispose of unused pharmaceuticals.	
Flush prescription drugs down the toilet only if the label or accompanying patient information specifically instructs doing so. The FDA advises that the following drugs be flushed down the toilet instead of thrown in the trash.	
Actiq (fentanyl citrate)	Tequin Tablets (gatifloxacin)
Daytrana Transdermal Patch (methylphenidate)	Zerit for Oral Solution (stavudine)
Duragesic Transdermal System (fentanyl)	Meperidine HCl Tablets
OxyContin Tablets (oxycodone)	Percocet (oxycodone and acetaminophen)
Avinza Capsules (morphine sulfate)	Xyrem (sodium oxybate)
Baraclude Tablets (entecavir)	Fentora (fentanyl buccal tablet)
Reyataz Capsules (atazanavir sulfate)	

Note: Patients should always refer to printed material accompanying their medication for specific instructions.

Note: From "Proper Disposal of Prescription Drugs: Federal Guidelines," n.d., Drug Facts: Office of National Drug Control Policy Guidelines. Retrieved April 18, 2008, from http://www.whitehousedrugpolicy.gov/drugfact/factsht/proper_disposal.html

and sometimes the phone number and address, are required. The prescription is always dated. Pharmacies have policies that allow them to refuse a prescription if the order is more than a few months old.

The body of the prescription includes the drug name, dosage, and amount to be dispensed. Tablets or capsules usually include the # symbol, which indicates the number to be dispensed. The body also includes patient instructions on the label, including how and when to take the drug. Abbreviations are usually used when prescribing drugs. Common abbreviations associated with medication administration are shown in Table 3.2. Certain abbreviations are to be avoided because they have been shown to cause frequent medication errors (see Chapter 7).

The most important feature of the closing of a prescription is the prescriber's signature. A Drug Enforcement Administration (DEA) number is required if the prescription is for a controlled substance. The closing may also include blanks or boxes, which indicate the number of refills permitted and whether a generic equivalent may be substituted.

Name Jane Cleary Age 36

Address 3376 W. 141st St., Scottsdale Date Nov 1, 2009

This prescription will be filled generically unless physician signs on line stating "Dispense as written."

℞

Tetracycline 250 mg PO

Disp. #30

Sig. 1 qid take on an empty stomach

F. March

Dispense as Written — Substitution Permissible

Frances March, M.D. 120 Madison Road Scottsdale, NY

DEA # ER639524 Ph. No. 685-9533

Figure 3.1

Sample prescription.

PharmFACT

From 1997 to 2007, the number of prescriptions purchased increased 72% (from 2.2 billion to 3.8 billion), compared to a U.S. population growth of only 11%. The average number of prescriptions per capita increased from 8.9 to 12.6. *Source:* Henry J. Kaiser Family Foundation, 2008.

CONNECTION *Checkpoint* 3.1

From what you learned in Chapter 2, explain why patients often prefer to take OTC drugs over prescription medications. See Answer to Connection Checkpoint 3.1 in Appendix A.

Dosing Intervals

3.4 For maximum effectiveness, drugs must be administered at the proper dosing intervals.

Drugs are administered by a dosing schedule that is largely determined by the physical and biologic characteristics of the

TABLE 3.2 Medication Administration Abbreviations

Abbreviation	Meaning
ac	before meals
ad lib	as desired/as directed
AM	morning
bid	twice per day
cap	capsule
gtt	drop
h or hr	hour
IM	intramuscular
IV	intravenous
no	number
pc	after meals; after eating
PO	by mouth
PM	afternoon
prn	when needed/necessary
q	every
qh	every hour
qid	four times per day
q2h	every 2 hours
q4h	every 4 hours
q6h	every 6 hours
q8h	every 8 hours
q12h	every 12 hours
Rx	take
STAT	immediately; at once
tab	tablet
tid	three times per day

Note: The Institute for Safe Medication Practices recommends that the following abbreviations be avoided because they can lead to medication errors: qd: instead use "daily" or "every day"; qhs: instead use "nightly"; qod: instead use "every other day."

drug. As a general rule, drugs that remain longer in the body are administered less frequently than those that are quickly metabolized or eliminated by the body. Normal dosing intervals for oral drugs range from one to four times daily. For the past 20 years, the trend has been to develop drugs that require less frequent dosing because it is more convenient to take a drug once daily and adherence is increased. Patients tend to forget doses when they must be taken more than twice daily, which leads to lower and less consistent levels of the drug in the bloodstream. Dosing intervals are very important to pharmacotherapy and are discussed in detail in Chapters 4 and 5.

In the hospital setting, drugs are often administered at specific times of the day, set by agency protocol, that are convenient for the patient and nurse. Some drugs are administered at specific times because this improves their effectiveness or reduces the risk of adverse effects. For example, if a drug causes stomach upset it is often administered with meals in order to reduce epigastric pain, nausea, or vomiting. Certain other medications should be administered between meals because food interferes with their absorption. Some central nervous system (CNS) drugs and antihypertensives are best taken at bedtime, because they may cause daytime drowsiness. Drugs such as sildenafil (Viagra) are unique in that they should be taken 30 to 60 minutes prior to expected sexual intercourse in order to achieve an effective erection. Patients must be taught the importance of proper dose scheduling to enhance the potential for therapeutic success.

Some medications are given only once or by irregular scheduling. For example, a "stat" order refers to a medication that is needed immediately, usually because of an emergency or life-threatening situation. Although not as urgent, an "ASAP" (as soon as possible) order should be available for administration to the patient within 30 minutes of the written order. A "prn" order (Latin: *pro re nata*) is administered as required by the patient's condition. The nurse makes the judgment, based on patient assessment, as to when such a medication is to be administered. The prescriber may qualify the time frame of prn orders. For example, prn q4h would direct the nurse to administer the drug only once every 4 hours.

When self-administering medications, it is not unusual for a patient to forget a dose. This is especially true for patients taking multiple prescription drugs and those who have some degree of mental impairment. In most cases, taking a missed dose several hours late will not affect the outcomes of pharmacotherapy; thus patients should be urged to take their medication as soon as they discover the error. Some drugs, however, have a more rigid dosing schedule and forgetting a dose can result in serious effects. For example, taking multiple doses of the anticoagulant warfarin (Coumadin) too close together can cause bleeding. If the patient discovers a missed dose at a time very close to when the next dose is to be taken, the patient should skip the missed dose. Patients should be reminded never to take a double dose (or skip a dose), unless advised by their health care provider. Some drugs, such as oral contraceptives, come with very specific patient instructions on the procedure to follow if a dose is missed.

Measurement of Drug Doses

3.5 The primary system of measurement used in pharmacology is the metric system.

Every OTC drug label and prescription must indicate the dose to be administered. Dosages are labeled and dispensed according to their weight (for solid drugs) or volume (for liquid drugs). Three systems of measurement are used in pharmacology: metric, household, and apothecary. Although health care providers and pharmacies primarily use the metric system, the apothecary and household systems are still encountered. Until the metric system totally replaces these other systems, the nurse must recognize dosages based on all three systems of measurement. Approximate equivalents between metric, household, and apothecary units of volume and weight are listed in Table 3.3.

By far, the most common system of drug measurement in pharmacology uses the **metric system of measurement.** The

TABLE 3.3 Metric, Apothecary, and Household Approximate Measurement Equivalents

Metric	Apothecary	Household
1 mL	15–16 minims	15–16 drops
4–5 mL	1 fluid dram	1 teaspoon or 60 drops
15–16 mL	4 fluid drams	1 tablespoon or 3–4 teaspoons
30–32 mL	8 fluid drams or 1 fluid ounce	2 tablespoons
240–250 mL	8 fluid ounces (1/2 pint)	1 glass or cup
500 mL	1 pint	2 glasses or 2 cups
1 L	32 fluid ounces or 1 quart	4 glasses or 4 cups or 1 quart
1 mg	1/60 grain	—
60–64 mg	1 grain	—
300–325 mg	5 grains	—
1 g	15–16 grains	—
1 kg	—	2.2 pounds

Note: To convert grains to grams, divide grains by 15 or 16. To convert grams to grains, multiply grams by 15 or 16. To convert minims to milliliters, divide minims by 15 or 16.

volume of a medication is expressed in terms of the liter (L) or milliliter (mL). The cubic centimeter (cc) is a common measurement of volume that is equivalent to 1 milliliter of fluid. Although cc is commonly used in clinical practice, it should be noted that mL is preferred because it results in fewer medical errors (see Table 3.2). The metric weight of a drug is stated in terms of kilograms (kg), grams (g), milligrams (mg), or micrograms (mcg or μg). Although scientists use the symbol μ for "micro," it is strongly recommended that mcg be used in prescription writing: When poorly written (as many prescriptions are), the symbol μ can be misinterpreted as "m" and cause medication errors.

Although not used very frequently in the health care setting, the **household system of measurement** is familiar to most Americans. Because patients understand the teaspoon, tablespoon, and cup, it is important for the nurse to be able to convert between the household and metric systems of measurement. For example, an 8-ounce glass of water is 240 mL (cc). If a patient being discharged is ordered to drink 2,400 mL of fluid per day, the nurse may instruct the patient to drink 10, 8-ounce glasses or 10 cups of fluid per day. Likewise, when a child is to be given a drug that is administered in elixir form, the nurse should explain that 5 mL of the drug is the same as 1 teaspoon. The nurse should encourage the use of accurate medical dosing devices at home, such as oral dosing syringes, oral droppers, cylindrical spoons, and medication cups. These are preferred over the traditional household measuring spoon because they are more accurate. Eating utensils that are commonly referred to as teaspoons or tablespoons often do not hold the volume that their names imply.

The **apothecary system of measurement** was developed in ancient Greece. The system became popular in England in the 1600s and came to America with the colonists. In early U.S. history, apothecaries performed many of the same duties as physicians, including preparing and administering drugs, and performing medical procedures, including surgery. Until the 1970s, apothecary units were still widely used when measuring pharmaceuticals. The basic unit, the grain (gr), was defined as the weight of one grain of wheat. It is now rare to find the apothecary system in use, although occasionally an aspirin tablet is referred to as being 5 grains (325 mg).

Dosage calculation is a skill used less frequently today than in previous times. In many cases, doses are packaged by the pharmacy for unit dispensing, making dosage calculations unnecessary. Doses of solid drugs are often ordered in multiples of the prescribed dose, such as 1 or 2 pills per dose. The most complex dosage calculations, flow rates for IV medications, are simplified by the use of modern delivery devices.

The fact that dosage calculations are less commonly performed does not decrease their importance to the nurse or patient. Errors in simple calculations can have devastating consequences for the patient and bring litigation against the nurse. The nurse is responsible for checking that the dose packaged by the pharmacy is correct.

Documenting Drug Administration

3.6 Medication administration should be properly recorded as soon as possible after the drug is administered.

Once a drug is administered, the nurse must correctly document on the **medication administration record (MAR)** that it has been given to the patient. Delay in documentation could result in a second dose being administered. It is not permissible to document medication before it is administered, because an emergency or other distraction could result in the medication not being distributed. Because the patient's chart is a medicolegal document, any errors, falsifications, or omissions in documenting drug administration could have legal consequences.

It is necessary to include on the MAR the drug's name, dosage, time administered, any assessments related to drug administration, and the nurse's signature. Drugs that are refused or omitted must be recorded on the appropriate form within the MAR. It is customary to document the reason for the nonmedication whenever possible. Patient concerns or complaints about the drug are also included. Documentation includes the signature or initials of the nurse who administered the drug.

Routes of Drug Administration

The three broad categories of routes of drug administration are enteral, topical, and parenteral. Each route has characteristics that offer both advantages and disadvantages. Whereas some drugs are formulated to be given by several routes, others are specific to only one route. Pharmacokinetic considerations, such as how the route of administration affects drug absorption and distribution, are discussed in Chapter 4. Certain general protocols and techniques common to all methods of drug administration are shown in Table 3.4.

3.7 Enteral drugs are administered by the oral route or through gastrostomy or nasogastric tubes.

The **enteral route** includes drugs delivered to the gastrointestinal (GI) tract, either orally or through nasogastric or gas-

TABLE 3.4 General Drug Administration Guidelines
Verify the medication order for accuracy.
Check the allergy history on the chart.
Identify any conditions that may result in a change in dosage, such as cardiac, renal, or hepatic impairment or potential drug–drug interactions. Notify the prescriber of any discrepancies.
Wash hands and apply gloves, if indicated (e.g., parenteral, rectal, vaginal routes).
Use aseptic technique when preparing and administering parenteral medications.
Identify the patient by asking the person to state his or her full name (or by asking the parent or guardian), checking the identification band, and comparing this information with the MAR.
Ask the patient about known allergies.
Inform the patient of the name of the drug, the expected actions and adverse effects, and how it will be administered.
Position the patient for the appropriate route of administration.
For enteral drugs, assist the patient to a sitting position.
If the drug is prepackaged (unit dose), remove it from the packaging at the bedside when possible.
Unless specifically instructed to do so in the orders, do not leave drugs at the bedside.
Document the medication administration and any pertinent patient responses on the MAR.
Evaluate the patient's response to the drug, reporting any adverse effects.

trostomy tubes. Oral medication administration is the most common, most convenient, and usually the least costly of all routes. It is also considered the safest route because the skin barrier is not compromised. In cases of overdose, drugs remaining in the stomach can be retrieved by inducing vomiting or by pumping out the stomach contents.

Most medications administered by the enteral route are intended for absorption to the general circulation, taking advantage of the combined absorptive surfaces of the oral mucosa, stomach, and small intestine. A few enteral medications are administered for local effects, such as infections of the GI tract. Oral preparations are available in tablet, capsule, and liquid forms.

Tablets and Capsules

Tablets and capsules are the most common forms of oral medications. Most patients prefer tablets or capsules because of their ease of use. In some cases, tablets may be scored, allowing for one-half or one-quarter dosing.

The strongly acidic stomach contents can present a destructive obstacle to some medications. To overcome this barrier, tablets may have a hard, waxy coating that enables them to resist acidity. These **enteric-coated** tablets are designed to dissolve in the alkaline environment of the small intestine. Some drugs are enteric coated because the agents will irritate the stomach mucosa if they are dissolved in the stomach.

Studies have clearly demonstrated that patient adherence declines as the number of doses per day increases. **Extended release** (XR, XL) tablets or capsules are designed to dissolve very slowly, resulting in a longer duration of action for the medication. Also called long-acting (LA) or sustained release (SR) medications, these forms allow for the convenience of once or twice a day dosing.

Some patients, particularly children, have difficulty swallowing tablets and capsules. Crushing tablets or opening capsules and sprinkling the medication over food or mixing it with juice may make the drug more palatable and easier to swallow. The nurse should not crush tablets or open capsules, however, unless the manufacturer specifically states this is permissible. The following type of drugs should not be chewed, crushed, or opened:

- **Extended release formulations.** These drugs contain a higher amount of medication that is intended to be released over an extended period. Opening the capsule or crushing the tablet will release the entire drug immediately, possibly resulting in a toxic effect.
- **Enteric-coated drugs.** When crushed or opened, these drugs are exposed to stomach acid, which may destroy them. In addition, the drugs may irritate the stomach mucosa and cause nausea or vomiting.
- **Oral cavity effects.** Drugs that have a bitter taste are often coated with a very thin layer of glucose or inert material to mask their taste. If crushed or opened, the bitter taste is experienced. Other drugs stain the teeth or cause an anesthetic-like effect on the tongue if crushed and exposed to the oral cavity. In addition, some drugs irritate the oral mucosa.

Selected drugs that should not be crushed are shown in Table 3.5. The student should refer to a current drug guide for a more comprehensive list.

As an alternative to crushing, some drugs are available in liquid form for patients who have difficulty swallowing tablets or capsules. Liquid forms include elixirs, syrups, and suspensions. Liquid drugs are usually heavily flavored and sweetened to mask their bitter taste. A few drugs are formulated as disintegrating tablets, lozenges, or **troches,** which are allowed to slowly dissolve in the mouth. Most patients are familiar with OTC throat lozenges, which are used to dampen a cough or ease a sore throat. One of the most common prescription troches is clotrimazole (Mycelex Troche), a drug for treating fungal infections of the oral cavity. The nurse should teach patients to allow the troche to slowly dissolve and not to swallow it whole.

Tablets, liquids, and capsules have certain disadvantages. The patient must be conscious and able to swallow properly. Certain types of drugs, including proteins such as insulin, are inactivated by the digestive enzymes in the stomach and small intestine. Furthermore, drugs absorbed from the stomach and small intestine first travel to the liver, where they may be inactivated before they ever reach their target organs—a process called first-pass metabolism (see Chapter 4). There is also significant variation among patients in the motility of the GI tract and in its ability to absorb medications. In addition, children and some adults have an aversion to swallowing large tablets and capsules or to taking oral medications that taste bad.

TABLE 3.5 Selected Drugs That Should Not Be Crushed or Opened

Trade Name	Generic Name	Dosage Form	Comments
Accutane	isotretinoin	Capsule	Mucous membrane irritant
Adalat CC	nifedipine	Tablet	Sustained release
Adderall XR	amphetamine	Capsule	Sustained release
Ambien CR	zolpidem	Tablet	Controlled release
Augmentin XR	amoxicillin	Tablet	Sustained release
Bayer Caplet	aspirin, enteric coated	Caplet	Enteric coated
Bisacodyl	bisacodyl	Tablet	Enteric coated
Calan SR	verapamil	Tablet	Sustained release
Cardizem LA, Cardizem CD, Cardizem SR	diltiazem	Tablet Capsule Tablet	Sustained release; capsules may be opened and contents taken without chewing or crushing
Cipro XR	ciprofloxacin	Tablet	Sustained release
Compazine Spansule	prochlorperazine	Capsule	Sustained release; capsules may be opened and contents taken without chewing or crushing
Cotazym S	pancrelipase	Capsule	Enteric coated; capsules may be opened and contents taken without chewing or crushing
Covera-HS	verapamil	Tablet	Sustained release
Cymbalta	duloxetine	Capsule	Sustained release
Depakene	valproic acid	Capsule	Sustained release; mucous membrane irritant
Depakote ER	valproate	Tablet	Sustained release
Dilacor XR	diltiazem	Capsule	Sustained release
Dilatate SR	isosorbide dinitrate	Capsule	Sustained release
Ecotrin	aspirin	Tablet	Enteric coated
Eryc	erythromycin	Capsule	Enteric coated; capsules may be opened and contents taken without chewing or crushing
Eskalith CR	lithium	Tablet	Sustained release
Feosol	ferrous sulfate	Tablet	Enteric coated
Glucotrol XL	glyburide	Tablet	Sustained release
Inderal LA	propranolol	Capsule	Sustained release
Indocin SR	indomethacin	Capsule	Sustained release; capsules may be opened and contents taken without chewing or crushing
Isoptin SR	verapamil	Tablet	Sustained release
Isosorbide dinitrate SR	isosorbide dinitrate	Tablet	Sustained release
Kaon CL, Klor-Con, Klotrix, K-Tab, Slow-K	potassium chloride	Tablet	Sustained release
Morphine sulfate extended release	morphine	Tablet	Sustained release
Nexium	esomeprazole	Capsule	Sustained release
Nicotinic acid	niacin	Tablet, capsule	Sustained release
Nitrostat	nitroglycerin	Tablet	Sublingual
OxyContin	oxycodone	Tablet	Sustained release
Pancrease	pancrelipase	Capsule	Enteric coated
Plendil	felodipine	Tablet	Sustained release
Prevacid	lansoprazole	Capsule	Sustained release; capsules may be opened and contents taken without chewing or crushing
Prilosec	omeprazole	Capsule	Sustained release
Procardia XL	nifedipine	Tablet	Sustained release
Pronestyl SR	procainamide	Tablet	Sustained release
Ritalin SR	methylphenidate	Tablet	Sustained release
Sinemet SR	levodopa, carbidopa	Tablet	Sustained release; tablet is scored and may be broken in half
Tessalon Perles	benzonatate	Capsule	Will anesthetize tongue and mouth if chewed
Toprol XL	metoprolol	Tablet	Sustained release
Trental	pentoxifylline	Tablet	Sustained release
Wellbutrin SR, XL	bupropion	Tablet	Sustained release

Sublingual and Buccal Drug Administration

Sublingual and buccal administrations are enteral routes in which the tablets are not swallowed, but instead are kept in the mouth. Unlike troches, which are slowly dissolved in the mouth to treat a local condition (sore throat or oral infections), sublingual and buccal drugs are intended to be absorbed. The mucosa of the oral cavity contains extensive capillaries that provide an excellent absorptive surface for certain drugs. Medications given by this route are not subjected to destructive stomach acid, and they do not undergo hepatic first-pass metabolism (see Chapter 4).

For the sublingual route, the medication is placed under the tongue and allowed to slowly dissolve. Because of the rich blood supply to this region, the sublingual route results in a rapid onset of drug action. Sublingual dosage forms are most often formulated as rapidly disintegrating tablets or as soft gelatin capsules filled with liquid drug.

When multiple medications are ordered, the sublingual preparations should be administered after oral medications have been swallowed. The patient should be instructed not to move the drug with the tongue or to eat or drink anything until the medication has completely dissolved. The sublingual mucosa is not suitable for extended release formulations because it is a relatively small area and is constantly being bathed by a substantial amount of saliva that will remove these drugs from the region. Figure 3.2a illustrates sublingual drug administration.

To administer drugs by the buccal route, the tablet is placed in the oral cavity between the gum and cheek. The patient must be instructed not to manipulate the drug with the tongue; otherwise it could get displaced to the sublingual area, where it will be more rapidly absorbed, or to the back of the throat, where it could be swallowed. The buccal mucosa is thicker and less permeable to medications than the sublingual area, providing for slower absorption. The buccal route is preferred over the sublingual route for sustained release delivery because of its greater mucosal surface area. For example, testosterone, a drug normally given by injection, is available in a buccal form (Striant). Buccal testosterone releases the drug over 12 hours and gives a more consistent, sustained drug level than does the transdermal patch delivery system for testosterone (see Chapter 72). Drugs formulated for buccal administration generally do not cause irritation and are small enough to not cause discomfort to the patient. Like the sublingual route, drugs administered by the buccal route avoid first-pass metabolism by the liver and the enzymatic processes of the stomach and small intestine. Figure 3.2b illustrates buccal drug administration.

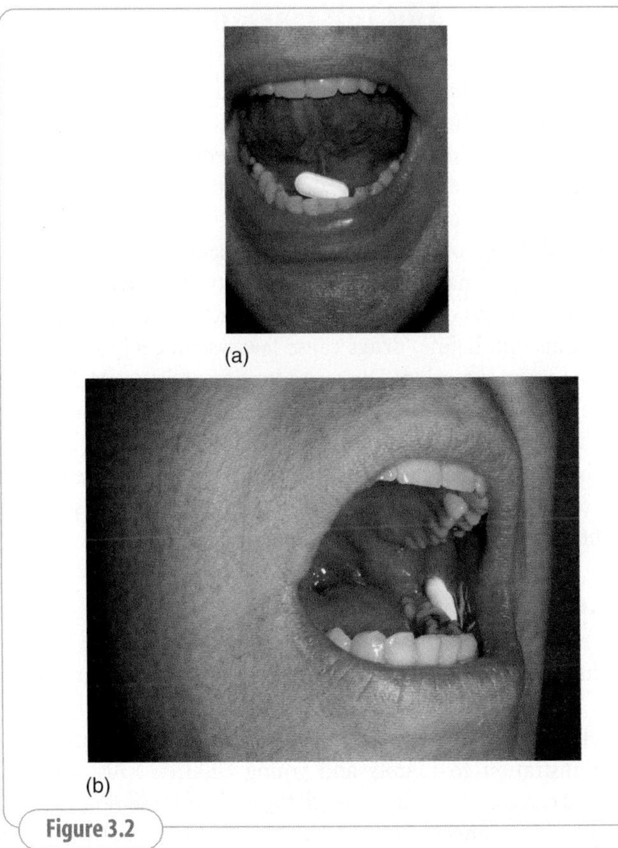

(a)

(b)

Figure 3.2

(a) Sublingual medical administration; (b) buccal medication administration.

Nasogastric and Gastrostomy Drug Administration

Patients with a nasogastric (NG) tube or an enteral feeding mechanism, such as a gastrostomy (G) tube, may have their medications administered through these devices. An NG tube is a soft, flexible tube inserted by way of the nasopharynx with the tip lying in the stomach. A G tube is surgically placed directly into the patient's stomach. Generally, an NG tube is used for short-term treatment, whereas the G tube is inserted for patients requiring long-term care. Drugs administered through these tubes are usually in liquid form. Although solid drugs can be crushed or dissolved, they tend to clog the tubes. Sustained release medications should not be crushed and administered through NG or G tubes. Drugs administered by these routes are exposed to the same physiological processes as those given orally. NG and G tubes should be flushed according to agency policy to maintain patency before and after administration of medications.

3.8 Topical medications are applied to the skin or mucous membranes.

The **topical route** of drug administration includes medications applied to the skin or the membranous linings of the eye, ear, nose, respiratory tract, urinary tract, vagina, and rectum. Types of topical applications include the following:

- Dermatologic preparations are drugs applied to the skin. Skin is the topical route most commonly used. Formulations include creams, lotions, ointments, gels, powders, and sprays.
- Instillations and irrigations are drugs applied into body cavities or orifices. These include the eyes, ears, nose, urinary bladder, rectum, and vagina.
- Inhalations are drugs applied to the respiratory tract by inhalers, nebulizers, or positive pressure breathing machines. The most common indication for inhaled drugs is bronchoconstriction caused by asthma. However, a number of illegal, abused drugs are taken by this route because it provides a very rapid onset of drug action. Additional details on inhalation drug administration can be found in Chapter 73.

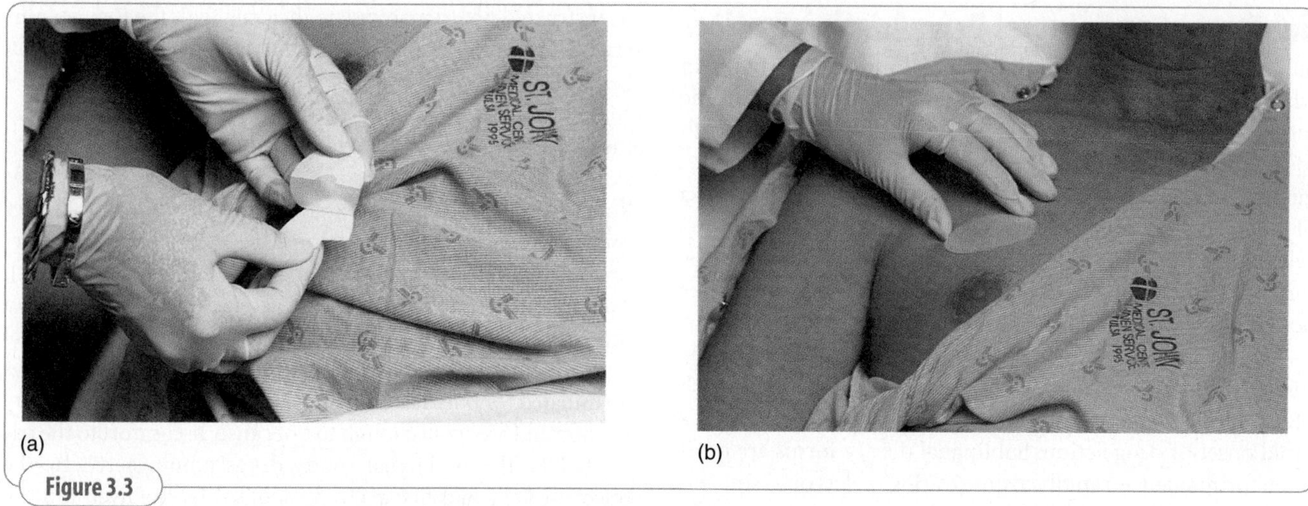

Figure 3.3

Transdermal patch administration: (a) Protective coating is removed from the patch. (b) The patch is immediately applied to clean, dry, and hairless skin and labeled with the date, time, and initials.

Many drugs are applied topically to produce a local effect. For example, antibiotics are applied topically to treat skin infections. Antineoplastic agents may be instilled into the urinary bladder via catheter to treat localized tumors of the bladder mucosa. Corticosteroids are sprayed into the nostrils to reduce inflammation of the nasal mucosa due to allergic rhinitis. Topical delivery produces fewer adverse effects compared to the same drug given orally or parenterally. This is because, when given topically, drugs are absorbed more slowly and the amount of the drug reaching the general circulation is minimal. The most common adverse events resulting from topical administration are transient burning, stinging, or redness of the area where they are applied.

Some drugs are given topically to provide for slow release and absorption of the drug to the general circulation. These agents are given for their systemic effects. For example, a nitroglycerin patch is not applied to the skin to treat a local skin condition but to treat a systemic condition such as coronary artery disease. Likewise, prochlorperazine (Compazine) suppositories are inserted rectally not to treat a disease of the rectum but to alleviate nausea.

The distinction between topical drugs given for local effects and those administered for systemic effects is an important one for the nurse. In the case of local drugs, absorption is undesirable and may result in adverse effects if the drug reaches the systemic circulation. For systemic drugs, absorption across the skin or mucous membrane is essential for the therapeutic action of the drug. With either type of topical agent, medication should not be applied to abraded or denuded skin because this could affect drug absorption.

Transdermal Delivery System

The use of **transdermal patches** provides an effective means of delivering certain medications. Examples include nitroglycerin to treat angina pectoris, testosterone for hypogonadism, and scopolamine (Transderm Scop) for motion sickness. Transdermal patches contain a specified amount of medication, although the rate of delivery and the actual dose received can vary. Patches are changed on a regularly scheduled basis using a site rotation routine, which should be documented in the MAR. Before applying a transdermal patch, the nurse should verify that the previous patch has been removed and disposed of appropriately. Medications administered by this route avoid the first-pass effect in the liver and bypass digestive enzymes. Figure 3.3 illustrates the application of a transdermal drug.

Ophthalmic Administration

The ophthalmic route is used to treat local conditions of the eye and surrounding structures. Common indications include excessive dryness, eye infections, glaucoma, and dilation of the pupil during eye examinations. Ophthalmic medications are available in the form of eye irrigations, drops, ointments, and medicated disks. Ophthalmic drugs are absorbed into the systemic circulation via drainage of the drug into the nasolacrimal ducts and subsequently to the nasopharynx and the GI tract. Generally this is a slow process and only small amounts reach the general circulation; thus ophthalmic drugs cause few systemic adverse effects. Infants are an exception: The concentration of drugs reaching the systemic circulation is higher than in an adult, giving a greater chance for adverse drug events. With a child, it is advisable to enlist the help of an adult caregiver to better immobilize the patient to prevent accidental injury to the eye during administration. Ophthalmic administration is shown in Figure 3.4a.

Otic Administration

The otic route is used to treat local conditions of the ear, including infections and accumulations of earwax in the auditory canal. Otic medications include eardrops and irrigations, which are usually ordered for cleaning purposes, as shown in Figure 3.4b. Administration to infants and young children must be performed carefully to avoid injury to the tympanic membrane. Systemic adverse effects from otic preparations are not observed unless the drug is applied to areas of open abrasions or injury, such as a ruptured tympanic membrane.

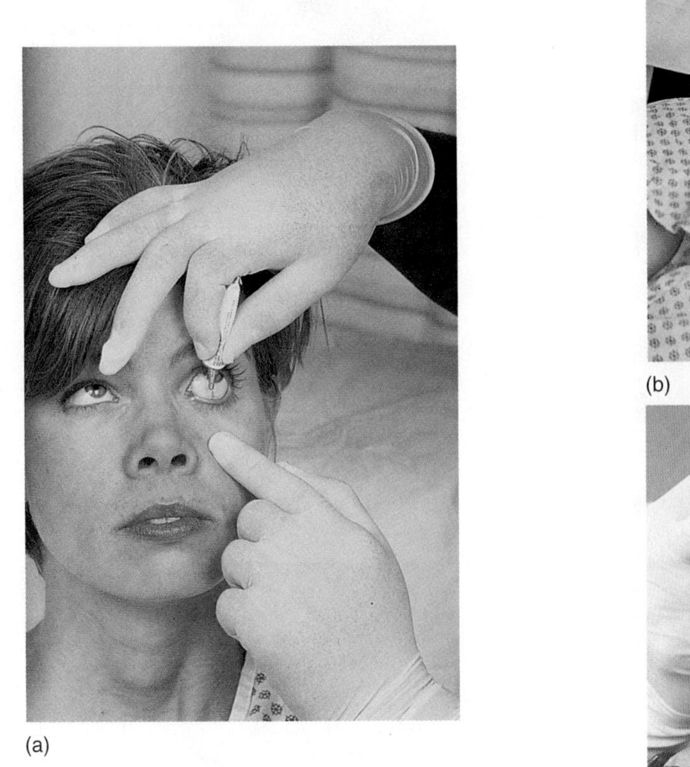

(a)

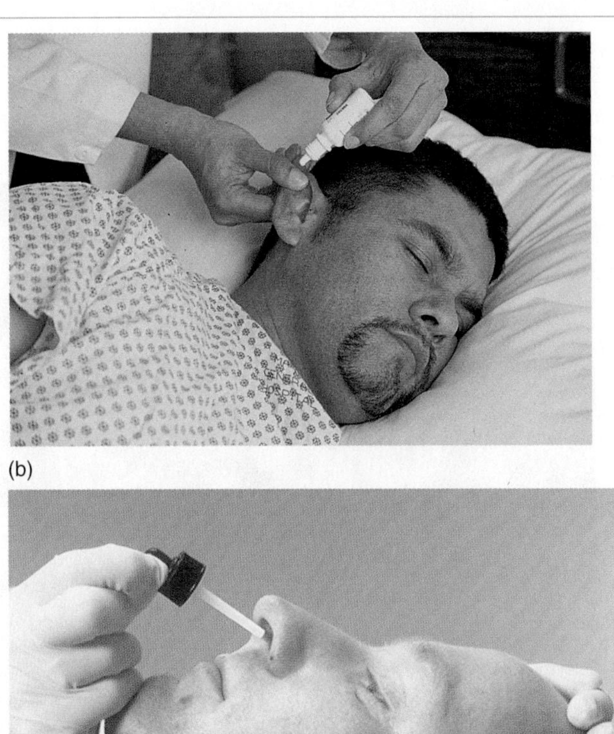

(b)

(c)

Figure 3.4

(a) Ophthalmic administration; (b) otic administration; and (c) intranasal administration.

Source: (a) *Photographer:* Jenny Thomas Photography; (b) *Photographer:* Elena Dorfman

Intranasal Administration

Drugs are applied by the intranasal route for their local effects on the nasal mucosa or for systemic absorption. Advantages of this route include convenience and rapid onset of action. Local indications include the application of drops or sprays for shrinking swollen nasal mucous membranes, or for loosening secretions and facilitating drainage. For example, decongestant nasal sprays bring immediate relief from the nasal congestion caused by the common cold (see Chapter 74). Intranasal formulations of corticosteroids have revolutionized the treatment of allergic rhinitis due to their effectiveness and high safety margin when administered by this route.

The nasal mucosa also provides an excellent absorptive surface for certain medications to produce systemic actions. Advantages of this route include avoidance of the first-pass effect and digestive enzymes. For example, an intranasal form of vitamin B_{12} is available that is used for patients lacking intrinsic factor, a substance required for the absorption of this vitamin in the GI tract. Intranasal calcitonin is available to treat osteoporosis. Being a protein, calcitonin would be destroyed by stomach enzymes if given orally (see Chapter 75).

Although the nasal mucosa provides an excellent surface for drug delivery, there is a potential for damage to the ciliated cells within the nasal cavity, and mucosal irritation is common. Mucus secretion is unpredictable and may inhibit drug absorption from this site. Figure 3.4c illustrates the nasal administration of drugs.

Vaginal Administration

The **vaginal route** is used to treat local conditions such as vaginal infections, pain, and itching. The vagina has a rich blood supply, and drugs inserted into it may be absorbed across the mucosa and produce systemic effects. For example, vaginal creams containing estrogen not only produce local effects on the vagina, but also result in significant levels of this hormone in the circulation. The contraceptive NuvaRing, inserted into the vagina, contains estrogen and progestin, which are rapidly absorbed to produce serum levels sufficient to prevent ovulation for a week. Intravaginal administration of NuvaRing is shown in Figure 3.5.

Vaginal medications are inserted as suppositories, creams, jellies, or foams. It is important that the nurse explain the purpose of treatment and provide for privacy during vaginal administration. Before inserting vaginal medications, the patient should be instructed to empty the bladder so there will be less discomfort during treatment and less possibility of irritating or injuring the vaginal lining.

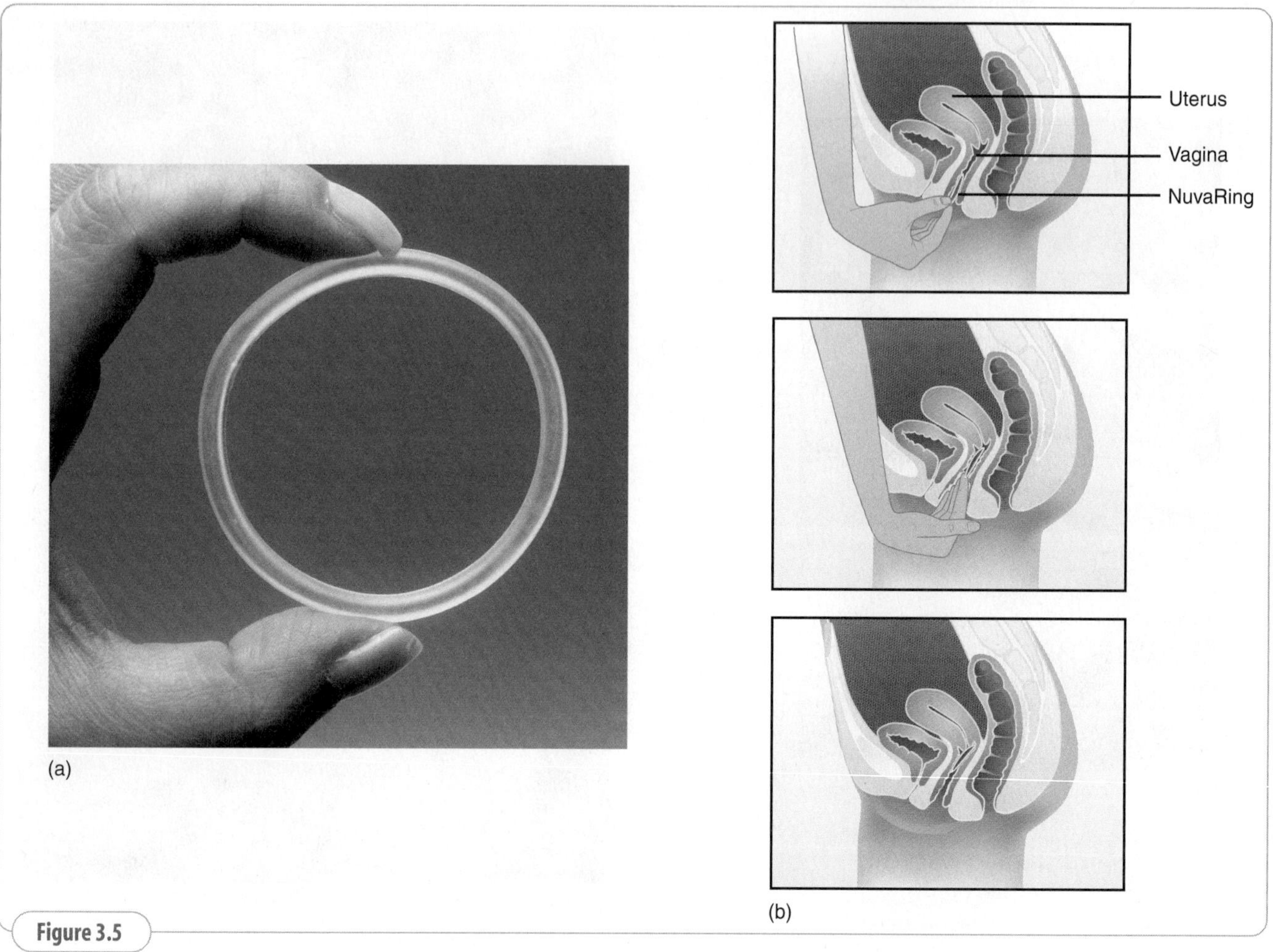

Figure 3.5

Vaginal medication administration: (a) The NuvaRing® contraceptive; (b) proper insertion of the NuvaRing.
Source: (a) *Photographer:* Joel Gordon/Joel Gordon Photography

Rectal Administration

The **rectal route** may be used for either local or systemic drug delivery. It is a safe and effective means of delivering medications to comatose patients or to those who are experiencing nausea and vomiting. Rectal medications are normally in suppository form, although a few laxatives and diagnostic agents are given via enema. Although absorption is slower than by other routes, it is steady and reliable provided the medication can be retained by the patient. Venous blood from the lower rectum is not transported to the circulation by way of the liver; thus the first-pass effect is avoided as are the digestive enzymes of the upper GI tract.

CONNECTION *Checkpoint* 3.2

Pharmaceutical companies are always exploring novel methods of drug delivery so they may be granted exclusivity. From what you learned in Chapter 1, why is exclusivity important to the pharmaceutical company? See Answer to Connection Checkpoint 3.2 in Appendix A.

3.9 Parenteral administration is the dispensing of medications via a needle, usually into the skin layers, subcutaneous tissue, muscles, or veins.

The parenteral route refers to the administration of drugs by routes other than enteral or topical. A needle is used to deliver drugs into the skin layers, subcutaneous tissue, muscles, or veins. Less common parenteral delivery methods include administration into arteries (intra-arterial), bone (intraosseous), body cavities (intrathecal), or organs (intracardiac). Parenteral drug administration is more invasive than topical or enteral because of the potential for introducing pathogenic microbes directly into the blood or body tissues. Specialized equipment and techniques are employed in the preparation and administration of injectable products. The nurse must know the correct anatomic locations for parenteral administration, proper administration technique, and safety procedures regarding disposal of hazardous equipment. Injectable medications are frequently supplied in prefilled unit dose systems from the pharmacy.

Intradermal and Subcutaneous Administration

Injection into the skin delivers drugs to the blood vessels that supply the various layers of the skin. Medications may be injected either intradermally or subcutaneously. The major difference between these methods is the depth of injection. An advantage of both methods is that they offer a means of administering drugs to patients who are unable to take medications orally. Drugs administered by these routes avoid digestive enzymes and the hepatic first-pass effect. However, only small volumes can be administered by these routes, and injections can result in pain and swelling at the injection site.

The intradermal (ID) route administers drugs into the dermis layer of the skin. Because the dermis contains more blood vessels than the deeper subcutaneous layer, drugs are more readily absorbed. This route is usually employed for allergy and disease screening or for local anesthetic delivery prior to venous cannulation. ID injections are limited to very small volumes of medication, usually only 0.1 to 0.2 mL. The usual sites for ID injections are the nonhairy skin surfaces of the upper back, over the scapulae, the high upper chest, and the inner forearm. An ID injection is illustrated in Figure 3.6 .

The subcutaneous route delivers drugs to the deepest layers of the skin. Insulin, heparin, vitamins, some vaccines, and other medications are given in this area because the sites are easily accessible and provide for rapid absorption. Body sites that are ideal for subcutaneous injections include the following:

- Outer aspect of the upper arms, in the area above the triceps muscle
- Middle two thirds of the anterior thigh area
- Subscapular areas of the upper back
- Upper dorsogluteal and ventrogluteal areas
- Abdominal areas, above the iliac crest and below the diaphragm, 1½ to 2 inches out from the umbilicus

Subcutaneous doses are small in volume, usually ranging from 0.5 to 1 mL. The needle size varies with the patient's quantity of body fat. The length is usually one half the size of a pinched/bunched skin fold that can be grasped between the thumb and forefinger. It is important to rotate injection sites in an orderly and documented manner to promote absorption, lessen tissue damage, and minimize discomfort. For insulin, rotation should be within an anatomical area to promote reliable absorption and to maintain consistent blood glucose levels. When performing subcutaneous injections, it is not necessary to aspirate prior to the injection. Figure 3.7 illustrates subcutaneous drug administration.

Intramuscular Administration

The intramuscular (IM) route delivers drugs directly into large muscles. Because muscle tissue has a rich blood supply, drug molecules quickly move into blood vessels to produce a more rapid onset of action than with oral, ID, or subcutaneous administration. In a few cases, the drug is formulated in an oily, viscous base that promotes slow and continuous absorption from the muscle.

The anatomic structure of muscle permits this tissue to receive a larger volume of drug than the subcutaneous region. An adult with well-developed muscles can safely tolerate up to 4 mL of medication in a large muscle, although only 2 to 3 mL is recommended. The deltoid and triceps muscles should receive a maximum of 1 mL.

A major consideration for the nurse regarding IM drug administration is the selection of an appropriate injection site. Injection sites must be located away from bone, large blood

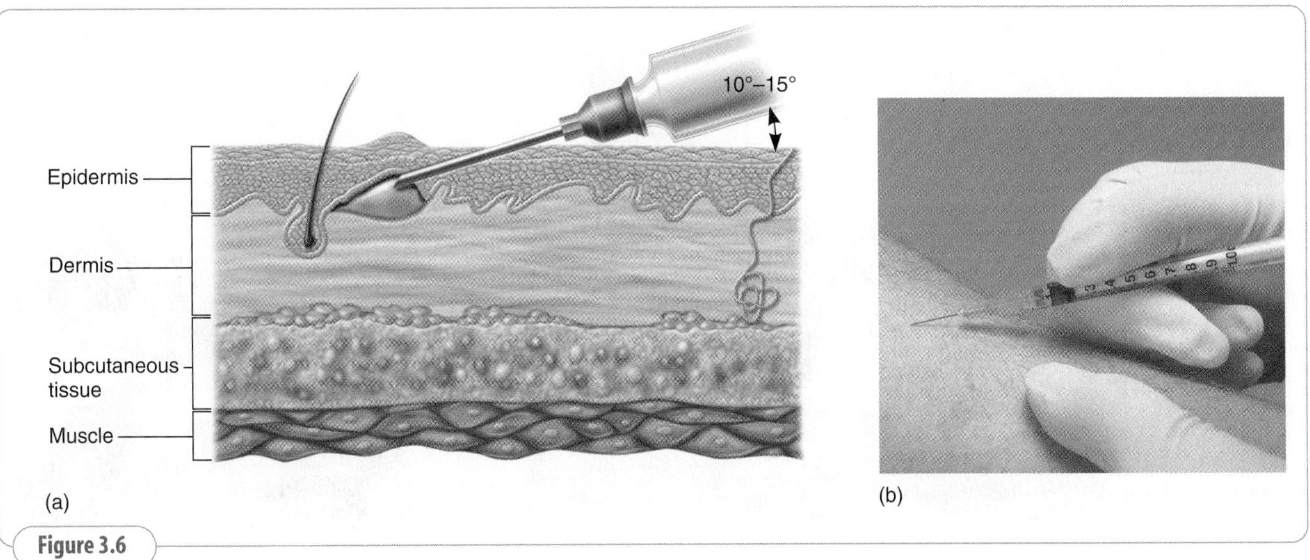

Figure 3.6

Intradermal drug administration: (a) Cross section of skin showing the depth of needle insertion. (b) The needle is inserted with the bevel up at 10–15°.

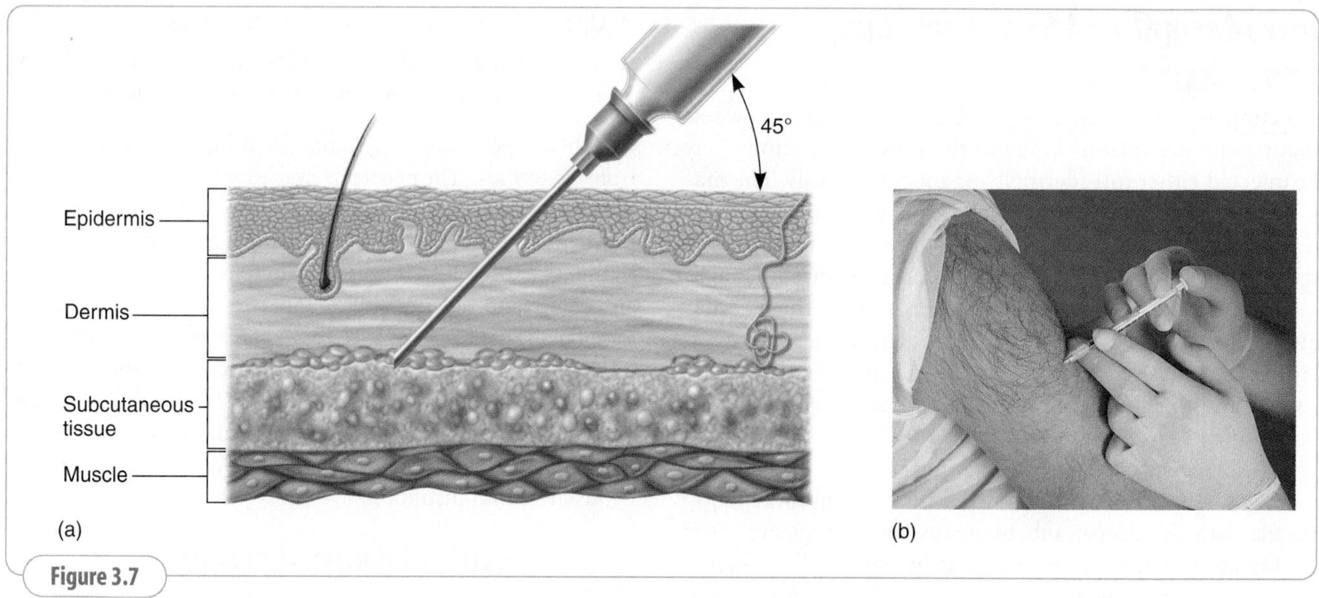

Figure 3.7

Subcutaneous drug administration: (a) Cross section of skin showing the depth of needle insertion. (b) The needle is inserted at a 45° angle.

vessels, and nerves. The size and length of the needle are determined by body size and muscle mass, the specific drug to be administered, the amount of adipose tissue overlying the muscle, and the age of the patient. Figure 3.8 illustrates IM injections. The four common sites for IM injections are given in Table 3.6.

Intravenous Administration

The intravenous (IV) route delivers drugs and fluids directly into the bloodstream, which immediately distributes them throughout the body. The IV route is used when a very rapid onset of action is desired. Unlike other routes in which absorption may be unpredictable, an exact level of drug in the bloodstream can be attained by fine adjustments to the IV flow rate. Like other parenteral routes, IV drugs bypass the enzymatic processes of the alimentary canal and avoid the first-pass effect of the liver. The IV route is useful for patients who are comatose or otherwise unable to take oral medications. The three basic types of IV administration include the following:

- **Large volume infusion.** For fluid maintenance, replacement, or supplementation. Compatible medications may be mixed into a large-volume IV container with fluids such as normal saline or Ringer's lactate, as shown in Figure 3.9a.
- **Intermittent infusion.** Small amount of IV solution that is arranged tandem or piggy-backed to the primary large-volume infusion. This is used to instill adjunct medications, such as antibiotics or analgesics over a short period.
- **IV bolus (push) administration.** Concentrated dose delivered directly to the circulation via syringe to administer single-dose medica-

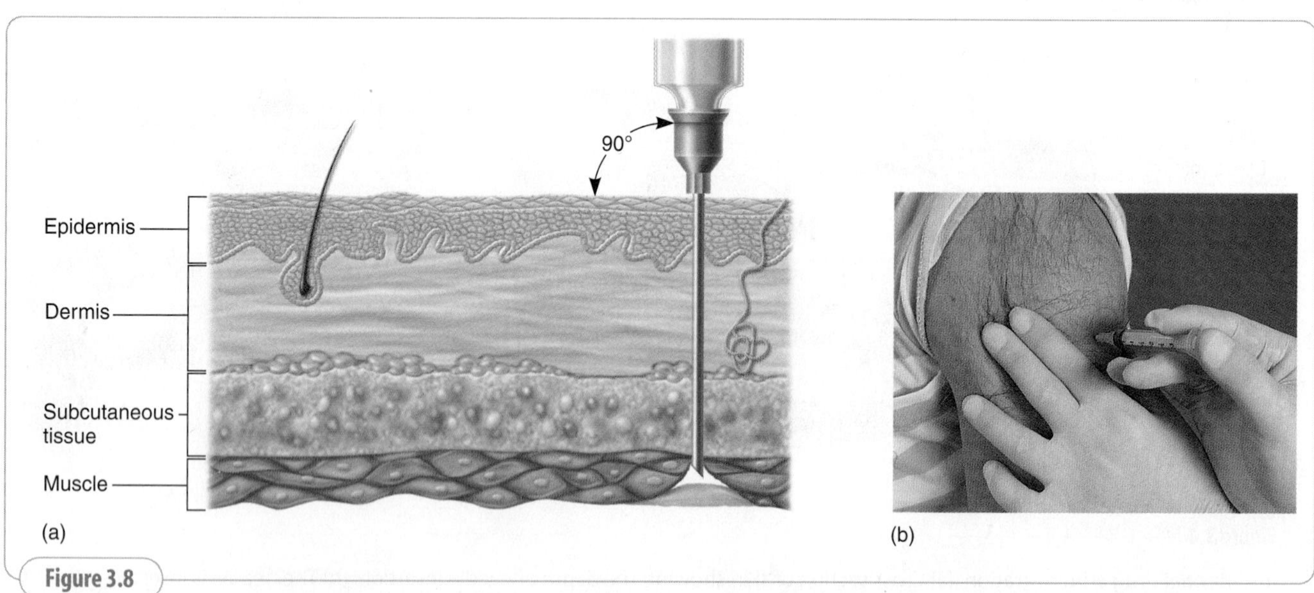

Figure 3.8

Intramuscular drug administration: (a) Cross section of skin showing the depth of needle insertion. (b) The needle is inserted at a 90° angle.

TABLE 3.6 Sites for Intramuscular Injections

Site	Description
Deltoid	Used in well-developed teens and adults for volumes of medication not to exceed 1 mL. Because the radial nerve lies in close proximity, the deltoid is not generally used except for small volume vaccines, such as for hepatitis B in adults.
Dorsogluteal	Used for adults and for children who have been walking for at least 6 months. The site is rarely used due to the potential for damage to the sciatic nerve.
Vastus lateralis	Usually thick and well developed in both adults and children, the middle third of the muscle is the site for IM injections. Sometimes this is considered the site of choice for infants 12 months and younger.
Ventrogluteal	A common site for IM injections. This area provides the greatest thickness of gluteal muscles, contains no large blood vessels or nerves, is sealed off by bone, and contains less fat than the buttock area, thus eliminating the need to determine the depth of subcutaneous fat. It is a suitable site for children and infants older than 7 months of age.

tions. Bolus injections may be given through an intermittent injection port or by direct IV push for treating emergencies. The bolus method of administration is illustrated in Figure 3.9b.

Although the IV route offers the fastest onset of drug action, it is also the most dangerous. Once injected, the medication cannot be retrieved. If the drug solution or the needle is contaminated, pathogens have a direct route to the bloodstream and body tissues. Patients receiving IV injections must be closely monitored for adverse reactions. Although some adverse reactions occur immediately after injection, others may take hours or days to appear. Antidotes for drugs that can cause potentially dangerous or fatal reactions must always be readily available.

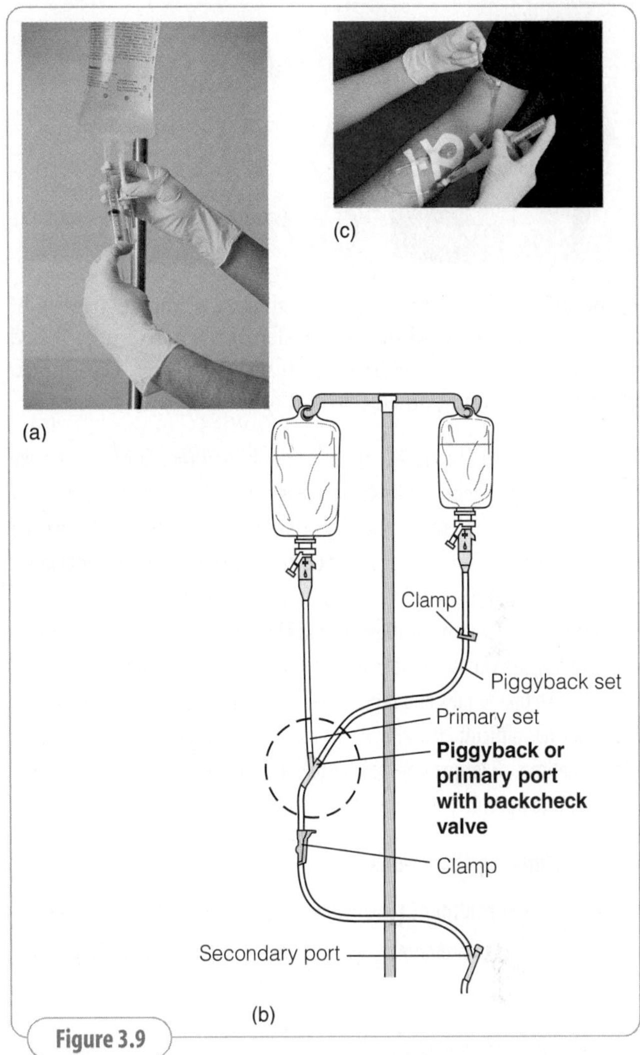

Figure 3.9

Intravenous drug administration: (a) A tandem intravenous alignment. (b) An intravenous piggyback (IVPB) alignment. (c) The drug is administered through the port using a needleless syringe.

Source: (a) *Photographer:* Elena Dorfman

UNDERSTANDING THE CHAPTER

Key Concepts Summary

3.1 Achieving patient adherence with pharmacotherapy is a major challenge for the nurse.

3.2 Drugs should be stored properly and never used past their expiration date.

3.3 Prescriptions must be clearly written and include a heading, a body, and a closing.

3.4 For maximum effectiveness, drugs must be administered at the proper dosing intervals.

3.5 The primary system of measurement used in pharmacology is the metric system.

3.6 Medication administration should be properly recorded as soon as possible after the drug is administered.

3.7 Enteral drugs are administered by the oral route or through gastrostomy or nasogastric tubes.

3.8 Topical medications are applied to the skin or mucous membranes.

3.9 Parenteral administration is the dispensing of medications via a needle, usually into the skin layers, subcutaneous tissue, muscles, or veins.

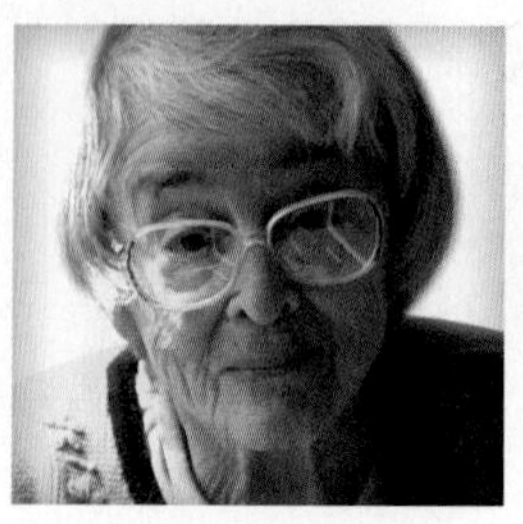

Making the PATIENT *Connection*

Remember the patient "Lavenia Deberry" at the beginning of the chapter? Now read the remainder of the case study. Based on the information presented within this chapter, respond to the critical thinking questions that follow.

Eighty-seven-year-old Lavenia Deberry lives in an assisted living facility. She is quite capable of caring for herself and is strongly independent. Today, she has come to her health care provider's office with fever and a productive cough that she has had for the last 10 days. She admits to self-medicating with various "leftover" antibiotics. She had hoped that one of the antibiotics would cure her infection.

Levenia is also on a medication for high blood pressure and diabetes. However, she has been known to take her medications inconsistently. She says she does not like taking pills and most of the time she feels pretty good without them. She has difficulty remembering to take medications. Ms. Deberry states that sometimes, "I forget whether I've taken the medication or not. Besides, I don't want to become dependent on any medications."

Critical Thinking Questions

1. What factors contribute to nonadherence with medication regimens?
2. Identify ways to promote patient adherence with medication regimens.
3. Prepare a list of concepts to teach the patient about taking medications.
4. What factors influence effective patient teaching related to drug therapy?

Case Study

Albert Lewis, a 52-year-old hospitalized patient, is receiving multiple medications. While in the hospital, Albert receives the following drugs:

- Nitroglycerin tablet sublingual prn for chest pain
- Nifedipine Extended Release (ER) orally every 6 hours
- Mycelex Troche twice a day
- Clorafan 500 mg intravenously (IV)
- Insulin subcutaneous injections every morning
- Garamycin optic solution, 2 drops to each eye, 3 times per day
- Fentanyl transdermal patch every 12 hours

1. How would you respond when the patient asks you, "Why can't I take all my medications orally?"
2. Discuss the advantages and disadvantages of each route for each of the medications listed above.
3. What special precautions should you take with drugs with enteric coating and those that are extended release?

NCLEX-RN® Review

1 The client who received a prescription for an antibiotic 2 weeks ago now presents with the same symptoms of bacterial infection. The nurse should suspect:

1. Faulty and low-quality medication.
2. Toxic adverse effects of the drug.
3. Excessive dosage of the prescription.
4. Nonadherence to the prescribed therapy.

2 Prior to administering a liquid medication to a client, the nurse notices that the medication color looks different than usual. Based on this observation the nurse should:

1. Administer the medication.
2. Consult the hospital pharmacist.
3. Notify the health care provider.
4. Call the poison control center.

3 The client is to receive a vaginal suppository. Which of the following should the nurse include in the instructions to the client concerning the drug's administration?

1. Remove the suppository 5 minutes after insertion.
2. Cleanse the perineal area with soap and water before insertion.
3. Insert the suppository only in the morning.
4. Urinate before insertion of the suppository.

4 Pronestyl SR has been prescribed for a client with a gastrostomy tube. Which of the following is the appropriate nursing action for this medication?

1. Crush the medication and dilute it in tepid tap water.
2. Instruct the client to take the medication with only sips of water.
3. Request the hospital pharmacist to send a substitute drug.
4. Notify the health care provider and request that another form of the drug be prescribed.

5 The health care provider orders Lasix 40 mg intravenous stat to a client with heart failure. Which of the following describes the correct response of the nurse to this medication order?

1. Give the medication at the next meal.
2. Administer the medication immediately.
3. Dispense the medication when the client requests it.
4. Oversee the self-administration of the medication.

6 Identify the missing or incorrect element in the following prescription. Select all that apply.

1. DEA number
2. Date of issuance
3. Signature of prescriber
4. Drug name and dose
5. Dosage form and amount to be taken
6. Refill instructions

Fast Pace Medical Emergency Clinic
5678 Getwell Road • Ailing Center,
Kentucky • (319) 678-5555

Name Arabella Rossi **Date** July 13th
Address 8292 South Street **Age** ______

RX
Lortab 7.5 mg
Disp #14
Sig: Take every 6-8 hrs prn pain

______________ John W Masters, MD, PC
Dispense as Written **Substitution Permissible**

Refills ______

See Answers to Critical Thinking Questions, Case Study, and NCLEX-RN® Review in Appendix A.

PEARSON
EXPLORE mynursingkit™

MyNursingKit is your one stop for online chapter review materials and resources. Prepare for success with additional NCLEX®-style practice questions, interactive assignments and activities, web links, animations and videos, and more!

Register your access code from the front of your book at
www.mynursingkit.com

References

Christensen, J. M. (2009). *Dosage forms and drug delivery systems.* New York: McGraw-Hill Medical.

Costantino, H. R., Illum, L., Brandt, G., Johnson, P. H., & Quay, S. C. (2007). Intranasal delivery: Physicochemical and therapeutic aspects. *International Journal of Pharmacology, 337*(1-2), 1–24.

Dunbar-Jacob, J., Erlen, J. A., Schlenk, E. A., Ryan, C. M., Sereika, S. M., & Doswell, W. M. (2000). Adherence in chronic disease. *Annual Review of Nursing Research, 18*, 48–90.

Henry J. Kaiser Foundation. (2008). *Prescription drug trends.* Retrieved November 11, 2008, from http://www.kff.org/rxdrugs/upload/3057_07.pdf

Institute for Safe Medication Practices. (2008). The *ISMP's list of error-prone abbreviations, symbols, and dose designations.* Retrieved November 11, 2008, from http://www.ismp.org/Tools/errorproneabbreviations.pdf

Kripalani, S., Yao, X., & Haynes, R. B. (2007). Interventions to enhance medication adherence in chronic medical conditions: A systematic review. *Archives of Internal Medicine, 167*(6), 540–550.

Magnuson, B. L., Clifford, T. M., Hoskins, L. A., & Bernard, A. C. (2005). Enteral nutrition and drug administration: Interactions and complications. *Nutrition in Clinical Practice, 20*(6), 618–624.

Myers, T. M., Wallace, D. K., & Johnson, S. M. (2005). Ophthalmic medications in pediatric patients. *Comprehensive Ophthalmology Update, 6*(2), 85–101.

Porter, C. J., Trevaskis, N. L., & Charman, W. N. (2007). Lipids and lipid-based formulations: Optimizing the oral delivery of lipophilic drugs. *Nature Reviews. Drug Discovery, 6*(3), 231–248.

Smith, D. (2004). Compliance packaging: A patient education tool. *American Pharmacy, NS29*(2).

Tabor, P. A., & Lopez, D. A. (2004). Comply with us: Improving medication adherence. *Journal of Pharmacy Practice, 17*(3), 167–181.

Wang, B., Sjahaan, T. J., & Soltero, R. A. (2005). Drug delivery: Principles and applications. Hoboken, NJ: Wiley-Interscience.

Wertheimer, A. I., & Santella, T. M. (2003). Medication compliance research: Still so far to go. *Journal of Applied Research, 3*(3), 254–261.

CHAPTER

I'm terribly worried about my father, John Kessler. He's been chronically ill for so long and now he has suffered a stroke. I don't know if his body can take much more.

Patient's daughter,
"Emily Kessler Myers"

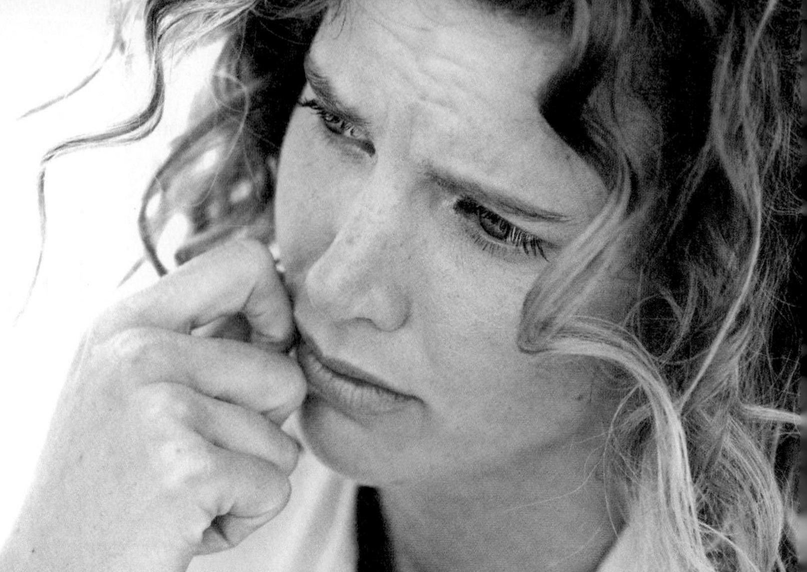

4 Pharmacokinetics

Learning Outcomes

After reading this chapter, the student should be able to:

1. Identify the four primary processes of pharmacokinetics.
2. Explain mechanisms by which drugs cross plasma membranes.
3. Discuss factors affecting drug absorption.
4. Discuss how drugs are distributed throughout the body.
5. Describe how plasma proteins affect drug distribution.
6. Explain the metabolism of drugs and its applications to pharmacotherapy.
7. Identify major processes by which drugs are excreted.
8. Explain how enterohepatic recirculation affects drug activity.
9. Explain how a drug reaches and maintains its therapeutic range in the plasma.
10. Explain the applications of a drug's plasma half-life ($t_{1/2}$) to pharmacotherapy.
11. Differentiate between loading and maintenance doses.

Chapter Outline

Introduction to Pharmacokinetics

Primary Processes of Pharmacokinetics

Absorption

Distribution

Metabolism

Excretion

Time–Response Relationships

Drug Plasma Levels

Drug Half-Life

Loading and Maintenance Doses

Key Terms

absorption, 43
affinity, 45
blood–brain barrier, 46
diffusion, 42
distribution, 45
drug-protein complexes, 45
enterohepatic recirculation, 49
enzyme induction, 47
excretion, 48
fetal–placental barrier, 46
first-pass effect, 48
hepatic microsomal enzyme system, 46
isozyme, 46
loading dose, 52
maintenance dose, 52
metabolism, 46
minimum effective concentration, 50
pharmacokinetics, 41
plasma half-life ($t_{1/2}$), 50
prodrugs, 46
substrate, 47
therapeutic range, 50
toxic concentration, 50

To produce a therapeutic effect, a drug must reach its target cells in sufficient quantities. For many medications, such as topical agents used to treat superficial skin conditions, this is an easy task. For most medications, however, the process of reaching target cells to cause a physiological change is challenging. Drugs are exposed to a myriad of different barriers and destructive processes after they enter the body. The purpose of this chapter is to examine factors that act on the drug as it attempts to reach its target cells.

Introduction to Pharmacokinetics

4.1 Pharmacokinetics focuses on what the body does to drugs after they are administered.

The term **pharmacokinetics** is derived from the root words *pharmaco,* which refers to medicines, and *kinetics,* which means "movement" or "motion." Pharmacokinetics is thus the study of drug movement throughout the body. In practical terms, it describes what the body does to the medication after it is administered. Pharmacokinetics is a core subject in pharmacology, and a firm grasp of this topic allows nurses to better understand and predict the actions and adverse effects of medications in their patients.

Drugs face numerous obstacles in reaching their target cells. For most medications, the greatest barrier is crossing the many membranes that separate the drug from its target cells. A drug taken by mouth, for example, must cross the plasma membranes of the mucosal cells of the gastrointestinal (GI) tract and the endothelial cells of the capillaries to enter the bloodstream. To leave the bloodstream, it must again cross capillary cells, travel through interstitial fluid, and perhaps enter target cells by passing through their plasma membranes. Depending on the mechanism of action, the drug may also need to enter cellular organelles such as nuclei, which are surrounded by additional membranes. Some of the membranes and barriers that many drugs must successfully penetrate before they can elicit a response are illustrated in Figure 4.1.

While seeking their target cells and attempting to pass through the various membranes, drugs are subjected to numerous physiological processes. For medications given by the enteral route, stomach acid and digestive enzymes often break down the drug molecules. Enzymes in the liver and other organs may chemically change the drug molecule, making it less active. If seen as foreign by the body, phagocytes may attempt to remove the drug, or an immune response may be triggered. The kidneys, large intestine, and other organs attempt to excrete the drug from the body.

The preceding examples all illustrate pharmacokinetic processes: how the body handles drugs. The many processes of pharmacokinetics are grouped into four categories: absorption, distribution, metabolism, and excretion, which are illustrated in Figure 4.2. All four of these processes have drug movement in common. Whether it involves movement to its target site or movement out of the body, kinetics is certainly an appropriate name for this important branch of pharmacology.

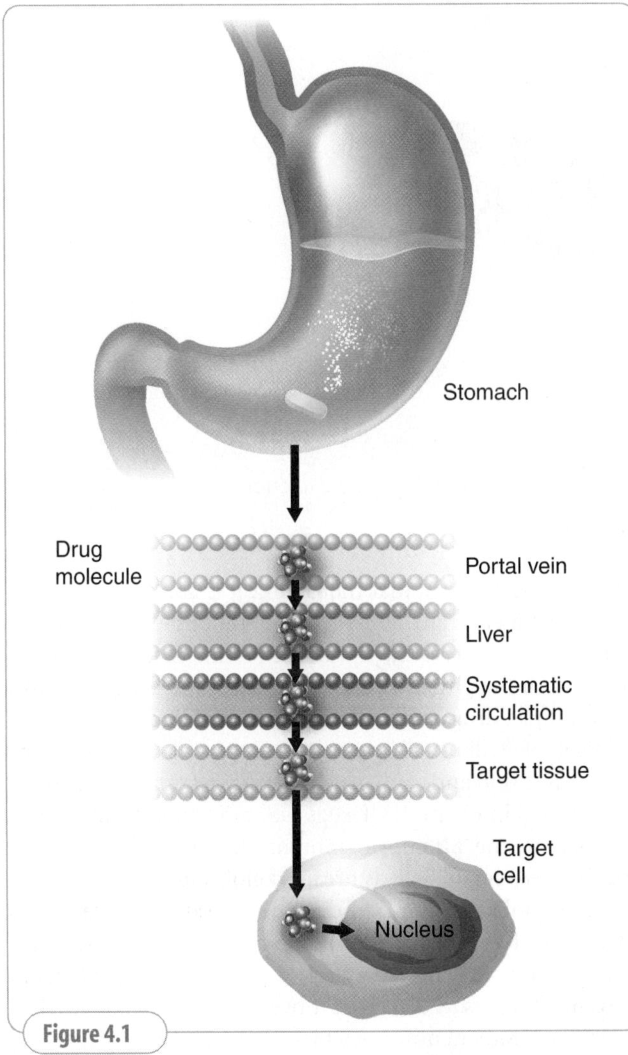

Figure 4.1

Barriers a drug must cross before interacting with a target cell.

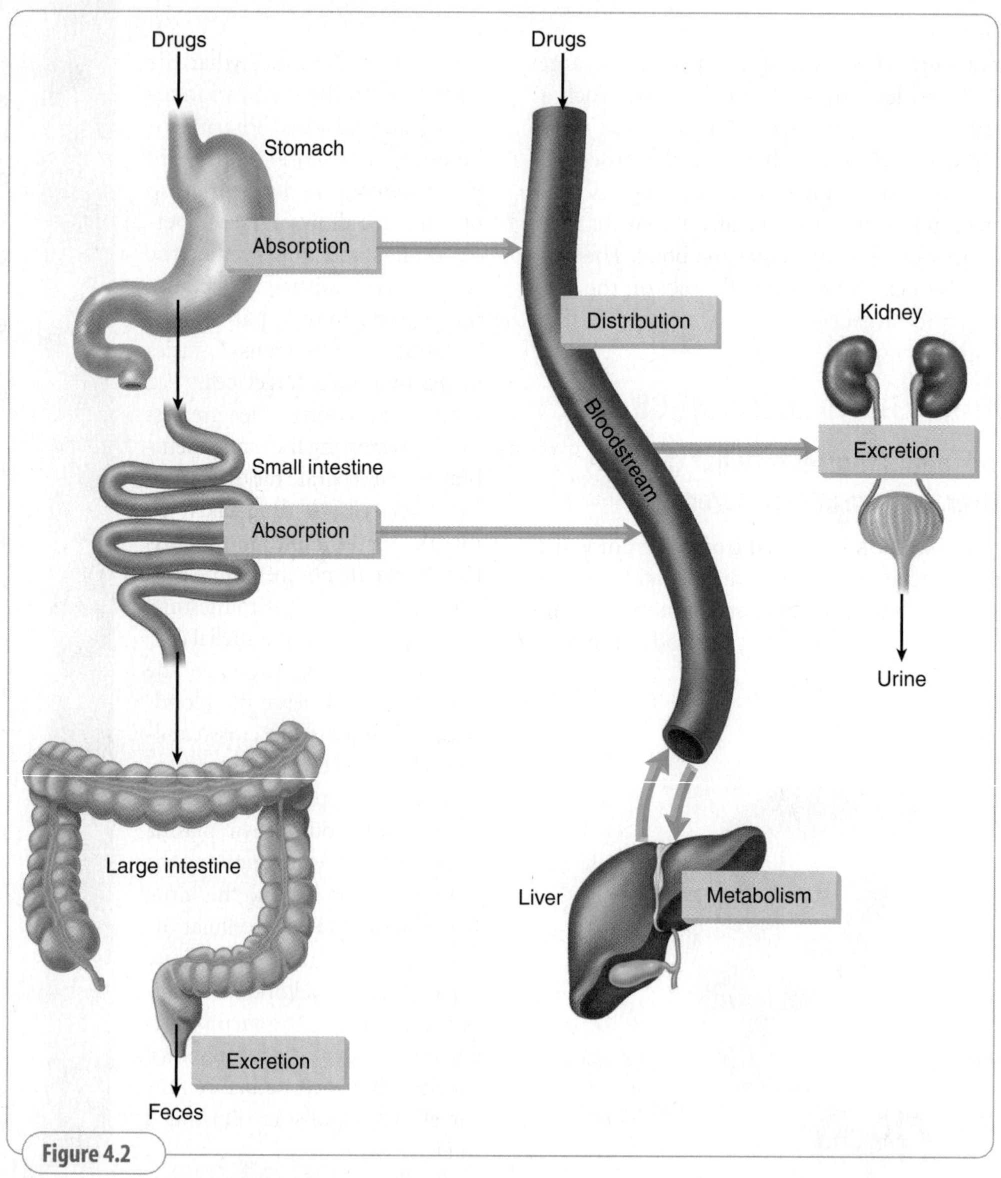

Figure 4.2

The four processes of pharmacokinetics: absorption, distribution, metabolism, and excretion.

4.2 Drugs use diffusion and active transport to cross plasma membranes to reach their target cells.

With few exceptions, drugs must penetrate plasma membranes to produce their effects. Plasma membranes are composed of a lipid bilayer, with proteins and other molecules interspersed in the membrane. Like other chemicals, drugs use two primary processes to cross membranes: diffusion and active transport.

Simple **diffusion** or passive transport is the movement of a chemical from an area of higher concentration to an area of lower concentration. This is best explained by the use of an example. When first administered, a drug given by the intravenous (IV) route is in high concentration in the blood but has not yet entered the tissues. The drug will move quickly by passive diffusion from its region of high concentration (blood) to a region of low concentration (tissues) to produce its action. With time the drug will be inactivated (metabolized) by the tissue and more doses of the drug may be administered, creating a continual concentration gradient from blood to tissue.

Diffusion assumes that the chemical is able to freely cross the plasma membrane. This, however, is not the case for many drugs. Passage across the lipid-rich plasma membrane is dependent on the physical characteristics of the drug molecule. For example, drug molecules that are small, nonionized, and lipid soluble will usually pass through plasma membranes by simple diffusion and easily reach their target cells. This process is illustrated in Figure 4.3. Drugs may also enter through open channels in the plasma membrane; however, the molecule must be very small, such as urea, alcohol, and water.

Large molecules, ionized drugs, and water-soluble agents have difficulty crossing plasma membranes by simple diffusion. These agents may use carrier, or transport, proteins to cross membranes. A drug that moves into a cell along its concentration gradient utilizing a membrane carrier protein is using the process of facilitated diffusion. This process does not require energy expenditure from the cell, but it does require that a specific carrier protein be present on the plasma mem-

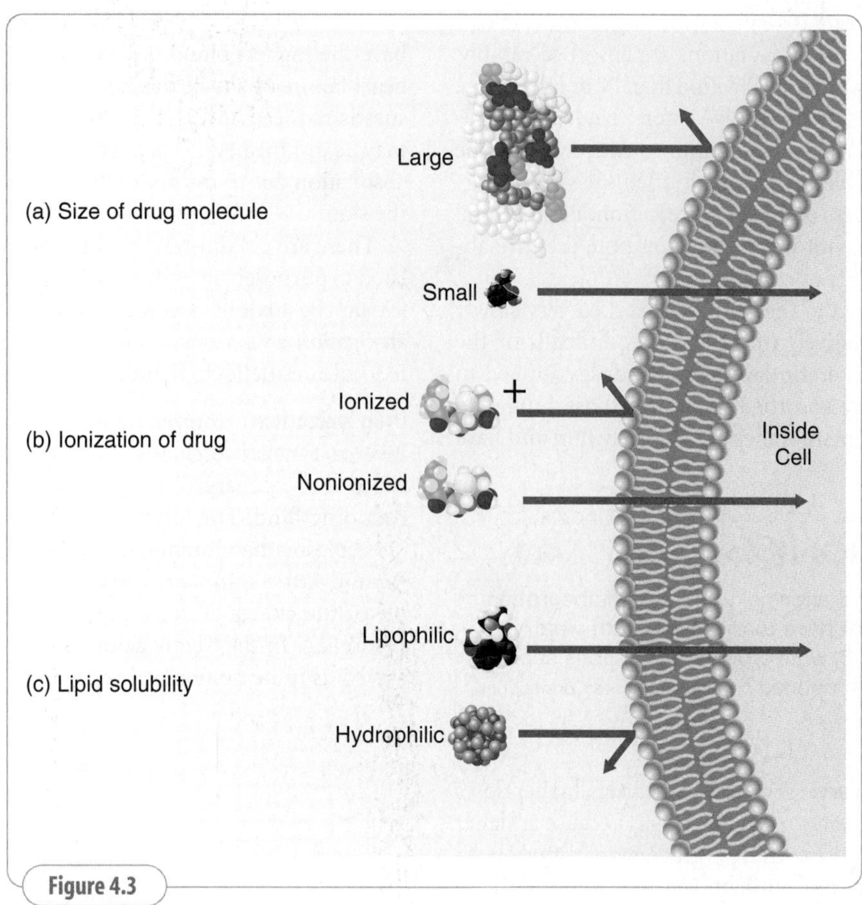

Figure 4.3

Passage of drugs across plasma membranes: (a) small drugs; (b) nonionized drugs; and (c) lipophilic drugs, which are more likely to cross membranes.

brane. Transport proteins are selective and only carry molecules that have specific structures.

Some drugs cross membranes against their gradient, from low concentration to high concentration, through the process of active transport. This requires expenditure of energy on the part of the cell and a carrier protein. Carrier proteins that assist in active transport are sometimes called pumps.

Primary Processes of Pharmacokinetics

4.3 Absorption is the process of moving a drug from the site of administration to the bloodstream.

For most medications the first step toward reaching target cells is **absorption,** the process by which drug molecules move from their site of administration to the blood. Topical drugs may be absorbed across the skin or associated mucous membranes lining the vagina, the respiratory tract, or the nasal passages. Enteral drugs are absorbed across membranes lining the GI tract to enter the blood. Drugs administered parenterally by the intradermal (ID) or subcutaneous routes are absorbed by blood vessels in the skin; intramuscular (IM) drugs cross membranes to enter the rich blood supply serving skeletal muscle. With the exception of a few topical medications, GI anti-infectives, and some radiologic contrast agents, the majority of drugs must be absorbed in order to produce an effect. Of course, drugs administered directly into blood vessels by IV or intra-arterial routes are not absorbed because they are already in the bloodstream.

Absorption is the primary pharmacokinetic factor determining the onset of drug action—the length of time it takes a drug to produce its effect. In general, the more rapid the absorption, the faster will be the onset of drug action. Drugs used in critical care are designed to be absorbed within seconds or minutes, or they are given intravenously. At the other extreme are drugs such as the contraceptive Mirena, which is a polyethylene tube placed in the uterus. The drug inside Mirena, levonorgestrel, is absorbed slowly from the tube and provides contraceptive protection for up to 5 years.

In addition to onset time, absorption determines the intensity of drug action. For any given drug, a specific percentage of the drug is absorbed, ranging from 0% to 100%. Everything else being equal, drugs with higher absorption rates produce a more effective response than those with lower absorption rates. The degree of absorption is conditional on many factors.

Route of administration: The different routes of drug administration are presented in Chapter 3. Because drugs administered by the IV route bypass absorption entirely, they have the most rapid onset of action. Inhalation also produces a very rapid response because the membrane separating the inhaled drug from the bloodstream is very thin, making absorption easier. Subcutaneous and IM formulations are absorbed rapidly, though they have a slower onset of action than IV or inhalation.

Tablets and capsules must dissolve before the drug is available for absorption, thus their onset time is relatively slow. The dissolution rate of a tablet or capsule is often the slowest part of the absorption process of an oral medication. Because oral liquid formulations do not undergo dissolution, they are absorbed faster than tablets or capsules.

Topical drugs applied to the skin are absorbed very slowly because the skin is relatively thick, and it is difficult for the drug to penetrate the keratin layer. Topical drugs applied to mucous membranes are absorbed faster than those applied to the skin because these membranes are relatively thin and have a rich blood supply.

CONNECTION *Checkpoint* 4.1

Crushing a tablet enhances a drug's rate of absorption because it does not have to dissolve. From what you learned in Chapter 3, what type of medications should not be crushed or opened? See Answer to Connection Checkpoint 4.1 in Appendix A.

Drug concentration and dose: For almost all drugs, higher doses produce a faster and greater response. This is because a higher dose produces a greater concentration gradient for diffusion. As an example, consider the antihypertensive drug diltiazem (Cardizem) given as a 100-mg tablet, which is about 50% absorbed. Half of the drug (50 mg) will reach the bloodstream for distribution to target cells. If the dose of diltiazem is doubled to 200 mg, greater amounts of the drug (100 mg) will be absorbed in the bloodstream. Although the percentage absorbed remains the same (50%), the higher dose results in a greater quantity of drug in the blood, and subsequently more available to produce an action at its target cells.

GI tract environment: For drugs given by mouth, the physical and chemical conditions within the GI tract play a significant role in drug absorption. Most drug absorption occurs in the small intestine, because this portion of the GI is longer, and the absorptive surfaces of the microvilli are much more extensive as compared to the stomach. Furthermore the time spent by food and drugs in the stomach is brief, and the thick mucous layer in the organ discourages absorption.

Digestive motility is variable among patients; very rapid motility may speed the drug through the GI tract too quickly before complete absorption occurs. Abnormally slow motility may cause the drug to be retained in the stomach, where it is exposed for a longer time to destructive enzymes and high acidity. Fatty foods in the stomach nearly always slow drug absorption. With few exceptions, absorption is most complete when the drug is taken between meals; the presence of food in the stomach may lessen the incidence of nausea and vomiting but it also slows absorption. All these factors contribute to wide patient variability with regard to absorption, as well as to drug action when drugs are administered orally.

Blood flow to the absorption site: For a drug to be absorbed there must be adequate blood flow to the site of administration. IM injections are placed into large muscles because they have the highest blood flow to maximize absorption. During heart failure or shock, the amount of blood flow to certain tissues is reduced and absorption from the GI tract or IM sites may be diminished. Topical drugs placed on the skin have slow absorption due to the poor blood supply to the upper layers of the skin.

There are circumstances where blood flow can be manipulated to purposely slow absorption. For example, local anesthetics can be toxic if absorbed too quickly. To purposely slow absorption, a vasoconstrictor (epinephrine) is sometimes added to local anesthetics to reduce blood flow to the treated region.

Drug ionization: Ionized molecules are those that carry a positive or a negative charge. Most drugs can exist in either a charged or uncharged state, depending on the pH of the surrounding fluid. The ionization of a drug affects its ability to cross plasma membranes and to be excreted by the body (see Section 4.6). Aspirin, or acetylsalicylic acid, provides an example of the effects of ionization on absorption, as depicted in Figure 4.4. In the highly acidic environment of the stomach, aspirin is in its nonionized form and is thus readily absorbed

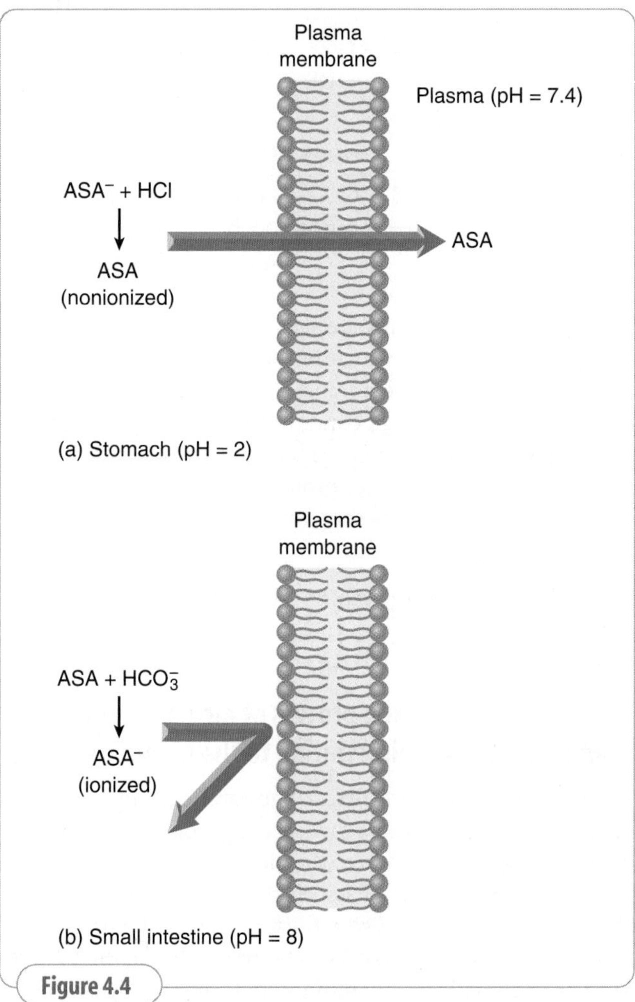

Figure 4.4

Effect of pH on drug absorption: (a) a weak acid such as aspirin (ASA) is in a nonionized form in an acidic environment and absorption occurs; (b) in a basic environment, aspirin is mostly in an ionized form and absorption is prevented.

and distributed in the bloodstream. As aspirin enters the alkaline environment of the small intestine, however, it becomes ionized. In its ionized form, the aspirin molecule is less likely to be absorbed and distributed to target cells. Unlike acidic drugs such as aspirin, medications that are weakly basic are in their nonionized form in an alkaline environment; therefore, basic drugs are much more likely to be absorbed in alkaline environments such as the small intestine. In simplest terms, it may help the student to remember the following:

- Acids are absorbed in acids because they are nonionized.
- Bases are absorbed in bases because they are nonionized.

Drug interactions: Many examples of drug–drug and food–drug interactions that influence absorption have been discovered. For example, administering oral tetracyclines with food or drugs containing calcium, iron, or magnesium can significantly delay absorption of the antibiotic. High-fat meals can slow stomach motility significantly and delay the absorption of oral medications taken with the meal. The mechanisms and types of drug interactions are presented in detail in Chapter 6.

Surface area: Other factors being equal, drugs will be absorbed faster when applied to regions of the body having a larger surface area. This is one reason why the small intestine is such an important organ for drug absorption. Relative to the oral cavity and stomach, the small intestine has a vast surface area richly supplied with blood vessels. Another region with an enormous surface area is the lung. Inhaled substances such as bronchodilators or crack cocaine act almost instantaneously due the large absorptive surface provided by terminal bronchioles and alveoli.

CONNECTION *Checkpoint* 4.2

From what you learned in Chapter 3, classify the following routes of administration as topical, enteral, or parenteral: buccal, subcutaneous, intravaginal, sublingual, and rectal. See Answer to Connection Checkpoint 4.2 in Appendix A.

4.4 Distribution describes how drugs are transported throughout the body.

Distribution is the branch of pharmacokinetics describing the transport of pharmacologic agents throughout the body after they are absorbed. Drugs are not simply passive agents, being swept along an inert path to their target tissues. Rather, drugs may interact with blood components and may be chemically and physically changed before they reach their targets. Like absorption, there are several key factors influencing drug distribution.

Blood flow to tissues: The simplest factor determining drug distribution is the amount of blood flow to body tissues. Because the heart, liver, and kidneys receive a great percentage of the blood supply, these organs receive the highest exposure to drugs. Skin, bone, and adipose tissue receive a meager blood flow; therefore, it is more difficult to deliver high concentrations of drugs to these areas.

Blood flow should also be considered at the local level. For example, after traumatic injury, the blood supply to a fractured bone may be reduced owing to broken blood vessels, or blocked by cellular debris from the inflammatory process. Antibiotics may have difficulty reaching the injured area until blood flow can be restored. To deliver high concentrations of drugs to injured, necrotic, or abscessed areas that have inadequate perfusion is always challenging.

Drug solubility: The physical properties of a drug greatly influence how it moves throughout the body after administration. Lipid solubility is an important characteristic because it determines how quickly a drug is absorbed, mixes within the bloodstream, crosses membranes, and becomes localized in body tissues. Lipid-soluble agents are not limited by the barriers that normally stop water-soluble drugs; thus, they are more completely distributed to body tissues.

Tissue storage: Some tissues have the ability to accumulate and store drugs in high concentrations relative to other tissues. The bone marrow, teeth, eyes, and adipose tissue have an especially high **affinity,** or attraction, for certain medications. Examples of agents that are stored in adipose tissue are thiopental (Pentothal), diazepam (Valium), and lipid-soluble vitamins. Tetracycline binds to calcium salts and accumulates in bones and teeth. Once stored in tissues, drugs may remain in the body for many months and be released very slowly back to the circulation.

Drug-protein binding: Many drugs bind reversibly to plasma proteins, particularly albumin, to form **drug-protein complexes.** Drug-protein complexes are too large to cross capillary membranes; the drugs continue circulating in the bloodstream and are unavailable for distribution to their target tissues. Drugs will remain "trapped" in the bloodstream bound to plasma proteins until they are released or displaced from the drug-protein complex. Only unbound, or free, drugs can reach their target cells or be excreted by the kidneys. This concept is illustrated in Figure 4.5. Some drugs, such as the anticoagulant warfarin (Coumadin), are very highly bound; 99% of the drug in the plasma exists in drug-protein complexes and only 1% exists as a free drug available to reach target cells.

Drugs and other chemicals compete with one another for plasma protein binding sites, and some agents have a greater affinity (attraction) for these binding sites than other agents. Drug–drug and drug–food interactions may occur when one agent displaces another from plasma proteins. The displaced medication can quickly reach high levels in the blood and produce adverse effects. For example, drugs such as aspirin or cimetidine (Tagamet) will displace warfarin from the drug-protein complex, thus raising blood levels of free warfarin and dramatically increasing the risk of hemorrhage. Most drug guides give the percentage of the drug bound to plasma proteins; when giving multiple medications that are highly bound, the nurse should carefully monitor for adverse effects. This topic is further discussed in Chapter 6.

Special barriers to drug distribution: Most capillaries in the body are relatively porous owing to spaces between the endothelial cells. Many drugs can exit the bloodstream by traveling

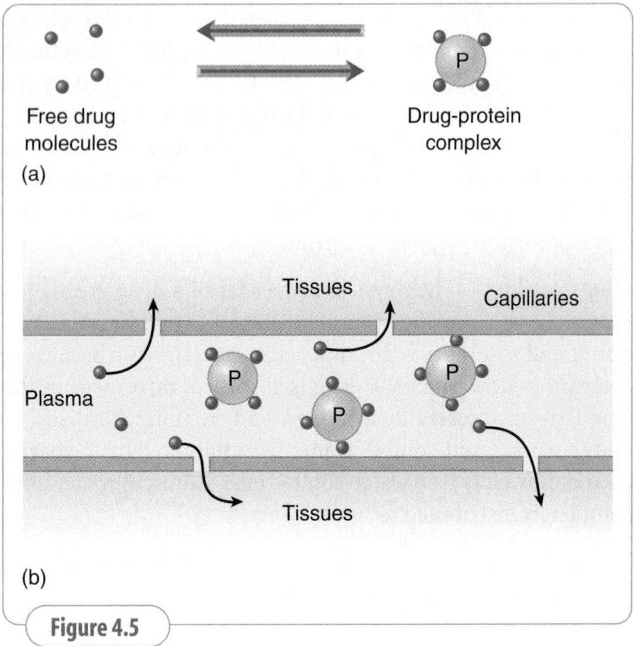

Figure 4.5

Plasma protein binding and drug availability: (a) the drug exists in a free state or is bound to plasma protein; (b) drug-protein complexes are too large to cross membranes.

through the spaces and enter the interstitial fluid with relative ease. The brain and placenta, however, possess special anatomic barriers that inhibit many chemicals and drugs from exiting the blood. These barriers are referred to as the **blood–brain barrier** and **fetal–placental barrier.**

Unlike other capillaries, those in the brain have endothelial cells that are sealed by tight junctions and a thick basement membrane. Brain cells known as astrocytes press firmly against the basement membrane, secreting chemicals that adjust the capillary permeability. The purpose of the blood–brain barrier is obvious: to protect the brain from pathogens and toxic substances. Some highly lipid-soluble agents such as general anesthetics, sedatives, antianxiety agents, and anticonvulsant drugs readily cross the blood–brain barrier to produce their actions on the central nervous system (CNS). In contrast, most antitumor medications and antibiotics do not easily cross this barrier, making brain cancers and infections difficult to treat. The blood–brain barrier is not fully developed in neonates, and the barrier becomes more permeable when it is inflamed due to infections such as meningitis.

The series of membranes that separate the maternal blood from the fetal blood serve as a fetal–placental barrier that prevents potentially harmful substances from passing from the mother's bloodstream to the fetus. In reality, the placenta is an ineffective barrier because many substances are able to cross it. Substances such as alcohol, cocaine, caffeine, and certain prescription medications easily cross the placental barrier and can potentially harm the fetus. Consequently, no prescription medication, over-the-counter (OTC) drug, or herbal therapy should be taken by a pregnant patient without first consulting a health care provider or nurse practitioner. The nurse should always question female patients in the childbearing years regarding their pregnancy status before a drug is prescribed. Substances that cause birth defects, or teratogens, are presented in Chapter 6. Chapter 10 presents special concerns related to pharmacotherapy of pregnant and lactating patients.

4.5 Metabolism is a process that changes the activity of a drug and makes it more likely to be excreted.

Drug **metabolism,** also called biotransformation, is the process used by the body to chemically change a drug molecule. Metabolism involves hundreds of complex biochemical pathways and reactions that alter the structure and function of drugs, nutrients, vitamins, and minerals. The liver is the primary site of drug metabolism, although the kidneys and cells of the intestinal tract also have high metabolic rates. To survive, all cells must undergo metabolism to some extent. The types of metabolic reactions, however, are specific to each type of cell: Reactions occurring in liver cells are very different from those in skin cells or brain cells.

In most cases, metabolic reactions change the structure of a drug so that it can be more easily excreted by the body. This often changes the drug from lipid soluble (easily absorbed and distributed) to water soluble, which is more easily excreted by the kidneys. In addition, once the molecule has been changed to water soluble, it is less able to enter tissues. This serves as a detoxifying effect for drugs and other substances entering the body.

Chemical changes to drugs always result in functional changes. The products of drug metabolism, or metabolites, usually have less pharmacologic activity than the original molecule. On rare occasions a metabolite may have greater activity than the original drug. This is the case for codeine. Although 90% of codeine is changed to inactive metabolites by the liver, 10% is converted to morphine, which has significantly greater ability to relieve severe pain. In a few cases, the metabolite has greater toxicity than the original drug. Probably the most common example of this is acetaminophen (Tylenol), which is converted to a metabolite that is highly toxic to the liver.

In a few cases, the drug administered to the patient has no pharmacologic activity until it undergoes metabolism. Agents that require metabolism to produce their action are called **prodrugs.** For example, the antihypertensive enalapril (Vasotec) is converted in the liver to enaliprat, which has considerably more ability to lower blood pressure than the original drug. Examples of other prodrugs include benazepril (Lotensin) and losartan (Cozaar).

Hepatic microsomal enzymes: Most metabolism in the liver is accomplished by the **hepatic microsomal enzyme system.** This enzyme complex is known as the P-450 system, named after cytochrome P450 (CYP), which is a key component of the system. Although this system is complex, a key point to remember is that CYP is simply an enzyme that metabolizes drugs as well as nutrients and other endogenous substances.

It was once thought that a single CYP was responsible for all drug metabolism, but scientists have since identified more than 50 CYPs. These different forms are called **isozymes** of

TABLE 4.1 Isozymes of Cytochrome P450: Selected Substrates, Inducers, and Inhibitors

Isozyme	Substrates	Inducers	Inhibitors
CYP1A2	acetaminophen, amitriptyline, caffeine, dantrolene, diazepam, estradiol, haloperidol, imipramine, lidocaine, methadone, ondansetron, ritonavir, tacrine, tamoxifen, verapamil, warfarin	omeprazole, phenobarbital, phenytoin, rifampin, ritonavir	cimetidine, ciprofloxacin, erythromycin, grapefruit juice, isoniazid, ketoconazole, levofloxacin, paroxetine
CYP2C9	amiodarone, amitriptyline, dapsone, ethosuximide, ibuprofen, imipramine, naproxen, nifedipine, omeprazole, phenytoin, progesterone, propranolol, ritonavir, sulfonamides, tamoxifen, testosterone, tricyclic antidepressants, valproic acid, warfarin	barbiturates, carbamazepine, ethanol, phenobarbital	cimetidine, disulfiram, fluconazole, fluoxetine, fluvastatin, ketoconazole, omeprazole, ritonavir, sertraline
CYP2C19	diazepam, omeprazole	none	
CYP2D6	amitriptyline, captopril, chlorpromazine, citalopram, codeine, fluoxetine, haloperidol, imipramine, lidocaine, loratadine, meperidine, methamphetamine, metoprolol, mexiletine, odansetron, oxycodone, paroxetine, propranolol, ritonavir, tamoxifen, tramadol, trazodone, venlafaxine	carbamazepine, phenobarbital, phenytoin, rifampin, ritonavir	amiodarone, cimetidine, citalopram, fluoxetine, haloperidol, methadone, paroxetine, ritonavir, sertraline
CYP3A4	alprazolam, amiodarone, carbamazepine, chlorpromazine, cocaine, cortisol, cyclosporine, diltiazem, erythromycin, ketoconazole, lidocaine, lovastatin, nifedipine, omeprazole, prednisone, ritonavir, sertraline, tamoxifen, venlafaxine, verapamil	dexamethasone, ethosuximide, nevirapine, phenobarbital, phenytoin, prednisone	clotrimazole, diltiazem, erythromycin, fluconazole, fluoxetine, ketoconazole, metronidazole, nifedipine, norfloxacin, omeprazole, fluoxetine, ritonavir, sertraline, verapamil, zafirlukast

cytochrome P450. Although very similar, each isozyme performs slightly different metabolic functions. CYPs are named by assigning numbers to indicate their subfamily, such as CYP1, CYP2, CYP3, and so on. Additional letters and numbers are added to further identify the specific gene, such as CYP1A1, CYP3A4, and CYP26C1. Fortunately for nursing students, there are only a handful of isozymes responsible for metabolizing the majority of drugs, as shown in Table 4.1.

The CYPs are very important to drug therapy because they determine the speed at which most drugs are metabolized and they contribute significantly to drug–drug interactions. Changes in the function of the hepatic microsomal enzymes can have significant effects on drug metabolism. There are three major consequences of the CYP system that have importance to pharmacotherapy.

- **Drugs as substrates.** When a drug is metabolized by a CYP, it is said to be a **substrate** for the enzyme. For example, naproxen and warfarin are substrates for CYP2C9. Codeine and amphetamine are substrates for a different isozyme, CYP2D6. Each CYP isozyme can metabolize dozens of different drugs. Furthermore, drugs are not specific for a single isozyme. Naproxen is metabolized by both CYP2C9 and CYP1A2, although the reactions occur at different rates. In other words, each isozyme of CYP can metabolize many different drugs, and a drug may be metabolized by multiple CYPs. Because of this overlap, drugs often compete for binding sites on the CYP isozymes, and drug–drug interactions are frequent.
- **Drugs as enzyme inhibitors.** Some drugs are able to inhibit the action of hepatic CYP isozymes. The inhibition may affect all hepatic microsomal enzymes or it may be specific to a single isozyme. For example, ciprofloxacin (Cipro) inhibits CYP1A2. What effect might this inhibition have on a drug that is a substrate metabolized by CYP1A2? Recall that in most cases, drugs are inactivated by metabolism. Thus, giving Cipro concurrently with naproxen (a substrate for CYP1A2) could result in less inactivation of naproxen, higher amounts of naproxen in the blood, and a prolonged drug effect. Because naproxen is a relatively safe drug, this higher level may not produce noticeable toxicity. However, giving Cipro with a more toxic drug such as warfarin (also a substrate for CYP1A2) has the potential for a serious drug interaction. The dose of warfarin would need to be adjusted downward to avoid toxicity.
- **Drugs as enzyme inducers.** A few drugs have the ability to increase metabolic activity in the liver, a process called **enzyme induction.** For example, phenobarbital causes the liver to synthesize greater amounts of microsomal enzymes, including CYP3A4, CYP2C19, and CYP2C9. By doing so, phenobarbital accelerates the metabolism (inactivation) of most drugs metabolized in the liver. In fact, with continued therapy phenobarbital increases the rate of its own destruction. In these patients, because drugs will be inactivated at a much faster rate, higher doses may be required to achieve an optimum therapeutic effect.

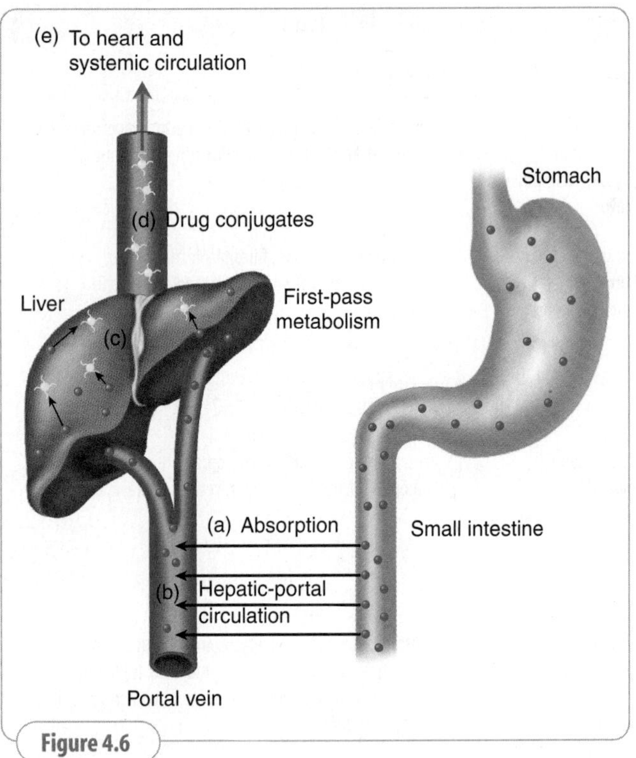

Figure 4.6

First-pass effect: (a) the drug is absorbed; (b) the drug enters the hepatic portal circulation and goes directly to the liver; (c) hepatic microsomal enzymes metabolize the drug to an inactive form; (d) the drug conjugates, leaving the liver; (e) the drug is distributed to the general circulation.

Metabolism has a number of additional therapeutic consequences. As illustrated in Figure 4.6, drugs absorbed after oral administration cross directly into the hepatic-portal circulation, which carries blood to the liver before it is distributed to other body tissues. Some drugs can be completely metabolized to an inactive form on their first trip through the liver before they even reach the general circulation. This **first-pass effect** is important to pharmacology, because a large number of oral drugs are rendered inactive by hepatic metabolic reactions. Alternate routes of delivery that bypass the first-pass effect, such as the sublingual, rectal, or parenteral routes, may need to be considered for these drugs. Remember, however, that even drugs administered by parenteral routes may be rapidly inactivated when passing through the liver.

Patient variation in metabolism: Certain patients have diminished hepatic metabolic activity, which may result in altered drug action. Infants do not develop a mature microsomal enzyme system until at least 1 year of age. Hepatic enzyme activity is generally reduced in older adults; thus these patients may require lower doses. Patients with liver impairment will require reductions in drug dosage because of the decreased metabolic activity. The nurse should pay careful attention to laboratory values that may indicate liver disease so that drug doses may be adjusted accordingly.

The baseline functions of hepatic microsomal enzyme systems are genetically determined. Genetic differences in the function of CYP enzymes may cause people to metabolize drugs at widely different rates. Some patients metabolize at a faster rate, others at a slower rate. Certain genetic disorders have been recognized in which patients lack specific metabolic enzymes. In these "slow metabolizers" normal drug doses may cause toxicity. Genetic differences are not always predictable, although some occur at a higher rate in certain ethnic populations (see Chapter 5).

4.6 Excretion processes remove drugs from the body.

Drugs will continue to act on the body until they are either metabolized to an inactive form, or they are removed from the body by **excretion**. The rate at which a drug is excreted determines its concentration in the blood and, ultimately, its duration of action. Pathologic states, especially liver or kidney disease, often increase the duration and intensity of drug action in the body because they interfere with natural excretion mechanisms.

Renal excretion: Although drugs are removed from the body by numerous organs and tissues, the primary site of excretion is the kidney. In an average size person, the kidneys filter approximately 180 L of blood each day. Unbound (free) drugs,

CONNECTIONS

Treating the Diverse Patient One Size Does Not Fit All

One of the difficult challenges of modern pharmacology is to develop medications that produce an optimal result with minimal adverse effects for all users. Because humans vary in their individual response to medications, drugs target the "average" person, a one-size-fits-all approach, when the "average person" does not exist. A solution to this dilemma may come in the near future with pharmacogenomics, the science that predicts when a patient will have a positive or an adverse response to a drug based on inherited genes.

Scientists have determined that the way a person responds to a medication depends on certain traits found in the genes: small variations in the sequence of their nucleotide bases. Without knowing the specific genes involved in the drug response, one cannot predict the individual response to a medication.

Gene variation diagnostic tools called SNPs (pronounced snips) are expensive to access. However, DNA microarrays (DNA chips) are part of an evolving technology that will open the door to a targeted drug response for a group of patients. Review of gene susceptibility prior to prescribing the drug may be a possibility in the future.

This technology would also be beneficial in clinical trials. By predetermining patients' responses, those with known adverse reaction to a drug would be excluded. Clinical trials would be conducted to smaller groups, resulting in less expense and, ultimately, in reduced cost of drugs to the consumer. The health care provider could prescribe in confidence, unlike the current method in which the prescriber gives the patient a medication that may or may not be effective or have adverse effects based on the individual response.

water-soluble agents, electrolytes, and small molecules easily pass through the pores of Bowman's capsule and enter the filtrate. Proteins, blood cells, and drug-protein complexes are not filtered because of their large size.

After filtration at the renal corpuscle, drugs may undergo reabsorption in the renal tubule. Mechanisms of reabsorption are the same as absorption elsewhere in the body. Nonionized and lipid-soluble drugs cross renal tubular membranes more easily and return to the circulation; ionized and water-soluble drugs generally remain in the filtrate.

Drug-protein complexes and other substances too large to be filtered in Bowman's capsule are sometimes secreted into the distal tubule of the nephron. For example, only 10% of a dose of penicillin G is filtered in Bowman's capsule; 90% is secreted into the renal tubule. As with metabolic enzyme activity, secretion mechanisms are less active in infants and in older adults.

The renal excretion of drugs is dependent on the pH of the filtrate in the renal tubule. Weak acids like aspirin are excreted more efficiently when the filtrate is slightly alkaline. This is because aspirin is ionized in an alkaline environment, and the ionized drug will remain in the filtrate to be excreted in the urine. Weakly basic drugs such as diazepam (Valium) are excreted more quickly if the filtrate is slightly acidic because they are ionized in that environment. The pH of the filtrate may be intentionally manipulated to speed up renal excretion. For example, following an overdose of an acidic drug such as aspirin, nurses may administer sodium bicarbonate. Sodium bicarbonate makes the urine more basic, which ionizes the aspirin molecule, facilitating its urinary excretion. The excretion of diazepam, on the other hand, can be enhanced by giving ammonium chloride, which acidifies the filtrate and ionizes the diazepam molecule.

Impairment of kidney function can dramatically affect pharmacokinetics. Patients with renal failure will have diminished ability to excrete medications and may retain drugs for extended periods. Doses for these patients must be reduced to prevent drug toxicity. Because small to moderate changes in renal function can cause rapid increases in serum drug levels, kidney function must be constantly monitored in patients receiving nephrotoxic drugs or medications that have a narrow margin of safety.

Pulmonary excretion: Drugs delivered by gaseous or volatile liquid forms are especially suited for excretion by the respiratory system. The rate of respiratory excretion is dependent on factors that affect gas exchange, including diffusion, gas solubility, and blood flow to the lungs. The elimination of gaseous and volatile anesthetics following surgery is primarily dependent on respiratory activity: The faster the breathing rate, the greater the excretion. On the other hand, the respiratory removal of water-soluble agents such as alcohol is more dependent on blood flow to the lungs. The greater the blood flow through lung capillaries, the greater the pulmonary excretion. In contrast with other methods of excretion, the lungs excrete most drugs in their original unmetabolized form.

Glandular secretion: Glandular activity is another elimination mechanism. Water-soluble drugs may be secreted into the saliva, sweat, or breast milk. The "funny taste" that patients experience when given certain drugs is an example of the secretion of medications into saliva. Another example is the garlic smell that can be detected when standing next to a perspiring person who has recently eaten garlic. Excretion into breast milk is of considerable importance for basic drugs such as morphine or codeine, because these can achieve high concentrations and potentially affect the nursing infant. Nursing mothers should always check with their health care provider before taking any prescription medication, OTC drug, or herbal supplement. Drugs of special concern to the pregnant or breast-feeding patient are discussed in Chapter 10.

Fecal and biliary excretion: Certain oral drugs travel through the GI tract without being absorbed and are excreted in the feces. Examples include mebendazole (Vermox), a drug used to kill intestinal worms, and barium sulfate, a radiologic contrast agent.

Some drugs are secreted in bile, a process known as biliary excretion. Drugs secreted into bile will enter the duodenum via the common bile duct and eventually leave the body in the feces. However, most bile is circulated back to the liver by **enterohepatic recirculation**, as illustrated in Figure 4.7. Drugs may be recirculated numerous times with the bile, thus extending their stay in the body; biliary excretion is influential in prolonging the activity of digoxin (Lanoxin), certain antibiotics and phenothiazines. Recirculated drugs are eventually metabolized by the liver and may be excreted by the kidneys. Recirculation and elimination of drugs through biliary excretion may continue for several weeks after therapy has been discontinued.

Time–Response Relationships

4.7 The therapeutic response of most drugs depends on their concentration in the plasma.

The therapeutic response from most drugs is directly related to their concentration in the plasma. Although the concentration of the drug at its target tissue is more predictive of drug action, this quantity is impossible to measure. For example, it is possible to conduct a laboratory test that measures the serum level of the drug lithium carbonate (Eskalith) by taking a blood sample; it is a far different matter to measure the quantity of this drug in neurons within the brain. It is common practice to monitor the plasma levels of certain drugs that have a low safety profile and to use these data to predict drug action or toxicity. It should always be remembered, however, that individual responses to drugs are highly variable and patients may experience toxic effects (or no effects) even if the serum concentration of the drug lies in the normal range.

A number of important pharmacokinetic principles can be illustrated by measuring the drug plasma level following a single dose administered by the oral route. These pharmacokinetic

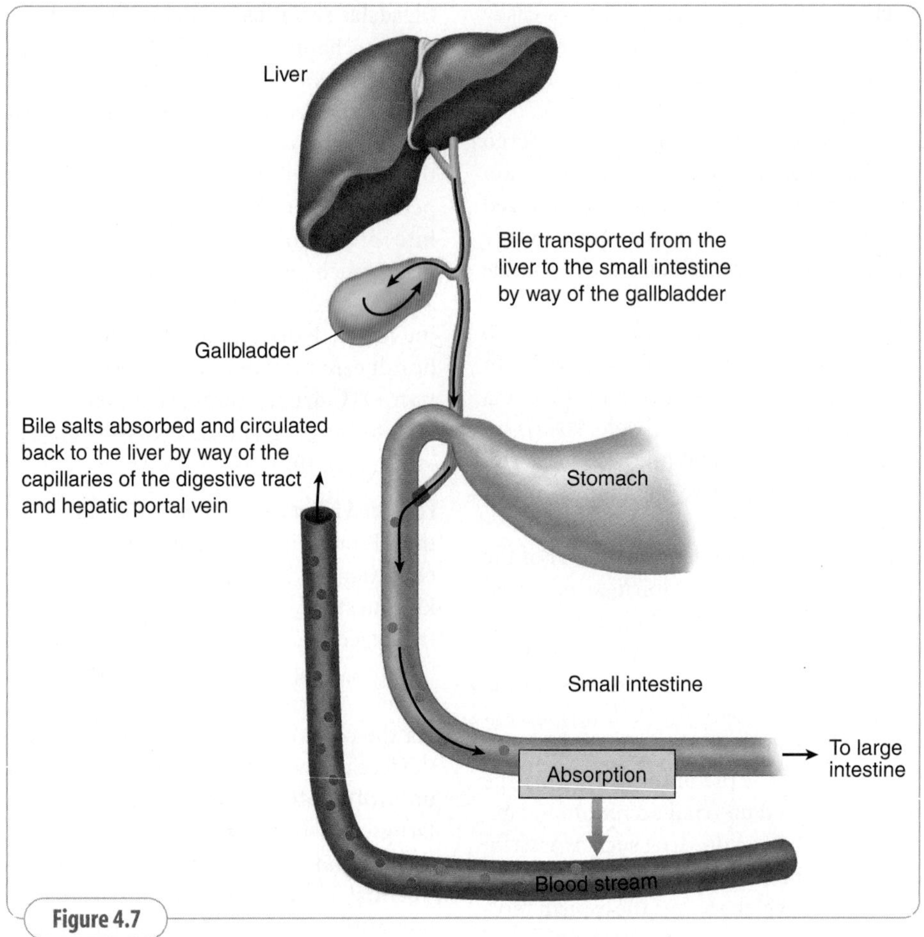

Figure 4.7

Enterohepatic recirculation.

values are shown graphically in Figure 4.8. In this example, the plasma drug level slowly increased and took about 2 hours before the **minimum effective concentration** was reached. The minimum effective drug plasma concentration, that amount of drug required to produce a therapeutic effect, is 6 mcg/mL. The level of drug then entered the **therapeutic range** of the drug, which in this case lies between 6 and 12 mcg/mL. In this range, the drug produced its desired therapeutic action. After peaking, the drug plasma level slowly began to fall out of the therapeutic range due to excretion processes. A higher dose might have caused the drug plasma level to reach a **toxic concentration,** that level of drug that results in serious adverse effects. The goal of pharmacotherapy is to reach and maintain a plasma drug level in the therapeutic range while avoiding the toxic concentration.

These values have great clinical significance. For example, if the patient has a severe headache and is given half of an aspirin tablet, the plasma drug level will remain below the minimum effective concentration, and the patient will not experience pain relief. Two or three tablets will increase the plasma level of aspirin into the therapeutic range, and the pain will subside. Taking six or more tablets may result in adverse effects, such as GI bleeding or tinnitus. For each drug administered, the nurse's goal is to keep its plasma concentration in the therapeutic range. For some drugs, this therapeutic range is quite wide. For other medications, the difference between a minimum effective dose and a toxic dose can be extremely narrow.

4.8 The drug half-life estimates the duration of action for most medications.

Figure 4.8 shows that the drug concentration reached a peak and then fell back below the therapeutic range. The length of time a drug concentration remains in the therapeutic range is its duration of action. In this example, the duration of action was 6 hours. The duration of action is an important pharmacokinetic variable that is determined by how rapidly the drug is metabolized and excreted.

The most common description of a drug's duration of action is its **plasma half-life ($t_{1/2}$)**: the length of time required for the plasma concentration of a drug to decrease by one half after administration. Some drugs have a half-life of only a few minutes, whereas others have a half-life of several hours or days. A few drugs have exceptionally long half-lives; for example, amiodarone (Cordarone) has a $t_{1/2}$ of 40 to 55 days.

Is it better to administer a drug with a short or long half-life? The answer depends on the patient's condition and the treatment goal. Drugs with short half-lives are ideal for conditions and procedures having a brief duration. For example, during a dental procedure, local anesthesia may only be needed for 15 to 20 minutes; thus procaine (Novocain), with a half-life of 8 minutes, may be sufficient. Giving a drug with a long duration of action could cause adverse effects after the patient leaves the office. As another example, a simple headache can be relieved with a short-acting

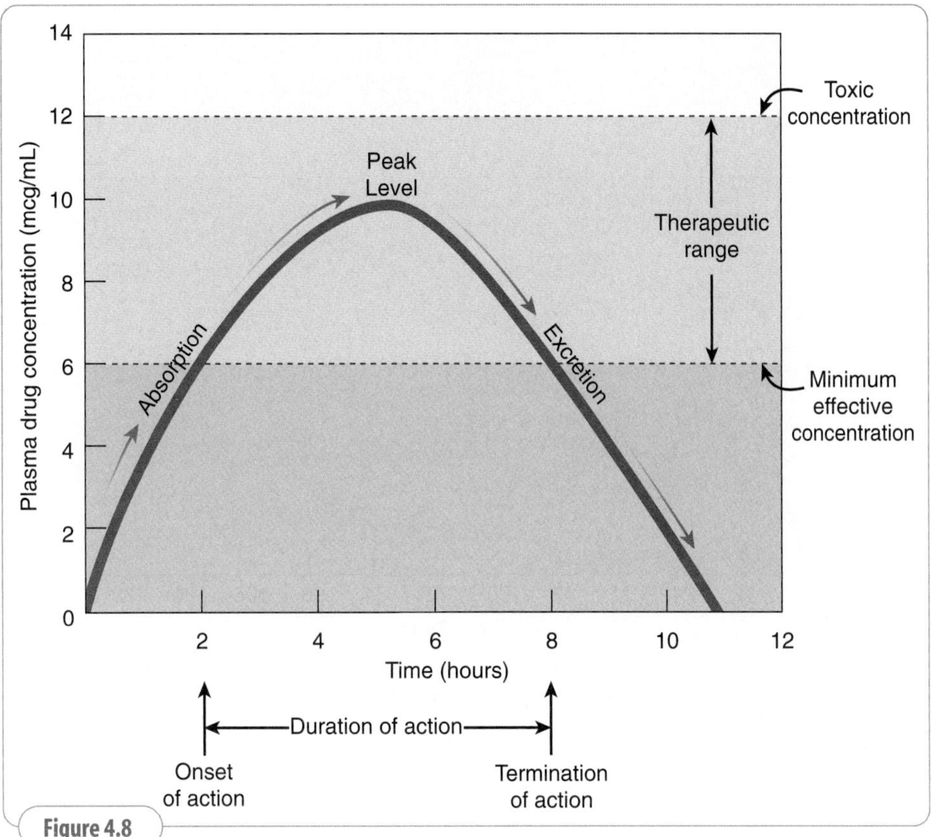

Figure 4.8

Single-dose drug administration: pharmacokinetic values for this drug are as follows: onset of action = 2 hours; duration of action = 6 hours; termination of action = 8 hours after administration; peak plasma concentration = 10 mcg/mL; time to peak drug effect = 5 hours; $t_{1/2}$ = 4 hours.

drug such as aspirin ($t_{1/2}$ = 15–20 minutes), rather than a drug with a 10- or 12-hour duration. Because short-acting drugs are rapidly excreted, the risk of long-term adverse effects is less.

Long duration drugs also have certain advantages. In the preceding example, procaine would not be suitable for a dental procedure that lasts 2 hours because multiple injections would be necessary. Long duration drugs are beneficial in treating chronic conditions such as heart failure or hypertension and for the prevention of conditions such as migraine headaches, seizures, or pregnancy. Short-acting drugs such as aspirin must be given every 3 to 4 hours, whereas medications with longer half-lives, such as felodipine ($t_{1/2}$ = 10 hours), need to be given only once a day. As drugs stay in the body for prolonged periods, however, the risk for long-term adverse effects increases. This can become particularly serious for patients with significant renal or hepatic impairment; diminished metabolism and excretion will cause the plasma half-life of a drug to increase, and the concentration may reach toxic levels. In these patients, medications must be given less frequently, or the dosages must be reduced.

As a rule of thumb, when a drug is discontinued it takes approximately four half-lives before the agent is considered "functionally" eliminated. After four half-lives, 94% of the drug has been eliminated. In the case of procaine with a half-life of only 8 minutes, the drug is considered eliminated in 32 minutes. Although some drug remains, it is likely too small an amount to produce any beneficial or toxic effect. In the example of felodipine ($t_{1/2}$ = 10 hours), the drug would take 40 hours to be eliminated. It must be noted that this is a "rule of thumb" and does not apply to all drugs; it certainly does not apply to medications administered to patients with renal or hepatic impairment.

4.9 Repeated dosing allows a plateau drug plasma level to be reached.

Few drugs are administered as a single dose. When drugs are taken in multiple doses for extended periods, the goal is to keep the drug plasma level continuously within the therapeutic range. In other words, the next dose should be administered before the drug plasma level falls below the minimum effective concentration.

Multiple doses result in an accumulation of drug in the bloodstream, as shown in Figure 4.9. If doses are timed correctly, a plateau drug plasma level will be reached and maintained within the therapeutic range. From a pharmacokinetic perspective, at the plateau level the amount of drug administered equals the amount of drug being excreted, resulting in a steady therapeutic level of drug being distributed to body tissues. Theoretically, it takes approximately four half-lives to reach this equilibrium. If the medication is given as a continuous infusion, the plateau can be reached very quickly and maintained with little or no fluctuation in drug plasma levels.

Note that in Figure 4.8, plasma drug levels are not necessarily smooth and continuous: There are peaks as well as troughs.

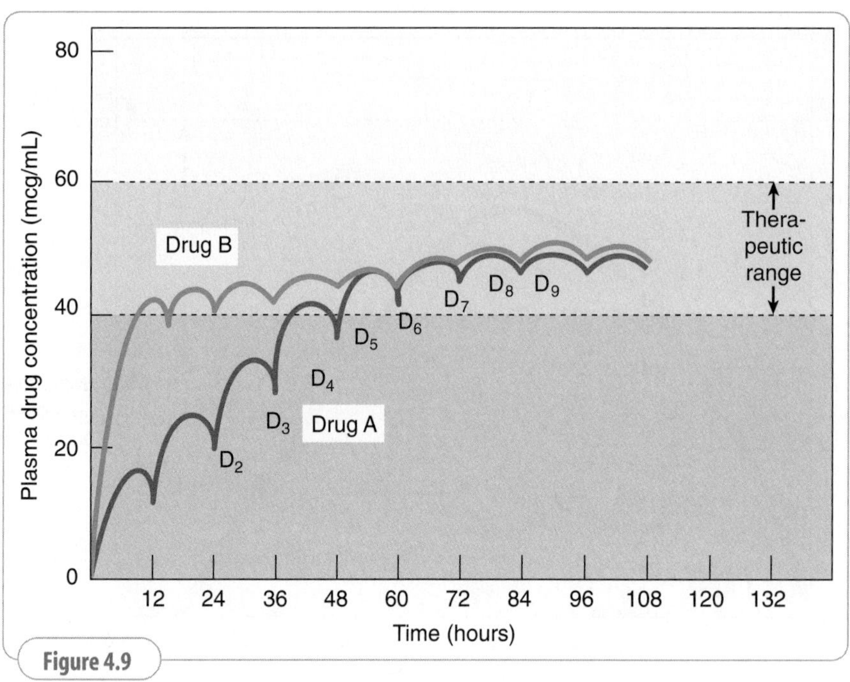

Figure 4.9

Multiple-dose drug administration: Drug A and drug B are administered every 12 hours. Drug B reaches the therapeutic range faster, because the first dose is a loading dose.

When giving oral drugs, there is always some degree of fluctuation in peak concentration and trough concentration levels. A key point is that the peak should not rise into the toxic range, nor should the trough fall below the therapeutic range. Sustained or extended release formulations are designed to slowly release the drug so peak and trough fluctuations are minimized. Changing the dosing schedule can also reduce fluctuations. For example, rather than giving 60 mg of codeine once daily, it may be given 30 mg bid or 20 mg tid to reduce wide variation in the peak and trough levels.

The plateau may be reached faster by administration of loading doses followed by regular maintenance doses. A **loading dose** is a higher amount of drug, often given only once or twice, that is administered to "prime" the bloodstream with a level sufficient to quickly induce a therapeutic response. Before plasma levels drop back toward zero, intermittent **maintenance doses** are given to keep the plasma drug concentration in the therapeutic range. Although blood levels of the drug fluctuate with this approach, the equilibrium state can be reached almost as rapidly as with a continuous infusion. Loading doses are particularly important for drugs with prolonged half-lives and for situations in which it is critical to raise drug plasma levels quickly, as might be the case when administering an antibiotic for a severe infection. In Figure 4.9, it took almost five doses (48 hours) before a therapeutic level was reached using a routine dosing schedule. With a loading dose, a therapeutic level was reached within 12 hours.

UNDERSTANDING THE CHAPTER

Key Concepts Summary

4.1 Pharmacokinetics focuses on what the body does to drugs after they are administered.

4.2 Drugs use diffusion and active transport to cross plasma membranes to reach their target cells.

4.3 Absorption is the process of moving a drug from the site of administration to the bloodstream.

4.4 Distribution describes how drugs are transported throughout the body.

4.5 Metabolism is a process that changes the activity of a drug and makes it more likely to be excreted.

4.6 Excretion processes remove drugs from the body.

4.7 The therapeutic response of most drugs depends on their concentration in the plasma.

4.8 The drug half-life estimates the duration of action for most medications.

4.9 Repeated dosing allows a plateau drug plasma level to be reached.

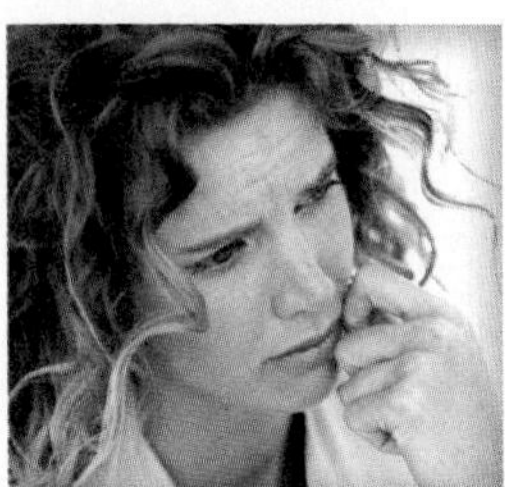

Making the PATIENT Connection

Remember the patient "John Kessler" at the beginning of the chapter? Now read the remainder of the case study. Based on the information presented within this chapter, respond to the critical thinking questions that follow.

Mr. Kessler has been ill for a long time and his prognosis is poor. He is 84 years old with multiple debilitating and chronic conditions. John, a patient with uncontrolled diabetes for more than 20 years, has experienced many complications due to this condition. Three years ago, he developed chronic renal failure and requires dialysis three times a week. Consequently, his heart has progressively weakened and no longer functions properly. To further complicate his condition, John has continued to consume alcohol every day and smokes one pack of cigarettes per day. He has a long history of alcoholism.

Five days ago, the patient suffered a massive stroke, which rendered him unconscious with respiratory insufficiency. Once admitted to the hospital, he was placed in the neurointensive care unit. As his respiratory status declined, he was placed on a mechanical ventilator. A chest x-ray this morning revealed bilateral pneumonia. Mr. Kessler is receiving multiple medications through both the intravenous and inhalation routes.

Critical Thinking Questions

1. What factors may influence drug metabolism in this patient?
2. Discuss why drug elimination for this patient may complicate the pharmacotherapy.
3. How will the IV or inhalation drug therapy affect the absorption of his medications?
4. John will receive a loading dose of IV antibiotic and then be placed on maintenance doses every 6 hours. What is the purpose of this regimen? Why would this patient be a candidate for a loading dose?

Case Study

Janice Albertson is a student nurse caring for this patient on the unit in which you are the RN. She has researched every drug her patient will be receiving and is familiar with the dose, mechanism of action, and possible adverse effects. Now she comes to you and asks, "Why is the drug's plasma half-life listed in the drug reference book? What's the value of this information?"

1. How would you respond to Janice's questions?
2. When are drugs with short half-lives indicated?
3. List the indications for the use of a drug with a long half-life.

NCLEX-RN® Review

1 The nurse is teaching the client about a newly prescribed medication. Which of the following statements made by the client would indicate the need for further medication education?

1. "The liquid form of the drug will be absorbed faster than the tablets."
2. "The higher the dose of the drug, the greater the response."
3. "Taking this drug with food will increase the absorption rate."
4. "I can consult my health care provider if I experience unexpected adverse effects."

2 The nurse is caring for several clients. With which of the following clients will the nurse most likely anticipate an alteration in drug metabolism?

1. A 3-day-old premature infant
2. A 22-year-old pregnant female
3. A 32-year-old man with kidney stones
4. A 50-year-old executive with hypertension

3 The client is receiving multiple medications, including one drug specifically used to stimulate gastric peristalsis. The nurse knows that this drug could have what influence on additional oral medications?

1. Increased absorption
2. Reduced excretion
3. Decreased absorption
4. Enhanced distribution

4 A client is being discharged from the hospital with a nebulizer for self-administration of inhalation medication. The nurse determines that client education has been successful when the client states:

1. "Inhaled medications should only be taken in the morning."
2. "Doses for inhaled medication are larger than those taken orally."
3. "Medicines taken by inhalation produce a very rapid response."
4. "Inhaled drugs are often rendered inactive by hepatic metabolic reactions."

5 The nurse is caring for a client with renal failure. The nurse would expect the duration of action for most medications to:

1. Decrease.
2. Improve.
3. Be unaffected.
4. Increase.

6 In which of the following anatomical structures would the nurse suspect high drug affinity? Select all that apply.

1. Bone marrow
2. Teeth
3. Blood
4. Eyes
5. Adipose tissue

See Answers to Critical Thinking Questions, Case Study, and NCLEX-RN® Review in Appendix A.

References

Alcorn, J., & McNamara, P. J. (2003). Pharmacokinetics in the newborn. *Advanced Drug Delivery Reviews, 55*(5), 667–686.

Buxton, I. L. (2006). Pharmacokinetics and pharmacodynamics: The dynamics of drug absorption, distribution, action and elimination. In L. L. Brunton, J. S. Lazo, & K. L. Parker (Eds.), *The pharmacological basis of therapeutics* (11th ed., pp. 1–39). New York: McGraw-Hill.

Cusak, B. J. (2004). Pharmacokinetics in older persons. *American Journal of Geriatric Pharmacotherapy, 2*(4), 274–302.

Eichelbaum, M., Ingelman-Sundberg, M., & Evans, W. E. (2006). Pharmacogenomics and individualized drug therapy. *Annual Review of Medicine, 57*, 119–137.

Ito, S., & Lee, A. (2003). Drug excretion into breast milk—Overview. *Advanced Drug Delivery Reviews, 55*(5), 617–627.

Mahato, R. I., Narang, A. S., Thoma, L., & Miller, D. D. (2003). Emerging trends in oral delivery of peptide and protein drugs. *Critical Reviews in Therapeutic Drug Carrier Systems, 20*(2-3), 153–214.

Yengi, L. G., Leung, L., & Kao, J. (2007). The evolving role of drug metabolism in drug discovery and development. *Pharmaceutical Research, 24*(5), 842–858.

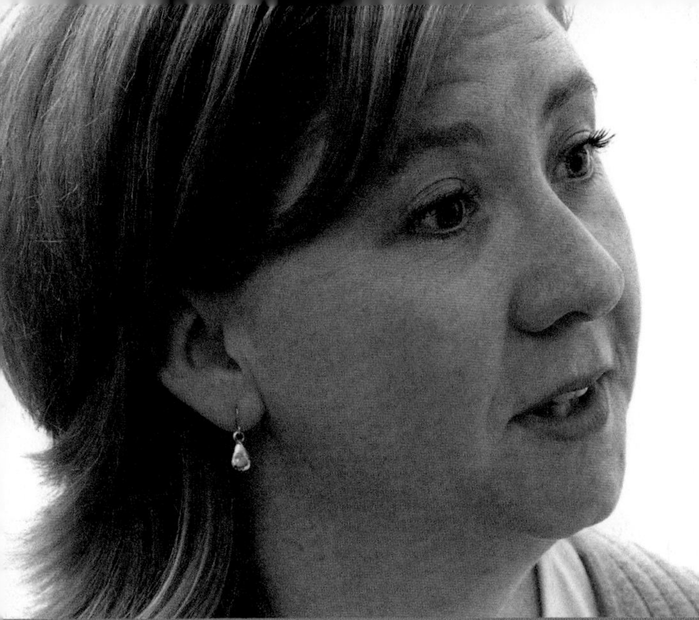

I am totally confused by all the antacid commercials on television. Some say their medication is the most efficient and others claim their brand is the most potent. What does it all mean?

Patient, "Katherine Hunter"

CHAPTER

Pharmacodynamics 5

Chapter Outline

Interpatient Variability

Therapeutic Index

Dose–Response Relationship

Potency and Efficacy

Receptor Theory

Agonists and Antagonists

Pharmacogenetics

Learning Outcomes

After reading this chapter, the student should be able to:

1. Employ principles of pharmacodynamics to explain variations in drug response in a population.
2. Use frequency distribution curves to explain interpatient variability in medication response.
3. Explain the importance of the median effective dose (ED_{50}) to clinical practice.
4. Compare and contrast median lethal dose (LD_{50}) and median toxicity dose (TD_{50}).
5. Relate a drug's therapeutic index to its margin of safety.
6. Identify the significance of the dose–response relationship to clinical practice.
7. Compare and contrast the terms *potency* and *efficacy*.
8. Describe the relationship between receptors and drug action.
9. Distinguish between an agonist, partial agonist, and antagonist.
10. Explain possible future developments in the field of pharmacogenetics.

Key Terms

agonist, 61
antagonist, 61
dose–response relationship, 57
efficacy, 58
frequency distribution curve, 56
idiosyncratic response, 62
intrinsic activity, 60
median effective dose (ED_{50}), 56
median lethal dose (LD_{50}), 57
median toxicity dose (TD_{50}), 57
partial agonist, 61
pharmacodynamics, 56
pharmacogenetics, 62
potency, 58
receptor, 60
second messenger, 60
therapeutic index, 57

The term *pharmacodynamics* is comprised of the root words *pharmaco*, which refers to medicines, and *dynamics*, which means "change." In simplest terms, pharmacodynamics refers to how a drug changes the body. A more complete definition explains **pharmacodynamics** as the branch of pharmacology concerned with the mechanisms of drug action and the relationships between drug concentration and responses in the body. This chapter examines the mechanisms by which drugs affect patients, and how the nurse can apply these principles to clinical practice.

Interpatient Variability

5.1 Patients have widely different responses to drugs, which can be depicted on a frequency distribution curve.

The principles of pharmacodynamics have important clinical applications. Health care providers and nurse practitioners must be able to predict whether a given dose of medication will produce a significant change in their patients. Why does the "average" dose obtained from a drug guide sometimes produce a hyperresponse and at other times no response at all? Knowledge of dose–response relationships, therapeutic indexes, and drug-receptor interactions—all topics of pharmacodynamics—helps nurses provide a safer and more effective treatment.

The interpatient variability observed during drug therapy can best be illustrated by examining a frequency distribution curve. Shown in Figure 5.1, a **frequency distribution curve** is a graphic representation of the actual number of patients responding with a particular drug action at different doses. On the horizontal axis, notice the wide range in doses that produced the patient responses shown on the curve. A few patients responded to the drug at very low doses (10–20 mg). As the dose was increased, more and more patients responded. The peak of the curve (50 mg) indicates the largest number of patients responding to the drug. Some patients required very high doses (80–90 mg) to elicit the desired response. The curve does not show the magnitude of the response, only whether or not a measurable response occurred among the patients. As an example, think of the given response to an antihypertensive drug as defined by a reduction of 20 mm in systolic blood pressure. A few patients experienced the desired 20-mm reduction at a drug dose of only 10 mg; a 50-mg dose gave the largest number of patients the 20-mm reduction in blood pressure. However, a few patients needed as much as 90 mg of the drug to produce the same 20-mm reduction.

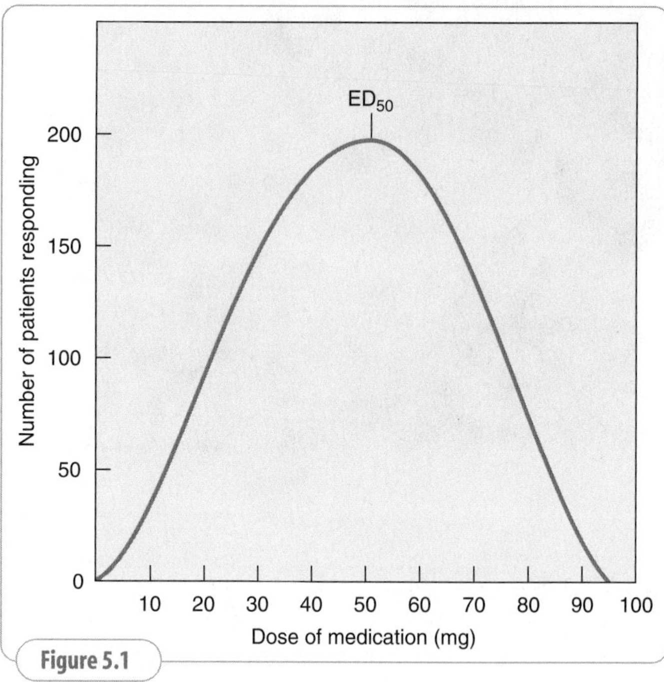

Figure 5.1

Frequency distribution curve: interpatient variability in drug response.

The dose in the middle of the frequency distribution curve represents the drug's **median effective dose (ED_{50})**. The ED_{50} is the dose required to produce a specific therapeutic response in 50% of a group of patients. Drug guides usually use the ED_{50} as the "average" or standard dose for a drug.

The interpatient variability shown in Figure 5.1 has important clinical implications. First, the nurse should realize that the standard or average dose predicts a satisfactory therapeutic response for only half the population. But what about responses in the rest of the patients? Many patients will require more or less than the average dose for optimum pharmacotherapy. Using the systolic blood pressure example, assume that a large group of patients is given the average dose of 50 mg. Some of these patients will experience toxicity at this level because they only need 10 mg to achieve blood pressure reduction. Other patients in this group will probably have no reduction in blood pressure at all. By monitoring the patient, taking vital signs, and interpreting any associated laboratory data, the nurse is critical in determining whether the average dose is effective for the patient. It is not enough to simply memorize an average dose for a drug; the nurse must have the skills to know when and how to adjust this dose to obtain the optimum therapeutic response.

Therapeutic Index

5.2 The therapeutic index describes a drug's margin of safety.

Selecting a dose that produces an optimum therapeutic response for each individual patient is certainly important, but the nurse must also be able to predict whether that dose is safe for that patient. Frequency distribution curves can also be used to illustrate the safety of a drug.

The **median lethal dose (LD_{50})** is a value often determined in laboratory animals in preclinical experiments as a part of the drug development process discussed in Chapter 1. The LD_{50} is the dose of drug that will kill 50% of a group of animals. Just as with ED_{50}, a population of animals will exhibit considerable variability in lethal dosage; what may be a nontoxic dose for one animal may kill another.

To examine the safety of a particular drug, the LD_{50} is compared to ED_{50}, as shown in Figure 5.2a. In this example, 10 mg of drug is the average effective dose, and 40 mg is the average lethal dose. The ED_{50} and LD_{50} are used to calculate one of the most important values in pharmacology, a drug's **therapeutic index.** The therapeutic index is defined as the ratio of a drug's LD_{50} to its ED_{50}.

$$\text{Therapeutic index} = \frac{\text{median lethal dose } (LD_{50})}{\text{median effective dose } (ED_{50})}$$

The larger the difference between the two doses, the greater the therapeutic index. In Figure 5.2a, the therapeutic index is 4 (40 mg ÷ 10 mg). Essentially, this means that it would take an error in magnitude of approximately four times the average dose to be lethal to a patient. In terms of dosage, this is a relatively safe drug and small to moderate medication errors or changes in the drug's bioavailability would likely not be fatal. Thus, the therapeutic index is a measure of a drug's safety margin: the higher the value, the safer the medication.

As another example, the therapeutic index of a second drug is shown in Figure 5.2b. Drug Z has the same ED_{50} as Drug X but shows a different LD_{50}. The therapeutic index for Drug Z is only 2 (20 mg ÷ 10 mg). The difference between an effective dose and a lethal dose is very small for Drug Z; thus the drug has a narrow safety margin. Small medication errors or changes in the drug's metabolism or excretion could have lethal consequences. The therapeutic index offers the nurse practical information on the safety of a drug and a means to compare one drug to another.

In Figure 5.2b, notice that the two curves overlapped. Some patients required a dose of 15 to 20 mg to produce the desired effect, yet this same dose was lethal in other patients. This type of drug would require careful assessment of hepatic and renal function prior to the initiation of therapy. With drugs exhibiting a low therapeutic index, it is prudent to begin with the lowest dose possible, then increase the amount of drug with careful monitoring.

Because the LD_{50} cannot be experimentally determined in humans, the **median toxicity dose (TD_{50})** is a much more practical value for clinical practice. The median toxicity dose is the dose that will produce a given toxicity in 50% of a group of patients. The TD_{50} value may be extrapolated from animal data or based on adverse effects recorded in patient clinical trials.

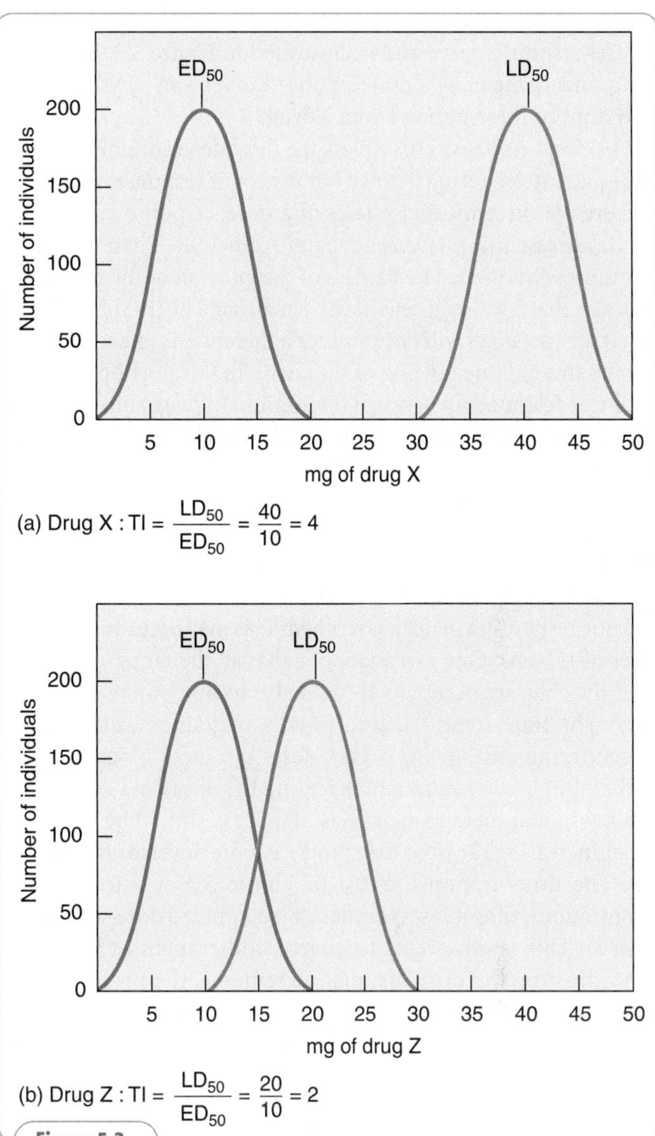

Figure 5.2

Therapeutic index: (a) drug X has a therapeutic index of 4; (b) drug Z has a therapeutic index of 2.

CONNECTION *Checkpoint* 5.1

From what you learned in Chapter 2, before a pharmaceutical company tests a drug in patients after preclinical trials are completed, what document must be submitted to the FDA? See Answer to Connection Checkpoint 5.1 in Appendix A.

Dose–Response Relationship

5.3 The dose–response relationship describes how the actions of a drug change with increasing dose.

In the examples in the preceding section, frequency distribution curves were used to graphically visualize interpatient differences in responses to medications in a population. Pharmacodynamics is also used to study the variability in responses in a single patient.

How does a patient respond to varying doses of a drug? Common sense would indicate that a larger dose would produce more drug effect. For example, an antibiotic would kill more bacteria if the dose was increased from 10 mg to 20 mg. An antihypertensive drug would cause a greater reduction in blood pressure if the dose was increased from 50 mg to 100 mg. These simple examples describe the **dose–response relationship,** one of the most fundamental concepts in pharmacology.

The graphic representation of this relationship is called a dose–response curve and is illustrated in Figure 5.3. Examining and comparing dose–response curves can yield a large amount of information about a drug.

A dose–response curve plots the drug dose administered to the patient versus the intensity or degree of response obtained. There are three distinct phases of a dose–response curve that indicate essential pharmacodynamic principles. Phase 1 occurs at the lowest doses. The flatness of this portion of the curve indicates that few target cells have been affected by the drug; doses that are too small will not produce a therapeutic effect. Phase 2 is the straight line portion of the curve. In this portion, there is a linear relationship between the amount of drug administered and the degree of response obtained from the patient. For example, if the dose is doubled, twice as much response may be obtained. This is the most desirable range of doses for pharmacotherapeutics, because giving more drug results in proportionately more effect; a lower drug dose gives less effect. In phase 3 increasing the drug dose produces no additional therapeutic response; a plateau is reached. This may occur for a number of reasons. One explanation is that all the target receptors for the drug are occupied. It could also mean that the drug has brought 100% relief, such as when a migraine headache has been terminated; giving higher doses produces no additional relief. In phase 3, although increasing the dose does not result in additional therapeutic effects, the nurse should be mindful that increasing the dose may produce more adverse effects.

The dose–response curve in Figure 5.3 is smooth and continuous; thus it is sometimes called a graded dose–response curve. This is important to pharmacotherapeutics because, by adjusting the dose in small increments, the prescriber is able to attain virtually any degree of therapeutic response (0% to 100%) within the linear range of drug doses. This is especially true when using the intravenous (IV) route, during which the nurse can adjust the infusion rate in very small increments.

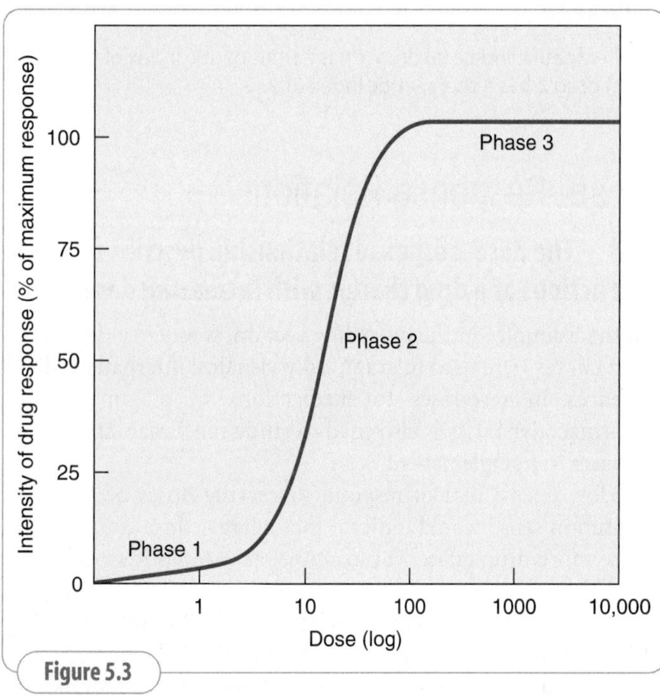

Figure 5.3

Dose–response relationship.

Many types of adverse effects also follow a graded dose–response relationship: the higher the dose, the more intense the adverse effect. By adjusting the dose lower, while still keeping it within the therapeutic range, adverse effects may be lessened. Some adverse effects, such as anaphylaxis, are independent of dose in that even the smallest amount of drug may trigger a serious adverse response (see Chapter 6).

Potency and Efficacy

5.4 Potency and efficacy are fundamental concepts of pharmacodynamics that describe a drug's activity.

Within a pharmacologic class, not all drugs are equally effective at treating a disorder. For example, some antineoplastic drugs kill more cancer cells than others; some antihypertensive agents lower blood pressure to a greater extent than others; and some analgesics are more effective at relieving severe pain than others in the same class. Furthermore, drugs in the same class are effective at different doses: One antibiotic may be effective at a dose of 1 mg/kg, whereas another is most effective at 100 mg/kg. Nurses need a method to compare one drug to another, so that they can administer treatment effectively.

There are two fundamental ways to compare medications within therapeutic and pharmacologic classes. First is the concept of **potency.** A drug that is more potent will produce its therapeutic effect at a lower dose, compared to another drug in the same class. As an example, consider two calcium channel blockers used for hypertension: amlodipine (Norvasc) and nifedipine (Procardia). Amlodipine produces its decrease in blood pressure at 10 mg (maximum dose) and nifedipine at 180 mg. Amlodipine is clearly more potent than nifedipine because it took a lower dose (18 times less) to produce its antihypertensive effect.

Thus, potency is a way to compare the doses of two independently administered drugs in terms of how much is needed to produce a particular response. A useful way to visualize the concept of potency is by examining dose–response curves. When comparing the two drugs shown in Figure 5.4a, Drug A is more potent because it requires a lower dose to produce the same response.

A second method used to compare drugs is called **efficacy,** which is defined as the greatest maximal response that can be produced from a particular drug. In the example in Figure 5.4b, Drug A is more efficacious because it produces a higher maximal response.

Which is more important to the outcomes of pharmacotherapy: potency or efficacy? Perhaps the best way to understand these important concepts is to use the specific example of headache pain. Two common over-the-counter (OTC) analgesic therapies are ibuprofen, 200 mg, and aspirin, 650 mg. The fact that ibuprofen relieves pain at a lower dose indicates that this agent is more potent than aspirin. At the given doses, however, both are equally effective at relieving headaches; thus they have the same efficacy. If

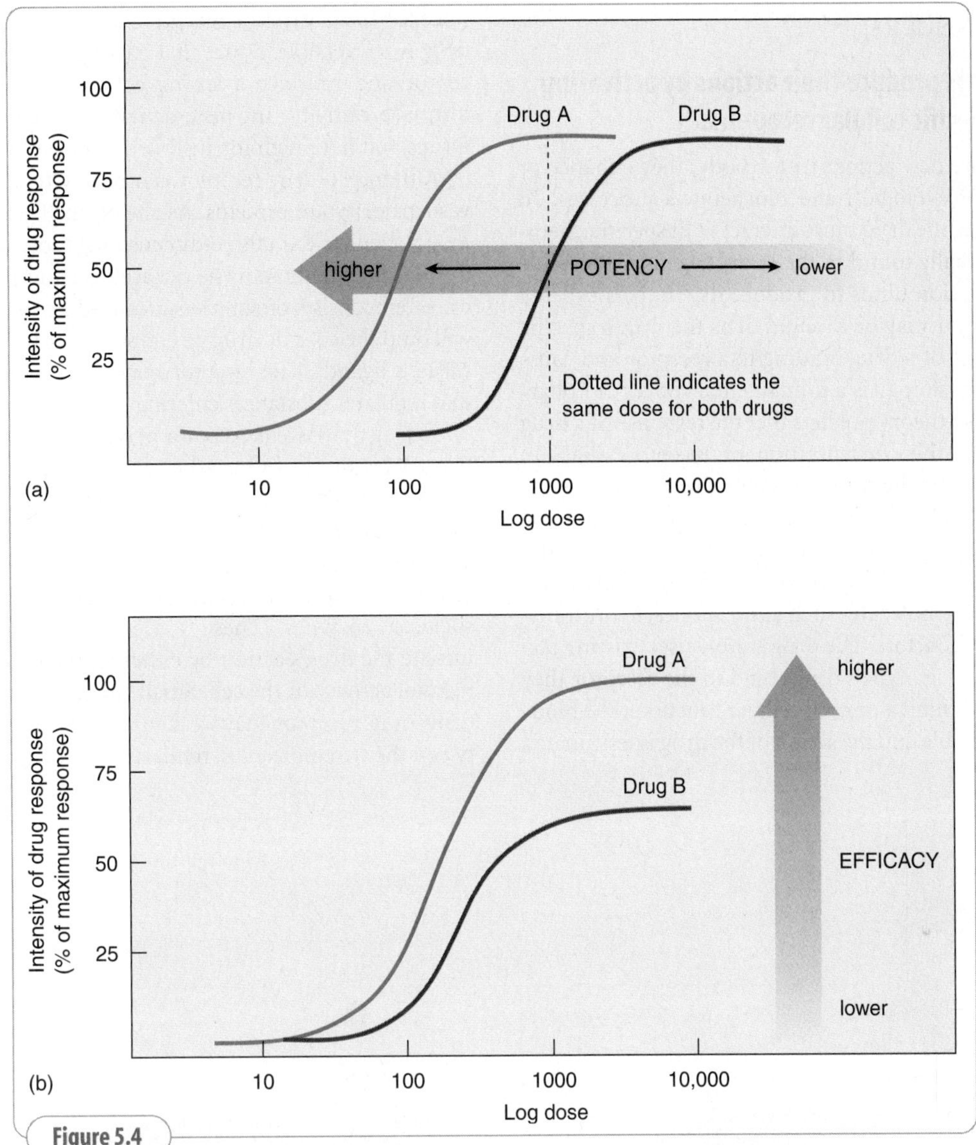

Figure 5.4

Potency and efficacy: (a) drug A has a higher potency than drug B; (b) drug A has a higher efficacy than drug B.

the patient is experiencing severe pain, however, neither aspirin nor ibuprofen has sufficient efficacy to bring relief. Narcotic analgesics such as morphine have a greater efficacy than aspirin or ibuprofen and could effectively treat this type of pain. From a pharmacotherapeutic perspective, efficacy is almost always more important than potency. In the preceding example, the average dose is unimportant to the patient, but headache relief is essential. As another comparison, the patient with cancer is much more concerned with how many cancer cells have been killed (efficacy) than with the dose the nurse administered (potency). In the comparison of Norvasc to Procardia, although Norvasc is clearly more potent, both drugs reduce blood pressure to the same degree; thus they have the same efficacy. Although the nurse will often hear claims that one drug is more potent than another, a more compelling concern is which drug is more efficacious.

A word of caution is necessary at this point. In Section 5.4, it is stated that many adverse effects are related to dose—that higher doses produce more intense adverse effects. This is true only when comparing doses of the same drug. For example, a therapeutic dose for amlodipine is 10 mg/day. Giving 20 mg or 30 mg of amlodipine will most certainly increase the risk of experiencing an adverse effect. Can the dose of amlodipine be compared to a dose of nifedipine, which is 180 mg/day? The answer is absolutely not. In fact, 10 mg of amlodipine gives roughly the same risk of adverse effects as 180 mg of nifedipine. The point is that when two different drugs are compared, one cannot assume that the drug with the lower dose gives fewer adverse effects.

An additional word of caution is necessary. In clinical practice the term *potency* is often misused to indicate a more effective drug. The nurse should remember the correct definitions of the words *potency* and *efficacy* and try to incorporate them into clinical practice.

Receptor Theory

5.5 Most drugs produce their actions by activating or inhibiting specific cellular receptors.

Drugs rarely create new actions in the body; they enhance or inhibit existing physiological and biochemical processes. To cause such changes the drug must interact with specific chemicals that are normally found in the body. A cellular molecule to which a medication binds to produce its effects is called a **receptor.** A receptor may be thought of as the drug's specific target. The concept of a drug binding to a receptor and causing a change in physiology is a fundamental concept in pharmacology. Receptor theory predicts that the response of a drug is proportional to the concentration of receptors that are bound or occupied by the drug. Receptor theory explains the mechanisms by which most drugs produce their effects.

It is important to understand, however, that receptors do not exist in the body solely to bind drugs; their normal function is to bind endogenous molecules such as hormones, neurotransmitters, and growth factors. The drug simply uses existing targets to cause its effects. When drugs bind to the receptor they either enhance or inhibit a normal cellular function. The binding is usually reversible and the action of the drug is terminated once the drug leaves its receptor. In a few cases, binding of the drug is irreversible. Drugs that have the ability to bind to a receptor and produce a strong action are said to have high **intrinsic activity.** Intrinsic activity and efficacy are related. Drugs that have high intrinsic activity have high efficacy.

Although a drug receptor can be any type of molecule, the vast majority are proteins. As shown in Figure 5.5, a receptor may be depicted as a three-dimensional protein spanning across the plasma membrane. The extracellular component of a receptor often consists of subunits arranged in a specific shape that will bind the specific drug or endogenous chemical (sometimes called a ligand). The receptor may form a membrane channel that regulates substances entering and leaving the cell.

A drug binds to its receptor in a very specific manner, much like a lock and key. Once the receptor is occupied, a series of **second messenger** events are triggered within the cell such as the conversion of adenosine triphosphate (ATP) to cyclic adenosine monophosphate (cyclic AMP), the release of intracellular calcium, or the activation of specific G proteins and associated enzymes. These cascades of biochemical events initiate the drug's action by either stimulating or inhibiting a normal activity of the cell. Small changes to the structure of a drug, or its receptor, may weaken or even eliminate binding between the two molecules, rendering the drug ineffective.

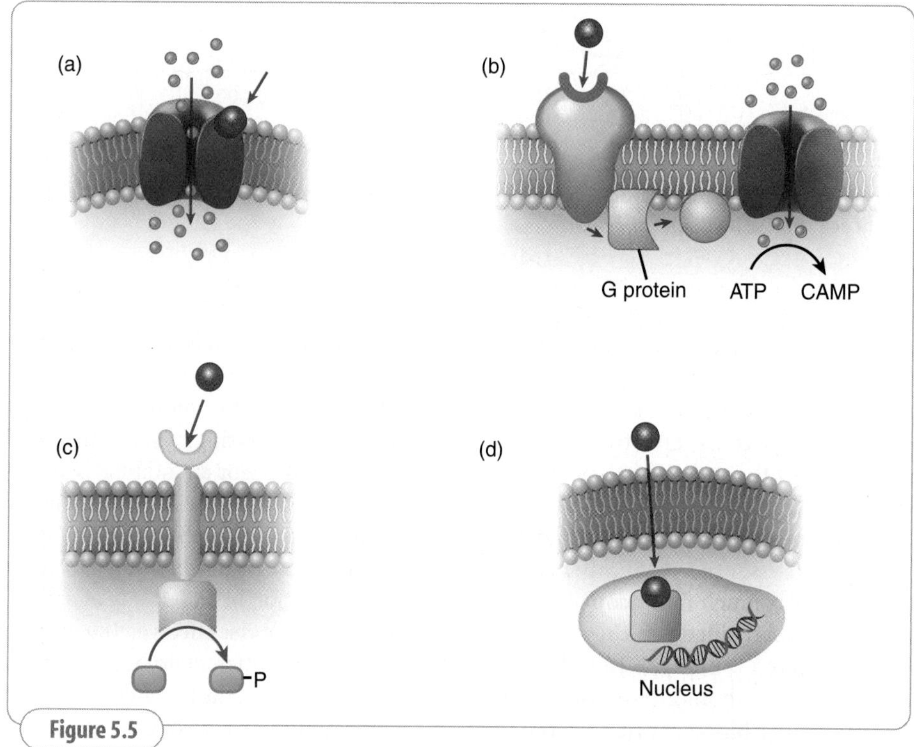

Figure 5.5

Types of cellular receptors: (a) Drug binds to the receptor opening channel. (b) Drug binds to the receptor, causing a G protein–mediated reaction in the cell. (c) Drug binds to the transmembrane receptor to signal a change inside the cell. (d) Drug enters the cell nucleus to increase synthesis of specific proteins.

Not all receptors are proteins bound to the plasma membrane: Some are intracellular molecules such as DNA or enzymes in the cytoplasm. By interacting with these types of receptors, medications are able to inhibit protein synthesis or regulate events such as cell division and metabolism. Examples of agents that bind intracellular components include steroid hormones and certain vitamins.

Receptor subtypes have been discovered that permit the "fine-tuning" of pharmacotherapy. For example, the first drugs affecting the autonomic nervous system affected all types of autonomic receptors. It was discovered that two basic receptor types existed in the body, alpha and beta, and drugs were then developed that affected only one type. Still later, several subtypes of alpha and beta receptors, including alpha-1, alpha-2, beta-1, and beta-2, were discovered that allowed even more specificity in pharmacotherapy. In recent years, researchers have further divided and refined various drug receptor subtypes. It is likely that research will continue to result in the development of new medications that activate very specific receptors to cause therapeutic responses while avoiding some adverse effects.

Some drugs act independently of cellular receptors. These agents are associated with other mechanisms, such as changing the permeability of cellular membranes, depressing membrane excitability, or altering the activity of cellular pumps. Actions such as these are often described as nonspecific cellular responses. Ethyl alcohol, general anesthetics, and osmotic diuretics are examples of agents that act by nonspecific mechanisms.

Agonists and Antagonists

5.6 Agonists, partial agonists, and antagonists compete for cellular receptors and can modify drug action.

When a drug binds to a receptor, several possible consequences can result. In simplest terms, some specific activity of the cell is either enhanced or inhibited. The actual biochemical mechanism underlying the therapeutic effect, however, may be extremely complex. In some cases, the mechanism of action is not known.

When a drug binds to its receptor, it may produce a response that mimics the effect of the endogenous regulatory molecule. For example, when the drug bethanechol is administered, it binds to acetylcholine receptors in the autonomic nervous system and produces the same actions as acetylcholine. A drug that activates a receptor and produces the same type of response as the endogenous substance is called an **agonist.** Agonists sometimes produce a greater maximal response than the endogenous chemical. The term **partial agonist** is used to describe a medication that produces a weaker, or less efficacious, response than an agonist.

A second possibility is that a drug will occupy a receptor and prevent the endogenous chemical from binding to produce its action. This type of drug, an **antagonist,** often competes with agonists for receptor binding sites. For example, the drug atropine competes with acetylcholine for certain receptors in the autonomic nervous system. If the dose is high enough, atropine may completely block the effects of acetylcholine because acetylcholine cannot reach its receptors. Antagonists may be used as medications when the body is producing too much of a response from an endogenous chemical or from a drug overdose, such as high blood pressure, fast heart rate, secretion of excess stomach acid, or sedation. Giving an antagonist in these situations may reverse the adverse effects. An antagonist has no intrinsic activity; the actions observed after administering an antagonist are caused by lack of agonist action.

Not all antagonism is associated with receptors, as in the previous example. Functional antagonists inhibit the effects of an agonist, not by competing for a receptor but by changing pharmacokinetic factors. For example, antagonists may slow the absorption of an agonist, resulting in less pharmacologic effect. An antagonist may change the pH of the surrounding fluid and neutralize the agonist before it is even absorbed. By speeding up metabolism or excretion, an antagonist can enhance the removal of an agonist from the body. The relationships that occur between agonists and antagonists explain many of the drug–drug and drug–food interactions that occur in the body and which are described in Chapter 6. Figure 5.6 illustrates the concept of agonist and antagonist drug action.

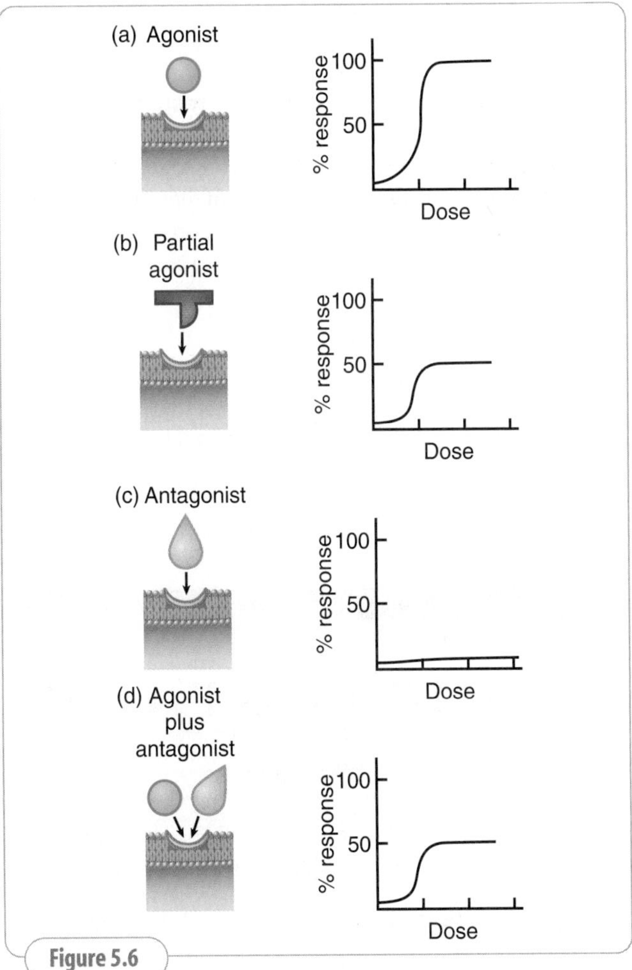

Figure 5.6

Agonists, partial agonists, and antagonists: (a) an agonist results in maximum response; (b) a partial agonist results in less than maximum response; (c) an antagonist results in little or no response; (d) an agonist plus antagonist results in diminished response.

CONNECTION *Checkpoint* 5.2

From what you learned in Chapter 4, phenytoin is an inducer of CYP1A2, the enzyme that metabolizes acetaminophen. Would phenytoin be considered a functional agonist or an antagonist to acetaminophen? See Answer to Connection Checkpoint 5.2 in Appendix A.

Pharmacogenetics

5.7 In the future, pharmacogenetics may allow customization of drug therapy.

Until quite recently, it was thought that drugs provided safe and effective treatment to every patient in the same manner. Unfortunately, a significant portion of the population either develops unacceptable adverse effects to certain drugs or is unresponsive to them. Some scientists and clinicians are now discarding the "one size fits all" approach to drug therapy, which was designed to treat the entire population without addressing important interpatient variation.

With the advent of the Human Genome Project and other advances in medicine, pharmacologists are hopeful that future drugs can be customized for patients with specific genetic similarities. In the past, any unpredictable and unexplained drug reaction has been labeled **idiosyncratic response.** It is now hoped that, by analyzing a DNA test before receiving a drug, these idiosyncratic adverse effects can someday be avoided.

Pharmacogenetics is the branch of pharmacology that examines the role of genetics in drug response. The most important advances in pharmacogenetics so far have been the identification of subtle genetic differences in drug-metabolizing enzymes. Genetic differences in these enzymes are responsible for a significant portion of drug-induced toxicity. It is hoped that the use of pharmacogenetic information may someday allow for drug therapy customized to a patient's individual molecules. Although therapies based on a patient's genetically based response may not be cost-effective at this time, pharmacogenetics may radically change the way pharmacotherapy will be practiced in the future.

CONNECTIONS

Treating the Diverse Patient

Enzyme Deficiencies in Ethnic Populations

Pharmacogenetics has identified ethnic populations of people, such as males of Mediterranean and African descent, who are deficient in glucose-6-phosphate dehydrogenase (G6PD), an enzyme that is essential in carbohydrate metabolism. G6PD deficiency is the most common enzyme deficiency with about 400 million people affected worldwide. Caused by mutations in the DNA structure that encode for G6PD, the disorder results in one or more amino acid changes in the enzyme molecule. When certain oxidative drugs are given, such as primaquine, sulfonamides, or nitrofurantoin (Macrobid), an acute hemolysis of red blood cells (RBCs) occurs due to the breaking of chemical bonds in the hemoglobin molecule, with up to 50% of the circulating RBCs being destroyed. Genetic typing does not always predict toxicity. Patients may report a history of severe "allergy" to fava beans, which induce the hemolytic symptoms. The role of the nurse is critical in observing patients carefully for 24 to 72 hours following administration of these medications. Prevention is the best treatment. Fortunately, good alternative choices for these medications are available (Frank, 2005).

UNDERSTANDING THE CHAPTER

Key Concepts Summary

5.1 Patients have widely different responses to drugs, which can be depicted on a frequency distribution curve.

5.2 The therapeutic index describes a drug's margin of safety.

5.3 The dose–response relationship describes how the actions of a drug change with increasing dose.

5.4 Potency and efficacy are fundamental concepts of pharmacodynamics that describe a drug's activity.

5.5 Most drugs produce their actions by activating or inhibiting specific cellular receptors.

5.6 Agonists, partial agonists, and antagonists compete for cellular receptors and can modify drug action.

5.7 In the future, pharmacogenetics may allow customization of drug therapy.

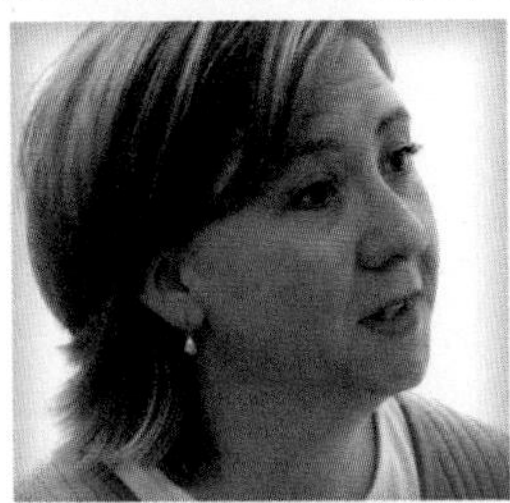

Making the PATIENT Connection

Remember the patient "Katherine Hunter" at the beginning of the chapter? Now read the remainder of the case study. Based on the information presented within this chapter, respond to the critical thinking questions that follow.

Katherine Hunter prides herself on being a wise consumer and cautiously examines the claims by manufacturers for all her purchases. She researches everything she buys, such as automobiles, household appliances, and medications. Recently, she has begun to seriously consider assertions made by the advertisements for various types of antacids. Most brands claim to be the most efficient in relieving the symptoms of indigestion. Others say that their brand is the most potent antacid available without a prescription. Some products claim that they not only relieve heartburn, but also supply the body with needed vitamins and minerals. When purchasing an over-the-counter (OTC) medication, all Katherine wants is something that will work quickly with few adverse effects.

Critical Thinking Questions

1. How would you teach Katherine the difference between potency and efficacy?
2. Which of the two concepts (potency and efficacy) would be most important for selecting a drug? Why?
3. What are the drawbacks of comparing two different medications?

Case Study

As the nurse practicing in a middle school, you have been asked to speak to the eighth-grade pre-health professionals' class. The topic for today's discussion is "how drugs work in the body." The teacher has provided you with an outline of concepts that you will need to address.

1. Describe the link between a drug's action and drug receptors.
2. Why do people respond differently to medication?
3. What are drug agonists and drug antagonists?

NCLEX-RN® Review

1 What parameters would the nurse use to determine whether the average dose of a medication is effective for a client? Select all that apply.

1. Physical examination
2. Vital signs
3. Laboratory values
4. Dosage time
5. Efficacy

2 The nurse knows that a drug with a high therapeutic index is:

1. Safe.
2. Often dangerous.
3. Frequently risky.
4. Most likely effective.

3 While reviewing a drug manufacturer package insert, the nurse reads about the dose–response curve. The purpose of the dose–response curve is to illustrate the relationship between:

1. The amount of a drug administered and the degree of response it produces.
2. The prevalence of toxic effects in a given population.
3. The degree of response and the total duration of action of the drug.
4. The peak serum drug level when half the dose is administered.

4 A research nurse is discussing the TD_{50} of a drug with the other members of the investigation team. The discussion is focused on:

1. Effectiveness.
2. Dose response.
3. Receptor subtypes.
4. Toxicity.

5 The nurse knows that an antagonist is a type of drug that:

1. Has maximal efficacy.
2. Has affinity for a receptor but little efficacy.
3. Binds to a receptor and activates it.
4. Has efficacy but low affinity.

6 When considering pharmacodynamic principles for a client's drug therapy, the nurse is aware that affinity for a receptor is most closely associated with a drug's:

1. Potency.
2. Efficacy.
3. Metabolism.
4. First-pass effect.

See Answers to Critical Thinking Questions, Case Study, and NCLEX-RN® Review in Appendix A.

References

Anderson, G. D. (2005). Sex and racial differences in pharmacological response: Where is the evidence? Pharmacogenetics, pharmacokinetics, and pharmacodynamics. *Journal of Women's Health, 14*(1), 19–29.

Becquemont, L. (2003). Clinical relevance of pharmacogenetics. *Drug Metabolism Review, 35*(4), 277–285.

Bjornsson, T. D., Wagner, J. A., Donahue, S. R., Harper, D., Karim, A., Khouri, M. S., et al. (2003). A review and assessment of potential sources of ethnic differences in drug responsiveness. *Journal of Clinical Pharmacology, 43*(9), 943–967.

Buaer, L. A. (2005). Clinical pharmacokinetics and pharmacodynamics. In J. T. DiPiro, R. L. Talbert, C. Y. Yee, G. R. Matzke, B. G. Wells, & L. M. Posey (Eds.), *Pharmacotherapy: A pathophysiologic approach* (6th ed., pp. 51–73). New York: McGraw-Hill.

Buxton, I. L. O. (2006). Pharmacokinetics and pharmacodynamics: The dynamics of drug absorption, distribution, action, and elimination. In L. L. Brunton, J. S. Lazo, & K. L. Parker (Eds.), *The pharmacological basis of therapeutics* (11th ed., pp. 1–40). New York: McGraw-Hill.

Frank, J. E. (2005). Diagnosis and management of G6PD deficiency. *American Family Physician 72*(7), 1277–1284.

Gandhi, M., Aweeka, F., Greenblatt, R. M., & Blaschke, T. F. (2004). Sex differences in pharmacokinetics and pharmacodynamics. *Annual Review of Pharmacology and Toxicology, 44*, 499–523.

Tobias, D. (2004). Age-related changes in pharmacokinetics and pharmacodynamics: A review. *The Consultant Pharmacist, 19*(8), 736–739.

Zineh, I., Pebanco, G. D., Aquilante, C. L., Gerhard, T., Beitelshees, A. L., Beasley, B. N., et al. (2006). Discordance between availability of pharmacogenetics studies and pharmacogenetics-based prescribing information for the top 200 drugs. *Annals of Pharmacotherapy, 40*(4), 639–644.

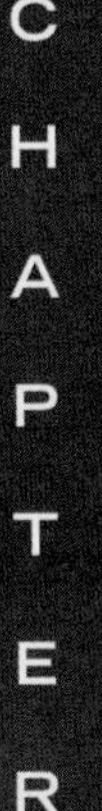

I was told to watch for drug reactions. But with all the drugs I take, how would I ever know if I'm having a reaction or not?

Patient "Elizabeth Edwards"

CHAPTER 6

Adverse Drug Effects and Drug Interactions

Chapter Outline

Adverse Effects

The Role of the Nurse in Managing Adverse Effects

Allergic Reactions

Idiosyncratic Responses

Carcinogenicity and Teratogenicity

Organ-Specific Drug Toxicity

Drug Interactions

Pharmacokinetic Drug Interactions

Pharmacodynamic Drug Interactions

Drug Interactions with Food and Dietary Supplements

Learning Outcomes

After reading this chapter, the student should be able to:

1. Differentiate between adverse effects and side effects.
2. Create a plan to minimize or prevent adverse drug events in patients.
3. Describe the incidence and characteristics of drug allergies.
4. Explain how idiosyncratic reactions differ from other types of adverse effects.
5. Explain why certain drugs with carcinogenic or teratogenic potential are used in pharmacotherapy.
6. Report the characteristic signs, symptoms, and treatment for each of the following organ-specific adverse events: nephrotoxicity, neurotoxicity, muscle toxicity, hepatotoxicity, dermatologic toxicity, and bone marrow toxicity.
7. Use examples to explain the importance of drug interactions to pharmacotherapy.
8. Describe the mechanisms of drug interactions that alter absorption, distribution, metabolism, or excretion.
9. Differentiate among additive, synergistic, and antagonistic drug interactions.
10. Identify examples of drug-food interactions that may impact pharmacotherapeutic outcomes.

Key Terms

additive effect, 73
adverse drug effect, 66
antagonistic effect, 74
drug allergy, 67
drug interaction, 70
idiosyncratic response, 67
risk-benefit ratio, 68
side effects, 66
synergistic effect, 74
teratogen, 68

Drugs are administered with the goal of producing a therapeutic effect. All drugs, however, produce both intended therapeutic effects as well as unintended effects. An **adverse drug effect** is an undesirable and potentially harmful action caused by the administration of medication. Adverse effects, also called adverse events, are a significant component of pharmacotherapy and, when severe, may cause treatment to be discontinued or result in permanent harm to the patient. Because they may significantly impact therapeutic outcomes, adverse drug effects must be minimized to the greatest extent possible. The purpose of this chapter is to examine the different types of adverse effects and drug interactions, so that the nurse may minimize their impact on treatment outcomes.

Adverse Effects

6.1 The nurse plays a key role in preventing and managing adverse drug effects.

Although every drug has the potential to produce adverse events, most pharmacotherapy can be conducted without significant undesirable effects. Indeed, drugs that produce serious adverse effects are screened and removed from consideration during the drug development and approval process, or are restricted for treating serious health conditions such as cancer. Patients expect that their drugs, including over-the-counter (OTC) agents, herbal products, and dietary supplements, will be free from serious adverse effects when taken as directed. Although the majority of drugs are very safe, adverse effects cannot be entirely avoided.

Side effects are types of adverse effects that are predictable and which may occur even at therapeutic doses. Side effects are less serious than adverse effects. Patients are often willing to tolerate annoying side effects if they believe the drug will improve their condition or prevent a disease. The distinction between an adverse effect and a side effect, however, is often unclear. For example, is headache a side or an adverse effect? What about nausea? The answer lies in the severity of the symptoms. Headache or nausea may be minor (side effects) or they may become intense and disabling (adverse effects). The U.S. Food and Drug Administration (FDA) defines serious drug effects as those that:

- Result in a patient's death, hospitalization, or disability.
- Cause a congenital abnormality.
- Cause a life-threatening event.
- Require an intervention to prevent permanent damage.

Adverse drug events may be specific to a single type of tissue or affect multiple organ systems. The most common adverse events are nausea and vomiting, which may occur when drugs are administered by any route. Headache and changes in blood pressure are also very common. Some adverse effects, though rare, are serious enough to warrant regular or continuous monitoring. Examples of serious events include impairment or failure of entire organs, such as cardiac, hepatic, or renal failure or loss of vision or hearing. Anaphylaxis, Stevens–Johnson syndrome (SJS), cancer, and birth defects are additional rare, though possible, adverse drug events that may occur with certain drugs.

Many adverse effects are extensions of a drug's pharmacologic actions. These types of events are considered dose dependent: As the drug dose increases, the risk for adverse effects also increases. For example, antihypertensive drugs are given to lower blood pressure, but high doses may cause hypotension, which may manifest as dizziness or fainting. Drugs for treating insomnia or anxiety may depress brain activity too much at higher doses, resulting in drowsiness or daytime sedation. Knowing the therapeutic actions of the drug enables the nurse to predict the signs and symptoms of many of the adverse effects that may occur during treatment. It is important for nurses and their patients to understand that the difference between a substance being a beneficial drug or a poison is simply a matter of dose.

A word of caution is necessary regarding the reporting of adverse drug events. The placebo effect predicts that a certain percentage of patients will respond with positive therapeutic outcomes to a treatment, even if the medication is inert and has no pharmacologic properties (essentially a "sugar pill"). The same holds true for side and adverse effects. A certain percentage of patients will experience headache, nausea and vomiting, rash, fall in blood pressure, or pain following the administration of a placebo. Thus when examining drug information, the nurse should always examine the incidence of adverse effects over and above that caused by a placebo. It is important to understand that the patient is not "faking" symptoms that result from placebo administration; they truly believe, and may be visibly experiencing, side effects. However, the drug itself may not be responsible for the effects.

Can adverse effects be prevented? Although nurses play a key role in minimizing the number and severity of adverse events in their patients, some adverse effects simply cannot be predicted or prevented. Skilled health care providers and nurses, however, have multiple ways to minimize or prevent adverse effects, from having expert knowledge of how a drug acts to obtaining a comprehensive medical history from their patients. The following are means that health care providers use to prevent adverse drug events in their patients.

- **Take a thorough medical history.** The medical history of the patient may reveal drug allergies or conditions that contraindicate the use of certain drugs. The history may also identify other drugs taken by the patient that could negatively interact with the prescribed medication.
- **Thoroughly assess the patient and all diagnostic data.** Assessment may reveal underlying hepatic or renal impairment that will affect the way the drug is handled by the body. The very young and the elderly are most susceptible to drug reactions because metabolism and excretion of drugs in these populations are less predictable. Average drug doses should be adjusted based on careful patient assessment to prevent adverse effects.

- **Prevent medication errors.** Administering the incorrect dose or giving the drug to the wrong patient may cause unnecessary adverse effects. Methods of preventing medication errors are described in detail in Chapter 7.
- **Monitor pharmacotherapy carefully.** Monitor patient signs and symptoms regularly after initial drug doses or when doses are increased, especially when giving parenteral agents and for very ill patients. Patients receiving drugs that have frequent or potentially severe adverse effects should be monitored continuously until the baseline effects of the drug have been established.
- **Know the drugs.** It is essential that nurses know the most frequent and most serious adverse effects for every drug administered. A comprehensive knowledge of the drugs, herbal products, and supplements taken by their patients helps nurses to monitor for and identify adverse effects and provide the necessary interventions before they become serious.
- **Be prepared for the unusual.** Anaphylaxis may occur immediately and unpredictably (see Section 6.2). Other adverse effects may be delayed, occurring days, weeks, or months after therapy is initiated. Some drugs produce actions opposite to those expected (see Section 6.3). Patients may be reluctant to report certain adverse effects (such as impotence) without prompting by the nurse.
- **Question unusual orders.** If the nurse suspects that the wrong dose has been ordered or the pharmacy has filled the order incorrectly, the drug should not be administered until the prescriber or the pharmacy has been contacted.
- **Teach patients about adverse effects.** The patient is the nurse's ally in identifying and preventing adverse effects. Teaching patients what therapeutic and adverse effects to expect from the drug and which types of symptoms to report to their health care provider are important in preventing serious adverse effects. In addition, inadequate teaching may result in poor patient adherence to the drug regimen and suboptimal treatment outcomes.

Pharm*FACT*

Approximately 28% of all adverse drug effects are preventable. Preventable reactions include allergic reactions, dose-related reactions, documented idiosyncratic reactions, drug interactions, nonadherence, inappropriate prescribing, and inappropriate administration.

Source: Gurwitz et al., 2003.

6.2 Allergic reactions are caused by a hyperresponse of the immune system.

Drug allergies are common events, comprising 6% to 10% of all adverse drug effects. Although drug allergies may elicit a diverse range of patient symptoms, all are caused by a hyperresponse of body defenses. Depending on the type of allergic response, basophils, mast cells, eosinophils, or lymphocytes secrete chemical mediators that trigger the allergic response. Specific chemical mediators of allergy include histamine, serotonin, leukotrienes, prostaglandins, and complement.

There are several characteristics that define drug allergy. Allergies typically occur with very small amounts of drug; in other words, the severity of allergy symptoms is usually not proportional to the dose. The symptoms of allergy are unrelated to the pharmacologic actions of the drug. In fact, the symptoms of allergy are nonspecific to the drug itself; anaphylaxis has the same symptoms regardless of the drug that induces it. Patients often exhibit cross-allergy, an allergic reaction to all drugs with a similiar structure, such as those from the same pharmacologic class. Drug allergies require a previous exposure to the drug (or a very similar drug). This sensitizes the patient to subsequent exposures, during which a hyperresponse is rapidly mounted upon reexposure to the drug.

The signs and symptoms of drug allergy are variable and range from minor to life threatening. Symptoms may appear within minutes after the drug is administered or they may develop after prolonged pharmacotherapy. Because the signs and symptoms of drug allergy are nonspecific, it is sometimes difficult to attribute an allergy symptom to any given drug, especially in patients receiving multiple drugs. Complicating an accurate diagnosis is that symptoms of drug allergy are the same as those of allergy to other substances, such as certain foods, or environmental triggers, such as animal dander or dust mites. It is important to determine the source of allergy, especially in patients with severe reactions, so that the offending drug or environmental substance can be avoided in the future. The pharmacologic treatment of allergy is presented in Chapter 74.

Although allergic reactions are possible with most drugs, some agents exhibit a relatively higher incidence. The drugs or drug classes most likely to cause allergic reactions include penicillins and related antibiotics (monobactams and cephalosporins), radiologic contrast media containing iodine, insulin, nonsteroidal anti-inflammatory drugs ([NSAIDs], including aspirin), sulfonamides, cancer chemotherapy agents, preservatives (sulfites and paraben), and certain antiseizure agents.

Patients are usually unaware of the true definition of allergy and often report any adverse effect they have experienced as a drug allergy. For example, many patients experience acute nausea and vomiting with narcotic analgesics such as codeine and will report that they have an allergy to codeine during a drug history. In fact, these symptoms are not caused by an overactive immune response and are thus not a "true" allergy. Inaccurate reporting of allergies may lead to the health care provider avoiding the use of entire drug classes and prescribing less effective or more expensive "second-choice" agents.

6.3 Idiosyncratic reactions are unusual drug responses often caused by genetic differences among patients.

An **idiosyncratic response** is an adverse drug effect that produces an unusual and unexpected response that is not related to the pharmacologic action of the drug. Idiosyncratic reactions are not classified as allergies because they are not immune related. They are rare, unpredictable, and vary from patient to patient.

Many, though not all, idiosyncratic reactions are due to unique, individual genetic differences among patients. For example, mutations involving specific metabolic enzymes may cause certain patients to be extremely sensitive to the effects of a drug or to be resistant. The drug may be handled by a different metabolic pathway, resulting in the accumulation of a metabolite that gives a different and unexpected response from the original drug.

Historically, the term *idiosyncratic* has been used to denote any drug effect that could not be explained. With advances in the understanding of drug mechanisms, there are fewer and fewer drug responses that are not understood, at least to some extent. With improved reporting of adverse drug events, rare "unexpected" events are now documented and may be "expected." Thus use of the term *idiosyncratic*, although still common in clinical practice, will likely continue to diminish with time.

PharmFACT

Between 3% and 11% of hospital admissions are caused by adverse drug effects.

TABLE 6.1 Drugs That Cause Cancer in Humans

Class	Drug	Type of Cancer
Antineoplastic	chlorambucil cyclophosphamide doxorubicin etoposide nitrosoureas teniposide	Leukemia, urinary bladder
Hormones and hormone antagonists	anabolic steroids estrogen replacement therapy and oral contraceptives tamoxifen	Uterus, breast, hepatic
Immunosuppressants	azathioprine cyclosporine	Lymphoma, skin

6.4 Some drugs have the ability to induce cancer or cause birth defects.

Most adverse effects occur within minutes or hours after a drug is administered; some develop after several days or weeks of pharmacotherapy. In a few instances, the adverse effect may occur years or even decades after the drug was administered. Such is the case with drug-induced cancer.

Why would a drug be approved by the FDA if it was known to cause cancer in humans? In most cases, drugs that produce cancer in laboratory animals during preclinical trials are not submitted for approval to the FDA. However, there are a few conditions that may warrant the approval of a drug with carcinogenic potential. The answer lies in the **risk-benefit ratio.** If a patient has a condition that will likely cause premature death if left untreated, the benefits of taking a drug with carcinogenic potential may outweigh the long-term risks. This assumes, of course, that effective, safer alternatives are not available.

The best examples of the risk-benefit ratio are the drugs used to treat cancer. If a patient has cancer, aggressive pharmacotherapy with antineoplastic drugs may slow tumor growth and prolong the patient's life. For a few types of cancer, pharmacotherapy combined with surgery and radiation therapy can produce a total cure.

Chemical carcinogens, including some antineoplastics, damage deoxyribonucleic acid (DNA), resulting in mutations. Although much of the DNA damage may be repaired by cellular enzymes, some mutations persist and accumulate in cells as a person ages, increasing the risk of cancer. The initial damage done by the drug may take decades to manifest as cancer. The patient may never develop cancer; indeed, the large majority of patients receiving antineoplastic drugs do not develop the disease. Furthermore, the patient may have benefited from decades of life he or she would never have experienced had it not been for treatment with these drugs. In other words, the benefit outweighed the small risk of developing cancer later in life.

Of the thousands of drugs and drug combinations approved for pharmacotherapy, only a few increase the risk of acquiring cancer. These drugs, which are shown in Table 6.1, fall into three primary classes. Many antineoplastic drugs are toxic to both cancer cells and normal cells. Leukemia is probably the greatest cancer risk due to these agents. The second category consists of immunosuppressive agents, which are administered to dampen the immune system for patients receiving transplanted tissues or who have serious inflammatory disorders. Because the immune system is responsible for removing cancer cells when they form in the body, any drug that inhibits this system would be expected to have some degree of cancer risk. Lymphoma is likely the greatest type of cancer risk from immunosuppressants. The third group of drugs that may cause cancer consists of hormones or hormone antagonists. Little is known about the mechanisms by which hormone imbalances lead to cancer, and the topic is a subject of ongoing research. In some cases, hormones protect the patient from cancer, or they may reduce the incidence against one type of cancer but increase the risk of another type. Cancers from hormones or hormone antagonists tend to affect reproductive organs, such as the vagina, uterus, or breast.

A similar question might be asked regarding drugs that cause birth defects, or **teratogens.** Why would a drug be approved by the FDA if it was shown to produce birth defects in laboratory animals during the preclinical stage of drug testing? The answer to this question is very different.

Teratogens affect a smaller percentage of the population: those who are pregnant. In most cases these drugs do not affect males, and they are also safe to use in elderly patients. Thus, known teratogens may be approved for indications in patients who do not have the potential to become pregnant. When approved for females with reproductive potential, however, these drugs have increased risks. Although a pregnancy test may be performed prior to pharmacotherapy and the nurse may warn the patient to discontinue the drug if pregnancy is suspected, the potential still remains for exposing an embryo or fetus to a toxic agent. In females of reproductive age, teratogenic drugs are not used unless they have clear benefits that outweigh the potential risk of birth defects. The

TABLE 6.2 Drugs with Teratogenic Potential

Class	Example Drugs
Androgen	testosterone
Angiotensin converting enzyme (ACE) inhibitors	benazepril, captopril, enalapril, fosinopril, lisinopril, quinapril, ramipril
Antiacne drug	isotretinoin
Antibiotics	doxycycline, streptomycin, tetracycline
Anticoagulant	warfarin
Antileprosy agent	thalidomide
Antineoplastics	methotrexate, mytomycin, leuprolide, and many others
Antirheumatic agent	penicillamine, ralaxiphene
Antiseizure agents	carbamazepine, phenytoin, valproic acid
Antithyroid agents	methimazole, propylthiouracil
Bipolar agent	lithium carbonate
Ethanol/alcohol	beer, spirits, and wine

health care practitioner must carefully assess patient compliance with instructions against this potential risk.

It should be remembered that drugs are not tested in pregnant humans before FDA approval, and that animal testing cannot predict with great accuracy the effects on the human fetus. In some cases, the risks to a human embryo or fetus have been determined after a drug has been approved. The FDA has established pregnancy categories, which gauge the risk of a drug causing birth defects (see Chapter 10). All drug use should be assumed dangerous during pregnancy, unless data have otherwise demonstrated the drug to be safe. No patient should take a drug, herbal product, or dietary supplement during pregnancy unless approved by the patient's health care practitioner. Drugs with known teratogenic potential in humans are listed in Table 6.2.

6.5 Many types of drug toxicity are specific to certain organs.

Few drugs produce adverse effects in every organ system; these drugs would be too toxic for safe pharmacotherapy. Instead, adverse effects are often organ specific, targeting one or a few organs. It is important that the nurse learn these specific toxicities so that appropriate signs, symptoms, and lab tests can be carefully monitored. Selected organ-specific toxicities are summarized in Table 6.3.

Nephrotoxicity: The kidneys are one of the most common organ systems affected by drugs. This is because these organs filter large volumes of blood, and most drugs are excreted by the renal route. Some drugs are reabsorbed or secreted by the kidney, exposing renal tubule cells to high concentrations of these agents. Others obstruct the urinary system by causing crystalluria in the urinary tract. Nephrotoxic drugs may cause acute symptoms that appear after one or several doses, or result in chronic symptoms that manifest only after several months of pharmacotherapy.

TABLE 6.3 Organ-Specific Toxicity

Toxicity	Example Drugs and Classes
Bone marrow	ACE inhibitors, antimalarials, antineoplastics, antiseizure agents (phenytoin, carbamazepine), antithyroid drugs, cephalosporins, chloramphenicol, chlorpropamide, chlorpromazine, cimetidine, furosemide, methyldopa, NSAIDs, phenylbutazone, sulfonamides
Dermatologic	antiseizure agents (phenobarbital, phenytoin, carbamazepine), cephalosporins, erythromycin, NSAIDs, penicillin, radiologic contrast media, sulfonamides, tetracyclines
Hepatotoxicity	carbamazepine, chlorpromazine, halothane
Muscle toxicity	statins (HMG CoA reductase inhibitors)
Nephrotoxicity	ACE inhibitors, acyclovir, aminoglycosides, amphotericin B, cisplatin, cocaine, cyclosporine, NSAIDs, radiologic contrast agents, sulfonamides, tacrolimus
Neurotoxicity	aminoglycosides, cisplatin, ethanol, loop diuretics, methyldopa, salicylates, vincristine

It is critical that the health care provider identify at-risk patients and attempt to prevent nephrotoxicity. Means for prevention include providing proper hydration, monitoring urinary lab values, and adjusting doses appropriately for patients with renal impairment. Patients with serious renal impairment should not receive nephrotoxic drugs unless other therapeutic options have been exhausted.

Neurotoxicity: Although the blood–brain barrier prevents many drugs from reaching the brain, neurotoxicity is a relatively common adverse effect of certain drug classes. This is because the brain receives a large percentage of the blood supply and is especially sensitive to small amounts of toxic substances. For sedatives, antidepressants, antianxiety agents, antiseizure agents, and antipsychotic drugs the difference between a therapeutic dose and one that produces adverse effects may be very small. Indeed, drowsiness is seen in a majority of patients receiving these drugs when therapy is initiated. Signs and symptoms of toxicity in the central nervous system (CNS) include depression, mania, sedation, behavioral changes, hallucinations, and seizures. The special senses may be affected, including visual changes, loss of balance, and hearing impairment.

Effective patient teaching is essential when patients are beginning therapy with potentially neurotoxic drugs. The nurse should warn patients not to drive vehicles or perform other hazardous tasks until they are certain of the effects of these drugs. Caregivers should be taught to report changes in patient behavior, because the patient may have difficulty recognizing these signs. The nurse should be aware that neurotoxic drugs can significantly worsen preexisting CNS disease. Serious symptoms such as seizures, delirium, or significant visual or hearing impairment should be immediately reported to the prescriber.

Muscle toxicity: Muscle tissue is relatively resistant to the effects of drugs, despite its extensive blood supply. In skeletal muscle the incidence of drug-induced myopathy is low but may be serious when it does occur. A few drugs are toxic to cardiac muscle, resulting in impairment of the ability of the heart to pump blood to the tissues. Although a large number of drugs affect heart rate or the electrical conductivity in the heart, this is not because they are exhibiting cardiotoxicity: These drugs generally act by changing the autonomic nervous system activation to the heart (see Chapter 16).

To prevent skeletal muscle toxicity, the nurse should assess for unexplained muscle soreness or pain during therapy. Laboratory tests such as creatine kinase should be evaluated regularly during therapy with drugs that have muscle toxicity. For cardiotoxic drugs, the nurse should regularly monitor electrocardiograms and lab tests measuring possible cardiac muscle damage.

Hepatotoxicity: A major function of the liver is to detoxify foreign chemicals that enter the body; thus it should not be surprising that hepatotoxicity is one of the most common adverse effects. Effects of hepatotoxic drugs range from minor, reversible symptoms to fatal hepatitis.

The nurse should regularly monitor liver enzyme tests when administering hepatotoxic drugs, because these show the earliest signs of liver toxicity. Symptoms of liver impairment are vague and nonspecific and include right upper quadrant pain, anorexia, and nausea or vomiting. In serious cases, the liver will be unable to metabolize other drugs, resulting in high serum drug levels. Extreme care must be taken when administering potentially hepatotoxic drugs to patients with preexisting liver disease.

Dermatologic toxicity: Drug reactions affecting the skin are some of the most common types of adverse effects. These reactions may be caused by a hypersensitivity response or by nonimmune-type responses. Rash, the most common cutaneous drug reaction, usually occurs within 1 to 2 weeks of initiation of drug therapy and resolves without serious complications. Drug-induced rash is sometimes accompanied by itching (pruritus). Although almost any drug can cause rash, antibiotics are the most frequent drug class causing this condition. Urticaria (hives) are raised welts that are often accompanied by intense pruritus and, although less common than rash, are a symptom of a potential allergic reaction that could lead to anaphylaxis.

Drug-induced dermatologic toxicity may be serious. In angioedema, swelling occurs in the dermis, periorbital region, and around the mouth and throat. Angioedema is considered a severe drug reaction because the swelling may impair breathing and may be fatal. SJS is another drug-induced condition that can be fatal. This syndrome causes severe blistering of the skin, usually accompanied by mucous membrane involvement and fever.

Phototoxicity is a type of drug-induced dermatologic toxicity in which certain drugs cause the skin to absorb excess ultraviolet radiation from the sun or heat lamps. Symptoms resemble sunburn and are best prevented by advising patients to avoid direct sunlight. Phototoxicity resolves when the drug is discontinued.

Most types of drug-induced dermatologic toxicity do not require pharmacotherapy. If pruritus is prominent, an antihistamine or corticosteroid may be administered. In all cases of serious drug-induced hypersensitivity, the nurse should discontinue the drug until the cause of the skin condition can be diagnosed.

Bone marrow toxicity: Drugs affecting the bone marrow are of great concern due to the possibility of serious and perhaps fatal outcomes. The bone marrow serves as a nursery for the production of red blood cells, white blood cells, and platelets. Drugs may affect only one of these types of cells or all three. When all three groups are affected, drug-induced pancytopenia or aplastic anemia occurs and the patient is at great risk for serious illness. Loss of white blood cells may cause agranulocytosis or neutropenia, which places the patient at risk for serious infections. The drug class most likely to cause bone marrow toxicity is the antineoplastics class. Bone marrow toxicity is the dose-limiting factor with these drugs (see Chapter 58).

The role of the nurse in preventing bone marrow toxicity is to carefully monitor laboratory data and recognize changes that suggest impending toxicity, such as decreases in red cells, white cells, or platelets. In many cases, bone marrow toxicity is quickly reversible if the condition is recognized early and the drug is discontinued. Furthermore, the nurse should carefully monitor the therapeutic regimen of patients who have preexisting blood cell disorders because adding a drug with bone marrow toxicity may worsen these conditions.

Drug Interactions

6.6 Drug interactions may significantly affect pharmacotherapeutic outcomes.

A **drug interaction** occurs when a medication interacts with another substance and the drug's actions are affected. The "other substance" causing the drug interaction may be another drug, a dietary supplement, an herbal product, or food. The substance participating in the drug interaction must be external to the body and is usually taken concurrently with the medication. Although substances that are naturally found in the body (endogenous substances) routinely interact with drugs, these are not considered drug interactions because this is considered part of the body's "normal" response to the drug.

Because patients often take multiple drugs concurrently, drug interactions occur continually. Even if only one drug is taken, the potential for a drug–food interaction still exists. Drug interactions are impossible to totally eliminate and should be considered an important component of pharmacotherapy. In the large majority of cases, the drug interaction goes unnoticed and treatment outcomes are unaffected. Indeed, it is likely that most drug interactions have yet to be documented or researched because they do not cause clinically noticeable effects or harm to the patient.

Some drug interactions are important to pharmacology because they are known to cause adverse effects or otherwise affect treatment outcomes. By studying the mechanisms of potential drug interactions, the nurse can sometimes prevent adverse effects or optimize treatment outcomes. For example, if the patient is receiving gentamicin, the nurse should use caution when administering acyclovir, because the drug combination can cause higher than normal levels of acyclovir in the blood. The nurse may suggest that the prescriber order a lower dose or substitute a different drug. Understanding drug interactions can have a direct effect on the success of pharmacotherapy.

Drug interactions occur by dozens of different mechanisms. To simplify their study, it may be helpful to remember that drug interactions can have three basic effects on the action of a drug.

- The actions of the drug can be inhibited, resulting in less therapeutic action. For example, milk interferes with the absorption of tetracycline, causing a lower serum level of antibiotic, thus diminishing its therapeutic action.
- The actions of the drug may be enhanced, causing a more effective therapeutic response. For example, coadministration of the two antiviral drugs lopinavir and ritonavir causes a greater reduction in levels of HIV than occurs when either drug is used alone.
- The actions of the drug may be changed and a new response produced. For example, when used alone disulfiram (Antabuse) causes no pharmacologic effects. When taken with alcohol, however, the combination produces dramatic, new actions such as severe headache, flushing, dyspnea, palpitations, and blurred vision (see Chapter 8).

6.7 Pharmacokinetic drug interactions include changes in the absorption, distribution, metabolism, or excretion of medications.

Recall from Chapter 5 that pharmacokinetics is the branch of pharmacology dealing with how the body acts on a drug after it is administered. Many drug interactions involve some aspect of the pharmacokinetics of the medication. When studying drug interactions, it is convenient to use the same categories for pharmacokinetics that are presented in Chapter 4. The general types of pharmacokinetic interactions are illustrated in Figure 6.1.

Absorption: Most drugs need to be absorbed to produce their actions. Any substance that affects absorption has the potential to influence drug response. If fact, this is one of the most common mechanisms of drug interactions. By interfering with normal absorption, drug action may be inhibited or enhanced. Increasing absorption will raise drug serum levels and produce an enhanced effect; substances inhibiting absorption have the opposite effect.

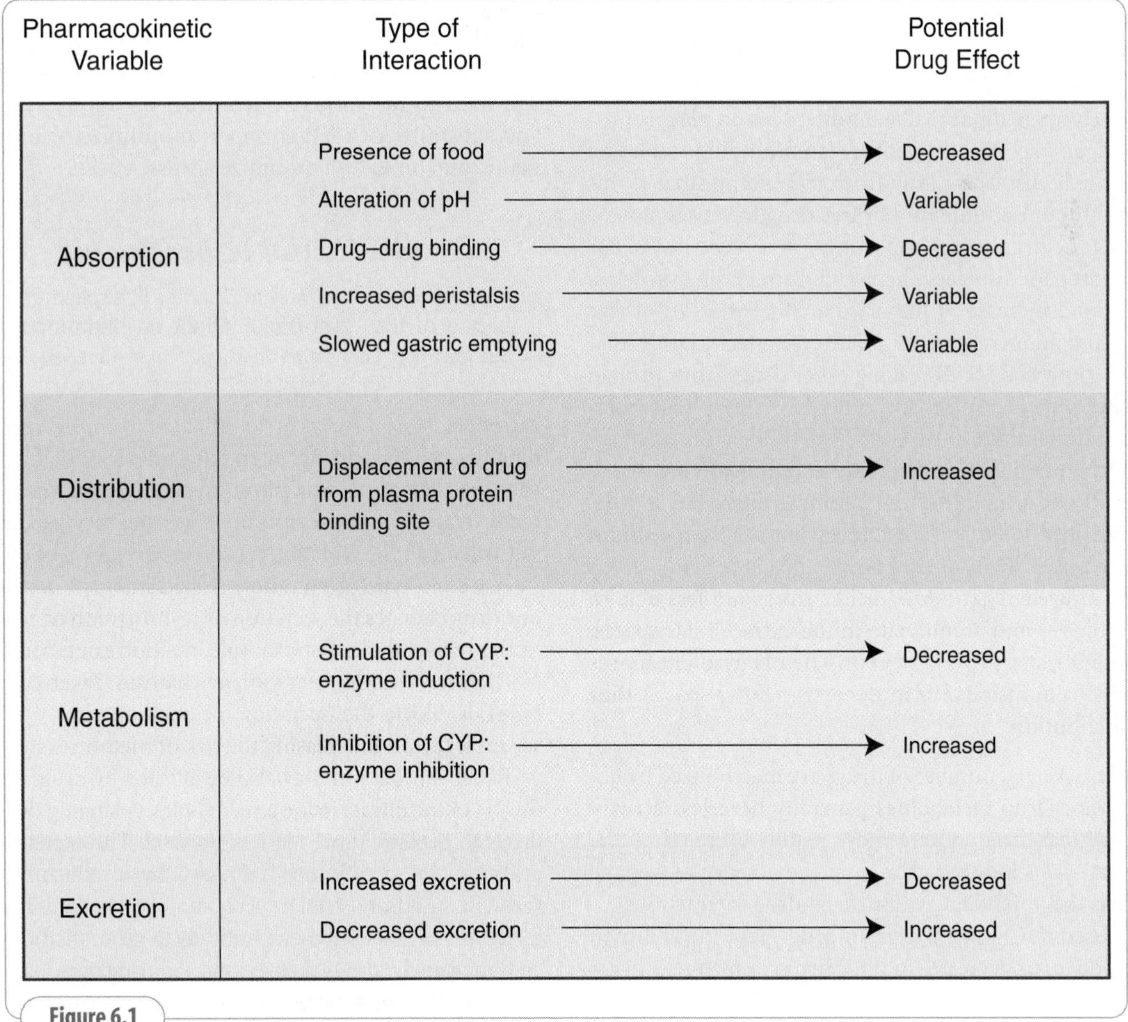

Figure 6.1

Types of pharmacokinetic drug–drug interactions.

The simplest way to affect absorption is to change the speed of substances moving through the gastrointestinal (GI) tract. Opioids such as morphine or heroin will slow peristalsis, giving drugs additional time for absorption. Laxatives and drugs that stimulate the parasympathetic nervous system will speed substances through the GI tract, diminishing the absorption time of drugs concurrently administered. The bile acid resins such as cholestyramine (Questran) bind other drugs and prevent their absorption.

Many drug–drug interactions caused by changes in absorption may be prevented by taking the two drugs at least 2 to 3 hours apart. In the case of drug–food interactions, the interacting food should be avoided, or the drug may be taken on an empty stomach. Taking drugs on an empty stomach, however, may increase the incidence of nausea or vomiting, which could result in loss of the drug before complete absorption occurs. The nurse must teach patients with drug-induced nausea not to take drugs with antacids or milk unless approved by the prescriber. Antacids are alkaline (basic) substances that raise the pH of the GI contents and have the potential to change the percentage of ionized drug. Ionized forms of drugs are less able to cross the intestinal mucosa than nonionized forms.

Distribution: Distribution is the movement of a drug from its site of absorption to its target tissue. Many drugs travel through the blood bound to plasma proteins and, when bound, the drug is unable to leave the blood to reach its target. Drugs may compete for available binding sites on plasma proteins; one drug may prevent another from binding to plasma proteins or may displace a drug from its binding sites. If this occurs, the amount of unbound or free drug increases, potentially raising the drug serum concentration to toxic levels. For example, diazepam displaces phenytoin from plasma proteins, causing a rapid increase in the plasma concentration of free phenytoin and an increased risk of adverse effects. Drugs that have a high potential for displacing other drugs from protein binding sites include aspirin and other NSAIDs, phenylbutazone, and sulfonamides.

A second potential drug–drug interaction involving distribution can occur if the pH of the plasma is altered by a drug. For example, infusions of an alkaline substance such as sodium bicarbonate raise the pH of the plasma and cause acidic drugs to become ionized. The ionized acidic drugs are less able to cross membranes and accumulate in the extracellular spaces, creating an ionization (pH) gradient. The pH gradient moves acidic drugs from inside cells to the extracellular spaces, thus altering distribution.

Metabolism: A large number of drugs are metabolized by hepatic enzymes. Drug metabolites generally have less activity than the original drug and are more readily excreted by the kidneys. Any drug-induced change in the activity of hepatic enzymes has the potential to cause drug–drug interactions.

As discussed in Chapter 5, certain drugs have the ability to increase (induce) or decrease (inhibit) hepatic enzyme activity. Inducers such as phenobarbital will increase drug metabolism, thus promoting the inactivation and excretion of drugs administered concurrently. Clinically, this will be observed as diminished drug effectiveness. For example, if phenobarbital is administered concurrently with the antihypertensive drug nifedipine, less blood pressure reduction will result. The dose of nifedipine will need to be increased to produce an optimal therapeutic effect. However, care must be taken if the inducer is discontinued because hepatic enzymes will return back to baseline levels in a few days or weeks. Once hepatic enzymes return to normal, the dose of nifedipine will have to be adjusted downward to avoid toxicity. Also, remember that a few drugs (prodrugs) are activated by metabolism. Increasing the metabolism of prodrugs will cause an increase, rather than a decrease, in therapeutic response.

Inhibitors of hepatic metabolism will cause drug interactions that are opposite to those of inducers. For example, ritonavir inhibits the hepatic enzyme CYP3A4 and will decrease the metabolism of other drugs that are substrates for this enzyme. Giving ritonavir concurrently with nifedipine causes an increased blood pressure reduction owing to diminished metabolism of the antihypertensive. The nifedipine dose must be lowered to avoid toxicity. After ritonavir is discontinued, hepatic enzyme levels return to baseline and the nifedipine dose must be adjusted once again to maintain blood pressure control.

Drug interactions involving hepatic metabolism are some of the most complex in pharmacology. Although many of these interactions are not clinically significant; others clearly have the potential to affect therapeutic outcomes. The nurse will need to remember which drugs are inducers, inhibitors, and substrates of CYP enzymes to optimize pharmacotherapeutic outcomes and minimize adverse effects.

CONNECTION *Checkpoint* 6.1

From what you learned in Chapter 5, explain the significance of the "first-pass" effect on pharmacotherapy.

See Answer to Connection Checkpoint 6.1 in Appendix A.

Excretion: Most drugs are eliminated from the body through renal excretion. A drug interaction may occur if a substance changes the glomerular filtration rate (GFR). The GFR is directly related to cardiac output; drugs that increase cardiac output will affect the GFR and hasten the excretion of other drugs.

A second type of excretion-related interaction may occur if one drug changes the secretion or reabsorption of another drug in the renal tubule. For example, methotrexate competes with NSAIDs for the same secretion mechanism. Taken concurrently, NSAIDs block the secretion of methotrexate, raising drug serum levels and increasing the risk of methotrexate toxicity.

Renal elimination may also be affected by drugs that change the pH of the filtrate in the renal tubules. Changing the pH causes drugs to become more (or less) ionized. The excretion of weak acids can be significantly increased by alkalinizing the urine through the administration of sodium bicarbonate. This drug interaction may be used therapeutically to promote more rapid excretion of acidic drugs such as aspirin during overdose situations. Similarly, excretion of weak bases can be increased by acidifying the urine through the administration of ammonium chloride.

Not all excretion-related drug interactions involve the kidneys. Some drugs are extensively excreted by the biliary system and two drugs may interact through this mechanism. For example, pravastatin and cyclosporine use the same carrier protein to move the drug molecules from the liver to bile. Giving the two drugs concurrently will slow the biliary excretion of pravastatin and raise its serum concentration to potentially toxic levels. Because biliary excretion is not the dominant form of elimination for most drugs, this type of drug–drug excretion interaction is far less common than those involving the kidneys.

6.8 Pharmacodynamic drug interactions include additive, synergistic, or antagonistic effects.

Recall from Chapter 5 that pharmacodynamics is the branch of pharmacology examining the mechanisms of drug action, meaning how a drug changes the body. Many drugs produce their actions by binding to specific receptors (see Section 5.5). When two drugs compete for the same receptor, or activate receptors that produce opposite effects, drug interactions are possible. Many common interactions encountered in clinical practice are pharmacodynamic in nature.

In simplest terms, two possible events can occur during a pharmacodynamic drug interaction: Drug action may be enhanced or inhibited. "Drug action" in the context of a drug interaction may be a therapeutic effect or an adverse effect. Thus, the drug interaction may be desirable (increased therapeutic response/decreased adverse effect) or undesirable (decreased therapeutic response/increased adverse effect). The basic pharmacodynamic drug–drug interactions are illustrated in Figure 6.2.

The pharmacodynamic drug interaction that is easiest to visualize is the **additive effect.** In this interaction, two drugs from a similar therapeutic class produce a combined summation response. This is used extensively in treating hypertension. For example, a diuretic may be used to lower systolic blood pressure by 10 mmHg, and a beta blocker may be added to the regimen to produce another 15-mmHg reduction. Combined, the two drugs produce a 25-mmHg reduction. Why would two drugs be prescribed (with more expense to the patient), rather than a single drug? There are two rationales. First, to produce a 25-mmHg reduction using only the diuretic, the dose would have to be increased. Keeping the doses of both the diuretic and

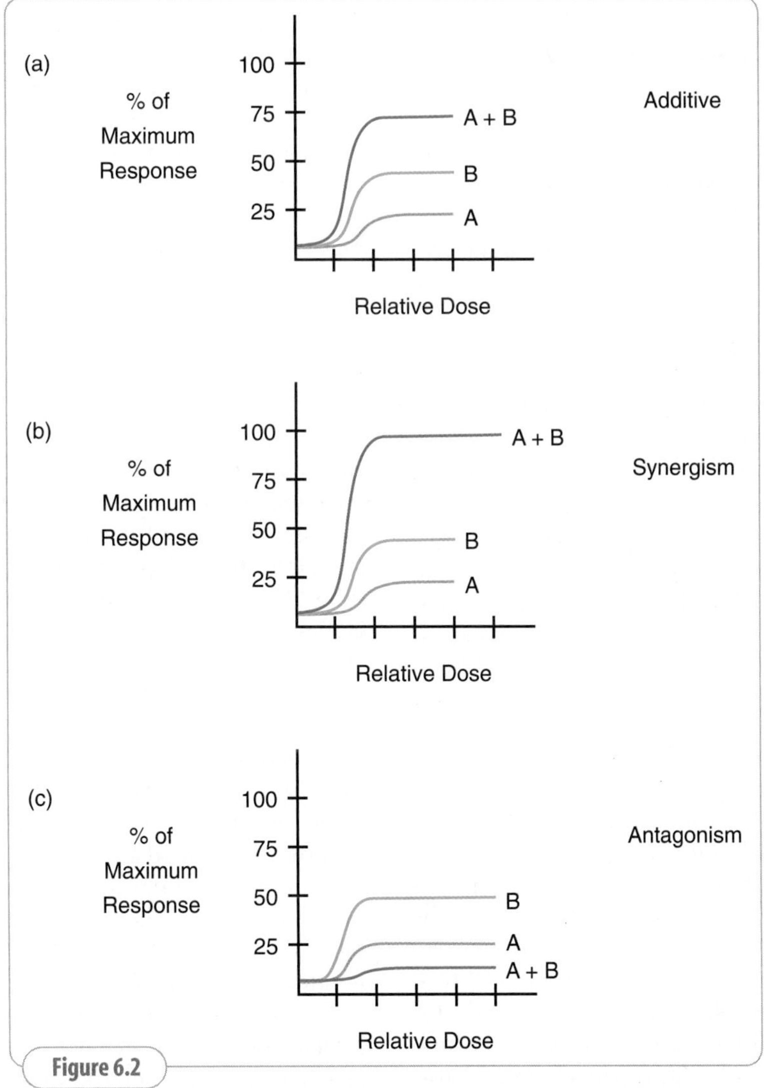

Figure 6.2

Additive, synergistic, and antagonistic drug interactions: (a) additive response; (b) synergistic response; (c) antagonistic response.

beta blocker low and taking advantage of their additive effect reduces the potential for adverse drug events. Second, some drugs have low efficacy and it may not be possible to achieve a 25-mmHg reduction with a single drug. The maximum effect from the diuretic may have been a 10-mmHg reduction, and another drug would need to be added to the regimen to achieve a greater response. In this example, the two drugs act at very different types of receptors to produce the additive therapeutic response: beta blockers in cardiac muscle and diuretics in the renal tubules.

Another pharmacodynamic drug interaction that produces an enhanced response is a **synergistic effect.** In this interaction, the effect of the two drugs is greater than would be expected from simply adding the two individual drugs' responses. This type of interaction is used extensively in treating infections. For example, Synercid is a combination drug that contains quinupristin and dalfopristin, two antibiotics that are effective against resistant *Staphylococcus* infections. Both drugs bind to the bacterial ribosome and produce greater killing than would be predicted from adding the two individual drugs' effects. Another example is the combination antibiotic Bactrim, which combines trimethoprim and sulfamethoxazole to produce a synergistic effect on bacterial cell killing.

A third type of pharmacodynamic interaction occurs when adding a second drug results in a diminished pharmacologic response. This **antagonistic effect** can result in drug actions being "cancelled." For example, drugs activating the sympathetic nervous system such as epinephrine will increase the heart rate and dilate the bronchi. A drug such as carvedilol (Coreg) will have the opposite effects: slowed heart rate and bronchoconstriction. Thus, carvedilol is considered an antagonist to epinephrine and may cancel its actions, depending on the doses of the two drugs. Why would a nurse administer drugs with opposite actions? This is generally done to reduce the adverse effects of a drug. For example, if a drug given to treat hypertension has an expected adverse effect of increasing heart rate, an antagonist may be given to slow the heart rate and keep it within normal limits. When given intentionally, an antagonist does not necessarily reverse all actions of the first drug: It may selectively inhibit an undesirable action.

In some cases, antagonists are used to treat symptoms of drug overdose. For example, patients taking an overdose of narcotics such as morphine or heroin experience coma and life-threatening CNS depression. The administration of naloxone (Narcan), a specific narcotic antagonist, can quickly reverse some of the serious adverse effects of morphine.

Pharmacodynamic interactions can be indirect and complex. The well-documented drug interaction between digoxin (Lanoxin) and diuretics such as furosemide (Lasix) is an excellent example of an indirect effect. Furosemide enhances the excretion of potassium ion (hypokalemia), which increases the cardiotoxicity of digoxin. This can be a life-threatening interaction. Another example is the inhibition of vitamin K production in the intestine caused by antibiotics. If the patient is also taking warfarin (Coumadin), bleeding may occur because the liver is prevented from producing certain clotting factors. Again, the antibiotic did not directly interact with warfarin, yet the combination produced a serious adverse effect.

CONNECTION *Checkpoint* 6.2

The types of curves shown in Figure 6.2 are called dose–response curves. From what you learned in Chapter 5, explain the three phases of these curves.

See Answer to Connection Checkpoint 6.2 in Appendix A.

PharmFACT

It is estimated that over 2 million serious drug interactions occur annually in hospitalized patients, resulting in 100,000 deaths. *Source:* Lazarou, Pomeranz, & Corey, 1998.

6.9 Food, nutrients, and dietary supplements may interact with medications and affect their actions.

Historically, interactions between drugs and food, dietary supplements, and herbal products have been largely dismissed as clinically unimportant. Although a few interactions, such as tetracyclines with calcium products, have been documented for decades, only since the late 1980s have drug–food interactions been recognized as important to maximizing pharmacotherapeutic outcomes. The interaction that prompted the increased interest in this topic was that of a benign and healthy substance: grapefruit juice. The interaction was discovered by chance in a research study designed to examine the effects of alcohol on felodipine, a calcium channel blocker. The researchers used grapefruit juice incidentally to disguise the taste of the alcohol.

Patients often take medications with juice because it covers up the bitter taste of many drugs and provides a plentiful source of vitamins and minerals. Unfortunately, grapefruit juice also contains substances that increase the absorption of certain oral drugs. This occurs because grapefruit juice inhibits the enzyme CYP3A4 in the wall of the intestinal tract. As drugs are absorbed, they are not inactivated by CYP3A4 and higher amounts reach the circulation. Surprisingly, the inhibition from grapefruit juice may last up to 3 days after drinking the juice. The substances in the juice inhibiting CYP3A4 enzymes are called furanocoumarins. Fortunately, only a few drug classes interact with grapefruit juice. These include benzodiazepines, certain calcium channel blockers, and statins (HMG CoA reductase inhibitors).

Most of the drug–food interactions discovered thus far act by either increasing or decreasing the absorption or bioavailability of the drug. Some of these interactions are shown in Table 6.4. Drug–food interactions are easily avoided by timing the drug dose appropriately with the food or supplement. In most cases, there should be a 2-hour time gap between ingestion of the food and drug. In a few cases, the drug should be administered with food to increase its absorption.

Interactions of drugs with herbal products have also largely been undocumented. As more patients take these products, research is emerging to demonstrate that certain drug–herb combinations have a significant impact on pharmacotherapy. Because patients view herbal products as "natural," they do not

TABLE 6.4 Selected Drug–Food and Drug–Herbal Interactions

Drug	Interaction
antiplatelet and anticoagulant drugs	Feverfew can increase the risk of bleeding.
azithromycin (Zithromax)	Food reduces absorption.
atovaquone (Malarone)	Fatty food enhances absorption.
calcium channel blockers and cyclosporine	Grapefruit juice enhances absorption.
cholestyramine (Questran)	Drug binds iron, folic acid, and vitamin A to decrease their absorption.
CNS depressants	Kava can increase drowsiness and sedation.
etidronate (Didronel)	Milk, calcium, and iron bind the drug and decrease absorption.
fluoroquinolones	Calcium, iron, and other metal ions bind the drug and decrease absorption.
lovastatin (Mevacor)	Food increases absorption.
MAO inhibitors	Food containing tyramine can cause hypertensive crisis.
penicillin G	Food (milk) and metal ions reduce absorption.
orlistat (Xenical)	Drug binds fat-soluble vitamins and reduces their absorption.
serotonin reuptake inhibitors (SSRIs)	St. John's wort and grapefruit juice increase risk of adverse effects (serotonin syndrome).
sucralfate (Carafate)	Food protein binds the drug to decrease absorption.
tetracyclines	Dairy products and iron reduce absorption.
warfarin (Coumadin)	Vitamin K antagonizes the action of warfarin; ginkgo, garlic, and St. John's wort may increase risk of bleeding.
zidovudine (AZT)	Food reduces bioavailability.

usually mention them when recording their drug history; thus the health care provider must ask specific questions about their use.

Perhaps the most widely studied herb is St. John's wort, which is taken by patients as a complementary therapy for depression. The herb induces hepatic metabolic enzymes, which can reduce the effectiveness of certain prescription medications, including antidepressants, warfarin, and benzodiazepines. A second herb that has been extensively studied is ginkgo biloba, which is taken by patients to improve circulation and memory. Ginkgo may produce additive anticoagulant effects when taken with warfarin or antiplatelet drugs. It can also antagonize the effects of anti-seizure drugs, thus increasing the risk for seizures. Other effects of herbal products are presented in Chapter 15.

CONNECTIONS

To the Community Food–Drug Interactions

The nurse has a critical role in patient education related to food–drug interactions. One of the common questions a patient will ask is, "Do I take this drug with food?" Most medications can be administered with food, so of greater importance is what foods the patient should avoid when taking the drug.

Foods may contain naturally occurring substances or be fortified with vitamins that do not mix well with medications. The drug ingredients may not work as well as they should when certain foods are taken concurrently. Food nutrients can affect absorption, metabolism, or elimination of the drug by binding with ingredients in the medication. One common food–drug interaction is taking grapefruit juice with selected statins, calcium channel blockers, estrogen containing birth control pills, tricyclic antidepressants, the antiarrhythmic drug amiodarone, or the immunosuppressant tacrolimus or Prograf.

Caffeine's effect may be increased when taken with ciprofloxacin and other fluoroquinolones. Other food–drug interactions can occur with dairy and other calcium products, antacids, protein-rich foods, high-fat meals, fiber, vitamin C, cranberry and other fruit juices, tyramine-containing foods, alcohol, leafy green vegetables, soy milk, and dietary supplements. Fad diets may include foods that interact with medications. In short, the safest way to take a medication is with a glass of water.

Here is what to teach the patient:

- Always read the prescription label because the pharmacist will indicate if the medication must be taken with food. If not, take with just a glass of water.
- Read drug handouts carefully because these give more detail about possible food–drug interactions. The same is true for OTC medications. Read all inserts for warnings.
- Drink a full 8-ounce glass of water with the medication.
- Avoid taking herbal supplements and vitamins at the same time as prescription medications to avoid interactions.
- Avoid taking a drug with a hot drink or opening the pill to stir in liquid. Both can affect the effectiveness of the drug.
- Avoid drinking alcohol while taking medication.
- Share a list of current prescription and nonprescription medications taken with pharmacist. Filling the prescription at the same store will assist the pharmacist in comparing your current and new medications for possible interactions.
- Seek information from your pharmacist or health care provider if uncertain about medications. A phone call can clear up any questions and support an improved therapeutic outcome.

UNDERSTANDING THE CHAPTER

Key Concepts Summary

6.1 The nurse plays a key role in preventing and managing adverse drug effects.

6.2 Allergic reactions are caused by a hyperresponse of the immune system.

6.3 Idiosyncratic reactions are unusual drug responses often caused by genetic differences among patients.

6.4 Some drugs have the ability to induce cancer or cause birth defects.

6.5 Many types of drug toxicity are specific to certain organs.

6.6 Drug interactions may significantly affect pharmacotherapeutic outcomes.

6.7 Pharmacokinetic drug interactions include changes in the absorption, distribution, metabolism, or excretion of medications.

6.8 Pharmacodynamic drug interactions include additive, synergistic, or antagonistic effects.

6.9 Food, nutrients, and dietary supplements may interact with medications and affect their actions.

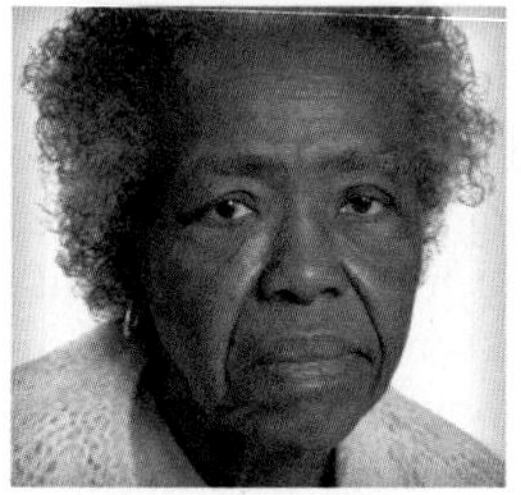

Making the PATIENT *Connection*

Remember the patient "Elizabeth Edwards" at the beginning of the chapter? Now read the remainder of the case study. Based on the information presented within this chapter, respond to the critical thinking questions that follow.

The more medication an individual takes, the more likely it is that an adverse reaction may occur. For Elizabeth Edwards this is a real possibility because she takes multiple medications for various physical problems. Ms. Edwards is a 77-year-old African American woman with several chronic conditions that require pharmacotherapy, including diabetes, heart failure, arthritis, and depression. She has been wheelchair bound since her stroke 2 years ago and has lost functional ability of her left side.

Unfortunately, she does not have a regular health care provider. Elizabeth obtains all her health care from a clinic operated for lower income individuals. The primary health care providers in the clinic are medical residents and interns who rotate every month as part of their medical training. Therefore, it is unlikely that she will see the same prescriber more than a couple of times. Her medical record is quite extensive and spans her health history for the last 15 years. Because her medical history record is so lengthy, Elizabeth fears that the new doctors will not take the time to read the entire chart before prescribing the newest treatment or therapy.

Critical Thinking Questions

1. Identify ways that you can minimize or prevent adverse drug events in this patient.
2. What existing conditions make Elizabeth more susceptible to a drug reaction?
3. Discuss how drug reactions can affect pharmacokinetics.
4. Differentiate among additive, synergistic, and antagonist drug effects.

Case Study

As the triage nurse in the emergency department, you determine the patient's chief complaint, obtain vital signs, collect past medical history information, and ask about drug and food allergies. While assessing a patient with a suspected ankle fracture, she tells you that she is allergic to codeine because it makes her nauseated and sleepy.

1. What further questions would you ask the patient about drug allergies?
2. Differentiate among adverse effect, side effect, and drug allergy.
3. Is this patient experiencing an idiosyncratic reaction? Explain.

NCLEX-RN® Review

1 Prior to the administration of an antibiotic, the client informs the nurse that 4 years ago the client experienced an allergic reaction. Based on this information what should the nurse do first?

1. Ask the client to describe the reaction further.
2. Notify the health care provider on call about the client's statements.
3. Administer the dose and observe the client for a reaction.
4. Check the medical administration record for documented allergies.

2 The nurse is researching a new drug prior to administration. The drug handbook states that the adverse effects are "dose related." The nurse is aware that this means that:

1. As the dose increases, the risk of adverse effects also increases.
2. The adverse effects should be expected after the first dose.
3. Oral preparations will produce the most adverse effects.
4. The timing of each dose should be correlated with the presence of adverse effects.

3 The client is receiving a medication that may cause nephrotoxicity. To prevent this adverse reaction the nurse should encourage the client to:

1. Avoid sunbathing and exposure to direct sunlight.
2. Increase the intake of potassium-enriched foods.
3. Abstain from alcoholic beverages.
4. Increase fluid intake to promote adequate hydration.

4 On physical examination, the nurse observes raised hive-like welts covering the client's trunk and arms. The client also complains of intense itching after receiving a new medication. The nurse will suspect what dermatologic adverse effect?

1. Angioedema
2. Stevens–Johnson syndrome
3. Urticaria
4. Phototoxicity

5 When observing a client for bone marrow toxicity, the nurse would monitor for:

1. Increased complaints of muscle and bone pain in the lower extremities.
2. Decrease in red blood cells, white blood cells, and platelets.
3. Decrease in the range of motion of the upper and lower extremities.
4. Increase in hepatic enzymes.

6 The client is receiving a medication that causes hepatotoxicity. What symptoms would alert the nurse that this drug-related toxicity has occurred?

1. Black furry tongue and vaginal yeast infection
2. A sudden reduction in blood pressure on rising
3. Right upper quadrant pain and anorexia
4. Uncontrollable movements in the face, arms, and legs

See Answers to Critical Thinking Questions, Case Study, and NCLEX-RN® Review in Appendix A.

References

Akamine, D., Filho, M. K., & Peres, C. M. (2007). Drug-nutrient interactions in elderly people. *Current Opinion in Clinical Nutrition and Metabolic Care, 10*(3), 304–310.

Boullata, J. (2005). Natural health product interactions with medication. *Nutrition in Clinical Practice, 20*(1), 33–51.

Boulatta, J., & Armenti, V. T. (2004). *Handbook of drug-nutrient interactions.* Totowa, NJ: Humana Press.

Gurwitz, J. H., Field, T. S., Harrold, L. R., Rothschild, J., Debellis, K., Seger, A. C., et al. (2003). Incidence and preventability of adverse drug events among older persons in the ambulatory setting. *Journal of the American Medical Association, 289*(9), 1107–1116.

Herr, S. M. (2005). *Herb-drug interaction handbook* (3rd ed.). Castleton, NY: Church Street Books.

Hu, Z., Yang, X., Ho, P. C., Chan, S. Y., & Heng, P. W. (2005). Herb-drug interactions: A literature review. *Drugs, 65*(9), 1239–1282.

Lazarou, J., Pomeranz, B., & Corey, P. N. (1998). Incidence of adverse drug reactions in hospitalized patients: A meta-analysis of prospective studies. *Journal of the American Medical Association, 279,* 1200–1205.

Liebler, D. C., & Guengerich, F. P. (2005). Elucidating mechanisms of drug-induced toxicity. *Nature Reviews. Drug Discovery, 4,* 410–420.

Obach, R. S. (2003). Drug-drug interactions: An important negative attribute in drugs. *Drugs Today, 39*(5), 301–338.

Osterberg, L., & Blaschke, T. (2006). Medication compliance and avoiding adverse drug reactions. Clinical review. *Medscape Today.* Retrieved April 20, 2008, from http://www.medscape.com/viewprogram/5912

Pronsky, Z. (2006). *Food-medication interactions handbook* (15th ed.). Pottstown, PA: Food Medication Interactions.

Twigger, M. (2006). A weighty problem: Monitoring the side effects of medications. *Learning Disability Practice, 9*(10), 28–31.

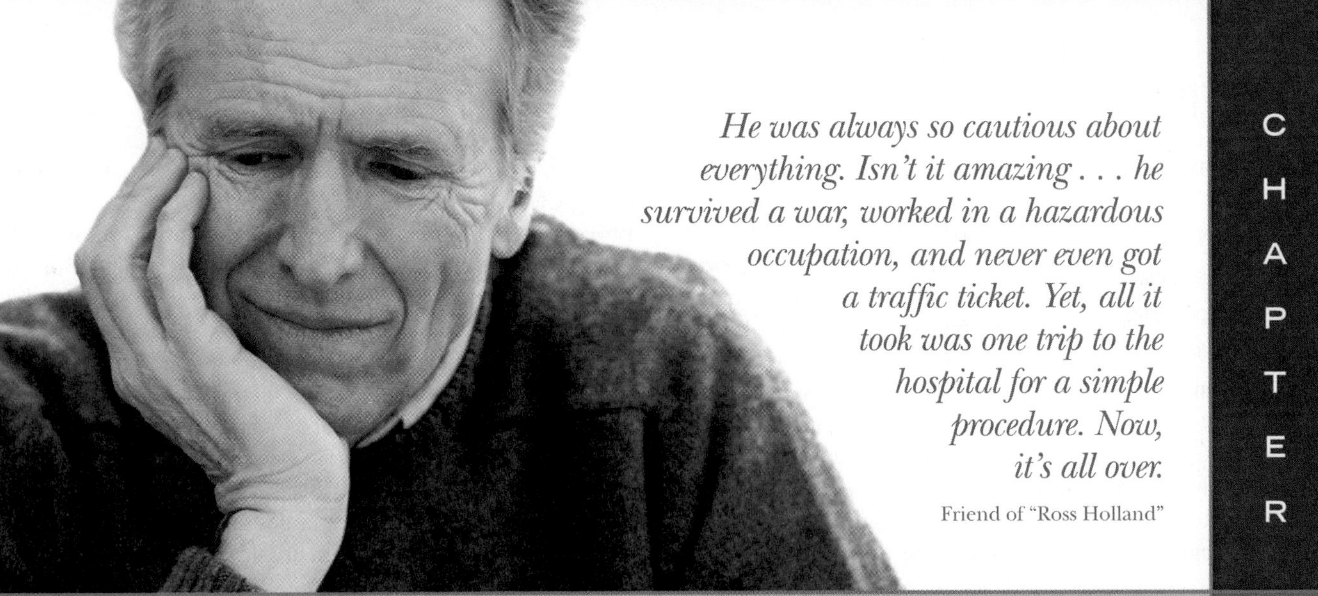

He was always so cautious about everything. Isn't it amazing . . . he survived a war, worked in a hazardous occupation, and never even got a traffic ticket. Yet, all it took was one trip to the hospital for a simple procedure. Now, it's all over.

Friend of "Ross Holland"

CHAPTER 7

Medication Errors and Risk Reduction

Chapter Outline

Medication Errors and Their Impact on Health Care

Factors Contributing to Medication Errors

Drug Names and Medication Errors

Reporting Medication Errors

Strategies for Reducing Medication Errors

Learning Outcomes

After reading this chapter, the student should be able to:

1. Critique the following statement: "All medication errors can be prevented."
2. Describe the impact of a medication error on all aspects of an institution, including patients, staff nurses, administrative personnel, and departments.
3. Using specific examples analyze major types of medication errors and how they can be prevented.
4. Describe procedures for reporting and documenting medication errors and incidents.
5. Explain how rules, policies, and procedures can help prevent medication errors.
6. Develop a list of strategies that the nurse can implement to reduce medication errors.
7. Explain how medication reconciliation can lead to a reduction in medication errors.
8. Design patient teaching information that can be used to reduce medication errors.
9. Identify efforts recommended by health care agencies to monitor medication errors and provide information to health care providers.

Key Terms

medication administration record (MAR), 87
medication error, 80
medication error index, 80
medication reconciliation, 88
polypharmacy, 88
risk management, 88

In their clinical practice, nurses maximize patient safety by striving to be 100% accurate when administering medications. Drug administration, however, requires multiple complex steps by physicians, pharmacists, nurses, and patients and can never be 100% error-free. Occasionally medication errors are made that can significantly impact treatment outcomes. The purpose of this chapter is to examine the reasons for medication errors and explore strategies that nurses may use to prevent them.

PharmFACT

It is estimated that 1.5 million medication errors occur in the United States each year, costing more than $3.5 billion in medical expenses annually. *Source:* The National Academies, 2006.

Medication Errors and Their Impact on Health Care

7.1 Medication errors are preventable events that may significantly impact treatment outcomes.

According to the National Coordinating Council for Medication Error Reporting and Prevention (NCC MERP), a **medication error** is "any preventable event that may cause or lead to inappropriate medication use or patient harm while the medication is in the control of the health care professional, patient, or consumer." The NCC MERP also classifies medication errors and has developed the **medication error index.** This index categorizes medication errors by evaluating the extent of harm an error can cause, as shown in Figures 7.1 and 7.2.

Although medication errors are the most common cause of morbidity and preventable death within hospitals, they do not always result in patient harm. A study of 154,816 medication errors over a 3-year period found that 97% of the actual errors did not result in harm to the patient (Santell, Hicks, McMeekin, & Cousins, 2003). Thirty-six percent of the errors were intercepted before they reached the patient. Of the errors that caused harm, 0.47% resulted in death. The most frequent drug class resulting in death due to medication error is opiates (narcotic analgesics).

When a medication error occurs, the repercussions can be emotionally devastating for the nurse and extend beyond the particular nurse and patient involved. A medication error can extend the patient's length of hospitalization, which increases medical costs. Undue harm to the patient due to medication errors is a cause of expensive legal challenges for the health care industry, physicians, and nurses. If frequent medication errors or serious errors are publicized, the reputation of the facility may suffer because the agency may be perceived as unsafe or delivering substandard care. Administrative personnel may also be penalized for errors within their departments or the hospital as a whole.

There is no acceptable incidence rate for medication errors. The goal of every health care organization should be to improve medication administration systems to prevent harm to patients due to medication errors. All errors, whether or not they affect the patient, should be investigated with the goal of identifying procedures that can improve the medication administration process to prevent future errors. The investigation should be conducted in a nonpunitive manner that encourages staff to report errors, thereby building a culture of safety within an organization. Medication errors, especially those types that occur repeatedly, can alert nurses and health care administrators that a new policy or procedure needs to be implemented to maximize patient safety.

Factors Contributing to Medication Errors

7.2 Medication errors may be caused by human factors, inadequate communication, or confusing labels, packaging, or drug names.

A large number of different factors contribute to medication errors. In a review by the U.S. Food and Drug Administration (FDA), the largest percentage of medication errors (42%) was the result of human factors such as performance and knowledge deficits and dose miscalculation (Thomas, Holquist, & Phillips, 2001). Lack of adequate oral or written communication, especially misinterpretation of the order, resulted in 19% of the errors. Inadequate or mislabeled products caused 20% of the errors. Name confusion involving similar sounding drugs resulted in 13% of the errors. Finally, poor or incorrect labeling, packaging, and design were responsible for 6% of the errors.

Studying the types and causes of medication errors allows agencies and facilities to design ways to prevent them. Once a common source of error is identified, the FDA works with health care agencies to determine changes that may be made to prevent that error in the future. For example, if two drug names sound too similar and are causing medication errors, the FDA may mandate a change in name. The FDA may request pharmaceutical companies to more clearly label or package a drug to avoid confusion. Other forms of intervention include educating health care professionals and consumers about common errors and how to prevent them.

The specific types of medication errors and their incidence reported to the FDA are shown in Table 7.1. Factors contributing to medication errors by health care providers include, but are not limited to, the following:

- Omitting one of the following rights of drug administration
  - Right dose
  - Right medication
  - Right patient
  - Right route of administration
  - Right time of delivery
- Failing to perform an agency system check. Both pharmacists and nurses must collaborate on checking the accuracy

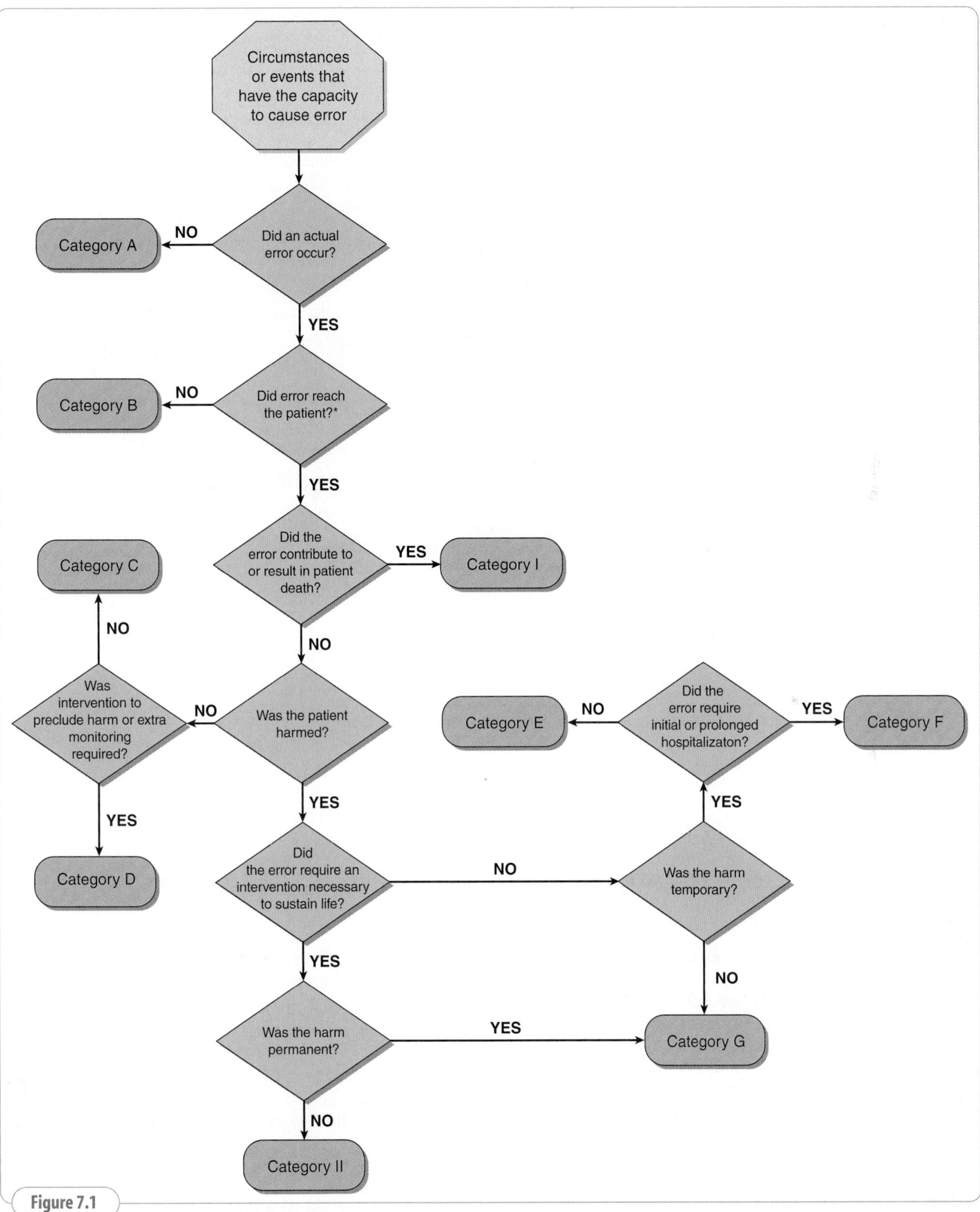

Figure 7.1

NCC MERP Index for categorizing medication errors algorithm.
Source: From National Coordinating Council for Medication Error Reporting and Prevention, © 2001. All rights reserved.

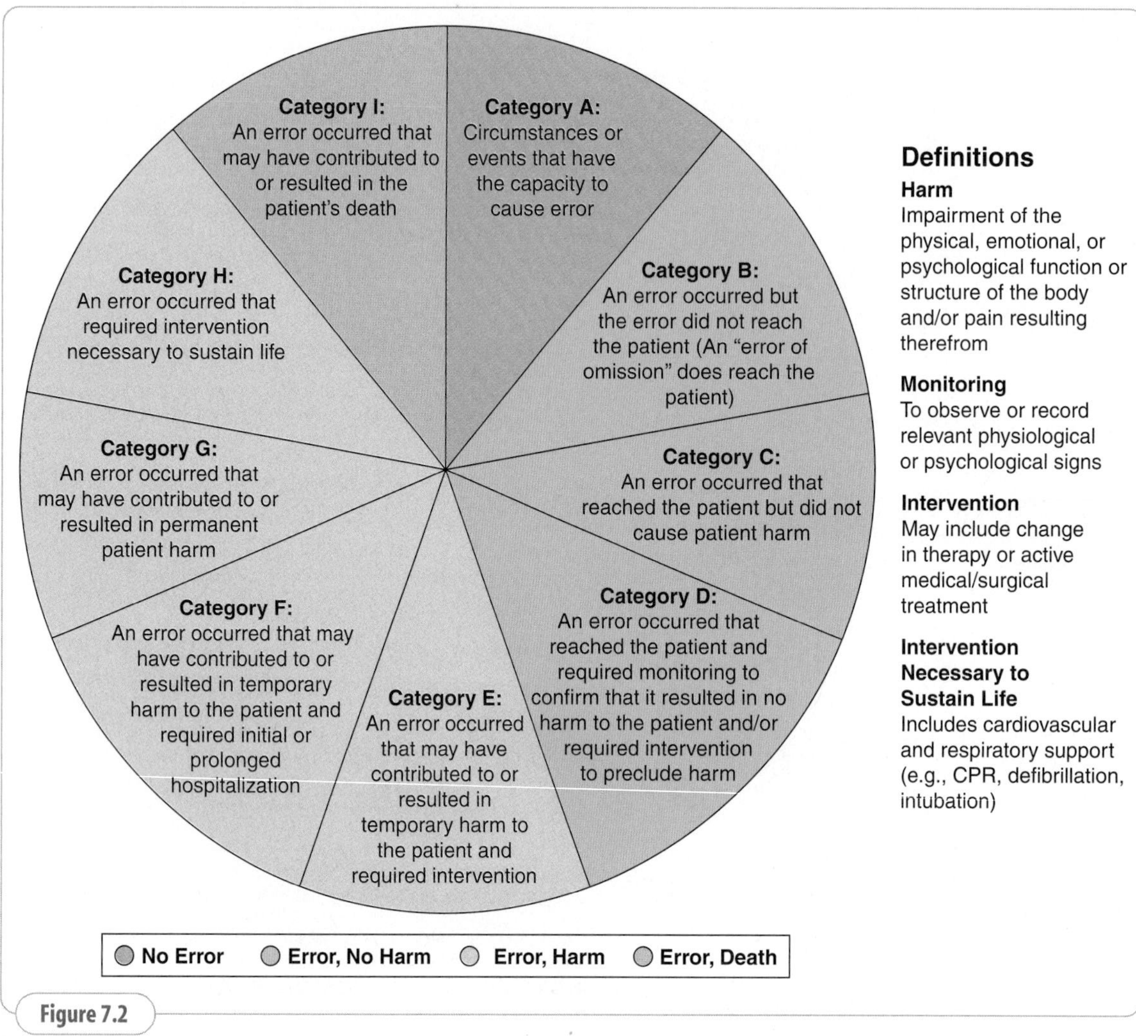

Figure 7.2

NCC MERP index for categorizing medication errors.
Source: From National Coordinating Council for Medication Error Reporting and Prevention, © 2001. All rights reserved.

CONNECTIONS

Lifespan Considerations — Parents' Role in Preventing Medication Errors: Ask Before You Act

The primary action that parents or guardians can take to safeguard their children against medication errors is to be active participants in their children's health care plan. Parents should ask for additional information and clarification about their child's disease or illness as well as any medications prescribed. They should request the child's complete treatment plan. Sources of information include discussions with the health care provider and reading the most recent scientific research or information from reputable sources in books, magazines, or the Internet.

A proactive parent can work with the health care provider by:

- Making a complete list of the child's current prescribed medications, over-the-counter (OTC) drugs, and any herbal supplements or vitamins.
- Noting the child's known allergies.
- Reading the prescription before leaving the health care provider's office and asking questions.
- Knowing the child's current weight because medication is based on weight.
- Reading the label on the medication bottle, comparing it with what is on the original prescription, and asking any questions before giving it to the child.

This is not the time to be silent. Parents should ask questions and write down answers. Some to consider are:

- What is the common name of this medication?
- Why is the child prescribed this medication? What is it for?
- Is this the appropriate dose for the child's weight?
- What are possible adverse effects? What should one do if any of these are noted?
- How often does the child receive this dose of medication and for how long?
- Is this drug safe with the other medications and vitamin supplements the child takes?
- What foods or drinks should the child avoid to have the best outcome?
- When can the parent or guardian expect to see improvement in the child's condition?
- What tool is best to administer any liquid medication? Cup? Spoon? Syringe?
- Where can one call for clarification of any future questions?

It must be remembered that the best way to protect the child is to ask, ask, and ask before one acts.

TABLE 7.1 Types of Medication Errors

Type of Error	Frequency (%)
Wrong drug	22
Overdosage	17
Wrong route of administration	8
Noncompliance	7
Wrong strength/concentration	7
Wrong technique	7
Monitoring error	7
Extra dose	3
Underdosage	2.5
Wrong time	2
Wrong duration	1
Wrong rate	1
Wrong patient	1
Dose omission	1
Deteriorated drug	1
Wrong dosage form	0.5
Other	12

Note: From "Med Error Reports to FDA Show a Mixed Bag," by M. Thomas, C. Holquist, & J. Phillips, October 10, 2001, FDA Safety Page. Retrieved April 20, 2008, from http://www.fda.gov/cder/drug/MedErrors/mixed.pdf

and appropriateness of drug orders prior to administering drugs to patients.

- Failing to account for patient variables such as age, body size, and renal or hepatic function. Nurses should always review recent laboratory data and other information in the patient's chart before administering medications, especially for those drugs that have a narrow margin of safety.
- Giving medications based on verbal orders or phone orders, which may be misinterpreted or go undocumented. Nurses should remind the prescriber that medication orders must be in writing before the drug can be administered.
- Giving medications based on an incomplete or an illegible order when the nurse is unsure of the correct drug, dosage, or administration method. Incomplete orders should be clarified with the prescriber before the medication is administered. A leading zero should precede a decimal smaller than 1 (e.g., 0.5 mg). Certain abbreviations that are sources of medication errors should be avoided in written orders, as listed in Table 7.2.
- Practicing under stressful work conditions. Studies have correlated an increased number of errors with the stress level of nurses. Studies have also indicated that the rate of medication errors may increase when individual nurses are assigned to patients who are the most acutely ill.

TABLE 7.2 Abbreviations to Avoid in Medication Administration

Abbreviation	Intended Meaning	Common Error	Correction
µg	Micrograms	Mistaken for "mg" (milligrams), resulting in an overdose	Use "mcg"
AU, AS, AD	Latin abbreviation for both ears, left ear, and right ear, respectively	Misinterpreted as the Latin abbreviation "OU" (both eyes); "OS" (left eye); "OD" (right eye)	Use "right ear," "left ear," or "each ear"
cc	Cubic centimeters	Mistaken as "U" (units) when poorly written	Use "mL"
D/C	Discharge; also discontinue	Patients' medications have been prematurely discontinued when D/C (intended to mean "discharge") was misinterpreted as "discontinue," because it was followed by a list of drugs	Use "discharge" and "discontinue"
HS	Half-strength At bedtime, hours of sleep	Mistaken as bedtime Mistaken as half-strength	Use "half-strength" or "bedtime"
IN	Intranasal	Mistaken as IV or IM	Use "intranasal" or "NAS"
IU	International unit	Mistaken as IV (intravenous) or 10 (ten)	Use "international units"
MS, MSO_4, $MgSO_4$	Confused for one another	Can mean morphine sulfate or magnesium sulfate	Use complete drug name
Q.D.	Latin abbreviation for every day	The period after the "Q" has sometimes been mistaken for an "I" and the drug has been given "QID" (four times daily) rather than daily	Use "every day"
Q.O.D.	Latin abbreviation for every other day	Misinterpreted as "QD" (daily) or "QID" (four times daily); if the "O" is poorly written, it looks like a period or an "I"	Use "every other day"
SC or SQ	Subcutaneous	Mistaken as "SL" (sublingual) when poorly written	Use "subcutaneous"
T I W or tiw	Three times a week	Misinterpreted as "three times a day" or "twice a week"	Use "three times weekly"
U	Units	Mistaken as a zero or a four (4), resulting in overdose; also mistaken for "cc" (cubic centimeters) when poorly written	Use "unit"

Note: Data from *The ISMP's List of Error-Prone Abbreviations, Symbols, and Dose Designations,* Institute for Safe Medication Practices, 2006. Retrieved August 12, 2008, from http://www.ismp.org/Tools/errorproneabbreviations.pdf

Patients, or their home caregivers, may also contribute to medication errors by:

- Taking drugs ordered by several health care providers without informing each prescriber about all their prescribed medications. This practice can lead to drug interactions such as additive, synergistic, or antagonistic effects (see Chapter 6).
- Getting prescriptions filled at more than one pharmacy. The pharmacist is a key member of the health care team who may recognize potential drug interactions and adverse effects.
- Not filling or refilling prescriptions. A large percentage of patients do not fill their prescriptions and are reluctant to admit this to their health care provider.
- Taking medications incorrectly. Taking the wrong amount of medication or at the wrong time of day are some of the most common medication errors in the home setting.
- Taking medications left over from a previous illness or that were prescribed for something else. The nurse must emphasize the importance of completing the entire treatment regimen and remind the patient never to "trade" drugs with others.

CONNECTION *Checkpoint* 7.1

From what you learned in Chapter 6, describe the similarities and differences between a synergistic effect and an additive effect and how they might contribute to a medication error. See Answer to Connection Checkpoint 7.1 in Appendix A.

Drug Names and Medication Errors

7.3 Certain drugs have higher rates of medication errors.

Some types of medication errors are independent of the drug being administered. For example, failure to perform a system check, forgetting to give a dose, or administering the medication to the wrong patient can occur with any medication. Some drugs, however, have higher error rates than others. Furthermore, when an error does occur, certain medications have greater potential to cause harm. Learning which drugs have the highest error rates and produce the most serious consequences can help the nurse to be more vigilant when administering these agents.

With thousands of generic and brand names for drugs, it is inevitable that some will sound similar; for example, hydroxyzine and hydralazine or Novalin and Novalog. It is easy to understand how a verbal order given in a hurry over a cell phone could result in the wrong drug. It is likely that hundreds of medication errors occur each year because of soundalike drugs. This is a primary reason why verbal drug orders should always be confirmed in writing before being administered. A partial listing of drugs with soundalike names is included in Table 7.3.

Many drugs also have names that look alike when written as a prescription and differ by only a few letters. When handwritten, the nurse may have difficulty determining the correct drug; for example, clonidine and Klonopin or taxol and paxil. With these types of names, it is often helpful to write both the generic and

TABLE 7.3 Look-Alike and Sound-Alike Drug Names

Abelcet	amphotericin B
Accupril	AcipHex
acetazolamide	acetohexamide
AcipHex	Aricept
Activase	TNKase
Actos	Actonel
Adderall	Inderal
Advicor	Altocor
Aldara	Alora
Alkeran	Leukeran or Myleran
Allegra	Viagra
Amaryl	Reminyl
amphotericin B	AmBisome
antacid	Atacand
Antivert	Axert
Anzemet	Avandamet
argatroban	Aggrastat
aripiprazole	rabeprazole
Asacol	Os-Cal
Atrovent	Natru-Vent
Avandia	Prandin
Avinza	Invanz
Avinza	Evista
BayHep B	BayRab or BayRho-D
Bicillin C-R	Bicillin L-A
Brethine	Methergine

TABLE 7.3 *Continued*

camphorated tincture of opium (paregoric)	opium tincture
carboplatin	cisplatin
Cedax	Cidex
Celexa	Zyprexa
chlorpromazine	chlorpropamide
Claritin-D	Claritin-D 24
Clozaril	Colazal
Colace	Cozaar
colchicine	Cortrosyn
Comvax	Recombivax HB
Cozaar	Zocor
dactinomycin	daptomycin
Darvon	Diovan
daunorubicin	idarubicin
Denavir	Indinavir
Depakote	Depakote ER
Depo-Medrol	Solu-Medrol
Diabinese	Diamox
DiaBeta	Zebeta
Dilacor XR	Pilocar
Dioval	Diovan
Diovan	Zyban
Diprivan	Ditropan
dobutamine	dopamine
doxorubicin hydrochloride	liposomal doxorubicin (DOXIL)
Duricef	Ultracet

TABLE 7.3 *Continued*

Enbrel	Levbid
Endocet	Indocid
Engerix-B adult	Engerix-B pediatric/adolescent
ephedrine	epinephrine
Estratest	Estratest H.S.
ethambutol	Ethmozine
Femara	Femhrt
fentanyl	sufentanil
folic acid	folinic acid (leucovorin calcium)
Foradil	Toradol
gentamicin	gentian violet
Granulex	Regranex
Healon	Hyalgan
heparin	Hespan
Humalog	Humulin
Humalog Mix 75/25	Humulin 70/30
hydromorphone	morphine
infliximab	rituximab
iodine	Lodine
Isordil	Plendil
isotretinoin	tretinoin
K-Phos Neutral	Neutra-Phos-K
Kaletra	Keppra
Ketalar	ketorolac
Lamisil	Lamictal
lamivudine	lamotrigine
Lanoxin	levothyroxine
Lantus	Lente
Lasix	Luvox
leucovorin calcium	Leukeran
Lexapro	Loxitane
Lotronex	Protonix
Lupron Depot-3 Month	Lupron Depot-Ped
Maxzide	Microzide
Metadate ER	methadone
methadone	Metadate
Micronase	Microzide
mifepristone	misoprostol
MiraLax	Mirapex
morphine, oral liquid concentrate	morphine, nonconcentrated oral liquid
MS Contin	OxyContin
Mucinex	Mucomyst
Narcan	Norcuron
Navane	Norvasc
Neulasta	Neumega
Neumega	Neupogen
Neurontin	Noroxin
Neutra-Phos-K	K-Phos Neutral
Novolin 70/30	NovoLog Mix 70/30
Occlusal-HP	Ocuflox
oxycodone	OxyContin
Pamelor	Panlor DC
Patanol	Platinol
Paxil	Taxol

TABLE 7.3 *Continued*

Paxil	Plavix
Percocet	Procet
Pilocar	Dilacor XR
pneumococcal 7-valent vaccine	pneumococcal polyvalent vaccine
Precare	Precose
Prilosec	Prozac
probenecid	Procanbid
Procardia XL	Protain XL
propylthiouracil	Purinethol
protamine	Protonix
quinine	quinidine
Reminyl	Robinul
Retrovir	ritonavir
Rifater	Rifidin
Ritalin	ritodrine
Ritalin LA	Ritalin SR
Roxanol	Roxicodone Intensol
Roxanol	Roxicet
saquinavir (free base)	saquinavir mesylate
saquinavir	Sinequan
Sarafem	Serophene
Seroquel	Serzone
sertraline	Soriatane
sumatriptan	zolmitriptan
Taxol	Taxotere
Tegretol	Tequin
Tequin	Ticlid
Testoderm	Testoderm w/ Adhesive
tiagabine	tizanidine
Tiazac	Ziac
TNKase	t-PA
TobraDex	Tobrex
Topamax	Toprol XL
Tracleer	TriCor
tramadol hydrochloride	trazodone hydrochloride
Tylenol	Tylenol PM
valacyclovir	valganciclovir
Valcyte	Valtrex
Varivax	VZIG
Vexol	Vosol
vinblastine	vincristine
Viracept	Viramune
Xeloda	Xenical
Zantac	Zyrtec
Zebeta	Zetia
Zestril	Zetia
Zostrix	Zovirax
Zovirax	Zyvox
Zyprexa	Celexa
Zyrtec	Zyprexa

Note: Modified from *ISMP Medication Safety Alert! Acute Care Edition,* January 1996–September 2004, © 2005, by Institute for Safe Medication Practices. This material is used with permission of ISMP.

trade names on the prescription so that the correct drug may be better identified. When picking up drugs at a pharmacy, patients should be encouraged to counsel with their pharmacist about the drug and to read the literature supplied by the pharmacy to be sure that the drug and its indications apply to their condition.

The Joint Commission on Accreditation of Healthcare Organizations (JCAHO) identifies and reviews look-alike and soundalike drugs as part of its national patient safety goals. For these drugs, JCAHO recommends specific safety strategies for reducing potential medication errors and their consequences. In addition, the Institute for Safe Medication Practices (ISMP) is a nonprofit agency devoted to promoting medication safety and reducing medication errors. The ISMP maintains an error-reporting program and provides newsletters and educational programs for health care professionals.

Drugs that have a narrow therapeutic index are more likely to cause serious consequences should a medication error occur. These drugs are not necessarily more "error-prone" than others but the nurse should give extra care when administering them due to their toxicity. Agencies may build additional safeguards with these medications such as independent double-checks or automated alerts. Listing of high-alert medications depends on the unit. For example, high-alert drugs on cancer units or a pediatric unit will differ from those on a medical–surgical unit. A selected list of high-alert drugs is shown in Table 7.4.

PharmFACT

A study of hospitalized pediatric patients found that 5.7% of their prescriptions contained medication errors and that 1.1% of the patients had potential adverse drug events. The potential adverse drug event rate was three times higher than in hospitalized adult patients. *Source:* Kaushal et al., 2001.

TABLE 7.4 Selected High-Alert Medications

Class	Drug Examples
Antibiotics	vancomycin, cefazolin
Anticoagulants	warfarin, heparin
Antineoplastics	Most drugs in this class
Cardiovascular agents (when given parenterally)	amiodarone, lidocaine, nitroprusside, digoxin, milrinone, epinephrine, propranolol
Electrolytes and fluid expanders	potassium chloride (IV concentrate), sodium chloride (hypertonic, more than 0.9%), dextrose (20% or greater)
General anesthetics	Most drugs in this class
Hypoglycemics	All insulins
Neuromuscular blockers	succinylcholine
Opiates	morphine and others
Sedatives (when given IV or for children)	chloral hydrate, midazolam

Note: From *ISMP's List of High-Alert Medications,* The Institute of Safe Medication Practices, 2008. Retrieved August 12, 2008, from http://www.ismp.org/Tools/highalertmedications.pdf. Adapted with permission.

Reporting Medication Errors

7.4 Medication errors must be properly documented and reported.

Although some medication errors go unreported, it is always the nurse's legal and ethical responsibility to document all occurrences. In severe cases, adverse reactions caused by medication errors may require the initiation of lifesaving interventions for the patient, including available antidotes. After such an incident, the patient may require close supervision, and additional medical treatments may be warranted.

The FDA has coordinated the reporting of medication errors at the federal level. The FDA Safety Information and Adverse Event Reporting Program, known as MedWatch, provides important and timely clinical information about safety issues involving medical products, including prescription and OTC drugs, biologics, medical- and radiation-emitting devices, and special nutritional products. The FDA encourages nurses and other health care providers to report medication errors for its database, which is used to assist other professionals in avoiding similar mistakes. Medication errors, or situations that can lead to errors, may be reported anonymously directly to the FDA by telephone or online. Since 1992, the FDA has received over 30,000 reports of medication errors. The number of actual errors is likely much higher.

The ISMP, a nonprofit agency comprised of 23 national health care organizations, was founded in 1994 to help standardize medication error reporting systems, examine interdisciplinary causes of medication errors, and promote medication safety. In conjunction with the *United States Pharmacopeia* (USP), the ISMP operates the voluntary Medication Error Reporting Program (MERP), which accepts reports from consumers and health care professionals related to medication safety. Medication errors from the MERP voluntary reporting system are shared with the FDA. The MERP has resulted in dozens of medication-related patient safety changes, including nationwide hazard alerts; packaging, labeling, and nomenclature changes; and health care system changes. The ISMP also publishes *Medication Safety Alert*, newsletters for health professionals, and *Safe Medicine*, a consumer newsletter about medication errors.

The USP also offers MEDMARX, a national, Internet-accessible database that hospitals and health care systems use to track adverse drug events and medication errors. Agencies participate in MEDMARX voluntarily and subscribe to it on an annual basis. MEDMARX is operated as a quality improvement tool, which facilitates productive and efficient documentation, reporting, analysis, tracking, trending, and prevention of adverse drug events.

All medical facilities have policies and procedures that provide guidance to the nurse on reporting medication errors. Documentation of the error should occur in a factual manner and must include specific nursing interventions that were implemented following the error to protect patient safety, such as monitoring vital signs and assessing the patient for possible complications. Documentation does not simply record that a medical error occurred. Failure to document nursing actions could be interpreted as either negligence or failure to acknowledge that the incident occurred. The nurse should also record the names of all individuals who were notified of the error. The **medication administration record (MAR)** is another source that should contain information about what medication was given or omitted.

In addition to documenting in the patient's medical record, the nurse who made or observed the medication error should complete a written incident report. The incident report allows the nurse an opportunity to identify factors that contributed to the medication error. The incident report, however, is not always included in the patient's medical record.

Accurate documentation in the medical record and on the incident report is essential for legal reasons. These documents verify that the patient's safety was protected and serve as a tool to improve medication administration processes. Legal issues may worsen if there is an attempt to hide a mistake or delay corrective action, or if the nurse forgets to document interventions in the patient's chart.

CONNECTION *Checkpoint* 7.2

Other important functions of the *United States Pharmacopeia* (USP) are presented in Chapter 2. What is the role of the USP in drug regulation? See Answer to Connection Checkpoint 7.2 in Appendix A.

Strategies for Reducing Medication Errors

7.5 Nurses use multiple strategies for reducing medication errors.

What can the nurse do in the clinical setting to avoid medication errors and promote safe drug administration? The nurse can begin by adhering to the four steps of the nursing process:

1. Assessment: Ask the patient about food or medication allergies, current health concerns, and use of OTC medications and herbal supplements. Ensure that the patient is receiving the right drug at the right dose, at the right time, and by the right route. Assess renal and hepatic functions, and determine if other body systems are impaired and could affect pharmacotherapy. Identify areas of needed patient education with regard to medications.

2. Planning: Minimize factors that contribute to medication errors: Avoid using abbreviations that could be misunderstood, question unclear orders, do not accept verbal orders, and follow specific facility polices and procedures related to medication administration. Have the patient restate dosing directions, including the correct dose of medication and the right time to take it. Ask the patient to demonstrate an understanding of the goals of pharmacotherapy.

3. Implementation: Be aware that stressful situations and distractions during medication administration increase the risk for a medication error. When engaged in a medication-related task, focus entirely on the task. Noise, other events, and talking coworkers can distract the nurse's attention and result in a medication error. Keep the following points in mind as well:

   - Positively verify the identity of each patient before administering the medication, according to facility policy and procedures.
   - Use the correct procedures and techniques for all routes of administration. Use sterile materials and techniques when administering parenteral medications.
   - Calculate medication doses correctly and measure liquid drugs carefully. Some medications, such as heparin, have a narrow safety margin for producing serious adverse effects. When giving these medications, ask a colleague or a pharmacist to check the calculations to make certain the dosage is correct. Always double-check pediatric calculations prior to administration.
   - Open medication packages or bottles immediately prior to administering the drug and in the presence of the patient.
   - Record the medication and all dosing information on the MAR immediately after administration.
   - Always confirm that the patient has swallowed an oral medication. Do not leave the medication at the bedside unless there is a specific order that it may be left there.
   - Be alert for long-acting oral dosage forms with indicators such as SR, LA, XL, and XR. These tablets or capsules usually must remain intact for the extended release feature to remain effective. Instruct the patient not to crush, chew, or break the medication in half, because doing so could cause an overdose.

4. Evaluation: Assess the patient for expected outcomes and determine if any adverse effects have occurred. The nurse should be especially vigilant in observing for adverse effects if this is the first time the patient has ever taken the drug, or if the dosage is being increased. Because antibiotics have the highest rate of drug allergy, the nurse must be especially observant for signs and symptoms of allergy following administration of these agents.

Nurses must be zealous in keeping up to date on pharmacotherapeutics and should never administer a medication unless they are familiar with its uses and adverse effects. There are many venues by which nurses can obtain updated medication knowledge. Each nursing unit should have current drug references available. Nurses can also call the pharmacy to obtain information about the drug or, if available, look it up on the Internet using reliable sources. Many nurses are now relying on personal digital assistants (PDAs) to provide current information. These devices can be updated daily or weekly by downloading information so that the information is current. A word of caution is necessary: Drug references can sometimes give incorrect information. Nurses must rely on common sense and good judgment. If a dose appears to be inaccurate in a reference source, nurses should always check with the prescriber or pharmacist before administering. Nurses have a duty to contact the publisher of the inaccurate data, so that future medication errors may be prevented.

7.6 Medication reconciliation is an important means of reducing medication errors.

Many older adults have several chronic medical disorders concurrently, each of which may be treated by individual specialists. It is common for patients to receive multiple prescriptions, sometimes for the same condition, that have conflicting pharmacologic actions, a condition termed **polypharmacy.** Although not unique to older patients, polypharmacy is most often seen in this age group. Keeping track of multiple medications, their doses, indications, routes, and frequency of administration is a major challenge for both patients and health care providers. Failure to properly record medication information, and to communicate that information to health care providers, is a potential cause of medication errors.

Medication reconciliation is a process of "keeping track" of a patient's medications as their care proceeds from one health care provider to another. Reconciliation accurately lists all medications a patient is taking in an attempt to reduce duplication, omissions, dosing errors, or drug interactions. For example, when a patient is admitted to care, the nurse records all medications that the patient has been taking at home, including their dose, route, and frequency. This list is checked against admission orders and is transferred to other practitioners whenever the patient is moved to different units within the hospital. It is also checked at discharge. These "interfaces of care" are the most likely places that medication reconciliation errors have been found to occur.

In 2004, JCAHO identified hundreds of serious medication errors attributed to medication reconciliation and developed recommendations for their prevention. In 2006, JCAHO recommendations included the following:

- Implementing a process for obtaining and documenting a complete list of the patient's current medications on the patient's admission. This process includes a comparison of the medications the organization provides to those on the list. Medications should include prescription medications, OTC medications, vitamins, and herbal products.
- Communicating a complete list of the patient's medications to the next provider of service when a patient is referred or transferred to another setting, service, practitioner, or level of care within or outside the organization.
- On discharge from the facility, providing the patient with the complete list of medications to be taken as well as instructions on how to take any newly prescribed medications.

7.7 Proper patient education is essential for safe medication usage.

In the hospital setting, the physician, nurse, and pharmacist are largely responsible for preventing medication errors. In the home setting, this responsibility relies on proper patient adherence to drug therapy. An essential strategy for avoiding medication errors in the home setting is to educate the patient by providing written handouts or audiovisual teaching aids about the medication and contact information about whom to notify in the event of an adverse reaction. All teaching materials must be age appropriate and in a language the patient can understand.

To minimize the potential for medication errors, the nurse should teach patients or their home caregivers the following:

- Know the names of all medications they are taking, the uses, the doses, and when and how they should be taken.
- Know which side or adverse effects need to be immediately reported.
- Read the label prior to each drug administration and use the medication device that comes with liquid medications rather than household measuring spoons.
- Carry a list of all medications, including OTC drugs and herbal and dietary supplements that are being taken. If possible, use one pharmacy for all prescriptions.
- Ask questions about drug safety. Health care providers should be enlisted as partners in maintaining safe medication principles.
- Consult with the pharmacist about any medications that look unfamiliar or that have changed color or shape since the last prescription.

PharmFACT

About 50% of the 2 billion prescriptions filled each year are not taken correctly. One third of patients take only some of their medication and one third never fill their prescription. *Source:* Patient Compliance and Medication Adherence Statistics and References: Prescriptions, n.d.

7.8 Health care agencies are actively involved in reducing medication errors.

There is a trend for health care agencies to use automated, computerized, locked cabinets for medication storage on patient care units. Each nurse on the unit has a code for accessing the cabinet and removing a medication dose. These automated systems also maintain an inventory of drug supplies.

Larger health care agencies often have **risk management** departments to examine risks and minimize the number of medication errors. Risk management personnel investigate incidents, track data, identify problems, and provide recommendations for improvement. Nurses collaborate with the risk management committees to seek means of reducing medication errors by modifying policies and procedures within the institution. Examples of institutional policies and procedures include:

- Storing medications under proper conditions (light and temperature control) and separating medications that have look-alike names or packaging
- Reading the drug label to avoid the administration of time-expired medications
- Avoiding the transfer of doses from one container to another
- Avoiding overstocking of medications
- Monitoring adherence with prohibited prescription abbreviations
- Removing outdated reference books

UNDERSTANDING THE CHAPTER

Key Concepts Summary

7.1 Medication errors are preventable events that may significantly impact treatment outcomes.

7.2 Medication errors may be caused by human factors, inadequate communication, or confusing labels, packaging, or drug names.

7.3 Certain drugs have higher rates of medication errors.

7.4 Medication errors must be properly documented and reported.

7.5 Nurses use multiple strategies for reducing medication errors.

7.6 Medication reconciliation is an important means of reducing medication errors.

7.7 Proper patient education is essential for safe medication usage.

7.8 Health care agencies are actively involved in reducing medication errors.

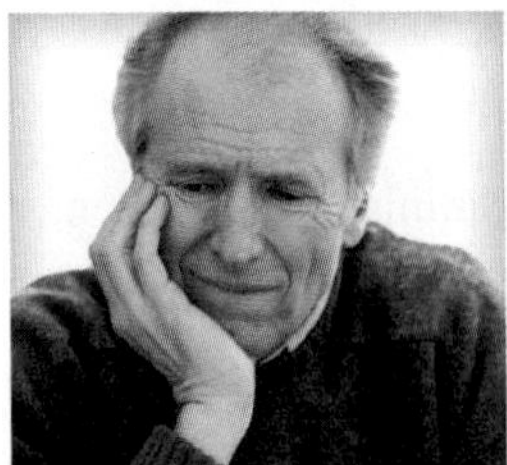

Making the PATIENT *Connection*

Remember the patient "Ross Holland" at the beginning of the chapter? Now read the remainder of the case study. Based on the information presented within this chapter, respond to the critical thinking questions that follow.

What happened to Ross Holland was truly a tragedy. He entered the hospital for simple sinus surgery and never recovered. Ironically, Ross was a super vigilant man. As a Vietnam veteran, he had seen the worst of combat for 4 years. During the last 6 months of the conflict, he survived in a prisoner of war camp. When he returned home, he took a job as a safety inspector in the automobile industry.

From a previous physical exam, Ross knew that he had a slightly irregular heartbeat, but he never really took it seriously. In fact, he never mentioned it when the nurse was admitting him to the hospital. However, the condition became a problem soon after surgery. The nurse caring for him noticed a series of cardiac irregularities on the monitor and contacted the physician. The physician ordered Ross to receive a cardiac medicine stat to correct the problem. In haste, the nurse never clarified the route that the medication was to be given. Additionally, the nurse was not familiar with the medication's usual dose or any precautions that needed to be taken. As a result, the medication was given by direct intravenous administration without being diluted as directed on the medication bottle. Ross was given 100 times the normal dose. Consequently, he experienced seizure activity that lasted 5 minutes followed by respiratory arrest. All efforts to resuscitate him were unsuccessful.

Critical Thinking Questions

1. Ultimately, who was responsible for this medication error? Ross? The physician? The nurse? Why?
2. Identify the contributing factors that resulted in the error.
3. What strategies should a nurse use to prevent medication errors?
4. What policy could health care facilities implement to avoid medication errors?

Case Study

You are the health nurse in an elementary school. One day, a student's mother tells you, "Medications frighten me. Both my children have asthma and frequently require medications. When I give any of my children medications, I worry that I will make an error. There is so much that can go wrong."

1. How would you respond to this mother's concern?
2. Create a list of strategies that parents can use to prevent medication errors.
3. What referral resources could help reduce her anxiety?

NCLEX-RN® Review

1 It is 2:45 a.m. and the nurse has telephoned the prescriber to report an acute episode of postoperative pain. How can the nurse avoid medication errors when receiving a telephone order from a prescriber?

1. Decline to accept the telephone order.
2. Refuse to call the prescriber but attempt to comfort the client.
3. Instruct the client's family to call the prescriber.
4. Repeat the order verbally to ensure accuracy.

2 The nurse cannot read the number of milligrams (mg) to be administered in a drug order written by the health care provider. It is questionable whether 125 mg, 1.25 mg, or 12.5 mg should be administered. What action would be most appropriate to prevent a medication error?

1. Telephone the health care provider about the illegible medication order.
2. Ask another nurse to read the questionable medication order.
3. Contact the pharmacist about the medication order.
4. Consult a drug handbook and administer the normal dose.

3 The nurse is counseling the client on the medication taken daily. Which of the following is a strategy that the nurse should include in this teaching session that might prevent a medication error? Instruct the client to:

1. Insist on brand-name drugs rather than generic drugs.
2. Have all prescriptions filled at one pharmacy.
3. Request all prescriptions be placed in easily opened containers.
4. Consult the Internet about possible adverse effects.

4 When given a medication, the client tells the nurse, "I've never seen this pill before. It's not like the others I take." The most appropriate action taken by the nurse would be to:

1. Instruct the client that different brands are frequently used.
2. Administer the medication in the existing form.
3. Verify the order and double-check the drug label.
4. Advise the client to talk with the health care provider and give the drug.

5 While administering medication to several clients, the nurse suddenly realizes that the wrong medication has been given to a client. Which of the following would be the first priority action taken by the nurse?

1. Assess the client and monitor for adverse effects.
2. Call the health care provider and report the error.
3. Complete the hospital's drug error form.
4. Report the medication error to MedWatch.

6 As the nurse enters the room to administer medication, the client states, "I'm in the bathroom. Please leave the medication on my bedside table, and I will take it when I come out." Which of the following would be the appropriate response by the nurse?

1. "I will leave the medication and follow up with you in 30 minutes."
2. "You must take the medication now or refuse the dose."
3. "Let me know when you are ready, and I will then return with your medicine."
4. "I've given the drug to your visitors. Take it when you come out of the bathroom."

See Answers to Critical Thinking Questions, Case Study, and NCLEX-RN® Review in Appendix A.

References

Committee on Drugs and Committee on Hospital Care. (2003). Prevention of medication errors in the pediatric inpatient setting. *Pediatrics, 112,* 431–436.

Ellenbecker, C., Frazier, S., & Verney, S. (2003). Nurses' observations and experiences of problems and adverse effects of medication management in home care. *Geriatric Nursing, 25*(3), 164–170.

Force, M. V., Derring, L., Hubbe, J., Andersen, M., Hagemann, B., Cooper-Hahn, M., et al. (2006). Effective strategies to increase reporting of medication errors in hospitals. *Journal of Nursing Administration, 36*(1) 34–41.

Fortescue, E. B., Kaushal, R., Landrigan, C. P., McKenna, K. J., Clapp, M. D., Federico, F., et al. (2003). Prioritizing strategies for preventing medication errors and adverse drug events in pediatric inpatients. *Pediatrics, 111*(4), 722–729.

Goldman, E. (2006, May 1). PDA-based drug dose calculator slashes NICU med errors. *Family Practice News,* 55.

Hoffman, J. M., & Proulx, S. M. (2003). Medication errors caused by confusion of drug names. *Drug Safety, 26*(7), 445–452.

Institute for Safe Medication Practices. (2005). *ISMP medication safety alert! Acute care edition, January 1996–September 2004.* Author.

Joanna Briggs Institute. (2006). Strategies to reduce medication errors with reference to older adults. *Nursing Standard, 20,* 53–57.

Kane-Gill, S., & Weber, R .J. (2006). Principles and practices of medication safety in the ICU. *Critical Care Clinics, 22,* 273–290.

Kaushal, R., Bates, D. W., Landrigan, C., McKenna, K. J., Clapp, M. D., Federico, F., et al. (2001). Medication errors and adverse drug events in pediatric inpatients. *Journal of the American Medical Association, 285,* 2114–2120.

Koczmara, C., Jelincic, V., & Perri, D. (2006). Communication of medication orders by telephone—"writing it right." *Dynamics, 17,* 20–24.

National Coordinating Council for Medication Error and Reporting (NCC MERP). (2005, June 2). *Recommendations to enhance accuracy in prescription writing* (Adopted September 4, 1996). Retrieved July 18, 2006, from http://www.nccmerp.org/council/council1996-09-04.html

Page, K., & McKinney, A. (2007, July 11). Addressing medication errors: The role of undergraduate nurse education. *Nurse Education Today, 27*(3), 219–224.

Patient compliance and medication adherence statistics and references: Prescriptions. (n.d.). Retrieved March 29, 2008, from http://www.epill.com/statistics.html

Phillips, J., Beam, S., Brinker, A., Holquist, C., Honig, P., Lee, L. Y., et al. (2001). Retrospective analysis of mortalities associated with medication errors. *American Journal of Health-System Pharmacy 58*(19), 1835–1841.

Preston, R. M. (2004). Drug errors and patient safety: The need for a change in practice. *British Journal of Nursing, 13*(2), 72–78.

Santell, J. P., Hicks, R. W., McMeekin, J., & Cousins, D. D. (2003). Medication errors: Experience of the *United States Pharmacopeia* (USP) MEDMARX reporting system. *Journal of Clinical Pharmacology, 43*(7), 760–767.

Shuttleworth, A. (2006). How to keep up to date with practice. *Nursing Times, 102,* 54–55.

The Joint Commission. (2006). Addendum to *Sentinal Event Alert, 35.* Using medication reconciliation to prevent errors. Retrieved December 29, 2008, from http://www.jointcommission.org/SentinelEvents/SentinelEventAlert/sea_35.htm

The National Academies. (2006, July 20). *Report offers comprehensive strategies for reducing drug-related mistakes.* Retrieved March 30, 2008, from http:// www8.nationalacademies.org/onpinews/newsitem.aspx?RecordID=11623

Thomas, M., Holquist, C., & Phillips, J. (2001, October 10). *Med error reports to FDA show a mixed bag.* FDA Safety Page. Retrieved April 20, 2008, from http://www.fda.gov/cder/drug/MedErrors/mixed.pdf

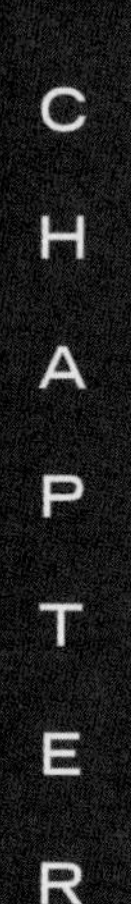

I have been getting high since I was 14 years old. Do I need to stop just because I am pregnant?

Patient "J. C. Wilkins"

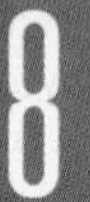

Pharmacology of Substance Abuse

Learning Outcomes

After reading this chapter, the student should be able to:

1. Describe the types of substances abused by individuals.
2. Identify the five drug schedules of controlled substances and give examples of drugs at each level.
3. Explain major legislation regulating controlled substances in the United States.
4. Identify factors contributing to addiction.
5. Compare and contrast psychological and physical dependence.
6. Compare and contrast withdrawal syndromes for the different classes of abused substances.
7. Discuss the significance of drug tolerance to pharmacology.
8. Explain the major characteristics of abuse, dependence, and tolerance resulting from the following substances: sedatives, opioids, alcohol, marijuana, hallucinogens, club drugs, amphetamines, methylphenidate, cocaine, caffeine, nicotine, inhalants, and anabolic steroids.
9. Identify the role of the nurse in recognizing, preventing, and treating substance abuse.

Chapter Outline

Fundamental Concepts of Substance Abuse

Legislation of Controlled Substances

Addiction and Dependence

Tolerance

Central Nervous System Depressants

Sedatives and Related Agents

Barbiturate and Nonbarbiturate Sedative–Hypnotics

Benzodiazepines

Opioids

Alcohol (Ethanol)

Cannabinoids—Marijuana

Hallucinogens

LSD and Similar Hallucinogens

Club Drugs and Miscellaneous Hallucinogens

Central Nervous System Stimulants

Amphetamines and Methylphenidate

Cocaine

Caffeine

Nicotine

Inhalants

Anabolic Steroids

Key Terms

addiction, 94
anterograde amnesia, 98
attention deficit/hyperactivity disorder (ADHD), 106
club drug, 105
controlled substances, 94
cross-tolerance, 97
delirium tremens, 102
hallucinogens, 103
opioids, 98
physical dependence, 96
psychological dependence, 95
rebound effects, 96
reticular formation, 106
scheduled drugs, 94
sedatives, 98
substance abuse, 93
tachyphylaxis, 97
tetrahydrocannabinol (THC), 102
tolerance, 97
withdrawal syndrome, 96

Substance abuse is the self-administration of a drug in a manner that does not conform to the norms within the person's given culture or society. The term *substance abuse* is preferred over the term *drug abuse*, because some of these agents are not considered to be drugs by the users. A more expanded definition of substance abuse is given in Table 8.1.

Throughout history individuals have consumed both natural substances and therapeutic drugs to increase performance, to assist with relaxation, to induce spiritual visions, or to simply fit in with the crowd. Substance abuse has a tremendous economic, social, and public health impact on society. The purpose of this chapter is to introduce the scope of the substance abuse problem and the individual drugs that may be abused by patients.

Fundamental Concepts of Substance Abuse

8.1 A wide variety of different substances may be abused by patients.

At first thought, substance abuse appears to be a societal or behavioral problem rather than a topic to be included in a pharmacology text. Nurses, however, play key roles in multiple aspects of substance abuse. During assessment, nurses may be the first members of the health care team to recognize symptoms and signs of substance abuse. In their role as educators, nurses distribute important information on substance abuse prevention and the proper use of prescription drugs. Some are involved in the pharmacotherapy of overdose or detoxification. Patients often turn to nurses to obtain the medical assistance needed to overcome their addiction or for referral advice to human service agencies that can help resolve personal or family issues related to the substance abuse.

Abused substances belong to a large number of diverse chemical classes. Although they have few structural similarities, most have in common an ability to affect the brain. Many of these drugs produce euphoria by enhancing the secretion of dopamine in the "pleasure center" of the brain called the nucleus acumens. The exception is the anabolic steroids, which are used for their effects on the muscular system rather than the nervous system.

Although the public associates substance abuse with illegal drugs, this is not necessarily the case. Alcohol and nicotine are the two most commonly abused drugs and both are legal for adults. In addition, legal prescription drugs such as oxycodone (OxyContin), methamphetamine, and alprazolam (Xanax) have become frequent drugs of abuse. Marijuana is the most frequently abused illegal drug. Other illegal substances that are frequently abused include hallucinogens such as lysergic acid diethylamide (LSD) and club drugs such as ecstasy.

Several drugs that were once used therapeutically are now illegal due to their high potential for

TABLE 8.1 *DSM-IV-TR* Criteria for Substance Dependence

Definition: A maladaptive pattern of substance use, leading to clinically significant impairment or distress, as manifested by three (or more) of the following, occurring at any time in the same 12-month period:
1. tolerance, as defined by either of the following: (a) a need for markedly increased amounts of the substance to achieve intoxication or desired effect (b) markedly diminished effect with continued use of the same amount of the substance
2. withdrawal, as manifested by either of the following: (a) the characteristic withdrawal syndrome for the substance (b) the same (or a closely related) substance is taken to relieve or avoid withdrawal symptoms
3. the substance is often taken in larger amounts or over a longer period than was intended
4. there is a persistent desire or unsuccessful efforts to cut down or control substance use
5. a great deal of time is spent in activities necessary to obtain the substance (e.g., visiting multiple doctors or driving long distances), use the substance (e.g., chain-smoking), or recover from its effects
6. important social, occupational, or recreational activities are given up or reduced because of substance use
7. the substance use is continued despite knowledge of having a persistent or recurrent physical or psychological problem that is likely to have been caused or exacerbated by the substance (e.g., current cocaine use despite recognition of cocaine-induced depression, or continued drinking despite recognition that an ulcer was made worse by alcohol consumption)
The diagnosis should specify "With Physiological Dependence" (either item 1 or 2 is present) or "Without Physiological Dependence" (neither item 1 nor 2 is present).

Note: From *Diagnostic and Statistical Manual of Mental Disorders*, Text Revision, 2000, American Psychiatric Association, Washington, DC.

abuse. Cocaine was once used as a local anesthetic, but today nearly all the cocaine acquired by users is obtained illegally from South America. LSD is now illegal although it was briefly used in psychotherapy in the 1940s and 1950s. Phencyclidine was popular back in the early 1960s as an anesthetic but was withdrawn from the market in 1965 due to patients reporting serious adverse effects while recovering from anesthesia. Many amphetamines once used for bronchodilation were discontinued in the 1980s after psychotic episodes were reported.

PharmFACT

Since the peak years of drug abuse in the mid-1990s, there have been significant decreases in illicit drug use among teens. Based on 2006 data, past year use has fallen by 37% among 8th graders since the peak year in 1996. The peak year for past year use among 10th and 12th graders was 1997; since then, past year use has fallen by 25% among 10th graders and by 14% among 12th graders. Combining all three grades, past month abuse for any illicit drug has dropped by 23% since 2001. *Source:* National Institute of Drug Abuse, 2007.

Legislation of Controlled Substances

8.2 Drugs with a potential for abuse are restricted by the Controlled Substances Act and are categorized into schedules.

It is not surprising that drugs with abuse potential are regulated. Many of these substances can cause significant harm to the user and those surrounding the user when memory or performance become impaired. A significant percentage of motor vehicle and other accidents result from substance abuse. The government clearly has a role in protecting individuals and the public from such dangerous drugs.

A major source of certain abused substances is diversion from legal medical use. Because of this, legislation has been enacted to closely track potential drugs of abuse from manufacturer to consumer. Prescription drugs may be stolen from pharmacies, physician offices, or patients, and sold illegally, sometimes at a very high profit. In some cases, health care workers who have the responsibility of dispensing or administering the medications conduct the theft.

Patients are also responsible for much of the diversion. For example, patients sometimes fake or exaggerate their symptoms to obtain prescriptions for pain medication or sedatives. Some patients obtain the same prescription from several health care providers, commonly referred to as "doctor shopping," and sell their pills to substance abusers. Because there are multiple levels where legal drugs may be diverted to the drug abuse culture, the tracking of drugs with abuse potential is closely monitored.

Some substances have such a high potential for abuse that they are not approved as therapeutic drugs by the United States Food and Drug Administration (FDA). Others have a strong potential for abuse but have therapeutic applications important enough to approve them as medications under conditions that restrict their use to situations of medical necessity.

In the United States, a **controlled substance** is defined as a drug whose use is restricted by the Comprehensive Drug Abuse Prevention and Control Act of 1970 and later revisions. Title II of this law, known as the Controlled Substances Act (CSA), is the legal basis for regulating drugs of abuse. The CSA created five categories or schedules for drugs of abuse. These **scheduled drugs** are classified according to their potential for abuse and toxicity. Schedule I drugs have the highest potential for abuse and have limited or no therapeutic value. Drugs in the other four schedules may be dispensed, but only in cases where therapeutic value has been clearly established. Schedule V is the only category wherein some drugs may be dispensed without a prescription. This is because the quantities of the controlled drug are so low that the possibility of causing dependence is extremely remote. Table 8.2 shows the five drug schedules with examples. Not all drugs with an abuse potential are regulated or placed into schedules. Tobacco, beer, wine, spirits, and caffeine are specifically exempt from regulation by the CSA.

The CSA created many other restrictive conditions for the possession, manufacture, sale, and distribution of controlled substances. Hospitals and pharmacies must register with the Drug Enforcement Administration (DEA) and use their registration numbers to purchase scheduled drugs. They must maintain complete records of all quantities purchased and sold. Drugs with higher abuse potential have additional restrictions. For example, practitioners must use a special order form to obtain Schedule II drugs, and orders must be written and signed by the practitioner. Telephone orders to a pharmacy are not permitted. Automatic refills for Schedule II drugs are not permitted; patients must visit their health care provider first. Those convicted of unlawful manufacturing, distributing, and dispensing of controlled substances face severe penalties.

CONNECTION *Checkpoint* 8.1

Prior to the CSA, other attempts were made to legislate narcotics. From what you learned in Chapter 2, name the first major law in the United States that was passed in 1914 to control narcotic use and explain its major provisions. See Answer to Connection Checkpoint 8.1 in Appendix A.

Addiction and Dependence

8.3 Addiction is an overwhelming compulsion to continue repeated drug use.

Addiction is an overwhelming compulsion that drives someone to repeat drug-taking behavior, despite serious health and social consequences. Why would someone continue to abuse drugs even when he or she is aware of its compelling negative consequences? The drug experience is highly personal for each user, and it is difficult to generalize reasons for continued substance abuse. It may be summarized that the drug experience brings some degree of pleasure or satisfaction to the user. Whether it be euphoria, sedation, hallucinations, or feelings of well-being or excitement, the substance abuser finds the drug experience reinforcing and worth repeating.

TABLE 8.2 U.S. Drug Schedules and Examples

Drug Schedule	Abuse Potential	Physical Dependence	Psychological Dependence	Examples	Therapeutic Use
I	Highest	High	High	Heroin, LSD, GHB, marijuana, MDMA, psilocybin, peyote, mescaline, and methaqualone	Limited or no therapeutic use in the United States; no prescriptions may be written
II	High	High	High	Potent opioids (morphine, oxycodone, meperidine, fentanyl), phencyclidine (PCP), cocaine, methadone, methamphetamine, methylphenidate, short-acting barbiturates	Used therapeutically with prescription; some drugs are no longer used; no refills, but a few exceptions
III	Moderate	Moderate	High	Anabolic steroids, ketamine, codeine, and hydrocodone when compounded with aspirin or acetaminophen (Vicodin, Tylenol 3), buprenorphine and intermediate-acting barbiturates	Used therapeutically with prescription; five refills allowed in a 6-month period
IV	Lower	Lower	Lower	Dextropropoxyphene, pentazocine, meprobamate, benzodiazepines (alprazolam, diazepam, flunitrazepam), zolpidem, long-acting barbiturates	Used therapeutically with prescription; five refills allowed in a 6-month period
V	Lowest	Lowest	Lowest	Over-the-counter (OTC) cough medicines with codeine, antidiarrheal medicines with small amounts of opioids	Some are used therapeutically without prescription

Addiction depends on multiple, complex, and interacting variables. These variables focus on the following categories:

- **Agent or drug factors.** Cost, availability, dose, mode of administration (e.g., oral, intravenous [IV], inhalation), speed of onset, duration of drug action, and length of drug use
- **User factors.** Genetic factors (e.g., metabolic enzymes, innate tolerance), risk-taking behavior, prior experiences with drugs, pathologic state (such as severe pain) that may indicate a drug with abuse potential
- **Environmental factors.** Social and community norms, role models, peer influences, educational opportunities

In the case of legal prescription drugs, addiction may begin with a legitimate need for pharmacotherapy. For example, narcotic analgesics may be indicated for pain relief or sedatives for a sleep disorder. These drugs may result in a favorable experience, such as pain relief or sleep, and patients will want to repeat these positive experiences. If pharmacotherapy is not carefully monitored, patients may take these drugs at high doses for prolonged periods, thus increasing the risk of addiction.

It is a common misunderstanding, even among some health professionals, that the therapeutic use of scheduled drugs creates large numbers of patients with addiction. In fact, prescription drugs rarely cause addiction when used according to accepted medical protocols. The risk of addiction for prescription medications is primarily a function of the dose and the length of therapy. Because of this, medications having a potential for abuse are prescribed at the lowest effective dose and for the shortest time necessary to treat the medical problem. Nurses should administer these medications as prescribed for the relief of patient symptoms without undue fear of producing dependency.

PharmFACT

In 2006, an estimated 20.4 million Americans aged 12 or older were current (past month) illicit drug users. This estimate represents 8.3% of the population aged 12 years old or older. *Source:* Substance Abuse and Mental Health Services Administration, 2007.

8.4 Physical and psychological dependence lead to continued drug-seeking behavior despite negative health and social consequences.

Whether or not a drug is addictive is related to how easily an individual can stop taking the substance on a repetitive basis. Substance dependence occurs when a person has an overwhelming craving to take a drug and cannot stop. Substance dependence is classified by two distinct categories: physical dependence and psychological dependence.

Physical dependence occurs when the body adapts to repeated use of the substance by altering normal physiology. Over time, the body's cells are tricked into believing that it is normal to have the drug present in the body. These alterations in physiology are reversible and when the agent is discontinued, uncomfortable symptoms known as withdrawal result (see Section 8.5). Opioids, such as morphine and heroin, may produce physical dependence relatively quickly with repeated doses, particularly when taken IV. Alcohol, central nervous system (CNS) depressants, some stimulants, and nicotine are other examples of substances that may produce physical dependence relatively easily with extended use.

It is important to understand that physical dependence is not the same as addiction. Physical dependence may occur during the normal course of therapy, such as in patients receiving high doses of narcotic analgesics during cancer treatment. A patient with cancer may be physically dependent, that is, withdrawal symptoms may occur on discontinuing the drug but should not be considered addicted. Addiction implies destructive, compulsive substance use. Although physical dependence does indeed occur in patients who are addicted, it is important to understand that the two terms have different meanings.

In contrast, **psychological dependence** produces no signs of physical discomfort after the agent is discontinued. The user, however, has an intense desire to continue despite obvious negative economic, physical, or social consequences. This intense craving may be associated with the patient's unsupportive home environment or social contacts. Strong psychological craving for a substance is often responsible for relapses during substance abuse therapy and often causes a return to drug-seeking behavior. The development of psychological dependence usually requires relatively high doses for a prolonged time, such as with marijuana and antianxiety drugs. However, psychological dependence may also develop quickly, perhaps after only one use, such as with crack, which is a potent, inexpensive form of cocaine. Whereas physical dependence is often overcome within a few days or weeks after discontinuing the drug, psychological dependence may persist for months, years, or even an entire lifetime.

8.5 The withdrawal syndrome is a set of characteristic symptoms that occurs when an abused substance is discontinued.

Once a patient becomes physically dependent and the substance is abruptly discontinued, a **withdrawal syndrome** will occur. Some classes of substances exhibit severe and prolonged withdrawal symptoms, whereas others cause barely noticeable symptoms. Because the withdrawal syndrome may be particularly acute for patients dependent on alcohol and sedatives, the process of withdrawal from these agents is best accomplished in a substance abuse treatment facility. Examples of the types of withdrawal syndromes experienced with the different abused substances are shown in Table 8.3. In patients who are physically dependent, a withdrawal syndrome may also be induced by rapid dosage reduction or by the administration of an antagonist drug.

In general, symptoms of withdrawal are opposite to those of the drug's effects. For example, a person may use alprazolam to reduce anxiety, but withdrawal may cause intense anxiety symptoms. A person may abuse methamphetamine as a stimulant to stay awake, but during withdrawal the person will experience lethargy and fatigue. Once these **rebound effects** become in-

TABLE 8.3 Withdrawal Symptoms and Treatment for Selected Drugs of Abuse

Drug Class	Symptoms	Treatment
Alcohol	Tremors, fatigue, anxiety, abdominal cramping, hallucinations, confusion, seizures, delirium	Benzodiazepines, antiseizure agents; disulfiram and naltrexone after withdrawal is over
Anabolic steroids	Mood swings, fatigue, restlessness, anorexia, insomnia, reduced sex drive, depression, and psychological craving for steroids	Behavioral therapy, symptomatic treatment such as antidepressants
Barbiturates and other sedative-hypnotics	Insomnia, anxiety, weakness, abdominal cramps, tremor, anorexia, seizures, hallucinations, and delirium	Same as alcohol
Benzodiazepines	Insomnia, irritability, abdominal pain, nausea, sensitivity to light and sound, headache, fatigue, and tremors	Gradual tapering of dosage over several weeks or months; for acute benzodiazepine intoxication, flumazenil (Romazicon) is administered by rapid IV infusion (15–20 seconds)
Cocaine and amphetamines	Mental depression, anxiety, agitation, irritability, extreme fatigue, hunger, disturbed sleep, psychological craving	Behavioral therapy; no specific pharmacologic treatment available
Hallucinogens	Dependent on the specific drug; may include anxiety, mental depression, insomnia, paranoid delusions, panic attacks, lethargy	Treatment usually is not necessary; symptoms resolve in about 12 h; PCP excretion is very pH dependent and acidification of the urine increases the clearance rate of PCP by about 100-fold. Thus, if urine acidification is thought to be safe for the patient, treatment with vitamin C or ammonium chloride may be helpful
Marijuana	Irritability, restlessness, insomnia, tremor, chills, weight loss	No treatment
Nicotine	Irritability, anxiety, restlessness, headaches, increased appetite, insomnia, inability to concentrate, decrease in heart rate and blood pressure	Nicotine replacement therapy or bupropion (Zyban)
Opioids	Excessive sweating, restlessness, dilated pupils, agitation, goose bumps, tremor, violent yawning, increased heart rate and blood pressure, nausea, vomiting, abdominal cramps and pain, muscle spasms with kicking movements, weight loss	Methadone/buprenorphine therapy; Clonidine/lofexidine—may reduce the severity of some withdrawal symptoms; oxazepam reduces muscle spasms and insomnia; antiemetics for nausea and vomiting; detoxification can be completed in 2–3 days; withdrawal may be done more rapidly using naltrexone in combination with propofol anesthetic, the antiemetic ondansetron, the antidiarrheal octreotide, and clonidine and benzodiazepines for other symptoms

tense, the person is often driven to take additional doses of the abused substance because that will cause the withdrawal symptoms to disappear. For some patients, avoidance of withdrawal symptoms is the major motivator for continuing drug use. Thus, the cycle of continued substance abuse is perpetuated.

Prescription drugs may be used to reduce the severity of withdrawal symptoms. For example, alcohol withdrawal can be treated with a short-acting benzodiazepine such as oxazepam (Serax), and opioid withdrawal can be treated with methadone. Symptoms of nicotine withdrawal may be relieved by nicotine replacement therapy in the form of patches or chewing gum. No specific pharmacologic intervention is indicated for withdrawal from CNS stimulants, hallucinogens, marijuana, or inhalants.

With chronic substance abuse, a patient will often associate the drug use with his or her conditions and surroundings, including social contacts with other users. Users tend to revert back to drug-seeking behavior when they return to the company of other substance abusers. Counselors often encourage users to refrain from associating with past social contacts or relationships with other substance abusers to lessen the possibility for relapse. The formation of new social contacts, including association with self-help groups such as Alcoholics Anonymous, helps some patients transition to a drug-free lifestyle.

It is important to note that there are some classes of prescription drugs that cause significant symptoms when discontinued, but these agents are not considered drugs of abuse. For example, patients taking beta-blockers, antidepressants, anticonvulsants, or corticosteroids for prolonged periods should never abruptly discontinue their medications because serious adverse effects may occur. In essence, these patients have become physically dependent on the drugs during therapy, and the adverse effects observed following discontinuation are evidence of withdrawal syndromes. Because these drugs do not meet the definition of an abused substance (self-administration of a drug in a manner that does not conform to the norms within the patient's given culture), these patients are not considered addicted.

Tolerance

8.6 Tolerance occurs when the body adapts to a drug and larger doses are needed to produce a therapeutic effect.

Tolerance is a biologic condition that occurs when the body adapts to a substance after repeated administration. Over time, larger doses of the agent are required to produce the same initial effect. For example, at the start of pharmacotherapy a patient may find that 2 mg of a sedative is effective at inducing sleep. After taking the medication for several months, the patient may require 4 or perhaps 6 mg to fall asleep. Development of drug tolerance is common for drugs that affect the nervous system. Tolerance should be considered a natural consequence of continued drug use: Development of tolerance is not evidence of addiction or drug abuse. Indeed, tolerance is an expression of natural homeostasis—the body's attempt to return systems to normal.

Tolerance does not develop at the same rate for all actions of a drug. For example, patients usually develop tolerance to the nausea and vomiting produced by narcotic analgesics after only a few doses. Tolerance to the mood-altering effects of these drugs and to their ability to reduce pain develops more slowly but eventually may be complete. Tolerance never develops to the drug's ability to constrict the pupils. Patients will often endure annoying side effects of drugs, such as the sedation caused by antihistamines, if they know that tolerance will develop quickly to these effects. Thus knowing details regarding the development of tolerance helps the nurse to deliver essential patient information that may enhance adherence.

Tolerance may lead to serious consequences for patients abusing hazardous substances. As a patient self-administers higher and higher doses to obtain a desired effect such as euphoria or sedation, the risk of overdose escalates. In some cases, the drug abuser may reach a daily dose that would be lethal for a nonaddicted person. Tolerance fades after the patient discontinues the abused drug, often after 10 to 14 days. If the patient should return to drug-taking behavior with the same high dose, it may be fatal.

The rapid development of tolerance, called **tachyphylaxis**, occurs with drugs such as cocaine and amphetamines but is not unique to abused substances. For example, patients with coronary artery disease will exhibit acute tachyphylaxis to the therapeutic effects of organic nitrates, such as nitroglycerin. Tachyphylaxis can occur to virtually any action of a drug, adverse effects as well as therapeutic effects. Tachyphylaxis is beneficial when it occurs to an adverse effect of a drug, such as nausea, vomiting, or dizziness.

Cross-tolerance occurs between closely related drugs. The more two drugs are similar chemically, the greater the possibility of cross-tolerance between them. This occurs frequently between drugs in the same class, such as among different barbiturates or among various opioids. It sometimes occurs between dissimilar drugs that have the same pharmacologic action. For example, patients who are physically dependent on ethanol exhibit cross-tolerance to other CNS depressant drugs such as benzodiazepines and barbiturates. Ethanol-dependent patients will require higher doses of these drugs to produce a therapeutic effect. Ethanol will not exhibit cross-tolerance to drugs in very different pharmacologic classes, such as amphetamines or LSD.

The terms *immunity* and *resistance* are often confused with tolerance. These terms more correctly refer to the immune system and infections and should not be used interchangeably with tolerance. For example, microorganisms may become resistant to the effects of an antibiotic: They do not become tolerant. Patients may become tolerant to the effects of pain relievers: They do not become resistant.

Central Nervous System Depressants

8.7 Central nervous system depressants, which include sedatives, opioids, and alcohol, decrease the activity of the central nervous system.

CNS depressants form a diverse group of drugs that cause patients to feel sedated or relaxed. Drugs in this group include sedatives, antianxiety agents, alcohol, and opioids. Although the majority are legal substances, these classes of drugs are strictly controlled due to their abuse potential.

PharmFACT

In 2006, seven million persons aged 12 or older (2.8% of the population) abused prescription psychotherapeutic drugs in the past month. Of these, 5.2 million used pain relievers. Among persons who abused analgesics, 56% reported that the source of the drug was a friend or relative for free. Another 19% reported that they got the drug from one health care provider. Only 4% got the pain relievers from a drug dealer or other stranger, and 0.1% reported buying the drug on the Internet. *Source:* Substance Abuse and Mental Health Services Administration, 2007.

MyNursingKit | National Institute of Drug Abuse and the Office of Applied Studies, Substance Abuse, and Mental Health Statistics

Sedatives and Related Agents

Sedatives, also known as sedative–hypnotics and tranquilizers, are primarily prescribed for sleep disorders and certain forms of epilepsy. The two general classes of sedatives are the barbiturates and the nonbarbiturate sedative–hypnotics. The actions, indications, safety profiles, and addictive potential of the two classes are roughly equivalent.

Physical and psychological dependence develop when high doses of barbiturates are taken for extended periods. Doses may be three or more times above normal due to the development of tolerance. Sedative abusers often obtain these drugs by faking prescriptions or by sharing their medication with friends and commonly combine them with other drugs of abuse, such as stimulants or alcohol. Addicts often alternate between amphetamines (uppers), which keep them awake for several days, and barbiturates (downers), which are needed in order to relax and fall asleep.

Sedatives may have a long duration of action in the body, sometimes lasting an entire day, depending on the specific drug. Patients may appear dull or apathetic. Reactions to higher doses resemble alcohol intoxication with slurred speech and motor incoordination. Abused barbiturates include pentobarbital (Nembutal), amobarbital (Amytal), secobarbital (Seconal), and a combination of secobarbital and amobarbital (Tuinal). The medical use of barbiturates and nonbarbiturate sedative–hypnotics has declined markedly over the past two decades because safer alternatives with lower abuse potential are now available. With the decline in therapeutic use, fewer cases of illicit barbiturate use have been reported. The use of the barbiturates in treating sleep disorders is discussed in Chapter 22, and their use in epilepsy is presented in Chapter 26.

Overdoses of sedatives are extremely dangerous because the drugs suppress the respiratory centers in the brain and the user may stop breathing or lapse into a coma. Very high doses are often fatal. In the 1960s to 1970s, barbiturates were the drugs most commonly used to commit suicide. The withdrawal syndrome from these drugs resembles that of alcohol and may be life threatening.

Benzodiazepines are another group of CNS depressants that have potential for abuse. They are one of the most widely prescribed classes of drugs, and the last decade has seen a sharp rise in their abuse among teens and college students. Their primary indication is anxiety (see Chapter 22), although they may be used as sedatives for patients with sleep disorders. Benzodiazepines are also used to treat seizure disorders (see Chapter 26) and as muscle relaxants (see Chapter 27). Benzodiazepines include alprazolam (Xanax), clonazepam (Klonopin), diazepam (Valium), temazepam (Restoril), triazolam (Halcion), and midazolam (Versed).

Flunitrazepam (Rohypnol) is an infamous benzodiazepine of abuse because it causes **anterograde amnesia,** a type of short-term memory loss where the user cannot remember events that occur while under the influence of the drug. Effects begin 30 minutes after oral administration and last for 8 hours or longer. The abuser is conscious during this time but is unable to transfer thoughts from short-term to long-term memory. Flunitrazepam is called a "date-rape" drug because sexual predators can expose an unknowing person to the drug and perform an assault with assurance that the victim will not remember the event. Flunitrazepam is not approved by the FDA for any medical condition. Most of the drug in the United States originates from Mexico, although it can be obtained legally in several other countries.

Despite their enormous popularity, benzodiazepines are not frequently abused in high doses. However, users may combine these agents with alcohol, cocaine, or heroin to augment their "high." High doses cause patients to appear detached, sleepy, or disoriented. Often, patients will appear carefree and without worry. In terms of acute toxicity, benzodiazepines are safer than barbiturates: Serious respiratory depression does not occur and death due to overdose is rare, even with extremely high doses. However, if combined with alcohol, cocaine, or heroin, overdose may be lethal. Withdrawal symptoms are less severe than with barbiturates.

Another popular abused CNS depressant is a substance that occurs naturally in the body called gamma-hydroxybutyric acid (GHB). The drug is approved by the FDA as sodium oxybate (Xyrem) to treat patients with narcolepsy who experience excessive daytime sleepiness or cataplexy (weak or paralyzed muscles). Although Xyrem is regulated as a Schedule III drug, its active ingredient GHB is classified as Schedule I. It is very unusual for the FDA to classify a drug in two schedules. It is distributed to prescribers and patients only through a single centralized pharmacy (see Chapter 28).

Once sold in health food stores as a dietary supplement to enhance athletic performance, GHB is now abused by recreational users for its ability to produce euphoria at low doses. Like flunitrazepam, GHB is called a date-rape drug because it induces retrograde amnesia in the user and has been used in sexual assaults. Most illegal GHB is obtained through home laboratories in the United States, with batches varying widely in purity and potency. The drug is usually dissolved in liquid and doses are difficult to estimate. The same enzyme as ethanol metabolizes GHB; concurrent use, which is common, leads to prolonged effects of GHB and an increased risk of overdose. Overdose may cause severe respiratory depression, seizures, coma, and death. Death from GHB overdose is sometimes caused by the aspiration of vomitus, because the patient may experience coma, vomiting, and seizures simultaneously. There is no antidote for overdose.

Opioids

Opioids, also known as opiates or narcotic analgesics, are prescribed for severe pain, anesthesia, persistent cough, and life-threatening diarrhea. The opioid class includes natural substances obtained from the seeds of the poppy plant such as opium, morphine, and codeine, and synthetic drugs such as propoxyphene (Darvon), meperidine (Demerol), oxycodone (OxyContin), fentanyl (Duragesic, Sublimaze), methadone (Dolophine), and heroin. The therapeutic effects of the opioids are discussed in detail in Chapter 29.

The effects of oral opioids begin within 30 minutes and may last over a day. Injecting or smoking opium produces immediate effects, including the brief, intense rush of euphoria sought by heroin addicts. Individuals experience a range of emotions from extreme pleasure to slowed body activities and profound sedation. Other symptoms include slurred speech, constricted pupils (miosis), an increase in the pain threshold, and respiratory depression. Tolerance develops rapidly to most effects of opioids, and the patient may eventually require 10 times the initial dose to achieve their desired effects.

Opioid dependence can occur rapidly and withdrawal can produce very intense and unpleasant symptoms that occur within a few hours after discontinuation of parenteral agents and within 3 to 5 days for those dependent on oral opiates. Withdrawal symptoms include dysphoria, diaphoresis, violent yawning, lacrimation, rhinorrhea, pupil dilation (mydriasis), fever, diarrhea, goose bumps, and muscle cramping and tremor. Although extremely unpleasant, withdrawal from opioids is not life threatening, compared to barbiturate or alcohol withdrawal, and the person is not delirious. The withdrawal syndrome is self-limiting, peaking within 36 to 72 hours after discontinuation of parenteral opioids, and individual symptoms are treated as necessary. For patients dependent on low to moderate doses, withdrawal symptoms are relatively mild and resemble a case of the flu. Babies born to pregnant opioid users will experience withdrawal symptoms following birth.

Methadone is a narcotic that has been the conventional treatment of choice for opioid addiction. Although methadone has addictive properties of its own, it does not produce the same degree of euphoria as other opioids; it may be taken orally and its effects last 24 hours. Heroin addicts are switched to methadone during the detoxification phase of treatment to prevent unpleasant withdrawal symptoms. Methadone is an antagonist to heroin. If the patient decides to take heroin during methadone therapy, most of the euphoric rush will be blocked. During maintenance therapy, patients must report to the methadone clinic daily for their dose and to receive counseling. In some cases, patients who have remained heroin-free may be trusted with several doses for home administration. Patients sometimes remain on methadone maintenance the remainder of their lives, although most patients eventually choose to detoxify altogether and discontinue methadone use. Gradual dose reduction occurs over a period of about 6 months. Withdrawal from methadone is more prolonged than with heroin or morphine, but the symptoms are less intense.

Newer treatments for opioid dependence, approved in 2003, include buprenorphine (Subutex) as monotherapy or buprenorphine combined with naloxone (Suboxone). These are Schedule III drugs intended for office management of opioid dependence. Outpatient management is more convenient for the patient and less expensive for the health care system. Buprenorphine is given sublingually only three to four times per week and produces less physical dependence than methadone; thus detoxification can be more rapid. One problem with buprenorphine is that substance abusers may crush the pills, dissolve the medication, and take it intravenously. To discourage this possibility, naloxone may be added. Naloxone is an opioid antagonist that will block any euphoric effects of buprenorphine and induce withdrawal symptoms if the patient tries to crush the drug and inject it. Although not yet approved in the United States, buprenorphine is also available as a transdermal patch.

Oxycodone is an opioid that deserves special attention because the incidence of substance abuse of this drug has escalated in the past decade. Oxycodone was approved by the FDA in 1976 and has been widely prescribed for moderate pain when combined with aspirin (Percodan) and acetaminophen (Percocet). In 1995, oxycodone (OxyContin) was formulated in a slow, timed release preparation for the purpose of bringing long-duration relief from chronic pain. Whereas Percocet and Percodan contain only 2.5 to 10 mg per tablet, OxyContin contains 10 to 160 mg per tablet. Drug abusers soon discovered that when OxyContin tablets are crushed, dissolved, and injected, the drug delivers a rush of euphoria similar to morphine or heroin. Crushing the tablet destroys the timed release feature of the drug. Most of the drug in the United States is obtained through diversion from medical sources such as fake prescriptions, patients selling their drug to make a profit, and people stealing the drug from patients or pharmacies. The steep rise in OxyContin abuse among teens and college students is of particular concern. Pharmacologically, OxyContin has the same actions, dependence potential, toxicity, and withdrawal syndrome as other potent opiates.

Alcohol (Ethanol)

One of the most commonly abused drugs is alcohol, which is the pharmacologically active agent in beer, wine, and liquor. Although there are many types of alcohol, the only one having widespread medical significance is ethanol or ethyl alcohol. Therefore, in this text, the terms *ethanol* and *alcohol* are used interchangeably. The economic, social, and health consequences of alcohol abuse are staggering. Small quantities of alcohol consumed on a daily basis, however, have been found to reduce the risk of stroke and heart attack.

Alcohol is readily absorbed across the gastrointestinal (GI) tract, primarily from the small intestine. Food slows the absorption of alcohol by delaying gastric emptying time and diluting the alcohol, thus delaying its onset of action. Once it enters the blood, alcohol is immediately distributed to the tissues. The drug easily crosses the blood–brain barrier so its effects on the brain are observed quickly, within 5 to 30 minutes after consumption.

MyNursingKit | Cirrhosis Animation

Alcohol is metabolized and excreted at a constant rate, depending primarily on the activity of two hepatic enzymes, alcohol dehydrogenase and aldehyde dehydrogenase. Metabolism is a two-step process, first yielding acetaldehyde and then acetic acid, or acetate, as shown in Pharmacotherapy Illustrated 8.1. There is wide variability in the amounts of these enzymes in different people. Asians exhibit a high incidence of deficiency of aldehyde dehydrogenase, resulting in an accumulation of acetaldehyde and severe flushing and other uncomfortable symptoms when consuming alcohol. Patients who are alcohol dependent and those who drink alcoholic beverages regularly have higher amounts of these enzymes and thus are able to drink greater quantities of alcohol without becoming intoxicated.

The elimination of alcohol from tissues occurs at a constant rate, which is independent of the concentration of alcohol in the blood. The blood alcohol level declines at about 15 mg/hour and there is no food or drug that can be given to speed up the rate of alcohol excretion once it has reached the blood. Eating pizza or drinking strong coffee following an alcohol binge does nothing to speed up excretion of the drug. It is a simple fact that if one drinks alcohol at a faster rate than it can be metabolized, intoxication will occur and will continue until the body eventually metabolizes the alcohol accumulated in the blood. The "average" rate of metabolism is one drink per hour. Because alcohol is vaporized and excreted by the lungs, breath testing can be used to estimate the amount of alcohol in the blood, a common practice in law enforcement.

Alcohol is classified as a CNS depressant because it has the ability to slow the region of the brain controlling alertness and wakefulness. Effects of alcohol include sedation, relaxation, loss of motor coordination, reduced judgment, and decreased inhibition. Alcohol intoxication may cause partial or total

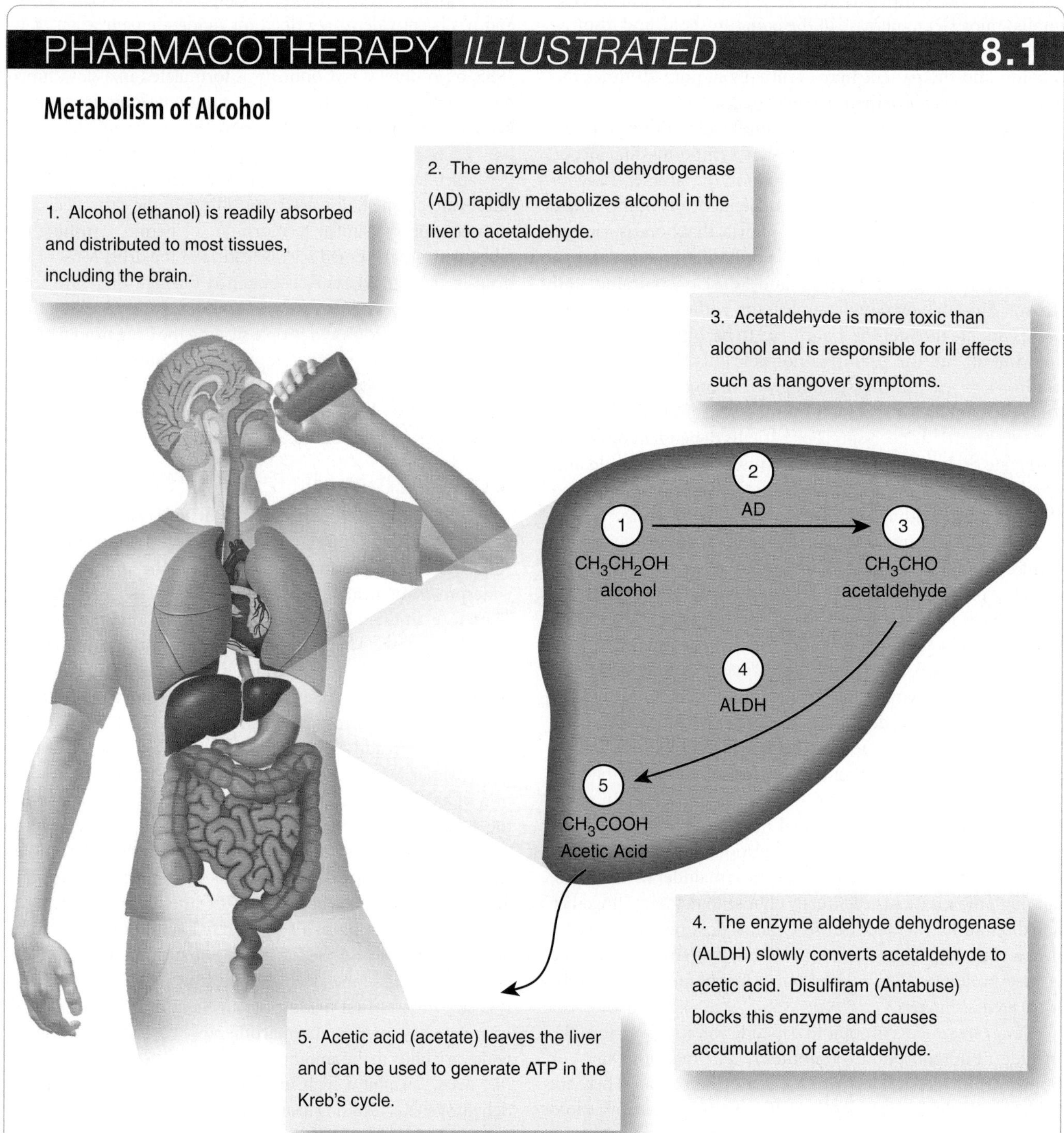

amnesia, resulting in an inability to remember details during an alcohol binge. Alcohol also increases blood flow in certain areas of the skin, causing a flushed face, pink cheeks, or red nose. Like most drugs, effects of alcohol are directly related to the amount consumed. Acute overdoses of alcohol produce vomiting, severe hypotension, respiratory failure, and coma. Death due to alcohol poisoning is not uncommon.

Chronic alcohol consumption produces both psychological and physiological dependence and results in a large number of adverse health effects. Not surprisingly, the organ most affected by chronic alcohol abuse is the liver, which is responsible for metabolizing and detoxifying alcohol. Hepatitis occurs in up to 90% of heavy users. Alcoholism is a common cause of cirrhosis, a debilitating and often fatal failure of the liver to perform its vital functions. Liver impairment results in abnormalities in blood clotting and nutritional deficiencies and makes the patient very sensitive to the effects of medications. Chronic alcohol use also damages the brain, impairing memory and cognitive function.

Drug doses for patients with alcoholism should generally be decreased to avoid toxicity: The patient is more susceptible to adverse drug effects and drug interactions. Combining alcohol with nonsteroidal anti-inflammatory agents (NSAIDs) such as aspirin can promote serious GI bleeding. Combining alcohol with acetaminophen can increase the risk of fatal hepatic injury. Alcohol should never be combined with other CNS depressants, because their effects are cumulative and profound sedation or coma may result. Combining alcohol with barbiturates, benzodiazepines, or opioids may be fatal. Selected drug interactions involving alcohol are shown in Table 8.4.

TABLE 8.4 Drug–Drug Interactions with Alcohol

Class	Example Drug(s)	Interaction	Consequences
Acetaminophen	—	Increased acetaminophen metabolism to toxic metabolites	Severe, possibly fatal liver damage
Anesthetics	Propofol (Diprivan), enflurane (Ethrane), and halothane (Fluothane)	Cross-tolerance	Larger anesthetic doses needed to induce anesthesia
		Additive hepatic toxicity	Increased risk of liver damage
Antianginal medications	Nitroglycerin, isosorbide dinitrate (Isordil)	Additive effects on blood pressure	Hypotension, dizziness, possible fainting
Antibiotics	Furazolidone (Furoxone), griseofulvin, metronidazole (Flagyl), and quinacrine (Atabrine)	Additive toxicity	Nausea, vomiting, headache, possible seizures, reduced antibiotic effectiveness
Anticoagulants	Warfarin (Coumadin)	Acute consumption enhances warfarin bioavailability; chronic consumption reduces its availability	Modification of coagulation: bleeding disorders, hemorrhage
Antidepressants	Amitriptyline (Elavil), paroxetine (Paxil), sertraline (Zoloft), fluoxetine (Prozac)	Additive CNS depression/sedation	Drowsiness, lethargy
Antihistamines	Diphenhydramine (Benadryl and others), loratadine (Claritin), cetirizine (Zyrtec)	Additive CNS depression	Drowsiness, lethargy, dizziness
Antipsychotics	Chlorpromazine (Thorazine)	Additive CNS depression	Drowsiness, lethargy
		Additive hepatotoxicity	Increased risk of liver damage
Antiseizure medications	Phenytoin (Dilantin)	Chronic alcohol use may decrease phenytoin bioavailability	Increased risk of seizures
Antituberculars	Isoniazid and rifampin	Decreased bioavailability	Decreased effectiveness in eliminating tuberculosis
Beta blockers	Propranolol (Inderal)	Additive effects on blood pressure	Hypotension, dizziness, possible fainting
HMG-CoA reductase inhibitors (statins)	Atorvastatin (Lipitor), simvastatin (Zocor)	Additive hepatotoxicity	Liver damage
NSAIDs	Aspirin, ibuprofen, naproxen, others	Additive GI toxicity	Increased risk of GI bleeding
Opioids	Morphine, codeine, propoxyphene (Darvon), and meperidine (Demerol)	Additive CNS depression and sedation	Drowsiness, lethargy
Sedatives and antianxiety agents	Diazepam (Valium), lorazapam (Ativan), alprazolam (Xanax), phenobarbital (Luminal)	Additive CNS depression and sedation	Drowsiness, lethargy
Miscellaneous	Sulfonylureas, metronidazole (Flagyl), isoniazid (INH)	Disulfiram-like reaction	Facial flushing, nausea, vomiting

CONNECTION *Checkpoint* 8.2

Alcohol induces CYP3A and increases the formation of a toxic metabolite of acetaminophen. From what you learned in Chapter 4, what is CYP3A and what is its importance to pharmacotherapy? See Answer to Connection Checkpoint 8.2 in Appendix A.

One of the major adverse effects of alcohol consumption occurs not in the patient, but in the fetus of a pregnant alcohol user. These effects, known as fetal alcohol syndrome, include birth defects and major health challenges for the child. There is no safe "dose" for alcohol consumption during pregnancy; thus consumption of this drug must be strictly avoided. Additional details on alcohol as a teratogen are presented in Chapter 10.

Alcohol withdrawal is severe and may be life threatening. About 5% to 10% of withdrawal cases proceed to **delirium tremens,** a syndrome of intense agitation, confusion, terrifying hallucinations, uncontrollable tremors, panic attacks, and paranoia. Without treatment, 35% of the patients with delirium tremens will die. Prevention of seizures and delirium tremens is a top priority and may be accomplished by administering a benzodiazepine such as lorazepam (Ativan) or diazepam (Valium). Hallucinations may require the administration of an antipsychotic agent such as haloperidol (Haldol).

MyNursingKit | Alcohol Poisoning and Toxicity

Long-term therapy for alcohol dependence includes behavioral counseling and self-help groups such as Alcoholics Anonymous. Pharmacologic management of alcohol dependence includes disulfiram and naltrexone. Disulfiram (Antabuse) is given to discourage relapses. By itself, disulfiram produces few effects. If alcohol is consumed while taking disulfiram, however, the patient becomes violently ill with headache, palpitations, chest pain, shortness of breath, nausea,vomiting, and other unpleasant symptoms. Symptoms begin within 5 to 10 minutes after alcohol consumption and continue for several hours. Disulfiram irreversibly inhibits the enzyme acetaldehyde dehydrogenase, causing the toxic substance acetaldehyde to build up in the blood. Acetaldehyde is sometimes called the "hangover" chemical because it is responsible for causing miserable symptoms following a night of high alcohol consumption. It is important to note that the use of disulfiram requires a motivated patient because the drug only prevents impulsive drinking as long as the patient chooses to take it. The "protective" action of disulfiram may last for 2 weeks after the drug is discontinued. Because the disulfiram reaction can be serious and even fatal, disulfiram therapy should not be initiated in patients at high risk for returning to alcohol abuse.

Naltrexone (ReVia, Vivitrol) is an opioid antagonist that is used in the management of alcoholism because it reduces the psychological craving for alcohol. Why does a drug that blocks opiate receptors have an effect on alcohol dependence? Although the mechanism is unclear, endogenous opioids appear to be involved in "reward pathways" for alcohol. Blocking the reward pathways with naltrexone affects the psychological experience or craving characteristic of alcohol dependence. Naltrexone does not produce a "hangover" reaction when a person consumes alcohol, as does disulfiram. Oral naltrexone may be given once daily for several months up to a year. An intramuscular (IM) suspension of naltrexone (Vivitrol) was approved in 2006 that offers the convenience of once a month injections. Naltrexone is also approved to treat opiate dependence and may be used off-label to treat nicotine withdrawal. Severe opioid withdrawal may occur if the drug is administered to a patient who has received opioids within 5 to 7 days prior to naltrexone dosing; thus the drug is contraindicated in these patients.

Cannabinoids—Marijuana

8.8 Marijuana is the most frequently abused illicit substance.

Cannabinoids are natural products obtained from the hemp plant *Cannabis sativa,* which thrives in tropical climates. Cannabinoids include marijuana, hashish, and hash oil. Hashish is a solid, dried resin of the plant that is extremely potent. Hash oil is made by dissolving hashish or marijuana in a solvent such as alcohol, then allowing the liquid to evaporate to form a thick, oily concentrated form of cannabis.

Although over 70 natural cannabinoid substances have been identified, the ingredient responsible for most of the psychoactive properties is **tetrahydrocannabinol (THC).** Selective breeding and cultivation of *Cannabis* has produced varieties of the plant that produce much higher concentrations of THC than in previous decades. The THC content of marijuana varies from 5% to 25%; hashish from 20% to 60%; and hash oil from 30% to 80%.

Humans, as well as many other mammals, fish, and birds, produce small amounts of endogenous cannabinoids. These substances, known as endocannabinoids, are types of internal messengers that allow for intercellular communication. The exact purpose of the endocannabinoids has yet to be discovered, although they have some of the same characteristics as neurotransmitters and can modulate neuronal function. The endocannabinoids have some structural similarities to THC and bind to the same receptors, known as CB1 and CB2 receptors. Agonists and antagonists to CB1 and CB2 have been discovered, with the hope that the research may lead to new pharmacologic agents.

Marijuana, also known as grass, pot, weed, reefer, or dope, is the most commonly used illicit drug in the United States; over 40% of the population age 12 or older has used the drug at least once. Marijuana is usually smoked as cigarettes (joints), but it may be used in pipes, brewed as teas, or added to food. Oral absorption results in a lower serum blood level of the drug than does inhalation.

When inhaled, marijuana produces effects that occur within minutes and last 1 to 3 hours. Use of marijuana slows motor activity, decreases coordination, and causes disconnected thoughts and euphoria. The experience is nearly always pleasant and involves laughter and an increase in the subjective perception of sounds, colors, and thoughts. The subjective experience is dependent on the social surroundings during drug use. Positive, friendly, happy surroundings produce a more favorable drug experience than taking the drug alone. Time appears to pass more slowly. It increases thirst and craving for food, particularly chocolate and other candies. One hallmark symptom of marijuana use is red or bloodshot eyes, caused by dilation of blood vessels.

Following feelings of euphoria, the person may become sleepy or depressed or experience paranoia. Driving is sometimes impaired, particularly when the drug is combined with alcohol. Because marijuana smoke is inhaled more deeply and held within the lungs for a longer period than cigarette smoke, marijuana smoke introduces four times more particulates (tar) into the lungs than does tobacco smoke. Smoking marijuana on a daily basis may increase the risk of lung cancer and other respiratory disorders. Chronic use is associated with apathy and a lack of motivation in achieving or pursuing life goals, and very high doses may cause hallucinations. THC accumulates in reproductive tissues, particularly the gonads and has been reported to cause amenorrhea and decreased spermatogenesis.

Unlike most drugs of abuse, marijuana produces very little physical dependence or tolerance. At usual doses, withdrawal symptoms are mild, if they are experienced at all. After chronic abuse of high doses, patients may experience irritability, restlessness, and insomnia. Psychological dependence occurs when the drug is taken on a chronic basis. Metabolites of THC remain in the body for months to years, allowing laboratory specialists to easily determine whether someone has taken marijuana. For 3 to 5 days after a single use, THC can be detected in the urine.

Medical marijuana is a controversial topic; physicians and politicians are reluctant to endorse a drug that impairs judgment and may harm users. THC appears to reduce the pressure in the eyeball, a condition called glaucoma. Patients receiving antineoplastic agents have reported that THC reduces the severe nausea and vomiting associated with these drugs. The ability of THC to reduce muscle spasticity may lead to applications for patients with multiple sclerosis and other spasticity disorders. In nearly all cases, current drugs for these conditions have been demonstrated to be more effective and safer. Despite numerous attempts to demonstrate therapeutic applications for marijuana, the medical value of the drug remains to be conclusively proven. Marijuana remains a Schedule I drug, with no approved uses by the FDA.

Hallucinogens

8.9 Hallucinogens and club drugs cause an altered state of thought and perception.

Hallucinogens are a diverse class of chemicals that have in common the ability to produce an altered, dreamlike state of consciousness. These drugs sometimes produce a profound emotional experience, allowing the user to feel enhanced interconnectedness with others and experience a higher, spiritual plane of consciousness. Sometimes called "psychedelics," the prototype drug for this class is lysergic acid diethylamide (LSD). More recently, some drugs in this class have become closely associated with the nightclub scene and are abused by those seeking a drug-induced experience from the music, dancing, and social contact; thus the name "club drugs."

For nearly all drugs of abuse, predictable symptoms occur in every user. Effects from hallucinogens, however, are highly variable and depend on the mood and expectations of the user and the surrounding environment in which the substance is used. Two patients taking the same agent will report completely different experiences, and the same patient may report different symptoms with each use. All hallucinogens are Schedule I drugs: They have no medical use.

Historically, the use of hallucinogens has ancient origins, being used in religious rituals of native cultures to create visions. Past and current use is sporadic. People do not take them continuously; they are reserved for particular occasions, events, or ceremonies.

MyNursingKit | The History of LSD

LSD and Similar Hallucinogens

LSD, also called acid, the beast, blotter acid, and California sunshine, is derived from a fungus that grows on rye and other grains. LSD is nearly always administered orally and can be manufactured in capsule, tablet, or liquid form. A common and inexpensive method for distributing LSD is to place drops of the drug on paper, often containing the images of cartoon characters or graphics related to the drug culture, as shown in

CONNECTIONS

Treating the Diverse Patient Nurses and Substance Abuse

When patients are admitted to the hospital, they assume that their caregivers are credentialed, competent, and clear headed. Unfortunately, the overall statistics for substance abuse in nurses are similar to those in the general population—10%. However, this percentage may be higher in critical care and emergency department nurses who are about three times as likely to abuse narcotics. In fact, the *American Journal of Public Health* reported that oncology nurses have the highest percentage, 42%, due to binge drinking. Psychiatry nurses have a substance abuse rate of about 40%.

Contributing factors to substance abuse in nurses are diverse but key ones may be easy access, availability, or opportunities to self-medicate as well as personal and work-related stress. Denial by the nurse is high and because substance abuse is seen as a weakness or failure, nurses are not likely to self-report. Peers may choose to ignore the problem adopting a "don't ask, don't tell" approach until an adverse outcome occurs.

Staff and managers must confront the issue of substance abuse for reasons of patient safety. Nurses must be proactive and learn about the personal dangers of substance abuse. Nurses should know the signs of potential problems such as absenteeism, slurred speech, ongoing crises, excuses, missing medications, inaccurate narcotic counts, lack of alertness, or forgetfulness. These do not necessarily indicate substance abuse but further investigation and observation may be appropriate if several signs occur. Nurses must know the procedure to report impairment issues to management and perhaps how to confront a peer or provide intervention. Remember, nurses, like all people, face life stresses, losses, and temptations. Combined with opportunity and access, nurses may become threats to themselves and others. Treatment programs are available. In this time of nursing shortages, health care facilities need competent and high-functioning professional nurses unencumbered with the many problems of substance abuse.

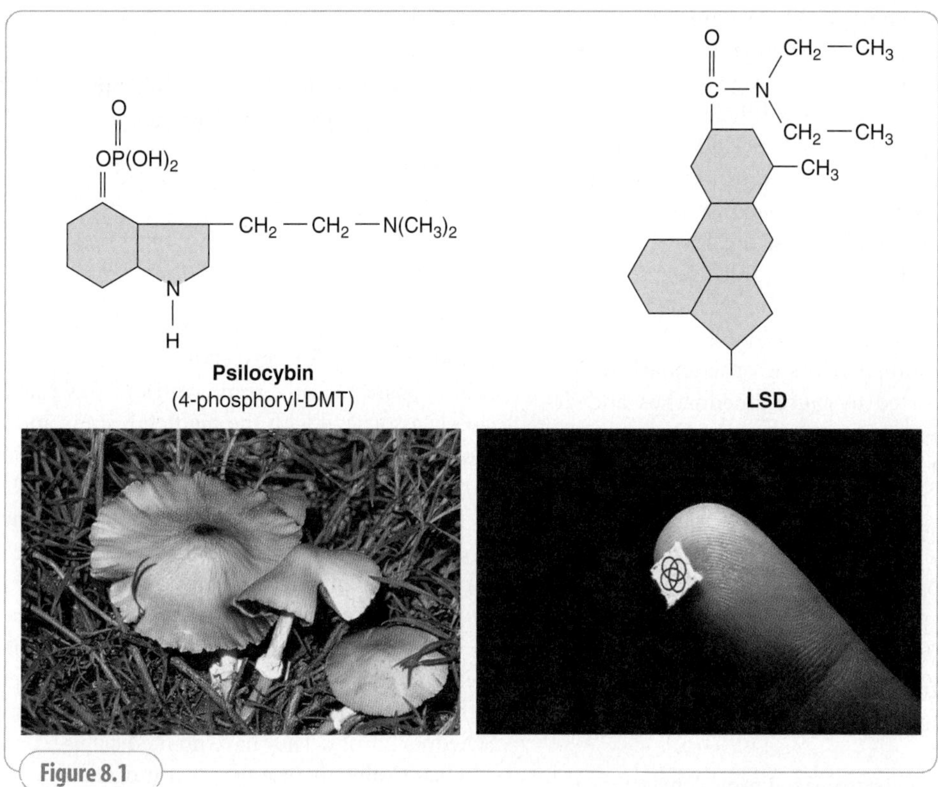

Figure 8.1

Comparison of the chemical structures of psilocybin and LSD. Psilocybin (left) is derived from a mushroom.

Source: (left) *Photographer:* James Beveridge/Visuals Unlimited; (right) Custom Medical Stock Photo, Inc.

Figure 8.1 After drying, the paper is then cut into small squares to be ingested, with each square representing a "dose." The drug is extremely potent, with doses as low as 25 mcg producing an effect.

Immediately after use, LSD is widely distributed throughout the body, including the brain. Effects begin within an hour and may last from 6 to 12 hours. Although the exact mechanism of action of the drug is unclear, it affects the central and autonomic nervous systems, increasing blood pressure, elevating body temperature, dilating pupils, causing dry mouth, and increasing the heart rate.

LSD and other hallucinogens are used for their psychoactive, rather than their physical, effects. LSD users may experience symptoms such as laughter, visions, religious revelations, or deep personal insights. Common occurrences are hallucinations and after-images being projected onto people as they move. Users also report extremely bright lights and vivid colors. Some users hear voices; others report seeing sounds and hearing colors. Many experience a profound sense of truth and deep directed thoughts. The user's sense of time is altered.

Unpleasant experiences of LSD, known as "bad trips," can be terrifying and may include acute anxiety, panic attacks, confusion, severe depression, and paranoia. Repeated use may impair memory and the ability to reason. In extreme cases, patients may develop psychoses. One common adverse effect is flashbacks, in which the user experiences the effects of the drug again, sometimes weeks, months, or years after the drug was initially taken. Flashbacks may occur without warning.

LSD is considered a recreational drug: Users rarely become dependent on the drug, and there are no withdrawal symptoms. Continuous users will experience tolerance very quickly, sometimes after only 2 to 3 days.

The following drugs are considered similar to LSD and produce equivalent biologic and psychoactive effects. They are generally less potent and less commonly abused, although certain geographical areas report a high incidence.

- **Psilocybin.** The primary psychoactive substance in over 100 species of psilocybin mushrooms found in Mexico and Central America (Figure 8.1). Known as "magic mushrooms" or "shrooms," psilocybin is a prodrug that is metabolized to its active metabolite psilocin. Possession of these mushroom species is illegal. Psilocybin and psilocin are listed as Schedule I drugs, although the fungi are easily cultivated indoors. The drug is taken by eating fresh psilocybin mushrooms, or by ingesting dried extracts.
- **Mescaline.** Found in the peyote cactus and several other cacti species of Mexico and Central America, as shown in Figure 8.2. The drug is usually taken in capsules consisting of dried cactus. The cactus, which grows very slowly, has become quite rare due to overharvesting. In the United States, peyote use is illegal for all but members of the Native American Church, who use the drug in religious ceremonies.
- **Dimethyltryptamine (DMT).** A natural substance found in very small amounts in humans but in much larger amounts in many species of plants in Central and South America and the Caribbean Islands. Like some of the other hallucinogens, DMT was used by native cultures in their spiritual ceremonies to induce visions. The drug is usually smoked

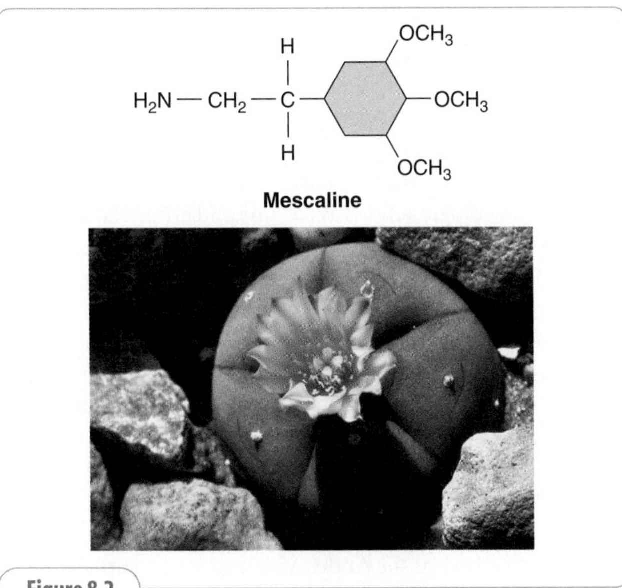

Figure 8.2

The chemical structure of mescaline, derived from the peyote cactus.

Source: Photographer: R. Konig/Jacana/Photo Researchers, Inc.

but may be snuffed (snorted through the nostrils), injected, or taken orally. A closely related hallucinogenic substance is 5-MeO-DMT.

Club Drugs and Miscellaneous Hallucinogens

Club drug is a relatively new term that refers to substances taken by people at dance clubs, all-night parties, and raves. It is a vague term that refers to a diverse group of abused substances that includes ecstasy, GHB, methamphetamine, Rohypnol, ketamine, and other agents, usually ingested with significant amounts of alcohol. Use of club drugs has escalated over the past decade. Not all club drugs are hallucinogens, and some of these are covered in other sections of this chapter. The following are descriptions of several major club drugs and some miscellaneous hallucinogens.

- **MDMA (3,4-methylenedioxymethamphetamine, XTC, or ecstasy).** A synthetic amphetamine originally synthesized for research purposes but has since become extremely popular among teens and young adults. Taken orally, its effects last 3 to 6 hours. The drug is unique because it produces both stimulant and hallucinogenic effects simultaneously. MDMA enhances emotions and awareness, increases social and extroversion behaviors, and allows the user to stay awake and physically active for long periods. Chronic users exhibit behavioral disorders such as depression, anxiety, sleeplessness, and hostility. It has a narrow therapeutic index and overdoses may be fatal.
- **MDA (3,4-methylenedioxyamphetamine).** Called the love drug due to a belief that it enhances sexual desires. This drug is sometimes a component of ecstasy.
- **DOM (2,5 dimethoxy-4-methylamphetamine).** A recreational drug often linked with rave parties as a drug of choice having the name STP. The drug has effects similar to LSD but with a longer duration.
- **Phencyclidine (PCP, crystal, angel dust).** Produces a trancelike state without loss of consciousness that may last for days. Once available as an anesthetic, the substance was removed from the market in 1965 because patients experienced delirium and panic attacks as they recovered from anesthesia. The powdered drug is sometimes sprinkled on marijuana and smoked, or it may be snorted or taken as tablets. Typical effects include slurred speech, detachment from reality, time distortion, and a sensation of floating in space. It does not produce the same types of hallucinations seen with LSD. Phencyclidine is probably the most dangerous of the hallucinogens because high doses can cause severe and violent panic attacks, seizures, coma, and death. With continuous use, tolerance develops.
- **Ketamine (K, kitkat, or special K).** Closely related to phencyclidine, it has been used historically as an anesthetic but is now rarely used for that purpose. The most common source of the drug is diversion from veterinary offices. Liquid ketamine may be added to drinks, injected, or evaporated to a solid form, which is snorted or taken as pills. Ketamine has become more popular than phencyclidine as a club drug. Effects are similar to those of phencyclidine, although they only last 35 to 40 minutes. Unconsciousness and amnesia may occur at high doses, and psychoses can be induced with continued use.
- **Dextromethorphan (DXM, robo).** A substance included in over-the-counter (OTC) cold remedies for its cough suppressant properties. Of the drugs of abuse, it is one of the only substances that can readily and legally be purchased by teens. Abusers will purchase extra-strength remedies and consume large quantities to achieve dissociative effects similar to those of phencyclidine and ketamine. Effects include slurred speech, dizziness, drowsiness, euphoria, and lack of motor coordination, Overdose can cause brain damage, seizures, cerebrovascular accident, hypothermia, and death. Because cold medicines also contain ingredients such as antihistamines, aspirin, or acetaminophen, abusers of dextromethorphan may experience toxicity due to overdose from these agents. Pure dextromethorphan is also available on the black market in high-dosage tablet form.

Central Nervous System Stimulants

8.10 Stimulants such as amphetamines and cocaine increase the activity of the central nervous system.

The stimulants include a diverse family of drugs known for their ability to increase the activity of the CNS. Some are available by prescription for use in the treatment of narcolepsy and attention deficit/hyperactivity disorder (ADHD). As drugs of abuse, stimulants are taken to produce a sense of exhilaration, improve mental and physical performance, reduce appetite, or prolong wakefulness. Stimulants include the amphetamines, methylphenidate, and cocaine. Some CNS stimulants are club drugs (see Section 8.9). Caffeine is also included as a CNS stimulant although it does not have the same negative health characteristics as the other drugs in this group.

Amphetamines and Methylphenidate

Amphetamines produce their effects by increasing the activity of the endogenous neurotransmitters norepinephrine, serotonin

(5-HT), and dopamine (see Chapter 16): norepinephrine affects awareness and wakefulness by activating neurons in a part of the brain called the **reticular formation.** High doses of amphetamines give the user a feeling of self-confidence, elevated mood, euphoria, and empowerment. Fatigue is diminished and the person can perform at a high level of alertness for an extended time. Appetite is suppressed.

By increasing the activity of norepinephrine, many physiological actions of amphetamines resemble those of sympathetic nervous system activation (see Chapter 19). Cardiovascular and respiratory activities are significantly affected, resulting in increased heart rate, high blood pressure, and increased breathing rate. Other symptoms include dilated pupils, sweating, and tremors. Overdoses of some stimulants lead to seizures, dysrhythmias, cerebrovascular accident (CVA), and cardiac arrest.

Although short-term use of amphetamines induces pleasurable feelings, long-term use results in feelings of restlessness, anxiety, defensiveness, and fits of rage, especially when the user is coming down from a prolonged drug experience. Chronic use can lead to a psychosis that closely resembles paranoid schizophrenia, although this condition usually resolves within several days after discontinuation of the drug. Tolerance to the pleasurable effects of amphetamines occurs very quickly, especially if the drugs are injected.

MyNursingKit | Cocaine Animation

Amphetamines and dextroamphetamines were once widely prescribed for depression, weight loss, drowsiness, and congestion. Because of their ability to enhance alertness, pilots, students, and health care workers on long shifts have historically abused amphetamines. In the 1970s it was recognized that the adverse effects and abuse potential of amphetamines outweighed their legitimate medical uses. Due to the development of safer medications, current therapeutic applications of these drugs are extremely limited. Most substance abusers obtain these agents from illegal laboratories, which can produce some of the amphetamines using readily available chemicals and make tremendous profits. Physical dependence to amphetamines is unusual, and withdrawal symptoms are not serious. The only potentially serious symptom of amphetamine withdrawal is depression.

Dextroamphetamine (Dexedrine) may be used for short-term weight loss, when all other attempts to reduce weight have been exhausted, and to treat narcolepsy, a rare disease in which patients fall asleep unexpectedly. Methamphetamine, commonly called ice, is often used as a recreational drug for users who like the rush of euphoria that it gives them. It is usually administered in powder or crystal form (crystal meth) but it may also be smoked. Methamphetamine is a Schedule II drug marketed under the trade name Desoxyn, although most abusers obtain it from illegal methamphetamine laboratories. Methamphetamine can be easily synthesized from pseudoephedrine, a common OTC decongestant. This has led to nearly all states placing pseudoephedrine behind the pharmacist counter and has motivated pharmaceutical manufacturers to find a replacement drug for pseudoephedrine in their cold and flu remedies. A structural analog of methamphetamine, methcathinone (street name Cat) is made illegally and snorted, taken orally, or injected IV. Methcathinone is a Schedule I agent.

Methylphenidate (Ritalin) is a CNS stimulant widely prescribed for children diagnosed with **attention deficit/hyperactivity disorder (ADHD)** because the drug exerts a calming effect in children who are inattentive or hyperactive. The drug stimulates the alertness center in the brain and the child is able to focus on complex tasks for longer periods. The therapeutic applications of methylphenidate are discussed in Chapter 28.

Methylphenidate is a Schedule II drug that has many of the same pharmacologic actions as cocaine and amphetamines. It is sometimes abused by adolescents and adults seeking euphoria, increased alertness, or appetite suppression. Tablets are crushed and snorted or dissolved in liquid and injected IV. Ritalin is sometimes mixed with heroin, a combination called a "speedball." Most Ritalin is obtained by diversion from legal prescriptions, by theft, or by patients selling or sharing their drugs.

Cocaine

Cocaine is a natural substance obtained from leaves of the coca plant, which grows in the Andes Mountains of South America. Natives in this region chew the coca leaves, or make teas of the substance. Much of the cocaine entering the United States comes from Columbia and other South American countries. It was once used as an anesthetic for eye, nose, and throat surgery but is no longer used for this purpose.

Cocaine is a Schedule II drug that produces psychoactive and physiological actions similar to the amphetamines, although its effects can be much more rapid and intense. It is the second most commonly used illicit drug in the United States. Routes of administration include snorting, smoking, inhaling vapors, and injecting. Injection or inhalation of cocaine produces an instantaneous euphoria that lasts 10 to 20 seconds. In small doses, cocaine produces feelings of intense euphoria, a decrease in hunger and pain, illusions of physical strength, and increased sensory perception. Larger doses will increase these effects and cause rapid heartbeat, dysrhythmias, sweating, dilation of the pupils, and an elevated body temperature. The half-life of cocaine is short, 60 to 90 minutes when injected, and tolerance rapidly develops to the pleasurable aspects of the drug. Because of the short half-life, addicts may take cocaine at intervals of 10 to 45 minutes, sometimes for several consecutive days. Unfortunately, tolerance develops slowly to the cardiovascular actions of cocaine. As the abuser escalates the doses to produce a desired level of euphoria, cardiovascular damage may be progressive. Hair analysis can reveal cocaine use for 2 to 6 months after the last dose.

Cocaine readily crosses the placenta to produce marked effects on the fetus. The fetus does not have the hepatic enzymes necessary to metabolize cocaine; thus drug effects are prolonged. Reports of cocaine-related changes include increased risk of miscarriage, preterm labor, low birth weight, and, possibly, birth defects. Newborns have increased irritability, feeding difficulties, and are easily startled.

Adverse effects of cocaine use are essentially the same as amphetamines. Metabolism by the liver forms an active metabolite that is more toxic than cocaine itself. After the feelings of euphoria diminish, the cocaine user may be left with a sense of irritability, exhaustion, insomnia, depression, and extreme distrust. Some users report the sensation that insects are crawling under the skin. Users who snort cocaine develop a runny nose, a crusty redness around the nostrils, and deterioration of the nasal cartilage. Overdose can result in dysrhythmias, seizures, CVA, or death due to respiratory arrest. Psychological dependence often leads to intense craving for the drug.

Caffeine

Caffeine is a natural substance found in the seeds, leaves, or fruits of more than 63 plant species throughout the world. Significant amounts of caffeine are consumed in chocolate, coffee, tea, soft drinks, and ice cream. Caffeine is sometimes added to OTC pain relievers and stimulants because it has been shown to increase the effectiveness of these medications. Caffeine is rapidly distributed to almost all parts of the body after ingestion, and several hours are needed to metabolize and eliminate the drug. Caffeine has a pronounced diuretic effect.

Caffeine is considered a CNS stimulant because it produces increased mental alertness, restlessness, nervousness, irritability, and insomnia. The physical effects of caffeine include dilation of the respiratory passages, increased blood pressure, increased production of stomach acid, and changes in blood glucose levels. Repeated use of caffeine may result in physical dependence and tolerance. Withdrawal symptoms include severe headaches, fatigue, depression, and impaired performance of daily activities.

Nicotine

8.11 Nicotine is a powerful and highly addictive cardiovascular and central nervous system stimulant.

Although nicotine is sometimes considered a CNS stimulant because it enhances alertness, its actions and long-term consequences place it into a class by itself. Nicotine is unique among abused substances in that it is legal, strongly addictive, and highly carcinogenic. Furthermore, tobacco use can cause harmful effects to those in the immediate area due to secondhand smoke. Patients often do not consider tobacco use as substance abuse. It is the most heavily used, legal, addictive drug in the United States, affecting over 29% of the population. Although statistics suggest that tobacco use is declining, over 50% of teens report trying cigarettes.

PharmFACT

In 2006, an estimated 72.9 million Americans aged 12 or older were current users of a tobacco product. This represents 29.6% of the population in that age range. *Source:* Substance Abuse and Mental Health Services Administration, 2007.

The most common method by which nicotine enters the body is through the inhalation of cigarette, pipe, or cigar smoke. Tobacco smoke contains several thousand chemicals, a significant number of which are carcinogens. The primary addictive drug present in cigarette smoke is nicotine, which reaches the brain in only 15 seconds, with effects that last from 30 minutes to several hours. Although nicotine has a half-life of only 2 to 3 hours, it accumulates in the body and is slowly released from the tissues, giving the patient virtually a 24-hour exposure to the drug.

Nicotine affects many body systems, including the nervous, cardiovascular, and endocrine systems. Nicotine promotes the release of epinephrine and has a direct stimulatory effect on the reticular activating system of the brain, causing symptoms that range from increased alertness and ability to focus to feelings of relaxation or light-headedness. The psychoactive effects of smoking are generally described as pleasurable. The cardiovascular effects of nicotine include an accelerated heart rate and increased blood pressure, caused by activation of nicotinic receptors located throughout the autonomic nervous system (see Chapter 16). The cardiovascular effects of nicotine are particularly serious in patients taking oral contraceptives: The risk of a fatal heart attack is five times greater in smokers than in nonsmokers. Muscular tremors may occur with moderate doses of nicotine, and convulsions result from very high doses. Nicotine produces lower body weight by reducing appetite and increasing body metabolism. Chronic use leads to emphysema, heart disease, and lung cancer. There is clear evidence that tobacco use affects the reproductive system. Smokers are much more likely to be infertile, and smoking during pregnancy can cause birth defects and lower birth weight.

Both psychological and physical dependence occur relatively quickly with nicotine. Once started on tobacco, patients tend to continue their drug use for many years, despite overwhelming medical evidence that the quality of their life will be adversely affected and their life span shortened. Furthermore, a large majority of smokers try to quit each year and are unsuccessful and state that they wish they had never started the habit. Only 25% of those who attempt to stop smoking remain tobacco-free 1 year later.

Discontinuation of tobacco results in a withdrawal syndrome that includes agitation, impaired concentration, weight gain, anxiety, headache, and an extreme craving for the drug. The syndrome peaks at 24 to 48 hours after the last dose and may continue over several weeks. Symptoms vary in intensity among patients and are not related to dose or duration of use; those who are light smokers or who have smoked for a shorter length of time do not necessarily have less intense withdrawal symptoms. Approximately 90% of individuals who successfully stop smoking do so without any treatment.

MyNursingKit | Do Nicotine Patches Work?

Nicotine replacement therapy (NRT) is based on the assumption that the blood level of nicotine is what drives people to continue smoking. When blood nicotine levels fall, the person begins to experience early symptoms of withdrawal, which are quickly eliminated by smoking another cigarette. Indeed, blood nicotine levels have clearly been shown to influence smoking behavior. For example, if a smoker is switched to low nicotine cigarettes, he or she will take longer and more frequent puffs. NRT delivery systems include transdermal patches (see Figure 8.3), nasal sprays, and chewing gum that raise serum nicotine levels and help patients to deal with the unpleasant withdrawal symptoms. Tobacco use, however, has a strong psychological component and simply replacing nicotine with patches or gum is ineffective for a large number of patients.

A second approach to encouraging smoking cessation is the use of bupropion (Zyban), a drug classified as an antidepressant. This drug reduces cravings for nicotine and has been found to double the likelihood of becoming tobacco-free if it

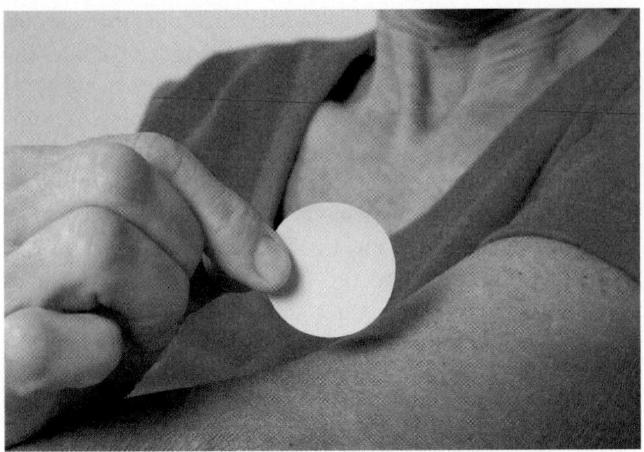

Figure 8.3 Nicotine replacement therapy: transdermal patch.
Source: © T & L/Comet Standard/CORBIS. All Rights Reserved.

is taken for 3 to 6 months. Approximately 44% to 51% of patients will be tobacco-free at week 10 of therapy, compared to 19% of those receiving a placebo. Therapy generally begins 1 to 2 weeks before smoking cessation to lessen the severity of withdrawal symptoms. Bupropion is sometimes given concurrently with NRT. When used for depression, bupropion is marketed by the trade name of Wellbutrin.

In 2006, varenicline (Chantix) was approved to manage nicotine withdrawal in patients seeking smoking cessation. Doses are gradually increased over an 8-day period and maintained for 12 to 24 weeks. Varenicline activates nicotine receptors in the brain to reduce withdrawal symptoms and cravings for smoking. It also blocks nicotine from reaching its receptors, thus blocking some of the pleasurable sensations should the person relapse and start smoking again. Nausea and vomiting are the most common side effects. In 2008, the FDA issued an alert to warn patients of the potential for changes in behavior, agitation, depressed mood, suicidal ideation, and attempted or completed suicide.

Inhalants

8.12 Inhalant abuse occurs when patients breathe the fumes of vaporized substances.

MyNursingKit | The Temptation of Steroids

Inhalants are a diverse group of substances that have in common the ability to vaporize or form a gas at room temperature. Some are already in gaseous form, whereas others are liquids that have the property of volatility—rapid evaporation when exposed to air. Sometimes the liquids are heated to increase the speed or extent of vaporization. Most drugs in this class are placed in a paper or plastic bag or soaked on a cloth and deeply inhaled. Inhaling the fumes is known as huffing.

Inhalants differ greatly in their chemical structures and include nearly any chemical that can be vaporized. Products abused as inhalants include adhesives and glues, aerosols, cleaning agents, solvents, and fuels. These products are readily available and can be purchased at hardware or office supply stores. The highest use of inhalants is found among teens and preteens, probably because these agents can be found in nearly every household. Often, parents are unaware that their children are huffing because they do not understand the symptoms of inhalant abuse or the potential dangers of these household products. Legal anesthetics such as nitrous oxide that are sometimes abused by medical personnel are also classified as inhalants and are presented in Chapter 30.

The inhalation route affords almost instantaneous drug action and, because most of the inhalants are lipid soluble, the substances quickly enter the brain. The specific psychoactive effects depend on the inhalant used but generally include light-headedness, drowsiness, exhilaration, and euphoria. Hallucinations are common. Symptoms of inhalant abuse often resemble alcohol intoxication. Because most psychoactive effects of inhalants are transient and disappear within minutes, the user may repeat the drug use multiple times over a period of several hours. Coma and death are possible with repeated exposure or high doses.

Because most inhalant abuse is sporadic, physical dependence is not observed, and it is unknown whether tolerance develops. Some of the inhalants cause hangover-like symptoms after the psychoactive effects wear off. When chronic abuse does occur, it is generally in adult males. Chronic effects can be serious and permanent, with the most obvious effects on the nervous system. Cognitive impairment, tremors, loss of coordination, hallucinations, psychosis, and dementia may be observed. Nephrotoxicity is common with certain inhalants. The breathing reflex may be diminished and patients may suffocate from placing a plastic bag over their heads.

Treatment for inhalant abuse is symptomatic. Long-term behavioral therapy may be needed to reinforce to the patient that permanent damage will result from chronic, continued abuse.

Anabolic Steroids

8.13 Anabolic steroids are abused for their ability to increase muscle strength.

All of the drugs presented thus far in this chapter have in common the ability to affect the CNS and produce psychoactive effects. Many produce euphoria, some induce relaxation, whereas others enhance alertness. In most cases, the user views the drug experience as pleasurable and the drug effects are experienced soon after it is taken, sometimes within seconds. Anabolic steroids, however, are not taken for their CNS actions and their desirable effects may be delayed for weeks or months. In this respect they are different from other abused substances.

Anabolic steroids are very similar to testosterone, the primary male sex hormone or androgen. The term *anabolic* means "growth" or "building up." Because these substances can add to skeletal muscle mass and increase strength, they are usually abused in an attempt to enhance athletic performance. Do these drugs actually boost performance? The answer is a qualified yes. The most important aspects of athletic performance are skill, training, and confidence. If these factors are equal among performers, anabolic steroids may indeed provide an extra boost in performance. It must be remembered that in some competitive sports such as track, downhill skiing, and swimming, a few hundredths of a second may be the difference between first and sixth place. On the other hand, no amount of steroid is able to overcome lack of athletic skill or inadequate training. Most sports organizations have banned the use of these drugs and athletes may be eliminated from competition if they test positive for anabolic steroids. Some abusers take anabolic steroids to enhance their appearance and self-confidence, rather than for athletic competition.

Anabolic steroids have legitimate medical uses as replacement therapy for men who secrete deficient quantities of testosterone (see Chapter 72) and they are occasionally used to treat certain cancers (see Chapter 58). Doses used by abusers, however, are 10 to 100 times higher than those required for therapeutic use.

Abusers obtain anabolic steroids through diversion from prescription medications or from illicit labs. These drugs may be taken as tablets, as IM injections, or applied as ointments or as a transdermal patch. Abusers may take two or more different types of steroids concurrently, sometimes by different routes, a practice called "stacking." The drugs may be taken in a cyclic pattern called "pyramiding" in which the dose is progressively increased over 6 to 12 weeks, then slowly decreased to zero. Abusers believe that this is a safer and more effective way to obtain benefits from the drugs. The safety and performance-enhancing effects of stacking and pyramiding have not been demonstrated.

One of the ironies of steroid abuse is that the very drug that is being taken to enhance appearance and performance eventually produces serious consequences that have the opposite effect. Men may believe that anabolic steroids make them appear more masculine, but the drugs can cause infertility, impotence, testicular atrophy, and breast enlargement (gynecomastia). Women taking anabolic steroids will develop masculine characteristics, excessive growth of body hair (hirsutism), shrinking of breast size, menstrual irregularities, and deepening of the voice. The most serious adverse effects, in both men and women, include hepatic cysts, elevated cholesterol, myocardial infarction, and CVA. Personality changes include aggression, violent behavior, depression, insomnia, anorexia, and decreased libido.

Anabolic steroids are classified as Schedule II drugs due to their abuse potential. In an attempt to stem the rising abuse of these drugs, Congress passed the Anabolic Steroid Control Act of 2004 to control 26 different steroid precursors, such as androstenedione (Andro). Some companies were legally selling these precursors as dietary supplements, despite the fact that these agents are metabolized to steroids in the body and essentially carry the same risks. It is interesting to note that one of the most popular supplements, dehydroepiandrosterone (DHEA), was specifically and intentionally omitted from that list and remains legal. DHEA is a natural steroid precursor secreted by the adrenal gland that is claimed to have "antiaging" and performance-enhancing properties. Some believe that the exclusion was due to powerful lobbying from the dietary supplement industry, whereas others claim that DHEA is safer than other steroid precursors.

8.14 The nurse has a pivotal role in recognizing and treating substance abuse.

The nurse serves a key role in the prevention, diagnosis, and treatment of substance abuse. A thorough medical history must include questions about substance abuse. In the case of IV drug users, the nurse must consider the possibility of HIV infection, hepatitis, tuberculosis, and associated diagnoses. Patients are often reluctant to report their drug use for fear of embarrassment or being arrested. The nurse must be knowledgeable about the signs and symptoms of substance abuse and develop a keen sense of perception during the assessment process. A trusting nurse–patient relationship is essential to helping patients deal with their dependence.

It is often difficult for a practitioner not to condemn or stigmatize a patient for his or her substance abuse. Nurses, especially those in large cities, are all too familiar with the devastating medical, economic, and social consequences of drug abuse. The nurse must be firm in disapproving substance abuse, yet compassionate in trying to help the patient receive treatment. A list of social agencies dealing with dependency should be readily available to provide to patients. Whenever possible, the nurse should attempt to involve family members and other close contacts in the treatment regimen.

UNDERSTANDING THE CHAPTER

Key Concepts Summary

8.1 A wide variety of different substances may be abused by patients.

8.2 Drugs with a potential for abuse are restricted by the Controlled Substances Act and are categorized into schedules.

8.3 Addiction is an overwhelming compulsion to continue repeated drug use.

8.4 Physical and psychological dependence lead to continued drug-seeking behavior despite negative health and social consequences.

8.5 The withdrawal syndrome is a set of characteristic symptoms that occurs when an abused substance is discontinued.

8.6 Tolerance occurs when the body adapts to a drug and larger doses are needed to produce a therapeutic effect.

8.7 Central nervous system depressants, which include sedatives, opioids, and alcohol, decrease the activity of the central nervous system.

8.8 Marijuana is the most frequently abused illicit substance.

8.9 Hallucinogens and club drugs cause an altered state of thought and perception.

8.10 Stimulants such as amphetamines and cocaine increase the activity of the central nervous system.

8.11 Nicotine is a powerful and highly addictive cardiovascular and central nervous system stimulant.

8.12 Inhalant abuse occurs when patients breathe the fumes of vaporized substances.

8.13 Anabolic steroids are abused for their ability to increase muscle strength.

8.14 The nurse has a pivotal role in recognizing and treating substance abuse.

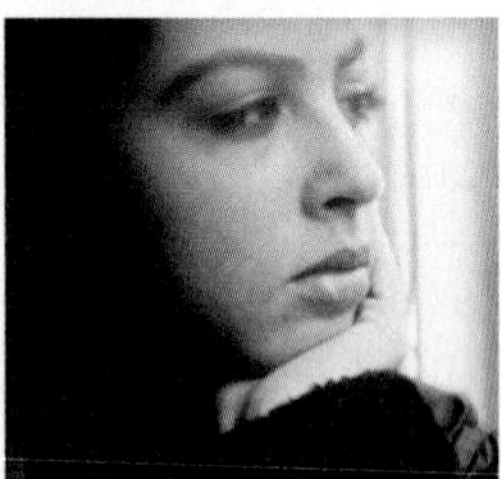

Making the PATIENT *Connection*

Remember the patient "J. C. Wilkins" at the beginning of the chapter? Now read the remainder of the case study. Based on the information presented within this chapter, respond to the critical thinking questions that follow.

J. C. Wilkins has come to the counseling clinic to get information and advice about her pregnancy and drug use. She is a 19-year-old woman who has been living with her boyfriend for the past 18 months. Since she moved in, she has been a daily user of heroin.

J. C. has a long history of substance abuse. When she was 14 years old, her stepfather sexually abused her on a regular basis. To cope with the guilt and shame, J. C. began using alcohol and marijuana. On her 16th birthday, J. C. ran away from home and never returned. Since then she has done anything and everything possible to survive, including selling herself for sex.

To support herself and her heroin addiction, J. C. has become a prostitute. She states that she usually drinks at least 4 to 5 beers before she walks the streets at night. If she cannot score enough heroin, she will smoke crack or take Valium just to "mellow out." J. C. says that her drug abuse is only to calm her nerves and get her through the night. In periods when she was not able to obtain drugs, she states she felt sick with trembling and perfuse sweating. However, she is convinced that she can stop any time she wishes.

J. C. reports that she has not had a menstrual period in 2 months and her breasts are swollen and tender. She is certain she is pregnant, although she has not been tested, and is confused about what to do. She is hopeful that her unemployed boyfriend is the father but is not totally sure. She believes that if she stops working he will abandon her and there will be no means to support herself or a baby.

Critical Thinking Questions

1. How would you classify J. C.'s substance abuse? Physical dependence or psychological dependence, or both? Explain.
2. Create a list of abuse substances reported by J. C. What symptoms of withdrawal would you expect with each?
3. What effect will J. C.'s substance abuse have on her unborn baby? Should J. C. stop using drugs while pregnant? Why or why not?
4. As the nurse, describe your approach in dealing with this patient.
5. Addiction depends on multiple variables such as drug factors, user factors, and environmental factors. Considering the case study, describe how each variable attributes to J. C.'s substance abuse.

Case Study

A neighbor reports that patient Martin Thomas was discovered wandering the halls in his apartment building in a confused state. The neighbor states that Martin called him by the wrong name even though they have known each other for several years. Martin was agitated about not being able to find the bus stop. In the emergency department, Martin appears apprehensive, diaphoretic, and trembling. His nose and cheeks are red with spider veins, and his abdomen is noticeably distended. He tells you that up until 3 days ago, he consumed alcohol daily. However, because he has no money, he cannot buy any liquor and has not been drinking.

1. Define *delirium tremens*. What is the treatment priority for this condition?
2. Discuss how food or beverages can increase the excretion rate of alcohol.
3. Describe the effects of alcohol on the central nervous system. Is alcohol a stimulant or a depressant?

NCLEX-RN® Review

1 The client returned from major surgery 3 hours ago and requests medication for pain. In considering the best action for this client, the nurse knows that:

1. Prescription drugs rarely cause addiction when used according to accepted medical protocol.
2. All drugs should be withheld until the client's past substance abuse history is evaluated.
3. It is best to wait until the client can no longer tolerate the pain to avoid addiction problems.
4. Clients often request analgesia when it is not really needed.

2 Which of the following statements made by the recovering substance abuse client would indicate high potential for relapse?

1. "I need the help of a support system to stop using."
2. "After I stop using, I will no longer have a desire to use drugs."
3. "Who I hang out with doesn't make any difference in whether or not I use drugs."
4. "Talking with other recovering addicts will help me cope."

3 A nurse monitoring the client for drug tachyphylaxis would watch for the development of which of the following?

1. Slow onset of psychological dependence
2. Prompt reversal of all narcotic agents
3. Gradual activation of psychological dependence
4. Rapid development of drug tolerance

4 Which of the following assessment parameters is most critical when a nurse is observing a client with an overdose of sedatives?

1. Cardiac stimulation
2. Respiratory suppression
3. Hepatic dysfunction
4. Depression of consciousness

5 A 22-year-old heroin addict is exhibiting withdrawal symptoms. Which of the following are symptoms of withdrawal that the nurse expects?

1. Somnolence, lethargy, and fatigue
2. Dry skin, rash, and itching
3. Paranoia, hallucinations, and delusions
4. Chills, runny nose, and muscle spasms

6 Disulfiram (Antabuse) is prescribed for the client. While teaching the client about this drug, the nurse should instruct the client to avoid:

1. Mouthwash, alcoholic beverages, and over-the-counter cold medications.
2. Dairy products such as milk, cream, and yogurt.
3. Foods high in iron such as green leafy vegetables.
4. Driving or operating machinery while taking this medication.

See Answers to Critical Thinking Questions, Case Study, and NCLEX-RN® Review in Appendix A.

References

American Psychological Association. (2000). *Diagnostic and statistical manual of mental disorders* (4th ed., Text Revision). Washington, DC: Author.

Anstey, K. J., Christensen, H., & Low, L. (2006). Prevalence, risk factors and treatment for substance abuse in older adults. *Current Opinion Psychiatry, 19*(6), 587–592.

Barangan, C. J., & Alderman, E. M. (2002). Management of substance abuse. *Pediatric Review, 23*(4), 123–131.

Bryner, J. K., Wang, U. K., Hui, J. W., Bedobo, M., MacDougall, C., & Anderson, I. B. (2006). Dextromethorphan abuse in adolescence. An increasing trend: 1999–2004. *Archives of Pediatrics & Adolescent Medicine, 60,* 1217–1222.

Chychula, N. M., & Sciamanna, C. (2002). Help substance abusers attain and sustain abstinence. *Nurse Practitioner, 27*(11), 30–47.

Fraschini, F., Demartini, G., & Esposti, D. (2002). Pharmacology of silymarin. *Clinical Drug Investigation, 22*(1), 51–65.

Freese, T. E., Miotto, K., & Reback, C. J. (2002). The effects and consequences of selected club drugs. *Journal of Substance Abuse Treatment, 23*(2), 151–156.

Gable, R. (2006). The toxicity of recreational drugs. *American Scientist, 94*(3), 206.

Goff, M. (2007). Perinatal care of women maintained on methadone. *Journal of Midwifery & Women's Health, 52*(3), e23–e26.

Hardie, T. L. (2002). The genetics of substance abuse. *AACN Clinical Issues, 13*(4), 511–522.

Kandel, D. B. (2003). Does marijuana use cause the use of other drugs? *Journal of the American Medical Association, 289*(4), 482–483.

Loth, C. (2007). Enhancing the quality of nursing care in methadone substitute clinics using action research: A process evaluation. *Journal of Advanced Nursing, 57*(4), 422–431.

Mann, K. (2004). Pharmacotherapy of alcohol dependence: A review of the clinical data. *CNS Drugs, 18*(8), 485–504.

McGuinness, T. (2006). Emergency methamphetamine abuse. *American Journal of Nursing, 106*(12), 54–59.

McKim, W. A. (2007). *Drugs and behavior: An introduction to behavioral pharmacology* (6th ed.). Upper Saddle River, NJ: Prentice Hall.

Naegle, M. A., & D'Avanzo, C. E. (2001). *Addictions and substance abuse: Strategies for advanced practice nursing.* Upper Saddle River, NJ: Prentice Hall.

National Institute of Drug Abuse. (2007). *NIDA InfoFacts: Science-based facts on drug abuse and addiction.* Retrieved April 18, 2008, from http://www.nida.nih.gov/Infofacts/Infofaxindex.html

Pirskanen, M. (2007). A formative evaluation to develop a school health nursing early intervention model for adolescent substance use. *Public Health Nursing, 24*(3), 256–264.

Schuckit, M. A. (2006). *Drug and alcohol abuse: A clinical guide to diagnosis and treatment* (6th ed.). New York: Springer.

Song, Z., Deaciuc, I., Song, M., Lee, D. Y., Liu, Y., Ji, X., et al. (2006). Silymarin protects against acute ethanol-induced hepatotoxicity in mice. *Alcoholism, Clinical and Experimental Research, 30*(3), 407–413.

Substance Abuse and Mental Health Services Administration. (2007). *Results from the 2006 national survey on drug use and health; National findings* (Office of Applied Studies, NSDUH Series H-32, DHHS Publication No. SMA 07-4293). Rockville, MD. Retrieved April 28, 2008, from http://www.drugabusestatistics.samhsa.gov/NSDUH/2k6NSDUH/2k6results.cfm#Ch2

Tuttle, J., Melnyk, B. M., & Loveland-Cherry, C. (2002). Adolescent drug and alcohol use. Strategies for assessment, intervention, and prevention. *Nursing Clinics of North America, 37*(3), 443–460.

Van Hook, S. (2007). The six T's barrier to screening teens for substance abuse in primary care. *Journal of Adolescent Health, 40*(5), 456–461.

Vega, C. (2007). Stimulant abuse may increase stroke among young adults. *Medscape Medical News.* Retrieved April 28, 2008, from http://www.medscape.com/viewarticle/555229

UNIT 2

Pharmacology and the Nurse–Patient Relationship

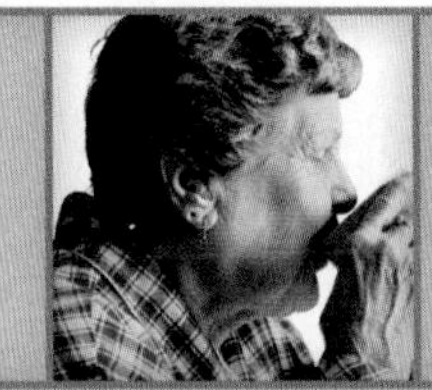
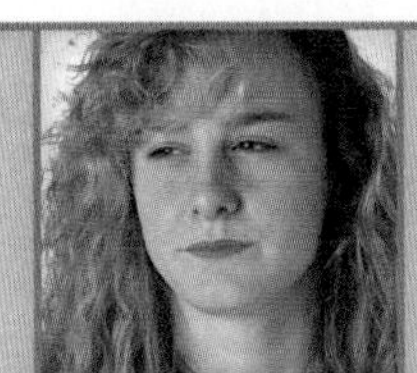
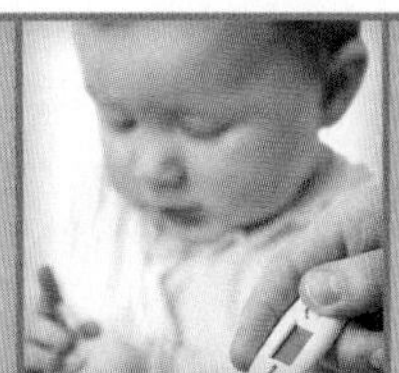
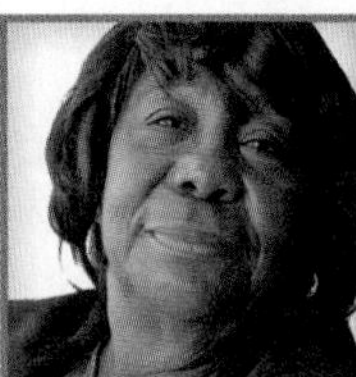

CHAPTER 9 Pharmacology and the Nursing Process

CHAPTER 10 Pharmacotherapy During Pregnancy and Lactation

CHAPTER 11 Pharmacotherapy of the Pediatric Patient

CHAPTER 12 Pharmacotherapy of the Geriatric Patient

CHAPTER 13 Psychosocial, Gender, and Cultural Influences on Pharmacotherapy

CHAPTER 14 Pharmacotherapy in the Community

CHAPTER 15 The Role of Complementary and Alternative Therapies in Pharmacotherapy

CHAPTER

I woke up twice last night because I was having trouble breathing; I remembered to take all my medicine, but this morning my feet and ankles are swollen, and I just feel so tired.

Patient "Mary Richards"

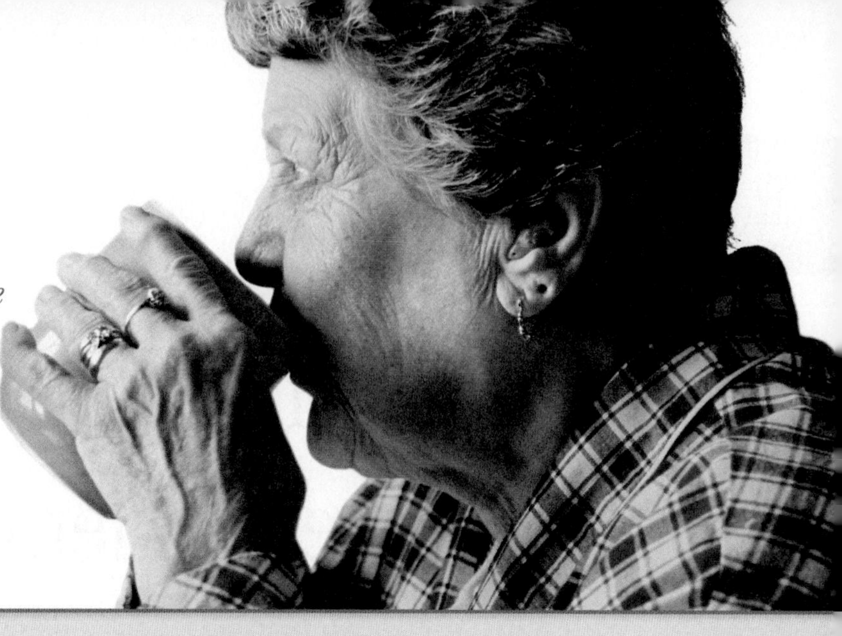

9 Pharmacology and the Nursing Process

Learning Outcomes

After reading this chapter, the student should be able to:

1. Compare and contrast the different phases of the nursing process.
2. Describe how the nursing process is used in pharmacology.
3. Identify the purposes of collecting data in the assessment phase of the nursing process.
4. Explain how nursing diagnoses are identified and worded.
5. Describe the steps in the planning phase of the nursing process.
6. Identify specific pharmacology topics employed in the implementation phase of the nursing process.
7. Explain the purpose of the evaluation phase in the nursing process.
8. Explain what actions follow the evaluation phase of the nursing process.

Chapter Outline

Assessment

Diagnosis

Planning

Implementation

Evaluation

Key Terms

assessment, 115
etiologies, 115
evaluation, 119
evaluation criteria, 117
evidence-based nursing practice, 117
goal, 117
implementation, 118
interventions, 116
nursing diagnosis, 115
nursing process, 115
outcome, 117
planning, 117

The **nursing process** is a systematic, rational method of planning and providing nursing care (Berman, Snyder, Kozier, & Erb, 2008). Its purpose is to identify a patient's actual or potential health problems, to establish plans to meet the identified needs, to deliver specific nursing interventions to address those needs, and to evaluate the success of those interventions. The nursing process follows a logical sequence, but several components may be involved simultaneously. If the established goals are achieved at the end of the first cycle, care may be terminated; or the cycle may continue with reassessment and modification of the plan of care. Pharmacotherapy is often integrated into the phases of the nursing process with the goals of enhancing therapeutic drug effects and minimizing or preventing adverse drug events. Use of the nursing process also helps ensure safe self-administration of medications through the provision of patient drug teaching.

The nursing process is an ongoing activity involving five distinct phases: assessment, diagnosis, planning, implementation, and evaluation (ADPIE). In this chapter, each phase is briefly reviewed, and each phase's use in pharmacology is emphasized. A summary of the phases is shown in Figure 9.1.

Assessment

9.1 The first phase of the nursing process is the assessment phase.

The **assessment** phase of the nursing process is the systematic collection, organization, validation, and documentation of patient data. The assessment phase serves two purposes. The first is to gather data that will enable the nurse to identify current patient health challenges and problems that the patient is at particular risk for developing. These data are used in developing nursing diagnoses and the plan of care.

The second purpose of the assessment phase is to gather initial baseline data on the patient that will be compared to subsequent data during the evaluation phase of the nursing process. These comparisons will indicate to what extent the treatment goals have been achieved. When applying the nursing process to pharmacology, baseline data are necessary for the nurse to be able to evaluate therapeutic drug effects, adverse drug effects, and the capacity for self-care. For example, a common adverse effect of many antibiotics is the risk for allergic reaction, often identified by a skin rash. To determine that the rash was due to a particular drug, the nurse must first have assessed that a rash was not present prior to initiating drug therapy. As another example, if a patient is exhibiting elevated liver enzymes during hospitalization, the nurse will use the baseline assessment data to determine whether the patient had this condition on admission, or whether it may be a sign of a recent adverse drug event.

Data collected in the assessment phase can come from many sources. These include the patient, caregivers, medical records, and other health care professionals. Subjective data include what the patient says or perceives, such as pain, anxiety, or nausea. Whenever possible, the subjective data are verified by objective data that were gathered through physical examination, medical history, laboratory tests, and other diagnostic sources.

Assessment must always include a comprehensive medical history that includes use of prescription drugs, over-the-counter (OTC) agents, dietary supplements, and herbal products. The nurse should inquire about tobacco and alcohol use, as well as past or current history of drug abuse because these may influence treatment outcomes. Any allergic or unusual reactions to drugs should be documented, including serious drug events that may have occurred to close family members.

The medical history gathered during the assessment phase is used to determine whether the patient has a contraindication that would present a risk for drug therapy. For example, the nurse may discover during assessment that the patient is pregnant and should not receive isotretinoin (Accutane) for acne because it is a pregnancy category X drug. During assessment a drug history may reveal that a patient is taking nitroglycerin, which should never be taken concurrently with vardenafil (Levitra), a drug for erectile dysfunction. The nurse may discover that the patient has a history of allergy to penicillin and should not be prescribed ampicillin due to the potential for cross-allergy. A thorough assessment is the best way to prevent adverse drug effects.

> **CONNECTION *Checkpoint* 9.1**
>
> A nurse administers a drug to a patient who has a contraindication for the medication. From what you learned in Chapter 7, is this considered a medication error? See Answer to Connection Checkpoint 9.1 in Appendix A.

Diagnosis

9.2 Nursing diagnoses are based on the data gathered in the assessment phase.

During the diagnosis phase of the nursing process, the nurse analyzes assessment data, identifies health problems, and formulates diagnostic statements. A **nursing diagnosis** is a clinical judgment of an actual or potential health problem of the patient that is within the nurse's scope of practice to address.

Nursing diagnoses differ from medical diagnoses, which are determined by physicians. Whereas the medical diagnosis remains constant during a patient's hospital stay, nursing diagnoses are in constant flux as the patient responds to treatments. Nursing diagnoses address changes in the patient's condition; for example, impaired mobility, nutritional intake, urinary elimination, knowledge, ability for self-care, and risk for injury. These nursing diagnoses are used to set goals and plan care.

Nursing diagnoses are often stated as a problem, or the risk for a problem, followed by "related to," which identifies the **etiologies,** or those conditions that have caused or contributed to the problem. By altering one or more of these etiologies, nurses are able to effect improvements in the diagnosed problem. This is

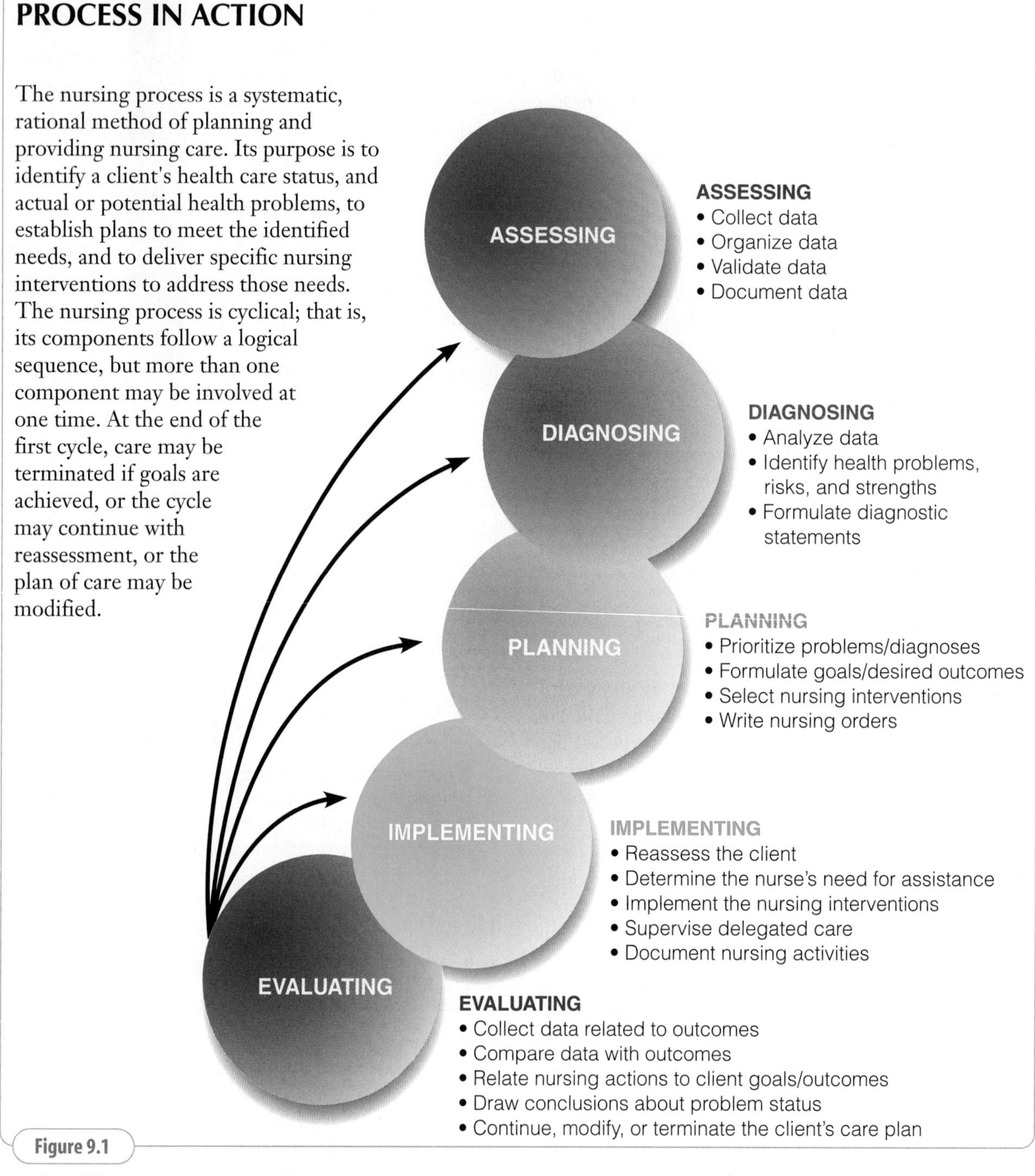

Figure 9.1

The nursing process in action.

Source: From *Kozier and Erb's Fundamentals of Nursing: Concepts, Process, and Practice* (8th ed.), by A. Berman, S. Snyder, B. Kozier, and G. Erb, 2008, Upper Saddle River, NJ: Pearson Education, Inc.

accomplished by planning and implementing **interventions,** which are actions that the nurse takes to achieve the patient goals. The nurse chooses interventions that are patient focused and target the etiologies of the problem. For example, a nursing diagnosis may be *Activity Intolerance,* related to acute knee pain. The nurse designs interventions to address the etiology (acute knee pain) that may include the administration of pain medications, heat, or ice packs.

Nursing diagnoses are prioritized by their level of importance and immediacy to the patient's clinical condition. For example, alterations in breathing would likely take precedence over the potential for skin breakdown. A primary nursing role is to enable patients to become active participants in their own care. Patients need to vocalize, to the extent possible, their priorities for care, which should be considered by the nurse when diagnoses are prioritized. By including patients when identifying needs, the nurse encourages them to take a more active role in working toward meeting the identified goals.

The North American Nursing Diagnosis Association (NANDA) has developed standard wording for identifying actual and potential patient health problems. With its Taxonomy II (NANDA, 2001), these diagnoses have become more precise. For example, instead of stating a diagnosis as "alteration in nutrition," the more precise wording has been changed to *Nutrition Imbalance: More than Body Requirements*, or *Nutrition Imbalance, Less than Body Requirements.* The American Nurses Association (ANA, 2007) has formally recognized the use of the language proposed by NANDA, Nursing Intervention Classification (NIC), and Nursing Outcome Classification (NOC). NANDA International continues to add new diagnoses and continues to revise existing nursing diagnoses, and these are now being used in many countries around the world (NANDA International, 2008).

The problem statement, also called the diagnostic label, needs to be specific. When a NANDA label is followed by the word *Specify*, the area in which the problem occurs must be included. An example would be *Deficient Knowledge (Medications).*

When applied to pharmacotherapy, the diagnosis phase of the nursing process addresses three main areas of concern.

- Promoting therapeutic drug effects
- Minimizing adverse drug effects and toxicity
- Maximizing the ability of the patient for self-care, including the knowledge, skills, and resources necessary for safe and effective drug administration

Patient teaching is one of the basic roles of nursing, and careful attention to drug teaching can promote therapeutic outcomes as well as minimize adverse effects. Examples of nursing diagnoses that intimately involve drug teaching include *Deficient Knowledge*, related to new drug therapy and *Noncompliance with Pharmacotherapy*, related to adverse effects. Patient teaching is discussed further in the planning phase. See Table 9.1 for selected nursing diagnoses for pharmacotherapy. For a complete list, the student should refer to a nursing fundamentals textbook.

TABLE 9.1 Nursing Diagnoses in Pharmacotherapy
Acute Confusion, related to drug effects
Disturbed Sensory Perception (Visual), related to drug effects
Deficient Fluid Volume, related to drug effects
Excess Fluid Volume, related to drug effects
Noncompliance (Drug Therapy), related to lack of knowledge
Risk for Infection, related to adverse drug effects
Risk for Injury, related to drug effects
Disturbed Sleep Pattern, related to drug effects
Imbalanced Nutrition, Less than Body Requirements, related to drug-induced nausea
Ineffective Health Maintenance, related to knowledge deficit
Activity Intolerance, related to drug effects
Deficient Knowledge, related to new drug therapy

Note: From *NANDA: Nursing Diagnoses: Definitions & Classification 2007–2008*, by North American Nursing Diagnosis Association, 2008, Philadelphia: Author.

Planning

9.3 In the planning phase, the nurse creates an individualized plan of care for a patient, based on the identified nursing diagnoses and etiologies.

After a nursing diagnosis has been established, the nurse begins to plan ways to assist the patient to return to, or maintain an optimum level of wellness as defined by that diagnosis. The **planning** phase of the nursing process prioritizes diagnoses, formulates desired outcomes, and selects nursing interventions.

There are two main steps of the planning phase. The first step is to identify the desired **goal,** or **outcome,** to be achieved, and the specific **evaluation criteria** that will be used to determine if that goal has been met. The outcome may be a short-term or a long-term goal, should include the time frame whenever possible, and must be realistic for the patient to achieve. The evaluation criteria should be specific and measurable. These criteria are often indicated by AEB (as evidenced by). The outcome should directly address the problem identified in the nursing diagnosis. For example, if the nursing diagnosis is *Risk for Constipation,* related to opioid analgesic use, a goal might be: the absence of constipation, as evidenced by (AEB) regular bowel evacuation, absence of difficulty passing stool, and absence of abdominal bloating or discomfort. Notice how this plan includes a clear goal as well as specific evaluation criteria.

The second step of the planning phase is to develop a list of interventions. The interventions are specific nursing actions designed to help move the patient toward the desired goal. These interventions should not include assessment or monitoring activities. Although it is important to assess and monitor, these activities belong in the assessment or evaluation phases.

Basing nursing practice, especially interventions, on research evidence is an important concept that has been added to the nursing process. By doing this, **evidence-based nursing practice** is promoted. Care decisions are made by evaluating the quality of existing research, patient preferences, costs, clinical expertise of the nurse, and clinical setting characteristics.

The interventions that make up the plan of care should be tailored to the individual patient. Interventions may be classified as follows:

- Independent: those the nurse can implement autonomously based on knowledge, experience, and the nurse's scope of practice
- Dependent: those ordered by another medical discipline
- Interdependent: those done collaboratively with other medical disciplines

When planning interventions the nurse should consider the specific health problem and etiologies, current practice guidelines, the evidence basis for the intervention, acceptability to the patient, and the nurse's own capabilities. In addition, the chosen nursing interventions should be safe and appropriate for the patient's age, health, and condition, congruent with the patient's values, beliefs, and culture, and appropriate to the other ordered therapies (Berman et al., 2008). The choice of nursing interventions will also depend on what is realistic and practical to the situation in terms of equipment availability, financial status of the patient, and available resources, including staff, agency, family, or community resources (LeMone & Burke, 2008). NIC "priority interventions" are research-based actions that are considered the treatments of choice for a particular diagnosis (Wilkinson, 2009).

With respect to pharmacotherapy, the planning phase involves two main issues: drug administration and patient teaching. For the first issue, the nurse must plan how and when to administer the drug. For oral medication, does it need to be given with food or on an empty stomach? Is it more effective if administered at a certain time of day? Can it be crushed or split? For intravenous (IV) medication, does it need to be diluted and, if so, with how much of what type of solution? Over how much time should it be given? Is it compatible with other substances in the IV line? For all medications, the nurse will plan interventions to enhance therapeutic outcomes and minimize or prevent adverse drug effects.

When planning patient drug teaching, the amount and type of teaching provided by the nurse are determined by the projected length of pharmacotherapy. Is the drug to be given for a short time during an acute care hospitalization, or is pharmacotherapy going to be long term and self-administered following discharge? If a drug is to be given short term, the patient should be told the name of the drug, its basic actions, why the patient is receiving it, and some of the most common and major adverse effects, including any that should be promptly reported to the nurse or health care provider.

For drugs that will be taken after discharge, patient teaching should be more comprehensive and be provided both orally and in writing. This teaching should include the drug name (both generic and trade), the drug class and its major effects, why the drug is being prescribed, the therapeutic effects and when they should occur, how and when to take the drug, common and major adverse effects and which ones should be reported to the prescriber, the types of follow-up monitoring needed, potential drug interactions, the duration of drug therapy, activities to avoid while taking the drug, and what to do if a dose is missed or forgotten. Refer to Chapter 14 for more information on patient teaching in community settings.

Implementation

9.4 The implementation phase puts the plan of care into action.

The **implementation** phase is when the nurse applies the knowledge, skills, and principles of nursing care to help move the patient toward the desired goal and optimal wellness. Implementation involves action on the part of the nurse or patient: administering a drug, providing patient teaching, and initiating other specific actions identified by the nursing diagnoses and plan of care. When applied to pharmacotherapy, the implementation phase involves administering the drug and carrying out the interventions developed in the planning phase to maximize a therapeutic response and prevent adverse events.

It must be remembered that implementation of the plan of care is subject to modification, based on the patient's evolving condition. In implementing pharmacotherapy, an important decision that must be made by the nurse is if it is appropriate to administer the drug at the planned time. To make this decision, the nurse needs to understand the drug's therapeutic and adverse effects well enough to know the circumstances under which it is appropriate, or not appropriate, to give the drug. After assessing a current vital sign, laboratory result, new health problem, or physical assessment finding, it may be appropriate for the nurse to not administer an ordered drug. For example, if the patient's current serum potassium level is below the normal range, and the nurse has an order to administer furosemide (Lasix) by IV push, it would be an error for the nurse to administer the drug. Carrying out the order would cause serum potassium to fall, which could trigger cardiac dysrhythmias. Likewise, a patient who has a scheduled dose of morphine for pain relief but currently has a respiratory rate of less than 8 should not receive the drug because it may cause respiratory failure.

As pharmacotherapy progresses, the nurse must be aware of circumstances that might require modification of the implementation phase. The patient may develop new symptoms that

CONNECTIONS

Lifespan Considerations Teaching Throughout the Life Span

Patient teaching is an essential component of the nursing process. To be effective, oral and written teaching must be age appropriate. The following are some tips for effective teaching.

Children

- Use family-centered approaches when providing drug teaching for children and adolescents.
- Engage young children and toddlers by using interactive strategies.
- Use simple, nonthreatening language.
- Provide a developmentally appropriate environment when teaching adolescents.
- Encourage problem solving to help adolescents make choices.

Adults

- Adult learners are independent; the nurse should facilitate learning.
- Adults learn best when the topic is of immediate value, and new material is connected to previous experiences.
- Adults vary widely in their learning styles and preferences; learning is enhanced when these things are considered.
- Consider the literacy level of learners; it is recommended that written materials be on a fifth-grade reading level.
- Employ multiple methods of delivering information; combinations of verbal and written material are beneficial.

Older Adults

- Time needed for learning often increases; plan several, short learning sessions; repeat and review material covered.
- Relate new learning to the patient's actual experiences.
- Provide printed material, videotapes, or pictures or diagrams that the patient can refer to at a later time.
- Modify teaching methods to sensory-perceptual deficits or cognitive decline. Ensure that the patient has the necessary aids (glasses, magnifying glass, hearing aid) to maximize learning experience.
- Offer opportunities for practice of psychomotor skills.

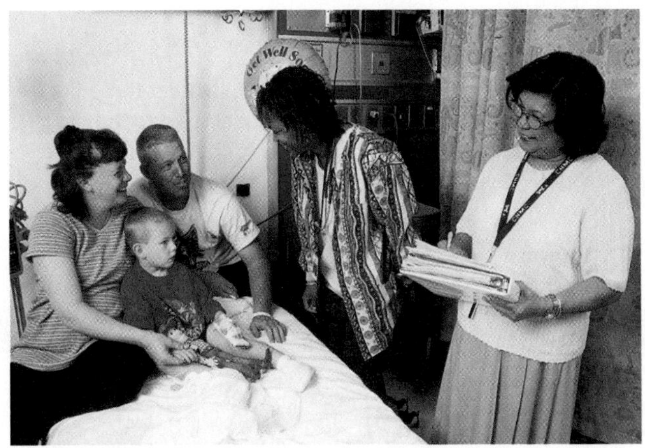

Figure 9.2 Effective patient teaching is a vital component of the nursing process.

contraindicate the use of the drug being administered. For example, the patient may begin to show signs of a developing rash, changes in blood pressure, or alterations in mental status that call for discontinuation of the drug. These examples help illustrate the cyclic nature of the nursing process: the importance of continuous assessment and the revision of the planning and implementation phases.

Implementation also includes providing patient teaching (Figure 9.2). Patient drug teaching should start with what the patient already knows about a drug and build from there. The specific topics to include in this teaching are developed in the planning phase. When preparing to carry out the teaching, other factors that the nurse should consider are the patient's readiness to learn, and whether or not it is an appropriate time for teaching. Patients who are in pain, sleepy, anxious, or distracted are less likely to understand instructions. Drug teaching should be tailored to the patient's developmental level, learning capacity, and preferred learning style. Patients may prefer that a family member or caregiver be present for the teaching. This is especially important for pediatric patients, elderly adults with cognitive deficits, and patients with mental illnesses who may be incapable of safe self-administration. The patient teaching is sometimes a collaborative effort, requiring coordination with other medical disciplines as part of the sessions. Often a registered dietician, physical therapist, or diabetic educator collaborates with the patient teaching. When teaching, sufficient time must always be allotted to address any areas of concern for the patient.

Finally, documentation is an essential part of the implementation phase. This includes a thorough reporting of the interventions carried out, the drugs that were given (or withheld), the teaching that took place, and the patient's responses to the interventions.

Evaluation

9.5 In the evaluation phase, the nurse obtains data to determine if the goal or outcome has been achieved.

The **evaluation** phase compares the patient's current health status with the desired outcome to determine if the plan of care is appropriate or if it needs revision. The evaluation phase is used to determine if the goal/outcome has been met. If it has been met, the plan of care was appropriate, and the problem or risk has been resolved. The next highest priority problem can then be addressed. If the goal was partially met, the patient is moving toward the goal, but the interventions may need to be continued for a longer time or somehow modified to completely resolve the problem.

As it relates to pharmacotherapy, evaluation is used to determine whether the therapeutic effects of the drug have been achieved, as well as whether adverse effects have been prevented or kept to acceptable levels. If the evaluation data show no improvement over the baseline data, the interventions may require revision. The drug dose may need to be increased, more time may be needed to achieve therapeutic drug levels, a different or additional drug may be needed, or other changes in nursing interventions may be necessary. The data gathered on the evaluation criteria form part of the assessment data for a continuation of the process as outcomes and interventions are revised or reformulated. These evaluation data need to be documented in the client's record to ensure proper communication of the client's response to the nursing interventions.

In an outpatient setting, lack of drug response determined during the evaluation phase may be caused by patient nonadherence to the drug regimen. During the assessment phase, the nurse

CONNECTIONS

Treating the Diverse Patient **Providing Culturally Appropriate Teaching**

Effective teaching requires the nurse to be sensitive and respect ethnic and cultural diversity. The following are some multicultural patient teaching considerations.

- Show respect; acknowledge racial and ethnic differences.
- Assess the patient for the influence of cultural health beliefs, norms, and values.
- Provide information in the patient's native language for those with limited English proficiency; arrange for the presence of a translator for teaching sessions.
- Assess for cultural and ethnic self-care practices that may interact with medications or treatment, such as folk or home remedies and dietary practices.
- Consider possible differences in family structure and decision making for health care concerns.

must determine if the patient is taking the drug as prescribed. If nonadherence is discovered, the nurse must plan and implement strategies for increasing adherence. This always includes addressing the reasons for nonadherence. Additional patient teaching is important to obtaining maximum adherence: The nurse must help the patient to value pharmacotherapy as important to health improvement.

CONNECTION Checkpoint 9.2

From what you learned in Chapter 3, identify three factors that may prompt a patient to not adhere to the drug therapy regimen prescribed by the health care provider. See Answer to Connection Checkpoint 9.2 in Appendix A.

UNDERSTANDING THE CHAPTER

Key Concepts Summary

9.1 The first phase of the nursing process is the assessment phase.

9.2 Nursing diagnoses are based on the data gathered in the assessment phase.

9.3 In the planning phase, the nurse creates an individualized plan of care for a patient, based on the identified nursing diagnoses and etiologies.

9.4 The implementation phase puts the plan of care into action.

9.5 In the evaluation phase, the nurse obtains data to determine if the goal or outcome has been achieved.

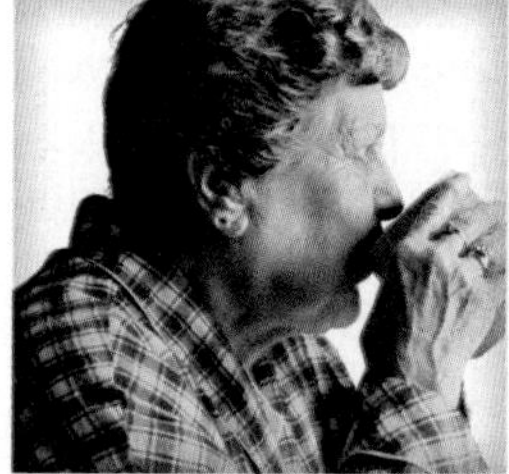

Making the PATIENT Connection

Remember the patient "Mary Richards" at the beginning of the chapter? Now read the remainder of the case study. Based on the information presented within this chapter, respond to the critical thinking questions that follow.

Mary Richards, who is 70 years old, sees her health care provider later that morning, who diagnoses her with an acute exacerbation of heart failure. She is sent to the local hospital's progressive care unit.

The nurse preparing for the admission of Ms. Richards turns to the nursing process to organize and develop a plan of care. Once the patient arrives, the nurse completes a patient history, including a complete drug history, noting the patient's current medications as well as OTC drugs and herbal remedies, and any drug allergies. Information about the patient's current problems is obtained, and a complete physical assessment is performed. This assessment reveals the following: blood pressure, 150/92 mmHg; heart rate, 96, regular; 2+ to 3+ dependent, pitting edema bilateral feet and ankles; bibasilar lung crackles anteriorly and posteriorly; weight, 70.8 kg (156 lb) (usual weight, 64.4 kg (142 lb)).

The nurse reports these findings to the prescriber and receives the following order: furosemide (Lasix) 40 mg by IV push, times one, now. The nurse knows that furosemide is a potent diuretic that acts in the loop of Henle to prevent reabsorption of sodium and chloride, and as these are being flushed out in the urine, water follows. This results in profound diuresis as well as loss of potassium. The nurse also knows that furosemide carries the risk for dehydration, ototoxicity with hearing loss, and allergic reaction.

Critical Thinking Questions

1. Identify a nursing diagnosis, the goal, evaluation criteria, nursing interventions, and evaluations to promote the therapeutic effects of this patient's drug therapy.
2. Identify a nursing diagnosis, the goal, evaluation criteria, nursing interventions, and evaluations to minimize adverse drug effects of this patient's drug therapy.
3. The patient is now being prepared for discharge and is to continue taking furosemide 20 mg/day by mouth at home. Identify a nursing diagnosis, the goal, evaluation criteria, nursing interventions, and evaluations to provide patient drug teaching for this patient.

Case Study

The nurse is caring for a 32-year-old woman who is being treated for pneumonia. The prescriber has ordered an antibiotic to be started today.

1. What elements need to be included in the assessment phase of the nursing process for this patient?
2. Identify two to three appropriate nursing diagnoses for this patient.
3. What are appropriate goals and outcome criteria for the identified nursing diagnoses?
4. List several interventions for each identified nursing diagnosis.

NCLEX-RN® Review

1 The nurse reviews a client record for drug allergies, current medications, and disease states that could affect drug responses. These actions are part of which phase of the nursing process?

1. Assessment
2. Planning
3. Implementation
4. Evaluation

2 What are the two main steps of the planning phase of the nursing process?

1. ____________________
2. ____________________

3 The implementation phase of the nursing process involves two main activities related to pharmacology. These are:

1. Developing and performing nursing interventions.
2. Providing and evaluating client teaching.
3. Administering drugs and providing client drug teaching.
4. Assessing and evaluating adverse drug effects.

4 Which of the following would be most important for the nurse to evaluate in the evaluation phase of the nursing process?

1. Client satisfaction with drug therapy
2. Evidence of therapeutic drug effects
3. Development of minor adverse drug effects
4. The possibility of nonadherence with drug therapy

5 Which of the following is appropriate information to gather in the assessment phase of the nursing process? Select all that apply.

1. Drug allergies
2. Therapeutic response to the drug
3. History of renal or hepatic disease
4. Baseline physical assessment data
5. Adverse effects have been prevented

6 Which of the following is a properly worded nursing diagnosis?

1. *Skin Integrity,* related to diabetes
2. *Risk for Injury* and *Deficient Knowledge (Medication)*
3. *Pneumonia,* related to retained secretions
4. *Fatigue,* related to sleep deprivation and physical deconditioning

See Answers to Critical Thinking Questions, Case Study, and NCLEX-RN® Review in Appendix A.

References

American Nurses Association. (2007). *Scope of nursing informatics practice.* ANA Nursing World: Nursing Practice Download Library. Retrieved April 29, 2008, from http://nursingworld.org/practice/

Berman, A., Snyder, S., Kozier, B., & Erb, G. (2008). *Kozier & Erb's fundamentals of nursing: Concepts, process, and practice* (8th ed.). Upper Saddle River, NJ: Pearson Education.

LeMone, P., & Burke, K. (2008). *Medical-surgical nursing: Critical thinking in client care* (4th ed.). Upper Saddle River, NJ: Pearson Education.

NANDA International. (2007). *Strategic plan 2004–2010.* Retrieved April 28, 2008, from http://www.nanda.org/docs/NANDA-I_StrategicPlan.pdf

North American Nursing Diagnosis Association. (2008). *NANDA: Nursing diagnoses: Definitions & classification 2007–2008.* Philadelphia: Author.

Potter, P., Wolf, L., Boxerman, S., Grayson, D., Sledge, J., Dungam, C., et al. (2005) Understanding the cognitive work of nursing in the acute care environment. *Journal of Nursing Administration, 35*(7–8), 327–335.

Wilkinson, J. M. (2009). *Nursing process and critical thinking* (4th ed.). Upper Saddle River, NJ: Prentice Hall Health.

Wilkinson, J. M., & Ahern, N. (2009). *Nursing diagnosis handbook with NIC interventions and NOC outcomes* (9th ed.). Upper Saddle River, NJ: Prentice Hall Health.

CHAPTER

I've been so nauseated every morning over the past 3 weeks and I'm late with my period. Please tell me I'm not pregnant. I just can't deal with a child right now.

Patient "May David"

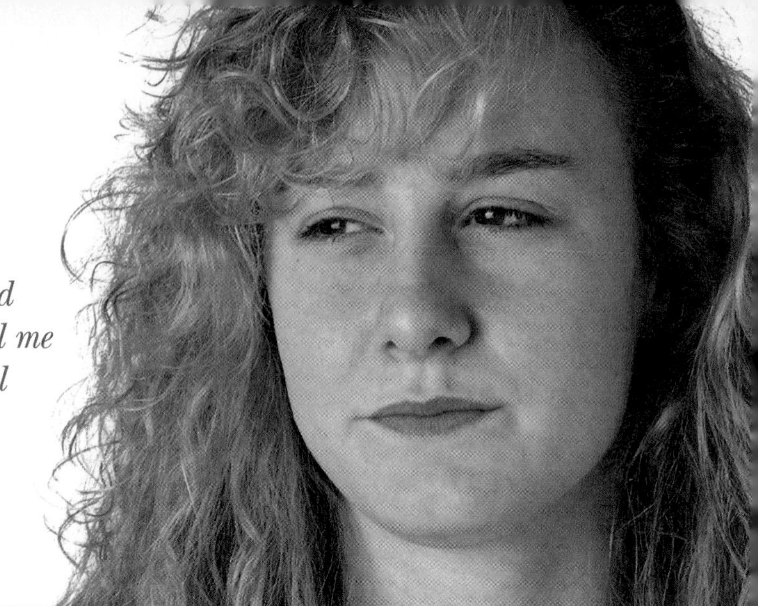

10 Pharmacotherapy During Pregnancy and Lactation

Learning Outcomes

After reading this chapter, the student should be able to:

1. Justify the rationale for using drugs during pregnancy and lactation.
2. Describe physiological changes during pregnancy that may affect the absorption, distribution, metabolism, and excretion of drugs.
3. Describe the placental transfer of drugs from mother to infant.
4. Differentiate among the United States Food and Drug Administration pregnancy risk categories.
5. Explain how drugs administered during the different stages of fetal development affect the potential for teratogenic effects.
6. Identify factors that influence the transfer of drugs into breast milk.
7. Describe signs of adverse drug reactions in the breast-feeding infant.
8. Outline important points in the patient and family education regarding drug use during pregnancy and lactation.

Chapter Outline

Rationale for Drug Use During Pregnancy and Lactation

Pharmacotherapy During Pregnancy

Changes in Pharmacokinetic Variables During Pregnancy

Placental Transfer of Drugs from Mother to Infant

FDA Fetal Risk Categories

Adverse Drug Effects During Pregnancy

Pharmacotherapy During Lactation

Transfer of Drugs into Breast Milk

Drug Adverse Effects During Lactation

Key Terms

placenta, 124
pregnancy categories, 125
teratogen, 126

To give appropriate patient care, the nurse must be aware of the physiological changes occurring in the pregnant woman along with the developmental stage of the fetus. The nurse must also be able to identify potential adverse drug events occurring in both the mother and the fetus. This chapter describes the pharmacokinetic changes occurring during pregnancy, and explains the importance of carefully monitoring the pharmacotherapy of pregnant and lactating women. Emphasis is placed on drugs to avoid or use cautiously, efforts to prevent adverse effects, and the importance of family and patient education.

Rationale for Drug Use During Pregnancy and Lactation

10.1 Women frequently use drugs during pregnancy and lactation.

The nurse caring for the pregnant or lactating woman faces the challenge of concurrently being responsible for the health and safety of two persons, knowing that most medications cross the placenta and are secreted in breast milk. Despite potential risks to the fetus, about 46% of women in childbearing years use prescription and over-the-counter (OTC) medications (Kaufman, Kelly, Rosenberg, Anderson, & Mitchell, 2002). About 59% of pregnant women are prescribed a medication other than vitamins or mineral supplements (Andrade et al., 2004), and up to 13% of pregnant women take a dietary or herbal supplement other than multivitamins and folic acid (Tsui, Dennehey, & Tsourounis, 2001). If nicotine and alcohol are included, more than 90% of women use drugs during pregnancy.

Health care providers exercise great caution when initiating pharmacotherapy during pregnancy or lactation. When possible, drug therapy is postponed until after pregnancy and lactation, and safer nonpharmacologic alternatives are implemented. There are certain acute and chronic conditions, however, that must be managed during pregnancy. These include the following:

- Treatment of preexisting illnesses. For example, if the patient has epilepsy, asthma, hypertension, or a psychiatric disorder prior to the pregnancy, it would be unwise to discontinue therapy during pregnancy or lactation.
- Treatment of complications related to pregnancy. For example, thromboembolic disorders, gestational diabetes, and gestational hypertension commonly occur during pregnancy, and must be treated for the safety of both the mother and growing fetus.
- Treatment of conditions unrelated to pregnancy. For example, antibiotics may be necessary to treat infections during pregnancy. Acute urinary tract infections and sexually transmitted infections are relatively common and can harm the fetus.

The goal of pharmacotherapy in pregnant patients is to treat the mother without causing ill effects for the fetus. Often, pharmacotherapy can be safely conducted with the same drugs and dosage levels as in nonpregnant patients. In other cases, a medication may need to be discontinued, changed to a lower dose, or replaced with a safer drug. In all patients, health care providers must balance the therapeutic value of a given medication against its potential adverse effects.

Pharmacotherapy During Pregnancy

10.2 Physiological changes during pregnancy can alter normal pharmacokinetic responses.

Most body systems in a woman undergo predictable changes during pregnancy. Some organs increase in size. Some physiological activities speed up while others slow down, altering the pharmacokinetic responses to drugs. The health care provider must understand these changes in maternal physiology when prescribing drugs for the pregnant woman (Figure 10.1).

Absorption: Drug absorption is affected during pregnancy by changes in gastric tone and motility and increased hydrochloric acid production. Increased levels of progesterone cause a decrease in gastric tone and intestinal motility, resulting in delayed gastric emptying. Drugs remain longer in the gastrointestinal (GI) tract, leading to extended time for absorption of oral drugs. High estrogen levels in the pregnant woman cause increased hydrochloric acid production in the stomach, which may affect the absorption of certain acid labile drugs. Furthermore, as the enlarging uterus rises into the abdomen it presses up against the stomach, leading to slower gastric emptying. Medications may take a longer time to be absorbed and distributed, thus prolonging their onset and durations of action. Some women suffer from nausea and vomiting and are unable to take oral medications during early pregnancy.

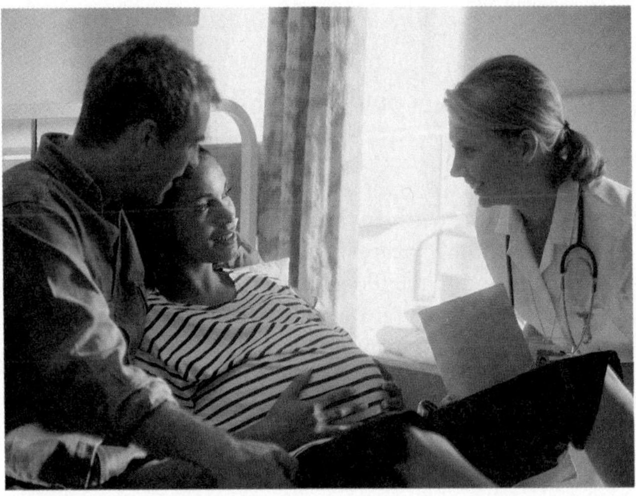

Figure 10.1 Teaching women about the safety of drug use during pregnancy is an essential component of nursing care.
Source: Photographer: C/L Fountain Group/Getty Images, Inc.

Progesterone also increases pulmonary blood flow, respiratory tidal volume, and minute volume by 40%. As a result, respiratory agents such as cromolyn (Intal) are absorbed in larger quantities, leading to higher serum drug levels.

Distribution: Distribution of drugs during pregnancy is affected by changes in total body water, which may increase by over 50%. This increase leads to greater hemodilution of plasma proteins and drugs. Because the plasma proteins are diluted, fewer are available to bind with drugs, thus causing a higher concentration of "free" drug in the plasma. This results in more drug molecules being available for transfer across the placenta or to be secreted in breast milk. Highly lipophilic drugs are distributed into the lipid-rich breast milk and are ultimately passed to the lactating infant. A woman's heart rate may increase up to 15 beats per minute during pregnancy, leading to greater drug distribution.

Metabolism: Of the pharmacokinetic variables, metabolism is least affected by pregnancy. CYP450 and other metabolic enzymes are present in the placenta and likely contribute somewhat to drug metabolism. Because the placenta and fetal liver contribute to overall drug metabolism, the metabolism of certain drugs may increase during pregnancy. Drugs such as nicotine can increase the amounts of placental metabolic enzymes, possibly affecting drug metabolism. In such cases, dose modification may be necessary.

Excretion: Excretion of drugs during pregnancy is enhanced by increases in renal plasma flow, glomerular filtration rate, creatinine clearance, and renal tubular reabsorption. Because these changes result in the increased renal elimination of drugs, doses of many medications must be adjusted.

CONNECTION *Checkpoint* 10.1

From what you learned in Chapter 8, what types of effects would you predict nicotine would have on the fetus in a mother who smokes? See Answer to Connection Checkpoint 10.1 in Appendix A.

10.3 Many drugs pass from mother to infant via the placenta.

The **placenta** is a temporary organ that allows for nutrition and gas exchange between the mother and fetus. As much as 10% of the mother's cardiac output circulates through the placenta. Although the blood of the mother does not circulate through the fetus, capillary-like structures in the placenta allow an extensive exchange of substances. The placenta offers a degree of protective filtration of the maternal blood, preventing certain harmful substances from reaching the fetus. Nutritional substances such as vitamins, fatty acids, glucose, and electrolytes freely pass from mother to fetus. The placenta also has a high degree of metabolic activity; it can detoxify certain harmful substances before they reach the fetus.

Most drugs cross the placenta and pass from mother to fetus by simple diffusion. A few drugs cross by way of active transport. It should be understood that drugs may cause fetal harm without crossing the placenta or entering the fetal blood. For example, certain drugs may cause constriction of placental blood vessels, impairing nutrient exchange. Other drugs can alter maternal physiology to such an extent that the fetus is affected.

There are multiple factors that impact the transfer of drugs across the placenta. These variables are the same as those affecting the movement of substances across other biologic membranes (see Chapter 4).

- **Plasma drug level in the mother.** In general, the higher the dose taken by the mother, the greater will be the amount of drug available to circulate through the placenta and have the potential to affect the fetus. This is the rationale for prescribing the lowest effective doses of drugs during pregnancy.
- **Solubility of the drug.** Highly lipid-soluble drugs will cross the placental barrier more easily than water-soluble drugs.
- **Molecular size.** Small molecules such as alcohol with molecular weights (MW) less than 300 easily cross the placental barrier; those with MW greater than 500 are slower to cross. Large drugs such as heparin, with MW greater than 1,000, do not generally cross the placenta to the fetus.
- **Protein binding.** When drugs are highly bound to plasma proteins, the molecules are too large to cross the placental membrane to enter the fetus.
- **Drug ionization.** Unionized drugs cross the placenta more easily than ionized drugs. The maternal serum pH is slightly higher than that of the fetus. Upon reaching the relatively acidic environment of the fetus, drugs that are weak bases become ionized. This effectively traps them on the fetal side of the placenta, because ionized drugs cannot recross the placental membrane back to the mother (ion trapping). An example is nicotine (a weak base), which can appear in higher concentrations in the fetus than in the mother due to ion trapping.
- **Blood flow to the placenta.** Decreased uterine blood flow may cause substances, including drugs, to remain trapped in the fetus for extended periods, resulting in fetal adverse effects. During labor the patient is usually instructed to remain in the lateral position during active uterine contractions to prevent pressure on the aorta and vena cava. Pressure on these vessels will obstruct uterine blood flow and may cause drug accumulation in the fetus.

Pharm*FACT*

Pregnancy predisposes women to depression. The most common antidepressants, the selective serotonin reuptake inhibitors (SSRIs), when taken by pregnant women, may cause withdrawal symptoms in newborns that include agitation, irritability, trouble feeding, and sleep disturbances. Physicians have been advised to taper dosages of SSRIs during the third trimester so that the fetus receives no drug through the placenta for at least 7 to 10 days prior to birth. *Source:* Rosack, 2004.

10.4 The United States Food and Drug Administration pregnancy risk categories are used as guides in prescribing medications during pregnancy.

In an effort to protect an unborn child from negative drug effects, the U.S. Food and Drug Administration (FDA) has developed drug **pregnancy categories** that rate medications as to their risks during pregnancy. Table 10.1 shows the five pregnancy categories, which guide the health care team and the patient in selecting drugs that are least hazardous for the fetus. Nurses who treat pregnant women must be knowledgeable of the drug pregnancy categories for all medications commonly prescribed for their patients.

Testing drugs to determine their ability to cause birth anomalies in human subjects is unethical and prohibited by law. Although drugs are tested in pregnant laboratory animals, the structure of the human placenta is unique among mammals. The FDA pregnancy drug categories are extrapolated from these animal data and may only be crude approximations of the actual risk to a human fetus. In a few cases, human data are available to show pregnancy risks. Regardless of the pregnancy category, no prescription drug, OTC medication, or herbal product should be taken during pregnancy unless the health care provider verifies that the therapeutic benefits to the mother clearly outweigh the potential risks for the unborn.

In a few cases, drugs are encouraged during pregnancy because they improve the health of the mother. For example, women are encouraged to take multivitamins and iron due to the increased metabolic demands placed on the mother during pregnancy. Vitamin B_9 (folic acid) has been found to prevent fetal spinal cord defects. These agents are designated as pregnancy category A drugs and are safe for use during pregnancy. The category B agents are also considered safe. For example, the penicillin and macrolide antibiotics are category B agents that may be safely used to treat infections during pregnancy.

The category C drugs make up to two thirds of all prescription medications. The primary reason for a category C designation is that sufficient data are simply not available to decide whether the drug is safe or whether it may cause birth defects. Category C agents should be avoided during pregnancy because there is a possibility they may cause fetal abnormalities.

All category D and X drugs should be avoided during pregnancy due to their potential for causing serious birth defects. For example, angiotensin-converting enzyme (ACE) inhibitors, a classification of drugs used to treat hypertension, are known to impede intrauterine growth and increase the risk of fetal demise. Use of certain other antihypertensive drugs can result in renal atrophy. Certain antibiotics such as tetracyclines cause permanent staining of deciduous teeth. A Class X such as isotretinoin (Accutane), which is commonly used for acne, can result in brain damage. Other category X drugs such as misoprostol (Cytotec), a GI protective agent, may lead to abortion, and thalidomide (Thalomid), an immunosuppressant, has been known to cause fetal limb abnormalities. Additionally, alcohol, nicotine, and certain illicit

TABLE 10.1 Current FDA Pregnancy Category Ratings with Examples

Risk Category	Interpretation	Drugs
A	Adequate, well-controlled studies in pregnant women have not shown an increased risk of fetal abnormalities to the fetus in any trimester of pregnancy.	Prenatal multivitamins, insulin, thyroxine, folic acid
B	Animal studies have revealed no evidence of harm to the fetus; however, there are no adequate and well-controlled studies in pregnant women. OR Animal studies have shown an adverse effect, but adequate and well-controlled studies in pregnant women have failed to demonstrate risk to the fetus in any trimester.	Penicillins, cephalosporins, azithromycin, acetaminophen, ibuprofen in the first and second trimesters
C	Animal studies have shown an adverse effect and there are no adequate and well-controlled studies in pregnant women. OR No animal studies have been conducted and there are no adequate and well-controlled studies in pregnant women.	Most prescription medicines; antimicrobials such as clarithromycin, fluoroquinolones, and Bactrim; selective serotonin reuptake inhibitors (SSRIs); corticosteroids; and most antihypertensives
D	Adequate well-controlled or observational studies in pregnant women have demonstrated a risk to the fetus. However, the benefits of therapy may outweigh the potential risk. For example, the drug may be acceptable if needed in a life-threatening situation or serious disease for which safer drugs cannot be used or are ineffective.	ACE inhibitors, angiotensin receptor blockers (ARBs) in the second and third trimesters, gentamicin, ibuprofen in the third trimester, tetracyclines, Premarin, alcohol, and nicotine
X	Adequate well-controlled or observational studies in animals or pregnant women have demonstrated positive evidence of fetal abnormalities or risks. The use of the product is contraindicated in women who are or may become pregnant. There is no indication for use in pregnancy.	Accutane, misoprostol, and thalidomide

TABLE 10.2 Drugs of Abuse and Their Potential Effects During Pregnancy

Drug	Potential Effects
Amphetamines/methamphetamine	Increased risk of pregnancy complications, such as premature birth and placental problems Possible birth defects, including heart defects and cleft lip or palate After birth, the infant may have withdrawal-like symptoms such as jitteriness, drowsiness, and breathing problems
Cannabis/marijuana	Reduced fertility in both men and women Slowed fetal growth Slightly decreased length of pregnancy After birth, the infant may have withdrawal-like symptoms such as excessive crying and trembling
Club drugs such as PCP, ketamine, and LSD	After birth, the infant may have withdrawal symptoms Increased risk of learning and behavioral problems
Cocaine	Increased risk of miscarriage or premature birth Low birth weight with increased risk of health problems such as mental retardation and cerebral palsy, and even death Increased risk of birth defects involving the urinary tract and possibly other birth defects May cause an unborn baby to have a stroke, which can result in irreversible brain damage or a heart attack, and sometimes death Placental problems, including placental abruption, which can lead to heavy bleeding that can be life threatening for both mother and baby After birth, the infant may have mild behavioral disturbances, jitteriness, and irritability; may startle and cry at the gentlest touch or sound Increased risk of SIDS
Heroin	Increased risk of serious pregnancy complications, including poor fetal growth, premature rupture of the membranes, premature birth and stillbirth Low birth weight often combined with breathing problems and possibility of lifelong disabilities Increased risk of birth defects After birth, the infant may have withdrawal symptoms such as fever, sneezing, trembling, irritability, diarrhea, vomiting, continual crying, and, occasionally, seizures Increased risk of sudden infant death syndrome (SIDS)
Inhalants, glues, and solvents	Miscarriage, slow fetal growth, preterm birth, and birth defects

Note: Adapted from "Illicit Drug Use During Pregnancy, March of Dimes Professionals and Researchers Quick Reference," 2006. Retrieved April 28, 2008, from http://www.marchofdimes.com/professionals/14332_1169.asp

drugs such as cocaine may negatively affect the unborn child. Selected abused substances and their effects on the fetus are listed in Table 10.2.

There are several problems associated with the current classification system used to determine drug safety in the pregnant patient. For example, the current A, B, C, D, and X pregnancy labeling system gives no specific clinical information to help guide nurses or their patients as to whether a medication is truly safe. Furthermore, the system does not indicate how the dose should be adjusted during pregnancy or lactation. To address these issues the FDA is updating these categories to provide more descriptive information on the risks and benefits of taking each medication. The new labels will include pharmacokinetic and pharmacodynamic information that will suggest optimum doses for the childbearing patient. To gather this information, the FDA is encouraging all pregnant women who are taking medications to join a pregnancy registry that will survey drug effects on both the patient and the fetus or newborn. Evaluation of a large number of pregnancies is needed to determine the effects of medicine on babies.

10.5 The stage of development has an important influence on adverse drug effects in the embryo and fetus.

The effects of drugs on the fetus depend on the dosage received by the fetus and stage of fetal development. Lo and Friedman (2002) reported that 90% of medications approved by the FDA between 1998 and 2000 had insufficient information about the safety risk when taken during pregnancy. Lack of knowledge does not mean they are safe; these drugs have the potential for causing adverse drug reactions in the fetus and, in some cases, may cause fetal malformations.

A **teratogen** is a substance, organism, or physical agent to which an embryo or fetus is exposed that produces a permanent abnormality in structure or function, causes growth retardation, or causes death (Gardella & Hill, 2000). The word derives from the Greek "gennan" (to produce) and "terata" (monster). The baseline incidence of teratogenic events is approximately 3% of all pregnancies. Potential fetal consequences of drug use include intrauterine fetal death, physical malformations, growth impairment, behavioral abnormalities, and neonatal toxicity.

There are no "absolute" teratogens. Whether or not a drug produces a teratogenic effect depends on multiple, complex factors. Like other effects of drugs, there is a dose–response relationship, with risk increasing with higher doses. The timing of drug therapy and the stage of fetal development critically affect the risk for possible fetal consequences. Because of the constant changes that occur during fetal development, the specific risk is dependent on when during gestation the drug is administered. A well-known example is the drug thalidomide, which causes its fetal effects from day 35 to day 48 after the last menstrual period. The specific malformation is linked to the time of exposure: 35 to 37 days, no ears; 39 to 41 days, no arms; 41 to 43 days, no uterus; 45 to 47 days, no tibia; and 47 to 49 days, triphalangeal thumbs.

Preimplantation period: Weeks 1 to 2 of the first trimester are known as the preimplantation phase. Before implantation, the developing embryo has not yet established a blood supply with the mother. This is sometimes called the "all-or-none" period because exposure to a teratogen either causes death of the embryo or has no effect. Drugs are less likely to cause congenital malformations during this period because the baby's organ systems have not yet begun to form. Drugs such as nicotine, however, can create a negative environment for the embryo and potentially cause intrauterine growth retardation.

Embryonic period: During the embryonic period, from 3 to 8 weeks postconception, there is rapid development of internal structures. This is the period of maximum sensitivity to teratogens. Teratogenic agents taken during this phase can lead to structural malformation and spontaneous abortion. The specific abnormality depends on which organ is forming at the time of exposure.

Fetal period: The fetal phase is from 9 to 40 weeks postconception or until birth. During this time there is continued growth and maturation of the baby's organ systems. Blood flow to the placenta increases and placental vascular membranes become thinner. Such alterations maximize the transfer of substances from the maternal circulation to the fetal blood. As a result, the fetus may receive larger doses of medications and other substances taken by the mother. Because the fetus lacks mature metabolic enzymes and efficient excretion mechanisms, medications will have a prolonged duration of action within the unborn child. Exposure to teratogens during the fetal period is more likely to produce slowed growth or impaired organ function, rather than gross structural malformations.

The nurse caring for the pregnant woman must differentiate adverse drug effects from the normal symptoms of pregnancy. Nausea, vomiting, abdominal cramps, flushed skin, or diaphoresis may indeed be either normal symptoms of pregnancy or adverse drug effects. Fetal tachycardia may be due to drugs being taken by the mother or a fetal cardiac anomaly. During all stages of pregnancy, the nurse should help the mother assess medications and dietary supplements to determine if they are necessary and if adjustments are required. Impairments in the functioning of the mother's liver or kidneys may have a profound impact on maternal and fetal safety. Health care providers must consider these factors, so as to minimize the risk of toxicity to the mother and child. Through careful assessments, the nurse contributes greatly to this risk–benefit analysis, which is essential for protecting both the mother and her baby.

CONNECTION *Checkpoint* 10.2

From what you learned in Chapter 6, explain why the FDA might approve a drug, even though it is a known teratogen and can cause fetal abnormalities. See Answer to Connection Checkpoint 10.2 in Appendix A.

Pharmacotherapy During Lactation

10.6 Transfer of drugs from mother to infant may occur through breast milk.

According to the 2004 National Immunization Survey conducted by the Centers for Disease Control and Prevention (CDC) almost 74% of mothers breast-feed their infants and 42% continue to breast-feed for at least 6 months. Breast-feeding is highly recommended as a means of providing nutrition, emotional bonding, and immune protection to the neonate (Figure 10.2).

The majority of drugs are secreted into breast milk to some extent. Fortunately, there are relatively few instances in which breast-feeding must be discontinued due to drug use. For the few drugs that are absolutely contraindicated during lactation, equally effective, safer alternatives are usually available. Some of these agents are shown in Table 10.3. Although most medications probably cause no harm to the breast-feeding baby, their effects have not been fully studied. The American Academy of Pediatrics (AAP) Committee on Drugs provides guidance on which drugs should be avoided during breast-feeding to protect the child's safety.

Drugs enter breast milk primarily by passive diffusion. In the first week of life the alveolar cells in the breast have large gaps between them, allowing drugs and other substances to penetrate the milk. By the second week of life the alveolar cells swell, closing the intracellular gaps and limiting the drug's access to the milk.

Pharm*FACT*

Human milk has antibacterial properties: About 80% of the cells in breast milk are macrophages, cells that kill bacteria, fungi, and viruses. Breast-fed babies are protected, in varying degrees, from a number of illnesses, including pneumonia, botulism, bronchitis, staphylococcal infections, influenza, ear infections, and German measles. *Source:* U.S. Department of Health and Human Services, 2005.

It is important that the nurse understand factors that influence the amount of drug secreted into breast milk. This allows the nurse to aid the patient in making responsible choices regarding lactation and in reducing exposure of her newborn to potentially harmful substances. The amount of drug that passes to the infant during lactation depends on multiple factors.

- Plasma drug level in the mother. The higher the dose taken by the mother, the more will be secreted into breast milk. It is therefore

TABLE 10.3 Selected Drugs Compatible with Breast-Feeding

Class	Compatible Drugs	Drugs to Be Avoided
Analgesics (opioids)	codeine and morphine in occasional doses	—
Analgesics (nonopioid)	acetaminophen, aspirin, ibuprofen	—
Antiseizure agents	carbamazepine, diazepam (single dose), valproic acid, phenytoin	ethosuximide
Anti-infectives	penicillins, trimethoprim, sulfisoxazole (over 1 month of age), macrolides, aminoglycosides, cephalosporins, isoniazid, fluconazole, acyclovir	chloramphenicol, ciprofloxacin, tetracyclines, metronidazole
Antimigraine agents	propranolol	ergotamine
Cytotoxic agents and immunosuppressants	—	all drugs in this class should be avoided
Cardiovascular agents	iron salts, heparin, warfarin, verapamil, lidocaine, digoxin, prazosin, nifedipine, spironolactone, furosemide	atenolol, ACE inhibitors, statins, hydrochlorothiazide
Gastrointestinal agents	aluminum hydroxide, magnesium hydroxide, promethazine (single dose)	cimetidine, metoclopramide
Hormones	prednisone, hydrocortisone (single dose), insulin, thyroid hormone, oxytocin (short term)	oral contraceptives, estrogens, testosterone
Central nervous system agents	tricyclic antidepressants	lithium carbonate

Note: From "Breastfeeding and Maternal Medication: Recommendations for Drugs in the Eleventh WHO Model List of Essential Drugs," World Health Organization, 2002. Retrieved April 30, 2008, from http://whqlibdoc.who.int/hq/2002/55732.pdf

standard practice that if a drug must be prescribed for a lactating patient, the lowest effective dose should be ordered.

- **Solubility of the drug.** Highly lipid-soluble drugs penetrate the milk at higher concentrations. Milk at the end of a feed contains considerably more fat and may have a higher concentration of fat-soluble drugs. Furthermore the percentage of lipids in milk increases progressively from day 1 to day 84 of lactation. Drugs that act on the central nervous system (CNS) are usually lipophilic and have a tendency to penetrate milk at higher concentrations.
- **Molecular size and protein binding.** Some drugs, such as heparin and insulin, are simply too large to pass membranes by passive diffusion. In addition when drugs are highly protein bound, they are less likely to enter the milk than those that are free. The health care provider may choose drugs with greater protein binding capacity for the lactating mother to limit the amount secreted in milk.
- **Drug ionization.** Milk is slightly more acidic than plasma; the pH of milk is 7.2 and plasma 7.4. This pH gradient allows weakly basic drugs to transfer more readily into breast milk and accumulate due to ion trapping (see Chapter 5).
- **Drug half-life.** Drugs with short half-lives will be metabolized and eliminated quickly by the mother. This results in smaller amounts secreted into milk.

Once ingested by the infant, a drug is subjected to the usual pharmacokinetic influences. The infant's stomach content is quite acidic and, therefore, some drugs may be destroyed and have reduced bioavailability. Additionally some drugs are inactivated when ingested with calcium and protein-rich nutrients in mother's milk. Some drugs by their nature are removed by the infant's liver during first-pass metabolism and never get to the plasma. It is important to remember that the baby's organs responsible for metabolizing and eliminating the drugs are immature and will not be able to perform all the functions of adult organs.

Considering the many variables, it is not surprising that it is difficult to accurately predict the amount of maternal drug that will transfer to the infant plasma during lactation. Estimates of drug transference to breast milk range from less than 1% to 3%. Regardless of the amount, it is imperative for the nurse to teach the mother that many prescription medications, OTC drugs, and herbal products are secreted in breast milk and have the potential to affect her child. The same guidelines for drug use during pregnancy apply during lactation—drugs should only be taken if the benefits to the mother clearly outweigh the potential risks to the infant (Figure 10.2).

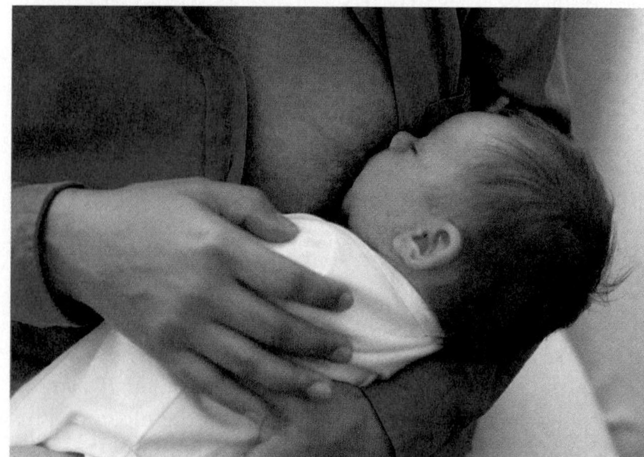

Figure 10.2 Nurses should teach lactating women to avoid all drugs, herbal products, or dietary supplements unless approved by their health care provider.
Source: Ruth Jenkinson © Dorling Kindersley

CONNECTIONS

Complementary and Alternative Therapies

Herbal Remedies as Galactogogues

A main concern of breast-feeding women is whether or not they have an adequate supply of milk for their infant. This concern leads women to take galactogogues, which are substances used to initiate or augment maternal milk supply. Galactogogues may be herbal preparations or prescription medications.

Fenugreek is the most commonly recommended herbal product. Other herbal galactogogues are alfalfa, goat's rue, and blessed thistle. The safety and efficacy of these substances have not been thoroughly researched and, therefore, their use in clinical practice should be limited. The nurse caring for a lactating woman who believes her milk supply is low should first offer guidance in proper feeding techniques, nutrition intake, and milk expression. If all fails the mother should be referred to a health care provider for further evaluation.

Source: From *Use of Galactogogues in Initiating or Augmenting Maternal Milk Supply,* (Protocol #9), Academy of Breastfeeding Medicine, 2004. Retrieved April 29, 2008, from http://www.bfmed.org/ace-files/protocol/prot9galactogoguesEnglish.pdf

10.7 Drugs present in breast milk may cause adverse effects in the breast-feeding infant.

Although the concentration of drugs in breast milk is often very low (less than 3%), their effects on the infant can be serious. Common drug effects seen in breast-feeding infants are nonspecific and include diarrhea, constipation, sedation, and irritability. The nurse has an important responsibility to monitor for adverse drug effects in breast-feeding infants and to teach new mothers to do the same. Selected drugs that enter the breast milk and have been shown to produce adverse effects are shown in Table 10.4.

The nurse must inform the mother that all drugs of abuse are contraindicated during both pregnancy and breast-feeding. If she takes such drugs, her infant may experience withdrawal symptoms and test positive for the drug for several weeks to months following exposure.

In general, topical medications applied to the mother's skin are safe to use during lactation. The nurse must remind the mother, however, that the breast-feeding infant may ingest substances like vitamins E, A, or D in creams that are rubbed on her nipples to soften them.

More recently, Hale (2006) developed lactation risk categories as guidelines for the health care provider to identify safe and contraindicated drugs during lactation. Table 10.5 summarizes Hale's categories.

CONNECTION *Checkpoint* 10.3

From what you learned in Chapter 4, how long would it take a 600-mg dose of a drug with a t ½ of 8 hours to reach five half-lives and be safe for a lactating patient? How much drug would be left at that time? See Answer to Connection Checkpoint 10.3 in Appendix A.

TABLE 10.4 Selected Drugs Associated with Adverse Effects During Breast-Feeding

Drug	Reported Effect or Reasons for Concern
acebutolol (Sectral)	Hypotension; bradycardia; tachypnea
amiodarone (Cordarone)	Hypothyroidism
amphetamine	Irritability, poor sleeping pattern
aspirin (salicylates)	Metabolic acidosis
atenolol (Tenormin)	Cyanosis; bradycardia
bromocriptine (Parlodel)	Suppresses lactation; may be hazardous to the mother
cocaine	Cocaine intoxication: irritability, vomiting, diarrhea, tremulousness, seizures
ergotamine (Ergostat)	Vomiting, diarrhea, convulsions (doses used in migraine medications)
fluoxetine (Prozac)	Feeding and sleeping disorders, reduced weight gain, colic
haloperidol (Haldol)	Decline in developmental scores
lithium (Eskalith)	One-third to one-half therapeutic blood concentration in infants
phenindione	Anticoagulant: increased prothrombin and partial thromboplastin time
phenobarbital (Luminal)	Sedation; infantile spasms after weaning from milk containing phenobarbital, methemoglobinemia
primidone (Mysoline)	Sedation, feeding problems
sulfasalazine (Azulfidine)	Bloody diarrhea

Note: From "The Transfer of Drugs and Other Chemicals into Human Breast Milk" by American Academy of Pediatrics, Committee on Drugs, 2001, *Pediatrics, 3,* pp. 776–782. Reprinted by permission.

TABLE 10.5 Summary of Hale's Lactation Risk Categories

Category	Explanation	Examples
L1 Safest	Controlled studies in breast-feeding women demonstrate remote possibility of harm to the infant.	Acetaminophen, penicillins, Depo-Provera greater than 1 month after birth
L2 Safer	Studies in limited number of breast-feeding women show no increased adverse effect in the infant. Risk to the infant is remote.	Macrolides, cephalosporins, second-generation antihistamines, prednisone, SSRIs
L3 Moderately Safe	No controlled studies are available; risk to the infant is possible. Drugs should be prescribed only if the benefit outweighs the risk to the infant.	Bactrim, first-generation antihistamines, doxycycline
L4 Possibly Hazardous	Positive evidence of risk to the infant exists. Benefits of the drug to the mother may be acceptable despite the risk to the infant. May be needed in a life-threatening situation for a serious disease for which no other drug can be used.	Lithium, ergot preparations, corticosteroids
L5 Contraindicated	Documentation of significant risk or potential for risk to the infant. The risk of using the drug far outweighs the benefit from breast-feeding. The drug is contraindicated in the breast-feeding woman.	Radioactive isotopes, cocaine, heroin

Note: From *Medications and Mother's Milk*, 12th ed., by T. W. Hale, 2006, Amarillo, TX: Hale Publishing Co. Adapted with permission.

UNDERSTANDING THE CHAPTER

Key Concepts Summary

10.1 Women frequently use drugs during pregnancy and lactation.

10.2 Physiological changes during pregnancy can alter normal pharmacokinetic responses.

10.3 Many drugs pass from mother to infant via the placenta.

10.4 The United States Food and Drug Administration pregnancy risk categories are used as guides in prescribing medications during pregnancy.

10.5 The stage of development has an important influence on adverse drug effects in the embryo and fetus.

10.6 Transfer of drugs from mother to infants may occur through breast milk.

10.7 Drugs present in breast milk may cause adverse effects in the breast-feeding infant.

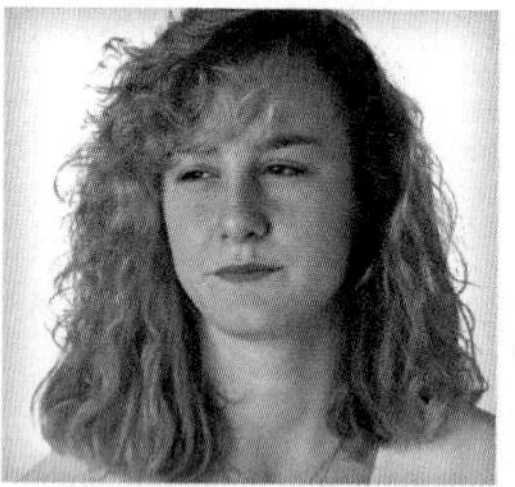

Making the PATIENT *Connection*

Remember the patient "May David" at the beginning of the chapter? Now read the remainder of the case study. Based on the information presented within this chapter, respond to the critical thinking questions that follow.

May David, a 22-year-old woman, comes to the clinic to obtain a pregnancy test. She has not had her menstruation for the past 6 weeks but claims that infrequent menses are not unusual for her. She feels nauseous in the mornings but the feeling is only temporary. You ask May, "Is it possible that you might be pregnant?" May's response is, "I doubt it, since we have always used a condom during intercourse." She goes on to explain to you that she has been taking an antiseizure medication for several years to control her epilepsy and is taking some herbal medicines for a feeling of well-being.

May's vital signs are: temperature, 98°F; pulse, 68 beats/minute; respiration, 18/minute; and blood pressure, 110/70 mmHg. She is 1.7m (5 feet 6 inches) tall and is surprised that she has gained 2.3 kg (5 lb) in the past 4 weeks, bringing her weight to 65.8 kg (145 lb). A urine specimen is sent to the laboratory for human chorionic gonadotropin (HCG). A complete physical examination is performed, followed by a vaginal examination via speculum. All physical findings were within normal limits except for the urine qualitative HCG, which is positive and quantitative HCG = 550, indicating pregnancy. The patient smokes approximately a half pack of cigarettes per day.

Critical Thinking Questions

1. What are some key points to discuss with Ms. David regarding her condition and the medication she is taking?
2. What education should you provide for Ms. David regarding the use of medication during pregnancy?
3. As the nurse caring for this client, you must consider FDA pregnancy risk categories. In your own words explain these categories.
4. What effect does May's tobacco use possibly have on her unborn fetus?

Case Study

You are caring for Irina, an 18-year-old mother of a 6-month-old baby boy. She confides in you that she has experienced postpartum depression since her child was born. She tries to take care of herself but just does not feel very good most of the time. Her husband insists that she continue with the breast-feeding but she is now having doubts. After a lengthy discussion Irina states, "The only time I feel good is when I smoke a 'joint' (marijuana) before feeding my son."

1. What is your response to Irina?
2. What teaching should you carry out at this time?

NCLEX-RN® Review

1 A client in her first trimester of pregnancy asks the nurse which medications should be avoided during pregnancy. The nurse's response is based on the knowledge that during pregnancy:

1. Most over-the-counter medications are safe.
2. When possible, drug therapy is postponed until after pregnancy and lactation.
3. It is wise to discontinue all drugs used in treating medical conditions.
4. The decision whether or not to take medication is the responsibility of the woman.

2 The nurse is preparing to discuss drug use during pregnancy with a group of nursing students. The main topic is the FDA drug classifications. Which of the following drugs should the nurse inform the students are the most detrimental to the fetus?

1. Category A
2. Category B
3. Category C
4. Category X

3 A pregnant client asks the nurse what factors determine if a drug will transfer across the placenta. The nurse's response will be based on which of the following principles?

1. Highly lipid-soluble drugs cross the placental membrane more easily than low lipids.
2. The lower the lipid content, the easier it crosses the placental membrane.
3. Drugs with large molecular weight pass rapidly through the placental membrane.
4. Highly protein bound drugs pass rapidly through the placental membrane.

4 The nurse is administering medication to a group of pregnant women. At which stage of fetal development will congenital malformations least likely occur?

1. 1 to 2 weeks
2. 3 to 4 weeks
3. 5 to 6 weeks
4. 7 to 8 weeks

5 The community health nurse is visiting a postpartum mother who is breast-feeding her 3.2 kg (7-lb) infant daughter. Which of the following statements, if made by the mother, indicates that further teaching is necessary?

1. "When using over-the-counter medication, I should take only the lowest effective dose."
2. "The higher the dose of medication, the more likely it will be secreted into breast milk."
3. "Drugs that work on the nervous system have a tendency to penetrate into the breast milk."
4. "Medication in liquid form should be avoided since it more readily enters the breast milk."

6 The nurse is administering medications to a client who is 32 weeks pregnant. Which of the following normal physiological principles associated with pregnancy will affect drug absorption?

1. Medications are absorbed and distributed more quickly in pregnant women.
2. There is greater hemoconcentration of drugs in pregnant clients.
3. Drugs remain longer in the gastrointestinal tract, leading to extended time for absorption.
4. Drug metabolism is highly affected by pregnancy.

See Answers to Critical Thinking Questions, Case Study, and NCLEX-RN® Review in Appendix A.

References

The Academy of Breastfeeding Medicine. (2004). *Protocol #9: Use of galactogogues in initiating or augmenting maternal milk supply.* Retrieved April 29, 2008, from http://www.bfmed.org/ace-files/protocol/prot9galactogoguesEnglish.pdf

American Academy of Pediatrics, Committee on Drugs. (2001). Transfer of drugs and other chemicals into human milk. *Pediatrics, 108*(3), 776–789.

Andrade, S. E., Gurwitz, J. H., Davis, R. L. Chan, K. A., Finkelstein, J. A., Fortman, K., et al. (2004). Prescription drug use in pregnancy. *American Journal of Obstetrics and Gynecology, 191*(2), 398–407.

Anwar, A. (2007). Prescribing in pregnancy and lactation: Factors to consider. *Nurse Prescribing, 5*(6), 245–249.

Briggs, G. G., Freeman, R. K., & Yaffe, S. J. (2005). *Drugs in pregnancy and lactation* (7th ed.). Philadelphia: Lippincott Williams & Wilkins.

Cardonick, E., & Iacobucci, A. (2004). Use of chemotherapy during human pregnancy. *Lancet Oncology, 5*(5), 283–291.

Centers for Disease Control and Prevention, U.S. Department of Health and Human Services. (2005). *Folic acid basics.* Retrieved April 28, 2008, from http://www.cdc.gov/ncbddd/folicacid/basics.htm

Centers for Disease Control and Prevention, U.S. Department of Health and Human Services. (2005). *National immunization survey.* Retrieved April 28, 2008, from http://www.cdc.gov/breastfeeding/data/NIS_data/data_2004.htm

Duley, L., Henderson-Smart, D. J., & Meher, S. (2006). Drugs for treatment of very high blood pressure during pregnancy. *Cochrane Database of Systematic Reviews, 3.* Art. No.: CD001449. DOI: 10.1002/14651858.CD001449.pub2.

Gardella, J. R., & Hill, J. A., III. (2000). Environmental toxins associated with recurrent pregnancy loss. *Seminar Reproductive Medicine, 18*(4), 407–424.

Hale, T. (2006). *Medications and mother's milk* (12th ed.). Amarillo, TX: Hale.

Hale, T. W. (2005). Drug therapy and breastfeeding: Antibiotics, analgesics, and other medications. *NeoReviews, 6*(5).

Källén, B. (2007). The safety of antidepressant drugs during pregnancy. *Expert Opinion on Drug Safety, 6*(4), 357–370.

Kaufman, D. W., Kelly, J. P., Rosenberg, L., Anderson, T. E., & Mitchell, A. (2002). Recent patterns of medication use in the ambulatory adult population of the United States: The Slone Survey. *Journal of the American Medical Association, 287*(3), 337–348.

Lee, K. (2007). Lactation and drugs. *Paediatrics and Child Health, 17*(2), 68–71.

Lo, W. Y., & Friedman, J. M. (2002). Teratogenicity of recently introduced medications in human pregnancy. *Obstetrics and Gynecology, 100*(3), 465–473.

March of Dimes Professionals and Researchers Quick Reference. (2006). *Illicit drug use during pregnancy.* Retrieved April 28, 2008, from http://www.marchofdimes.com/professionals/14332_1169.asp

Marcus, D. M., & Snodgrass, W. R. (2005). Do no harm: Avoidance of herbal medicines during pregnancy. *Obstetrics and Gynecology, 105,* 1119–1122.

McCarter-Spaulding, D. E. (2005). Medications in pregnancy and lactation. *MCN, American Journal of Maternal Child Nursing, 30*(1), 10–17.

McKenna, L., & McIntyre, R. M. (2006). What over-the-counter preparations are pregnant women taking? A literature review. *Journal of Advanced Nursing, 56*(6), 636–645.

Ostrea, E. M., Jr., Mantaring, J. B., III, & Silvestre, M. A. (2004). Drugs that affect the fetus and newborn infant via the placenta or breast milk. *Pediatric Clinics of North America, 51*(3), 539–579.

Rosack, J. (2004). FDA committee urges new warning on antidepressants for pregnancy. *Psychiatric News, 39*(14), 33.

Syme, M. R., Paxton, J. W., & Keelan, J. A. (2004). Drug transfer and metabolism by the human placenta. *Clinical Pharmacokinetics, 43*(8), 487–514.

Tsui, B., Dennehey, C. E., & Tsourounis, C. (2001). A survey of dietary supplement use during pregnancy at an academic medical center. *American Journal of Obstetrics and Gynecology, 185*(2), 433–437.

U.S. Department of Health and Human Services, Office of Women's Health. (2005). *Benefits of breastfeeding.* Retrieved April 30, 2008, from http://www.4woman.gov/breastfeeding/index.cfm?page=227

Weiner, C. P., & Buhimschi, C. (2005). *Drugs for pregnant and lactating women.* New York: Churchill Livingstone.

World Health Organization. (2002). *Breastfeeding and maternal medication: Recommendations for drugs in the eleventh WHO model list of essential drugs.* Retrieved April 30, 2008, from http://whqlibdoc.who.int/hq/2002/55732.pdf

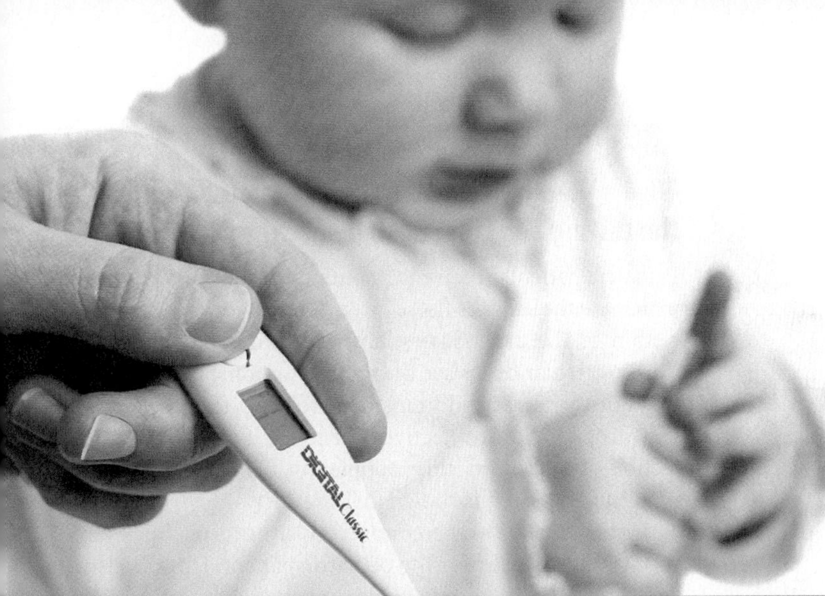

Last evening my Timmy suddenly started vomiting and refused to eat. This morning he had two large loose green stools. Please help him.

Patient "Timmy's" mother, Ms. Thomas

CHAPTER 11

Pharmacotherapy of the Pediatric Patient

Chapter Outline

Testing and Labeling of Pediatric Drugs

Pharmacokinetic Variables in Pediatric Patients

Pharmacologic Implications Associated with Growth and Development

Medication Safety for Pediatric Patients

Determining Pediatric Drug Dosages

Adverse Drug Reactions in Children and Promoting Adherence

Learning Outcomes

After reading this chapter, the student should be able to:

1. Identify the purposes of the Food and Drug Administration Modernization Act of 1997 and the Best Pharmaceuticals for Children Act of 2002.
2. Explain how differences in pharmacokinetic variables can impact drug response in pediatric patients.
3. Discuss the nursing and pharmacologic implications associated with each of the pediatric developmental age groups.
4. Describe safe methods and techniques appropriate for administering medications to pediatric patients.
5. Explain several methods for accurately calculating drug doses in pediatric patients.
6. Describe nursing interventions for minimizing adverse effects during pediatric pharmacotherapy.
7. Propose appropriate teaching strategies to enhance medication adherence in pediatric patients.

Key Terms

adherence, 143
Best Pharmaceuticals for Children Act, 135
blood–brain barrier, 136
body surface area (BSA) method, 140
body weight method, 140
directly observed therapy (DOT), 143
Food and Drug Administration (FDA) Modernization Act, 134
nomogram, 140
Pediatric Research Equity Act of 2003, 136

Beginning with conception, and continuing throughout the life span, the organs and systems within the body undergo predictable physiological changes that influence the absorption, metabolism, distribution, and elimination of medications. A child's body systems are in a constant state of development; therefore, the effects of drugs can often be unpredictable. Health care providers must recognize such changes to ensure that drugs are delivered in a safe and effective manner to patients of all ages.

The purpose of this chapter is to examine how principles of developmental physiology and life span psychology apply to drug administration. Emphasis is placed on drug dosage determination, maximizing therapeutic effects, and minimizing adverse effects. There is strong focus on patient and family education as well as on the importance of promoting adherence with pharmacotherapy.

Testing and Labeling of Pediatric Drugs

11.1 Recent legislation has attempted to improve the testing and labeling of pediatric drugs.

Pediatric patients receive large numbers of drugs, nearly all of which are the same as those given to adult patients. The distribution of the drug classes, however, is different in children. Cardiovascular drugs are the most commonly prescribed class in adults, whereas children are more likely to receive respiratory drugs and anti-infectives due to the high incidence of infectious diseases in this population. The drug utilization pattern in children is shown in Table 11.1.

Until the 1990s there was very little drug information specifically targeted for the pediatric patient. Drug trials with pediatric patients were virtually unheard of, and data regarding the pharmacokinetics and adverse effects of most drugs were not well documented in this population. Most pediatric drugs were not available in dosage and delivery forms compatible with neonates or infants. Few drugs contained labeling information specifically for pediatric patients. Drugs that were found to be effective in adults were assumed to also be effective in children.

In 1997, the U.S. **Food and Drug Administration (FDA) Modernization Act** was passed, which gave financial incentives for

TABLE 11.1 Drug Utilization Pattern in Children

Drug Category	% of Prescriptions	Frequently Used Drug Classes
Respiratory system	30	Drugs for obstructive airway disease
		Nasal preparations
		Cough and cold preparations
		Antihistamines for systemic use
General anti-infectives, systemic	28	Antibacterials for systemic use
Dermatologic	12	Antifungals for dermatologic use
		Emollients and protectives
		Corticosteroids, dermatologic preparations
Sensory organs	7	Eyedrops and eardrops
Central nervous system	4	Analgesics/antipyretics
		Psychostimulant agents used for attention deficit/hyperactivity disorder (ADHD)
		Antiepileptics
Hormones	3	Corticosteroids, for systemic use
Blood and blood-forming organs	3	Vitamin K
Alimentary tract and metabolism	2	Drugs for peptic ulcer and gastroesophageal reflux disease
		Insulin and analogues
Musculoskeletal system	2	Anti-inflammatory and antirheumatic products, nonsteroids
Genitourinary system and sex hormones	2	Hormonal contraceptives for systemic use
Cardiovascular system	1	Diuretics
Total	105% (exceeds 100% due to rounding)	

Note: From "Stimulation Programs for Pediatric Drug Research—Do Children Really Benefit?" by I. Boots, R. Sukhai, R. Klein, R. Holl, J. Wit, A. Cohen, et al., 2007, *European Journal of Pediatrics, 166*(8), 849–855.

pharmaceutical companies to conduct pediatric research in pharmacology. In exchange for providing pediatric labeling, the legislation provides drug companies with an additional 6 months of exclusivity, giving them the ability to market the drug with no competition. It is estimated that the additional 6 months generates an average of $35 million for the drug company sponsoring the pediatric study (Tufts Center for the Study of Drug Development, 2005). In some cases, the pharmaceutical company gained significantly more: $1.4 billion for Prilosec, $974 million for Claritin, and $831 million for Prozac (Hammer-Breslow, 2003). From 1998 to 2006, 135 drugs were granted pediatric exclusivity by the FDA. The most frequent drug classes were antidepressants and mood stabilizers, ACE inhibitors, lipid-lowering preparations, HIV antivirals, nonsteroidal anti-inflammatory drugs (NSAIDs), and antirheumatic drugs (Boots et al., 2007).

Several flaws in the FDA Modernization Act were quickly noted. Many of the medications studied by the drug companies were chosen not for their potential value in children, but instead to extend their exclusivity and generate higher profits. The act gave no incentives for studying off-patent (generic) drugs or those that have smaller markets. In 2002, Congress passed the **Best Pharmaceuticals for Children Act,** which authorizes the FDA to contract for the testing of already approved pediatric drugs, or when the pharmaceutical company declines the option of exclusivity. Table 11.2 shows some of the labeling changes that

TABLE 11.2 Examples of Labeling Changes

Potential Risks Hazards	Drug Name	Disease or Condition Treated	Summary of New Information Contained in Drug Labeling
Unnecessary exposure to ineffective therapies	sumatriptan (Imitrex)	Migraines	Five studies did not establish safety and effectiveness, and postmarketing experience showed that children were having serious adverse effects, such as stroke and vision loss. The product is not recommended for children under 18 years old.
	tolterodine (Detrol)	Overactive bladder and urge incontinence	The drug was not shown to be effective for children and appeared to show a possible increase in aggressive, hyperactive, and abnormal behavior.
	irinotecan (Camptosar)	Tumors	Children had more rapid disease progression and died more quickly. The labeling states that the drug should not be used to treat children with a particular kind of tumor.
	temozolomide (Temodar)	Astrocytoma	Effectiveness in children is not demonstrated.
Ineffective dosing	oxcarbazepine (Trileptal)	Partial seizures	Dose for children aged 2 to 4 and weighing less than 44 pounds is twice the dose per body weight compared to adults.
	methylphenidate (Ritalin)	Attention-deficit/hyperactivity disorder	Children aged 13 to 17 eliminated the drug from their bodies faster than the comparison age group. Therefore, the dosing regimen may be increased to prevent ineffective dosing.
Overdosing	leflunomide (Arava)	Juvenile rheumatoid arthritis	Children weighing less than 88 pounds require a lower-than-expected dose. Overdosing on leflunomide, which has significant toxicity, could make the drug's risks to children outweigh its benefits.
Previously unlabeled adverse effects, including effect on growth and development	venlafaxine (Effexor)	Depression; generalized anxiety disorder	This drug is associated with an increased risk of suicidal thinking and behavior.
	ciprofloxacin (Cipro)	Complicated urinary tract infection or kidney infection	This drug is associated with increased adverse effects to joints or surrounding tissues for children.
	fentanyl (Duragesic)	Chronic pain	This drug should be used only by children who are 2 years of age or older and are opioid tolerant. Use by others can lead to life-threatening respiratory depression and death.
	budesonide (Pulmicort Respules)	Asthma	This drug is now labeled with safety information in patients as young as 6 months. Drug can cause growth suppression and pneumonia.
	fluoxetine (Prozac)	Depression, obsessive-compulsive disorder (OCD)	Effectiveness established in ages 7 to 17 with OCD and ages 8 to 17 with depression. Drug can cause height and weight suppression. It also has a possible link to suicide ideation.
	fluticasone	Flonase: Allergic rhinitis Intranasal	Effectiveness and safety have been established in ages 3 to 9 years with no effect on bone function.
		Cutivate: Dermatoses Topical	Subnormal adrenal function was noted. Drug is not recommended for children.

Note: From *Pediatric Drug Research: Studies Conducted Under Best Pharmaceuticals for Children Act,* from the General Accounting Office, 2007. Retrieved April 30, 2008, from http://www.gao.gov/new.items/d07557.pdf

have resulted from research studies conducted under the FDA Modernization Act and the Best Pharmaceuticals for Children Act. The **Pediatric Research Equity Act of 2003** authorized the FDA to require research of pediatric uses for new drugs.

Today, based on ongoing research, there is more information available to guide the pharmacotherapy of the pediatric patient. Drugs such as vaccines and antibiotics have adequate pediatric labeling. Unfortunately, steroids and drugs for treating HIV, gastrointestinal (GI) disorders, pain, and hypertension still have very little information regarding use in pediatric patients.

PharmFACT

Seventy-five percent of all medications marketed today do not contain approved labels for pediatric use. Of the 80 drugs most frequently prescribed for newborns and infants, only 5 are labeled for pediatric use. *Source:* Lanski, Greenwald, Perkins, & Simon, 2003.

Pharmacokinetic Variables in Pediatric Patients

11.2 Pharmacokinetic responses in children differ from those in adults.

As discussed in Chapters 4 and 5, most drugs must reach their target cells in sufficient quantities to produce therapeutic effects. This depends on what the body does to the medication after it is administered (pharmacokinetics) and the mechanisms by which a drug changes the body (pharmacodynamics). The normal physiological changes of growth and development markedly affect pharmacokinetics and pharmacodynamics. The nurse must understand the unique actions of drugs in pediatric patients to deliver safe and effective pharmacotherapy.

Absorption: Two primary factors have the potential to influence the oral absorption of drugs in pediatric patients: increased gastric pH and delayed gastric emptying. Low gastric acid production may enhance the absorption of acid-labile drugs such as ampicillin and penicillin and slow the absorption of weak acids like phenobarbital. This is especially true for premature infants and neonates. Gastric acid production usually stabilizes by 2 months of age.

Slowed gastric motility in very young children will keep the drug longer in the stomach. This will increase the absorption of drugs that are absorbed across the stomach lining, but slow the rate of drug absorption for those that rely on the intestine for absorption. The rate of bile salt secretion is diminished in premature infants and neonates, which will delay the absorption of lipid-soluble drugs and vitamins.

In the infant, relatively low blood flow to skeletal muscles leads to slow and erratic absorption of drugs administered by the intramuscular (IM) and subcutaneous routes. Weak muscle contractions may also contribute to the delayed absorption and distribution of IM drugs. IM injections are generally avoided due to their unpredictable absorption rates and their associated pain.

The skin of infants is thin and highly permeable, allowing lotions and topical drugs to be absorbed at a more rapid rate than adults. For example, use of topical corticosteroids in infants has been found to cause systemic effects such as adrenal insufficiency, hyperglycemia, and glaucoma (Hengge, Ruzicka, Schwartz, & Cork, 2006). Care must be taken to prevent accidental overdose.

CONNECTION *Checkpoint* 11.1

From what you learned in Chapter 4, what effect does food in the stomach have on drug absorption? What effect might this have on neonates who are given frequent feedings? See Answer to Connection Checkpoint 11.1 in Appendix A.

Distribution: Three main factors affecting drug distribution in children are the proportion of water to fat, immature liver function, and the underdeveloped blood–brain barrier.

Approximately 80% of a newborn's body weight is due to water. This gradually decreases to 60%, that of an adult, during the first year. The higher proportion of water dilutes water-soluble drugs such as furosemide (Lasix). In addition, water-soluble drugs will move out of the serum to other areas of the infant's body where water concentration is high. The overall effect is lower serum drug levels; higher doses may be needed to maintain adequate serum levels of the drug.

What about lipid-soluble drugs? Infants have a low percentage of body fat compared to adults. Lipid-soluble drugs that would normally be distributed to fat tend to stay in the blood, raising serum drug levels.

Prior to age 6 months, the child's immature liver produces very small amounts of plasma proteins. Drugs that normally bind to plasma proteins will now be present as "free" drug in the serum. Drugs and endogenous substances such as bilirubin compete for the few available protein-binding sites. In some cases, previously bound substances or drugs may be displaced into the serum, leading to potential toxicity. Drugs with high levels of protein binding include ampicillin, morphine, phenytoin (Dilantin), and propranolol (Inderal).

The **blood–brain barrier** is a network of capillaries in the central nervous system (CNS) that form tight junctions, which prevent the passage of certain medications into the brain. Because the child's blood–brain barrier is not fully developed at birth, drugs and other chemicals can easily penetrate the CNS, resulting in heightened responses. The nurse caring for neonates taking drugs such as barbiturates that affect CNS functions should assess for potential toxicity. It is also possible that some drugs not intended for CNS penetration may access the brain, causing CNS adverse effects such as seizures, drowsiness, or dizziness.

Metabolism: The rate at which drugs are metabolized in children is impacted by the immaturity of the hepatic cytochrome P450 (CYP450) enzyme system. Metabolism is significantly slower in children, leading to reduced clearance rates and extended half-lives for drugs extensively metabolized by the liver. To avoid toxicity, drug doses must be accurately determined and administered at adequately spaced intervals to allow sufficient time for metabolic handling of the drug. The metabolic rate reaches adult levels by ages 3 to 5 years. Until then, the nurse should remain vigilant for signs of toxicity in patients taking drugs such as salicylates that are metabolized primarily in the liver.

The enzyme alcohol dehydrogenase is markedly reduced at birth, gradually increasing until age 5. This enzyme is responsible for detoxifying benzyl alcohol, a preservative found in parenteral drug formulations. Newborns are especially sensitive to the effects of benzyl alcohol and can develop "gasping syndrome" that can lead to respiratory and cardiovascular failure. The nurse must ensure that neonates do not receive products containing benzyl alcohol.

Excretion: The child's ability to effectively excrete most drugs depends on the maturity and function of the kidneys. For drugs to be excreted efficiently the kidneys must have an adequate glomerular filtration rate and active tubular secretion and reabsorption functions. Young children have immature renal systems with slower renal clearance, resulting in accumulation of drugs excreted by the kidneys. Signs of nephrotoxicity include oliguria, urinary frequency, hematuria, cloudy urine, rising blood urea nitrogen (BUN) and creatinine, and fever. Although standard pediatric doses can be administered at approximately 3 to 5 months of age when the infant is able to concentrate urine, serum levels of drugs such as theophylline and gentamicin must be monitored closely to prevent adverse reactions.

Pharmacologic Implications Associated with Growth and Development

11.3 The role of the nurse in administering medications changes with each developmental age group.

The nurse responsible for administering pediatric medications must take into consideration the age, weight, and developmental level of the child. For the purposes of medication administration, the pediatric patient is defined as being any age from birth to 16 years and weighing less than 50 kg (110 lb). Additionally, children are classified as neonates, infants, toddlers, preschool, school age, and adolescent.

Growth is a term that characterizes the progressive increase in physical (body) size. *Development* refers to the functional evolution of the physical, psychomotor, and cognitive capabilities of a living being. Stages of growth and physical development usually go hand in hand in a predictable sequence, whereas psychomotor and cognitive development have a tendency to be more variable in nature.

From birth through adolescence, the growth and development of the pediatric patient mandate adjustments in pharmacotherapeutics above and beyond the calculation of doses. The child's ability to become an active (and willing) partner in his or her own wellness has important implications to nursing care and pharmacotherapeutics.

Pharmacotherapy of the infant: Infancy is the period from birth to 12 months of age. The first 28 days of life are referred to as the neonatal period. During this time, nursing care and pharmacotherapy are directed toward safety of the infant, proper dosing of prescribed drugs, and teaching parents how to administer medications properly. A primary goal is to have the child ingest the entire dose of medication without spitting it out because it is difficult to estimate the amount lost. If the child vomits immediately after taking the drug, the dose may be reordered. The following specific nursing interventions and parental teaching points are important for this age group.

- The infant should be held and cuddled while administering medications and offered a pacifier if the infant is on fluid restrictions caused by vomiting or diarrhea.
- Medications are often administered to infants via droppers into the eyes, ears, nose, or mouth. Oral medications should be directed to the inner cheek and the child given time to swallow the drug to avoid aspiration. If rectal suppositories are administered, the buttocks should be held together for 5 to 10 minutes to prevent expulsion of the drug before absorption has occurred.
- In very young infants the medication may be given via a nipple. Some believe this is controversial because the infant may associate the nipple with medication and refuse feedings.
- Special considerations must be observed when administering IM or intravenous (IV) injections to infants. Unlike adults, infants lack well-developed muscle masses, so the smallest needle appropriate for the drug should be used. For volumes less than 1 mL a tuberculin syringe is appropriate. The vastus lateralis is a preferred site for IM injections, because it has few nerves and is relatively well developed in infants. The gluteal site is usually contraindicated because of potential damage to the sciatic nerve, injury to which may result in permanent disability.
- Because of the lack of choices for injection sites, the nurse must rotate injection sites from one leg to the next to avoid overuse and to prevent inflammation and excessive pain.
- For IV sites, the feet and scalp veins may provide good venous access.

Pharmacotherapy of the toddler: Toddlerhood ranges from 1 to 3 years of age. By age 1 most of the pharmacokinetic responses are similar to that of the adult. The 2-year-old is able to metabolize drugs at a very rapid rate; therefore, the health care provider must adjust drug doses accordingly to maintain therapeutic levels.

During this period, a toddler displays a tremendous sense of curiosity. The child begins to explore, wants to try new things, and tends to place everything in the mouth. This becomes a major concern for medication and household product safety. Toddlers can swallow liquids and may be able to chew solid medications. When prescription drugs are supplied as flavored elixirs, it is important to teach parents that the child not be given access to the medications. Poisoning is extremely common at this age. Some of the most common poisonous substances involved in the exposure of children less than 6 years are analgesics, cough and cold preparations, topical ointments, and vitamins.

Administering medications to toddlers can be challenging for the nurse. At this stage, the child is rapidly developing increased motor ability and learning to assert independence but has extremely limited ability to reason or understand the relationship of medicines to health. Giving long, detailed explanations to the toddler will prolong the procedure and create additional anxiety. Short, concrete explanations followed by immediate drug administration are best for this age group. Physical comfort in the form of touching, hugging, or verbal praise following drug administration is important.

- Pharmaceutical companies often formulate pediatric medicines in sweet syrups to facilitate drug administration. The nurse should mix unpleasant tasting oral medications with more appetizing food such as jam, syrup, or fruit puree, if possible. The medication may be followed with a carbonated beverage or mint-flavored candy. Nurses should teach parents to avoid placing medicine in milk, orange juice, or cereals because children may associate these healthy foods with unpleasant tasting medications.
- IM injections for toddlers may be given into the vastus lateralis muscle. For IV injections the nurse may choose the scalp or feet veins. Additional peripheral site options become available in late toddlerhood.
- Suppositories may be difficult to administer due to the child's resistance. For these invasive administration procedures, having a parent in close proximity will usually reduce the toddler's anxiety and increase cooperation.

Pharmacotherapy of preschoolers: The preschool child ranges in age from 3 to 5 years. In general, principles of medication administration that pertain to the toddler also apply to this age group. Preschoolers tend to cooperate better in taking oral medications if they are crushed or mixed with food or flavored beverages.

- After a child has been walking for about a year, the ventrogluteal site may be used for IM injections because it causes less pain than the vastus lateralis site. Use of the dorsogluteal site has declined due to the risk of affecting the sciatic nerve. The scalp veins can no longer be used for IV access; peripheral veins are used for IV injections.
- Like the toddler, the preschooler often physically resists medication administration. A brief explanation followed immediately by medication administration is usually the best method. Uncooperative children may need to be restrained, and patients over 4 years of age may require two adults to administer the medication.
- Before and after medication procedures, the child may benefit from opportunities to play-act troubling experiences with dolls. When the child plays the role of doctor or nurse by giving a "sick" doll a pill or injection, comforting the doll, and explaining that the doll will now feel better, the little actor feels safer and more in control of the situation.

CONNECTIONS

Evidence-Based Practice Acute Otitis Media

Clinical Question

Acute otitis media (AOM) is an inflammatory or infective process of the middle ear that may be bacterial, fungal, or viral in origin and is often associated with upper airway infection. It is common among young children, especially those exposed to cigarette smoking. In the United States, 93% of all children are reported to have at least one episode of AOM by age 7 years (Sarrell, Cohen, & Kahan, 2003). There is an ongoing debate as to whether or not health care providers should routinely order antibiotic treatment for this condition or if there should be a period of watchful waiting instead of immediate treatment.

Evidence

AOM is responsible for most outpatient antimicrobial treatment in the United States. It is a condition of high morbidity and low mortality. The most common bacterial causes for AOM are *Streptococcus pneumoniae* and *Haemophilus influenzae*. According to McCormick et al. (2005) the widespread use of antibiotics for treatment of AOM has resulted in the emergence of multidrug-resistant pathogens that are difficult to treat. These authors carried out a clinical trial study to compare outcomes of "watchful waiting" versus immediate antibiotic treatment. The objective of the study was to evaluate the safety, efficacy, and acceptability of a nonantibiotic intervention for children with nonsevere AOM. The overall conclusion was that 66% of subjects completed the study without the need for antibiotics. Subjects who were placed on immediate antibiotic therapy had decreased numbers of treatment failures but increased adverse effects from antibiotics treatment, including diarrhea. Subjects without antibiotics were administered higher numbers of pain relievers but were found to have a less multidrug resistant strain of *S. pneumoniae* in the nasopharynx after 12 days of treatment (McCormick et al., 2005). The authors believe that with proper symptom management, "watchful waiting" may be an acceptable alternative to antibiotic treatment for some children with nonsevere AOM. If antibiotics are withheld, the condition can go on to become more inflammatory. High fevers and earaches are presenting signs for this condition. Amoxicillin/clavulanic acid (Augmentin) and erythromycin (Erythrocin) are commonly prescribed for this condition. These antibiotics increase the risk of vomiting, diarrhea, and rashes.

Implications

Nurses are responsible for monitoring children for signs of infection. AOM may be present with or without symptoms; therefore, a careful history from the parents can help avoid unnecessary testing of the infant. Infants with AOM often present with extremely high fevers, vomiting, diarrhea, pallor, dehydration, and irritability. Based on the evidence, the nurse should take a careful history to determine when the condition started and what previous treatment has been given. Parents should be given information regarding the option of "watchful waiting" and immediate antibiotic treatment.

Critical Thinking Question

Based on the research, what are some of the factors to be taken into consideration when deciding whether to treat AOM with antimicrobials versus management of AOM symptoms?

See Answers to Critical Thinking Questions in Appendix A.

Pharmacotherapy of the school-age child: The school-age child is between 6 and 12 years of age. Some refer to this period as the middle childhood years. Rapid physical, mental, and social development occur and early ethical–moral development begins to take shape. During this time, most children remain relatively healthy, with respiratory infections and GI upsets being the most common complaints. When serious illness occurs at this age, the child may become confused and depressed because it is important for the child to be like his peers during this developmental age. When caring for an ill child the nurse must be aware of possible nonadherence to treatment regimens.

The nurse is usually able to gain considerable cooperation from school-age children. More detailed explanations of the effects and importance of medications in maintaining wellness may be of value, because the child has developed some reasoning ability and can understand the relationship between receiving the medicine and feeling better. When children are old enough to welcome choices, they can be offered limited dosing alternatives to provide a sense of control and encourage cooperation. The option of taking one medication before another or the chance to choose which drink will follow a chewable tablet helps to distract children from the issue of whether they will take the medication at all. It also makes an otherwise strange or unpleasant experience a little more enjoyable.

- Allowing children to feel that they are willing participants, rather than victims, in medication administration is an important foundation for adherence.
- Praise for cooperation is appropriate for any pediatric patient and will set the stage for successful medication administration in the future.
- School-age children can take chewable tablets and may be able to swallow tablets or capsules. Many still resist injections; however, an experienced pediatric nurse can usually administer parenteral medications quickly and compassionately without the need for restraining the child.
- The ventrogluteal site is preferred for IM injections, although the muscles of older children are developed enough for the nurse to use other sites.

Pharmacotherapy of the adolescent: Adolescence occurs between ages 13 and 16 years. Rapid physical growth and psychological maturation have a great impact on personality development. The adolescent strongly relates to peers, wanting and needing their support, approval, and presence. Physical appearance and conformity with peers in terms of behavior, dress, and social interactions is important. The strong sense of independence leads teens to self-medicate, either with or without their parents' knowledge. Treatment objectives for the nurse should include teaching parents to keep their medications safely stowed out of sight from inquisitive, experiment-minded adolescents. Parents should also be taught the signs and symptoms of drugs commonly abused by teens such as marijuana, inhalants, and methamphetamine.

The most common needs for the pharmacotherapy of teens are for skin problems, headaches, menstrual symptoms, sex-related concerns, eating disorders, contraception, alcohol and tobacco use, and sports-related injuries.

- Of primary concern to the adolescent are the initiation of sexual intercourse and the avoidance of pregnancy and sexually transmitted infections. The nurse must be prepared to address a variety of topics related to sexuality, including the importance of responsible sexual practices, condom use, and other contraceptive methods.
- Eating disorders commonly occur in this population. The nurse should carefully question adolescents about their eating habits and their use of over-the-counter (OTC) appetite suppressants or laxatives that may be contributing to bulimia or anorexia.
- Alcohol, tobacco use, and other illicit drug experimentation are prevalent in this population. Teenage athletes may use amphetamines to delay the onset of fatigue as well as anabolic steroids to enhance performance. The nurse assumes a key role in educating adolescent patients about the hazards of tobacco use and illicit drugs.
- The adolescent has a need for privacy and control in drug administration. The nurse should communicate with the teen more in the manner of an adult rather than as a child. Teens usually appreciate thorough explanations of their treatment, and ample time should be allowed for them to ask questions.
- Despite their need to have independence and the desire to self-medicate, teens have a very poor understanding of medication information (Buck, 2007). Adolescents are reluctant to admit their lack of knowledge, so the nurse should carefully explain important information regarding their medications and expected adverse effects, even if these patients claim to understand.

CONNECTION *Checkpoint* 11.2

The nurse writes the following in the chart of a toddler receiving morphine: *Risk for Constipation*, related to opioid analgesic use. From what you learned in Chapter 9, what type of statement is this and what part of the nursing process is being utilized? See Answer to Connection Checkpoint 11.2 in Appendix A.

Medication Safety for Pediatric Patients

11.4 The nurse is a key member of the health care team in ensuring medication safety in pediatric patients.

The nurse is often the one responsible for administering medications to children. The importance of accurate drug dosage calculations, proper administration techniques, proper efforts to minimize adverse effects, and the need for overall safety cannot be overemphasized.

Principles of safe medication practice for pediatric patients are identical to those of adult patients (see Chapter 7). Medication safety is a team approach. Every level of responsibility is involved, including hospitalwide (or corporationwide) policies, prescriber actions, pharmacy guidelines, nursing interventions, and patient and family adherence. Responsibility for preventing medication errors in pediatric patients is shared by every member of the team.

The safety and effectiveness of a medication regimen depends on proper procurement, storage, and administration of the drug. In the hospital setting, nurses are ultimately responsible for adherence to the basic rules of drug administration: right patient, right drug, right route, right dose, at the right time. Younger pediatric patients may not be able to accurately identify themselves; thus it is imperative that the nurse use precautions to ensure that the right patient receives the prescribed medication. The nurse must check the child's identification band against the medication record. Most hospitals' policies require that drugs such as digoxin, heparin, insulin, chemotherapeutic agents, opioid analgesics, and barbiturates be double-checked with another nurse prior to administration. If the nurse suspects that a dose of medication ordered by the prescriber is outside the normal range, it is the nurse's responsibility to question the order because some drugs can be lethal to pediatric patients. The nurse should regularly check a drug handbook or *Physician's Desk Reference* (PDR) for updated information on pediatric drugs and their adverse effects.

The American Academy of Pediatrics (2003) has established guidelines to prevent pediatric medication errors in the inpatient setting. The guidelines that directly affect the nurse are as follows.

Nursing Actions and Guidelines

- Check medication calculations with another professional member of the health care team.
- Confirm patient identity before administration of each dose.
- Be familiar with medication ordering and dispensing systems.
- Verify drug orders before medication administration.
- Verify unusually large or small volumes or dosage units for a single patient dose.
- When a patient, a parent, or a caregiver questions whether a drug should be administered, listen attentively, answer questions, and double-check the medication order.
- Remain familiar with the operation of medication administration devices and the potential for errors with such devices, particularly patient-controlled analgesia (PCA) or infusion pumps.

Nursing Education and Communication

- Develop and maintain continuous education programs for nursing competencies in devices used for pediatric medication administration, particularly PCA and infusion pumps.
- Develop and maintain a pediatric medications knowledge base.
- Discuss medication orders with the prescriber whenever possible.
- Integrate and provide education for the patient and caregiver regarding the medication regimen.
- Record and verify patient identity, weight, allergies, and previous medication use.
- Be aware of and be involved in ongoing error-tracking systems and pharmacy programs. Encourage blame-free error reporting. Ensure that all staff members understand the method of reporting and are knowledgeable about the Joint Commission on Accreditation for Healthcare Organization's (JCAHO) reporting rules.

Determining Pediatric Drug Dosages

11.5 The nurse must be accurate in calculating drug dosages of pediatric patients.

Nurses must consistently update their skills in calculating pediatric doses because errors in drug administration may have serious consequences. Drug dosage calculation for pediatric patients should be individualized and nurses should take into consideration the children's age, height, weight, maturational state, and body surface area (BSA). All drug calculations for pediatric patients in critical care settings should be double-checked by the pharmacist and another nurse prior to administration.

Two common procedures of calculating pediatric dosages are the body weight method and body surface area method. Utilization of the **body weight method** requires a calculation of the number of milligrams of drug, based on the child's weight in kilograms (mg/kg). A unit of time is usually included; for example, gentamicin 5 mg/kg/24 h. The body weight method is simple and a dose can be calculated quickly. However, the serum concentrations of many drugs are not proportional to body weight, and body weight does not take into consideration pharmacokinetic variables such as changes in metabolism and elimination rates discussed in Section 11.2.

The **body surface area (BSA) method** uses an estimate of the child's BSA. This method is believed to be the most valid basis for dosage, because it is related to certain physiological functions that account for the pharmacokinetic differences in pediatric patients. The BSA method better estimates blood volume, metabolism, and the effects of drugs. Measurements of the fluid volume compartment and the serum concentrations of drugs also correlate well with the BSA.

Using the BSA method, the child's height and weight are plotted on a **nomogram** (Figure 11.1) and a line is drawn between the two points. The point at which the line intersects the surface area line is the child's BSA. The dose is calculated as: BSA $\div$ 1.73 $\times$ adult dose $=$ pediatric dose.

Other methods, including electronic calculators, are used to estimate pediatric doses. Each method has specific advantages and disadvantages. The student should refer to a medication mathematics text for practice calculation examples.

Adverse Drug Reactions in Children and Promoting Adherence

11.6 Pediatric patients are more susceptible than adults to adverse drug effects.

Because of their smaller size and immature or developing organ systems, pediatric patients are more susceptible to adverse effects. The nurse may find it challenging to identify adverse effects because infants and young children often do not have the maturity or verbal skills to accurately describe

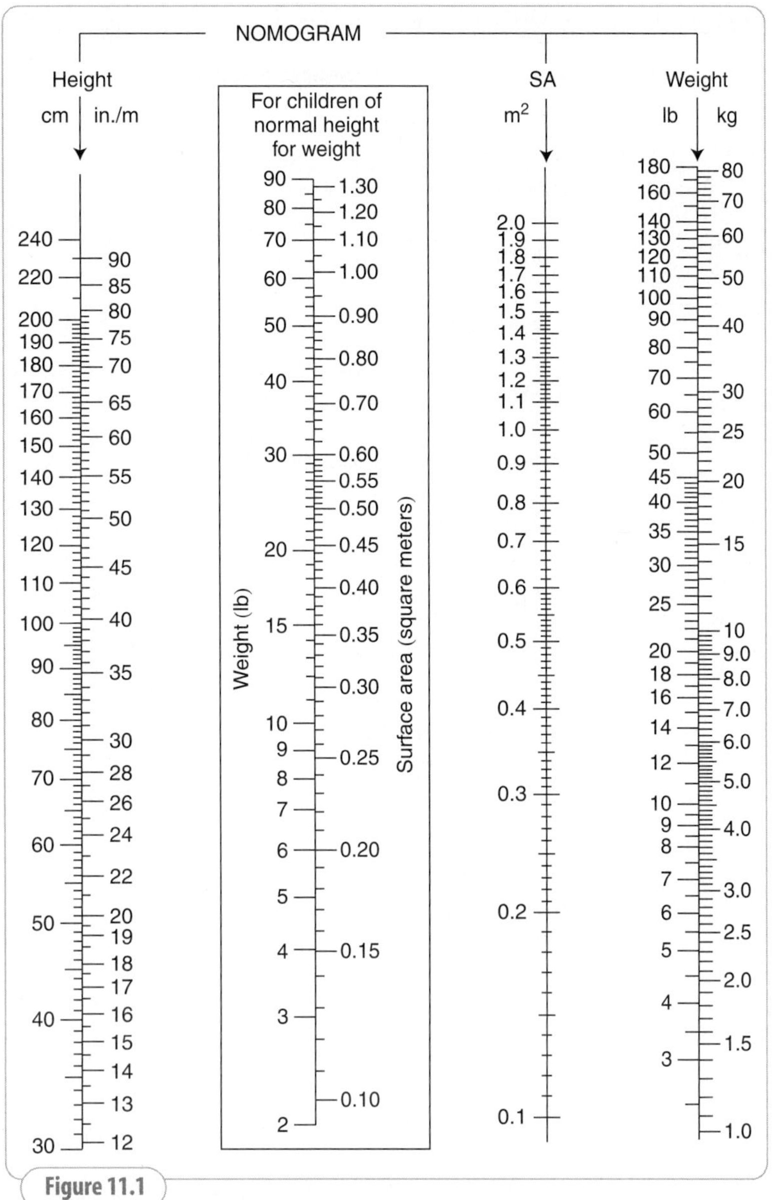

Figure 11.1

West nomogram for estimation of surface areas.

Source: From *Nelson Textbook of Pediatrics,* 18th ed., by R. E. Behrman, R. M. Kliegman, & H. B. Jenson, Eds., 2007, Philadelphia, PA: W. B. Saunders.

their feelings following the medication administration. Identifying pediatric adverse effects will depend on the skill and ability of the nurse in assessing subtle changes in patient response. For example, a child on diuretics should have strict intake and output measurements to help determine if the drug is working properly. Excessive weight gain could be caused by edema resulting from poor kidney excretion, or weight loss might be due to excessive diuresis. Signs of ototoxicity may go unnoticed for a long time unless someone checks that the child no longer responds to verbal commands. It may be necessary to consult a psychologist to identify signs of suicidal ideation from antidepressant use in adolescents.

Most types of adverse effects that occur in children age 1 or older are the same as those in adults. Like adults the majority of adverse effects are dose related; thus the nurse must pay close attention to the proper dose and frequency of drug administration. Knowing specific drugs and their adverse effects in the adult population will help the nurse quickly identify signs and symptoms in pediatric patients. For example, antibiotics such as amoxicillin frequently result in diarrhea in both adults and children. Antianxiety agents, antidepressants, and antipsychotic drugs that cause CNS depression will cause drowsiness in both adults and children.

A few types of adverse effects are specific to children. Often these are the result of immature or developing organs and tissues. For example, tetracycline must be avoided in the neonate because of the potential for permanent staining of the teeth. Sulfonamides can cause jaundice in neonates, and aspirin is contraindicated in children with fever due to the potential for Reye's syndrome. Glucocorticoids can inhibit growth. Table 11.3 illustrates a list of commonly used drugs and their adverse effects on the pediatric patient.

TABLE 11.3 Selected Pediatric Drugs for Which Specific Indications and Dosage Guidelines Exist

Drug	Dosage/Route (maximum dose where indicated)	Adverse Effects
acetaminophen (Tylenol)	PO: 10–15 mg/kg every 8 h	Methemoglobinemia, hepatotoxicity
acyclovir (Zovirax)	PO: 200 mg 5 times daily for genital herpes	*Diarrhea, nausea* Renal failure, seizures
amoxicillin (Amoxil, Trimox, Larotid) or amoxicillin/clavulanate (Augmentin)	PO: 20–40 mg/kg/day	*Diarrhea* Anaphylaxis
ampicillin (Omnipen, Polycillin, Principen)	PO: 50–100 mg/kg/day	*Diarrhea* Anaphylaxis
azithromycin (Zithromax)	PO: 5–10 mg/kg/day	*Diarrhea* Hepatotoxicity
budesonide (Rhinocort)	Intranasal: 2 sprays in each nostril 2 times a day for allergies	*Headache, fatigue* Paresthesia
ceftriaxone (Rocephin)	IV/IM: 50–100 mg/kg/day	*Diarrhea* Colitis
cephalexin (Keflex)	PO: 25–50 mg/kg/day every 6 h	*Diarrhea* Anaphylaxis, angioedema
clarithromycin (Biaxin)	PO: 15 mg/kg/day	*Vomiting, diarrhea* Colitis
diphenoxylate and atropine (Lomotil)	PO: ½–1 tsp, up to 4 doses/day	*Dizziness, sedation* Paralytic ileus
erythromycin (Erythrocin, Pediamycin)	PO: 30–50 mg/kg/day	*Nausea, vomiting* Hepatotoxicity
ferrous sulfate (Feosol, Fergon, others)	PO: 0.5–1 mg/kg/day maintenance	*Nausea, black stools* Shock
fluconazole (Diflucan)	PO: 6 mg/kg/day first dose, then 3 mg/kg/day	*Headache, nausea* Hepatotoxicity
fluticasone (Flonase)	Intranasal: 1 spray in each nostril once a day; may increase to 2 sprays daily	*Nasal dryness* Epistaxis
gentamicin (Garamycin)	Eyedrops: 1–2 drops in conjunctival sac, 2–6 times daily	*Ocular irritation*
ibuprofen (Advil, Motrin)	PO: 5–10 mg/kg/dose given every 6–8 h	*Nausea, heartburn* GI bleeding
imipramine (Tofranil)	PO: 25–50 mg/day for nocturnal enuresis	*Urinary retention* Angioedema
loracarbef (Lorabid)	PO: 15–30 mg/kg/day	*Nausea, rash*
methylphenidate (Ritalin)	PO: 5–10 mg/kg/day	*Nervousness, insomnia* Palpitations
minocycline (Minocin)	4 mg/kg/day bid	*Dizziness, nausea*
nystatin (Mycostatin)	PO: 1–6 mL (100,000–600,000 units) qid	*Nausea, vomiting* Diarrhea
oxcarbazepine (Trileptal)	PO: 8–10 mg/kg/day initial dose	*Fatigue* Somnolence
penicillin VK (Pen Vee K, V-Cillin K)	PO: 25–50 mg/kg/day every 3–4 h	*Diarrhea* Anaphylaxis
trimethoprim-sulfamethoxazole (Bactrim, Septra)	8 mg/kg/day trimethoprim/ 40 mg/kg/day sulfamethoxazole every 12 h	*Nausea, rash, anemia* Exfoliative dermatitis
valproic acid (Depakene, Depakote)	PO: 15 mg/kg/day	*Drowsiness, nausea* Bone marrow suppression

Note: *Italics* indicate common adverse effects. Underline indicates serious adverse effects.

CONNECTION Checkpoint 11.3

The nurse gives a preschooler a sedative but, rather than sleep, the child becomes excited and experiences insomnia. From what you learned in Chapter 3, this is most likely classified as what type of effect? See Answer to Connection Checkpoint 11.3 in Appendix A.

Like adults, children may also experience drug interactions. Drugs that are most likely to participate in drug interactions in pediatric patients are those with high potency, narrow therapeutic index, and extensive protein binding, and those that affect vital organ functions or hepatic metabolism.

Often parents' first response to their child's illness is to provide home remedies. OTC and herbal treatments are extremely common in some households, and research suggests that they are on the rise among a large segment of the population. The nurse must become aware of commonly used OTC and herbal remedies in order to advise the families about the pros and cons. Parents must understand that OTC and herbal therapies may have adverse effects of their own and may interact with prescription medications. Herbal remedies commonly used in homes include St. John's wort, echinacea, ginseng, licorice, and sassafras.

PharmFACT

In a study of pediatric emergency visits, the following data were obtained regarding the use of herbal therapies by caregivers:

- **45% gave their child an herbal product in the past year, the most common being aloe and echinacea.**
- **27% gave their child three or more herbal products.**
- **80% reported that friends or relatives were their primary source of herbal information.**
- **Only 45% discussed the herbal products with their pediatrician.** *Source:* Lanski et al., 2003.

A drug will fail to achieve optimum therapeutic outcomes if it is not taken properly. **Adherence,** also called compliance, is taking the drug according to the instructions on the label or as provided by the prescriber. Maximizing medication adherence is a major goal of the pediatric nurse. The nurse must assess the patient and family to determine factors that will affect the family's ability to assist the child with the medication regimen, and develop strategies that will enhance medication adherence. The more complex, expensive, and inconvenient the medication regimen, the less likely will the child and family adhere. Children are most likely to adhere to their medication regimen if the following conditions exist:

- High expectations of successful outcomes of the therapy
- Supportive family members who are able to communicate with the prescriber
- Positive interactions with the nurse and caregivers
- Minimal adverse effects from the medications
- Simple, short-term, inexpensive regimen with minimum disruption to daily routine

The nurse works with the child and family to enhance adherence by applying direct measures. The patient and family should be asked directly whether or not they have doubts about their ability to adhere. If there is doubt, the nurse should explore the areas of concerns with the family and start by teaching the importance of the drug, route of administration, expected outcomes, and possible adverse effects. In long-term drug therapy the nurse may have to arrange for follow-up appointments to assess drug responses or to administer the oral drug(s) to the child and observe the drug being swallowed. This technique is known as **directly observed therapy (DOT).** In extreme cases when the child does not appear to be responding appropriately to the prescribed regimen, periodic measurement of plasma drug levels can help determine the amount of drug ingested, and whether it has been taken as prescribed.

UNDERSTANDING THE CHAPTER

Key Concepts Summary

11.1 Recent legislation has attempted to improve the testing and labeling of pediatric drugs.

11.2 Pharmacokinetic responses in children differ from those in adults.

11.3 The role of the nurse in administering medications changes with each developmental age group.

11.4 The nurse is a key member of the health care team in ensuring medication safety in pediatric patients.

11.5 The nurse must be accurate in calculating the drug dosages of pediatric patients.

11.6 Pediatric patients are more susceptible to adverse drug effects than adults.

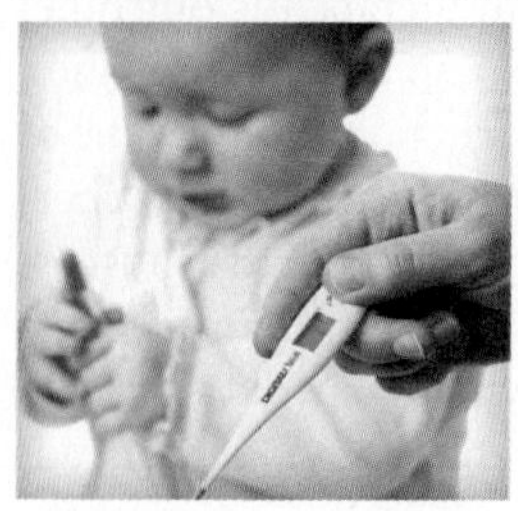

Making the PATIENT Connection

Remember 11-month-old "Timmy," the patient introduced at the beginning of the chapter? Now read the remainder of the case study. Based on the information presented within this chapter, respond to the critical thinking questions that follow.

Ms. Thomas reports that Timmy has not been eating well for the past 72 hours. Last night he vomited three times after drinking sips of water and also had several very loose green foul-smelling bowel movements. He voided only once in the past 12 hours. For the past 5 days Timmy has been taking amoxicillin for an ear infection. Timmy lies still on the examination table but responds to his mother's commands. The nurse prepares Timmy for examination.

Timmy's preliminary diagnosis is gastroenteritis with mild dehydration. His vital signs are as follows: temperature, 38.9°C (102°F); heart rate, 160 beats/minute; respiration, 38/minute; blood pressure, 100/57 mmHg; and weight, 8.6 kg (19 lb.) His skin is dry and warm to touch, and there is slight tenting. The following laboratory studies were performed: serum electrolytes, complete blood count, blood urea nitrogen, creatinine, urinalysis, and stool for culture and sensitivity. Electrolytes were as follows: sodium, 136; potassium, 4.2 mEq/L; chloride, 114 mEq/L; bicarbonate, 9 mEq/L.

An IV line was inserted immediately and a solution of D_5W in 1/3 NSS was started to infuse at 30 mL/hour. Timmy was put on NPO and was given an acetaminophen (Tylenol) suppository 45 mg stat.

Critical Thinking Questions

1. What factors contribute mostly to this risk for deficit in fluid balance?
2. What are some physical signs to look for when evaluating dehydration in this infant?
3. What would best explain the cause for diarrhea in this patient?
4. What are some key points to pay special attention to while monitoring the infant's IV fluid?
5. Why was Timmy given an acetaminophen (Tylenol) suppository?

Case Study

Snead, a 3-year-old girl, arrives at the emergency department in status asthmaticus. Her mother informs you that she was diagnosed as an asthmatic 9 months ago and since then has been back to the emergency department for treatment twice. Two hours prior to admission Snead started coughing and wheezing and then an hour ago started having difficulty breathing. Her mother attempted to relieve the symptoms by giving steam and fluids but the condition only worsened. Snead has audible expiratory wheeze, nasal flaring, and inter- and substernal retractions.

1. What nursing actions would take priority?
2. What nursing assessment should you carry out immediately?
3. What medications would you prepare to administer and how would this be determined?
4. What immediate outcomes could be expected from this treatment?

NCLEX-RN® Review

1 The nurse is preparing to administer medication to the pediatric client. Which of the following factors will affect the oral absorption of drugs?

1. Decreased gastric pH
2. Increased gastric emptying
3. High gastric acid production
4. Delayed gastric emptying

2 The nurse is preparing to give an intramuscular (IM) injection to a 7-month-old infant. Which of the following is the preferred site?

1. Vastus lateralis
2. Deltoid
3. Dorsogluteal
4. Ventrogluteal

3 The experienced pediatric nurse is teaching a new nursing student about injections in the pediatric population. Which of the following statements by the student would indicate that teaching was effective?

1. "Intramuscular (IM) injections in infants are absorbed slowly."
2. "Children experience rapid absorption of IM medications."
3. "IM injections are encouraged due to their predictable absorption rate."
4. "Strong muscle contractions result in delayed absorption of IM medication."

4 It is time to give a 3-year-old oral medication. Which comment by the nurse is most therapeutic?

1. "This is the medicine that makes you better."
2. "If you don't take your medicine you can't go home."
3. "Would you like to take your medicine with water or juice?"
4. "See how easily your roommate has taken his medicine?"

5 Drugs that are most likely to participate in drug interactions in pediatric clients are those with:

1. Low potency.
2. Wide therapeutic index.
3. Extensive protein binding.
4. Effects on the skin.

6 The health care provider knows that the pediatric client and parents will most likely adhere with the medication regimen if the:

1. Regimen is simple and inexpensive.
2. Medications are costly but well known.
3. Medications are prescribed for a long period.
4. Medications are taken at different times each day.

See Answers to Critical Thinking Questions, Case Study, and NCLEX-RN® Review in Appendix A.

References

American Academy of Pediatrics. (2003). Policy statement: Prevention of medication errors in the pediatric inpatient setting (Reaffirmed May 1, 2007). *Pediatrics, 112,* 431–436.

Behrman, R. E., Kliegman, R. M., & Jenson, H. B. (Eds.). (2007). *Nelson textbook of pediatrics* (18th ed.). Philadelphia: W. B. Saunders.

Boots, I., Sukhai, R., Klein, R., Holl, R., Wit, J., Cohen, A., et al. (2007). Stimulation programs for pediatric drug research—Do children really benefit? *European Journal of Pediatrics, 166*(8), 849–855.

Buck, M. L. (2007). Self-medication by adolescents. *Pediatric Pharmacology, 13*(5), 1–4.

Cohen, H. A., Versano, I., Kahan, E., Sarrell, E. M., & Uziel, Y. (2004). Effectiveness of an herbal preparation containing echinacea, propolis, and vitamin C in preventing respiratory tract infections in children: A randomized, double-blind, placebo controlled multicenter study. *Archives of Pediatric Adolescent Medicine, 158,* 217–221.

General Accounting Office. (2007). *Pediatric drug research: Studies conducted under Best Pharmaceuticals for Children Act.* Retrieved April 30, 2008, from http://www.gao.gov/new.items/d07557.pdf

Hammer-Breslow, L. (2003). The Best Pharmaceuticals for Children Act of 2002: The rise of the voluntary incentive structure and congressional refusal to require pediatric testing. *Harvard Journal on Legislation, 40*(1), 133–192.

Hengge, U. R., Ruzicka, T., Schwartz, R. A., & Cork. M. J. (2006). Adverse effects of topical glucocorticosteroids. *Journal of American Academy of Dermatology, 54*(1), 1–15.

Lanski, S. L., Greenwald, M., Perkins, A., & Simon, H. K. (2003). Herbal therapy use in a pediatric emergency department population: Expect the unexpected. *Pediatrics, 111*(5), 981–985.

McCormick, D. P., Chonmaitree, T., Pittman, C., Saeed, K., Friedman, N. R., Uchida, T., et al. (2005). Nonsevere acute otitis media: A clinical trial comparing outcomes of watchful waiting versus immediate antibiotic treatment. *Journal of Family Practice, 54*(9), 754.

Newman, T. B., Bernzweig, J. A., Takayama, J. I., Finch, S. A., Wasserman, R. C., & Pantell, R. H. (2002). Urine testing and urinary tract infections in febrile infants seen in office settings: The Pediatric Research in Office Settings' Febrile Infant Study. *Archives of Pediatric Adolescent Medicine, 156*(1), 6–7.

Pandolfini, C., & Bonati, M. (2005). A literature review on off-label drug use in children. *European Journal Pediatrics, 164*(9), 552–558.

Roberts, R., Rodriguez, W., Murphy, D., & Crescenzi, T. (2003). Pediatric drug labeling: Improving the safety and efficacy of pediatric therapies. *Journal of the American Medical Association, 290*(7), 905–911.

Sarrell, E. M., Cohen, H. A., & Kahan, E. (2003). Naturopathic treatment for ear pain in children. *Journal of Family Practice, 52*(9), 673, 676.

Tufts Center for the Study of Drug Development. (2005). U.S. pediatric studies incentive led to new labeling for nearly 100 drugs. *Impact Report, 4*(7).

U.S. Food and Drug Administration. (2008). *Safety alerts for drugs, biologics, medical devices and dietary supplements.* Retrieved May 1, 2008, from http://www.fda.gov/medwatch/SAFETY.htm

U.S. Food and Drug Administration, Department of Health and Human Services. (2005). *Regulations requiring manufacturers to assess the safety and effectiveness of new drugs and biological products in pediatric patients.* Retrieved May 1, 2008, from http://www.fda.gov/cder/guidance/pedrule.htm

CHAPTER

Mary Smith, 80 years old, is being transported via ambulance to the emergency department. She looks pale and thin with sunken eyes and extremely dry lips. "I'm so relieved my neighbor came by to check on me. I have not been able to get out of bed for 2 days."

Patient "Mary Smith"

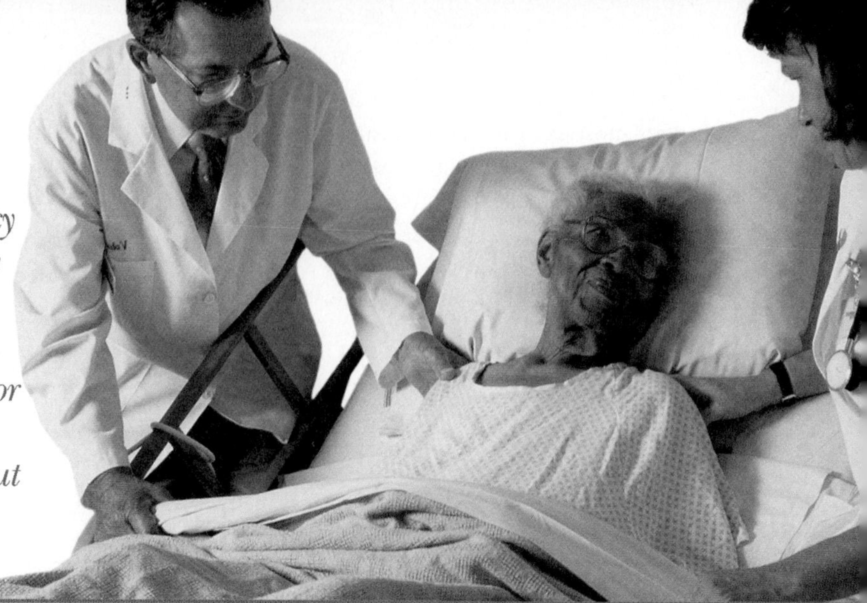

12 Pharmacotherapy of the Geriatric Patient

Learning Outcomes

After reading this chapter, the student should be able to:

1. Describe factors that lead to polypharmacy in older adults.
2. Identify age-related physiological changes in the older adult.
3. Explain how age-related physiological changes alter pharmacokinetics and pharmacodynamics and affect drug response in the older adult.
4. Explain strategies that the nurse may implement to improve adherence with drug therapy in geriatric patients.
5. Explain why older adults are more likely to experience adverse drug reactions and interactions.
6. Identify specific drugs that are particularly hazardous for use in older patients.
7. Differentiate medication responses that result from age-related alterations in specific body systems from those that occur in younger individuals.
8. Develop nursing interventions that maximize pharmacotherapeutic outcomes in the older adult.
9. Generate key points for family and patient education regarding drug therapy for the older adult.

Chapter Outline

Polypharmacy

Physiological Changes Related to Aging

Pharmacokinetic and Pharmacodynamic Changes in the Older Adult

Adherence and Drug Misuse Among Older Adults

Adverse Drug Reactions in Older Adults

Key Terms

adherence, 150
Beers criteria, 152
drug misuse, 150
polypharmacy, 147

Older adults are persons who are 65 years of age and older. Of this age group, those older than 84 years are the fastest growing segment of the population. The average age of the population has increased significantly over the last few decades because of improved access to health care, people choosing healthier lifestyles, and more effective treatment of diseases. With the increase in life span, however, has come an increased reliance on medications to maintain health. This chapter focuses on aspects of pharmacology unique to geriatric patients, and provides steps that the nurse can take to provide safe, effective pharmacotherapy for this population.

PharmFACT

The elderly population will grow rapidly when 76 million baby boomers reach age 65 years and older between 2010 and 2030. By 2030 it is expected that older adults will account for 20% of the total population, according to the U.S. Bureau of the Census *Source:* Goldstein & Damon, 1993.

Polypharmacy

12.1 Older adults take more medications than any other segment of the population.

The pharmacotherapy of older adults is more challenging than that of their middle-age or younger counterparts. To deliver safe and effective pharmacotherapy for patients in this age group, the nurse must consider many age-related variables that affect pharmacotherapy. Failure to recognize these variables may lead to suboptimal therapeutic outcomes and possibly endanger patient safety.

Giving an "average dose" of a drug to an older adult may produce a very different response than when the same dose is given to a younger patient, even if the two patients have the same weight. The pharmacologic action of the drug in older adults may be enhanced or diminished. The adverse effects may be more severe or entirely different from those observed in younger patients. The older patient may experience more drug interactions. What factors are responsible for this wide variation in drug response in the geriatric population?

Longevity inevitably leads to increased illnesses, which, in turn, necessitate the use of increased numbers of medications. Comorbidity, the presence of several chronic medical disorders concurrently, is common among older adults. By about age 65, half the elderly population has two or more chronic disorders, the most prevalent being a combination of hypertension and arthritis. Other comorbidities that occur in a significant number of older adults are heart disease with arthritis, hypertension with diabetes, and depression with nearly any other chronic disorder.

Comorbidities call for use of multiple drugs, a condition termed **polypharmacy.** Although not unique to older patients, polypharmacy is prevalent in this age group because of these comorbidities. The higher the number of drugs taken by a patient, the greater is the possibility of experiencing adverse effects and drug interactions. As presented in Chapter 6, drugs that may be safe when used as monotherapy can have additive adverse effects when combined with other drugs. For example, taking multiple drugs that cause central nervous system (CNS) depression can lead to excessive sedation, thus increasing the risk for accidents or injury due to falls. Taking two or more drugs that cause renal or liver impairment can result in additive organ damage in older adults who may already have some degree of impaired function due to normal aging processes.

Polypharmacy may also occur when the patient takes over-the-counter (OTC) drugs, herbal products, and dietary supplements in conjunction with prescribed medications. For example, older adults frequently seek OTC medications to treat constipation and minor aches and pains. Many also take vitamins, alternative therapies, and dietary supplements. Most patients are unaware that these agents can interact with prescription medications.

Patients who visit multiple physicians and use different pharmacies may experience polypharmacy because each doctor or pharmacist may not be aware of all the drugs ordered by

CONNECTIONS

To the Community — Reducing Medication Errors in Older Adults

Most older adults take multiple prescription drugs. It is common for older adults with some degree of cognitive impairment to forget to take medicines or to take double doses. In the home setting there are certain strategies that should be implemented to avoid these types of medication errors. Nurses should teach geriatric patients (or their caregiver) to follow some or all of the following strategies:

- Set a schedule whereby medicines are taken at the same time each day.
- Keep a written daily record of drugs taken that includes drug name, dose, date, and time taken.
- Use a memory aid such as pill holders that have compartments for each day of the week and each time of day (morning, noon, or night).
- For visually impaired patients, clearly color code the medication bottles so they are easily recognized.
- Keep an up-to-date written record of all drugs taken, the doses, and the prescriber's name. Bring this to all health care provider appointments.
- Keep a record of all OTC drugs, herbal product dietary supplements, and vitamins taken. Bring this to all health care provider appointments.
- If possible, learn medicines by name, and understand why each is being prescribed.
- Use one pharmacy to fill all prescriptions.

other prescribers. Nurses should urge patients to report all prescription and OTC products on each office visit and teach them to use one pharmacy for their prescription needs.

PharmFACT

Prescription drugs account for the single largest component of out-of-pocket spending on health care after premium spending. A report by Families USA, *Cost Overdose: Growth in Drug Spending for the Elderly 1992–2010*, indicates that annual spending for elderly persons for prescription drugs rose from $559 in 1992 to $1,205 in 2000—a 116% increase. *Source:* McCloskey, 2000.

In addition to polypharmacy, many other factors can alter a geriatric patient's response to medication. These include physiological changes associated with aging (see Section 12.2), changes in pharmacokinetics and pharmacodynamics (see Section 12.3), and patient adherence with the therapeutic regimen (see Section 12.4).

CONNECTION *Checkpoint* 12.1

From what you learned in Chapter 6, state the differences among additive, synergistic, and antagonistic effects. See Answer to Connection Checkpoint 12.1 in Appendix A.

Physiological Changes Related to Aging

12.2 Anatomic and physiological changes associated with aging may alter the patient's response to medications.

With advancing age, certain anatomic and physiological changes occur. These predictable changes should be considered a normal part of the aging process, rather than as diseases or pathologic conditions. Awareness of the normal physiological changes that occur during the life span is critically important in properly assessing and caring for the older adult.

In general, physiological processes slow down with advancing age. For example, the rate of absorption of nutrients from the gastrointestinal (GI) system slows due to the decrease in GI motility and reduced GI blood flow. Metabolism also diminishes due to decreased liver size and reduced blood flow to this organ. Additionally, as a person ages the production of serum albumin by the liver declines. The older adult has a decreased volume of total body water, leading to higher concentrations of substances in the serum.

Cardiovascular system changes in the older adult are related to weakened cardiac muscle and increased peripheral resistance (hypertension). These physiological changes lead to decreased contractile force, which diminishes cardiac output and slows the circulation of nutrients and drugs.

In the nervous system, conduction velocity slows and sensory functions such as vision, hearing, and smell begin to diminish. Brain mass begins to decline, resulting in a progressive loss of cognitive ability. Additionally, as one ages the efficiency of the blood–brain barrier declines, allowing more substances to enter the CNS and affect the brain.

Older adults undergo a progressive decline in renal function as a result of decreased renal blood flow, decreased glomerular filtration rate, and decreased numbers of nephrons. The kidneys begin to lose their ability to effectively excrete creatinine and other wastes from the body. The body retains drugs and other substances for longer periods.

Normal, age-related physiological changes in organ systems can greatly affect responses to medications. Selected changes, and their effects on drug response, are shown in Table 12.1.

Pharmacokinetic and Pharmacodynamic Changes in the Older Adult

12.3 Normal aging processes can alter pharmacokinetic and pharmacodynamic responses to drugs.

To produce therapeutic effects, most drugs must reach their target cells in sufficient quantities. To a large extent, this depends on what the body does to the medications after they are administered, or pharmacokinetics. Drug response also is dependent on pharmacodynamic factors: the mechanisms by which drugs change the body. The normal physiological changes of aging affect pharmacokinetics and pharmacodynamics. Knowing these changes in the handling of medications helps the nurse to understand the unique actions of drugs in geriatric patients and to predict (and prevent) adverse effects.

Absorption: Overall, drug absorption tends to slow with aging. Fortunately, although the rate of absorption of most drugs is slower in the older adult, absorption is usually complete.

Because of the increased gastric pH that occurs with normal aging, oral tablets and capsules that require high levels of acid for absorption may take longer to dissolve and, therefore, take longer to reach their target tissues. Furthermore, decreased blood flow to and from the GI tract in the aging adult delays the absorption and subsequent distribution of medications. Slowed motility allows drugs to remain longer in the GI tract, increasing the length of time for absorption and raising the risk for adverse effects such as nausea and vomiting. Physiological changes that lead to alterations in the rate and quantity of drug absorption are listed in Table 12.1.

Distribution: The extent to which drug distribution is affected in the older adult depends on whether the drug is fat soluble or water soluble. Age-related increases in fat storage cause lipid-soluble drugs such as diazepam (Valium), phenobarbital (Luminal), and haloperidol (Haldol) to be stored in the body for extended periods, leading to lower plasma levels and increased drug concentrations in the tissues. The longer a drug remains in the tissues, the more significant will be the response to the drug and the greater the potential for adverse effects. Age-related decreases in total body water result in water-soluble drugs such as gentamicin (Garamycin) and hydrochloro-

TABLE 12.1 Physiological Factors Affecting Medication Responses in Older Adults

Body System	Changes in Physiological Factors	Effect on Medication Response
Cardiovascular System	• Decreased force of contractions, contractile efficiency, and stroke volume • Decreased oxygen uptake by tissues • Decreased serum albumin and serum-binding capacity	• Reduced cardiac output and slowed distribution • Decreased metabolism • Changed drug distribution, producing unpredictable and toxic levels of highly protein-bound drugs such as phenytoin
Central Nervous System	• Decreased brain size, number of neurons, and peripheral nerve function • Declining efficiency of blood–brain barrier	• Decreased drug distribution • Increased penetration of drug in the brain
Endocrine System	• Alterations in carbohydrate metabolism • Decreased growth hormone production and altered glucocorticoid activity, leading to increased body fat, decreased muscle, and bone mass	• Reduced insulin secretion and increased insulin resistance, manifesting as type 2 diabetes mellitus • Increased absorption of fat-soluble drugs
Gastrointestinal System `	• Decreased GI motility • Decreased emptying of gastric contents • Reduced gastric acid production • Increased gastric pH • Decreased blood flow to the GI tract • Decreased thirst perception, leading to risk for dehydration, electrolyte imbalance, and poor nutritional intake	• Slowed rate of absorption • Increased potential for adverse effects
	• Decreased liver size • Decreased blood flow to the liver • Decreased ability of the liver to metabolize drugs	• Slowed metabolism • Prolonged drug half-life, increasing the potential for adverse effects
Musculoskeletal System	• Decreased lean muscle mass and increased and redistributed body fat	• Extended and increased effect of fat-soluble drugs such as diazepam
Respiratory System	• Decreased muscle strength and endurance	• Decreased chest and lung expansion and response to hypoxia, resulting in altered rate of absorption and excretion of some respiratory drugs
Urinary System	• Decreased fluid volume • Decreased renal blood flow, glomerular filtration, and tubular secretory function • Decreased creatinine clearance	• Higher concentrations of water-soluble drugs • Reduced rate of excretion and decreased drug clearance • Decreased drug excretion

thiazide (HCTZ) having less total body fluid for dilution. Therefore, water-soluble drugs have higher serum concentrations and may produce more intense actions. To prevent toxicity, the peak and trough levels of drugs with a low safety index such as gentamicin are checked periodically, and drug dosages are adjusted accordingly.

Another factor that may alter drug distribution in the older adult is the change in plasma protein levels. Because of declining liver function, plasma protein levels are reduced up to 13% in the older adult. This decrease leads to fewer binding sites for certain drugs, resulting in higher concentration of free drug, which may lead to toxicity. In older adults taking highly protein-bound drugs such as phenytoin (Dilantin) and warfarin (Coumadin), the nurse must carefully assess for signs of toxicity, even when the patient is receiving therapeutic doses.

Higher levels of drugs are able to enter the brain in older adults due to the inefficient blood–brain barrier. Patients taking drugs such as benzodiazepines, antipsychotic agents, antiepileptic drugs, or tranquilizers that affect the CNS must be assessed for signs of adverse effects that often manifest as reduced cognitive function, drowsiness, confusion, and even hallucinations and psychoses.

Metabolism: Although most tissues metabolize drugs to some extent, the liver is by far the most important organ performing this function. Age-related changes in the liver include reduced hepatic function, decreased liver mass, diminished blood flow, and alteration in the activity of some hepatic enzymes.

The liver is a complex organ, and age-related changes are often unpredictable. The level of some metabolic enzymes may be reduced with aging, whereas others remain unchanged. In general, reduced metabolism means that drugs will have extended durations of action. Drugs with a long half-life such as gentamicin, digoxin (Lanoxin), and acetaminophen (Tylenol) remain longer in the body with the potential for accumulation in tissues. Such drugs should be prescribed less frequently or in reduced dosages, and the patient should be monitored closely.

CONNECTION *Checkpoint* 12.2

From what you learned in Chapter 5, what are CYP enzymes? State the differences between a substrate and an inducer of CYP enzymes. See Answer to Connection Checkpoint 12.2 in Appendix A.

Excretion: The kidneys excrete the majority of drugs. The rate of drug excretion in older adults decreases proportionately to age-related decrease in renal function. The half-life of drugs is increased and the dosages or frequency of administration should be decreased to avoid toxicity due to drug accumulation. Patients who are taking drugs that are excreted primarily by the kidneys should receive periodic serum creatinine tests to determine renal function. Creatinine clearance levels tend to decrease from about 140 mL/minute at ages 17 to 24 years to around 96 mL/minute at ages 75 to 84. Dosages of drugs must be adjusted periodically in patients with impaired renal function.

Pharmacodynamic changes: Pharmacodynamic changes are usually associated with drug receptors. Evidence suggests that older adults have decreased numbers of receptors and, possibly, changes in receptor sensitivity. In assessing the older adult, the nurse will find that there is a decreased response to beta-adrenergic agonists and antagonists and, at the same time, an increased response to anticholinergics, CNS depressants, and drugs such as warfarin. There is limited information on how pharmacodynamic alterations actually occur in older adults.

Adherence and Drug Misuse Among Older Adults

12.4 Adherence with the therapeutic regimen is a major challenge for many older adults.

Drug **adherence** or compliance is the willingness and ability to take medication as prescribed. Health care providers often assume that patients leaving the clinic or hospital will be adherent, fill their prescriptions, and take their medicines as directed. It may be surprising to learn that over a third of patients report they are often nonadjerent with drug therapy. Reasons for nonadherence are many and varied but include the following patient responses (Harris Interactive, 2005):

- "I had no symptoms or the symptoms went away" (36%).
- "I wanted to save money" (35%).
- "I didn't believe the drugs were effective" (33%).
- "I didn't think I needed to take them" (31%).
- "I had painful or frightening adverse effects" (28%).
- "The drugs prevented me from doing other things I wanted to do" (25%).

CONNECTIONS

Lifespan Considerations

Drug Monitoring in the Older Adult

To avoid toxicity, a number of drug dosage changes should be made for the older adult.

- The older adult should be started on the smallest effective dose of medication and then be titrated upward.
- Observe the older patient for signs of drug accumulation about 3 to 5 days after new drug initiation. Consider any change in physical or emotional behavior as possible drug intoxication.
- Monitor hydration especially among older patients because dehydration is one of the main causes of drug toxicity in this age group.

Although nonadherence is not unique to older adults, this population is especially vulnerable. Geriatric patients are more likely to have visual impairment, functional disabilities, and cognitive dysfunction that may be sources of medication errors and nonadherence. This population has more hearing disabilities that may prevent them from understanding verbal instructions from the health care provider. The large number of drugs taken by some geriatric patients makes for a complicated dosing schedule that can be confusing for patients of any age.

Successful management of medical problems depends on a patient's adherence with the regimen. One of the main responsibilities of the nurse is to assess barriers to medication adherence in the older adult. Studies suggest that nonadherence is affected by three factors: the individual patient, the health care provider, and the patient's social support network.

Adherence at the patient level requires the patient's comprehension and commitment to the treatment. The patient must be able to afford the medication, believe in its efficacy, appropriately self-administer, and adjust to lifestyle changes that may be required. The health care provider must be able to effectively instruct the patient regarding a medication's efficacy, prescribe cost-effective medication, decrease the complexity of the regimen, and provide manageable and understandable instructions.

Pharm*FACT*

Adults older than 65 years make up 12% to 13% of the population and are known to consume up to 33% of all prescribed medications and up to 85% of OTC drugs.

Source: McCloskey, 2000.

The nurse should provide the older adult's spouse or caregiver with adequate information regarding the patient's medication regimen, expected lifestyle changes, and the need for emotional support and monitoring. Table 12.2 lists reasons that patients give for nonadherence and provides suggestions for the nurse to promote adherence.

Drug misuse is a specific form of nonadherence that is common among older patients. Misuse includes overuse, underuse, or, in some cases, erratic use. Older patients sometimes misuse drugs accidentally, inappropriately, or deliberately. Self-adjusting the medication dose is a common practice: Patients change their dose level depending on how they feel. Some believe that taking extra

TABLE 12.2 Promoting Adherence in Geriatric Patients

Reasons for Nonadherence	• Unpleasant adverse effects • Forgetfulness • Cognitive or physical impairment • Poor or misunderstood instructions • Complicated regimens • Inability or downright refusal to purchase the medication • Health beliefs about medications
Ways the Nurse Can Promote Adherence	• Assist the older adult in comprehending and committing to the drug treatment regimen. • Communicate the instructions in such a manner that the older patient fully understands the purpose of the treatment. • Provide the elderly patient with social support services to obtain the medications. • Work with a pharmacist to ensure that the medication is dispensed in containers that are easily opened and in formulations that are easily taken. • Make sure all drugs are clearly labeled with instructions. • Simplify the regimen to reduce the number of drugs and doses per day. • Suggest that the older patient use a daily or weekly pill counter. • Provide the patient with a check-off calendar to document each time a medication is taken. • Engage family members or friends in supporting the elderly patient in efforts to comply. • Encourage the elderly patient to report signs of adverse effects. • Schedule periodic tests to determine plasma drug levels. • Place follow-up calls to high-risk patients.

doses will speed their recovery. Uninsured or underinsured patients who cannot afford their medications may try to make the medications last longer by splitting doses. Patients rarely report such practices to their health care provider. Drug misuse may have serious consequences: Many elderly visits to emergency departments are drug related, with nonadherence accounting for a substantial percentage (Malhotraa, Karana, Pandhia, & Jain, 2001).

CONNECTION *Checkpoint* 12.3

From what you learned in Chapter 2, describe some of the benefits to older adults created by the Medicare Prescription Drug Improvement and Modernization Act of 2003. See Answer to Connection Checkpoint 12.3 in Appendix A.

Adverse Drug Reactions in Older Adults

12.5 Older adults are at high risk for experiencing adverse drug reactions and interactions.

An adverse effect is an undesirable and potentially harmful action caused by the administration of medications (see Chapter 6). Older adults have many factors that predispose them to an increased risk of adverse effects. One of the most important factors is the number of drugs prescribed. The risk of an adverse effect greatly increases with the number of drugs taken. The average person over age 65 takes four prescription medications and three OTC drugs every day and fills prescriptions for more than 28 different medications each year (Duxbury, 2007). To minimize adverse effects, prescribers should order drugs only when they are needed and for the shortest length of time necessary to produce a therapeutic effect. Medications and doses should be reviewed on a regular basis to ensure that the intervention is still necessary.

Age-related physiological changes in renal and hepatic function are especially important in placing geriatric patients at greater risk for adverse effects. As the ability of the kidney to excrete drugs diminishes, serum drug levels may rise to cause toxicity. Loss of the ability of the liver to metabolize drugs can also raise serum drug levels and cause adverse effects. The nurse must be vigilant in assessing laboratory results of renal and hepatic function in elderly patients. Doses of most drugs must be adjusted in older adults with renal or hepatic impairment to prevent adverse effects.

As a patient ages it often becomes difficult for the nurse to differentiate between behaviors that may be a natural part of aging and symptoms caused by adverse effects. For example, a frail older person who walks with an ataxic gait might be wrongly suspected of having an adverse effect from benzodiazepines or phenytoin, although the condition might be caused

CONNECTIONS

Lifespan Considerations Reducing the Cost of Medications for Older Adults

Because the cost of prescription drugs may be a major cause for nonadherence in the elderly, nurses should teach these patients ways to cut pharmacy costs, such as the following:

- For a new prescription, do not buy a whole bottle; instead ask for just a few pills. Adverse effects may require a change in medication.
- For ongoing conditions, buy medications in large quantities.
- Call around for the lowest price because pharmacy prices can vary greatly. Try to use the same pharmacy for all drugs.
- Ask for a senior citizen discount.
- Ask for a generic equivalent.
- Ask the health care provider for a supply of free drug samples.
- Buy store brand or discount brand OTC products.
- Find out about drug discount or assistance programs.
- If less expensive, try using mail order from a reputable pharmacy.

Source: From "Medications and Older People," (2003). U.S. Food and Drug Administration, *FDA Consumer Magazine Sept-Oct 1997* (Updated in 2003). Pub. No. FDA 03-1315C .Retrieved May 5, 2008, from http://www.fda.gov/fdac/features/1997/697_old.html

by normal aging. Older adults are more likely to experience CNS drug adverse effects such as dizziness, drowsiness, and confusion, which are also symptoms that are often associated with normal aging processes. Medications should be considered as an underlying cause of the following symptoms in older patients:

- Sudden change in mental status
- Rapid weight loss
- Dehydration
- Restlessness
- Anorexia
- Urinary retention or fluid retention
- Change in bowel habits
- Major change in functional status of any organ system

Physicians have compiled a list of drugs of special concern for older adults. Known as the **Beers criteria,** health care providers should avoid prescribing these drugs to older adults because they have been found to produce a high incidence of adverse effects in this population (Fick et al., 2007). Table 12.3 provides a list of commonly used drugs among older adults and their specific toxic responses. Nurses should review the Beers criteria periodically and become familiar with these high-risk drugs.

A drug interaction occurs when a medication interacts with another substance and the drug's actions are affected. The "other substance" causing the drug interaction may be another drug, a dietary supplement, or an herbal product or food (see Chapter 6). The large number of prescription drugs and OTC products taken by older adults predisposes this population to a high risk for drug interactions.

Another factor contributing to the increased risk for drug interactions is the presence of comorbidities (see Section 12.2). For example, the patient with both arthritis and heart disease may be using nonsteroidal anti-inflammatory drugs (NSAIDs) for pain and warfarin (Coumadin) to prevent blood clots. The NSAID may increase the effect of the warfarin, thus raising the potential for bleeding. The patient with both diabetes and hypertension may be taking thiazides and insulin. The thiazides reduce the effectiveness of insulin, thus affecting glycemic control.

The nurse plays a key role in optimizing pharmacotherapy outcomes in geriatric patients, including addressing adverse effects, drug interactions, and issues of polypharmacy. One of the primary nursing responsibilities is to make a connection between the patient and family and the medication regimens. This entails assessing the level of comprehension, cultural beliefs, dietary practices, and physiological conditions of the patient and family. Advanced age does not negate the patient's right to know the names of the prescribed medications, the reasons they are being prescribed, and the potential adverse effects. Table 12.4 highlights nursing responsibilities and rationales regarding adverse effects and drug–drug interactions in older patients.

PharmFACT

The chance of an adverse effect or drug interaction increases with the number of drugs a patient is taking. The risk is estimated to be 6% when two medications are taken, 50% with five medications, and almost 100% with eight or more concurrent medications.
Source: Terrie, 2004.

TABLE 12.3 Selected High-Risk Drugs for Older Adults

Drug	Adverse Response
antihistamines (e.g., chlorpheniramine, diphenhydramine, hydroxyzine)	Sedation, confusion, anticholinergic effects
benzodiazepines (e.g., alprazolam, lorazepam, oxazepam)	Confusion, depression, anticholinergic effects
cimetidine (Zantac)	Confusion, depression
digoxin (Lanoxin)	Reduced renal clearance can cause serious toxicity
muscle relaxants (e.g., carisoprodol, cyclobenzaprine, oxybutynin)	Sedation, weakness, anticholinergic effects
nonsteroidal anti-inflammatory drugs (NSAIDs) (e.g., Naprosyn, Naproxen, oxaprozin)	Photosensitivity, nephrotoxicity, fluid retention
phenytoin (Dilantin)	Confusion, ataxia, slurred speech, diplopia
ranitidine (Zantac)	Liver dysfunction, blood dyscrasias
tricyclic antidepressants (e.g., amitriptyline, doxepin, imipramine)	Hallucinations, confusion, anticholinergic effects

TABLE 12.4 Nursing Responsibilities Related to Adverse Drug Reactions and Drug Interactions in Older Adults

Nursing Responsibilities	Rationales
• Review the patient's medications to determine the potential for adverse effects and drug interactions. Consider cultural and dietary issues.	• Adverse effects are common in older patients because of physiological changes in body composition, multiple illnesses, polypharmacy, and nonadherence. • Some dietary practices may lead to adverse effects and interactions (e.g., low-salt intake may lead to lithium toxicity).
• Instruct the patient about potential adverse effects.	• A well-informed patient is better able to notify the health care provider as early as possible to minimize the effect of adverse effects.
• If the patient is taking sulfa drugs, teach ways to avoid sunburn.	• Sulfa drugs are photosensitizing and may lead to rapid sunburn in some patients.
• Assess the patient's fluid volume.	• Alteration in fluid volume could lead to increased sensitivity to alpha antagonists and other drugs.
• Instruct the patient about the proper time to administer medications.	• Taking medications at the proper time will ensure optimum effectiveness and lower the chance for adverse effects.
• Ensure that the fewest number and lowest doses of medications with the simplest regimens have been prescribed for the patient.	• Polypharmacy may lead to drug toxicity.
• Monitor the patient for expected responses and any changes from normal.	• Adverse effects may not always be predictable because they may arise from sudden changes in the patient's condition.
• Discard all unused and expired medications, and instruct the patient to do the same.	• Drug effects diminish after the expiration date.
• Assess and monitor the patient's mental status for any alterations that may be caused by adverse effects.	• Delirium or confusion may be caused by adverse effects of psychoactive drugs.
• Periodically review the patient's OTC medications, nutritional supplements, and prescribed medications.	• Review of all drugs and alternative therapies can reduce the chances of adverse effects.
• Counsel the patient who is taking cardiac drugs about the drug's effect on sexual activity.	• Cardiac drugs may lead to sexual dysfunction.

UNDERSTANDING THE CHAPTER

Key Concepts Summary

12.1 Older adults take more medications than any other segment of the population.

12.2 Anatomic and physiological changes associated with aging may alter the patient's response to medications.

12.3 Normal aging processes can alter pharmacokinetic and pharmacodynamic responses to drugs.

12.4 Adherence with the therapeutic regimen is a major challenge for many older adults.

12.5 Older adults are at high risk for experiencing adverse drug reactions and interactions.

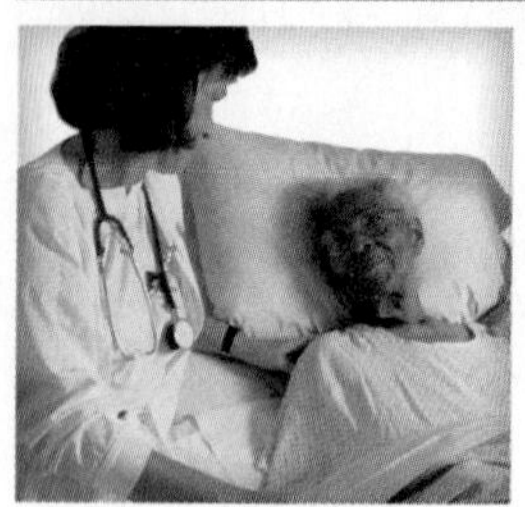

Making the PATIENT Connection

Remember the patient "Mary Smith" at the beginning of the chapter? Now read the remainder of the case study. Based on the information presented within this chapter, respond to the critical thinking questions that follow.

Ms. Smith has an IV solution of normal saline infusing in her left arm and oxygen by mask at 2 liters/minute. Last week she heard that her older cousin passed away, and since then she has become extremely depressed. She refuses to eat or drink but continues to take her medications on a regular basis. This 80-year-old woman is dehydrated and somewhat confused. Her neighbor provides the history. The nurse finds that Ms. Smith has been taking hydrochlorothiazide, phenothiazine, atenolol, and multivitamins daily.

Vital signs are: temperature, 38.6°C (101.4°F); pulse, 100 beats/minute; respiratory rate, 32/minute; and blood pressure, 100/62 mmHg. Her skin is dry and warm to the touch, and her lips are pale, dry, and chapped. She weighs 51.3 kg (113 lb) and her height is 1.7m (5' 7"). Her speech is quiet and slurred. Ms. Smith has not eaten anything during the past 24 hours and has only taken sips of water during the past 12 hours. She has voided once in 12 hours.

The following laboratory tests are completed: urinalysis, BUN/creatinine, CBC, and basal metabolic panel (BMP). Ms. Smith is prescribed IV rehydration fluid and is stabilized in the emergency department before being admitted to the hospital unit.

Critical Thinking

1. What are some potential predisposing factors that could lead to this patient's condition?
2. What preparations for treatment are priorities for the nurse?
3. What are some critical assessment points for the nurse?
4. What are some of the expected patient outcomes following management of dehydration?

Case Study

Ms. Brown, 88 years of age, has mild dementia and was admitted to the hospital where she began treatment for pneumonia with penicillin. She routinely takes insulin, atenolol (Tenormin), cimetidine (Tagamet), and atorvastatin (Lipitor). On day 3 she developed a diffuse maculopapular rash that was diagnosed as an adverse reaction to the penicillin. Her antibiotic order was changed to erythromycin and she was given diphenhydramine (Benadryl) 25 mg four times daily for the allergy. The next day, Ms. Brown became confused and anxious. She was given lorazepam (Ativan) 1 mg every 4 hours prn for confusion.

1. Which of the medications most likely was causing Ms. Brown's delirium?
2. What nonmedication factors noted in the case study could have contributed to Ms. Brown's condition?
3. What teaching regarding medications should the nurse have provided Ms. Brown?

NCLEX-RN® Review

1 Overall, drug absorption in the older adult is somewhat slowed. One of the main reasons attributed to this change is:

1. Increased gastric pH.
2. Increased rate of blood flow.
3. Increased gastrointestinal motility.
4. Increased body surface area.

2 The nurse completes an initial home assessment of an 82-year-old woman recently diagnosed with type 2 diabetes mellitus. She lives at home with her 50-year-old daughter. The woman is able to function independently in all areas of activities of daily living. The most appropriate nursing action for insulin administration for this client is to:

1. Teach the daughter how to administer the insulin to her mother.
2. Instruct the client how to administer the insulin.
3. Recommend daily visits by a home health aide to give the insulin.
4. Ask the health care provider to change the order to an oral hypoglycemic medication.

3 Age-related changes make it necessary to reduce drug dosages in elderly clients due to the:

1. Decrease in total body fat.
2. Increase in lean muscle mass.
3. Decrease in lean muscle mass.
4. Decrease in serum hemoglobin.

4 Older adults experience adverse effects more frequently than young adults due to which of the following? Select all that apply.

1. Excessive prescribing
2. Multiple-drug therapy
3. Increased drug sensitivity
4. Increased body mass
5. Lack of consistent exercise

5 One third of clients report that they are often nonadherent with drug therapy. Which of the following responses is given most frequently for nonadherence?

1. The drugs prevented me from doing other things I wanted to do.
2. I had no symptoms, or, the symptoms went away.
3. I wanted to save money.
4. I didn't believe the drugs were effective.

6 Which of the following statements by the client would inform the nurse that more teaching is necessary prior to discharge?

1. "It doesn't matter if the medication works as long as the doctor prescribed it."
2. "This medication is fully covered by my health insurance."
3. "I have been taking my medications by myself all my life."
4. "I don't mind making changes to my lifestyle while I am on this drug."

See Answers to Critical Thinking Questions, Case Study, and NCLEX-RN® Review in Appendix A.

References

Duxbury, A. S. (2007). *Geropharmacy: Preventing adverse drug effects.* Retrieved May 3, 2008, from http://www.uabhealth.org/32087/

Fick, D. M., Cooper, J. W., Wade, W. E., Waller, J. L., Maclean, J. R., & Beers, M. H. (2007). Updating the Beers criteria for potentially inappropriate medication use in older adults: Results of a US consensus panel of experts. *Archives of Internal Medicine, 163,* 2716–2724.

Fontaine, K. L. (2005). *Complementary and alternative therapies for nursing practice.* Upper Saddle River, NJ: Prentice Hall.

Glasziou, P. P., Del Mar, C. B., Sanders, S. L., & Hayem, M. (2003). Antibiotics for acute otitis media in children. *The Cochrane Database of Systematic Reviews 2003, 4.* Art No: CD000219.

Goldstein, A., & Damon, B. (1993). *We, the American elderly.* U.S. Department of Commerce, Economic and Statistics Administration, Bureau of the Census. Retrieved May 5, 2008, from http://www.census.gov/apsd/wepeople/we-9.pdf

Harris Interactive. (2005). *Prescription drug compliance a significant challenge for many patients, according to new national survey.* Retrieved May 3, 2008, from http://www.harrisinteractive.com/news/allnewsbydate.asp?NewsID=904

Hayes, B., Klein-Schwartz, W., & Barrueto, F., Jr. (2007). Polypharmacy and the geriatric patient. *Clinics in Geriatric Medicine, 23*(2), 371–390.

Kuijpers, M. A. J., van Marum, R. J., Egberts, A. C. G., & Jansen, P. A. F. (2008). Relationship between polypharmacy and underprescribing. *British Journal of Clinical Pharmacology, 65*(1), 130–133.

Malhotraa, S., Karana, R. S., Pandhia, P., & Jain, S. (2001). Drug-related medical emergencies in the elderly: Role of adverse drug reactions and non-compliance. *Postgraduate Medicine Journal, 77,* 703–707.

McCloskey, A. (2000). *Cost overdose: Growth in drug spending for the elderly 1992–2010.* Washington, DC: Families USA. Retrieved May 5, 2008, from http://www.familiesusa.org/assets/pdfs/drugod852b.pdf

Mezey, M., Fulmer, T., Abraham, I., & Zwicker, D. (2003). *Geriatric nursing protocols for best practices* (2nd ed.). New York: Springer.

Olsen, C. G., Tindall, W. N., & Clasen, M. E. (2007). *Geriatric pharmacotherapy: A guide for the helping professional.* Washington, DC: American Pharmacists Association.

Patel, R. (2003). Polypharmacy and the elderly. *Journal of Infusion Nursing, 26*(3), 166–169.

Scott, G. N., & Elmer, G. W. (2002). Update on natural product-drug interactions. *American Journal Health Systems Pharmacy, 59*(4), 339.

Terrie, Y. (2004, December). Understanding and managing polypharmacy in the elderly. *Pharmacy Times.* Retrieved May 5, 2008, from http://www.pharmacytimes.com/issues/articles/2004-12_1812.asp

CHAPTER

It was so humiliating. When I was in the hospital, no one ever called me by name. I overheard someone refer to me as the Hindu woman in room 425. No one really tried to communicate with me.

Patient "Chakreshwari Bhavana"

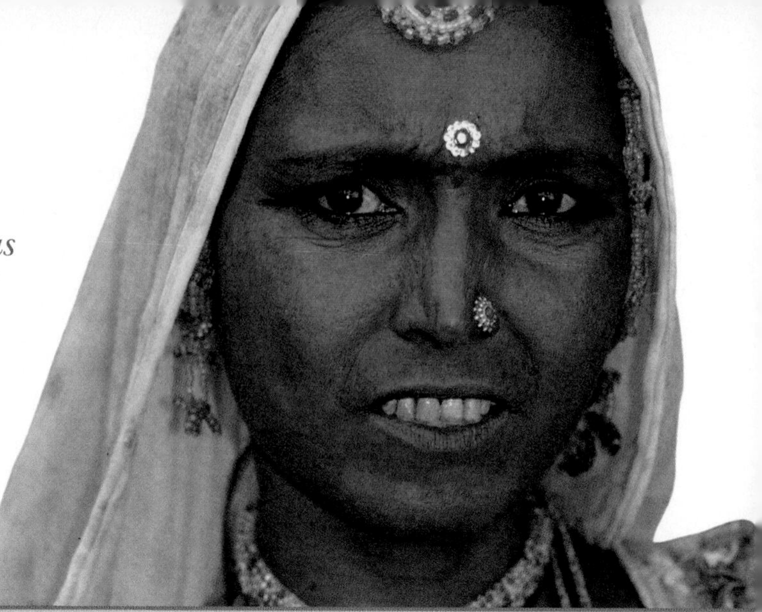

13 Psychosocial, Gender, and Cultural Influences on Pharmacotherapy

Learning Outcomes

After reading this chapter, the student should be able to:

1. Describe the fundamental concepts underlying a holistic approach to patient care and their importance to pharmacotherapy.
2. Describe the components of the human integration pyramid model.
3. Identify psychosocial and spiritual factors that can affect pharmacotherapeutics.
4. Explain how ethnicity can affect pharmacotherapeutic outcomes.
5. Identify examples of how cultural values and beliefs can influence pharmacotherapeutic outcomes.
6. Convey how genetic polymorphisms can influence pharmacotherapy.
7. Relate the implications of gender to the actions of certain drugs.

Chapter Outline

Holistic Pharmacotherapy

Psychosocial Influences

Cultural and Ethnic Variables

Genetic Influences

Gender Influences

Key Terms

allopathy, 157
cultural competence, 158
culture, 158
ethnicity, 158
genetic polymorphism, 159
holistic, 157
pharmacogenetics, 160
psychosocial, 157

Since the days of Florence Nightingale, nurses have been concerned with the well-being of the whole patient. In her conceptual framework of nursing care, Nightingale proposed a new theory in caring for the soldiers at Scutari. She believed that for soldiers to survive traumatic injury, nurses should promote positive physical environments (such as fresh air, clean water, good nutrition, and dry temperate space) for healing. This clearly demonstrates how Nightingale recognized that human health is dependent on multiple factors, and that nurses could improve health by addressing these diverse factors.

Holistic Pharmacotherapy

13.1 The concept of holistic pharmacotherapy is critical to effective therapy.

Pharmacotherapy would indeed be simplified if the "average" dose given in a drug guide produced the same response in every patient. However, as presented in Chapter 5, there is wide interpatient variability to drug administration. For example, the same dose of an antihypertensive drug can result in a desired therapeutic effect in one patient but produce no effect or profound hypotension in other patients. The skilled nurse can predict some of this variability by understanding how biologic, social, and environmental factors influence drug action.

Providing health care requires nurses to be fully aware that optimal patient outcomes can only be achieved if the patient is addressed as an integrated whole person. In health care the term **holistic** can have several definitions. In this text, holistic means treating the whole person rather than just the symptoms of a disease. Using this approach, the nurse assesses the entire person when developing pharmacotherapy outcomes. Only by recognizing the synergy of the individuality and totality of the patient can high-quality health care be delivered. When each person is viewed as an integrated biologic, psychological, social, and cultural whole, one can better understand the variables that influence pharmacotherapy.

Considering the entire person (holism) is not always easy. Traditional Western medicine, or **allopathy,** is a system of therapeutics in which diseases are treated by producing a condition opposite to the illness to be cured. In a more modern context, allopathy refers to conventional, Western medicine that is focused on treating symptoms of the patient without addressing the underlying causes. For example, research clearly indicates that stressful lifestyles contribute to disease. However, health care providers commonly treat the symptoms, such as hypertension, instead of the stress. To care for patients holistically, nurses should assess underlying etiologies and address solutions in the plan of care.

The human integration model, shown in Figure 13.1, serves as a conceptual framework in dealing with patients' problems holistically. This model provides a useful approach to addressing the nursing and pharmacologic needs of patients within the health care delivery system. All levels of the pyramid are interconnected and interdependent. As nurses address pharmacologic needs, each level of the pyramid is considered in relationship to the therapy. Consideration of these levels helps to ensure that the pharmacotherapy is not only treating the symptoms, but also is addressing the related issues of the entire patient.

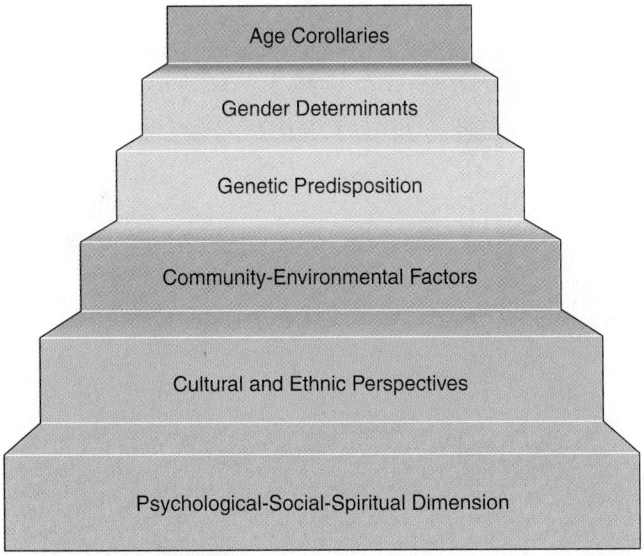

Figure 13.1

The human integration pyramid care model.

CONNECTION *Checkpoint* 13.1

The frequency dose–response curve can be used to depict interpatient variability to drug response. From what you learned in Chapter 5, draw a typical frequency dose–response curve, labeling the axes and the median effective dose (ED_{50}). See Answer to Connection Checkpoint 13.1 in Appendix A.

Psychosocial Influences

13.2 Many psychosocial influences impact pharmacotherapy.

The term **psychosocial** is often used in health care to describe one's psychological development in the context of one's social environment. This involves both the social and psychological aspects of a person's life. For example, women who undergo mastectomies for breast cancer often report that the surgery affects their self-confidence to the point that they may isolate themselves from others or may fear rejection from their mates.

Psychosocial also includes the spiritual nature of a person. *Psycho-social-spiritual* is a term that appears in the health care literature. Studies have established that these factors have a tremendous impact on health and well-being. Health care providers recognize that the close relationship among the psychological, social, and spiritual nature of individuals strongly influences their illness.

Critical to effective pharmacotherapy is the psychosocial history of the patient, which is often collected during the initial assessment between the patient and the nurse. This interaction collects in-depth information about the psychosocial dynamics affecting the patient. A well-performed psychosocial assessment reveals the relationship between the patient and his or her physical and social environment.

Other assessment parameters include developmental needs, environmental stressors, and life transitions that require major adaptation by the patient. The nurse might also consider the patient's motivation to correct the health issue because nonadherence to medication regimens is a frequent problem impeding the success of pharmacotherapy. A thorough psychosocial assessment provides the health care provider with a clear picture of the patient's living arrangements, family involvement and interaction, financial resources, emotional condition, physical condition, and cognitive functioning. All of this information is important to developing effective pharmacotherapeutic outcomes.

PharmFACT

Native Americans and Alaska Natives have an infant death rate almost double the rate of Caucasians. They are twice more likely to have diabetes than Caucasians.

Source: U.S. Department of Health and Human Services (USDHHS), 2008.

Cultural and Ethnic Variables

13.3 Cultural and ethnic variables can influence pharmacotherapy.

Although used interchangeably, culture and ethnicity differ in their exact definitions. An ethnic group is a community of people who share a common ancestry and similar genetic heritage. **Ethnicity** implies that people have biologic and genetic similarities. **Culture** is a set of beliefs, values, and norms that provide meaning for an individual or group. People within a culture have common rituals, religious beliefs, language, and certain expectations of behavior. Cultural and ethnic variables are important aspects of patient care that directly relate to pharmacotherapy. Both have a profound influence on patient outcomes and the occurrence of specific drug effects as perceived and interpreted by the user.

Advancement in drug therapy has led to numerous effective therapies for a wide variety of medical conditions. Though non-Caucasians comprise about 25% of the U.S. population, modern clinical pharmacology has been based largely on research and clinical experiences with Caucasians. Research has determined a biologic basis for variations or differences in metabolic response to agents among various ethnic groups. Scientists have identified specific regions on various chromosomes that influence hepatic metabolism. For example, certain drugs, such as antidysrhythmics, antidepressants, and opioids, are metabolized differently in individuals of African, Native American, and Asian descent (see Chapter 4). As technology advances, nurses will likely begin to see variations in the prescribed amounts and forms of medication based on the ethnicity of the patient.

Certainly there are many more cultures and subcultures than ethnic groups. To have complete knowledge about the many variations in culture among a population of patients is impossible. However, nurses can strive to understand the significance of the cultural traditions and their potential impact on the patients' pharmacologic regimens. Patients bring cultural beliefs (religious or ideological) that may challenge or conflict with what the health care provider believes to be in their best interests. How illness is defined is sometimes based on the cultural beliefs of an individual. One example that illustrates this point is the difference in belief systems between age groups—each with its own unique culture.

Cultural competence in health care is the ability of health care providers to provide care to people with diverse values, beliefs, and behaviors, including the ability to adapt delivery of care to meet the needs of these patients. Cultural competence requires knowledge of this diversity, as well as an attitude of awareness, openness, and sensitivity (Figure 13.2). Understanding and respecting the beliefs of patients are keys to establishing and maintaining positive therapeutic relationships in culturally sensitive nursing care. Therapeutic communication mandates that all health care providers bear in mind the cultural, racial, and social factors that make up each person, and how these affect behavior. Nurses can instill trust by being attentive to individual patient beliefs and by supporting patients to seek adequate medical care when it is needed. Culture and ethnicity can affect pharmacotherapy in many ways.

The nurse must keep in mind the following variables when treating patients from different ethnic groups.

- Dietary considerations. Cultures vary in their dietary preferences and practices, with diets that include some foods and exclude others. Patients need to understand that foods can increase or decrease the effectiveness of a medication. Spices and herbs can be important to a patient's culture but may affect pharma-

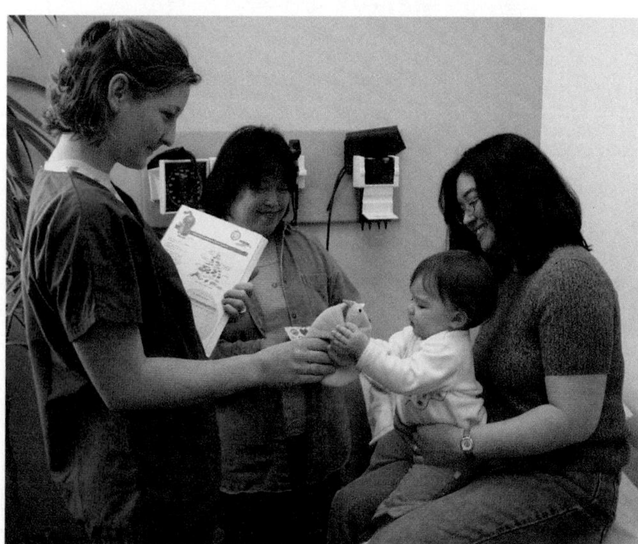

Figure 13.2 To be effective, nurses must be able to deliver culturally competent care to their patients.

cologic therapies. For example, some cultures include a diet high in foods such as cheese, pickled fish, or wine that can interact with medications to cause adverse events. Certain herbs can affect anticoagulants and beta blockers, or antidepressants. Assessing the primary foods of a patient's culture is an important component of the patient's psychosocial history.

- **Alternative therapies.** Various cultural groups believe in using alternative therapies, such as vitamins, herbs, or acupuncture, either along with or in place of modern medicines. Some folk remedies and traditional treatments have existed for thousands of years and helped form the foundation for modern medical practice. For example, Chinese patients may consult with herbalists to treat diseases, whereas Native Americans may collect, store, and use herbs to treat and prevent disease. Certain Hispanic cultures use spices and herbs to maintain a balance of hot and cold to promote wellness. The nurse can assess the treatments used and interpret the effect of these herbal and alternative therapies on the prescribed medications to maximize positive outcomes. The nurse can explain that certain herbs or supplements may cause potential health risks when combined with prescribed drugs.
- **Beliefs about health and disease.** Cultures view health and illness in different ways. Individuals may seek assistance from people in their own community whom they believe have healing powers. Native Americans may consult with a tribal medicine man, whereas Hispanics seek a folk healer. African Americans sometimes practice healing through the gift of laying-on-of-hands. The nurse's understanding of the patient's trust in alternative healers is important. The more nurses know about the various cultural beliefs, the better support and guidance they can provide to patients.

Pharm*FACT*

Many ethnic minorities are uninsured and are thus less likely to seek health care. Of black, non-Hispanic Americans, 10.5% are uninsured in comparison to 6.3% of white, non-Hispanic Americans. Hispanics are more than four times as likely as non-Hispanic whites and approximately 2.5 times as likely as non-Hispanic blacks to have been uninsured for more than 1 year.

Source: Cohen, Hao, & Coriaty, 2004.

Genetic Influences

13.4 Genetic polymorphisms can affect drug action.

Although 99.8% of human deoxyribonucleic acid (DNA) sequences are alike, the remaining 0.2% may result in significant differences in patients' ability to handle certain medications. Some of these differences arise when a mutation occurs in the DNA that encodes for a certain protein. This creates a **genetic polymorphism**—two or more versions of the same protein. In pharmacology, the best characterized genetic polymorphisms have been discovered in enzymes that metabolize drugs and in proteins that serve as receptors for drugs.

How can a genetic polymorphism affect drug action? In the case of enzymes, the "mutated" form of the enzyme has a changed structure. The structure of an enzyme is intimately related to its function; even a single base mutation in DNA can cause an amino acid change in the enzyme, altering its function. The mutated version of the enzyme may increase or decrease the speed of drug metabolism and excretion, depending on the specific genetic polymorphism.

As a specific example, polymorphism has been discovered in the enzyme acetyl transferase, which metabolizes isoniazid (INH), a drug prescribed for tuberculosis. Essentially, the mutated form of the enzyme performs its metabolic process, known as acetylation, more slowly. The reduced hepatic metabolism and diminished clearance by the kidney in patients with this polymorphism can cause INH to accumulate in the blood to toxic levels. These patients, who are usually Caucasians, are known as slow acetylators. However, fast acetylation is found in many patients of Japanese descent. These patients will inactivate the drug so quickly that it will not produce a therapeutic effect.

Several other enzyme polymorphisms have importance to pharmacotherapy. Asian Americans are less able to metabolize codeine or morphine due to an inherent absence of the enzyme debrisoquin, a defect that interferes with the analgesic properties of codeine. Some African Americans have decreased effects from beta-adrenergic antagonist drugs such as propranolol (Inderal) because of genetically influenced variances in plasma renin levels. Another set of oxidation enzyme polymorphisms has been found that alters the response to drugs such as warfarin (Coumadin) and diazepam (Valium).

A second type of genetic polymorphism affects protein receptors. Receptors are proteins that have a specific structure that

CONNECTIONS

Treating the Diverse Patient: Providing Culturally Competent Care

Understanding a patient's cultural beliefs is critical to effective pharmacotherapy. Health care providers should continually strive to understand various cultural differences in patients. Following are a few suggestions that will help the nurse to become more competent when dealing with culturally diverse patients:

- Use casual conversation to establish a personal relationship.
- Learn about the traditions, culture, rules of interaction, family and social roles, health and illness beliefs, and practices of various groups within the practice geographic area.
- Avoid profiling or stereotyping.
- Ask the patient about their beliefs related to disease causation, treatment, and cure.
- Show acceptance of the patient's beliefs and listen to any advice or alternative treatments the patient may have been given by a nontraditional healer.
- Respect religious or cultural rules prohibiting touch or treatment by a person of the opposite sex.
- Learn and respect, as much as legally possible, patient health decision-making practices and preferences.
- Negotiate a treatment plan that is acceptable to the patient's belief system and lifestyle as well as Western medical standards.

TABLE 13.1 Polymorphisms of Importance to Pharmacotherapy

Type	Result of Polymorphism	Drugs Affected
Enzymes		
Acetyltransferase	Slow acetylation in Scandinavians, Jews, North African Caucasians; fast acetylation in Japanese	Isoniazid, hydralazine, procainamide, caffeine
Debrisoquin hydroxylase	Poorly metabolized in Asians and African Americans	Amitriptyline, imipramine, perphenazine, haloperidol, propranolol, metoprolol, codeine, morphine
Mephenytoin hydroxylase	Poorly metabolized in Asians and African Americans	Diazepam, imipramine, barbiturates, warfarin
Receptors or Drug Targets		
Angiotensinogen	Blood pressure reduction	Angiotensin-converting enzyme (ACE) inhibitors
Dopamine receptor	Dyskinesias	Levodopa, antipsychotics
Beta_2-adrenergic receptor	Bronchodilation	Beta_2 agonists

accepts the drug (or other endogenous molecule), in a lock-and-key-type interaction. Small changes in the structure of the protein may result in a defective receptor that no longer "accepts" the drug. An active area of current research, receptor polymorphisms have been associated with an increased risk of schizophrenia, prostate cancer, breast cancer, and many other disorders. Relative to impacting drug therapy, a few receptor polymorphisms have been shown to impact drug action, as shown in Table 13.1.

Genetic polymorphisms often occur in specific ethnic groups because members have settled in the same geographic area and have married mates within the same ethnic group for hundreds of generations. This practice results in amplified genetic polymorphisms expressed within that specific group. **Pharmacogenetics** is the study of genetic variations that give rise to differences in the way patients handle medications.

CONNECTION *Checkpoint* 13.2

The best known genetic polymorphisms are those involving hepatic CYP enzymes. From what you learned in Chapter 4, explain the type of drug–drug interaction that might occur if Drug A induced CYP enzymes and Drug B was inactivated by the same enzymes. See Answer to Connection Checkpoint 13.2 in Appendix A.

Gender Influences

13.5 Males and females may respond differently to drugs.

There are well-established differences in the patterns of disease between males and females. Women tend to pay more attention to changes in health patterns and seek health care earlier than their male counterparts. However, many women do not seek medical attention for potential cardiac problems, because heart disease has traditionally been considered to be a "man's disease." Alzheimer's disease affects both men and women, but studies in various populations have shown that 1.5 to 3 times as many women suffer from the disease. Alzheimer's disease is now recognized as a primary "woman's health issue," along with osteoporosis, breast cancer, and fertility disorders.

Adherence to the medication regimen of a particular drug class may be influenced by gender because the adverse effects affect only one gender. A common example is certain antihypertensive agents that produce male impotence. Males can suffer strokes if they abruptly stop taking their medication to avoid impotence. Many drugs can cause gynecomastia, an increase in breast size, which can be embarrassing for males. Similarly, certain drugs can cause masculine adverse effects such as increased hair growth, which can be a cause of nonadherence in women taking these medications. Also in females, the estrogen contained in oral contraceptives causes an elevated risk of thromboembolic disorders.

Research has found many examples of differences in drug response between men and women. If males and females contain nearly all the same genes, how can these differences be explained? Recent studies have shown that although they may have identical genes, the "expression" of the genes differs greatly. For example, both males and females possess the same genes for hepatic metabolic enzymes, but one gender may produce more of a certain enzyme, thus producing a different degree of drug action. An example of a gender difference in a pharmacologic outcome is aspirin in that it is more effective at preventing heart attacks in men than in women.

Some of the gender differences in drug response may be explained by differences in body composition, such as the fat-to-muscle ratio. Cerebral blood flow variances in genders can alter patient response to specific analgesics. An example is the benzodiazepines given for anxiety; women experience slower elimination rates and this difference becomes more significant if a woman is concurrently taking oral contraceptives.

In the past, the majority of drug research studies were conducted using only male subjects. These studies assumed that there were no differences between genders and that conclusions would apply to both males and females. In 1993, the FDA formalized policies requiring that research studies for drug development include both genders. Gender consideration is necessary in the analyses of clinical data and assessment of potential pharmacokinetic and pharmacodynamic differences; in some situations, studies are targeted to women's health.

UNDERSTANDING THE CHAPTER

Key Concepts Summary

13.1 The concept of holistic pharmacotherapy is critical to effective therapy.

13.2 Many psychosocial influences impact pharmacotherapy.

13.3 Cultural and ethnic variables can influence pharmacotherapy.

13.4 Genetic polymorphisms can affect drug action.

13.5 Males and females may respond differently to drugs.

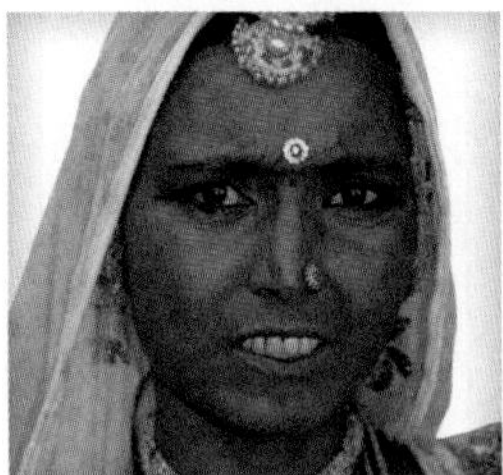

Making the PATIENT *Connection*

Remember the patient "Chakreshwari Bhavana" at the beginning of the chapter? Now read the remainder of the case study. Based on the information presented within this chapter, respond to the critical thinking questions that follow.

While traveling with her husband in the United States, Chakreshwari Bhavana became ill and was hospitalized. Once examined in the emergency department, she was diagnosed with appendicitis and underwent an emergency appendectomy. Mrs. Bhavana has been to the United States many times in the past. In fact, she has traveled to many countries. Although her native language is Hindi, she speaks several languages. She is well educated and speaks broken English.

Mrs. Bhavana willingly accepts Western medical treatments. However, when she is home in India, she also uses some remedies that come from the Ayurveda tradition. As the nurse caring for this patient, you are curious about her culture and health practices. However, you do not want to appear nosy or intrusive.

Critical Thinking Questions

1. Do you believe that nurses should discuss cultural beliefs with patients?
2. Describe how you could learn about Mrs. Bhavana's culture.
3. Do you believe that health care workers are culturally competent? Why? Why not?

Case Study

Marjorie, a 30-year-old woman, is a single parent with three small children. She works as a self-employed housekeeper and earns the minimum wage. Her annual income is $15,600, which pays for her family's housing, groceries, bus transportation, and clothing. Marjorie needs a job that pays benefits such as medical insurance. However, she fears that she will not be able to secure one because she never finished high school. She is constantly trying to save money. She has just been diagnosed with diabetes and requires insulin therapy.

1. Is it likely that Marjorie will be able to adequately care for her diabetes?
2. List the psychosocial factors that will influence this patient's ability to adhere to the therapy for her diabetes.
3. What can you do to help this patient?

NCLEX-RN® Review

1 The nurse is working with a client who has chronic headaches. In initiating holistic care, the nurse would:

1. Tell the client to take Tylenol as directed on the label.
2. Ask the client what he or she believes may be contributing to the problem.
3. Monitor the client's pupil response to light.
4. Refer the client to an ophthalmologist for an eye exam.

2 Which of the following, if reported by the client, would the nurse consider a psychosocial variable that may influence nonadherence to pharmacotherapy? The prescribed drug:

1. Produces an unpleasant aftertaste.
2. Is a very large tablet and difficult to swallow.
3. Is too expensive for the client to afford.
4. Potentially causes hepatotoxicity.

3 A Native American client states, "I will only take medications that are approved by the Shaman." The nurse understands that this statement reflects the client's:

1. Ethnicity.
2. Cultural belief.
3. Genetic polymorphisms.
4. Health-related bias.

4 The nurse knows that clients characterized as slow acetylators:

1. Are more prone to drug toxicity.
2. Require more time to absorb enteral medications.
3. Must be given liquid medications only.
4. Should be advised to decrease protein intake.

5 Which of the following is considered a gender factor that may influence effective pharmacotherapy? Select all that apply.

1. Fat-to-muscle ratio
2. Cerebral blood flow
3. Limited drug research on females
4. Health beliefs
5. Dietary considerations

See Answers to Critical Thinking Questions, Case Study, and NCLEX-RN® Review in Appendix A.

References

Cohen, R. A., Hao, C., & Coriaty, N. Z. (2004). *Health insurance coverage: Estimates from the National Health Interview Survey, January–June 2004.* Retrieved May 5, 2008, from http://www.cdc.gov/nchs/data/nhis/earlyrelease/insur200412.pdf

Edlin, M. (2006). Complex issues of compliance continue to make an impact: Cost saving from compliance can happen with education, collaboration, buy-in from patients and creative design plan. *Managed Care Executive, 16*(9), 42–46.

Eichelbaum, M., Ingelman-Sundberg, M., & Evans, W. E. (2006). Pharmacogenomics and individualized drug therapy. *Annual Review of Medicine, 57,* 119–137.

Elliott, V. S. (2000). Precision prescribing: The impact of genetics on drug effectiveness. *American Medical News, 43*(33), 33.

Franconi, F., Brunelleschi, S., Steardo, L., & Cuomo, V. (2007). Gender differences in drug responses. *Pharmacological Research, 55*(2), 81–85.

Greenspan, J., Craft, R., LeResche, L., Arendt-Nielsen, L., Berkley, K., Fillingim, R., et al. (2007). Studying sex and gender differences in pain and analgesia: A consensus report. *Pain, 132,* S26–S45.

Salimbene, S. (2005). *What language does your patient hurt in? A practical guide to culturally competent patient care* (2nd ed.). Amherst, MA: Diversity Resources.

Shuttleworth, A. (2004). Improving drug concordance in patients with chronic conditions. *Nursing Times, 100*(24), 28–29.

Simpson, R. J. (2006). Challenges for improving medication adherence. *Journal of the American Medical Association, 296*(21), 2614–2616.

Snelgrove, S. (2006). Factors contributing to poor concordance in healthcare. *Nursing Times, 102*(2), 28–30.

U.S. Department of Health & Human Services, The Office of Minority Health. (2008). *American Indian, Alaska Native profile.* Retrieved May 5, 2008, from http://www.omhrc.gov/templates/browse.aspx?lvl=2&lvlid=52

U.S. Department of Health and Human Services, The Office of Minority Health. *Cultural competency.* Retrieved August 18, 2008, from http://www.omhrc.gov/templates/browse.aspx?lvl=1&lvlID=3

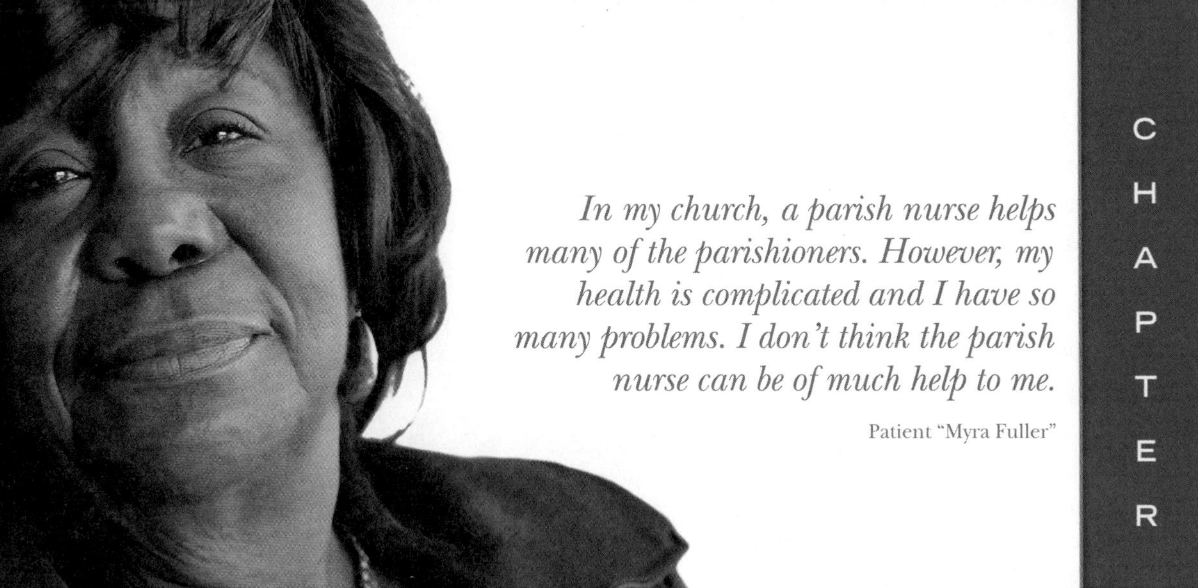

In my church, a parish nurse helps many of the parishioners. However, my health is complicated and I have so many problems. I don't think the parish nurse can be of much help to me.

Patient "Myra Fuller"

CHAPTER 14

Pharmacotherapy in the Community

Chapter Outline

Roles of the Nurse in the Community

- **Home Health Care**
- **Hospice**
- **Assisted Living**
- **Parish Nursing**
- **School Health**
- **Occupational Health**
- **Public Health**

Nurses as Community Resources

Learning Outcomes

After reading this chapter, the student should be able to:

1. Analyze why the role of the nurse in community health has expanded in recent years.
2. Identify key professional roles of nurses in the community and the importance of knowledge about pharmacology in professional nursing practice.
3. Discuss specific community settings where knowledge of pharmacology is critical to nursing practice.
4. Discuss how the nurse can serve as a pharmacology resource in the community.

Key Terms

home care nurse, 164
hospice nursing, 164
occupational health nurse (OHN), 166
parish nursing, 165
public health nurse, 167

Nurses have more choices of practice settings than ever before. Much of health care today is delivered in community clinics, physician offices, and outpatient centers as well as in the home and in independent or assisted living facilities. Nurses today can choose to practice as clinicians, educators, or administrators, or as a blend of these roles. Each role requires a working knowledge and understanding of pharmacology. This chapter describes ways that nurses can positively affect health care outcomes in the community with adequate knowledge of pharmacology.

Roles of the Nurse in the Community

14.1 More patients are being cared for in their home settings.

The community offers diverse opportunities for professional nursing practice. One expanding practice setting is home care. The National Association for Home Care reports that in 2007 approximately 7.6 million residents in the United States with acute and chronic illnesses, disabilities, and terminal illness received home health care services. Some 20,000 agencies provide these services.

The **home care nurse** monitors the patient's condition, including medication adherence and reports any adverse reactions. The nurse works with the health care provider and pharmacist to achieve optimal therapeutic outcomes. Patients receive oral medications, suppositories, injections, and parenteral drugs in the home. Antibiotics such as vancomycin, antivirals, or total parenteral nutrition (TPN) can also be provided in the home. Some home care agencies offer parenteral services such as intravenous (IV) blood components, dobutamine, immunoglobulin, antiemetics, anticoagulation therapy, or red and white blood cell growth stimulators. Respiratory drugs and nebulizers are part of patient care at home. As technology evolves, the home care nurse will continue to be a key player in providing safe and effective pharmacotherapy for the patient.

Home care nurses are in key positions to observe the use of tobacco, alcohol, or vitamins and dietary supplements in the home. Nurses in this setting need to recognize that negative drug interactions can occur with the use of these substances. For example, alcohol can adversely affect the patient when taken with analgesics, antidepressants, aspirin, antihypertensives, antihistamines, barbiturates, tranquilizers, or anticoagulants. With as many as 40% of the American population taking herbal supplements and vitamins, another concern for home care nurses is supplement–drug interactions. For example, a common natural supplement for depression is St. John's wort, which is contraindicated for patients taking digoxin (Lanoxin), antineoplastic agents, tricyclic antidepressants, or oral contraceptives. Tobacco smoke can affect the effectiveness of insulin, theophylline, alprazolam (Xanax), and heparin to name a few.

The home care nurse is also responsible for providing teaching regarding drug safety in the home. For example, medications must be stored in areas inaccessible to children and placed in child-resistant containers. In addition, if narcotics are prescribed, the drugs should be stored in locations safe from criminals who sometimes break into homes and steal to support their drug habit. The nurse can assess the ability of the patient or caregiver to safely administer the drugs (Figure 14.1).

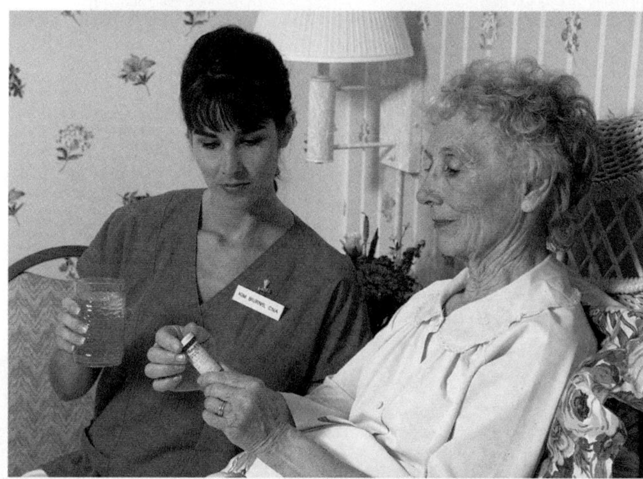

Figure 14.1 Home health care provides an opportunity for nurses to interact with patients and their caregivers in their home environment.

14.2 Hospice nursing presents the challenge of providing the patient with a dignified and comfortable death.

Hospice nursing is the care of terminally ill patients in their homes or in a health care facility and focuses on effective pain management. Nurses play a critical part in teaching patients and families about the many medication options available for pain management. Nurses must understand the indicators for changing the drug regimen for better control of pain and for working with the prescriber to reach the desired therapeutic outcomes. Opioid drugs such as codeine, hydromorphone (Dilaudid), levorphanol (Levo-Dromoran), methadone (Dolophine), morphine, oxycodone (Percodan), or oxymorphone (Numorphan) may be prescribed. For moderate pain or pain from bone metastasis, the patient in hospice may also take nonsteroidal anti-inflammatory drugs (NSAIDs) such as ibuprofen (Motrin).

Pain medications can cause serious adverse effects such as respiratory depression, sedation, lethargy, nausea, and vomiting so the hospice nurse must understand the toxic effects of overmedication. The nurse must teach the patient and family the synergistic effect of alcohol, sedatives, opioids, antihistamines, or antidepressants and that respiratory depression, confusion, excessive drowsiness, or even death can occur with overuse. Safety measures must be observed when taking these drugs because falls or injuries can result from dizziness. As a primary health care provider, the hospice nurse is in the critical role of supporting the comfort of the patient in hospice while maintaining safety through knowledge of pharmacology.

Pain management using opioids in hospice patients often includes dealing with tolerance and dependence. The nurse and prescriber should collaborate to ensure that the patient is not suffering from excess pain during the final days or weeks of life. For example, as cancer progresses, escalating doses of opioids may be necessary to relieve intractable pain. Although the patient may become physically dependent on these drugs due to the high doses, this is not a concern for patients facing the end of life. The nurse should counsel concerned patients and family members that this is a natural consequence of opioid use and that these drugs will be used safely to make their loved one comfortable.

PharmFACT

The number of Medicare-certified hospices increased from 31 in 1984 to over 3,000 in 2006. *Source:* Simms, 2007.

14.3 Assisted living facilities provide patients and their families with another alternative.

Nurses working in independent, assisted living, and skilled nursing homes have many challenges. Most of their patients are older adults with chronic mental and physical illnesses. Studies estimate that two thirds of older adults take one or more prescription drugs daily and one fourth take four or more daily. Those over 65 years of age represent about 15% of the population, yet they consume about one third of the drugs. These patients need the watchful assessment of the skilled nurse to achieve therapeutic goals without experiencing serious adverse effects from the medications. Nurses in these settings need to fully understand the implications of pharmacology in older adults. For example, with aging comes slower metabolism, which affects the amount of drug that is needed to reach and maintain a therapeutic level. Also, renal function may be diminished so that over time a drug may not be excreted as efficiently and may accumulate in the patient's bloodstream, causing adverse effects (see Chapter 12).

Over-the-counter (OTC) drugs taken by older adults can interact with prescription medications, causing adverse drug reactions. Vitamins and supplements should be assessed as well. When a new health problem presents in an older adult, the nurse should evaluate the medication regimen first to discern if drug adverse effects might be the root cause. Common symptoms experienced by the older adult that may be drug related are dizziness, blurred vision, nausea, constipation, incontinence, diarrhea, mood changes, sleep disturbances, loss of energy, memory disturbances, or rash.

Because sleep disorders are common in older adults, sedatives present another challenge to nurses in assisted living facilities. Because many patients have a sedative ordered at bedtime, safety measures should be implemented to prevent injury due to falls. Sedatives can also produce cognitive impairment in the older adult. Nurses must recognize the signs and symptoms associated with sedative toxicity so they can notify the prescriber if these occur. Common drugs prescribed for the older adult include antidepressants and muscle relaxants.

CONNECTION *Checkpoint* 14.1

From what you learned in Chapter 12, list at least five age-related changes in physiology that can affect drug response in older adults. See Answer to Connection Checkpoint 14.1 in Appendix A.

14.4 Congregational health focuses on the spiritual as well as physical needs of parishioners.

Parish nursing is recognized by the American Nursing Association as a specialty practice that emphasizes health and healing within a faith community. The philosophy of parish nursing embraces the spiritual dimension as central to nursing practice and the idea that caring for self and others is an expression of faith. The parish nurse collaborates with the pastoral staff and community health partners in providing members of the congregation with a holistic approach to health and healing. Parish nursing is endorsed by many different religious denominations. Courses and classes preparing registered nurses for parish nursing are available online throughout the United States.

Parish nurses work within faith communities as advocates, educators, and counselors. Parish nurses may form support groups within their congregation to help people deal with medical issues and refer members to agencies providing medical resources. The parish nurse may assist with health screening programs and teach the faith community members about medications used in chronic diseases such as diabetes, heart disease, and hypertension. For example, various medications are prescribed for people with diabetes so the nurse should be familiar with the most common ones and their appropriate use. The parish nurse needs to understand the main types of diabetic drugs, why each is prescribed, and how she or he can teach and support church members to have better control of their disease. Knowledge and understanding of commonly prescribed drugs for chronic disease are helpful when working in this community setting. Vaccination programs may be established to ensure that the children of congregation members are afforded the benefits of immunization.

14.5 Nurses in the school systems serve as valuable resources to students and educators.

School health nurses work within the school system to address the special health needs of students and to provide resources to meet those needs (Figure 14.2). The National Association of School Nurses (1999) defines this community practice as follows:

> "School nursing is a specialized practice of professional nursing that advances the well being, academic success, and life-long achievement of students. To that end, school nurses facilitate positive student responses to normal development; promote health and safety; intervene with actual and potential health problems; provide case management services; and actively collaborate with others to build student and family capacity for adaptation, self management, self advocacy, and learning."

School nurses are key to the case management of children with chronic health conditions and support the health education of children, parents, and school staff. School nurses ensure that immunizations are current in school-age children and monitor the safety and administration of medications that students need during school hours. One growing chronic illness among school-age children is childhood asthma, which affects between 3 and 8 million youth under age 17. School nurses must know that short-acting beta agonists work within minutes to open the airway

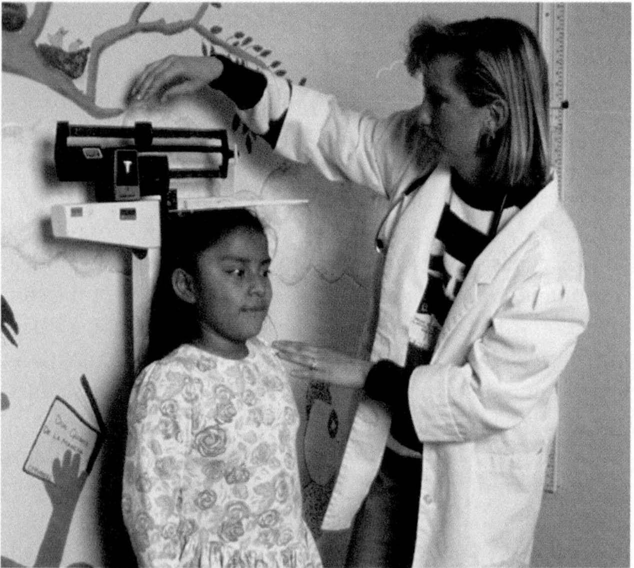

Figure 14.2 The school nurse provides care for pupils as well as information for healthy habits and lifestyles.
Source: Photographer: Michael Newman/PhotoEdit Inc.

during an asthma attack. These bronchodilators, such as albuterol (Proventil, Ventolin), can cause restlessness, headache, rapid heart rate, or muscle tremors, which can interfere with the student's ability to learn or participate in traditional school activities. Likewise, attention deficit/hyperactivity disorder (ADHD) is a frequent school-age health challenge that often requires medications such as methylphenidate (Ritalin) to improve learning. Besides these prescription drugs, the school nurse must understand drug-related interactions when providing OTC drugs such as acetaminophen, ibuprofen, or antihistamine for headaches, menstrual cramps, or toothaches.

One important aspect of the school nurse is to recognize symptoms of substance abuse (see Chapter 8). To adequately perform this function, the school nurse must be aware of community and school trends in substance abuse and associated symptoms. Adolescents may abuse virtually any substance because they are highly experimental at that stage in life. Student athletes present a special case of substance abuse due to the high incidence of anabolic steroid use in this population. Referrals to substance abuse counselors may be necessary.

The school nurse is often called on to teach classes in health education. Young people who are sexually active may have questions for the school nurse about contraception. Depending on school guidelines, the nurse may be able to either discuss contraceptive options or refer the student to a local clinic for further information. The nurse may also receive questions regarding signs, symptoms, and treatment of sexually transmitted infections (STIs). A strong knowledge of reproductive system pharmacology is required of school nurses.

CONNECTION *Checkpoint* 14.2

Because dextromethorphan is available OTC, school-age children frequently abuse it. From what you learned in Chapter 8, describe the symptoms of dextromethorphan abuse. See Answer to Connection Checkpoint 14.2 in Appendix A.

14.6 The occupational health nurse aids in ensuring a safe and healthy work environment for workers in the workplace.

The **occupational health nurse (OHN)** addresses the health and safety of workers on the job. The American Association of Occupational Health Nurses (n.d.) defines this specialty practice as follows:

> "Occupational and environmental health nursing is the specialty practice that provides for and delivers health and safety programs and services to workers, worker populations and community groups. The practice focuses on promotion and restoration of health, prevention of illness and injury and protection from work related and environmental hazards."

OHNs can treat job-related injuries and illnesses on site and help employers assess the workplace for potential hazards to worker health. Injuries that require treatment with medications may include burns, puncture or stab wounds, cuts, or allergic reactions to fumes, chemicals, or latex gloves.

Workers come to the job each day with various illnesses and diseases. Many are already taking drugs or may need medications in the course of their day's work. One example of a poten-

CONNECTIONS

Lifespan Considerations School Nurses and Medication Administration Guidelines

One of the many functions of the school nurse is administration of medications. The school setting requires defined policies that are shared with students, parents, and school staff. Each school system's policies may vary somewhat, but basic key guidelines are as follows:

1. Administer medications only with written permission from the parent, who provides the name of the drug, dose, the time to be given, and the diagnosis or reason for the medication.
2. Make sure prescription drugs are prescribed and authorized by a physician or nurse practitioner.
3. Check that each prescribed medication is in a separate container labeled by the pharmacy.
4. Store medications in a dark, clean cabinet with a secured lock.
5. Record the administration of all medicine.
6. Make a plan for times when the nurse is not present to give medications or when students go on field trips.
7. Establish a policy for self-medication by older students for OTC drugs or inhalers for asthma.
8. Notify parents that they are responsible for any medical devices needed for medication administration.
9. Establish policies for emergency drug treatments and a log for documenting each occurrence.
10. Maintain student confidentiality.

tially dangerous situation is when workers take medications such as antihistamines or muscle relaxants and then operate heavy machinery, drive an automobile, or fly an airplane. OHNs can provide education and alternatives for workers who could potentially harm themselves and others by taking their medications. Other common diagnoses that can present dangerous conditions on the job are diabetes, hypertension, and glaucoma, which can require medications with associated adverse effects. OHNs must have a thorough knowledge of implications and adverse effects of common medications to maintain a safe environment as they counsel workers. By supporting workers, OHNs help maintain wellness for the community at large.

14.7 Public health nursing provides care to the population in the community.

Many nurses work as primary clinicians in the national public health system. The following defines the role of the **public health nurse.**

> "'Public health nurse' designates a nursing professional with educational preparation in public health and nursing science with a primary focus on population-level outcomes. The primary focus of public health nursing is to promote health and prevent disease for entire population groups. This may include providing care to patients and identification of individuals who may not request care but who have health problems that put themselves and others in the community at risk, such as those with infectious diseases. Public health nurses work with other providers of care to plan, develop, and support systems and programs in the community to prevent problems and provide access to care" (American Public Health Association, 1996).

In the U.S. Department of Health and Human Services nurses are typically employed in the area of disease identification and prevention. Here nurses practice in departments dedicated to disease screening and prevention, mental health, clinical trials, genetics, alcohol and tobacco use, substance abuse, complementary and alternative medicine, organ donor and transplantation, and emerging infectious diseases. Public health nurses work in collaboration with the Centers for Disease Control and Prevention (CDC) in areas such as STI prevention and treatment through drug therapy.

Public health nurses may staff methadone maintenance programs where users of heroin, oxycodone (OxyContin), hydromorphone (Dilaudid), or hydrocodone (Vicodin), can reduce or stop their abuse of opioids and learn to lead healthier lifestyles. Nurses also work in public health to prevent and manage communicable diseases. For example, although the tuberculosis (TB) rate is declining, the disease remains a public health concern in America with over 13,700 cases reported in 2006 and 646 deaths in 2005. Nurses who work with patients with TB must understand the pharmacologic therapies and encourage patient adherence for treatment success. Nurses teach their patients common adverse effects of antitubercular drugs, including those that are considered minor and require no intervention and those that are major, requiring immediate action. In all areas of public health, pharmacology plays a major role in successful treatment outcomes.

Nurses as Community Resources

14.8 All nurses are community resources for drug therapy information.

Regardless of the setting, nurses are educators for both their patients and the community in which they live. Nurses have both formal and informal opportunities to teach preventive health strategies to minimize illness and disease. On those occasions they educate their patients, family, and friends about medication use, adherence, and drug interactions. Many people use prescribed medications, or OTC drugs, or a combination of both. Due to the time limitations of their health care provider or pharmacist, they often receive inadequate teaching. These people may ask the nurse at their church or the nurse whose son plays soccer with their children about their personal health conditions and medications. Nurses are never really off duty because they serve as resources and advocates within the community at all times.

For example, nurses can teach about the storage of medications in the home. Although most people keep their medication in the bathroom, this is not recommended due to the increased risk of damaging or degrading the drug due to moisture. This process can make the medication ineffective, lowering the therapeutic value of the patient's costly drug. Medications should be stored in a cool, dry place away from light, windows, or the stove, such as in a drawer or kitchen cabinet. Also, nurses can share that if the drug comes with cotton in the bottle, it should be removed because it may serve as a wick to bring moisture into the container. Keeping the bottle tightly closed will help retain the drug's potency by minimizing exposure to air and moisture. Practical information such as this can make a difference in the effectiveness of the drug.

Administering medications to infants and children can be stressful for parents and caregivers. Nurses can provide education and support to improve pharmacologic outcomes in the home. Parents need to be taught the adverse effects of any medication prescribed for their children and when to report them. They need to be reminded that continuing the prescribed dosage frequency is important to maintain a therapeutic blood level.

Community nurses can teach medication safety by warning against mixing different medications in the same bottle. Keeping the drug in its original container with directions can prevent accidental misuse. Nurses can also discourage taking a medication prescribed for someone else or sharing prescribed drugs with others. They can teach patients that outdated medicine may be ineffective or even harmful and that patients should clean their medicine cabinets regularly. Nurses can teach how limiting accessibility of medications to children can help minimize the chance of accidental poisoning by drugs.

Nurses can teach that for optimal benefit the medication should be taken at the times and frequency prescribed and in accordance with any dietary limitation or interactions listed in the information provided by the pharmacy. Patients should be encouraged to take all the medicine prescribed and not keep some for a later illness. Nurses can explain that an incomplete therapeutic regimen may result in a relapse or rehospitalization. Understanding drug adverse effects and knowing when to report them can maximize treatment options and minimize life-threatening dangers.

Working with different age groups is important when teaching medication usage and safety in the community. With older adults, the nurse may assist by providing bottles that will open easily for them. Polypharmacy is common in seniors, so the nurse may assist the older adult by reviewing the drugs taken, the way they are taken, and the reasons for use. Perhaps the nurse can set up a pill box that contains the medication needed for a week and allow the senior to be more independent. Most people will readily show a nurse their medications and ask for advice and support.

An educated nurse who is well versed in pharmacology is an asset to both the professional work setting and his or her community. This "expert" role provides the unique opportunity to teach appropriate information about drugs and to support the proper adherence to the prescribed regimen. The more knowledgeable nurses can be about pharmacology, the more they can contribute to positive health care outcomes for those in their community and sphere of influence.

UNDERSTANDING THE CHAPTER

Key Concepts Summary

14.1 More patients are being cared for in their home settings.

14.2 Hospice nursing presents the challenge of providing the patient with a dignified and comfortable death.

14.3 Assisted living facilities provide patients and their families with another alternative.

14.4 Congregational health focuses on the spiritual as well as physical needs of parishioners.

14.5 Nurses in the school systems serve as valuable resources to students and educators.

14.6 The occupational health nurse aids in ensuring a safe and healthy work environment for workers.

14.7 Public health nursing provides care to the population in the community.

14.8 All nurses are community resources for drug therapy information.

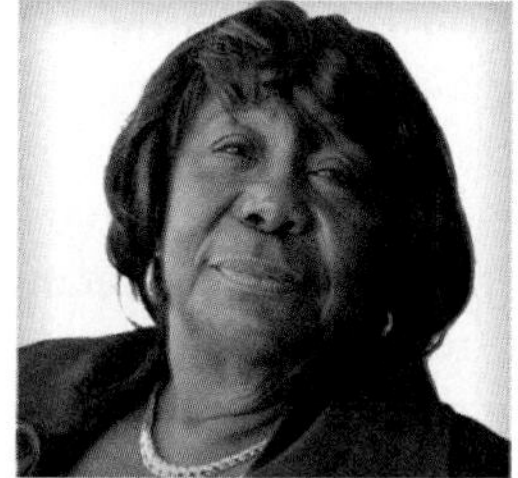

Making the PATIENT *Connection*

Remember the patient "Myra Fuller" at the beginning of the chapter? Now read the remainder of the case study. Based on the information presented within this chapter, respond to the critical thinking questions that follow.

Myra is a 71-year-old widow who has been active in her church all of her life. Until recently Myra was involved in the church choir, outreach ministries, and women's prayer groups. However, her involvement has diminished recently due to her health problems. After Myra was diagnosed with diabetes, it seemed that one health problem followed another. She was soon diagnosed with irritable bowel syndrome and arthritis. In addition to daily insulin injections, she was prescribed medications for chronic diarrhea as well as corticosteroids and other anti-inflammatory drugs for arthritis. Because Myra lives alone and does not drive, she has difficulty in picking up the needed medication at the local drugstore.

Critical Thinking Questions

1. Based on the case study, list the problems that may affect Myra's well-being.
2. How can a parish nurse aid Myra with her medications?
3. Identify ways that a parish nurse could ensure that Myra maintains her church relationships.

Case Study

Camden Industries is a moderately sized paper company in northwest Texas. The company employs approximately 350 employees and has been in operation for the last 40 years. One of the benefits offered to Camden employees is health insurance. However, over the last 5 years the cost of the insurance premiums has dramatically increased. Red Starr Healthcare Insurance Incorporated (the provider) claims that Camden's insurance usage has increased due to its aging workforce. Employees are using the insurance benefits more than ever before, especially in the area of pharmaceuticals. In an effort to reduce health care cost, executives at Camden are considering hiring occupational health nurses (OHNs).

1. Discuss the role of the OHN in reducing the health care costs of Camden's workforce.
2. If you were the OHN in this situation, describe how you would assess and implement an occupational health program.
3. Describe ways in which the OHN may help to reduce the company's pharmaceutical costs.

NCLEX-RN® Review

1 A primary area of pharmacologic expertise required by the hospice nurse is:

1. Analgesia therapies.
2. Antihypertensive modalities.
3. Diuretic treatments.
4. Nutritional support.

2 Which of the following would likely be performed by a school health nurse? Select all that apply.

1. Teaching students about the hazards of substance abuse
2. Prescribing antibiotic therapy to a student with strep throat
3. Assessing the respiratory status of a student with asthma
4. Administering prescribed medication for attention deficit/hyperactivity disorder
5. Checking that each student's medications are together in one container

3 The community health nurse is preparing a brochure about medication storage in the home. Which of the following concepts would be inappropriate to include in the written material?

1. Keep all medications in the bathroom for quick access.
2. Medication should be stored away from light such as in a drawer.
3. Remove cotton from the medication bottle because it can wick moisture.
4. Keep the medication bottle tightly closed to minimize exposure to air.

4 While making a home visit, the home care nurse assesses for client behavior that may produce a negative drug interaction. Which of the following could potentially affect pharmacotherapy? Select all that apply.

1. Smokes one pack of cigarettes per day
2. Drinks two to three glasses of wine per night
3. Uses herbal therapies for common ailments
4. Knits clothing from natural fibers
5. Sits in a chair by the window

5 The client in hospice is receiving around-the-clock narcotics for pain relief. Which of the following observations by the hospice nurse would prompt immediate modifications in the home environment?

1. Absence of address numbers on the residence
2. Presence of throw rugs and a foot stool
3. Mouse droppings and roach infestation
4. Poor ventilation in the client's sleeping room

See Answers to Critical Thinking Questions, Case Study, and NCLEX-RN® Review in Appendix A.

References

American Association of Occupational Health Nurses, Inc. (n.d.). *Occupational and environmental health nursing profession factsheet.* Retrieved May 5, 2008, from www.aaohn.org/press_room/fact_sheets/profession.cfm

American Public Health Association. (1996). *The definition and role of public health nursing. A statement of the APHA public health nursing section.* Retrieved May 5, 2008, from http://www.dhss.mo.gov/LPHA/PHNursing/DefinitionPHN_%20R_04.htm

Carson, M. D. (2007). Hospice care: What services do patients and their families receive? *Health Services Research, 42*(4), 1672–1690.

Fitzpatrick, C. (2008). Explore occupational health nursing. *Nursing Career Directory, 8*, 10.

Kendall, M. (2007). Being an exemplary hospice nurse. *Beginnings, 27*(4), 24–25.

Lashley, R. M. (2006). Teaching community based nursing in a parish nurse faculty practice. *Nurse Education in Practice, 6*(4), 232–236.

Lukes, E. (2007). Creating new career opportunities in occupational health nursing. *American Association of Occupational Health Nurses, 55*(8), 301–302.

National Association for Home Care and Hospice. (2007). *Basic statistics about home care.* Retrieved May 5, 2008, from http://www.nahc.org/facts/07HC_Stats.pdf

National Association of School Nurses. (1999). *Definition of school nursing.* Definition adopted at the NASN Board of Directors meeting in Providence, Rhode Island, in June 1999. Retrieved May 5, 2008, from http://www.nasn.org/Default.aspx?tabid=57

Redmond, G. M. (2006). Developing programs for older adults in a faith community. *Journal of Psychosocial Nursing & Mental Health Services, 44*(11), 15–18.

Rubingh. R. (2007). School nursing: More than just BAND-AID®s. *Journal of Christian Nursing, 24*(3), 148–151.

Simms, T. J. (2007). A perspective on the end of life: Hospice care. *Topics in Advanced Practical Nursing eJournal.* Retrieved May 5, 2008, from http://www.medscape.com/viewarticle/549702_1

Thobaben, M. (2007). Noncompliance: A challenge for home health nurses. *Home Health Care Management & Practice, 19*(5), 404–406.

Van Dover, L., & Pfeiffer, J. B. (2007). Spiritual care in Christian parish nursing. *Journal of Advanced Nursing, 57*(2), 213–221.

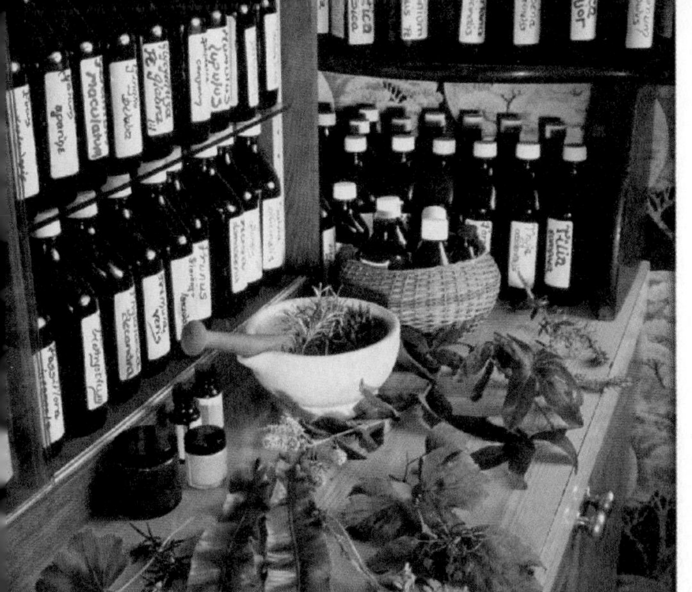

My daughter is getting so frustrated with me. It seems that I can't remember anything. Just last week I forgot to take my medications twice and failed to pick up my grandson at his weekly tae kwon do lesson.

Patient "Larry Bunch"

CHAPTER 15

The Role of Complementary and Alternative Therapies in Pharmacotherapy

Chapter Outline

Types of Complementary and Alternative Therapies

History of Herbal Therapies

Standardization of Herbal Products

Dietary Supplement Regulation

Herb–Drug Interactions

Specialty Supplements

Learning Outcomes

After reading this chapter, the student should be able to:

1. Explain the role of complementary and alternative medicine in patient wellness.
2. Analyze why herbal and dietary supplements have increased in popularity.
3. Identify the parts of an herb that may contain active ingredients and the types of formulations made from these parts.
4. Compare and contrast the strengths and weaknesses of the Dietary Supplement Health and Education Act of 1994 (DSHEA).
5. Describe specific adverse effects that may be caused by herbal preparations.
6. Discuss the role of the nurse in teaching patients about complementary and alternative therapies.
7. Identify common herb-drug interactions.
8. Explain why it is important to standardize herbal products based on specific active ingredients.

Key Terms

botanical, *172*
complementary and alternative medicine (CAM), *172*
dietary supplements, *175*
Dietary Supplement and Nonprescription Drug Consumer Protection Act, *176*
Dietary Supplement Health and Education Act of 1994 (DSHEA), *175*
herb, *172*
specialty supplements, *179*
USP Verification Program, *176*

Complementary and alternative medicine represents a multibillion dollar industry. Sales of dietary supplements alone now exceed $17 billion annually, with over 158 million consumers using them. Despite the fact that these therapies have not been subjected to the same scientific scrutiny as prescription medications, consumers have turned to these treatments for a wide variety of reasons. Many people have the impression that natural substances have more healing power than synthetic medications. The ready availability of herbal supplements at a reasonable cost has convinced many consumers to try them. This chapter focuses on the role of complementary and alternative therapies in the prevention and treatment of disease.

Types of Complementary and Alternative Therapies

15.1 Complementary and alternative therapies are used by a large number of people to prevent and treat disease.

Complementary and alternative medicine (CAM) comprises an extremely diverse set of therapies and healing systems that are considered to be outside of mainstream health care. Although diverse, the major CAM systems have certain common characteristics:

- Focus on treating the individual person
- Consideration of the health of the whole person
- Integration of mind and body
- Emphasis on disease prevention, self-care, and self-healing
- Recognition of the role of spirituality in health and healing

Because of its popularity, the scientific community has begun to examine the effectiveness, or lack of effectiveness, of CAM therapies. Although research into these alternative systems has begun to appear worldwide, few CAM therapies have been subjected to rigorous, controlled clinical and scientific studies. It is likely that some of these therapies will be found ineffective, whereas others will become mainstream treatments. The definition of a complementary therapy as being "outside the mainstream" is somewhat ambiguous because the line between an alternative therapy and a conventional therapy is constantly changing. Increasing numbers of health care providers are now recommending CAM therapies to their patients. Table 15.1 lists the most common CAM therapies.

Nurses have long known the value of CAM in preventing and treating disease. Prayer, meditation, massage, and yoga have been used to treat both body and spirit for centuries. From a pharmacologic perspective the value of CAM therapies lies in their ability to reduce the need for medications. For example, if a patient can find anxiety relief through massage or biofeedback therapy, the use of antianxiety drugs may be reduced or eliminated. Reduction of drug dose leads to fewer adverse effects.

Despite the fact that not all CAM therapies are beneficial, the nurse should be sensitive to the patient's beliefs about and need for alternative treatment and not be judgmental. Both the advantages and the limitations must be presented to patients so they may make rational and informed decisions on their treatment. Both pharmacotherapy and alternative therapies can play complementary roles in healing.

History of Herbal Therapies

15.2 Natural products from plants have been used as medicines for thousands of years.

An **herb** is technically a **botanical** without any woody tissue such as stems or bark. Over time, the terms *botanical* and *herb*

TABLE 15.1 Complementary and Alternative Therapies

Healing Method	Examples
Biologic-based therapies	Herbal therapies
	Nutritional supplements
	Special diets
Alternate health care systems	Naturopathy
	Homeopathy
	Chiropractic
	Native American medicine (e.g., sweat lodges, medicine wheel)
	Chinese traditional medicine (e.g., acupuncture, Chinese herbs)
Manual healing	Massage
	Pressure-point therapies
	Hand-mediated biofield therapies
Mind–body interventions	Yoga
	Meditation
	Hypnotherapy
	Guided imagery
	Biofeedback
	Movement-oriented therapies (e.g., music, dance)
Spiritual	Shamans
	Faith and prayer
Others	Bioelectromagnetics
	Detoxifying therapies
	Animal-assisted therapy

have come to be used interchangeably to refer to any plant product with some useful application either as a food enhancer, such as flavoring, or as a medicine.

The use of botanicals has been recorded for thousands of years. One of the earliest recorded uses of plant products was a prescription for garlic written in 3000 BC. Eastern and Western medicine have recorded thousands of herbs and herb combinations reputed to have therapeutic value. Over time, the popularity of specific herbs and remedies has varied, depending on the availability of the botanical (i.e., geographical region) and perceived effectiveness. The most popular herbals in the United States and their primary uses are shown in Table 15.2.

With the birth of the pharmaceutical industry in the late 1800s, the interest in herbal medicine began to wane. Synthetic drugs could be standardized and produced more cheaply than natural herbal products. Regulatory agencies required that products be safe and effective. The focus of health care was on diagnosing and treating specific diseases, rather than promoting wellness and holistic care. Most alternative therapies were no longer taught in medical or nursing schools. These healing techniques were criticized as being unscientific relics of the past.

Beginning in the 1970s and continuing to current times, however, alternative therapies and herbal medicine have experienced a remarkable resurgence, such that the majority of adult Americans are either currently taking botanicals on a regular basis or have taken them in the past. Why would people turn to folk remedies and products with uncertain effectiveness

TABLE 15.2 Best-Selling Herbal Supplements

Rank	Herb	Medicinal Part	Primary Use(s)	Herb Feature (Chapter)
1	Soy	Beans	Source of protein, vitamins, and minerals; relief of menopausal symptoms, prevent cardiovascular disease, anticancer	58
2	Cranberry	Berries/juice	Prevent urinary tract infection	51
3	Garlic	Bulbs	Reduce blood cholesterol, reduce blood pressure, anticoagulation	40
4	Ginkgo	Leaves and seeds	Improve memory, reduce dizziness	25
5	Saw palmetto	Berries	Treatment of benign prostatic hyperplasia	72
6	Echinacea	Entire plant	Enhance immune system, anti-inflammatory	45
7	Black cohosh	Roots	Relief of menopausal symptoms	71
8	Milk thistle	Seeds	Antitoxin, protection against liver disease	—
9	Ginseng	Root	Relieve stress, enhance immune system, decrease fatigue	37
10	St. John's wort	Flowers, leaves, stems	Reduce depression, reduce anxiety, anti-inflammatory	23
11	Green tea	Leaves	Provide antioxidant therapy; lower LDL cholesterol; prevent cancer; relieve stomach problems, nausea, vomiting	—
12	Evening primrose	Seeds/oil	Source of essential fatty acids, relief of premenstrual or menopausal symptoms, relief of rheumatoid arthritis and other inflammatory symptoms	—
13	Valerian	Roots	Relieve stress, promote sleep	—
14	Horny goat weed	Leaves and roots	Enhance sexual function	—
15	Bilberry	Berries/leaf	Terminate diarrhea, improve and protect vision, antioxidant	77
16	Grape seed	Seeds/oil	Source of essential fatty acids, antioxidant, restore microcirculation to tissues	36
17	Yohimbe	Bark	Treatment for impotence	—
18	Red clover	Flowers	Treatment of menopausal symptoms, sedation, asthma, skin conditions (topical)	—
19	Horse chestnut	Seeds	Treatment of edema and inflammation	—
20	Ginger	Root	Antiemetic, antithrombotic, diuretic, promote gastric secretions, anti-inflammatory, increase blood glucose, stimulation of peripheral circulation	60

Note: Adapted from "Herbal Supplement Sales in United States Show Growth in All Channels," 2008, *HerbalGram: The Journal of the American Botanical Council, 78*, 60–63, Retrieved August 28, 2008, from http://content.herbalgram.org/wholefoodsmarket/herbalgram/articleview.asp?a=3263

when effective prescription medications are available? This increase in popularity has been due to a number of factors:

- Herbal products and dietary supplements were once available only in specialty health food stores but can now be purchased in virtually all supermarkets and pharmacies.
- Complementary therapies are aggressively marketed by the herbal and supplement industry as viable and natural alternatives to conventional medicine. The increased availability of the Internet as a marketing tool has led to sites with misleading information about the effectiveness of herbal and dietary supplements.
- The "baby-boom" generation has demonstrated a renewed interest in natural alternatives and preventive medicine.
- The gradual aging of the population has led people to seek therapeutic alternatives for chronic conditions such as pain, arthritis, anxiety, depression, hormone-replacement therapy, and prostate difficulties.
- Several high-profile drugs such as Vioxx have been removed from the market or their use severely restricted due to "unexpected" adverse effects. People have the impression that natural substances are safer than synthetic pharmaceuticals.
- The high cost of prescription medicines has driven people to seek less expensive alternatives.
- Nurses and other health care providers have been more proactive in promoting self-care and recommending alternative therapies for their patients.

Numerous surveys have been conducted to determine the extent of alternative therapy use in the United States. Results of these studies agree that there is widespread and progressively increasing use of these therapies. One of the largest studies of Americans' use of complementary therapies conducted by the National Center for Health Statistics surveyed over 31,000 people (Barnes, Powell-Griner, McFann, & Nahin, 2004). Findings of this study included the following:

- Thirty-six percent of adults are currently using complementary therapies. If megavitamin therapy and prayer specifically for health reasons are included in CAM, the number increases to 62%.
- Women and those with higher educational levels are most likely to use CAM.
- Of those who take natural products, the most commonly used are echinacea (40%), ginseng (24%), ginkgo biloba (21%), garlic (20%), and glucosamine (15%).
- The most frequent conditions treated with CAM are back pain (17%), head cold (10%), joint pain/arthritis (10%), neck pain (7%), and anxiety or depression (5%).
- Twenty-eight percent of people use CAM because they think conventional treatments would not help their condition. Thirteen percent feel that conventional medicine is too expensive.
- Most people use CAM in addition to conventional medicine, rather than as a replacement.
- Twenty-six percent of those who tried alternatives did so on the recommendation of a doctor or nurse.

This pharmacology text emphasizes CAM by the use of features appearing throughout the chapters. The inclusion of these therapies is not an endorsement, nor does it imply their effectiveness. They are included because the nurse will frequently need to teach specific natural therapies, and because some of them have the potential to impact pharmacotherapy (see Section 15.5). The student should refer to the current medical literature for complete dosing and safety information. Several excellent sources of reliable information are available. The National Center for Complementary and Alternative Medicine (NCCAM), a branch of the National Institutes of Health (NIH) offers current information on research involving these products. Although somewhat dated, another extensive source of reliable information is *The Complete German Commission E Monographs: Therapeutic Guide to Herbal Medicines*, which evaluates the safety and effectiveness of over 380 herbs licensed for medical prescribing in Germany.

Standardization of Herbal Products

15.3 Herbal products are available in a variety of formulations, some containing standardized extracts and others containing whole herbs.

The pharmacologically active chemicals in an herbal product may be present in only one specific part or in all parts of the plant. For example, the active chemicals in chamomile are in the aboveground portion such as the leaves, stems, or flowers. For other herbs, such as ginger, the underground rhizomes and roots are used for their healing properties. It is, therefore, essential to know which portion of the plant contains the active chemicals if growing or collecting herbs for home use.

Most prescription drugs contain only one active chemical. This chemical can be standardized and measured, so that the amount of drug received by the patient is precisely known. Herbs, however, may contain dozens of active chemicals, many of which have not yet been isolated, studied, or even identified. It is possible that some of these substances work together synergistically and may not have the same activity if isolated. Furthermore, the strength of an herbal preparation can vary from batch to batch, depending on where it was grown and how it was collected, stored, and preserved.

Some attempts have been made to standardize herbal extracts, using a marker substance such as the percent flavones in ginkgo or the percent lactones in kava kava. Some of these standardizations are shown in Table 15.3. Until science can better characterize these substances, however, it is best to conceptualize the active ingredient of an herb as being the entire herb. An example of the ingredients and standardization of ginkgo biloba using a marker substance is shown in Figure 15.1. It should not be assumed that an herb is safe or effective simply because it contains the standard amount of marker substance.

The two basic formulations of herbal products are solid and liquid. Solid products include pills, tablets, and capsules made from the dried herbs. Other solid products are salves and ointments that are administered topically. Liquid formulations are made by extracting the active chemicals from

TABLE 15.3 Standardization of Selected Herb Extracts

Herb	Standardization	Percent
Black cohosh rhizome	Triterpene glycosides	2.5
Cascara sagrada bark	Hydroxyanthracenic heterosides	20
Echinacea purpurea, whole herb	Phenolics	4
Ginger rhizome	Pungent compounds	>10
Ginkgo leaf	Flavoglycosides	24–25
	Lactones	6
Ginseng root	Ginseosides	20–30
Kava kava rhizome	Kavalactones	40–45
Milk thistle root	Silymarin	80
St. John's wort, whole herb	Hypericins	0.3–0.5
	Hyperforin	3–5
Saw palmetto berries	Total fatty acids	80–90

TABLE 15.4 Liquid Formulations of Herbal Products

Product	Description
Tea	Fresh or dried herbs are soaked in hot water for 5–10 min before ingestion; convenient
Infusion	Fresh or dried herbs are soaked in hot water for long periods, at least 15 min; stronger than teas
Decoction	Fresh or dried herbs are boiled in water for 30–60 min until much of the liquid has boiled off; very concentrated
Tincture	Active ingredients are extracted using alcohol by soaking the herb; alcohol remains as part of the liquid
Extract	Active ingredients are extracted using organic solvents to form a highly concentrated liquid or solid form; solvent may be removed or be part of the final product

the plant using solvents such as water, alcohol, or glycerol. The liquids are then concentrated in various strengths and ingested. The types of liquid herbal formulations are described in Table 15.4. Figure 15.2 illustrates some of the formulations of ginkgo biloba, one of the most popular herbals.

Dietary Supplement Regulation

15.4 Herbal products and dietary supplements are regulated by the Dietary Supplement Health and Education Act of 1994.

Since the passage of the Food, Drug, and Cosmetic Act in 1936, Americans have come to expect that all approved prescription and over-the-counter (OTC) drugs have passed rigid standards of safety prior to being marketed. Furthermore, it is expected that these drugs have been tested for effectiveness and that they truly provide the medical benefits claimed by the manufacturer. Americans cannot and should not expect the same quality standards, however, for herbal products. These products are regulated by a far less rigorous law, the **Dietary Supplement Health and Education Act of 1994 (DSHEA).**

According to the DSHEA, dietary supplements are exempted from the Food, Drug, and Cosmetic Act that regulates prescription drugs. **Dietary supplements** are defined as products intended to enhance or supplement the diet such as botanicals, vitamins, minerals, or any other extract or metabolite that is not already approved as a drug by the FDA (as of 1994). A major strength of the legislation is that it gives the FDA the authority to remove from the market any product that

(a)

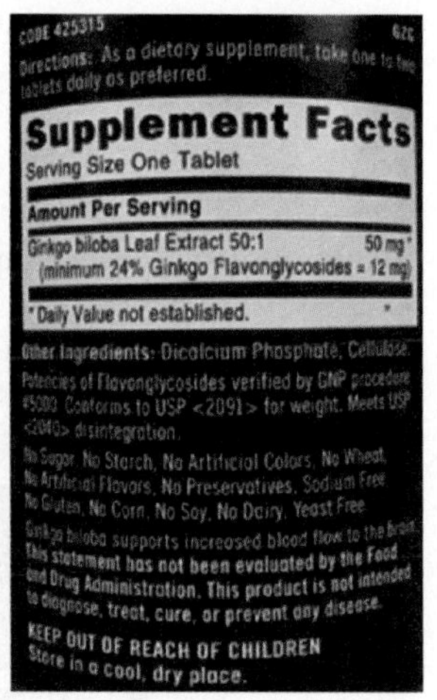

(b)

Figure 15.1 Two ginkgo biloba labels. Note the lack of standardization: (a) 60 mg of extract, 24% Ginkgo Flavone Glycosides and 6% Terpene Lactones; and (b) 50:1 Ginkgo Biloba Leaf Extract, 24% Ginkgo Flavinoglycosides.

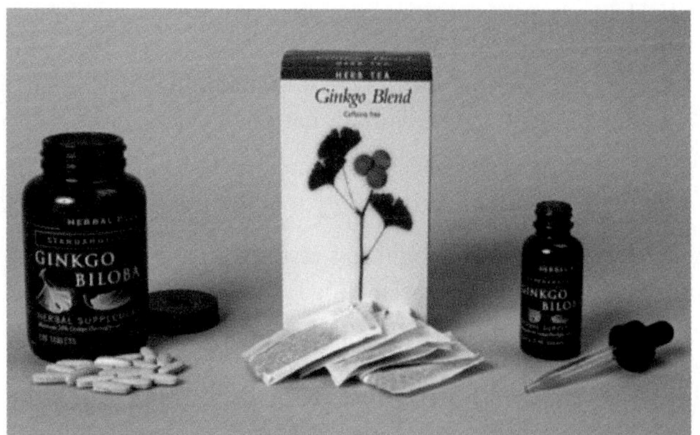

Figure 15.2 Three different ginkgo formulations: tea bags, liquid extract, and tablets.

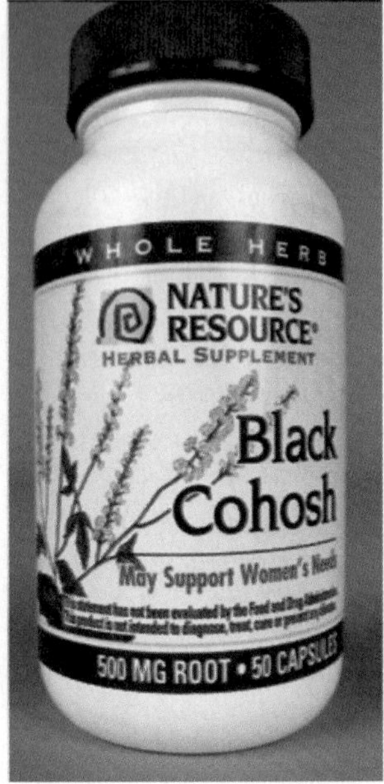

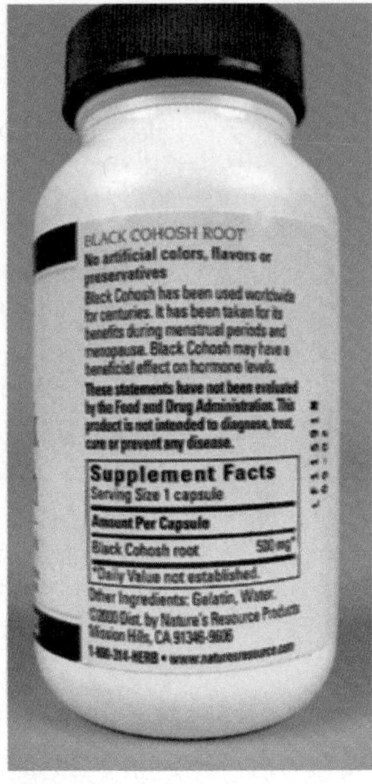

(a) (b)

Figure 15.3 Labeling of black cohosh: (a) Front label with general health claim; and (b) back label with more health claims and FDA disclaimer.

poses a "significant or unreasonable" risk to the public. It also requires these products to be clearly labeled as "dietary supplements." An example of an herbal label for black cohosh is shown in Figure 15.3.

Unfortunately, the DSHEA has several significant flaws that lead to a lack of standardization in the dietary supplement industry and, ultimately, to less protection for the consumer, such as:

- The manufacturer does not have to test the safety of the dietary supplement prior to marketing. If it is to be removed from the market, the FDA has the burden of proving that the dietary supplement is harmful.
- Effectiveness does not have to be demonstrated by the manufacturer.
- Dietary supplements must state that the product is not intended to diagnose, treat, cure, or prevent any disease; however, the label may make claims about the product's effect on body structure and function, such as the following:
  - Helps promote healthy immune systems
  - Reduces anxiety and stress
  - Helps to maintain cardiovascular function
  - May reduce pain and inflammation
- The accuracy of the label is not regulated; the product may or may not contain the product listed in the amounts claimed.

Lax government oversight has resulted in a lack of quality and sometimes blatant mislabeling of herbal and supplement products. For example, testing of more than 1,200 dietary supplement products has determined that 25% did not contain the correct amount of labeled ingredients. In some cases, the products contained none of the ingredients claimed on the label, and others were contaminated with potentially dangerous heavy metals such as cadmium and lead.

PharmFACT

In the year the DSHEA was passed, 4,000 dietary supplement products were on the market. It is estimated that about 1,000 products have been added every year since then to total at least 29,000 products on the market in 2005. *Source:* Atwater, Montgomery-Salguero, & Roll, 2005.

Several steps have been taken to address the lack of purity and mislabeling of herbal and dietary supplements. The United States Pharmacopoeia (USP) is a nonprofit public health organization that has attempted to raise the standards and quality of pharmaceuticals and dietary supplements (see Chapter 1). The USP has developed a voluntary process by which a manufacturer may submit a product for the **USP Verification Program.** Using a multistep approach, the USP examines the manufacturing processes used to create a supplement and tests the product to see if it contains the ingredients specified on the label and whether the product will break down and release its ingredients in the body (bioavailability). If the product meets the stringent standards of the USP, it may then carry the USP verified dietary supplement mark on the label. The verification mark, shown in Figure 15.4, indicates to consumers that the product has been manufactured under acceptable standards of purity, has been tested for active ingredients stated on the label, and is free of harmful contaminants. However, it does not indicate that the product is safe or effective.

In another attempt to protect consumers, Congress passed the **Dietary Supplement and Nonprescription Drug Consumer Protection Act,** which took effect in 2007. Companies that market herbal and dietary supplements are now required to include their contact information (address and phone number) on the product labels so consumers can report adverse events. Companies must notify the FDA of any serious adverse event reports within 15 days of receiving such reports. Under this act, a "serious adverse event" is defined as any adverse reaction resulting in death, a life-threatening experience, inpatient hospitalization, a persistent or significant disability or incapacity, or a congenital anomaly or birth defect, as well as any event requiring a medical or surgical intervention to prevent one of these conditions based on reasonable medical judgment. Companies must keep records of such events for at least 6 years, and the records are subject to inspection by the FDA.

Also in 2007, the FDA announced a final rule that requires the manufacturers of dietary supplements to evaluate the identity,

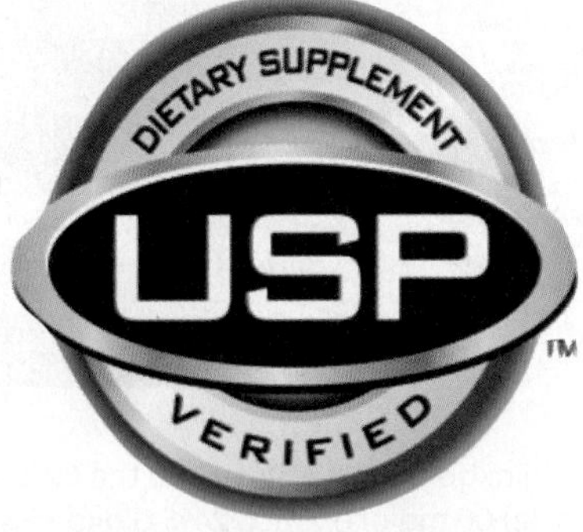

Figure 15.4 USP verified dietary supplement mark.
Source: U.S. Pharmacopeia

purity, potency, and composition of their products. The labels must accurately reflect what is in the products, which must be free of contaminants such as pesticides, toxins, glass, or heavy metals. The rule is scheduled to be phased in over a 3-year period.

CONNECTION *Checkpoint* 15.1

From what you learned in Chapter 2, what is a pharmacopeia? What function does it serve in the United States? See Answer to Connection Checkpoint 15.1 in Appendix A.

Herb–Drug Interactions

15.5 Natural products may have pharmacologic actions and can interact with conventional drugs.

A key concept to remember when learning about alternative therapies is that "natural" is not synonymous with "better" or "safe." It is likely that some botanicals do indeed contain active chemicals that are as powerful as, and perhaps more effective than, some currently approved medications. Thousands of years of experience, combined with current scientific research, have shown that some of these herbal remedies have therapeutic actions. Just because a substance comes from a natural product, however, does not make it safe or effective. For example, poison ivy is natural but it certainly is not safe or therapeutic. The dried seed pods of the poppy plant yield opium, which has therapeutic effects but can also kill if taken inappropriately. Some natural products may not offer an improvement over conventional therapy in treating certain disorders and, indeed, may be of no value whatsoever. Furthermore, a patient who substitutes an unproven alternative therapy for an established, effective medical treatment may delay healing and suffer irreparable harmful effects.

Some herbal products contain ingredients that may cause additive, synergistic, or antagonistic interactions with prescription or OTC drugs. For example, ginkgo biloba and ginger have the ability to increase bleeding time. If used concurrently with anticoagulants, these herbs may increase the potential for adverse bleeding events. St. John's wort, kava, and valerian cause relaxation and may result in excessive sedation if taken concurrently with central nervous system (CNS) depressants. A few herbals have organ-specific toxicity. The herb comfrey given concurrently with large doses of acetaminophen may increase the patient's risk of hepatotoxicity. Herbals such as psyllium, aloe, and flaxseed may bind to drugs in the gastrointestinal (GI) tract, thus slowing their absorption.

The true extent of herb–drug interactions is unknown. Most reports in the medical literature are anecdotal, often given as a case report on a single patient. It is often impossible to know the exact amount of herb taken because there is such a wide variation in the quality of products on the market (see Section 15.6), or even to know what chemical within the herb (either active ingredients or contaminants) may have caused the reported interaction. Few controlled scientific studies of herb–drug or dietary supplement–drug interactions have been conducted. The majority of the information regarding these interactions is theoretical, rather than clinical, based.

CONNECTIONS

Lifespan Considerations

Older Adults at Risk for Polyherbacy

One of the most important health issues affecting older adults is the excessive or inappropriate use of medications. Although health care providers consider polypharmacy in older adults, elderly patients may not divulge the use of herbs and supplements when talking to health care providers. With the increased use of herbs and supplements by older adults, a new health care dilemma—polyherbacy—may be present in older patients.

There are many issues related to the use of herbals and nutritional supplements that should be considered with older adults. For example, there may be:

- Inadequate data that examine the effects and impact that supplements have on the natural physiological changes that occur during the aging process. Older adults experience diminished kidney and liver function and are at greater risk for toxicity.
- Altered pharmacokinetic processes that would increase the older adult's incidence of serious adverse effects.
- Unknown chemicals in the preparation that could interact with other medications.

Health care providers should always inquire about herbal use and should also be aware of the adverse effects that may result from such products.

When obtaining medical histories nurses should include questions on the use of herbal and dietary supplements because these products are contraindicated for certain patients. Patients taking medications with potentially serious adverse effects such as insulin, warfarin (Coumadin), antiepileptic drugs, antineoplastic agents, or digoxin (Lanoxin) should be warned never to take any herbal product or dietary supplement without first discussing their needs with a health care provider. As presented in Chapter 10, pregnant or lactating women should not take these products without approval of their health care provider. The nurse should also remember that the potential for any drug interaction increases in older adults, especially those with hepatic or renal impairment. Potential drug interactions with selected herbs are shown in Table 15.5.

Another warning that must be heeded with natural products is to beware of allergic reactions. It is not unusual to find dozens of different chemicals in teas and infusions made from the flowers, leaves, or roots of a plant. Patients who have known allergies to food products or medicines should seek medical advice before taking a new herbal product. It is always wise to take the smallest amount possible when starting herbal therapy, even less than the recommended dose, to see if allergies or other adverse effects occur.

Nurses have an obligation to seek the latest medical information on herbal products, because there is a good possibility that their patients are using them to supplement traditional medicines. Each patient who takes an herbal product does so for a reason. The nurse needs to listen, assess, and understand the patient's goals for taking the supplement. Does the patient have an accurate understanding of the actions of the herb? Are there more effective therapies, either pharmacologic or nonpharmacologic, for the

TABLE 15.5 Documented Herb–Drug Interactions

Common and (Scientific) Name	Interacts with	Effects of Interaction
Echinacea (*Echinacea purpurea*)	amiodarone, anabolic steroids, ketoconazole, methotrexate	Possible increased hepatotoxicity
Feverfew (*Tanacetum parthenium*)	aspirin and other NSAIDs; heparin; warfarin	Increased bleeding risk
Flaxseed (*Linum usitatissimum*)	most drugs	Binds to drugs; decreased absorption
Garlic (*Allium sativum*)	aspirin and other NSAIDs; warfarin	Increased bleeding risk
	insulin; oral hypoglycemic agents	Additive hypoglycemic effects
	saquinavir	Induces CYP3A4 enzymes; decreased drug effectiveness
Ginger (*Zingiber officinale*)	aspirin and other NSAIDs; heparin; warfarin	Increased bleeding risk
Ginkgo (*Ginkgo biloba*)	anticonvulsants	Decreased drug effectiveness
	tricyclic antidepressants	May decrease seizure threshold
	omeprazole	Induces CYP2C19 enzymes; decreased drug effectiveness
	trazodone	Increased drug effects
Ginseng (*Panax quinquefolius/ Eleutherococcus senticosus*)	CNS depressants	Potentiates sedation
	digoxin	Increased toxicity
	diuretics	May attenuate diuretic effects
	insulin; oral hypoglycemic agents	Increased hypoglycemic effects
	MAO inhibitors	Hypertension, manic symptoms, headaches, nervousness
	warfarin	Decreased anticoagulant effects
Goldenseal (*Hydrastis canadensis/ Eleutherococcus senticosus*)	diuretics	May attenuate diuretic effects
Green tea	warfarin	Decreased anticoagulant effects
Kava kava (*Piper methysticum*)	barbiturates; benzodiazepines; alcohol and other CNS depressants	Potentiates sedation
	levodopa/carbidopa	Worsens Parkinson's symptoms
	phenothiazines	Increased risk and severity of dystonic reactions
St. John's wort (*Hypericum perforatum*)	opioids, alcohol, and other CNS depressants	Potentiates sedation
	cyclosporine	May decrease cyclosporine levels
	efavirenz, indinavir	Decreased antiretroviral activity
	MAO inhibitors	May cause hypertensive crisis
	oral contraceptives	Decreased drug effectiveness
	selective serotonin reuptake inhibitors; tricyclic antidepressants	Increases risk of serotonin syndrome
	warfarin	Decreased anticoagulant effects
Soy	warfarin	Decreased anticoagulant effects
Valerian (*Valeriana officinalis*)	barbiturates; benzodiazepines and other CNS depressants	Potentiates sedation

patient's condition? Is there a potential for harmful effects from the product due to high doses or herb–drug interactions? Establishing a supportive attitude toward the use of CAM is important. Nurses often need to educate their patients on the role of alternative therapies in the treatment of their disorder and discuss which treatment or combination of treatments will best meet their patients' health goals. Patients should be advised to be skeptical of marketing claims for herbal products and to seek health information from reputable sources.

CONNECTION *Checkpoint* 15.2

St. John's wort induces hepatic CYP metabolic enzymes. From what you learned in Chapter 6, how could this herb affect therapy with antidepressants or benzodiazepines that are substrates for CYP enzymes? See Answer to Connection Checkpoint 15.2 in Appendix A.

Specialty Supplements

15.6 Specialty supplements are nonherbal dietary products that are widely used to promote wellness.

Specialty supplements are nonherbal dietary products used to enhance a wide variety of body functions. These supplements form a diverse group of products obtained from plant and animal sources. They are more specific in their action than herbal products and are generally targeted for one condition or a smaller group of related conditions. The most popular specialty supplements are listed in Table 15.6.

In general, specialty supplements have a legitimate rationale for their use. For example, chondroitin and glucosamine are natural substances in the body necessary for cartilage growth and maintenance. Amino acids are natural building blocks of muscle protein. Flaxseed and fish oils contain omega fatty acids that have been shown to reduce the risk of heart disease in certain patients.

As with herbal products, the link between most specialty supplements and their claimed benefits is unclear. In most cases, the body already has sufficient quantities of the substance; thus taking additional amounts may be of no benefit. In other cases, the supplement is marketed for conditions for which the supplement has no proved effect. The good news is that these substances are generally not harmful unless taken in large amounts. The bad news, however, is that they can give patients false hopes of an easy cure for chronic conditions such as heart disease or the pain of arthritis. As with herbal products, the health care provider should advise patients to be skeptical about the health claims regarding the use of these supplements.

TABLE 15.6 Selected Specialty Supplements

Name	Primary Uses	Supplement Feature (Chapter)
Amino acids	Build protein, muscle strength, and endurance	—
Carnitine	Enhance energy and sports performance, heart health, memory, immune function, and male fertility	38
Chromium	Treatment of diabetes; hyperglycemia	67
Coenzyme Q10	Prevent heart disease, provide antioxidant therapy	32
DHEA	Boost immune and memory functions	—
Fish oil	Reduce cholesterol levels, enhance brain function, increase visual acuity owing to the presence of the omega-3 fatty acids	69
Flaxseed oil	Reduce cholesterol levels, enhance brain function, increase visual acuity owing to the presence of the omega-3 fatty acids	—
Glucosamine and chondroitin	Alleviate arthritis and other joint problems	75
Lactobacillus acidophilus	Maintain intestinal health	61
Methyl sulfonyl methane (MSM)	Reduce allergic reactions to pollen and foods, relieve pain and inflammation of arthritis and similar conditions	—
Selenium	Reduce the risk of certain types of cancer	57
Vitamin C	Prevention of colds	74

UNDERSTANDING THE CHAPTER

Key Concepts Summary

15.1 Complementary and alternative therapies are used by a large number of people to prevent and treat disease.

15.2 Natural products from plants have been used as medicines for thousands of years.

15.3 Herbal products are available in a variety of formulations, some containing standardized extracts and others containing whole herbs.

15.4 Herbal products and dietary supplements are regulated by the Dietary Supplement Health and Education Act of 1994.

15.5 Natural products may have pharmacologic actions and can interact with conventional drugs.

15.6 Specialty supplements are nonherbal dietary products that are widely used to promote wellness.

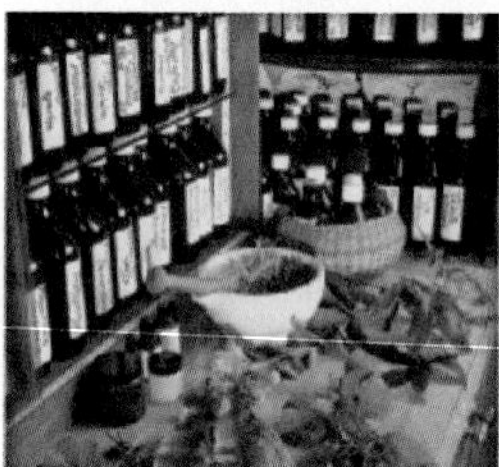

Making the PATIENT *Connection*

Remember the patient "Larry Bunch" at the beginning of the chapter? Now read the remainder of the case study. Based on the information presented within this chapter, respond to the critical thinking questions that follow.

Sixty-nine-year old Larry Bunch was not only frustrating his daughter, but his forgetfulness was annoying him as well. Since the death of his wife 2 years ago, his forgetfulness seemed to be worsening. To remedy the situation, Larry purchased a bottle of ginkgo biloba at the health food store and began taking the supplement about 6 months ago.

Larry was hospitalized 3 years ago for a cardiac condition (atrial fibrillation). When he was discharged from the hospital, he was placed on an anticoagulant therapy to prevent blood clots from forming in his heart. Today, Larry comes to his health care provider's office for a scheduled blood test to determine the effectiveness of his anticoagulant.

When the results from the blood test return, it is noted that Larry's coagulation time is abnormally high. Based on the test, Larry is at high risk of hemorrhaging. As the nurse, you note that his vital signs are within normal limits, and he states he feels well. However, you also observe some large bruises on Larry's arms, which he cannot explain.

Critical Thinking Questions

1. What is the relationship between this patient's use of ginkgo and the laboratory results?
2. What instructions should this patient receive about taking the supplement?
3. Discuss the hazards that patients face with using complementary and alternative therapies.
4. What should the health care provider do concerning Larry's forgetfulness?

Case Study

"It must be safe, after all, it is sold in the grocery store!" exclaimed Linda. As you, the nurse, talk with the patient, Linda Thomas, she explains to you that she takes multiple over-the-counter dietary supplements. Because the bottle states that the ingredients are "all natural," she knows it must be good for her.

1. What are the hazards associated with believing that all medication-type substances sold in the supermarket are safe?
2. Discuss how the words "all natural ingredient" can be confusing.
3. Identify the nurse's role in working with patients who participate in complementary and alternative therapies.

NCLEX-RN® Review

1 A client asks why all health care providers do not rely on complementary and alternative medicine. When talking to this client the nurse knows that many complementary and alternative therapies:

1. Have not been subjected to rigorous clinical studies.
2. Consist only of old wives' tales and fables.
3. Only provide a placebo effect.
4. Are costly and not worth the risk.

2 Which of the following health teaching concepts should be included in the instructions for a client taking echinacea?

1. Dosage can be doubled if symptoms fail to resolve in 48 hours.
2. Limit fluid intake while taking this supplement.
3. Take the smallest amount possible when starting herbal therapy.
4. Allergic reactions are not possible with natural supplements.

3 Which of the following clients is most likely to experience drug toxicity while taking herbal supplements? A(n):

1. 80-year-old female with cirrhosis
2. 58-year-old male with cardiac irregularities
3. 30-year-old female with pneumonia
4. 18-year-old male with chronic acne

4 The client asked the nurse, "Why are herbal supplements so popular?" The nurse's answer is based on which factors? (Select all that apply.) Herbal supplements:

1. Can now be purchased in virtually all supermarkets.
2. Are aggressively marketed by the herbal and supplement industry.
3. Cost less than prescription medicines.
4. Are safer than synthetic pharmaceuticals.
5. Appeal to the aging population.

5 The nurse is teaching at a community wellness seminar when one participant asks, "How can I be sure that my herbal supplement is pure?" Which of the following labeling marks indicates that the product meets acceptable standards of purity?

1. USP verified dietary supplement mark
2. DEA prescriber number
3. FDA identification and regulation code
4. U.S. Customs Service integers

See Answers to Critical Thinking Questions, Case Study, and NCLEX-RN® Review in Appendix A.

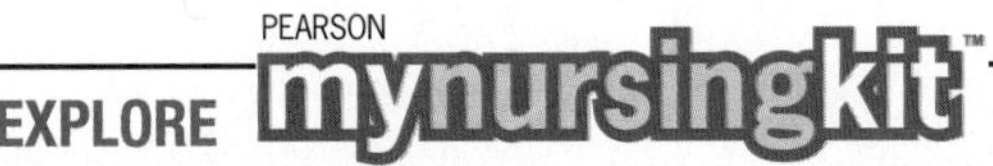

MyNursingKit is your one stop for online chapter review materials and resources. Prepare for success with additional NCLEX®-style practice questions, interactive assignments and activities, web links, animations and videos, and more!

Register your access code from the front of your book at **www.mynursingkit.com**

References

Atwater, J., Montgomery-Salguero, J., & Roll, D. B. (2005). The USP dietary supplement verification program: Helping pharmacists and consumers select dietary supplements. *U.S. Pharmacist, 30*(6), 61–64.

Barnes, P., Powell-Griner, E., McFann, K., & Nahin, R. (2004). *Complementary and alternative medicine use among adults: United States, 2002* (CDC Advance Data Report No. 343). Hyattsville, MD: National Center for Health Statistics.

Blumenthal, M. (Ed.). (2000). *Herbal medicine: Expanded Commission E monographs.* Austin, TX: American Botanical Council.

Blumenthal, M. (Ed.). (1988). *The complete German Commission E monographs: Therapeutic guide to herbal medicines.* Austin, TX: American Botanical Council.

Chavez, M. L. (2005). Herbal-drug interactions. *InetCE, 9*(10), 2–30.

Facts and Comparisons™. (n.d.). *The review of natural products* (4th ed.). St. Louis: Wolters Kluwer Health.

Fontaine, K. L. (2009). *Complementary and alternative therapies for nursing practice* (3rd ed.). Upper Saddle River, NJ: Prentice Hall.

Gagnier, J. J., van Tulder, M., Berman, B., & Bombardier, C. (2007). Herbal medicine for low back pain: A Cochrane review. *Spine, 32*(1), 82–92.

Gardiner, P., Graham, R., Legedza, A. T., Ahn, A. C., Eisenberg, D. M., & Phillips, R. S. (2007). Factors associated with herbal therapy use by adults in the United States. *Alternative Therapies Health Medicine, 13*(2), 22–29.

Haynes, L. C., Martin, J. H., & Endres, D. (2003). Use of nontraditional therapies—Implications for older adults. *Association of Perioperative Registered Nurses Journal, 77*(5), 913–921.

Herbal supplement sales in United States show growth in all channels. *HerbalGram, The Journal of the American Botanical Council, 78,* 60–63. Retrieved August 28, 2008, from http://content.herbalgram.org/wholefoods market/herbalgram/articleview.asp?a=3263

Marcus, D. M., & Snodgrass, W. R. (2005). Do no harm: Avoidance of herbal medicines during pregnancy. *Obstetrics & Gynecology, 105,* 1119–1122.

Medical Economics Staff (Ed.). (2007). *PDR for herbal medicines* (4th ed.). Montvale, NJ: Thomson Healthcare.

Ness, J., Cirillo, D. J., Weir, D. R., Nisly, N. L., & Wallace, R. B. (2002). Use of complementary medicine in older Americans: Results from the health and retirement study. *Gerontologist, 45*(4), 516–525.

Saving wild ginseng, goldenseal, and other native plants from mountain top removal. (2007). *HerbalGram, 73*(50).

Snyder, M., & Lundquist, R. (2006). *Complementary/alternative therapies in nursing.* New York: Springer.

U.S. Department of Health and Human Services, U.S. Food and Drug Administration. (1994). Dietary Supplement Health and Education Act of 1994, Pub. L. No. 103-417. Retrieved May 8, 2008, at http://www.fda.gov/opacom/laws/dshea.html#sec3

White House commission on complementary and alternative medicine policy, final report. (2002, March). Retrieved May 8, 2008, at http://govinfo.library.unt.edu/whccamp/

UNIT 3

Pharmacology of the Autonomic Nervous System

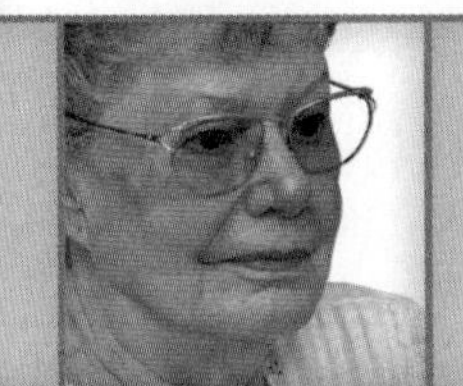
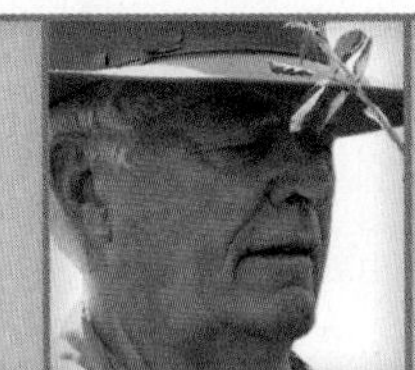
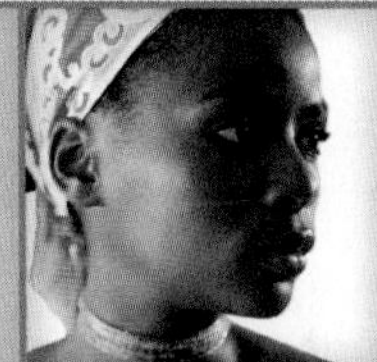
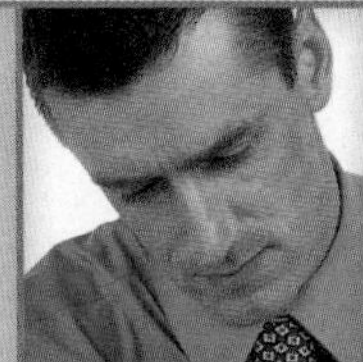

CHAPTER 16 Review of Neurotransmitters and the Autonomic Nervous System

CHAPTER 17 Cholinergic Agonists

CHAPTER 18 Cholinergic Antagonists

CHAPTER 19 Adrenergic Agonists

CHAPTER 20 Adrenergic Antagonists

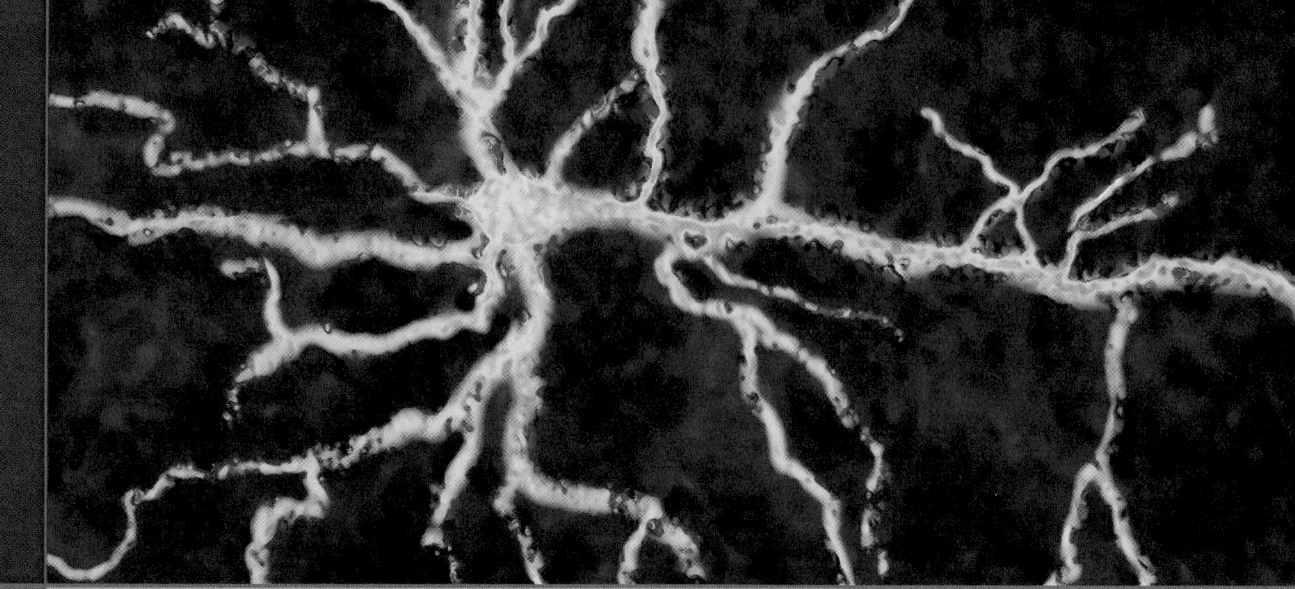

16 Review of Neurotransmitters and the Autonomic Nervous System

Learning Outcomes

After reading this chapter, the student should be able to:

1. Distinguish between the central and peripheral nervous systems.
2. Compare and contrast the two divisions of the peripheral nervous system.
3. Compare and contrast the actions of the sympathetic and parasympathetic divisions of the autonomic nervous system.
4. Explain the process of synaptic transmission.
5. Explain the basic mechanisms by which drugs affect synaptic transmission.
6. Describe the actions of acetylcholine at cholinergic synapses.
7. Describe the actions of norepinephrine at adrenergic synapses.
8. Assess how the actions of the adrenal medulla compare to those of other sympathetic effector organs.
9. Explain how higher centers in the brain can influence autonomic function.
10. Design a method for classifying autonomic drugs based on which receptors are affected.

Chapter Outline

Basic Structure of the Nervous System

Structure and Function of the Autonomic Nervous System

Synaptic Transmission

Cholinergic Transmission

Cholinergic Receptors and Neurotransmitters

Adrenergic Transmission

Adrenergic Receptors and Neurotransmitters

Adrenal Medulla Hormones

Regulation of Autonomic Functions

Classifying Autonomic Drugs

Key Terms

acetylcholine (Ach), 188
acetylcholinesterase (AchE), 192
adrenergic, 192
autonomic nervous system (ANS), 185
autonomic tone, 187
catecholamine, 192
catechol-O-methyltransferase (COMT), 194
cholinergic, 190
fight-or-flight response, 186
ganglia, 188
monoamine oxidase (MAO), 194
muscarinic, 191
neuroeffector junction, 188
neurotransmitter, 188
nicotinic, 191
norepinephrine (NE), 188
parasympathetic nervous system, 186
rest-and-digest response, 186
somatic nervous system, 185
sympathetic nervous system, 186
synapse, 188
synaptic cleft, 188

Neuropharmacology represents one of the largest, most complicated, and least understood branches of pharmacology. Nervous system drugs are used to treat a large and diverse set of conditions, including pain, anxiety, depression, schizophrenia, insomnia, and seizures. Through their action on nerves, these medications are used to treat disorders affecting other body systems such as abnormalities in heart rate and rhythm, hypertension, glaucoma, asthma, and even a runny nose.

Traditionally, the study of neuropharmacology begins with the autonomic nervous system. This is because autonomic physiology lays the foundation for understanding nervous, cardiovascular, and respiratory pharmacology. This chapter serves two purposes. First, it is a comprehensive review of autonomic nervous system physiology, a subject that is sometimes covered superficially in anatomy and physiology classes. Second, it introduces the four fundamental classes of autonomic medications, which are presented in depth in Chapters 17 through 20.

Basic Structure of the Nervous System

16.1 The two major subdivisions of the nervous system are the central nervous system and the peripheral nervous system.

The nervous system is considered the master controller of most activities occurring within the body. Compared to the other major regulator, the endocrine system, cells of the nervous system act instantaneously to promote homeostasis and make the adjustments necessary to maintain vital functions. The brain, spinal cord, and peripheral nerves act as a smoothly integrated whole to accomplish minute-to-minute changes in essential functions such as heart rate, blood pressure, pupil size, and intestinal movement. The basic functions of the nervous system are to:

- Recognize changes in the internal and external environments.
- Process and integrate the environmental changes that are perceived.
- Respond to the environmental changes by producing an action or response.

The nervous system has two major divisions: the central nervous system (CNS) and the peripheral nervous system. The CNS is made up of the brain and spinal cord, whereas the peripheral division consists primarily of nerves that carry messages to and from the CNS. Drugs used to treat disorders and conditions of the CNS are discussed in Chapters 22 through 30. Figure 16.1 illustrates the functional divisions of the nervous system.

16.2 The peripheral nervous system is divided into somatic and autonomic components.

With its immense potential and complexity, the human brain requires a continuous flow of information to accomplish its functions. In addition, the brain would be useless without a means to carry out its commands. The peripheral nervous system provides the brain the means to communicate with and receive sensory messages from the outside world.

Neurons in the peripheral nervous system either recognize changes to the environment (sensory division) or respond to those changes by moving muscles or secreting chemicals (motor division). The sensory division consists of specialized nerves that recognize touch, pain, heat, body position, light, or specific chemicals in body fluids.

The motor division is divided into two components. The **somatic nervous system** consists of nerves that provide voluntary control of skeletal muscle. The nerves of the **autonomic nervous system (ANS)** provide involuntary control of vital functions of the cardiovascular, digestive, respiratory, and genitourinary systems. The ANS controls vital life activities without people being aware of its functions. The three main activities of the ANS include the following:

- Contraction of smooth muscle of the bronchi, blood vessels, gastrointestinal (GI) tract, eye, and genitourinary tract
- Contraction of cardiac muscle
- Secretion of salivary, sweat, and gastric glands

The ANS is particularly important to pharmacology because a large number of medications affect autonomic nerves. Some of these drug actions produce desirable, therapeutic effects, whereas others produce adverse effects. The remainder of this chapter introduces the structure and function of this complex system.

Structure and Function of the Autonomic Nervous System

16.3 The autonomic nervous system is divided into two mostly opposing components: the sympathetic and parasympathetic branches.

The ANS has two distinct divisions: the sympathetic nervous system and the parasympathetic nervous system. Most organs and glands receive nerves from both branches, and the two divisions have opposing actions. For example, one branch may cause smooth muscle to contract; the other may cause it to

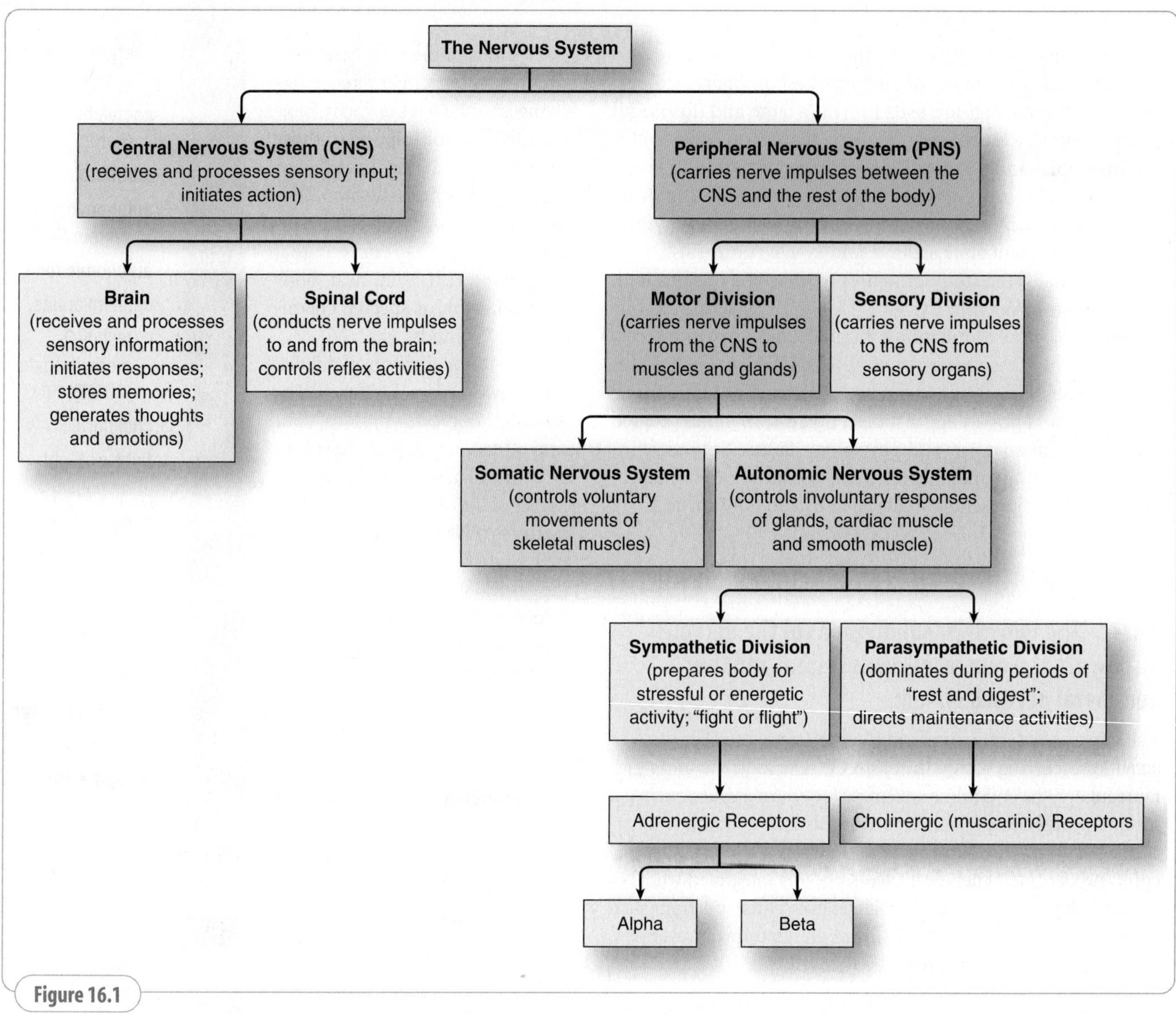

Figure 16.1

Functional divisions of the nervous system.

relax. The ultimate action of the smooth muscle or gland depends on which branch is sending the most signals at a given time. The major actions of the two divisions are shown in Figure 16.2. It is essential that the student learn these actions early in the study of pharmacology because knowledge of autonomic effects is used to predict the actions and adverse effects of many drugs.

The **sympathetic nervous system** is activated under emergency conditions or stress and produces a set of actions called the **fight-or-flight response.** Activation of this branch prepares the body for heightened activity and for an immediate response to a threat. The brain experiences an increase in alertness and readiness. Heart rate and blood pressure increase and blood is shunted to skeletal muscles, thus preparing the body for sudden, intense physical activity. The liver immediately produces more glucose for energy. The bronchi dilate to allow maximum airflow into the lungs, and breathing becomes faster and deeper. The pupils dilate to provide better vision for dealing with the emergency. The body warms and perspiration increases. At the same time the body is preparing for the threat, nonemergency maintenance functions such as peristalsis and urine formation are temporarily suspended.

The **parasympathetic nervous system** is activated under nonstressful conditions and produces a set of symptoms known as the **rest-and-digest response.** These nerves promote relaxation and body maintenance activities. Digestive secretions increase, peristalsis propels substances along the alimentary canal, and defecation is promoted. Heart rate and blood pressure decline. Because less air is needed, the bronchi constrict and respiration slows. The student should notice that the actions of the parasympathetic division are opposite to those of the sympathetic division.

Under most conditions, the two branches of the ANS cooperate to achieve a balance of readiness and relaxation. Because they have opposite effects, homeostasis may be achieved by changing one or both branches. For example, heart rate can be increased by either increasing the firing of

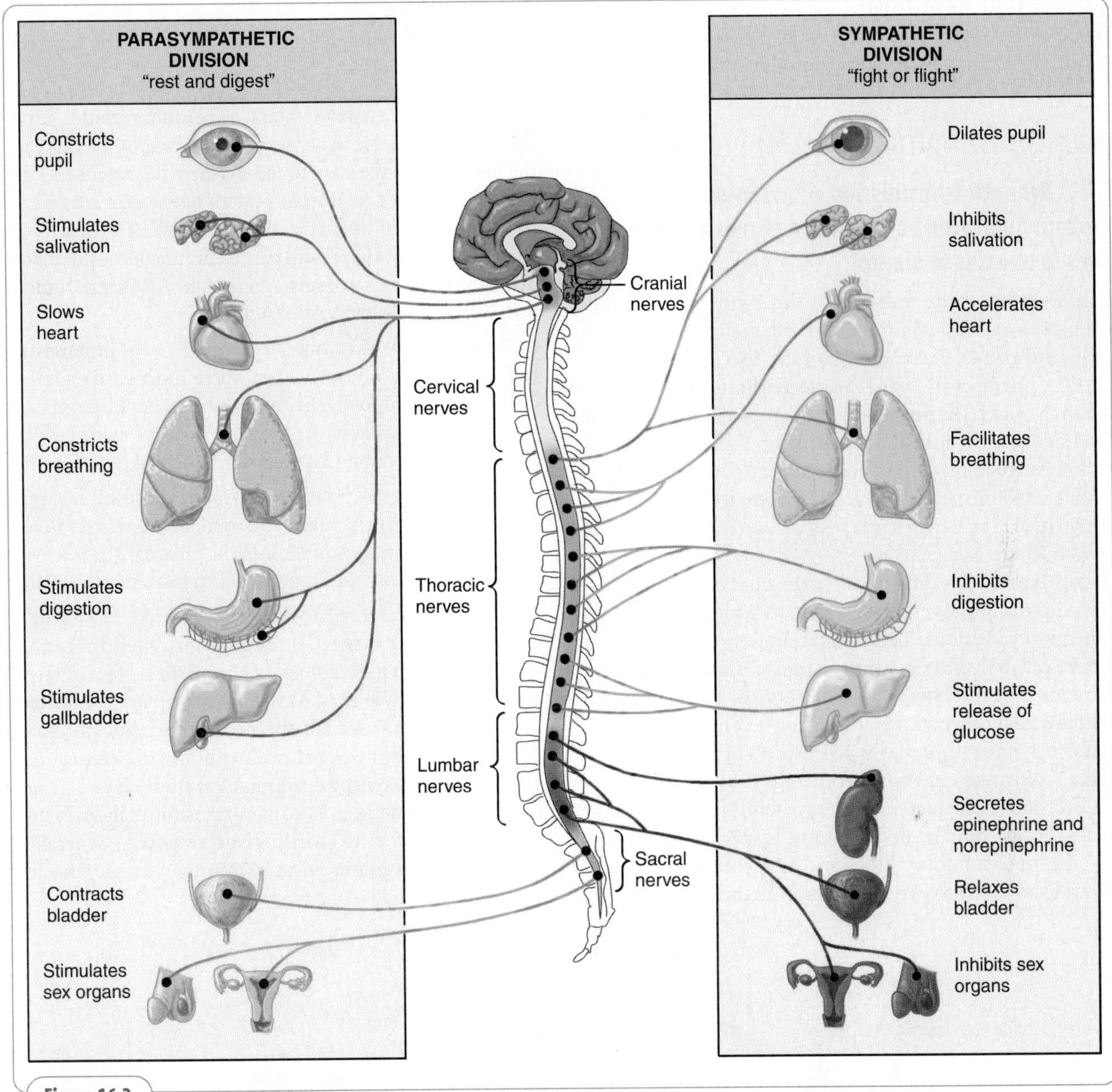

Figure 16.2

Effects of the sympathetic and parasympathetic nervous systems.

Source: From *Biology: A Guide to the Natural World* (4th ed.), by D. Krogh, 2009, Upper Saddle River, NJ: Prentice Hall. Reprinted with permission.

sympathetic nerves or by decreasing the firing of parasympathetic nerves. This allows the body a means of fine-tuning its essential organ systems.

There is always some degree of autonomic activity even in the absence of stimuli. This background level of activity is known as **autonomic tone.** For example, sympathetic nerves are constantly firing, keeping arterioles in a constant state of constriction. This sympathetic tone allows for faster changes in blood pressure because the vessels are in a constant state of readiness. On the other hand, parasympathetic tone on the smooth muscle of the alimentary and urinary tracts maintains continuous contractions and keeps intestinal peristalsis and urine flow steady. With the important exception of the vascular system, the predominant tone of autonomic tissues is from the parasympathetic nervous system.

The sympathetic and parasympathetic divisions do not always have opposite effects. For example, the constriction of arterioles is controlled entirely by the sympathetic branch. Sympathetic stimulation causes constriction of arterioles, whereas lack of stimulation causes vasodilation. Only sympathetic nerves control the adrenal medulla and the sweat glands. The sympathetic division is also solely responsible for the release of renin by the kidneys, an action that increases blood pressure. Metabolic effects such as increases in blood glucose and mobilization of lipids for energy are uniquely sympathetic functions.

In the male reproductive system, the roles are complementary. Erection of the penis is a function of the parasympathetic division, and the sympathetic branch controls ejaculation.

Synaptic Transmission

16.4 Synaptic transmission allows information to be communicated between two nerves or from nerves to muscles or glands.

For information to be transmitted throughout the nervous system, neurons must communicate with each other and with muscles and glands. The basic unit of the ANS is a two-neuron chain. The first neuron, called the preganglionic neuron, originates in the CNS. The preganglionic neuron connects with the second nerve outside the CNS in structures called **ganglia.** A ganglion (singular of *ganglia*) contains the neuron cell body of the postganglionic neuron, which is waiting to receive the action potential. The basic structure of an automatic pathway is shown in Figure 16.3.

Before the message can be transferred from one nerve to another, however, it must cross the **synapse,** a physical space between the two neurons. The communication of the message from one cell to another, or synaptic transmission, utilizes special chemicals called **neurotransmitters.** It is important to study the details of synaptic transmission because a large number of drugs affect this process. The process of synaptic transmission is illustrated in Pharmacotherapy Illustrated 16.1.

The second (postganglionic) neuron terminates on smooth muscle, cardiac muscle, or a gland at a specialized synapse called the **neuroeffector junction.** As mentioned earlier a neurotransmitter conveys the message from the second neuron to the muscle or gland. The movement of the nerve impulse from the CNS to the ganglia to the neuroeffector junction occurs in several steps.

1. **Synthesis of the neurotransmitter.** The neurotransmitter, or chemical messenger in the synapse, is synthesized in the cell body of the neuron or in the axon terminal where the synapse is located. Over 50 different neurotransmitters have been identified, the most common of which are shown in Table 16.1. Each neurotransmitter is associated with particular functions and responses. The two primary neurotransmitters of the ANS are **norepinephrine (NE)** and **acetylcholine (Ach).**

2. **Storage of the neurotransmitter.** Because nerve impulses travel rapidly from neuron to neuron, there must be an ample and continuous supply of the neurotransmitter. At the terminal ends of each axon lie millions of granules or vesicles loaded with neurotransmitters, waiting for an action potential to release them.

3. **Release of the neurotransmitter.** When the nerve impulse reaches the end of the axon, it stimulates some of the vesicles to release their stored neurotransmitter into the synapse. The neurotransmitter enters the **synaptic cleft,** which must be crossed for the impulse to reach the postganglionic neuron or effector tissue.

4. **Binding to the receptor.** The neurotransmitter diffuses across the synaptic cleft to receptors that lie on the surface of the postsynaptic cell. There is a brief delay in impulse conduction of about 0.2 to 0.5 msec for the neurotransmitter to cross the synapse. Once the neurotransmitter binds, the message is conveyed to the postsynaptic cell, which is a muscle cell, glandular cell, or another neuron. The neurotransmitter induces the target tissue to elicit its characteristic response. Generally, the more neurotransmitter released into the synapse, the greater and longer lasting will be the response.

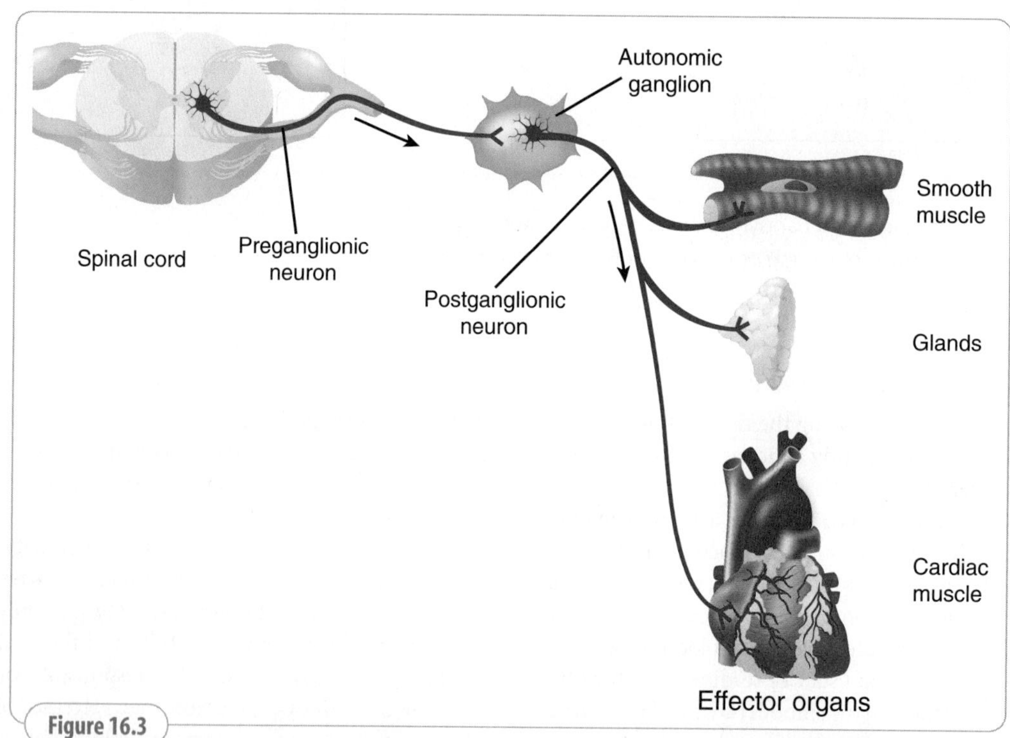

Figure 16.3

Basic structure of an autonomic pathway.

PHARMACOTHERAPY ILLUSTRATED 16.1

Synaptic Transmission

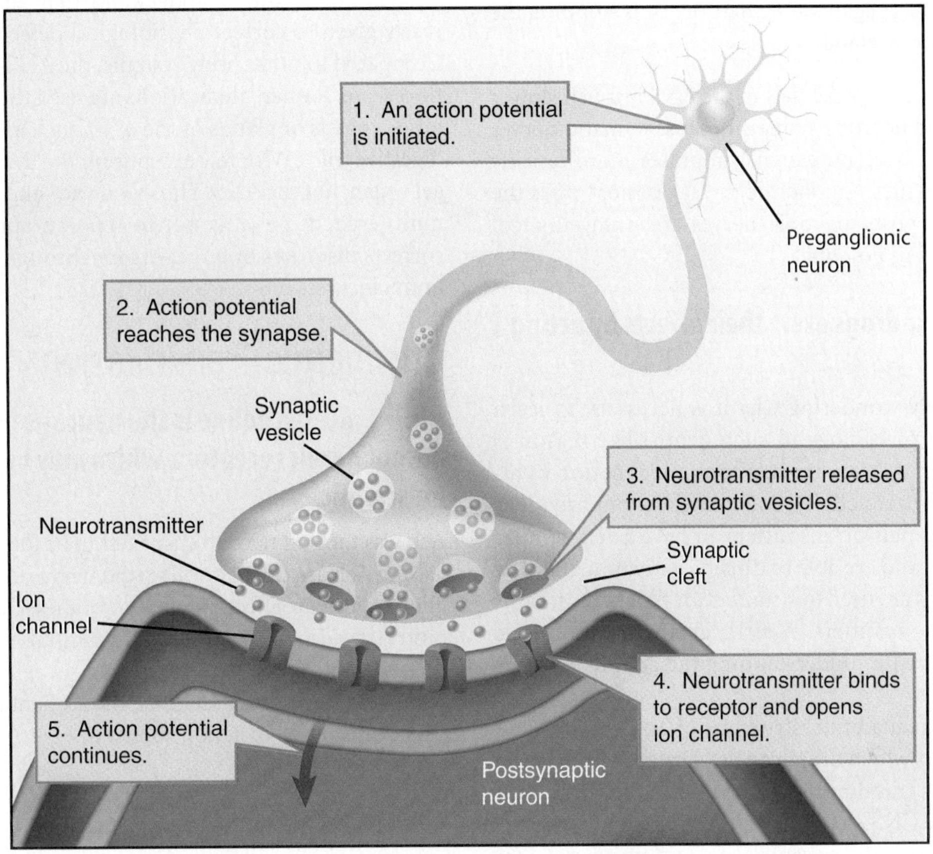

TABLE 16.1 Selected Neurotransmitters, Their Effects and Clinical Applications

Neurotransmitter	Primary Location	Clinical Application (Chapter Number)
Acetylcholine	Synapses throughout the CNS; preganglionic neurons ending in the ganglia in both the sympathetic and parasympathetic nervous systems (nicotinic); postganglionic neurons ending in neuroeffector target tissues in the parasympathetic nervous system (muscarinic)	Myasthenia gravis (17); Alzheimer's disease (25)
Dopamine	Limbic system and hypothalamus; some sympathetic ganglia	Attention deficit/hyperactivity disorder (28); Parkinson's disease (25); psychoses (24)
Gamma aminobutyric acid (GABA)	Cerebellum, cerebral cortex; interneurons throughout the CNS	Anxiety (22); seizures (26)
Glutamate	Throughout the CNS	Seizures (26)
Nitrous oxide	CNS, adrenal gland, and nerves to the penis	Impotence (72)
Norepinephrine	Throughout the CNS; most neuroeffector target junctions in the sympathetic nervous system	Attention deficit/hyperactivity disorder (28); cocaine and amphetamine abuse (8); depression (23)
Serotonin (5-HT)	Limbic system and hypothalamus; primary neurotransmitter in the extrapyramidal system; GI tract	Anxiety (22); depression (23); nausea and vomiting (61); psychoses (24)
Substance P	Pain pathways in the spinal cord; brain and sensory neurons	Analgesia (29)

5. **Termination of neurotransmitter action.** Once the message is transmitted, the two cells must return to baseline conditions and ready themselves for future messages. This is accomplished by removal of the neurotransmitter. The neurotransmitter is either degraded in the synaptic cleft by enzymes, or it diffuses back into the preganglionic neuron, thus stopping the action of the muscle or gland.

Conduction of action potentials in the ANS is much slower than in the somatic nervous system. Because somatic nerves are myelinated and have no ganglia, impulses more quickly reach their target tissues. Autonomic messages must cross the synaptic cleft, and postganglionic nerves are unmyelinated, which slows the action potential.

16.5 Autonomic drugs exert their effects by acting at synapses.

The student is likely wondering why it is necessary to learn ANS anatomy and physiology to such depth. The reason is that a large number of drugs affect autonomic function by altering neurotransmitter activity. Some medications are identical to endogenous neurotransmitters, or have a very similar chemical structure, and are able to directly activate a gland or muscle. Other drugs are used to stimulate or block the actions of natural neurotransmitters. A firm grasp of autonomic physiology is essential to understanding the actions of hundreds of drugs.

The two-neuron anatomic structure of the ANS allows multiple locations at which drugs can act. Drugs can affect the outflow of impulses traveling along the preganglionic neuron at their source—the CNS. A second site is in the ganglia, which is at the synapse where the preganglionic and postganglionic neurons meet. Yet a third site is at the end of the chain, at the target tissues of the postganglionic neuron.

Despite the complexity of the ANS, actions of drugs affecting this system can be grouped into just a few categories. The following are the five general mechanisms by which drugs affect synaptic transmission.

- Medications may affect the synthesis of the neurotransmitter in the preganglionic nerve. Drugs that decrease neurotransmitter synthesis inhibit autonomic responses. Those that increase neurotransmitter synthesis have the opposite effect.
- Medications can prevent the storage of the neurotransmitter in vesicles within the preganglionic nerve. Prevention of neurotransmitter storage inhibits autonomic actions.
- Medications can influence the release of the neurotransmitter from the preganglionic nerve. Promoting neurotransmitter release stimulates autonomic responses, whereas preventing neurotransmitter release has the opposite effect.
- Medications can bind to the neurotransmitter receptor site on the postganglionic cell. Drugs that bind to postganglionic receptors and stimulate the cell will increase autonomic responses. Those that attach to the postganglionic cell and prevent the natural neurotransmitter from reaching its receptors will inhibit autonomic actions.
- Medications can prevent the normal destruction or reuptake of the neurotransmitter. These drugs cause the neurotransmitter to remain in the synapse for a longer time and will stimulate autonomic actions.

It is important to understand that autonomic drugs are rarely given to correct physiological defects in the ANS itself. Compared to other body systems, the ANS has remarkably little disease. Rather, medications are used to stimulate or inhibit target organs or glands of the ANS, such as the heart, lungs, or digestive tract. With few exceptions, the disorder lies in the target organ, not the ANS. Thus when an "autonomic drug" is administered, the goal is not to treat an autonomic disease; it corrects disorders of target organs through its effects on autonomic nerves.

Cholinergic Transmission

16.6 Acetylcholine is the neurotransmitter released at cholinergic receptors, which may be nicotinic or muscarinic.

Ach was the first neurotransmitter to be identified. Neurons releasing Ach are called **cholinergic** nerves. Located on postganglionic or neuroeffector cell membranes, cholinergic receptors bind Ach and either continue the impulse (at the ganglia) or cause an autonomic action (at the neuroeffector tissue). When reading the following sections, the student should refer to the sites of Ach and NE action shown in Figure 16.4.

PharmFACT

Sir Henry Dale identified acetylcholine as a neurotransmitter in 1914, and Otto Loewi demonstrated its physiology. The pair was awarded the Nobel Prize in Physiology or Medicine in 1936 for their work. Dale also is responsible for creating the terminology "ergic" when naming synapses, such as cholinergic or adrenergic.
Source: Nobelprize.org, 2008.

Ach is synthesized in the preganglionic nerve terminal and stored in synaptic vesicles. A preganglionic neuron may contain 300,000 vesicles, each housing as many as 50,000 Ach molecules. When an action potential reaches the nerve terminal, a brief burst of Ach is released into the synaptic cleft, where it diffuses across to attach to its receptors on the postganglionic cell.

Cholinergic Receptors and Neurotransmitters

There are two types of cholinergic receptors that bind Ach. They are named after certain chemicals that bind to them.

- **Nicotinic receptors.** Located at preganglionic neurons ending in the ganglia in both the sympathetic and parasympathetic nervous systems
- **Muscarinic receptors.** Located at postganglionic neurons ending in neuroeffector target tissues in the parasympathetic nervous system

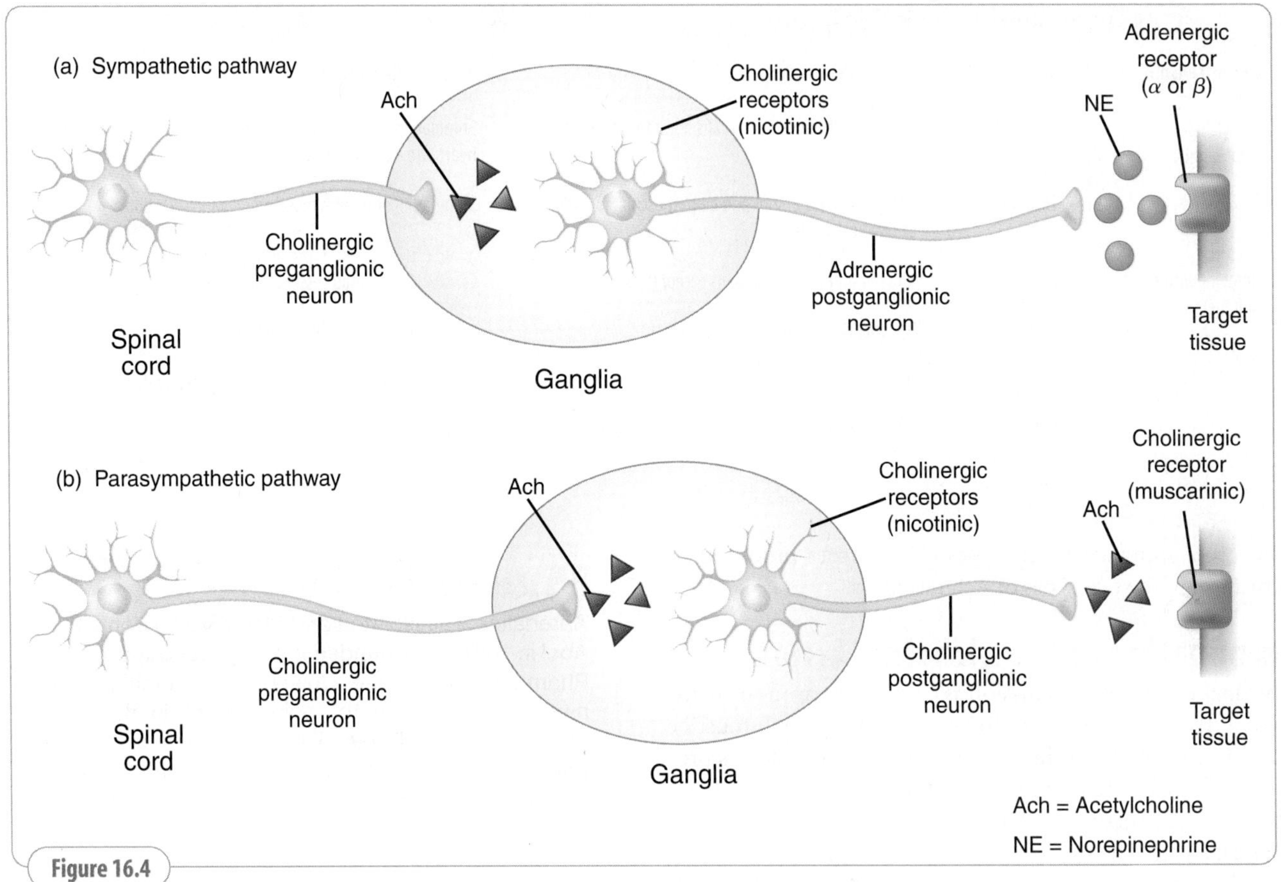

Figure 16.4

Receptors in the autonomic nervous system: (a) Sympathetic pathway: Ach is released at the ganglia (nicotinic receptor) and NE at the effector organ (adrenergic receptor); (b) Parasympathetic pathway: Ach is released at both the ganglia (nicotinic receptor) and effector organ (cholinergic receptor).

Early research on laboratory animals found that the actions of Ach at the ganglia resemble those of nicotine, the active chemical in tobacco products. Because of this similarity, receptors for Ach in the ganglia are called **nicotinic** receptors. Nicotinic receptors are also found in skeletal muscle, which is controlled by the somatic nervous system, and in the adrenal medulla. Because nicotinic receptors are present in so many locations, drugs affecting these receptors produce profound effects on both the ANS and somatic nervous system. Activation of Ach nicotinic receptors causes tachycardia, hypertension, and increased tone and motility in the digestive tract. Although nicotinic receptor blockers were some of the first drugs used to treat hypertension, they are rarely used for this purpose today due to the discovery of safer drugs. The primary current therapeutic application of these agents is to produce skeletal muscle relaxation (a somatic effect) during surgical procedures. A complete discussion of nicotinic blockers can be found in Chapter 18.

CONNECTION *Checkpoint* 16.1

Nicotine is presented in Chapter 8 as an addictive drug. Describe the effects that nicotine has on the body. See Answer to Connection Checkpoint 16.1 in Appendix A.

Activation of Ach receptors at postganglionic nerve endings in the parasympathetic nervous system results in the classic symptoms of parasympathetic stimulation shown in Figure 16.2. Early research determined that these actions closely resemble those produced after eating the poisonous mushroom *Amanita muscaria.* The active substance in this mushroom is the chemical muscarine; thus, these Ach receptors were named **muscarinic** receptors. Muscarinic receptors are also found in most sweat glands and in blood vessels serving skeletal muscles. The locations of nicotinic and muscarinic receptors are illustrated in Figure 16.5.

When Ach binds to nicotinic receptors, the action is always stimulatory. Examples include increased sweat production, increased release of adrenal medullary hormones, and enhanced nerve conduction in the ganglia. Ach action at muscarinic receptors, however, may be stimulatory or inhibitory, depending on the target tissue. Examples include decreased heart rate and increased peristalsis. Muscarinic receptors are affected by a larger number of drugs that have more pharmacologic applications than the nicotinic agents. Drugs that block muscarinic receptors are used during ophthalmic procedures, as preanesthetic agents, and in the pharmacotherapy of asthma and bradycardia (see Chapter 20).

Although Ach itself can stimulate both muscarinic and nicotinic receptors, some drugs are selective to only one type.

TABLE 16.2 Types of Autonomic Receptors

Neurotransmitter	Receptor	Primary Locations	Selected Responses
Acetylcholine (cholinergic)	Muscarinic	Parasympathetic target: organs other than the heart	Stimulation of smooth muscle and gland secretions; decreased heart rate and force of contraction
	Nicotinic	Postganglionic neurons and neuromuscular junctions of skeletal muscle	Stimulation of smooth muscle and gland secretions
Norepinephrine (adrenergic)	$Alpha_1$	All sympathetic target organs except the heart	Constriction of blood vessels; dilation of pupils
	$Alpha_2$	Presynaptic adrenergic nerve terminals	Inhibition of norepinephrine release
	$Beta_1$	Heart and kidneys	Increased heart rate and force of contraction; release of renin
	$Beta_2$	All sympathetic target organs except the heart	Inhibition of smooth muscle contraction

Table 16.2 summarizes the types of responses produced by activation of the two types of Ach receptors.

Termination of Acetylcholine Action

The goal of nerve transmission is to produce an immediate, though transient, response. To accomplish this, Ach must be rapidly removed from the synaptic cleft after its effect is produced. The enzyme that resides in the synaptic cleft and catalyzes the destruction of Ach is called **acetylcholinesterase (AchE).** (Note: The suffix "erase" can be thought of as "wiping out" the Ach.) AchE is quite efficient at performing its task. It is estimated that over half the Ach molecules released from the vesicles are destroyed before they have a chance to reach their receptors. Following the breakdown of Ach, choline is reformed and is taken up by the preganglionic neuron, where it is used to synthesize more Ach. The life cycle of Ach in the neuron is shown in Figure 16.5.

Pseudocholinesterase, also known as plasma cholinesterase, is another enzyme that destroys Ach. Found primarily in the liver, pseudocholinesterase rapidly inactivates Ach and drugs with a chemical structure similar to Ach as they circulate in the plasma. Some people are born with a genetic deficiency of this enzyme and are unable to inactivate plasma Ach or succinylcholine, a surgical drug structurally similar to Ach. These patients are particularly sensitive to the effects of succinylcholine because they are unable to inactivate the drug (see Chapter 30).

Adrenergic Transmission

16.7 Norepinephrine is the primary neurotransmitter released at adrenergic receptors, which may be alpha or beta.

In the sympathetic nervous system, NE is the neurotransmitter released at almost all postganglionic nerves. NE belongs to a class of endogenous hormones called **catecholamines,** all of which are involved in neurotransmission. Other catecholamines include epinephrine (adrenaline) and dopamine. The receptors at the ends of postganglionic sympathetic neurons are called **adrenergic,** which is derived from the word *adrenaline.*

PharmFACT

Adrenaline was isolated and identified by John Jacob Abel in 1897, who founded the very first Department of Pharmacology at the University of Michigan. The name was changed to "epinephrine" in the United States because Parke, Davis, and Co. owned the trademark rights to the word *adrenalin* (without a final "e"). It is still known as adrenaline in the rest of the world. *Source:* Aronson, 2000.

NE is synthesized in the nerve terminal and stored in vesicles until an action potential triggers its release into the synaptic cleft. NE then diffuses across the cleft to bind to its receptors on the effector cell.

Adrenergic receptors are of two basic types: alpha (α) and beta (β). These receptors are further divided into the subtypes $beta_1$, $beta_2$, $alpha_1$, and $alpha_2$. Activation of each type of subreceptor results in a characteristic set of physiological responses, which are summarized in Table 16.2.

Alpha-Adrenergic Receptors

When alpha receptors are stimulated, enzymes on the inside of the plasma membrane are activated and a cascade of changes occurs within the cell. These changes occur due to the production of a second messenger, the G-protein, which initiates the cascade. In $alpha_1$ receptors intracellular calcium stores are released, causing excitatory effects such as smooth muscle contraction or sphincter closure. Drugs affecting $alpha_1$ receptors are primarily used for their effects on vascular smooth muscle in the treatment of hypertension (see Chapter 20).

Stimulation of $alpha_2$ receptors causes different effects due to the activation of a separate cascade of events. By increasing cyclic adenosine monophosphate (cAMP) within the cell, activation of $alpha_2$ receptors causes mostly inhibitory actions. Activation of the $alpha_2$ receptor will inhibit NE release from sympathetic nerve endings. In addition, activation of $alpha_2$ receptors in the CNS can suppress the outflow of sympathetic activity from the brain. Indeed, as discussed in Chapter 19, drugs that affect $alpha_2$ receptors are usually used for their ability to decrease blood pressure due to their effects on the CNS, not the ANS.

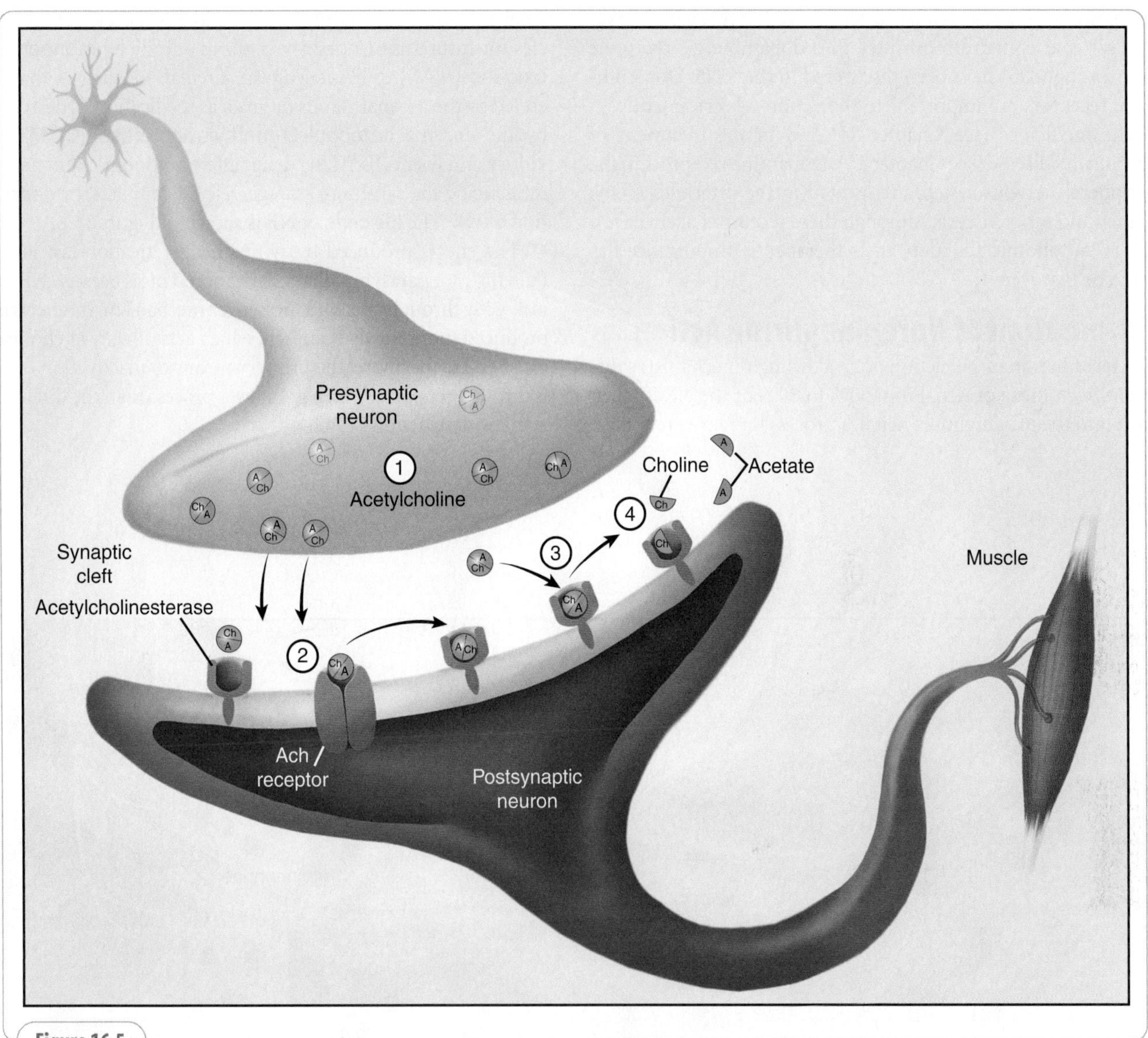

Figure 16.5

Life cycle of acetylcholine (Ach): (1) Ach is released into the synaptic cleft; (2) Ach binds to receptors on the postsynaptic membrane; (3) Ach binds to the acetycholinesterase enzyme; (4) Ach is broken down into acetate and choline.

Beta-Adrenergic Receptors

Three subtypes of beta-adrenergic receptors have been identified, although only beta$_1$ and beta$_2$ have pharmacologic importance. Beta receptors act by increasing the second messenger cAMP in target cells. The specific response caused by activation of the beta receptor depends on its location.

The primary tissues served by beta$_1$ receptors are the heart and coronary vessels. Activation of these receptors increases the heart rate and strength of contraction and dilates the coronary arteries, thus preparing the heart for fight or flight. Beta$_1$ receptors in the kidney respond by releasing renin, which helps to maintain blood pressure.

Beta$_2$ receptors are more widely distributed than beta$_1$ receptors, with locations in the smooth muscle in blood vessels, the GI tract, and the lung. Activation of these receptors will inhibit vasoconstriction (thus causing vasodilation), dilate bronchioles, slow peristalsis, and decrease urine production.

The significance of adrenergic receptor subtypes to pharmacology cannot be overstated. Some drugs are selective and activate only one type of adrenergic receptor, whereas others affect all of them. Furthermore, a drug may activate one type of receptor at low doses and begin to affect other receptor subtypes as the dose is increased. Committing the receptor types and their responses to memory is an essential step in learning autonomic pharmacology.

Other types of adrenergic receptors exist. Although the functional role of dopamine was once thought to be only a chemical precursor to NE, research has determined that this agent serves a larger role as neurotransmitter. Five dopaminergic receptors (D1 through D5) have been discovered in the CNS. Dopaminergic receptors are important to the action of certain antipsychotic medicines (see Chapter 24) and in the treatment of Parkinson's disease (see Chapter 25). Dopamine receptors in the peripheral nervous system are located in the arterioles of the kidney and other viscera. Although these receptors likely have a role in autonomic function, their therapeutic importance has yet to be discovered.

Termination of Norepinephrine Action

The termination of NE action occurs through mechanisms different from those of Ach. From 50% to 80% of the NE is taken back into the preganglionic nerve, a process known as reuptake. After reuptake, NE in the nerve terminal is repackaged in vesicles for future use or destroyed enzymatically by **monoamine oxidase (MAO).** NE entering the circulation, such as that secreted by the adrenal glands or given as medication, is destroyed by the enzyme **catechol-O-methyltransferase (COMT)** in kidney and liver cells. Many drugs affect autonomic function by influencing the synthesis, storage, release, reuptake, or destruction of NE. The life cycle of NE is shown in Figure 16.6.

The effects produced by sympathetic activation last longer than those of parasympathetic activation. This is because NE acts indirectly through a second messenger mechanism. Its effects are produced more slowly than Ach, which acts directly at cholinergic sites. Furthermore, the primary means of inactivation of NE is through reuptake, which is a slower process than the direct enzymatic destruction of Ach.

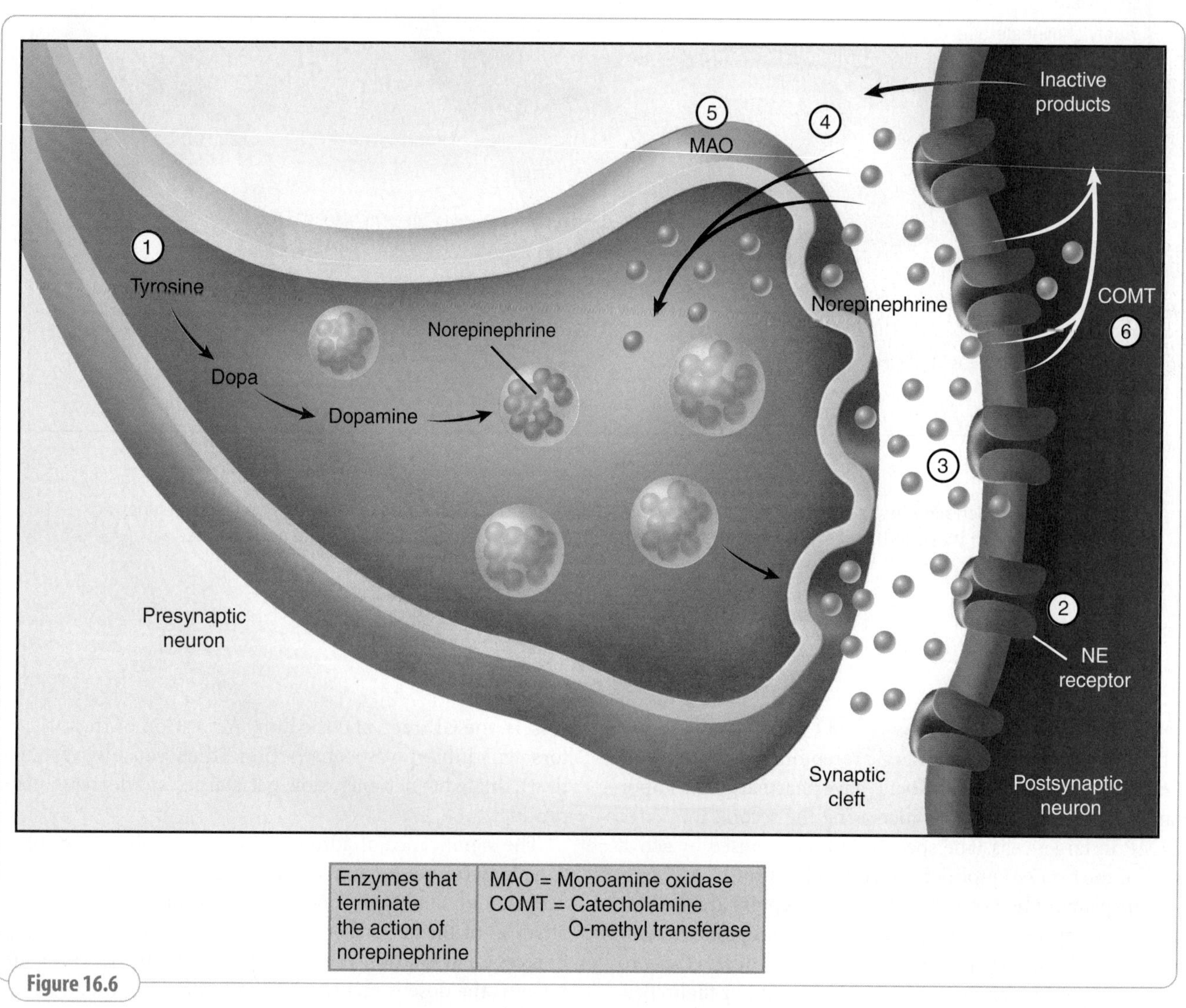

Enzymes that terminate the action of norepinephrine	MAO = Monoamine oxidase COMT = Catecholamine O-methyl transferase

Figure 16.6

Life cycle of norephinephrine (NE): (1) NE is synthesized from the amino acid tyrosine; (2) NE is released into the synaptic cleft; (3) NE binds to receptors on the postsynaptic membrane; (4) NE is taken back into the presynaptic neuron; (5) NE is degraded by MAO; (6) Small amounts of NE enter the postsynaptic cell and are degraded by COMT.

16.8 The adrenal medulla is a specialized type of sympathetic nervous system tissue that secretes epinephrine and norepinephrine.

The adrenal medulla is closely associated with the sympathetic nervous system but has a different anatomic and physiological arrangement than the rest of the sympathetic branch. Early in embryonic life, the adrenal medulla is part of the neural tissue that is destined to become the sympathetic nervous system. The primitive tissue splits, however, and the adrenal medulla becomes its own functional division. Preganglionic neurons from the spinal cord terminate in the adrenal medulla and release the neurotransmitters epinephrine and NE directly into the blood. Approximately 80% of the secretion is epinephrine, with the other 20% being NE. Once released, these agents are widely distributed to target organs, where they elicit the classic fight-or-flight symptoms.

When released into the systemic circulation, the effects of epinephrine and NE are more diffuse and longer lasting than those produced by activation of postganglionic sympathetic neurons in the ANS. In addition, when released into the bloodstream, these agents are distributed to most body cells, not just those innervated by the ANS. Significant concentrations of epinephrine and NE may persist for as long as 30 seconds, and their effects on the tissues may continue for several minutes until the liver deactivates the hormones. It is estimated that 25% to 50% of all sympathetic nervous system responses at any given time are due to circulating hormones from the adrenal medulla.

Regulation of Autonomic Functions

16.9 The autonomic nervous system is influenced by higher levels of control in the cerebral cortex and hypothalamus.

Although it is often stated that control of the ANS is involuntary, this is an oversimplification. For example, strong emotions such as rage are seated in the brain, but they trigger the heart to race, the blood pressure to rise, and the respiration rate to increase. Mental depression can have the opposite effects. The smell of steak or chicken cooking on the grill can increase peristalsis, resulting in "grumbling" of the stomach and increased salivation. Clearly, autonomic actions can be modified by higher brain centers.

The roles of higher centers in regulating the ANS are shown in Figure 16.7. The hypothalamus is thought to be the main integration center of the ANS. This tissue receives signals from the cerebrum and sensory input, such as emotions, from the limbic system of the brain. The hypothalamus

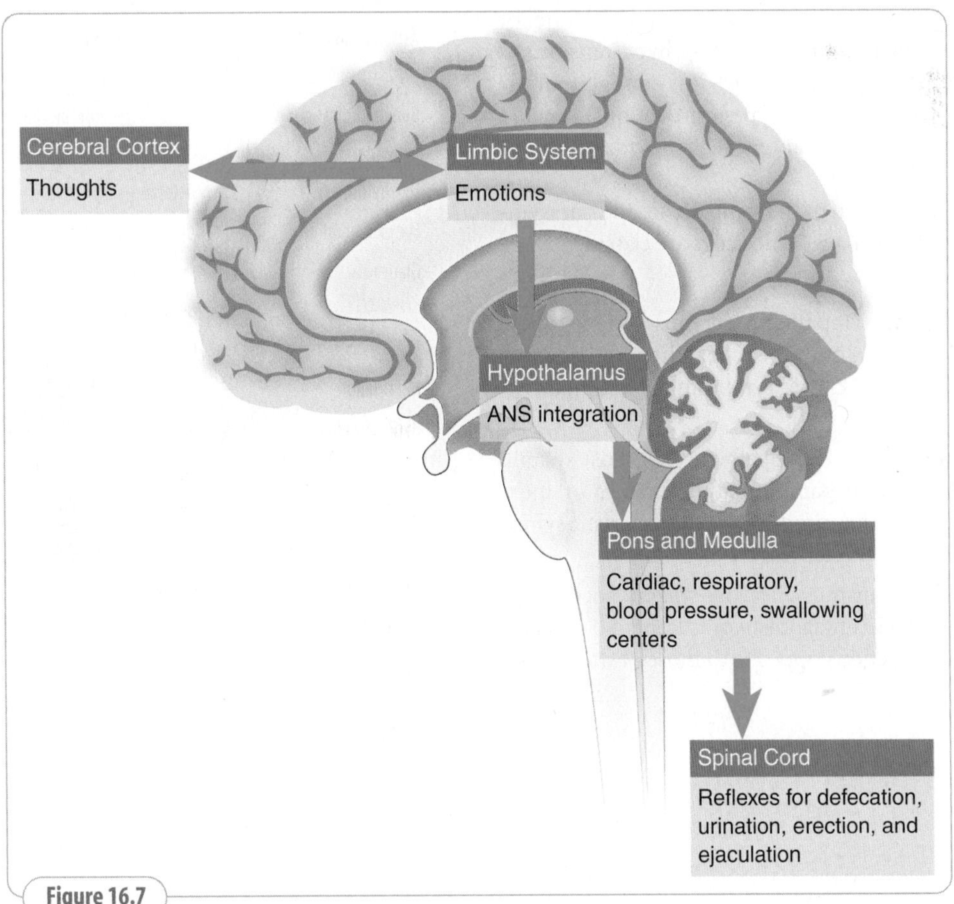

Figure 16.7

Higher centers influencing autonomic function.

interprets the information and responds by sending messages to the various portions of the ANS, such as increasing peristalsis and salivation when the sights, sounds, and smells of the grilled steak are experienced. Messages from the hypothalamus travel along the medulla oblongata, the brainstem, and the spinal cord.

Drugs can affect the ANS by influencing these higher centers. For example, drugs that decrease anxiety or diminish the incidence of panic attacks can slow the heart rate and lower blood pressure through their ability to affect conscious thought. It is important to understand that these drugs do not necessarily act on autonomic receptors. Nor does the patient consciously lower their blood pressure or heart rate. The autonomic effect is indirect, caused by a reduction of stress, and it is at a subconscious level. Controlling autonomic activity through conscious thought is the principle underlying biofeedback therapy.

Classifying Autonomic Drugs

16.10 Autonomic drugs are classified by which receptors they stimulate or block.

At this point of the chapter, it is normal for students to feel overwhelmed by the complexity of the various autonomic receptors and their actions. It is the existence of these different receptors, however, that allows drugs to cause very specific therapeutic actions. For example, it is desirable to have drugs that affect blood pressure without increasing heart rate, or drugs that dilate bronchi without causing hypertension. At this stage in the study of pharmacology, it is enough that the student memorizes the receptor types and actions, because applications in the coming chapters will provide clarity to this subject.

Given the opposite actions of the sympathetic and parasympathetic nervous systems, autonomic drugs are classified based on one of four possible actions.

1. Stimulation of the sympathetic nervous system. These drugs are called sympathomimetics or adrenergic agonists and they produce the classic symptoms of the fight-or-flight response.
2. Stimulation of the parasympathetic nervous system. These drugs are called parasympathomimetics or muscarinic agonists and they produce the characteristic symptoms of the rest-and-digest response.
3. Inhibition of the sympathetic nervous system. These drugs are called adrenergic antagonists or adrenergic blockers and they produce actions opposite to those of the sympathomimetics.
4. Inhibition of the parasympathetic nervous system. These drugs are called anticholinergics, parasympatholytics, or muscarinic blockers and they produce actions opposite to those of the parasympathomimetics.

There is a method for simplifying the learning of autonomic pharmacology. On examining the preceding four drug classes, it is evident that only one group need be learned because the others are logical extensions of the first. If the fight-or-flight symptoms of the sympathomimetics are learned, the other three groups are either the same or opposite. For example, both the sympathomimetics and the anticholinergics increase heart rate and dilate the pupils. The other two groups, the parasympathomimetics and the adrenergic antagonists, have the opposite effects of slowing heart rate and constricting the pupils. Although this is an oversimplification and exceptions exist, it is a timesaving means of learning the basic actions and adverse effects of dozens of drugs affecting the ANS. It should be emphasized again that mastering the actions and terminology of autonomic drugs early in the study of pharmacology will reap rewards later in the course when these drugs are applied to various systems. Table 16.3 shows the many applications of autonomic drugs in medicine.

TABLE 16.3 Indications for Autonomic Agents

Indication	Autonomic Class	Chapter
Angina pectoris	Beta-adrenergic blockers	37
Asthma and COPD	Beta-adrenergic agonists Anticholinergics	73
Benign prostatic hyperplasia	Alpha-adrenergic blockers	72
Dysrhythmias	Beta-adrenergic blockers	39
Eye examinations	Anticholinergics	77
Glaucoma	Alpha-adrenergic blockers Beta-adrenergic blockers Cholinergic agonists	77
Heart failure	Beta-adrenergic blockers	38
Hypertension	$Alpha_1$-adrenergic blockers $Alpha_2$-adrenergic agonists Beta-adrenergic blockers	36
Myocardial infarction	Beta-adrenergic blockers	37
Parkinson's disease	Anticholinergics	25
Peptic ulcer disease	Anticholinergics	60
Shock	Beta-adrenergic agonists	38

UNDERSTANDING THE CHAPTER

Key Concepts Summary

16.1 The two major subdivisions of the nervous system are the central nervous system and the peripheral nervous system.

16.2 The peripheral nervous system is divided into somatic and autonomic components.

16.3 The autonomic nervous system is divided into two mostly opposing components: the sympathetic and parasympathetic branches.

16.4 Synaptic transmission allows information to be communicated between two nerves or from nerves to muscles or glands.

16.5 Autonomic drugs exert their effects by acting at synapses.

16.6 Acetylcholine is the neurotransmitter released at cholinergic receptors, which may be nicotinic or muscarinic.

16.7 Norepinephrine is the primary neurotransmitter released at adrenergic receptors, which may be alpha or beta.

16.8 The adrenal medulla is a specialized type of sympathetic nervous system tissue that secretes epinephrine and norepinephrine.

16.9 The autonomic nervous system is influenced by higher levels of control in the cerebral cortex and hypothalamus.

16.10 Autonomic drugs are classified by which receptors they stimulate or block.

References

Aronson, J. K. (2000). Where name and image meet—the argument for "adrenaline." *British Medical Journal, 320*, 506–509.

Bear, M. F., Connors, B. W., & Paradiso, M. A. (2007). *Neuroscience, exploring the brain* (3rd ed.). Philadelphia: Lippincott Williams & Wilkins.

Krogh, D. (2009). *Biology: A guide to the natural world* (4th ed.). Upper Saddle River, NJ: Benjamin Cummings.

Martini, F. H. (2009). *Fundamentals of human anatomy and physiology* (8th ed.). San Francisco: Benjamin Cummings.

McCorry, L. K. (2007). Physiology of the autonomic nervous system. *American Journal of Pharmacy Education, 71*(4), 78.

Nobelprize.org. (2008). *The Nobel prize in physiology or medicine 1936.* Retrieved May 9, 2008, from http://nobelprize.org/nobel_prizes/medicine/laureates/1936/

Silverthorn, D. U. (2009). *Human physiology: An integrated approach* (4th ed.). Upper Saddle River, NJ: Pearson Education/Benjamin Cummings.

Westfall, T. C., & Westfall, D. P. (2006). Neurotransmission: The autonomic and somatic motor nervous systems. In L. L. Brunton, J. S. Lazo, & K. L. Parker (Eds.), *Goodman and Gilman's: The pharmacological basis of therapeutics* (11th ed.). New York: McGraw Hill.

C H A P T E R

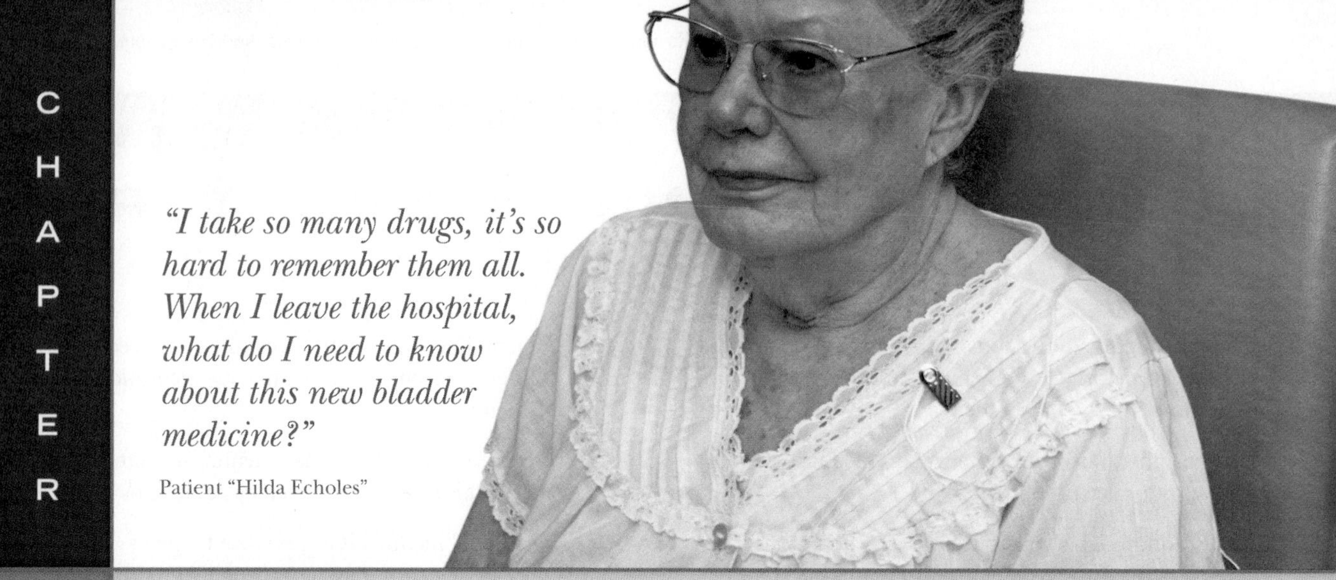

"I take so many drugs, it's so hard to remember them all. When I leave the hospital, what do I need to know about this new bladder medicine?"

Patient "Hilda Echoles"

17 Cholinergic Agonists

Learning Outcomes

After reading this chapter, the student should be able to:

1. Identify the physiological responses that occur when a drug activates cholinergic receptors.
2. Compare and contrast the mechanisms of action for direct- and indirect-acting cholinergic agonists.
3. Differentiate among the following types of cholinergic drugs: direct muscarinic agonists, indirect muscarinic agonists, and nicotinic agonists.
4. Differentiate between the pharmacotherapy of cholinergic crisis and myasthenic crisis.
5. Describe the pharmacotherapy of myasthenia gravis.
6. For each of the classes shown in the chapter outline, identify the prototype and representative drugs and explain the mechanism(s) of drug action, primary indications, contraindications, significant drug interactions, pregnancy category, and important adverse effects.
7. Apply the nursing process to care for patients receiving drug therapy with cholinergic agonists.

Chapter Outline

Cholinergic Receptors

Muscarinic Agonists

Direct-Acting Muscarinic Agonists

PROTOTYPE **Bethanechol Chloride (Duvoid, Urecholine)** *p. 203*

Indirect-Acting Muscarinic Agonists (acetylcholinesterase inhibitors)

Pharmacotherapy of Myasthenia Gravis

PROTOTYPE **Neostigmine (Prostigmin)** *p. 206*

Nicotinic Agonists

Key Terms

acetylcholinesterase (AchE) inhibitor, *204*
cholinergic agonist, *199*
cholinergic crisis, *205*
muscarinic agonist, *199*
myasthenia gravis (MG), *205*
myasthenic crisis, *206*
nicotinic agonist, *199*
reflex tachycardia, *202*
Sjögren's syndrome, *201*
xerostomia, *201*

Of the four classes of autonomic drugs, the cholinergic agonists comprise the smallest and least prescribed group. Because cholinergic synapses are so widely dispersed throughout the central and peripheral nervous systems, drugs affecting these receptors will have multiple and diverse effects. A few have specific applications in ophthalmology and in the treatment of myasthenia gravis.

Cholinergic Receptors

17.1 Drugs can activate cholinergic receptors either directly or indirectly.

Recall from Chapter 16 that cholinergic receptors are located throughout the peripheral nervous system. To understand the effects of cholinergic drugs, it is important to review these locations. In the autonomic nervous system:

- At the neuroeffector junctions in the parasympathetic division
- At the ganglia in both the parasympathetic and sympathetic divisions

In the somatic nervous system:

- At the neuromuscular synapses, which are responsible for skeletal muscle contraction

In addition, cholinergic synapses are present throughout the central nervous system (CNS). These locations are summarized in Figure 17.1.

The degree of activation at a cholinergic synapse is dependent on the amount of acetylcholine (Ach) interacting with its receptors. Drugs and chemicals that increase the action of Ach at cholinergic receptors will promote rest-and-digest responses. These substances are called **cholinergic agonists,** or parasympathomimetics.

Also recall from Chapter 16 that there are two basic types of cholinergic receptors: muscarinic and nicotinic. Although Ach itself stimulates both types of receptors, drugs may be selective for only one type. For example, bethanechol is selective for muscarinic receptors and thus it is called a **muscarinic agonist.** On the other hand, nicotine is selective for nicotinic receptors and therefore is classified as a **nicotinic agonist.** Note that both bethanechol and nicotine are considered cholinergic agonists: The terms *muscarinic* and *nicotinic* are used to specify which cholinergic synapses are activated. If the student has not yet memorized the differences between muscarinic and nicotinic receptors, then Section 16.6 should be reviewed before continuing. A summary of the differences is provided in Table 17.1.

Based on their mechanism of action, cholinergic agonists are classified as direct acting or indirect acting. Some direct-acting drugs, such as bethanechol, enter the synaptic cleft and bind to cholinergic receptors to produce the rest-and-digest response. In this respect, they act by the same mechanism as Ach itself. A second type of direct mechanism is caused by drugs, such as carbachol, that stimulate the release of Ach from nerve terminals, thus permitting more Ach to reach its receptors and cause a

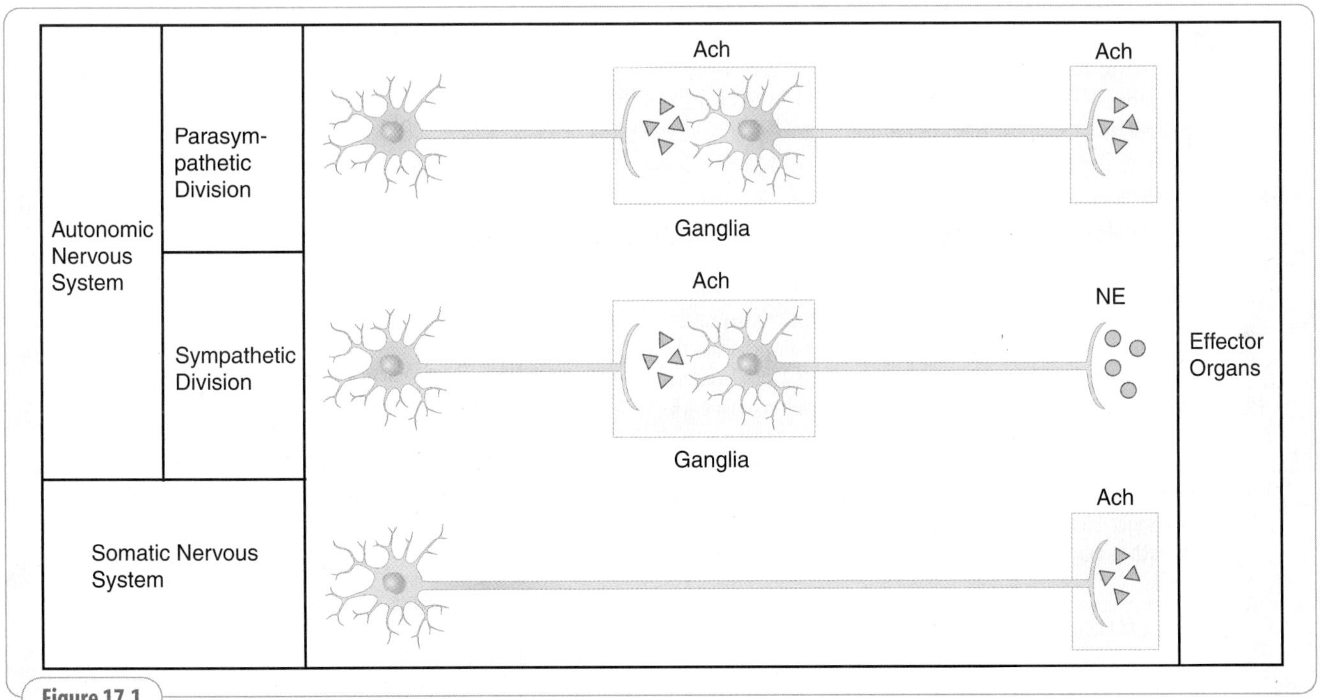

Figure 17.1

Locations of cholinergic synapses. Acetylcholine is released at the ganglia in both the parasympathetic and sympathetic divisions, at the neuroeffector junctions in the parasympathetic division, and in the somatic nervous system at neuromuscular synapses.

TABLE 17.1 Types of Cholinergic Receptors and Their Actions

	Muscarinic	Nicotinic
Receptor location	Glands, smooth muscle, cardiac muscle	Skeletal muscle, autonomic ganglia, brain, adrenal gland*
General actions	Pupil constriction Decreased accommodation of the eye Increased GI motility Decreased heart rate Decreased blood pressure Increased glandular secretions (salivary, lacrimal, and sweat) Constriction of bronchial smooth muscle	Skeletal muscle contraction Initial stimulation of glandular secretion, followed by inhibition Increased heart rate Increased blood pressure
Antagonists	Atropine, scopolamine	Mecamylamine, succinylcholine, tubocurarine

*Some effects of nicotinic activation are caused by the release of epinephrine from the adrenal gland. The epinephrine subsequently activates the adrenergic receptors.

greater effect. Note that although direct activation can occur by two different mechanisms, the result is the same: activation of cholinergic receptors. Direct mechanisms of cholinergic activation are shown in Figure 17.2.

Indirect-acting drugs block the destruction of Ach, allowing the neurotransmitter to accumulate and remain in the synaptic cleft for a longer time. The mechanism by which indirect agents act is by inhibiting acetylcholinesterase (AchE), the enzyme in cholinergic synapses that destroys Ach. Some of these agents bind to AchE for a brief period and thus have short durations of action. These drugs are called reversible inhibitors. Some insecticides and nerve gas agents are considered irreversible inhibitors because they bind to AchE for prolonged periods. These irreversible inhibitors have no therapeutic applications and can cause significant mortality if ingested or absorbed. Again, it should be noted that physiologically it does not matter whether the cholinergic synapse was stimulated directly or indirectly: The parasympathetic responses are the same. There are some important differences, however, as will be discussed in Section 17.3. Indirect mechanisms are shown in Figure 17.2.

Muscarinic Agonists

17.2 Muscarinic agonists produce their effects by directly stimulating cholinergic receptors.

Muscarinic agonists are drugs that activate cholinergic receptors located at the neuroeffector junctions in the parasympathetic nervous system. Although Ach is the classic muscarinic agonist, it has little therapeutic value as a drug because it is rapidly destroyed both in the bloodstream and in synapses (by AchE) and produces many adverse effects. The other drugs in this class are relatively resistant to destruction by AchE; thus they have a longer duration of action than Ach. Muscarinic agonists are poorly absorbed across the gastrointestinal (GI) tract and generally do not cross the blood–brain barrier. They have minimal effects on Ach nicotinic receptors in the ganglia. Because of the potential for serious adverse effects, few muscarinic agonists are used in pharmacotherapy. Available drugs are listed in Table 17.2.

CONNECTIONS

Complementary and Alternative Therapies Lecithin

Description: Lecithin is a mixture of phospholipids that occurs naturally in nervous tissue and is a primary component of pulmonary surfactant. Lecithin contains about 10% to 20% phosphatidylcholine, the agent that is responsible for lecithin's biological effects. When lecithin is taken, the GI tract breaks down the phosphatidylcholine to choline, a B-vitamin. As its name implies, choline is essential to the nervous system as a metabolic precursor of the neurotransmitter acetylcholine. Lecithin protects cells from oxidation. In nature, it is found in high amounts in certain vegetables, such as peanuts, cauliflower, and cabbage, and in fruits, such as oranges. Commercial sources are primarily soybeans and egg yolks.

History and Claims: Lecithin has been used primarily to lower serum cholesterol. More recently, however, lecithin has been claimed to benefit patients with Alzheimer's disease, in whom Ach is deficient in certain regions of the brain. Phosphatidylcholine is also marketed in Germany as a treatment for liver disorders, including protecting the liver from alcohol damage. In addition to its purported role in the nervous system and the liver, choline is widely marketed as a dietary supplement to increase muscle strength and stamina and to promote weight loss.

Standardization: There are several forms of lecithin supplements. Typical supplements contain 20% to 30% phosphatidylcholine. The U.S. Food and Drug Administration (FDA) recommended intake of choline for adults is 550 mg/day for men and 425 mg/day for women. Although quite safe, the most serious adverse effect from high intake of choline is hypotension with possible cholinergic adverse effects (e.g., sweating and diarrhea) and fishy body odor. The upper intake level for adults is 3.5 g/day.

Evidence: The best evidence for lecithin has been from clinical trials showing a hepatoprotective effect in patients suffering from liver damage due to alcohol or viral hepatitis. Clinical trials of lecithin on cholesterol levels have given mixed results and no clear benefit has been established. Research has not demonstrated a clear benefit of treating memory loss or other neurologic disorders with lecithin. Until further research indicates so, patients should not consume more than the recommended FDA intake.

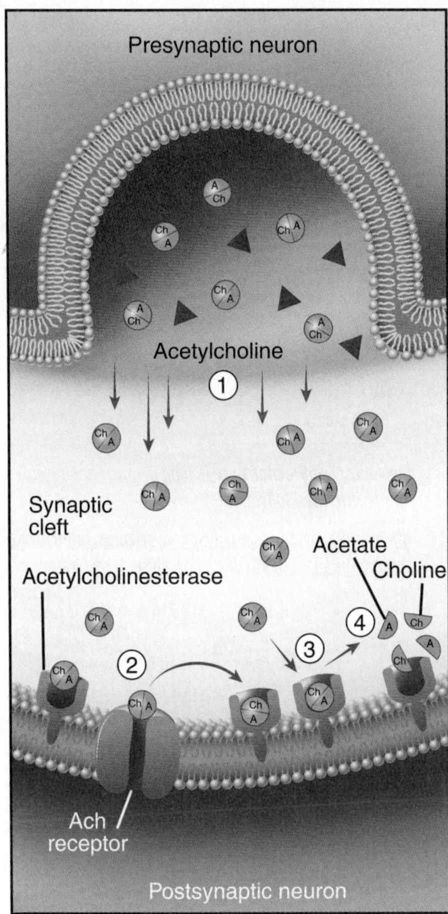

(a) Direct Cholinergic Agonists. Drug (▲) releases more Ach (●) into synapse or binds directly to the Ach receptor.

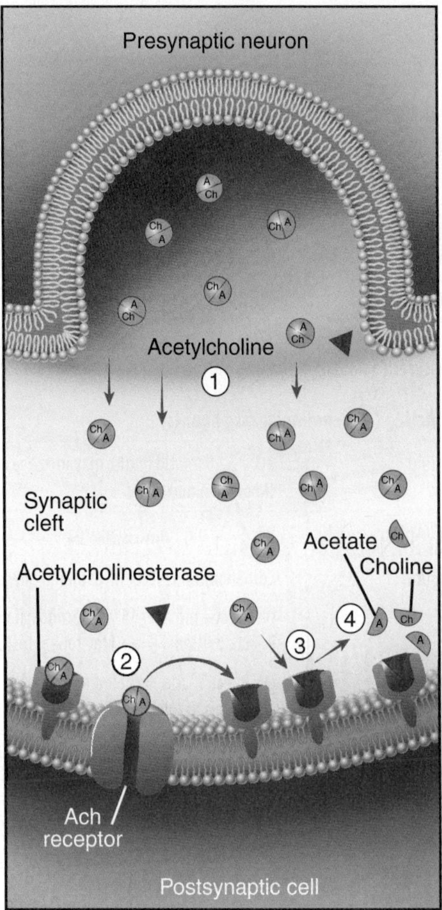

(b) Indirect Cholinergic Agonists. Drug (▲) blocks destruction of Ach (●) allowing more to remain in synapse.

Figure 17.2

Mechanisms of action of cholinergic agonists: (a) Direct cholinergic agonists: (1) Drug causes more acetylcholine (Ach) to be released into the synaptic cleft. (2) Additional Ach occupies Ach receptors, enhancing the action potential on the postsynaptic neuron. (3) Ach binds to acetylcholinesterase. (4) Ach action is terminated by acetylcholinesterase.
(b) Indirect cholinergic agonists: (1) Acetylcholine (Ach) is released into the synaptic cleft. (2) Ach occupies Ach receptors, causing an action potential on the postsynaptic neuron. (3) The drug binds to acetylcholinesterase, preventing the Ach from binding to the enzyme. (4) Ach action is prolonged because it is not destroyed as quickly by acetylcholinesterase.

Muscarinic agonists have widespread effects on the body, nearly all of which are due to parasympathetic activation. All of these drugs can increase the degree of smooth muscle tone and contractions of the GI tract. When administered before meals, stomach emptying is promoted due to increased peristalsis of the alimentary canal. Muscarinic agonists should never be administered to patients with suspected obstructive disease of the GI tract because the increased peristaltic contractions could lead to injury or rupture to the mucosa.

CONNECTION *Checkpoint* 17.1

From what you learned in Chapter 16, would you expect the cholinergic agonists to have similar or opposite effects to the following: adrenergic agonists, adrenergic antagonists, cholinergic antagonists? See Answer to Connection Checkpoint 17.1 in Appendix A.

Muscarinic agonists also stimulate the smooth muscle of the urinary tract, and thus increase ureteral peristalsis and promote emptying of the bladder. These are therapeutic actions in patients with urinary retention. Care must be taken not to administer muscarinic agonists when obstructive uropathy is present, however, because the increased smooth muscle contractions of the ureters and bladder could aggravate pain and bleeding.

Muscarinic agonists stimulate most exocrine glands, increasing lacrimal, sweat, digestive, and salivary secretions. This action has been used to advantage in treating patients with **xerostomia** (dry mouth) or those with **Sjögren's syndrome,** a chronic autoimmune disorder characterized by excessive dryness of mucous membranes, which is associated with rheumatoid arthritis in menopausal women. In addition to creating discomfort for the patient, xerostomia can promote dental caries, periodontal disease, oral ulcers, and candidiasis.

TABLE 17.2 Cholinergic Agonists

Drug	Route and Adult Dose (maximum dose where indicated)	Adverse Effects
Direct Acting (Muscarinic Agonists)		
bethanechol chloride (Duvoid, Urecholine)	PO: 10–50 mg tid or qid (max: 200 mg/day) Subcutaneous: 2.5–5 mg tid or qid (max: 40 mg/day)	*Increased salivation, abdominal cramping, sweating, flushing of the skin, miosis, blurred vision, nausea, vomiting* Orthostatic hypotension with possible syncope, bradycardia, reflex tachycardia, complete heart block, acute bronchospasm
carbachol (Miostat, Isopto Carbachol)	Topical: 1–2 drops of 0.75–3% solution tid in lower conjunctival sac every 4–8 h	
cevimeline HCl (Evoxac)	PO: 30 mg tid (max: 90 mg/day)	
pilocarpine (Isopto-Carpine, Ocusert, Salagen)	Topical: 1–2 drops in affected eye tid or qid for chronic glaucoma PO: 5–10 mg tid for xerostomia (max: 10 mg/dose, 30 mg/day)	
Indirect Acting (Anticholinesterase Agents)		
ambenonium (Mytelase)	PO: 2.5–5 mg tid or qid; may increase every 1–2 days to 50–75 mg tid or qid if necessary	*Involuntary contraction or twitching of muscles, nausea/vomiting, miosis, increased salivation* Bradycardia, hypotension, dyspnea, seizures, bronchospasm, cholinergic crisis, death due to paralysis of respiratory muscles
donepezil (Aricept)	PO: 5–10 mg (max: 10 mg/day)	
edrophonium (Tensilon)	Edrophonium test for myasthenia gravis IV: Inject 2 mg over 15–30 seconds; if no reaction after 45 seconds, inject additional 8 mg. May repeat test in 30 min IM: Inject 10 mg; if cholinergic reaction occurs, retest after 30 min with 2 mg to rule out false-negative reaction	
galantamine hydrobromide (Razadyne)	PO: 4 mg bid for 4 weeks; may increase by 4 mg bid every 4 weeks to target dose of 12 mg bid as tolerated (max: 24 mg/day)	
neostigmine (Prostigmin)	PO: Start 15 mg every 8 h and increase as necessary IM/IV/subcutaneous: every 2–3 hours (max: 375 mg/day PO or 10 mg/day IM/IV/subcutaneous)	
physostigmine salicylate	IM/IV: 0.5–2 mg (IV not faster than 1 mg/min); repeat as needed	
pyridostigmine (Mestinon)	PO: 60 mg–1.5 g/day; sustained release: 180–540 mg 1–2 times/day at intervals of at least 6 hours IM/IV: Approximately 1/30 of PO dose	
rivastigmine (Exelon)	PO: 1.5 mg bid; may increase by 1.5 mg bid every 2 weeks to target dose 3–6 mg bid (max: 12 mg/day) Transdermal: Start 4.6 mg/24 h, can increase to 9.5 mg/24 h	
tacrine (Cognex)	PO: 10 mg qid; increase in 40 mg/day increments not sooner than every 4 weeks (max: 160 mg/day)	

Note: *Italics* indicate common adverse effects. Underline indicates serious adverse effects.

In the eye, muscarinic agonists cause the iris sphincter to contract, producing pupillary constriction, or miosis. Miosis has no therapeutic application and is considered an adverse effect of muscarinic agonists. A second effect on the eye is contraction of the ciliary muscle, which causes loss of ability to focus for near vision. Although this loss of ability to focus may result in blurred vision, ciliary muscle contraction has an indirect, beneficial effect: It allows fluid to drain from the anterior chamber of the eye, reducing intraocular pressure. When applied locally to the eye, cholinergic agonists, such as pilocarpine, can be of value in treating primary open-angle glaucoma, and prior to surgery in patients with acute angle closure glaucoma as discussed in Chapter 78.

Muscarinic agonists contract bronchial smooth muscle, causing the airways to narrow. In patients with respiratory disease, bronchoconstriction may trigger episodes of breathlessness or an asthma attack. This is why muscarinic agonists are contraindicated in patients with a history of asthma.

When activated, muscarinic receptors in the cardiovascular system reduce the heart rate and lower blood pressure. Baroreceptors in the carotid arteries and aortic arch, however, recognize the falling blood pressure and signal the vasomotor center in the medulla to increase the heart rate. This phenomenon, known as **reflex tachycardia,** may result when any drug that causes blood pressure to fall is administered. When administering cholinergic agonists by the oral (PO) or parenteral routes, the patients' heart rate must be closely monitored to avoid bradycardia, and blood pressure to prevent serious hypotension, particularly in those with preexisting cardiovascular disease. Patients with hyperthyroidism may experience atrial fibrillation. Serious heart disease is a contraindication to therapy with cholinergic agonists.

Occasionally, patients suffer acute poisoning from eating certain species of mushrooms containing high amounts of muscarine, the original cholinergic agonist isolated from the mushroom *Amanita muscaria. A. muscaria* itself has only small amounts of muscarine, but several other species of fungi possess significant amounts of this toxin that can cause severe illness if ingested. Symptoms of acute poisoning appear 30 to 90 minutes after ingestion and resemble an overdose of cholinergic agonists: an exaggerated parasympathetic response. Symptoms may persist for 24 hours. Amanita species are sometimes intentionally ingested to obtain psychotic effects, reportedly to expand or alter spatio-temporal awareness.

Pharm*FACT*

Muscarinic receptors are named after muscarine, which is obtained from the mushroom *Amanita muscaria.* When ingested, the patient experiences alternating CNS depression and excitement, seizures, hallucinations, and confusion. Death from mushroom poisoning is rare. *Source:* Fest & Bianchi, 2001.

Symptoms of parasympathetic stimulation, whether caused by medications or mushroom poisoning, may be reversed by administering an anticholinergic drug (see Chapter 18). Atropine is considered the specific antidote for these conditions. Acute symptoms of parasympathetic stimulation will begin to resolve within minutes after an intravenous (IV) injection of atropine.

PROTOTYPE DRUG Bethanechol chloride (Duvoid, Urecholine)

Classification: **Therapeutic:** Drug to restore peristalsis or treat urinary retention

Pharmacologic: Cholinergic agonist, muscarinic agonist (direct acting)

Therapeutic Effects and Uses: Approved in 1948, bethanechol is an older drug that is available in tablet form or as a subcutaneous injection. The oral dose is significantly higher than the subcutaneous dose because the drug is poorly absorbed across the GI tract. Effects of bethanechol are most noted in the digestive and urinary tracts, where it stimulates smooth muscle contraction. These actions can restore smooth muscle tone and peristalsis following general anesthesia. Off-label uses include the treatment of adynamic ileus and gastric atony.

In the urinary tract, bethanechol relaxes the sphincters and causes the detrusor muscle of the bladder to contract. These combined actions result in voiding; thus it is used to treat nonobstructive urinary retention in patients with atony of the bladder. Subcutaneous injection of bethanechol can rapidly stimulate micturition.

Mechanism of Action: Structurally similar to Ach, bethanechol interacts directly with muscarinic receptors to cause body responses typical of parasympathetic stimulation. This drug is selective for muscarinic receptors. Bethanechol is not destroyed by AchE; therefore, its actions are more prolonged than those of Ach.

Pharmacokinetics:

Route(s)	PO, subcutaneous
Absorption	Poorly absorbed PO, well-absorbed subcutaneous
Distribution	Widely distributed; does not cross the blood–brain barrier
Primary metabolism	Unknown
Primary excretion	Renal
Onset of action	PO: 30 minutes; subcutaneous: 5–15 minutes
Duration of action	PO: 1–6 h; subcutaneous: 2 h

Adverse Effects: The adverse effects of bethanechol are predicted from its parasympathetic actions. Common adverse effects include increased salivation, abdominal cramping, sweating, flushing of the skin, miosis, blurred vision, nausea, and vomiting. Serious effects include orthostatic hypotension with possible syncope, bradycardia, reflex tachycardia, complete heart block, and acute bronchospasm.

Contraindications/Precautions: Bethanechol should be used with extreme caution in patients with disorders that could be aggravated by increased contractions of the GI tract, such as suspected bowel obstruction, recent GI surgery, an active ulcer, or an inflammatory disease. Patients with suspected urinary obstruction or those who have had recent bladder surgery should not receive this drug, because the increased smooth muscle contractions could worsen these conditions. Patients with cystitis should not be given bethanechol because contractions of the bladder may force urine up the ureters to the kidneys if the sphincter fails to open. Because of the possibility of bronchoconstriction, administration of bethanechol to patients with asthma or chronic obstructive pulmonary disease (COPD) is contraindicated. Muscarinic agonists such as bethanechol can slow the heart rate; thus they are contraindicated in patients with recent myocardial infarction (MI), severe bradycardia, hypotension, or hypertension. Patients with hyperthyroidism can experience dysrhythmias with bethanechol use. Other contraindications include peritonitis, epilepsy, and Parkinson's disease.

Drug Interactions: Concurrent therapy with AchE inhibitors should be avoided because this class also stimulates muscarinic receptors, and excessive parasympathetic activity will result. Procainamide, quinidine, atropine, and epinephrine antagonize the effects of bethanechol. Concurrent administration of bethanechol with ganglionic blockers may result in a rapid fall in blood pressure. **Herbal/Food:** Unknown.

Pregnancy: Category C.

Treatment of Overdose: Overdose will result in serious cholinergic symptoms such as nausea, vomiting, abdominal cramping, salivation, and hypotension. Administration of atropine quickly reverses most symptoms.

Nursing Responsibilities:

- Monitor blood pressure and pulse, and observe for adverse effects for at least 1 hour following subcutaneous administration.

- Monitor for early signs of overdose, which include salivation, sweating, flushing, abdominal cramps, and nausea.
- Observe and record the patient's response to bethanechol and notify the prescriber of the drug's failure to relieve urinary retention or increase gastric peristalsis.
- Closely monitor respiratory status when the medication is administered parenterally. Promptly report dyspnea or any other symptom of respiratory distress to the prescriber.
- When ambulating, supervise the patient because this drug may cause blurred vision.

Patient and Family Education:

- Make position changes slowly when moving from a lying to a standing position to prevent dizziness and possible fainting.
- Do not stand still for prolonged periods; sit or lie down at first indication of faintness.
- Do not drive or perform other hazardous activities until the effects of the drug are known because this drug may cause drowsiness or dizziness.
- Do not breast-feed without approval of the health care provider.

Drugs Similar to Bethanechol Chloride (Duvoid, Urecholine)

Other direct-acting cholinergic agonists include carbachol, cevimeline, and pilocarpine.

Carbachol (Isopto Carbachol, Miostat): Carbachol is a direct-acting cholinergic agonist. Carbachol intraocular (Miostat) is a solution for injection into the anterior chamber of the eye to promote miosis during surgery. Carbachol topical (Isopto Carbachol) is an ophthalmic solution used to lower intraocular pressure in certain types of glaucoma. Vision may be clouded due to pupillary constriction. Should absorption occur, adverse effects would be those of parasympathetic stimulation. This drug is pregnancy category C.

Cevimeline (Evoxac): Cevimeline is a newer, direct-acting cholinergic agent whose only indication is the treatment of xerostomia in patients with Sjögren's syndrome. Given orally, cevimeline increases saliva flow, relieving dry mouth. The most common adverse effect is excessive sweating, although this occurs less frequently than with pilocarpine. Other signs of parasympathetic stimulation are possible, such as diarrhea, runny nose, miosis, and bradycardia. This drug is pregnancy category C.

Pilocarpine (Isopto-Carpine, Ocusert, Salagen): Pilocarpine is a direct cholinergic agonist that is administered as an ophthalmic solution in the pharmacotherapy of certain types of glaucoma, and to counteract the effects of mydriatics and cycloplegics following eye examinations. Ocusert is an ocular system that continuously releases pilocarpine, thus providing for less frequent dosing for glaucoma. Pilocarpine is a prototype antiglaucoma agent and is discussed in Chapter 78. Salagen is an oral preparation of pilocarpine given for xerostomia due to its ability to stimulate salivary flow. When given orally, the adverse effects of pilocarpine are those expected of parasympathetic stimulation, which include diarrhea, runny nose, miosis, and bradycardia. Excessive sweating occurs in 30% to 60% of the patients taking oral pilocarpine. This drug is pregnancy category C.

17.3 Acetylcholinesterase inhibitors may be used to treat Alzheimer's disease, glaucoma, or myasthenia gravis.

The indirect-acting cholinergic agonists do not produce their effects by binding to Ach receptors. Instead, these drugs inhibit the action of the enzyme AchE, allowing Ach to avoid rapid destruction and to remain on cholinergic receptors for a longer time, thus prolonging its actions. Unlike the direct-acting agonists, the **acetylcholinesterase (AchE) inhibitors** are nonselective and affect all Ach synapses located at the autonomic ganglia, muscarinic receptors, neuromuscular junctions, and Ach synapses in the CNS.

The muscarinic actions of the AchE inhibitors are identical to those described for the direct-acting agents in Section 17.2. These drugs increase peristalsis in the GI and urinary tracts, and some have the ability to contract the ciliary muscle of the eye and decrease intraocular pressure. Primary indications for the AchE inhibitors are limited due to their adverse effects and include Alzheimer's disease, glaucoma, prophylaxis of nerve gas poisoning, and myasthenia gravis. The agents used to treat myasthenia gravis are described in Section 17.4.

Alzheimer's disease: AchE inhibitors used to treat mild to moderate Alzheimer's disease include galantamine (Reminyl), donepezil (Aricept), rivastigmine (Exelon), and tacrine (Cognex). These agents increase the amount of Ach in cholinergic synapses in the brain which improves memory and cognitive function. The AchE inhibitors do not cure or slow the progress of Alzheimer's disease: Improvement is limited and short-lived. Donepezil is presented as a prototype drug for Alzheimer's disease in Chapter 25.

Glaucoma: Physostigmine (Antilirium) and echothiophate (Phospholine Iodide) are available as ophthalmic solutions. These drugs are called miotics because they cause pupillary constriction by contracting the iris sphincter. They reduce intraocular pressure in the eye by contracting the ciliary muscle; thus they are used to treat glaucoma. The ophthalmic AchE inhibitors have largely been replaced by safer and more effective antiglaucoma agents (see Chapter 77).

Prophylaxis of nerve gas poisoning: A relatively new use of the AchE inhibitors is to protect military and public service personnel in the event of a bioterrorist attack with nerve gases. In the U.S.-Iraq Persian Gulf War in 1990, American soldiers were given 30 mg tid of oral pyridostigmine for several weeks. Theoretically, the pyridostigmine would cover the active site of AchE so that a toxic nerve agent would be unable to bind to the enzyme. Unfortunately, the pyridostigmine given during this war has been implicated as a potential cause of Persian Gulf War syndrome, a disorder characterized by a vague collection of neuromuscular and nervous system symptoms. Interestingly, subsequent research discovered that pyridostigmine, which usually does not enter the CNS, may cross the blood–brain barrier in the presence of stress. In any event, it is unlikely that pyridostigmine alone is responsible for this syndrome, because patients with myasthenia gravis take 10 to 50 times higher doses of this drug and do not display the same syndrome.

Cholinergic Crisis

Research conducted under secrecy during World War II resulted in the discovery of highly toxic substances with actions similar to those of the AchE inhibitors. These compounds have potent neurologic effects and have the potential to be used as chemical warfare agents. This class of agents now includes widely used organophosphate insecticides, such as Malathion, and toxic nerve gases, such as Sarin. The use of nerve gases as a bioterrorist threat is discussed in Chapter 78.

Overdosage with AchE inhibitors or poisoning with organophosphate insecticides or toxic nerve gases causes a **cholinergic crisis,** which is characterized by signs of intense parasympathetic stimulation such as miosis, nausea, vomiting, urinary incontinence, increased exocrine secretions, and abdominal cramping. As the crisis progresses, signs of sympathetic and nicotinic stimulation appear, including tachycardia, hyperglycemia, and muscle twitching, with progressive muscle weakness. In massive overdoses, mechanical ventilation may be required and paralysis of respiratory muscles may cause death. CNS effects are prominent with the organophosphates and include headache, blurred vision, anxiety, delirium, convulsions, and coma. Poisoning may occur by oral or dermal exposure or inhalation. In general, overdose with AchE drugs produces less severe and shorter duration effects than does poisoning with organophosphates.

The treatment of cholinergic crisis includes administration of atropine, the specific antidote that reverses muscarinic effects. When given IV, atropine can act within minutes. Because some insecticides have long-lasting effects, atropine therapy may continue for several weeks. Pralidoxime (Protopam) is an alternative to atropine that has antimuscarinic and antinicotinic action, which can reverse muscle twitching and increase muscle strength. It is a specific antidote for poisoning by organophosphate insecticide compounds and is not effective in treating overdoses due to other AchE inhibitors. Although intramuscular (IM) and subcutaneous forms of pralidoxime are available, the usual route of administration is by IV infusion over 15 to 30 minutes. To be most effective, pralidoxime must be given as soon as possible after the suspected poisoning.

Pharmacotherapy of Myasthenia Gravis

17.4 Acetylcholinesterase inhibitors are used in the pharmacotherapy of myasthenia gravis to increase the strength of muscular contraction.

Myasthenia gravis (MG), which literally means "grave muscular weakness," first appeared in medical reports in 1672 and afflicts about 125 per million people in the United States. It is one of the best understood autoimmune diseases of the nervous system. The disease occurs when antibodies attack nicotinic synapses on skeletal muscles, resulting in symptoms of extreme fatigue, double vision, speech impairment, and difficulty chewing or swallowing. The most visible symptom is an obvious drooping of the eyelids (ptosis) due to muscular weakness. The ocular muscles may become so fatigued that the patient is unable to open the eyelids. Muscle fatigue worsens after exercise, or late in the day. MG is considered a progressive disease, although the severity of symptoms fluctuates over time.

> **PharmFACT**
>
> **Myasthenia gravis affects females more often than males. The disorder has a peak incidence from age 20 to 30 and again after age 50. In rare cases, pregnancy can trigger the onset of MG.** *Source:* Newton & Testa, 2007.

MG is diagnosed by clinical symptoms and the presence of antibodies to AchE. If the diagnosis is unclear, the edrophonium test may be performed. A small amount of edrophonium (Tensilon), an anticholinesterase inhibitor, is administered by rapid IV infusion. An immediate, dramatic improvement in muscle strength, posture, and respiratory function following the injection supports a diagnosis of MG. The most useful measurement is the degree of ptosis of the eyelids. If ptosis diminishes or a completely closed eyelid opens after the edrophonium injection, diagnosis of MG is confirmed. Patients often exhibit adverse effects from the edrophonium injection, including bradycardia, bronchospasm, or lightheadedness; however, they resolve within a few minutes due to the very short half-life of the drug. Atropine should be available as an antidote in the event that more severe symptoms develop.

For patients with suspected MG, it is important to perform an accurate baseline physical assessment of neuromuscular and respiratory function. The patient's swallowing ability should be assessed prior to medication administration due to decreased muscle strength caused by the disease process. Subsequent assessments are used to monitor the progress of pharmacotherapy.

Pharmacotherapy of MG begins with AchE inhibitors, usually pyridostigmine. These drugs are effective for mild symptoms, act rapidly, and produce few serious adverse effects at low to moderate doses. Muscarinic effects such as diarrhea and abdominal cramps are common, and muscle twitching can occur. High doses should not be used because AchE inhibitors can affect Ach nicotinic receptors, worsening the degree of muscle weakness.

As MG progresses, AchE inhibitors alone may not be effective and immunosuppressant drugs such as corticosteroids may be added to the regimen to bring additional relief to these patients. Although their mechanism in treating MG is not completely known, corticosteroids reduce AchE receptor antibody levels and result in symptomatic improvement. Prednisone is the corticosteroid frequently used for MG. Care must be taken when initiating corticosteroid therapy because patient symptoms may dramatically worsen during the first few days of therapy. Doses of prednisone are gradually increased until the desired therapeutic effect is obtained. Unfortunately, improvement may take weeks or even months, and corticosteroids can exhibit considerable toxicity when given on a long-term basis (see Chapter 69). Therapy with corticosteroids is limited to the shortest time necessary, although some patients may require these drugs for the rest of their life. Other immunosuppressants such as azathioprine (Imuran), cyclosporine (Sandimmune), or mycophenolate mofetil (CellCept) may be administered as alternatives to corticosteroids. Occasionally, these alternatives are administered concurrently with prednisone to allow for lower doses of the corticosteroid. Immunosuppressants are presented in Chapter 45.

A **myasthenic crisis** may occur if a patient with MG abruptly discontinues the medication. This leads to extreme muscular weakness and symptoms similar to those of a cholinergic crisis, as described in Section 17.3. Rapid, correct diagnosis is essential, however, because antidotes for the myasthenic crisis and the cholinergic crisis are very different. To distinguish between the two, the edrophonium test is used, administering the smallest amount possible. If symptoms improve, this indicates that the patient is experiencing a myasthenic crisis, and intensive AchE inhibitor therapy is indicated. If symptoms worsen after giving edrophonium, this indicates a cholinergic crisis; all cholinergic drugs are withdrawn and pharmacotherapy with an anticholinergic such as atropine is immediately initiated.

It should be clearly understood that MG is a disease affecting skeletal muscle; it is not a disorder of the autonomic nervous system. It is presented in this chapter dealing with the autonomic nervous system because the primary pharmacotherapy for the disease is AchE inhibitors. Although these drugs provide symptomatic relief, they do not cure or slow the progression of MG. With treatment, however, patients may experience a near-normal life expectancy.

PROTOTYPE DRUG Neostigmine (Prostigmin)

Classification: **Therapeutic:** Agent for MG
Pharmacologic: Indirect-acting cholinergic agonist, AchE inhibitor

Therapeutic Effects and Uses: Approved in 1939, neostigmine is available by both oral and parenteral routes for the symptomatic treatment of MG. Affecting the neuromuscular synapses, neostigmine increases the strength of skeletal muscle contraction and delays fatigue. A major disadvantage of neostigmine is that it has a short half-life that requires the drug to be taken as often as every 2 to 4 hours. If using large doses of neostigmine to treat MG, atropine (an anticholinergic) is sometimes administered concurrently to reverse the muscarinic adverse effects of neostigmine.

In addition to its effects on nicotinic receptors, neostigmine also affects muscarinic receptors. At muscarinic synapses, neostigmine will enhance the parasympathetic response, resulting in increased peristasis, bronchoconstriction, bradycardia, and hypotension. These effects are used to advantage in relieving postoperative abdominal distension and urinary retention and in reversing the effects of nondepolarizing muscle relaxants. The drug is usually administered by the IM or subcutaneous routes for these indications.

Mechanism of Action: Neostigmine inhibits the action of AchE at cholinergic synapses, which allows Ach to accumulate and cause a greater effect. Its use in treating MG is due to its effects on nicotinic Ach synapses in skeletal muscle.

Pharmacokinetics:

Route(s)	PO, IM, IV, and subcutaneous
Absorption	PO: only 1–2% is absorbed. The oral dose is about 30 times higher than the parenteral dose
Distribution	Does not appear to cross the placenta; is not secreted in breast milk; 15–25% bound to plasma protein
Primary metabolism	Hepatic, by cholinesterases
Primary excretion	Kidneys
Onset of action	PO: 2–4 h; IM/IV: 10–30 minutes
Duration of action	Half-life: 50–90 minutes

Adverse Effects: The adverse effects of neostigmine are due to its ability to stimulate the parasympathetic nervous system. Common adverse effects include involuntary contraction or twitching of muscles, nausea, vomiting, miosis, and increased salivation. Potentially serious adverse effects include bradycardia, hypertension, dyspnea, and death due to paralysis of respiratory muscles.

Contraindications/Precautions: Neostigmine should be used with caution in patients with disorders that could be aggravated by increased contractions of the GI tract, such as suspected bowel obstruction or active ulcers. Patients with suspected urinary obstruction should not receive this drug because the increased smooth muscle contractions could worsen this condition. Because of the potential for bronchoconstriction, patients with asthma or COPD should be treated cautiously with cholinergic agonists. Cholinergic agonists such as neostigmine can cause bradycardia; thus they are contraindicated in patients with recent MI or heart failure. Other contraindications include hyperthyroidism, peritonitis, and epilepsy.

Drug Interactions: Because of the potential for additive effects, other cholinergic agonists should not be administered concurrently with neostigmine. Drugs that interfere with neuromuscular transmission such as local anesthetics, some general anesthetics, and antidysrhythmic agents should be used cautiously in patients with MG because severe muscular weakness may result. If administered to patients with MG, the dose of neostigmine should be increased. Cholinergic drugs increase gastric acid secretion and should be used with caution with other ulcer-promoting drugs such as corticosteroids or nonsteroidal anti-inflammatory drugs (NSAIDs). **Herbal/Food:** Unknown.

Pregnancy: Category C.

Treatment of Overdose: Overdose with neostigmine is life threatening because the drug can cause a cholinergic crisis leading to respiratory failure. The administration of atropine reverses most overdose symptoms.

Nursing Responsibilities:

- Monitor pulse, respiration, and blood pressure regularly during the initial therapy period of dosage adjustment in the treatment of myasthenia gravis. If below 60 per minute or other established parameter, notify the prescriber.

- Ensure that atropine is always available to restore heart rate or treat cholinergic crisis.
- Report the onset of myasthenic symptoms (ocular motor disturbances, ptosis, diplopia, oropharyngeal muscle weakness, difficulty chewing, swallowing, or talking) and drug adverse effects in relation to the last dose in order to assist the prescriber in determining the lowest effective dosage schedule.
- To determine whether the patient is in cholinergic or myasthenic crisis, note the time of muscular weakness onset. Weakness that appears approximately 1 hour after drug administration typically suggests cholinergic crisis (overdose) and is treated by prompt withdrawal of neostigmine and immediate administration of atropine. Weakness that occurs 3 hours or more after drug administration is more likely due to myasthenic crisis (underdose or drug resistance) and is treated by more intensive AchE therapy.

Patient and Family Education:

- Take this drug with milk or food to minimize gastric irritation.
- Be aware that regulation of dosage interval is extremely difficult. Dosages must be adjusted for each patient.
- Take larger portions of the total dose at times of greater fatigue, such as late afternoon and at mealtimes.
- Certain factors may require an increase in size or frequency of dose (e.g., physical or emotional stress, infection, menstruation, surgery), whereas remission requires a decrease in dosage.
- Keep a diary of "peaks and valleys" of muscle strength. An accurate record of the patient's response to the drug will assist the health care provider in the regulation of the medication.
- Notify the health care provider of any other prescription or over-the-counter (OTC) medications, and use of caffeine, alcohol, or tobacco because these may affect the drug's actions.
- Immediately report any of the following: difficulty breathing, dizziness, difficulty moving, muscle cramps or spasms, slow or irregular heartbeat, or vomiting. Modify the dosage regimen or administer atropine according to instructions provided by the health care provider.
- Wear a medic-alert bracelet or other device describing your disease and the details of your medications.

Drugs Similar to Neostigmine (Prostigmin)

Other AchE inhibitors for MG include ambenonium, edrophonium, and pyridostigmine.

Ambenonium (Mytelase): Ambenonium is an older oral drug approved in 1956 that is six times more potent than neostigmine. Its only indication is in the pharmacotherapy of MG. It is not a first-line agent for this disorder because it tends to produce more muscarinic adverse effects than other agents. This drug is pregnancy category C.

Edrophonium (Tensilon): The primary use of edrophonium is to diagnose MG, although it may be used to periodically assess the progress of AchE therapy (see discussion of the edrophonium test earlier in this section). It was approved in 1951. This drug is pregnancy category C.

Pyridostigmine (Mestinon): Pyridostigmine exhibits a longer duration of action and fewer adverse effects than neostigmine and is a drug of choice in the oral pharmacotherapy of mild MG. The adverse effects and contraindications are the same as neostigmine's. Because of its short half-life, pyridostigmine regular-release tablets must be taken every 3 to 4 hours. A slow release form, Mestinon Timespan, is available that allows for dosing once or twice daily. The drug is also used to reverse the actions of neuromuscular blockers following surgery. In 2003, the FDA approved pyridostigmine for military personnel with potential exposure to certain nerve gases. Pyridostigmine is only effective if administered several hours prior to nerve gas exposure. If exposure occurs, pyridostigmine is discontinued and the antidotes (atropine and pralidoxime) are administered. The drug is pregnancy category C.

CONNECTION *Checkpoint* 17.2

Ambenonium is six times more potent than neostigmine. Does this mean it is six times more effective? From what you learned in Chapter 4, clearly explain the difference between efficacy and potency. See Answer to Connection Checkpoint 17.2 in Appendix A.

NURSING PROCESS APPLICATION

Patients Receiving Cholinergic Agonists

Assessment Data	Potential Nursing Diagnoses
Prior to administration: • Obtain a complete health history including vital signs, allergies, and drug history for possible drug interactions. • Assess the reason for drug administration. • Assess for contraindications of drug administration. • Assess for urinary retention and urinary patterns initially and throughout therapy (direct acting). • Assess muscle strength and neuromuscular status, ptosis, diplopia, and chewing.	• *Urinary Retention,* related to direct acting agents • *Impaired Urinary Elimination,* related to direct actingagents • *Impaired Physical Mobility,* related to indirect acting agents • *Deficient Knowledge (Therapeutic Regimen),* related to drug administration and adverse effects • *Risk for Injury,* related to adverse effects

(continued)

NURSING PROCESS APPLICATION *(continued)*

Planning: Patient Goals and Expected Outcomes

The patient will (depending on the reason the drug therapy is prescribed):

- Exhibit increased bowel/ bladder function and tone by regaining normal pattern of elimination.
- Exhibit decrease in myasthenia gravis symptoms such as muscle weakness, ptosis, and diplopia.
- Demonstrate understanding of the drug's action by accurately describing drug adverse effects and precautions.

Implementation

Interventions and (Rationales)	Patient and Family Education
All Cholinergic Agonists	
• Monitor for adverse effects. (Abdominal cramping, diarrhea, excessive salivation, difficulty breathing, and muscle cramping are common adverse effects and should be reported to the prescriber.)	• Instruct the patient to report nausea, vomiting, diarrhea, rash, jaundice, or change in the color of stool, or any other adverse reactions to the drug for immediate treatment of the antidote for atropine.
• Monitor liver enzymes with initiation of therapy and weekly for 6 weeks (for possibility of hepatotoxicity).	• Instruct the patient to adhere to laboratory testing regimen for serum blood level tests of liver enzymes as directed.
• Assess and monitor for appropriate self-care administration to prevent complications. (These medications may be prescribed to patients after discharge from the health care facility and need health teaching for effective self-care management.)	Instruct the patient to: • Take the drug as directed on a regular schedule to maintain serum levels and to control symptoms. • Not chew or crush sustained-release tablets. • Take oral parasympathomimetics on an empty stomach to lessen the incidence of nausea and vomiting and to prevent decreased absorption.
• Evaluate concurrent use of other medications and herbs. (Many OTC medications, when mixed with these drugs, can cause serious adverse drug reactions.)	• Instruct the patient to report use of any other medication or herbal supplement.
Direct Acting	
• Monitor intake and output ratio. Palpate the abdomen for bladder distention. (Drugs used for treatment of urinary retention have an onset of action within 60 minutes due to binding of the drug to cholinergic receptors on the smooth muscle of the bladder, which relaxes the bladder to stimulate urination.)	• Advise the patient to be near bathroom facilities after taking the drug.
• Monitor for visual impairment related to drug therapy. (These drugs may cause miosis and blurred vision.)	Instruct the patient: • That blurred vision is a possible adverse effect and to take appropriate precautions. • To not drive or engage in potentially hazardous activities until response to the drug is known.
• Monitor for blood pressure fluctuations during sudden changes in body position. (Cholinergic agonists may cause orthostatic hypotension.)	• Instruct the patient to make position changes slowly and in stages, particularly from lying down to standing. Instruct the patient to avoid prolonged standing in one place.
Indirect Acting	
• Monitor muscle strength and neuromuscular status. (Ptosis, diplopia, and chewing will determine if the therapeutic effect is achieved.)	• Instruct the patient to report difficulty with vision or swallowing.
• Schedule medication administration around mealtimes. (Mastication may be affected with myasthenia gravis. Medication administered near mealtime will reduce the risk of choking.)	• Instruct the patient to take the medication about 30 minutes before a meal to achieve its therapeutic effect and to aid in chewing and swallowing.
• Schedule activities to maximize the effects of drug therapy. (This avoids fatigue associated with neuromuscular disease.)	Instruct the patient to: • Plan activities according to muscle strength and fatigue. • Take frequent rest periods to avoid fatigue.
• Monitor muscle strength at regular intervals. (Changes in muscle strength, depending on time onset, indicate cholinergic crisis or myasthenic crisis.)	Instruct the patient to: • Report any severe muscle weakness that occurs 1 hour after administration of the medication. • Report any muscle weakness that occurs 3 or more hours after medication administration, because this is a major symptom of myasthenic crisis (underdose).

Evaluation of Outcome Criteria

Evaluate the effectiveness of drug therapy by confirming that patient goals and expected outcomes have been met (see "Planning").

CONNECTIONS

To the Community Myasthenia Gravis—Medications and Nutrition

Although all people need good nutrition for optimal health, persons with chronic disease may have special needs. Persons with myasthenia gravis (MG) may face certain nutritional challenges due to difficulty related to fatigue, chewing, swallowing, and medications.

If possible, meals should be planned for times when the person's strength is best. If the person gets fatigued later in the day, smaller, more frequent feedings may help. Modifications such as the consistency of food or body position at meals can help improve tolerance of meals.

When taking an anticholinergic drug like Mestinon, the person should eat a meal about an hour after taking the medicine. Sometimes these drugs can cause diarrhea or cramping. The person should notify the health care provider and not take OTC medications. Foods with high-fat content, spicy foods, or dairy products can aggravate diarrhea. Coffee, tea, or chocolate can stimulate the intestinal system because they contain caffeine.

Diarrhea can result in loss of body fluid and minerals. Therefore, easy to digest foods that are high in minerals should be added to the person's diet. Foods such as applesauce, ripe bananas, white rice, and baked or broiled chicken or fish may help. Light nutritious soups are good choices as well.

When a person takes corticosteroids such as prednisone for an extended time, bone thinning may result. Taking adequate amounts of calcium and vitamin D is important. Foods to include are milk products, cooked dark green vegetables, salmon, dried beans, and calcium-fortified juices and cereals. Because corticosteroids can cause fluid retention, salt substitutes or spices may be healthy alternatives to table salt. Avoid cured or smoked meats, canned vegetables and soups, salty snacks, and pickled foods.

Nicotinic Agonists

17.5 Nicotine acts by activating Ach receptors at the ganglia.

Very few drugs are used for their effects on Ach nicotinic receptors located in the autonomic ganglia. These ganglia synapse with neurons leading to skeletal muscles (nicotinic receptors) as well as those leading to effector organs (muscarinic receptors). Drugs affecting the ganglia have the potential to produce widespread, nonselective effects on the body.

The only drug in widespread use that activates ganglionic receptors is nicotine. The most active component of tobacco smoke, nicotine is well absorbed from the GI and respiratory mucosa as well as from the skin. Because nicotine acts at the ganglia, both parasympathetic and sympathetic responses are stimulated. Although responses are variable, stimulation of organ activity generally occurs first with low doses. Activation of the CNS increases alertness. The heart rate and blood pressure increase, although these parameters may subsequently decrease due to the baroreceptor reflex. The emetic center in the CNS is triggered, causing a feeling of nausea. As the level of nicotine in the blood falls, these same organ systems may become depressed.

Nicotine is an extremely dangerous substance. Acute toxicity, which can occur due to the accidental ingestion of insecticides containing nicotine, may cause death due to paralysis of the respiratory muscles. The chronic effects of nicotine in tobacco smokers such as lung cancer and emphysema are well documented and presented in Chapter 8.

As a drug, nicotine is used as nicotine replacement therapy (NRT) in tobacco cessation programs. Delivery systems include chewing gum (Nicorette), transdermal patches (Habitrol, NicoDerm), and nasal spray (Nicotrol NS). Use of these products reduces the uncomfortable symptoms of nicotine withdrawal, such as difficulty sleeping, lack of concentration, depression, headaches, and food cravings. As tobacco use diminishes over an 8- to 12-week period, these products are gradually withdrawn.

The goal of NRT is to gradually reduce the patient's physical dependence on nicotine. The nurse should remember, however, that psychological dependence also occurs with nicotine and that most successful smoking cessation programs include behavioral modification therapy such as self-help groups. The consistent use of NRT roughly doubles a patient's chances of quitting smoking, but a great deal of persistence and motivation is required (Stead, Perera, Bullen, Mant, & Lancaster, 2008).

CONNECTION *Checkpoint* 17.3

Some cholinergic agonists activate both muscarinic and nicotinic receptors. From what you learned in Chapter 16, give the locations where each of these receptors may be found. See Answer to Connection Checkpoint 17.3 in Appendix A.

UNDERSTANDING THE CHAPTER

Key Concepts Summary

17.1 Drugs can activate cholinergic receptors either directly or indirectly.

17.2 Muscarinic agonists produce their effects by directly stimulating cholinergic receptors.

17.3 Acetylcholinesterase inhibitors may be used to treat Alzheimer's disease, glaucoma, or myasthenia gravis.

17.4 Acetylcholinesterase inhibitors are used in the pharmacotherapy of myasthenia gravis to increase the strength of muscular contraction.

17.5 Nicotine acts by activating Ach receptors at the ganglia.

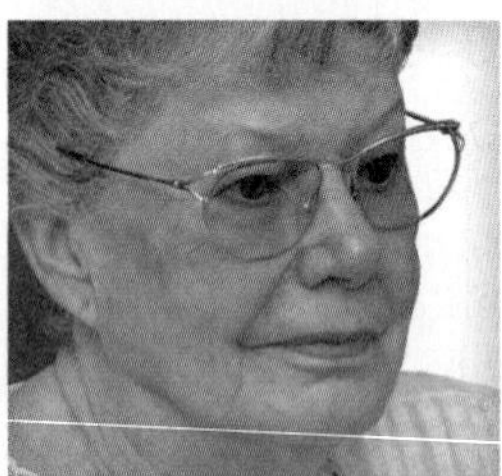

Making the PATIENT Connection

Remember the patient "Hilda Echoles" at the beginning of the chapter? Now read the remainder of the case study. Based on the information presented within this chapter, respond to the critical thinking questions that follow.

Hilda Echoles is an 82-year-old patient who lives alone in a two-story house. Recently, she fell down her front door steps and fractured her right femur. She was taken to the nearest hospital and underwent a total hip replacement 2 weeks ago. As she nears the time for her discharge, the urinary catheter, which was inserted during surgery, was removed. Since that time, Hilda has experienced urinary retention and required intermittent catheterization.

To aid in urinary elimination the health care provider has ordered bethanechol (Urecholine) 20 mg three times per day. Because the medication has demonstrated some effectiveness in achieving bladder emptying, Hilda will be discharged on this medication until she sees the health care provider 2 weeks after discharge.

Critical Thinking Questions

1. As Hilda's nurse, you will be reviewing her discharge medications before she leaves the hospital. What pertinent information should she receive about bethanechol?
2. The patient states, "Sometimes, my memory is not so good and I often forget to take my medication." What should she do if she forgets a dose? List suggestions that you could provide this patient to help remember her medication times.
3. What parameters would you use to determine the effectiveness of this drug therapy?

Case Study

The patient has smoked cigarettes for the past 25 years. She tells the nurse that she has been using the nicotine replacement therapy (Nicorette), as prescribed, for the past week. However, she continues to think about cigarettes, especially when she is with a group of her coworkers who smoke.

1. What should the nurse tell this patient about her obsession with cigarettes?
2. Identify two websites with helpful tips that might aid this patient with smoking cessation.

NCLEX-RN® Review

1 The nurse is discussing the adverse effects associated with a muscarinic agonist. The nurse knows that reflex tachycardia occurs with this drug because:

1. Baroreceptors acknowledge transient hypotension and signal to the medulla to increase the heart rate.
2. This agent simulates the sinoatrial node in the right atrium.
3. Aortic receptors identify episodes of systolic hypertension and simulate heart rhythms.
4. This agent stimulates bronchial smooth muscle contraction and a narrowing of the airway.

2 The nurse is preparing a plan of care for a client with myasthenia gravis. Which of the following outcome statements would be appropriate for a client receiving cholinergic agonists such as pyridostigmine (Mestinon) for this condition? The client will exhibit:

1. An increase in pulse rate, blood pressure, and respiratory rate.
2. Enhanced urinary elimination.
3. A decrease in muscle weakness, ptosis, and diplopia.
4. Prolonged muscle contractions and proprioception.

3 The nurse is discussing the therapeutic effects of bethanechol (Urecholine) with a client who is receiving this drug for urinary retention. The nurse would explain that bethanechol:

1. Diminishes the size of structural defects that inhibit urinary elimination.
2. Augments glomerular filtration in the kidneys, thereby increasing urine production.
3. Improves blood flow to the kidney and reduces reabsorption of electrolytes.
4. Increases ureteral peristalsis and promotes urinary bladder elimination.

4 The nurse is monitoring the client for the common adverse effects associated with bethanechol (Urecholine), including which of the following? Select all that apply.

1. Abdominal discomfort
2. Sweating
3. Flushed skin
4. Constipation
5. Blurred vision

5 A health care provider has ordered neostigmine for each of these clients. A nurse should question the order for which client? A client:

1. With postoperative abdominal distension.
2. Experiencing urinary retention.
3. Suffering from chronic obstructive pulmonary disease.
4. Who has received nondepolarizing muscle relaxants.

6 The provider orders neostigmine for a client who has not urinated in the last 16 hours. The nurse collaborates with the prescriber about which of the following data related to this drug therapy?

1. Heart rate less than 60 beats per minute
2. Change in pupillary size
3. Increased salivation and thirst
4. Respiratory rate of 16 per minute

See Answers to Critical Thinking Questions, Case Study, and NCLEX-RN® Review in Appendix A.

References

Brown, J. H., & Taylor, P. (2006). Muscarinic receptor agonists and antagonists. In L. L. Brunton, J. S. Lazo, & K. L. Parker (Eds.), *The pharmacological basis of therapeutics* (11th ed., pp. 183–200). New York: McGraw-Hill.

Fest, F., & Bianchi, A. (2001). Amanita muscaria: *Mycopharmacological outline and personal experiences.* Retrieved May 28, 2008, from http://leda.lycaeum.org/ ?ID=16317

Giacobini, E. (2004). Cholinesterase inhibitors: New roles and therapeutic alternatives. *Pharmacology Research, 50*(4), 433–440.

Meenakshisundaram, S. (2006). Myasthenia gravis in older patients. *Age & Ageing, 35*(5), 542.

Newton, E., & Testa, N. (2007). Myasthenia gravis. *emedicine.* Retrieved May 28, 2008, from http://www.emedicine.com/emerg/TOPIC325.HTM

Racké, K., Juergens, U. R., & Matthiesen, S. (2006). Control by cholinergic mechanisms. *European Journal of Pharmacology, 533*(8), 57–68.

Schwendimann, R., Burton, E., & Minagar, A. (2005). Management of myasthenia gravis. *American Journal of Therapeutics, 12*(3), 262–268.

Sieb, J. P. (2005). Myasthenia gravis: Emerging new therapy options. *Current Opinion in Pharmacology, 5*(3), 303–307.

Silman, I., & Sussman, J. L. (2005). Acetylcholinesterase: "Classical" and "non-classical" functions and pharmacology. *Current Opinion in Pharmacology, 5*(3), 293–302.

Stead, L. F., Perera, R., Bullen, C., Mant, D., & Lancaster, T. (2008). Nicotine replacement therapy for smoking cessation. *Cochrane Database of Systematic Reviews,* Issue 1. Art. No.: CD000146. DOI: 10.1002/14651858.CD000146.pub3.

Taylor, P. (2006). Anticholinesterase agents. In L. L. Brunton, J. S. Lazo, & K. L. Parker (Eds.), *The pharmacological basis of therapeutics* (11th ed., pp. 217–236). New York: McGraw-Hill.

Thanvi, B. R., & Lo, T. C. (2004). Update on myasthenia gravis. *Postgraduate Medical Journal, 80*(950), 690–700.

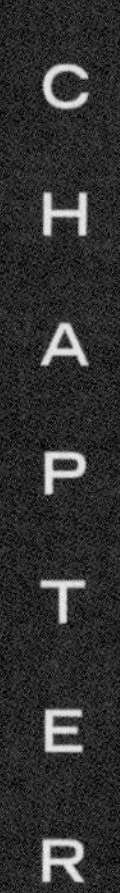

I felt fine 2 days ago while working in the garden. How did I end up in this emergency room?

Patient "Pete Elbertson"

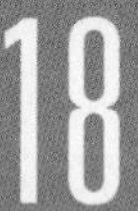

Cholinergic Antagonists

Learning Outcomes

After reading this chapter, the student should be able to:

1. Identify the physiological responses that occur when a drug blocks cholinergic receptors.
2. Differentiate among the following terms: *cholinergic antagonists, muscarinic antagonists, nicotinic antagonists, ganglionic blockers,* and *neuromuscular blockers*.
3. Explain how the therapeutic actions and adverse effects of the cholinergic antagonists can be explained by their blockade of muscarinic or nicotinic receptors.
4. Compare and contrast the actions of the depolarizing and nondepolarizing neuromuscular blockers.
5. Compare and contrast the indications for drugs that block nicotinic receptors at the ganglia versus those that block nicotinic receptors at the neuromuscular junction.
6. For each of the classes shown in the chapter outline, identify the prototype and representative drugs and explain the mechanism(s) of drug action, primary indications, contraindications, significant drug interactions, pregnancy category, and important adverse effects.
7. Use the nursing process to care for patients receiving drug therapy with cholinergic antagonists.

Chapter Outline

Classification of Cholinergic Antagonists

Muscarinic Antagonists

PROTOTYPE **Atropine** *p. 216*

Nicotinic Antagonists

Ganglionic Blockers

PROTOTYPE **Mecamylamine (Inversine)** *p. 218*

Neuromuscular Blockers (depolarizing type)

PROTOTYPE **Succinylcholine (Anectine)** *p. 222*

Neuromuscular Blockers (nondepolarizing type)

PROTOTYPE **Tubocurarine** *p. 223*

Key Terms

belladonna, 214
cholinergic crisis, 216
curare, 223
ganglionic blockers, 214
malignant hyperthermia, 222
motor end plate, 220
muscarinic antagonists, 213
neuromuscular blockers, 214
nicotinic antagonists, 213
nondepolorizing neuromuscular blocker, 223
pseudocholinesterase, 222

Cholinergic antagonists or anticholinergics are drugs that inhibit the action of acetylcholine (Ach) at cholinergic synapses. Because cholinergic synapses may be muscarinic or nicotinic, the actions and therapeutic uses of these drugs are dependent on their site of action. Though not as widely used as the adrenergic antagonists, several anticholinergics are important to pharmacotherapy.

Classification of Cholinergic Antagonists

18.1 Cholinergic antagonists act by blocking the effects of acetylcholine at muscarinic or nicotinic receptors.

As discussed in Chapter 16, cholinergic receptors in the autonomic nervous system are found in three anatomic locations, illustrated in Figure 18.1. This results in two primary classes of cholinergic antagonists.

- **Muscarinic antagonists** are drugs that block receptors at cholinergic synapses in the parasympathetic nervous system and at a few target organs in the sympathetic nervous system.
- **Nicotinic antagonists** are drugs that block receptors at cholinergic synapses in the ganglia or in the somatic nervous system at the neuromuscular junction.

Agents that block the action of Ach at muscarinic receptors have more therapeutic applications than those that block nicotinic receptors. These drugs are known by a number of names, including anticholinergics, cholinergic blockers, muscarinic antagonists, and parasympatholytics. Although the term *anticholinergic* is commonly used in clinical practice, the most accurate term for this group of drugs is *muscarinic antagonists.* This is because these drugs are selective for Ach muscarinic receptors at therapeutic doses and have little effect on nicotinic receptors. The muscarinic antagonists are shown in Table 18.1.

The muscarinic antagonists compete with Ach for binding at muscarinic receptors. Because less Ach binds to its receptors, the parasympathetic response is diminished at the neuroeffector organs. Suppressing the effects of Ach at muscarinic receptors will allow symptoms of sympathetic nervous system activation to predominate. Most therapeutic uses of the muscarinic antagonists are predictable extensions of

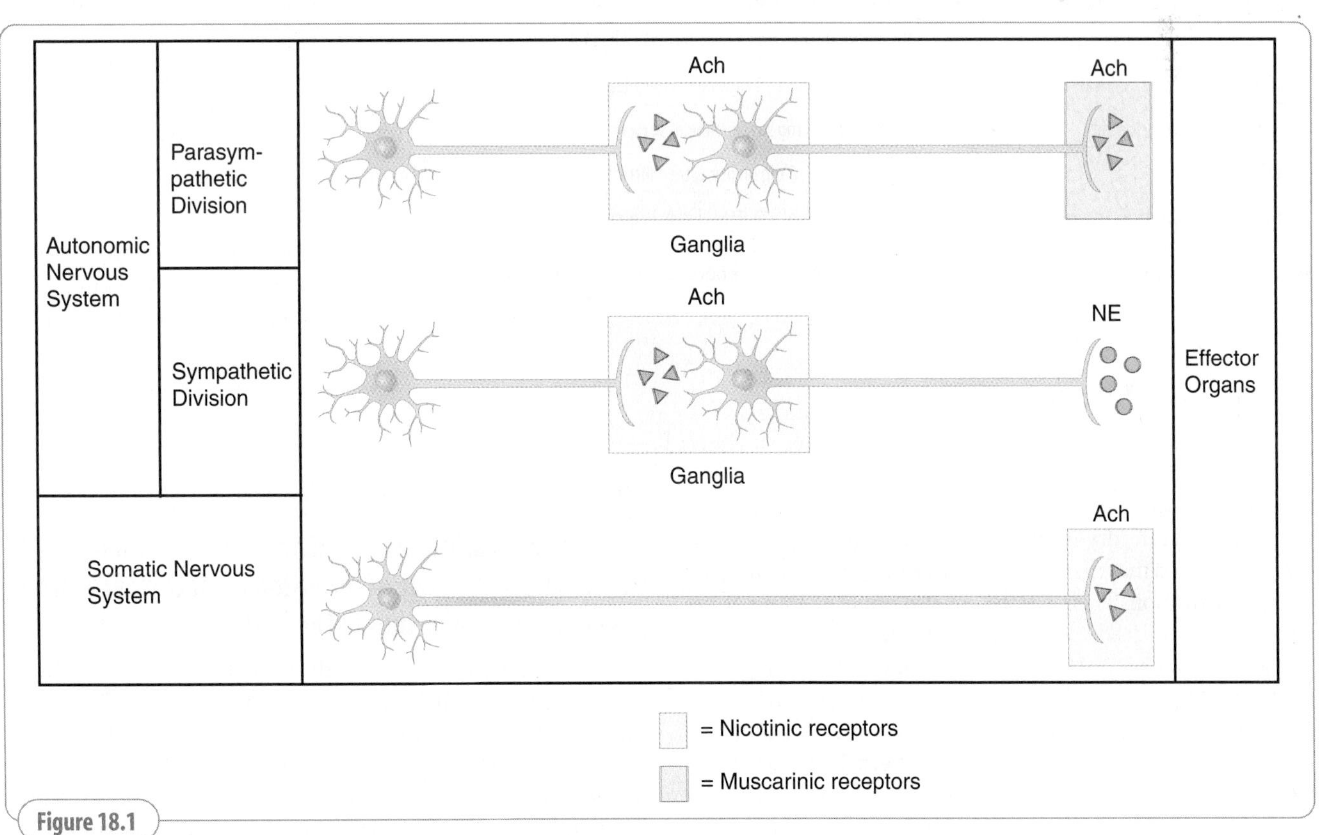

Figure 18.1

Sites of cholinergic antagonist actions. Muscarinic antagonists block cholinergic receptors in the parasympathetic nervous system. Nicotinic antagonists block cholinergic receptors at ganglia, or in the somatic nervous system at the neuromuscular junction.

TABLE 18.1 Muscarinic Antagonists (Anticholinergics)

Drug	Route and Adult Dose (maximum dose where indicated)	Adverse Effects
atropine	Preanesthesia: IV/IM/subcutaneous: 0.4–0.6 mg 30–60 min before surgery Dysrhythmias: IV/IM; 0.5–1 mg every 1–2 h prn (max: 3 mg) Cholinergic crisis: IV; 1–2 mg, repeated every 20–30 min	*Headache, cough, dry mouth, blurred vision, mydriasis, constipation, insomnia, urinary retention, burning or stinging (eyedrop formulations)* <u>Worsening of glaucoma, tachycardia, paradoxical bradycardia, dysrhythmias, paralytic ileus, urinary retention; inhalation forms can cause sinusitis, pharyngitis, and oropharyngeal candidiasis</u>
benztropine (Cogentin)	PO: 0.5–1 mg/day; may gradually increase to 6 mg/day	
cyclopentolate (Cyclogyl)	Topical: 1 drop of 0.5–2% solution in the eye 40–50 min before the procedure, followed by 1 drop in 5 min	
dicyclomine (Bentyl, others)	PO: 20–40 mg qid IM: 20 mg qid	
glycopyrrolate (Robinul)	PO: 1–2 mg tid–bid (max: 8 mg/day) IM/IV: 0.1–0.2 mg tid–qid	
homatropine hydrobromide	Topical: 1–2 drops of 2–5% solution in each eye	
ipratropium (Atrovent)	Metered-dose inhaler (MDI): 2 inhalations qid (max: 12 inhalations/day) Nebulizer: 500 mcg every 6–8 h	
methscopolamine (Pamine)	PO: 2.5 mg tid	
oxybutynin chloride (Ditropan, Oxytrol)	PO: 5 mg bid–tid (max: 20 mg/day) or 5 mg sustained release daily (max: 30 mg/day) Transdermal: Apply 1 patch twice weekly	
propantheline (Pro-Banthine)	PO: 7.5–15 mg tid–qid	
scopolamine (Hyoscine, Transderm-Scop)	Preanesthetic: PO: 0.4–0.8 mg Motion sickness: IM/subcutaneous /IV: 0.3–0.6 mg Transdermal: 1 patch every 72 h starting 12 h before travel	
tiotropium bromide (Spiriva)	Inhalation/Handihaler: 1 capsule inhaled/day	
tolterodine tartrate (Detrol)	PO: 2 mg bid, or 4 mg sustained release daily	
trihexyphenidyl	PO: 1 mg on day 1, 2 mg on day 2, then increase to 6–10 mg/day (max: 15 mg/day)	
tropicamide (Mydriacyl, Tropicacyl)	Topical: 1–2 drops of 0.5–1% solution in each eye	

Note: *Italics* indicate common adverse effects. <u>Underline</u> indicates serious adverse effects.

their parasympathetic-blocking actions: dilation of the pupil, increase in heart rate, drying of secretions, and bronchodilation. It should be noted that these are symptoms of fight-or-flight sympathetic activation. Their actions are also opposite those of the cholinergic agonists discussed in Chapter 17.

Nicotinic antagonists can act at two locations. **Ganglionic blockers** inhibit transmission at the ganglia in the sympathetic and parasympathetic nervous systems, thus affecting both autonomic divisions. **Neuromuscular blockers** do not act on the autonomic nervous system at all but instead inhibit transmission at the neuromuscular junctions on skeletal muscles in the somatic nervous system. The therapeutic uses of nicotinic antagonists are more limited than those of muscarinic antagonists due to their widespread and diverse actions on body function.

Muscarinic Antagonists

18.2 Muscarinic antagonists have been used for a diverse number of conditions, but they are rarely the drugs of choice due to their adverse effects.

Anticholinergics are very old drugs that have been used for a large number of disorders over many centuries. The deadly nightshade plant, *Atropa belladonna,* grows throughout the world and has been a natural source of alkaloids with anticholinergic activity. References to the use of **belladonna** date back to the ancient Hindus, the Roman Empire, and the Middle Ages. The name *belladonna* is Latin for "pretty woman." Roman women applied extracts of belladonna to the face and to the eyes to create the preferred female attributes of that era—pink cheeks and dilated doe-like eyes. Because of its extreme toxicity, extracts of belladonna were sometimes used for intentional poisoning, including suicide.

Although once widely prescribed, the development of safer and more effective medications has greatly decreased the current usage of muscarinic antagonists. Most muscarinic antagonists are now used as second-line agents when the drug of choice is not well tolerated. Potential therapeutic applications of these agents include the following:

- **Gastrointestinal (GI) disorders.** Muscarinic antagonists suppress the secretion of gastric acid and were once widely used to treat peptic ulcer disease (see Chapter 60). These agents also slow intestinal motility and have been used to reduce cramping and diarrhea associated with irritable bowel syndrome (IBS) (see Chapter 61).
- **Ophthalmic procedures.** Topical application of muscarinic antagonists to the eye causes mydriasis and cycloplegia, which may be beneficial during ophthalmic examinations (see Chapter 77).
- **Cardiac rhythm abnormalities.** Muscarinic antagonists accelerate the heart rate, which is beneficial for patients experiencing bradycardia.
- **Adjuncts to anesthesia.** Combined with drugs from other classes, muscarinic antagonists can decrease excessive salivary and respiratory secretions and reverse the bradycardia caused by general anesthetics (see Chapter 30).
- **Asthma:** The muscarinic antagonists ipratropium (Atrovent) and tiotropium (Spiriva) are useful in treating asthma due to their ability to dilate the bronchi (see Chapter 73).
- **Antidotes for poisoning or overdose.** Anticholinergics are administered as antidotes for overdoses with muscarinic agonists or for poisoning with muscarinic mushrooms or organophosphate insecticides (see Chapter 17).
- **Urge incontinence.** A few muscarinic antagonists such as oxybutynin (Ditropan, Oxytrol) are used to prevent involuntary voiding due to their effects of the smooth muscle of the bladder and detrusor muscle (see Chapter 72).
- **Parkinson's disease.** Some muscarinic antagonists such as benztropine (Cogentin) are used for their effects on the central nervous system (CNS) and are prescribed to treat mild symptoms of Parkinson's disease (see Chapter 25).

CONNECTION *Checkpoint* 18.1

From what you learned in Chapter 17, describe the symptoms of a cholinergic crisis and explain why muscarinic antagonists are drugs of choice in treating this condition. See Answer to Connection Checkpoint 18.1 in Appendix A.

Muscarinic antagonists exhibit a relatively high incidence of adverse effects, most of which are predictable because they are associated with inhibition of the parasympathetic nervous system. Adverse effects that limit their usefulness include tachycardia and CNS stimulation. Men with prostate disorders should avoid muscarinic antagonists due to the increased risk of urinary retention. Adverse effects such as xerostomia and dry eyes occur in many patients due to the blockade of muscarinic receptors on the salivary glands and lacrimal glands, respectively. Blockade of muscarinic receptors can inhibit sweating, which may lead to hyperthermia. Photophobia can occur due to the pupil being unable to constrict in response to bright light. In addition, muscarinic antagonists can increase intraocular pressure by causing paralysis of the iris muscle and thus are usually avoided in patients with glaucoma.

PharmFACT

- **Atropine derives its name from Greek mythology: Atropos was the fiercest of the three fates who chose how a person was to die.**
- **Atropine extracts from henbane were used by Cleopatra to dilate her pupils, so she would appear more alluring.**
- **In Scotland, an entire army of invading Danes led by King Sven of Norway were poisoned and defeated by belladonna in 1035. The Danes were poisoned by eating a meal or drinking liquor that had been mixed with belladonna.** *Source:* University of Iowa Hospitals and Clinics, 2006.

CONNECTIONS

To the Community Avoiding Accidental Insecticide Poisoning

Although pesticides can be beneficial to society, they can be dangerous if used carelessly, or if they are not stored properly. Providing the patient with information to avoid accidental poisoning is a teaching opportunity that nurses should pursue once it is known that the patient is at risk of pesticide contamination. Following are some patient teaching tips that should be covered.

To avoid accidental poisoning:

- Leave the area where the chemical was released, and move to fresh air.
- Remove clothing that may contain the chemical. If possible, any clothing that has to be pulled over the head should be cut off the body instead, so the chemical does not get near the eyes, mouth, or nose. If helping other people to remove their clothing, try to avoid touching any contaminated areas.
- Wash any chemical from the skin with lots of soap and water.
- Rinse the eyes with plain water for 10 to 15 minutes, if the eyes are burning or vision is blurred.
- Remove contact lenses and put them with the contaminated clothing. Do not put the contacts back into the eyes. If eyeglasses are worn, wash them with soap and water. Eyeglasses can be put back on after they are washed.
- Wash jewelry with soap and water. Jewelry can be put back on after they are washed.
- Place the clothing and any other contaminated items inside a plastic bag. Avoid touching contaminated areas of the clothing. Anything that touches the contaminated clothing should also be placed in the bag.
- Seal the bag, and then seal that bag inside another plastic bag.

Accidental poisoning with belladonna alkaloids has occurred in children who eat the colorful, purple berries of the deadly nightshade plant, mistaking them for cherries. Symptoms of acute overdose from muscarinic antagonists, called a **cholinergic crisis,** include fever, visual changes, difficulty swallowing, psychomotor agitation, or hallucinations. (The nurse can easily recall the signs of cholinergic crisis by memorizing the following simile: "Hot as Hades, blind as a bat, dry as a bone, mad as a hatter.") Drugs from several other classes have cholinergic-blocking effects and can also trigger a cholinergic crisis. These include antihistamines, phenothiazine, and tricyclic antidepressants. Because anticholinergic effects are additive, concurrent use of multiple drugs that block cholinergic receptors should be avoided.

PROTOTYPE DRUG Atropine

Classification: **Therapeutic:** Agent for bradycardia, antidote for muscarinic agonist overdose

Pharmacologic: Anticholinergic, muscarinic antagonist

Therapeutic Effects and Uses: Atropine has been used for centuries for a wide variety of disorders; however, it remains a drug of choice for very few conditions because adverse effects are so common. The actions of atropine are predictable based on its ability to block muscarinic receptors.

One of the most important actions of atropine is to increase the heart rate, which can be used to advantage when the drug is administered to patients with bradycardia. However, this increase in heart rate is considered an adverse effect when atropine is administered for other indications. The drug should be used with caution in patients with dysrhythmias because it can cause tachycardia.

Like other muscarinic antagonists, atropine can relax smooth muscle in the GI, genitourinary (GU), and respiratory tracts. This action has led to its use in treating hypermotility or spastic disorders of the GI tract including dysentery, abdominal cramping, and IBS. Slowing peristalsis too much, however, can lead to constipation. In the urinary tract, decreased smooth muscle tone can lead to urinary retention.

Because atropine decreases the quantity of exocrine secretions, the drug has been used to suppress secretions of the salivary glands and respiratory tract during surgical procedures. Excessive drying and thickening of bronchial secretions, however, can worsen asthma. Once widely used to produce bronchodilation in patients with asthma, atropine is now rarely prescribed for this disorder due to the development of safer agents.

Topical administration of atropine to the eye will cause mydriasis and paralyze the ciliary muscle, causing cycloplegia. This may be used to advantage in ophthalmic examinations. When used for other indications, however, these actions on the eye are considered adverse effects and can result in blurred vision and photophobia.

Atropine is an antidote used to reverse symptoms of toxicity due to overdose of cholinergic agonists, including organophosphate insecticides and ingestion of mushrooms containing muscarine. AtroPen is an intramuscular (IM) autoinjection delivery system for atropine for poisonings due to toxic nerve agents or insecticides. Improvement in symptoms is usually noted within minutes.

Mechanism of Action: By occupying muscarinic receptors, atropine blocks the parasympathetic activation by Ach and induces symptoms of the fight-or-flight response. At therapeutic doses, atropine is specific for muscarinic receptors. At high doses, the drug may block nicotinic receptors in the ganglia and on skeletal muscle.

Pharmacokinetics:

Route(s)	PO, IV, IM, subcutaneous, inhalation, or ophthalmic
Absorption	Well absorbed by all routes
Distribution	Completely distributed; crosses the blood–brain barrier and placenta; small amounts are secreted in breast milk
Primary metabolism	Hepatic
Primary excretion	Renal
Onset of action	Subcutaneous/IM: 15 minutes; PO: 30 minutes; IV: 2–4 minutes
Duration of action	Half-life: 2–3 h

Adverse Effects: Common adverse effects include drying of the oral and nasal mucosa, constipation, urinary retention, increased heart rate, blurred vision, and photophobia. Serious adverse effects include ventricular fibrillation, delirium, and coma.

Contraindications/Precautions: Atropine is contraindicated in patients with acute angle-closure glaucoma because the drug may cause paralysis of the iris muscle, which can increase intraocular pressure. Safety has not been established for pregnancy and lactating mothers. Anticholinergics may cause fetal tachycardia.

Atropine should be used with caution in patients with preexisting cardiopulmonary conditions such as chronic obstructive pulmonary disease (COPD), myocardial infarction (MI), heart failure, and hypertension (HTN). Blockade of cardiac muscarinic receptors can accelerate heart rate and exacerbate these conditions. Patients with hyperthyroidism should not be given atropine because the heart rate in these patients is generally high and administration of anticholinergics can cause dysrhythmias. Serious GI conditions such as ulcerative colitis and ileus are contraindicated because blockade of muscarinic receptors can decrease the tone and motility of intestinal smooth muscle, which can exacerbate intestinal conditions. Patients with gastrointestinal reflux disease (GERD) and hiatal hernia experience decreased muscle tone in the lower esophageal sphincter and delayed stomach emptying. Atropine exacerbates these symptoms, increasing the risk of esophageal injury and aspiration. Patients with Down syndrome are more sensitive to the effects of atropine due to structural differences in the CNS caused by the trisomy chromosomal abnormality. Patients with Down syndrome also tend to have disorders such as GERD and heart disease, which may be adversely affected by anticholinergics.

Drug Interactions: Care must be taken when administering atropine concurrently with other drugs with anticholinergic actions, such as antihistamines, tricyclic antidepressants, quinidine, and phenothiazines, because their anticholinergic effects will be additive. Because atropine slows GI motility, the absorption of orally administered drugs may be altered. **Herbal/Food**: Some herbal supplements have atropine-like effects that potentiate the medication and can be harmful to the patient. For example, aloe, senna, buckthorn, and cascara sagrada may increase the effect of atropine, particularly if the herbs are used chronically.

Pregnancy: Category C.

Treatment of Overdose: Overdose with atropine is serious, with signs of parasympathetic blockade that include respiratory depression and circulatory collapse. Central signs such as hallucinations, seizures, and mania may be evident. Treatment is mostly supportive and may include drugs to control seizures and to increase respirations and heart rate.

Nursing Responsibilities:

- Monitor vital signs. Assess heart rate for changes in rate, rhythm, and quality as an indicator of the patient's response to atropine. Be alert to changes in respiration and to changes in blood pressure and temperature. Initial paradoxical bradycardia following intravenous (IV) administration of atropine usually lasts only 1 to 2 minutes. This usually occurs when the IV drug is administered slowly (more than 1 min) or when small doses (less than 0.5 mg) are used. Use caution because orthostatic hypotension can occur when the patient ambulates too soon after parenteral administration.
- Observe for systemic effects with frequent use or overuse of eye medications. Some deaths of children have resulted from systemic absorption following ocular atropine administration. Children and older adults may be more sensitive.
- Monitor intake and output, especially in older adults and patients who have had surgery because atropine may contribute to urinary retention. Ask the patient to void before administering atropine. Observe for abdominal distention. Palpate the lower abdomen for bladder distention and auscultate for bowel sounds.
- Assess CNS status. Older and debilitated patients can manifest drowsiness or CNS stimulation (excitement, agitation, confusion) with usual doses of atropine or other belladonna alkaloids. Adjust the dosage and use side rails plus supervision when the patient ambulates.
- Monitor for signs and symptoms of atropine fever (hyperpyrexia due to suppression of perspiration and heat loss) in small children and in older adults, which increases the risk of heatstroke.
- Determine the intraocular tension and depth of the anterior chamber before and during therapy with ophthalmic preparations to avoid worsening of glaucoma.
- Observe for mild CNS stimulation in patients receiving atropine via inhalation in doses in excess of 5 mg, and mental depression and other mental disturbances with larger doses.

Patient and Family Education:

- Prevent or relieve dry mouth by drinking plenty of water; use small, frequent mouth rinses; practice meticulous mouth and dental hygiene; chew sugarless gum or suck on hard candy or sourballs.
- Use lubricating eyedrops if eyes become dry or irritated.
- Increase dietary fiber and fluids to prevent or correct constipation.
- Avoid driving and other activities requiring visual acuity and mental alertness because this drug can cause drowsiness, sensitivity to light, blurring of near vision, and can temporarily impair the ability to judge distance.
- Discontinue use of ophthalmic preparations if eye pain, conjunctivitis, palpitation, rapid pulse, or dizziness occurs, and notify the health care provider.
- Do not breast-feed while taking this drug without approval of the health care provider.
- Immediately notify the health care provider of any known or suspected pregnancy.

Drugs Similar to Atropine

Other muscarinic antagonists include benztropine, cyclopentolate, dicyclomine, glycopyrrolate, hyoscyamine, ipratropium, mepenzolate, methscopolamine, oxybutynin, propantheline, scopolamine, tolterodine, trihexyphenidyl, and tropicamide.

Antisecretory agents: Glycopyrrolate (Robinul), mepenzolate (Cantil), methscopolamine (Pamine), and propantheline (Pro-Banthine) are called antisecretory agents because they reduce gastric acid secretions in patients with peptic ulcer disease. Drugs with greater effectiveness and fewer adverse effects have replaced the anticholinergics for the first-line therapy of peptic ulcer disease. Rarely, some of these agents may be used off-label to treat IBS. An IV form of glycopyrrolate is available to reverse neuromuscular blockade following surgery.

Antispasmodic agents: Although all anticholinergics slow motility in the GI tract, only two drugs in this class, hyoscyamine and dicyclomine, are FDA approved for slowing GI motility. Hyoscyamine (Cystospaz, others) is a belladonna alkaloid with potent antispasmodic activity that is available by the oral (PO), sublingual, or IM routes. It is used for hypermotility disorders including IBS, spastic colitis, infant colic, renal and biliary colic, and spastic bladder. It has been used as a preanesthetic medication to dry secretions. Although not a first-line agent, it has been used to reduce the muscle rigidity and tremors characteristic of Parkinson's disease. Dicyclomine (Bentyl, others) is given for its ability to relax bowel spasms in patients with IBS. Hyoscyamine and dicyclomine should never be administered to patients with suspected obstructive disease of the GI or GU tracts because the decreased motility and tone caused by the drugs can worsen these conditions.

Asthma agents: Ipratropium (Atrovent) and tiotropium (Spiriva) are relatively new anticholinergics used for patients with COPD. The primary action of these drugs is relaxation of bronchial smooth muscle, which dilates the airways. Delivered via aerosol spray, these drugs produce more localized action with fewer systemic adverse effects than atropine.

Centrally acting agents: Benztropine (Cogentin) and trihexyphenidyl (Artane, others) are prescribed to reduce the muscular tremor and rigidity associated with Parkinson's disease. They may be used alone for mild forms of the disease or in combination with other agents for advanced Parkinson's symptoms. Benztropine tends to produce less CNS stimulation than does trihexyphenidyl. A parenteral form of benztropine is available for treating symptoms of acute parkinsonism associated with the use of certain antipsychotic medications. Their use is limited by adverse effects such as sedation and confusion.

Ophthalmic agents: Anticholinergics may be applied topically to the eye to block the responses of the iris sphincter muscle and the ciliary body muscle to cholinergic stimulation, thus producing cycloplegia and mydriasis during ophthalmic procedures. Agents used for this purpose include tropicamide (Mydriacyl), cyclopentolate (Cyclogyl), and scopolamine.

Scopolamine (Hyoscine, Transderm-Scop): Scopolamine is a belladonna alkaloid available for a number of indications. It is very similar to atropine, although scopolamine crosses the blood–brain barrier and is more likely to cause sedation at therapeutic doses. Scopolamine hydrobromide (Isopto hyoscine) is an ophthalmic solution applied topically to produce mydriasis and cycloplegia. Scopolamine is the most effective drug available for preventing motion sickness. For this indication, a transdermal patch containing scopolamine is applied to the skin, usually behind the ear, for slow release of the drug. The most common adverse effect from the transdermal product is dry mouth, although sedation may be a problem in some patients. This drug is pregnancy category C.

Urge incontinence agents: Oxybutynin (Ditropan) and tolterodine (Detrol) are anticholinergics used for their ability to relax smooth muscle in the urinary bladder in patients with urge incontinence. This action limits smooth muscle spasms in the bladder, thus diminishing incidences of involuntary voiding. Oxybutynin is a drug of choice for this condition. Formulations include immediate release and extended release (XL) tablets and a transdermal patch (Oxytrol). The slower release formulations tend to cause fewer autonomic-related adverse effects. Tolterodine is an alternative to oxybutynin and is also available in an extended release (LA) formulation.

CONNECTION *Checkpoint* 18.2

From what you learned in Chapter 16, which of the following classes would give physiological responses similar to the muscarinic antagonists: adrenergic agonists, adrenergic antagonists, or cholinergic agonists? See Answer to Connection Checkpoint 18.2 in Appendix A.

Nicotinic Antagonists: Ganglionic Blockers

18.3 Ganglionic blockers act at the autonomic ganglia to lower blood pressure in emergency situations.

Ganglionic blockers are drugs that interrupt the transmission of nerve impulses at the nicotinic receptors at the autonomic ganglia. As discussed in Chapter 16, both the sympathetic and parasympathetic nervous systems have ganglia. This means that, unlike the muscarinic antagonists that selectively block parasympathetic actions, nicotinic antagonists nonselectively inhibit the entire autonomic nervous system. If parasympathetic and sympathetic actions are both inhibited, what types of effects will be observed?

In most cases, inhibiting the ganglia in both systems will affect the parasympathetic system more than the sympathetic. This is because the predominant, baseline autonomic tone to most organs is from the parasympathetic nervous system. When ganglionic blockers block parasympathetic tone, symptoms characteristic of anticholinergic drugs, such as urinary retention, constipation, blurred vision, increased heart rate, and dry mouth, occur.

Although they affect all autonomic organs, the ganglionic blockers' only action that has therapeutic usefulness is vasodilation. By reducing sympathetic vasomotor tone at the arterioles, ganglionic blockers are capable of causing profound hypotension. Emergency kits must be readily available so that a vasoconstrictor such as epinephrine may be administered if blood pressure falls to a dangerous level.

Because of their potential toxicity only one ganglionic blocker, mecamylamine (Inversine), is approved for use. Trimethaphan (Arfonad), an IV agent, is no longer available in the United States. Dosage information for mecamylamine is given in Table 18.2.

PROTOTYPE DRUG Mecamylamine (Inversine)

Classification: **Therapeutic:** Antihypertensive
Pharmacologic: Ganglionic blocker, nicotine receptor antagonist

Therapeutic Effects and Uses: Mecamylamine was originally used to reduce blood pressure in patients with severe or malignant HTN. The drug is rarely prescribed for this purpose today due to the development of safer antihypertensives. New indications for mecamylamine began to emerge in the late 1990s. Mecamylamine was approved by the U.S. Food and Drug Administration (FDA) as an orphan drug for the treatment of nicotine-responsive psychiatric disorders in 1998. Research has suggested that mecamylamine may be of benefit in treating Tourette's syndrome and for treating cocaine and nicotine addictions. It has been approved by the FDA as an orphan drug to treat Tourette's syndrome that is unresponsive to other medications.

TABLE 18.2 Nicotinic Antagonists

Drug	Route and Adult Dose (maximum dose where indicated)	Adverse Effects
Ganglionic Blocker		
mecamylamine (Inversine)	PO: 2.5 mg, increased by increments of 2.5 mg until desired blood pressure response is attained	*Orthostatic hypotension, blurred vision, anorexia, nausea, vomiting, constipation, diarrhea, dry mouth* Adynamic ileus
Neuromuscular Blockers		
Ultrashort Acting		
succinylcholine (Anectine)	IV: 0.3–1.1 mg/kg over 10–30 sec, may repeat prn IM: 2.5–4 mg/kg (max: 150 mg)	*Transient flushing of the face, neck, or chest; rash, weakness, increased salivation* Respiratory depression, prolonged apnea, cardiac arrest, bradycardia or tachycardia, dysrhythmias, hypotension, increases and decreases in heart rate, malignant hyperthermia, muscle paralysis
Short Acting		
mivacurium (Mivacron)	IV loading dose: 0.15 mg/kg given over 5–15 sec IV maintenance dose: 0.1 mg/kg generally every 15 min IV continuous infusion: initial infusion of 9–10 mcg/kg/min, then 6–7 mcg/kg/min	
Intermediate Acting		
atracurium (Tracrium)	IV: 0.4–0.5 mg/kg initial dose, then 0.08–0.1 mg/kg 20–45 min after the first dose if necessary; reduce doses if used with general anesthetics	
cisatracurium (Nimbex)	IV: 0.15 or 0.20 mg/kg for intubation; 0.03 mg/kg every 20 min prn or 1–2 mcg/kg/min for maintenance	
pancuronium (Pavulon)	IV: 0.04–0.1 mg/kg initial dose, may give additional doses of 0.01 mg/kg at 30–60 min intervals	
rocuronium (Zemuron)	IV: 0.6 mg/kg initially followed by continuous infusion of 0.01–0.012 mg/kg/min	
vecuronium (Norcuron)	IV: 0.04–0.1 mg/kg initially, then after 25–40 min, 0.01–0.15 mg/kg every 12–15 min or 0.001 mg/kg/min by continuous infusion	
Long Acting		
tubocurarine chloride	IV: 6–9 mg followed by 3–4.5 mg in 3–5 min if necessary	

Note: *Italics* indicate common adverse effects. Underline indicates serious adverse effects.

Mechanism of Action: Mecamylamine is a potent, long-acting nicotinic receptor antagonist that blocks neurotransmission at both sympathetic and parasympathetic ganglia by competing with Ach for cholinergic receptor sites on postsynaptic membranes. In addition, the drug readily crosses the blood–brain barrier and inhibits the release of dopamine and norepinephrine, which is thought to be responsible for its effects on nicotine-responsive psychiatric disorders. At low doses, mecamylamine produces its beneficial effects in the CNS without causing major parasympathetic adverse effects.

Pharmacokinetics:

Route(s)	PO
Absorption	Almost completely absorbed from the GI tract
Distribution	Crosses the blood–brain barrier and placenta; secreted in breast milk
Primary metabolism	Hepatic
Primary excretion	Renal
Onset of action	30 minutes–2 h
Duration of action	6–12 h

Adverse Effects: Common adverse effects include weakness, fatigue, sedation, headache, mydriasis, blurred vision, decreased libido, impotence, and urinary retention. Serious adverse effects include orthostatic hypotension, precipitation of angina, choreiform movement, and adynamic ileus. Effects may last hours to days after the drug is discontinued.

Contraindications/Precautions: Mecamylamine must be used with caution in patients with impaired renal function because the drug can build to toxic levels. Other contraindications include coronary insufficiency, pyloric stenosis, glaucoma, recent MI, mild labile HTN, and unreliable uncooperative patients. **Herbal/Food:** None known.

Drug Interactions: Alcohol, bethanechol, and other antihypertensive agents including thiazide diuretics may potentiate hypotensive effects. Acetazolamide and sodium bicarbonate increase mecamylamine toxicity because they decrease its elimination.

Pregnancy: Category C.

Treatment of Overdose: Overdose will produce profound hypotension, which may be treated with vasopressors. Other anticholinergic symptoms such as blurred vision, dry mouth, palpitations, nausea, and vomiting are treated symptomatically.

Nursing Responsibilities:

- Monitor vital signs such as blood pressure and pulse rate. Take blood pressure readings in the standing position at the time of maximal drug effect. Assess for symptoms of orthostatic hypotension such as faintness, dizziness, and light-headedness.
- Assess for partial tolerance by monitoring blood pressure. This can develop in select patients and requires a dosage adjustment.
- Assess and report constipation, frequent loose stools with abdominal distension, or decreased bowel sounds because these first signs of paralytic ileus may occur.

Patient and Family Education:

- Make position changes slowly when moving from a lying to a standing position to prevent dizziness and possible fainting.
- Lie down immediately if dizzy or light-headed.
- Note that seasonal variations may alter the hypotensive effect so smaller doses may be required in summer than in winter.
- Do not drive or perform other hazardous activities until the effects of the drug are known because this drug may cause drowsiness or dizziness.
- Use various methods to relieve dry mouth such as rinsing mouth frequently with water or sucking on hard candy.
- Do not breast-feed while taking this drug without approval of the health care provider.
- Immediately notify the health care provider of any known or suspected pregnancy.
- Never discontinue this drug abruptly because this can result in severe rebound HTN.

Nicotinic Antagonists: Neuromuscular Blockers

18.4 Muscle contraction occurs when the motor end plate is depolarized.

The neuromuscular junction is a specialized cholinergic synapse that allows for communication between the nervous system and skeletal muscle. This synapse on the muscle, known as a **motor end plate,** receives an action potential from the axon of a motor neuron. Like other cholinergic synapses, the action potential causes the release of Ach, which travels across the synaptic cleft to its receptors on skeletal muscle. Anatomically, the neuromuscular junction is part of the somatic nervous system (not the autonomic).

Binding of Ach to its receptors changes the permeability of the muscle cell membrane and opens sodium channels, allowing sodium ions to rush in. Being a positive ion, sodium causes the inside of the muscle cell to depolarize and acquire a positive charge. This depolarization at the motor end plate triggers the release of calcium ions from internal storage areas within the muscle cell. The intense, though brief, release of calcium is quickly followed by skeletal muscle contraction.

As presented in Chapter 16, destruction of Ach by the enzyme acetylcholinesterase (AchE) removes the neurotransmitter from the motor end plate, allowing the muscle cell membrane to repolarize. Calcium returns to its internal storage depots, and muscle relaxation occurs. This process by which the action potential causes muscular contraction is known as excitation-contraction coupling.

When multiple action potentials arrive at a specific motor end plate, the muscle cell undergoes a series of repeated depolarizations and repolarizations. This results in a continuous depolarized state in which calcium does not return to its storage depots, and a sustained, muscle contraction may be achieved. This contraction, however, can only be sustained by a continuous cycle of depolarizations and repolarizations. If the cell is simply depolarized (without undergoing repolarization), calcium will return to its storage areas and contraction will totally cease, resulting in a flaccid muscle. This paralyzed condition is necessary when performing certain surgical procedures. The depolarization of the motor end plate is illustrated in Figure 18.2.

18.5 Depolarizing neuromuscular blockers are given to produce muscle paralysis during short medical–surgical procedures.

The nicotinic synapse at the neuromuscular junction can be affected by drugs that can act by two distinct mechanisms. One group of agents acts on the synapse to produce a constant depolarized state. The second group produces similar effects without causing depolarization of the muscle cells. The depolarizing and nondepolarizing neuromuscular blockers both produce the same result: skeletal muscle relaxation or muscle paralysis.

Succinylcholine is the sole member of the class of drugs known as the depolarizing neuromuscular blockers. This drug competes with Ach for cholinergic receptors on the motor end plate. Once bound to Ach receptors, succinylcholine produces muscle contraction by the same mechanism as Ach. Unlike Ach, however, succinylcholine is not destroyed by AchE, and the drug causes a prolonged and continuous depolarization of the muscle cell. Without repolarization, calcium returns to its internal storage depots and the muscle relaxes. The mechanism of action of succinylcholine is illustrated in Figure 18.3a.

It is important to note that succinylcholine does not enter the CNS. Although the drug causes muscle paralysis, it does not produce anesthesia or loss of consciousness. The patient is still able to feel pain and is aware of his or her surroundings. Thus succinylcholine is only one component of balanced anesthesia, as discussed in Chapter 30.

CONNECTION *Checkpoint* 18.3

Pyridostigmine also affects nicotinic receptors in skeletal muscle. From what you learned in Chapter 17, would you expect this drug to interact with neuromuscular blockers? What is the primary indication for pyridostigmine? See Answer to Connection Checkpoint 18.3 in Appendix A.

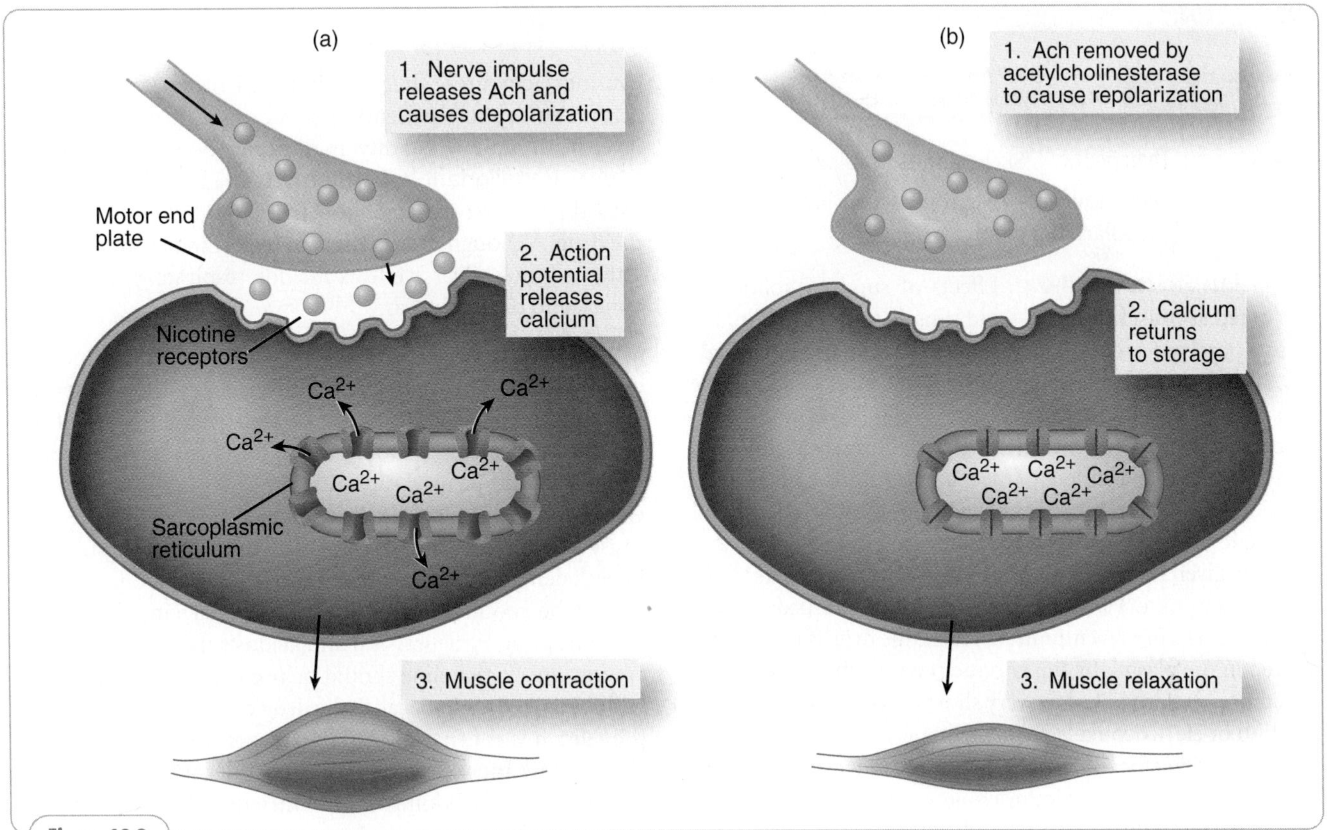

Figure 18.2

Depolarization of the motor end plate: (a) depolarization: Ach causes calcium to be released from storage, resulting in muscle contraction; (b) repolarization: Ach is destroyed by acetylcholinesterase, calcium returns to storage, and muscle relaxation results.

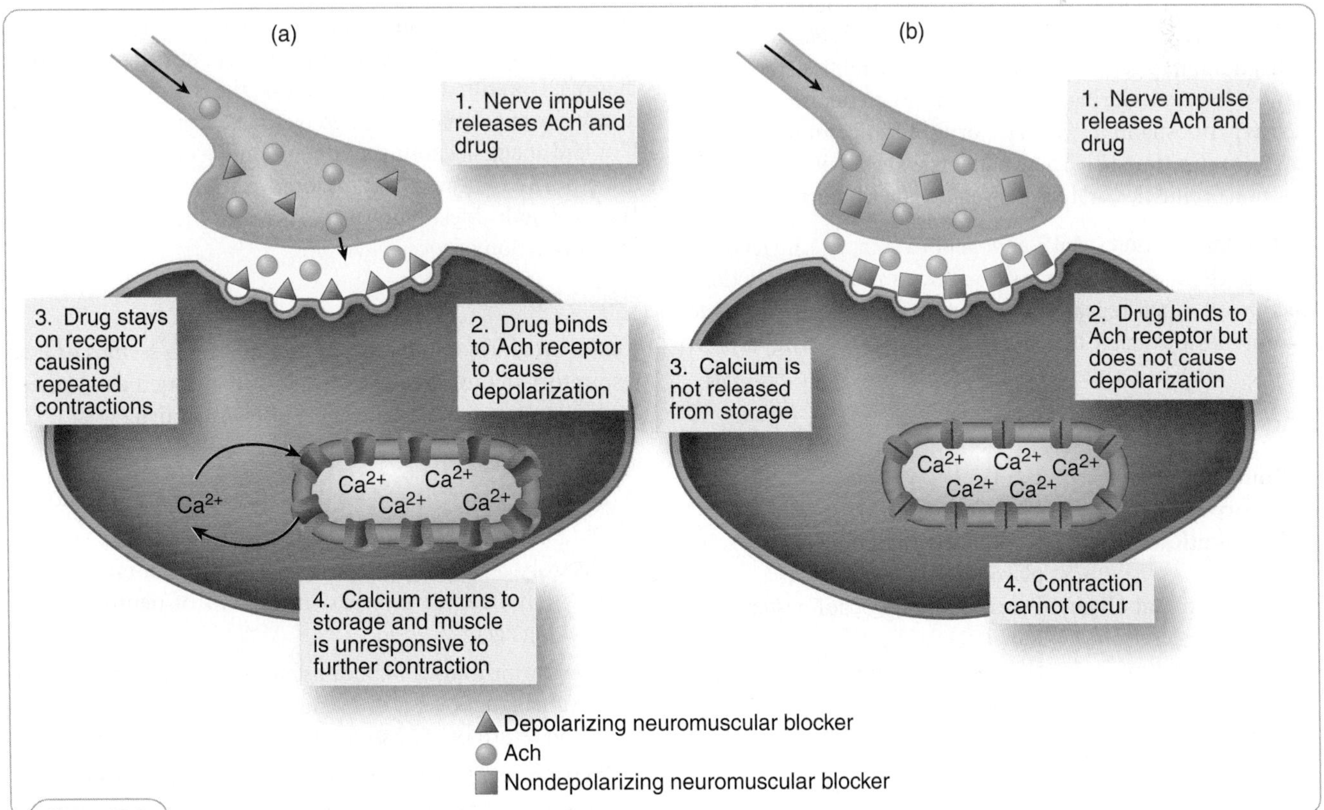

Figure 18.3

Mechanism of action of neuromuscular blockers: (a) depolarizing neuromuscular blocker occupies Ach receptors and causes depolarization and muscle paralysis; (b) nondepolarizing neuromuscular blocker occupies Ach receptors and causes muscle paralysis without depolarization.

PROTOTYPE DRUG Succinylcholine (Anectine)

Classification: Therapeutic: Skeletal muscle relaxant
Pharmacologic: Neuromuscular blocker (depolarizing type)

Therapeutic Effects and Uses: Effects of succinylcholine are first noted as muscle weakness and muscle spasms. Eventually muscle paralysis occurs. The drug is primarily used as an adjunct to surgical anesthesia to cause complete skeletal muscle relaxation of the abdominal muscles. It may also be used to relax muscles during the insertion of an endotracheal tube and to assist in the management of mechanical ventilation. Administration of succinylcholine reduces the amount of general anesthetic needed for surgical procedures.

When given IV, succinylcholine induces muscle relaxation in less than a minute. When the infusion is discontinued, muscle control returns in a few minutes, because the drug is rapidly destroyed in the plasma by the enzyme **pseudocholinesterase.** This makes the drug ideal for very short procedures, such as intubation or electroconvulsive shock therapy.

Some patients have a genetic deficiency in plasma cholinesterase. In these patients, succinylcholine will have an unusually prolonged duration of action, and paralysis may persist for hours. Because there is no specific antidote for succinylcholine overdose, the patient must receive supportive treatment until the drug is metabolized and removed by the body. This adverse effect may be avoided by assessing pseudocholinesterase levels prior to surgery. If low, succinylcholine may be contraindicated, or the dose lowered to prevent prolonged muscle paralysis.

In addition to genetic deficiency, pseudocholinesterase levels may be decreased during therapy with cholinesterase inhibitors such as pyridostigmine, which is a drug of choice for myasthenia gravis (see Chapter 17). These patients will exhibit a prolonged duration of muscle paralysis if given succinylcholine.

Mechanism of Action: Like endogenous Ach, succinylcholine binds to cholinergic receptor sites at neuromuscular junctions (nicotinic). After repeated contractions the skeletal muscle membranes are unable to repolarize as long as the drug stays on the receptor. The result is total muscle relaxation or paralysis.

Pharmacokinetics:

Route(s)	IM, IV
Absorption	Well-absorbed IM
Distribution	Completely, including crossing the placenta
Primary metabolism	Plasma by pseudocholinesterase
Primary excretion	Renal
Onset of action	IV: less than 1 minute; IM: 2–3 minutes
Duration of action	IV: 2–3 minutes; IM: 10–30 minutes

Adverse Effects: Succinylcholine can cause complete paralysis of the diaphragm and intercostal muscles; thus mechanical ventilation is necessary during surgery. If doses are high, succinylcholine will also inhibit nerve transmission at the ganglia, causing tachycardia, hypotension, and urinary retention. In certain susceptible patients, a rapid onset of extremely high fever with muscle rigidity may occur, a serious condition known as **malignant hyperthermia.** The high temperature is caused by excessive metabolic activity in muscles, triggered by the drug. Although rare, malignant hyperthermia may be fatal. Other serious adverse effects include respiratory depression, apnea, and dysrhythmias.

Contraindications/Precautions: Because succinylcholine is an essential component of balanced surgical anesthesia, there are few absolute contraindications. Patients with a history of malignant hyperthermia should not receive this drug. Succinylcholine should be used cautiously in patients with preexisting electrolyte imbalances or heart failure because this drug can cause a sudden release of intracellular potassium, resulting in hyperkalemia. Patients with pulmonary or metabolic disorders should be monitored carefully because succinylcholine can cause respiratory depression and acidosis. Due to its renal excretion, succinylcholine should be used cautiously in patients with kidney disease. Because the drug can increase intraocular pressure, it is contraindicated in patients with glaucoma. Succinylcholine must be used with extreme caution in children because acute rhabdomyolysis, ventricular dysrhythmias, and cardiac arrest have occurred in pediatric patients.

Drug Interactions: Additive skeletal muscle inhibition will occur if succinylcholine is given concurrently with clindamycin, phenothiazine, aminoglycosides, furosemide, lithium, quinidine, or lidocaine. If succinylcholine is given concurrently with the anesthetics halothane or nitrous oxide, there is an increased risk of dysrhythmias, sinus arrest, apnea, and malignant hyperthermia. Use with digoxin can increase the risk of dysrhythmias due to the hyperkalemia caused by the neuromuscular blocker. If opioid analgesics are given concurrently with succinylcholine, there is an increased risk of bradycardia and sinus arrest. **Herbal/Food:** Melatonin may increase the neuromuscular blocking action of succinylcholine.

Pregnancy: Category C.

Treatment of Overdose: Overdose can lead to serious or fatal respiratory depression. The drug is discontinued and assisted ventilation is provided until the effects of the drug wear off.

Nursing Responsibilities:

- Monitor vital signs and keep the airway free of secretions.
- Obtain baseline laboratory tests such as serum electrolytes. Electrolyte imbalance (particularly potassium, calcium, magnesium) can potentiate the actions of neuromuscular blocking agents.
- Monitor for transient apnea usually occurring at the time of maximal drug effect (1 to 2 minutes); spontaneous respiration should return in a few seconds or, at most, 3 or 4 minutes.
- Prepare for emergency endotracheal intubation, artificial respiration, and assisted or controlled respiration with oxygen.

Patient and Family Education:

- Muscle stiffness and pain that may last for as long as 24 to 30 hours will persist after the procedure.

- Understand that sore throat and hoarseness are common even when the pharyngeal airway has not been used.
- Report persistent muscle weakness.

Drugs Similar to Succinylcholine chloride (Anectine)

Succinylcholine is the only depolarizing neuromuscular blocker.

CONNECTION *Checkpoint* 18.4

From what you learned in Chapter 17, explain why a patient with myasthenia gravis might be particularly susceptible to the actions of neuromuscular blockers. See Answer to Connection Checkpoint 18.4 in Appendix A.

18.6 Nondepolarizing neuromuscular blockers are given to produce muscle paralysis during longer surgical procedures.

The first neuromuscular blocker was **curare,** which was initially extracted from several different plant species native to the rainforests of South America. Indians of the region cooked the roots and stems to produce a thick, tarry substance that could be rubbed on the tips of arrows. Once shot into the muscle of an animal, curare would rapidly cause muscle weakness, allowing the Indians to overcome and kill the game. It is these same properties that allowed medical science to use curare to reduce muscle spasms and to cause skeletal muscle paralysis during operative procedures. The active chemical extracted from curare, and which is used for medical procedures, is called tubocurarine.

Like succinylcholine, tubocurarine is a nicotinic antagonist that binds to Ach receptors at motor end plates in skeletal muscle. However, tubocurarine does not cause depolarization of the muscle cell; it acts by preventing Ach from reaching its receptors. Thus tubocurarine is classified as a **nondepolarizing neuromuscular blocker.** Since the discovery of tubocurarine, a number of other natural and synthetic neuromuscular blockers in this class have been found to have clinical utility. Nine other drugs, shown in Table 18.2, have a mechanism of action similar to that of tubocurarine. The mechanism of action of the nondepolarizing neuromuscular blockers is illustrated in Figure 18.3b.

All nondepolarizing neuromuscular blockers have identical actions, with their primary application being to relax skeletal muscles during operative procedures. These agents may also be used to facilitate management of mechanical ventilation by suppressing contractions of respiratory muscles, eliminating resistance to mechanical ventilation. Suppressing muscular reflexes allows smoother insertion of an endotracheal tube, which is an additional indication for the use of these agents. For patients undergoing electroconvulsive shock therapy or those suffering from tetanus, neuromuscular blockers can reduce the intensity and pain of severe muscle contractions.

The nondepolarizing neuromuscular blockers are charged molecules that do not readily cross membranes. Thus, they are almost always administered IV. Because they do not cross the blood–brain barrier, they do not induce sedation, analgesia, or loss of consciousness. This allows for complete skeletal muscle paralysis without loss of consciousness. Administration of an anesthetic is necessary when diminished consciousness or analgesia is desired, such as during surgical anesthesia.

The 10 nondepolarizing neuromuscular blockers differ in their durations of action. This is a critical difference because the muscular relaxation induced by the drug must last long enough to complete the specific surgical procedure. The shortest acting agent mivacurium lasts only 12 to 18 minutes, whereas the longer acting doxacurium may last up to 2 hours. All nondepolarizing neuromuscular blockers have a very rapid onset of action, inducing paralysis within minutes.

The most serious concern when using neuromuscular blockers is paralysis of respiratory muscles leading to apnea and possible respiratory arrest. Excessive respiratory depression caused by nondepolarizing blockers can be treated by administration of an AchE inhibitor such as neostigmine (Prostigmin). In this respect, the nondepolarizing blockers differ from the depolarizing blockers. Administration of an AchE inhibitor will not reverse the respiratory depression caused by succinylcholine.

Hypotension is another potentially serious adverse effect of these agents. Hypotension results when these agents trigger the release of histamine and at higher doses when nicotinic receptors at the ganglia are activated. Some neuromuscular blockers, including metocurine, pipecuronium, pancuronium, and vecuronium, cause less histamine release and have little effect on the ganglia, thus posing less risk of hypotension. An antihistamine may be administered to lessen the hypotension caused by those neuromuscular blockers that induce histamine release.

PROTOTYPE DRUG Tubocurarine

Classification: **Therapeutic:** Skeletal muscle relaxant
Pharmacologic: Neuromuscular blocker (nondepolarizing type)

Therapeutic Effects and Uses: The primary therapeutic effect of tubocurarine is skeletal muscle relaxation or paralysis. It is used as an adjunct to anesthesia to cause complete skeletal muscle relaxation of the abdominal muscles during operative procedures. It may also be used to relax muscles during the insertion of an endotracheal tube, to assist in the management of mechanical ventilation, and to reduce the intensity of acute muscle contractions.

Given by the IV route, tubocurarine can produce total muscle paralysis within minutes. It has a longer duration of action than succinylcholine, with effects lasting 20 to 30 minutes. Because it does not enter the CNS, other drugs must be used when loss of consciousness or analgesia is required for a surgical procedure.

Mechanism of Action: Tubocurarine competes with Ach for nicotinic receptor sites at motor end plates in skeletal muscle. Blocking nerve transmission to skeletal muscle prevents the muscles from contracting. Unlike succinylcholine, tubocurarine produces its effects without depolarizing the muscle cell membrane. Tubocurarine will block Ach synapses at the ganglia at higher doses.

Pharmacokinetics:

Route(s)	IV
Absorption	N/A
Distribution	Completely distributed; does not cross the blood–brain barrier; crosses the placenta
Primary metabolism	Hepatic
Primary excretion	Renal, with smaller amounts in bile and feces
Onset of action	1 minute
Duration of action	Half-life: 1–3 h

Adverse Effects: Tubocurarine has the potential to cause serious adverse effects and death due to paralysis of the respiratory muscles. Mechanical ventilation must always be available when the drug is administered. Like succinylcholine, malignant hyperthermia is a rare, though serious, adverse effect. Among the drugs in this class, tubocurarine has the greatest potential to release histamine, causing bronchospasm and hypotension. Common adverse effects include muscle weakness, hypotension, and increased salivation.

Contraindications/Precautions: Due to the risk of malignant hyperthermia, patients with preexisting hyperthermia or who have a history of this condition should not receive tubocurarine. Because neuromuscular blockers can release intracellular potassium resulting in hyperkalemia, patients with preexisting electrolyte imbalances or heart failure should not receive tubocurarine. The drug is contraindicated in patients with acidosis because tubocurarine slows respirations, which can cause carbon dioxide to build up and worsen acidosis. Due to its renal excretion, tubocurarine should be used cautiously in patients with kidney disease.

Drug Interactions: Other skeletal muscle relaxants and inhaled anesthetics can cause additive muscle relaxation when given concurrently with tubocurarine. Drugs that block calcium channels or otherwise deplete calcium, including aminoglycoside and tetracycline antibiotics and calcium channel blockers, will have synergistic effects with tubocurarine. Other drugs that potentiate the muscle relaxation caused by tubocurarine include procainamide, quinidine, clindamycin, amphotericin B, and diuretics. **Herbal/Food**: Unknown.

Pregnancy: Category C.

Treatment of Overdose: Overdose can lead to serious or fatal respiratory depression. The drug is discontinued and assisted ventilation is provided until the effects of the drug wear off. Neostigmine may be administered to more rapidly reverse the neuromuscular blockade. Supportive therapy may be used to treat symptoms caused by histamine release.

Nursing Responsibilities:

- Monitor vital signs, including blood pressure, and assess for patent airway until patient recovery from drug effects is confirmed. Specific adverse effects of this drug include hypotension (ganglionic blockade), increased salivation and bronchospasm (histamine release), and respiratory depression (neuromuscular blockade).
- Obtain baseline laboratory tests, including kidney function and serum electrolytes. Electrolyte imbalances, especially potassium and magnesium, can potentiate the effects of nondepolarizing neuromuscular blocking agents.
- Note that selective muscle paralysis following drug administration occurs in the following sequence: jaw muscles, levator eyelid muscles and other muscles of the head and neck, limbs, intercostals and diaphragm, abdomen, trunk. Recovery occurs as follows: Facial and diaphragm muscles, followed in order by legs, arms, shoulder girdle, trunk, larynx, hands, feet, pharynx. Muscle function is usually restored within 90 minutes.
- Measure and record intake and output ratio during the day of drug administration. Patients with renal impairment may experience prolonged drug action.
- Check for bowel sounds because peristaltic action may be suppressed.

Patient and Family Education:

- Report residual muscle weakness to the health care provider. Drug effects can remain in the body for some time after the procedure.

Drugs Similar to Tubocurarine

The nine other neuromuscular blockers have the same indications and adverse effects as tubocurarine but differ in their duration of action (see Table 18.2). Choice of a specific blocker will depend on the length of the surgical procedure and the clinical experience of the anesthesiologist.

Short-acting agent: Mivacurium (Mivacron) is the shortest acting nondepolarizing blocker. Its duration of action is 15 to 20 minutes. A continuous infusion may be used to maintain the neuromuscular block.

Intermediate-acting agents: Atracurium (Tracrium), cisatracurium (Nimbex), pancuronium (Pavulon), rocuronium (Zemuron), and vecuronium (Norcuron) have durations of action of 20 to 45 minutes. Cisatracurium and atracurium are not eliminated by the liver or kidneys and may be better choices for patients with hepatic or renal disease. Vecuronium has the advantage of causing no histamine release.

NURSING PROCESS APPLICATION

Patients Receiving Anticholinergic Drug Therapy

Assessment	Potential Nursing Diagnoses
Prior to administration: • Obtain a complete health history, including drug history, to determine possible drug interactions and allergies. • Assess the reason for drug administration. • Assess for heart rate, blood pressure, temperature, and elimination patterns (initially and throughout therapy).	• *Deficient Knowledge (Drug Therapy)* • *Decreased Cardiac Output,* related to drug therapy • *Risk for Imbalanced Body Temperature,* related to inhibited sweat gland secretions • *Impaired Oral Mucous Membrane,* related to decrease in exocrine secretions • *Constipation,* related to adverse drug effects • *Urinary Retention,* related to adverse effects of anticholinergic therapy

Planning: Patient Goals and Expected Outcomes

The patient will:

- Exhibit a decrease in symptoms for which the medication is prescribed.
- Demonstrate an understanding of the drug's action by accurately describing drug adverse effects and precautions.
- Verbalize techniques to avoid hazardous adverse effects associated with anticholinergic therapy.

Implementation

Interventions and (Rationales)	Patient and Family Education
• Monitor for signs of anticholinergic crisis: fever, tachycardia, difficulty swallowing, ataxia, reduced urine output, psychomotor agitation, confusion, hallucinations. (Anticholinergic crisis results from overdosage of these medications.) • Report significant changes in heart rate and blood pressure or the development of dysrhythmias. (Many anticholinergic antagonists may cause tachycardia.)	• Instruct the patient to report adverse effects related to therapy such as shortness of breath, cough, dysphagia, syncope, fever, anxiety, right upper quadrant pain, extreme lethargy, or dizziness. • Instruct patients to monitor vital signs, ensuring proper use of home equipment.
• Observe for adverse effects such as drowsiness, blurred vision, tachycardia, dry mouth, urinary hesitancy, and decreased sweating. (Adverse effects may negatively impact some activities.)	Instruct the patient to: • Report adverse effects. • Avoid driving and hazardous activities until the effects of the drugs are known. • Wear sunglasses to decrease sensitivity to bright light.
• Provide comfort measures for dryness of mucous membranes, such as applying lubricant to moisten lips and the oral mucosa, or assisting in rinsing the mouth. Use artificial tears for dry eyes, as needed. (Anticholinergics such as atropine decrease the quantity of exocrine secretions.)	• Instruct the patient to use oral rinses, sugarless gum, or candy and practice frequent oral hygiene to help relieve dry mouth. Avoid alcohol-containing mouthwashes that can further dry oral tissue.
• Minimize exposure to heat or cold and strenuous exercise. (Anticholinergics can inhibit sweat gland secretions due to direct blockade of the muscarinic receptors on the sweat glands. Sweating is necessary for patients to cool down and this can increase their risk for hyperthermia.)	• Instruct the patient to limit outside activity when the temperature is hot to prevent heatstroke.
• Monitor intake and output ratio. Palpate the abdomen for bladder distention. (Urinary retention is a common adverse effect of anticholinergic therapy.)	• Instruct the patient to notify the health care provider if difficulty in voiding occurs.
• Monitor patients routinely for abdominal distention and auscultate for bowel sounds. (Constipation is one adverse effect associated with anticholinergic drugs.)	• Instruct the patient to increase fluid and add bulk to their diet, if constipation becomes a problem.

Evaluation of Outcome Criteria

Evaluate the effectiveness of drug therapy by confirming that patient goals and expected outcomes have been met (see "Planning").

UNDERSTANDING THE CHAPTER

Key Concepts Summary

18.1 Cholinergic antagonists act by blocking the effects of acetylcholine at muscarinic or nicotinic receptors.

18.2 Muscarinic antagonists have been used for a diverse number of conditions, but they are rarely drugs of choice due to their adverse effects.

18.3 Ganglionic blockers act at the autonomic ganglia to lower blood pressure in emergency situations.

18.4 Muscle contraction occurs when the motor end plate is depolarized.

18.5 Depolarizing neuromuscular blockers are given to produce muscle paralysis during short medical–surgical procedures.

18.6 Nondepolarizing neuromuscular blockers are given to produce muscle paralysis during longer surgical procedures.

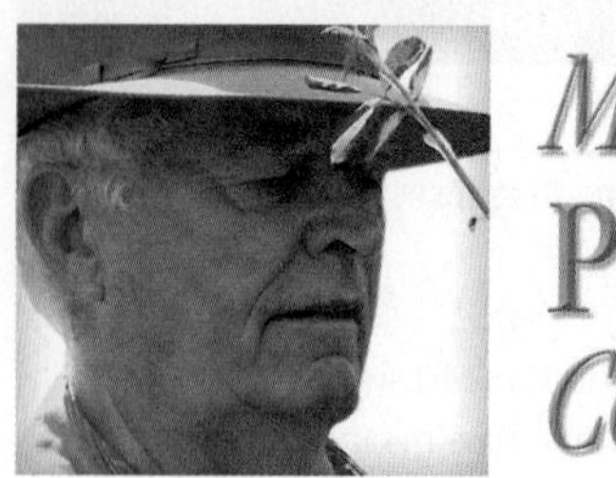

Making the PATIENT Connection

Remember the patient "Pete Elbertson" at the beginning of the chapter? Now read the remainder of the case study. Based on the information presented within this chapter, respond to the critical thinking questions that follow.

Pete Elbertson is a 60-year-old man who enjoys working in his large vegetable garden. Two days ago, while working with his tomatoes, Pete noticed that insects had infested the plants. To avoid further damage, he powdered the plants with some insecticide. In his rush to finish, he accidentally contaminated himself with the insecticide and kept working for several hours before showering.

Now, Pete presents to the local emergency department with nausea, dizziness, sweating, excessive salivation, weepy eyes, and a runny nose. He reports intermittent twitching of his upper extremities and uncoordinated movement.

His initial assessment reveals an 84-kg (185 lb) Caucasian male with a past medication history of HTN diagnosed 5 years ago. He is married and has two adult children. He smokes one pack of cigarettes per day and does not use alcohol. His vital signs are blood pressure, 158/94 mmHg; heart rate, 58; respiratory rate, 30; and temperature, 37.3°C (99.2°F). His skin is pale and moist. He exhibits copious lacrimation and rhinorrhea. Both pupils are constricted. Bilaterally, the patient's lung sounds reveal wet and crackly on inspiration. Since admission to the emergency department he has vomited twice and had one large diarrhea stool.

Pete is diagnosed with acute organophosphate poisoning. The patient is started on oxygen therapy, and the nurse will observe him closely for further respiratory distress. Atropine 2 mg is administered IV every 15 minutes over the next hour.

Critical Thinking Questions

1. Discuss the mechanism of action associated with atropine.
2. Why is this drug being given to Pete?
3. What adverse effects should you expect for the patient from the administration of atropine?

Case Study

You are caring for Nick, a 56-year-old man, in the intensive care unit. Over the last 2 hours, you have been closely monitoring this patient due to increased respiratory distress. When the health care provider arrives, he informs you that Nick will need to be placed on a mechanical ventilator. The patient will be given a neuromuscular blocking agent to assist with the insertion of an endotracheal tube.

1. Describe the mechanism of action associated with this drug classification.
2. What is the rationale for the administration of neuromuscular blocking drugs for this patient?
3. Identify the problems associated with the administration of neuromuscular blocking agents.

NCLEX-RN® Review

1 Which of the following health teaching concepts should the nurse review with a client receiving anticholinergic drug therapy? The client should be taught to:

1. Exercise daily to avoid muscle atrophy.
2. Increase dietary fiber and water intake to avoid constipation.
3. Consume foods high in iron to increase red blood cell production.
4. Monitor the heart rate for bradycardia.

2 The nurse is aware that the therapeutic uses for muscarinic antagonists include: (Select all that apply.)

1. Ophthalmic procedures.
2. Cardiac rhythm abnormalities.
3. Asthma.
4. Poisonings.
5. Urinary retention.

3 Which of the following factors in the client's history would cause the nurse to question a medication order for atropine?

1. A 42-year-old woman with a history of drug abuse
2. An 85-year-old man with benign prostatic hyperplasia
3. An 18-year-old man with irritable bowel syndrome
4. A 22-year-old woman on the second day of her menstrual cycle

4 Muscarinic agents, such as benztropine (Cogentin), are most often contraindicated in glaucoma because these drugs can:

1. Increase intraocular pressure.
2. Promote ocular infections.
3. Cause miosis, which leads to blindness.
4. Detach the retina.

5 The client will be taking cholinergic antagonists following discharge from the acute care hospital. Which of the following statements, made by the client, would indicate that additional teaching is needed?

1. "To relieve dry mouth, I should drink plenty of water."
2. "I will avoid activities requiring mental alertness until I know the effects of this drug."
3. "The use of lubricating eyedrops should be avoided. I should see an eye doctor for dry eyes."
4. "I will not breast-feed while taking this drug without consulting my health care provider."

6 The nurse administering succinylcholine knows that this drug causes:

1. Muscle paralysis; it does not produce anesthesia or loss of consciousness.
2. Loss of consciousness, along with muscle paralysis and anesthesia.
3. Deep muscle relaxation and relief from pain.
4. Increased mental alertness with muscle paralysis.

See Answers to Critical Thinking Questions, Case Study, and NCLEX-RN® Review in Appendix A.

References

Barnes, P. J. (2004). The role of anticholinergics in chronic obstructive pulmonary disease. *The American Journal of Medicine, 20*(117, Suppl. 12A), 24S–32S.

Betten, D. P. (2006). Antidote use in the critically ill poisoned patient. *Journal of Intensive Care Medicine, 21*(5), 255–277.

Bowman, W. C. (2006). Neuromuscular block. *British Journal of Pharmacology, 147*(Suppl. 1), S277–S286.

Cope, T. M., & Hunter, J. M. (2003). Selecting neuromuscular-blocking drugs for elderly patients. *Drugs Aging, 20*(2), 125–140.

Hogan, M. A. (2005). *Pharmacology reviews and rationales.* Upper Saddle River, NJ: Prentice Hall.

Katz, K., Brooks, D., Furtado, M., & Chan, L. (2008). Toxicity, organophosphate. *emedicine.* Retrieved May 31, 2008, from http://www.emedicine.com/med/TOPIC1677.HTM

Mertes, P. M., & Laxenaire, M. C. (2004). Adverse reactions to neuromuscular blocking agents. *Current Allergy and Asthma Reports, 4*(1), 7–16.

Pic, L. C. (2005). Novel pharmacological approaches for the antagonism of neuromuscular blockade. *American Association of Nurse Anesthetists Journal, 73*(1), 37–40.

Sheridan, R. D., Smith, A. P., Turner, S. R., & Tattersall, J. E. (2005). Nicotinic antagonists in the treatment of nerve agent intoxication. *Journal of the Royal Society of Medicine, 98*(3), 114–115.

Simmons, R. (2005). Conservative and surgical approaches to the treatment of overactive bladder. *Professional Nurse, 20*(6), 31–33.

Spinks, A. B., Wasiak, J., Villanueva, E. V., & Bernath, V. (2007). Scopolamine for preventing and treating motion sickness. *Cochrane Database of Systematic Reviews, 3,* CD002851.

Thomas, D. R. (2004). Pharmacologic management of urinary incontinence. *Clinics in Geriatric Medicine, 20*(3), 511–523.

University of Iowa Hospitals and Clinics. (2006). *Deadly nightshade: Atropa belladonna.* Retrieved May 31, 2008, from http://www.uihealthcare.com/depts/medmuseum/galleryexhibits/naturespharmacy/nightshadeplant/nightshade.html

Westfall, T. C., & Westfall, D. P. (2006). Neurotransmission: The autonomic and somatic motor nervous systems. In L. L. Brunton, J. S. Lazo, and K. L. Parker (Eds.), *The pharmacological basis of therapeutics* (11th ed., pp. 137–182). New York: McGraw-Hill.

CHAPTER

I woke this morning having difficulty breathing. I think my asthma is acting up again.

Patient "Alexia Howard"

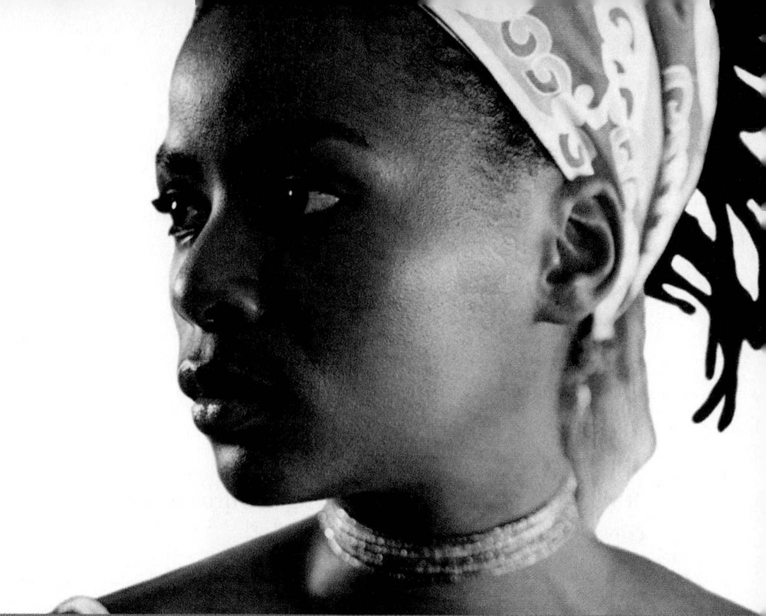

19 Adrenergic Agonists

Learning Outcomes

After reading this chapter, the student should be able to:

1. Identify the physiological responses that occur when a drug activates adrenergic receptors.
2. Explain the direct and indirect mechanisms by which adrenergic agonists act.
3. Compare and contrast the characteristics of catecholamines and noncatecholamines.
4. Identify indications for pharmacotherapy with adrenergic agonists.
5. Compare and contrast the types of responses that occur when a drug activates alpha$_1$, alpha$_2$, beta$_1$, or beta$_2$-adrenergic receptors.
6. For each of the classes shown in the chapter outline, identify the prototype and representative drugs and explain the mechanism(s) of drug action, primary indications, contraindications, significant drug interactions, pregnancy category, and important adverse effects.
7. Use the nursing process to care for patients receiving drug therapy with adrenergic agonists.

Chapter Outline

Actions of Adrenergic Agonists

Mechanisms of Action of Adrenergic Agonists

Classification of Adrenergic Agonists

Nonselective Adrenergic Agonists

PROTOTYPE **Epinephrine (Adrenalin)** *p. 233*

Alpha-Adrenergic Agonists

PROTOTYPE **Phenylephrine (Neo-Synephrine)** *p. 236*

Beta-Adrenergic Agonists

PROTOTYPE **Isoproterenol (Isuprel)** *p. 239*

Key Terms

adrenergic agonists, 229
cardiotonic drugs, 238
catecholamine, 230
catechol-O-methyltransferase, 231
ephedra, 235
inotropic agents, 239
monoamine oxidase (MAO), 231
sympathomimetic, 229
tocolytic, 239

Adrenergic agonists activate the sympathetic nervous system and induce symptoms of the fight-or-flight response. The pharmacology of adrenergic drugs is more complex than their cholinergic counterparts, due to the existence of the receptor subtypes alpha and beta. Drugs that activate these subtypes have applications to the pharmacotherapy of shock, hypotension, and asthma.

As discussed in Chapter 16 the actions produced by cholinergic (muscarinic) antagonists are similar to those of adrenergic agonists. This is because blocking muscarinic receptors in the parasympathetic nervous system produces similar effects to activating the sympathetic nervous system. However, because the sympathetic nervous system has alpha- and beta-receptor subtypes, the actions of many adrenergic agonists are more specific, which allows for wider therapeutic applications due to a lower incidence of side adverse effects.

Actions of Adrenergic Agonists

19.1 Adrenergic agonists activate the sympathetic nervous system to produce fight-or-flight symptoms.

Adrenergic agonists, also known as **sympathomimetics**, are agents that activate adrenergic receptors in the sympathetic nervous system. Drugs in this class include endogenous substances such as norepinephrine (NE), epinephrine, and dopamine. NE is the major neurotransmitter in the sympathetic nervous system, whereas epinephrine is the primary hormone released by the adrenal medulla. Dopamine is the immediate biochemical precursor to NE and is a key neurotransmitter in certain regions of the central nervous system (CNS). In addition to their natural physiological roles in the body, NE, epinephrine, and dopamine are available as prescription drugs. A number of synthetic adrenergic agonists that mimic the effects of these natural neurotransmitters are also available.

The physiological actions of the adrenergic agonists are those of the fight-or-flight response. As drugs, their most important therapeutic actions are on the cardiovascular and respiratory systems. Heart rate and cardiac output increase due to activation of adrenergic receptors in the myocardium. Constriction of vascular smooth muscle causes a rapid increase in blood pressure. Administration by the parenteral or inhalation routes immediately relaxes bronchial smooth muscle, resulting in bronchodilation. Activation of adrenergic receptors in the smooth muscle of the gastrointestinal (GI) and urinary tracts slows peristalsis and may cause constipation and urine retention. Metabolic effects include increased oxygen consumption and increased blood glucose and lactate levels. Other adrenergic actions include reduction of glandular secretory activity and mydriasis.

It is important to remember that the symptoms of the fight-or-flight response elicited by the adrenergic agonists may be considered as therapeutic or adverse, depending on the condition of the patient and the goals of pharmacotherapy. For example, if the patient is in shock, increased blood pressure is a key therapeutic effect. However, if the patient is taking an adrenergic agonist for nasal congestion, an increase in blood pressure is an adverse effect. Furthermore a therapeutic effect may become an adverse effect if taken to extreme, such as raising blood pressure too much or causing excessive drying of the nasal or oral mucosa.

CONNECTION *Checkpoint* 19.1

From what you learned in Chapter 16, where are most dopaminergic receptors located? Dopaminergic drugs would most likely be prescribed for what disorders?

See Answer to Connection Checkpoint 19.1 in Appendix A.

Pharm*FACT*

Pheochromocytomas are tumors of the adrenal medulla that secrete large amounts of adrenergic agonists, including dopamine, epinephrine, and norepinephrine. As expected, signs and symptoms are those of sympathetic nervous system hyperactivity: increased heart rate, blood pressure, and anxiety resembling that of a panic attack. Treatment includes pharmacotherapy with antihypertensives until surgery can be performed to remove the tumor. *Source:* Sweeney, Blake, & Einhorn, 2007.

Mechanisms of Action of Adrenergic Agonists

19.2 Adrenergic agonists may act directly by binding to adrenergic receptors, or indirectly by increasing the amount of norepinephrine at synapses.

Sympathomimetics exert their effects by two distinct mechanisms. Most act directly by binding to and activating adrenergic receptors. Examples include the three endogenous hormones epinephrine, NE, and dopamine.

Some adrenergic agonists act indirectly by increasing the amount of NE available at adrenergic synapses. Any substance that increases the amount of NE in the synaptic cleft will produce

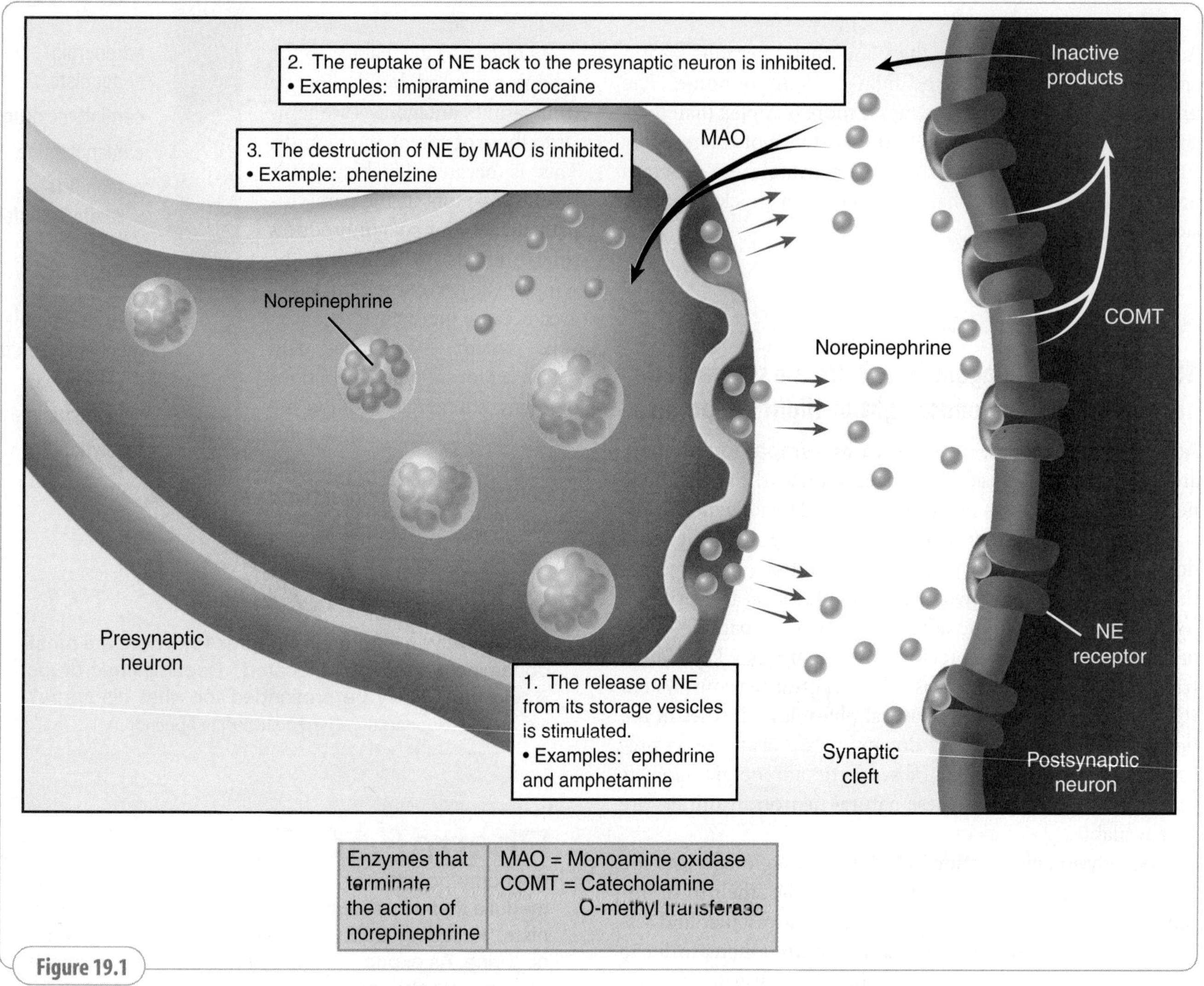

Figure 19.1

Mechanisms of action of adrenergic agonists: (1) stimulation of the release of NE; (2) inhibition of the reuptake of NE; (3) inhibition of the destruction of the NE by MAO..

a more intense and prolonged fight-or-flight response. A few agents, such as ephedrine, act by both direct and indirect mechanisms. The mechanisms of indirect-acting agents are shown in Figure 19.1. The three means by which NE can be increased at the synapse include the following:

- Stimulating the release of NE from its storage vesicles on the presynaptic neuron. Drugs that act by this mechanism include ephedrine and amphetamine.
- Inhibiting the reuptake of NE from the synaptic cleft back to the presynaptic neuron. Examples of drugs that inhibit reuptake of NE include the antidepressant imipramine (Tofranil) and cocaine.
- Inhibiting the destruction of NE by the enzyme monoamine oxidase (MAO). Phenelzine (Nardil) is an example of a MAO inhibitor (MAOI).

Indirect adrenergic agonists are less commonly prescribed than the direct agents due to a higher incidence of potentially serious adverse effects. Some indirect-acting agents such as amphetamine and cocaine are drugs of abuse and are used for their central effects on the brain rather than their autonomic effects.

Classification of Adrenergic Agonists

19.3 Adrenergic agonists may be classified as catecholamines or noncatecholamines.

The first adrenergic agonist to be identified, epinephrine, was isolated from extracts of the adrenal gland in the late 1890s. The chemical structure of epinephrine was found to have an aromatic ring with two OH groups, similar to a common organic chemical known as catechol. Because the molecule also has an NH or amino group, the term **catecholamine** was assigned to epinephrine by physiologists. Several other adrenergic agonists share this core chemical structure, including NE, dopamine, isoproterenol, and dobutamine. This has led to a simple chemical classification of adrenergic agonists as catecholamines or noncatecholamines. Examples of noncatecholamines include phenylephrine, terbutaline, and ephedrine. The fundamental chemical structure of a catecholamine is shown in Figure 19.2.

There are important pharmacokinetic differences between catecholamines and noncatecholamines. As discussed in Chapter 16 catecholamines have a short duration of ac-

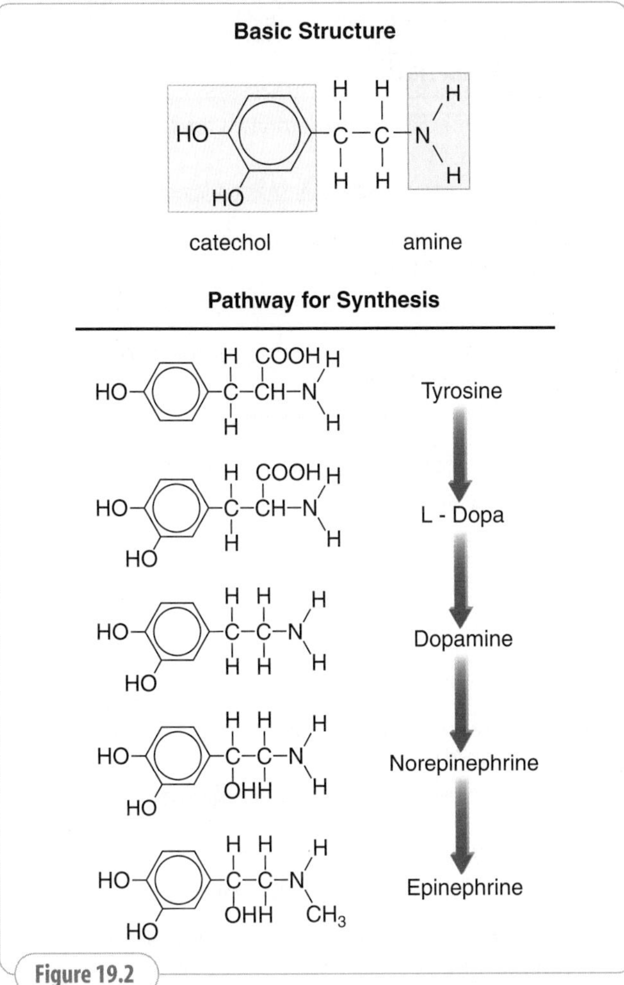

Figure 19.2

Basic chemical structure and synthesis of catecholamines. The synthesis of norepinephrine occurs in the neuron near the neuroeffector junction.

tion because they are destroyed rapidly by the enzymes **monoamine oxidase (MAO)** and **catechol-O-methyltransferase (COMT)**. Because these destructive enzymes are active in the mucosa of the intestinal tract, catecholamines cannot be given PO and must be administered parenterally or by inhalation. The OH groups on the catechol portion of the molecule make these drugs polar, preventing them from crossing the blood–brain barrier.

On the other hand, the noncatecholamines may be taken PO because they are not destroyed as readily by MAO or COMT. This also extends their duration of action. These drugs are less polar than the catecholamines, and they are better able to enter the brain and affect the CNS.

CONNECTION *Checkpoint* 19.2

From what you learned in Chapter 5, how does the polarity of a drug molecule affect its absorption? How does it affect its distribution to tissues? See Answer to Connection Checkpoint 19.2 in Appendix A.

Nonselective Adrenergic Agonists

19.4 The nonselective adrenergic agonists activate both alpha and beta receptors and are used to treat bronchospasm, cardiac arrest, and hypotension.

Although the general actions of adrenergic agonists are predictable, based on their activation of the sympathetic nervous system, the specific effects of each drug are dependent on which receptor subtypes are stimulated. As discussed in Chapter 16 adrenergic receptors include alpha$_1$, alpha$_2$, beta$_1$, and beta$_2$ subtypes. Because the receptor responses are very different and critical to understanding drug action, the student will need to remember the specific subclass(es) of receptors activated by each adrenergic agonist drug. Therapeutic applications for the different receptor activations are summarized as follows:

- Alpha$_1$-receptor agonists: Generally prescribed for the pharmacotherapy of nasal congestion and hypotension. These agents may also be used to produce mydriasis during ophthalmic examinations.
- Alpha$_2$-receptor agonists: These agents are prescribed for the treatment of hypertension (HTN). They act through nonautonomic (centrally acting) mechanisms.
- Beta$_1$-receptor agonists: These agents are critical care drugs used for cardiac arrest, heart failure, and shock due to their powerful effects on the heart.
- Beta$_2$-receptor agonists: These widely used drugs are for treating asthma and reducing preterm labor contractions of the uterus.

Some sympathomimetics are nonselective, stimulating two or more adrenergic receptor subtypes. For example, epinephrine and ephedrine stimulate all four types of adrenergic receptors. In doing so, these agents cause widespread activation of the sympathetic nervous system and an intense fight-or-flight response (and many adverse effects). One of the most important applications of the nonselective adrenergic agonists is for the pharmacotherapy of shock and other life-threatening cardiac disorders.

In certain types of shock, the most serious medical challenge facing the patient is hypotension, which may become so severe as to collapse the circulatory system. In the early stages of shock, the body compensates by activating the sympathetic nervous system; blood pressure is raised and the rate and force of myocardial contraction is increased. These compensatory measures maintain blood flow to vital organs such as the heart and brain, and decrease flow to "less vital" organs, including the kidneys and liver.

The body's ability to compensate for severe shock is limited, however, and profound hypotension may develop as the condition progresses. In minor to moderate shock, fluid replacement agents are agents of choice for raising blood pressure (see Chapter 42). Should fluid replacement agents prove ineffective, however, adrenergic agonists are administered to maintain blood pressure. When given intravenously (IV) these drugs immediately increase blood pressure. Because rapid, intense vasoconstriction can cause serious hypoperfusion of tissues with potential organ damage, these drugs are generally used as a last

TABLE 19.1 Selected Adrenergic Agonists

Drug	Route and Adult Dose (maximum dose where indicated)	Adverse Effects
albuterol (Proventil, Ventolin, Provox)	PO: 2–4 mg tid–qid	*Headache, dizziness, tremor, nervousness, throat irritation, drug tolerance* <u>Tachycardia, dysrhythmias, hypokalemia, hyperglycemia</u>
dobutamine (Dobutrex)	IV: infused at a rate of 2.5–20 mcg/kg/min (max: 40 mcg/kg/min)	*Headache, palpitations, nausea, vomiting, increased heart rate and blood pressure, anginal pain* <u>Dysrhythmias, gangrene, severe HTN</u>
dopamine (Dopastat, Intropin)	IV: 2–5 mcg/kg/min initial dose; may be increased to 20–50 mcg/kg/min	*Headache, palpitations, nausea, vomiting, changes in blood pressure (hypo- or hypertension)* <u>Dysrhythmias, gangrene, severe HTN</u>
ephedrine (Efedron)	For bronchodilation and decongestant: PO: 25–50 mg every 3–4 h prn (max: 150 mg/24 h) IM/IV/subcutaneous: 12.5–25 mg For hypotension: PO: 25 mg 1–4 times/day (max: 150 mg/24 h) IM/subcutaneous/IV: 10–50 mg IM/subcutaneous or 10–25 mg slow IV: may repeat in 5–10 min if necessary (max: 150 mg/24 h)	*Headache, nervousness, palpitations, nausea, vomiting* <u>Dysrhythmias, severe HTN</u>
epinephrine (Adrenalin)	Anaphylaxis: Subcutaneous: 0.1–0.5 mL of 1:1,000 every 10–15 min prn IV; 0.1–0.25 mL of 1:1,000 every 10–15 min	*Headache, palpitations, nausea, vomiting, changes in blood pressure (hypo- or hypertension)* <u>Dysrhythmias, gangrene, severe HTN, pulmonary edema</u>
isoproterenol (Isuprel)	IV: 0.01–0.02 mg prn	*Headache, nervousness, palpitations, tachycardia* <u>Ventricular dysrhythmias, unstable blood pressure</u>
levalbuterol (Xopenex)	Nebulizer: 0.63 mg tid Metered-dose inhaler (MDI): 90 mcg (2 inhalations) every 4–6 h (max: 3.75 mg/day via nebulizer; 12 inhalations [0.54 mg]/day via MDI)	*Headache, dizziness, tremor, nervousness, throat irritation, drug tolerance* <u>Tachycardia, dysrhythmias, hypokalemia, hyperglycemia</u>
midodrine (ProAmatine)	PO: 10 mg tid (max: 20 mg/dose)	*Paresthesia, pruritus* HTN, urinary retention
norepinephrine (Levarterenol, Levophed)	IV: Initial 0.5–1 mcg/min, titrate to response; usual range 8–30 mcg/min	*Restlessness, anxiety, palpitations, nausea, vomiting, headache* <u>Tachycardia or bradycardia (overdose), HTN, hepatic necrosis, cerebral hemorrhage</u>
phenylephrine (Neo-Synephrine, others)	IV: 0.1–0.18 mg/min until blood pressure stabilizes, then 0.04–0.06 mg/min for maintenance	*Palpitations, tingling or coldness of extremities, nervousness* <u>Severe peripheral vasoconstriction, tachycardia or bradycardia (overdose), HTN, dysrhythmias, necrosis at injection site</u>

Note: *Italics* indicate common adverse effects. <u>Underline</u> indicates serious adverse effects.

resort, when safer alternatives have failed to produce the desired therapeutic outcome. Epinephrine, NE, and dopamine are nonselective agents for shock or anaphylaxis when blood pressure and heart rate need to be quickly restored to normal levels. The nonselective adrenergic agonists are shown in Table 19.1.

The nonselective adrenergic agonists generally cause more autonomic-related adverse effects than the selective agents, which are presented in Sections 19.5 through 19.7. Most adverse effects of adrenergic agonists are extensions of their autonomic actions. Cardiovascular effects such as tachycardia, HTN, and dysrhythmias are particularly troublesome and may limit therapy. Blood pressure and heart rate must be monitored continuously during parenteral administration of these agents. Large doses can induce CNS excitement and seizures. Patients with diabetes may experience an increase in blood glucose levels due to an increased breakdown of glycogen in the liver and skeletal muscle. Other adverse effects associated with sympathetic activation include dry mouth, nausea, and vomiting.

Amphetamine is a nonselective adrenergic agonist with a marked CNS stimulant effect. Amphetamine also causes anorexia, which has led its historical use as an appetite suppressant. Because of prominent cardiovascular adverse effects and the risk of physical dependence, the drug is no longer prescribed for weight loss. Additional details on amphetamine may be found in Chapters 8 and 28.

PROTOTYPE DRUG Epinephrine (Adrenalin)

Classification: **Therapeutic:** Antishock and antianaphylaxis agent, bronchodilator

Pharmacologic: Nonselective adrenergic agonist, catecholamine

Therapeutic Effects and Uses: Epinephrine has several therapeutic applications, all of which result from adrenergic receptor activation. It can be administered parenterally, topically, by inhalation, or by instillation.

Epinephrine is a drug of choice in cardiopulmonary resuscitation. Given as an IV infusion or by intracardiac injection, the drug has the ability to restore cardiac rhythm almost immediately. Epinephrine also constricts arterioles, raising cerebral and cardiac perfusion pressure, which discourages cardiovascular collapse. The intracardiac route is used only under extreme conditions, usually during open cardiac massage, or when no other route is possible.

Epinephrine can reverse many of the distressing symptoms of anaphylaxis within minutes. Almost immediately after injection, blood pressure increases due to stimulation of $alpha_1$ receptors. Activation of $beta_2$ receptors in the bronchi dilates the airways to relieve shortness of breath. Epinephrine can also be administered by inhalation, which can terminate acute bronchospasm almost immediately.

Epinephrine is sometimes added to cartridges of local anesthetics to cause vasoconstriction of local vessels. This forces the anesthetic to remain localized in the tissues for a longer period, prolonging analgesia and slowing the absorption of anesthetic. Epinephrine can also be applied topically to control superficial bleeding along a surgical incision. Repeated injection or application to the same site can result in tissue necrosis due to the diminished blood supply to the area.

Ophthalmic administration of epinephrine causes mydriasis and the outflow of fluid from the anterior chamber of the eye, making the drug an adjunct to the pharmacotherapy of open-angle glaucoma. Intranasal administration can be used to reduce nasal congestion.

Mechanism of Action: Epinephrine is a nonselective adrenergic agonist, stimulating both alpha- and beta-adrenergic receptors throughout the body. Actions typical of the fight-or-flight response are induced.

Pharmacokinetics:

Route(s)	Subcutaneous, IV, intramuscular (IM), inhalation, topical, ophthalmic
Absorption	Not absorbed PO; minimal absorption by inhalation; rapidly absorbed by IM and subcutaneous routes
Distribution	Widely distributed; does not cross the blood–brain barrier; crosses the placenta; secreted in breast milk
Primary metabolism	Rapidly metabolized by MAO and COMT in the liver and most tissues
Primary excretion	Small amount excreted unchanged in the kidneys
Onset of action	Subcutaneous: 3–5 minutes; IM: 5–10 minutes; inhalation: 1 minute (for local respiratory effects); and IV: immediate onset
Duration of action	1–4 h

Adverse Effects: The most common adverse effects of epinephrine are nervousness, tremors, palpitations, tachycardia, dizziness, headache, and stinging at the site of application. Serious adverse effects include HTN, dysrhythmias, pulmonary edema, and cardiac arrest. Intense CNS stimulation may occur in patients with preexisting psychiatric disorders, including hallucinations, panic attacks, and aggression. Extravasation of epinephrine can produce an injection site reaction, causing severe tissue damage and necrosis.

Contraindications/Precautions: Contraindications for epinephrine include hypersensitivity to other adrenergic agonists, closed-angle glaucoma, severe shock (other than anaphylaxis), and dysrhythmias. The drug should be used with caution in patients with coronary artery disease because intense angina symptoms may result. Due to its ability to relax uterine smooth muscle, epinephrine will delay labor. Patients with hyperthyroidism or HTN are more sensitive to the effects of administered epinephrine (and other catecholamines). In life-threatening conditions such as anaphylaxis or cardiac arrest, there are no absolute contraindications for the use of epinephrine. Special precautions regarding the administration of epinephrine are given in Table 19.2.

Drug Interactions: Epinephrine may result in hypotension if used with phenothiazines or oxytocin. There may be additive cardiovascular effects if epinephrine is concurrently used with other sympathomimetics. MAO inhibitors, tricyclic antidepressants, and alpha- and beta-adrenergic agents inhibit the actions of epinephrine. Epinephrine will decrease the effects of beta blockers. Digoxin and some general anesthetics may sensitize the heart to the effects of epinephrine. Two drugs used for Parkinson's disease, entacapone and tolcapone, are inhibitors

TABLE 19.2 Precautions for Administering Epinephrine

Route of Administration	Precautions
Inhalation	Keep the patient sitting upright when using an aerosol medication. This allows administration of a fine mist and minimizes the risk of overdose from large droplets that can occur when the patient reclines.
	Advise the patient to rinse the mouth and throat with water immediately after inhalation to avoid swallowing any residual medication. Ingesting this drug could result in both epigastric pain and systemic effects.
	Avoid administration of isoproterenol concurrently with epinephrine. Allow at least a 4-hour interval between drug usage.
Instillation	Prevent the drug from entering the throat by instilling nose drops with the head in lateral, head-low position.
	Teach the patient to prevent contamination of the drug solution with nasal secretions by rinsing the spray tip or dropper with hot water after each use.
Ophthalmic	Remove contact lenses before using eyedrops.
	Teach the patient how to apply gentle pressure against the nasolacrimal duct with the finger for at least 1 or 2 min immediately after using the eyedrops. This will help prevent excessive systemic absorption.
	Teach the patient that if using separate solutions of epinephrine and a topical miotic, the miotic should be instilled 2–10 min before epinephrine because the conjunctival sac has limited capacity.
Subcutaneous	Use a tuberculin syringe to accurately measure parenteral doses.
	Protect the epinephrine injection from exposure to light at all times. Keep the ampule or vial in the carton until ready to use.
	Mix the drug particles in the suspension by vigorously shaking the vial or ampule before withdrawing epinephrine into a syringe. Inject promptly.
	Aspirate carefully before injecting epinephrine because IV injection of usual subcutaneous doses can cause sudden HTN and even cerebral hemorrhage.
	Rotate injection sites and observe for blanching. Tissue necrosis can result from vascular constriction with repeated injections in one site.
Intravenous	Verify with the prescriber the accurate rate of intravenous injection to neonates, infants, and children.
	Understand dosages: 1:1,000 solution contains 1 mg/1 mL; 1:10,000 solution contains 0.1 mg/1 mL.

of COMT, the enzyme that degrades epinephrine; concurrent use may cause increased effects of epinephrine on the heart and blood pressure. **Herbal/Food:** None known.

Pregnancy: Category C.

Treatment of Overdose: Overdose of epinephrine is life-threatening and the immediate administration of an alpha- or beta-adrenergic blocker is indicated. If blood pressure remains high, a direct vasodilator may be administered.

Nursing Responsibilities:

- Determine the reason the patient is receiving the medication and focus nursing assessments on the underlying problem prompting the administration of the drug.
- Assess the patient for preexisting conditions that may warrant cautious use of epinephrine, which include HTN, angina, and other cardiovascular conditions.
- Establish baseline vital signs, including heart rate, respiratory rate, and blood pressure.
- If patient is receiving epinephrine to circumvent anaphylactic or hypersensitivity reaction, closely monitor the respiratory status for impending signs of distress such as wheezing, air hunger, dyspnea, or orthopnea. Administer oxygen as indicated.
- Use a cardiac monitor with patients receiving epinephrine by the IV route. Keep full resuscitation equipment readily available for emergencies.
- Monitor blood pressure closely during the first 5 minutes of IV administration of epinephrine, and continue to take measurements every 3 to 5 minutes until stable.
- Inform the prescriber of marked changes in intake and output ratio.
- When epinephrine is administered to patients with diabetes, monitor for hypoglycemia.
- Examine ocular and nasal mucosa when epinephrine solution is used. Do not administer if excoriation is present.

Patient and Family Education:

- Expect slight stinging or burning with intranasal application.
- Take ophthalmic drugs at bedtime to minimize blurred vision and sensitivity to light, especially if you have glaucoma.
- Expect some transitory stinging after beginning ophthalmic administration. Headache and brow ache are frequent early

adverse effects but will usually subside with continued use. Notify the health care provider if symptoms persist.

- If prone to severe hypersensitivity reactions due to insect stings or other allergens, give epinephrine subcutaneously. Always keep medication and equipment available for home emergency and consult the health care provider as needed.
- Observe for signs of hypersensitivity and discontinue epinephrine eyedrops if itching, discharge, swelling of eyelids, or crusted eyelids occur.
- When inhaled epinephrine is administered for hypersensitivity reactions, report symptoms that are not relieved within 20 minutes or that become worse following inhalation.
- Inhaled epinephrine can reduce bronchial secretions, making removal of mucus more difficult.

Drugs Similar to Epinephrine (Adrenalin)

Other nonselective adrenergic agonists include dopamine, ephedrine, and NE.

Dopamine (Dopastat, Intropin): Approved as a drug in 1974, dopamine is a naturally occurring catecholamine that has both alpha- and beta-agonist activity. At low doses (1–5 mcg/kg/minute), the drug selectively stimulates dopaminergic receptors, especially in the kidneys, leading to vasodilation, increased renal blood flow, and enhanced urine output. This makes dopamine of particular value in hypovolemic and cardiogenic shock. Whenever possible, hypovolemia is corrected with fluid expanding agents before starting a dopamine infusion. At higher doses (more than 10 mcg/kg/minute), dopamine stimulates $beta_1$-adrenergic receptors, causing the heart to beat more forcefully, thus increasing cardiac output. Also at higher doses, dopamine stimulates $alpha_1$-adrenergic receptors, thus causing vasoconstriction and increased blood pressure. It is administered by the IV route and has a brief 10-minute duration of action. Doses are slowly increased until the desired therapeutic effects have been achieved; vital signs should be monitored continuously during the infusion. Headache, nausea, and vomiting are common adverse effects. High doses can produce ventricular tachycardia. Severe necrosis or gangrene can result if extravasation occurs. Phentolamine is the antidote for extravasation of dopamine and should be readily available. Dopamine is pregnancy category C.

Ephedrine (Efedron): Although approved by the U.S. Food and Drug Administration (FDA) in 1939, ephedra has been used to treat various ailments for thousands of years. Ephedrine is a noncatecholamine, originally obtained from the **ephedra** plant species, that activates both alpha and beta receptors. The drug acts by two mechanisms: directly, by binding to adrenergic receptors, and indirectly, by causing the release of NE from storage vesicles. Ephedrine has been used for its ability to relieve respiratory congestion caused by allergies and to prevent bronchospasm in patients with asthma. It is available by the PO, topical, and parenteral routes, readily absorbed from the GI tract, and crosses the blood–brain barrier. Once in the brain, ephedrine exhibits prominent stimulatory effects, keeping patients alert and awake. This CNS action has been used to treat patients with narcolepsy, a disease characterized by sudden, unexpected sleep attacks. The CNS stimulation has also been used to alleviate the CNS depression caused by opioid or barbiturate overdose. This stimulatory effect of ephedrine is also the cause of the major adverse effects of the drug such as nervousness, insomnia, palpitations, and tachycardia. Like the closely related drug pseudoephedrine, ephedrine is highly regulated because it can be used to make methamphetamine. This drug is pregnancy category C.

Norepinephrine (Levarterenol, Levophed, Noradrenaline): Approved in 1938, NE is a nonselective catecholamine that has effects similar to epinephrine, except that is does not activate $beta_2$ receptors. Approved to treat shock and hypotension, NE acts directly on alpha-adrenergic receptors in vascular smooth muscle to immediately raise blood pressure. It also stimulates $beta_1$ receptors in the heart to increase cardiac output. It is given by the IV route and has a duration of only 1 to 2 minutes after the infusion is terminated. Because NE is a powerful vasoconstrictor, continuous monitoring of blood pressure is required to avoid HTN. When first administered, reflex bradycardia is sometimes experienced, and the drug has the ability to produce various dysrhythmias. Blurred vision and photophobia are signs of overdose. Like other drugs in this class, NE produces symptoms of CNS stimulation such as nervousness, insomnia, and confusion. Severe tissue necrosis can result if extravasation occurs; thus phentolamine should be readily available. The primary indications for NE are acute shock and cardiac arrest. This drug is pregnancy category C.

CONNECTIONS

Patient Safety

Proper Use of the EpiPen®

The EpiPen® is an autoinjector containing epinephrine that is used to prevent and treat anaphylaxis and severe allergic reactions to insect stings, foods, or drugs. The device is easy to operate, although the word *auto* sometimes gives people a false sense of security. An Australian study in 2007 reported that of 100 hospital-based pediatricians, only 2 were able to demonstrate the correct way to administer the drug using the EpiPen® (Mehr, Robinson, & Tang, 2007). Even after reading instructions, only 40% got most of the steps right. In 37% of cases, epinephrine would not have reached the patient's circulation.

The nurse has a key responsibility in teaching parents and older children the correct use of the EpiPen®. The following is important safety information regarding this device.

- Exert sufficient pressure to activate the EpiPen®.
- Hold the device in place for 5 to 10 seconds.
- The EpiPen® is designed for a single injection; discard after use, preferably in a hospital emergency department or health care provider's office.
- The EpiPen® is not a replacement for proper medical care; seek emergency treatment as soon as possible.
- Check the expiration date often and replace when needed.
- Keep the EpiPen® in a cool, dark place; refrigeration is not recommended.

CONNECTIONS

To the Community Methamphetamine: When a Good Drug Goes Bad

For years consumers have relied on over-the-counter (OTC) medications containing pseudoephedrine. Typically this nasal decongestant relieved sneezing and runny noses for people with allergies and colds. Now this medication has found a new place in the community: in methamphetamine (meth) laboratories.

Drug dealers and addicts have discovered that they can combine pseudoephedrine with drain cleaner, iodine crystals, and the strike pad on a matchbox to "cook" methamphetamine, commonly known as "crystal meth." Supplies for a meth laboratory can cost as little as $50.

Though useful to allergy sufferers, pseudoephedrine faces removal from the market due to its use in meth laboratories. The Drug Enforcement Administration (DEA) reported 5,456 arrests for methamphetamine violations in 2004. Senator Craig Estes proposed Senate Bill 107 to prohibit OTC sales of medications containing single-entity forms of pseudoephedrine such as Sudafed. When pseudoephedrine is not the single active ingredient, such as in liquid and gel capsule forms, sales will be permitted OTC because pseudoephedrine is not extractable from non–starch-based drugs. Keeping pseudoephedrine behind the counter limits illegitimate use in meth laboratories.

Methamphetamine, a strongly addictive and destructive drug, has great potential for abuse. Nurses need to be aware of the widespread incidence of meth addiction as related to pseudoephedrine. Symptoms include physical deterioration with increased heart rate and blood pressure. Users have increased confidence, sex drive, talkativeness, and energy. Many negative physical and psychological effects occur. Over time addiction may result in brain damage and emaciation, tooth decay, and psychosis.

Another community concern is that the toxic fumes from a meth laboratory can cause asphyxiation and even death due to explosion and fire. Families and children in the neighborhood can be adversely affected. Cleanup of toxic meth laboratories presents an environmental challenge and is expensive. When the toxic by-products are poured down the home drain or onto soil in the home yard, severe and far-reaching environmental damage can occur.

Alpha-Adrenergic Agonists

19.5 Alpha-adrenergic agonists are used to relieve nasal decongestion and elevate blood pressure.

Activation of alpha-adrenergic receptors causes a number of important physiological responses, most of which relate to contraction of vascular smooth muscle. Like the nonselective adrenergic agonists, several of the selective alpha agonists are used to treat hypotension associated with shock and other critical care conditions. Alpha agonists may also be administered to treat patients who are susceptible to orthostatic hypotension. The alpha-adrenergic agonists are shown in Table 19.2.

A second application of alpha-adrenergic agonists is for the treatment of nasal congestion. During upper respiratory infections or allergic rhinitis, arterioles in the nose dilate and produce excess mucus. Alpha$_1$ agonists relieve nasal congestion by causing vasoconstriction of vessels serving the nasal mucosa. Intranasal agents such as phenylephrine work within minutes and are highly effective at clearing the nasal passages of mucus. Oral decongestants such as ephedrine take longer to act but are less damaging to the nasal mucosa. The pharmacotherapy of upper respiratory congestion is presented in Chapter 74.

Topical instillation of alpha$_1$ agonists to the eye has two applications. Alpha$_1$-adrenergic receptors are present on the radial muscle of the iris. When these receptors are activated, the radial muscle contracts and the pupil dilates, allowing the health care provider to better examine the interior structures of the eye. Although the alpha$_1$ agonists are effective at producing mydriasis, they are generally not drugs of choice for ophthalmic exams. Another ophthalmic application of alpha$_1$ agonists is to relieve conjunctival congestion and redness. The mechanism behind this effect is through alpha$_1$-receptor activation of arterioles in the eye, causing vasoconstriction. Tetrahydrozoline (Tyzine) is the primary drug in this class used for minor eye irritation and redness. The pharmacotherapy of ophthalmic conditions is discussed in detail in Chapter 77.

Most adverse effects of the apha$_1$-adrenergic agonists are extensions of their autonomic actions. Should extravasation occur, intense local vasoconstriction can lead to tissue necrosis. Systemically, their intense vasoconstrictive effect can lead to HTN. In addition, the increase in blood pressure caused by the alpha$_1$ agonists can activate the baroreceptor reflex, causing reflex bradycardia. If necessary, bradycardia can be prevented or reversed by administration of an anticholinergic agent such as atropine. Major adverse effects or overdose with drugs in this class may be treated by administering a specific alpha-adrenergic antagonist such as phentolamine. Because of the potential for cardiovascular adverse effects, patients should be continuously monitored when receiving high doses or infusions of these drugs.

Activation of alpha$_2$-adrenergic receptors produces very different responses than alpha$_1$ activation. The most important responses to alpha$_2$-receptor agonists occur in the brain rather than the peripheral nervous system. Unlike alpha$_1$ agonists, which increase sympathetic nervous system activity, alpha$_2$ agonists that act in the CNS decrease sympathetic activity. Because they decrease blood pressure, their primary therapeutic application is for the treatment of HTN. The alpha$_2$-adrenergic agonists are discussed in greater detail in Chapter 20, because they produce actions and therapeutic effects similar to adrenergic antagonists.

PROTOTYPE DRUG Phenylephrine (Neo-Synephrine)

Classification: **Therapeutic:** Antihypotensive, nasal decongestant
Pharmacologic: Alpha-adrenergic agonist

Therapeutic Effects and Uses: Approved in 1938, the actions and indications of phenylephrine are predictable extensions of its sympathetic activation. Parenteral administration can prevent or reverse acute hypotension caused by spinal anesthesia or vascular shock. Its longer duration of activity and lack of significant cardiac adverse effects gives phenylephrine some advantages over epinephrine or NE in treating acute hypotension. Unlike epinephrine, which markedly increases the heart rate, phenylephrine tends to slow the heart rate probably due to reflex bradycardia. In situations in which reflex bradycardia is undesirable, this action may be blocked by the administration of atropine.

In addition to its use in critical care and surgical situations, phenylephrine is available as ophthalmic and nasal solutions. Applied topically to the eye during ophthalmic examinations, phenylephrine can dilate the pupil, without causing significant cycloplegia. When applied intranasally by spray or drops, it reduces nasal congestion by constricting small blood vessels in the nasal mucosa.

One advantage of phenylephrine is that this drug cannot be used as a precursor molecule to synthesize methamphetamine. Because of this, phenylephrine has begun to replace pseudoephedrine in OTC cold and sinus remedies. Formulations containing phenylephrine are exempt from regulations in most states that require pseudoephedrine products to be kept behind the pharmacy counter.

Mechanism of Action: Phenylephrine directly activates alpha$_1$-adrenergic receptors in the peripheral nervous system. It has weak beta-adrenergic activity at high doses, but this is usually not of clinical significance.

Pharmacokinetics:

Route(s)	Intramuscular (IM), subcutaneous, IV, intranasal, and ophthalmic solutions
Absorption	Not absorbed in the GI tract; well absorbed when given IM or subcutaneous
Distribution	Unknown
Primary metabolism	Hepatic by monoamine oxidase (MAO)
Primary excretion	Unknown
Onset of action	Subcutaneous/IM: 10–15 minutes; IV: immediate
Duration of action	Subcutaneous/IM: 30–120 minutes; IV: 15–20 minutes

Adverse Effects: Phenylephrine causes few serious adverse effects when taken by the PO, intranasal, or ophthalmic routes. Common adverse effects with intranasal phenylephrine use include stinging of the nasal mucosa, sneezing, and rebound congestion. Ophthalmic use can cause narrow-angle glaucoma or photophobia. Parenteral use can lead to symptoms of CNS stimulation such as anxiety, restlessness, and tremor. Serious adverse effects include reflex bradycardia and reduced blood flow to peripheral tissues due to severe vasoconstriction. OTC cough and cold products containing phenylephrine or pseudoephedrine should not be given to children under age 2 because overdose has caused serious illness and several infant deaths.

Contraindications/Precautions: Phenylephrine is contraindicated in patients with severe HTN, because the drug will raise blood pressure to dangerous levels. Because it causes reflex bradycardia, patients with preexisting bradycardia should not receive phenylephrine. Phenylephrine causes vasoconstriction, which can reduce coronary blood flow in patients with advanced coronary artery disease, causing angina attacks. Phenylephrine also reduces the effectiveness of nitrates such as nitroglycerin that are taken to prevent anginal episodes. Because of its effects on the eye, it should not be administered to patients with narrow-angle glaucoma. Phenylephrine should be used with caution in patients with hyperthyroidism or diabetes because these patients are more sensitive to the potential cardiac adverse effects.

Drug Interactions: Phenylephrine will reduce the effectiveness of antihypertensive medications. A hypertensive crisis may occur in patients receiving MAOIs; phenylephrine should not be administered within 21 days of a MAOI. Increased effects of phenylephrine may occur in patients taking ergot alkaloids and tricyclic antidepressants. Additive effects may occur if phenylephrine is given concurrently with other adrenergic agonists, including amphetamines or cocaine. Concurrent administration with oxytocin during the postpartum period may cause persistent HTN. Concurrent use with halothane or digoxin may increase the risk of dysrhythmias. **Herbal/Food**: Phenylephrine should be used with caution with St. John's wort because this herb has MAO-like activity. Ingestion of substances with high amounts of caffeine will worsen the CNS stimulation caused by phenylephrine.

Pregnancy: Category C.

Treatment of Overdose: When given by the parenteral route, overdose will result in HTN and possible dysrhythmias. Phentolamine is a specific alpha antagonist that can be used to lower blood pressure, and antidysrhythmic agents may be indicated.

Nursing Responsibilities:

- Determine the reason the patient is receiving the medication and focus nursing assessments on the underlying problem prompting the administration of the drug.
- Assess the patient for preexixting conditions that may warrant cautious use of phenylephrine, which include HTN, angina, and other cardiovascular conditions, as well as hyperthyroidism and glaucoma.
- Establish baseline vital signs, including heart rate, respiratory rate, and blood pressure.
- Examine IV sites frequently to assess for extravasation because parenteral administration can cause tissue necrosis.
- Monitor vital signs frequently during parenteral administration and report HTN (systolic blood pressure higher than 140 mmHg) or bradycardia (heart rate less than 60 beats per minute) to the prescriber.
- Advise the patient to remove contact lenses before ophthalmic administration because phenylephrine may damage soft contact lenses.
- Advise the patient to wear dark eye protection after ophthalmic administration to avoid pain due to pupillary dilation.

Patient and Family Education:

- Carefully read and follow the instructions provided with the drug, if using OTC products that contain phenylephrine.
- Do not give the drug to infants and children unless directed by a health care provider because children are especially sensitive to the effects of phenylephrine.

- Do not use OTC products containing this drug unless specifically prescribed by the health care provider if you have cardiovascular disease or hyperthyroidism.
- Do not share the nasal spray container with other people to prevent spread of infection.
- Do not use decongestant nasal sprays for longer than 3 days without approval of the health care provider. Do not use more of it and do not use it more often than directed.
- Report symptoms of excessive use of this drug, such as rapid, irregular, or pounding heartbeat, nervousness, or insomnia.
- Limit or eliminate the use of caffeine-containing foods and beverages because these can cause excessive nervousness, insomnia, and tremors.

Drugs Similar to Phenylephrine (Neo-Synephrine)

Most agents with predominant alpha-adrenergic agonist activity can be grouped into subclasses based on their indications: intranasal or ocular decongestants. Midodrine is an alpha agonist that does not fit into these subclasses. Another drug in this class, methoxamine (Vasoxyl), is no longer available in the United States.

Intranasal decongestants: Oxymetazoline (Afrin), pseudoephedrine (Sudafed), xylometazoline (Neo-Synephrine II, Long-acting), and tetrahydrozoline (Tyzine) are given by the intranasal route to diminish nasal congestion due to allergies and the common cold. Use of these agents is generally limited to 3 to 5 days. With continued use of these drugs congestion may worsen, a phenomenon known as rebound congestion. Although these drugs may also have some beta-adrenergic activity, they are only used for their effects on alpha-adrenergic receptors in the nasal mucosa. Pharmacotherapy with these agents is presented in Chapter 74.

Pseudoephedrine is an intranasal decongestant that deserves special attention because of its potential for misuse. Pseudoephedrine is the starting chemical for the synthesis of illegal methamphetamine by drug traffickers. Most states have enacted laws to regulate the sale of solid tablet formulations containing pseudoephedrine, requiring that pseudoephedrine be placed behind the pharmacy counter so that only pharmacists can provide the product. Most states also require the pharmacist to record the name and address of the buyer. It should be noted that these precautions are not being taken because pseudoephedrine itself is a dangerous drug, but to limit the availability of the drug to illicit makers of methamphetamine. A prototype feature for pseudoephedrine can be found in Chapter 74.

Ocular decongestants: Naphazoline (Naphcon, ClearEyes), oxymetazoline (Afrin 12 hour), and tetrahydrozoline (Visine) are available as ophthalmic solutions to relieve redness due to minor eye irritations, such as those caused by the common cold, swimming, allergies, or contact lenses. These agents act by constricting arteries in the conjunctiva. Other than local stinging, they rarely cause adverse effects. Pharmacotherapy with these agents is presented in Chapter 77.

Midodrine (ProAmatine): Approved in 1996, midodrine is an $alpha_1$ agonist given PO for the symptomatic treatment of orthostatic hypotension. The drug increases standing, sitting, and supine systolic and diastolic blood pressure. The most common adverse effects are paresthesia, goosebumps, dysuria, and pruritus of the scalp. Supine HTN can occur in as many as 13% of the patients taking the drug. The nurse should monitor for signs of supine HTN, including pounding sensations in the ears or chest, blurred vision, and headache. Because of its marked effects on the cardiovascular system, midodrine is contraindicated in patients with heart failure, severe cardiac disease, or excessive supine HTN. The drug is pregnancy category C.

CONNECTION *Checkpoint* 19.3

Parenteral phenylephrine can cause reflex bradycardia. From what you learned in Chapter 18, would the administration of an anticholinergic such as atropine improve or worsen this condition? See Answer to Connection Checkpoint 19.3 in Appendix A.

Beta-Adrenergic Agonists

19.6 Beta-adrenergic agonists are used to treat asthma, shock, heart failure, and other cardiac disorders.

Activation of beta-adrenergic receptors can produce a wide variety of physiological responses, depending on the location of the receptor and which subtype is stimulated. Some beta-adrenergic agonists affect both receptor subtypes, whereas others are selective for either $beta_1$ or $beta_2$. The indications for the $beta_1$ activators are very different from those of the $beta_2$ activators. Because of these differences, the receptor subtypes are considered separately.

$Beta_1$-adrenergic agonists: $Beta_1$-adrenergic receptors are more limited in distribution throughout the body than $alpha_1$ receptors. Pharmacologically, the most significant site having $beta_1$ receptors is cardiac muscle. Activation of $beta_1$ receptors results in cardiac actions typical of the fight-or-flight response: heart rate, force of contraction, and velocity of impulse conduction through the myocardium all increase. These cardiac effects may be considered beneficial or adverse, depending on the condition of the patient and the therapeutic goals.

Most drugs with $beta_1$-agonist activity are nonselective and have the ability to activate other receptor subtypes. For example, although epinephrine affects all receptor subtypes, its $beta_1$ activation is crucial in stimulating the heart to regain sinus rhythm following cardiac arrest. Similarly, although NE also activates alpha receptors, its $beta_1$-agonist effects are useful in treating cardiac arrest. Dopamine is somewhat unique in that its effects are dose-dependent. At low doses the drug activates dopamine receptors, and at moderate doses it stimulates both $beta_1$ and dopamine receptors. At high doses dopamine activates all three receptor types: dopamine, alpha, and $beta_1$.

Drugs used for their $beta_1$-agonist actions are sometimes called **cardiotonic drugs** because they increase the force of contraction of the heart. In the treatment of cardiac failure or shock, they are administered to increase cardiac output. Another name applied to these drugs is **inotropic agents,** because they reverse the cardiac symptoms of shock by increasing the strength of myocardial contraction.

Drugs with significant $beta_1$-adrenergic agonist activity include dobutamine and isoproterenol. Epinephrine, dopamine, and NE have significant $beta_1$-agonist activity, in addition to alpha-agonist activity. These drugs are presented in Section 19.4.

$Beta_2$-adrenergic agonists: $Beta_2$-adrenergic receptors are more widely distributed than $beta_1$ receptors. Pharmacologically, the most important site is in the lung, where activation of $beta_2$ receptors leads to relaxation of bronchial smooth muscle. $Beta_2$-adrenergic agonists, commonly referred to as bronchodilators, are used extensively in the treatment of asthma and other pulmonary disorders. The following discussion is limited to autonomic bronchodilators; information on other classes of drugs used in the pharmacotherapy of asthma is presented in Chapter 73.

Autonomic drugs used as bronchodilators include nonselective adrenergic agonists, as well as those that are selective for $beta_2$ receptors. Epinephrine is the best example of a nonselective agent that is an effective bronchodilator. Unfortunately, epinephrine exhibits a high incidence of adverse effects, such as HTN and dysrhythmias, due to its stimulation of multiple receptor subtypes throughout the body. Likewise, isoproterenol is an effective bronchodilator; however, it also affects $beta_1$ receptors, which increases its potential for producing cardiovascular adverse effects. Selective $beta_2$ agonists were developed to minimize these adverse effects. Selective $beta_2$ agonists such as albuterol and salmeterol have become first-line drugs in the pharmacotherapy of asthma and other conditions characterized by bronchospasm. A drug prototype feature for albuterol can be found in Chapter 73.

When given for asthma, $beta_2$ agonists are administered by either the inhalation or PO route. Inhalation administration of these agents relieves acute bronchospasm within minutes. Some of the inhaled $beta_2$ agonists, such as albuterol and pirbuterol, have a rapid onset; however their duration of action is only 3 to 5 hours. Others such as salmeterol have somewhat longer onsets of action, but their effects can last up to 12 hours. The specific agent of choice and dosage schedule is individualized for the particular pattern of asthma exhibited by each patient.

Only two $beta_2$ agonists, albuterol and terbutaline, are available by the PO route. An extended release form of albuterol (Proventil Repetabs) allows for the convenience of twice a day dosing. Terbutaline (Brethine) is given 3 or 4 times per day. Because the oral (PO) forms take up to 30 minutes to act, they are not indicated for the relief of acute bronchospasm.

A second therapeutic application of $beta_2$ agonists is for the treatment of preterm labor contractions. Activation of $beta_2$ receptors in uterine smooth muscle relaxes uterine smooth muscle, leading to a delay in labor. This delay allows for additional maturation of the organ systems of the fetus, which increases the probability of neonatal survival. Terbutaline and ritodrine are the only beta agonists used for this purpose. Drugs used to delay preterm labor are called **tocolytics** and are discussed in Chapter 71.

Adverse effects of the $beta_2$ agonists are predictable extensions of their autonomic activation. Tachycardia, palpitations, flushing, insomnia, and tremor are possible adverse effects with all $beta_2$ agonists. The oral forms have some $beta_1$ activity; thus systemic adverse effects are more common than the inhaled drugs, which act locally and produce few systemic adverse effects. Beta agonists should be used cautiously in patients with dysrhythmias or heart failure. These drugs will antagonize the actions of beta-adrenergic blockers.

PROTOTYPE DRUG Isoproterenol (Isuprel)

Classification: **Therapeutic:** Bronchodilator
Pharmacologic: Nonselective beta-adrenergic agonist

Therapeutic Effects and Uses: Isoproterenol is a catecholamine that has been available for over 50 years. It is available by the inhalation, sublingual, or IV routes, activating both $beta_1$- and $beta_2$-adrenergic receptors, but with little effect on alpha receptors. When given IV, isoproterenol immediately activates $beta_1$ receptors to increase the strength of myocardial contraction and improve cardiac output. The cardiac actions of isoproterenol are used to advantage in the pharmacotherapy of cardiogenic or bacteremic shock, cardiac arrest, Adams-Stokes syndrome, and certain types of ventricular dysrhythmias. Dobutamine has largely replaced isoproterenol as a cardiac agent, because it is more specific to $beta_1$ receptors in the heart.

Isoproterenol was once a drug of choice for asthma pharmacotherapy due to its bronchodilation effects caused by activation of $beta_2$ receptors in the airways. The development of selective $beta_2$ agonists with fewer cardiac adverse effects has led to a significant decline in the use of isoproterenol as an antiasthmatic agent. This drug is no longer available via inhalation devices. Other types of acute bronchospasm, such as that caused by anesthesia, may be reversed by IV isoproterenol.

Mechanism of Action: Isoproterenol is a potent activator of both $beta_1$- and $beta_2$-adrenergic receptors throughout the body.

Pharmacokinetics:

Route(s)	IV
Absorption	N/A
Distribution	Distributed to most tissues; it is unknown if it crosses the placenta or is secreted in breast milk
Primary metabolism	Hepatic by COMT and MAO
Primary excretion	Renal: 40–50% unchanged
Onset of action	Immediate
Duration of action	Less than 1 h

Adverse Effects: Adverse effects of isoproterenol are predictable based on its activation of beta-adrenergic receptors. Common adverse effects include headache, nausea, vomiting, and symptoms of CNS stimulation such as tremors, anxiety, and insomnia. Adverse effects affecting the heart include serious dysrhythmias.

Contraindications/Precautions: Because isoproterenol increases the myocardial workload, it should be used with extreme caution in patients with severe cardiac disease, dysrhythmias, or HTN. The drug should be used with caution in patients with hyperthyroidism or diabetes because these patients are more sensitive to the potential cardiac adverse effects.

Drug Interactions: Concurrent administration with a beta-adrenergic blocker diminishes the bronchodilation effect of isoproterenol and may induce bronchospasm in patients with asthma. Use with other bronchodilators or adrenergic agonists such as epinephrine or dopamine may result in additive effects. MAOIs and tricyclic antidepressants should be discontinued at least 2 weeks prior to isoproterenol therapy to avoid possible hypertensive crisis. Isoproterenol should not be concurrently administered with potassium-wasting diuretics because hypokalemia may result. Isoproterenol may lower serum levels of digoxin and induce dysrhythmias.

Pregnancy: Category C.

Treatment of Overdose: Overdose with isoproterenol will cause tachycardia and other dysrhythmias. Blood pressure usually falls. Due to the relatively short half-life of the drug, discontinuing the infusion is often enough to reverse symptoms, although supportive cardiac drugs may be necessary.

Nursing Responsibilities:

- Determine the reason the patient is receiving the medication and focus nursing assessments on the underlying problem prompting the administration of the drug.
- Assess the patient for preexisting conditions that may warrant cautious use of isoproterenol, which include cardiac disease, dysrhythmias, HTN, hyperthyroidism, or diabetes mellitus.
- Assess for therapeutic effectiveness through improvement in vital signs and urine flow, perfusion of vital organs as evidenced by improved skin color, warming of extremities, adequate nail bed capillary filling and return, and the return of mental clarity with decreased confusion.
- Establish baseline vital signs, including heart rate, respiratory rate, and blood pressure.
- Check the pulse before and during IV administration. A rate greater than 110 usually indicates a need to slow the infusion rate or the discontinue the infusion. Consult the prescriber for guidelines.
- Monitor for drug tolerance to the bronchodilation effect and cardiac stimulant effect with prolonged use.

Patient and Family Education:

- Notify the health care provider of any of the following diseases: asthma, diabetes mellitus, overactive thyroid, and pheochromocytoma.
- Notify the health care provider of all of the medications that you are currently taking, including nutritional supplements and OTC medicines.
- Notify the health care provider because these chemicals may interfere with the effectiveness of isoproterenol, if a frequent user of caffeinated beverages, alcohol, or illegal drugs.
- Report the following adverse effects immediately because the dosage may require adjustment: palpitations; a disproportionate rise in diastolic pressure (marked decrease in pulse pressure); decreased urine output in the absence of hypotension; signs of peripheral ischemia such as coldness, pallor or cyanosis, mottling, numbness, tenderness, pain, or burning sensation.
- Do not breast-feed while taking this drug without approval of the health care provider.
- Immediately notify the health care provider of any known or suspected pregnancy.

Drugs Similar to Isoproterenol (Isuprel)

Beta-adrenergic agonists may be grouped into two primary subclasses: bronchodilators and tocolytics.

Bronchodilators: Bitolterol (Tornalate), levalbuterol (Xopenex), and pirbuterol (Maxair) are short-acting beta-adrenergic agonists given by inhalation to terminate acute bronchospasm. They are drugs of choice for controlling acute asthma attacks. Patients can be dosed every 20 to 30 minutes until control is achieved. Formoterol (Foradil) and salmeterol (Serevent) are also given by inhalation, but these agents have a somewhat longer duration of action. These longer-acting drugs are used in combination with inhaled corticosteroids in the pharmacotherapy of chronic asthma.

Albuterol (Proventil, Ventolin, VoSpire ER) and terbutaline (Brethaire) are available in tablet form. Because the PO route results in more delayed onset of action, these drugs should not be used to terminate an asthma attack in progress. When given 15 minutes before exercise, albuterol may be used for the prophylaxis of exercise-induced bronchospasm. A complete discussion of bronchodilators may be found in Chapter 73.

Dobutamine (Dobutrex): Dobutamine is a selective beta$_1$-adrenergic agonist that has value in the short-term treatment of certain types of shock due to its ability to cause the heart to beat more forcefully. Dobutamine is especially beneficial in cases where the primary cause of shock is related to heart failure, not hypovolemia. In fact, hypovolemia should be corrected before administering adrenergic agonists such as dobutamine. The resulting increase in cardiac output assists in maintaining blood flow to vital organs; renal blood flow is enhanced, and urine output increased. Dobutamine has a brief half-life of 2 minutes and is only given as an IV infusion. The patient should be monitored continuously during the infusion for abnormal changes in heart rate or rhythm. Dobutamine is a pregnancy category C drug.

Tocolytics: Terbutaline and ritodrine are beta$_2$ agonists that relax uterine smooth muscle. The FDA removed oral ritodrine from the U.S. market in 1992; however, it is still available by the IV route. Although not approved by the FDA as a tocolytic, terbutaline is used off-label for this purpose. It may be administered as an IV infusion, subcutaneous injection, or by a portable infusion pump programmed to deliver small amounts of the drug at prescribed intervals. Tocolytics may cause the fetus to experience transient tachycardia. Tocolytics are presented in greater detail in Chapter 72.

CONNECTION *Checkpoint* 19.4

A patient is suffering from severe bronchoconstriction due to an acute allergic attack. From what you learned in Chapter 4, which route of administration—oral, subcutaneous, or inhalation—would likely give the fastest onset of drug action for this patient? See Answer to Connection Checkpoint 19.4 in Appendix A.

NURSING PROCESS APPLICATION

Patients Receiving Adrenergic Agonists Therapy

Assessment

Prior to administration:

- Determine the reason for drug administration.
- Assess the patient for preexisting conditions that may warrant cautious use of adrenergic agents, such as HTN, angina, diabetes, and hyperthyroidism.
- Monitor vital signs, urinary output, and cardiac output, initially and throughout therapy.
- For treatment of nasal congestion, assess the nasal mucosa for changes such as excoriation or bleeding.
- Obtain a complete health history, including allergies, drug history, and possible drug interactions.

Potential Nursing Diagnoses

- *Deficient Knowledge (Drug Therapy)*
- *Decreased Cardiac Output,* related to disorder
- *Ineffective Tissue Perfusion (Cardiopulmonary)*
- *Risk for Injury,* related to adverse effect of drug therapy
- *Ineffective Breathing Pattern,* related to nasal congestion
- *Sleep Deprivation,* related to adrenergic stimulation and drug induced excitation

Planning: Patient Goals and Expected Outcomes

The patient will:

- Exhibit a decrease in the symptoms for which the drug is being given.
- Demonstrate an understanding of the drug's action by accurately describing drug adverse effects and precautions.
- Return demonstrate proper nasal or ophthalmic medication instillation technique.

Implementation

Interventions and (Rationales)	Patient and Family Education
• Closely monitor for excessive peripheral nervous system stimulation. (Adrenergic drugs stimulate heart rate and elevate blood pressure.) Notify the prescriber if heart rate or blood pressure exceeds established criteria.	• Instruct the patient to report palpitations, dizziness, shortness of breath, or headache to the health care provider.
• Closely monitor IV insertion sites for extravasation with IV administration. Use an infusion pump to deliver the medication. (Extravasation into the tissue can cause severe necrosis.) • Use a tuberculin syringe when administering subcutaneously. (Doses are extremely small and require accurate measurement.) • For metered-dose inhalation, shake the container well and wait at least 2 minutes between medications. (This allows for pulmonary absorption.) • Instill only the prescribed number of drops when using ophthalmic solutions. (Instillation of too much medication may cause toxicity.)	Instruct the patient to: • Use the drug as prescribed, and not to "double up" on doses. • Take the medication early in the day to avoid insomnia.
• Monitor the patient for adverse effects. (Adverse effects of adrenergic agonists may be serious and limit therapy.)	Instruct the patient to: • Immediately report shortness of breath, palpitations, dizziness, chest or arm pain or pressure, or other angina-like symptoms. • Consult the health care provider before attempting to use adrenergic agonists to treat nasal congestion or eye irritation. • Monitor blood pressure, pulse, and temperature, ensuring proper use of home equipment.
• Monitor breathing patterns and observe for shortness of breath or audible wheezing. (When medication is given for bronchodilation effect, the patient's breath sounds should improve and shortness of breath will lessen.)	Instruct the patient: • To immediately report any difficulty breathing. • If a history of asthma, consult the health care provider before using OTC drugs to treat nasal stuffiness.
• Observe the patient's responsiveness to light. Provide eye comfort by reducing exposure to direct bright light in the environment; shield the eyes with a rolled washcloth or eye bandages for severe photosensitivity. (Some adrenergic agonists cause photosensitivity by affecting the pupillary light accommodation/response.)	• Instruct patients using ophthalmic sympathomimetics that transient stinging and blurred vision on instillation is normal. Headache or brow pain may also occur. • Instruct the patient to avoid driving and other activities requiring visual acuity until blurring subsides.
• For patients receiving nasal adrenergic agonist solutions, observe the nasal cavity. (Rhinorrhea and epistaxis are potential adverse effects.)	Instruct the patient to: • Observe the nasal cavity for signs of excoriation or bleeding before instilling nasal spray or drops; review the procedure for safe instillation of nasal sprays or eyedrops. • Limit OTC usage of sympathomimetics; inform the patient about rebound nasal congestion.

Evaluation of Outcome Criteria

Evaluate the effectiveness of drug therapy by confirming that patient goals and expected outcomes have been met (see "Planning").

UNDERSTANDING THE CHAPTER

Key Concepts Summary

19.1 Adrenergic agonists activate the sympathetic nervous system to produce fight-or-flight symptoms.

19.2 Adrenergic agonists may act directly by binding to adrenergic receptors, or indirectly by increasing the effect of norepinephrine at synapses.

19.3 Adrenergic agonists may be classified as catecholamines or noncatecholamines.

19.4 The nonselective adrenergic agonists activate both alpha and beta receptors and are used to treat bronchospasm, cardiac arrest, and hypotension.

19.5 Alpha-adrenergic agonists are used to relieve nasal decongestion and elevate blood pressure.

19.6 Beta-adrenergic agonists are used to treat asthma, shock, heart failure, and other cardiac disorders.

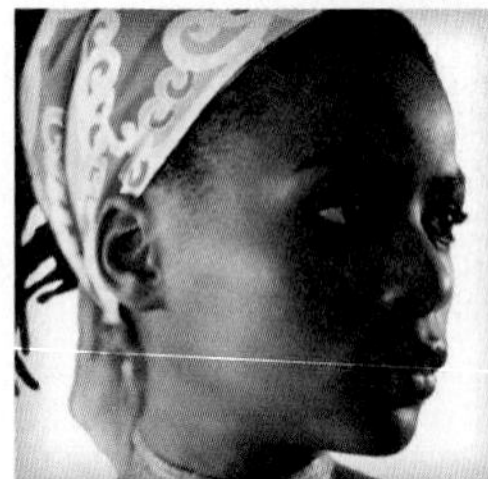

Making the PATIENT *Connection*

Remember the patient "Alexia Howard" at the beginning of the chapter? Now read the remainder of the case study. Based on the information presented within this chapter, respond to the critical thinking questions that follow.

Alexia Howard is a 22-year-old African American woman with a history of asthma since childhood. She is presently a student at the local university where she lives in a dormitory. Since the beginning of the semester, Alexia has experienced tremendous stress trying to manage school and part-time employment. Her roommate, an animal lover, has brought stray dogs and cats into their room several times over the past few months until she could find them good homes.

Today Alexia arrives at the University Health Center with tachypnea and acute shortness of breath with audible wheezing. She has not consistently taken her prescribed medications to avoid asthma attacks. A physical exam revealed a heart rate of 110 and a respiratory rate of 40 with signs of accessory muscle use. Auscultation revealed decreased breath sounds with inspiratory and expiratory wheezing. The patient was coughing up small amounts of white sputum. Her saturated oxygen is 93% on room air.

An aerosol treatment with albuterol (Proventil) was ordered, using a small-volume nebulizer for 15 minutes. Peak flow measures after the treatment showed marked improvement of airflow. On auscultation there was clearing of bilateral breath sounds. Alexia's respiratory rate at the time of discharge was 20 and her heart rate was 108. The patient verbalized that she felt much better but a little nervous.

Alexia was discharged from the University Health Center. She was given a prescription for inhaled steroids and instructed to resume her home medications and use them consistently.

Critical Thinking Questions

1. Discuss the mechanism of action associated with albuterol (Proventil).
2. Why is albuterol being given to Alexia, and why is this route of administration being used?
3. What adverse effects is Alexia demonstrating as a result to the administration of albuterol (Proventil)?

Case Study

Bill Jennings, a 55-year-old man, has been using an epinephrine inhaler for asthma for several months. He is attending a community health fair at a local church, and you are the nurse screening his blood pressure.

When you take Bill's blood pressure, you discover it is 172/94 mmHg. As you talk with him, the patient reveals that he is also self-medicating with OTC pseudoephedrine 60 mg three times per day for seasonal allergies. Bill says his blood pressure is usually 120/80 mmHg.

1. Explain why the increased blood pressure might be related to the drug combination.
2. What patient teaching should occur in this situation?

NCLEX-RN® Review

1 The client, who uses phenylephrine (Neo-Synephrine) nasal spray, asks the nurse how the medication works. The nurse's response would be based on which of the following physiological concepts? This drug:

1. Activates $alpha_1$ adrenergic receptors in the peripheral nervous system.
2. Deactivates beta adrenergic receptors in the peripheral nervous system.
3. Activates alpha adrenergic receptors in the central nervous system.
4. Deactivates beta adrenergic receptors in the central nervous system.

2 The nurse is teaching the client about the use of an adrenergic agonist nasal spray at home. What client teaching is needed related to this medication? (Select all that apply.)

1. Do not share the nasal spray with another person.
2. Only use this drug for 3 days unless directed by a health care provider.
3. Symptoms of excessive use of this drug will result in lethargy and fatigue.
4. Infants and children should not use this medication unless directed by a health care provider.
5. This drug can be safely used by individuals with diabetes.

3 The health care provider prescribes epinephrine (adrenalin) to a client who was stung by several wasps 30 minutes ago. The nurse knows that the primary purpose of this medication for this client is to:

1. Stop the systemic release of histamine produced by the mast cells.
2. Counteract the formation of antibodies in response to an invading antigen.
3. Increase the number of white blood cells produced to fight the primary invader.
4. Increase a declining blood pressure and dilate constricting bronchi associated with anaphylaxis.

4 Which finding, if present, in a client who took a $beta_2$-adrenergic agonist prior to bedtime would the nurse consider normal?

1. Insomnia
2. Sleepiness
3. Urticaria
4. Tinnitus

5 To evaluate the effectiveness of high-dose dopamine hydrochloride (Dopa Stat), the nurse would assess the:

1. Pupillary response.
2. Blood pressure.
3. Level of consciousness.
4. Gag reflex.

6 A beta-adrenergic agonist is prescribed for each of the following conditions. A nurse should question the order for which client? Select all that apply.

1. Hyperthyroidism
2. Asthma
3. Shock
4. Dysrhythmias
5. Heart failure

See Answers to Critical Thinking Questions, Case Study, and NCLEX-RN® Review in Appendix A.

References

Brown, S. G. (2005). Cardiovascular aspects of anaphylaxis: Implications for treatment and diagnosis. *Current Opinion in Allergy and Clinical Immunology, 5*(4), 359–364.

Courtney, A. U., McCarter, D. F., & Pollart, S. M. (2005). Childhood asthma: Treatment update. *American Family Physician, 71*(10), 1959–1968.

Crompton, G. (2006). A brief history of inhaled asthma therapy over the last fifty years. *Primary Care Respiratory Journal, 15*(6), 326–331.

Ephedra: A step backwards. (2005). *American Medical News, 48*(1), 31.

Hogan, M. A. (2005). *Pharmacology reviews & rationales.* Upper Saddle River, NJ: Prentice Hall.

Kelly, H. W. (2005). What is new with the beta$_2$-agonists: Issues in the management of asthma. *Annals of Pharmacotherapy, 39*(5), 931–938.

Lam, F., & Gill, P. (2005). Beta-agonist tocolytic therapy. *Obstetrics and Gynecology Clinics of North America, 32*(3), 457–484.

Leone, M., & Martin, C. (2008). Vasopressor use in septic shock: An update. *Current Opinion in Anaesthesiology, 21*(2), 141–147.

Maule, S., Papotti, G., Naso, D., Magino, C., Testa, E., & Veglio, F. (2007). Orthostatic hypotension: Evaluation and treatment. *Cardiovascular & Hematological Disorders Drug Targets, 7*(1), 63–70.

Mehr, S., Robinson, M., & Tang, M. (2007). Doctor—how do I use my EpiPen? *Pediatric Allergy and Immunology, 18*(5), 448–452

Murray, J. J. (2005). Cardiovascular risks associated with beta-agonist therapy. *Chest, 127*(6), 2283–2285.

Sweeney, A. T., Blake, M. A., & Einhorn, D. (2007). Pheochromocytoma. *emedicine.* Retrieved May 24, 2008, from http://www.emedicine.com/med/topic1816.htm

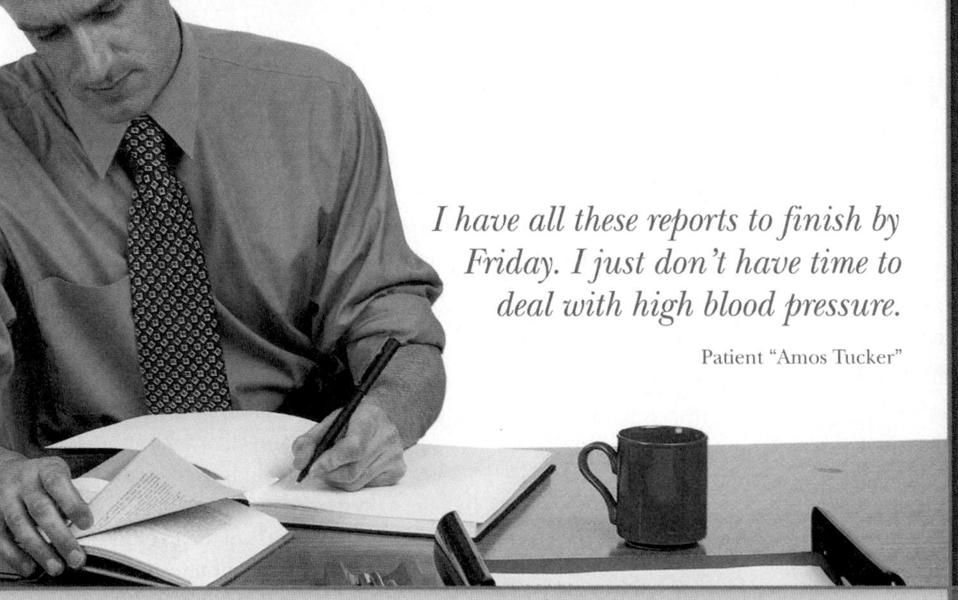
I have all these reports to finish by Friday. I just don't have time to deal with high blood pressure.
Patient "Amos Tucker"

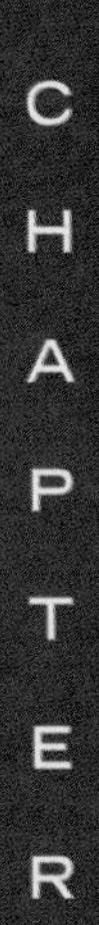
CHAPTER

Adrenergic Antagonists 20

Chapter Outline

Actions of Adrenergic Antagonists

Alpha-Adrenergic Antagonists

PROTOTYPE **Prazosin (Minipress)** *p. 249*

Beta-Adrenergic Antagonists

Nonselective Beta-Adrenergic Antagonists

PROTOTYPE **Propranolol (Inderal)** *p. 253*

Selective Beta$_1$ Adrenergic Antagonists

PROTOTYPE **Metoprolol (Lopressor, Toprol)** *p. 256*

Learning Outcomes

After reading this chapter, the student should be able to:

1. Identify the physiological responses that occur when a drug blocks adrenergic receptors.
2. Compare and contrast the types of physiological responses that occur when a drug blocks alpha$_1$, alpha$_2$, beta$_1$, and beta$_2$-adrenergic receptors.
3. Identify indications for pharmacotherapy with adrenergic antagonists.
4. Describe the first-dose phenomenon and how it may be prevented.
5. Explain the advantages of selective beta antagonists versus nonselective beta antagonists.
6. Explain why beta-adrenergic antagoinists should never be abruptly discontinued.
7. For each of the classes shown in the chapter outline, identify the prototype and representative drugs and explain the mechanism(s) of drug action, primary indications, contraindications, significant drug interactions, pregnancy category, and important adverse effects.
8. Apply the nursing process to care for patients receiving drug therapy with adrenergic antagonists.

Key Terms

adrenergic antagonists, 246
alpha-adrenergic antagonists, 246
beta-adrenergic antagonists, 251
first-dose phenomenon, 248
intrinsic sympathomimetic activity (ISA), 251
orthostatic hypotension, 248
pheochromocytoma, 248
Raynaud's disease, 248

Adrenergic antagonists inhibit the sympathetic nervous system and produce many of the same rest-and-digest symptoms as the cholinergic agonists. They have wide therapeutic application in the treatment of hypertension (HTN) and a limited role in the pharmacotherapy of benign prostatic hyperplasia.

Actions of Adrenergic Antagonists

20.1 Adrenergic antagonists act by blocking the effects of norepinephrine at the adrenergic receptors.

As discussed in Chapter 16 the adrenergic receptor binds norepinephrine (NE) to induce symptoms typical of the fight-or-flight response. Drugs that activate these receptors to enhance the sympathetic response for patients experiencing shock or asthma are discussed in Chapter 19. If the student is not yet thoroughly familiar with these actions, Chapters 16 and 19 should be reviewed before continuing.

Adrenergic antagonists are drugs that compete with NE for adrenergic receptors, as shown in Figure 20.1. By blocking NE from reaching its receptors, symptoms of the fight-or-flight response are prevented. With reduced sympathetic activation, nerve impulses from the parasympathetic nervous system will predominate. In fact, most of the symptoms produced by adrenergic antagonists are those of parasympathetic activation. In other words, adrenergic antagonists and cholinergic agonists produce many of the same symptoms.

CONNECTION *Checkpoint* 20.1

Although cholinergic agonists and adrenergic antagonists may produce similar physiological actions, their indications are very different. From what you learned in Chapter 17, what are the primary indications for pharmacotherapy with cholinergic agonists? See Answer to Connection Checkpoint 20.1 in Appendix A.

The presence of the alpha- and beta-adrenergic receptor subtypes in the sympathetic nervous system allows for more specific pharmacologic responses. For example, with the adrenergic agonists, epinephrine activates both alpha and beta receptors, whereas albuterol activates only beta$_2$ receptors. The same type of division occurs with adrenergic antagonists. Actions of these agents are specific to either alpha blockade or beta blockade. Beta blockade is further divided into those drugs that inhibit both beta$_1$ and beta$_2$ receptors and those that selectively inhibit only beta$_1$ receptors. The therapeutic uses and adverse effects of each drug are dependent on which receptor subtype is activated.

Adrenergic antagonists have wide therapeutic application: They are the most frequently prescribed class of autonomic drugs. With few exceptions, these applications relate to the cardiovascular system.

Alpha-Adrenergic Antagonists

20.2 Alpha$_1$-adrenergic antagonists are used to treat hypertension and benign prostatic hyperplasia.

Alpha-adrenergic receptors are primarily located on smooth muscle, and their activation results in contraction. Most blood vessels, including those serving the heart, genitourinary (GU) system, gastrointestinal (GI) system, and brain, have alpha receptors. Because of their key locations on arterial smooth muscle, the most important effects of **alpha-adrenergic antagonists,** or alpha blockers, are on the cardiovascular system. Blockade of alpha receptors will dilate blood vessels, thus lowering blood pressure.

The specific actions of each alpha-adrenergic antagonist depend on its degree of selectivity for alpha$_1$ or alpha$_2$ receptors. Drugs selective for alpha$_1$ receptors have greater therapeutic application and are listed in Table 20.1. The selective alpha$_1$ blockers doxazosin (Cardura), prazosin (Minipress), and terazosin (Hytrin) have very similar actions, indications, and adverse effects.

Phentolamine (Regitine) and phenoxybenzamine (Dibenzyline) are the only currently available drugs that are nonselective, activating both alpha$_1$ and alpha$_2$ receptors. These agents have very limited usefulness because they exhibit a high incidence of adverse effects, such as hypotension, tachycardia, nausea, vomiting, and diarrhea.

Selective alpha$_1$ antagonists are primarily used to treat HTN. Alpha$_1$-receptor antagonists block the peripheral vascular effects of endogenous catecholamines. Their most significant action is blocking vasoconstriction in arterioles and veins, which results in decreased peripheral resistance and a reduction in blood pressure. Their ability to block alpha$_1$ receptors on arterial smooth muscle lowers blood pressure directly. Their ability to dilate veins lowers blood pressure indirectly by decreasing venous return to the heart. This reduces cardiac output, which causes a reduction in systemic blood pressure. When used to treat HTN, the alpha blockers are usually used concurrently with other classes of antihypertensives, such as diuretics (see Chapter 35).

In addition to dilating vascular smooth muscle, alpha$_1$ blockers relax smooth muscle in the trigone and sphincter muscles at the base of the urinary bladder and in the prostate. Relaxation of these muscles promotes an increase in urine flow in patients who have difficulty voiding due to strictures in this region. This action has resulted in the use of alpha blockers in the treatment of benign prostatic hyperplasia (BPH), a nonmalignant condition in which the prostate gland enlarges to restrict urine flow through the urethra. These agents increase urine flow and decrease residual urine volume in patients with BPH. Two selective alpha$_1$ antagonists, alfuzosin (Uroxatral) and tamsulosin (Flomax), are approved only for BPH. Alpha$_1$ blockers do not cure this disorder, and patients with moderate to severe BPH usually require surgery to correct the restriction in urinary flow. A complete discussion on the pharmacotherapy of BPH is found in Chapter 72.

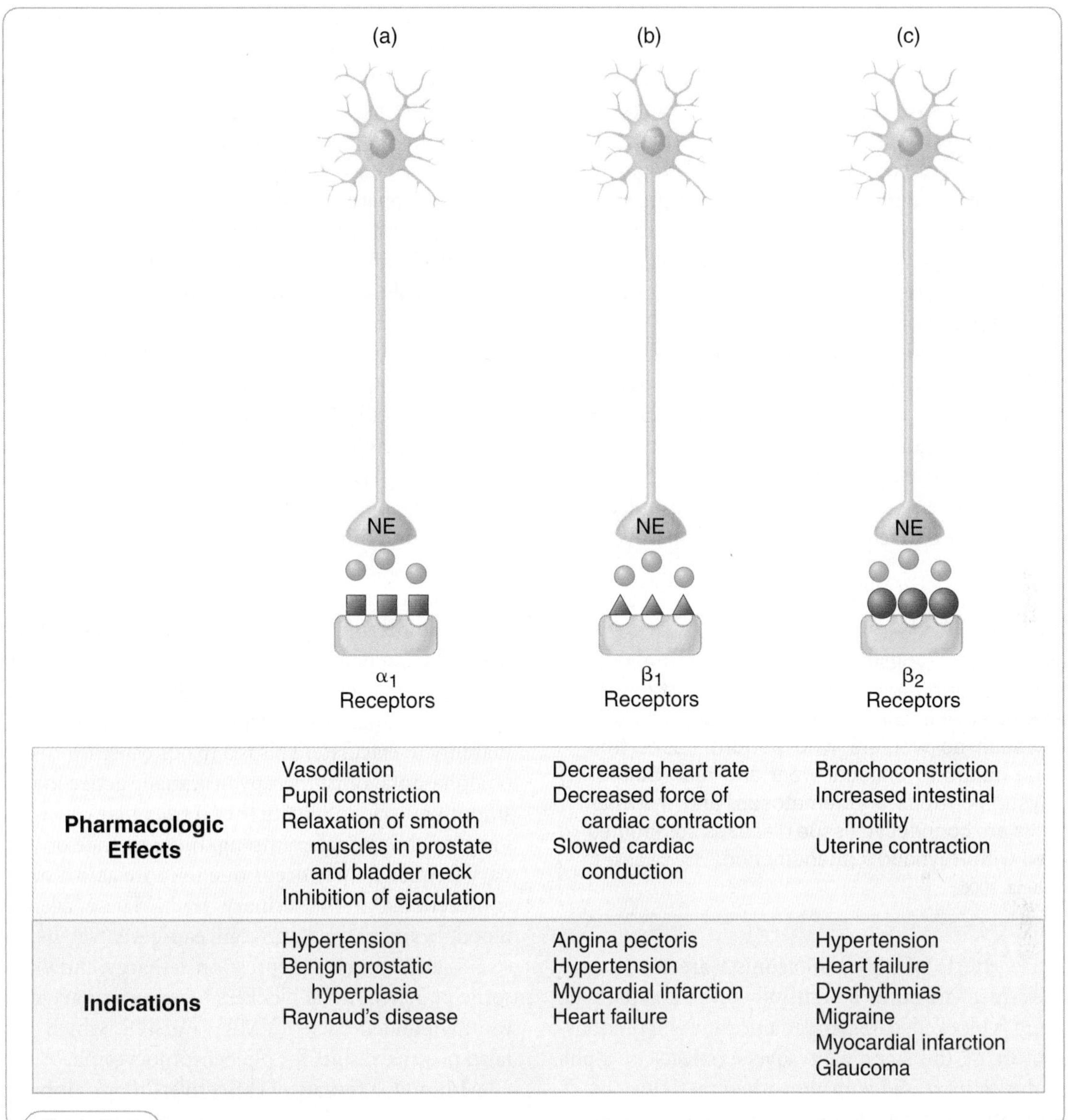

Figure 20.1

Pharmacologic effects and indications of adrenergic antagonists: (a) blockade of $alpha_1$ receptors; (b) blockade of $beta_1$ receptors; (c) blockade of $beta_2$ receptors.

TABLE 20.1 Alpha-Adrenergic Antagonists

Drug	Route and Adult Dose (maximum dose where indicated)	Adverse Effects
alfuzosin (Uroxatral)	Oral (PO): 10 mg once daily	*Orthostatic hypotension, dizziness, headache, fatigue* <u>First-dose phenomenon, tachycardia, dyspnea</u>
doxazosin (Cardura)	PO: 1 mg/day; may increase to 16 mg/day in one to two divided doses (max: 16 mg/day)	
phenoxybenzamine (Dibenzyline)	PO: Initially 10 mg bid, may increase by 10 mg at 4-day intervals to 20–40 mg bid or tid	
phentolamine	IV/IM: 5 mg 1–2 h prior to surgery; repeat as needed Intradermal: 5–10 mg diluted in 10 mL of normal saline injected into the affected area within 12 h of catecholamine extravasation	
prazosin (Minipress)	PO: 1 mg/day; may increase to 1 mg bid–tid (max: 20 mg/day)	
tamsulosin (Flomax)	PO: 0.4–0.8 mg/day after a meal (max: 0.8 mg/day)	
terazosin (Hytrin)	PO: 1 mg/day; may increase 1–5 mg/day (max: 20 mg/day)	

Note: *Italics* indicate common adverse effects. <u>Underline</u> indicates serious adverse effects.

Alpha$_1$ antagonists are occasionally used to treat pheochromocytoma and Raynaud's disease. **Pheochromocytoma** is a tumor, usually benign, arising from the adrenal medulla that is characterized by excessive secretion of catecholamines. A patient with a pheochromocytoma will exhibit extreme HTN, palpitations, dyspnea, anxiety, and profuse sweating. All are signs of catecholamine (sympathetic) overdose. Alpha$_1$ blockers are administered to reduce the profound HTN caused by inoperable pheochromocytomas. They may also be given preoperatively to lower the risk of hypertensive crisis during surgical removal of the tumor.

In **Raynaud's disease,** vasospasms of vessels leading to the fingers and toes can lead to intermittent pain and cyanosis of the digits. Emotional stress or cold temperatures usually exacerbate the disorder. Alpha$_1$ antagonists can diminish the vasospasm and bring some relief to patients who suffer from Raynaud's disease. Calcium channel blockers (see Chapter 33) such as nifedipine (Procardia) are also used to relieve Raynaud's vasospasms.

PharmFACT

Raynaud's disease typically occurs between the ages of 15 and 40; women account for over 75% of cases. Raynaud's disease is linked to certain occupations or activities, such as workers who perform tasks that subject the hands to unusual wear and tear. Scleroderma, systemic lupus erythematosus, and rheumatoid arthritis are connective tissue diseases sometimes associated with Raynaud's phenomenon. *Source:* Lisse & Oberto-Medina, 2006.

The adverse effects of alpha antagonists are predictable based on their mechanism of action. When the sympathetic nervous system is blocked, parasympathetic tone will predominate; thus most of the significant adverse effects of alpha blockers are due to increased parasympathetic activity.

The most limiting adverse effect of pharmacotherapy with all alpha$_1$ antagonists is hypotension. The vasodilation effect of alpha$_1$ blockers is more intense when the patient is upright, as compared to recumbent. Significant **orthostatic hypotension** can occur when the patient abruptly changes from a supine to an upright position, resulting in diminished blood flow to the brain. Much of this effect is caused by blockade of alpha$_1$ receptors in the veins. As the patient moves to an upright position, blood accumulates in the veins, cardiac output decreases, and blood pressure falls. Orthostatic hypotension is especially pronounced at the beginning of pharmacotherapy and when increasing the dose. Because this **first-dose phenomenon** can lead to syncope due to reduced blood flow to the brain, initial therapy is begun with low doses, usually administered at bedtime.

The fall in blood pressure during alpha$_1$-antagonist therapy may be accompanied by reflex tachycardia, which occurs when the baroreceptor reflex is triggered. Reflex tachycardia can be particularly troublesome in patients who are susceptible to dysrhythmias. A beta-adrenergic antagonist is sometimes concurrently administered with alpha blockers to reduce the possibility of reflex tachycardia. A less serious, though annoying, adverse effect of alpha antagonists is vasodilation of blood vessels serving the nasal mucosa, resulting in nasal congestion.

A number of noncardiovascular adverse effects may also occur during pharmacotherapy with alpha$_1$ blockers. Because smooth muscle contraction is inhibited in the vas deferens and ejaculatory ducts, these drugs can cause impotence due to an inability to ejaculate. This is a major cause for discontinuation of alpha-antagonist therapy in sexually active males. Increased smooth muscle activity in the GI tract may cause nausea, vomiting, or abdominal cramping. Incontinence or increased urinary frequency may occur due to more active smooth muscle contractions in the urinary tract. These agents cross the blood–brain barrier and can cause central nervous system (CNS) effects such as depression, lethargy, and vivid dreams in some patients. Alpha blockers increase urinary metabolites of vanillylmandelic acid (VMA) and NE, which can result in false-positive results for pheochromocytoma.

Although a few agents selectively block alpha$_2$-adrenergic receptors, they are used for research purposes and have no clinical application. Yohimbine is the only drug thought to selectively block alpha$_2$ receptors, although it also acts by other mechanisms. Approved in 1938 for the treatment of

CONNECTIONS — To the Community: Lifestyle Modifications for Hypertension

Hypertension is prevalent in the U.S. and Canada and is treatable with medications. However, patients should be encouraged to adopt healthy lifestyle changes to assist in management of this disease. Changing some basic daily habits can help control HTN and improve quality of life. Nurses can play a major role in helping patients to manage their HTN. Following are some ideas that the nurse should discuss with patients with HTN:

- Begin a weight loss program if overweight.
- Limit alcohol intake to 24 oz of beer, 10 oz of wine, or 2 oz of hard liquor per day for men and one half that amount per day for women and smaller built men.
- Participate in physical activity for 30 to 45 minutes, 4 to 6 days per week.
- Eat a balanced diet with fruits, vegetables, grains and grain products, and low-fat or nonfat dairy foods.
- Lower the amount of sodium ingested to a moderate level. Avoid adding salt to foods and minimize eating salty foods.
- Monitor and reduce saturated fat and cholesterol in the diet.
- Stop smoking or using tobacco products.
- Have blood pressure checked regularly, at least once every year.
- Monitor blood pressure at home and record daily to track your progress.
- Take the prescribed medicine every day.
- Talk to your health care provider if you are concerned about your progress. Communication is the key to success.
- Make and keep appointments every 3 to 6 months with the health care provider even if your blood pressure is under control.

CONNECTIONS

To the Community Sodium Restrictions: How Much Is Too Much?

Often, individuals who suffer from HTN are instructed to reduce intake of sodium in the diet. However, the patient may not understand the extent of their salt limitation. The American Heart Association recommends that healthy adults limit sodium intake to no more than 2,300 milligrams per day. This equals about 1 teaspoon of salt (sodium chloride). The following illustrates the sodium content of various foods in the average diet:

2 tablespoons peanut butter	= 120 mg sodium
1/2 cup peas	= 390 mg sodium
2 tablespoons salsa	= 220 mg sodium
8 graham crackers	= 160 mg sodium
1 ounce (13) corn chips	= 120 mg sodium

To reduce the amount of sodium in the diet, one must be aware of both natural and added sodium content. Table salt, sodium chloride, is 40% sodium by weight. Always read labels when buying and preparing packaged foods. Sodium may be listed as "soda" (referring to sodium bicarbonate, or baking soda), "sodium," and the symbol "Na."

erectile dysfunction, this drug is rarely, if ever, prescribed for this purpose today due to the availability of safer and more effective drugs. Yohimbe (converted to yohimbine in the body) is a natural product obtained from the bark of a West African tree and may be purchased over-the-counter (OTC) as an herbal supplement. Claims that this herb is a sexual stimulant or aphrodisiac have not been supported by controlled research studies.

PROTOTYPE DRUG Prazosin (Minipress)

Classification: **Therapeutic:** Antihypertensive

Pharmacologic: Selective alpha$_1$-adrenergic antagonist

Therapeutic Effects and Uses: The primary therapeutic action of prazosin is a rapid decrease in peripheral resistance that reduces blood pressure. The drug has very little effect on cardiac output or heart rate and it causes less reflex tachycardia than some other drugs in this class. Approved in 1976, its most common use is in combination with other agents, such as beta blockers or diuretics, in the pharmacotherapy of HTN. Optimum therapeutic effects may require 4 to 6 weeks of therapy. Off-label indications include symptomatic BPH, prevention of Raynaud's disease, and hypertensive emergencies associated with pheochromocytoma.

One disadvantage of prazosin is its relatively short half-life, which requires it to be administered two to three times per day. Patients should be taught to be alert for dizziness, light-headedness, fatigue, and palpitations at the beginning of therapy. These symptoms may disappear after the first few doses but can persist in some patients throughout therapy.

Mechanism of Action: Prazosin competes with NE at alpha-adrenergic receptors on vascular smooth muscle in arterioles and veins. It is selective for alpha$_1$-adrenergic receptors and has no activity at alpha$_2$- or beta-adrenergic receptors.

Pharmacokinetics:

Route(s)	PO
Absorption	Well absorbed
Distribution	Completely distributed; small amounts secreted in breast milk
Primary metabolism	Hepatic
Primary excretion	Primarily bile and feces, with small amounts by the kidneys
Onset of action	2 h
Duration of action	Less than 24 h

Adverse Effects: The most common adverse effects of prazosin include dizziness, drowsiness, fatigue, weakness, palpitations, orthostatic hypotension, and headache. Nausea, vomiting, and other GI effects occur in about 5% of patients. Most patients develop tolerance to these adverse effects as therapy progresses. The first-dose phenomenon may cause syncope. Erectile dysfunction, including priapism, is rare but can present a barrier to patient adherence.

Contraindications/Precautions: The only contraindication to the use of prazosin is prior sensitivity to the drug. The drug should be used with caution in older patients and those with renal impairment because these groups tend to exhibit more pronounced orthostatic hypotension and syncope. Patients with coronary artery disease should be treated with caution because prazosin may worsen angina symptoms in these patients.

Drug Interactions: Additive hypotensive effects may occur when prazosin is used concurrently with other antihypertensives and diuretics. This additive effect is used to advantage in the pharmacotherapy of HTN, in which the dose of each individual agent may be lower than if a single drug were used as monotherapy. Ingestion of alcohol or use with erectile dysfunction agents such as sildenafil (Viagra) may cause increased hypotension. Use with sympathomimetics having alpha-agonist activity will antagonize the therapeutic effects of prazosin. **Herbal/Food:** Hawthorn may cause an additive drop in blood pressure when used with antihypertensive drugs such as prazosin.

Pregnancy: Category C.

Treatment of Overdose: Overdose will lead to hypotension; thus it is important to keep the patient supine because of the possibility of syncope. Vasopressors such as levarterenol or dopamine may be necessary to increase blood pressure. Fluid expanders may be administered to raise blood pressure, and renal function should be monitored. Drowsiness may also be prominent.

Nursing Responsibilities:

- Establish baseline vital signs prior to administration. Withhold medication and notify the prescriber if systolic blood pressure is less than 100 mmHg.
- Assess for conditions for which the drug is indicated such as HTN, Raynaud's disease, or BPH.
- Determine whether any other drugs are being taken concurrently to identify significant potential drug interactions.
- Administer the initial dose of medication at bedtime to minimize adverse effects such as postural hypotension and syncope. If the initial dose must be taken during the day, advise the patient not to perform hazardous activities for at least 4 hours after taking the drug.
- Monitor for drug-related adverse effects, which include dizziness, fatigue, weakness, palpitations, orthostatic hypotension, and headache.
- Give medication with food to decrease the occurrence of possible faintness and dizziness; food may delay the absorption rate but it does not affect the extent of absorption.
- Assess for first-dose phenomenon (rare adverse effect in 0.15% of patients), which results in a rapid decline in blood pressure, bradycardia, and syncope within 90 to 120 minutes of the initial dose of prazosin. Recovery is usually within several hours. Increased risk occurs with preexisting low plasma volume from diuretic therapy or salt restriction, beta-adrenergic therapy, or dehydration.
- Monitor blood pressure and notify the prescriber if it falls below the set established value.
- Assess for full therapeutic effect, which should occur within 4 to 6 weeks of initiation of therapy.

Patient and Family Education:

- Avoid situations that could result in injury if fainting should occur, particularly during initial therapy, when dose is increased, or if another antihypertensive drug is added to the medication regimen.
- Sit or lie down immediately if you feel dizzy, feel lightheaded, have blurred vision, or feel faint. Do not attempt to stand or walk until the sensation passes.
- Make position changes slowly when moving from a lying to a standing position to prevent dizziness and possible fainting.
- Do not drive or perform other hazardous activities until the effects of the drug are known because this drug may cause drowsiness and dizziness.
- Take the drug at the same time(s) each day. Record daily blood pressure, when medication was taken, which arm was used, and your position such as standing or sitting. Take the record to the health care provider at follow-up appointment.
- Consult the health care provider before taking OTC products, especially cold, cough, or allergy remedies, because these may alter the effectiveness of prazosin.
- Expect adverse effects to diminish with continued therapy.

Drugs Similar to Prazosin (Minipress)

Other alpha-adrenergic blockers used for HTN include doxazosin, phenoxybenzamine, phentolamine, and terazosin. Two alpha-adrenergic blockers, alfuzosin and tamsulosin, are indicated only for BPH.

Alfuzosin (Uroxatral): Approved in 2003, alfuzosin is one of the newer alpha blockers approved to treat BPH. It is available as an extended release tablet that permits once-daily dosing. Both tamsulosin and alfuzosin relax smooth muscle in the bladder and prostate gland, which reduces pressure on the urethra, thus enhancing urine flow. The drug is well tolerated, with the most common adverse effects being dizziness, fatigue, headache, and upper respiratory infection. Hypotension may be a serious problem in patients taking antihypertensive drugs or erectile dysfunction agents such as sildenafil. This drug is rated as pregnancy category B but it is not indicated for women or children.

Doxazosin (Cardura): Approved in 1990, doxazosin is an oral drug approved for both HTN and BPH. It has the longest duration of action of the selective alpha$_1$ blockers, allowing for once-daily dosing. The most frequent adverse effects are dizziness, fatigue, headache, and edema. Orthostatic hypotension occurs in about 10% of patients taking the drug, especially when therapy is initiated or with changes in dose. Patients who ingest alcohol or use this drug with erectile dysfunction agents such as sildenafil (Viagra) may experience increased hypotension. The drug should be used cautiously in older adults because they tend to experience more hypotension-related adverse effects. Doxazosin should be taken at bedtime to avoid the first-dose phenomenon. This drug is pregnancy category B.

Phenoxybenzamine (Dibenzyline): Phenoxybenzamine is an older drug, approved in 1954, that blocks both alpha$_1$- and alpha$_2$-adrenergic receptors. The drug has a very prolonged duration of action, and its effects may last up to a week after the drug is discontinued. Because it has the potential to cause extended alpha blockade and serious cardiovascular adverse effects, its use is limited to treating pheochromocytoma. Off-label indications include symptomatic BPH, Raynaud's disease, and frostbite. The drug is pregnancy category C.

Phentolamine: Like phenoxybenzamine, phentolamine blocks both alpha$_1$ and alpha$_2$ receptors. Approved in 1952, it is the only alpha blocker that is given parenterally. During surgery, phentolamine may be administered to treat or prevent hypertensive crises during removal of pheochromocytomas. Phentolamine is considered an antidote for treating hypertensive emergencies caused by catecholamine overdose. The drug may be injected subcutaneously to prevent or treat dermal necrosis or sloughing caused by extravasation of catecholamines such as NE and dopamine. Although the drug has been used in the past to diagnose pheochromocytoma, safer measures such as urinary or blood assays of catecholamines levels are more accurate indicators of this disease. This drug is pregnancy category C.

Terazosin (Hytrin): Approved in 1987, terazosin has a longer duration of action than prazosin and is approved for both HTN and symptomatic BPH. Given orally, its prolonged half-life permits once-daily dosing. Approximately 16% of the patients taking terazosin will experience headache. Other common adverse effects include dizziness and fatigue. Tolerance develops to most of these adverse effects as therapy progresses. Like other drugs in this class, terazosin should be taken at bedtime to avoid the first-dose phenomenon. Older adults are more sensitive to the hypotensive and adverse effects of terazosin, such as dry mouth and drowsiness. The drug is pregnancy category C.

Tamsulosin (Flomax): Like alfuzosin, tamsulosin has only one indication: BPH. It is administered orally and should always be taken with food to reduce the incidence of orthostatic hypotension. The drug is generally well tolerated and exhibits adverse effects similar to other alpha blockers. It is extensively metabolized by hepatic CYP enzymes and may interact with drugs that are inducers or substrates of these enzymes. This drug is pregnancy category B.

Beta-Adrenergic Antagonists

20.3 Nonselective beta-adrenergic antagonists affect both beta$_1$ and beta$_2$ receptors and are prescribed for HTN, angina, and other cardiovascular disorders.

Beta-adrenergic antagonists, or beta blockers, are grouped as nonselective or selective. Nonselective beta-adrenergic antagonists, such as propranolol, block both beta$_1$ and beta$_2$ receptors. Selective drugs that block only beta$_1$ receptors are sometimes called cardioselective agents and are discussed in Section 20.4.

Some beta blockers, such as carvedilol (Coreg), also have some alpha-antagonist activity, which adds to their ability to lower blood pressure. A few beta blockers such as pindolol (Visken) exhibit mixed beta-antagonist and beta-agonist activity. This low level of beta-agonist activity is called **intrinsic sympathomimetic activity (ISA).** Theoretically, the agonist action of these agents may result in fewer adverse effects in patients who have bradycardia, congestive heart failure, or compromised pulmonary function. Regardless of their receptor specificity, most therapeutic applications of the beta blockers relate to their effects on the cardiovascular system (Table 20.2).

Because their mechanism of action is to antagonize the effects of endogenous catecholamines, all beta blockers have the potential to reduce the heart rate, decrease the force of myocardial contraction, and slow conduction velocity through the atrioventricular node. These effects are modest when the heart is at rest. During periods of stress or exercise, however, beta blockers tend to prevent the normal increase in sympathetic stimulation to the heart. In some cases, this results in an undesirable short-term decrease in cardiac output, because the drug prevents the heart from responding adequately to the need for increased blood flow. During this time, the sympathetic nervous system responds by activating alpha receptors and raising blood pressure. In time, peripheral resistance returns to normal, or below normal levels, particularly in patients with HTN, and blood pressure falls.

The primary use of beta-adrenergic antagonists is the treatment of HTN. Although the exact mechanism by which beta blockers reduce blood pressure is not completely understood, it is thought that part of their hypotensive effect is due to the decreased cardiac output resulting from diminished myocardial contractility. A second mechanism for the blood pressure reduction is that beta blockers antagonize the release of renin by the kidney, which is normally stimulated by catecholamines. Nonselective adrenergic antagonists, such as carvedilol (Coreg), also block alpha$_1$-adrenergic receptors, which directly contributes to their antihypertensive action. An additional possible mechanism is that beta blockers may act centrally to reduce sympathetic output from the vasomotor center in the brain. The student should refer to Chapter 36 for additional details on the use of beta blockers in HTN management.

Beta-adrenergic antagonists have several other important applications, although they are not always drugs of choice for these conditions. By decreasing cardiac workload and oxygen demands, beta blockers can ease the acute chest pain characteristic of angina pectoris (see the prototype feature for atenolol in Chapter 37). Because they slow cardiac conduction, beta blockers are used in the pharmacotherapy of certain types of dysrhythmias (see Chapter 39). Some nonselective beta blockers have the ability to reduce intraocular pressure when given as ophthalmic solutions in the pharmacotherapy of glaucoma. (See the prototype feature for timolol in Chapter 77). Other therapeutic uses include the treatment of heart failure (see Chapter 38), myocardial infarction (MI) (see Chapter 37), and migraine prophylaxis (see Chapter 29).

Due to the presence of beta-adrenergic receptors throughout the body, pharmacotherapy with nonselective beta antagonists usually produces more adverse effects than treatment with selective beta$_1$ antagonists. Because of this, the use of the nonselective agents has declined over the past few decades. One of the more serious adverse effects with the nonselective beta blockers is that inhibition of beta$_2$ receptors in the lung can cause bronchoconstriction, which may be particularly acute in patients with chronic obstructive pulmonary disease (COPD) or asthma.

The metabolic effects of beta-adrenergic antagonists can be important for patients with diabetes mellitus. Under normal conditions, catecholamines break down glycogen, which frees glucose to enter the blood to be used as an energy source for fight-or-flight actions. Many body tissues, particularly skeletal muscles, must receive a continuous source of glucose, especially during prolonged physical activity such as running or heavy exercise. Beta blockers prevent this hyperglycemic effect of the catecholamines and patients may develop hypoglycemia. In addition, beta blockers will prevent tachycardia, an important warning sign of impending hypoglycemia. Beta-blocker therapy in patients with diabetes must be carefully monitored.

A second metabolic effect of nonselective beta-adrenergic antagonists relates to lipid metabolism. Catecholamines

TABLE 20.2 Beta-Adrenergic Antagonists

Drug	Route and Adult Dose (maximum dose where indicated)	Adverse Effects
Selective $Beta_1$-Adrenergic Antagonists		
acebutolol (Sectral)	PO: 400–800 mg/day (max: 1200 mg/day) for HTN PO: 200 mg bid increased to 600–1200 mg/day for dysrhythmias	*Fatigue, insomnia, diarrhea, constipation, drowsiness, impotence or decreased libido, hypotension, bradycardia, confusion* Agranulocytosis, bronchospasm, laryngospasm, Stevens-Johnson syndrome, anaphylaxis; if the drug is abruptly withdrawn, palpitations, rebound. HTN, dysrhythmias, MI
atenolol (Tenormin)	PO: 25–50 mg daily (max: 100 mg/day for HTN or MI; 200 mg/day for angina)	
betaxolol (Betoptic, Kerlone)	PO: 5–10 mg daily (max: 20 mg/day) Ophthalmic solution: 1–2 drops of 0.5% solution bid (max: 4 drops/day)	
bisoprolol (Zebeta, Ziac)	PO: 2.5–5 mg daily (max: 20 mg/day)	
esmolol (Brevibloc)	IV: 500 mcg/kg loading dose followed by 50 mcg/kg/min, may increase dose every 5–10 min prn (max: 200 mcg/kg/min)	
metoprolol (Lopressor, Toprol)	PO: 50–100 mg once daily or bid (max: 450 mg/day)	
nebivolol	PO: 5 mg once daily (max: 40 mg)	
$Alpha_1$ and Beta Blockers (Centrally Acting)		
carteolol (Ocupress)	Ophthalmic solution: 1 drop of 1% solution bid (max: 2 drops/day)	*Headache, dizziness, fatigue, drowsiness, anxiety, depression, lethargy, impotence, peripheral vascular insufficiency* Agranulocytosis, bradycardia, bronchospasm, laryngospasm, respiratory disturbances, may worsen heart failure and mask symptoms of hypoglycemia, Stevens-Johnson syndrome (propranolol), toxic epidermal necrolysis (propranolol), exfoliative dermatitis (propranolol), dysrhythmias (sotalol)
metipranolol (OptiPranolol)	Ophthalmic solution: 1 drop of 0.3% solution bid (max: 2 drops/day)	
nadolol (Corgard)	PO: Begin with 40 mg/day and increase by 40–80 mg every 3–7 days as needed (max: 240–320 mg/day)	
penbutolol (Levatol)	PO: 20–40 mg/day (max: 80 mg/day)	
pindolol (Visken)	PO: 5 mg bid, may increase by 10 mg/day every 2–3 weeks as needed (max: 60 mg/day)	
propranolol (Inderal, InnoPran XL)	PO: 40 mg bid, up to 160–480 mg/day for HTN or 80–120 mg at bedtime (extended release) PO: 10–20 mg bid or tid, may need 160–320 mg/day in divided doses for angina IV: 0.5–3 mg every 4 h prn for dysrhythmias	
sotalol (Betapace)	PO: Initial dose of 80–160 mg/day ac, may increase every 3–4 days in 40–160 mg increments (max: 640 mg/day for life-threatening dysrhythmias)	
timolol (Blocadren)	PO: 10 mg bid (max: 60 mg/day for HTN) Ophthalmic solution: 1 drop of 0.25% solution bid (max: 2 drops/day)	
Mixed $Alpha_1$- and Beta-Adrenergic Antagonists		
carvedilol (Coreg)	PO: Start with 3.125 mg bid for 2 weeks; may double dose every 2 weeks up to 25 mg bid (max: 50 mg/day)	Same as the above two classes
labetalol (Normodyne, Trandate)	PO: 100 mg bid; may increase to 200–400 mg bid (max: 2,400 mg/day)	

Note: *Italics* indicate common adverse effects. Underline indicates serious adverse effects.

normally stimulate lipolysis, the breakdown of stored lipid in adipose tissue, resulting in the release of free fatty acids into the blood. Like glucose, these fatty acids serve as an essential energy source for skeletal muscle. By blocking the actions of catecholamines, beta antagonists will decrease the amount of free fatty acids available during periods of metabolic stress. Nonselective beta blockers may also increase serum triglycerides and decrease high-density lipoproteins. During the course of therapy with beta blockers, patients with preexisting hyperlipidemia should have their lipid profiles monitored periodically to prevent hyperlipidemia.

Treatment of overdose with a nonselective beta blocker involves restoring cardiovascular function. Patients may experience excessive bradycardia. An anticholinergic such as atropine or a beta-adrenergic agonist such as isoproterenol may be administered to reverse severe bradycardia and cause bronchodilation. Cardiac failure caused by beta-antagonist overdose may be treated by administering digoxin (Lanoxin) or diuretics. Severe hypotension may require the administration of a vasopressor such as epinephrine or NE.

Beta blockers should be withdrawn gradually over several weeks. If withdrawn abruptly, the heart displays hypersensitivity to catecholamines and sweating, palpitations, headache, and tremulousness may occur. This phenomenon is called rebound cardiac excitation. Patients with coronary artery disease may experience a worsening of angina symptoms, and MIs have been recorded in some patients.

PROTOTYPE DRUG Propranolol (Inderal)

Classification: **Therapeutic:** Antihypertensive, antidysrhythmic
Pharmacologic: Nonselective beta-adrenergic blocker

Therapeutic Effects and Uses: Approved in 1967, propranolol reduces heart rate and slows conduction velocity through the AV node by blocking $beta_1$ receptors in cardiac muscle. The decrease in cardiac output, as well as its suppression of renin activity, results in a reduction in blood pressure. Cardiac workload and myocardial oxygen demand are decreased due to the slower heart rate and decreased cardiac output. Propranolol is approved for a wide variety of indications, including the following:

- **Hypertension.** For the treatment of HTN, propranolol has largely been replaced by angiotensin-converting enzyme (ACE) inhibitors and calcium channel blockers, which have been found to be more effective at preventing long-term consequences of HTN such as cerebrovascular accident and MI. It is still widely used in patients with HTN who have angina, prior MI, or heart failure.
- **Angina pectoris.** Beta blockers are the drugs of choice for treating chronic angina. The nonselective drugs such as propranolol are less frequently used than the cardioselective agents.
- **Dysrhythmias.** Until 1978, propranolol was the only beta-adrenergic antagonist approved to treat dysrhythmias. As an antidysrhythmic, propranolol is most effective against tachycardia caused by excessive sympathetic stimulation.
- **Migraine prophylaxis.** Propranolol has been one of the most frequently prescribed drugs for the prevention of migraines.
- **Prophylaxis of MI.** When given following an MI, propranolol has been found to reduce cardiovascular mortality and the risk of reinfarction.

Propranolol has a number of off-label indications. By reducing venous pressure, it may be useful in reducing portal HTN and bleeding due to esophageal varices. It has been used to treat panic attacks, chronic agitation, and aggressive behavior. Lastly, it has been used to manage involuntary, rhythmic movements of essential tremor.

A long-acting form of the drug, InnoPran XL, was approved in 2003. InnoPran XL has a timed delivery system that is designed for bedtime dosing, with a peak effect in the morning.

Mechanism of Action: Propranolol is a nonselective beta-adrenergic antagonist, affecting both $beta_1$ receptors in the heart, and $beta_2$ receptors in the lung and other locations throughout the body. It has no ISA.

Pharmacokinetics:

Route(s)	Usually PO; IV for severe dysrhythmias
Absorption	Completely absorbed
Distribution	Widely distributed, including the CNS and placenta; secreted in breast milk; 90% bound to plasma protein
Primary metabolism	Hepatic
Primary excretion	90–95% renal
Onset of action	PO: 1–2 h; IV: immediate
Duration of action	Half-life: 3–5 h

Adverse Effects: Propranolol is well tolerated and common adverse effects such as nausea, vomiting, and diarrhea generally diminish as therapy progresses. Other common adverse effects include fatigue, insomnia, drowsiness, bradycardia, and confusion. Impotence or loss of libido may occur in a small percentage of patients. Serious adverse effects include agranulocytosis, bronchospasm, Stevens-Johnson syndrome, and anaphylaxis. If the drug is abruptly withdrawn, palpitations, rebound HTN, life-threatening dysrhythmias, or myocardial ischemia may occur.

Contraindications/Precautions: Because of its depressive effects on the heart, propranolol is contraindicated in cardiogenic shock, sinus bradycardia, greater than first-degree heart block, and severe heart failure. Patients with cardiac impairment must be monitored carefully to prevent worsening of their condition. Due to its constriction of smooth muscle in the airways, the drug is contraindicated in patients with COPD or asthma. Propranolol should be used cautiously in patients with diabetes because it interferes with glucose metabolism and can cause hypoglycemia. The drug can also mask signs of impending hypoglycemia such as tachycardia and tremors. Propranolol should be used with caution in patients with reduced renal output, because the drug may accumulate to toxic levels in the blood and cause dysrhythmias.

Drug Interactions: Propranolol interacts with many other drugs. When given with other beta blockers, effects on the cardiovascular system may be additive and bradycardia or hypotension may result. Because both propranolol and calcium channel blockers such as verapamil (Calan) and diltiazem (Cardizem) suppress myocardial contractility, concurrent use may lead to additive bradycardia. Use with antidysrhythmic drugs that slow conduction through the AV node such as amiodarone may lead to AV block. Phenothiazines can add to the hypotensive effects of propranolol. Because MAO inhibitors deplete endogenous catecholamines, concurrent administration with propranolol could result in severe bradycardia and hypotension.

Use of ethanol or antacids containing aluminum hydroxide gel will slow the absorption of propranolol and reduce its therapeutic effects. Administration of beta-adrenergic agonists such as albuterol (Proventil) will antagonize the antihypertensive action of propranolol. **Herbal/Food:** Hawthorn may cause an additive drop in blood pressure when used with antihypertensive drugs such as propranolol. Large doses of vitamin C may reduce the absorption of propranolol.

MyNursingKit | Mechanism of Action Animation: Propranolol

Pregnancy: Category C.

Treatment of Overdose: Overdose will cause bradycardia, hypotension, and bronchospasm. Treatment may require the use of plasma volume expanders or vasopressors to raise blood pressure to normal levels and atropine to counteract the bradycardia. Isoproterenol (a beta agonist) may be administered to reverse bronchospasm.

Nursing Responsibilities:

- Monitor vital signs, especially apical pulse, respirations, blood pressure, and circulation to extremities during initial therapy dosage adjustment. Withhold the drug if systolic blood pressure is less than 100 mmHg or apical pulse rate is less than 60 per minute.
- Obtain thorough medical history to assess for allergies, asthma, and COPD because drugs in this class can cause bronchiolar constriction even in patients without respiratory compromise.
- Evaluate response to therapy for HTN by checking blood pressure near the end of the dosage interval or before administration of the next dose.
- Monitor for drug-related adverse effects, which include nausea, vomiting, dizziness, and palpitations.
- Assess laboratory tests for kidney, liver, hematologic, and cardiac functions during prolonged pharmacotherapy.
- Remember that adverse reactions most often occur following IV administration soon after therapy initiation. Adverse reactions are most likely to occur in the older adult and in patients with impaired renal function.
- Monitor intake and output ratio and take daily weights to detect fluid retention and possibly heart failure.
- Consult with the prescriber regarding salt restrictions. Drug plasma volume may increase with risk of congestive heart failure if dietary sodium is not restricted in patients who are not receiving concurrent diuretic therapy.
- Examine the patient for impaired circulation if he or she complains of cold, painful, or tender feet or hands. Peripheral pulses may still be present even with impaired circulation.

Patient and Family Education:

- Take radial pulse before each dose and report irregular pulse, or if pulse drops below the value recommended by your health care provider.
- If you have diabetes, remember that the drug suppresses signs of hypoglycemia such as increased pulse rate and changes in blood pressure. Monitor blood glucose frequently and report other possible signs of hypoglycemia such as sweating, fatigue, hunger, or lack of concentration.
- Take medication exactly as prescribed and do not omit, increase or decrease dosage, or change the dosage interval.
- Do not abruptly discontinue this drug because you may experience tremors, sweating, palpitation, malaise, headache, rebound HTN, and life-threatening dysrhythmias (in patients with angina pectoris or MI).
- Make position changes slowly when moving from a lying to a standing position to prevent dizziness and possible fainting.
- Avoid prolonged exposure of arms or legs to cold.
- Do not drive or perform other hazardous activities until the effects of the drug are known because this drug may cause drowsiness and dizziness.
- Do not take any other prescription or nonprescription drugs, dietary supplements, or herbal products without approval of the health care provider.
- Inform the dentist, ophthalmologist, surgeon, and other health care providers that you are taking a beta blocker.
- Do not breast-feed while taking this drug without approval of the health care provider.
- Immediately notify the health care provider of any known or suspected pregnancy.

Drugs Similar to Propranolol (Inderal)

There are many beta blockers available. All nonselective beta-adrenergic blockers have the same actions but differ in their pharmacokinetics and therapeutic applications.

Carteolol (Cartrol, Ocupress): Approved in 1988, carteolol is a nonselective beta-adrenergic blocker with a long duration of action. The oral form of carteolol (Cartrol) was indicated for the treatment of HTN; however, the drug is no longer available in the United States. As a 1% ophthalmic solution, carteolol (Ocupress) reduces intraocular pressure and is used for chronic open-angle glaucoma. Transient local irritation, burning, tearing, and conjunctival hyperemia may occur in 25% of patients. The ophthalmic solution can be absorbed and cause systemic adverse effects. This drug is pregnancy category C.

Carvedilol (Coreg): Approved in 1995, carvedilol is an oral medication indicated for the management of HTN and heart failure. It also has been found to reduce mortality in patients who have survived the acute phase of an MI. It may be used off-label to treat angina. In addition to being a nonselective beta-receptor blocker, carvedilol blocks alpha$_1$-adrenergic receptors. Because of its alpha-antagonist action, carvedilol shares similar adverse effects, such as orthostatic HTN, with the alpha$_1$ blockers. Like most beta blockers, fatigue and dizziness are common adverse effects. Patients with asthma or chronic lung disorders may experience dyspnea or wheezing due to the bronchoconstriction effects of the drug. This drug is pregnancy category C. Carvedilol is presented as a prototype drug for heart failure in Chapter 38.

Labetalol (Normodyne, Trandate): Like carvedilol, labetalol has nonselective beta-blocking action as well as the ability to selectively block alpha$_1$-adrenergic receptors. Approved in 1984, it is available by both the oral and IV routes for the therapy of HTN. When treating HTN, the drug may be given concurrently with a thiazide diuretic. The most common adverse effects are generally mild and include insomnia, drowsiness, fatigue, decreased libido, and tingling of the scalp. Orthostatic hypotension is greatest 2 to 4 hours after the drug is administered. When given by the IV route for hypertensive emergencies, as many as 60% of patients will experience orthostatic hypotension. This drug is pregnancy category C.

Metipranolol (OptiPranolol): Approved in 1989, metipranolol is only administered as a 0.3% ophthalmic solution for glaucoma. Metipranolol reduces aqueous humor production, which decreases intraocular pressure. It has minimal effect on pupil size or lens accommodation. Adverse effects are limited to the eye and include transient local burning. This drug is pregnancy category C.

Nadolol (Corgard): Approved in 1989, nadolol is a nonselective beta-adrenergic blocker that is used to treat HTN and for the long-term management of angina. Off-label uses of nadolol include suppression of ventricular dysrhythmias, migraine prophylaxis, treatment of essential tremor, and anxiety. Given by the oral route, it has a long half-life of 20 to 24 hours, which offers the benefit of once-daily dosing. Unlike many beta blockers, it is not metabolized by the liver and is excreted mostly unchanged by the kidneys. Adverse effects are generally mild and similar to those of propranolol and include drowsiness, fatigue, and decreased libido. This drug is pregnancy category C.

Penbutolol (Levatol): Penbutolol is a nonselective beta-adrenergic antagonist that has a long duration of action, which offers the benefit of once-daily dosing. Approved in 1987, it is used in the pharmacotherapy of HTN as monotherapy, or in combination with other antihypertensives. Treatment of chronic stable angina is an off-label use of penbutolol. Penbutolol has higher lipid solubility than most other drugs in its class and thus has a greater potential for causing CNS adverse effects such as dizziness and fatigue. Other common adverse effects include nausea, vomiting, and diarrhea. The drug is pregnancy category C.

Pindolol (Visken): Approved in 1982, pindolol is an oral, nonselective beta blocker that is used in the pharmacotherapy of HTN, usually in combination with a thiazide diuretic. It is used off-label for the management of chronic stable angina. Pindolol has the highest degree of ISA of any beta blocker, which gives it some beta-agonist action in addition to antagonist activity. Adverse effects are generally mild and temporary and include nausea, vomiting, insomnia, fatigue, and dizziness. Maximum antihypertensive action may take up to 2 weeks to achieve. This drug is pregnancy category B.

Sotalol (Betapace): Although all nonselective beta blockers affect heart rate and rhythm, sotalol is one of the few drugs in this class used excusively as an antidysrhythmic. By slowing the action potential crossing the myocardium, the heart is able to regain normal rhythm. Therapy with sotalol is always begun in a setting where the electrocardiogram (ECG) can be continuously monitored for a minimum of 3 days because this drug can cause or worsen certain dysrhythmias. Adverse effects are those typical of beta blockers but occur more frequently. For example, fatigue may occur in 20% of patients, dyspnea in 21%, and sinus bradycardia in 16%. Patients with a history of dysrhythmias are more likely to experience serious adverse effects. Abrupt discontinuation of the drug can cause dysrhythmias and MI. Other adverse effects include insomnia, nausea, vomiting, and drowsiness. Approved in 1992, details of the pharmacotherapy of dysrhythmias are presented in Chapter 39. This drug is pregnancy category B.

Timolol (Blocadren, Timoptic): In its oral formulation, timolol (Blocadren) is indicated for HTN, migraine prophylaxis, and reduction of mortality following an acute MI. Chronic, stable angina is an off-label indication for the drug. Timolol (Timoptic) is available as a 0.25% and 0.5% ophthalmic solution to treat glaucoma. When used topically on the eye, adverse effects include localized stinging and transient blurred vision. Systemic adverse effects are generally mild and transient and include nausea, vomiting, diarrhea, bradycardia, fatigue, and dizziness. Abrupt discontinuation of timolol can cause dysrhythmias and MI. Approved in 1978, timolol (Timoptic) is presented as a prototype for glaucoma in Chapter 78.

20.4 Beta$_1$-adrenergic antagonists are selective for beta$_1$ receptors in the myocardium and are used to treat HTN and other cardiovascular disorders.

Because of their specificity for beta$_1$ receptors in the myocardium, the beta$_1$-adrenergic antagonists exert fewer noncardiac adverse effects than nonselective agents such as propranolol. This selectivity is not absolute, however; some of these agents affect beta$_2$ receptors at higher doses, and a few have intrinsic sympathomimetic activity.

The primary indication for selective beta$_1$ antagonists is HTN. Some are also used in the pharmacologic management of chronic angina pectoris and heart failure. Although used for the same indications as the nonselective agents, the beta$_1$ blockers have certain advantages. The major advantage is that they have little effect on beta$_2$ receptors in bronchial smooth muscle. This allows the beta$_1$ blockers to be safely administered to most patients with asthma or COPD with less possibility of bronchospasm. Because their selectivity for beta$_1$ receptors is not absolute, bronchospasm is still a potential adverse effect in susceptible patients with these disorders. The beta$_1$ blockers also have less effect on glucose and lipid metabolism than the nonselective agents.

Beta blockers must be used with great caution in patients with a history of heart failure because both the nonselective and selective beta$_1$ blockers depress the myocardium. In patients with healthy hearts, this effect is a clinical problem only at high doses. In patients with diseased hearts, however, this depression can worsen cardiac impairment and lead to heart failure. Cardiac failure may develop gradually in patients taking beta blockers for prolonged periods; therefore, the patient should receive regular assessments of cardiac function during therapy. Generally, beta blockers are discontinued or their doses adjusted as soon as heart failure is suspected.

Overdose with beta$_1$ antagonists is treated in a manner similar to the nonselective beta blockers. An anticholinergic agent such as atropine or a beta agonist such as isoproterenol may be given to promote bronchodilation and increase the heart rate. Digoxin (Lanoxin) or diuretics may be indicated if heart failure develops. Severe hypotension may require the administration of an emergency vasopressor such as dopamine (a beta agonist).

CONNECTION *Checkpoint* 20.2

Dopamine is a catecholamine. From what you learned in Chapter 19, identify other catecholamines that are used to quickly raise blood pressure in acute care situations.

See Answer to Connection Checkpoint 20.2 in Appendix A.

PROTOTYPE DRUG Metoprolol (Lopressor, Toprol)

Classification: **Therapeutic:** Antihypertensive
Pharmacologic: Selective $beta_1$-adrenergic antagonist

Therapeutic Effects and Uses: Approved in 1978, the primary indication for metoprolol is HTN, as monotherapy or in combination with other antihypertensives. The therapeutic effects of metoprolol include decreases in heart rate (both resting and during exercise), cardiac output, and blood pressure (both systolic and diastolic). Fixed-dose combination formulations are available: Lopressor HCT combines metoprolol with the diuretic hydrochlorothiazide in a single tablet. Because it slows the rate and force of myocardial contraction, metoprolol can reduce oxygen demands on the heart and benefit patients with chronic stable angina. Off-label uses include stable, symptomatic heart failure, essential tremor, migraine prophylaxis, and the control of heart rate in patients with atrial dysrhythmias.

Recent research has determined that metoprolol reduces the mortality associated with recent MI. Following an acute MI, metoprolol is infused slowly until a target heart rate between 60 and 90 beats per minute is reached. This reduces myocardial oxygen demand at a time when the heart is at great risk for a subsequent MI or life-threatening dysrhythmias. On hospital discharge, patients continue metoprolol therapy by switching to the PO form of the drug.

Mechanism of Action: Metoprolol is a selective $beta_1$-adrenergic antagonist that competes with endogenous catecholamines at adrenergic receptors in cardiac muscle. At high doses, it may affect $beta_2$ receptors in bronchial smooth muscle.

Pharmacokinetics:

Route(s)	Usually PO; IV for MI
Absorption	Well absorbed
Distribution	Completely, including CNS and placenta; secreted in breast milk; 12% bound to plasma protein
Primary metabolism	Hepatic
Primary excretion	Renal
Onset of action	PO: 15 minutes; IV: immediate
Duration of action	13–19 h

Adverse Effects: Metoprolol is well tolerated and adverse effects generally diminish as therapy progresses. Nausea and vomiting are the most common adverse effects. Other common adverse effects include dizziness, fatigue, insomnia, bradycardia, heartburn, and dyspnea. Serious adverse effects include agranulocytosis, laryngospasm, complete heart block, and thyroid storm in patients with thyrotoxicosis. Dysrhythmias, severe HTN, or MI may occur if the drug is abruptly withdrawn. Bronchospasm and dyspnea are rare because the drug has little effect on $beta_2$ receptors in bronchial smooth muscle.

Contraindications/Precautions: Because of its multiple effects on the heart, patients with preexisting cardiac disease such as heart failure should be carefully monitored. This agent is contraindicated in cardiogenic shock, severe bradycardia, and heart block greater than first degree. Metoprolol should be used with caution in patients with severe hepatic disease because its major route of excretion is the liver. Metoprolol should be used with caution in patients with asthma and those with a history of bronchospasm because the drug may affect $beta_2$ receptors at high doses.

Drug Interactions: $Beta_1$ blockers such as metoprolol have the potential to interact with many different drugs. The nurse should always be cautious when administering a beta blocker with any other medication that affects the heart, particularly those that depress AV node conduction. Because certain calcium channel blockers such as verapamil suppress myocardial contractility, concurrent use with metoprolol can lead to additive bradycardia and even heart block. Use with other antihypertensive drugs has the potential to cause additive hypotension. Certain drugs, including cimetidine and oral contraceptives, can also add to the hypotensive effect of metoprolol. Metoprolol should not be given with sympathomimetics because the actions of the drugs will cancel each other out. Metoprolol can reduce the clearance of lidocaine and cause lidocaine toxicity.

Pregnancy: Category C.

Treatment of Overdose: Overdose of metoprolol will cause bradycardia, hypotension, and bronchospasm. Treatment may require the use of plasma volume expanders or vasopressors to raise blood pressure to normal levels and atropine to counteract the bradycardia. Isoproterenol may be administered for bronchospasm.

Nursing Responsibilities:

- Assess vital signs, especially the apical pulse and blood pressure, before administering the drug. Report significant changes in rate, rhythm, or quality of pulse or blood pressure. Withhold the drug if systolic blood pressure is less than 100 mmHg or the apical pulse rate is less that 60/minute.
- Monitor blood pressure, heart rate, and ECG carefully during IV drug administration.
- Monitor laboratory tests by establishing a baseline and intermittent blood cell counts, liver and kidney function, and blood glucose.
- Assess blood pressure readings close to the end of a 12-hour dosing interval to evaluate adequacy of dosage for patients with HTN and those on twice-daily doses. Some patients may require doses three times a day to maintain satisfactory blood pressure control.
- Maximal drug effect on blood pressure usually occurs after 1 week of therapy.
- Monitor hypertensive patients with congestive heart failure for symptoms of impending heart failure such as dyspnea on exertion, night cough, edema, orthopnea, and distended neck veins.
- Discontinue the drug if the patient develops symptoms of mental depression, such as disinterest in food, personal hygiene, people, and surroundings, as well as withdrawal, insomnia, apathy, sadness, or difficulty concentrating.
- This drug masks hyperthyroidism in patients with thyrotoxicosis. Abrupt withdrawal could precipitate thyroid storm.

- Record intake and output and daily weight, and monitor bilateral breath sounds for adventitious lung sounds such as pulmonary rales.

Patient and Family Education:

- Take the radial pulse before each dose and report irregular pulse or if the pulse drops below the value recommended by your health care provider.
- Immediately report any changes in vision to the health care provider.
- Avoid late evening dosing to decrease insomnia or increased dreaming.
- If you have diabetes, remember that the drug suppresses signs of hypoglycemia such as increased pulse rate and changes in blood pressure. Monitor blood glucose frequently and report other possible signs of hypoglycemia such as sweating, fatigue, hunger, or lack of concentration.
- Do not drive or perform other hazardous activities until the effects of the drug are known because this drug may cause drowsiness and dizziness.
- Take the medication exactly as prescribed and do not omit, increase or decrease dosage, or change the dosage interval.
- Report cold, painful, or tender feet or hands or other symptoms of Raynaud's disease such as cyanosis, intermittent pallor, redness, or paresthesias. The health care provider may prescribe a vasodilator for these symptoms.
- Discontinue beta blockers slowly over a period of 1 to 2 weeks. Sudden withdrawal can result in anginal attacks and MIs in patients diagnosed with angina pectoris or thyroid storm in patients with hyperthyroidism.
- Use measures to relieve dry mouth such as rinsing the mouth frequently with water, chewing sugarless gum, or sucking on hard candy.
- Relieve dry eyes with sterile artificial tears available OTC.
- Do not breast-feed while taking this drug without approval of the health care provider.
- Immediately noify the health care provider of any known or suspected pregnancy.

Drugs Similar to Metoprolol (Lopressor, Toprol)

Other $beta_1$-adrenergic antagonists include acebutolol, atenolol, betaxolol, bisoprolol, esmolol, and nebivolol. The $beta_1$-adrenergic antagonists are very similar but differ in their pharmacokinetics and specific indications.

Acebutolol (Sectral): Approved in 1984, acebutolol is an oral cardioselective $beta_1$ antagonist similar to metoprolol that is used for HTN and recurrent ventricular dysrhythmias. An unlabeled indication is chronic stable angina. In addition to being a selective $beta_1$ blocker, it has mild intrinsic sympathomimetic activity. Because of its 3- to 4-hour half-life, it is usually administered twice daily. Common adverse effects include CNS effects such as fatigue, dizziness, and headache. Higher doses can produce hypotension and bradycardia. Like other beta blockers care must be taken when using acebutolol with other drugs that depress myocardial conduction because bradycardia and hypotension may result. This drug is pregnancy category B.

Atenolol (Tenormin): Approved in 1981, atenolol is available by the oral route for HTN and for the long-term management of chronic stable angina. It is also given by the IV route to reduce the risk of sudden death in patients with an acute MI. Off-label indications include migraine prophylaxis and the prevention of symptoms in patients undergoing ethanol withdrawal. Atenolol has a longer half-life than metoprolol, which allows for once-daily dosing. Common adverse effects are the same as those of other drugs in this class, such as nausea, vomiting, fatigue, dizziness, and headache. The risk of bradycardia is low at normal doses. Like other beta blockers, care must be taken to avoid abrupt discontinuation of therapy, especially in patients with coronary artery disease. Atenolol is presented as a prototype drug for angina in Chapter 37. This drug is pregnancy category D and is not recommended during pregnancy or lactation.

Betaxolol (Betoptic, Kerlone): Approved in 1985, betaxolol (Kerlone) is available in tablet form for the pharmacotherapy of HTN, sometimes given concurrently with thiazide diuretics. The drug is one of the most potent and selective of the beta blockers; it is nine times more potent than atenolol. It has no ISA, and it inhibits $beta_2$-adrenergic receptors in the lung only at very high doses. When given PO, adverse effects such as nausea, vomiting, dizziness, fatigue, and headache are typical of the beta blockers. The risk of bradycardia increases with higher doses. Like other beta blockers, care must be taken to avoid abrupt discontinuation of therapy, especially in patients with coronary artery disease because myocardial ischemia, MI, HTN, or dysrhythmias may result.

Betaxolol (Betoptic) is also available as a 0.25% ophthalmic suspension for chronic open-angle glaucoma. Like other beta blockers, Betoptic reduces intraocular pressure. Adverse effects are limited to the eye and include burning and transient blurred vision. This drug is pregnancy category C.

Bisoprolol (Zebeta, Ziac): Approved in 1992, bisoprolol is approved only for HTN, although heart failure and chronic stable angina are off-label indications. Given orally, bisoprolol has a longer half-life than metoprolol, which allows for less frequent dosing. The cardioselective nature of bisoprolol action only applies to low doses; at higher doses it also blocks $beta_2$ receptors to cause dyspnea and wheezing. Common adverse effects are the same as those of other drugs in this class, such as fatigue, dizziness, and headache. Like other beta blockers, care must be taken to avoid abrupt discontinuation of therapy, especially in patients with coronary artery disease. Ziac combines bisoprolol with the diuretic hydrochlorothiazide in a single tablet. The drug is pregnancy category C.

Esmolol (Brevibloc): Approved in 1986, esmolol is very different from other $beta_1$-adrenergic blockers. It is administered by continuous IV infusion in emergency situations, usually postoperative or perioperative, to rapidly correct supraventricular tachycardia or severe HTN. It has a very short half-life of only

8 minutes, and the patient must be monitored for hypotension and bradycardia during the infusion. Although it has the same actions and adverse effects as other beta blockers, the actions of esmolol begin to diminish within minutes after discontinuation of the infusion. Esmolol should be used with extreme caution in patients with severe bradycardia, AV block, or cardiogenic shock. Hypotension occurs in about 40% of the patients receiving the drug but resolves quickly following completion of the infusion. The drug is pregnancy category C.

Nebivolol (Bystolic): Approved in 2007, nebivolol is a selective $beta_1$-adrenergic blocker that is indicated for the treatment of HTN, either as monotherapy or in combination with other antihypertensives. Nebivolol is highly cardioselective but may activate $beta_2$ receptors at higher doses. It appears to have equal effectiveness to other drugs in its class, but it produces fewer adverse effects. The drug is well tolerated, with the most frequently observed adverse effects being headache, fatigue, paresthesia, dizziness, hypotension, and bradycardia. This drug is pregnancy category C.

NURSING PROCESS APPLICATION

Patients Receiving Adrenergic Antagonist Therapy

Assessment	Potential Nursing Diagnoses
Prior to administration: • Obtain a complete health history, including allergies, drug history, and possible drug interactions. • Assess vital signs, urinary output, and cardiac output initially and throughout therapy. • Assess the reason for drug administration. • Withhold the medication if systolic blood pressure less than 100 mmHg or heart rate is less than 60 beats/minute. • Assess for conditions for which the drug is contraindicated.	• *Deficient Knowledge (Drug Therapy)* • *Disturbed Sensory Perception,* related to hypotensive action of drug • *Risk for Injury,* related to dizziness, syncope • *Impaired Urinary Elimination,* related to adverse effects • *Sexual Dysfunction,* related to drug therapy

Planning: Patient Goals and Expected Outcomes

The patient will:

- Exhibit a decrease in blood pressure with few adverse effects.
- Report a decrease in urinary symptoms such as hesitancy and difficulty voiding.
- Demonstrate an understanding of the drug's action by accurately describing drug adverse effects and precautions, and the importance of follow-up care.

Implementation

Interventions and (Rationales)	Patient and Family Education
• For prostatic hyperplasia, monitor for urinary hesitancy, feeling of incomplete bladder emptying, or interrupted urinary stream. (These drugs potentially impair urinary elimination.)	• Instruct the patient to report increased difficulty with urinary voiding to the health care provider.
• Monitor for syncope. (Alpha-adrenergic antagonists produce first-dose syncope phenomenon and may cause loss of consciousness.)	Instruct the patient to: • Take this medication at bedtime, and to take the first dose immediately before getting into bed. • Avoid abrupt changes in position. • Be aware of the first-dose phenomenon; reassure that this effect diminishes with continued therapy.
• Monitor vital signs, level of consciousness, and mood. (Adrenergic antagonists can exacerbate existing mental depression.)	• Instruct the patient to immediately report any feelings of dysphoria. Interview the patient regarding suicide potential.
• Monitor carefully for dizziness, drowsiness, or light-headedness. (These are signs of decreased blood flow to the brain due to the drug's hypotensive action.)	Instruct the patient: • To monitor vital signs, especially blood pressure, ensuring proper use of home equipment. • Regarding the normotensive range of blood pressure, instruct the patient to consult the nurse regarding "reportable" blood pressure readings. • To report dizziness or syncope that persists beyond the first dose, as well as paresthesia and other neurologic changes.
• Observe for adverse effects, which may include blurred vision, tinnitus, epistaxis, and edema. (Adverse effects may be serious and limit therapy.)	Instruct the patient: • That nasal congestion may be a adverse effect. • To report any adverse reactions to the health care provider. • About the potential danger of concomitant use of OTC nasal decongestants.
• Monitor liver function. (Liver impairment may cause toxic levels of the drug to build up in the blood.)	Instruct the patient: • To adhere to a regular schedule of laboratory testing for liver function as ordered by the health care provider. • To report signs and symptoms of liver toxicity, such as nausea, vomiting, diarrhea, rash, jaundice, abdominal pain, tenderness or distention, or change in the color of stool. • Of the importance of ongoing medication adherence and follow-up.

Evaluation of Outcome Criteria

Evaluate the effectiveness of drug therapy by confirming that patient goals and expected outcomes have been met (see "Planning").

UNDERSTANDING THE CHAPTER

Key Concepts Summary

20.1 Adrenergic antagonists act by blocking the effects of norepinephrine at the adrenergic receptors.

20.2 Alpha$_1$-adrenergic antagonists are used to treat hypertension and benign prostatic hyperplasia.

20.3 Nonselective beta-adrenergic antagonists affect both beta$_1$ and beta$_2$ receptors and are prescribed for HTN, angina, and other cardiovascular disorders.

20.4 Beta$_1$-adrenergic antagonists are selective for beta$_1$ receptors in the myocardium and are used to treat HTN and other cardiovascular disorders.

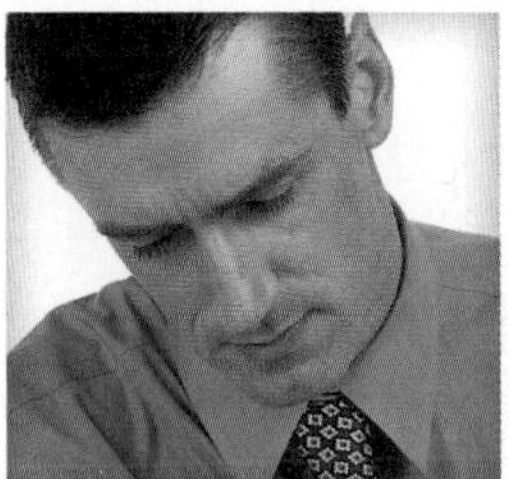

Making the PATIENT *Connection*

Remember the patient "Amos Tucker" from the beginning of the chapter? Now read the remainder of the case study. Based on the information presented within this chapter, respond to the critical thinking questions that follow.

Amos Tucker is a 48-year-old executive who lives a very active life. He has a wife and two teenage children. His job requires frequent travel for up to 2 weeks at a time. Every year, Amos's company recommends a complete health physical as part of the executive benefits package. Amos has not taken advantage of this opportunity in the past. However, this year his wife has insisted that he have a checkup.

Amos arrives at the employee health clinic for the physical exam. On arrival he is visibly anxious and has accepted three calls on his cell phone since entering the clinic. During the initial health history session, Amos reveals that he smokes one pack of cigarettes per day and does not drink alcohol. He states that he has no time for exercise and has gained weight over the past year. Most nights Amos sleeps 4 to 6 hours. He states that he frequently wakes up during the night with thoughts of what he needs to do the next day. He finds it difficult to return to sleep after waking.

His past medical and family history indicate that both his parents died within the last 10 years. His father died of a stroke and his mother died of a heart attack. Amos states that he has been prescribed prazosin (Minipress) in the past but he stopped taking it. When questioned about why he chose not to take the medication, Amos reluctantly confides in you that he suspected that the medication was causing "sexual" adverse effects.

The physical examination reveals that Amos is 1.9 m (6′2″) tall and weighs 119 kg (262 lb). His body temperature is 37°C (98.6°F), heart rate is 88 beats/minute, respiratory rate is 18/minute, and blood pressure is 160/90 mmHg. During the examination an ECG and laboratory test results were all within normal limits.

Critical Thinking Questions

1. Identify the mechanism of action associated with prazosin (Minipress).
2. Discuss the physiology of sexual disorders associated with alpha-adrenergic antagonists.
3. As this patient's nurse, how would you approach the topic of medication-induced sexual dysfunction?

Case Study

Richard Perry is a 64-year-old patient who has been successfully treated for HTN for over 15 years with propranolol (Inderal). Mr. Perry is allergic to cats. However, he recently visited his grandson who has a new kitten. He now has weepy eyes and a running nose. He is considering taking the OTC medication pseudoephedrine (Sudafed) to relieve the allergic symptoms.

1. Is it safe for Mr. Perry to take this OTC medication? Why? Why not?
2. Is there another OTC medication that would be safer for this patient?

NCLEX-RN® Review

1 The client is started on propranolol (Inderal). The most important action to be included in the plan of care for this client related to this medication includes which of the following?

1. Monitor apical pulse and blood pressure.
2. Elevate the head of the bed during meals.
3. Take the medication after meals.
4. Consume foods high in potassium.

2 A nurse should instruct a client with diabetes who is prescribed a beta-adrenergic blocker for the treatment of hypertension to:

1. Increase insulin intake by 2 to 3 units daily each morning.
2. Decrease the intake of carbohydrates while on the antihypertensive medications.
3. Elevate the lower extremities to promote venous drainage.
4. Monitor blood glucose levels frequently and report hypoglycemia.

3 To avoid the first-dose phenomenon, the nurse knows that the initial dose of prazosin (Minipress) should be:

1. Very low and given at bedtime.
2. Doubled and given before breakfast.
3. The usual dose and given before breakfast.
4. Doubled and given immediately after breakfast.

4 A client who is taking an adrenergic antagonist for hypertension complains of dizziness when first getting out of bed in the morning. The nurse should advise the client to:

1. Move slowly from the recumbent to the upright position.
2. Drink a full glass of water before rising to increase vascular circulatory volume.
3. Avoid sleeping in a prone position.
4. Stop taking the medication.

5 A health care provider has ordered an alpha$_1$-adrenergic antagonist for each of these clients. A nurse should question the order for the client with which of the following disorders?

1. Benign prostatic hyperplasia
2. Pheochromocytoma
3. Raynaud's disease
4. Tachycardia

6 The nurse is caring for a client with chronic hypertension. The client is receiving a beta-adrenergic blocker daily. Which client manifestations would the nurse conclude are adverse effects of this medication? (Select all that apply.)

1. Anorexia
2. Increased serum triglycerides
3. Hypoglycemia
4. Decreased libido
5. Thrombocytopenia

See Answers to Critical Thinking Questions, Case Study, and NCLEX-RN® Review in Appendix A.

References

Bers, D. M. (2005). Beyond beta blockers. *Nature Medicine, 11*(4), 379–380.

Burger, P. C., & Brunner-La Rocca, H. (2005). Pharmacotherapy of congestive heart failure in elderly patients. *Journal of Cardiovascular Pharmacology and Therapeutics, 10*(2), 85–94.

Egan, B. M., Basile, J., Chilton, R. J., & Cohen, J. D. (2005). Cardioprotection: The role of beta-blocker therapy. *Journal of Clinical Hypertension (Greenwich), 7*(7), 409–416.

Foody, J. M., Farrell, M. H., & Krumholz, H. M. (2002). Beta-blocker therapy in heart failure: Scientific review. *The Journal of the American Medical Association, 287*(7), 883–889.

Ghali, J. K. (2005). Beta-blockers in selected heart failure populations. *Current Heart Failure Reports, 2*(2), 100–105.

Harvard Health Publications. (2006). *New drugs for the prostate.* Retrieved May 29, 2008, from http://body.aol.com/conditions/new-drugs-for-the-prostate

Lisse, J. R., & Oberto-Medina, M. (2006). *Raynaud phenomenon.* Retrieved June 3, 2008, from http://www.emedicine.com/med/TOPIC1993.HTM

Messerli, F. H., Bangalore, S., & Julius, S. (2008). Risk/benefit assessment of β-blockers and diuretics precludes their use for first-line therapy in hypertension. *Circulation, 117*(20), 2706–2715.

Rossnagel, L. K. (2004). Propranolol for migraine prophylaxis. *Cochrane Database of Systematic Reviews, 2.* Art. No.: CD003225. DOI: 10.1002/14651858.CD003225.pub2.

Sauls, J. L., & Rone, T. (2005). Emerging trends in the management of heart failure: Beta blocker therapy. *The Nursing Clinics of North America, 40*(1), 135–148.

Schumann, S. A., & Hickner, J. (2008). When not to use beta-blockers in seniors with hypertension. *Journal of Family Practice, 57*(1), 18–21.

Staessen, J. A., Thijs, L., Wang, J., & Li, Y. (2005). Cardiovascular outcomes and antihypertensive drug treatment in older women. *The Journal of the American Medical Association, 293*(13), 1588.

Tefera, L., Perry, C. M., Sharma, A., & Roth, B. (2007). *Toxicity, beta-blocker.* Retrieved June 3, 2008, from http://www.emedicine.com/emerg/TOPIC59.HTM

Westfall, T. C., & Westfall, D. P. (2006). Adrenergic agonists and antagonists. In L. L. Brunton, J. S. Lazo, and K. L. Parker (Eds.), *The pharmacological basis of therapeutics* (11th ed., pp. 237–296). New York: McGraw-Hill.

UNIT 4

Pharmacology of the Central Nervous System

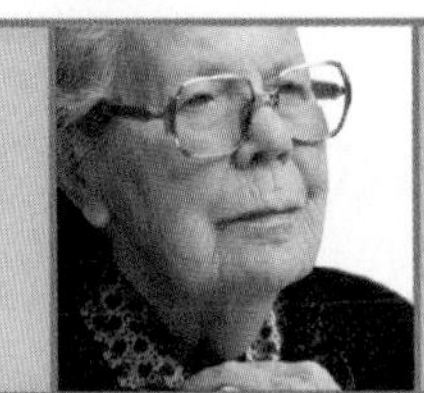
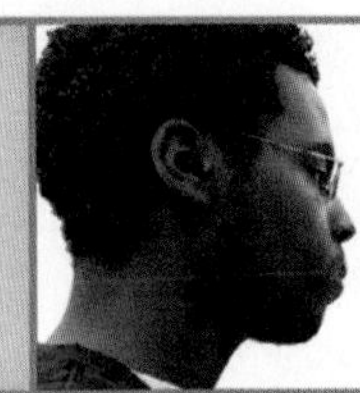
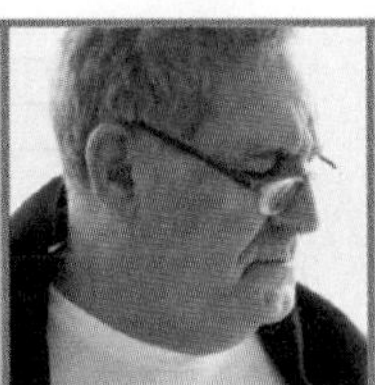
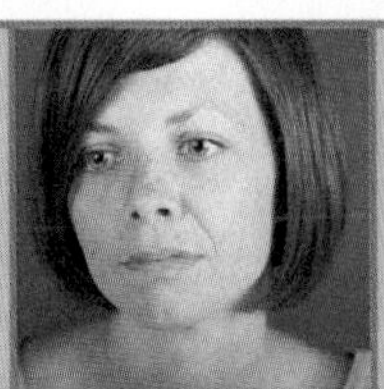

CHAPTER 21 Review of the Central Nervous System

CHAPTER 22 Pharmacotherapy of Anxiety and Insomnia

CHAPTER 23 Pharmacotherapy of Mood Disorders

CHAPTER 24 Pharmacotherapy of Psychoses

CHAPTER 25 Pharmacotherapy of Degenerative Diseases of the Central Nervous System

CHAPTER 26 Pharmacotherapy of Seizures

CHAPTER 27 Pharmacotherapy of Muscle Spasms and Spasticity

CHAPTER 28 Central Nervous System Stimulants and Drugs for Attention Deficit/Hyperactivity Disorder

CHAPTER 29 Pharmacotherapy of Severe Pain and Migraines

CHAPTER 30 Anesthetics and Anesthesia Adjuncts

CHAPTER

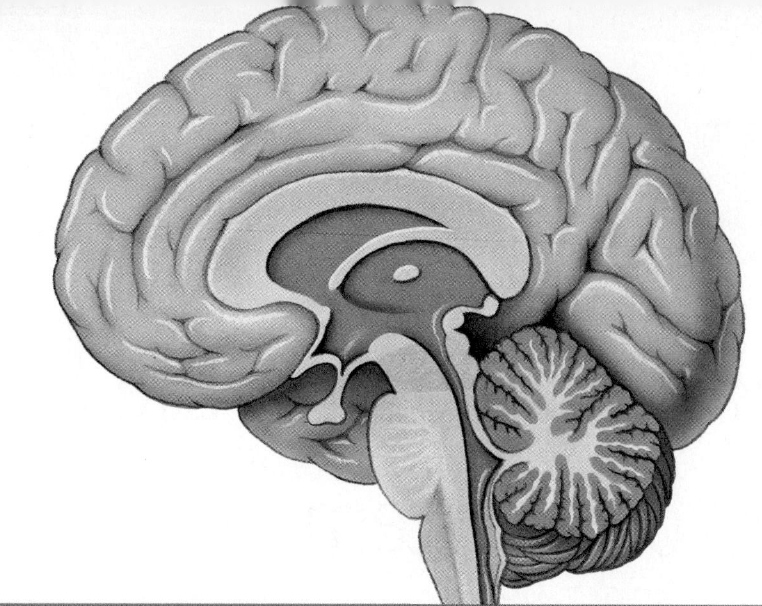

21 Review of the Central Nervous System

Learning Outcomes

After reading this chapter, the student should be able to:

1. Explain why the mechanisms of action of central nervous system drugs are incompletely understood.
2. Identify types of conditions for which central nervous system drugs are prescribed.
3. Diagram the major components of a synapse within the central nervous system.
4. Identify the major neurotransmitters in the central nervous system and their functions.
5. Describe the major structural regions of the brain and their primary functions.
6. Explain the major functional systems of the brain and their primary functions.

Chapter Outline

Scope of Central Nervous System Pharmacology

Neurons and Neurotransmission

Major Structural Components of the Central Nervous System

Functional Systems of the Central Nervous System

Key Terms

acetylcholine (Ach), 266
basal ganglia, 270
dopamine, 266
extrapyramidal system, 270
gamma aminobutyric acid (GABA), 266
glutamate, 267
limbic system, 270
neuron, 266
norepinephrine (NE), 266
reticular activating system (RAS), 270
serotonin, 267
synapses, 266

Chapters 16 through 20 introduce the student to the autonomic nervous system (ANS)—the system that gives involuntary control over vital functions of the cardiovascular, digestive, respiratory, and genitourinary systems. This chapter launches Unit 4, which examines the pharmacology of the central nervous system (CNS). The two components of the CNS, the brain and spinal cord, are collectively responsible for interpreting sensory information and formulating appropriate responses. Typical responses may include thinking (deciding if the sensory information is harmful or pleasurable), emotions (anger, depression, euphoria), or movement (running away, pounding a fist, or hugging). The purpose of this chapter is to provide a brief review of those concepts of CNS anatomy and physiology that are relevant to neuropharmacology.

PharmFACT

The adult human brain weighs about 3 pounds. The brains of males are about 10% larger than those of females due to their larger body size. *Source:* Martini & Nath, 2009.

Scope of Central Nervous System Pharmacology

21.1 Pharmacology of the central nervous system is complex and many drug mechanisms are incompletely understood.

CNS pharmacology is one of the most important divisions in medicine, encompassing 10 chapters in this textbook. Medications may be administered to treat specific neurologic or psychiatric conditions of the CNS. Many drugs cause CNS adverse effects during pharmacotherapy, whereas some are self-administered to produce pleasurable psychoactive effects (see Chapter 8). At high doses, a large number of drugs affect the brain, and CNS toxicity is a dose-limiting factor in the pharmacotherapy of many diseases.

Of all divisions of pharmacology, CNS drug mechanisms are probably the least understood. For some conditions pharmacologists know that the drug acts on the CNS, but its mechanism of action remains largely unknown. There are two primary reasons for this lack of understanding about how CNS drugs produce their effects: the uniqueness of the human brain and the complexity of the disorders affecting it.

The human brain is truly unique, with no other species having the same complexity. It is not known if animals suffer from the same types of mental disorders as humans, and measurement of hallucinations, euphoria, or depression is difficult, if not impossible, in most species. If a drug does induce changes in animal behavior such as depression or anxiety, it is not known whether these data apply to humans because of the enormous differences in brain physiology as well as human social networks that can profoundly influence mental health conditions. Pharmacologists are certainly able to measure changes in brain activity or in the amounts of neurotransmitters in specific regions of the brain, but these do not adequately explain changes in complex behaviors. Without good animal models, pharmacologists must rely largely on empirical observations—evidence derived from giving the drugs to patients and determining what works rather than how it works.

Also complicating the study of CNS pharmacology is that mental disorders themselves are incompletely understood. The physiological basis for conditions such as schizophrenia, major depression, bipolar disorder, panic attacks, or post-traumatic stress disorder is not well established. There is great patient variability in symptoms and disease progression with these conditions, and social factors play important roles. Without a complete understanding of the etiology and pathophysiology of mental disorders, pharmacotherapy of these conditions and the development of new drug therapies for CNS disorders will remain challenging.

The next nine chapters present the major classes of drugs whose pharmacotherapeutic goal is to modify the activity of some portion of the CNS. In a few cases, these drugs affect the function of very specific regions of the brain. Most CNS drugs, however, are nonspecific and affect multiple brain regions.

In simplest terms, CNS drugs have two basic actions: they either stimulate (activation) or suppress (inhibition) the firing of neurons. In some cases, CNS drugs may have both actions: activation of some neurons and inhibition of others. The pharmacologic effects of a CNS drug observed in a patient are the result of which neurons are affected, and how many are affected. As a result of neuron modification, the following beneficial effects of CNS drugs are observed and are studied in this unit.

- Reduction in anxiety
- Improved sleep patterns
- Elevated mood
- Management of psychotic symptoms
- Reduction in seizure frequency
- Slowing the progression of chronic degenerative disease of the brain
- Reduction of hyperactivity and mania
- Reduction in pain
- Induction of anesthesia

CONNECTION *Checkpoint* 21.1

From what you learned in Chapter 16, what are the two divisions of the peripheral nervous system and what are their primary functions? See Answer to Connection Checkpoint 21.1 in Appendix A.

Neurons and Neurotransmission

21.2 Neurons in the central nervous system communicate with each other and with body tissues, using neurotransmitters.

The **neuron** is the primary functional cell in all portions of the nervous system. It is estimated that over 100 billion neurons make up the brain. The function of these cells is to communicate messages through conduction of an action potential. In the CNS, the vast majority of neurons are communicating with other neurons. These neuronal pathways or circuits, are extremely complex and provide the basis for the higher level functions of the brain such as thinking, memory, and intelligence. Although a single neuron serves no practical function, the interconnections among 100 billion neurons are a major part of what distinguishes the human brain from that of all other species.

Communication between neurons in the brain, as well as that between the brain and other organs, is provided through **synapses.** Synapses in the ANS are presented in detail in Chapter 16. The student should review that chapter before proceeding.

Synapses within the CNS operate by the same basic principles as those in the ANS. An electrical impulse releases a neurotransmitter that then moves across a physical space to activate a receptor on the neuron on the opposite side (postsynaptic), as illustrated in Figure 21.1. In some cases, the electrical impulse inhibits the neurotransmitter from being released, or it causes the release of an inhibitory neurotransmitter that suppresses neuronal conduction. All interconnections in the CNS depend on synaptic transmission of the action potential from one neuron to another neuron, or to multiple neurons.

As discussed in Chapter 16, two neurotransmitters account for nearly all synaptic transmission in the ANS: **acetylcholine (Ach)** and **norepinephrine (NE).** Although these two chemicals also are found in the CNS, more than 30 additional substances have been identified as neurotransmitters in the brain, making the study of neuronal communication in this organ very complex. Some neurotransmitters such as glutamate are primarily stimulatory, whereas others such as gamma aminobutyric acid (GABA) inhibit neuronal activity. NE can activate or inhibit neuronal activity, depending on its location in the brain. A summary of the better understood brain neurotransmitters is shown in Table 21.1.

Adrenergic synapses: Adrenergic synapses utilize NE as the neurotransmitter. Adrenergic synapses in the CNS are abundant in the hypothalamus, the limbic system, and the reticular activating system (RAS). NE activates parts of the brain to heighten alertness and is prominent during waking hours. Adrenergic neurons likely play a role in mood disorders such as depression and anxiety.

Cholinergic synapses: Cholinergic synapses utilize Ach as the neurotransmitter. In the brain, these synapses are most often stimulatory. Cholinergic synapses are abundant in the motor cortex and basal ganglia but are uncommon in other areas. Cholinergic synapses are especially important in the pathophysiology of Parkinson's disease and Alzheimer's disease (see Chapter 25). Ach is also a major neurotransmitter in the ANS (see Chapter 16).

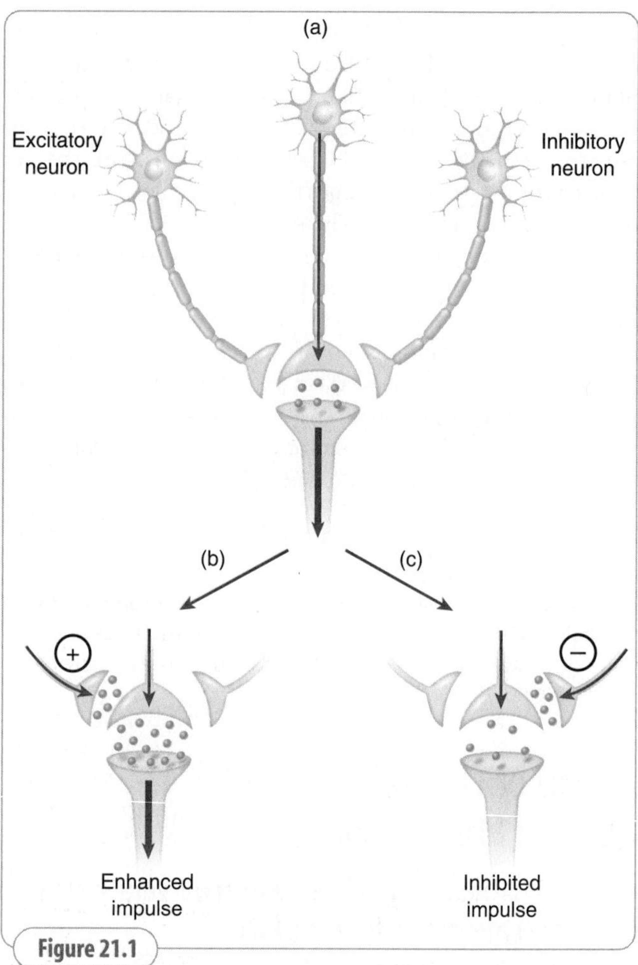

Figure 21.1

Synapses in the central nervous system: (a) normal impulse; (b) enhanced impulse due to firing of excitatory neuron; (c) suppressed impulse due to firing of inhibitory neuron.

Dopaminergic synapses: These synapses utilize dopamine as the neurotransmitter. **Dopamine** is a chemical precursor in the synthesis of NE and, like epinephrine and NE, is classified chemically as a catecholamine. Dopaminergic synapses are generally excitatory and affect arousal and wakefulness. However, two major receptor subtypes exist: D1 is stimulatory, and D2 is inhibitory. Dopamine receptors are important in the pharmacotherapy of psychosis and Parkinson's disease. Cocaine and amphetamines produce their stimulatory actions by affecting dopamine receptors; marijuana is also thought to exert some of its psychoactive effects by increasing dopaminergic activity.

Endorphins and enkephalins: Endorphins and enkephalins are small peptides secreted by neurons in the hypothalamus, pituitary, limbic system, and spinal cord. The receptor for these molecules is the opioid receptor, which is involved in pain transmission. Endorphins and enkephalins are sometimes called natural opiates because they produce effects very similar to morphine and other opioid drugs. Opioids and their receptors are presented in detail in Chapter 29.

Gamma aminobutyric acid synapses: These synapses utilize **gamma aminobutyric acid (GABA)** as a neurotransmitter. GABA synapses are the second most common type in the CNS, accounting for 30% to 40% of all brain synapses. GABA is the

TABLE 21.1 Selected Central Nervous System Neurotransmitters and Their Functions

Neurotransmitter	Abundance	Effect	Clinical Significance
Acetylcholine	Widely distributed in the CNS; a major transmitter in the ANS	CNS: May be excitatory or inhibitory; controls voluntary skeletal muscle movement. ANS: Activates the parasympathetic nervous system	Myasthenia gravis, Alzheimer's disease
Dopamine	Basal ganglia and limbic system	Usually excitatory; locomotion, attention, learning, and the reinforcing effects of abused drugs	Parkinson's disease; psychoses; motivation, pleasure
Endorphins and Enkephalins	Widely distributed in the CNS and peripheral nervous system (PNS)	Usually inhibitory; reduction of pain	Opioids bind to endorphin receptors
Gamma aminobutyric acid (GABA)	Widely distributed in the CNS	Most common inhibitory CNS neurotransmitter	Seizure and anxiety disorders
Glutamate	Widely distributed in the CNS	Most common excitatory CNS neurotransmitter	Memory
Norepinephrine	Widely distributed in the CNS; a major transmitter in the ANS	CNS: May be excitatory or inhibitory. ANS: Activates the sympathetic nervous system	Depression, memory, panic attacks
Serotonin	Common in the brainstem but also found in the limbic system	Usually inhibitory	Anxiety, bipolar disorder, and depression

primary inhibitory neurotransmitter in the CNS and is found throughout the brain, with greatest abundance in the basal ganglia and hypothalamus. GABA receptors are the primary site of action for several classes of drugs, including the benzodiazepines, which are used to treat anxiety. Several GABA receptor subtypes have been identified.

Glutamate synapses: Glutamate synapses utilize the amino acid **glutamate** (glutamic acid) as a neurotransmitter. Glutamate is the most common neurotransmitter in the CNS, and its synapses are always excitatory in nature. It is found in nearly all regions of the brain. Several glutamate receptor subtypes have been identified, with the N-methyl D-aspartate (NMDA) receptor being particularly important. In addition to glutamate, zinc, magnesium, glycine, and even phencyclidine (a hallucinogen) bind to the NMDA receptor, thus modulating neuronal activity. High amounts of glutamate can cause death of neurons and may be the mechanism responsible for certain types of neurotoxicty.

Serotonergic synapses: Serotonergic synapses utilize **serotonin,** also known as 5-hydroxytryptamine (5-HT), as a neurotransmitter. Although some serotonergic synapses are located in the CNS, 98% of the serotonergic receptors are found outside the CNS in platelets, mast cells, and other peripheral cells. Serotonergic receptors are found throughout the limbic system of the brain, often in close association with adrenergic synapses. Low serotonin levels in the CNS are associated with anxiety and impulsive behavior, including suicidal ideation. Serotonergic receptors play an important role in the mechanism of action of antidepressant drugs. Serotonin is used by the body to synthesize the hormone melatonin in the pineal gland.

CONNECTION *Checkpoint* 21.2

The neurotransmitter dopamine is also available as a drug. From what you learned in Chapter 19, what are the indications for dopamine therapy? See Answer to Connection Checkpoint 21.2 in Appendix A.

Pharm*FACT*

There are an estimated 1 quadrillion (1,000,000,000,000,000) synapses in the human brain. *Source:* U.S. Public Health Service, 2008.

Major Structural Components of the Central Nervous System

21.3 The central nervous system is divided into several major structural components.

The brain consists of dozens of structural divisions that serve common functions. Identification of the many anatomic components in the CNS is complex and beyond the scope of this text. This section focuses on regions of the CNS that have applications to neuropharmacology. For a more complete discussion of CNS anatomy, the student should consult anatomy and physiology textbooks. Basic brain structures are illustrated in Figure 21.2.

Cerebrum: The cerebrum is the "thinking" part of the brain responsible for perception, speech, conscious motor movement,

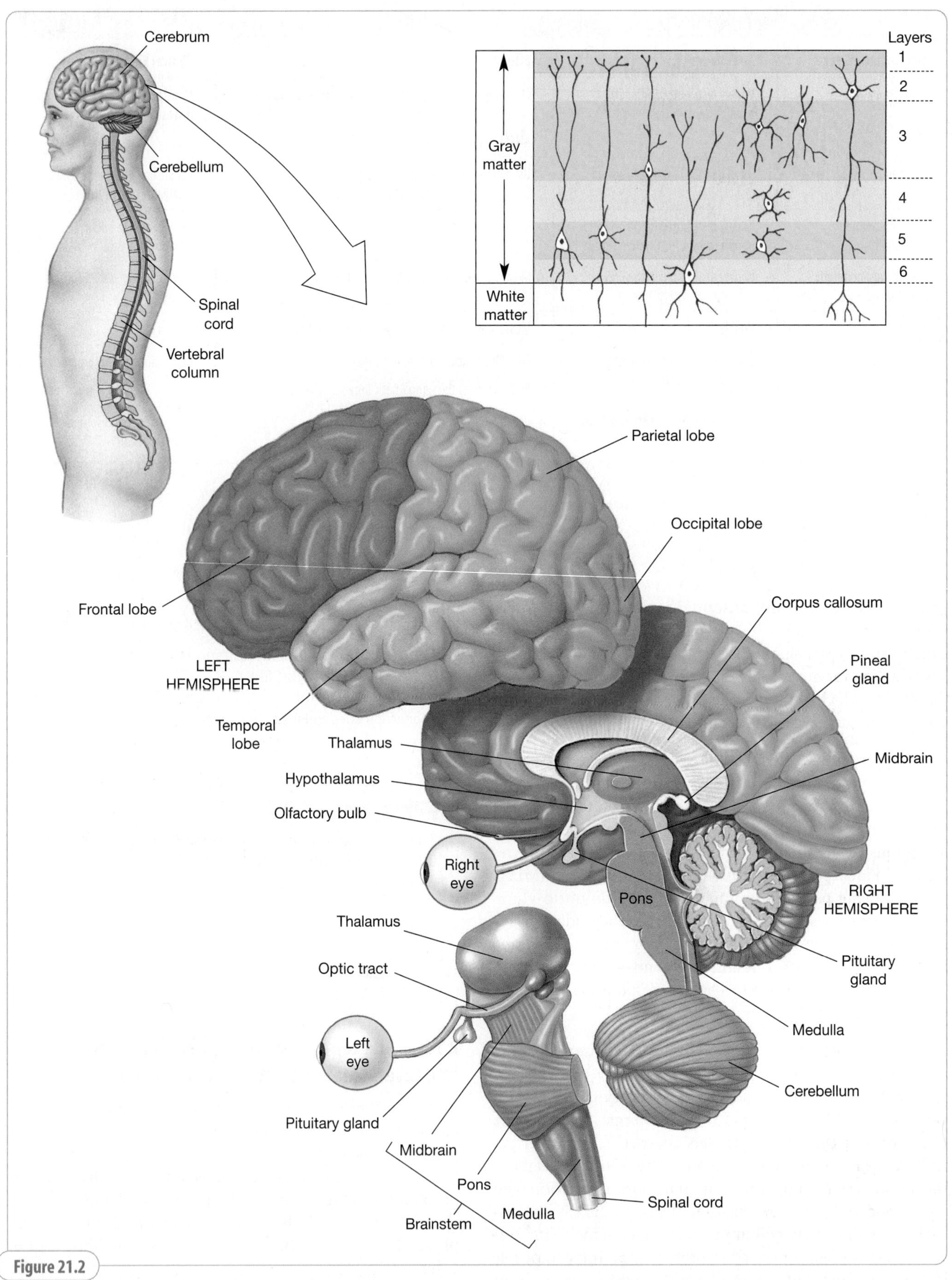

Figure 21.2

Basic anatomy of the brain.

Source: From *Human Physiology: An Integrated Approach* (2nd ed., p. 256) by D. Silverthorn, 2001. Reprinted by permission of Pearson Education, Inc., Upper Saddle River, NJ.

movement of skeletal muscles, memory, and smell. It is the largest part of the brain, by weight, and the most advanced. Portions of the cerebrum are organized for specialized functions. For example, the occipital lobe is associated with vision and the frontal lobes are concerned with reasoning and planning. Other areas are specific to language, hearing, motor, or sensory functions.

Disorders of the cerebrum may be focal or generalized. Focal abnormalities, often the result of cerebrovascular accidents (CVA), occur in specific regions and may affect a single brain function such as vision, hearing, or movement of a particular limb. Generalized disorders of the cerebrum affect widespread areas or multiple regions and can produce drowsiness, coma, hallucinations, depression, or generalized anxiety.

Thalamus: The thalamus is the major relay center in the brain that sends sensory information such as sounds, sights, pain, touch, and temperature to the cerebral cortex for analysis. To reach the cerebrum, all sensory information must travel through the thalamus. Portions of the thalamus comprise the limbic system, an area that controls mood and motivation (see Section 21.4). Abnormalities of the thalamus have been associated with diverse mood disorders such as obsessive-compulsive disorder, bipolar disorder, anxiety, and panic disorder.

Hypothalamus: The hypothalamus is the major visceral control center in the body. Regulation of hunger, thirst, water balance, and body temperature are functions of this region. The hypothalamus is also part of the limbic system, which is associated with emotional balance (see Section 21.4). Some neurons in the hypothalamus connect to the brainstem to affect vital centers such as heart rate, respiratory rate, blood pressure, and pupil size. These responses are associated with the fight-or-flight response of the ANS. The many endocrine functions of the hypothalamus are discussed in Chapter 65. Disorders of the hypothalamus may affect some or all of these essential functions.

CONNECTION *Checkpoint* 21.3

From what you learned in Chapter 16, describe the symptoms of the fight-or-flight response. See Answer to Connection Checkpoint 21.3 in Appendix A.

Cerebellum: The cerebellum controls muscle movement, balance, posture, and tone. It is involved in learning fine motor skills that make muscular movements smooth and continuous. The cerebellum receives sensory information, including vision, position, equilibrium, and touch, and calculates the strength and extent of muscle movement needed to maintain posture and coordinate complex tasks such as walking, driving, or playing a musical instrument. Injury to this region results in uncoordinated, jerky body movements.

Brainstem: The brainstem, consisting of the medulla oblongata, pons, and midbrain, connects the spinal cord to the brain. Because of its critical location, it serves as the major relay center for messages traveling to and from the brain. In addition, it contains major reflex and control centers involving breathing, heart rate, vision, swallowing, coughing, and vomiting. Injury to the brainstem can be fatal if vital centers are disrupted. The brainstem contains clusters of scattered neurons known as the reticular formation, which help maintain alertness (see Section 21.4).

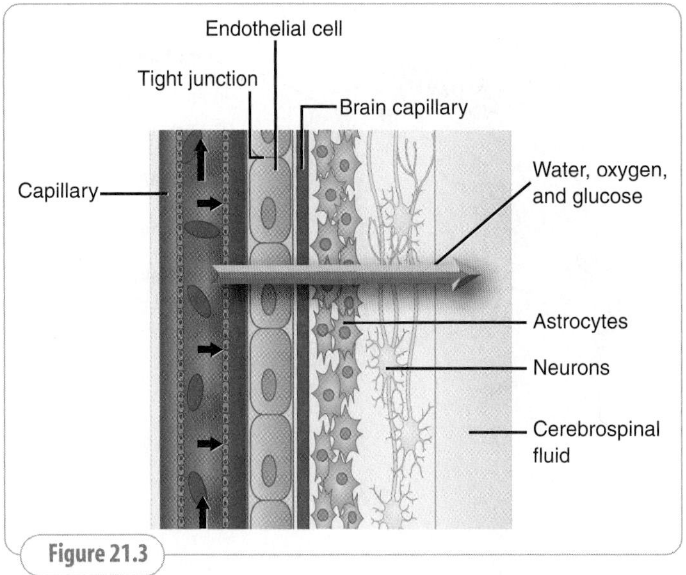

Figure 21.3

Blood–brain barrier.

Spinal cord: The spinal cord is essentially a conduction pathway to and from the brain. Disruptions of these pathways will prevent transmission of nerve impulses and cause loss of sensory (paresthesia) or motor (paralysis) function.

Blood–brain barrier: The brain must receive a continuous supply of oxygen and glucose; interruptions for even brief periods may cause loss of consciousness. At the same time it needs large quantities of nutrients, the brain must also protect itself from pathogens or toxins that may have entered the blood. Capillaries in most regions of the brain are not as porous as those in other organs; the endothelial cells form tight junctions, creating a seal or barrier to many substances. This is important to pharmacology because CNS drugs must be designed with the capability of penetrating the blood–brain barrier to produce their effects. The blood–brain barrier is illustrated in Figure 21.3.

Functional Systems of the Central Nervous System

21.4 Several functional divisions of the central nervous system are important to pharmacotherapy.

Functional brain systems are clusters of neurons that work together to perform a common function. These clusters are physically located far apart in the CNS but form a communication network to act as a coordinated unit. Some of these systems are important to pharmacotherapy because drugs produce their effects by modifying their functions.

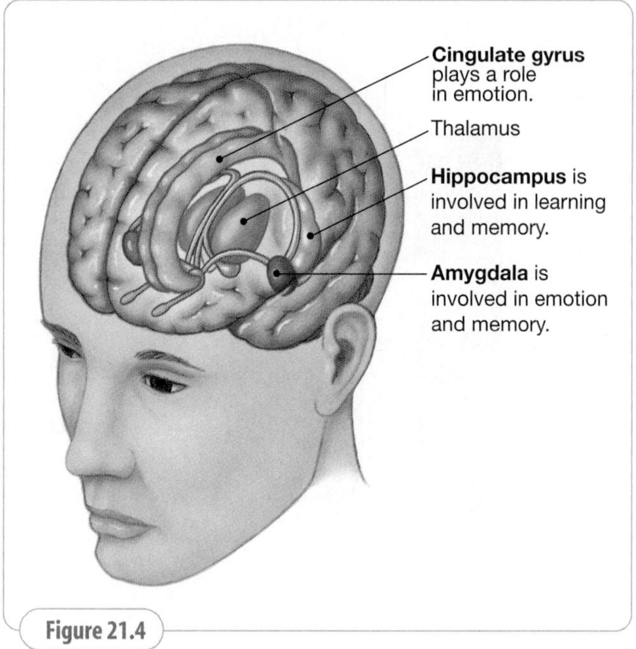

Figure 21.4

Limbic system.
Source: From *Human Physiology: An Integrated Approach* (4th ed., p. 308), by D. Silverthorn, 2007. Reprinted by permission of Pearson Education, Inc., Upper Saddle River, NJ.

Limbic system: The **limbic system** is a group of structures deep in the brain that are responsible for emotional expression, learning, and memory. Emotional states associated with this system include anxiety, fear, anger, aggression, remorse, depression, sexual drive, and euphoria. Signals routed through the limbic system ultimately connect with the hypothalamus (see Section 21.3). Through its connection with the hypothalamus, autonomic actions such as rapid heart rate, high blood pressure, or peptic ulcers are associated with intense emotional states. The limbic system also communicates with the cerebrum, which allows people to think and reflect on their emotional states. The connection to the cerebrum allows one to use logic to "override" emotional reactions that might be inappropriate or harmful. Parts of the limbic system also allow one to remember emotional responses. The components of the limbic system are illustrated in Figure 21.4.

Reticular activating system: The reticular formation, a network of neurons found along the entire length of the brainstem, is shown in Figure 21.5. Stimulation of the reticular formation causes heightened alertness and arousal of the brain as a whole. Inhibition causes general drowsiness and the induction of sleep.

The larger area in which the reticular formation is found is called the **reticular activating system (RAS).** This structure projects from the brainstem to the thalamus. The RAS is responsible for sleeping and wakefulness and performs an alerting function for the cerebral cortex. It also acts as a filter, allowing one to ignore weak, repetitious, or unimportant sensory stimuli and to focus attention on individual tasks by transmitting information to higher brain centers. This is important in busy, noisy environments when a person must concentrate on a specific task, such as studying or reading. In any given situation, as much as 99% of all sensory information may be filtered and never reach consciousness.

The RAS has particular importance to pharmacology because many drugs act by decreasing neuronal activity in this system to cause drowsiness or sleep. Examples include alcohol and sedative–hypnotics. Lysergic acid diethylamide (LSD) interferes with portions of the RAS, causing unusual sensory experiences such as seeing odors or hearing colors.

Basal ganglia: The **basal ganglia** are a cluster of neurons in the brain that help regulate the initiation and termination of skeletal muscle movement. They also help initiate and terminate certain cognitive functions such as memory, learning, planning, and attention. Connections between the basal ganglia and the limbic system are thought to be associated with psychoses, attention deficit/hyperactivity disorder and obsessive-compulsive disorder. Reduced dopaminergic transmission through the basal ganglia is the most common etiology for Parkinson's disease. The basal ganglia are illustrated in Figure 21.6.

Extrapyramidal system: Messages controlling the voluntary movement of skeletal muscle originate in the cerebrum and travel down the CNS in tracts or pathways. The two motor pathways, traveling through the brain, brainstem, and spinal cord, are called pyramidal (direct) and extrapyramidal (indirect). The pyramidal tracts are voluntary tracts involved with the movement of skeletal muscles. The **extrapyramidal system** controls locomotion, complex muscular movements, and posture. The extrapyramidal system has particular importance to pharmacology because it is adversely affected by certain medications, especially the conventional antipsychotic agents (see Chapter 24). Adverse extrapyramidal symptoms include jerking motions, muscular spasms of the head, face, and neck, and akathisia, an inability to remain at rest. Some extrapyramidal symptoms resemble those of Parkinson's disease (see Chapter 25).

PharmFACT

There are some postsynaptic neurons that connect with and receive information from as many as 10,000 presynaptic neurons. *Source:* Silverthorn, 2009.

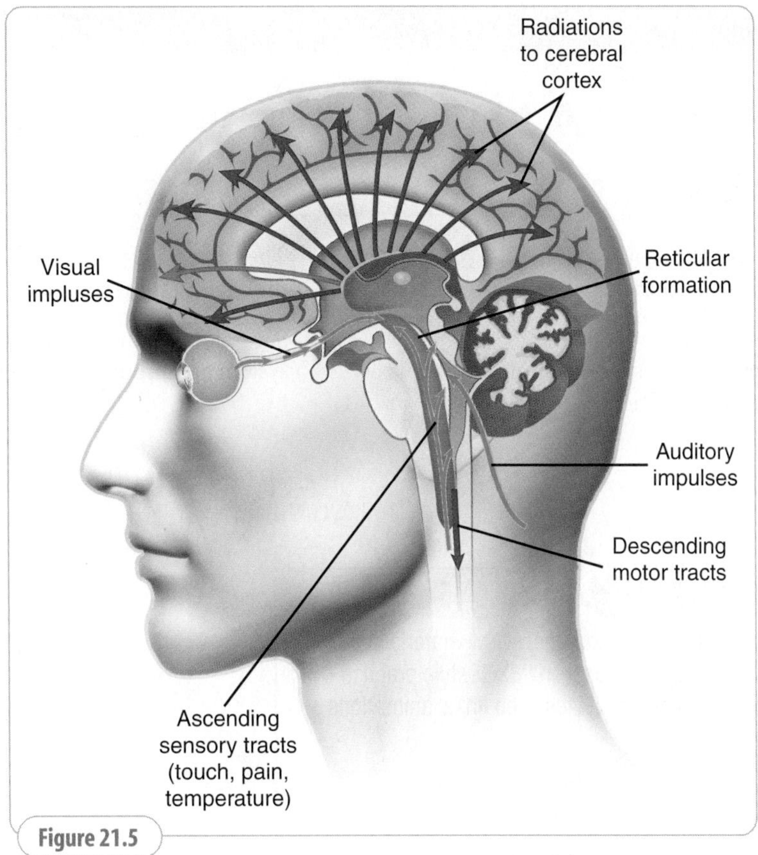

Figure 21.5

With input from sensory neurons, activation of the reticular activating system (RAS) causes arousal of the cerebral cortex, thus maintaining the awake-and-alert state.

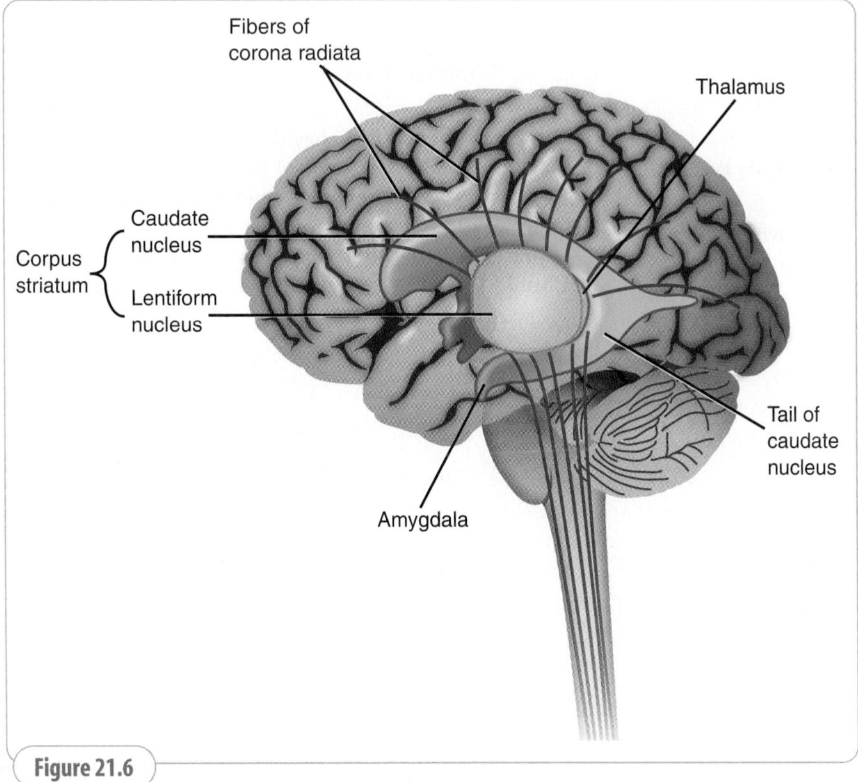

Figure 21.6

The basal ganglia are clusters of gray matter that control learned movement and are involved with the subconscious control of skeletal muscle tone.

UNDERSTANDING THE CHAPTER

Key Concepts Summary

21.1 Pharmacology of the central nervous system is complex and many drug mechanisms are incompletely understood.

21.2 Neurons in the central nervous system communicate with each other and with body tissues, using neurotransmitters.

21.3 The central nervous system is divided into several major structural components.

21.4 Several functional divisions of the central nervous system are important to pharmacotherapy.

References

Krogh, D. (2009). *Biology: A guide to the natural world* (4th ed.). San Francisco: Pearson Benjamin Cummings.

Martini, F. H., & Nath, J. L. (2009). *Fundamentals of human anatomy and physiology* (8th ed.). San Francisco: Pearson Benjamin Cummings.

Rice, J. (2005). *Medical terminology with human anatomy* (5th ed.). Upper Saddle River, NJ: Prentice Hall.

Silverthorn, D. U. (2009). *Human physiology: An integrated approach* (4th ed.). San Francisco: Pearson Benjamin Cummings.

U.S. Public Health Service. (2008). The fundamentals of mental health and mental illness. In *Mental health: A report of the surgeon general.* Retrieved June 5, 2008, from http://www.surgeongeneral.gov/library/mentalhealth/chapter2/sec1.html

von Bohlen und Halbach, O., & Dermietzel, R. (2006). *Neurotransmitters and neuromodulators: Handbook of receptors and biological effects.* Weinheim, Germany: Wiley-VCH.

Westfall, T. C., & Westfall, D. P. (2006). Neurotransmission: The autonomic and somatic nervous systems. In L. L. Brunton, J. S. Lazo, & K. L. Parker (Eds.). *The pharmacological basis of therapeutics* (11th ed., pp. 137–181). New York: McGraw-Hill.

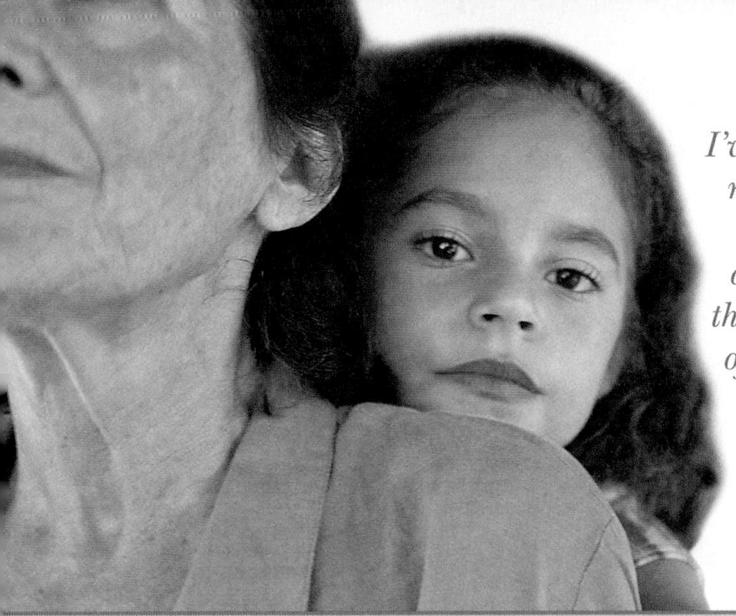

I've always worked hard and enjoyed my work, whether it was helping Joe establish our home, raising our children, or teaching school. Lately, though, it takes all I've got to get out of bed, deal with my family, and get to work. I just don't understand why my life has taken this turn, and I don't see when, if ever, things will improve.

Patient "Seraphina Alvarez"

CHAPTER 22

Pharmacotherapy of Anxiety and Insomnia

Chapter Outline

Anxiety Disorders

Sleep Disorders

Management of Anxiety and Insomnia

Pharmacotherapy of Anxiety and Insomnia

Benzodiazepines

PROTOTYPE **Lorazepam (Ativan)** *p. 284*

Nonbenzodiazepine anxiolytics and miscellaneous agents

PROTOTYPE **Zolpidem (Ambien, Tovalt)** *p. 287*

Antidepressants

Barbiturates

PROTOTYPE **Phenobarbital (Luminal)** *p. 291*

Learning Outcomes

After reading this chapter, the student should be able to:

1. Explain why it is important to obtain an accurate diagnosis of anxiety.
2. Compare and contrast the five major types of anxiety disorders.
3. Identify the regions and systems of the brain associated with anxiety, sleep, and wakefulness.
4. Describe the normal stages of sleep and explain how they are affected by anxiety and stress.
5. Identify sleep disorders that may benefit from pharmacotherapy.
6. Explain the association between insomnia and anxiety.
7. Describe nonpharmacologic methods for managing anxiety and insomnia.
8. Identify the major classes of medications used to treat anxiety and sleep disorders.
9. Describe the nurse's role in the pharmacologic and nonpharmacologic management of anxiety and insomnia.
10. For each of the classes shown in the chapter outline, identify the prototype and representative drugs and explain the mechanism(s) of drug action, primary indications, contraindications, significant drug interactions, pregnancy category, and important adverse effects.
11. Use the nursing process to care for patients receiving drug therapy for anxiety and insomnia.

Key Terms

agoraphobia, *275*
amygdala, *276*
anxiety, *274*
anxiolytic, *281*
cataplexy, *279*
circadian rhythm, *278*
generalized anxiety disorder (GAD), *275*
hypnagogic hallucinations, *279*
insomnia, *279*
locus coeruleus, *276*
narcolepsy, *279*
non–rapid eye movement (NREM) sleep, *277*
obsessive–compulsive disorder (OCD), *276*
panic disorder, *275*
phobia, *275*
post-traumatic stress disorder (PTSD), *276*
rapid eye movement (REM) sleep, *278*
rebound insomnia, *280*
sedative–hypnotic, *281*
situational anxiety, *275*
social anxiety disorder, *275*

Anxiety occurs when a person perceives a threat to his or her well-being or security. This threat, such as an upcoming divorce or pharmacology test, may be clearly identifiable, or it may be a diffuse, general feeling of worry or dread. Anxiety is a normal, adaptive response that prepares a person to deal, both physically and emotionally, with the perceived danger. When the anxiety response occurs continuously or without a genuine threat, however, the patient's quality of life may become seriously affected and there will be an increased risk of developing chronic gastrointestinal (GI) and cardiovascular conditions. Anxiety disorders are the most common mental health conditions encountered in clinical practice. This chapter deals with medications that treat anxiety, cause sedation, or help patients sleep.

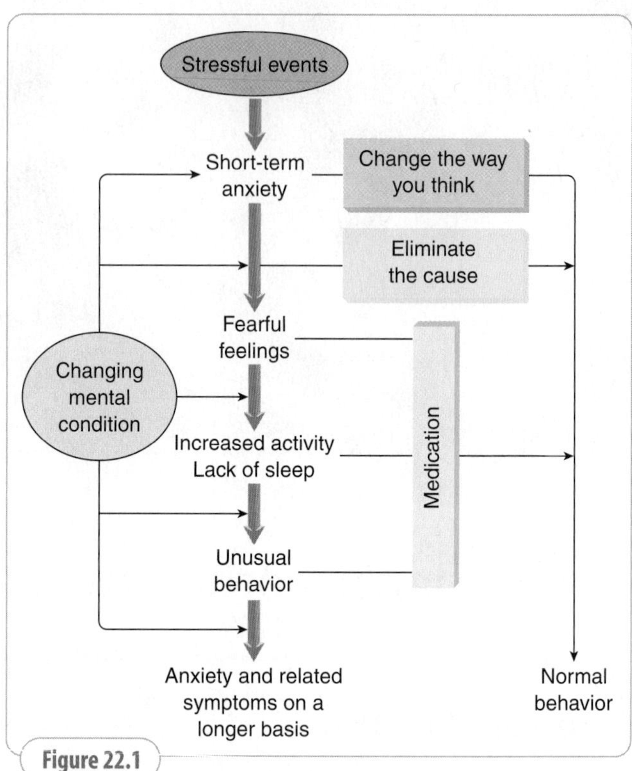

Figure 22.1

A model of anxiety in which stressful events or a changing mental condition can produce unfavorable symptoms, some of which may be controlled by medication.

Anxiety Disorders

22.1 Proper diagnosis of anxiety disorders is important to identifying the most effective treatment option.

The International Classification of Diseases, 10th edition (ICD-10), is an official list of categories of diseases compiled by the World Health Organization. According to the ICD-10, **anxiety** is a state of "apprehension, tension, or uneasiness that stems from the anticipation of danger, the source of which is largely unknown or unrecognized."

In the clinical setting, most patients with anxiety will present with multiple symptoms and describe their condition in diverse ways. Patients often describe their feelings using terms such as *apprehension, dread, fear,* or *worry* and report physical symptoms such as palpitations, shortness of breath, heartburn, pounding in the ears, excessive sweating, or dry mouth. Most people realize that their feelings of anxiety are disproportionate to any real threats or dangers. A diagram of how people typically deal with stressful events is shown in Figure 22.1.

It is often challenging for the nurse to sort through the many diverse and subjective patient symptoms to determine the etiology of the anxiety. Patients may be unaware of the source of their symptoms, or they may be reluctant to discuss their causes because they may be deeply personal. The health care provider must accurately diagnose the condition, however, because treatment differs among the various types of anxiety disorders. In some cases pharmacotherapy may not be the best option. Anxiety is a disorder that responds well to complementary and alternative medicine (CAM), and the nurse is a key person to recommend and teach patients nonpharmacologic stress-reduction techniques. Some patients benefit from individual or group psychotherapy, which can help to identify and overcome the root causes of their worry and fear. Some anxiety disorders, however, are debilitating and require effective pharmacotherapy.

When obtaining a comprehensive medication history during the initial patient assessment, the nurse should notice any substances that the patient is taking that may worsen or cause anxiety symptoms. Sometimes discontinuing or substituting alternate drugs for these "anxiety-promoting" medications can lessen patient symptoms. A simple example is substituting decaffeinated beverages for those containing caffeine. In addition, there are many medical conditions associated with anxiety symptoms. For example, knowing that one has cancer or has a high risk for myocardial infarction (MI) certainly creates high stress for a patient. In these cases, the anxiety is considered secondary and may resolve once the underlying medical condition is treated. Drugs and medical conditions associated with anxiety disorders are shown in Table 22.1.

TABLE 22.1 Medications and Medical Conditions Associated with Anxiety

Medications
Antibiotics: isoniazid, fluoroquinolones
Antidepressants: Selective serotonin reuptake inhibitors (SSRIs), tricyclic antidepressants (TCAs), bupropion
Antihypertensives: felodipine, methyldopa
Antiseizure drugs: carbamazepine
Bronchodilators: albuterol, theophylline
Hallucinogens: LSD, Ecstasy
Hormones: prednisone, thyroid hormone
Nonsteroidal anti-inflammatory drugs (NSAIDs): ibuprofen
Stimulants: amphetamines, caffeine, cocaine, methylphenidate
Sympathomimetics: pseudoephedrine
Medical Conditions
Cardiovascular: angina, cerebrovascular accident (CVA), dysrhythmias, heart failure, MI, pulmonary embolus
Endocrine: Cushing's disease, hyperthyroidism, hypoglycemia
Neurologic: dementia, epilepsy, Parkinson's disease, severe or chronic pain
Others: anemias, cancer, impotence, nausea, withdrawal from abused substances, vertigo
Respiratory: asthma, chronic obstructive pulmonary disease (COPD), pneumonia

PharmFACT

About 40 million Americans are affected by anxiety disorders every year. Illnesses that commonly coexist with anxiety include depression, eating disorders, and substance abuse. *Source:* Anxiety Disorders Association of America, 2008.

22.2 Anxiety disorders may be divided into five major categories.

The anxiety experienced by people faced with a temporary stressful environment is called **situational anxiety.** Situational anxiety is not considered a major anxiety disorder because it is not disabling or persistent. To a degree, situational anxiety is beneficial because it motivates people to accomplish tasks in a prompt manner—if for no other reason than to eliminate the source of nervousness. All persons experience situational stress at some time in their lives and, although it may be intense, it does not generally require pharmacotherapy.

According to the *Diagnostic and Statistical Manual of Mental Disorders,* Fourth Edition, Text Revision *(DSM-IV-TR),* anxiety may require treatment when it becomes chronic and interferes with activities of daily living. This handbook published by the American Psychiatric Association lists the official diagnostic classifications of mental disorders. The latest complete revision was made in 1994 (with "text revisions" in 2000) and divides anxiety disorders into several major categories: generalized anxiety disorder, panic disorder, social anxiety disorder (phobia), obsessive–compulsive disorder, and post-traumatic stress disorder. Not all anxiety experienced by patients is easily classified, and it is common for people to present with multiple types of anxiety, such as generalized anxiety disorder along with panic attacks.

PharmFACT

For three anxiety disorders, women are twice as likely to be affected as men. These disorders include generalized anxiety disorder, panic disorder, and specific phobias. *Source:* Anxiety Disorders Association of America, 2008.

Generalized anxiety disorder (GAD) is excessive anxiety that persists for 6 months or longer. GAD has a gradual onset and is most prevalent in the 20 to 35 age group. The characteristic feature of GAD is excessive worry or fear regarding life events or activities, frequently focusing on family, money, or health. It is by far the most common type of clinical stress disorder and the one most frequently encountered by the nurse. Symptoms include restlessness, fatigue, muscle tension, nervousness, inability to focus or concentrate, an overwhelming sense of dread, and sleep disturbances. Signs of sympathetic nervous system activation that accompany GAD include blood pressure elevation, heart palpitations, varying degrees of respiratory change, and dry mouth. Parasympathetic responses may consist of abdominal cramping, diarrhea, fatigue, and urinary urgency. Women are slightly more likely to experience GAD than men. Some patients experience symptoms for over a decade before seeking help for their condition.

Panic disorder is a type of anxiety characterized by intense feelings of immediate apprehension, fearfulness, terror, or impending doom, accompanied by increased autonomic nervous system activity such as sweating, racing heart rate, shortness of breath, and trembling. To be diagnosed with panic disorder the patient must present with at least 1 month of ongoing concern or worry about experiencing subsequent episodes. Panic attacks typically last only 1 to 10 minutes, although one attack may quickly follow another and patients may describe the episode as seemingly endless. Up to 5% of the population will experience one or more panic attacks during their lifetime, with women being affected about twice as often as men. Patients with panic disorder usually modify their behavior to try to avoid another attack. Some develop **agoraphobia,** an extreme avoidance of closed places where a panic attack might occur such as airplanes, public meetings, or elevators. Panic attacks are often associated with major depression.

MyNursingKit | Panic Disorder Videos

Social anxiety disorder, also called social phobia, is an unreasonable and persistent fear of crowds or of being ridiculed or embarrassed in public. Performing and speaking in public are two common examples of activities that may trigger social anxiety disorder. Patients will either avoid the situation entirely or tolerate it with great discomfort. Symptoms include sweating, blushing, tachycardia, trembling, and bowel cramping or diarrhea. The average age of onset is the mid teens, and the disorder may persist for decades before the person seeks treatment. Social anxiety disorder is a type of **phobia,** a fearful feeling attached to situations or objects. In addition to social anxiety disorder, specific phobias include fear of snakes, spiders, high altitudes, or exposure to blood. Panic attacks may occur when the person encounters his or her phobia; for example, the person sees blood or is forced to speak or perform in public.

MyNursingKit | Obsessive–Compulsive Disorder Videos

Obsessive–compulsive disorder (OCD) involves recurrent, intrusive thoughts or repetitive behaviors. To be diagnosed with OCD, the behavior or thought must occupy more than 1 hour each day and negatively impact the patient's normal daily activities or relationships. The obsession portion of this behavior involves thoughts, whereas the compulsion portion involves actions. Most patients with this disorder have both obsessions and compulsions. One common example is repetitive thoughts about the fear of exposure to germs. The patient may think about the presence of germs constantly and what can be done to decrease exposure (obsession). The person may engage in repetitive hand washing, possibly to the point of doing damage to the skin of the hands (compulsion). This repetitive activity can occur so frequently that it severely intrudes on the person's ability to do any other activity during the day, including work or school. Other obsessions or compulsions include viewing sexually explicit pictures, doubting whether the iron or stove was turned off, repeating the same words silently, or repetitive counting. Most commonly, the age of onset is the teen years or early adulthood.

Post-traumatic stress disorder (PTSD) is a type of situational anxiety that develops in response to reexperiencing a previous life event. Witnessing or experiencing traumatic events such as war, physical or sexual abuse, torture, natural disasters, or murder may lead to a sense of helplessness and reexperiencing of the event. Hurricanes Katrina and Rita, as well as witnessing the terrorist attack on September 11, 2001, are examples of situations that may trigger PTSD. The reexperience may take the form of nightmares, hallucinations, or flashbacks, accompanied by uncomfortable physical signs such as tachycardia and extreme nervousness or panic attacks. If the reaction occurs immediately and resolves within 1 month of the event, it is classified by the *DSM-IV-TR* as acute stress disorder. To be diagnosed with PTSD the patient must be experiencing distressing symptoms for more than 1 month. PTSD may occur at any age and 80% of patients with PTSD have comorbid depression or another anxiety disorder. Approximately 20% of patients with serious PTSD attempt suicide because they feel they lack a future.

22.3 Specific regions of the brain that are responsible for anxiety have been identified.

Research has clearly demonstrated that the modulation of anxiety is accomplished in specific brain regions and by multiple neurotransmitter systems. Neuroimaging studies show that the different types of anxiety disorders activate distinct areas of the brain. Neural pathways associated with GAD, social anxiety disorder, and panic disorder are different.

Neural systems in the brain that are associated with anxiety include the limbic system and the reticular activating system. These are illustrated in Pharmacotherapy Illustrated 22.1. The student should read Section 21.4 in Chapter 21 for a brief review of these two systems before proceeding.

The limbic system is a cluster of structures in the middle of the brain that is responsible for governing emotions, behavior, and long-term memory. A key part of the limbic system that is involved in the pathogenesis of anxiety is the **amygdala,** the center of human emotions (Silverthorn, 2009). The amygdala helps determine the emotional significance of the conscious and subconscious signals received from the cerebral cortex. Once activated the amygdala generates feelings of anxiety and fear and stimulates several regions of the brain that begin the stress response. For example, the midbrain and brainstem may be activated, resulting in stress symptoms related to the autonomic nervous system, such as high blood pressure, elevated breathing rate, and dilated pupils.

Signals routed through the amygdala ultimately connect with the hypothalamus, an important center responsible for modulating the fight-or-flight response of the autonomic nervous system. Emotional states associated with this connection include anxiety, fear, anger, aggression, remorse, depression, sexual drive, and euphoria. The hypothalamus may respond by secreting corticotropin-releasing factor (CRF), which eventually causes the release of corticosteroids from the adrenal glands. Corticosteroids are major modulators of the stress response (see Chapter 69). The hypothalamus also regulates essential somatic functions, including sleep, appetite, and body temperature.

An area in the anterior hypothalamus, called the suprachiasmatic nucleus, receives input from the retina, providing information about light and dark. This structure controls the production of melatonin, which influences the induction of sleep. Melatonin is available as a dietary supplement and is often taken to treat jet lag and sleeplessness. A melatonin agonist, ramelteon (Rozerem), is approved by the U.S. Food and Drug Administration (FDA) for treating insomnia (see Section 22.9).

Within the brainstem, an area in the pons known as the **locus coeruleus** has been associated with fear responses and panic attacks. The locus coeruleus monitors internal and external signals and is a major location for norepinephrine in the brain. Release of norepinephrine from the locus coeruleus causes the brain to become activated for fight or flight. Certain medications act on this area of the brain.

The hypothalamus connects with the reticular formation, a collection of neurons found along the core of the brainstem. The reticular formation receives input from nearly all sensory organs as well as from the cerebrum and cerebellum. Ascending fibers project to the cerebrum to form the reticular activating system (RAS). The RAS is responsible for sleeping, wakefulness, and the ability to respond to stimuli, and performs an alerting function for the entire cerebral cortex. Drugs that stimulate the RAS cause heightened alertness and arousal; inhibitory drugs cause general drowsiness and the induction of sleep. Neurotransmitters within the RAS regulate the sleep–wake cycle by shifting the balance from one neurotransmitter to another.

If signals are prevented from passing through the RAS there is a reduction in general brain activity. If signals coming from the hypothalamus are allowed to proceed, then those signals are further routed through the RAS and on to higher brain centers. This is the neural mechanism thought to be responsible for feelings such as anxiety and fear. It is also the mechanism associated with restlessness and an interrupted sleeping pattern.

PHARMACOTHERAPY ILLUSTRATED 22.1

Regions of the Brain Affected by Antianxiety Medications

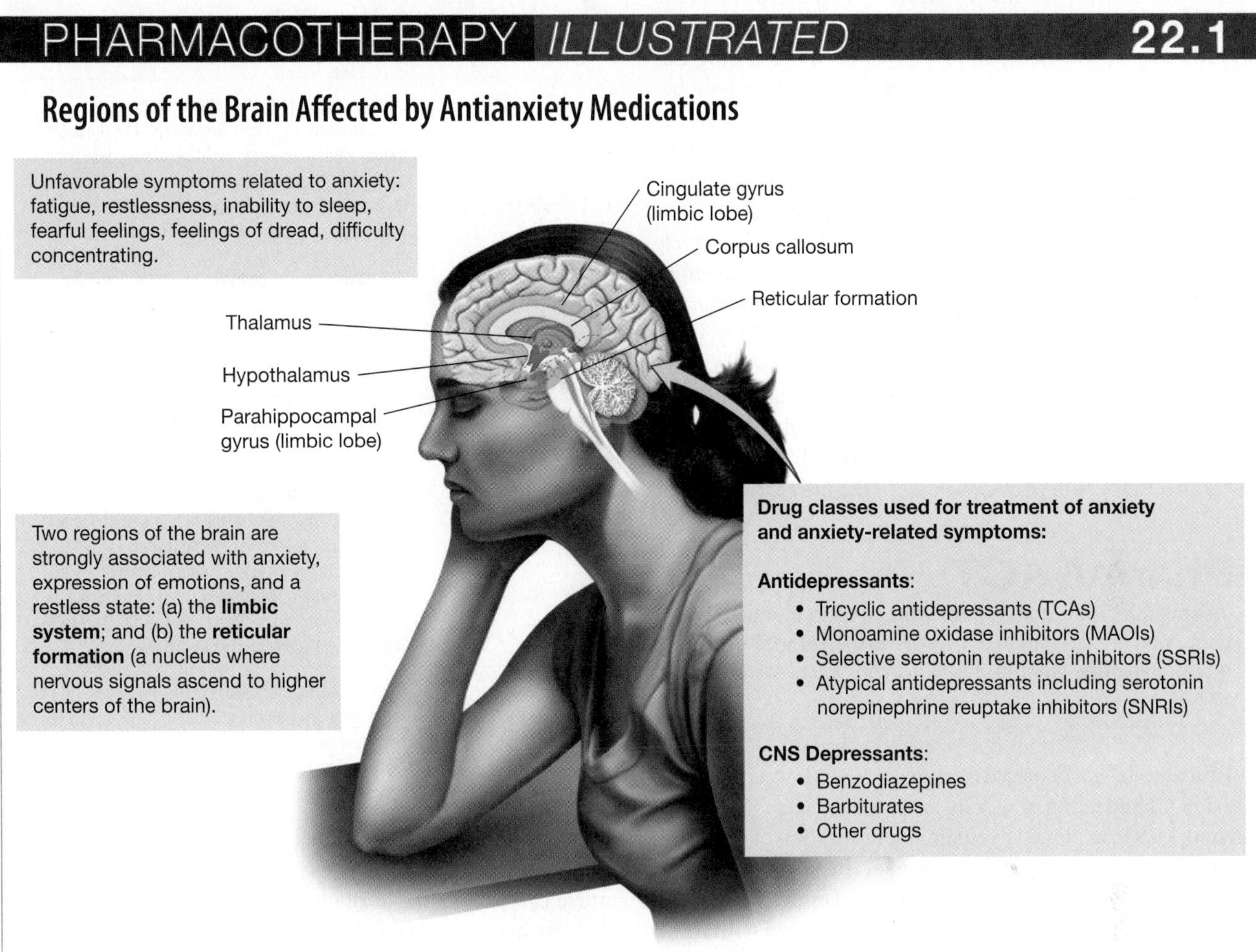

Sleep Disorders

22.4 Sleep occurs in distinct stages.

The process of sleep has been well studied. It has been established that all people need an adequate amount of sleep to function optimally, although the amounts change throughout the life span. For middle-aged adults, 7 to 8 hours of sleep appear to be adequate. Most older adults sleep less than 8 hours, and infants and babies require much more sleep. Although it is known that sleep is essential for wellness, scientists are unsure of its function or how much is needed to maintain optimum health. Following are some theories:

1. Inactivity during sleep gives the body time to repair itself.
2. Sleep is a function that evolved as a protective mechanism. Throughout history, night-time was the safest time of day for resting.
3. Sleep involves "electrical" charging and discharging of the brain. The brain needs time for processing and filing new information collected throughout the day. When this is done without interference from the outside environment, these vast amounts of data can be later retrieved through memory.

Sleep occurs in two basic phases: rapid eye movement (REM) sleep and non–rapid eye movement (NREM) sleep. NREM sleep is further subdivided into four distinct stages based the depth of sleep. Drugs may affect the length of time spent in the different stages of sleep. Decreases in the neurotransmitters acetylcholine, norepinephrine, and serotonin signal the change from wakefulness to **non–rapid eye movement (NREM) sleep.** During this phase, respirations slow, heart rate and blood pressure decrease, oxygen consumption by muscles decreases, and urine formation decreases. NREM accounts for about 75% to 85% of total sleep time. The four stages of NREM sleep are:

- **Stage I.** This is very light sleep during which respirations begin to slow and muscles relax. During this stage many persons do not even realize or believe they were asleep. They may describe their condition as drowsiness rather than sleep. Muscle twitches and jerks are normal during this stage.
- **Stage II.** This is also light sleep but deeper than stage I. The person loses conscious awareness in this stage. As much as one half of the time spent in sleep is in stages I and II.
- **Stage III.** Considered deep sleep, this is the period in which a person may experience nightmares, bedwetting, or sleep walking.
- **Stage IV.** This is the deepest NREM sleep, being very similar to stage III.

MyNursingKit | National Center on Sleep Disorders Research Website

Rapid eye movement (REM) sleep is considered the active dreaming stage of sleep, although dreams may also occur in NREM sleep. As the name implies, the eyes move during this stage. Muscle tone diminishes and heart rate and breathing become irregular. Penile erections and clitoral enlargement may occur. Although adults spend about 25% of their sleep in REM, newborns may spend as much as 80% of their sleep in this phase.

Sleep occurs in cycles, alternating between REM and NREM sleep about four to five times each night, with each sleep cycle lasting approximately 90 minutes. There is more time spent in NREM in early cycles, with REM sleep increasing in the later cycles. When the person moves from NREM to REM sleep, there is an increase of acetylcholine and further decreases in serotonin and norepinephrine. As REM sleep continues, the body progressively increases the levels of serotonin and norepinephrine until the amounts are adequate to stop REM sleep. For a brief time, the person may awaken until the next cycle begins.

Pharm*FACT*

Insomnia is more common in women than in men. Patients who are older than 65 sleep less than any other age group, whereas infants sleep more. *Source:* Winkelman, 2005.

TABLE 22.2 Stages of Sleep

Stage of Sleep	Description
NREM Stage I	At the onset of sleep, the patient experiences drowsiness for 1 to 7 min. During this time, the patient can be easily awakened. This stage of sleep is so light that when awakened from it, persons often deny that they were asleep. Respirations slow, muscles relax. This stage lasts for about 4–5% of total sleep time.
NREM Stage II	The patient can still be easily awakened. This stage constitutes the greatest amount of total sleep time, 45–55%.
NREM Stage III	The patient may move into or out of a deeper sleep. Heart rate and blood pressure fall; GI activity rises. This stage lasts for about 4–6% of total sleep time.
NREM Stage IV	The deepest stage of sleep, this stage lasts a little longer than stage 1 or stage 3 sleep—about 12–15%. Dreams that occur are usually thoughtlike and revolve around current concerns or recent events with little story line. This is the stage during which nightmares occur in children. Sleepwalking is also a common behavior for this stage. Heart rate and blood pressure remain low; GI activity remains high.
REM Sleep	This stage is characterized by eye movement and a loss of muscle tone. Eye movement occurs in bursts of activity. Dreaming takes place in this stage; dreams are vivid, emotional, storylike, and frequently bizarre. The mind is very active and resembles a normal waking state.

Patients who are deprived of stage IV NREM experience depression and a feeling of apathy and fatigue. Stage IV NREM sleep appears to be linked to repair and restoration of the physical body, whereas REM sleep is associated with learning, memory, and the capacity to adjust to changes in the environment. The body requires the dream state associated with REM sleep to keep the psyche functioning normally. When deprived of REM sleep, people experience a sleep deficit and become frightened, irritable, paranoid, and even emotionally disturbed. Judgment is impaired, and reaction time is slowed. It is speculated that to make up for their lack of dreaming, these persons experience far more daydreaming and fantasizing throughout the day. The stages of sleep are shown in Table 22.2.

There is a wide variation in sleep patterns among adults. Some people do very well with less sleep, whereas others require above average amounts to feel refreshed and mentally alert. Most people, even young adults, awaken at least once during the night; the elderly awaken more frequently. The nurse can be a valuable ally to the patient experiencing sleep disturbances by explaining these normal variations and by assisting the patient to reach a desirable sleep pattern.

The acts of sleeping and waking are synchronized with many different bodily functions. Body temperature, blood pressure, hormone levels, and respiration all fluctuate on a cyclic basis throughout the 24-hour day, known as the **circadian rhythm.** Even without realizing it, people who are "day persons" or "night persons" structure their activities, even their occupations, around what they recognize as their best individual pattern of sleep and wakefulness. *Circadian dysrhythm* refers to the psychological and biologic stress a person undergoes when traveling rapidly through several time zones, such as during a long airplane journey. "Jet lag" is a very real, and sometimes disabling,

CONNECTIONS

Lifespan Considerations Sleep–Wake Patterns

Normal sleep–wake patterns vary dramatically as a person moves from infancy to old age. An infant will sleep as much as 20 hours in a 24-hour period. This sleep may not occur during the normal day–night periods; an infant may sleep through the day but be awake during the night-time hours. As a child moves into toddlerhood and school-age, sleep requirements will be lessened, but this age child still requires as much as 12 hours of sleep, even though in the United States few school-age children receive this much sleep. The normal adult requires 7 to 8 hours of sleep a night. Adults also are frequently sleep-deprived and report receiving only 4 to 5 hours of sleep per night. Aging adults receive less quality sleep than younger adults. It takes them longer to fall asleep, they have more incidents of night-time wakefulness, and they often feel sleepy during the day. Stage IV sleep and REM sleep decrease; the time spent in stage I sleep increases. The length of time it takes to fall asleep and to get back to sleep after awakening also increases. Other issues affect normal sleep, including health problems, the need to void, a partner whose sleep pattern is the opposite, external stimulation such as that encountered when a person is hospitalized, and worries and concerns.

phenomenon although not a permanent dysfunction. When this cycle becomes impaired, pharmacologic or other interventions may be needed to readjust it. Circadian rhythms are based on many complex variables, including light–dark cycles and secretion of hormones such as melatonin. Biologic rhythms likely exist in all living things and have even been identified in bacteria.

CONNECTION Checkpoint 22.1

Patients abusing amphetamine will often experience sleep disorders. From what you learned in Chapter 8, describe some symptoms of amphetamine abuse that may lead you to suspect this type of sleep disorder. See Answer to Connection Checkpoint 22.1 in Appendix A.

22.5 Sleep disorders affect a large percentage of the population.

A sleep disorder is a disturbance in the normal pattern, quality, or quantity of sleep. It is estimated that 40 million Americans suffer from sleep disorders. Examples of common sleep disorders include insomnia, narcolepsy, sleep apnea, nightmares (night terrors), sleepwalking, excessive daytime drowsiness, and bedwetting (enuresis). Although there are dozens of different types of sleep disorders, pharmacotherapy is beneficial in treating only a few of them.

Insomnia is the most common sleep disorder and the one that is the most frequent indication for pharmacotherapy. Insomnia can be simply defined as the lack of adequate sleep; however, the disorder can be better explained by the following terms:

- Sleep-onset insomnia. Inability to fall asleep within a reasonable time, usually more than 30 minutes
- Sleep-maintenance insomnia. Frequent awakenings during the night or the inability to fall back asleep
- Sleep-offset insomnia. Premature, early morning awakenings
- Nonrestorative sleep. Persistent sleepiness during the day, despite adequate sleep duration

According to *DSM-IV-TR* the diagnosis of chronic insomnia requires that the condition persist for 30 days or longer and interfere with activities of daily living. The most frequent symptom reported by patients is excessive daytime drowsiness. The severity of the disorder is normally determined by its duration and the degree to which it affects daytime activities.

Insomnia has multiple causes and often presents secondary to an underlying disorder. Examples of conditions causing secondary insomnia are shown in Table 22.3. The best approach to resolving secondary insomnia is to treat the underlying disorder. Insomnia not associated with another medical, psychiatric, or medication-related cause is considered to be *primary*.

A good medical history can sometimes distinguish between primary and secondary insomnia; however, objective testing such as polysomnography and actigraphy are referred to sleep disorder specialists. Polysomnography is a series of tests that record physiological changes occurring during sleep, including eye movement, muscle tension, respiration, cardiac rhythm, and brain wave activity. Polysomnography can also determine the amount of REM and NREM sleep. Brain wave activity is measured using an electroencephalogram (EEG). Actigraphy is another frequently used diagnostic test that measures the motor activity of a patient during waking and sleeping hours. The results of these comprehensive tests can be used to diagnose most sleep disorders.

TABLE 22.3 Causes of Secondary Insomnia

Cause	Description
Drugs	Amphetamines, cocaine, caffeinated beverages, corticosteroids, sympathomimetics, antidepressants, alcohol use, nicotine or tobacco use
Medical Disorder	Dementia, anxiety disorder, epilepsy, Parkinson's disease, Tourette's syndrome, psychosis, mania, migraines, asthma, sleep apnea, chronic or severe pain, COPD, gastroesophageal reflux, hyperthyroidism
Poor Sleep Hygiene	Noisy environment; too much light in the bedroom; large meals; working or exercise just prior to sleeping; partner who snores, talks, or moves frequently during sleep
Stressful Situation	Major life event such as marriage, divorce, death of a loved one, chronic or terminal disease, stressful job

Treatment is indicated if the insomnia interferes significantly with normal daily activities. Insomnia is not only distressing for the individual, but it also affects society in terms of lost productivity of workers and an increased number of accidents due to daytime drowsiness.

In addition to insomnia, **narcolepsy** is a sleep disorder that may respond to pharmacotherapy. Narcolepsy is characterized by severe daytime sleepiness such that the patient is unable to stay awake and may fall asleep quickly and at inappropriate times. An episode of narcolepsy may last from a few seconds to about 30 minutes and the disorder may start anytime between ages 5 and 50. Four "classic" symptoms are observed in some patients with narcolepsy. In addition to the sleep attack, patients may exhibit one or more of the following:

- **Cataplexy** is a sudden loss of muscle strength manifested as slurred speech, sagging of the jaw, head nodding, or even complete collapse of the body. The condition is triggered by strong emotions.
- **Hypnagogic hallucinations** are vivid, fearful illusions that may be experienced at the onset of sleep or on awakening.
- Muscular paralysis may result in the temporary inability to move or speak on awakening.
- Automatic behavior may include actions such as talking or repetitive movements during the sleep episode. The person has no memory of the behavior on awakening.

Pharmacologic treatment for narcolepsy includes stimulants such as amphetamines, methylphenidate, and modafinil (Provigil), which is considered a drug of choice for the disorder. Modafinil is well tolerated and adverse effects such as headache, nausea, nervousness, and anxiety are generally mild. This drug is a Schedule IV controlled substance due to its stimulant properties; however, it has a low potential for abuse.

Stimulants such as modafinil are not effective for cataplexy symptoms. Older therapies for cataplexy include antidepressants such as tricyclic antidepressants (TCAs) or selective serotonin reuptake inhibitors (SSRIs). A newer therapy approved in 2002 utilizes sodium oxybate (gamma hydroxybutyrate [GHB], Xyrem). This drug appears to be effective in managing symptoms of both narcolepsy and cataplexy. GHB has a significant potential for abuse.

Management of Anxiety and Insomnia

22.6 There is a link between insomnia and anxiety.

The student may be wondering why two seemingly different conditions, anxiety and insomnia, are being presented in the same chapter. There are two fundamental reasons. First, there is a pathophysiologic link between sleep and anxiety, and, second, many of the drugs used to treat anxiety are also effective for treating insomnia.

MyNursingKit | National Institute of Mental Health Website

Research has shown a high incidence of serious insomnia in patients with comorbid mental health conditions such as depression and anxiety. Patients with insomnia are more likely to report symptoms of nervousness and anxiety. But which comes first, the anxiety or insomnia? In some patients, insomnia can lead to anxiety and worry about lack of restful sleep. In other patients, anxiety and worry can cause someone to lie awake and experience insomnia. Thus, it is not a matter of which came first or which caused the other. Anxiety and insomnia should be recognized as a continuous, destructive cycle with each "feeding" on the other. Recognizing this link makes insomnia therapy more than just a night-time problem. It involves treating anxiety during the day while improving sleep at night. The nurse should assess patients for anxiety when they report sleeplessness, and vice versa.

There are three classes that contain drugs of choice for treating both anxiety and insomnia: the benzodiazepines, nonbenzodiazepine antianxiety and miscellaneous agents, and antidepressants. The benzodiazepines are used for the intermittent, short-term therapy of anxiety. They are indicated for the treatment of patients who are unable to fall asleep due to excessive worrying at bedtime. Some of the nonbenzodiazepines and the newer antidepressants are effective for the longer term therapy of insomnia and anxiety. A second approach is to use combined therapy for the two disorders. Treating both conditions concurrently may result in better sleep outcomes than treating insomnia only (Nierengarten, 2007).

Long-term use of sleep medications is likely to worsen insomnia, and many of these medications cause physical or psychological dependence. Patients may experience a phenomenon referred to as **rebound insomnia.** This condition occurs when a sedative drug is discontinued abruptly after it has been taken for several months or longer. Symptoms of sleeplessness, anxiety, and daytime drowsiness become markedly worse for a few days before the original insomnia symptoms return.

22.7 Management of anxiety and sleep disorders utilizes a combination of pharmacologic and nonpharmacologic therapies.

There are a variety of possible treatments for anxiety and insomnia, and choice of therapy depends primarily on the severity of the symptoms. In some cases, several therapies may be combined to achieve optimum results. The three types of therapies include complementary and alternative therapies, nonprescription drugs, and prescription drugs.

Complementary and alternative therapies: In mild cases of anxiety or insomnia, patients should be encouraged to explore and develop nonpharmacologic coping strategies to deal with the underlying causes. Such strategies may include cognitive–behavioral therapy, counseling, biofeedback techniques, yoga, and meditation. A list of complementary and alternative treatments that may be useful in reducing anxiety and enhancing sleepiness is shown in Table 22.4.

Many natural products and supplements are claimed to promote relaxation and sleep. The best studied natural remedy is melatonin. Research studies have demonstrated that melatonin supplementation may improve both sleep onset and sleep duration. Melatonin is a natural hormone; however, taking too much can disrupt homeostasis and cause adverse effects such as headaches, mental impairment, and nightmares.

Two herbal products with demonstrated efficacy in promoting relaxation are valerian and kava. Although research has confirmed their effectiveness at promoting sleep, high doses of kava can damage the liver and the herb has the potential to interact with prescription sleep medications. Kava should not be used unless recommended by a health care provider. Valerian, featured as a complementary and alternative therapy in Chapter 28, has not been shown to cause liver damage. Other herbs are claimed to have relaxation and sleep-promoting properties (often by those marketing the products), but research has not proved their validity or safety in treating anxiety or insomnia.

Nonprescription drugs: Antihistamines are drugs used to treat cold or allergy symptoms. One of the adverse effects of antihistamines is drowsiness. This is used to advantage in over-the-counter (OTC) sleep aid products such as Sominex and Nytol. In addition, products indicated as "P.M." or "night-time" contain antihistamines that promote sleep. The two antihistamines most frequently used to produce drowsiness are diphenhydramine and doxylamine.

Antihistamines can have a long duration of action (up to 12 hours) and may leave the patient feeling drowsy the next day. They also cause drying of the nose and mouth, which is the reason they are included in cold and flu remedies. Some patients experience dizziness and blurred vision. Antihistamines

TABLE 22.4 Complementary and Alternative Treatments for Anxiety and Insomnia*

Alternative Therapies	Acupuncture, aromatherapy, yoga, prayer, massage, meditation, biofeedback therapy, hypnosis, guided imagery, music therapy
Exercise and Nutrition	Exercise therapy, nutrition therapy, deep breathing
Herbal Therapies	Kava, valerian, chamomile, catnip, ginseng, lemon balm, passionflower, hops, lavender

*Safety and effectiveness have not been demonstrated for most complementary and alternative therapies.

should not be taken for prolonged periods for insomnia because patients become tolerant to the drowsiness effect of the drugs. The use of antihistamines in treating allergic rhinitis and the common cold is presented in Chapter 74.

Prescription drugs: The remainder of this chapter examines the classes of prescription drugs used to treat anxiety and insomnia. These agents are used when the anxiety or sleep disorder is severe or when the condition is unresponsive to nonpharmacologic therapies.

The first drugs to treat anxiety and insomnia were general central nervous system (CNS) depressants. Ethanol and opium were the two general CNS depressants most widely used for treating anxiety and insomnia until the discovery of the barbiturates in the early 1900s. Other nonselective CNS depressants such as chloral hydrate, methaqualone (Quaalude), and meprobamate (Miltown) were also widely prescribed in the mid-20th century. Because general CNS depressants suppress most neuronal functions, they have serious adverse effects and are very dangerous in overdose situations. Methaqualone was removed from the U.S. market in 1984 because of its addictive potential and widespread illegal use in the 1960s and 1970s. Starting in the 1960s and continuing until present day, selective CNS depressants have been developed that more specifically target areas of the brain controlling anxiety and sleep, without causing the serious adverse effects of the older drugs.

The terminology used to describe these drugs can be confusing to nurses who are treating patients with anxiety or insomnia. An **anxiolytic** is any drug that has the ability to relieve anxiety. In the broadest definition, anxiolytics include drugs from a large number of different pharmacologic classes. In clinical practice, however, the term *anxiolytic* is often more narrowly defined to include just the benzodiazepine and nonbenzodiazepine antianxiety drugs.

A sedative is a CNS depressant that produces relaxation, calmness, and a reduction in anxiety and excitement. *Tranquilizer* is an older term, though still often used, to describe a sedative. A hypnotic is a drug that produces sleep. A sedative is most often administered during the day to induce a feeling of calm or relaxation without causing sleep, whereas hypnotics are used during the night to induce sleep. The term **sedative–hypnotic** is used to describe a drug with the ability to produce a calming effect at lower doses and sleep at higher doses. Very high doses of sedative–hypnotics may produce anesthesia, as in the case of thiopental sodium (Pentobarbital), an ultra-short-acting barbiturate. All of these drugs—anxiolytics, tranquilizers, sedatives, and hypnotics—are considered CNS depressants.

The overlap in meaning can easily be seen with the preceding definitions. Some medications may be used as an anxiolytic, a sedative, or a hypnotic, depending on the dose administered. This is because CNS depression is a continuum ranging from relaxation to sedation to the induction of sleep and anesthesia. To avoid this confusion in terminology, drugs for anxiety and insomnia are usually referred to by their chemical or pharmacologic classifications. The four general classifications of drugs used for patients experiencing anxiety or sleep disorders are as follows:

- Benzodiazepines
- Nonbenzodiazepine anxiolytics and miscellaneous agents
- Antidepressants
- Barbiturates

Many CNS depressants have the potential to cause physical and psychological dependence and most are controlled substances. The withdrawal syndrome for some CNS depressants such as the barbiturates can cause life-threatening neurologic reactions (see Chapter 8). CNS agents for treating anxiety and insomnia are listed in Table 22.5.

CNS depressants are very effective drugs. If patients do not respond to these agents with relaxation or sleep, this may indicate a serious underlying psychiatric or medical condition that requires further assessment by behavioral specialists. This is especially true if the drug worsens insomnia or produces bizarre thinking or unusual behaviors. Examples of such

MyNursingKit | National Institute of Mental Health Website

CONNECTIONS

Complementary and Alternative Therapies Melatonin

Description: Melatonin is a natural hormone (N-acetyl-5-methoxytryptamine) produced during the night by the pineal gland.

History and Claims: The secretion of melatonin is stimulated by darkness and inhibited by light. As melatonin production rises, alertness decreases, and body temperature starts to fall, both of which make sleep more inviting. Melatonin production is related to age. Children manufacture more melatonin than older adults; however, melatonin production begins to drop at puberty. Supplemental melatonin, 0.5 to 3 mg at bedtime, is alleged to decrease the time required to fall asleep and to produce a deep and restful sleep.

Standardization: Melatonin is commonly marketed as 1- to 3-mg tablets. Melatonin is one of only two hormones not regulated by the FDA and sold over-the-counter without a prescription (dehydroepiandrosterone [DHEA] is the other).

Evidence: The Agency for Healthcare Research and Quality (AHRQ), 1 of 12 agencies within the Department of Health and Human Services, examined the research regarding melatonin. Melatonin appears to have some effect on sleep onset latency, especially for people who have delayed sleep onset syndrome (those who cannot fall asleep until late at night and feel tired in the morning). It is believed that melatonin helps to "reset" the circadian rhythm for these patients, rather than cause drowsiness. Melatonin was not found to have any significant effect in treating insomina or those with jet lag. Melatonin appears to be safe for short-term use.

Source: From *Melatonin for Treatment of Sleep Disorders. Summary, Evidence Report/Technology Assessment No. 108* (AHRQ Publication No. 05-E002-2), by N. Buscemi, B. Vandermeer, R. Pandya, N. Hooton, L. Tjosvold, L. Hartling, et al., 2004, Rockville, MD: Agency for Healthcare Research and Quality.

TABLE 22.5 Central Nervous System Agents for Anxiety and Insomnia

Drug	Route and Adult Dose (maximum dose where indicated)	Adverse Effects
Benzodiazepines for Anxiety		
alprazolam (Xanax)	Anxiety: PO: 0.25–0.5 mg tid (max: 10 mg/day of extended release tablets) Panic attacks: PO: 1–2 mg tid	*Drowsiness, sedation, lethargy, ataxia, dizziness, headache* Confusion, paradoxical excitation, tachycardia, vivid dreams, hypotension, dyspnea, blurred vision, birth defects, respiratory depression, cardiovascular collapse (diazepam), laryngospasm (diazepam), agranulocytosis (estazolam)
chlordiazepoxide (Librium)	PO: 5–25 mg tid or qid; IM/IV 50–100 mg 1 h before a medical procedure	
clonazepam (Klonopin)	PO: 1–2 mg/day in divided doses (max: 4 mg/day)	
clorazepate (Tranxene)	PO: 15 mg/day at bedtime (may increase to 60 mg/day in divided doses)	
diazepam (Valium)	PO: 2–10 mg bid to qid or 15–30 mg/day sustained release IM/IV: 2–10 mg, repeat if needed in 3–4 h	
lorazepam (Ativan)	PO: 2–6 mg/day in divided doses (max: 10 mg/day)	
oxazepam (Serax)	PO: 10–30 mg tid or qid	
Benzodiazepines for Insomnia		
estazolam (ProSom)	PO: 0.5–2 mg at bedtime	
flurazepam (Dalmane)	PO: 15–30 mg at bedtime	
quazepam (Doral)	PO: 7.5–15 mg at bedtime	
temazepam (Restoril)	PO: 7.5–30 mg at bedtime	
triazolam (Halcion)	PO: 0.125–0.25 mg at bedtime (max: 0.5 mg/day)	
Nonbenzodiazepine Anxiolytics and Miscellaneous Agents		
buspirone (BuSpar)	PO: 7.5–15 mg in divided doses; may increase by 5 mg/day every 2–3 days if needed (max: 60 mg/day)	*Dizziness, headache, nausea, vomiting, drowsiness, fatigue, dry mouth, headache, dream disturbances, unpleasant taste (eszopiclone, ramelteon)* Paradoxical excitation, mood changes, tachycardia, blurred vision, confusion, myalgia
eszopiclone (Lunesta)	PO: 1–3 mg/day at bedtime	
ramelteon (Rozerem)	PO: 8 mg/day at bedtime (max: 8 mg/day)	
zaleplon (Sonata)	PO: 5–10 mg at bedtime (max: 20 mg/day)	
zolpidem (Ambien, Tovalt)	PO: immediate release: 5–10 mg at bedtime for 7–10 days (max: 10 mg/day); 12.5 mg extended release at bedtime	
Antidepressants Approved for Anxiety and Insomnia		
duloxetine (Cymbalta)	PO: 30–60 mg once daily (max: 60 mg/day)	*Insomnia, nausea, vomiting, somnolence, agitation, dry mouth, GI disturbances, nervousness, dizziness, fatigue, anorexia, hot flashes, rash, pruritus, anorexia (fluvoxamine)* Tachycardia, orthostatic, hypotension, agitation, tremor, decreased libido, impotence sedation, viral infections, rash, pruritus, serotonin syndrome
escitalopram (Lexapro)	PO: 10 mg/day; may increase to 20 mg/day if needed after 1 week	
fluoxetine (Prozac)	PO: 20 mg/day in a.m.; may increase by 20 mg/day at weekly intervals (max: 80 mg/day); when stable may switch to 90-mg sustained release capsule per week (max: 90 mg/week)	
fluvoxamine (Luvox)	PO: start with 50 mg/day; may increase slowly up to 300 mg/day given at bedtime or divided bid	
paroxetine (Paxil)	PO: start with 10 mg/day; may increase by 10 mg/day at weekly intervals to reach the target dose of 40 mg/day (max: 60 mg/day)	
sertraline HCl (Zoloft)	PO: start with 50 mg/day; gradually increase every few weeks according to response (max: 200 mg)	
venlafaxine (Effexor)	PO: 75 mg extended release once daily (max: 375 mg/day immediate release; 225 mg/day extended release)	
Selected Barbiturates		
butabarbital (Butisol)	Sedative: PO: 15–30 mg tid or qid Hypnotic: PO: 50–100 mg at bedtime	*Somnolence, hangover, confusion, nausea, vomiting, rebound insomnia* CNS depression, coma, death, bradycardia, liver damage, hypocalcemia, Stevens–Johnson syndrome, severe respiratory depression, birth defects
pentobarbital	Preoperative sedation: IM: 150–200 mg in two divided doses Hypnotic: IM: 150–200 mg; IV: 100 mg every 1–3 min up to 500 mg dose	
phenobarbital (Luminal)	Sedative: PO: 30–120 mg/day IV/IM/subcutaneous: 100–320 mg/day	
secobarbital (Seconal)	Sedative: PO: 100–300 mg/day in three divided doses Hypnotic: PO: 100–200 mg	

Note: *Italics* indicate common adverse effects. Underline indicates serious adverse effects.

behaviors that should be immediately reported to the health care provider include aggressiveness, hallucinations, suicidal thinking, and unusual extroversion or depersonalization.

Pharmacotherapy of Anxiety and Insomnia

22.8 Benzodiazepines are drugs of choice for generalized anxiety disorder and the short-term therapy of insomnia.

The benzodiazepines are versatile drugs used for a diverse collection of medical conditions that include anxiety, seizure disorders (see Chapter 26), muscle spasms (see Chapter 27), premedication for medical procedures and anesthesia (see Chapter 30), and alcohol withdrawal (see Chapter 8). Diazepam (Valium) is featured as a prototype drug in Chapter 26 for its use in treating acute seizure disorders.

The benzodiazepines are drugs of choice for GAD and for the short-term management of insomnia. Since the introduction of the first benzodiazepines—chlordiazepoxide (Librium) and diazepam (Valium)—in the 1960s, the class has become one of the most widely prescribed in medicine. Benzodizapines account for approximately three fourths of all prescriptions for anxiety because they are effective, have a low incidence of drug interactions, and have less abuse potential compared to other drugs for anxiety and insomnia. In addition, there is a wide margin of safety between therapeutic and lethal doses.

Although about 15 benzodiazepines are available, all have very similar actions and adverse effects; the various benzodiazepines differ primarily in their onset and duration of action. Some, such as midazolam (Versed), have a rapid onset time of 15 to 30 minutes; others, such as halazepam (Paxipam), take 1 to 3 hours to reach peak serum levels. The benzodiazepines are categorized as Schedule IV drugs; they produce considerably less physical dependence and result in less tolerance than the barbiturates. Although their actions are similar, they have different indications, which are shown in Table 22.6.

Benzodiazepines bind to the gamma-aminobutyric acid (GABA) receptor and intensify the effect of GABA, the natural inhibitory neurotransmitter found throughout the brain. Most are metabolized in the liver to active metabolites and are excreted primarily in urine. One major advantage of the benzodiazepines is that they do not produce life-threatening respiratory depression or coma if taken in excessive amounts. Death due to overdose is unlikely unless the benzodiazepines are taken in extreme quantities in combination with other CNS depressants, or if the patient suffers from sleep apnea.

Most benzodiazepines are given orally (PO). Those that can be given parenterally, such as diazepam (Valium) and lorazepam (Ativan), the prototype drug in this category, should be monitored carefully owing to their rapid onset of CNS effects and possible respiratory depression. Benzodiazepines are given parenterally for serious conditions such as status epilepticus or severe symptoms of acute schizophrenia. Midazolam (Versed) is administered parenterally because it can act within minutes to produce conscious sedation in patients undergoing minor medical–surgical procedures.

The benzodiazepines have replaced the barbiturates for the short-term treatment of insomnia caused by anxiety because of their greater margin of safety. Benzodiazepines shorten the

MyNursingKit | Mechanism of Action Animation: Zolpidem

TABLE 22.6 Indications for Benzodiazepines

Drug	GAD	Panic Disorder	Insomnia	Seizures	Alcohol Withdrawal	Preanesthetic Medication	Other
alprazolam (Xanax)	A	A	O				Premenstrual dysphoric disorder
chlordiazepoxide (Librium)	A				A		
clonazepam (Klonopin)	O	A	O	A			
clorazepate (Tranxene)	A		O	A	A		
diazepam (Valium)	A		O	A	A	A	Muscle spasms
estazolam (ProSom)	O		A				
flurazepam (Dalmane)	O		A				
lorazepam (Ativan)	A	O	O	O	O	A	
midazolam (Versed)	A			O		A	
oxazepam (Serax)	A		O		A		
quazepam (Doral)	O		A				
temazepam (Restoril)			A				
triazolam (Halcion)			A				

Note: A = FDA-approved for this indication; O = Off-label use.

Note: Off-label uses are highly dependent on the presciber and change frequently. The student should refer to current reference sources for updated information on approved and off-label indications.

length of time it takes to fall asleep and reduce the frequency of interrupted sleep. Initially, patients will report an increase in refreshed, deep sleep. Although most benzodiazepines increase total sleep time, some reduce stage IV sleep, and some affect REM sleep. With chronic use, the patient will experience a gradual increase of REM sleep as tolerance develops to the REM suppressant effects of the medication.

The benzodiazepines approved to treat short-term insomnia are different from those indicated for GAD (see Table 22.6). These anti-insomnia benzodiazepines are administered as hypnotics to induce sleep. Like other benzodiazepines tolerance develops to their therapeutic effects, and all have the potential for physical and psychological dependence. Most produce excessive daytime drowsiness, although this diminishes after a few days of therapy. They are indicated for short-term therapy of insomnia, approximately 4 weeks, although in clinical practice they may be used for longer periods. Rebound insomnia may be significant if these agents are used for prolonged therapy.

Sedative–hypnotic medications such as the benzodiazepines have the potential to cause sleep-related behaviors that the patient does not remember. These include sleepwalking, sleep-eating, and even making phone calls or driving a car (sleep-driving) while not fully awake. Patients often deny that these events occurred.

Flumazenil (Romazicon) is an antidote for benzodiazepine overdose. Given by rapid IV injection, flumazenil competes with benzodiazepines for the GABA receptor and reverses benzodiazepine-induced sedation within minutes. It has a very short duration of action and multiple doses, given every 30 to 45 seconds, may be necessary. If there is no response after the maximum dose (3 mg/h) has been administered, the patient's sedation was likely caused by a drug other than a benzodiazepine. Flumazenil must be used cautiously because the patient may awaken abruptly with dysphoria, agitation, and even seizures. Flumazenil does not reverse the depressed respiration characteristic of benzodiazepine overdose and it is not an antidote for the serious CNS depression caused by barbiturates or opioids. It does, however, reverse the CNS effects of benzodiazepine-like drugs such as zolpidem and eszopiclone.

PROTOTYPE DRUG Lorazepam (Ativan)

Classification: **Therapeutic:** Antianxiety agent, sedative–hypnotic, antiseizure agent

Pharmacologic: Benzodiazepine, GABA receptor agonist

Therapeutic Effects and Uses: Approved in 1977, lorazepam is administered as oral tablets, concentrated oral solution, or by the intramuscular (IM) or intravenous (IV) routes. It is well absorbed by all routes. Lorazepam is approved for the routine management of GAD and to reduce anxiety prior to surgical or medical procedures. As a preanesthetic drug, it is administered by the IV route 15 to 20 minutes prior to surgery or by the IM route 2 hours prior to the procedure. Mechanically ventilated patients may receive lorazepam infusions to manage excessive anxiety and agitation that are characteristic of being connected to this device.

Lorazepam is also used for several off-label indications, including insomnia, seizures, and the prevention or control of acute symptoms associated with ethanol withdrawal. Although used off-label, it is a drug of choice for treating life-threatening status epilepticus. For this indication it is administered by slow IV injection over a 2- to 4-minute period.

Mechanism of Action: Lorazepam potentiates the actions of GABA, an inhibitory neurotransmitter in the CNS. It is capable of causing all levels of CNS depression, from simple relaxation, to the induction of sleep, to coma.

Pharmacokinetics:

Route(s)	PO, IM, IV
Absorption	Readily absorbed
Distribution	91% bound to plasma proteins; widely distributed, including crossing the placenta; secreted in breast milk
Primary metabolism	Hepatic
Primary excretion	Renal
Onset of action	Peak effect: PO: 1–6 h; IM: 1–1.5 h; IV: unknown
Duration of action	Half-life: 14 h

Adverse Effects: The most frequently reported adverse effects, such as dizziness, ataxia, drowsiness, blurred vision, vertigo, sedation, and confusion, are CNS related. These effects are dose related and tolerance to them may develop as therapy progresses. Less common adverse effects include hepatotoxicity (including jaundice), alopecia, anaphylaxis, orthostatic hypotension, cardiac changes (tachycardia, hypotension, cardiac arrest following rapid IV administration), constipation, dry mouth, nausea, vomiting, diarrhea, and anorexia. Paradoxical CNS stimulation can occur in psychiatric patients, the elderly, and hyperactive children. Patients may experience nightmares, talkativeness, mania, sleep disorders, acute rage reactions, anxiety, restlessness, and euphoria.

Contraindications/Precautions: Like other benzodiazepines, use of lorazepam may cause fetal malformations; thus this drug is contraindicated during pregnancy unless the patient's condition is life threatening. It is also contraindicated in lactating women because the drug is secreted in breast milk. Those with a hypersensitivity to benzodiazepines or have narrow-angle glaucoma, psychosis, or chronic obstructive pulmonary disease (COPD) should not take lorazepam. Precautions must be taken in older adults, those who are debilitated, or those who have hepatic or renal dysfunction. Safe use in children has not been established. Lorazepam is a Schedule IV controlled substance and can cause both physical and psychological dependence. Those with a history of drug abuse should not receive lorazepam.

Drug Interactions: There are many potential drug interactions with lorazepam. Most notably additive CNS depression will occur if the drug is given concurrently with other CNS depressants, such as alcohol, opiates, or other sedative–hypnotics. Oral contraceptives inhibit the metabolism of benzodiazepines that undergo oxidation (e.g., alprazolam, chlordiazepoxide, diazepam, and others); thus the effectiveness of these antianxiety drugs may be increased. On the other hand, oral contraceptives increase the metabolism of benzodiazepines that undergo conjugation (e.g., lorazepam, oxazepam, and temazepam); thus the antianxiety effects of these drugs may be reduced. There may be increased sedation if lorazepam is taken concurrently with disulfiram. Valproic acid may decrease the effects of lorazepam. **Herbal/Food:** Kava, melatonin, and valerian may cause excessive drowsiness if taken with lorazepam. Excessive ingestion of caffeinated food and drinks may decrease the effectiveness of lorazepam.

Pregnancy: Category D.

Treatment of Overdose: Overdose will cause sedation, lethargy, and coma. Supportive care should be provided while the patient is recovering. Gastric lavage and activated charcoal may be administered. The benzodiazepine antagonist flumazenil may be administered to reverse sedation.

Nursing Responsibilities:

- When administering benzodiazepines by the parenteral route, aspirate prior to injection. Injection into an artery may cause vasospasm and gangrene.
- Assess for paradoxical CNS excitement and discontinue therapy should this occur.
- Assess vital signs, heart rate, complete blood count (CBC), and liver function tests.
- Assess patient needs for antianxiety drugs, including intensity and duration of symptoms; factors that worsen anxiety or insomnia such as physical symptoms, excessive daytime drowsiness; or too little exercise or activity.
- Assess for a history of smoking because patients who smoke heavily may require a larger dose of benzodiazepines.
- Assess for therapeutic response.
- Assess for signs and symptoms of overdose or abuse, such as somnolence, confusion, decreased reflexes, and coma.
- Teach the patient nonpharmacologic measures for improving relaxation and sleep.

Patient and Family Education:

- Store this medication in a secure place because benzodiazepines are often used illegally for recreation.
- Do not take any other prescription or nonprescription drugs, dietary supplement, or herbal product without the approval of the health care provider because these may interact and cause excessive drowsiness.
- Do not breast-feed while taking this drug without approval of the health care provider.
- Never consume alcoholic beverages with this medication because this may cause sedation.
- Do not drive or perform other hazardous activities until the effects of the drug are known because this drug may cause drowsiness and dizziness.
- Immediately notify the health care provider of any known or suspected pregnancy because this drug has the potential to cause birth defects.
- Make position changes slowly when moving from a lying to a standing position, to prevent dizziness and possible fainting.
- Incorporate measures to enhance sleep, including avoiding caffeinated drinks within 6 hours of bedtime; avoiding eating a heavy meal right before bedtime; decreasing stimulation (TV, loud conversation, bright lights); forming a habit of using the bed for sleeping, not for reading or watching TV; and establishing a regular bedtime and rising time.

Drugs Similar to Lorazepam (Ativan)

Benzodiazepines for anxiety: Benzodiazepines that are primarily used to treat anxiety are discussed next and include alprazolam, chlordiazepoxide, clorazepate, diazepam, and oxazepam. Benzodiazepines that are used to treat seizures (see Chapter 26) and those that are used as adjuncts to anesthesia (see Chapter 30) are presented in their respective chapters.

Alprazolam (Xanax): Approved in 1981, alprazolam is available in several oral formulations and is indicated for the management of GAD and panic disorder. It is used off-label for the short-term treatment of insomnia and for premenstrual dysphoric disorder that is unresponsive to nonpharmacologic therapies. An extended release form (Xanax XR) is available for once-daily dosing. The drug is well tolerated, with drowsiness being the most common adverse effect. Patients are encouraged to refrain from consuming grapefruit and grapefruit juice while taking alprazolam, because the combination may inhibit the metabolism of the drug. Older adults should receive a small dose, which can then be gradually increased as indicated, to prevent ataxia or excessive sedation. Care must be taken when treating women of childbearing age because alprazolam is a pregnancy category D drug.

Chlordiazepoxide (Librium): Chlordiazepoxide is a long-acting benzodiazepine that has been available in the United States for almost 50 years. It is available as capsules for oral administration: The parenteral formulations are no longer marketed in the United States. It is approved to manage GAD, acute anxiety situations, and symptoms associated with acute alcohol withdrawal. Experimental uses include treatment of panic disorder, tremors, and tension headaches. The use of chlordiazepoxide has markedly declined in favor of the shorter-acting drugs in this class such as lorazepam and alprazolam. Drowsiness is the most common adverse effect. Precautions should be used in those with impaired hepatic or renal function. Children and older adults are more likely to experience adverse effects and should be started with a low dose, which may then be gradually increased as needed. Chlordiazepoxide is a pregnancy category D drug and is secreted in breast milk.

Clorazepate (Tranxene): Approved in 1972, clorazepate is available by the oral route to treat GAD, partial seizures, and symptoms associated with ethanol withdrawal. It may be used off-label for the short-term management of insomnia. Clorazepate is essentially a prodrug that is converted into the same active metabolites as diazepam; thus these drugs share the same actions and adverse effects. They are both pregnancy category D drugs.

Diazepam (Valium): Diazepam is an older benzodiazepine that is available for PO, IM, and IV administration. It is FDA approved to treat GAD, seizures, and muscle spasms and for the relief of symptoms associated with acute alcohol withdrawal. It is also approved to produce relaxation or sedation prior to medical procedures. Off-label uses include reduction of agitation in intensive care patients, acute chloroquine overdose, and treatment of withdrawal symptoms associated with benzodiazepine abuse. Diazepam has the same actions and adverse effects as other drugs in its class. A drug prototype feature for diazepam is included in Chapter 26.

Oxazepam (Serax): Approved in 1965, oxazepam is approved to manage the symptoms of acute alcohol withdrawal and for the treatment of mild to moderate GAD associated with depression. It may be used off-label for the short-term management of insomnia associated with situational anxiety. It is available only by the oral route. Actions and adverse effects are the same as other benzodiazepines.

Benzodiazepines primarily for insomnia: Benzodi-azepines primarily used as hypnotics to treat insomnia include estazolam, flurazepam, quazepam, temazepam, and triazolam.

Estazolam (ProSom): Approved in 1990, estazolam is an intermediate duration benzodiazepine approved as a hypnotic in the short-term management of insomnia. This drug should be given at bedtime because it causes significant drowsiness and promotes sleep. Adverse effects include headache, asthenia, and dizziness. Estazolam appears to produce a lower incidence of adverse effects than flurazepam. After several weeks of therapy, patients may exhibit tolerance to the sedative effects of the drug and will experience difficulty sleeping during the early morning hours. Estazolam is a pregnancy category X drug.

Flurazepam (Dalmane): Flurazepam is the oldest benzodiazepine hypnotic and was approved in 1970. This drug is only available orally and should be taken at bedtime because it quickly produces significant drowsiness. Flurazepam has a longer duration of action than some drugs in this class because it is converted to long-acting active metabolites in the liver. Its longer duration has the potential to extend drowsiness into the morning hours. Because of the development of tolerance to the sedative effects of this drug and the potential for physical and psychological dependence, therapy is usually limited to 4 weeks. Flurazepam is a pregnancy category X drug.

Quazepam (Doral): Approved in 1985, quazepam is a benzodiazepine hypnotic drug available only by the oral route. It is administered just before bedtime because it quickly produces significant drowsiness. This drug has a long duration of action because it is converted to several active metabolites in the liver that extend the drug's half-life. Patients may experience daytime sedation, although tolerance develops to this adverse effect after a few days. Therapy is usually limited to 4 weeks because of the development of tolerance and the potential for dependence. Quazepam is a pregnancy category X drug.

Temazepam (Restoril): Approved in 1981, temazepam is indicated for the short-term therapy of insomnia. It is administered orally and should be taken at bedtime due to its rapid onset of action. Unlike flurazepam and quazepam, the metabolism of temazepam does not result in active metabolites; thus the drug may be safer for use in patients with hepatic impairment. Like the other benzodiazepine hypnotics, however, temazepam is a pregnancy category X drug.

Triazolam (Halcion): Approved in 1982, triazolam is very similar to other benzodiazepine hypnotics. It has a relatively short half-life and has no active metabolites. Because of its rapid onset, it must be taken immediately prior to sleep. Daytime drowsiness is less of a problem with triazolam because of its relatively short half-life. Anterograde amnesia may occur more frequently with triazolam than with other benzodiazepine hypnotics. Triazolam is a pregnancy category X drug.

Pharm*FACT*

Chronic lack of sleep may make people more prone to developing type 2 (non–insulin-dependent) diabetes. Healthy adults who average about 5 hours of sleep per night over eight consecutive nights secrete 50% more insulin than those who average 8 hours of sleep per night. Those who sleep less are 40% less sensitive to insulin than those who get more sleep. *Source:* Ferrie et al., 2007.

CONNECTION *Checkpoint* 22.2

Differences in sleep patterns and ability to sleep may be apparent in different age groups. From what you learned in Chapter 10, should sleeping difficulties in the pregnant or lactating woman be treated with medications? See Answer to Connection Checkpoint 22.2 in Appendix A.

22.9 Several nonbenzodiazepine anxiolytics and miscellaneous agents are used successfully to treat anxiety and sleep disorders.

Several CNS depressants are used for anxiety and sleep disorders that are chemically unrelated to benzodiazepines or barbiturates. These agents come from multiple classes and are grouped together as nonbenzodiazepine anxiolytics and miscellaneous CNS depressants.

Older CNS depressants, such as paraldehyde (Paracetaldehyde), ethchlorvynol (Placidyl), chloral hydrate, meprobamate (Equanil), and glutethimide (Doriglute), have only historic interest because they are so rarely prescribed owing to their potential for serious adverse effects. The student should refer to drug guides or older pharmacology references for information on these agents.

A few miscellaneous drugs are primarily prescribed for indications other than anxiety but have antianxiety properties. For example, valproic acid (Depakote) is a commonly prescribed antiseizure medication that is used off-label to treat elderly patients with agitation, or anxiety in patients with bipolar disorder. Atenolol (Tenormin), metoprolol (Toprol), and propranolol (Inderal) are beta blockers that reduce the autonomic nervous system symptoms of anxiety such as nervousness, tremor, and tachycardia. Similarly, clonidine (Catapres) is an adrenergic antagonist that can block the autonomic symptoms that accompany anxiety. Diphenhydramine (Benadryl) and hydroxyzine (Vistaril) are antihistamines that produce drowsiness and may be beneficial in calming patients. They offer the advantage of not causing dependence, although their use is often limited by their anticholinergic adverse effects. Diphenhydramine is a common component of OTC sleep aids and medications used to treat seasonal allergies (see Chapter 74).

The most frequently prescribed miscellaneous agents are newer drugs that produce more selective CNS depression. Buspirone (BuSpar) is commonly prescribed for its anxiolytic effect. Zolpidem (Ambien), ramelteon (Rozerem), zaleplon (Sonata), and eszopiclone (Lunesta) are used for their hypnotic effects. These agents are discussed individually next.

PROTOTYPE DRUG Zolpidem (Ambien, Tovalt)

Classification: **Therapeutic:** Sedative–hypnotic
Pharmacologic: Nonbenzodiazepine anxiolytic, miscellaneous CNS depressant

Therapeutic Effects and Uses: Approved in 1993, zolpidem is an oral drug approved only for the short-term (7 to 10 days) treatment of insomnia. Zolpidem decreases sleep onset time and the number of night-time awakenings and improves the length and quality of sleep. Muscle relaxation and anticonvulsant effects occur at doses much higher than the hypnotic dose. Immediate release (Ambien), extended release (Ambien CR), and disintegrating tablet (Tovalt) forms are available.

Zolpidem should be administered just prior to expected sleep owing to its rapid onset of action. Its lack of active metabolites and short half-life reduce the incidences of excessive daytime drowsiness and rebound insomnia.

Mechanism of Action: Zolpidem has a similar mechanism of action as the benzodiazepines: enhancing the action of GABA, the inhibitory neurotransmitter. Whereas the benzodiazepines bind nonselectively to all three known subtypes of the GABA receptors, zolpidem only binds to one specific type (omega-1). This explains why the drug shares some actions of the benzodiazepines (sedation) but not others (antianxiety, antiseizure, or muscle relaxation).

Pharmacokinetics:

Route	PO
Absorption	70% absorbed
Distribution	Widely distributed; unknown if it crosses the placenta; small amounts are secreted in breast milk; 92% bound to plasma protein
Primary metabolism	Hepatic
Primary excretion	Renal, small amounts in bile and feces
Onset of action	7–27 minutes; peak effect: 90 minutes
Duration of action	Duration: 6–8 h; half-life: 1.4–4.5 h

Adverse Effects: Adverse reactions to zolpidem are usually mild and include nausea, dizziness, diarrhea, and daytime drowsiness. Other adverse effects include vomiting, depression, confusion, sleepwalking, sleep-eating, and amnesia. Very high doses may cause severe ataxia, bradycardia, altered vision, severe nausea, vomiting, drowsiness, difficulty breathing, and coma. Zolpidem is a Schedule IV controlled substance; dependency may occur with long-term, high-dose use. Abrupt withdrawal after long-term use may result in asthenia, diaphoresis, vomiting, tremor, or facial flushing.

Contraindications/Precautions: There are no known contraindications to the use of zolpidem. As with other CNS depressants it should be used cautiously in patients with respiratory impairment and in older adults, who are generally more sensitive to the depressive effects of the drugs; lower dosages may be necessary. Because zolpidem is metabolized in the liver and excreted by the kidneys, impaired liver or kidney function can increase serum drug levels and doses should be lowered. Zolpidem should be used with caution in individuals with depression and suicidal ideation because there is a potential for intentional overdose in these patients. The safety and effectiveness in patients under age 18 have not been established.

Drug Interactions: Zolpidem is a substrate for hepatic CYP3A4 enzymes and thus may interact with drugs that induce or inhibit this enzyme system. Concurrent use with other CNS depressants, including alcohol, will cause additive sedation. When given concurrently with certain SSRIs, disorientation or worsening of depression may occur. **Herbal/Food:** The presence of food will reduce absorption of the drug; thus it should be taken on an empty stomach. St. John's wort may cause confusion and, rarely, hallucinations. Valerian, kava, and melatonin supplements may cause additive sedation.

Pregnancy: Category B (immediate release) or C (extended release).

Treatment of Overdose: Overdose with zolpidem can cause serious impairment of consciousness and may be fatal. The benzodiazepine antagonist flumazenil will reverse the sedative effects of zolpidem but may precipitate seizures. Other treatment involves supportive care, such as gastric lavage.

Nursing Responsibilities:

- Assess patient needs for sedative–hypnotic drugs, including intensity and duration of symptoms and factors that worsen insomnia such as physical symptoms, excessive daytime drowsiness, or too little exercise or activity.
- Assess for correct and incorrect use of the medication.
- Teach the patient nonpharmacologic measures for improving relaxation and sleep.
- Inform caregivers to observe for night-time behavioral activities such as sleepwalking, sleep-eating, or sleep-driving and to report these activities immediately. The patient may not remember or be aware of these activities.

Patient and Family Education:

- Do not open, chew, or crush extended release tablets (Ambien CR); swallow them whole with plenty of water.

- Take this drug immediately prior to expected sleep.
- Never consume alcoholic beverages with this medication because it may cause excessive drowsiness.
- Do not take any other prescription drugs, nonprescription drugs, dietary supplements, or herbal products without approval of the health care provider because these may interact and cause excessive drowsiness.
- Do not drive or perform other hazardous activities until the effects of the drug are known because this drug may cause drowsiness and dizziness.
- Immediately notify the health care provider of any known or suspected pregnancy.

Drugs Similar to Zolpidem (Ambien, Tovalt)

Other drugs in this category include buspirone, eszopiclone, ramelteon, and zaleplon.

Buspirone (BuSpar): Buspirone is a nonbenzodiazepine anxiolytic approved in 1986 for the short-term management (up to 1 month) of GAD. Available as an oral tablet, it should be taken consistently either with or without food because food affects its absorption. Grapefruit juice may increase the effects of the drug and should be avoided. The mechanism of action for buspirone is unclear but appears to involve two pathways: enhancing D_2 dopamine receptors and suppressing serotonin receptors in the brain. It is less likely to affect cognitive and motor performance than benzodiazepines and rarely interacts with other CNS depressants. The most common adverse effects include dizziness, drowsiness, nausea, vomiting, and headache. When switching from a benzodiazepine to buspirone, the patient may experience withdrawal symptoms or anxiety; therefore, the dose of benzodiazepine should be gradually tapered while buspirone is increased. Safety and efficacy have not been established in children. Dependence and withdrawal problems are less of a concern with buspirone than with many other CNS depressants. Therapy may take several weeks to achieve optimal results. It is a pregnancy category B drug.

Eszopiclone (Lunesta): Although structurally unrelated to other drugs used to treat insomnia, eszopiclone shares certain properties with zolpidem and the benzodiazepines. Approved in 2004, eszopiclone has a long elimination half-life, about twice as long as that of zolpidem, which may give it an advantage in maintaining sleep and decreasing early-morning awakening. On the other hand, the long half-life is more likely to cause daytime sedation. Adverse effects are mild and include headache, dizziness, dry mouth, and an unpleasant taste that may persist into the following day. It is only available PO and should be taken immediately before bedtime due to its rapid onset of action. Eszopiclone is metabolized by hepatic CYP3A4 enzymes; thus potential drug–drug and drug–herb interactions exist for substances that induce or inhibit these enzymes. The onset of action may be reduced if taken with or immediately following a high-fat meal. Older adults with impaired hepatic or renal function may need a lower dose. Eszopiclone may be used for the long-term treatment of insomnia. However, tolerance develops to the sedative effects after a few weeks of therapy and rebound insomnia may occur on withdrawal. Eszopiclone is a Schedule IV controlled substance. It is a pregnancy category C drug.

Ramelteon (Rozerem): Approved in 2005, ramelteon is a new hypnotic that has FDA approval to treat chronic insomnia in people who have problems falling asleep. It appears to be safe for long-term use. Ramelteon has a unique mechanism of action: It activates melatonin receptors, specifically MT1 and MT2, which are mediators of the normal sleep–wake cycle. Ramelteon is the first FDA-approved hypnotic that is not a controlled substance; there is no evidence that it leads to abuse or physical dependence. With an onset of action of 30 minutes and a short duration of action, it is helpful in treating sleep onset but it does not maintain sleep. It is less effective if taken with or immediately after a high-fat meal. There is little next-day residual drowsiness owing to its short half-life. Adverse effects of ramelteon are mild and include dizziness, fatigue, and somnolence. Ramelteon is contraindicated in persons with severe hepatic impairment. Ramelteon can affect the levels of sex hormones in the body, so the patient may experience amenorrhea, decreased libido, galactorrhea, and problems with fertility. Alcohol should be avoided because it may cause additive CNS depression. Fluvoxamine (Luvox), if used concurrently, can greatly increase (more than 50 times) the levels of ramelteon so it should be avoided. Ramelteon is a pregnancy category X drug.

Zaleplon (Sonata): Approved in 1999, zaleplon is an oral nonbenzodiazepine sedative–hypnotic whose only indication is for the short-term treatment (7 to 10 days) of insomnia. It is the first drug in a new class called pyrazolopyrimidines. Like zolpidem, it binds specifically to the omega-1 GABA receptor but it has a faster onset and shorter duration of action than zolpidem. Zaleplon decreases sleep onset time and may be useful for patients who awaken early in the morning, for example, 2:00 a.m. or 3:00 a.m. It is sometimes used for treatment of "jet lag" and has been advertised by pharmaceutical companies for this purpose. Zaleplon should be taken immediately before bedtime due to its rapid onset of action. Administration immediately following a high-fat meal slows the absorption of zaleplon and reduces its effectiveness. The drug is well tolerated and causes few adverse effects. High doses produce symptoms characteristic of other sedative–hypnotics such as drowsiness, confusion, dizziness, and lethargy. Long-term use does not result in tolerance and, although it is a Schedule IV drug, dependence potential appears to be low. It is a pregnancy category C drug.

22.10 Antidepressants are widely prescribed for anxiety disorders.

Until the 1980s, antidepressants were used mainly to treat mental depression. Over the past 20 years, however, pharmacologists have discovered the value of these drugs in treating other disorders, including anxiety. Today, antidepressants are frequently used to treat various anxiety disorders and are the drugs of choice in some cases. Given the effectiveness of antidepressants for these conditions, many believe that in the future, anxiolytics and antidepressants will eventually merge into a single drug class.

Antidepressants have the ability to reduce anxiety symptoms by altering the levels of two important neurotransmitters in the brain: norepinephrine and serotonin. Restoration of neurotransmitter imbalances may reduce symptoms associated with depression, panic attacks, obsessive–compulsive behavior, PTSD, and phobias. More detailed treatment of these drugs and their mechanisms of action are covered in Chapter 23. The following section focuses on their applications to treating anxiety disorders and insomnia.

For most patients, panic attacks and other intense anxiety symptoms come in two stages. The first stage is termed anticipatory anxiety in which the patient begins to think about an upcoming challenge and starts to experience feelings of dread. The second stage is when physical symptoms such as shortness of breath, accelerated heart rate, and muscle tension start to emerge as a consequence of activation of the autonomic nervous system. For panic attacks or phobias, the most useful therapy is to help motivate the patient to face his or her fear and to suppress symptoms in one or both of these stages. If drugs can reduce the negative thoughts associated with the anticipatory component of panic, then there is less likelihood that the patient will become stressed. Drugs can also be used to reduce neuronal activity and suppress the autonomic nervous system, helping the patient to remain calm. The patient can then use self-help coping skills to control the negative behavior.

The antidepressants used to reduce symptoms of panic and anxiety are the SSRIs, atypical antidepressants, TCAs, and monoamine oxidase inhibitors (MAOIs). The newer SSRIs treat symptoms of panic attacks, OCD, and phobias. Indications for these agents are shown in Table 22.7. Following is a brief summary of additional important considerations for each antidepressant class. Individual drug information, patient teaching, and nursing responsibilities are presented in Chapter 23.

Selective serotonin reuptake inhibitors: This is the most widely prescribed antidepressant class because these drugs are safer than those from other classes and cause fewer sympathomimetic effects (increased heart rate and hypertension) and anticholinergic effects. SSRIs can, however, cause weight gain and sexual dysfunction. Overdoses can cause confusion, anxiety, restlessness, hypertension, tremors, sweating, fever, and lack of muscle coordination.

Five SSRIs are approved for anxiety disorders although other drugs in this class are often used off-label. The indications for each drug are given in Table 22.7.

- Generalized anxiety disorder. Paroxetine (Paxil) and escitalopram (Lexapro) are drugs of choice for patients with GAD and anxiety that is associated with depressive disorders. Unlike the benzodiazepines that act immediately, the antianxiety effects of the SSRIs may take several weeks.
- Panic disorder. The two SSRIs approved for panic attacks, paroxetine (Paxil) and sertraline (Zoloft), are drugs of choice for this disorder. Both frequency and intensity of panic attacks are reduced.
- Obsessive–compulsive disorder. Four SSRIs are approved to treat OCD, although others in this class may be used off-label. Paroxetine (Paxil), fluvoxamine (Luvox), fluoxetine (Prozac), and sertraline (Zoloft) are drugs of choice for this disorder. Optimum therapeutic effects may take several months to achieve.
- Social anxiety disorder. Paroxetine (Paxil) and sertraline (Zoloft) are two SSRIs approved for the long-term therapy of social anxiety disorder. Because several months may be necessary for optimum therapeutic benefit, the benzodiazepines are better choices for acute symptoms of social anxiety disorder.
- Post-traumatic stress disorder. Paroxetine (Paxil) and sertraline (Zoloft) are the only two drugs approved for the therapy of PTSD. Therapy should be initiated as soon after the traumatic event as possible, and several months may be necessary for optimum results.

Atypical antidepressants: These include serotonin–norepinephrine reuptake inhibitors (SNRIs). Adverse effects include insomnia, abnormal dreams, sweating, constipation, dry mouth, loss of appetite, weight loss, tremor, abnormal vision, headaches, nausea, vomiting, dizziness, and loss of sexual desire. Two atypical antidepressants are used for anxiety disorders.

- Duloxetine (Cymbalta). Approved in 2007 for GAD, duloxetine has the potential to become a first-line drug for this disorder due to its safety and effectiveness, especially in patients with accompanying depression.
- Venlafaxine (Effexor). This was the first antidepressant approved for GAD. It is also beneficial in treating panic attacks and social anxiety disorder. It is widely used for anxiety disorders that are accompanied by depression.

Tricyclic antidepressants (TCAs): TCAs are older drugs that are not recommended in patients with a history of heart attack, heart block, or dysrhythmia. Patients often have annoying anticholinergic effects such as dry mouth, blurred vision, urine retention, and hypertension (see Chapter 18). Most TCAs are pregnancy category C or D. Concurrent use with alcohol or other CNS depressants should be avoided, and patients with asthma, GI disorders, alcoholism, schizophrenia, or bipolar disorder should take TCAs with extreme caution. Two TCAs are approved for anxiety disorders.

- Clomipramine (Anafranil). The only TCA approved for OCD, clomipramine is very effective but tends to cause more adverse effects than drugs in the SSRI class. It is considered an alternative for patients who are unable to tolerate SSRIs.
- Doxepin (Sinequan). Approved for anxiety associated with depressive disorders, doxepin produces a rapid antianxiety effect. Because of significant anticholinergic adverse effects, it is not a drug of first choice for anxiety.

Monoamine oxidase inhibitors (MAOIs): Once commonly prescribed, it is rare to find these drugs used today due to their high incidence of potential adverse effects. No MAOIs are FDA-approved for anxiety disorders, although some may be occasionally used off-label when other therapies fail to produce

TABLE 22.7 Antidepressants for Anxiety or Insomnia

Drug	Anxiety	Insomnia
Atypical Antidepressants, Including the SNRIs		
duloxetine (Cymbalta)	A (GAD)	
trazodone HCl (Desyrel)	0 (GAD, panic)	0
venlafaxine HCl (Effexor)	A (GAD, panic, social anxiety disorder)	
Monoamine Oxidase Inhibitors (MAOIs)		
isocarboxazid (Marplan)	0 (GAD, panic, social anxiety disorder)	
phenelzine sulfate (Nardil)	0 (GAD, OCD, panic, social anxiety disorder)	
tranylcypromine sulfate (Parnate)	0 (GAD, panic, social anxiety disorder)	
Selective Serotonin Reuptake Inhibitors (SSRIs)		
citalopram (Celexa)	0 (GAD, OCD, panic, PTSD, social anxiety disorder)	
escitalopram (Lexapro)	A (GAD) 0 (panic, social anxiety disorder)	
fluoxetine (Prozac)	A (OCD) 0 (GAD, PTSD, panic)	
fluvoxamine (Luvox)	A (OCD) 0 (panic, GAD, social anxiety disorder, PTSD)	
paroxetine (Paxil)	A (OCD, PTSD, social anxiety disorder, GAD, panic)	
sertraline (Zoloft)	A (OCD, PTSD, social anxiety disorder, panic) 0 (GAD)	
Tricyclic Antidepressants (TCAs)		
amitriptyline (Elavil)	0 (panic, social anxiety disorder)	0
clomipramine (Anafranil)	A (OCD)	
desipramine (Norpramin)	0 (panic, GAD)	
doxepin (Sinequan)	A (GAD)	0
imipramine (Tofranil)	0 (panic, social anxiety disorder)	
nortriptyline (Aventyl)	0 (panic, social anxiety disorder)	

Note: A = FDA-approved for this indication; O = Off-label use.

Note: Off-label uses are highly dependent on the prescriber and change frequently. The student should refer to current reference sources for updated information on approved and off-label indications.

MyNursingKit | Mechanism of Action Animation: Escitalopram

CONNECTIONS

To the Community Treating Childhood Anxiety with Antidepressants

Children and adolescents may experience intense fear and worry that can lead to the same types of anxiety disorders experienced by adults. Signs may include excessive worrying about ordinary school activities; physical symptoms such as sweating, headaches, trembling, palpitations; or social withdrawal. If not recognized and treated, childhood anxiety disorders may lead to low self-esteem, poor interpersonal relationships, drug or alcohol use, or repeated school absences. The incidence is believed to be 13% of all children age 9 to 17, with girls being affected more than boys.

Treatment of childhood anxiety usually begins with cognitive–behavioral therapy and relaxation techniques. If medication is indicated, the SSRIs are the drugs of choice for children. Although Prozac is the only SSRI approved for pediatric anxiety by the FDA, other drugs in this class may be prescribed off-label. The use of antidepressants in children must be carefully monitored. In 2004, the FDA issued an advisory warning, pointing out the potential warning signs of suicide in adults and children at the beginning of antidepressant treatment and when doses are changed. Parents and caregivers must be diligent in monitoring for signs of potential suicidal thoughts in children taking SSRIs, including unusual changes in behavior, sleeplessness, agitation, or social withdrawal.

Source: From "Children's Mental Health Facts," in *Mental Health: A Report of the Surgeon General*, by U.S. Department of Health and Human Services, Substance Abuse and Mental Health Services Administration, 1999, Rockville, MD. Retrieved June 7, 2008, from http://mentalhealth.samhsa.gov/publications/allpubs/ca-0007/default.asp

satisfactory results. Patients must strictly avoid foods containing tyramine, a form of the amino acid tyrosine, to avoid a hypertensive crisis and should refrain from caffeine intake. MAOIs potentiate the effects of insulin and other diabetic drugs. Common adverse effects include orthostatic hypotension, headache, and diarrhea.

CONNECTION *Checkpoint* 22.3

Fluvoxamine, fluoxetine, and duloxetine have similar sounding names and may look alike when written as prescriptions. From what you learned in Chapter 7, describe means that you should implement to avoid these types of medication errors. See Answer to Connection Checkpoint 22.3 in Appendix A.

22.11 Barbiturates are effective sedative–hypnotics but have potentially serious adverse effects that limit their use.

Barbiturates are a class of drugs derived from barbituric acid. They are powerful CNS depressants prescribed for their sedative, hypnotic, and antiseizure effects that have been employed in pharmacotherapy since the early 1900s.

Until the discovery of the benzodiazepines, barbiturates were the drugs of choice for patients with anxiety and insomnia. Although barbiturates are still indicated for several conditions, they are rarely prescribed for anxiety or insomnia because of their significant adverse effects and because of the availability of more effective medications. When barbiturates are used as sedative–hypnotics, their use should be limited to a 14-day maximum. The risk of psychological and physical dependence is high—several are Schedule II drugs. If a patient does become physically dependent on barbiturates, the withdrawal syndrome is extremely severe and can be fatal. Overdose results in profound respiratory depression, hypotension, and shock. Barbiturates have frequently been used to commit suicide, and death due to overdose was common when these drugs were frequently prescribed in the 1960s and 1970s.

Barbiturates are capable of depressing CNS function at all levels. Like benzodiazepines, barbiturates act by binding to GABA receptor–chloride channel molecules, intensifying the effect of GABA throughout the brain. At low doses they reduce anxiety and cause drowsiness. At moderate doses they inhibit seizure activity (see Chapter 26) and promote sleep, presumably by inhibiting brain impulses traveling through the limbic system and the RAS. At higher doses, some barbiturates can induce anesthesia (see Chapter 30). Barbiturates are classified by their duration of action: short acting, intermediate acting, or long acting.

When taken for prolonged periods, barbiturates induce the production of hepatic CYP450 enzymes and can stimulate their own metabolism as well as that of hundreds of other drugs that use these enzymes for their breakdown. After 2 weeks, tolerance begins to develop to the sedative effects of barbiturates; this includes cross-tolerance to other CNS depressants such as the opioids. Tolerance does not develop, however, to the respiratory depressant effects. Thus the patient may take higher and higher doses to produce sleep while approaching dangerous and even lethal dosage levels.

PROTOTYPE DRUG Phenobarbital (Luminal)

Classification: **Therapeutic:** Sedative–hypnotic, antiepileptic drug

Pharmacologic: Barbiturate, GABA receptor agonist

Therapeutic Effects and Uses: A Schedule IV drug, phenobarbital is available as tablets or elixir for PO doses and as injection for IM or IV administration. By the IV route, phenobarbital is reserved for emergency situations such as status epilepticus and should be administered slowly. It is effective for treating all types of seizures except absence seizures. The drug is FDA approved for the short-term treatment of insomnia, although there are many safer and equally effective medications available for this indication. Therapeutic serum phenobarbital concentrations range from 15 to 40 mcg/mL.

As a sedative–hypnotic, phenobarbital decreases time to sleep onset and lengthens total sleep time. The number of night-time awakenings diminishes. Significant rebound insomnia occurs when the drug is discontinued.

Mechanism of Action: Phenobarbital binds to GABA receptors, where it enhances the activity of GABA.

Pharmacokinetics:

Route(s)	PO, IM, and IV
Absorption	Well absorbed by all routes
Distribution	Rapidly and widely distributed; may cross the placenta; secreted in breast milk; 20–45% bound to protein
Primary metabolism	Hepatic
Primary excretion	Renal
Onset of action	IV drug level peaks in 30 minutes; PO: 8–12 h
Duration of action	Half-life: 53–118 h

Adverse Effects: There are many adverse effects reported with phenobarbital. Serious ones include coma, Stevens–Johnson syndrome, angioedema, and thrombophlebitis. Many adverse reactions are related to CNS depression, mainly oversedation, "hangover" effect, lethargy, and hallucinations. Other adverse effects can include blood dyscrasias, hypocalcemia, hepatic disease, nausea, vomiting, diarrhea, or constipation. Deficiency in folic acid, calcium, and vitamin D may result in osteomalacia. Phenobarbital can cause paradoxical excitation in older adults or children, especially during the first 2 weeks of treatment. If abruptly discontinued after prolonged use, the patient may suffer nightmares, insomnia, tremor, hallucinations, nausea, and vomiting.

Contraindications/Precautions: Phenobarbital is contraindicated in patients with hypersensitivity to barbiturates, suicidal ideation or previous suicide attempt, preexisting CNS depression, severe respiratory disease, severe pain, hyperthyroidism, or porphyria. Patients with impaired hepatic, renal, and cardiovascular function should not receive phenobarbital, or the dose should be lowered to prevent toxicity. Patients with COPD may experience profound respiratory depression, even at therapeutic doses, and should not receive phenobarbital. A patient who has a familial history of porphyria should not be administered phenobarbital. Porphyria is a metabolic disorder in which neurologic disturbances are noted. Phenobarbital should be used cautiously in patients with hyperthyroidism, diabetes mellitus, and severe anemia. Phenobarbital can cause birth defects and physical dependence in the neonate, and thus it is contraindicated during pregnancy. Phenobarbital is secreted in breast milk and can cause profound effects on the neonate; thus it should not be administered during lactation.

Drug Interactions: Phenobarbital induces CYP450 enzymes and has the potential to interact with drugs that are metabolized by the liver such as corticosteroids, oral contraceptives, and anticonvulsants. Use with other CNS depressants, including alcohol, will cause additive sedation. Valproic acid may increase the risk of toxicity of phenobarbital. Phenobarbital may decrease the effectiveness of digoxin, TCAs, metronidazole, quinidine, or oral anticoagulants. **Herbal/Food:** St. John's wort may lead to decreased barbiturate effect. Use of kava, chamomile, eucalyptus, lemon balm, or valerian may increase additive CNS depression.

Pregnancy: Category D.

Treatment of Overdose: Overdosage of phenobarbital is a medical emergency and may be fatal. Activated charcoal is administered followed by gastric lavage. Alkalinization of the urine with sodium bicarbonate increases the renal elimination of phenobarbital.

Nursing Responsibilities:

- Monitor vital signs and monitor for respiratory depression, bradycardia, mental status, level of consciousness (LOC), and memory during therapy.
- Assess the patient who has been administered IV barbiturates every 15 minutes for bradycardia and hypotension.
- Monitor for signs of blood dyscrasias such as fever, sore throat, rash, jaundice, and bruising.
- When administering by the parenteral route, aspirate prior to injection. Injection into an artery may cause vasospasm, and extravasation may cause tissue necrosis.
- Monitor therapeutic serum concentrations of the drug and report all values outside the established range to the prescriber.
- Teach the patient nonpharmacologic measures for improving relaxation and sleep.
- Assess baseline hepatic and renal function and monitor during therapy.

Patient and Family Education:

- Take this medication exactly as instructed and do not discontinue the medication without consulting the health care provider because seizures may result.
- Do not drive or perform other potentially hazardous activities until the effects of the drug are known because this drug may cause drowsiness and dizziness.
- Consume plenty of foods high in vitamins D and K.
- Never consume alcoholic beverages with this medication because this may cause excessive drowsiness.
- Store this medication in a secure place because benzodiazepines are often used illegally for recreation.
- Do not breast-feed while taking this drug without approval of the health care provider.
- For women of childbearing age, barbiturates decrease the effectiveness of oral contraceptives; therefore, a second form of birth control should be used.
- Immediately notify the health care provider of any known or suspected pregnancy.

Drugs Similar to Phenobarbital (Luminal)

The barbiturates are classified by duration of action, and all have the same actions and adverse effects as phenobarbital. None are in common use.

Ultra-short acting: With a half-life of less than 10 minutes, thiopental (Pentothal) and methohexital (Brevital) are used by the IV route to induce or maintain anesthesia, as preoperative sedation, or in the emergency management of seizures.

Short acting: With half-lives of 15 to 40 minutes, secobarbital (Seconal) and pentobarbital are oral agents that have been used to treat insomnia and as preoperative medications. These are Schedule II drugs and have been the most widely abused barbiturates.

Intermediate acting: With slightly longer half-lives, amobarbital (Amytal) and butabarbital (Butisol) are oral agents that have been used as sedative–hypnotics and to provide preanesthesia sedation.

Long acting: Mephobarbital (Mebaral) and phenobarbital are the two long-acting agents. Mephobarbital is metabolized to phenobarbital in the liver and may be used as a sedative–hypnotic or, rarely, for seizures.

NURSING PROCESS APPLICATION

Patients Receiving Therapy for Anxiety or Sleep Disorders

Assessment

Prior to administration:

- Obtain a complete health history (both physical and mental), including allergies and drug history for possible drug interactions.
- Identify factors that precipitate anxiety or insomnia.
- Identify factors, both positive and negative, that have been previously tried by the patient to decrease anxiety or insomnia.
- Assess for the presence and degree of depression; monitor for suicidal ideation.
- Assess the likelihood of drug abuse and dependence.
- Establish baseline vital signs and LOC.

Potential Nursing Diagnoses

- *Anxiety,* related to health status
- *Noncompliance (Medication)*
- *Deficient Knowledge (Medication)*
- *Sleep Deprivation,* related to adverse effects of medication
- *Risk for Activity Intolerance*, related to sedative effects of medication
- *Interrupted Family Processes,* related to dysfunctional family dynamics
- *Ineffective Role Performance,* related to inability to perform activities of daily living
- *Situational, Low Self-Esteem,* related to anxiety-induced fear and selfdoubt

Planning: Patient Goals and Expected Outcomes

The patient will:

- Report absence or decrease of physical and behavioral manifestations of anxiety or insomnia.
- Demonstrate an understanding of the drug's action by accurately describing drug adverse effects and precautions.
- Verbalize the need to discuss with the health care provider any intention to discontinue the drug and the importance of not withdrawing the drug abruptly.

Implementation: Anxiolytics, Sedatives, and Hypnotics

Interventions and (Rationales)	Patient and Family Education
• Monitor vital signs. Observe respiratory patterns, especially during sleep, for evidence of apnea or shallow breathing. (Benzodiazepines and barbiturates can reduce the respiratory drive in susceptible patients.)	• Instruct the patient to consult the health care provider before taking this drug if snoring is a problem. Snoring may indicate an obstruction in the upper respiratory tract, resulting in hypoxia.
• Monitor the patient's neurologic status, especially LOC. (Confusion or lack of response may indicate overmedication.)	• Instruct the patient to monitor vital signs at home, especially respirations, and LOC and presence of confusion.
• Ensure patient safety. (Drug may cause excessive drowsiness and increase the risk for injury.)	• Instruct the patient about safety measures, including changing position slowly, accompanied walking until the effects of the medication are known, and no driving or other potentially hazardous activities until the effects of the medication are known.
• Monitor the patient's intake of stimulants, including caffeine (in beverages such as coffee, tea, cola and other soft drinks, and OTC analgesics such as Excedrin), nicotine from tobacco products, and nicotine patches. (These products can reduce the drug's effectiveness.)	Instruct the patient: • Which common products contain caffeine and other stimulants, including coffee, tea, cola drinks, chocolate, and tobacco products. • That products containing stimulants may negate effectiveness of medications used for anxiety or insomnia.
• Monitor affect and emotional status. (This drug may increase risk of mental depression, especially in patients with suicidal tendencies.)	Instruct the patient: • To be aware of symptoms of depression or suicidal ideation, including changes in normal activity level, decreased attention to personal hygiene, lack of interest in normal activities including work or school, and isolating self from family and friends. • That the patient may not be aware of the presence of these symptoms, or may not want to admit their presence. • To report appearance of any of these symptoms immediately.
• Avoid abrupt discontinuation of therapy. (Withdrawal symptoms, including rebound anxiety and sleeplessness, are possible with abrupt discontinuation after long-term use.)	• Instruct the patient not to abruptly discontinue the medication but to contact the prescriber if the patient wishes to discontinue the medication so that the dose can be tapered.

Evaluation of Outcome Criteria

Evaluate the effectiveness of drug therapy by confirming that patient goals and expected outcomes have been met (see "Planning").

UNDERSTANDING THE CHAPTER

Key Concepts Summary

22.1 Proper diagnosis of anxiety disorders is important to identifying the most effective treatment option.

22.2 Anxiety disorders may be divided into five major categories.

22.3 Specific regions of the brain that are responsible for anxiety have been identified.

22.4 Sleep occurs in distinct stages.

22.5 Sleep disorders affect a large percentage of the population.

22.6 There is a link between insomnia and anxiety.

22.7 Management of anxiety and sleep disorders utilizes a combination of pharmacologic and nonpharmacologic therapies.

22.8 Benzodiazepines are drugs of choice for generalized anxiety disorder and the short-term therapy of insomnia.

22.9 Several nonbenzodiazepine anxiolytics and miscellaneous agents are used successfully to treat anxiety and sleep disorders.

22.10 Antidepressants are widely prescribed for anxiety disorders.

22.11 Barbiturates are effective sedative–hypnotics but have potentially serious adverse effects that limit their use.

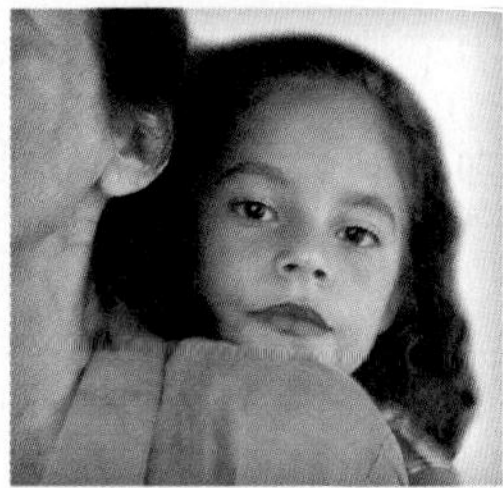

Making the PATIENT *Connection*

Remember the patient "Seraphina Alvarez" at the beginning of the chapter? Now read the remainder of the case study. Based on the information presented within the chapter, respond to the critical thinking questions that follow.

Mrs. Seraphina Alvarez, age 65, is an elementary school teacher who has planned on retiring at the end of this academic year. She is the married mother of seven adult children, six of whom live within a 15-mile radius and see her often. Her husband, Joe, has been retired for 3 years. He receives social security and a small pension from his former employment as a construction worker. Seraphina and Joe's oldest daughter's two children and two dogs came to live with them approximately 10 months ago because their daughter is unable to provide a home for them. The children, Joseph, age 15, and Mariah, age 12, are "good kids." They are good students who are active in school and church activities. They resent having to move from their long-time home and school and are acting-out some. Seraphina also resents having to raise her grandchildren. It interferes with plans that she and her husband had made to travel after she retired. In fact, she may not be able to retire as planned because they need the extra income to meet the children's needs. She loves the children and tries very hard not to let her resentment show. She also has guilt feelings that she did not do all she could or should have done to raise her daughter to be a responsible parent. As a result, she is unable to sleep well and suffers from anxiety. Seraphina first turned to herbal remedies common in her culture and to prayer. Neither of these interventions has helped, but she is reluctant to discuss her problems with anyone else. She sees her parish priest on a regular basis. He is very supportive of her and understanding of her feelings of resentment but does not realize that she is suffering from anxiety and insomnia.

Seraphina, whose health has always been good, has begun having some health issues, including hypertension, diarrhea, and weight loss. She finds herself becoming more anxious, and her family has noticed that she is decreasing time spent with family and friends and does not leave her home other than to go to work and to go to church. She has lost 35 pounds in 2 months and appears to have lost her "zest" for living. Her diet consists of black coffee and fresh fruit. Joe frequently finds her sitting in a rocking chair on their front porch during the night, rather than being in bed. She also has begun missing work, saying "I just don't feel up to facing the kids today."

Critical Thinking Questions

1. What factors in her life currently are interfering with Seraphina's ability to get a good night's sleep?
2. What medications may Seraphina's health care provider order on a short-term or longer-term basis?
3. What part do herbal remedies play in anxiety control and sleep induction in the Latino culture? What specific herbs is Seraphina probably using?

Case Study

Seraphina finally agrees to see her health care provider at Joe's insistence. He accompanies her to her appointment. Her health care provider diagnoses Seraphina with an anxiety disorder, which is causing her insomnia. Seraphina is prescribed lorazepam (Ativan) for her anxiety.

1. What adverse effects are associated with this drug therapy?
2. What information should Seraphina have received about this medication?
3. What nonpharmacologic measures can the nurse recommend to Seraphina to assist her in feeling better about her current situation?

NCLEX-RN® Review

1 A nurse should advise a client who is receiving lorazepam (Ativan) about the adverse effects of this medication, which include:

1. Tachypnea.
2. Astigmatism.
3. Ataxia.
4. Euphoria.

2 The client with insomnia is being treated with temazepam (Restoril). The nurse monitors for therapeutic effectiveness by noting which of the following?

1. Sleeping in 3-hour intervals, awaking for a short time, and then returning to sleep
2. Feeling less anxiety during activities of daily living
3. Having fewer episodes of panic attacks when stressed
4. Sleeping 7 hours without awakening

3 Which of these statements, if made by a client, would indicate that further instruction is needed about alprazolam (Xanax)?

1. "I will stop smoking by undergoing hypnosis."
2. "I will not drive immediately after I take this medication."
3. "I will stop the medicine when I feel less anxious."
4. "I will take my medication with food if my stomach feels upset."

4 The nurse should question a health care provider's order of phenobarbital for the client with which of the following conditions?

1. Seizure disorder
2. Panic disorder
3. Prior to a bronchoscopy
4. Prior to receiving a general anesthetic

5 The nurse is caring for a client receiving a sedative–hypnotic. Which of the following adverse effects associated with this drug therapy is the highest priority for the nurse?

1. Urinary incontinence
2. Activity intolerance
3. Risk for falls
4. Poor nutritional intake

6 The client, who is receiving benzodiazepines, is a two-pack per day cigarette smoker. The nurse expects to administer a(an) ______________ dose of this medication.

1. Larger
2. Smaller
3. Extra
4. Half

See Answers to Critical Thinking Questions, Case Study, and NCLEX-RN® Review in Appendix A.

References

American Psychiatric Association. (2000). *Diagnostic and statistical manual of mental disorders* (4th ed., Text revision). Washington, DC: Author.

Antai-Otlong, D. (2006). Patient education guide: Anxiety disorders. *Nursing, 36*(3), 48–49.

Anxiety Disorders Association of America. (2008). *Statistics and facts about anxiety disorders.* Retrieved June 7, 2008, from http://www.adaa.org/AboutADAA/PressRoom/Stats&Facts.asp

Baldessarini, R. J. (2006). Drug therapy of depression and anxiety disorders. In L. L. Brunton, J. S. Lazo, & K. L. Parker (Eds.). *The pharmacological basis of therapeutics* (11th ed., pp. 429–460). New York: McGraw-Hill.

Buscemi, N., Vandermeer, B., Pandya, R., Hooton, N., Tjosvold, L., Hartling, L., et al. (2004). *Melatonin for treatment of sleep disorders. Summary, evidence report/technology assessment, No. 108* (AHRQ Publication No. 05-E002-2). Rockville, MD: Agency for Healthcare Research and Quality.

Charney, D. S., Mihic, J., & Harris, A. (2006). Hypnotics and sedatives. In L. L. Brunton, J. S. Lazo, & K. L. Parker (Eds.). *The pharmacological basis of therapeutics* (11th ed., pp. 401–428). New York: McGraw-Hill.

Ernst, E. (2006). Herbal remedies for anxiety—A systematic review of controlled clinical trials. *Phytomedicine, 13*(3), 205–208.

Ferrie, J. E., Shipley, M. J., Cappuccio, F. P., Brunner, E., Miller, M. A., Kumari, M., et al. (2007). A prospective study of change in sleep pattern: Associations with mortality in the Whitehall II cohort. *Journal of Sleep, 30*(12), 1659–1666.

Goldsmith, C. (2007, February). Insomnia: Sleepless in America. *Nursing Spectrum,* 16–18.

Kennedy, D., Little, W., Haskell, C., & Scholey, A. (2006). Anxiolytic effects of a combination of *Melissa officinalis* and *Valeriana officinalis* during laboratory induced stress. *Phytotherapy Research, 20*(2), 96–102.

Martin, G.N. (2006). *Human neuropsychology* (2nd ed.). Upper Saddle River, NJ: Pearson Prentice-Hall.

Nierengarten, M. B. (2007). Better sleep and daytime functioning with combined therapy for insomnia and anxiety. *Medscape Medical News.* Retrieved June 8, 2008, from http://www.medscape.com/viewarticle/558233

Olfson, M., Marcus, S. C., & Shaffer, D. (2006). Antidepressant drug therapy and suicide in severely depressed children and adults: A case-control study. *Archives of General Psychiatry, 63*(8), 865–872.

Pittler, M., & Ernst, E. (2003). Kava extract versus placebo for treating anxiety. *Cochrane Database of Systematic Reviews, 1.* Art. No.: CD003383. DOI: 10.1002/14651858.CD003383.

Silverthorn, D. U. (2009). *Human physiology: An integrated approach* (4th ed.). Upper Saddle River, NJ: Pearson Education/Benjamin Cummings.

U.S. Department of Health and Human Services, Substance Abuse and Mental Health Services Administration. (1999). Children's mental health facts. In *Mental health: A report of the surgeon general.* Rockville, MD: Author. Retrieved June 7, 2008, from http://mentalhealth.samhsa.gov/publications/allpubs/ca-0007/default.asp

U.S. Food and Drug Administration. (2004). FDA launches a multi-pronged strategy to strengthen safeguards for children treated with antidepressant medications. *FDA News.* Retrieved June 8, 2008, from http://www.fda.gov/bbs/topics/news/2004/new01124.html

Winkelman, J. W. (2005). A primary care approach to insomnia management. *Medscape Pharmacists.* Retrieved June 8, 2008, from http://www.medscape.com/viewprogram/3807

World Health Organization. (1994/2006). *International statistical classification of diseases and related health problems, 10th revision, version for 2006.* Geneva: WHO/DIMDI.

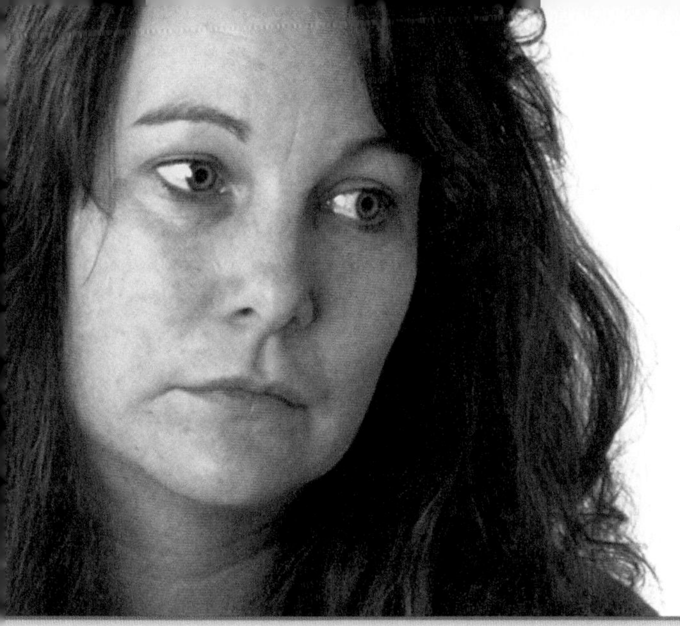

For the past 4 to 5 weeks my wife, Jane, has been having problems. She doesn't get up to see that the children are off to school, dinner is not started when I get home from work at 6:00 p.m., no housework or laundry has been done, she is frequently still in pajamas with her hair uncombed, and obviously has not showered or brushed her teeth. Her friends say that Jane has not returned their calls in weeks now.

"Charlie Albright," Jane's husband

CHAPTER 23

Pharmacotherapy of Mood Disorders

Chapter Outline

Types of Mood Disorders

Major Depressive Disorder

Pathophysiology of Depression

Assessment of Depression

Nonpharmacologic Therapies for Depression

Pharmacotherapy of Depression

Tricyclic Antidepressants

PROTOTYPE **Imipramine (Tofranil)** *p. 306*

Selective Serotonin Reuptake Inhibitors

PROTOTYPE **Fluoxetine (Prozac, Sarafem)** *p. 308*

Atypical Antidepressants

PROTOTYPE **Venlafaxine (Effexor)** *p. 311*

Monoamine Oxidase Inhibitors

PROTOTYPE **Phenelzine (Nardil)** *p. 314*

Bipolar Disorder

Drugs for Bipolar Disorder

PROTOTYPE **Lithium Carbonate (Eskalith, Lithobid)** *p. 318*

Learning Outcomes

After reading this chapter, the student should be able to:

1. Compare and contrast the major categories of mood disorders and their symptoms.
2. Explain the pathophysiology of major depression and bipolar disorder.
3. Discuss the nurse's role in the assessment of patients with mood disorders.
4. Identify the relationship between suicide and depression.
5. Describe the nurse's role in the pharmacologic and nonpharmacologic management of mood disorders.
6. For each of the classes shown in the chapter outline, identify the prototype and representative drugs and explain the mechanism(s) of drug action, primary indications, contraindications, significant drug interactions, pregnancy category, and important adverse effects.
7. Use the nursing process to care for patients receiving drug therapy for mood disorders.

Key Terms

antidepressants, *303*
atypical antidepressant, *311*
bipolar disorder, *317*
depression, *298*
electroconvulsive therapy (ECT), *302*
hypomania, *318*
major depressive disorder, *298*
mania, *317*
monoamine oxidase inhibitor (MAOI), *313*
mood disorder, *298*
mood stabilizer, *318*
phototherapy, *301*
postpartum onset depression, *299*
seasonal affective disorder (SAD), *299*
serotonin, *307*
serotonin syndrome (SES), *308*
suicide, *301*
tricyclic antidepressants (TCA), *303*
tyramine, *314*

Inappropriate or unusually intense emotions are among the leading mental health disorders. Although mood changes are a normal part of life, when they become prolonged and severe and impair functioning within the family, work environment, or interpersonal relationships, a patient may be diagnosed as having a mood disorder. The purpose of this chapter is to explain the role of pharmacotherapy in treating the two primary categories of mood disorders: major depression and bipolar disorder.

PharmFACT

Clinical depression affects more than 19 million Americans each year, and fewer than 50% seek medical treatment. There is no common age, sex, or ethnic factor related to depression—it can happen to anyone. *Source:* National Education Association Health Information Network, n.d.

Types of Mood Disorders

23.1 The two primary types of mood disorders are depression and bipolar disorder.

Mood disorders form a cluster of mental health conditions that are very common in the population. They affect all cultures and occur throughout the life span. Mood disorders are a major cause of disability and can significantly strain social relationships. They are a leading cause of absenteeism and diminished productivity in the workplace.

Defining and diagnosing mood disorders is sometimes difficult; the line between normal emotion and a mood disorder is often unclear. Because health care providers see patients for such brief periods, they must rely on patient self-reports or caregiver information, which can be unreliable. As a working definition, a **mood disorder** is a change in emotion that impairs the patient's ability to effectively deal with normal activities of daily living.

The American Psychiatric Association's *Diagnostic and Statistical Manual of Mental Disorders,* Fourth Edition, Text Revision *(DSM-IV-TR)* provides the criteria for a wide variety of mental illnesses. According to this manual, mood disorders may be classified by the following:

- Major depressive disorder. When people use the word *depression,* they are most often referring to major depressive disorder.
- Dysthymic disorder. This is mild, chronic depression that persists for at least 2 continuous years.
- Bipolar disorder. Formerly called manic depression, the patient alternates between intense excitement (mania) and major depressive disorder.
- Manic and hypomanic episodes. Includes mania symptoms that last for at least 1 week and significantly impact social functioning. Hypomania is less intense, lasting only 4 days and has less impact on social or work functioning.
- Cyclothymic disorder. A mild form of bipolar disorder in which the patient alternates between hypomania and mild depression. Largely undiagnosed, 33% of these patients will eventually develop bipolar disorder.

Mood disorders often coexist with other conditions. For example, about 50% of patients diagnosed with major depression also meet the criteria for an anxiety disorder (see Chapter 22). Of those patients with mood disorder 25% to 40% have a comorbid substance abuse condition. Those with chronic medical conditions such as hypertension (HTN) or arthritis have a higher incidence of depression. The most serious of the comorbid conditions is completed or attempted suicide (see Section 23.5).

Major Depressive Disorder

23.2 Major depressive disorder is characterized by a depressed mood, with accompanying symptoms, that lasts at least 2 weeks.

Depression is a disorder characterized by a sad or despondent mood that becomes out of proportion to actual life events. Depression can manifest as an extremely diverse set of symptoms, including lack of energy, sleep disturbances, abnormal eating patterns, or feelings of despair, guilt, and hopelessness. Depression is the most common mental health disorder, affecting approximately 10% to 20% of the population. Although women between the ages of 25 and 45 are more likely to have a depressive disorder than any other group, depression in men more frequently results in suicide. Many persons who are depressed never seek or receive care for their depression.

The *DSM-IV-TR* describes **major depressive disorder** as a depressed mood lasting for a minimum of 2 weeks that is present for most of the day, every day, or almost every day. In addition, at least five of the symptoms shown in Table 23.1 must be present. Depressed moods caused by general medical conditions or by substances such as alcohol or other central nervous system (CNS) depressants do not warrant a diagnosis of major depressive disorder. For the purposes of this text, the terms *depression* and *major depressive disorder* are considered the same unless otherwise specified.

The *DSM-IV-TR* also states that the current mood of the patient who is depressed must represent a change from previous functioning. For example, some people who might appear depressed to a health care provider may be exhibiting the exact same functioning level that they have exhibited their entire lives; these people would not fit the *DSM-IV-TR* classification of depression.

TABLE 23.1 Symptoms of Depression

CNS Symptoms	Behavioral Symptoms	General Symptoms
Feelings of despair, lack of self-worth, guiltiness, and misery	Staying in bed most of the day and night	Extremely tired; without energy
Obsessed with death; expresses desire to die or to commit suicide	Neglecting usual household chores	Vague physical symptoms (GI pain, joint or muscle pain, or headaches)
Delusions or hallucinations	Not going to work, or if the person goes he or she is not able to function effectively	Physiological depression (constipation, sleep disorders, decreased heart rate, etc.)
	Abnormal eating patterns (eating too much or not enough)	
	Lack of interest in personal appearance or sex	
	Avoiding psychosocial and interpersonal interactions	

Once a diagnosis of a mood disorder is made, more detailed information about it may be provided by the health care provider in the form of "specifiers." The use of specifiers gives mental health professionals additional information about the disorder and its treatment. Specifiers are best thought of as subcategories of major depressive disorder and bipolar disorder. Some of the specifiers used with depression include with or without psychotic features, single episode or recurrent, melancholic features, atypical features, and catatonic features. Two important specifiers are postpartum onset and seasonal onset.

Up to 80% of women experience brief "baby blues" or **postpartum onset depression** during the first 2 weeks after the birth of a baby. About 10% of new mothers will experience major depression within the first 6 months postdelivery, which is related to the dramatic hormonal shifts that occur during that period. Along with the hormonal changes, additional situational stresses such as changing responsibilities at work and at home, single parenthood, and caring for children and for aging parents may contribute to the onset of symptoms. Because of the potentially serious consequences of postpartum onset depression, some states mandate that all new mothers receive information about these mood disorders prior to their discharge after giving birth. All levels of health care providers in obstetricians' offices, pediatric outpatient settings, and family medicine centers are encouraged to conduct routine screening for symptoms of perinatal mood disorders.

During the dark winter months, some patients experience a type of depression known as **seasonal affective disorder (SAD).** SAD is more common in areas such as Alaska, where the days are very short during the winter months and there is little natural sunlight. This type of depression is associated with a reduced release of the brain neurohormone melatonin. The condition is generally self-limiting and resolves when spring arrives. Exposing patients on a regular basis to specific wavelengths of light may relieve SAD depression and prevent future episodes.

PharmFACT

The lifetime risk for major depression for women is 20% to 30%, and for men 7% to 12%; overall, 25% of patients who have had a major depressive episode will have chronic, recurrent depression. *Source:* Ikezu & Gendelman, 2008.

Pathophysiology of Depression

23.3 The pathophysiology of depression has biologic, genetic, and environmental components.

Depression is one of the oldest known mental health conditions and one of the most frequently diagnosed. Despite this the etiology of depression is not well understood. Several theories have been proposed to explain the causes of depression and why some people are predisposed to developing the disease. The etiology and pathogenesis are likely influenced by multiple, complex variables.

Research attempting to identify the biologic causes of depression has focused on the levels and function of neurotransmitters in the limbic system of the brain. The limbic system is the region that regulates emotions (see Chapters 21 and 22). Major depression has been associated with abnormally low levels of neurotransmitters such as norepinephrine, serotonin, and dopamine in the limbic system. Although it is well known that some of the antidepressant medications act by increasing the levels of these neurotransmitters, scientists are many years from discovering what role each specific neurotransmitter plays in the development of major depressive disorder. Does having depression deplete the brain of these neurotransmitters, or does a loss of neurotransmitters cause depression? The answers remain elusive.

Certain hormonal abnormalities are associated with depression, suggesting that the endocrine system also plays an important physiological role in the pathogenesis of the disease. About half of depressed persons have excessive serum cortisol levels. Cortisol mobilizes the body for stress situations and is thought to reduce serotonin levels in the brain, bringing about symptoms of depression. Hypothyroidism is also strongly linked to depression. In some patients, therapy with thyroid hormone (T_3) results in a marked improvement in depression symptoms.

It is well established that depression has a genetic component. Major depression is 1.5 to 3 times more common in persons who have a first-degree relative (parent or sibling) with depression compared to the general population. In identical twins, when one twin is diagnosed with depression, the other twin has a 50% probability of acquiring the disorder. This relationship holds true whether the twins were raised together or separately. Even fraternal twins have a 19% chance of developing depression when the other twin is diagnosed, which is a percentage higher than that of the general population.

Many environmental causes of depression have been identified and include prolonged stress at work or at home, loss of a loved one, and other traumatic life events. Various childhood events have been associated with an increased risk of adult depression, including sexual or physical abuse, and death of, separation from, or mental illness of a parent.

CONNECTION *Checkpoint* 23.1

From what you learned in Chapter 21, what are the connections between the limbic system, the hypothalamus, and the cerebrum and how can these connections be used to explain symptoms of depression? See Answer to Connection Checkpoint 23.1 in Appendix A.

Assessment of Depression

23.4 Assessment and diagnosis of depression are a collaborative effort among health care providers.

The majority of people who are depressed are not found in psychiatric hospitals but in mainstream everyday settings. For proper diagnosis and treatment to occur, the recognition of depression must be a collaborative effort among health care providers. Because people who are depressed are present in multiple settings and in all areas of practice, every nurse should be proficient in the assessment and nursing care of patients afflicted with this disorder.

The first step in implementing appropriate treatment for depression is a complete medical examination; the diagnosis of depression begins by ruling out other medical conditions. Certain drugs such as corticosteroids, beta blockers, levodopa, antipsychotic agents, oral contraceptives, and CNS depressants can cause symptoms of clinical depression, and the health care provider must rule out this possibility. Depression may be mimicked by a variety of medical and neurologic disorders, ranging from B-vitamin deficiencies to thyroid gland malfunction to early Alzheimer's disease. If medical causes for the depression are discovered, proper treatment of the underlying disorder may be enough to resolve symptoms of depression. If causes for the depression cannot be identified, a psychiatrist or psychologist may be consulted to perform a comprehensive psychological evaluation to confirm the diagnosis.

Because they are comorbid with depression in a significant number of patients, inquiries should be made about alcohol and drug use and any thoughts about suicide. The initial exam should also include questions about any family history of depressive illness. If other family members have been treated, the nurse should document what therapies they may have received and which were effective. The manifestation of depression that is most obvious to those surrounding a depressed person is a change in attitude toward usual daily activities. The patient loses interest in work, school, or other hobbies or activities that he or she previously enjoyed.

Severe depressive illness, particularly that which is recurrent, will require both medication and psychotherapy to achieve optimum outcomes. Daily outpatient visits to a treatment facility may be necessary when beginning treatment, then tapered to a less frequent schedule as improvement is noted. Some patients, especially those at high risk for suicide, will require an initial period of hospitalization where continuous monitoring is provided.

Depression remains greatly underdiagnosed among older adults despite the fact that as many as 6 million Americans over the age of 65 suffer from the disorder. Of this group, only about 10% receive treatment. Too often elderly patients are reluctant to admit to depression, seeing this as a sign of weakness or an

CONNECTIONS

Treating the Diverse Patient Cultural Influences and the Treatment of Depression

To fully understand any patient who is suffering from depression, sociocultural factors must be considered. Depression (and other mental illness) is often ignored in many Asian communities because of the tremendous amount of stigma attached to it. Emotions are largely suppressed. Asian patients tend to come to the attention of mental health workers late in the course of their illness and often have feelings of hopelessness. A noteworthy point, according to Spector (2004), is the importance that is placed on the family in caring for the mentally ill in Asian culture. It should be noted that Asians and African Americans generally metabolize antidepressants more slowly than other subgroups; therefore, initial doses should be reduced to avoid drug toxicity.

Alternative therapies such as ethnopharmacologic teas are often used to treat emotional illnesses within some Hispanic American groups; thus, medical help may not be sought for treatment of depression. Specific teas that may be used by persons of Hispanic origin include *manzanilla* or chamomile, used to cure fright; *yerba buena* or spearmint, used to treat nervousness; *té de naranja* or orange leaves, used as a sedative or to treat nervousness. There is often a stigma attached to mental health problems along with the belief that religious practices will solve them. Hispanics metabolize antidepressants about the same as other subgroups, although there are reports of greater susceptibility to anticholinergic effects.

Among Native American people, the family frequently is nuclear with large numbers of extended family. One mental health problem affecting American Indians is termed "ghost sickness" and involves being preoccupied with death and the deceased. Many of the symptoms are the same as those of depression such as anorexia, confusion, nightmares, and physical weakness. Suicide secondary to depression and other mental health issues ranks higher among Native Americans than for the population at large. There are documented instances of variations in drug metabolism and excretion rates between American Indians and peoples of other ethnic groups.

Some people of European origin deny that mental illness exists and therefore believe that depression will subside on its own. Higher doses of antidepressants are tolerated in this subgroup.

inability to continue to care for themselves. Depression in the older adult may be manifested as difficulty making decisions and as a growing reluctance to leave the home. Feelings of despair, lack of self-worth, and guilt are common. In some cases the person may overuse alcohol or combine alcohol with other CNS depressants, resulting in further depression.

Some people incorrectly believe that the symptoms of depression are a normal part of aging and therefore need no special attention. Factors that contribute to depression in the older adult include loss of spouse or children; the need to move from a long-term residence to a smaller home or in with other family or to assisted living of some type; loss of friends and other support systems; being unmarried; living alone; having multiple health challenges; the expense of polypharmacy; decreased finances; and worry about end-of-life issues.

23.5 The majority of patients who attempt suicide have major depression.

Suicide is defined as the intentional act of ending one's life. The Centers for Disease Control and Prevention (CDC) lists suicide as the 11th cause of death in the United States; almost 30,000 people every year take their own lives. Suicide is the third leading cause of death, behind accidents and homicide, among Americans between the ages of 15 and 24. No age group, income level, educational level, race, religion, or other demographic group is exempt from it. Almost 95% of all persons who turn to suicide, whether successful or not, have a diagnosed mental disorder (Sadock & Sadock, 2003). Comorbid conditions include mood disorders, psychoses, personality disorder, anxiety disorders, severe insomnia, chronic alcohol or substance use, chronic disabling or painful disease, and family history, especially in the same-sex parent.

The majority of persons who commit suicide have been diagnosed with major depression. Unfortunately, depending on the drug and the individual patient's response, 6 or more weeks of antidepressant pharmacotherapy may be required before the patient begins to feel less depressed. Suicide may occur early in treatment during the period a patient is being stabilized on the antidepressant. Some theories have proposed that antidepressant medications actually increase the risk of suicide. This prompted the U.S. Food and Drug Administration (FDA) to issue a black box warning in 2004 indicating that antidepressant medications are associated with an increased risk of suicidal thinking and behavior in children and adolescents. This black box warning was expanded in 2007 to include patients 18 to 24 years of age.

A recent study of over 100,000 patients on antidepressant drugs disputed this theory; the patterns of suicide attempts before and after starting antidepressant therapy were the same (Simon & Savarino, 2007). The highest risk of suicide was in the month before pharmacotherapy, and attempts declined after pharmacotherapy was initiated. Another recent study of patients in the Veterans Administration (VA) system came to similar conclusions; the highest rate of suicide was in depressed patients without pharmacotherapy, and the suicide rate significantly declined in those receiving antidepressants (Gibbons et al., 2007). The relationship between antidepressants and suicide will likely be a continuing topic of research.

So what interventions can the nurse implement to reduce the potential for suicidal behavior during antidepressant therapy? Careful monitoring of the patient is the simplest yet most important intervention. Weekly and even daily patient contact may be necessary until the antidepressant begins to effectively elevate mood, which would typically be 4 to 12 weeks. A patient who has had a previous suicide attempt is at higher risk and must be more carefully monitored. If a person verbalizes about committing suicide, the talk must be taken seriously. It is a myth that a person who talks about suicide will not actually act. The person may be so depressed that suicide seems like the only option, and talking about it to a friend or nurse may be a last attempt for help or intervention. The nurse must judiciously monitor all prescribed drugs because suicidal patients often take overdoses of their medications. Therapy with multiple CNS depressants such as for pain, anxiety, insomnia, and depression is strongly discouraged because these agents produce additive sedation. Worsening symptoms of depression must be reported immediately because these may indicate that the drug is not working or that the patient is not compliant with pharmacotherapy. Switching to a different antidepressant or even hospitalization may be necessary.

Nonpharmacologic Therapies for Depression

23.6 Depression is sometimes treated with nonpharmacologic therapies.

Although pharmacotherapy is the standard treatment for patients with serious depression, other therapies may be beneficial for patients with mild to moderate depression or for those whose condition is refractory to conventional treatment. Indeed, psychotherapy is often the treatment of choice when the patient is willing to participate and the depressive state is mild to moderate in severity. Other nonpharmacologic therapies for depression are shown in Table 23.2.

Counseling therapies help patients gain insight into and resolve mental health issues through verbal "give-and-take" with the therapist. Behavioral therapies help patients learn how to obtain more satisfaction and rewards through their own actions and how to unlearn the behavioral patterns that contribute to or result from their depression. Interpersonal therapy focuses on a patient's disturbed personal relationships that both cause and exacerbate the depression. Cognitive–behavioral therapies help patients change negative styles of thought and behavior that are often associated with their depression. Psychodynamic therapies focus on resolving the patients' internal conflicts by looking at the influence of past experiences on current behavior and how behavior is influenced by emotional factors. These therapies are sometimes postponed until the acute depressive symptoms have improved.

Light therapy or **phototherapy** is a type of therapy especially useful for persons suffering from SAD. Phototherapy uses artificial lighting approximately 5 to 20 times brighter than normal indoor lighting while the patient sits with eyes open about 3 feet away from and at eye level with the light source. Normal activities can be pursued during the treatment which can be conducted in the patient's home.

CONNECTIONS

Lifespan Considerations Depression in Children and Adolescents

Depression has become a major issue with children and adolescents. It is estimated that almost 20% of preadolescents have a major depressive disorder. Children as young as 3 years old have been diagnosed with depression. Most studies on depression in children and adolescents have been conducted within the last 4 to 5 years, and available scientific literature is much less extensive than what is available on depression in adults. One large study, titled "Treatment for Adolescents with Depression Study (TADS)," was conducted between 2000 and 2003 (March et al., 2004). A total of 439 adolescents with major depression were studied in 13 sites across the nation. The results showed that a combination of medication and psychotherapy was most effective. The medication used in the study was fluoxetine (Prozac), which at the time of the study was the only FDA-approved antidepressant to treat adolescents. One result of the TADS was the determination that large treatment trials are necessary to determine which treatments work best for which children and adolescents. It went on to say that studies are also needed on how to best incorporate these treatments in primary care practice. There is an increased risk for physical illness and intrapersonal and psychosocial difficulties that are much more long-lasting than the depressive episode itself. In adolescents, there is also an increased risk for substance abuse and suicide.

Depression in children and adolescents manifests itself differently than depression in adults. Common symptoms include boredom; talk of or attempts to run away from home; frequent vague, nonspecific physical complaints (headache, muscle aches, stomach aches, fatigue, etc.); social isolation; poor communication skills; lack of interest in playing with friends; reckless behavior; fear of death; or alcohol or substance abuse. The depressed teen may demonstrate irritability, hostility, and anger. These may be misdiagnosed as normal rebellious adolescent behavior, and the depression does not get correctly diagnosed.

Studies of depression in young people have demonstrated that selective serotonin reuptake inhibitors (SSRIs) are safe and effective for the short-term treatment of severe and persistent depression. Studies have found that both fluoxetine and paroxetine are effective. Tricyclic antidepressants (TCAs) are not recommended treatments for depressed youth.

One consequence of untreated or undertreated depression in children and adolescents is suicide. The method of suicide appears to be what is convenient and readily available. Preventive measures should be tailored to address trends in a localized area, rather than throughout the United States. Shaw, Fernandes, and Rao (2005) reported on a 10-year study of suicide in adolescents done in Canada. Results showed that more than twice as many males as females in the age group 15 to 19 committed suicide. The most common method used by males was hanging, with firearms, poisoning, drowning, and blunt force vehicular trauma following on the list. No trend was identified for females. Similar results are available in studies conducted in other countries.

The major result of all of the studies is that depression alone, and depression leading to suicide, are major health issues among children and adolescents. Steps must be taken to better and earlier diagnose depressed youths, then institute appropriate treatments.

In patients with serious and life-threatening mood disorders that are unresponsive to pharmacotherapy and psychotherapy, **electroconvulsive therapy (ECT)** continues to be a useful treatment. ECT induces a brief convulsion (grand mal seizure) by passing an electric current into the brain through electrodes applied to one or both temples. The patient is anesthetized and given a muscle relaxant prior to the treatment and therefore is unaware of the convulsion as it is occurring. Although ECT has been found to be safe, there are still deaths (1 in 10,000 patients) and other serious complications related to seizure activity and anesthesia caused by ECT. Some patients receive repeated courses of ECT over a period of years, because their depressive episodes cannot be improved with either pharmacotherapy or psychotherapy. Adverse effects of ECT include transient short-term memory loss and confusion immediately after the procedure. If the patient is aware of these before beginning treatment, there is much less anxiety when one or both of them occur.

TABLE 23.2 Types of Therapy for Major Depression

Type	Definition
Cognitive–Behavioral Therapy	Therapy that helps patients change the negative styles of thought and behavior that are often associated with their depression.
Electroconvulsive Therapy (ECT)	The induction of a brief convulsion by passing an electric current through the brain as therapy for affective disorders, especially in patients who have not responded to pharmacotherapy.
Interpersonal Therapy	Therapy focusing on the patient's disturbed personal relationships that both cause and exacerbate the depression.
Light Therapy or Phototherapy	Therapy that uses artificial lighting that is 5 to 20 times brighter than usual indoor lighting; it is used to simulate natural sunlight in areas where there is little natural sunlight for several months of the year, such as Alaska and other areas near the North Pole.
Psychodynamic Therapy	Therapy focusing on resolving a patient's internal conflicts.
Repetitive Transcranial Magnetic Stimulation (rTMS) Therapy	An effective somatic therapy, experimental in the United States, that involves a device that administers a train of multiple stimuli per second. The device is a metal coil that is placed on or near the patient's head, allowing the magnetic field to pass through the skull and into specific target areas of the brain.
Vagus Nerve Stimulation (VNS)	Somatic therapy that involves placing a small generator into a patient's chest; it is attached to an electrode with ends wrapped around the left vagus nerve on the patient's neck; the generator is programmed for frequency and intensity of stimulus. The electrical current stimulates the vagus nerve.

Recent studies suggest that repetitive transcranial magnetic stimulation (rTMS) is an effective somatic treatment for major depression. rTMS is a noninvasive procedure that passes a high electric current through a wire stimulation coil placed on or close to a specific area of the head. Treatments are generally administered daily; the length of treatment varies according to patient response. This treatment may require surgical implant of the device. In contrast with ECT, rTMS has minimal effects on memory, does not require general anesthesia, and produces its effects without a generalized seizure. The major concern with this type of therapy is the possibility of inducing seizures.

Another somatic therapy currently under investigation is vagus nerve stimulation (VNS). VNS involves the surgical implantation of a small generator, about 3 to 4 inches in diameter, into the patient's chest. An electrode is threaded through the subcutaneous tissue from the generator to the vagus nerve on the left side of the patient's neck. The left vagus connects to the brainstem and deep brain structures thought to be involved in epilepsy and some psychiatric disorders. Stimulating these fibers may cause changes in the functions of some structures and affect the concentration of the neurotransmitter gamma aminobutyric acid (GABA) and other neurotransmitters in that area. Once implanted, the generator is programmed via computer to adjust both the intensity and frequency of the stimulus according to the patient's needs. At this time, VNS is approved in the United States only for use in treating epilepsy, although it appears to be successful in treating the symptoms of depression. Adverse effects have been mild and mostly involve hoarseness, which is thought to be secondary to the vagal stimulation.

PharmFACT

Approximately 22% of female and 12% of male students in grades 9 through 12 seriously consider suicide each year. Over 8% state that they actually attempted suicide. Among people ages 15 to 24, suicide accounts for 13% of all deaths annually. *Source:* Centers for Disease Control and Prevention, 2007.

Pharmacotherapy of Depression

23.7 The mechanism of action of antidepressants involves modulation of neurotransmitter levels in the brain.

Antidepressants are drugs used to enhance, elevate, or stabilize mood. In the treatment of depression they are used to treat all symptoms of major depressive disorder as well as the depressive phases of bipolar disorder. They are ineffective against the manic phases of bipolar disorder, and other drugs must be used to control those symptoms (see Section 23.12).

The antidepressants act by restoring normal neurotransmitter balances in certain regions of the brain. Depending on the medication, the primary neurotransmitters affected are norepinephrine, serotonin, and, to a lesser degree, dopamine. The two basic mechanisms of action of antidepressants are blocking the enzymatic breakdown of norepinephrine and slowing the reuptake of serotonin into neurons. Although antidepressants may not be able to completely restore chemical balance, they help to manage depressive symptoms while the patient develops effective strategies for coping.

In addition to elevating mood, changing the neurotransmitter balance has a number of other effects on the brain. Some of the antidepressants have become major drugs in the treatment of anxiety disorders such as phobia, obsessive–compulsive behavior, panic disorder, and generalized anxiety disorder (see Chapter 22). Certain antidepressants are also beneficial as adjuvant analgesics in the pharmacotherapy of pain (see Chapter 29). Antidepressants are beneficial in treating depression that is often associated with painful, chronic conditions such as fibromyalgia or muscle spasticity (see Chapter 27).

Once patients begin to "feel better" they sometimes want to discontinue drug therapy due to the expense of the medication or because they are experiencing uncomfortable adverse effects. Nurses must be aware that many patients taking antidepressants will stop taking their medication. About half of these patients, however, will relapse within 6 months of discontinuing antidepressant therapy; the percentage increases to 85% after 3 years. It is important to teach patients that antidepressant therapy may extend for many years and that adherence to the health care provider's instructions is essential for the long-term maintenance of mental health. In general, antidepressant therapy should continue for a minimum of 6 months after the depressive symptoms resolve.

When administered at comparable doses, all antidepressants have similar effectiveness; therefore, the choice of drug is not usually based on this factor. The treatment of depression, however, is highly individualized and patients who are unresponsive to one class of medications may respond favorably to drugs from a different class. In fact, patients may respond differently to drugs within the same class. Furthermore the spectrum of adverse effects differs among the classes and patients may find that drugs from one class are more tolerable than another. Overall, about 65% of patients will respond favorably to antidepressant pharmacotherapy. Success rates improve to 85% when psychotherapy or alternative or adjunctive medicine is used along with antidepressant medications. The five primary classes of antidepressants, shown in Table 23.3, are as follows:

- Tricyclic antidepressants (TCAs)
- Selective serotonin reuptake inhibitors (SSRIs)
- Serotonin–norepinephrine reuptake inhibitors (SNRIs)
- Atypical antidepressants
- Monoamine oxidase inhibitors (MAOIs)

Tricyclic Antidepressants

23.8 Tricyclic antidepressants have been the mainstay for the treatment of depression but have many adverse effects.

The **tricyclic antidepressants (TCAs)** have been available in the United States for over 50 years, and they are still prescribed for many patients with major depressive disorder. Imipramine

TABLE 23.3 Antidepressant Drugs

Drug	Route and Adult Dose (maximum dose where indicated)	Adverse Effects
Tricyclic Antidepressants (TCAs)		
amitriptyline (Elavil)	PO: 75–100 mg/day (max: 300 mg/day)	*Drowsiness, sedation, dizziness, orthostatic hypotension, dry mouth, constipation, urinary retention, constipation, blurred vision, mydriasis, tachycardia* Bone marrow depression, seizures, dysrhythmias, heart block, MI, hepatitis, acute renal failure
desipramine (Norpramin)	PO: 75–100 mg/day; may increase to 150–300 mg/day	
clomipramine (Anafranil)	PO: 25 mg once daily (max: 250 mg/day)	
doxepin (Sinequan)	PO: 30–150 mg/day at bedtime (max: 300 mg/day)	
imipramine (Tofranil)	PO: 75–150 mg/day (max: 300 mg/day) IM: 50–100 mg/day in divided doses	
maprotiline (Ludiomil)	PO: 25 mg tid (max: 225 mg/day)	
nortriptyline (Aventyl, Pamelor)	PO: 25 mg tid or qid (max: 150 mg/day)	
protriptyline (Vivactil)	PO: 15–40 mg/day in 3–4 divided doses (max: 60 mg/day)	
trimipramine (Surmontil)	PO: 75–100 mg/day in divided doses (max: 300 mg/day)	
Selective Serotonin Reuptake Inhibitors (SSRIs)		
citalopram (Celexa)	PO: start at 20 mg once daily; may increase to 40 mg after 1 week (max: 60 mg/day)	*Nausea, vomiting, dry mouth, insomnia, somnolence, headache, nervousness, anxiety, diarrhea, dizziness, anorexia, fatigue, sexual dysfunction, weight changes* SJS, serotonin syndrome
escitalopram (Lexapro)	PO: 10 mg once daily; may increase to 20 mg after 1 week (max: 20 mg/day)	
fluoxetine (Prozac)	PO: 20 mg/day in the a.m., may increase by 20 mg/day at weekly intervals (max: 80 mg/day); when stable may switch to 90-mg sustained release capsule once weekly (max: 90 mg/week)	
fluvoxamine (Luvox)	PO: start with 50 mg/day and increase every 4–7 days as needed (max: 300 mg/day)	
paroxetine (Paxil, Pexeva)	PO (Immediate release): start with 20 mg once daily and increase by 10 mg each week as needed (max: 60 mg/day for immediate release form)	
	PO (Sustained release): 25 mg daily and increase by 12.5-mg intervals (max: 62.5 mg/day)	
sertraline (Zoloft)	PO: start with 50 mg once daily and increase at weekly intervals as needed (max: 200 mg/day)	
Atypical Antidepressants		
amoxapine	PO: start with 50 mg bid–tid and increase to 100 mg bid–tid by the end of the first week (max: 400 mg/day)	*Insomnia, nausea, dry mouth, constipation, increased blood pressure and heart rate, dizziness, sweating, agitation, blurred vision, headache, dizziness, tremor, vomiting, drowsiness, somnolence, increased appetite, orthostatic hypotension, increased blood glucose level (duloxetine)* Stevens-Johnson syndrome (SJS), seizures, vaginal, uterine or anal hemorrhage, suicidal ideation, priapism, neuroleptic malignant syndrome (amoxapine), parkinsonism (amoxapine), elevated hepatic enzymes (duloxetine, mirtazapine), bone marrow suppression (mirtazapine), liver failure (nefazodone)
bupropion HCl (Wellbutrin, Zyban)	PO: start with 100 mg bid (immediate release) or 150 mg once daily (extended release) and increase gradually as needed (max: 450 mg/day for immediate release, 400 mg/day for extended release, or 300 mg/day for Zyban)	
desvenliafaxine (Prestiq)	PO: 50 mg once daily (max: 100 mg/day)	
duloxetine (Cymbalta)	PO: 40–60 mg/day in 1–2 divided doses (max: 60 mg/day)	
mirtazapine (Remeron)	PO: 15 mg/day in a single dose at bedtime; may increase every 1–2 weeks (max: 45 mg/day)	
nefazodone	PO: 50–100 mg bid (max: 600 mg/day)	
trazodone (Desyrel)	PO: 150 mg/day in divided doses; may increase by 50 mg/day every 3–4 days (max: 400 mg/day)	
venlafaxine (Effexor)	PO: start with 75 mg/day and increase slowly at 4–7-day intervals as needed (max: 375 mg/day for regular release; 225 mg/day for extended release)	
MAO Inhibitors (MAOIs)		
isocarboxazid (Marplan)	PO: 10–30 mg/day (max: 30 mg/day)	*Drowsiness, insomnia, orthostatic hypotension, blurred vision, nausea, constipation, anorexia, dry mouth, urinary retention, sexual dysfunction, overactivity* Hypertensive crisis, circulatory collapse, dysrhythmias
phenelzine (Nardil)	PO: 15 mg tid rapidly increase to at least 60 mg/day tid or qid (max: 90 mg/day)	
selegiline (Emsam)	Transdermal: one patch (6 mg)/day	
tranylcypromine (Parnate)	PO: 30 mg/day; may increase by 10 mg/day at 3-week intervals (max: 60 mg/day)	

Note: *Italics* indicate common adverse effects. Underline indicates serious adverse effects.

(Tofranil), the prototype drug for this class, was the first TCA available. This group of medications is named after its molecular structure, which has a nucleus that consists of three rings. This arrangement is very similar to the structure of the phenothiazine antipsychotics. Thus these two classes of drugs share similar adverse effects (see Chapter 24).

The TCAs act by blocking the reuptake of norepinephrine and serotonin in neurons, as shown in Figure 23.1. This blockade results in more neurotransmitters being available in the synaptic space, thus a more intensified action. Some TCAs such as desipramine, maprotiline, and protriptyline are specific to blocking the reuptake of norepinephrine, whereas the other drugs in this class affect both norepinephrine and serotonin. In general, all TCAs have similar effectiveness and exhibit the same types of adverse effects.

The advantages of TCAs are that they are inexpensive and their effectiveness in treating depression has been well established for many decades. They are rapidly absorbed when given orally (PO) and widely distributed throughout the body. Frequent adverse effects, however, have limited their use. Many health care providers prefer to prescribe drugs in the SSRI class because they are better tolerated by most patients.

Blockade of muscarinic receptors by TCAs is responsible for causing a high incidence of anticholinergic adverse effects with symptoms such as dry mouth, blurred vision, constipation, urinary retention, and tachycardia. Orthostatic hypotension is frequently reported and may be serious enough to cause injury due to falls. One of the most serious adverse effects is the ability of TCAs and some of their metabolites to accumulate in cardiac tissue and depress the myocardium. They can cause life-threatening cardiac dysrhythmias, especially if the patient receives an overdose.

A few of the TCAs have central effects that cause sedation, which can usually be managed by taking the drugs at bedtime. Sedation is worsened by the concurrent use of other CNS depressants such as alcohol. Confusion, dizziness, and fatigue are other possible dose-limiting effects of TCAs. At high doses some cause seizures.

Compared to other classes of antidepressants, TCAs exhibit a relatively high incidence of sexual dysfunction, including impotence and delayed ejaculation in men; breast enlargement and impaired orgasm occur in women. Weight gain is possible. In addition, some patients quickly change mood from depression to hypomania or mania and may begin to display symptoms of bipolar disorder. These patients require a dosage adjustment or a change to a different antidepressant.

Tolerance and psychological dependence are usually not major problems when using TCAs. Therapy may often be conducted for years without requiring a dosage adjustment. Unlike many CNS depressants, antidepressants such as the TCAs are not drugs of abuse. Patients on high doses for prolonged periods, however, may exhibit a mild withdrawal syndrome on discontinuation and experience symptoms such as irritability, nausea, sleep impairment, muscle aches, and fatigue. To avoid unpleasant symptoms, and to ensure that depression does not quickly return, these drugs are usually withdrawn gradually.

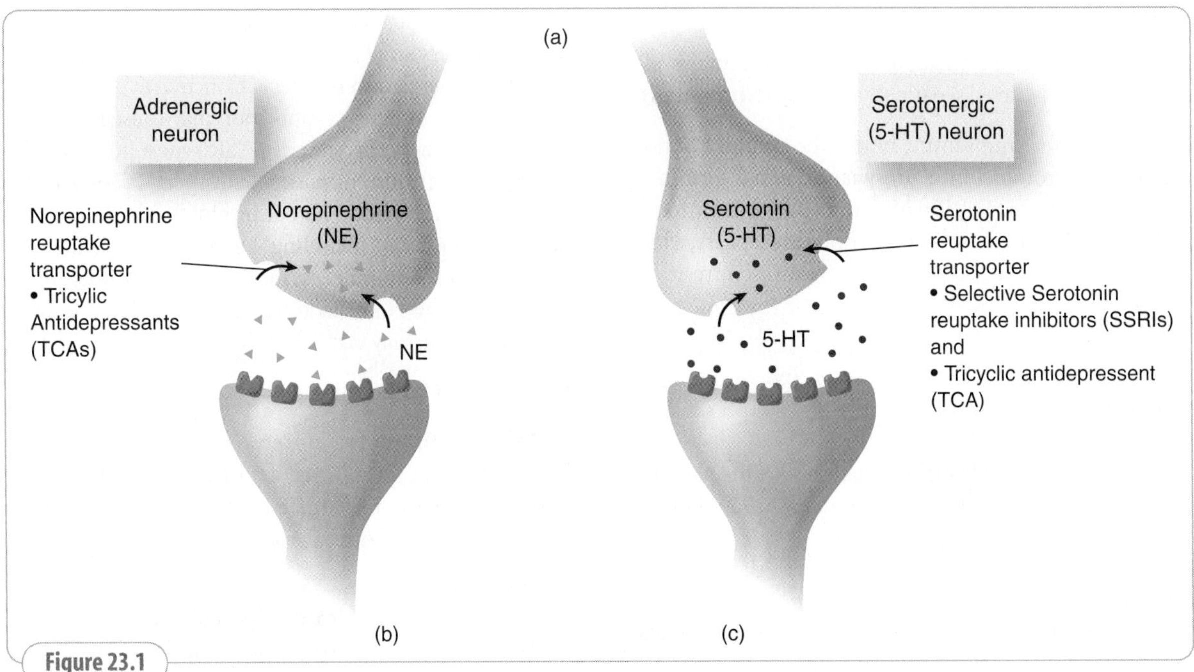

Figure 23.1

Mechanisms of action of antidepressants: (a) in adrenergic and serotonergic neurons the activity of the neurotransmitter is terminated by reuptake; (b) tricyclic antidepressants produce their effects by inhibiting the reuptake of neurotransmitters at both the norepinephrine and serotonin transporters; (c) selective serotonin reuptake inhibitors produce their effects by inhibiting the reuptake of neurotransmitters at only serotonin transporters.

CONNECTION Checkpoint 23.2

Anticholinergic effects are common with TCAs and some other antidepressants. From what you learned in Chapter 18, name the prototype anticholinergic drug. If anticholinergic effects become prominent in a patient, what class of drugs can be used to counteract the adverse effects? See Answer to Connection Checkpoint 23.2 in Appendix A.

PROTOTYPE DRUG Imipramine (Tofranil)

Classification: **Therapeutic:** Tricyclic antidepressant
Pharmacologic: Norepinephrine reuptake inhibitor

Therapeutic Effects and Uses: Approved in 1959, imipramine is an older drug that is effective in treating major depressive disorder. Like other TCAs, it is given PO and is well absorbed from the GI tract. Although very effective, a drawback to the use of imipramine is that it takes 2 to 6 weeks to achieve full therapeutic effect. During the initial weeks of therapy when blood levels of imipramine have not yet produced their full therapeutic effects, suicide risks may increase, especially in children and adolescents. This is true for other antidepressants as well. Imipramine is one of only two drugs approved for enuresis, or bedwetting, in children. The urge to urinate is diminished by the anticholinergic (urinary retention) effects of the drug.

Like other TCAs, imipramine has a number of off-label indications. These include the adjuvant treatment of cancer or neuropathic pain, overactive bladder, attention deficit/hyperactivity disorder (ADHD), and bulimia. The use of TCAs in treating social anxiety disorder (social phobia) and panic disorder are presented in Chapter 22. The active metabolite of imipramine is desipramine, which is marketed separately as a drug (Norpramin).

Mechanism of Action: Imipramine blocks the reuptake of norepinephrine and serotonin into presynaptic nerve terminals. This results in an increased action of both neurotransmitters in neurons. Imipramine also blocks acetylcholine receptors, which is likely responsible for its effectiveness in treating enuresis.

Pharmacokinetics:

Route(s)	PO, IM (rare)
Absorption	Well absorbed from the GI tract and muscle
Distribution	Widely distributed; crosses the placenta; secreted in breast milk; 85–95% bound to plasma protein
Primary metabolism	Hepatic; metabolized to the active metabolite desipramine
Primary excretion	Renal; small amounts in bile and feces
Onset of action	1–2 h for peak serum level; mood elevation requires 2–3 weeks
Duration of action	Not known

Adverse Effects: Frequent adverse reactions with imipramine include orthostatic hypotension (the most common adverse effect), dizziness, confusion, drowsiness, diarrhea, dry mouth, increased appetite, jaundice, urinary retention, rash, pruritus, and photosensitivity. Serious adverse reactions include seizures, hepatitis, acute renal failure, paralytic ileus, leukopenia, agranulocytosis, thrombocytopenia, or eosinophilia. Serious adverse reactions occur with acute doses when imipramine accumulates in cardiac tissue; dysrhythmias, heart failure, or myocardial infarction (MI) can occur.

Contraindications/Precautions: Imipramine should not be used by patients with seizure disorders because it lowers the seizure threshold. It must be used with caution in persons with suicidal tendencies, urinary retention, prostatic hyperplasia, cardiac or hepatic disease, increased intraocular pressure, or hyperthyroidism. Use in patients with Parkinson's disease will induce or worsen parkinsonism symptoms. Patients with cardiac disease such as heart failure, QT prolongation, or history of MI should be carefully monitored during therapy; use in patients recovering from MI has resulted in sudden death. Imipramine should not be used during pregnancy or lactation. This drug is a pregnancy category D drug.

Drug Interactions: Like other TCAs, imipramine is metabolized by hepatic P450 enzymes and is highly protein bound; thus there is a high potential for drug–drug interactions. Increased sedation can occur when imipramine is given concurrently with alcohol, barbiturates, benzodiazepines, direct-acting sympathomimetics, and other CNS depressants. Drug interactions causing decreased effects of imipramine include oral contraceptives, clonidine, carbamazepine, and indirect-acting sympathomimetics. Concurrent use with thyroid hormone may induce dysrhythmias. Imipramine should not be given concurrently with other drugs that prolong the QT interval, such as the Class IA antidysrhythmics, because of the potential for serious cardiac toxicity. Phenothiazines and TCAs are structurally very similar and concurrent use will likely cause additive anticholinergic adverse effects. Concurrent use of MAOIs must be avoided because this combination may cause hypertensive crisis, seizures, or hyperpyretic crisis. SSRIs must not be used concurrently; this can cause increased toxicity of TCAs. **Herbal/Food:** Several commonly used herbal products may lead to increased imipramine effects, including kava, hops, lavender, valerian, skullcap, and chamomile. An increased anticholinergic effect can occur with the use of belladonna, jimsonweed, or henbane. Serotonin syndrome may occur with the use of St. John's wort.

Pregnancy: Category D.

Treatment of Overdose: Overdoses with TCAs may be life threatening with symptoms that include mixed mania and depression followed by coma. Medical management includes treating possible seizures, hypotension, and dysrhythmias.

Nursing Responsibilities:

- Obtain a complete history, especially for presence of cardiovascular disease, epilepsy, prostatic hypertrophy, narrow-angle glaucoma, or urinary retention.
- Assess for hepatic and renal impairment, cardiovascular dysfunction, orthostatic hypotension, urinary and bowel functions, and presence of diabetes mellitus prior to and during treatment.

- Monitor for suicidal ideation, especially during the first few weeks of therapy.
- Be sure that the patient swallows each dose; a depressed patient may stockpile medications for a suicide attempt.
- Evaluate for signs of therapeutic response, which includes decreased depression and melancholia.
- Encourage the patient to continue taking the drug even if no benefits are felt for several weeks.
- Monitor for urinary retention or constipation, which may require a dosage reduction.

Patient and Family Education:

- The full therapeutic effects of the medication will take 2 to 6 weeks (or more) to appear.
- Immediately report any of the following to the health care provider: thoughts of suicide, difficulty passing urine, yellowing of the skin or whites of the eyes, or unusual bleeding or bruising.
- Take this drug exactly as prescribed and do not discontinue the medication without approval of the health care provider.
- Make position changes slowly when moving from a lying to a standing position to prevent dizziness and possible fainting.
- Do not take any other prescription or nonprescription drugs, dietary supplements, or herbal products without approval of the health care provider.
- Maintain all recommended follow-up appointments with mental health professionals.
- Immediately notify the health care provider of any known or suspected pregnancy because this drug may cause birth defects. Oral contraceptives may be less effective, so barrier contraception must be used.
- Anticholinergic effects such as dry mouth may occur; some simple ways to decrease symptoms are to increase fluids, suck on sugarless hard candy, chew sugarless gum, or take frequent sips of water.

Drugs Similar to Imipramine (Tofranil)

There are nine TCAs available. Desipramine is an active metabolite of imipramine, and the two drugs have the same actions and adverse effects as described previously.

Amitriptyline (Elavil) and nortriptyline (Aventyl, Pamelor): Amitriptyline has been available by the PO route since 1961 for the therapy of major depression. It has been used for a large number of off-label indications, including neuropathic pain syndromes such as fibromyalgia, and nocturnal enuresis, social anxiety disorder, ADHD, migraines, persistent hiccups, insomnia, or bulimia. It produces more sedation than most other TCAs and is thus taken at bedtime. It is metabolized in the liver to nortriptyline, which is marketed as a separate drug. Both amitriptyline and nortriptyline produce significant anticholinergic adverse effects. Like other TCAs, cardiac toxicity is a major concern at high doses. These drugs are pregnancy category D.

Clomipramine (Anafranil): Approved in 1991, the only FDA-approved indication for clomipramine is obsessive–compulsive disorder (OCD). Depression is an off-label indication. Other off-label uses are premature ejaculation and childhood autism. The drug produces significant anticholinergic effects and orthostatic hypotension; thus it is not a first-line drug for depression. This drug is pregnancy category C.

Doxepin (Sinequan): Approved in 1969 to treat major depression, doxepin is also FDA-approved to treat anxiety. A topical form of doxepin (Zonalon) is available for pruritus associated with eczema. Off-label uses include insomnia and migraine prophylaxis. The PO dosages produce drowsiness and anticholinergic effects similar to other drugs in the class. Topical application can cause intense burning sensations on the skin in a significant number of patients. In addition, because doxepin is absorbed through the skin, topical applications can result in systemic adverse effects. This drug is pregnancy category C.

Maprotiline (Ludiomil): Maprotiline does not have a tricyclic chemical structure but it is included with the TCAs because it has very similar therapeutic and adverse effects. It was approved to treat depression in 1980. Off-label indications include ADHD and enuresis. It has the same adverse effects as other drugs in this class and offers no specific advantages over other TCAs. This drug is pregnancy category D.

Protriptyline (Vivactil): Protriptyline is an oral antidepressant that was approved in 1967. It has the same adverse effects as other TCAs except that it tends to produce CNS stimulation rather than sedation. It is the only TCA that has respiratory stimulant activity. These respiratory effects have led to its occasional off-label use for treating chronic obstructive pulmonary disease or sleep apnea. This drug is pregnancy category C.

Trimipramine (Surmontil): Trimipramine was approved in 1979 for major depression. Off-label indications include anxiety, schizophrenia, and rheumatoid arthritis. Drowsiness is a serious problem; however, the incidence of anticholinergic effects is one of the lowest of any drug in its class. It offers no major benefits over other TCAs. This drug is pregnancy category C.

Selective Serotonin Reuptake Inhibitors

23.9 Selective serotonin reuptake inhibitors are the drugs of choice for treating depression due to their low incidence of serious adverse effects.

Serotonin is a natural neurotransmitter in the CNS that is found in high concentrations in certain neurons in the hypothalamus, limbic system, medulla, and spinal cord. It is essential for several body activities, including the cycling between NREM and REM sleep (see Chapter 22), pain perception, and emotions. Lack of adequate serotonin in the limbic regions of the CNS can lead to depression. The actions of serotonin are terminated when it is metabolized to a less active substance by the enzyme monoamine oxidase (MAO). This mechanism is illustrated in Figure 23.2. In the scientific literature, serotonin is commonly referred to by its chemical name, 5-hydroxytryptamine (5-HT).

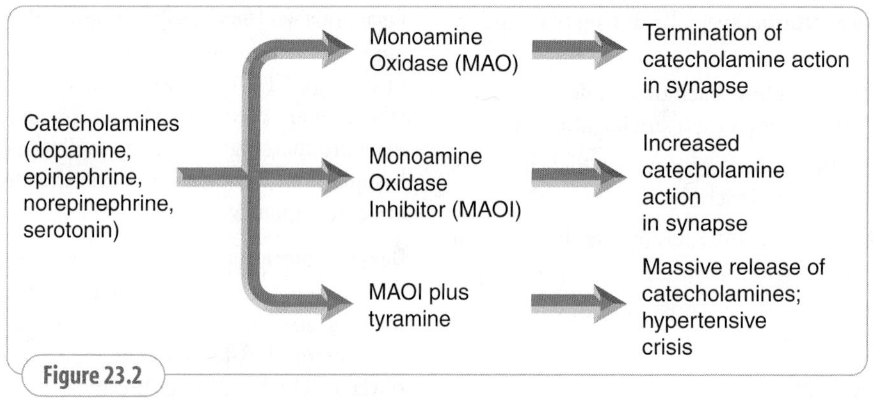

Figure 23.2

Catecholamines and monoamine oxidase.

In the 1970s, it became increasingly clear that serotonin had a more substantial role in depression than once thought. Clinicians knew that the TCAs altered the sensitivity of serotonin to certain receptors in the brain, but they did not know how this change connected to depression. Ongoing efforts to find antidepressants with fewer adverse effects than TCAs and monoamine oxidase inhibitors (MAOIs) led to the development of the selective serotonin reuptake inhibitors (SSRIs), which were first introduced in 1987. Whereas the TCAs inhibit the reuptake of both norepinephrine and serotonin into presynaptic nerve terminals, the SSRIs selectively target serotonin. Increased levels of serotonin in the synaptic spaces induce complex neurotransmitter changes in presynaptic and postsynaptic neurons in the brain. Essentially, presynaptic receptors become less sensitive, and postsynaptic receptors become more sensitive.

SSRIs are as effective in treating depression as the TCAs but exhibit fewer significant adverse effects. Sympathomimetic effects (increased heart rate and HTN) and anticholinergic effects (dry mouth, blurred vision, urinary retention, and constipation) are less common with this drug class. Sedation occurs less frequently, and cardiotoxicity is not observed. The greater safety profile of the SSRIs has led to their becoming the drugs of choice for depression.

MyNursingKit | Mechanism of Action Animation: Fluoxetine

One of the most common adverse effects of SSRIs relates to sexual dysfunction. Up to 70% of both men and women can experience decreased libido and lack of ability to reach orgasm. In men, delayed ejaculation and impotence may occur. For patients who are sexually active, these adverse effects may be serious enough to cause nonadherence with pharmacotherapy, and a different antidepressant may be indicated. The SSRIs can cause weight gain, which may also lead to discontinuation. Other common adverse effects include nausea, headache, nervousness, and insomnia.

All drugs in the SSRI class have equal effectiveness and similar adverse effects. In general, SSRIs produce elevations in mood more quickly than TCAs, which can be a major advantage when treating serious depression disorders. Like the TCAs, the SSRIs are used for a wide variety of other mental health disorders, including OCD, social anxiety disorder, panic disorder, generalized anxiety disorder, PTSD, and premenstrual dysphoric disorder. They are one of the most widely prescribed drug classes in the United States.

Serotonin syndrome (SES) is a serious medical condition that can occur when a patient is taking multiple medications that affect the metabolism, synthesis, or reuptake of serotonin, causing this neurotransmitter to accumulate in neurons in the CNS. These drugs include SSRIs, MAOIs, TCAs, lithium, St. John's wort, opioids, and triptans. SES sometimes occurs as a result of illicit drug use because amphetamines, cocaine, MDMA or Ecstasy, and opioids also affect serotonin levels. Symptoms of SES include mental status changes (confusion, anxiety, restlessness), HTN, tremors, sweating, hyperpyrexia, and ataxia. Symptoms can begin as early as 2 hours after taking the first dose or as late as several weeks after initiating pharmacotherapy. Conservative treatment is to discontinue the drugs responsible for causing the syndrome and to provide supportive care; the condition usually resolves in 24 hours. In severe cases, mechanical ventilation and muscle relaxants such as benzodiazepines may be necessary. If left untreated, death may occur.

PROTOTYPE DRUG Fluoxetine (Prozac, Sarafem)

Classification: **Therapeutic:** Antidepressant, antianxiety agent
Pharmacologic: Selective serotonin reuptake inhibitor (SSRI)

Therapeutic Effects and Uses: Approved in 1987, fluoxetine was the first SSRI marketed in the United States. Fluoxetine was subsequently approved to treat bulimia nervosa, the first medication ever approved for this condition. It is the only SSRI approved for the treatment of pediatric depression. In 2002, it received FDA approval for the treatment of panic attacks. Fluoxetine is available as tablets, capsules, oral solution, and delayed release capsules. Sarafem is a formulation of fluoxetine specifically marketed for premenstrual dysphoric disorder in a pulvule—a gelatin-based capsule. It is taken daily or for just the 2 weeks prior to an expected menses. Prozac Weekly is a capsule containing enteric-coated granules. Patients who have stabilized on daily fluoxetine can be switched to Prozac Weekly, which offers the convenience of once-a-week dosing. Symbyax is a fixed-dose combination of fluoxetine and olanzapine that is indicated for bipolar disorder. Olanzapine, an antipsychotic agent, is marketed by itself as Zyprexa for schizophrenia and the manic phase of bipolar disorder.

Fluoxetine is used off-label to treat many other disorders involving multiple body systems. Off-label indications include anorexia nervosa, obesity, alcohol dependence in patients with alcoholism, fibromyalgia, autism, refractory orthostatic hypotension, premature ejaculation, premenstrual dysphoric disorder, and menopausal hot flashes. Although patients gradually begin to feel less depressed after about 2 weeks of therapy, optimal response may take 8 weeks or longer.

Fluoxetine is extensively metabolized in the liver to norfluoxetine, which has about the same pharmacologic activity as the parent drug. Fluoxetine and norfluoxetine have long half-lives; it takes 30 to 60 days after discontinuing the drug for them to be eliminated by the body. This duration is even more prolonged in patients with liver disease.

Mechanism of Action: As with other serotonin reuptake inhibitors, fluoxetine blocks the uptake of the neurotransmitter serotonin (but not norepinephrine) at the neuronal presynaptic membrane. This increases the amount of neurotransmitter available at the postsynaptic receptor sites, thus enhancing the actions of serotonin.

Pharmacokinetics:

Route	PO
Absorption	Readily absorbed
Distribution	Widely distributed, including the cerebrospinal fluid; likely crosses the placenta; secreted in breast milk; 94% bound to plasma protein
Primary metabolism	Hepatic
Primary excretion	Renal, small amounts in feces
Onset of action	Peak plasma level: 6–8 h
Duration of action	Half-life: 2–3 days

Adverse Effects: Fluoxetine is better tolerated than drugs from either the TCA or the MAOI classes. The most common adverse effects are nausea and vomiting, which diminish as therapy progresses. Other common GI effects include diarrhea, anorexia, cramping, and flatulence. Fluoxetine does not cause sedation; in fact, insomnia may occur in as many as 25% of patients receiving the drug. Fluoxetine also does not cause the serious cardiotoxicity, orthostatic hypotension, or anticholinergic effects seen with the TCAs. Fluctuations in weight are common. Significant anorexia and weight loss occurs in 10% to 15% of patients, whereas others experience a weight gain of as much as 20 pounds or more. Patients may experience various types of sexual dysfunction, including delayed ejaculation, impotence, anorgasmia, decreased libido, and priapism. The drug may induce seizures in patients with preexisting seizure disorders or during overdoses. Other adverse effects include cramping, constipation, poor concentration, diarrhea, hot flashes, palpitations, and nervousness. Serotonin syndrome can occur. Pediatric patients may experience personality disorders or hyperkinesia. In 2004, the FDA required expanded warning statements for fluoxetine and other antidepressant medications, detailing the increased risk of suicidality in children and adolescents with major depressive disorder and other psychiatric conditions.

Abrupt withdrawal of fluoxetine or other SSRIs can result in a withdrawal syndrome; the patient may experience dizziness, headache, tremor, anxiety, dysphoria, and sensory disturbances. These symptoms usually begin 1 to 7 days after the last dose and may continue for 1 to 3 weeks. Because fluoxetine has such an extended half-life and serum levels diminish gradually, withdrawal symptoms are generally less serious than those of the shorter-acting SSRIs. Tapering the dose over 2 weeks or longer can prevent withdrawal symptoms.

Contraindications/Precautions: Hypersensitivity to fluoxetine is a contraindication to using the drug. The drug should not be administered to patients with bipolar disorder because it may precipitate a manic episode. It must be used cautiously in persons with cardiac dysfunction, diabetes, or seizure disorders. Pediatric patients must be carefully observed, especially during the first few months of therapy, for possible suicidal behavior. Children or adults with a history of attempted suicide should not receive fluoxetine. There are no known age-related precautions for use in the elderly, but children may experience more behavioral adverse effects such as restlessness and insomnia.

Caution must be used when fluoxetine is administered late in pregnancy. The neonate may exhibit symptoms of withdrawal, including irritability, respiratory distress, tremors, abnormal crying, and, possibly, seizures. With supportive care, symptoms of withdrawal in the neonate will disappear in a few days. In most cases, the benefits of treating pregnant women who have major depression with fluoxetine are greater than the potential risks to the neonate.

Drug Interactions: Fluoxetine inhibits multiple CYP450 isozymes and has the potential to interact with many other drugs and herbal products. Drugs that are metabolized by CYP450 may build to toxic levels due to their impaired metabolism. Some drugs affected by diminished metabolism include TCAs, phenothiazines, most atypical antipsychotics, certain antidysrhythmics, and benzodiazepines. Excessive sedation may occur if fluoxetine is given concurrently with other CNS depressants, including opioids, sedative–hypnotics, or alcohol. Taken concurrently with or within 14 days of MAOIs can result in serotonin syndrome or neuroleptic malignant syndrome (NMS). Concurrent use with warfarin, aspirin, or other nonsteroidal anti-inflammatory drugs (NSAIDs) may increase the risk of bleeding. Fluoxetine may cause an increased risk of toxicity to phenytoin, digoxin, or carbamazepine. Concurrent use with certain antipsychotic agents may lead to increased extrapyramidal symptoms such as akathisia, dystonia, tardive dyskinesia, and pseudoparkinsonism. Fluoxetine can increase the half-life of diazepam. Caution must also be used if the patient is taking lithium because fluoxetine may increase plasma levels of the drug. **Herbal/Food:** Increased CNS effects may occur if fluoxetine is given concurrently with lavender, kava, or hops. There is an increased risk of serotonin syndrome with the concurrent use of St. John's wort. Increased anticholinergic effects may result from the use of jimsonweed or corkwood.

Because grapefruit juice may cause elevated serum levels of fluoxetine, it should be avoided during therapy.

Pregnancy: Category C.

Treatment of Overdose: Overdose can result in seizures, somnolence, and, rarely, death. Supportive treatment is indicated, including gastric lavage and activated charcoal.

Nursing Responsibilities:

- Assess for depression before initiating therapy and reassess regularly.
- Obtain a comprehensive medical history, including previous episodes of major depression, factors leading to depression, need for antidepressants, history of cardiovascular disorders, seizure disorders, sexual dysfunction and use of other drugs (including illicit drugs), or herbal products.
- Monitor for suicidal ideation, especially in pediatric and adolescent patients, during the first few weeks of therapy.
- Encourage the patient to continue taking the drug even if no benefits are felt for several weeks.
- Assess for signs and symptoms of adverse reactions such as nausea, vomiting, insomnia, or restlessness.
- Evaluate for symptoms of therapeutic response to fluoxetine.
- Monitor for weight loss, especially in underweight patients.

Patient and Family Education:

- Take exactly as prescribed and do not discontinue the medication without approval from the health care provider.
- Do not take any other prescription or nonprescription drugs, dietary supplements, or herbal products without approval of the health care provider.
- The full therapeutic effects of the medication will take 2 to 6 weeks or more to appear.
- Do not drive or perform other hazardous activities until the effects of the drug are known because this drug may cause drowsiness or dizziness.
- Do not consume alcoholic beverages with this medication because this may cause sedation.
- If unpleasant adverse effects occur, contact the health care provider but continue taking the medication until adjustments can be made.
- Immediately notify the health care provider of any known or suspected pregnancy.
- Take the last dose before 4 p.m. to avoid insomnia.
- Immediately report any of the following to the health care provider: suicidal thoughts, palpitations, major changes in sexual function, and excessive drowsiness.

Drugs Similar to Fluoxetine (Prozac, Sarafem)

Other SSRIs include citalopram, escitalopram, fluvoxamine, paroxetine, and sertraline.

Citalopram (Celexa): Citalopram was approved by the FDA in 1998 for the treatment of major depressive disorder in adults. All of its antianxiety uses are off-label. These include all five major antianxiety categories: generalized anxiety disorder, SAD, OCD, panic disorder, and post-traumatic stress disorder (PTSD). Other off-label uses include schizophrenia, premenstrual dysphoric disorder, and menopausal hot flashes. Citalopram is available as regular tablets, as oral disintegrating tablets, or as an oral solution. It is almost identical structurally to escitalopram but is very different from other SSRIs. The elderly are more susceptible to the anticholinergic effects of citalopram than to other SSRIs. There are fewer drug interactions than with fluoxetine. All other actions and adverse effects are the same as those of fluoxetine and escitalopram. This drug is pregnancy category C.

Escitalopram (Lexapro): Escitalopram was approved in 2002 to treat major depressive disorder in adults, which is its major indication. Since its approval, it has become one of the most frequently prescribed drugs in the United States. Escitalopram is also FDA-approved for the treatment of generalized anxiety disorder and is used off-label to treat SAD and panic attacks. It is nearly identical structurally to citalopram although it is more potent; 20 mg of escitalopram is bioequivalent to 40 mg of citalopram. It is available as a tablet or solution. Escitalopram has the same spectrum of adverse effects as fluoxetine and other SSRIs. It appears to elevate mood relatively quickly, in 1 to 2 weeks. Its safety and effectiveness in children have not been established. This drug is pregnancy category C.

Fluvoxamine (Luvox): Approved in 1994, fluvoxamine is available as oral tablets. Fluvoxamine is FDA approved as a treatment for OCD, although it is also used off-label to treat depression, anxiety disorders in children, social anxiety disorder, generalized anxiety disorder, PTSD, bulimia nervosa, and panic disorder. In 2007, the FDA approved an extended release capsule of Luvox (Luvox CR) for the treatment of OCD and social anxiety disorder. Adverse reactions are the same as with fluoxetine except that fluvoxamine causes sedation rather than CNS excitement. This drug is pregnancy category C.

Paroxetine (Paxil, Pexeva): Approved in 1992, paroxetine is available as oral tablets, oral suspension, or controlled release tablets (Paxil CR). It is approved to treat major depression, OCD, social anxiety disorder, panic disorder, generalized anxiety disorder, PTSD, and premenstrual dysphoric disorder. Off-label indications include hot flashes and premature ejaculation. Adverse effects are mild, dose dependent, and similar to other SSRIs. They usually diminish or disappear completely in time. The elderly may need dosage adjustments. Precautions are similar to other SSRIs except that paroxetine is a pregnancy category D drug.

Sertraline (Zoloft): Approved in 1991, sertraline is one of the most frequently prescribed SSRIs. It is available as tablets or as an oral concentrate that must be diluted before use. Approved indications include major depressive disorder, OCD, PTSD, social anxiety disorder, or premenstrual dysphoric disorder. Contraindications and precautions are the same as with escitalopram. The main difference between sertraline and fluoxetine is that sertraline blocks the uptake of dopamine in addition to blocking the uptake of serotonin. Adverse effects, uses, and drug interactions are the same as those of fluoxetine.

The oral concentrate contains 12% alcohol, which is contraindicated in patients taking disulfiram (Antabuse). This drug is pregnancy category C.

Atypical Antidepressants

23.10 Atypical antidepressants are alternatives to the selective serotonin reuptake inhibitors that are prescribed for depression and anxiety disorders.

Atypical antidepressants are a diverse class of newer drugs that act by mechanisms other than those of the SSRIs, TCAs, and MAOIs. In effect, this is a "miscellaneous" class of drugs because they have very little in common with each other except their ability to alleviate symptoms of depression. They act by preventing the reuptake of specific neurotransmitters in the CNS or by blocking neurotransmitter receptors. Mechanisms include the following:

- Serotonin–norepinephrine reuptake inhibitors (SNRIs): desvenlafaxine (Prestiq) venlafaxine (Effexor) and duloxetine (Cymbalta)
- Norepinephrine and dopamine reuptake inhibitors (NDRIs): bupropion (Wellbutrin)
- Norepinephrine reuptake inhibitors (NRIs): reboxetine (Edronax, Vestra)
- Combined reuptake inhibitor and receptor blocker: trazodone (Desyrel), nefazodone, and mirtazapine (Remeron)

As a group, the atypical antidepressants have similar pharmacologic actions to the SSRIs and exhibit fewer adverse effects than the TCAs and MAOIs. Each drug in the class has certain specific adverse effects, as described next. Like other antidepressants some are used for indications other than depression, such as neuropathic pain and anxiety disorders. Although some are quite effective, they are generally not superior to other, well-established antidepressants.

PROTOTYPE DRUG Venlafaxine (Effexor)

Classification: **Therapeutic:** Atypical antidepressant
Pharmacologic: Serotonin–norepinephrine reuptake inhibitor (SNRI)

Therapeutic Effects and Uses: Venlafaxine is a newer antidepressant approved by the FDA in 1993 to treat major depression. Later, its approved indications were extended to include panic disorder, generalized anxiety disorder, and social anxiety disorder. It has been used off-label to treat a large number of other conditions, including neuropathic pain, premenstrual dysphoric disorder, menopausal hot flashes, migraines, and fibromyalgia. Venlafaxine XR is an extended release capsule that permits once-daily dosing. It is metabolized to an active metabolite in the liver. Venlafaxine has pharmacologic effects, drug interactions, and adverse effects very similar to those of the SSRIs.

Like other antidepressants, there is little potential for psychological dependence with venlafaxine—it is not a drug of abuse. Abrupt discontinuation, however, can cause mild to moderate withdrawal symptoms similar in nature to those resulting from SSRI withdrawal. Gradual tapering of the dose is a means of preventing withdrawal symptoms.

Mechanism of Action: Venlafaxine inhibits the presynaptic neuronal reuptake of both norepinephrine and serotonin in the CNS.

Pharmacokinetics:

Route(s)	PO
Absorption	92% absorbed from the GI tract
Distribution	Widely distributed; crosses the placenta; secreted in breast milk; 27% bound to protein
Primary metabolism	Hepatic, including substantial first-pass effect
Primary excretion	Renal
Onset of action	Peak serum level: 5.5 h but the antidepressant action may take 2–3 weeks
Duration of action	Half-life: 5–7 h (9–11 h for the active metabolite)

Adverse Effects: The most common adverse effect of venlafaxine is nausea, which can occur in 37% of patients. Tolerance may develop to the nausea as therapy progresses. The nausea, combined with anorexia, sometimes leads to weight loss. Pediatric patients taking venlafaxine have been shown to have a decrease in overall height as well as weight. Venlafaxine has structural similarities to amphetamines and can cause CNS stimulation, nervousness, and insomnia. Other patients, however, exhibit sedative effects from venlafaxine. Other CNS adverse effects include headache, emotional lability, dizziness, and asthenia. Sustained elevations, 10 to 15 mmHg, of blood pressure may occur. Types of sexual dysfunction seen with venlafaxine include impotence, abnormal ejaculation, and delayed or absent orgasm in women. Life-threatening adverse reactions could include rectal, vaginal, or uterine hemorrhage. Like other antidepressants, venlafaxine has a black box warning about the potential for an increased risk of suicide in children and adolescents taking the drug.

Contraindications/Precautions: Venlafaxine is contraindicated if the patient has hypersensitivity to venlafaxine or an SSRI, if a MAOI is being used concurrently, or during lactation. Caution must be used when administered to patients with cardiac, hepatic, or renal impairment; recent MI; seizure disorder; anorexia; or suicidal ideation. Venlafaxine is not administered to patients with bipolar disorder or with a history of mania because it can trigger manic episodes. Safety in children under age 18 has not been established. The elderly may require a reduced dose and patients with hepatic impairment may require as much as 50% reduction in dose. Venlafaxine should be discontinued by tapering doses gradually because abrupt discontinuation can result in uncomfortable withdrawal symptoms such as nervousness, headache, agitation, fatigue, drowsiness, tremor, and sweating.

Drug Interactions: Venlafaxine is primarily metabolized by the hepatic CYP2D6 isozyme; drugs that inhibit CYP2D6 may cause venlafaxine serum levels to rise. Serotonin syndrome may

MyNursingKit | Mechanism of Action Animation: Venlafaxine

occur if venlafaxine is given concurrently with SSRIs, MAOIs, lithium, or other drugs that act by increasing serotonin levels. If switching from venlafaxine to an MAOI, venlafaxine must be withdrawn at least 7 days before beginning the MAOI. Alcohol, opioids, sedatives, hypnotics, or antihistamines can cause additive CNS depression. Cimetidine, haloperidol, fluoxetine, sertraline, or phenothiazine can lead to increased toxicity. **Herbal/Food:** No food interactions have been reported, but there are several possible interactions with herbal products. St. John's wort and SAM-e may increase the risk of SES. CNS depression may occur with concurrent use of chamomile, kava, hops, lavender, valerian, or skullcap. Jimsonweed or corkwood may cause increased anticholinergic effects. Yohimbe may increase the risk for HTN.

Pregnancy: Category C.

Treatment of Overdose: Overdoses are generally not fatal but can cause serious symptoms such as CNS depression, seizures, altered level of consciousness, hypotension, and dysrhythmias. General measures include inducing emesis and administering activated charcoal and gastric lavage. The ECG must be monitored and antiseizure drugs administered as necessary.

Nursing Responsibilities and Patient and Family Education: These are the same as for the SSRIs, listed on page 310.

Drugs Similar to Venlafaxine (Effexor)

Other atypical antidepressants include amoxapine, bupropion, desvenlafaxine, duloxetine, mirtazapine, nefazodone, reboxetine, and trazodone.

Amoxapine (Asendin): Approved in 1980, amoxapine is chemically related to older TCAs and phenothiazines. The drug exhibits potentially serious adverse effects, which limit its use to patients who have major depression with psychotic symptoms. Adverse effects resemble those of TCAs (blood dyscrasias, orthostatic hypotension, sedation, anticholinergic effects, sexual dysfunction, and cardiac toxicity) and phenothiazines (neuroleptic malignant syndrome and parkinsonism symptoms). There is cross hypersensitivity between amoxapine and TCAs. Amoxapine must be used cautiously in those with suicidal ideation. This drug is pregnancy category C.

Bupropion HCl (Wellbutrin, Zyban): Approved in 1985, bupropion is similar in structure to amphetamines and unrelated to other antidepressants. It is approved to treat major depression as well as being the first approved therapy for persistent SAD. Bupropion is also marketed as Zyban for the management of nicotine withdrawal during smoking cessation. Off-label uses include neuropathic pain and ADHD. It is available as immediate release tablets and in an extended release formulation (Wellbutrin XL). In 2008 a new salt form, bupropion hydrobromide (Aplenzin) was approved as a once daily tablet for depression.

Bupropion not only inhibits the reuptake of serotonin, but it may also affect the activity of norepinephrine and dopamine. Like amphetamine, bupropion has stimulant actions and suppresses the appetite. It does not cause weight gain or sexual dysfunction, which makes it appealing to women who suffer from hypoactive sexual disorder. It is sometimes used to counteract the sexual dysfunction that occurs in patients taking SSRIs. Antidepressant action begins in 1 to 3 weeks and is equal to that of the TCAs. Because bupropion has a greater potential for causing seizures than other antidepressants, it should be used with caution in patients with seizure disorders. The risk for seizures is dose dependent and increased for patients drinking alcohol or taking other drugs that lower the seizure threshold. Seizures have been reported in infants receiving breast milk from mothers taking bupropion. Common adverse reactions include CNS stimulation (agitation, insomnia, and restlessness), weight loss, headache, dry mouth, constipation, and GI upset. About 20% of patients taking this drug will develop tremors. It is an alternative to SSRIs in those persons who cannot tolerate their adverse effects. This drug is pregnancy category C.

Desvenlafaxine: Desvenlafaxine (Prestiq) is a new SNRI approved in 2008 for the treatment of major depression. It is available as an extended release tablet that is taken once daily. Common adverse effects include nausea, dizziness, sweating, constipation, and decreased appetite. This drug is pregnancy category C.

Duloxetine (Cymbalta): Like venlafaxine, duloxetine is an atypical antidepressant that is classified as an SNRI. First approved for major depression in 2004, it has since received FDA approval to treat neuropathic pain in people with diabetes, generalized anxiety disorder, and fibromyalgia. Off-label indications include fibromyalgia and urinary stress incontinence. Abnormal vision is the most frequently reported adverse effect, and nausea is a common reason for discontinuation of therapy. Other adverse events include photosensitivity, bruising, anorexia, thrombophlebitis, constipation, diarrhea, dry mouth, insomnia, and anxiety. No life-threatening adverse effects have been identified. Postmarketing incidences of liver injury suggest that the drug should be used with great caution in patients with preexisting hepatic impairment or in alcoholics. Caution must be exercised when administered to persons with mania, seizures, HTN, cardiac, renal or hepatic disease, the elderly, children, or lactating women. When discontinuing therapy, the dose should be tapered slowly to prevent withdrawal symptoms. Patients may begin feeling the antidepressant effects of duloxetine within 2 weeks of beginning treatment. This drug is pregnancy category C.

Mirtazapine (Remeron): Classified as a tetracyclic compound, this drug was approved in 1996 for major depression in adults. It blocks presynaptic serotonin and norepinephrine receptors, thereby enhancing release of these neurotransmitters from nerve terminals. Unlike the TCAs, it has few anticholinergic actions. It does carry a higher risk of seizure activity in patients with no previous seizure history. Serious adverse reactions include acute renal failure, hepatitis, jaundice, thrombocytopenia, leukopenia, eosinophilia, or agranulocytosis. Other adverse reactions include dizziness, orthostatic hypotension, ECG changes, sedation (which may be a positive effect in those having insomnia secondary to depression), tachycardia, HTN, or extrapyramidal symptoms in the elderly. Mirtazapine should not be used in patients with hypersensitivity to TCAs, seizure disorders, prostatic hypertrophy, serious hepatic or renal impairment, or who are recovering from MI. Mirtazapine usually elevates mood within 2 to 4 weeks after the initiation of therapy. This drug is pregnancy category C.

Nefazodone: Chemically similar to trazodone, nefazodone causes minimal cardiovascular effects, fewer anticholinergic effects, less sedation, and less sexual dysfunction than some of the other antidepressants. The most common adverse effects are xerostomia, drowsiness, nausea, vomiting, dizziness, and constipation. Although approved only for major depression, off-label indications include anxiety, panic attacks, premenstrual dysphoric disorder, PTSD, and social anxiety disorder. Nefazodone acts by blocking serotonin receptors and inhibiting serotonin reuptake. It also has some blocking effect on norepinephrine reuptake. Originally approved in 1994, a brand name form of the drug, Serzone, was removed from the market in 2004, due to a possibility of liver damage; generic nefazodone is still available. Hepatic laboratory values should be regularly monitored during therapy and the drug should not be used in patients with serious liver impairment. This drug is pregnancy category C.

Reboxetine (Vestra): Reboxetine was the first approved drug in a newer class of antidepressants known as the SNRIs. Its effects are limited almost exclusively to enhancing transmission at norepinephrine receptors, and it is not related chemically to any other class of antidepressants. Although approved in 1999, the FDA withdrew its approval until additional studies could be conducted by the pharmaceutical company. It is available in 60 countries but has yet to be marketed in the United States.

Trazodone (Desyrel): Approved in 1981, trazodone works by producing a moderate, selective blockade of serotonin reuptake. It is not very effective when used alone as an antidepressant, but its sedative properties are especially useful in patients who have antidepressant-induced insomnia. In fact, trazodone is most frequently used off-label as a sleep aid, rather than as an antidepressant. Other off-label indications include generalized anxiety disorder, panic disorder, and as an adjuvant to reduce cravings for alcohol in patients with alcohol dependency. It causes little cardiac toxicity and very few anticholinergic effects so it may be useful for elderly patients and other persons for whom either of these may be intolerable. Common adverse effects include orthostatic hypotension, nausea, sedation, and dry mouth. Sexual adverse reactions include priapism, anorgasmia, and ejaculation dysfunctions. Overdose with trazodone is considered to be safer than overdose from MAOIs or TCAs, and there have been no reports of death from trazodone use alone. However, death can occur from overdose when the patient combines trazodone with other CNS depressants. This drug is pregnancy category C.

CONNECTION *Checkpoint* 23.3

Atypical antidepressants are sometimes used to treat anxiety when other agents are not effective. From what you learned in Chapter 22, what class of drugs is the traditional choice for the short-term therapy of generalized anxiety disorder? See Answer to Connection Checkpoint 23.3 in Appendix A.

Monoamine Oxidase Inhibitors

23.11 Monoamine oxidase inhibitors are effective antidepressants but are seldom used due to potentially serious adverse effects.

MAO is a key enzyme located in the liver, intestinal wall, and adrenergic neurons. It is responsible for inactivating monoamines: substances that contain one $-NH_2$ (amine) group. Not only does MAO inactivate natural monoamines such as norepinephrine, dopamine, and serotonin, it also acts on those present in food and drugs. The **monoamine oxidase inhibitors (MAOIs)** are antidepressants that block the actions of MAO.

In adrenergic neurons, MAOIs slow the destruction of norepinephrine, dopamine, and serotonin. This creates higher levels and enhances the activity of these neurotransmitters in the brain. Through mechanisms incompletely understood, this increase in neurotransmitters creates an antidepressant action.

Although they are as effective in treating depression as the SSRIs or TCAs, serious adverse reactions limit their use. Because of their low safety margin, these drugs are reserved for patients with refractory depression that has not responded to TCAs, atypical antidepressants, or SSRIs. They are rarely used in clinical practice.

CONNECTIONS

Complementary and Alternative Therapies St. John's Wort for Depression

Description: St. John's wort (*Hypericum perforatum*) is an herb found throughout Great Britain, Asia, Europe, and North America.

History and Claims: The herb gets its name from a legend that red spots once appeared on its leaves on the anniversary of St. John's beheading. The word *wort* is a British term for "plant." Use of the plant dates to ancient Greece, and Native Americans used the herb as an antiseptic or anti-inflammatory agent. Modern uses have focused on the antidepressant properties of the herb.

Standardization: The active agents in St. John's wort are believed to be hyperforin and hypericin. There is no standard dosage; however, some manufacturers are beginning to report dose by the percentage of hypericin in the extract. For example, one commonly used dose is 300 mg tid of St. John's wort standardized to 0.3% hypericin. Some studies use 5% hyperforin.

Evidence: Scientists once thought that St. John's wort produced its effects by the same mechanism as MAOIs, by increasing the levels of serotonin, norepinephrine, and dopamine in the brain. More recent evidence suggests that it may selectively inhibit serotonin reuptake. Some claim that it is just as effective as fluoxetine, paroxetine, or sertraline and with fewer adverse effects (Gastpar, Singer, & Zeller, 2006). St. John's wort induces hepatic P450 enzymes and has been reported to interact with many medications, including oral contraceptives, warfarin, digoxin, and cyclosporine (National Center for Complementary and Alternative Medicine, 2007). It should not be taken concurrently with antidepressant medications.

An active ingredient in St. John's wort is a photoactive compound that when exposed to light produces substances that can damage myelin. Patients have reported feeling stinging pain on the hands after sun exposure while taking the herbal remedy. Patients who take this herb should be advised to apply sunscreen or to wear protective clothing when outdoors.

Many researchers, including Cott and Fugh-Berman (1998) state that although St. John's wort is a safe antidepressant, large studies about its efficacy as an adjunct to conventional antidepressants are lacking.

TABLE 23.4 Foods High in Tyramine

Category of Food	Specific Foods
Meats	Beef or chicken liver, pate Hot dogs, bologna Pepperoni, salami, sausage
Dairy Products	Aged cheese Sour cream Yogurt
Fruits	Avocados Bananas, in large amounts Canned figs Papaya products, including meat tenderizers Raisins
Vegetables	Pods of fava beans Fermented soybeans, soybean paste
Fish	Dried or cured fish Fermented, smoked, aged fish Pickled or kippered herring
Alcohol	Beer Wine, especially red wine
Miscellaneous	Protein dietary supplements Soups (may contain protein extract) Shrimp paste Soy sauce Yeast, Brewers or extracts

A serious adverse reaction with MAOIs is their ability to cause a hypertensive crisis if combined with foods that contain **tyramine.** Widely found in nature, tyramine is a type of monoamine that is formed by the metabolism of tyrosine, an amino acid. When a patient is taking an MAOI, the drug blocks the breakdown of dietary tyramine, causing it to accumulate to high levels. In turn, tyramine causes the release of norepinephrine stored in adrenergic neurons. Rapid vasoconstriction occurs with a potential rise of blood pressure of 30 mmHg or more. Table 23.4 contains a list of tyramine-rich foods that must be avoided by patients taking MAOIs. Products containing tyramine are sometimes marketed as dietary supplements to increase fat loss from the body. There is no valid scientific evidence to support this claim, and these supplements must be strictly avoided by patients taking MAOIs.

PROTOTYPE DRUG Phenelzine (Nardil)

Classification: Therapeutic: Antidepressant

Pharmacologic: Monoamine oxidase inhibitor

Therapeutic Effects and Uses: An older drug approved in 1959, phenelzine was once widely used to treat major depression. It has also been used off-label to treat OCD, panic disorder, and social anxiety disorder and for migraine prophylaxis. Although very effective in treating these disorders, phenelzine interacts with tyramine in foods and with many other drugs to produce potentially serious interactions.

Like other antidepressants, phenelzine may take up to 4 to 8 weeks to produce a maximum antidepressant response. This drug is changed to active metabolites in the liver.

Mechanism of Action: Phenelzine produces its effects by binding irreversibly to MAO. This intensifies the actions of endogenous epinephrine, norepinephrine, serotonin, and dopamine in the CNS. Increased concentrations of these neurotransmitters result in elevated mood.

Pharmacokinetics:

Route(s)	PO
Absorption	Well absorbed
Distribution	Widely distributed; crosses the placenta
Primary metabolism	Hepatic
Primary excretion	Renal
Onset of action	Peak level: 2–4 h (antidepressant action takes 2 to 8 weeks)
Duration of action	Half-life: 11 h

Adverse Effects: The most serious adverse effect of phenelzine is hypertensive crisis precipitated by foods containing tyramine, which can induce fatal intracranial bleeding. Dizziness and orthostatic hypotension are common during therapy. Other frequent adverse reactions include drowsiness, sexual dysfunction, and anorexia. Life-threatening adverse reactions include dysrhythmias and a syndrome of inappropriate antidiuretic hormone-like symptoms.

Contraindications/Precautions: Patients with schizophrenia, cardiovascular or cerebrovascular disease, hepatic or renal impairment, or pheochromocytoma should not take phenelzine. Caution should be used when prescribing phenelzine to a person with epilepsy, severe or frequent headaches, HTN, dysrhythmias, or suicidal tendencies.

Drug Interactions: Phenelzine interacts with many other drugs. The nurse should consult a current drug guide for a comprehensive list of drug–drug interactions. Other CNS depressants, including alcohol, may lead to additive CNS depression. Concurrent administration with buspirone may increase blood pressure. Use with opioid analgesics may lead to immediate excitation, rigidity, severe HTN or hypotension, and, occasionally, severe respiratory distress, vascular collapse, seizures, coma, and death. CNS stimulants and sympathomimetics may increase the cardiac stimulant and vasopressor effects of phenelzine. Phenelzine may increase the effects of insulin or oral antidiabetic medications. SES may occur if phenelzine is administered with other drugs such as SSRIs, lithium, or dextromethorphan that potentiate the actions of serotonin. **Herbal/Food:** Patients who are taking phenelzine or any MAOI must avoid tyramine-containing foods (Table 23.4) because these foods may precipitate a hypertensive crisis. Medications containing caffeine, including OTC products, should be avoided because they may increase the risk of HTN and dysrhythmias. An increased sympathomimetic effect may occur when phenelzine is combined with capsicum peppers, large amounts of green tea, butcher's broom, and others. Ginkgo, nutmeg, and yohimbe can result in increased effects. Ginseng use can lead to irritability, hallucinations, mania, and increased tension headaches. Decreased effects can occur with the use of valerian. Serotonin syndrome may occur with the use of St. John's wort.

Pregnancy: Category C.

Treatment of Overdose: Overdosage with phenelzine is serious and can result in death if untreated. Symptoms may include either CNS stimulation (seizures) or depression (coma). Induction of gastric lavage with activated charcoal may be beneficial. Electrolytes and vital signs must be monitored and the appropriate intervention administered to keep values within normal ranges.

Nursing Responsibilities:

- Obtain a comprehensive history, including previous episodes of major depression, major factors leading to depression, need for antidepressants, and history of cardiovascular disorders, especially HTN.
- Assess for suicidal ideation, especially in pediatric and adolescent patients, during the first few weeks of therapy.
- Obtain a complete drug history, especially for hypersensitivity to MAOIs, drugs that may interact with MAOIs, and those drugs that cannot be taken within 14 days of an MAOI.
- Monitor caffeine intake. Excessive amounts of caffeine can potentiate hypertensive reactions.
- Encourage the patient to continue the drug even if no benefits are felt for several weeks.
- Assess for withdrawal symptoms (headache, nausea, vomiting, weakness, muscle pain), which may occur if the drug is abruptly discontinued.

Patient and Family Education:

- Avoid high-protein foods that have undergone protein breakdown by aging, fermentation, pickling, smoking, or bacterial contamination, such as cheeses (especially aged varieties), pickled herring, beer, wine, liver, yeast extract (including brewer's yeast in large quantities), dry sausage (including Genoa salami, hard salami, pepperoni, and Lebanon bologna), pods of broad beans (fava beans), and yogurt.
- Do not take any other prescription or nonprescription drugs, dietary supplements, or herbal products without approval of the health care provider.
- The full therapeutic effects of MAOIs may take 2 to 6 weeks or more to appear.
- Avoid alcohol and other CNS depressants.
- Wear or carry identification stating that you are taking an MAOI.
- If sedation occurs take the medication at bedtime.
- Make position changes slowly when moving from a lying to a standing position to prevent dizziness and possible fainting.
- Take exactly as prescribed and do not discontinue the medication without approval of the health care provider.
- Report headache, palpitations, neck stiffness, dizziness, rash, insomnia, changes in urinary pattern, color of urine, change in strength, or constriction in the chest or throat.
- Anticholinergic effects such as dry mouth may occur. Simple ways to decrease symptoms are to increase fluids, suck on sugarless hard candy, chew sugarless gum, or take frequent sips of water.

Drugs Similar to Phenelzine (Nardil)

There are two other MAOIs available: isocarboxazid and tranylcypromine.

Isocarboxazid (Marplan): Like phenelzine, isocarboxazid was initially approved by the FDA for depression in the 1950s. Off-label indications include refractory panic disorder and social anxiety disorder. It is only used when other therapies have failed to produce satisfactory outcomes. The drug has the same precautions and potential interactions as phenelzine, including the possibility of a hypertensive crisis occurring when taken with tyramine-containing products. This drug is pregnancy category C.

Selegiline (Emsam): Approved in 2006 for major depression, selegiline is a transdermal patch that delivers a controlled amount of the MAOI over 24 hours. Absorption across the skin bypasses MAO in the intestine; thus there is less risk of a hypertensive

NURSING PROCESS APPLICATION

Patients Receiving Antidepressant Therapy

Assessment	Potential Nursing Diagnoses
Prior to administration: • Obtain a complete health history (allergies, drug history, potential drug,food,and herb interactions). • Obtain a history of previous illnesses, especially cardiac, hepatic, and renal disorders. • Obtain a history of previous or concurrent psychiatric disorders. • Assess neurologic status, including seizure history, behavior, mood, and the risk for suicide.	• *Disturbed Thought Processes,* related to depression • *Ineffective Coping,* related to inadequate level of confidence in ability to cope • *Risk for Self-Directed Violence,* related to disease process • *Deficient Knowledge, (Disease Process)* • *Risk for Injury,* related to adverse effects of medications

Planning: Patient Goals and Expected Outcomes

The patient will:

- Report reduction of symptoms related to depression.
- Report understanding of and adherence to the therapeutic regimen.
- Report increased social interactions with others.
- Report increased involvement in activities of daily living.
- Report an absence of suicidal thought and an improvement in thought processes.

(continued)

Implementation: Tricyclic Antidepressants

Interventions and (Rationales)	Patient and Family Education
• Monitor vital signs, especially blood pressure and pulse. (TCAs may cause orthostatic hypotension.)	Instruct the patient: • That it may take 4–8 weeks to reach full therapeutic effectiveness. • To change position slowly to prevent injury from orthostatic hypotension.
• Monitor for suicidal ideation. (As serum levels increase but have not reached full therapeutic levels, risk for suicide increases.)	• Teach the patient and family signs of possible suicidal ideation, including decreased interest and participation in former activities, a sense of peace or of purpose (the patient may have decided to commit suicide), or giving away possessions.
• Carefully monitor the patient with epilepsy for any seizure activity. (TCAs lower the seizure threshold.)	Instruct the patient to: • Be aware of aura and to take precautions if aura occurs. • Take protective measures to decrease injury, including laying the patient on the floor or loosening clothing.
• Monitor for anticholinergic adverse effects, especially in patients with urinary retention, narrow-angle glaucoma, benign prostatic hyperplasia (BPH). (One adverse effect of TCAs is anticholinergic responses.)	Instruct the patient to: • That sweating may occur as well as anticholinergic adverse effects. • Measures to decrease discomfort from anticholinergic effects, including frequent sips of water, chewing sugarless gum, sucking on sugarless hard candy, increasing fiber and fluids in the diet, etc. • To report any changes in urinary function or in vision.
• Monitor weight. (Weight gain is a adverse effect of TCAs and frequently a reason for nonadherence with therapy.)	Instruct the patient to: • To monitor weight. • To decrease weight gain by increasing exercise and including low-calorie foods in the diet. • The importance of continuing the medication even if weight gain does occur.
• Monitor for pregnancy or the desire to become pregnant. (TCAs are pregnancy category C or D drugs, so they should be used only if absolutely necessary.)	Instruct the female patient to: • Use safe, effective birth control and not to breast-feed. • Notify the health care provider if she intends to become pregnant.
• Monitor for use of other medications. (Significant drug interactions may occur with TCAs.)	• Instruct the patient and family the importance of not taking any other medications, including OTC medications or herbal products, without the approval of the health care provider.
• Monitor the amount of sedation that occurs. (Some patients will experience significant sedation, especially at the beginning of therapy.)	• Instruct the patient to take the medication at bedtime if sedation occurs.
• Monitor alcohol use. (Alcohol is a CNS depressant; concurrent use may lead to excessive sedation.)	Instruct the patient to: • Refrain from alcohol use. • Be aware of signs of alcohol consumption or unusual or excessive sedation. • Attend appropriate appointments with Alcoholics Anonymous or other support group.

Implementation: Selective Serotonin Reuptake Inhibitors (SSRIs)

Interventions and (Rationales)	Patient and Family Education
• Assess the intensity and duration of symptoms. (Symptoms should begin to decrease in a few weeks but the drug may take 8 weeks to reach full therapeutic effects.)	• Instruct the patient that the SSRI may take up to 8 weeks to reach full therapeutic benefits.
• Obtain baseline liver function tests and blood studies. (SSRIs are metabolized in the liver, and hepatic dysfunction can result in higher serum levels; abnormal blood studies can result.)	• Instruct the patient the importance of having routine blood studies performed.
• Obtain a baseline body weight. (SSRIs can cause weight gain, which may lead to nonadherence with the medication regimen.)	Instruct the patient to: • Monitor weight. • Decrease weight gain by increasing exercise and including low-calorie foods in the diet. • Continue the medication even if weight gain occurs.
• Assess for other drugs the patient may be taking. (Many other drugs can interact with SSRIs; other CNS depressants and alcohol can cause excessive sedation; MAOIs can cause serotonin syndrome.)	• Instruct the patient not to take any other prescription, OTC, or herbal preparations without consulting the health care provider.
• Assess suicidal ideation. (SSRIs may take several weeks to be fully therapeutic. Some patients may feel better so they can now act on suicidal thoughts, where previously they did not have enough energy to do this.)	• Instruct the patient and family signs of suicidal thoughts, including lack of interest in previously enjoyed activities, decreased attention to personal hygiene, giving away possessions, and sudden happiness or a sense of peace.
• Monitor alcohol use. (Alcohol is a CNS depressant; concurrent use can cause excessive sedation.)	Instruct the patient to: • Refrain from alcohol use. • Be aware of signs of alcohol consumption and unusual or excessive sedation. • Attend appropriate appointments with Alcoholics Anonymous or other support group.
• Monitor urinary retention or constipation (may occur with use of SSRIs).	Instruct the patient and family to: • Report any changes in urinary or bowel function. • Prevent constipation by increasing fiber and fluids in the diet.
• Monitor for sexual dysfunction. (This is one of most common adverse effects of SSRIs and may lead to nonadherence to medications.)	Instruct the patient: • That sexual dysfunction is common, but that the medication must be continued. • To report sexual dysfunction.

Implementation: Atypical Antidepressants	
Interventions and (Rationales)	**Patient and Family Education**
• Monitor vital signs, especially blood pressure. (Medications may cause orthostatic hypotension.)	Instruct the patient and family: • To keep all follow-up appointments. • That orthostatic hypotension may occur, and safety measures should be incorporated to prevent injury.
• Monitor blood laboratory values. (This drug may cause abnormalities, especially leukocytosis and cardiac enzymes.)	• Instruct the patient to keep all follow-up appointments.
• Assess the medical history. (Patients with seizure disorder or eating disorders cannot take atypical antidepressants; caution must be taken for patients with a history of renal or hepatic disease, recent MI, or cranial trauma.)	• Instruct the patient to take the drug exactly as prescribed because the risk of seizures may increase if the dose is exceeded.
• Monitor other medications that the patient is taking. (Several possible drug interactions can occur.)	Instruct the patient to: • Avoid alcohol, caffeine, or other CNS depressants. • Notify the health care provider of all medications and dietary supplements taken.
• Assess mental status. (Symptoms, suicide ideation, mood, sensorium, affect, or depression can all worsen.)	• Instruct the patient and family signs of adverse effects and to report them immediately.

Implementation: Monoamine Oxidase Inhibitors (MAOIs)	
Intervention and (Rationales)	**Patient and Family Education**
• Monitor for suicide ideation (MAOIs may take 1–4 weeks to reach full therapeutic effects.)	• Instruct the patient that full therapeutic effects may take up to 1 month to obtain.
• Monitor hepatic function. (MAOIs are metabolized in the liver; decreased liver function can lead to toxicity.)	Instruct the patient and family: • The importance of routine laboratory studies. • To recognize signs of potential decreased liver function, including pale stools, yellowing of the sclera of the eyes, yellowing of the skin, etc.
• Monitor vital signs, especially blood pressure. (MAOIs may cause orthostatic hypotension; hypertensive crisis can also occur.)	Instruct the patient and family: • How to monitor blood pressure. • The importance of keeping all appointments for routine follow-up. • Safety measures to decrease injury if orthostatic hypotension occurs.
• Assess cardiovascular functioning. (Phenelzine is contraindicated in preexisting cardiac disease; MAOIs may lead to ECG changes, dysrhythmias, inhibit platelet function.)	• Teach the patient and family the importance of keeping all follow-up appointments.
• Assess for pregnancy or the desire to become pregnant or for lactation. (MAOIs are pregnancy category C drugs and are secreted in breast milk.)	Instruct the female patient to: • Use safe, effective birth control and not to breast-feed. • Notify the health care provider if she intends to become pregnant.
• Monitor the diet. (Persons taking MAOIs must avoid foods containing tyramine to prevent hypertensive crisis.)	• Instruct the patient to avoid foods high in tyramine, including aged cheese, beer, red wine, sardines, liver, raisins, avocado, chocolate, meat tenderizer, and yogurt.
• Monitor for the presence of adverse reactions (headache, palpitations, dizziness, nuchal rigidity, chest or throat congestion, rash, insomnia, weakness, or changes in urinary pattern or in the color of urine).	• Instruct the patient to report headache, palpitations, dizziness, neck stiffness, chest or throat congestion, rash, insomnia, weakness, or changes in urinary pattern or in the color of urine.

Evaluation of Outcome Criteria

Evaluate the effectiveness of drug therapy by confirming that patient goals and expected outcomes have been met (see "Planning").

crisis when eating foods containing tyramine. Common adverse effects include skin irritation at the site of the patch application, headache, sleep disorders, diarrhea, and dry mouth. This drug is pregnancy category C.

Tranylcypromine (Parnate): Tranylcypromine was approved in 1961 for the therapy of depression. Off-label indications include refractory panic disorder and social anxiety disorder. The drug binds reversibly to MAO. This results in a more rapid onset of antidepressant action than phenelzine or isocarboxazid and a more rapid return to normal MAO levels after the drug is discontinued. However, it has the same precautions and potential interactions as phenelzine and is rarely used due to its adverse effects. This drug is pregnancy category C.

Bipolar Disorder

23.12 Bipolar disorder is a serious psychiatric disorder characterized by extreme mood swings from depression to euphoria.

Bipolar disorder, once known as manic-depression, is a common and serious psychiatric disorder. Suicide risk is high and many patients stop taking their medication during the course of pharmacotherapy. The etiology of the disorder is unknown, and symptoms may persist throughout the patient's life span.

Mania is characterized by symptoms that are generally the opposite of depressive symptoms. The excessive CNS stimulation that is characteristic of mania can be recognized by the following symptoms:

- Inflated self-esteem or grandiosity; the belief that one's ideas are far superior to anyone else's
- Decreased need for sleep or food
- Distractibility; racing thoughts with attention too easily drawn to irrelevant external stimuli
- Increased psychomotor or goal-directed activity (either socially, at work or school, or sexually)
- Excessive pursuit of pleasurable activities without consideration of the negative consequences, such as shopping sprees, sexual indiscretions, or unsound business investments
- Increased talkativeness or pressure to keep talking
- With severe disease, delusions, paranoia, hallucinations, and bizarre behavior

To be diagnosed with bipolar disorder, these symptoms must persist for at least 1 week and evidence of impaired functioning must be present. Suicide is a major risk in patients who have bipolar disorder; up to 50% of these patients attempt suicide, and 10% to 20% succeed in taking their lives. **Hypomania** is characterized by the same symptoms, but they are less severe and do not cause impaired functioning. In some cases, patients may experience a mixed episode where depression and mania are experienced simultaneously.

MyNursingKit | Bipolar Disorder Videos

Although the pathophysiology of bipolar disorder is incompletely understood, mania and hypomania likely result from abnormal functioning of neurotransmitters in the brain. Mania may involve an excess of excitatory neurotransmitters (such as glutamate or norepinephrine) or a deficiency of inhibitory neurotransmitters (such as GABA). It is important to distinguish bipolar disorder from drug abuse, severe anxiety disorders, schizophrenia, dementia, or electrolyte disturbances, which can all produce symptoms similar to those of bipolar disorder.

Nonpharmacologic interventions play important roles in the treatment of patients with bipolar disorder. Lack of sleep, excessive stress, and poor nutrition are triggers for manic episodes and should be addressed in the plan of care. Support groups and psychotherapy are helpful for many patients. ECT is very effective at treating acute manic and depressive episodes.

Like the treatment of major depression, nonadherence with drug therapy is a serious problem in patients with bipolar disorder; as many as 50% of patients discontinue their medication during the first year of therapy. Lack of awareness is the single most common reason for nonadherence; mania is simply not viewed as abnormal by the person experiencing it. In fact, people with mania are often able to work tirelessly on projects and accomplish many work- and home-related tasks. Surprisingly, the second most common reason for nonadherence is the presence of a comorbid substance abuse disorder, usually alcoholism. Psychotherapy and family support may be necessary to achieve proper adherence.

Drugs for Bipolar Disorder

23.13 Lithium is the conventional therapy for the treatment of bipolar disorder.

Drugs for bipolar disorder are called **mood stabilizers**, because they have the ability to moderate extreme shifts in emotion and relieve symptoms of mania and depression during acute episodes. The traditional treatment for bipolar disorder is lithium carbonate (Eskalith), a mood stabilizer prescribed as monotherapy or in combination with other drugs. In recent years, valproic acid (Depakene) has begun to replace lithium as the first-line therapy for bipolar disorder due to its improved safety profile. Valproic acid and other miscellaneous drugs for bipolar disorder are discussed in Section 23.14. Drugs used to treat bipolar disorder are shown in Table 23.5.

PROTOTYPE DRUG Lithium carbonate (Eskalith, Lithobid)

Classification: **Therapeutic:** Antimanic, agent for bipolar disorder
Pharmacologic: Alkali metal ion salt

Therapeutic Effects and Uses: Lithium was approved in the United States in 1970. Its benefit in treating bipolar disorder had been established since the 1950s; however, its therapeutic safety had not been proved. Lithium is a simple inorganic element that is found in the same group as sodium and potassium. It is available for PO administration, as tablets, syrup, and controlled release and slow release tablets. Onset of action may take 1 to 3 weeks. Dosing is highly individualized and is based on serum drug levels and clinical response. Serum lithium levels are monitored regularly during therapy and should be maintained within the narrow range of 0.8 to 1.4 mEq/L at the start of therapy and 0.4 to 1 mEq/L during maintenance therapy. Lithium has a short half-life and must be taken in multiple doses each day.

Lithium is a drug of choice in controlling the acute manic episodes characteristic of bipolar disorder and in preventing the recurrence of mania or depression. In the patient with mania, lithium decreases euphoria, hyperactivity, and other symptoms without causing sedation. Previously lithium was used for all patients with mania; at the present time it is used primarily for those patients with classic euphoric mania. Lithium, rather than valproic acid, appears to be more effective in reducing suicide risk in persons diagnosed with bipolar disorder. Lithium is also used for off-label indications, including alcoholism, bulimia, neutropenia, schizophrenia, prevention of vascular headaches, and hyperthyroidism.

Mechanism of Action: The precise mechanism of action of lithium is not known. It likely acts by changing neurotransmitter balance in specific brain regions. Lithium increases the synthesis of serotonin.

TABLE 23.5 Drugs for Bipolar Disorder

Drug	Route and Adult Dose (maximum dose where indicated)	Adverse Effects
lithium carbonate (Eskalith, Lithobid)	PO: initially 600 mg tid or 900 mg sustained release bid or 30 mL (48 mEq) of solution tid Maintenance: 300 mg tid or qid or 15–20 mL (24–32 mEq) in two to four divided doses (max: 2.4 g/day)	*Headache, lethargy, fatigue, recent memory loss, nausea, vomiting, anorexia, abdominal pain, diarrhea, dry mouth, muscle weakness, nephrogenic diabetes insipidus, fine hand tremors, reversible leukocytosis* <u>Peripheral circulatory collapse</u>
Antiseizure Drugs		
carbamazepine (Tegretol)	PO: 200 mg bid, gradually increased to 800–1,200 mg/day in three to four divided doses	*Dizziness, ataxia, somnolence, headache, nausea, diplopia, blurred vision, sedation, drowsiness, nausea, vomiting, prolonged bleeding time, transient leukopenia* <u>Heart block, aplastic anemia, agranulocytosis, respiratory depression, exfoliative dermatitis, SJS, toxic epidermal necrolysis, deep coma, death (with overdose), liver failure, pancreatitis, bone marrow depression</u>
lamotrigine (Lamictal)	PO: 50 mg/day for 2 weeks, then 50 mg bid for 2 weeks; may increase gradually up to 300–500 mg/day in two divided doses (max: 700 mg/day)	
valproic acid (Depakene)	PO: 250 mg tid (max: 60 mg/kg/day)	
Atypical Antipsychotic Drugs		
aripiprazole (Abilify)	PO: 30 mg daily; may decrease to 15 mg (max: 30 mg daily)	*Tachycardia, sedation, dizziness, headache, light-headedness, somnolence, anxiety, nervousness, agitation, hostility, insomnia, nausea, vomiting, transient fever, constipation, akathisia, parkinsonism* <u>Agranulocytosis, neuroleptic malignant syndrome (risperidone, rare), risk of stroke in elderly with dementia-related psychosis (aripiprazole)</u>
olanzapine (Zyprexa)	PO: start with 10 mg once daily; may increase or decrease in 5 mg/day increments	
quetiapine (Seroquel)	PO: start with 25 mg bid and increase by 25–50 mg bid to tid to target dose of 300–400 mg/day divided bid or tid (max: 800 mg/day)	
risperidone (Risperdal)	PO: start with 2–3 mg daily, may increase dose at intervals of 1 mg/day (max: 6 mg/day)	
ziprasidone (Geodon)	PO: 40 mg bid with food, may increase every 2 days up to 80 mg bid	

Note: *Italics* indicate common adverse effects. <u>Underline</u> indicates serious adverse effects.

Pharmacokinetics:

Route(s)	PO
Absorption	Completely absorbed
Distribution	Distributed to all tissues and body fluids; crosses the blood–brain barrier and placenta; secreted in breast milk; not bound to plasma protein
Primary metabolism	Not metabolized
Primary excretion	Renal
Onset of action	Peak levels: 4–12 h (tablets) or 15–60 minutes (solutions)
Duration of action	Unknown

Adverse Effects: There are many possible adverse effects associated with the use of lithium. These are sometimes divided into those that occur at the initiation of therapy and those that occur with long-term therapy. Initial adverse effects are muscle weakness, lethargy, nausea, vomiting, polyuria, nocturia, headache, dizziness, drowsiness, tremors, and confusion. Many of the initial adverse effects are transient or may be easily managed. Long-term therapy can produce serious toxicity, including kidney impairment (proteinuria, albuminuria, or glycosuria), dysrhythmias, circulatory collapse, and leukocytosis. Lithium interferes with the synthesis of thyroid hormone and can cause hypothyroidism and goiter.

Contraindications/Precautions: Contraindications to the use of lithium include serious cardiovascular or renal impairment and severe dehydration or sodium depletion. Older adults and debilitated patients must be carefully monitored. Caution must be used when the drug is given to patients with cardiovascular disease, thyroid disease, history of a seizure disorder, diabetes, urinary retention, or a systemic infection. Lithium produces an increased incidence of congenital defects, especially those involving the heart, and is normally not used during pregnancy. Its use should be discouraged during lactation.

Drug Interactions: There are many potential drug interactions, some of which can be serious. Diuretics can increase the risk of lithium toxicity by promoting sodium loss; the body replaces lost sodium with lithium, which is also a salt. NSAIDs and thiazide diuretics can increase lithium levels by increasing the renal reabsorption of lithium. A decreased lithium effect can occur if theophylline or urinary alkalizers are used. Lithium may cause an increased hypothyroid effect of antithyroid drugs or drugs containing iodine. Concurrent administration with haloperidol may cause increased neurotoxicity. SES may result if lithium is administered with other drugs, such as SSRIs or dextromethorphan, or MAOIs that potentiate the actions of serotonin. **Herbal/Food:** An increased lithium effect may be found with the use of dandelion, goldenrod, juniper, parsley, nettle, or horsetail. Black or green tea, cola nut, plantain, guarana, or yerba may lead to a decreased lithium effect. Significant changes in sodium intake from foods will alter lithium excretion.

Pregnancy: Category D.

Treatment of Overdose: Overdose of lithium is treated with supportive measures such as emesis or lavage, maintaining airway and respiratory function, and dialysis, if lithium intoxication is severe.

Nursing Responsibilities:

- Assess for symptoms of bipolar disorder before initiating therapy and reassess regularly.
- Assess for lithium hypersensitivity.
- Obtain baseline thyroid, kidney, and cardiac function and electrolyte levels.
- Monitor serum lithium levels every 1 to 3 days at the outset of therapy and every 2 to 3 months thereafter, and report values outside the normal range.
- Monitor for symptoms of minor lithium toxicity (vomiting, diarrhea, weakness, lassitude, poor coordination, fine motor tremors) and major lithium toxicity (severe thirst, tinnitus, dilute urine, coarse tremors).
- Assess daily for weight changes, presence of edema, and changes in skin turgor.
- Monitor sodium intake.
- Assess neurologic status, level of consciousness (LOC), gait, hand tremors, and motor reflexes.
- Monitor urine for albuminuria, glycosuria, and uric acid levels frequently during early treatment, then every 2 months thereafter.
- Monitor for mood swings because these may indicate that the drug is ineffective or the patient is not taking the medication.
- Monitor GI, metabolic, and electrolyte status.

Patient and Family Education:

- Immediately report any significant changes in mood or behavior to the health care provider.
- Use effective contraception to prevent pregnancy. Immediately notify the health care provider of any known or suspected pregnancy.
- Monitor and maintain a stable intake of sodium and fluids.
- The full therapeutic effects of the medication will take 1 to 3 weeks to appear.
- Do not take other prescription or nonprescription drugs, dietary supplements, or herbal products, without approval of the health care provider.
- Take lithium with food if GI upset occurs, but do not break, crush, or chew tablets.
- Limit caffeine and alcohol intake.

Drugs Similar to Lithium Carbonate (Eskalith, Lithobid)

There are no drugs similar to lithium carbonate.

23.14 Antiseizure and atypical antipsychotic agents are used to control symptoms of bipolar disorder.

Although lithium is well established as an effective treatment for bipolar disorder, pharmacologists have searched for safer alternatives. Several drugs have been found to be effective for this disorder and have received FDA approval. A number of others are prescribed off-label for bipolar disorder. All of these agents have other primary indications and are presented in other chapters of this textbook. The other classes include antiseizure agents, atypical antipsychotics, and antidepressants.

Antiseizure agents: The antiseizure drugs for bipolar disorder are classified as mood stabilizers. These agents have pharmacologic actions similar to lithium: relieving symptoms and preventing the recurrence of mania and depression.

Valproic acid (Depakene) and divalproex sodium (Depakote ER) are FDA approved for mood stabilization and mania suppression. Valproic acid has replaced lithium as the drug of choice for many patients because it has far fewer adverse effects, a higher therapeutic index, and a more rapid onset of action. The only area in which it does not compare favorably with lithium is in the ability to prevent suicide. Valproic acid is well tolerated in most patients but can occasionally cause serious toxicity. Rare cases of thrombocytopenia, pancreatitis, and liver failure have occurred and signs of any of these adverse events require immediate withdrawal of the drug. As with lithium, valproic acid is teratogenic and should not be used during pregnancy. It is secreted in breast milk and therefore should not be used during lactation. A prototype feature for this drug is included in Chapter 26.

Carbamazepine (Tegretol) was one of the initial drugs studied as a lithium alternative, but it was not until 2005 that it was approved for that indication. It reduces the symptoms of both manic and depressive phases of bipolar disorder and can reduce recurrence of the condition. It is preferred over lithium for patients who have mixed mania or rapid-cycling bipolar disorder. Neurologic adverse effects such as vertigo, headache, unsteadiness, and ataxia are common during early therapy but usually subside with continued use. Oral contraceptives may be less effective, and pregnant women should not take carbamazepine. This is a pregnancy category D drug. Increased CNS toxicity can result if carbamazepine is used concurrently with lithium. Carbamazepine is one of the most frequently prescribed antiseizure drugs, and a prototype feature is included in Chapter 26.

Approved for treating bipolar disorder in 2003, the antiepileptic drug lamotrigine (Lamictal) is indicated for long-term maintenance therapy to prevent or delay relapses. It may be used alone or in combination with other mood stabilizers. The drug is well tolerated by most patients, with the most common adverse events being drowsiness, dizziness, ataxia, headache, diplopia, blurred vision, nausea, vomiting, and rash. Because rare cases of Stevens–Johnson syndrome (SJS) have been documented, any appearance of rash calls for discontinuation of the drug. To minimize the risk of serious skin rashes, the dose of lamotrigine is increased gradually. Lamotrigine is a pregnancy category C drug and should be used cautiously in lactating women.

Other antiseizure drugs have been used off-label for bipolar disorder but they do not appear to be more effective than existing medications. These include oxcarbazepine (Trileptal), gabapentin (Neurontin), and topiramate (Topamax). Clonazepam (Klonopin) and lorazepam (Ativan) are benzodiazepines used for seizures that have been used off-label for bipolar disorder in combination with other agents.

Atypical antipsychotics: Antipsychotic drugs are used to control acute symptoms during episodes of mania and as long-term mood stabilizers. They benefit patients with or without psychotic symptoms. These agents are usually used in combination with lithium or valproic acid, but they are effective if used as monotherapy. The atypical antipsychotics are preferred over the conventional antipsychotics because of a much lower risk of developing extrapyramidal adverse effects. Five atypical antipsychotics have been approved for use in treating bipolar disorder. They include aripiprazole (Abilify), olanzapine (Zyprexa), quetiapine (Seroquel), risperidone (Risperdal), and ziprasidone (Geodon). All of these drugs are effective against manic episodes, but only olanzapine is approved for long-term maintenance therapy. For specific information on typical and atypical antipsychotics, refer to Chapter 24.

Antidepressants: Antidepressants may be used to treat the depressed stage of bipolar disorder. These agents must be used with caution because they have a tendency to cause hypomania or mania in depressed patients with bipolar disorder. Because of this potentially serious adverse effect, antidepressants are always administered concurrently with a mood stabilizer. The antidepressants of choice for treating patients with bipolar disorder are the SSRIs, venlafaxine (Effexor), and bupropion (Wellbutrin). The antidepressant medications are discussed earlier in this chapter.

NURSING PROCESS APPLICATION

Patients Receiving Therapy for Bipolar Disorder

Assessment	Potential Nursing Diagnoses
Prior to administration: • Obtain a complete health history, including allergies, drug history, and possible drug interactions. • Assess mental and emotional status, including any suicidal ideation. • Obtain cardiac history and history of renal or hepatic disorders.	• *Disturbed Thought Processes,* related to mania • *Ineffective Coping,* related to inadequate level of confidence in ability to cope • *Risk for Self-Directed Violence,* related to disease process • *Deficient Knowledge (Disease Process)* • *Risk for Injury,* related to adverse effects of medications

Planning: Patient Goals and Expected Outcomes

The patient will:

- Experience mood stabilization with no or few episodes of either depression or mania.
- Experience improved interpersonal relationships.
- Engage in normal activities of daily living.
- Report subjective improvement in mood.
- Demonstrate understanding of medication regimen.

Implementation: Drugs to Treat Bipolar Disorder

Interventions and (Rationales)	Patient and Family Education
• Monitor mental and emotional status, mania, or depression. (Drugs should prevent mood swings.)	• Instruct the patient how to keep a symptom log to document response to medication.
• Monitor electrolyte balance, especially if taking lithium. (Lithium is a salt; changes in sodium levels can affect excretion of lithium.)	• Instruct the patient how to ensure adequate sodium intake; increase sodium during periods of excessive exercise or hot weather, or other activities leading to heavy sweating.
• Measure intake and output; do daily weights. (Weight fluctuations and intake–output imbalances are indicators of fluid retention, which increase the risk of heart failure or of polyuria.)	Instruct the patient to: • Increase fluid intake to 1–1.5 L daily, if not contraindicated. • Decrease or eliminate caffeine from the diet. • Report weight changes or signs of edema.
• Monitor cardiac status. (Toxicity may lead to dysrhythmias or angina.)	Instruct the patient: • To immediately report chest pain, palpitations, or other signs of possible MI. • The proper use of home blood pressure monitoring equipment.
• Monitor renal status. (Decreased renal function can lead to toxicity.)	• Instruct the patient and family to immediately report decreased urinary output, especially if accompanied by lower abdominal tenderness, flank pain, distention, headache, diaphoresis, or changes in quality of urine (hematuria, proteinuria, etc.)
• Monitor laboratory tests. (Report abnormal values to the health care provider; lithium must be used cautiously if abnormal results appear.)	• Instruct the patient and family to report any unusual symptoms such as vital sign changes, lethargy, agitation, or headache.

Evaluation of Outcome Criteria

Evaluate the effectiveness of drug therapy by confirming that patient goals and expected outcomes have been met (see "Planning").

UNDERSTANDING THE CHAPTER

Key Concepts Summary

23.1 The two primary types of mood disorders are depression and bipolar disorder.

23.2 Major depressive disorder is characterized by a depressed mood, with accompanying symptoms, that lasts at least 2 weeks.

23.3 The pathophysiology of depression has biologic, genetic, and environmental components.

23.4 Assessment and diagnosis of depression are a collaborative effort among health care providers.

23.5 The majority of patients who attempt suicide have major depression.

23.6 Depression is sometimes treated with nonpharmacologic therapies.

23.7 The mechanism of action of antidepressants involves modulation of neurotransmitter levels in the brain.

23.8 Tricyclic antidepressants have been the mainstay for the treatment of depression but have many adverse effects.

23.9 Selective serotonin reuptake inhibitors are the drugs of choice for treating depression due to their low incidence of serious adverse effects.

23.10 Atypical antidepressants are alternatives to the selective serotonin reuptake inhibitors that are prescribed for depression and anxiety disorders.

23.11 Monoamine oxidase inhibitors are effective antidepressants but are seldom used due to potentially serious adverse effects.

23.12 Bipolar disorder is a serious psychiatric disorder characterized by extreme mood swings from depression to euphoria.

23.13 Lithium is the conventional therapy for the treatment of bipolar disorder.

23.14 Antiseizure and atypical antipsychotic agents are used to control symptoms of bipolar disorder.

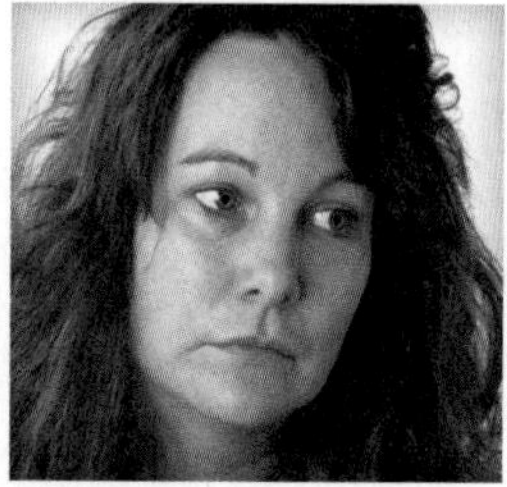

Making the PATIENT *Connection*

Remember the patient "Jane Albright" at the beginning of the chapter? Now read the remainder of the case study. Based on the information presented within this chapter, respond to the critical thinking questions that follow.

Jane is a 37-year-old mother of three young children. Before the children were born she was employed as a corporate attorney, but she and her husband decided prior to the birth of their first child that she would stay at home until the children completed high school. They are financially stable. Jane has been a soccer coach, Boy Scout leader, president of the ladies' group at her church, and involved in various other community organizations. Within the last month, she has not participated in any of her previous activities and she has not explained why. Jane is in good physical health and had her annual physical exam the previous month. She takes no routine medications or herbal products.

Critical Thinking Questions

1. What first step must Charlie take to aid his wife with her depression?
2. When Jane is evaluated by a mental health professional, they begin talking about how antidepressant drug therapy works. Provide a brief explanation of antidepressant therapy.
3. How can a nurse determine if a therapeutic effect from the antidepressant medication is being achieved with Jane?

Case Study

It is recommended that Jane be hospitalized in the local mental health facility for further evaluation of her depression and for self-protection as well as for stabilization on an antidepressant medication.

1. What is the priority assessment that the nurse must make on Jane's admission to the treatment facility?
2. What classification of antidepressant medications is most likely to be ordered for Jane?
3. What teaching will be included for patients prescribed antidepressant therapy?

NCLEX-RN® Review

1 A health care provider has ordered imipramine (Trofanil) for each of these clients. A nurse should question the order for the client with:

1. Seizure disorders.
2. Depression.
3. Enuresis.
4. Neuropathic pain.

2 The nurse determines that the client understands an important principle in self-administration of fluoxetine (Prozac) when the client makes which of the following statements?

1. "I should not decrease my sodium or water intake."
2. "This drug can be taken concurrently with an MAOI."
3. "It may take up to 1 month to reach full therapeutic effects."
4. "There are no problems associated with concurrent use of other depressants."

3 The nurse is monitoring the client for early lithium carbonate (Eskalith) toxicity. Which of the following symptoms, if manifested by the client, would indicate that toxicity may be developing? Select all that apply.

1. Persistent gastrointestinal upset
2. Confusion
3. Polyuria
4. Convulsions
5. Ataxia

4 Which statement made by the client who is taking lithium carbonate (Eskalith) indicates that further teaching is necessary?

1. "I will be sure to remain on a low sodium diet."
2. "I will have blood levels drawn every 2 to 3 months, even when I have no symptoms."
3. "Lithium has a narrow margin of safety, so toxicity is a very real concern."
4. "I will not be able to breast-feed my baby."

5 The client who has been taking imipramine (Tofranil) for 3 weeks calls the nurse to report that there is no improvement in the depression. The nurse's best response is:

1. "Call your health care provider and see if he or she will change the order to a different medication."
2. "Are you sure that you are taking it as it is ordered? Perhaps you should consider increasing the dosage gradually."
3. "The medication may take up to 8 weeks to be effective. Continue taking the medication as ordered."
4. "Add an over-the-counter antianxiety agent to your daily medications."

6 The nurse knows that the most commonly prescribed antidepressant classification in the United States today is:

1. Monoamine oxidase inhibitors.
2. Tricyclic antidepressants.
3. Selective serotonin reuptake inhibitors.
4. Serotonin–norepinephrine reuptake inhibitors.

See Answers to Critical Thinking Questions, Case Study, and NCLEX-RN® Review in Appendix A.

References

American Psychiatric Association. (2000). *Diagnostic and statistical manual of mental disorders* (4th ed., Text revision). Washington, DC: Author.

Centers for Disease Control and Prevention. (2007). *Suicide facts at a glance.* Retrieved June 12, 2008, from http://www.cdc.gov/ncipc/dvp/Suicide/SuicideDataSheet.pdf

Cott, J. M., & Fugh-Berman, A. (1998). Is St. John's wort (*Hypericum perforatum*) an effective antidepressant? *Journal of Nervous and Mental Disease, 186*(8), 500–501.

Gaster, B., & Holroyd, J. (2006). St. John's wort in depression. *Archives of Internal Medicine, 160*(2), 152–156.

Gastpar, M., Singer, A., & Zeller, K. (2006). Comparative efficacy and safety of a once-daily dosage of hypericum extract STW3-VI and citalopram in patients with moderate depression: A double-blind, randomised, multicentre, placebo-controlled study. *Pharmacopsychiatry, 39*(2), 66–75.

Gibbons, R. D., Brown, C. H., Hur, K., Marcus, S. M., Bhaumik, D. K., & Mann, J. J. (2007). Relationship between antidepressants and suicide attempts: An analysis of the Veterans Health Administration data sets. *American Journal of Psychiatry, 164,* 1044–1049.

Goldsmith, D. R., Wagstaff, A. J., Ibbotson, T., & Perry, C. M. (2004). Spotlight on lamotrigine in bipolar disorder. *CNS Drugs, 18*(1), 63–67.

Ikezu, T., & Gendelman, H. E. (2008). *Neuroimmune pharmacology.* New York: Springer.

Janicak, P. (2002). *Research report: rTMS vs. ECT in depressed patients.* Chicago: University of Illinois.

Kramer, T. A. M. (2003). New generation of antipsychotics and bipolar disorder. *Medscape Psychiatry & Mental Health, 8*(1). Retrieved June 12, 2008, from http://www.medscape.com/viewarticle/455436

March, J., Silva, S., Petrycki, S., Curry, J., Wells, K., Fairbank, J., et al. (2004). Fluoxetine, cognitive-behavioral therapy, and their combination for adolescents with depression: Treatment for adolescents with depression study (TADS) randomized control trial. *Journal of the American Medical Association, 292,* 807–820.

Nardi, D. (2007). Depression in school-aged children: Assessment and early interventions. *Journal of Psychosocial Nursing and Mental Health Services, 45*(3), 48–53.

National Center for Complementary and Alternative Medicine. (2007). *Get the facts: St. John's wort and depression.* Retrieved June 13, 2008, from http://nccam.nih.gov/health/stjohnswort/sjwataglance.htm

National Education Association Health Information Network. (n.d.). *Clinical depression factsheet.* Retrieved June 11, 2008, from http://www.neahin.org/resources/Images/docs/Clinical_Depression_Fact.pdf

Price, L. H., Tyrka, A. R., Henry, C., Demotes-Mainard, J., Leboyer, M., El-Mallakh, R. S., et al. (2007). Adjunctive antidepressant treatment for bipolar depression. *New England Journal of Medicine, 357,* 614–615.

Sadock, V., & Sadock, B. R. (2003). *Kaplan & Sadock's concise textbook of clinical psychiatry* (2nd ed.). Washington, DC: American Psychiatric Press.

Shaw, D., Fernandes, J., & Rao, C. (2005). Suicide in children and adolescents: A 10-year retrospective review. *American Journal of Forensic Medicine and Pathology, 26*(4), 309–315.

Simon, G. E., & Savarino, J. (2007). Suicide attempts among patients starting depression treatment with medications or psychotherapy. *American Journal of Psychiatry, 164,* 1029–1034.

Spector, R. (2004). *Cultural diversity in health and illness* (6th ed.). Upper Saddle River, NJ. Pearson Education.

Strakowski, S. M. (2007). Approaching the challenge of bipolar depression: Results from STEP-BD. *American Journal of Psychiatry, 164,* 1301–1303.

Tishler, C., Reiss, N., & Rhodes, A. (2007). Suicidal behavior in children younger than twelve: A diagnostic challenge for emergency department personnel. *Academic Emergency Medicine Journal, 14*(9), 810–818.

U.S. Food and Drug Administration. (2004). *FDA launches a multi-pronged strategy to strengthen safeguards for children treated with antidepressant medications* (FDA Publication No. P04-97). Washington, DC: U.S. Government Printing Office.

U.S. Food and Drug Administration Center for Drug Evaluation and Research. (2006). *Clinical review: Relationship between antidepressant drugs and suicidality in adults.* Retrieved November 1, 2007, from http://www.fda.gov/ohrms/dockets/ac/06/briefing/2006-4272b1-01-FDA.pdf

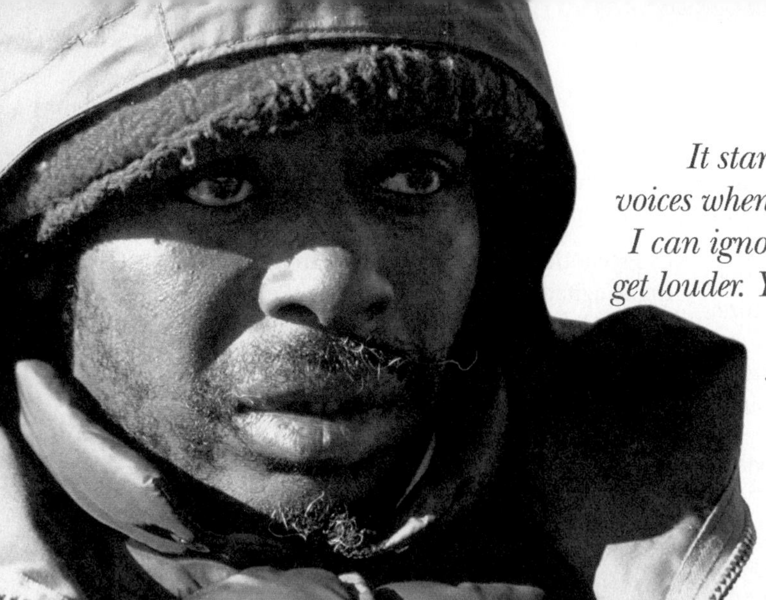

It started when I was a teenager. I hear voices when there is nobody there. Sometimes, I can ignore them, but other times the voices get louder. You have to watch out because the neighbors may try to steal your soul. You can't let that happen to you. That's not going to happen to me. Don't let it happen to you.

Patient "George Watkins"

CHAPTER 24

Pharmacotherapy of Psychoses

Chapter Outline

Characteristics of Psychoses

Symptoms of Schizophrenia

Etiology of Schizophrenia

Management of Psychoses

Antipsychotic Drugs

First-Generation Antipsychotics

PROTOTYPE **Chlorpromazine** *p. 333*

PROTOTYPE **Haloperidol (Haldol)** *p. 335*

Second-Generation (Atypical) Antipsychotics

PROTOTYPE **Risperidone (Risperdal)** *p. 336*

Dopamine System Stabilizer (DSS)

PROTOTYPE **Aripiprazole (Abilify)** *p. 340*

Learning Outcomes

After reading this chapter, the student should be able to:

1. Describe the general symptoms of psychosis.
2. Compare and contrast the positive and negative symptoms of schizophrenia.
3. Explain theories for the etiology of schizophrenia.
4. Describe the initial and maintenance pharmacotherapy of schizophrenia.
5. Explain the importance of patient drug adherence in the pharmacotherapy of psychoses.
6. Explain how antipsychotic drugs are classified.
7. Discuss the rationale for selecting a specific antipsychotic drug for the treatment of schizophrenia.
8. Identify the symptoms associated with the extrapyramidal symptoms of antipsychotic drugs.
9. Describe the nurse's role in the pharmacologic management of schizophrenia.
10. For each of the classes shown in the chapter outline, identify the prototype and representative drugs and explain the mechanism(s) of drug action, primary indications, contraindications, significant drug interactions, pregnancy category, and important adverse effects.
11. Use the nursing process to care for patients receiving drug therapy for psychosis.

Key Terms

acute dystonia, *331*
akathisia, *331*
basal ganglia, *328*
basal nuclei, *328*
delusions, *326*
dopamine system stabilizers (DSS), *340*
dopamine type 2 (D_2) receptors, *328*
extrapyramidal symptoms (EPS), *331*
hallucinations, *326*
negative symptoms, *327*
neuroleptic malignant syndrome (NMS), *332*
parkinsonism, *331*
positive symptoms, *327*
psychosis, *326*
schizoaffective disorder, *327*
schizophrenia, *326*
tardive dyskinesia (TD), *331*

Severe mental illness can be incapacitating for the patient and intensely frustrating for caregivers and those dealing with the patient on a regular basis. Schizophrenia, the most common of the severe psychotic disorders, has been misdiagnosed, misunderstood, and mysterious, according to Vaughan (2004). Vaughan went on to say that treatment of schizophrenia has been challenging to patients and health care providers because of the often severe adverse effects of the antipsychotic drugs used to treat it. This chapter examines the nature of psychotic illness and the pharmacotherapy currently utilized to treat this illness.

Characteristics of Psychoses

24.1 Psychoses are severe mental disorders characterized by the inability to recognize reality.

Psychosis is a general term used in medicine to describe a loss of contact with reality. A psychosis is a symptom of a mental illness and is not considered a disease in itself. Characteristics of psychosis are relatively easy to recognize and include the following:

- Delusions. **Delusions** are firm ideas and beliefs that are false and not founded in reality. Delusions sometimes are religious in nature, with the individual believing he is Jesus, or a messenger sent from God. Delusions may be grandiose, with the person believing he is a king or great leader. Some patients with psychosis exhibit paranoid delusions, an extreme suspicion that they are being followed, and that others are trying to harm them.
- Hallucinations. **Hallucinations** involve seeing, hearing, or feeling something that is not really there. Hallucinations most often are auditory; patients may hear voices telling them to harm themselves or others, that they are worthless or ugly, or that their behavior is unacceptable. Some patients may have visual hallucinations, seeing persons or objects that are not present.
- Lack of insight and judgment. Patients are often unaware of their bizarre behavior and truly believe that the voices they hear and the delusions they experience are real. Some patients have normal insight and do understand that their experiences are not based on reality.
- Mood and affect. During psychotic episodes, the patient's mood and affect may vary widely and be inappropriate. The patient may laugh at sad events or show no emotion at all. The patient may rapidly shift between happy and sad moods for no apparent reason.

Psychotic behavior may range from total inactivity to extreme agitation and combativeness. Because patients are unable to distinguish what is real from what is illusion, they are often labeled as insane.

Psychoses may be classified as acute or chronic. Acute psychotic episodes occur over hours or days, whereas chronic psychoses develop over months or years. Sometimes a specific cause may be attributed to the psychosis, such as brain tumors, overdoses of certain medications, extreme depression, electrolyte disorders, chronic alcoholism, or psychoactive drugs (see Chapter 8). Treating the underlying disorder may cause the psychosis to disappear.

Unfortunately, the vast majority of psychoses have no identifiable cause. These include psychoses associated with schizophrenia, bipolar disorder, and severe clinical depression.

PharmFACT

Approximately 3 million Americans have schizophrenia. The probability of developing schizophrenia is 1 in 100 for the general population. *Source:* Gerstein, 2007.

Prior to the 1950s, patients with severe mental illness were institutionalized as soon as symptoms appeared and often remained that way for their entire lives, with little or no hope of ever improving to the point of being able to function in society. The introduction of chlorpromazine (Thorazine) in the 1950s, and the subsequent development of newer agents, revolutionized the treatment of mental illness. Many people with schizophrenia and other serious mental illnesses can now lead normal or near-normal lives as functioning members of society, as long as their health care provider successfully manages their condition.

To function in society, patients with chronic psychoses require long-term pharmacotherapy. Patients must see their health care provider at regular intervals, and medication must be taken for life. Family members and social support groups are important sources of help for patients who cannot function normally in society without continuous drug therapy. One major difficulty is that family relationships may be fractured secondary to the symptoms of psychosis, the length of time symptoms have been evident, and the tendency for the patients to become nonadherent to drug therapy. If these patients stop taking the antipsychotic medications, then symptoms of psychosis will most assuredly promptly reappear.

Symptoms of Schizophrenia

24.2 Schizophrenia, the most common psychosis, has both positive and negative symptoms.

Schizophrenia is the most common psychotic disorder, affecting 1% to 2% of the population. Symptoms generally begin to appear in early adulthood, with a peak incidence in men

TABLE 24.1 Common Symptoms of Schizophrenia

Mental Symptoms	Behavioral Symptoms	Interpersonal Symptoms
Hallucinations	Strange behavior, such as communicating in rambling statements or made-up words	Marked withdrawal from social interactions and interpersonal relationships
Delusions	Rapid alternation between extreme hyperactivity and stupor	
Illusions	Strange or irrational actions Deterioration of personal hygiene and job or academic performance	Stopping attendance at work or school
Paranoia	Constant hypervigilance, worry, and vocalizations that everyone is "out to get me"	Obvious lack of trust in anyone, even those persons with whom the patient has a positive relationship when disease is under control
Attitude of indifference or detachment toward life activities	Not appearing to care if someone else (or self) is in danger; not moving to help in a crisis situation; not moving self out of harm's way	Showing a complete lack of concern for self or another's well-being or even safety

15 to 24 years of age and women 25 to 34 years of age. It is present in all cultures and ethnic groups.

Patients with schizophrenia experience a variety of diverse symptoms that may change over time. The disorder is characterized by abnormal thoughts and thought processes, disordered communication, withdrawal from people and the outside environment, an inability to independently perform activities of daily living (ADLs), and a high risk for suicide. Patients have a marked impairment in their ability to work or attend school. Many people with schizophrenia demonstrate all of these symptoms at some time during their illness, whereas others exhibit only one or two. Several subtypes of schizophrenia have been identified based on clinical presentation. Table 24.1 gives examples of symptoms frequently observed in patients with schizophrenia.

Symptoms of schizophrenia are classified as either positive or negative. **Positive symptoms** are those associated with an excess or distortion of normal function. These include hallucinations, delusions, disorganized thought or speech pattern, and movement disorders. **Negative symptoms** are those associated with a loss of normal functioning. These symptoms include a lack of interest in social activities, reduced or repetitious speech, loss of desire to perform personal hygiene measures, lack of emotion, unresponsiveness, or lack of pleasure in daily activities. Negative symptoms are characteristic of the indifferent personality exhibited by many patients with schizophrenia. Negative symptoms are harder to associate with schizophrenia and may be mistaken for depression or even laziness. Table 24.2 lists the different categories of schizophrenia symptoms.

Proper diagnosis of positive and negative symptoms is important for selection of the appropriate antipsychotic drug. Positive symptoms are easily recognized and more likely to motivate the patient or caregiver to seek treatment. Indeed, the positive symptoms respond more favorably to pharmacotherapy with antipsychotic drugs. The negative symptoms, however, often prevent a patient with schizophrenia from living independently, holding down a job, and enjoying life. When selecting outcomes for pharmacotherapy, the health care provider must address both positive and negative symptoms (see Table 24.2).

A third and more recently recognized category of symptoms exhibited during schizophrenia is called cognitive symptoms. These include thinking difficulties, decreased attentiveness or ability to concentrate, and significant learning and memory problems. A retrospective look at the patient diagnosed with schizophrenia will usually discover that these cognitive symptoms were present for some time but were not recognized as part of schizophrenia until the more obvious positive and negative symptoms appeared.

Schizoaffective disorder is a condition in which the patient exhibits symptoms of both schizophrenia and mood disorder. An

MyNursingKit | Schizophrenia: Hallucinations Video

TABLE 24.2 Categories of Symptoms of Schizophrenia

Positive Symptoms	Negative Symptoms	Cognitive Symptoms
Hallucinations	Apathy	Deficits in long-term memory
Delusions	Withdrawal from other persons and the social environment	Inability to focus attention
Illusions	Lack of ability to perform ADLs	Disorganized thoughts
Paranoia	Diminished or missing affect	Difficulty following instructions
Agitation, anxiety	Poor judgment	Difficulty following the thread of a conversation
Disorganized thoughts and speech	Lack of awareness or insight	
Aggressiveness, combativeness	Little or no functional speech	

acute schizoaffective reaction may include distorted perceptions, hallucinations, and delusions, followed by extreme depression. Over time both positive and negative psychotic symptoms usually appear.

Many conditions can cause bizarre behavior, and these should be distinguished from schizophrenia. Chronic use of amphetamines or cocaine can create a paranoid syndrome. Certain complex partial seizures can cause unusual symptoms that are sometimes mistaken for psychosis (see Chapter 26). Brain neoplasms, infections, or hemorrhage can also cause bizarre, psychotic-like symptoms.

MyNursingKit | Schizophrenia: Hearing Voices Video

Etiology of Schizophrenia

24.3 The precise etiology of schizophrenia remains unknown.

The cause of schizophrenia has not been determined, although several theories have been proposed. The etiology and pathogenesis is complex and likely involves multiple factors. Schizophrenia is best understood as a cluster of distinct disorders, each having a different etiology rather than as a single disease.

Early theories of the etiology of schizophrenia focused on specific disturbances in child rearing, such as poor communication between parents and offspring with schizophrenia. This view has been rejected in favor of biologic theories. It should be understood, however, that environmental factors such as family dynamics can affect coping skills, which can influence the onset of psychosis, drug response, and adherence with treatment.

There is a definite genetic component to schizophrenia. People have 5 to 10 times greater risk of getting schizophrenia if they have a first-degree relative with the disorder. In identical twins, if one twin has schizophrenia, the other has nearly a 50% risk of having the disorder. If both parents have schizophrenia, there is a 40% risk that their offspring will have the disorder.

Whether caused by genetics or the environment, schizophrenia is likely the result of neurotransmitter imbalances in specific areas of the brain. This theory suggests the possibility of overactive dopaminergic pathways in the **basal nuclei (basal ganglia),** an area of the brain responsible for starting and stopping synchronized motor activity such as leg and arm motions during walking. Symptoms of schizophrenia seem to be associated with **dopamine type 2 (D_2) receptors.** The basal nuclei are particularly rich in D_2 receptors, whereas the cerebrum contains very few. Most antipsychotic drugs act by entering dopaminergic synapses and competing with dopamine for receptors. By blocking D_2 receptors, antipsychotic drugs reduce the symptoms of schizophrenia. Pharmacotherapy Illustrated 24.1 shows antipsychotic drug action at the dopaminergic receptor.

PharmFACT

Schizophrenia occurs with approximately equal frequency in men and women. The disease symptoms usually start earlier in men, and men experience more negative symptoms than women. *Source:* Internet Mental Health, 2008.

Management of Psychoses

24.4 Medical management of psychosis is challenging because patients often lack insight into their disease and believe their behavior is normal.

The medical management of severe mental illness is extremely challenging. Many patients do not view their behavior as abnormal and have difficulty understanding the need for drug therapy. When a medication produces undesirable adverse effects, such as severe muscle twitching or sexual dysfunction, patients stop taking it and relapse to experience their former symptoms. Agitation, distrust, and extreme frustration are common because patients cannot comprehend why others are unable to think as they do or see the same things that they see.

The primary goal in treating psychosis is to manage symptoms such that the patient can function independently and accomplish ADLs with minimum assistance. This includes obtaining and holding employment and maintaining satisfactory interpersonal relationships. This level of success in treatment requires setting many small, realistic benchmarks that the patient, caregiver, and health care provider can achieve. These subgoals nearly always involve pharmacotherapy as well as establishing effective psychological and social support.

Initial treatment: The first psychotic episode may occur suddenly or it may be preceded by a long period of subacute symptoms such as depression or withdrawal from normal activities. If the patient is exhibiting agitation or aggressiveness or presenting a physical danger to others, the first doses of the antipsychotic drug may be higher than normal. High doses produce sedation, which is normally viewed as an adverse effect but which is therapeutic in combative patients. Although most antipsychotics are given orally (PO), a few are available by the intramuscular (IM) route if the patient is uncooperative or if it is suspected that the patient is "cheeking" the medicine—hiding it in the mouth until the nurse leaves the room. Benzodiazepines such as lorazepam (Ativan) may be administered IM during the initial treatment period to relax or provide sedation for agitated patients. Lorazepam produces fewer serious adverse effects than antipsychotic agents and allows the dose of the antipsychotic drug to be reduced. Acute symptoms usually resolve in 3 to 7 days, at which time the patient is switched to maintenance therapy.

Maintenance treatment: The pharmacotherapy of psychosis is a long-term process, with symptoms resolving gradually. Some symptoms resolve faster than others, depending on the patient and specific drug used. A patient or caregiver may notice improvement in acute symptoms after less than a week of therapy. After 2 to 4 weeks, there is usually improvement in mood, socialization, and the ability to provide self-care. By 6 to 8 weeks, definite improvement should be noted in most symptoms. Patients who have experienced untreated schizophrenia for many years are slower to respond than those experiencing their first episode. As long as symptoms continue to gradually improve, the patient is maintained on a stable dosage.

If substantial improvement is not observed after 8 to 12 weeks of therapy, the health care provider must explore reasons for the

PHARMACOTHERAPY ILLUSTRATED 24.1

Mechanism of Action of Antipsychotic Drugs

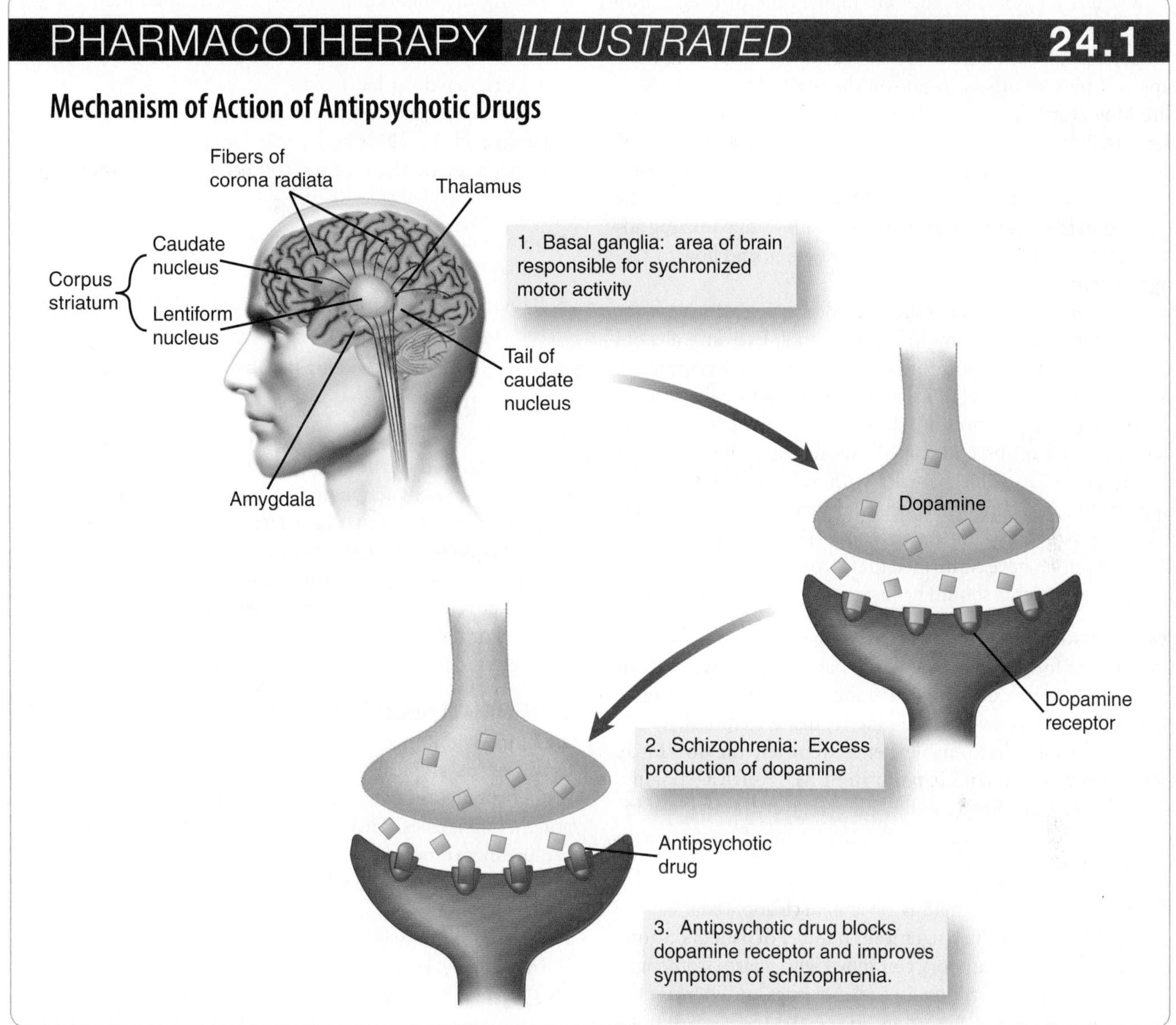

lack of response. For example, the patient may not be taking the medication, or the original diagnosis may have been incorrect. If the patient has been taking the medication at average doses or higher, the health care provider will generally not increase the dose because doing so increases the potential for serious adverse effects. Instead of increasing dosage, a different antipsychotic drug may be substituted. The nurse, patient, and caregivers must understand that drug therapy is not a cure; in some cases, medications simply will not eliminate all psychotic symptoms.

How long does drug maintenance therapy continue? The answer to this is highly individualized, but the most common answer is for the lifetime of the patient. In patients experiencing their first acute episode, health care providers may slowly taper the dose after a year of successful therapy. Abrupt cessation of some antipsychotics can cause serious withdrawal symptoms, including nightmares, nausea, vomiting, salivation, sweating, and nervousness. When discontinuation is attempted, the patient should be monitored carefully and the drug restarted at the first sign of relapse. Approximately 15% to 25% of patients with psychoses can successfully stop drug therapy without returning to their former symptoms. Discontinuation is not usually attempted in patients with long-standing chronic psychosis.

Nonadherence: Patients with serious mental illness have a very high nonadherence rate. Unless they are deemed overtly dangerous to themselves or other people, patients cannot be held for long periods of hospitalization against their wishes. Once the patient returns to the community he or she may discontinue taking the drug and not return for follow-up appointments.

Reasons for nonadherence are many. Lack of insight into their illness causes patients with psychosis to view their behavior as normal. Patients with paranoia may feel that drug therapy is a plot by others to poison them and keep them from thinking clearly. Adverse effects are common and sometimes serious. Even motivated patients who understand the need for continuous drug therapy may have difficulty tolerating the adverse effects. The nurse member of the treatment team must be diligent in teaching caregivers about means of maximizing adherence to the pharmacotherapeutic regimen and how to recognize signs of nonadherence.

Another factor causing nonadherence with medications for schizophrenia is the desire to drink alcohol. Excessive alcohol use is considered a comorbid condition with schizophrenia. Some patients use alcohol in an attempt to elevate their mood or to decrease symptoms of schizophrenia. Alcohol can interact with some antipsychotic medications and cause a suboptimal response. In some patients with schizophrenia, alcohol appears to cause euphoric effects and patients may exhibit increased positive psychotic symptoms (D'Souza et al., 2006). Because studies have confirmed that alcohol worsens psychotic symptoms, patients should be instructed to avoid alcohol use.

MyNursingKit | National Association of Mental Illness

Nonpharmacologic therapies: Psychotherapy is an essential component for the total care of the patient with psychosis. In addition to individual supportive therapy, occupational therapy is initiated to give patients the requisite technical, social, and behavioral skills to enable them to return to the workforce. Some patients need skills in performing ADLs such as cooking, cleaning, and dressing. Family and caregiver training are included in the plan of care for the treatment of patients with schizophrenia whenever feasible.

Prognosis: Although there is no cure, schizophrenia can be successfully managed in a significant number of patients. Strong family and caregiver support, combined with pharmacotherapy, can decrease hospitalization and relapse rates and increase the potential for recovery. According to the World Fellowship for Schizophrenia and Allied Disorders (2007) the prognosis for schizophrenia after 10 years of the disease is as follows:

- 25% completely recovered
- 25% much improved, relatively independent
- 25% improved, but require extensive support network
- 15% hospitalized, unimproved
- 10% deceased (mostly suicide)

Antipsychotic Drugs

24.5 Selection of an antipsychotic drug depends on its spectrum of adverse effects and the experience of the health care provider.

The pharmacotherapy of psychosis has undergone two major "generations." The first generation appeared in the early 1950s when the original drugs for treating severe mental illnesses were discovered. These drugs include conventional antipsychotics such as chlorpromazine. This essentially ended the era of placing all patients in insane asylums for their lifetimes. Unfortunately, first-generation drugs came with adverse effects that were sometimes as serious as the symptoms of the patient's original disorder.

The second-generation or atypical antipsychotic agents were discovered in the 1970s and 1980s. "Atypical" refers to several characteristics of these drugs compared to the conventional agents.

- Significantly fewer adverse effects related to the extrapyramidal system
- Better patient adherence due to reduced adverse effects and less cognitive impairment
- More effective at resolving negative psychotic symptoms

Two older terms are occasionally used to describe antipsychotic drugs. *Major tranquilizer* was the term used following the introduction of the first-generation agents because sedation is a prominent action of these agents. *Neuroleptic* is a term used to denote drugs that have effects on the nervous system, especially those that have parkinson-like adverse effects on posture and body movement. Although the student will still encounter reference sources that refer to these drugs as tranquilizers or neuroleptics, *antipsychotic* is more accurate and is the preferred term.

Classification of antipsychotics: There are two means of classifying antipsychotic medications. The older system uses the conventional versus atypical distinction. The conventional group is further subdivided by chemical classes into phenothiazines and nonphenothiazines. This older classification scheme has flaws because there is not always a clear distinction between a drug that is "conventional" and one that is "atypical." Furthermore, some antipsychotics have an adverse effect profile that appears as if it is atypical at low doses but becomes conventional at high doses.

In recent years, a new system for classification has emerged. This system divides these agents by potency levels: low potency (drugs that require higher doses), moderate potency (drugs that require middle range dosing), and high potency (drugs able to control symptoms of schizophrenia with low doses). This categorization was made based on the amount of medication necessary to produce an equivalent effect as compared to other drugs in the same category. As an example, 100 mg of chlorpromazine is approximately equivalent to 2 mg of haloperidol (Haldol). According to the categories, haloperidol is a high-potency drug, whereas chlorpromazine is a low-potency drug (although both are conventional antipsychotics). The nurse must not confuse potency with efficacy or effectiveness. Potency refers to a quantity, whereas efficacy refers to therapeutic response. Unfortunately, the potency classification method does not give any indication of a drug's effectiveness, mechanism of action, or chemical class.

So for the antipsychotic drugs, which classification should the student learn and use? Because the conventional and atypical and potency methods of drug classification are used in clinical practice, the student must be aware of both schemes.

Drug selection: In terms of effectiveness, there is no single drug of choice for the long-term therapy of schizophrenia. Selection of a specific drug is based on clinician experience, the occurrence of adverse effects, and the therapeutic response of each individual patient. For example, patients with psychosis and Parkinson's disease need an antipsychotic with minimal extrapyramidal symptoms. Those who operate machinery need a drug that does not cause sedation. Men who are sexually active may adhere better to a regimen with a drug that does not cause sexual dysfunction.

Clearly, the second-generation atypical antipsychotics result in lower incidence of serious adverse effects and have become drugs of choice for many patients. They are also considerably more expensive. The experience and skills of the health care provider and mental health nurse are particularly valuable in achieving successful psychiatric pharmacotherapy.

CONNECTION *Checkpoint* 24.1

From what you learned in Chapter 5, explain why it is more important to receive an antipsychotic drug that has greater effectiveness versus one that has higher potency. See Answer to Connection Checkpoint 24.1 in Appendix A.

Managing adverse effects: From a pharmacologic perspective, antipsychotic drug therapy has both a positive and a negative effect. Although many symptoms of psychosis can be controlled with drugs, adverse effects are common and often serious.

Extrapyramidal symptoms (EPS) are a particularly serious set of adverse reactions to antipsychotic drugs. The term *extrapyramidal* refers to locations in the central nervous system (CNS) outside the cerebrospinal pyramidal tracts of the brain. Whereas the pyramidal system controls visible, voluntary movements, the extrapyramidal system is associated with postural and automatic movements that are not usually noticeable. EPS include the following:

- **Acute dystonia** occurs early in the course of pharmacotherapy with antipsychotics and involves severe muscle spasms, particularly of the back, neck, tongue, and face. In rare cases, acute dystonia can be so severe as to dislocate joints and impair respiration due to laryngospasm. The risk of acute dystonia is greater with high-potency antipsychotics. Administration of anticholinergic drugs such as biperiden (Akineton) or procyclidine (Kemadrin) or an antihistamine such as diphenhydramine or benztropine can reverse acute dystonia symptoms within minutes when administered parenterally.
- **Akathisia,** the most common EPS, is an inability to rest or relax. The patient paces, has trouble sitting or remaining still, and has difficulty sleeping. Repetitive movements such as rocking while standing or sitting and crossing and uncrossing legs may be evident. Beta-adrenergic blockers such as propranolol (Inderal) and benzodiazepines have been treatments of choice for akathisia.
- **Parkinsonism** induced by antipsychotic drugs may include tremor, loss of fine motor skills, muscle rigidity, stooped posture, and a shuffling gait. The treatment of antipsychotic drug-induced parkinsonism includes anticholinergic drugs and amantadine (Symmetrel) (see Chapter 25).
- **Tardive dyskinesia (TD)** is characterized by involuntary, unusual tongue and face movements such as lip smacking, rapid eye blinking, and wormlike motions of the tongue. They generally occur during long-term therapy, and symptoms may persist for months or years after the drug is discontinued. In fact, symptoms of TD may worsen when the antipsychotic drug is withdrawn. Because there are no established medicines to treat TD, the best approach is prevention.

When EPS are reported early, the drug is withdrawn or the dosage reduced, and the symptoms can be reversible. With higher doses given for prolonged periods, EPS symptoms may become permanent. The nurse must be vigilant in observing and reporting EPS, because prevention is the best treatment. Table 24.3 contains further information on the EPS of antipsychotic medications.

MyNursingKit Extrapyramidal Side Effects Video

MyNursingKit Tardive Dyskinesia Videos

TABLE 24.3 Extrapyramidal Symptoms of Antipsychotic Medications

Type of Symptom	Time of Onset	Manifestations	Treatment
Acute Dystonia	Several hours to 5 days	Severe spasms of the muscles of the tongue, face, neck, or back; involuntary upward deviation of the eyes; arching forward of the trunk while the head and legs are thrust backward	Immediately administer an anticholinergic such as diphenhydramine or benztropine IV or IM. Symptoms usually resolve within 5–20 min.
Akathisia	Within first 2 months of treatment	Pacing, squirming, inability to sit still, uncontrollable need to be moving	Anticholinergics (Benadryl, etc.), benzodiazepines (diazepam or alprazolam, etc.), or beta blockers (atenolol, labetalol, etc.).
Antipsychotic-Induced Parkinsonism	5–30 days	Tremor, rigidity, shuffling gait, masklike facies, drooling, cogwheeling, stooped posture, bradykinesia. Symptoms cannot be distinguished from true Parkinson's disease.	Anticholinergics (benztropine, diphenhydramine, etc.), amantadine. Treatment should not need to be continued for more than a few months, because symptoms should resolve.
Tardive Dyskinesia	During long-term therapy	Involuntary, unusual movements of the tongue and face, lip-smacking movements; later may be involuntary movements of the arms and legs, fingers, toes, and trunk.	For some patients, there is nothing that can be done. For some patients, decreased doses of antipsychotics, administration of benzodiazepines, or gradual withdrawal of anticholinergics may help. Some patients may benefit from switching to an atypical antipsychotic.

A potentially fatal adverse reaction to antipsychotic medications is **neuroleptic malignant syndrome (NMS).** Symptoms include high fever, diaphoresis, muscle rigidity, tachycardia, and blood pressure fluctuations. Although rare, without quick, aggressive treatment the condition can rapidly deteriorate to stupor or coma. Treatment includes antipyretics, electrolytes, and muscle relaxants.

Adverse effects on the reproductive system are a major cause of nonadherence to the drug regimen in some patients. Up to 50% to 60% of men taking antipsychotics may experience ejaculation and erectile dysfunction. In women, decreased libido and inability to reach orgasm may occur. Many antipsychotics increase serum levels of the hormone prolactin, which can cause secretion of breast milk (galactorrhea) and breast enlargement (gynecomastia). These events may occur in both men and women. Most women will also experience menstrual dysfunction due to the high prolactin levels.

Unlike many CNS drugs, antipsychotic medications do not cause physical or psychological dependence. They also have a wide safety margin between a therapeutic and a lethal dose; deaths due to overdoses of antipsychotic drugs are uncommon. They should be gradually discontinued, however, to avoid withdrawal symptoms.

First-Generation Antipsychotics

24.6 The phenothiazines are effective at treating schizophrenia symptoms but exhibit a high incidence of adverse effects.

The first-generation or conventional antipsychotics are classified as phenothiazines or nonphenothiazines (see Section 24.7). *Phenothiazine* is a chemical term that refers to compounds with three rings that are joined together by nitrogen and sulfur atoms. Originally developed as a yellow dye in the 1800s, phenothiazine became the starting molecule for a series of drugs, which are recognized by the "–zine" suffix. The student will encounter the term *phenothiazine* in other chapters because several drug classes produce "phenothiazine-like" adverse effects. The phenothiazine agents are listed in Table 24.4.

At equivalent doses, all phenothiazines have the same effectiveness in treating psychoses, and all produce a similar spectrum of adverse effects. Selection of a specific phenothiazine is determined by the severity and extent of expected adverse effects. For example, if EPS are a major concern, thioridazine may be selected because it gives the lowest incidence of EPS in the class. If the patient is driving or working, fluphenazine may

TABLE 24.4 First-Generation Antipsychotic Drugs

Drug	Route(s) and Adult Dose (maximum dose where indicated)	Adverse Effects
Phenothiazines		
chlorpromazine	PO: Hydrochloride: 25–100 mg tid or qid (max: 1,000 mg/day) IM/IV: 25–50 mg (max: 600 mg every 4–6 h) Subcutaneous/IM: Decanoate12.5–25 mg every 1 to 4 weeks	*Sedation, drowsiness, dizziness, EPS, constipation, photosensitivity, orthostatic hypotension, anticholinergic effects, seizures* <u>agranulocytosis, pancytopenia, anaphylaxis, TD, NMS, hypothermia, adynamic ileus, sudden unexplained death</u>
fluphenazine	PO: 0.5–10 mg/day in one to four divided doses (max: 20 mg/day)	
perphenazine	PO: 4–16 mg bid to qid (max: 64 mg/day)	
prochlorperazine	PO: 5–10 mg tid or qid IM: 10–20 mg initially, may repeat every 1–4 h	
thioridazine (Mellaril)	PO: 50–100 mg tid (max: 800 mg/day)	
trifluoperazine	PO: 1–2 mg bid (max: 20 mg/day)	
Nonphenothiazines		
haloperidol (Haldol)	PO: 0.2–5 mg bid or tid IM: 2–5 mg every 4 h prn	*Akathisia, sedation, transient drowsiness, EPS, tremor, orthostatic hypotension, weight changes, anticholinergic effects* <u>TD, NMS, acute renal failure, respiratory depression, laryngospasm, hepatotoxicity, sudden unexplained death, agranulocytosis</u>
loxapine (Loxitane)	PO: start with 20 mg/day and rapidly increase to 60–100 mg/day in divided doses (max: 250 mg/day)	
molindone (Moban)	PO: 50–75 mg/day in three to four divided doses (max: 225 mg/day)	
pimozide (Orap)	PO: 1–2 mg/day (max: 10 mg/day)	
thiothixene (Navane)	PO: 2 mg tid (max: 60 mg/day)	

Note: *Italics* indicate common adverse effects. <u>Underline</u> indicates serious adverse effects.

be selected because it produces less sedation and fewer anticholinergic effects than other phenothiazines.

It should be clearly understood at the outset of conventional antipsychotic therapy that it is not always possible to control the disabling symptoms of schizophrenia without producing some degree of EPS or anticholinergic adverse effects. Adjunct drug therapy may be warranted to treat expected adverse effects. For example, concurrent pharmacotherapy with an anticholinergic drug (see Chapter 18) may prevent some of the EPS. For acute dystonias, benztropine (Cogentin) may be given parenterally. Levodopa (Dopar, Larodopa) is usually avoided because its ability to increase dopamine function antagonizes the mechanism of action of the phenothiazines. Beta-adrenergic blockers and benzodiazepines are sometimes given to reduce signs of akathisia.

Some phenothiazines have indications beyond psychiatry. These indications include:

- **Nausea and vomiting.** The phenothiazines reduce nausea and vomiting by blocking dopamine receptors in the chemoreceptor trigger zone in the medulla. They are most often used for treating the severe nausea and vomiting associated with cancer chemotherapy.
- **Tourette's syndrome.** This condition is characterized by tics: sudden, loud vocalizations, often cursing, and muscle movements such as twitches, kicking, or hitting. The patient feels a premonitory urge, a type of warning, that a tic is forthcoming, and the tics may be consciously suppressed for limited periods. Drugs from a large number of classes have been used to suppress tics, including phenothiazines. There is no cure for Tourette's syndrome.
- **Organic brain syndrome (OBS).** *OBS* is a general term that refers to decreased mental function due to physical disorders rather than psychiatric disorders. OBS can cause symptoms similar to those of schizophrenia, including delirium, amnesia, and agitation. OBS is a common diagnosis in elderly patients and is associated with a large number of conditions, including head trauma, brain tumors, cerebrovascular accident (CVA), shock, drug interactions, adverse effects, and renal or hepatic failure. Chronic OBS is known as dementia. Although historically the phenothiazines were the drugs of choice for treating symptoms of OBS, haloperidol and second-generation antipsychotics are more commonly prescribed.

PROTOTYPE DRUG Chlorpromazine

Classification: Therapeutic: Antipsychotic (first generation)
Pharmacologic: Phenothiazine, dopamine antagonist

Therapeutic Effects and Uses: Approved in 1954, chlorpromazine is a low-potency antipsychotic that blocks several types of receptors within and outside the CNS, including dopamine, histamine, norepinephrine, and acetylcholine receptors. The therapeutic effects in a patient with schizophrenia appear to be due to the blocking of dopamine receptors. Peak antipsychotic effects may take as long as 6 weeks to several months. IM dosing is available for acutely agitated patients. Thorazine was once a popular brand name for this drug, but chlorpromazine is now only available in generic form.

The major use of chlorpromazine is to treat the symptoms of schizophrenia and other psychotic disorders. The drug can effectively suppress symptoms of acute psychotic episodes and can greatly decrease the incidence of relapse if it is used consistently. Although once widely prescribed for psychosis, chlorpromazine is rarely used today because of the potential for serious adverse effects. Other approved uses for chlorpromazine include treating schizoaffective disorder, the manic phase of bipolar disorder, as an antiemetic, as an adjunct in the treatment of tetanus, and for intractable hiccups. It is important to understand that chlorpromazine, and the other phenothiazines, do not change the underlying pathology of psychotic disease, but rather deal only with the symptoms.

Mechanism of Action: Chlorpromazine acts by blocking postsynaptic dopamine receptors. Decreases in the function of this neurotransmitter are associated with diminished psychotic symptoms. Decreased dopamine in the chemoreceptor trigger zone in the medulla results in an antiemetic effect.

Pharmacokinetics:

Route(s)	PO, rectal, IM, intravenous (IV) (only for severe conditions)
Absorption	Variable PO; well-absorbed IM
Distribution	Widely distributed; crosses the placenta; secreted in breast milk; 92–97% bound to plasma protein
Primary metabolism	Hepatic; some active metabolites
Primary excretion	Renal
Onset of action	½–12 h, depending on route; optimum results will take several months
Duration of action	Half-life: 30 h

Adverse Effects: Common adverse effects of chlorpromazine include headache, anticholinergic symptoms (dry mouth, anorexia, nausea, vomiting, and constipation), weight gain, anemia, phototoxicity, blurred vision, dry eyes, and glaucoma. Of all the antipsychotics, phenothiazines are the most likely to produce EPS. Serious or life-threatening adverse effects include tachycardia, cardiac arrest, laryngospasm, respiratory depression, seizures, agranulocytosis, leukopenia, leukocytosis, and NMS. Abrupt withdrawal can induce symptoms such as nausea, vomiting, and tremors.

Contraindications/Precautions: There are many contraindications to the use of chlorpromazine; these are coronary artery disease, severe hypertension or hypotension, blood dyscrasias, coma, brain damage, bone marrow depression, alcohol or barbiturate withdrawal, glaucoma, hepatic dysfunction, and children under age 6 months. The drug should be used with caution in patients with cardiovascular disease because it may cause orthostatic hypotension (especially in older adults), increase the heart rate, and prolong the QT interval on the electrocardiogram (ECG). Patients with severe hepatic impairment

MyNursingKit | Schizophrenia: When Did It Begin Video

may experience excessive CNS depression. The drug decreases the seizure threshold; thus patients with preexisting epilepsy must be carefully monitored. Chlorpromazine may produce drowsiness and lethargy in breast-feeding newborns; thus use is not recommended during lactation. The elderly are very sensitive to the EPS effects of phenothiazines; thus the drug must be used with caution in this population. Patients with benign prostatic hyperplasia (BPH) should use this drug with caution because it may cause urinary retention.

Drug Interactions: Many drug interactions are possible with chlorpromazine. Use with other CNS depressants, including alcohol, will cause additive sedation. Use with tricyclic antidepressants or anticholinergic drugs will result in additive anticholinergic adverse effects. Decreased absorption and thus lower serum levels of chlorpromazine will occur if used with antacids, barbiturates, or lithium. Increased serum levels and possible hypotension may occur if administered concurrently with epinephrine. Use with warfarin can lead to decreased anticoagulant effects. Phenothiazines inhibit the therapeutic effects of levodopa and may cause excessive sedation if used concurrently. **Herbal/Food**: Increased action of chlorpromazine may occur with nutmeg, hops, nettle, and cola tree. Increased anticholinergic effects can occur with henbane leaf, kava, and betel palm.

Pregnancy: Category C.

Treatment of Overdose: Overdose will cause profound CNS depression, seizures, hypotension, and EPS. Treatment is supportive and may include vasopressors and antiseizure drugs. Airway and gastric lavage are provided if taken orally. Epinephrine should not be administered and vomiting should not be induced.

Nursing Responsibilities:

- Complete a comprehensive health history, including any long-term physical problems (e.g., seizure disorders, cardiovascular or pulmonary disease), medication use, allergies, and lifestyle information such as the use of alcohol, illegal drugs, or caffeine, smoking, or use of herbal preparations.
- Monitor for impaired liver and kidney functions because these may cause drug toxicity.
- Monitor for changes in vision because chlorpromazine accumulates in the eye. There is a risk of blindness as well as other ocular defects such as color blindness from continued use of chlorpromazine.
- Assess for the patient's use of other CNS depressants because they may cause excessive sedation.
- Assess the age of the patient (typical antipsychotics cannot be used in very young children; extra caution must be taken if used by the child or the elderly).
- Monitor for appearance of EPS such as acute dystonia, akathisia, and TD.
- Monitor for signs of NMS such as high fever, fluctuations in blood pressure, and muscle rigidity. Immediately notify the prescriber if these occur.
- Monitor safety of the patient in performing normal ADLs.
- If the patient is a child, assess for hyperexcitability, dehydration, or gastroenteritis as well as chickenpox or measles.

Patient and Family Education:

- Take the drug exactly as prescribed and do not discontinue use without approval of the health care provider.
- Immediately report to the health care provider any of the following: worsening of psychosis symptoms; uncontrollable movements of the eyes, mouth, head, arms, legs; seizure activity; unusual bleeding or bruising; or changes in vision.
- Document on a calendar that each dose has been taken daily.
- Refrain from drinking alcoholic beverages because this may cause excessive drowsiness.
- If excessive drowsiness occurs, take the dose at bedtime.
- Maintain all scheduled follow-up appointments.
- Wear adequate skin protection when exposure to the sun is likely because this drug can sensitize the skin to sunburn.
- Do not drive or perform other hazardous activities until the effects of the drug are known because this drug may cause drowsiness and dizziness.
- Immediately notify the health care provider of any known or suspected pregnancy.

Drugs Similar to Chlorpromazine

Similar drugs include fluphenazine, perphenazine, thioridazine, and trifluoperazine. Mesoridazine (Serentil), thiethylperazine (Torecan), and promazine (Sparine) are first-generation phenothiazines that have been discontinued in the United States. Promethazine (Phenergan) is chemically classified as a phenothiazine but the drug has no antipsychotic action and its primary use is as an antihistamine (see Chapter 74).

Fluphenazine: Approved in 1959, fluphenazine is a high-potency phenothiazine approved to treat psychotic disorders, including schizophrenia. The drug is most often given as fluphenazine decanoate, a newer long-acting depot formulation approved in 1987, that is given either subcutaneously or IM. Administered at 1- to 4-week intervals, fluphenazine decanoate is advantageous for those patients who are not adherent to taking their oral medications daily. Oral and injectable preparations (fluphenazine hydrochloride) are also available. A stable dose of oral fluphenazine is generally achieved before placing the patient on the depot preparation. The injectable preparations are not recommended for children under age 12. Fluphenazine produces less sedation and fewer anticholinergic effects than chlorpromazine, but EPS are a major concern. This drug is pregnancy category C.

Perphenazine: Approved in 1959, perphenazine is a medium-potency agent used to treat schizophrenia, nausea, and vomiting. EPS are prominent. The drug has the same actions and adverse effects as chlorpromazine. This drug is pregnancy category C.

Prochlorperazine: Approved in 1956, prochlorperazine, once marketed as Compazine, is a phenothiazine rarely used as an antipsychotic. Its primary use is for the management of severe nausea and vomiting. For this purpose, it may be administered PO, rectally, IM, or IV. When used as an antiemetic doses are low and phenothiazine-like adverse effects are rare. Pharmacotherapy with antiemetics is presented in Chapter 61. This drug is pregnancy category C.

Thioridazine (Mellaril): Thioridazine, a low-potency phenothiazine, is approved to treat psychotic disorders, including schizophrenia, behavioral problems in children, major depression, anxiety, organic brain syndrome, dementia in the elderly, or as an adjunct in the treatment of alcohol withdrawal. Because of the possibility of fatal dysrhythmias, thioridazine should be used only to treat conditions that have not responded to safer drugs. Approved in 1959, thioridazine is available PO and has one of the lowest incidences of EPS of the phenothiazines. This drug is pregnancy category C.

Trifluoperazine: Trifluoperazine is a high-potency phenothiazine approved to treat psychotic disorders. Approved in 1958, it is available in oral form. Trifluoperazine causes less sedation than chlorpromazine but EPS is prominent. All other information is the same as with chlorpromazine, except that it cannot be used in children under age 6. Trifluoperazine was formerly available as Stelazine, but this brand name is no longer marketed. This drug is pregnancy category C.

24.7 The nonphenothiazine first-generation antipsychotics have the same therapeutic applications and similar adverse effects as the phenothiazines.

The nonphenothiazine conventional antipsychotic class consists of drugs whose chemical structures are dissimilar to the phenothiazines. Introduced shortly after the phenothiazines, the nonphenothiazines were initially expected to produce fewer serious adverse events. Unfortunately, this is not the case. The spectrum of adverse effects for the nonphenothiazines is identical to that for the phenothiazines, although the degree to which a particular effect occurs depends on the drug utilized.

In general, the nonphenothiazine agents cause less sedation and fewer anticholinergic adverse effects than chlorpromazine but exhibit an equal or greater incidence of EPS. Concurrent therapy with other CNS depressants must be carefully monitored because of potential additive sedation.

Drugs in the nonphenothiazine class have the same therapeutic effects and efficacy as the phenothiazines. They are also believed to act by the same mechanism as the phenothiazines; that is, by blocking postsynaptic D_2 dopamine receptors. As a class, they offer no significant advantages over phenothiazines in the treatment of schizophrenia and have largely been replaced by the second-generation, atypical antipsychotics. Doses of the nonphenothiazine antipsychotics are shown in Table 24.4.

PROTOTYPE DRUG Haloperidol (Haldol)

Classification: **Therapeutic:** Antipsychotic (first generation)
Pharmacologic: Nonphenothiazine, dopamine antagonist

Therapeutic Effects and Uses: Haloperidol, a high-potency antipsychotic approved in 1967, is effective in treating both acute and chronic psychotic disorders. It may also be used off-label to treat Tourette's syndrome, persistent hiccups, autism, children with severe behavioral problems (short term) and organic brain syndrome with psychotic features, and for the emergency sedation of severely agitated or delirious patients. It may be administered PO or IM but should not be given IV.

Haloperidol decanoate (Haldol LA) is a long-acting IM formulation that is administered once a month. This is an excellent formulation for patients who cannot be independent in their drug regimen, who may become nonadherent to the drug regimen, or who have no family members to assist them in taking their medication on a regular basis. The medication can be administered either in a clinic setting or by a home health nurse in the patient's own residence.

Mechanism of Action: Haloperidol depresses the cerebral cortex, hypothalamus, and limbic system, which are parts of the brain controlling activity and aggression. It blocks neurotransmission at postsynaptic dopamine D_2 receptors and exhibits alpha$_1$-adrenergic blocking and anticholinergic effects.

Pharmacokinetics:

Route(s)	PO, IM
Absorption	Variable PO; well-absorbed IM
Distribution	Widely distributed; may cross the placenta; secreted in breast milk and 92% bound to plasma protein
Primary metabolism	Hepatic; significant first-pass metabolism
Primary excretion	Renal; small amounts biliary with extensive enterohepatic recycling
Onset of action	Erratic if given PO; 15–30 minutes IM; decanoate form reaches peak plasma level in 7 days
Duration of action	Half-life: 24 h (PO); 21 h (IM)

Adverse Effects: Haloperidol exhibits an adverse effect profile similar to other first-generation antipsychotics. Common adverse effects include drowsiness and EPS. Life-threatening adverse effects include TD, NMS, agranulocytosis, respiratory depression, and laryngospasm. Like chlorpromazine, thioridazine, and pimozide, haloperidol increases the QT interval and can pose a risk for dysrhythmias.

Contraindications/Precautions: Contraindications for use of haloperidol include Parkinson's disease, seizure disorders, coma, alcoholism, severe mental depression, CNS depression, or lactation. The elderly or debilitated patients, those with urinary retention, glaucoma, or severe cardiovascular disorders must be given haloperidol cautiously. The drug lowers the seizure threshold; thus patients with preexisting epilepsy must be carefully monitored.

Drug Interactions: Haloperidol is metabolized by hepatic CYP enzymes and can inhibit some isozymes (CYP2D6). Thus interactions are possible with other drugs affecting these enzymes. For example, carbamazepine, an inducer of CYP enzymes, can reduce the serum level of haloperidol by up to 50%. Increased CNS depression can occur if given concurrently with other CNS depressants, including alcohol, tricyclic antidepressants, or opioids. Anticholinergics that are given concurrently may increase intraocular pressure. Use with methyldopa may precipitate dementia. Haloperidol may increase the QT interval and should be used with caution with other agents that increase this interval due to the potential for additive cardiotoxicity. A few patients who were taking haloperidol and lithium concurrently experienced irreversible brain damage; thus the two drugs should not be combined. Haloperidol inhibits the therapeutic effects of levodopa and may cause excessive sedation if used concurrently. **Herbal/Food**: Increased action of haloperidol may occur if chamomile, cola tree, hops, kava, nettle, nutmeg, skullcap, or valerian is used concurrently. An antagonist action may occur with the use of scopolia or jimsonweed. Increased EPS may occur if betel palm or kava is used concurrently.

Pregnancy: Category C.

Treatment of Overdose: Overdose will result in sedation, respiratory depression, coma, hypotension, and severe EPS. Treatment is supportive. Antidysrhythmic and vasopressor agents may be necessary to maintain cardiovascular function.

Nursing Responsibilities and Patient and Family Education: The phenothiazine and nonphenothiazine drug classes are both first-generation antipsychotics with very similar pharmacologic actions and adverse effects. The nursing care and teaching for these two drug classes are the same and are shown on page 334.

Drugs Similar to Haloperidol (Haldol)

Similar drugs include loxapine, molindone, pimozide, and thiothixene.

Loxapine (Loxitane): Approved in 1975, loxapine is a medium-potency antipsychotic given by the PO route. It is approved to treat schizophrenia, psychotic depression, and other psychotic disorders, and it is used off-label to treat severe behavioral disturbances associated with Parkinson's and Alzheimer's diseases. Use of loxapine is restricted to treating mental illness refractory to treatment from safer drugs. The adverse effect profile of loxapine is the same as that of haloperidol, and EPS frequently occur during therapy. An active metabolite of loxapine is amoxapine, a drug marketed separately as an antidepressant. This drug is pregnancy category C.

Molindone (Moban): Approved in 1974, molindone is another medium-potency agent that is indicated only for treating schizophrenia. Its high incidence of EPS limits its use. Adverse events and other actions are the same as those of haloperidol. This drug is pregnancy category C.

Pimozide (Orap): Approved in 1984, pimozide is an oral, high-potency antipsychotic medication used for treating motor and vocal tics associated with Tourette's syndrome. It may be used off-label to treat schizophrenia. The drug has little sedative action and should not be used to control acute psychosis characterized by agitation or hyperexcitability. EPS occur frequently with pimozide. Although effective, the drug exhibits a higher degree of cardiotoxicity than others in its class and is thus only used when other therapies fail to achieve their designated outcomes. This drug is pregnancy category C.

CONNECTIONS

Treating the Diverse Patient

Genetic Lack of Enzyme

Many Asian patients have a genetic lack of the enzyme debrisoquine hydroxylase, which is used by the body to metabolize certain antipsychotic agents and antidepressants. These people, sometimes called "poor metabolizers," may have up to 50% higher serum levels of haloperidol and other drugs than Caucasians. It is prudent to reduce the starting dose in Asian patients in order to decrease the chances of serious adverse reactions.

Thiothixene (Navane): Thiothixene, a high-potency antipsychotic, is approved to treat psychotic disorders, including schizophrenia, and acute agitation. Approved in 1967, it is available as an oral preparation and has adverse effects that are characteristic of those of other first-generation antipsychotics. It is not a drug of first choice for psychosis. This drug is pregnancy category C.

Second-Generation (Atypical) Antipsychotics

24.8 Second-generation antipsychotics have become drugs of choice for the treatment of schizophrenia.

The second-generation, or atypical, antipsychotics have become drugs of choice in the pharmacotherapy of severe mental illness. Available since the early 1990s, the members of this group are diverse and have little in common with each other, except that they all cause a lower incidence of adverse effects, especially EPS, than the first-generation drugs.

The exact mechanisms of action of the various second-generation antipsychotics are mostly unknown. It is known that atypical antipsychotics target more specific dopamine receptors than the first-generation agents, which may explain the relatively low incidence of EPS with these drugs. Some inhibit different subtypes of dopamine receptors, D_1 and D_4, which are especially prominent in the limbic system of the brain. Some also inhibit serotonin (5-HT) receptors in the CNS. Like the first-generation drugs, some atypical antipsychotics have prominent anticholinergic adverse effects. Doses of the second-generation antipsychotics are listed in Table 24.5.

PROTOTYPE DRUG Risperidone (Risperdal)

Classification: **Therapeutic:** Antipsychotic (second-generation, atypical)
Pharmacologic: Dopamine antagonist

Therapeutic Effects and Uses: Risperidone is an atypical antipsychotic available for oral or IM use that has become one of the most frequently prescribed drugs in this class. It was initially approved in 1993 to treat negative psychotic symptoms in persons with schizophrenia and related psychoses. In 2003,

TABLE 24.5 Second-Generation (Atypical) Antipsychotics

Drug	Route and Adult Dose (maximum dose where indicated)	Adverse Effects
aripiprazole (Abilify)	PO: 10–15 mg/day (max: 30 mg/day)	*Sedation, headache, akathisia, confusion, insomnia, depression, tachycardia, transient fever, dizziness, light-headedness, anxiety, nervousness, hostility, nausea, vomiting, constipation, parkinsonism, somnolence, dyspepsia, EPS, asthenia, dry mouth, weight gain, tremor, restlessness, sleep disorders* Agranulocytosis (clozapine), NMS, bone marrow suppression, seizures, suicidal tendencies (aripiprazole), TD, diabetes mellitus, ischemia
clozapine (Clozaril)	PO: start at 12.5–25 mg/day and increase 25–50 mg/day every 3–7 days; (max: 900 mg/day)	
olanzapine (Zyprexa)	Adult: PO: start with 5–10 mg/day; may increase by 2.5–5 mg every week (max: 20 mg/day)	
paliperidone (Invega)	PO: 6 mg/day (max: 12 mg/day)	
quetiapine fumarate (Seroquel)	PO: start with 25 mg bid; increase up to 300–400 mg/day in divided doses by day 4; then adjust by 25–100 mg/day every 2 days (max: 800 mg/day)	
risperidone (Risperdal)	PO: start at 1–2 mg/day then, increase by 0.5–1 mg/day every 3–7 days (max: 16 mg/day)	
ziprasidone (Geodon)	PO: 20 mg bid (max: 80 mg bid)	

Note: *Italics* indicate common adverse effects. Underline indicates serious adverse effects.

approved indications were extended to include acute mania associated with bipolar disorder. In 2006, risperidone became the first drug approved to treat irritability associated with autism in pediatric patients. Off-label uses include the pharmacotherapy of Tourette's syndrome, attention deficit/hyperactivity disorder, severely disruptive behavior in children with developmental disabilities, dementia, and psychotic depression. The IM depot form of Risperdal (Risperdal Consta) requires three weeks to produce a therapeutic response: the patient is usually placed on PO antipsychotics during this 3 week period. Subsequent IM injections are administered every two weeks. Risperidone is also available as PO disintegrating tablets (Risperdal M-TAB), which are especially beneficial when treating patients suspected of "cheeking" the drug.

Mechanism of Action: The precise mechanism for risperidone is unknown. It is believed that the drug acts by blocking the binding of dopamine to its receptors in various brain regions. It has highest affinity for type D_2 and has less effect on D_1 receptors. It also blocks 5-HT receptors, alpha$_1$-adrenergic receptors and histaminergic receptors.

Pharmacokinetics:

Route	PO, IM
Absorption	Well absorbed PO; slowly absorbed IM
Distribution	Widely distributed; crosses both the blood-brain and placental barriers; secreted in breast milk; 90% bound to plasma protein
Primary metabolism	Extensive hepatic metabolism by CYP2D6; changed to the active metabolite 9-hydroxyrisperidone
Primary excretion	Renal, with small amounts in feces
Onset of action	Peak action = 1-3 h (optimum antipsychotic effects may take several months)
Duration of action	Half-life = 20 h

Adverse Effects: Adverse effects of risperidone therapy are similar to other atypical antipsychotics. The incidence of anticholinergic adverse effects is low, and the drug does not cause agranulocytosis. GI effects such as drowsiness, nausea, vomiting, constipation and increased salivation are common. Symptoms of parkinsonism may occur in 5% to 10% of patients. Risperidone elevates serum prolactin levels, which can result in galactorrhea, impotence, gynecomastia and menstrual irregularities. Hyperglycemia, including some rare cases of diabetic ketoacidosis has been reported in patients taking this drug. Orthostatic hypotension is common at the initiation of therapy. Excessive weight gain occurs in children taking risperidone. Adverse effects for the PO and IM depot formulations are the same, except the parenteral form may cause pain and local injection site reactions.

Contraindications/Precautions: Hypersensitivity to risperidone is a contraindication. The drug contains a black box warning that it should not be used in elderly patients with dementia-related psychosis due to an increased risk of death. The drug should be used with caution in patients with severe CNS depression, seizures, dysrhythmias, hypotension, diabetic ketoacidosis, and suicidal ideation. Patients with renal impairment should be treated with caution. Use during lactation is contraindicated because the drug and its active metabolite are secreted in breast milk.

Drug Interactions: Risperidine is a substrate for hepatic CYP2D6 enzymes; thus it may interact with drugs that inhibit or induce these enzymes. For example, many of the selective serotonin reuptake inhibitors (SSRIs) inhibit CYP2D6, which reduces the metabolism of risperidone and raises serum drug levels. Concurrent use with alcohol, benzodiazepines or other CNS depressants can cause severe CNS depression. Antihypertensives and nitrates may potentiate hypotension. Decreased risperidone levels may occur with the use of phenobarbital, rifampin, omeprazole, or carbamazepine. Increased risperidone levels may occur with the use of verapamil, azole antifungal

CONNECTIONS

Evidence-Based Practice Weight Gain with Use of Atypical Antipsychotics

Clinical Question

Why might patients be reluctant to, or even refuse to, take one of the atypical antipsychotic medications, even if the health care provider believes that it will help them gain control of the symptoms of schizophrenia more than any other medication?

Evidence

Some patients who take atypical antipsychotic drugs (AAPDs), especially clozapine, olanzapine, and quetiapine, experience substantial weight gain. One patient gained 100 pounds in a short time after beginning an atypical antipsychotic. The weight gain effects do not appear to be related to the medication's therapeutic effects. The study showed that these drugs stimulate the appetite. The study found that clozapine, olanzapine, and quetiapine stimulate hypothalamic AMP-activated protein kinase (AMPK) within brain tissue. Because of this, they are termed orexigenic AAPDs. They act via histamine H_1 receptors and AMPK, an enzyme that is important in maintaining energy homeostasis. The study went on to say that AMPK has been linked to the regulation of food intake. A related fact is that persons who take antihistamines to treat allergies or other disorders for a long period also experience weight gain. Risperidone, ziprasidone, and aripiprazole did not stimulate the AMPK within brain tissue and are termed less orexigenic AAPDs. Hampton (2007) went on to report that researchers are continuing their study of this problem, and hope they will find ways to get around the patient's likelihood of weight gain while being able to continue taking the orexigenic AAPDs.

Implications

Many patients with schizophrenia who would benefit from treatment with an atypical antipsychotic medication may not want to take it because they are aware of the possibility of significant weight gain. Weight gain can lead to depression, decreased self-image, nonadherence with the medication regime, and a return of symptoms with probable rehospitalization.

Critical Thinking Question

What can the nurse do to help the patient who is beginning to take one of the orexigenic AAPDs?

Source: From "Antipsychotics Link to Weight Gain Found," by T. Hampton, 2007, *Journal of the American Medical Association, 297*(12), pp. 1305–1306.

agents, and lamotrigine. Risperidone antagonizes the actions of levodopa and dopamine agonists. Risperidone should be used with caution with drugs known to prolong the QT intervals, such as amiodarone, droperidol and pimozide. **Herbal/Food:** Increased CNS depression may occur if used with St. John's wort or valerian. Food does not affect the absorption of risperidone.

Pregnancy: Category C.

Treatment of Overdose: Symptoms of overdose include confusion, sedation, hypotension, and dysrhythmias. Treatment is supportive and includes gastric lavage and maintenance of cardiovascular function.

Nursing Responsibilities:

- Complete a comprehensive assessment, including past medical and psychiatric history, drug allergies, previous and current medications and previous adverse drug reactions.
- Assess for contraindications for atypical antipsychotics, including Parkinson's disease, CNS depression, alcoholism, seizure disorders, and blood dyscrasias.
- Assess elderly patients carefully because unusual adverse reactions such as confusion, depression, and hallucinations are more likely to occur in this population.
- Complete a baseline assessment, including a complete blood count (CBC), liver function tests, renal function tests, and vision screening. Reassess at regular intervals.
- Assess for the presence of diabetes mellitus; periodically monitor blood glucose.
- Assess mental status (orientation, affect, cognition).
- Monitor for signs of NMS such as high fever, fluctuations in blood pressure, and muscle rigidity.
- For the IM formulation, administer by deep gluteal injection, using the diluent and safety needle enclosed in the pack provided by the manufacturer. The entire dose pack should be refrigerated and protected from light.

Patient and Family Education:

- If excessive drowsiness occurs with the drug, take the dose at bedtime.
- Do not drive or perform other hazardous activities until the effects of the drug are known because this drug may cause drowsiness or dizziness.
- Make position changes slowly when moving from a lying to standing position to prevent dizziness and possible fainting.
- Take exactly as prescribed and do not discontinue the medication without approval of the health care provider.
- Immediately report symptoms of NMS: fever, unstable blood pressure, lung congestion, incontinence, paleness, or restlessness.
- Maintain all scheduled follow-up appointments.
- Immediately report any of the following: worsening of psychosis symptoms; uncontrollable movements of the eyes, mouth, head, arms, or legs; seizure activity; unusual bleeding or bruising.
- Report symptoms of hyperglycemia, which may include thirst, urinary frequency, and unusual hunger.
- If taking the oral solution, mix the exact amount of drug with water, coffee, orange juice or low-fat milk. Do not mix with cola or tea.
- Do not chew or swallow the oral disintegrating tablets. Allow them to dissolve in the mouth before swallowing.

- Report any suspected or known pregnancy to the health care provider.
- Do not drink alcohol while taking this drug because it may cause excessive drowsiness.
- Do not breast-feed while taking this drug without approval of the health care provider.

Drugs Similar to Risperidone (Risperdal)

Other drugs classified as atypical antipsychotics include clozapine, olanzapine, paliperidone, quetiapine, and ziprasidone. Aripiprazole (Abilify) is an atypical antipsychotic that is a prototype for a new pharmacologic class (see Section 24.8).

Clozapine (Clozaril): In 1989, clozapine (Clozaril) was the first atypical antipsychotic approved for use in the United States. Clozapine is approved for the management of schizophrenia in patients resistant to standard therapies and to reduce the risk of recurrent suicidal behavior in patients with schizophrenia. Off-label indications include treatment of bipolar disorder, severe obsessive-compulsive disorder and dementia related behavioral disorders. Clozapine is available as regular tablets or as oral disintegrating tablets (Fazaclo). Because of potentially severe adverse effects, it is generally reserved for schizophrenia symptoms that have not responded favorably to other drugs. The most serious and limiting adverse effect of clozapine is agranulocytosis, a white blood cell (WBC) count below 500/mm^3. Although it occurs in less than 1% of patients taking the drug, agranulocytosis can be fatal. To avoid toxicity, clozapine therapy requires special monitoring and surveillance requirements. WBC and absolute neutrophil counts (ANC) are performed weekly for the first 6 months of treatment, and reduced in frequency to every 2 weeks for the next 6 months. CNS effects such as sedation, dizziness, confusion, fatigue, and headache are common at the initiation of therapy but may diminish with continued therapy. Clozapine lowers the seizure threshold and can precipitate seizures in 5% of patients taking high doses. Although the incidence of EPS is less than with first-generation agents, akathisia, tremor, and agitation can still occur. Orthostatic hypotension is common at the initiation of therapy and during dosage changes. Other warnings on the drug label include an increased risk of hyperglycemia leading to diabetic ketoacidosis, increased risk of fatal myocarditis, and a public health advisory stating that the unapproved use of atypical antipsychotics in older adults has been associated with a higher death rate compared to a placebo. This drug is pregnancy category B.

Olanzapine (Zyprexa): A newer antipsychotic approved in 1996, olanzapine is a second-generation antipsychotic available in several preparations, such as regular tablets, oral-disintegrating tablets, and powder for IM administration with reconstitution. It is used to treat both the positive and negative symptoms of schizophrenia, and it is also approved to treat acute agitation and mania associated with bipolar disorder (see Chapter 23). A single IM dose can usually calm patients presenting with acute agitation in 15 minutes. Off-label, it is used to treat severe behavioral symptoms associated with the dementia of Alzheimer's disease. It is also being used experimentally to treat nausea and vomiting in patients with cancer.

Like other second-generation antipsychotics, the incidence of EPS with olanzapine is low, with drowsiness being the most frequent adverse effect. Weight gain has been reported in up to 25% of patients and is a frequent cause for discontinuation of the drug. Other common adverse effects include dizziness, nervousness, insomnia, headache, and hostility. Use with other CNS depressants may cause additive CNS depression. The risk of patients developing type 2 diabetes mellitus is greater with the use of olanzapine than with other atypical agents. A major advantage of olanzapine is that it does not cause neutropenia or agranulocytosis, which are major drawbacks to clozapine therapy. Safety and effectiveness in children under age 18 has not been established. This drug is pregnancy category C.

Paliperidone (Invega): Approved in 2006, paliperidone is one of the newest antipsychotics approved for the acute and maintenance therapy of schizophrenia. Paliperidone can improve both the positive and negative symptoms of schizophrenia. It is available only as an extended release tablet. Paliperidone is the principal active metabolite of risperidone, an agent also marketed as an antipsychotic (see later).

The incidence of serious adverse events with paliperidone is very low. The drug is not extensively metabolized in the liver; thus it has less potential for drug–drug interactions than many other antipsychotics. The most common reported adverse effects include restlessness, akathisia, tachycardia, orthostatic hypotension, syncope, increased sensitivity to environmental heat, and sleepiness. NMS or TD may occur with the use of paliperidone. Like olanzapine, increased appetite and weight gain are possible. It does not cause neutropenia or agranulocytosis and does not appear to lower the seizure threshold. Like other drugs in this class, paliperidone should not be used to treat dementia-related psychoses in elderly patients because it increases the risk of death due to CVA, heart failure, or infections, especially pneumonia. This drug is pregnancy category C.

Quetiapine (Seroquel): Approved to treat both positive and negative symptoms of schizophrenia in 1997, indications were later extended to include the short-term therapy of acute mania associated with bipolar disorder. In 2007, the drug was also approved to treat depression associated with bipolar disorder. It is sometimes used off-label to treat obsessive-compulsive disorder that is unresponsive to other therapies. Quetiapine is available only in tablet form. An extended release formulation (Seroquel XR) was approved in 2007.

Like other atypical antipsychotics, the incidence of EPS and other serious adverse effects with quetiapine is low. Unlike clozapine, agranulocytosis has not been reported. Sedation is commonly experienced during the initial stages of therapy. Cautious use is recommended in patients who have a history of cardiovascular disease, seizures, history of suicide attempts, persons with Alzheimer's disease, those who are taking other CNS depressants, and those who are elderly or debilitated. Lens changes have occurred during quetiapine use; thus it is recommended that baseline and 6-month eye examinations be conducted. Other common adverse reactions include weight gain, constipation, postural hypotension, dyspepsia, and xerostomia. This drug is pregnancy category C.

Ziprasidone (Geodon): Approved in 2001, ziprasidone is available in PO or IM formulations to treat schizophrenia and acute mania associated with bipolar disorder. The IM formulation is used to treat acute symptoms of schizophrenia because it can reduce major symptoms in 15 minutes. Ziprasidone may be used off-label to treat Tourette's syndrome. Ziprasidone causes fewer EPS than most other antipsychotics but has the possibility of prolonging the QT interval and thereby causing potentially fatal dysrhythmias; it should not be administered concurrently with other medications that increase the QT interval. It must also be used cautiously in patients with seizure history, Alzheimer's disease, cardiovascular or hepatic disease, or who are being treated with antihypertensives. Additive CNS depression will occur if used concurrently with antianxiety agents, sedative–hypnotics, alcohol, or opiate preparations. Ziprasidone causes less weight gain than other atypical antipsychotics and does not cause agranulocytosis. This drug is pregnancy category C.

CONNECTION *Checkpoint* 24.2

When atypical antipsychotic drugs are used to treat bipolar disorder, they are usually combined with drugs from other classes. From what you learned in Chapter 23, what two drugs are usually combined with the atypical antipsychotics? See Answer to Connection Checkpoint 24.2 in Appendix A.

24.9 Dopamine system stabilizers are the newest class of atypical antipsychotics.

Dopamine system stabilizers (DSS) are so named because they exhibit both antagonist and partial agonist activities on dopamine receptors. The balance between these two activities appears to account for the decrease in observed adverse effects, relative to other antipsychotic agents. Aripiprazole (Abilify) is the only approved drug in this class at the current time. It is hoped that this new class will have the same efficacy as other antipsychotic classes, with fewer serious adverse effects. So far this appears to be the case, although the drug is too new and long-term studies are needed.

PROTOTYPE DRUG Aripiprazole (Abilify)

Classification: **Therapeutic:** Atypical antipsychotic
Pharmacologic: Dopamine system stabilizer (DSS)

Therapeutic Effects and Uses: First approved in 2002, aripiprazole controls both the positive and negative symptoms of schizophrenia and improves cognition with only minimal risk of EPS. It is available in regular tablet and disintegrating tablet forms. An IM formulation was approved in 2006 for the treatment of agitation associated with schizophrenia or bipolar disorder.

An advantage over other atypical agents is that there is little or no weight gain, hypotension, dysrhythmias, anticholinergic effects, or prolactin release with aripiprazole. It does not appear to lower the seizure threshold. Aripiprazole is generally classified with the atypical antipsychotics because of its ability to control both negative and positive symptoms. Aripiprazole is as effective as other atypical antipsychotics but safer.

Mechanism of Action: Aripiprazole is thought to act through a combination of partial agonist activity at dopamine type 2 (D_2 and D_3) and serotonin type 2 (5-HT_{1A}) receptors and antagonist activity at 5-HT_{2A} receptors.

Pharmacokinetics:

Route(s)	PO, IM
Absorption	Well absorbed
Distribution	Widely distributed; unknown if crosses the placenta or is secreted in breast milk
Primary metabolism	Hepatic; metabolized to active metabolite
Primary excretion	Feces, some in urine
Onset of action	Peak effect: 3–5 h (PO); 1–3 h (IM)
Duration of action	Half-life: 75–146 h

Adverse Effects: Although aripiprazole was specifically formulated to eliminate many of the adverse effects of other antipsychotic medications, adverse events may still occur. Frequently reported adverse effects include drowsiness, insomnia, agitation, hyper- or hypotension, light-headedness, anxiety, headache, akathisia, nausea, vomiting, or constipation. Life-threatening adverse effects include seizures, NMS, and tachycardia. Like other atypical antipsychotics, elderly persons with dementia-related psychosis have an increased risk of death due to CVA and other cardiovascular disorders.

Contraindications/Precautions: Lactation, seizure disorders, or hypersensitivity are contraindications to the use of aripiprazole. Precautions must be taken when administering aripiprazole to persons with cardiovascular or cerebrovascular disease or any condition that predisposes them to hypotension. The drug must be used with caution in those with suicide ideation. Safe use has not been established in patients under age 18.

Drug Interactions: Aripiprazole is a substrate for several hepatic CYP enzymes and induces others; thus it may interact with drugs that undergo hepatic metabolism. For example, many of the SSRIs inhibit CYP2D6, which can cause reduced metabolism of aripiprazole, raised serum levels, and possible toxicity. Concurrent use of other antipsychotics or lithium may increase the incidence of EPS. Alcohol and other CNS depressants will cause increased CNS depression. Decreased excretion of aripiprazole may occur with the use of drugs such as fluoxetine or paroxetine. **Herbal/Food:** Grapefruit juice may increase the serum levels of aripiprazole and cause toxicity.

Pregnancy: Category C.

Treatment of Overdose: Overdose can cause vomiting, tremor, and drowsiness, but fatalities have not been reported. There is no specific treatment for overdose.

Nursing Responsibilities:

- Complete a comprehensive assessment, including past medical and psychiatric history, drug allergies, previous and current medications, previous adverse drug reactions, and age of the patient.
- Assess mental status prior to administration of the first dose and at regular intervals during therapy.
- Assess for contraindications for this drug, including hypersensitivity, seizure disorders, QT prolongation, dementia in the elderly, and lactation.
- Complete a baseline assessment, including laboratory results (especially CBC, liver function tests, and renal function tests), cardiovascular status, body temperature, and other vital signs.
- Assess for the presence of diabetes mellitus; routinely monitor blood sugar if diabetes is present.
- Monitor for adverse effects of the drug, including orthostatic hypotension, somnolence, insomnia, agitation, headache, blurred vision, or skin rash.
- Assess for alcohol and illegal drug use, which causes an increased CNS depressant effect when used with antipsychotic drugs.

Patient and Family Education:

- Immediately report the following symptoms of NMS to the health care provider: fever, unstable blood pressure, lung congestion, incontinence, paleness, or restlessness.
- Make position changes slowly when moving from a lying to a standing position, to prevent dizziness and possible fainting.
- Avoid hot baths or showers and hot tubs to decrease the chance of hypotension.
- Avoid any activity that may cause overheating, especially in hot weather.
- Do not take any other prescription or nonprescription drugs, dietary supplements, or herbal products without approval of the health care provider.
- Avoid beverages and products containing caffeine because caffeine used with these drugs will increase anxiety.
- Do not drive or perform other hazardous activities until the effects of the drug are known because this drug may cause drowsiness and dizziness.
- Immediately report vision impairment, tremors, muscle twitching, or urinary retention.
- Immediately notify the health care provider of any known or suspected pregnancy.

Drugs Similar to Aripiprazole (Abilify)

There are no other dopamine system stabilizers.

CONNECTIONS

Evidence-Based Practice The Clinical Antipsychotic Trials of Intervention Effectiveness (CATIE) Study

Clinical Question

Although this study was not exclusively conducted by nurses, why does its conclusion have a far-reaching impact on nursing practice?

Evidence

The effectiveness of olanzapine, quetiapine, and risperidone in patients with chronic schizophrenia who recently discontinued the use of perphenazine was studied. The study was initiated and funded by the National Institute of Mental Health (NIMH) to determine the comparative effectiveness of antipsychotics in typical clinical settings and situations. This study was unique in that it allowed patients to discontinue one antipsychotic that was part of the study and continue in the study with a different drug. The researchers believed that allowing the participants to do this made the study more like real life, where patients want to discontinue their antipsychotic medications because they are not getting the desired results in a short time. The study was conducted over 3 full years at 57 different clinical sites throughout the United States. The only criteria for participants were that they had to meet the *DSM-IV-TR* criteria for a diagnosis of schizophrenia, be between the ages of 18 and 65, and be appropriate for oral antipsychotics. Results of the study concluded that quetiapine and olanzapine were more effective than risperidone in the group of patients who had recently discontinued perphenazine; olanzapine was at least as effective in symptom control as other comparable drugs, despite substantial weight gain and adverse effects on lipid metabolism; individual variations in response to medications are likely due to multiple factors that may be difficult to identify, including the individual patient's ability to tolerate adverse effects. Another conclusion is that the CATIE study may help patients and health care providers find an effective medication sooner than might otherwise be possible. In 2007, the NIMH prepared a press release as an addendum to the information published in the *American Journal of Psychiatry*, which stated that sometimes multiple medications must be tried for a single patient before the most effective one is found. Dr. T. S. Stroup, who took part in the CATIE study, stated that the variables exist, and that clinicians must be responsive to an individual patient's needs and preferences in regard to an antipsychotic medication.

Implications

All of the parties involved in successful pharmacologic management of psychoses—health care providers, nurses, patients, and families—must realize and accept the fact that the first medication tried may not be the best one for a particular patient. Sometimes several medications must be tried before the "ideal" antipsychotic is found. This in no way indicates failure on the part of anyone of the involved parties. When one medication does not achieve the desired effect, there are other medications that can be tried until the best one is found for a particular patient.

Critical Thinking Question

What nursing implications are there in the results of this study for the older patient who took perphenazine for several years before switching to an atypical antipsychotic?

Source: From "Effectiveness of Olanzapine, Quetiapine, and Risperidone in Patients with Chronic Schizophrenia after Discontinuing Perphenazine: A CATIE Study," by T. Stroup, J. Lieberman, J. McEvoy, M. Swartz, S. Davis, and G. Capuano, et al., for the CATIE Investigators, 2007, *American Journal of Psychiatry, 164*(3), pp. 41–54; and *New Details in Schizophrenia Treatment Trial Emerge* [Press Release], by National Institute of Mental Health, March 1, 2007. Retrieved June 16, 2008, from http://www.nimh.nih.gov/science-news/2007/new-details-in-schizophrenia-treatment-trial-emerge.shtml

NURSING PROCESS APPLICATION

Patients Receiving Antipsychotic Therapy

Assessment

Prior to administration:

- Complete a thorough physical exam. Determine any physical problems or drug allergies the patient may have.
- Assess cardiac status. Four conventional antipsychotics—chlorpromazine, thioridazine, haloperidol, and pimozide—carry a risk of serious dysrhythmias occurring as a result of prolongation of the QT interval.
- Obtain baseline vital signs and laboratory studies: CBC, electrolytes, liver and renal function tests.
- Complete a thorough mental status exam. Determine whether or not the patient is out of contact with reality and how severe; and whether or not the patient is a danger to self or others.
- Assess for suicide risk so that measures can be taken to protect the patient who is at high risk.
- Monitor behavior. Determine if the patient is overactive, agitated, restless, pacing, or depressed, so appropriate steps can be taken to assist and protect the patient.
- Complete a thorough family history. It is important to know if anyone else in the family has been diagnosed with schizophrenia, has committed or attempted suicide, or abuses alcohol or illegal drugs, and any positive and negative coping mechanisms used by family members.
- Complete a social history. Determine the patient's usual and current functioning level.

Potential Nursing Diagnoses

- *Disturbed Thought Processes,* related to disease process
- *Ineffective Coping,* related to perception of inadequate level of control
- *Ineffective Role Performance,* related to depression and social isolation
- *Risk for Suicide,* related to impaired cognitive function
- *Ineffective Therapeutic Regimen Management: Family,* related to complexity and length of therapy

Planning: Patient Goals and Expected Outcomes

The patient will:

- Report a reduction of psychotic symptoms, including delusions, paranoia, irrational behavior, hallucinations.
- Demonstrate an understanding of the drug's action by accurately describing drug adverse effects and precautions.
- Immediately report adverse effects or adverse reactions.
- Adhere to recommended treatment regimen.
- Report more positive interactions with others.

Implementation: Conventional Antipsychotics

Interventions and (Rationales)	Patient and Family Education
• Monitor vital signs. (Abnormalities must be recognized immediately so potential problems can be handled.)	• Instruct the patient to change positions slowly and avoid sudden movements to prevent orthostatic hypotension.
• Monitor cardiac status. (Abnormalities must be detected immediately, and measures taken to correct them.)	• Instruct the patient to take medications exactly as ordered and not to skip doses or double up.
• Monitor for EPS. (Parkinsonism, acute dystonia, and akathisia occur early in treatment and can be managed with an additional medication; TD occurs late in therapy and is without effective treatment.)	• Instruct the patient to report any of the following: severe, sudden spasms of the neck, face, or back; involuntary upward deviation of the eyes; masklike faces, bradykinesia, shuffling gait, rigidity, stooped posture, drooling, tremor; an inability to sit still with an uncontrollable need to be constantly moving; involuntary face and tongue movements (tongue thrusting, lip-smacking, etc.); sudden high fever with rigidity, sweating, dysrhythmias, blood pressure fluctuations, confusion, seizures, or coma.
• Monitor skin condition. (Photosensitivity may occur as well as contact dermatitis in anyone handling antipsychotics.)	Instruct the patient to: • Avoid excessive exposure to sunlight. • Use sunscreen and protective clothing when outside. • Use care when self-administering medication, or if a family member is administering the medication.
• Monitor seizure activity. (Seizure threshold may be decreased by antipsychotics.)	• Instruct the patient or caregiver to notify the health care provider if seizure activity occurs.
• Monitor laboratory results, especially WBC counts. (Agranulocytosis is a serious adverse reaction that compromises the immune system.)	Instruct the patient to: • Keep all follow-up appointments. • Stay away from persons with known infectious diseases if the WBC count is low. • Eat a well-balanced diet to protect the immune system and to get adequate rest.
• Monitor sexual function. (Antipsychotics can interfere with libido, the ability to achieve orgasm, and may cause erectile and ejaculatory dysfunction.)	Instruct the patient to: • Report sexual dysfunction to the health care provider if it does occur. A change in dose or of medication may help decrease or eliminate the problem. • Continue taking the medication as ordered.
• Monitor for anticholinergic adverse effects. (Dry mouth, blurred vision, urinary hesitancy, tachycardia, constipation, and photophobia are very likely to occur with antipsychotics.)	Instruct the patient to: • Suck on sugarless hard candy, take frequent sips of water, protect against falls, and increase fluids and fiber to decrease constipation. • Notify the health care provider if symptoms worsen.

Implementation: Atypical Antipsychotics

Interventions and (Rationales)	Patient and Family Education
Prior to administration: • Obtain a complete health history (medical and psychological), including allergies, drug history, and possible drug interactions. (In case anything abnormal occurs during therapy, there will be baseline comparisons.)	• Instruct the patient to report any changes in medication regimen or in health condition in response to medications.
• Obtain baseline laboratory studies, especially red blood cell and white blood cell counts. (In case anything abnormal occurs during therapy, there will be baseline comparisons; clozapine produces a potentially fatal agranulocytosis in a small percent of patients.)	Instruct the patient to: • Keep all follow-up appointments, especially routine laboratory appointments. • Stay away from persons with known infectious diseases, avoid crowds, get adequate rest, and eat a well-balanced diet if WBC is low.
• Monitor for diabetes mellitus, history of abnormal fasting blood glucose readings, and family history of diabetes mellitus. (All atypical antipsychotics have the possibility of causing new-onset diabetes mellitus.)	Instruct the patient to: • Monitor glucose levels routinely. • Have fasting blood glucose test performed with other routine laboratory studies. • Report any polyuria, polydipsia, and polyphagia.
• Assess for hallucinations, mental status, and level of consciousness. (Baseline data will be important in determining whether or not prescribed antipsychotic is effective.)	• Instruct the patient to report any changes in mental status, level of consciousness, behavior, any hallucinations, illusions, or delusions.
• Assess patient support system(s). (A patient with a support system will have better adherence to the medical regimen, plus he or she will have someone close to monitor adherence and the presence of adverse reactions.)	• Encourage the family or significant others to maintain contact with the patient; provide them with information regarding support groups for family members of persons with schizophrenia.
• Assess weight. (Baseline information will be useful when determining if the patient is experiencing weight gain, which is common with atypical antipsychotics.)	• Instruct the patient to eat a well-balanced diet of low-calorie foods, avoid high-calorie foods and snacks, and increase exercise levels.
• Monitor vision. (Quetiapine use can lead to cataract formation or other lens changes.)	Instruct the patient to: • Report any decreased vision, blurring, or distortion of objects. • Have an annual ophthalmologic examination.
• Assess cardiovascular status. (Atypical antipsychotics except for aripiprazole may lead to prolongation of the QT interval, leading to serious, sometimes fatal, dysrhythmias.)	Instruct the patient to: • Keep all appointments for routine ECG studies. • Report any unusual heart rates, palpitations, or skipped beats.
• Assess the age of the patient. (Elderly patients may need lower doses of atypical antipsychotics.)	• Instruct the patient to report any changes in responses to medication as the patient ages.

Evaluation of Outcome Criteria

Evaluate the effectiveness of drug therapy by confirming that patient goals and expected outcomes have been met (see "Planning").

UNDERSTANDING THE CHAPTER

Key Concepts Summary

24.1 Psychoses are severe mental disorders characterized by the inability to recognize reality.

24.2 Schizophrenia, the most common psychosis, has both positive and negative symptoms.

24.3 The precise etiology of schizophrenia remains unknown.

24.4 Medical management of psychosis is challenging because patients often lack insight into their disease and believe their behavior is normal.

24.5 Selection of an antipsychotic drug depends on its spectrum of adverse effects and the experience of the health care provider.

24.6 The phenothiazines are effective at treating schizophrenia symptoms but exhibit a high incidence of adverse effects.

24.7 The nonphenothiazine first-generation antipsychotics have the same therapeutic applications and similar adverse effects as the phenothiazines.

24.8 Second-generation antipsychotics have become drugs of choice for the treatment of schizophrenia.

24.9 Dopamine system stabilizers are the newest class of atypical antipsychotics.

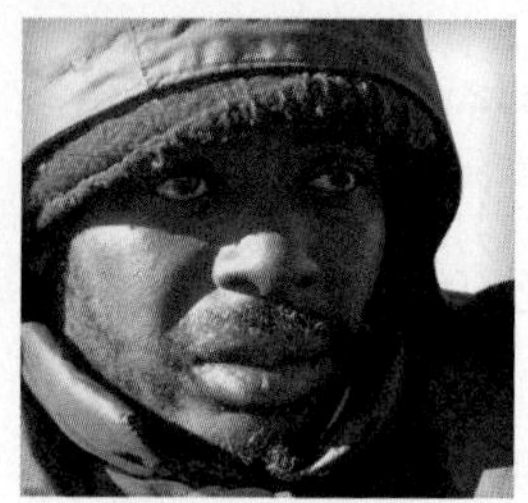

Making the PATIENT *Connection*

Remember the patient "George Watkins" at the beginning of the chapter? Now read the remainder of the case study. Based on the information presented within the chapter, respond to the critical thinking questions that follow.

George Watkins is a 37-year-old African American male who was admitted to the psychiatric unit this morning. He was diagnosed with schizophrenia at age 20. He is disheveled looking, with long, dirty, stringy hair. His clothes are mismatched and dirty. Although it is summer, he is wearing an overcoat and a winter hat pulled down over his ears. This is George's fourth hospitalization for out-of-control schizophrenia. The last severe episode occurred 4 years ago.

Sheri Watkins, George's wife, states that he quit his job as an assembly line supervisor about 2 weeks ago. He has also quit coaching softball and soccer games. Sheri and George have been married since they were both 18. Their marriage is basically strong but has had its difficult times, especially when George's schizophrenia is active. About 3 to 4 weeks before each hospitalization for psychosis, he stopped taking his antipsychotic medication. He has taken different antipsychotic medications over the course of his schizophrenia, but none have proven to be successful over a long period.

George and Sheri have two children: Toby, who is 14, and Felecia, who is 10. Both children do well in school, have many friends, and are active in several organizations and sports. As the children get older, they realize that "something is not quite right" with their father. They have never been told of their father's mental illness. The children worry that they will catch whatever it is that causes their father's erratic behavior. George's parents and four siblings live in the same town. George, his father, and two brothers work at the same manufacturing plant. His other two siblings are teachers in the local school system, as is Sheri.

Mr. and Mrs. Watkins, George's parents, tell you that their son had a "normal" childhood. He was active in sports, starred on the high school football team, was an honor student, was a Boy Scout, and had many friends. They have always enjoyed many social occasions with their large extended family. George is always welcome at family gatherings, but relatives tend to avoid him when his behavior becomes bizarre. They all know he has schizophrenia but do not fully understand the implications of the diagnosis.

Critical Thinking Questions

1. What are the most likely reasons George gives for discontinuing his medication?
2. What clues do his family and friends have that would indicate that his schizophrenia may be getting out of control?
3. What can be done to prevent George's schizophrenia from getting out of control in the future?

Case Study

George is oriented to the unit, and his family returns home. There are 20 other patients with various psychiatric diagnoses currently on the unit. George paces back and forth in the day room until he is called for dinner. He is heard muttering to himself, "I don't know why they put me here. They just don't want me to get my inheritance. Maybe it's because they know I'll leave them all when I get the money. I'll be real rich and can start a new life for myself." He demonstrates no overt threatening behavior toward any of the other patients or toward the staff. His agitation escalates until he cannot calm himself down and will not listen to staff. He begins hitting his fist into the wall and shouting. There is an order for haloperidol (Haldol), 4 mg IM every 1 to 4 hours prn for agitation.

1. What is the main use of haloperidol (Haldol) in this situation?
2. As the nurse caring for George, what adverse effects would you monitor for?
3. How long would you expect George to remain hospitalized? Why?

NCLEX-RN® Review

1 The client states that he has not taken his antipsychotic drug for the past 2 weeks because it was causing sexual dysfunction. The nurse is aware that the name *antipsychotic* indicates that continuing the medication as prescribed is important because:

1. Hypertensive crisis may occur with abrupt withdrawal.
2. Muscle twitching may occur with abrupt withdrawal.
3. Parkinson-like symptoms will occur with withdrawal.
4. Symptoms of psychosis are likely to return if the medication is withdrawn.

2 Prior to discharge, the nurse provides teaching related to adverse effects of phenothiazines to the client and caregivers. Which of the following should be included?

1. The client may experience social withdrawal and slowed activity.
2. Severe muscle spasms may occur early in therapy.
3. Tardive dyskinesia is likely early in therapy.
4. Medications should be taken as prescribed to prevent adverse effects.

3 The nurse expects that the client experiencing extrapyramidal symptoms during therapy with phenothiazines will be prescribed:

1. Benztropine (Cogentin).
2. Diazepam (Valium).
3. Haloperidol (Haldol).
4. Lorazepam (Ativan).

4 Nursing implications of the administration of haloperidol (Haldol) to a client exhibiting psychotic behavior include which of the following? Select all that apply.

1. Take 1 hour before or 2 hours after antacids.
2. The incidence of extrapyramidal symptoms is high.
3. It is therapeutic if ordered on an as-needed basis.
4. Haldol is contraindicated in Parkinson's disease, seizure disorders, alcoholism, and severe mental depression.
5. Crush the sustained release form for easier swallowing.

5 Which statement made by the client who is taking chlorpromazine indicates that further teaching is necessary?

1. "I'll monitor my weight every month."
2. "I'll call my doctor if I notice a decreased ability to see clearly."
3. "I'll have my blood pressure monitored regularly."
4. "There is no problem if I want to drink alcohol on the weekends."

6 The development of which symptom(s) in a client taking an antipsychotic must be reported immediately?

1. Fever, tachycardia, stupor, and incontinence
2. Suddenly occurring muscle spasms, especially in the neck and back
3. Sexual dysfunction
4. Leg pains, pacing, an inability to sit still

See Answers to Critical Thinking Questions, Case Study, and NCLEX-RN® Review in Appendix A.

References

D'Souza, D. C., Gil, R. B., Madonick, S., Perry, E. B., Forselius-Bielen, K., Braley, G., et al. (2006). Enhanced sensitivity to the euphoric effects of alcohol in schizophrenia. *Neuropsychopharmacology, 31*(12), 2767–2775.

Emsley, R., Oosthuizen, P., & vanRensburg, S. (2003). Clinical potential of omega-3 fatty acids in the treatment of schizophrenia. *CNS Drugs 17*(15), 1081–1091.

Ernst, E. (2006). Herbal remedies for anxiety—A systematic review of controlled clinical trials. *Phytomedicine, 13*(3), 205–208.

Gerstein, P. S. (2007). Schizophrenia. *Emedicine.* Retrieved June 13, 2008, from http://www.emedicine.com/emerg/TOPIC520.HTM

Hampton, T. (2007). Antipsychotics link to weight gain found. *Journal of the American Medical Association, 297*(12), 1305–1306.

Internet Mental Health. (2008). *Schizophrenia.* Retrieved June 12, 2008, from http://www.mentalhealth.com/

Joy, C., Mumby-Croft, R., & Joy, L. (2006). Polyunsaturated fatty acid supplementation for schizophrenia. *Cochrane Database of Systematic Reviews 2006, 3.* Art. No.: CD001257.DOI: 10.1002/14651858.CD001257.pub2.

National Institute of Mental Health. (2007, March). *New details in schizophrenia treatment emerge* [Press release]. Retrieved June 16, 2008, from http://www.nimh.nih.gov/science-news/2007/new-details-in-schizophrenia-treatment-trial-emerge.shtml

Rathbone, J., Zhang, L., Zhang, M., Xia, J., Liu, X., Yang, Y., et al. (2007). Chinese herbal medicine for schizophrenia: Cochrane systematic review of randomized trials. *British Journal of Psychiatry, 190,* 379–384.

Stroup, T., Lieberman, J., McEvoy, J., Swartz, M., Davis, S., Capuano, G., et al. (2007). Effectiveness of olanzapine, quetiapine, and risperidone in patients with chronic schizophrenia after discontinuing perphenazine: A CATIE Study for the CATIE investigators. *American Journal of Psychiatry, 164*(3), 41–54.

Vaughan, D. (2004). Schizophrenia: New drugs new promise. *Nurseweek.* Retrieved September 12, 2008, from http://www.nurseweek.com/news/Features/04-11/Clinical_Schizophrenia.asp

World Fellowship for Schizophrenia and Allied Disorders. (2007). *Schizophrenia.* Retrieved June 14, 2008, from http://www.world-schizophrenia.org/disorders/schizophrenia.html

Zuardi, A., Crippa, J., Hallak, F., & Moreira, F. (2006). Cannabidiol, a *cannabis sativa* constituent, as an antipsychotic drug. *Brazilian Journal of Medical and Biological Research, 39,* 421–429.

CHAPTER

I just don't understand what's happening. I drove to the beauty shop—it's only three blocks—but forgot I had driven there, and walked home. I walked around and around, until I finally saw our house. Then I couldn't get in because my key wouldn't work, so I paced around the yard until Robert got home. Why did he change the lock on the front door?

Patient "Mary Lee"

25 Pharmacotherapy of Degenerative Diseases of the Central Nervous System

Learning Outcomes

After reading this chapter, the student should be able to:

1. Identify the most common degenerative diseases of the central nervous system.
2. Distinguish between idiopathic Parkinson's disease and secondary Parkinson's disease.
3. Describe symptoms of Parkinson's disease.
4. Explain the neurochemical basis for Parkinson's disease, focusing on the roles of dopamine and acetylcholine in the brain.
5. Describe symptoms of Alzheimer's disease and explain theories about why these symptoms develop.
6. Describe the nurse's role in the pharmacologic management of Parkinson's disease and Alzheimer's disease.
7. Discuss the pharmacologic goals for the management of Parkinson's disease, Alzheimer's disease, and other neurodegenerative disorders.
8. For each of the classes shown in the chapter outline, identify the prototype and representative drugs and explain the mechanism(s) of drug action, primary indications, contraindications, significant drug interactions, pregnancy category, and important adverse effects.
9. Use the nursing process to care for patients receiving drug therapy for degenerative diseases of the central nervous system.

Chapter Outline

Degenerative Diseases of the Central Nervous System

Parkinson's Disease

Etiology and Pathogenesis of Parkinson's Disease

Pharmacotherapy of Parkinson's Disease

Dopamine Replacement Therapy

PROTOTYPE DRUG **Levodopa (L-Dopa, Dopar, Larodopa)** *p. 350*

Dopamine Agonists

PROTOTYPE DRUG **Pramipexole (Mirapex)** *p. 353*

Miscellaneous Dopaminergic Agents

Anticholinergic Drugs

PROTOTYPE DRUG **Benztropine (Cogentin)** *p. 355*

Alzheimer's Disease

Pharmacotherapy of Alzheimer's Disease

Cholinesterase Inhibitors

Reversible Cholinesterase Inhibitors

NMDA Receptor Antagonist

PROTOTYPE DRUG **Donepezil (Aricept)** *p. 361*

Multiple Sclerosis

Amyotrophic Lateral Sclerosis

Key Terms

Alzheimer's disease (AD), 358
basal ganglia, 348
bradykinesia, 348
cholinesterase inhibitors, 359
COMT inhibitors, 355
dementia, 358
extrapyramidal symptoms (EPS), 349
glutamate, 361
immunomodulator, 364
muscle rigidity, 348
neurodegenerative disease, 347
neurofibrillary tangles, 358
on-off syndrome, 349
Parkinson's disease (PD), 348
pill rolling, 348
striatum, 348
substantia nigra, 348
wearing off effect, 349

Degenerative diseases of the central nervous system (CNS) are difficult to treat pharmacologically. In nearly all cases, medications are unable to cure or reverse the progressive nature of these disorders, and the symptomatic relief provided by the drugs is only temporary. The focus of this chapter is on four debilitating and progressive conditions categorized as degenerative diseases of the CNS: Parkinson's disease, Alzheimer's disease, multiple sclerosis, and amyotrophic lateral sclerosis.

Degenerative Diseases of the Central Nervous System

25.1 Degenerative diseases of the central nervous system are characterized by irreversible and progressive loss of neuronal function.

Degenerative diseases of the CNS **(neurodegenerative disease)** include a diverse set of disorders differing in their causes and outcomes. Each involves a progressive and irreversible loss of neuron function in the brain or spinal cord, or both. Neuron loss is sometimes isolated to specific regions of the CNS, and symptoms will vary by the region(s) most affected by the disorder.

Alzheimer's disease and Parkinson's disease are neurodegenerative disorders that present major health care challenges for older adults as well as for the health care industry, which must be prepared to provide services for the vast numbers of patients with these disorders. Although less common, Huntington's disease, multiple sclerosis, and amyotrophic lateral sclerosis are equally devastating to patients and their families. The various neurodegenerative diseases can affect any age group. These disorders are described in Table 25.1.

The etiology of most neurodegenerative diseases is unknown, although the loss of neurons appears to have both genetic and environmental components. Huntington's disease is clearly the result of an autosomal dominant genetic defect. Alzheimer's disease and Parkinson's disease also tend to occur more commonly within families but this does not account for the majority of cases. It is likely that exposure of neurons to various toxins, genetic predisposition, and normal aging all have important roles in the etiology of these disorders.

Most neurodegenerative diseases progress from very subtle signs and symptoms early in the course of the disease to profound neurologic and cognitive deficits. Because of this, neurodegenerative disorders are quite difficult to diagnose in their early stages. With some of them, diagnosis is made only after other neurologic, infectious, cardiovascular, or traumatic etiologies have been ruled out.

With the exception of Parkinson's disease, pharmacotherapy provides only minimal benefit to patients with neurodegenerative disease. Currently, medications are unable to cure or significantly alter the clinical course of any of the degenerative diseases of the CNS.

Pharm*FACT*

More than 1.5 million Americans have Parkinson's disease. Approximately 60,000 new cases are diagnosed each year. *Source:* National Parkinson Foundation, n.d.

TABLE 25.1 Major Degenerative Diseases of the Central Nervous System

Disease	Description
Alzheimer's Disease	A chronic, progressive disease that leaves the patient totally disoriented and dependent on others for all aspects of care; usually affects persons over age 60.
Amyotrophic Lateral Sclerosis (Lou Gehrig's Disease)	A degenerative disease of the motor neurons characterized by weakness and atrophy of the muscles of the hands, forearms, and legs, spreading to involve most of the body and face; symptoms usually begin during the middle years, with death occurring within 2–5 years.
Huntington's Disease (formerly called Huntington's chorea)	A rare hereditary condition characterized by progressive chorea and mental deterioration resulting in dementia; symptoms usually begin in the 30s–50s with death occurring within 15 years.
Myasthenia Gravis	A chronic debilitating autoimmune disease characterized by fatigue and weakness, especially in muscles innervated by the cranial nerves; symptoms usually begin in the 20s–30s; women are three times more often afflicted than men (see Chapter 17).
Parkinson's Disease (may also be called paralysis agitans)	A debilitating disease characterized by resting tremor, muscle rigidity, hypokinesia, masklike faces, and a slow, shuffling gait; symptoms usually appear in the 60s.

Parkinson's Disease

25.2 Parkinson's disease is a progressive neurodegenerative disorder characterized by abnormal motor movement.

Named after British physician James Parkinson who identified the condition in 1817, **Parkinson's disease (PD)** is the second most common degenerative disease of the nervous system and the third most common neurologic disorder of older adults. As the average age of the population continues to rise, increasing numbers of persons will likely be diagnosed with PD. The usual age of onset is 40 to 70, with a peak between 58 and 62 years of age; however, even teenagers can develop the disorder. Men are affected slightly more often than women. The disease is progressive, with the expression of full symptoms developing over many years.

The two etiologies of PD are called idiopathic and secondary. Idiopathic PD, the most common type, has no known cause and is characterized by a progressive destruction of neurons in specific regions of the brain. Some patients with idiopathic parkinsonism have a family history of the disorder, and a genetic link is highly probable.

Secondary PD is caused by medical conditions such as head trauma, brain infections, brain tumors, and exposure to neurotoxins. The most frequent cause of secondary PD is treatment with antipsychotic drugs (see Chapter 24). Once a patient on antipsychotic therapy shows signs of parkinsonism, the drug is normally discontinued. Symptoms of drug-induced PD are usually reversible but may become permanent if pharmacotherapy is prolonged.

PD begins with subtle symptoms. The patient complains of feeling tired and seems to move more slowly, often demonstrating a slight tremor along with fatigue. There are no definitive tests for PD; diagnosis is based on clinical findings after the presence of other neurologic diseases has been ruled out. Once the disease progresses, the symptoms of PD are quite characteristic and can be easily recognized. The four cardinal signs of PD, or parkinsonism, are summarized as follows:

- **Tremor.** The hands and head develop a palsy-like, continuous motion or shaking when at rest. The tremors may be so pronounced that the person cannot hold a glass or eating utensils and successfully bring them to his or her mouth. **Pill rolling** is a common behavior in progressive states, in which patients rub the thumb and forefinger together in a circular motion, resembling the motion of rolling a tablet between two fingers.
- **Muscle rigidity.** Resistance to passive movements of the arms and legs develops. The **muscle rigidity** or stiffness may resemble symptoms of arthritis. Patients often have difficulty bending over and moving limbs. Changes in facial expression, or a lack of facial expression, are due to rigidity of the facial muscles. This rigidity can lead to chewing and swallowing difficulties if the pharyngeal muscles are involved. Uncontrollable drooling may also be evident. A noticeable symptom of PD is a lack of arm swinging while walking; the patient walks with the arms close to the side. Muscle rigidity is present early in the disease process. Although the symptoms may be less noticeable at first, they progress and become obvious in later years.
- **Bradykinesia.** An involuntary slowness of voluntary movement and speech, **bradykinesia** is one of the most noticeable of all symptoms and is marked by difficulty chewing, swallowing, or speaking. Patients with PD have difficulties initiating movement and controlling fine muscle movements. Patients shuffle their feet without taking normal strides, making walking difficult.
- **Postural instability.** Patients may be stooped over and easily lose their balance. Stumbling results in frequent falls with associated injuries.

Although PD is a progressive neurologic disorder primarily affecting muscle movement, other health problems often develop in these patients, including anxiety, sleep disturbances, dementia, and disturbances of the autonomic nervous system such as difficulty urinating and sexual dysfunction. Over half of these patients present with clinical depression. Many develop thought disturbances, and dementia may occur, especially in those over age 70. These associated health problems often require pharmacologic intervention, which increases the possibility of drug interactions and adverse effects in these patients.

25.3 Parkinson's disease is caused by a lack of sufficient amounts of dopamine produced by the substantia nigra.

Although the precise etiology of PD is incompletely understood, much is known about the effects of the disease on the CNS. Defects in the amounts of neurotransmitters in specific regions of the brain are closely associated with the disease.

Involuntary muscle movements are controlled by the **basal ganglia** (also called basal nuclei). The basal ganglia consist of clusters of interconnected neurons in several distinct regions of the brain and are responsible for regulating the flow of information from the cerebral cortex to the motor neurons in the spinal cord. Two of the basal ganglia that are important to the pathogenesis of PD are the substantia nigra and the striatum. The student should review the functions of the basal ganglia and associated structures in Chapter 21.

The **substantia nigra,** a dark band of gray matter in the midbrain, is a primary producer of the neurotransmitter dopamine. The dopamine travels through axons along the nigrostriatal pathway to the **striatum** (also called corpus striatum), where the neurotransmitter is released. In the striatum, dopamine encounters its receptors and produces multiple actions. One function that is important to the pathogenesis of PD is the planning and modulation of motor pathways responsible for unconscious muscle movement. Dopamine serves an inhibitory function, slowing the flow of impulses down spinal neurons.

When dopamine is present, the normal flow of motor impulses from the striatum helps to produce coordinated, unconscious muscle movement. Should levels of dopamine fall because of the loss of dopamine-producing neurons in the substantia ni-

MyNursingKit | The American Parkinson Disease Association

gra, symptoms of parkinsonism may develop. Remarkably, the body can function normally even when as many as 50% of the neurons stop producing dopamine. When 60% to 80% lose their function, however, parkinsonism develops.

A second neurotransmitter modulates the effects of neuronal outflow from the striatum. Acetylcholine (Ach) serves an excitatory function. Under normal conditions, the inhibitory effects of dopamine and the excitatory effects of Ach balance one another and produce smooth, coordinated muscle movement. If dopamine levels decline, Ach has a more dramatic stimulatory effect in this area and the abnormal muscular movements characteristic of PD are observed.

CONNECTION *Checkpoint* 25.1

Dopamine belongs to a class of natural hormones called catecholamines. From what you learned in Chapter 16, what are the other two major catecholamines found in the nervous system? See Answer to Connection Checkpoint 25.1 in Appendix A.

Pharmacotherapy of Parkinson's Disease

25.4 The drugs used for Parkinson's disease help to alleviate symptoms but do not cure the disease.

The balance of the two neurotransmitters, dopamine and Ach, offers several means by which drug therapy may be used to improve the symptoms of PD. Antiparkinson agents are given to restore the balance between dopamine and Ach in specific regions of the brain.

- **Dopamine agonists.** These drugs increase the levels of dopamine in the striatum. This may be accomplished by directly replacing dopamine, decreasing the breakdown of dopamine, increasing the release of dopamine from neurons, or activating dopamine receptors.
- **Anticholinergic agents.** These agents block the excitatory actions of Ach in the striatum.

The goal of pharmacotherapy for PD is to increase the ability of the patient to perform normal activities of daily living (ADLs) such as eating, walking, dressing, and bathing, and decrease the chances of falls that could cause serious injury. Pharmacotherapy is an essential part of the management of PD; drugs decrease symptoms and allow the patient to provide at least some self-care, have some degree of self-worth, and improve his or her quality of life. Although pharmacotherapy does not cure this disorder, symptoms are dramatically reduced in many patients.

Patients receiving prolonged antiparkinson pharmacotherapy may periodically experience a loss of drug effect. A **wearing off effect** appears gradually near the end of a dosing interval. Symptoms become worse near the end of the cycle because the concentration of the drug has fallen below the therapeutic level. Adjusting the dosing interval to provide for more frequent dosing may help to reduce this effect.

Another type of loss of drug effect occurs abruptly. The **on-off syndrome** occurs when the patient alternates between symptom-free periods (on) and times when the drugs stop working and symptoms abruptly reappear (off). The on-off time intervals range from just a few minutes to several hours. Off periods may occur even when the serum level of the drug is high. The on-off syndrome is difficult to control. Scheduling doses closer together or using a second, adjunct medication during the off period are strategies used to reduce the on-off syndrome.

Symptoms of parkinsonism are major adverse effects of several classes of antipsychotic drugs (see Chapter 24). These dyskinesias are referred to as **extrapyramidal symptoms (EPS).** The term *extrapyramidal* refers to locations in the CNS associated with postural and automatic movements. Recall from Chapter 24 that antipsychotic drugs act through a blockade of dopamine receptors. Thus EPS develop for the same neurochemical reasons as PD: deficiency of dopamine in the striatum. Antiparkinson drugs may be used to treat these symptoms.

If drug therapy becomes ineffective, there are other treatments that can be tried. Again, these treatments may help control symptoms, but they will not cure or prevent the disease from progressing. There are four accepted nonmedication treatments for PD: stereotactic pallidotomy, thalamotomy, fetal tissue transplantation, and deep brain stimulation (DBS). Table 25.2 describes each of these nonpharmacologic therapies.

MyNursingKit | Parkinson's Disease Video

25.5 Replacement therapy with levodopa is the most effective therapy for treating Parkinson's disease.

Drug therapy attempts to restore the functional balance of dopamine and Ach in the striatum of the brain. Dopamine replacement agents are used to directly increase dopamine levels in this region. Dopamine itself cannot be used for this purpose because it is unable to cross the blood–brain barrier after it is administered.

The drug of choice for PD is levodopa (L-Dopa, Larodopa), a dopaminergic drug that has been prescribed more extensively than any other medication for this disorder. As shown in Pharmacotherapy Illustrated 25.1, levodopa is a precursor in the synthesis of dopamine. Unlike dopamine, however, levodopa can easily cross the blood–brain barrier. Administration of levodopa directly leads to increased biosynthesis of dopamine within the nerve terminals.

Levodopa is nearly always combined with carbidopa because the combination "boosts" the effectiveness of levodopa. Carbidopa has no therapeutic effects of its own because it cannot cross the blood–brain barrier. However, carbidopa inhibits the breakdown of levodopa in the intestine and peripheral tissues, which makes more levodopa available to reach the CNS. Without carbidopa, only 1% of the dose of levodopa reaches the CNS. One of the biggest advantages to this combination drug (Sinemet) is that it allows for much lower doses of levodopa to be prescribed than when levodopa is used alone; 25 mg of levodopa is used as a combination drug versus 125 mg of levodopa when delivered as monotherapy. Carbidopa also decreases dopamine production in the periphery, leading to reduced nausea and vomiting as well as fewer cardiovascular responses to levodopa. Doses for these drugs are listed in Table 25.3.

MyNursingKit | Mechanism of Action Animation: Levodopa

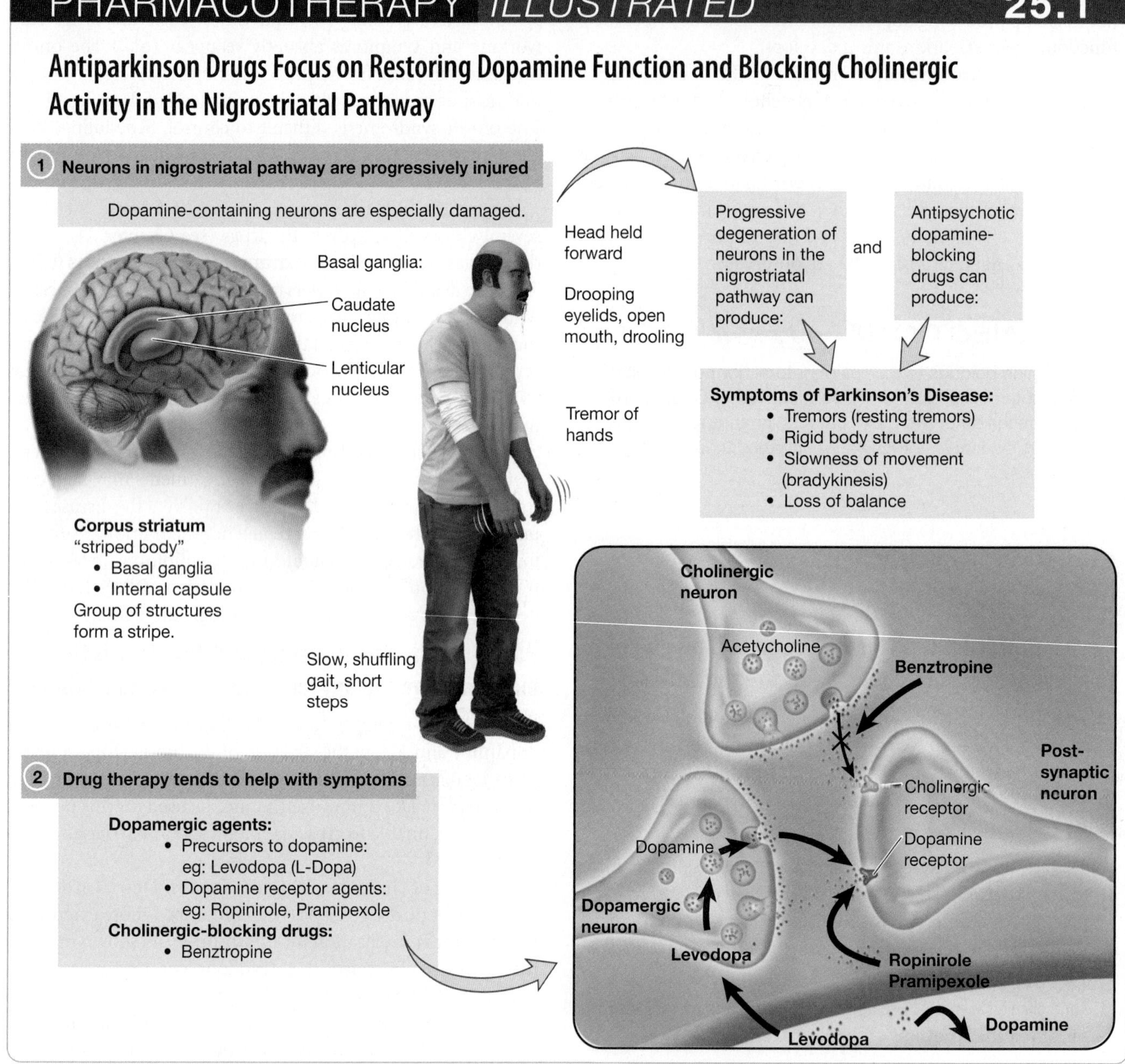

Carbidopa has no significant adverse effects; the adverse effects of Sinemet are due to the levodopa component of the drug. Sinemet is available as an immediate release tablet or a sustained release tablet. Paracopa is a preparation of levodopa and carbidopa that dissolves on the tongue and is swallowed with saliva, which is a distinct advantage for patients with swallowing difficulties. Stalevo is a combination of levodopa, carbidopa, and the COMT inhibitor, entacapone (see Section 25.7). The addition of entacapone is believed to create a more consistent level of levodopa in the blood, which can minimize the extent and duration of the wearing off effect.

Although the dystonias characteristic of PD are treated with levodopa and carbidopa, this drug combination also causes dystonias. Some dystonias such as head-bobbing or jaw clenching may be minor adverse effects of levodopa therapy, whereas others such as quick jerking movements may be serious. These dystonias may occur just as the optimum dosage level of levodopa is reached, which is extremely discouraging for patients and their caregivers. To reduce the severity of these dystonias, the dose of levodopa and carbidopa must be reduced. This, of course, often causes the symptoms of PD to return.

PROTOTYPE DRUG Levodopa (L-Dopa, Dopar, Larodopa)

Classification: Therapeutic: Antiparkinson agent

Pharmacologic: Dopamine replacement agent

Therapeutic Effects and Uses: Approved in 1970, levodopa is an oral (PO) drug indicated for the treatment of idiopathic and secondary PD. The drug restores normal dopamine levels

TABLE 25.2 Nondrug Treatments for Parkinson's Disease

Name of Treatment	Type of Treatment	Procedure
Deep Brain Stimulation (DBS)	Electrical stimulation	An electrode is implanted in the thalamus or subthalamus. It is connected to a pacemaker-like device that delivers electric currents to interfere with cells that cause tremors. An implantable generator is inserted under the patient's skin in much the same way as a cardiac pacemaker. The patient can adjust the settings by using a special magnet placed over the implanted generator. DBS is used when medications are no longer controlling symptoms.
Fetal Tissue Transplantation	Surgical	Fetal tissue from either humans or pigs is transplanted into the caudate nucleus of the brain. Expected outcome is that the patient will show a substantial decrease of motor symptoms. This is very controversial and considered experimental at this time. No long-term results are available.
Stereotactic Pallidotomy	Surgical and electrical stimulation	The target area is identified with a computed tomography (CT) scan or magnetic resonance imaging (MRI). When the patient has been sedated, a burr hole is made into that area into which an electrode is inserted. A mild electrical current is passed through the electrode. The patient is closely observed for the desired effects of decreased tremor and rigidity. If the desired effect is not seen, or if untoward effects occur, the probe is repositioned until desired effects occur. A temporary lesion is made. If it is successful, a permanent lesion is made.
Thalamotomy	Surgical	Lesions are surgically produced within the thalamus, which are thought to decrease tremor and rigidity. This is done only to benefit the side of the body that is most affected because there have been surgical complications from bilateral thalamotomy.

TABLE 25.3 Drugs for Parkinson's Disease

Drug	Route and Adult Dose (maximum dose where indicated)	Adverse Effects
Dopamine Replacement Agents		
levodopa/carbidopa (Sinemet)	PO: 1 tablet containing 10 mg carbidopa/100 mg levodopa or 25 mg carbidopa/100 mg levodopa tid (max: 6 tabs/day)	*Involuntary movements (dyskinetic, dystonic, choreiform), orthostatic hypotension, anorexia, nausea, vomiting*
levodopa (L-Dopa, Larodopa)	PO: 500 mg–1 g/day; may be increased by 100–750 mg every 3–7 days (max: 800 mg/day)	Neuroleptic malignant syndrome, agranulocytosis, depression with suicidal tendencies
Dopamine Agonists		
apomorphine	Subcutaneous: 2–4 mg (max: 4 mg)	*Nausea and vomiting, bruising, dyskinesias, frequent penile erections, hallucinations* Acute circulatory failure
bromocriptine (Parlodel)	PO: 1.25–2.5 mg/day up to 100 mg/day in divided doses	*Nausea, orthostatic hypotension* Shock, acute myocardial infarction (MI)
pramipexole (Mirapex)	PO: start with 0.125 mg tid for 1 week; double this dose for the next week; continue to increase by 0.25 mg/dose tid every week to a target dose of 1.5 mg tid	*Dizziness, somnolence, insomnia, dyskinesia, postural hypotension, nausea, constipation* EPS, asthenia, sleep attacks, hallucinations
ropinirole (Requip)	PO: start with 0.25 mg tid; may increase by 0.25 mg/dose tid every week to a target dose of 1 mg tid (max: 24 mg/day)	*Fatigue viral infection, dizziness, somnolence, nausea, vomiting, dyspepsia* Sleep attacks, syncope
rotigotine (Neupro)	Transdermal Patch: 1 patch/day, equivalent to 2–6 mg/day (max: 6 mg/day)	*Nausea, redness, and rash at application site, drowsiness, dizziness, headache* Vision changes, asthenia, syncope
COMT Inhibitors		
entacapone (Comtan)	PO: 200 mg administered with each dose of levodopa/carbidopa up to 8 times/day	*Urine discoloration, hyperkinesia, nausea, diarrhea, dystonia, excessive dreaming, sleep disorder*
tolcapone (Tasmar)	PO: 100 mg tid (max: 600 mg/day)	Dyskinesia, liver failure (tolcapone)
Miscellaneous Agents		
amantadine (Symmetrel)	PO: 100 mg 1–2 times/day	*Dizziness, light-headedness, difficulty concentrating, anxiety, headache, fatigue, nausea, vomiting, orthostatic hypotension* Dysrhythmias, leukopenia (rare), heart failure
selegiline (Carbex, Eldepryl, L-Deprenyl, Zelapar)	PO: 5 mg/dose bid; doses greater than 10 mg/day are potentially toxic	*Nausea* Dyskinesias, hallucinations

Note: *Italics* indicate common adverse effects. Underline indicates serious adverse effects.

in the striatum of the brain. Levodopa is also used to treat symptoms of PD that occur in patients with manganese and carbon monoxide poisoning. Some symptoms of PD, such as tremor, bradykinesia, gait, and muscle rigidity, respond well to levodopa treatment. Others, such as imbalance, sensory problems, sexual dysfunction, and constipation, do not respond as well. Dosing is highly individualized to deliver the least amount of drug that will resolve the patient's symptoms.

Two to three weeks of therapy are needed before improvement is observed, and many patients require several months of therapy for optimum therapeutic outcomes to be achieved. Dramatic improvement in symptoms is often noted early in therapy. As therapy progresses, however, the beneficial effects of the drug tend to diminish. In addition, the on-off syndrome tends to worsen with continued use of the drug.

Mechanism of Action: Levodopa is a metabolic precursor of dopamine. When metabolized through decarboxylation to dopamine, dopamine levels in the brain increase. If given alone, 99% of a dose is decarboxylated to dopamine before it ever enters the CNS. If given with carbidopa, peripheral metabolism is diminished and more levodopa reaches the brain to produce its therapeutic effect.

Pharmacokinetics:

Route(s)	PO
Absorption	Well absorbed from the gastrointestinal (GI) tract; absorption is decreased when given with meals
Distribution	Widely distributed throughout the body
Primary metabolism	Stomach, intestines, and liver
Primary excretion	Renal
Onset of action	1–3 h
Duration of action	Half-life: 1 h

Adverse Effects: There are many potential adverse effects of levodopa. Common adverse effects include orthostatic hypotension, nausea, vomiting, anorexia, flatulence, dysphagia, abdominal distress, choreiform and involuntary movements, hand tremors, fatigue, headache, anxiety, twitching, numbness, confusion, agitation, nightmares, and insomnia. Life-threatening adverse effects include agranulocytosis, leukopenia, and hemolytic anemia. Other potential adverse effects are related to the anticholinergic properties of levodopa, including urinary retention and dry mouth. Psychosis develops in up to 20% of patients taking levodopa, and drug therapy with an antipsychotic agent such as clozapine (Clozaril) or quetiapine (Seroquel) may be necessary to control hallucinations and paranoid feelings.

Contraindications/Precautions: Levodopa is contraindicated in persons with hypersensitivity to the drug and those with narrow-angle glaucoma, undiagnosed skin lesions, acute psychoses, severe psychoneuroses, or within 2 weeks of use of a monoamine oxidase inhibitor (MAOI). Caution must be taken if administering levodopa to persons with cardiac, respiratory, endocrine, renal, or hepatic disease; MI with dysrhythmias; seizure disorder; lactation; peptic ulcer; psychiatric disorders; or hypertension on antihypertensives. The drug should not be abruptly discontinued due to the possibility of the development of neuroleptic malignant syndrome (NMS), such as tachycardia, muscular rigidity, fever, mental status changes, diaphoresis, and tachypnea.

Drug Interactions: Although antipsychotic drugs may be used to control psychosis associated with parkinsonism, conventional antipsychotic drugs block dopamine receptors in the brain and can decrease the therapeutic effects of levodopa. MAOIs can lead to a hypertensive crisis. Increased postural hypotension may occur if used with tricyclic antidepressants. Concurrent use with antihypertensives may cause additive hypotension. Decreased levodopa effects can occur with use of anticholinergics, hydantoins, papaverine, or pyridoxine. Antacids may increase the effects of levodopa. **Herbal/Food:** Food, especially high-protein foods and vitamin-fortified foods containing vitamin B_6, decreases the rate and extent of levodopa absorption; however, many persons must take levodopa with food to decrease the nausea and vomiting that may occur. Kava may worsen symptoms of PD. Indian snakeroot will decrease levodopa action while increasing EPS.

Pregnancy: Category C.

Treatment of Overdose: No specific treatment.

Nursing Responsibilities:

- Obtain a comprehensive health history, including any long-term physical problem (e.g., seizure disorders, cardiovascular or pulmonary disease), medication use, and allergies and lifestyle information such as the use of alcohol, illegal drugs, or caffeine, smoking, or the use of herbal preparations.
- Monitor for impaired liver and kidney functions because metabolism and excretion abnormalities could lead to toxic levels of the drug.
- Assess the patient for symptoms associated with parkinsonism, which include tremor, muscle rigidity, bradykinesia, and postural instability.
- Determine if the patient has narrow-angle glaucoma, undiagnosed skin lesions, or history of hypersensitivity; any of these are contraindications.
- Monitor the patient for severe cardiac, renal, liver, or endocrine diseases; mood disorders; history of seizures or ulcers; or pregnancy or lactation. Extra caution must be taken when these patients are given a dopamine agonist.
- Obtain baseline and periodic blood tests, including a complete blood count (CBC) and liver and renal function studies.
- Fully evaluate all other medications taken by the patient for compatibility with dopamine agonists.
- During initial treatment, closely monitor blood pressure, pulse, and respirations; these drugs may cause orthostatic hypotension and tachycardia.
- Monitor the patient for excessive daytime sleepiness, eye twitching, involuntary movements, hand tremors, fatigue, anxiety, mood changes, confusion, agitation, nausea, vomiting, anorexia, dry mouth, and constipation.
- Assist the patient with drug administration and ADLs, including ambulation, at the initiation of therapy and until effects of the medication are known.

Patient and Family Education:

- Do not crush or chew sustained release tablets.
- Immediately report muscle twitching, spasmodic winking, involuntary muscle movements, and mood changes because these may be signs of toxicity.
- Urine and perspiration may darken in color; this is a normal response to the medication.
- Make position changes slowly when moving from a lying to a standing position to prevent dizziness or possible fainting.
- Increase fiber and fluid intake to prevent constipation.
- Avoid foods high in protein or pyridoxine (vitamin B_6) such as beef, liver, ham, pork, egg yolks, sweet potatoes, and oatmeal because they will decrease the effects of the medications.
- Do not take other prescription or nonprescription drugs, dietary supplements, or herbal products without approval of the health care provider.
- Do not breast-feed while taking this drug without approval of the health care provider.
- Immediately notify the health care provider of any known or suspected pregnancy.
- Do not abruptly discontinue the drug because symptoms may become more severe.
- The full therapeutic effects of the medication will take several months to appear.
- Report any periods during which the drug stops working.

25.6 Dopamine agonists may be used as monotherapy for early symptoms of Parkinson's disease or as adjuncts to levodopa in patients with advanced disease.

Dopamine agonists (also called dopaminergic agonists) directly activate dopamine receptors in the CNS. They are less effective than levodopa at reducing symptoms of PD. They are used as monotherapy for patients with mild to moderate symptoms of PD and may be used as adjuncts to levodopa in patients with advanced disease. Doses of these agents are listed in Table 25.3.

Dopamine agonists have certain advantages over levodopa. The drugs do not have to be metabolized to be effective and they are not converted to potentially toxic metabolites. Dietary protein does not interfere with their absorption, so a low-protein diet is not necessary. With long-term use they have a lower incidence of the wearing off effect and are less likely to cause dyskinesias.

Certain adverse effects of dopamine agonists may be more serious than those of levodopa. These include postural hypotension, daytime sleepiness, and hallucinations. This group of drugs is generally reserved for younger patients, who tend to tolerate adverse effects better than elderly patients.

The dopamine agonists are divided into two subclasses. Bromocriptine (Parlodel) is an ergot alkaloid derived from the ergot fungus that grows on rye wheat. Another use of ergot alkaloids is in the treatment of migraine headaches (see Chapter 29). The nonergot alkaloids include apomorphine (Apokyn), pramipexole (Mirapex), ropinirole (Requip), and rotigotine (Neupro).

PROTOTYPE DRUG Pramipexole (Mirapex)

Classification: **Therapeutic:** Antiparkinson agent
Pharmacologic: Dopamine receptor agonist, nonergot

Therapeutic Effects and Uses: Pramipexole is an oral drug indicated for the treatment of PD. It is used as monotherapy in early PD and in combination with levodopa in advanced stages of the disease. It can produce significant motor improvement in early PD and decreases fluctuations in motor performance in late disease. Many patients are able to lower their doses of levodopa when they take pramipexole concurrently. It is also approved for treating moderate to severe symptoms of restless leg syndrome. Several weeks of therapy are necessary for the patient to obtain maximum benefits from pramipexole.

Mechanism of Action: Pramipexole is a selective agonist of the D_2 subfamily of dopamine receptors at both presynaptic and postsynaptic sites in the striatum. The binding helps to restore the balance of dopaminergic effects in the striatum. Binding at D_3 receptors contributes to the antiparkinson effects.

Pharmacokinetics:

Route(s)	PO
Absorption	Rapid absorption
Distribution	Widely distributed, especially to red blood cells; 15% bound to plasma proteins
Primary metabolism	Hepatic (minimal)
Primary excretion	Renal, mostly unchanged
Onset of action	2 h
Duration of action	Half-life: 8 h; in the elderly, 12–14 h

Adverse Effects: There are many possible adverse effects with the use of pramipexole. The most common are hallucinations, dizziness, drowsiness, and nausea. The incidence of hallucinations increases with age and may cause discontinuation of therapy in older patients. Orthostatic hypotension occurs in over half the patients taking the drug and may contribute to injury due to falls. Life-threatening adverse effects include sleep attacks, hemolytic anemia, agranulocytosis, and leukopenia. Sleep attacks can occur without warning, regardless of current activity level, and cause accidents. Agitation, insomnia, hypotension, constipation, anorexia, and dyskinesias are other adverse effects.

Contraindications/Precautions: Pramipexole should not be used in a person who has hypersensitivity to the drug or to ropinirole. The drug should be used cautiously if the patient has renal, hepatic, or cardiac disease; is taking CNS depressants; or has psychosis, dyskinesia, or affective disorders.

Drug Interactions: Dopamine antagonists that may decrease pramipexole levels include phenothiazines, metoclopramide, and the butyrophenones. Drugs that may increase pramipexole levels include levodopa, cimetidine, ranitidine, diltiazem, verapamil, and quinidine. Pramipexole may worsen dyskinesias when used concurrently with levodopa. **Herbal/Food:** Kava may decrease the effects of pramipexole.

Pregnancy: Category C.

Treatment of Overdose: No specific treatment is available for overdose. General supportive measures should be implemented.

Nursing Responsibilities

- Assess baseline vital signs, especially blood pressure, and symptoms of PD.
- Monitor for presence of orthostatic hypotension, especially when the dose is increased.
- Monitor for presence of tardive dyskinesia, which is associated with the long-term high-dose use of dopamine antagonists. Tardive dyskinesia is characterized by repetitive, involuntary, purposeless movements.
- Assess mental status, including affect, mood, depression, and behavioral changes at regular intervals during therapy.
- Alert the patient and caregivers about the possibility of sleep attacks, which can occur without warning.

Patient and Family Education:

- Change positions slowly to prevent dizziness, fainting, or falls.
- Take exactly as prescribed and do not discontinue the medication without approval of the health care provider.
- Do not drive or perform other hazardous activities until the effects of the medication are known because this drug may cause drowsiness or dizziness.
- Avoid alcohol, CNS depressants, and OTC sleep medications because these may cause excessive drowsiness.
- The full therapeutic effects of the medication will take several months to appear.
- Immediately report any hallucinations or uncontrollable muscle movements to the health care provider.

Drugs Similar to Levodopa (L-Dopa, Dopar, Larodopa) and Pramipexole (Mirapex)

Other dopamine agonists used to treat PD include apomorphine, bromocriptine, and ropinirole. Pergolide (Permax) is a dopamine agonist that was discontinued in the United States due to the possible development of valvular heart disease.

Apomorphine (Apokyn): Apomorphine, available as a subcutaneous injection, is a nonergot dopamine agonist used as a single dose to treat severe "off" episodes in patients who have advanced PD. It is not intended for use as routine management of PD symptoms. Apomorphine is structurally related to morphine, but it does not bind to opioid receptors or cause morphine-like effects (see Chapter 29). Life-threatening adverse effects include sleep attacks or acute circulatory failure. Sleep attacks are more serious than the general drowsiness or sleepiness that occurs frequently with dopaminergic agonists. They can occur during any activity, including driving and other potentially dangerous activities. The drug causes significant nausea and vomiting, and the manufacturer recommends the administration of trimethobenzamide (Tigan), an antiemetic agent, 3 days prior to the apomorphine injection. Common adverse effects are orthostatic hypotension, anorexia, and agitation. The drug can produce erections and is approved to treat erectile dysfunction in some countries (but not in the United States). This drug is pregnancy category C.

Bromocriptine (Parlodel): Approved in 1978, bromocriptine, available as a tablet, is an ergot alkaloid that has a variety of uses. In addition to being a dopamine agonist for the adjunctive treatment with levodopa for PD, it is approved for pituitary adenoma, acromegaly, and for women with amenorrhea and infertility caused by excessive prolactin secretion. Off-label indications include alcoholism, cocaine withdrawal, mastalgia, NMS, and premenstrual syndrome.

When used concurrently, bromocriptine allows a significant dose reduction of levodopa. Life-threatening adverse reactions may be seizures, shock, or MI. The most common dose-limiting adverse effects are psychological reactions, including confusion, agitation, hallucinations, paranoid delusions, or nightmares. Other adverse effects include orthostatic hypotension, headache, nausea, vomiting, anorexia, or rash on the face and arms. This drug is pregnancy category B.

Ropinirole (Requip): Approved for PD in 1997, ropinirole is an oral nonergot dopamine receptor agonist used as monotherapy for the treatment of early PD, or in combination with levodopa in more advanced disease. The most common adverse effects are syncope, fatigue, drowsiness, nausea and vomiting, and viral infections. A major advantage of ropinirole is that it causes a much lower rate of dyskinesias than levodopa. In addition, the patient taking ropinirole rarely experiences sleep attacks. In 2005, the U.S. Food and Drug Administration (FDA) approved ropinirole to treat restless leg syndrome. This drug is pregnancy category C.

Rotigotine (Neupro): One of the newest of the dopamine agonists, rotigotine was approved in 2007 for early stage Parkinson's Disease. It offers the convenience of once daily dosing using a transdermal patch. The drug is well tolerated with application site reaction, nausea, dizziness, and drowsiness being the most common adverse effects. Some patients have reported falling asleep unexpectedly while performing daily routine tasks. This drug is pregnancy category C.

25.7 Several miscellaneous dopaminergic agents are used as adjuncts to levodopa therapy.

In addition to levodopa and dopaminergic agonists, several other drugs may be used to increase dopamine levels in the striatum. These drugs act on neurons by either increasing the release of dopamine or by reducing its destruction. Doses of these drugs are listed in Table 25.3.

Amantadine (Symmetrel): Amantadine is the only FDA-approved drug that acts by increasing the release of dopamine from storage sites in the presynaptic neurons. It also blocks the reuptake of dopamine into the presynaptic neurons. Both of these mechanisms result in increased dopamine action. Given PO, the drug produces a rapid reduction in parkinsonism symptoms but its effects begin to diminish after several months of therapy. Adverse effects are primarily CNS related and include confusion, dizziness, irritability, and headache. Amantadine should be used with caution in patients with mental illness because it can exacerbate psychoses and cause hallucinations and suicidal ideation. Amantadine is an antiviral agent used for the prophylactic and symptomatic treatment of influenza A virus infections. A prototype feature may be found in Chapter 55. This drug is pregnancy category C.

Catecholamine O-methyl transferase inhibitors: Catecholamine O-methyl transferase, or COMT, is the enzyme responsible for metabolizing levodopa to its inactive intermediate 3-O-methyldopa. The **COMT inhibitors** are drugs that prevent the destruction of levodopa in peripheral tissues, thus increasing the amount of levodopa available to enter the brain. This results in a longer half-life and more consistent serum levels of levodopa.

There are only two drugs in this category approved for use in the United States. Approved in 1999, entacapone (Comtan) is available as a tablet and is recommended as an adjunct to levodopa/carbidopa. Entacapone can significantly reduce the "off" time experienced during levodopa therapy. It is contraindicated for pregnant patients (this drug is pregnancy category D) and during lactation. Approved in 1998, tolcapone (Tasmar) is also available as a tablet as an adjunct to levodopa and carbidopa. Tolcapone has a longer duration of action than entacapone and acts on COMT both peripherally and centrally. Tolcapone is a pregnancy category C drug.

The adverse effects of the COMT inhibitors are the same as those of excessive amounts of levodopa: nausea, vomiting, dyskinesias, postural hypotension, and psychiatric symptoms. In addition, tolcapone has caused fatal liver failure in some patients; therefore, regular monitoring of hepatic status must be performed during therapy.

Monoamine oxidase inhibitors (MAOIs): Monoamine oxidase (MAO) is an enzyme found in synaptic spaces that metabolizes catecholamines to inactive compounds. MAO-A acts on norepinephrine and serotonin, whereas MAO-B inactivates dopamine. Approved in 1989 for PD, selegiline (Eldepryl) is the only MAO-B inhibitor. It is available as a tablet, an orally disintegrating tablet (Zelapar), or a capsule. Although MAOs are distributed throughout the body, most of the MAO in the brain is type B. Selegiline may slow the progression of PD by delaying the degeneration of neurons; however, the effectiveness of the drug in this regard has not been clearly established. Some health care providers treat newly diagnosed patients with selegiline concurrently with levodopa or levodopa/carbidopa, hoping to delay disease progression. Selegiline is used off-label to treat Alzheimer's disease. A selegiline transdermal patch (Emsam) was approved by the FDA in 2006 for the treatment of depression.

The most frequent adverse effects during selegiline therapy are those that are also associated with levodopa: nausea, vomiting, confusion, orthostatic hypotension, bradykinesia, dyskinesias, and emotional lability. With most MAOIs, the patient must strictly avoid food containing tyramine and certain medications that could result in hypertensive crisis. Because selegiline selectively inhibits MAO-B, this is not a major concern. It is a pregnancy category C drug.

CONNECTION *Checkpoint* 25.2

From what you learned in Chapter 23, what is the other major indication for MAO inhibitors? What food nutrient must be strictly avoided in patients taking these drugs? See Answer to Connection Checkpoint 25.2 in Appendix A.

25.8 Anticholinergic drugs are the oldest of the antiparkinson agents and are effective at reducing tremor.

Anticholinergic drugs comprise the oldest category of drugs used to treat PD, having been used for over 150 years. They help to restore the balance between Ach and dopamine by blocking Ach (muscarinic) receptors in the striatum of the brain. This inhibits the effects of Ach, allowing dopamine to have greater influence.

Anticholinergics are of most benefit to the patients whose primary symptom is tremor; they are less effective at reducing bradykinesia. Overall, they exhibit fewer serious adverse effects than levodopa but they are less effective. Anticholinergics are not recommended for older adults because this population often has difficulty with the CNS adverse effects, including confusion, delusion, and hallucinations. The two anticholinergic drugs used most often to treat PD are benztropine (Cogentin) and trihexyphenidyl (Artane). The student should refer to Chapter 18 for a complete discussion on the indications, actions, and adverse effects of the anticholinergics. Doses of selected anticholinergics used to treat Alzheimer's disease are listed in Table 25.4.

PROTOTYPE DRUG Benztropine (Cogentin)

Classification: Therapeutic: Antiparkinson agent
Pharmacologic: Cholinergic antagonist

Therapeutic Effects and Uses: Benztropine is frequently used as combination therapy with trihexyphenidyl or levodopa/carbidopa in the management of PD symptoms. It is also used

TABLE 25.4 Anticholinergic Drugs and Drugs with Anticholinergic Activity Used for Parkinsonism

Drug	Route and Adult Dose (maximum dose where indicated)	Adverse Effects
benztropine (Cogentin)	PO: 0.5–1 mg/day; gradually increase as needed (max: 6 mg/day)	*Sedation, nausea, constipation, dry mouth, blurred vision, drowsiness, dizziness, tachycardia, hypotension, nervousness* <u>Paralytic ileus, cardiovascular collapse, anaphylactic shock (diphenhydramine)</u>
biperiden (Akineton)	PO: 2 mg 1–4 times/day	
diphenhydramine (Benadryl)	PO: 25–50 mg tid–qid (max: 300 mg/day)	
procyclidine (Kemadrin)	PO: 2.5 mg tid after meals; may be increased to 5 mg tid if tolerated, with an additional 5 mg at bedtime (max: 45–60 mg/day)	
trihexyphenidyl (Artane)	PO: 1 mg on day 1; 2 mg on day 2; then increase by 2 mg every 3–5 days up to 6–10 mg/day (max: 15 mg/day)	

Note: *Italics* indicate common adverse effects. <u>Underline</u> indicates serious adverse effects.

to treat drug-induced EPS. Although it suppresses tremor and rigidity, it is not effective at alleviating tardive dyskinesia. The patient may notice decreased symptoms after only 2 to 3 days of therapy with benztropine. It is an older medication approved in 1954 that is available by PO and parenteral routes. An unlabeled indication is to treat hypersalivation in patients who are developmentally disabled.

Mechanism of Action: Benztropine acts by reducing the excess cholinergic effect associated with dopamine deficiency and restores neurotransmitter balance in the striatum.

Pharmacokinetics:

Route(s)	PO, intramuscular (IM), intravenous (IV)
Absorption	Very rapid absorption if given IV; rapid with PO administration
Distribution	Wide distribution
Primary metabolism	Hepatic
Primary excretion	Renal
Onset of action	1–2 h PO; within minutes if given IM or IV
Duration of action	Half-life: 6–10 h

Adverse Effects: Common adverse reactions of benztropine are related to its anticholinergic effects and include sedation, constipation, blurred vision, dry mouth, decreased sweating, urinary retention, and confusion. Paralytic ileus is the only identified life-threatening adverse reaction.

Contraindications/Precautions: Contraindications to the use of benztropine include closed-angle glaucoma, myasthenia gravis, tardive dyskinesia, GI or urinary obstruction, prostatic hypertrophy, peptic ulcers, tachycardia, and children under age 3. Caution must be taken when benztropine is given to persons with psychiatric diagnoses because it may worsen these conditions.

Drug Interactions: Additive toxicity can occur when benztropine is taken with other drugs that exhibit anticholinergic effects, including antihistamines, tricyclic antidepressants, phenothiazines, MAOIs, or quinidine. Alcohol and other CNS depressants will have an additive sedative effect. Antidiarrheals will slow GI motility and decrease absorption of the medication. **Herbal/Food:** Kava or jaborandi will cause a decreased benztropine effect. Jimsonweed or butterbur may lead to increased benztropine effects. Black catechu can cause increased constipation.

Pregnancy: Category C.

Treatment of Overdose: Overdose can cause circulatory collapse, respiratory depression, shock, and coma. Physostigmine, 1–2 mg subcutaneous or IV, will reverse symptoms of anticholinergic intoxication. If needed, it may be repeated in 2 hours. Other treatment is supportive, according to symptoms being experienced.

Nursing Responsibilities:

- Assess mental status, including affect, mood, CNS depression or stimulation, and worsening of mental symptoms at the beginning of therapy.
- Assess therapeutic response to the medication, which should include reduced tremor and muscle rigidity but not bradykinesia.
- Monitor input and output ratio and pattern because anticholinergic drugs can produce urinary retention.
- Monitor for muscle weakness or inability to move muscle groups.
- Monitor for symptoms of impending paralytic ileus because it is the only identified life-threatening adverse reaction.
- Monitor bowel status, especially the presence of constipation.

Patient and Family Education:

- Avoid alcohol, CNS depressants, and over-the-counter sleep medications because these may cause excessive drowsiness.
- Do not take any other prescription or nonprescription drugs, dietary supplements, or herbal products without approval of the health care provider.
- Do not abruptly discontinue this drug because symptoms of parkinsonism will worsen.
- Avoid excessive manual labor, strenuous exercise, or other activities that may lead to heat stroke because this drug will decrease sweating.
- Make position changes slowly when moving from a lying to a standing position to prevent dizziness and possible fainting.
- Use good oral hygiene; take frequent sips of water, chew sugarless gum, or suck on sugarless candy to prevent dry mouth.
- Tablets may be crushed and mixed with food.
- Increase fluid and bulk in the diet and increase exercise to prevent constipation.
- Do not drive or perform other hazardous activities until the effects of the drug are known because this drug may cause drowsiness or dizziness.

Drugs Similar to Benztropine (Cogentin)

The only other anticholinergic used for PD is trihexyphenidyl (Artane).

Trihexyphenidyl (Artane): Approved in 1949, trihexyphenidyl is available in several PO formulations, in both regular and extended release forms. Its actions and adverse effects are very similar to those of benztropine. It is useful in decreasing involuntary movements and salivation, which are two problems experienced by many persons with PD. The only life-threatening adverse effect is paralytic ileus. Other adverse effects include typical anticholinergic effects such as constipation, dryness of the mouth, nausea, blurred vision, urinary retention, dizziness, and nervousness. It must not be given to patients with hypersensitivity to the drug, closed-angle glaucoma, severe cardiac impairment, myasthenia gravis, or GI or urinary obstruction. This drug should be used with caution in elderly males due to the potential for developing prostatic hyperplasia. This drug is pregnancy category C.

NURSING PROCESS APPLICATION

Patients Receiving Therapy for Parkinson's Disease

Assessment	Potential Nursing Diagnoses
Prior to administration: • Obtain a complete health history, including allergies and drug history. • Obtain information regarding symptoms, including when they began; severity; what, if anything, decreases; and the patient's response to symptoms. • Complete a mental status questionnaire. • Weigh the patient; compare current weight to usual weight. • Obtain laboratory studies.	• *Activity Intolerance,* related to consequences of disease • *Impaired Verbal Communication,* related to consequences of disease • *Constipation,* related to adverse effects of medications • *Risk for Falls,* related to physical instability, secondary to disease • *Fatigue,* related to consequences of disease • *Deficient Knowledge (Disease and Treatments)* • *Impaired Physical Mobility,* related to consequences of disease • *Total Self-Care Deficit,* related to disease progression

Planning: Patient Goals and Expected Outcomes

The patient will:

- Report a decrease of symptoms related to PD.
- Demonstrate an understanding of medications used by relating dosing schedule, desired actions, and adverse reactions.
- Know which adverse effects must be reported immediately.
- Take medications as recommended.
- Keep all follow-up appointments.

Implementation: Drugs to Treat Parkinson's Disease

Interventions and (Rationales)	Patient and Family Education
• Monitor vital signs. (Medications may cause hypo- or hypertension; hypotension may lead to falls and injuries.)	Instruct the patient and family to: • Monitor vital signs and report changes. • Report any dizziness or falls.
• Monitor for decrease or increase of symptoms. (If medications are working properly, symptoms should decrease. An increase of symptoms may mean that the medication is no longer effective, and changes in dose or medication may be necessary.)	Instruct the patient: • To be aware of any changes in symptoms. • To report any increase in symptoms. • That medication dose or medication itself may need to be changed if symptoms worsen; reassure the patient that usually changes can be made that will improve functioning.
• Monitor the diet. (The patient may not be eating enough secondary to fatigue, difficulty chewing, or swallowing. Levodopa must not be taken with high-protein foods, or with large quantities of foods containing pyridoxine.)	Instruct the patient: • To eat low-volume, high-calorie nutritious foods, and to eat six small meals daily instead of three larger ones. • Taking levodopa preparations to avoid high-protein foods, and avoid foods with high concentrations of pyridoxine (green vegetables, bananas, whole grain cereals, and legumes).
• Monitor fluid intake. (The patient may have decreased fluid consumption secondary to difficulty managing a cup or glass, a desire to decrease urine production, or not wanting to ask family members for assistance.)	Instruct the patient to: • Drink 2 L of fluids every day to help decrease renal disease and constipation, unless contraindicated by other medical diagnosis. • Locate adaptive equipment so the patient can be independent in taking fluids.
• Monitor medication regimen and adherence. (The patient may be depressed, discouraged, lack finances, or simply not understand the importance of taking medications as prescribed.)	• Instruct the patient to take all medications exactly as prescribed. • Assist the patient and family in locating financial assistance to obtain medications, if necessary.
• Monitor for adverse reactions. (Adverse reactions can be life threatening, or they can be simply irritating; the patient needs to be able to recognize them.)	Instruct the patient and family on: • Possible adverse reactions specific to the medication being taken. • Which adverse reactions must be reported immediately. • Measures to take to decrease adverse effects such as dry mouth or constipation.
• Monitor for muscle twitching and winking spasmodically. (These symptoms may indicate an overdose.)	• Instruct the patient to report immediately if muscle twitching or spasmodic winking is noted.
• Monitor for any signs of on-off phenomenon. (These may indicate the need for a dose adjustment.)	• Instruct the patient and family to be aware of incidences of symptom reappearance followed by periods of decreased symptoms, and to report them immediately.
• Monitor for changes in mental status. (Antiparkinson drugs can induce neuropsychiatric adverse reactions.)	• Instruct the patient and family to be alert for mental status or behavioral changes, such as irritability, somnolence, or violence.

Evaluation of Outcome Criteria

Evaluate the effectiveness of drug therapy by confirming that patient goals and expected outcomes have been met (see "Planning").

Alzheimer's Disease

25.9 Alzheimer's disease, the most common dementia, leads to a progressive loss of cognitive function.

Dementia is a chronic, degenerative disorder characterized by progressive memory loss, confusion, and inability to think or communicate effectively. It is usually associated with cerebral atrophy or other degenerative structural changes within the brain. Loss of short-term memory is an early sign. Patients have difficulty finding their way around familiar places and forget where they leave items. Mood swings and changes in behavior or personality eventually develop as patients become angry and frustrated with their condition. They forget how to perform normal ADLs such as bathing, cooking, or toileting and may not comprehend instructions. They often have an altered sense of time and place. Psychosis occurs in about 10% of patients and 15% to 20% develop major depression as comorbid conditions. Late changes include the inability to walk or feed themselves, incontinence, and inability to swallow.

PharmFACT

Over 5 million Americans have Alzheimer's disease. Approximately 50% of all residents admitted to nursing homes have AD as a diagnosis. *Source:* Alzheimer's Association, 2008.

The etiology of most dementia is unknown. Known causes of dementia include multiple small cerebral infarcts (vascular dementia), toxins (lead), severe infections, metabolic disorders (hypothyroidism and vitamin B_{12} deficiency), and brain tumors. Infection with the human immunodeficiency virus (HIV) causes dementia late in the progress of the disease. Alzheimer's disease is the most common type of dementia.

It should be emphasized that dementia is not a normal consequence of aging. Although cognitive changes such as memory impairment and a decline in the speed of information recall do occur with aging, these rarely interfere with ADLs and are not considered dementia.

Alzheimer's disease (AD) is a neurodegenerative disease that involves a chronic, progressive, loss of cognitive function. The disorder generally begins after age 60, and affects as many as 50% of the population over age 85. The patient generally lives 5 to 10 years following diagnosis. AD is the fourth leading cause of death. A summary of the major symptoms of AD is shown in Table 25.5.

AD leads to loss of productivity and wages (both for the patient and the caregivers), and often the patient must be placed in a long-term care facility. It is the third most expensive disease in the United States. In addition to the economics of caring for a person with AD, there are the psychological and emotional costs to families and caregivers. Cotter (2006) states that the challenge in AD is in identifying those persons with symptoms who may have decreased capacity to recognize their disorder, or blame whatever symptoms they do recognize on aging or on chronic illness. Pharmacotherapy has limited success in improving the cognitive function of patients with AD.

Despite many attempts at identifying the etiology of AD, the causes remain largely unknown. Although the cause has been elusive, structural damage in the brains of patients with AD has been well documented. Beta-amyloid protein and **neurofibrillary tangles** are found at autopsy in the brains of nearly all patients with AD. The neurofibrillary tangles are composed of insoluble proteins (Figure 25.1) and their abundance is proportional to the amount of cognitive impairment observed in the patient. It is suspected that these structural changes are caused by chronic inflammatory or oxidative cellular damage to the surrounding neurons. Environmental, immunologic, and nutritional factors, as well as viruses, are considered possible sources of brain damage. There are losses in both the numbers and functions of neurons.

TABLE 25.5 Symptoms of Alzheimer's Disease

Early (2–4 years duration)	Middle (2–12 years duration)	Late (2–4 years duration and longer)
Depression	Lack of ability to recall names of acquaintances	Lack of ability to recognize family members
Loss of ability to concentrate	Recent memory loss	Loss of ambulation ability
Increased anxiety and agitation	Loss of orientation to time, person, or place	Loss of ability to perform any ADLs
Irritability	Changes in personal habits (may become loud, use profane language; undesirable personality characteristics may become pronounced)	Loss of sphincter control
Weight loss	Increasing difficulty with self-care	Loss of ability to recognize self (e.g., does not recognize self in the mirror)
Forgetting the location of common items (car keys, home, etc.); blaming others for moving or "stealing" items		"Sundowning" syndrome (worsening of symptoms in the evening)
Forgetting important dates (family birthdays, health care provider appointments, etc.)		
Not paying bills		

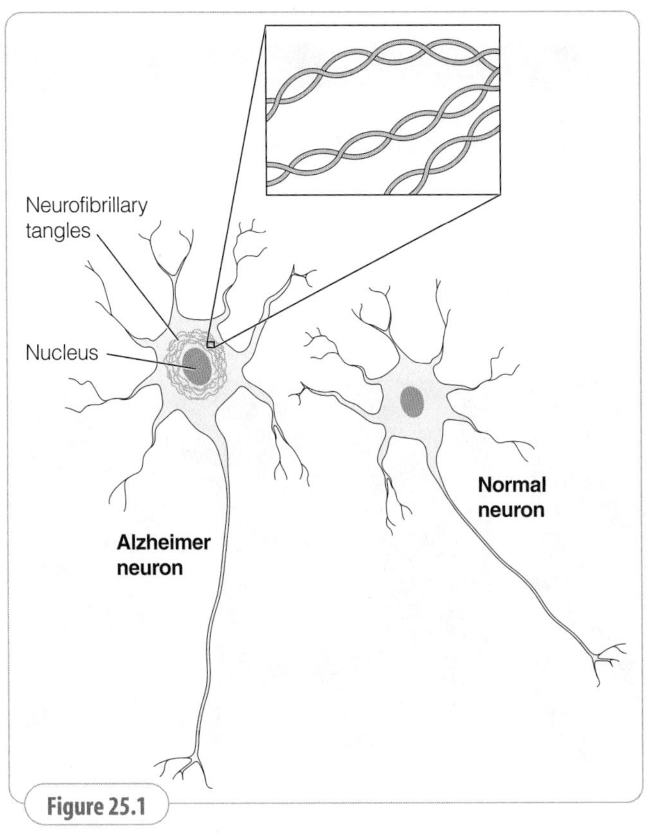

Figure 25.1

Neuron with neurofibrillary tangles seen in Alzheimer's disease.

In addition to structural changes, there are abnormalities in the balance of neurotransmitters in the brains of patients with AD. The best documented change is a deficiency of Ach, which is likely caused by brain atrophy and destruction of neurons. This loss of cholinergic activity is thought to be responsible for decreased cognition, loss of recent memory, and the inability to retain new information. Deficiencies in other brain neurotransmitters are also likely to contribute to the complex symptoms of AD.

Genetic factors appear to play a large part in the development of AD; genetic defects on chromosomes 14, 19, and 21 have been identified and may be factors leading to the development of the neurofibrillary tangles. About 5% to 15% of patients with AD show a family history of the disorder.

It is important to assess the degree of cognitive impairment in patients with dementia. Various assessment tools are used to determine a baseline degree of cognition to make decisions on whether pharmacotherapy should be implemented. During pharmacotherapy, these tools are used to determine the progression of dementia and to gauge the effectiveness (or ineffectiveness) of therapy. One very common exam is the Mini-Mental State Exam (MMSE), which is very simple and takes only 5 to 10 minutes to administer.

Pharmacotherapy of Alzheimer's Disease

25.10 Pharmacotherapy of Alzheimer's disease produces only modest results and is ineffective at stopping the progress of the disorder.

Drugs are used to slow memory loss and other progressive symptoms of dementia. In most cases, the pharmacologic treatment of dementia is the same regardless of its cause. In addition, pharmacotherapy is often necessary to treat common comorbid conditions such as depression, anxiety, or psychosis.

The FDA has approved only a few drugs for AD. The medications available do not cure or prevent AD; at best, they may slow progression of the dementia. Agents used to treat AD are listed in Table 25.6. The pharmacotherapy of AD is shown in Pharmacotherapy Illustrated 25.2.

The reversible **cholinesterase inhibitors** are the most widely prescribed drug class for treating AD. Patients treated with these drugs may demonstrate stabilization or show modest improvement of symptoms in the mild to moderate stages of AD.

Ach is naturally degraded in the synaptic cleft by the enzyme cholinesterase. When cholinesterase is inhibited, Ach levels become elevated and produce a more profound effect on Ach receptors. They are similar to the peripheral cholinesterase inhibitors such as neostigmine but appear to demonstrate more CNS activity. As described in Chapter 17, the cholinesterase inhibitors are indirect-acting parasympathomimetics.

The goal of pharmacotherapy with reversible cholinesterase inhibitors is to improve function in three domains: ADLs,

MyNursingKit | Alzheimer's Disease Video

TABLE 25.6 Drugs to Treat Alzheimer's Disease

Drug	Route and Adult Dose (maximum dose where indicated)	Adverse Effects
memantine (Namenda)	PO: initiate with 5 mg once daily; increase dose by 5 mg/week over a 3-week period to target dose of 10 mg bid	*Headache, confusion, dizziness, cough, hypertension* No serious reactions
Cholinesterase Inhibitors		
donepezil (Aricept)	PO: 5–10 mg at bedtime	*Nausea and vomiting, anorexia, diarrhea, abdominal pain, dizziness, headache, weight loss, muscle cramps* Hallucinations, depression, confusion, hepatotoxicity, increased mortality in patients with mild cognitive impairment (galantamine)
galantamine (Reminyl)	PO: initiate with 4 mg bid for at least 4 weeks; if tolerated, may increase by 4 mg bid every 4 weeks to target dose of 12 mg bid (max: 8–16 mg bid)	
rivastigmine (Exelon)	PO: start with 1.5 mg bid with food; may increase by 1.5 mg bid every 2 weeks if tolerated; target dose 3–6 mg bid (max: 12 mg bid)	
tacrine (Cognex)	PO: 10 mg qid; increase in 40 mg/day increments not sooner than every 6 weeks (max: 160 mg/day)	

Note: *Italics* indicate common adverse effects. Underline indicates serious adverse effects.

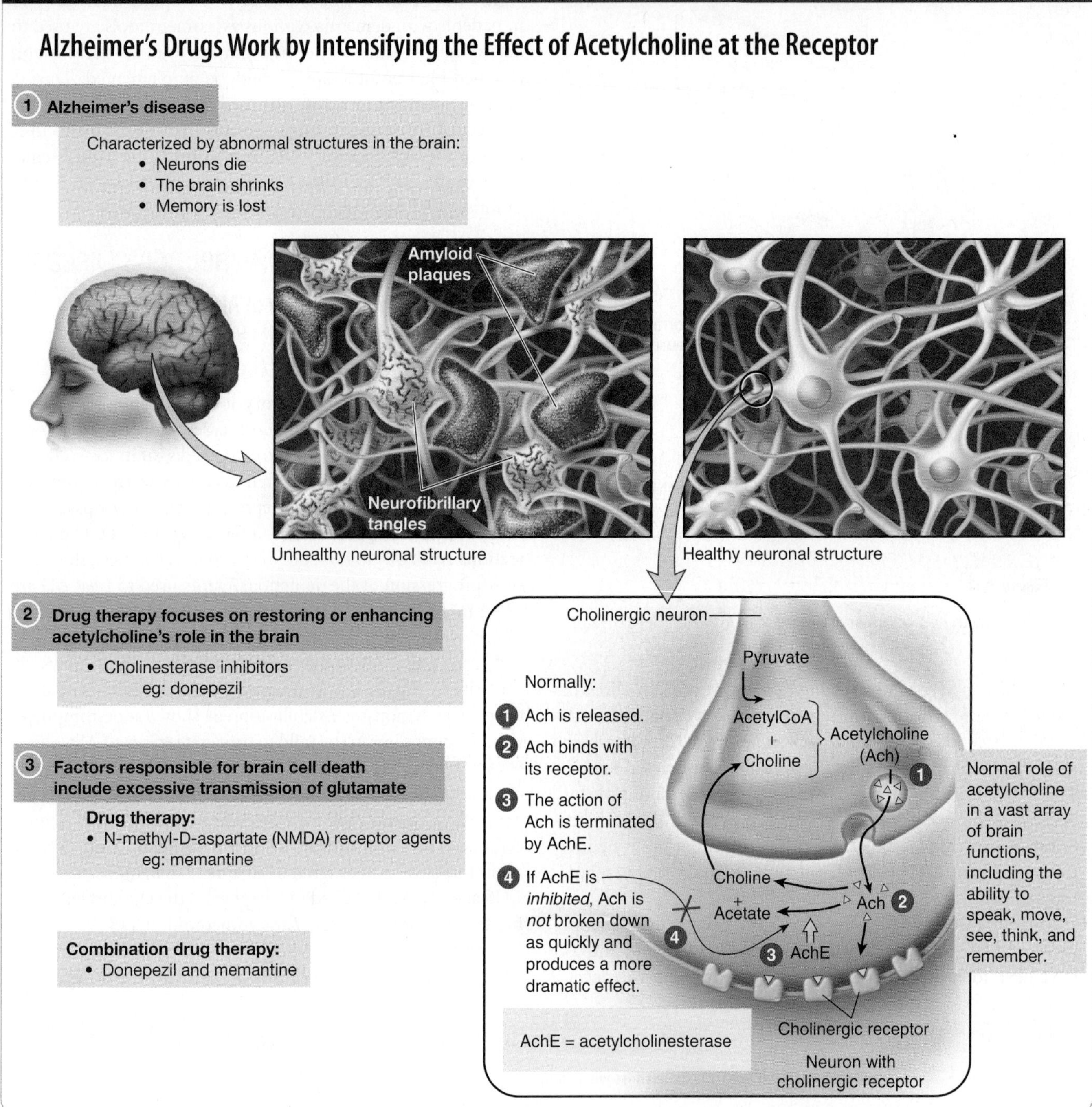

behavior, and cognition. Although the cholinesterase inhibitors improve all three domains, their effectiveness is modest at best. Therapy is begun as soon as the diagnosis of AD is established. These agents are ineffective in treating the severe stages of this disorder, probably because too many neurons have died; increasing the level of Ach is effective only if functioning neurons are present. As the disease progresses and fewer neurons are present, drug effects diminish and the cholinesterase inhibitors are discontinued; their therapeutic benefit may not outweigh their expense or the risks of adverse effects.

All cholinesterase inhibitors used to treat AD have equal efficacy. Adverse effects are those expected of drugs that enhance the parasympathetic nervous system (see Chapter 17). The GI system is most often affected, with nausea, vomiting, and diarrhea being frequent adverse events. Tacrine (Cognex) is associated with hepatotoxicity, and rivastigmine (Exelon) is associated with weight loss, which is a potentially serious adverse effect in some elderly patients. When therapy is discontinued, doses of the cholinesterase inhibitors should be tapered gradually.

CONNECTIONS

Complementary and Alternative Therapies Ginkgo Biloba for Treatment of Dementia

Description: Ginkgo biloba is one of the oldest species of trees in the world, with fossils of the tree dating back to the dinosaurs. Ginkgo seeds and leaves have been used in traditional Chinese medicine for thousands of years. The tree is now planted throughout the world, including the United States.

History and Claims: In Chinese medicine, ginkgo was used to treat asthma, tinnitus, hypertonia, and angina. In Western medicine, the focus has been on treating depression and memory loss. In Germany, an extract of ginkgo biloba is approved for the treatment of dementia.

Standardization: Ginkgo biloba extract is often standardized to contain 24% ginkgo flavonoids and 6% terpenoids. A typical dose is 120 mg/day.

Evidence: In U.S. studies, 120 mg of ginkgo taken daily has been shown to improve mental functioning and stabilize AD. The mechanism of action seems to be related to increasing the blood supply to the brain by dilating blood vessels, decreasing the viscosity of the blood, modifying the neurotransmitter system, and decreasing the density of oxygen-free radicals (Birks & Grimley, 2007). Studies concluded that cognitive performance and behavior stabilized or improved for a period of 6 to 12 months in patients with uncomplicated AD. These are the same results as those seen with tacrine (Cognex). However, not all evidence for ginkgo has been positive. A six-year study involving over 3,000 elderly adults concluded that the administration of ginkgo does not delay or prevent the progression of AD. (Dekosky, Williamson, Fitzpatrick, et al., 2008)

Patients should consult with their health care provider before taking this herb. Although most persons can take ginkgo without problems, those persons who are also taking anticoagulants, aspirin, or NSAIDs may have an increased risk for bleeding. Because the FDA does not approve herbal products, ginkgo and other herbs have not undergone the same scrutiny given to newly developed medications.

CONNECTION *Checkpoint* 25.3

The cholinesterase inhibitors for Alzheimer's disease are used for their central actions. From what you learned in Chapter 17, what are the indications for cholinesterase inhibitors that act peripherally? What drug is the prototype peripheral cholinesterase inhibitor? See Answer to Connection Checkpoint 25.3 in Appendix A.

Memantine (Namenda) is a newer drug that was approved in October 2003 for the treatment of patients with moderate to severe AD. It acts by a different mechanism than the centrally acting cholinesterase inhibitors. Memantine reduces the abnormally high levels of **glutamate,** which is the major excitatory neurotransmitter of the CNS. Chronic, high levels of brain glutamate have been associated with the pathogenesis of AD and cell death. Glutamate exerts its neural effects through interaction with the N-methyl-D-aspartate (NMDA) receptor. Memantine binds to the NMDA receptor, preventing glutamate from causing its excitatory actions and, theoretically, slowing nerve damage.

The only contraindication to the use of memantine is renal failure. Caution is indicated when given to older adults or those with renal impairment or seizure disorder. No life-threatening adverse effects have been identified. Occasional adverse effects have been reported, including nausea, vomiting, diarrhea, anorexia, anemia, coughing, conjunctivitis, and urinary incontinence. Because memantine and cholinesterase inhibitors act by different mechanisms, they may be taken in combination. When taken together, these drugs do not interfere with each other's absorption, distribution, metabolism, or elimination.

Several other agents have been investigated for their possible benefit in delaying the progression of AD. Some of these agents include various vitamins, statins, nonsteroidal anti-inflammatory drugs (NSAIDs), estrogen, and ginkgo biloba. These agents have not been found to produce any reliable effects on the progression of dementia.

Other classes of drugs frequently prescribed for symptoms associated with AD include antipsychotics, antidepressants, and antianxiety agents. Agitation occurs in the majority of patients with AD, which may be accompanied by delusions, paranoia, hallucinations, or other psychotic symptoms. Atypical antipsychotic agents such as risperidone (Risperdal) and olanzapine (Zyprexa) may be used to control these episodes. Conventional antipsychotics such as haloperidol (Haldol) are occasionally prescribed, although EPS often limit their use. The antipsychotic medications are presented in detail in Chapter 24.

Although not as common as agitation, anxiety and depression occur in many patients with AD. Anxiolytics such as buspirone (BuSpar) or benzodiazepines are used to control anxiety. Mood stabilizers such as sertraline (Zoloft), citalopram (Celexa), or fluoxetine (Prozac) are given when major depression interferes with daily activities. The student should refer to Chapters 22 and 23 for information on these drugs.

PROTOTYPE DRUG Donepezil (Aricept)

Classification: Therapeutic: Anti-Alzheimer's agent
Pharmacologic: Reversible cholinesterase inhibitor

Therapeutic Effects and Uses: Originally approved to treat mild to moderate symptoms of AD in 1996, the indication was extended to the treatment of severe AD in 2006. The drug is available in tablet, PO solution, and PO disintegrating tablet (Aricept ODT) forms. It has an extended duration of action that allows for once-daily dosing.

There is no evidence that donepezil stops the destruction of neurons or that it alters the course of the underlying dementia. It may, however, prolong the time between diagnosis and the institutionalization of the patient. A caregiver must be present to assist the patient in adhering to the medication regimen.

Mechanism of Action: Donepezil raises Ach concentrations in the brain. Because the drug is moderately selective for cholinesterase in the CNS, it produces fewer peripheral adverse effects than tacrine.

Pharmacokinetics:

Route(s)	PO
Absorption	Well absorbed
Distribution	Well distributed; crosses the blood–brain barrier; 96% bound to plasma proteins
Primary metabolism	Hepatic; metabolized to active metabolites
Primary excretion	Renal (73%); feces (15%)
Onset of action	3–4 h
Duration of action	Half life: 10 h, if single dose; 70 h if multiple dose

Adverse Effects: Common adverse effects of donepezil that cause discontinuation of therapy are diarrhea, nausea, and vomiting. Other frequent adverse effects are anorexia, muscle cramps, syncope, ecchymosis, fatigue, arthralgia, abnormal dreams, and headache. Many of these adverse events will diminish with continued therapy or by using a lower dose of the drug. Potential life-threatening adverse effects include atrial fibrillation, sinus bradycardia, and seizures. Unlike tacrine, donepezil is not associated with hepatotoxicity. Abrupt discontinuation of the drug results in a sudden decline of cognitive function and an increase in behavioral disturbances.

Contraindications/Precautions: The only contraindications to the use of donepezil are hypersensitivity to the drug or to tacrine. Donepezil exhibits typical cholinergic effects, which can worsen preexisting conditions such as bradycardia, sick sinus syndrome, asthma, chronic obstructive pulmonary disorder, ulcers or GI bleeding, urinary tract or intestinal obstruction, or hypotension. It should be used with caution in patients with hyperthyroidism or hepatic dysfunction, or who are lactating. Increased numbers of seizures have been recorded in patients taking donepezil, especially in those patients with a history of seizures.

MyNursingKit | Alzheimer's Disease Information

Drug Interactions: Donepezil is metabolized by CYP 450 enzymes (CYP2D6 and CYP3A4), and drugs that enhance or inhibit these enzymes have the potential to interact with donepezil. Decreased effects of donepezil will occur with concurrent administration of phenytoin, phenobarbital, rifampin, dexamethasone, and carbamazepine. Concurrent use of NSAIDs may lead to GI ulceration and bleeding. Synergistic effects will occur with cholinergic agonists, cholinesterase inhibitors, and succinylcholine. Because it is a cholinergic agonist, donepezil will decrease the effects of anticholinergic drugs. Metabolism of donepezil may be inhibited by quinidine and ketoconazole. **Herbal/Food:** None known.

Pregnancy: Category C.

Treatment of Overdose: Overdosage will result in signs of cholinergic crisis, such as nausea, vomiting, bradycardia, respiratory depression, hypotension, and seizures. Anticholinergic agents such as 1 to 2 mg IV atropine may be administered to reverse some of the overdose symptoms.

Nursing Responsibilities:

- Determine the patient's level of cognitive functioning, ability to self-administer medication, and ability to perform ADLs.
- Determine what symptoms of AD the patient is demonstrating, when they began, and if there is anything that makes the symptoms worse or better.
- Obtain baseline laboratory tests, especially CBC, liver and renal function tests, vital signs, weight, and vision checks.
- Determine if safety issues are present, such as the inability to function independently, the inability to be left alone, or the inability to drive. Alert the caregiver of any safety concerns.
- Determine the degree of depression, agitation, or anxiety that may be present.
- Periodically evaluate the need for alternate living arrangements, such as assisted living or a nursing home.
- Encourage participation in a support group for the patient in early stages of AD and for family members with a patient in any stage of AD.

Patient and Family Education:

- Be aware that medications may decrease some symptoms of AD but they will not cure or reverse the disease. The drug will become ineffective at some point as AD progresses.
- Immediately report any of the following signs of GI system bleeding such as blood in vomit or stools, or black, tarry stools, palpitations or slowed heart rate, changes in vision, fainting, falls, or loss of appetite.
- Take the drug with food or milk to decrease GI upset.
- Take the drug exactly as prescribed because abruptly discontinuing the medication may cause symptoms to worsen.
- Report any changes in mental status or mood to the prescriber because symptoms may be indicative of worsening of AD.
- Use good oral hygiene, take frequent sips of water, chew sugarless gum, or suck on sugarless candy to prevent dry mouth.
- To prevent constipation, increase fluid and bulk in the diet and increase exercise.

Drugs Similar to Donepezil (Aricept)

Other cholinesterase inhibitors used to treat the symptoms of AD are galantamine, rivastigmine, and tacrine.

Galantamine (Reminyl, Razadyne): Galantamine is an oral cholinesterase inhibitor that has the same uses and actions as donepezil. Approved in 2001, it is indicated for mild to moderate symptoms of dementia. Like other AD medications, it does not alter the progression of the disease. It is available in immediate and extended release forms.

The most frequent adverse effects are nausea and vomiting: The drug may be administered with food or with an antiemetic to reduce this effect. Other adverse reactions include diarrhea, bradycardia, chest pain, fatigue, anemia, syncope, vertigo, headache, insomnia, or tremor. Anorexia and weight loss are possible, which may be serious effects in debilitated patients. In addition, it is not recommended for use in persons with severe hepatic or renal dysfunction or in children or a lactating woman. It must be used cautiously in persons with respiratory disease, bradycardia, cardiac conduction disorders, seizure history, history of GI bleeding, peptic ulcer disorder, or asthma. It is a pregnancy category B drug.

Rivastigmine (Exelon): Like other drugs in this class, rivastigmine inhibits brain cholinesterase more than heart or skeletal muscle cholinesterase. Approved in 2000, it is used to treat mild to moderate symptoms of dementia associated with AD and PD. It has similar effectiveness to donepezil and tacrine. Rivastigmine is given PO with food to prevent nausea and vomiting. Liquid preparations should be mixed only with water, soda, or juice. In 2007, a once-daily transdermal patch of rivastigmine was approved by the FDA for moderate to severe AD.

Rivastigmine is contraindicated in patients with hypersensitivity to rivastigmine or carbamate. Nausea, vomiting, anorexia, and diarrhea occur in a significant number of patients. The transdermal patch form of the drug causes a lower incidence of GI adverse effects. Other common adverse effects include headache, vertigo, abdominal pain, and confusion. Cautious use is indicated when given to patients with a hypersensitivity to cholinesterase inhibitors, including tacrine, cardiac, pulmonary, renal or hepatic disease, diabetes, GI disorders, concurrent use of other cholinergic agents or anticholinergic agents, PD, seizure history, or concurrent use of NSAIDs. No potential life-threatening adverse effects have been identified. It is a pregnancy category B drug.

Tacrine (Cognex): Tacrine is the oldest of the cholinesterase inhibitors for AD and other dementias, being approved in 1993. It is very similar to donepezil in its uses and actions. A major disadvantage of tacrine is that it must be administered four times daily. In addition, the drug tends to cause a higher incidence of adverse events than others in this class. The most serious disadvantage of tacrine is hepatotoxicity. Serum transaminase (ALT) levels may become elevated in half of the patients taking the

NURSING PROCESS APPLICATION

Patients Receiving Therapy for Alzheimer's Disease

Assessment	Potential Nursing Diagnoses
Prior to administration: • Obtain a complete health history, including other medical conditions, allergies, and drug history. • Complete a mental status assessment. • Obtain information regarding symptoms: when they began, severity, and so on. • Obtain information regarding current functional status, including whether or not the patient is able to perform ADLs independently. • Obtain information regarding caregivers.	• *Total Self-Care Deficit,* related to cognitive changes • *Disturbed Sensory Perception (Visual),* related to cognitive changes • *Disturbed Thought Processes,* related to cognitive changes • *Ineffective Health Maintenance,* related to inability to recognize signs and symptoms of illness • *Ineffective Therapeutic Regimen Management,* related to cognitive changes • *Risk for Compromised Human Dignity,* related to disease process • *Risk for Injury,* related to disease process

Planning: Patient Goals and Expected Outcomes

The patient will:

- Experience a period of status quo, during which symptoms do not worsen for as long as possible.
- Remain safe from injury.
- Participate in ADLs to the maximum extent for as long as is possible.
- Not experience adverse effects of medications.
- Maintain a positive relationship with family members for as long as possible.

Implementation: Drugs Used to Treat Alzheimer's Disease

Interventions and (Rationales)	Patient and Family Education
• Monitor symptoms of AD. (Symptoms help determine the stage of the disease.)	• Instruct the patient and family to report an increase of symptoms or decrease in the patient's ability to perform self-care activities.
• Monitor adherence to medication regimen. (Symptom worsening may be delayed if medications are taken on a regular basis.)	Instruct the patient and family: • To administer medications exactly as ordered. • Not to add any medications or herbal products without discussing with the health care provider.
• Monitor the patient's safety. (If the patient's disease is worsening, injury may occur; medication may cause dizziness with subsequent falls.)	• Instruct the patient and family to monitor the patient's ability to perform previously safe activities, such as cooking, driving, and walking alone, and report if deterioration is noted. • Instruct the family to supervise ambulation until the effects of the medication are known.
• Monitor the caregiver's status. (Caring for a patient with AD can be wearing on family as well as expensive. If the caregiver is overstressed with providing care, harm may come to the patient.)	• Instruct family members on the signs of caregiver strain and to report if any of them appear. • Instruct family members of available caregiver support groups and agencies that may provide financial aid or respite care assistance.
• Instruct the patient and caregiver that medication will not cure AD. (Medication may delay worsening of symptoms but cannot effect a cure.)	• Have the patient and family verbalize the purpose of medication use in AD.
• Monitor for follow-up appointments. (Appointments must be kept so progression of the disease can be monitored and medications changed as necessary.)	• Instruct the patient and family to keep all appointments for laboratory work and health care provider follow-up.
• Monitor for GI bleeding, especially if the patient is also taking NSAIDs. (GI bleeding may occur if NSAIDs and AD are taken concurrently.)	• Instruct the patient and family to be alert for signs of GI bleeding: black, tarry stools; hematemesis; weakness; or fatigue; and to report them immediately.

Evaluation of Outcome Criteria

Evaluate the effectiveness of drug therapy by confirming that patient goals and expected outcomes have been met (see "Planning").

drug and must be monitored regularly during therapy. High ALT levels or the development of jaundice may indicate serious liver damage and are causes for discontinuation of the drug. Like other drugs in this class, common adverse effects include nausea and vomiting, diarrhea, dyspepsia, and anorexia. Food taken with tacrine will significantly slow the drug's absorption. Precautions and other adverse effects are similar to the other cholinesterase inhibitors. It is a pregnancy category C drug.

Multiple Sclerosis

MyNursingKit | Multiple Sclerosis Animation

25.11 Multiple sclerosis is a chronic, neurodegenerative disease that is treated with immunomodulator drugs.

Multiple sclerosis (MS) is a neurodegenerative disease characterized by demyelination, the destruction or removal of the myelin sheath from a nerve or nerve fiber. The destruction is secondary to an inflammatory response that leads to random areas of demyelination, known as plaques, in the white matter of the CNS. The exact cause of MS is unknown. It is believed that a pathogen, such as a latent virus, may trigger an abnormal autoimmune response in patients who are genetically susceptible. MS is a leading cause of neurologic disability in the 20 to 40 age group, although it may affect persons of any age (Figure 25.2).

PharmFACT

Although it most commonly occurs in adults, it is estimated that 8,000 to 10,000 children have MS in the United States. Children have similar symptoms but present with a higher incidence of seizures and mental status changes. *Source:* National Multiple Sclerosis Society, n.d.

MS has a typical pattern of progression that is characterized by periods of symptom exacerbation alternating with periods of remission during which symptoms completely disappear. Remissions may last several months or even years. Less commonly, progression may be continuous without any clear remission periods.

Diagnosis of MS is often difficult because its symptoms mimic those of other neurologic disorders. The early symptoms are frequently vague and nonspecific and include weakness, visual disturbances, paresthesias, mild affective disturbances, and difficulty with bladder control. Cognitive impairment is common. It should be determined if the symptoms are worsening or are intermittent. Also of note is whether the activity level of the patient has decreased, along with worsening fatigue, things that aggravate the symptoms (e.g., hot showers or baths, overexertion, stress), and any changes in personality or behavior. A diagnosis is made after other neurologic disorders have been ruled out. Imaging studies such as magnetic resonance imaging are useful in identifying the areas of demyelination in the brain.

Like other neurodegenerative disorders, there are no drugs available that can cure MS or reverse the progressive demyelination of nerves. Existing drugs for MS are only partially effective and some have serious adverse effects. In general, pharmacotherapy has three goals: to modify the disease process, to treat exacerbations and to manage symptoms.

Although the exact etiology of the disorder remains unknown, MS is considered an autoimmune disease. The body has mounted an immune attack against its own tissues, in this case, the myelin surrounding nerves. Strategies for treating MS have therefore focused on modifying the abnormal immune response of these patients through the application of immunomodulators. **Immunomodulator** is a general term that

CONNECTIONS

To the Community Living with Alzheimer's or Parkinson's Disease

Both Alzheimer's and Parkinson's diseases are progressive, degenerative neurologic disorders. It is because of these progressive symptoms that patients need all the help and support that caregivers can give. Although nonpharmacologic management such as providing a safe environment can help, medications are available to slow the progression and minimize symptoms. Caregivers need to provide assistance with ADLs, including making sure that these patients receive their medications.

Family members of patients with either diagnosis must be taught that neither they nor the patient did anything to cause the disease. They must also understand that at the present time there are no scientifically proven measures that can be taken to prevent the disease or slow progression. Disease progression will occur, despite excellent care being provided. Unscrupulous persons may try to take advantage of patient and caregiver vulnerability by trying to sell them magic "cures" or treatments, none of which have been proven to work. They need to be warned against this and strongly advised to consult their health care provider before agreeing to any new therapy.

A major consideration for persons with either diagnosis is to assist them to maintain as much independence as possible for as long as possible. Medications will help with this, but the caregivers and the community can do a lot to ensure this. Keeping routines the same; avoiding introducing too many new people, especially at the same time; and assisting the patient to continue to attend church, restaurants, and important family functions will aid in maintaining the patient's self-concept.

One of the community issues for the person diagnosed with AD is wandering or forgetting where they live. In a small community, everyone knows who has this disorder and looks out for the person. In a larger community, this is not the case. Unfortunately, people with AD may leave their homes undetected by their caregivers and then not know where they are, where they live, or even in some cases, who they are. This can lead to accidents or to criminal acts against them.

The caregivers of patients with either an AD or a PD diagnosis need to be cared for, too. They need to know that there is someone who will listen to their concerns who may have suggestions for how to make things easier and to share important issues such as nursing home placement. Many communities have caregiver support groups and the nurse should encourage caregivers to participate. Many organizations provide respite care, either a few hours at a time or 2 to 3 days at a time, so the primary caregiver can have a break. Caregivers must be encouraged to use these services without feeling guilty about trying to care for themselves. A caregiver who is rested, both emotionally and physically, will be able to provide better care to the patient than one who is not rested.

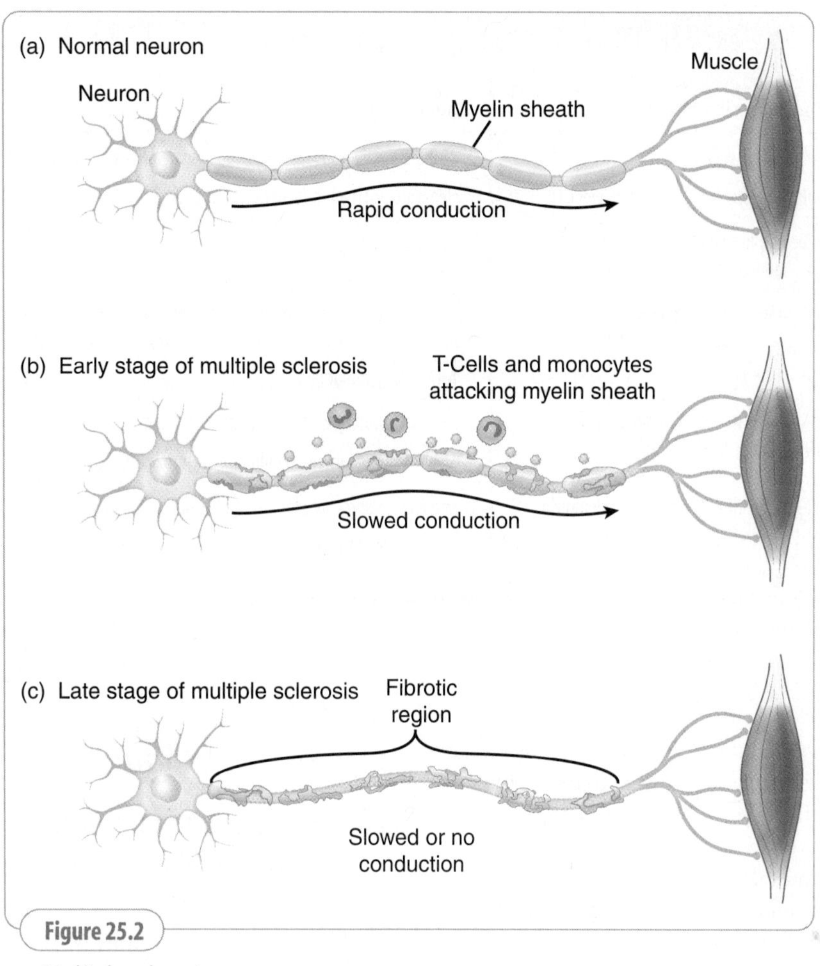

Figure 25.2

Multiple sclerosis.

refers to drugs that affect body defenses. There are two basic types of immunomodulators: those that stimulate or boost the immune response and those that suppress some aspect of immune function. Both types are used in MS pharmacotherapy. For detailed information on the immunomodulators, the student should refer to Chapter 45.

The immunomodulators are used to prevent exacerbations. They can decrease the number of new plaques being formed within the CNS, delay future disability, and help patients maintain their present quality of life. Immunomodulators should be initiated as soon as the diagnosis of MS is confirmed. The earlier treatment is begun, the better chance the patient has of avoiding or delaying permanent neurologic deficits. Treatment should continue indefinitely and only be stopped if toxicity develops or there is no apparent benefit. Doses of these drugs are listed in Table 25.7. There are four immunomodulators available in this category as first-line therapy to treat persons with MS:

- Interferon beta-1a (Avonex): IM, once weekly
- Interferon beta-1b (Betaseron): subcutaneous, every other day
- Interferon beta-1a (Rebif): subcutaneous, three times a week
- Glatiramer (Copaxone): subcutaneous, once daily

The four immunomodulators have equal efficacy in treating MS. Selection is frequently based on the clinical experiences of the health care provider and patient tolerance. They all are expensive, with monthly costs exceeding $1,000. The interferon beta preparations may cause flulike symptoms, liver impairment, leukopenia, depression, and thyroid dysfunction. Glatiramer may cause a systemic reaction that resembles myocardial ischemia. All four drugs require frequent self-administration, which increases the risk for injection site reactions or abscess formation.

Two other immunomodulators are FDA approved for patients with MS but are second-line agents due to potential toxicities. Mitoxantrone (Novantrone) is an immunomodulator that is primarily used to treat acute myelogenous leukemia and other malignancies. In 2000, indications for the drug were extended to include MS but only for patients with chronic, progressive relapses of the disorder. In treating MS, mitoxantrone acts by suppressing certain cells of the immune system, which can slow the worsening disability associated with MS. The most serious toxicities are myelosuppression and cardiomyopathy, which can result in heart failure. It is only administered by IV infusion.

Another immunomodulator, natalizumab (Tysabri), is a monoclonal antibody that acts by preventing white blood cells from migrating to the CNS. This inhibition reduces the inflammation

TABLE 25.7 Drugs Used to Treat Multiple Sclerosis

Drug	Route and Adult Dose (maximum dose where indicated)	Adverse Effects
interferon beta-1a (Avonex, Rebif)	IM: 30 mcg/week Subcutaneous: 44 mcg 3 times/week	*Myalgia, upper respiratory tract infection, flulike symptoms, local reactions, depression, headache* Hepatotoxicity, anemia, myelosuppression
interferon beta-1b (Betaseron)	Subcutaneous: 0.25 mg (8 million international units) every other day	
glatiramer (Copaxone)	Subcutaneous: 20 mg daily	*Local reactions, arthralgia, back pain, flulike symptoms, infection, anxiety, vasodilation, chest pain, palpitations, rash, pruritus, diarrhea, nausea, dyspnea, rhinitis* Asthenia, lymphadenopathy
mitoxantrone (Novantrone)	IV: 12 mg/m^2 every 3 months (max: lifetime dose 140 mg/m^2)	*Nausea, vomiting, diarrhea, cough, headache, abdominal pain, fever, alopecia* Myelosuppression, renal failure, hepatotoxicity, cardiotoxicity (heart failure, MI, fetal harm)
natalizumab (Tysabri)	IV: 300 mg infused over 1 h every month	*Headache, depression, fatigue, menstrual dysfunction* Anaphylaxis (rare), infections

Note: *Italics* indicate common adverse effects. Underline indicates serious adverse effects.

and demyelination of nerves in the brain. It is administered by IV infusion. Although natalizumab is thought to be the most effective drug for treating MS, its use is severely restricted due to a small risk of progressive multifocal leukoencephalopathy (PML), a rare and sometimes fatal demyelinating disease of the CNS. The drug was briefly removed from the market in 2005 but has since been reapproved with restrictions that limit the prescribers to those who have special training in PML. Only patients of these "approved" health care providers may take the drug. In addition, only certain pharmacies can distribute the drug. Considerable research is ongoing to identify safer monoclonal antibodies that are equally effective in treating MS. Additional details on the monoclonal antibody class of drugs may be found in Chapter 45.

Acute exacerbations of the disease are treated with high-dose corticosteroid therapy with prednisone or methylprednisolone. The recommended length of treatment is no longer than 3 weeks and no more than three times a year. Although very high doses are administered, the short-term use of corticosteroids does not usually cause significant adverse effects (see Chapter 69). Another drug that can be used to treat an acute exacerbation is IV gamma globulin. This has proven to be a successful treatment for patients who are unresponsive or unable to tolerate corticosteroids.

Other categories of drugs may be ordered to manage symptoms of MS. These symptomatic medications are used to treat other conditions and are discussed in length in other chapters of this text. The patient may suffer from physical symptoms such as muscle spasticity or bladder or bowel dysfunction. Depression is very common; it may be the emotional response to a diagnosis of a chronic, progressive, potentially debilitating disease, or it may be secondary to damage to mood-regulating neurons as the disease progresses. Chronic pain may require the use of analgesics.

Amyotrophic Lateral Sclerosis

25.12 The pharmacotherapy of amyotrophic lateral sclerosis is limited to a single drug.

Amyotrophic lateral sclerosis (ALS), commonly known as Lou Gehrig's disease, is the most common degenerative disease of the motor neurons. Its symptoms include weakness and atrophy of the muscles of the legs, hands, and forearms that spread to all muscles of the body. Sensory and cognitive functions are not affected. It usually occurs in middle age and progresses rapidly to death in 2 or 3 years due to respiratory failure or pneumonia. There is no known cause or curative treatment for the disease. About 10% of cases have a familial history of the disorder.

There is only one drug with FDA approval for treating patients with ALS. Approved in 1995, riluzole (Rilutek) cannot cure the disease, but it has been proven to extend survival by reducing the degeneration of neurons. It is estimated that survival is prolonged by only 3 months. Riluzole is a tablet that is given every 12 hours on an empty stomach. The patient should avoid high-fat meals immediately before or after taking riluzole because it interferes with medication absorption. Seizures are the only life-threatening adverse effect. Common adverse effects include headache, dizziness, poor concentration, confusion, anxiety, hypotension, and edema.

The patient with ALS suffers from painful muscle spasticity. Treatment with muscle relaxants such as baclofen (Lioresal) may bring some relief (see Chapter 27). An anticholinergic agent such as trihexyphenidyl or benztropine may be administered to decrease saliva production. Opioids may be necessary to treat severe pain late in the progress of the disease.

UNDERSTANDING THE CHAPTER

Key Concepts Summary

25.1 Degenerative diseases of the central nervous system are characterized by irreversible and progressive loss of neuronal function.

25.2 Parkinson's disease is a progressive neurodegenerative disorder characterized by abnormal motor movement.

25.3 Parkinson's disease is caused by a lack of sufficient amounts of dopamine produced by the substantia nigra.

25.4 The drugs used for Parkinson's disease help to alleviate symptoms but do not cure the disease.

25.5 Replacement therapy with levodopa is the most effective therapy for treating Parkinson's disease.

25.6 Dopamine agonists may be used as monotherapy for early symptoms of Parkinson's disease or as adjuncts to levodopa in patients with advanced disease.

25.7 Several miscellaneous dopaminergic agents are used as adjuncts to levodopa therapy.

25.8 Anticholinergic drugs are the oldest of the antiparkinson agents and are effective at reducing tremor.

25.9 Alzheimer's disease, the most common dementia, leads to a progressive loss of cognitive function.

25.10 Pharmacotherapy of Alzheimer's disease produces only modest results and is ineffective at stopping the progress of the disorder.

25.11 Multiple sclerosis is a chronic, neurodegenerative disease that is treated with immunomodulator drugs.

25.12 The pharmacotherapy of amyotrophic lateral sclerosis is limited to a single drug.

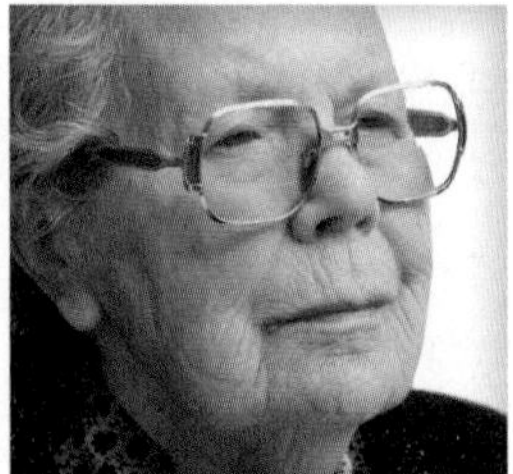

Making the PATIENT *Connection*

Remember the patient "Mary Lee" at the beginning of the chapter? Now read the remainder of the case study. Based on the information presented within this chapter, respond to the critical thinking questions that follow.

Mary Lee is a 73-year-old retired high school principal with a PhD in educational administration. She has been married to Robert for almost 50 years, and they have three grown children who live within 25 miles of them. Mary's physical health has been good. She has mild hypertension and had colon cancer successfully removed 20 years ago. She has an annual physical and cancer screenings as recommended for her age. Robert makes an appointment with Mary's health care provider, because he has noticed signs of decreasing mental acuity over the past year. Mary's physical exam is negative, but the health care provider suspects that she is experiencing the early stage of Alzheimer's disease (AD). Mary is started on donepezil (Aricept), 5 mg at bedtime.

Critical Thinking Questions

1. What information should be included in the initial assessment in order to determine a diagnosis for Mary?
2. What recommendations will the health care provider most likely make to Mary and her husband?
3. What should Robert be alert for with regard to the donepezil?

Case Study

Michael, at 45 years of age, could not believe his ears when the health care provider told him he had Parkinson's disease (PD). "Isn't that an old person's disease?" he asked. However, he knew something had been very wrong for about 3 months. At first he felt more tired than usual, and he noticed a slight tremor, especially when he became fatigued. Michael's wife pointed out that his "hand shakes" were getting worse. Like many people first diagnosed with a degenerative nervous system disease, Michael has many questions and concerns. Following are just a few of his questions. As his nurse, how would you respond?

1. What is the physiological problem that causes PD and what is the etiology of this disease?
2. Eventually, Michael is prescribed carbidopa/levodopa (Sinemet) for his parkinsonism. How does this medication work? What is the advantage of combining the two medications?
3. What drug-related adverse effects would you discuss with Michael?

NCLEX-RN® Review

1 The client is receiving levodopa (Larodopa) for parkinsonism. Which of the following drugs would the nurse expect to be added to the client's drug regimen to help control tremors?

1. Amantadine (Symmetrel)
2. Benztropine (Cogentin)
3. Haloperidol (Haldol)
4. Donepezil (Aricept)

2 Which statement, if made by the client, would alert the nurse that the antiparkinson medication is effective?

1. "I'm sleeping a lot more, especially during the day."
2. "My appetite has improved."
3. "I'm able to shower by myself."
4. "My skin doesn't itch anymore."

3 The nurse is counseling the caregivers of a client with Alzheimer's disease. Which of the following statements, if made by a caregiver, would indicate that the session had been effective?

1. "I should give this medication as symptoms of AD become noticeable."
2. "If constipation occurs, I will notify the health care provider immediately."
3. "The medication may improve symptoms but will not cure the disease."
4. "I will take the client's vital signs before every dose of the medication."

4 The nurse knows that a major disadvantage for the use of tacrine (Cognex) to treat the symptoms of early Alzheimer's disease is that it: (Select all that apply.)

1. Must be administered four times per day.
2. Causes weight gain.
3. May cause vision difficulties.
4. May cause serious hepatic damage.
5. Can be purchased over-the-counter.

5 The nurse knows that an advantage to rivastigmine (Exelon) over other cholinesterase inhibitors is that it:

1. Has no significant drug interactions.
2. Does not cause cholinergic adverse effects.
3. Is absorbed best on an empty stomach.
4. Does not alter glucose control in clients with diabetes.

6 The family of a client diagnosed with early stage Alzheimer's disease confides in the nurse about the client's depression. Which of the following responses provided by the nurse would be appropriate?

1. "Don't worry; the depression will go away by itself."
2. "Soon the client won't be able to remember anything, so won't be depressed."
3. "The health care provider can order a trial with an antidepressant medication."
4. "You can get some OTC estrogen cream; it will help delay the symptoms."

See Answers to Critical Thinking Questions, Case Study, and NCLEX-RN® Review in Appendix A.

References

Alzheimer's Association. (2008). *Alzheimer's disease facts and figures.* Retrieved June 14, 2008, from http://www.alz.org/national/documents/report_alzfactsfigures2008.pdf

Birks, J., & Grimley, E. J. (2007). Ginkgo biloba for cognitive impairment and dementia. *Cochrane Database of Systematic Reviews, 2.* Art. No.: CD003120. DOI: 10.1002/14651858.CD003120. pub2.

Cotter, V. (2006). Alzheimer's disease: Issues and challenges in primary care. *Nursing Clinics of North America, 41,* 83–93.

Dekosky, S. T., Williamson, J. D., Fitzpatrick, A. L., Kronmal, R. A., Ives, R. G., Saxton, J. A., et al. (2008). Ginkgo biloba for dementia. *Journal of the American Medical Association, 300*(19), 2253–2262.

Kleinschnitz, C., Meuth, S. G., Stüve, O., Kieseier, B., & Wiendl, H. (2007). Multiple sclerosis therapy: An update on recently finished trials. *Journal of Neurology, 254*(11), 1473–1490.

National Multiple Sclerosis Society. (n.d.). *Pediatric (child) MS.* Retrieved June 13, 2008, from http://www.nationalmssociety.org/about-multiple-sclerosis/who-gets-ms/pediatric-ms/index.aspx

National Parkinson Foundation. (n.d.). *About Parkinson disease.* Retrieved June 13, 2008, from http://www.parkinson.org/NETCOMMUNITY/Page.aspx?pid=225&srcid=201

Onega, L. (2006). Assessment of psychoemotional and behavioral status in patients with dementia. *Nursing Clinics of North America, 41*(1), 23–41.

Qiu, C., De Ronchi, D., & Fratiglioni, L. (2007). The epidemiology of dementias: An update. *Current Opinion in Psychiatry, 20*(4), 380–385.

Reese, R. (2005). The long trip home. *Nursing 2005, 35,* 46–47.

Scatena, R., Martorana, G. E., Bottoni, P., Botta, G., Pastore, P., & Giardina, B. (2007). An update on pharmacological approaches to neurodegenerative diseases. *Expert Opinion on Investigational Drugs, 16*(1), 59–72.

Schutte, D. (2006). Alzheimer disease and genetics: Anticipating the questions. *The American Journal of Nursing, 106*(12), 40–48.

Schutte, D. (2004). The evolving role of genomics in shaping care for persons with dementia. *Nursing Clinics of North America, 39*(3), 582–592.

Shumaker, S. A., Legault, C., Kuller, L., Rapp, S. R., Thal, L., Lane, D. S., et al. (2004). Conjugated equine estrogens and incidence of probable dementia and mild cognitive impairment in postmenopausal women: The Women's Health Initiative Memory Study. *Journal of the American Medical Association, 291,* 2947–2958.

Torrisi, D. (2005). My dad has Parkinson disease. And my mother has boundless love. *The American Journal of Nursing, 105,* 39.

Vega, C. (2006). New guidelines address care of patients with Alzheimer's dementia. *American Journal of Geriatric Psychiatry, 14,* 561–572.

C H A P T E R

I'm not sure I can cope with my child having a seizure disorder. The schedule for giving the medicines seems daunting to me. I am not sure I will remember all of the steps to watch for when he has a seizure. Also, I am not sure I understand all the aspects of the medications and how they work.

Patient "Jorge Alvarez's" mother

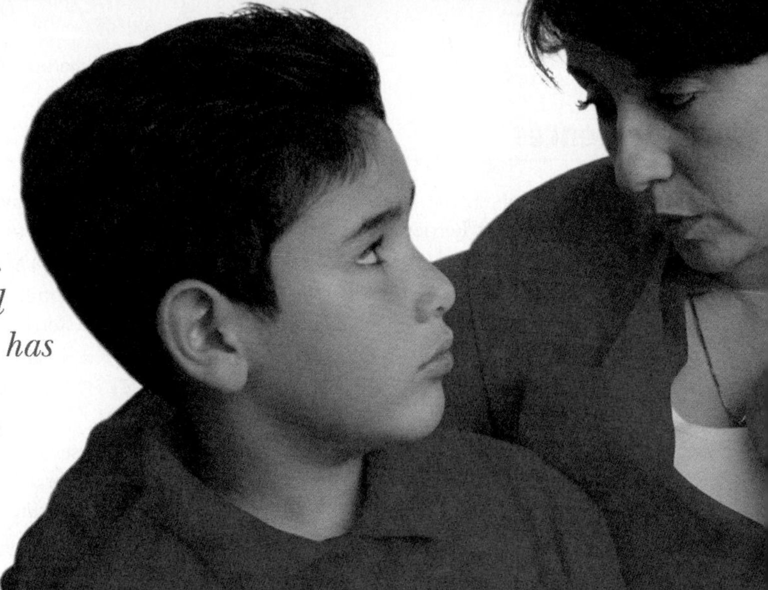

26 Pharmacotherapy of Seizures

Learning Outcomes

After reading this chapter, the student should be able to:

1. Differentiate among the following terms: *epilepsy, seizures,* and *convulsions*.
2. Understand the causes of epilepsy.
3. Describe how the presentation and pharmacotherapy of epilepsy change throughout the life span.
4. Differentiate the signs, symptoms, and pharmacotherapy of the different types of seizure disorders.
5. Compare and contrast the pharmacotherapy of generalized and partial seizures.
6. Describe the nurse's role in the pharmacologic management of seizures.
7. For each of the classes shown in the chapter outline, identify the prototype and representative drugs and explain the mechanism(s) of drug action, primary indications, contraindications, significant drug interactions, pregnancy category, and important adverse effects.
8. Use the nursing process to care for patients receiving antiseizure drugs.

Chapter Outline

Characteristics of Seizure Disorders

Classification of Seizure Disorders

Antiseizure Drugs

Barbiturates

Benzodiazepines

PROTOTYPE DRUG **Diazepam (Valium)** *p. 382*

Hydantoins

PROTOTYPE DRUG **Phenytoin (Dilantin, Phenytek)** *p. 384*

Iminostilbenes

PROTOTYPE DRUG **Carbamazepine (Tegretol, Tegetrol XR, Carbatrol, Others)** *p. 386*

Succinimides

PROTOTYPE DRUG **Ethosuximide (Zarontin)** *p. 388*

Miscellaneous Antiepileptics

PROTOTYPE DRUG **Gabapentin (Neurontin)** *p. 389*

PROTOTYPE DRUG **Valproic Acid (Depacon, Depakene, Depakote)** *p. 390*

The word *epilepsy* is derived from the Greek word "epilepsia," meaning to take hold or seize. Epilepsy is a neurologic condition characterized by recurrent seizures that affects approximately 2 million Americans. Research in the past two decades has resulted in the development of new drugs to treat epilepsy and other seizure disorders. In this chapter the student will study the current medications for seizures and understand the nurse's role in the administration and patient education associated with the medication regimen.

Characteristics of Seizure Disorders

26.1 Epilepsy is characterized by recurrent seizures caused by disturbances in the electrical activity of the brain.

According to the National Institute of Neurological Disorders and Stroke, **epilepsy** is a disruption of the neuronal activity of the brain characterized by two or more seizures. A **seizure** is a disturbance of the brain's electrical activity that may result in loss of consciousness and sensation and an alteration in motor activity. The many diverse symptoms of seizure are caused by abnormal neuronal discharges within the different regions of the brain. Abnormal neuronal discharges can be measured as sharp spikes or waves on an electroencephalogram (EEG), which is a valuable tool in diagnosing seizure disorders. Figure 26.1 compares normal and abnormal EEG recordings.

It is important to identify the cause of seizure activity so that the appropriate treatment regimen may be implemented. Epileptic seizures are sometimes symptoms of an underlying disorder such as a brain tumor, head trauma, brain aneurysm, cerebrovascular accident (CVA), alcoholism, or infectious disease of the brain. The diagnosis of epilepsy always begins with a search for an underlying disorder that could explain the seizures. Table 26.1 lists common etiologies for seizure disorders. Seizures that result from acute, temporary conditions generally do not reoccur once the underlying medical condition has been successfully treated. If a brain abnormality exists after the acute situation resolves, recurrent seizures are likely.

CONNECTION *Checkpoint* 26.1

Seizures often occur during alcohol withdrawal. From what you learned in Chapter 8, describe other signs and symptoms of withdrawal that a patient may exhibit to lead you to conclude that a seizure might be alcohol related. See Answer to Connection Checkpoint 26.1 in Appendix A.

In 50% to 70% of cases, the etiology of a seizure is idiopathic; no specific cause can be identified. These patients may have a lower tolerance to environmental triggers, and seizures may occur when they are sleep deprived, are exposed to strobe or flickering lights, or have a fluid and electrolyte imbalance. Diagnostic tests such as complete blood count (CBC), serum lead levels, and blood glucose are important in excluding the systemic causes of seizures. Virtually anything that changes the homeostatic environment of brain neurons has the potential to cause seizures, thus complicating the diagnosis and treatment of epilepsy.

It is important to distinguish between the terms *convulsion* and *seizure*. Most often, patients associate epilepsy with **convulsions,** which are involuntary, violent spasms of the large skeletal muscles of the face, neck, arms, and legs. Convulsions are a characteristic sign of tonic–clonic seizures. Epilepsy, however, is a diverse disease that includes nearly 20 different seizure disorders, only some of which involve convulsions. For example, absence seizures do not involve any dramatic movement of the limbs and may be barely noticeable by those observing the affected person. Thus, it may be stated that all convulsions are seizures, but not all seizures are convulsions. Because of this difference, agents used to treat epilepsy are best described as antiepileptic drugs (AEDs) or antiseizure medications, rather than anticonvulsants.

Key Terms

absence seizures, 374
atonic seizures, 374
automatisms, 375
complex partial seizures, 375
convulsions, 371
eclampsia, 373
epilepsy, 371
febrile seizures, 376
generalized seizures, 374
infantile spasm, 376
Lennox-Gestaut syndrome, 376
myoclonic seizures, 375
partial (focal) seizures, 375
postictal state, 374
preeclampsia, 373
seizure, 371
simple partial seizures, 375
status epilepticus, 376
tonic–clonic seizures, 374

Pharm*FACT*

Older adults over age 60 have the highest incidence of new-onset seizures. If untreated, the recurrence rate of seizures in the elderly is estimated at 90%.

Source: Ossemann et al., 2006.

Seizures have the potential to significantly impact one's quality of life. They may cause serious injury if they occur while a person is driving a vehicle or performing a dangerous activity. Without pharmacotherapy, epilepsy can severely limit participation in school, employment, and social activities and affect self-esteem. Chronic depression may accompany poorly controlled seizures. Proper treatment, however, can reduce or completely eliminate seizures in many patients. Important considerations in nursing care include identifying patients at risk for seizures, documenting the pattern and type of seizure activity, and implementing safety precautions. In collaboration with the patient, health care provider, and pharmacist, the nurse is instrumental in achieving positive therapeutic outcomes during AED therapy. The nurse must educate patients that effective seizure control can be achieved by the majority of patients through a combination of pharmacotherapy and support from family and caregivers.

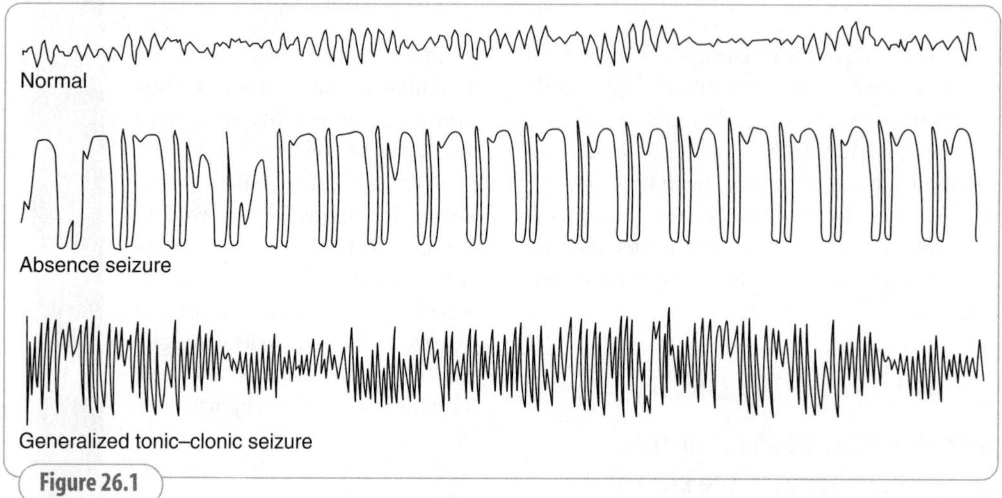

Figure 26.1

EEG readings showing the differences among normal, absence seizure, and generalized tonic–clonic seizure tracings.

26.2 Seizure disorders differ throughout the life span.

Seizure disorders occur throughout the life span. Of those who experience seizures, about half will experience their first seizure before age 10. Because of this, epilepsy is considered a major disorder of childhood. Fortunately, many patients who have childhood epilepsy experience a reduction in symptoms as they age, and some will no longer require pharmacotherapy as adults. In addition to childhood, epilepsy manifests with higher frequency during pregnancy and in older adults. Treatment differs somewhat throughout the life span.

Women, pregnancy, and lactation: The pharmacotherapy of epilepsy in women with childbearing potential can be challenging. These patients require special education to either prevent conception or to safely prevent seizures during pregnancy.

Some AEDs interact with oral contraceptives, diminishing the effectiveness of birth control pills. AEDs that are inducers of CYP450 enzymes will increase the metabolism of contraceptive hormones, thus decreasing their ability to prevent conception. Antiseizure drugs that induce CYP450 include phenobarbital, carbamazepine, oxcarbazepine, topiramate, and phenytoin. To prevent an unplanned pregnancy the patient should receive a higher dose of oral contraceptive and be instructed to use additional methods of birth control. Therapy with antiseizure drugs that do not induce CYP450 enzymes, such as valproic acid or gabapentin, should be considered for these women.

Pregnancy is a major concern for women with seizure disorders. Women with epilepsy have a higher baseline risk for delivering a child with congenital abnormalities, and many of the AEDs have the potential to produce teratogenic effects. The

TABLE 26.1 Etiology of Seizure Disorders

Etiology	Pathophysiology
Fever	Rapid increase in body temperature may result in febrile seizure. This is particularly noted in infants and toddlers.
Infectious Disease	Meningitis and encephalitis, which are infections of the brain, result in brain inflammation and seizure development.
Metabolic Disorders	Alteration in the fluid and electrolyte levels can result in seizure development. Hypoglycemia, hyponatremia, and water intoxication contribute to the alteration in electrical impulse transmission at the cellular level.
Miscellaneous Causative Agents	Medication used to treat mood disorders and psychotic episodes and local anesthetics produce increased levels of stimulatory neurotransmitters or toxicity. Drug abuse, such as cocaine addictions, alter the neurotransmitters in the brain and produce seizures. Alcohol and sedative–hypnotic drug withdrawal can result in seizure activity.
Neoplastic Disorders	Both benign and malignant brain lesions, particularly those that possess rapid growth, prevent adequate oxygenated blood supply to the brain tissue and contribute to increased intracranial pressure, which results in seizure development.
Trauma	Head injuries may result in increased intracranial pressure, which results in seizure development. Exposure to toxic fumes or substances, or ingestion of poisons can result in trauma to brain tissue and resultant seizures.
Vascular Disorders	Hypoxia of brain tissue disrupts the electrical transmission of impulses contributing to seizure development. Carbon monoxide poisoning reduces the oxygen carrying ability of the blood and results in cerebral hypoxia. The related ischemia of brain tissue alters the electrical transmission of impulses and contributes to seizure development. Other vascular causes of seizures include hypotension, CVAs, shock, and cardiac dysrhythmias.

risk of birth defects is further increased because some AEDs cause folic acid (folate) deficiency, a condition that has been associated with increased risk of neural tube defects in the embryo. Folic acid supplements (0.4 to 4 mg per day) should always be recommended for women who are considering pregnancy and those who become pregnant. The use of vitamin supplementation will also contribute to the prevention of cardiac abnormalities and the development of cleft lip or palate. Single drug therapy should be used whenever possible because therapy with multiple AEDs results in a higher risk of birth defects. Doses are reduced to the lowest possible level that effectively controls the seizures. Newer AEDs such as lamotrigine, gabapentin, and zonisamide should be considered because they appear to have less teratogenicity.

Women who suffer from epilepsy have a significantly reduced rate of fertility. Epilepsy and AEDs disrupt the hypothalamus–pituitary axis, causing menstrual irregularities. The length of the menstrual cycle in these patients may vary from 23 to 35 days, and 40% of women with epilepsy have polycystic ovaries. Many women suffering from epilepsy do not ovulate. Genital blood flow is diminished and libido is reduced, likely contributing to a reduction in the frequency of intercourse.

Vitamin K deficiency in neonates has been noted as a result of AED therapy during pregnancy. According to the American Academy of Neurology, it is recommended that prenatal vitamin K be prescribed to women who are taking AEDs during pregnancy to prevent hemorrhagic disease in the newborn; 10 mg of vitamin K should be administered daily beginning on the 36th week of gestation and continuing until delivery.

Gestational epilepsy is a rare condition in which the patient experiences her first seizure during pregnancy. Seizures in a pregnant patient who has never been diagnosed with epilepsy may indicate the development of preeclampsia or eclampsia. **Preeclampsia** occurs during pregnancy when blood pressure increases to 140/90 mmHg or higher on two separate occasions, and 300 mg of protein is found in the urine over a 24-hour period. Abnormal swelling of the hands and feet may be observed. The rate of preeclampsia in the United States is approximately 5% to 7% of all pregnancies, affecting about 1 in every 2,000 to 3,000 deliveries.

Eclampsia occurs if hypertension (HTN) continues to worsen during pregnancy. Eclampsia is associated with seizures and a high risk of cerebral edema, which can result in coma. If the baby is of proper gestational age, delivery is the treatment of choice for eclampsia. When the pregnant woman is diagnosed with preeclampsia or eclampsia and delivery is not imminent, intravenous (IV) magnesium sulfate may be administered to prevent or terminate seizures. Magnesium sulfate acts by decreasing the amount of acetylcholine liberated from the motor nerve terminals and produces a peripheral neuromuscular blockade. It also has the therapeutic effect of increasing uterine blood flow. Because seizures may extend beyond labor and delivery, magnesium sulfate therapy may continue for 24 hours postpartum or until the HTN resolves.

Because the amounts of AEDs secreted in breast milk are low, breast-feeding may be allowed during AED therapy. The benefits of breast-feeding outweigh the potential adverse effects caused by the drugs (American Academy of Neurology, 2008). AEDs that have the most protein binding are least likely to appear in high concentration in breast milk. Those with the highest degree of protein binding include phenytoin, tiagabine, and valproic acid. The nurse should instruct mothers taking sedating antiepileptic drugs how to monitor neonates for sedation.

Childhood: Seizures in children are either idiopathic or acquired. Children with idiopathic seizures often have a family history of epilepsy or have an associated serious neurologic abnormality, such as mental retardation or cerebral palsy. Febrile seizures are another form of idiopathic seizure that occurs in children under the age of 2 years. Seizures represent the most common serious neurologic problem affecting children, with an overall incidence of approximately 1% for idiopathic epilepsy.

MyNursingKit | Epilepsy Video

Acquired seizure disorders may result from injury to the brain during the prenatal, antenatal, or postpartum periods. Infants whose mothers have been exposed to cytomegalovirus during pregnancy are at increased risk of developing an acquired seizure disorder. Other causes of acquired seizures include head trauma, metabolic imbalances, exposure to toxins, and infection.

Seizure treatment for infants and children is usually accomplished with pharmacotherapy. The most commonly prescribed pediatric AEDs include phenobarbital, valproic acid, phenytoin, carbamazepine, felbamate, lamotrigine, and topiramate. To maintain optimum seizure control, the dosage of AEDs should be increased during periods of rapid growth and development.

Nonpharmacologic treatments for epilepsy are available. One such alternative therapy is the ketogenic diet. The beneficial effects of this diet occur when ketones are eliminated from the body, thus decreasing seizure activity. Other forms of seizure treatment include surgical intervention with an excision of a circumscribed area of the brain affected by the seizure activity. The implantation of a vagal nerve stimulator in the brain is a type of therapy that delivers electrical signals to the vagus nerve to reduce the frequency of seizures.

Older adults: Seizure disorders in the older adult are most often associated with an underlying comorbid condition. Cerebrovascular disease, especially CVA, accounts for one third of all cases and is the most common risk factor for the development of epilepsy after age 60. Other conditions associated with epilepsy in the aging patient include progressive Alzheimer's disease, subdural hematoma from a head injury due to falling, central nervous system (CNS) infection, and brain tumors.

MyNursingKit | Preeclampsia Video

Older adults often take multiple medications that can contribute to seizure activity. It is vital to regularly monitor the liver and kidney functions of the elderly patient when administering multiple medications because impairment may lead to toxic serum drug levels and possible seizures.

The nurse needs to assess the patient's therapeutic response to the AEDs as well as the serum drug level. The clinical response should be used to guide the needed dosage changes. When possible, only a single AED is prescribed because the use of multiple AEDs increases the risk of adverse drug events. In most patients, therapy with AEDs begins

CONNECTIONS

Complementary and Alternative Therapies The Ketogenic Diet

Description: The ketogenic diet is used when seizures cannot be controlled through pharmacotherapy or when there are unacceptable adverse effects to the medications. Before antiepileptic drugs were developed, this diet was a primary treatment for epilepsy.

History and Claims: The ketogenic diet may be used for babies, children, or adults. With adults, however, it is harder to develop the ketones that are necessary for the diet.

Standardization: The ketogenic diet is a stringently calculated diet that is high in fat and low in carbohydrates and protein. It limits water intake to avoid ketone dilution and carefully controls caloric intake. Each meal has the same ketogenic ratio of 4 g of fat to 1 g of protein and carbohydrate. Extra fat is usually given in the form of cream. The diet works rapidly in some children, with improvement noted in an average of 5 days (Kossoff et al., 2008).

Evidence: Research suggests that the diet produces success rates similar to those of medication use, with one third of the children using it becoming seizure free, one third having their seizures reduced, and one third not responding. The diet appears to be equally effective for every seizure type, although those with drop attacks (atonic seizures) may be the most rapid responders. It also helps children with Lennox-Gastaut syndrome and shows promise in babies with infantile spasms. Adverse effects include hyperlipidemia, constipation, vitamin deficiencies, kidney stones, acidosis, and, possibly, slower growth rates. Those interested in trying the diet must consult with their health care provider. This is not a do-it-yourself diet and may be harmful if not carefully monitored by skilled professionals. Recent studies have examined the possibility that the ketogenic diet could provide symptomatic benefit for patients with Alzheimer's disease (Gasior, Rogawski, & Hartman, 2006).

with low doses followed by careful monitoring for drug effectiveness. Gradual dosage changes are made based on clinical outcomes.

Older patients with memory deficits may have difficulty remembering to take their AEDs. The nurse should teach these patients and their caregivers that these medicines must be taken on a regular basis, at the same time each day, for the most effective seizure prevention. If a dose is forgotten, the nurse should teach these patients never to take a double dose of an AED because this may cause serious CNS toxicity. Furthermore, patients need to understand that waiting until the first sign of a seizure before taking their AED is ineffective at stopping the seizure because the drug will not be absorbed quickly enough.

Classification of Seizure Disorders

26.3 Most seizures are classified as generalized or partial.

Seizures begin with the firing of hyperexcitable neurons in the brain. The area where the abnormal electrical activity starts is known as an abnormal focus (plural = foci). As these neurons discharge impulses, the patient begins to exhibit the characteristic signs and symptoms of epilepsy. The specific symptoms depend on the nature of the discharge: the location of the abnormal focus in the brain and the extent of the discharge. Because symptoms vary widely from patient to patient, there are many ways to classify seizures. It is important to identify and classify the type of seizure experienced by the patient because this determines which drugs will be prescribed. There are two broad categories of seizure activity: generalized and partial.

Generalized Seizures

In **generalized seizures,** multiple foci spread abnormal neuronal discharges across both hemispheres of the brain simultaneously. The patient often experiences loss of consciousness, and the seizure may occur with or without convulsions. The four primary types of generalized seizures are tonic–clonic seizures, absence seizures, atonic seizures, and myoclonic seizures.

Tonic–clonic seizures, also referred to as grand mal seizures, are the type of seizure most associated by the public with epilepsy. It is the most common type of seizure in every age group. The seizure may be preceded by an aura, a warning that a seizure is imminent, that some patients describe as a spiritual feeling, flash of light, or special noise. Neurologists consider the aura as part of the actual seizure. Loss of consciousness and intense muscle contractions indicate the tonic phase. A hoarse cry may occur at the onset of the seizure due to air being forced out of the lungs, and patients may temporarily lose bladder or bowel control. Breathing may become shallow and even stop momentarily. The clonic phase is characterized by alternating contraction and relaxation of muscles that are characteristic of convulsions. The seizure usually lasts 1 to 2 minutes, after which the patient becomes drowsy and disoriented and sleeps deeply. The period following the seizure is known as the **postictal state.**

Absence seizures, formerly known as petit mal seizures, most often occur in children and last only a few seconds. Approximately half of the patients with absence seizures may also experience at least one tonic–clonic seizure. Absence seizures involve a reduction of normal brain activity. Staring and transient loss of responsiveness are the most common signs, but there may be slight motor activity with eyelid fluttering or muscular jerking movements. These episodes are subtle and can be mistaken for daydreaming or inattention, such as seen in attention deficit/hyperactivity disorder (ADHD). Children with absence seizures may experience poor academic performance because these episodes can occur several times per day. These children are also at risk for accidental injury. Most children who experience absence seizures will "outgrow" the disorder and become seizure free in adulthood.

Atonic seizures are sometimes known as drop attacks, due to the fact that the patient will stumble and fall for no apparent

CONNECTIONS

Evidence-Based Practice Seizures in the Older Adult

Clinical Question

When should older adults be treated with pharmacotherapy for partial seizures?

Evidence

Seizures and recurrent seizures (epilepsy) occur more frequently in patients older than 60 years because they are often secondary to conditions that occur more commonly in this age group. Such conditions include strokes, hemorrhages, infections, and degenerative disorders such as dementia. Acute symptomatic seizures or provoked seizures occur in the context of metabolic disturbances or at the time of an acute insult to the CNS. Epilepsy, repeated unprovoked seizures, is commonly a long term complication from a CNS lesion. One obstacle in the treatment of epilepsy in older adults is misdiagnosis. Patients older than 60 years are more likely to experience seizures of partial rather than generalized onset, but the manifestations of these seizures differ in older patients compared with younger patients. Older patients are more likely to have seizure recurrence compared to younger patients. As a general guideline any patient who has had a seizure and has a structural cortical lesion has a higher risk of seizure recurrence and would benefit from AED treatment" (Sirven, 2001, pp. 175–185).

Implication

The nurse caring for older patients in the period following a seizure must be advocates for their care. Understanding this research enhances patient care. The older adult must be educated on the medication regimen for the prevention of further seizure activity.

Critical Thinking Question

How would you differentiate between simple partial seizures and complex partial seizures?

See Answers to Critical Thinking Questions in Appendix A.

Source: From "Acute and Chronic Seizures in Patients Older than 60 Years," by J. Sirven, 2001, *Mayo Clinic Proceedings, 76*(2), pp. 175–183.

reason. The episode is short and lasts only a few seconds. The patient loses control of muscle function throughout the body. During the episode of weakness the patient's head will droop forward or the trunk muscles will not support the patient, thus causing the drop attack. Although the seizure itself causes no serious harm, the patient is at risk of injury due to falls.

Myoclonic seizures are generalized seizures characterized by jerking body movements, usually involving the muscles of the neck, shoulders, and upper arms. Major muscle groups contract quickly, usually for only a few seconds, and patients appear unsteady and clumsy. These patients do not lose consciousness but may fall or drop whatever they might be holding. These seizures occur most frequently in the morning, on awakening, and are worsened by sleep deprivation. Most patients with myoclonic seizures also exhibit tonic–clonic or absence seizures, or both. Myoclonic seizures usually begin around puberty and comprise 5% to 10% of all epilepsies. Although these seizures continue for the life of the patient, they can be controlled with pharmacotherapy. Valproic acid has been the traditional drug of choice for myoclonic seizures but newer AEDs such as topiramate and lamotrigine are being increasingly prescribed.

Partial Seizures

Partial (focal) seizures involve a limited portion of the brain, with the abnormal neuronal discharges starting on one side and traveling only a short distance before they stop. Many partial seizures do not involve loss of consciousness or convulsions, although discharge may begin as a partial seizure and become a generalized seizure. Some symptoms are subtle and reflect the simple nature of neuronal misfiring in limited areas of the brain, whereas other symptoms may be more complex. Medications administered for the management of partial seizures are listed in Table 26.2.

Simple partial seizures have an onset that may begin as a small, regional focus, and subsequently progress to a generalized seizure. Patients with simple partial seizures experience a wide array of symptoms depending on the specific region of the brain affected. If the motor cortex is affected, jerky, rhythmic contractions of a specific muscle group are noted. Seizures affecting the sensory cortex are less noticeable to an observer. Patients may feel for a brief moment that their precise location is vague, they may hear or see things that are not present, or they may have an upset stomach. Senses of hearing, taste, smell, or sensation may be affected. Other patients become emotional and experience a sense of joy, fear, or grief. Consciousness is retained during the seizure, although the patient may express amnesia about the event. Numerous AEDs are available to treat simple partial seizures.

Complex partial seizures (formerly known as psychomotor or temporal lobe seizures) originate from a single focus, usually in the temporal lobe of the brain. Patients exhibit sensory, motor, or autonomic symptoms with some degree of altered or impaired consciousness. Total loss of consciousness may not occur during a complex partial seizure, but a brief period of somnolence or confusion may follow the episode. Complex partial seizures are usually preceded by an aura that may be described as an unpleasant odor or taste, colored spots, unexplained fear, or tingling. Seizures may start with a blank stare and proceed to repetitive arm movements, leg movements, head rolling, chewing, lip-smacking, or swallowing. These repetitive movements are called **automatisms.** Other patients may fumble with their clothes or even undress. Most patients will be unresponsive to verbal commands and act as if they are having hallucinations. Complex partial seizures occur in about 35% of patients with epilepsy. Numerous AEDs are available to treat complex partial seizures.

MyNursingKit | The Epilepsy Foundation of America (EFA)
MyNursingKit | Tonic-Clonic Seizure
MyNursingKit | Complex Partial Seizure Video

TABLE 26.2 Drugs Used for the Management of Seizures

Type of Seizure	Drugs of Choice*	Alternative Drugs
Generalized Seizures		
Absence	ethosuximide, lamotrigine, valproic acid	clonazepam
Atonic	clonazepam, valproic acid	lamotrigine, levetiracetam, topiramate
Myoclonic	valproic acid	clonazepam, lamotrigine, phenobarbital, topiramate
Tonic–Clonic	carbamazepine, lamotrigine, valproic acid	clonazepam, diazepam, oxcarbazepine, levetiracetam, phenobarbital and other barbiturates, phenytoin, topiramate, zonisamide
Partial Seizures		
Complex Partial	carbamazepine, lamotrigine, phenobarbital, phenytoin	gabapentin, oxcarbazepine, pregabalin, tiagabine, topiramate, zonisamide
Simple Partial	carbamazepine, lamotrigine, phenobarbital, phenytoin, valproic acid	clorazepate, diazepam, felbamate, gabapentin, levetiracetam, oxcarbazepine, pregabalin, tiagabine, topiramate, zonisamide
Other Seizures		
Febrile	acetaminophen for prophylaxis	diazepam, phenytoin
Infantile Spasms	adrenocorticotropic hormone (ACTH)	None
Lennox-Gastaut	valproic acid, benzodiazepines	felbamate
Status Epilepticus	lorazepam	diazepam, phenobarbital or other barbiturate, midazolam, phenytoin, valproic acid

*Drugs of choice vary by patient age and comorbid conditions, prescriber experiences, institution, and geographical region.

26.4 Some types of seizures are called special epileptic seizures or are unclassified.

Not all seizure disorders can be classified neatly into the two broad categories of generalized and partial. These "other" types of seizures are referred to as special or unclassified epileptic seizures.

Febrile seizures are most likely to occur in the 3-month to 5-year age group. As many as 5% of children experience febrile seizures. These seizures are associated with fever in the child and are characterized by tonic–clonic motor activity lasting 1 to 2 minutes with rapid return of consciousness. They usually occur only once during any given illness. Febrile seizures may be generalized (occur once and quickly resolve) or complex partial (occur multiple times in 24 hours and are prolonged). Pharmacotherapy with AEDs is not necessary with most febrile seizures. Prevention of the onset of fever with acetaminophen is the best method for controlling this disorder.

Status epilepticus is a medical emergency that occurs when a seizure continues for more than 30 minutes or when two or more sequential seizures occur without full recovery of consciousness between seizures. Status epilepticus is sometimes classified as a generalized form of epilepsy because tonic–clonic symptoms are usually exhibited. However, some forms of this disorder do not involve convulsions and may resemble simple partial or complex partial seizures. When generalized tonic–clonic seizures are prolonged or continuous, the time in which breathing is affected by muscle contraction is lengthened and hypoxia may develop. The continuous muscle contraction also can lead to hypoglycemia, acidosis, and hypothermia due to increased metabolic needs, lactic acid production, and heat loss during contraction. If untreated, status epilepticus could lead to brain damage and death. Medical treatment involves administration of AEDs by the IV route. In the home setting, valproic acid or diazepam can be administered by the rectal route.

Infantile spasm, also called West syndrome, usually occurs in the first year of life and is characterized by a sudden bending forward, body stiffening, or arching of the torso. Infantile spasms may occur in clusters, often with several dozens separated by 5 to 30 seconds. Infants who experience infantile spasms often have some degree of mental and developmental delays. Adrenocorticotropic hormone (ACTH) and prednisone are drugs of choice in the treatment of infantile spasms.

Lennox-Gastaut syndrome is considered a mixed seizure that has characteristics of tonic–clonic, atonic, and atypical absence seizures. The cause of this syndrome is unknown. This seizure disorder has a mean age of onset of 26 to 28 months and is often associated with mental retardation and mood instability. In older children, this type of epilepsy is associated with personality disorders and psychotic episodes. The drugs of choice for Lennox-Gastaut syndrome include benzodiazepines and valproic acid, although newer AEDs are being increasingly prescribed. Seizures of Lennox-Gastaut syndrome are often resistant to pharmacotherapy.

26.5 The choice of antiepileptic drug therapy is dependent on seizure type and characteristics.

The choice of AED therapy is highly individualized for each patient and is dependent on many factors, including the type of seizure; the patient's medical history, including the characteristics and length of the seizure; the results of the EEG and other diagnostic laboratory studies; and the presence of comorbid medical conditions. To prevent adverse drug effects, it is important that the prescriber initially choose the lowest, effective dose of AED and increase it as necessary. Serum drug levels may be obtained to assist the health care provider in determining the most effective drug concentration. To prevent adverse effects and possible seizure onset, the discontinuation of an AED or significant dose reductions should always be extended over 6 to 12 weeks. The drugs of choice for the different types of seizure are listed in Table 26.2.

In most cases, effective seizure management can be obtained by using a single AED. If seizure activity continues, the initial drug is gradually discontinued and replaced by another drug from a different class. Some patients require multiple AEDs for effective seizure control. However, certain AED drug combinations have the potential to increase the incidence of seizures; thus it is important that the nurse consult current literature for drug compatibility and administration guidelines. At the initiation of pharmacotherapy, the patient must be carefully assessed for adverse effects, particularly increased CNS depression, and advised not to drive or engage in hazardous activities until the drug levels have stabilized.

Patients who remain symptom free for prolonged periods often believe that they have "outgrown" their seizures and therefore no longer require medication. Although this may indeed be the case, the nurse should teach patients to never stop taking AEDS without the guidance of their health care provider. In general, withdrawal of antiepileptic medications is attempted only after the patient is seizure free for at least 3 years. The withdrawal of medications requires close monitoring by the patient's health care provider, and doses must be reduced slowly, one medication at a time, over a period of several months. If seizures recur during the withdrawal process, pharmacotherapy is resumed with the same medication previously prescribed. The nurse must educate the patient and family to maintain strict adherence to the pharmacotherapy regimen. Periodic serum drug levels can assist the nurse in assessing adherence: Low serum drug levels in a patient claiming to be taking his or her medication may indicate nonadherence to therapy.

The use of alternative therapies alone for the treatment of epilepsy is not considered effective and should be discouraged by the nurse. However, the implementation of complementary therapies combined with antiepileptic medications is acceptable. The National Society for Epilepsy in the United Kingdom and the Epilepsy Foundation of America encourage the use of complementary therapy when used as a component of an effective pharmacotherapeutic regimen. The nurse should educate the patient on the use of relaxation techniques to reduce stress because stress can affect the development of seizures. The implementation of the ketogenic diet can produce positive effects in some patients by decreasing seizure activity.

PharmFACT

Contrary to popular belief, it is impossible to swallow the tongue during a seizure, and one should never force an object into the mouth of someone who is having a seizure. *Source:* Epilepsy Foundation of America, n.d.

26.6 Antiseizure drugs act by suppressing abnormal neuronal discharges.

Antiepileptic medications suppress neuron discharges, thus preventing the abnormal focus from forming or spreading across the cerebrum. These drugs act by controlling the movement of electrolytes across neuronal membranes or by affecting the neurotransmitter balance in the brain. These mechanisms are shown in Pharmacotherapy Illustrated 26.1. It is important to know that the mechanisms of action of AEDs are incompletely understood, and that most of these drugs act by multiple mechanisms.

MyNursingKit | Epilepsy Canada

Control of electrolyte movement: In the resting state, neurons are surrounded by a higher extracellular concentration of sodium, calcium, and chloride ions. Potassium levels are higher inside the cell. An influx of sodium or calcium into the neuron enhances neuronal activity, whereas an influx of chloride ions has an inhibitory effect. This affords several mechanisms.

The primary target for many AEDs is the sodium channel. The sodium channel on the neuron plasma membrane must open, allowing sodium to rush into the cell, for an action potential to be generated and propagated. Phenytoin, lamotrigine, and carbamazepine bind to the sodium channel, keeping it in an inactivated state, which prevents sodium ion flow. This slows the excitability of neurons, essentially reducing the flow of abnormal, repetitive discharges.

MyNursingKit | National Institute of Neurological Disorders and Stroke

The role of calcium channels in slowing neuronal discharges is less understood. Calcium channels are found at the synaptic terminals. When opened, calcium enters the presynaptic neuron, causing the release of stored neurotransmitter into the cleft. Blocking these calcium channels prevents the release of the neurotransmitter. Several AEDs are thought to affect calcium channels, including ethosuximide, gabapentin, pregabalin, and lamotrigine.

Neurotransmitter balance: Drugs that enhance or inhibit neurotransmitter activity in the CNS have the ability to affect neuronal firing. Over 30 different neurotransmitters have been identified in the CNS (see Chapter 21).

The neurotransmitter most affected by AEDs is gamma aminobutyric acid (GABA), the primary inhibitory neurotransmitter in the brain. Increasing the activity of GABA in the CNS will decrease neuronal firing, thus suppressing seizure activity. There are several mechanisms by which this

PHARMACOTHERAPY *ILLUSTRATED* 26.1

Model of the GABA Receptor-Chloride Channel Molecules in Relationship to Epilepsy Pharmacotherapy

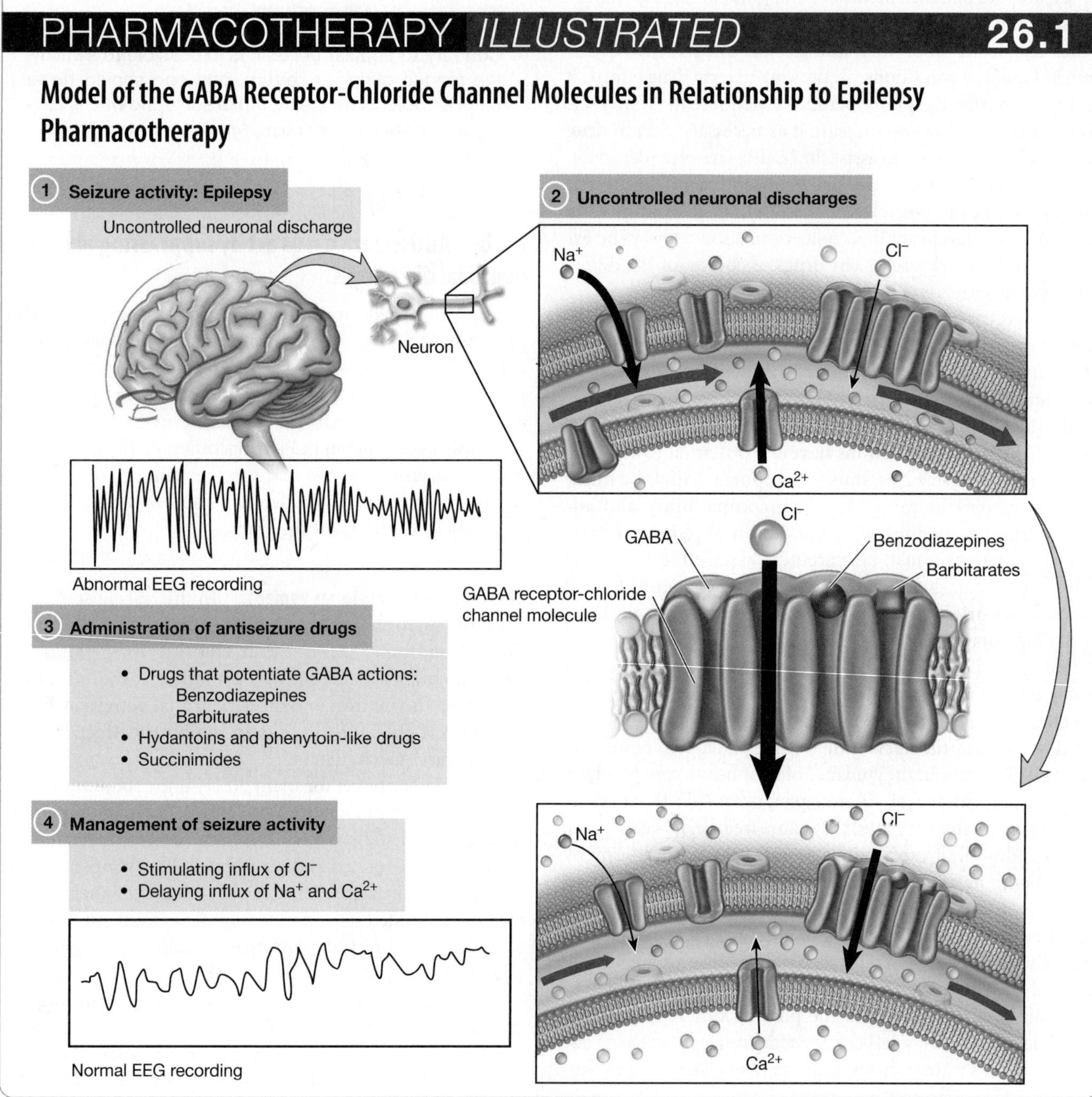

may be accomplished by AEDs, and they are illustrated in Figure 26.2.

- **Increased synthesis or amount of GABA in the presynaptic nerve terminal.** Some drugs block the metabolic breakdown of GABA or enhance its formation. An example is valproic acid.
- **Blocked reuptake of GABA.** After GABA produces its action at the synapse, it is normally taken back into the presynaptic neuron, which terminates its action. Drugs that block the reuptake will keep GABA on its receptors for a longer period, thus causing more neuronal inhibition. An example is tiagabine.
- **Activation of GABA receptors.** Some drugs mimic GABA and occupy its receptor on the postsynaptic membrane. These cause the same inhibitory effect as GABA and act by stimulating an influx of chloride ion into the neuron. Examples include barbiturates, benzodiazepines, topiramate, and felbamate.

A second neurotransmitter affected by AEDs is glutamate, the primary stimulatory neurotransmitter in the brain. By blocking glutamate receptors (known as NMDA receptors), these drugs serve as antagonists to glutamate and suppress neuronal firing. Examples include topiramate and felbamate.

Antiepileptic medications can be classified in many different ways. One method is by mechanism of action; however, some AEDs act by multiple means or have unknown mechanisms. Another classification scheme groups these drugs into "newer" and "older" generations, but there is no clear distinction between the groups. Grouping by type of seizure is not

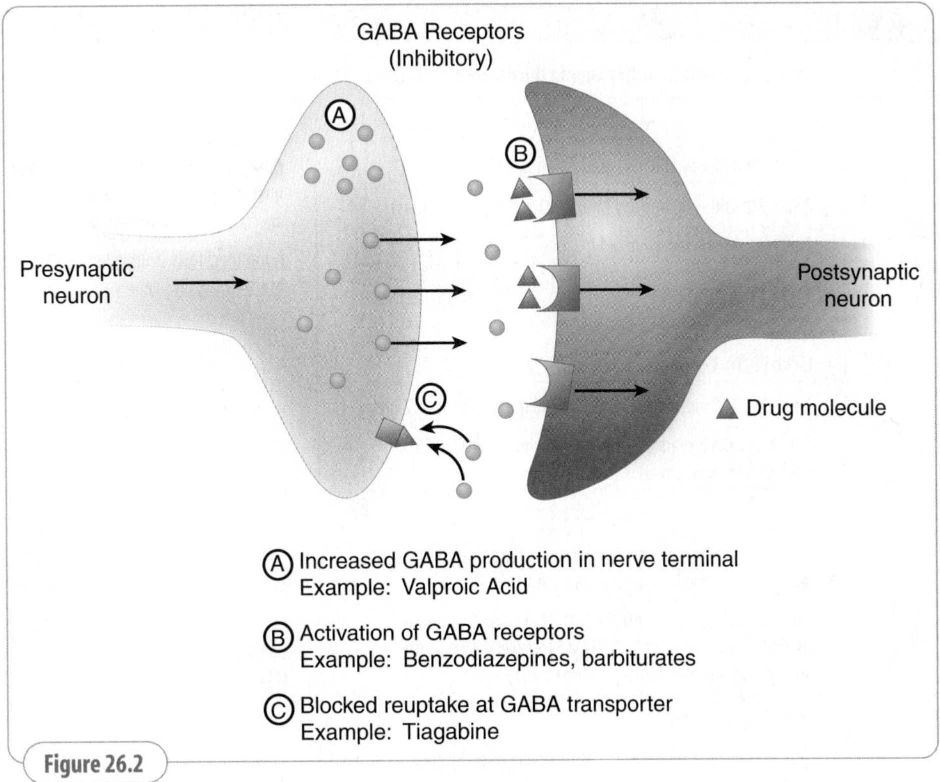

Figure 26.2

Mechanisms of action of antiepileptic drugs that affect GABA.

possible because most drugs are useful against more than one type. This textbook uses a combination of chemical classes and mechanisms of action. The student should be aware, however, that other classifications will be encountered in clinical practice. The AEDs are listed in Table 26.3.

Antiseizure Drugs

26.7 Barbiturates are traditional drugs for tonic–clonic seizures but have been replaced by newer and safer medications.

The barbiturates have been used to treat seizures for almost 100 years. The antiseizure properties of phenobarbital (Luminal) were discovered in 1912. Barbiturates act biochemically in the brain by enhancing the action of GABA, which is responsible for suppressing the abnormal neuronal discharges that can cause seizure activity.

Although barbiturates are still prescribed for epilepsy, newer drugs have largely replaced them as first-line drugs for this indication. Barbiturates have several major disadvantages. As a class, they have a low margin of safety and cause profound CNS depression, including sedation, coma, and death. The extent of CNS depression is related to the dosage, route of administration, and patient tolerance to the medication. Barbiturates will yield significant sedation when combined with alcohol, antidepressants, and other CNS depressants. Children may exhibit hyperkinesis rather than sedation. The main cardiovascular and respiratory adverse effects include respiratory depression, bradycardia, syncope, and hypotension. Patients with impaired hepatic, respiratory, renal, and cardiovascular function should not receive barbiturates, or the doses should be lowered to prevent toxicity. Barbiturates also possess a high potential for drug dependence, and the nurse must be certain that this factor is included as part of patient and caregiver teaching.

This section highlights only the antiseizure properties of barbiturates. These drugs are also classified as sedative–hypnotics, and a prototype feature for phenobarbital can be found in Chapter 22. Nursing responsibilities and patient and family education for this drug class may also be found in Chapter 22.

Amobarbital (Amytal): Amobarbital is an intermediate-acting barbiturate that produces CNS depression by interfering with the transmission of impulses from the reticular activating system to the cerebral cortex. This increases the seizure threshold of the motor cortex. It is approved for preoperative sedation induction, insomnia, and seizures. The primary use of amobarbital in the pharmacotherapy of epilepsy is to control seizures related to status epilepticus or eclampsia when administered parenterally. The parenteral administration must take place within a 30-minute period after the vial is opened because the medication quickly becomes unstable. Adverse effects are similar to those of phenobarbital. Administration of amobarbital places the patient at risk for Stevens–Johnson syndrome (SJS). The drug was approved in 1938 but is rarely used today. It is pregnancy category D.

Mephobarbital (Mebaral): Mephobarbital is a long-acting antiepileptic agent administered orally for preventing tonic–clonic and

TABLE 26.3 Drugs for Seizures

Drug	Route and Adult Dose (maximum dose where indicated)	Adverse Effects
Barbiturates		
amobarbital (Amytal)	Adult/child IV: 65–500 mg (max: 500 mg/day)	*Drowsiness, dizziness, nausea, vomiting, sedation, confusion, unsteady gait, lethargy, paradoxical excitement, pain at the injection site, hypotension with IV administration* Agranulocytosis, angioedema, SJS, respiratory depression, bradycardia, CNS depression, coma
mephobarbital (Mebaral)	Adult: PO: 400–600 mg/day (max: 600 mg/day for seizures) Child: PO: 16–64 mg tid or qid	
phenobarbital (Luminal)	Adult: PO: 100–300 mg/day IV/IM: 200–600 mg (max: 20 mg/kg) Child: PO/IV: 3–8 mg/kg or 125 mg/m²/day	
primidone (Mysoline)	Adult: PO: 250 mg/day increased by 250 mg/week (max: 2 g/day) Child less than 8 years: PO: 125 mg/day increased by 125 mg/week (max: 2 g/day)	
Benzodiazepines		
clonazepam (Klonopin)	Adult: PO: 1.5 mg/day, increased by 0.5–1 mg every 3 days until seizures are controlled (max: 20 mg/day) Child: less than10 years: PO: 0.01–0.03 mg/kg/day in three divided doses; increased by 0.25–0.5 mg every 3 days until seizures are controlled (max: 0.2 mg/kg/day)	*Sedation, headache, drowsiness, weakness, vertigo, ataxia, paradoxical excitement, short-term amnesia* Coma, respiratory depression, cardiac arrest, suicidal ideation, blood dyscrasias, physical dependence, cardiovascular collapse (diazepam)
clorazepate (Tranxene)	Adult: PO: 7.5 mg tid Child 9–12 years: PO: 3.75–7.5 mg bid; increased by 3.75 mg/week (max: 60 mg/day)	
diazepam (Valium)	Status epilepticus: Adult: IV/IM: 5–10 mg, repeat if needed at 10- to 15-min intervals up to 30 mg, repeat if needed every 2–4 h Children: IV/IM: 0.2–1 mg slowly every 2–5 min up to 5–10 mg. Repeat if needed every 2–4 h	
lorazepam (Ativan)	Adult: IV: 4 mg injected slowly at 2 mg/min; may repeat dose once if inadequate response after 10 min (max: 8 mg during any 12 h period) Status epilepticus: Child: IV: 0.1 mg/kg slow IV over 2–5 min; may repeat with 0.05 mg in 10–15 min if needed (max: 4 mg/dose)	
midazolam (Versed)	Child older than 2 months: IV loading dose: 0.15 mg/kg; IV maintenance dose: 1 mcg/kg/min infusion; may adjust dose upward as needed every 5 min	
Hydantoins		
fosphenytoin (Cerebyx)	Adult: IV loading dose: 15–20 mg phenytoin equivalents/kg administered at 100–150 mg phenytoin equivalents/min Maintenance IV dose: 4–6 mg PE/kg/day	*Nystagmus, ataxia, lethargy, confusion, slurred speech, dizziness, nervousness, headache, nausea, vomiting, gingival hyperplasia, rash, somnolence, drowsiness* Seizures, blood dyscrasias, lymphadenopathy, systemic lupus, erythematosus, cardiac arrest, cardiovascular collapse, coma, toxic epidermal necrolysis, SJS
phenytoin (Dilantin)	Adult: PO: 20 mg/kg or 1 g loading dose; then 300 mg/day; may increase 100 mg/week until seizures are controlled IV: 10–15 mg/kg or 1 g loading dose then 100 mg tid Child: IV/PO: 15–20 mg/kg loading dose then 5 mg/kg in two to three divided doses	
Iminostilbenes		
carbamazepine (Tegretol)	Adult: PO: 200 mg bid; may be increased to 800–1,200 mg/day Child: PO: younger than 6 years of age 10–20 mg/kg/day with gradual increase weekly (max: 35 mg/kg/day) 6–12 years: PO: 100 mg, gradually increase to 400–800 mg	*Dizziness, headache, ataxia, fatigue, rash, pruritus, dry mouth, nausea, vomiting, diplopia, abnormal gait* SJS, aggravated seizures, hallucinations, aplastic anemia, agranulocytosis, heart block, respiratory depression, exfoliative dermatitis
oxcarbazepine (Trileptal)	Adult: PO: 300 mg increase by 600 mg/day every week (max: 2,400 mg/day when used for monotherapy, 1,200 mg/day with other AEDs) Child: PO: 4–16 years, 8–10 mg/kg/day (max: 600 mg/day)	

TABLE 26.3 *Continued*

Drug	Route and Adult Dose	Adverse Effects
Succinimides		
ethosuximide (Zarontin)	Adult and child older than 6 years: PO: 250 mg bid; may increase dosage every 4–7 days as needed (max: 1.5 g/day) Child age 3–6: PO: 250 mg/day may increase every 4–7 days (max: 1.5 g/day)	*Drowsiness, headache, euphoria, restlessness, irritability, anxiety, hyperactivity, aggressive behavior, inability to concentrate, night tremors, abdominal pain, epigastric distress* <u>Anorexia, SJS, weight loss, blood dyscrasias</u>
methsuximide (Celontin)	PO: 150–300 mg/day (max: 1.2 g/day)	
phensuximide (Milontin)	PO: 0.5–1 g bid or tid	
Miscellaneous Antiepileptic Drugs		
felbamate (Felbatol)	Adult: PO: 1,200 mg/day; may increase by 600 mg/day every 2 weeks (max: 3,600 mg/day) Child: PO: 15 mg/kg/day (max: 45 mg/kg/day)	*Headache, dizziness, blurred vision, nausea and vomiting, anorexia* <u>Liver failure, aplastic anemia</u>
gabapentin (Neurontin)	Adult/child older than12 years: PO: 300 mg gradually increased to 400 mg tid; may increase to 1,800–2,400 mg/day based on patient response Child: age 3–12 years: PO: 10–15 mg/kg/day in divided doses, may increase every 3 days to target dose of 40 mg/kg/day	*Dizziness, drowsiness, fatigue, weight gain, ataxia, diplopia, nystagmus, tremor, peripheral edema, impaired concentration, dry mouth, flulike syndrome* <u>Increased frequency of partial seizures, blurred vision, accidental injury</u>
lamotrigine (Lamictal)	Adult: PO: 25–50 mg/day for 2 weeks then increase gradually to 150–500 mg/day (max: 700 mg/day without concurrent valproic acid, 200 mg/day with valproic acid) Child age 2–16 years: PO: 0.2–1 mg/kg/day for 2 weeks then gradually increase to 1–5 mg/kg/day (max: 15 mg/kg/day without valproic acid, 5 mg/kg/day or 250 mg/day with concurrent valproic acid)	*Dizziness, headache, ataxia, drowsiness, insomnia, tremor, rash, diplopia, blurred vision, flulike symptoms, infection, nausea, vomiting, back pain* <u>SJS, toxic epidermal necrolysis, emotional lability (children), suicidal ideation</u>
levetiracetam (Keppra)	Adult: PO: 500 mg bid; may increase by 500 mg bid every 2 weeks (max: 3 g/day) Child age 4–16: PO: 20 mg/kg/day; may increase by 20 mg/kg/day every 2 weeks up to 60 mg/kg/day	*Drowsiness, headache, dizziness, nervousness, flulike symptoms, vomiting, anorexia, asthenia* <u>Emotional lability and personality disorder (children), accidental injury, suicidal ideation, blood dyscrasias</u>
pregabalin (Lyrica)	Adult: PO: 75 mg bid or 50 mg tid; may be increased to 150–300 mg bid or 100–200 mg tid	*Dizziness, drowsiness, fatigue, weight gain, ataxia, diplopia, nystagmus, tremor, peripheral edema, impaired concentration, dry mouth, flulike syndrome* <u>Increased frequency of partial seizures, blurred vision, accidental injury</u>
tiagabine (Gabitril)	Adult: PO: start with 4 mg/day and increase dose by 4–8 mg/day every week (max: 56 mg/day) Adolescent age 12–18: PO: start with 4 mg every day and increase doses by 4–8 mg/day every week (max: 32 mg/day)	*Dizziness, asthenia, tremor, somnolence, nervousness, difficulty concentrating* <u>Vasodilation, HTN, palpitations, tachycardia, syncope, peripheral edema</u>
topiramate (Topomax)	PO: 50 mg/day (max 1600 mg/day)	*Paresthesia, drowsiness, weight loss* <u>Depression, difficulty with memory, psychomotor slowing</u>
valproic acid (Depakene, Depakote, Depacon)	Adult/child: PO/IV: 10–15 mg/kg/day; may increase every week by 5–10 mg/kg/day until seizures are controlled (max: 60 mg/kg/day)	*Nausea, vomiting, abdominal cramps, anorexia, dyspepsia, drowsiness, dizziness, asthenia, insomnia, weight gain* <u>Deep coma, hallucinations, hyperammonemia, thrombocytopenia, blurred vision, hepatotoxicity, pancreatitis, bone marrow depression, prolonged bleeding time</u>
zonisamide (Zonegran)	Adult: PO: 100 mg/day; may increase dose to 200 mg/day after 2 weeks, then increase every 2 weeks as needed (max: 400 mg/day)	*Dizziness, ataxia, drowsiness, fatigue, anorexia, speech abnormalities and difficulty in concentrating or remembering, flulike symptoms, headache, abnormal gait, gingivitis, rhinitis* <u>Severe rash including SJS, kidney stones, depression, psychosis</u>

Note: *Italics* indicate common adverse effects. <u>Underline</u> indicates serious adverse effects.

absence seizures. It is also approved for preoperative sedation induction. Both amobarbital and mephobarbital produce adverse hematologic effects such as agranulocytosis, leukopenia, and thrombocytopenia. Both medications should be administered cautiously and the patient should be assessed for signs and symptoms of hypotension and CNS depression. Mephobarbital is converted to phenobarbital in the liver and offers no significant advantages over phenobarbital. It is pregnancy category D.

Phenobarbital (Luminal): For epilepsy, phenobarbital is effective for long-term management of tonic–clonic seizures and partial seizures. It can be administered in patients with status epilepticus or febrile seizures or to treat eclampsia. It is relatively ineffective in treating absence seizures. Oral administration of phenobarbital may take several weeks for an optimal level of antiseizure activity to be achieved. The advantages of phenobarbital are that it is relatively inexpensive and long acting, and it can suppress seizures without causing major sedation with careful selection of dosage.

Phenobarbital is a major inducer of hepatic CYP450 enzymes and will markedly increase the metabolism of other drugs metabolized by these enzymes. This results in a significant potential for drug interactions with other medications metabolized in the liver. Phenobarbital also increases its own metabolism, which leads to significant tolerance as therapy progresses. Phenobarbital is pregnancy category D. Women of childbearing potential who are taking barbiturates should use two methods of birth control.

Primidone (Mysoline): Primidone is a barbiturate that is metabolized in the liver to phenobarbital, which is responsible for many of its pharmacologic effects. It is effective for treating all types of seizures except absence seizures. It has no approved indications other than seizure. The actions and adverse effects of primidone are similar to those of phenobarbital. It is pregnancy category D.

PharmFACT

Twenty to thirty percent of children with mental retardation also have epilepsy. The success rate of pharmacotherapy is lower in children with mental retardation (50%) than in children without mental retardation (60–70%). *Source:* Alvarez, 2007.

26.8 Benzodiazepines are important drugs in the treatment of status epilepticus.

Benzodiazepines are the drugs of choice for the treatment of anxiety disorders and are one of the most widely prescribed drug classes in the United States. Detailed information about the benzodiazepines used for anxiety and a prototype feature for lorazepam (Ativan) are included in Chapter 22. The remainder of this section focuses on the antiseizure properties of drugs in this class.

Benzodiazepines control seizures by acting in the limbic, thalamic, and hypothalamic regions of the CNS. All drugs in this class act by enhancing the inhibitory action of GABA. They accomplish this by increasing the affinity of GABA for its receptors.

The applications of benzodiazepines in the treatment of seizure disorders are limited. The parenteral benzodiazepines diazepam (Valium) and lorazepam are utilized in the treatment of status epilepticus. Clonazepam (Klonopin), clorazepate (Tranxene), and midazolam (Versed) are used for specific types of seizures, usually when other drugs have not proven effective.

When giving these medications by the IV route the patient should be administered oxygen, and resuscitation equipment should be readily available. IV administration of diazepam or lorazepam for status epilepticus should be given in a large vein and they should not be mixed with other drugs or IV fluid additives. These drugs have a tendency to precipitate from solution and are irritating to veins. Close monitoring of the respiratory and cardiovascular systems is necessary for the early recognition of adverse effects associated with respiratory depression or cardiovascular collapse.

PROTOTYPE DRUG Diazepam (Valium)

Classification: **Therapeutic:** Antiepileptic drug, antianxiety agent, skeletal muscle relaxant
Pharmacologic: Benzodiazepine, GABA receptor agonist

Therapeutic Effects and Uses: Diazepam was originally approved in 1963. In antiseizure therapy, the primary indication for diazepam is status epilepticus. It may also be used to prevent seizures in patients who have received toxic substances or during the acute phase of alcohol or benzodiazepine withdrawal. Oral diazepam may be combined with other AEDs in the treatment of refractory seizures. A newer indication for diazepam is the oral prophylaxis of febrile seizures in children age 6 months to 5 years.

Diazepam has a large number of other indications. It was once widely prescribed for the management of anxiety disorders, although it has largely been replaced by other drugs such as alprazolam (Xanax) (see Chapter 22). It is administered prior to procedures such as cardioversion or endoscopy to provide relaxation or sedation. Oral or parenteral diazepam may be administered for muscle relaxation in patients with acute inflammation, trauma, tetanus, or spasticity.

Mechanism of Action: Diazepam enhances the action of GABA in the brain, thus inhibiting the abnormal neuronal discharges characteristic of seizures.

Pharmacokinetics:

Route(s)	IV, IM, PO, rectal
Absorption	Rapidly absorbed by the GI tract; erratic absorption with IM administration
Distribution	Widely distributed; crosses the blood–brain barrier and the placenta; 99% bound to protein
Primary metabolism	Hepatic
Primary excretion	Renal
Onset of action	IV: 1–5 minutes; IM: 15–30 minutes; PO: 30–60 minutes
Duration of action	Half-life: 20–50 h

Adverse Effects: The most serious adverse effect of diazepam is cardiovascular collapse. The nurse should assess for hypotension, tachycardia, and edema, which are precursors to cardiovascular collapse. CNS adverse effects include drowsiness, fatigue, ataxia, dizziness, and vertigo. Diazepam can cause urinary retention and menstrual irregularities. The major respiratory adverse effect is laryngeal spasm and cough. Benzodiazepines are Schedule IV drugs and possess a risk for substance abuse in susceptible individuals (see Chapter 8).

Contraindications/Precautions: Diazepam should not be administered to patients with depressed vital signs, those in shock, or those with acute alcohol intoxication. It is also contraindicated in the presence of narrow-angle glaucoma because it can increase intraocular pressure. Diazepam should be used cautiously in patients with depression and myasthenia gravis, and a reduced dose should be administered in patients with impaired hepatic or renal function. Patients suffering from respiratory disorders such as chronic obstructive pulmonary disease (COPD) should be monitored closely due to the risk of respiratory depression. After prolonged therapy, abrupt discontinuation of diazepam may precipitate withdrawal symptoms, including seizures in patients with epilepsy. The drug can cause birth defects and should not be administered to pregnant patients unless benefits clearly outweigh the potential risks. Diazepam is not recommended during lactation because the drug is secreted in breast milk and may cause CNS depression in the neonate.

Drug Interactions: Diazepam is metabolized by hepatic CYP450 enzymes and may interact with drugs that inhibit these enzymes. Other CNS depressants, including alcohol, will intensify the sedative effects of diazepam. Concurrent administration with cimetidine will increase the plasma levels of diazepam. Administration of diazepam with antiparkinsonism medications may worsen the severity of Parkinson's disease symptoms. Diazepam when administered with phenytoin will result in increased phenytoin levels and possible toxicity. Diazepam should never be administered within 14 days of a monoamine oxidase inhibitor (MAOI) due to the risk of hypertensive crisis. **Herbal/Food:** Kava and valerian administered with diazepam will result in additive sedative effects. Echinacea may lower the serum levels of diazepam. Grapefruit juice increases the peak serum concentrations of diazepam as much as two times.

Pregnancy: Category D.

Treatment of Overdose: Flumazenil (Romazicon) is administered for overdosage of diazepam. This medication is a specific benzodiazepine receptor antagonist that reverses the CNS depression from diazepam.

Nursing Responsibilities

- Educate all members of the health care team on the effect of the medication and the signs and symptoms of respiratory depression and cardiovascular collapse.
- Assess for decrease in seizure activity.
- Maintain patient safety by keeping the side rails of the bed elevated and padded and by assisting with ambulation.
- Assess the patient for a history of smoking because patients who smoke heavily require a larger dose of benzodiazepine medications.
- Assess for urinary retention.
- When administering parenterally do not mix diazepam with any other drug and give slowly by direct IV injection.

Patient and Family Education

- Take precautions for safe storage of the medication because benzodiazepines are often used illegally for recreation.
- Do not drive or perform other hazardous activities until the effects of the drug are known because this drug may cause drowsiness or dizziness.
- Do not consume alcoholic beverages with this medication because this may cause sedation.
- Immediately notify the health care provider of any known or suspected pregnancy because benzodiazepines have the potential to cause birth defects.
- Take this medication exactly as instructed and do not discontinue the drug without consulting the health care provider because seizures may result.
- Check with the health care provider before taking any over-the-counter (OTC) medications or herbal products.
- If taking oral contraceptives, a second form of birth control should be used because benzodiazepines may decrease their effectiveness.
- Do not breast-feed while taking this drug without approval of the health care provider.

Drugs Similar to Diazepam (Valium)

Clonazepam, clorazepate, lorazepam, and midazolam are benzodiazepine antiepileptic medications.

Clonazepam (Klonopin): Approved in 1975, clonazepam is an oral benzodiazepine with strong antiseizure capabilities. It is approved for the prophylaxis of absence seizures, Lennox-Gastaut syndrome, akinetic and myoclonic seizures, and nocturnal myoclonus. Its primary use as an AED is to treat refractory myoclonic seizures. It is occasionally prescribed off-label for anxiety disorders, insomnia, and restless legs syndrome.

Like other drugs in the class, the most common adverse effect is sedation. Hyperactivity, restlessness, irritability, and cardiovascular or respiratory depression are possible. If given for an extended period, the patient may require an increase in dose due to the development of tolerance. Tolerance also develops to the sedative side effects of the drug. Therapeutic serum levels are 20 to 80 mg/mL. Clonazepam is pregnancy category C and a Schedule IV controlled substance.

MyNursingKit Mechanism of Action Animation: Diazepam

Clorazepate (Tranxene): Approved in 1972, clorazepate is approved for the pharmacotherapy of anxiety, partial seizures, and seizures associated with acute ethanol withdrawal. It may be used off-label to treat insomnia. Clorazepate is only administered orally, is rapidly absorbed, and has a long duration of action. The actions of clorazepate are the same as those of diazepam because the two drugs form the same active metabolite. It is not a first-line drug for epilepsy but it may be used as an adjunct to control partial seizures. Most adverse effects are CNS related and include mental depression, confusion, fatigue, tremor, and vertigo. Like diazepam, clorazepate is a Schedule IV drug and is pregnancy category D.

Lorazepam (Ativan): Approved in 1977, lorazepam is the drug of choice for status epilepticus because it persists in the cerebrospinal fluid (CSF) longer than diazepam. Whereas diazepam remains active in the brain for 30 to 60 minutes, lorazepam may prevent seizures for up to 12 hours. It is also used to prevent or treat seizures associated with acute ethanol withdrawal. It is the most potent of the benzodiazepines and has the ability to produce skeletal muscle relaxation, sedation, and a hypnotic state.

Oral, IM, and IV forms are available. Lorazepam is pregnancy category D and a Schedule IV controlled substance. A prototype feature for lorazepam is presented in Chapter 22.

Midazolam (Versed): Approved in 1985, the primary use of midazolam is to provide conscious sedation, anesthesia, or relaxation prior to minor dental, surgical, or medical procedures. It is administered parenterally for status epilepticus in children older than age 2 months, usually after other drugs have failed to control the seizures. It has a very rapid onset of action and is available PO, IV, IM, or intranasally. Midazolam is pregnancy category D and a Schedule IV controlled substance.

CONNECTION *Checkpoint* 26.2

In addition to epilepsy, what are other indications for benzodiazepines? See Answer to Connection Checkpoint 26.2 in Appendix A.

26.9 Hydantoins are effective in the management of most types of seizures but have many adverse effects.

First used in 1938, phenytoin (Dilantin) became a drug of choice for many types of epilepsy because it provides effective seizure prevention without the serious CNS depression and abuse potential associated with barbiturates such as phenobarbital. Despite having many drawbacks, phenytoin remains an important drug in the pharmacotherapy of seizures.

Hydantoins act by delaying the influx of sodium ions across neuronal membranes in the brain. Sodium ion movement is the major factor determining the initiation and propagation of a neuron action potential. Hydantoin medications do not block the sodium channels but instead desensitize them. Total blockage of sodium channels would cause neuronal activity to cease as is seen with the administration of local anesthetic agents. At high doses, the hydantoins begin to exert excitatory CNS effects and can induce seizures.

PROTOTYPE DRUG Phenytoin (Dilantin, Phenytek)

Classification: **Therapeutic:** Antiepileptic drug
Pharmacologic: Hydantoin, neuronal sodium channel modulator

Therapeutic Effects and Uses: Phenytoin, the most commonly prescribed hydantoin, is approved for the prophylactic therapy of all types of seizures except absence seizures. Phenytoin has been used to prevent seizures that might occur during neurosurgery or eclampsia. The IV form of phenytoin is effective in treating generalized convulsions due to status epilepticus. The action of IV phenytoin is not immediate; therefore, an IV benzodiazepine should be administered prior to, or concurrently with, IV phenytoin to achieve faster seizure control. Phenytoin injections must always be performed slowly to prevent cardiovascular collapse. Phenytoin (Phenytek) is an extended release form of the drug approved in 2001 for once-daily dosing.

Patients who are prescribed phenytoin must be monitored very closely and the dosage adjusted based on clinical response and laboratory results. The therapeutic serum range is narrow, 10 to 20 mcg/mL, and small increases in dose can produce large changes in the serum concentration. Thus, the patient should be educated on the importance of maintaining a strict schedule for administration of the medication and for keeping all laboratory appointments. The brand of phenytoin should not be changed without approval of the health care provider because differences in bioavailability among brands have been noted.

Phenytoin is a Class 1B antidysrhythmic and may be used to treat ventricular tachycardia (especially those induced by digoxin) or paroxysmal atrial tachycardia, although it is not approved for these indications (see Chapter 39). Other off-label indications for phenytoin include the treatment of migraine headaches, diabetic neuropathy, and neuropathic pain.

Mechanism of Action: Phenytoin inhibits seizure activity by delaying the influx of sodium ions in neurons, thus slowing the propagation and spread of abnormal discharges. Unlike some AEDs, phenytoin does not elevate the seizure threshold.

Pharmacokinetics:

Route(s)	PO, IV
Absorption	Slowly but completely absorbed in the GI tract
Distribution	Enters the CSF; crosses the placenta; secreted in breast milk; 95% bound to protein
Primary metabolism	Hepatic
Primary excretion	Renal
Onset of action	PO: 30–120 minutes
Duration of action	Half-life is highly variable, ranging from 7 to 42 h with an average of 24 h

Adverse Effects: Phenytoin can be a very toxic drug and patients must be monitored carefully during therapy. CNS adverse effects are relatively common and include lethargy, headache, drowsiness, and dizziness, which may occur even at therapeutic doses. High doses can cause nystagmus, confusion, ataxia, coma, and seizures. Cardiovascular adverse effects include bradycardia, ventricular fibrillation, hypotension, and phlebitis. Gastrointestinal (GI) adverse effects include gingival hyperplasia (swelling of the gums), weight loss, and liver necrosis. Hematologic adverse effects include agranulocytosis, leukopenia, thrombocytopenia, and aplastic anemia. Rashes and serious dermatologic conditions occur in 5% to 10% of patients taking the drug. Abrupt discontinuation of phenytoin can induce status epilepticus.

Contraindications/Precautions: Patients who have developed a rash, sore throat, fever, oral ulcers, or other hypersensitivity reactions to a hydantoin should not receive phenytoin. This medication is contraindicated in patients who have experienced seizures caused by hypoglycemia. Phenytoin should be administered cautiously to patients with impaired liver or kidney function because these may increase the serum concentration of phenytoin to toxic levels. Patients with serious cardiovascular signs and symptoms such as dysrhythmias, bradycardia, and heart failure must be monitored carefully during therapy. Patients with blood dyscrasias should not receive phenytoin because this drug can worsen these conditions. Phenytoin is a known teratogen and should not be administered to pregnant patients unless the seizures cannot be managed by safer drugs. The drug is secreted in breast milk, although it may be used during lactation, if necessary, to control serious seizures.

Drug Interactions: Because phenytoin induces CYP450 enzymes, the metabolism of many other drugs will be affected, and drug–drug interactions are common. Phenytoin increases the metabolism of corticosteroids, warfarin, and oral contraceptives, thus rendering these drugs less effective. Chronic alcohol ingestion, carbamazepine, and barbiturates can increase the metabolism of phenytoin, thus decreasing the antiseizure effects of phenytoin. Amiodarone, chloramphenicol, diazepam, valproic acid, isoniazid, omeprazole, and ticlopidine will increase phenytoin levels when administered concurrently. **Herbal/Food:** The administration or consumption of foods that contain folic acid, calcium, and vitamin D will decrease the absorption of phenytoin. Ginkgo may decrease the antiseizure effectiveness of phenytoin.

Pregnancy: Category D.

Treatment of Overdose: Overdoses of phenytoin are treated with activated charcoal with gastric lavage.

Nursing Responsibilities:

- Shake the suspension to mix well prior to administration.
- Monitor and maintain serum therapeutic concentration at 10 to 20 mcg/mL. The toxic level is 30 to 50 mcg/mL and the lethal level is 100 mcg/mL.
- Monitor CBC with differential, platelet count, calcium and magnesium levels, and liver function tests. Cardiovascular and respiratory function should be continuously monitored.
- Assess for neurologic adverse effects such as drowsiness, dizziness, and ataxia.
- Patients with diabetes who are prescribed phenytoin are at risk for loss of glycemic control; therefore, monitor blood glucose in these patients.
- Assess for folic acid deficiency and recommend supplementation as indicated.
- Discontinue the medication and immediately notify the prescriber if signs of hypersensitivity develop.
- Use extra caution when administering phenytoin by the IV route because extravasation can cause tissue injury.

Patient and Family Education:

- Because this drug can cause gingival hyperplasia, it is very important to maintain routine dental examinations and the provision of excellent mouth care.
- Take this medication with food if nausea occurs.
- Never chew or crush sustained release tablets.
- Do not drive or perform other hazardous activities until the effects of the drug are known because this drug may cause drowsiness or dizziness.
- The medication may change the color of urine to pink or red-brown but this is not harmful.
- Take this medication exactly as instructed and do not discontinue the drug without consulting the health care provider because seizures may result.
- Never change brands of phenytoin without the approval of the health care provider.
- Never consume alcoholic beverages with this medication because this may cause sedation.
- The administration of the flu vaccine may increase seizure activity.
- Immediately notify the health care provider of any suspected or known pregnancy because this drug has the potential to cause birth defects.
- Do not breast-feed while taking this drug without the approval of the health care provider.
- Report skin rash or jaundice immediately.

Drugs Similar to Phenytoin (Dilantin, Phenytek)

Fosphenytoin is the only other hydantoin. A third drug in this class, mephenytoin (Mesantoin), was removed from the market due to an unacceptable incidence rate of fatal blood dyscrasias.

Fosphenytoin (Cerebyx): Approved in 1996, fosphenytoin is a prodrug that is converted to phenytoin following metabolism. Given only by the parenteral route, it is considered functionally equivalent to phenytoin; their actions and adverse effects are the same. Doses on the label are indicated as phenytoin equivalents (PE). Indications for fosphenytoin include tonic–clonic seizures, status epilepticus, and seizure prophylaxis during neurosurgery. Because the drug is converted to phenytoin, therapeutic serum levels of phenytoin are monitored during therapy. Advantages of fosphenytoin over phenytoin include more rapid IV administration (important during status epilepticus), ability to be administered by the IM route, and less pain and phlebitis at the injection site. The drug is considerably more expensive than phenytoin.

26.10 Carbamazepine is a drug of choice for many tonic–clonic and partial seizures.

The iminostilbenes are a small class of two drugs, that have important applications to seizure management. These drugs have three rings in their structures, which makes them chemically related to the tricyclic antidepressants (see Chapter 23). The iminostilbenes, carbamazepine (Tegretol) and oxcarbazepine (Trileptal), have a similar pharmacologic activity.

The mechanisms of action of the iminostilbenes are incompletely understood. Like phenytoin, they affect the sodium channels in cortical neurons, slowing the propagation and spread of repetitive action potentials. These drugs have other actions, however, that are unexplained by the sodium channel mechanism, including analgesic, anticholinergic, antidysrhythmic, antidepressant, and sedative effects. They also have muscle relaxant and neuromuscular-blocking properties. The iminostilbenes are listed in Table 26.3 on page 381.

CONNECTIONS

Evidence-Based Practice Role of the School Nurse in Treating Epilepsy

Clinical Question

How do seizure disorders affect children psychosocially?

Evidence

Lew, Lewis, Owen, and West (2006) suggest that one contributory cause to the psychosocial problems in children with seizure disorders is the lack of understanding of the thoughts and intentions of others in interpersonal relationships. The problems encountered by children with seizures with regard to communication and social understanding are well documented. There is, however, a lack of research with regard to the children who are symptomatic. The researchers utilized questionnaires to determine the clinically relevant communication problems, including the specific language impairment and autistic spectrum disorder. The results revealed that clinicians and educators need to be aware that children with focal seizures may be particularly vulnerable to problems of social understanding and communication, irrespective of whether there is seizure control.

Implication

The school nurse plays a significant role in the life of each student in the school. It is the role of the nurse to educate the faculty and staff of the school about the signs and symptoms of all childhood diseases. It is very easy for the faculty to observe behaviors and classify them incorrectly. Thus the nurse must provide the school personnel with the information to guide them in finding health care professionals who can support them in the care of their students.

Critical Thinking Question

Imagine that you are the school nurse where some of the students suffer from seizure disorder. Describe how you could be most effective while addressing the psychosocial issues of these students.

See Answers to Critical Thinking Questions in Appendix A.

Source: From "Psychosocial Problems and Seizure-Related Factors in Children with Epilepsy," by A. R. Lew, C. Lewis, L. Owen, and S. West, 2006, *Developmental Medicine and Child Neurology, 48*(8), p. 704.

PROTOTYPE DRUG Carbamazepine (Tegretol, Tegretol XR, Carbatrol, others)

Classification: Therapeutic: Antiepileptic drug

Pharmacologic: Iminostilbene, neuronal sodium channel modulator

Therapeutic Effects and Uses: Approved by the U.S. Food and Drug Administration (FDA) in 1968, carbamazepine is one of the most widely prescribed AEDs in the world because of its effectiveness and relative safety. Approved to treat tonic–clonic seizures and partial seizures (simple and complex), carbamazepine may be administered alone or in combination with other AEDs. Carbamazepine is also approved for the treatment of acute mania associated with bipolar disorder, either as monotherapy or in combination with lithium (see Chapter 23). Extended release forms are available (Tegretol XR and Carbatrol), and a multiphasic extended release form (Equetro) was marketed for bipolar disorder in 2004.

Off-label uses of carbamazepine include the symptomatic treatment of neuropathic pain associated with diabetic neuropathy, trigeminal neuralgia, or postherpetic pain. The drug is also used off-label to treat hiccups and for the management of severe symptoms of dementia such as aggression and agitation, which are seen in some patients with Alzheimer's disease.

Although carbamazepine is structurally similar to the tricyclic antidepressants it does not produce the antidepressant effects of drugs in that class (see Chapter 23). The medication is metabolized in the liver to an active metabolite and is a potent inducer of CYP450 enzymes that will increase its own metabolism. Long-term administration of carbamazepine will result in the need to increase the dose because its half-life becomes shortened.

For all indications, therapy with carbamazepine must be monitored carefully and the dosage adjusted based on clinical outcomes and drug serum levels. The therapeutic serum concentrations usually range from 4 to 12 mcg/mL. Several weeks of therapy may be required before the optimum dose is determined and the effective plasma drug concentration is achieved.

Mechanism of Action: Carbamazepine inhibits sodium channels, blocking the repetitive, sustained firing of neurons that is characteristic of epilepsy. Other mechanisms are likely but are incompletely understood.

Pharmacokinetics:

Route(s)	PO
Absorption	Slowly absorbed through the GI tract
Distribution	Widely distributed; enters the CSF; crosses the placenta; secreted in breast milk; 75–85% bound to protein
Primary metabolism	Hepatic
Primary excretion	Renal and GI
Onset of action	Slow and variable
Duration of action	Half-life: 14–16 h

Adverse Effects: Carbamazepine is well tolerated; adverse effects are usually transient and will diminish as therapy progresses. The most frequently observed adverse effects include drowsiness, dizziness, ataxia, and nausea and vomiting. Transient sedation is common at the onset of therapy or after dosage increases. Other CNS effects include confusion, blurred vision, lethargy, and visual disturbances, although the patient usually develops tolerance to these effects. Other possible adverse effects include myalgia, leg cramps, carbamazepine-induced systemic erythematosus, heart block, aplastic anemia, agranulocytosis, and respiratory depression. Various types of dermatologic toxicity have been reported, including exfoliative dermatitis, phototoxicity, urticaria, alopecia, and SJS. Elevated hepatic enzymes occur during therapy, although the patient is usually asymptomatic for hepatic disease. A few rare cases of serious hepatic impairment have been documented. Some patients have reported urinary retention and frequency, and male patients may experience impotence.

Contraindications/Precautions: Patients who are hypersensitive to tricyclic antidepressants should not take carbamazepine. Patients who have been diagnosed with increased intraocular pressure, systemic lupus erythematosus, cardiac disease, hepatic disease, and liver disease should not take carbamazepine. This medication is contraindicated with HTN. Older adults should be monitored closely if they possess a history of cardiac disease because a major adverse effect is heart block. Carbamazepine causes multiple birth defects in laboratory animals. If used during pregnancy, monotherapy is recommended because the use of two or more AEDs increases the risk of teratogenesis.

Drug Interactions: Carbamazepine has the ability to increase the activity of hepatic CYP450 enzymes, which can result in decreased serum concentrations of AEDs and other drugs metabolized by the liver. Increased carbamazepine levels have been noted when the drug is administered with verapamil, erythromycin, ketoconazole, or nefazodone. Patients who take carbamazepine with anticoagulants will experience decreased hypoprothrombinemic effects. Carbamazepine may decrease the effectiveness of oral contraceptives. **Herbal/Food:** Ginkgo may decrease the antiepileptic effectiveness of carbamazepine. Grapefruit juice and St. John's wort induce CYP enzymes and can decrease serum carbamazepine levels.

Pregnancy: Category D.

Treatment of Overdose: Activated charcoal and gastric lavage are administered with carbamazepine overdose.

Nursing Responsibilities:

- Do not administer carbamazepine within 14 days of an MAOI.
- Do not administer the elixir formulation with any other medication because precipitates may form.
- Assess periodic CBC, platelets, electrolytes, aspartate transaminase (AST), alanine transaminase (ALT), serum iron, and urinalysis.
- Assess serum carbamazepine levels and immediately report levels outside the prescribed range to the prescriber.
- Assess for adverse CNS effects such as dizziness, lethargy, light-headedness, and ataxia.
- Assess for gastric distress.
- Withhold the medication if signs and symptoms of myelosuppression are noted: red blood cells less than 4 million/mm^3; hematocrit less than 32%; hemoglobin less than 11; and platelet count less than 100,000/mm^3.
- Assess for dysrhythmias if doses exceed 600 mg/day.
- Assess intake and output and vital signs.

Patient and Family Education:

- Take this medication with food if nausea occurs. Do not take this drug with grapefruit juice.
- Take this medication exactly as instructed and do not discontinue the drug without consulting the health care provider because seizures may result.
- If taking the chewable tablet form of the drug, chew the tablets well before swallowing.
- If taking Tegretol XR, swallow the drug whole and do not open or chew it.
- If taking Carbatrol or Equetro, the capsule may be opened and spread over soft food. Do not chew the beads of medication.
- Immediately report any of the following symptoms: lack of coordination, anorexia, fever, sore throat, dry mouth, malaise, bruising, or bleeding.
- Do not drive or perform other hazardous activities until the effects of the drug are known because this drug may cause drowsiness or dizziness.
- Avoid direct sunlight and apply sunscreen to prevent rash or sunburn.
- Do not change medication brands unless directed to do so by the prescriber.
- Immediately notify the health care provider of any suspected or known pregnancy because this drug has the potential to cause birth defects.
- Do not breast-feed while taking this drug without the approval of the health care provider.

Drugs Similar to Carbamazepine (Tegretol, Tegretol XR, Carbatrol, Others)

Oxcarbazepine is the only other iminostilbene.

Oxcarbazepine (Trileptal): Like carbamazepine, oxcarbazepine is similar to the tricyclic antidepressants and does not possess antidepressant activity. The two drugs act by the same mechanism and have similar actions. Approved in 2000, oxcarbazepine can be administered alone or in combination with other medications in the treatment of partial seizures, with or without secondary generalization. Off-label uses include the treatment of neuropathic pain and bipolar disorder. A major advantage of oxcarbazepine over carbamazepine is that drug interactions appear less significant and monitoring of drug plasma levels and hematologic values is generally not necessary. Although it induces CYP450 enzymes, it is not as strong an inducer as carbamazepine and it does not induce its own metabolism. For checking adherence with the drug regimen or in overdose situations, the therapeutic serum concentration of the drug is 12 to 30 mcg/mL. Adverse effects are similar to those of carbamazepine, with dizziness, drowsiness, headache, and ataxia being the most common effects. It is important to monitor renal function when administering this medication because it is excreted through the kidneys. This drug is pregnancy category C.

26.11 Succinimides are often the drugs of choice for the pharmacotherapy of absence seizures.

Succinimides form a small group of AEDs that suppress the influx of calcium into neurons during neuronal transmission. This is believed to increase the electrical threshold of the neuron, which reduces the likelihood of abnormal action potentials. Recent research has questioned this mechanism of action, and the actual mechanism of antiepileptic activity of this group remains largely unknown. Despite the small size of the class and their unknown mechanism of action, these drugs have important roles in the pharmacotherapy of absence seizures.

PROTOTYPE DRUG Ethosuximide (Zarontin)

Classification: **Therapeutic:** Antiepileptic drug
Pharmacologic: Succinimide, neuronal calcium channel modulator

Therapeutic Effects and Uses: Ethosuximide is the only drug in this class that is commonly prescribed. Approved in 1960, it is the drug of choice for managing absence seizures. Because ethosuximide is ineffective in treating simple or complex partial seizures and tonic–clonic seizures, combination pharmacotherapy is needed to manage mixed seizures.

Ethosuximide is only administered by the oral route. Therapeutic serum concentrations range from 40 to 100 mcg/mL, although dosing is usually based on clinical response rather than serum levels. It may take 4 to 7 days before optimum therapeutic levels are attained.

Mechanism of Action: Ethosuximide depresses the motor cortex by delaying the calcium influx into the neuron.

Pharmacokinetics:

Route(s)	PO
Absorption	Readily and completely absorbed
Distribution	Widely distributed; not bound to plasma proteins; crosses the placenta and is secreted in breast milk
Primary metabolism	Hepatic
Primary excretion	Primarily renal, with some in feces and bile
Onset of action	Peak: 4 h
Duration of action	Half-life: 30 h in children; 60 h in adults

Adverse Effects: The most common adverse effects of ethosuximide are GI related, including anorexia, nausea, vomiting, abdominal pain, and diarrhea. Adverse CNS events include drowsiness, dizziness, ataxia, confusion, aggressiveness, and night terrors. Hematologic toxicity may include agranulocytosis, pancytopenia, and aplastic anemia. Dermatologic effects include rash, pruritus, and exfoliative dermatitis.

Contraindications/Precautions: Ethosuximide is contraindicated in patients who have a known sensitivity to succinimides. It should be administered with caution to patients with liver or kidney impairment. Administration of ethosuximide may increase the frequency of tonic–clonic seizures. Patients with blood dyscrasias or bone marrow suppression should not receive this drug because it can worsen these conditions. Safety has not been established for the administration of this medication during pregnancy. Although only small amounts of the drug are secreted in breast milk, the American Academy of Pediatrics considers the use of the drug compatible with breast-feeding.

Drug Interactions: Ethosuximide can participate in many drug–drug interactions. When used in combination therapy with other AEDs, serum drug levels should be regularly monitored. CNS depressants and ethanol may cause additive sedation. Use of ethanol may also reduce the effectiveness of the antiseizure medication. Ethosuximide administered concurrently with phenobarbital, phenothiazines, or tricyclic antidepressants can increase seizure frequency. Isoniazid administered in combination with ethosuximide can result in increased serum ethosuximide levels. Carbamazepine will cause a decrease in ethosuximide serum levels. Concurrent use of valproic acid will inhibit the metabolism of ethosuximide, leading to possible toxicity. **Herbal/Food:** Unknown.

Pregnancy: Category C.

Treatment of Overdose: Activated charcoal and gastric lavage are administered with ethosuximide overdose.

Nursing Responsibilities:

- Obtain baseline and periodic renal and hepatic function tests.
- Monitor for adverse effects, including drowsiness, headache, fatigue, dizziness, nausea, vomiting, diarrhea, weight loss, and suicidal ideations.
- Assess periodic blood counts to prevent the development of blood dyscrasias.
- Assess seizure activity to determine drug effectiveness.
- Assess serum drug levels, which should be 40 to 100 mcg/mL.

Patient and Family Education:

- Take this medication with food if nausea occurs.
- The medication may change the color of urine to pink or red-brown but this is not harmful.
- Report the development of flulike symptoms, worsening of mood (including thoughts of suicide), unusual bleeding, redness or blistering of the skin, or any weight loss or diminished appetite.
- Take this medication exactly as instructed and do not discontinue the drug without consulting the health care provider because seizures may result.
- Do not drive or perform other hazardous activities until the effects of the drug are known because this drug may cause drowsiness or dizziness.
- Never consume alcoholic beverages with this medication because this will cause excessive sedation.
- Immediately notify the health care provider of any known or suspected pregnancy because this drug has the potential to cause birth defects.
- Do not breast-feed while taking this drug without approval of the health care provider.

Drugs Similar to Ethosuximide (Zarontin)

Methsuximide is the only other drug in the succinimide class.

Methsuximide (Celontin): This drug is rarely used in clinical practice because it is less effective and more toxic than ethosuximide. It has the same indications and adverse effects as ethosuximide. This drug is pregnancy category C.

26.12 Several miscellaneous drugs are important in treating epilepsy.

As explained in Section 26.6, it is difficult to classify AEDs because many act by multiple mechanisms, whereas others are unique and are the only drug in a class. Several of these "miscellaneous" drugs are widely used. Following the two prototypes, other miscellaneous drugs and their indications are described.

PROTOTYPE DRUG Gabapentin (Neurontin)

Classification: Therapeutic: Antiepileptic drug
Pharmacologic: GABA analog

Therapeutic Effects and Uses: Gabapentin consists of a molecule of the neurotransmitter GABA with an attached side chain. The side chain makes the molecule lipid soluble so that it readily crosses the blood–brain barrier. Approved in 1993, gabapentin is used in combination with other AEDs to control partial seizures with or without secondary generalization. Doses are based on therapeutic response, making it unnecessary to measure serum drug levels during therapy. It is available as capsules, as tablets, and as an oral solution.

Therapy with gabapentin has been found to benefit a number of other conditions. It is FDA approved for the treatment of postherpetic neuralgia and is used off-label for other conditions with neuropathic pain such as diabetic neuropathy. In fact, the drug is likely prescribed more often for the treatment of neuropathic pain than for epilepsy. Hot flashes are reduced in approximately 50% of the women taking the drug. It has been designated as an orphan drug for the treatment of amyotrophic lateral sclerosis (ALS). Some research has suggested that gabapentin is useful in treating trigeminal neuralgia, paresthesia, spasticity, and ocular ataxia in patients with multiple sclerosis.

Mechanism of Action: The exact mechanism of action of gabapentin is unknown. Although closely related structurally to GABA, it does not appear to bind to GABA receptors or to prevent endogenous GABA from binding. It does not appear to affect the binding of other neurotransmitters such as serotonin, dopamine, glutamate, or histamine. It likely affects calcium channels, but its exact mechanism remains to be determined.

Pharmacokinetics:

Route(s)	PO
Absorption	50–60% is absorbed from the GI tract
Distribution	Crosses the blood–brain barrier and the placenta; readily passes into the CSF; secreted in breast milk; not bound to plasma proteins
Primary metabolism	Not metabolized
Primary excretion	Excreted unchanged by the kidneys
Onset of action	1 h
Duration of action	Half-life: 5–6 h

Adverse Effects: Gabapentin is well tolerated, with CNS symptoms such as drowsiness, fatigue, nystagmus, and dizziness being the primary adverse effects. The administration of gabapentin can lead to increased frequency of viral infections, weight gain, and gastric upset. Behavioral problems such as hostility, emotional lability, impaired cognition, aggressiveness, and hyperkinesia have been reported in the pediatric population age 3 to 12.

Contraindications/Precautions: Gabapentin should not be administered during pregnancy or lactation unless the benefits of pharmacotherapy outweigh the risks. It should not be administered in patients who have experienced a hypersensitivity reaction to GABA-related medications. It should be used cautiously with status epilepticus, renal impairment, and with older adults. Gabapentin should be used with caution in patients with renal impairment because the drug could accumulate to toxic levels. The drug should be discontinued gradually to prevent withdrawal-associated seizures.

Drug Interactions: A major advantage of gabapentin is that it does not induce CYP450 enzymes, and thus it exhibits fewer drug interactions than many other AEDs. No interactions with carbamazepine, phenobarbital, phenytoin, or valproic acid have been observed. Morphine and hydrocodone may cause additive CNS depression when administered with gabapentin. **Herbal/Food:** The administration of ginkgo with gabapentin may result in decreased anticonvulsant effects.

Pregnancy: Category C.

Treatment of Overdose: Overdose results in dyspnea, sedation, double vision, and slurred speech. Renal dialysis can be utilized to treat gabapentin overdose.

Nursing Responsibilities:

- Assess renal function prior to therapy to determine if excretion is adequate to prevent drug toxicity.
- Monitor for signs and symptoms of CNS depression.
- Monitor the effects of the medication carefully if dosage is changed.
- Monitor pediatric patients for CNS adverse effects and unusual behavioral problems.

Patient and Family Education:

- Notify the health care provider immediately of any suspected or known pregnancy because this drug has the potential to cause birth defects.
- If nausea occurs, take this medication with food.
- Report any visual changes, suicidal thoughts, bruising or bleeding, swelling of the feet or ankles, or increased seizure activity.
- Do not drive or perform other hazardous activities until the effects of the drug are known because this drug may cause drowsiness or dizziness.
- Do not consume alcoholic beverages with this medication because this may cause excessive sedation.
- Do not breast-feed while taking this drug without the approval of the health care provider.
- Take this medication exactly as instructed and do not discontinue the drug without consulting the health care provider because seizures may result.

PROTOTYPE DRUG Valproic acid (Depacon, Depakene, Depakote)

Classification: Therapeutic: Antiepileptic drug, antimanic agent
Pharmacologic: GABA agonist

Therapeutic Effects and Uses: Valproic acid has been an important drug in treating epilepsy since 1978. Valproic acid has several trade names and formulations, which sometimes causes confusion when studying this drug.

- Valproic acid (Depakene) is the standard form of the drug given by the oral route.
- Valproate sodium is the sodium salt of valproic acid given orally or IV (Depacon).
- Divalproex sodium (Depakote ER) is a sustained release combination of valproic acid and its sodium salt in a 1:1 mixture. It is given orally and is available in an enteric-coated form.

All three formulations of the drug form valproate after absorption or on entering the brain. The pharmacokinetics of each form varies, and they are not interchangeable. In this text, the name "valproic acid" is used to describe all forms of the drug, unless specifically stated otherwise.

Valproic acid is administered alone or in combination with other AEDs to treat absence seizures and complex partial seizures. It is also approved for the prevention of migraine headaches and mania associated with bipolar disorder. Off-label indications include severe behavioral disturbances such as agitation due to dementia, Alzheimer's disease, or explosive temper in patients with ADHD; persistent hiccups; and status epilepticus refractory to IV diazepam. Dosage adjustments for valproic acid are usually based on patient response; normal serum drug levels for epilepsy are 50 to 100 mcg/mL. In 2007, the FDA approved Stavzor, a soft gelatin capsule of valproic acid. The capsule dissolves in the small intestine, rather than the stomach, thus reducing nausea and vomiting, which are common adverse effects of the drug.

Mechanism of Action: Valproic acid increases concentrations of the inhibitory neurotransmitter GABA in the brain. Abnormal neuron discharges are suppressed, leading to decreased seizure activity.

Pharmacokinetics:

Route(s)	IV, PO
Absorption	Rapidly absorbed in the GI tract
Distribution	Crosses the placenta; and is secreted in breast milk; 80–90% bound to protein
Primary metabolism	Hepatic
Primary excretion	Renal and GI tract
Onset of action	15–30 minutes
Duration of action	Half-life: 5–20 h

Adverse Effects: Valproic acid is well tolerated in most patients and adverse effects rarely cause discontinuation of therapy. The most common adverse effects are GI related, such as nausea, vomiting, diarrhea, abdominal pain, and diminished appetite. An enteric-coated formulation of valproic acid can be used to reduce these uncomfortable effects. These effects are usually transient and not severe. CNS adverse effects such as headache, tremor, dizziness, and sedation occur in about 25% of patients. High doses of valproic acid cause diminished platelet aggregation, which can result in prolonged bleeding and clotting times. Bone marrow depression, photosensitivity, and pulmonary edema are rare potential adverse effects. Valproic acid may cause hyperammonemic encephalopathy, especially in combination with topiramate, which requires discontinuation of valproic acid therapy. Life-threatening pancreatitis can occur as a result of valproic acid administration. Serious hepatotoxicity has been reported in infants younger than age 2 taking valproic acid.

Contraindications/Precautions: Patients with hypersensitivity to any formulation of valproic acid should not be administered this drug. Other contraindications include bleeding disorders, cirrhosis, congenital metabolic disorders, and autoimmune deficiency syndrome. Patients with known or suspected pancreatitis should not receive this drug because life-threatening pancreatitis has been reported. Valproic acid should be administered cautiously in patients with a low serum albumin and renal impairment. Extreme caution should be used in treating patients under age 2 because fatal hepatotoxicity has been reported. The drug should not be administered to patients with known hepatic impairment. Abrupt discontinuation may cause status epilepticus. This drug is a known teratogen and should only be used during pregnancy when benefits of therapy clearly outweigh the risk of birth defects.

Drug Interactions: Valproic acid administered concurrently with alcohol and other CNS depressants may result in additive sedation. Patients taking enzyme-inducing AEDs such as carbamazepine, phenytoin, and phenobarbital will metabolize valproic acid more rapidly, and dosage adjustment will be necessary. Valproic acid may increase the serum levels of tricyclic antidepressants, requiring a reduction in antidepressant dosage. Aspirin increases the serum drug levels of valproic acid and should not be administered concurrently. Isoniazid will elevate serum valproic acid levels. Cholestyramine will decrease absorption of valproic acid. Cimetidine will increase valproic acid levels and will place the patient at risk for hepatotoxicity. Valproic acid should not be administered with topiramate due to an increased risk of hyperammonemic encephalopathy. **Herbal/Food:** Ginkgo may decrease the antiepileptic effects of valproic acid.

Pregnancy: Category D.

Treatment of Overdose: The effects from overdose of valproic acid may be serious and include sedation, heart block, deep coma, and death. Naloxone (Narcan) is utilized to reverse the CNS depression, and hemodialysis can lower drug serum levels. Caution must be used when administering naloxone because this drug may also reverse the antiseizure action of valproic acid.

Nursing Responsibilities:

- Monitor for seizure activity to determine drug effectiveness.
- Assess the serum level of valproic acid, which should be 50 to 100 mcg/mL.
- When changing dosages, monitor the patient carefully for increased adverse effects.

- Obtain baseline platelet counts before beginning therapy and assess bleeding and clotting times during therapy to prevent abnormal bleeding.
- Monitor for signs of hyperammonemia, such as lethargy, anorexia, nausea, and vomiting.
- Obtain baseline and periodic hepatic function tests to prevent hepatotoxicity; monitor for signs of liver impairment.

Patient and Family Education:

- Do not change brands of valproic acid without approval of the health care provider.
- Take this medication exactly as instructed and do not discontinue the drug without consulting the health care provider because seizures may result.
- Do not crush or chew the extended release forms of this drug.
- Check with the health care provider before taking any OTC medications or herbal products.
- Inform dentists and other health care providers that you are taking valproic acid because excessive bleeding may result.
- Do not drive or perform other hazardous activities until the effects of the drug are known because this drug may cause drowsiness or dizziness.
- Immediately report signs of unusual bleeding or bruising, increase in seizure frequency, extreme fatigue, suicidal thoughts, or yellowing of the skin or whites of the eyes.
- Immediately notify the health care provider of any suspected or known pregnancy because this drug has the potential to cause severe birth defects.
- Do not breast-feed while taking this drug without approval of the health care provider.

Other Miscellaneous Drugs

Felbamate (Felbatol): Approved in 1993, felbamate is an oral agent that is effective against most types of seizures. Serious adverse effects, however, limit its use to severe partial seizures and the treatment of partial and generalized seizures associated with Lennox-Gastaut syndrome in children who have not responded to other therapies. Fatal aplastic anemia and fatal hepatic failure have been associated with felbamate use. Although the incidence of these adverse effects is rare, they occurred frequently enough for the FDA to place restrictive conditions on the use of this drug in 1994. More common adverse effects include nausea, vomiting, anorexia, drowsiness, dizziness, insomnia, and vision changes. This drug is pregnancy category C.

Lamotrigine (Lamictal): Approved in 1994, lamotrigine is an oral agent indicated for the adjunctive therapy of partial seizures, Lennox-Gastaut syndrome, absence seizures, and tonic–clonic seizures in adults and pediatric patients (2 years of age or older). It is also used to treat bipolar disorder. The mechanism of antiseizure action is largely unknown but likely relates to this drug's ability to inhibit flow through sodium ion channels and probably calcium channels as well. Lamotrigine is rapidly absorbed, 55% bound to plasma proteins, and almost entirely excreted by the kidneys.

Lamotrigine does not induce or inhibit hepatic metabolic enzymes. Lamotrigine is metabolized by CYP450 enzymes, however, and patients who are taking potent inducers of CYP450 enzymes (e.g., carbamazepine, phenytoin, and phenobarbital) will metabolize the drug more rapidly. Doses of lamotrigine will need to be increased in these patients to produce an optimal antiseizure response. On the other hand, valproic acid will reduce the elimination of lamotrigine, and the dose of lamotrigine should be reduced to prevent toxicity. Oral contraceptives reduce serum levels of lamotrigine, and the dosage of the AED will need to be adjusted when therapy with the hormones is initiated or discontinued and during the "pill-free" week of the month.

Lamotrigine is generally well tolerated by patients. The most commonly adverse effects associated with lamotrigine therapy are drowsiness, dizziness, ataxia, headache, diplopia, blurred vision, nausea, vomiting, and rash. Over 10% of patients taking this AED will develop a rash. Although rare, serious dermatologic toxicity, including SJS, has been reported with this drug, especially in children. Therefore, lamotrigine should be discontinued at the first sign of any type of rash. Lamotrigine has not been shown to be teratogenic and thus is one of the preferred drugs for managing epilepsy in pregnant patients. This drug is pregnancy category C.

Levetiracetam (Keppra): Levetiracetam is an AED available by both oral and IV routes that is utilized in the therapy of the following seizures: adjunctive therapy for partial seizures in adults and children age 4 years and older, adjunctive therapy for myoclonic seizures in adults and adolescents age 12 years and older, and adjunctive therapy of primary generalized tonic–clonic seizures in adults and children age 6 years and older. Approved in 1999, the mechanism of its antiseizure activity is unknown. Levetiracetam is rapidly absorbed and only 10% is bound to plasma proteins. It is excreted unchanged by the kidneys; thus dosage should be reduced in patients with renal impairment. No significant drug interactions have been recorded.

Levetiracetam is well tolerated, with the most common adverse effects being drowsiness, dizziness, infections, headache, and asthenia. The nurse must teach the patient to exercise care in performing tasks because an increase in accidental injuries is associated with levetiracetam use. Pediatric patients exhibit a relatively high incidence of behavioral effects, including agitation, nervousness, hyperkinesia, hostility, depression, and emotional lability. Levetiracetam is pregnancy category C.

MyNursingKit Mechanism of Action Animation: Valproic Acid

Pregabalin (Lyrica): Approved in 2004, pregabalin is an oral AED that is very similar to gabapentin. For epilepsy management, pregabalin is indicated for the adjunctive therapy of adult patients with partial onset seizures. Like gabapentin, it is also indicated for the management of neuropathic pain associated with diabetic peripheral neuropathy and postherpetic neuralgia. Off-label uses include the therapy of anxiety and social phobia. The safety of pregabalin in pediatric patients has not been established. Although its mechanism of action has not been clearly demonstrated, it is thought to act by increasing GABA levels by reducing the calcium channel function of neurons in the brain. This drug does not affect CYP450 enzymes; thus it has fewer drug–drug interactions than many other AEDs. Pregabalin is not bound to plasma proteins and is excreted in an unmetabolized

NURSING PROCESS APPLICATION

Patients Receiving Antiepileptic Medications

Assessment	Potential Nursing Diagnoses
Prior to administration: • Obtain a complete health history, including allergies and drug history, to determine drug interactions. • Assess neurologic status, including identification of recent seizure activity. • Assess growth and development, including an accurate weight.	• *Risk for Injury*, related to drug adverse effects and potential falls during seizure • *Deficient Knowledge (Antiepileptic Medication)*, related to purpose, precautions, and adverse effects of drug therapy • *Noncompliance (Medication Regimen)*

Planning: Patient Goals and Expected Outcomes

The patient will:

- Experience the absence of, or reduction in, the number or severity of seizures.
- Avoid physical injury related to seizure activity or medication-induced sensory changes.
- Demonstrate an understanding of the drug's action by accurately describing adverse effects and precautions.

Implementation of Antiepileptic Medication Therapy

Interventions and (Rationales)	Patient and Family Education
• Monitor neurologic status, especially changes in level of consciousness and/or mental status. (Sedation may indicate impending toxicity.)	Instruct the patient to: • Report any significant change in sensorium, such as slurred speech, confusion, hallucinations, or lethargy. • Report any changes in seizure quality or unexpected involuntary muscle movement, such as twitching, tremor, or unusual eye movement. • Avoid driving and other hazardous activities until the effects of the drug are known. • Request assistance to get out of bed and abulate until the effect of the drug is known. • Be aware that some medications may cause initial drowsiness, which may decrease with continued treatment.
• Monitor vital signs, especially blood pressure and depth and rate of respirations. (Barbiturates can cause severe respiratory depression.)	• Instruct the patient to withhold medications if any difficulty in breathing is experienced or if respirations are less than 12 breaths per minute.
• Monitor the effectiveness of drug therapy (Drug effectiveness must be individualized for each patient.) • Monitor children for paradoxical response to barbiturates. (Hyperactivity may occur.)	Instruct the patient to: • Keep a seizure diary to chronicle symptoms phase, or during dose adjustment. • Take the medication exactly as ordered, including the same manufacturer's drug, each time the prescription is refilled. (Switching brands may result in alterations in seizure control.) • Take a missed dose as soon as it is remembered, but not to take double doses. • Not to discontinue barbiturates abruptly, because this can cause increased seizure activity. • Notify the health care provider if hyperactive behavior is experienced.
• Monitor for adverse effects. Observe for hypersensitivity, nephrotoxicity, and hepatotoxicity. (Most antiseizure medications are metabolized by the liver and excreted by the kidneys.)	Instruct the patient to: • Report adverse effects specific to the drug regimen. • Report signs of toxicity such as nausea, vomiting, rash, diarrhea, jaundice, abdominal pain, change in color of stool, flank pain, or blood in urine. • Adhere to the regular schedule for laboratory testing for liver and kidney function as ordered by the prescriber.
• Monitor oral health. Observe for signs of gingival hyperplasia, bleeding, or inflammation. (These signs are specific adverse effects of phenytoin.)	Instruct the patient to: • Use a soft toothbrush and oral rinses as prescribed by the dentist. • Avoid mouthwash containing alcohol. • Report any changes in oral health such as excessive bleeding or inflammation of the gums. • Visit the dentist regularly.
• Monitor GI status. (Valproic acid is a GI irritant and anticoagulant.)	• Instruct the patient to take the drug with food to reduce GI upset.
• Conduct guaiac stool testing for occult blood. (CNS effects of phenytoin decrease GI motility, producing constipation.)	• Immediately report severe or persistent heartburn, upper GI pain, or nausea or vomiting. • Increase exercise and fluid and fiber intake to facilitate stool passage.
• Monitor nutritional status. (Phenytoin may cause decreased absorption of folic acid, vitamin D, magnesium, calcium, leading to anemia and osteoporosis. Barbiturates may cause deficiencies in vitamin D, vitamin K, folate, and other B vitamins. Valproic acid may cause an increase in appetite and weight.)	Instruct the patient to: • Immediately report signs of vitamin K deficiency: bleeding tendency, tarry stools, bruising, and pallor. • Immediately report signs of vitamin D deficiency: skin changes, dandruff, peripheral neuropathy, fatigue. • Report significant changes in appetite or weight gain.

Evaluation of Outcome Criteria

Evaluate the effectiveness of drug therapy by confirming that patient goals and expected outcomes have been met (see "Planning").

form by the kidneys. Dose reduction in patients with renal impairment is necessary to avoid toxicity.

Pregabalin is well tolerated by most patients. Dizziness and drowsiness are the most common adverse effects and these may affect 20% to 40% of the patients, especially at high doses. Other common adverse effects of pregabalin are blurred vision, lethargy, dry mouth, peripheral edema, weight gain, and difficulty with concentration or attention. Concurrent administration with other CNS depressants can lead to increased sedation. Because pregabalin is a Schedule V controlled substance that may cause physical and psychological dependence, it should be used with caution in patients with a known or suspected history of substance abuse. Pregabalin is pregnancy category C.

Tiagabine (Gabitril): Tiagabine is given by the oral or IV routes for the adjunctive treatment of partial seizures in patients older than 12 years. Safety in patients under age 12 has not been established. Approved in 1997, it acts by inhibiting GABA reuptake into the presynaptic neuron. Tiagabine is extensively metabolized by CYP3A enzymes. Patients who are taking potent inducers of CYP450 enzymes (e.g., carbamazepine, phenytoin, and phenobarbital) will metabolize tiagabine more rapidly. Doses of tiagabine will need to be increased in these patients to produce an optimal antiseizure response. Tiagabine itself does not induce CYP enzymes; thus it has fewer drug–drug interactions than many other AEDs. Tiagabine is 98% bound to plasma proteins and is eliminated in both the urine and feces.

Approximately 10% to 20% of patients taking tiagabine experience an adverse effect that requires discontinuation of therapy. The most common adverse effects are dizziness, lethargy, somnolence, nausea, irritability, tremor, asthenia, abdominal pain, and difficulty with concentration or attention. As with other AEDs the nurse should teach patients to avoid injury due to possible sedative effects. Although tiagabine suppresses seizures in patients with epilepsy, it has been found to increase seizure activity in patients given the drug for off-label indications. Because of this, the FDA and the manufacturer have issued a warning not to administer tiagabine for any indication other than partial seizures. Patients with hepatic impairment will exhibit higher serum levels of the drug; thus dosage must be reduced. Tiagabine is pregnancy category C.

Zonisamide (Zonegran): Approved in 2000, zonisamide (Zonegran) is an oral sulfonamide that is effective in combination with other AEDs for partial seizures in adults. Safety in patients under age 16 has not been established although the drug is sometimes used off-label in children. It produces antiepileptic effects by inhibiting sodium and calcium channels in brain neurons. Zonisamide has a long half-life and 2 weeks may be required before optimum antiseizure activity is achieved.

Zonisamide is well tolerated by most patients. The most common adverse effects are dizziness, ataxia, drowsiness, fatigue, anorexia, speech abnormalities, and difficulty in concentrating or remembering. Because many patients are allergic to sulfonamides, it is important to assess these patients for sulfonamide hypersensitivity prior to the administration of the medication. Sulfonamides can cause fatal skin reactions, including SJS. Other adverse effects include flulike symptoms, weight gain, headache, abnormal gait, gingivitis, rhinitis, kidney stones, and heat stroke. The medication should be administered cautiously in patients who are receiving drugs that inhibit or reduce CYP3A4 enzymes; phenytoin, carbamazepine, phenobarbital, and valproic acid will decrease the half-life of zonisamide. Doses of zonisamide will need to be increased in these patients to produce an optimal antiseizure response. Zonisamide itself does not induce CYP enzymes; thus it has fewer drug–drug interactions than many other AEDs. Zonisamide is pregnancy category C.

UNDERSTANDING THE CHAPTER

Key Concepts Summary

26.1 Epilepsy is characterized by recurrent seizures caused by disturbances in the electrical activity of the brain.

26.2 Seizure disorders differ throughout the life span.

26.3 Most seizures are classified as generalized or partial.

26.4 Some types of seizures are called special epileptic seizures or are unclassified.

26.5 The choice of antiepileptic drug therapy is dependent on seizure type and characteristics.

26.6 Antiseizure drugs act by suppressing abnormal neuronal discharges.

26.7 Barbiturates are traditional drugs for tonic–clonic seizures but have been replaced by newer and safer medications.

26.8 Benzodiazepines are important drugs in the treatment of status epilepticus.

26.9 Hydantoins are effective in the management of most types of seizures but have many adverse effects.

26.10 Carbamazepine is a drug of choice for many tonic–clonic and partial seizures.

26.11 Succinimides are often the drugs of choice for the pharmacotherapy of absence seizures.

26.12 Several miscellaneous drugs are important in treating epilepsy.

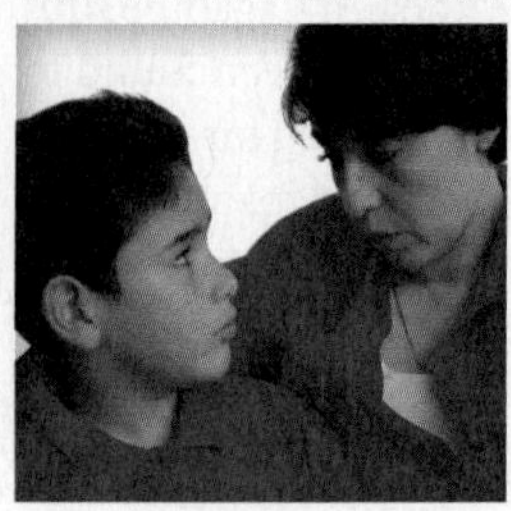

Making the PATIENT Connection

Remember the patient "Jorge Alvarez" at the beginning of the chapter? Now read the remainder of the case study. Based on the information presented within this chapter, respond to the critical thinking questions that follow.

Jorge Alvarez is an 8-year-old boy who has been hospitalized following his seizure. Since being admitted 2 days ago he has experienced three subsequent tonic–clonic seizures lasting 2 to 2½ minutes each. Prior to having a seizure Jorge notices a flash of light. He then loses consciousness, emits a hoarse cry, and has intense muscle contractions. During the clonic phase he is incontinent of bowel and bladder. His postictal phase is characterized by drowsiness, disorientation, and deep sleep.

On admission Jorge was scheduled for a sleep-and-awake EEG. His EEG revealed a high-voltage spike discharge, which is diagnostic of a tonic–clonic seizure. The laboratory studies performed on Jorge included a lead level to rule out lead intoxication and a blood glucose to rule out hypoglycemia. Both the lead level and blood glucose were in the normal range.

Jorge has been started on the following medications to assist in controlling his tonic–clonic seizures: carbamazepine (Tegretol) 300 mg PO tid and phenytoin (Dilantin) 120 mg PO tid.

Critical Thinking Questions

1. Jorge's mother expresses concern about what to do if he has a seizure. Create a list of home safety tips that could be given to her.
2. What will you instruct Jorge's mother with regard to his medication administration?

Case Study

Matt has suffered from epilepsy since childhood. It seems that his current medications are no longer keeping him "seizure free." Valproic acid (Depakene) is being added to Matt's medication regimen. How would you respond to the following questions from Matt about this new medication?

1. How does valproic acid (Depakene) work to prevent seizures?
2. What adverse effects are associated with this drug?
3. Why should Matt inform his dentist that he is now on valproic acid?

NCLEX-RN® Review

1 A 10-year-old child is being medically evaluated for a learning disability. However, with the presenting symptoms, the health care provider wants to rule out absence seizures. What diagnostic test would the nurse expect to be performed before initiating any drug therapy?

1. Blood glucose
2. Echocardiogram
3. Electroencephalogram
4. Computed tomography (CT) scan

2 The nurse is caring for an infant who was recently diagnosed with West syndrome. Which of the following drug therapies would the nurse expect to be ordered?

1. Valproic acid (Depakote)
2. Diazepam (Valium)
3. Phenytoin (Dilantin)
4. Adrenocorticotropic hormone (ACTH)

3 An 80-year-old client is prescribed phenobarbital (Luminal) for a newly diagnosed seizure disorder. The client is at risk for which disorder with the administration of this drug?

1. Hyperkinetic behavior disorder
2. Sleep apnea
3. Cerebrovascular accident
4. Osteomalacia

4 A client has been taking phenobarbital for many years. To enhance coagulation, which type of food would the nurse recommend that the client eat?

1. Green leafy vegetables and organ meats
2. Dairy products such as milk and cream
3. Whole wheat products such as breads and cereal
4. Cultured foods such as buttermilk and yogurt

5 The nurse, who is monitoring a client taking phenytoin (Dilantin), has noted symptoms of nystagmus, confusion, and ataxia. Considering these findings, the nurse would suspect that the dose of the drug should be:

1. Reduced.
2. Increased.
3. Maintained.
4. Discontinued.

6 Ethosuximide (Zarontin) is prescribed for each of the following clients. A nurse should question the order for the client with: (Select all that apply.)

1. Absence seizures.
2. Simple partial seizures.
3. Tonic–clonic seizures.
4. Simple complex seizure.
5. Febrile seizure.

See Answers to Critical Thinking Questions, Case Study, and NCLEX-RN® Review in Appendix A.

References

Alvarez, N. (2007). Epilepsy in children with mental retardation. *eMedicine.* Retrieved June 20, 2008, from http://www.emedicine.com/neuro/TOPIC550.HTM

American Academy of Neurology. (2008). *Breastfeeding while taking seizure medicine does not appear to harm children.* Retrieved June 20, 2008, from http://www.aan.com/press/index.cfm?fuseaction=release.view&release=603

Begley, C. E., Famulari, M., Annegaers, J. F., Lairson, D. R., Reynolds, T. F., Coan, S., et al. (2000). The cost of epilepsy in the United States: An estimate from population-based clinical survey data. *Epilepsia, 41*(3), 342–351.

Caplin, D., Austin, J. K., Dunn, D. W., Shen, J., & Perkins, S. (2002). Development of a self-efficacy scale for children and adolescents with epilepsy. *Children's Health Care, 31*(4), 295–309.

Duncan, J. S., Josemir, W. S., Sisodiya, S., & Walker, M. (2006). Adult epilepsy. *The Lancet, 367*(9516), 1087–1100.

Epilepsy Foundation of America. (n.d.). *First aid for epilepsy.* Retrieved June 21, 2008, from http://www.epilepsyfoundation.org/about/firstaid/

Gasior, M., Rogawski, M. A., & Hartman, A. L. (2006). Neuroprotective and disease-modifying effects of the ketogenic diet. *Behavioral Pharmacotherapy, 17*(5), 431–439.

Herzog, A. G., Farina, E. L., & Blum, A. S. (2005). Serum valproate levels with oral contraceptive use. *Epilepsia, 46*(6), 970–971.

Kossoff, E. H., Laux, L. C., Blackford, R., Morrison, P. F., Pyzik, P. L., Hamdy, R. M., et al. (2008). When do seizures usually improve with the ketogenic diet? *Epilepsia, 49*(2), 329–333.

Lew, A. R., Lewis, C., Owen, L., & West, S. (2006). Psychosocial problems and seizure-related factors in children with epilepsy. *Developmental Medicine and Child Neurology, 48*(8), 704.

Morantz, C. A. (2004). Recommendations for prescribing new antiepileptic drugs. *American Family Physician, 70*(6), 1167–1168.

Morris, A. A. M. (2005). Cerebral ketone body metabolism. *Journal of Inherited Metabolic Disease, 28*(2), 109–121.

Ossemann, M., Bruls, E., de Borchgrave, V., De Cock, C., Delcourt, C., Delvaux, V., et al. (2006). Guidelines for the management of epilepsy in the elderly. *Acta Neurologica Belgica, 106*(3), 111–116.

Sirven, J. (2001). Acute and chronic seizures in patients older than 60 years. *Mayo Clinic Proceedings, 76*(2), 175–183.

Small, M. J., Kershaw, T., Frederic, R., & Blanc, C. (2005). Characteristics of preeclampsia and eclampsia related maternal death in rural Haiti. *Journal of Maternal-Fetal and Neonatal Medicine, 18*(5), 343–348.

Velez, L., & Selwa, L. (2003). Seizure disorders in the elderly. *American Family Physician, 67*(2), 325–332.

CHAPTER

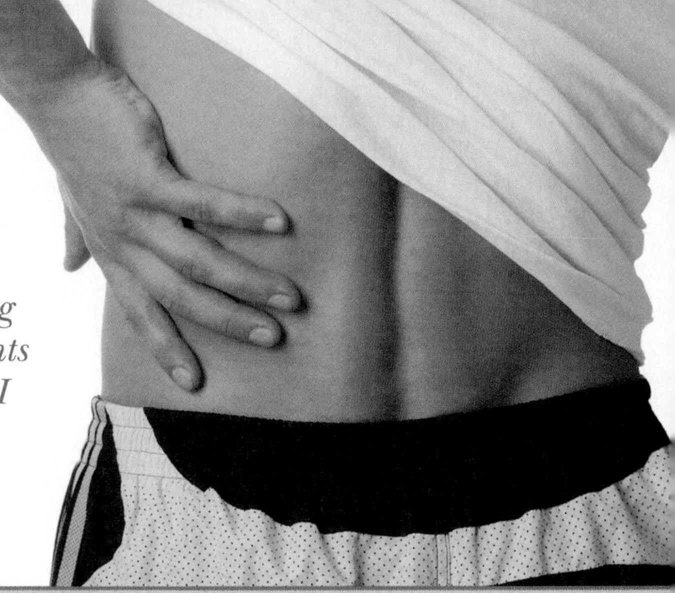

I was lifting concrete blocks to build a landscaping wall in my front yard yesterday. When I woke up this morning I couldn't bend down to put on my pants after my shower. My back hurts so bad I can hardly walk.

Patient "Andrew Eskew"

27 Pharmacotherapy of Muscle Spasms and Spasticity

Learning Outcomes

After reading this chapter, the student should be able to:

1. Compare and contrast the etiology and pathophysiology of muscle spasm and muscle spasticity.
2. Describe the pharmacologic and nonpharmacologic management of muscle spasms and muscle spasticity.
3. Compare and contrast the actions of the centrally acting and direct-acting skeletal muscle relaxants.
4. Explain the role of skeletal muscle relaxants as surgical adjuncts.
5. Describe the nurse's role in the pharmacologic management of muscle spasms and muscle spasticity.
6. For each of the classes shown in the chapter outline, identify the prototype and representative drugs and explain the mechanism(s) of drug action, primary indications, contraindications, significant drug interactions, pregnancy category, and important adverse effects.
7. Use the nursing process to care for patients receiving pharmacotherapy for muscle spasms and spasticity.

Chapter Outline

Etiology and Pathophysiology of Muscle Spasms

Nonpharmacologic Therapies for Muscle Spasms

Pharmacotherapy of Muscle Spasms

Centrally Acting Skeletal Muscle Relaxants

PROTOTYPE DRUG **Cyclobenzaprine (Amrix, Flexeril)** *p. 399*

Etiology and Pathophysiology of Muscle Spasticity

Nonpharmacologic and Pharmacologic Therapies for Muscle Spasticity

Direct-Acting Skeletal Muscle Relaxant Agents

PROTOTYPE DRUG **Dantrolene Sodium (Dantrium)** *p. 403*

Skeletal Muscle Relaxants as Surgical Adjuncts

Key Terms

clonic spasms, 397
dystonia, 403
malignant hyperthermia, 404
muscle spasms, 397
muscle spasticity, 402
tonic spasm, 397

The administration of drugs to relieve muscle spasms and musculoskeletal pain dates back to the early 19th century with the discovery and use of curare, a substance once used as a poison on arrows by Amazon Indians. The search for new medications to relax muscles and relieve painful muscle spasms and spasticity continues today. This chapter examines how these drugs produce their actions and their applications to the pharmacotherapeutics of muscle conditions.

Etiology and Pathophysiology of Muscle Spasms

27.1 Muscle spasms are involuntary contractions most commonly caused by injury or overuse of skeletal muscle.

Depending on the extent of the condition and the muscles affected, abnormal or intense skeletal muscle contractions can cause severe pain and disability. Abnormal contractions may be classified as spasms or spasticity. Each has different etiologies. Although they may both occur in the same patient, pharmacologic treatments differ somewhat. The pathogenesis and treatment of spasticity are presented in Sections 27.4 and 27.5.

Muscle spasms are involuntary contractions of muscles that are usually localized to a specific muscle group. As the muscles contract and tighten, the spasm causes sudden, intense pain, which slowly diminishes after a few minutes. If it occurs in the leg, patients may refer to the condition as a charley horse or cramp. A single, prolonged contraction is a **tonic spasm;** multiple, rapidly repeated contractions are called **clonic spasms** or clonus. Chronic or severe spasms can impair joint mobility.

The etiology of muscle spasms may involve many body systems, including the nervous, musculoskeletal, endocrine, and cardiorespiratory systems. The most common etiology of muscle spasm is injury to a skeletal muscle: Spasms often occur when a muscle is overused or suffers trauma. Electrolyte imbalances, hypocalcemia, and dehydration can also cause muscles to spasm. Multiple sclerosis (MS), epilepsy, muscular dystrophy, fractures, and chronic low back pain are pathologies associated with significant muscle spasm.

Nonpharmacologic Therapies for Muscle Spasms

27.2 Nonpharmacologic interventions are often successful at decreasing the pain caused by muscle spasms.

The therapeutic goals of treating a patient with muscle spasms are to decrease discomfort and enhance mobility so that the patient is better able to perform activities of daily living (ADLs). In many cases, these goals may be achieved using nonpharmacologic, complementary, and alternative therapies. When the spasms are particularly disabling, pharmacotherapy may be initiated. A combination of drug therapy and alternative therapies is often the most effective treatment.

The implementation of complementary and alternative interventions may enhance the patient's mobility and decrease the intensity of muscle spasms caused by injury. Nonpharmacologic interventions that might be ordered by the health care provider or physical therapist include the application of heat or cold, hydrotherapy, therapeutic ultrasound, assisted exercise, massage, traction, and manipulation. The application of heat or cold to the affected site will reduce or relieve the muscle spasm and pain. A source of heat applied to the area will work best to reduce cramping and relieve localized pain. The application of cold to the site has the ability to slow the transmission of pain impulses and is more effective for pain relief than heat. The implementation of hydrotherapy increases blood circulation to the site of the muscle spasm in an effort to relieve pain. The patient should be encouraged to exercise the muscle group during the bath to enhance movement and circulation. Therapeutic ultrasound applies low-frequency sound waves to the muscle. The waves generate heat deep in the muscle mass to reduce pain and inflammation. The application of touch, massage, and gentle pressure are effective at promoting musculoskeletal relaxation. Patients who suffer from bone fractures will experience muscle spasms associated with interrupted alignment of bones. The application of traction provides a pulling force on the bone to return it to normal anatomic alignment and decrease the accompanying spasm.

The use of herbal remedies in the care of patients with muscle spasms has become popular. Herbal remedies that may be administered orally (PO) or topically for muscle spasms include kava, black cohosh, castor oil packs, and capsaicin. Kava is taken PO and has antianxiety effects, which may aid in muscle relaxation. Black cohosh was first used for neuralgia and muscular pain in the 1840s. The tincture is applied topically to produce relaxation of the muscles. Castor oil packs can be applied to the site of pain and muscle spasm. The castor oil should be warmed, soaked into a flannel cloth, and then applied to the tonic muscle. Capsaicin, derived from cayenne pepper, is applied topically as a cream four times per day to increase mobility and reduce pain. It is important that the patient be instructed to apply the cream with gloves to prevent irritation of the skin on the hands. Although topical herbal therapies are generally safe, not all of them have been proven effective.

CONNECTIONS

Evidence-Based Practice Low-Back Pain and Antidepressants

Clinical Question

Are antidepressants indicated as an adjunct therapy in the management of low-back pain?

Antidepressants are commonly used in the management of low-back pain. However, their use is controversial. A group of researchers examined a series of randomized controlled trials described in the scientific literature that compared antidepressant medication and placebos for patients with nonspecific low-back pain. Ten trials that compared antidepressants with placebos were included in this review.

Evidence

The results showed no difference in pain relief or depression between antidepressant and placebo treatments. The qualitative analyses found conflicting evidence for the effect of antidepressants on pain intensity in chronic low-back pain and no clear evidence that antidepressants reduce depression in patients with chronic low-back pain. Two pooled analyses showed no difference in pain relief between different types of antidepressants and placebos. There is no clear evidence that antidepressants are more effective than placebos in the management of patients with chronic low-back pain. These findings do not imply that severely depressed patients with back pain should not be treated with antidepressants; furthermore, there may be evidence for their use in other forms of chronic pain.

Implication

Based on these findings, routinely prescribing antidepressant therapy as an adjunct therapy for low-back pain is clearly not indicated for all patients. However, nurses must understand that chronic pain is a subjective experience having both physiological and emotional components. Chronic pain can be both physically and emotionally exhausting. Furthermore, chronic back pain may lead to feelings of despair, hopelessness, and other symptoms of a major depression or clinical depression.

For this reason, health care providers must avoid the attitude that pharmacotherapy can always treat both of these two very real problems. The treatment of depression should include psychological interventions such as counseling and relaxation training. Additional treatment for the chronic pain might include such things as physical rehabilitation aimed at restoration of function, trying to "normalize" one's life as much as possible even with the pain, and appropriate medication management. Multidisciplinary treatment of the chronic back pain and major depression will ultimately give the patient more of a sense of control over the pain and start a "positive spiral" toward physical and mental reconditioning.

Critical Thinking Question

List nonpharmacologic interventions that may enhance the patient's mobility and decrease low-back pain.

See Answers to Critical Thinking Questions in Appendix A.

Source: From "Antidepressants for Non-specific Low Back Pain," by D. M. Urquhart, J. L. Hoving, W. J. Assendelft, M. Roland, and M. W. van Tulder, 2008, *Cochrane Database of Systematic Reviews, 1.* Art. No.: CD001703. DOI: 10.1002/14651858.CD001703.pub3.

Pharmacotherapy of Muscle Spasms

27.3 Nonsteroidal anti-inflammatory drugs and skeletal muscle relaxants are used to treat muscle spasms.

Muscle spasms, especially those caused by injury, are painful and sometimes associated with inflammation. Nonsteroidal anti-inflammatory drugs (NSAIDs) such as aspirin, naproxen, and ibuprofen have the ability to relieve muscle pain and reduce inflammation around the injury site. Relieving inflammation can take pressure off the surrounding nerves, thus promoting increased mobility. The pharmacology of NSAIDs is presented in Chapter 44.

Muscle relaxants are prescribed for moderate to severe muscle spasms. Although these drugs are not analgesics, they can promote pain relief by relaxing tight, contracted muscles at the site of injury without interfering with normal muscle function. When skeletal muscle relaxants are used in combination with NSAIDs, pain relief is greater than when either agent is used alone.

Centrally Acting Skeletal Muscle Relaxants

27.4 Centrally acting skeletal muscle relaxants are the drugs of choice for treating muscle spasms.

The centrally acting skeletal muscle relaxants relieve muscle spasms by their actions in the central nervous system (CNS). They do not have any direct effect on the neuromuscular junction or on the muscles themselves. The precise mechanism of action of centrally acting skeletal muscle relaxants is unclear but it is believed that much of the muscle relaxation is caused by the general sedative properties of these medications. This sedative action may produce significant drowsiness, especially if the relaxants are combined with alcohol or other CNS depressants. Thus the patient should be protected from injury and fall potential when administering these medications. The sedative effects may be beneficial in helping patients with muscle spasms to obtain needed sleep. Doses of the centrally acting muscle relaxants are listed in Table 27.1

The centrally acting skeletal muscle relaxants include cyclobenzaprine (Amrix, Flexeril) baclofen (Lioresal), and tizanidine (Zanaflex). Some drugs in this class are used for both muscle spasm and spasticity.

The benzodiazepines are drugs primarily used for their antianxiety effects (see Chapter 22). Diazepam (Valium) is a drug in this class that acts centrally to relax skeletal muscle. It may be used as an adjunct to relieve skeletal muscle spasm associated with cerebral palsy, paraplegia, and tetanus. In general, diazepam is only used when medications such as baclofen and tizanidine fail to produce adequate muscle relaxation. The most common adverse effects associated with diazepam are drowsiness and ataxia. For dosing and additional information on the antianxiety and antiseizure actions of benzodiazepines, the student should refer to Chapters 22

CONNECTIONS

Complementary and Alternative Therapies Kava

Description: Kava root contains starch and has 3% to 20% kavalactones, which have the ability in high doses to produce peripheral nerve paralysis. Kava produces muscle relaxant effects related to the kavalactones called dihydrokavain and dihydromethysticin, which affect muscle contractility. Studies on animals indicate that kava produces relaxation of the muscles by binding with GABA receptors in the brain. The roots and lower stem of the plant contain the most effective active ingredients.

History and Claims: The plant *Piper methysticum* is a member of the pepper family and is very important in the Pacific Island cultures, particularly the countries of Micronesia. It is used as a sacred drink and cash crop. It is the belief of these cultures that kava acts to transport those who ingest it to the realm of the gods. It promotes peace and goodwill in the culture. The kava cup is clearly identifiable on the official flag for the state of Pohpei in Micronesia. In Germany kava is approved for treating anxiety, stress, and restlessness.

Standardization: The standardized extract of kava is called Kavatrol. Kavatrol is administered twice daily with 60 mg of kavalactones in each capsule. It is administered for 4 weeks to reduce stress and promote relaxation. The standardized extract is 70 mg of kavalactones given two to three times per day.

Evidence: The U.S. Food and Drug Administration (FDA) has advised consumers of the risk of severe liver failure with dietary supplements containing kava. At least four individuals have required a liver transplant. Studies have shown that the administration of kava lowered the scores on the Hamilton Anxiety Scale. German studies on kava were begun in the 1950s and have produced evidence of muscle relaxant properties.

Source: From *Kava-Containing Dietary Supplements May Be Associated with Severe Liver Injury, 2002* (Consumer advisory), by U.S. Food and Drug Administration, Center for Food Safety and Applied Nutrition. Retrieved June 23, 2008, from http://www.cfsan.fda.gov/~dms/addskava.html

and 26, respectively. Diazepam is a prototype drug for seizures in Chapter 26.

CONNECTION *Checkpoint* 27.1

Benzodiazepines are some of the most widely prescribed drugs. From what you learned in Chapter 22, what are the major indications for drugs in this class? See Answer to Connection Checkpoint 27.1 in Appendix A.

PROTOTYPE DRUG Cyclobenzaprine (Amrix, Flexeril)

Classification: **Therapeutic:** Skeletal muscle relaxant
Pharmacologic: Centrally acting norepinephrine-releasing agent

Therapeutic Effects and Uses: Cyclobenzaprine is indicated for the short-term therapy of acute musculoskeletal conditions that are unrelated to CNS disease. The drug promotes skeletal muscle relaxation, thus decreasing muscle spasms and increasing joint mobility. Cyclobenzaprine is much less effective in treating muscle spasm due to spinal cord injury or cerebral palsy. The manufacturer recommends that treatment not extend beyond 3 weeks. Fibromyalgia is an off-label indication for the drug.

Cyclobenzaprine is chemically related to the TCAs and it exhibits some antidepressant effects. In 2007, an extended release capsule form (Amrex) was approved by the United States Food and Drug Administration (FDA). Cyclobenzaprine is occasionally abused as a recreational drug owing to its sedative actions.

Mechanism of Action: The action of cyclobenzaprine is thought to occur at the brainstem and spinal cord levels. The drug increases norepinephrine activity by blocking its synaptic reuptake to produce an anticholinergic effect. Cyclobenzaprine acts centrally and thus has no direct action on skeletal muscle.

Pharmacokinetics:

Route(s)	PO
Absorption	Well absorbed in the gastrointestinal (GI) tract
Distribution	It is unknown whether the drug crosses the placenta or is secreted in breast milk; 93% bound to protein
Primary metabolism	Extensive hepatic metabolism to inactive metabolites
Primary excretion	Renal
Onset of action	1 h
Duration of action	12–24 h

Adverse Effects: The commonly reported adverse effects of cyclobenzaprine are drowsiness, dizziness, and xerostomia. Sedation can be a limiting effect with the first few doses. Other adverse effects of cyclobenzaprine include edema of the tongue and face with sweating, myalgia, hepatitis, and alopecia. Potential cardiovascular adverse events include orthostatic hypotension, tachycardia, syncope, palpitations, and vasodilation. The patient may complain of an unpleasant taste, a coated tongue with discoloration, vomiting, anorexia, diarrhea with flatulence, or paralysis.

Contraindications/Precautions: Cyclobenzaprine should be used with great caution in patients older than age 65 because this population is more likely to experience confusion, hallucinations, and adverse cardiac events from the drug. Cyclobenzaprine also should be used cautiously in patients who suffer from increased intraocular pressure, prostatic hyperplasia, urinary retention, and seizures. Patients with hypersensitivity to tricyclic antidepressants (TCAs) should not receive this drug. Like the TCAs cyclobenzaprine can adversely affect the heart and therefore should be used with caution in patients with cardiovascular disease, including those with congestive heart failure or dysrhythmias with heart

TABLE 27.1 Centrally Acting Skeletal Muscle Relaxants

Drug	Route and Adult Dose (maximum dose where indicated)	Adverse Effects
baclofen (Lioresal)	PO: start with 5 mg tid and increase slowly every 3 days, as needed, to control spasms (max: 80 mg/day) Intrathecal: 50 mcg bolus	*Drowsiness, dizziness, weakness, fatigue, headache, confusion, altered mental status, nausea, and vomiting, constipation, urinary frequency* <u>QT prolongation, dysrhythmias</u>
carisoprodol (Soma)	Adult: PO: 350 mg tid	*Drowsiness, confusion, postural hypotension, nausea, vomiting, hiccups, vertigo, ataxia, tremor, headache, syncope, insomnia, pruritus* <u>Anaphylactic shock, physical dependence</u>
chlorzoxazone (Paraflex, Parafon Forte)	PO: 250–500 mg tid or qid (max: 3 g/day)	*Drowsiness, dizziness, anorexia, heartburn, nausea, vomiting, constipation, diarrhea, abdominal pain, light-headedness, overstimulation, rash, pruritus, urticaria, discoloration of urine* <u>Hepatotoxicity, jaundice, anemia, neutropenia</u>
cyclobenzaprine (Amrix, Flexeril)	PO: 5–10 mg tid for tablets; 15 mg once daily for extended release capsules (max: 30 mg/day)	*Drowsiness, xerostomia, dizziness, fatigue, asthenia, nausea and vomiting, constipation, dyspepsia, dysgeusia, blurred vision, headache, nervousness, confusion* <u>Tongue edema, potential for QT prolongation, hallucinations</u>
metaxalone (Skelaxin)	PO: 800 mg tid–qid	*Nausea, vomiting, GI upset, drowsiness, dizziness, headache, anxiety* <u>Hemolytic anemia, jaundice, hepatotoxicity, anaphylaxis</u>
methocarbamol (Robaxin)	PO: 1.5 g qid for 2–3 days then 4–4.5 g/day in divided doses IV/IM: 1–3 g once daily for 3 days. Repeat after a drug-free interval of 48 h if necessary. Do not exceed 3 mL/min	*Drowsiness, dizziness, light-headedness, fever, pruritus, rash, syncope, thrombophlebitis, pain, blurred vision, headache, tachycardia, syncope* <u>Anaphylactic shock, sloughing of skin with extravasation</u>
orphenadrine (Banflex, Myophen, Norflex)	PO: 100 mg bid; IM or IV: 60 mg every 12 h (max: 250 mg/day)	*Dry mouth, drowsiness, weakness, dizziness, agitation, tachycardia, syncope, palpitations, increased ocular tension, blurred vision, nausea, vomiting, abdominal cramps, pruritus, urticaria* <u>Anaphylactic shock, hallucinations</u>
tizanidine (Zanaflex)	PO: 4–8 mg every 6–8 h as needed (max: 36 mg/day)	*Asthenia, somnolence, dizziness, dry mouth, flulike symptoms, fever, myasthenia, back pain, infection, dyskinesia, depression, anxiety, urinary frequency, speech alterations, blurred vision, abdominal pain, nausea, dyspepsia, pharyngitis, rhinitis, urinary frequency* <u>Hepatotoxicity, hypotension, bradycardia, urinary tract infection</u>

Note: *Italics* indicates common adverse effects. <u>Underline</u> indicates serious adverse effects.

block. It is contraindicated in patients who have QT interval prolongation on the electrocardiogram (ECG), or who are in the recovery phase of a myocardial infarction (MI). The drug is metabolized in the liver and thus should be administered cautiously to patients with hepatic impairment. Patients with a history of hyperthyroidism should not be administered cyclobenzaprine.

Drug Interactions: Cyclobenzaprine should not be administered with alcohol, opioids, barbiturates, or any other CNS depressants because significant sedation may occur. Phenothiazines and anticholinergic agents will enhance the anticholinergic adverse effects and are contraindicated with cyclobenzaprine. Use with TCAs may result in additive CNS depression and increased anticholinergic effects. A potentially fatal hypertensive crisis can occur if cyclobenzaprine is used within 14 days of a monoamine oxidase inhibitor. **Herbal/Food:** Additive CNS depression may occur if cyclobenzaprine is administered concurrently with valerian or kava.

Pregnancy: Category B.

Treatment of Overdose: Signs of overdose include CNS depression and tachycardia. Physostigmine (Antilirium) may be administered to reverse serious anticholinergic adverse effects. Overdose is generally not fatal.

Nursing Responsibilities:

- Obtain a complete physical examination that includes baseline vital signs. Notify the prescriber of any preexisting cardiovascular condition that may preclude the use of cyclobenzaprine.
- Establish baseline neurologic status, specifically the level of consciousness.
- Assess for pain using a pain scale and limitation of range of motion.
- Evaluate for the therapeutic effects of the medication.
- Protect the patient from injury related to falls due to excessive drowsiness.

- Assess for urticaria, rash, or pruritus. Withhold the medication if symptoms appear because this may indicate a hypersensitivity reaction.

Patient and Family Education:

- Do not use alcohol when taking this medication because excessive sedation may result.
- Do not crush or chew the extended release capsule.
- Do not drive or perform other hazardous activities until the effects of the drug are known because this drug may cause drowsiness or dizziness.
- Use gum or hard candy to reduce symptoms of dry mouth.
- This drug may be taken with food or milk if gastric upset occurs.
- Inform the health care provider if improvement is not noted within 1 to 2 weeks.
- Immediately report rapid heartbeat, palpitations, or excessive drowsiness.
- Do not breast-feed while taking the medication without the approval of the health care provider.
- Take the medication exactly as prescribed; the drug is more effective if taken at regular intervals.
- Do not take any other prescription or nonprescription drugs, dietary supplements, or herbal products without approval of the health care provider.

Drugs Similar to Cyclobenzaprine (Amrix, Flexeril)

The following medications are other centrally acting skeletal muscle relaxants: baclofen, carisoprodol, chlorzoxazone, metaxalone, methocarbamol, orphenadrine, and tizanidine. Chlorphenesin (Maolate) is a centrally acting muscle relaxant that was removed from the market in the United States.

Baclofen (Lioresal): Approved in 1977, baclofen is used to reduce muscle spasm and muscle spasticity in patients with injury or disease of upper motor neurons such as that associated with MS, cerebral palsy, amyotrophic lateral sclerosis (ALS), and spinal cord trauma. Off-label indications include the treatment of tardive dyskinesia related to long-term pharmacotherapy with antipsychotic agents, persistent hiccups, and for management of neuropathic pain. The drug resembles the inhibitory neurotransmitter GABA and acts by inhibiting neuronal activity within the brain and spinal cord. Baclofen is usually administered PO, but it can be administered by intrathecal infusion through a lumbar puncture for severe spasm or spasticity that cannot be managed through PO dosing. Several months of therapy may be required to achieve full therapeutic benefit from baclofen. Adverse effects related to the administration of baclofen include drowsiness, dizziness, weakness, and fatigue. Abrupt discontinuation following prolonged therapy may cause high fever, seizures, severe rebound muscle spasticity, and hallucinations. This drug is pregnancy category C.

Carisoprodol (Soma): An older drug approved by the FDA in 1959, carisoprodol is administered PO for skeletal muscle spasms. It is also effective in relieving the pain, muscle spasms, and spasticity associated with cerebral palsy. The drug produces significant sedation in 40% of patients taking it and may cause significant CNS and respiratory depression if taken with alcohol or other CNS depressants. The general sedative nature of the drug is likely responsible for its ability to relieve the pain associated with muscle spasms. Although not a controlled substance, carisoprodol can cause physical dependence and has been abused by recreational drug users. The active metabolite of carisoprodol is meprobamate, a rarely used antianxiety agent and a Schedule IV drug. The development of newer drugs and increased levels of carisoprodol abuse in recent years has led to less frequent prescribing of the drug. This drug is pregnancy category C.

Chlorzoxazone (Paraflex, Parafon Forte): Chlorzoxazone is an oral centrally acting skeletal muscle relaxant administered for the symptomatic treatment of muscle spasm and pain related to musculoskeletal conditions. It is ineffective in the treatment of spasticity related to neurodegenerative disorders such as cerebral palsy. The actions of the drug may be largely due to its sedative effects. It should not be combined with alcohol or other CNS depressants. Chlorzoxazone is hepatotoxic and should not be used in patients with liver impairment. Other adverse effects include anorexia, nausea, vomiting, rash, and red-orange discoloration of urine. Older adults may experience more adverse CNS effects than younger patients. This drug is pregnancy category C.

Metaxalone (Skelaxin): Approved in 1962, metaxalone is administered PO and is indicated for the symptomatic relief of muscle spasm and pain related to musculoskeletal conditions. It is ineffective in the treatment of spasticity-related neurologic disorders. The therapeutic effects of metaxalone are likely due to its ability to depress the CNS. Like chlorzoxazone, metaxalone may cause liver injury and is contraindicated in patients with hepatic impairment. It should not be administered to patients over age 65 due to significant anticholinergic effects. Drowsiness, nausea and vomiting, and anxiety are common adverse effects. The pregnancy status of this drug has not been determined; this drug should not be used during pregnancy or lactation unless its benefits outweigh the potential risks.

Methocarbamol (Relaxin, Robaxin): Approved in 1957, methocarbamol has central sedative effects that likely are responsible for its ability to reduce muscle spasms. It is used as an adjunct to physical therapy interventions. It can be administered intravenously (IV) for the treatment of tetanus or other acute musculoskeletal conditions. Methocarbamol may cause significant dizziness and sedation and should not be taken with alcohol or other CNS depressants. It is contraindicated in patients with significant renal impairment. It should not be administered to patients over age 65 due to significant anticholinergic effects. This drug is pregnancy category C.

MyNursingKit | Mechanism of Action Animation: Cyclobenzaprine

Orphenadrine (Banflex, Myophen, Norflex): Orphenadrine is an older drug that was approved in 1959. It is administered PO or parenterally to relax skeletal muscles and reduce pain. The drug has analgesic properties and may be administered parenterally to produce local anesthetic effects. It may be used off-label as an adjunct in the treatment of the muscular rigidity associated with Parkinson's disease. The most common side effect of orphenadrine is xerostomia. Orphenadrine is structurally very similar to diphenhydramine (Benadryl) and can cause prominent anticholinergic effects. It should not be used with other anticholinergic drugs due to its additive effects. Orphenadrine produces a mild to moderate euphoria effect that has led to its abuse. This drug is pregnancy category C.

Tizanidine (Zanaflex): A newer drug in this class approved in 1996, tizanidine is a centrally acting alpha$_2$-adrenergic agonist that inhibits motor neurons mainly at the spinal cord level. It is most effective in patients who have significantly diminished muscle tone, including spasticity related to brain or spinal cord injury or MS. Tizanidine is as effective as baclofen in treating muscle spasticity and is considered a drug of choice by some health care providers. The most common adverse effects include xerostomia, fatigue, weakness, dizziness, and drowsiness. Hypotension is common at higher doses; the drug is closely related to clonidine (Catapres), which is an antihypertensive agent. Hallucinations are uncommon but patients with a history of psychosis should be carefully monitored for this adverse effect. Tizanidine is hepatotoxic and should not be used in patients with liver impairment. Older adults, especially those with some degree of renal impairment, may experience frequent adverse effects such as drowsiness, dizziness, dry mouth, and asthenia. This drug is pregnancy category C.

CONNECTION *Checkpoint* 27.2

Cyclobenzaprine is very similar to the tricyclic antidepressants. From what you learned in Chapter 23, describe the major indications (approved and off-label) for the tricyclics. See Answer to Connection Checkpoint 27.2 in Appendix A.

Etiology and Pathophysiology of Muscle Spasticity

27.5 Spasticity is a condition in which certain muscle groups remain in a continuous state of contraction.

Muscle spasticity is a condition caused by damage to the CNS in which certain muscle groups remain in a continuous state of contraction. The affected muscles will have increased muscle tone accompanied by mild to severe pain. The patient may experience irritable deep tendon reflex activity, muscle spasms, scissoring movements of the lower extremities, and fixed joint movement. Patients with muscle spasticity are unable to voluntarily relax their limbs. Spasticity, also referred to as hypertonia, causes pain that is more intense than muscle spasm and produces greater impairment of mobility.

Pharm*FACT*

More than 12 million people worldwide suffer from muscle spasticity. *Source:* American Association of Neurological Surgeons, 2006.

Whereas muscle spasms occur most often with injury or overuse, muscle spasticity is associated with neuromuscular diseases that are the result of damage to the motor region in the cerebral cortex, the region of the brain that controls muscle movements. Conditions most commonly associated with muscular spasticity include severe head or spinal cord trauma, MS, cerebrovascular accident (CVA), cerebral palsy, trauma, and ALS.

Acute spasticity may begin only a few days following brain or spinal cord injury. Spasticity that results from a spinal cord injury is associated with the loss of both facilitory and inhibitory effects on the neurons below the level of the spinal cord injury. Facilitory neurons send messages for the muscle to contract; inhibitory neurons send a message to not contract. The area that is distal to the spinal cord injury or lesion becomes disassociated from the inhibitory area of the brain,

CONNECTIONS

To the Community The Intrathecal Baclofen Pump

Intrathecal baclofen (Lioresal) therapy has been approved by the FDA to treat spasticity related to MS. Patients who are candidates for intrathecal baclofen therapy must have severe spasticity with severe impairment and disability that cannot be improved through oral baclofen. Intrathecal baclofen therapy improves quality of life, controls painful spasms, improves transfers, and allows for the patient to better perform ADLs.

This drug is delivered in the intrathecal space, using a small catheter and a pump. This provides a direct route for the baclofen to reach its target sites in the spinal cord. Because the baclofen is delivered continuously at its site of action, very small amounts are needed to produce a therapeutic effect.

The pump consists of a small metal disk that is surgically placed under the skin at the waistline. The health care provider determines the amount of drug to be released by the pump and the dosing schedule. The pump must be refilled every 1 to 3 months and the battery lasts 5 to 7 years.

Source: From "Intrathecal Baclofen Therapy: Challenges in Patients with Multiple Sclerosis," by B. Ridley, 2006, *Rehabilitation Nursing, 31*(4), pp. 158–164; and *Intrathecal Baclofen Therapy (for MS)*, by Cleveland Clinic, 2008. Retrieved June 23, 2008, from http://my.clevelandclinic.org/devices/Intrathecal_Baclofen_Pump_System/hic_Intrathecal_Baclofen_Therapy_for_MS.aspx

and the facilitory impulses dominate at the site of the muscle. The muscles involved may go into spastic paralysis; flexor muscles become tight, and the muscles can be extended only with great difficulty. Once extended, the muscles tend to immediately flex back.

In the advanced stages of MS, muscle spasticity is due to the interruption of the main motor pathways of the spinal cord. This is caused by the destruction of the myelin sheath, which covers the nerves of the spinal cord, brain, and optic nerve. Spasticity results in a stiff, unbalanced gait and may eventually confine these patients to a wheelchair. Patients with MS are treated with a combination of medications, including muscle relaxants, corticosteroids, and immunosuppressants (see Chapter 25).

Approximately 35% of patients suffer from spasticity following CVA. If the brain area affected by the CVA is able to effectively reestablish communication with the muscle, the spasticity may be reversible and voluntary movement may be restored. In many cases, the spasticity becomes permanent and can be recognized by a clenched fist, permanently flexed elbow, or pointed toes.

Cerebral palsy is a neurologic disorder that affects movement and posture. A major symptom of cerebral palsy is that of severe muscular spasticity, which can affect facial muscles, cause an unsteady, scissoring gait, and result in painful joint contractures and deformities. The primary cause of spasticity associated with cerebral palsy is trauma to the brain or spinal cord at birth. Pharmacologic options for treating cerebral palsy are limited. Intrathecal baclofen may be beneficial in reducing severe spasticity.

Muscle spasms, spasticity, and twitching are also characteristic of ALS, also known as Lou Gehrig's disease. ALS is caused by the functional degeneration and loss of lower and upper motor neurons. The disorder is progressive and fatal. Muscle relaxants may bring some pain relief during periods of intense muscle spasticity.

Dystonia is a chronic neurologic disorder that is characterized by involuntary muscle contraction that forces body parts into abnormal, painful movements or postures. This affects the muscle tone of the arms, legs, trunk, neck, eyelids, face, or vocal cords. The condition may affect the entire body (generalized dystonia), or it may be localized to a single body part (focal dystonia). Dystonia may occur secondary to other neurologic diseases such as MS, CVA, or cerebral palsy. Patients who experience dystonia are greatly affected both due to discomfort and altered body image, resulting in diminished quality of life. The alteration in mobility and pain produced by muscle spasms and spasticity inhibits the patients' ability to effectively perform ADLs. Generalized dystonias are treated with high doses of anticholinergic drugs such as benztropine, benzodiazepines, and baclofen. Patients with focal dystonia may obtain some relief with botulinum toxin type A.

Pharm*FACT*

Cerebral palsy is usually not diagnosed until age 2 or 3. Premature babies who weigh less than 3.3 pounds are 30 times more likely to develop cerebral palsy. *Source:* Nemours Foundation, 2006.

Pharm*FACT*

Dystonia affects about 250,000 people in the United States and is the third most common movement disorder, following essential tremor and Parkinson's disease. It can affect someone at any stage of the life span. *Source:* American Association of Neurological Surgeons, 2005.

Nonpharmacologic and Pharmacologic Therapies for Spasticity

27.6 Direct-acting skeletal muscle relaxants are often used to relieve muscle spasticity.

Effective therapies for spasticity include the administration of medications and the implementation of physical therapy. Medications alone are not adequate in reducing the complications of spasticity. Routine and consistent physical therapy exercises provide the patient with increased muscle movement and decreased severity of symptoms. Effective physical therapy exercises include muscle stretching, which assists in the prevention of contractures. The implementation of muscle group strengthening and repetitive motion exercises improve accuracy. In extreme cases, surgery may be necessary to release tendons or to sever the nerve–muscle pathway.

Medications effective in the treatment of spasticity include muscle relaxants that act at the level of the CNS, neuromuscular junction, or muscle tissue. Baclofen (Lioresal) and tizanidine (Zanaflex) are centrally acting muscle relaxants that also are effective in treating spasticity. These agents are discussed in Section 27.4.

Dantrolene (Dantrium), botulinum toxin type A (Botox), and botulinum toxin type B (Myobloc) act directly on skeletal muscle to relieve spasticity. These are called direct-acting muscle relaxants or antispasticity agents. Dantrolene is the prototype for direct-acting agents. Doses of these agents are listed in Table 27.2. The mechanism of action of direct-acting antispasmodics is shown in Pharmacotherapy Illustrated 27.1.

PROTOTYPE DRUG Dantrolene sodium (Dantrium)

Classification: **Therapeutic:** Direct-acting skeletal muscle relaxant, antispasticity agent

Pharmacologic: Calcium release blocker (muscle cells)

Therapeutic Effects and Uses: Approved in 1974, dantrolene is a direct-acting skeletal muscle relaxant indicated for spasticity, especially for spasms of the head and neck muscles. Dantrolene is indicated for muscle spasms that occur following a spinal cord injury or CVA, in cases of cerebral palsy or MS, and occasionally for the treatment of pain following heavy exercise.

Dantrolene produces a 50% decrease in the degree of contraction of skeletal muscle without producing effects on the cardiac or smooth muscle. It is administered PO to produce

TABLE 27.2 Direct-Acting Muscle Relaxants

Drug	Route and Dose (maximum dose where indicated)	Adverse Effects
botulinum toxin type A (Botox)	Cervical dystonia: IM:198–300 units, in divided doses Frown wrinkles: IM: 25 units, divided among affected muscles, may be repeated every 3–4 months Other wrinkles: Subcutaneously: 1–2 units, at the site of the wrinkle Axillary hyperhydrosis: IM: 50 units per site every 4 months as needed	*Injection reactions, headache dysphagia, muscle weakness, pain, tenderness, bruising, flulike symptoms, dry mouth, upper respiratory infections, ptosis of eyelids* <u>Few serious adverse effects</u>
botulinum toxin type B (Myobloc)	IM: 2,500–5,000 units divided among affected muscles	*Dysphagia, dyspepsia, injection site pain, xerostomia, headache, infection, flulike symptoms* <u>Few serious adverse effects</u>
dantrolene sodium (Dantrium)	Spasticity: PO: 25 mg once daily; may increase to 25 mg bid–qid (max: 100 mg bid–qid) Malignant hyperthermia: IV push: 1 mg/kg; repeat as needed (max: 10 mg/kg); may continue PO at 1–2 mg/kg qid for 1–3 days	*Hypersensitivity, drowsiness, dizziness, light-headedness, fatigue, speech disturbance, insomnia, mental depression, blurred vision, diplopia, photophobia, vomiting, anorexia, GI upset, crystalluria, urinary frequency, urinary retention, nocturia, enuresis, difficult erection* <u>Muscle weakness, diarrhea, hepatic necrosis</u>

Note: *Italics* indicates common adverse effects. <u>Underline</u> indicates serious adverse effects.

relaxation in the skeletal muscle. When administered parenterally it relieves symptoms of malignant hyperthermia related to general anesthesia.

Dantrolene is the drug of choice for treating **malignant hyperthermia**, a very rare condition that is an adverse effect of succinylcholine (Anectine) and some general anesthetics. A patient with malignant hyperthermia will experience a sudden onset of tachycardia, ventricular dysrhythmia, and hypotension. This is due to the rapid release of calcium ions in muscle cells, which produces hypermetabolism and intense muscle rigidity. The muscle metabolic rate becomes so elevated that it quickly raises the body temperature to a dangerous level. Dantrolene is administered IV at a rate of 1 mg/kg and repeated as needed up to 10 mg/kg. It is important that the anesthesia provider and circulating nurse have phentolamine (Regitine) available in the event of extravasation of dantrolene. There is a strong genetic predisposition to malignant hyperthermia, and patients with a family history of the disorder should not receive drugs that have the potential to cause this adverse effect.

Mechanism of Action: Dantrolene is a hydantoin derivative structurally related to phenytoin (Dilantin), an antiepileptic drug. Dantrolene directly relaxes spastic muscles by interfering with the release of calcium ions that have been stored in the sarcoplasmic reticulum of skeletal muscle.

Pharmacokinetics:

Route(s)	PO, IV
Absorption	Approximately 35% is slowly and incompletely absorbed from the GI tract
Distribution	Crosses the placenta; highly bound to plasma protein
Primary metabolism	Hepatic
Primary excretion	Renal
Onset of action	Peak concentration: 5 h
Duration of action	Half-life: 8.7 h (PO) or 4–8 h (IV)

Adverse Effects: Muscle weakness and drowsiness are the most common adverse effects of dantrolene therapy. The most serious adverse effect is hepatotoxicity; deaths due to hepatic failure have occurred in patients taking this drug. Other adverse effects include xerostomia, dizziness, nausea, photosensitivity, diarrhea, tachycardia, erratic blood pressure, and urinary retention.

Contraindications/Precautions: There are no contraindications to the use of dantrolene in treating malignant hyperthermia because this is a fatal condition if left untreated. For spasticity, dantrolene is contraindicated in patients with preexisting hepatic disease, and liver function should be monitored regularly in all patients during therapy. Because it can cause muscle weakness, dantrolene should not be used when spasticity is necessary to sustain an upright position or balance when standing or walking. Dantrolene should be used cautiously in the presence of impaired cardiac or pulmonary function. The risk of dantrolene-induced hepatotoxicity is greatest in women over the age of 35; thus it should be administered cautiously in these patients.

Drug Interactions: Dantrolene interacts with other CNS depressants, including alcohol, to cause additive sedation. The combination of estrogen and dantrolene in women can result in hepatotoxicity. Calcium channel blockers such as verapamil (Calan) place the patient at increased risk of ventricular fibrillation and cardiovascular collapse when dantrolene sodium is administered intravenously. **Herbal/Food:** Use of kava or valerian may result in additive sedation.

Pregnancy: Category C.

Treatment of Overdose: Overdose with dantrolene results in muscle weakness, lethargy, and coma. General supportive measures are administered until the effects of the drug diminish.

PHARMACOTHERAPY ILLUSTRATED 27.1

Mechanism of Action of Direct-Acting Antispasmodics

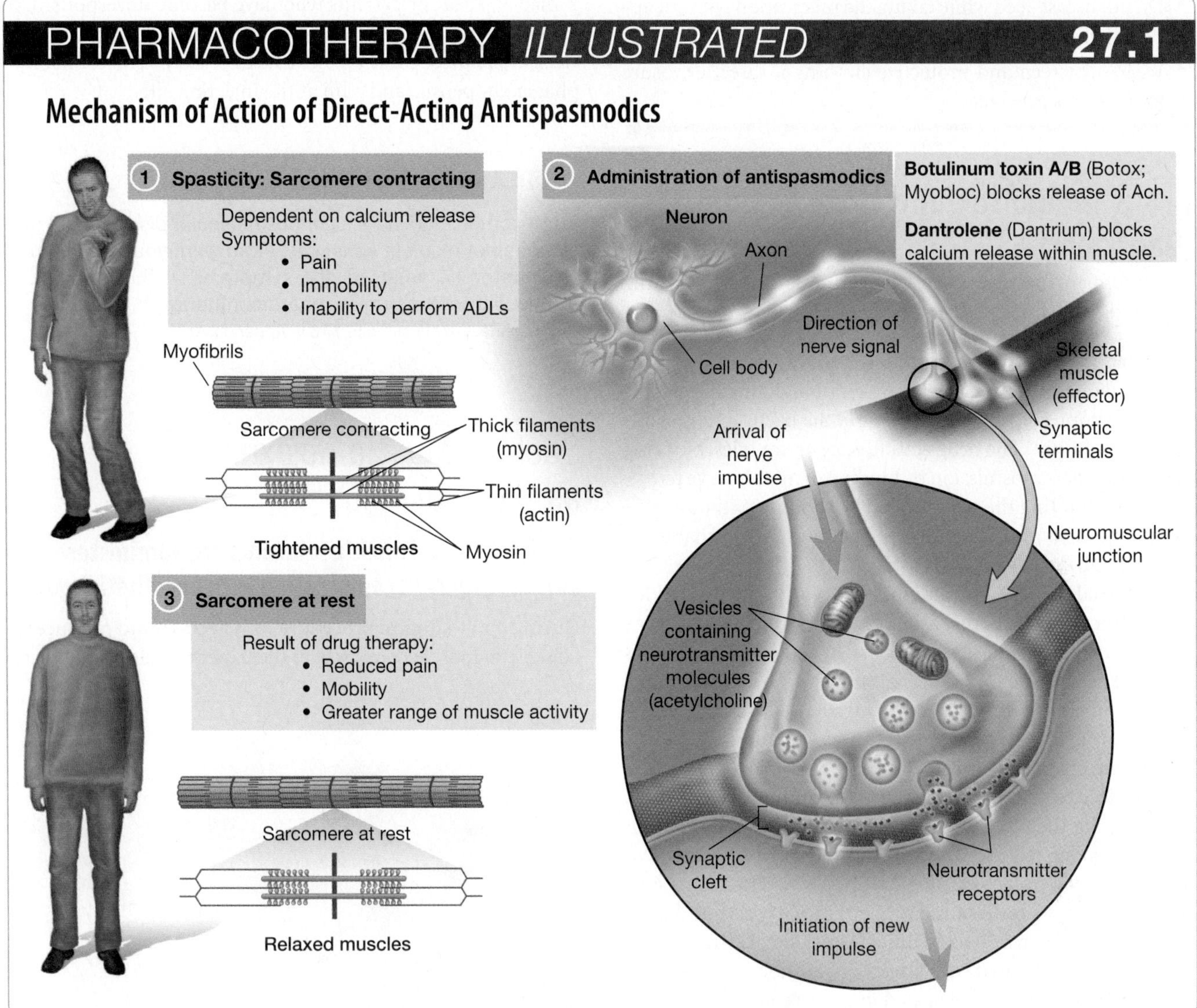

Nursing Responsibilities:

- Obtain a complete physical examination that includes baseline vital signs
- Establish baseline neurologic status, specifically level of consciousness.
- Assess for pain using a pain scale and limitation of range of motion and degree of spasticity.
- Assess the patient for therapeutic effects of the medication.
- Assess vital signs closely during IV administration because the drug may cause tachycardia and erratic blood pressure.
- Assess the patient with impaired cardiac or pulmonary function for cardiopulmonary changes during medication administration.
- Monitor breath sounds and heart sounds because dantrolene may cause pleural effusion and pericarditis.
- Monitor liver function tests (aspartate transaminase [AST] and alanine transaminase [ALT], total bilirubin, and alkaline phosphatase) and assess for hepatotoxicity.
- Assess bowel function, particularly uncontrolled diarrhea.
- Assess for severe constipation, which may indicate an intestinal obstruction.

Patient and Family Education:

- Be aware that the therapeutic effects of dantrolene may not be seen for 1 week.
- Immediately report signs of jaundice, yellowing of the whites of the skin or eyes, clay-colored stools, itching, abdominal distention, sensations of suffocation, and excessive muscle weakness.
- Do not drive or perform other hazardous activities until the effects of the drug are known because this drug may cause drowsiness or dizziness.
- Do not consume alcohol or take mood-altering medications because this may intensify the sedative effects of the drug.
- Do not take any other prescription or nonprescription drugs, dietary supplements, or herbal products without approval of the health care provider.

- Do not breast-feed while taking the medication without approval of the health care provider.
- Wear sunscreen and protective clothing if direct exposure to the sun is expected.

Drugs Similar to Dantrolene Sodium (Dantrium)

Botulinum toxins type A and type B are also direct-acting muscle relaxants.

Botulinum toxin type A (Botox): Botulinum toxin is an unusual drug because it acts as a poison in high quantities. It is obtained from *Clostridium botulinum*, the bacterium responsible for botulism. The drug acts directly on muscles, blocking neuromuscular transmission by binding to motor nerve terminals and inhibiting the release of acetylcholine. Without sufficient amounts of acetylcholine, the muscle is unable to contract and flaccid paralysis occurs.

Approved in 1989, botulinum toxin type A is indicated for the treatment of blepharospasm, cervical dystonia, facial wrinkles (Figure 27.1), and severe axillary hyperhydrosis, which is excessive axillary perspiration. This medication can be administered by the intramuscular (IM), intradermal (ID), or subcutaneous routes. The therapeutic dosage administered is dependent on the diagnosis. Cervical dystonia requires the highest dose, which is 198 to 300 units administered IM divided among the patient's affected muscles. The treatment of frown wrinkles requires the administration of 25 units IM, whereas other wrinkles should be treated with 1 to 2 units subcutaneously per site. Treatment of spasticity with botulinum toxin type A requires 20 to 50 units IM per site. Lastly, axillary hyperhydrosis is treated with an administration of botulinum 50 units ID per site and repeated every 4 months as needed. Blepharospasm is treated with an ID injection of 1.25 to 2.5 units per site.

Because of the extreme weakness associated with botulinum, therapies may be needed to improve muscle strength. To circumvent major problems with mobility or posture, administration of botulinum toxin is often limited to the small muscle groups. Sometimes this drug is administered with centrally acting PO medications to increase the functional mobility range of muscle groups.

Drawbacks to botulinum therapy are its delayed and limited effects. The treatment is mostly effective within 6 weeks and lasts for only 3 to 6 months. Another drawback is the pain experienced by patients when it is injected directly into the muscle. The severity of pain experienced can be blocked by the administration of a local anesthetic. This drug is pregnancy category C.

Botulinum toxin type B (Myobloc): Botulinum toxin type B was approved in 2000 for the treatment of neck pain in patients with cervical dystonia. The drug may be used off-label to treat sialorrhea (drooling) in patients with neurologic disorders such as Parkinson's disease. It is administered by local IM injection and acts by the same mechanism as type A. Type B may be used for patients who have become unresponsive to injections of type A. The duration of action is from 12 to 16 weeks. The most common adverse effects are xerostomia, dysphagia, dyspepsia, and pain at the injection site.

CONNECTION *Checkpoint* 27.3

Myasthenia gravis is a serious muscular disorder, but it does not result in spasticity. From what you learned in Chapter 17, what are the symptoms of this disorder and what is the primary pharmacotherapy? See Answer to Connection Checkpoint 27.3 in Appendix A.

Skeletal Muscle Relaxants as Surgical Adjuncts

27.7 Skeletal muscle relaxants are administered during surgery in combination with anesthetic agents.

During many surgical procedures it is necessary to produce total skeletal muscle relaxation in the patient. Skeletal muscle re-

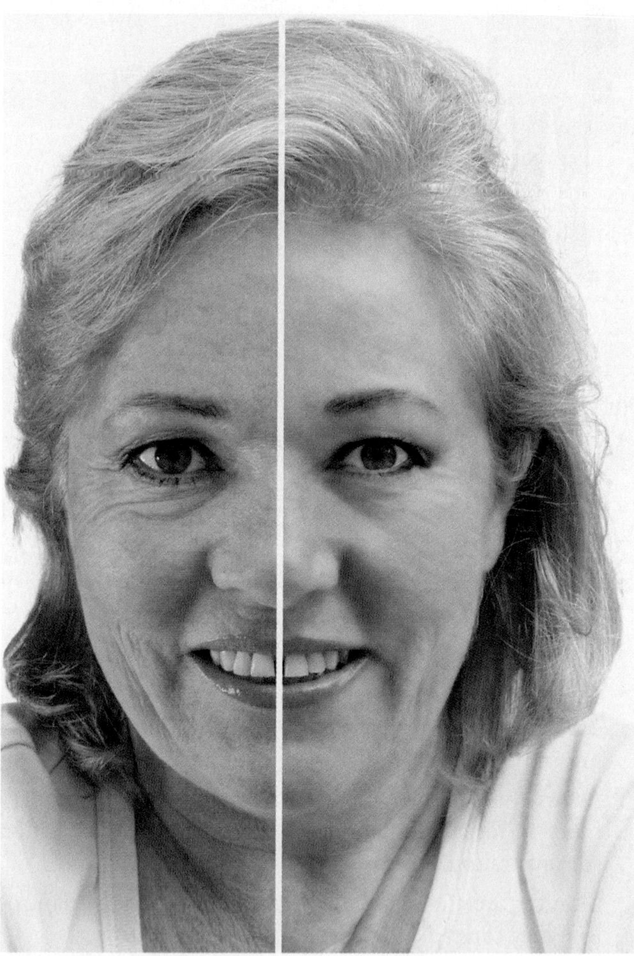

Figure 27.1 Botox therapy: (left) before treatment; (right) after treatment.

Source: JoAnn Snover/Shutterstock

NURSING PROCESS APPLICATION

Patients Receiving Pharmacotherapy for Muscle Spasms and Spasticity

Assessment	Potential Nursing Diagnoses
Prior to administration: • Obtain a complete health history, including allergies, drug history, and possible drug interactions. • Obtain laboratory data, which include electrolytes, particularly potassium, calcium, and renal and liver function. • Obtain a complete physical examination that includes baseline vital signs, especially pulse and blood pressure. • Establish baseline level of consciousness.	• *Chronic Pain,* related to muscle spasms • *Impaired Mobility, Physical,*, related to decreased muscle strength, control, or mass • *Risk for Injury,* related to altered level of consciousness • *Deficient Knowledge (Analgesic Therapy)*

Planning: Patient Goals and Expected Outcomes

The patient will

- Report a decrease in pain, increase in mobility, and reduction in muscle spasms.
- Report no incidences of falls or injury.
- Report any difficulty with diminished or impaired respirations.
- Demonstrate an understanding of the drug's action by accurately describing drug adverse effects and precautions.

Implementation

Interventions and (Rationales)	Patient and Family Education
• Monitor level of consciousness and vital signs. (Skeletal muscle relaxants alter consciousness, diminish respirations, and lower blood pressure.)	Instruct the patient to: • Avoid driving and the tasks that require mental alertness. • Report changes in sensorium, such as slurred speech, confusion, hallucinations, or lethargy. • Report palpitations, chest pain, dyspnea, fatigue, weakness, flaccidity, and visual changes. • Abstain from alcohol while taking this medication, including any OTC medication that contains alcohol (liquid cough and cold products).
• Monitor pain and determine the location, duration, and precipitating factors. (Drugs should diminish the patient's pain.)	Instruct the patient to: • Report the development of new sites of muscle pain. • Use relaxation techniques, deep breathing, and meditation methods to facilitate relaxation and reduce pain.
• Monitor for withdrawal reactions. (Abrupt withdrawal of baclofen may cause visual hallucinations, paranoid ideations, and seizures.)	• Instruct the patient not to abruptly discontinue medication.
• Provide additional pain relief measures such as positional support, gentle massage, and application of heat or cold. (Medications alone may not be sufficient in the provision of pain relief.)	• Instruct the patient in complementary pain interventions such as positioning, gentle massage, and the application of heat or cold to the painful area.
• Monitor for adverse effects such as drowsiness, dizziness, nausea, vomiting, headache, nervousness, diplopia, and urinary retention. (These adverse effects occur with certain drugs in this class.)	Instruct the patient to: • Report adverse effects. • Take with food to decrease GI effects. • Void before administration. • Report urinary bladder fullness, distended abdomen, and discomfort.

Evaluation of Outcome Criteria

Evaluate the effectiveness of drug therapy by confirming that patient goals and expected outcomes have been met (see "Planning").

laxants such as succinylcholine (Anectine) and tubocurarine are administered in combination with anesthetic agents to induce skeletal muscle relaxation, which aids in intubation and other invasive procedures. These agents are also administered to facilitate endoscopy, to enhance the management of mechanical ventilation, and to control the severity of muscle contractions resulting from electroshock therapy.

The skeletal muscle relaxants used as surgical adjuncts have the capability of producing complete muscle paralysis; thus mechanical ventilation may be necessary. Continuous monitoring is required. Most of these drugs have very rapid onsets of action and brief half-lives; drug effects rapidly diminish following the surgical procedure.

The skeletal muscle relaxants used as surgical adjuncts are presented in Chapter 30. Prototype features for succinylcholine and tubocurarine are found in that chapter.

UNDERSTANDING THE CHAPTER

Key Concepts Summary

27.1 Muscle spasms are involuntary contractions most commonly caused by injury or overuse of skeletal muscle.

27.2 Nonpharmacologic interventions are often successful at decreasing the pain caused by muscle spasms.

27.3 Nonsteroidal anti-inflammatory drugs and skeletal muscle relaxants are used to treat muscle spasms.

27.4 Centrally acting skeletal muscle relaxants are the drugs of choice for treating muscle spasms.

27.5 Spasticity is a condition in which certain muscle groups remain in a continuous state of contraction.

27.6 Direct-acting skeletal muscle relaxants are often used to relieve muscle spasticity.

27.7 Skeletal muscle relaxants are administered during surgery in combination with anesthetic agents.

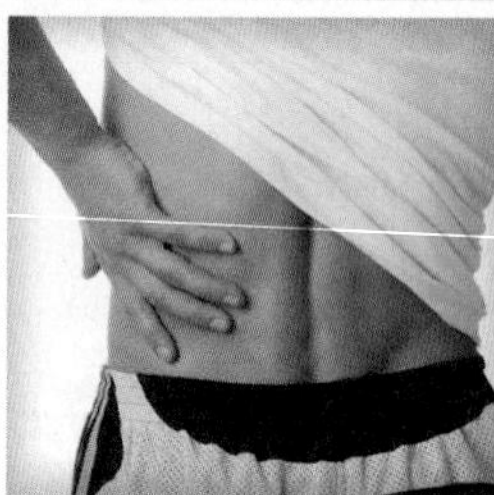

Making the PATIENT *Connection*

Remember the patient "Andrew Eskew" at the beginning of the chapter? Now read the remainder of the case study. Based on the information presented within this chapter, respond to the critical thinking questions that follow.

Andrew Eskew is a 48-year-old landscaper who was building a landscaping wall yesterday. His job requires lifting, bending, and twisting. On arising today he stated that his back hurts and he cannot move from side to side. The nurse has performed a physical assessment on Andrew, which revealed tightened muscles in the lumbosacral region and limited mobility. The patient describes his pain as a level 7 on a scale of 1 to 10.

Critical Thinking Questions

1. What are the etiology and pathophysiology of muscle spasms?
2. Mr. Eskew has been prescribed cyclobenzaprine (Flexeril) to relieve his back spasms. What is the action of this medication and why has it been prescribed?
3. What should the patient be instructed regarding the administration of this medication?

Case Study

A 46-year-old woman is diagnosed with cervical dystonia. She has difficulty maintaining normal head position and reports neck pain. She is to start on botulinum therapy.

1. What is the action of and rationale for administering botulinum toxin type A?
2. Create a list of adverse effects that this patient may experience due to botulinum therapy.

NCLEX-RN® Review

1 A client who is a body builder has been administered a general anesthetic to allow for the repair of a radial fracture. Following the administration of the anesthesia the client begins to spike a high fever of 104°F. The circulating nurse is alerted to obtain which medication?

1. Botulinum toxin type A
2. Carisoprodol (Soma)
3. Dantrolene sodium
4. Phenytoin (Dilantin)

2 A client is being treated for painful muscle spasms with cyclobenzaprine (Flexeril). The client should be instructed on which of the following? Select all that apply.

1. Void before administration.
2. Increase foods rich in calcium.
3. Do not operate machinery.
4. Utilize hard candy to decrease dry mouth.
5. Consume a diet low in fiber.

3 A client has been taught to apply capsaicin to increase mobility and relieve pain. Which of the following educational interventions is most important for the client to learn?

1. Apply the medication liberally above and below the site of pain.
2. Apply with a gloved hand only to the site of pain.
3. Apply to areas of redness and irritation.
4. Apply with a bare hand liberally.

4 A client has been treated for 20 years with antipsychotic agents. The extended therapy of antipsychotic medications has caused the client to suffer from tardive dyskinesia. Which of the following centrally acting skeletal muscle relaxants possesses a structure that is similar to the inhibitory neurotransmitter GABA and will decrease the symptom of tardive dyskinesia?

1. Baclofen (Lioresal)
2. Tizanidine (Zanaflex)
3. Dantrolene (Dantrium)
4. Botulinum toxin type A

5 A client has been taking cyclobenzaprine (Amrix, Flexeril) for muscle spasms. The client is admitted to the emergency department with severe central nervous system depression. Which of the following medications will the nurse expect to be ordered and administered?

1. Naloxone (Narcan)
2. Meperidine (Demerol)
3. Diazepam (Valium)
4. Physostigmine (Antilirium)

6 A client is receiving dantrolene sodium (Dantrium) after a spinal cord injury. The nurse will include in the care plan to monitor the client for which of the following adverse effects?

1. Muscle tension
2. Muscle weakness
3. Muscle tremors
4. Muscle pain

See Answers to Critical Thinking Questions, Case Study, and NCLEX-RN® Review in Appendix A.

References

American Association of Neurological Surgeons. (2006). *Spasticity.* Retrieved June 22, 2008, from http://www.neurosurgerytoday.org/what/patient_e/spasticity_06.asp

American Association of Neurological Surgeons. (2005). *Dystonia.* Retrieved June 22, 2008, from http://www.neurosurgerytoday.org/what/patient_e/dystonia.asp

Ball, C., & Westhorpe, R. N. (2006). Muscle relaxants-reversal agents. *Anaesthesia and Intensive Care, 34*(4), 415.

Cleveland Clinic. (2008). *Intrathecal baclofen therapy (for MS).* Retrieved June 23, 2008, from http://my.clevelandclinic.org/devices/Intrathecal_Baclofen_Pump_System/hic_Intrathecal_Baclofen_Therapy_for_MS.aspx

Donnes, I., Nazzi, V., & Broggi, G. (2006). The guidelines for the diagnosis and treatment of spasticity. *Journal of Neurosurgical Sciences, 50*(4), 101–105.

Hirayama, J., Yamagata, M., Ogata, S., Shimizu, K., Ikeda, Y., & Takahashi, K. (2006). Relationship between low-back pain, muscle spasm and pressure pain thresholds in patients with lumbar disc herniation. *European Spine Journal, 15,* 41–47.

Lemone, P., & Burke, K. (2008). *Medical surgical nursing: Critical thinking in client care* (4th ed.). Upper Saddle River, NJ: Pearson Education.

Nemours Foundation. (2006). *Cerebral palsy.* Retrieved June 22, 2008, from http://kidshealth.org/parent/medical/brain/cerebral_palsy.html

Pathak, M. S., Nguyen, H. T., Graham, H. K., & Moore, A. P. (2006). Management of spasticity in adults: Practical application of botulinum toxin. *European Journal of Neurology, 13*(Suppl. 1), 42–50.

Rice, J., O'Donnell, M., & Armstrong, R. (2006). Intrathecal baclofen use in children with spasticity—A physician's survey. *Developmental Medicine and Child Neurology, 48*(12), 1006–1008.

Ridley, B. (2006). Intrathecal baclofen therapy: Challenges in patients with multiple sclerosis. *Rehabilitation Nursing, 31*(4), 158–164.

Urquhart, D. M., Hoving, J. L., Assendelft, W. J., Roland, M., & van Tulder, M. W. (2008). Antidepressants for non-specific low back pain. *Cochrane Database of Systematic Reviews, 1.* Art. No.: CD001703. DOI: 10.1002/14651858.CD001703.pub3.

U.S. Food and Drug Administration, Center for Food Safety and Applied Nutrition. (2002). *Kava-containing dietary supplements may be associated with severe liver injury* (Consumer advisory). Retrieved June 22, 2008, from http://www.cfsan.fda.gov/~dms/addskava.html

van Tulder, M. W., Touray, T., Furlan, A. D., Solway, S., & Bouter, L. M. (2003). Muscle relaxants for nonspecific low back pain: A systematic review within the framework of the Cochrane Collaboration. *Spine, 28*(17), 1978–1992.

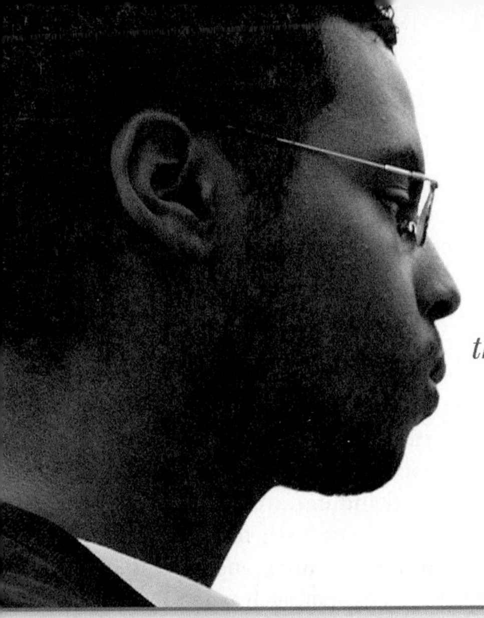

The nursing school I am applying to is an evening program. I am concerned about being at school in the evening because I take medication for attention deficit/hyperactivity disorder.

Patient "Jonathon Hogan"

CHAPTER 28

Central Nervous System Stimulants and Drugs for Attention Deficit/Hyperactivity Disorder

Chapter Outline

Characteristics of Central Nervous System Stimulants

Etiology and Pathophysiology of Attention Deficit/Hyperactivity Disorder

Pharmacotherapy of Attention Deficit/Hyperactivity Disorder

Amphetamines and Amphetamine-Like Drugs

PROTOTYPE **Amphetamine Sulfate (Racemic Amphetamine, Adderall)** *p. 415*

Nonstimulants

PROTOTYPE **Atomoxetine (Strattera)** *p. 418*

Pharmacotherapy of Narcolepsy

PROTOTYPE **Modafinil (Provigil, Alertec)** *p. 420*

Methylxanthines

PROTOTYPE **Caffeine** *p. 421*

Learning Outcomes

After reading the chapter, the student should be able to:

1. Describe the action, adverse effects, uses, and therapeutic effects of central nervous system stimulants.
2. Identify the signs and symptoms of attention deficit/hyperactivity disorder and narcolepsy.
3. Compare and contrast the central nervous system stimulants and nonstimulants in treating attention deficit/hyperactivity disorder.
4. Compare and contrast the different pharmacotherapies available for narcolepsy.
5. Describe the nurse's role in the pharmacologic management of attention deficit/hyperactivity disorder and narcolepsy.
6. For each class shown in the chapter outline, identify the prototype and representative drugs and explain the mechanism(s) of drug action, primary indications, contraindications, significant drug interactions, pregnancy category, and important adverse effects.
7. Apply the nursing process to care for patients receiving central nervous system stimulants.

Key Terms

anorexiants, 415
attention deficit/hyperactivity disorder (ADHD), 413
cataplexy, 419
central nervous system (CNS) stimulants, 412
euphoria, 412
hyperkinetic disorder (HKD), 413
hypnagogic hallucinations, 420
methylxanthine, 421
narcolepsy, 419
sleep attacks, 419
sleep paralysis, 419

The central nervous system (CNS) stimulants are a small group of drugs that have limited pharmacotherapeutic applications. Attention deficit/hyperactivity disorder (ADHD) and narcolepsy are conditions that diminish mental alertness and that may benefit from treatment with these medications. Some of the CNS stimulants such as cocaine and methamphetamine are widely abused. The purpose of this chapter is to examine the actions and pharmacotherapeutic applications of the CNS stimulants.

Characteristics of Central Nervous System Stimulants

28.1 Central nervous system stimulants increase alertness, enhance the ability to concentrate, and delay the symptoms of fatigue.

The **central nervous system (CNS) stimulants** consist of a diverse group of pharmacologic agents. The stimulants range from widely accessible agents (caffeine) to Schedule I controlled substances (Ecstasy). All CNS stimulants have the common action of raising the general alertness level of the brain. Wakefulness and the ability to focus or concentrate are increased. Mood is often elevated and the person may temporarily become unaware of physical fatigue. For some of the controlled substances, mood elevation may progress to **euphoria,** an intense sense of happiness and well-being.

Because people generally view the sensations associated with CNS stimulation as desirable, many are driven to repeat the pleasurable experience. With continued use, physical and psychological dependence occur with these agents. Because of this, many CNS stimulants are highly regulated and are scheduled drugs (Table 28.1).

Not all effects of these drugs on the CNS are pleasurable. Stimulants have the potential to cause adverse effects due to excessive excitation. Nervousness, dizziness, and irritability are common, and convulsions may occur at higher doses. Most of the stimulants also affect the cardiovascular system and can increase heart rate and cause dysrhythmias. Loss of appetite, or anorexia, occurs with some of the agents.

Some drugs are not classified as CNS stimulants but may produce CNS excitation as a adverse effect. For example, antihistamines are prescribed to treat allergy symptoms but may cause CNS stimulation and insomnia in some patients. Albuterol (Proventil) inhalers are used for asthma but the drug may cause nervousness, tremors, and anxiety. Drugs that normally cause CNS depression, such as antidepressants, may cause paradoxical CNS excitement especially in the very young or very old. Occasionally, drugs are purposefully taken in large amounts for their CNS stimulation adverse effects. For example, the primary over-the-counter (OTC) drug for treating cough, dextromethorphan, is abused by teenagers and can cause dizziness, restlessness, hallucinations, and seizures in very high amounts. Additional information on the substance abuse aspects of the CNS stimulants is presented in Chapter 8.

The therapeutic applications of the CNS stimulants are limited. These include the following:

- ADHD
- Narcolepsy
- Weight management
- Respiratory stimulation
- Migraine headaches

If CNS stimulants elevate mood, why are they not used to treat major depression? In fact, CNS stimulants have been used in the past to treat major depression. CNS stimulants, however, are nonselective in their CNS actions; the excitement produced by these drugs affects all parts of the brain. They produce many potentially serious adverse effects, including physical and psychological dependence. The tricyclic antidepressants and the selective serotonin reuptake inhibitors (SSRIs) have been demonstrated to be more effective and safer than stimulants in the treatment of depression.

TABLE 28.1 Central Nervous System Stimulants That Are Scheduled Drugs

Schedule	Central Nervous System Stimulants
I	aminoxaphen (Aminorex), cathinone, fenethylline, methcathinone, methylaminorex, amphetamine variants (including MDMA—Ecstasy)
II	biphetamine, cocaine, dextroamphetamine (Dexedrine), methamphetamine (Desoxyn), methylphenidate (Ritalin), phenmetrazine (Preludin)
III	benzphetamine (Didrex), chlorphentermine, clortermine, phendimetrazine (Plegine, Prelu 2)
IV	armodafinil (Nuvigil), diethylpropion (Tenuate), fencamfamin, fenproporex, mazindol (Sanorex, Mazanor), mefenorex, modafinil (Provigil), norpseudoephedrine, pemoline (Cylert), phentermine (Fastin, Apipex), pipradrol, sibutramine (Meridia)
V	pyrovalerone

Note: From "Stimulants," by K. Divadeenam, 2008, *emedicine*. Retrieved June 24, 2008, from http://www.emedicine.com/med/topic3094.htm

Etiology and Pathophysiology of Attention Deficit/Hyperactivity Disorder

28.2 Attention deficit/hyperactivity disorder is characterized by inattention, hyperactivity, and impulsive behavior.

Attention deficit/hyperactivity disorder (ADHD) is a neuropsychiatric condition that presents in children before age 7 and can extend into adulthood. It is characterized by symptoms of impulsive behavior, lack of attention, and hyperactivity. The patient diagnosed with ADHD must have six of nine symptoms of inattention and six of nine symptoms of hyperactivity, with some degree of symptom presentation in more than one setting, as shown in Table 28.2. In Canada the diagnosis of ADHD is referred to as **hyperkinetic disorder (HKD).**

ADHD occurs in approximately 3% to 5% of all children. The condition is more common in males: 9% of males versus 3% of females. However, the diagnosis of ADHD has tripled among girls according to the United States population-adjusted rate of office visits (Robison, Skaer, Sclar, & Galin, 2002). Girls with ADHD have been noted to have less aggressive behavior than boys but have greater anxiety and mood swings. They often withdraw socially and may experience cognitive and language delays. The diagnosis in females is usually later than age 7.

Symptoms of ADHD such as impulsive behavior, distractibility, lack of attention, and hyperactivity during the school-age years can lead to poor performance and lack of interest in school activities. The symptoms of inattention and hyperactivity also contribute to difficulty with peer and family relationships. Hyperactive children usually have increased motor activity with impulsivity and a tendency to interrupt at inappropriate times. This behavior can result in disciplinary action by teachers and parents. Some additional symptoms noted include difficulty remembering details and the placement of personal items, changing tasks without completing prior tasks, and disturbances in sleep.

Considerable attention has focused on the causes of ADHD, and it is clear that the etiology is complex and involves multiple variables. Studies on twins have indicated that genetics is an important contributor to the development of ADHD. An identical twin has a 92% probability of presenting with ADHD if his or her twin has been diagnosed with the disorder. According to the National Institute of Mental Health (NIMH), 25% of families with a member diagnosed with ADHD will have other relatives also diagnosed. This percentage is significantly higher than the general population, which is approximately 5%.

Brain injury has been studied as a contributing factor in the development of ADHD because some children suffering from head trauma will exhibit symptoms of the disorder. The percentage of brain injuries that lead to a diagnosis of ADHD is small but remains relevant in assessing the patient in future years.

TABLE 28.2 Diagnosis of Attention Deficit/Hyperactivity Disorder

I. Either A or B:

A. Six or more of the following symptoms of inattention have been present for at least 6 months to a point that is disruptive and inappropriate for developmental level:

Inattention

1. Often does not give close attention to details or makes careless mistakes in schoolwork, work, or other activities.
2. Often has trouble keeping attention on tasks or play activities.
3. Often does not seem to listen when spoken to directly.
4. Often does not follow instructions and fails to finish schoolwork, chores, or duties in the workplace (not due to oppositional behavior or failure to understand instructions).
5. Often has trouble organizing activities.
6. Often avoids, dislikes, or doesn't want to do things that take a lot of mental effort for a long period of time (such as schoolwork or homework).
7. Often loses things needed for tasks and activities (e.g., toys, school assignments, pencils, books, or tools).
8. Is often easily distracted.
9. Is often forgetful in daily activities.

B. Six or more of the following symptoms of hyperactivity-impulsivity have been present for at least 6 months to an extent that is disruptive and inappropriate for developmental level:

Hyperactivity

1. Often fidgets with hands or feet or squirms in seat.
2. Often gets up from seat when remaining in seat is expected.
3. Often runs about or climbs when and where it is not appropriate (adolescents or adults may feel very restless).
4. Often has trouble playing or enjoying leisure activities quietly.
5. Is often "on the go" or often acts as if "driven by a motor."
6. Often talks excessively.

Impulsivity

1. Often blurts out answers before questions have been finished.
2. Often has trouble waiting one's turn.
3. Often interrupts or intrudes on others (e.g., butts into conversations or games).

II. Some symptoms that cause impairment were present before age 7 years.

III. Some impairment from the symptoms is present in two or more settings (e.g., at school/work and at home).

IV. There must be clear evidence of significant impairment in social, school, or work functioning.

V. The symptoms do not happen only during the course of a pervasive developmental disorder, schizophrenia, or other psychotic disorder. The symptoms are not better accounted for by another mental disorder (e.g., mood disorder, anxiety disorder, dissociative disorder, or a personality disorder).

Note: From *Diagnostic and Statistical Manual of Mental Disorders, Fourth Edition, Text Revision,* by American Psychiatric Association, 2000, Washington, DC: Author.

CONNECTIONS

Treating the Diverse Patient Attention Deficit/Hyperactivity Disorder Increase in Girls

In 1998 the Council on Scientific Affairs of the American Medical Association reported that the criteria used to diagnose children and adolescents with ADHD had broadened. This change was related to the broadened awareness of the condition and its progression into the adult years. The estimated rate of office visits among children increased from 947,208 in 1990 to 3,234,180 in 1998. The mean number of girls diagnosed with ADHD tripled from 1991 through 1998. The United States population-adjusted rate of office visits with a patient's diagnosis of ADHD among girls increased 2.7-fold from 1991 to 1998. The rate of girls prescribed with stimulant pharmacotherapy increased 2.8-fold. Based on these data it is important that research that focuses on the diagnosis and treatment of ADHD among the female population be conducted.

Source: From "Is Attention Deficit Hyperactivity Disorder Increasing Among Girls in the US? Trends in Diagnosis and the Prescribing of Stimulants," by L. M. Robison, T. Skaier, D. A. Sclar, and R. S. Galin, 2002, *CNS Drugs, 16*(2), pp. 129–137.

Environmental agents such as lead can contribute to the development of ADHD in children. Children living in buildings built prior to 1972 have a higher risk of developing lead poisoning. Other environmental agents that contribute to the development of ADHD include alcohol and cigarette smoking by the mother during pregnancy. Food additives and sugar intake by the child have been implicated as causes of ADHD, but research studies have failed to find a strong link.

There are differences in the anatomy and physiology of children with ADHD and control subjects. Recent studies conducted by the NIMH have shown that children with a known diagnosis of ADHD possess a 3% to 4% smaller brain volume in the frontal lobes, temporal gray matter, caudate nucleus, and cerebellum. Children who are affected by ADHD have a deficiency in the catecholamines, dopamine and norepinephrine. The brain of a child with ADHD also has decreased development in the area of self-regulation. This factor yields the development of symptoms such as irritability, aggression, learning disability, and motor disorders when the child is stimulated.

The symptoms of ADHD can cause functional impairment in the child and be challenging for parents and teachers. The goal of pharmacotherapy for ADHD is to reduce inattention and promote the child's ability to focus and concentrate on tasks. CNS stimulants have been the mainstay of drug therapy for ADHD for decades. The primary types of medications used to treat ADHD include amphetamines, and non–central nervous system stimulants. Successful treatment of ADHD usually requires a combination of pharmacotherapy and behavioral therapies.

PharmFACT

Symptoms of ADHD continue into adulthood in 35% to 55% of persons with childhood ADHD. Symptoms in adults include workaholic tendencies, being overscheduled and overwhelmed, talking excessively, low frustration tolerance, short temper, quitting jobs abruptly, ending relationships, driving too fast, and "addictive" personality. *Source:* Busko, 2008.

Pharmacotherapy of Attention Deficit/Hyperactivity Disorder

28.3 Amphetamines are central nervous system stimulants indicated for the treatment of attention deficit/hyperactivity disorder and narcolepsy.

The most frequently prescribed medications for ADHD are amphetamines and amphetamine-like agents. During the

CONNECTIONS

Evidence-Based Practice Controlling Symptoms of Attention Deficit/Hyperactivity Disorder

Clinical Question

What role does pharmacotherapy play in reducing the symptoms of ADHD in children, adolescents, and adults?

Evidence

ADHD is a CNS disorder that is characterized by developmentally inappropriate behavior with inattention. Pharmacotherapy plays an important role in controlling the symptoms of ADHD. The literature supports the premise that compounds that possess dopaminergic and norepinephrine properties are the most effective in treating ADHD. The literature possesses a great deal of research on pharmacologic effects among children and adolescents but research remains limited among the adult population. Stimulant therapy is still considered the first-line treatment for ADHD among the adult population.

Implication

Data support that atomoxetine in adults is useful in treating ADHD. It has also been proven effective in the treatment of ADHD and accompanying anxiety reactions. Tricyclic antidepressants and bupropion have not been studied but appear to be effective in patients who do not respond to stimulant therapy.

Critical Thinking Question

Atomoxetine is useful in treating ADHD in adults. What is the action of this medication? What client education should be provided to the client prescribed this medication?

See Answers to Critical Thinking Questions in Appendix A.

Source: From "Drug Therapy for Adults with Attention Deficit Hyperactivity Disorder," by T. C. Wilens, 2003, *Drugs, 63*(22), pp. 2395–2411.

1920s, amphetamines were used to treat asthma, hay fever, and the common cold. Later, amphetamines came into widespread use in World War II because these drugs were able to keep soldiers alert and delay fatigue during combat. Amphetamines were not listed as scheduled substances until 1970. Amphetamine sulfate has been used to make several other salts that have psychoactive properties, including methamphetamine and Ecstasy (methylenedioxymethamphetamine or MDMA).

CONNECTION *Checkpoint* 28.1

MDMA is known as a club drug. From what you learned in Chapter 8, define *club drug* and explain the signs and symptoms of MDMA abuse. See Answer to Connection Checkpoint 28.1 in Appendix A.

Amphetamine exists in two closely related but distinct chemical forms: d-amphetamine (dextroamphetamine) and l-amphetamine (levoamphetamine). When using the term *amphetamine* it is understood that the drug is a 50:50 mixture of the d- and l- forms. To be more precise, this 50:50 mixture is sometimes called racemic amphetamine. Dextroamphetamine is marketed separately as Dexedrine. Doses of these drugs are listed in Table 28.3.

Amphetamines increase attention and alertness and enhance the child's ability to focus and learn. When used appropriately, amphetamines used for ADHD do not cause euphoria, and dependence has not been a serious problem. In fact at least one study found that teens taking amphetamines for ADHD had a lower incidence of later substance abuse, compared to those who were not on amphetamines (Wilens, Faraone, Biederman, & Gunawardene, 2003). These agents are effective in reducing the symptoms of ADHD in 70% to 90% of the children treated with the drugs.

Amphetamines have actions on both the autonomic nervous system and CNS. Amphetamines are sympathomimetics and activate alpha- and beta-adrenergic receptors by promoting the release of norepinephrine in the autonomic nervous system (see Chapter 19). Typical symptoms of sympathetic activation caused by amphetamines include vasoconstriction, hypertension (HTN), and tachycardia.

The CNS stimulant actions of amphetamines are the result of increased release of dopamine due to inhibition of the reuptake of this neurotransmitter in presynaptic neurons. At very high doses, amphetamines enhance the release of the neurotransmitter serotonin (5-hydroxytryptamine or 5-HT) in the brain, which is responsible for serious psychotic behaviors. Amphetamines also are **anorexiants,** which means that they diminish the appetite. This effect is produced by direct inhibition of the appetite center in the hypothalamus. The application of the amphetamines to the pharmacotherapy of obesity is presented in Chapter 64.

Almost from the time they were discovered, amphetamines have been abused for their stimulant effects. These drugs are often abused by those who wish to delay fatigue; for example, truck drivers, students, and health care workers working long shifts. Athletes may take amphetamines to increase their energy level and enhance performance. Long-term amphetamine abuse may lead to tolerance, dependence, and serious adverse effects, as presented in Chapter 8. Amphetamine and methamphetamine are Schedule II drugs.

Cocaine is an illicit drug that has similar sympathomimetic, CNS stimulant, and anorexiant effects to amphetamine. In fact, the signs and symptoms of cocaine abuse are indistinguishable from those of amphetamine abuse. Cocaine has a much shorter half-life, which leads to more frequent repeated doses.

PROTOTYPE DRUG Amphetamine sulfate (Racemic amphetamine, Adderall)

Classification: **Therapeutic:** ADHD agent
Pharmacologic: CNS stimulant, anorexiant, sympathomimetic

Therapeutic Effects and Uses: Amphetamine increases motor activity, alertness, and wakefulness, and elevates the patient's mood. In children who suffer from ADHD the medication produces a paradoxical sedation effect. The mechanism of this effect is unclear. The drug affects the satiety center in the hypothalamus, causing anorexiant effects that lead to loss of appetite and weight.

Amphetamines are used to treat ADHD and narcolepsy. Although an effective appetite suppressant, amphetamine is rarely used for weight loss therapy because its inhibition of appetite is short term, and dependence results from long-term use. Amphetamine was approved by the U.S. Food and Drug Administration (FDA) in 1939 and is available in tablet form. Illegal forms of amphetamine may be smoked, inhaled, or injected.

Mechanism of Action: Amphetamine produces sympathomimetic effects as well as central stimulation actions on the cerebral cortex and the reticular activating system (RAS). The actions of the medication are due to the release of norepinephrine and dopamine. The benefits of the drug in treating ADHD may also be due to its effects on the neurotransmitter serotonin in the brain.

Pharmacokinetics:

Route(s)	Oral (PO)
Absorption	Rapid
Distribution	Widely distributed to all tissues, including the CNS; secreted in breast milk
Primary metabolism	Hepatic
Primary excretion	Renal
Onset of action	Peak effect: 1–5 h
Duration of action	Up to 10 h

Adverse Effects: Symptoms of excessive CNS and peripheral stimulation by amphetamine include irritability, insomnia, nervousness, palpitations, elevated blood pressure, and tachycardia.

TABLE 28.3 Central Nervous System Stimulants and Drugs for Attention Deficit/Hyperactivity Disorder and Narcolepsy

Drug	Route and Adult Dose (maximum dose where indicated)	Adverse Effects
Amphetamines and Amphetamine-Like Drugs		
amphetamine sulfate (Racemic, Amphetamine, Adderall)	ADHD: Child 6 years: PO: 5 mg 1–2 times per day; may increase by 5 mg/week (max: 40 mg/day) Adolescents/adults: PO: 10 mg 0 extended release, once daily in the morning; may increase dosage by 5 mg/day (max: 30 mg/day) Narcolepsy: Child 6–12 years: PO: 5 mg/day; may increase by 5 mg/week Older than 12 years: PO: 10 mg/day; may increase by 5–10 mg/week Adult: PO: 5–60 mg/day every 4–6 h in two to three divided doses	*Irritability, dizziness, palpitations, euphoria, insomnia, tachycardia, weight loss* <u>Sudden death, dependence, psychosis</u>
benzphetamine (Didrex)	PO: 25–50 mg 1–3 times per day (max: 150 mg/day)	
dexmethylphenidate (Focalin)	Child older than 6 years: PO: 2.5 mg bid may increase by 2.5–5 mg/week (max: 20 mg/day); 5 mg/day extended release may increase by 5 mg/week Adult: PO: 2.5 mg bid; may increase by 2.5–5 mg/day at weekly intervals (max: 20 mg/day)	
lisdexamfetamine (Vyvanse)	PO: 30 mg once daily in the a.m. (max: 70 mg/day)	
methylphenidate (Concerta, Metadate, Methylin, Ritalin)	Narcolepsy: Adult: PO: 10 mg bid–tid ADHD: Child: PO: 5–10 mg before breakfast and lunch; gradually increase by 5–10 mq/week (max: 60 mg/day); Adult: 20–30 mg immediate release bid-tid (max: 60 mg)	
Nonstimulant for ADHD		
atomoxetine (Strattera)	Child less than 70 kg: PO: start with 0.5 mg/kg/day; may increase after 3 days to target dose of 1.2 mg/kg/day (max: 1.4 mg/kg or 100 mg) Adult: PO: start with 40 mg; may increase after 3 days to target dose of 80 mg/day (max: 100 mg/day)	*Headache, palpitations, decreased appetite, insomnia, irritability, fatigue, somnolence, dry mouth, upper abdominal pain, nausea, vomiting, constipation, urinary retention, cough* <u>Suicidal ideation, severe liver injury</u>
Drugs for Narcolepsy		
armodafinil (Nuvagil)	PO: 150–250 mg/day given as a single dose in the a.m.	*Dizziness, nausea, insomnia, headache, anxiety* <u>Stevens-Johnson syndrome (SJS), hypersensitivity, mania</u>
modafinil (Provigil, Alertec)	PO: 200 mg/day	*Chest pain, headache, nervousness, dizziness, insomnia, syncope, diarrhea, pharyngitis, rhinitis, dyspnea, SJS, anxiety* <u>Hypersensitivity reaction</u>
sodium oxybate (Xyrem)	PO: Two doses of 2.25 g, the first given at bedtime, the second given 2.5 to 4 h later (max: 9 g/day)	*Headache, nausea, dizziness, neopharyngitis, drowsiness* <u>Disorientation, irritability, paresthesia</u>
Methylxanthine		
caffeine	Neonatal apnea: PO or IV: 20–30 mg/kg as a loading dose; maintenance dose: 5 mg/kg citrate for 10–12 days Mental alertness: PO: 100–200 mg tid–qid as needed	*Tachycardia, flushing, restlessness, insomnia, irritability, tremor, palpitations, polyuria* <u>Kernicterus in neonates, seizures</u>

Note: *Italics* indicate common adverse effects. <u>Underline</u> indicates serious adverse effects.

Weight loss is noted with the medication. Impotence and change in libido may occur with high doses. Long-term use of amphetamines has been reported to cause growth inhibition in children; however, discontinuation of the drug often results in rebound growth. Psychiatric symptoms associated with amphetamine abuse include euphoria, hallucinations, delusions, paranoia, delirium, and depression. The most severe adverse effect is sudden death, which has been reported in children with structural heart anomalies.

Long-term users of amphetamine will experience tolerance to the mood-elevating effects of the drug. This results in abusers requiring higher and higher doses to achieve the same stimulant effect. Over time, physical and psychological dependence will develop.

Contraindications/Precautions: Patients with hypersensitivity to sympathomimetic amines (e.g., epinephrine or norepinephrine), or who have a history of drug abuse, should not be prescribed amphetamine. The following disorders are contraindicated with amphetamine because the conditions may worsen: diabetes, hyperthyroidism, HTN, cardiac disorders, and Gilles de la Tourette disorder. Patients with bipolar disorder may exhibit signs of mania when administered amphetamines. Amphetamines should be discontinued gradually to prevent withdrawal symptoms such as severe depression, anxiety, agitation, hypersomnia, dysphoric mood, or suicidal ideation.

Drug Interactions: Alkaline drugs such as acetazolamide and sodium bicarbonate decrease the elimination of amphetamine from the body and prolong its half-life. On the other hand, acidic drugs such as ammonium chloride and ascorbic acid increase the elimination of amphetamine from the body. The administration of amphetamine with furazolidone can cause an increase in blood pressure effects. Guanethidine and guanadrel antagonize antihypertensive effects in combination with amphetamine. Selegiline administered with amphetamine can precipitate hypertensive crisis, which may be fatal. **Herbal/Food:** Foods and fluids containing caffeine can cause additive CNS stimulation and increase insomnia, nervousness, and anxiety. Melatonin should be avoided because it may enhance the CNS stimulation from amphetamine.

Pregnancy: Category C.

Treatment of Overdose: The treatment of overdosage of amphetamine and amphetamine-related medications includes gastric lavage and the administration of chlorpromazine. Chlorpromazine contains strong alpha-adrenergic blocking actions that counteract the effects of amphetamine. In the event that overdosage results in severe HTN, phentolamine is administered intravenously (IV). Acidification of the urine can speed the renal elimination of the drug.

Nursing Responsibilities:

- Before starting therapy, perform a comprehensive cardiovascular examination. Sudden cardiac death, strokes, and myocardial infarction (MI) have occurred in patients with serious cardiac disease or those with structural abnormalities of the heart.
- Assess for psychiatric illness that may contraindicate use of the drug, such as aggressiveness, bipolar disorder, or psychoses.
- Assess for history of glaucoma, drug abuse, and moderate to severe HTN because these are contraindications for the use of this drug.
- Assess for the effectiveness of treatment and symptom control.
- Assess for insomnia, increased blood pressure, or anorexia.
- Evaluate growth in children and compare to normal heights and weights using standardized growth charts.

Patient and Family Education:

- Keep the medication in a secure location and take exactly as prescribed because this drug has abuse potential.
- Do not take any other prescription or nonprescription drugs, dietary supplements, or herbal products without approval of the health care provider.
- Immediately report any of the following: palpitations, persistent increases in blood pressure, insomnia, seizures, blurred vision.
- If loss of appetite occurs, eat small frequent meals.
- Do not open, crush, or chew the extended release forms of the drug.
- Take the dose in the morning because taking it late in the day may cause insomnia.
- Perform frequent mouth care and chew gum or eat hard candy to prevent dry mouth.
- Avoid foods or fluids containing caffeine or other stimulants.
- Do not abruptly discontinue the drug.
- Do not breast-feed while taking this drug without approval of the health care provider.

Drugs Similar to Amphetamine Sulfate (Racemic Amphetamine, Adderall)

CNS stimulants that are similar to amphetamine include benzphetamine, dexmethylphenidate, and methylamphetamine. Pemoline (Cylert), an amphetamine-like drug used for ADHD and narcolepsy, was removed from the market in 2005 due to incidences of fatal hepatic failure.

Benzphetamine (Didrex): Approved in 1960, benzphetamine is an oral drug that is metabolized in the liver to amphetamine and methamphetamine. Its actions and adverse effects are the same as those of amphetamine. Benzphetamine has been used for the short-term, 8- to 12-week management of obesity. The drug loses its anorexiant properties when used for longer than 12 weeks. For optimum weight loss, use of the drug should be combined with lifestyle changes, including diet management and exercise. The drug has a high potential for abuse and is a Schedule III substance. HTN, dizziness, restlessness, insomnia, and euphoria may be experienced at the beginning of therapy. This drug is pregnancy category X.

Dexmethylphenidate (Focalin): Approved in 2001, dexmethylphenidate has effects identical to methylphenidate and the amphetamines. The drug blocks the reuptake of norepinephrine and dopamine in presynaptic neurons. It is used to manage symptoms of ADHD. In 2005, a once-daily extended release capsule (Focalin XR) was approved by the FDA. The most common adverse effects are abdominal pain, nausea, fever, and decreased appetite. Although not common, twitching (vocal or motor tics) is a reported reason for discontinuation of therapy. Inhibition of growth is a potential long-term adverse effect of the use of stimulants in children. Dexmethylphenidate should not be administered to patients who have primary psychiatric disorders because the drug may worsen these conditions. The drug has a high potential for abuse and is a Schedule II substance. This drug is pregnancy category C.

Lisdexamfetamine (Vyvanse): Approved in 2007, lisdexamfetamine is a prodrug of dextroamphetamine approved for the treatment of ADHD. Because the drug is rapidly metabolized to dextroamphetamine, the actions and adverse effects are identical to those of dextroamphetamine. This drug is a schedule II controlled substance and is pregnancy category C.

MyNursingKit | Mechanism of Action Animation: Methylphenidate

Methylphenidate (Concerta, Metadate, Methylin, Ritalin): Although structurally dissimilar to amphetamine, the two drugs share the same mechanism of action, pharmacologic actions, and adverse effects. Methylphenidate is approved for the treatment of ADHD and narcolepsy. Rarely, it may be used off-label for major depression refractory to more traditional therapies. In treating ADHD, it is as effective as the amphetamines. The patient's condition should be regularly assessed and drug-free periods may be ordered during prolonged therapy. The drug is available in several extended release forms for once-daily dosing. A transdermal patch (Daytrana) was approved by the FDA in 2006 for children aged 6 to 12. The long duration forms are beneficial to children because they do not require the school nurse to administer a dose during the school day. It is important to note that this medication is contraindicated in children under the age of 6.

Methylphenidate is well tolerated and produces fewer peripheral adverse effects than amphetamine. Physical dependence is uncommon at therapeutic doses, although it may occur with the illicit parenteral or inhaled forms of the drug. Withdrawal symptoms are uncommon when the drug is discontinued. Nervousness, loss of appetite, and insomnia are the most common adverse effects. Methylphenidate should not be used in patients with severe anxiety, psychoses, or bipolar disorder because it may worsen these conditions. Sudden unexplained cardiac death has occurred in some people taking this drug; therefore, all patients should be screened for preexisting cardiac disease, especially structural abnormalities or ventricular dysrhythmias. This drug is pregnancy category C.

28.4 Atomoxetine (Strattera) is a newer drug for treating attention deficit/hyperactivity disorder that does not stimulate the central nervous system.

In 2002 the FDA approved atomoxetine (Strattera), a nonstimulant for the treatment of ADHD. Because atomoxetine does not appear to have any abuse potential, it is not classified as a controlled substance. The drug offers an alternative for parents who are hesitant to place their children on CNS stimulants. The dose for atomoxetine (Strattera) is listed in Table 28.3.

Antidepressants have been used to treat ADHD, but these agents are generally less effective than the CNS stimulants. Tricyclic antidepressants (TCAs) that have been used off-label for ADHD include imipramine (Tofranil), desipramine (Norpramin), and nortriptyline (Aventyl). The TCAs can cause significant anticholinergic adverse effects such as dry mouth and constipation and are cardiotoxic when taken in very high doses. Bupropion (Wellbutrin) is a non-TCA antidepressant that has been used off-label for treating ADHD. Antidepressants are considered second-line therapy for ADHD and are usually only used when the patient has not responded adequately to CNS stimulants or has a comorbid condition such as depression or anxiety.

CONNECTION *Checkpoint* 28.2

From what you learned in Chapter 23, what class of antidepressants contains the drugs of choice for major depressive disorder? To what antidepressant class does bupropion belong? See Answer to Connection Checkpoint 28.2 in Appendix A.

PROTOTYPE DRUG Atomoxetine (Strattera)

Classification: **Therapeutic:** ADHD agent
Pharmacologic: Nonstimulant, norepinephrine reuptake inhibitor

Therapeutic Effects and Uses: Atomoxetine (Strattera) is administered to improve attentiveness and the ability to follow tasks in patients with ADHD. The medication decreases distraction and forgetfulness. It has the ability to diminish symptoms of ADHD in children and adults, and it is approved for patients aged 6 years and older. Unlike the stimulants that have an onset of action of 1 hour, atomoxetine takes 2 to 4 weeks for optimal reduction of ADHD symptoms.

Mechanism of Action: Atomoxetine is a selective norepinephrine reuptake inhibitor (SNRSI), which allows for increased concentration of the neurotransmitter in the prefrontal cortex. This region of the brain is associated with control of social behavior, personality expression, and short-term memory.

Pharmacokinetics:

Route(s)	PO
Absorption	Rapidly absorbed
Distribution	Distributed to most tissues; unknown if secreted in breast milk; 98% bound to protein
Primary metabolism	Hepatic, by cytochrome P450 (CYP2D6)
Primary excretion	Renal
Onset of action	2–4 weeks for ADHD symptoms
Duration of action	Half-life: 5.2 h

Adverse Effects: The most serious adverse effect of atomoxetine is suicidal ideation. Other CNS adverse effects include mood swings, irritability, and agitation. Because rare incidences of liver injury have been reported, patients with elevated hepatic enzymes or symptoms such as jaundice, nausea, vomiting, or anorexia should immediately discontinue the drug. Cardiovascular adverse effects include orthostatic hypotension, tachycardia, HTN, and palpitations. The patient may experience cough due to rhinorrhea, nasal congestion, and sinusitis. Weight loss and anorexia, along with urinary retention, urinary hesitancy, impotence, delayed menses, and menstrual irregularities, have been reported. In 2005, the FDA issued a public health advisory to closely monitor for suicidal ideation in patients taking this medication.

Contraindications/Precautions: If the patient has received a monoamine oxidase inhibitor (MAOI) in the last 14 days the administration of atomoxetine should be delayed due to the risk of neuroleptic malignant syndrome or hypertensive crisis. Administration of the medication to any patient who has jaundice or elevated liver enzymes should be delayed until enzyme levels are in the normal range. Atomoxetine is also contraindicated in patients who have been diagnosed with narrow-angle glaucoma. It is important to administer atomoxetine cautiously in patients with HTN, tachycardia, moderate to severe hepatic insufficiency, and cardiovascular disease.

Drug Interactions: The elimination of atomoxetine is prolonged if it is administered with fluoxetine, paroxetine, or quinidine. Concurrent administration of albuterol with atomoxetine can result in increased heart rate and HTN. Drugs that activate the sympathetic nervous system should be used cautiously with atomoxetine due to the possibility of HTN. Some common sympathomimetics include amphetamines, pseudoephedrine, ephedrine, phenylephrine, dopamine, and norepinephrine. **Herbal/Food:** It is recommended that the patient not consume any herbal supplements while taking atomoxetine.

Pregnancy: Category C.

Treatment of Overdose: Overdose with atomoxetine will cause agitation, abnormal behavior, and signs of sympathetic stimulation such as mydriasis, dry mouth, and tachycardia. The patient should receive supportive treatment for cardiopulmonary effects. Gastric lavage and repeated applications of activated charcoal may prevent systemic absorption.

Nursing Responsibilities:

- Assess for personal or family history of bipolar disorder because these patients have a higher suicide risk while on this medication.
- Perform a comprehensive cardiovascular examination. Sudden cardiac death, strokes, and MI have occurred in patients with serious cardiac disease or those with structural abnormalities of the heart.
- Assess the patient for the effectiveness of treatment and symptom control.
- Assess cardiovascular status such as blood pressure and heart rate because HTN and tachycardia may occur.
- Monitor aspartate transaminase (AST) and alanine transaminase (ALT) levels periodically during medication administration and assess for hepatotoxicity.
- Monitor for abnormal behavior or increased anxiety, agitation, and aggression, which may indicate the need to discontinue the medication or adjust the dosage.

Patient and Family Education:

- Immediately report signs and symptoms of chest pain, palpitations, urinary retention, appetite loss, weight loss, thoughts of suicide, yellowing of the eyes or skin, or insomnia.
- Make position changes slowly when moving from a lying to a standing position to prevent dizziness and possible fainting.
- Do not drive or perform other hazardous activities until the effects of the drug are known because this drug can cause drowsiness or dizziness.
- Do not breast-feed while taking this drug without approval of the health care provider.

Drugs Similar to Atomoxetine (Strattera)

There are no drugs similar to atomoxetine (Strattera).

Pharmacotherapy of Narcolepsy

28.5 Narcolepsy is characterized by excessive daytime sleepiness and is treated with central nervous system stimulants and antidepressants.

Narcolepsy is a chronic neurologic disorder in which the patient suffers from excessive daytime sleepiness. The disorder affects 1 in 2,000 Americans and usually begins in childhood, although it may not be diagnosed until adulthood. Narcolepsy is caused by a deficiency in certain neurotransmitters in the neurons in the hypothalamus, a region responsible for controlling sleep patterns. The patient experiences an abnormal pattern of rapid eye movement (REM) sleep during the night, which causes the patient to have a "deficit" of restful sleep. There is a genetic predisposition to acquiring the disorder.

Narcolepsy is characterized by four symptoms, which separate it from other types of sleep disorders. Patients with narcolepsy may not experience all four symptoms.

- Sleep attacks. **Sleep attacks** are sudden bouts of sleep that last 10 to 30 minutes and may occur during the daytime without warning.
- Cataplexy. Approximately 90% of patients who suffer from narcolepsy experience **cataplexy,** a bilateral loss of muscle tone and emotion. The cataplexy may last from several seconds to minutes, and symptoms range from clumsiness to complete collapse.
- Sleep paralysis. Approximately 60% of patients diagnosed with narcolepsy suffer from **sleep paralysis,** which is the temporary inability to move after waking up from sleep.

- Hypnagogic hallucinations. **Hypnagogic hallucinations** are vivid, dreamlike sensations, sometimes of a frightening nature, that occur with sleep paralysis.

Severe narcolepsy can be disabling and interfere with normal activities such as employment or success at school. To accommodate their disorder, the patient may require a schedule that includes several 15-minute daytime naps.

PharmFACT

After obstructive sleep apnea and restless legs syndrome, narcolepsy is the third most frequently diagnosed primary sleep disorder found in patients seeking treatment at sleep clinics. Up to 10% of patients diagnosed with narcolepsy and cataplexy together report having a close relative with the same symptoms. *Source:* National Institute of Neurological Disorders and Stroke, 2008.

The goal of narcolepsy pharmacotherapy is to reduce the incidence of daytime drowsiness and other symptoms associated with the disorder. Traditional therapies have focused on CNS stimulants. Dextroamphetamine and methylphenidate are approved to treat narcolepsy (see Section 28.3). The CNS stimulants are effective at reducing daytime drowsiness but may cause nervousness, insomnia, and dependence. A newer stimulant, modafinil, has become widely used in the treatment of narcolepsy and is the prototype for this disorder. The dose of modafinil is listed in Table 28.3.

CNS stimulants are not effective at treating cataplexy. Antidepressants such as selegiline (Eldepryl), imipramine (Tofranil), and fluoxetine (Prozac) have been used off-label to treat cataplexy and are effective at treating this disorder in about 80% of patients. The only agent specifically approved by the FDA for treating cataplexy is sodium oxybate (gamma-hydroxybutyrate, GHB, Xyrem). Sodium oxybate reduces daytime sleepiness as well as episodes of cataplexy, sleep paralysis, and hypnagogic hallucinations.

PROTOTYPE DRUG Modafinil (Provigil, Alertec)

Classification: **Therapeutic:** Narcolepsy agent
Pharmacologic: CNS stimulant

Therapeutic Effects and Uses: Approved in 1998, modafinil is an oral drug used to treat patients with narcolepsy and to treat excessive sleepiness associated with shift work (circadian rhythm disruption). The drug increases daytime alertness and locomotor activity. Modafinil may also be prescribed to treat fatigue related to Parkinson's disease, obstructive sleep apnea, and multiple sclerosis.

Similar to amphetamines, modafinil can induce euphoria and psychoactive symptoms. Although the abuse potential for modafinil is less than other CNS stimulants, it is still classified as a Schedule IV controlled substance. It does not appear to suppress appetite or promote weight loss.

Mechanism of Action: The mechanism by which modafinil exerts its wake-promoting effects is unknown.

Pharmacokinetics:

Route(s)	PO
Absorption	Rapid
Distribution	Distributed to most tissues; unknown if secreted in breast milk; approximately 60% bound to protein
Primary metabolism	Hepatic
Primary excretion	Renal
Onset of action	Peak: 2–4 h
Duration of action	Half-life: 15 h

Adverse Effects: Serious adverse effects from modafinil are infrequent. The primary CNS adverse effects are headache, nervousness, insomnia, cataplexy, and paresthesia. Cardiovascular adverse effects include increased and decreased blood pressure, vasodilation, and syncope. Nausea, vomiting, diarrhea, and dry mouth are frequent gastrointestinal (GI) adverse effects. Pulmonary effects include pharyngitis, rhinitis, and dyspnea. Cases of Stevens–Johnson syndrome (SJS) have been reported.

Contraindications/Precautions: Modafinil should not be administered to patients who suffer from acute MI, valvular heart disease, and hypersensitivity to modafinil. The safety of the medication has not been established in patients younger than age 16. The drug should be discontinued at the first sign of rash because SJS has been reported with the use of modafinil. The drug should be used with caution in patients with schizophrenia because it may worsen symptoms of patients with psychotic disorders and may cause suicide ideation. The drug should be used with caution in those with a history of substance abuse. Severe hepatic impairment may increase serum modafinil levels as much as 50%; doses in these patients must be reduced to prevent toxicity.

Drug Interactions: CYP450 enzymes metabolize modafinil, and the drug can inhibit and induce different isozymes. For example, modafinil inhibits CYP2C19, the primary metabolic enzyme for phenytoin, diazepam, and propranolol; levels of these drugs increase when given concurrently with modafinil. When modafinil is administered with cyclosporine, the therapeutic levels of cyclosporine decrease. Modafinil may increase the levels of clomipramine and warfarin. TCA levels increase with modafinil. Modafinil may decrease the effectiveness of oral contraceptives and cause unplanned pregnancies. **Herbal/Food:** Foods and beverages containing caffeine can increase insomnia.

Pregnancy: Category C.

Treatment of Overdose: Overdose causes agitation, insomnia, anxiety, aggressiveness, palpitations, and confusion. Overdoses are usually not fatal. The patient should receive supportive treatment and gastric lavage.

Nursing Responsibilities:

- Assess for improved daytime wakefulness.
- Assess blood pressure and cardiovascular status; patients may require a new or increased dose of antihypertensive medication.

- Monitor for signs and symptoms of psychosis, especially in patients with a history of psychiatric illness.
- Monitor aspartate transaminase (AST) and alanine transaminase (ALT) levels periodically during medication administration and assess for hepatotoxicity.
- Assess international normalized ratio (INR) in patients receiving warfarin (Coumadin) to determine abnormalities in coagulation time.
- Assess for signs of rash. Immediately discontinue the drug at the first indication of rash and notify the prescriber.

Patient and Family Education:

- Take the dose in the morning because taking it late in the day may cause insomnia.
- Do not breast-feed while taking this drug without approval of the health care provider.
- Do not drive or perform other hazardous activities until the effects of the drug are known because this drug may cause drowsiness or dizziness.
- Do not drink alcohol because this will interfere with the beneficial effects of the medication.
- Do not discontinue the drug abruptly because excessive sleepiness may occur.
- Immediately report signs and symptoms of an allergic reaction such as rash, hives, or shortness of breath.
- Do not take any other prescription or nonprescription drugs, dietary supplements, or herbal products without approval of the health care provider.
- Use barrier methods of birth control because this drug may decrease the effectiveness of oral contraceptives.
- Immediately report psychiatric symptoms such as suicidal thoughts, depression, hallucinations, or excessive excitement.

Drugs Similar to Modafinil (Provigil, Alertec)

Antidepressants used to treat narcolepsy are presented in Chapter 23, and the amphetamines are discussed in Section 25.3. Sodium oxybate is the only other drug specifically indicated for narcolepsy.

Armodafinil (Nuvagil): Approved in 2007, armodafinil is very closely related to modafinil. It is approved to treat narcolepsy, shift work sleep disorder, and to improve wakefulness in patients with obstructive sleep apnea who often experience daytime drowsiness. It has the same adverse effects as modafinil and is a Schedule IV controlled substance. This drug is pregnancy category C.

Sodium oxybate (Xyrem): Sodium oxybate is a very unusual drug because it is the sodium salt of a Schedule I controlled substance, known as gamma hydroxybutyrate (GHB). GHB can produce euphoria, sedation, and amnesia and is known as a "date rape" drug (see Chapter 8). Classified as a Schedule III controlled substance, sodium oxybate is only available from a centralized pharmacy to approved health care providers due to its abuse potential. Sodium oxybate is approved for excessive daytime sleepiness associated with narcolepsy and for symptoms of cataplexy. The drug is sometimes administered with CNS stimulants in the management of narcolepsy. The most frequently reported adverse effects are headache, nausea, vomiting, dizziness, depression, and drowsiness. This drug is pregnancy category B.

CONNECTION *Checkpoint* 28.3

From what you learned in Chapter 22, describe the four stages of normal sleep. During which stage does most of the active dreaming occur? See Answer to Connection Checkpoint 28.3 in Appendix A.

Methylxanthines

28.6 Methylxanthines are central nervous system stimulants used for their ability to increase alertness or their effects on the respiratory system.

Methylxanthines are agents similar to xanthine, a chemical produced during the breakdown of deoxyribonucleic acid (DNA). Unlike the other CNS stimulants discussed in this chapter, the methylxanthines are not used for their effects on the brain. Instead, the methylxanthines are associated with treating patients with chronic obstructive pulmonary disease (COPD), asthma, and other restrictive lung diseases due to their ability to relax bronchial smooth muscle. The methylxanthines include caffeine, theophylline, and theobromine. Caffeine is the prototype drug for the methylxanthines. The dose of caffeine is listed in Table 28.3.

Theophylline and theobromine are formed by the metabolic breakdown of caffeine in the liver. Although rarely used, theophylline is still available as a drug to treat asthma that is resistant to other therapies. Theobromine is a natural substance found in chocolate that once was used as a drug to treat HTN and other vascular disorders. Although similar to caffeine, it has very little CNS stimulant activity.

PROTOTYPE DRUG Caffeine

Classification: **Therapeutic:** CNS and respiratory stimulant
Pharmacologic: Methylxanthine

Therapeutic Effects and Uses: Caffeine is a methylxanthine naturally found in over 60 plant species. Most consumption in the United States is from coffee, tea, soft drinks, chocolate, and energy beverages. Caffeine has potent psychoactive properties. When taken orally it quickly restores mental alertness and aids in wakefulness. In addition to its consumption in beverages and food, caffeine is also available in OTC products designed to increase alertness and delay fatigue.

The only FDA-approved indication for caffeine is as a respiratory stimulant in the management of apnea in premature infants. For this indication, caffeine (Cafcit) may be administered IV or by the oral route, added to formula feedings.

Caffeine also has a number of off-label indications. In patients who suffer from asthma, orally administered caffeine will produce bronchodilation and smooth muscle relaxation. Caffeine produces a mild diuresis due to increased blood flow to the glomerulus and has been used as an OTC diuretic product. Caffeine can be administered IV to relieve headache associated with lumbar puncture.

Caffeine itself has no analgesic properties. However, it enhances pain relief when administered with a narcotic analgesic. Caffeine is also combined with ergotamine (Cafergot) in the treatment of migraine headaches. It may be administered parenterally in emergency situations to treat circulatory collapse.

Mechanism of Action: Caffeine is metabolized in the liver to theobromine and theophylline, both of which are active metabolites that enhance the CNS and respiratory stimulant effects of caffeine. When higher doses are administered the medulla, respiratory center, and vagus nerve are stimulated and produce a relaxation of smooth muscle, which is particularly evident in the bronchi and coronary and systemic blood vessels.

Pharmacokinetics:

Route(s)	PO, intramuscular (IM), IV
Absorption	Rapidly absorbed
Distribution	Widely distributed; crosses the blood–brain barrier and the placenta: secreted in breast milk; 36% bound to plasma proteins
Primary metabolism	Hepatic
Primary excretion	Renal
Onset of action	15–45 minutes
Duration of action	Half-life: 3–5 h in adults; 36–144 h in neonates

Adverse Effects: Caffeine may cause adverse effects at therapeutic doses, many of which are extensions of its pharmacologic actions. Excessive CNS stimulation may cause nervousness, insomnia, tremors, and restlessness. The cardiovascular effects of caffeine include tingling of the face, palpitations, tachycardia, bradycardia, and ventricular ectopic beats. GI effects noted with the administration of caffeine are related to the stimulation of the vagus nerve and include nausea, vomiting, epigastric pain, hematemesis, and kernicterus in neonates. Clonic seizures can result in rare instances. Caffeine withdrawal can produce symptoms of irritability, headache, lethargy, or anxiety.

Contraindications/Precautions: Caffeine should not be administered during acute MI or to patients with cardiac dysrhythmias because the drug increases the workload of the heart. Caffeine increases the secretion of gastric acid; therefore, patients who suffer from peptic ulcer disease should limit their caffeine intake. Patients with anxiety disorders, insomnia, or panic attacks should not be administered caffeine because it may worsen these conditions. It should be used cautiously in patients with diabetes mellitus, hiatal hernia, HTN, and heart disease. Patients with hepatic or renal impairment should receive lower doses because the drug may accumulate to toxic levels.

Drug Interactions: Caffeine administered with cimetidine will increase the effect of cimetidine. Beta-adrenergic agonists administered with caffeine will result in increased cardiovascular stimulation. Additive effects are likely if the drug is taken concurrently with other CNS stimulants. Patients taking drugs for insomnia or anxiety should limit their intake of caffeine. Caffeine is a substrate of hepatic cytochrome CYP1A2. Drugs that enhance or inhibit this enzyme may interact with caffeine. **Herbal/Food:** Food and fluids that contain caffeine will increase the insomnia or restlessness that is normally noted with methylxanthines.

Pregnancy: Category B (Cafcit is labeled as category C).

Treatment of Overdose: Caffeine overdose can potentially cause dysrhythmias, insomnia, delirium, and seizures. The patient is supported through symptom management. High serum levels of caffeine can be dialyzed with peritoneal or hemodialysis.

Nursing Responsibilities:

- Assess vital signs during IV medication administration.
- Assess for improvement of the breathing pattern of neonates.
- Assess children for adverse effects due to the increased susceptibility to CNS effects.
- Assess blood glucose in patients with diabetes because this drug may increase or decrease glucose tolerance.
- Assess for signs and symptoms of excessive CNS stimulation.

Patient and Family Education:

- Limit consumption of food or beverages that contain large amounts of caffeine because this may cause anxiety, irritability, headache, and nervousness.
- If the patient has diabetes, take frequent blood glucose measurements and immediately report significant changes.
- Immediately report seizures, palpitations, or tremor.

Drugs Similar to Caffeine

Theophylline is the only other methylxanthine used as a drug.

Theophylline: Theophylline is not used to treat ADHD, but it is administered to produce bronchodilation in patients suffering from acute bronchospasm. It decreases wheezing and obstructed airways in asthma and bronchitis. It is important to note that the medication is a CNS stimulant that can produce restlessness, insomnia, and irritability. Close monitoring is required to prevent drug toxicity. Once widely prescribed, theophylline use has declined due to the development of safer drugs for patients with asthma (see Chapter 73).

NURSING PROCESS APPLICATION

Patients Receiving Pharmacotherapy for Attention Deficit/Hyperactivity Disorder and Narcolepsy

Assessment

Prior to administration:

- Obtain a complete health history, including allergies, drug history, and possible drug interactions.
- Obtain a history of neurologic, cardiac, renal, biliary, and mental disorders, including blood studies such as liver enzymes and renal function.
- Assess neurologic status, including identification of recent behavioral patterns.
- Assess growth and development.

Potential Nursing Diagnosis

- *Risk for Delayed Development,* related to growth retardation, secondary to cerebral stimulants.
- *Delayed Growth and Development,* related to increased motor activity, and growth retardation, secondary to cerebral stimulants and unsuccessful interpersonal relationships.
- *Imbalanced Nutrition: Less than Body Requirements,* related to adverse effects of drug therapy
- *Deficient Knowledge (Drug Therapy)*

Planning: Patient Goals and Expected Outcomes

The patient will:

- Experience subjective improvement in attention and concentration and reduction in impulsivity and psychomotor symptoms.
- Demonstrate an understanding of the drug's action by accurately describing drug adverse effects and precautions.

Implementation

Interventions and (Rationales)	Patient and Family Education
• Monitor mental status and observe for changes in level of consciousness and adverse effects. (Medication may cause persistent drowsiness, psychomotor agitation, anxiety, dizziness, trembling, or seizures.)	• Instruct the patient to report any significant increase in motor behavior, changes in sensorium, or feelings of dysphoria.
• Use caution in the administration of cerebral stimulants with seizure disorders. (Medication may lower the seizure threshold.)	Instruct the patient to: • Discontinue medication immediately if seizures occur. • Notify the health care provider of onset of seizure activity.
• Monitor GI and nutritional status. (CNS stimulants cause anorexia and increase basal metabolic rate, producing weight loss. Other GI effects include nausea, vomiting, and abdominal pain.)	Instruct the patient to: • Immediately report rapid heart rate, palpitations, or dizziness. • Take blood pressure and pulse rate regularly and report significant changes.
• Monitor the effectiveness of drug therapy. (Dosage may be modified if symptoms continue.)	Instruct the patient to: • Report any GI adverse effects. • Take medication with meals to reduce GI upset and to counteract anorexia; eat frequent, small nutritious and high-calorie snacks. • Assess weight weekly and report losses of over 1 lb.
• Monitor growth and development. (Growth may be stalled in response to nutritional deficiency related to anorexia.)	• Instruct the patient that reductions in growth rate are associated with drug usage. (Washout periods or drug holidays decrease this effect.)
• Monitor laboratory tests such as liver and renal function. (Some drugs in this class are toxic to the liver and kidneys.)	Instruct the patient to: • Report shortness of breath, fatigue, pallor, or bleeding. • Report nausea, vomiting, diarrhea, rash, jaundice, abdominal pain, or changes in stool. • Obtain periodic liver and renal function testing.
• Monitor sleep–wake cycle. (CNS stimulants may disrupt normal sleep patterns.)	Instruct the patient that: • Insomnia is an adverse effect. • Sleeplessness can sometimes be counteracted by taking the last dose no later than 4 p.m. • Medication is not intended to treat fatigue. Fatigue may accompany the washout period.

Evaluation of Outcome Criteria

Evaluate the effectiveness of drug therapy by confirming that patient goals and expected outcomes have been met (see "Planning").

UNDERSTANDING THE CHAPTER

Key Concepts Summary

28.1 Central nervous system stimulants increase alertness, enhance the ability to concentrate, and delay the symptoms of fatigue.

28.2 Attention deficit/hyperactivity disorder is characterized by inattention, hyperactivity, and impulsive behavior.

28.3 Amphetamines are central nervous system stimulants indicated for the treatment of attention deficit/hyperactivity disorder and narcolepsy.

28.4 Atomoxetine (Strattera) is a newer drug for treating attention deficit/hyperactivity disorder that does not stimulate the central nervous system.

28.5 Narcolepsy is characterized by excessive daytime sleepiness and is treated with central nervous system stimulants and antidepressants.

28.6 Methylxanthines are central nervous system stimulants used for their ability to increase alertness or their effects on the respiratory system.

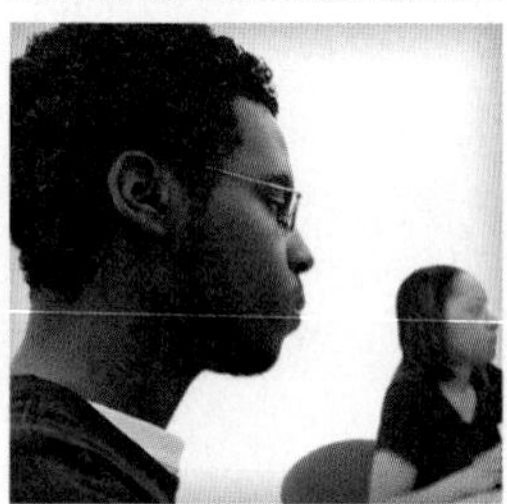

Making the PATIENT *Connection*

Remember the patient "Jonathon Hogan" at the beginning of the chapter? Now read the remainder of the case study. Based on the information presented within this chapter, respond to the critical thinking questions that follow.

Jonathon Hogan was diagnosed with ADHD at the age of 12. Now at the age of 22 years, he is taking atomoxetine (Strattera) 80 mg PO daily. Jonathon has adhered to the drug therapy since it was prescribed. He states that he is concerned about entering an evening nursing program.

Critical Thinking Questions

1. What is ADHD and why would Jonathon be concerned about entering an evening nursing program?
2. What assessments would the nurse want to make regarding his medications and the nursing care for ADHD?
3. What patient education would be appropriate regarding atomoxetine (Strattera)?

Case Study

Anna Steinmetz has graduated from nursing school and is working nights. She is having difficulty adjusting to her night schedule. Her health care provider suggested she utilize a medication to assist with her adjustment to shift work. She has been prescribed modafinil (Provigil, Alertec).

1. What effect does modafinil (Provigil, Alertec) have on the patient's ability to maintain alertness during shift work?
2. What patient teaching will you provide to the patient regarding this medication?
3. The patient complains of feelings of light-headedness with position changes. What interventions will assist in maintaining patient safety?

NCLEX-RN® Review

1 An elementary school nurse is providing education to the faculty on the use of cerebral stimulants. Of the following, which is most important for the nurse to convey to the faculty?

1. Provide an environment that is active and overly stimulating.
2. Use low-calorie snacks for students on cerebral stimulants.
3. Position the child at the back of the classroom.
4. Be aware that a student needs a period without the stimulants.

2 Which of the following outcomes would the nurse consider most significant in evaluating a client who started atomoxetine (Strattera) 6 months ago?

1. Decrease in attention
2. Decrease in hyperactivity
3. Development of mydriasis
4. Elevated liver enzymes

3 A client who has overdosed on amphetamine sulfate (Adderall XR) is admitted to the emergency department. The nurse would anticipate which of the following medications to be administered to assist in counteracting the effects of the overdosage?

1. Chlorpromazine
2. Phenytoin (Dilantin)
3. Sodium pentothal (Pentothal)
4. Dexamethasone (Decadron)

4 A high school student visits the school nurse's office and states, "I am so depressed. The world would be better off without me." Which of the following medications would have the greatest effect on the development of suicidal ideations?

1. Atomoxetine (Strattera)
2. Amphetamine sulfate (Adderall XR)
3. Modafinil (Provigil, Alertec)
4. Caffeine

5 While the nurse is taking a health history, the client falls asleep suddenly and becomes flaccid. Within a few minutes the client wakes up and appears somewhat confused. What condition might the nurse suspect?

1. Hyperkinetic disorder
2. Narcolepsy
3. Tonic–clonic seizure
4. Transient ischemia attack

6 A client who is taking atomoxetine (Strattera) for attention deficit/hyperactivity disorder complains of insomnia. Which of the following interventions will assist in the promotion of sleep?

1. Have a glass of wine with dinner.
2. Eat a chocolate bar at bedtime.
3. Drink a high-energy drink at 4 p.m.
4. Switch to decaffeinated coffee.

See Answers to Critical Thinking Questions, Case Study, and NCLEX-RN® Review in Appendix A.

References

American Psychiatric Association. (2000). *Diagnostic and statistical manual of mental disorders* (4th ed., Text revision). Washington, DC: Author.

Ball, J. W., & Bindler, R. C. (2006). *Child health nursing: Partnering with children and families.* Upper Saddle River, NJ: Pearson Education.

Biederman, J., & Faraone, S. V. (2005). Attention-deficit hyperactivity disorder. *The Lancet, 366,* 237–248.

Buck, M. L. (2003). Atomoxetine: A new alternative for the treatment of attention deficit/hyperactivity disorder. *Pediatric Pharmacology, 9*(2). Retrieved June 24, 2008, from http://www.medscape.com/viewarticle/452714_print

Busko, M. (2008). Adult ADHD is common among patients in anxiety-disorders clinics. *Medscape Medical News.* Retrieved June 24, 2008, from http://www.medscape.com/viewarticle/571537

Dauvilliers, Y., Arnulf, I., & Mignot, E. (2007). Narcolepsy with cataplexy. *The Lancet, 369*(9560), 499–511.

Department of Health and Human Services, Centers for Disease Control and Prevention. (2001). *Attention-deficit/hyperactivity disorder—A public health perspective.* Retrieved June 24, 2008, from http://www.cdc.gov/ncbddd/factsheets/ADHD_public_health.pdf

Devinsky, O. (2004). Therapy for neurobehavioral disorders in epilepsy. *Epilepsia, 45*(2), 34–40.

Divadeenam, K. (2008). Stimulants. *emedicine.* Retrieved June 24, 2008, from http://www.emedicine.com/med/topic3094.htm

Dodson, W. W. (2005). Pharmacotherapy of adult ADHD. *Journal of Clinical Psychology/In Session, 61*(5), 589–606.

Lesesne, C., Abramowitz, A., Perou, R., & Brann, E. (2000). *Attention deficit/hyperactivity disorder(ADHD): ADHD research agenda.* Retrieved June 24, 2008, from http://www.cdc.gov/ncbddd/adhd/dadagenda.htm

Markowitz, J. S., Straughn, A. B., & Patrick, K. S. (2003). Advances in the pharmacotherapy of attention-deficit-hyperactivity disorder: Focus on methylphenidate formulations. *Pharmacotherapy, 23*(10), 1281–1299.

Retrieved June 24, 2008, from http://www.medscape.com/viewarticle/462703_print

National Institute of Mental Health. (2006). *Attention deficit hyperactivity disorder.* Retrieved June 24, 2008, from http://www.nimh.nih.gov/health/publications/adhd/complete-publication.shtml

National Institute of Neurological Disorders and Stroke. (2008). *Narcolepsy fact sheet.* Retrieved June 24, 2008, from http://www.ninds.nih.gov/disorders/narcolepsy/detail_narcolepsy.htm

Robison, L. M., Skaer, T., Sclar, D. A., & Galin, R. S. (2002). Is attention deficit hyperactivity disorder increasing among girls in the US? Trends in diagnosis and the prescribing of stimulants. *CNS Drugs, 16*(2), 129–137.

Rushton, J. L., Fant, K. E., & Clark, S. J. (2004). Use of practice guidelines in the primary care of children with attention deficit hyperactivity disorder. *Pediatrics, 114*(1), 23–28.

Shireman, T. I., Reichard, A., & Rigler, S. K. (2005). Psychotropic medications use among Kansas Medicaid youths with disabilities. *Journal of Child and Adolescent Psychopharmacology, 15*(1), 107–115.

Wilens, T. E. (2003). Drug therapy for adults with attention-deficit disorder. *Drugs 2003, 63*(22), 2395–2411.

Wilens, T. E., Biederman, J., & Spencer, T. J. (2002). Attention deficit/hyperactivity disorder across the lifespan. *Annual Review of Medicine, 53,* 113–131.

Wilens, T. E., Faraone, S. V., Biederman, J., & Gunawardene, S. (2003). Does stimulant therapy of attention-deficit/hyperactivity disorder beget later substance abuse? A meta-analytic review of the literature. *Pediatrics, 111*(1), 179–185.

Wolkove, N., Elkholy, O., Baltzan, M., & Palayew, M. (2007). Sleep and aging: Management of sleep disorders in older people. *Canadian Medical Association Journal, 176*(10), 1449–1454.

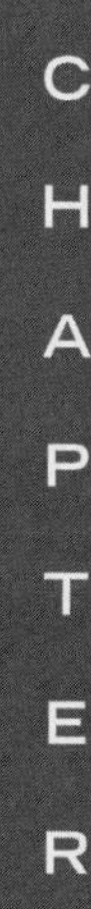

I'm having urological surgery tomorrow and I am worried about pain. I've taken pain medicine daily for years because of chronic pain from back problems and numerous back surgeries. Will I experience severe pain after this procedure?

Patient "Larry Smith"

Pharmacotherapy of Severe Pain and Migraines

29

Chapter Outline

General Principles of Pain Management

Pharmacotherapy of Acute and Chronic Pain

Opioid Analgesics

PROTOTYPE **Morphine Sulfate (Astramorph PF, Duramorph RF, Roxanol, Others)** *p. 437*

Mixed Agonist-Antagonist Opioids

Nonopioid Analgesics

Nonsteroidal Anti-Inflammatory Drugs (NSAIDs) and Acetaminophen

Centrally Acting Analgesics

PROTOTYPE **Tramadol (Ultram)** *p. 442*

Adjuvant Analgesics

Pharmacotherapy with Opioid Antagonists

PROTOTYPE **Naloxone (Narcan)** *p. 447*

Pharmacotherapy of Migraines

PROTOTYPE **Sumatriptan (Imitrex)** *p. 451*

Learning Outcomes

After reading this chapter, the student should be able to:

1. Identify changes that have occurred in pain management over the past two decades.
2. Differentiate the types and classifications of pain.
3. Refute the common pain myths, using objective evidence.
4. Explain the phases of pain physiology: transduction, transmission, modulation, and perception.
5. Describe the role of nonpharmacologic therapies in pain management.
6. Describe the nursing assessment of pain.
7. Identify the classes of drugs used for minor, moderate, and severe pain.
8. Compare and contrast the actions of opioid agonists, mixed opioid agonists-antagonists, and opioid antagonists.
9. Describe the advantages of combining opioid, nonopioid, and adjuvant analgesics in the treatment of pain.
10. Compare and contrast the actions and adverse effects of the opioids and nonopioids for analgesia.
11. For each of the classes shown in the chapter outline, identify the prototype and representative drugs and explain the mechanism(s) of drug action, primary indications and contraindications, significant drug interactions, pregnancy category, and important adverse effects.
12. Explain the role of opioid antagonists in the diagnosis and treatment of acute opioid toxicity.
13. Compare the pharmacotherapeutic approaches of preventing migraines to those of aborting migraines.
14. Use the nursing process to care for patients receiving drug therapy for pain.

Key Terms

addiction, *429*
adjuvant analgesics, *444*
analgesics, *429*
auras, *449*
endorphins, *431*
gate control theory, *430*
kappa receptors, *434*
migraine, *449*
mu receptors, *434*
narcotic, *434*
neuropathic pain, *429*
nociceptors, *428*
nociceptor pain, *429*
nonopioid analgesics, *442*
opiates, *434*
opioids, *434*
opium, *434*
tension headache, *449*

Pain is a subjective experience that has both physiological and emotional components. Usually associated with trauma or disease, pain may be viewed as a natural defense mechanism that helps people avoid potentially damaging situations and encourages them to seek medical help. Pain medications are some of the most frequently prescribed drugs in medicine. This chapter examines the drug classes used in pain management and for the pharmacotherapy of migraines.

General Principles of Pain Management

29.1 Strategies for pain management have changed over the past two decades.

In recent years health care professionals have come to realize that accurate pain assessment and treatment are essential for quality patient care. To this end, the American Pain Society coined the phrase "Pain: The Fifth Vital Sign" to elevate the awareness of pain treatment among health care providers. Many health care agencies now include assessment of pain as part of the process of monitoring vital signs.

The perception of pain can clearly be influenced by comorbid conditions such as anxiety, fatigue, and depression. For example, knowing that health care providers and caregivers are attentive and actively engaged in pain management lowers patients' anxiety associated with pain, thus reducing pain perception and increasing pain tolerance. Furthermore, culture and ethnicity can also influence pain perception and expression. Listening, showing respect, and allowing patients to help develop and choose treatment options consistent with their beliefs and customs are the most culturally sensitive approaches to attain optimum pain relief.

Beginning in the early 1990s, groups such as the American Pain Society established guidelines for the management of pain in different populations. The Agency for Health Care Policy and Research of the Public Health Service published *Guidelines for Clinicians*, summarizing research and recommendations for operative and procedure pain in adults, infants, children, and adolescents. Guidelines for the management of cancer pain and nonmalignant chronic pain followed. These guidelines have been updated regularly as research has determined optimum strategies for pain management. Current guidelines are periodically updated based on evidence-based practice research summaries.

An important and effective advance in pain management was the adoption of the guidelines on pain published by the Joint Commission on Accreditation of Healthcare Organizations (JCAHO) in 2001. Its standards required appropriate assessment and management of pain as an integral component of health care, essentially "guaranteeing" every patient the right to effective pain management. As a result of the guidelines, most institutions have implemented the practice of assessing every patient's pain from the time of admission, ensuring staff competency regarding pain management, and educating patients and their families about pain.

Pharm*FACT*

Pain in America

- Over 50 million Americans suffer from chronic pain, and nearly 25 million experience acute pain each year due to injuries or surgery.
- Back pain is the leading cause of disability in Americans under 45 years old.
- Pain costs an estimated $100 billion each year, including over 50 million lost workdays per year.
- At least 70% of those with cancer experience significant pain during their illness, yet fewer than half receive adequate pain relief. *Source:* American Pain Foundation, n.d.

29.2 Pain is classified by its duration and its source.

The purpose of classifying pain is to guide appropriate treatment rationales based on the type of pain reported by the patient. A simple classification is to group types of pain as either acute or chronic. Acute pain is of brief duration, usually from injury; it subsides as healing takes place or the stimulus ceases. Examples of acute pain include that associated with surgical incisions, labor and delivery, sprained joints, or myocardial infarction (MI). Although it may be severe, acute pain is often self-limiting; high doses of pain medication may be necessary but therapy is usually limited to several weeks. There is little risk of chronic drug adverse effects or dependence because of the relatively short length of the treatment period.

Chronic pain persists longer than 6 months, can interfere with daily activities, and is sometimes associated with feelings of helplessness or hopelessness. Chronic pain can be further classified as either nonmalignant or malignant (cancer) pain. Chronic nonmalignant pain is not life threatening and usually responds favorably to a consistent, stable dose of pain medication as part of a treatment regimen. The most common example is low back pain. Cancer pain ends with control of the disease or death. Although the majority of patients with cancer experience pain during the advanced stages of the disease, 90% of the cancer pain can be controlled with oral (PO) drugs, using around-the-clock dosing, with prn doses or augmentation as needed for breakthrough pain.

Pain can also be classified as to its source. **Nociceptors** are the sensory nerve receptors strategically located throughout

CONNECTIONS

Evidence-Based Practice Best Practices in Acute and Cancer Pain Management

Clinical Question

What are the best approaches for managing acute and cancer pain?

Pain is a phenomenon that causes most individuals to seek health care. It is estimated that one in four Americans suffers an episode of pain lasting longer than 24 hours annually. Additionally, each year cancer-related pain afflicts approximately 9 million people worldwide. Treatment approaches for pain are numerous and range from pharmacotherapy to guided imagery and meditation.

Evidence

The American Pain Society set out to revise and expand its 1995 Quality Improvement (QI) Guidelines for the Treatment of Acute Pain and Cancer Pain, based on current research literature. Eleven multidisciplinary experts (nurses, physicians, psychologists, and pharmacists) comprised the Quality of Care task force. MEDLINE and CINAHL databases were searched for the years 1999 to 2004 for articles on pain quality measurement and quality improvement that were published after the development of the 1995 guidelines. The task force systematically reviewed the 51 research reports that met the selection criteria (of 617 citations). Then 3,000 members of the American Pain Society provided input, and the task force synthesized the final set of recommendations.

Based on the research reviewed, as well as expert input, the task force developed five recommendations:

1. Recognize and treat pain promptly.
2. Involve patients in the pain management plan.
3. Improve treatment patterns; eliminate inappropriate practices and provide multimodal therapy.
4. Reassess and adjust the pain management plan as needed.
5. Monitor the process and outcomes of pain management.

Critical Thinking Question

Select two or three of the preceding recommendations and develop strategies that the nurse can incorporate in the care of a patient suffering from acute or cancer pain.

See Answers to Critical Thinking Questions in Appendix A.

Source: From "American Pain Society Recommendations for Improving the Quality of Acute and Cancer Pain Management," by D. B. Gordon, J. L. Dahl, C. Miakowski, B. McCarberg, K. H. Todd, J. A. Paice, et al., July 25, 2005, *Archives of Internal Medicine, 165,* 1574–1580.

the body that initiate pain transmission when stimulated. Injury to tissues stimulates those receptors, producing **nociceptor pain.** This type of pain may be further subdivided into somatic pain, which produces sharp, localized sensations usually experienced in muscles and joints, or visceral pain, which is described as a generalized dull, throbbing, or aching pain usually located in internal organs. In contrast, **neuropathic pain** is caused by injury to nerves rather than stimulation of nerves by injury and typically is described as burning, shooting, or numbing pain. Nociceptor pain responds quite well to **analgesics,** which are medications that relieve pain. Analgesic treatment of neuropathic pain is less successful. However, adding nonanalgesic drugs, or adjuvant analgesics, concurrently with complementary and alternative therapies (CATs) may provide some degree of pain relief for these patients. CAT and adjuvant analgesics are discussed in Sections 29.5 and 29.12, respectively.

29.3 Health care providers and patients sometimes hold myths about pain that impede optimum pain management.

Commonly held but untrue beliefs by both patients and health care professionals often interfere with pain management. For example, health care providers may undertreat pain because of common misconceptions about pain. Furthermore, patients may not report their pain accurately or may refuse pain medications because of similar misconceptions.

A pervasive myth is that health care professionals can successfully recognize pain, independent of the patient's report. The nurse must understand that patients are the authorities on their own pain. Pain is whatever the patient says it is, existing whenever the patient says it does. Patient self-report of pain is sufficient for a nursing diagnosis of pain.

A closely related myth is that a person in pain must look and act like he or she is in pain. Some patients do not show or report pain accurately because they feel it is a sign of weakness. In addition, vital signs are sometimes unreliable indicators of pain. Although they may be elevated during the initial experience of acute pain owing to sympathetic arousal, vital signs return to normal as the body adapts. A related misconception is the belief that if a person is able to sleep, he or she must not be experiencing much pain. Although it is certainly true that pain can interfere with sleep quality and quantity, social withdrawal and excessive sleep may be indicators of coping mechanisms for some people with severe or chronic pain.

Both patients and health care providers may share the myth that the use of potent analgesics will lead to addiction. **Addiction** is an intense psychological drug craving accompanied by drug-seeking behavior (see Chapter 8). The incidence of addiction to opioids, which are used in the treatment of severe pain, is less than 1% in patients with no previous history of drug abuse. Related to this myth is the belief that patients experiencing chronic pain overreport pain because they are addicted to opioids.

A contradictory myth is the belief that the more pain a person experiences, the more he or she is likely to tolerate it. In fact, the opposite is more likely to occur. Unrelieved pain creates anxiety and fatigue, both of which increase pain perception and decrease tolerance. A related myth is that there is no physiological basis for the moderating effects of emotions of pain perception.

29.4 Pain transmission processes allow multiple targets for pharmacologic intervention.

Pain physiology has four phases: transduction, transmission, perception, and modulation. These phases are illustrated in Figure 29.1.

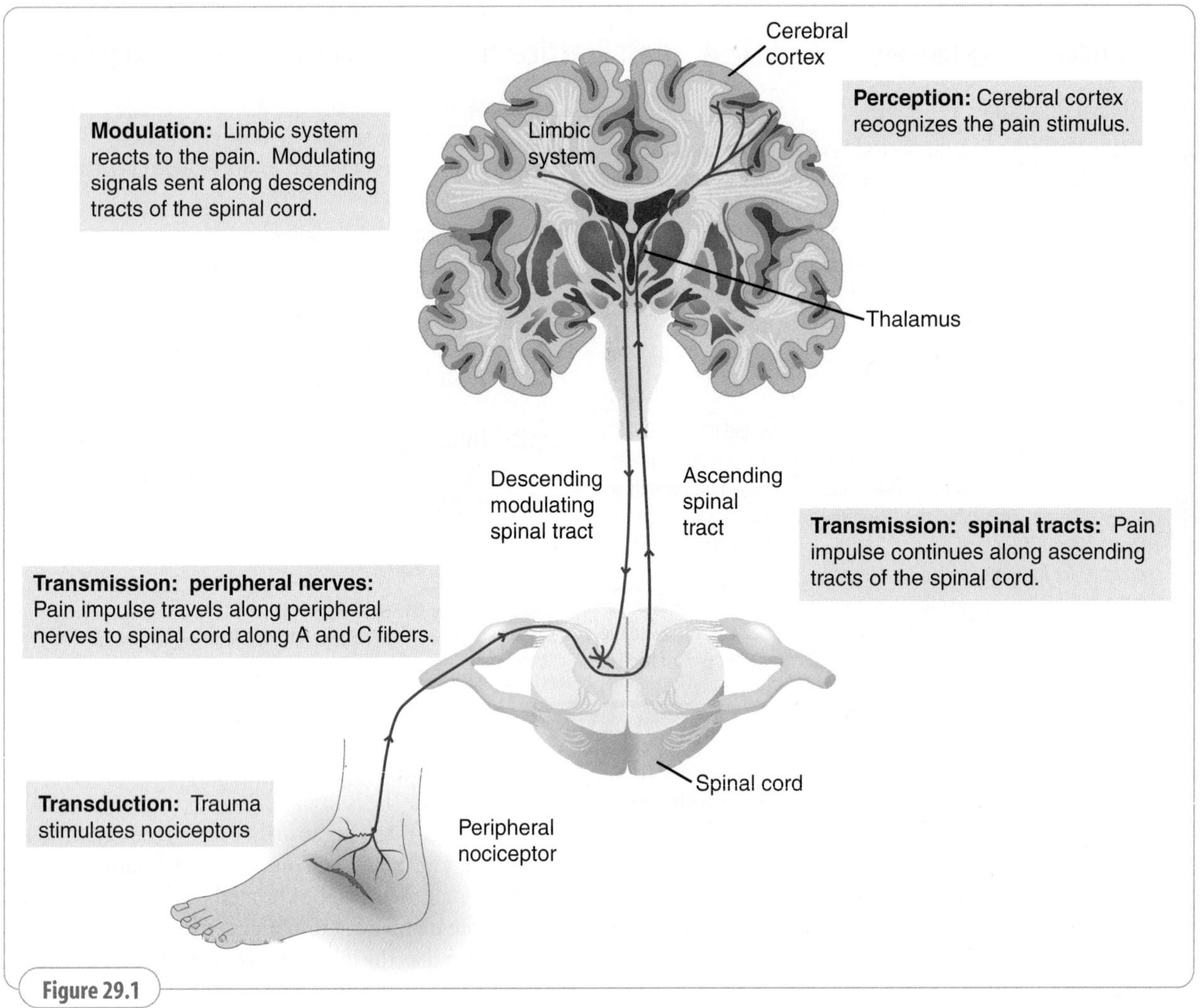

Figure 29.1

Phases of pain physiology.

Pain transduction: Pain transduction begins when nociceptor nerve endings in the peripheral nervous system are stimulated. This occurs when local tissue injury causes the release of chemical mediators of inflammation, including prostaglandins, leukotrienes, histamine, bradykinin, and substance P. These substances sensitize peripheral nociceptors, making them easier to activate.

Pain transmission: The nerve impulse signaling the pain travels from the nociceptor to the spinal cord along two types of sensory neurons called A and C fibers. A fibers are wrapped in myelin, a lipid substance that speeds nerve transmission, and carrry signals for intense, well-defined pain. On the other hand, C fibers are unmyelinated and thus carry information more slowly and conduct poorly localized pain, which is often perceived as burning or a dull ache.

There are three subtypes of A fibers: alpha (α), beta (β), and delta (Δ). Aα fibers have the fastest transmission and respond to touch and pressure on muscle; Aβ fibers are slower and respond to touch and pressure on skin. Finally, AΔ fibers are the slowest of the A fibers and respond to tissue injury, producing the sensation of sharp pain.

The sensory nerve fibers enter the dorsal horn of the spinal cord and have adjacent synapses in an area called the substantia gelatinosa. The **gate control theory** proposes a gating mechanism for the transmission of pain in the spinal cord. Signals from faster Aα or Aβ fibers reach the spinal cord and close the gate before those of C fibers reach the region (or gate), in effect blocking the transmission of these types of pain impulses. The gate control theory, proposed in 1965, has withstood the test of time and has been found to be more complex than originally proposed. The "gates" can also be closed when flooded with nonnociceptor impulses. Gate control explains the effectiveness of massage, transcutaneous electrical nerve stimulation, and possibly acupuncture in reducing pain.

Once a pain impulse reaches the spinal cord, neurotransmitters are responsible for passing the message along to the next neuron. At the spinal cord, glutamate is the neurotransmitter for A fibers, whereas both glutamate and substance P are neurotransmitters for C fibers. Impulse transmission from the spinal cord to the brain is moderated by both excitatory and inhibitory neurotransmitters. The activity of substance P may be affected by other neurotransmitters released from neurons in the central nervous system (CNS). One group of neurotransmitters functions as endogenous opioids, or natural pain modifiers; these include **endorphins** and enkephalins.

Pain perception: Perception, the conscious experience of pain, occurs in the brain. Numerous cortical structures and pathways are involved in perception, including the reticular activating system, the somatosensory system, and the limbic system (see Chapter 21). When the pain impulse reaches the brain, it may respond to the sensation with a wide variety of possible actions, ranging from signaling the skeletal muscles to jerk away from a sharp object to mental depression in those suffering from chronic pain.

Pain modulation: Modulation involves descending nervous impulses traveling down the spinal cord that inhibit afferent pain transmission via a feedback mechanism. Neurotransmitters such as serotonin, norepinephrine, and endogenous opioids (endorphins and enkephalins) inhibit pain transmission.

The four phases of pain physiology allow for multiple targets for the pharmacologic intervention of pain impulse transmission. The two primary classes of analgesics act at different locations: The nonsteroidal anti-inflammatory drugs (NSAIDs) act at the peripheral level, whereas the opioids act on the CNS. Drugs that affect or mimic the inhibitory neurotransmitters are used as adjuvant analgesics.

29.5 Nonpharmacologic interventions are often utilized to reduce and augment analgesic use.

Although drugs are quite effective at relieving pain in most patients, they can have significant adverse effects. For example, high doses of aspirin cause gastrointestinal (GI) bleeding, and the opioids can cause significant drowsiness and respiratory depression. Nonpharmacologic techniques may be used to attain adequate pain relief in place of drugs, or they may serve as adjuncts to analgesics. When used concurrently with medication, nonpharmacologic techniques may allow for improved comfort, lower doses, and the potential for fewer drug-related adverse events. Nondrug interventions should routinely be considered in the nursing plan of care for patients with pain. Some CATs used for reducing pain include the following:

- Relaxation and imagery
- Meditation
- Distraction, including art or music therapy, or laughter
- Application of cold or heat
- Massage
- Transcutaneous electrical nerve stimulation (TENS)
- Acupressure and acupuncture
- Therapeutic touch
- Energy therapies such as Reiki
- Biofeedback therapy

Some of these interventions are part of standard nursing practice and can be performed by nurses; for example, massage, relaxation, and heat and cold packs. Additional training is needed for therapeutic touch, Reiki, and acupressure or acupuncture. Some of these techniques appear to act by increasing endogenous endorphin release. Others use gate control as the probable physiological mechanism to reduce the perception of pain.

Patients with intractable cancer pain require more invasive techniques because rapidly growing tumors often press on vital tissues and nerves. Furthermore, chemotherapy and surgical treatments for cancer can cause severe pain. Radiation therapy may provide pain relief by shrinking solid tumors that may be pressing on nerves. Surgery may be used to reduce pain by removing part of or the entire tumor. Injection of alcohol or another neurotoxic substance into neurons is occasionally performed to cause nerve blocks. Nerve blocks irreversibly stop impulse transmission along the treated nerves and have the potential to provide total pain relief. Injection of local anesthetics or steroid hormones as nerve blocks can provide relief for months and is used for pain resulting from pressure on spinal nerves.

29.6 The overall goal of pain management is to maintain a patient pain level that allows self-care and activities of daily living.

Nursing management of pain involves all phases of the nursing process, including the use of both drug and nondrug interventions. The effectiveness of those interventions is regularly evaluated, and appropriate revisions are made to the plan of care based on therapeutic outcomes. Nursing process applications for patients receiving opioid therapy and patients receiving nonopioid therapy, are included later in this chapter.

Pain assessment: Pain is assessed as a baseline and regularly during analgesic therapy as the fifth vital sign (see Section 29.1). Pain assessment includes documenting the location, intensity, and quality (sharp, dull, burning) of the pain and any precipitating or relieving factors. For most adults, the 0 to 10 numeric rating scale is the standard for rating pain intensity, with 0 being no pain and 10 being the greatest pain imaginable. Alternative rating scales include the 0 to 10 Visual Analog scale and the Wong-Baker FACES pain rating scale for children 3 years of age and older as well as for adults with language difficulties. Rating scales such as the FLACC scale have been tested with children 3 months to 7 years (University of Michigan Health Systems, 2006). Each category (face, legs, activity, cry, consolability) is scored 0 to 2 and then added to get a 1 to 10 rating.

The patient's level of pain should be reassessed at appropriate time intervals following pharmacotherapy and nondrug interventions. The pain rating is used as a reference point, initially as a baseline level of pain and later as an indicator of effectiveness as to how well the treatment is achieving the patient's goals. Assessment needs to include the patient's ability to perform activities of daily living (ADLs) such as eating, sleeping, self-care, and ambulation—especially for chronic pain.

Goals and principles of pain management: The immediate goal of pain management is to reduce pain to a level that allows for reasonable ADLs. An acceptable level of pain is one that

MyNursingKit | The American Holistic Nurses Association

CONNECTIONS

Lifespan Considerations

Pain Assessment in the Very Young

Behavioral rating scales such as the FLACC scale have been tested with children 3 months to 7 years of age. Developed by the University of Michigan Health System, FLACC stands for the five categories assessed: face, legs, activity, cry, and consolability. Each category is scored 0 to 2 and then added to get a 0 to 10 rating. For example, an infant with a pain rating of 0 would have no particular facial expression (F), legs relaxed (L), be lying quietly (A), without crying (C), and relaxed (C). On the other extreme, a rating of 10 would be seen as an infant crying steadily, with a rigid body and drawn up or kicking legs, clenched jaw or quivering chin, and who is difficult to console or comfort.

Source: From *Pain Management Staff Development & Education: Part 4: Adult Pain Management Staff Education*, University of Michigan Health System, 2006. Retrieved September 19, 2008, from http://www.med.umich.edu/pain/apainmgt.htm

enables the patient to sleep, eat, and perform other required or desired physical activities. For acute pain the primary goal is to reduce pain during the healing process until the source of the pain is eliminated. For chronic pain the long-term goal is to reduce pain to a level that allows for self-care and ADLs. The patient should understand that the total elimination of chronic pain may not be a realistic goal, or that it may require a long period of treatment. Several key principles underlie the nursing management of pain:

- The patient must be considered the expert on his or her own pain; the nurse should always believe the patient's self-assessment of pain.
- Pain management is a patient right and should be based on the patient's goals. The rule is to "assess, treat, reassess, and continue to treat until the patient is comfortable or adverse effects prevent further treatment." If pain cannot be effectively managed, then a pain management specialist should be consulted.
- Nondrug interventions should routinely be utilized in pain management. A combination of therapies is optimum because different modalities work by different mechanisms, thus improving the effectiveness of pain management.
- Dosing should be individualized and titrated to produce the desired effect.
- Adverse effects should be actively and proactively managed.
- Preventive around-the-clock dosing for moderate to severe pain should be implemented. It is much easier to maintain a comfort level than to eliminate existing or escalating pain. A fixed dosing schedule avoids the unnecessary discomfort and anxiety sometimes associated with prn dosing.

Pharmacologic therapies: There are dozens of over-the-counter (OTC) and prescription pain medications available, and the selection of a specific medication depends on many factors. Foremost is the severity of the pain. The drug selected must be capable of providing adequate pain relief. Secondarily, the choice of analgesic depends on potential adverse events and drug interactions and contraindications. A key point is that every analgesic, even an OTC pain reliever, has the potential to cause serious adverse effects in susceptible patients. This reinforces the need to utilize nonpharmacologic therapies for pain relief whenever possible.

The two broad categories of analgesics are the opioids and nonopioids. A third category of drugs for the management of pain are the adjuvant analgesics. The adjuvant analgesics have no pain relief activity when used alone but they are able to enhance the analgesic action of opioids and nonopioids.

The drug class of choice for severe pain is the opioids. Minor to moderate pain is treated with nonopioids such as NSAIDs, centrally acting agents, or acetaminophen. There are dozens of opioids and NSAIDs to choose from and it is difficult for beginning students, and even experienced health care providers, to learn the subtle differences of drugs within each class. Although the large number of analgesics appears overwhelming, many of them are quite similar and prescribers most often use only a few drugs in each class. The various drugs used for analgesia and the levels at which they act are shown in Pharmacotherapy Illustrated 29.1.

The pharmacologic management of acute and chronic pain is based on the Analgesic Ladder proposed by the World Health Organization, shown in Figure 29.2. Pain ratings less than 4 are treated with nonopiod analgesics, CATs, or a combination of the two. When pain ratings become moderate (4 to 6), PO opioids are added to the baseline treatment. When pain is severe (7 to 10), parenteral opioids are used. If chronic pain has neuropathic qualities, adjuvant analgesics are added.

Opioid and nonopioid combinations: It is common practice to use opioid and nonopioid analgesics concurrently in the pharmacotherapy of pain. For convenience, these combinations are available as single, fixed-dose tablets or capsules. The two classes of analgesics work synergistically to relieve pain, and the dose of opioid can be kept small to avoid dependence and opioid-related adverse effects. Use of these combinations in chronic pain management has a dose ceiling due to the toxicities of the nonopioid analgesic. For example, patients taking a combination product containing acetaminophen need to have their liver enzyme levels monitored regularly and take care not to exceed the maximum daily dosages for acetaminophen. Common combination analgesics include:

- Vicodin or Lortab (hydrocodone, 5 mg; acetaminophen, 500 mg)
- Vicodin ES (hydrocodone, 7.5 mg; acetaminophen, 750 mg)
- Norco (hydrocodone, 5 to 10 mg; acetaminophen, 325 mg)
- Percocet (oxycodone HCl, 5 mg; acetaminophen, 325 mg)
- Percodan (oxycodone HCl, 4.5 mg; oxycodone terephthalate, 0.38 mg; aspirin, 325 mg)
- Darvocet-N (propoxyphene 50 to 100 mg; acetaminophen, 325 to 650 mg)

Patient-controlled analgesia: Patient-controlled analgesia (PCA) is a method of drug delivery that uses an infusion pump to de-

PHARMACOTHERAPY ILLUSTRATED 29.1

Sites of Analgesic Action

Cerebral cortex

Limbic system

4. Perception
- opiods
- alpha$_2$ adrenergic agonists

Thalamus

5. Modulation
- antidepressants
- antiepileptic agents

Descending modulating spinal tract

Ascending spinal tract

3. Transmission: spinal tracts
- opiods
- alpha$_2$ adrenergic agonists
- NSAIDs

2. Transmission: peripheral nerves
- local anesthetics

1. Transduction
- NSAIDS

Spinal cord

Peripheral nociceptor

1) Trauma stimulates nociceptors which generate a pain signal that is blocked by NSAIDs; 2) The pain impulse travels along afferent peripheral nerve to the spinal cord and is blocked by local anesthetics; 3) the pain impulse continues along ascending tracts of the spinal cord and is blocked by NSAIDs, opioids and alpha$_2$ agonists; 4) The cerebral cortex perceives pain that is blocked by opioids and alpha$_2$ agonists; 5) the limbic system sends modulating impules along descending tracts of the spinal cord that are blocked by antiepileptic and antidepressant drugs.

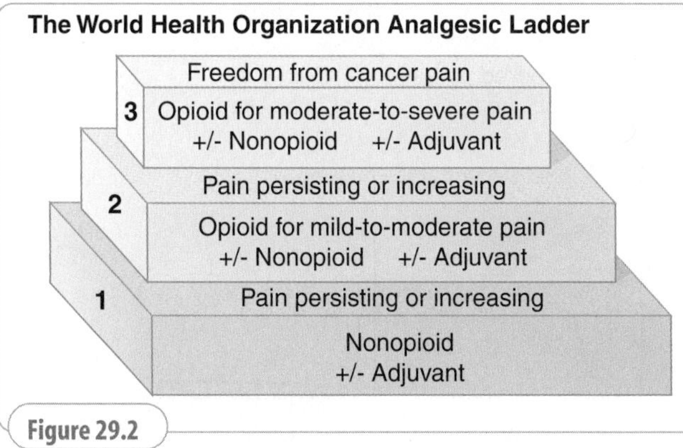

Figure 29.2

The World Health Organization Analgesic Ladder.

Source: From *Cancer Pain Relief*, 2nd ed., by World Health Organization, 1996, Geneva: Author.

liver a prescribed amount of opioid whenever a patient feels the need for pain relief. By pressing a button, the patient can self-administer the opioid, thus relieving the anxiety of waiting for a prn drug administration. The patient does not have unlimited access to the drug; the infusion pump is programmed by the nurse to deliver a prescribed amount of drug over a designated time period. If the patient attempts to self-administer the drug too often, the patient is locked out until the next dose interval. The program is adjusted depending on the patient's response to the drug. Morphine is the opioid usually used for PCA.

PCA allows patients to participate in their own care. Frequent, small doses of analgesics give a more consistent serum drug level than would be obtained by administering larger doses three to four times per day. PCA requires that the patient be conscious and capable of understanding the operation of

MyNursingKit | Oxford Pain Internet Site

the pump. Patients should be taught not to be overly concerned about activating the pump because the program is set to prevent the possibility of overdose.

Pharmacotherapy of Acute and Chronic Pain

29.7 Opioid analgesics exert their effects by interacting with specific receptors in the central nervous system.

Opium is one of the oldest known natural remedies; it has been used to relieve pain for thousands of years. Extracted from the unripe seeds of the poppy plant, *Papaver somniferum*, **opium** is a milky substance that contains over 20 different chemicals having pharmacologic activity. Opium contains 9% to 14% morphine and 0.8% to 2.5% codeine. Natural substances obtained from opium (such as morphine and codeine) are called **opiates.**

In the late 1800s, scientists began to create synthetic and semisynthetic substances with morphine-like properties. There are now over a dozen different synthetic drugs with morphine-like activity. **Opioid** is a general term referring to any of these substances, natural or synthetic, and is often used interchangeably with the term *opiate.*

Pharmacotherapy with opioids is predominately used to relieve moderate to severe pain. With proper dosing, opioids can relieve any degree of pain; they are most effective in treating constant, dull types of pain. In large quantities opioids produce euphoria and severe CNS depression that can lead to stupor, coma, or death. When used consistently, opioids cause physical and psychological addiction.

Narcotic is another term commonly used to describe morphine-like drugs that produce analgesia and CNS depression. In clinical practice, a narcotic analgesic is the same as an opioid, and the terms may be used interchangeably. In the context of law enforcement, however, the term *narcotic* is often used to describe a much broader range of abused illegal drugs such as hallucinogens, cocaine, amphetamines, and marijuana.

Opioids exert their actions by interacting with at least six types of receptors in the CNS; mu, kappa, and delta are the three major receptor types. From the perspective of pain management, the **mu** and **kappa receptors** are the most important, as shown in Figure 29.3. Activation of the mu receptor is responsible for the analgesic properties of the opioids as well as some of the adverse effects such as respiratory depression and physical dependence (see Chapter 8). Drugs that activate opioid receptors are called opioid agonists; those that block these receptors are called opioid antagonists. Because there are multiple opioid receptors, three general types of drug–receptor interactions are possible.

- **Opioid agonist.** Drugs that activate both mu and kappa receptors; for example, morphine and codeine (see Section 29.8)
- **Mixed opioid agonist-antagonist.** Drugs that occupy one receptor and block (or have no effect) on the other; for example, penta-

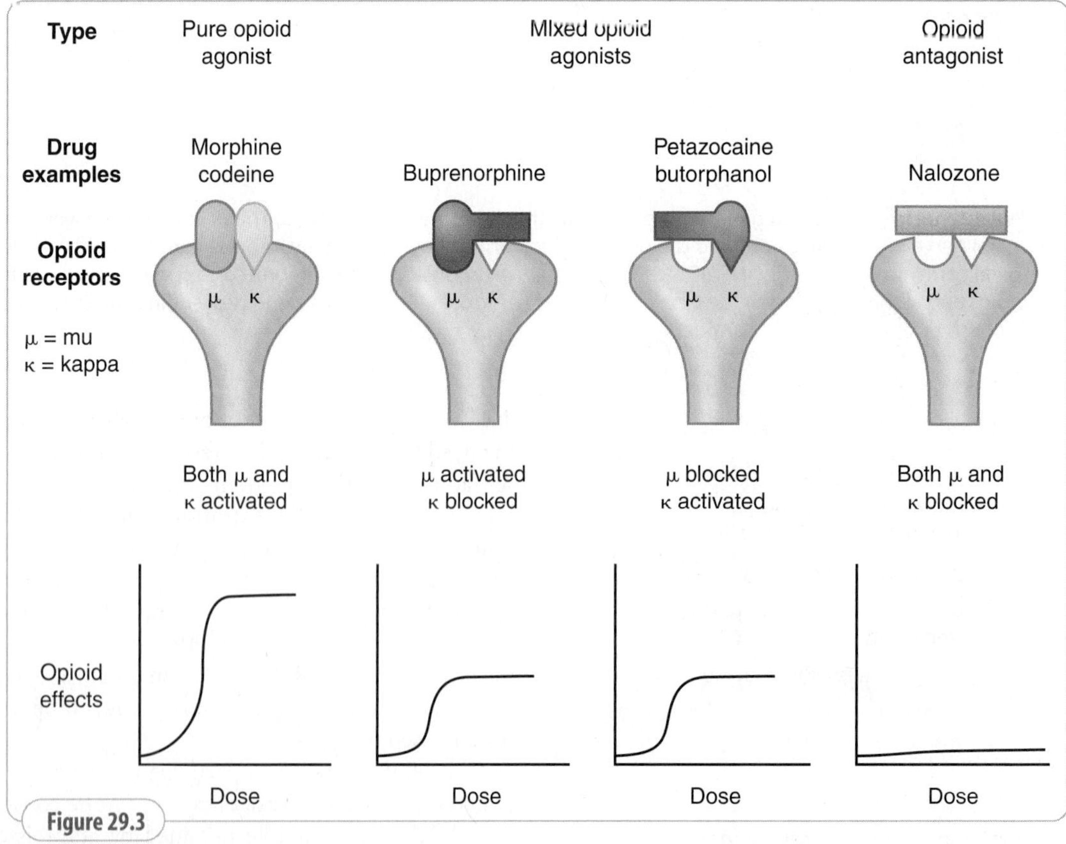

Figure 29.3

Opioid receptors.

zocine (Talwin), butorphanol (Stadol), and buprenorphine (Buprenex) (see Section 29.9)

- **Opioid antagonist.** Drugs that block both mu and kappa receptors; for example, naloxone (Narcan) (see Section 29.10)

The types of agonist actions produced by activating the mu and kappa receptors are shown in Table 29.1. Analgesia is obviously the desired response in pain management. The other responses constitute adverse effects of opioid therapy and must be assessed, prevented, or managed as part of the plan of care for a patient receiving opioid therapy (see Nursing Process Application: Care of the Patient Receiving Opioid Analgesics on page 441).

Opioids do not lower the threshold for pain at the nociceptors and they do not slow or block the transmission of the pain impulse. It is the perception and emotional response to pain that is altered. Essentially the patient knows that the pain still exists, but it does not cause concern or anxiety.

29.8 Opioids are the drugs of choice for moderate to severe pain that cannot be controlled with other classes of analgesics.

Over 20 different opioids are available as medications. This large group is split into subclasses by similarities in their chemical structures, mechanisms of action, and effectiveness. Each method of classification is useful in explaining some of the similarities and differences among the opioids. The most basic method is by effectiveness, which places opioids into the two basic categories of strong or moderate analgesic activity. The opioids are listed in Table 29.2. The opioids that have very short durations of action are used primarily as anesthesia adjuncts and are presented in Chapter 30.

Opioids produce many important physiological actions in addition to analgesia. They are effective at suppressing the cough reflex and at slowing the motility of the GI tract in patients with severe diarrhea. Opioids are powerful CNS depressants and can cause sedation, which may be considered a therapeutic effect or an adverse effect, depending on the patient's disease state. Some patients experience euphoria and intense relaxation, which are reasons why these drugs are frequently abused.

Opioids have the potential to produce many serious adverse effects, including respiratory depression, sedation, nausea, vomiting, and constipation. Table 29.2 compares the major adverse effect potentials of the individual opioids. The greater number of marks indicates a higher incidence of that adverse effect.

Management of opioid adverse effects is summarized in Table 29.3. Through activation of primarily the mu receptors, opioids can cause profound respiratory depression, which is the most serious adverse effect of drugs in this class. Respiratory depression is most problematic during the initial period of drug administration and with patients who have not previously taken these drugs (opiate naive). Patients at greatest risk include those with preexisting respiratory impairment or those concurrently taking other respiratory depressant drugs. A current medication history is very important, especially alcohol and other CNS depressants, because these drugs will cause additive respiratory depression and sedation. Tolerance to respiratory depression usually occurs within 48 to 72 hours of initiation of therapy.

Respirations should be monitored before initiating therapy and regularly throughout opioid pharmacotherapy. The drugs should be withheld if respirations fall below 12 per minute. Narcotic antagonists such as naloxone (Narcan) should be readily available if respirations fall below 10 per minute (see Section 29.13). If opioids are administered by continuous epidural or intravenous (IV) routes, interventions should be taken to reduce the risk of respiratory depression. These include frequent monitoring of vital signs, level of consciousness (LOC), and pain rating as well as proper body positioning. Airway equipment and narcotic antagonists are usually kept at the bedside.

Opioids can cause orthostatic hypotension by inhibiting the baroreceptor reflex and by causing peripheral vasodilation. Dizziness and fainting are possible; assistance may therefore be needed with ambulation. Hydromorphone and meperidine are especially prone to cause hypotension. Patients with hypovolemia are more sensitive to this hypotensive effect; therefore, volume deficiencies should be corrected before initiating opioid therapy.

Increased intracranial pressure (ICP) is a severe adverse reaction that can occur as an indirect result of respiratory depression. When respiration is suppressed, the CO_2 content of the blood increases. The result is vasodilation of cerebral blood vessels and rising ICP. This is of particular concern in patients with conditions that might cause elevated ICP, such as those with head injury, intracranial bleeding, or brain tumors. Narcotic analgesics are usually contraindicated in these patients.

Opioids promote urinary retention by increasing the tone in the bladder sphincter and through suppression of stimuli that normally signal bladder fullness. If the patient has not voided within 6 hours, especially after surgery, insertion of a urinary catheter may be necessary. Patients prone to urinary hesitancy, such as those with benign prostatic hyperplasia, must be carefully monitored.

Constipation, nausea, and vomiting frequently occur during opioid administration. Constipation occurs because the drugs suppress intestinal peristalsis, increase the tone of the anal sphincter, and inhibit secretion of fluids into the intestine. Bowel function should be closely monitored, especially after surgery or with long-term use. The plan of care for these patients should include a bowel program to prevent or manage constipation. A baseline program would include increased dietary fiber, adequate fluid intake, and a stool softener such as docusate. More

TABLE 29.1 Responses Produced by Activation of Specific Opioid Receptors

Response	Mu Receptor	Kappa Receptor
Analgesia	Yes	Yes
Decreased GI motility	Yes	Yes
Euphoria	Yes	No
Miosis	No	Yes
Physical dependence	Yes	No
Respiratory depression	Yes	No
Sedation	Yes	Yes

TABLE 29.2 Selected Opioid Analgesic Comparison

Drug	Route and Dose (maximum dose where indicated)	Equivalent Dose	Analgesic Duration	Respiratory Depression	Emesis	Constipation	Dependence Potential
Opioid Agonists with High Effectiveness							
fentanyl (Sublimaze)	IM: 0.05–0.1 mg Transdermal: 25–100 mcg every 72 h	0.1–0.2 mg 25 mcg/h	1–2 h 3 days	Y	Y	?	Y
hydromorphone (Dilaudid)	PO: 1–4 mg every 4–6 h Subcutaneous/ IM/IV: 1–4 mg every 4–6 h	7.5 mg 1.5 mg	4–5 h	YY	Y	Y	YYY
levorphanol (Levo-Dromoran)	PO: 2–3 mg tid/qid Subcutaneous/IV: 1–2 mg every 6–8 h	4 mg 2 mg	4–8 h	YY	Y	YY	YY
meperidine (Demerol)	PO: 50–150 mg every 3–4 h IM: 50–100 mg every 3–4 h IV: 1–1.5 mg/kg every 3–4 h	300 mg 75 mg 50 mg	2–4 h	YY		Y	YYY
methadone (Dolophine)	PO: 20 mg every 6–8 h	20 mg	4–8 h	YY	Y	YY	Y
morphine	PO: 30 mg every 4 h Sustained release IM: 10 mg every 4 h IV: 2–10 mg every 2–4 h; 0.1–1 mg/mL continuous	30 mg 30 mg SR 10 mg 10 mg	4–5 h 8–12 h 4–5 h 4–5 h	YY	YY	YY	YYYY
Opioids with Moderate Effectiveness							
codeine	PO: 15–60 mg qid IM: 15–30 mg every 4–6 h	200 mg 120 mg	4–6 h				
hydrocodone (Hycodan)	PO: 5–10 every 4–6 h	30 mg	4–6 h	Y		Y	Y
oxycodone (OxyContin)	PO: 5–10 mg qid Controlled release: 10–20 mg every 12 h	20 mg 20 mg	4–6 h 8–12 h	YY	YY	YY	YY
propoxyphene (Darvon) propoxyphene napsylate (Darvon-N)	PO: 65 mg every 4 h PO: 100 mg napsylate forms every 4 h	130 mg	4–6 h	Y	Y		YY
Opioids with Mixed Agonist-Antagonist Effects							
buprenorphine (Buprenex)	IM/IV: 0.3 mg every 6 h	0.3 mg	6 h	YY	Y		YY
butorphanol (Stadol)	IM: 1–4 mg every 3–4 h IV: 0.5–2 mg IV every 3–4 h	2 mg 1 mg	3–4 h	YYY	Y		YY
nalbuphine (Nubain)	Subcutaneous/IM/IV: 10–20 mg every 3–6 h	10 mg	3–6 h	Y	Y		YY
pentazocine (Talwin)	PO: 50–100 every 3–4 h Subcutaneous/IM: 30 mg every 3–4 h	25 mg 50 mg	2–3 h	Y	YY		YY

TABLE 29.3 Management of Opioid Adverse Effects

Adverse Effect	Management
Respiratory depression	Monitor respiratory status frequently—especially initially and with dosing increases. Use coughing, deep breathing, and incentive spirometry. If the patient is unresponsive and the respiratory rate is less than 12/min, administer naloxone per protocol.
Orthostatic hypotension	Assess blood pressure before ambulation; change positions slowly; assist with ambulation if needed.
Constipation	Assume it will occur and initiate preventive measures: Increase dietary fiber and fluid intake; use stool softeners and mild laxatives if needed.
Nausea	Usually transient. Antiemetics are administered, as needed.
Sedation	Common with initiation or dosage increase. Tolerance develops in several days. Use safety precautions, especially with ambulation.
Urinary retention	Monitor for bladder distension. More common in elderly men. Tolerance usually develops with long-term dosing. Monitor; if receiving epidural administration, use an indwelling catheter.

active interventions are implemented if the patient does not resume or maintain normal bowel elimination. The constipation-promoting effect of the opioids is used to advantage in the treatment of severe diarrhea (see Chapter 61).

Opioids directly stimulate the chemoreceptor trigger zone in the medulla to cause intense nausea and vomiting in certain patients. An antiemetic such as promethazine (Phenergan) or ondansetron (Zofran) may be indicated. Orders for prn antiemetics should be made available whenever parenteral opioids are used.

Prolonged use of opioids results in tolerance. Typically, tolerance is noted when patients report that the duration of analgesia is decreasing or admit to taking the drug more frequently as therapy progresses. Higher and higher doses will be needed to produce the same degree of analgesia. Tolerance does not develop equally for all opioid actions. Whereas tolerance to respiratory depression, sedation, and euphoria develop rapidly, tolerance never develops to the constipation or miosis effects. It should be remembered that as doses of opioids are increased to more effectively manage pain, the incidence of adverse effects will also increase.

All of the narcotic analgesics have the potential to cause physical and psychological dependence, as previously discussed in Chapter 8. Dependence is most likely to occur when high doses are taken for extended periods. Many health care providers and nurses are hesitant to administer the proper amount of opioid analgesics for fear of causing patient dependence or of producing serious adverse effects such as sedation or respiratory depression. Undermedication, however, results in patients not receiving adequate pain relief. When used according to accepted medical practice, patients can and indeed should, receive the pain relief they need without fear of dependence or serious adverse effects.

Opioids are frequently abused for nonmedical purposes. The risk of abuse is especially high in patients with a history of substance abuse. Opioids are frequently diverted from medical sources (e.g., patients, pharmacies, hospitals), either stolen or sold for criminal intent. Opioids are even stolen from family members, especially the elderly. Illicit users may "doctor shop" and obtain opioids from different prescribers then sell the pills for profit.

Many patients who experience an adverse reaction to an opioid will report that they are allergic to these drugs. For example, patients who experience nausea, vomiting, or severe dizziness will often state they are allergic to narcotics. True allergic reactions to opioids, however, are actually rare. When hypersensitivity does occur, it often extends to other drugs in the opioid class.

Equianalgesic use in pain management: Table 29.2 includes a column labeled Equivalent Dose. It is often necessary to change the route of a patient's pain medication or even the drug itself. The most frequently occurring scenario is the transition from IV medications after surgery to PO analgesics prior to discharge. Using relative potency information (equivalent dose), the primary health care provider can determine the appropriate new dose. The nurse can use these same equivalencies in choosing the drug and dose when a range of analgesic options are ordered, as happens frequently following surgery. It is not unusual to have orders for a parenteral opioid with a dosage range for severe pain, an oral opioid for moderate pain, and a combination opioid and nonopioid for mild pain. The oral drugs may also be ordered with a dosage range.

CONNECTION *Checkpoint* 29.1

A common abbreviation for morphine sulfate is MS or MSO_4. From what you learned in Chapter 7, why should this abbreviation be avoided and what can you do to prevent this type of medication error? See Answer to Connection Checkpoint 29.1 in Appendix A.

PROTOTYPE DRUG Morphine sulfate (Astramorph PF, Duramorph RF, Roxanol, others)

Classification: **Therapeutic:** Narcotic analgesic
Pharmacologic: Opioid agonist

Therapeutic Effects and Uses: Morphine sulfate is the narcotic analgesic of choice for the management of most types of acute and severe chronic pain. Morphine is a drug of choice for relieving acute chest pain associated with MI. The drug was in use for thousands of years prior to its approval by the U.S. Food and Drug Administration (FDA) in 1939 and is still obtained from unripe seeds of the poppy plant.

In addition to relieving severe pain, morphine is used off-label to treat several other conditions. Its CNS depressant action may be used to provide preanesthetic sedation and to calm severely agitated patients. In terminally ill patients, its respiratory depressant action may be used to relieve shortness of breath associated with end-stage cancer, heart failure, or pulmonary edema.

MyNursingKit | Mechanism of Action: Morphine

The advantages of morphine therapy, especially in the treatment of chronic cancer pain where dosing increases over time, are that morphine has no upper end dose limit, and that patients develop tolerance to all the adverse effects except constipation. Extended release tablets (MS Contin, Oramorph SR) or capsules (Kadian, Avinza) are available. Initiation of therapy is usually begun with shorter-acting agents. Once the correct dose has been titrated, the patient may be switched to extended release formulations. In 2004, the FDA approved an extended release liposome injection (DepoDur), which is given by a single epidural injection for postsurgical pain.

Mechanism of Action: Morphine occupies mu and kappa receptor sites in the brain and dorsal horn of the spinal cord that alter the release of afferent neurotransmitters. The dominant effect alters the perception of and emotional response to pain, producing analgesia and euphoria. The drug mimics the actions of endogenous endorphins.

Pharmacokinetics:

Routes(s)	PO, IV, subcutaneous, intramuscular (IM), rectal, epidural, intrathecal
Absorption	PO variable, 30%; subcutaneous or IM may be erratic or delayed
Distribution	Widely distributed; crosses the placenta; is secreted in breast milk
Primary metabolism	Hepatic; significant first-pass metabolism
Primary excretion	Renal; 7–10% in bile and feces
Onset of action	PO: 30–60 minutes; IV: rapid; epidural: 15–30 minutes
Duration of action	PO: 4–7 h; IV: 4–5 h; epidural: 4–24 h

Adverse Effects: Morphine depresses the CNS, causing sedation, dizziness, anxiety, and a feeling of floating or disorientation. Tolerance often develops to these CNS effects after a few days of therapy. Hallucinations and seizures may occur at high doses. Morphine reduces the sensitivity of the respiratory center to CO_2, thus decreasing tidal volume and rate and producing respiratory depression. The resulting increase in CO_2 produces cerebral vasodilation and increases cerebrospinal fluid (CSF) pressure. Morphine stimulates the chemoreceptor trigger zone in the medulla, producing nausea and vomiting, which may require the administration of an antiemetic drug during the first few days of therapy. The drug delays digestion, increases smooth muscle tone in the intestinal tract, and slows peristalsis in the colon, leading to constipation. Morphine also causes spasm of the sphincter of Oddi, which can result in intense pain (biliary colic) and potential obstruction of bile flow. Urinary retention may occur due to increasing bladder sphincter tone. Peripheral vasodilation may cause orthostatic hypotension. Morphine is a Schedule II controlled substance with a high potential for physical and psychological dependence. Pruritus is more common when morphine is given by the IV and epidural routes and is not considered a sign of hypersensitivity in the absence of skin rash.

Contraindications/Precautions: Morphine is contraindicated in patients with hypersensitivity to opioids. Premature infants are especially sensitive to the effects of morphine; thus the drug should not be used during pregnancy or during the delivery of premature infants. It should be used with caution in the elderly and in those with undiagnosed abdominal pain, hepatic or renal impairment, shock, CNS depression, head injury or increased ICP, chronic obstructive pulmonary disease (COPD), or other conditions with decreased respiratory reserve, including severe obesity. Mothers should wait 4 to 6 hours after a dose of morphine before breast-feeding; withdrawal symptoms have been noted in nursing infants whose mothers abruptly discontinue opioid use. Morphine should never be withdrawn abruptly because this will precipitate symptoms of acute opioid withdrawal. Discontinuation should be conducted gradually over several days.

Drug Interactions: When used with other CNS depressants, including alcohol, skeletal muscle relaxants, and monoamine oxidase inhibitors (MAOIs), increased sedation will result. Administration of an opioid antagonist such as naloxone will reverse the effects of morphine and may produce immediate withdrawal symptoms. Concurrent use with antidiarrheal drugs such as loperamide will cause additive constipation. **Herbal/Food:** Use of kava, valerian, or chamomile can increase CNS depression. St. John's wort may decrease the analgesic action of morphine.

Pregnancy: Category C.

Treatment of Overdose: Morphine overdose can cause coma and life-threatening respiratory depression and requires immediate treatment. Naloxone is a specific antidote for morphine intoxication (see Section 29.13).

Nursing Responsibilities:

- Prior to administration assess for allergies, LOC, vital signs, and the time since last administration.
- Assess the patient's response when asked to rate pain on a scale of 0 (no pain) to 10 (worst possible pain).
- Administer the dose that is individually adjusted according to severity of pain, patient response, and patient size.
- Provide around-the-clock dosing for optimum pain management. Treat pain before it becomes severe.
- Use with great caution in patients with severe respiratory disorders, increased ICP, and liver or renal disease. Assess these patients closely for baseline function and monitor for changes in patient condition.
- Monitor vital signs at regular intervals after administration. Report respiratory rate that is less than 10 per minute before administration.
- Closely monitor elderly patients who are at highest risk for hypotension, respiratory depression, and increased incidence of adverse CNS effects.
- Monitor for orthostatic hypotension and supervise ambulation. Patients with less severe pain or hypovolemia are more sensitive to the hypotensive effect.

- Monitor for bowel function after surgery and with long-term use. Institute a bowel program to prevent or manage constipation.
- Monitor input and output and voiding pattern, especially during IV use or after surgery. If no voiding occurs in 6 hours, assess for bladder distention and urinary retention.
- Monitor for the development of tolerance by noting the frequency of dosing and the effectiveness of analgesia.
- When giving IV, dilute with at least 5 mL sterile water or IV solution. Administer by IV push over 4 to 5 minutes with the patient supine. Morphine may be added to the IV solutions (0.1–1 mg/mL) and given by titrated drip with an infusion controller or continuous PCA.
- Evaluate the effectiveness of the drug. Supplement analgesia with positional and psychological variables such as elevation of the painful extremity, guided imagery, and relaxation techniques.

Patient and Family Education:

- Inform the health care provider if pain increases above the selected goal rating.
- Follow label instructions carefully: Never take a double dose or take the drug more frequently than indicated.
- Immediately report difficulty breathing, shortness of breath, persistent nausea, vomiting, dizziness on standing, difficulty in voiding, constipation, skin rash, or nonrelief of pain.
- Make position changes slowly when moving from a lying to a standing position to prevent dizziness and possible fainting.
- Do not drive or perform other hazardous activities until the effects of the drug are known because this drug may cause drowsiness or dizziness.
- Avoid alcohol or other CNS depressants because they may cause intense drowsiness.
- Store the medication in a safe place away from children. Be aware that these drugs are often the target of criminal activity and may be stolen. Do not disclose the use of opioids to those who do not need to know.
- Increase dietary fiber and fluid intake, and use a stool softener such as docusate as recommended by the health care provider.
- Do not take any other prescription or nonprescription drugs, dietary supplements, or herbal products without approval of the health care provider.

Drugs Similar to Morphine Sulfate (Astramorph PF, Duramorph RF, Roxanol, Others)

Other opioids used for pain management are shown in Table 29.2. The following are descriptions of opioids with pure agonist activity. All these agents have the same actions and adverse effects as morphine. All are controlled substances.

Codeine: Approved by the FDA in 1939, codeine can be administered by the PO, subcutaneous, or IM routes. Because it has stronger antitussive action than morphine, it is often used for suppression of severe cough. At the low doses needed for cough suppression, codeine does not produce the serious adverse effects characteristic of morphine. Doses required to produce analgesia are much higher than those needed for cough suppression. Analgesic use is in combination with acetaminophen and is often limited by nausea and vomiting. During the metabolism of codeine in the CNS, about 10% is converted to morphine, which is responsible for its analgesic effects. Codeine may also be used off-label to treat serious diarrhea. This drug is pregnancy category C; the category changes to D if used in high doses or close to term.

Hydrocodone (Hycodan, others): Approved in 1957, hydrocodone is used for analgesia, most often combined with acetaminophen, aspirin, or ibuprofen in fixed dose combinations such as Vicodin, Lortab, and Norco. Acetaminophen has a dose ceiling that limits the use of such combinations in chronic pain management. Hydrocodone is an effective antitussive and is combined with decongestants or antihistamines for severe cold and flu symptoms. Although it is slightly more effective than codeine as an antitussive, it causes more sedation. This drug is pregnancy category C; the category changes to D if used in high doses or close to term.

Hydromorphone (Dilaudid): Approved in 1984, hydromorphone is available by the PO, rectal, and parenteral routes. Its primary application is analgesia, including PCA. Hydromorphone produces less nausea but more orthostatic hypotension than morphine. It has a more rapid onset of action and a shorter duration of activity than morphine, requiring PO dosing every 3 to 6 hours. An extended duration formulation of the drug (Palladone) was approved in 2004 but was quickly removed from the market due to a potentially fatal interaction with alcohol. This drug is pregnancy category C.

Levorphanol (Levo-Dromoran): Approved in 1953, levorphanol is a pure opioid agonist available by the PO and parenteral routes for severe pain. At equianalgesic doses, levorphanol exhibits the same actions and adverse effects as morphine. It offers no advantages over the use of other drugs in this class. This drug is pregnancy category B; the category changes to D if used in high doses or close to term.

Meperidine (Demerol): Approved in 1942, meperidine is available by both the PO and parenteral routes for the treatment of severe pain. Toxicity can occur due to its active metabolite, called normeperidine, which is a CNS stimulant with a half-life of 15 to 30 hours. Accumulation of this metabolite can result from doses greater than 400 to 600 mg per day or administration longer than 48 hours. Normeperidine can cause tremors and seizures, which are not reversed with narcotic antagonists (naloxone). For this reason, meperidine is not recommended for use longer than 48 hours, for chronic pain, or for use in PCA. When meperidine is used in high doses or longer than 48 hours, the nurse needs to consult with the prescriber and report any incidences of tremors and irritability before giving the next dose. Because of these adverse effects, meperidine is considered a second-line agent that is used when other opioids are contraindicated. The drug has a short half-life that requires dosing every 3 to 4 hours. This drug is pregnancy category C; the category changes to D if used in high doses or close to term.

Methadone (Dolophine): Approved in 1947, methadone is an oral preparation with similar pharmacologic effects as those of morphine; adverse effects are similar with lower incidence. Methadone is the most frequently prescribed agent in the management of opiate dependency (see Chapter 8) and is increasingly used for management of chronic pain. Methadone has a very long duration of action and can be dosed once daily. Oral liquid (Methadose) and dispersible tablets (Diskets) are available in treating opiate withdrawal symptoms because they offer less risk for abuse than regular tablets. IV methadone is used for the short-term therapy of hospitalized patients. This drug is pregnancy category C.

MyNursingKit | Mechanism of Action: Oxycodone

Oxycodone (OxyContin, others): Approved in 1976, oxycodone is an oral opioid that is most often combined with acetaminophen as Percocet or with aspirin as Percodan. Oxycodone causes less nausea, vomiting, and hallucinations than morphine. The immediate release forms of this drug have a short duration of action, requiring dosing every 3 to 4 hours. The controlled release form (OxyContin) can be dosed twice a day. OxyContin has become a popular drug of abuse (see Chapter 8). This drug is pregnancy category B; the category changes to D if used in high doses or close to term.

Propoxyphene (Darvon): Approved in 1957, propoxyphene is an oral drug that is used for its analgesic effects. Compared to other pure opiate agonists, it has less potency and effectiveness; its use is limited to treating mild to moderate pain. It is combined with acetaminophen (Darvocet) and aspirin (Darvon Compound). At therapeutic doses, propoxyphene produces few adverse effects, but in overdose situations, however, typical opioid adverse events are evident. The adverse effects of propoxyphene overdosage are difficult to reverse with naloxone owing to the long half-life of its metabolites. Because of its low effectiveness and the potential for serious overdosage effects, the use of propoxyphene has declined. Because it rarely causes dependence, it is one of the few pure opioid agonists classified as a Schedule IV drug. This drug is pregnancy category C; the category changes to D if used in high doses or close to term.

29.9 Mixed agonist and antagonist opioids exhibit moderate analgesia with less risk of dependence than morphine.

The mixed agonist-antagonist opioids are narcotic analgesics that were developed with the intention of producing drugs with strong analgesia that have fewer adverse effects than morphine and other pure opioid agonists. The four drugs in this class are used to treat moderate pain but are not as effective as morphine in treating severe pain. Their advantage is that they cause less respiratory depression and have a lower potential for dependence. These drugs have some abuse potential but less so than the pure opioid agonists. The types of adverse effects, contraindications, and nursing responsibilities are similar to those of the pure opioid agonists (see Section 29.8).

With both agonist and antagonist actions, what would happen if a person addicted to morphine or heroin takes one of the drugs in this class? Blocking opioid receptors will cause the patient to experience opioid withdrawal symptoms. In fact, some of the mixed agonist-antagonist drugs are indicated for the induction of opioid withdrawal and the maintenance of opioid dependence (see Chapter 8).

Buprenorphine (Buprenex, Suboxone, Subutex): Approved in 1981, buprenorphine is a partial agonist at the mu receptors and an antagonist at the kappa receptors. It is indicated for the relief of moderate to severe pain when given by the parenteral route (Buprenex). The sublingual form (Suboxone, Subutex) is reserved for treatment of opioid withdrawal and dependence. Suboxone is a combination drug that also contains the narcotic antagonist naloxone. Abuse of buprenorphine has been reported but is uncommon because the drug is unable to produce the degree of euphoria observed with the pure opioid agonists. Furthermore, withdrawal symptoms from this drug are generally mild and its onset may be delayed 1 to 2 weeks. Buprenorphine is a Schedule III drug. Respiratory depression can be a serious adverse effect at high doses. This drug is pregnancy category C.

Butorphanol (Stadol): Approved in 1978, butorphanol is an agonist at the kappa receptors and is a weak antagonist at the mu receptors. Delivered by the IV or IM route, it is approved for moderate to severe pain and as a preanesthesia or general anesthesia adjunct. A nasal spray form of the drug is used for the treatment of obstetric pain or migraines. Drowsiness and dizziness are experienced by a large number of patients. Like buprenorphine, the drug is not commonly abused and withdrawal symptoms are mild. This drug is pregnancy category C.

Nalbuphine (Nubain): Approved in 1979, nalbuphine is an agonist at the kappa receptors and a weak antagonist at the mu receptors. Given by the IV, IM, or subcutaneous route, it is approved for moderate to severe pain and as a preanesthesia or general anesthesia adjunct. Drowsiness is the most common adverse effect. The risk for dependence is low, and nalbuphine is not a scheduled drug. Abrupt discontinuation, however, can precipitate mild opioid withdrawal symptoms. This drug is pregnancy category B (category D with prolonged use or high doses at term).

Pentazocine (Talwin): Approved in 1967, pentazocine was the first of the agonist-antagonist opioids marketed. Available by both the PO and parenteral routes, it is approved to treat moderate to severe pain. The drug acts as an agonist at the kappa receptors and a weak antagonist at the mu receptors. Pentazocine causes less nausea, vomiting, and respiratory depression than morphine. Like other drugs in this class, drowsiness and dizziness are common adverse effects. Also like other

NURSING PROCESS APPLICATION

Patients Receiving Opioid Analgesics

Assessment

Prior to administration:

- Assess pain: location, quality, intensity (use a standard scale).
- Monitor vital signs and ability to perform ADLs.
- If chronic pain, assess the impact of pain on daily life.
- Establish a mutually acceptable pain management goal using the pain rating scale.

Potential Nursing Diagnoses

- *Acute Pain*
- *Chronic Pain*
- *Risk for Falls,* related to drug-induced level of consciousness changes
- *Deficient Knowledge (Analgesic),* related to purpose, precautions, and adverse effects of drug therapy

Planning: Patient Goals and Expected Outcomes

The patient will:

- Rate pain less than the goal level (typically less than 3 on a 0 to 10 pain rating scale).
- Have a relaxed posture and facial expression.
- Be able to accomplish desired ADLs.
- Evidence no signs of constipation, urinary retention, or nausea.
- Maintain vital signs within baseline for the individual.

Interventions and (Rationales)	Patient and Family Education
• Monitor vital signs before and at regular intervals after administration. Monitor respiratory status (rate and tidal volume), especially in patients with compromised respiratory capacity or postsurgery. Report respiratory rate less than 12/minute before parenteral administration. Use nursing measures to prevent atelectasis: coughing and deep breathing, incentive spirometry. Initiate agency protocol for epidural or PCA use. Oxygen, respiratory resuscitation equipment, and narcotic antagonist should be available. (Opioids depress the respiratory center and increase hypotension.)	• Instruct the patient to report breathing difficulty, shortness of breath, persistent nausea, vomiting, dizziness on standing, constipation, skin rash, or nonrelief of pain.
• Monitor orthostatic blood pressure and supervise ambulation. (Patients with less severe pain or hypovolemia are more sensitive to hypotensive effect. Hypotension is a common adverse effect of opioid drugs.)	Instruct the patient to: • Change position or stand slowly. • Know the drug response before driving or operating machinery due to the possibility of drowsiness or blurred vision. • Avoid alcohol or other CNS depressants.
• Monitor for bowel function after surgery and with long-term use. Institute a bowel program to prevent or manage constipation. Encourage intake of at least eight 240-mL glasses of fluid daily. Encourage exercise, unless contraindicated, to increase abdominal muscle tone and increase peristalsis. (Constipation is a very common adverse effect of opioid drugs due to slowed peristalsis.)	• In ongoing use, increase dietary fiber and fluid, and use a stool softener such as docusate. If you do not have soft, regular bowel movements, use a mild laxative as recommended.
• Monitor the character, location, and intensity of pain on a regular basis. Report nonrelief of pain to the health care provider. Medicate around the clock to maintain a consistent blood level. (Less medication is needed to control pain when dosed around-the-clock, rather than the peaks and valleys of prn dosing. Pain ratings are used as a baseline and an indicator of treatment effectiveness.)	• Instruct the patient to inform the nurse if pain is not relieved or increases.
• Reduce factors that may increase pain, such as anxiety and fatigue. Encourage the patient to rest and control environmental factors such as noise and lighting when possible. (Feeling rested increases pain tolerance and knowing that pain is being treated increases the ability to cope.)	• Instruct the patient to report factors that are interfering with the ability to rest.
• Monitor intake and output ratios and voiding patterns, especially during IV use, or after surgery. If voiding has not occurred in 6 hours, scan the bladder for urinary retention and insert a urinary catheter prn. Maintain the indwelling catheter during epidural use. (Urinary retention is a common adverse effect of opioid drugs.)	• Instruct the patient to report difficulty voiding.
• Obtain an order for antiemetics to control nausea, a possible opioid adverse effect. (Controlling nausea improves tolerance of opioids. Dose separately from opioids.)	• Instruct the patient to report nausea when it starts.
Use a combination of nondrug pain control strategies: • Positioning: cushion and elevate the painful area if possible. (Cushioning increases comfort, whereas elevation reduces edema.) • Massage or applications of cold or heat. (Stimulating nonpain fibers inhibits ascending pain pathways [gate control].) • Relaxation techniques such as guided imagery, rhythmic breathing, meditation, or distraction. (These techniques divert attention from the pain, promote a sense of self-control, and may stimulate endorphin release.)	• Instruct the patient in the use of nondrug pain control strategies.
• For IV push: dilute with at least 5 mL sterile water and give over 4–5 minutes. The patient should be supine; monitor for dizziness or hypotension. (Dilution of IV dosages avoids accidental overdoses.)	• Instruct the patient to remain supine for at least 15 minutes after IV administration.
• In pancreatitis, space opioid administration and laboratory tests for amylase and lipase as much as possible. Record the time and amount of the last opioid used in relation to the blood sample. (Opioid administration may produce false elevations for 24 hours after the last dose.)	• Instruct the patient to keep all laboratory appointments for pancreatic and blood testing.

Evaluation of Outcome Criteria

Evaluate the effectiveness of drug therapy by confirming that patient goals and expected outcomes have been met (see "Planning").

mixed agonists-antagonists, pentazocine does not produce euphoria and has a low potential for abuse (Schedule IV). Withdrawal symptoms are similar to those of other opioids but milder. A major advantage is that overdose with pentazocine does not result in the high mortality observed with morphine. This drug is pregnancy category C.

29.10 Nonsteroidal anti-inflammatory drugs are the medications of choice for mild to moderate pain.

The **nonopioid analgesics** include NSAIDs, acetaminophen, and a few centrally acting agents. NSAIDs, such as aspirin and ibuprofen, are the drugs of choice for mild to moderate pain, especially for pain associated with inflammation. Nonopioids have many advantages over the opioids. Acetaminophen, aspirin, and many NSAIDs are available OTC and are inexpensive. They are available in many different formulations, including those designed for children. For most patients, they are safe and produce adverse effects only at high doses. NSAIDs have antipyretic and anti-inflammatory activities as well as analgesic properties. Some NSAIDs are used primarily for their anti-inflammatory properties. The doses and roles of NSAIDs in the treatment of inflammation and fever are discussed in Chapter 44. Prototype features for ibuprofen and aspirin are also included in Chapter 44.

NSAIDs act at peripheral sites by inhibiting pain mediators at the nociceptor level. When tissue is damaged, chemical mediators, including histamine, potassium ion, hydrogen ion, and bradykinin, are released locally. Also released during tissue damage is arachidonic acid, which is metabolized into chemical mediators of inflammation and pain such as prostaglandins. Prostaglandins can induce pain through the formation of free radicals.

NSAIDs inhibit cyclooxygenase, an enzyme responsible for the formation of prostaglandins. Because they act by a different mechanism than opioids, NSAIDs do not produce the severe adverse effects of NSAIDs observed with the narcotic analgesics. The most prominent effects are GI related and include nausea, vomiting, anorexia, dyspepsia, and ulceration of the GI mucosa. At high doses, the ulceration can be severe, resulting in bleeding and even perforation. Other common adverse events include dizziness, headache, and rash. These drugs do not cause physical or psychological dependence. When combined with opioids in fixed dose combinations, NSAIDs produce a synergistic analgesic effect that allows the dose of opioid to be lowered.

It is important to note that several important nonopioid analgesics are not classified as NSAIDs. Acetaminophen is a nonopioid analgesic whose effectiveness is equal to aspirin and ibuprofen in relieving pain and reducing fever. Acetaminophen is featured as a prototype antipyretic in Chapter 44. Clonidine (Catapres) and tramadol (Ultram) are nonopioid analgesics that act centrally, rather than at the nociceptors. These agents are presented in the following section.

29.11 A few miscellaneous analgesics reduce pain by acting on the central nervous system.

Three analgesics suppress pain by acting on the CNS but are not classified as opioids. Clonidine (Catapres), tramadol (Ultram), and ziconotide (Prialt) act by unique mechanisms and are described next. Of the three drugs in this small class, only tramadol is widely prescribed. The doses of the three centrally acting agents are listed in Table 29.4.

PROTOTYPE DRUG Tramadol (Ultram)

Classification: **Therapeutic:** Analgesic
Pharmacologic: Centrally acting nonopioid analgesic

Therapeutic Effects and Uses: Tramadol is approved for the treatment of moderate pain. Although widely prescribed in other countries since the 1970s, the FDA approved tramadol only in 1995. It is available as an immediate release formulation for acute pain and as an extended release form for chronic pain. Off-label uses of tramadol include treatment of neuropathic pain and restless leg syndrome.

Tramadol has gained in popularity as an alternative to NSAIDs and opioids. It does not exhibit the GI ulceration typical of high-dose NSAID therapy, and it does not cause severe respiratory depression characteristic of opioids. Ultracet is a fixed dose combination of tramadol and acetaminophen.

Mechanism of Action: Tramadol has a unique mechanism that involves both opioid and nonopioid actions. The drug and one of its metabolites bind to the opioid mu receptor. This opioid

CONNECTIONS — Lifespan Considerations: Influence of Age on Pain Expression and Perception

Pain control in the elderly can be challenging. Knowledge of the aging process, behavioral cues, subtle signs of discomfort, and verbal and nonverbal responses to pain are a must when it comes to effective pain management. Older patients may have a decreased perception of pain or simply ignore pain as a natural consequence of aging. Because these patients frequently go undermedicated, a thorough assessment is a necessity. Older adults may have difficulty with numerical rating scales and may respond to the Wong-Baker Faces scale.

When administering opioids for pain relief, the nurse should always monitor patients closely. Aging decreases both hepatic metabolism and renal excretion; smaller doses are usually indicated and adverse effects may be heightened. Initial doses should be 25% to 50% lower with frequent reassessment. The nurse should closely monitor decreased respirations, LOC, and dizziness. Body weight should be taken prior to the start of opioid administration and doses calculated accordingly. Bed rails should be kept raised and the bed in a low position at all times to prevent injury from falls. Some opioids, such as meperidine (Demerol) or hydromorphone (Dilaudid), should be used cautiously due to orthostatic hypotension. Many elders take multiple drugs (polypharmacy); therefore, it is important to obtain a complete list of all medications taken and to check for interactions.

TABLE 29.4 Nonopioid Centrally Acting Analgesics

Drug	Adult Dose for Pain (maximum dose where indicated)	Adverse Effects
clonidine (Duraclon)	Epidural: 30–40 mcg/h by continuous infusion or 100–900 mcg bolus	*Drowsiness, orthostatic hypotension, dry mouth, anxiety, constipation* Severe hypotension, dysrhythmias
tramadol (Ultram)	PO: 25–100 mg every 4–6 h prn (max: 400 mg/day)	*Dizziness, nausea, vomiting, constipation, lethargy* Hallucinations, emotional lability, respiratory depression
ziconotide (Prialt)	Intrathecal: 0.1 mcg/h via infusion; may increase as needed up to 0.1 mcg/h no more than every 2–3 days (maximum of 0.8 mcg/h)	*Dizziness, nausea, diarrhea, somnolence, asthenia* Confusion, memory impairment, hallucinations

Note: *Italics* indicate common adverse effects. Underline indicates serious adverse effects.

agonist activity is weak: approximately 10 times less than codeine. In addition to its central opioid action, tramadol inhibits norepinephrine and serotonin reuptake in spinal neurons, which inhibits the transmission of pain impulses.

Pharmacokinetics:

Routes(s)	PO
Absorption	75% absorbed
Distribution	Widely distributed; crosses the placenta; small amounts secreted in breast milk; 20% bound to protein
Primary metabolism	Hepatic; significant first-pass metabolism
Primary excretion	Renal
Onset of action	30–60 minutes
Duration of action	3–7 h

Adverse Effects: Tramadol is well tolerated, and its most common adverse effects are vertigo, dizziness, headache, nausea, vomiting, constipation, and lethargy. Because it acts centrally, symptoms of CNS stimulation such as nervousness, tremor, anxiety, agitation, confusion, visual impairment, and hallucinations are possible. Some patients experience drowsiness or depression rather than CNS excitation. Seizures have been reported. Although respiratory depression can occur, it is much less than that caused by opioids. Physical dependence is possible although at much less risk than morphine; tramadol is not a controlled substance. Symptoms of opioid withdrawal, such as anxiety, sweating, tremors, panic attacks, and paresthesias, may occur if the drug is abruptly discontinued.

Contraindications/Precautions: Patients with a hypersensitivity to tramadol should not be given the drug. Caution should be exercised in patients allergic to codeine and other opioid agonists because cross-hypersensitivity has been reported. Although the risk for dependence is low, the drug should be used with caution in patients with a history of substance abuse. Tramadol should not be administered to patients with a history of depression or suicide ideation because the drug can be fatal in overdose situations, especially if combined with alcohol or other CNS depressants. Because tramadol causes some degree of respiratory depression, it should be used cautiously in patients with COPD. The drug should be used with caution in patients with renal or hepatic impairment or in those with increased ICP. Because tramadol lowers the seizure threshold, it should be used with caution in patients with a history of seizures. Tramadol should be avoided during pregnancy and lactation because its chronic use can cause physical dependence and postpartum withdrawal symptoms in the newborn.

Drug Interactions: Use of tramadol concurrently with carbamazepine or certain antidepressants increases the risk of seizures. Carbamazepine also has additive CNS depressant effects and may reduce the analgesic activity of tramadol. Ethanol combined with tramadol may result in death. When used with other CNS depressants, the dose of tramadol should be reduced. Concurrent use of tramadol with MAOIs can result in seizures or serotonin syndrome. Tramadol is changed to an active metabolite by the hepatic CYP2D6 enzyme. If inhibitors of this enzyme (e.g., amiodarone, chloroquine, haloperidol, ritonavir, quinidine) are given concurrently with tramadol, a reduced analgesic effect may result. **Herbal/Food:** Food significantly affects the absorption of the extended release form of tramadol. St. John's wort is contraindicated due to the possibility of serotonin syndrome. Caution should be observed when using herbs such as valerian or kava that may have an additive CNS depressant effect.

Pregnancy: Category C.

Treatment of Overdose: Overdose with tramadol will result in serious CNS depression, respiratory depression, and perhaps death. Administration of naloxone will reduce some, but not all, of the symptoms of tramadol overdose and may precipitate convulsions.

Nursing Responsibilities:

- Prior to administration assess allergies, LOC, vital signs, and time since last analgesia administration.
- Assess the patient's response when asked to rate pain on a scale of 0 (no pain) to 10 (worst possible pain).

- Assess for history, signs, and symptoms of substance abuse; withhold the drug and notify the prescriber if noted.
- Monitor for bowel function after surgery and with long-term use. Institute a bowel program to prevent or manage constipation.
- Evaluate the effectiveness of the drug. Supplement analgesia with positional and psychological variables such as elevation of painful extremity, guided imagery, and relaxation techniques.

Patient and Family Education:

- Take the drug on a consistent schedule before the pain level becomes too high.
- Do not drive or perform other hazardous activities until the effects of the drug are known because this drug may cause drowsiness or dizziness.
- Do not break, crush, or chew the extended release tablets; swallow them whole.
- Do not use alcohol when taking this drug because the combination can cause extreme drowsiness and possibly death.
- Do not abruptly discontinue the drug because symptoms of withdrawal may occur.
- Store the medication in a safe place away from children.
- Follow label instructions carefully. Never take a double dose or take the drug more frequently than indicated.
- Immediately report any of the following: difficulty breathing, continued nausea, vomiting, fainting, seizures, or confusion.

Drugs Similar to Tramadol (Ultram)

The two other centrally acting, nonopioid analgesics are clonidine and ziconotide. These drugs act by very different mechanisms than tramadol and are much less frequently prescribed.

Clonidine (Catapres, Duraclon): Originally approved as an oral drug for hypertension (Catapres) in 1974, clonidine has been used off-label for a large number of other indications, including hot flashes, Tourette's syndrome, attention deficit/hyperactivity disorder, and withdrawal from ethanol, nicotine, and opioids. It has a very limited role in treating severe, intractable cancer pain that is refractory to other drugs, including opioids. For this indication, it is administered as an epidural infusion, usually in combination with opioids. Clonidine prevents pain signals from reaching the brain by blocking pain transmission at the presynaptic and postjunctional alpha$_2$-adrenergic receptors in the spinal cord. Because this drug is absorbed into the circulation, the most serious adverse effects from the epidural use of clonidine are the same as those from PO administration: severe hypotension and bradycardia. Clonidine is also available as a transdermal therapeutic system (clonidine TTS), which consists of a patch that releases the drug over 7 days. The antihypertensive actions of clonidine are discussed in Chapter 36. Clonidine is pregnancy category C.

Ziconotide (Prialt): Ziconotide is a relatively new drug approved in 2004 that was obtained from a species of saltwater snail. Like clonidine, its use is limited to patients whose pain is refractory to all other analgesics, including morphine. It is only administered by intrathecal infusion. An off-label use is for severe muscle spasticity due to spinal cord injury. The drug provides analgesia by blocking N-type calcium channels at the presynaptic nerve terminals in the spinal cord. This prevents neurotransmitter release, thus blocking pain transmission. Ziconotide has the potential for frequent and serious adverse effects. The drug labeling carries a warning regarding the potential for severe psychiatric symptoms and neurologic impairment, including impaired cognition, decreased consciousness, and hallucinations. Dizziness, nausea, and vomiting occur in about half the patients receiving the drug. Although these adverse effects are serious, the student should remember that cancer patients receiving this agent are terminally ill and pain relief is often the primary therapeutic goal. This drug is pregnancy category C.

29.12 Adjuvant analgesics have primary indications other than pain but can enhance analgesia.

Some types of pain are not adequately relieved by analgesics alone. **Adjuvant analgesics** are a diverse group of drugs that are used to enhance analgesia for specific indications. All of these drugs have other primary classifications, such as antidepressant, antiseizure, tranquilizer, or anti-inflammatory. The use of adjuvant analgesics includes two primary indications:

- Pain that is refractory to opioids, such as intractable cancer pain
- Neuropathic pain, which is caused by damage to the nerve itself, and pain caused by swelling in the CNS putting pressure on nerves

In patients with intractable cancer pain, adjuvant analgesics are used in combination with analgesics to enhance the level of pain relief. It is important to understand that these agents supplement pain relief; they do not substitute for proper dosing of opioid analgesics in patients with severe pain. Adjuvant analgesics are generally not used if the pain is well managed with opioids, because these drugs have additional adverse effects and drug interactions that can complicate therapy.

Neuropathic pain is difficult to control with analgesics. The most common cause of neuropathic pain is diabetes, but herpes zoster infections, acute trauma, cancer, and certain autoimmune conditions can also cause this type of pain. Neuropathic pain is commonly described as steady burning, electric shock, or "pins and needles" sensations. Rather than treat with high doses of opioids, several adjuvant analgesics have been found to be effective at relieving neuropathic pain. These drugs may be used alone or in combination with opioids.

Adjuvant analgesics can be added at any step in the pain management ladder; they are usually dosed routinely as opposed to

NURSING PROCESS APPLICATION

Patients Receiving Nonopioid Analgesics

Assessment	Potential Nursing Diagnoses
Prior to administration: • Assess pain: location, quality, intensity (use standard scale). • Monitor vital signs and the ability to perform ADLs. • Assess for history of GI or bleeding disorders. • Establish a mutually acceptable pain management goal using the pain rating scale.	• *Acute Pain,* related to inflammation • *Chronic Pain*, related to inflammation • *Risk for Injury,* related to adverse effects of medication • *Deficient Knowledge* (*Analgesic*), related to purpose, precautions, and adverse effects of drug therapy

Planning: Patient Goals and Expected Outcomes

The patient will:

- Rate pain less than the goal level (typically less than 3 on a 0 to 10 pain rating scale).
- Have a relaxed posture and facial expression.
- Be able to accomplish desired ADLs.
- Evidence no signs of abnormal bleeding, GI or other source.

Interventions and (Rationales)	Patient and Family Education
• Monitor closely for GI bleeding in patients with previous history, long-term use, and the elderly. (NSAIDs irritate the GI tract and interfere with platelet activity via their effect on thromboxane A_2. Incidence is increased with use and is more pronounced in the elderly.)	Instruct the patient to: • Report skin rash, dizziness, persistent GI or abdominal pain, tarry stools, unusual bruising or bleeding, difficulty breathing, unusual tiredness, cloudy or bloody urine, confusion or depression, ankle swelling, or unexplained weight gain, or persistent headache. • Take the drug with food or milk to reduce GI upset.
• With high doses or long-term use, periodically monitor hepatic function and hemoglobin (Hgb) and hematocrit (Hct). (Abnormal liver function may occur, possibly leading to toxic hepatitis. Decreasing Hgb and Hct may indicate occult bleeding.)	• Instruct the patient to avoid the use of alcohol with long-term NSAID or aspirin therapy due to increased chance of GI bleeding.
• Monitor for fluid retention: ankle swelling, weight gain, or increased blood pressure. (Some NSAIDs are sodium salts and promote fluid retention.)	• Instruct the patient to report ankle swelling, unexplained weight gain, or increases in blood pressure.
• Monitor for signs of hypersensitivity or salicylism: rash, dizziness, and tinnitus. (These are signs of salicylate toxicity.)	• Aspirin: Instruct the patient to report skin rash, dizziness, ringing in the ears, difficulty hearing, persistent GI or abdominal pain, tarry stools, need to use the drug longer than 10 days (5 days in children). • Discontinue use if allergic to aspirin or other NSAIDs, or in children less than 12 years of age.
• Monitor the character, location, and intensity of pain on a regular basis. Report nonrelief of pain to the prescriber. (Pain management may require multiple modalities for relief.)	Instruct the patient to: • Notify the health care provider if pain lasts more than 10 days, fever lasts more than 3 days, or symptoms worsen.
• Monitor intake of OTC products that may contain aspirin or other NSAIDs. (Aspirin decreases NSAIDs blood level and excretion and increases GI adverse effects; do not use together.)	• Instruct the patient to not take OTC medications without the health care provider's approval because many contain acetaminophen or salicylates.
• Monitor closely for bleeding when taken with PO anticoagulants and thrombolytic agents (due to risk of bleeding complications.)	• Report any signs of bleeding or bruising.
Use a combination of nondrug pain control strategies: • Positioning: Cushion and elevate the painful area if possible. (Cushioning increases comfort while elevation reduces edema.) • Massage or applications of cold or heat. (Stimulating nonpain fibers inhibits the ascending pain pathways [gate control.]) • Relaxation techniques such as guided imagery, rhythmic breathing, meditation, or distraction. (These techniques divert attention from the pain, promote a sense of self-control, and may stimulate endorphin release.)	• Instruct the patient in the use of nondrug pain control strategies.
• Do not give to women who are in the last trimester of pregnancy. (Some of these drugs are pregnancy category D.)	• Instruct the patient to not take the drug during the last 3 months of pregnancy.
• Do not leave drug at the bedside. (Nonopioid analgesics are the most common cause of accidental poisoning and death in small children.)	Instruct the patient to: • Keep the drug out of the reach of children. • Do not give more than five doses per day to children.
• Do not use in children with influenza symptoms (due to the possibility of developing Reye's syndrome.)	• Instruct the patient to not use aspirin in children younger than 16 years old with influenza or chickenpox.
• If female clients are menstruating, use acetaminophen rather than aspirin. (Aspirin has the potential for increasing bleeding during menstrual flow.)	Instruct the patient that: • If taken for menstrual cramps, it is more effective to begin taking the drug 1–2 days before the period begins. • If menstrual flow is heavy, use acetaminophen rather than aspirin.

Evaluation of Outcome Criteria

Evaluate the effectiveness of drug therapy by confirming that patient goals and expected outcomes have been met (see "Planning").

prn. The use of specific adjuvant analgesics and their doses are often guided by experience, rather than controlled clinical trials, and the majority of these drugs are prescribed off-label for their analgesic effects. Table 29.5 summarizes the effects and uses of selected adjuvant analgesics.

Antidepressants: Some of the most commonly prescribed adjuvant analgesics come from the antidepressant drug class. Both of the common classes of antidepressants, tricyclics and selective serotonin reuptake inhibitors (SSRIs), are used as adjuncts in the management of neuropathic pain. Although the tricyclics seem to be more effective, the SSRIs cause fewer serious adverse effects. These drugs increase the levels of the inhibitory neurotransmitters serotonin and norepinephrine in the CNS, resulting in increased pain modulation and decreased pain perception. Patients experiencing neuropathic pain may need trials with different antidepressants until the right combination of effectiveness and tolerable adverse effects is found. Doses of these drugs are generally lower than those used to treat depression, and the drugs act quickly to relieve pain (5 to 7 days). If improvement in pain relief is not noted within 1 week, the drug is discontinued. Examples include amitriptyline (Elavil), imipramine (Tofranil), doxepin (Sinequan), paroxetine (Paxil), and venlafaxine (Effexor).

CONNECTION *Checkpoint* 29.2

Use of tricyclic antidepressants has declined in recent decades due to a higher incidence of adverse effects compared to drugs in the SSRI class. From what you learned in Chapter 23, what type of adverse effects would likely be observed in patients taking tricyclics for migraines? See Answer to Connection Checkpoint 29.2 in Appendix A.

Antiseizure drugs: Antiseizure drugs commonly prescribed for neuropathic pain include gabapentin (Neurontin), valproic acid (Depakene), phenytoin (Dilantin), and carbamazepine (Tegretol). Gabapentin is considered a drug of choice for treating neuropathic pain. The drugs act by suppressing neuronal discharges and reducing the hyperexcitability that occurs after nerve injury. The drugs may cause nausea, vomiting, sedation, confusion, or dizziness.

Corticosteroids: Corticosteroids are used as adjuvants in pain management because they reduce inflammatory swelling and pressure on the brain, spinal cord, and spinal nerves in the CNS. Dexamethasone (Decadron) is the drug of choice when given parenterally to reduce either cerebral or spinal cord edema; oral prednisone (Deltasone) may follow for a period of

TABLE 29.5 Adjuvant Analgesics

Drug Class	Examples	Effect	Use
Antiseizure agent	carbamazepine (Tegretol) clonazepam (Klonopin) gabapentin (Neurontin)	Decrease nerve impulse transmission and spontaneous neuron firing (Phantom pain is theorized as a type of sensory seizure.)	Reduce peripheral nerve pain in neuropathy and phantom pain after amputation
Benzodiazepine	diazepam (Valium) lorazepam (Ativan)	Potentiate effects of gamma aminobutyric acid (GABA) and other inhibitory neurotransmitters	Relax skeletal muscle in muscle spasm, reduce anxiety in terminal dyspnea
Bisphosphonate	etidronate (Didronel) pamidronate (Aredia)	Inhibit bone resorption	Reduce cancer-related bone pain
Corticosteroids	dexamethasone (Decadron) prednisone (various)	Reduce cerebral and spinal edema via various mechanisms in prostaglandin cascade	Reduce swelling and pain in CNS cancer, spinal cord compression, postspinal surgery
Selective serotonin reuptake inhibitor (SSRI)	citalopram (Celexa) fluoxetine (Prozac) fluvoxamine (Luvox) sertraline (Zoloft)	Increase concentrations of inhibitory neurotransmitters (serotinin and norepinephrine) in the CNS	Reduce neuropathic pain
Tricyclic antidepressant	amitriptyline (Elavil) amoxapine desipramine (Norpramin) doxepin (Sinequan) imipramine (Tofranil) nortriptyline (Aventyl) protriptyline (Vivactil)	Increase concentrations of inhibitory neurotransmitters (serotonin and norepinephrine) in the CNS	Reduce neuropathic pain

time. Steroids can also be injected into joint capsules in refractory arthritis, or epidural/spinal tracts for chronic musculoskeletal pain. Their effects are discussed in Chapter 69.

Local anesthetics: Mexiletine (Mexitil) is an antidysrhythmic drug with anesthetic properties that is given PO for neuropathic pain refractory to other analgesics. Caution must be used when giving this drug to patients with heart disease or dysrhythmias. Short IV infusions of lidocaine (Xylocaine) may also provide temporary relief for some patients.

Muscle relaxants: Muscle relaxants such as the benzodiazepines may be used effectively as adjuvant analgesics when muscle spasm is a component of the pain. Muscle spasm can be present following orthopedic injury or with musculoskeletal disease or degenerative nervous system conditions. Benzodiazepines can also be used to reduce anxiety in the terminal dyspnea of heart failure or end-stage respiratory disease. Examples include diazepam (Valium), lorazepam (Ativan), and oxazepam (Serax).

Bone-specific agents: Patients with bone cancer or metastases may experience severe pain. For palliative care, the administration of calcitonin, either subcutaneously or intranasally, may provide some relief for bone pain. The adjuvant analgesic activity of the bisphosphonates such as pamidronate (Aredia) and zoledronic acid (Zometa) has been well established. The use of calcitonin and bisphosphonates in treating bone disorders is presented in Chapter 75.

Pharmacotherapy with Opioid Antagonists

29.13 The primary indication for an opioid antagonist is opioid-induced respiratory depression.

Opioid overdose can occur as a result of overly zealous pain therapy or attempted suicide or from substance abuse. Any opioid may be abused for its psychoactive effects; however, morphine, meperidine, and heroin are preferred by abusers due to their potency. Although heroin is currently available as a legal analgesic in many countries, it is deemed too dangerous for therapeutic use by the FDA, and it is a major drug of abuse. Once injected or inhaled, heroin rapidly crosses the blood–brain barrier to enter the brain, where it is metabolized to morphine. Thus, the effects of heroin administration are actually caused by activation of the mu and kappa receptors from its morphine metabolite. The initial effect is an intense euphoria, or rush, followed by several hours of deep relaxation.

Acute opioid intoxication is a medical emergency, with respiratory depression being the most serious medical challenge. Infusion with the opioid antagonist naloxone (Narcan) may be used to reverse respiratory depression and other acute symptoms. In cases when the patient arrives unconscious and the health care provider is unclear what drug has been taken, small amounts of opioid antagonists may be given to diagnose the overdose. If an opioid antagonist fails to quickly reverse the acute symptoms, the overdose was likely due to a nonopioid substance. Doses for the opioid antagonists are listed in Table 29.6.

When abusing an opioid, the user usually develops tolerance to the euphoric effects of the drug and quickly escalates the dose. Following therapy with an opioid antagonist, however, the patient will become much more sensitive to the effects of opioids. If the patient returns to drug-taking behavior at the same dose used prior to opioid antagonist therapy, death may result.

Another indication for opioid antagonists is for the treatment of opioid-induced constipation or postoperative ileus. Alvimopan (Entereg) and methylnaltrexone (Rellstar), both approved in 2008, act as mu receptors in the GI tract. Because they do not cross the blood-brain barrier, these drugs do not interfere with the central effects of opioids such as analgesia.

PROTOTYPE DRUG Naloxone (Narcan)

Classification: Therapeutic: Opioid (narcotic) antagonist
Pharmacologic: Opioid overdose agent

Therapeutic Effects and Uses: Naloxone was approved in 1971 to reverse the respiratory depression caused by opioid overdose. It is also used postoperatively to reverse the effects of opioids given prior to or during surgery. It has no pharmacologic actions in the absence of opioids. Off-label uses include the

TABLE 29.6 Opioid Antagonists

Drug	Adult Dose (maximum dose where indicated)	Adverse Effects
nalmefene (Revex)	Subcutaneous/IM/IV: use 1 mg/mL concentration Nonopioid dependent: 0.5 mg/70 kg Opioid dependent: 0.1 mg/70 kg	*Muscle and joint pains, difficulty sleeping, anxiety, headache, nervousness, withdrawal symptoms, vomiting* <u>Hepatotoxicity</u>
naloxone (Narcan)	IV: 0.4–2 mg; may be repeated every 2–3 min up to 10 mg if necessary	
naltrexone (ReVia)	PO: 25 mg followed by another 25 mg in 1 h if no withdrawal response (max: 800 mg/day)	

Note: *Italics* indicate common adverse effects. <u>Underline</u> indicates serious adverse effects.

management of nausea, vomiting, urinary retention, or constipation induced by opioid therapy. It has also been used to reverse the effects of benzodiazepines and ethanol.

In administering naloxone, small doses are usually used and repeated until the patient gradually exhibits opioid withdrawal symptoms. The patient must be constantly monitored to ensure that the effects of the drug are sufficiently long to outlast the respiratory depression caused by the opioid overdose; IV doses of naloxone only last 1 hour. Maintenance of a patent airway is essential and resuscitation equipment should be immediately available. The IV route is preferred owing to its more rapid onset of action.

It is important to understand that naloxone will reverse both the toxic and therapeutic effects of opioids. Thus if the patient was using the opioid for analgesia, naloxone will reverse this effect and pain will quickly return.

Mechanism of Action: Naloxone competes with opioid agonists for the mu and kappa receptors, thus antagonizing all the effects of morphine and other opioids and reversing respiratory depression and coma.

Pharmacokinetics:

Routes(s)	Subcutaneous, IM, IV
Absorption	Inactivated after absorption
Distribution	Widely distributed; crosses the placenta; may be secreted in breast milk
Primary metabolism	Hepatic
Primary excretion	Renal
Onset of action	IV: 1–2 minutes; subcutaneous/IM: 2–5 minutes
Duration of action	IV: 1 h; IM: up to 4 h

Adverse Effects: Naloxone has no common adverse effects. Serious adverse effects result from abrupt reversal of opioid depression and include tachycardia, dysrhythmia, hypertension, nausea, and vomiting.

Contraindications/Precautions: Naloxone is contraindicated in patients with hypersensitivity to the drug. Opioid antagonists should be used cautiously in patients who have chronic physical dependence on opioids, because drug-induced withdrawal may be more intense than spontaneous opioid withdrawal. Naloxone should be used with caution in patients with cardiovascular disease. Naloxone may precipitate seizures in patients with seizure disorders.

Drug Interactions: When given concurrently, naloxone reverses all the effects of opioids. Use with tramadol can increase the risk for seizures.

Pregnancy: Category C.

Treatment of Overdose: Overdose with naloxone is rare.

Nursing Responsibilities:

- Assess the patient's respiratory status and administer the opioid antagonist if respirations are below 10 breaths per minute.
- Ensure that resuscitation equipment is immediately available. Be aware that the administration of this drug is an emergency situation to prevent opioid-induced respiratory arrest.
- Monitor for signs of opioid withdrawal such as cramping, vomiting, hypertension, and anxiety.
- Assess the patient's pain level before drug administration and during therapy.
- Monitor vital signs and pupil size every 3–5 minutes. The duration of action of many opioids is longer than the duration of naloxone: repeated doses may be necessary.
- Give IV push undiluted at a rate of 0.4 mg/15 seconds; or dilute and infuse via microdrip and IV pump, titrated to response.
- Use in known or suspected opioid dependency (including in neonates) produces immediate severe withdrawal symptoms. With a mother who is an addict, administration to the infant immediately postdelivery is preferred to maternal administration during labor.

Patient and Family Education:

- Inform the patient and family why the administration of the drug is necessary.

Drugs Similar to Naloxone (Narcan)

Two additional opioid antagonists, nalmefene and naltrexone, have actions similar to those of raloxone.

Nalmefene (Revex): Approved in 1995, nalmefene is given parenterally with similar effects to naloxone but with a longer duration of action that equals that of most opioids. Like the other opioid antagonists, nalmefene will precipitate withdrawal symptoms in opioid-dependent patients within minutes after IV administration. The drug has no serious toxicity associated with it. It is a pregnancy category C drug.

Naltrexone (Depade, ReVia, Vivitrol): Approved in 1984, naltrexone has similar effects to naloxone but is administered by the PO route. An IM form is available for patients who are unable to take the drug by the PO route. Naltrexone prevents the euphoric effects of opioids and is used primarily in drug abuse rehabilitation programs. Successful use of naltrexone in opioid rehabilitation programs is entirely dependent on patient adherence; if the patient stops taking naltrexone, the euphoric effects of opioid abuse will return. If given to opioid-dependent patients, naltrexone will precipitate withdrawal symptoms. Naltrexone is also used to inhibit reward pathways associated with alcoholism (see Chapter 8). When it was approved for alcohol dependence in the 1990s, the trade name Trexan was changed to ReVia. Naltrexone has been awarded orphan drug status by the FDA to treat symptoms of childhood autism. Patients with serious hepatic impairment should not receive naltrexone because the drug is hepatotoxic. This drug is pregnancy category C.

CONNECTION *Checkpoint* 29.3

From what you learned in Chapter 8, describe the symptoms of a patient undergoing acute withdrawal from opioids. How are these symptoms treated? See Answer to Connection Checkpoint 29.3 in Appendix A.

Pharmacotherapy of Migraines

29.14 Migraines are a severe type of headache related to specific triggers.

Headaches are some of the most common complaints of patients. The pain and inability to concentrate causes a significant number of work-related absences and can interfere with activities of daily life. When the headaches are persistent, or manifest as migraines, drug therapy is warranted.

Why does a headache hurt? Although the skull and the brain lack pain receptors, the muscles of the scalp, face, and neck are abundantly supplied with nociceptors. These receptors can be stimulated by muscle tension, dilated blood vessels, and other headache triggers.

Of the several varieties of headaches, the most common type is the **tension headache.** This occurs when muscles of the head and neck become tight due to stress, causing a steady and lingering pain. Although quite painful, tension headaches are self-limiting and more of an annoyance than an emergency. Tension headaches can be effectively treated with OTC analgesics such as aspirin, acetaminophen, or ibuprofen. Table 29.7 differentiates the two common types of headaches.

The most painful type of headache is the **migraine,** which is characterized by throbbing or pulsating pain, sometimes preceded by an aura. **Auras** are sensory warnings of an imminent migraine attack. Examples include flashing lights, visual blind spots, and arm or leg tingling. Nausea, vomiting, and extreme sensitivity to light and sound accompany most migraines. A positive family history is present in the majority of migraine sufferers.

Patients who get migraines appear to have blood vessels that overreact to various triggers. Triggers for migraines include foods containing nitrates or MSG, alcohol (especially red wine), perfumes, food additives, caffeine, chocolate, aspartame, and hormonal, and environmental changes. Some patients can prevent or reduce the frequency of migraine attacks by avoiding known triggers.

The neurotransmitter serotonin (5-hydroxytryptamine or 5-HT) appears to be a key factor (although not the only factor) in the pathogenesis and treatment of migraines. What is the connection between serotonin levels and migraines? Although not precisely understood, the migraine "trigger" creates a spasm in the arteries at the base of the brain, reducing blood flow to the brain. During a migraine, the amount of serotonin in the brain declines and the vessels dilate; nerves surrounding the dilated vessels become inflamed. The expansion of these vessels and associated inflammation are believed to be responsible for the throbbing nature of migraine pain. As neurons in the brain generate additional serotonin, or serotonin agonist drugs are administered, the vessels dilate and pain diminishes.

PharmFACT

Migraine Statistics

- About 20% of the population experiences migraines.
- Before puberty, more boys have migraines than girls; after puberty, women are three times more likely to have migraines than men.
- Headaches and migraines appear mostly among people in their 20s and 30s.
- Migraines are rare after age 50, and their presence in this age group suggests intracranial pathology.

Source: Blanda & Wright, 2008.

29.15 Analgesics and triptans are the primary classes of drugs used to abort acute migraine pain.

There are two primary goals for migraine pharmacotherapy: to terminate an acute migraine in progress and to prevent or reduce the frequency of the disorder. Drugs used to stop a migraine in progress are different from those used for prophylaxis. The prophylactic agents are discussed in Section 29.16.

Migraine pharmacotherapy is most effective if begun before the pain has reached a severe level. Drug therapy is conducted in stages based on the severity of the migraine.

- Mild migraine (occasional headaches with no other functional impairment): NSAIDs offer the safest and least expensive therapy; thus they are tried initially. Acetaminophen is generally not effective alone but offers additive

TABLE 29.7 Differentiation of Major Headache Types

Characteristics	Vascular (Migraine) Headache	Tension Headache
Pain quality	Pulsating or throbbing	Steady pressure or tightness
Pain location	Unilateral (more often) or bilateral	Bilateral (head-band or ice tongs) pattern
Pain severity	Moderate to severe	Mild to moderate
Duration	4–72 hours	Usually several hours
Precursors or triggers	Hormonal changes in women; stress or heightened emotions; bright or flickering lights; change in weather or altitude Foods: alcohol, aged cheeses, chocolate, caffeine, fermented or pickled foods, aspartame, MSG	Stress or anxiety
Associated symptoms	May be preceded by aura, nausea, vomiting, extreme sensitivity to light or sound; aggravated by physical activity	Uncommon

pain relief when combined with an NSAID and caffeine. Oral serotonin (5-HT) agonists (triptans or ergot alkaloids) are initiated in persistent mild migraines that are refractory to NSAIDs.

- Moderate migraine (moderate headaches, nausea, and some functional impairment): Oral, intranasal, or subcutaneous serotonin (5-HT) agonists are the drugs of choice. If serotonin agonists are contraindicated or ineffective, dopamine agonists such as metoclopramide (Reglan) or prochlorperazine (Compazine) may be prescribed.
- Severe migraine (severe headaches more than three times per month, marked nausea or vomiting, and functional impairment): Subcutaneous, IM, or IV serotonin agonists may be indicated. A secondary choice would be a parenteral dopamine agonist, either as monotherapy or in combination with a serotonin agonist. Narcotic analgesics are effective at terminating pain from migraines that have proven to be refractory to other therapies.

The two major drug classes used to terminate migraines, the triptans and the ergot alkaloids, are both serotonin receptor agonists. About 90% of the serotonin receptors (also called serotonergic) are found in the intestine, with the remaining 10% occurring throughout the CNS and in platelets. In the CNS, serotonin is responsible for moderating diverse responses such as anger, anxiety, depression, sleep, appetite, and vomiting. At least seven receptor subtypes have been identified. Other drugs acting at serotonin receptors include certain antianxiety agents, antidepressants, antiemetics, and various hallucinogens. Doses for the triptans and ergot alkaloids are listed in Table 29.8.

TABLE 29.8 Drugs Used to Terminate Acute Migraines

Drug	Adult Dose (maximum dose where indicated)	Adverse Effects
Triptans		
almotriptan (Axert)	PO: 6.25–12.5 mg, may repeat in 2 h (max: 2 doses/24 h)	*Asthenia, tingling, warming sensation, dizziness, vertigo* Coronary artery vasospasm, MI, cardiac arrest
eletriptan (Relpax)	PO: 20–40 mg, may repeat in 2 h (max: 80 mg/24 h)	
frovatriptan (Frova)	PO: 2.5 mg, may repeat in 2 h (max: 3 doses/24 h)	
naratriptan (Amerge)	PO: 1–2.5 mg, may repeat in 4 h (max: 5 mg/24 h)	
rizatriptan (Maxalt)	PO: 5–10 mg, may repeat in 2 h (max: 30 mg/24 h) Use with propranolol: reduce dose to 5 mg (max: 15 mg/24 h)	
sumatriptan (Imitrex)	PO: 25–100 mg, may repeat in 2 h (max: 200 mg/24 h) Nasal: 5–20 mg, may repeat once (max: 40 mg/24 h) Subcutaneous: 6 mg, may repeat in 1 h, once in 24 h	
zolmitriptan (Zomig)	PO: 2.5 mg or less, may repeat in 2 h (max: 10 mg/24 h) Nasal: 5 mg, may repeat once after 2 h (max: 10 mg/24 h)	
Ergot Alkaloids		
dihydroergotamine (DHE 45, Migranal)	Nasal: 1 spray (0.5 mg) each nostril, may repeat once in 15 min (max: 3 mg/24 h, 4 mg/week) IM/subcutaneous: 1 mg, repeat at 1 h intervals for total 3 mg (max: 6 mg/week)	*Weakness, nausea, vomiting, abnormal pulse, throat irritation, nasal irritation, or dysgeusia* Delirium, seizures, cerebrovascular events (hemorrhage), intermittent claudication, birth defects, inhibition of lactation or cause infant vomiting, physical dependence, withdrawal resembles migraine
ergotamine (Ergostat; with caffeine: Cafergot; with caffeine, belladonna, pentobarbital: Cafergot P-B)	Sublingual: 2 mg, may repeat in 30 min for total 3 doses/24 h or 5 doses/week PO: 2 tablets (2 mg), 1 additional tablet repeated every 30 min (max: 6 mg/attack or 10 mg/week) Rectal: 2 mg, may repeat once in 1 h	

Note: *Italics* indicate common adverse effects. Underline indicates serious adverse effects.

Triptans: The first of the triptans, sumatriptan (Imitrex), was marketed in the United States in 1992. This drug was quickly followed by the introduction of the "second-generation" triptans with improved pharmacokinetic profiles; more thorough absorption, faster onset of action, and longer duration. Although all triptans have very similar actions and adverse effects, individual patients may respond more favorably, and with fewer adverse effects, to one triptan over another. The longer duration triptans are believed to be better at preventing the headache from recurring following its termination.

Triptans are selective for the 5-HT_1 receptor subtype, and they are thought to act by constricting certain intracranial vessels. They are effective in aborting migraines with or without auras. Although the PO forms of the triptans are most convenient, patients who experience nausea and vomiting during the migraine may require an alternate dosage form. Intranasal formulations are available and prefilled syringes of triptans may be used for patients who are able to self-administer the medication.

Triptans are not effective at preventing migraines. Other drugs, accompanied by lifestyle changes, must be used for prophylaxis (see Section 29.16).

Ergot alkaloids: For patients who are unresponsive to triptans, the ergot alkaloids may be used to abort migraines. They should be separated from triptan use by at least 24 hours. The first purified alkaloid, ergotamine (Ergostat), was isolated from the ergot fungus in 1920, although the actions of the ergot alkaloids had been known for thousands of years. Ergotamine is an inexpensive drug that is available in PO, sublingual, and suppository forms. Modification of the original molecule has produced a number of other pharmacologically useful drugs, such as dihydroergotamine (Migranal), which is available parenterally and as a nasal spray. Because the ergot alkaloids interact with adrenergic, dopaminergic, and serotonergic receptors, they produce multiple actions and adverse effects. The ergot alkaloids promote vasoconstriction, which terminates a migraine in progress. Adverse effects may include nausea, vomiting, weakness in the legs, myalgia, numbness and tingling in fingers and toes, angina-like pain, and tachycardia. Toxicity may be evidenced by constriction of peripheral arteries: cold, pale, numb extremities and muscle pain. Other possible adverse effects include dizziness, drowsiness, vasoconstriction, warming sensations, tingling, lightheadedness, weakness, and neck stiffness.

Ergot alkaloids, which constrict both arteries and veins, are contraindicated in peripheral vascular disease, coronary artery disease, and severe hypertension because they decrease blood flow. Metoclopramide or prochlorperazine may be administered concurrently with ergot alkaloids to reduce or prevent nausea and vomiting. Many ergot alkaloids are pregnancy category X drugs and should not be used by women who may become pregnant. These drugs may inhibit lactation or cause vomiting in breast-fed infants. Regular daily use can cause physical dependence. Withdrawal symptoms of headache, nausea, and vomiting resemble the symptoms of migraines. Dosing and duration of use need to be restricted. Dangers of overuse and dependence should be included in patient and family teaching.

PROTOTYPE DRUG Sumatriptan (Imitrex)

Classification: **Therapeutic:** Antimigraine agent
Pharmacologic: Serotonin (5-HT_1) receptor agonist

Therapeutic Effects and Uses: Available by the PO, intranasal, and subcutaneous routes, sumatriptan is used to relieve acute migraine headaches. It was the first triptan approved by the FDA in 1992. It is not effective for long-term prophylaxis of migraines; other drugs must be used for this purpose. In 2006 the FDA approved Imitrex STATdose, a system that consists of a 4-mg subcutaneous dose of sumatriptan with an autoinjector pen. Treximet is a fixed dose combination of sumatriptan and naproxen that was approved in 2008 for the treatment of acute migraines.

Mechanism of Action: Sumatriptan is structurally similar to serotonin. Sumatriptan activates the 5-HT_1 serotonin receptors on intracranial and extracerebral blood vessels, resulting in cranial vessel constriction and reduced transmission in trigeminal pain pathways. It has no intrinsic analgesic activity.

Pharmacokinetics:

Routes(s)	PO, intranasal, subcutaneous
Absorption	Limited bioavailability PO (14%)
Distribution	Widely distributed; crosses the placenta; secreted in breast milk; less than 21% bound to plasma protein
Primary metabolism	Hepatic
Primary excretion	60% renal; 40% feces
Onset of action	PO: 30–60 minutes; intranasal: 15–20 minutes; subcutaneous: 10–15 minutes
Duration of action	PO: 6–8 h; intranasal: unknown; subcutaneous: 4–6 h

Adverse Effects: Sumatriptan has infrequent adverse effects that include mild and transient dizziness or nausea, diarrhea, myalgia, and inflammation and pain at the subcutaneous injection site. Headache recurrence occurs in a large percentage of patients taking sumatriptan. Although rare, serious cardiac events have been documented with sumatriptan use. These events include coronary artery vasospasm, myocardial ischemia, dysrhythmias, and MI. These serious events are more likely to occur in patients with preexisting cardiac disease.

Contraindications/Precautions: Sumatriptan is contraindicated in patients with coronary artery disease, cerebrovascular disease, or peripheral vascular disease. This drug is not recommended for patients with uncontrolled hypertension, hypercholesterolemia, or who have a strong family history of cardiovascular disease. Sumatriptan is contraindicated in patients with serious renal or hepatic impairment. Patients with a history of epilepsy have an increased risk for seizures when taking sumatriptan. The drug is associated with fetal deformities and demise in animal studies; it should be avoided in pregnant women. Overuse of abortive therapies for migraine headaches can lead to rebound headaches.

Drug Interactions: Sumatriptan is metabolized by monoamine oxidase and should not be used within 2 weeks of MAOIs or SSRIs. Use of sumatriptan should be avoided within 24 hours of ergot alkaloids or any other 5-HT_1 agonist due to risk of vasospastic reactions. Serotonin syndrome is possible when giving sumatriptan with other drugs that increase serotonin levels or activity, including buspirone (BuSpar), other triptans, amphetamines, sibutramine, trazodone (Desyrel), tricyclic antidepressants (TCAs), lithium, duloxetine (Cymbalta), venlafaxine (Effexor), or meperidine (Demerol). **Herbal/Food**: St. John's wort and feverfew should be avoided during therapy with sumatriptan.

Pregnancy: Category C.

Treatment of Overdose: Few overdoses have been recorded. Treatment of overdose is supportive.

Nursing Responsibilities:

- Assess the patient's neurologic status, including reduced level of consciousness, blurred vision, nausea, vomiting, and tingling in the extremities. These may indicate that a migraine is beginning.
- Administer the drug as soon as possible during the prodromal phase or after the first symptoms of vascular headache occur; then have the patient lie in a quiet, calm environment with decreased noise and subdued lighting.
- Organize care to limit disruptions and decrease neural stimulation.
- Monitor for chest or jaw pain or tightness: If present, contact the health care provider for differentiation from angina or MI.
- Monitor laboratory tests for renal and liver function; impaired organ function can increase serum drug levels.
- Because migraines may be stress related, investigate the patient's stress level and coping mechanisms.
- If using the subcutaneous form, instruct on the use and disposal of the autoinjector. If the migraine returns, a second injection may be used at least an hour after the first; no more than two injections may be given in 24 hours.
- Do not administer antidepressants such as MAOIs or SSRIs within 2 weeks of a triptan.

Patient and Family Education:

- Recognize, avoid, or eliminate factors that trigger a migraine, such as fatigue, anxiety, and alcohol.
- Immediately report any of the following: chest pain or tightness; wheezing; swelling of the eyelids, face, or lips; skin rash; or hives.
- Do not drive or perform other hazardous activities until the effects of the drug are known because this drug may cause drowsiness or dizziness.
- If using the nasal spray, use a single spray in one nostril. A second dose may be used after 2 hours.
- Be aware that this drug only stops a migraine in progress; these drugs do not prevent migraines.
- Take as soon as possible after experiencing an aura or the first symptom of a migraine. Then lie down in a quiet darkened room and apply cold packs to help lessen the pain.
- Do not use this drug if you are pregnant or plan to become pregnant, and use contraception while taking this drug. Triptans are associated with birth defects in animals.
- Do not crush or chew tablets because they have an unpleasant taste.
- Do not breast-feed while using this drug without the approval of the health care provider.
- Use this drug exactly as prescribed because overuse can lead to rebound headaches.

Drugs Similar to Sumatriptan (Imitrex)

Other triptans include almotriptan, eletriptan, frovatriptan, naratriptan, rizatriptan, and zolmitriptan. All the triptans have the same therapeutic effects and spectrum of adverse effects. All the drugs in this class are pregnancy category C.

Almotriptan (Axert): Almotriptan was approved as an oral antimigraine drug in 2001. The drug is well absorbed and has an onset of action of 1 to 3 hours. The drug is extensively metabolized to inactive metabolites by CYP450 enzymes, and 75% is excreted via the kidneys. Drug–drug interactions with agents metabolized in the liver may occur.

Eletriptan (Relpax): Approved in 2002, eletriptan is a newer triptan with improved GI absorption and a more rapid onset of action than sumatriptan. It also has a longer duration. Less than 10% is excreted via the kidneys, making the drug safer to use in patients with renal impairment. The drug is extensively metabolized by CYP450 enzymes and thus has the potential for drug–drug interactions with agents metabolized in the liver.

Frovatriptan (Frova): Frovatriptan has the same effects as sumatriptan but has a slow onset and a very long duration. The 26-hour half-life results in less headache recurrence with this drug. This drug is extensively metabolized by hepatic CYP450 enzymes, and the majority is eliminated in the feces.

Naratriptan (Amerge): Approved in 1998, this drug has a relatively slow onset of action (3 to 4 hours) but with a longer duration of action than sumatriptan. This drug is extensively metabolized to inactive metabolites by CYP450 enzymes and is excreted by the kidneys.

Rizatriptan (Maxalt): Approved in 1998, rizatriptan is absorbed more quickly than sumatriptan, with an onset of 60 to 90 minutes. It is available as PO disintegrating tablets (Maxalt-MLT), which are allowed to dissolve on the tongue and be swallowed with saliva. Hepatic CYP450 enzymes do not significantly metabolize the drug.

Zolmitriptan (Zomig): Zolmitriptan is an oral drug that has the same effects as sumatriptan but is available in additional formulations as a nasal spray and as dissolvable tablets for sublingual (SL) use without water. This drug is metabolized to an active metabolite in the liver, which is responsible for some of its antimigraine activity. Although most adverse effects are mild and transient, zolmitriptan has the highest incidence of adverse effects in the triptan class.

29.16 Many drug therapies are used for migraine prophylaxis.

Prior to initiation of migraine prophylaxis, patients should attempt lifestyle changes and nonpharmacologic therapies to reduce the frequency of their condition. First and foremost, the patient needs to identify personal triggers for migraines. Here the nurse can be helpful in guiding the patient through the process of assessing and identifying those personal migraine triggers. Foods are a common culprit, especially those containing nitrates or MSG. Omitting common migraine triggers from the diet is a first step in migraine prophylaxis. Other lifestyle changes that may help include regular sleep patterns and meals, aerobic exercise (start slowly because sudden intense activity may cause headaches), avoiding alcohol (especially red wine), and smoking cessation. Other helpful self-care measures include keeping a diary that notes when headaches start, how long they last, what provides relief, what the response is to the medication, and food intake or stress in the past 24 hours. Relaxation exercises, meditation, yoga, or progressive muscle relaxation may help. Nontraditional therapies may also be useful in preventing migraines in some patients.

Drugs for migraine prophylaxis include various classes of drugs that are discussed in other chapters of this textbook. These include beta-adrenergic blockers, calcium channel blockers, antidepressants, and antiseizure drugs. Because all of these drugs have the potential to produce adverse effects, prophylaxis is only initiated if the incidence of migraines is high and the patient is unresponsive to the drugs used to abort migraines. Example prophylactic antimigraine agents are shown in Table 29.9. Doses for these drugs are found in the chapters where their primary indication is presented.

Preventive treatment is recommended for headaches that occur three or more times a month. Of the various drugs, the beta-adrenergic blocker propranolol (Inderal) is one of the most commonly prescribed, although other drugs in this class have similar effectiveness. The use of beta blockers is particularly beneficial in patients with comorbid conditions such as hypertension or angina.

TABLE 29.9 Drugs Used for Migraine Prophylaxis

Drug Class	Examples
Antiseizure Drugs	gabapentin (Neurontin)
Beta-Adrenergic Blockers	atenolol (Tenormin)
	metoprolol (Lopressor)
	propranolol (Inderal)
	timolol (Blocadren)
Calcium Channel Blockers	nifedipine (Procardia)
	nimodipine (Nimotop)
	verapamil (Isoptin)
Tricyclic Antidepressants	amitriptyline (Elavil)
	imipramine (Tofranil)
	protriptyline (Vivactil)
	topiramate (Topamax)
	valproic acid (Depakene, Depakote)
Miscellaneous	methysergide (Sansert)

TCAs, especially amitriptyline (Elavil), have been used for decades to prevent migraines and are preferred for patients who may have a mood disorder or suffer from insomnia in addition to their migraines. The antimigraine action of these drugs is independent of their antidepressant action. SSRIs such as fluoxetine (Prozac) have been prescribed off-label for migraines because they exhibit fewer adverse effects than the tricyclics.

Other classes of drugs used for migraine prevention include calcium channel blockers, certain antiseizure drugs, estrogens for menstrual migraines, and miscellaneous agents such as methysergide (Sansert). A recent finding requiring further research is reflected in the use of botulinum toxin type A (Botox) (Mayo Clinic, 2007). Some people receiving Botox injections for facial wrinkles have noted improvement of their headaches. The relationship of Botox to migraines is unclear.

CONNECTIONS

Complementary and Alternative Therapies Natural Therapies for Migraines

- Biofeedback and relaxation training can be learned and used to abort or relieve migraine pain. Patients who learn to consciously raise hand temperature can reduce the number and intensity of migraines. While learning thermal biofeedback, patients wear a device that transmits the temperature to a monitor, which displays temperature or emits a sound as temperature increases. The goal is to wean the patient from the machine so that biofeedback can be used anywhere at the first sign of a headache.
- Massage has proven to be useful in reducing tension headaches. As a stress reduction technique, it may be useful for migraine prevention.
- Riboflavin (vitamin B_2) can reduce migraine attacks, but effects develop slowly, up to 3 months for maximum effect. Doses of 400 mg per day produce few adverse effects.
- Feverfew (*Tanacetum parthenium*) is an herb whose name is derived from its antipyretic properties. The leaves contain the active ingredients, the most prevalent of which is a lactone known as parthenolide. In clinical trials, feverfew was associated with a reduction in number and severity of migraine attacks, as well as decreased vomiting. The most common adverse effect is mouth ulceration (10%).
- Butterbur *(Petasites hybridus)* is an herbal root that may reduce migraine attacks. The preparation Petadolor removes an alkaloid that is toxic to the liver. Adverse effects include mild GI upset.

Source: From *Migraine Headache*, by Mayo Clinic, 2007. Retrieved June 26, 2008, from http://www.mayoclinic.com/health/migraine-headache/DS00120

UNDERSTANDING THE CHAPTER

Key Concepts Summary

29.1 Strategies for pain management have changed over the past two decades.

29.2 Pain is classified by its duration and its source.

29.3 Health care providers and patients sometimes hold myths about pain that impede optimum pain management.

29.4 Pain transmission processes allow multiple targets for pharmacologic intervention.

29.5 Nonpharmacologic interventions are often utilized to reduce and augment analgesic use.

29.6 The overall goal of pain management is to maintain a patient pain level that allows self-care and activities of daily living.

29.7 Opioid analgesics exert their effects by interacting with specific receptors in the central nervous system.

29.8 Opioids are the drugs of choice for moderate to severe pain that cannot be controlled with other classes of analgesics.

29.9 Mixed agonist and antagonist opioids exhibit moderate analgesia with less risk of dependence than morphine.

29.10 Nonsteroidal anti-inflammatory drugs are the medications of choice for mild to moderate pain.

29.11 A few miscellaneous analgesics reduce pain by acting on the central nervous system.

29.12 Adjuvant analgesics have primary indications other than pain but can enhance analgesia.

29.13 The primary indication for an opioid antagonist is opioid-induced respiratory depression.

29.14 Migraines are a severe type of headache related to specific triggers.

29.15 Analgesics and triptans are the primary classes of drugs used to abort acute migraine pain.

29.16 Many drug therapies are used for migraine prophylaxis.

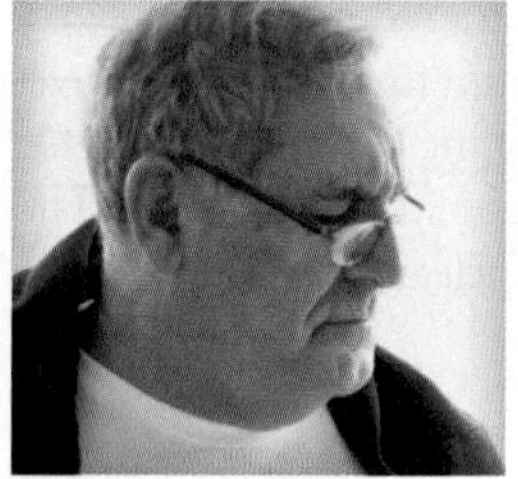

Making the PATIENT *Connection*

Remember the patient "Larry Smith" at the beginning of the chapter? Now read the remainder of the case study. Based on the information presented within this chapter, respond to the critical thinking questions that follow.

Larry Smith was being seen for outpatient presurgery work-up the evening before scheduled urologic surgery. As a registered nurse in the clinic, you conduct a thorough history and examination related to his back pain and current pain management. His anticipated hospital stay is 2 days postsurgery.

Mr. Smith is a 64-year-old male. Vital signs are: blood pressure, 108/64 mmHg; pulse, 88 beats/minute; respirations, 16/minute. He has a well-healed midline scar on his back from lumbar vertebrae surgery, with a shorter scar over his right iliac crest. He moves a bit slowly with some limited lumbar range of motion. He also uses a cane for ambulating any distance. He describes his pain as a constant dull ache in the lower back, which increases with prolonged standing or walking. Mr. Smith also reports a feeling of "cold electricity" down both legs, with the left greater than the right, which increases with standing and walking, as well as numbness of the middle toes on his left foot. He has been using mixed opioid and nonopioid analgesics for the last 8 years and previously had used SSRI antidepressants as adjuvant for his pain. His current health care provider weaned him off Vicodin ES about a year ago. He now takes methadone 20 mg twice a day. When the pain is not relieved he uses Norco for breakthrough pain. His use of Norco is 1 to 2 per day. Constipation is an ongoing problem, requiring stool softeners and occasional laxatives.

Critical Thinking Questions

1. How should Mr. Smith's postoperative pain be managed? Is there a referral you can make to facilitate effective pain management?
2. How could you best communicate Mr. Smith's needs to the postoperative nursing staff?
3. What should the nurse plan be for postoperative management of analgesic adverse effects?

Case Study

Rita Manson presents to the emergency department with vomiting, severe abdominal and back pain, and jaundice. Her jaundice is recent but the pain and vomiting have continued for a couple of months. Her diagnostic work-up reveals advanced pancreatic cancer with metastasis to the spine.

1. What is the drug of choice for Rita's pain management? Which route would you expect to see used initially?
2. Her prescribed pain medication is morphine sulfate 2–10 mg IV every 2 hours as needed for pain. Outline your approach to pain management for the first 24 hours.
3. What adverse effects would you expect?
4. As part of the patient's pain management, dexamethasone (Decadron) 5 mg IV is prescribed every 6 hours for 2 days. Explain the use of corticosteroids in pain management.
5. After several days, Rita expresses her concern about "becoming hooked on that narcotic." How would you respond?

NCLEX-RN® Review

1 The nurse is monitoring the client for adverse effects associated with morphine. Which of the following adverse effects would be the expected? Select all that apply.

1. Respiratory depression
2. Hypertension
3. Urinary retention
4. Constipation
5. Nausea

2 Several days postoperative bowel surgery, the client is eating soft food, ambulating regularly, and using hydromorphone (Vicodin) for pain. The nursing care plan should include:

1. Monitoring vital signs for respiratory depression.
2. Inserting a urinary catheter for urinary retention.
3. Weaning pain medication to prevent addiction.
4. Increasing dietary fiber and fluids and administering a stool softener.

3 A female client, who suffers from migraine headaches, self-administered sumatriptan (Imitrex) for the first time yesterday. Today, the client informs the nurse that after taking the medication she began to experience chest pain. She further states that the drug was effective in relieving the headache. The nurse should:

1. Encourage the client to continue using the drug because it was effective.
2. Advise the client to tell her health care provider about the chest pain on her next visit.
3. Caution the client to contact her health care provider to report the chest pain today and to not use the sumatriptan until she talks to her health care provider.
4. Encourage the client to lie down in a quiet room and use cold packs during the next migraine.

4 A client with diabetes reports increasing pain and numbness in his legs. "It feels like pins and needles all the time, especially at night." Which drug would the nurse expect to be prescribed for this client?

1. Ibuprofen (Motrin)
2. Gabapentin (Neurontin)
3. Naloxone (Narcan)
4. Methadone

5 The emergency department nurse is caring for a client with a migraine headache. Which of the following drugs would the nurse anticipate administering to abort the client's migraine attack?

1. Morphine
2. Dihydroergotamine (Migranal)
3. Propranolol (Inderal)
4. Ibuprofen (Motrin)

6 The nurse is caring for several clients who are receiving opioids for pain relief. Which client is at the highest risk of developing hypotension, respiratory depression, and mental confusion?

1. A 23-year-old female, post delivery of a 6-lb baby
2. A 16-year-old male, post motorcycle injury with lacerations
3. A 54-year-old female, post myocardial infarction
4. An 86-year-old male postoperative femur fracture

See Answers to Critical Thinking Questions, Case Study, and NCLEX-RN® Review in Appendix A.

References

American Pain Foundation. (n.d.). *Fast facts about pain.* Retrieved June 26, 2008, from www.painfoundation.org/page.asp?file=Library/FastFacts.htm

Blanda, M., & Wright, J. T. (2008). Headache, migraine. *eMedicine.* Retrieved June 26, 2008, from http://www.emedicine.com/emerg/TOPIC230.HTM

Brennan, F., Carr, D. B., & Cousins, M. (2007). Pain management: A fundamental human right. *Anesthesia and Analgesia, 105,* 205–221.

Drug Facts & Comparisons (60th ed.). (2006). St. Louis: Facts & Comparisons.

Drug Information 2006. (2006). Bethesda, MD: American Hospital Formulary Service.

Fine, P. G., & Low, C. M. (2007). *Principles of effective pain management at the end of life.* Retrieved June 26, 2008, from http://www.medscape.com/viewprogram/6079

Glickman-Simon, R. (2006). *Persistent pain and palliative care.* Proceedings of the American College of Physicians 2006 Annual Session, April 6–8, 2006, Philadelphia.

Gordon, D. B., Dahl, J. L., Miaskowski, C., McCarberg, B., Todd, K. H., Paice, J. A., et al. (2005, July 25). American Pain Society recommendations for improving the quality of acute and cancer pain management. *Archives of Internal Medicine, 165,* 1574–1580.

LeMone, P., & Burke, K. M. (2008). *Medical surgical nursing care: Critical thinking in client care* (4th ed.). Upper Saddle River, NJ: Prentice-Hall.

Lussier, D., Huskey, A. G., & Portenoy, R. K. (2004). Adjuvant analgesics in cancer pain management. *The Oncologist, 9*(5), 571–591.

Mayo Clinic. (2007). *Migraine headache.* Retrieved June 26, 2008, from http://www.mayoclinic.com/health/migraine-headache/DS00120

Pasternak, G. W., Inturrisi, C. E., Porreca, F., & Rowbotham, M. C. (2008). Signal transduction of pain: Implications for opioid therapy. *Medscape Today.* Retrieved June 26, 2008, from http://www.medscape.com/viewprogram/8437

Sinatra, R. (2006). Opioid analgesics in primary care: Challenges and new advances in the management of noncancer pain. *Journal of the American Board of Family Medicine, 19*(2), 165–177.

University of Michigan Health System. (2006). *Pain management staff development & education; Part 4: Adult pain management staff education.* Retrieved September 19, 2008, from www.med.umich.edu/pain/apainmgt.htm

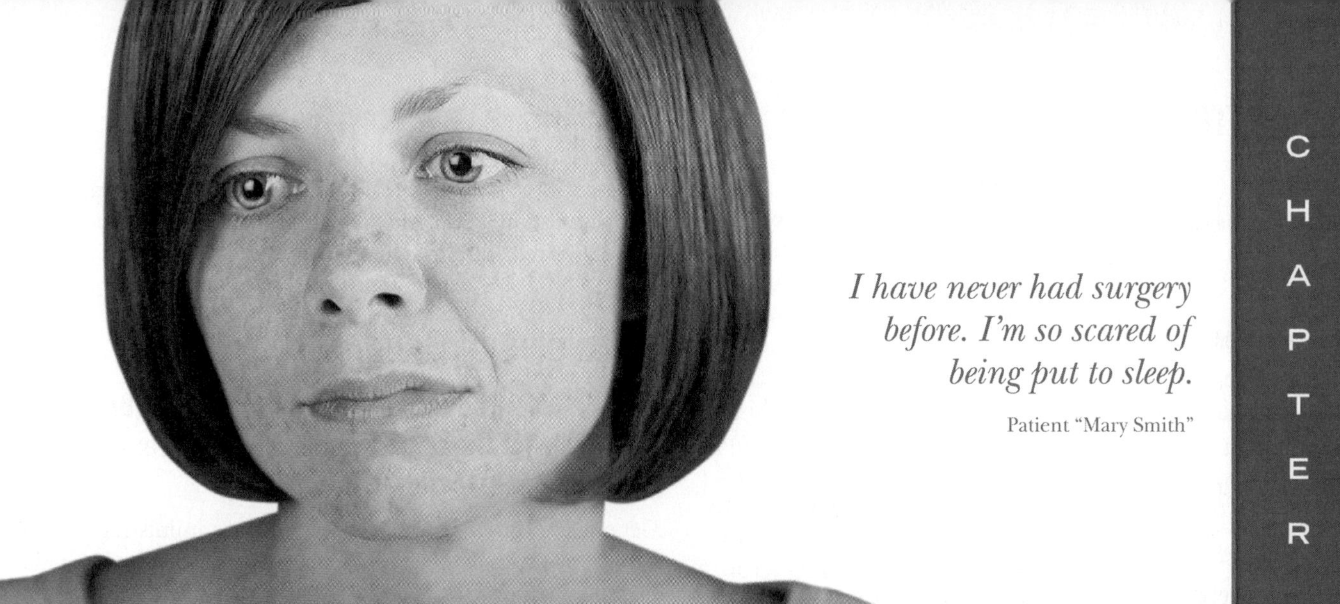

I have never had surgery before. I'm so scared of being put to sleep.

Patient "Mary Smith"

CHAPTER 30

Anesthetics and Anesthesia Adjuncts

Chapter Outline

Types of Anesthesia

Principles of General Anesthesia

Intravenous Anesthetic Agents

Barbiturate Anesthetics

PROTOTYPE **Thiopental Sodium (Pentothal)** *p. 459*

Opioid Anesthetics

PROTOTYPE **Fentanyl (Actiq, Duragesic, Sublimaze)** *p. 461*

Benzodiazepine Anesthetics

PROTOTYPE **Midazolam (Versed)** *p. 463*

Miscellaneous Intravenous Anesthetic Agents

PROTOTYPE **Ketamine (Ketalar)** *p. 464*

Inhalation General Anesthetic Agents

Gaseous Anesthetics

PROTOTYPE **Nitrous Oxide** *p. 466*

Volatile Liquid Anesthetics

PROTOTYPE **Isoflurane (Forane)** *p. 468*

Local Anesthetics

Classification of Local Anesthetic Agents

Esters

PROTOTYPE **Procaine (Novocaine)** *p. 472*

Amides

PROTOTYPE **Lidocaine (Anestacon, Dilocaine, Xylocaine, Others)** *p. 474*

Adjuncts to Anesthesia

Learning Outcomes

After reading this chapter, the student should be able to:

1. Compare and contrast the four basic types of anesthesia.
2. Understand the effects of regional and general anesthetic agents.
3. Explain the five general purposes of balanced anesthesia.
4. Compare and contrast the four stages of general anesthesia.
5. For each of the classes shown in the chapter outline, identify the prototype and representative drugs and explain the mechanism(s) of drug action, primary indications, contraindications, significant drug interactions, pregnancy category, and important adverse effects.
6. Describe the nursing care associated with the administration of regional and general anesthesia.
7. Explain the rationale for using adjunct agents during general anesthesia.
8. Use the nursing process to care for patients receiving local or general anesthesia.

Key Terms

amide, 474
balanced anesthesia, 458
dissociative anesthesia, 464
ester, 472
general anesthesia, 458
local anesthesia, 458
minimum alveolar concentration, 465
monitored anesthesia care (MAC), 458
narcoanalysis, 459
neurolept analgesia, 461
regional anesthesia, 458
surgical anesthesia, 459

Throughout history, the induction of anesthesia has allowed patients to experience a temporary loss of sensation, resulting in comfort during surgical intervention. The use of opium as an anesthetic was recorded as far back as 4200 BC, and the ancient Chinese recorded acupuncture as a form of anesthesia. The modern implementation of anesthesia dates back to 1856 when Dr. John C. Warren performed a surgical procedure using ether. Modern anesthesia has progressed and now offers safer and more effective drugs. This chapter introduces the student to the general and regional anesthetic agents along with the adjuvant medications administered during medical procedures that require anesthesia.

Types of Anesthesia

30.1 Anesthesia is used to produce a controlled loss of sensation during a diagnostic or surgical procedure.

Certain medical procedures produce a significant degree of anxiety or pain, or both, and some of these procedures would not be possible without anesthesia. There are four types of anesthesia. The type of anesthesia selected depends on the degree of sedation and analgesia needed to conduct the procedure.

General anesthesia is the loss of sensation throughout the entire body, accompanied by the loss of consciousness (LOC). General anesthesia is necessary for major surgical procedures.

The induction of **local anesthesia** results in loss of sensation to a limited body region without the LOC. It affects only the immediate area that surrounds where the anesthetic is administered. **Regional anesthesia** is similar, except that it encompasses a larger body area, such as an entire limb. Local and regional anesthesias produce fewer adverse effects than general anesthesia and are thus the methods of choice where applicable.

A fourth type of anesthesia is **monitored anesthesia care (MAC),** which uses sedatives, analgesics, and other low-dose drugs that allow patients to remain responsive and breathe without assistance. This type of anesthesia is used during diagnostic procedures and minor surgeries to supplement local and regional anesthesias. Subtypes of MAC are based on the degree of sedation produced.

- Minimal sedation (anxiolysis). Patients respond to verbal commands. Airway, ventilation, and cardiovascular functions are normal.
- Moderate (conscious) sedation. Patients respond to verbal or light tactile prompting. Airway, ventilation, and cardiovascular functions are usually adequate.
- Deep sedation/analgesia. Patients are aroused by repeated or painful stimulation. Airway and ventilation intervention may be required. Cardiovascular functions are usually adequate.

Principles of General Anesthesia

30.2 Balanced anesthesia uses multiple drugs to provide for the safe induction and maintenance of general anesthesia.

General anesthesia is accomplished by the administration of a variety of drugs. The general purposes of general anesthesia include the following:

- Analgesia: blocking the sensation of pain
- Relaxation: relieving the intense anxiety associated with medical procedures
- Hypnosis: production of unconsciousness to block awareness of the procedure
- Amnesia: blocking memory of the events associated with the procedure
- Loss of reflexes: blocking autonomic and other reflexes that may be affected by the procedure

No single drug can safely accomplish these five general purposes. **Balanced anesthesia** is the use of a combination of medications to produce general anesthesia. Agents administered to achieve balanced anesthesia include neuromuscular blockers, short-acting barbiturates, opioids, and general anesthetics. The purpose of the combination of these medications is to provide sedation, rapid induction of unconsciousness, muscle relaxation, and analgesia. The use of multiple drugs reduces the need for large amounts of inhaled anesthetics, which increases patient safety.

The process of balanced general anesthesia involves the administration of intravenous (IV) agents prior to the inhalation agents. The IV medications produce relaxation of the muscles, diminish pain, and promote sleep. After the patient loses consciousness, inhaled agents are administered to maintain the anes-

TABLE 30.1 Stages of General Anesthesia

Stage	Characteristics
1	Analgesia: The patient loses general sensation but may remain awake. This stage progresses until the patient loses consciousness.
2	Excitement and hyperactivity: The patient may become delirious and attempt to resist treatment. The heart rate and respiratory rate may become irregular. The patient's blood pressure may increase. The administration of IV agents may calm the patient.
3	Surgical anesthesia: The patient's skeletal muscles become relaxed and delirium stabilizes. The cardiopulmonary effects stabilize. The patient becomes still with diminished eye movements. The surgical procedure is begun. The patient remains in stage three until the procedure ends.
4	Paralysis of the medulla: If breathing and cardiac function cease, death could result. This stage of general anesthesia is avoided.

thetized state. For short procedures, lower amounts of anesthesia are administered, or parenteral agents alone may be sufficient.

General anesthesia is a progressive process that occurs in distinct phases, which are described in Table 30.1. The most effective medications can quickly induce all four stages, whereas others are able to induce only stage 1. Major surgical procedures require the patient to be maintained in stage 3, which is referred to as **surgical anesthesia.** In the event of major surgery the patient should progress from stage 2 to stage 3 anesthesia rapidly. Stage 2 produces excitement and hyperactivity and resistance to treatment. Because of these symptoms, it is important to move the patient through stage 2 as rapidly as possible. During stage 2 the patient is monitored closely for heart rate irregularities and increases in blood pressure.

PharmFACT

The most common type of anesthesia for pain relief during labor is epidural anesthesia. About 50% of women giving birth in hospitals receive epidural anesthesia. *Source:* American Pregnancy Association, 2007.

Intravenous Anesthetic Agents

30.3 Intravenous general anesthetic agents include barbiturates, opioids, and benzodiazepines.

IV anesthetics are important supplements to general that provide the patient with the ability to rapidly progress through stages 1 and 2. They are on occasion used alone during minor diagnostic and surgical interventions. Concurrent administration of IV agents and inhaled anesthetics allows the dose of the inhaled anesthetic to be reduced. The lowered dosage of inhaled anesthetic agents produces a better surgical outcome and lowers the risk of serious adverse effects from the anesthesia. The combined use of IV and inhaled anesthesia allows for a greater degree of analgesia and muscle relaxation than when inhalation anesthetics are used alone.

Approximately 12 agents are used as IV general anesthetics. Some of these drugs also have nonanesthetic indications. Drugs from the following classes are used for IV anesthesia.

- Barbiturates
- Benzodiazepines
- Opioids
- Miscellaneous agents

30.4 Barbiturates induce rapid general anesthesia but their duration of action is very brief.

Barbiturates have been used as drugs since the early 1900s. These agents have a powerful sedative–hypnotic effect that led to their widespread use in treating anxiety and insomnia for many decades. Although they have been replaced by safer agents for most indications, barbiturates are still used as IV anesthetics. Details on the mechanisms of action of barbiturates and their applications as sedatives may be found in Chapter 22.

Barbiturates are classified by their duration of action. Because the two IV anesthetic drugs in this class have very short durations of action, they are employed for procedures that have approximately 15 minutes duration. In the event that the surgical procedure lasts longer than 15 minutes barbiturates can be administered as a supplement to other anesthetic agents. The degree of analgesia produced by barbiturates is poor; thus other drugs must be used concurrently if pain is an expected part of the procedure. Barbiturates produce little or no vomiting and they do not produce obstructive secretions. Table 30.2 lists doses for barbiturate IV agents.

PROTOTYPE DRUG Thiopental sodium (Pentothal)

Classification: **Therapeutic:** General anesthetic agent
Pharmacologic: Barbiturate, GABA receptor agonist

Therapeutic Effects and Uses: Thiopental is an older drug, having been administered first for anesthesia in the 1930s. Thiopental is administered IV to induce hypnosis and anesthesia during brief surgical procedures lasting 15 minutes or less. It can also be administered prior to inhalation anesthesia or given intermittently during a surgical procedure to maintain anesthesia. It is an ultra-short-acting barbiturate that produces brief anesthesia without analgesia. It is a Schedule III controlled substance.

In addition to its use as an anesthetic, thiopental has been approved by the U.S. Food and Drug Administration (FDA) to treat status epilepticus, a severe condition involving repetitive seizures. It may be used as a bolus injection to reduce intracranial pressure during intraoperative procedures and in patients with head trauma. In the past, thiopental was administered as a "truth serum" during psychoanalysis to encourage patients to freely share information. During this procedure, called **narcoanalysis,** the patient is placed in a hypnotic state but is able to answer questions or explore painful memories. Evidence gathered during narcoanalysis is often inadmissible in court because studies have shown that people can indeed be untruthful under the influence of the drug. Narcoanalysis remains an FDA-approved indication for thiopental.

MyNursingKit | Virtual Anesthesia Textbook

Mechanism of Action: Thiopental sodium depresses the central nervous system (CNS), reduces cardiac output, and produces vasodilation. This medication is rapidly redistributed out of the brain, reducing the level of anesthesia. Thiopental sodium produces slight muscle relaxation and poor control of reflexes.

Pharmacokinetics:

Route(s)	IV
Absorption	Rapid: 30–60 seconds
Distribution	Distributed in muscle and liver; crosses the placenta and is secreted in breast milk
Primary metabolism	Hepatic
Primary excretion	Renal
Onset of action	30–60 seconds
Duration of action	10–30 minutes

TABLE 30.2 Intravenous General Anesthetic Agents

Drug	Route and Adult Dose (maximum dose where indicated)	Adverse Effects
Barbiturates		
methohexital	IV: 5–120 mg at a rate of 5 mg every 5 min; then 20–40 mg every 4–7 min as needed	*Myocardial depression, postoperative psychomotor impairment, retrograde amnesia, hypothermia, sloughing with extravasation, skeletal muscle hyperactivity* Circulatory depression, respiratory depression, respiratory arrest, apnea, anaphylaxis
thiopental (Pentothal)	IV test dose: 25–75 mg then 50–75 mg at 20–40-second intervals, an additional 50 mg as needed	
Opioids		
alfentanil (Alfenta)	IV: 8–20 mcg/kg for surgery lasting longer than 30 min Maintenance anesthesia: 3–5 mcg/kg in incremental doses Continuous infusion: 0.5–1 mcg/kg/min Total dose: 8–40 mcg/kg	*Skeletal muscle rigidity, nausea, vomiting, postoperative drowsiness, shivering, hypertension (HTN), bradycardia, prolonged QT interval, constipation* Apnea, respiratory depression, laryngospasm, bronchospasm, circulatory depression, cardiac arrest, respiratory depression, respiratory arrest, anaphylactoid reaction
fentanyl with droperidol	Droperidol: 2.5 mg IV; additional doses of 1.25 mg as needed Fentanyl: 2–20 mcg/kg IV; additional doses of 25–100 mcg as needed	
morphine sulfate	IV: 2.5–15 mg/70 kg	
remifentanil (Ultiva)	IV: 0.5 mcg/kg/min or 1 mcg/kg IV bolus	
sufentanil (Sufenta)	IV: 1–8 mcg/kg; may give additional doses of 10–50 mcg if needed Primary anesthetic: 1–30 mcg/kg IV administered with 100% oxygen	
Benzodiazepines		
diazepam (Valium)	IV: 5–10 mg, repeat every 10–15 min as needed	*Drowsiness, hypotension, tachycardia, retrograde amnesia* Cardiovascular collapse, respiratory arrest, laryngospasm
midazolam (Versed)	Premedication: 0.15–0.25 mg/kg IV over 20–30 seconds Nonpremedicated: 0.3–0.35 mg/kg IV over 20–30 seconds	
Miscellaneous IV General Anesthetics		
ketamine (Ketalar)	IV: 1–4 mg/kg IM: 6.5–13 mg/kg	*Respiratory depression, laryngospasm, apnea, nausea, vomiting* HTN, tachycardia, emergence phenomena
propofol (Diprivan)	IV: 2–2.5 mg/kg every 10 seconds until induction onset	*Jerking, thrashing, bucking, clonic or myoclonic movements* Ventricular systole

Note: *Italics* indicate common adverse effects. Underline indicates serious adverse effects.

Adverse Effects: Thiopental sodium is a dangerous drug that is only administered by trained health care personnel in a controlled setting with continuous monitoring. Severe adverse reactions include respiratory depression, laryngospasm, and hypotension. CNS effects may persist for 24 hours and include confusion, delirium, somnolence, anxiety, and seizures. Other adverse events include shivering, nausea, vomiting, and anaphylaxis. Immediate access to resuscitative drugs and equipment must be provided.

Contraindications/Precautions: Patients with a known hypersensitivity to barbiturates should not be administered thiopental. The patient who does not have adequate IV access should not be administered thiopental due to the risk of extravasation and resultant arteritis, neuritis, and sloughing of the skin. Thiopental sodium is also contraindicated in status asthmaticus, hepatic porphyrias, and pregnancy. It should be used cautiously in patients who have been diagnosed with coronary artery disease, liver or kidney disease, myxedema, and Addison's disease.

Drug Interactions: The administration of thiopental with phenothiazines increases the risk of hypotension. Probenecid administered with thiopental will result in prolonged anesthesia. Use during ethanol intoxication or with other sedating drugs may cause additive CNS depression. **Herbal/Food:** The administration of thiopental with kava or valerian may result in increased sedation.

Pregnancy: Category C.

Treatment of Overdose: In the event of overdosage of thiopental sodium the patient should be ventilated to prevent hypoxia. If the patient is experiencing a laryngospasm, a muscle relaxant should be administered and endotracheal intubation is indicated.

Nursing Responsibilities:

- Assess the patient's vital signs every 3 to 5 minutes before, during, and after administration and until recovery.
- Ensure a patent airway and place the patient in a side-lying position (unless contraindicated) to prevent pulmonary aspiration.
- Report increases in pulse rate or drops in blood pressure to the prescriber.
- Assess the patient for shivering, excitement, and muscle twitching in the recovery period if the patient is in pain.

Patient and Family Education:

- Know that the onset of drug action is rapid, with loss of consciousness in 30 to 60 seconds.
- Following recovery, immediately report dizziness, palpitations, numbness, or tingling in hands or feet; pain or swelling at the injection site; skin rash; or difficulty breathing.
- For 24 hours after recovery, change positions slowly to avoid dizziness.
- Do not drive or perform other hazardous activities requiring mental alertness, and do not drink alcohol.

Drugs Similar to Thiopental Sodium (Pentathol)

The only other barbiturate used for anesthesia is methohexital.

Methohexital (Brevital): Methohexital is a barbiturate general anesthetic agent that can be used to induce general anesthesia or administered as a continuous IV infusion. Compared to thiopental sodium, it is more potent, has less cumulative effect, and has a more rapid onset and a shorter duration of action. The recovery from this medication is more rapid than that of thiopental sodium. Intramuscular (IM) and rectal forms are available for use in children. Approved in 2001, the adverse effects and contraindications are the same as those for thiopental. This drug is pregnancy category B.

PharmFACT

About half of the 26 million anesthetics given each year are administered by a nurse anesthetist. *Source:* American Association of Nurse Anesthetists, 2008.

30.5 Opioids are used as intravenous anesthetics to provide analgesia and to accomplish neurolept anesthesia.

Opioids, or narcotic analgesics, are the most effective drugs available for pain relief, and they have been used for perioperative pain management for many decades. To produce deep anesthesia, however, opioids must be combined with other anesthetics. Combinations allow lower doses to be used and provide the necessary analgesia for painful procedures.

Alfentanil (Alfenta), fentanyl (Sublimaze), remifentanil (Ultiva), and sufentanil (Sufenta) are opioids used as IV general anesthetic agents. These medications are opioid receptor agonists that provide a rapid onset of action with a short duration of 10 to 30 minutes. Their primary disadvantage is respiratory depression. Muscle rigidity may occur, which can impair ventilation further. A complete discussion of mechanisms, actions, and adverse effects of the opioids is included in Chapter 29. A prototype feature for morphine can be found in that chapter. Doses for the opioid general anesthetic agents are listed in Table 30.2.

The combination of droperidol and fentanyl produces a type of anesthesia called **neurolept analgesia.** Neurolept analgesia produces feelings of indifference to the patient's surroundings. The patient appears to be asleep but does not lose consciousness. Fentanyl is a potent opioid agonist with pharmacologic action that is similar to morphine. Droperidol is an antipsychotic agent related to haloperidol. It has the ability to reduce the nausea and vomiting adverse effects of opioids and produces sedation by reducing anxiety and motor activity.

PROTOTYPE DRUG Fentanyl (Actiq, Duragesic, Sublimaze)

Classification: **Therapeutic:** Analgesic, anesthetic
Pharmacologic: Opioid agonist

Therapeutic Effects and Uses: Fentanyl is an opioid analgesic that is administered IV for short duration analgesia as part of premedication, balanced anesthesia, induction, and maintenance of anesthesia, and in the postoperative period for pain. It may be administered with droperidol to produce neurolept analgesia. As an anesthetic agent it may be administered with oxygen in high-risk patients, such as those undergoing open heart surgery or certain complicated neurologic or orthopedic procedures.

Transdermal fentanyl (Duragesic) is a patch for treating severe, chronic pain. Before receiving the fentanyl patch, patients should be opioid tolerant (received oral [PO] or parenteral opiates for at least a week). Patients may require short-term administration of other opioids for breakthrough pain until the correct patch dose has been titrated. A transmucosal form of fentanyl (Actiq) is used for breakthrough pain in opiate-tolerant patients. The patient places the transmucosal tablet between the cheek and gum until it is entirely dissolved. Fentora is a form of fentanyl administered as a buccal tablet.

Opioids such as fentanyl will result in tolerance if taken in high drug dosages over an extended time. Doses need to be adjusted periodically for adequate pain management. Physical and psychological dependence may occur with continued use. Abrupt discontinuation of the drug may cause intense withdrawal symptoms (see Chapter 8). Fentanyl is a Schedule II controlled substance. When taken illegally, fentanyl gives the same effects as heroin.

Mechanism of Action: Fentanyl is an opioid agonist at the mu and kappa receptors. The mechanism of action is the same as morphine and other opioids. Fentanyl has a more rapid onset of action than morphine.

Pharmacokinetics:

Route(s)	IV, transdermal, transmucosal, epidural
Absorption	Rapid
Distribution	Crosses the placenta; secreted in breast milk; 80% bound to protein
Primary metabolism	Hepatic (CYP3A4)
Primary excretion	Renal
Onset of action	IV: immediate; IM: 7–15 minutes; transdermal: 24–72 h peak; transmucosal: 20–30-minute peak; epidural: 10–15 minutes
Duration of action	IV: 0.5–1 h; IM: 1–2 h; transdermal: 17 h half-life; transmucosal: unknown; epidural: 2–3 h

Adverse Effects: The most common adverse effects of fentanyl include respiratory depression, apnea, skeletal muscle rigidity, and bradycardia. The respiratory depression may occur postoperatively and outlast the analgesic effects of the drug. Nausea, vomiting, and constipation are common adverse effects produced by most opioids. Transdermal patches can cause localized pain, irritation, ulceration, and bleeding.

Contraindications/Precautions: Patients with respiratory impairment should be administered fentanyl with caution due to the respiratory depression caused by the drug. Patients with hepatic or renal impairment should receive lower doses. The drug may worsen bradydysrhythmia. Patients with head trauma should not receive fentanyl because intracranial pressure may increase. Fentanyl is secreted in breast milk and can cause sedation and respiratory depression in the neonate; thus it should not be administered during lactation.

Drug Interactions: Caution should be used when administering fentanyl with other CNS depressants due to additive sedation. Fentanyl is metabolized by CYP450 enzymes (CYP3A4) in the liver and intestinal mucosa and has the potential to interact with other drugs that induce or inhibit this enzyme. Cardiovascular depression may occur if nitrous oxide is used with high doses of fentanyl. **Herbal/Food:** St. John's wort may intensify or prolong the effects of fentanyl anesthesia and may induce the metabolism of fentanyl via CYP3A4. Use of valerian or kava may cause additive CNS depression.

Pregnancy: Categories B (parenteral) and C (transdermal and transmucosal forms).

Treatment of Overdosage: In the event of overdosage the patient is supported with mechanical ventilation until the drug is metabolized and the effects diminish. The patient may be administered a narcotic antagonist such as naloxone (Narcan).

Nursing Responsibilities:

- Monitor for signs of respiratory depression, such as respiratory rates less than 10, poor breath sounds, or shallow respiratory effort.
- Monitor the electrocardiogram (ECG) throughout medication administration and examine for signs of cardiac dysrhythmias.
- Monitor for adverse effects such as hypotension and tachycardia.
- Monitor for signs and symptoms of dystonia, such as muscle tremors, cramps, and spasms.
- Assess for therapeutic effect of the drug if given for pain. Solicit the patient's rating of pain on a pain scale (0 to 10).

Patient and Family Education:

- Do not drive or perform other hazardous activities because this drug may cause drowsiness or dizziness. All three drugs are pregnancy category C.
- Apply fentanyl patches to clean, dry skin. Press firmly on the patch for 30 seconds to ensure proper skin contact.
- Do not split, chew, or swallow the transmucosal or buccal forms of fentanyl.
- Immediately report palpitations, shortness of breath, chest pain, muscle rigidity, or pain that does not go away or worsens to the health care provider.
- Take this medication exactly as instructed and do not take extra doses without approval of the health care provider.
- Add extra fiber and fluid to the diet because this drug will cause constipation.
- Do not breast-feed while taking this drug without approval of the health care provider.
- Store the medication out of reach of children and animals because accidental overdoses may be fatal.

Drugs Similar to Fentanyl (Actiq, Duragesic, Sublimaze)

Additional opioid IV general anesthetics include alfentanil, remifentanil, and sufentanil.

Alfentanil (Alfenta): Approved in 1996, alfentanil is an opiate agonist that has a more rapid onset and a shorter duration of action than fentanyl. It is administered IV to provide analgesia as a component of balanced anesthesia. Uses include assisting in intubation, promoting the induction of anesthesia, and as an infusion for the maintenance of anesthesia. A labeled indication is for the management of severe postoperative pain when given by the epidural route. The most common adverse effects are respiratory depression, nausea, vomiting, and muscle rigidity. Respiratory depression may be delayed; thus the patient should be monitored for some time after surgery. Alfentanil must be used with caution with other CNS depressants. Other actions and adverse effects are the same as those for fentanyl.

Remifentanil (Ultiva): Approved in 1996, remifentanil is an IV opioid that is similar to fentanyl. It is rapidly metabolized, which allows for a shorter duration of respiratory depression than fentanyl. Recovery from anesthesia occurs 5 to 10 minutes after discontinuation of the drug. This agent is administered during the induction and maintenance of general anesthesia to provide analgesia during the postoperative period. Although it does not produce deep anesthesia, remifentanil may be used alone or in combination with midazolam in monitored anesthesia care. Hypotension is greater with remifentanil than with fentanyl. Respiratory depression, pruritus, sweating, nausea, and vomiting are other adverse effects. Other actions and adverse effects are the same as those for fentanyl.

Sufentanil (Sufenta): Approved in 1984, sufentanil is an IV opioid used as a component of balanced anesthesia or as a primary anesthetic agent. As a primary anesthetic the patient should be administered 100% oxygen. During IV use, the onset of action is immediate and recovery time is comparable to that of fentanyl. It is sometimes administered with bupivacaine as an epidural anesthesia adjunct during labor and delivery. During epidural use, the onset of action is about 10 minutes and recovery time is 1.7 hours. Sufentanil is 5 to 10 times more potent than fentanyl. The most common adverse effects are respiratory depression and muscle rigidity, and the drug must be used with caution with other CNS depressants.

CONNECTION *Checkpoint* 30.1

In pain management, opioids are often available in fixed dose combinations with nonopioids. From what you learned in Chapter 29, what is the rationale for using a nonopioid analgesic with an opioid? What specific nonopioid analgesic is most frequently found in these combination drugs? See Answer to Connection Checkpoint 30.1 in Appendix A.

30.6 Benzodiazepines are used in anesthesia to produce relaxation, sedation, and amnesia.

The primary indication for benzodiazepines is to treat symptoms of anxiety (see Chapter 22). When used in high doses, however, these drugs can cause sedation and induce unconsciousness. For anesthesia, benzodiazepines are most often administered in combination with inhalation anesthetics, allowing the patient to feel less anxious and experience amnesia. They may be administered orally as a premedication to relax the patient prior to minor medical procedures. The most commonly utilized benzodiazepine for surgical procedures is midazolam (Versed). Diazepam (Valium) and lorazepam have a slower onset and longer duration than midazolam and are occasionally used as anesthesia adjuncts. A detailed discussion of benzodiazepines is found in Chapter 26, along with a prototype feature for diazepam. Doses for the two benzodiazepines used as IV anesthetics are listed in Table 30.2.

PROTOTYPE DRUG Midazolam (Versed)

Classification: **Therapeutic:** Antianxiety agent, anesthetic
Pharmacologic: Benzodiazepine, GABA receptor agonist

Therapeutic Effects and Uses: Approved in 1985, midazolam is administered to reduce the anxiety and stress associated with surgery. It is FDA approved for the induction of amnesia, induction and maintenance of general anesthesia, and sedation prior to short diagnostic procedures such as an endoscopy. Off-label uses include status epilepticus that is refractory to other agents and for sedation of mechanically ventilated patients.

Midazolam is a Schedule IV controlled substance. It has abuse potential similar to that of other benzodiazepines.

Mechanism of Action: Midazolam acts at the limbic, thalamic, and hypothalamic regions of the brain to produce CNS depression and skeletal muscle relaxation. This is the same mechanism of action as other benzodiazepines.

Pharmacokinetics:

Route(s)	IV, IM, PO
Absorption	Rapid absorption
Distribution	Widely distributed; crosses the blood–brain barrier and the placenta; secreted in breast milk; 97% protein bound
Primary metabolism	Hepatic
Primary excretion	Renal
Onset of action	IV: immediate; IM: 5–15 minutes; PO: 10–30 minutes
Duration of action	IV/IM/PO: 2–6 h

Adverse Effects: Respiratory depression and apnea are potentially serious adverse events. CNS adverse effects include drowsiness, fatigue, ataxia, slurred speech, and tremor. Potentially serious cardiovascular effects include hypotension, tachycardia, and cardiovascular collapse. Laryngospasm is the most severe pulmonary complication noted with the administration of midazolam.

Contraindications/Precautions: Patients who suffer from glaucoma should not be administered midazolam. Any patient who has been prescribed monoamine oxidase inhibitors (MAOIs) should not be administered midazolam. It is important that the patient not have MAOIs for 14 days prior to the administration of benzodiazepines. Patients who suffer from shock, coma, or depressed vital signs should not be administered benzodiazepines.

Drug Interactions: The administration of benzodiazepines with any medication that depresses the CNS, including alcohol, increases the patient's risk for sedation. Use of benzodiazepines and phenytoin (Dilantin) will result in an increased serum phenytoin level and additive CNS depression. Midazolam is metabolized by hepatic CYP3A4 enzyme, and inhibitors or inducers of this enzyme may interact with midazolam. Melatonin should be avoided because it may increase the actions of benzodiazepines. **Herbal/Food:** Increased sedation may occur if benzodiazepines are administered with kava or valerian. Grapefruit juice may increase the serum concentration of midazolam.

Pregnancy: Category D.

Treatment of Overdose: Overdose with midazolam causes sedation, confusion, diminished reflexes, and coma. General supportive measures should be taken, and the patient may be treated with flumazenil, which is a specific benzodiazepine antagonist. The patient's breathing should be supplemented mechanically.

Nursing Responsibilities:

- Assess vital signs every 3 to 5 minutes before, during, and after administration of midazolam and until recovery.
- Monitor for signs of respiratory depression, such as respiratory rates less than 10, poor breath sounds, or shallow respiratory effort.
- Ensure a patent airway and place the patient in a side-lying position (unless contraindicated) to prevent pulmonary aspiration.
- Monitor for adverse effects, particularly hypotension, muscle weakness, tachycardia, and respiratory depression.
- Assess the patient for a history of smoking because users of tobacco may require higher dosages.

Patient and Family Education:

- Request assistance when walking or getting out of bed to prevent falls and potential injury.
- Do not drive or perform other hazardous activities until the effects of the drug are known, because this drug may cause drowsiness or dizziness.
- Take this medication exactly as instructed, and do not discontinue its use without consulting the health care provider.
- Avoid alcohol and other CNS depressants because increased sedation may result.
- Make position changes slowly when moving from a lying to a standing position to prevent dizziness and possible fainting.

Drugs Similar to Midazolam (Versed)

The only other benzodiazepine administered to produce anesthesia is diazepam.

Diazepam (Valium): Diazepam has been widely prescribed as an antianxiety agent and as an adjunct in seizure management. In the surgical suite it may be used for induction of amnesia or to reduce anxiety prior to surgery or short medical procedures. Administered parenterally, it has an onset of action of 1 to 5 minutes and produces short-acting effects. Diazepam decreases the patient's anxiety and relaxes the skeletal muscles. Diazepam impairs the patient's ability to remember the perioperative events. A prototype feature for diazepam may be found in Chapter 26.

CONNECTION *Checkpoint* 30.2

Benzodiazepines are sometimes used for seizure control. From what you learned in Chapter 26, what are the indications for lorazepam and diazepam in treating seizures? See Answer to Connection Checkpoint 30.2 in Appendix A.

30.7 Ketamine and propofol are intravenous general anesthetics used to induce and maintain anesthesia.

Ketamine (Ketalar) and propofol (Diprivan) are IV anesthetics that are grouped together as a "miscellaneous" category because they are not barbiturates, opioids, or benzodiazepines. The two drugs are not related chemically, but both have shorter durations and can induce anesthesia rapidly. Doses for ketamine and propofol are listed in Table 30.2.

PROTOTYPE DRUG Ketamine (Ketalar)

Classification: **Therapeutic:** General anesthetic
Pharmacologic: N-methyl-D-aspartate (NMDA) receptor agonist

Therapeutic Effects and Uses: Approved in 1970, ketamine is a general IV anesthetic that was initially used in veterinary medicine. It is a rapid-acting anesthetic agent that produces a trance-like feeling of being separated from the environment called **dissociative anesthesia.** As a single anesthetic agent ketamine is used during surgeries and brief diagnostic procedures that do not require skeletal muscle relaxation. It is also used prior to the administration of other general anesthetic agents. Ketamine is used extensively with pediatric patients due to its rapid induction of general anesthesia and the fact that it lasts up to 25 minutes.

Ketamine has strong analgesic actions and immediately increases blood pressure and skeletal muscle tone. The patient's eyes may be open during the procedure. Ketamine is a common drug of abuse that is known under the names of jet, super acid, Special "K," green K, and cat Valium. It is a club drug that is similar to phencyclidine (PCP), which is popular among teens and young adults. It is easily added to drinks or administered through injection to cause temporary amnesia and is sometimes referred to as a date rape drug (see Chapter 8).

Mechanism of Action: Ketamine produces dissociative anesthesia by interrupting the pathways of the brain prior to producing somesthetic sensory blockade. It depresses the function of the reticular activating and limbic systems.

Pharmacokinetics:

Route(s)	IM, IV
Absorption	Rapid
Distribution	Body tissues with highest concentration in the fat, liver, lung, and brain
Primary metabolism	Hepatic
Primary excretion	Renal
Onset of action	IV: immediate; IM: 3–4 minutes
Duration of action	IV: 5–10 minutes; IM: 12–25 minutes

Adverse Effects: Potentially serious cardiovascular adverse effects of ketamine include HTN and tachycardia. Respiratory depression occurs with the administration of IV ketamine. Laryngospasm has also been noted with periods of apnea.

Anorexia, nausea, and vomiting can occur during the postoperative phase. The most serious neurologic adverse effect is emergence phenomena in adult patients, which can occur for 24 hours postoperatively. Emergence phenomena include delirium, hallucinations, confusion, excitement, and irrational behavior.

Contraindications/Precautions: Patients who have significant HTN, intracranial bleeding, suspected intracranial pressure, or hypersensitivity to ketamine should not be administered this drug. Ketamine should be used with caution in patients with cardiac pathology because this drug increases myocardial oxygen consumption. Ketamine may exacerbate psychosis and should be used with caution in patients with schizophrenia.

Drug Interactions: Ketamine should not be administered with barbiturates and opioids due to prolonged recovery time in the postoperative phase. Use with other CNS depressants can cause additive CNS and respiratory depression. **Herbal/Food:** St. John's wort may potentiate the actions of general anesthetics and should be discontinued 2 to 3 weeks prior to ketamine administration.

Pregnancy: Category C.

Treatment of Overdose: The treatment of overdosage includes mechanical ventilation of the patient.

Nursing Responsibilities:

- Monitor for signs of respiratory depression such as respiratory rates less than 10, poor breath sounds, or shallow respiratory effort.
- Ensure a patent airway and place the patient in a side-lying position (unless contraindicated) to prevent pulmonary aspiration.
- Protect the patient from injury that could occur due to dissociative anesthesia.
- Monitor blood pressure, heart rate, and respiratory status. Report episodes of HTN and tachycardia to the prescriber.
- Monitor mental status, especially in patients with a history of psychiatric illness.
- Administer IV ketamine slowly (over at least 60 seconds) to prevent respiratory depression.

Patient and Family Education:

- Do not drive or perform other hazardous activities for at least 24 hours after the administration of ketamine because this drug may cause drowsiness or dizziness.
- Immediately report dizziness, fainting, slow heart rate, hallucinations, and involuntary muscle movements to the health care provider.
- Do not consume alcohol or take CNS depressants within 24 hours of anesthesia administration.

Drugs Similar to Ketamine (Ketalar)

Propofol is the only other miscellaneous IV general anesthetic agent.

Propofol (Diprivan): A newer anesthetic approved in 1989, propofol is an IV sedative–hypnotic agent indicated for the induction and maintenance of general anesthesia. It has a rapid onset of action and is used effectively for conscious sedation. Emergence from anesthesia is 10 times faster compared to thiopental, and few adverse effects occur during recovery. Propofol is contraindicated in patients who have a known hypersensitivity reaction to the medication or its emulsion, which contains soybean and egg phosphatide. Apnea and hypotension are common adverse effects. Obstetric patients and those with increased intracranial pressure should not be administered propofol. The medication should be administered under strict aseptic conditions due to the fact that the emulsion supports rapid microorganism growth; unused portions must be discarded. Unlike other anesthetics that cause nausea and vomiting, propofol has an antiemetic effect that can prevent nausea and vomiting in patients receiving chemotherapy. Off-label uses include refractory migraines, refractory status epilepticus, and the treatment of agitation associated with alcohol withdrawal. This drug is pregnancy category C.

Inhalation General Anesthetic Agents

30.8 Inhalation anesthetics used to produce loss of consciousness are classified as gases or volatile liquids.

Following the administration of IV agents, inhalation anesthetics are given to rapidly produce unconsciousness and total analgesia. Inhaled general anesthetic agents are supplied as gases or volatile liquids. These agents produce their effects on the CNS by inhibiting the flow of sodium into neurons, which delays the nerve impulses and dramatically reduces the activity of the neurons. Although the mechanism of action is incompletely understood, inhibitory gamma-aminobutyric acid (GABA) receptors in the brain become active and are thought to be responsible for the anesthetic action. This action is similar to that of the antiepileptic medications described in Chapter 26. Other CNS neurotransmitters likely contribute to the sedative effects of the inhalation anesthetics.

The first general anesthetic was the gas diethyl ether, which was discovered in the 1840s. Although popular for over 100 years, gaseous anesthetics were explosive and presented a danger to the surgical team members, who were exposed to fumes from the drugs. Furthermore, the gases produced a very high incidence of nausea and vomiting following the procedure. The only gaseous anesthetic in use today is nitrous oxide.

The potency of inhalation anesthetics is described by the **minimum alveolar concentration:** the concentration of drug vapor in the alveoli that prevents a motor response in 50% of subjects when exposed to a painful stimulus. A low value of minimum alveolar concentration indicates that a very small amount of anesthetic is needed to immobilize the patient. Inhalation anesthetics have low minimum alveolar concentrations and are thus very potent. The exception is nitrous oxide, which is a low-potency anesthetic with a high minimum alveolar concentration value. The minimum alveolar concentration changes with the age of the patient: It is lowest in newborns, peaks in infants, and gradually declines with age.

CONNECTIONS

Evidence-Based Practice Malignant Hyperthermia and Anesthetic Agents

Clinical Question

Does a patient's genetic mapping play a role in the response to general anesthesia?

Evidence

To date, the bulk of pharmacogenetic research has focused on finding genetic causes of adverse reactions to anesthetic agents. A well-documented example of how genetic mapping results in adverse effects of anesthesia is noted in patients who suffer from malignant hyperthermia syndrome. Malignant hyperthermia was an unknown condition until approximately 1960. The disease was documented in Australia when a young man from Melbourne suffered a fracture and the family history revealed deaths under anesthesia. It was the beginning of research on malignant hyperthermia. According to the article by Ball (2007) during the next 20 years the cause of deaths related to general anesthesia was discovered and effective treatment was found. Pharmacogenetic studies on malignant hyperthermia have revealed associations with variations in the ryanodine receptor (RYR1). It is estimated that 50% of cases involved mutations within this gene.

Implication

It is important that the nurse in the preoperative phase of patient assessment investigates whether the patient's family has a history of sudden unexplained death during general anesthesia. This investigation is pivotal in decreasing the risk of development of malignant hyperthermia during the surgical procedure.

It is also imperative that the surgical team recognizes the signs and symptoms of malignant hyperthermia early during the operative procedure. The initial symptoms of the disorder include tachycardia, which is noted when the heart rate is above 150 beats per minute. The patient also suffers from hypotension. The last sign exhibited by the patient is that of increased body temperature and ultimate cardiac arrest. At the onset of the symptoms the patient should be administered dantrolene sodium, a skeletal muscle relaxant, and sodium bicarbonate.

Critical Thinking Question

Why is it important for the nurse to ask about a patient's family surgical history before the administration of anesthesia?

See Answers to Critical Thinking Questions in Appendix A.

Source: From "Pharmacogenetics of Anesthetic and Analgesic Agents," by S. Palmer, N. Giesecke, S. C. Body, S. Shernan, A. Fox, and C. Collard, 2005, *Anesthesia, 102*(3), pp. 663–671; "Unraveling the Mystery of Malignant Hyperthermia," by C. Ball, June 2007, *Anaesthesia and Intensive Care, 35*, pp. 26–31; and "Malignant Hyperthermia: Update 2000," by N. Fortunato-Phillips, 2000, *Critical Care Nursing Clinics of North America, 12*(2), pp. 192–210.

Anesthetics are rapidly absorbed from the alveoli into the general circulation. The anesthesiologist can control the length and depth of anesthesia by delivering the exact concentration of drug needed to maintain a desirable degree of immobility. These drugs are very lipid soluble and quickly distribute to the brain and other organs. Because nerve cells have high lipid content, the anesthetic agent can more readily cross the blood–brain barrier to produce sedating effects. Metabolism of inhalation anesthetics is minimal and elimination of the drug is mostly by exhalation. Modern anesthetics are designed to have a fast recovery time so that the patient regains consciousness soon after the infusion is stopped. Because anesthetics are lipid soluble, they are stored in fat and slowly released, which explains why obese patients may take longer to recover from anesthesia.

PROTOTYPE DRUG Nitrous oxide

Classification: **Therapeutic:** Gaseous general anesthetic
Pharmacologic: GABA-receptor agonist, opioid agonist

Therapeutic Effects and Uses: Nitrous oxide is an odorless, nonirritating, inorganic gas used for a large number of medical and surgical procedures. When administered alone it is one of the least potent anesthetics and is unable to induce deep anesthesia at therapeutic doses. Because of its low potency, the use of nitrous oxide is either limited to minor surgical procedures or combined with the IV anesthetic agents for more complex procedures. The majority of patients requiring sedation for dental, diagnostic, and surgical procedures are administered nitrous oxide.

One major advantage of nitrous oxide is that it has strong analgesic properties. At a concentration of 20%, nitrous oxide delivers analgesic efficiency equaling that of morphine. This agent has a low potency and does not produce LOC or profound skeletal muscle relaxation.

Nitrous oxide is always combined with oxygen (25% to 30%) and is administered in a semi-closed method. The patient may be administered an IV anesthetic to produce sedation. When drowsy or asleep, the patient inhales the nitrous oxide through a tube or by mask. Nitrous oxide is also used for dental procedures in which the mask is placed over the nose. Other procedures in which nitrous oxide is administered include those related to obstetrics and surgery. Nitrous oxide lowers the minimum alveolar concentration of other anesthetics, essentially making them more potent. This permits a decrease in the dosages required for IV and inhalation anesthetics.

Nitrous oxide has been used illegally to produce relaxation, euphoria, and hallucinations. Abusers may steal the nitrous oxide tanks from medical facilities. The gas has also been used as a propellant in whipped cream canisters and cooking sprays, and abusers can obtain small amounts from those sources. Long-term abuse can lead to anemia, depletion of vitamin B_{12}, tinnitus, and peripheral neuropathy.

Mechanism of Action: The mechanism of action of nitrous oxide is not fully known. Its analgesic effects are believed to be due to activation of opioid receptors in the midbrain. The relaxation properties of the drug are likely due to activation of GABA receptors, which inhibits neuronal firing.

Pharmacokinetics:

Route(s)	Inhalation
Absorption	Rapid
Distribution	Crosses the blood–brain barrier to concentrate in the nerve cells
Primary metabolism	Not metabolized
Primary excretion	100% through the lungs, unchanged
Onset of action	2–5 minutes
Duration of action	Half-life is variable; peak effect: less than 10 minutes

Adverse Effects: When administered in low to moderate doses, nitrous oxide produces few adverse effects. When administered in higher doses, patients exhibit some adverse effects of stage 2 anesthesia such as anxiety, excitement, and combativeness. Lowering the inhaled dose quickly reverses these adverse effects. Because nitrous oxide is exhaled the patient may temporarily have some difficulty breathing at the end of the procedure.

Rapid diffusion of the gas from the bloodstream back into the lungs causes alveolar hypoxia, with symptoms that include nausea, vomiting, lethargy, and dizziness. Some patients describe these symptoms as equivalent to a "hangover" from too much alcohol consumption. Alveolar hypoxia can be prevented by breathing 100% oxygen for several minutes following the conclusion of nitrous oxide therapy.

Contraindications/Precautions: Because patients must be awake and follow the instructions of the physician or dentist, nitrous oxide is contraindicated in those with an impaired LOC or an inability to comply with instructions. Because the diffusion of nitrous oxide may lead to expansion of closed spaces, conditions such as undiagnosed abdominal pain, abdominal distention, bowel obstruction, head injury, and pneumothorax are contraindicated. Patients who suffer from hypotension, shock, chronic obstructive pulmonary disease, cyanosis, or chest pain should not be administered nitrous oxide.

Drug Interaction: The administration of adrenergic agonists (such as epinephrine) or caffeine with nitrous oxide may exacerbate dysrhythmias. Use with CNS depressants may cause additive sedation and respiratory depression. Excessive hypotension may result if amiodarone or antihypertensive drugs are used concurrently with nitrous oxide. **Herbal/Food:** Milk thistle taken before and after anesthesia may lower the potential risk of liver damage. St. John's wort should be discontinued 2 to 3 weeks prior to administration of general anesthetics due to possible hypotension risk.

Pregnancy: Category C.

Treatment of Overdose: Effects of the drug usually diminish quickly after the gas is discontinued. Metoclopramide (Reglan) or another antiemetic agent may be administered to reduce the nausea and vomiting associated with nitrous oxide.

Nursing Responsibilities:

- Monitor the preoperative status of the patient for anxiety, pulmonary function, and cardiac function.
- Assess LOC and assess the patient's ability to follow instructions.
- Prior to administering the drug, assess for contraindications such as pneumothorax, bowel obstruction, or head injury.

Patient and Family Education:

- Report any nausea or vomiting after the procedure to the health care provider.
- Immediately report palpitations or labored breathing to the health care provider.
- Call the nurse for assistance when changing positions in the postoperative phase.
- Do not drive or perform other hazardous activities for at least 24 hours after administration of anesthesia because this drug may cause drowsiness or dizziness.

Drugs Similar to Nitrous Oxide

Nitrous oxide is the sole gaseous general anesthetic agent.

30.9 Volatile liquid general anesthetic agents are used to induce and maintain deep anesthesia.

Several liquid anesthetics have a low vapor pressure that allows them to vaporize (form a gas) at low temperatures and pressures. An anesthesia machine is used to vaporize the liquid, mix the vapors with oxygen and air, and deliver them to patients in precisely controlled amounts. The anesthesia machine also establishes a partial pressure gradient that ensures the anesthetic will continue to flow from the machine to the alveoli, to the blood, and eventually to the brain. The inhalation anesthetics are lipid soluble and will freely cross the blood–brain barrier.

Desflurane (Suprane), isoflurane (Forane), and sevoflurane (Ultane) are the most widely used of the volatile liquid anesthetics. Halothane (Fluothane), the traditional prototype of the inhalation anesthetics for many decades, has been replaced by these safer drugs. All of these agents have a rapid onset of action.

The minimum alveolar concentrations of the volatile inhaled anesthetic agents are very low. For example, halothane has the lowest minimum alveolar concentration at 0.75% concentration in alveolar air. This factor contributes to the ability of the agents in this class to rapidly produce unconsciousness at low doses. Although they have the ability to produce deep anesthesia, they produce little analgesia and are usually used in combination with nitrous oxide and opioids as part of balanced anesthesia.

Some general anesthetics sensitize the heart to the action of catecholamines such as epinephrine, norepinephrine, and dopamine and can cause serious dysrhythmias. These agents also depress cardiovascular and pulmonary function, placing the patient at risk for laryngospasm, or respiratory arrest. The gaseous and volatile liquid general anesthetic agents are listed in Table 30.3.

TABLE 30.3 Inhalation General Anesthetic Agents

Drug	Adult Concentration	Adverse Effects
Gas		
nitrous oxide	20–40% with oxygen 70% with 30% oxygen	*Anxiety* <u>Malignant hyperthermia, nausea, vomiting</u>
Volatile Liquids		
desflurane (Suprane)	7.3% concentration	<u>Laryngospasm, hypotension, apnea, increased secretions, vasodilation, respiratory depression, tachycardia, malignant hyperthermia, nausea, vomiting, hepatotoxicity (halothane)</u>
enflurane (Ethrane)	0.5–3% concentration	
isoflurane (Forane)	0.1–2% concentration	
sevoflurane (Ultane)	0.5–3% concentration	

Note: *Italics* indicate common adverse effects. <u>Underline</u> indicates serious adverse effects.

PROTOTYPE DRUG Isoflurane (Forane)

Classification: Therapeutic: Inhaled general anesthetic
Pharmacologic: GABA and glutamate receptor agonist

Therapeutic Effects and Uses: Approved in 1979, isoflurane has become an inhalation general anesthetic of choice due to its effectiveness and safety profile. Isoflurane provides the patient with smooth and rapid induction of general anesthesia with a low degree of metabolism by the body. It is almost entirely eliminated through respirations. The drug provides excellent muscle relaxation. It is FDA approved for the induction and maintenance of general anesthesia and may be used off-label as adjuvant therapy in the treatment of status asthmaticus.

Isoflurane does not sensitize the myocardium for dysrhythmias, and it produces fewer cardiovascular effects than other general anesthetics. Isoflurane does not cause the hepatotoxicity observed with halothane.

Mechanism of Action: The exact mechanism of action of isoflurane is unknown. It interacts with multiple receptors in the brain, including glutamate and GABA receptors.

Pharmacokinetics:

Route(s)	Inhalation
Absorption	Rapidly absorbed by the lungs
Distribution	Crosses the blood–brain barrier to concentrate in neurons; unknown if it is secreted in breast milk
Primary metabolism	Minimal metabolism
Primary excretion	95% pulmonary
Onset of action	7–10 minutes for surgical anesthesia
Duration of action	Patient begins to regain consciousness less than 1 h after drug is discontinued

Adverse Effects: Mild nausea, vomiting, and tremor are common adverse effects. The drug produces a dose-dependent respiratory depression and a reduction in blood pressure. Malignant hyperthermia with elevated temperature and unstable blood pressure has been reported, although the incidence is rare.

Contraindications/Precautions: Patients with a known history or genetic predisposition to malignant hyperthermia should not use isoflurane. Caution should be used when treating patients with head trauma or brain neoplasms due to possible increases in intracranial pressure. Safety has not been established in patients under age 18. Elderly patients are more susceptible to the cardiovascular effects of the drug. Patients with a prolonged QT interval should be administered isoflurane with caution.

Drug Interactions: Coughing, breath holding, or laryngospasm may occur when used concurrently with nitrous oxide. Skeletal muscle weakness, respiratory depression, or apnea may occur if isoflurane is administered concurrently with systemic polymyxin or aminoglycosides. Additive effects can occur if isoflurane is administered with other skeletal muscle relaxants. Additive hypotension may result if used concurrently with antihypertensive medications such as beta-adrenergic blockers. Epinephrine, norepinephrine, dopamine, and other adrenergic agonists should be administered with caution because of the possibility of dysrhythmias. Levodopa should be discontinued 6 to 8 hours before isoflurane administration. Isoflurane should be administered with caution with other drugs that prolong the QT interval, such as amiodarone, ibutilide, droperidol, and phenothiazines. **Herbal/Food:** St. John's wort should be discontinued 2 to 3 weeks prior to administration of general anesthetics due to possible hypotension risk.

Pregnancy: Category C.

Treatment of Overdose: Isoflurane is a profound respiratory depressant. The patient is treated symptomatically until the effects of the drug diminish.

Nursing Responsibilities:

- Assess vital signs every 3 to 5 minutes before, during, and after administration and until complete recovery.

- During postanesthesia ensure a patent airway and place the patient in side-lying position unless contraindicated to prevent pulmonary aspiration.
- Provide warmth with blankets in the postoperative period to reduce drug-induced shivering.
- Administer antiemetic agents as needed for nausea and vomiting.
- Monitor for signs of respiratory depression such as respiratory rates less than 10, poor breath sounds, or shallow respiratory effort.
- Ensure that resuscitation equipment is available during administration and in the postoperative phase.
- Instruct on alterations in sensation and perception during anesthesia administration and in the postoperative phase.

Patient and Family Education:

- Report postoperative nausea, vomiting, and pain to the health care provider.
- After surgery, request assistance when changing positions or walking postoperatively.
- Do not drive or perform other hazardous activities for at least 24 hours after administration of anesthesia because this drug may cause drowsiness or dizziness.

Drugs Similar to Isoflurane (Forane)

Volatile liquid general anesthetic agents similar to isoflurane include desflurane, enflurane, and sevoflurane. Halothane (Fluothane), the historical prototype for this class, was voluntarily removed from the market due to a small incidence of fatal hepatitis associated with the drug.

Desflurane (Suprane): Desflurane, approved in the 1990s, produces a rapid induction of general anesthesia. It is administered to induce and maintain anesthesia in adults. When administered to children it is used to maintain anesthesia. Adverse effects of desflurane are laryngospasm, apnea, and increased pulmonary secretions. The drug produces a dose dependent reduction in blood pressure, and malignant hyperthermia has been reported. Desflurane must be used with IV anesthetics because it may cause coughing and excitation during induction. It does not sensitize the myocardium for dysrhythmias. This is a pregnancy category B drug.

Enflurane (Ethrane): Approved in 1972, enflurane is administered for induction and maintenance of general anesthesia, usually in conjunction with other agents as a component of balanced anesthesia. It is approved for obstetric anesthesia. It has strong muscle relaxant properties. It does not sensitize the myocardium for dysrhythmias and postanesthesia nausea, vomiting, and CNS stimulation are uncommon. When administered in high concentrations, however, it can cause seizures and is thus contraindicated in patients with a history of seizure disorders. Rare cases of malignant hyperthermia have been reported, and enflurane is contraindicated in patients with a history of this disorder. This is a pregnancy category B drug.

Sevoflurane (Ultane): Approved in 1995, sevoflurane is a volatile liquid general anesthetic agent that is administered to induce and maintain sedation. It has a faster uptake, distribution, and elimination than isoflurane. It also does not cause the cardiovascular reactions commonly encountered with some of the other general anesthetics, and it is safer to use in patients with coronary artery disease. Sevoflurane does not cause respiratory irritation and is safe for administration with children. Furthermore, this drug does not cause coughing and excitation during induction and can thus be used without IV anesthetics. Sevoflurane produces a dose dependent reduction in blood pressure, and malignant hyperthermia has been reported. This is a pregnancy category B drug.

PharmFACT

Malignant hyperthermia is a dominantly inherited disorder. Those who have had previous anesthetics without adverse effects cannot be certain they are safe. Malignant hyperthermia-related deaths have occurred even after patients have undergone prior uneventful surgeries. Muscle biopsy is the only way to definitively determine malignant hyperthermia susceptibility status. *Source:* Malignant Hyperthermia Association of the United States, 2005.

CONNECTIONS

Treating the Diverse Patient Exposure to Anesthesia and the Risk of Alzheimer's Disease

A case control study on Alzheimer's disease (AD) and the exposure to anesthesia was conducted between January 1, 1990 and June 30, 1997. The study consisted of 115 patients with probable AD, 230 nondemented patients with Parkinson's disease, and 230 patients affected by nondegenerative neurologic diseases. The three study groups revealed that in the 1-year period preceding disease onset the patients had been exposed to general anesthesia. It should be noted that the AD group had a higher mean age than the other study groups. The study revealed that exposure to anesthesia does not increase the risk of AD. It suggested that other causes, such as the relationship between anesthetic agents and endogenous variables, could be of epidemiologic relevance. Patients can show a cognitive decline in the postsurgical period due to a linkage of the genotype APOEe4. Patients with this genotype have been shown to be at risk for the development of AD. Thus, patients who have the genotype and are exposed to general anesthesia may be at increased risk of developing AD.

Source: From "A Case-Control Study on Alzheimer's Disease and Exposure to Anesthesia," by M. Gasparini, N. Vanacore, C. Schiaffini, L. Brusa, M. Panella, G. Talarico, et al., 2002, *Neurological Science, 23*, pp. 11–14.

NURSING PROCESS APPLICATION

Patients Receiving General Anesthesia

Assessment

Prior to administration:

- Obtain a complete health history, including allergies, drug history, and possible drug interactions.
- Assess for presence or history of severe respiratory, cardiac, renal, or liver disorders.
- Assess for genetic predisposition to malignant hyperthermia or sudden death of a family member during surgery.
- Obtain baseline vital signs.
- Obtain blood work, including complete blood count and chemistry panel.
- Assess the patient's knowledge of the surgical or diagnostic procedure.
- Ensure that written informed consent is signed according to institution policy.
- Assess the patient's level of anxiety.

Potential Nursing Diagnoses

- *Anxiety*, related to surgical procedure
- *Deficient Knowledge (Anesthesia Agents),* related to purpose, precautions, and adverse effects of drug therapy
- *Nausea*, related to anesthesia agents
- *Disturbed Sensory Perception*, related to altered sensorium produced by anesthesia
- *Ineffective Breathing Pattern,* related to depressed respirations, secondary to anesthesia agent

Planning Patient Goals and Expected Outcomes

Patient will:

- Maintain effective breathing status in spite of anesthesia-induced respiratory depression as evidenced by a respiratory rate of more than 12 per minute and normal breathing pattern.
- Remain free of sensory and perception alterations through repeated reorientation to surroundings.
- Not experience adverse effects related to general anesthesia.
- Verbalize an understanding of the anesthesia process as well as the postoperative recovery period.

Implementation

Interventions and (Rationales)	Patient and Family Education
• Preoperatively assess the knowledge level of preoperative and postoperative procedures. Ensure that the patient has accurate information and that questions are answered. (Patient teaching reduces anxiety.)	Instruct the patient on: • Preoperative and postoperative instructions. • All aspects of the surgical experience. • The postanesthesia experience. • What the patient and family will see and hear postoperatively. • The surgical facilities and equipment.
• Preoperatively assess emotional status. (Patients who are fearful or extremely anxious may be more difficult to induce and maintain under anesthesia.)	• Instruct the patient on relaxation techniques such as deep breathing, imagery, and distraction.
• Monitor preoperative status. (Nonadherence with preoperative instructions may result in serious problems for the patient.)	Instruct the patient to: • Not ingest food or beverages prior to surgery to prevent aspiration, nausea, and vomiting. • Stop taking medications 24 hours prior to surgery as ordered by the health care provider. • Refrain from drinking alcohol 24 hours prior to surgery. • Stop taking herbal supplements 2–3 weeks prior to surgery.
• Preoperatively, monitor for respiratory difficulty and adequate oxygen and carbon dioxide exchange. (Anesthetics will cause respiratory depression.)	• Inform the patient to report shortness of breath, difficulty breathing, or dizziness.
• Monitor recovery from anesthesia. Evaluate LOC, nausea, vomiting, and pain. (Failure to control pain, nausea, and vomiting can result in a longer recovery period.)	• Instruct the patient to report all adverse effects of medications and anesthesia.
• Monitor vital signs. (Respiratory status may be impaired, leading to prolonged apnea, respiratory depression, and cyanosis. Blood pressure may decrease, leading to impending shock.)	• Instruct the patient to report heart palpitations, dizziness, difficulty breathing, or faintness.

Evaluation of Outcome Criteria

Evaluate the effectiveness of drug therapy by confirming that patient goals and expected outcomes have been met (see "Planning").

Local Anesthetics

30.10 Local anesthetic agents block pain transmission in peripheral nerves and are grouped in two major classes.

Local anesthesia results in the loss of sensation to a small, limited area of the body. The primary advantage of local anesthesia is that pain relief can be provided without causing generalized depression of the CNS and respiratory systems. Nausea, vomiting, tremors, and anxiety associated with general anesthetic recovery are avoided. The types of adverse events associated with local anesthesia are relatively minor relative to the potential risks of general anesthesia.

Several techniques are used to deliver local and regional anesthesia. The method employed is dependent on the location and extent of the desired anesthesia (Figure 30.1).

- **Surface anesthesia.** The drug is applied or sprayed directly on the surface of the skin or mucous membrane. The anesthesia does not penetrate into deeper skin layers. This is used to provide relief for minor skin irritations or prior to needlesticks.
- **Infiltration anesthesia.** The drug is injected into deeper skin layers and travels to surrounding regions. This provides relief from minor skin surgeries or dental procedures, or prior to deep needlesticks.
- **Nerve block.** The drug is injected surrounding a peripheral nerve and all regions innervated by the nerve lose sensation. This is used for dental procedures or for regional anesthesia.
- **Epidural anesthesia.** The drug is injected into the epidural space surrounding the spinal cord. The anesthetic blocks sensation to multiple nerve roots supplying limited regions of the chest, pelvis, abdomen, or limbs. It is used for urologic and obstetric procedures.
- **Spinal anesthesia.** The drug is injected into the cerebrospinal fluid, usually in the lumbar region. This procedure is used to block sensation to larger areas of the lower abdomen or pelvis.

Although safer than general anesthetics, the health care provider has less control over the onset and duration of drug action. The onset of local anesthesia is dependent on the drug's ability to diffuse from the application site to the surrounding nerves. In general, local anesthetics are small, lipid-soluble molecules that can move quickly through tissues and spaces to enter neurons. Local anesthetics are nonselective; they will block transmission at all types of sensory nerves. The sense of sharp pain is usually affected first, followed by other senses such as warmth, cold, touch, and pressure. Motor fibers are also affected by local anesthetics.

Termination of local anesthetic action depends on blood flow to the region. Local blood vessels carry the drug away

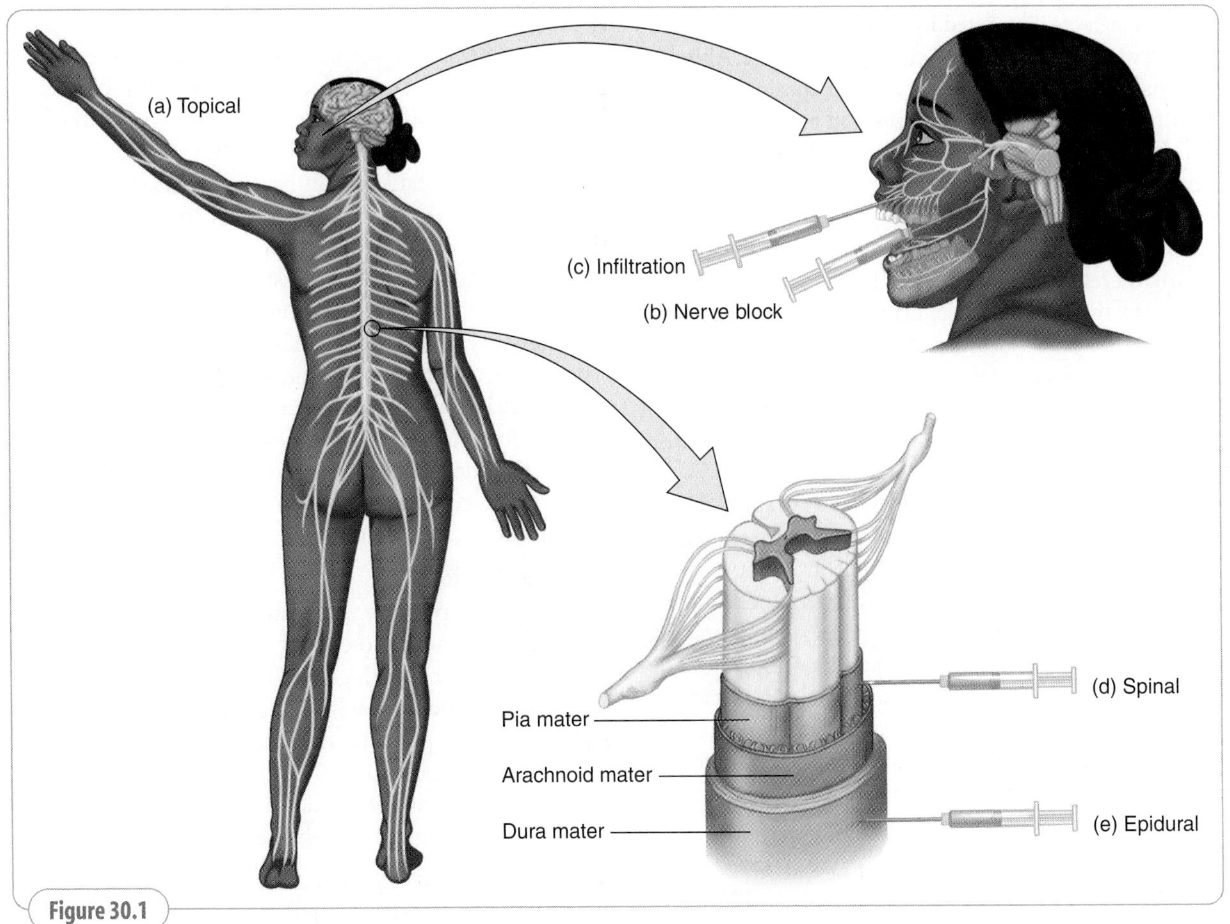

Figure 30.1

Techniques for applying local anesthesia: (a) topical; (b) nerve block; (c) infiltration; (d) spinal; and (e) epidural.

from the application site to the systemic circulation, where it is metabolized and excreted. Usually no systemic effects result because absorption into the general circulation is slow and the drug is sufficiently diluted by the blood.

The duration of anesthetic action may be extended by injecting a vasoconstrictor such as epinephrine in combination with the local anesthetic. The epinephrine reduces blood flow to the region and slows absorption of the anesthetic. This not only extends the anesthetic duration but it also prevents the anesthetic from reaching the circulation too quickly, which could cause systemic toxicity. Although epinephrine itself has toxic effects, the amount used in local anesthesia is very small and it is released very slowly into the systemic circulation. Adverse effects from epinephrine use in local anesthesia are rare.

The two major classes of local anesthetic agents are named by their chemical structures: esters and the amides. The two classes differ primarily by their incidence of allergic reactions, with the amide type having the lower incidence. Although they vary in time of onset and duration of action, most local anesthetics have equivalent effectiveness. The local anesthetics are listed in Table 30.4.

30.11 Ester-type local anesthetics have been widely used as topical and spinal anesthetics.

Cocaine was the first local anesthetic agent to be widely used for medical procedures. Cocaine is a natural ester found in the leaves of the *Erythroxylum coca,* a plant native to the Andes Mountains in Peru. Cocaine was discovered by a German chemist in 1855 and ultimately used in 1884 as a topical eye anesthetic. Although still approved by the FDA as a local anesthetic, cocaine is a Schedule II controlled substance and is rarely used because of its high potential for abuse. In 1904 a German chemist named Einhorn discovered procaine (Novocaine), which soon came into widespread use, especially in dental offices.

Esters act by decreasing the amount of sodium that enters the neuron, thereby depressing depolarization and preventing conduction of the pain impulse. Esters may be administered with epinephrine as a vasoconstrictor to limit blood loss at the surgical site and to decrease the amount of anesthetic agent absorbed systemically. The local anesthetic effect of an ester is rapid, occurring in 1 to 8 minutes. The duration ranges from 15 to 60 minutes.

Ester-type anesthetics are generally safe when applied as directed. All can cause serious CNS and cardiac toxicity, however, if they reach the blood in high concentrations. The first CNS symptoms may be stimulatory: anxiety, nervousness, dizziness, tremor, or seizures. Subsequent CNS depression may cause the patient to become drowsy, experience respiratory depression, and enter a coma. High amounts can cause dysrhythmias, QT prolongation, hypotension, and cardiac arrest. Care must be taken that the drug is administered correctly to prevent serious adverse effects.

PROTOTYPE DRUG Procaine (Novocaine)

Classification: Therapeutic: Local anesthetic
Pharmacologic: Ester, sodium channel blocker

Therapeutic Effects and Uses: Procaine is used for spinal, epidural, and peripheral nerve blocks through injection or infiltration. It produces local anesthesia with loss of sensation close to the injection or application site. It has a short duration of action. An off-label use is for the treatment of severe pain due to cancer, herpes, or burns. Once used widely in dentistry, it has largely been replaced by other local anesthetics.

Procaine causes vasodilation, which could potentially increase its rate of absorption from tissues and cause systemic toxicity. Epinephrine may be added to counteract the vasoconstriction and prolong the anesthetic effect. The drug is rapidly metabolized to inactive metabolites by esterase, an enzyme found in the plasma. Once it reaches the plasma, the half-life of procaine is only 40 seconds.

Mechanism of Action: Procaine decreases the influx of sodium into the neuron, which increases the threshold for depolarization and prevents the conduction of the nerve impulse.

Pharmacokinetics:

Route(s)	Subcutaneous
Absorption	Rapid
Distribution	Not distributed; highly bound to plasma proteins
Primary metabolism	Metabolized by plasma esterase
Primary excretion	Renal: 80% as metabolites
Onset of action	2–5 minutes
Duration of action	1 h

Adverse Effects: With therapeutic doses, adverse effects are rare. Adverse events may occur, however, if multiple doses of procaine are administered or if it is injected intravascularly. The most severe adverse effects include respiratory arrest and anaphylaxis. A patient who has experienced an allergic reaction to procaine will likely be allergic to other esters. Myocardial depression may result in atrioventricular (AV) block dysrhythmias or cardiac arrest. CNS effects are stimulatory and usually transient; nervousness, dizziness, confusion, and tremor may occur. Spinal anesthesia with procaine can cause headache, palsies, spinal nerve paralysis, and meningism (nuchal rigidity, photophobia, and headache). Cutaneous lesions can occur in a delayed time frame. The caudal or epidural administration of procaine in the obstetric patient can result in urinary incontinence, loss of perineal sensation, slowing of labor, and increased incidence of forceps delivery.

Contraindications/Precautions: Patients who have experienced hypersensitivity to any ester anesthetic or agent containing para-aminobenzoic acid (PABA) should not receive procaine. Patients with generalized septicemia, inflammation, or sepsis should not be injected with procaine. It is also contraindicated in patients with heart block, hypotension, HTN, or altered coagulation. It should be used cautiously in elderly and acutely ill patients. Patients who have increased abdominal pressure should be administered procaine cautiously.

Drug Interactions: Ester anesthetics such as procaine may antagonize the antimicrobial effects of sulfonamides. There is an increased risk of hypotension when administered with antihypertensives. Procaine is incompatible with aminophylline,

TABLE 30.4 Local Anesthetics

Drug	Route and Adult Dose (maximum dose where indicated)	Adverse Effects
Ester Type		
benzocaine (Americaine, Anbesol, Solarcaine, others)	Topical: 5% spray, cream, ointment 6% cream 8% lotion 20% spray, ointment, gel, liquid, otic solution	Topical applications: *erythema, dermatitis, burning* Anaphylaxis Infiltration, nerve block, epidural applications: *Postspinal headache, sedation, paresthesia, blurred vision, urinary retention* Myocardial depression, anaphylactic reactions, cardiac arrest, respiratory arrest, seizures, fetal bradycardia
chloroprocaine (Nesacaine)	Infiltration and nerve block: 1–2% solution (max: 800 mg without epinephrine, 1 g with epinephrine) Caudal and epidural block (without preservatives): 2–3% solution (max: 800 mg without epinephrine, 1 g with epinephrine)	
procaine (Novocain)	Spinal anesthesia: 10% solution diluted in normal saline at 1 mL/5 seconds subcutaneous Infiltration anesthesia orperipheral nerve block: 0.25–0.5% solution subcutaneous	
tetracaine (Pontocaine)	Topical: 1–2 drops of 0.5% solution or 1.25–2.5 cm of ointment in the lower conjunctival fornix or 0.5% solution or ointment to the nose or throat Spinal: 1% solution diluted with equal volume of 10% dextrose injected in the subarachnoid space	
Amide Type		
articaine (Septocaine, Zorcaine)	Infiltration: 0.5–2.5 mL (20–100 mg) Nerve block: 0.5–3.4 mL (20–136 mg) Oral surgery: 1–5.1 mL (40–204 mg)	Topical applications: *Erythema, dermatitis, burning* Infiltration, nerve block, epidural applications: *Hypersensitivity, dizziness, drowsiness, urinary retention, fecal incontinence, slowing of labor, numbness of lips or tongue, hypotension, blurred or double vision* Laryngeal edema, bradycardia, anaphylactoid reaction, respiratory arrest, seizures, rectal bleeding (dibucaine)
bupivacaine (Marcaine, Sensorcaine)	Local infiltration, sympathetic block: 0.25% solution Lumbar epidural block: 0.25%, 0.5%, 0.75% solutions Caudal block, peripheral nerve block: 0.25%, 0.5% solutions Retrobulbar block: 0.75% solution	
dibucaine (Nupercainal)	Topical: Apply to skin 1 ounce every 24 h	
lidocaine (Anestacon, Dilocaine, Xylocaine, others)	Infiltration: 0.5–1% solution Nerve block: 1–2% solution Epidural: 1–2% solution Caudal: 1–1.5% solution Spinal: 5% solution with dextrose Saddle block: 1.5% with dextrose Topical: 2.5–5% jelly, ointment, cream, or solution	
prilocaine	Subcutaneous: 1–2 mL (40–80 mg) of a 4% solution	
ropivacaine (Naropin)	Surgical anesthesia: Intrathecal administration: Epidural: 25–200 mg (0.5–1% solution) Nerve block: 5–250 mg (0.5–0.75% solution) Labor pain: 20–40 mg (0.2% solution) Postoperative pain management: Epidural: 12–20 mg/h (0.2% solution) Infiltration: 2–200 mg (0.2–0.5% solution)	

Note: *Italics* indicate common adverse effects. Underline indicates serious adverse effects.

amobarbital, chlorothiazide, magnesium sulfate, phenobarbital, phenytoin, secobarbital, and sodium bicarbonate. **Herbal/Food:** Unknown.

Pregnancy: Category C.

Treatment of Overdose: The effects of procaine overdosage are treated symptomatically. Rapid systemic absorption will affect the cardiovascular system and could require cardiopulmonary resuscitation.

Nursing Responsibilities:

- Assess for history of allergy to ester-type anesthetics.
- Monitor the patient for headaches, palpitations, tachycardia, HTN, and dizziness.
- Monitor the site of injection for limited blood supply, which could present with pallor, decreased temperature at the site, and sensitivity of the skin.
- Monitor the blood pressure closely during the first 30 minutes after spinal anesthesia induction. Hypotension is the most common and severe complication.
- If injecting, perform the procedure slowly, frequently aspirating to ensure that the drug is not being injected into a blood vessel.
- Evaluate the patient for lack of sensation to pain before starting the procedure.

Patient and Family Education:

- Do not consume hot foods or beverages or chew gum following a dental procedure until sensation returns.
- Report any symptoms such as hypotension, difficulty breathing, anxiety, palpitations, or dizziness to the health care provider.
- Notify the health care provider if numbness does not begin to diminish after a few hours.

Drugs Similar to Procaine (Novocaine)

Other local anesthetic esters include benzocaine, chloroprocaine, and tetracaine.

Benzocaine (Americaine, Anbesol, others): Approved in 1938, benzocaine is an over-the-counter (OTC) local anesthetic ester applied topically as a lotion, cream, ointment, spray, gel, or otic solution. Chemically it is almost identical to procaine, but it has a prolonged duration of anesthetic action. It provides temporary relief of pain and discomfort due to sunburn, minor wounds, pruritus, serous otitis media, swimmer's ear, otitis externa, canker sores, sore throat, hemorrhoids, and anal fissures. It can be applied to the penis as a male desensitizer to slow the onset of ejaculation. Benzocaine preparations are commonly used as an anesthetic for the passage of catheters and endoscopic tubes. Onset of anesthetic action occurs in less than a minute and because absorption of benzocaine is minimal, systemic effects are rare. Contact dermatitis can occur and is more common with benzocaine than with some of the other topical anesthetics. Although rare, benzocaine sprays have been associated with serious methemoglobinemia, a condition in which hemoglobin is unable to bind sufficient oxygen. This drug is pregnancy category C.

Chloroprocaine (Nesacaine): Approved in 1957, chloroprocaine is a short-acting local anesthetic ester that is used for infiltration, epidural, and caudal anesthesia. It is not effective as a topical agent. Anesthesia occurs in 6 to 12 minutes and can last up to 90 minutes if epinephrine is added to the injection. A test dose is given before epidural use to assess for intravascular or subarachnoid injection. In the event of intravascular injection, the patient would experience an epinephrine response with tachycardia, circumoral pallor, palpitations, and nervousness. Signs of subarachnoid injection include motor paralysis and extensive sensory anesthesia. Like other ester anesthetics, allergic reactions such as rash, pruritus, and anaphylaxis are possible. This drug is pregnancy category C.

Tetracaine (Pontocaine): Tetracaine is a local anesthetic ester that is used in spinal anesthesia and topically. It may be used to anesthetize the conjunctiva during eye surgery and in the nose and throat to eliminate the laryngeal and esophageal reflexes. It is administered on the skin to relieve pruritus, pain, and burning. An OTC preparation (Viractin) is available for topical treatment of pain associated with cold sores and fever blisters. Onset of action is rapid for topical use (3 to 10 minutes) but longer following spinal administration (15 minutes). Of the topical anesthetics, tetracaine is the most likely to cause skin sensitivity, including rash, erythema, pruritus, burning, and edema. Systemic absorption can cause significant CNS and cardiac toxicity. Tetracaine is contraindicated in patients who are hypersensitive to ester-type anesthetics, sulfites, or PABA. This drug is pregnancy category C.

30.12 Local anesthetic agents from the amide class have a lower incidence of adverse effects than those from the ester class.

Amide-type local anesthetics have largely replaced the administration of agents from the ester class. The amides produce less effect on myocardial contractility, and the incidence of allergic reactions is lower. Amides and esters have the same mechanism of action: decreasing the sodium flux into the neuron, thus inhibiting the initial depolarization and conduction of the nerve impulse. Whereas the esters are inactivated by the enzyme esterase in the plasma, the amides are metabolized by hepatic CYP450 enzymes. Caution should be exercised when administering large amounts of amide anesthetics to patients with hepatic impairment.

PROTOTYPE DRUG Lidocaine (Anestacon, Dilocaine, Xylocaine, others)

Classification: **Therapeutic:** Local anesthetic
Pharmacologic: Amide, sodium channel blocker

Therapeutic Effects and Uses: Lidocaine is a local anesthetic agent that has a prompt onset of action of 2 to 5 minutes. It has a longer duration of action than procaine, lasting 10 to 90 minutes, depending on its route of administration. It may be administered as a surface and infiltration anesthetic agent to block the nerve. It is also used in caudal and spinal block anesthesia to relieve local discomfort of the skin and mucous membranes. Lidocaine patches are administered to relieve pain related to postherpetic neuralgia (Lidoderm) or dental procedures (DentiPatch). Parenteral lidocaine is administered to treat life-threatening ventricular dysrhythmias (see Chapter 39). In 2007 the FDA approved Zingo (lidocaine hydrochloride monohydrate), which is a needle-free intradermal injection system. Zingo is indicated for rapid local anesthesia for procedures such as IV insertions or blood draw.

Mechanism of Action: Lidocaine blocks the conduction of action potentials by reducing the sodium permeability, thus decreasing the action potential and slowing nerve conduction.

Pharmacokinetics:

Route(s)	Subcutaneous, IM, IV, IV bolus; topical
Absorption	Topical absorption: 3% through intact skin
Distribution	Crosses the blood–brain barrier and the placenta; secreted in breast milk
Primary metabolism	Hepatic via CYP3A4 and 2D6
Primary excretion	Renal
Onset of action	IV: 45–90 seconds; IM: 5–15 minutes; topical: 2–5 minutes
Duration of action	IV: 10–20 minutes; IM: 60–90 minutes; topical: 30–60 minutes Half-life: 1.5–2 h

Adverse Effects: When used topically, adverse reactions to lidocaine are uncommon. Mild and transient reactions at the site of application include erythema, pruritus, dermatitis, and burning. The transoral DentiPatch may cause alterations in taste, headache, and gingivitis. Should the drug be accidentally injected intravascularly, CNS adverse effects will be those of stimulation (anxiety, tremors, shivering, and seizures) followed by depression (drowsiness, respiratory depression, and coma). Cardiovascular effects include hypotension, dysrhythmias, cardiovascular collapse, and cardiac arrest.

Contraindications/Precautions: Patients who have experienced a hypersensitivity reaction to amide-type local anesthetics should not be administered lidocaine. Topical lidocaine should not be applied to seriously damaged skin from trauma, burns, or eczema.

Other precautions apply to patients receiving parenteral lidocaine, although these also apply to situations in which the drug is accidentally injected intravascularly. Patients who have been diagnosed with Stokes-Adams syndrome, untreated sinus bradycardia, sinoatrial, atrioventricular, and intraventricular heart block should not be administered lidocaine. The medications should be used cautiously in the presence of liver or kidney disease, myasthenia gravis, and hypovolemia as well as in debilitated patients and the elderly or when there is a family history of malignant hyperthermia.

Drug Interactions: Lidocaine patches can cause toxic effects with tocainide and mexiletine. Barbiturates decrease lidocaine activity. Increased pharmacologic effects of lidocaine will be noted if it is administered with cimetidine, beta blockers, or quinidine. **Herbal/Food:** After receiving transoral lidocaine, patients should not eat or drink until the effects of the anesthesia have worn off.

Pregnancy: Category B.

Treatment of Overdose: Overdose may occur if the drug is injected intravascularly. The patient is treated through symptom management.

Nursing Responsibilities:
- Assess for history of allergy to amide-type anesthetics.
- Monitor the blood pressure, heart rate, and respiratory rate following the administration of the anesthetic.
- Monitor for CNS toxicity such as anxiety, tremors, shivering, seizures, respiratory depression, and coma.
- Evaluate the patient for lack of sensation to pain before starting the procedure.

Patient and Family Education:
- Lidocaine solution for throat or mouth pain should be swished and spat out.
- Do not consume hot foods or beverages or chew gum following a dental procedure until sensation returns.
- Report any symptoms such as hypotension, difficulty breathing, anxiety, seizures, palpitations, or dizziness to the health care provider.
- Discard lidocaine patches safely: The amount of drug left on the patch may cause serious effects in pets or children.

MyNursingKit | Mechanism of Action Animation: Lidocaine

Drugs Similar to Lidocaine (Anestacon, Dilocaine, Xylocaine, Others)

Other local anesthetic amides include articaine, bupivacaine, dibucaine, mepivacaine, prilocaine, and ropivacaine. Levobupivacaine (Chirocaine) and etidocaine (Duranest) are amides that have been removed from the U.S. market.

Articaine (Septocaine, Zorcaine): A newer local anesthetic approved in 2000, articaine is approved for administration by infiltration or by nerve block for dental procedures. It is unique because it has both an amide and an ester group. Anesthesia is rapid, occurring in 1 to 6 minutes, and lasts up to an hour. Articaine appears to diffuse through soft tissue and bone better than other local anesthetics. It is combined with epinephrine, which provides vasoconstriction and prolongs the duration of action. The adverse effects are the same as those of other amide anesthetics. This drug is pregnancy category C.

Bupivacaine (Marcaine, Sensorcaine): Approved in 1972, bupivacaine is an amide local anesthetic that is used for infiltration anesthesia, peripheral sympathetic nerve, and epidural block. Bupivacaine in dextrose solution is administered for spinal anesthesia. All forms are available with epinephrine as a vasoconstrictor. Its 3- to 9-hour duration of action is one of the longest of any local anesthetic. Adverse effects are similar to those of other amide anesthetics. This drug is pregnancy category C.

Dibucaine (Nupercainal): Approved in 1947, dibucaine is administered to relieve pain and itching related to hemorrhoids and other anorectal disorders. It is also administered to relieve discomfort from insect bites, sunburn, minor burns, cuts, and scratches. It is a long-acting amide anesthetic that inhibits the initiation and conduction of nerve impulses by reducing the permeability of nerve cells to sodium ions. This drug is pregnancy category C.

Mepivacaine (Carbocaine, Isocaine, Polocaine): Approved in 1960, mepivacaine is an amide anesthetic used for infiltration, transtracheal anesthesia, and epidural nerve blocks in surgical and dental procedures. Onset of action is very rapid; it is less than a minute for the upper and lower jaws. Epidural onset is 7 to 15 minutes. This drug has an intermediate duration of action of 60 to 100 minutes for soft tissue and 115 to 150 minutes for epidural. Mepivacaine is sometimes combined with levonordefrin, a vasoconstrictor that prolongs the duration of action of the local anesthetic. The adverse effects are the same as those of other amide anesthetics. This drug is pregnancy category C.

Prilocaine (Citanest): Approved in 1965, prilocaine is used primarily for dental anesthesia via infiltration or nerve block. Onset of action is 2 minutes and its duration is 1 to 2 hours. The adverse effects are the same as those of other amide anesthetics. This drug is pregnancy category B.

Ropivacaine (Naropin): Ropivacaine is a newer local anesthetic agent approved in 1996 that is used in epidural anesthesia and postoperative pain management. It has an onset of action of 1 to 30 minutes and a duration of anesthetic action of 2 to 6 hours. It is important that disinfecting agents with heavy metal content not be used to disinfect the skin prior to the insertion of the epidural catheter. Also, the container of ropivacaine should not be cleaned with a heavy metal disinfecting agent. Unlike most local anesthetics, the presence of

NURSING PROCESS APPLICATION

Patients Receiving Local Anesthesia

Assessment	Potential Nursing Diagnoses
Prior to administration: • Obtain a complete health history, including allergies or amide- or ester-type local anesthetic agents. • Assess for the presence of broken skin, infection, burns, and wounds where medication is to be applied. • Assess for character, duration, location, and intensity of pain where medication is applied.	• *Risk for Injury,* related to loss of sensation and function of anesthetized area or region • *Deficient Knowledge,* related to purpose, precautions, and adverse effects of drug therapy • *Decreased Cardiac Output,* related to drug toxicity

Planning: Patient Goals and Expected Outcomes

Patient will:

- Experience no pain during the surgical procedure.
- Refrain from activity that may cause injury due to paresthesia.
- Experience no adverse effects from anesthesia.

Implementation

Interventions and (Rationales)	Patient and Family Education
• Monitor for cardiovascular adverse effects. (These may occur if local anesthetic is absorbed.)	• Instruct the patient to report any unusual heart palpitations. If medication is being used on a regular basis, instruct the patient to see a health care provider regularly.
• Monitor the skin or mucous membranes for infection or inflammation. (Condition could be worsened by the drug.)	• Instruct the patient to report any irritation or increase in discomfort in areas where medication is administered.
• Monitor for length of effectiveness. (Local anesthetic agents are effective for 1 to 3 hours.)	• Instruct the patient to report any discomfort during the procedure.
• Obtain information and monitor use of other medications. (There is always the potential for severe drug interactions.)	• Instruct the patient to report use of any medications to the health care provider.
• Provide for patient safety. (There is a potential for injury related to lack of sensation in the area being treated.)	• Instruct the patient that having no feeling in the anesthetized area requires taking extra caution to avoid injury, including heat-related injury.
• Monitor for gag reflex. (Xylocaine viscous may interfere with swallowing reflex.)	Instruct the patient to: • Not eat within 1 hour of administration. • Not chew gum while any portion of the mouth or throat is anesthetized to prevent biting injuries.

Evaluation of Outcome Criteria

Evaluate the effectiveness of drug therapy by confirming that patient goals and expected outcomes have been met (see "Planning").

epinephrine does not affect the systemic absorption of ropivacaine. Like other amide anesthetics, high serum concentrations may cause serious CNS and cardiac toxicity; care must be taken not to accidentally inject the drug intravascularly or intrathecally. This drug is pregnancy category B.

Adjuncts to Anesthesia

30.13 Adjunctive agents are used during the perioperative phase to enhance anesthesia or to treat the potential adverse effects of the anesthetics.

Surgery is often a stressful and painful procedure for patients. In addition, anesthetics dampen vital reflexes, which can lead to aspiration pneumonia. Diminished autonomic function can have serious adverse effects on the cardiovascular and gastrointestinal (GI) systems. Adjunctive medications are those used to enhance anesthesia or to make the procedure safer and less unpleasant for patients.

Preoperative medications: The most common preoperative symptom is anxiety. Oral benzodiazepines may be given for several days prior to a major procedure to lessen anxiety. Just prior to surgery, midazolam (Versed) may be administered parenterally to sedate the patient and to cause perioperative amnesia (see Section 30.6).

Aspiration pneumonia is a potentially serious problem during a surgical procedure because the patient may lose protective airway reflexes. Histamine (H_2) receptor antagonists such as ranitidine (Zantac) or famotidine (Pepcid) can reduce the possibility of aspiration pneumonia by decreasing gastric fluid volume and reducing acidity. For aspiration prophylaxis, the H_2 receptor antagonist may be given PO the night prior to surgery and by IV infusion an hour before the procedure. A drug prototype feature for ranitidine is found in Chapter 60.

Anticholinergic drugs such as atropine may be administered prior to surgery to reduce salivary and airway secretions. Atropine also blocks the bradycardia caused by some anesthetics. The drug is given by the IM route 45 to 60 minutes prior to anesthesia. A prototype feature for atropine is presented in Chapter 18.

Pain management: Pain reduction is an important component of preanesthesia and postanesthesia care. Opioids are used when the pain is expected to be severe, but these agents can cause significant respiratory depression. If the pain level is moderate or mild, nonsteroidal anti-inflammatory drugs (NSAIDs) are administered because they cause fewer serious adverse reactions than the opioids. Clonidine (Catapres, Duraclon) is a centrally acting alpha$_2$-adrenergic agonist that has been used to reduce severe pain associated with surgery. When administered epidurally Duraclon allows the dosages of the anesthetic and opioids to be reduced. The primary indication of clonidine is HTN (Catapres), but it has largely been replaced by safer antihypertensives (see Chapter 36).

Neuromuscular blockers: Skeletal muscle relaxation is an important component of general anesthesia. Insertion of an endotracheal tube would be difficult and painful without muscle relaxation, and contraction or spasticity of muscles during a surgical procedure could render some operations impossible. Complete paralysis of muscle is necessary for major surgical procedures. Although some of the general anesthetics do have mild to moderate ability to relax skeletal muscles, most are incapable of causing the degree of relaxation necessary for surgery.

The nondepolarizing neuromuscular blocking agents such as atracurium (Tracrium) and cisatracurium (Nimbex) have a short duration of action and bind competitively with acetylcholine to produce skeletal muscle relaxation. The depolarizing neuromuscular blocking agents such as succinylcholine (Anectine) are ultra-short acting and possess a high affinity for the acetylcholine receptor sites.

The neuromuscular blocking agents are very dangerous; the diaphragm and intercostal muscles are paralyzed and breathing requires a mechanical ventilator. Serious cardiovascular adverse effects are possible. Details of the actions, indications, and adverse effects of the neuromuscular blockers are included in Chapter 18. A prototype feature for succinylcholine is included in that chapter.

CONNECTION *Checkpoint* 30.3

Atropine and succinylcholine are both cholinergic blockers but they produce very different effects. From what you learned in Chapter 18, explain the mechanisms for the differences in pharmacologic actions. (Hint: One drug affects the muscarinic receptor and the other the nicotinic receptor.) See Answer to Connection Checkpoint 30.3 in Appendix A.

Postoperative medications: Because many anesthetics induce severe nausea and vomiting in the postanesthesia phase, the administration of antiemetic drugs is indicated for prophylaxis in high-risk patients or for treatment. Several drugs have been used as antiemetics. Promethazine (Phenergan) is an older antiemetic that may be administered pre- or postoperatively. It has the advantage of also being a sedative; thus it can be used in the induction phase of anesthesia. Also an older medication, metoclopramide (Reglan) may be administered near the end of the surgical procedure for prophylaxis of postanesthetic nausea and vomiting. The newest antiemetic, and perhaps the most effective, is ondansetron (Zofran). Commonly used to treat the acute nausea and vomiting caused by cancer chemotherapeutic agents, ondansetron may be injected just prior to surgery or postoperatively.

UNDERSTANDING THE CHAPTER

Key Concepts Summary

30.1 Anesthesia is used to produce a controlled loss of sensation during a diagnostic or surgical procedure.

30.2 Balanced anesthesia uses multiple drugs to provide for the safe induction and maintenance of general anesthesia.

30.3 Intravenous general anesthetic agents include barbiturates, benzodiazepines, and opioids.

30.4 Barbiturates induce rapid general anesthesia but their duration of action is very brief.

30.5 Opioids are used as intravenous anesthetics to provide analgesia and to accomplish neurolept anesthesia.

30.6 Benzodiazepines are used in anesthesia to produce relaxation, sedation, and amnesia.

30.7 Ketamine and propofol are intravenous general anesthetics used to induce and maintain anesthesia.

30.8 Inhalation anesthetics used to produce loss of consciousness are classified as gases or volatile liquids.

30.9 Volatile liquid general anesthetic agents are used to induce and maintain deep anesthesia.

30.10 Local anesthetic agents block pain transmission in peripheral nerves and are grouped in two major classes.

30.11 Ester-type local anesthetics have been widely used as topical and spinal anesthetics.

30.12 Local anesthetic agents from the amide class have a lower incidence of adverse effects than those from the ester class.

30.13 Adjunctive agents are used during the perioperative phase to enhance anesthesia or to treat the potential adverse effects of the anesthetics.

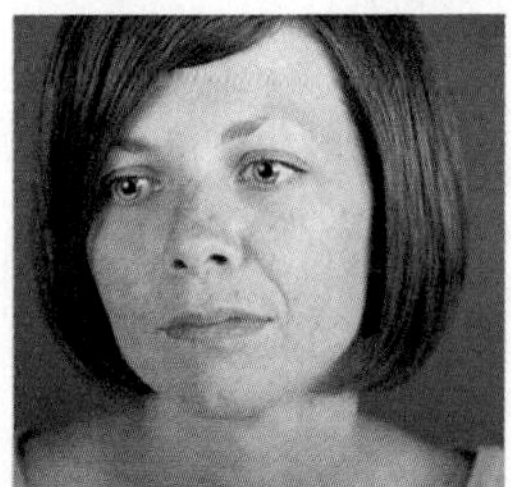

Making the PATIENT *Connection*

Remember the patient "Mary Smith" at the beginning of the chapter? Now read the remainder of the case study. Based on the information presented within this chapter, respond to the critical thinking questions that follow.

Mary Smith is a 42-year-old woman who is scheduled for a vaginal hysterectomy. While in the holding area of the operating room suite, she states that she is fearful of general anesthesia. As the preoperative nurse caring for this patient you notice that she is very anxious. Upon further assessment and conversation, she states that her mother died of breast cancer when she was young.

The patient's vital signs are as follows: Blood pressure 138/88 mmHg, Temperature 36.3°C (97.4°F), Pulse 94 beats/minute, and R 20/minute. She denies pain and states that she is concerned she will wake up during the surgery. She is to receive balanced anesthesia.

Critical Thinking Questions:

1. In your own words, how would you describe balanced anesthesia to Mary?
2. How does nitrous oxide differ from intravenous anesthetic agents?
3. How would you educate a patient regarding the use of intravenous propofol?

Case Study

Anthony Holiday is a 28-year-old steelworker for a heating and cooling company. While on the job he cuts his right hand with a piece of steel for an air-conditioning vent. He is admitted to the emergency department for sutures to the right middle finger and palm. The laceration will be anesthetized prior to suturing.

1. What is the action of lidocaine?
2. Why is lidocaine preferred over procaine?

NCLEX-RN® Review

1 The surgical nurse becomes alerted that the client who is receiving general anesthesia has become excitable and hyperactive with irregular heart and respiratory rates. The nurse knows that the client has entered which stage of general anesthesia?

1. Stage one
2. Stage two
3. Stage three
4. Stage four

2 The nurse should question the administration of thiopental sodium (Pentothal) for which of the following clients? An individual with:

1. A seizure disorder.
2. Lung cancer.
3. Kidney disease.
4. Addison's disease.

3 During the administration of thiopental sodium (Pentothal) the client develops a laryngospasm. The nurse would anticipate that which of the following medications would be ordered?

1. Lidocaine (Xylocaine)
2. Morphine sulfate (Astramorph)
3. Succinylcholine (Anectine)
4. Atropine sulfate

4 The nurse is providing the client, who will be receiving ketamine (Ketalar), with preoperative instructions. Which of the following statements, if made by the client, indicates that teaching is successful?

1. "The medication will decrease anxiety during surgery."
2. "I will experience increased energy due to this drug."
3. "I may experience a feeling of being separated from the environment."
4. "The drug will cause me to have dry mouth after the operation."

5 The client who is having a scalp laceration sutured will be receiving local anesthesia with lidocaine (Xylocaine) that contains epinephrine. The nurse knows that the purpose of this drug combination is to:

1. Decrease bleeding at the site of trauma.
2. Increase vasodilation at the site of the laceration.
3. Decrease blood pressure in individuals who are hypertensive.
4. Ensure that infection at the wound site will not occur.

6 Identify the general anesthetic agents that are parenteral opioid agents. Select all that apply.

1. Nitrous oxide
2. Alfentanil (Alfenta)
3. Sufentanil (Sufenta)
4. Regimental (Ultiva)
5. Succinylcholine (Anectine)

See Answers to Critical Thinking Questions, Case Study, and NCLEX-RN® Review in Appendix A.

References

American Association of Nurse Anesthetists. (2008). *Anesthesia options for labor and delivery.* Retrieved June 30, 2008, from http://www.aanadc.com/forpatients.aspx?ucNavMenu_TSMenuTargetID=68&ucNavMenu_TSMenuTargetType=4&ucNavMenu_TSMenuID=6&id=291

American Pregnancy Association. (2007). *Epidural anesthesia.* Retrieved June 30, 2008, from http://www.americanpregnancy.org/labornbirth/epidural.html

Anaesthesia UK. (2005). *Mechanism of action of inhaled anaesthetic agents.* Retrieved June 30, 2008, from http://www.frca.co.uk/article.aspx?articleid=100341

Ball, C. (2007, June). Unraveling the mystery of malignant hyperthermia. *Anaesthesia and Intensive Care, 35,* 26–31.

Bloomington Hospital. (n.d.). *Types of anesthesia and your anesthesiologist.* Retrieved June 30, 2008, from http://www.bloomingtonhospital.org/Content.asp?PageID=P01391

Darden, K., & Hewitt, C. (2004). Benchmarking in post-anesthetic care. *Nursing Standard, 18*(42), 42–44.

Fortunato-Phillips, N. (2000). Malignant hyperthermia: Update 2000. *Critical Care Nursing Clinics of North America, 12*(2), 192–210.

Gasparini, M., Vanacore, N., Schiaffini, C., Brusa, L., Panella, M., Talarico, G., et al. (2002). A case-control study on Alzheimer's disease and exposure to anesthesia. *Neurological Sciences, 23(1),* 11–14.

Jaffer, A., Barsoum, W., Krebs, V., Hurbanek, J., Morra, N., & Brotman, D. (2005). Duration of anesthesia and venous thromboembolism after hip and knee arthroplasty. *Mayo Foundation for Medical Education and Research, 80*(6), 732–738.

Jenson, M. G. (2006). Early use of regional and local anesthesia in a combat environment may prevent the development of complex regional pain syndrome in wounded combatants. *Military Medicine, 171(5),* 396–398.

Lemone, P., & Burke, K. (2004). *Medical surgical nursing: Critical thinking in client care* (4th ed.). Upper Saddle River, NJ: Pearson Prentice Hall.

Malignant Hyperthermia Association of the United States. (2005). *Drugs and MH susceptibility.* Retrieved June 30, 2008, from http://patients.mhaus.org/index.cfm/fuseaction/Content.Display/PagePK/SusceptFAQ.cfm

Nordin, P., Zetterstrom, H., Gunnarsson, U., & Nisson, E. (2003). Local, regional, or general anaesthesia in groin hernia repair: Multicentre randomised trial. *Lancet, 362*(9387), 853–858.

Palmer, S., Giesecke, N., Body, S., Shernan, S., Fox, A., & Collard, C. (2005). Pharmacogenetics of anesthetic and analgesic agents. *Anesthesiology, 102*(3), 663–671.

Paparella, S. (2005). Topical anesthetic sprays directly associated with serious, sometimes fatal adverse drug reactions: Methemoglobinemia. *Journal of Emergency Nursing, 31*(5), 468–469.

Sice, P. (2005). Depth of anaesthesia. *Update in Anaesthesia, 19*(10). Retrieved June 30, 2008, from http://www.nda.ox.ac.uk/wfsa/html/u19/u1910_01.htm

University of Wisconsin. (n.d.). *Local anesthesia and regional anesthetics.* Retrieved June 30, 2008, from http://www.anesthesia.wisc.edu/med3/localanes/localhandout.html

U.S. Drug Enforcement Administration. (n.d.). *Drug information: K, ketamine/khat.* Retrieved July 2, 2008, from http://www.usdoj.gov/dea/concern/k.html

UNIT 5

Pharmacology of the Cardiovascular System

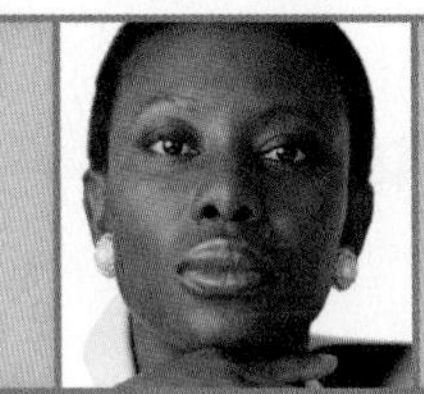
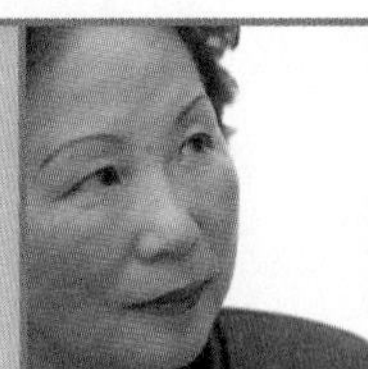
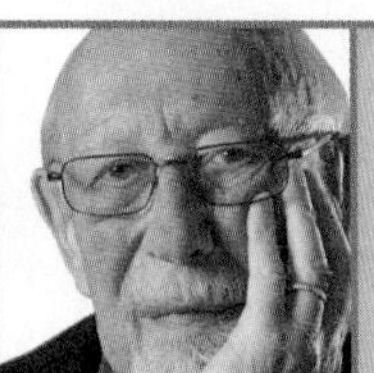
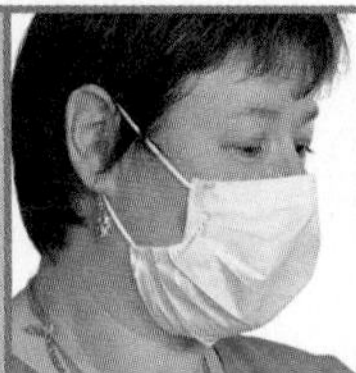

CHAPTER 31	Review of the Cardiovascular System
CHAPTER 32	Pharmacotherapy of Hyperlipidemia
CHAPTER 33	Calcium Channel Blockers
CHAPTER 34	Drugs Affecting the Renin-Angiotensin-Aldosterone System
CHAPTER 35	Diuretic Therapy and the Pharmacotherapy of Renal Failure
CHAPTER 36	Pharmacotherapy of Hypertension
CHAPTER 37	Pharmacotherapy of Angina Pectoris and Myocardial Infarction
CHAPTER 38	Pharmacotherapy of Heart Failure
CHAPTER 39	Pharmacotherapy of Dysrhythmias
CHAPTER 40	Pharmacotherapy of Coagulation Disorders
CHAPTER 41	Pharmacotherapy of Hematopoietic Disorders
CHAPTER 42	Pharmacotherapy of Fluid, Electrolyte, and Acid–Base Disorders

CHAPTER

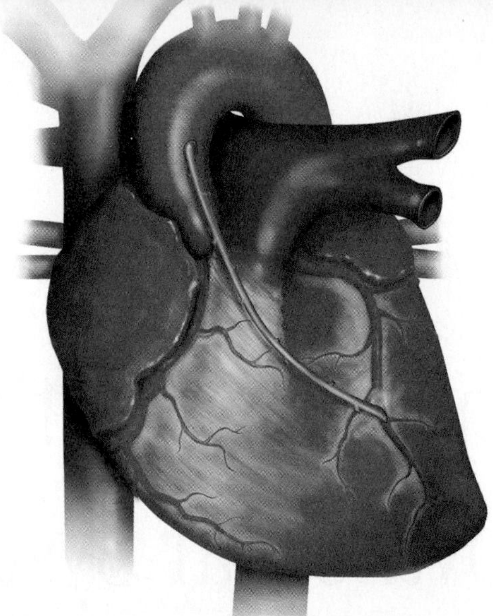

31 Review of the Cardiovascular System

Learning Outcomes

After reading this chapter, the student should be able to:

1. Describe the major structures of the cardiovascular system.
2. Identify each of the components of blood and their functions.
3. Construct a flow chart diagramming the primary steps of hemostasis.
4. Describe the structure of the heart and the function of the myocardium.
5. Describe the role of the coronary arteries in supplying the myocardium with oxygen.
6. Illustrate the flow of electrical impulses through the normal heart.
7. Explain the major factors affecting cardiac output.
8. Explain the effects of cardiac output, peripheral resistance, and blood volume on hemodynamics.
9. Discuss how the vasomotor center, baroreceptors, chemoreceptors, and hormones regulate blood pressure.

Chapter Outline

Structure and Function of the Cardiovascular System

Functions and Properties of Blood

Components of Blood

Hemostasis

Cardiac Structure and Function

Cardiac Muscle

Coronary Arteries

Cardiac Conduction System

Cardiac Output

Hemodynamics and Blood Pressure

Hemodynamic Factors Affecting Circulation

Regulation of Blood Pressure and Blood Flow

It is likely that the nurse will administer more cardiovascular drugs than any other class of medications. Why is this the case? First, health care providers have discovered the huge benefits in keeping blood pressure and blood lipid values within normal limits and how to prevent heart attacks and strokes. Secondly, the heart and vessels simply weaken over time and, as the average life span of the population increases, more pharmacotherapy will be needed to treat the cardiovascular diseases of older adults. These two goals of cardiovascular pharmacotherapeutics, prevention and treatment, are used routinely on nearly all people at some stage during their life span.

A comprehensive knowledge of cardiovascular anatomy and physiology is essential to understanding cardiovascular pharmacology, which encompasses the next 11 chapters of this book. The purpose of this chapter is to offer a brief review of the components of the structure and function of the cardiovascular system that are important to pharmacotherapy. For more comprehensive treatments of these topics, the student should refer to an anatomy and physiology textbook.

Structure and Function of the Cardiovascular System

31.1 The cardiovascular system consists of the blood, heart, and blood vessels.

The three major components of the cardiovascular system are the blood, heart, and blood vessels, as shown in Figure 31.1. These three components work as an integrated whole to transport various substances throughout the body, providing the necessary life substances essential to all cells. Disruption of this flow for even brief periods can have serious, if not mortal, consequences. The functions of the cardiovascular system are diverse and include the following:

- Transport of nutrients and wastes
- Pumping of blood
- Regulation of blood pressure
- Regulation of acid–base balance
- Regulation of fluid balance
- Regulation of body temperature
- Protection against invasion by microbes

It must be clearly understood that the cardiovascular system can only function with the cooperation of other body systems. For example, the role of the autonomic nervous system in controlling heart rate and blood vessel diameter is presented in Chapter 16. The kidneys are intimately involved in assisting the cardiovascular system with fluid and acid–base balance, as discussed in Chapter 42. The respiratory system must bring oxygen to the blood and remove carbon dioxide from it. The student should view the cardiovascular system as an important part of the overall homeostasis of the human body.

Functions and Properties of Blood

31.2 Blood consists of formed elements and plasma.

Blood is a fluid tissue that consists of solid, formed elements suspended in plasma. The solid, formed elements of the blood are the erythrocytes, leukocytes, and platelets. When combined, the formed elements comprise about 45% of the composition of blood.

The most numerous blood cells are erythrocytes, which comprise 99.9% of the formed elements. Carrying the iron-containing protein hemoglobin, the erythrocytes are responsible for transporting oxygen to the tissues and carbon dioxide from the tissues to the lungs. Without a nucleus, a single erythrocyte can carry as many as one billion molecules of oxygen. Erythrocyte homeostasis is controlled by **erythropoietin**, a hormone secreted by the kidney in response to low oxygen levels in the blood. Once secreted, erythropoietin stimulates the body's production of erythrocytes. Insufficient numbers of erythrocytes or structural defects such as sickle shapes lead to anemia, which is a common indication for pharmacotherapy (see Chapter 41).

Although small in number, leukocytes serve an essential role in the body's defense against infection. Unlike erythrocytes, which are all identical, there are several types of leukocytes, each serving a different function. For example, neutrophils are the most common leukocyte and they respond to bacterial infections through phagocytosis of the microbes. The second most common leukocyte, the lymphocyte, is the key cell in the immune response that responds by secreting antibodies (B lymphocytes) or secreting cytokines (T lymphocytes) that rid the body of the microbe. Homeostasis of leukocytes is controlled by different **colony-stimulating factors (CSF)**. Once secreted, CSFs activate existing white blood cells to

Key Terms

- **action potentials**, *487*
- **afterload**, *490*
- **antidiuretic hormone (ADH)**, *493*
- **atrial natriuretic peptide (ANP)**, *493*
- **atrial reflex**, *492*
- **automaticity**, *487*
- **baroreceptors**, *492*
- **cardiac output (CO)**, *489*
- **chemoreceptors**, *492*
- **coagulation**, *485*
- **colony-stimulating factors (CSF)**, *483*
- **contractility**, *490*
- **ectopic foci**, *489*
- **erythropoietin**, *483*
- **extrinsic pathway**, *486*
- **fibrin**, *486*
- **fibrinogen**, *486*
- **hemopoiesis**, *484*
- **hemostasis**, *485*
- **inotropic agents**, *490*
- **intrinsic pathway**, *486*
- **myocardium**, *487*
- **peripheral resistance**, *491*
- **preload**, *490*
- **prothrombin**, *486*
- **reflex tachycardia**, *492*
- **renin-angiotensin-aldosterone system (RAAS)**, *493*
- **sinus rhythm**, *487*
- **stroke volume**, *489*
- **thrombin**, *486*
- **thrombopoietin**, *484*
- **vasomotor center**, *492*
- **venous return**, *490*

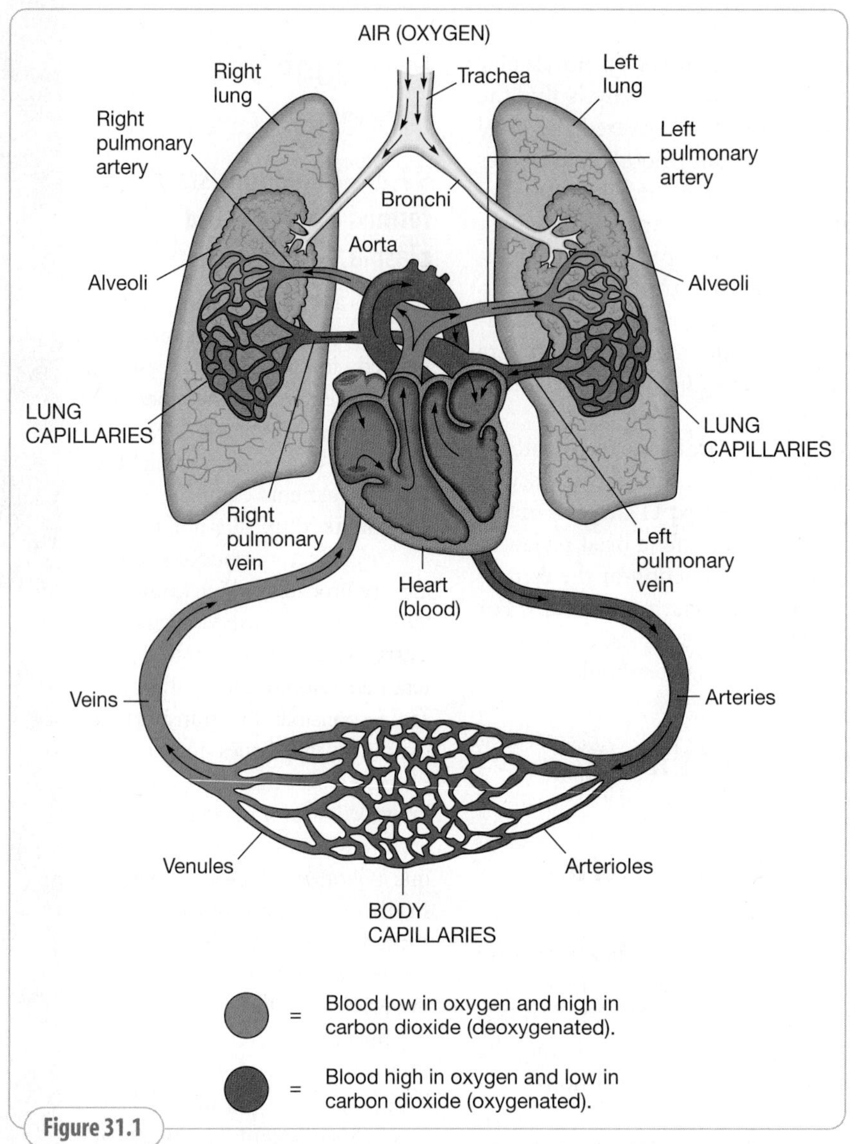

Figure 31.1

The cardiovascular system.
Source: From *Anatomy and Physiology for Health Professions: An Interactive Journey* (p. 271), by B. Colbert, J. Ankney, & K. Lee, 2007. Reprinted by permission of Pearson Education, Inc., Upper Saddle River, NJ.

fight an infection and increase the production of leukocytes. Too few leukocytes, called leukopenia, will make the patient susceptible to infection. Too many leukocytes, called leukocytosis, is a sign of infection, inflammation, or perhaps leukemia. Lymphocyte activation, CSFs, and enhancing body defenses are important topics in pharmacology and are presented in Chapters 43 through 46.

The final formed elements of the blood are thrombocytes or platelets, which are actually fragments of larger cells called megakaryocytes. Platelets stick to the walls of damaged blood vessels to begin the process of blood coagulation, which prevents excessive bleeding from sites of injury. Abnormally low numbers of platelets, or thrombocytopenia, can result in serious delays in blood clotting. Platelet homeostasis is controlled by the hormone **thrombopoietin,** which promotes the formation of additional platelets. The role of platelets and thrombopoietin in blood coagulation is a major topic in Chapter 40, which discusses the pharmacotherapy of blood coagulation.

The production and maturation of blood cells, called **hemopoiesis,** occurs in red bone marrow. It is here that primitive stem cells of the blood, which have the capacity to develop into any blood cell type, become committed to becoming an erythrocyte, leukocyte, or platelet. This process occurs continuously throughout the life span and is subject to various homeostatic controls as well as chemical and physical agents. For example, ionizing radiation and a large number of drugs have the potential to adversely affect bone marrow and cause myelosuppression. Myelosuppression is a very serious adverse effect that reduces the number of erythrocytes, leukocytes, and thrombocytes, leaving patients susceptible to anemia, infection, and abnormal clotting. Many agents used to treat cancer and those given to reduce the possibility of transplant rejection can produce profound myelosuppression as a dose-limiting adverse effect.

Plasma is the fluid portion of blood that consists of water and various proteins, electrolytes, lipoproteins, carbohydrates, and other regulatory substances. The primary proteins in plasma are albumins (54%), globulins (38%), and fibrinogen (7%). Albumin is the primary regulator of blood osmotic pressure, which determines the movement of fluids among the vascular, interstitial, and cellular compartments or spaces. Globulins, also known as immunoglobulins or antibodies, are important in protecting the body from foreign agents such as bacteria or viruses. Fibrinogen is a critical protein in the coagulation of blood. The liver synthesizes over 90% of the plasma proteins; therefore, patients with serious hepatic impairment will have deficiencies in coagulation and in maintaining body defenses.

Normal fluid balance in the body is achieved by maintaining the proper amount of plasma in the blood. Too little water in plasma results in dehydration, whereas too much causes edema and hypertension. Various organs help to maintain normal fluid balance, including the kidneys, gastrointestinal (GI) tract, and skin. The pharmacotherapy of fluid and electrolyte imbalances is an important topic in pharmacology and is discussed in Chapter 42.

CONNECTION *Checkpoint* 31.1

From what you learned in Chapter 4, what role does plasma protein play in the distribution of drugs? See Answer to Connection Checkpoint 31.1 in Appendix A.

Pharm*FACT*

To maintain homeostasis, the body must make 3 million erythrocytes every second. Red blood cells are so numerous that they comprise approximately one third of all cells in the body. *Source:* Martini, 2009.

31.3 Hemostasis is a complex process involving multiple steps and a large number of enzymes and factors.

The process of **hemostasis** is complex, involving 13 different clotting factors that contribute to the stoppage of blood flow. Hemostasis occurs in a series of sequential steps, sometimes referred to as a cascade. Hemostasis is an essential mechanism that the body uses to prevent excessive bleeding following injury. Medications can be used to modify several of these steps, either to speed up or delay the clotting process (see Chapter 40).

When a blood vessel is injured, the clotting process is initiated. The vessel spasms, causing constriction, which slows blood flow to the injured area. Platelets have an affinity to the damaged vessel: They become sticky and adhere to each other and to the injured area. The clumping of platelets, or aggregation, is facilitated by adenosine diphosphate (ADP), the enzyme thrombin, and thromboxane A_2. Platelet receptor sites and von Willebrand's factor make adhesion possible. The aggregated platelets disintegrate to initiate a platelet binding cascade. Blood flow is further slowed, thus allowing the process of **coagulation,** which is the formation of an insoluble clot, to occur. The basic steps of hemostasis are shown in Figure 31.2.

When collagen is exposed at the site of injury, the damaged cells initiate the coagulation cascade. Coagulation itself occurs when fibrin threads create a meshwork that fortifies the blood constituents so that clots can develop. During the cascade, various plasma proteins that are circulating in an inactive state are converted to their active forms. Two separate pathways, along

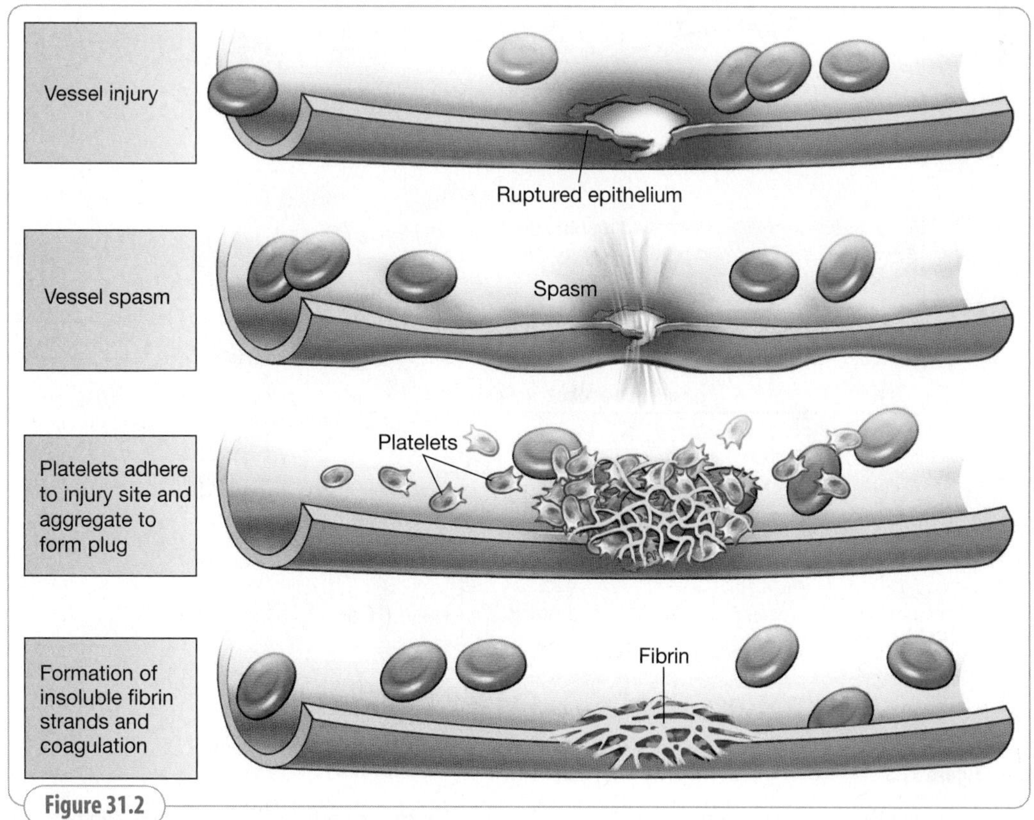

Figure 31.2

The basic steps in hemostasis.
Source: From *Medical Terminology: A Word-Building Approach* (6th ed., p. 301), by J. Rice, 2008. Reprinted by permission of Pearson Education, Inc., Upper Saddle River, NJ.

with numerous biochemical processes, lead to coagulation. The **intrinsic pathway** is activated in response to injury and takes several minutes to complete. The **extrinsic pathway** is activated when blood leaks out of a vessel and enters tissue spaces. The extrinsic pathway is less complex and is completed within seconds. There are common steps between the two pathways and the outcome is the same—the formation of the fibrin clot. The steps in each pathway are shown in Figure 31.3.

Near the end of the common pathway, a chemical called prothrombin activator or prothrombinase is formed. The prothrombin activator converts the clotting factor **prothrombin** to an enzyme called **thrombin.** Thrombin then converts **fibrinogen,** a plasma protein, to long strands of **fibrin.** The fibrin strands provide a framework to anchor the clot. Thus two of the factors essential to clotting, thrombin and fibrin, are only formed after injury to the vessels. The fibrin strands form an insoluble web over the injured area to stop blood loss. Normal blood clotting occurs in about 6 minutes.

It is important to note that several clotting factors, including thromboplastin and fibrinogen, are proteins made by the liver, which are constantly circulating through the blood in an inactive form. Vitamin K, which is made by bacteria residing in the large intestine, is required for the liver to make four of the clotting factors. Because of the crucial importance of the liver in creating these clotting factors, patients with serious hepatic disorders often have abnormal coagulation.

Cardiac Structure and Function

31.4 The heart is responsible for pumping blood throughout the circulatory system.

The heart is the hardest working organ in the body, pumping blood from before birth to the last minute of life. With the massive, continuous workload, it is not surprising that this organ weakens over time and that heart disease is one of the most

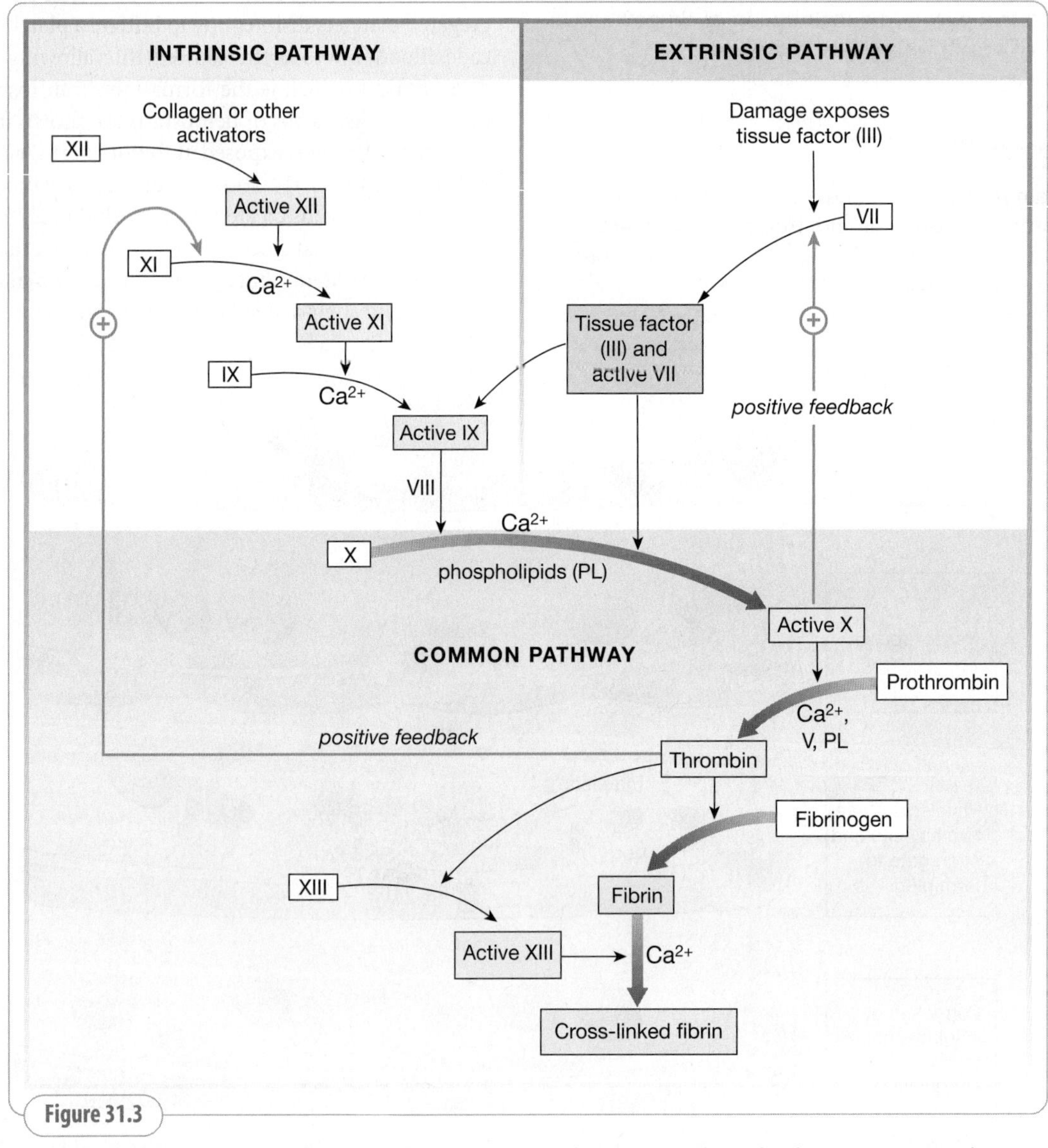

Figure 31.3

The coagulation cascade. Both the intrinsic pathway and extrinsic pathway lead to a common pathway and eventually a dense fibrin clot.

Source: From *Human Physiology: An Integrated Approach* (4th ed., p. 552), by D. Silverthorn, 2007. Reprinted by permission of Pearson Education, Inc., Upper Saddle River, NJ.

common causes of death. The heart is a frequent target for pharmacotherapy.

The heart may be thought of as a thick, specialized muscle. The muscular layer, called the **myocardium,** is the thickest of the heart layers and is responsible for the physical pumping action of the heart. The thickness of the myocardium varies throughout the different regions of the heart in proportion to its function. Because the ventricles perform the most work, the myocardium is thickest there. Cardiac muscle is a highly specialized tissue that is unlike either skeletal muscle or smooth muscle. Extensive branching networks of cellular structures connect cardiac muscle cells to each other, allowing the entire myocardium to contract as a coordinated whole.

Should cardiac cells, or myocytes, die the body is unable to replace them with new cardiac muscle cells. If a large area becomes deprived of oxygen and undergoes necrosis, the cells are replaced by fibrotic scar tissue and cardiac function may be impaired. The different regions of the heart may not contract in a coordinated manner, and conduction of the electrical potential across the heart may encounter "dead spots" where no conduction occurs. This can result in heart failure or dysrhythmias, which are frequent indications for pharmacotherapy (see Chapters 38 and 39).

The heart has four chambers that receive blood prior to being pumped, as illustrated in Figure 31.4a. These chambers differ in size, depending on their function. The left ventricle is the largest, because it must hold enough blood to pump to all body tissues. The size of the left ventricle and the thickness of the myocardial layer in this chamber can increase in size in patients with heart failure, which is a condition known as left ventricular hypertrophy.

Pharm*FACT*

The heart pumps up to 100,000 times in a single day, 35 million times every year. Each year, the heart pumps 2.6 million gallons of blood. *Source:* Martini, 2009.

31.5 The coronary arteries bring essential nutrients to the myocardium.

Working continuously around the clock, the heart requires a bountiful supply of oxygen and other nutrients. These are provided by the right and left coronary arteries and their branches, as shown in Figure 31.4b. The coronary arteries must have the ability to rapidly adapt to the heart's needs for oxygen. For example, during exercise the heart rate and strength of contraction markedly increase, and the coronary arteries must be able to quickly dilate to meet this increased workload placed on the myocardium.

As critical vessels, the coronary arteries serve a major role in maintaining body health. Should these arteries be unable to deliver essential nutrients, the myocardium will be affected either immediately, such as during intense exercise, or slowly, over a period of many years. The coronary arteries are subject to atherosclerosis, a buildup of fatty plaque, which narrows the lumen and restricts the amount of blood supply reaching the myocardium. If allowed to progress, the narrowing results in chest pain on exertion, a condition known as angina pectoris.

The coronary arteries are important targets for pharmacotherapy. Chapter 32 explains how reducing lipid levels in the blood can decrease the risk of atherosclerosis of the coronary arteries (and other arteries). Chapter 37 discusses how drugs can be used to reduce angina pain and decrease the risk of mortality following a heart attack. Chapter 39 introduces drugs that reduce the cardiac workload in patients with heart failure so that the heart does not require as much oxygen from the coronary arteries.

31.6 The cardiac conduction system keeps the heart beating in a synchronized manner.

For the heart to function properly, the atria must contract simultaneously, sending their blood into the ventricles. Following atrial contraction, the right and left ventricles then must contract simultaneously. Lack of synchronization of the atria and ventricles or of the right and left sides of the heart may have profound consequences. Proper timing of chamber contractions is made possible by the cardiac conduction system, a branching network of specialized cardiac muscle cells that sends a synchronized, electrical signal across the myocardium. These electrical impulses, or **action potentials,** carry the signal for the cardiac muscle cells to contract and must be coordinated precisely for the chambers to beat in a synchronized manner. The cardiac conduction system is illustrated in Figure 31.5.

Control of the cardiac conduction system begins in a small area of tissue in the wall of the right atrium known as the sinoatrial (SA) node or cardiac pacemaker. The SA node has the property of **automaticity,** which is the ability to spontaneously generate an action potential. The SA node generates a new action potential approximately 75 times per minute under resting conditions. This is referred to as the normal **sinus rhythm.** The SA node is greatly influenced by the activity of the sympathetic and parasympathetic divisions of the autonomic nervous system.

Upon leaving the SA node, the action potential travels quickly across both atria and through internodal pathways to the atrioventricular (AV) node. The AV node also has the property of automaticity, although less so than the SA node. Should the SA node malfunction, the AV node has the ability to spontaneously generate action potentials and continue the heart's contraction at a rate of 40 to 60 beats per minute. Compared to other areas in the heart, impulse conduction through the AV node is slow. This allows the atria sufficient time to completely contract and empty their blood before the ventricles receive their signal to contract. If the ventricles should contract prematurely, the AV valves will close and the atria will be prevented from completely emptying their contents.

As the action potential leaves the AV node it travels rapidly to the AV bundle or bundle of His. The pathway between the AV node and the bundle of His is the only electrical connection between the atria and the ventricles. The impulse is conducted down the right and left bundle branches to the Purkinje fibers, which rapidly carry the action potential to all regions of the ventricles almost simultaneously. Should the SA and AV nodes become nonfunctional, cells in the AV bundle and Purkinje

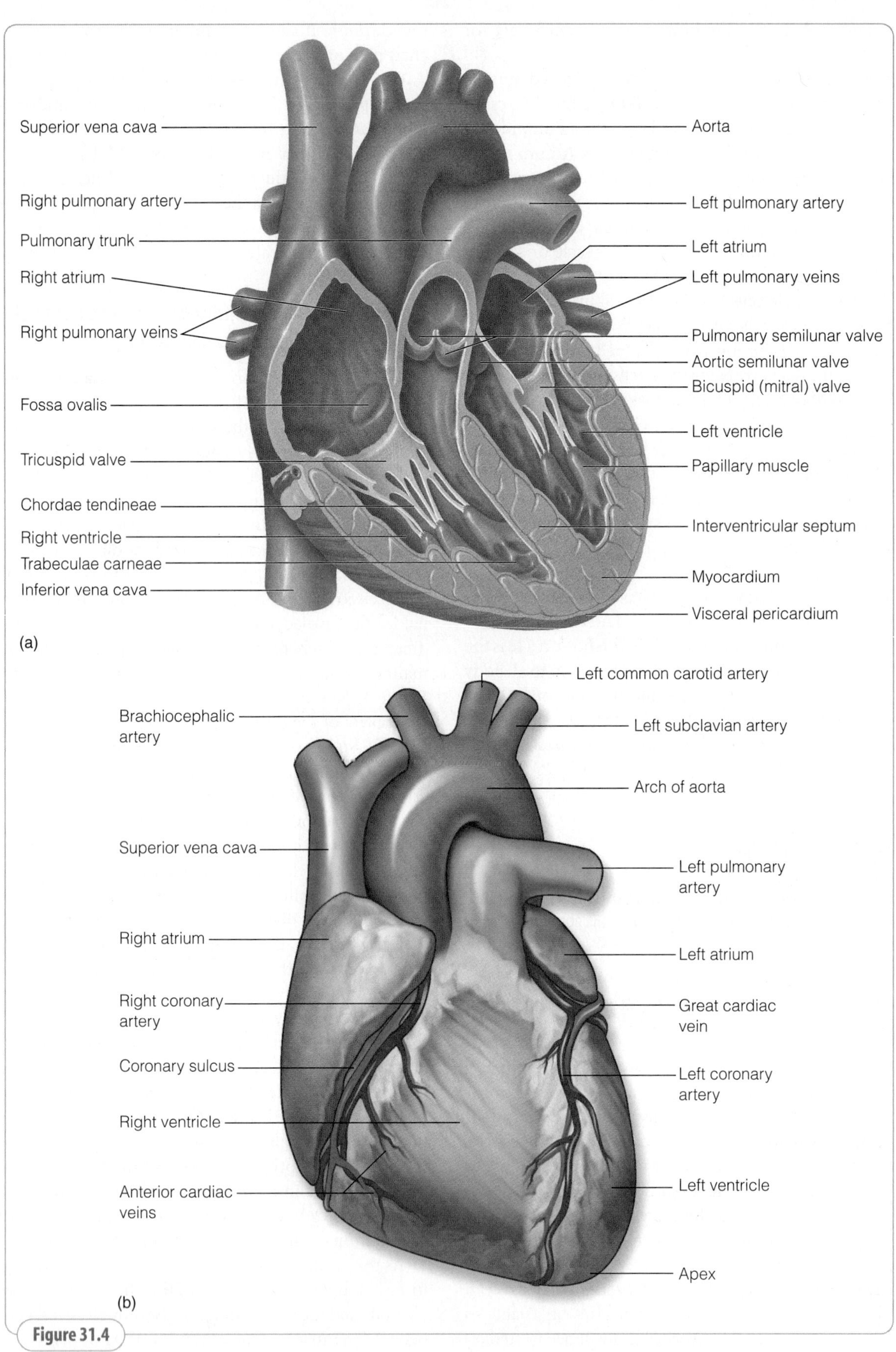

Figure 31.4

(a) The heart, showing chambers. (b) The heart, showing coronary arteries.

Source: From *Health and Physical Assessment in Nursing* (p. 428), by D. D'Amico & C. Barbarito, 2007. Reprinted by permission of Pearson Education, Inc., Upper Saddle River, NJ.

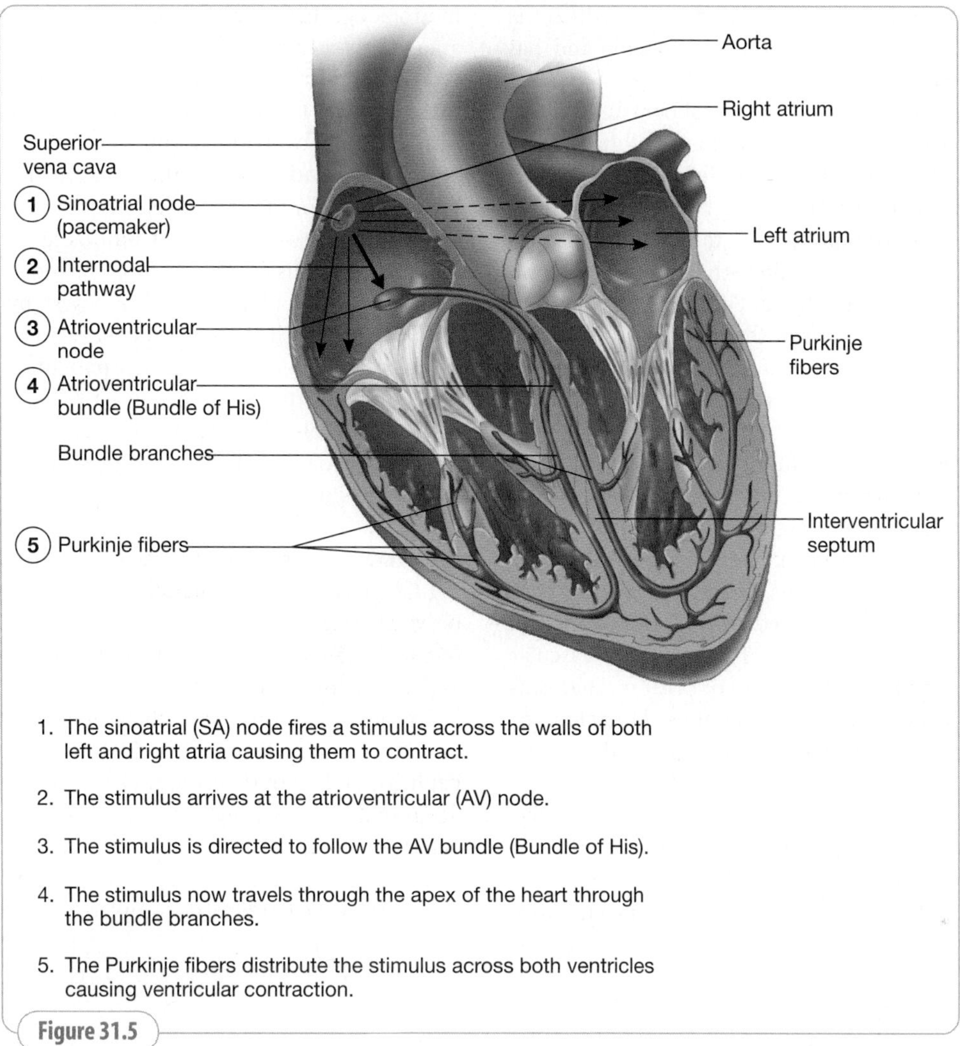

1. The sinoatrial (SA) node fires a stimulus across the walls of both left and right atria causing them to contract.
2. The stimulus arrives at the atrioventricular (AV) node.
3. The stimulus is directed to follow the AV bundle (Bundle of His).
4. The stimulus now travels through the apex of the heart through the bundle branches.
5. The Purkinje fibers distribute the stimulus across both ventricles causing ventricular contraction.

Figure 31.5

The cardiac conduction system.
Source: From *Anatomy and Physiology for Health Professions: An Interactive Journey* (p. 278), by B. Colbert, J. Ankney, & K. Lee, 2007. Reprinted by permission of Pearson Education, Inc., Upper Saddle River, NJ.

fibers can continue to generate myocardial contractions at a rate of about 30 beats per minute.

Although action potentials normally begin at the SA node and spread across the myocardium in a coordinated manner, other regions of the heart may also initiate beats. These areas, known as **ectopic foci** or ectopic pacemakers, may send impulses across the myocardium that competes with those from the normal conduction pathway. The timing and synchronization of atrial and ventricular contractions may be affected. Although healthy hearts occasionally experience an extra beat without incident, ectopic foci in diseased hearts have the potential to cause dysrhythmias, or disorders of cardiac rhythm. The events associated with the cardiac conduction system are recorded on the electrocardiogram (ECG).

It is important to understand that the underlying purpose of the cardiac conduction system is to keep the heart beating in a regular, synchronized manner so that cardiac output can be maintained. Dysrhythmias that profoundly affect cardiac output have the potential to produce serious, if not mortal, consequences. These types of dysrhythmias require pharmacologic intervention, as discussed in Chapter 39.

31.7 Cardiac output is determined by stroke volume and heart rate.

To understand how medications act on the heart and to predict the consequences of pharmacotherapy, it is essential to have a comprehensive knowledge of normal cardiac physiology. This includes a thorough understanding of factors that determine the amount of blood pumped by the heart and the forces acting on the chambers.

The amount of blood pumped by each ventricle per minute is the **cardiac output (CO).** The average CO is 5 L/minute. CO may be calculated by multiplying stroke volume by the heart rate.

$$\text{CO} = \text{stroke volume (mL/beat)} \times \text{heart rate (beats/minute)}$$

Stroke volume is the amount of blood pumped by a ventricle in a single contraction. What types of factors might cause the ventricle to eject more blood in a contraction? To understand these factors, a simple comparison to a rubber band is useful. If you stretch a small rubber band 2 inches, it will snap back with a certain force. Stretching the band 4 inches will cause it to snap back with greater force. The force of the snap will continue to increase up to a certain limit, after which the rubber band has been stretched as far as possible and has reached maximum force (or it breaks!).

Cardiac muscle fibers are analogous to rubber bands. If you fill the chambers with more blood, the fibers will have more stretch and will "snap back" with greater force. This is known as Starling's law of the heart: The strength of contraction, or **contractility,** is proportional to the muscle fiber length (stretch). The contractility determines the amount of blood ejected per beat, or the stroke volume. The degree to which the ventricles are filled with blood and the myocardial fibers are stretched just prior to contraction is called **preload.** Up to a physiological limit, drugs that increase preload and contractility will increase the CO.

What causes the chambers to fill up with more blood, become stretched (more preload), and contract with greater force? Although there are several factors that affect preload, the most important is **venous return:** the volume of blood returning to the heart from the veins. Giving a drug that constricts veins will increase venous return to the heart, as will simply increasing the total amount of blood in the vascular system (increased blood volume). Drugs or other mechanisms that constrict veins or increase blood volume will therefore increase stroke volume and CO. Conversely, drugs that dilate veins or reduce blood volume will lower CO.

Drugs that increase contractility are called positive **inotropic agents.** Examples of positive inotropic agents include epinephrine, norepinephrine, thyroid hormone, and dopamine. Drugs that decrease contractility are called negative inotropic agents. Examples include quinidine and beta-adrenergic antagonists such as propranolol.

A second primary factor affecting stroke volume is afterload. In order for the left ventricle to pump blood out of the heart, it must overcome a substantial "back pressure" in the aorta. **Afterload** is the systolic pressure in the aorta that must be overcome for blood to be ejected from the left ventricle. As afterload increases, the heart pumps less blood, and stroke volume (and thus CO) decreases. The most common cause of increased afterload is an increase in systemic blood pressure, or hypertension (HTN). HTN creates an increased workload on the heart, which explains why patients with chronic HTN are more likely to experience heart failure. Antihypertensive drugs create less afterload, increase stroke volume, and result in less workload for the heart. Preload and afterload are illustrated in Figure 31.6.

Heart rate: Heart rate is the second primary factor determining CO. Heart rate is generally controlled by the autonomic nervous system, which makes the minute-by-minute adjustments demanded by the circulatory system. Both sympathetic and parasympathetic fibers are found in the SA node, and heart rate is determined by which fibers are firing at a greater rate at any given moment. Circulating hormones such as epinephrine and thyroid hormone also affect heart rate. In theory, drugs that increase heart rate will increase CO, although compensatory mechanisms may prevent this effect (see Section 31.8). In addition, a very rapid heart rate may not give the chambers sufficient time to completely fill, thus reducing CO.

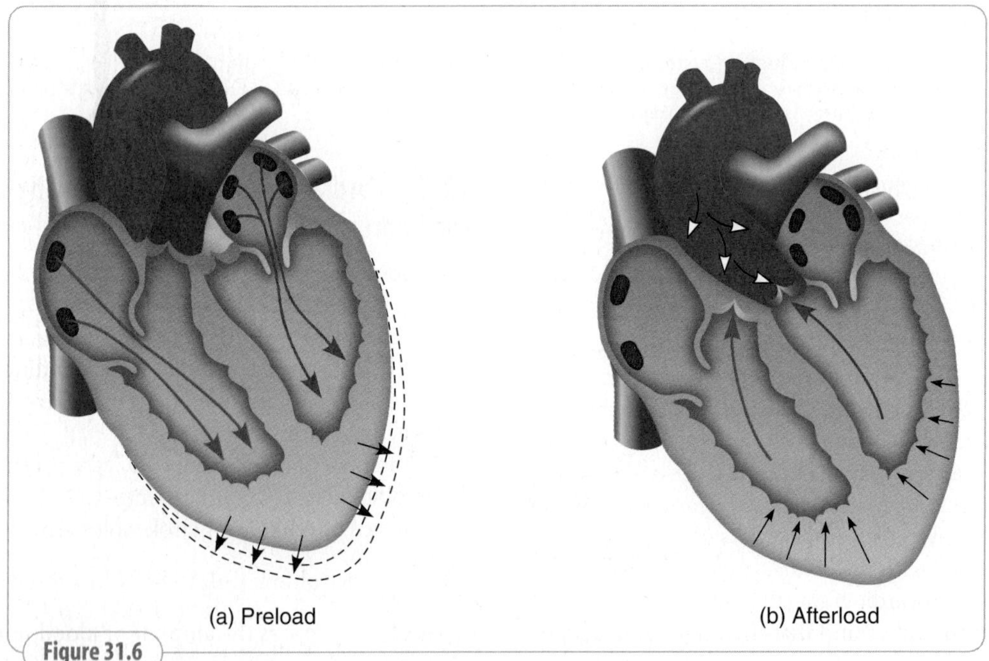

Figure 31.6

(a) Preload is the degree to which the ventricles are filled with blood and the myocardial fibers are stretched just prior to contraction. (b) Afterload is the systolic pressure in the aorta that must be overcome for blood to be ejected from the left ventricle.

Source: From *Health and Physical Assessment in Nursing* (p. 441), by D. D'Amico & C. Barbarito, 2007. Reprinted by permission of Pearson Education, Inc., Upper Saddle River, NJ.

CONNECTION *Checkpoint* 31.2

From what you learned in Chapter 16, predict what effect the following would have on heart rate: sympathomimetics, parasympathomimetics, adrenergic agonists, and anticholinergics. See Answer to Connection Checkpoint 31.2 in Appendix A.

Hemodynamics and Blood Pressure

31.8 The primary factors responsible for blood pressure are cardiac output, peripheral resistance, and blood volume.

The homeostatic regulation of blood pressure is a key topic in pharmacology because HTN is so prevalent in the population. Regulation of blood pressure is complex with many diverse factors, both local and systemic, interacting to maintain adequate blood flow to the tissues. The three primary factors that regulate arterial blood pressure—CO, peripheral resistance, and blood volume—are shown in Figure 31.7. The following simple formula should be memorized (as well as understood) because it will help the student predict the actions and adverse effects of many classes of cardiovascular medications.

$$\text{Blood Pressure} = \text{CO} \times \text{peripheral resistance}$$

CO is determined by heart rate and stroke volume as discussed in Section 31.7. From the preceding equation, it is easy to see that as CO increases, blood pressure also increases. This is important to pharmacology because medications that change the CO, stroke volume, or heart rate have the potential to influence a patient's blood pressure.

As blood flows at high speeds through the vascular system, it exerts force against the walls of the vessels, or friction. Although the endothelial lining of the blood vessel is extremely smooth, friction reduces the velocity of blood flow. Further friction is encountered as the stream of fast-moving blood narrows to enter smaller vessels, divides into two channels (arteries), or encounters fatty deposits on the vessel walls (plaque). Blood flow may become turbulent, which is a chaotic, tumbling motion that greatly increases friction. The friction that blood encounters in the arteries is called **peripheral resistance.** Arteries have smooth muscle in their walls, which can control the total peripheral resistance. For example, if arteries constrict, their inside diameter or lumen will become smaller and create more resistance and higher blood pressure. A large number of medications affect vascular smooth muscle. Some of these agents cause vessels to constrict, thus raising blood pressure, whereas others relax smooth muscle, thereby opening the lumen and lowering blood pressure.

An additional factor responsible for blood pressure is the total amount of blood in the vascular system, or blood volume. Although the average person maintains a relatively constant blood volume of approximately 5 L, this can change due to many regulatory factors, certain disease states, and pharmacotherapy. More fluid in the vascular system increases venous pressure and venous return to the heart, thus increasing CO and arterial blood pressure. Drugs are frequently used to adjust blood volume. For example, infusion of intravenous (IV) fluids quickly increases blood volume and raises blood pressure. This is used to advantage when treating hypotension due to shock. On the other hand, diuretics cause fluid loss through urination, thus decreasing blood volume and lowering blood pressure.

Pharm*FACT*

If all blood vessels in the body were placed end to end it is estimated that they would extend for 25,000 miles. *Source:* Martini, 2009.

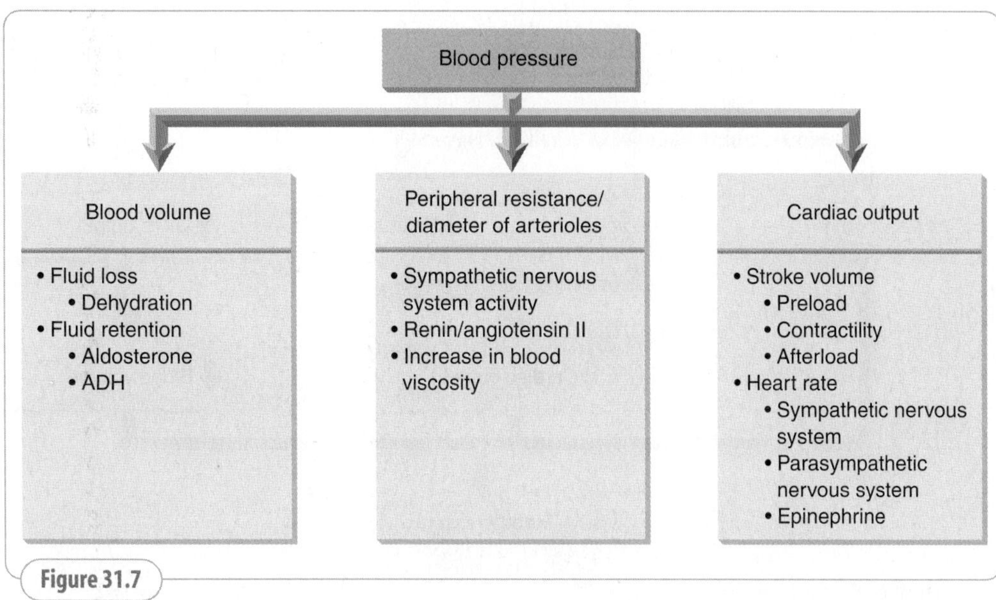

Figure 31.7

The primary factors affecting blood pressure.

31.9 Neural regulation of blood pressure includes baroreceptor and chemoreceptor reflexes.

It is critical that the body maintains a normal range of blood pressure, and that it has the ability to safely and rapidly change pressure as it proceeds through daily activities such as sleep and exercise. Hypotension can cause dizziness and lack of adequate urine formation, whereas extreme HTN can cause vessels to rupture and result in ischemia of critical organs. Figure 31.8 illustrates how the body maintains homeostasis during periods of blood pressure change.

The central and autonomic nervous systems are intimately involved in regulating blood pressure. On a minute-to-minute basis, blood pressure is regulated by a cluster of neurons in the medulla oblongata called the **vasomotor center.** Sensory receptors in the aorta and the internal carotid artery provide the vasomotor center with vital information on conditions in the vascular system. **Baroreceptors** have the ability to sense pressure within large vessels, whereas **chemoreceptors** recognize levels of oxygen, carbon dioxide, and the acidity or pH in the blood. The vasomotor center reacts to information from baroreceptors and chemoreceptors by raising or lowering blood pressure accordingly. Nerves travel from the vasomotor center to the arteries, where the smooth muscle is directed to either constrict (raise blood pressure) or relax (lower blood pressure). As discussed in Chapter 16, sympathetic outflow from the vasomotor center stimulates alpha$_1$-adrenergic receptors on arterioles, causing vasoconstriction. Alpha$_2$-adrenergic agonists can also decrease blood pressure by their central effects on the vasomotor center.

The baroreceptor reflex is an important mechanism used by the body for making rapid adjustments to blood pressure. If pressure in the vascular system increases, the baroreceptors in the aortic arch and carotid sinus trigger reflexes that constrict the arterioles and veins and accelerate the heart rate. Together, these actions return blood pressure to normal levels within seconds.

Drugs that raise or lower blood pressure can trigger the baroreceptor reflex. For example, antihypertensives administered by the IV route cause an immediate reduction in blood pressure that is recognized by the baroreceptors. The baroreceptors respond by attempting to return blood pressure back to the original levels. The resulting accelerated heart rate, or **reflex tachycardia,** may cause the patient to experience palpitations. The baroreceptors are not able to offer a continuous or sustained reduction in blood pressure. Continued administration of an antihypertensive drug will "overcome" the reflex. In addition, with aging or certain disease states such as diabetes, the baroreceptor response may be diminished.

Another example of the baroreceptor reflex occurs when baroreceptors in the right atrium are triggered. These receptors recognize excess stretching of the right atrium, such as might occur when large amounts of IV fluids are administered. The **atrial reflex** causes the heart rate and CO to increase until the backlog of venous blood (or IV fluid) is distributed throughout the body.

The chemoreceptor reflex can also significantly affect blood pressure. Sensors in the carotid sinus and near the aortic arch recognize levels of oxygen and carbon dioxide and the acidity (pH) in the blood. Triggering these chemoreceptors activates the sympathetic nervous system and causes heart rate and CO to increase. The purpose of this reflex is to circulate blood faster so that the respiratory system can remove excess carbon dioxide (which returns pH to normal levels) and add more oxygen to the blood.

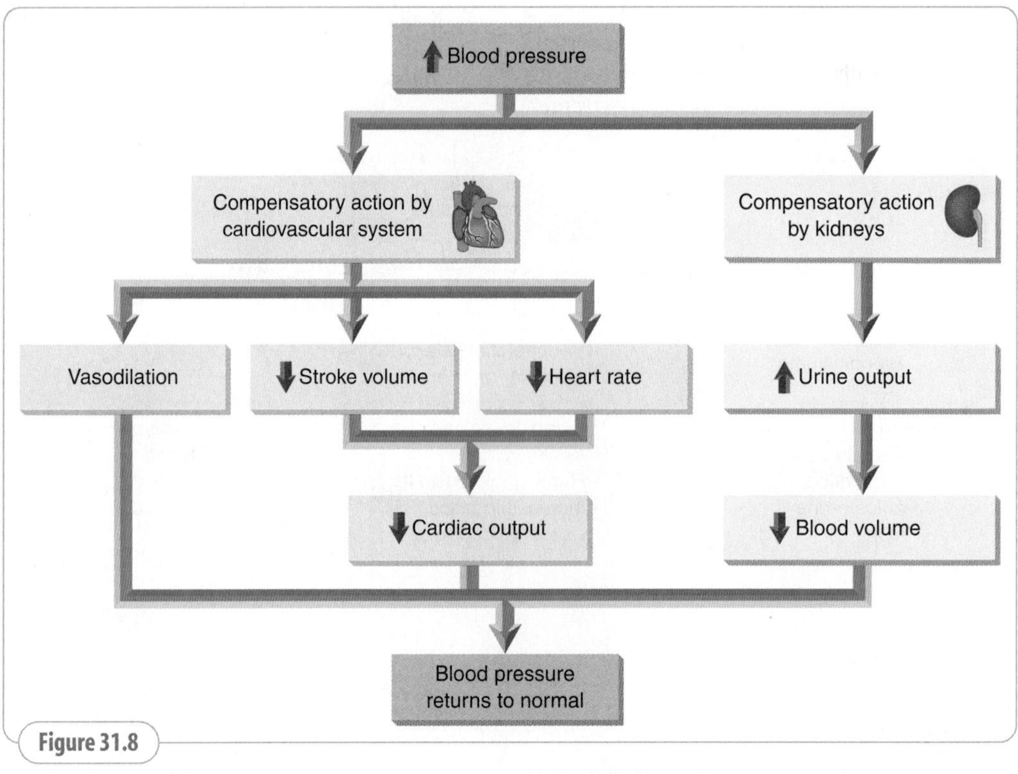

Figure 31.8

Blood pressure homeostasis.

CONNECTION Checkpoint 31.3

Many autonomic drugs dilate or constrict blood vessels. From what you learned in Chapter 16, which class of autonomic drugs is most commonly prescribed for HTN? See Answer to Connection Checkpoint 31.3 in Appendix A.

31.10 Hormones may have profound effects on blood pressure.

Several hormones affect blood pressure, and certain classes of medications are given to either enhance or block the actions of these hormones. For example, injection of the catecholamines epinephrine or norepinephrine will immediately raise blood pressure, which is essential for patients experiencing shock.

Antidiuretic hormone (ADH) is a hormone released by the posterior pituitary gland when blood pressure falls or when the osmotic pressure of the blood increases. ADH is a potent peripheral vasoconstrictor that quickly increases blood pressure. The hormone also acts on the kidneys to conserve water and increase blood volume, thereby causing blood pressure to increase. The pharmacotherapy of ADH and related hormones is discussed in Chapter 67.

The **renin-angiotensin-aldosterone system (RAAS)** is particularly important in the drug therapy of HTN. As blood pressure falls, the enzyme renin is released by the kidneys. Through a two-step pathway, angiotensin II is formed, which subsequently increases CO and constricts arterioles to return blood pressure to original levels. Angiotensin II also promotes the release of aldosterone from the adrenal gland, which causes sodium and water retention. Drugs that block the RAAS are key drugs in the treatment of HTN and are presented in Chapter 34.

Atrial natriuretic peptide (ANP) is a hormone that is secreted by specialized cells in the right atrium when large increases in blood volume produce excessive stretch on the atrial wall. ANP has multiple effects, all of which attempt to return blood pressure to original levels. Sodium ion transport in the kidney is affected, resulting in enhanced sodium and water excretion. The release of ADH and aldosterone is suppressed by ANP. In addition, ANP reduces sympathetic outflow from the CNS, resulting in dilation of peripheral arteries. A summary of the various nervous and hormone factors influencing blood pressure is shown in Figure 31.9.

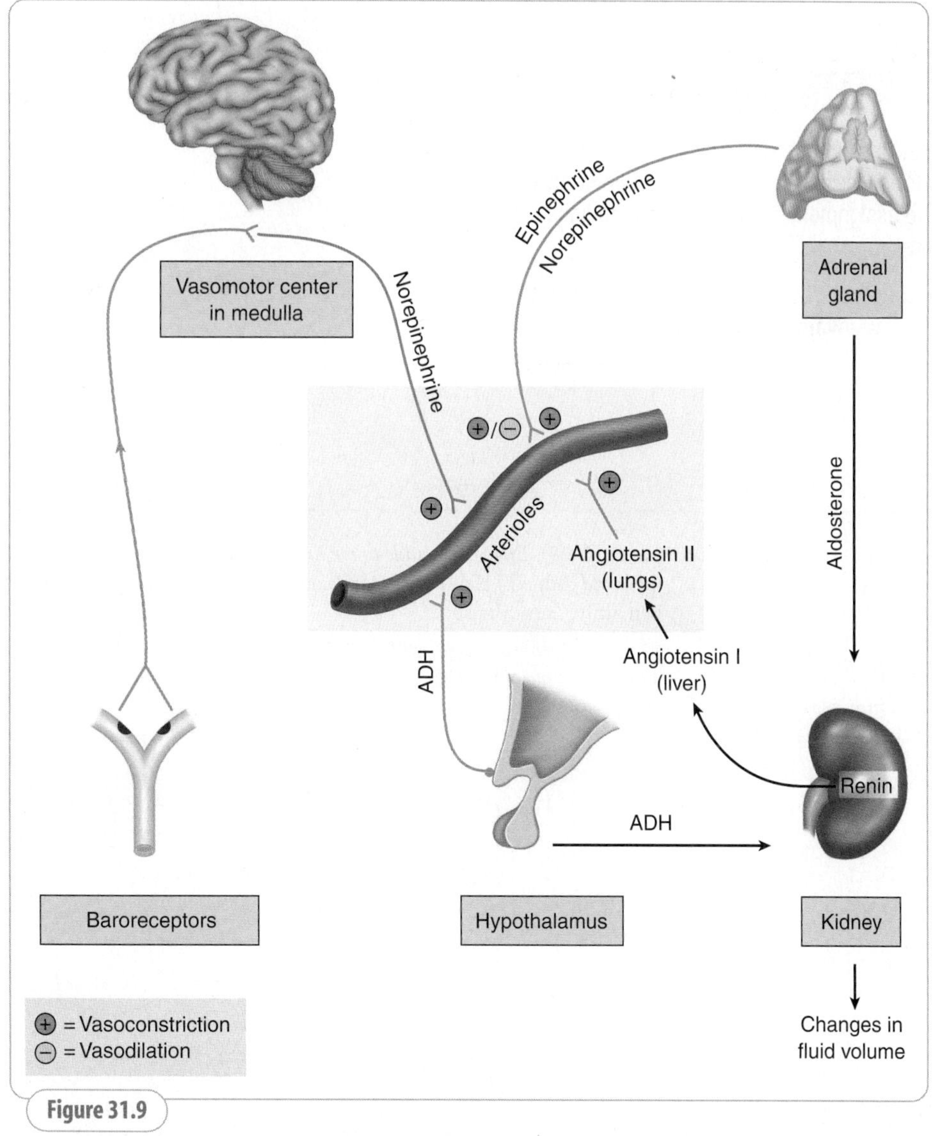

Figure 31.9

Hormonal and neural factors influencing blood pressure.

UNDERSTANDING THE CHAPTER

Key Concepts Summary

31.1 The cardiovascular system consists of the blood, heart, and blood vessels.

31.2 Blood consists of formed elements and plasma.

31.3 Hemostasis is a complex process involving multiple steps and a large number of enzymes and factors.

31.4 The heart is responsible for pumping blood throughout the circulatory system.

31.5 The coronary arteries bring essential nutrients to the myocardium.

31.6 The cardiac conduction system keeps the heart beating in a synchronized manner.

31.7 Cardiac output is determined by stroke volume and heart rate.

31.8 The primary factors responsible for blood pressure are cardiac output, peripheral resistance, and blood volume.

31.9 Neural regulation of blood pressure includes baroreceptor and chemoreceptor reflexes.

31.10 Hormones may have profound effects on blood pressure.

References

Colbert, B. J., & Mason, B. J. (2008). *Integrated cardiopulmonary pharmacology* (2nd ed.). Upper Saddle River, NJ: Pearson Prentice Hall.

D'Amico, D., & Barbarito, C. (2007). *Health and physical assessment in nursing.* Upper Saddle River, NJ: Pearson Prentice Hall.

Krogh, D. (2009). *Biology: A guide to the natural world* (4th ed.). San Francisco: Pearson Benjamin Cummings.

Martini, F. H. (2009). *Fundamentals of human anatomy and physiology* (8th ed.). San Francisco: Pearson Benjamin Cummings.

Silverthorn, D. U. (2006). *Human physiology: An integrated approach* (4th ed.). San Francisco: Pearson Benjamin Cummings.

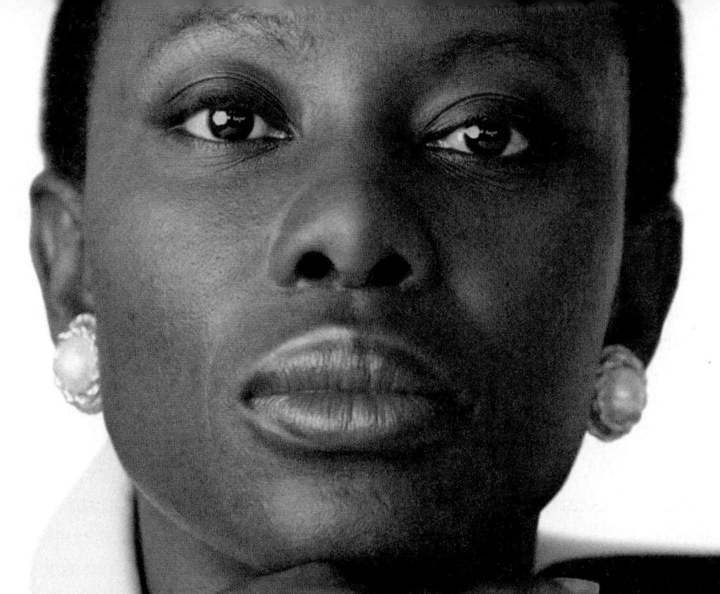

My mother had it and my grandmother had it too. Now, I'm told that I have it. My doctor says my cholesterol level is too high.

Patient "Belinda Cummings"

CHAPTER

Pharmacotherapy of Hyperlipidemia 32

Chapter Outline

Types of Lipids and Lipoproteins

Measurement and Control of Serum Lipids

Drugs for Dyslipidemias

HMG-CoA Reductase Inhibitors

PROTOTYPE **Atorvastatin (Lipitor)** *p. 504*

Bile Acid Sequestrants

PROTOTYPE **Cholestyramine (Questran)** *p. 507*

Nicotinic Acid

Fibric Acid Agents

PROTOTYPE **Gemfibrozil (Lopid)** *p. 509*

Cholesterol Absorption Inhibitors

Learning Outcomes

After reading this chapter, the student should be able to:

1. Summarize the link between high blood cholesterol, low-density lipoprotein levels, and atherosclerosis.
2. Compare and contrast the different types of lipids.
3. Illustrate how lipids are transported through the blood.
4. Compare and contrast the clinical importance of the different types of lipoproteins.
5. Give examples of how cholesterol and low-density lipoprotein levels can be controlled with nonpharmacologic means.
6. For each of the classes shown in the chapter outline, identify the prototype and representative drugs and explain the mechanism(s) of drug action, primary indications, contraindications, significant drug interactions, pregnancy category, and important adverse effects.
7. Categorize antihyperlipidemic drugs based on their classification and mechanism of action.
8. Explain the nurse's role in the safe administration of drugs for lipid disorders.
9. Use the nursing process to care for patients receiving drug therapy for lipid disorders.

Key Terms

apoprotein, *496*
atherosclerosis, *496*
dyslipidemia, *498*
high-density lipoprotein (HDL), *496*
HMG-CoA reductase, *501*
hypercholesterolemia, *498*
hyperlipidemia, *498*
hypertriglyceridemia, *498*
lecithins, *496*
lipoprotein, *496*
low-density lipoprotein (LDL), *496*
phospholipids, *496*
reverse cholesterol transport, *498*
rhabdomyolysis, *502*
steroids, *496*
sterol nucleus, *496*
triglycerides, *496*
very low-density lipoprotein (VLDL), *496*

Research during the 1970s and 1980s brought about a nutritional revolution as new knowledge about lipids and their relationships to obesity and cardiovascular disease allowed people to make more intelligent lifestyle choices. Since then advances in the diagnosis of lipid disorders have helped to identify those people at greatest risk for cardiovascular disease and those most likely to benefit from pharmacologic intervention. As a result of this knowledge and from advancements in pharmacology, the incidence of death due to most cardiovascular diseases has been declining, although cardiovascular disease remains the leading cause of death in the United States.

PharmFACT

The incidence of high blood cholesterol increases until age 65. Prior to age 50, high blood cholesterol occurs more frequently in men, but after age 55 the disease is more common in women. *Source:* Isley, 2006.

MyNursingKit | How Can I Lower My Cholesterol by Changing My Diet?

Types of Lipids and Lipoproteins

32.1 Lipids are classified as triglycerides, phospholipids, or sterols.

There are three types of lipids that are important to human physiology, and these are illustrated in Figure 32.1. The most common types are **triglycerides** or neutral fats, which form a large family of different lipids, all having three fatty acids attached to a chemical backbone of glycerol. Triglycerides are the major storage form of fat in the body and the only type of lipid that serves as an important energy source. They account for 90% of the total lipids in the body.

A second class, the **phospholipids,** is formed when a phosphorous group replaces one of the fatty acids in a triglyceride. This class of lipids is essential to building plasma membranes. The best known phospholipids are **lecithins,** which are found in high concentration in egg yolks and soybeans. Once promoted as a natural treatment for high cholesterol levels, controlled studies have not shown lecithin to be of benefit for this disorder. Likewise, lecithin has been proposed as a remedy for nervous system diseases such as Alzheimer's disease and bipolar disorder, but there is no definitive evidence to support these claims.

The third class of lipids, the **steroids,** is a diverse group of substances having a common **sterol nucleus** or ring structure. Cholesterol is the most widely known of the steroids, and its role in promoting **atherosclerosis** has been clearly demonstrated. Atherosclerosis is the presence of plaque—a fatty, fibrous material within the walls of the coronary arteries. Unlike the triglycerides that provide fuel for the body, cholesterol is a vital component of plasma membranes and serves as a building block for essential biochemicals, including vitamin D, bile acids, cortisol, estrogen, and testosterone. Although clearly essential for life, the body needs only minute amounts of cholesterol because the liver is able to synthesize adequate amounts from other chemicals. It is not necessary, nor desirable, to provide excess cholesterol in the diet. The dietary sources of cholesterol are obtained solely from animal products; humans do not absorb the sterols produced by plants. The American Heart Association recommends less than 300 mg of dietary cholesterol per day.

32.2 Lipoproteins are important predictors of cardiovascular disease.

Because lipid molecules are not soluble in plasma, they must be specially packaged for transport through the blood. To accomplish this, the body forms complexes called **lipoproteins,** which consist of various amounts of cholesterol, triglycerides, and phospholipids bound to carrier proteins. The protein component is called an **apoprotein** (*apo-* means "separated from" or "derived from"). The four apoproteins important to lipid transport are known as A-I, A-II, A-IV, and B-100.

Lipoproteins are classified according to their composition, size, and weight or density, which come primarily from the amount of apoprotein present in the complex. Each type varies in lipid and apoprotein makeup and serves a different function in transporting lipids from the sites of synthesis and absorption to the sites of utilization. For example, **high-density lipoprotein (HDL)** contains the most apoprotein, up to 50% by weight. The highest amount of cholesterol is carried by **low-density lipoprotein (LDL).** Figure 32.2 illustrates the three basic lipoproteins and their compositions.

To understand the pharmacotherapy of lipid disorders, it is important to know the functions of the major lipoproteins and their roles in transporting cholesterol. LDL transports cholesterol from the liver to the tissues and organs, where it is used to build plasma membranes or to synthesize other steroids. Once in the tissues it can also be stored for later use. Storage of cholesterol in the lining of blood vessels, however, is not desirable because it contributes to plaque buildup. LDL is often called "bad" cholesterol because this lipoprotein contributes significantly to plaque deposits and coronary artery disease (CAD). Sixty to seventy percent of the cholesterol circulating in the blood is found in LDL.

Very low-density lipoprotein (VLDL) is the primary carrier of triglycerides in the blood. VLDLs account for virtually all triglycerides being transported from the liver to storage in adipose tissue. Through a series of steps, VLDL is reduced in

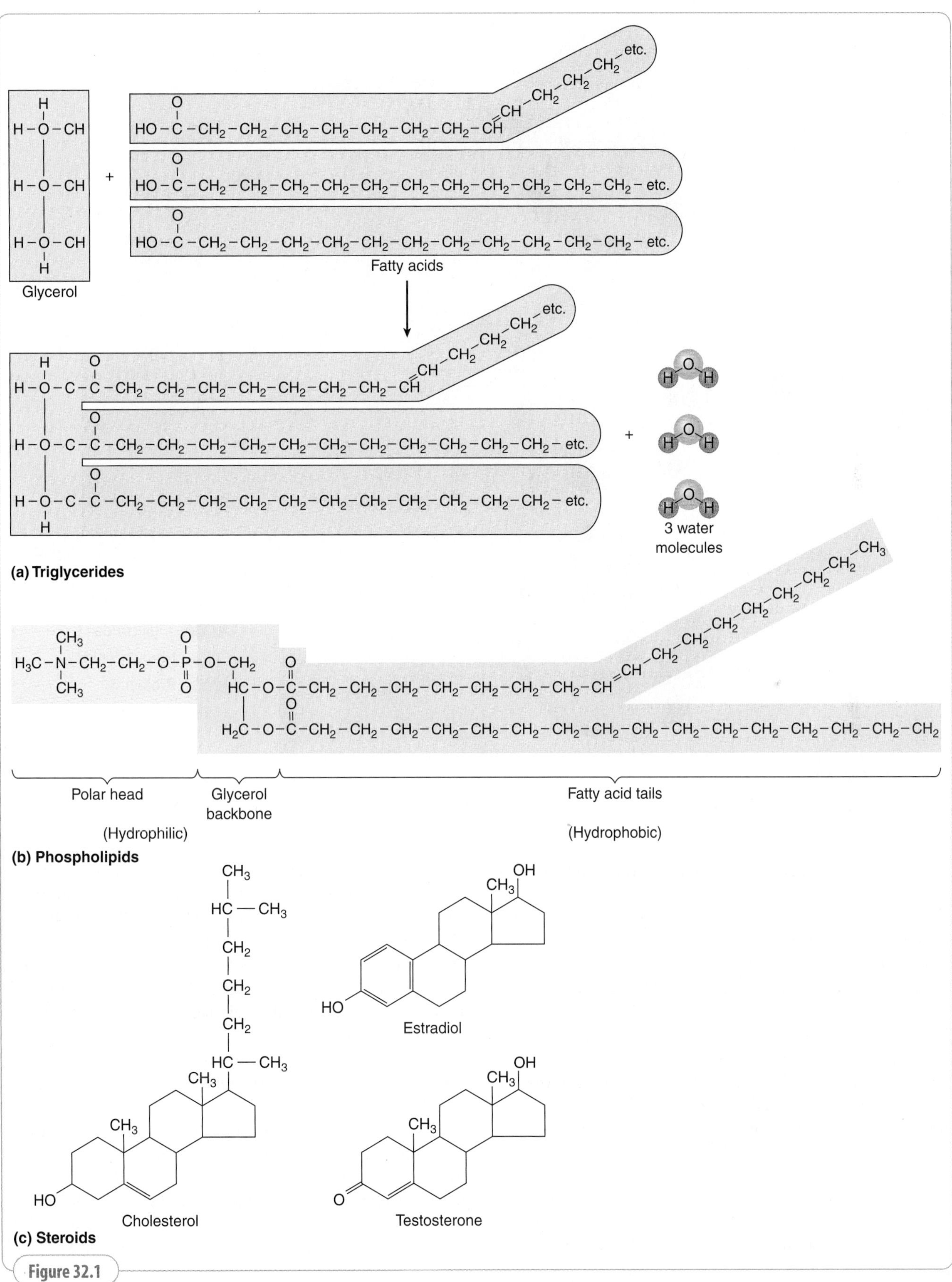

Figure 32.1

Chemical structure of lipids.

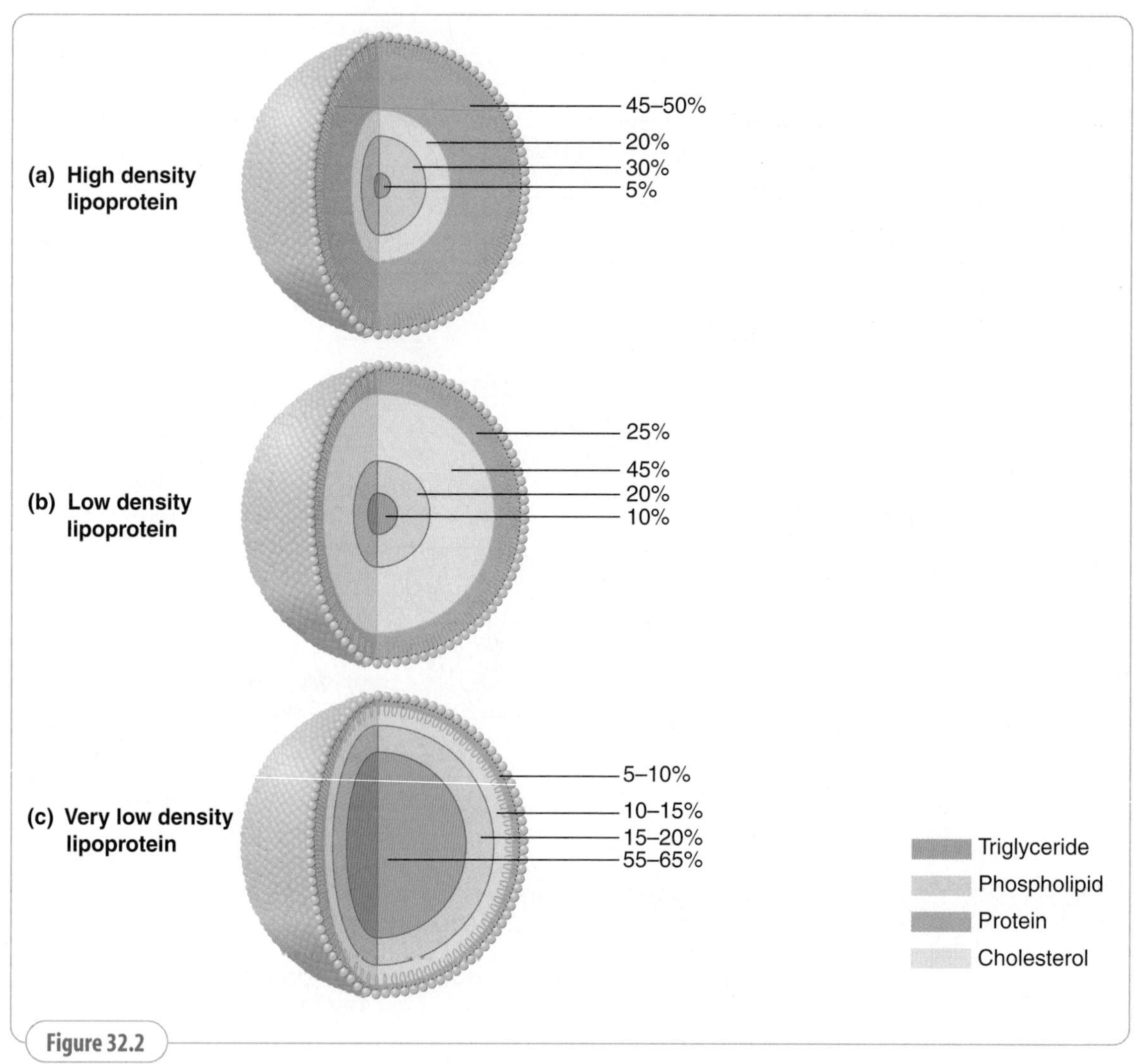

Figure 32.2

Composition of lipoproteins: (a) HDL; (b) LDL; and (c) VLDL.

size to become LDL. Lowering LDL levels in the blood has been shown to decrease the incidence of CAD.

HDL is manufactured in the liver and small intestine and assists in the transport of excess cholesterol away from the body tissues and back to the liver for metabolism in a process known as **reverse cholesterol transport.** The cholesterol component of the HDL is then broken down to unite with bile, which is subsequently excreted in the feces. Excretion via bile is the only route the body uses to remove cholesterol. Because HDL transports cholesterol for destruction and removes it from the body, it is considered "good" cholesterol. Patients with insufficient amounts of HDL are at risk for atherosclerosis, even if their total cholesterol levels are normal.

Several terms are used to describe lipid disorders. **Hyperlipidemia** is the general term meaning high levels of lipids in the blood. The term *hyperlipidemia* does not specify which lipid is elevated. Elevated blood cholesterol, or **hypercholesterolemia,** is the type of hyperlipidemia that is most familiar to the general public. **Dyslipidemia** is the term that refers to abnormal (excess or deficient) levels of lipoproteins. Some patients exhibit an increase in triglyceride levels known as **hypertriglyceridemia.**

Patients with lipid disorders are asymptomatic and often do not seek medical intervention until cardiovascular disease produces symptoms such as chest pain or signs of hypertension. Research suggests that over half the adult population in the United States has total cholesterol levels above 200 mg/dL and that two thirds of these patients are unaware of their hyperlipidemia. Nurses will likely face challenges getting their patients to adhere to the antihyperlipidemic drug regimen. It is often difficult to convince patients to spend money for medications and to continue taking them when they do not feel ill.

Hyperlipidemia may be inherited or acquired. Certainly, diets high in saturated fats and lack of exercise contribute greatly to the development of hyperlipidemia and resulting cardiovascular diseases. However, genetics determines one's ability to metabolize lipids and contributes to high lipid levels in substantial numbers of patients. Some genetic dyslipidemias can be so severe as to cause CAD in early childhood and death due to myocardial infarction (MI) by age 32. For most patients, dyslipidemias are the result of a combination of genetic and environmental (lifestyle) factors.

CONNECTIONS

To the Community Teaching Patients About a Lipid Profile

Patients taking drugs to lower LDL and cholesterol levels will be required to routinely have a lipid profile test to determine the effectiveness of their therapy. Nurses can aid in their patients' understanding of this information by stressing the importance of adherence to the therapeutic regimen. Here are some questions and answers that you might face in a patient situation.

What Is a Lipid Profile Laboratory Test?

The group of laboratory tests that the health care providers may use to determine risk for coronary heart disease is called a lipid profile. The results from these tests may be indicators of a high risk for a heart attack or stroke due to blood vessel blockage, often called hardening of the arteries.

How Is a Lipid Profile Used in Determining My Care?

Tests included in the lipid profile include total cholesterol, triglycerides, HDL cholesterol (good cholesterol), and LDL cholesterol (bad cholesterol). Other indicators such as the ratio of HDL to cholesterol may be determined, as well as the risk based on the results of the lipid profile, age, sex, and other factors for treatment.

What Results Are Reported in a Lipid Profile Test?

Health care providers may use the results of the lipid profile as a guide for prescribing a plan of care for persons at risk for coronary heart disease. They will also consider other known risk factors in defining the treatment plan. In some cases the health care provider may recommend a low-fat diet combined with exercise. This may be sufficient to bring lipid levels back to normal ranges. In other cases, drug therapy may be needed. In all cases, a sensible weight management program and exercise should be included in the plan of care.

Measurement and Control of Serum Lipids

32.3 Blood lipid profiles are important diagnostic tools in guiding the therapy of dyslipidemias.

Although high levels of cholesterol in the blood are associated with cardiovascular disease, it is not enough to simply measure total cholesterol in the blood. Because some cholesterol is being transported for destruction, a more accurate profile is obtained by measuring the LDL and HDL. The goal in maintaining normal cholesterol levels is to maximize the HDL and minimize the LDL. This is sometimes stated as a ratio of LDL to HDL. If the ratio is greater than 5 (five times more LDL than HDL), the male patient is considered at risk for cardiovascular disease. The normal ratio in women is slightly lower at 4.5.

Scientists have further divided LDL into subclasses of lipoproteins. For example, one variety found in LDL called lipoprotein (a) has been strongly associated with plaque formation and heart disease. It is likely that further research will find other varieties with the expectation that drugs will be designed to be more selective toward the "bad" lipoproteins. Table 32.1 gives the desirable, borderline, and high laboratory values for each of the major lipids and lipoproteins.

TABLE 32.1 Standard Laboratory Lipid Profiles

Type of Lipid	Laboratory Value (mg/dL)	Standard
Total Cholesterol	Less than 200	Desirable
	200–239	Borderline high risk
	Greater than 239	High risk
LDL Cholesterol	Less than 100	Optimal
	100–129	Near or above optimal
	130–159	Borderline high risk
	160–189	High risk
	Greater than 190	Very high risk
HDL Cholesterol	Less than 40	High risk
	40–59	Borderline high risk
	Greater than 60	Desirable
Triglycerides	Less than 150	Normal
	150–199	Borderline high risk
	200–499	High risk
	Greater than 500	Very high risk

Establishing treatment guidelines for dyslipidemia has been difficult because the condition itself has no symptoms and the progression to cardiovascular disease may take decades. Based on many years of research, the National Cholesterol Education Program (NCEP), a panel of experts of the National Heart, Lung, and Blood Institute, has published the recommended treatment guidelines for dyslipidemia. The guidelines are based on accumulated evidence that reducing "borderline" high cholesterol levels can result in fewer heart attacks and decreased mortality. It is estimated that for every 1% reduction in LDL, there is a 1% reduction in the possibility of an acute coronary event such as an MI. For example, lowering LDL levels by 25%, which is possible through lifestyle changes and medications, can reduce the risk of heart attack by 25%. Changes in HDL are claimed to be even more protective; each 1% increase in HDL may decrease the risk of MI by as much as 2%.

Based on this research, optimal levels of LDL cholesterol have been lowered from 130 mg/dL to 100 mg/dL. HDL cholesterol is now at least 40 mg/dL compared to 35 mg/dL in the past. In addition, the NCEP guidelines recommend that high cholesterol levels be treated more aggressively in patients with diabetes because it is the most common systemic disease associated with dyslipidemia. These guidelines will likely lead to more widespread use of antihyperlipidemics, which are already the most widely prescribed drug class in the United States.

Blood lipid profiles are used to classify the different patterns of hyperlipidemias observed in clinical practice. These patterns are shown in Table 32.2. The specific type of dyslipidemia exhibited by patients is considered when planning therapy. For example, Type I requires dietary restrictions and does not respond well to pharmacotherapy. Whereas the remaining types respond to the statins, the hypertriglyceridemias may respond better to therapy with fibric acid agents.

MyNursingKit | Natural Methods for Lowering Blood Cholesterol

32.4 Lipid levels can often be controlled through therapeutic lifestyle changes.

Therapeutic lifestyle changes (TLCs) should always be included in any treatment plan for reducing blood lipid levels. Many patients with borderline high-risk laboratory values can control their dyslipidemia entirely through nonpharmacologic means. It is important to note that all the TLCs for reducing blood lipid levels also apply to cardiovascular disease in general. Because many patients who take lipid-lowering drugs have underlying cardiovascular disease, these lifestyle changes are particularly important.

Patients should be taught that all drugs used for hyperlipidemia have adverse effects and that maintaining normal lipid values without pharmacotherapy should be a therapeutic goal. Pharmacotherapy should only be initiated after attempts to lower lipid levels with TLCs fail. Following are the most important lipid-reduction lifestyle interventions:

- Monitor blood lipid levels regularly, as recommended by the health care provider.
- Maintain weight at an optimal level.
- Implement a medically supervised exercise plan.
- Reduce dietary saturated fats and cholesterol.
- Increase soluble fiber in the diet, as found in oat bran, apples, beans, grapefruit, and broccoli.
- Eliminate tobacco use.

The single most important lifestyle factor contributing to dyslipidemia is a high amount of saturated fat in the diet. Nutritionists recommend that the intake of dietary fat be limited to less than 30% of the total caloric intake. Cholesterol intake should be reduced as much as possible and not exceed 200 mg/day. It is interesting to note that restriction of dietary cholesterol alone will not result in a significant reduction in blood cholesterol levels. In fact, cutting back on cholesterol consumption may actually increase the amount of circulating cholesterol. How is this possible? The liver reacts to a low cholesterol diet by making more cholesterol and by inhibiting its excretion whenever saturated fats are present. Saturated fats are the building blocks that the liver uses for making cholesterol. Patients must therefore reduce saturated fat in their diet to less than 7% of total calories, in addition to reducing cholesterol consumption, in order to control the amount made by the liver and to ultimately lower blood cholesterol levels.

The NCEP recommends a dietary intake of plant sterols as a means to reduce blood cholesterol levels. Plant sterols, also called phytosterols or stanols, are lipids used by plants to con-

TABLE 32.2 Types of Dyslipidemias

Name	Laboratory Findings	Features
Type I Exogenous hyperlipidemia	Triglycerides increased three times Chylomicrons increased Cholesterol normal	Rare condition, usually occurring in childhood
Type IIa Familial hypercholesterolemia	LDL and cholesterol increased Triglycerides and VLDL normal	Common condition, may occur at any age
Type IIb Combined familial hyperlipidemia Carbohydrate-induced hypertriglyceridemia	LDL, VLDL, cholesterol, and triglycerides increased	May occur at any age but more commonly in adults
Type III Dysbetalipoproteinemia	Chylomicrons, VLDL, cholesterol, and triglycerides increased	Uncommon condition, occurs in middle-aged adults
Type IV Endogenous hyperlipidemia Carbohydrate-induced hypertriglyceridemia	VLDL and triglycerides increased Cholesterol normal or elevated Glucose intolerance Hyperuricemia	Most common dyslipidemia, occurs in middle-aged adults; associated with obesity, excessive alcohol intake, tobacco use, and other lifestyle factors
Type V Mixed hyperlipidemia Carbohydrate and fat-induced hypertriglyceridemia	LDL, VLDL, cholesterol, and chylomicrons increased Triglycerides increased three times Glucose intolerance Hyperuricemia	Uncommon type, may begin in childhood and manifest in adults

CONNECTIONS

To the Community Teaching Patients About Dietary Measures to Lower Cholesterol

Nurses can be instrumental in providing patients and families with information regarding mechanisms to reduce cholesterol. Because hyperlipidemia is an epidemic in the United States, nurses have multiple venues to present these health facts to promote a healthier community.

Oat Products for Soluble Fiber

Soluble dietary fiber can be effective in lowering the bad LDL without lowering the good HDL. The U.S. Food and Drug Administration (FDA) authorized a public claim that beta-glucan soluble fiber, which can be found in oat products, can reduce the risk of heart disease. Some common dietary options for lowering LDL include whole oat flour, oat bran, and rolled oats or oatmeal. A dietary intake of 5 to 10 grams of soluble fiber per day can decrease LDL cholesterol by a minimum of 5% to 23%, depending on the research study. Choices for dietary intake of soluble fiber include oatmeal, apples, kidney beans, pears, barley, and psyllium laxatives.

Fish for Omega-3 Fatty Acids

Fish provides a good source of omega-3 fatty acids, which can lower LDL cholesterol and triglycerides, and raise HDL cholesterol,. The American Heart Association (AHA) recommends a minimum of two servings of fish per week to add omega-3 fatty acids to the diet. Choices include mackerel, herring, trout, sardines, and salmon. The AHA also recommends 2 to 4 grams of the dietary supplements eicosapentaenoic acid (EPA) and docosahexaenoic acid (DHA), which are types of omega-3 oils and which should be taken under the supervision of a health care provider.

Nuts for Healthy Fats

Nuts provide many dietary nutrients, including fiber and the antioxidants vitamin E and selenium. Nuts contain high plant sterols and fat, which are mostly monounsaturated and polyunsaturated fats, and which have been shown to lower LDL (bad) cholesterol. The FDA recognized the claim for the benefits of nuts in their role in heart disease prevention. Almonds, hazelnuts, peanuts, pecans, pine nuts, pistachios, and walnuts are known for their heath advantages. However, nuts are high in calories so intake should be limited to 1.5 ounces per day. Replacing meat and meat products with nuts can decrease high triglyceride levels.

Soy

Soy products can be a healthy substitute for animal products. In the past, the FDA recognized the health benefits of soy in heart disease by approving a soy health claim. However, a large research study no longer recommends eating soy to lower cholesterol because it decreases LDL levels by only 3%.

Foods with Plant Sterols

Plant sterols or stanols naturally occur in plants and can block cholesterol absorption. Research demonstrates that a person can experience a decrease in LDL cholesterol by 10% to 15% by consuming two servings of sterols-fortified foods per day. Plant sterols are not appropriate for everyone but are recommended for persons with high LDL cholesterol. People diagnosed with high cholesterol should eat 2 grams of plant sterols or stanols per day. Choices include salad dressings, orange juice, and margarine.

struct their cell membranes. The structure of plant sterols is very similar to that of cholesterol. When ingested, the plant sterols compete with cholesterol for absorption in the digestive tract. When the body absorbs the plant sterols, cholesterol is excreted from the body, less cholesterol is delivered to the liver, and serum LDL (the "bad" cholesterol) levels fall. Rich sources of plant sterols include wheat, corn, rye, oats, and rice, as well as nuts and olive oil. Commercially they are available in products fortified with Reducol, which is found in margarines, salad dressings, certain cereals, and some fruit juices.

To be of benefit in reducing high serum cholesterol, nutritionists recommend a daily intake of plant sterols of 2 to 3 grams. Cholesterol levels can be reduced by 10% to 15% after just a couple of months of sufficient plant sterol intake.

Drugs for Dyslipidemias

32.5 The statins are the most effective drugs for reducing blood lipid levels.

In the late 1970s substances were isolated from various species of fungi that were found to inhibit cholesterol production in human cells in the laboratory. This class of drugs, known as the statins, has revolutionized the treatment of lipid disorders. Statins can produce a dramatic 20% to 40% reduction in LDL cholesterol levels. In addition to dropping the LDL cholesterol level in the blood, statins can lower triglyceride and VLDL levels and raise the level of "good" HDL cholesterol. These effects have been shown to reduce the incidence of serious cardiovascular-related events by 25% to 30%.

Cholesterol is manufactured in the liver by a series of more than 25 metabolic steps, beginning with acetyl CoA, a two-carbon unit that is produced from the breakdown of fatty acids (Figure 34.3). Of the many enzymes involved in this complex pathway, **HMG-CoA reductase** (3-hydroxy-3-methylglutaryl coenzyme A reductase) serves as the primary regulatory enzyme for cholesterol biosynthesis. Under normal conditions, this enzyme is controlled through negative feedback. High levels of LDL cholesterol in the blood will shut down production of HMG-CoA reductase, thus turning off the cholesterol synthesis pathway. Pharmacotherapy Illustrated 32.1 shows some of the steps in the biosynthesis of cholesterol and the importance of HMG-CoA reductase.

The statins act by inhibiting HMG-CoA reductase, resulting in less cholesterol biosynthesis. As the liver makes less cholesterol, it responds by making more LDL receptors on the surface of liver cells. The greater number of LDL receptors on liver cells removes additional LDL from the blood. Blood levels of both

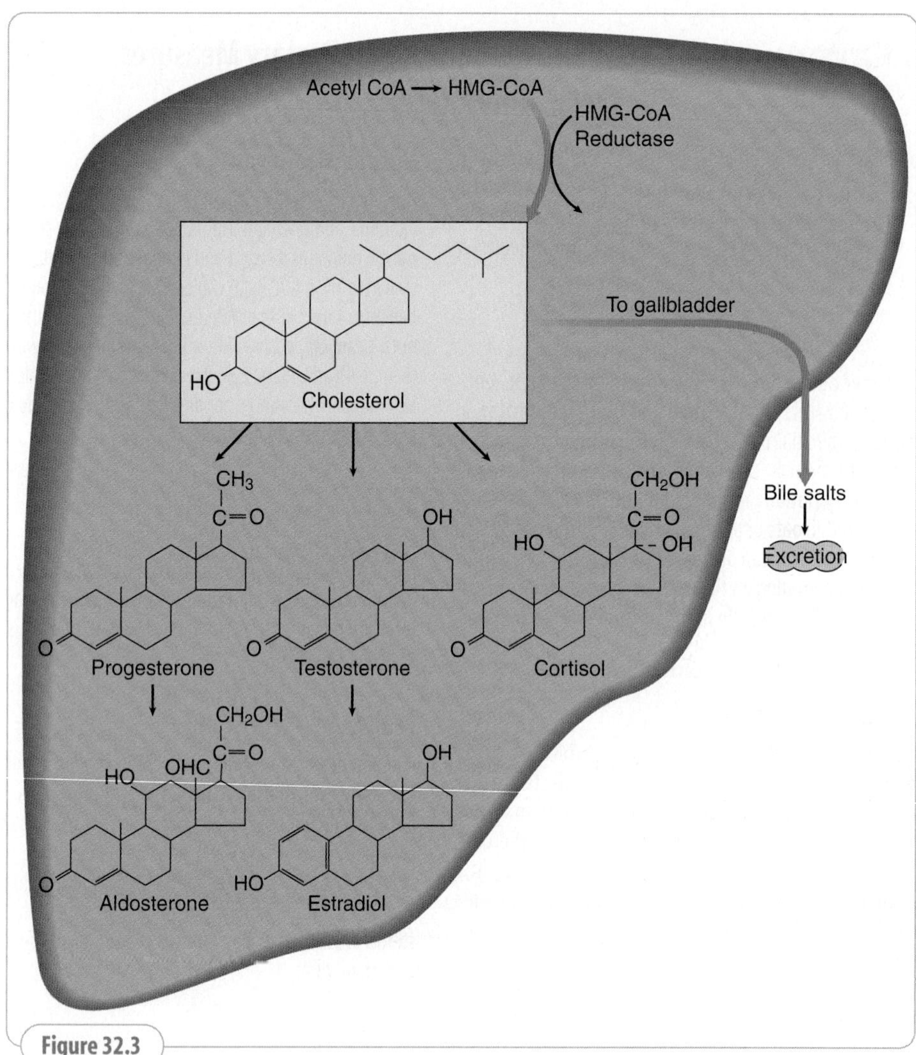

Figure 32.3

Cholesterol biosynthesis and excretion.

LDL and cholesterol are reduced. The drop in lipid levels is not permanent, however, so patients must continue these drugs for the remainder of their lives or until their hyperlipidemia can be controlled through dietary or lifestyle changes. Statins have been shown to slow the progression of CAD and to reduce mortality from cardiovascular disease. Currently, six statins are available for treating various types of dyslipidemias and these are listed in Table 32.3.

Although differences among the statins exist, their actions and adverse effects are similar. Lovastatin, pravastatin, and simvastatin are natural agents derived from fungi and have a different chemical structure than the synthetic statins. There are also differences in potency among the drugs. For example, the maximum daily dose for rosuvastatin is 40 mg, whereas the dose is 80 mg for atorvastatin. The half-lives of the statins vary from 20 hours (rosuvastatin) to less than an hour (fluvastatin). Whereas pravastatin is eliminated by the renal route, the other statins are metabolized by hepatic P450 enzymes. In patients with renal disease, dosage adjustment is required for lovastatin, pravastatin, simvastatin, and rosuvastatin but not for fluvastatin or atorvastatin. Despite these pharmacokinetic differences, in clinical practice the choice of statin is often guided by the experience of the prescriber and the response of each individual patient.

All the statins are given orally (PO) and are tolerated well by most patients. Adverse effects are rarely severe enough to cause discontinuation of therapy. Minor adverse effects include headache, abdominal cramping, diarrhea, muscle or joint pain, and heartburn.

Severe myopathy and rhabdomyolysis are rare, although they are serious adverse effects of the statins. **Rhabdomyolysis** is a breakdown of muscle fibers usually due to muscle trauma or ischemia. The mechanism by which statins cause this disorder is unknown. During rhabdomyolysis, contents of muscle cells spill into the systemic circulation, causing potentially fatal acute renal failure. Macrolide antibiotics such as erythromycin, azole antifungals, fibric acid agents, and certain immunosuppressants should be avoided during statin therapy, because these interfere with statin metabolism and increase the risk of severe myopathy. Levels of creatine kinase (CK), an enzyme released during muscle injury, should be obtained if myopathy is

PHARMACOTHERAPY ILLUSTRATED 32.1

Mechanisms of Action of Lipid-Lowering Drugs

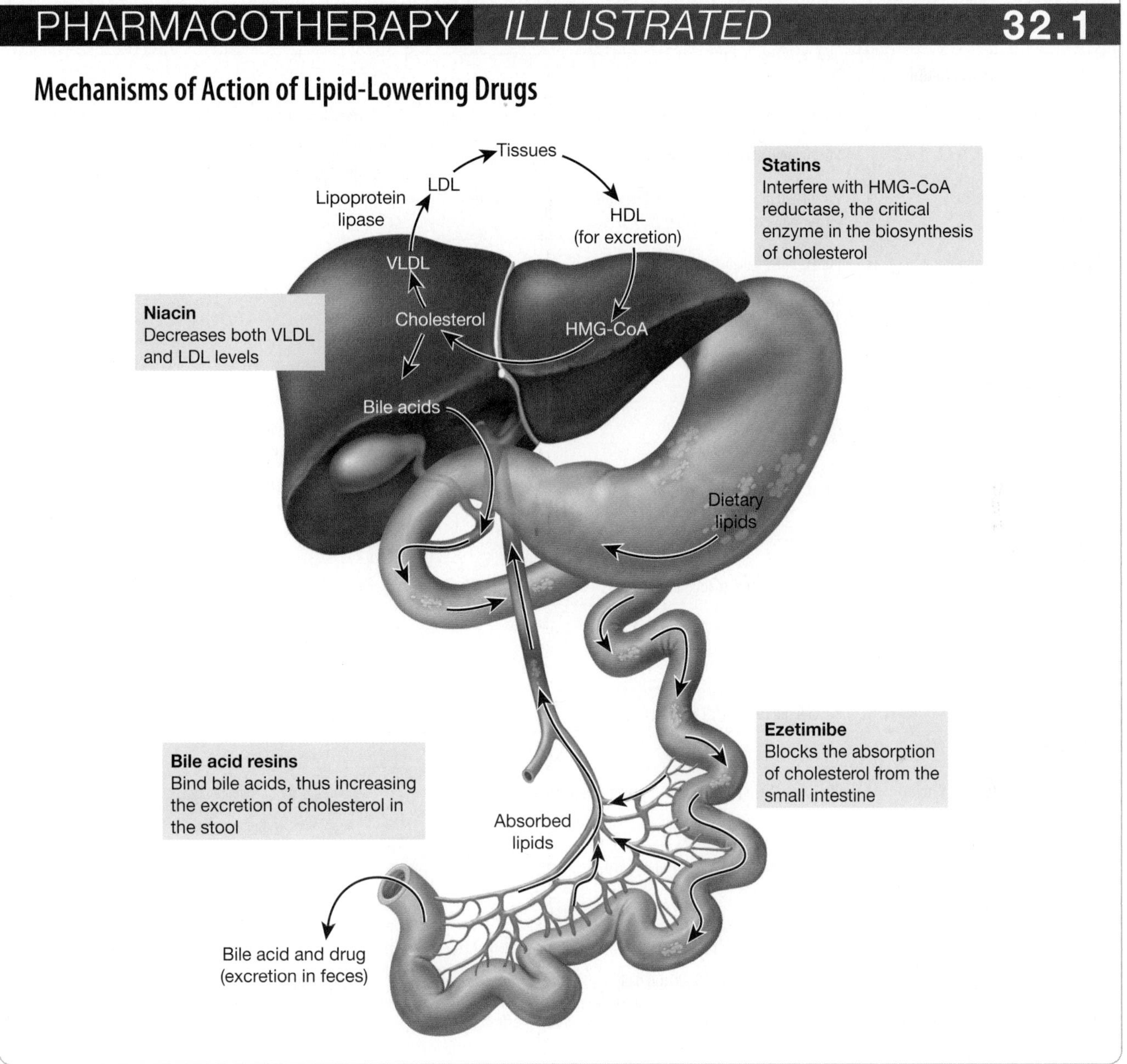

suspected. If CK levels become elevated during therapy, the drug should be immediately discontinued. Statins may be discontinued if muscle weakness persists even without CK elevation. Nurses should urge all patients who develop unexplained muscle or joint pain during statin therapy to immediately report this to the prescriber.

Statins are pregnancy category X drugs because teratogenic effects have been reported in laboratory animals exposed to these agents. Statins should not be used in patients who may become pregnant, are pregnant, or who are breast-feeding.

Because cholesterol biosynthesis in the liver is higher at night, statins with short half-lives such as lovastatin should be administered in the evening. The other statins have longer half-lives and are effective regardless of the time of day they are taken.

Much research is ongoing to determine the other therapeutic effects of the drugs in the statin class. For example, statins block the vasoconstrictive effect of the A-beta protein, a significant chemical associated with Alzheimer's disease. Cholesterol and A-beta protein had very similar effects on blood vessels, both causing vasoconstriction. Preliminary research suggests that the statins may protect against dementia by inhibiting this protein, thus slowing dementia caused by blood vessel constriction. Research also suggests that the statins may have the ability to lower the incidence of colorectal cancer. The mechanism of this effect is unknown. Several attempts have been made to move low doses of certain statins to over-the-counter (OTC) status; however, the FDA has not approved these applications.

TABLE 32.3 Drugs for Dyslipidemias

Drug	Route and Adult Dose (maximum dose where indicated)	Adverse Effects
HMG-CoA Reductase Inhibitors		
atorvastatin (Lipitor)	PO: 10–20 mg once daily (max: 80 mg/day)	*Headache, dyspepsia, abdominal cramping, myalgia, rash, or pruritus* <u>Rhabdomyolysis, severe myositis</u>
fluvastatin (Lescol)	PO: 20 mg daily (max: 80 mg/day)	
lovastatin (Mevacor)	PO: 10–20 mg once daily (max: 80 mg/day immediate release; 60 mg/day extended release)	
pravastatin (Pravachol)	PO: 10–40 mg daily (max: 80 mg/day)	
rosuvastatin (Crestor)	PO: 5–40 mg daily (max: 80 mg/day)	
simvastatin (Zocor)	PO: 5–40 mg daily (max: 80 mg/day)	
Bile Acid Sequestrants		
colesevelam (WelChol)	PO: 1.9 g bid (max: 4.4 g/day)	*Constipation, nausea, vomiting, abdominal pain, bloating, dyspepsia* <u>Gastrointestinal (GI) tract obstruction, vitamin deficiencies due to poor absorption</u>
colestipol (Colestid)	PO: 5–20 g/day in divided doses (30 g/day granules or 16 g/day tablets)	
Fibric Acid Agents		
clofibrate (Atromid-S)	PO: 2 g/day in two to four divided doses	*Abdominal pain, rash, myalgia, fatigue, flulike symptoms, dyspepsia, nausea, vomiting, asthenia* <u>Cholelithiasis, pancreatitis</u>
fenofibrate (TriCor)	PO: 54 mg daily (max: 160 mg/day)	
fenofibric acid (Triplix)	PO: 45–135 mg once daily	
gemfibrozil (Lopid)	PO: 600 mg bid (max: 1,500 mg/day)	
Other Agents		
ezetimibe; simvastatin (Vytorin)	PO: 10 mg/10 mg or 10 mg/20 mg every evening (max: 10 mg/80 mg)	*Arthralgia, fatigue, abdominal pain, diarrhea* <u>Anaphylaxis, rhabdomyolysis</u>
ezetimibe (Zetia)	PO: 10 mg daily (max: 10 mg/day)	*Arthralgia, fatigue, abdominal pain, diarrhea* <u>Anaphylaxis, rhabdomyolysis</u>
niacin (Niac, Nicobid, others)	Hyperlipidemia: PO: 1.5–3 g daily in divided doses (max: 6 g/day) Niacin deficiency: PO: 10–20 mg daily	*Flushing, nausea, pruritus, headache, bloating, diarrhea* <u>Dysrhythmias</u>

Note: *Italics* indicate common adverse effects. <u>Underline</u> indicates serious adverse effects.

PROTOTYPE DRUG Atorvastatin (Lipitor)

Classification: **Therapeutic:** Antihyperlipidemic
Pharmacologic: HMG-CoA reductase inhibitor, statin

Therapeutic Effects and Uses: Approved in 1996, atorvastatin was initially approved to treat hypercholesterolemia. Following several years of use it became evident that the drug also prevents cardiovascular events in high-risk patients. After 2 to 4 weeks of therapy, atorvastatin lowers LDL and VLDL cholesterol as well as triglycerides. It appears to lower LDL cholesterol levels greater than most other statins—as much as 60%. Atorvastatin may also be prescribed for the treatment of familial hypercholesterolemia. All patients receiving this drug should be placed on a cholesterol-lowering diet, because this will enhance the drug's therapeutic effects. The primary goal in atorvastatin therapy is to reduce the risk of MI and stroke.

To decrease gastrointestinal (GI) discomfort, atorvastatin may be administered with food. It produces the same degree of LDL cholesterol reduction regardless of the time of day it is taken. Because atorvastatin is not excreted by the kidneys, no adjustment in dosage is necessary in patients with renal impairment. Extensive metabolism to active metabolites gives atorvastatin a long duration of action.

Mechanism of Action: Atorvastatin acts by inhibiting HMG-CoA reductase, the primary regulatory enzyme in cholesterol biosynthesis. As the liver makes less cholesterol, it responds by making more LDL receptors, removing LDL cholesterol from the blood. Blood levels of both LDL and cholesterol are reduced.

Pharmacokinetics:

Route(s)	PO
Absorption	Rapidly absorbed but only 30% reaches the circulation; food reduces absorption
Distribution	Widely distributed; crosses the placenta and is secreted in breast milk; 98% bound to plasma proteins
Primary metabolism	Hepatic; extensively metabolized to active metabolites
Primary excretion	Biliary
Onset of action	2 weeks for lipid-lowering effect; peak plasma level: 1–2 h
Duration of action	Half-life: 14 h (20–30 h for active metabolites)

Adverse Effects: Most patients tolerate atorvastatin well and only 2% or less discontinue the drug due to adverse effects. Common adverse effects include headache, intestinal cramping, diarrhea, and constipation. The most serious adverse effect is rhabdomyolysis. Therapy is generally discontinued in patients reporting unexplained muscle pain, weakness, fever, or fatigue due to the potential for rhabdomyolysis.

Contraindications/Precautions: Patients with hepatic impairment should be monitored carefully, because the liver extensively metabolizes atorvastatin and the drug has been associated with a small risk of liver failure. Liver enzyme tests may become elevated during therapy, although this does not necessarily indicate liver damage. Because atorvastatin is pregnancy category X, pregnancy testing should be conducted prior to treatment in women of childbearing years, and these patients should be advised to take precautions to prevent pregnancy during therapy. Atorvastatin is contraindicated during lactation because the drug is secreted in breast milk.

Drug Interactions: Because atorvastatin is a substrate for hepatic CYP3A4, it has the potential to interact with many other drugs. For example, it may increase digoxin levels by 20% as well as increase levels of norethindrone and ethinyl estradiol (oral contraceptives). Erythromycin may increase atorvastatin levels as much as 40%. Risk of rhabdomyolysis increases with concurrent administration of atorvastatin with macrolide antibiotics, cyclosporine, and azole antifungals. The risk of myopathy increases when atorvastatin is administered concurrently with fibric acid agents or niacin. Atorvastatin may increase serum transaminase and CK levels. **Herbal/Food:** Grapefruit juice inhibits the metabolism of statins, allowing them to reach high serum levels. Because HMG-CoA reductase inhibitors decrease the synthesis of Coenzyme Q10, patients may benefit from CoQ10 supplements.

Pregnancy: Category X.

Treatment of Overdose: No specific therapy is available; patients are treated symptomatically.

Nursing Responsibilities:

- Obtain baseline laboratory lipid values, including total cholesterol, LDL, HDL, and triglycerides.
- Complete a thorough physical examination and history to identify individuals at high risk for CAD or who have conditions that cause drug therapy to be contraindicated such as liver disease or alcoholism.
- Monitor therapeutic effectiveness by evaluating LDL cholesterol levels.
- Assess lipid laboratory tests levels within 2 to 4 weeks of therapy initiation or after any change in dosage. Monitor liver function test levels at 6 and 12 weeks after initiation or elevation of dose and then periodically.
- Assess for muscle pain, tenderness, or weakness and monitor the CK level. If the CK level is high or myopathy is present, discontinue the medication and immediately notify the prescriber.
- Observe for digoxin (Lanoxin) toxicity when using this drug.

Patient and Family Education:

- Take this medication in the evening time with food or before going to bed because cholesterol biosynthesis in the liver is higher at night.
- The most common adverse effects are gas, constipation, stomach pain, and heartburn, which tend to decrease over time.
- Immediately report the following symptoms to the health care provider: unexplained muscle pain, weakness, or tenderness, especially with fever; yellowing of skin or eyes; stomach pain with nausea, loss of appetite, or vomiting; or skin rash or hives.
- Maintain a cholesterol-lowering diet during drug therapy.
- Avoid grapefruit and grapefruit juice because these may lead to an interaction with potentially dangerous effects.
- Consult with the health care provider when using statins with erythromycin, cyclosporine, antifungals, niacin, cholestyramine, or birth control pills.
- Immediately notify the health care provider of any known or suspected pregnancy because statins can cause birth defects. Discontinue use if confirmed pregnant.
- Do not breast-feed while taking statins, unless approved by the health care provider.
- Restrict or eliminate alcohol intake while taking statins.

MyNursingKit | Mechanism of Action Animation: Atorvastatin

Drugs Similar to Atorvastatin (Lipitor)

Other statins include fluvastatin, lovastatin, pravastatin, rosuvastatin, and simvastatin.

Fluvastatin (Lescol): Approved in 1993, fluvastatin is a synthetic statin that has the shortest half-life of all the drugs in this class. Because the kidneys excrete less than 5% of an oral (PO) dose, dosage adjustment for patients with renal impairment is not necessary. Fewer drug interactions are expected with fluvastatin because it is not metabolized through the hepatic P450 system. It is approved for hypercholesterolemia and several other types of dyslipidemia. In 2003, the indications were expanded to include prevention of major cardiac events such as cardiac death and nonfatal MI. An extended release formulation, called Lescol-XL, is available. The drug may be administered without regard to meals. Fluvastatin is well tolerated and its adverse effects are similar to those of atorvastatin. It is contraindicated in patients with severe hepatic impairment and in patients who are pregnant. Fluvastatin is a pregnancy category X drug.

Lovastatin (Mevacor): Approved in 1987, lovastatin, a natural substance derived from fungi, was the first HMG-Co reductase inhibitor marketed. Lovastatin is a prodrug with no intrinsic activity of its own, but the liver converts it to several active metabolites. This drug may achieve a 20% to 40% reduction in LDL cholesterol. Lovastatin is more effective if administered in the evening and should be taken on an empty stomach to maximize absorption. Although only 10% of this drug is excreted by the kidneys, dosage adjustment for patients with renal impairment is recommended. Lovastatin was originally approved for hypercholesterolemia; however, its indications have been expanded to include slowing the progression of coronary atherosclerosis and prevention of MI and cerebrovascular accident (CVA). An extended release form is available (Altoprev), as is a fixed-dose combination product with lovastatin and niacin (Advicor). Adverse effects are the same as those of other drugs in this class. It is contraindicated in patients with severe hepatic impairment and in patients who are pregnant. Lovastatin is a pregnancy category X drug.

Pravastatin (Pravachol): Like lovastatin, pravastatin is a natural substance derived from fungi. Twenty percent of the drug is excreted by the kidneys, and dosage adjustment for patients with renal impairment is recommended. Like fluvastatin, it is not metabolized through the hepatic P450 system; thus fewer drug interactions are expected. The drug may be taken without regard to meals and is slightly more effective if administered in the evening. Approved in 1991, pravastatin is approved for primary hypercholesterolemia, slowing the progression of coronary atherosclerosis and the prevention of MI and CVA. Unlabeled uses include other types of dyslipidemias. Pravigard PAC is a copackage that contains separate aspirin and pravastatin tablets in various dosage strengths. Adverse effects are the same as those of other drugs in this class. It is contraindicated in patients with hepatic impairment and in those who are pregnant. Pravastatin is a pregnancy category X drug.

Rosuvastatin (Crestor): Approved in 2003, rosuvastatin is a "second-generation" statin that contains a sulfur group. This drug is the most potent, has the longest half-life in its class (20 hours), and is capable of lowering LDL cholesterol by as much as 65%. Rosuvastatin is not a prodrug and it undergoes minimal hepatic metabolism. This drug may be administered with or without food and without regard to time of day. It is approved for hypercholesterolemia, hypertriglyceridemia, and for slowing the progression of coronary atherosclerosis. Adverse effects are the same as those of other drugs in this class. Rosuvastatin is a pregnancy category X drug.

Simvastatin (Zocor): Approved in 1991, simvastatin is a natural substance derived from fungi. Like lovastatin, simvastatin is an inactive prodrug that is changed to active metabolites by the liver. The drug can lower LDL cholesterol levels by as much as 47%. Although the kidneys excrete only 13% of the drug, dosage adjustment for patients with significant renal impairment is recommended. The drug may be taken with or without food but should be administered in the evening for maximum effectiveness. It is approved for hypercholesterolemia, hypertriglyceridemia, slowing the progression of coronary atherosclerosis, and prevention of MI and CVA. Adverse effects are the same as those of other drugs in this class. Simvastatin is contraindicated in patients with hepatic impairment and in those who are pregnant. This is a pregnancy category X drug.

CONNECTION *Checkpoint* 32.1

Several of the statins are prodrugs. From what you learned in Chapter 4, what type of dosage adjustment should be made if these statin prodrugs are prescribed for a patient with hepatic cirrhosis? If a dosage adjustment is not made, what types of adverse effects might you observe? See Answer to Connection Checkpoint 32.1 in Appendix A.

PharmFACT

About 10% of adolescents aged 12 through 19 are estimated to have total blood cholesterol levels of 200 mg/dL or above. Female adolescents have significantly higher "bad" cholesterol levels than do boys of the same age. *Source:* American Heart Association, n.d.

32.6 Bile acid sequestrants are often combined with statins to reduce LDL cholesterol levels.

Bile acids contain a high concentration of cholesterol and are secreted by the liver to emulsify fats in the small intestine. After performing their digestive function, bile acids are reabsorbed in the ileum and sent back to the liver to again become part of bile. This mechanism is known as enterohepatic circulation. In effect, the cholesterol in bile acids is recycled, with only small amounts leaving the body in the feces.

Prior to the discovery of the statins, the primary means of lowering blood cholesterol was through the use of bile acid sequestrants or resins. The bile acid sequestrants bind to bile acids, forming a large complex that cannot be reabsorbed from the small intestine. The enterohepatic circulation of cholesterol is interrupted and the bound bile acids and cholesterol are eliminated in the feces. The liver responds to the loss of cholesterol by making more LDL receptors, which removes LDL cholesterol from the blood in a mechanism similar to that of the statins.

CONNECTIONS

Complementary and Alternative Therapies Coenzyme Q10

Description: Coenzyme Q10 (CoQ10) is a lipid-soluble vitamin-like substance found in most animal cells. It is an essential component in the cell's mitochondria for producing adenosine triphosphate (ATP) energy. Because the heart requires high levels of ATP, a sufficient level of CoQ10 is especially important to that organ.

History and Claims: The applications of CoQ10 to treating disease are relatively recent, with the agent being claimed to be an antioxidant and having benefited patients with heart failure in the mid-1960s. Subsequent reports have claimed that CoQ10 may be beneficial in angina pectoris, dysrhythmias, periodontal disease, immune disorders, neurologic disease, obesity, diabetes mellitus, and cancers.

Standardization: The dose of CoQ10 varies widely. Typical doses range from 100 to 200 mg/day.

Evidence: As with most dietary supplements, controlled research studies with CoQ10 are often lacking and give conflicting results. Supplementation with CoQ10 may be important to patients taking the HMG-CoA reductase inhibitors (statins) because these drugs significantly lower blood levels of CoQ10 (Rundek, Naini, Sacco, Coates, & DiMauro, 2004). Coenzyme Q10 and cholesterol share the same metabolic pathways. Inhibition of the enzyme HMG-CoA reductase concurrently decreases CoQ10 levels. Many of the adverse effects of statins, including muscle weakness and rhabdomyolysis, are due to the decrease in CoQ10 levels; supplementation with CoQ10 may improve myopathy symptoms (O'Riordan, 2005).

Foods richest in this substance are pork, sardines, beef heart, salmon, broccoli, spinach, and nuts. Elderly people appear to have an increased need for CoQ10. Although CoQ10 can be synthesized by the body, many amino acids and other substances are required for this synthesis; thus patients having nutritional deficiencies may need supplementation.

The bile acid resins are capable of producing a 20% drop in LDL cholesterol, which is generally less response than can be obtained from the statins. They are no longer considered first-line drugs for dyslipidemia, although they are sometimes combined with statins for patients who are unable to achieve sufficient response from the statins alone.

The bile acid sequestrants tend to cause more frequent adverse effects than statins. Because they are not absorbed into the systemic circulation, adverse effects are limited to the GI tract, causing symptoms such as abdominal pain, bloating, diarrhea, steatorrhea, and constipation. In addition to binding bile acids, these agents can bind drugs such as digoxin and warfarin and increase the potential for drug–drug interactions. Bile acid sequestrants also interfere with the absorption of vitamins and minerals, and nutritional deficiencies may occur with extended use. Other medications and vitamins should be taken at least 1 hour before or 4 hours after taking a bile acid sequestrant to avoid drug interactions.

Bile acid sequestrants may cause a transient increase in triglyceride levels. This effect is particularly prominent and often sustained in patients with preexisting hypertriglyceridemia. Because of this, the bile acid sequestrants are generally not prescribed for patients with elevated triglycerides.

PROTOTYPE DRUG Cholestyramine (Questran)

Classification: **Therapeutic:** Antihyperlipidemic
Pharmacologic: Bile acid sequestrant

Therapeutic Effects and Uses: Approved in 1966, cholestyramine is used to treat hypercholesterolemia, especially elevated LDL cholesterol. It is available as a powder that is mixed with fluid before being taken once or twice daily. The drug should be mixed with 60 to 180 mL water, noncarbonated beverages, highly liquid soups, or pulpy fruits (applesauce, crushed pineapple) to prevent esophageal irritation. The patient should swallow the medication immediately after stirring. If taken with too small a fluid volume or if not completely swallowed, the drug can swell in the throat or esophagus to cause an obstruction.

It may take 30 days or longer for cholestyramine to produce its maximum effect. To avoid interference with absorption, cholestyramine should not be taken at the same time as vitamins or other medications. An off-label indication for cholestyramine is diarrhea caused by *Clostridium difficile*, although antibiotics are the drugs of first choice.

MyNursingKit | Psyllium: A Natural Bile Acid Binder

Mechanism of Action: Cholestyramine binds to bile acids, forming an insoluble complex containing cholesterol that is excreted in the feces. Cholestyramine lowers LDL cholesterol levels by increasing LDL receptors on hepatocytes.

Pharmacokinetics:

Route(s)	PO
Absorption	Not absorbed
Distribution	Not distributed; drug acts locally in the alimentary canal
Primary metabolism	Not metabolized
Primary excretion	Feces
Onset of action	1–2 days
Duration of action	2–4 weeks

Adverse Effects: Cholestyramine is not absorbed or metabolized once it enters the intestine; thus it does not produce systemic adverse effects. Common GI-related adverse effects include constipation, bloating, belching, and nausea. Serious adverse effects include obstruction of the GI tract, hyperchloremic acidosis, and malabsorption syndrome.

Contraindications/Precautions: Cholestyramine should be used cautiously in patients with GI disorders such as peptic ulcer disease, hemorrhoids, inflammatory bowel diseases or chronic constipation, as bile acid sequestrants may worsen or aggravate these conditions. This drug should not be used in patients with complete biliary obstruction. Bile acid resins should be used with caution in patients with hypertriglyceridemia because they may increase serum triglyceride concentrations. They are absolutely contraindicated if serum triglycerides rise above 400 mg/dL. Although cholestyramine use is safe during pregnancy because it is not absorbed, precautions must be taken to ensure that this drug is not interfering with vitamin absorption, especially folic acid.

Drug Interactions: Cholestyramine can bind to other drugs and interfere with their absorption, causing reduced effects. This interaction has been reported for digoxin, penicillins, iron supplements, thyroid hormone, and thiazide diuretics, although it has the potential to occur with any drug administered by the oral route. Cholestyramine may indirectly increase the effects of warfarin by binding to vitamin K, decreasing its absorption and lowering the levels of vitamin K in the body. The absorption of raloxifene can be reduced as much as 60% if coadministered with cholestyramine. To reduce the possibility of absorption interference, cholestyramine should be administered 4 hours before or 2 hours after other oral medications. **Herbal/Food:** Cholestyramine may block the absorption of iron and fat-soluble vitamins in food.

Pregnancy: Category B.

Treatment of Overdose: No specific therapy is available; patients are treated symptomatically.

Nursing Responsibilities:

- Obtain baseline laboratory values, including total cholesterol, LDL, HDL, and triglyercides.
- Completely dissolve cholestyramine powder before administration because it is irritating to mucous membranes and may cause esophageal impaction if administered dry.
- Monitor for therapeutic effectiveness by determining if serum cholesterol levels have been reduced within 24 to 48 hours after treatment begins. After withdrawal of the medication, cholesterol levels usually return to the previous baseline level in 2 to 4 weeks.
- Assess for early signs of hypoprothrombinemia such as ecchymoses, petechiae, tarry stools, or abnormal bleeding from mucous membranes. Report these immediately to the prescriber. Long-term use of this medication may increase bleeding tendency.
- Monitor laboratory tests for periodic complete blood count (CBC), platelet count, serum electrolytes, and lipid profile.
- Consult the prescriber to determine if supplemental vitamins A and D and folic acid are required for patients on long-term therapy.

Patient and Family Education:

- Mix powdered drug or granules thoroughly in liquid such as water or fruit juice.
- Take other medications 1 hour before or 4 hours after administration of bile sequestrants.
- Report symptoms such as severe gastric distress with nausea or vomiting, unexplained weight loss, black stools, severe hemorrhoids, unusual bleeding, or sudden back pain to the health care provider.
- Do not omit doses because sudden cessation can promote the absorption of other drugs, possibly leading to toxicity or overdose.
- Consult with the health care provider about taking vitamin supplements because this drug can reduce the absorption of vitamins.
- Increase intake of oral fluids and maintain a high-fiber diet to prevent constipation. Report constipation to the health care provider. GI symptoms usually subside after the first month of therapy.

Drugs Similar to Cholestyramine (Questran)

Other bile acid sequestrants include colesevelam and colestipol.

Colesevelam (WelChol): The newest of the bile acid-binding agents, colesevelam, is claimed to have more bile acid-binding capacity than the older resins. The drug has the capacity to reduce LDL cholesterol by as much as 20%. It may be administered concurrently with statins to achieve greater efficacy. Approved in 2000, it is formulated in smaller tablets, which are easier to swallow, and fewer tablets per day are required as compared to other drugs in this class. At least 2 weeks of therapy may be necessary before maximum therapeutic response is achieved. In 2008, colesevelam was approved as an adjunct to diet, exercise, and antidiabetic drugs to improve glycemic control in patients with type 2 diabetes. Colesevelam can interfere with the absorption of other oral medications although considerably less so than cholestyramine. Like cholestyramine, colesevelam can increase serum triglyceride levels and is contraindicated in patients with triglyceride levels greater than 500 mg/dL. This drug is pregnancy category B.

Colestipol (Colestid): Approved in 1977, colestipol acts by the same mechanism as cholestyramine, has the same effectiveness in lowering LDL cholesterol, and exhibits the same adverse effects. Other drugs should be administered at least 1 hour before or 4 to 6 hours after a dose of colestipol to prevent interference with absorption. Maximum therapeutic effects may take as long as a month to appear. Because the drug can increase serum triglycerides, it should not be administered to patients with hypertriglyceridemia. Colestipol is rarely used as monotherapy. In addition to its use in treating elevated HDL cholesterol, colestipol may be used off-label to treat digoxin overdose, diarrhea, and pruritus associated with biliary obstruction. This drug is pregnancy category B.

PharmFACT

Familial hypercholesterolemia affects 1 in 500 people and is a genetic disease that predisposes people to premature CAD. *Source:* Citkowitz, 2007.

32.7 Nicotinic acid can reduce triglycerides and LDL cholesterol levels, but adverse effects limit its usefulness.

Nicotinic acid, or niacin, is a B-complex vitamin (B_3). Its ability to lower lipid levels, however, is unrelated to its role as a vitamin because much higher doses are needed to produce its antihyperlipidemic effects. For lowering cholesterol, the usual dose is 2 to 3 g per day. When taken as a vitamin, the dose is only 25 mg per day.

The primary action of nicotinic acid is to decrease the production of VLDL, which lowers serum triglyceride levels. Because LDL is synthesized from VLDL, the patient also experiences a reduction in LDL cholesterol levels. In addition, it has the desirable effect of increasing HDL levels. As with other lipid-lowering drugs, maximum therapeutic effects may take a month or longer to achieve.

Although effective at reducing LDL cholesterol by 20%, nicotinic acid produces more adverse effects than the statins. Intense flushing and hot flashes occur in almost every patient. Taking one aspirin tablet 30 minutes prior to niacin administration can reduce uncomfortable flushing in many patients. In addition, a variety of uncomfortable GI effects such as nausea, excess gas, and diarrhea are commonly reported.

More serious adverse effects such as hepatotoxicity and gout are possible but uncommon. Patients with elevated liver enzymes or a history of liver disease should use an alternate drug to lower lipids. In patients predisposed to gout, nicotinic acid may increase uric acid levels and precipitate acute gout.

Niacin is not usually prescribed for patients with diabetes mellitus because the drug can raise fasting glucose levels. When beginning therapy, patients with diabetes should monitor their blood glucose levels more frequently until the effect of nicotinic acid is determined.

Because of the high incidence of adverse effects, nicotinic acid is most often used in lower doses in combination with a statin or bile acid sequestrant; the beneficial effects of these drugs are additive. Combining nicotinic acid with lovastatin can reduce LDL cholesterol by as much as 45%. The two drugs are combined in a fixed-dose formulation marketed as Advicor. In 2008 the United States Food and Drug Administration (FDA) approved Simcor, a combination of nicotine acid and simvastatin to lower LDL levels.

Because supplemental niacin is available without a prescription, patients should be instructed not to attempt self-medication with this drug. One form of niacin that is available OTC as a vitamin supplement, called nicotinamide, has no lipid-lowering effects. If nicotinic acid is to be used to lower cholesterol, it should be done under medical supervision.

32.8 Fibric acid agents lower triglyceride levels but have little effect on LDL cholesterol.

The first fibric acid agent, clofibrate (Atromid-S), was widely prescribed until a 1978 study determined that it did not reduce mortality from cardiovascular disease. In fact, clofibrate was found to increase overall mortality, compared to a control group. Although this drug is no longer marketed in the United States, two other fibric acid agents, fenofibrate (Tricor) and gemfibrozil (Lopid), are sometimes indicated for patients with excessive triglyceride (VLDL) levels. They are the drugs of choice for treating severe hypertriglyceridemia (Types IV and V hyperlipidemia), although they have little effect on LDL cholesterol. Combining a fibric acid agent with a statin results in greater decreases in triglyceride levels than either drug used alone. The mechanism of action of the fibric acid agents is largely unknown. Doses for the fibric acid agents are listed in Table 32.3.

The most common adverse effects of the fibrates are abdominal pain, nausea, and vomiting. Taking these medications with meals usually diminishes GI distress. Clofibrate has a tendency to concentrate bile and cause gallbladder disease. This increase in gallbladder disease has not been seen with other fibric acid agents, but drugs in this class are generally not used in patients with preexisting gallbladder or biliary disease.

PROTOTYPE DRUG Gemfibrozil (Lopid)

Classification: Therapeutic: Antihyperlipidemic
Pharmacologic: Fibric acid agent (fibrate)

Therapeutic Effects and Uses: Approved in 1981, gemfibrozil lowers serum triglycerides and LDL cholesterol. It is most effective in patients who present with hypertriglyceridemia and VLDL. Effects of gemfibrozil include up to a 50% reduction in VLDL with an increase in HDL. It is less effective than the statins at lowering LDL; thus it is not used as monotherapy. It is considered a second-line therapy that is used when statins are ineffective or not well tolerated.

Mechanism of Action: The exact mechanism of action of gemfibrozil is unknown. The drug inhibits the breakdown of stored fat, or lipolysis, in adipose tissue. By inhibiting the uptake of free fatty acids by the liver, hepatic production of triglycerides is decreased. The drug may also increase the excretion of cholesterol in the feces.

Pharmacokinetics:

Route(s)	PO
Absorption	Well absorbed
Distribution	Unknown; distribution across the placenta or secretion in breast milk is unknown; 99% bound to plasma protein
Primary metabolism	Hepatic; undergoes enterohepatic recirculation
Primary excretion	Primarily renal, 6% in feces
Onset of action	1–2 h
Duration of action	Half-life: 1.5 h

Adverse Effects: The most common adverse effects of gemfibrozil are GI related, such as abdominal cramping, diarrhea, nausea, and dyspepsia. Nervous system effects include headache, dizziness, peripheral neuropathy, and diminished libido. Serious adverse effects include cholelithiasis, anemia, and eosinophilia.

Contraindications/Precautions: Gemfibrozil may worsen or cause biliary disease; thus it is contraindicated in patients with preexisting gallbladder disease or serious liver impairment. Because it is excreted by the kidneys, the drug should be used cautiously in patients with renal impairment.

Drug Interactions: Although antihyperlipidemic agents from different drug classes are sometimes combined to produce an enhanced effect, the use of gemfibrozil with certain statins increases the risk of myositis and rhabdomyolysis. CK levels should be regularly monitored during combined therapy and the combination immediately discontinued if myopathy is suspected. In most cases the risk of rhabdomyolysis, which may be fatal, outweighs the potential benefits of combined statin and gemfibrozil therapy.

Concurrent use of gemfibrozil with oral anticoagulants may increase the risk of bleeding because the fibrate displaces warfarin from its plasma protein binding sites. If a patient is taking warfarin, dosages should be lowered. More frequent monitoring of prothrombin time (PT) and international normalized ratio (INR) is necessary until stabilization occurs.

Gemfibrozil may enhance the hypoglycemic effects of antidiabetic agents. Serum glucose levels must be carefully monitored because the dosage of the antidiabetic drug may require adjustment. **Herbal/Food:** No significant interactions.

Pregnancy: Category C.

Treatment of Overdose: No specific therapy is available; patients are treated symptomatically.

Nursing Responsibilities:

- Obtain baseline laboratory values, including total cholesterol, LDL, HDL, and triglycerides.
- Complete a thorough physical examination and history to identify individuals at high risk for CAD, liver disease, or gallbladder disease.
- Monitor laboratory tests for serum LDL and VLDL, triglycerides, total cholesterol, CBC, blood glucose, and liver function tests. Establish baseline values and reevaluate at regular intervals. Mild decreases in white blood cell count (WBC), hemoglobin, and hematocrit may occur early in treatment but stabilizes with continued therapy.
- Consult with the prescriber if the lipid response is inadequate after 3 months of therapy.
- Notify the prescriber if the patient demonstrates signs and symptoms that might indicate cholelithiasis or cholecystitis such as severe, steady upper abdominal pain or biliary colic, upper right-sided abdominal pain, nausea, vomiting, or flatulence. Confirm with gallbladder testing.

Patient and Family Education:

- Immediately report unexplained bleeding, such as easy bruising, nosebleeds, or blood in the urine; yellowing of the skin or eyes; or muscle pain to the health care provider.
- Consult with the health care provider when using this drug concurrently with anticoagulants (blood thinners) or statins, which may worsen muscle or kidney problems.
- Inform the health care provider if you have other medical problems such as gallbladder disease, gallstones, kidney disease, or liver disease.
- Do not drive or perform other hazardous activities until the effects of the drug are known because this drug may cause drowsiness or dizziness.
- Follow the low-cholesterol diet prescribed by the health care provider. Limit both carbohydrates and alcohol intake. Alcohol can increase serum triglyceride levels.
- If the patient has diabetes, monitor blood glucose levels frequently and report abnormal values.
- Do not breast-feed while taking this drug without approval of the health care provider.

Drugs Similar to Gemfibrozil (Lopid)

The only other fibrate currently available is fenofibrate.

Fenofibrate (Antara, TriCor, others): Like gemfibrozil, fenofibrate is most effective in treating patients presenting with very high serum triglycerides and VLDL. Approved in 1993, fenofibrate may reduce serum triglycerides by as much as 30%. The only advantage of the fenofibrate formulations over gemfibrozil is that they may be taken once daily rather than twice a day. Several fenofibrate formulations, which vary in strength, bioavailability, and whether the drug should be administered with a meal, are available. These forms are not interchangeable. The most frequent adverse effects are GI related, such as nausea, vomiting, dyspepsia, constipation, flatulence, and abdominal pain. Rash and photosensitivity are other adverse effects. This drug is pregnancy category C.

CONNECTION *Checkpoint* 32.2

From what you learned in Chapter 12, what changes in physiology occur with aging that may require decreased starting dosages for antihyperlipidemic agents? See Answer to Connection Checkpoint 32.2 in Appendix A.

Cholesterol Absorption Inhibitors

32.9 Cholesterol absorption inhibitors are the newest class of drugs for hyperlipidemia.

In the early 2000s, a new class of drugs was discovered that inhibits the absorption of cholesterol. Ezetimibe is the only drug in this class.

Cholesterol is absorbed from the intestinal lumen by cells in the jejunum of the small intestine. Ezetimibe blocks this absorption by as much as 50%, causing less cholesterol to enter the blood. Unfortunately the body responds to this lack of absorption by making more cholesterol; the drug has no effect on cholesterol synthesis in the liver. To prevent the liver from compensating and making additional cholesterol, a statin may be administered concurrently.

NURSING PROCESS APPLICATION

Patients Receiving Drugs for Hyperlipidemia

Assessment	Potential Nursing Diagnoses
Prior to administration: • Obtain a complete health history, including allergies, drug history, and possible drug interactions. • Obtain baseline liver function tests, lipid studies, and pregnancy tests in women of childbearing age.	• *Deficient Knowledge (Need for Altered Lifestyle)* • *Noncompliance (Dietary and Drug Regimen)* • *Chronic Pain,* related to drug-induced myopathy • *Ineffective Health Maintenance,* related to insufficient knowledge of actions and effects of prescribed drug therapy

Planning: Patient Goals and Expected Outcomes

Patient will:

- Immediately report skeletal muscle pain, unexplained muscle soreness, or weakness.
- Demonstrate adherence with appropriate lifestyle changes.
- Demonstrate understanding of the drug's action by accurately describing drug adverse effects and precautions.
- Exhibits a reduction in serum LDL and triglyceride levels.

Implementation

Interventions and (Rationales)	Patient and Family Education
• Monitor blood cholesterol and triglyceride levels at intervals during therapy. (This helps to determine the effectiveness of therapy.)	• Advise the patient about the importance of keeping appointments with the health care provider.
• Monitor patient adherence to the dietary regimen. (Maintenance of controlled saturated fat diet is essential to the effectiveness of medications.)	• Provide the patient with information needed to maintain a low-saturated fat, low-cholesterol diet.
• Monitor the patient for alcohol abuse. (Excessive alcohol intake may result in liver damage and interfere with drug effectiveness.)	• Instruct the patient to avoid or limit alcohol use.
• Monitor the creatine phosphokinase (CPK) level. (Elevated CPK may be indicative of an impending myopathy.)	• Instruct the patient to report symptoms of leg or muscle pain to the health care provider.
• Obtain the patient's smoking history. (Smoking increases the risk of cardiovascular disease and may decrease HDL levels.)	• Encourage smoking cessation if appropriate.

Evaluation of Outcome Criteria

Evaluate the effectiveness of drug therapy by confirming that patient goals and expected outcomes have been met (see "Planning").

When given as monotherapy, ezetimibe produces a modest reduction in LDL of about 20%. Adding a statin to the therapeutic regimen reduces LDL by an additional 15% to 20%. The drug produces a slight drop in serum triglycerides. Ezetimibe is available as a single tablet with a once-daily dosing regimen. Vytorin is a fixed-dose combination tablet containing ezetimibe and simvastatin.

Adverse effects from ezetimibe are uncommon. Abdominal pain, back pain, diarrhea, and arthralgia are the most common adverse effects, although these rarely require discontinuation of therapy. Because it is extensively metabolized in the liver, patients with significant hepatic impairment should receive other antihyperlipidemic agents. Ezetimibe is pregnancy category C.

Because bile acid sequestrants inhibit the absorption of ezetimibe, these drugs should not be taken together. In addition, ezetimibe and statins should not be given concurrently to patients with serious hepatic impairment or with elevated serum transaminase levels.

UNDERSTANDING THE CHAPTER

Key Concepts Summary

32.1 Lipids are classified as triglycerides, phospholipids, or sterols.

32.2 Lipoproteins are important predictors of cardiovascular disease.

32.3 Blood lipid profiles are important diagnostic tools in guiding the therapy of dyslipidemias.

32.4 Lipid levels can often be controlled through therapeutic lifestyle changes.

32.5 The statins are the most effective drugs for reducing blood lipid levels.

32.6 Bile acid sequestrants are often combined with statins to reduce LDL cholesterol levels.

32.7 Nicotinic acid can reduce triglycerides and LDL cholesterol levels, but adverse effects limit its usefulness.

32.8 Fibric acid agents lower triglyceride levels but have little effect on LDL cholesterol.

32.9 Cholesterol absorption inhibitors are the newest class of drugs for hyperlipidemia.

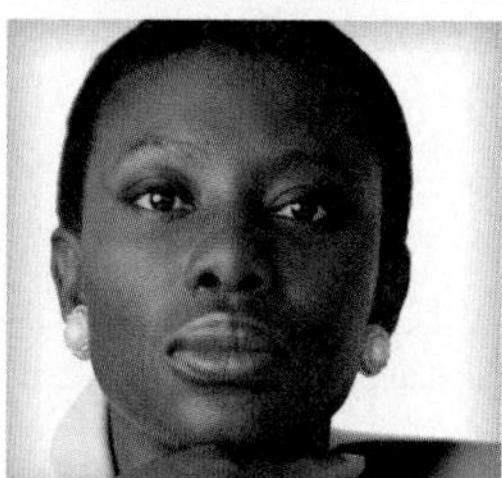

Making the PATIENT *Connection*

Remember the patient "Belinda Cummings" at the beginning of the chapter? Now read the remainder of the case study. Based on the information presented within this chapter, respond to the critical thinking questions that follow.

Belinda Cummings is a 39-year-old black female who feels fine. However, she recently had her cholesterol level checked at her church's health fair where she was told that it exceeded the normal value. As directed, she made an appointment and saw her health care provider for a checkup.

During the office visit, the nurse collects Belinda's social and health history. Belinda's vital signs are within normal limits, except her blood pressure is slightly elevated (142/90 mmHg). She is also slightly overweight and has been on a low-carbohydrate diet for 1 week. Her favorite foods are potato chips and all dairy products, especially cheese. She admits to smoking less than a pack of cigarettes per day and occasionally drinks beer. Belinda is divorced and has one teenage son.

A series of laboratory and diagnostic tests are completed during the visit. Belinda's physical exam is normal, and there are no ECG abnormalities. The blood tests are unremarkable with the exception of the lipid profile.

	Patient Value	Standard
Total Cholesterol	240 mg/dL	Less than 200
Triglycerides	199 mg/dL	Less than 150
HDL Cholesterol	30 mg/dL	Greater than 60
LDL Cholesterol	184	Less than 100
Cholesterol-to-HDL Ratio	6.6	Less than 4.5

The patient is placed on a standard cholesterol-lowering diet and prescribed atorvastatin (Lipitor) 10 mg daily. Belinda is instructed to return to the office in 1 month for a follow-up visit.

Critical Thinking Questions

1. How would you respond to Belinda when she asks you, "Is high cholesterol due to heredity or from what I eat?"
2. What health teaching should you provide the patient about ways to reduce high blood lipid levels?
3. Describe the mechanism of action associated with atorvastatin.
4. Create a list of potential adverse effects that this patient should be taught to watch for related to the medication.

Case Study

David Hamilton has been taking cholestyramine (Questran) for elevated blood lipid levels for 2 years. He presents today in your clinic for a routine follow-up visit that will include a lipid profile test. He states that he has been somewhat consistent with his cholesterol-lowering diet and attempting to get "a little more" exercise. You are the nurse caring for David.

1. Outline key concepts related to health promotion activities that you would want to be sure David understands.
2. What adverse effects related to Questran should David watch for?
3. How would you explain the laboratory values associated with a lipid profile to a patient such as David?

NCLEX-RN® Review

1 The client taking atorvastatin (Lipitor) reports decreased urine output, edema, and weight gain. The nurse initially assesses the client for which of the following conditions?

1. Rhabdomyolysis
2. Rhabdomyoma
3. Rhabdomyosarcoma
4. Rhinorrhea

2 A client is receiving cholestyramine (Questran) for elevated low-density lipoprotein levels. Which of the following adverse effects did the nurse include in the care plan to monitor the client?

1. Orange-colored urine
2. Abdominal pain
3. Sore throat and fever
4. Decreased capillary refill

3 The provider orders a bile acid sequestrant for a client with elevated low-density lipoprotein levels. The nurse collaborates with the prescriber about which of the following data related to the client?

1. Past history of peptic ulcer disease
2. Recent myocardial infarction
3. Laboratory value of serum sodium 136 mEq/L
4. Allergies to foods high in tyramine

4 Which of the following assessment findings discovered by the nurse would be an expected adverse effect associated with nicotinic acid therapy?

1. Fever and chills
2. Intense flushing and hot flashes
3. Tingling of the fingers and toes
4. Dry mucous membranes

5 The community health nurse visits a client who has been prescribed atorvastatin (Lipitor). Which of the following statements, if made by the client, indicates that further teaching is necessary concerning this drug therapy?

1. "I should try to maintain my body weight at an optimal level."
2. "Most clients with lipid disorders have chest pain or shortness of breath."
3. "The best time for me to take this medication is before I go to bed."
4. "I will avoid beverages that contain grapefruit juice."

6 The nurse is caring for a client receiving bile acid sequestrants for hyperlipidemia. Which of the following statements concerning this drug therapy are accurate? Bile acid sequestrants: (Select all that apply.)

1. Are absorbed into the circulation and cause fewer adverse effects than statins.
2. Cause adverse effects, including bloating, abdominal pain, diarrhea, and steatorrhea.
3. Bind drugs such as digoxin and warfarin, increasing the potential for toxic interactions.
4. Interfere with the absorption of vitamins and minerals, causing nutritional deficiencies.
5. Can be taken at the same time as other medications and vitamins.

See Answers to Critical Thinking Questions, Case Study, and NCLEX-RN® Review in Appendix A.

References

American Heart Association. (n.d.). *Youth and cardiovascular diseases—Statistics.* Retrieved July 3, 2008, from http://www.americanheart.org/downloadable/heart/1059110431975FS11YTH3REV7-03.pdf

Ballantyne, C. M., O'Keefe, J. H., Jr., & Gotto, A. M., Jr. (2005). *Dyslipidemia essentials.* Royal Oak, MI: Physician's Press.

Citkowitz, E. (2007). Hypercholesterolemia, familial. *emedicine.* Retrieved July 3, 2008, from http://www.emedicine.com/med/TOPIC1072.HTM

Florentin, M., Liberopoulos, E. N., Mikhailidis, D. P., & Elisaf, M. S. (2008). Fibrate-associated adverse effects beyond muscle and liver toxicity. *Current Pharmaceutical Design, 14*(6), 574–587.

Insull, W., Jr. (2006). Clinical utility of bile acid sequestrants in the treatment of dyslipidemia: A scientific review. *Southern Medical Journal, 99*(3), 257–273.

Isley, W. L. (2006). Hypercholesterolemia, polygenic. *emedicine.* Retrieved July 3, 2008, from http://www.emedicine.com/med/TOPIC1073.HTM

Law, M., & Rudnicka, A. (2006). Statin safety: A systematic review. *American Journal of Cardiology, 97*(8), S52–S60.

Mahley, R. W., & Bersot, T. P. (2006). Drug therapy for hypercholesterolemia and dyslipidemia. In L. L. Brunton, J. S. Lazo, & K. L. Parker (Eds.), *The pharmacological basis of therapeutics* (pp. 933–964). New York: McGraw-Hill.

Marcoff, L., & Thompson, P. (2007). The role of coenzyme Q10 in statin-associated myopathy: A systematic review. *Journal of the American College of Cardiology, 49*(23), 2231–2237.

McLoughlin, C. (2004). Statins. *Professional Nurse, 19*(11), 51–52.

Nichols, N. (2004). Clinical practice guidelines for the management of dyslipidemia. *Canadian Journal of Cardiovascular Nursing, 14*(2), 7–10.

O'Riordan, M. (2005). Coenzyme Q10 improves myopathic pain in statin-treated patients. *Medscape Medical News.* Retrieved July 3, 2008, from http://www.medscape.com/viewarticle/538168

Rundek, T., Naini, A., Sacco, R., Coates, K., & DiMauro, S. (2004). Atorvastatin decreases the coenzyme Q10 level in the blood of patients at risk for cardiovascular disease and stroke. *Archives of Neurolology, 61,* 889–892.

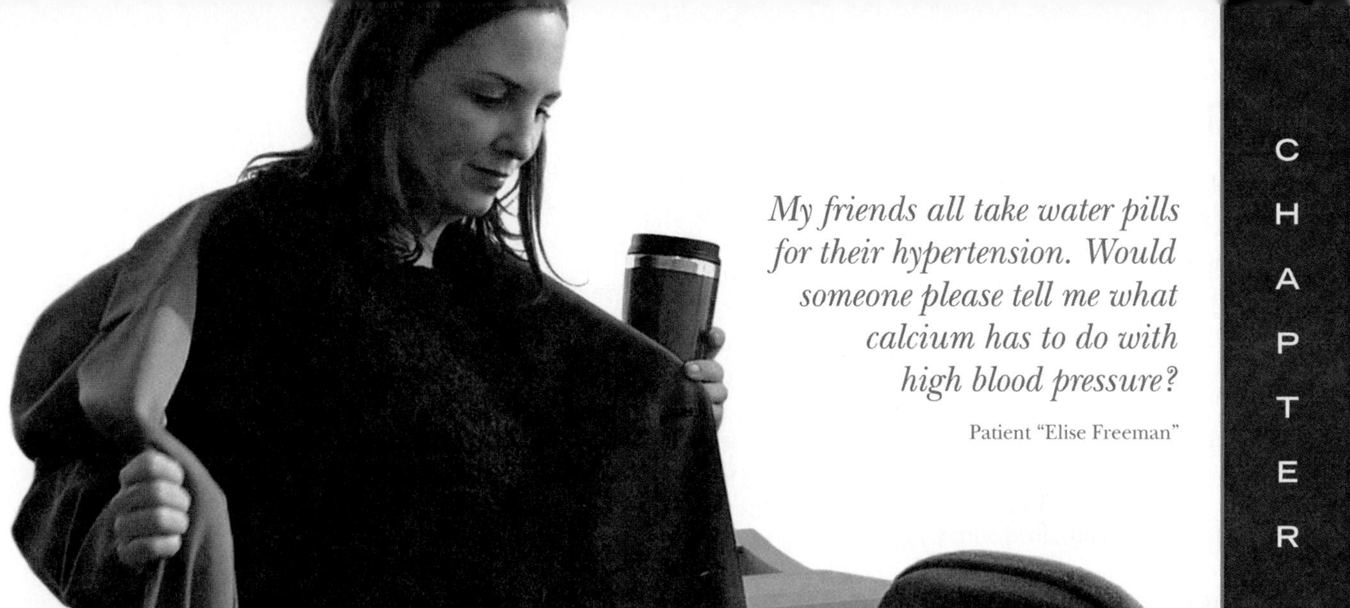

My friends all take water pills for their hypertension. Would someone please tell me what calcium has to do with high blood pressure?

Patient "Elise Freeman"

CHAPTER 33

Calcium Channel Blockers

Chapter Outline

Physiological Role of Calcium Channels in Muscle Contraction

Types of Calcium Channels

Consequences of Calcium Channel Blockade

Classification of Calcium Channel Blockers

Dihydropyridine

PROTOTYPE **Nifedipine (Adalat, Procardia XL)** *p. 520*

Nondihydropyridine

PROTOTYPE **Verapamil (Calan, Isoptin)** *p. 523*

Learning Outcomes

After reading this chapter, the student should be able to:

1. Describe the role of calcium ions in the contraction of smooth and cardiac muscle.
2. Explain why the actions of the $beta_1$-adrenergic antagonists are similar to those of the calcium channel blockers.
3. Describe how calcium channel blockers interact with the L-type calcium channel.
4. Identify the physiological effects of calcium channel blockers on arterial smooth muscle and cardiac muscle.
5. Explain the classification of calcium channel blockers.
6. Compare and contrast the action of dihydropyridine versus nondihydropyridine calcium channel blockers.
7. For each of the classes shown in the chapter outline, identify the prototype and representative drugs and explain the mechanism(s) of drug action, primary indications, contraindications, significant drug interactions, pregnancy category, and important adverse effects.
8. Apply the nursing process to care for patients receiving calcium channel blockers.

Key Terms

calcium channel, *516*
dihydropyridine, *518*
negative chronotropic effect, *518*
negative inotropic effect, *518*
sarcolemma, *516*
sarcoplasmic reticula, *516*

Since the approval of the first calcium channel blocker (CCB) almost 20 years ago, this class of drug has become one of the most widely prescribed in medicine. One reason for their widespread use is that these drugs treat two chronic diseases that affect millions of patients: hypertension (HTN) and coronary artery disease (CAD). Their success, however, is also due to their effectiveness combined with a highly favorable safety profile.

CCBs are also known as calcium channel antagonists. These drugs do not physically block calcium channels; therefore, *antagonist* is a more accurate term. Because both terms are used interchangeably in clinical practice, they are used as synonyms throughout this text.

Physiological Role of Calcium Channels in Muscle Contraction

33.1 Calcium channels facilitate contraction in cardiac and smooth muscles.

Recall from muscle physiology that the signal for contraction is an action potential traveling across the muscle membrane, or **sarcolemma.** The action potential causes a depolarization of the sarcolemma that opens voltage-gated channels in the membrane, allowing ions to enter and leave. In skeletal muscle, like nervous tissue, the primary ion channels facilitate Na^+ and K^+ movement. The importance of sodium and potassium channels in depolarizing neuronal cell membranes is discussed in Chapter 19. In cardiac muscle and smooth muscles a third type of voltage-gated channel, called the **calcium channel,** is of particular importance to physiology and the pharmacotherapy of cardiovascular disease.

Contraction of smooth and cardiac muscles requires the movement of calcium ions (Ca^{2+}). Under resting conditions, the concentration of free Ca^{2+} in the cytoplasm of a muscle cell is very low. Depolarization of the muscle cell membrane, however, changes the amount of free Ca^{2+} in two ways. First, calcium channels in the sarcolemma open, allowing calcium to rush into the cell. Secondly, depolarization releases large amounts of calcium ions stored inside the cell in structures called **sarcoplasmic reticula.** This huge increase in cytoplasmic Ca^{2+} removes the inhibition of actin and myosin filaments by the proteins calmodulin (smooth muscle) or troponin C (cardiac muscle) through a cascade of complex reactions. Actin and myosin are then free to slide, and muscle contraction occurs. This process is illustrated in Figure 33.1.

Muscle contraction is terminated when the amount of free cytoplasmic Ca^{2+} is reduced, by either pumping to the outside of the cell or by returning to the sarcoplasmic reticulum.

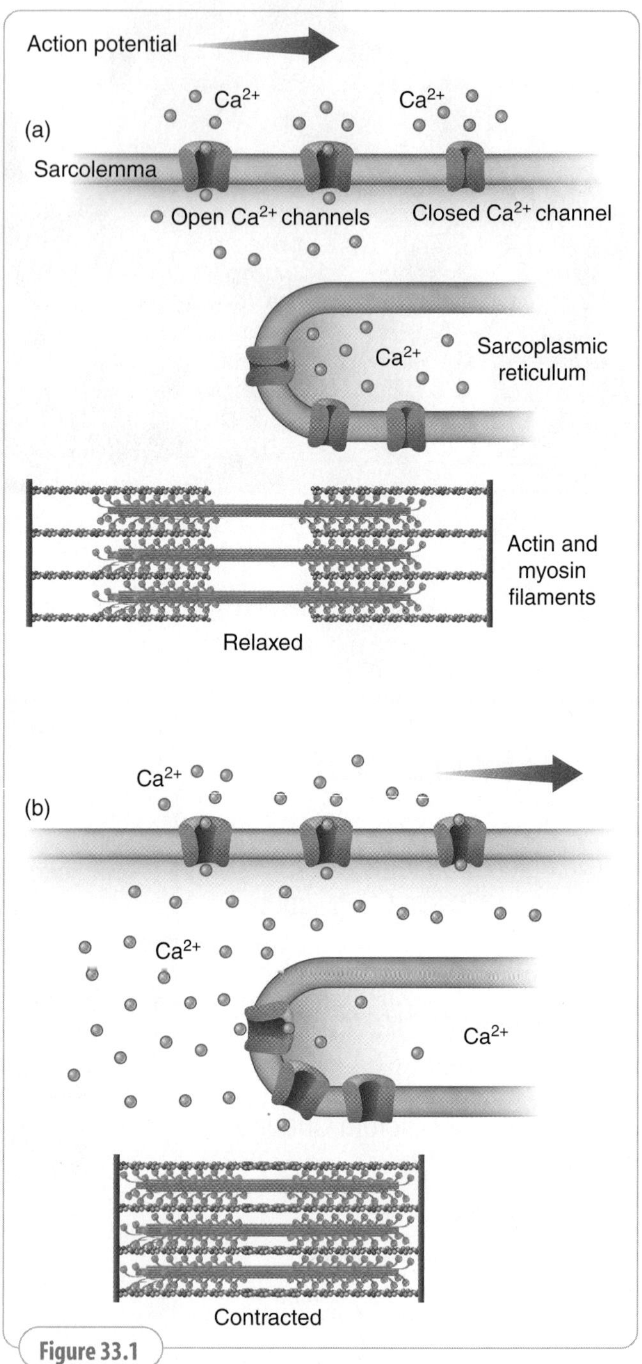

Figure 33.1

Calcium channels and muscle contraction: (a) Calcium channels open as the action potential travels along the sarcolemma. (b) Large amounts of calcium are released from storage in the sarcoplasmic reticula causing actin and myosin filaments to slide and muscle contraction to occur.

Recall from Chapter 19 that activation of beta$_1$-adrenergic receptors in cardiac muscle increases heart rate and contractility. This is because, in myocardial cells, the signal for opening calcium channels is linked to activation of the sympathetic nervous system. In effect, calcium channels open when the sympathetic nervous system supplies the action potential, depolarizing the sarcolemma. This has important implications to pharmacology. Blocking cardiac beta$_1$ receptors with adrenergic blockers will prevent the opening of calcium channels. Thus the cardiac effects of beta$_1$-adrenergic blockers, and their pharmacotherapeutic indications and adverse effects, are similar to those of CCBs.

CONNECTION Checkpoint 33.1

Adrenergic antagonists have the same effect on the cardiovascular system as calcium channel antagonists. From what you learned in Chapters 19 and 20, what type of drug-drug interaction would you expect between a CCB and (a) an anticholinergic such as atropine and (b) a sympathomimetic such as epinephrine? See Answer to Connection Checkpoint 33.1 in Appendix A.

Types of Calcium Channels

33.2 The calcium channel consists of multiple subunits and is present in many tissues.

Research has discovered different types of calcium ion channels, which are named by the letters *L, T,* and *N.* Differences in the structures and locations of the channels are important to drug action.

Pharmacologically, the most important calcium channels are the L type, because they are the ones that bind CCBs. L-type calcium channels are found on the sarcolemma of cardiac and smooth muscles. The channel spans across the membrane and consists of three main parts. An extracellular portion serves as a receptor to bind CCBs. A central portion serves as a pore through which calcium ions travel. An intracellular portion serves as a second messenger capable of initiating a cascade of events that signal the cell to perform specific functions.

The L-type calcium channel is regulated by voltage changes or depolarization across the sarcolemma. When an action potential depolarizes the membrane the channel opens, allowing Ca^{2+} to rush in. The L-type channels are relatively slow, allowing for a sustained flow of Ca^{2+} into the cell. When a CCB is present, the channel changes shape. Although the drug does not physically block the opening, the change in shape of the channel is enough to prevent Ca^{2+} from entering the muscle cell. The L-type calcium channel is illustrated in Figure 33.2.

L-type calcium channels are widespread in the cardiovascular system, and these channels bind all current CCBs. L-type calcium channels are also present in other tissues, particularly in neurons, endocrine, and sensory cells. This leads to other potential uses of these drugs, a topic discussed later in this chapter.

T-type calcium channels are present in vascular smooth muscle as well as the sinoatrial (SA) node where they are involved in pacemaker functions of the heart. Like the L-type channels, they are also located in other tissues throughout the body. The drug mibefradil was developed as a selective T-channel blocker but was removed from the market after serious drug interactions were discovered. At this time, there are no drugs approved by the U.S. Food and Drug Administration (FDA) that act by blocking T-type calcium channels.

N-type calcium channels are found throughout the nervous system. Their primary role appears to be to control neurotransmitter release at synapses. They also are involved in the transmission of pain impulses in the spinal cord. Although a great deal of research is currently being conducted on drugs that target N-type channels in the nervous system, none are currently approved for use in the United States.

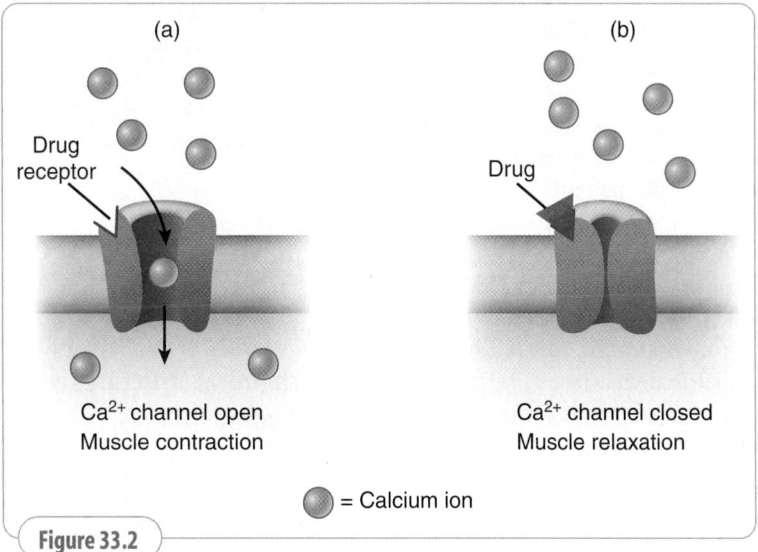

Figure 33.2

L-type calcium channel: (a) Calcium channel opens when an action potential passes across the sarcolemma. Calcium enters the cell and muscle contraction occurs. (b) Calcium channel antagonist binds to the receptor, changing its shape; channel closes and muscle relaxation occurs.

CONNECTIONS

To the Community White Coat Hypertension

White coat HTN syndrome occurs when patients have elevated blood pressure in the health care provider's office only. These patients may have occasional high blood pressure when taken at home, but it is notably high when taken in the health care provider's office. Some patients who have sustained high blood pressure will have even higher readings in the office. The mechanism may be manifested at the subconscious level, without the patients feeling anxiety.

Occasional high blood pressure may not be as dangerous as consistent high blood pressure. When high blood pressure occurs exclusively in the health care provider's office, many will not prescribe any treatment at all. Some studies have shown that white coat HTN may convert to sustained high blood pressure, particularly as one responds to other stresses in daily life.

The main dangers with this condition are:

- The tendency for patients to believe they do not need treatment because it occurs intermittently.
- Assuming that the high reading taken in the health care provider's office is the patient's usual blood pressure and overtreating it.

The most prudent plan of action is to:

- Explain to the patient the phenomenon of white coat HTN.
- Instruct patients with white coat HTN syndrome to obtain a blood pressure cuff and record blood pressures on multiple occasions at home and to take the record to the health care provider for review.
- Measure blood pressure through a monitoring device for a 24-hour period. This will record when, how long, and under what conditions blood pressure becomes elevated.
- Maintain normal body weight, avoid overuse of salt and sodium, and follow an effective exercise program.

Consequences of Calcium Channel Blockade

33.3 Blocking calcium channels has significant physiological effects on the heart and vascular smooth muscle.

The therapeutic applications of CCBs are the result of actions of the drugs on vascular smooth muscle, cardiac muscle, and the conduction system in the heart. Some CCBs have greater effect on the heart, whereas others have more effect on arteriolar smooth muscle. None of the CCBs affect serum calcium levels.

Effects on vascular smooth muscle: The influx of calcium ions into smooth muscle cells is essential for contraction. Because the degree of contraction of arterioles controls peripheral resistance, the blockade of calcium channels has significant physiological effects on blood pressure. CCBs prevent contraction of peripheral arterioles, resulting in vasodilation and a fall in systemic blood pressure. Afterload is reduced, resulting in lower myocardial oxygen demand and less workload for the heart. This is particularly important for patients with angina, who will experience less chest pain due to the decrease in cardiac workload (see Chapter 37).

Another important group of vessels affected by CCBs are the coronary arteries. Dilation of the coronary arteries by the CCBs brings more blood to the myocardium, which is beneficial for patients with myocardial ischemia (see Chapter 37). One group of vessels not affected by CCBs is veins. Cardiac preload is not affected by drugs in this class.

CONNECTION *Checkpoint* 33.2

From what you learned in Chapter 31, define afterload. If a drug increases afterload, what effect would this likely have on cardiac output? See Answer to Connection Checkpoint 33.2 in Appendix A.

Effects on the myocardium: Most CCBs reduce the force of myocardial contraction. This **negative inotropic effect** occurs because these drugs reduce the inward movement of Ca^{2+} during the plateau phase of the action potential. This delayed entry of Ca^{2+} prevents the timely release of Ca^{2+} from its storage depots in the sarcoplasmic reticulum, resulting in fewer actin–myosin cross bridges being formed and a diminished force of contraction.

Effects on cardiac conduction: In general, CCBs exhibit a **negative chronotropic effect:** the property of slowing the speed of electrical conduction across the myocardium. Under normal conditions, the SA node automatically generates an action potential because of an inward movement of Ca^{2+} through calcium channels. Blocking calcium entry causes the SA node to generate fewer action potentials, thus decreasing automaticity and slowing heart rate. Similarly, some of the CCBs block calcium channels in the atrioventricular (AV) node, reducing conduction velocity through this region of the heart and further slowing the spread of the action potential across the myocardium. Not all CCBs affect cardiac conduction: Some are selective for vascular smooth muscle.

Classification of Calcium Channel Blockers

33.4 Calcium channel blockers are classified by their chemical structures as dihydropyridines or nondihydropyridines.

Despite the fact that all CCBs affect L-type calcium channels, there are differences in actions and adverse effects among the specific drugs. This is because the drugs interact with different subunits of the calcium channel. This gives rise to a classification of calcium channel antagonists based on their chemical structures.

The **dihydropyridines** are the largest class of CCBs, which includes amlodipine (Norvasc), felodipine (Plendil), isradipine (DynaCirc), nicardipine (Cardene), nifedipine (Adalat,

Procardia), and nisoldipine (Nisocor). The dihydropyridines bind reversibly to closed-type (inactivated) calcium channels to change the channels' structure to make them unresponsive to depolarization. Because closed-type channels are found in greater numbers in vascular smooth muscle than in cardiac muscle, dihydropyridines are primarily used for their vasodilation effect on arterial smooth muscle.

The remaining CCBs are chemically dissimilar to the dihydropyridines and bind to different subunits of the L-type calcium channel. Although they are chemically different from each other, diltiazem (Cardizem, Dilacor) and verapamil (Calan, Isoptin, Veralin) have quite similar pharmacologic properties and may be grouped together as nondihydropyridines. These drugs bind to open-type calcium channels, causing them to revert to their inactivated or closed state. In addition these drugs delay reactivation of the calcium channel, thus slowing repolarization of the muscle cell membrane. This effect is particularly noticeable in cardiac muscle, where the nondihydropyridines slow the speed of myocardial conduction. Like the dihydropyridines, the nondihydropyridines have a vasodilation effect on vascular smooth muscle. Indications for the various CCBs that have been approved by the FDA are shown in Table 33.1.

33.5 The dihydropyridines are selective for vascular smooth muscle and are used to treat hypertension and angina pectoris.

The six dihydropyridines are very similar in their actions and adverse effects. They are well absorbed after oral (PO) administration, and most are highly protein bound, excreted by the liver, and undergo extensive first-pass metabolism. Because of this, dosage adjustments are necessary in patients with significant hepatic impairment.

Drugs in this class are highly selective for calcium channels located in vascular smooth muscle. At high doses, however, the dihydropyridines lose their selectivity and also affect calcium channels in the heart. All dihydropyridines are equivalent in effectiveness and safety for treating HTN and angina. Some are available in extended release formulations that allow for once-daily dosing. Doses for the dihydropyridines are listed in Table 33.2.

The dihydropyridines are well tolerated in most patients. Common adverse effects include flushed skin, headache, dizziness, peripheral edema, light-headedness, nausea, and diarrhea, although these are usually not severe enough to warrant discontinuation of therapy. The vasodilation caused by the blockade of

TABLE 33.1 FDA-Approved Indications for Calcium Channel Blockers

Drug	Hypertension	Chronic Stable Angina	Vasospastic Angina	Unstable Angina	Dysrhythmias	Subarachnoid Hemorrhage
Dihydropyridines						
amlodipine (Norvasc)	X	X				
felodipine (Plendil)	X					
isradipine (DynaCirc)	X					
nicardipine (Cardene)	X	X				
nicardipine SR (Cardene SR)	X					
nifedipine (Adalat, Procardia)	X	X	X			
nifedipine SR (Adalat, Procardia XL)	X		X			
nimodipine (Nimotop)						X
nisoldipine (Nisocor, Sular)	X					
Nondihydropyridines						
diltiazem (Cardizem, Dilacor)		X				
diltiazem SR (Cardizem SR, Dilacor XR)	X	X	X			
diltiazem injection (Cardizem)					X	
verapamil (Calan, Verelan)	X	X	X	X	X	
verapamil injection (Isoptin)					X	

TABLE 33.2 Calcium Channel Blockers

Drug	Route and Adult Dose (maximum dose where indicated)	Adverse Effects
Dihydropyridines		
amlodipine (Norvasc)	PO: 5–10 mg once daily (max: 10 mg/day)	*Flushed skin, headache, dizziness, peripheral edema, light-headedness, nausea, diarrhea, constipation* <u>Hepatotoxicity, MI, CHF, confusion, mood changes, gingival hyperplasia</u>
felodipine (Plendil)	PO: 5–10 mg daily (max: 20 mg/day)	
isradipine (DynaCirc)	PO: 1.25–10 mg bid (max: 20 mg/day)	
nicardipine (Cardene)	PO: 20–40 mg tid or 30–60 mg Cardene SR bid (max: 120 mg/day)	
nifedipine (Adalat, Procardia)	PO: 10–20 mg tid (max: 180 mg/day) Extended release forms: 30–90 mg once daily	
nisoldipine (Nisocor, Sular)	PO, extended release: 17 mg once daily (max: 34 mg/day)	
Nondihydropyridines		
clevidipine (Cleviprex)	IV: 1–2 mg/hr initital dose; maintenance dose 4–6 mg/hr.	
diltiazem (Cardizem, Dilacor, Tiamate)	PO: 30 mg 4 times daily (max: 480 mg/day) or 60–120 mg bid sustained release (max: 540 mg/day)	
verapamil (Calan, Isoptin, Verelan)	PO: 80–160 mg tid (max: 480 mg/day)	

Note: *Italics* indicate common adverse effects. <u>Underline</u> indicates serious adverse effects.

calcium channels in vascular smooth muscle may cause reflex tachycardia. This is generally transient and clinically important only in patients with preexisting myocardial ischemia or dysrhythmias. If a CCB must be used for these patients, extended release formulations are selected because they produce a more gradual change in blood pressure with less reflex tachycardia.

PROTOTYPE DRUG Nifedipine (Adalat, Procardia XL)

MyNursingKit | Mechanism of Action Animation: Nifedipine

Classification: **Therapeutic:** Antihypertensive
Pharmacologic: Calcium channel blocker, dihydropyridine type

Therapeutic Effects and Uses: Approved in 1981, nifedipine is a CCB with several indications. For HTN it may be given alone or in combination with drugs from other antihypertensive classes. Its ability to dilate the coronary arteries makes it an important drug in the treatment of chronic stable or variant angina (see Chapter 37). When used as an antianginal, a beta-adrenergic blocker may be administered concurrently to prevent reflex tachycardia. It may be used off-label to treat hypertensive emergency, persistent hiccups, or premature labor contractions, or to prevent migraines.

Nifedipine is available as capsules (immediate release) and as extended release tablets. At high doses, the immediate release form of nifedipine should be used with great caution because its use has been associated with an increased risk for myocardial infarction (MI).

Mechanism of Action: Nifedipine acts by selectively blocking calcium channels in vascular smooth muscle, including those in the coronary arteries, causing a decrease in the amount of intracellular calcium available for muscle contraction. This results in a fall in blood pressure and a diminished myocardial oxygen demand due to the reduced afterload. Nifedipine has no effect on myocardial conduction except at toxic doses.

Pharmacokinetics:

Route(s)	PO
Absorption	Well absorbed (90%)
Distribution	Widely distributed; secreted in breast milk; 92–98% bound to plasma protein
Primary metabolism	Hepatic; extensive first-pass metabolism
Primary excretion	Renal (80%) with small amounts in feces (15%)
Onset of action	30–60 minutes (immediate release capsules); 6 h (extended release tablet)
Duration of action	4–8 h (24 h for extended release; half-life: 2–5 h

Adverse Effects: Nifedipine is well tolerated and serious adverse effects are not common. Most adverse effects such as hypotension, dizziness, headache, and flushing are related to the vasodilation action of the drug. The most common cardiovascular-related adverse effect is peripheral edema, which occurs more commonly with nifedipine than with other CCBs. Other severe, though rare, adverse effects include hepatotoxicity, MI, congestive heart failure (CHF), severe hypotension, and confusion.

Contraindications/Precautions: The only contraindication is hypersensitivity to nifedipine or other dihydropyridines. Caution must be observed when using nifedipine in patients with bradycardia or CHF because this drug has negative inotropic effects that can worsen these conditions. The immediate release form is contraindicated in patients with acute MI or cardiogenic shock. Because nifedipine causes blood pressure to fall, it should be used cautiously in patients with preexisting hypotension. Any signs of worsening pulmonary edema call for discontinuation of the drug. Patients with significant hepatic impairment are at risk for drug accumulation and toxicity. Older adults are at much greater risk of nifedipine toxicity and experience a higher overall mortality when treated with this drug.

Drug Interactions: Nifedipine is a substrate for hepatic CYP3A4 and may interact with drugs that induce or inhibit this enzyme. When given concurrently with nifedipine, other antihypertensive drugs have additive effects on blood pressure. These additive hypotensive effects are used to advantage in the pharmacotherapy of HTN (see Chapter 36). Concurrent use of nifedipine with a beta-adrenergic blocker increases the risk of CHF due to additive negative inotropic and chronotropic effects. Nifedipine may increase the serum levels of digoxin by as much as 45%, leading to bradycardia and digoxin toxicity. Alcohol potentiates the vasodilation action of nifedipine and could lead to syncope caused by a rapid drop in blood pressure. **Herbal/Food**: Grapefruit juice may enhance the absorption of nifedipine. Melatonin may reduce the effectiveness of nifedipine by increasing blood pressure and heart rate. St. John's wort can induce CYP3A4 and increase the metabolism of nifedipine and reduce the plasma level of this drug.

Pregnancy: Category C.

Treatment of Overdose: Overdosage will result in hypotension, which is treated with rapid-acting vasopressors such as dopamine or dobutamine. Calcium infusions may also be indicated.

Nursing Responsibilities:

- Obtain a complete health history, including data on recent cardiac events, allergies, drug history, and possible drug interactions.
- Inform the prescriber if the patient has preexisting kidney or liver impairment or cardiovascular disease such as sick sinus syndrome, hypotension, aortic stenosis, CAD, or CHF.
- Monitor blood pressure before administration of this drug and 30 minutes to 1 hour after.
- Monitor blood pressure carefully during the titration period. Patients may experience severe hypotension if taking other drugs known to lower blood pressure. Withhold this drug and notify the prescriber if systolic blood pressure drops below 90.
- Monitor patients with diabetes for blood glucose because CCBs may have diabetogenic properties.
- For chronic HTN, use only the sustained release form swallowed whole with a full glass of water.
- Discontinue CCBs gradually, with close medical supervision, to prevent rebound HTN and other adverse effects.
- Report gingival hyperplasia promptly. It is a rare but serious adverse effect.

Patient and Family Education:

- Monitor blood pressure regularly as directed by the health care provider. Maintain a written log of blood pressure readings and present it at follow-up visits.
- Immediately report palpitations, weight gain, swelling of ankles and feet, or rashes to the health care provider.
- Do not abruptly stop taking this drug because serious withdrawal symptoms such as chest pain, palpitations, or heart attack may occur.
- Take a missed dose as soon as remembered, unless it is almost time for the next scheduled dose. Never take a double dose of this medicine.
- Refrain from ingesting grapefruit or grapefruit juice during treatment because it may result in a drug-food interaction.
- Inspect gums daily for changes such as bleeding or enlargement, which can be gradual. If noted, seek prompt treatment.
- Note that occasionally the nonabsorbable shell of this drug may be seen in the stool. This is normal.
- Discontinue smoking because this decreases the effectiveness of this drug and can have adverse effects on the heart.
- Do not drink alcohol while taking this drug because this can cause low blood pressure and fainting.
- Do not breast-feed while taking this drug without approval of the health care provider.

Drugs Similar to Nifedipine (Adalat, Procardia XL)

Other dihydropyridines include amlodipine, felodipine, isradipine, nicardipine, and nisoldipine.

Amlodipine (Norvasc): Amlodipine is indicated for the treatment of HTN, chronic stable angina, and Prinzmetal's variant angina. Approved in 1992, amlodipine has the longest half-life (35 hours) of the dihydropyridines, which allows for once-daily dosing. Like other dihydropyridines, amlodipine affects mainly arteriolar smooth muscle, including that in the coronary arteries, and has no significant effect on cardiac conduction. The drug is well tolerated, with headache, dizziness, and peripheral edema being frequent adverse effects. Reflex tachycardia rarely occurs because the drug has a very gradual onset. In the treatment of HTN, several weeks may be required to achieve optimal outcomes. This drug is pregnancy category C.

Felodipine (Plendil): Approved in 1991, felodipine is a dihydropyridine that has greater selectivity for vascular smooth muscle than nifedipine and is approved only for the pharmacotherapy of HTN. It exerts no significant effects on the heart. Its elimination half-life of 11 to 16 hours allows for once-daily dosing. Typical adverse effects are facial flushing, headache, peripheral edema, and reflex tachycardia. Lexxel is a fixed-dose combination of enalapril (an angiotensin-converting enzyme [ACE] inhibitor) and felodipine. This drug is pregnancy category C.

Isradipine (DynaCirc): Approved in 1990, isradipine is the most potent of the dihydropyridines and is approved for the pharmacotherapy of HTN, either alone or in combination with a thiazide diuretic (see Chapter 36). Chronic stable angina is an off-label indication for the drug. The physiological actions of isradipine are selective to arterioles, and the drug has no appreciable effect on the heart. Reflex tachycardia is usually not significant. A sustained release form (DynaCirc CR) is available for once-daily dosing. Optimum response may require 2 to 4 weeks of therapy. Headache, facial flushing, and dizziness are the most common adverse effects. This drug is pregnancy category C.

Nicardipine (Cardene): Approved in 1988, nicardipine is indicated for the pharmacotherapy of chronic stable angina and HTN. Beta-adrenergic blockers or sublingual nitrates may be administered concurrently to reduce the possibility of reflex tachycardia in patients with angina pectoris. A sustained release form (Cardene SR) allows for once-daily dosing, and an intravenous (IV) form (Cardene IV) is available for initiation of therapy in patients with severe HTN. An off-label use of nicardipine is for migraines. The actions, contraindications, and adverse effects are similar to those of nifedipine. Peripheral edema, dizziness, headache, and facial flushing are the most common adverse effects. This drug is pregnancy category C.

Nisoldipine (Nisocor, Sular): Approved in 1995, nisoldipine is selective for vascular smooth muscle and has no significant effect on the myocardium. It is approved only for HTN but may be used off-label for angina. The extended release form, Sular, allows for once-daily dosing. Peripheral edema and headache are relatively common in patients taking this drug. Reflex tachycardia may cause angina pain in patients with myocardial ischemia. Like other CCBs, it should be used with caution in patients with hypotension, peripheral edema, or heart failure. This drug is pregnancy category C.

PharmFACT

It is estimated that 10% to 20% of patients taking calcium channel antagonists will develop gingival hyperplasia. This condition can be successfully managed by professional dental care and oral antiseptic rinses such as chlorohexidene (Peridex). *Source:* Vacharotayangul & Lozada-Nur, 2006.

33.6 The nondihydropyridines act on both vascular smooth muscle and the myocardium.

The nondihydropyridine group of CCBs consists of two drugs. Although they belong to different chemical classes, both have common physiological actions, adverse effects, and indications. A third drug in this class, bepridil (Vascor), is no longer sold in the United States because it was found to produce dysrhythmias, especially in patients who had experienced a recent MI. Current nondihydropyridines include the following:

- Phenylalkylamine: Verapamil (Calan, Isoptin)
- Benzodiazepine: Diltiazem (Cardizem, Dilacor, Tiazac)

Like the dihydropyridines, drugs in this class block L-type calcium channels in vascular smooth muscle, causing vasodilation. As expected from this physiological action, the nondihydropyridines are used in the pharmacotherapy of HTN and angina. Thus the dihydropyridines and nondihydropyridines share these two indications. Doses for the nondihydropyridines are listed in Table 33.2.

It is important to note that verapamil and diltiazem have actions on the heart that the dihydropyridines do not possess. These drugs block calcium channels in the myocardium, causing a negative inotropic effect. In addition, the nondihydropyridines decrease the speed of myocardial conduction, resulting in a slower heart rate.

These cardiac effects of the nondihydropyridines may be viewed as either therapeutic or adverse, depending on the patient and the reasons for administering the drugs. For example, by slowing conduction across the heart, verapamil and diltiazem can suppress abnormal cardiac rhythms. They are indicated for specific types of dysrhythmias, such as atrial flutter or fibrillation (see Chapter 39). In certain patients, however, slowing the speed of conduction may result in serious adverse effects. For example, slowing the heart rate can diminish cardiac output in patients with moderate or severe heart failure and worsen this condition. Slowing impulse conduction may cause partial or complete heart block in patients with bradycardia or second-degree or third-degree AV block. Concurrent treatment with a beta-adrenergic agonist may be necessary to counteract these adverse cardiac effects.

Other adverse effects from the nondihydropyridines include constipation, flushed skin, headache, dizziness, edema of the ankles and feet, and light-headedness. Gingival hyperplasia is an uncommon adverse effect that occurs with long-term therapy and usually reverses after the drugs are discontinued. Most patients tolerate the nondihydropyridine CCBs well and experience few serious adverse effects.

CONNECTIONS

Lifespan Considerations High Blood Pressure in Children

Though HTN is often perceived as an adult health problem, children and even babies can have high blood pressure. The American Heart Association recommends that all children age 3 and older have their blood pressure taken yearly. Early detection can improve the health of children and their transition into adulthood.

When childhood HTN is caused by other diseases, such as heart or kidney disease, secondary HTN may be diagnosed by the health care provider. If the primary disease is treated, high blood pressure often returns to normal. Likewise when medications cause high blood pressure, discontinuance of the drug results in a normal blood pressure. Primary HTN of unknown origin can also occur in children.

Children who are overweight usually have higher blood pressure than those who are not overweight. Children can inherit the tendency toward high blood pressure. HTN occurs more frequently in African Americans than in Caucasians. Overweight children have higher blood pressure than normal weight children. Healthy diet and regular exercise are advised for overweight children to lower blood pressure and improve general well-being.

PROTOTYPE DRUG Verapamil (Calan, Isoptin)

Classification: **Therapeutic:** Antihypertensive, antianginal, antidysrhythmic

Pharmacologic: Calcium channel blocker; phenylalkylamine type

Therapeutic Effects and Uses: Verapamil was the first CCB approved by the FDA in 1981. The drug is a class IV antidysrhythmic (see Chapter 39) because it slows myocardial conduction velocity, especially through the AV node, and stabilizes certain types of abnormal heart rhythms. In the vasculature, calcium channel blockade causes vasodilation of arterioles, which lowers blood pressure and reduces cardiac workload. Verapamil also dilates the coronary arteries, an action that is important when the drug is used to treat angina. It is approved to treat variant, unstable, and chronic angina (see Chapter 37). Off-label indications include migraine prophylaxis and acute mania.

Verapamil is available in PO, oral extended release, and IV formulations. Covera-HS is a unique formulation that delays the release of verapamil until 4 to 5 hours after ingestion and then releases it slowly. Covera-HS should be taken at night so that the drug is in the bloodstream on awakening. The inert shell of the drug is sometimes found in the stool. The therapeutic serum level of verapamil is 0.08 to 0.3 mcg/mL.

Mechanism of Action: Verapamil acts by inhibiting the flow of calcium ions into both cardiac muscle cells and vascular smooth muscle cells. Blocking calcium entry causes vasodilation of peripheral arterioles and reduced contractility of the myocardium.

Pharmacokinetics:

Route(s)	PO and IV
Absorption	Well absorbed
Distribution	Widely distributed; crosses the placenta; secreted in breast milk
Primary metabolism	Hepatic; extensive first-pass metabolism
Primary excretion	Renal (70%) with small amounts in feces (16%)
Onset of action	PO: 1–2 h; IV: 1–5 minutes
Duration of action	PO: 3–7 h (extended release: 24 h); IV: 2 h Half-life: 2–8 h

Adverse Effects: Most adverse effects of verapamil are extensions of its actions on the cardiovascular system. Peripheral vasodilation may cause flushed skin, headache, dizziness, light-headedness, and peripheral edema. High doses and IV administration may cause serious hypotension. The most serious adverse effects of verapamil are cardiac related, including worsening of CHF, bradycardia, reflex tachycardia, and AV block. Central nervous system (CNS) effects such as confusion, drowsiness, and mood changes have been reported, though they are uncommon. Constipation is relatively common.

Contraindications/Precautions: Verapamil is contraindicated in patients with AV heart block, sick sinus syndrome, severe hypotension, bleeding aneurysm, or those undergoing intracranial surgery. Because verapamil can cause bradycardia and pulmonary edema, patients with heart failure should be carefully monitored, especially when the drug is administered IV. The drug should be used with caution in patients with renal or hepatic impairment because this can delay clearance of verapamil and its metabolites.

Drug Interactions: Verapamil is metabolized by hepatic P450 enzymes and exhibits many drug–drug interactions. Verapamil has the ability to elevate blood levels of digoxin. Because digoxin and verapamil both slow conduction through the AV node, their concurrent use must be carefully monitored to avoid bradycardia. Use with other antihypertensive drugs, including ACE inhibitors or beta-adrenergic blockers, may cause additive hypotension or bradycardia. Concurrent administration of verapamil with buspirone can triple the plasma concentration of buspirone. Verapamil should not be administered with statins (see Chapter 32) because the risk of myopathy increases significantly. Carbamazepine serum concentration may increase during concurrent therapy with verapamil, causing adverse effects such as diplopia, ataxia, or dizziness. Use with alcohol can raise serum levels of the CCB and prolong its effects. **Herbal/Food:** Grapefruit juice may increase verapamil levels. Use with caution with herbal supplements, such as hawthorn, which may have additive hypotensive effects. High does of calcium supplements may diminish the effects of CCBs and should not be used without consulting the health care provider.

Pregnancy: Category C.

Treatment of Overdose: Treatment of overdose is aimed at reversing hypotension with vasopressors such as dopamine or dobutamine. Atropine or isoproterenol may be administered to treat bradycardia. Calcium salts may be administered to increase calcium available to the myocardium and arterioles.

Nursing Responsibilities:

- Obtain a complete health history, including data on recent cardiac events, allergies, drug history, and possible drug interactions.
- Notify the prescriber of patient history of liver or kidney impairment, cardiovascular disease such as sick sinus syndrome, heart failure or block, muscular dystrophy, CAD, or hypotension.
- Monitor blood pressure before administration of this drug and 30 minutes to 1 hour after. Withhold the drug and notify the prescriber if systolic blood pressure drops below 90.
- Establish baseline vital signs and periodically monitor blood pressure and pulse.
- Monitor for pedal and ankle edema and report incidences to the prescriber.
- Establish baseline laboratory test values for liver and kidney functions.
- Keep the patient in recumbent position for at least 1 hour after a dose is given to avoid transient asymptomatic hypotension that may accompany IV infusion.
- Monitor therapeutic effectiveness by noting decreased anginal frequency or reduced blood pressure.

- Monitor for heart block or excessive bradycardia when infusion is given concurrently with digoxin (Lanoxin).
- Monitor the intake and output ratio during IV and early oral maintenance therapy. Renal impairment prolongs the duration of action and increases the potential for toxicity and incidence of adverse effects. Report gradual weight gain and edema.
- Monitor the electrocardiogram (ECG) continuously during IV administration because the drug's action may be prolonged. The incidence of adverse reactions is highest during IV administration in older adults, patients of short stature, and those with impaired kidney function.
- Check blood pressure shortly before administration of the next dose to evaluate the degree of blood pressure control during the early treatment for HTN.

Patient and Family Education:

- Take with food and a full glass of water to reduce gastric irritation.
- Monitor blood pressure regularly as directed by the prescriber. Maintain a written log of blood pressure readings and present it at follow-up visits.
- Immediately report palpitations, weight gain, or swelling of ankles and feet to the health care provider.
- Do not stop taking this medication without consulting the health care provider or the condition could worsen.
- Take a radial pulse before each dose and notify the health care provider if it is irregular or if slow pulse occurs.
- Do not crush, chew, or break the extended release forms of this drug
- Discuss all current medications, dietary supplements, and herbal products with the health care provider to avoid adverse interactions.
- Maintain established guidelines for an exercise program.
- Do not drive or perform other hazardous activities until the effects of the drug are known because this drug may cause drowsiness or dizziness.
- Refrain from ingesting grapefruit or grapefruit juice during treatment because it may result in a drug–food interaction.
- Decrease intake of caffeinated beverages, such as coffee and tea, and foods such as chocolate.
- Do not drink alcohol because this may lower blood pressure and increase drowsiness and dizziness.
- Make position changes slowly when moving from a lying to a standing position to prevent dizziness and possible fainting until tolerance to reduced blood pressure is established.
- Notify the health care provider of easy bruising or unexplained bleeding.
- Avoid over-the-counter drugs, especially aspirin, unless approved by the health care provider.
- Do not breast-feed while taking this drug without approval of the health care provider.

Drugs Similar to Verapamil (Calan, Isoptin)

The only other nondihydropyridine is diltiazem.

Diltiazem (Cardizem, Dilacor, others): Like other nondihydropyridines, diltiazem has the ability to relax both coronary and peripheral blood vessels. Approved in 1982, diltiazem reduces heart rate, blood pressure, and cardiac workload. The drug slows electrical conduction through the AV node. It is useful in the treatment of atrial dysrhythmias and HTN as well as stable and vasospastic angina. Migraine prophylaxis is an off-label indication. When given as extended release capsules (CardizemLA, DilacorXR), it is administered once daily. An IV formulation is available to treat atrial fibrillation. The drug is well tolerated and serious adverse effects are uncommon and similar to those of verapamil. Like verapamil, diltiazem should be used cautiously in patients with bradycardia, AV block, CHF, or serious hypotension.

CONNECTION *Checkpoint* 33.3

A patient with major depression is taking amitriptyline (Elavil), a drug with prominent anticholinergic-like adverse effects. From what you learned in Chapters 18 and 23, predict what effect adding verapamil to the regimen would have on these adverse effects. See Answer to Connection Checkpoint 33.3 in Appendix A.

NURSING PROCESS APPLICATION

Patients Receiving Calcium Channel Blocker Therapy

Assessment

Prior to administration:

- Obtain a complete health history, including data on recent cardiac events, allergies, drug history, and possible drug interactions.
- Monitor blood pressure utilizing the correct technique, appropriate cuff size, and properly maintained and calibrated equipment.
- Obtain an ECG and vital signs; assess in the context of the patient's baseline values.
- Assess the neurologic status and level of consciousness (LOC).
- Auscultate chest sounds for rales or rhonchi indicative of pulmonary edema.
- Assess the lower limbs for edema; note the character and level. Report its presence to the prescriber.

Potential Nursing Diagnoses

- *Ineffective Health Maintenance,* related to uncontrolled blood pressure
- *Deficient Knowledge (Calcium Channel Blocker Therapy),* related to purpose, precautions, and adverse effects of drug therapy
- *Decreased Cardiac Output,* related to the disease process
- *Ineffective Tissue Perfusion (Cardiopulmonary),* related to drug therapy

Planning: Patient Goals and Expected Outcomes

The patient will:

- Exhibit a reduction in blood pressure or a decrease in the number of anginal attacks.
- Demonstrate an understanding of the drug's action by accurately describing drug adverse effects and precautions.

Implementation

Interventions and (Rationales)	Patient and Family Education
• Monitor vital signs. • Monitor the ECG during initial therapy. (CCBs dilate the arteries, reducing blood pressure, thereby producing cardiac irregularities.) • Obtain blood pressure readings in the sitting, standing, and supine positions to monitor fluctuations in blood pressure. (Measuring blood pressure in various positions helps to determine if the patient is experiencing drug-induced orthostatic hypotension.)	Instruct the patient to: • Monitor blood pressure and ensure the proper use of home equipment. • Withhold the medication if blood pressure falls below the target blood pressure and notify the health care provider. • Immediately report palpitations or sensation of rapid heartbeat or shortness of breath.
• Observe for changes in LOC, dizziness, fatigue, and orthostatic hypotension. (The vasodilation effect of the drug produces these symptoms.)	Instruct the patient to: • Rise slowly from prolonged periods of sitting or lying down. • Report dizziness or light-headedness.
• Observe for paradoxical increase in chest pain or angina symptoms. (These symptoms are produced by drug-induced hypotension.)	• Instruct the patient to report chest pain or other angina-like symptoms.
• Monitor for signs of heart failure. (CCBs can decrease myocardial contractility, increasing the risk of heart failure.)	• Instruct the patient to immediately report any severe shortness of breath, frothy sputum, profound fatigue, or swelling of the extremities. These may be signs of heart failure or fluid accumulation in the lungs.
• Measure intake and output and daily weights. (Edema is an adverse effect of some CCBs.)	• Instruct the patient to weigh daily at the same time each day and to report weight gain of more than 2 pounds in 24 hours.
• Observe for skin rash or other signs of allergy. (Some patient may have a hypersensitivity reaction to CCBs.)	• Instruct the patient to immediately seek medical attention for difficulty breathing, throat tightness, hives or rash, muscle cramps, or tremors.
• Monitor liver and kidney function. (CCBs are metabolized in the liver and excreted by the kidneys.)	Instruct the patient to: • Report signs of liver toxicity such as nausea, vomiting, anorexia, bleeding, severe abdominal pain, heartburn, jaundice, or a change in the color or character of stools. • Report signs of renal toxicity such as fever; flank pain; changes in urine output, color, or character (such as cloudiness or sediment). • Adhere to laboratory testing regimens as ordered by the health care provider.
• Assess for constipation. (CCBs may cause constipation.)	Instruct the patient to: • Maintain adequate fluid and fiber intake to facilitate stool passage. • Use a bulk laxative or stool softener as recommended by the health care provider.
• Monitor for safe ambulation until response to the drug is known. (CCBs may cause orthostatic hypotension.)	• Instruct the patient to avoid driving or other activities requiring mental alertness or physical coordination until the effects of the drug are known.

Evaluation of Outcome Criteria

Evaluate the effectiveness of drug therapy by confirming that patient goals and expected outcomes have been met (see "Planning").

UNDERSTANDING THE CHAPTER

Key Concepts Summary

33.1 Calcium channels facilitate contraction in cardiac and smooth muscles.

33.2 The calcium channel consists of multiple subunits and is present in many tissues.

33.3 Blocking calcium channels has significant physiological effects on the heart and vascular smooth muscle.

33.4 Calcium channel blockers are classified by their chemical structures as dihydropyridines or nondihydropyridines.

33.5 The dihydropyridines are selective for vascular smooth muscle and are used to treat hypertension and angina pectoris.

33.6 The nondihydropyridines act on both vascular smooth muscle and the myocardium.

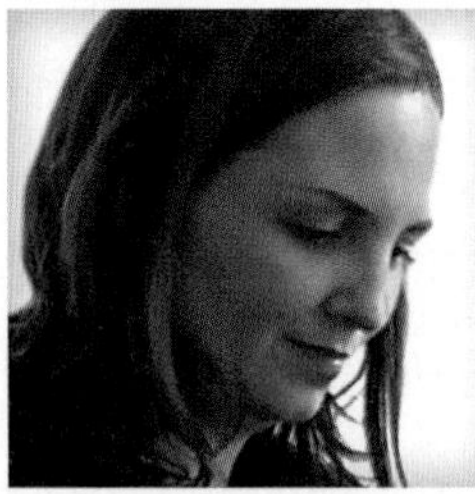

Making the PATIENT *Connection*

Remember the patient "Elise Freeman" at the beginning of the chapter? Now read the remainder of the case study. Based on the information presented within this chapter, respond to the critical thinking questions that follow.

Elise Freeman, a 40-year-old interior designer, had no idea that her blood pressure was elevated. One day at the shopping mall she saw an automatic blood pressure machine and thought she would try it. She could hardly believe the machine's reading when it revealed her blood pressure was 150/92. She was certain that there must be something wrong with the machine. After all, she felt fine. In fact, she never misses work and is rarely ill.

Just to be certain, Elise made an appointment with her doctor for a checkup. During her first clinic visit, her blood pressure was 146/90 mmHg, heart rate was 78 beats/minute, respiratory rate was 16/minute, and temperature was 36.8°C (98.2°F). Elise was instructed on lifestyle modifications for HTN and told to return to the clinic in 1 week. The next week, Elise's blood pressure remained elevated. Multiple diagnostic studies, which included an ECG and serum chemistry levels, were completed. Her health care provider prescribed a low-dose diuretic and instructed her to return in 1 week.

All of this has caused Elise to be concerned and worried about her health. She has accessed the Internet to learn as much about HTN as possible. Although she has not been prescribed a calcium channel blocker, she has discovered that sometimes these drugs are used to reduce elevated blood pressure. With all the information about high blood pressure, she is even more confused and anxious.

Critical Thinking Questions

1. Describe how calcium channel blockers control HTN.
2. The patient wants to know all the consequences of untreated HTN. How would you answer this question?
3. Elise asks you if calcium channel blockers can cure HTN. How would you respond?
4. Are there any adverse effects with calcium channel blockers? What are they?

Case Study

Mabel Hillside was prescribed verapamil (Calan) 80 mg three times per day. However, Mabel's health insurance does not cover prescription drug cost and she will be required to self-pay for the drug. As you are talking with this patient, she says, "Why should I take this medicine? After all, I feel just fine and it is very expensive. Plus I keep forgetting to take it."

1. How would you respond to Mabel's remark about feeling "just fine"?
2. What adverse effects related to verapamil might cause the patient to stop taking the medication?
3. List strategies that Mabel can use to remember to take her hypertensive medication.
4. What about the cost? Is this a problem that you, as the nurse, should be concerned about?

NCLEX-RN® Review

1 Nifedipine (Procardia) is being initiated for a client with an elevated blood pressure. What health teaching would be most appropriate? The client should:

1. Weigh daily at the same time each day.
2. Avoid crowds while taking this medication.
3. Increase intake of calcium-containing foods.
4. Take this medication only when feeling the blood pressure is elevated.

2 A client is receiving a calcium channel antagonist for hypertension. The nurse included in the care plan to monitor the client for which of the following adverse effects?

1. Rash and chills
2. Increased urinary output
3. Weight loss
4. Changes in level of consciousness

3 A client with primary hypertension has started therapy with verapamil (Calan). The nurse performs what important intervention during the initial course of this treatment?

1. Uses an electric razor to shave the client
2. Monitors the client for increased thrombocyte levels
3. Administers the medication only during waking hours
4. Measures intake and output ratio

4 The nurse determines that the client understands an important principle in self-administration of nifedipine (Procardia) when the client makes which of the following statements?

1. "The use of antacids when taking the medication will enhance absorption."
2. "Grapefruit juice may enhance the absorption of nifedipine."
3. "If I miss a dose, I should take two nifedipine capsules when I remember."
4. "This drug will make my birth control pills ineffective."

5 Health teaching provided by the nurse for a client receiving calcium channel blockers should include: (Select all that apply.)

1. Avoid driving or performing other activities requiring mental alertness until the effects of the drug are known.
2. Maintain adequate fluid and fiber intake to facilitate stool passage.
3. Report weight gain of 2 pounds per week.
4. Rise slowly from prolonged periods of sitting or lying down.
5. Immediately stop taking the medication if sexual dysfunction is noted.

6 A health care provider has ordered nifedipine (Procardia XL) for each of these clients. A nurse will most closely monitor which client for drug-related problems?

1. A client who is admitted for an appendectomy in the morning
2. A client who is receiving renal dialysis three times per week
3. A client who develops pulmonary edema in the intensive care unit
4. A client who receives psychotropic drugs for bipolar disease

See Answers to Critical Thinking Questions, Case Study, and NCLEX-RN® Review in Appendix A.

References

Chojnowski, D. (2006). Managing systolic heart failure. *Nursing, 36*(7), 36–42.

Davis, G. (2006). Blood pressure: Anatomy and physiology in relation to drug therapies. *Nurse Prescribing, 4*(9), 358–364.

McCallum, C. (2007). An update on managing hypertension. *Practice Nursing, 18*(2), 73–75.

Oceandy, D., Mamas, M. A., & Neyses, L. (2007). Targeting the sarcolemmal calcium pump: A potential novel strategy for the treatment of cardiovascular disease. *Cardiovascular & Hematological Agents in Medicinal Chemistry, 5*(4), 300–304.

Sica, D. A. (2006). Pharmacotherapy review: Calcium channel blockers. *Journal of Clinical Hypertension, 8*(1), 53–56.

Sylvain, R. (2005). Vascular effects of calcium channel antagonists: New evidence. Review article. *Drugs, 6*(Suppl. 2), 1–10.

Tfelt-Hansen, J., & Brown, E. (2005). The calcium-sensing receptor in normal physiology and pathophysiology: A review. *Critical Reviews in Clinical Laboratory Sciences, 42*(1), 35– 70.

Tulip, S. (2006). Medicines management in hypertension. *Practice Nursing, 17*(4), 184–188.

Vacharotayangul, P., & Lozada-Nur, F. (2006). *Drug-induced gingival hyperplasia.* Retrieved July 6, 2008, from http://www.emedicine.com/DERM/topic645.htm

CHAPTER

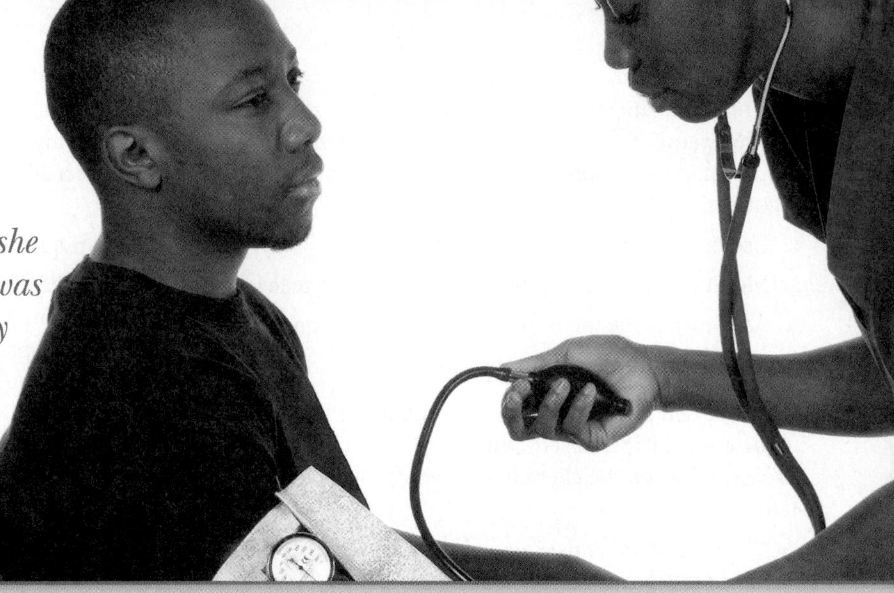

When I saw my doctor, she said my blood pressure was still high. I'm taking my medicine as directed. So what's the problem?

Patient "Carlos McKay"

34 Drugs Affecting the Renin-Angiotensin-Aldosterone System

Learning Outcomes

After reading this chapter, the student should be able to:

1. Illustrate the steps in the pathway leading to the formation of angiotensin II.
2. Identify primary physiological factors that control renin secretion.
3. Explain the two primary functions of angiotensin-converting enzyme.
4. Describe the multiple mechanisms by which angiotensin II raises blood pressure.
5. Explain how the actions of aldosterone can lead to high blood pressure.
6. Identify the specific steps in the renin-angiotensin-aldosterone system that can be blocked by medications.
7. For each of the classes shown in the chapter outline, identify the prototype and representative drugs and explain the mechanism(s) of drug action, primary indications, contraindications, significant drug interactions, pregnancy category, and important adverse effects.
8. Apply the nursing process to care for patients receiving drugs affecting the renin-angiotensin-aldosterone system.

Chapter Outline

Components of the Renin-Angiotensin-Aldosterone System

Physiological Effects of the Renin-Angiotensin-Aldosterone System

Drugs Affecting the Renin-Angiotensin-Aldosterone System

Angiotensin-Converting Enzyme (ACE) Inhibitors

PROTOTYPE **Lisinopril (Prinivil, Zestril)** *p. 534*

Angiotensin II Receptor Blockers (ARBs)

PROTOTYPE **Losartan (Cozaar)** *p. 539*

Aldosterone Antagonists

Key Terms

angioedema, 534
angiotensin I, 529
angiotensin II, 529
angiotensinogen, 529
bradykinin, 531
cardiac remodeling, 532
juxtaglomerular (JG) cells, 530
macula densa, 530
renin, 530
renin-angiotensin-aldosterone system (RAAS), 529

The **renin-angiotensin-aldosterone system (RAAS)** is a key homeostatic mechanism controlling blood pressure and fluid balance. The RAAS is presented early in the study of cardiovascular pharmacology because the drugs affecting this pathway are frequently used to treat hypertension (HTN) and heart failure. This chapter examines components of the RAAS and describes how drugs affecting this system are used for therapeutic benefit.

Components of the Renin-Angiotensin-Aldosterone System

34.1 The formation of angiotensin II requires two enzymatic steps.

In the mid-1900s, scientists discovered a peptide circulating in the blood that caused profound vasoconstriction. Named angiotensin (*angio* = blood vessel; *tensin* = pressure), high levels of this substance were found in people with HTN. Thus began the search for components of what is now called the renin-angiotensin-aldosterone system.

We now know that there are several forms of angiotensin. **Angiotensin II** is the vasopressor substance originally isolated by scientists in the 1900s. The formation of angiotensin II requires two key enzymatic steps, and an understanding of these steps is critical to learning the pharmacology of drugs affecting the RAAS. The RAAS is illustrated in Figure 34.1.

Step 1: Formation of angiotensin I: **Angiotensinogen** is a protein synthesized by the liver that is continuously circulating in the bloodstream. In the blood, angiotensinogen is split by the enzyme renin to form **angiotensin I**. Neither angiotensinogen nor angiotensin I has any significant biologic activity; they simply serve as precursors to angiotensin II.

Step 2: Formation of angiotensin II: Angiotensin I travels through the circulation until it encounters angiotensin-converting enzyme (ACE), which cleaves two amino acids to form angiotensin II. ACE is located on the membrane surface of the blood vessel endothelium. Because the lung possesses such an extensive number of capillaries, it is the primary organ responsible for converting angiotensin I to angiotensin II. Angiotensin II is one of the most potent natural vasoconstrictors known; it is approximately 40 times more potent at raising blood pressure than norepinephrine.

34.2 Renin secretion is controlled by the juxtaglomerular cells of the kidney and the sympathetic nervous system.

Because renin is responsible for the first step in the RAAS pathway, it is a major factor in determining the amount of angiotensin II produced in the body. Therefore, factors affecting the secretion of renin are important to understanding the pharmacotherapy associated with this system.

CONNECTIONS

To the Community: Teaching Patients About Dietary Sodium, Hypertension, and Food Labels

Evidence from randomized controlled trials provides overwhelming support for a causal relationship between dietary sodium intake and elevated blood pressure. However, it seems that salt metabolism, and its effects on HTN, are extremely complex and are not well understood. The American Heart Association (AHA) strongly supports the reduction of sodium intake for individuals with HTN. According to the AHA, reducing the amount of sodium consumed may help to reduce or avoid high blood pressure.

Many people do not realize that most foods (in their natural state) contain sodium. Furthermore, most sodium in the average diet is added to food while it is being commercially processed or prepared at home. That is why patients who are trying to lower sodium intake need to be aware of both natural and added sodium content when choosing foods. Individuals with documented HTN or coronary valve disease are instructed to limit sodium intake to less than 2,400 mg/day in most cases. It is also highly recommended that when individuals with HTN are buying prepared and prepackaged foods that they read the labels on the products.

However, food labels can be somewhat confusing to everyone, especially with terms such as *low sodium, reduced sodium,* and *salt free.* Virtually all processed foods are loaded with sodium, including breakfast cereal and ketchup. The chart that follows helps to clarify some of the terminology used on food labels. During patient teaching sessions, the nurse can be instrumental in providing the patient with this helpful information. Here is how the U.S. Department of Agriculture defines sodium content:

Label Term	What Does It Mean?
Sodium free	Less than 5 milligrams sodium per serving
Very low sodium	35 milligrams or less sodium per serving
Low sodium	140 milligrams or less sodium per serving
Reduced sodium	At least 25% less sodium as compared with a standard serving size
Light sodium	50% less sodium; restricted to foods with more than 40 calories per serving or more than 3 grams of fat per serving
Salt free	Less than 5 milligrams sodium per serving
Unsalted or no salt added	No salt added during processing does not necessarily mean sodium free

Source: From *Dietary Guidelines for Americans*, by U.S. Department of Health and Human Services, 2005. Retrieved July 8, 2008, from www.health.gov/DietaryGuidelines/

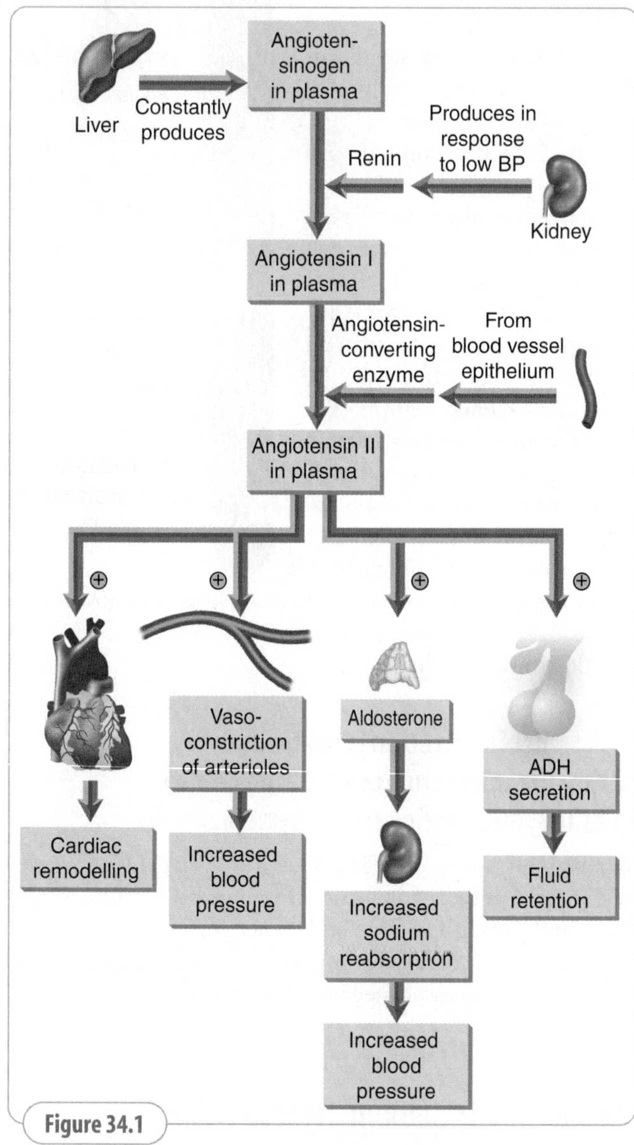

Figure 34.1

The renin-angiotensin-aldosterone pathway.

Renin is an enzyme that is synthesized, stored, and secreted by specialized cells in the kidney known as **juxtaglomerular (JG) cells.** Found in the afferent arteriole that supplies blood to the glomerulus, JG cells are specialized smooth muscle cells that act as pressure sensors. As blood pressure falls, there is less pressure on the JG cells, which respond by releasing renin to the circulation. The increase in renin ultimately leads to larger amounts of circulating angiotensin II, which returns blood pressure to normal. The release of renin may be caused by anything that lowers blood pressure, such as a loss of blood volume due to dehydration or hemorrhage. Through negative feedback, increased blood pressure is sensed by the JG cells, which turn off renin secretion.

Several other important factors control the release of renin. Adjacent to the JG cells in the distal convoluted tubule of the nephron is a specialized cluster of cells called the **macula densa.** The macula densa is in a perfect location to sense the flow rate and the concentration of sodium ions (osmolality) in the filtrate. As blood pressure falls, blood flow through the kidney diminishes and the flow rate of renal tubular filtrate slows. The macula densa recognizes the slow flow rate (and less sodium) and sends a chemical message to the JG cells to release more renin. The renin release forms more angiotensin II and blood pressure rises.

Anatomically, the JG cells and the macula densa are in close proximity, as shown in Figure 34.2. The JG cells and the macula densa are sometimes considered a single anatomic unit called the juxtaglomerular apparatus.

CONNECTION *Checkpoint* 34.1

Substances that lower blood pressure may trigger reflex tachycardia. From what you learned in Chapter 31, explain the mechanism involved in this reflex. See Answer to Connection Checkpoint 34.1 in Appendix A.

A third mechanism for controlling the release of renin is more direct: activation of the sympathetic nervous system. JG cells contain beta$_1$-adrenergic receptors, which are activated by the classic fight-or-flight response of the sympathetic nervous system (see Chapter 16). The release of renin helps to raise blood pressure when dealing with a stressful or harmful situation.

To summarize, the factors that promote the release of renin by JG cells will raise blood pressure. The three primary factors causing an increase are decreased pressure in blood flowing through the kidney, decreased tubular flow rate (or fewer sodium ions) sensed by the macula densa, and activation of the sympathetic nervous system. Conversely, the factors that decrease renin secretion lower blood pressure. These factors are illustrated in Figure 34.3.

Increasing renin secretion will not always cause an increase in blood pressure. Remember that RAAS is a two-step pathway, and both steps are essential to produce a physiological response. Section 34.3 examines this second step.

CONNECTION *Checkpoint* 34.2

From what you learned in Chapter 16, other than JG cells, in what organ are beta$_1$-adrenergic receptors predominately located? What is the response of that organ when these receptors are activated? See Answer to Connection Checkpoint 34.2 in Appendix A.

34.3 Angiotensin-converting enzyme is responsible for the formation of angiotensin II.

Once angiotensin I is formed, its conversion to angiotensin II by ACE is almost instantaneous. This is because ACE lies on the membranes of blood vessels and has immediate access to angiotensin I as soon as it is formed. A single pass of the blood through lung capillaries can convert most of the circulating angiotensin I to angiotensin II.

In addition to its role in the formation of angiotensin II, ACE has a second function important to homeostasis and

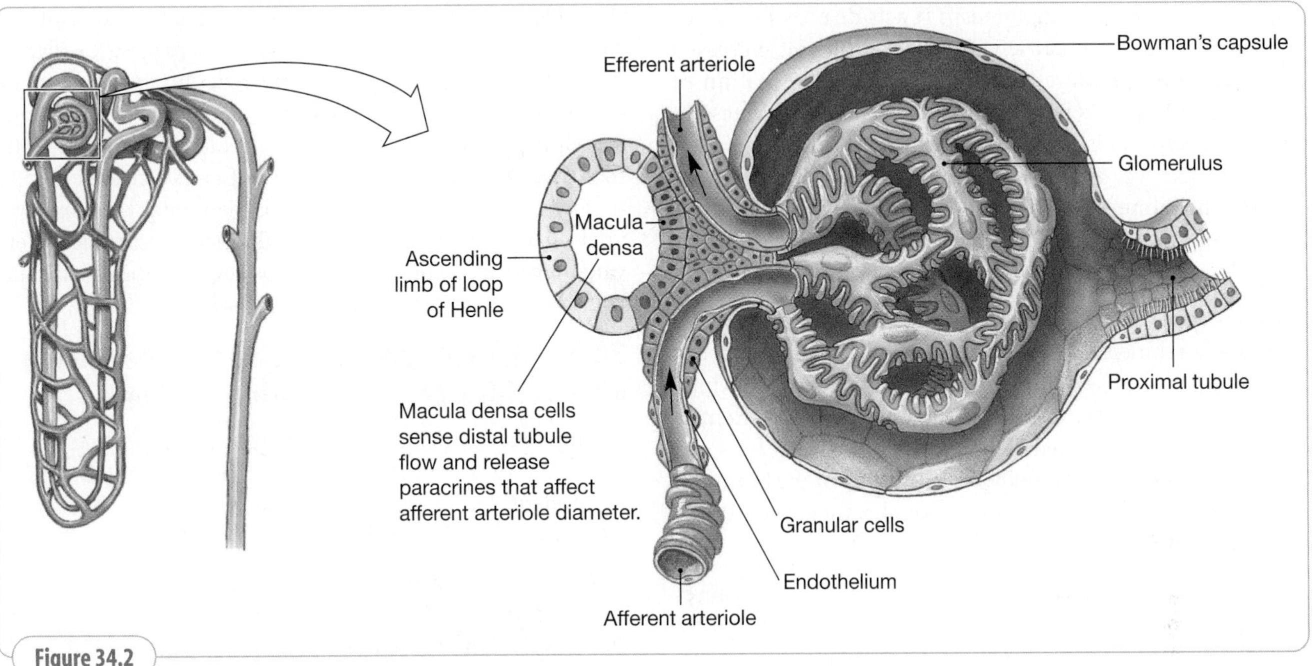

Figure 34.2

The macula densa and the juxtaglomerular (JG) cells. Osmoreceptors in the macula densa sense low sodium levels, which signals the JG cells to release renin.

Source: From *Human Physiology: An Integrated Approach* (4th ed.), by D. U. Silverthorn, 2006, San Francisco: Pearson/Benjamin Cummings.

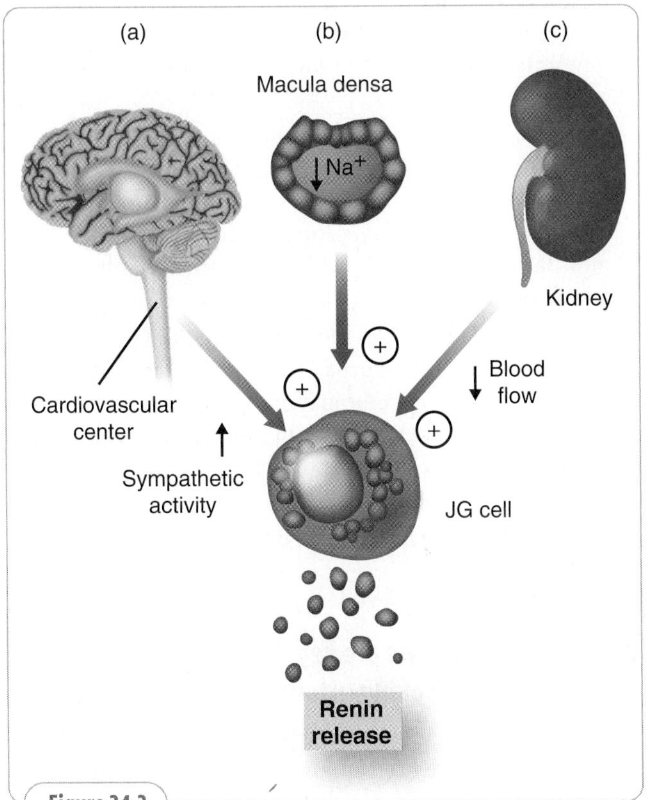

pharmacotherapy. ACE is one of several enzymes that break down **bradykinin**, a natural mediator of inflammation and pain. Bradykinin has many of the same effects as histamine (see Chapter 44), including increasing arteriolar vasodilation and vascular permeability, and is likely responsible for some of the adverse effects of the ACE inhibitor medications. When referring to its actions on bradykinin, ACE is sometimes called kinase II; *kinase* is the general term for an enzyme that breaks down kinins. ACE and kinase II refer to the identical enzyme.

Pharmacologically, ACE is an important enzyme in the RAAS because it serves as a target molecule for drugs in the ACE inhibitor class of medications. Inhibition of ACE will prevent the formation of angiotensin II, thus interrupting the RAAS pathway. These medications also inhibit kinase II, thus preventing the breakdown of bradykinin. Accumulation of bradykinin in certain tissues can cause several adverse effects of ACE inhibitors, such as angioedema and cough.

Physiological Effects of the Renin-Angiotensin-Aldosterone System

34.4 Angiotensin II has multiple effects on the cardiovascular system that raise blood pressure and affect cardiac function.

The final product of the two-step renin-angiotensin pathway is angiotensin II. Angiotensin II has several important physiological effects important to homeostasis and to pharmacotherapy.

Figure 34.3

Overview of factors affecting renin release: (a) activation of the sympathetic nervous system; (b) low osmolarity in the macula densa; (c) low blood flow through the kidney.

Direct vasoconstriction: Angiotensin II acts directly on vascular smooth muscle to cause vasoconstriction and increased systemic blood pressure. This effect is rapid; formation of angiotensin II results in nearly an instantaneous increase in blood pressure. This vasopressor action of angiotensin II is much greater on arterioles compared to veins; arterioles serving the kidneys are especially sensitive to this vasopressor action.

Increased sympathetic nervous system activity: Angiotensin II activates the sympathetic nervous system by causing the release of norepinephrine from sympathetic nerve terminals. The adrenal medulla is also affected by angiotensin II, which responds by releasing additional epinephrine to the circulation. Furthermore, through largely unknown mechanisms, angiotensin II increases sympathetic outflow from the brain. All three of these actions increase peripheral resistance and raise blood pressure.

Alteration of cardiovascular structure: Angiotensin II causes hypertrophy of myocardial cells (myocytes) and promotes collagen deposits in the cardiac matrix, essentially forming scar-like tissue in the heart. These changes are known as **cardiac remodeling.** The hypertrophy, fibrosis, and remodeling of cardiac structure has been correlated to increased morbidity and mortality associated with heart disease. In blood vessels, angiotensin II causes the release of multiple chemical mediators of atherosclerosis, accelerating the deposition of fatty plaque deposits on the walls of the vessels. Increased plaque deposits lead to an increased risk for myocardial infarction (MI) and cerebrovascular accident (CVA).

CONNECTION *Checkpoint* 34.3

From what you learned in Chapter 31, what effect would you expect angiotensin II formation to have on cardiac output and afterload? See Answer to Connection Checkpoint 34.3 in Appendix A.

Release of aldosterone and effects on the renal tubule: Angiotensin II has two primary effects on the kidney that promote an increase in blood pressure. First, angiotensin II has a direct effect on the nephron that increases Na^+ and Cl^- reabsorption in the proximal tubule. Second, angiotensin II indirectly affects sodium reabsorption by stimulating the adrenal cortex to synthesize and secrete additional amounts of the hormone aldosterone. Aldosterone acts on the distal and collecting tubules of the nephron to increase Na^+ reabsorption and K^+ and H^+ excretion. The enhanced sodium reabsorption from both direct and indirect actions of angiotensin II causes the body to retain water, thus increasing blood volume and raising blood pressure. Aldosterone is an essential component of the RAAS.

Unlike its immediate and direct effects on sympathetic nerves, the actions of angiotensin II on the kidney develop more slowly. This slow vasopressor response is believed to be responsible for producing a sustained elevation of blood pressure and a gradual decline of renal function.

Students often think of angiotensin II as a "bad actor" because it can create HTN and result in damaging cardiac remodeling. It must be remembered, however, that the cardiovascular and renal effects of angiotensin II serve an essential homeostatic function. Should blood pressure fall, the increased synthesis and production of angiotensin II help return blood pressure to normal levels to maintain blood flow to vital organs. When the body is subjected to chronically elevated levels of angiotensin II, however, the once vital reflex pathway becomes a detriment to the body.

34.5 The renin-angiotensin-aldosterone pathway offers multiple points for drug intervention.

Having learned details of the different components in the short pathway leading from angiotensinogen to angiotensin II, the student should recognize several potential mechanisms by which drugs could intervene.

- **ACE inhibitors.** These are the first and, thus far, the largest and most important class of agents modifying the RAAS. ACE inhibitors block the conversion of angiotensin I to angiotensin II.
- **Angiotensin receptor blockers.** After angiotensin II is formed, it must interact with its receptors on target cells to cause its biologic actions. There are two receptor subtypes, known as AT_1 and AT_2 receptors. Blocking AT_1 receptors prevents angiotensin from raising blood pressure and from causing cardiac remodeling. Angiotensin receptor blockers are medications that intervene at this step in the RAAS by blocking the AT_1 receptor. The role of the AT_2 receptor in physiology is largely unknown but is an area of active research.
- **Aldosterone antagonists.** Much of the blood pressure increase resulting from the formation of angiotensin II is caused by its stimulation of aldosterone secretion. Two drugs are available that block receptors for aldosterone in the kidney, thus preventing the aldosterone-induced increase in blood pressure.
- **Renin inhibitors.** In 2007, the FDA approved the first renin inhibitor. Aliskiren (Tekurna) is approved to treat HTN as monotherapy or in combination with other antihypertensives. It is likely that other renin inhibitors will be submitted for FDA approval in the future.

Drugs Affecting the Renin-Angiotensin-Aldosterone System

34.6 ACE inhibitors are key drugs in the pharmacotherapy of hypertension and heart failure.

First detected in the venom of pit vipers in the 1960s, inhibitors of ACE have been approved for HTN since the 1980s. Since then drugs in this class have become first-line agents in the treatment of HTN and heart failure. Doses for the ACE inhibitors are listed in Table 34.1

ACE inhibitors block the conversion of angiotensin I to angiotensin II. The decline in angiotensin II levels causes blood

CONNECTIONS

To the Community

Body Weight and Hypertension

Hypertension (HTN) is often associated with body weight and changes in body weight over time. Overweight people are more likely to have high-normal to mild high blood pressure. Even moderately obese adults have an increased risk of HTN. Weight gain can mean elevated blood pressure in older adults, and obesity in children and youth can result in high blood pressure in adulthood.

If a patient is overweight or has gained weight over time, the nurse should counsel the patient to reduce calorie intake, incrementally increase physical activity, and lose weight gradually. Reduced caloric intake alone seldom results in weight loss for most people. The health care provider may prescribe an appropriate diet for the patient, considering other health concerns. The patient should reduce alcohol intake, because alcoholic drinks are high in empty or nonnutritious calories. Often when one loses weight and gradually increases physical activity, the blood pressure drops as well.

Thin people can have HTN and be at risk for heart attacks and stroke as well. Thin people with HTN may have other health concerns such as an enlarged heart. Low-birth-weight babies, especially females, may have high blood pressure in childhood and adulthood.

pressure to decrease because there is less sympathetic activation, thus lowering peripheral resistance. In addition, the decreased aldosterone secretion reduces blood volume, which also contributes to blood pressure reduction.

CONNECTION *Checkpoint* 34.4

Knowing that ACE inhibitors decrease sympathetic activation, what type of interaction (additive or antagonistic) would you expect from the autonomic drugs atropine, epinephrine, and propranolol? See Answer to Connection Checkpoint 34.4 in Appendix A.

Research studies have clearly demonstrated that ACE inhibitors can slow the progression of heart failure and reduce mortality from this disease. This is likely due to both the reduction in systemic blood pressure and a reversal of the angiotensin II-induced structural changes in the heart. Because of their relative safety, they have replaced digoxin (Lanoxin) as the first-line drugs for the treatment of chronic heart failure. Indeed, unless specifically contraindicated, all patients with heart failure should receive an ACE inhibitor, as discussed in Chapter 38.

Research has also indicated a clear benefit for administering ACE inhibitors to patients who have suffered a recent MI. If therapy is begun immediately after the infarction and continued for several weeks, these drugs lower the mortality associated with an acute MI. The mechanism by which these drugs improve the outcome following an acute MI involves reduced peripheral vascular resistance, improved perfusion, and a direct action on the myocardium that reduces the cardiac workload.

ACE inhibitors may also be prescribed as prophylaxis therapy in patients at high risk for an adverse cardiovascular event. ACE inhibitors can reduce the incidence of a CVA or MI in these high-risk patients. They may also prevent or delay the progression of renal disease and retinopathy in patients with diabetes.

At least 11 ACE inhibitors have been approved and all have very similar indications and adverse effect profiles. All drugs in this class are approved to treat HTN, although only a few are approved for heart failure and acute MI and for prophylaxis of cardiovascular disease. With the exception of enalaprilat, ACE inhibitors are administered orally (PO), and nearly all offer the convenience of once-daily dosing. Many of the ACE inhibitors are prodrugs, which are converted to active metabolites by enzymes in the liver. Most ACE inhibitors are excreted by the kidneys; thus dose reductions may be required in patients with significant renal impairment.

TABLE 34.1 ACE Inhibitors

Drug	Route and Adult Dose (maximum dose where indicated)	Adverse Effects
benazepril (Lotensin)	PO: 10–40 mg in one to two divided doses (max: 40 mg/day)	*Headache, dry cough, dizziness, orthostatic hypotension, rash* Angioedema, acute renal failure, first-dose phenomenon
captopril (Capoten)	PO: 6.25–25 mg tid (max: 450 mg/day)	
enalapril (Vasotec)	PO: 5–40 mg in one to two divided doses (max: 40 mg/day)	
fosinopril (Monopril)	PO: 5–40 mg daily (max: 40 mg/day)	
lisinopril (Prinivil, Zestril)	PO: 10 mg daily (max: 80 mg/day)	
moexipril (Univasc)	PO: 7.5–30 mg daily (max: 30 mg/day)	
perindopril (Aceon)	PO: 4 mg once daily (max: 16 mg/day for HTN; 4 mg/day for heart failure)	
quinapril (Accupril)	PO: 10–20 mg daily (max: 80 mg/day)	
ramipril (Altace)	PO: 2.5–5 mg daily (max: 20 mg/day)	
trandolapril (Mavik)	PO: 1–4 mg daily (max: 8 mg/day)	

Note: *Italics* indicate common adverse effects. Underline indicates serious adverse effects.

The low incidence of serious adverse effects is a major contributing factor to the widespread use of the ACE inhibitors. Orthostatic hypotension following the first few doses of the drug can be severe in patients who are on low sodium diets or who have heart failure. Drug therapy is sometimes begun with very low doses and increased gradually to avoid orthostatic hypotension. Hyperkalemia may occur during ACE inhibitor therapy; however, this is a major concern only for patients with diabetes, those with renal impairment, and those who are taking potassium supplements or potassium-sparing diuretics. Persistent, dry cough is an annoying adverse effect that occurs in 5% to 20% of patients taking ACE inhibitors. This adverse effect is likely due to a buildup of bradykinin in the lung. Drugs in this class have minimal or no effect on serum glucose or uric acid levels.

Though rare, the most serious adverse effect of ACE inhibitors is the development of **angioedema**, a rapid swelling of the throat, face, larynx, and tongue that can lead to airway obstruction and death. When it does occur, angioedema most often develops within a few hours after the first dose, although it may occur after several days of ACE inhibitor therapy. Accumulation of bradykinin is thought to be responsible. Treatment of angioedema is to discontinue the drug immediately and maintain the airway until the effects of the drug wear off.

Pharm*FACT*

Ninety-four percent of all angioedema cases are drug induced, and ACE inhibitors are the most frequent medication causing this disorder. Although the incidence of angioedema in patients taking ACE inhibitors is only 0.1% to 0.2%, the mortality rate is 11%. African Americans have an almost five times greater risk of experiencing angioedema than do Caucasians. *Source:* Reid & Eurle, 2005.

PROTOTYPE DRUG Lisinopril (Prinivil, Zestril)

Classification: **Therapeutic:** Antihypertensive
Pharmacologic: ACE inhibitor

Therapeutic Effects and Uses: Approved for the treatment of heart failure, HTN, and acute MI, lisinopril is one of the most frequently prescribed medications. Approved in 1987, it may be used as monotherapy or it may be combined with other agents: The fixed-dose combination of lisinopril and hydrochlorothiazide (a diuretic) is marketed for HTN as Zestoretic. Unlike many drugs in this class, lisinopril is active itself; it is not a prodrug. Treatment of migraines is an off-label indication for lisinopril.

Although captopril was the first drug that was marketed in this class, lisinopril is more widely prescribed because it has a longer duration of action that allows for once-daily dosing. Like other ACE inhibitors, 2 to 3 weeks of therapy may be required to achieve maximum therapeutic outcomes.

Mechanism of Action: Lisinopril binds to and inhibits the action of ACE, thus preventing the conversion of angiotensin I to angiotensin II. The decrease in serum angiotensin II reduces aldosterone secretion, which results in less sodium and water retention. In patients with HTN, blood pressure is reduced with minimal effect on heart rate, stroke volume, or cardiac output.

Pharmacokinetics:

Route(s)	PO
Absorption	25–30% absorbed from the gastrointestinal (GI) tract
Distribution	Small amount crosses the blood–brain barrier; crosses the placenta; limited amounts are secreted in breast milk; not bound to plasma protein
Primary metabolism	Not metabolized
Primary excretion	Renal
Onset of action	1 h; peak effect: 6–8 h
Duration of action	24 h; half-life: 12 h

Adverse Effects: Lisinopril is well tolerated and adverse effects are uncommon and transient. The most common adverse effects are cough, headache, dizziness, orthostatic hypotension, and rash. Hyperkalemia occurs in about 2% to 4% of patients taking ACE inhibitors, although this usually resolves during therapy. Patients with congestive heart failure (CHF) or renal impairment, or who are taking potassium supplements or potassium-sparing diuretics are at highest risk for hyperkalemia. Rare, though serious adverse effects include angioedema, agranulocytosis, and hepatotoxicity.

Contraindications/Precautions: Lisinopril should be used with extreme caution in patients with hyperkalemia because they may experience serious and even fatal dysrhythmias. Patients with a history of angioedema should not receive lisinopril. Serious fetal and neonatal injury may occur when ACE inhibitors are taken during the second and third trimesters; thus lisinopril should not be used during pregnancy. Caution should be used in treating patients with serious renal impairment: Dosage should be reduced.

Drug Interactions: Indomethacin and other nonsteroidal anti-inflammatory drugs (NSAIDs) interact with lisinopril to decrease antihypertensive activity. The combination of lisinopril and NSAIDs may also worsen preexisting renal disease. Because of synergistic hypotensive action, concurrent therapy with diuretics and other antihypertensives such as ACE inhibitors should be carefully monitored. When taken with potassium supplements or potassium-sparing diuretics, hyperkalemia may result. Lisinopril may increase lithium levels and toxicity. **Herbal/Food:** Hawthorn should not be taken concurrently with lisinopril due to the possibility of additive hypotensive action.

Pregnancy: Categories C (first trimester) and D (second and third trimesters).

Treatment of Overdose: Overdose will cause hypotension, which may be treated with normal saline or a vasopressor. The drug may also be removed by hemodialysis.

Nursing Responsibilities:

- Obtain a complete health history, including data on recent cardiac events, allergies, drug history, and possible drug interactions.
- Notify the prescriber if the patient has kidney disease (or is on dialysis), liver disease, CHF, diabetes, or connective tissue disease such as lupus, scleroderma, or rheumatoid arthritis.
- Monitor blood pressure before administration of the drug and 30 minutes to 1 hour after. Withhold the drug and notify the prescriber if systolic blood pressure drops below 90.
- Keep the patient in the supine position and notify the prescriber if sudden and severe hypotension occurs within the first 1 to 5 hours of the initial drug dose. Closely monitor patients who are taking diuretic therapy who have hyponatremia or are volume depleted.
- Evaluate the antihypertensive effect of the drug. Consult with the prescriber if HTN is not controlled by the drug.
- Discontinue the drug and immediately notify the prescriber if there is any evidence of angioedema of the extremities, face, lips, tongue, glottis, and larynx. Assess for airway obstruction.
- Monitor serum sodium and serum potassium levels for hyponatremia and hyperkalemia, respectively.
- Although a rare complication, monitor patients with renal impairment, systemic lupus, or scleroderma for drug-induced neutropenia. Determine the white blood cell (WBC) count prior to initiation of treatment every month for the first 3 to 6 months of therapy and at regular intervals. Withhold therapy and notify the health care provider if the neutrophil count falls below 1,000/mm^3.
- Monitor kidney function tests regularly in patients with severe volume or sodium replacement or those with advanced CHF.
- Monitor lithium levels frequently if the patient is receiving lithium therapy because ACE inhibitors contribute to lithium accumulation.

Patient and Family Education:

- Monitor blood pressure regularly as directed by the health care provider. Maintain a written log of blood pressure readings and present it at follow-up visits.
- Immediately report any swelling of the face, mouth, hands, or feet; hoarseness; sudden trouble breathing; or any sign of infection such as fever or sore throat to the health care provider.
- Proper diet, including sodium and potassium restrictions, is important to the management of hypertension and heart failure. Avoid salt substitutes that contain potassium.
- Report vomiting, diarrhea, or heavy sweating to the health care provider because these can cause dehydration, leading to low blood pressure, electrolyte disorders, or kidney failure.
- Take a missed dose as soon as remembered, unless it is almost time for the next scheduled dose. Never take a double dose of this medicine.
- Do not drive or perform other potentially hazardous activities until the effects of the drug are known because this drug may cause adverse effects that impair thinking and reaction time.
- Make position changes slowly when moving from a lying to a standing position because this drug may cause drowsiness and possible fainting.
- Drink at least 6 to 8 glasses of water per day when taking this drug.
- Do not drink alcohol because this can cause low blood pressure and fainting.
- Avoid over-the-counter (OTC) NSAIDs such as aspirin, ibuprofen, and naproxen because these drugs can reduce the effectiveness of ACE inhibitors.
- Keep all scheduled appointments with the health care provider for checkups.
- Immediately inform the health care provider of any known or suspected pregnancy because these drugs can cause birth defects.
- Do not breast-feed while taking this drug without approval of the health care provider.

MyNursingKit | Mechanism of Action Animation: Lisinopril

Drugs Similar to Lisinopril (Prinivil, Zestril)

There are 11 ACE inhibitors on the market. All have very similar actions and adverse effects.

Benazepril (Lotensin): Approved in 1991, benazepril is approved only for HTN, although an off-label indication is heart failure. It is a prodrug that is metabolized by hepatic enzymes to its active form, benazeprilat. It has a long duration of action that allows for once-daily dosing and is excreted by the kidneys. Orthostatic hypotension is the most common adverse effect, especially after the first dose. Other adverse effects, contraindications, and indications are the same as lisinopril. Lotensin HCT is a fixed-dose combination of benazepril and hydrochlorothiazide. This drug is pregnancy category C (first trimester) and D (second and third trimesters).

Captopril (Capoten): Captopril, the first ACE inhibitor marketed in 1981, is approved for HTN, heart failure, left ventricular dysfunction after an acute MI, and diabetic nephropathy. It has a short half-life, which requires multiple daily doses for some patients. The drug should be taken on an empty stomach, because food reduces its bioavailability. Adverse effects, contraindications, and indications are the same as those of lisinopril. Capozide is a fixed-dose combination of captopril and hydrochlorothiazide. This is a pregnancy category D drug.

Enalapril (Vasotec): Approved in 1985, enalapril is approved for HTN, heart failure, and asymptomatic left ventricular dysfunction in post-MI patients. Like most drugs in this class, it has an extended half-life and is excreted by the kidneys. It has a shorter half-life than some ACE inhibitors and may require twice-daily dosing. Enalapril is a prodrug, being converted by hepatic enzymes to enalaprilat, which is its active form. The most frequent adverse effect is hypotension, which can be especially troublesome in patients with CHF. Adverse effects, contraindications, and indications are the same as lisinopril. Enalaprilat (Vasotec IV) is available as a drug for severe HTN and is the only ACE inhibitor administered parenterally. Vaseretic is a fixed-dose combination of enalapril and hydrochlorothiazide. Both enalapril and enalaprilat are pregnancy category D drugs.

Fosinopril (Monopril): Approved in 1991, fosinopril is approved for HTN and heart failure. It is a prodrug that is metabolized by hepatic enzymes to its active form, fosinoprilat. An extended half-life allows for once-daily dosing, and it may be taken without regard to meals. It is excreted by both the liver and kidneys and does not require a dosage adjustment in patients with renal impairment. The most common adverse effects of fosinopril are orthostatic hypotension, dizziness, and headache. Monopril HCT is a fixed-dose combination of Monopril and hydrochlorothiazide. This drug is pregnancy category C (first trimester) and D (second and third trimesters).

Moexipril (Univasc): Approved in 1995 moexipril is indicated only for HTN. It is a prodrug that is metabolized to its active form, moexiprilat, by hepatic enzymes. An extended half-life allows for once-daily dosing. This drug should be taken on an empty stomach, because food reduces its bioavailability by 40% to 50%. It is excreted by the kidneys, and dosage should be reduced in patients with renal impairment. Dizziness is one of the most common adverse effects. Adverse effects, contraindications, and indications are the same as lisinopril. Uniretic is a fixed-dose combination of moexipril and hydrochlorothiazide. Moexipril is a pregnancy category D drug.

Perindopril (Aceon): Approved in 1993, perindopril is approved for HTN and the prophylaxis of cardiovascular events such as MI in patients with coronary artery disease. Heart failure is an off-label use. It is a prodrug that is metabolized by hepatic enzymes to its active form, perindoprilat. It is excreted by the kidneys and its long half-life allows for once- or twice-daily dosing. Food may reduce the bioavailability of the drug by as much as 35%. Cough and dizziness are the most frequent adverse effects of perindopril. Other adverse effects, contraindications, and indications are the same as those of lisinopril. This is a pregnancy category D drug.

Quinapril (Accupril): Approved in 1991, quinapril is indicated for HTN and heart failure. It is a prodrug that is metabolized by hepatic enzymes to its active form, quinaprilat, and may be dosed either once or twice daily. Because the kidney contributes to about 96% of the excretion of the drug, doses should be reduced in patients with renal impairment. Adverse effects are generally mild and transient and include dizziness, cough, and diarrhea. Other adverse effects, contraindications, and indications are the same as those of lisinopril. Accuretic is a fixed-dose combination of quinapril and hydrochlorothiazide. This is a pregnancy category D drug.

Ramipril (Altace): Approved in 1991, ramipril is indicated for HTN and heart failure following an MI, and to reduce mortality and CVA in high-risk patients with left ventricular dysfunction after an acute MI. It is a prodrug that is metabolized by hepatic enzymes to its active form, ramiprilat. Excretion is predominantly renal, and dosage should be reduced in patients with serious renal impairment. It may be administered without regard to meals. The most common adverse effects are orthostatic hypotension, dizziness, and headache. Other adverse effects, contraindications, and indications are the same as those of lisinopril. This is a pregnancy category D drug.

Trandolapril (Mavik): Approved in 1996, trandolapril is indicated for HTN and heart failure following an MI, and to reduce the mortality in high-risk patients with left ventricular dysfunction after an acute MI. It is a prodrug that is metabolized by hepatic enzymes to trandolaprilat, its active form. It has an extended half-life that permits once-daily dosing and may be administered without regard to meals. Unlike other ACE inhibitors, a large amount of trandolapril (66%) is excreted in the feces. Dosages should be lowered in patients with hepatic or renal impairment. The most common adverse effects are cough, dizziness, and fatigue. Other adverse effects, contraindications, and indications are the same as those of lisinopril. Tarka is a fixed-dose combination of trandolapril and the calcium channel blocker verapamil SR, which is prescribed for HTN. This is a pregnancy category D drug.

34.7 Angiotensin II receptor blockers act by inhibiting the AT_1 receptor and are used for hypertension and heart failure.

While pharmacologists were examining the mechanism of action of the ACE inhibitors in the 1980s and developing drugs in this class, research continued on the other enzymes and components of the RAAS. The receptors for angiotensin II in smooth muscle, known as AT_1 and AT_2, were identified and a new class of drugs, called the angiotensin II receptor blockers (ARBs), was developed. The ARBs are selective for AT_1-type receptors. Unlike the ACE inhibitors, ARBs do not prevent the formation of angiotensin II, but they do effectively prevent it from activating their target receptors. Doses for the ARBS are listed in Table 34.2.

The ARBs cause vasodilation, with a resultant reduction in peripheral resistance and fall in blood pressure, by blocking angiotensin II receptors in arteriolar smooth muscle, The ARBs' blockade of AT_1 receptors in the adrenal gland prevents secretion of aldosterone and promotes increased Na^+ and excretion of water by the kidneys. Blockade of AT_1 receptors in the heart prevents the destructive effects of angiotensin-induced cardiac remodeling. Although they act by a different mechanism, ARBs essentially produce the same pharmacotherapeutic actions as the ACE inhibitors.

NURSING PROCESS APPLICATION

Patients Receiving Angiotensin-Converting Enzyme (ACE) Inhibitor Therapy

Assessment	Potential Nursing Diagnoses
Prior to administration: • Obtain a complete health history, including data on recent cardiac events and any incidence of angioedema, allergies, drug history, and possible drug interactions. • Obtain an ECG and vital signs; assess in the context of the patient's baseline values. • Assess neurologic status and level of consciousness. • Obtain blood and urine specimens for laboratory analysis. • Determine pregnancy status in women who are within the childbearing age group.	• *Risk for Injury,* related to orthostatic hypotension and electrolyte imbalance (hyperkalemia) • *Deficient Knowledge (Drug Therapy)*

Planning: Patient Goals and Expected Outcomes

The patient will:

- Exhibit a reduction in systolic/diastolic blood pressure.
- Maintain normal serum electrolyte levels during drug therapy.
- Demonstrate an understanding of the drug's action by accurately describing drug adverse effects and precautions.

Implementation

Interventions and (Rationales)	Patient and Family Education
• Monitor for profound hypotension. (ACE inhibitors can cause "first-dose phenomenon" with initial doses.)	• Warn the patient about the first-dose phenomenon; reassure that this effect diminishes with continued therapy. Instruct the patient: • That changes in consciousness may occur due to rapid reduction in blood pressure; immediately report feelings of faintness. • To rest in the supine position beginning 1 hour after administration and for 3 to 4 hours after the first dose. • To always arise slowly, avoiding sudden position changes.
• Observe for hypersensitivity reaction, particularly angioedema. (Angioedema may occur at any time during ACE inhibitor therapy but is generally expected shortly after initiation of therapy.)	• Instruct the patient: • To immediately seek medical attention for difficulty breathing, throat tightness, muscle cramps, hives or rash, or tremors. These symptoms can occur on the first dose or much later as a delayed reaction. • That angioedema can be life threatening and to call emergency medical services if severe dyspnea or hoarseness is accompanied by swelling of the face or mouth.
• Monitor for neutropenia and signs of infection. (ACE inhibitors can lower white blood cell count and decrease the ability to fight infection.)	• Instruct the patient to immediately report any flulike symptoms such as fever, sore throat, malaise, and joint pain.
• Monitor for changes in level of consciousness, dizziness, drowsiness, or light-headedness. (ACE inhibitors can cause decreased circulation to the brain due to vasodilation.)	Instruct the patient to: • Report dizziness or fainting that persists beyond the first dose as well as unusual sensations such as numbness and tingling or other changes in the face or limbs. Sudden collapse is possible. • Contact the health care provider before the next scheduled dose of the drug if fainting occurs.
• Monitor for persistent dry cough. (ACE inhibitors affect the proinflammatory action of bradykinin.) • Monitor changes in cough pattern. (This may indicate another disease process.)	Instruct the patient to: • Report persistent dry cough to the prescriber. • Report any change in the character or frequency of cough. Any cough accompanied by shortness of breath, fever, or chest pain should be reported immediately because it may indicate MI. • Sleep with the head elevated if cough becomes troublesome when in the supine position. • Use nonmedicated sugar-free lozenges or hard candies to relieve cough.
• Monitor for hyperkalemia. (May occur due to reduced aldosterone levels, especially in patients with CHF, impaired kidney function, and diabetes.)	Instruct the patient to: • Immediately report signs of hyperkalemia such as nausea, irregular heartbeat, profound fatigue or muscle weakness, and slow or faint pulse. • Avoid consuming electrolyte-fortified snacks or sports drinks that may contain potassium. • Avoid using salt substitute (KCl) to flavor foods. • Consult the health care provider before taking any nutritional supplements containing potassium.

(continued)

NURSING PROCESS APPLICATION *(continued)*

• Monitor liver and kidney function. (ACE inhibitors are metabolized by the liver and excreted by the kidneys.)	Instruct the patient to: • Report signs of liver toxicity such as nausea, vomiting, anorexia, diarrhea, rash, jaundice, abdominal pain, tenderness or distention, or change in the color or character of stools. • Discontinue the drug immediately and contact the health care provider if jaundice occurs. • Adhere to laboratory testing regimen as ordered by the health care provider.
• Monitor for safe ambulation until response to the drug is known. (ACE inhibitors may cause orthostatic hypotension and/or dizziness.)	Instruct the patient to: • Obtain help prior to getting out of bed or attempting to walk alone. • Avoid driving or performing other activities that require mental alertness or physical coordination until the effects of the drug are known.

Evaluation of Outcome Criteria

Evaluate the effectiveness of drug therapy by confirming that patient goals and expected outcomes have been met (see "Planning").

The indications for ARBs are the same as those for the ACE inhibitors. All are approved to treat HTN, and they are often combined with drugs from other classes. Valsartan (Diovan) and candesartan (Atacand) were also approved to treat heart failure in 2005. Some are approved to treat MI and are used for the prophylaxis of CVA. All are administered orally and have prolonged half-lives that permit once-daily dosing. A few are prodrugs and most are extensively bound to plasma proteins.

Are the ARBs identical to the ACE inhibitors? Not exactly. Unlike the ACE inhibitors, they do not cause cough, and angioedema is less common with ARBs. This is because ARBs do not promote the accumulation of bradykinin, as is the case of the ACE inhibitors. ARBs can, however, cause dizziness, hypotension, and hyperkalemia, especially in patients with renal impairment or who are concurrently taking potassium supplements or potassium-sparing diuretics.

TABLE 34.2 Angiotensin II Receptor Blockers, Aldosterone Antagonists, and Renin Inhibitors

Drug	Route and Adult Dose (maximum dose where indicated)	Adverse Effects
Angiotensin II Receptor Blockers		
candesartan (Atacand)	PO: start at 16 mg/day for HTN and 4 mg/day for heart failure (max: 32 mg/day)	*Headache, dizziness, orthostatic hypotension, rash* <u>Angioedema, acute renal failure, first-dose phenomenon</u>
eprosartan (Teveten)	PO: 600 mg/day or 400 mg PO qid–bid (max: 800 mg/day)	
irbesartan (Avapro)	PO: 150–300 mg/day (max: 300 mg/day)	
losartan (Cozaar)	PO: 25–50 mg in one to two divided doses (max: 100 mg/day)	
olmesartan medoxomil (Benicar)	PO: 20–40 mg/day	
telmisartan (Micardis)	PO: 40 mg/day (max: 80 mg/day	
valsartan (Diovan)	PO: 80 mg/day (max: 320 mg/day)	
Aldosterone Antagonists		
eplerenone (Inspra)	PO: start with 25–50 mg/day; (max: 100 mg/day for HTN; 50 mg/day for heart failure)	*Minor hyperkalemia, headache, fatigue, gynecomastia (spironolactone)* <u>Dysrhythmias (from hyperkalemia), dehydration, hyponatremia, agranulocytosis and other blood dyscrasias</u>
spironolactone (Aldactone)	PO: 50–100 mg/day in single or divided doses (max: 400 mg/day)	
Renin Inhibitor		
aliskiren (Tekurna)	PO: 150 mg/day (max: 300 mg/day)	*Diarrhea, hypotension, cough* <u>Angioedema</u>

Note: *Italics* indicate common adverse effects. <u>Underline</u> indicates serious adverse effects.

If ARBs have the same pharmacologic actions and an improved safety profile, why have they not replaced the ACE inhibitors? The answer is because the ACE inhibitors are generally less expensive, and health care providers have much more clinical experience prescribing them. Because the ARBs are newer, a significant body of research has not yet accumulated that demonstrates clear benefits over the ACE inhibitors. Because of these factors, the ARBs are usually reserved for patients unable to tolerate the adverse effects of ACE inhibitors.

PROTOTYPE DRUG Losartan (Cozaar)

Classification: Therapeutic: Antihypertensive
Pharmacologic: Angiotensin II receptor blocker

Therapeutic Effects and Uses: Approved for the treatment of HTN, CVA prophylaxis in patients with left ventricular hypertrophy, and the prevention of diabetic nephropathy, losartan was the first ARB marketed in 1995. An off-label use is for heart failure. Although losartan undergoes extensive first-pass metabolism and has a short half-life, it is metabolized to an active intermediate that exerts more prolonged action, allowing for once-daily dosing. Its actions include vasodilation and reduced blood volume, due to the drug blocking the release of aldosterone by angiotensin II. Hyzaar is a fixed-dose combination of losartan and hydrochlorothiazide.

Mechanism of Action: Losartan selectively blocks angiotensin AT_1 receptors, resulting in a decline in blood pressure. The blockade of angiotensin II receptors prevents cardiac remodeling and deterioration of renal function in patients with diabetes.

Pharmacokinetics:

Route(s)	PO
Absorption	Well absorbed from the GI tract
Distribution	Does not appear to cross the blood–brain barrier or the placenta, or to be secreted in breast milk; approximately 99% bound to protein
Primary metabolism	Hepatic: extensive first-pass metabolism; converted to active metabolite
Primary excretion	35% renal, 60% in feces
Onset of action	Peak effect: 6 h
Duration of action	Half-life: 1.5–2 h (losartan), 6–9 h (active metabolite)

Adverse Effects: The incidence of adverse effects of losartan is very low. The most common adverse effects are headache, dizziness, nasal congestion, fatigue, and insomnia. Serious adverse effects include angioedema and acute renal failure.

Contraindications/Precautions: Losartan is contraindicated in patients with prior hypersensitivity to the drug. Because ARBs exhibit the same teratogenic effects as ACE inhibitors, they should not be used during pregnancy and lactation. Caution should be used in treating patients with serious renal or hepatic impairment and dosage may need to be reduced. Patients with a history of angioedema should be monitored carefully. Patients with hypovolemia are at high risk of symptomatic hypotension during therapy. Hypovolemia should be corrected prior to administration of losartan.

Drug Interactions: The drug interactions of losartan and other ARBs are similar to those of the ACE inhibitors. Indomethacin and other NSAIDs may decrease the antihypertensive activity of losartan. When taken concurrently with potassium supplements or potassium-sparing diuretics, care must be taken to avoid hyperkalemia. Concurrent use of losartan with diuretics and other antihypertensives may cause additive hypotensive effects. Use with alcohol may also add to the hypotensive effects of losartan. Losartan may increase lithium levels and toxicity. **Herbal/Food:** Hawthorn should not be taken concurrently with losartan due to the possibility of additive hypotensive action.

Pregnancy: Categories C (first trimester) and D (second and third trimesters).

Treatment of Overdose: Overdose will cause hypotension, which may be treated with an infusion of normal saline or a vasopressor. The drug is not removed by hemodialysis.

Nursing Responsibilities:

- Obtain a complete health history, including data on recent cardiac events, allergies, drug history, and possible drug interactions.
- If evident, any volume depletion should be corrected prior to initiating therapy.
- Notify the prescriber if the patient has serious renal or hepatic impairment, history of angioedema, or hypovolemia.
- Monitor blood pressure at drug trough (prior to a scheduled dose).
- Evaluate the antihypertensive effect of the drug. Consult with the prescriber if HTN is not controlled by the drug. Monitor drug effectiveness, especially in African Americans, when this drug is used as monotherapy.
- Monitor lab tests such as complete blood count (CBC), electrolytes, and liver and kidney function with long-term therapy.

Patient and Family Education:

- Monitor blood pressure regularly as directed by the health care provider. Maintain a written log of blood pressure readings and present it at follow-up visits.
- Avoid OTC medications for colds, sinus or fever, asthma, or appetite control because they may increase blood pressure.
- Proper diet, including sodium and potassium restrictions, is important to the management of HTN or heart failure. Avoid salt substitutes that contain potassium.
- Report symptoms of hypotension such as dizziness or fainting to the health care provider.

CONNECTIONS

Complementary and Alternative Therapies Hawthorn

Description: Hawthorn (*Crataegus*) is a thorny shrub or small tree that is widespread in North America, Europe, and Asia. Leaves, flowers, and berries of the plant are dried or extracted in liquid form.

History and Claims: Hawthorn, sometimes called May bush, was used in ancient Greece. In traditional Chinese medicine, hawthorn is used as a digestive aid. European and American interest in the herb began in the late 1800s. It has been widely used in European countries to treat HTN and CHF. The berries may be consumed raw or made into jellies, juices, and alcoholic beverages. Some cultures believe that the shrub is magical, and it is used with religious rites to ward off evil spirits.

Standardization: Active ingredients in hawthorn include flavonoids and procyanidins. A typical dose is 4.5 to 6 g of dried leaves or flowers or 160 to 900 mg of extract per day.

Evidence: Hawthorn has been well studied. Positive inotropic action, improved exercise tolerance, and vasodilation have been documented. Some studies also report its ability to lower blood lipids. Hawthorn has been used to lower blood pressure but is slow in onset, taking 4 weeks or longer before a small effect is experienced. Hawthorn may work by inhibition of ACE or reduction of cardiac workload. Hawthorn has few adverse effects at normal doses. This product should be used with caution in patients taking cardiac glycosides and other prescription medications for cardiovascular disease. Because hypotension may occur, frequent blood pressure measurements should be taken when using this therapy.

Source: From *Herbs at a Glance: Hawthorn,* by the National Center for Complementary and Alternative Medicine, 2008. Retrieved July 7, 2008, from http://nccam.nih.gov/health/hawthorn/; *Herbal Medicine: Expanded Commission E Monographs* (pp. 182–191), by M. Blumenthal, A. Goldberg, and J. Brinckmann (Eds.), 2000, Newton, MA: Lippincott Williams & Wilkins; and "Hawthorn: Pharmacology and Therapeutic Uses," by J. M. Rigelsky and B. V. Sweet, 2002, *American Journal of Health Systems Pharmacy, 59*(5), pp. 417–422.

- Do not drive or perform other hazardous activities until the effects of the drug are known because this drug may cause drowsiness or dizziness.
- Report vomiting, diarrhea, or heavy sweating to the health care provider because the drug may cause dehydration, leading to low blood pressure, electrolyte disorders, or kidney failure.
- Keep regularly scheduled follow-up appointments with the health care provider.
- Avoid alcohol because it can lower blood pressure and lead to dizziness and faintness.
- Avoid heavy exercise and sweating in hot weather because these can lead to fluid loss.
- Immediately report any swelling of the face, mouth, hands, or feet; hoarseness; sudden trouble breathing; or any sign of infection such as fever or sore throat to the health care provider.
- Immediately inform the health care provider of any known or suspected pregnancy because these drugs can cause birth defects.
- Do not breast-feed while taking this drug without approval of the health care provider.

Drugs Similar to Losartan (Cozaar)

At this time there are seven ARBs available.

Candesartan (Atacand): Approved in 1998, candesartan is indicated for HTN and heart failure. It is a prodrug that is metabolized to its active form during its absorption from the GI tract. Optimal therapeutic effects may take up to 4 weeks. The drug is 99% protein bound and is primarily excreted in the bile (66%). Adverse effects are generally mild and include headache and dizziness. Other adverse effects, contraindications, and indications are the same as those of losartan. Atacand HCT is a fixed-dose combination of candesartan and hydrochlorothiazide. This drug is pregnancy category D.

Eprosartan (Teveten): Approved in 1997, eprosartan is indicated only for HTN. It is mostly unmetabolized and primarily excreted in the feces (90%). Optimum blood pressure reduction may require 2 to 3 weeks of therapy. The most common adverse effects are headache, dizziness, arthralgia, and fatigue. Other adverse effects, contraindications, and indications are the same as those of losartan. Teveten HCT is a fixed-dose combination of eprosartan and hydrochlorothiazide. This drug is pregnancy category D.

Irbesartan (Avapro): Approved in 1997, irbesartan is indicated for HTN and diabetic nephropathy. The drug is 90% protein bound and is primarily excreted in the feces (80%). Adverse effects are generally mild and include diarrhea, dyspepsia, arthralgia, and fatigue. Other adverse effects, contraindications, and indications are the same as those of losartan. Avalide is a fixed-dose combination of irbesartan and hydrochlorothiazide. This drug is pregnancy category D.

Olmesartan medoxomil (Benicar): Approved in 2002, olmesartan is indicated only for HTN. It is a prodrug that is metabolized to its active form during its absorption from the GI tract. Olmesartan is 99% protein bound and excreted equally in urine and the feces. The drug is administered once daily and optimal blood pressure reduction may require 2 weeks of therapy. The drug exhibits few adverse effects, with dizziness being the most common complaint. Other adverse effects, contraindications, and indications are the same as those of losartan. Benicar HCT is a fixed-dose combination of olmesartan and hydrochlorothiazide. This drug is pregnancy category D.

Telmisartan (Micardis): Approved in 1998, telmisartan is indicated only for HTN. An off-label use is for the treatment of renal dysfunction in patients with diabetic nephropathy. It is mostly unmetabolized, 99% protein bound, and excreted primarily in the feces. Initial doses should be reduced in patients with hepatic impairment. The drug is well tolerated and serious adverse effects are uncommon. Adverse effects, contraindications, and indications are the same as those of losartan. Micardis HCT is a fixed-dose combination of telmisartan and hydrochlorothiazide. This drug is pregnancy category D.

Valsartan (Diovan): Approved in 1996, valsartan is indicated for HTN, heart failure, and MI when the patient is unable to tolerate an ACE inhibitor. It undergoes hepatic metabolism, is 95% protein bound, and is eliminated in the feces. Because food can reduce drug absorption by as much as 40%, the drug should be given on an empty stomach. Headache and dizziness are the two most common adverse effects. Other adverse effects, contraindications, and indications are the same as those of losartan. Diovan HCT is a fixed-dose combination of valsartan and hydrochlorothiazide. This drug is pregnancy category D.

34.8 Aldosterone antagonists block the biologic effects of aldosterone in the renal tubule.

As described in Section 34.3, angiotensin II causes the release of aldosterone, which subsequently contributes to increased blood pressure due to sodium and water retention. Receptors for aldosterone are located in the distal tubule and collecting ducts of the nephron. Two drugs are available that block these receptors in the kidney, thus inhibiting the physiological actions of aldosterone. Both spironolactone (Aldactone) and eplerenone (Inspra) are used to treat edema and HTN. Doses for these drugs are listed in Table 34.2.

Spironolactone is an aldosterone antagonist that has been used for its diuretic action for many decades. By binding to aldosterone receptors, spironolactone produces a mild diuresis by promoting Na^+ and Cl^- excretion. Because it has little or no effect on the excretion of potassium, spironolactone is also classified as a potassium-sparing diuretic and is featured as a prototype diuretic in Chapter 35. Spironolactone produces only a mild diuresis; it is often combined with drugs from other diuretic classes when used for HTN. It is also useful in treating primary aldosteronism, a rare condition in which the body produces an overabundance of aldosterone, usually due to a tumor of the adrenal gland. Spironolactone has been shown to reduce morbidity, mortality, and dysrhythmias associated with heart failure.

The primary concern with spironolactone is potassium retention, which can result in serious hyperkalemia. Some patients experience GI-related adverse effects such as nausea, vomiting, and diarrhea. Because spironolactone has a similar chemical structure to steroid hormones, it sometimes causes endocrine adverse effects in males, such as gynecomastia and erectile dysfunction. Females may experience menstrual irregularities, hirsutism, and breast tenderness.

Eplerenone (Inspra) is a newer aldosterone antagonist that has a very different chemical structure than spironolactone. It is more selective for aldosterone receptors and has a very low incidence of endocrine-related adverse effects. Like spironolactone, hyperkalemia is a potentially serious adverse effect. Headache and dizziness are common adverse effects. Eplerenone is approved to treat HTN and heart failure and to reduce morbidity and mortality associated with post-MI in patients with left ventricular dysfunction.

For additional information on aldosterone antagonists, see Chapter 35.

UNDERSTANDING THE CHAPTER

Key Concepts Summary

34.1 The formation of angiotensin II requires two enzymatic steps.

34.2 Renin secretion is controlled by the juxtaglomerular cells of the kidney and the sympathetic nervous system.

34.3 Angiotensin-converting enzyme is responsible for the formation of angiotensin II.

34.4 Angiotensin II has multiple effects on the cardiovascular system that raise blood pressure and affect cardiac function.

34.5 The renin-angiotensin-aldosterone pathway offers multiple points for drug intervention.

34.6 ACE inhibitors are key drugs in the pharmacotherapy of hypertension and heart failure.

34.7 Angiotensin II receptor blockers act by inhibiting the AT_1 receptor and are used for hypertension and heart failure.

34.8 Aldosterone antagonists block the biologic effects of aldosterone in the renal tubule.

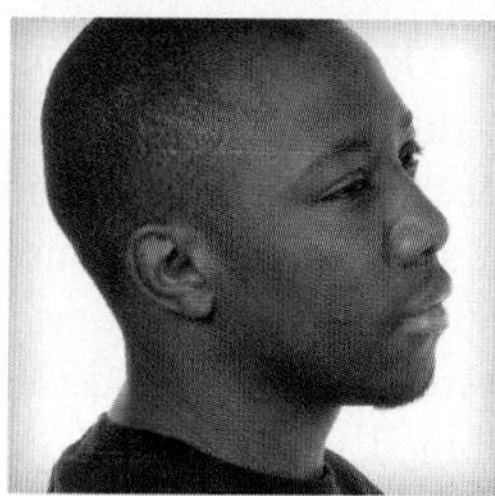

Making the PATIENT Connection

Remember the patient "Carlos McKay" at the beginning of the chapter? Now read the remainder of the case study. Based on the information presented within this chapter, respond to the critical thinking questions that follow.

Carlos McKay is a 30-year-old bachelor who was diagnosed with primary HTN 4 months ago. Carlos has been taking losartan (Cozaar) 50 mg daily PO and has been faithful in taking the medication as prescribed. When Carlos was told that his blood pressure was still elevated during this clinic visit, he was obviously distressed and concerned.

The health care team begins to investigate external factors that may be causing his blood pressure to remain elevated. Carlos has never smoked or used alcohol. He does not like to exercise but participates in a weekly game of basketball at the nearby community center. He denies being overly stressed with work or home life. Furthermore, he claims that he rarely salts his food.

The nurse asks Carlos to describe a typical day. During the description the nurse notices a concerning pattern. Because Carlos lives alone, he frequently cooks for himself. He admits that he enjoys salty foods such as pretzels and popcorn. He denies having consumed either prior to the visit to the clinic. However, to Carlos, cooking a meal involves preparing canned processed foods and frozen dinners. He never reads food labels.

Without recording a complete dietary history, the nurse is able to determine that Carlos's intake of sodium-rich foods is quite extensive. For example, within that last 24 hours, the patient has eaten a sandwich with Canadian bacon and a large bowl of canned cream of potato soup for lunch. For his dinner he consumed three slices of cured, canned ham and 3 cups of canned chow mein vegetables.

Critical Thinking Questions

1. In your own words, how would you describe how losartan (Cozaar) works to reduce blood pressure?
2. Considering the adverse effects of losartan (Cozaar), when would you instruct Carlos to notify the prescriber?
3. What is the connection between dietary sodium and HTN?

Case Study

Ella Daniels, a middle-aged African American woman, takes spironolactone (Aldactone) for HTN. As the nurse responsible for providing her with health information, you plan to talk with her about this drug.

1. How does the mechanism of action of spironolactone differ from that of lisinopril (Prinivil, Zestril)?
2. What are the main precautions specific to Aldactone that should be included in the teaching plan?

NCLEX-RN® Review

1 The community health nurse teaches a client at home. The nurse teaches the client about lisinopril (Prinivil), which has been prescribed for the client. Which of the following statements, if made by the client, indicates that further teaching is necessary?

1. "I should notify my health care provider of symptoms of hypotension such as dizziness or fainting."
2. "I should avoid the use of salt substitute containing potassium."
3. "If a dose is missed, I will take it as soon as possible but not too close to the next dose."
4. "Too much calcium in my diet will elevate my blood pressure."

2 The client states, "I always keep my lisinopril (Prinivil) on my kitchen window sill. It helps me to remember to take it." The nurse's response would be based on which of the following pharmacologic concepts? Heat and moisture may:

1. Cause the medicine to break down.
2. Enhance the strength of the drug.
3. Crystallize the medication.
4. Convert the medicine to toxic metabolites.

3 A client is hospitalized for uncontrolled hypertension and is receiving angiotensin-converting enzyme (ACE) inhibitors. The nurse should notify the health care provider if the client exhibits:

1. Dry mucous membranes.
2. A decline in systolic blood pressure.
3. Nonproductive cough.
4. A reduction of diastolic blood pressure.

4 The nurse is caring for a client with chronic hypertension. The client is receiving losartan (Cozaar) daily. Which of the following client manifestations would the nurse conclude is an adverse effect of this medication?

1. Irritability and insomnia
2. Headache and dizziness
3. Sleepiness and slurred speech
4. Pruritus and rash

5 Losartan (Cozaar) is prescribed for each of the following clients. A nurse should question the order for which client? A client who has:

1. Severe dehydration from diuretic therapy.
2. Long-term diabetes mellitus.
3. A systolic blood pressure of 162.
4. A 5-year history of heart failure.

6 The nurse determines that the client does not understand an important principle in self-administration of losartan (Cozaar) when the client makes which of the following statements?

1. "I will learn to monitor my own blood pressure and write down all my daily measurements."
2. "While taking this medication, I should avoid over-the-counter medications for colds, sinus, or appetite control."
3. "This drug will not impair thinking and reaction time. I don't need to wait to start driving my car."
4. "Drinking alcohol while on this medication can lower my blood pressure and lead to dizziness and faintness."

See Answers to Critical Thinking Questions, Case Study, and NCLEX-RN® Review in Appendix A.

References

Blumenthal, M., Goldberg, A., & Brinckmann, J. (Eds.). (2000). *Herbal medicine: Expanded Commission E Monographs.* Newton, MA: Lippincott Williams & Wilkins.

Brugts, J. J., Danser, A. H. J., de Maat, M. P. M., den Uil, C. A., Boersma, E., Ferrari, R., et al. (2008). Pharmacogenetics of ACE inhibition in stable coronary artery disease: Steps towards tailored drug therapy. *Current Opinion in Cardiology, 23*(4), 296–301.

Casas, J., Chua, W., Loukogeorgakis, S., Vallance, P., Smeeth, L., Hingorani, A., et al. (2005). Effect of inhibitors of the renin-angiotensin system and other antihypertensive drugs on renal outcomes: Systematic review and meta-analysis. *The Lancet, 366*(9502), 2026–2033.

Kaplan, N., & Opie, L. (2006). Controversies in hypertension. *The Lancet, 367*(9505), 168–176.

Kaufman, J. S., & Flack, J. M. (2005). Angiotensin-converting enzyme inhibitors in black patients. *Annals of Internal Medicine, 142*(52), 589.

Linus, S. L. (2008). Are two better than one? Angiotensin-converting enzyme inhibitors plus angiotensin receptor blockers for reducing blood pressure and proteinuria in kidney disease. *Clinical Journal of the American Society of Nephrology, 3*(Suppl. 1), S17–S23.

National Center for Complementary and Alternative Medicine. (2008). *Herbs at a glance: Hawthorn.* Retrieved July 7, 2008, from http://nccam.nih.gov/health/hawthorn/

Parfrey, P. S. (2008). Inhibitors of the renin angiotensin system: Proven benefits, unproven safety. *Annals of Internal Medicine, 148*(1), 76–77.

Reid, M., & Eurle, B. (2005). *Angioedema.* Retrieved July 7, 2008, from http://www.emedicine.com/med/TOPIC135.HTML

Rigelsky, J. M., & Sweet, B. V. (2002). Hawthorn: Pharmacology and therapeutic uses. *American Journal of Health Systems Pharmacy, 59*(5), 417–422.

Silverthorn, D. U. (2006). *Human physiology: An integrated approach* (4th ed.). San Francisco: Pearson/Benjamin Cummings.

United States Department of Health and Human Services. (2005). *Dietary guidelines for Americans.* Retrieved July 7, 2008, from http://www.health.gov/DietaryGuidelines/

C H A P T E R

I feel terrible. I have no energy and I feel as weak as a kitten. Lately, I don't even feel like getting out of bed in the mornings. I try to take my medications just as I was told to do.

Patient "Katherine Crosland"

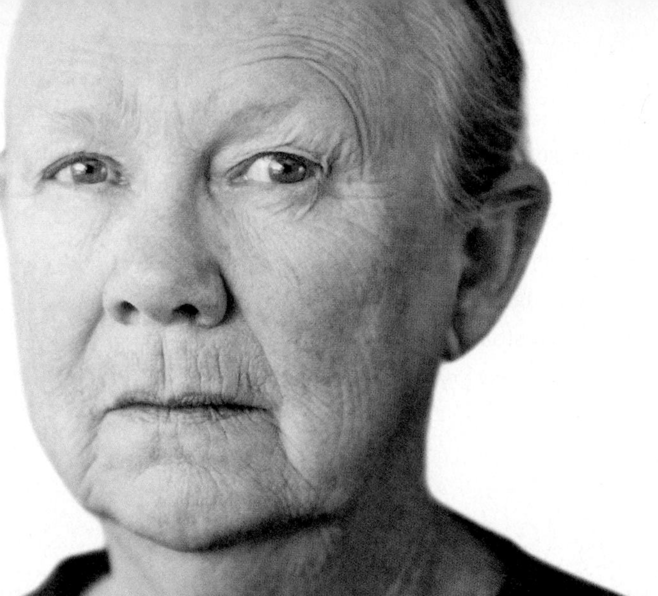

35 Diuretic Therapy and the Pharmacotherapy of Renal Failure

Learning Outcomes

After reading this chapter, the student should be able to:

1. Explain the role of the urinary system in maintaining fluid, electrolyte, and acid–base homeostasis.
2. Explain the processes that change the composition of filtrate as it travels through the nephron.
3. Describe the adjustments in pharmacotherapy that must be considered in patients with renal failure.
4. Identify indications for diuretics.
5. Compare and contrast the loop, thiazide, potassium-sparing, osmotic, and carbonic anhydrase inhibitor diuretics.
6. Describe the nurse's role in the pharmacologic management of renal failure and in diuretic therapy.
7. For each of the classes shown in the chapter outline, identify the prototype and representative drugs and explain the mechanism(s) of drug action, primary indications, contraindications, significant drug interactions, pregnancy category, and important adverse effects.
8. Use the nursing process to care for patients who are receiving diuretics and drug therapy for renal failure.

Chapter Outline

Review of Renal Physiology

Pharmacotherapy in Patients with Renal Failure

Diuretic Therapy

Loop (High-Ceiling) Diuretics

PROTOTYPE **Furosemide (Lasix)** *p. 551*

Thiazide and Thiazide-Like Diuretics

PROTOTYPE **Hydrochlorothiazide (HydroDIURIL, HCTZ)** *p. 553*

Potassium-Sparing Diuretics

PROTOTYPE **Spironolactone (Aldactone)** *p. 556*

Osmotic Diuretics

PROTOTYPE **Mannitol (Osmitrol)** *p. 559*

Carbonic Anhydrase Inhibitors

PROTOTYPE **Acetazolamide (Diamox)** *p. 560*

Key Terms

carbonic anhydrase, *560*
diuretic, *555*
filtrate, *545*
glomerular filtration rate (GFR), *547*
glomerulus, *545*
natriuresis, *548*
nephrons, *545*
osmotic pressure, *558*
reabsorption, *546*
renal failure, *546*
secretion, *546*
symporter, *549*

The kidneys serve an amazing role in maintaining proper homeostasis. By filtering a volume equivalent to all of the body's extracellular fluid every 100 minutes, the kidneys are able to make immediate adjustments to fluid volume, electrolyte composition, and acid–base balance. Failure of the kidneys to adjust to changing internal conditions of the body may result in dire consequences, and pharmacotherapy is often used to correct these imbalances. This chapter examines diuretics, agents that increase urine output, and other drugs used to treat patients with renal dysfunction.

PharmFACT

More than 16,000 kidney transplants are performed annually. Approximately 10,000 of these patients received organs from deceased donors, and 6,000 received organs from living donors. *Source:* The Organ Procurement and Transplantation Network, 2008.

Review of Renal Physiology

35.1 The kidneys are major organs of excretion and body homeostasis.

When most people think of the kidneys, they think of excretion. Although this is certainly true, the kidneys have many other essential homeostatic functions. The kidneys are the primary organs for regulating fluid balance, electrolyte composition, and the pH of body fluids. They also secrete the enzyme renin, which helps to regulate blood pressure (see Chapter 34), and erythropoietin, a hormone that stimulates red blood cell production (see Chapter 41). In addition, the kidneys are responsible for the production of calcitriol, the active form of vitamin D, which helps maintain bone homeostasis (see Chapter 75). It is not surprising that our overall health is strongly dependent on the proper functioning of the kidneys.

The urinary system consists of two kidneys, two ureters, one urinary bladder, and a urethra. Blood enters the kidneys through the large renal arteries, bringing 25% of the total cardiac output to the kidneys each minute. After a series of branches, blood enters the **nephrons,** the functional units of the kidney. Once in the nephron, the artery forms the **glomerulus,** a specialized capillary containing pores. Each kidney contains over 1 million nephrons.

As blood travels at high pressure through the glomerulus, the fluid portion of the blood is filtered through the glomerular pores and collected by Bowman's capsule, the first portion of the collecting system of the nephron. Together, the glomerulus and Bowman's capsule are called the renal corpuscle. During filtration, not all substances in the blood reach Bowman's capsule. Plasma proteins and the formed elements of the blood—the erythrocytes, leukocytes, and platelets—are too large to pass through the pores of the glomerulus and thus continue circulating through the bloodstream. Water and other small molecules in plasma, however, readily pass through the glomerular pores and enter the next section of the nephron.

The fluid filtered into Bowman's capsule is called **filtrate.** Essentially, the initial composition of filtrate may be thought of as plasma minus proteins. After leaving Bowman's capsule, the filtrate enters the proximal tubule, travels through the loop of Henle and, subsequently, the distal tubule. The proximal and distal tubules are twisted and highly convoluted, which greatly increases the length of the nephron, allowing for enhanced processing of substances in the filtrate. The filtrate eventually reaches common collecting ducts, which empty into larger and larger collecting structures inside the kidney. Fluid leaving the collecting ducts and entering subsequent portions of the kidney is called urine. Approximately 1 mL of urine is produced each minute. Parts of the nephron and their functions are illustrated in Figure 35.1.

Many drugs are small enough to pass through the glomerulus and enter the filtrate. If the drug is bound to plasma proteins, however, it will be too large and will continue circulating in the blood. Plasma proteins such as albumin are also too large to pass through the filter and will not be present in the filtrate or in the urine of healthy patients.

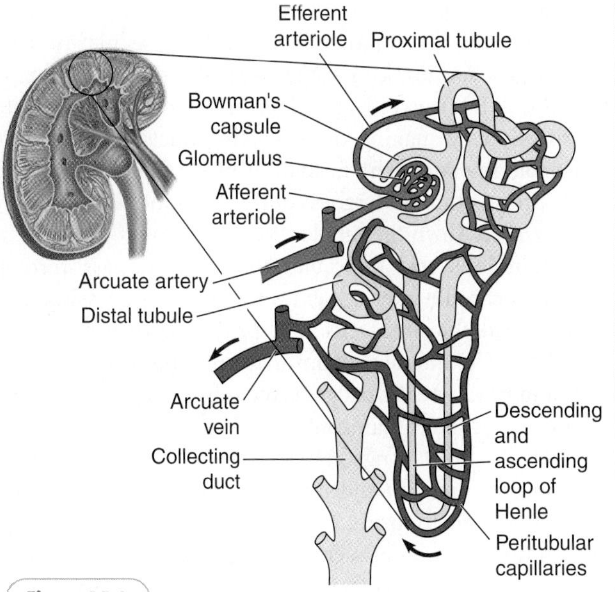

Figure 35.1

The nephron.
Source: From *Anatomy and Physiology for Health Professions: An Interactive Journey*, by B. J. Colbert, J. Ankney, and K. T. Lee, 2007, Upper Saddle River, NJ: Pearson Prentice Hall.

MyNursingKit | Renal Function Animation

The appearance of plasma proteins in urine (proteinuria or albuminuria) is a sign of kidney pathology. For example, during glomerulonephritis the glomeruli become inflamed and the size of the pores increases, allowing larger substances such as proteins to enter the filtrate.

CONNECTION Checkpoint 35.1

From what you learned in Chapter 4, explain how plasma protein binding markedly affects the pharmacokinetic properties of a drug. See Answer to Connection Checkpoint 35.1 in Appendix A.

35.2 The composition of filtrate changes dramatically as a result of the processes of reabsorption and secretion.

The filtrate's composition changes dramatically as it makes its long journey through the nephron. Some substances in the filtrate cross the tubule walls to reenter the blood; this process is known as tubular **reabsorption.** Water is the most important molecule reabsorbed in the tubule. For every 180 L of water entering the filtrate each day, approximately 178.5 L are reabsorbed, leaving only 1.5 L to be excreted in the urine. Over 65% of the filtered sodium is reabsorbed in the proximal tubule, and 25% in the loop of Henle. Glucose, amino acids, and essential ions such as chloride, calcium, and bicarbonate are also reabsorbed.

Hormones can markedly affect the degree of reabsorption in the renal tubule. This is important to pharmacology because many drugs either enhance or block the effects of hormones on tubular processes. Aldosterone, for example, exerts a major effect on the tubule by stimulating sodium reabsorption in the distal portions of the nephron. Under the influence of aldosterone, potassium excretion is increased because this ion is "exchanged" for sodium ions, which are reabsorbed. Antidiuretic hormone (ADH) also affects kidney function, increasing water reabsorption by making the collecting ducts become more permeable to water. The formation of urine is indeed a dynamic process that undergoes continuous modification as the filtrate travels down the tubule.

MyNursingKit | Nephrology Channel

Certain ions and molecules too large to pass through Bowman's capsule may still enter the urine by crossing from the blood to the filtrate using a process known as tubular **secretion.** The tubule contains molecular pumps for organic acids and bases. Acidic drugs secreted in the proximal tubule include penicillin G, ampicillin, sulfisoxazole, nonsteroidal anti-inflammatory drugs (NSAIDs), and furosemide. Basic drugs include procainamide, epinephrine, dopamine, neostigmine, and trimethoprim. Potassium, phosphate, hydrogen, and ammonium ions also enter the filtrate through active secretion. The amounts of selected substances reabsorbed, secreted, and excreted are shown in Table 35.1.

Reabsorption and secretion are critical to the pharmacokinetics of drugs. Some drugs are reabsorbed, whereas others are secreted into the filtrate. For example, approximately 90% of a dose of penicillin G enters the urine through secretion. When the kidney is diseased, reabsorption and secretion mechanisms are impaired and serum drug levels may be dramatically affected. Figure 35.2 illustrates the possible fates of drugs entering the glomerulus.

TABLE 35.1 Substances Filtered, Reabsorbed, and Excreted by the Kidneys

Substance	Filtered	Reabsorbed	Excreted
Water	180 L	178–179 L	1–2 L
Glucose	162 g	162 g	0 g
Proteins	2 g	1.9 g	0.1 g
Ions			
Sodium	579 g	575 g	4 g
Potassium	29.6 g	29.6 g	2 g
Bicarbonate	275 g	274.97 g	0.03 g
Metabolic Waste Products			
Creatine	1.6 g	0 g	1.6 g
Urea	54 g	24 g	30 g
Uric acid	8.5 g	7.7 g	0.8 g

CONNECTION Checkpoint 35.2

From what you learned in Chapter 34, explain the relationship between angiotensin II and the release of aldosterone by the adrenal gland and its significance to pharmacology. See Answer to Connection Checkpoint 35.2 in Appendix A.

Pharmacotherapy in Patients with Renal Failure

35.3 Renal failure may significantly impact the success of pharmacotherapy.

Renal failure is a condition characterized by a decrease in the kidneys' ability to maintain electrolyte and fluid balance and excrete waste products. Renal failure may be intrinsic to the kidney itself or result from disorders of other body systems. The primary treatment goals for a patient with renal failure are to maintain blood flow through the kidneys and adequate urine output.

PharmFACT

More than 485,000 Americans are treated for kidney failure each year, and about 86,000 die annually from causes related to the disease. Type 2 diabetes is the leading cause of chronic kidney failure, accounting for 30% to 40% of all new cases each year. Hypertension (HTN) is the second leading cause. *Source:* National Kidney Foundation, 2008.

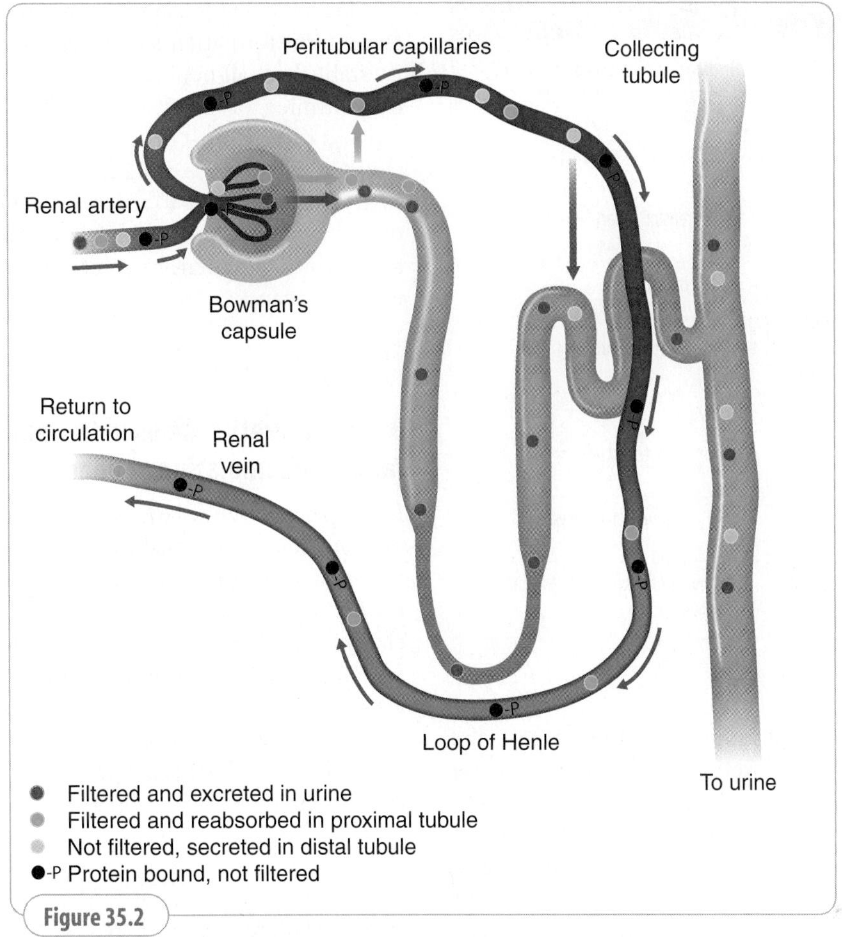

Figure 35.2

Fates of drugs entering the glomerulus: filtration, reabsorption, secretion, and excretion.

The most basic diagnostic test of kidney function is a urinalysis, which examines urine for the presence of blood cells, proteins, pH, specific gravity, ketones, glucose, and microorganisms. The urinalysis can detect proteinuria and albuminuria, which are the primary measures of structural kidney damage. Although easy to perform, the urinalysis is nonspecific: Many diverse diseases and conditions can cause abnormal urinalysis values. Serum creatinine is an additional measure for detecting kidney disease. To provide a more definitive diagnosis, diagnostic imaging such as computed tomography, sonography, or magnetic resonance imaging may be necessary. Renal biopsy may be performed to obtain a more specific diagnosis.

The best marker for estimating kidney function is the **glomerular filtration rate (GFR),** which is the volume of water filtered through the Bowman's capsules per minute. The GFR can be used to predict the onset and progression of kidney failure and it indicates the ability of the kidneys to excrete drugs from the body. A progressive decline in GFR indicates a reduction in the number of functioning nephrons. As nephrons "die," however, the remaining healthy ones have the ability to compensate by increasing their filtration capacity. Because of this, patients with significant kidney damage may be asymptomatic until 50% or more of the nephrons have become nonfunctional and the GFR has fallen to less than half its normal value.

Renal failure may be classified as acute or chronic, depending on its onset. Acute renal failure requires immediate treatment because retention of nitrogenous waste products in the body such as urea and creatinine can result in death if untreated. The most common cause of acute renal failure is renal hypoperfusion, the lack of sufficient blood flow through the kidneys. Hypoperfusion can lead to permanent destruction to kidney cells and nephrons. To correct this type of renal failure, the cause of the hypoperfusion must be quickly identified and corrected. Potential causes include heart failure, dysrhythmias, hemorrhage, toxins, and dehydration. Pharmacotherapy with nephrotoxic drugs can also lead to either acute or chronic renal failure. It is good practice for the nurse to remember common nephrotoxic drugs, which are listed in Table 35.2, so that kidney function may be continuously monitored during therapy with these agents.

Chronic renal failure occurs over a period of months or years. Over half of the patients with chronic renal failure have long-standing hypertension (HTN) or diabetes mellitus. Due to the long, gradual development of chronic renal failure and its nonspecific symptoms, the condition may go undetected for many years. By the time the disease is diagnosed, the renal impairment may be irreversible. In end-stage renal disease (ESRD), dialysis and kidney transplantation become treatment alternatives.

TABLE 35.2 Nephrotoxic Drugs

Drug or Class	Indication/Classification
Aminoglycosides	Antibiotics
amphotericin B (Amphotec, AmBisome)	Systemic antifungal
Angiotensin-converting enzyme (ACE) inhibitors	Hypertension, heart failure
cisplatin (Platinol), carboplatin (Paraplatin)	Antineoplastic
cyclosporine (Neoral, Sandimmune), tacrolimus (Prograf)	Immunosuppressant
foscarnet (Foscavir)	Antiviral
Nonsteroidal anti-inflammatory drugs (NSAIDs)	Inflammation and pain
pentamidine (Pentacarinat, Pentam)	Anti-infective (*Pneumocystis*)
Radiographic intravenous (IV) contrast agents	Diagnosis of kidney and vascular disorders

Pharmacotherapy of renal failure attempts to cure the cause of the dysfunction. Diuretics are given to increase urine output, and cardiovascular drugs are administered to treat underlying HTN or heart failure. Dietary management is often necessary to prevent worsening of renal impairment. Depending on the stage of the disease, dietary management may include restriction of protein and reduction of dietary sodium, potassium, phosphorous, and magnesium intake. For patients with diabetes, control of blood glucose through intensive insulin therapy may reduce the risk of renal damage. A summary of selected pharmacologic agents used to prevent and treat the complications of renal failure is given in Table 35.3.

The nurse serves a key role in assessing and providing interventions for patients with renal failure. Once a diagnosis is established, all nephrotoxic medications should be either discontinued or used with extreme caution. Because the kidneys excrete most drugs or their metabolites, many medications will require a significant dosage reduction in patients with moderate to severe renal failure. The importance of this cannot be overemphasized: Administering the "average" dose to a patient in severe renal failure can have mortal consequences.

Diuretic Therapy

35.4 Diuretics are used to treat hypertension, heart failure, accumulation of edema fluid, and renal failure.

By simple definition, a **diuretic** is a drug that increases the rate of urine flow. When used therapeutically for HTN, heart failure, renal failure, or removal of edema fluid, however, diuretics do much more than increase urine flow. These drugs change the rate of excretion of specific electrolytes, most importantly sodium and chloride. The goal of most diuretic therapy is to reduce extracellular fluid volume, so that abnormal fluid retention by the body may be reversed. Excretion of excess fluid in the body is particularly desirable in the following conditions:

- HTN
- Heart failure
- Renal failure
- Liver failure or cirrhosis
- Pulmonary edema

The most common mechanism by which diuretics act is by blocking sodium ion (Na^+) reabsorption in the nephron, thus sending more Na^+ to the urine **(natriuresis).** The human

TABLE 35.3 Pharmacologic Management of Renal Failure

Complication	Pathogenesis	Selected Therapies
Anemia	Kidneys are unable to synthesize sufficient erythropoietin for red blood cell production.	epoetin alfa (Procrit, Epogen)
Hyperkalemia	Kidneys are unable to adequately excrete potassium.	Dietary restriction of potassium; polystyrene sulfate (Kayexalate) with sorbitol
Hyperphosphatemia	Kidneys are unable to adequately excrete phosphate.	Dietary restriction of phosphate; phosphate binders such as calcium carbonate (Os-Cal 500, others), calcium acetate (Calphron, PhosLo), lanthanum carbonate (Fosrenol), or sevelamer (Renagel)
Hypervolemia	Kidneys are unable to excrete sufficient sodium and water, leading to water retention.	Dietary restriction of sodium; loop diuretics in acute conditions, thiazide diuretics in mild conditions
Hypocalcemia	Hyperphosphatemia leads to loss of calcium.	Usually corrected by reversing the hyperphosphatemia, but additional calcium supplements may be necessary
Metabolic acidosis	Kidneys are unable to adequately excrete metabolic acids.	Sodium bicarbonate or sodium citrate

CONNECTIONS

Lifespan Considerations Diuretic Therapy

Children

The use of diuretics in children is typically for the treatment of milder degrees of heart failure. There is no indication that the risk of adverse effects from diuretics is different in children than in adults. Dosages are lower for children and the dosage interval may be longer. Children who are taking potassium-sparing diuretics are more prone to developing calcium deficiencies than are adults. Safety of diuretic use in children has not been scientifically established for all diuretics, and parents are encouraged to discuss the potential risks and benefits with a board-certified pediatric cardiologist before their child begins taking these drugs.

Geriatric Patients

Diuretics are one of the most common classes of drugs prescribed for older adults. Older adults have a higher frequency and intensity of adverse effects from diuretics, such as light-headedness, dizziness, and fainting (syncope). They are also more susceptible to dehydration, hypovolemia (decrease in circulating blood volume), and deficiencies of calcium, potassium, sodium, and magnesium. The more potent loop diuretics may cause urge incontinence that may interfere with the ability or desire to participate in social activities in which restroom facilities are not nearby. Generally, older patients require lower doses of diuretics and require close observation.

body is particularly sensitive to sodium imbalances and dietary intake must be balanced with excretion mechanisms. For example, a 1% increase in sodium reabsorption could potentially cause a 1.8-L net gain of water each day, which is equivalent to 4 pounds of body weight. This example illustrates the need for patients to monitor their weight daily when taking these drugs.

Natriuresis results in two other important effects. Chloride ions (Cl^-) follow sodium, resulting in a net loss of chloride from the body and possible hypochloremia. Because water molecules travel passively with sodium ions, blocking the reabsorption of Na^+ increases the total volume of urination, or diuresis. The amount of diuresis produced by a diuretic is directly related to the amount of sodium reabsorption that is blocked: Those that block the most sodium are the most effective at increasing urine output. Diuretics also affect the renal excretion of ions such as magnesium, potassium, phosphate, calcium, and bicarbonate. It is important to remember that imbalances may occur in virtually any electrolyte during diuretic therapy.

Diuretics are classified into five major groups, based on differences in their chemical nature and mechanism of action. The sites in the nephron at which the various diuretics act are shown in Pharmacotherapy Illustrated 35.1.

- **Loop or high-ceiling.** These drugs prevent the reabsorption of Na^+ in the loop of Henle; thus, they are called loop diuretics. Because there is an abundance of Na^+ in the filtrate within the loop of Henle, drugs in this class are capable of producing large increases in urine output.
- **Thiazides.** The largest diuretic class, the thiazides act by blocking Na^+ in the distal tubule. Because most Na^+ has already been reabsorbed from the filtrate by the time it reaches this part of the nephron, the thiazides produce less diuresis than loop diuretics.
- **Potassium-sparing.** The third major class is named potassium-sparing, because these diuretics have minimal effect on potassium ion (K^+) excretion. These agents produce a mild diuresis.
- **Osmotic.** These agents are relatively inert drugs that change the osmolality of filtrate, causing water to remain in the nephron for excretion. These drugs are very effective but are rarely prescribed because they can produce potentially serious adverse effects.
- **Carbonic anhydrase inhibitors.** These agents block the enzyme in the nephron responsible for bicarbonate reabsorption. They produce a weak diuresis and are rarely used.

It is common practice to combine two or more drugs in the pharmacotherapy of HTN and fluid retention disorders. Diuretics are often a component of fixed-dose combinations with drugs from other classes. The primary rationales for combination therapy are that the incidence of adverse effects is decreased and the pharmacologic effects (such as diuresis or blood pressure reduction) may be enhanced. For patient convenience, some of these drugs are available in single tablet formulations. Examples of single tablet diuretic combinations include the following:

- **Aldactazide.** Hydrochlorothiazide and spironolactone
- **Apresazide.** Hydrochlorothiazide and hydralazine
- **Dyazide.** Hydrochlorothiazide and triamterene
- **Moduretic.** Hydrochlorothiazide and amiloride

Loop (High-Ceiling) Diuretics

35.5 The most effective diuretics are the loop diuretics that block sodium reabsorption in the loop of Henle.

The most effective diuretics, the loop or high-ceiling diuretics, act by blocking the reabsorption of sodium and chloride in the loop of Henle. This occurs when the drug inhibits the molecule responsible for transporting sodium and chloride from the filtrate to the blood, known as the Na^+-K^+-$2Cl^-$ symporter. A **symporter** is a membrane protein that transports two molecules at the same time. When the loop diuretics

MyNursingKit | National Kidney and Urologic Diseases Clearinghouse

PHARMACOTHERAPY *ILLUSTRATED* 35.1

Sites of Action of the Diuretics

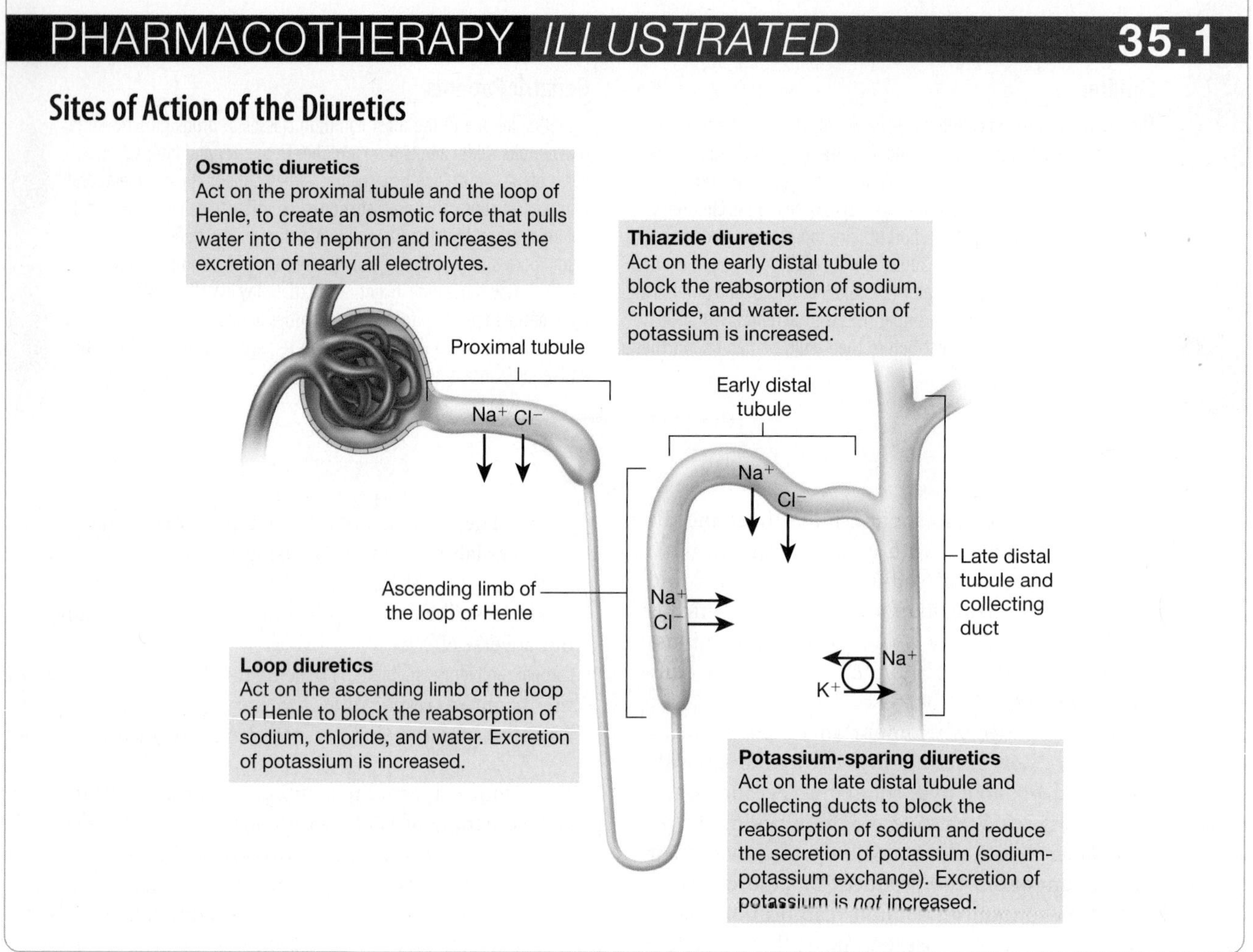

block this symporter, sodium and chloride are prevented from being reabsorbed, and diuresis is increased. All loop diuretics have an additional action that is responsible for a major adverse effect of drugs in this class: increasing potassium excretion. An illustration showing the effects caused by inhibiting this symporter is shown in Figure 35.3.

All loop diuretics are available for either oral (PO) or parenteral administration and are extensively bound by plasma proteins. They have relatively short half-lives, and extended release preparations are not available. When given intravenously (IV), loop diuretics have the ability to cause large amounts of fluid to be excreted by the kidney in a very short time. Loop diuretics are used to reduce the edema associated with heart failure, hepatic cirrhosis, or chronic renal failure. Furosemide and torsemide are also approved for HTN, although their short half-lives make them less suitable for this indication than thiazide diuretics. Occasionally, loop diuretics are given to speed the renal excretion of a drug that has been overdosed or a toxin that has been accidentally ingested. Doses of the loop diuretics are listed in Table 35.4.

The rapid excretion of large amounts of fluid has the potential to produce serious adverse effects, including dehydration and electrolyte imbalances. Signs of dehydration include thirst, dry mouth, weight loss, and headache. Dizziness and fainting can result from the fall in blood pressure caused by the rapid fluid loss. Potassium depletion can be serious and result in dysrhythmias. Potassium supplements are often prescribed concurrently with these diuretics to prevent hypokalemia. Potassium loss is of particular concern to those concurrently taking digoxin (Lanoxin), because hypokalemia predisposes these patients to dysrhythmias. Significant loss of sodium, magnesium, and calcium is also possible, especially with large doses. Continuous use of loop diuretics in postmenopausal women may affect bone metabolism due to excessive calcium loss. Loop diuretics can cause gout in some patients due to hyperuricemia—the accumulation of uric acid in the blood.

Although rare, loop diuretics may cause ototoxicity, which may manifest as tinnitus, vertigo, or deafness. Use of other ototoxic drugs such as the aminoglycoside antibiotics should be avoided during loop diuretic therapy due to the potential for additive hearing impairment. Because of the potential for serious adverse effects, the loop diuretics are normally prescribed for patients with moderate to severe fluid retention such as acute pulmonary edema, or when thiazide diuretics have failed to achieve therapeutic goals.

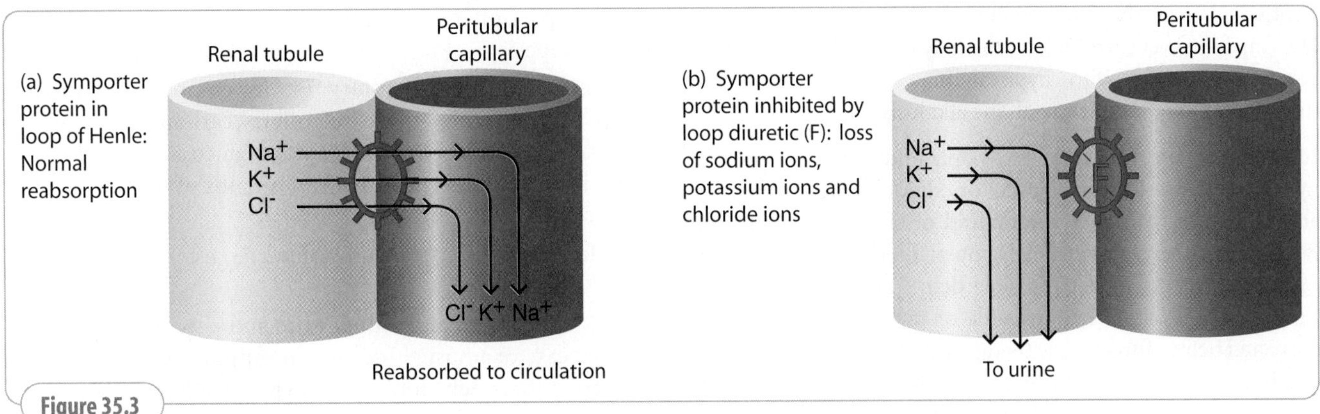

Figure 35.3

Symporter protein in the loop of Henle: (a) normal reabsorption of inhibition of the Na^+, K^+, and Cl^-; (b) inhibition of symporter by furosemide causes excretion of Na^+, K^+, CL^-.

PROTOTYPE DRUG Furosemide (Lasix)

Classification: **Therapeutic:** Antihypertensive
Pharmacologic: Loop- or high-ceiling-type diuretic

Therapeutic Effects and Uses: Approved in 1966, furosemide is frequently used in the treatment of acute edema associated with liver cirrhosis, renal impairment, or heart failure because it has the ability to remove large amounts of edema fluid from the patient in a short time. When given IV, diuresis begins within 5 minutes, providing patients quick relief from their distressing symptoms. Unlike the thiazide diuretics, furosemide is able to increase urine output even when blood flow to the kidneys is diminished, which makes it of particular value in patients with low cardiac output or renal failure. It is also approved for HTN, although it is not generally a drug of choice for this indication because of its short half-life and potential for serious adverse effects.

Mechanism of Action: Furosemide prevents the reabsorption of sodium and chloride by blocking the Na^+-K^+-$2Cl^-$ symporter in the loop of Henle. Because this is the region of the nephron that normally filters the bulk of sodium, furosemide can exert a profound diuresis. The extensive diuresis results in the increased urinary excretion of sodium, chloride, potassium, and hydrogen ions.

Pharmacokinetics:

Route(s)	PO, IV, intramuscular (IM)
Absorption	60% absorbed PO
Distribution	Distributes to most tissues; crosses the placenta; secreted in breast milk; 95% bound to plasma protein
Primary metabolism	Hepatic (small amounts)
Primary excretion	Renal
Onset of action	PO: 30–60 minutes; IV: 5 minutes
Duration of action	PO: 6–8 h; IV: 2 h; half-life: 30–60 minutes

Adverse Effects: The greatest concerns during furosemide therapy are excessive fluid loss and electrolyte imbalances. Hypovolemia may cause orthostatic hypotension and syncope. Imbalances may occur in any or all electrolytes, causing symptoms such as tachycardia, dysrhythmias, nausea, and vomiting.

TABLE 35.4 Loop Diuretics

Drug	Route and Adult Dose (maximum dose where indicated)	Adverse Effects
bumetanide (Bumex)	PO: 0.5–2 mg/day, may repeat at 4–5 h intervals if needed (max: 10 mg/day) IV/IM: 0.5–1 mg over 1–2 min, repeated every 2–3 h prn (max: 10 mg/day)	*Minor hypokalemia, orthostatic hypotension, tinnitus, nausea, diarrhea, dizziness, fatigue* Serious hypokalemia, blood dyscrasias, dehydration, ototoxicity, electrolyte imbalances, circulatory collapse
ethacrynic acid (Edecrin)	PO: 50–100 mg one to two times/day; may increase by 25–50 mg prn (max: 400 mg/day) IV: 0.5–1 mg/kg or 50 mg (max: 100 mg/dose)	
furosemide (Lasix)	PO: 20–80 mg in one or more divided doses (max: 600 mg/day) IV/IM: 20–40 mg in one or more divided doses (max: 600 mg/day)	
torsemide (Demadex)	PO/IV: 10–20 mg/day (max: 200 mg/day)	

Note: *Italics* indicate common adverse effects. Underline indicates serious adverse effects.

MyNursingKit | Mechanism of Action Animation: Furosemide

Ototoxicity is rare but may result in permanent hearing deficit. Hyperuricemia caused by the drug may cause exacerbations of gout. In patients with hypokalemia and hypochloremia, furosemide may induce metabolic alkalosis.

Contraindications/Precautions: Contraindications include hypersensitivity to furosemide or sulfonamide antibiotics, anuria, hepatic coma, or severe fluid or electrolyte depletion. Because furosemide is extremely potent, fluid loss must be carefully monitored to avoid possible dehydration and hypotension. Any preexisting hypovolemia or hypotension should be corrected before furosemide therapy is initiated. Loop diuretics can impair glucose tolerance: Serum glucose levels should be assessed in patients with diabetes mellitus.

Drug Interactions: Hypokalemia from the use of furosemide may cause dysrhythmias in patients taking digoxin; therefore, combination therapy with furosemide and digoxin should be avoided or carefully monitored. Concurrent use with corticosteroids, amphotericin B, or other potassium-depleting drugs can result in hypokalemia. When given with lithium, elimination of lithium is decreased, causing a higher risk of toxicity. Furosemide may diminish the hypoglycemic effects of sulfonylureas and insulin. Concurrent use with NSAIDs can result in a diminished diuretic effect. Additive hypotension will occur if furosemide is given concurrently with antihypertensives, including thiazide diuretics. Use of ethanol should be restricted because it may add to the hypotensive and diuretic actions of furosemide. **Herbal/Food:** Oral aloe can decrease the levels of potassium and should not be used concurrently with loop diuretics. Use with hawthorn could result in additive hypotensive effects. Ginseng may decrease the effectiveness of loop diuretics. High sodium intake can reduce the effectiveness of diuretics; patients should be placed on a sodium-restricted intake of 8 g or less per day.

Treatment of Overdose: Overdose with furosemide can cause serious hypotension, fluid loss, and electrolyte imbalances. Treatment is supportive, with replacement of fluids and electrolytes and the possible administration of a vasopressor.

Pregnancy: Category C.

Nursing Responsibilities:

- Obtain a complete health history, including data on recent surgeries or trauma, nicotine and alcohol consumption, and use of complementary and alternative therapies to determine possible drug allergies and interactions.
- Carefully monitor patients receiving parenteral loop diuretics, especially vital signs.
- Monitor blood pressure frequently during periods of diuresis and through periods of dosage adjustment.
- Establish safety precautions if central nervous system (CNS) effects or orthostatic hypotension occurs. Consider measurement of blood pressure (reclining, sitting, and standing) prior to ambulation if fluid volume deficit is suspected.
- Observe older adults closely during periods of brisk diuresis. Sudden alteration in fluid and electrolyte balance may precipitate significant adverse reactions, including syncope.
- Obtain frequent laboratory tests for complete blood count (CBC), serum and urine electrolytes, carbon dioxide (CO_2), blood urea nitrogen (BUN), serum glucose, and serum uric acid values during the first few months of therapy and periodically thereafter.
- Monitor serum potassium values and assess for symptoms of hypokalemia.
- Monitor intake and output ratio and pattern, and report a decrease or unusual increase in output. Excessive diuresis can result in dehydration and hypovolemia, circulatory collapse, and hypotension.
- Ensure ready access to restroom facilities. Keep the urinal, bedpan, or bedside commode readily available for patients with limited mobility.
- Monitor urine and blood glucose and glycosylated hemoglobin (HbA_{1C}) closely in patients with diabetes and those with decompensated hepatic cirrhosis. Loop diuretics may cause hyperglycemia in patients with diabetes.
- Close monitoring of patients with dehydration is warranted. Excessive dehydration is most likely to occur in older adults, those with chronic cardiac disease on prolonged salt restriction, or those receiving adrenergic blockers.
- Assess results of audiometry tests and immediately report any hearing deficits to the prescriber.
- Administer diuretics early in the day (whenever possible) so sleep will not be disturbed by frequent urination.

Patient and Family Education:

- Monitor blood pressure regularly. Maintain a written log of blood pressure readings and present it at follow-up visits.
- Weigh daily and report gains or losses of greater than 2 pounds in 2 days.
- Report swelling in the ankles or hand, unusual bleeding or bruising, palpitations, or muscle cramps to the health care provider.
- Follow the health care provider's instructions carefully regarding allowable salt and fluid intake.
- Eat potassium-rich foods daily (e.g., bananas, oranges, peaches, or dried dates) to reduce or prevent potassium depletion. Learn symptoms of low potassium levels; report muscle cramps or weakness.
- Make position changes slowly when moving from a lying to standing position to prevent dizziness and possible fainting.
- Avoid prolonged exposure to direct sun because furosemide may cause the skin to be more sensitive to sunlight.
- Report any changes in hearing immediately.
- If diabetic, monitor blood glucose levels frequently at the beginning of therapy and during dosage adjustments.
- Do not breast-feed while taking this drug without approval of the health care provider.

Drugs Similar to Furosemide (Lasix)

Furosemide is the most commonly prescribed drug in this class. Other loop diuretics include bumetanide, ethacrynic acid, and torsemide.

Bumetanide (Bumex): Approved in 1983, bumetanide is indicated for ascites and the treatment of peripheral edema, usually associated with heart failure or renal failure. This drug is available by the PO, IV, and IM routes and is 40 times more potent than furosemide but has a shorter duration of action. It may be used in acute clinical situations when furosemide has proven ineffective in patients with severe renal impairment. Like furosemide, bumetanide can cause electrolyte imbalances, hypotension, and dehydration. Unlike furosemide and torsemide, bumetanide is not approved for HTN, although it may be used off-label for that indication. This drug is pregnancy category C.

Ethacrynic acid (Edecrin): Approved in 1967, ethacrynic acid is indicated for the treatment of edema, usually associated with heart, liver, or renal failure. Given by either the oral or IV route, ethacrynic acid is the only loop diuretic that does not contain a sulfur group in its structure; thus it can safely be used in patients allergic to sulfonamides. Of the loop diuretics, ethacrynic acid causes the most severe hearing loss, which may be irreversible. The patient must be carefully monitored to prevent excessive electrolyte and fluid losses. Although ethacrynic acid is not approved for HTN, it may be prescribed off-label for this indication. This drug is pregnancy category B.

Torsemide (Demadex): Approved in 1993, torsemide is indicated for the treatment of HTN and edema, usually associated with heart, liver, or renal failure. Given by either the oral or IV route, torsemide is twice as potent as furosemide and has a longer half-life, which offers the advantage of once-a-day dosing. The incidence of ototoxicity with torsemide is very low, and the risk of hypokalemia is less than other drugs in this class. At higher doses, however, torsemide carries the same potential risks as furosemide and other loop diuretics, including electrolyte imbalances and hypovolemia. Torsemide is contraindicated in patients with sensitivity to sulfonylureas. This drug is pregnancy category B.

Thiazide and Thiazide-Like Diuretics

35.6 The thiazides are the most commonly prescribed class of diuretics.

The thiazides comprise the largest and most commonly prescribed class of diuretics. Like the loop diuretics, the thiazides block a symport protein in the renal tubule wall that is responsible for reabsorbing sodium and chloride ions from the filtrate. However, the thiazides block a different symport protein, and in a different location than the loop diuretics. The thiazides act on the Na^+Cl^- symporter in the distal tubule to block Na^+ reabsorption and increase K^+ and water excretion. The thiazides are less effective than the loop diuretics because over 90% of the Na^+ has already been reabsorbed by the time the filtrate reaches the distal tubule. There are simply fewer Na^+ to block; thus the maximum diuresis produced by thiazides is less than the loop diuretics.

The primary indication for thiazide diuretics is the treatment of mild to moderate HTN. Mild HTN can often be controlled with only a thiazide diuretic, whereas moderate to severe HTN requires two or more antihypertensive agents. Thiazides are also indicated for edema due to mild to moderate heart, liver, and renal failure. They are not effective in patients with severe organ impairment because their ability to produce a diuresis diminishes as blood flow through the kidneys is reduced. Doses of the thiazide diuretics are listed in Table 35.5.

Thiazides are available only by the PO route with the exception of chlorothiazide (Diuril, Diurigen), which is also available parenterally. All the thiazide diuretics have equivalent effectiveness and safety profiles. They differ, however, in their potency and duration of action. For example, metolazone (Zaroxolyn) is 10 times more potent than hydrochlorothiazide (HCTZ). At therapeutic doses all thiazides produce the same level of diuresis.

Three drugs in Table 35.5, chlorthalidone (Hygroton), indapamide (Lozol), and metolazone (Zaroxolyn), are not true thiazides because they do not contain the two-ring structure that chemically defines a thiazide. However, these drugs block the same symport protein and have the same pharmacologic effects as thiazides. They are sometimes called "thiazide-like" and are always considered along with the true thiazides because of their similar mechanism of action, indications, and adverse effects.

The adverse effects of thiazides are similar to those of the loop diuretics, though their frequency is less and they do not cause ototoxicity. Dehydration and excessive loss of sodium, potassium, or chloride ions may occur with overtreatment: Hypokalemia and hypochloremia can cause metabolic alkalosis. Concurrent therapy with digoxin requires careful monitoring to avoid dysrhythmias caused by excessive potassium loss. Potassium supplements are sometimes prescribed during thiazide therapy to prevent hypokalemia. Patients with diabetes should be aware that thiazide diuretics sometimes raise blood glucose levels. Like the loop diuretics, thiazides can increase serum levels of uric acid, although this is only clinically significant in patients with a history of gout.

PROTOTYPE DRUG Hydrochlorothiazide (HydroDIURIL, HCTZ)

Classification: **Therapeutic:** Antihypertensive
Pharmacologic: Thiazide-type diuretic

Therapeutic Effects and Uses: Approved in 1959, hydrochlorothiazide is the most widely prescribed diuretic for HTN. Like many diuretics, it produces few adverse effects and is effective at producing a 10- to 20-mmHg reduction in blood pressure. Patients with severe HTN or a compelling condition

TABLE 35.5 Thiazide and Thiazide-Like Diuretics

Drug	Route and Adult Dose (maximum dose where indicated)	Adverse Effects
Short Acting		
chlorothiazide (Diuril)	PO: 250 mg–1 g/day once or twice daily in divided doses. IV: 250 mg–1 g/day in one to two divided doses (max: 2 g/day)	*Minor hypokalemia, fatigue* <u>Serious hypokalemia, electrolyte depletion, dehydration, hypotension, hyponatremia, hyperglycemia, coma, blood dyscrasias</u>
hydrochlorothiazide (HydroDIURIL, HCTZ)	PO: 25–100 mg/day as single or divided dose (max: 50 mg/day for HTN; 100 mg/day for edema)	
Intermediate Acting		
bendroflumethiazide and nadolol (Corzide)	PO: 1 tablet/day (40–80 mg nadolol and 5 mg bendroflumethiazide)	
metolazone (Zaroxolyn)	PO: 2.5–10 mg once daily (max: 5 mg/day for HTN; 20 mg/day for edema)	
Long Acting		
chlorthalidone (Hygroton)	PO: 50–100 mg/day (max: 50 mg/day for HTN; 200 mg/day for edema)	
indapamide (Lozol)	PO: 1.25–2.5 mg once daily (max: 5 mg/day)	
methyclothiazide (Enduron)	PO: 2.5–5 mg once daily (max: 5 mg/day for HTN; 10 mg/day for edema)	

Note: *Italics* indicate common adverse effects. <u>Underline</u> indicates serious adverse effects.

such as heart failure, postmyocardial infarction (post-MI), high risk for coronary artery disease, diabetes, chronic kidney disease, or recurrent stroke prevention may require the addition of a second drug from a different class to control the disease (see Chapter 36).

Hydrochlorothiazide is approved to treat ascites, edema, heart failure, HTN, and nephrotic syndrome. Off-label indications include premenstrual syndrome (PMS), diabetes insipidus, hypercalciuria, and nephrolithiasis. Hydrochlorothiazide is the most common agent found in fixed-dose combination drugs for HTN.

Mechanism of Action: Hydrochlorothiazide acts on the distal tubule to decrease the reabsorption of Na^+. This results in less water reabsorption, increased diuresis, and removal of edema fluid. Blood volume decreases and blood pressure falls. Increasing the amount of sodium in the distal tubule also increases potassium excretion via a sodium–potassium exchange mechanism.

Pharmacokinetics:

Route(s)	PO
Absorption	Variable; incompletely absorbed
Distribution	Distributed to most tissues; crosses the placenta and is secreted in breast milk
Primary metabolism	Not metabolized
Primary excretion	Renal
Onset of action	2 h; peak effect: 4 h
Duration of action	6–12 h; half-life: 45–120 minutes

Adverse Effects: Hydrochlorothiazide is generally well tolerated and exhibits few serious adverse effects. Hypotension may cause dizziness or headache. Electrolyte imbalances such as hypochloremia, hypomagnesemia, hypokalemia, and hyponatremia may occur. Dysrhythmias due to hypokalemia may be serious if not prevented by maintaining normal serum potassium levels, usually by the administration of potassium supplements during therapy. Hydrochlorothiazide may precipitate gout attacks due to its tendency to cause hyperuricemia. Blood dyscrasias such as leukopenia, agranulocytosis, and aplastic anemia are rare, though serious, adverse effects.

Contraindications/Precautions: Contraindications include anuria and prior hypersensitivity to thiazide diuretics or sulfonamide antibiotics. Because hydrochlorothiazide can cause glycosuria and hyperglycemia, serum glucose levels must be carefully monitored in patients with diabetes. Preexisting hypovolemia or hypotension should be corrected before thiazide therapy is initiated because diuretics can worsen these conditions. Hydrochlorothiazide should not be used in jaundiced neonates because it can cause hyperbilirubinemia.

Drug Interactions: When given concurrently with other antihypertensives, additive effects on blood pressure usually occur. Thiazides may reduce the effectiveness of anticoagulants, sulfonylureas, and antidiabetic drugs, including insulin. Cholestyramine and colestipol bind to and decrease the absorption of HCTZ, thus reducing its effectiveness. Hydrochlorothiazide increases the risk of renal toxicity from NSAIDs. Corticosteroids and amphotericin B increase potassium loss when given with HCTZ. Hypokalemia caused by HCTZ may increase digoxin toxicity and the possibility of dysrhythmias. Hydrochlorothiazide decreases the excretion of lithium and can lead to lithium toxicity. Because thiazides decrease the renal excretion of calcium, concurrent administration with calcium supplements may lead to hypercalcemia. **Herbal/Food:** Ginkgo biloba may produce a paradoxical increase in blood pressure. Oral aloe can decrease levels of potassium and should not be used concurrently with thiazide diuretics. Use with hawthorn could result in additive hypotensive effects. High sodium intake can reduce the effectiveness of diuretics; patients should be placed on a sodium-restricted diet of 8 g or less per day.

Treatment of Overdose: Overdose is manifested as electrolyte depletion, which is treated with infusions of fluids containing electrolytes. Infusion of fluids also prevents dehydration and hypotension.

Pregnancy: Category B.

Nursing Responsibilities:

- Obtain a complete health history, including data on recent surgeries or trauma, nicotine and alcohol consumption, and use of complementary and alternative therapies, to determine possible drug allergies or interactions.
- Obtain baseline and periodic determinations of serum electrolytes, CBCs, BUN, serum glucose, serum uric acid, and CO_2.
- Measure blood pressure before initiation of therapy and at regular intervals.
- Monitor intake and output ratio and check for edema.
- Monitor for therapeutic effectiveness. Antihypertensive effects may be noted in 3 to 4 days; maximal effects may require 3 to 4 weeks.
- Monitor serum potassium values and assess for symptoms of hypokalemia.
- Establish safety precautions if CNS effects or orthostatic hypotension occurs. Consider blood pressure measurement (reclining, sitting, and standing) prior to ambulation if fluid volume deficit is suspected.
- Monitor for hyperglycemia and loss of glycemic control in patients with diabetes.
- Ensure ready access to restroom facilities. Keep the urinal, bedpan, or bedside commode readily available for patients with limited mobility.

Patient and Family Education:

- Monitor blood pressure regularly as directed by the health care provider. Maintain a written log of blood pressure readings and present it at follow-up visits.
- Consult the health care provider before using over-the-counter (OTC) drugs. Many contain significant amounts of sodium as well as potassium that could interfere with the effectiveness of drug therapy.
- Weigh daily and report gains or losses of greater than 2 pounds in 2 days.
- If diabetic, monitor blood glucose levels frequently at the beginning of therapy and during dosage adjustments.
- Eat potassium-rich foods daily (e.g., bananas, oranges, peaches, or dried dates) to reduce or prevent potassium depletion. Learn the symptoms of low potassium levels; report muscle cramps or weakness.
- Make position changes slowly when moving from a lying to a standing position because this drug may cause dizziness and possible fainting.
- Avoid direct contact with sunlight because photosensitivity may occur 10 to 14 days after initial sun exposure.
- Do not breast-feed while taking this drug without the approval of the health care provider.

Drugs Similar to Hydrochlorothiazide (HydroDIURIL, HCTZ)

There are many thiazide and thiazide-like diuretics available. They may be grouped into subclasses based on their relative duration of action.

Short-acting thiazides: This group includes chlorothiazide (Diuril) and hydrochlorothiazide (HydroDIURIL, HCTZ). These drugs have a rapid onset of 1 to 2 hours with a duration of action of 6 to 12 hours. Chlorothiazide is available by the IV route for patients who are unable to take PO thiazides.

Intermediate-acting thiazides: This group includes metolazone (Zaroxolyn) and Corzide, a fixed-dose combination of bendroflumethiazide (a thiazide) with nadolol (a beta-adrenergic blocker). These drugs have an onset time of about 2 hours with a duration of action of 12 to 24 hours.

Long-acting thiazides: This group includes chlorthalidone (Hygroton), indapamide (Lozol), and methyclothiazide (Aquatensen, Enduron). These agents have a 2-hour onset with a duration of action ranging from 24 to 72 hours.

CONNECTION *Checkpoint* 35.3

The use of lithium is often contraindicated when a patient is taking diuretics. From what you learned in Chapter 23, identify the indications for lithium and explain how the use of a diuretic can lead to lithium toxicity. See Answer to Connection Checkpoint 35.3 in Appendix A.

Potassium-Sparing Diuretics

35.7 Potassium-sparing diuretics have low effectiveness but can help prevent hypokalemia.

As discussed in Sections 35.5 and 35.6, hypokalemia is a potentially serious adverse effect of the loop and thiazide diuretics. The therapeutic advantage of the potassium-sparing diuretics is that increased diuresis can be obtained without affecting blood potassium levels. The potassium-sparing diuretics are listed in Table 35.6. There are two distinct subclasses of potassium-sparing diuretics: sodium channel inhibitors and aldosterone antagonists.

Sodium ion channel inhibitors: In the distal tubule, Na^+ is reabsorbed from the filtrate through sodium ion channels. As the sodium ion in the filtrate travels across the renal tubule cell and returns to the bloodstream, potassium ion moves in the opposite direction. In other words, as sodium ion is reabsorbed, potassium ion is secreted.

Triamterene (Dyrenium) and amiloride (Midamor) block the Na^+ channel, causing sodium to stay in the filtrate. Because water always follows sodium ions, additional water remains in the filtrate and ultimately leaves in the urine. When the sodium ion channel is blocked, another important action occurs: Potassium ion is not secreted to the filtrate. The body, therefore, does not lose potassium, as is the case with the thiazide and loop diuretics. Because most of the sodium ion has already been removed before the filtrate reaches the distal tubule, these potassium-sparing diuretics produce only a mild diuresis. Drugs in this class are rarely prescribed alone, but they may be used in combination with thiazide or loop diuretics to minimize loss of potassium ions in the pharmacotherapy of HTN or edema.

Aldosterone antagonists: Aldosterone is the primary mineralocorticoid hormone secreted by the adrenal gland. The physiological targets, or membrane receptors (MRs), for aldosterone are located in the distal tubule and collecting ducts of the nephron. Once bound to its receptors, the MR–aldosterone complex causes the renal tubule cells to synthesize more Na^+ channels, thereby allowing for more reabsorption of Na^+ from the filtrate. Simply stated, aldosterone increases sodium reabsorption.

Spironolactone (Aldactone) and eplerenone (Inspra) prevent the formation of the MR–aldosterone complex and are called aldosterone antagonists. By blocking the actions of aldosterone, these drugs enhance the excretion of sodium and the retention of potassium. Like the sodium ion channel inhibitors, spironolactone and eplerenone produce only a weak diuresis, and they are normally combined with drugs from other classes when treating HTN or edema. Spironolactone, however, has also been found to significantly reduce mortality in patients with heart failure (see Chapter 38) and, because of this important beneficial effect, its use has been increasing. The aldosterone antagonists are also used to treat hyperaldosteronism, a rare disorder in which a tumor of the adrenal gland secretes large amounts of aldosterone.

Using potassium supplements or adding potassium-rich foods to the diet when taking these medications may lead to life-threatening hyperkalemia. Signs and symptoms of hyperkalemia include muscle weakness, ventricular tachycardia, or fibrillation. Other minor adverse effects of the drugs include headache, dizziness, nausea, and vomiting. Spironolactone binds to progesterone and androgen receptors, resulting in a small incidence of adverse effects such as gynecomastia, menstrual abnormalities, and impotence. Gynecomastia appears to be related to dosage level and duration of therapy; it may persist in some after the drug is discontinued. The incidence of adverse reproductive system effects is lower with eplerenone.

PROTOTYPE DRUG Spironolactone (Aldactone)

Classification: **Therapeutic:** Antihypertensive
Pharmacologic: Potassium-sparing diuretic/aldosterone antagonist

Therapeutic Effects and Uses: Approved in 1960, spironolactone is the most commonly prescribed potassium-sparing diuretic. The most common indication for spironolactone is mild HTN. Because it does not cause potassium depletion, the drug is particularly useful in patients who are at high risk for hypokalemia. However, spironolactone does such an efficient job of retaining potassium that hyperkalemia may develop, especially if the patient is taking potassium supplements or is concurrently receiving angiotensin-converting enzyme (ACE) inhibitors. When serum potassium levels are monitored carefully and maintained within normal values, serious adverse effects from spironolactone are uncommon.

Spironolactone is frequently used as maintenance therapy to reduce the edema and sodium retention associated with

TABLE 35.6 Potassium-Sparing Diuretics

Drug	Route and Adult Dose (maximum dose where indicated)	Adverse Effects
Sodium Channel Inhibitors		
amiloride (Midamor)	PO: 5–10 mg/day (max: 20 mg/day)	*Minor hyperkalemia, headache, fatigue, gynecomastia (spironolactone)* Dysrhythmias (from hyperkalemia), dehydration, hyponatremia, agranulocytosis, and other blood dyscrasias
triamterene (Dyrenium)	PO: 50–100 mg bid (max: 300 mg/day)	
Aldosterone Antagonists		
eplerenone (Inspra)	PO: 25–50 mg once daily (max: 100 mg/day for HTN; 50 mg/day for heart failure)	
spironolactone (Aldactone)	PO: 25–100 mg one to two times/day (max: 400 mg/day)	

Note: *Italics* indicate common adverse effects: Underline indicates serious adverse effects.

congestive heart failure (CHF), nephrotic syndrome, or liver disease. It is particularly useful in treating edema or ascites in patients with hepatic cirrhosis, because it counteracts the large amount of aldosterone secreted by these patients. Spironolactone may also be used for the short-term, preoperative treatment of primary hyperaldosteronism. An off-label indication is to improve survival and reduce hospitalizations in patients with severe heart failure. Other off-label indications include treatment of minor edema associated with PMS, polycystic ovary, and hirsutism in females. It is available in tablet form and as a fixed-dose combination with hydrochlorothiazide.

Mechanism of Action: Spironolactone acts by inhibiting the actions of aldosterone in the distal tubule and collecting ducts of the nephron. When the actions of aldosterone are blocked by spironolactone, sodium, chloride, and water excretion are increased and the body retains potassium.

Pharmacokinetics:

Route(s)	PO
Absorption	Rapid absorption; 73% absorbed
Distribution	Distributed to most tissues; crosses the placenta; secreted in breast milk; more than 90% bound to plasma protein
Primary metabolism	Hepatic and renal; converted to active metabolites
Primary excretion	Renal (40–57%) and biliary (35–40%)
Onset of action	2–3 days; may take 2 weeks for maximum effect
Duration of action	2–3 days; half-life: 1.3–2.4 h for parent compound, and 18–23 h for active metabolites

Adverse Effects: Hyperkalemia induced by spironolactone can cause life-threatening cardiac dysrhythmias. Signs and symptoms associated with spironolactone-induced hyperkalemia include muscle weakness, paresthesia, fatigue, bradycardia, flaccid paralysis of the extremities, and shock. In men, spironolactone can cause gynecomastia, impotence, and diminished libido. Women may experience menstrual irregularities, hirsutism, and breast tenderness. Fertility may decrease during therapy. Agranulocytosis and other blood dyscrasias are rare adverse effects.

Contraindications/Precautions: Contraindications include anuria, significant renal impairment, pregnancy, and hyperkalemia. Older patients and those with renal insufficiency or diabetes mellitus are at greatest risk for hyperkalemia. At high doses, spironolactone produces teratogenic effects in laboratory animals; thus it should not be used during pregnancy. A major metabolite of spironolactone is secreted in breast milk; thus this drug should not be given to lactating patients.

Drug Interactions: When combined with ammonium chloride, acidosis may occur. Aspirin and other salicylates may decrease the diuretic effect of the medication. Concurrent use with digoxin may decrease the effects of digoxin. When taken with potassium supplements, ACE inhibitors, angiotensin-receptor blockers, or the potassium salts of other drugs (such as penicillin G potassium), severe hyperkalemia and possible dysrhythmias may result. Concurrent use with other antihypertensives will result in an additive hypotensive effect. **Herbal/Food:** Licorice extract contains a substance with aldosterone-like actions and should be avoided. Use with hawthorn could result in additive hypotensive effects.

Treatment of Overdose: The most serious symptoms of spironolactone overdose are related to hyperkalemia. If severe, therapies are administered to counteract the hyperkalemia. These include IV calcium chloride, IV sodium bicarbonate, or the administration of glucose with rapid-acting insulin. Cationic exchange resins such as sodium polystyrene sulfonate (Kayexalate) may be administered.

Pregnancy: Category D.

Nursing Responsibilities:

- Obtain a complete health history, including data on recent surgeries or trauma, nicotine and alcohol consumption, and the use of complementary and alternative therapies to determine possible drug allergies or interactions.
- Obtain baseline and periodic determinations of serum electrolytes, CBCs, BUN, blood glucose, uric acid, and CO_2.
- Check blood pressure before the initiation of therapy and at regular intervals.
- Assess for signs of fluid and electrolyte imbalance, especially potassium levels.
- Concurrent use with digoxin may decrease the effects of digoxin. Monitor the patient for signs of heart failure (edema, shortness of breath, or sensorium changes) or cardiac dysrhythmias.
- Monitor daily intake and output and check for edema. Report lack of diuretic response or development of edema; both may indicate tolerance to this drug.
- Weigh the patient under standard conditions before therapy begins and daily throughout therapy. Weight is a useful index of need for dosage adjustment. For patients with ascites, the prescriber may want measurements of abdominal girth.
- Observe for and immediately report the onset of mental changes, lethargy, or stupor in patients with liver disease to the prescriber.

Patient and Family Education:

- Monitor blood pressure regularly. Maintain a written log of blood pressure readings and present it at follow-up visits.
- Be aware that diuretic effects may not occur until several days of therapy, and that diuresis may continue for 2 to 3 days after the drug is withdrawn.
- Learn symptoms of potassium imbalances (hyperkalemia) and immediately report nausea, fatigue, muscle weakness, or tingling, should they occur. More serious signs include slow heartbeat and weak pulse.
- Weigh two to three times each week. Report gains or losses of greater than 2 pounds in 2 days.

MyNursingKit | Mechanism of Action Animation: Spironolactone

- Do not drive or perform other hazardous activities until the effects of the drug are known because this drug may cause drowsiness or dizziness.
- Avoid excessive intake of high-potassium foods or salt substitutes (these contain potassium). Never take OTC potassium supplements without approval of the health care provider.
- Do not breast-feed while taking this drug without approval of the health care provider.

Drugs Similar to Spironolactone (Aldactone)

The three other potassium-sparing diuretics include amiloride, eplerenone, and triamterene.

Amiloride (Midamor): Approved in 1981, amiloride is an oral Na^+ channel inhibitor with weak diuretic activity whose major indication is HTN. It is also used to treat peripheral edema due to heart failure and to reverse hypokalemia. When combined with a thiazide diuretic, additive hypotensive action is achieved, and potassium balance is maintained. It should not be used as monotherapy or in combination with other potassium-sparing diuretics because hyperkalemia may develop. Contraindications and adverse effects are similar to those of spironolactone, including the risk of severe hyperkalemia in patients receiving other potassium-containing drugs. Moduretic is a fixed-dose combination of amiloride and hydrochlorothiazide. Amiloride is pregnancy category B.

Eplerenone (Inspra): Approved in 2002, eplerenone is an aldosterone antagonist administered by the oral route that was initially approved for HTN. Later, post-MI management of heart failure was added as an indication. Research has not shown eplerenone to be more effective than spironolactone, but it is considerably more expensive. Two to four weeks of therapy are required to achieve maximum therapeutic effects. Eplerenone is more selective for the aldosterone receptor than spironolactone, and it has the advantage of producing a lower incidence of endocrine-related adverse effects such as gynecomastia, impotence, or menstrual irregularities. Like other drugs in this class, the development of hyperkalemia is a potentially serious adverse effect of this drug. Eplerenone is sometimes referred to as a selective aldosterone receptor antagonist. This drug is pregnancy category B.

Triamterene (Dyrenium): Approved in 1964, triamterene is an oral drug that acts by the same mechanism as amiloride and has the same indications and adverse effects. It is a relatively weak diuretic and is sometimes used to manage hypokalemia in patients who are unable to tolerate potassium supplements. Triamterene is rarely used as monotherapy and should not be used concurrently with other potassium-sparing diuretics due to the potential for hyperkalemia. Dyazide is a fixed-dose combination of triamterene and hydrochlorothiazide. This drug is pregnancy category C.

CONNECTION Checkpoint 35.4

From what you learned in Chapter 34, explain why patients who are taking an ACE inhibitor should probably not receive an aldosterone antagonist. See Answer to Connection Checkpoint 35.4 in Appendix A.

Osmotic Diuretics

35.8 Osmotic diuretics cause diuresis by increasing the osmolality of the filtrate.

The osmotic diuretics, shown in Table 35.7, are a small class of drugs that are reserved for very specific indications. Unlike the thiazides and loop diuretics that block transport proteins, osmotic diuretics are mostly inert and act by raising the osmolality, or **osmotic pressure,** of body fluids. Osmotic diuretics cause water to shift compartments by creating a difference in osmotic pressure across a membrane or between two body compartments.

When given IV, osmotic diuretics are filtered at the glomerulus and readily enter the renal filtrate. Once in the tubule, they remain unchanged. As normal sodium and water reabsorption progresses in the proximal tubule, the diuretic remains behind, and its concentration in the tubule begins to increase. The osmolality of the filtrate increases due to the presence of the osmotic diuretic in the tubule. This osmotic force draws water into the filtrate, resulting in increased diuresis. The influence of osmotic pressure on water movement is presented in greater detail in Chapter 42.

A second action of osmotic diuretics is their ability to raise the osmolality of the plasma. This creates an osmotic force that moves water from the intracellular and extravascular spaces to the plasma. The increased volume of water in the plasma is filtered by the kidney, resulting in enhanced diuresis. This action is used to advantage in the treatment of two conditions where fluid has accumulated in extravascular spaces. For example, following a traumatic head injury, fluid accumulates in the brain, causing dangerously high intracranial pressure. Osmotic diuretics create an osmotic force that promotes the fluid to leave the brain and enter the blood, thus reducing cerebral edema. A second example is high intraocular pressure caused by excess fluid accumulation in the eye (glaucoma). Osmotic diuretics can cause the fluid to leave the eye and enter the blood, thus relieving the high intraocular pressure.

Osmotic diuretics are rarely the drugs of first choice due to their potential toxicity. Mannitol and urea are given by the IV route under controlled conditions where the patient can be closely monitored. Although as diuretics they are useful in increasing urine output, they are contraindicated in patients with severe renal impairment. The rapid movement of water from the extravascular spaces to the blood can result in severe dehydration in the tissues, and cause a serious fluid overload in patients with severe heart failure. Electrolyte imbalances, especially hyponatremia, may occur with these agents.

TABLE 35.7 Miscellaneous Diuretics

Drug	Route and Adult Dose (maximum dose where indicated)	Adverse Effects
Carbonic Anhydrase Inhibitors		
acetazolamide (Diamox)	PO: 250–375 mg/day (max: 1,500 mg/day) IM/IV: 250–375 mg/day	*Electrolyte imbalances, fatigue, nausea, vomiting, dizziness* Dehydration, blood dyscrasias, pancytopenia, flaccid paralysis, hemolytic anemia, aplastic anemia
methazolamide (Neptazane)	PO: 50–100 mg bid–tid (max: 300 mg/day)	
Osmotic Type		
glycerin (Colace, Osmoglyn)	PO: 1–1.8 g/kg, 1–2 h before ocular surgery	*Electrolyte imbalances, fatigue, nausea, vomiting, dizziness* Hyponatremia, edema, convulsions, tachycardia
mannitol (Osmitrol)	IV: 100 g infused over 2–6 h	
urea (Ureaphil)	IV: 1–1.5 g/kg over 1–2.5 h	

Note: *Italics* indicate common adverse effects. Underline indicates serious adverse effects.

PROTOTYPE DRUG Mannitol (Osmitrol)

Classification: Therapeutic: Drug for renal failure
Pharmacologic: Osmotic diuretic

Therapeutic Effects and Uses: Approved in 1944, mannitol is a parenteral diuretic primarily used to increase urine output in patients experiencing oliguria from acute renal failure. In addition, by its ability to increase the osmolality of plasma, this drug is able to "pull" fluid out of extravascular spaces; thus it is used to reduce intracranial pressure following head trauma and to lower intraocular pressure in patients with acute glaucoma. Reduction in the amount and pressure of cerebrospinal fluid can occur as quickly as 15 minutes after initiating the infusion; intraocular pressure reduction may take up to an hour. Mannitol may be administered concurrently with nephrotoxic drugs such as cisplatin (an antineoplastic drug) to speed them through the kidney and reduce damage to the walls of the renal tubules.

Mannitol has nondrug uses as a sweetener and food stabilizer. When taken orally, it is absorbed so slowly that it has no effect on insulin levels, making it an alternative sweetener in foods for patients with diabetes. The drug has a laxative effect when taken in large quantities.

Mechanism of Action: Administered by the IV route, mannitol is filtered by the glomerulus of the kidney but is incapable of being reabsorbed from the renal tubule. This creates an osmotic gradient, resulting in decreased water and Na^+ reabsorption and increased diuresis.

Pharmacokinetics:

Route(s)	IV
Absorption	Does not cross biologic membranes
Distribution	Remains in extracellular space; does not cross the blood–brain barrier
Primary metabolism	Hepatic (small amounts)
Primary excretion	Renal
Onset of action	1–3 h
Duration of action	4–6 h; half-life: 100 minutes

Adverse Effects: Electrolyte imbalances, either deficiencies or excesses, can occur during mannitol therapy. For example, as mannitol draws fluid from the intravascular spaces, hyperkalemia or hypernatremia may occur. However, mannitol also increases the excretion of sodium and potassium ions, which can result in hypokalemia or hyponatremia. The same holds true for fluid balance. As mannitol draws fluid into the extracellular spaces, peripheral edema, CHF, or pulmonary edema may occur. As diuresis progresses, the patient may become hypovolemic and dehydrated. Other adverse effects include fatigue, nausea, vomiting, dizziness, convulsions, and tachycardia.

Contraindications/Precautions: Contraindications include anuria, severe CHF, organic CNS disease or intracranial bleeding, severe dehydration, and shock. A test dose may be given to patients with oliguria to determine renal function. Function is considered satisfactory if urine flow is at least 30 to 50 mL/h over 2 to 3 hours following an IV test dose of 0.2 g/kg. If this response is not achieved, the kidneys are too impaired to administer a full dose of mannitol.

There is evidence that high doses of mannitol may open the blood–brain barrier by temporarily shrinking the endothelial cells that line the barrier. Should this happen, mannitol will enter the brain (bringing water with it) and increase intracranial pressure. Extreme precautions must be taken when treating patients with high intracranial pressure. Experimentally, mannitol is used to intentionally open the blood–brain barrier to deliver higher doses of various drugs, such as antineoplastic agents, directly to the brain.

Drug Interactions: Because of its intense diuretic effect, mannitol can increase the excretion of many drugs. This results in a decreased effect for drugs such as lithium, imipramine, salicylates, barbiturates, and potassium supplements. **Herbal/Food:** Unknown.

Pregnancy: Category C.

Treatment of Overdose: Overdose will result in a shift of fluid to the vascular compartment, resulting in CHF and pulmonary edema. Intense diuresis may cause significant electrolyte imbalances, especially hyponatremia. There is no specific antidote and treatment is supportive to the presenting symptoms.

Nursing Responsibilities:

- Take care to avoid extravasation. Observe the injection site for signs of inflammation or edema.
- Closely monitor serum and urine electrolytes and kidney function during therapy.
- Measure daily intake and output accurately and record to achieve proper fluid balance. Assess for signs of CHF and pulmonary edema.
- Monitor vital signs closely and report significant changes in blood pressure.
- Monitor for possible indications of fluid and electrolyte imbalance such as thirst, muscle cramps or weakness, and paresthesias.
- Be alert to the possibility that a rebound increase in intracranial pressure sometimes occurs about 12 hours after drug administration. The patient may complain of headache or confusion.
- Weigh the patient under standard conditions before therapy begins and daily throughout therapy. Weight is a useful index of the need for dosage adjustment.

Patient and Family Education:

- Report increased thirst; muscle cramps or weakness; shortness of breath; swelling of the hands, feet, or ankles; or headache to the health care provider.
- Family members should immediately report any evidence of confusion to the health care provider.
- Do not breast-feed while taking this drug without approval of the health care provider.

Drugs Similar to Mannitol (Osmitrol)

Other osmotic diuretics include glycerin and urea. Drugs in this class are infrequently used.

Glycerin (Colace, Osmoglyn): Also known as glycerol, glycerin is an osmotic diuretic given for a large number of indications. When given by the oral route, glycerin creates an osmotic gradient like mannitol that can reduce intraocular and intracranial pressure. As a laxative suppository (Colace), glycerin draws water into the colon, creating more bulk and promoting defecation. It is used in a variety of OTC products as an emollient or lubricant, including toothpaste, shaving cream, hair products, soaps, and skin care products. Like mannitol, it tastes sweet and is used as a food additive to sweeten and keep products moist. Contraindications for oral use include hypovolemia, CHF, or intestinal obstruction. This drug is pregnancy category C.

Urea (Ureaphil): Urea is a small molecule that is a natural waste product of nitrogen metabolism in the body. Approved in 1966 as a drug, it is given IV to create an osmotic gradient that reduces cerebral edema and intraocular pressure. Contraindications and adverse effects are similar to those of mannitol. It is also available topically to rehydrate the skin or to remove excess keratin. Urea has a large number of industrial uses, including its use in fertilizer, hair products, deicing agents, and bath oils, and even as a flavor enhancer in cigarettes. This drug is pregnancy category C.

Carbonic Anhydrase Inhibitors

35.9 Carbonic anhydrase inhibitors are weak diuretics that have specific indications.

Carbonic anhydrase is an essential enzyme that helps regulate the acid–base balance in the body. Carbonic anhydrase converts CO_2 to carbonic acid (H_2CO_3), which immediately dissociates to bicarbonate ion (HCO_3^-). Note that these reactions are reversible.

$$CO_2 + H_2O \longleftrightarrow H_2CO_3 \longleftrightarrow HCO_3^- + H^+$$

Carbonic acid is present in multiple tissues. In red blood cells, it converts CO_2 (an acidic, poorly soluble gas) to bicarbonate, which can be transported to the lungs, reconverted to CO_2, and exhaled. In the mucosa of the stomach, carbonic anhydrase is responsible for forming gastric acid (H^+). For this chapter, the most important action of carbonic anhydrase occurs in the renal tubule cells.

In the kidney tubules, carbonic anhydrase is necessary for the formation and reabsorption of bicarbonate ion, which is essential for maintaining proper acid–base balance. Sodium ions are reabsorbed with bicarbonate ion in the proximal tubule using a symporter protein.

Several drugs that inhibit CA are available. Blocking the CA enzyme prevents bicarbonate formation and reabsorption in the renal tubule. Without bicarbonate ion, sodium reabsorption does not occur, more water remains in the filtrate, and diuresis is promoted. The reduction in plasma bicarbonate eventually causes metabolic acidosis, which tends to reverse the diuretic action of this drug.

Although once used as diuretics, the carbonic anhydrase inhibitors are now rarely prescribed for that purpose because they produce only a weak, short-lived diuresis and can contribute to metabolic acidosis. Carbonic anhydrase inhibitors that are given by the oral route include acetazolamide (Diamox) and methazolamide (Neptazane). Methazolamide is only approved for reducing intraocular pressure in patients with open-angle glaucoma. Acetazolamide (Diamox), also used to decrease intraocular fluid pressure, has several other indications. Two drugs in this class, dorzolamide (Trusopt) and brinzolamide (Azopt), are administered topically to the eye for open-angle glaucoma. The antiglaucoma drugs in this class are discussed in Chapter 77.

PROTOTYPE DRUG Acetazolamide (Diamox)

Classification: **Therapeutic:** Drug for edema, antiglaucoma agent
Pharmacologic: Carbonic anhydrase inhibitor

Therapeutic Effects and Uses: Given by either the oral or parenteral route, acetazolamide produces a mild diuresis and is occasionally used to reduce edema fluid in patients with CHF. An older drug approved in 1953, it has largely been replaced by thiazide diuretics.

Acetazolamide also has applications as an anticonvulsant for treating absence seizures and in treating motion sickness. It has been used to acclimatize people to high altitudes to prevent or treat acute mountain sickness. It accomplishes this by increasing the renal excretion of bicarbonate, which accumulates in the body because of the hyperventilation that occurs at high altitude. Acetazolamide is effective in treating open-angle glaucoma and for preoperative treatment of acute closed-angle glaucoma, although it is not a drug of first choice for these disorders.

Mechanism of Action: Acetazolamide produces its diuretic effect by inhibiting carbonic anhydrase activity in the proximal renal tubule, causing increased excretion of sodium and bicarbonate. In the eye, the inhibition of carbonic anhydrase reduces the rate of aqueous humor formation and consequently lowers intraocular pressure.

Pharmacokinetics:

Route(s)	PO, IV, IM
Absorption	75% absorbed when given with food
Distribution	Distributed to most tissues; crosses the placenta, and is secreted in breast milk
Primary metabolism	Not metabolized
Primary excretion	Renal
Onset of action	PO: 90 minutes; IV: 2 minutes
Duration of action	PO: 8–12 h; PO sustained release: 18–24 h; IV: 15 minutes; half-life: 2.4–5.8 h

Adverse Effects: Acetazolamide can cause various electrolyte imbalances, including hyperchloremia and hypokalemia. Gastrointestinal adverse effects include nausea, vomiting, diarrhea, and anorexia. CNS effects may occur, such as dizziness, fatigue, and numbness in the extremities, lips, or facial muscles. Metabolic acidosis may result from excess bicarbonate loss.

Contraindications/Precautions: Acetazolamide is contraindicated in patients who have hypersensitivity to sulfonamides and similar drugs such as thiazide diuretics. Other contraindications include severe renal or hepatic impairment and adrenocortical insufficiency. Patients with preexisting electrolyte imbalances such as hyponatremia, hypokalemia, or hypochloremic acidosis should be treated with caution because acetazolamide may worsen these conditions.

Drug Interactions: The potential for hypokalemia is greatest early in the course of acetazolamide therapy and is accelerated by amphotericin B and corticosteroids. Because acetazolamide alkalinizes the urine, the renal excretion of many drugs may be decreased, including tricyclic antidepressants, procainamide, amphetamines, ephedrine, and quinidine. Renal excretion of lithium and phenobarbital may be increased. High-dose aspirin therapy can compete with tubular secretory mechanisms with acetazolamide, causing the CA inhibitor to accumulate to toxic levels. **Herbal/Food:** Unknown.

Pregnancy: Category C.

Treatment of Overdose: Overdose with acetazolamide results in metabolic acidosis, which may be treated by administering sodium bicarbonate. Electrolyte depletion and dehydration are treated with infusions of fluids containing electrolytes.

Nursing Responsibilities:

- Establish a baseline weight before initial therapy and weigh daily thereafter when this drug is used to treat edema.
- Monitor for symptoms of mild to severe metabolic acidosis and potassium loss, which are greatest early in therapy.
- Monitor daily intake and output, especially when used concurrently with other diuretics.
- Obtain baseline and periodic determinations of blood pH, blood gases, urinalysis, CBC, and serum electrolytes.

Patient and Family Education:

- Maintain adequate fluid intake (1.5–2.5 L/24 h; 1 liter is approximately equal to 1 quart) to reduce risk of kidney stones.
- Immediately report numbness, tingling, burning, drowsiness, visual problems, sore throat or mouth, unusual bleeding, fever, and skin or urinary problems to the health care provider.

CONNECTIONS

Complementary and Alternative Therapies Dandelion

Description: The common dandelion, *Taraxacum officinale*, is found worldwide and is considered a weed by homeowners and gardeners. The plant has both culinary and medicinal uses.

History and Claims: Medicinal applications of dandelion have been recorded as early as the 10th century by Arab health care providers, and the plant was introduced by the Celts when Roman legions invaded Britain. Native Americans used the plant to treat heartburn and kidney disease. Leaves of the plant are rich in vitamin A, potassium, minerals, and fiber and have been eaten raw in salads or cooked like spinach as a major nutritional source. The dandelion root has been dried and used to treat a large variety of conditions, including constipation, liver ailments, bronchitis, gout, and arthritis. The plant is also sold as a diuretic to ease premenstrual fluid retention. The *German Commission E Monographs* authorize the use of combination products containing dandelion root for biliary disease, anorexia, and dyspepsia, and to stimulate diuresis.

Standardization: Dandelion is available in tea, liquid, or tablet form. Standardization is generally based on the amount of dandelion in grams (2 to 12 grams/day).

Evidence: Research evidence to support most uses of dandelion is lacking, and data regarding the use of dandelion as a diuretic are conflicting. When taken in moderation, dandelion is safe and is a significant source of vitamins and minerals. High doses of dandelion should be discouraged due to potential interactions with prescription medications.

Source: From *Herbs at a Glance: Dandelion*, by the National Center for Complementary and Alternative Medicine, 2008. Retrieved July 8, 2008, from http://nccam.nih.gov/health/dandelion/; *Herbal Medicine: Expanded Commission E Monographs* (pp. 182–191), by M. Blumenthal, A. Goldberg, & J. Brinckmann, Eds., 2000, Newton, MA: Lippincott Williams & Wilkins; "Taraxacum—A Review on Its Phytochemical and Pharmacological Profile," by K. Schütz, R. Carle, & A. Schieber, 2006, *Journal of Ethnopharmacology, 107*(3), pp. 313–323.

NURSING PROCESS APPLICATION

Patients Receiving Diuretic Therapy

Assessment

Prior to administration:

- Obtain a complete health history (mental and physical), including data on recent surgeries or trauma.
- Obtain vital signs; assess in the context of the patient's baseline values.
- Obtain the patient's medication history, including nicotine and alcohol consumption and use of herbal supplements or alternative therapies, to determine possible drug allergies or interactions.
- Obtain blood and urine specimens for laboratory analysis.

Potential Nursing Diagnoses

- *Excess Fluid Volume,* related to disease process
- *Risk for Deficient Fluid Volume,* related to diuretic response
- *Impaired Urinary Elimination,* related to diuretic use and frequent urination
- *Risk for Injury,* related to fluid and electrolyte imbalances and orthostatic hypotension

Planning: Patient Goals and Expected Outcomes

The patient will:

- Exhibit normal fluid balance and maintain electrolyte levels within normal limits during drug therapy.
- Demonstrate an understanding of the drug by accurately describing the drug's action, adverse effects, and precautions.
- Immediately report symptoms of hyperkalemia or hypokalemia and hypersensitivity.

Implementation

Interventions and (Rationales)	Patient and Family Education
• Monitor for fluid overload by measuring intake, output, and daily weights. (Intake, output, and daily body weight are indications of the effectiveness of diuretic therapy.)	Instruct the patient to: • Immediately report any severe shortness of breath, frothy sputum, profound fatigue, edema in the extremities, potential signs of heart failure, or pulmonary edema. • Accurately measure intake, output, and body weight, and report weight gain of 2 or more pounds within 2 days, or a decrease in output. • Avoid excessive heat, which contributes to fluid loss through perspiration. • Consume adequate amounts of plain water.
• Monitor laboratory values, especially potassium and sodium. (Diuretics can cause electrolyte imbalances.)	• Instruct the patient to inform laboratory personnel of diuretic therapy when providing blood or urine samples.
• Monitor vital signs, especially blood pressure. (Diuretics reduce blood volume, resulting in lowered blood pressure.)	Instruct the patient to: • Monitor blood pressure as specified by the health care provider and ensure proper use of home equipment. • Stop the medication if severe hypotension exists, as specified by the health care provider (e.g., "hold for levels below 88/50 mmHg").
• Observe for changes in level of consciousness (LOC), dizziness, fatigue, and orthostatic hypotension. (Reduction in blood volume due to diuretic therapy may produce changes in LOC or syncope.)	Instruct the patient to: • Immediately report any change in consciousness, especially feeling faint. • Make position changes slowly. • Obtain blood pressure readings in the sitting, standing, and lying positions.
• Monitor potassium intake. (Potassium is vital to maintaining proper electrolyte balance and can become depleted with thiazide or loop diuretics.)	• For patients receiving loop or thiazide diuretics, instruct the patient to eat foods high in potassium. • For patients receiving potassium-sparing diuretics, instruct the patient to avoid foods high in potassium and consult with the health care provider before using vitamin or mineral supplements or electrolyte-fortified sports drinks.
• Observe for signs of hypersensitivity reaction. (Allergic responses may be life threatening.)	Instruct the patient or caregiver to report: • Difficulty breathing, throat tightness, hives or rash, or bleeding. • Flulike symptoms, such as shortness of breath, fever, sore throat, malaise, joint pain, or profound fatigue.
• Monitor hearing and vision. (Loop diuretics are ototoxic. Thiazide diuretics increase serum digoxin levels; elevated levels produce visual changes.)	• Instruct the patient to report any changes in hearing or vision such as ringing or buzzing in the ears; becoming "hard of hearing"; or experiencing dimness of sight, seeing halos, or having "yellow vision."
• Monitor reactivity to light exposure. (Some diuretics cause photosensitivity.)	Instruct the patient to: • Limit exposure to the sun. • Wear dark glasses and light-colored loose-fitting clothes when outdoors.

Evaluation of Outcome Criteria

Evaluate the effectiveness of drug therapy by confirming that patient goals and expected outcomes have been met (see "Planning").

- Eat potassium-rich foods and take a potassium supplement when taking this drug in high doses or for prolonged periods.
- Do not breast-feed while taking this drug without approval of the health care provider.

Drugs Similar to Acetazolamide (Diamox)

The other oral carbonic anhydrase inhibitor is methazolamide (Neptazane), which is used as a systemic antiglaucoma agent (see Chapter 77) rather than a diuretic.

UNDERSTANDING THE CHAPTER

Key Concepts Summary

35.1 The kidneys are major organs of excretion and body homeostasis.

35.2 The composition of filtrate changes dramatically as a result of the processes of reabsorption and secretion.

35.3 Renal failure may significantly impact the success of pharmacotherapy.

35.4 Diuretics are used to treat hypertension, heart failure, accumulation of edema fluid, and renal failure.

35.5 The most effective diuretics are the loop diuretics that block sodium reabsorption in the loop of Henle.

35.6 The thiazides are the most commonly prescribed class of diuretics.

35.7 Potassium-sparing diuretics have low effectiveness but can help prevent hypokalemia.

35.8 Osmotic diuretics cause diuresis by increasing the osmolality of the filtrate.

35.9 Carbonic anhydrase inhibitors are weak diuretics that have specific indications.

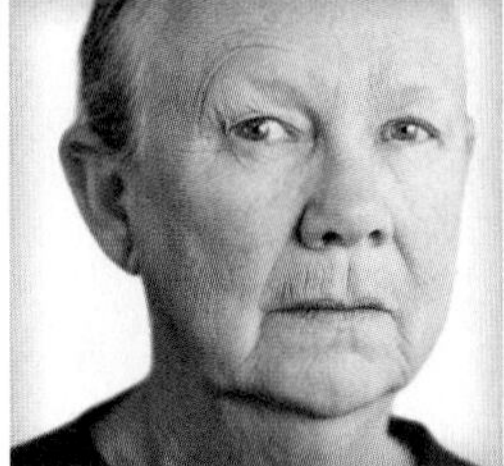

Making the PATIENT *Connection*

Remember the patient "Katherine Crosland" at the beginning of the chapter? Now read the remainder of the case study. Based on the information presented within this chapter, respond to the critical thinking questions that follow.

Katherine Crosland, a 79-year-old widow, has lived alone for the past 5 years. Although her son and daughters all reside in distant locations, they check on her at least weekly by telephoning. Katherine is fairly independent; however, she does not drive and is dependent on a neighbor to get her groceries and medications.

Three years ago, Katherine was hospitalized for an MI, which resulted in heart failure. She is adherent with her medications, which include digoxin (Lanoxin) 0.125 mg daily, furosemide (Lasix) 20 mg/day, and potassium supplements (K-Dur) 20 mEq daily.

Recently Katherine's neighbor went on an extended, out-of-town trip. Katherine was certain that she had enough of her medicine to last through that time. However, before the neighbor returned, Katherine discovered she had miscalculated her potassium supplement and only had enough for 10 days. Katherine figured that because the potassium was only a "supplement," she would be able to wait until her neighbor returned to get the medication refilled.

Today, she presents to the clinic with generalized weakness and fatigue. She has lost 3.6 kg (8 lb) since her last clinic visit 6 weeks ago. Her blood pressure is 104/62 mmHg, heart rate is 98 beats/minute, and slightly irregular, respiratory rate is 20/minute, and body temperature is 36.2°C (97.2°F). The blood specimen collected for diagnostic studies showed several outstanding findings such as a serum sodium level of 150 mEq and potassium level of 3.2 mEq. Katherine is diagnosed with dehydration and hypokalemia induced by diuretic therapy.

Critical Thinking Questions

1. Discuss fluid and electrolyte imbalances related to the following diuretic therapies:
   a. Loop diuretics
   b. Thiazide diuretics
   c. Potassium-sparing diuretics
   d. Osmotic diuretics
2. What relationship exists between this patient's diuretic therapy, digoxin therapy, and hypokalemia?
3. What patient education should the nurse provide about diuretic therapy?

Case Study

During a recent visit to the clinic, Miles Davenport learned that his antihypertensive medication was not maintaining his blood pressure at the desired level. The nurse practitioner prescribed spironolactone (Aldactone) 50 mg twice daily in addition to his regular antihypertensive medications.

1. Discuss the mechanism of action for spironolactone.
2. Prepare a list of foods that should be eaten sparingly while taking spironolactone.
3. List the symptoms of hyperkalemia that Miles needs to know to manage his disease and medications.

NCLEX-RN® Review

1 The nurse is talking with a group of clients with cardiac conditions who are taking diuretic therapy. The nurse explains that individuals prescribed furosemide (Lasix) should:

1. Avoid consuming large amounts of cabbage, cauliflower, and kale.
2. Rise slowly from sitting or lying positions.
3. Count their pulse for 1 full minute before taking the medication.
4. Inject the medication subcutaneously around the umbilicus.

2 The client who is receiving a high-ceiling diuretic is instructed to watch for symptoms associated with electrolyte imbalances. Of the following conditions, which would the client most likely expect?

1. Hyponatremia
2. Hypokalemia
3. Hyperkalemia
4. Hypocalcemia

3 While preparing a client for discharge, which of the following statements should the nurse include in the instructions regarding the client's new prescription of furosemide (Lasix)?

1. "There are no limitations on the amount of salt and fluid intake."
2. "Ingest vitamin K-rich foods daily, such as green, leafy vegetables and broccoli."
3. "Report muscle cramps or weakness to the health care provider."
4. "Antihypertensive drugs taken concurrently may produce sleepiness."

4 Clients prescribed spironolactone (Aldactone) are often at risk for electrolyte imbalance. The nurse assesses for this adverse effect because this drug:

1. Retains potassium.
2. Releases magnesium.
3. Excretes potassium.
4. Binds calcium.

5 Which of the following nursing measures should be included in the therapeutic management of a client receiving spironolactone (Aldactone)? Select all that apply.

1. Keep the urinal or bedpan available for clients with limited mobility.
2. Assess for hypokalemia and encourage foods high in potassium.
3. Monitor intake and output ratio, and weigh the client daily.
4. Monitor blood pressure and assess for orthostatic hypotension.
5. Instruct the client to use salt substitutes in food preparation.

6 The nurse is monitoring a client receiving acetazolamide (Diamox). Which of the following acid–base imbalance is at potential risk for this client?

1. Metabolic acidosis
2. Metabolic alkalosis
3. Respiratory acidosis
4. Respiratory alkalosis

See Answers to Critical Thinking Questions, Case Study, and NCLEX-RN® Review in Appendix A.

References

Blumenthal, M., Goldberg, A., & Brinckmann, J. (Eds.). (2000). *Herbal medicine: Expanded Commission E Monographs.* Newton, MA: Lippincott Williams & Wilkins.

Charlesworth, J. A., Gracey, D. M., & Pussell, B. A. (2008). Adult nephrotic syndrome: Non-specific strategies for treatment. *Nephrology, 13*(1), 45–50.

Colbert, J. B., Ankney, J., & Lee, K. T. (2007). *Anatomy and physiology for health professions: An interactive journey.* Upper Saddle River, NJ: Pearson Hall.

Gallagher, M., Perkovic, V., & Chalmers, J. (2006). Diuretics: A modern day treatment option? *Nephrology, 11*(5), 419–427.

Grossman, E., & Messerli, F. (2006). Long-term safety of antihypertensive therapy. *Progress in Cardiovascular Diseases, 49*(1), 16–25.

Gu, Q., Paulose-Ram, R., Dillon, C., & Burt, V. (2006). Antihypertensive medication use among U.S. adults with hypertension. *Circulation, 113*(1), 213–221.

Jackson, E. K. (2006). Diuretics. In L. L. Brunton, J. S. Lazo, & K. L. Parker (Eds.), *The pharmacological basis of therapeutics* (11th ed., pp. 737–770). New York: McGraw-Hill.

National Center for Complementary and Alternative Medicine. (2008). *Herbs at a glance: Dandelion.* Retrieved July 8, 2008, from http://nccam.nih.gov/health/dandelion/

National Kidney Foundation. (2008). *End stage renal disease in the United States.* Retrieved July 8, 2008, from http://www.kidney.org/news/newsroom/fsitem.cfm?id=38

Schiffrin, E. L., Lipman, M. L., & Mann, J. F. E. (2007). Chronic kidney disease: Effects on the cardiovascular system. *Circulation, 116*(1), 85–97.

Schütz, K., Carle, R., & Schieber, A. (2006). Taraxacum—A review on its phytochemical and pharmacological profile. *Journal of Ethnopharmacology, 107*(3), 313–323.

Sica, D., Gehr, T., & Frishman, W. (2006). Use of diuretics in the treatment of heart failure in the elderly. *Heart Failure Clinics, 3*(4), 455–464.

The Organ Procurement and Transplantation Network. (2008). *Data.* Retrieved July 8, 2008, from http://www.optn.org/latestData/rptData.asp

Zillich, A. J., Garg, J., Basu, S., Bakris, G. L., & Carter, B. L. (2006). Thiazide diuretics, potassium, and the development of diabetes: A quantitative review. *Hypertension, 48*(10), 219–224.

C H A P T E R

I am doing everything my doctor has advised me to do to control my hypertension. My physician has prescribed several different types of drugs over the last few months. My blood pressure is still elevated. What else can I do? Having this problem is very distressing and I have been quite depressed lately.

Patient "Elmer Foley"

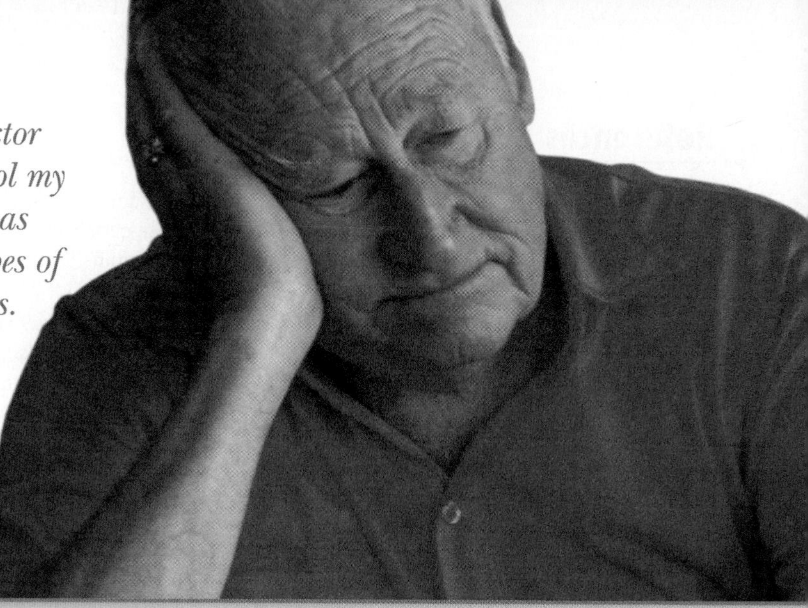

36 Pharmacotherapy of Hypertension

Learning Outcomes

After reading this chapter, the student should be able to:

1. Explain how hypertension is classified.
2. Summarize the long-term consequences of untreated hypertension.
3. Compare and contrast the roles of nonpharmacologic and pharmacologic methods in the management of hypertension.
4. Describe general principles guiding the pharmacotherapy of hypertension.
5. Identify drug classes used in the primary and alternate management of hypertension.
6. Describe the pharmacologic management of hypertensive emergencies.
7. For each of the classes shown in the chapter outline, identify the prototype and representative drugs and explain the mechanism(s) of drug action, primary indications, contraindications, significant drug interactions, pregnancy category, and important adverse effects.
8. Use the nursing process to care for patients receiving antihypertensive drugs.

Chapter Outline

Definition and Classification of Hypertension

Etiology and Pathogenesis of Hypertension

Nonpharmacologic Management of Hypertension

Pharmacologic Management of Hypertension

Drug Classes for Hypertension

Diuretics

Calcium Channel Blockers

Drugs Affecting the Renin-Angiotensin-Aldosterone System

Angiotensin-Converting Enzyme (ACE) Inhibitors

Angiotensin II Receptor Blockers

Adrenergic Antagonists

Beta-Adrenergic Antagonists

Alpha$_1$-Adrenergic Antagonists

Centrally Acting Agents (Alpha$_2$-Adrenergic Agonists)

PROTOTYPE **Methyldopa (Aldomet)** *p. 577*

Adrenergic Neuron–Blocking Agents

Direct Vasodilators

PROTOTYPE **Hydralazine (Apresoline)** *p. 579*

Management of Hypertensive Emergency

PROTOTYPE **Nitroprusside Sodium (Nipride, Nitropress)** *p. 582*

Key Terms

angiotensin-converting enzyme (ACE), 575
first dose phenomenon, 576
hypertension (HTN), 567
hypertensive emergency (HTN-E), 581
hypertensive urgency, 581
hypertrichosis, 581
primary hypertension, 568
reflex tachycardia, 579
secondary hypertension, 568

Diseases affecting the heart and blood vessels are the most frequent causes of death in the United States. Hypertension (HTN) or high blood pressure is the most common of the cardiovascular diseases. According to the American Heart Association, chronic HTN affects one in every three Americans and is responsible for over 50,000 deaths in the United States each year (American Heart Association, 2008). Although mild HTN can be controlled with lifestyle modifications, moderate to severe HTN requires pharmacotherapy.

Because nurses encounter so many patients with this disease, it is critical for the nurse to understand the underlying principles of antihypertensive therapy. By improving public awareness of HTN and teaching the importance of early intervention, the nurse can contribute significantly to reducing cardiovascular mortality.

PharmFACT

Among people with HTN, about one third do not know they have the disorder. African Americans have the highest rate of HTN; 44% of adult African Americans have high blood pressure. *Source:* American Heart Association, 2008.

When most people use the word "hypertension," they are referring to systemic HTN, that which is measured routinely by a conventional blood pressure cuff on the upper arm over the brachial artery. Systemic HTN is a general measurement of arterial blood pressure in the body. Localized HTN may also occur. For example, patients with cirrhosis of the liver often develop portal HTN, which occurs in the portal vein and its branches serving the liver. Pulmonary HTN occurs in the pulmonary artery and its branches and is most often observed in patients with left heart failure. These localized types of HTN respond to many of the same antihypertensive drugs used for systemic HTN.

To develop guidelines for treatment, many attempts have been made to further define HTN. In 2003, the National High Blood Pressure Education Program Coordinating Committee of the National Heart, Lung, and Blood Institute at the National Institutes of Health determined the need for new guidelines that addressed the relationship between blood pressure and the risk of cardiovascular disease. This committee issued The Seventh Report of the Joint National Committee on Prevention, Detection, Evaluation, and Treatment of High Blood Pressure (JNC-7), which has become the standard for treating HTN. The recommendations from the JNC-7 report are summarized in Table 36.1.

In addition to classifying HTN into three categories (prehypertension, Stage 1, and Stage 2), the JNC-7 report issued remarkable data regarding the disease.

- The risk of cardiovascular disease beginning at 115/75 mmHg doubles with each additional increment of 20/10 mmHg.

Definition and Classification of Hypertension

36.1 Hypertension is classified by stages, based upon the degree of elevation of systolic and diastolic blood pressure.

Hypertension (HTN) is defined as the consistent elevation of systemic arterial blood pressure. The diagnosis of chronic HTN is made after repeated blood pressure measurements. A patient with a sustained systolic blood pressure of greater than 140 mmHg or diastolic pressure of greater than 90 to 99 mmHg after multiple assessments are conducted over several clinic visits is said to have HTN.

TABLE 36.1 Recommendations for Treating Hypertension

CLASSIFICATION OF HYPERTENSION		INITIAL ANTIHYPERTENSIVE THERAPY	
Blood Pressure Classification	**Systolic/Diastolic Blood Pressure (mmHg)**	**Without Compelling Indication***	**With Compelling Indication***
Normal	119/79 or less	No antihypertensive indicated	No antihypertensive indicated
Prehypertension	120–139/80–89		
Stage 1 Hypertension	140–159/90–99	Thiazide diuretic (for most patients)	Other antihypertensives, as needed
Stage 2 Hypertension	160 or higher/100 or higher	Two-drug combination antihypertensive (for most patients)	

*Compelling indications include: heart failure, post myocardial infarction, high risk for coronary artery disease, diabetes, chronic kidney disease and recurrent stroke prevention.

Note: From *JNC-7 Express: The Seventh Report of the Joint National Committee on Prevention, Detection Evaluation and Treatment of High Blood Pressure,* by U.S. Department of Health and Human Services, National Institute of Health, National Heart, Lung, and Blood Institute, National High Blood Pressure Education Program, 2003, Bethesda, MD: Author. Retrieved July 11, 2008, from http://www.nhlbi.nih.gov/guidelines/hypertension/express.pdf

TABLE 36.2 Variation in Blood Pressure Throughout the Life Span

Age (Years)	Male	Female
1	96/66	95/65
5	92/62	92/62
10	103/69	103/70
20–24	123/76	116/72
30–34	126/79	120/75
40–44	129/81	127/80
50–54	135/83	137/84
60–64	142/85	144/85
70–74	145/82	159/85
80–84	145/82	157/83

- Individuals with a systolic blood pressure of 120 to 139 mmHg or a diastolic blood pressure of 80 to 89 mmHg should be considered as prehypertensive. These patients should be strongly encouraged by the nurse to adopt health-promoting lifestyle modifications to prevent cardiovascular disease.
- Patients with prehypertension are at increased risk for progression to HTN; those in the 130 to 139/80 to 89 mmHg blood pressure range are at twice the risk to develop HTN as those with lower values.

Average blood pressure changes throughout the lifespan, gradually and continuously rising from childhood through adulthood. Normal blood pressure at one age may be considered abnormal in someone older or younger. Table 36.2 shows the normal variation in blood pressure in patients that occurs throughout the life span. HTN affects approximately 30% of those over 50 years old, 64% of men over age 65, and 75% of women over age 75.

Etiology and Pathogenesis of Hypertension

36.2 Failure to properly manage hypertension can lead to cerebrovascular accident, heart failure, or myocardial infarction.

Hypertension is a complex disease that is caused by a combination of genetic and environmental factors. Approximately 30% to 40% of HTN is thought to be due to genetic factors. Scientists have discovered specific genes that appear to predispose a patient to HTN. These genes control critical activities such as renal sodium and water transport and the renin-angiotensin-aldosterone system. As discussed in Section 36.3, environmental factors related to diet and exercise also play an important role in the development of HTN.

For the large majority of hypertensive patients, no specific cause can be identified. HTN having no identifiable cause is called **primary,** idiopathic, or essential **hypertension,** and accounts for 90% of all cases. Although patients with primary HTN may not be cured, the disease can be managed such that the risk of serious, long-term consequences can be reduced.

In some cases, a specific cause of the HTN can be identified. This type, called **secondary hypertension,** accounts for 10% of all patients with HTN. Certain diseases, such as Cushing's syndrome, hyperthyroidism, chronic renal impairment, pheochromocytoma, and arteriosclerosis are associated with elevated blood pressure. Certain drugs are also associated with HTN, including corticosteroids, oral contraceptives, estrogen, erythropoietin, and sibutramine. The therapeutic goal for secondary HTN is to treat or remove the underlying condition that is causing the blood pressure elevation. In many cases, correcting the comorbid condition will cure the associated HTN.

Research has clearly demonstrated that failure to control HTN can result in serious consequences. Prolonged or improperly controlled HTN damages blood vessels, particularly small arteries and arterioles. As HTN progresses, the walls of the arteries gradually thicken, in an attempt to protect the vessels against

CONNECTIONS

To the Community Blood Pressure Self-Measurement

Many patients choose to monitor their own blood pressure. Patients can benefit from documenting their responses to antihypertensive medication by improved adherence to the therapeutic regimen. For accurate measurement, home devices should be checked at the beginning of therapy and intermittently for accuracy. Upper-arm cuff blood pressure monitors are best, while wrist and finger devices are less accurate. Home monitoring should not substitute for ambulatory care monitoring or follow-up assessments with the health care provider.

When teaching a patient to monitor blood pressure, the nurse should remember these concepts:

- Measure blood pressure after a resting period of 5 minutes.
- Measure at different times of the day to determine the effectiveness of the antihypertensive medications.
- For at least 30 minutes before taking the blood pressure reading, avoid eating, smoking, exercising, or taking medications known to raise blood pressure such as certain nasal decongestant sprays.
- When measuring blood pressure, keep the cuffed arm at heart level.
- Maintain a detailed record of blood pressure measurements.
- If available, choose measurement devices that have memory to store readings.
- Measure blood pressure with the oversight of health care provider and reevaluate technique yearly.
- Discourage patients with physical or mental disabilities from self-monitoring their blood pressure.

injury from the increased pressure. The injured vessel walls become inflamed, increasing the permeability of the vessels and causing additional thickening of their walls. Eventually, the lumen of the artery permanently narrows, reducing blood flow to vital tissues. HTN accelerates atherosclerosis, and will worsen conditions such as coronary artery disease (CAD).

Hypertension may exist for years, indeed decades, before becoming symptomatic. As the disease progresses, however, the risk of target-organ damage increases. Because sustained HTN may affect any artery in the body, damage may be widespread and symptoms vary greatly according to which vessels are affected.

The heart is a primary organ damaged by chronic HTN. Hypertension increases afterload, forcing the heart to work harder to pump blood to the tissues. The heart is subjected to chronic pressure overload, resulting in left ventricular hypertrophy. If untreated, this excessive workload eventually causes the heart to fail and the lungs to fill with fluid, a condition known as congestive heart failure (CHF). Drug therapy for CHF is covered in Chapter 38.

CONNECTION *Checkpoint* 36.1

From what you learned in Chapter 31, define afterload and explain its relationship to stroke volume and cardiac output. See Answer to Connection Checkpoint 36.1 in Appendix A.

Further damaging the heart is the effect of HTN on the coronary vessels. Hypertension accelerates the deposition of atherosclerotic plaque, creating or worsening CAD. This places the patient at greater risk of dysrhythmias, angina pectoris, and myocardial infarction (MI). Heart failure and MI are the most common causes of death in hypertensive patients.

The brain is also a major target organ for hypertensive damage. Occlusion of the small vessels supplying blood and oxygen to the brain can cause transient ischemic attacks and cerebrovascular accident (CVA). These neurologic events are common in hypertensive patients and are a major cause of disability.

Because a large percentage of blood pumped per minute circulates through the kidneys, chronic HTN creates major stress on these organs. As the small arteries supplying the kidney become injured, inflamed, and atherosclerotic, the patient's renal function gradually declines. Poorly managed HTN is an important contributor to kidney failure and end-stage kidney disease.

Hypertension is a major cause of visual impairment, which can occur when vessels in the eye become atherosclerotic. Although patients may remain asymptomatic for many years, small hemorrhages that affect vision may occur. Symptoms of retinal damage range from subtle vision changes to blindness. Retinopathy is particularly serious in patients who present with diabetes as a comorbid condition with HTN.

The importance of treating this disorder in the prehypertensive stage cannot be overstated. The long-term damage to target organs caused by HTN may be irreversible if the disease is allowed to progress unchecked. This is especially critical in diabetics and those with chronic kidney disease, as these patients are particularly susceptible to the long-term consequences of HTN.

Nonpharmacologic Management of Hypertension

36.3 Therapeutic lifestyle changes can reduce blood pressure and lessen the need for antihypertensive medications.

When a patient is first diagnosed with HTN, a comprehensive medical history is necessary to determine if the disease can be controlled by nonpharmacologic means. Therapeutic lifestyle changes should be recommended for all patients with prehypertension or HTN. Of greatest importance is maintaining optimum weight, since obesity is closely associated with dyslipidemia (abnormal serum lipid levels) and HTN. A 5–9 kg (10 to 20 lb) weight loss often produces a measurable decrease in blood pressure, even in obese patients. Combining a medically supervised

CONNECTIONS

Complementary and Alternative Therapies Grape Seed Extract

Description: Grape seed extract is obtained from the seeds of the types of grapes that are usually used in the process of winemaking.

History and Claims: Grapes and grape seeds have been used for thousands of years. The primary use of the extract has been for cardiovascular conditions such as HTN, high blood cholesterol, atherosclerosis, and to generally improve circulation. Some claim that it improves wound healing, prevents cancer, and lowers the risk for the long-term consequences of diabetes. The drug is being examined for its effects on Alzheimer's disease.

Standardization: The grape seeds are crushed and placed into tablet, capsule, or liquid forms. Typical doses are 50–300 mg/day. Standardization is based on percentage of polyphenols. The seeds also contain a high concentration of essential fatty acids and vitamin E.

Evidence: Thousands of studies have been conducted on the polyphenols contained in this supplement. Grape seed extract has antioxidant properties. In general, antioxidants improve wound healing and repair cellular injury. Preliminary evidence suggests it may have some benefit in repairing blood vessel damage that could lead to atherosclerosis and HTN. Controlled, long-term studies on the effects of grape seed extracts on HTN have not been conducted. It has few adverse effects. Caution should be used if taking anticoagulant drugs, because increased bleeding may result. Overall, the benefits of grape seed extract are no different than those of a diet balanced with natural antioxidants (and an occasional glass of red wine).

Source: From *Herbs at a Glance: Grape Seed Extract,* by National Center for Complementary and Alternative Medicine, 2008. Retrieved July 11, 2008, from http://nccam.nih.gov/health/grapeseed/; "Polyphenols and Prevention of Cardiovascular Diseases," by C. Manach, A. Mazur, & A. Scalbert, 2005, *Current Opinion in Lipidology, 16*(1), pp. 77–84; and *Grape Seed Extract,* by Drug Digest, 2007. Retrieved June 11, 2008, from http://www.drugdigest.org/DD/DVH/HerbsWho/0,3923,552554%7CGrape%2BSeed%2BExtract,00.html

CONNECTIONS

To the Community

Public Health Challenges and Community Programs

Public health approaches such as reducing calorie intake, as well as intake of saturated fat and salt in processed foods, can help improve public health. Increasing diverse community and school opportunities for physical activity can achieve a difference in the public's blood pressure and reduce morbidity, mortality, and lifetime risk of people becoming hypertensive. With the epidemic increase in BMI of Americans now at 122 million overweight adults, hypertension and related health concerns are widespread. The American Heart Association has published a resolution that food manufacturers and restaurants reduce sodium in the food by 50% over the next decade. However, the public health intervention strategies must address the diversity of racial, ethnic, cultural, linguistic, religious, and social factors in the delivery of their services if public acceptance is expected. Public health approaches can provide an attractive opportunity to help prevent the costly cycle of managing hypertension and its related complications.

CONNECTIONS

To the Community

The DASH Diet

DASH is the acronym for Dietary Approaches to Stop Hypertension and has proved so healthy that it has been recommended for all Americans, not just those diagnosed with HTN. The DASH diet emphasizes replacing animal protein, saturated and animal fats, and refined sugars with more simple nutrients such as beans and lentils, fresh fruits and vegetables, and small amounts of meat, fish, poultry, low-fat dairy products, and nuts. The DASH diet suggests a maximum of two portions of meat, poultry, or fish, and three portions of low-fat or nonfat dairy food per week. The DASH diet can lower blood pressure among hypertensive people. It is recommended for all Americans especially at-risk groups such as African Americans, who have higher occurrences of HTN, kidney failure, and stroke.

weight loss program with proper nutrition can delay the progression from prehypertension to HTN.

In some cases, implementing positive lifestyle changes may eliminate the need for pharmacotherapy altogether. Even if medication is required to manage the HTN, positive lifestyle changes may allow dosages to be minimized, thus lowering the potential for drug adverse effects. The nurse plays a vital role in educating patients about controlling their HTN. Because all blood pressure medications have potential adverse effects, it is important that patients attempt to control their disease though nonpharmacologic means, to the greatest extent possible. Nonpharmacologic methods for controlling HTN include the following:

- Limit intake of alcohol.
- Restrict sodium consumption.
- Reduce intake of saturated fat and cholesterol, and increase consumption of fruits and vegetables.
- Increase aerobic physical activity.
- Discontinue use of all tobacco products.
- Explore measures for dealing with excessive stress.
- Maintain optimum weight.

MyNursingKit | Dietary Modifications for the Hypertensive Patient

Pharmacologic Management of Hypertension

36.4 The choice of antihypertensive medication is determined by the degree of hypertension and the presence of other medical conditions.

The goal of antihypertensive therapy is to reduce the morbidity and mortality associated with chronic HTN. Research has confirmed that keeping blood pressure within normal limits reduces the risk of hypertension-related target-organ damage.

The pharmacologic management of HTN is individualized to the patient's risk factors, comorbid medical conditions, and degree of blood pressure elevation. Patient responses to antihypertensive medications vary widely because of the many complex genetic and environmental factors affecting blood pressure.

There are nine different drug classes used to treat HTN. Each class has specific benefits and characteristic adverse effects. The mechanisms of action of these agents are summarized in Figure 36.1. Although there are many effective drugs available, and the data supporting the benefits of therapy are strong, HTN remains a challenging disorder to treat successfully. Choice of therapy is often based on the clinician's experience. Although antihypertensive treatment varies, there are several principles that guide pharmacotherapy.

Initial Drug of Choice

The JNC-7 report recommends thiazide diuretics as drugs of choice for mild to moderate HTN. Clinical research has clearly demonstrated that thiazide diuretics reduce HTN-related morbidity and mortality. Patients with a compelling condition, however, may benefit from a second drug, either in combination with the thiazide or in place of the thiazide. The JNC-7 report lists the following as compelling conditions: heart failure, post-myocardial infarction, high risk for CAD, diabetes, chronic kidney disease, and recurrent stroke prevention.

In most cases, low doses of the initial drug are prescribed and the patient is reevaluated after an appropriate time period. As therapy continues, dosage is adjusted to maintain optimum blood pressure. The following drug classes are considered primary antihypertensive agents.

- Diuretics
- Angiotensin-converting enzyme (ACE) inhibitors
- Angiotensin II receptor blockers (ARBs)
- Calcium channel blockers (CCBs)
- Beta-adrenergic antagonists

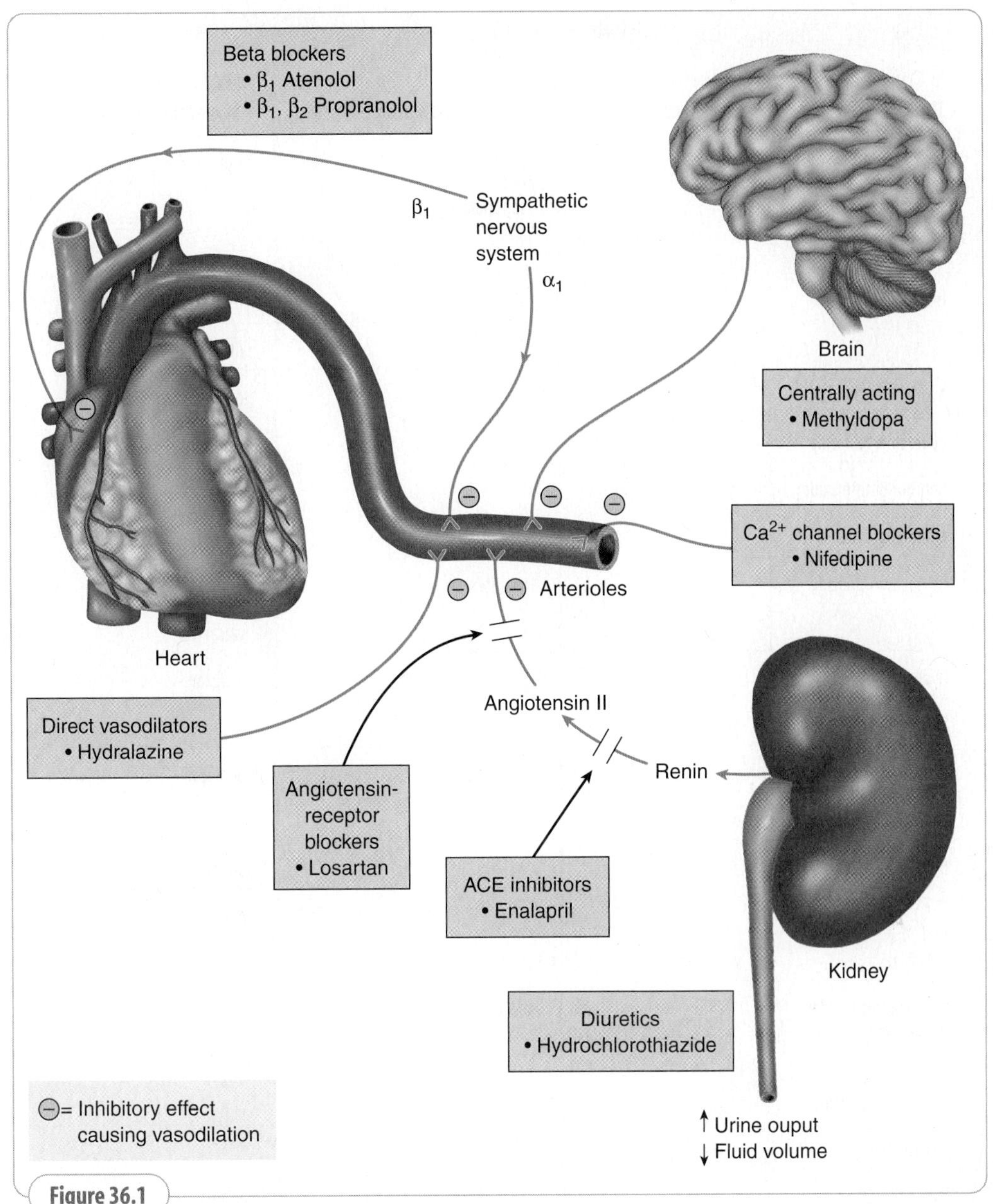

Figure 36.1

Mechanism of action of antihypertensive drugs.

Adding Drugs to the Antihypertensive Regimen

If the patient does not respond to the initial medication, a drug from a different antihypertensive class may be added to the regimen. Prescribing two antihypertensives concurrently results in additive or synergistic blood pressure reduction, and is common practice when managing resistant HTN. This is often necessary when the patient has a compelling condition, or when sustained blood pressure is particularly high. The advantage of using two drugs is that lower doses of each may be used, resulting in fewer adverse effects and better patient adherence. Drug manufacturers sometimes combine two drugs into a single pill or capsule for dosing convenience and to improve patient adherence. The majority of these combinations include a thiazide diuretic, usually hydrochlorothiazide (HCTZ). Selected combination antihypertensives are shown in Table 36.3.

Certain antihypertensive classes cause more adverse effects and are generally prescribed when first-line agents do not produce a satisfactory response. In some cases, research studies have not demonstrated a firm link between drug use and lowered morbidity or mortality. The alternative antihypertensive drug classes include the following:

- Alpha$_1$-adrenergic antagonists
- Alpha$_2$-adrenergic agonists
- Direct-acting vasodilators
- Peripheral adrenergic antagonists

TABLE 36.3 Combination Medications Commonly Used for Hypertension

Trade Name	Thiazide Diuretic	Adrenergic Agent	Potassium-Sparing Diuretic	ACE Inhibitor or Angiotensin II Blocker	Other
Accuretic	hydrochlorothiazide			quinapril	
Aldactazide	hydrochlorothiazide		spironolactone		
Aldoril	hydrochlorothiazide				methyldopa
Avalide	hydrochlorothiazide			irbesartan	
Azor				olmesartan	amlodipine
Benicar HCT	hydrochlorothiazide			olmesartan	
Capozide	hydrochlorothiazide			captopril	
Corzide	bendroflumethiazide	nadolol			
Diovan HCT	hydrochlorothiazide			valsartan	
Dyazide	hydrochlorothiazide		triamterene		
Exforge				valsartan	amlodipine
Hyzaar	hydrochlorothiazide			losartan	
Inderide	hydrochlorothiazide	propranolol			
Lexxel				enalapril	felodipine
Lopressor HCT	hydrochlorothiazide	metoprolol			
Lotensin HCT	hydrochlorothiazide			benazepril	
Lotrel				benazepril	amlodipine
Minizide	polythiazide	prazosin			
Moduretic	hydrochlorothiazide		amiloride		
Tarka				trandolapril	verapamil
Tekturna HCT	hydrochlorothiazide				aliskiren
Tenoretic	chlorthalidone	atenolol			
Teveten HCT	hydrochlorothiazide			eprosartan	
Timolide	hydrochlorothiazide	timolol			
Uniretic	hydrochlorothiazide			moexipril	
Vaseretic	hydrochlorothiazide			enalapril	
Zestoretic	hydrochlorothiazide			lisinopril	
Ziac	hydrochlorothiazide	bisoprolol			

Promoting Patient Adherence

Because chronic HTN may produce no identifiable symptoms for as long as 10 to 20 years, many people are not aware of their condition. Convincing patients to change established lifestyle habits, spend money on medication, and take drugs on a regular basis when they are feeling healthy is a difficult task for the nurse. Patients with limited income or who do not have health insurance are at high risk for not purchasing the drugs after receiving a prescription. The prescriber should consider generic forms of these drugs, to reduce cost and increase adherence.

Further reducing adherence to the regimen is the occurrence of adverse drug effects. Some of the antihypertensive drugs cause embarrassing adverse effects such as impotence, which may go unreported. Others cause fatigue and generally make the patient feel sicker than they were before therapy was initiated. The nurse should teach the patient the importance of treating the disease to avoid serious long-term consequences. Furthermore, the nurse should teach patients to report drug adverse effects so that dosage can be adjusted, or the drug changed, so the treatment may continue without interruption. Simple adjustments to the dosage or changing the selected drug can often eliminate the adverse effects causing nonadherence.

Antihypertensives in African Americans

The incidence of HTN is significantly higher in African Americans than in other ethnic groups. As expected from this high incidence, African Americans experience greater target-organ damage than other populations. In an effort to reduce the high morbidity and mortality risks, aggressive antihypertensive therapy may be necessary to overcome resistant HTN in African Americans.

Some studies have suggested that certain antihypertensive drug classes are less effective in African Americans. For example monotherapy with ACE inhibitors, angiotensin II receptor blockers, or beta-adrenergic antagonists does not reduce blood pressure as much in African Americans compared to other ethnic groups. Thiazide diuretics and calcium channel blockers seem to provide the greatest blood pressure reduction in this population. Some health care providers recommend initiating therapy with two drugs to ensure an adequate response.

Although African Americans present a special challenge in controlling HTN, the fundamental principles and guidelines for effective clinical practice apply to all ethnic groups: early treatment of HTN, therapeutic lifestyle changes, and keeping blood pressure within established limits.

Drug Classes for Hypertension

36.5 Diuretics are often drugs of first choice for treating mild to moderate hypertension.

Diuretics were the first class of medications used to treat HTN in the 1950s. Despite the many advances in drug therapy, diuretics are still considered first-line drugs for this disease because they are very effective at controlling mild to moderate HTN with few serious adverse effects. Although sometimes used as monotherapy, they are frequently prescribed with other antihypertensive medications to enhance their effectiveness. Because this class of drugs was presented in detail in Chapter 35, the following section is a brief summary of their application to the treatment of HTN.

Although dozens of diuretics are available for the treatment of HTN, all produce a similar result: the reduction of blood volume through the urinary excretion of water and electrolytes. Reducing blood volume places less pressure on the arterial walls, thereby decreasing peripheral resistance and lowering systemic blood pressure. The mechanism by which diuretics increase the excretion of water and electrolytes, specifically where and how the kidney is affected, differs among the various classes of diuretics.

Whenever a medication changes urine flow or composition, dehydration and electrolyte depletion are possible. Dehydration may manifest as increased thirst or poor skin turgor. Excessive sodium loss (hyponatremia) is a concern for all diuretics. Potassium loss (hypokalemia) is of particular concern for loop and thiazide diuretics. The potassium-sparing diuretics such as triamterene (Dyrenium) have fewer tendencies to cause hypokalemia. Drug classes for HTN are shown in Table 36.4.

Thiazide and thiazide-like diuretics: Thiazide and thiazide-like diuretics have been the mainstay for the pharmacotherapy of HTN for decades. The thiazide diuretics are inexpensive, and most are available in generic formulations. They are safe drugs, with excessive urinary potassium loss being the primary adverse effect. Because hypokalemia can induce serious dysrhythmias in susceptible patients, careful laboratory monitoring of serum potassium is necessary. Patients should increase their amount of dietary potassium, and potassium supplements may be prescribed. These diuretics may also cause hyperglycemia and hyperuricemia. Because thiazides may increase blood lipids, these agents should be used cautiously in patients with existing hyperlipidemia. Hydrochlorothiazide (HCTZ) is featured as the prototype drug in this class in Chapter 35.

Potassium-sparing diuretics: Although potassium-sparing diuretics such as spironolactone (Aldactone) and triamterene (Dyrenium) produce only a modest diuresis, their primary advantage is they do not cause potassium depletion. They are especially beneficial when the patient is at risk to developing hypokalemia due to their medical condition, or the use of thiazide or loop diuretics. The primary concern when using potassium-sparing diuretics is the possibility of retaining too much potassium, which can cause serious dysrhythmias. Diabetic patients and those with renal impairment are particularly susceptible to hyperkalemia. Patients should be instructed to avoid excess potassium in their diet, including salt substitutes containing KCl, and not to use potassium supplements during therapy. Concurrent use with an ACE inhibitor or angiotensin II receptor blocker significantly increases the potential for development of hyperkalemia. Spironolactone is presented as a prototype drug for this class in Chapter 35.

Loop (high-ceiling) diuretics: The loop diuretics such as furosemide (Lasix) and bumetanide (Bumex) cause greater diuresis, and have the potential to produce a higher reduction in blood pressure than the thiazides or potassium-sparing diuretics. Although this makes them very effective at reducing blood pressure, they are not ideal agents for maintenance therapy. The risk of adverse effects such as hypokalemia and dehydration is great because of their ability to remove large amounts of fluid from the body in a short time period. Loop diuretics are ototoxic, an effect more likely to occur in patients with renal insufficiency or when high doses are administered. Because of their greater toxicity, loop diuretics are sometimes reserved for patients with resistant HTN. Furosemide, the only loop diuretic in widespread use, is presented as a prototype drug in Chapter 35.

MyNursingKit | Herbal Therapies for Hypertension

TABLE 36.4 Drug Classes for Hypertension

Diuretics	**Angiotensin II Receptor Blockers**	***Alpha$_1$ Blockers***
Potassium-Sparing Type	candesartan (Atacand)	doxazosin (Cardura)
amiloride (Midamor)	eprosartan (Teveten)	prazosin (Minipress)
eplerenone (Inspra)	irbesartan (Avapro)	terazosin (Hytrin)
spironolactone (Aldactone)	losartan (Cozaar)	***Alpha$_2$-Adrenergic Agonists***
triamterene (Dyrenium)	olmesartan (Benicar)	clonidine (Catapres)
Thiazide and Thiazide-Like	telmisartan (Micardis)	methyldopa (Aldomet)
chlorothiazide (Diuril)	valsartan (Diovan)	***Alpha and Beta Blockers (Centrally Acting)***
chlorthalidone (Hygroton)		carvedilol (Coreg)
hydrochlorothiazide (Microzide)	**Calcium Channel Blockers**	labetalol (Trandate, Normodyne)
indapamide (Lozol)	amlodipine (Norvasc)	***Adrenergic Neuron Blockers (Peripherally Acting)***
methyclothiazide (Enduron)	clevidipine (Cleviprex)	guanethidine (Ismelin)
metolazone (Diulo, Mykrox, others)	diltiazem (Cardizem, Dilacor, others)	reserpine (Serpasil)
Loop/High-Ceiling Type	felodipine (Plendil)	
bumetanide (Bumex)	isradipine (DynaCirc)	**Direct-Acting Vasodilators**
ethacrynic acid (Edecrin)	nicardipine (Cardene)	diazoxide (Hyperstat IV)
furosemide (Lasix)	nifedipine (Procardia, Adalat)	minoxidil (Loniten)
torsemide (Demadex)	nisoldipine (Nisocor, Sular)	nitroprusside (Nitropress)
	verapamil (Calan, Isotopic, Verelan)	
ACE Inhibitors		**Direct Renin Inhibitor**
benazepril (Lotensin)	**Adrenergic Agents**	Aliskiren (Tekturna)
captopril (Capoten)	***Beta Blockers***	
enalapril (Vasotec)	atenolol (Tenormin)	
fosinopril (Monopril)	betaxolol (Kerlone)	
lisinopril (Prinivil, Zestril)	bisoprolol (Zebeta)	
moexipril (Univasc)	metoprolol (Toprol, Lopressor)	
perindopril (Aceon)	nadolol (Corgard)	
quinapril (Accupril)	propranolol (Inderal)	
ramipril (Altace)	timolol (Betimol and others)	
trandolapril (Mavik)		

MyNursingKit | Mechanism of Action Animation: Doxazosin

CONNECTION Checkpoint 36.2

From what you learned in Chapter 35, why must the thiazide diuretics be used with great caution in patients taking digoxin (Lanoxin)? See Answer to Connection Checkpoint 36.2 in Appendix A.

36.6 Calcium channel blockers have emerged as important drugs in the treatment of hypertension.

Calcium channel blockers (CCBs) are widely used in the treatment of HTN, angina pectoris, and dysrhythmias, as presented in Chapter 33. The following section summarizes their application to the treatment of HTN.

CCBs exert beneficial effects on the heart and blood vessels by blocking calcium ion channels in cardiac and arteriolar smooth muscle. The flow of calcium ions into muscle cells is inhibited, limiting the degree of muscular contraction. At low doses, CCBs relax arterial smooth muscle, thus decreasing peripheral resistance and lowering blood pressure. Some CCBs such as nifedipine (Procardia) are selective for arterioles while others such as verapamil (Calan) affect channels in both arterioles and the myocardium. CCBs vary in potency and in the frequency and types of adverse effects produced. Nifedipine and verapamil are highlighted as drug prototypes in Chapter 33.

Due to their potent vasodilating effects, CCBs can cause reflex tachycardia, which is worse with those CCBs that are selective for arterioles. Because CCBs can slow myocardial conduction, they are contraindicated in patients with certain types of heart conditions such as sick sinus syndrome or third-degree AV block without the presence of a pacemaker. The CCBs that reduce myocardial contractility can worsen heart failure.

CCBs are usually not used as monotherapy for chronic HTN. They are, however, useful in combination therapy for treating certain populations such as the elderly and African Americans who are sometimes less responsive to drugs in other antihypertensive classes.

CONNECTION Checkpoint 36.3

Verapamil and nifedipine are both calcium channel blockers used for HTN. From what you learned in Chapter 33, why would a beta blocker be used concurrently with nifedipine, but be contraindicated with verapamil? See Answer to Connection Checkpoint 36.3 in Appendix A.

36.7 Blocking the renin-angiotensin-aldosterone system leads to a decrease in blood pressure.

As discussed in Chapter 34, the renin-angiotensin-aldosterone system (RAAS) is one of the primary homeostatic mechanisms controlling blood pressure and fluid balance. Drugs inhibiting the RAAS are widely used in the treatment of cardiovascular disease. Clinical research suggests ACE inhibitors are as effective as the diuretics in reducing HTN-related morbidity and mortality. The following section summarizes their applications to HTN pharmacotherapy.

Angiotensin-converting enzyme (ACE) inhibitors block the formation of angiotensin II, decreasing blood pressure through two mechanisms. First, ACE inhibitors block the intense vasoconstriction of arterioles caused by angiotensin II, which decreases blood pressure due to diminished peripheral resistance. Second, these drugs block the effects of angiotensin II on the secretion of aldosterone, which lowers blood pressure by decreasing blood volume. Through their inhibition of aldosterone secretion, ACE inhibitors enhance the effects of the thiazide diuretics; thus drugs from these two classes may be used concurrently in the management of HTN. Enalapril (Vasotec), lisinopril (Prinivil, Zestril), and captopril (Capoten) are three widely prescribed ACE inhibitors. Lisinopril is the prototype drug for the ACE inhibitors in Chapter 34.

Adverse effects of ACE inhibitors are usually minor and include persistent cough and orthostatic hypotension, particularly following the first few doses of the drug. Hyperkalemia may occur, and can be a major concern for diabetics, those with renal impairment, and patients taking potassium-sparing diuretics. Though rare, the most serious adverse effect of ACE inhibitors is the development of angioedema. When it does occur, angioedema most often develops within days after beginning ACE inhibitor therapy. Cough and angioedema arise more frequently in African Americans than in other ethnic groups.

The angiotensin II receptor blockers (ARBs) afford a second method for altering the RAAS pathway. ARBs such as losartan (Cozaar) block receptors for angiotensin II in arteriolar smooth muscle and in the adrenal gland, thus causing blood pressure to fall. Their actions are similar to those of the ACE inhibitors.

Angiotensin II receptor blockers have the lowest incidence of serious adverse effects of any of the antihypertensive classes. Most ARB adverse effects are related to hypotension. Unlike the ACE inhibitors, they do not cause cough, and angioedema is rare. Medications in this class are often combined with drugs from other classes in the management of HTN. A drug prototype feature for losartan (Cozaar) is included in Chapter 34.

Aliskiren (Tekturna) was the first in a new class of antihypertensives called direct renin inhibitors approved in 2007. In 2008 the United States Food and Drug Administration (FDA) approved the combination of aliskiren with hydrochlorothiazide (Tekturna ACT) for treating HTN. The most common adverse effects of aliskiren are diahrrhea, cough, flulike symptoms, and rash.

MyNursingKit | The National Heart, Blood, and Lung Institute

36.8 Adrenergic antagonists are commonly used to treat hypertension.

The adrenergic antagonists, or blockers, are used for a wide variety of cardiovascular disorders, including HTN, angina pectoris, dysrhythmias, and MI prophylaxis (see Chapter 20). Blocking adrenergic receptors in the sympathetic nervous system has a number of beneficial effects on the heart and vessels. For example, by blocking the "fight-or-flight" responses, heart rate slows, blood pressure declines, and the bronchi dilate.

Adrenergic blockers affect the sympathetic division through a number of distinct mechanisms, although all have in common the effect of lowering blood pressure. These mechanisms include the following:

- Blockade of beta$_1$-adrenergic receptors
- Blockade of alpha$_1$-adrenergic receptors
- Nonselective blockade of both alpha$_1$ and beta-adrenergic receptors
- Stimulation of centrally acting alpha$_2$-adrenergic receptors in the brainstem
- Blockade of peripheral adrenergic neurons

The earliest drugs for HTN were nonselective agents that blocked nerve transmission at the ganglia or at both alpha- and beta-adrenergic receptors. Although the nonselective agents revolutionized the treatment of HTN, they caused significant adverse effects. These drugs are rarely used today because selective agents are more efficacious and better tolerated by patients. Of the five subclasses of adrenergic antagonists, only the beta-adrenergic antagonists are considered first-line drugs for the pharmacotherapy of HTN.

Beta-adrenergic antagonists: In this section, the discussion of beta-adrenergic antagonists is limited to their use in treating HTN. The student should refer to Chapter 20 for a detailed discussion of the basic pharmacology of this drug class. Other important therapeutic applications of the beta blockers include angina pectoris and MI (see Chapter 37), dysrhythmias (see Chapter 39), heart failure (see Chapter 38), and migraines (see Chapter 29).

Beta adrenergic antagonists may be cardioselective (beta$_1$) or nonspecific (beta$_1$ and beta$_2$). Cardioselective beta blockers decrease heart rate, myocardial contractility, and cardiac conduction. Nonspecific beta blockers produce the same effects, but also act on the respiratory system to cause bronchoconstriction. Decreasing the heart rate and contractility also reduces cardiac output and lowers systemic blood pressure. Some of their antihypertensive effect is also caused by the blockade of beta$_1$ receptors in the juxtaglomerular apparatus, which inhibits the secretion of renin and the formation of angiotensin II (see Chapter 34). The beta-adrenergic antagonists have been some of the most widely used drugs in the treatment of HTN.

At low doses, beta blockers are well tolerated and serious adverse events are uncommon. As the dosage is increased, however, adverse effects can become numerous and potentially serious in certain patients. Because nonselective beta blockers will slow the heart rate and cause bronchoconstriction, they should be used with caution in patients with asthma or heart failure. Heart rate and rhythm should be regularly monitored during beta-blocker therapy. Many patients report fatigue and activity intolerance at higher doses because the reduction in heart rate causes the heart to become less responsive to exertion. Diabetics should be warned that symptoms of hypoglycemia (diaphoresis, nervousness, and palpitation) may become less observable while on beta-blocker therapy. Beta blockers have been reported to cause or worsen the symptoms of erectile dysfunction more than many other antihypertensive classes. Some drugs in this class are associated with clinical depression. Abrupt cessation of beta-blocker therapy can result in rebound HTN, angina, MI, and even death in patients with CAD. When discontinuing a beta blocker, drug doses should be tapered over a several week period.

Prototype features for beta-adrenergic antagonists can be found for propranolol (Inderal) and metoprolol (Lopressor) in Chapter 20, atenolol (Tenormin) in Chapter 37, and timolol (Timoptic) in Chapter 78.

CONNECTION *Checkpoint* 36.4

From what you learned in Chapter 20, should a hypertensive patient with asthma receive a selective beta$_1$ blocker or a nonselective beta blocker for HTN? See Answer to Connection Checkpoint 36.4 in Appendix A.

Alpha$_1$-adrenergic antagonists: The alpha$_1$-adrenergic antagonists have several clinical applications, which were presented in Chapter 20. In addition to their use in HTN, they are prescribed for benign prostatic hyperplasia (BPH) because their ability to relax smooth muscle in the prostate and bladder neck reduces urethral resistance. A prototype drug feature for prazosin (Minipress) is included in Chapter 20 and the use of tamsulosin (Flomax) in treating BPH is discussed in Chapter 72.

The alpha$_1$-adrenergic antagonists lower blood pressure directly by blocking sympathetic receptors in arterioles, causing the vessels to dilate. They also dilate veins, which lowers blood pressure indirectly by decreasing venous return to the heart and reducing cardiac output. The alpha blockers are not first-line drugs for HTN. Although they are effective in reducing blood pressure, long-term clinical trials have shown them to be less effective at reducing the incidence of serious HTN-related cardiovascular events than diuretics. When used to treat HTN, the alpha blockers are used concurrently with other classes of antihypertensives, such as diuretics.

The alpha$_1$-adrenergic blockers may cause significant orthostatic hypotension. It is particularly serious with the initial doses of these medications and is referred to as the **first dose phenomenon,** although orthostatic hypotension may persist throughout treatment. In severe cases, syncope can occur. Blood pressure should be assessed regularly during therapy to maintain patient safety. Other common adverse effects include weakness, dizziness, dry mouth, headache, and gastrointestinal (GI) complaints such as nausea and vomiting. The elderly are especially prone to orthostatic hypotension and to hypothermic effects related to vasodilation caused by these drugs. Less common, though sometimes a major cause for nonadherence, are adverse effects on male sexual function that include decreased libido and erectile dysfunction.

Nonselective alpha$_1$- and beta-adrenergic antagonists: Carvedilol (Coreg) and labetalol (Normodyne) are unique in that they block both alpha$_1$- and beta-adrenergic receptors. These drugs act by a combination of effects: reducing cardiac output, inhibiting renin secretion, and blocking vasoconstriction of arterioles and veins. As expected, their adverse effects are a combination of alpha and beta blockade and include orthostatic hypotension, bradycardia, and bronchoconstriction. The applications of carvedilol in treating heart failure are presented in Chapter 38.

CONNECTION *Checkpoint* 36.5

Patients with pheochromocytoma often present with severe HTN. From what you learned in Chapter 20, why would this HTN be controlled more effectively with alpha blockers than with beta blockers? See Answer to Connection Checkpoint 36.5 in Appendix A.

Alpha$_2$ agonists: If an alpha antagonist such as prazosin (Minipress) lowers blood pressure, it might be predicted that the administration of an alpha$_2$-adrenergic agonist would raise blood pressure. This is not the case. The answer to this contradiction lies in the different locations of the two subtypes of alpha receptors. The alpha$_1$ receptors blocked by prazosin lie in the peripheral nervous system (PNS), at arterioles. The alpha$_2$ receptors reside in the central nervous system (CNS).

When alpha$_2$ receptors are activated, the outflow of sympathetic nerve impulses from the CNS to the heart and arterioles is inhibited. In effect, this produces the same responses as inhibition of the alpha$_1$ receptor: slowing the heart rate and conduction velocity, and dilating the arterioles. Thus, activating alpha$_2$ receptors (in the CNS) produces similar actions as inhibiting alpha$_1$ receptors (in the PNS).

Although the two drug classes have similar actions and are both used for HTN, the centrally acting alpha$_2$ agonists are used less frequently than the alpha$_1$ antagonists. The alpha$_2$ agonists have a tendency to cause sedation, depression, and other potentially serious CNS adverse effects. The incidence of dizziness and orthostatic hypotension is higher compared to other antihypertensives, and is especially troublesome in elderly patients. Extended use results in sodium and water retention, which increases blood volume and counteracts the antihypertensive action of these drugs. Diuretics must be administered concurrently with alpha$_2$ agonists to diminish this adverse effect. Alpha$_2$ agonists are usually reserved for treating resistant HTN that is unable to be managed by safer medications.

PROTOTYPE DRUG Methyldopa (Aldomet)

Classification: Therapeutic: Antihypertensive
Pharmacologic: Alpha$_2$-adrenergic agonist

Therapeutic Effects and Uses: Methyldopa is an older drug approved in 1962. Its only indication is HTN that has not responded adequately to safer antihypertensives. The drug is normally administered by the oral (PO) route, although an intravenous (IV) form known as methyldopate is available for hypertensive crises. Compared to other antihypertensives given by the IV route, methyldopa has a relatively slow onset of action because it must first be metabolized inside neurons to an active metabolite, methyl norepinephrine. Methyldopa is sometimes a preferred agent for treating HTN occurring during pregnancy because it maintains stable blood flow to the uterus, and its safety to the fetus has been demonstrated in long-term studies.

Unlike many of the alpha$_1$- and beta-adrenergic blockers, methyldopa has very little effect upon the heart, and cardiac output remains unaffected. It also has no significant effect upon plasma renin levels or activity. Orthostatic hypotension may occur, but it is less severe than that produced by the alpha$_1$ antagonists. Because tolerance develops after 3 to 4 months of therapy, a dosage increase may be required to manage HTN.

Mechanism of Action: Methyldopa is converted to a "false" neurotransmitter in the brainstem, thus causing a shortage of the "real" neurotransmitter and inhibition of the sympathetic nervous system. This creates less peripheral resistance, and blood pressure declines.

Pharmacokinetics:

Route(s)	PO, IV
Absorption	50% absorbed from the GI tract
Distribution	Completely, including crossing the blood–brain barrier and the placenta; secreted in breast milk
Primary metabolism	Liver and GI tract
Primary excretion	Renal
Onset of action	Peak effect: 4–6 h
Duration of action	Half-life: 1.7 h

Adverse Effects: Because it is a centrally acting agent, CNS effects such as drowsiness, depression, headache, sedation, and bizarre dreams are relatively common. CNS changes are most prominent during the first 72 hours of therapy, and when dosages are adjusted. Decreased libido and impotence are possible. Peripheral edema due to sodium retention may occur, which can be managed by administration of a thiazide diuretic. Hepatic function should be regularly monitored, as rare cases of hepatotoxicity have been reported. Methyldopa can increase the production of prolactin, resulting in numerous endocrine effects that may include decreased libido, inability to ejaculate, menstrual irregularities, or gynecomastia.

A significant number of patients develop a positive Coombs test, which detects antibodies against the patient's own red blood cells. In a small number of patients, the positive Coombs test is associated with hemolytic anemia. The drug should be discontinued if signs of anemia develop.

Contraindications/Precautions: Methyldopa is contraindicated in patients with serious liver disease, as the drug is hepatotoxic in some patients. Patients with blood dyscrasias should not receive the drug because methyldopa can cause granulocytopenia, hemolytic anemia, and other blood disorders. Patients with renal impairment should be treated with caution because metabolites of methyldopa have prolonged half-lives and may accumulate to toxic levels.

Drug Interactions: Methyldopa interacts with many drugs. It should be used with caution with other antihypertensives or ethanol, as additive hypotension could result. Use of lithium should be avoided, as methyldopa can increase the risk of lithium toxicity. Several drug classes reduce the antihypertensive actions of methyldopa, including phenothiazines, tricyclic antidepressants, and nonsteroidal anti-inflammatory Drugs (NSAIDs). Methyldopa should be administered several hours before iron salts to prevent interference with drug absorption. Concurrent use of methyldopa with levodopa may cause psychosis. **Herbal/Food**: Hawthorn should be avoided because it may cause additive hypotensive effects.

Pregnancy: Category B.

Treatment of Overdose: Treatment includes gastric lavage, dialysis, and administration of a sympathomimetic such as epinephrine to maintain blood pressure and reverse bradycardia.

Nursing Responsibilities:

- Obtain a complete health history including medications to determine possible drug interactions and allergies; identify any recent cardiac or pulmonary events.
- Obtain a baseline electrocardiogram (ECG) and vital signs, including blood pressure.
- Auscultate heart and chest sounds for adventitious sounds.
- Assess neurologic status and level of consciousness (LOC).
- Check blood pressure and pulse at least every 30 minutes until stabilized during IV infusion. Assess for adequate urinary output.
- Assess baseline and periodic laboratory tests for blood counts, serum electrolytes, and liver function tests. This is especially important the first 6 to 12 weeks of treatment or when the patient has fever of unknown origin.
- Minimize daytime sedation by changing medication dosages at night. Some patients reach adequate blood pressure control with a single evening dose.
- Monitor fluid and electrolyte balance along with intake and output. Report changes in intake and output, and oliguria. Weigh patient daily and check for edema that can result from sodium and water retention.
- Note that when the dose is initiated or increased, transient symptoms such as sedation, drowsiness, headache, weakness, and mental depression commonly occur. These tend to disappear as treatment continues.
- Supervise ambulation in older adults and patients with impaired kidney function during any dose adjustment as these groups may experience orthostatic hypotension with resulting dizziness and light-headedness. Caution patients that hot baths and showers, prolonged standing in one position, and strenuous exercise may worsen orthostatic hypotension.
- Assess for symptoms of drug-induced mental depression such as withdrawal, anorexia, or insomnia.
- Obtain baseline blood laboratory values prior to methyldopa therapy to rule out preexisting anemia. Obtain periodic Coombs tests and blood counts and discontinue the drug if signs of anemia develop.
- Discontinue the drug if persistent elevation of serum hepatic transaminase or alkaline phosphatase values occurs, because these may signal the onset of hepatitis.

Patient and Family Education:

- Shake the suspension well before measuring a dose. To get a correct dose, measure the liquid form of methyldopa with a special dose-measuring spoon, not with a regular tablespoon. Ask the pharmacist where you can get one.
- If a dose is missed, take it as soon as possible, unless it is close to the time for the next dose. Do not take a double dose.
- Do not take any other prescription or nonprescription drugs, dietary supplements, or herbal products without the approval of the health care provider.
- Make position changes slowly, when moving from a lying to a standing position to prevent dizziness and possible fainting.
- Do not drive or perform other hazardous activities until the effects of the drug are known because this drug may cause drowsiness or dizziness.
- Do not abruptly stop taking this drug because severe high blood pressure, anxiety, and nervousness can result.
- Do not breast-feed without approval of the health care provider.

Drugs Similar to Methyldopa (Aldomet)

Clonidine is the only other $alpha_2$ agonist.

Clonidine (Catapres, Duraclon): Approved in 1974, clonidine activates $alpha_2$-adrenergic receptors in the cardiovascular control centers in the brainstem. The reduced sympathetic outflow causes vasodilation and slows the heart rate. As an antihypertensive, it is available as oral tablets or a transdermal patch that releases the drug at a constant rate over 7 days. A second approved indication for clonidine (Duraclon) is intractable pain in cancer patients that is not relieved by opiates. Pain control is achieved by a continuous epidural infusion of the drug. To assist in pain management, transdermal clonidine may be used to provide some degree of analgesia so that the dose of opiate can be reduced.

Clonidine has many off-label indications. These include dysmenorrhea, menopausal flushing, migraine prophylaxis, smoking cessation, opiate and benzodiazepine withdrawal, attention deficit/hyperactivity disorder, and Tourette's syndrome.

The most common adverse effect of clonidine is dry mouth, which occurs in about 40% of the patients taking the drug. Like methyldopa, CNS adverse effects such as sedation, drowsiness, and dizziness are common. Transdermal clonidine produces fewer serious adverse effects, although the patches can cause skin irritation and itching. The patient should be warned not to abruptly discontinue the drug, as severe rebound HTN, agitation, nervousness, and anxiety may result.

Adrenergic neuron–blocking agents: The adrenergic neuron–blocker class consists of two drugs that inhibit the synthesis or release of norepinephrine (NE) in sympathetic neurons. With less NE available to cross the synapse, sympathetic activity is diminished at both alpha- and beta-adrenergic receptors. In effect, the actions of these drugs are the same as the nonselective $alpha_1$- and beta-adrenergic antagonists: reduced heart rate and cardiac output (beta effects) combined with dilation of arterioles (alpha effect).

The adrenergic neuron–blocking agents have mostly historical interest, as they are rarely prescribed today due to the availability of safer medications. Reserpine (Serpalan), isolated from the shrub *Rauwolfia serpentina* in 1952, was one of the earliest drugs used for HTN. It is an ancient drug, used for centuries in India as an herbal tea to produce sedation and calm the nerves. Reserpine lowers blood pressure by irreversibly binding to NE storage vesicles, causing depletion of NE and other neurotransmitters in both the central and peripheral nervous systems. The drug may take 2 to 6 weeks to deplete NE and produce an optimal antihypertensive effect.

Unfortunately, reserpine can cause profound depression and sedation, and cardiovascular adverse effects such as bradycardia and orthostatic hypotension can be severe. Effects are often prolonged because once depleted of NE, neurons may take several weeks to synthesize adequate amounts of the neurotransmitter. Reserpine is only prescribed when patients are unable to tolerate safer antihypertensives. Although it was once used to treat psychotic disorders, it is no longer used for this purpose because more effective drugs are available.

Guanethidine (Ismelin) is also an adrenergic neuron–blocking drug. It acts by preventing the storage and release of NE in nerve terminals. As with reserpine, depletion of NE causes the heart rate to slow, and blood pressure to fall. The limiting adverse effects of guanethidine are severe diarrhea and orthostatic hypotension, which occur frequently and can be serious enough to cause syncope. Guanethidine is rarely prescribed due to the potential for serious adverse effects. A third drug in this class, guanadrel (Hylorel) has similar actions and adverse effects to guanethidine, but its use has been discontinued in the United States.

36.9 Direct-acting vasodilators lower blood pressure by relaxing arteriolar smooth muscle.

The ability to cause vasodilation is a property shared by many different classes of drugs, as shown in Figure 36.1. Most vasodilators are used to treat HTN, and some are used for the pharmacotherapy of heart failure, angina pectoris, and MI. Some of the drugs presented in previous sections of this chapter produce vasodilation indirectly by affecting autonomic nerves or by influencing the renin-angiotensin-aldosterone pathway. The agents presented in this section affect the vascular smooth muscle itself; thus, they are called direct vasodilators.

Direct relaxation of arteriolar smooth muscle is an effective way to reduce blood pressure. Indeed, sodium nitroprusside (Nitropress) and diazoxide (Hyperstat IV) are used in hypertensive emergencies and can lower blood pressure almost instantaneously. Unfortunately, the medications in this class have the potential to produce serious adverse effects. This limits their applications in the pharmacotherapy of HTN to hypertensive emergencies, and for HTN unresponsive to medications from safer drug classes.

All direct vasodilators cause **reflex tachycardia,** a compensatory increase in heart rate due to the sudden decrease in blood pressure. The baroreceptor reflex is an essential component of the normal physiologic control of blood pressure. However, when reflex tachycardia occurs as the result of vasodilator agents, the heart is forced to work harder and the resultant blood pressure increase counteracts the effect of the antihypertensive drug. Patients with CAD may experience an acute angina attack due to the sudden increase in cardiac workload. Fortunately, reflex tachycardia can be prevented by administering a beta-adrenergic blocker, such as propranolol (Inderal). Beta blockers are often administered concurrently with direct vasodilators for this reason.

A second potentially serious adverse effect of direct vasodilator therapy is salt and water retention. The reduction in blood pressure from the vasodilator causes a compensatory increase in aldosterone secretion by the adrenal gland. The increased aldosterone level signals the kidney to retain more sodium and water. Blood volume increases, thus raising blood pressure and canceling the antihypertensive action of the vasodilator. A diuretic may be administered concurrently with a direct vasodilator in order to prevent fluid retention.

Other adverse effects are drug specific. Hydralazine can induce a lupuslike syndrome characterized by myalgia, arthralgia, fever, and the presence of antinuclear antibodies. Although rare, symptoms may persist for 6 months or longer and antinuclear antibodies may be present for 9 years. The occurrence of this lupuslike syndrome is more common in Caucasians who are slow acetylators (see Chapter 5). Antinuclear antibody titers should be determined prior to initiating therapy, and periodically thereafter to identify the development of this syndrome.

PROTOTYPE DRUG Hydralazine (Apresoline)

Classification: **Therapeutic:** Antihypertensive
Pharmacologic: Direct vasodilator

Therapeutic Effects and Uses: In 1952, hydralazine was one of the first oral antihypertensive medications marketed in the United States. It is most commonly administered in tablet form for moderate to severe HTN, usually in combination with other antihypertensives. Apresazide is a fixed-dose combination of hydralazine with hydrochlorothiazide. When given orally, hydralazine is administered 2 to 4 times per day, usually with food because this increases its bioavailability. Therapy is generally begun with low doses, which are gradually increased until the desired therapeutic response is obtained. After several months of therapy, tolerance to the drug develops and a dosage increase may be necessary. Although it produces an effective reduction in blood pressure, drugs in other antihypertensive classes have largely replaced hydralazine.

Hydralazine is also available by the intramuscular (IM) and IV routes for hypertensive emergencies, especially those associated with preeclampsia, although it is not a drug of choice for this indication. It is sometimes administered to patients with acute heart failure because the drug reduces the workload on the heart due to its antihypertensive action. ACE inhibitors have largely replaced the drug for patients with heart failure (see Chapter 38). A fixed-dose combination therapy of isosorbide dinitrate and hydralazine (BiDil) is available for the treatment of heart failure in African American patients.

Mechanism of Action: By causing peripheral vasodilation, hydralazine acts directly to relax arterial smooth muscle. The decreased peripheral resistance is accompanied by an increase in heart rate and cardiac output. The overall result is a reduction in afterload. Because the drug is selective for arterioles and does not cause dilation of veins, orthostatic hypotension is not a major adverse effect.

Pharmacokinetics:

Route(s)	PO, IM, IV
Absorption	Rapidly absorbed PO and well absorbed IM
Distribution	Widely distributed; crosses the placenta and is secreted in breast milk; 87% bound to plasma protein
Primary metabolism	GI mucosa and liver; extensive first-pass metabolism
Primary excretion	90% renal, 10% feces
Onset of action	PO: 20–30 minutes; IM: 10–30 minutes; IV: 5–20 minutes
Duration of action	2–6 h; half-life: 3–7 h

Adverse Effects: Hydralazine may cause several adverse events that have the potential to prompt discontinuation of therapy. Headache, tachycardia, palpitations, flushing, nausea, and diarrhea are common, but may resolve as therapy progresses. Orthostatic hypotension, fluid retention, and peripheral edema may also occur. Patients who are "slow acetylators" and those with renal impairment or who are receiving high doses of hydralazine are susceptible to experiencing a lupuslike syndrome. Symptoms may include rash, urticaria, myalgia, fever, chills, and fatigue. Blood dyscrasias such as agranulocytosis and leucopenia are rare, though potentially serious, adverse effects.

Contraindications/Precautions: Patients with lupus should not receive hydralazine, as the drug can worsen symptoms. The drug is contraindicated in patients with cerebrovascular disease or rheumatic heart disease. Patients should discontinue hydralazine gradually because abrupt withdrawal may cause severe rebound HTN and anxiety. Because it is excreted primarily by the kidneys, the drug should be used with caution in patients with renal impairment. Caution must be used when administering hydralazine to patients who are known slow acetylators because plasma drug levels will be significantly higher in these patients. Caution should be used when treating patients with CAD, because hydralazine can precipitate angina attacks and an acute MI.

Drug Interactions: Administering hydralazine with other antihypertensives or monoamine oxidase inhibitors (MAOIs) may cause severe hypotension. This includes all drug classes used as antihypertensives. NSAIDs may decrease the antihypertensive action of hydralazine. Beta blockers are usually used concurrently with hydralazine to block reflex tachycardia, and heart rate should be carefully monitored to avoid bradycardia. Hydralazine may produce false-positive Coombs tests. **Herbal/Food:** Hawthorn should be avoided because it may cause additive hypotensive effects.

Pregnancy: Category C.

Treatment of Overdose: Treatment includes gastric lavage, activated charcoal and administration of a plasma volume expander to raise blood pressure. Tachycardia may require treatment with a beta blocker.

Nursing Responsibilities:

- Obtain a complete health history including medications to determine possible drug interactions and allergies; identify any recent cardiac or pulmonary events.
- Obtain baseline ECG and vital signs, including blood pressure.
- Auscultate heart and chest sounds for adventitious sounds.
- Assess neurologic status and LOC.
- Report history to health care provider if the patient has kidney disease, systemic lupus erythematosus (SLE), stroke or transient ischemic attack, pulmonary HTN, or high cholesterol or triglycerides. A lower dose or special monitoring may be needed.
- Monitor laboratory tests to determine antinuclear antibody titer before initiation of therapy and periodically during prolonged therapy.
- Establish baseline and periodic assessment of blood urea nitrogen (BUN), creatinine clearance, uric acid, serum potassium, blood glucose, and ECG. Monitor blood pressure and heart rate closely during a hypertensive crisis, checking every 5 minutes until stabilized, then every 15 minutes until crisis passes.
- Monitor intake and output with parenteral drug administration and in patients with renal dysfunction.

Patient and Family Education:

- Do not abruptly stop taking this drug because it could result in dangerously high blood pressure and anxiety.
- Headache and palpitations may occur within 2 to 4 hours after the first oral dose but these symptoms usually subside.
- Check for swelling of feet and ankles and weight gain. If present, report to the health care provider.
- Make position changes slowly when moving from a lying to a standing position to prevent dizziness and possible fainting.
- Avoid alcohol because alcohol intake could result in dizziness.
- Do not drive or perform other hazardous activities until the effects of the drug are known, because this drug may cause drowsiness and dizziness.
- Take the drug with a full glass of water.
- Do not breast-feed without approval of the health care provider.

Drugs Similar to Hydralazine (Apresoline)

Other direct vasodilators used for HTN include diazoxide, minoxidil, and nitroprusside. Nitroprusside is a drug of choice for hypertensive emergencies and is presented as a prototype drug in Section 36.10.

Diazoxide (Hyperstat IV, Proglycem): Acting in 30 to 60 seconds, Hyperstat IV is one of the most effective and rapid-acting antihypertensive drugs available for the management of hypertensive emergencies. Approved in 1973, hypotensive actions may persist for 2 to 12 hours after the infusion is discontinued. The drug is administered as a rapid IV push, with doses repeated at 5 to 15 minute intervals until the desired therapeutic response is achieved. Like hydralazine, the drug is selective for arterioles and has no effect on veins.

As expected of any drug that causes a rapid drop in blood pressure, reflex tachycardia is prominent with Hyperstat IV and a beta blocker may be required to slow the heart rate. The patient should be kept recumbent during the infusion and for at least 30 minutes following an injection to avoid symptoms of orthostatic hypotension. Hyperstat IV can result in significant sodium and water retention; thus, the presence of edema should be monitored. Diuretics may be used to counteract this effect. Diazoxide is chemically related to the thiazide diuretics: Patients hypersensitive to thiazides should not receive this drug. It is a pregnancy category C drug.

Proglycem is an oral form of diazoxide that is used to treat various hypoglycemic states, usually caused by the presence of excessive insulin (hyperinsulinism). Proglycem reduces the secretion of insulin from the pancreas, causing blood glucose to increase. Caution must be used when administering any form of diazoxide to patients with diabetes, as hyperglycemia may result. Unlike Hyperstat IV, Proglycem has little effect on blood pressure.

Minoxidil (Loniten): Minoxidil is a direct vasodilator with profound vasodilation activity that is selective for arterioles: It does not dilate veins. It is administered by the oral route for severe HTN that is unresponsive to drugs from other classes. Because of its efficacy and the potential for serious effects on the cardiovascular system, initial doses are very low, and the amount is increased gradually. It is a pregnancy category C drug.

Minoxidil is considerably more toxic than hydralazine. The most serious adverse effects are cardiovascular in nature, including reflex tachycardia and plasma volume expansion due to sodium and water retention. Beta blockers are usually administered concurrently to minimize tachycardia, and diuretics to prevent fluid retention. Although rare, pericardial effusion has been reported with minoxidil use. Minoxidil causes **hypertrichosis:** the elongation, thickening, and increased pigmentation of body hair. This is normal and will reverse when the drug is discontinued. The drug's effect on hair growth is used to the patient's advantage in Rogaine, a topical form of minoxidil used to stimulate hair growth in patients with male-pattern baldness. The topical form of the drug is not absorbed into the systemic circulation, thus Rogaine produces none of the serious cardiovascular effects observed with Loniten.

Management of Hypertensive Emergency

36.10 Hypertensive crisis is a medical emergency that is treated by the intravenous administration of antihypertensive medications.

A **hypertensive emergency (HTN-E)**, also called hypertensive crisis, is defined as a diastolic pressure of greater than 120 mmHg, with evidence of target-organ system damage. HTN-E requires aggressive treatment, usually within minutes to hours, to prevent further organ damage. A related condition, **hypertensive urgency,** is when a patient presents with severe HTN, but has no evidence of target-organ damage.

Target-organ damage from extreme HTN most often occurs in the cardiovascular system, the kidneys, or the CNS. In the cardiovascular system, the increased workload on the heart leads to acute left heart failure with pulmonary edema, sometimes accompanied by myocardial ischemia or infarction. Chest pain and dyspnea are the most common symptoms in patients with HTN-E. Renal function is diminished, as evidenced by oliguria, hematuria, and proteinuria. Acute renal failure may occur, or preexisting chronic renal failure may worsen. In the brain, thrombotic or hemorrhagic stroke may occur. The capillaries in the brain become leaky, producing hypertensive encephalopathy, with resulting headache, paralysis, seizures, or coma. In addition, retinal hemorrhages and edema of the retina (papilledema) are signs of severe HTN.

The most common cause of HTN-E is untreated or poorly controlled essential HTN. In some cases, the patient has abruptly discontinued their antihypertensive medication. There are, however, a large number of possible secondary causes of HTN-E, including the following conditions:

- Renovascular hypertension
- Pheochromocytoma
- Cocaine use
- Eclampsia or preeclampsia
- Head injuries
- Primary hyperaldosteronism
- Coarctation of the aorta
- Hyperthyroidism or thyroid storm

In the management of HTN-E, the therapeutic goal is to lower blood pressure quickly. Care must be taken, however, to not decrease blood pressure too quickly because rapid and intense vasodilation can result in serious hypoperfusion of the cerebral, coronary, or renal vascular capillaries. This can cause ischemia or infarction, worsening target-organ damage to the brain, heart, kidneys, or retina. It is recommended that the pretreatment blood pressure be progressively reduced by 20% to 25%, over 30 to 60 minutes. Additional, gradual reductions are made over a 12- to 48-hour period until blood pressure is reduced to a value within the normal range. Parenteral antihypertensives are agents of choice due to their rapid onset of action and because infusions offer more precise control during the gradual pressure reduction.

In patients with hypertensive urgencies, target-organ damage has not yet developed. These patients are treated more conservatively by increasing the dose of their current antihypertensive drug, or by adding a second drug to the regimen. Oral medications are used to lower blood pressure because these drugs are less toxic than parenteral antihypertensives. Oral agents with a relatively rapid onset of action that may be used for hypertensive urgency include clonidine (Catapres), captopril (Capoten), or labetalol (Normodyne). The patient should be monitored for several hours, and doses may be repeated at frequent intervals, as needed, to lower pressure to acceptable levels. All patients with hypertensive urgency should receive follow-up assessments after 1 to 3 days on the new regimen.

PROTOTYPE DRUG Nitroprusside sodium (Nipride, Nitropress)

Classification: **Therapeutic:** Drug for hypertensive emergency
Pharmacologic: Direct vasodilator

Therapeutic Effects and Uses: Nitroprusside is a drug of choice for patients with aggressive, life-threatening HTN because it has the ability to lower blood pressure almost instantaneously upon IV administration. The drug has a short half-life, and the hypotensive effects disappear approximately 3 minutes after the infusion is discontinued. Unlike most direct vasodilators, nitroprusside causes very little reflex tachycardia. Although discovered in 1850, the drug was not approved by the FDA until 1974.

Patients must be continuously monitored while receiving nitroprusside to prevent hypotension due to over treatment. Therapy is limited to 72 hours because the drug is metabolized to toxic thiocyanate and cyanide compounds. This is of special concern to patients with renal impairment who are unable to excrete the cyanide. If serum thiocyanate exceeds 12 mg/dL, the nitroprusside infusion should be discontinued. As a general rule, patients are switched from nitroprusside to an oral antihypertensive as soon as blood pressure has stabilized.

Mechanism of Action: Nitroprusside dilates both arteries and veins; therefore, the hypotensive action of nitroprusside is due to direct relaxation of arteriolar smooth muscle and to blood pooling in the veins. In most patients, heart rate is mildly increased, while cardiac output is decreased. In patients with severe left ventricular hypertrophy, however, cardiac output may increase.

Pharmacokinetics:

Route(s)	IV
Absorption	N/A
Distribution	Unknown
Primary metabolism	Metabolized to thiocyanates in erythrocytes and other tissues
Primary excretion	Renal
Onset of action	1–2 minutes
Duration of action	1–10 minutes

Adverse Effects: Signs and symptoms of vasodilation such as hypotension, headache, dizziness, and flushing of the skin are expected adverse effects. With extended therapy, thiocyanate toxicity may manifest. Thiocyanate poisoning is characterized by hypotension, lethargy, blurred vision, metabolic acidosis, faint heart sounds, and loss of consciousness. Irritation may occur at the infusion site

Contraindications/Precautions: Patients with inadequate cerebral circulation or who have compensatory HTN should not receive nitroprusside. Because the kidneys excrete the toxic thiocyanate metabolite of the drug, patients with serious renal impairment should be treated cautiously. Nitroprusside is contraindicated in patients with high intracranial pressure because the drug may worsen this condition.

Drug Interactions: Antihypertensive agents, ethanol, general anesthetics, and ganglionic blockers should be used with caution with nitroprusside because additive hypotension could result. Sympathomimetics such as epinephrine will block the antihypertensive actions of nitroprusside. Dobutamine (Dobutrex) and nitroprusside are sometimes administered concurrently because this interaction results in a beneficial synergistic increase in cardiac output and decrease in pulmonary capillary wedge pressure. **Herbal/Food:** Hawthorn may cause additive hypotensive effects.

Pregnancy: Category C.

Treatment of Overdose: Extreme hypotension may be treated with a vasopressor. Cyanide toxicity caused by the overdose may require the use of a Cyanide Antidote Kit, which contains amyl nitrate, sodium nitrite and sodium thiosulfate. The purpose of these drugs is to convert toxic cyanide into nontoxic thiocyanate.

Nursing Responsibilities:

- Obtain a complete health history including medications to determine possible drug interactions and allergies; identify any recent cardiac or pulmonary events.
- Obtain baseline ECG and vital sign readings, including blood pressure.
- Auscultate heart and chest sounds for adventitious sounds.
- Titrate (adjust) the IV infusion rate to blood pressure response with constant hemodynamic monitoring.
- Slow or stop the infusion if serious adverse effects (hypotension) are noted. Keep patient supine to lessen hypotension-related adverse effects.
- Notify the prescriber if blood pressure rises after the drug infusion rate is decreased or the infusion is discontinued.
- Monitor intake and output ratio.
- Monitor laboratory tests for blood thiocyanate level when the patient receives prolonged treatment or has severe kidney dysfunction. Determine plasma cyanogen level following 1 or 2 days of therapy in patients with impaired liver function.
- Nitroprusside is chemically unstable and exceptionally light sensitive. Check the drug solution periodically and discard if the color turns dark brown.

Patient and Family Education:

- Be aware that therapy is short term and will be discontinued when blood pressure is controlled.
- Report headache, which can be treated with over-the-counter (OTC) analgesics, to the health care provider.

Drugs Similar to Nitroprusside Sodium (Nipride, Nitropress)

Other vasodilators for HTN-E include clevidipine, diazoxide, enalaprilat, esmolol, fenoldopam, hydralazine, labetalol, nicardipine, and phentolamine. Table 36.5 summarizes their applications to the pharmacotherapy of hypertensive crisis.

PharmFACT

Hypertensive crisis is a common condition, affecting 1% of the patients with primary HTN. The most common presentation, occurring in 25% of patients, is CVA. If left untreated, 79% of the patients with hypertensive crisis will die within 12 months. *Source:* McCowan, 2007.

NURSING PROCESS APPLICATION

Patients Receiving Direct Vasodilators

Assessment	Potential Nursing Diagnoses
Prior to drug administration: • Obtain complete health history; identify any recent cardiac or pulmonary events. • Obtain drug history to determine possible drug interactions and allergies. • Obtain ECG and vital signs, including blood pressure. • Auscultate heart and chest sounds. • Assess neurologic status and LOC. • Obtain blood and urine specimens for laboratory analysis.	• *Ineffective Tissue Perfusion (Cardiopulmonary),* related to sustained elevated blood pressure • *Ineffective Health Maintenance,* related to inability to modify lifestyle • *Impaired Skin Integrity,* related to intravenous infusion of medications • *Deficient Knowledge* (Effects of prescribed treatment)

Planning: Patient Goals and Expected Outcomes

The patient will:

- Exhibit a reduction in systolic/diastolic blood pressure not to exceed a systolic reading of 150 and a diastolic reading of 90.
- Incorporate lifestyle changes (dietary changes, smoking cessation, and exercise) to manage hypertension.
- Demonstrate understanding of the drug's action by accurately describing drug adverse effects and precautions.

Implementation

Interventions and (Rationales)	Patient and Family Education
IV nitroprusside requires special handling during preparation and administration. Follow hospital policy regarding administration (Nipride is extremely light sensitive and must be protected from light)	• Instruct the patient that the infusion will lower the blood pressure rapidly. Explain the health facility's protocol for administration of nitroprusside.
With IV nitroprusside monitor vital signs every 5 –15 minutes and titrate the infusion based on prescribed parameters. (Blood pressure reduction occurs very rapidly with this drug. Life threatening hypotension can occur within minutes.)	• Inform the patient of the necessity of frequent vital sign monitoring and titration protocol.
Assess the IV site for swelling or signs of infiltration (Nitropresside may cause tissue damage if extravasation occurs)	• Instruct the patient to report any burning or stinging pain, swelling, warmth, redness, or tenderness at the IV insertion site. These may signal phlebitis or drug seepage into soft tissues.
Use with caution with impaired cardiac or cerebral circulation. (The drop in blood pressure produced by vasodilators may further compromise individuals who already suffer from ischemia).	Instruct the patient to: • Report angina-like symptoms: chest, arm, back and or neck pain, or palpitations. • Report faintness, dizziness, drowsiness, any sensation of cold, numbness, or tingling, or a pale or dusky look to the hands and feet. • Report headache or signs of stroke: facial drooping, visual changes, or limb weakness or paralysis.
Monitor for dizziness and orthostatic hypotension. (These symptoms occur due to insufficient blood flow to the CNS.)	Instruct the patient: • That drug therapy may cause extreme dizziness and light-headedness with sudden position changes. • To always arise slowly, allowing blood pressure to adjust with movement.
Observe for signs and symptoms of lupus, such as the classic "butterfly rash" over the nose and cheeks, or muscle aches and fatigue when taking hydralazine.(Lupus is an adverse effect of this drug therapy)	• Instruct patient to report unusual rashes or changes in skin color, muscle aches, or atypical fatigue.
Assess lifestyle factors that may contribute to a hypertensive state such as obesity, smoking, or tobacco use, and poor dietary patterns. (Modification in lifestyle and habits may aid in the reduction of blood pressure)	• Instruct the patient to adhere to additional interventions for hypertension such as weight reduction, modification of sodium intake, smoking cessation, exercise, and stress management.
Discontinue vasodilators gradually. (Abrupt withdrawal of drug may cause rebound hypertension.)	• Instruct patient to not stop taking the medication suddenly.

Evaluation of Outcome Criteria

Evaluate the effectiveness of drug therapy by confirming that patient goals and expected outcomes have been met (see "Planning").

TABLE 36.5 Drugs for Hypertensive Emergency

Drug	Class	Applications
clevidipine (Cleviprex)	Calcium channel blocker	Newer drug, approved in 2008; very rapid onset and short duration
diazoxide (Hyperstat IV, Proglycem)	Direct vasodilator	Rarely used due to serious adverse effects such as reflex tachycardia, fluid retention, hyperglycemia
enalaprilat (Enalapril IV)	ACE inhibitor	Onset of action is 15–30 min; useful in HTN-E associated with heart failure or high plasma levels of angiotensin II
esmolol (Brevibloc)	Beta-adrenergic antagonist	Onset of action is 1–5 min; useful for patients with severe left ventricular dysfunction or with peripheral vascular disease
fenoldopam (Corlopam)	Dopamine agonist	Onset of action is 5 min; useful for patients with renal impairment, as the drug increases renal blood flow
hydralazine (Apresoline)	Direct vasodilator	Onset of action is 5–20 min; useful in HTN-E due to eclampsia and preeclampsia because it increases uterine blood flow
labetalol (Normodyne)	Alpha- and beta-adrenergic antagonist	Onset of action is 2–5 min; reduces incidences of MI and death
nicardipine (Cardene IV)	Calcium channel blocker	Onset of action is 1 min; rapid and effective for most HTN-E, with fewer adverse effects than some other HTN-E drugs
nitroprusside sodium (Nipride)	Direct vasodilator	Onset of action is 1 min; drug of choice for many HTN-E
phentolamine (Regitine)	Alpha-adrenergic antagonist	Onset of action is 1–5 min; rarely used due to high incidence of reflex tachycardia and myocardial ischemia; useful for HTN-E due to pheochromocytoma

UNDERSTANDING THE CHAPTER

Key Concepts Summary

36.1 Hypertension is classified by stages, based upon the degree of elevation of systolic and diastolic blood pressure.

36.2 Failure to properly manage hypertension can lead to cerebrovascular accident, heart failure, or myocardial infarction.

36.3 Therapeutic lifestyle changes can reduce blood pressure and lessen the need for antihypertensive medications.

36.4 The choice of antihypertensive medication is determined by the degree of hypertension and the presence of other medical conditions.

36.5 Diuretics are often drugs of first choice for treating mild to moderate hypertension.

36.6 Calcium channel blockers have emerged as important drugs in the treatment of hypertension.

36.7 Blocking the renin-angiotensin-aldosterone system leads to a decrease in blood pressure.

36.8 Adrenergic antagonists are commonly used to treat hypertension.

36.9 Direct-acting vasodilators lower blood pressure by relaxing arteriolar smooth muscle.

36.10 Hypertensive crisis is a medical emergency that is treated by the IV administration of antihypertensive medications.

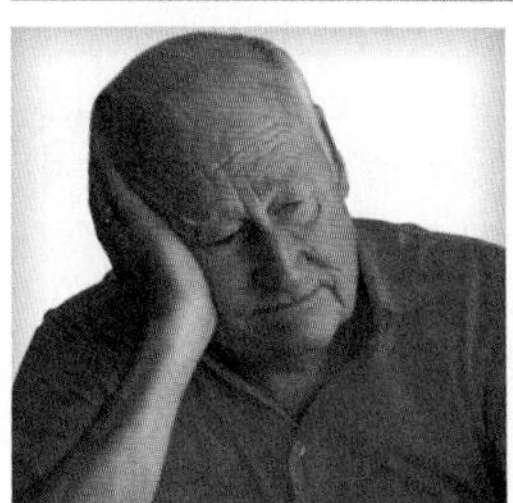

Making the PATIENT Connection

Remember the patient "Elmer Foley" at the beginning of the chapter? Now read the remainder of the case study. Based on the information presented within this chapter, respond to the critical thinking questions that follow.

Elmer Foley is a 72-year-old Caucasian male with a 10-month history of uncontrolled HTN. Initially, Elmer was prescribed the thiazide diuretic hydrochlorothiazide (HydroDIURIL). However, after 1 week of therapy his blood pressure has remained at 168/102 mmHg. Next, Elmer's health care provider added an angiotensin-converting enzyme inhibitor, captopril (Capoten), to the regimen. Still, Elmer's blood pressure remained above normal limits. Lastly, the health care provider discontinued the captopril and started Elmer on hydralazine (Apresoline). With this visit, his blood pressure is 146/90 mmHg.

When Elmer was first told he had HTN, he began many of the suggested lifestyle changes encouraged by his health care provider. He has lost a total of 15 kg (32 lb) since starting his diet 10 months ago. Elmer started walking daily for exercise and can now walk up to 1 mile without fatigue. He avoids all salty foods and diligently checks food labels for fat and salt content. Elmer occasionally drinks a glass of wine, although never more than 1 to 2 glasses per month. Although it was difficult for Elmer to stop smoking totally, he proudly claims he has been smokeless for 8 months.

Critical Thinking Questions

1. How would you respond to Elmer's question, "What else can I do?" Is there anything else he can do to reduce his blood pressure?
2. What factors would you contribute to Elmer's depression? Is the drug therapy possibly a causative factor?
3. Elmer wants to know why the previous therapies were unsuccessful. What would you say as his nurse?
4. As the nurse, how can you support Elmer before he leaves the clinic?

Case Study

Helen Edwards is a 44-year-old African American woman who presents to the emergency department with headache and shortness of breath. Helen has a long-standing history of HTN. She has never consistently adhered to any HTN management strategies and has been nonadherent with her medication regimen for the past 8 months. Upon arrival at the emergency department her blood pressure is 192/126 mmHg.

When you assess the patient, it is noted that she is approximately 1.7 m (5′6″) in height and the self-reported weight is 107 kg (236 lb). She is slightly lethargic and complains of left arm numbness and tingling. Other physical assessment parameters are normal.

Helen is started on an infusion of nitroprusside (Nipride) 50 mg in 250 mL in D_5W. The dose will be titrated between 0.5 to 10 mcg/kg/minute to maintain the patient's diastolic pressure at less than 100 mmHg.

1. Describe the mechanism of action related to nitroprusside (Nipride).
2. For what adverse effects should you monitor in patients receiving this drug therapy?
3. What factors does this patient have that predisposes her to hypertensive crises?

NCLEX-RN® Review

1 Methyldopa (Aldomet) is being initiated for a client with hypertension. Which of the following health teaching would be most appropriate for this drug?

1. Avoid hot baths and showers, and prolonged standing in one position.
2. This drug may discolor the urine a pinkish-brown color.
3. You may experience bloating and weight gain.
4. The tablet should be taken only with food or milk.

2 A client is receiving a direct vasodilator for elevated blood pressure levels. The nurse would include in the care plan to monitor the client for which of the following adverse effects?

1. Atelectasis
2. Crystalluria
3. Photosensitivity
4. Orthostatic hypotension

3 The nurse determines that the client understands an important principle in self-administration of hydralazine (Apresoline) when the client makes which of the following statements?

1. "I should not drive until the response to drug therapy is determined."
2. "I can stop taking this medication once I begin to feel better."
3. "If I experience dizziness, I should take only half the dose."
4. "I should avoid air travel while taking this medication."

4 A client with hypertensive crisis is started on nitroprusside (Nipride) therapy. The nurse would perform what priority intervention during the course of this treatment?

1. Monitor for the presence or absence of bowel sounds.
2. Obtain urine samples for specific gravity measurements and glucose levels.
3. Observe skin pressure points for turgor and integrity.
4. Titrate intravenous infusion rate according to the blood pressure response.

5 The nurse knows that the primary factors responsible for blood pressure are: (Select all that apply.)

1. Number of red blood cells.
2. Cardiac output.
3. Peripheral resistance.
4. Blood volume.
5. Skin elasticity.

6 The client, who is receiving a daily dose of methyldopa (Aldomet), informs the nurse that the medication is causing severe drowsiness during the day. Which of the following responses would be best when addressing this complaint?

1. "You should drink at least 1 to 2 cups of caffeinated beverages such as coffee daily."
2. "You can minimize daytime sedation by changing medication dosages to nighttime."
3. "A midday nap each day will be most effective immediately after lunch."
4. "Daytime sleepiness is not an expected adverse effect. Stop taking the medication."

See Answers to Critical Thinking Questions, Case Study, and NCLEX-RN® Review in Appendix A.

References

American Heart Association. (2008). *Heart disease and stroke statistics.* Retrieved July 11, 2008, from http://www.americanheart.org/downloadable/heart/1200078608862HS_Stats%202008.final.pdf

Burnier, M. (2006). Medication adherence and persistence as the cornerstone of effective antihypertensive therapy. *American Journal of Hypertension, 19*(11), 1190–1196.

Colbert, B. J., & Mason, B. J. (2008). *Integrated cardiopulmonary pharmacology* (2nd ed.). Upper Saddle River, NJ: Prentice Hall.

Drug Digest. (2007). *Grape seed extract.* Retrieved June 11, 2008, from http://www.drugdigest.org/DD/DVH/HerbsWho/0,3923,552554%7CGrape%2BSeed%2BExtract,00.html

Feldman, P. H., & McDonald, M. V. (2006). Clinical guidelines and recent research on hypertension and heart failure. *Home Healthcare Nurse, 24*(1), 50–53.

Grossman, E., & Messerli, F. (2006). Long-term safety of antihypertensive therapy. *Progress in Cardiovascular Diseases, 49*(1), 16–25.

Gu, Q., Paulose-Ram, R., Dillon, C., & Burt, V. (2006). Antihypertensive medication use among U.S. adults with hypertension. *Circulation, 113*(1), 213–221.

Hoffman, B. B. (2006). Therapy of hypertension. In L. Brunton, J. Lazo, & K. Parker (Eds.), *The pharmacological basis of therapeutics* (pp. 845–968). New York: McGraw-Hill.

Israili, Z. H., Hernandez-Hernandez, R., & Valasco, M. (2007). The future of antihypertensive treatment. *American Journal of Therapeutics, 14*(2), 121–134.

Kaplan, N., & Opie, L. (2006). Controversies in hypertension. *The Lancet, 367*(9505), 168–176.

Manach, C., Mazur, A., & Scalbert, A. (2005). Polyphenols and prevention of cardiovascular diseases. *Current Opinion in Lipidology, 16*(1), 77–84.

McCowan, C. (2007). Hypertensive emergencies. *eMedicine.* Retrieved July 11, 2008, from http://www.emedicine.com/emerg/TOPIC267.HTM

McLean, D. L. (2007). Nurses managing high blood pressure in patients with diabetes in community pharmacies. *Canadian Journal of Cardiovascular Nursing, 17*(2), 17–21.

National Center for Complementary and Alternative Medicine. (2008). *Herbs at a glance: Grape seed extract.* Retrieved July 11, 2008, from http://nccam.nih.gov/health/grapeseed/

Ong, K. L., Cheung, B. M. Y., Man, Y. B., Lau, C. P., & Lam, K. S. L. (2007). Prevalence, awareness, treatment, and control of hypertension among United States adults 1999–2004. *Hypertension, 49*(12), 69–75.

U.S. Department of Health and Human Services, National Institute of Health, National Heart, Lung, and Blood Institute, National High Blood Pressure Education Program. (2003). *JNC-7 Express: The seventh report of the Joint National Committee on Prevention, Detection Evaluation and Treatment of High Blood Pressure.* Bethesda, MD: Author. Retrieved July 11, 2008, from http://www.nhlbi.nih.gov/guidelines/hypertension/express.pdf

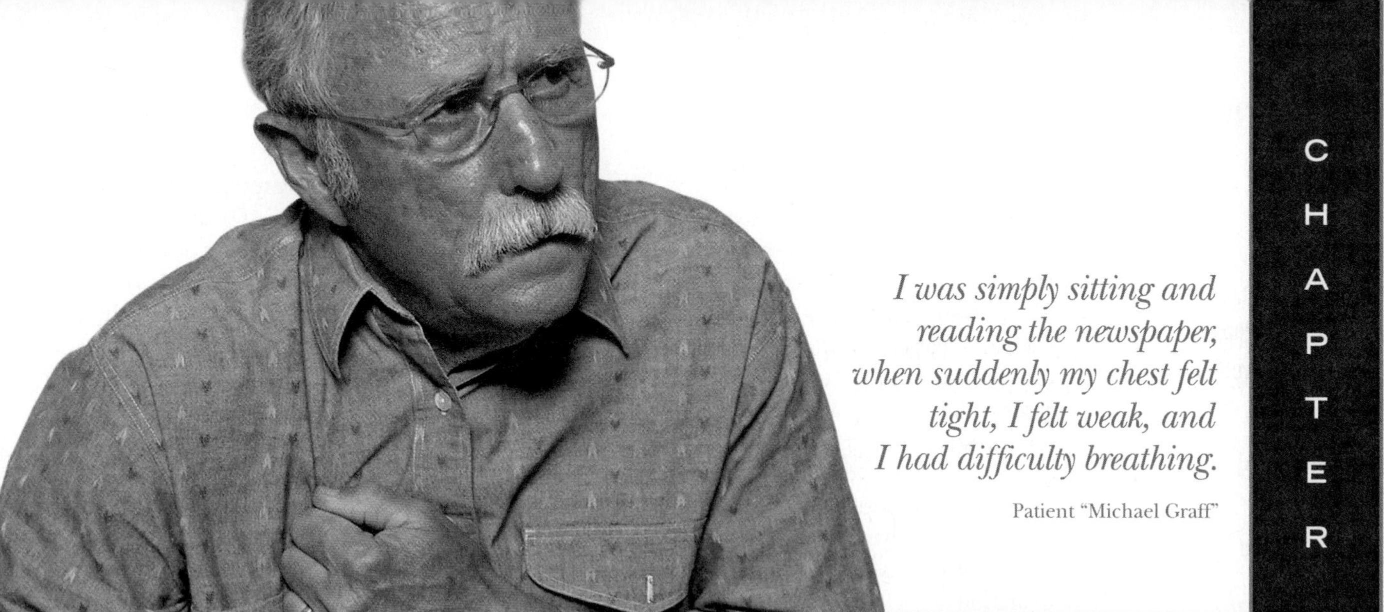

I was simply sitting and reading the newspaper, when suddenly my chest felt tight, I felt weak, and I had difficulty breathing.

Patient "Michael Graff"

CHAPTER 37

Pharmacotherapy of Angina Pectoris and Myocardial Infarction

Chapter Outline

Pathophysiology of Myocardial Ischemia

Etiology of Coronary Artery Disease

Pathophysiology of Angina Pectoris

Nonpharmacologic Therapy of Coronary Artery Disease

Pharmacologic Management of Angina Pectoris

Drug Classes for Angina Pectoris

Organic Nitrates

PROTOTYPE Nitroglycerin (Nitrostat, Nitro-Bid, Nitro-Dur, Others) *p. 593*

Beta-Adrenergic Blockers (Antagonists)

PROTOTYPE Atenolol (Tenormin) *p. 597*

Calcium Channel Blockers

Pathophysiology of Myocardial Infarction

Pharmacologic Management of Myocardial Infarction

Thrombolytics and Adjunct Medications for Myocardial Infarction

Learning Outcomes

After reading this chapter, the student should be able to:

1. Describe factors that affect myocardial oxygen supply and demand.
2. Explain the relationship between atherosclerosis and coronary artery disease.
3. Explain the pathophysiology of angina pectoris and myocardial infarction.
4. Discuss the role of therapeutic lifestyle changes in the management of coronary artery disease.
5. Describe the pharmacologic management of the different types of angina.
6. Describe the pharmacologic management of myocardial infarction.
7. For each of the classes shown in the chapter outline, identify the prototype and representative drugs and explain the mechanism(s) of drug action, primary indications, contraindications, significant drug interactions, pregnancy category, and important adverse effects.
8. Use the nursing process to care for patients receiving drugs for angina and myocardial infarction.

Key Terms

angina pectoris, 589
atherosclerosis, 588
coronary artery disease (CAD), 588
glycoprotein IIb/IIIa, 600
myocardial infarctions (MIs), 598
myocardial ischemia, 588
nitric oxide, 592
partial fatty-acid oxidation inhibitors, 591
plaque, 588
silent angina, 589
stable angina, 589
unstable angina, 589
vasospastic (Prinzmetal's) angina, 589

The tissues of the body depend upon a continuous supply of oxygen and vital nutrients to support life and health. The heart is particularly demanding of a steady source of oxygen. Insufficient arterial blood supply to cardiac muscle may result in angina pectoris, acute myocardial infarction (heart attack), and possibly death. This chapter focuses on the pharmacologic interventions related to angina pectoris and myocardial infarction (MI).

Pathophysiology of Myocardial Ischemia

37.1 Myocardial ischemia develops when there is inadequate blood supply to meet the metabolic demands of cardiac muscle.

Myocardial ischemia is a condition in which the heart is receiving an insufficient amount of oxygen to meet its metabolic demands. This occurs when there is an imbalance between oxygen supply and oxygen demand in myocardial cells. Knowledge of factors affecting myocardial oxygen supply and demand is necessary for understanding the pharmacotherapy of the diseases associated with myocardial ischemia.

Myocardial Oxygen Supply

The heart, from the moment it begins to function in utero until death, works to distribute oxygen and nutrients by means of its nonstop pumping action. It is the hardest working organ in the body, functioning continuously during both activity and rest. Because the heart is a muscle, it needs a steady supply of nourishment to sustain itself and maintain the systemic circulation in a balanced state of equilibrium. Any disturbance in blood flow to the myocardium—even for brief episodes—can result in life-threatening consequences. A review of the coronary circulation is provided in Section 31.5.

As with other arteries in the body, the amount of blood flow through the coronary arteries is dependent upon a number of hemodynamic factors. Of these, blood pressure is the most important. When systolic blood pressure falls, the quantity of blood flowing to the coronary arteries is diminished. If this occurs suddenly, it could be life threatening, as occurs in severe shock. Immediate restoration of blood pressure is required to reestablish adequate oxygen supply to the myocardium, as well as other vital tissues. Other important hemodynamic factors affecting the myocardial oxygen supply include changes in blood volume (e.g., hemorrhage) and disorders that reduce the oxygen content or carrying capacity of the blood (e.g., anemia).

The narrowing of a coronary artery resulting from atherosclerosis or coronary artery disease (CAD) deprives cells of needed oxygen and nutrients. If the narrowing develops over a long period of time, the heart compensates for its inadequate blood supply and the patient may be asymptomatic. Indeed, coronary arteries may be occluded as much as 50% or more and cause no symptoms.

Myocardial Oxygen Demand

As CAD progresses, cardiac muscle does not receive enough oxygen to meet the body's metabolic demands. The physiologic demands on the heart are highly variable and depend upon a large number of hemodynamic and lifestyle factors.

Basically, anything that increases the workload of the heart will increase myocardial oxygen demand. It is not difficult to think of the many daily activities that increase cardiac workload. Exercise, for example, will cause the heart to beat faster in order to pump more blood to muscles. This physical activity need not be extreme: Simply walking at a normal pace will increase cardiac workload over resting levels.

In some patients, the increased cardiac workload can be the result of mental, rather than physical, stressors. Think of the first time (or last time) you had to give a speech in front of a group, or became angry with a child, spouse, or coworker. These activities resulted in your heart pumping harder or faster, even though there was no physical activity involved. What factors do physical exercise and mental stress have in common that produced the increased cardiac workload?

The answer is simple. Anything that increases heart rate, contractility, or tension on the ventricular walls causes the heart to work harder. For example, if heart rate increases due to exercise or hyperthyroidism, it is easy to understand why the heart needs more oxygen because it must beat more times per minute. Similarly, the heart will need more oxygen if it beats more forcefully (increased contractility). A patient with heart failure has a thickened myocardium (increased tension) that will require more work to contract. The heart of a hypertensive patient will have to work harder to eject blood. It is important to remember that anything that makes the heart beat faster or contract with more force will increase myocardial oxygen demand. Drugs that diminish these factors are of value in the treatment of angina, MI, and heart failure.

Etiology of Coronary Artery Disease

37.2 Coronary artery disease is the major cause of myocardial ischemia.

Coronary artery disease (CAD) is one of the leading causes of mortality in the United States. The primary defining characteristic of CAD is narrowing or occlusion of one or more coronary arteries. Narrowing can result in symptoms of angina pectoris, whereas occlusion results in MI. The two disorders are closely related, as most patients who experience an MI have narrowing of the coronary vessels.

The most common etiology of CAD in adults is **atherosclerosis,** the presence of **plaque**—a fatty, fibrous

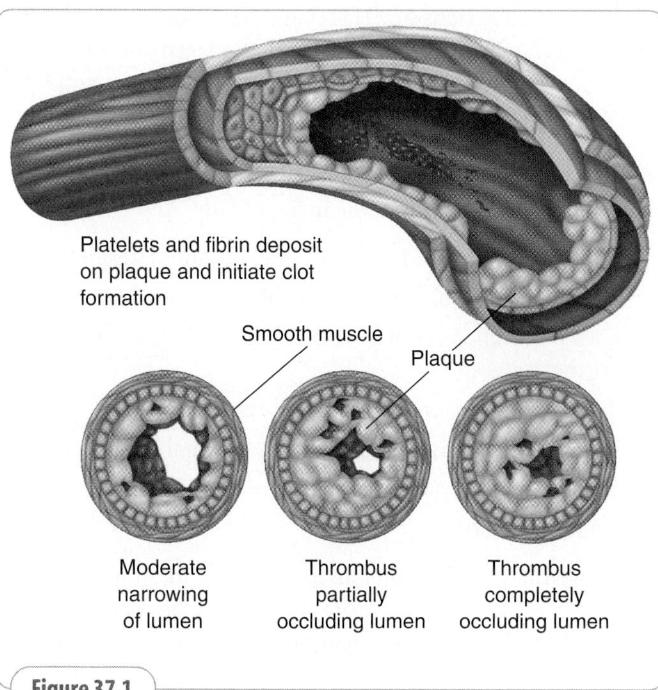

Figure 37.1

Atherosclerosis in the coronary arteries.

Source: From *Human Diseases: A Systematic Approach*, 6th ed. (p. 115), by M. Mulvihill, M. Zelman, P. Holdaway, E. Tompary, and J. Raymond, 2006. Reprinted with permission of Pearson Education, Inc., Upper Saddle River, NJ.

material—within the walls of the coronary arteries. Plaque develops progressively over time, producing varying degrees of intravascular narrowing, a situation that results in partial or total blockage of the vessel. During periods of rest, demands on the heart are less and a partially occluded artery may be able to provide adequate oxygen. During exercise (or a pharmacology test), however, workload on the heart increases, the cardiac muscle distal to the obstruction receives insufficient oxygen supply, and ischemia results.

A healthy heart responds to stress by changing the diameter of the coronary arteries. Thus, when the oxygen demands of the heart increase, the vessels respond immediately by dilating to bring more oxygen to the myocardium. Plaque impairs normal elasticity, and the coronary vessel is unable to dilate properly when the myocardium demands additional oxygen. Myocardial ischemia occurs when cardiac demands exceed the amount of oxygen that can be supplied through the narrowed, inelastic vessels characteristic of CAD.

Plaque accumulation occurs gradually, over periods of 40 to 50 years in some individuals, but actually begins to accrue very early in life. The development of atherosclerosis is illustrated in Figure 37.1.

CONNECTION *Checkpoint* 37.1

From what you learned in Chapter 31, predict what would happen to the cardiac workload when plasma volume is increased by an infusion of normal saline. What affect might this have on a patient with CAD? See Answer to Connection Checkpoint 37.1 in Appendix A.

Pathophysiology of Angina Pectoris

37.3 Angina pectoris is characterized by severe chest pain brought on by physical exertion or emotional stress.

Angina pectoris is acute chest pain caused by myocardial ischemia. The classic presentation of angina pectoris is steady, intense pain, sometimes with a crushing or constricting sensation in the anterior chest. Typically, the discomfort radiates to the left shoulder and proceeds down the left arm. It may also extend to the posterior thoracic region or move upward to the jaw, and in some patients the pain is experienced in the epigastrium or abdominal area. Accompanying the discomfort is severe emotional distress—a feeling of panic with fear of impending death. There is usually pallor, dyspnea with cyanosis, diaphoresis, tachycardia, and elevated blood pressure.

Anginal pain is usually precipitated by physical exertion or emotional excitement—events associated with increased myocardial oxygen demand. Angina pectoris episodes are of short duration. With physical rest and mental relaxation, the workload demands upon the heart diminish and the discomfort subsides within 5 to 10 minutes. Descriptions of the four basic types of angina follow.

When angina occurrences are fairly predictable in frequency, intensity, and duration, the condition is described as classic or **stable angina.** Rest usually relieves the pain associated with stable angina.

Vasospastic (Prinzmetal's) angina occurs when the decreased myocardial blood flow is caused by spasms of the coronary arteries. The vessels undergoing spasms may or may not contain atherosclerotic plaque. Thus, the primary cause of the narrowing and subsequent angina pain is vasoconstriction, rather than plaque buildup in the artery. Vasospastic angina pain occurs most often during periods of rest, although it may occur unpredictably, unrelated to rest or activity.

Although most people equate angina with chest pain, this is not always the case. When myocardial ischemia occurs in the absence of pain, it is called **silent angina.** Although one or more coronary arteries are occluded, the patient is asymptomatic. Some patients diagnosed with stable angina also experience silent angina. Although the mechanisms underlying silent angina are not completely understood, the condition is associated with a high risk for acute MI and sudden death.

Unstable angina occurs when episodes of angina occur suddenly, have added intensity, and occur during periods of rest. Unstable angina is a type of acute coronary syndrome in which an atherosclerotic plaque within a coronary artery ruptures. A thrombus quickly builds on the displaced plaque, and the artery becomes at serious risk of occlusion. This condition is a medical emergency requiring aggressive intervention because it is associated with an increased risk for MI.

Anginal pain often parallels the signs and symptomatology of MI. It is extremely important that the nurse be able to accurately identify the characteristics that differentiate the two conditions, since the pharmacologic interventions related to angina differ considerably from those of MI. Angina, while aggravating and uncomfortable, rarely leads to a fatal outcome and the chest pain is usually immediately relieved by nitroglycerin. MI, however, carries with it a high mortality rate if appropriate treatment is delayed (Section 37.9). In the event of MI, pharmacologic intervention must be immediately initiated and systematically maintained. When a patient presents with chest pain, the foremost objective for the health care provider is to quickly determine the cause of the pain so that proper, effective interventions can be delivered.

PharmFACT

Over 6 million Americans experience angina each year. The risk of angina increases with age, and is more common in women. Over 1 million new and recurrent cases of an acute coronary event occur annually, and more than 40% are fatal. *Source:* Alaeddini & Sharini, 2007.

Nonpharmacologic Therapy of Coronary Artery Disease

37.4 Therapeutic lifestyle changes can decrease the frequency of angina episodes and reduce the risk of coronary artery disease.

A combination of variables influences the development and progression of angina, including dietary patterns and lifestyle choices. The nurse is instrumental in teaching patients the means of preventing CAD, as well as how to lower the rate of recurrence of anginal episodes. Such support includes the formulation of a comprehensive plan of care that incorporates psychosocial support and an individualized teaching plan. The patient needs to understand the causes of angina, identify the conditions and situations that trigger it, and develop the motivation to modify behaviors associated with their disease.

Listing therapeutic lifestyle changes that modify the development and progression of cardiovascular disease (CVD) may seem repetitious, as these same factors have been included in chapters on hypertension (HTN) and heart disease. However, the importance of prevention and management of CVD through nonpharmacologic means cannot be overemphasized. Making healthy lifestyle choices can prevent CAD in many individuals, and slow the progression of the disease in those who have existing plaque. The following interventions have been shown to reduce the incidence of CAD:

- Limit alcohol consumption to small or moderate amounts.
- Eliminate foods high in cholesterol or saturated fats.
- Keep blood cholesterol and other lipid indicators within the normal ranges.
- Keep blood pressure within the normal range.
- Keep blood glucose levels within the normal range.
- Exercise regularly and maintain optimum weight.
- Do not use tobacco.

When the patient is unable or unwilling to adopt healthy lifestyle choices, preventive drug therapy may be used to lower CAD risk factors. For example, antihypertensives are often used to control blood pressure, statins to lower blood lipids, and insulin or oral hypoglycemics to keep blood glucose within the normal range. The nurse should teach patients that therapeutic lifestyle changes should be incorporated into their daily routine, even if medications are needed to control major risk factors.

Pharmacologic Management of Angina Pectoris

37.5 The pharmacologic management of angina includes beta-adrenergic blockers, organic nitrates, and calcium channel blockers.

There are several desired therapeutic outcomes for a patient receiving pharmacotherapy for angina. A primary goal is to reduce the frequency and intensity of angina episodes. Additionally, successful pharmacotherapy should improve exercise tolerance

CONNECTIONS

Complementary and Alternative Therapies Ginseng

Description: Ginseng is one of the oldest known herbal remedies, with at least six species being reported to have medicinal properties. *Panax ginseng* is distributed throughout China, Korea, and Siberia, whereas *Panax quinquefolius* is native to Canada and the United States. Because the plant's popularity has led to its extinction from certain regions, much of the available ginseng is now grown commercially.

History and Claims: Ginseng has been used for centuries to promote general wellness, boost immune function, and reduce fatigue. There are some claims that the herb lowers blood glucose and can help in the management of HTN.

Standardization: Standardization of ginseng focuses on a group of chemicals called ginsenosides, although there are many other chemicals in the root, which is the harvested portion of the plant. Dosages range from 100 to 600 mg/day. This value is sometimes reported as a percentage, with 5% being the standard amount of ginsenosides.

Evidence: Ginseng has received much research attention. Although some evidence shows that it may increase general wellness, studies have not been conclusive. There are differences in chemical composition among the various species of ginseng; American ginseng is not considered equivalent to Siberian ginseng. Ginseng is reported to be a calcium channel antagonist and has been shown to increase phagocytosis. By increasing the conversion of L-arginine to nitric oxide, ginseng improves blood flow to the heart in times of low oxygen supply, such as with myocardial ischemia. The nurse should caution clients who take ginseng, because herb–drug interactions are possible with warfarin and loop diuretics.

Source: From *Herbs at a Glance: Asian Ginseng*, National Center for Complementary and Alternative Medicine, National Institutes of Health, 2008. Retrieved July 13, 2008, from http://nccam.nih.gov/health/asianginseng/; "Ginseng Root," In: *Herbal Medicine: Expanded Commission E Monographs* (pp. 170–177), by M. Blumenthal, A. Goldberg, J. Brinckman, Eds., 2000, Newton, MA: Lippincott Williams & Wilkins; "Panax Ginseng," by D. Kiefer, & T. Pantuso, 2003, *American Family Physician*, *68*(8), pp. 1539–1544.

PHARMACOTHERAPY *ILLUSTRATED* 37.1

Mechanisms of Action of Drugs Used to Treat Angina

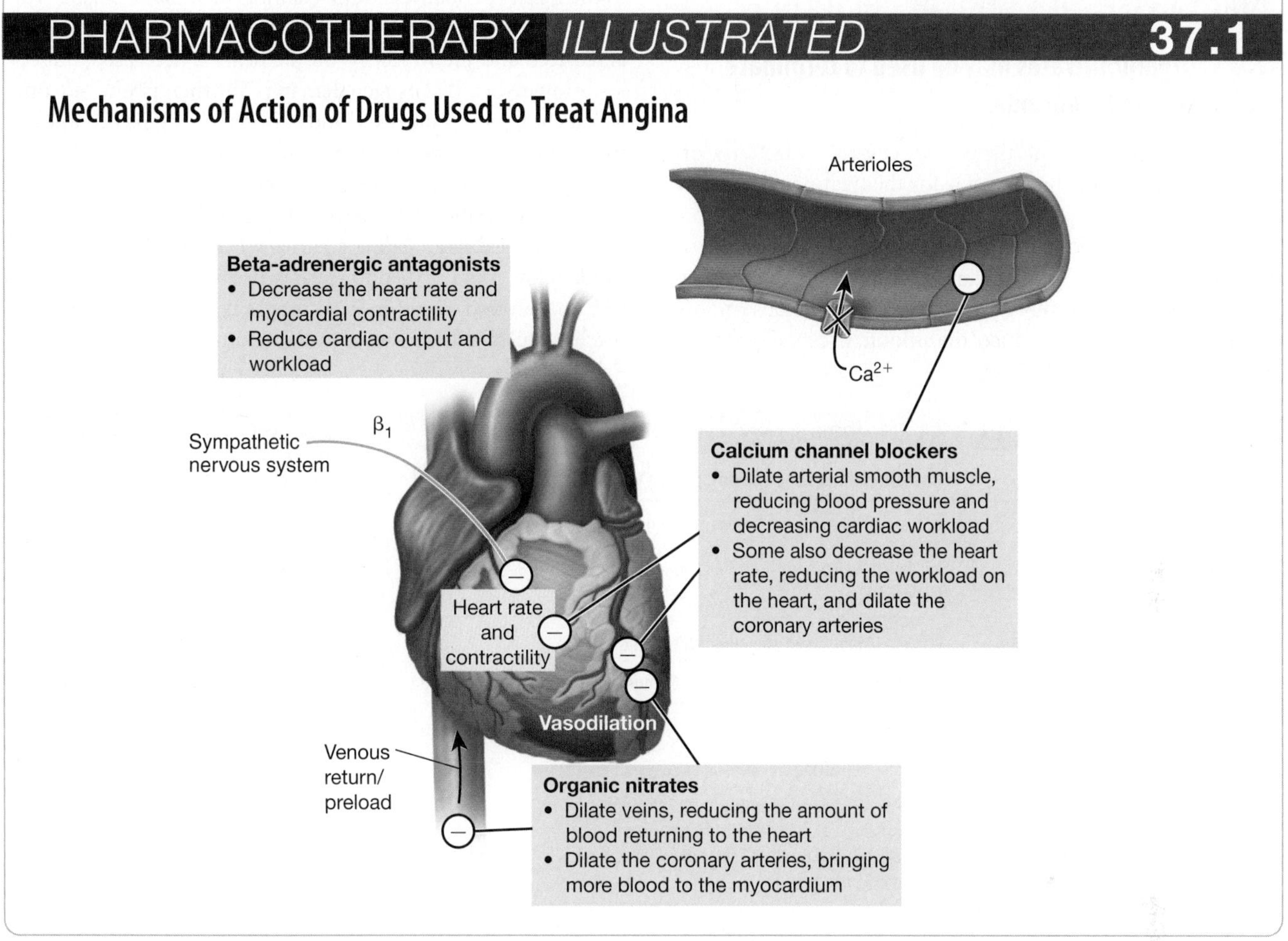

and allow the patient to more actively participate in activities of daily living. Long-term goals include extending the patient's lifespan by preventing serious consequences of ischemic heart disease such as dysrhythmias, heart failure, and MI. Pharmacotherapy alone, however, cannot usually achieve these outcomes; the patient must be willing to implement therapeutic lifestyle changes that promote a healthy heart.

Medications for angina are sometimes placed into two categories: those that terminate an acute angina episode in progress, and those that decrease the frequency of angina episodes. The primary means by which antianginal medications act is by reducing the myocardial demand for oxygen. This may be accomplished by the following mechanisms:

- Slowing the heart rate
- Dilating veins so that the heart receives less blood (reduced preload)
- Causing the heart to contract with less force (reduced contractility)
- Lowering blood pressure (reduced afterload)

The pharmacotherapy of angina uses three primary classes of drugs: organic nitrates, beta-adrenergic blockers, and calcium channel blockers (CCBs). Rapid-acting organic nitrates are drugs of choice for terminating an acute angina episode. Beta-adrenergic blockers are drugs of choice for prophylactic treatment. CCBs are used when beta blockers are not tolerated well by a patient. Long-acting nitrates, given by the oral (PO) or transdermal routes, are alternatives for prophylaxis. Persistent angina requires drugs from two or more classes, such as a beta blocker combined with a long-acting nitrate or a CCB. Pharmacotherapy Illustrated 37.1 illustrates the mechanisms of action of medications used to prevent and treat CAD.

Approved in 2006, ranolazine (Ranexa) is the first in a new class of drugs called **partial fatty-acid oxidation inhibitors.** Although its exact mechanism is not known, ranolazine is believed to act by shifting the metabolism of cardiac muscle cells so that they utilize glucose as the primary energy source rather than fatty acids. This decreases the metabolic rate and oxygen demands of myocardial cells. Thus, this is the only antianginal that acts through its metabolic effects, rather than hemodynamic effects. Effects on heart rate and blood pressure are minimal. The drug is only approved for chronic angina that has not responded to other agents.

CONNECTION *Checkpoint* 37.2

Many patients take HMG-CoA reductase inhibitors (statins) concurrently with antianginal medications. From what you learned in Chapter 32, what is the rationale for prescribing drugs from this class for a patient with CAD? See Answer to Connection Checkpoint 37.2 in Appendix A.

Drug Classes for Angina Pectoris

37.6 Organic nitrates may be used to terminate or prevent angina episodes.

After their medicinal properties were discovered in 1857, the organic nitrates became the mainstay for the treatment of angina for the next 100 years. Their mechanism of action results from the formation of **nitric oxide** in vascular smooth muscle. Nitric oxide is an important cell-signaling molecule and a potent vasodilator, causing relaxation of both arterial and venous smooth muscle. Dilation of veins reduces the amount of blood returning to the heart (preload), and the chambers contain a smaller volume. With less blood for the ventricles to pump, cardiac output is reduced and the workload on the heart is decreased, thereby lowering myocardial oxygen demand. The therapeutic outcome is that chest pain is alleviated and episodes of angina become less frequent. The organic nitrates are listed in Table 37.1.

Organic nitrates also have the ability to dilate coronary arteries, which was once thought to be their primary mechanism of action. It seems logical that dilating a partially occluded coronary vessel would allow more oxygen to reach ischemic tissue. While this effect does indeed occur, it is no longer considered the primary mechanism of nitrate action in the treatment of stable angina.

TABLE 37.1 Selected Drugs for Angina and Myocardial Infarction

Drug	Route and Adult Dose (maximum dose where indicated)	Adverse Effects
Organic Nitrates		
amyl nitrite	Inhalation: 1 ampule (0.18–0.3 mL) prn. May repeat dose in 3–5 min, if needed.	*Headache, orthostatic hypotension, flushing of the face, dizziness, rash (transdermal patch), tolerance* Anaphylaxis, circulatory collapse due to hypotension, syncope due to orthostatic hypotension
isosorbide dinitrate (Dilatate, Isordil)	PO: 2.5–30 mg 4 times daily (max: 480 mg/day) Sustained release: 40 mg daily (max: 160 mg/day)	
isosorbide mononitrate (Imdur, Ismo, Monoket)	PO: 20 mg qid Ismo, Monoket 20 mg bid (max: 40 mg/day) Imdur: 30–60 mg each morning (max: 240 mg/day)	
nitroglycerin (Nitrostat, Nitro-Dur, Nitro-Bid, others)	SL: 1 tablet (0.3–0.6 mg) or 1 spray (0.4–0.8 mg) every 3–5 min (max: 3 doses in 15 min)	
Beta-Adrenergic Antagonists		
atenolol (Tenormin)	PO: 25–50 mg daily (max: 100 mg/day)	*Fatigue, insomnia, drowsiness, impotence or decreased libido, bradycardia, and confusion* Agranulocytosis, laryngospasm, Stevens–Johnson syndrome, anaphylaxis; if the drug is abruptly withdrawn, palpitations, rebound HTN, life-threatening dysrhythmias or myocardial ischemia may occur
metoprolol (Lopressor, Toprol XL)	PO: 100 mg bid (max: 400 mg/day)	
propranolol (Inderal, Inderal LA)	PO: 10–20 mg bid tid (max: 320 mg/day)	
timolol maleate (Betimol, Timoptic, Timoptic XE)	PO: 15–45 mg tid (max: 60 mg/day)	
Calcium Channel Blockers		
amlodipine (Norvasc)	PO: 5–10 mg daily (max: 10 mg/day)	*Flushed skin, headache, dizziness, peripheral edema, light-headedness, nausea, diarrhea* Hepatotoxicity, MI, CHF, confusion, mood changes
bepridil (Vascor)	PO: 200 mg daily (max: 400 mg/day)	
diltiazem (Cardizem, Cartia XT Dilacor XR, Taztia XT, Tiazac)	PO regular release: 30 mg tid qid (max: 480 mg/day) Extended release: 20–240 mg bid (max: 540 mg/day)	
nicardipine (Cardene)	PO: 20–40 mg tid or 30–60 mg sustained release bid (max: 120 mg/day)	
nifedipine (Adalat, Procardia, others)	PO: 10–20 mg tid (max: 180 mg/day) Extended release: 30–90 mg once daily	
verapamil (Calan, Covera-HS, Isoptin SR, Verelan)	PO: 80 mg 3–4 times daily (max: 480 mg/day)	
Other Agents		
ranolazine (Ranexa)	PO: 500 mg bid (max: 2,000 mg/day)	*Dizziness, constipation, headache, nausea, and vomiting* QT interval prolongation

Note: *Italics* indicate common adverse effects. Underline indicates serious adverse effects.

Coronary artery vasodilation, however, is crucial in treating vasospastic angina, in which the chest pain is caused by coronary artery spasm. The organic nitrates relax these spasms, allowing more oxygen to reach the myocardium, thereby terminating the pain.

Organic nitrates are classified by their onset and duration of action. The short-acting nitrates, such as nitroglycerin, may be taken sublingually or as an oral spray or buccal tablet to quickly terminate an acute anginal episode. Long-acting nitrates, such as isosorbide dinitrate (Isordil), are taken orally or are absorbed slowly through a transdermal patch to decrease the frequency and severity of angina episodes. Long-acting organic nitrates are occasionally used to treat symptoms of heart failure; their role in the treatment of that disease is presented in Chapter 38.

Tolerance is a common and potentially serious problem with the long-acting organic nitrates. The magnitude of the tolerance depends upon the dosage and the frequency of drug administration. Although tolerance develops rapidly, as quickly as 24 hours after the initiation of therapy in some patients, it also disappears rapidly when the drug is withheld. Patients are often instructed to remove the transdermal patch for 6 to 12 hours each day or withhold a night-time dose of the oral medications in order to delay the development of tolerance. Because the oxygen demands of the heart during sleep are diminished, the patient with stable angina experiences few angina episodes during this drug-free interval.

Most adverse effects of the organic nitrates are extensions of their hypotensive action. Flushing of the face and headache are common effects, secondary to vasodilation. Orthostatic hypotension is a frequent adverse effect of this drug class, and patients should be advised to change positions gradually to prevent light-headedness. Blood pressure should be carefully monitored, and the nurse should hold nitrates and remove topical forms if serious hypotension is discovered. Taking organic nitrates concurrently with alcohol may cause severe hypotension and even cardiovascular collapse.

An additional adverse effect that can be limiting in some patients is reflex tachycardia. When the organic nitrates dilate vessels and blood pressure falls, the baroreceptor reflex is triggered. Sympathetic stimulation of the heart increases heart rate and contractility, which are undesirable effects in a patient with angina. This adverse effect is often transient and asymptomatic. Patients who report significant palpitations may be administered a beta blocker, which will prevent the reflex cardiac stimulation.

PROTOTYPE DRUG Nitroglycerin (Nitrostat, Nitro-Bid, Nitro-Dur, others)

Classification: **Therapeutic:** Antianginal drug
Pharmacologic: Organic nitrate, vasodilator

Therapeutic Effects and Uses: Nitroglycerin, the oldest and most widely used organic nitrate, can be delivered by a number of different routes: sublingual, lingual spray, PO, intravenous (IV), transmucosal, transdermal, topical, and extended release forms. The rapid-acting forms may be taken while an acute angina episode is in progress or just prior to physical activity. When given sublingually, it reaches peak plasma levels within minutes, thus quickly terminating angina pain. Chest pain that does not respond within 10 to 15 minutes after two or three doses of sublingual nitroglycerin may indicate MI, and emergency medical services (EMS) should be contacted. The transdermal and oral sustained release forms are for prophylaxis only, since they have a relatively slow onset of action. The long-acting forms should be discontinued gradually because vasospasm may result if they are abruptly withheld.

There are indications for nitroglycerin other than angina. When administered by the IV route, the drug is approved for controlled hypotension induction during anesthesia, and the treatment of acute congestive heart failure (CHF), acute pulmonary edema, acute MI, severe HTN, or hypertensive emergency. Off-label indications include use as a uterine relaxant to aid in the extraction of a retained placenta and for pain associated with anal fissures or hemorrhoids.

Mechanism of Action: Upon reaching vascular smooth muscle, nitroglycerin forms nitric oxide, which triggers a cascade resulting in the release of calcium ions in smooth muscle. Nitroglycerin relaxes both arterial and venous smooth muscle. The venous dilation decreases the amount of blood returning to the heart, reducing preload. With less blood for the ventricles to pump, myocardial oxygen demand is decreased. In addition, direct vasodilation of coronary arteries enhances the blood supply to the myocardium, and is partially responsible for its therapeutic effects.

Pharmacokinetics:

Route(s)	PO: sublingual tablets, sublingual spray, buccal tablets; transdermal patch, topical ointment
Absorption	Rapid
Distribution	Widely distributed; 60% bound to plasma protein
Primary metabolism	Hepatic; extensive first-pass metabolism
Primary excretion	Renal
Onset of action	Sublingual: 1–3 minutes; buccal: 2–5 minutes; transdermal patch: 40–60 minutes
Duration of action	Sublingual: 30–60 minutes; buccal: 2 h; transdermal patch: 18–24 h

Adverse Effects: Most patients experience flushing of the face and a throbbing, transient headache, which result from the drug's vasodilation action. Orthostatic hypotension and syncope may occur. Stinging and rash may occur with ointments and transdermal patches. Methemoglobinemia is a rare adverse effect that can cause shock and coma. Anaphylaxis leading to circulatory collapse due to severe hypotension is rare. Tolerance develops with continuous therapy or large doses of the drug.

Contraindications/Precautions: Nitrates are contraindicated in patients with preexisting hypotension, shock, head injury with increased intracranial pressure, or head trauma because additive vasodilation would worsen these conditions. Drugs in this class are contraindicated in pericardial tamponade and constrictive pericarditis because the heart is unable to increase cardiac output to maintain blood pressure when the drug causes vasodilation. Sustained release forms of the medicine should not be given to patients with glaucoma because the drug may increase intraocular pressure. Nitroglycerin should be used cautiously in patients with severe liver or renal disease, as the drug could build to toxic levels. Dehydration or hypovolemia should be corrected before nitroglycerin is administered; otherwise serious hypotension may result.

Drug Interactions: Concurrent use with sildenafil (Viagra) or other phosphodiesterase-5 inhibitors may cause life-threatening hypotension and cardiovascular collapse. Nitrates should not be taken within 24 hours before or after taking these drugs. Concurrent use with ethanol, CCBs, antidepressants, phenothiazines, or antihypertensive drugs may cause additive hypotension. Sympathomimetics such as epinephrine will antagonize the vasodilation effects of nitroglycerin. **Herbal/Food**: Use with hawthorn may result in additive hypotension.

Pregnancy: Category C.

Treatment of Overdose: During overdose, hypotension may be reversed with the IV administration of normal saline. If methemoglobinemia is suspected, methylene blue may be administered.

Nursing Responsibilities:

- Assess blood pressure and heart rate prior to administration. Hold medication if systolic blood pressure is less than 100 mmHg.
- Assess the location, duration, intensity of chest pain, and precipitating factors. Solicit patient's response to rate pain on a scale of zero (no pain) to 10 (worst possible pain).
- Evaluate the effectiveness of nitrate therapy by recording the frequency and duration of angina pain.
- Monitor for adverse effects related to nitrate therapy such as flushing of the face, throbbing, headache, orthostatic hypotension, and syncope.
- Nitroglycerin comes in varied formulations appropriate for angina prophylaxis such as ointment, transdermal unit, translingual spray, transmucosal tablet, and oral sustained release forms. Each form of the drug has specific nursing responsibilities, which are listed in Table 37.2.

Patient and Family Education:

- At the earliest sign of oncoming angina pain, sit or lie down and take the drug. Stop any activity that may have caused the onset of chest pain.
- When pain is totally relieved, spit out the remainder of the sublingual tablet, especially if experiencing headaches or unpleasant adverse effects. After taking the tablet, relax for 15 to 20 minutes to minimize dizziness or faintness.
- Pain unrelieved by 3 sublingual tablets over a 15-minute period (1 tablet every 5 minutes) may indicate a heart attack. Call the emergency response system within the community (911). If no 911 system is available, go directly to the closest emergency department.
- Take medication 5 to 10 minutes prior to exercise or other activity known to trigger angina attacks. The drug effects last 30 to 60 minutes.
- Tablets can cause a sweet-tasting, tingling feeling under the tongue, which is normal.
- Immediately report blurred vision, dry mouth, chest pain, or fainting to the health care provider because these symptoms may warrant discontinuing the drug.
- Remove nitro patches at bedtime and wash the area with soap and water to remove excess medication; replace in the morning.
- Report headaches to the health care provider and ask if acetaminophen is appropriate. Avoid use of aspirin or any other medication without approval of the health care provider.
- Keep a record of the number of angina attacks, amount of medication required for relief of each attack, and possible contributing factors to share with the health care provider. Report any increase in the frequency, duration, or severity of angina attacks.
- Sublingual tablets may be used to prevent or terminate angina attacks while the transdermal patch or ointment is in place.
- Make position changes slowly when moving from a lying to a standing position to prevent dizziness and possible fainting.
- Avoid alcohol use after taking a nitroglycerin tablet, because it can cause a sharp drop in blood pressure resulting in dizziness, fainting, flushing, or pallor.
- Keep medication out of the reach of children. Follow expiration dates on the container, and discard all nitroglycerine tablets that are more than 12 months old.
- If taking nitrates daily, do not abruptly stop taking the drug.
- Wear a medic-alert bracelet or identification.
- Do not breast-feed while taking this drug without approval of the health care provider.

Drugs Similar to Nitroglycerin (Nitrostat, Nitro-Bid, Nitro-Dur, Others)

Other organic nitrates include amyl nitrate, isosorbide dinitrate, and isosorbide mononitrate.

Amyl nitrate: Approved in 1938, amyl nitrate is a highly volatile liquid supplied in ampules to be given by the inhalation route. When the ampule is crushed, the drug acts within minutes to dilate coronary vessels. Although it is rarely used for angina, amyl nitrate is used for cyanide poisoning, and occasionally to relieve pain due to urinary or biliary colic. Amyl nitrate is abused as an inhalant because it is thought to produce a "rush" or "orgasmic" sensation. Those abusing the drug may experience dizziness and loss of consciousness. This drug is pregnancy category X.

Isosorbide dinitrate (Iso-Bid, Isordil, Dilatrate-SR, Sorbitrate): Approved in 1961, isosorbide dinitrate is an organic nitrate used to terminate anginal attacks (sublingual) and for the prophylaxis of angina (sustained release tablets). It is occasionally used to treat CHF. The dosing schedule must allow for a drug-free period of at least 14 hours to prevent tolerance to the drug's effects. The drug should not be used to terminate angina attacks in progress because it takes 20 to 90 minutes to reach therapeutic drug levels. Adverse effects are similar to those of nitroglycerin. A fixed dose

TABLE 37.2 Administration of Organic Nitrates

Route	Administration
Sublingual Tablet	• Give 1 tablet. If pain is unrelieved, may give additional tablets at 5-minute intervals up to 3 tablets in a 15-minute period. • Moisture on sublingual tissue is necessary for the sublingual tablet to dissolve. A patient may be unresponsive to sublingual nitroglycerin, as the anxiety caused by chest pain typically leads to dry mouth.
Sustained-Release Buccal Tablet	• Place 1 tablet between lip and gum above incisors or between cheek and gum. Allow to slowly dissolve over 3–5 hours. • Avoid touching tongue to tablet or drinking hot fluids, as these can increase dissolving of the tablet, decrease duration of the medicinal effect, and lead to the onset of angina pain. • Avoid chewing, crushing, or swallowing the tablet.
Sustained-Release Tablet or Capsule	• Give on an empty stomach with a full glass of water 1 hour before, or 2 hours after, meals. The tablet should be swallowed whole. • Note that the sustained-release form helps to prevent angina attacks but is not intended for immediate relief of angina. • Avoid chewing or crushing the tablet.
Translingual Spray	• Avoid shaking medicine canister. Spray on or under the tongue. Never inhale spray. • Repeat spray every 5 minutes if needed for a maximum of 3 metered doses. • Teach the patient to avoid swallowing for at least 10 seconds.
Transdermal Ointment	• Avoid touching ointment with fingers. Squeeze the prescribed dosage onto the dose-determining applicator (paper application patch) in the medication package. Spread ointment in a thin, even layer to pre-marked 5.5 by 9 cm (2 1/4 by 3 1/2 in.) square. Place patch with ointment side down onto nonhairy skin surface such as the forearm, chest, abdomen, or anterior thigh. Cover with transparent wrap and secure with tape. • Rotate application sites to prevent skin inflammation and sensitization. Remove any residual ointment before reapplication. • Keep medication container closed and stored in a cool place. • Contact with water, such as in swimming or bathing, does not affect the transdermal patch.
Transdermal Unit	• Apply transdermal patch at the same time each day to nonhairy or closely trimmed area without excessive movement. • Avoid application on irritated or scarred skin. • Rotate application site each application to prevent skin irritation and sensitization.
Intravenous (IV)	• Verify with health care provider the correct IV concentration and rate of infusion. • Remove any existing transdermal or ointment in place before starting IV infusion to prevent overdosage. • Note that IV nitroglycerin can cause hypotension, so give with extreme caution to patients with preexisting hypotension or hypovolemia. • Monitor patient closely for any change in levels of consciousness and for dysrhythmias, because IV nitroglycerin contains a substantial amount of ethanol as a diluent. Ethanol intoxication with symptoms of nausea, vomiting, coma, lethargy, and alcohol breath can occur with high doses of IV nitroglycerin. Stop infusion if intoxication occurs. The patient should recover immediately when drug administration is discontinued.

combination of isosorbide dinitrate with hydralazine (BiDil) was approved in 2005 to reduce morbidity and mortality associated with heart failure. This drug is pregnancy category C.

Isosorbide mononitrate (Imdur, Ismo, Monoket): Approved in 1991, isosorbide mononitrate is an active, long-acting metabolite of isosorbide dinitrate. The mononitrate is only used for prophylaxis: Its 1-hour onset of action makes it unacceptable for termination of acute anginal pain. The dosing schedule must allow for a drug-free period of at least 7 hours to prevent the development of tolerance to the drug's effects. It is available in tablet form only. Imdur is an extended release form of the drug that permits once daily dosing. Adverse effects are the same as the other organic nitrates. This drug is pregnancy category C.

37.7 Beta-adrenergic antagonists are often drugs of choice for stable angina.

Beta-adrenergic antagonists or blockers decrease cardiac workload by lowering blood pressure, slowing heart rate, and reducing contractility. These actions on the heart are particularly beneficial during exercise. Beta blockers are as effective as the organic nitrates in decreasing the frequency and severity of anginal episodes caused by exertion. For the pharmacotherapy of CAD, cardioselective $beta_1$ antagonists are preferred over nonselective beta antagonists because they are less likely to cause bronchoconstriction (a $beta_2$ response). Beta-adrenergic antagonists are not effective for treating vasospastic angina and may, in fact, worsen this condition.

Beta-adrenergic blockers offer several advantages over the organic nitrates. Tolerance does not develop to the antianginal effects of the beta blockers during prolonged therapy. They possess antidysrhythmic properties, which help prevent cardiac conduction abnormalities that are common complications of patients with ischemic heart disease. Beta blockers are ideal for patients who have both HTN and CAD due to their antihypertensive action. They have also been shown to reduce the incidence of MI. Because of these cardioprotective actions, beta blockers are considered drugs of choice for the prophylaxis of

NURSING PROCESS APPLICATION

Patients Receiving Nitroglycerin

Assessment	Potential Nursing Diagnoses
Prior to administration: • Obtain a complete health history including allergies, drug history, and possible drug interactions. • Assess vital signs, ECG, frequency and severity of angina, and alcohol use. • Obtain a history of cardiac disorders and blood testing including cardiac enzymes, complete blood count (CBC), blood urea nitrogen (BUN), creatinine, and liver function tests. • Assess if patient has taken sildenafil (Viagra) within last 24 hours.	• *Ineffective Tissue Perfusion* (*Cardiopulmonary*), related to hypotension from drug therapy • *Risk for Injury,* related to dizziness or fainting due to hypotension from drug therapy • *Acute Pain,* related to adverse effects of drug • *Deficient Knowledge (Drug Therapy)*

Planning: Patient Goals and Expected Outcomes

The patient will

- Experience relief or prevention of chest pain.
- Report immediately any chest pain unrelieved by nitroglycerin.
- Demonstrate an understanding of the drug's action by accurately describing drug adverse effects and precautions.

Implementation

Interventions and (Rationales)	Patient and Family Education
• Ask the patient to describe and rate the pain of the anginal episode prior to drug administration and document the response. (Establishment of baseline assessment will aid in determining the effectiveness of the medication.) • Obtain a 12-lead ECG to differentiate between angina and infarction. (Pharmacotherapy depends upon which disorder is presenting.)	Instruct the patient to: • Take one tablet every 5 minutes until pain is relieved, or for up to three doses during an acute angina attack. • Call EMS if chest pain is not relieved after three doses. • Place the sublingual tablet under the tongue or spray under the tongue; do not inhale the spray.
• Monitor blood pressure and pulse. Do not administer drug if patient is hypotensive or if systolic blood pressure is less than 100 mmHg. (Drug will further reduce blood pressure.)	• Instruct the patient to sit or lie down before taking medication and to avoid abrupt changes in position.
• Monitor alcohol use. (Extremely low blood pressure may result, which could cause death.)	• Emphasize the importance of avoiding alcohol while taking nitroglycerin.
• Monitor for headache in response to use of nitrates. (Vasodilation of cranial blood vessels related to drug activity may result in headache.)	Instruct the patient that: • Headache is a common adverse effect, that usually decreases over time. • Over-the-counter medications usually relieve the headache.
• Monitor for use of sildenafil (Viagra) concurrently with nitrates, because cardiovascular disease is a major cause of erectile dysfunction in men. (Life-threatening hypotension may result with concurrent use of sildenafil.)	Instruct the patient to: • Not take Viagra within 24 hours after taking nitrates. • Wait at least 24 hours after taking Viagra to resume nitrate therapy.
• Monitor need for prophylactic nitrates. (Determine what activities precipitate onset of angina.)	• Advise the patient to take medication prior to a stressful event or physical activity to prevent angina.

Evaluation of Outcome Criteria

Evaluate the effectiveness of drug therapy by confirming that patient goals and expected outcomes have been met (see "Planning").

chronic angina. The beta blockers used for angina are listed in Table 37.1. Beta blockers are widely used in medicine, and additional details may be found in chapters on adrenergic antagonists (see Chapter 20), HTN (see Chapter 36), heart failure (see Chapter 38), and dysrhythmias (see Chapter 39). A Nursing Process Application for patients receiving beta blockers is included in Chapter 20.

Beta-adrenergic antagonists are well tolerated by most patients. In some patients, fatigue, lethargy, and depression are reasons for discontinuation of beta-blocker therapy. At high doses, drugs in this class can cause shortness of breath and respiratory distress due to bronchoconstriction, and they should be used cautiously in patients with asthma or chronic obstructive pulmonary disease (COPD). Because beta blockers slow the heart rate and myocardial conduction velocity, they are contraindicated in patients with bradycardia and greater than first-degree heart block. Heart rate should be closely monitored so that it does not fall below 50 to 60 beats/minute at rest or 100 beats/minute during exercise. Beta blockers are also contraindicated in cardiogenic shock and overt cardiac failure.

Diabetic patients should be aware that the actions of beta blockers can obscure the initial symptoms of hypoglycemia (palpitations, diaphoresis, and nervousness). Because of this, blood glucose levels should be monitored more frequently, and insulin doses may need to be adjusted accordingly.

Beta-adrenergic antagonists should never be abruptly discontinued. With long-term beta blocker use, the heart becomes more sensitive to catecholamines, which are blocked by these medications. When withdrawn abruptly, adrenergic receptors are activated and rebound excitation occurs. In patients with CAD, this can exacerbate angina, precipitate tachycardia, or cause an MI.

PROTOTYPE DRUG Atenolol (Tenormin)

Classification: **Therapeutic:** Antianginal agent
Pharmacologic: Beta-adrenergic antagonist

Therapeutic Effects and Uses: Atenolol is one of the most frequently prescribed drugs in the United States, due to its relative safety and effectiveness in treating a number of chronic disorders, including heart failure, HTN, stable angina, and MI. Approved in 1981, it is given by the PO route and has a long duration of action that allows for once daily dosing. An IV form of the drug is no longer available in the United States. Off-label indications for atenolol include ethanol withdrawal, migraine prophylaxis, and unstable angina.

Mechanism of Action: Atenolol selectively blocks beta$_1$-adrenergic receptors in the heart. Its effectiveness in angina is attributed to its ability to slow the heart rate and reduce contractility, both of which lower myocardial oxygen demand.

Pharmacokinetics:

Route(s)	PO, IV
Absorption	50% absorbed from the gastrointestinal (GI) tract
Distribution	Distributed to most tissues including the placenta; secreted in breast milk; does not readily cross the blood–brain barrier; 5–15% bound to protein
Primary metabolism	Not metabolized
Primary excretion	Renal (50%), feces (50%)
Onset of action	PO: 1 h
Duration of action	Half-life: 6–7 h

Adverse Effects: Oral atenolol is well tolerated by most patients. Beta-blocking effects can result in bradycardia and hypotension. Fatigue, weakness, and dizziness are other potential adverse effects. Nausea and vomiting occur in some patients.

Contraindications/Precautions: Because atenolol slows heart rate, it should not be used by patients with severe bradycardia, advanced atrioventricular (AV) heart block, cardiogenic shock, or decompensated heart failure. Due to its vasodilation effects, it is contraindicated in patients with severe hypotension. Patients with severe renal impairment should receive reduced doses to prevent drug accumulation. Because atenolol reduces cardiac output, patients with stroke or low cerebrovascular blood flow should not receive this drug. Patients with major depression should not receive beta blockers because these drugs can worsen this condition.

Drug Interactions: Anticholinergics may decrease the absorption of atenolol from the GI tract. Use with digoxin or other antidysrhythmic agents that depress myocardial conduction may cause AV heart block. Concurrent use of atenolol with other antihypertensives may result in additive hypotension. Although CCBs are often used concurrently with beta blockers for their additive therapeutic actions, patients must be monitored carefully due to the possibility of excessive cardiac suppression. **Herbal/Food:** Use with hawthorn may result in additive hypotension.

Pregnancy: Category D.

Treatment of Overdose: The most serious symptoms of atenolol overdose are hypotension and bradycardia. Atropine or isoproterenol may be used to reverse bradycardia. Atenolol can be removed from the systemic circulation by hemodialysis.

Nursing Responsibilities:

- Assess blood pressure and heart rate before administration and monitor closely, particularly when administered with a CCB or similar agents.
- Monitor apical pulse, blood pressure, respirations, and peripheral circulation throughout dosage adjustment period. Consult the prescriber for acceptable parameters.
- Assess pulmonary status and breathing pattern for bronchospasm or bronchoconstriction.
- Hold dose and contact the prescriber when the patient's systolic blood pressure is less than 100 mmHg or the apical pulse is less than 60 beats/minute.
- Monitor diabetic patients for hypoglycemia when the drug is given concurrently with insulin or sulfonylureas.
- Monitor hypertensive patients with CHF for symptoms of impending heart failure such as dyspnea on exertion, night cough, edema, orthopnea, and distended neck veins.
- Discontinue the drug if patient develops symptoms of mental depression, such as disinterest in food, personal hygiene, people, or surroundings, as well as withdrawal, insomnia, apathy, sadness, or difficulty concentrating.
- This drug masks hyperthyroidism in patients with thyrotoxicosis. Abrupt withdrawal could precipitate thyroid storm.
- Discontinue beta blockers slowly over a period of 1–2 weeks. Sudden withdrawal can result in anginal attacks and heart attacks in patients diagnosed with angina pectoris, or thyroid storm in patients with hyperthyroidism.

Patient and Family Education:

- Do not drive or perform other hazardous activities until the effects of the drug are known because this drug may cause drowsiness or dizziness.
- Make position changes slowly when moving from a lying to a standing position because this drug may cause dizziness and possible fainting.
- If diabetic, remember that this drug suppresses signs of hypoglycemia such as increased pulse rate and changes in blood pressure. Monitor blood glucose frequently and report other possible signs of hypoglycemia such as sweating, fatigue, hunger, or lack of concentration.
- Do not breast-feed while taking this drug without approval of the health care provider.

Drugs Similar to Atenolol (Tenormin)

Atenolol, metoprolol, propranolol, and timolol are equally effective in treating chronic angina. Information on these beta-adrenergic antagonists is presented in other chapters. The student should review the general information on beta blockers in Chapter 19. Several are featured as prototype drugs: metoprolol (Lopressor, Toprol XL) and propranolol (Inderal) in Chapter 20, and timolol (Betimol, Blocadren, Timoptic, Timoptic XE) is featured as an antiglaucoma medication in Chapter 77.

37.8 Calcium channel blockers are effective at reducing myocardial oxygen demand and treating stable and vasospastic angina.

Blockade of calcium channels has a number of effects on the heart, most of which are similar to those of beta blockers. Although the first approved indication for CCBs was for the treatment of angina, these medications are also used for HTN (see Chapter 36) and dysrhythmias (see Chapter 39). The mechanisms of calcium channel blockade by drugs in this class are presented in detail in Chapter 33. The actions of CCBs relevant to ischemic heart disease are discussed in this section. The CCBs used for angina are listed in Table 37.2.

CCBs have several actions on the cardiovascular system that benefit the patient with angina. Most importantly, CCBs relax arteriolar smooth muscle, thus reducing blood pressure. This reduction in afterload decreases myocardial oxygen demand. Some of the CCBs also slow cardiac conduction velocity through the AV node, thereby decreasing heart rate and contributing to the reduced cardiac workload. An additional effect of the CCBs is their ability to dilate the coronary arteries, bringing more oxygen to the myocardium. This vasodilation is especially important in patients with vasospastic angina. CCBs are considered drugs of choice for that condition. For stable, exertional angina, they may be used as monotherapy in patients unable to tolerate beta blockers. In patients with persistent symptoms, CCBs may be administered concurrently with organic nitrates or beta blockers.

MyNursingKit | Sexual Relations After Heart Attacks

Adverse effects of CCBs are generally not serious and are related to vasodilation: headache, dizziness, and edema of the ankles and feet. CCBs should be used with caution in patients taking other cardiovascular medications that slow conduction through the AV node, particularly digoxin or beta-adrenergic blockers. The combined effects of these drugs may cause partial or complete AV heart block, heart failure, or dysrhythmias. Some CCBs worsen heart failure by reducing myocardial contractility.

CONNECTION *Checkpoint* 37.3

For patients with asthma, calcium channel blockers are generally the preferred antianginal agents, rather than beta-adrenergic antagonists. From what you learned in Chapter 20, why would calcium channel blockers be preferred for patients with this comorbid condition?

See Answer to Connection Checkpoint 37.3 in Appendix A.

Pathophysiology of Myocardial Infarction

37.9 The early diagnosis and pharmacotherapy of myocardial infarction increases chances of survival.

Myocardial infarctions (MIs) are responsible for a substantial number of deaths each year. Many patients die before reaching a medical facility for treatment, or within 48 hours following the initial MI, due to complications of the disorder. Clearly, MI is a serious and frightening disease and one responsible for a large percentage of sudden deaths.

The primary cause of MI is advanced CAD: atherosclerotic plaque accumulation in the endothelial wall of one or more branches of the coronary arteries. Pieces of unstable plaque in a coronary artery can ulcerate or rupture and lodge in a small vessel serving a portion of the myocardium. Exposed plaque activates the clotting cascade, resulting in platelet aggregation. A new clot quickly builds on the existing plaque, making obstruction of the vessel imminent. A detailed discussion of coagulation and clot formation is included in Chapter 40.

Deprived of adequate oxygen supply, the obstructed region of the myocardium becomes ischemic. The myocytes shift to anaerobic metabolism after only 8 to 10 seconds of oxygen loss. Anaerobic metabolism, however, is inefficient and cannot produce enough ATP to keep the heart beating efficiently for prolonged periods. Lactic acid accumulates, causing acidosis, which affects contractility and suppresses normal conduction across the myocardium. As contractility diminishes, the patient may experience heart failure. Myoctes will begin to die in about 20 minutes unless the blood supply is quickly restored. The necrosis of myocardial tissue, which may be irreversible, releases certain "marker" enzymes, such as creatine phosphokinase (CK) or cardiac-specific troponin (cTn), which can be measured in the blood to confirm the patient has experienced an MI.

Extreme chest pain is often the first symptom of MI, and the one that drives most patients to seek medical attention. An electrocardiogram (ECG) can give important clues as to the extent and location of the MI because the infarcted region of the myocardium is nonconducting, producing abnormalities of Q waves, T waves, and ST segments. Patients showing elevation of the ST segment on the ECG are at highest risk for death and require immediate treatment. Laboratory test results are used to aid in diagnosis and monitor progress after an MI. Table 37.3 describes some of these important laboratory values.

Early diagnosis and prompt pharmacotherapy of MI can significantly reduce the mortality and long-term disability associated with MI. The pharmacologic goals for treating a patient with an acute MI are as follows:

- If cardiac arrest has occurred, restart the heart and restore normal blood pressure with vasopressors.
- Restore blood supply (reperfusion) to the damaged myocardium as quickly as possible through the use of thrombolytics.
- Reduce myocardial oxygen demand with organic nitrates, beta blockers, or CCBs to lower the risk of additional infarctions.

TABLE 37.3 Changes in Blood Test Values with Acute Myocardial Infarction

Blood Test	Initial Elevation After MI	Peak Elevation After MI	Duration of Elevation	Normal Range
Cholesterol			4 or more weeks, during stress response	
CK = creatine kinase	3–8 hours	12–24 hours	2–4 days	Males: 12–80 units/L Females: 10–70 units/L
ESR	1st week		several weeks	Males: 1–13 mm/hr Females: 1–20 mm/hr
Glucose			duration of stress response	Fasting: 80–120 mg/dL
LDH = lactate dehydrogenase	8–72 hours	3–6 days	8–14 days	50–150 units/L
Myoglobin	1–3 hours	4–6 hours	1–2 days	0–85 mg/mL
Troponin I	2–4 hours	24–36 hours	7–10 days	<3.1 mcg/L
Troponin T	2–4 hours	24–36 hours	10–14 days	<0.2 mcg/L
WBC	few hours		3–7 days	4800–10,800 mcg/L

- Control or prevent MI-associated dysrhythmias with amiodarone (Cordarone), beta blockers, or other antidysrhythmics.
- Reduce post-MI mortality with aspirin, beta blockers, and ACE inhibitors.
- Manage severe MI pain and associated anxiety with narcotic analgesics.

Pharmacologic Management of Myocardial Infarction

37.10 Thrombolytic agents can restore perfusion to ischemic regions of the myocardium if administered soon after a myocardial infarction.

Thrombolytic therapy is administered to dissolve clots obstructing the coronary arteries in order to restore circulation to the ischemic region of the myocardium. Clinical research has confirmed that quick restoration of coronary circulation reduces mortality following an acute MI. After the clot is successfully dissolved, anticoagulant or antiplatelet therapy is initiated to prevent additional clot formation. Dosages and descriptions of the various thrombolytics are listed in Chapter 40. A Nursing Process Application for thrombolytics is also included in Chapter 40, where alteplase (Activase) is presented as a drug prototype for this class.

Thrombolytics are most effective when administered from 20 minutes to 12 hours after the onset of MI symptoms. Ideally, the time from presentation in the emergency department to administration of the thrombolytic agent should be 30 minutes or less. Research has demonstrated little or no therapeutic benefit if the drugs are administered 24 hours or more after the MI onset. In addition, research suggests that patients over age 75 do not experience reduced mortality from these drugs. Because thrombolytic therapy is expensive and has the potential to produce serious adverse effects, it is important to identify circumstances that contribute to successful therapy. The development of clinical practice guidelines for thrombolytic therapy remains an area of active research. Pharmacotherapy Illustrated 37.2 illustrates this reperfusion process.

Thrombolytics exhibit a narrow margin of safety between dissolving clots and producing serious adverse effects. Although therapy is usually targeted to a single thrombus in a specific artery, once infused in the blood the drugs travel to all vessels and may cause adverse effects anywhere in the body. The primary risk of thrombolytics is excessive bleeding from interference with the clotting process. Vital signs must be monitored continuously and signs of bleeding call for discontinuation of therapy. Because these medications have a brief half-life and are rapidly destroyed in the blood, stopping the infusion normally results in the rapid termination of adverse effects. Physical and laboratory assessment for the possibility of abnormal bleeding should continue for 2 to 4 days after therapy is discontinued.

Thrombolytic therapy is contraindicated for many conditions, including recent trauma or surgery, internal bleeding (other than menses), active peptic ulcer, postpartum (within 10 days), history of intracranial hemorrhage, suspected ischemic stroke within the past 3 months, bleeding disorders, severe liver disease, or thrombocytopenia. Caution should be used when administering thrombolytics to patients taking anticoagulants or antiplatelet drugs.

37.11 Drugs are used to treat the symptoms and complications of acute myocardial infarction.

The most immediate needs of the patient with MI are to ensure that the heart continues functioning, and that permanent damage from the infarction is minimized. In addition to restoring perfusion to the myocardium with thrombolytic

CONNECTIONS

To the Community Sexual Activity: Just Another Form of Exercise

Sexual activity is a normal desire for all humans. When someone has a heart attack, he or she may think that sex will stress the heart and be dangerous. Often, the fear of another heart attack or death will cause significant decline in sexual activity and even erectile dysfunction in men.

Actually, this fear is unfounded. After a reasonable recovery time, sex can be considered just another form of exercise. Nurses can reassure their patients that sex after a heart attack is normal, even healthy. This may be a difficult topic for some patients to discuss, and the nurse may avoid embarrassing the patient by including this topic in general education topics such as medications, exercise, diet, and other lifestyle changes. Nurses can assure the patient that studies show that only about 1% of heart attacks are related to sexual activity.

Sex can be viewed as a form of exercise, such as a 20-minute brisk walk, or climbing stairs. Tests will be done prior to hospital discharge to determine the extent of heart damage and a progressive exercise program can be initiated. This planned program is as important as weight loss, a low-salt diet, or smoking cessation. Within about 4–6 weeks after the heart attack, patients can be encouraged to resume exercise, including sexual activity, when no adverse symptoms such as chest pain or breathlessness occur on exertion. If these symptoms do occur, the patient should check with the health care provider. If a patient is anxious about having sex, medication may be prescribed. If symptoms continue, report these to the health care provider.

Medical school researchers at Deaconess Hospital report that there is little danger with sexual activity after a heart attack (Muller, 2000). Healthy people have a risk factor of 2 in 1 million, while a person with coronary disease has a risk factor of 20 in 1 million, or 1 in 50,000. The lowest risk is for those who exercise regularly. A previous research study described a risk for heart attack in a healthy 50-year-old man to be 1 in 1 million.

therapy, drugs from several other classes are administered soon after the onset of symptoms, to prevent reinfarction and to ultimately reduce mortality from the episode.

Aspirin

Unless contraindicated, 160 to 325 mg of aspirin is given as soon as an MI is suspected. Research has determined that aspirin use in the weeks following an acute MI dramatically reduces mortality. These effects from aspirin are believed to be due to several mechanisms. Clearly, aspirin has antiplatelet action that reduces platelet aggregation and thus the formation or enlargement of thrombi. Additionally, its anti-inflammatory properties decrease the formation of C-reactive protein, which is associated with an increased risk of MI.

The major concern over aspirin use is its tendency to promote GI bleeding in some patients. This could be a serious adverse effect, given that some post-MI patients receive anticoagulants. However the benefits of taking aspirin following an acute MI generally outweigh the risks for most patients. Aspirin maintenance therapy can cut the risk of death due to a subsequent MI by as much as 50% in some populations. Furthermore, the low doses used in maintenance therapy (75 to 150 mg/day) rarely cause GI bleeding. Additional discussion of aspirin may be found in Chapter 29, where it is featured as a prototype drug, and in Chapter 44.

ADP Receptor Blockers

Clopidogrel (Plavix) and ticlopidine (Ticlid) are effective antiplatelet agents that are approved for the prevention of thrombotic stroke and MI. Research has demonstrated that these agents reduce mortality associated with thromboembolic events. Because they are more expensive than aspirin, they are usually considered for antiplatelet therapy for patients allergic to aspirin or who are at high risk for GI bleeding from aspirin. Some protocols call for combination therapy with clopidogrel and aspirin. Additional details on the ADP receptor blockers are presented in Chapter 40. Clopidogrel is the more frequently used of the two drugs in the class, and is featured as a prototype in Chapter 40.

Glycoprotein IIb/IIIa Inhibitors

Glycoprotein IIb/IIIa is a receptor found on the surface of platelets. Drugs that occupy the glycoprotein IIb/IIIa receptor inhibit thrombus formation by a mechanism of action distinct from that of aspirin. The glycoprotein IIb/IIIa inhibitors used for myocardial ischemia are listed in Table 37.1.

Glycoprotein IIb/IIIa inhibitors are sometimes indicated for unstable angina or MI, or for those undergoing percutaneous coronary intervention (PCI) procedures such as angioplasty. The most common drug in this class, abciximab (ReoPro), is infused at the time of PCI, and continued for 12 hours after the procedure is completed to prevent reinfarction.

As with other drugs having an anticoagulant effect, glycoprotein IIb/IIIa inhibitors are contraindicated in the presence of active bleeding, recent surgery, or trauma. They may be used in combination therapy with aspirin and heparin, thus increasing the need for careful monitoring for bleeding. Additional details on glycoprotein IIb/IIIa inhibitors and a prototype feature for abciximab are found in Chapter 40.

Anticoagulants

Upon diagnosis of MI in the emergency department, patients may be placed on the anticoagulant heparin to prevent additional thrombi from forming. Unfractionated heparin therapy is sometimes continued for 48 hours, or until PCI is completed, at which time they are switched to warfarin (Coumadin) or clopidogrel (Plavix). An alternative is to administer a low molecular weight heparin, such as enoxaparin (Lovenox). A comparison of these different anticoagulants is presented in Chapter 40, along with prototype drug features for heparin, warfarin, and enoxaparin.

Some patients may remain on anticoagulant therapy on a chronic basis after hospital discharge. These include patients at

PHARMACOTHERAPY ILLUSTRATED 37.2

Thrombolytic Pharmacotherapy

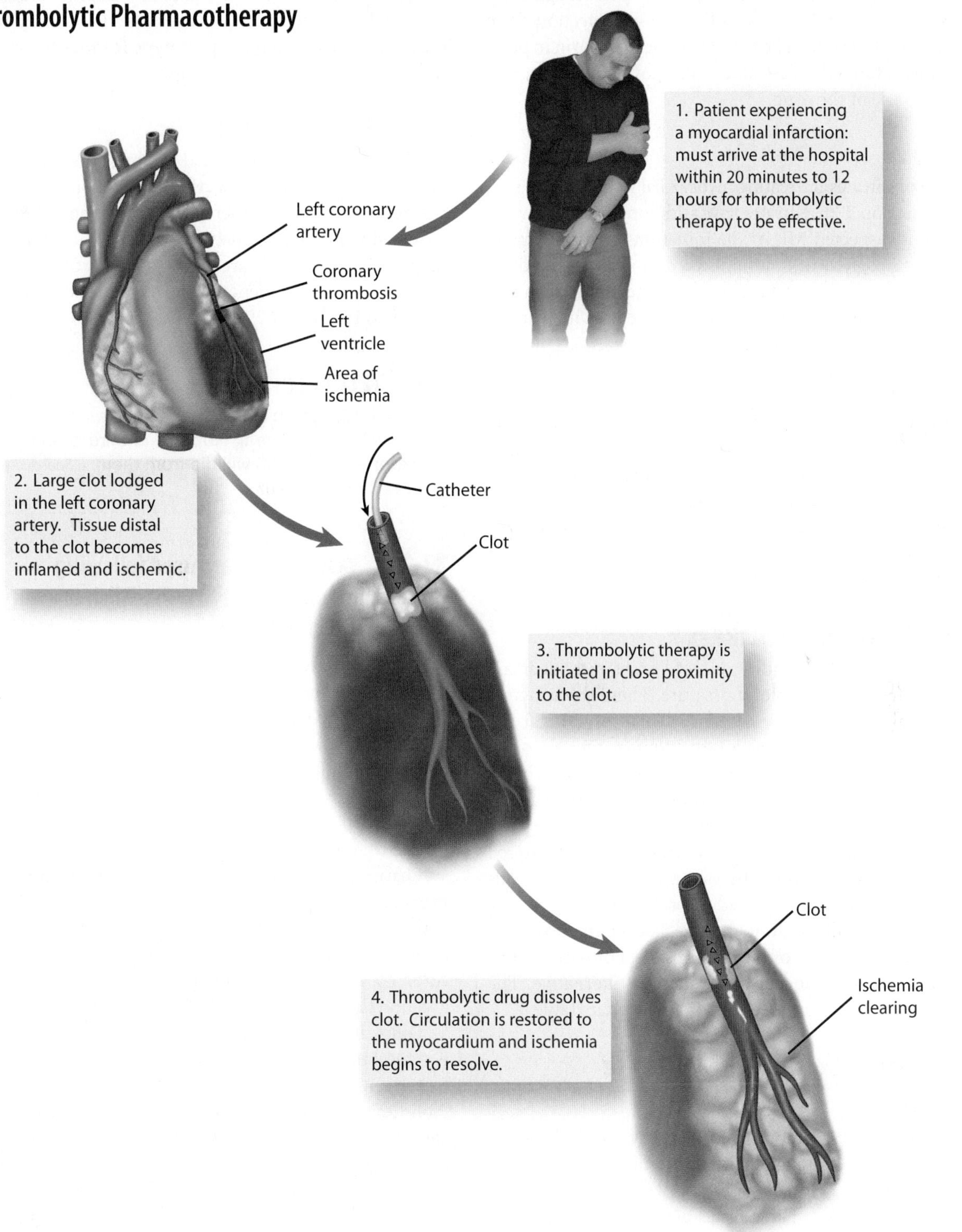

1. Patient experiencing a myocardial infarction: must arrive at the hospital within 20 minutes to 12 hours for thrombolytic therapy to be effective.

Left coronary artery

Coronary thrombosis

Left ventricle

Area of ischemia

2. Large clot lodged in the left coronary artery. Tissue distal to the clot becomes inflamed and ischemic.

Catheter

Clot

3. Thrombolytic therapy is initiated in close proximity to the clot.

Clot

Ischemia clearing

4. Thrombolytic drug dissolves clot. Circulation is restored to the myocardium and ischemia begins to resolve.

high risk to thromboembolic disease and those with chronic atrial fibrillation. Research has not shown that the use of warfarin lowers mortality in post-MI patients; however, it does increase the risk of bleeding. For most patients, anticoagulation with aspirin or clopidogrel is sufficient for protection from thromboembolic events. The long-term use of heparin in post-MI patients is limited unless other conditions are present that warrant the use of the drug.

Nitrates

The value of nitrates in treating myocardial ischemia was presented in Section 37.6. Nitrates have additional uses in the patient with a suspected MI. At the initial onset of chest pain, sublingual nitroglycerin is administered to assist in the diagnosis, and three doses may be taken 5 minutes apart. Pain that persists 5 to 10 minutes after the initial dose may indicate an MI, and the patient should seek medical assistance. Thus, nitrates serve a diagnostic role for MI patients.

Patients with persistent pain, heart failure, or severe HTN may receive IV nitroglycerin for 24 hours following the onset of pain. The arterial and venous dilation produced by the drug reduces myocardial oxygen demand. Organic nitrates also relieve coronary artery vasospasm, which may be present during the acute stage of MI. Upon discharge from the hospital, organic nitrates are discontinued, unless the patient needs them for relief of stable anginal pain.

Beta-Adrenergic Blockers

Beta blockers have the ability to slow heart rate, decrease contractility, and reduce blood pressure. These three factors reduce myocardial oxygen demand, which is critical for patients experiencing a recent MI. In addition, they slow impulse conduction through the heart, suppressing dysrhythmias, which are serious and sometimes fatal complications following an MI. Research has clearly demonstrated that beta blockers can reduce MI-associated mortality if administered within 8 hours of MI onset. These drugs may be initially administered IV, and then switched to oral dosing for chronic therapy. Unless contraindicated, beta-blocker therapy continues for the remainder of the patient's life. For patients unable to tolerate beta blockers, CCBs are an alternative. The beta blockers most often used for MI are listed in Table 37.1.

Angiotensin-Converting Enzyme Inhibitors

Clinical research has demonstrated increased survival for patients administered the angiotensin-converting enzyme (ACE) inhibitors captopril (Capoten) or lisinopril (Prinivil, Zestoretic) following an acute MI. These drugs are most effective when therapy is started within 24 hours after the onset of symptoms. Oral doses are normally begun after thrombolytic therapy is completed and the patient's condition has stabilized. IV therapy may be used during the early stages of MI pharmacotherapy.

The benefit of ACE inhibitors is believed to be due to their ability to prevent cardiac remodeling, and their ability to suppress dysrhythmias. Unless otherwise contraindicated, post-MI patients should receive an ACE inhibitor indefinitely to prevent heart failure and future ischemic development. The mechanisms of action and prototype features for several ACE inhibitors may be found in Chapter 34.

Pain Management

The pain associated with an MI can be debilitating and stressful, creating an increased workload for the myocardium. Pain control is essential in order to ensure patient comfort and to reduce stress. Narcotic analgesics such as morphine sulfate or meperidine (Demerol) are given to ease extreme pain and to sedate the anxious patient. Pharmacology of the analgesics was presented in Chapter 29.

PharmFACT

About 1.2 million Americans experience a new or recurrent MI each year. About one third of the patients experiencing an MI will die from them. *Source:* American Heart Association, 2007.

37.12 Vasopressors are used following cardiopulmonary arrest to reestablish coronary and cerebral blood flow.

Cardiopulmonary arrest is a complete stoppage of heart and lungs activity, usually resulting from a dysrhythmia such as ventricular fibrillation or pulseless ventricular tachycardia. Most patients who experience cardiopulmonary arrest have underlying CAD.

Cardiopulmonary resuscitation (CPR) must be initiated as quickly as possible to restore ventilation and blood circulation to avoid hypoxic injury to the tissues. Electrical defibrillation is used to restore normal cardiac rhythm.

Pharmacotherapy is an important component of CPR. The primary drugs used in the initial phase of resuscitation are sympathomimetics, and epinephrine is the drug of choice. Sympathomimetics cause vasoconstriction, immediately raising cerebral, coronary, and systemic blood pressure. Vasopressin, also called antidiuretic hormone, is an alternative therapy.

Following restoration of cardiac function and ventilation, it is critical that the heart maintain normal conduction in order to prevent the recurrence of ventricular fibrillation or the establishment of other serious dysrhythmias. Historically, lidocaine has been the agent of choice for ventricular dysrhythmias associated with MI. Clinical research, however, has shown that the administration of amiodarone (Cordarone) results in improved patient survival. If the risk of dysrhythmia is high, a loading dose of amiodarone is given by infusion, and the patient is switched to oral forms after a therapeutic plasma level of the drug has been achieved. Amiodarone is featured as an antidysrhythmic drug prototype in Chapter 39.

UNDERSTANDING THE CHAPTER

Key Concepts Summary

37.1 Myocardial ischemia develops when there is inadequate blood supply to meet the metabolic demands of cardiac muscle.

37.2 Coronary artery disease is the major cause of myocardial ischemia.

37.3 Angina pectoris is characterized by severe chest pain brought on by physical exertion or emotional stress.

37.4 Therapeutic lifestyle changes can decrease the frequency of angina episodes and reduce the risk of coronary artery disease.

37.5 The pharmacologic management of angina includes beta-adrenergic blockers, organic nitrates, and calcium channel blockers.

37.6 Organic nitrates may be used to terminate or prevent angina episodes.

37.7 Beta-adrenergic antagonists are often drugs of choice for stable angina.

37.8 Calcium channel blockers are effective at reducing myocardial oxygen demand and treating stable and vasospastic angina.

37.9 The early diagnosis and pharmacotherapy of myocardial infarction increases chances of survival.

37.10 Thrombolytic agents can restore perfusion to ischemic regions of the myocardium if administered soon after a myocardial infarction.

37.11 Drugs are used to treat the symptoms and complications of acute myocardial infarction.

37.12 Vasopressors are used following cardiopulmonary arrest to reestablish coronary and cerebral blood flow.

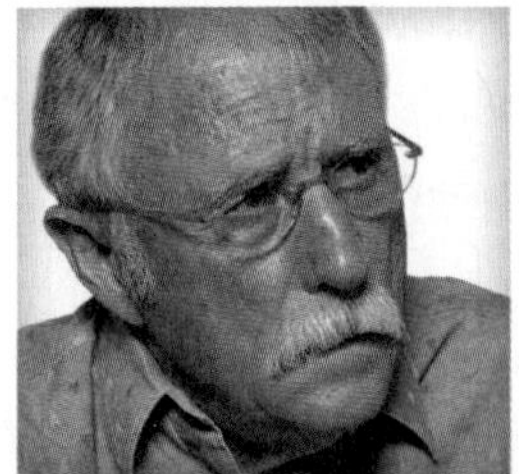

Making the PATIENT *Connection*

Remember the patient "Michael Graff" at the beginning of the chapter? Now read the remainder of the case study. Based on the information presented within this chapter, respond to the critical thinking questions that follow.

Early one morning, 60-year-old Michael Graff began to feel severe anterior "crushing" chest pain that lasted for 35 minutes. He experienced dizziness, cold sweats, and nausea. Although he considered driving to the local emergency department, his family insisted on calling an ambulance for emergency transport to the hospital.

Michael, a general contractor, is a 2-pack-per-day smoker and consumes alcohol (beer) two to three times per week. He has a family history of coronary artery disease, diabetes mellitus, and hyperlipidemia. It has been at least 10 years since his last physical examination.

Upon arrival at the emergency department, he presents with symptoms of anxiety, moderate chest pain, and cold extremities. Auscultation of the thorax revealed tachycardia and clear lung fields. Blood pressure was slightly above normal at 156/90 mmHg. He had no neck venous distention. His white blood cell count was 7,600/mm^3, hematocrit 43.8%, platelets 256,000/mm^3, creatine phosphokinase (CPK) 87 international units/L, and troponin-I <0.4 ng/mL. An ECG showed ST-segment elevation.

Once stabilized, Michael is transported to the coronary care unit with the admission diagnosis of unstable angina and to rule out MI. In the coronary care unit, he receives IV nitroglycerin 50 mg in D_5W 25 mL. The nurse begins the infusion at 10 mcg/minute and titrates the rate based upon his complaint of chest pain every 5 to 10 minutes (5 to 10 mcg/minute).

Critical Thinking Questions

1. Michael and his family ask you to explain what is occurring with his heart. How would you describe the pathophysiology of Michael's condition to them?
2. Discuss the reason Michael is receiving nitroglycerin.
3. What adverse effects should the nurse monitor with patients receiving IV nitroglycerin?
4. How do nitroglycerin infusions differ from other IV infusions?

Case Study

Bill Shackley, a 52-year-old man, is prescribed a nitroglycerin transdermal patch every 6 hours. While discussing his medications, Bill shares several of his concerns. How would you respond to the following questions?

1. "I heard that I can become 'tolerant' to this drug. What does this mean? How can it be avoided?"
2. "Sometimes, after applying the nitroglycerin patch, I get a throbbing headache. Is there anything I can do about this?"
3. "I was told to report episodes of dizziness when I stand up plus rapid heart rates. How does nitroglycerin cause these two adverse effects?"

NCLEX-RN® Review

1 Nitroglycerin topical ointment is being initiated for a client with angina. Which of the following health teachings would be most appropriate?

1. Keep the medication in the refrigerator.
2. Only take this medication when chest pain is severe.
3. Remove the old paste before applying the next dose.
4. Apply the ointment on the chest wall only.

2 A client with chest pain is receiving sublingual nitroglycerin. The nurse would include in the care plan to monitor the client for which of the following adverse effects?

1. Photosensitivity
2. Elevated blood pressure
3. Vomiting and diarrhea
4. Decreased blood pressure

3 The client states, "I always put my nitroglycerin patch in the same place so I do not forget to take it off." The nurse's response would be based on which of the following physiologic concepts?

1. Clients are more likely to remember to apply the patch if the same site is used daily.
2. Repeated use of the same application site will enhance medication absorption.
3. Rebound phenomenon is likely to occur when the same site is used more than once.
4. Skin irritation due to the nitroglycerin ointment can occur if the same site is used repeatedly.

4 The nurse is caring for a client with chronic angina pectoris. The client is receiving nitroglycerin. Which of the following client manifestations would the nurse conclude is a common adverse effect of this medication?

1. Flushing and headache
2. Tremors and anxiety
3. Syncope and dizziness
4. Sleepiness and lethargy

5 The client asks how atenolol (Tenormin) helps angina. The response provided by the nurse is based on which of the following concepts? This medication:

1. Slows the heart rate and reduces contractility.
2. Increases the heart rate and diminishes contractility.
3. Blocks sodium channels and elevates depolarization.
4. Decreases blood pressure and blocks the alpha$_2$ receptors.

6 Which of the following assessment findings, if discovered in a client receiving atenolol (Tenormin), would be cause for the nurse to withhold the medication? (Select all that apply.)

1. Bradycardia: heart rate of 40 beats/minute
2. Tachycardia: heart rate of 126 beats/minute
3. Hypotension: blood pressure 76/46 mmHg
4. Tinnitus with hearing loss
5. Hypertension: blood pressure 156/92 mmHg

See Answers to Critical Thinking Questions, Case Study, and NCLEX-RN® Review in Appendix A.

References

Alaeddini, J., & Sharini, J. (2007). *Angina pectoris.* Emedicine from WebMD. Retrieved July 13, 2008, from http://www.emedicine.com/med/topic133.htm

American Heart Association, American Stroke Association. (2007). *Learn and live, know the facts, get the stats 2007: Heart attack/Sudden cardiac death.* Retrieved July 13, 2008, from http://www.americanheart.org/downloadable/heart/1168615457098551041%20KnowTheFactsStats07_loRes.pdf

Aronow, W. S., Frishman, W. H., & Cheng-Lai, A. (2007). Cardiovascular drug therapy in the elderly. *Cardiology in Review, 15*(4), 195–215.

Blumenthal, M., Goldberg, A., Brinckman, J. (Eds.). (2000). *Herbal medicine: Expanded Commission E monographs* (pp. 170–177). Newton, MA: Lippincott Williams & Wilkins.

Decker, C., Garavalia, L., Chen, C., Buchanan, D. M., Nugent, K., Shipman, A., et al. (2007). Acute myocardial infarction: Patients' information needs over the course of treatment and recovery. *Journal of Cardiovascular Nursing, 22*(6), 459–465.

Gehi, A. K., Ali, S., Na, B., & Whooley, M. A. (2007). Self-reported medication adherence and cardiovascular events in patients with stable coronary heart disease: The heart and soul study. *Archives of Internal Medicine, 167*(16), 1798–1803.

Harvey, S. (2004). The nursing assessment and management of patients with angina. *British Journal of Nursing, 13*(10), 598–601.

Jackevicius, C. A., Li, P., & Tu, J. V. (2008). Prevalence, predictors, and outcomes of primary nonadherence after acute myocardial infarction. *Circulation, 117*(2), 1028–1036.

Kiefer, D., & Pantuso, T. (2003). Panax ginseng. *American Family Physician, 68*(8), 1539–1544.

Manfredini, R., Salmi, R., & Manfredini, F. (2008). Survival patterns with in-hospital cardiac arrest. *Journal of the American Medical Association, 299*(22), 2625–2626.

Michel, T. (2006). Treatment of myocardial ischemia. In L.L. Brunton, J. S. Lazo, & K. L. Parker (Eds.), *The pharmacological basis of therapeutics* (11th ed.) (pp. 823–844). New York: McGraw-Hill.

Muller, J. E. (2000). Triggering of cardiac events by sexual activity: Findings from a case-crossover analysis. *American Journal of Cardiology, 86*(2A), 14F–18F.

Mulvihill, M., Zelman, P., Holdaway, E., Tompary, E., & Raymond, J. (2006). *Human diseases: A systematic approach* (6th ed.) (p. 115). Upper Saddle River, NJ: Pearson Education.

National Center for Complementary and Alternative Medicine. (2008). *Herbs at a glance: Asian ginseng.* Retrieved July 13, 2008, from http://nccam.nih.gov/health/asianginseng/

Quinn, T. (2004). Managing acute myocardial infarction. *Emerging Nurse, 12*(3), 17–19.

Rasmussen, J. N., Chong, A., & Alter, D. A. (2007). Relationship between adherence to evidence-based pharmacotherapy and long-term mortality after acute myocardial infarction. *Journal of the American Medical Association, 297*(2), 177–186.

Vega, C. (2004). *Angina guidelines recommend treatment and follow-up.* Medscape Medical News. Retrieved June 13, 2008, from http://www.medscape.com/viewarticle/491419

CHAPTER

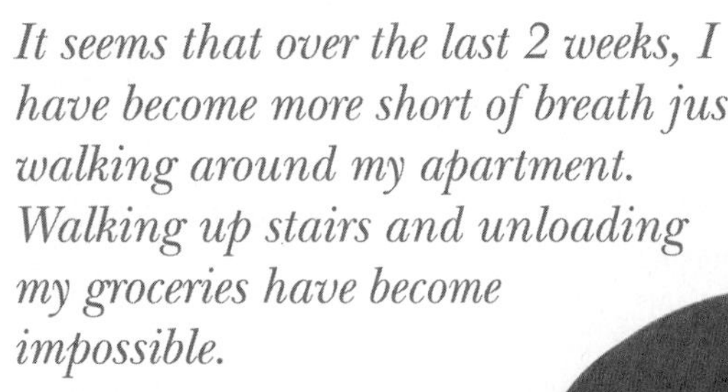

38 Pharmacotherapy of Heart Failure

Learning Outcomes

After reading this chapter, the student should be able to:

1. Identify the major diseases associated with heart failure.
2. Relate how the symptoms associated with heart failure may be caused by weakened heart muscle and diminished cardiac output.
3. Identify compensatory mechanisms used by the body to maintain cardiac output in patients with heart failure.
4. Describe how heart failure is classified.
5. Describe the nurse's role in the pharmacologic management of heart failure.
6. For each of the classes shown in the chapter outline, identify the prototype and representative drugs and explain the mechanism(s) of drug action, primary indications, contraindications, significant drug interactions, pregnancy category, and important adverse effects.
7. Use the nursing process to care for patients receiving drug therapy for heart failure.

Chapter Outline

Etiology of Heart Failure

Pathophysiology of Heart Failure

Pharmacologic Management of Heart Failure

Drugs for Heart Failure

Angiotensin-Converting Enzyme Inhibitors and Angiotensin Receptor Blockers

Diuretics

Beta-Adrenergic Antagonists

Vasodilators

Cardiac Glycosides

PROTOTYPE **Digoxin (Lanoxin, Lanoxicaps)** *p. 615*

Phosphodiesterase III Inhibitors and Other Inotropic Agents

Beta-Adrenergic Agonists

PROTOTYPE **Milrinone Lactate (Primacor)** *p. 618*

Key Terms

cardiac remodeling, 608
digitalization, 614
diuretic resistance, 613
heart failure (HF), 607
natriuretic peptides, 609
phosphodiesterase III, 618
reverse remodeling, 614

Heart failure is one of the most common and fatal of the cardiovascular diseases, and its incidence is increasing as the population ages. Although improved treatment of myocardial infarction and hypertension has led to declines in mortality due to heart failure, approximately one in five patients still dies within a year of diagnosis of heart failure, and 50% die within 5 years. Historically, this condition was called congestive heart failure; however, because not all incidences of this disease are associated with congestion, the more appropriate name is heart failure.

PharmFACT

The incidence of heart failure increases with age, and is especially high in African Americans, Hispanics, and Native Americans. The higher prevalence of heart failure in minorities is directly related to the higher incidence of HTN and diabetes in these populations.
Source: Zevitz, 2006.

Etiology of Heart Failure

38.1 Heart failure is closely associated with disorders such as chronic hypertension, coronary artery disease, and diabetes.

Heart failure (HF) is the inability of the heart to pump enough blood to meet the metabolic demands of the body. HF can be caused by any disorder that affects the heart's ability to receive or eject blood. While weakening of cardiac muscle is a natural consequence of aging, the process can be caused or accelerated by the following:

- Coronary artery disease (CAD)
- Mitral stenosis
- Myocardial infarction (MI)
- Chronic hypertension (HTN)
- Diabetes mellitus

The student should detect a common theme throughout the chapters on cardiovascular pharmacology. That theme is the ability to prevent major causes of morbidity and mortality through control of healthy lifestyle choices. Controlling lipid levels and keeping blood pressure within normal limits reduces the incidences of CAD and MI. Maintaining blood glucose within normal values reduces the consequences of uncontrolled diabetes. Thus, for many patients, HF is a preventable condition; controlling associated diseases will greatly reduce the risk of development and progression of HF.

Since there is no cure for HF, the treatment goals are to prevent, treat, or remove the underlying causes whenever possible and treat its symptoms, so that the patient's quality of life can be improved. Advances in understanding the pathophysiology of HF over the past two decades have lead to a change in pharmacotherapeutic goals. No longer is therapy of HF focused on end stages of the disorder. Pharmacotherapy is now targeted at prevention and slowing the progression of HF. This change in emphasis has lead to significant improvements in survival and quality of life in patients with HF.

Pathophysiology of Heart Failure

38.2 The body attempts to compensate for heart failure by increasing cardiac output.

HF is a general term used to describe several different types of cardiac dysfunction. The dysfunction may occur on the left side, the right side, or on both sides of the heart.

Left HF is called congestive heart failure (CHF) because it is characterized by an accumulation of fluid causing congestion in the pulmonary capillary beds. Although left HF is more common, the right side of the heart can also become weak, either simultaneously with the left side or independently from the left side. In right HF, the blood pools in the veins resulting in peripheral edema and engorgement of organs such as the liver.

Left HF is further subdivided into two types. Systolic HF occurs when cardiac output (CO) is diminished due to decreased contractility of the myocardium. Approximately 60% to 80% of left HF is the systolic type. Diastolic HF occurs when the lungs become congested even though cardiac output is normal. Diastolic HF is caused by a restriction in ventricular filling, resulting in higher-than-normal pressure in the ventricle. Although cardiac output is normal, the increased pressure in the ventricle creates higher pressure in the pulmonary capillaries, resulting in pulmonary edema. A patient may have both systolic and diastolic HF. Pharmacotherapy of the two types differs somewhat. For

CONNECTIONS

To the Community

Lifestyle Modifications to Control Heart Failure

Although heart failure can be acute and require immediate treatment, it is often considered a progressive, chronic disorder. In its early stages, many symptoms can be alleviated through nonpharmacologic intervention. With the following lifestyle changes, the patient can experience a higher quality of life either without drug therapy or with lower drug doses that have less risk for adverse effects:

- Stop using tobacco.
- Limit salt (sodium) intake and eat foods rich in potassium and magnesium.
- Limit alcohol consumption.
- Implement a medically supervised exercise plan.
- Learn and use effective ways to deal with stress.
- Reduce weight to an optimum level.
- Avoid consumption of caffeinated foods and beverages.

example, inotropic drugs that increase contractility are more successful with systolic HF than diastolic HF.

HF may progress slowly over many years, or it may have an acute onset. Once HF reaches the stage where cardiac output is affected, tissues receive inadequate perfusion and organ failure is possible. The body has developed a complex series of actions to compensate for HF. Knowledge of these compensatory mechanisms is important to understanding the pharmacotherapy of HF. Prior to continuing in this chapter, factors affecting cardiac output, stroke volume, afterload, and preload in Chapter 31 should be reviewed. The pathophysiology of HF is illustrated in Figure 38.1.

Ventricular Hypertrophy

In left HF, the left ventricle is forced to work harder due to the increased preload or afterload. Over time, the wall of the left ventricle thickens and enlarges (ventricular hypertrophy) in an attempt to compensate for the increased workload. Changes in the size, shape, and structure of the myocardial cells (myocytes) occur. These compensatory changes in structure benefit the heart by allowing it to better maintain adequate stroke volume and cardiac output. The term **cardiac remodeling** is sometimes used to describe these changes to myocyte structure and function.

The benefits of cardiac remodeling as a compensatory mechanism, however, are limited. Myocytes continuously die, likely due to workload injury, and fibrotic tissue fills the spaces between them. These tissue changes stiffen the myocardium, causing diminished contractility and reduced cardiac output. The heart responds with even more remodeling, continuing the destructive cycle. Without intervention, the abnormal structural changes can result in irreversible cardiac impairment.

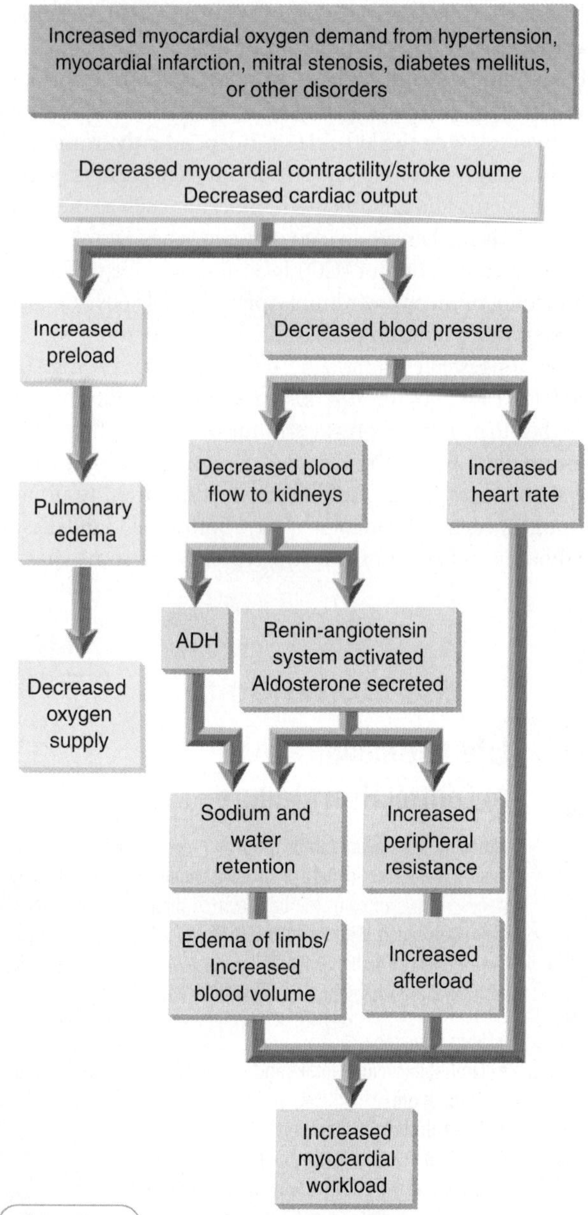

Increased myocardial oxygen demand from hypertension, myocardial infarction, mitral stenosis, diabetes mellitus, or other disorders

Decreased myocardial contractility/stroke volume
Decreased cardiac output

Increased preload

Decreased blood pressure

Pulmonary edema

Decreased blood flow to kidneys

Increased heart rate

ADH

Renin-angiotensin system activated
Aldosterone secreted

Decreased oxygen supply

Sodium and water retention

Increased peripheral resistance

Edema of limbs/ Increased blood volume

Increased afterload

Increased myocardial workload

Figure 38.1

Pathophysiology of heart failure.

Activation of the Sympathetic Nervous System

One of the fastest homeostatic responses to diminished cardiac output is activation of the sympathetic nervous system (SNS). The tachycardia caused by sympathetic activation is a normal compensatory mechanism to increase cardiac output.

The SNS, however, also constricts arteries and activates the renin-angiotensin-aldosterone (RAAS) system. Higher angiotensin II levels raise blood pressure and afterload, causing the heart to work harder. The stressed myocardium, which already has reduced contractility and is having difficulty maintaining cardiac output, is faced with even greater challenges by this additional workload. The diminished cardiac output caused by the high afterload produces an ongoing activation of the SNS. Patients with preexisting CAD may suffer an anginal attack from the increased SNS activity. Again, although there are certain compensatory benefits to activating the SNS to maintain cardiac output, a destructive cycle is created that can lead to or worsen HF.

CONNECTION *Checkpoint* 38.1

Propranolol (Inderal) is an example of a negative inotropic agent. From what you learned in Chapter 20, explain why this type of drug should be administered with caution to a heart failure patient who also has asthma. See Answer to Connection Checkpoint 38.1 in Appendix A.

Increased Plasma Volume and Preload

When cardiac output in a patient with HF is diminished, blood flow to the kidneys is reduced. The kidneys respond to the decreased perfusion by secreting renin and activating the RAAS. As a result of the action of angiotensin II, aldosterone secretion is increased, and the body retains sodium and water. This has the beneficial effect of increasing preload, stretching the myocardial fibers and increasing contractility, thus returning cardiac output to normal levels. This is an important compensatory mechanism in normal hearts.

However, the ability of the heart to increase contractility is limited. In a failing heart, the increased preload leads to volume overload and pulmonary congestion. In addition, the increased plasma volume increases blood pressure, which further adds to afterload and to the burden of an already weak heart.

Recent research has discovered additional detrimental effects related to activation of the RAAS. Angiotensin II has been found to promote ventricular hypertrophy, myocyte death, and fibrosis formation in the myocardium. Aldosterone also has direct effects on the myocardium, promoting fibrosis and stiffening of the ventricular wall. Angiotensin-converting enzymes (ACE) inhibitors have become drugs of choice for HF, in part, because they are able to block these detrimental effects of angiotensin II and aldosterone on cardiac remodeling.

Natriuretic Peptides and Neurohumoral Factors

Natriuretic peptides are substances secreted in response to increased pressure in the heart. Three types have been identified:

1. Atrial natriuretic peptide (ANP) is secreted by the atria.
2. B-type natriuretic peptide (BNP) is secreted by the ventricles.
3. C-type natriuretic peptide (CNP) is secreted by the brain.

The physiologic functions of ANP and BNP are to cause diuresis, vasodilation, and decreased aldosterone secretion, thus balancing the effects of the SNS and RAAS activation. Nesiritide (Natrecor), a drug structurally identical to BNP, has a limited role in the treatment of HF, as discussed in Section 38.11.

Research has identified several other substances as potential mediators in the progression of HF. Two proinflammatory substances, tumor necrosis factor (TNF) and interleukin, are found in high levels in patients with HF, and are associated with a poor prognosis. The hormone endothelin is a vasoconstrictor that also is associated with a poor prognosis in HF patients. Vasopressin (antidiuretic hormone), which is elevated in HF patients, causes fluid retention and worsens this condition. It is likely that research will identify additional mediators of HF, along with potential novel therapies for the disease.

38.3 Symptoms of heart failure occur when compensatory mechanisms fail to maintain adequate cardiac output.

The classic symptoms of HF are dyspnea on exertion, fatigue, pulmonary congestion, and peripheral edema. Lung congestion causes a cough and orthopnea (difficulty breathing when recumbent). If pulmonary edema occurs, the patient feels as if he or she is suffocating and extreme anxiety may result. The condition often worsens at night.

Through pharmacotherapy and lifestyle modifications, many patients with HF can be maintained in a symptom-free, compensated state for years. The most common reason patients experience decompensation is fluid overload due to nonadherence to sodium and water restrictions. The second most common reason is nonadherence to the pharmacotherapeutic regimen. The nurse must stress to patients the importance of sodium restriction and treatment adherence to maintain a properly functioning heart. Cardiac events such as MI or myocardial ischemia can also precipitate acute HF. Certain medications can worsen HF, and the nurse should use these drugs with caution in these patients. A list of selected drugs that may worsen HF is shown in Table 38.1.

MyNursingKit | The Beating Heart

TABLE 38.1 Drugs That May Worsen Heart Failure

Mechanism	Drug/Drug Class
Negative inotropic effect: Slow heart rate or reduce contractility	Antidysrhythmics Calcium channel blockers Itraconazole
Cardiotoxicity: Damage to the myocardium	Cyclophosphamide Daunomycin Doxorubicin
Increase blood volume: Cause sodium and water retention and fluid overload	Androgens Estrogens Glucocorticoids NSAIDs Rosiglitazone and pioglitazone

CONNECTIONS

Treating the Diverse Patient Women and Heart Failure

Although heart failure can occur in both genders, it is a significant factor in disability and death of women. Usually heart failure is the result of long-standing HTN or CAD. Many women with heart failure do not receive optimal treatment. Women may minimize their symptoms of heart failure, so that the health care provider is unaware of just how sick and disabled they are. This leads to inadequate treatment in women with heart failure. In fact, women do not fair as well as men in many aspects of heart disease.

- 38% of women and 25% of men will die within 1 year of a first recognized heart attack.
- 35% of women and 18% of men heart attack survivors will have another heart attack within 6 years.
- 46% of women and 22% of men heart attack survivors will be disabled with heart failure within 6 years.
- Women are almost twice as likely as men to die after bypass surgery.
- Women are less likely than men to receive beta blockers, ACE inhibitors, or even aspirin after a heart attack.
- More women than men die of heart disease each year, yet women receive only:
  - 33% of angioplasties, stents, and bypass surgeries;
  - 28% of implantable defibrillators; and
  - 36% of open-heart surgeries.
- Women comprise only 25% of participants in all heart-related research studies.

Diastolic heart failure is more common in women than in men and accounts for at least half the cases of heart failure in women. Furthermore, women develop acute stress cardiomyopathy more often than men.

Source: From *Women and Heart Disease Fact Sheet*, The National Coalition for Women with Heart Disease, 2008, Retrieved July 14, 2008, from http://www.womenheart.org/information/women_and_heart_disease_fact_sheet.asp

Pharmacologic Management of Heart Failure

38.4 The specific therapy for heart failure depends upon the clinical stage of the disease.

Several models are available to guide the pharmacologic management of HF. The New York Heart Association (NYHA) model has been widely used in clinical practice. This model classifies symptomatic HF into four functional classes:

- I: Patients with cardiac disease but with no symptoms during physical activity
- II: Patients with cardiac disease who have slight limitations on physical activity, with symptoms such as fatigue, palpitations, dyspnea, or angina
- III: Patients with cardiac disease who have marked limitations during physical activity
- IV: Patients with cardiac disease who are unable to perform physical activity, and who have symptoms at rest

A more recent model, proposed by the American College of Cardiology (ACC) and the American Heart Association (AHA), categorizes HF in four stages, shown in Table 38.2. Although similar to the NYHA model, the ACC/AHA model better illustrates the progressive nature of the disease and the role of risk factor modification.

Drugs for Heart Failure

Medications can relieve the symptoms of HF by a number of different mechanisms, including slowing the heart rate, increasing contractility, and reducing cardiac workload. These mechanisms are illustrated in Pharmacotherapy Illustrated 38.1.

38.5 Angiotensin-converting enzyme inhibitors are drugs of choice for heart failure.

Due to their effectiveness and relative safety, the ACE inhibitors have replaced digoxin as first-line drugs for the treatment of chronic HF. Indeed, unless specifically contraindicated, all patients with HF and many patients at high risk of HF should receive an ACE inhibitor. The student should refer to Chapter 34 for details on the pharmacology of the drugs in this class. The following section focuses on the benefits of these drugs for patients with HF.

Clinical research has clearly demonstrated that ACE inhibitors slow the progression of HF and reduce mortality from this disease. Although this is probably true for all ACE inhibitors, the largest body of research has been conducted using captopril (Capoten) and lisinopril (Prinivil, Zestril). Doses for the ACE inhibitors indicated for HF are listed in Table 38.3.

The two primary actions of the ACE inhibitors are to lower peripheral resistance through the inhibition of angiotensin II formation, and to reduce blood volume through inhibition of aldosterone secretion. The resultant reduction of arterial blood pressure diminishes afterload, and increases cardiac output. An additional effect of the ACE inhibitors is dilation of veins. This action, which is probably not directly related to their inhibition of angiotensin, lowers preload and reduces pulmonary congestion and peripheral edema. The combined reductions in preload, afterload, and blood volume from the ACE inhibitors substantially decrease the workload on the heart and allow it to work more efficiently for the patient with HF. Patients taking ACE inhibitors experience fewer HF-related symptoms, hospitalizations, and treatment failures. Exercise tolerance is improved.

Research has also demonstrated that several ACE inhibitors are effective in preventing HF following an acute MI (see Chapter 37). Furthermore, post-MI therapy with ACE inhibitors reduces mortality and decreases reinfarction rates. Although these effects are most prominent when therapy is initiated within 36 hours after the onset of the MI, benefits are also obtained when therapy is begun later and continued for several years.

Therapy with ACE inhibitors is generally begun at low doses, and the amount gradually increased until the desired therapeutic level is reached. Clinical research has not shown a significant difference in mortality between patients receiving low versus high doses. Because higher doses reduce HF symp-

TABLE 38.2 The Stages for Treating Heart Failure

Stage	Description	Treatment Examples
A	Patients are at high risk of developing HF.	Make lifestyle modifications. Treat and control associated conditions: HTN, dyslipidemia, and diabetes. If hypertensive, use ACE inhibitor.
B	Patients have structural evidence of heart disease, such as a previous MI or valvular disease, but no symptoms of HF.	Continue treatments for Stage A. Treat with ACE inhibitor, possibly combined with a beta blocker.
C	Patients have structural evidence of heart disease with symptoms of HF such as fatigue, fluid retention, or dyspnea.	Treat with ACE inhibitor and beta blocker. Add digoxin and spironolactone if needed to control symptoms. If symptoms do not improve, add a loop or thiazide diuretic, an angiotensin receptor blocker, a nitrate, or hydralazine.
D	Patients have symptoms at rest, despite optimal medical therapy; decompensated HF.	Treatment may include intravenous (IV) diuretics, dopamine, dobutamine, IV nitroglycerin, nesiritide, or phosphodiesterase inhibitors.

Note: From "ACC/AHA 2005 Guideline Update for the Diagnosis and Management of Chronic Heart Failure in the Adult." A Report of the American College of Cardiology/American Heart Association Task Force on Practice Guidelines (Writing Committee to Update the 2001 Guidelines for the Evaluation and Management of Heart Failure)", 2005, *Circulation, 112,* e154-e235. Retrieved October 9, 2008, from http://circ.ahajournals.org/cgi/content/full/112/12/e154

PHARMACOTHERAPY ILLUSTRATED 38.1

Mechanisms of Action of Drugs Used for Heart Failure

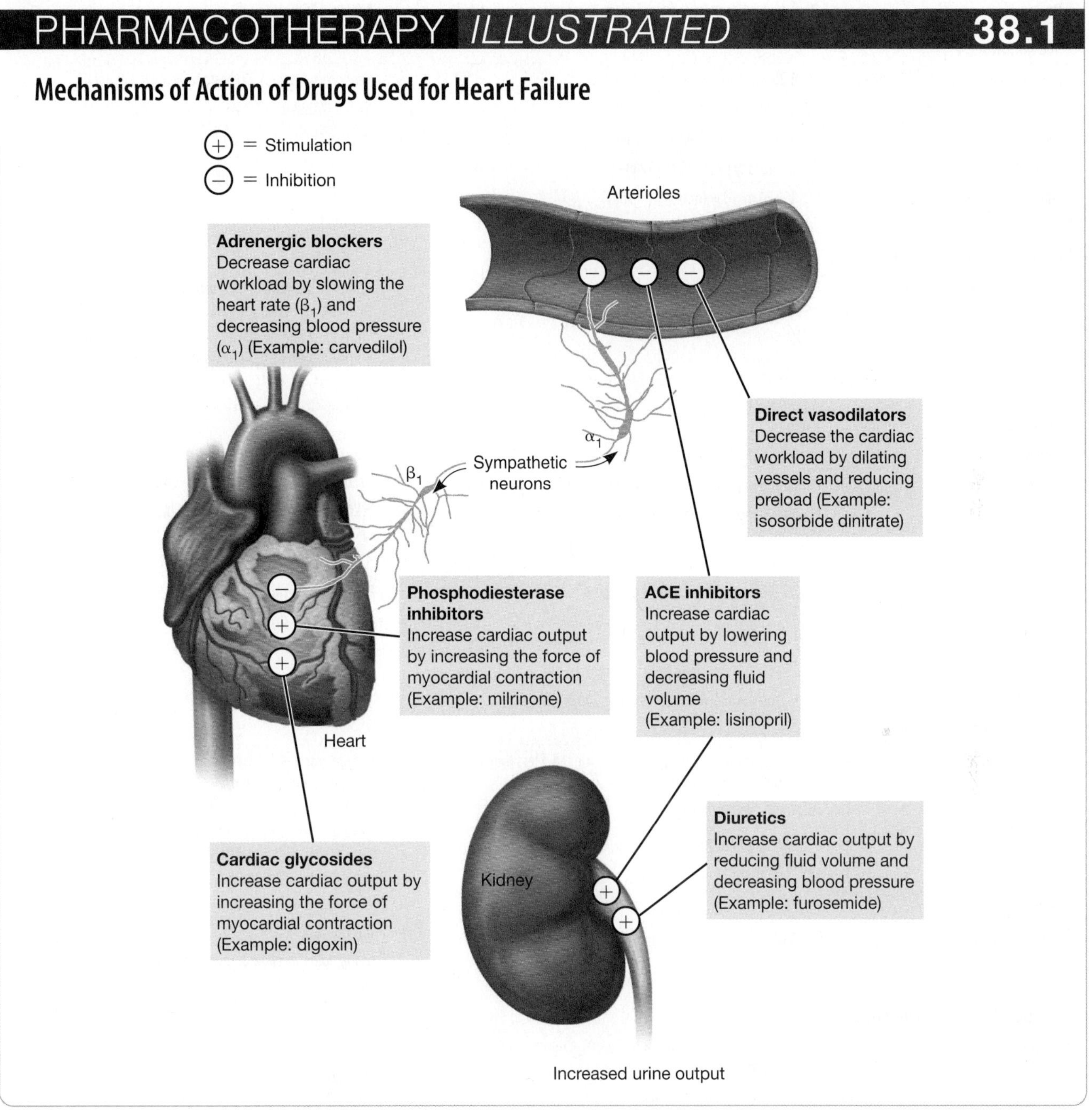

toms more effectively, however, these patients often receive doses in the higher range, as long as significant adverse effects do not interfere with therapy. Symptomatic relief from HF symptoms occurs within days of initiating therapy, but maximum benefits may take several weeks.

The ACE inhibitors are well tolerated by most patients with HF. Hypotension is the most common adverse effect, and the risk is increased when the patient is receiving other drugs that lower blood pressure such as diuretics and beta blockers. Hypotension is generally worse at the beginning of therapy or when dosage is increased. Multidrug therapy is common in these patients and the nurse serves a key role in teaching patients how to space drug administration times to minimize hypotensive adverse effects.

An additional concern during ACE inhibitor therapy is functional renal insufficiency. Patients with severe HF have high circulating levels of angiotensin II, which helps to maintain renal blood flow by constricting efferent arterioles in the kidney. When ACE inhibitors are administered, the level of angiotensin II declines rapidly, leading to reduced blood flow through the kidneys. During therapy with ACE inhibitors, renal insufficiency may also result from sodium depletion, often secondary to the concurrent use of diuretics. To avoid this potentially serious adverse effect, serum creatinine, serum electrolytes, and blood urea nitrogen (BUN) should be monitored during therapy. Should an assessment discover signs of renal impairment, the dose should be immediately decreased or the drug discontinued.

TABLE 38.3 Drugs for Heart Failure

Drug	Route and Adult Dose (maximum dose where indicated)	Adverse Effects
ACE Inhibitors		
captopril (Capoten)	PO: 6.25–12.5 mg tid (max: 450 mg/day)	*Headache, dizziness, orthostatic hypotension, cough* Severe hypotension (first-dose phenomenon), syncope, angioedema, blood dyscrasias
enalapril (Vasotec)	PO: 2.5 mg qid–bid (max: 40 mg/day)	
fosinopril (Monopril)	PO: 5–40 mg/day (max: 40 mg/day)	
lisinopril (Prinivil, Zestril)	PO: 10 mg/day (max: 80 mg/day)	
quinapril (Accupril)	PO: 10–20 mg/day (max: 40 mg/day)	
ramipril (Altace)	PO: 2.5–5 mg bid (max: 10 mg/day)	
Direct Vasodilators		
hydralazine with isosorbide dinitrate (BiDil)	PO; 1–2 tablets tid (max: 2 tablets/day)	*Headache, flushing of face, orthostatic hypotension, dizziness, reflex tachycardia* Fainting, severe headache, severe hypotension with overdose, lupus-like reaction (hydralazine)
Diuretics		
Loop or High Ceiling		
bumetanide (Bumex)	PO: 0.5–2 mg/day (max: 10 mg/day)	Loop and thiazides: *Electrolyte imbalances, orthostatic hypotension* Severe hypotension, dehydration, hypokalemia, hyponatremia, ototoxicity (loop diuretics)
furosemide (Lasix)	PO: 20–80 mg in one or more divided doses (max: 600 mg/day)	
torsemide (Demadex)	PO: 10–20 mg/day (max: 200 mg/day)	
Thiazide and Thiazide-Like		
hydrochlorothiazide (Microzide)	PO: 25–200 mg in one to three divided doses (max: 200 mg/day)	Potassium-sparing: *Hyperkalemia, gynecomastia in males, fatigue* Dysrhythmias due to hyperkalemia
Potassium-Sparing (Aldosterone Antagonist)		
eplerenone (Inspra)	PO: 25–50 mg once daily (max: 100 mg/day)	
spironolactone (Aldactone)	PO: 5–200 mg in divided doses (max: 200 mg/day)	
Beta-Adrenergic Blockers		
carvedilol (Coreg)	PO: 3.125 mg bid for 2 weeks (max: 25 mg bid if less than 85 kg or 50 mg bid if more than 85 kg) Sustained release: 10 mg/day (max: 80 mg/day)	*Fatigue, insomnia, drowsiness, impotence or decreased libido, bradycardia, confusion* Agranulocytosis, laryngospasm, Stevens–Johnson syndrome, anaphylaxis; if the drug is abruptly withdrawn, palpitations, rebound HTN, life-threatening dysrhythmias, or myocardial ischemia may occur
metoprolol extended release (Toprol-XL)	PO: 25 mg/day for 2 weeks; 12.5 mg/day for severe cases (max: 200 mg/day)	
Cardiac Glycoside		
digoxin (Digitek, Lanoxin, Lanoxicaps)	PO: 0.125–0.5 mg/day	*Nausea, vomiting, headache, and visual disturbances such as seeing halos, a yellow or green tinge, or blurring* Dysrhythmias, AV block
Phosphodiesterase Inhibitors		
inamrinone (Inocor)	IV: 0.75 mg/kg bolus given slowly over 2–3 min; then 5–10 mcg/kg/min (max: 10 mg/kg/day)	*Headache, hypotension* Dysrhythmias
milrinone (Primacor)	IV: 50 mcg/kg over 10 min; then 0.375–0.75 mcg/kg/min	
Beta-Adrenergic Agonists		
dobutamine (Dobutrex)	IV: Infused at a rate of 2.5–40 mcg/kg/min for a max of 72 h	*Headache, palpitations, nausea, vomiting, changes in blood pressure (hypo- or hypertension)* Dysrhythmias, gangrene, severe HTN
dopamine hydrochloride (Dopastat, Intropin)	IV: 1.5 mcg/kg/min initial dose; may be increased to 30 mcg/kg/min (max: 50 mcg/kg/min)	
epinephrine (Adrenalin)	Subcutaneous: 0.1–0.5 mL of 1:1,000 every 10–15 min prn IV: 0.1–0.25 mL of 1:1,000 every 10–15 min	
isoproterenol (Isuprel)	IV: 0.01–0.02 mg prn MDI: 1–2 inhalations 4–6 times/day (max: 6 inhalations in any hour during a 24-h period) Subcutaneous: 0.15–0.2 mg prn	
norepinephrine (Levarterenol, Levophed)	IV: Initially, 0.5–1 mcg/min until pressure stabilizes, then 2–4 mcg/min for maintenance (max: 30 mcg/min)	

Note: *Italics* indicate common adverse effects. Underline indicates serious adverse effects.

Other adverse effects of ACE inhibitors are angioedema, cough, and hyperkalemia. The student should refer to Chapter 34 for additional information on the adverse effects of ACE inhibitors and for a drug prototype feature for lisinopril (Prinivil, Zestril).

Another mechanism that blocks the effects of angiotensin II is the use of angiotensin receptor blockers (ARBs). Pharmacologically, the effects of the ARBs are very similar to those of the ACE inhibitors, as would be expected because both drug classes inhibit angiotensin II. In patients with HF, ARBs show equivalent efficacy to the ACE inhibitors. Clinical research, however, has suggested that combining ARBs with ACE inhibitors does not improve patient survival but does increase the risk of adverse effects. Because they show no clear advantage over other HF medications, the use of ARBs in the treatment of HF is usually reserved for patients who are unable to tolerate the adverse effects of ACE inhibitors. Losartan (Cozaar) is an ARB featured as a drug prototype in Chapter 34.

38.6 Diuretics relieve symptoms of heart failure by reducing fluid overload and decreasing blood pressure.

Diuretics are common medications for the treatment of patients with HF, since they are effective at reducing peripheral edema and pulmonary congestion and produce few adverse effects. By reducing blood volume and lowering blood pressure, the workload on the heart is reduced, and cardiac output increases. Diuretics are rarely used alone for HF, but are frequently prescribed in combination with ACE inhibitors, beta blockers, and other HF medications. Doses for selected diuretics are listed in Table 38.3.

Although diuretics are effective at relieving HF symptoms, clinical research has not demonstrated their effectiveness in slowing the progression of HF or in decreasing the mortality rate associated with the disease. Indeed, some of the actions of the diuretics, particularly effects on potassium balance, may increase the risk of adverse effects from other HF drugs. Because of this, diuretics are only indicated when there is evidence of fluid retention. In patients presenting with fluid retention, especially with symptoms of severe pulmonary congestion or peripheral edema, diuretics are essential medications.

Of the diuretic classes, the loop diuretics are most commonly prescribed for HF, due to their effectiveness in removing fluid from the body. Loop diuretics are also able to function in patients with renal impairment, an advantage for many patients with decompensated HF. Another major advantage in treating acute HF is that loop diuretics act quickly, within minutes for IV formulations. For chronic HF, therapy is begun with low doses of furosemide (Lasix), bumetanide (Bumex), or torsemide (Demadex), and gradually increased until the desired volume reduction is obtained.

As therapy continues with loop diuretics, some patients become less responsive, a phenomenon known as **diuretic resistance.** The loop diuretics exhibit a ceiling effect; once the "ceiling dose" is reached, increases in dosage will not produce additional diuresis. To obtain additional diuresis and volume reduction, the loop diuretic may be administered more frequently, or a diuretic from a different class may be added to the regimen.

Thiazide diuretics are also used in the pharmacotherapy of HF, sometimes combined with loop diuretics to achieve a more effective diuresis in patients with acute HF. Because they are less effective than the loop diuretics, thiazides are generally reserved for patients with mild-to-moderate HF.

In addition to being a potassium-sparing diuretic, spironolactone is also classified as an aldosterone antagonist. As a diuretic, spironolactone has a limited role in HF, due to its low efficacy. Clinical research, however, has demonstrated that the drug is able to block the deleterious effects of aldosterone on the heart. High levels of aldosterone promote cardiac remodeling and the deposition of fibrotic tissue in the myocardium of patients with HF. By blocking these cardiac effects, spironolactone decreases mortality due to sudden death, as well as progression to advanced HF.

At the low doses used for HF patients (25 mg daily), spironolactone produces few adverse effects. The most common adverse effect at this dose is gynecomastia in male patients. More serious, however, is the risk of hyperkalemia. Caution must be used when administering spironolactone concurrently with ACE inhibitors due to the possibility of additive hyperkalemia. Care must be taken to educate patients to limit potassium-rich foods in the diet and eliminate potassium supplements.

Diuretic use in HF patients should be carefully monitored to avoid dehydration or electrolyte imbalances. These adverse effects are more likely to occur in HF patients who have comorbid renal impairment. During maintenance therapy, patients are urged to weigh themselves frequently, and report significant changes to their health care provider. Frequent laboratory tests for blood electrolyte levels are obtained to prevent the development of hypokalemia during loop or thiazide diuretic therapy. This is especially important in patients who are also taking digoxin (Lanoxin), because hypokalemia may induce fatal dysrhythmias.

Hydrochlorothiazide, furosemide, and spironolactone are featured as drug prototypes in Chapter 35. The role of diuretics in the treatment of HTN is discussed in Chapter 36.

MyNursingKit | Support for Heart Failure Patients and Health Professionals

CONNECTION *Checkpoint* 38.2

Conn's syndrome is characterized by excess secretion of aldosterone. From what you learned in Chapter 34, what effect would you predict this syndrome would have on the heart, and what medication might be a drug of choice? See Answer to Connection Checkpoint 38.2 in Appendix A.

38.7 Beta-adrenergic antagonists can dramatically reduce hospitalizations and increase the survival of patients with heart failure.

Cardiac glycosides, beta-adrenergic agonists, and other medications that produce a positive inotropic effect serve important roles in reversing the diminished contractility that is the hallmark of HF. It may seem somewhat surprising, then, to find beta-adrenergic blockers—drugs that exhibit a negative inotropic effect—prescribed for this disease. Even though this class of drugs has the potential to worsen HF, beta-adrenergic blockers are standard therapy for many patients with this chronic disorder. Why is this the case?

In patients with HF, high levels of endogenous norepinephrine and other catecholamines cause excessive activation of the sympathetic nervous system, and are associated with cardiac remodeling and progression of the disease. Beta-adrenergic antagonists block the actions of these catecholamines, slowing the heart rate and reducing blood pressure, thus decreasing the cardiac workload. After several months of therapy, heart size, shape, and function return to normal in some patients, in essence producing a **reverse remodeling** of the heart. Extensive clinical research has demonstrated that the careful use of beta-adrenergic antagonists can dramatically reduce the number of HF-associated hospitalizations and deaths. They are effective in all stages of symptomatic HF. Doses for selected beta-adrenergic antagonists are listed in Table 38.3.

To benefit patients with HF, however, beta-adrenergic antagonists must be administered in a very specific manner. Initial doses must be 1/10 to 1/20 of the target dose. Doses are doubled every 2 weeks until the target dose is reached. If therapy is begun with the target dose, or the dose is increased too rapidly, beta blockers can worsen HF. Carvedilol and metoprolol are the two beta-adrenergic antagonists approved for HF, although bisoprolol has also been shown to be effective. When treating HF, beta blockers are almost always combined with other agents, especially the ACE inhibitors.

Adherence to beta-blocker therapy can be a major clinical challenge for some patients. The patient may not report symptomatic improvement with the drug and, in fact, may feel worse at the initiation of therapy. To achieve maximum patient adherence, the nurse must teach the patient the important long-term benefits of beta blockers.

Beta-adrenergic antagonists are contraindicated in patients with chronic obstructive pulmonary disease (COPD) and patients with severe bradycardia or heart block. These medications should be used with caution in patients with diabetes, peripheral vascular disease, and hepatic impairment. Caution is needed with older adults because these patients often require a reduced dose. Hepatic function tests should be performed periodically, and the prescriber notified if signs or symptoms of liver toxicity become apparent.

The basic pharmacology of the beta-adrenergic antagonists is presented in Chapter 20, where metoprolol is featured as a prototype for this class. Other applications of the beta-adrenergic blockers are discussed elsewhere in this text: HTN is discussed in Chapter 36, angina and MI in Chapter 37, and dysrhythmias in Chapter 39.

38.8 Vasodilators reduce symptoms of heart failure by reducing preload or afterload.

The direct vasodilators relax blood vessels and lower blood pressure, creating less workload on the heart. The two vasodilators that have been traditionally used for HF include hydralazine and isosorbide dinitrate. Both are used off-label for this indication for patients who have not responded well to drugs from other classes.

Hydralazine (Apresoline) acts on arterioles to decrease peripheral resistance, reduce afterload, and increase cardiac output. It is an effective antihypertensive drug, although it is not a drug of first choice for this indication because hypotension and reflex tachycardia are common, and may limit therapy. The drug must be taken 3 to 4 times daily, which places an extensive pill burden on HF patients, who often are taking multiple drugs.

Isosorbide dinitrate (Isordil) is a long-acting organic nitrate that reduces preload by directly dilating veins. The drug is not very effective as monotherapy, and tolerance develops to its actions with continued use. Isosorbide dinitrate is usually combined with hydralazine because the two drugs act synergistically when used in HF patients. The high incidence of adverse effects such as reflex tachycardia and orthostatic hypotension, however, limits their use to patients who cannot tolerate ACE inhibitors.

Hydralazine is presented as a prototype vasodilator for HTN in Chapter 36. The use of isosorbide dinitrate in the pharmacotherapy of angina pectoris is presented in Chapter 37.

CONNECTION *Checkpoint* 38.3

Isosorbide dinitrate is also used for angina. From what you learned in Chapter 37, why is nitroglycerin a preferred drug for acute angina, rather than isosorbide dinitrate? See Answer to Connection Checkpoint 38.3 in Appendix A.

38.9 Cardiac glycosides increase the force of myocardial contraction and were once drugs of choice for heart failure.

Once used as arrow poisons by African tribes and as medicines by the ancient Egyptians and Romans, the value of the cardiac glycosides in treating heart disorders has been known for over 2,000 years. Originally extracted from the beautiful flowering plants, *Digitalis purpura* (purple foxglove) and *Digitalis lanata* (white foxglove), the cardiac glycosides were the mainstay of HF treatment until the discovery of the ACE inhibitors. Over the past 20 years, the role of the cardiac glycosides in the pharmacotherapy of HF has become more limited. The two primary cardiac glycosides, digoxin and digitoxin, are quite similar in efficacy; the primary difference is that the latter has a more prolonged half-life. Digitoxin is no longer available in the United States. The dose for digoxin is listed in Table 38.3.

Because of its long historical use, the effectiveness of digitalis in the pharmacotherapy of HF remained unquestioned until the late 1980s, when a controlled study of 6800 patients with HF revealed no significant difference in mortality between patients who took digoxin, and those who received a placebo. The drug did, however, produce symptomatic benefit in patients. Based on this study, and the development of safer and more effective drug classes, cardiac glycosides are now limited to late-stage HF, in combination with other agents. Digoxin remains an important therapy in HF patients with supraventricular tachyarrhythmias, because the drug has antidysrhythmic activity that can stabilize these types of cardiac conduction abnormalities.

The margin of safety between a therapeutic dose and a toxic dose of cardiac glycosides is very narrow, and severe adverse effects may result from poorly managed therapy. **Digitalization** refers to the procedure by which the dose of digoxin is gradually increased until tissues become saturated with the medication, and the symptoms of HF diminish. If the patient is critically ill, digitalization can be done rapidly with IV doses in a controlled clinical environment, where adverse effects may be carefully monitored. As an outpatient, digitalization may be completed over a period of 7 days, using oral (PO) dosing. In either case, the goal is to determine the proper dose of medication to be administered, without undue adverse effects.

PROTOTYPE DRUG Digoxin (Lanoxin, Lanoxicaps)

Classification: Therapeutic: Drug for heart failure
Pharmacologic: Cardiac glycoside, inotropic agent

Therapeutic Effects and Uses: The primary benefit of digoxin is its ability to increase the strength of myocardial contraction, a positive inotropic action. By increasing myocardial contractility, digoxin directly increases cardiac output, which alleviates symptoms of HF and improves exercise tolerance. The higher cardiac output increases urine production and results in a desirable reduction in blood volume, relieving the distressing symptoms of pulmonary congestion and peripheral edema. In current clinical practice, digoxin use is usually limited to patients who are not responding adequately to ACE inhibitor therapy or to HF patients with atrial fibrillation.

In addition to its positive inotropic effect, digoxin also affects the speed of myocardial conduction. Through a mechanism not fully understood, digoxin decreases SNS activity and increases parasympathetic activity. This helps attenuate the excessive sympathetic activation that causes tachycardia and worsens HF (Section 38.2). Digoxin has the ability to suppress the sinoatrial node and slow electrical conduction through the atrioventricular node. The heart rate decreases, allowing greater diastolic filling of the ventricles. Because the heart rate may decline too much, health care providers establish parameters for each patient. As a general rule, if the apical pulse falls below 60 beats per minute, the medication is withheld and the health care provider notified. Digoxin is sometimes used to treat dysrhythmias, as discussed in Chapter 39.

Digoxin is available by the PO or IV route. The capsule formulation (Lanoxicaps) has a more predictable bioavailability than the tablet form, but it is more expensive. Because differences in bioavailability of digoxin formulations can potentially affect drug action and the potential for adverse effects, it is advisable to continue with the same brand name, unless otherwise changed by the prescriber.

Mechanism of Action: Digoxin inhibits Na^+-K^+ ATPase, the critical enzyme responsible for pumping sodium ions out of the myocardial cells in exchange for potassium ions. As sodium ions accumulate in myocytes, calcium ions are released from their storage areas in the cell to activate contractile elements. The release of calcium ions produces a more forceful contraction of myocardial fibers.

Pharmacokinetics:

Route(s)	PO, IV
Absorption	70–90% absorbed from the gastrointestinal (GI) tract
Distribution	Widely distributed; crosses the placenta; secreted in breast milk; 20–25% bound to protein
Primary metabolism	Hepatic, 14%
Primary excretion	Renal
Onset of action	PO: 30–90 minutes; IV: 5–30 minutes
Duration of action	Half-life: 3–4 days

Adverse Effects: Adverse effects of digoxin involve multiple body systems and can be severe. The most dangerous adverse effect is its ability to cause ventricular dysrhythmias, which may result in sudden cardiac death. The most common cause of digoxin-induced dysrhythmias is hypokalemia due to diuretic use. Other factors placing patients at risk to digoxin-induced dysrhythmias include hypomagnesemia, hypercalcemia, and impaired renal function. Additional serious adverse cardiac effects include atrioventricular (AV) block, atrial dysrhythmias, and sinus bradycardia. Frequent electrocardiograms (ECGs) should be obtained to assess for cardiotoxicity.

Noncardiac adverse effects include general malaise, dizziness, headache, anorexia, nausea, and vomiting. The drug may produce unusual visual effects such as halos, changes in color perception, and photophobia.

Frequent serum digoxin levels should be obtained during therapy, and the dosage adjusted based on the laboratory results and the patient's clinical response. Clinical research suggests that digoxin levels from 0.5 to 1 ng/mL give the most therapeutic benefit, with an acceptable risk of adverse effects. In some patients, raising the dose does not increase the therapeutic effect, but it does increase the risk of serious digoxin toxicity. For each patient, the health care provider should establish acceptable parameters for serum digoxin levels, and the drug should be discontinued should the level rise above the maximum. Digoxin levels higher than 1.8 ng/mL are considered toxic. However, the nurse should remember that toxicity should be based on patient symptoms rather than serum level. Levels should be taken 6 to 12 hours after a dose, because digoxin has a prolonged distribution time.

MyNursingKit | Mechanism of Action Animation: Digoxin

Contraindications/Precautions: Patients with AV block or ventricular dysrhythmias unrelated to HF should not receive digoxin, because the drug may worsen these conditions. Digoxin should be administered with caution to older adults because these patients experience a higher incidence of adverse effects. Patients with renal impairment should receive lower doses of digoxin, because the drug is excreted by this route. The drug should be used with caution in patients with MI, cor pulmonale, or hypothyroidism.

Drug Interactions: Digoxin interacts with many drugs. Concurrent use of digoxin with diuretics must be carefully monitored, since diuretics can cause hypokalemia and increase the risk of dysrhythmias. Use with ACE inhibitors, spironolactone, or potassium supplements can lead to hyperkalemia and reduce the therapeutic action of digoxin. Administration of digoxin with other positive inotropic agents can cause additive effects on myocardial contractility. Concurrent use with beta blockers may result in additive bradycardia. Antacids and cholesterol-lowering drugs can decrease the absorption of digoxin. If calcium is administered intravenously together with digoxin, it can increase the risk of dysrhythmias. Quinidine, verapamil, amiodarone, and alprazolam will decrease the distribution and excretion of digoxin, thus increasing the risk of digoxin toxicity. **Herbal/Food:** The drug should be used with caution with ginseng, which may increase the risk of digoxin toxicity.

Pregnancy: Category A.

Treatment of Overdose: Digoxin overdose can be fatal and the nurse should be prepared to administer digoxin immune Fab

(Digibind). Digoxin immune Fab consists of digoxin-specific antibodies, which form a complex with digoxin that prevents the drug from reaching the tissues, and is removed through renal excretion. Reversal of adverse effects occurs quickly: 90% of patients respond within an hour after IV administration. As digoxin is removed from the body, the inotropic effects of the drug will diminish, and the patient may be at risk of HF. The patient must be monitored continuously during the infusion.

Nursing Responsibilities:

- Obtain a complete health history including allergies, and drug history for possible drug interactions.
- Take apical pulse for 1 full minute noting rate, rhythm, and quality before administering the drug.
- Withhold medication and notify the prescriber if apical pulse falls below ordered parameters (e.g., less than 50 or 60/minute in adults and less than 60 or 70/minute in children).
- Monitor baseline data (e.g., quality of peripheral pulses, blood pressure, clinical symptoms, serum electrolytes, creatinine clearance) as a foundation for making comparative assessments.
- Monitor baseline and periodic serum digoxin, potassium, magnesium, and calcium levels, and notify the prescriber of abnormal values. Collect blood samples for determining plasma digoxin levels at least 6 hours after the daily dose and preferably just before the next scheduled daily dose.
- Monitor for symptoms of drug toxicity: In children, cardiac dysrhythmias are usually reliable signs of early toxicity. Early indicators in adults (anorexia, nausea, vomiting, diarrhea, visual disturbances) are rarely initial signs in children.
- Monitor intake and output ratio during digitalization, particularly in patients with impaired renal function. Monitor for edema daily and auscultate chest for sounds of crackles (fluid accumulation.)
- Observe patients closely when being transferred from one preparation (tablet, elixir, or parenteral) to another; when tablet is replaced by elixir the potential for toxicity increases because more than 30% of the drug is absorbed.

Patient and Family Education:

- Take radial pulse daily and immediately report values below 60 or above 110, or if skipped beats or other changes in rhythm are detected to the health care provider.
- Immediately report any of the following to the health care provider because they may indicate toxicity: loss of appetite, nausea, vomiting, diarrhea, or visual disturbances.
- Weigh each day under standard conditions and report weight gain of 1 kg (2 lb) over 2 days.
- Self-monitor for a decrease in urine output or an increase in swelling of the hands and feet.
- Take digoxin precisely as prescribed. Do not skip or double a dose or change dose intervals, and take it at same time each day.
- Do not take any over-the-counter (OTC) medications, especially those for coughs, colds, allergy, GI upset, or obesity, without approval of health care provider.
- Do not switch brands of digoxin originally prescribed, unless directed by the prescriber.
- Do not breast-feed while taking this drug without approval of the health care provider.

Drugs Similar to Digoxin (Lanoxin, Lanoxicaps)

Digoxin is the only cardiac glycoside available in the United States.

CONNECTIONS

Complementary and Alternative Therapies Carnitine (L-Carnitine)

Description: Carnitine is a natural substance structurally similar to amino acids. Its primary function in metabolism is to move fatty acids from the bloodstream into cells, where it assists in the breakdown of lipids in the mitochondria. This breakdown produces energy and increases the availability of oxygen, particularly in muscle cells. A congenital deficiency of carnitine leads to severe brain, liver, and heart damage. The best food sources of carnitine are organ meat, fish, muscle meats, and milk products.

History and Claims: Carnitine has been claimed to enhance energy and sports performance, heart health, memory, immune function, and male fertility. It is also being marketed as a "fat burner" for weight reduction.

Standardization: Carnitine is available as a supplement in several forms, including L-carnitine, D-carnitine, and L-acetylcarnitine. D-carnitine is associated with potential adverse effects, and should be avoided. Doses range from 2 to 6 g/day.

Evidence: Carnitine has been extensively studied. There is solid evidence to support supplementation in patients who are deficient in carnitine. Although a normal diet supplies 300 mg per day, certain patients may need additional amounts. Vegetarians are at risk for carnitine depletion, since plant protein supplies little or no carnitine.

Carnitine supplementation has been shown to improve exercise tolerance in patients with angina. The use of carnitine may prevent the occurrence of dysrhythmias in the early stages of heart disease. Carnitine has also been shown to decrease triglyceride levels while increasing HDL serum levels, thus helping to minimize one of the major risk factors associated with heart disease.

Research has not shown carnitine supplementation to be of significant benefit in enhancing sports performance, improving brain function in patients with Alzheimer's disease, or weight loss.

Source: From "Therapeutic Effects of l-Carnitine and Propionyl-l-Carnitine on Cardiovascular Diseases: A Review," by R. Ferrari, E. Merli, G. Cicchitelli, D. Mele, A. Fucili, and C. Ceconi, 2004, *Annals New York Academy of Science, 1033*(12), pp. 79–91; "Acetyl-L-Carnitine for Dementia," by S. Hudson and N. Tabet, 2003, *Cochrane Database of Systematic Reviews, Issue 2.* (Art. No. CD003158. DOI: 10.1002/14651858.CD003158); and "Supplemental Conditionally Essential Nutrients in Cardiovascular Disease Therapy," by B. S. Kendler, 2006, *Journal of Cardiovascular Nursing, 21*(1), pp. 9–16.

NURSING PROCESS APPLICATION

Patients Receiving Cardiac Glycosides

Assessment Data	Potential Nursing Diagnoses
Prior to administration: • Auscultate apical heart rate for 1 full minute. Hold medication for heart rate less than 60 beats/minute. • Assess vital signs, urinary output, and sensorium, initially and throughout therapy. (These are indicators of the effectiveness of adequate cardiac output.) • Determine the reason the medication is being administered. • Obtain a complete health history including allergies, drug history, and possible drug interactions.	• *Ineffective Tissue Perfusion (Cardiopulmonary)*, related to impaired cardiac status • *Decreased Cardiac Output,* related to impaired cardiac pumping ability • *Excess Fluid Volume,* related to poor perfusion to kidneys, secondary to heart failure • *Deficient Knowledge (Medication Regimen)*

Planning: Patient Goals and Expected Outcomes

The patient will:

- Report decreased symptoms of cardiac decompensation related to fluid overload, which may include edema, low urine output, shortness of breath, and mental confusion.
- Exhibit evidence of improved organ perfusion, including kidney, heart, and brain.
- Demonstrate understanding of the drug's action by accurately describing drug adverse effects and precautions.
- Immediately report adverse effects such as nausea, vomiting, diarrhea, heart rate below 60, and vision changes.

Implementation

Interventions and (Rationales)	Patient and Family Education
• Monitor ECG for rate and rhythm changes during initial digitalization therapy. (Digoxin decreases cardiac heart rate and the nurse should monitor for bradycardia.) • Monitor intake and output ratio during digitalization, particularly in patients with impaired renal function. (Low urinary output may be evidence of poor renal perfusion related to cardiac decompensation.)	Instruct patient to: • Count the pulse for a full minute and record with every dose. • Report if the pulse falls below 60 or rises above 110, or if skipped beats or other changes in rhythm are detected.
• Observe for adverse effects related to digoxin toxicity, such as nausea, vomiting, anorexia, or vision changes. (These salient signs of digoxin toxicity are often overlooked and should be reported promptly to the health care provider.)	• Instruct the patient to report adverse effects immediately to prevent toxicity.
• Weigh the patient daily. (Weight gain is a prime indicator of the heart's ability to adequately pump the circulatory volume. Weight gain of 2 or more pounds per 2 days may indicate inefficiency of the heart muscle.)	Instruct the patient to: • Weigh at the same time under the same conditions daily. • Report a weight gain of 2 or more pounds in 2 days.
• Administer precise ordered dose at same time each day. (Maintain therapeutic level of drug therapy.)	Instruct the patient to: • Take as directed; do not double dose. • Not discontinue without advice of health care provider. • Not change formulations of medication without consulting the health care provider.
• Monitor serum drug level to determine therapeutic concentration and toxicity. (Report serum drug levels greater than 1.8 ng/mL to health care provider. This indicates impending drug toxicity.) • Monitor levels of potassium, magnesium, calcium, BUN, and creatinine. (Hypokalemia and hypomagnesia predispose the patient to digoxin toxicity.)	Instruct the patient to: • Report to the laboratory as scheduled by health care provider for ongoing drug level determinations. • Immediately report visual changes, mental depression, palpitations, weakness, and loss of appetite, vomiting, and diarrhea to the health care provider. • Instruct the patient to consume foods high in potassium if appropriate and not contraindicated by other treatment modalities. Foods high in potassium include bananas, apricots, kidney beans, sweet potatoes, and peanut butter.

Evaluation of Outcome Criteria

Evaluate the effectiveness of drug therapy by confirming that patient goals and expected outcomes have been met (see "Planning").

CONNECTION *Checkpoint* 38.4

Cholestyramine reduces the bioavailability of digoxin, thus potentially decreasing the actions of the cardiac glycoside. From what you learned in Chapter 32, what is the primary indication for cholestyramine and what is the likely reason this drug causes a decrease in digoxin bioavailability? (See Answer to Connection Checkpoint 38.4 in Appendix A.)

38.10 Phosphodiesterase III inhibitors and other positive inotropic agents are used for acute decompensated heart failure.

Advanced or decompensated HF can be a medical emergency and prompt, effective treatment is necessary to avoid organ failure or death. In addition to high doses of loop diuretics, positive inotropic drugs are often necessary. The two primary classes of inotropic agents used for decompensated HF are beta-adrenergic agonists and phosphodiesterase inhibitors. Doses for these agents are listed in Table 38.3.

Beta-Adrenergic Agonists (Sympathomimetics)

Beta-adrenergic agonists used for HF include isoproterenol (Isuprel), epinephrine, norepinephrine, dopamine (Dopastat), and dobutamine (Dobutrex). Dobutamine has been a traditional drug of choice in this class because it has the ability to rapidly increase myocardial contractility, with minimal changes to heart rate or blood pressure. This is important because increases in heart rate or blood pressure will create greater oxygen demands on the heart and possibly worsen HF. Therapy with dobutamine is usually limited to 72 hours, as continuous infusion of the drug causes the heart to become tolerant to beta adrenergic activation, making the drug less effective. The two most common adverse effects with beta-agonists are tachycardia and dysrhythmias.

Patients who have both HF and hypotension benefit from dopamine, which not only increases myocardial contractility but also activates alpha-adrenergic receptors to increase blood pressure. However, tachycardia is more prominent with dopamine than with dobutamine. Patients who have been receiving a beta-adrenergic antagonist for their HF may require a higher initial dose of beta-agonist. The basic pharmacology of the beta-adrenergic agonists was presented in Chapter 18, where epinephrine and isoproterenol were featured as prototypes for this drug class.

Phosphodiesterase III Inhibitors

In the 1980s, two medications became available that block the enzyme **phosphodiesterase III** in cardiac and smooth muscle, which leads to increases in the amount of calcium available for myocardial contraction. The enzyme inhibition results in two main actions that benefit patients with HF: a positive inotropic action and vasodilation. Cardiac output is increased due to the increase in contractility and the decrease in left ventricular afterload. There is little effect on heart rate. Arterial pressure is either decreased or, in some patients, it remains unchanged.

Although the actions of the phosphodiesterase III inhibitors are very similar to dobutamine, they have a much longer half-life. This makes it more difficult to make rapid changes in dose when controlling acute HF. In addition, if adverse effects do occur, they are more prolonged than with dobutamine.

Phosphodiesterase inhibitors have serious toxicity that limits their use to patients with resistant HF who have not responded to ACE inhibitors, digoxin, or other therapies. Therapy is limited to 2 to 3 days and the patient is continuously monitored for ventricular dysrhythmias, including ectopic beats, supraventricular dysrhythmias, premature ventricular contractions, ventricular tachycardia, and ventricular fibrillation. If the patient presents with hypokalemia, this should be corrected before administering phosphodiesterase III inhibitors because this can increase the likelihood of dysrhythmias. These medications can cause hypotension. When using inamrinone, frequent laboratory blood tests should be conducted to assess for thrombocytopenia.

PROTOTYPE DRUG Milrinone lactate (Primacor)

Classification: **Therapeutic:** Drug for heart failure
Pharmacologic: Phosphodiesterase inhibitor; inotropic agent

Therapeutic Effects and Uses: Approved in 1987, milrinone is approved for the short-term treatment of patients with acute decompensated heart failure. Although inamrinone was the first drug in this class to be marketed, milrinone is generally preferred because it has a shorter half-life and fewer adverse effects. It is only given intravenously, and peak effects occur in 2 minutes. Immediate effects of milrinone include an increased force of contraction and an increase in cardiac output. Research has not yet demonstrated any decrease in mortality or morbidity with the use of milrinone infusions.

Mechanism of Action: Milrinone inhibits phosphodiesterase III, the enzyme responsible for the breakdown of cAMP to AMP, in cardiac and vascular smooth muscle. The rise in cAMP levels increases intracellular calcium, resulting in greater contractility. Cardiac output is increased and pulmonary capillary wedge pressure is decreased.

Pharmacokinetics:

Route(s)	IV
Absorption	N/A
Distribution	Unknown; 70% bound to plasma protein
Primary metabolism	Unknown; 83% is excreted unchanged
Primary excretion	Renal
Onset of action	2–10 minutes
Duration of action	Half-life: 3–6 h

Adverse Effects: The most serious adverse effect of milrinone is ventricular dysrhythmia, which can occur in more than 10% of patients taking the drug. The patient's ECG is monitored continuously during the infusion of the drug to prevent serious dysrhythmias. Blood pressure is also continuously monitored during the infusion to avoid hypotension. Less serious adverse effects include headache, nausea, and vomiting.

Contraindications/Precautions: Milrinone is contraindicated in patients with severe valvular heart disease. The drug should be used with caution in patients with preexisting dysrhythmias. Hypovolemia or electrolyte imbalances should be corrected before starting the infusion, and the dose should be reduced in patients with renal impairment.

Drug Interactions: Caution should be used when administering milrinone with digoxin, dobutamine, or other inotropic drugs, since their cardiac effects may be additive. Use with antihypertensive agents may cause additive hypotension. **Food/Herbal:** Ginger may contribute to the cardiac actions of milrinone.

Pregnancy: Category C.

Treatment of Overdose: Overdose of milrinone causes hypotension, which may be treated with the administration of normal saline or a vasopressor.

Nursing Responsibilities:

- Monitor cardiac status closely during, and for several hours following, infusion because supraventricular and ventricular arrhythmias may occur.
- Monitor blood pressure and promptly slow or stop the infusion if significant hypotension occurs. Closely monitor those patients who have been prescribed recent aggressive diuretic therapy for decreasing blood pressure.
- Monitor fluid and electrolyte status and immediately report impending hypokalemia to the prescriber.

Patient and Family Education:

- Immediately report chest pain (angina) to the health care provider should it occur during the infusion.
- This drug may cause a headache, which can be treated with analgesics.
- Do not take other prescription or nonprescription drugs, dietary supplements, or herbal products without approval of the health care provider.

Drugs Similar to Milrinone Lactate (Primacor)

The only other drug in the phosphodiesterase inhibitor class is inamrinone.

Inamrinone (Inocor): Approved in 1984, inamrinone has similar indications and inotropic actions as milrinone. Its only approved use is for the short-term therapy of serious or decompensated HF. Like milrinone it is administered by IV infusion with continuous monitoring to detect the possibility of dysrhythmias and to avoid hypotension. One difference is that inamrinone causes a higher incidence of thrombocytopenia. The nurse should assess for signs and symptoms of bleeding during therapy. In addition, the liver metabolizes inamrinone and caution must be used when treating patients with hepatic impairment. Prior to 2000, inamrinone was called amrinone. The name change was done to avoid medication errors. The name amrinone looked and sounded too similar to amiodarone, an antidysrhythmic drug. This drug is pregnancy category C.

38.11 Several novel approaches to therapy have resulted in new drugs for heart failure.

In 2001, the first new medication for HF in over 10 years was approved. Nesiritide (Natrecor) is a small peptide hormone, produced through recombinant deoxyribonucleic acid (DNA) technology that is structurally identical to endogenous beta-type natriuretic peptide (hBNP).

In healthy individuals, the atria secrete atrial natriuretic hormone (ANP), in response to increasing blood pressure. As a natural component of homeostasis, ANP acts on the kidney to increase the excretion of sodium and water and return pressure to normal levels. When HF occurs, the ventricles begin to secrete hBNP, in response to the increased stretch on the ventricular walls. hBNP has the same action as ANP: diuresis and renal excretion of sodium. In therapeutic doses, hBNP causes vasodilation, which also contributes to reduced preload. By reducing preload and afterload, hBNP compensates for diminished cardiac function.

Nesiritide is generally given by an initial IV bolus, immediately followed by a continuous IV infusion. The medication has limited uses due to its ability to cause severe hypotension, which can persist several hours after the infusion is discontinued. Patients require continuous monitoring. It is approved for patients with acute decompensated HF. Nesiritide is pregnancy category C.

UNDERSTANDING THE CHAPTER

Key Concepts Summary

38.1 Heart failure is closely associated with disorders such as chronic hypertension, coronary artery disease, and diabetes.

38.2 The body attempts to compensate for heart failure by increasing cardiac output.

38.3 Symptoms of heart failure occur when compensatory mechanisms fail to maintain adequate cardiac output.

38.4 The specific therapy for heart failure depends upon the clinical stage of the disease.

38.5 Angiotensin-converting enzyme (ACE) inhibitors are drugs of choice for heart failure.

38.6 Diuretics relieve symptoms of heart failure by reducing fluid overload and decreasing blood pressure.

38.7 Beta-adrenergic antagonists can dramatically reduce hospitalizations and increase the survival of patients with heart failure.

38.8 Vasodilators reduce symptoms of heart failure by reducing preload or afterload.

38.9 Cardiac glycosides increase the force of myocardial contraction and were once drugs of choice for heart failure.

38.10 Phosphodiesterase III inhibitors and other positive inotropic agents are used for acute decompensated heart failure.

38.11 Several novel approaches to therapy have resulted in new drugs for heart failure.

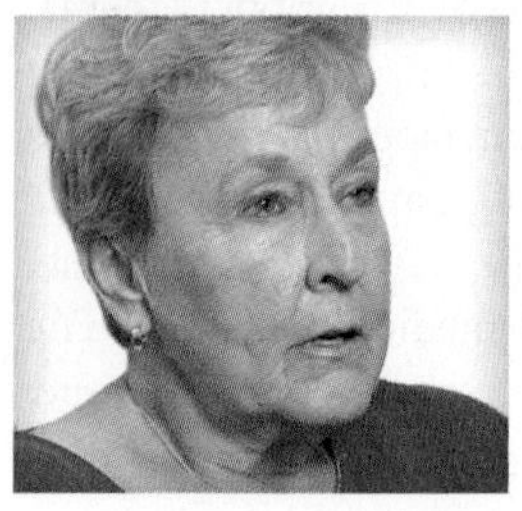

Making the PATIENT Connection

Remember the patient "Thelma Walters" at the beginning of the chapter? Now read the remainder of the case study. Based on the information presented within this chapter, respond to the critical thinking questions that follow.

Thelma Walters is a 77-year-old woman who presents to the emergency department complaining of increasing dyspnea for the past 2 days. She has also noticed swelling in her feet and ankles. Due to her onset of shortness of breath, she has had to sleep in a recliner and is unable to lay flat in bed at night. Her past medical history includes a myocardial infarction 3 years ago at which time she had a coronary artery bypass graft procedure. Her surgical history includes a hysterectomy 20 years ago. She has never used tobacco or alcohol. Thelma takes low-dose atenolol (Tenormin) for mild HTN.

As the nurse performs the initial physical assessment the following relevant findings are discovered. The patient's blood pressure is 112/62 mmHg, heart rate is 138 beats/minute and irregular, and respiratory rate is 32/minute and labored. The patient is 1.7 m (5′6″) tall and weighs 82 kg (180 lb). The neck veins of the patient are distended when she is placed at a 45-degree incline. The nurse notes scattered crackles bilaterally throughout the lung bases. The patient has a productive frothy cough. The examination of the extremities exhibits 4+ pitting edema of both hands and legs with the nail beds minimally cyanotic.

Immediately upon arrival to the emergency department, the patient received IV fluids and oxygen therapy. Blood is collected for initial laboratory data with the following abnormal results: serum sodium 128 mEq/L (normal 135–147 mEq/L), serum potassium 3.1 mEq/L (normal 3.5–5.2 mEq/L), and arterial blood gases on room air: pH 7.32, PaO_2 54, $PaCO_2$ 26, SaO_2 68%, indicating overall hypoxemia. Thelma is admitted to the intensive care with a diagnosis of heart failure. She will be receiving digitalization therapy.

Critical Thinking Questions

1. Discuss how each of the symptoms presented by the patient correlate with the condition of heart failure:
   - Irregular labored respirations
   - Neck vein distention
   - Scattered crackles throughout the lungs
   - 4+ pitting edema of both hands and legs
2. Describe how digoxin (Lanoxin) aids in treating heart failure.
3. What is digitalization?
4. What electrolyte imbalance must be corrected to avoid digoxin toxicity?

Case Study

Jim Mabry, a 77-year-old man, currently takes the following medications daily: digoxin (Lanoxin) 0.125 mg; furosemide (Lasix) 20 mg daily; and potassium supplementation (K-Dur) 20 mEq. As his nurse, you will be discussing Jim's medication regimen and his next health care provider office visit after discharge from the hospital.

1. Discuss the relationship among the three medications.
2. Jim will have a digoxin serum level collected during the health care provider office visit. What does he need to know about this procedure?
3. Jim asked you to compile a list of foods that are rich in potassium. Prepare the list.

NCLEX-RN® Review

1 Which of the following laboratory findings would cause the nurse to be concerned about digoxin (Lanoxin) toxicity?

1. Hypocalcemia
2. Hypermagnesemia
3. Hyperbilirubinemia
4. Hypokalemia

2 In providing the heart failure client with information prior to discharge, the nurse will discuss digoxin (Lanoxin) therapy. Which of the following would the nurse include in the client 's teaching?

1. Take the drug in the morning before rising.
2. Monitor the pulse daily prior to taking the drug.
3. Discontinue the drug if the pulse rate is 70 beats per minute.
4. Eat a diet high in bran fiber and calcium.

3 The nurse is evaluating the effects of a drug that causes a positive inotropic effect. The nurse knows that an agent with this property:

1. Increases the force of cardiac contractions.
2. Decreases the volume of the cardiac output.
3. Relaxes the myocardial muscle.
4. Inhibits cardiac irregularities.

4 The client is receiving milrinone (Primacor) infusion for heart failure. The nurse should monitor this client for:

1. Confusion and agitation.
2. Heart beat irregularities.
3. Tingling or cramping in the legs.
4. Brown discoloration in the skin creases.

5 The nurse is explaining the reason that angiotensin-converting enzyme (ACE) inhibitors are prescribed for heart failure to a group of clients in a cardiac rehabilitation session. The nurse's response is based on knowing that ACE inhibitors:

1. Slow the progression of heart failure and reduce mortality.
2. Reduce the incidence of renal toxicity associated with heart failure.
3. Impair coronary dilation and increase cardiac output.
4. Decrease the adrenergic effects that typically increase fatalities.

6 The nurse is caring for several clients with heart failure. Which of the following would the nurse consider appropriate pharmacologic therapy for a client with heart failure? (Select all that apply.)

1. Angiotensin-converting enzyme (ACE) inhibitors
2. Diuretics
3. Insulin therapy
4. Cardiac glycosides
5. Phosphodiesterase III inhibitors

See Answers to Critical Thinking Questions, Case Study, and NCLEX-RN® Review in Appendix A.

References

Albert, N. M. (2006). Evidence-based nursing care for patients with heart failure. *AACN Advanced Critical Care, 17*(2), 170–185.

Amabile, C. M., & Spencer, A. P. (2004). Keeping your patient with heart failure safe: A review of potentially dangerous medications. *Archives of Internal Medicine, 164*(7), 709–720.

American College of Cardiology/American Heart Association Task Force on Practice Guidelines. (2005). *ACC/AHA 2005 guideline update for the diagnosis and management of chronic heart failure in the adult.* A Report of the (Writing Committee to Update the 2001 Guidelines for the Evaluation and Management of Heart Failure). *Circulation, 112,* e154-e235. Retrieved October 9, 2008, from http://circ.ahajournals.org/cgi/content/full/112/12/e154

Ferrari, R., Merli, E., Cicchitelli, G., Mele, D., Fucili, A., & Ceconi, C. (2004). Therapeutic effects of l-carnitine and propionyl-l-carnitine on cardiovascular diseases: A review. *Annals New York Academy of Science, 1033*(12), 79–91.

Gislason, G. H., Rasmussen, J. N., Abildstrom, S. Z., Schramm, T. K., Hansen, M. L., Buch, P., et al. (2007). Persistent use of evidence-based pharmacotherapy in heart failure is associated with improved outcomes. *Circulation, 116*(10), 734–744.

Hudson, S., & Tabet, N. (2003). Acetyl-L-carnitine for dementia. *Cochrane Database of Systematic Reviews, Issue 2.* (Art. No. CD003158; DOI 10.1002/14651858.CD003158).

Kendler, B. S. (2006). Supplemental conditionally essential nutrients in cardiovascular disease therapy. *Journal of Cardiovascular Nursing, 21*(1), 9–16.

Lovlien, M., Schei, B., & Hole, T. (2006). Women with myocardial infarction are less likely than men to experience chest symptoms. *Scandinavian Cardiovascular Journal, 40*(6), 342–347.

McCarthy, P. M., & Young, J. B. (Eds.). (2007). *Heart failure: A combined medical and surgical approach.* Malden, MA: Blackwell.

National Coalition for Women with Heart Disease. (2008). *Women and heart disease fact sheet.* Retrieved July 14, 2008, from http://www.womenheart.org/information/women_and_heart_disease_fact_sheet.asp

Pauly, D. F. (2005). Cardiac function and heart failure. *Journal of the American College of Cardiology, 45*(11 Suppl B), 24B–29B.

Rocco, T. P., & Fang, J. C. (2006). Pharmacotherapy of congestive heart failure. In L. L. Brunton, J. S. Lazo, & K. L. Parker (Eds.), *The pharmacological basis of therapeutics* (11th ed., pp. 869–898). New York: McGraw-Hill.

Torpy, J. M., Lynm, C., & Glass, R. M. (2007). Heart failure. *Journal of the American Medical Association, 297*(22), 2548.

Tweed, V. (2006). Heart-warming nutrients. *Better Nutrition, 68*(9), 24–25.

Wagner, J. A. (2006). Top ten challenges in heart failure management. *Journal for Nurse Practitioners, 2*(8), 528–532.

Zevitz, M. E. (2006). *Heart failure.* eMedicine. Retrieved July 14, 2008, from http://www.emedicine.com/med/topic3552.htm

C H A P T E R

I will never forget the fear that overwhelmed me as I woke up in the emergency department. I had no idea what had happened. I only remember a strange sensation in my chest. It was like my heart was fluttering. Then I must have passed out.

Patient "Jada Chinn Nguyen"

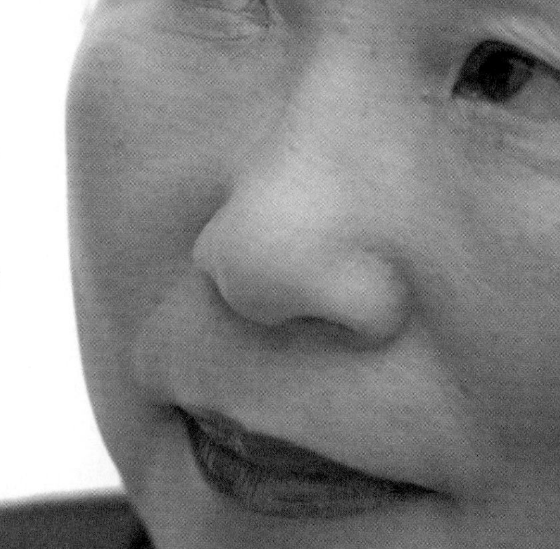

39 Pharmacotherapy of Dysrhythmias

Learning Outcomes

After reading this chapter, the student should be able to:

1. Identify disorders associated with an increased risk of dysrhythmias.
2. Explain how rhythm abnormalities can affect cardiac function.
3. Diagram a typical cardiac action potential and label the flow of potassium, sodium, and calcium ions during each phase.
4. Design a table that indicates the classification of dysrhythmias and the types of drugs used to treat them.
5. Describe general principles in the management of dysrhythmias.
6. Identify the primary mechanisms of action of antidysrhythmic drugs.
7. For each of the classes shown in the chapter outline, identify the prototype and representative drugs and explain the mechanism(s) of drug action, primary indications, contraindications, significant drug interactions, pregnancy category, and important adverse effects.
8. Use the nursing process to care for patients receiving drug therapy for dysrhythmias.

Chapter Outline

Etiology of Dysrhythmias

Phases and Measurement of the Cardiac Action Potential

Classification of Dysrhythmias

General Principles of Dysrhythmia Management

Drugs for Dysrhythmias

Sodium Channel Blockers: Class I

PROTOTYPE Procainamide (Procan SR, Pronestyl) *p. 630*

Beta-Adrenergic Antagonists: Class II

Potassium Channel Blockers: Class III

PROTOTYPE Amiodarone (Cordarone, Pacerone) *p. 634*

Calcium Channel Blockers: Class IV

Miscellaneous Antidysrhythmics

Key Terms

bradydysrhythmias, 625
cardioversion, 627
cinchonism, 632
defibrillation, 627
depolarization, 624
dysrhythmias, 623
electrocardiogram (ECG), 625
paroxysmal supraventricular tachycardia (PSVT), 626
polarized, 623
prodysrhythmic, 623
refractory period, 624
repolarization, 624
tachydysrhythmias, 626
threshold potential, 624
torsades de pointe, 627

Dysrhythmias are disorders of cardiac rhythm characterized by abnormal heart rate or irregular contractions. Also called arrhythmias, they encompass a number of different disorders that range from harmless to life threatening. Diagnosis is difficult and patients often must be connected to an electrocardiogram (ECG) and must be experiencing symptoms in order to determine the exact type of rhythm disorder. Proper diagnosis and optimum pharmacotherapy can significantly affect the frequency of dysrhythmias and their consequences.

PharmFACT

Although tachycardia in adults is usually defined as a heart rate greater than 100 beats/minute in adults, for pediatric patients the definition varies with age. The following are considered the normal ranges for heart rate:

- Newborns: 100 to 180 beats/minute
- Infants to 2 years: 80 to 130 beats/minute
- 2–6 years: 70 to 120 beats/minute
- 6–10 years: 70 to 110 beats/minute
- 10–16 years: 60 to 100 beats/minute *Source:* Ball & Bindler, 2006.

Etiology of Dysrhythmias

39.1 Some dysrhythmias produce no patient symptoms, while others may be life threatening.

Some dysrhythmias are asymptomatic and have no effect on cardiac function, while others require immediate treatment. Typical symptoms of dysrhythmias include dizziness, weakness, fatigue, decreased exercise tolerance, palpitations, dyspnea, and syncope. It is difficult to estimate the frequency of the disease, although it is likely that dysrhythmias are quite common in the population. Patients often wait until these symptoms occur more frequently or become acute before seeking medical intervention.

Dysrhythmias occur in all age groups, and in both healthy and diseased hearts. While the actual cause of most dysrhythmias is elusive, the majority are closely associated with certain conditions, primarily heart disease and myocardial infarction (MI): 90% of patients experiencing an MI will develop a dysrhythmia. Persistent dysrhythmias are associated with increased risk of cerebrovascular accident (CVA) and heart failure (HF), and severe dysrhythmias may result in sudden death. Conditions that promote the formation of cardiac rhythm abnormalities are called **prodysrhythmics.** Following are some of the diseases and conditions associated with dysrhythmias:

- Hypertension (HTN)
- Cardiac valve disease such as mitral stenosis
- Coronary artery disease (CAD)
- Low or high potassium levels in the blood
- Myocardial infarction (MI)
- Cerebrovascular accident (CVA)
- Diabetes mellitus
- Congestive heart failure (CHF)

In addition to the preceding list, a number of medications have been found to cause new dysrhythmias or worsen existing ones. Caution must be used when administering prodysrhythmic drugs to patients with preexisting cardiac impairment or who may have any of the above conditions. Table 39.1 lists selected drugs known to have prodysrhythmic properties.

Phases and Measurement of the Cardiac Action Potential

39.2 The phases of cardiac action potential include rapid depolarization, a long plateau, and repolarization.

Dysrhythmias are defects in the electrical properties of the heart. In some manner, the normal generation or conduction of the electrical impulse, or action potential, across the myocardium has been altered. Because antidysrhythmic drugs act by correcting or modifying impulse conduction, a firm grasp of cardiac electrical properties is essential for understanding drug mechanisms. Before proceeding, the student should review the normal pathway of impulse conduction in the heart presented in Section 31.6.

Action potentials occur in neurons and cardiac muscle cells due to the changes in the concentration of specific ions found inside and outside the cell. Under resting conditions, sodium ions (Na^+) and calcium ions (Ca^{2+}) are in higher concentrations outside of myocardial cells, while potassium ions (K^+) are found in higher concentration inside these cells. These imbalances are, in part, responsible for the inside of a myocardial cell membrane having a slightly negative charge (80 to 90 mV), relative to the outside of the membrane. A cell having this negative membrane potential is **polarized.**

TABLE 39.1 Selected Prodysrhythmic Drugs

Class of Medication	Example Drugs
Antidysrhythmic Drugs	amiodarone, disopyramide, dofetilide, flecainide, ibutilide, procainamide, propafenone, quinidine, sotalol
Autonomic Agents	atenolol, clonidine, methyldopa, nadolol, propranolol
Calcium Channel Blockers	diltiazem, nifedipine, verapamil
Cardiac Glycosides	digoxin
Miscellaneous Agents	amitriptyline, chloroquine, cimetidine, haloperidol, lithium carbonate, phenothiazines

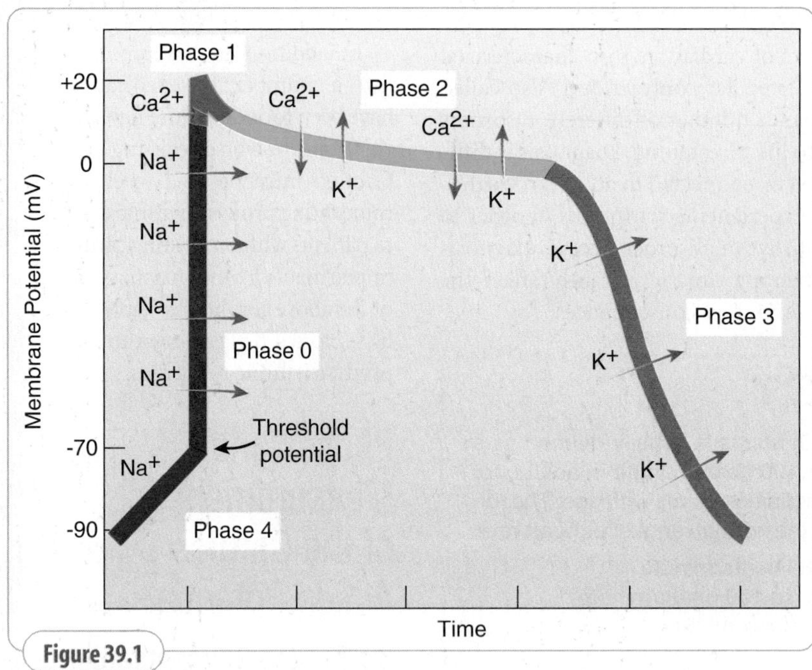

Figure 39.1

Phases of the myocardial action potential. Ion movements during each phase are shown.

An action potential illustrating the steps in electrical conduction is shown in Figure 39.1. The changes in ions, or fluxes, occurring during an action potential may be grouped into four phases.

Phase 4: It is easiest to begin with phase 4 because this is the period during which the cell is "resting" and the action potential has not yet occurred. Note in Figure 39.1, however, that during phase 4 the membrane potential is slowly increasing toward a potential that will trigger an action potential: the **threshold potential.** Sodium is slowly "leaking" into the cell during this period, causing the change in potential, which gives certain regions such as the sinoatrial (SA) node the property of automaticity, the ability to depolarize spontaneously, without input from the nervous system.

Phase 0: An action potential begins when the threshold potential is reached and gated sodium ion channels located in the plasma membrane become activated and open. Sodium ions rush into the cell producing a rapid **depolarization,** or loss of membrane potential. Because they open and close rapidly, these sodium channels are sometimes referred to as "fast" channels. During this period, Ca^{2+} also enters the cell through calcium ion channels, although the influx is slower than that of sodium. In cells located in the SA and atrioventricular (AV) nodes, it is the influx of Ca^{2+}, rather than Na^{+}, which generates the rapid depolarization of the membrane.

Phase 1: During depolarization, the inside of the plasma membrane temporarily reverses its charge, becoming positive. This is a brief, transient phase.

Phase 2: During phase 2, a plateau is reached in which depolarization is maintained. The entry of Ca^{2+} into the cells signals the release of additional calcium ions that had been held in storage inside the sarcoplasmic reticula. This large and sudden increase in intracellular Ca^{2+} is responsible for the contraction of cardiac muscle. Gated potassium ion channels open, causing an efflux of K^{+} from the cells. The plateau is maintained as long as the positive calcium ions entering the cell are balanced by the positive potassium ions leaving the cell. Action potentials in skeletal muscle lack this plateau phase.

Phase 3: During phase 3, the calcium channels close and additional potassium channels open, thus causing a net loss of positive ions from the cell. This **repolarization** returns the negative resting membrane potential to the cell.

MyNursingKit | Dysrhythmias Animation

The synchronized pumping action of the heart requires alternating periods of contraction and relaxation. There is a brief period of time following depolarization and most of repolarization, that the cell cannot initiate a subsequent action potential. This **refractory period** ensures that the myocardial cell finishes contracting before a second action potential begins.

While it may seem complicated to learn the different ions involved in an action potential, this is very important to cardiac pharmacology. Blocking potassium, sodium, or calcium ion channels is a pharmacologic strategy used to terminate or prevent dysrhythmias. In addition, the therapeutic effect of some antidysrhythmic agents is due to their prolongation of the refractory period. It is not possible to understand drug mechanisms without adequate knowledge of the normal electrical conduction properties of the heart. In general, most cardiac drugs:

- Increase impulse formation or automaticity
- Increase conduction velocity
- Increase both impulse formation or automaticity and conduction velocity

OR

- Decrease impulse formation or automaticity
- Decrease conduction velocity
- Decrease both impulse formation or automaticity and conduction

CONNECTION *Checkpoint* 39.1

From what you learned in Chapter 33, what are the three types of calcium channels? Which type is blocked by calcium channel blocker medications? See Answer to Connection Checkpoint 39.1 in Appendix A.

39.3 The electrocardiogram is used to measure electrical conduction across the myocardium.

The **electrocardiogram (ECG)** is a graphic recording of the wave of electrical conduction across the myocardium. The ECG is a primary tool in the diagnosis of dysrhythmias and other heart diseases. A normal ECG and its relationship to impulse conduction in the heart are shown in Figure 39.2.

Three distinct waves are produced by a normal ECG: the P wave, the QRS complex, and the T wave. Changes to the wave patterns or in their timing are associated with certain pathologies. The different classes of antidysrhythmic drugs also affect the ECG in characteristic manners. A summary of the different waves and their importance to cardiac physiology is shown in Table 39.2.

Classification of Dysrhythmias

39.4 Dysrhythmias are classified by the impulse origin and type of rhythm abnormality produced.

There are many types of dysrhythmias and classification is by a number of different methods. The two broad categories of rhythm abnormalities are those that affect impulse formation, and those that affect impulse conduction. Although a correct diagnosis of the type of dysrhythmia is sometimes difficult, it is essential for effective treatment.

Bradydysrhythmias are disorders characterized by a heart rate of less than 60 beats/minute. Bradysrhythmias are very common in older adults because the number of cells in the SA node declines progressively such that by age 75 about 90% of the cells are nonfunctional. Similar age-related changes occur

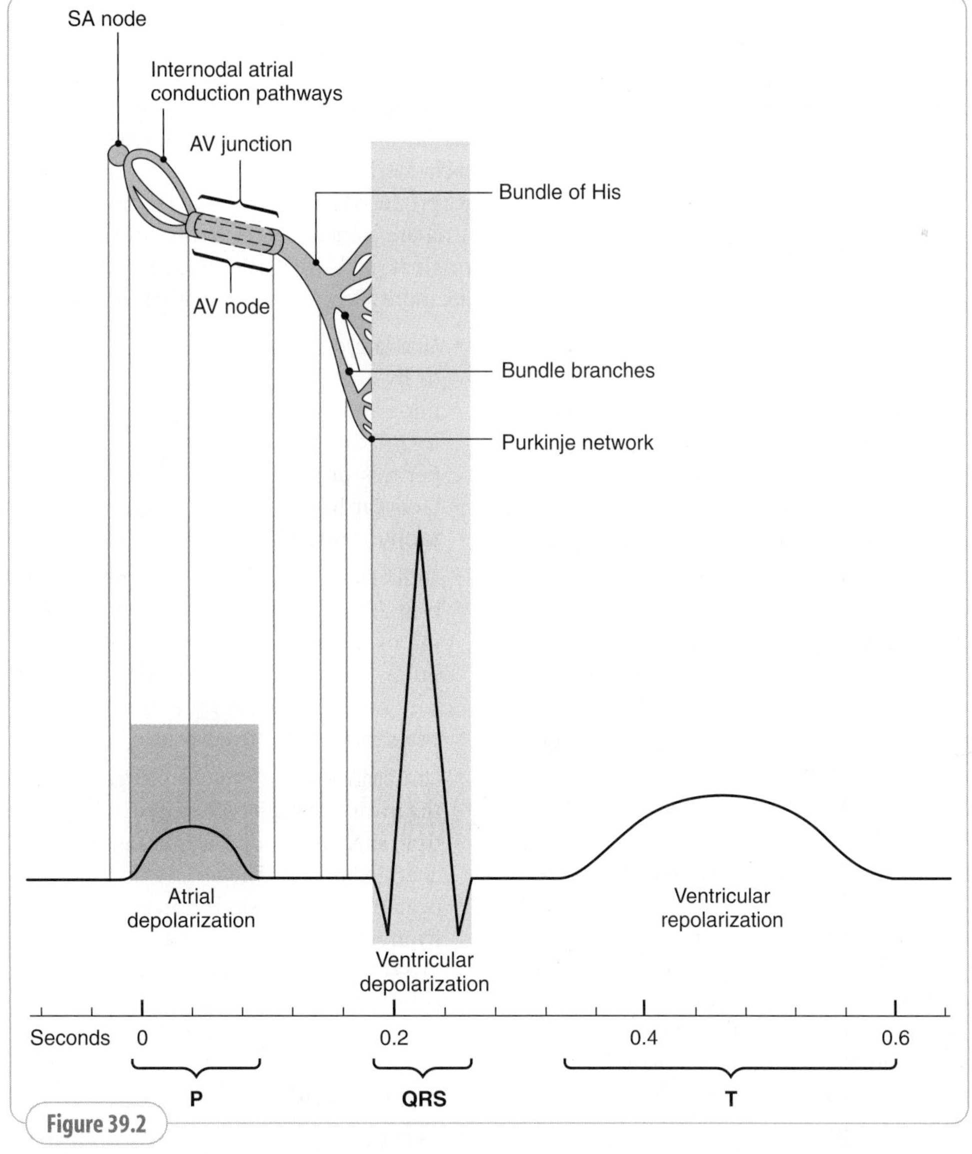

Figure 39.2

Relationship of the electrocardiogram to electrical conduction in the heart.

TABLE 39.2 ECG Waves and Intervals

Wave or Interval	Physiological Significance	Importance
P wave	Represents atrial depolarization.	A large P wave (voltage greater than 2.5 mm or 2 ½ small boxes) suggests the atria may be enlarged.
PQ segment	Represents the delay at the AV node; sometimes referred to as the PR segment.	This delay is vital so the ventricles can fill with blood. Prolonged PQ segments suggest slow or non-conducting fibrotic areas in the myocardium.
PQ interval	Represents all electrical activity prior to the impulse reaching the ventricles and contains the P wave and the PQ segment; Sometimes referred to as the PR interval.	Normal measurements range between 0.12–0.20 seconds. Slightly prolonged PQ intervals are common and considered harmless. More prolonged PQ intervals suggest a first degree heart block.
QRS complex	Represents ventricular depolarization.	An exaggerated R wave suggests enlargement of the ventricles. The QRS should not be longer than 0.11 seconds. Patients experiencing an MI may show QRS complexes that are abnormally high or that have extended durations.
T wave	Represents ventricular repolarization.	A flat T wave suggests ischemia to the myocardium.
ST segment	Represents the plateau phase of the action potential when the ventricles are depolarized.	Elevated ST segments are used to guide the pharmacotherapy of MI.
QT interval	Represents the time from the start of ventricular depolarization to the completion of ventricular repolarization.	Drugs that lengthen the QT interval have been linked to cardiac dysrhythmias, cardiac arrest, and sudden death. At the same time, prolongation of the action potential duration is a primary antidysrhythmic mechanism.

in the AV node, where normal cells progressively die and are replaced by fibrotic tissue. Bradydysrhythmias are the major indication for pacemaker implantation. Common bradydysrhythmias include the following:

- **Sinus bradycardia.** The most common slow heart rhythm. Sinus bradycardia generally does not require treatment unless the patient is experiencing syncope or dizziness due to lack of sufficient blood flow to the brain, or if the heart rate fails to increase during periods of exertion.
- **Sinoatrial node dysfunction (sick sinus syndrome).** The SA node fails to generate or transmit sufficient electrical impulses. Patients with this condition may experience severe bradycardia (less than 40 beats/minute resting), failure of the heart rate to increase with exercise, or significant sinus "pauses." Severe episodes of bradycardia may alternate with periods of abnormally rapid heart rates.
- **Atrioventricular conduction block.** The AV node fails to conduct impulses to the rest of the myocardium. AV blocks are classified by degree. In first-degree AV block, the AV node conducts the impulse slowly, and conduction is delayed but not prevented. In second-degree AV block, some, but not all, impulses are prevented (blocked) from leaving the AV node. Second-degree AV block results in nonconducted P waves. A third-degree AV block results in total stoppage of impulses through the AV node. None of the impulses originating in the atria can make their way through the block into the ventricles. Second- and third-degree blocks require pharmacotherapy or the insertion of a temporary or permanent pacemaker. Some AV blocks are temporary in origin, and can be due to cardiac drug toxicity. Any drug that slows AV conduction can cause a temporary form of AV block.

MyNursingKit | Childhood Dysrhythmias

Tachydysrhythmias are disorders exhibiting a heart rate greater than 100 beats/minute. The incidence of tachydysrhythmias increases in older adults and in patients with preexisting cardiovascular disease. The simplest method for categorizing tachydysrhythmias is according to the type of rhythm abnormality produced and its location. Dysrhythmias that originate in the atria are sometimes referred to as supraventricular. Those that originate in the ventricles are generally more serious because they are more likely to interfere with the normal function of the heart.

- **Atrial tachycardia.** May be caused by a rapidly firing SA node or by an ectopic focus in the atria that suppresses the SA node and establishes a rapid heart rate, often between 160 to 200 beats/minute. When these episodes alternate with periods of normal rhythm, it is called paroxysmal atrial tachycardia (PAT), or **paroxysmal supraventricular tachycardia (PSVT).**
- **Atrial flutter.** A rapid, regular heartbeat in which the atria may beat 250 to 350 times per minute. During atrial flutter, the job of the AV node is to selectively block some of the impulses coming from the atria, so the ventricular rate (pulse) is 125 to 175 beats/minute (usually two, three, or four atrial beats for each ventricular beat).
- **Atrial fibrillation.** A complete disorganization of rhythm, this is the most common type of dysrhythmia. It is caused by multiple sites of impulse formation in the atria, all firing in a chaotic fashion. The atrial rate can range from 300 to 600 beats/minute, causing an irregular ventricular rate ranging from 50 to 200 beats/minute. The rapid atrial rate causes a loss of organized atrial contraction, and results in quivering (fibrillation). This lack of contraction causes blood to lie dormant in parts of the atria and may give rise to clots. Because of the potential for clot formation, atrial fibrillation is a leading risk factor for stroke.
- **Ventricular tachycardia.** Usually recognized by regular, rapid, wide beats with a ventricular rate of 100 to 200 beats/minute.

Patients with sustained or symptomatic ventricular tachycardia must be treated immediately because this condition is associated with a high risk of sudden death. **Torsades de pointe** is a specific type of ventricular tachycardia that is characterized by rates between 200 and 250 beats/minute and "twisting of the points" of the QRS complex on the ECG.

- **Ventricular fibrillation.** A complete disorganization of rhythm in which the ventricles pump little or no blood, quickly starving the tissues of oxygen. Ventricular fibrillation is now considered cardiac arrest.

> **CONNECTIONS**
>
> **To the Community**
>
> **Dysrhythmias and Diet**
>
> Patients with dysrhythmias may benefit from education about certain foods that can increase cardiac problems. Basically, the patient should avoid foods and beverages that trigger an irregular heartbeat and should eat a healthy low-salt, low-fat diet. Alcohol, such as beer, wine, or hard liquor, can trigger dysrhythmias in some patients; atrial fibrillation can occur after an alcohol binge. Because food and drinks with caffeine can trigger this reaction as well, the nurse should advise the patient to avoid drinks such as coffee, tea, and some soft beverages, as well as chocolate. Another caution comes with herbal remedies, especially substances used to improve sports performance. In short, teach the patient to avoid salt and excessive fluids while eating a healthy, well-balanced diet.

General Principles of Dysrhythmia Management

39.5 Antidysrhythmic drugs are only used when there is a clear benefit to the patient.

Some antidysrhythmic drugs have the potential to produce serious adverse effects. The very drugs used to treat dysrhythmias may actually worsen or create new dysrhythmias. Furthermore, research suggests that mortality may actually increase when some of these drugs are used to treat or prevent dysrhythmias. The following guidelines are used in the management of the patient with dysrhythmias.

Asymptomatic dysrhythmias: Research has shown little or no benefit to the patient in treating asymptomatic dysrhythmias with medications. Antidysrhythmic drugs are normally reserved for patients experiencing overt symptoms or for those whose condition cannot be controlled by other means.

Acute dysrhythmias: Some types of dysrhythmias are very serious and may be life threatening. In these cases, pharmacotherapy or cardioversion is warranted. For example, ventricular dysrhythmias often interfere with cardiac output and have greater potential for harm than atrial dysrhythmias. Dysrhythmias that are sustained may worsen and affect cardiac function. Several antidysrhythmics available by the intravenous (IV) route have an immediate onset of action to terminate life-threatening dysrhythmias.

Prophylaxis of dysrhythmias: Patients who are afflicted with recurring dysrhythmias or who have a comorbid condition, such as preexisting heart disease, may benefit from prophylactic therapy with antidysrhythmics. These patients should be monitored regularly to assess for prodysrhythmic effects from the drugs. Drug combinations that have the potential to prolong the QT interval are avoided and doses are kept as low as possible to minimize risk. Prophylactic therapy should only be initiated for high-risk patients.

Nonpharmacologic treatment: Serious types of dysrhythmias are corrected through electrical shock of the heart, a treatment called **cardioversion** or **defibrillation.** The electrical shock momentarily stops all electrical impulses in the heart, both normal and abnormal. Under ideal conditions, the temporary cessation of electrical activity will allow the SA node to automatically return conduction to a normal sinus rhythm.

Other types of nonpharmacologic treatment include identification and destruction of the myocardial cells responsible for the abnormal conduction through a surgical procedure called catheter ablation. Cardiac pacemakers are sometimes inserted to correct the types of dysrhythmias that cause the heart to beat too slowly. Implantable cardioverter defibrillators (ICDs) are placed in a patient to restore normal rhythm by either pacing the heart or giving it an electric shock when dysrhythmias occur. In addition, the ICD is capable of storing information regarding the heart rhythm for the health care provider to evaluate.

Drugs for Dysrhythmias

39.6 Antidysrhythmic drugs are classified by their mechanism of action.

The therapeutic goals of antidysrhythmic pharmacotherapy are to terminate existing dysrhythmias or to prevent abnormal rhythms for the purpose of reducing the risks of sudden death, CVA, or other complications resulting from the disease. Antidysrhythmic drugs act by altering specific electrophysiologic properties of the heart. They do this through two basic mechanisms: blocking flow through ion channels (conduction) or altering autonomic activity (automaticity).

The most common method of classifying antidysrhythmic drugs is called the Vaughan Williams classification, which was begun in 1985. This classification scheme groups drugs as Classes I, II, III, and IV based on the stage they affect the action potential. A fifth group includes miscellaneous drugs not acting by one of the first four mechanisms. Although widely used, the Vaughan Williams classification method is simplistic because some of these drugs act by more than one mechanism and the drugs within each class have unique properties that distinguish them from each other. For example, the Class I drugs have three subclasses. The categories of antidysrhythmics and their mechanisms are shown in Table 39.3.

The use of antidysrhythmic drugs has significantly declined in recent years. The reason for this decline is that research studies determined that the use of antidysrhythmic medications for prophylaxis can actually increase patient mortality. Drugs affecting cardiac electrophysiology have a narrow margin of

TABLE 39.3 Classification of Antidysrhythmics

Class	Actions	Primary Indications
I: Sodium Channel Blockers		
IA Example: quinidine	Delays repolarization; slows conduction velocity; increases duration of the action potential	Atrial fibrillation, premature atrial contractions, premature ventricular contractions, tachycardia
IB Example: lidocaine	Accelerates repolarization; slows conduction velocity; decreases duration of action potential	Severe ventricular dysrhythmias
IC Example: flecainide	No significant effect on repolarization; slows conduction velocity	Severe ventricular dysrhythmias
II: Beta-Adrenergic Blockers		
Example: propranolol	Slows conduction velocity; decreases automaticity; prolongs refractory period	Atrial flutter and fibrillation, tachydysrhythmias, ventricular dysrhythmias
III: Drugs That Slow Repolarization		
Example: amiodarone	Slows repolarization; increases duration of action potential; prolongs refractory period	Severe atrial and ventricular dysrhythmias
IV: Calcium Channel Blockers		
Example: verapamil	Slows conduction velocity; decreases contractility; prolongs refractory period	Paroxysmal supraventricular tachycardia, supraventricular tachydysrhythmias

safety between a therapeutic effect and a toxic effect. They not only have the ability to correct dysrhythmias, but also to worsen or even create new dysrhythmias. These prodysrhythmic effects have resulted in less use of drugs in Class I; however, drugs in Class II and Class III (specifically amiodarone) have increased in usage.

Another reason for the decline in antidysrhythmic drug use is the success of nonpharmacologic techniques. Catheter ablation and implantable defibrillators are more successful in managing many types of dysrhythmias than is the prophylactic use of medications.

Sodium Channel Blockers: Class I

39.7 Class I antidysrhythmics act by blocking ion channels in myocardial cells.

Sodium channel blockers, the Class I drugs, are the largest group of antidysrhythmics. They are further divided into three subgroups (IA, IB, and IC) based on subtle differences in their mechanisms of action. Because initiation of the action potential is dependent upon the opening of gated sodium ion channels, a blockade of these channels will prevent depolarization of the myocardium. The spread of the action potential will slow, and areas of ectopic pacemaker activity will be suppressed. The sodium channel blockers are shown in Table 39.4 and Figure 39.3.

The sodium channel blockers are similar in structure and action to local anesthetics. In fact, the Class I antidysrhythmic lidocaine is a prototype local anesthetic in Chapter 30. This anesthetic-like action slows impulse conduction across the heart. Some, such as quinidine and procainamide, are effective against many types of dysrhythmias. The remaining Class I drugs are more specific, and indicated only for life-threatening ventricular dysrhythmias.

The adverse effects of the sodium blockers vary with each individual drug. All these agents can cause new dysrhythmias or worsen existing ones. The slowing of the heart rate can cause hypotension, dizziness, and fainting. During pharmacotherapy, the ECG should be monitored for signs of cardiotoxicity, such as increases in the PR and QT intervals and widening of the QRS complex. Some Class I drugs have significant anticholinergic adverse effects such as dry mouth, constipation, and urinary retention. Special precautions should be taken with older adults, as anticholinergic adverse effects may worsen urinary hesitancy in men with prostate enlargement.

Class IA: The class IA antidysrhythmics include quinidine (Quinidex, others), disopyramide (Norpace), and procainamide (Procan SR, Pronestyl). Although quinidine is the oldest and best known Class IA drug, procainamide is the prototype because it has been more widely used than quinidine in recent decades. All are available by the oral (PO) route and act by blocking sodium ion channels during phase 0 of the action potential.

The primary action responsible for the antidysrhythmic effects of the Class IA drugs is a slowing of conduction velocity. These agents also inhibit potassium channels, which delays repolarization and increases the refractory period. Subsequent action potentials must wait slightly longer before triggering the next electrical impulse. These actions allow the Class IA drugs to inhibit the formation of ectopic foci in both the atria and ventricles.

The effects of the Class IA agents can be recognized on the ECG. The QRS complex widens, owing to the slowed depolarization of the ventricles. The QT interval is increased due to the delay in repolarization of the ventricles.

TABLE 39.4 Antidysrhythmic Drugs

Drug	Route and Adult Dose (maximum dose where indicated)	Adverse Effects
Class IA: Sodium Channel Blockers		
disopyramide (Norpace)	PO: 100–200 mg qid (max: 1,200–1,600 mg/day)	*Nausea, vomiting, diarrhea, dry mouth, urinary retention, cinchonism (quinidine), anorexia, rash, photosensitivity* <u>May produce new dysrhythmias or worsen existing ones; hypotension, torsades de pointes, blood dyscrasias (quinidine), hepatotoxicity (quinidine), lupus (procainamide)</u>
procainamide (Pronestyl, others)	PO: 1 g loading dose followed by 250–500 mg every 3 h	
quinidine gluconate	PO: 200–600 mg tid qid (max: 3–4 g/day) IV: 0.25 mg/kg/min (max: 5-10 mg/kg)	
quinidine sulfate	PO: 200–400 mg tid qid (max: 3–4 g/day). Therapeutic serum drug level is 2–5 mcg/mL	
Class IB: Sodium Channel Blockers		
lidocaine (Xylocaine)	IV: 1–4 mg/min infusion (max: 3 mg/kg per 5–10 min)	*Nausea, vomiting, drowsiness, dizziness, lethargy, confusion (phenytoin)* <u>May produce new dysrhythmias or worsen existing ones; hypotension, bradycardia, CNS toxicity (lidocaine), malignant hyperthermia (lidocaine), cardiac arrest (lidocaine), status epilepticus if abruptly withdrawn (phenytoin), blood dyscrasias (phenytoin)</u>
mexiletine (Mexitil)	PO: 200–300 mg tid (max: 1,200 mg/day)	
phenytoin (Dilantin phenytek)	IV: 50–100 mg every 10–15 min until dysrhythmia is terminated (max: 1 g/day) PO: 100–200 mg tid (max: 625 mg/day)	
Class IC: Sodium Channel Blockers		
flecainide (Tambocor)	PO: 100 mg bid; increase by 50 mg bid every 4 days (max: 400 mg/day)	*Nausea, vomiting, fatigue, dizziness, headache, visual disturbances (flecainide)* <u>May produce new dysrhythmias or worsen existing ones; hypotension, bradycardia, cardiac arrest (flecainide), lupus (propafenone), HF (propafenone)</u>
propafenone (Rythmol)	PO: 150–300 mg tid (max: 900 mg/day)	
Class II: Beta-Adrenergic Antagonists		
acebutolol (Sectral)	PO: 200–600 mg bid tid (max: 1,200 mg/day)	*Fatigue, insomnia, drowsiness, impotence, decreased libido, dizziness, bradycardia, confusion* <u>Agranulocytosis, HF, bronchospasm, hypotension, Stevens–Johnson syndrome, anaphylaxis; if the drug is abruptly withdrawn, palpitations, rebound HTN, life-threatening dysrhythmias, or myocardial ischemia may occur</u>
esmolol (Brevibloc)	IV: 500 mcg/kg/min loading dose; maintenance dose 50–300 mcg/kg/min (maintenance max: 200 mcg/kg/min)	
propranolol (Inderal)	PO: 10–30 mg 3–4 times daily (max: 480 mg/day) IV: 0.5–3.1 mg every 4 h or prn	
Class III: Potassium Channel Blockers		
amiodarone (Cordarone, Pacerone)	PO: 400–600 mg/day in 1–2 divided doses (max: 1,600 mg/day as loading dose)	*Blurred vision (amiodarone), photosensitivity, nausea, vomiting, anorexia* <u>May produce new dysrhythmias or worsen existing ones; hypotension, HF, heart block, bradycardia, pneumonia-like syndrome (amiodarone), angioedema (dofetilide), CNS toxicity (ibutilide)</u>
dofetilide (Tikosyn)	PO: 125–500 mcg bid based on creatinine clearance	
ibutilide (Corvert)	IV: 1 mg infused over 10 min (for patients over 60 kg); 0.01 mg/kg (for patients under 60 kg); (max: 2 mg infused over at least 20 min)	
sotalol* (Betapace, Betapace AF, Sorine)	PO: 80 mg bid (max: 320 mg/day)	
Class IV: Calcium Channel Blockers		
diltiazem (Cardizem, Dilacor XR, Others)	IV: 5–10 mg/h continuous infusion for a maximum of 24 h (max: 15 mg/h)	*Flushed skin, headache, dizziness, peripheral edema, light-headedness, nausea, diarrhea, syncope* <u>Hepatotoxicity, MI, CHF, confusion, mood changes, hypotension</u>
verapamil (Calan, Isoptin, Others)	PO: 240–480 mg/day in divided doses; 5–10 mg IV direct over 2 min, may repeat in 15–30 min	
Miscellaneous Antidysrhythmics		
adenosine (Adenocard, Adenoscan)	IV: 6–12 mg given as a bolus injection every 1–2 min as needed (max: 12 mg/dose)	*Facial flushing, dyspnea, headache* <u>May produce new dysrhythmias or worsen existing ones, AV block</u>
digoxin (Digitek, Lanoxin, Lanoxicaps)	PO: 0.125–0.5 mg 4 times daily Therapeutic serum drug level: 0.8–2 ng/mL	*Nausea, vomiting, headache, diarrhea, visual disturbances* <u>May produce new dysrhythmias or worsen existing ones</u>

Note: *Italics* indicate common adverse effects. <u>Underline</u> indicates serious adverse effects.

*Sotalol is a beta blocker, but because its cardiac effects are more similar to amiodarone, it is considered in Class III. Adverse effects are those of Class II and Class III.

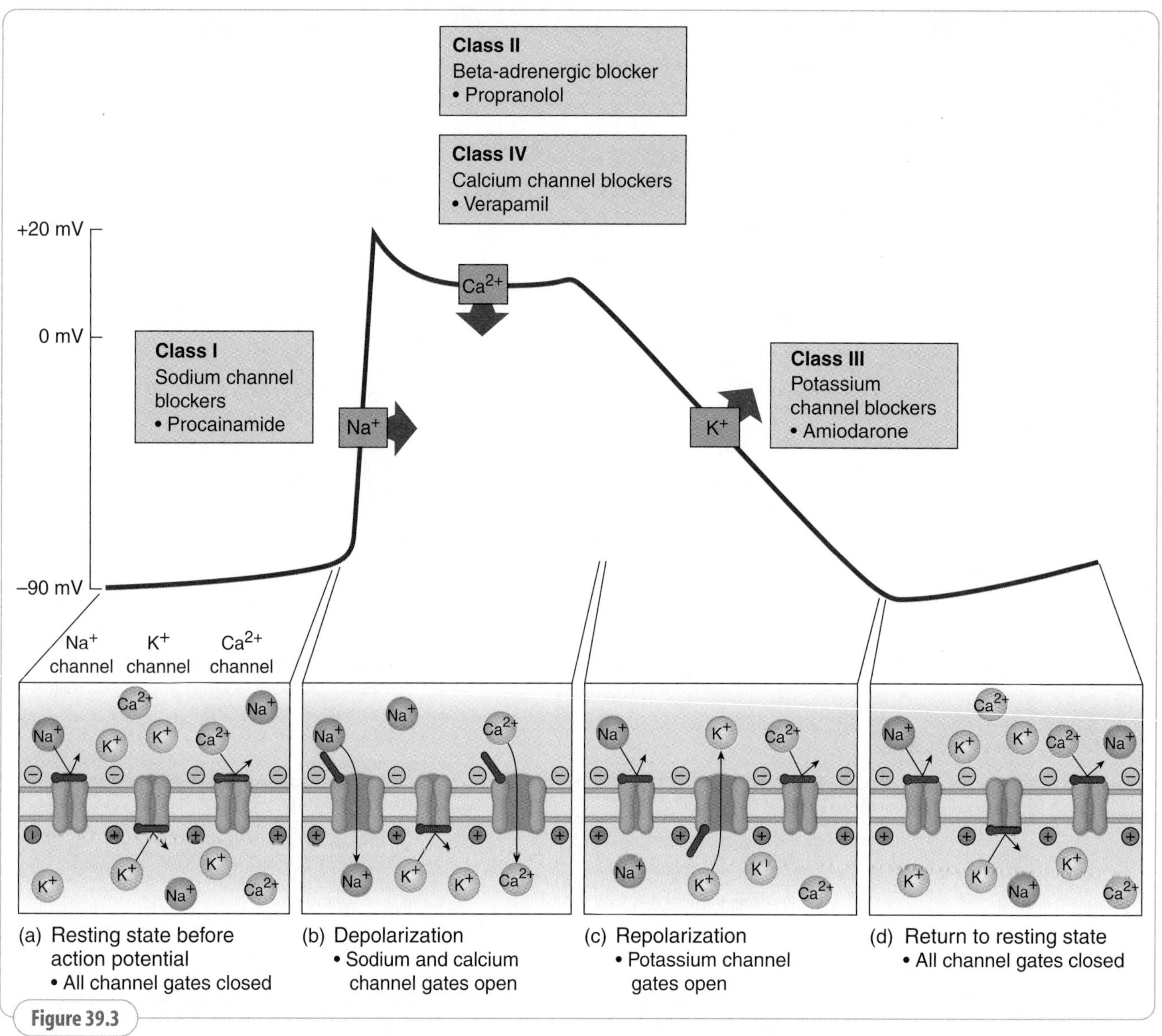

Figure 39.3

Ion channels in myocardial cells: (a) resting state before action potential (all channel gates closed); (b) depolarization (sodium and calcium channel gates open); (c) repolarization (potassium channel gates open); (d) return to resting state (all channel gates closed).

PROTOTYPE DRUG Procainamide (Procan SR, Pronestyl)

Classification: **Therapeutic:** Antidysrhythmic, Class IA
Pharmacologic: Sodium channel blocker

Therapeutic Effects and Uses: Approved in 1950, procainamide is a broad-spectrum antidysrhythmic chemically related to the local anesthetic procaine that has the ability to correct many different types of atrial and ventricular dysrhythmias. Indications include ventricular tachycardia during cardiopulmonary resuscitation (CPR); refractory ventricular fibrillation or pulseless ventricular tachycardia during CPR; conversion to sinus rhythm in patients with paroxysmal atrial tachycardia, atrial flutter, or atrial fibrillation; and treatment or prophylaxis of PSVT. Procainamide is now considered a drug of "last choice" for advanced cardiac life support due to its toxicity; it is used when other drugs have failed to reverse a severe dysrhythmia. The major hepatic metabolite of the drug, N-acetyl procainamide, also has antidysrhythmic activity. Because the rate of acetylation to the active metabolite is genetically determined, "slow acetylators" and "fast acetylators" will require adjustments in dosages to obtain optimum therapeutic results.

Procainamide is available in capsule, extended-release tablet, IV, and intramuscular (IM) formulations. The most common dosage form is the extended-release tablet because it allows for twice-daily dosing. Dosage is guided by periodic serum drug levels, which are maintained between 4 and 8 mcg/mL. The supine position should be used during IV administration because severe hypotension may occur during the infusion. Use of procainamide must be terminated if the QRS widens more that 50% of its original width.

Mechanism of Action: Procainamide blocks sodium ion channels in myocardial cells, thus reducing automaticity and slowing the velocity of the action potential across the myocardium.

This slight delay in conduction velocity prolongs the refractory period and can suppress dysrhythmias.

Pharmacokinetics:

Route(s)	PO, IV, and IM (if other routes are not possible)
Absorption	Readily absorbed
Distribution	Widely distributed; crosses the placenta; secreted in breast milk; 15% bound to plasma protein
Primary metabolism	Hepatic; metabolized to active metabolite
Primary excretion	Renal, 50–70% unchanged
Onset of action	PO: 30 minutes; IV: Immediate
Duration of action	3–4 h (sustained release tablets: 8–12 h); half-life: 3 h

Adverse Effects: Procainamide has a narrow therapeutic index and dosage must be monitored carefully to avoid serious adverse effects. Nausea, vomiting, abdominal pain, and headache are common during therapy. The drug can cause fever, accompanied by anorexia, weakness, nausea, and vomiting. High doses may produce central nervous system (CNS) effects such as confusion or psychosis. Like all antidysrhythmic drugs, procainamide has the ability to produce new dysrhythmias or worsen existing ones. Rapid IV administration of procainamide can cause severe hypotension. A lupus-like syndrome may occur in 30% to 50% of patients taking the drug over a year, including an increased titer of antinuclear antibodies (ANA).

Contraindications/Precautions: Procainamide is contraindicated in patients with second- or third-degree AV block (unless controlled by a pacemaker), severe HF, peripheral neuropathy, and myasthenia gravis. Because procainamide may activate or worsen lupus, the drug is only used in these patients when there is no safer alternative. Doses must be lowered in patients with renal impairment due to possible accumulation of the drug. Patients in shock or with severe hypotension should not receive this drug due to additive hypotension. Procainamide may worsen blood dyscrasias; thus, it should be used with caution in patients with preexisting bone marrow suppression.

Drug Interactions: Additive cardiac depressant effects may occur if procainamide is administered with other antidysrhythmics. Additive anticholinergic adverse effects will occur if procainamide is used concurrently with anticholinergic agents. Procainamide may increase plasma levels of amiodarone or quinidine. Use with antihypertensives may result in hypotension. **Herbal/Food:** Although no interactions have been well documented, the use of all herbal products or supplements should be avoided unless approved by the health care provider due to the toxicity of the drug.

Pregnancy: Category C.

Treatment of Overdose: No specific therapy is available for overdose. Supportive treatment is targeted to reversing hypotension with vasopressors and preventing or treating procainamide-induced dysrhythmias.

Nursing Responsibilities:

- Check apical and radial pulses before each dose during period of adjustment to the oral route. Withhold the medication and notify the prescriber if heart rate is less than 50 beats/minute.
- Provide continuous monitoring of ECG and blood pressure during IV administration.
- Assess for adverse effects such as fever, chills, urticaria, nausea, vomiting, psychoses, rapid drop in blood pressure, or polyarthralgia.
- Discontinue the IV drug temporarily when any of these occur: interrupted dysrhythmia, toxic adverse adverse effects, QRS complex widened greater than 50%, prolonged PR interval, or a drop in blood pressure of 15 mmHg or more. Document incidence with ECG (rhythm strip) and notify the prescriber.
- Assess for severe heart, liver, or kidney disease and hypotension because these conditions place a patient at risk for adverse effects.
- Report complaints of chest pain, dyspnea, and anxiety to the prescriber, as these may indicate a pulmonary embolus.
- Note that ventricular dysrhythmias will respond within a few minutes after an IV dose and within 1 hour after PO or IM drug administration.
- Monitor for therapeutic drug blood levels normally reached in 24 hours but delayed in the presence of renal dysfunction.
- Administer PO medication whole and with a full glass of water.

Patient and Family Education:

- Immediately report wheezing, chest pain, fever, sore throat or mouth, infection, excessive bruising or bleeding, fainting, hallucinations, severe dizziness, dark urine, or irregular heartbeat.
- Record weight at the same time each week and report a weight gain of 2 or more pounds with swelling in extremities to the health care provider.
- Do not drive or perform other hazardous activities until the effects of the drug are known because this drug may cause drowsiness or dizziness.
- Monitor pulse rates and report any changes to the health care provider.
- Avoid alcohol use when taking this drug.
- Report signs of reduced medication effectiveness such as weakness, irregular pulse, palpitations, chest pain, unexplained fatigue, or anxiety to the health care provider.
- Do not double the dose when a previous dose is missed. Medication should be taken around the clock in evenly spaced doses.
- Do not take any other prescription or nonprescription drugs, dietary supplements, or herbal products without approval of the health care provider.
- Carry identification (medic alert) and information about medication at all times.
- Attend all follow-up visits to the health care provider when taking this drug.

Drugs Similar to Procainamide (Procan SR, Pronestyl)

There are similar Class IA, IB, and IC antidysrhythmics. Other Class IA antidysrhythmics include quinidine and disopyramide.

Quinidine: Approved in 1938, quinidine is the oldest antidysrhythmic drug, originally obtained as a natural substance from the bark of the South American Cinchona tree. Like procainamide, quinidine is a broad-spectrum drug having the ability to correct many different types of atrial and ventricular dysrhythmias. The two salts of quinidine are sulfate which is given PO, and gluconate which is given PO and IV. Like other drugs in this class, quinidine blocks sodium ion channels in myocardial cells, thus reducing automaticity and slowing the velocity of the action potential across the myocardium. In addition to dysrhythmias, quinidine gluconate may be used to treat malaria and persistent hiccups. The most common adverse effect of quinidine is diarrhea, which occurs in approximately one third of patients, and may be intense. The drug can induce various types of dysrhythmias when serum levels rise above normal. High doses result in a syndrome called **cinchonism** with symptoms such as tinnitus, headache, blurred vision, hearing loss, and dysrhythmias. These symptoms are reversible once the drug is discontinued. Quinidine is contraindicated in patients with incomplete AV block because it can induce total blockage of conduction. This drug is pregnancy category C.

Disopyramide (Norpace): Approved in 1977, disopyramide has actions and indications similar to other Class IA agents. Available only by the PO route, the drug is used infrequently due to a high incidence of anticholinergic effects such as xerostomia and urinary retention in patients with benign prostatic hyperplasia. The anticholinergic effects cause an increase in heart rate, which may directly cancel out the therapeutic cardiac depressant effects of the drug. Disopyramide may worsen dysrhythmias or create new ones. Because of its toxicity, the use of disopyramide is usually restricted to patients with life-threatening dysrhythmias such as sustained ventricular tachycardia. Off-label uses include maintenance of, or conversion to, sinus rhythm in patients with atrial flutter or atrial fibrillation. This drug is pregnancy category C.

Class IB: The class IB antidysrhythmics include lidocaine, mexiletine, and phenytoin. Like other Class I drugs, these agents act by blocking gated sodium ion channels in cardiac muscle cells. Unlike the Class IA drugs, the Class IB agents shorten the refractory period and have little effect on conduction velocity. The Class IB drugs have minimal effects on the ECG and their primary indication is ventricular dysrhythmias. A fourth drug in this class, tocainide, was discontinued in 2003 due to a high incidence of adverse effects.

Lidocaine (Xylocaine): Lidocaine, the most frequently prescribed Class IB antidysrhythmic, was featured as a prototype local anesthetic in Chapter 30. It is an important treatment for life-threatening ventricular dysrhythmia, although amiodarone is sometimes considered the drug of choice for this indication. It is not effective in preventing or treating atrial dysrhythmias. Lidocaine decreases the refractory period of the action potential, especially in ischemic myocardial tissue. For acute conditions, lidocaine is administered by IV bolus or infusion; it is rarely given by the IM or subcutaneous routes. Serum lidocaine levels may be monitored and should be between 2 to 6 mcg/mL. The first signs of lidocaine toxicity usually involve the CNS and include confusion, anxiety, tremors, and paresthesias. As doses increase, the patient may become comatose and experience seizures or respiratory arrest. The correct lidocaine formulation must be used for IV infusions: local anesthetic lidocaine preparations may contain preservatives and epinephrine. This drug is pregnancy category B.

Mexiletine (Mexitil): Approved in 1985, mexiletine is chemically similar to lidocaine, has local anesthetic properties, and is used only for serious ventricular dysrhythmias. Mexiletine, however, is well absorbed orally. An off-label indication is for the treatment of neuropathic pain. The most common adverse effects are nausea and vomiting. CNS effects such as dizziness, tremor, and ataxia are common. Less common, though potentially serious adverse effects include blood dyscrasias, pulmonary fibrosis, and worsening of HF. The target range for serum mexiletine concentration is 0.5 to 2 mcg/mL. This drug is pregnancy category C.

Phenytoin (Dilantin): The primary use for phenytoin is to treat seizures, and it was presented in Chapter 26 as a prototype antiseizure medication. As an antidysrhythmic, phenytoin may be administered by the oral or IV routes. IV phenytoin must be pushed extremely slowly: 100 mg over 5 minutes. Phenytoin is rarely used for its antidysrhythmic properties and is not approved by the United States Food and Drug Administration (FDA) for this purpose. Historically, it has been used to treat dysrhythmias secondary to digoxin (Lanoxin) toxicity. If used for dysrhythmias, serum phenytoin levels should be carefully monitored to be 10 to 20 mcg/mL because the drug can have multiple serious adverse effects, including seizures, ataxia, coma, blood dyscrasias, and hepatotoxicity. This drug is pregnancy category D.

Class IC: The Class IC antidysrhythmics include two drugs: flecainide and propafenone. Like other Class agents, these drugs block gated sodium ion channels in cardiac muscle cells. The Class IC antidysrhythmics profoundly decrease conduction velocity. Thus the PR, QRS, and QT intervals are often prolonged. The refractory period may be shortened slightly, but is mostly unchanged by the Class IC drugs. Their primary indication is for life-threatening atrial dysrhythmias, although they can also prevent ventricular dysrhythmias. Research has shown these drugs to have a pronounced prodysrhythmic effect that has the potential to increase mortality in patients who have suffered a recent MI.

Flecainide (Tambocor): Flecainide is an oral drug used primarily to treat or prevent paroxysmal atrial fibrillation or atrial flutter due to its ability to markedly decrease conduction velocity. Unfortunately, the prodysrhythmic effects of the drug may generate new ventricular dysrhythmias in about 10% of the patients. It is indicated for the prophylaxis of life-threatening ventricular dysrhythmias, although it is rarely used for this purpose. The drug is contraindicated in patients with left ventricular dysfunction or who have experienced a recent MI. Serum flecainide

CONNECTIONS

Treating the Diverse Patient

Asian Patients' Sensitivity to Propranolol

Growing evidence from research studies has shown a differential drug response to propranolol among Asian Americans. These individuals typically lack a specific enzyme (mephenytoin hydroxylase) that is needed to metabolize propranolol. Because of this sensitivity to propranolol, the drug has a significantly greater effect on heart rate. In other words, individuals of Asian descent will develop signs of toxicity more quickly than non-Asians. The nurse should assess this population for signs and symptoms of early drug toxicity, possible overdosage, and adverse reactions due to high drug levels. Assessing for unique cultural sensitivity to drug therapies is necessary for safe drug administration of pharmacologic agents.

levels should be monitored, especially in patients with renal or hepatic impairment, and maintained between 0.2 to 1 mcg/mL. Other adverse effects include dizziness, headache, asthenia, tremor, and malaise. This drug is pregnancy category C.

Propafenone (Rythmol): Approved in 1989, propafenone is an oral drug similar to flecainide that is used primarily for atrial fibrillation and the prophylaxis of PSVT. Its prodysrhythmic activity limits its use in treating ventricular dysrhythmias. Unlike flecainide, propafenone exhibits clinically significant beta-adrenergic antagonist activity. This beta-blocker action may cause a negative inotropic effect that can worsen symptoms of CHF. Furthermore, the beta-blocking actions may cause bronchospasm in patients with asthma or chronic obstructive pulmonary disease (COPD). An extended release formulation (Rythmol SR) allows for twice-daily dosing. Propafenone is metabolized to active metabolites, which account for much of the drug's effects. In addition to exacerbating or creating new dysrhythmias, propafenone may cause dizziness and dysgeusia (altered sense of taste). This drug is pregnancy category C.

Other Class I agents: Moricizine (Ethmozine): Moricizine is a unique oral antidysrhythmic that possesses some properties attributed to all three Class I subclasses: IA, IB, and IC. The drug was discontinued in 2007 due to lack of market demand.

Beta-Adrenergic Antagonists: Class II

39.8 Beta-adrenergic antagonists reduce automaticity as well as slow conduction velocity in the heart.

Beta-adrenergic antagonists, or blockers, are used to treat HTN, MI, HF, and dysrhythmias. The basic pharmacology of beta-adrenergic blockers was explained in Chapter 20; the student should refer to that chapter for nursing responsibilities and patient and family education related to this drug class. Only the actions of these drugs that relate to dysrhythmias are discussed in this section.

As expected from their effects on the autonomic nervous system, beta-adrenergic antagonists slow the heart rate (negative chronotropic effect), and decrease conduction velocity. These effects are primarily caused by the blockade of calcium ion channels in the SA and AV nodes, although these drugs also block gated sodium ion channels in the atria and ventricles. The reduction in myocardial automaticity stabilizes many types of dysrhythmias. The main value of beta blockers as antidysrhythmic agents is to treat atrial dysrhythmias associated with HF. When administered to post-MI patients, beta blockers decrease the likelihood of sudden death due to fatal dysrhythmias. Tachydysrhythmias respond well to beta blockers, including those that are induced by exercise.

Only a few beta blockers are approved for dysrhythmias, due to potential adverse effects, and these are listed in Table 39.4. Unless a functioning pacemaker is present, these drugs are contraindicated in patients with severe bradycardia, sick sinus syndrome, or advanced AV block because they depress conduction through the AV node. Blockade of beta-adrenergic receptors in the heart causes bradycardia, which may not be well tolerated in patients with preexisting cardiac disease, and hypotension may cause dizziness and possible fainting. Nonselective beta blockers may affect $beta_2$ receptors in the lung, causing bronchospasm in patients with asthma or COPD. Higher doses may produce depression, as well as hallucinations and psychosis, especially in older adults. Abrupt discontinuation of beta blockers can lead to dysrhythmias and HTN.

CONNECTION *Checkpoint* 39.2

Both $alpha_1$ blockers and $beta_1$ blockers are used to treat HTN but only the $beta_1$ blockers are antidysrhythmics. From what you learned in Chapter 20, explain why the selective alpha blockers are not used to treat dysrhythmias. See Answer to Connection Checkpoint 39.2 in Appendix A.

Acebutolol (Sectral): Approved in 1984, acebutolol is a cardioselective $beta_1$-adrenergic antagonist available only by the oral route. Like other beta blockers, acebutolol reduces sympathetic activity to the heart, thus lowering heart rate. It also has a negative inotropic effect. As an antidysrhythmic, it is used to treat premature ventricular contractions and reduce exercise-induced tachycardia. Other indications include chronic, stable angina, and HTN. Adverse effects such as hypotension and bradycardia are extensions of its beta-blocking action. At high doses, the selectivity for $beta_1$ receptors diminishes and the drug may cause bronchoconstriction ($beta_2$ receptors). Because the negative inotropic effects of the drug may worsen symptoms of HF, it is usually contraindicated in these patients. This drug is pregnancy category B.

Esmolol (Brevibloc): Approved in 1986, esmolol differs from the other antidysrhythmic beta blockers in that it is has a very short half-life of 9 minutes and is only given by IV infusion. As an antidysrhythmic, esmolol is used for the immediate termination of atrial tachyarrhythmias and noncompensatory sinus tachycardia, and to control ventricular rate in patients with atrial flutter or fibrillation. When a loading dose is administered, peak plasma levels can be reached after only 5 minutes. Off-label indications include treatment of hypertensive emergencies, acute MI, and unstable angina. Hypotension and bradycardia are common adverse effects but they quickly resolve once the infusion is discontinued. At therapeutic doses, the drug is selective for $beta_1$-adrenergic receptors. This drug is pregnancy category C.

Propranolol (Inderal): Propranolol is a nonselective beta-adrenergic antagonist. Because it slows automaticity, propranolol is indicated for many types of dysrhythmias including suppression of exercise-induced tachycardia, atrial dysrhythmias, ventricular dysrhythmias, premature ventricular contractions, and digoxin-induced tachydysrhythmias. Propranolol exhibits few serious adverse effects at therapeutic doses. At high doses, patients may experience bradycardia, hypotension, HF, and bronchospasm. Propranolol is featured as a prototype beta-adrenergic antagonist in Chapter 20. This drug is pregnancy category C.

Potassium Channel Blockers: Class III

39.9 Potassium channel blockers prolong the refractory period of the heart.

The potassium channel blockers are a small but diverse class of drugs that have very important applications to the treatment of dysrhythmias. After the action potential has passed and the myocardial cell is in a depolarized state, repolarization depends upon removal of potassium from the cell. The drugs in Class III exert their actions by blocking potassium ion channels in myocardial cells. Although there are significant differences among the drugs, all have in common the ability to delay repolarization and prolong the refractory period. This action is reflected by an increase in the QT interval on the ECG. Automaticity is also reduced.

Most drugs in this class have multiple actions on the heart and also affect adrenergic receptors or sodium channels. For example, in addition to blocking potassium channels, sotalol (Betapace) is considered a beta-adrenergic blocker. The potassium channel blockers are shown in Table 39.4.

Drugs in this class have limited uses due to potentially serious toxicity. Like other antidysrhythmics, potassium channel blockers slow the heart rate, resulting in bradycardia and possible hypotension in a significant percentage of patients. These agents can create or worsen dysrhythmias, especially during the first few doses. Older adults with preexisting HF must be carefully monitored because these patients are at higher risk to the cardiac adverse effects of potassium channel blockers.

PROTOTYPE DRUG Amiodarone (Cordarone, Pacerone)

Classification: Therapeutic: Antidysrhythmic, Class III
Pharmacologic: Potassium channel blocker

Therapeutic Effects and Uses: Approved in 1985, amiodarone is the most frequently prescribed Class III antidysrhythmic. It is considered a broad-spectrum antidysrhythmic because it is effective in terminating both atrial and ventricular dysrhythmias. It is approved for the treatment of resistant ventricular tachycardia and recurrent fibrillation that may prove life threatening, and it has become a medication of choice for the treatment of atrial dysrhythmias in patients with HF.

Amiodarone is available as PO tablets and as an IV infusion. IV infusions are limited to short-term therapy, normally only 2 to 4 days. Although its onset of action may take several weeks when the medication is given PO, its effects can last 4 to 8 weeks after the drug is discontinued because it has an extended half-life that may exceed 100 days. Amiodarone is a structural analog of thyroid hormone. The therapeutic serum level for amiodarone is 1 to 2.5 mcg/mL.

Mechanism of Action: Amiodarone exerts multiple, complex actions on the heart, and its exact mechanism of action is not completely known. In addition to blocking potassium ion channels, some of this drug's actions relate to its blockade of sodium ion channels and inhibiting sympathetic activity to the heart. Repolarization is delayed, the refractory period prolonged, and automaticity reduced. In addition to prolonging the QT interval, amiodarone increases the PR interval and widens the QRS complex on the ECG.

Pharmacokinetics:

Route(s)	PO, IV
Absorption	Completely absorbed by the gastrointestinal (GI) tract
Distribution	Widely distributed; crosses the placenta; secreted in breast milk; concentrated in the lung, kidneys, spleen, and adipose tissue
Primary metabolism	Hepatic; some enterohepatic recirculation occurs
Primary excretion	Primarily biliary; some feces
Onset of action	2–3 days to 1–3 weeks
Duration of action	10–150 days

Adverse Effects: Potentially serious adverse effects limit the use of amiodarone. The most serious effects occur in the lung, with the drug causing a pneumonia-like syndrome. Because the pulmonary toxicity may be fatal, baseline and periodic assessment of lung function is essential. Amiodarone may cause nausea, vomiting, anorexia, fatigue, dizziness, and hypotension. Visual disturbances are common in patients taking this drug for extended periods and include blurred vision due to cornea deposits, photophobia, xerostomia, cataracts, and macular degeneration. Rashes, photosensitivity, and other skin reactions occur in 10% to 15% of patients taking the drug. Certain tissues concentrate this medication; thus, adverse effects may be slow to resolve, persisting long after the drug has been discontinued. Amiodarone has prodysrhythmic action and may cause bradycardia, cardiogenic shock, or AV block.

Contraindications/Precautions: Amiodarone is contraindicated in patients with severe bradycardia, cardiogenic shock, sick sinus syndrome, severe sinus node dysfunction, or third-degree AV block. Because amiodarone contains iodine in its chemical structure, patients who have hypersensitivity to this element should not receive the drug. It should be used with caution in patients with HF because it has a negative inotropic effect that can worsen symptoms. Electrolyte imbalances, especially hypokalemia and hypomagnesemia, should be corrected before administering amiodarone because these conditions predispose the patient to the development of dysrhythmias. Due to the drug's pulmonary toxicity, it is contraindicated in patients with COPD or respiratory insufficiency. Breast-feeding during amiodarone therapy may cause infant hypothyroidism; thus, the drug is contraindicated during lactation.

Drug Interactions: Amiodarone is metabolized by the cytochrome P450 enzymes and markedly inhibits the metabolism of many other drugs. This can raise the serum levels of these drugs and cause toxicity. For example, amiodarone can increase serum digoxin levels by as much as 70%. Amiodarone greatly enhances the actions of anticoagulants, thus the dose of warfarin must be cut by as much as half. Use with beta-adrenergic blockers or calcium channel blockers (CCBs) may potentiate sinus bradycardia, sinus arrest, or AV block. Amiodarone may increase phenytoin levels two- to threefold. Caution must be used during therapy with loop diuretics because hypokalemia can enhance the prodysrhythmic properties of amiodarone. Because of the large number of potential drug interactions, the nurse should regularly check current reference sources when patients are taking amiodarone concurrently with other medications. **Herbal/Food:** Use with echinacea may increase the risk of hepatotoxicity. Aloe may cause an increased effect of amiodarone. When the drug is administered PO, grapefruit juice can increase serum amiodarone levels by over 80%.

Pregnancy: Category D.

Treatment of Overdose: Overdose will cause bradycardia, hypotension, and life-threatening dysrhythmias. Supportive treatment is targeted to reversing hypotension with vasopressors and bradycardia with atropine or isoproterenol.

Nursing Responsibilities:

- Monitor blood pressure during IV infusions and slow the rate if hypotension or bradycardia develops; assess heart rate and rhythm and blood pressure until stabilized. Sustained monitoring is essential because this medication has a very long half-life.
- Assess for signs and symptoms of adverse effects such as conduction disturbances or dysrhythmias, especially in patients receiving concomitant antidysrhythmic therapy, pulmonary toxicity with progressive dyspnea, fatigue, cough, pleuritic pain, or fever.
- Perform baseline and intermittent laboratory tests to monitor liver, lung, thyroid, neurologic, and GI function.
- Obtain baseline and periodic thyroid function test results because amiodarone may cause either hyper- or hypothyroidism.
- Assess respiratory status by auscultating the chest and observing for complains of respiratory symptoms such as shortness of breath. Observe breathing patterns and listen for diminished breath sounds, crackles, or pleuritic friction rub to distinguish between drug-induced pulmonary function problems and CHF, or pneumonia.
- Supervise ambulation because proximal muscle weakness and tremors are common adverse effects.
- Obtain baseline ophthalmic exam and assess for symptomatic changes in vision as therapy progresses.

Patient and Family Education:

- Immediately report the following signs to the health care provider: coughing or spitting up blood, shortness of breath, chest pain, difficulty breathing, palpitations or fast or irregular heartbeats, unusual fatigue, or unusual weight gain or loss.
- Do not take this drug with grapefruit juice.
- Check pulse daily and report values less than 60 beats/minute.
- Take the oral drug consistently at the same time of day and with meals, to maintain therapeutic level,.
- Wear dark glasses to ease photophobia in daytime. Wear protective clothing and a barrier-type sunscreen to prevent itching or redness, which are signs of a photosensitivity reaction.
- Schedule regular ophthalmic exams.
- Do not take other prescription or nonprescription drugs, dietary supplements, or herbal products without approval of the health care provider.
- Immediately notify the health care provider of any known or suspected pregnancy.

Drugs Similar to Amiodarone (Cordarone, Pacerone)

Other Class III antidysrhythmics include dofetilide, ibutilide, and sotalol. A fourth drug in this class, bretylium, was discontinued in the United States due to the availability of safer and more effective antidysrhythmic drugs.

Dofetilide (Tikosyn): Approved in 1999, dofetilide is an oral drug indicated for conversion of symptomatic atrial flutter or fibrillation to normal sinus rhythm. Like other potassium channel blockers, dofetilide prolongs the refractory period and action potential duration, thus increasing the QT interval. Dofetilide does not exhibit a negative inotropic effect, as do amiodarone and sotalol. The drug has no effect on the PR interval and it does not widen the QRS complex. Dofetilide has many potentially serious adverse effects, thus therapy is generally begun in a clinical setting under continuous monitoring for several days. The drug exhibits significant dose-related prodysrhythmic effects, including heart block, ventricular tachycardia, and torsades de pointes. The risk for drug-induced dysrhythmias is increased when dofetilide is administered concurrently with other medications that prolong the QT interval, including Class I and Class III antidysrhythmics. Dofetilide may accumulate to toxic levels in patients with renal impairment. Therefore, serum creatinine levels are monitored frequently during therapy. Electrolyte imbalances. especially hypokalemia or hypomagnesemia, should be corrected before administering dofetilide because these conditions predispose the patient to developing dysrhythmias. This drug is pregnancy category C.

Ibutilide (Corvert): Approved in 1995, ibutilide is only administered as an IV infusion. Continuous ECG monitoring should be conducted for at least 4 hours following the infusion to identify the potential development of new or worsening dysrhythmias. Administered over 10 minutes, ibutilide is a drug of choice for rapidly converting atrial flutter or fibrillation to normal sinus rhythm. The

MyNursingKit | Mechanism of Action: Amiodarone

drug prolongs the duration of the cardiac action potential without affecting the PR interval or QRS complex. The infusion is stopped as soon as the dysrhythmia is terminated. Ibutilide is generally well tolerated, although it does have prodysrhythmic effects, including induction of ventricular tachycardia and torsades de pointes. Like other Class III agents, precautions must be taken when administering this drug concurrently with other medications that prolong the QT interval or if given to patients with hypokalemia or hypomagnesemia, as these conditions increase the risk of dysrhythmias. This drug is pregnancy category C.

Sotalol (Betapace, Betapace AF, Sorine): Approved in 1992, sotalol is unique in that the drug has both Class II and Class III antidysrhythmic properties. As a Class II agent, it is a nonselective beta blocker that slows conduction through the AV node. Its Class III actions delay repolarization and prolong the refractory period, thus widening the QT interval. Its mixed mechanisms are reflected in the diversity of indications for the drug.

Betapace and its generic equivalents are indicated for sustained ventricular fibrillation that is deemed to be life threatening. Betapace AF converts atrial fibrillation to normal sinus rhythm and is indicated for highly systematic atrial sysrhythmias. The drugs contain a black box warning stating that they are not interchangeable.

Because of its prodysrhythmic activity, the first 3 days of therapy with sotalol are usually conducted in a controlled clinical setting with continuous monitoring. The drug should be used with caution when taken concurrently with other medications that prolong the QT interval or if given to patients with hypokalemia or hypomagnesemia, as these conditions increase the risk of dysrhythmias. Other adverse effects and contraindications for beta-adrenergic antagonists are given in Chapter 20. This drug is pregnancy category B.

Calcium Channel Blockers: Class IV

MyNursingKit | Alternative Antidysrhythmic Drugs

39.10 Calcium channel blockers are used to treat atrial dysrhythmias.

Although about 10 CCBs are available to treat cardiovascular disease, only a limited number are approved for dysrhythmias. Chapter 33 should be reviewed for details regarding the mechanism of actions, indications, and nursing responsibilities for this drug class. Only actions relevant to dysrhythmias are discussed in this section. The antidysrhythmic CCBs are shown in Table 39.4.

Blockade of calcium ion channels has a number of effects on the heart, which are very similar to those of beta-adrenergic blockers. Effects include reduced automaticity in the SA node and slowed impulse conduction through the AV node. These effects are predictable, because nodal tissues are more dependent upon calcium channels than other areas of the myocardium. This slows the heart rate and prolongs the refractory period. On an ECG, the most prominent effect of CCBs is prolongation of the PR interval. Indications include the control of ventricular rate in cases of atrial flutter or fibrillation, and prophylaxis of PSVT. CCBs are only effective against atrial dysrhythmias.

CCBs are safe medications that are well tolerated by most patients. As with many other antidysrhythmics, patients should be carefully monitored for bradycardia and hypotension. Because their cardiac effects are almost identical to those of beta-adrenergic blockers, patients concurrently taking drugs from both classes are especially at risk for bradycardia and possible HF. Because older adults often have multiple cardiovascular disorders, such as HTN, HF, and dysrhythmias, it is not unusual to find elderly patients taking drugs from multiple classes.

> **CONNECTION *Checkpoint* 39.3**
>
> **Nifedipine (Procardia) is a prototype CCB discussed in Chapter 33. From what you learned in Chapter 33, why is this drug (and other dihydropyridines) not effective in treating dysrhythmias?** See Answer to Connection Checkpoint 39.3 in Appendix A.

Diltiazem (Cardizem, Dilacor, others): Like other CCBs, diltiazem inhibits the transport of calcium into myocardial cells. The actions and indications for diltiazem are the same as those of verapamil. The drug may be given by the IV route for rapid control of acute dysrhythmias, or orally for prophylaxis. In addition to its use in treating and preventing atrial dysrhythmias, it is indicated for HTN, as well as stable and vasospastic angina. Adverse effects of diltiazem are generally not serious and are related to vasodilation: headache, dizziness, and edema of the ankles and feet. Because of its profound depressant effects on nodal tissue, diltiazem is contraindicated in patients with severe bradycardia, AV block, or sick sinus syndrome. Concurrent use of diltiazem with digoxin or beta-adrenergic blockers may cause partial or complete heart block, HF, or dysrhythmias.

Verapamil (Calan, Isoptin, others): Verapamil was the first CCB approved by the FDA. In the heart, verapamil slows conduction velocity and stabilizes dysrhythmias. The drug may be given by the IV route for rapid control of acute dysrhythmias, or orally for prophylaxis. Because verapamil can cause bradycardia and AV block, patients with HF should be carefully monitored. The patient should notify their health care practitioner if their heart rate falls below 60 beats/minute or if systolic blood pressure falls below 90 mmHg. The therapeutic serum level is 0.08 to 0.3 mcg/mL. A prototype drug feature that describes other indications for verapamil is presented in Chapter 33.

> **Pharm*FACT***
>
> **Sudden cardiac arrest (SCA), also called sudden cardiac death, is usually caused by ventricular defibrillation. Although people with heart disease have a greater risk of SCA, it most frequently occurs in people with healthy hearts between ages 35 and 45. The mortality rate is 95%.** *Source:* National Heart, Lung, and Blood Institute, 2006.

Miscellaneous Antidysrhythmics

39.11 Adenosine and digoxin are used for specific dysrhythmias.

Two other medications, adenosine and digoxin, are occasionally used to treat specific dysrhythmias, but do not act by the mechanisms described above. These miscellaneous agents are shown in Table 39.4.

NURSING PROCESS APPLICATION

Patients Receiving Antidysrhythmic Therapies

Assessment	Potential Nursing Diagnoses
Prior to administration: • Obtain complete health history including allergies, drug history, and possible drug interactions. • Assess to determine if cardiac alteration is producing a symptomatic effect on cardiac output. Assessment should include vital signs, level of consciousness, urinary output, skin temperature, and peripheral pulses. • Obtain baseline ECG to compare throughout therapy.	• *Ineffective Tissue Perfusion (Cardiopulmonary)*, related to cardiac conduction abnormality • *Deficient Knowledge (Antidysrhythmic Drug)*, related to purpose, precautions, and adverse effects of drug therapy • *Risk for Injury*, related to adverse effects of drug • *Decreased Cardiac Output*, related to cardiac conduction abnormality

Planning: Patient Goals and Expected Outcomes

The patient will:

- Exhibit improved cardiac output as evidenced by stabilization of heart rate, heart rhythm, sensorium, urinary output, and vital signs.
- State expected outcomes of drug therapy.
- Demonstrate an understanding of the drug's action by accurately describing drug adverse effects and precautions.
- Be free of preventable adverse effects.

Implementation

Interventions and (Rationales)	Patient and Family Education
• Monitor cardiac rate and rhythm continuously if administering the drug IV. (IV route is used when rapid therapeutic effects are needed. Constant monitoring is needed to detect serious dysrhythmias.)	• Explain the need for continuous ECG monitoring when administering the medication intravenously.
• Monitor the IV site. Administer all parenteral medication via infusion pump. (Parenteral antidysrhythmia drugs have very narrow safety margin.)	• Instruct the patient to report any burning or stinging pain, swelling, warmth, redness, or tenderness at the IV insertion site.
• Investigate possible causes of the dysrhythmia such as electrolyte imbalances, hypoxia, pain, anxiety, caffeine ingestion, and tobacco use. (Treatment should be directed to underlying pathology contributing to dysrhythmia.)	Instruct patient to: • Maintain a diet low in sodium and fat with sufficient potassium. • Report illness such as flu, vomiting, diarrhea, and dehydration to health care provider to avoid adverse effects. • Restrict the use of caffeine and tobacco products.
• Observe for adverse effects specific to the antidysrhythmic used especially the appearance of ECG abnormalities. (Drugs in these classes are prodysrhythmic and require careful monitoring.)	Instruct the patient to: • Report adverse effects specific to prescribed antidysrhythmic. • Report palpitations, chest pain, dyspnea, unusual fatigue, weakness, and visual disturbances.
• Monitor for proper use of medication. (Improper use may result in dysrhythmias, hypotension, or bradycardia.)	Instruct the patient to: • Take the drug exactly as prescribed, even if feeling well. • Never discontinue the drug abruptly. • Take pulse prior to taking the drug. (Instruct patient regarding the normal range and rhythm of pulse; instruct to consult the health care provider regarding "reportable" pulse.)

Evaluation of Outcome Criteria

Evaluate the effectiveness of drug therapy by confirming that patient goals and expected outcomes have been met (see "Planning").

Adenosine (Adenocard, Adenoscan): Adenosine is a naturally occurring nucleoside that activates potassium channels in the SA and AV nodes, causing the potassium to leave cardiac muscle cells. When given as a rapid 1- to 2-second IV bolus, adenosine blocks reentry pathways in the AV node and terminates the tachycardia. It is usually followed by a 1- to 5-second period of asystole. Patients should be laid supine prior to adenosine use, and warned that they may feel faint. The IV site used to give adenosine should be antecubital or above, and an 18-gauge angio catheter or larger should be used. If the tachycardia has not been eliminated in 1 to 2 minutes, a second rapid bolus may be given. The primary indication for adenosine is PSVT, for which it is a drug of choice. It is also used to assist in the diagnosis of coronary artery disease of dysrhythmias in patients who are unable to undergo a cardiac exercise stress test. It is not effective in treating ventricular dysrhythmias. Although the drug has prodysrhythmic effects and dyspnea is common, adverse effects are generally self-limiting because of its 10-second half-life. This drug is pregnancy category C.

Digoxin (Lanoxin): Although digoxin is primarily used to treat HF, it is also prescribed for atrial flutter or fibrillation and PSVT because of its ability to decrease automaticity of the SA node and slow conduction through the AV node. The drug is not effective against ventricular dysrhythmias. Because excessive levels of digoxin can produce serious dysrhythmias, and interactions with other medications are common, patients must be carefully monitored during therapy. Additional information on the mechanism of action, adverse effects, and nursing responsibilities for digoxin may be found in Chapter 38, where the drug is featured as a prototype.

UNDERSTANDING THE CHAPTER

Key Concepts Summary

39.1 Some dysrhythmias produce no patient symptoms, while others may be life threatening.

39.2 The phases of the cardiac action potential include rapid depolarization, a long plateau, and repolarization.

39.3 The electrocardiogram is used to measure electrical conduction across the myocardium.

39.4 Dysrhythmias are classified by the impulse origin and type of rhythm abnormality produced.

39.5 Antidysrhythmic drugs are only used when there is a clear benefit to the patient.

39.6 Antidysrhythmic drugs are classified by their mechanism of action.

39.7 Class I antidysrhythmics act by blocking sodium ion channels in myocardial cells.

39.8 Beta-adrenergic antagonists reduce automaticity as well as slow conduction velocity in the heart.

39.9 Potassium channel blockers prolong the refractory period of the heart.

39.10 Calcium channel blockers are used to treat atrial dysrhythmias.

39.11 Adenosine and digoxin are used for specific dysrhythmias.

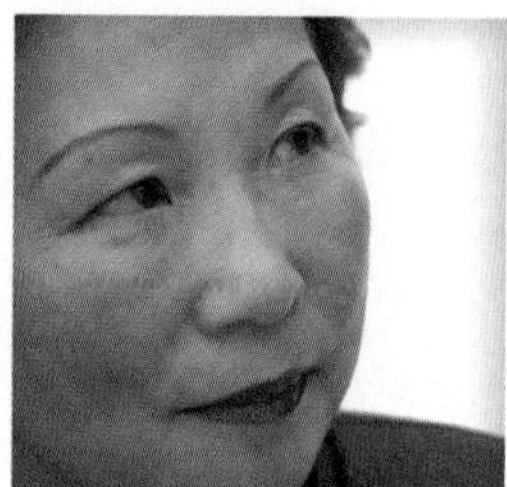

Making the PATIENT *Connection*

Remember the patient "Jada Chinn Nguyen" at the beginning of the chapter? Now read the remainder of the case study. Based on the information presented within this chapter, respond to the critical thinking questions that follow.

The day had been busy as Jada prepared for her daughter's upcoming wedding. There were so many arrangements to be made, and Jada felt overwhelmed. During the day she experienced heaviness in her chest, but she attributed it to the stress of the wedding and perhaps a touch of bronchitis. Nonetheless, she knew there was no time to stop and rest; there was too much to do.

Later that afternoon, she realized that she had to take it easy. Then she experienced that strange sensation once again. As she sat in a chair, Jada suddenly felt dizzy with extreme weakness and difficulty breathing. Her family members report that she became pale and unexpectedly collapsed. Emergency personnel were called to the scene, and Jada was taken to the nearest hospital.

In the emergency department, Jada's physical examination revealed the following findings: weak, middle-aged Asian female; vital signs: blood pressure 102/68 mmHg, heart rate 116 beats/minute, respiratory rate 18/minute, afebrile; weight 53 kg (116 lb). She has clear bilateral breath sounds and active bowel sounds heard in all four quadrants. Her ECG reveals atrial fibrillation with a ventricular rate of 116 beats/minute. She is admitted to the coronary care unit for further testing and observation.

Critical Thinking Questions

1. Jada's ECG shows atrial fibrillation. Trace the electrical conduction system through the heart. What part of the ECG complex would be most affected with this patient's medical diagnosis?
2. While in the coronary care unit, Jada will receive amiodarone (Cordarone) IV infusion. She wants to know how long she will need to receive the IV medication and how it works. How would you respond to this patient's questions?
3. The patient is being discharged on amiodarone 400 mg twice daily. What instructions should this patient receive?
4. List any drug–food interaction concerns you should discuss with Jada.

Case Study

Malcolm Hibbert is a 56-year-old man who was diagnosed with atrial dysrhythmia and placed on pharmacologic agents to control the condition. He has been surfing the Internet to find out more about his condition and drug therapy. When he returns to the clinic, he has multiple questions to ask you. How would you respond to each of the following?

1. "I read that some drugs are prodysrhythmic. What does that mean?"
2. "What does depolarization and repolarization have to do with my drug therapy?"
3. "Are there any foods that might cause an increase in dysrhythmias?"

NCLEX-RN® Review

1 A health care provider has ordered procainamide (Pronestyl) for each client. A nurse should question the order for a client with which of the following?

1. Ventricular tachycardia
2. Paroxysmal atrial tachycardia
3. Atrial fibrillation
4. Severe heart failure

2 A client is receiving intravenous procainamide (Pronestyl) for cardiac dysrhythmias. Which of the following nursing interventions is appropriate for this therapy?

1. Monitor the client for increased thrombolytic levels.
2. Place client in a supine position during administration.
3. Limit intake of foods high in calcium such as milk and cheese.
4. Encourage coughing and deep breathing to remove secretions.

3 The client with atrial dysrhythmia is being treated with a potassium channel blocker. The nurse would monitor for therapeutic effectiveness by noting which of the following?

1. Change in the blood pressure
2. Increase in the serum potassium level
3. Changes in the cardiac rhythm
4. Reduction in the urine output

4 A client who is receiving intravenous lidocaine (Xylocaine) for ventricular dysrhythmias exhibits confusion and anxiety. The appropriate response by the nurse would be to:

1. Withhold the drug and notify the health care provider immediately.
2. Increase the infusion rate and calm the client.
3. Discontinue the infusion and administer the antidote.
4. Decrease the infusion rate and monitor for confusion.

5 The client is prescribed a beta-adrenergic antagonist for the treatment of atrial dysrhythmias associated with heart failure. The nurse knows that this drug will have what physiologic effect?

1. Increased heart rate and reduced respiratory status
2. Decreased heart rate and conduction velocity
3. Elimination of phase 4 of the action potential
4. Flattened T wave on the ECG pattern

6 A client is being discharged with a diagnosis of dysrhythmias. The nurse is teaching the client about amiodarone (Cordarone). What client teaching is needed related to this medication?

1. Avoid crowds while taking this medication.
2. Avoid birth control pills and use an alternate form of birth control.
3. Wear protective clothing and a barrier-type sunscreen.
4. Use an electric razor to shave.

See Answers to Critical Thinking Questions, Case Study, and NCLEX-RN® Review in Appendix A.

References

American College of Cardiology, American Heart Association Task Force, European Society of Cardiology. (2006). ACC/AHA/ESC 2006 guidelines for management of patients with ventricular arrhythmias and the prevention of sudden cardiac death—Executive Summary. *Journal of the American College of Cardiology, 48*, 1064–1108. Retrieved July 15, 2008, from http://content.onlinejacc.org/cgi/content/full/48/5/1064

Ball, J. W., & Bindler, R. C. (2006). *Child health nursing: Partnering with children and families.* Upper Saddle River, NJ: Pearson Education.

Beattie, W. S., & Elliot, R. F. (2005). Magnesium supplementation reduces the risk of arrhythmia after cardiac surgery. *Evidence-Based Cardiovascular Medicine 9*(1), 82–85.

Berry, C., Rankin, A. C., & Brady, A. (2004). Bradycardia and tachycardia occurring in older people: An introduction. *British Journal of Cardiology, 11*(1), 61–64.

De Bruin, M. L., Langendijk, P. N. J., Koopmans, R. P., Wilde, A. A. M., Leufkens, H. G. M., & Hoes, A. M. (2007). In-hospital cardiac arrest is associated with use of non-antiarrhythmic QTc-prolonging drugs. *British Journal of Clinical Pharmacy, 63*(2), 216–223.

Laidlaw, D. W., Homoud, M. K., Weinstock, J., Mark Estes III, N. A., & Link, M. S. (2007). Prognosis and treatment of ventricular arrhythmias following myocardial infarction. *Current Cardiology Reviews, 3*(1), 23–33.

National Heart, Lung, and Blood Institute. (2006). *Sudden cardiac arrest.* Retrieved July 15, 2008, from http://www.nhlbi.nih.gov/health/dci/Diseases/scda/scda_whatis.html

Roden, D. M. (2006). Antiarrhythmic drugs. In L. L. Brunton, J. S. Lazo, and K. L. Parker (Eds.), *The pharmacological basis of therapeutics* (11th ed., pp. 899–932). New York: McGraw-Hill.

Somberg, J. C., Cao, W., Cvetanovic, I., Ranade, V. V., & Molnar, J. (2005). The effect of magnesium sulfate on action potential duration and cardiac arrhythmias. *American Journal of Therapeutics, 12*(3), 218–222.

Tong, G. M., & Rude, R. K. (2005). Magnesium deficiency in critical illness. *Journal of Intensive Care Medicine, 20*(1), 3–17.

Ueshima, K. (2005). Magnesium and ischemic heart disease: A review of epidemiological, experimental, and clinical evidences. *Magnesium Research, 18*(4), 275–284.

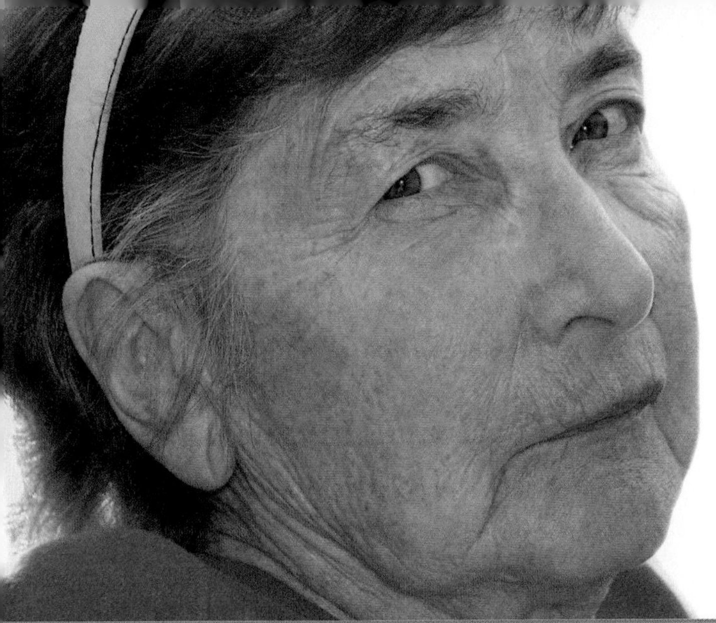

Ever since I returned from my trip to Bangkok, my right calf has really hurt. I first thought my arthritis was flaring up again, especially after sitting on the plane for so long.

Patient "Ruby Dwyer"

CHAPTER 40

Pharmacotherapy of Coagulation Disorders

Chapter Outline

Disorders of Hemostasis

Overview of Coagulation Modifiers

Parenteral Anticoagulants

Indirect Thrombin Inhibitors

PROTOTYPE **Heparin (Hep-Lock, Monoject)** *p. 646*

Direct Thrombin Inhibitors

PROTOTYPE **Lepirudin (Refludan)** *p. 648*

Oral Anticoagulants

PROTOTYPE **Warfarin (Coumadin)** *p. 650*

Antiplatelet Agents

Aspirin

Adenosine Diphosphate Receptor Blockers

PROTOTYPE **Clopidogrel (Plavix)** *p. 654*

Glycoprotein IIb/IIIa Receptor Inhibitors

PROTOTYPE **Abciximab (ReoPro)** *p. 655*

Thrombolytics

PROTOTYPE **Alteplase (Activase)** *p. 658*

Hemostatics

PROTOTYPE **Aminocaproic Acid (Amicar)** *p. 661*

Drugs for Hemophilia

Learning Outcomes

After reading this chapter, the student should be able to:

1. Describe primary risk factors for thromboembolic disorders.
2. Explain the etiology and symptoms of coagulation disorders.
3. Identify the primary mechanisms by which coagulation-modifier drugs act.
4. Explain how laboratory testing of coagulation parameters is used to monitor anticoagulant pharmacotherapy.
5. Describe the nurse's role in the pharmacologic management of patients with coagulation disorders.
6. For each of the classes shown in the chapter outline, identify the prototype and representative drugs and explain the mechanism(s) of drug action, primary indications, contraindications, significant drug interactions, pregnancy category, and important adverse effects.
7. Apply the nursing process to care for patients receiving drug therapy for coagulation disorders.

Key Terms

activated partial thromboplastin time (aPTT), *644*
anticoagulants, *642*
antithrombin III (AT-III), *645*
deep vein thrombosis (DVT), *642*
fibrinolysis, *657*
glycoprotein IIb/IIIa, *655*
hemophilia, *643*
hemostasis, *642*
plasminogen, *657*
procoagulants, *642*
prothrombin time (PT), *644*
pulmonary embolism, *642*
thrombocytopenia, *643*
thromboembolic disorder, *642*
venous thromboembolism (VTE), *642*
von Willebrand's disease (vWD), *664*

Everyone is familiar with the bleeding associated with simple cuts and scrapes, and we take for granted that bleeding will stop in a few minutes. The stoppage of blood flow, or **hemostasis,** is complex and essential to our well-being. The underlying mechanisms of hemostasis promote blood clotting that protects us from injuries that could lead to shock and perhaps death. Too much clotting, however, can be just as dangerous. The physiological processes of hemostasis must maintain a delicate balance between blood fluidity and coagulation.

Many common diseases and conditions affect hemostasis, including myocardial infarction (MI), cerebrovascular accident (CVA), venous or arterial thrombosis, valvular heart disease, and indwelling catheters. Because these conditions are so prevalent in clinical practice, nurses will have frequent occasions to administer and monitor coagulation-modifying medications. Drugs may be used to enhance coagulation, inhibit coagulation, or dissolve existing clots to restore blood flow.

Disorders of Hemostasis

40.1 Thromboembolic disorders are abnormalities of hemostasis that include deep vein thrombosis and pulmonary embolism.

Coagulation is regulated by a large number of natural substances circulating in the blood. Some of these are **procoagulants,** which favor the formation of clots, while others are **anticoagulants,** which inhibit clot formation. Coagulation, then, can be thought of as a delicate balance between procoagulants and anticoagulants. For example, injuries to blood vessels release procoagulants that tip the balance in favor of initiating coagulation. The student should review the coagulation cascade presented in Section 31.3 before proceeding.

Once a stationary clot, or thrombus, forms in a vessel it often grows larger as more fibrin is added. Pieces of the thrombus may break off and travel in the bloodstream to block other vessels. A traveling clot is called an embolus. Because these two conditions often occur concurrently in patients, the term **thromboembolic disorder** is used to describe conditions in which the body forms undesirable clots. Thromboembolic disorders may be classified as either venous or arterial.

Venous thromboembolism (VTE) is a common disease that occurs when blood flow through a vein is very slow (stasis). Venous stasis allows procoagulation factors to accumulate and overcome the natural anticoagulant substances in the blood. There are two manifestations of VTE: deep vein thrombosis and pulmonary embolism.

When thrombosis occurs in the legs it is called **deep vein thrombosis (DVT).** Because blood flow is slowest in the deep veins of the lower limbs, these vessels are the most common sites for VTE. Conditions associated with venous stasis and DVT include the following:

- **Extended immobility.** During major illness or following surgery, patients may be supine or otherwise immobile for extended periods of time. Because the movement of blood through the deep veins is entirely dependent upon the squeezing action from skeletal muscular contraction, blood in the deep veins of these patients has difficulty returning to the heart.
- **Major trauma.** Trauma often causes serious bleeding that activates procoagulation factors. In addition, stasis will likely occur surrounding the injured area, promoting the development of DVT. Trauma involving the lower extremities places the patient at high risk for DVT.
- **Major surgery.** Surgery of the lower extremities, especially knee and hip replacements, are common causes of DVT for the same reasons as trauma; bleeding activates procoagulation factors and stasis occurs around the surgical site.
- **Hypercoagulability states.** Malignancy, lupus, and pregnancy are examples of conditions associated with an increased risk of coagulation and DVT. Certain genetic disorders also produce hypercoagulability, the most common being a genetic deficiency of protein C, a natural anticoagulant.
- **Drug therapy.** High amounts of estrogen, prescribed as replacement therapy or as a component of oral contraceptives, have been associated with DVT in numerous studies. Selective estrogen receptor modulators (SERMS) such as raloxifene (Evista) are also associated with a higher risk of DVT.

The second primary thromboembolic disorder is **pulmonary embolism,** which occurs when a venous clot dislodges, migrates to the pulmonary vessels, and blocks arterial circulation to the lungs. Pulmonary emboli are the most serious consequence of VTE because death may occur within minutes after the onset of symptoms. The factors associated with an increased risk of pulmonary embolism are the same as those for patients with DVT: prolonged immobility, major trauma, lower extremity surgery, hypercoagulability states, and estrogen therapy. Prevention of pulmonary embolism is a primary goal for all patients with VTE, and a major indication for pharmacotherapy.

Patients with DVT are sometimes asymptomatic, or complain of nonspecific symptoms such as pain, swelling, or warmth of the legs. The disorder may be present for years, causing progressive damage to venous valves, thus worsening blood flow in the region and increasing the risk of an acute episode. A pulmonary embolism, however, produces a sudden onset of cough, chest pain, tachypnea, dyspnea, tachycardia, and hemoptysis. Symptoms of pulmonary embolism resemble an MI, and rapid diagnosis and treatment is essential.

PharmFACT

Approximately 1 person in 20 will develop a DVT in the course of his or her lifetime. The incidence in hospitalized patients, however, is much higher at 20–70% of all patients. *Source:* Schreiber, 2008.

Arterial thromboembolism may deprive an area of blood flow and is a medical emergency because tissue hypoxia and cellular death will result soon after blood stoppage. The most serious arterial thromboembolism disorders are MI and CVA.

Arterial thrombi and emboli commonly result from procedures involving arterial punctures such as angiography and stent placement. They may also originate from the heart. Emboli are common complications of mitral valve disease, prosthetic heart valves, and atrial dysrhythmias. Emboli originating from the left side of the heart may lodge in any organ in the body.

CONNECTION *Checkpoint* 40.1

Coagulation occurs by intrinsic and extrinsic pathways. From what you learned in Chapter 31, which pathway is activated when blood leaks from a vessel? Which is more complex and takes several minutes? Which results in the formation of fibrin? See Answer to Connection Checkpoint 40.1 in Appendix A.

40.2 Coagulation disorders are caused by decreased numbers of platelets or by deficiencies in specific clotting factors.

While thromboembolic disorders are caused by too much clotting, coagulation disorders result from too little clotting. Serious consequences result if the body does not form clots in a timely manner. The two most common etiologies of coagulation disorders are decreased numbers of platelets and deficiencies in one or more clotting factors.

Platelets are central to the process of coagulation. Recognizing a site of vessel injury, activated platelets release von Willebrand factor, which causes platelets to become "sticky" and adhere to the site. Following adhesion, platelets secrete substances such as adenosine diphosphate (ADP) and thromboxane A_2 that promote platelet aggregation and the formation of a platelet plug at the site. Procoagulation factors become activated on the platelets and a fibrin mesh clot results. Nearly every step of this pathway requires sufficient numbers of properly functioning platelets.

The most common coagulation disorder is a deficiency of platelets, or **thrombocytopenia,** which occurs when platelet counts fall below 150,000 mm^3. Thrombocytopenia is the result of either decreased platelet production or increased platelet destruction. Any condition or disease that suppresses bone marrow function has the potential to cause decreased platelet production. Other common causes of decreased platelet production are folic acid or vitamin B_{12} deficiencies, and decreased production of thrombopoietin by the liver during hepatic failure. Increased destruction of platelets may occur in patients with thrombocytopenic purpura, disseminated intravascular coagulation (DIC), or lupus.

Of special concern is thrombocytopenia caused by drug therapy. A large number of drugs have the potential to increase platelet destruction, either by direct toxic effects on bone marrow or by inducing the immune system to destroy them. When caring for patients receiving these drugs, the nurse must be vigilant in assessing blood laboratory test results and observing for signs of thrombocytopenia such as bleeding gums, nosebleeds, and extensive bruising. Selected drugs that cause thrombocytopenia are listed in Table 40.1. Heparin-induced thrombocytopenia, a particularly serious form of this disorder, is discussed in Section 40.4.

Deficiencies in specific clotting factors may prolong coagulation and lead to excess bleeding. Deficiencies in multiple coagulation factors occur frequently in patients with serious hepatic impairment, because the liver synthesizes most clotting factors. Deficiency in a single coagulation factor suggests **hemophilia:** a series of coagulation disorders caused by genetic deficiencies in specific clotting factors. Hemophilia disorders are typified by prolonged coagulation times, resulting in persistent bleeding that can be acute or chronic. Patients may experience various forms of the disease, with symptoms ranging from mild to severe. Approximately two thirds of patients with hemophilia will report a family history of the disease. The pharmacotherapy of hemophilia is described in Section 40.12.

MyNursingKit Immune Thrombocytopenic Purpura (ITP)

TABLE 40.1 Selected Drugs Causing Thrombocytopenia

Class	Examples
Analgesics	acetaminophen, aspirin, diclofenac, ibuprofen, indomethacin, morphine, naproxen
Anticoagulants and antiplatelets	heparin, clopidogrel, glycoprotein IIb/IIIa inhibitors
Anti-Infectives	acyclovir, amphotericin B, ampicillin, clarithromycin, ethambutol, fluconazole, indinavir, isoniazid, itraconazole, linezolid, oxacillin, piperacillin, rifampin, trimethoprim, sulfonamides, vancomycin
Antineoplastic and Immunotherapy Agents	carboplatin, interferon-alfa, methotrexate
Cardiovascular Agents	atorvastatin, captopril, digoxin, hydrochlorothiazide, inamrinone, nitroglycerin, procainamide, quinidine, simvastatin
Central Nervous System Agents	carbamazepine, chlorpromazine, diazepam, haloperidol, lithium, phenobarbital, phenytoin, valproic acid
Other Classes	cimetidine, MMR vaccine, isotretinoin, octreotide, ranitidine, sirolimus

To diagnose coagulation and thromboembolic disorders, a thorough medical history and physical examination is necessary. Laboratory tests measuring coagulation must be obtained. These usually include a whole-blood clotting time, **prothrombin time (PT),** thrombin time, **activated partial thromboplastin time (aPTT),** liver functions tests, platelet count, and, in some instances, a bleeding time. Additional tests, such as serum levels of specific clotting factors, may be indicated, based on the results of these laboratory analyses.

Overview of Coagulation Modifiers

40.3 The normal coagulation process can be modified by a number of different mechanisms.

Medications can be used to modify hemostasis in a number of ways. An overview of the basic mechanisms of coagulation-modifying drugs is presented in Table 40.2. These mechanisms are illustrated in Figure 40.1.

The most commonly prescribed coagulation modifiers are the anticoagulants, which are used to prevent clot formation. Patients usually call these drugs "blood thinners," which is an inaccurate description because they do not change the viscosity or thickness of the blood. Drugs may accomplish clot prevention by the following mechanisms:

- Inhibition of specific clotting factors in the coagulation cascade: examples include heparin and warfarin (Coumadin)
- Inhibition of the clotting action of platelets: examples include aspirin and clopidogrel (Plavix)

Regardless of the mechanism, all anticoagulant medications will increase the normal time the body takes to form clots. Anticoagulants are widely used for thromboembolic disease and are discussed in Sections 40.4–40.6.

Once an abnormal clot has formed, it may block blood vessels that serve critical tissues and it must be quickly removed to restore normal function. This is particularly important for vessels serving the heart, lungs, and brain. A specific class of drugs, the thrombolytics, has been developed to dissolve life-threatening clots. These agents are presented in Section 40.11.

TABLE 40.2 Overview of Coagulation Modifiers

Type of Modification	Mechanism	Drug Classification
Prevention of clot formation	Inhibition of specific clotting factors	Anticoagulants
	Inhibition of platelet actions	Antiplatelet agents
Removal of an existing clot	Clot dissolved by the drug	Thrombolytics
Promotion of clot formation	Inhibition of fibrin destruction	Hemostatics
	Administration of missing clotting factors	Clotting factor concentrates

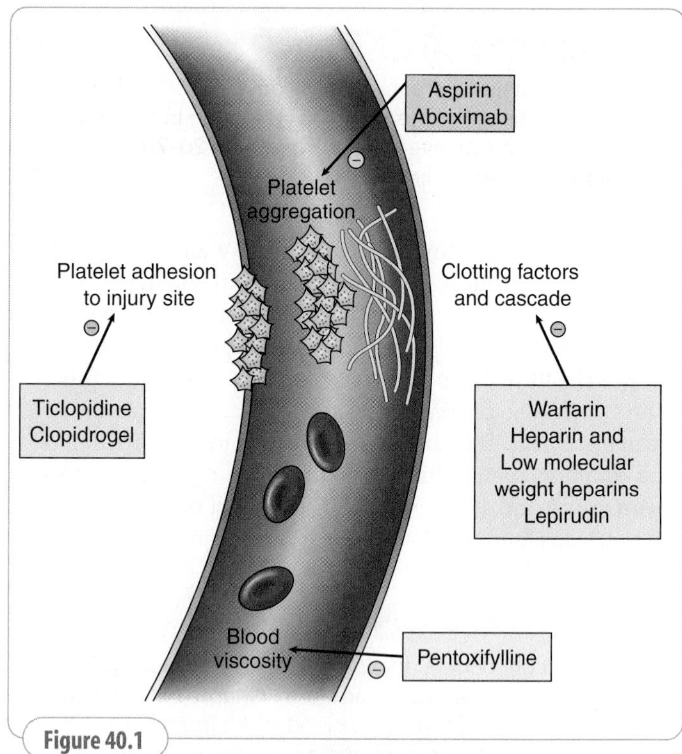

Figure 40.1 Mechanisms of action of antiplatelet drugs.

Coagulation modifiers are also used to promote the formation of clots. Drugs called hemostatics inhibit the normal removal of fibrin, thus keeping the clot in place for a longer period of time. These drugs are primarily used to speed clot formation to limit bleeding from a surgical site, and are discussed in Section 40.12. For patients with hemophilia, clotting factors may be administered to promote clotting by providing a missing or deficient component in the coagulation cascade, as presented in Section 40.13.

Since hemostasis involves a fine balance of factors favoring clotting versus those inhibiting clotting, pharmacotherapy with coagulation modifiers is individualized to each patient. Serious adverse effects may occur if the drugs are not used properly; therefore, these patients will require frequent assessment and monitoring to ensure the goal that normal coagulation is being achieved, without serious adverse events.

Parenteral Anticoagulants

40.4 Heparin, the most commonly used parenteral anticoagulant, acts by indirectly inhibiting thrombin.

Extensively used in the treatment of thromboembolic disease, anticoagulants lengthen clotting time and prevent thrombi from forming or growing larger. Since thromboembolic disease can be life threatening, therapy is often begun by administering anticoagulants parenterally to achieve the most rapid onset of action. As the disease stabilizes and the desired degree of anticoagulation has been achieved, the patient is gradually

TABLE 40.3 Anticoagulants

Drug	Route and Adult Dose (maximum dose where indicated)	Adverse Effects
fondaparinux (Arixtra)	Subcutaneous: 2.5 mg/day starting at least 6 h postop for 5–9 days (max: 10 mg/day)	*Minor bleeding, nausea, vomiting, transient thrombocytopenia (heparin), anemia (fondaparinux)* <u>Hemorrhage, anaphylaxis (heparin)</u>
heparin (Heplock)	IV Infusion: 5,000–40,000 units/day Subcutaneous: 15,000–20,000 units bid	
warfarin (Coumadin)	PO/IV: Dose based on target INR, which is usually within the range of 2–3	
Low Molecular Weight Heparins (LMWHs)		
dalteparin (Fragmin)	Subcutaneous: 2,500–5,000 units/day for 5–10 days (max: 18,000 international units/day)	*Minor bleeding, nausea, vomiting, hematoma, local pain, fever* <u>Hemorrhage, thrombocytopenia, pancytopenia, anaphylaxis</u>
enoxaparin (Lovenox)	Subcutaneous: 30 mg bid for 7–10 days	
tinzaparin (Innohep)	Subcutaneous: 175 units/kg daily for at least 6 days	
Direct Thrombin Inhibitors		
argatroban (Acova, Novastan)	IV: 2 mcg/kg/min (max: 10 mcg/kg/min)	*Fever, nausea, allergic skin reactions, hepatic impairment, pneumonia, fever, minor bleeding, back pain (bivalirudin)* <u>Serious internal hemorrhage, hemoptysis, hematuria, sepsis, heart failure</u>
bivalirudin (Angiomax)	IV: 0.75 mg/kg initial bolus followed by 1.75 mg/kg/h for 4 h. May continue at 0.2 mg/kg/h up to 20 h	
desirudin (Iprivask)	Subcutaneous: 15 mg bid for 9–12 days (max: 80 mg/day)	
lepirudin (Refludan)	IV: 0.4 mg/kg initial bolus (max: 44 mg) followed by 0.15 mg/kg/h (dose adjusted to an aPTT value 1.5–2.5 above baseline)	

Note: *Italics* indicate common adverse effects. <u>Underline</u> indicates serious adverse effects.

switched to oral anticoagulants, with careful monitoring of appropriate coagulation laboratory values. The most frequently prescribed parenteral anticoagulant is heparin; warfarin is the most common oral anticoagulant (Section 40.6). The anticoagulants are listed in Table 40.3.

Heparin is a natural chemical found in the liver and the lining of blood vessels. As a drug, heparin has been used for many decades and is one of the few agents still obtained from animal tissue, usually beef lung or pig intestine. Chemically, heparin is a special type of carbohydrate called a glycosaminoglycan that consists of repeated disaccharide units of differing lengths. Thus, heparin is actually a mixture of different molecules, varying in size. This drug is also called unfractionated heparin because it contains a mixture of different molecular "fractions." This mixture affects protein binding and drug bioavailability, and is partially responsible for the wide variation in patient responses to heparin.

Heparin produces its anticoagulant effects by binding to **antithrombin III (AT-III).** As its name implies, antithrombin inactivates thrombin (as well as several other clotting factors). The binding to heparin produces a structural change in AT-III that makes it 1,000 times more active in inhibiting thrombin, factor Xa, factor IXa, and other substances involved in coagulation. Within minutes after intravenous (IV) administration, the loss of these activated clotting factors prevents the formation of fibrin clots.

Because responses to heparin anticoagulation vary considerably among patients, regular monitoring of laboratory values during heparin therapy is essential to patient safety. aPTT is the conventional measurement guiding heparin therapy, with normal values ranging from 25 to 40 seconds. For therapeutic anticoagulation, the aPTT should be between 1.5 and 2 times the patient's baseline, or 60 to 80 seconds. Elevated aPTT values indicate the patient is at high risk for bleeding and that a reduction in heparin dose is necessary. aPTT values less than 60 seconds indicate the need for higher heparin doses. During continuous IV heparin therapy, the aPTT is measured daily and 6 to 8 hours after any changes in dosage.

Low molecular weight heparins: In recent years, the heparin molecule has been shortened and modified to create a new class of drugs called low molecular weight heparins (LMWHs). Given subcutaneously, the mechanism of action of these agents is very similar to that of heparin, except the shorter heparin molecules are unable to bind thrombin, making them more selective for factor Xa inhibition.

LMWHs possess the same anticoagulant activity as heparin but have several advantages. They produce a more predictable anticoagulant response than heparin because there is less binding of the drug to proteins and macrophages; therefore, less frequent laboratory monitoring is required. They are about 10 times less likely to cause thrombocytopenia, a potentially serious adverse effect of heparin. They also exhibit a half-life that is 2 to 4 times longer than heparin that permits once-daily dosing, and family members or the patient can be trained to give the necessary subcutaneous injections at home. Like heparin, the LMWHs do not cross the placenta. LMWHs have become the drugs of choice for a number of clotting disorders, including the prevention of DVT following surgery. One disadvantage is that LMWHs are considerably more expensive than heparin.

When using LMWHs, the aPTT laboratory value does not reflect the anticoagulant effects of the drugs because aPTT is insensitive to changes in factor Xa. Instead, dosage calculations with LMWHs are fixed and based upon the patient's weight. A given amount of subcutaneous LMWH results in a predictable plasma drug level. This is a major advantage over heparin, for which levels continually fluctuate and doses must be adjusted based on aPTT levels. In highly unstable patients or those with renal impairment, measurement of antifactor Xa activity may be used to gauge therapeutic response. Acceptable target values for antifactor Xa range from 0.5 to 1 unit/mL.

PROTOTYPE DRUG Heparin (Hep-Lock, Monoject)

Classification: **Therapeutic:** Anticoagulant
Pharmacologic: Indirect thrombin inhibitor

Therapeutic Effects and Uses: Heparin is the "gold standard" to which other parenteral anticoagulants are compared. Because it has an immediate onset of action when administered IV, heparin is a drug of choice for acute thromboembolic disorders where rapid anticoagulation is necessary. Subcutaneous heparin is injected into the deep fatty layers of the abdomen and may take up to 1 hour to achieve a therapeutic effect. A continuous IV infusion allows for better titration and finer management of aPTT values. Indications include DVT, pulmonary embolism, unstable angina, evolving MI, and prevention of thrombosis in high-risk patients. Heparin and LMWHs are preferred anticoagulants during pregnancy because heparin molecules are too large to cross the placenta. Heparin is also used to maintain the patency of peripheral catheters (heparin locks) and arterial lines.

MyNursingKit | Mechanism of Action: Heparin

Heparin prolongs coagulation time, thereby inhibiting excessive clotting within blood vessels. As a result, it prevents the enlargement of existing clots and the formation of new ones. It has no ability to dissolve existing clots. Clotting time is prolonged, although bleeding time is only affected at high doses.

Mechanism of Action: Heparin activates the enzyme antithrombin III, which in turn inhibits thrombin. To a lesser extent, and by a separate mechanism, heparin also inactivates factor Xa. Other clotting factors are affected by heparin, but these have little clinical significance. High doses interfere with platelet aggregation.

Pharmacokinetics:

Route(s)	Subcutaneous, IV bolus injection, or continuous infusion
Absorption	Heparin is poorly absorbed by the gastrointestinal (GI) mucosa because of rapid metabolism by the hepatic enzyme, heparinase
Distribution	Unknown; does not cross the placenta and is not secreted in breast milk
Primary metabolism	Hepatic and by reticuloendothelial system
Primary excretion	Reticuloendothelial system
Onset of action	IV: immediate; subcutaneous: 30–60 minutes
Duration of action	8–12 h; half-life: 90 minutes

Adverse Effects: Abnormal bleeding is common with heparin therapy, occurring in about 10% of patients, and is the most serious adverse effect. Bleeding may be major or minor, and involve any system in the body. The risk of bleeding is dose dependent; the higher the dose, the higher the risk. Should the aPTT become excessively prolonged or bleeding be observed, discontinuation of the drug will result in loss of anticoagulant activity within hours.

Heparin-induced thrombocytopenia (HIT) is a serious complication that occurs in up to 30% of patients taking the drug. Symptoms range from mild to severe. More severe symptoms usually appear after 5 to 10 days of therapy; thus, frequent blood laboratory testing should be conducted during this period. Although thrombocytopenia usually leads to excessive bleeding, HIT causes the opposite effect: an increase in adverse thrombotic events. HIT markedly increases platelet aggregation and the patient may experience serious and even life-threatening thrombosis. Although the half-life of heparin is brief, it may take a week after the drug is discontinued for platelets to recover. In addition HIT may not even become evident until several weeks after the drug is discontinued.

Because heparin is derived from animal sources, hypersensitivity reactions are possible. Mild allergic symptoms include fever, chills, and urticaria. Anaphylaxis is rare. Osteoporosis has been reported in patients taking the drug longer than 30 days, and may be severe enough to cause bone fractures. Skin lesions may develop, especially at the site of parenteral injections.

Contraindications/Precautions: Heparin should not be administered to patients with active internal bleeding, serious bleeding pathologies, severe hypertension (HTN), recent trauma, intracranial hemorrhage, or bacterial endocarditis. Some heparin products may contain sulfites and should not be administered to patients with sulfite sensitivity. Patients with severe thrombocytopenia or HIT should not be given heparin. Whenever possible, intramuscular (IM) injections of other medications should be avoided because they may cause serious bruising, bleeding, or hematomas. Although relatively safe during pregnancy, the drug should be used with caution during the peripartum period due to the risk of maternal hemorrhage. Caution must be used when administering heparin to patients with serious renal or hepatic impairment because the drug may rise to toxic levels.

Drug Interactions: Oral anticoagulants, including warfarin, potentiate heparin activity. Drugs that inhibit platelet aggregation (such as aspirin, indomethacin, and ibuprofen) may induce bleeding. Nicotine, digoxin, tetracyclines, or antihistamines may inhibit anticoagulation. **Herbal/Food:** Herbal supplements that may affect coagulation such as ginger, garlic, green tea, feverfew, or ginkgo should be avoided because they may increase the risk of bleeding.

Pregnancy: Category C.

Treatment of Overdose: If serious hemorrhage occurs, a specific antagonist, protamine sulfate, may be administered IV (1 mg for every 100 units of heparin) to neutralize the anticoagulant activity of heparin. Protamine sulfate has an onset of action of 5 minutes and a duration of 2 hours. Multiple doses may be necessary to control extensive hemorrhage. Protamine is also an antagonist to the LMWHs.

Nursing Responsibilities:

- Obtain a complete health history including recent surgeries or trauma, allergies, drug history, and possible drug interactions. Notify the prescriber if patient has history of active internal bleeding, serious bleeding disorders, severe HTN, or intracranial hemorrhage.
- Prior to drug therapy, obtain a baseline profile of blood coagulation tests, hematocrit (Hct), hemoglobin (Hgb), red blood cell (RBC), and platelet counts, and monitor laboratory values intermittently during therapy.
- Monitor the activated partial thromboplastin time (aPTT) levels, and adjust drug dosage to keep aPTT between 1.5 to 2.5 times baseline level.
- Collect blood for coagulation testing 30 minutes before each scheduled subcutaneous or intermittent IV dose and about every 4 hours in patients with continuous IV heparin during dosage adjustment periods. Test daily after this period is established.
- Monitor for signs of bleeding: excessive bruising, pallor, epistaxis, hemoptysis, hematemesis, menorrhagia, hematuria, melena, rectal bleeding, or excessive bleeding from wounds or in the mouth. Risk for hemorrhage is greatest in women, patients over 60 years of age, and those with liver or renal disease.
- Record vital signs and report fever, drop in blood pressure, rapid pulse, or signs and symptoms of hemorrhage.
- Apply firm but gentle pressure to a needlestick site for at least 10 minutes post-venipuncture. Observe all needle sites for hematoma and signs of inflammation (swelling, heat, redness, pain) on a daily basis.
- Maintain an environment to reduce risk for trauma and hemorrhage secondary from injury. Handle the patient gently to avoid injury and avoid parenteral injections.
- Keep the specific heparin antidote, protamine sulfate (1% solution), readily available.

Patient and Family Education:

- Avoid activities that may result in injury. Use a soft-bristle toothbrush or sponge tooth cleaners. Avoid dental floss and use only an electric razor for shaving. Avoid wearing clothing that is tight or rubs, and avoid blowing or picking the nose.
- Immediately report bleeding symptoms such as pink, red, dark brown, or cloudy urine; red or dark brown vomit that looks like coffee grounds; red or black stools; bleeding gums or mouth when brushing teeth; unexplained bruising, clotting, nose bleeds, or bloody sputum; chest pain; abdominal or lower back pain or swelling; joint pain or swelling; unusual increase in menstrual flow; pelvic pain; and severe or continuous headache, faintness, or dizziness.
- For female patients: Menstruation may be increased and prolonged but will not affect therapy unless bleeding becomes excessive.
- Avoid smoking and drinking alcohol because these may alter the response to heparin.
- Do not take other prescription or nonprescription drugs, dietary supplements, or herbal products without approval of the health care provider because these may interact with heparin.
- Learn subcutaneous injection techniques before hospital discharge if indicated.
- Inform the dentist that you are taking this drug, before dental procedures are performed.

Drugs Similar to Heparin (Hep-Lock, Monoject)

The LMWHs include dalteparin, enoxaparin, and tinzaparin. Two drugs in this class, ardeparin (Normiflo) and danaparoid (Orgaran), have been discontinued in the United States. Fondaparinux is similar to the LMWHs but has a few significant differences.

Dalteparin (Fragmin): As a LMWH, dalteparin has smaller glycosaminoglycan chains than unfractionated heparin. Approved in 1994, dalteparin is given by the subcutaneous route for the treatment and prophylaxis of DVT or pulmonary embolism. Other approved indications include thrombosis prophylaxis in patients at increased risk due to unstable angina, an acute MI, or cancer. It has a longer half-life than heparin, which allows for less frequent dosing. Like other LMWHs, bleeding is the most serious adverse effect and the drug should not be administered to patients with active bleeding. This drug is pregnancy category B.

Enoxaparin (Lovenox): Enoxaparin was the first LMWH approved by the U.S. Food and Drug Administration (FDA) in 1993. Indications include treatment and prophylaxis of DVT and pulmonary embolism. Following hip or lower extremity surgery, enoxaparin may be administered once daily for 7 to 10 days. Some orthopedic procedures such as repair of hip fractures require more prolonged therapy. Enoxaparin may also be administered for the prophylaxis of coronary artery thrombosis and the prevention of ischemic complications in patients with acute coronary syndrome, for patients with unstable angina, and patients having percutaneous coronary intervention. Bleeding is the most serious adverse effect and the drug should not be administered to patients with active bleeding. This drug is pregnancy category B.

Fondaparinux (Arixtra): Approved in 2001, fondaparinux is an anticoagulant used for many of the same indications as heparin and the LMWHs but has certain differences that make it unique. Fondaparinux is a synthetic agent that consists of only five saccharide units (a pentasaccharide) that is structurally identical to the region of the heparin molecule that binds AT-III. The pentasaccharide unit is able to selectively inhibit factor Xa without directly affecting thrombin. Fondaparinux is only given by the subcutaneous route, and is approved for the prophylaxis of VTE following orthopedic surgery and the treatment of DVT or pulmonary embolism. Off-label uses include the prophylaxis of coronary artery thrombosis and the prevention of ischemic complications in patients with unstable angina. Like the LMWHs, fondaparinux is administered as fixed doses based on the patient's weight, and routine laboratory monitoring is not required because aPTT and PT are not accurate measures of drug activity. Doses of fondaparinux are not interchangeable with heparin or the LMWHs. There is no specific antidote for overdose: Administration of protamine is ineffective. This drug is pregnancy category B.

Tinzaparin (Innohep): Tinzaparin is a newer LMWH, approved in 2000 for the therapy of acute, symptomatic DVT, with or without evidence of pulmonary embolism. Therapy is continued for 6 days, or until the patient has been switched to oral anticoagulation with warfarin. Therapy may be prolonged for 3 to 6 months in cancer patients at high risk to DVT or pulmonary embolism. Thrombosis prophylaxis is an off-label indication for tinzaparin. Bleeding is the most serious adverse effect and the drug should not be administered to patients with active bleeding. This drug is pregnancy category B.

40.5 The direct thrombin inhibitors are parenteral anticoagulants obtained from medical leeches that are used to treat or prevent venous thromboembolism.

The direct thrombin inhibitors have an interesting history; they were derived from chemicals found in leeches. Leeches are wormlike animals that survive by sucking and digesting blood from mammals. Medical leeches are an ancient treatment that dates back to early Egyptian and Greek civilizations. They were applied to the skin as a type of bloodletting, which was thought to remove harmful substances from the body. Known as hirudotherapy, the use of leeches was largely discontinued with the advent of modern medicine in the early 1900s. However, leeches are still an approved therapy for relieving venous congestion in transplanted or reattached fingers or limbs.

While studying leeches, scientists isolated a potent chemical called hirudin, which prevented blood from coagulating in the leech. Drugs in the direct thrombin inhibitor class were derived from the original hirudin molecule and are structurally very similar.

The direct thrombin inhibitors bind reversibly to thrombin, preventing the formation of fibrin. They are highly specific for thrombin and do not require AT-III as an intermediate in promoting anticoagulation as does heparin. They bind to circulating thrombin, as well as thrombin attached to fibrin clots. These drugs exhibit typical anticoagulant actions and are used for the same types of indications as heparin and the LMWHs. They are all administered parenterally.

CONNECTIONS

Treating the Diverse Patient

Pregnancy and Deep Vein Thrombosis

A rare but serious complication of pregnancy is deep vein thrombosis (DVT). Pregnancy is characterized by a hypercoagulation state which can be life threatening to the mother. In fact, thromboembolism is the most common cause of maternal morbidity in the United States and Great Britain.

Several risk factors for DVT may be present in pregnancy. Some include bed rest, obesity, or immobility as well as Cesarean section, preeclampsia, varicose veins, or thrombophilias such as Factor V Leiden. About 25% of women who experience DVT with pregnancy carry the Factor V Leiden. The drug of choice for DVT in pregnancy is low molecular weight heparin. Warfarin therapy is contraindicated. OB-GYN nurses should observe for the sign and symptoms of DVT and understand the therapeutic use and adverse effects of drug therapy.

CONNECTIONS

Patient Safety

Be Aware of Similar Packaging

The morning headlines read, "Fatal Overdose Given to Babies by Nurse." In the fall of 2006, the media reported a story about three premature infants who received fatal overdoses of heparin. Several other babies were affected but survived. Apparently, 1 mL heparin vials with 10,000 units/mL were placed in an automated dispensing unit where 10-unit/mL vials were usually kept. The packaging was similar so the nurse gave the wrong concentration to flush the umbilical line of the infants. What should be done to avoid this error in the future?

See Answers to Patient Safety Questions in Appendix A.

PROTOTYPE DRUG Lepirudin (Refludan)

Classification: Therapeutic: Anticoagulant
Pharmacologic: Direct thrombin inhibitor

Therapeutic Effects and Uses: Lepirudin is a protein that is nearly identical to hirudin, the natural substance isolated from leeches. It is approved to provide anticoagulation in patients with HIT and to prevent associated thromboembolic events. Lepirudin was the first drug approved in the United States for anticoagulation in patients with HIT in 1998.

Lepirudin is administered IV using a 15- to 20-second bolus or by continuous infusion. Patient monitoring involves daily aPTT values, to obtain an optimum aPTT ratio of 1.5 to 2.5 times the laboratory control.

Mechanism of Action: Lepirudin directly inhibits the action of thrombin without requiring the intermediate step of antithrombin III inhibition.

Pharmacokinetics:

Route(s)	IV
Absorption	NA
Distribution	Confined to extracellular fluids; unknown if it crosses the placenta, or is secreted in breast milk
Primary metabolism	Blood
Primary excretion	Renal 50%
Onset of action	Unknown
Duration of action	Unknown; half-life: 1.3 h

Adverse Effects: Like other anticoagulants, the most serious adverse effect of lepirudin is bleeding. Symptoms may include bleeding from puncture or wound sites, epistaxis, hematuria, vaginal bleeding, or GI bleeding. Hypersensitivity reactions, including anaphylaxis, have been reported.

Contraindications/Precautions: Lepirudin should not be administered to patients with active bleeding or those with an aPTT ratio of above 2.5. The drug should be used with caution in patients with severe HTN, recent trauma, recent surgery, intracranial hemorrhage, and bacterial endocarditis. Patients with renal impairment should receive a dose reduction because the drug may accumulate and cause bleeding in these patients.

Drug Interactions: Oral anticoagulants, including warfarin or heparin, may potentiate lepirudin activity. Drugs that inhibit platelet aggregation (such as aspirin, indomethacin, and ibuprofen) and thrombolytic drugs may induce bleeding. **Herbal/Food:** Herbal supplements that affect coagulation such as ginger, garlic, green tea, feverfew, or ginkgo may increase the risk of bleeding.

Pregnancy: Category B.

Treatment of Overdose: There are no specific antidotes for lepirudin overdose. Administration of protamine is not effective. Because of its relatively brief half-life, discontinuing the infusion results in an improvement in coagulation in a few hours.

Nursing Responsibilities:

- Obtain a complete health history including recent surgeries or trauma, allergies, drug history, and possible drug interactions. Notify the prescriber if the patient has a history of internal bleeding, serious bleeding disorders, severe HTN, or intracranial hemorrhage.
- Prior to drug therapy, assess and monitor baseline laboratory tests such as PT, international normalized ratio (INR), and aPTT. Withhold therapy and notify the prescriber if baseline aPTT ratio is greater than 2.5.
- Monitor aPTT 4 hours after start of therapy and at least once daily; monitor more frequently in patients with renal or hepatic impairment.
- Use extreme caution in administering this drug to patients with increased bleeding risk.
- Monitor for bleeding events such as from puncture wounds, hematoma, or hematuria, and report immediately to the prescriber.
- Do not give oral anticoagulants until lepirudin dose has been reduced and aPTT ratio has decreased to just above 1.5.

Patient and Family Education:

- Immediately report signs of unusual bleeding to the health care provider.
- Minimize the risk for hemorrhage by avoiding activities that may result in injury.
- Do not take other prescription or nonprescription drugs, dietary supplements, or herbal products without approval of the health care provider.
- Immediately notify the health care provider of any known or suspected pregnancy.
- Do not breast-feed while taking this drug without approval of the health care provider.

Drugs Similar to Lepirudin (Refludan)

Other direct thrombin inhibitors include argatroban, bivalirudin, and desirudin.

Argatroban (Acova, Novastan): Approved in 2000, argatroban is a synthetic thrombin inhibitor that is given by the IV route for HIT. It is also approved to treat or prevent thrombotic events associated with percutaneous coronary intervention. Unlike lepirudin, which is excreted by the kidneys, argatroban is metabolized and eliminated by the liver and therefore may be used in patients with renal impairment. Caution must be observed, however, when administering the drug to patients with hepatic impairment. Allergic reactions occur in up to 10% of patients receiving argatroban. Bleeding is the most serious adverse effect and the drug should not be administered to patients with active bleeding. This drug is pregnancy category C.

Bivalirudin (Angiomax): Approved in 2000, bivalirudin is a direct thrombin inhibitor very similar to lepirudin that is only available by the IV route. Bivalirudin is given concurrently with aspirin to reduce the incidence of thromboembolic events associated with HIT and to provide anticoagulation in patients undergoing percutaneous coronary intervention. Back pain is a common adverse effect of the drug, occurring in about 40% of patients. Nausea, vomiting, hypotension, and headache also occur in a significant number of patients. Bleeding is the most serious adverse effect and the drug should not be administered to patients with active bleeding. Bivalirudin is as effective as heparin and produces a lower incidence of serious bleeding, although it is very expensive. This drug is pregnancy category B.

Desirudin (Iprivask): Made through recombinant DNA technology, desirudin is nearly identical to hirudin and is the only direct thrombin inhibitor administered by the subcutaneous route. It acts by the same mechanism and has the same adverse effects and contraindications as lepirudin and other drugs in this class. The drug was approved in 2003 for DVT prophylaxis in patients undergoing hip replacement surgery. Off-label uses include prevention of thromboembolic events in patients with unstable angina and those undergoing percutaneous coronary intervention. Allergic reactions, including anaphylaxis, are rare. Bleeding is the most serious adverse effect and the drug should not be administered to patients with active bleeding. This drug is pregnancy category C.

Oral Anticoagulants

40.6 Warfarin is the most widely used drug for oral anticoagulant therapy.

Although parenteral anticoagulants have the advantage of an almost immediate onset of action, drugs given by this route require close medical supervision because adverse effects such as bleeding can rapidly ensue. When the patient's condition allows, oral anticoagulants are used due to their convenience and greater safety.

Warfarin (Coumadin) has been available as an anticoagulant for over 50 years and is the most frequently used drug in this class. Often, patients begin anticoagulation therapy with heparin and are switched to warfarin when their condition stabilizes. When transitioning, the two drugs must be administered concurrently for 2 to 3 days. This is because heparin has a brief half-life (90 minutes), and aPTT returns to normal within 2 to 3 hours following discontinuation of heparin. Warfarin, on the other hand, takes 1 to 3 days of therapy to achieve optimum anticoagulation. Thus, concomitant pharmacotherapy is necessary to ensure continuous anticoagulation. During this transition, there is increased risk of bleeding, due to the additive anticoagulant action of the two drugs.

Unlike heparin, which is monitored with aPTT values, PT is the standard laboratory test used to monitor the effectiveness of warfarin. The normal PT range is 12 to 15 seconds. During therapeutic anticoagulation, PT should increase to 1.5 to 2 times the patient's baseline. Because laboratory testing methods for PT vary, however, PT time is also reported as an international normalized ratio (INR) value; INR values averaging 2.5 are considered therapeutic for most indications. PT is measured daily until the desired level of therapeutic anticoagulation is achieved. Then, the frequency of laboratory testing is decreased to weekly or monthly as the patient's condition stabilizes. Home monitoring devices are available to provide convenient and reliable INR values, which can guide the patients to adjust their own medication amounts. Self-monitoring has its limitations, however. The devices are expensive and the patient or their caregiver must be capable of understanding how to properly adjust the dosage.

Warfarin is truly in a class by itself, with no other oral drugs acting by the same mechanism. The oral anticoagulant ximelagatran (Exanta) recently reached the final stages of clinical trials. Available as an anticoagulant in several countries, the primary advantages of this medication are that it may be given at a fixed dose, it requires little laboratory monitoring, and it has a low potential for drug–drug interactions. Unfortunately, several cases of serious liver injury were reported and the manufacturer has abandoned development of the drug in the United States. Several related drugs, however, remain in the development process in an attempt to find safer alternatives to warfarin.

Pentoxifylline (Trental) is a unique agent with anticoagulation properties, that works by a unique mechanism. Pentoxifylline acts on red blood cells to reduce their viscosity and increase their flexibility, thus allowing them to enter vessels that are partially occluded and prevent thrombi formation. It is given orally (PO) to increase the microcirculation in patients with intermittent claudication. Technically, it is classified as a hemorheologic drug, rather than an anticoagulant.

PROTOTYPE DRUG Warfarin (Coumadin)

Classification: **Therapeutic:** Anticoagulant
Pharmacologic: Vitamin K antagonist

Therapeutic Effects and Uses: Indications for warfarin therapy include the long-term prophylaxis of arterial thromboembolism, including prevention of CVA and MI. Other uses include the prophylaxis and treatment of DVT or pulmonary embolism in patients undergoing hip or knee surgery, or in those with long-term indwelling central venous catheters or prosthetic heart valves. The drug may be given to prevent thromboembolic events in high-risk patients following an MI or an atrial fibrillation episode.

Warfarin is well absorbed after oral administration but takes several days to produce an optimum therapeutic effect. Ninety-nine percent of absorbed warfarin is bound to plasma proteins and is not immediately available to produce its effect. This high level of protein binding is also responsible for some of the many drug–drug interactions that occur with warfarin.

There is wide variation in response to warfarin therapy. Dosage levels must be determined individually for each patient and carefully monitored. Patients stabilized on warfarin should not switch brands of the drug unless recommended by the health care provider, owing to differences in bioavailability. For most indications, the therapeutic range of serum warfarin levels varies from 1 to 10 mcg/mL, to achieve a target INR value of 2 to 3.

Mechanism of Action: Warfarin inhibits two enzymes involved in the formation of activated vitamin K, which is required for the synthesis of clotting factors II, VII, IX, and X. Warfarin inhibits the synthesis of new clotting factors but does not affect clotting factors that are already circulating in the blood. It takes 3 to 4 days for the plasma levels of existing clotting factors to fall, and for the anticoagulant effect of warfarin to appear. After discontinuing the drug, 3 to 4 days are needed for the body to make new clotting factors and return coagulation to baseline levels.

Pharmacokinetics:

Route(s)	PO, IV (rare)
Absorption	Well absorbed
Distribution	Widely distributed; crosses the placenta but is not secreted in breast milk; 99% bound to plasma protein
Primary metabolism	Hepatic
Primary excretion	Renal, small amounts in bile
Onset of action	2–7 days
Duration of action	3–5 days, half-life: 0.5–3 days

Adverse Effects: Like all anticoagulants, the most serious adverse effect of warfarin is abnormal bleeding, which may occur in any body system. Warfarin may release pieces of atheromatous plaque from vessel walls, resulting in systemic cholesterol microembolization that may occlude small vessels. For example, "purple-toe syndrome" is caused by cholesterol microembolization and severe cases may lead to gangrene or amputation.

Long-term use of warfarin may increase the risk of osteoporosis and bone fractures.

Contraindications/Precautions: Patients with recent trauma, active internal bleeding, serious bleeding disorders, intracranial hemorrhage, severe HTN, bacterial endocarditis, or severe hepatic or renal impairment should not take warfarin. When possible, warfarin should be discontinued or the dosage lowered before dental or elective surgical procedures. Patients with congestive heart failure may exhibit excessive anticoagulation with warfarin, which requires lower doses. Whenever possible, IM injections of other medications should be avoided because they may cause bruising, bleeding, or hematomas. Warfarin should not be taken during pregnancy because the drug has been shown to produce numerous fetal abnormalities, induce fatal bleeding, and can cause fetal death. Warfarin is believed to be safe for lactating women who are at risk to postpartum venous thrombus because very little of the drug enters breast milk. Studies have shown no change in the INR values of lactating infants whose mothers are receiving warfarin.

Drug Interactions: Drug–drug interactions with warfarin are numerous. Because the therapeutic index of warfarin is very low, drugs that interact with warfarin have the potential to affect coagulation time and cause harm. Concurrent use with other drugs with anticoagulant activity, including aspirin, heparin, and antiplatelet drugs, may produce additive effects and excessive bleeding. Extensive protein binding is responsible for numerous drug–drug interactions, some of which include: nonsteroidal anti-inflmmatory drugs (NSAIDs), diuretics, selective serotonin reuptake inhibitors (SSRIs) and other antidepressants, steroids, antibiotics, and vaccines or vitamins (e.g., vitamin K). NSAIDs increase bleeding risk. During warfarin therapy, the patient should not take any other prescription or OTC drugs or herbal products unless approved by the health care provider. A listing of selected drugs and supplements affecting warfarin therapy is given in Table 40.4. **Herbal/Food**: Herbal supplements such as green tea, ginkgo, feverfew, garlic, cranberry, chamomile, and ginger may increase the risk of bleeding.

Pregnancy: Category X.

TABLE 40.4 Drug–Drug Interactions with Warfarin

Interaction	Drug or Drug Class
Increased anticoagulant effect	acetaminophen, amiodarone, anabolic steroids, azole antifungals, aspirin, cephalosporins, cimetidine, clopidogrel, danazol, disulfiram, heparin, isoniazid, macrolides, metronidazole, nalidixic acid, NSAIDs, omeprazole, paroxetine, penicillin, propafenone, quinidine, tamoxifen, tetracyclines, thyroid hormone, ticlopidine, trimethoprim-sulfisoxazole, statins
Decreased anticoagulant effect	barbiturates, bile-acid sequestrants, carbamazepine, cyclosporine, dicloxacillin, oral contraceptives, rifampin
Mixed effect	allopurinol, corticosteroids, ethanol, phenytoin
Supplements and food	American ginseng, cranberry, feverfew, ginkgo, green tea, vitamin E, vitamin K

Treatment of Overdose: The specific treatment for warfarin overdose is oral or parenteral administration of vitamin K_1. When administered IV, vitamin K_1 can reverse the anticoagulant effects of warfarin within 6 hours.

Nursing Responsibilities:

- Obtain a complete health history including recent surgeries or trauma, allergies, drug history, and possible drug interactions. Notify the prescriber if the patient has a history of internal bleeding, serious bleeding disorders, severe HTN, recent trauma, or intracranial hemorrhage.
- Assess and monitor PT/INR prior to initiation of therapy and then daily until maintenance dosage is established. Adjust drug dose to maintain PT at 1.5 to 2.5 times the control (12 to 15 seconds), or 15% to 35% of normal prothrombin activity, or an INR of 2 to 4 depending on diagnosis.
- Monitor PT/INR determinations at 1- to 4-week intervals depending on the patient's response.
- Monitor periodic urinalyses, stool guaiac, and liver function tests. Blood samples should be drawn 12 to 18 hours after the last dose is taken.
- Monitor older adults, and psychotic, or alcoholic patients for possible nonadherence.
- Recognize that patients at greatest risk of hemorrhage include those whose PT/INR values are difficult to regulate, have an aortic valve prosthesis, are receiving long-term anticoagulant therapy, or are older adults or debilitated patients.

Patient and Family Education:

- Minimize the risk for hemorrhage by avoiding activities that may result in injury. Use soft-bristle toothbrush or sponge tooth cleaners. Avoid dental floss and use only an electric razor for shaving. Avoid wearing clothing that is tight or rubs against the skin, and avoid blowing or picking the nose.
- Report to the health care provider bleeding symptoms such as pink, red, dark brown, or cloudy urine; red or dark brown vomit that looks like coffee grounds; red or black stools; bleeding gums or mouth when brushing teeth; unexplained bruising, clotting, nose bleeds, or bloody sputum; chest pain; abdominal or lower back pain or swelling; joint pain or swelling; unusual increase in menstrual flow; pelvic pain; and severe or continuous headache, faintness, or dizziness.
- Stop the drug and immediately report symptoms of hepatitis such as dark urine, itchy skin, jaundice, abdominal pain, light stools, or hypersensitivity reaction to the health care provider.
- Use the same brand drug and take the dose at the same time each day (usually at night). Never skip a dose or take a double dose.
- For female patients: Report an unusual increase in menstrual bleeding. PT/INR should be checked at least monthly in menstruating women.
- Understand that fever, prolonged hot weather, malnutrition, and diarrhea can lengthen PT/INR, which enhances the anticoagulant effect.
- Avoid a high-fat diet with moderate intake of vitamin K–rich foods such as cabbage, cauliflower, brussels sprouts,

MyNursingKit | Mechanism of Action: Warfarin

broccoli, asparagus, lettuce, turnip greens, onions, spinach, kale, fish, beef liver, coffee, or green tea (with caffeine), soybean or canola oil, or by tube feedings with high vitamin K content, as these shorten PT/INR.

- Avoid excessive intake of alcohol.
- Inform the dentist and all health care providers of anticoagulant therapy.
- Use extra precautions such as barrier contraceptive measures because warfarin therapy while pregnant can cause birth defects. Avoid taking the drug between the 6th and 12th week of pregnancy.
- Do not take OTC drugs or herbal supplements without approval of the health care provider.
- Carry medical identification at all times that includes medical diagnosis, medication(s), health care provider's name, address, and telephone number.
- Use only low doses of acetaminophen for pain or discomfort. Avoid all OTC aspirin products and NSAIDs.

Drugs Similar to Warfarin (Coumadin)

There are no oral anticoagulants acting by the same mechanism as warfarin.

NURSING PROCESS APPLICATION

Patients Receiving Anticoagulant Therapy

Assessment	Potential Nursing Diagnoses
Prior to administration: • Obtain a complete health history including recent surgeries or trauma, allergies, drug history, and possible drug interactions. • Obtain vital signs; assess in context of patient's baseline values. • Determine patient's baseline bleeding studies (aPTT, PT, or INR).	• *Risk for Injury*, related to adverse effects of anticoagulant therapy • *Ineffective Tissue Perfusion (Peripheral)*, related to hemorrhage • *Deficient Knowledge (Anticoagulation Therapy)*, related to purpose, precautions, and adverse effects of drug

Planning: Patient Goals and Expected Outcomes

The patient will:

- Experience a decrease in blood coagulation as evidenced by laboratory values ordered by the health care provider.
- Be free of adverse effects such as hemorrhage related to anticoagulation therapy.
- Demonstrate an understanding of the drug's action by accurately describing drug adverse effects and precautions.

Implementation

Interventions and (Rationales)	Patient and Family Education
• Monitor for adverse clotting reaction(s). (Heparin can cause thrombus formation with thrombocytopenia, or "white clot syndrome." Warfarin may cause cholesterol microemboli, which result in gangrene, localized vasculitis, or "purple toes syndrome.")	• Instruct the patient to immediately report sudden dyspnea, chest pain, or temperature or color change in the hands, arms, legs, and feet.
• Observe for skin necrosis, and blue or purple mottling of the feet that blanches with pressure or fades when the legs are elevated. (Patients on anticoagulant therapy remain at risk for developing emboli resulting in CVA or pulmonary embolism.)	Instruct the patient to: • Check pulses in the ankle daily.
• Use with caution in patients with GI, renal, or liver disease, alcoholism, diabetes, HTN, hyperlipidemia, and in the elderly and premenopausal women. (Patients with coronary artery disease (CAD), diabetes, HTN, and hyperlipidemia are at increased risk for developing cholesterol microemboli.)	• Instruct elderly patients, menstruating women, and those with peptic ulcer disease, alcoholism, or kidney or liver disease that they have an increased risk of bleeding.
• Monitor for signs of bleeding: flulike symptoms, excessive bruising, pallor, epistaxis, hemoptysis, hematemesis, menorrhagia, hematuria, melena, rectal bleeding, or excessive bleeding from wounds or in the mouth. (Bleeding is a sign of anticoagulant overdose.) • Maintain the environment to reduce risk for trauma and hemorrhage secondary from injury. Handle the client gently to avoid injury. Avoid parenteral injections. (Patients are at high risk for bleeding.)	Instruct the patient to: • Immediately report flulike symptoms (dizziness, chills, weakness, pale skin); blood coming from a cough, the nose, mouth, or rectum; menstrual "flooding"; "coffee grounds" vomit; tarry stools; excessive bruising; bleeding from wounds that cannot be stopped within 10 minutes; all physical injuries. • Avoid all contact sports and other activities that cause intense or violent bumping or jostling. • Use a soft toothbrush and electric shaver.
• Monitor vital signs. (Increase in heart rate accompanied by low blood pressure or subnormal temperature may signal bleeding.)	• Instruct the patient to immediately report palpitations, fatigue, or feeling faint, which may signal low blood pressure related to bleeding.
• Monitor laboratory values: aPTT and PTT for therapeutic values. (Heparin may cause significant elevations of aspartate aminotransferase [AST] and alanine transaminase [ALT] because the drug is metabolized by the liver.)	Instruct the patient to: • Always inform laboratory personnel of heparin therapy when providing samples. • Carry a wallet card, or wear medical ID jewelry indicating heparin therapy.
• Monitor the complete blood count (CBC), especially in premenopausal women. (Changes in CBC may indicate excessive bleeding.)	• Instruct the patient to keep a "pad count" during menstrual periods to estimate blood losses.

Evaluation of Outcome Criteria

Evaluate the effectiveness of drug therapy by confirming that patient goals and expected outcomes have been met (see "Planning").

Antiplatelet Agents

40.7 Antiplatelet agents provide anticoagulation by reducing the aggregation properties of platelets.

Antiplatelet drugs modify coagulation primarily by interfering with platelet aggregation. Unlike the anticoagulants, which are used primarily to prevent thrombosis in veins, the primary indications for antiplatelet agents are to prevent clot formation in arteries. The antiplatelet agents are listed in Table 40.5.

Because platelets are a central component of blood hemostasis, reducing the number of platelets or their function can profoundly increase bleeding time. Three groups of drugs are classified as antiplatelet agents.

- Aspirin
- Adenosine diphosphate (ADP) receptor blockers
- Glycoprotein IIb/IIIa receptor blockers

Aspirin deserves special mention as an antiplatelet agent. Because it is available OTC, patients may not consider aspirin a potent medication; however, its anticoagulant activity is well documented. Aspirin acts by binding irreversibly to the enzyme cyclooxygenase (COX) in platelets. This binding inhibits the formation of thromboxane A_2, a powerful inducer of platelet aggregation. The anticoagulant effect of a single dose of aspirin may persist for as long as 1 week. Concurrent use of aspirin with other coagulation modifiers should be avoided, unless medically approved. The indications for aspirin are described in a number of places in this text: pain relief in Chapter 29, prevention of CVA and MI in Chapter 37, and reduction of inflammation in Chapter 44. Nursing responsibilities and a prototype feature for aspirin are in Chapter 44.

40.8 The adenosine diphosphate receptor blockers are antiplatelet agents prescribed for the prevention and treatment of arterial thrombosis.

Although platelets are simply fragments of cells that have no nucleus, they contain many receptors on their plasma membranes and their functions are complex. Chemicals such as epinephrine, thromboxane A_2, thrombin, serotonin, and fibrinogen can bind to these receptors and modify coagulation through their interaction with the platelets.

Following vessel injury, platelets become "sticky," bind to exposed collagen, and release substances that recruit additional platelets to the site. One of these chemicals is adenosine diphosphate (ADP), whose function is to promote platelet aggregation. The ADP receptor blockers comprise a small group of drugs that irreversibly alter the plasma membrane of platelets. For the remainder of their lifespan, the affected platelets are unable to recognize the chemical signals required for them to aggregate.

Ticlopidine (Ticlid) and clopidogrel (Plavix) are ADP receptor blockers given orally to prevent thrombi formation in patients who have experienced a recent thromboembolic event such as CVA or MI. Ticlopidine can cause life-threatening neutropenia and agranulocytosis in a small percentage of patients. Clopidogrel is safer, having a lower incidence of adverse GI, hematologic, and cutaneous adverse effects.

TABLE 40.5 Antiplatelet Agents

Drug	Route and Adult Dose (maximum dose where indicated)	Adverse Effects
aspirin (ASA, acetylsalicylic acid)	PO: 80 mg daily to 650 mg bid	*Nausea, vomiting, diarrhea, abdominal pain, dizziness, headache* Increased clotting time, GI bleeding (aspirin), central nervous system (CNS) effects (dipyridamole), anaphylaxis (aspirin)
dipyridamole (Persantine)	PO: 75–100 mg qid as adjunct to warfarin therapy	
ADP Receptor Blockers		
clopidogrel (Plavix)	PO: 75 mg/day (max: 300 mg/day for life-threatening cases)	*Minor bleeding, dyspepsia, abdominal pain, headache, rash and diarrhea* Increased clotting time, GI bleeding, blood dyscrasias, angina
prasugrel (Effient)	PO: 60 mg loading dose followed by 10 mg/day	
ticlopidine (Ticlid)	PO: 250 mg bid (max: 500 mg/day)	
Glycoprotein IIb/IIIa Receptor Antagonists		
abciximab (ReoPro)	IV: 0.25 mg/kg initial bolus over 5 min, then 0.125 mcg/kg/min for 12 h (max: 10 mcg/min)	*Dyspepsia, dizziness, pain at injection site, hypotension, bradycardia, minor bleeding* Major hemorrhage, thrombocytopenia
eptifibatide (Integrilin)	IV: 180 mcg/kg initial bolus over 1–2 min, then 2 mcg/kg/min for 24–72 h (max: 180 mcg/kg bolus, 2 mcg/kg/min infusion)	
tirofiban (Aggrastat)	IV: 0.4 mcg/kg/min for 30 min, then 0.1 mcg/kg/min for 12–24 h	
Agents for Intermittent Claudication		
cilostazol (Pletal)	PO: 100 mg bid	*Dyspepsia, nausea, vomiting, dizziness, myalgia, headache* Tachycardia and palpitations (cilostazol), CNS effects (pentoxifylline), heart failure, MI
pentoxifylline (Trental)	PO: 400 mg tid (max: 1200 mg/day)	

Note: *Italics* indicate common adverse effects; Underline indicates serious adverse effects.

CONNECTIONS

Complementary and Alternative Therapies Garlic

Description: Garlic (Allium sativum) is a perennial plant in the onion family that can be grown and cultivated worldwide.

History and Claims: Garlic has been used for centuries by most cultures as a flavoring and as a medicine. Historical uses have included curing deafness and earaches, and treating leprosy and scurvy. Modern claims have focused on cardiovascular uses: treatment of high blood lipid levels, atherosclerosis, and HTN. Other modern claims are that garlic reduces blood glucose levels and has antibacterial and antineoplastic activity.

Standardization: Substances called alliaceous oils have been isolated from garlic and shown to have pharmacologic activity. Dosage forms include eating prepared garlic oil or the fresh bulbs (cloves) from the plant. In tablet or capsule form, doses range from 1 to 4 g/day. Extracts may be standardized by percent allicin.

Evidence: Garlic is one of the best-studied herbs. Like most other herbal products, garlic likely has some health benefits, but controlled, scientific studies are often lacking and the results are mixed. It has been shown to decrease the aggregation or "stickiness" of platelets, thus producing an anticoagulant effect. There is some research to show that the herb has a small effect on lowering blood cholesterol, although the effects seem to be short term. Evidence on the effects of the herb on blood pressure is mixed. Evidence of antineoplastic or antibacterial effects of garlic is not strong.

Garlic is safe for consumption in small and moderate amounts. Patients taking anticoagulant medications should limit their intake of garlic to avoid bleeding complications. Diabetic patients should monitor their blood glucose levels closely if taking high doses of garlic.

Source: From *Garlic*, Drug Digest, 2007. Retrieved July 17, 2008, from http://www.drugdigest.org/DD/DVH/HerbsWho/0,3923,4041Garlic,00.html; "Garlic and Cardiovascular Disease: A Critical Review," by K. Rahman and G. M. Lowe, 2006, *Journal of Nutrition, 136*(3 Suppl), pp. 736S–740S; and "Complementary, Holistic, and Integrative Medicine: Garlic," by L. Shamseer, T. L. Charrois, and S. Vohra, 2006, *Pediatrics in Review, 27*(12), pp. e77–e80.

Drugs affecting platelet aggregation increase the risk of bleeding should the patient sustain trauma or undergo dental or surgical procedures. These drugs are sometimes given concurrently with anticoagulants, which can further increase bleeding risk. Prolonged direct pressure over injection or venipuncture sites may be required to control bleeding. Bleeding lasting more than 10 minutes may require special medical or nursing interventions, such as suturing or applying a sandbag to a venipuncture site that does not stop bleeding.

PROTOTYPE DRUG Clopidogrel (Plavix)

Classification: **Therapeutic:** Antiplatelet agent
Pharmacologic: ADP receptor blocker

Therapeutic Effects and Uses: Approved in 1997, clopidogrel is used for the prophylaxis of arterial thromboembolism to reduce the risk of CVA and MI. The drug has been shown to be more effective than aspirin in reducing thromboembolic events in patients with recent CVA or MI. It may also be given to prevent thrombi formation in patients with unstable angina or coronary artery stents, and to prevent postoperative deep vein thromboses. Clopidogrel has similar anticoagulant activity to aspirin but is much more expensive.

Clopidogrel is given orally and has the advantage of once-daily dosing. Inhibition of platelet function may persist for 7 to 10 days after the drug is discontinued. When possible, clopidogrel should be discontinued at least 5 days prior to surgery to avoid excessive bleeding.

Mechanism of Action: Clopidogrel inhibits ADP receptors on platelets and prolongs bleeding time by irreversibly inhibiting platelet aggregation. Clopidogrel itself has little activity; however, it is changed to a highly active metabolite in the liver through extensive first-pass metabolism.

Pharmacokinetics:

Route(s)	PO
Absorption	Rapidly absorbed
Distribution	Unknown; unknown if it crosses the placenta or is secreted in breast milk; 94–98% bound to plasma protein
Primary metabolism	Hepatic; metabolized to active metabolite
Primary excretion	Renal 50%; feces 50%
Onset of action	1–2 h
Duration of action	5 days

Adverse Effects: Clopidogrel has approximately the same tolerability as aspirin and adverse effects are rarely severe enough to cause discontinuation of therapy. Although excessive bleeding is a potential adverse effect, it only occurs in about 1% of patients. Older adults are more susceptible to bleeding during therapy and should be carefully monitored. The incidence of GI bleeding is less than that of aspirin. Common adverse effects are flulike syndrome, headache, diarrhea, dizziness, bruising, upper respiratory tract infection, and rash or pruritus. Clopidogrel does not exhibit the same degree of bone marrow toxicity as ticlopidine.

Contraindications/Precautions: Clopidogrel is contraindicated in patients with active bleeding and should be used with caution in patients at high risk to bleeding, including those with peptic ulcer disease. Severe hepatic disease may impair the ability of the liver to convert the drug to its active metabolite.

Drug Interactions: Use with anticoagulants, other antiplatelet agents, thrombolytic agents, or NSAIDs, including aspirin, will increase the risk of bleeding. Drugs that inhibit hepatic metabolic enzymes—such as the azole antifungals, protease inhibitors, erythromycin, verapamil, or zafirlukast—may diminish the antiplatelet actions of clopidogrel. Drugs that increase hepatic metabolic enzyme activity, such as barbiturates, rifampin, or carbamazepine may increase the anticoagulant activity of clopidogrel. **Herbal/Food**: Herbal supplements that affect coagulation such as feverfew, green tea, ginkgo, fish oil, ginger, or garlic may increase the risk of bleeding.

Treatment of Overdose: There is no specific therapy for clopidogrel overdose. Platelet transfusions may be beneficial in preventing hemorrhage.

Pregnancy: Category B.

Nursing Responsibilities:

- Assess current use of anticoagulants and NSAIDs including aspirin, prior to initiating therapy.
- Assess for increased bleeding or bruising tendencies before and during therapy. Bleeding is more likely to occur in older patients and those taking other drugs that affect coagulation.
- Monitor for signs and symptoms of bleeding and immediately report to the prescriber.
- Evaluate patients with unexplained fever or infection for myelotoxicity.

Patient and Family Education:

- Immediately report any unusual bleeding such as black, tarry stools; blood in urine; vomiting of material that looks like coffee grounds or blood; bleeding with tooth brushing; nosebleed; unusual bruising; bloody sputum; profuse menstrual bleeding; continuous headache; faintness; or dizziness.
- Know that it may take longer than usual to stop bleeding. Refrain from sports and activities that increase the risk of traumatic injury.
- Do not stop taking the drug unless approved by the health care provider.
- Do not use NSAIDs including aspirin, other OTC drugs, or herbal supplements unless approved by health care provider.
- Inform the dentist and all health care providers of antiplatelet therapy prior to dental or medical procedures.

Drugs Similar to Clopidogrel (Plavix)

Other antiplatelet agents include dipyridamole and ticlopidine. Aspirin also provides anticoagulation by this mechanism and is discussed in Section 40.7.

Dipyridamole (Persantine): Approved in 1961, the only currently approved use of dipyridamole is in combination with warfarin for postoperative prophylaxis of thromboembolic complications in patients with prosthetic heart valves. By itself, dipyridamole provides little antithrombotic protection, but it may be combined with aspirin or warfarin to produce an anticoagulant effect. Dipyridamole acts by a different mechanism than clopidogrel. Rather than blocking ADP receptors, dipyridamole elevates levels of cyclic AMP (cAMP), which is a potent inhibitor of platelet aggregation. Originally approved in 1961 for treating angina due to its vasodilation action on the coronary arteries, dipyridamole is no longer used for that indication. Dizziness, abdominal pain, and headache are the most common adverse effects. This drug is pregnancy category B.

Ticlopidine (Ticlid): Approved in 1991, ticlopidine is an ADP receptor blocker with antiplatelet effects very similar to those of clopidogrel. Ticlopidine is approved to prevent thrombotic CVA, and has been widely used to prevent thromboembolic events in those receiving coronary artery stents. The drug is administered PO, and may take up to 5 to 6 days of therapy to achieve optimum effects. Anticoagulant action may persist 1 to 2 weeks after the drug is withdrawn, because new platelets must be synthesized to replace those bound to the drug. The limiting factor for ticlopidine therapy is bone marrow toxicity, which may manifest as agranulocytosis, pancytopenia, thrombocytopenic purpura, or neutropenia. Although these cases are rare, they may be life threatening. Thus, ticlopidine is generally only used when other drugs such as aspirin and clopidogrel have failed to produce the desired therapeutic results. Common adverse effects include diarrhea, nausea, vomiting, and dyspepsia. This drug is pregnancy category B.

40.9 The glycoprotein IIb/IIIa receptor inhibitors are the most effective antiplatelet drugs for preventing coagulation.

Glycoprotein IIb/IIIa is a receptor found on the surface of platelets. The receptor contains two distinct protein chains: IIb and IIIa designate the two chains. Platelets contain a huge number of glycoprotein IIb/IIIa receptors: approximately 50,000 to 80,000 per cell. These receptors serve as "docking stations," waiting for signals from chemical messengers that indicate injury may have occurred.

Substances that may bind to and activate glycoprotein IIb/IIIa receptors include thrombin, von Willebrand factor, ADP, and thromboxane A_2. Following activation of the surface glycoprotein, the platelets change shape, bind fibrinogen, and become "sticky." Essentially, the platelets develop an enhanced ability to bind to each other, to fibrinogen, and to the exposed collagen of damaged vessels. This process is illustrated in Figure 40.2.

Glycoprotein IIb/IIIa receptor inhibitors are relatively new additions to the therapy of thromboembolic disease. Inhibition of the glycoprotein IIb/IIIa receptor prevents platelet activation and thrombus formation in patients with a recent MI, CVA, and percutaneous coronary intervention, with or without stent placement.

Although these medications are the most effective antiplatelet agents, they are very expensive. Another major disadvantage is that they are given only by the IV route. PO forms of these drugs recently entered clinical trials but proved less effective than aspirin in reducing thromboembolic events.

PROTOTYPE DRUG Abciximab (ReoPro)

Classification: **Therapeutic:** Antiplatelet agent
Pharmacologic: Glycoprotein IIb/IIIa inhibitor

Therapeutic Effects and Uses: Abciximab was the first glycoprotein IIb/IIIa inhibitor approved by the FDA in 1994. It is of value in decreasing the incidence of thromboembolic events in patients with acute coronary syndrome, and in conjunction

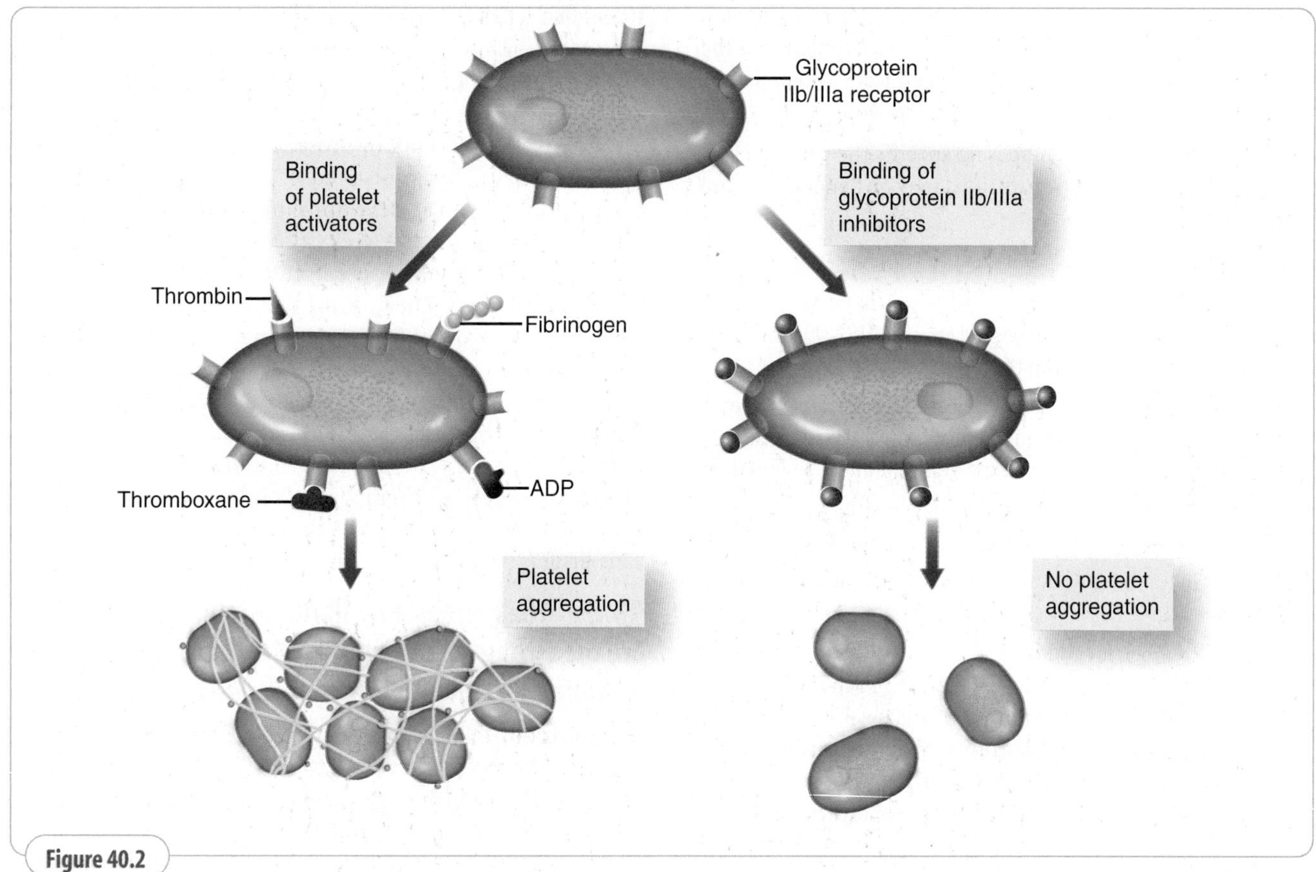

Figure 40.2

Glycoprotein IIb/IIIa receptor activation of platelet function.

with percutaneous coronary intervention, both before and after the procedure. Abciximab is only available by IV bolus injection and infusion. It is often given concurrently with aspirin, clopidogrel, or heparin to achieve optimum therapeutic results.

Glycoprotein IIb/IIIa receptor inhibitors act very rapidly: Platelet function is reduced by as much as 90% in just 2 hours. Effects may persist for more than 10 days following discontinuation of the drug.

Mechanism of Action: Abciximab is an antibody fragment that binds to glycoprotein IIb/IIIa receptors on platelets, thus preventing fibrinogen, von Willebrand factor (vWF), and other procoagulants from activating platelets.

Pharmacokinetics:

Route(s)	IV
Absorption	NA
Distribution	Mostly bound to platelets, with very little circulating free; unknown if the drug crosses the placenta or is secreted in breast milk
Primary metabolism	Rapidly destroyed by proteases in plasma
Primary excretion	Unknown
Onset of action	2 h
Duration of action	48 h; half-life: 10–30 minutes

Adverse Effects: The most common adverse effect of abciximab is abnormal bleeding, which may occur in any body system. Major bleeding occurs in about 10% of patients, with the most common bleeding occurring at the arterial access site. Hypotension may occur secondary to loss of blood. Thrombocytopenia occurs in more than 5% of the patients; thus, blood counts must be periodically monitored during therapy. Anaphylaxis is rare. Back pain and chest pain occur in 11% to 18% of patients taking the drug.

Contraindications/Precautions: Abciximab is contraindicated in patients with active bleeding, recent trauma or surgery, or serious bleeding disorders, or patients who have conditions that place them at high risk for bleeding. Patients with thrombocytopenia (less than 100,000 cells/mL) should not receive this drug. Patients who have received previous abciximab therapy have a higher risk of anaphylaxis and thrombocytopenia upon reexposure to the drug.

Drug Interactions: Concurrent administration of abciximab with heparin, other anticoagulants, or thrombolytics increases the risk of bleeding. Abciximab is contraindicated when IV dextran has been used before or during percutaneous coronary intervention because bleeding risk is increased. Oral anticoagulants should be discontinued at least 7 days prior to abciximab use, unless the PT is less than 1.2 times control. **Herbal/Food:** Herbal supplements, such as white willow, that contain salicylates may create an additive effect with antiplatelet drugs. Ginkgo and feverfew should also be avoided

Pregnancy: Category C.

Treatment of Overdose: There is no specific therapy for abciximab overdose. Platelet transfusions may be beneficial in preventing hemorrhage.

Nursing Responsibilities:

- Monitor laboratory tests for Hgb, Hct, platelet count, PT, aPTT, INR, and activated clotting time every 2 to 4 hours during the first 24 hours of therapy.
- Observe for signs and symptoms of bleeding at all potential sites such as catheter insertion, needle puncture, or IV cut-down sites or retroperitoneal sites.
- Stop infusion and notify the prescriber if hypersensitivity or bleeding occurs. Hypersensitivity may occur any time during drug administration.
- Minimize any unnecessary invasive procedures and devices to reduce the risk of bleeding.
- Elevate the head of the bed 30° or more and keep the limb straight when femoral artery access is used for drug administration.

Patient and Family Education:

- Immediately report to the health care provider any signs and symptoms of bleeding such as black, tarry stools; blood in urine; vomiting substances that look like coffee grounds or blood; bleeding with tooth brushing; nosebleed; bloody sputum; profuse menstrual bleeding; unusual bruising; continuous headache; faintness; or dizziness.
- Do not take any other prescription or nonprescription drugs, dietary supplements, or herbal products unless approved by health care provider.

Drugs Similar to Abciximab (ReoPro)

The two other glycoprotein IIb/IIIa inhibitors are eptifibatide and tirofiban.

Eptifibatide (Integrilin): Approved in 1998, eptifibatide is a synthetic drug administered by the IV route that is highly specific to binding the glycoprotein IIa/IIIb receptor. Unlike abciximab, the binding of eptifibatide is rapidly reversible and a large amount of unbound drug may circulate in the plasma. In overdose situations, platelet infusions may be of little benefit because the unbound drug will quickly occupy glycoprotein IIb/IIIa receptors on the new platelets to prevent their activation by procoagulants. The drug is indicated for the prevention of thromboembolic events in patients with acute coronary syndrome and those undergoing percutaneous coronary intervention. Aspirin or heparin are usually administered concurrently with eptifibatide. Should platelet count decrease to less than 100,000/mm^3, the aspirin or heparin is discontinued. The duration of action of eptifibatide is only 2 to 4 hours, compared to 24 to 48 hours for abciximab with eptifibatide. The kidneys primarily excrete the drug; thus, caution should be used in patients with renal impairment. Bleeding at the arterial access site is the most common adverse effect. This drug is pregnancy category B.

Tirofiban (Aggrastat): Like eptifibatide, tirofiban is an IV synthetic drug highly selective for binding the glycoprotein IIb/IIIa receptor in a rapid, reversible manner. The drug is indicated for the prevention of thromboembolic events in patients with acute coronary syndrome and those undergoing percutaneous coronary intervention. Aspirin or heparin are usually administered concurrently. It has a longer duration of action (4 to 8 hours) than eptifibatide, but still considerably less than abciximab. The kidneys primarily excrete the drug; thus, caution should be used in patients with renal impairment. Tirofiban is contraindicated in patients with platelet counts less than 100,000/mm^3. Bleeding secondary to the drug's antiplatelet effect is the most common adverse effect. This drug is pregnancy category B.

40.10 Fibrinolysis is a process that removes thrombi.

The goal of hemostasis has been achieved once a blood clot is formed and the body is protected from excessive hemorrhage. The process of hemostasis, however, is a positive feedback mechanism in which small amounts of clotting leads to additional clotting. Without an effective means of controlling the process, clotting would spread far beyond the zone of injury and, indeed, occur throughout the vascular system until existing clotting factors were used up. Furthermore, fibrin clots can prevent blood flow to the surrounding area. Circulation must eventually be restored so that the tissue can resume normal activities.

Fibrinolysis is the physiologic process that limits clot formation and removes existing clots. During the time a fibrin clot is forming, the surrounding damaged tissue secretes anticoagulant chemicals that limit the spread of the clot to the area of injury. Removal of the clot begins about 24 to 48 hours following clot formation and continues until it is dissolved.

Like hemostasis, fibrinolysis involves several cascading steps. The process is initiated by plasminogen activators. The two best studied plasminogen activators are tissue-plasminogen activator (tPA), which is secreted by the endothelium of blood vessels, and urokinase-plasminogen activator (uPA), secreted by the kidney. The function of tPA and uPA is to convert the inactive protein **plasminogen,** which is present in the fibrin clot, to its active form called plasmin. Plasmin is an enzyme that attacks the fibrin strands, breaking them into small fragments that are soluble and no longer able to hold the clot together. The procoagulation factors fibrinogen, prothrombin, and clotting factors V and XII are also inactivated by plasmin. The body normally regulates fibrinolysis such that unwanted fibrin clots are removed, while fibrin present in wounds is left to maintain hemostasis. The steps of fibrinolysis are shown in Figure 40.3.

Thrombolytics

40.11 Thrombolytics are used to dissolve existing intravascular clots in patients with myocardial infarction and cerebrovascular accident.

It is often mistakenly believed that the purpose of anticoagulants such as heparin or warfarin is to digest clots. This is not the case. A totally different type of drug is needed for this goal. The thrombolytics, shown in Table 40.6, are administered very differently from the anticoagulants and antiplatelet agents, and produce their effects by different mechanisms. Thrombolytics are prescribed for disorders in which an intravascular clot has already formed, such as acute MI, pulmonary embolism, acute ischemic CVA, and DVT.

Thrombolytics promote fibrinolysis by converting plasminogen to plasmin. The enzyme plasmin then digests fibrin,

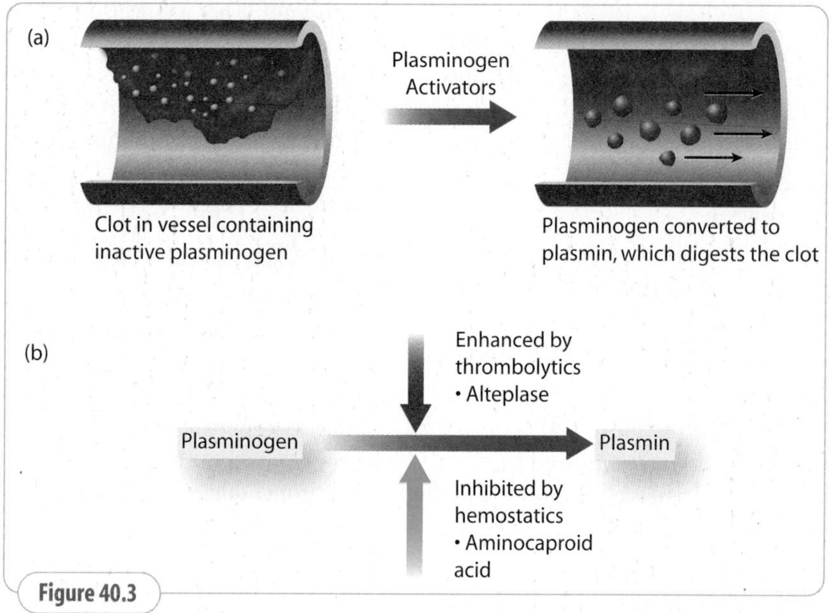

Figure 40.3

Steps in fibrinolysis: (a) Clot dissolves when plasminogen is converted to plasmin; (b) thrombolytics enhance fibrinolysis; hemostatics inhibit fibrinolysis.

breaking it into small soluble fragments. In essence, the thrombolytics simply accelerate the normal process of clot removal in the body. The thrombolytics are also called fibrinolytics, owing to their destructive effects on fibrin. The therapeutic outcomes of thrombolytic therapy are strongly dependent on the time frame in which they are administered. They are considerably more effective when given as soon as possible after the clot has formed—preferably within 4 hours. The mechanism of action of the thrombolytics was shown in Pharmacotherapy Illustrated 37.2 on page 601.

Thrombolytics are nonspecific and have a very narrow margin of safety between dissolving "normal" and "abnormal" clots. Vital signs must be monitored continuously and any signs of bleeding may call for discontinuation of therapy. Patients with recent trauma, active bleeding, or surgery may have "fresh" clots that could be disrupted by the action of these drugs. Thus, they may not be candidates for thrombolytic therapy due to the risk of bleeding.

The use of thrombolytics in elderly patients is controversial. Research has shown that thrombolytic therapy in patients older than age 75 does not decrease mortality from the MI or CVA the patient has suffered. The risks of serious bleeding following drug administration may outweigh the therapeutic benefits. Patients older than 75 must be carefully screened for contraindicated conditions, such as uncontrolled HTN, recent ischemic stroke, or current use of anticoagulants.

Because these medications are rapidly destroyed in the bloodstream, discontinuing the infusion quickly terminates their thrombolytic activity. After the clot is successfully dissolved with the thrombolytic, anticoagulant therapy with an anticoagulant is initiated to prevent the reformation of clots.

Since the discovery of streptokinase, the first drug in this class, there have been several subsequent generations of thrombolytics. The newer drugs such as tenecteplase (TNK-tPA) are more fibrin specific and are reported to have fewer adverse effects than streptokinase. tPA, marketed as alteplase (Activase), has replaced urokinase as the thrombolytic of choice in clearing thrombosed central IV lines.

PROTOTYPE DRUG Alteplase (Activase)

Classification: **Therapeutic:** None
Pharmacologic: Thrombolytic/fibrinolytic

TABLE 40.6 Thrombolytics

Drug	Route and Adult Dose (maximum dose where indicated)	Adverse Effects
alteplase (Activase, t-PA)	IV: Begin with 60 mg and then infuse 20 mg/h over next 2 h	*Superficial bleeding at injection sites, allergic reactions* <u>Serious internal bleeding, intracranial hemorrhage, HTN</u>
reteplase (Retavase)	IV: 10 units over 2 min; repeat dose in 30 min	
streptokinase (Kabikinase)	IV: 250,000–1.5 million units over 60 min	
tenecteplase (TNKase)	IV: 30–50 mg infused over 5 seconds	

Note: *Italics* indicate common adverse effects. <u>Underline</u> indicates serious adverse effects.

all pulses present equal and strong in all extremities; no respiratory distress—regular, clear, breath sounds; audible bowel sounds in all four quadrants. Her right mid-calf area has 3–4+ pitting edema, and is hot and painful to touch and she has a moderate amount of varicosities in lower extremities bilaterally.

Ruby had a hysterectomy 15 years ago, and does not drink alcohol or use tobacco. She takes occasional aspirin use for muscle aches, and has no known allergies. Her family history indicates that her father died from a stroke and her mother died of "old age." She has one sister who has diabetes.

Ruby was diagnosed with deep vein thrombosis (DVT) in her right leg. The treatment plan was to admit her into the hospital for anticoagulant therapy and pain control. In the hospital setting, Ruby will receive heparin therapy. You are the nurse caring for this patient.

Critical Thinking Questions

1. Ruby asks, "How soon will the heparin dissolve my blood clot?" How would you respond to this question?
2. What patient education should you provide Ruby about anticoagulation therapy?
3. What is an activated partial thromboplastin time? How will this test be used to direct heparin therapy?
4. What factors predisposed this patient to deep vein thrombosis?
5. What should Ruby be taught about taking aspirin for arthritis pain?

Case Study

You are attending your annual family reunion and begin talking to your favorite uncle Lewis about his recent hospitalization. Lewis Kinard, a 55-year-old man, was recently discharged from the hospital following an episode of atrial fibrillation. He returned home with instructions to take warfarin (Coumadin) 10 mg daily. He has many questions for you, his favorite relative.

1. Why would someone with atrial fibrillation be prescribed Coumadin?
2. What special precautions should Lewis take while on this drug?
3. Are there any foods that he should avoid or limit in his diet?
4. What laboratory testing will be done to determine this drug's effectiveness?

NCLEX-RN® Review

1 The client with deep vein thrombosis is being treated with a heparin infusion. The nurse would monitor for therapeutic effectiveness by noting which of the following?

1. Activated partial thromboplastin time (aPTT)
2. Prothrombin time (PT)
3. Platelet counts
4. International normalized ratio (INR)

2 Which of the following should not be included in the care plan for a client receiving subcutaneous heparin?

1. Inject medication in the deep fatty layer of the abdomen.
2. When assessing blood pressure, release cuff pressure as soon as possible.
3. Hold direct pressure on venipuncture sites for 10 minutes.
4. Instruct client on the importance of using dental floss daily.

3 A client who is taking an anticoagulant states, "I wake up every morning with arthritis pain and I always take aspirin or ibuprofen." The nurse's response would be based on which of the following physiologic concepts?

1. Aspirin and ibuprofen (Motrin) will counteract the therapeutic effects of many anticoagulants.
2. Anticoagulants will reduce the half-life of drugs such as aspirin and ibuprofen.
3. Many substances such as aspirin and ibuprofen will increase the risk of bleeding.
4. The combination of aspirin products with anticoagulants will worsen arthritis pain.

4 What should the nurse teach the client about the use of warfarin (Coumadin) at home?

1. Take one baby aspirin before your next international normalized ratio is collected.
2. Discontinue Coumadin prior to your next dental procedure.
3. Have your blood pressure and pulse checked at least monthly.
4. Adopt a low-fat, low-carbohydrate diet and begin exercising.

5 A client who is taking clopidogrel (Plavix) to prevent another stroke asks a nurse how the medication works. The nurse's response should be based upon an understanding that Plavix:

1. Prolongs the bleeding time by inhibiting platelet aggregation.
2. Activates antithrombin III and subsequently inhibits thrombin.
3. Inhibits enzymes involved in the formation of vitamin K.
4. Converts plasminogen to plasmin to dissolve fibrin clots.

6 A client will be receiving lepirudin (Refludan). Which of the following is true concerning this drug therapy? (Select all that apply.)

1. Ginger, garlic, and green tea may increase the risk of bleeding.
2. Vitamin B_{12} is used to augment this drug's response.
3. Refludan is used for heparin-induced thrombocytopenia.
4. Activated partial thromboplastin time is monitored to determine effectiveness.
5. This drug is contraindicated for clients with severe hypertension.

See Answers to Critical Thinking Questions, Case Study, and NCLEX-RN® Review in Appendix A.

References

Cooney, M. F. (2006). Heparin-induced thrombocytopenia: Advances in diagnosis and treatment. *Critical Care Nurse, 26*(6), 30–36.

Drug Digest. (2007). *Garlic.* Retrieved July 17, 2008, from http://www.drugdigest.org/DD/DVH/HerbsWho/0,3923, 4041Garlic,00. html

Eriksson, B. I., & Quinlan, D. J. (2006). Oral anticoagulants in development: Focus on thromboprophylaxis in patients undergoing orthopaedic surgery. *Drugs, 66*(11), 1411–1429.

Franchini, M., Zaffanello, M., & Veneri, D. (2005). Recombinant factor VIIa: An update on its clinical use. *Thrombosis and Haemostasis, 93*(6), 1027–1035.

Gallagher, D., & Rix, E. (2006). Understanding the implications of oral anticoagulants. *Nursing Times, 102*(25), 30–32.

Gómez-Moreno, G., Cutando-Soriano, A., Arana, C., & Scully, C. (2005). Hereditary blood coagulation disorders: Management and dental treatment. *Journal of Dental Research, 84*(11), 978–985.

Hairon, N. (2007). Prevention of venous thromboembolism in patients. *Nursing Times, 103*(18), 24–25.

Heit, J.A. (2008). The epidemiology of venous thromboembolism in the community. *Arteriosclerosis, Thrombosis and Vascular Biology, 28*(3), 370–372.

Hirsh, J., Guyatt, G., Albers, G. W., Harrington, R., & Shünemann, H. J. (2008). Antithrombotic and thrombolytic therapy: American College of Chest Physicians Guidelines (8th ed.). *Chest, 133,* 110S–112S. Retrieved July 17, 2008, from http://www.chestjournal.org/content/vol133/6_suppl/

Lambing, A. (2005). Clearing the way: Treating venous thromboembolism and deep vein thrombosis. *Advance for Nurse Practitioners, 13*(6), 24–30.

Lins, S., Guffey, D., VanRiper, S., & Kline-Rogers, E. (2006). Decreasing vascular complications after percutaneous coronary interventions: Partnering to improve outcomes. *Critical Care Nurse, 26*(6), 38–45.

National Hemophilia Association. (2008). *HIV/AIDS.* Retrieved July 17, 2008, from http://www.hemophilia.org/NHFWeb/MainPgs/MainNHF.aspx?menuid=43&contentid=39

Rahman, K., & Lowe, G. M. (2006). Garlic and cardiovascular disease: A critical review. *Journal of Nutrition, 136*(3 Suppl), 736S–740S.

Schreiber, D. (2008). *Deep venous thrombosis and thrombophlebitis.* Emedicine. Retrieved July 17, 2008, from http://www.emedicine.com/emerg/topic122.htm

Segal, J. B., Streiff, M. B., Hofmann, L. V., Thornton, K., & Bass, E. B. (2007). Management of venous thromboembolism: A systematic review for a practice guideline. *Annals of Internal Medicine, 146*(3), 211–222.

Shamseer, L., Charrois, T. L., & Vohra, S. (2006). Complementary, holistic, and integrative medicine: Garlic. *Pediatrics in Review, 27*(12), e77–e80.

Spader, C. (2006). Keeping a grip on anticoagulant therapy. *Nursing Spectrum, 18A*(12), 46–49.

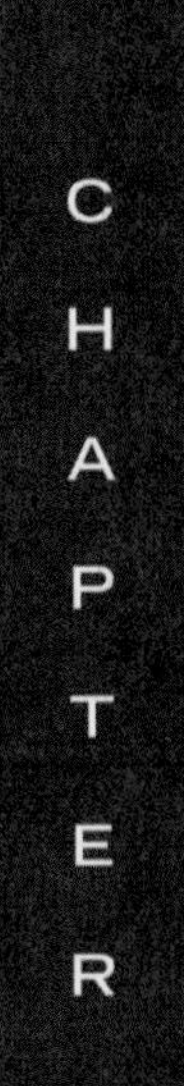

For me, the worst part is the isolation from people. It's almost unbearable. I feel so lonely. If I could just be with people, I know I would feel better.

Patient "Carl Guenther"

Pharmacotherapy of Hematopoietic Disorders

41

Chapter Outline

The Physiology of Hematopoiesis

Hematopoietic Growth Factors

Erythropoietin

PROTOTYPE **Epoetin Alfa (Epogen, Procrit)** *p. 669*

Colony-Stimulating Factors

PROTOTYPE **Filgrastim (Neupogen)** *p. 673*

Platelet Enhancer

PROTOTYPE **Oprelvekin (Neumega)** *p. 675*

Classification of Anemias

Antianemic Agents

Iron-Deficiency Anemia

PROTOTYPE **Ferrous Sulfate (Feosol, Feostat, Others)** *p. 678*

Megaloblastic Anemia

PROTOTYPE **Cyanocobalamin (Calomist, Nascobal)** *p. 682*

Learning Outcomes

After reading this chapter, the student should be able to:

1. Describe the process of hematopoiesis.
2. Explain how hematopoiesis is regulated.
3. Explain the functions of erythropoietin.
4. Explain the functions of colony-stimulating factors.
5. Classify types of anemia based on their causes.
6. Illustrate the metabolism, storage, and transfer of iron in the body.
7. Identify the role of intrinsic factor in the absorption of vitamin B_{12}.
8. Compare and contrast anemias caused by vitamin B_{12} and folate deficiency.
9. Describe the nurse's role in the pharmacologic management of hematopoietic disorders.
10. For each of the classes shown in the chapter outline, identify the prototype and representative drugs and explain the mechanism(s) of drug action, primary indications, contraindications, significant drug interactions, pregnancy category, and important adverse effects.
11. Use the nursing process to care for patients who are receiving drug therapy for hematopoietic disorders.

Key Terms

anemia, *675*
colony-stimulating factor (CSF), *671*
erythropoietin, *668*
ferritin, *677*
folate, *682*
folic acid, *682*
hematopoiesis, *668*
hemosiderin, *677*
intrinsic factor, *680*
pernicious anemia, *680*
pluripotent stem cell, *670*
thrombopoietin, *674*
transferrin, *677*

The blood serves all other cells in the body and is the only fluid tissue. Because of its diverse functions, diseases affecting blood constituents have widespread effects on the body. This chapter will examine medications used to enhance the functions of erythrocytes, leukocytes, and platelets. Pharmacology of the hematopoietic system is a small, though emerging, branch of medicine.

The Physiology of Hematopoiesis

41.1 Hematopoiesis is a dynamic process that is responsive to the changing demands of the body.

Blood is a highly dynamic tissue; over 200 billion new blood cells are formed every day. The process of blood cell formation is called **hematopoiesis,** or hemopoiesis. In adults, hematopoiesis occurs primarily in red bone marrow and requires B vitamins, vitamin C, copper, iron, and other nutrients. Before proceeding, the student should read the brief review of blood found in Chapter 31.

Hematopoiesis is responsive to the demands of the body. For example, the production of white blood cells (WBCs) can increase tenfold in response to infection. The number of red blood cells (RBCs) can increase as much as fivefold in response to anemia or hypoxia. Homeostatic control of hematopoiesis is influenced by a number of hormones and growth factors, which allow for points for pharmacologic intervention. The process of hematopoiesis is illustrated in Figure 41.1.

The process of hematopoiesis begins with a **pluripotent stem cell,** which is capable of maturing (differentiating) into any blood cell type. In theory, a single pluripotent stem cell has the potential to generate the entire hematopoietic system. What determines whether the stem cell produces RBCs, macrophages, lymphocytes, or perhaps platelets? The specific path taken by the pluripotent stem cell depends on the internal needs of the body. These needs are transmitted to pluripotent stem cells by regulatory substances that include various hormones and proteins. For example, high amounts of the hormone erythropoietin circulating through the blood signal the stem cells to differentiate into erythrocytes. Many types of cells secrete cytokines (interferons and interleukins) that signal the stem cells to increase or decrease the production of white blood cells. Through recombinant deoxyribonucleic acid (DNA) technology some of these regulatory agents are now available in sufficient quantities to be used as medications.

PharmFACT

The recommended dietary allowance of iron for a woman is 10 to 15 mg. However, during pregnancy, a woman's body needs 1 g of iron daily: 300 mg for the fetus, 500 mg for expansion of the maternal RBCs, and 200 mg due to excretion. *Source:* Lichtman et al., 2005.

The pharmacologic management of hematopoietic diseases often involves simply replacing a deficient substance that is essential to hematopoiesis. In some cases, the drug is identical, or very closely resembles, the deficient endogenous factor. For example, the drug epoetin alfa (Epogen, Procrit) is identical to the natural hormone erythropoietin and stimulates the production of RBCs in the same manner. As another common example, administration of antianemic agents such as ferrous sulfate or vitamin B_{12} supplies deficient factors that are essential to hematopoiesis.

Some of the hematopoietic drugs have become important adjunct medications in the pharmacotherapy of malignancies. For example, antineoplastic drugs often are toxic to bone marrow and cause neutropenia, a reduced number of WBCs. Neutropenia is a primary cause of patient morbidity and mortality in the treatment of cancer. Hematopoietic drugs can be used to boost the WBC counts in these patients.

Natural hormones that regulate some aspect of blood formation are called hematopoietic growth factors. These drugs and their doses are listed in Table 41.1.

CONNECTION *Checkpoint* 41.1

From what you learned in Chapter 31, name the three formed elements of blood. What percentage of blood do the formed elements comprise? See Answer to Connection Checkpoint 41.1 in Appendix A.

Hematopoietic Growth Factors

41.2 Erythropoietin stimulates production of red blood cells and is used to treat anemia.

The process of RBC formation, or erythropoiesis, is regulated primarily by the hormone **erythropoietin.** In adults, 90% of erythropoietin is secreted by the kidney and 10% is secreted by the liver.

The primary signal to increase the renal secretion of erythropoietin is a reduction in oxygen reaching the proximal tubule cells in the kidney. Once secreted, erythropoietin travels to the bone marrow where it interacts with receptors on stem cells and delivers the message to increase erythrocyte production. Just as important, erythropoietin also stimulates the production of hemoglobin, which is required for a functional erythrocyte. Hemorrhage, chronic obstructive pulmonary disease, anemia, or high altitudes may increase serum levels of erythropoietin as much as 1,000-fold in response to severe hy-

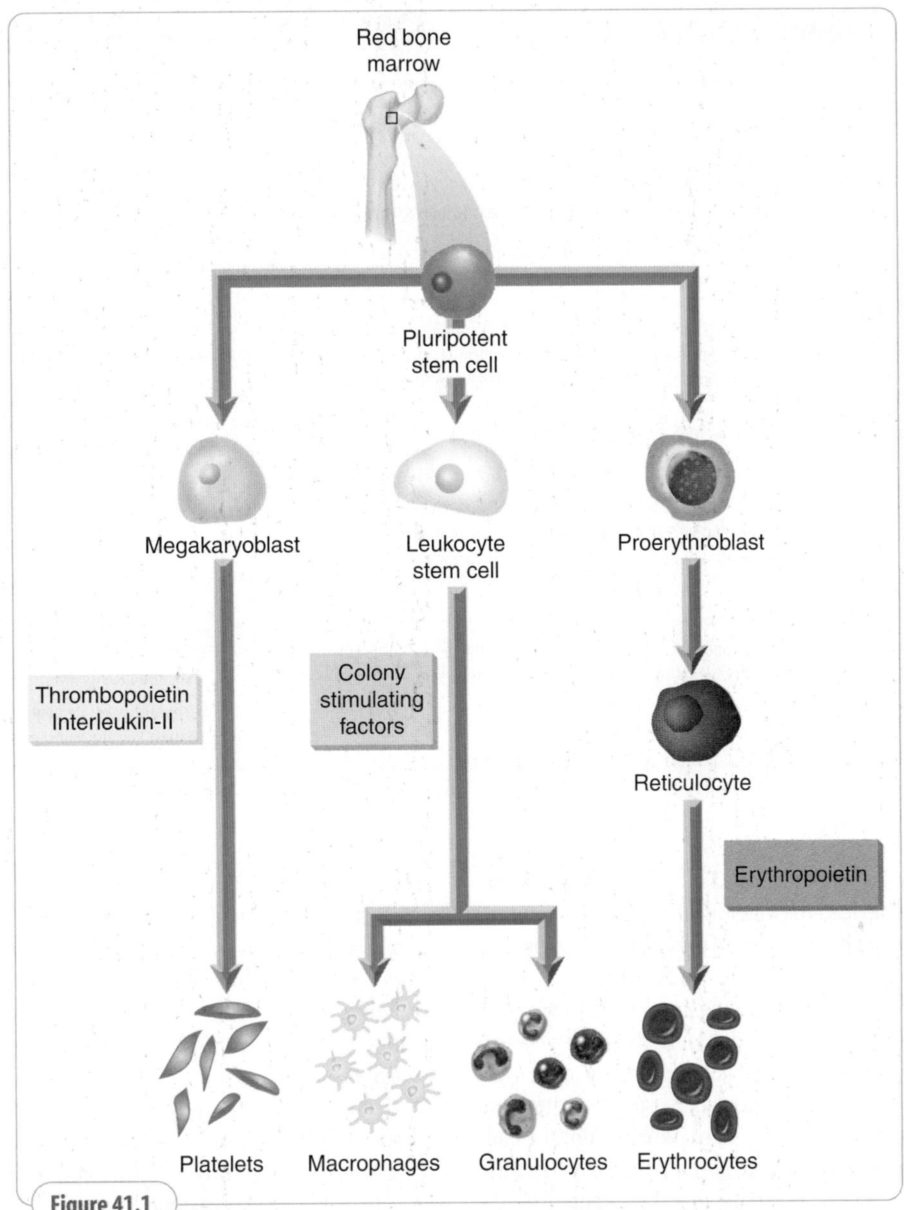

Figure 41.1

Hematopoiesis: Blood cells are formed from stem cells under the influence of hormones such as thrombopoietin, colony-stimulating factors, and erythropoietin.

poxia. Erythropoietin is marketed as the drug epoetin alfa (Epogen, Procrit). Darbepoetin alfa (Aranesp) is a newer agent that is closely related to epoetin alfa, but has a duration of action that is 2 to 3 times longer. These agents are sometimes called erythropoietic growth factors.

PROTOTYPE DRUG Epoetin alfa (Epogen, Procrit)

Classification: **Therapeutic:** Hematopoietic growth factor, drug for anemia

Pharmacologic: Erythropoietin

Therapeutic Effects and Uses: Approved in 1989, epoetin alfa is made through recombinant DNA technology and is functionally identical to human erythropoietin. Although the drug may be administered intravenously (IV), the subcutaneous route is generally preferred because lower doses are needed, absorption is slower, and a more sustained response can be achieved. The hematocrit increases 2% per week during the initial weeks of epoetin therapy. Some patients require 2 to 6 weeks of therapy for a change in hematocrit to occur. Most patients on epoetin therapy also receive iron supplements to meet the increased demands caused by the increased erythrocyte production. Although epoetin alfa does not cure any primary disease, it reduces anemia symptoms and dramatically improves the patient's ability to perform daily activities. A typical initial regimen for epoetin alfa requires 50 to 100 units/kg three times per week until a target hemoglobin level of 10 to 12 g/dL is achieved.

Although anemia may be caused by a large number of underlying disorders (see Section 41.5), certain patients are more prone to developing the condition. Patients with chronic renal failure often suffer from anemia because they are unable to secrete

TABLE 41.1 Hematopoietic Growth Factors

Drug	Route and Adult Dose (maximum dose where indicated)	Adverse Effects
darbepoetin alfa (Aranesp)	Subcutaneous/IV: 0.45 mcg/kg once per week (max: 74 mg/kg)	*Headache, fever, nausea, diarrhea, insomnia, cough, upper respiratory infection, edema* HTN, seizures, HF, MI
epoetin alfa (Epogen, Procrit): erythropoietin	Subcutaneous/IV: Start with 50–100 units/kg/dose and increase until target hematocrit range of 30–33% (max: 36%) is reached. Hematocrit should not increase by more than 4 points in any 2-week period.	
Colony-Stimulating Factors		
filgrastim (Neupogen): granulocyte-CSF	IV: 5 mcg/kg/day by 30 min infusion, may increase by 5 mcg/kg/day (max: 30 mcg/kg/day); 5 mcg/kg/day subcutaneous as single dose, may increase by 5 mcg/kg/day (max: 20 mcg/kg/day)	*Flulike syndrome, fever, dyspnea, nausea, vomiting, bone pain (sargramostim)* Bone pain, arthralgia, thrombocytopenia, cutaneous vasculitis, pericardial effusion (sargramostim), tachycardia (sargramostim)
pegfilgrastim (Neulasta)	Subcutaneous: 6 mg once per chemotherapy cycle at least 24 h after chemotherapy	
sargramostim (Leukine): GM-CSF	IV: 250 mcg/m²/day infused over 2 h for 14 days, begin 2–4 h after bone marrow transfusion and not less than 24 h after last dose of chemotherapy or 12 h after last radiation therapy	
Platelet Enhancer		
oprelvekin (Neumega)	Subcutaneous: 50 mcg/kg once daily starting 6–24 h after completing chemotherapy for 14–21 days or until platelet count is at least 50,000/mcL	*Edema, fever, headache, dizziness, dyspnea, fatigue, rash, nausea, vomiting* Tachycardia, febrile neutropenia, pleural effusion, anaphylaxis, dysrhythmias, candidiasis

Note: *Italics* indicate common adverse effects. Underline indicates serious adverse effects.

sufficient endogenous erythropoietin. The drug is occasionally prescribed to reduce the need for transfusions in anemic patients prior to elective surgery, if a significant blood loss is expected. HIV-infected patients who are receiving zidovudine may receive epoetin alfa to treat anemia caused by the antiretroviral agents.

Epoetin alfa is given to patients undergoing chemotherapy for non-myeloid malignancies, to counteract the anemia commonly caused by antineoplastic agents. It should be carefully noted that the anemia must be secondary to the chemotherapy, not the cancer itself. Research has shown that the administration of epoetin alfa does not benefit patients when the anemia is caused by the malignancy; in fact mortality is increased in these patients by the administration of the drug. Care must be taken not to administer epoetin alfa to patients with myeloid malignancies such as myelogenous leukemia, because the drug may increase tumor growth.

Mechanism of Action: Epoetin alfa stimulates the division and differentiation of stem cells in the bone marrow to become erythrocytes. Erythropoietin also promotes the synthesis of hemoglobin and causes a shift of marrow reticulocytes into the circulation.

Pharmacokinetics:

Route(s)	IV, subcutaneous
Absorption	Readily absorbed (subcutaneous)
Distribution	Unknown; unknown if the drug crosses the placenta or is secreted in breast milk
Primary metabolism	Plasma
Primary excretion	Mostly unknown; 10% renal
Onset of action	7–14 days
Duration of action	Unknown; half-life: 4–13 h

Adverse Effects: The most serious adverse effect of epoetin alfa is hypertension (HTN), which occurs in 30% of patients receiving the drug. An antihypertensive agent may be indicated. Some patients with chronic renal failure develop neutralizing antibodies to subcutaneous epoetin alfa, which can lead to a rapidly developing severe anemia known as pure red cell aplasia. Increased seizure activity may occur during the first 90 days of therapy. Common adverse effects include headache, fever, nausea, diarrhea, and edema.

The risk of thromboembolic events is increased with epoetin alfa therapy. Transient ischemic attacks (TIAs), myocardial infarctions (MIs), and cerebrovascular accidents (CVAs) have occurred in chronic renal failure patients on dialysis who are being treated with epoetin alfa. Seizures may occur during the first 90 days of therapy, especially if blood pressure and hematocrit rise rapidly.

Contraindications/Precautions: The drug should not be given to patients with uncontrolled HTN because epoetin alfa may increase blood pressure. The risk of thromboembolic events, CVA, and MI greatly increases when hemoglobin rises above 12 g/dL. Patients with known hypersensitivity to products derived from mammal cells, such as albumin, should not receive this drug.

Drug Interactions: Androgens can increase blood viscosity, resulting in an increased response from epoetin alfa. The effectiveness of epoetin alfa will be greatly reduced in patients with iron deficiency or other vitamin-depleted states. Whenever possible, such deficiencies should be corrected prior to initiating epoetin alfa therapy. Hemodialysis patients with preexisting heart disease who are taking epoetin may require increased doses of heparin. **Herbal/Food:** Unknown.

Pregnancy: Category C.

Treatment of Overdose: Overdose may lead to polycythemia (too many erythrocytes), which can be corrected by phlebotomy.

Nursing Responsibilities:

- Notify the prescriber prior to administration if the patient has history of uncontrolled HTN or hypersensitivity to products derived from mammal cells such as albumin.
- Determine the reason for drug administration such as presence or history of anemia secondary to chronic renal failure, malignancy, chemotherapy, autologous blood donation, and HIV-infected patients treated with zidovudine.
- Assess vital signs, especially blood pressure. Hypertension should be treated before initiating epoetin therapy. Be aware that blood pressure may rise during early therapy as the hematocrit increases. Notify the prescriber of a rapid increase greater than 4 points in 2 weeks. Dosage may need to be reduced because of the risk of serious HTN.
- Assess complete blood count (CBC), specifically hematocrit and hemoglobin levels, to establish baseline values. Monitor baseline laboratory tests such as transferrin and serum ferritin.
- Monitor CBC with differential and platelet count regularly. Monitor blood urea nitrogen (BUN), creatinine, phosphorus, and potassium regularly.
- Monitor for hypertensive encephalopathy in patients with chronic renal failure during a period of increasing hematocrit.
- Observe for premonitory neurologic symptoms such as aura, and report promptly to the health care provider. The potential for seizures exists during periods of rapid hematocrit increase.
- Monitor closely for thrombotic events such as MI, CVA, or TIA, especially in patients with chronic renal failure.

Patient and Family Education:

- Do not take any other prescription or nonprescription drugs, dietary supplements, or herbal products without approval of the health care provider.
- Stop the drug and immediately report allergic symptoms such as a rash over the entire body, shortness of breath or wheezing, itching, swelling around the mouth or eyes, profuse sweating, or rapid heart beat.
- Take antihypertensive medication and observe dietary restrictions as directed.
- Do not drive or perform other hazardous activities during the first 90 days of therapy and until the effect of the drug are known because this drug may cause drowsiness, dizziness, or possible seizure activity.
- Report excessive fatigue to the health care provider.
- Take acetaminophen for headache which is a common adverse effect of this drug. Report to the health care provider if the headache is severe or persistent because this may indicate developing HTN.
- For self-administration, follow the procedure demonstrated to prevent contamination of the vial, syringe, or medicine. Never touch the rubber stopper of the vial or the needle of the syringe with your fingers. Dispose of needles and syringes as directed by a health care provider.
- Immediately notify the health care provider of any known or suspected pregnancy.
- Do not breast-feed while taking this drug without approval of the health care provider.

Drugs Similar to Epoetin Alfa (Epogen, Procrit)

The only similar drug is darbepoetin alfa.

Darbepoetin alfa (Aranesp): Approved in 2001, darbepoetin alfa is a newer agent with a chemical structure that is closely related to epoetin alfa, differing only by two carbohydrate chains. It has the same mechanism of action, efficacy, and safety profile as epoetin alfa. However, it has an extended duration of action that allows it to be administered once weekly. Maximum response occurs in 2 to 4 weeks. Darbepoetin alfa is approved for the treatment of anemia associated with cancer chemotherapy or chronic renal failure. Like epoetin alfa, darbepoetin should only be administered to patients with anemia secondary to the chemotherapy, and not caused by the malignancy itself. In addition, hemoglobin levels should be maintained below 12 g/dL to reduce the risks of serious cardiovascular adverse events. It is administered by the subcutaneous or IV routes. Adverse effects are similar to those of epoetin alfa. This drug is pregnancy category C.

MyNursingKit | Mechanism of Action Animation: Epoetin Alfa

41.3 Colony-stimulating factors increase the production of leukocytes.

Regulation of WBC production, or leukopoiesis, is more complicated than erythropoiesis because there are different types of leukocytes in the blood. It is clearly established that a large number of substances modify the synthesis and activation of leukocytes. However, most of the processes of leukopoiesis regulation are poorly understood. Pharmacologically, the most important substances are **colony-stimulating factors (CSFs).** Also called leukopoietic growth factors, the CSFs comprise a small group of drugs that stimulate the growth and differentiation of one or more types of leukocytes. Doses for these agents are shown in Table 41.1.

CSFs are produced by a diverse group of cells that include endothelial cells, fibroblasts, macrophages, and T-lymphocytes. Normally present at undetectable or minute levels in the blood, the production of CSFs rapidly increases when the body receives a bacterial challenge. The leukopoietic growth factors are active at very low concentrations; each stem cell stimulated by these growth factors is capable of producing as many as 1,000 mature leukocytes. The CSFs not only increase the production of new leukocytes, but they also activate existing white blood cells. Examples of enhanced functions include increased migration of leukocytes to antigens, increased antibody toxicity, and increased phagocytosis.

CSFs are named according to the types of blood cells that they stimulate. For example, granulocyte colony-stimulating factor (G-CSF) increases the production of neutrophils, the most common type of granulocyte. Granulocyte-macrophage

NURSING PROCESS APPLICATION

Patients Receiving Epoetin Alfa

Assessment

Prior to administration:

- Obtain a complete health history including allergies, drug history, and possible drug reactions.
- Assess the reason for drug administration such as presence or history of anemia secondary to chronic renal failure, malignancy, chemotherapy, autologous blood donation, and HIV-infected patients treated with zidovudine.
- Assess vital signs, especially blood pressure.
- Assess CBC, specifically hematocrit and hemoglobin levels, to establish baseline values.

Potential Nursing Diagnoses

- *Ineffective Protection*, related to reduced production of endogenous erythropoietin
- *Risk for Injury*, related to weakness, dizziness, and syncope, caused by anemia
- *Risk for Injury*, related to seizure activity secondary to drug
- *Activity Intolerance*, related to red blood cell deficiency
- *Deficient Knowledge (Epoetin Alfa Therapy)*, related to purpose, precautions, and adverse effects of drug

Planning: Patient Goals and Expected Outcomes

The patient will:

- Exhibit an increase in hematocrit level and improvement in anemia-related symptoms.
- Immediately report effects such as severe headache, chest pain, confusion, numbness, or loss of movement in an extremity.
- Demonstrate an understanding of the drug's action by accurately describing drug adverse effects and precautions.

Implementation

Interventions and (Rationales)	Patient and Family Education
• Monitor vital signs, especially blood pressure. (The rate of HTN is directly related to the rate of rise of the hematocrit. Patients who have existing HTN are at higher risk for stroke and seizures. HTN is also much more likely in patients with chronic renal failure.)	• Instruct the patient to periodically monitor blood pressure using proper monitoring equipment. Consistent increases in blood pressure should be reported immediately.
• Monitor for adverse effects, especially symptoms of neurologic or cardiovascular events. (Headache, seizures, and HTN have been related to drug usage.)	• Instruct the patient to report adverse effects such as nausea, vomiting, constipation, redness or pain at injection site, confusion, numbness, chest pain, and difficulty breathing.
• Monitor the patient's ability to self-administer medication. (Inability to self-administer medication requires the nurse to arrange for someone else to administer the medication.)	• Instruct the patient in the technique for subcutaneous injection if patient is to self-administer the medication, and on the proper disposal of needles and syringes.
• Monitor laboratory values such as hematocrit and hemoglobin to evaluate effectiveness of treatment. (Increases in hematocrit and hemoglobin values indicate increased RBC production.)	• Instruct the patient to keep all laboratory appointments for testing and to adjust activities according to the latest hematocrit value.
• Monitor the patient for signs of seizure activity. (Seizures result in a rapid rise in the hematocrit, especially during first 90 days of treatment.)	• Instruct the patient to avoid driving or performing hazardous activities until the effects of the drug are known.
• Monitor the patient for signs of thrombus such as swelling, warmth, and pain in an extremity. (As hematocrit rises, there is an increased chance of thrombus formation particularly for patients with chronic renal failure.)	Instruct the patient to: • Report any increase in size, pain, or warmth in an extremity. • Monitor for signs and symptoms of blood clots. • Avoid rubbing or massaging calves and to report leg discomfort.
• Monitor dietary intake. Ensure adequate intake of all essential nutrients. (Response to this medication is minimal if blood levels of iron, folic acid, and vitamin B_{12} are deficient.)	Instruct the patient to: • Maintain adequate dietary intake of essential vitamins and nutrients. • Continue to follow necessary dietary restrictions if receiving renal dialysis.

Evaluation of Outcome Criteria

Evaluate the effectiveness of drug therapy by confirming that patient goals and expected outcomes have been met (see "Planning").

colony-stimulating factor (GM-CSF) stimulates both neutrophil and macrophage production. The process of identifying the many endogenous CSFs, determining their normal functions, and discovering their potential value as therapeutic agents is an emerging area of pharmacology.

Through recombinant DNA technology, three CSFs are now available as medications. The goal of CSF therapy is to produce a rapid increase in the number of neutrophils in patients who have suppressed immune systems (neutropenia). CSF therapy shortens the length of time patients are neutropenic and susceptible to life-threatening infections. The degree of increase in circulating neutrophils is dose related. Indications include patients undergoing chemotherapy or radiation therapy, receiving transplants, or who have certain malignancies. Neutropenia is a limiting adverse effect with many antineoplastic agents and may cause chemotherapy schedules to be delayed or abandoned. By raising neutrophil counts, CSFs can assist in keeping antineoplastic dosing regimens on schedule (and more effective).

It is often difficult to assess the adverse effects of CSF medications because the same types of patient symptoms may be caused by the condition or disease being treated. Nonspecific adverse effects include nausea, vomiting, fatigue, fever, and flushing. Therapy requires careful laboratory monitoring to avoid producing too many neutrophils. Several recent research studies have suggested that the risk of developing acute myeloid leukemia or myelodysplastic syndrome may be doubled when CSFs are administered to patients undergoing chemotherapy for breast cancer.

PROTOTYPE DRUG Filgrastim (Neupogen)

Classification: **Therapeutic:** Agent for increasing neutrophil production

Pharmacologic: Colony-stimulating factor

Therapeutic Effects and Uses: Produced through recombinant DNA technology, filgrastim is nearly identical to human G-CSF and has the same biologic activity. Its two primary actions are to:

- Increase neutrophil production in the bone marrow.
- Enhance the phagocytic and cytotoxic functions of existing neutrophils.

These effects are particularly important for patients with neutropenia, which often leads to severe bacterial and fungal infections. Administration of filgrastim shortens the length of time of neutropenia in cancer patients whose bone marrow has been suppressed by antineoplastic agents or in patients with recent bone marrow transplants. It may also be used to elevate neutrophil counts in patients with AIDS-related immunosuppression. The subcutaneous route is preferred, although filgrastim may also be administered by slow IV infusion. A typical regimen is 5 to 10 mcg/kg given once or twice daily. The dose is based on absolute neutrophil counts (ANC): The target range is 1,500 to 10,000 cells/mm^3.

Mechanism of Action: Filgrastim acts by the same mechanism as endogenous G-CSF. The drug causes an increase in neutrophil production in the bone marrow, resulting in higher levels of circulating neutrophils.

Pharmacokinetics:

Route(s)	IV, subcutaneous
Absorption	Rapidly absorbed (subcutaneous)
Distribution	Unknown; unknown if the drug crosses the placenta or is secreted in breast milk
Primary metabolism	Unknown
Primary excretion	Renal
Onset of action	4 h
Duration of action	Up to 1 week; half-life: 3.5 h

Adverse Effects: Although filgrastim is well tolerated, the drug is associated with potentially serious adverse effects and close monitoring is required. Bone pain may occur in up to 33% of patients receiving filgrastim. The pain may be diffuse or localized to bones with the greatest amount of bone marrow: long bones, sternum, ribs, and pelvis. The degree of pain is dose dependent and can usually be managed with nonopioid analgesics. Frequent laboratory tests are conducted to ensure that excessive numbers of neutrophils (leukocytosis) do not occur. Leukocyte counts higher than 100,000 cells/mm^3 increase the risk of serious adverse effects such as respiratory failure, intracranial hemorrhage or infarction, retinal hemorrhage, and MI. Hyperuricemia and elevated lactate dehydrogenase and alkaline phosphatase levels occur in a significant number of patients. Splenomegaly may occur in 30% of the patients receiving long-term therapy with filgrastim. Other common adverse effects include fatigue, rash, epistaxis, decreased platelet counts, neutropenic fever, nausea, and vomiting, which occur in over half the patients receiving the drug. Allergic reactions, including anaphylaxis, are rare.

Contraindications/Precautions: Patients with hypersensitivity to *E. coli* proteins should not receive filgrastim because this microbe is used to produce the recombinant drug. Patients with sickle-cell disease should be treated with caution because filgrastim may worsen this condition. Filgrastim should not be administered to patients with myeloid cancers.

Drug Interactions: Because antineoplastic drugs and CSFs produce opposite effects, filgrastim is not administered until at least 24 hours after a chemotherapy session. Lithium causes the release of neutrophils and may contribute to filgrastim-induced leukocytosis. **Herbal/Food:** Unknown.

Pregnancy: Category C.

Treatment of Overdose: Overdose can lead to leukocytosis and should be prevented by discontinuing the drug when ANC rises above 10,000 cells/mm^3. No specific therapy for overdose is available.

Nursing Responsibilities:

- Notify the prescriber if the patient has a history of hypersensitivity to proteins derived from *Escherichia* prior to administration.
- Prior to administering the drug, obtain baseline laboratory tests, including CBC with differential and platelet count. Obtain CBC twice weekly during therapy to monitor neutrophil count and leukocytosis. Monitor hematocrit and platelet count regularly.
- Monitor patients with preexisting cardiac conditions closely because MI and dysrhythmias have been associated with a small percent of patients receiving filgrastim.
- Monitor temperature every 4 hours. Incidence of infection should be reduced after administration of filgrastim.
- Assess the degree of bone pain if present. Consult the health care provider if nonnarcotic analgesics do not provide relief.
- Do not shake the medication vial or syringe because this may damage the drug.

Patient and Family Education:

- Stop the drug and immediately report allergic symptoms such as rash over entire body, shortness of breath or wheezing, swelling around mouth or eyes, profuse sweating, or rapid heart beat.
- Consult with the prescriber if signs of an infection develop such as fever; chills; rash; sore throat; diarrhea; or pain, redness, or swelling around a cut or a sore.
- Attend all follow-up appointments for laboratory testing because these are important to the success of pharmacotherapy and to avoid drug adverse effects.

- Report bone pain and request analgesics to control pain.
- For self-administration, follow the procedure demonstrated to prevent contamination of the vial, syringe, or medicine. Never touch the rubber stopper of the vial or the needle of the syringe with your fingers. Dispose of needles and syringes as directed by the health care provider.
- Immediately notify the health care provider of any known or suspected pregnancy.
- Do not breast-feed while taking this drug without approval of the health care provider.

Drugs Similar to Filgrastim (Neupogen)

The two other CSFs are pegfilgrastim and sargramostim.

Pegfilgrastim (Neulasta): Approved in 2002, pegfilgrastim is a form of filgrastim bonded to a molecule of polyethylene glycol (PEG). This delays the renal excretion of the molecule, allowing the drug to remain in the body with a sustained duration of action. The drug is only given by the subcutaneous route. Its only approved indication is prophylaxis of chemotherapy-induced neutropenia. Adverse effects, interactions, and contraindications are the same as filgrastim. This drug is pregnancy category C.

Sargramostim (Leukine): Sargramostim is structurally very similar to natural GM-CSF and has the same biologic activity. It may be administered IV, but subcutaneous is the preferred route. The drug has multiple effects that include increasing the number of circulating neutrophils, eosinophils, and monocytes; activating macrophages; increasing the cytotoxic activity of monocytes; and enhancing the bacteriocidal activity of other cells of the immune system. Indications include decreasing the period of neutropenia in patients treated for acute lymphocytic leukemia or Hodgkin's disease, and those having autologous bone marrow transplantation. Typically, therapy with sargramostim is initiated when ANC is less than 500 cells/mm^3 and continues until an ANC of 1,500 cells/mm^3 for 3 consecutive days is achieved. To prevent leukocytosis, sargramostim should be discontinued if the ANC rises above 10,000 cells/mm^3.

Like filgrastim, bone pain is a common adverse effect. A serious adverse effect of sargramostim is respiratory distress that occurs during the IV infusion the first time the drug is administered, which appears to be related to the trapping of granulocytes in the pulmonary circulation. The patient develops difficulty breathing, tachycardia, low blood pressure, and light-headedness. These symptoms usually call for discontinuing sargramostim therapy. This drug is pregnancy category C.

41.4 Platelet production can be increased by administering oprelvekin.

The production of platelets, or thrombocytopoiesis, begins when megakaryocytes in the bone marrow start shedding membrane-bound packets. These packets enter the bloodstream and become platelets. A single megakaryocyte can produce thousands of platelets.

Megakaryocyte activity is controlled by the hormone **thrombopoietin,** which is produced by the liver and bone marrow. Thrombopoietin is not available as a medication, although it has undergone clinical trials. The only hematopoietic growth factor available to enhance platelet production is oprelvekin (Neumega), which is functionally equivalent to endogenous interleukin-11 (IL-11). Interleukins are cytokines secreted by monocytes, lymphocytes, and other cell types that signal cells in the immune system to respond to an infection. Over 30 interleukins have been identified but only a few have been isolated and approved as drugs.

CONNECTIONS

To the Community Teaching Patients with Neutropenia

As more patients are treated with chemotherapy, more are living with the effects of neutropenia. Neutropenia is a reduction of neutrophils in the circulating blood. Neutrophils are part of the white blood cell defense team necessary to fight infections. Although this condition can arise from several sources, typical chemotherapy-induced neutropenia occurs 3 to 7 days after treatment and lasts for several days while the body recovers. During this time, the patient needs to take additional precautions to minimize infection as listed below:

- Wash hands often but especially after shaking hands, using the bathroom, and before eating. An antibacterial soap adds additional protection.
- Avoid disposable razors. Use a clean electric razor to minimize cuts and nicks.
- Bathe daily and pat skin dry.
- Avoid cutting nails during this time if possible. A hangnail should be clipped carefully to avoid a tear.
- Do not squeeze blemishes or acne. Any small scratch can be a portal for infection.
- Clean rectal area thoroughly after bowel movements. Women should clean perianal area from front to back to avoid urinary tract infections.
- Women should use sanitary napkins and avoid tampons to reduce the chance of infection.
- Avoid crowds and people with colds or open sores.
- Wear shoes to protect feet from scratches and cuts, thereby preventing the invasion of pathogenic microorganisms.
- When entering the home, change to a clean pair of house shoes, which will prevent bringing outdoor microorganisms into the living space. Also, ask guests to remove shoes when entering the home.
- Eat a healthy diet and avoid constipation by including adequate fiber.
- Use only a soft toothbrush and no dental floss. Do not schedule dental work during times of neutropenia.
- Clean and replace furnace and air conditioning filters frequently.
- Avoid rectal medications.
- Avoid contact with animal urine or stool and stagnant water where bacteria tend to breed.
- Exercise and get plenty of rest.
- Read and become knowledgeable about neutropenia.

PROTOTYPE DRUG Oprelvekin (Neumega)

Classification: Therapeutic: Platelet enhancer
Pharmacologic: Interleukin

Therapeutic Effects and Uses: Produced through recombinant DNA technology, oprelvekin is used to stimulate the production of platelets in patients who are at risk for severe thrombocytopenia caused by the chemotherapy of nonmyeloid cancers. The drug shortens the time that the patient is thrombocytopenic and most susceptible to adverse bleeding events. Dosing is initiated 6 to 24 hours after chemotherapy and continues daily until the platelet count is greater than 50,000/mm^3. Dosing beyond 21 days is not recommended. Platelet counts will remain elevated for about 7 days after the last dose. Therapy with oprelvekin decreases the need for platelet infusion. Oprelvekin is only given by the subcutaneous route.

Mechanism of Action: Oprelvekin is equivalent to interleukin-11 and stimulates the synthesis and maturation of megakaryocytes into platelets.

Pharmacokinetics:

Route(s)	Subcutaneous
Absorption	80% absorbed
Distribution	Well distributed to highly perfused organs; it is not known if the drug crosses the placenta or is secreted in breast milk
Primary metabolism	Not metabolized
Primary excretion	Renal
Onset of action	5–9 days
Duration of action	7 days; half-life: 6.9 h

Adverse Effects: Adverse effects from oprelvekin occur frequently but are reversible upon discontinuation of therapy. The primary adverse effect of oprelvekin is fluid retention, which occurs in about 60% of patients and can be a concern for patients with preexisting cardiovascular or renal disease. Adverse effects related to fluid retention may be severe, and include pulmonary edema, pericardial effusion, and ascites. Cardiovascular adverse effects include transient atrial dysrhythmias, sinus tachycardia, vasodilation, and peripheral edema. Visual impairment, including blurred vision, papilledema, and optic neuropathy may occur during therapy. Although not common, allergic reactions, including anaphylaxis, have been reported.

Contraindications/Precautions: Oprelvekin is contraindicated in patients who have shown hypersensitivity to the drug on a previous exposure. It should be used with caution in patients with cardiac disease, especially heart failure (HF), dysrhythmias, and left ventricular dysfunction since fluid retention is a common adverse effect that can worsen these conditions. The drug should be used with caution in patients with preexisting visual impairment; papilledema is a dose-limiting adverse effect in children receiving this drug.

Drug Interactions: Oprelvekin should not be administered within 24 hours of chemotherapy because the cytotoxic effects of the antineoplastic agents decrease the effectiveness of the drug. Concurrent use with thiazide or loop diuretics may cause serious hypokalemia. Herbal/Food: Unknown.

Pregnancy: Category C.

Treatment of Overdose: Overdose may result in serious adverse effects and close monitoring of cardiovascular and renal function is necessary. No specific therapy is available.

Nursing Responsibilities:

- Notify the prescriber prior to administration if the patient has a history of leukemia, multiple myeloma, or other myeloid malignancies.
- Monitor platelet counts until adequate recovery has occurred; periodically monitor CBC with differential and serum electrolytes.
- Monitor for and immediately report signs and symptoms of fluid overload, hypokalemia, and cardiac dysrhythmias.
- Monitor patients with preexisting fluid retention conditions carefully, such as congestive heart failure, pleural effusion, or ascites, for worsening of symptoms.

Patient and Family Education:

- Do not take any other prescription or nonprescription drugs, dietary supplements, or herbal products without the approval of the health care provider.
- Immediately report shortness of breath, swelling of feet or ankles, rapid weight gain, chest pain, unusual fatigue or weakness, irregular heartbeat, fever of 38°C (100.5°F) or higher, unusual bruising or bleeding, or blurred vision.
- For self-administration, follow the procedure demonstrated to prevent contamination of the vial, syringe, or medicine. Never touch the rubber stopper of the vial or the needle of the syringe with your fingers. Dispose of needles and syringes as directed by a health care provider.
- Do not drive or perform other hazardous activities until the effects of the drug are known because this drug may cause drowsiness or dizziness.
- Immediately notify the health care provider of any known or suspected pregnancy.
- Do not breast-feed while using this drug without approval of the health care provider.

Drugs Similar to Oprelvekin (Neumega)

There are no drugs similar to oprelvekin.

Classification of Anemias

41.5 Anemias may be caused by hemorrhage or a change in red blood cell production or destruction.

Anemia is a condition in which RBCs have a diminished capacity to deliver oxygen to tissues. Anemia is a serious health problem that can have a major impact on the quality of life; it is estimated that over 3.4 million Americans have the disorder.

TABLE 41.2 Classification of Anemia

Morphology	Description	Examples
Normocytic-normochromic	Destruction or depletion of normal erythroblasts or mature erythrocytes	Aplastic anemia, hemorrhagic anemia, sickle cell anemia, hemolytic anemia
Macrocytic-normochromic	Large, abnormally shaped erythrocytes with normal hemoglobin concentration	Pernicious anemia, folate deficiency anemia
Microcytic-hypochromic	Small, abnormally shaped erythrocytes with decreased hemoglobin concentration	Iron-deficiency anemia, thalassemia

Although there are dozens of possible causes of anemia, they fall into one of the following categories:

- Blood loss due to hemorrhage
- Increased erythrocyte destruction
- Decreased erythrocyte production

Anemia is considered a sign of an underlying disorder, rather than a distinct disease. For example, anemia is commonly associated with peptic ulcer, various malignancies, and chronic renal disease. For therapy to be successful, the underlying pathology must be identified and treated. Despite the fact it is often considered "secondary" to other diseases, proper treatment of anemia is necessary to improve the patient's ability to adequately perform activities of daily living.

Classification of anemia is generally based on a description of the erythrocyte's size and color. Sizes are described as normal (normocytic), small (microcytic), or large (macrocytic). Color is based on the amount of hemoglobin present and is described as normal red (normochromic) or light red (hypochromic). This classification is shown in Table 41.2. It is not unusual for patients to have more than one type of anemia concurrently.

Although each type of anemia has specific characteristics, all have common signs and symptoms. Assessment includes sources and causes of potential bleeding, as well as a thorough dietary history to rule out deficiencies in the intake of nutrients essential to RBC production, such as vitamin B_{12}, folic acid, or iron. Some types of anemia, including sickle cell and thalassemia, are hereditary, and discovered by family history. If the anemia occurs gradually, the patient may remain asymptomatic, except during periods of physical exercise. As the condition progresses, the patient often exhibits pallor, which is a paleness of the skin and mucous membranes due to hemoglobin deficiency. Decreased exercise tolerance, fatigue, and lethargy occur because of insufficient oxygen reaching muscles. Dizziness and fainting are common because the brain is not receiving enough oxygen to function properly. The respiratory and cardiovascular systems compensate for the oxygen depletion by increasing respiration rate and heart rate. Chronic or severe disease can result in HF. Because symptoms are nonspecific, laboratory tests such as complete blood count, hemoglobin, hematocrit, and serum iron are essential to making a diagnosis so that appropriate pharmacotherapy can be initiated.

Depending on the type of anemia, several vitamins and minerals may be given to enhance the oxygen-carrying capacity of blood. The most common antianemic agents are iron salts, cyanocobalamin (Crystamine, others), and folic acid (Folvite, others). Doses of these agents are listed in Table 41.3.

TABLE 41.3 Antianemic Agents

Drug	Route and Adult Dose (maximum dose where indicated)	Adverse Effects
cyanocobalamin (Calomist, Nascobal)	IM/deep subcutaneous: 30 mcg/day for 5–10 days, then 100–200 mcg/month	*Diarrhea, hypokalemia, rash* Anaphylaxis
ferumoxytol (Feraheme)	IV; single dose of 510 mg followed by a second 510 mg dose 3 to 8 days later	
folic acid (Folvite)	PO/IM/subcutaneous/IV: less than 1 mg/day	No adverse effects
Iron Salts		
ferrous fumarate (Feostat, others)	PO: 200 mg tid or qid	*Nausea, heartburn, constipation, dark stools* Cardiovascular collapse, aggravation of peptic ulcers or ulcerative colitis, hepatic necrosis, anaphylaxis (iron dextran), respiratory arrest (iron dextran), seizures (iron dextran)
ferrous gluconate (Fergon, others)	PO: 325–600 mg qid, may be gradually increased to 650 mg qid as needed	
ferrous sulfate (Feosol, others)	PO: 750–1,500 mg/day in one to three divided doses	
iron dextran (Dexferrum, others)	IM/IV: Dose is individualized and determined from a table supplied by the drug manufacturer that correlates body weight to hemoglobin values (max: 100 mg within 24 h)	

Note: *Italics* indicate common adverse effects. Underline indicates serious adverse effects.

Antianemic Agents

41.6 Administration of iron salts can rapidly reverse symptoms of iron-deficiency anemia.

Iron is a mineral essential to the function of several mitochondrial enzymes involved in metabolism and energy production in the cell. It is also a component of certain antioxidant enzymes that assist in clearing the body of free radicals. Most iron in the body, 60% to 80%, is associated with hemoglobin inside erythrocytes. Knowledge of iron balance and homeostasis is necessary to understanding the pharmacotherapy of iron-deficiency anemia. Factors affecting iron balance are illustrated in Figure 41.2.

The two basic forms of iron in biologic systems are ferrous (Fe^{2+}) and ferric (Fe^{3+}). Most food contains iron in the ferric state, which is not absorbed in the gastrointestinal (GI) tract. In the presence of stomach acid, however, the ferric form is converted to the ferrous form, which is readily absorbed in the duodenum. Iron absorption is dynamic; if the body senses a shortage of iron in the blood, GI absorption increases. When iron stores are plentiful, less iron is absorbed from food. Since adults only need about 8 mg of iron per day, a normal diet supplies sufficient amounts of the mineral for most people.

Other factors affect the absorption of iron. Iron in heme, which is found in meat, fish, and poultry, is three times more absorbable than the nonheme iron found in vegetables and grains. Thus meats are considered the best natural source of absorbable iron. Calcium inhibits the absorption of iron; thus, those who drink milk with meals are at greater risk for iron deficiency. Vitamin C increases iron absorption about 30%, while black tea will diminish absorption.

Because free iron is toxic, the body binds the mineral to the protein complexes **ferritin, hemosiderin,** and **transferrin.** Ferritin and hemosiderin maintain iron stores inside cells, whereas transferrin transports iron to sites throughout the body where it is needed, such as to the bone marrow for incorporation into hemoglobin. Serum ferritin levels are a reliable indicator of how much iron is being stored by the body. Low serum ferritin levels (less than 12 ng/mL) are characteristic of iron-deficiency anemia. In addition to hemoglobin, major storage depots for iron are the liver and myoglobin in skeletal muscle.

After erythrocytes die, nearly all of the iron in their hemoglobin is incorporated into transferrin and recycled for later use. Because of this efficient recycling, only about 1 mg of iron is excreted from the body per day, making daily dietary iron requirements in most individuals quite small. Vegetarians are at higher risk of iron-deficiency anemia because of a lack of heme intake from meat and must take care to select foods rich in iron. Iron requirements may double during growth, pregnancy, and menses; thus, intake of iron must be increased to maintain proper iron balance.

Iron deficiency is the most common cause of anemia worldwide. More than 50% of patients diagnosed with iron-deficiency anemia have GI bleeding, such as may occur from GI malignancies or chronic peptic ulcer disease (PUD). In the United States and Canada, iron deficiency most commonly occurs in women of childbearing age due to pregnancy, and blood losses during menses. Low-dose iron supplements are recommended during pregnancy to prevent this condition. Certain individuals have an increased demand for iron, including those who are on meat-free diets or undergoing intensive

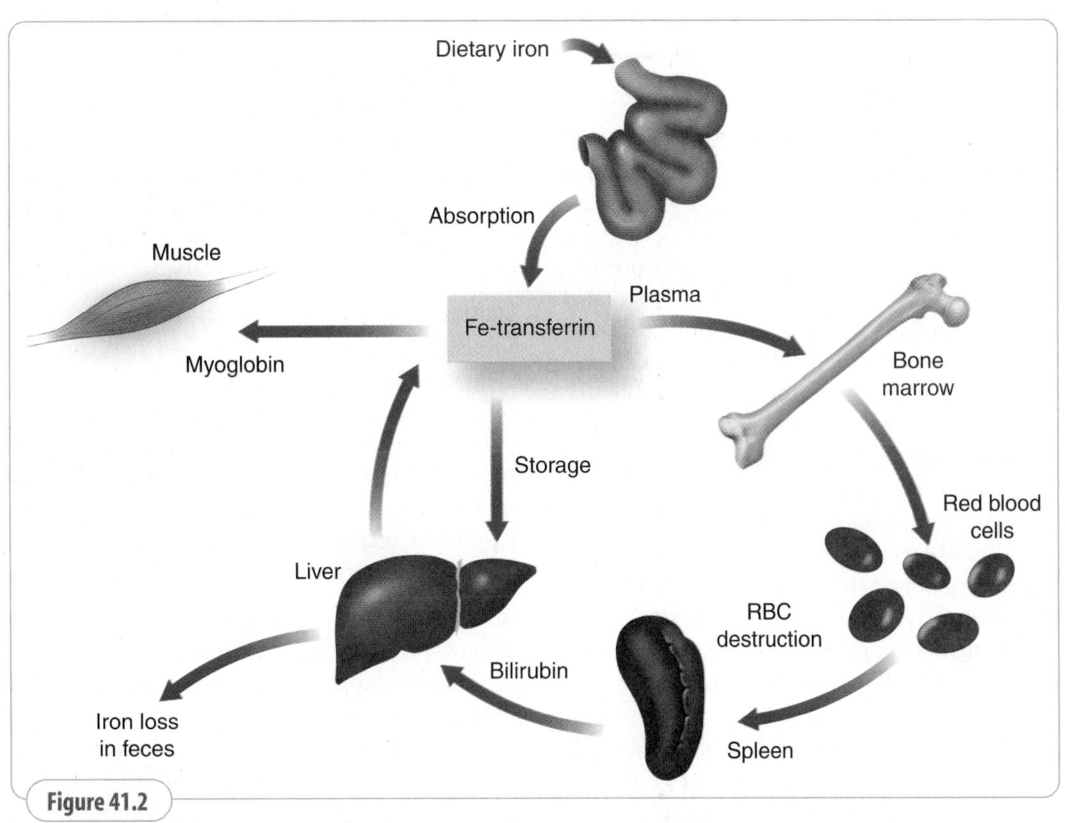

Figure 41.2

Iron metabolism.

CONNECTIONS

Patient Safety

Iron Overdose in Children

While talking with a group of young mothers the nurse becomes concerned about the remarks made by one of the group members. The mother states, "I insist that my children take iron fortified vitamins every day. My children really enjoy taking the cute little cartoon vitamins. They call the vitamins their 'morning candy.'" Should the nurse be concerned? How should the nurse respond?

See Answers to Patient Safety Questions in Appendix A.

athletic training. These conditions may require more than the recommended dietary allowance (RDA) of iron (see Chapter 62). In undeveloped countries, the primary cause of iron-deficiency anemia is the lack of meat or fresh fruits and vegetables in the diet. The most significant effect of iron deficiency is a reduction in erythropoiesis, resulting in symptoms of anemia.

Iron therapy is initiated to alleviate symptoms of anemia caused by blood loss or dietary deficiency. Once diagnosed, a primary goal is to identify the etiology of the disorder and treat the underlying pathology. Choice of therapy depends upon the etiology and severity of the deficiency.

- Mild anemia may be prevented or corrected in most patients by increasing the intake of iron-rich foods, such as fish, red meat, fortified cereal, and whole-grain breads.
- Moderate anemia is corrected by oral iron supplementation.
- Severe anemia, and that caused by iron malabsorption disorders, is corrected by parenteral iron therapy.

PROTOTYPE DRUG Ferrous sulfate (Feosol, Feostat, others)

Classification: **Therapeutic:** Agent for anemia
Pharmacologic: Iron supplement

Therapeutic Effects and Uses: Ferrous sulfate is an iron supplement containing about 20% elemental iron. Desiccated (dried) ferrous sulfate contains 30% elemental iron. It is inexpensive and available in a wide variety of dosage forms to prevent or rapidly reverse symptoms of iron deficiency anemia. Enteric-coated and extended release forms are available. If tolerated, the drug should be taken on an empty stomach, at least 1 hour before or 2 hours after a meal.

In general, patients with iron deficiency respond rapidly to the administration of ferrous sulfate. Although a positive therapeutic response may be achieved in 48 hours, therapy may continue for several months to replenish the storage depots for iron. As the deficiency is corrected, the body will absorb a smaller percentage of elemental iron in each dose until iron intake balances iron loss. This is assuming, of course, that the source of the iron imbalance, such as bleeding or dietary insufficiency, has been corrected. Laboratory evaluation of hemoglobin, transferrin, and hematocrit levels is conducted regularly to assess the progress of pharmacotherapy. Dosage is decreased as therapy progresses and the deficiency is corrected.

If rapid, symptomatic improvement is not experienced, the reasons for the treatment failure must be carefully explored. The patient may be experiencing continued bleeding or they may have a malabsorption disorder that prevents the iron from being absorbed. A common reason for treatment failure is lack of adherence to pharmacotherapy. Patients may stop taking the drug due to severe nausea and vomiting, or they may take the drug with food or other drugs that inhibit iron absorption. Excellent assessment and teaching skills of the nurse are key to achieving successful pharmacotherapeutic outcomes in these patients.

Mechanism of Action: After absorption, most iron is used by the body to make hemoglobin. Laboratory values of hemoglobin should increase 2 to 4 g/dL every 3 weeks until normal values are achieved. In addition, therapy is continued until serum ferritin levels return to normal, indicating that the iron storage depots are filled.

Pharmacokinetics:

Route(s)	PO
Absorption	5–30% absorbed
Distribution	Well distributed; crosses the placenta
Primary metabolism	Undergoes extensive enterohepatic recirculation
Primary excretion	Feces, urine, and skin
Onset of action	Unknown
Duration of action	Unknown

Adverse Effects: The most common adverse effects of ferrous sulfate are nausea and vomiting, which will occur to some degree in most patients. Taking the drug with food will diminish GI upset but can decrease the absorption of iron by 50% to 70%. The degree of nausea and vomiting is dose related and serious symptoms may require a dosage adjustment. Contact of liquid iron with teeth should be avoided because the drug can cause brown stains. Iron preparations will darken stools but this is a harmless adverse effect. Because constipation is common, especially in older adults, an increase in dietary fiber intake is indicated.

Contraindications/Precautions: Iron salts should not be administered for anemia other than that caused by iron deficiency, because iron will not correct these conditions and may build to toxic levels. The drug should not be administered to patients with hemochromatosis, a disease in which the patient has excess iron stores. Ferrous sulfate may irritate the stomach mucosa and increase bleeding in patients with PUD. The drug may cause diarrhea if administered to patients with regional enteritis or ulcerative colitis.

Drug Interactions: Absorption is reduced when oral iron salts are given concurrently with antacids, proton pump inhibitors, or calcium supplements. Iron decreases the absorption of tetracyclines, fluoroquinolones, levodopa, and etidronate. To prevent possible interactions, it is advisable to take iron supplements 1 to 2 hours before or after other medications. **Herbal/Food:** Food (especially dairy products), coffee, and tea will inhibit iron absorption. Vitamin C will increase absorption.

Pregnancy: Category A.

Treatment of Overdose: Iron is very toxic and most overdoses are accidental, occurring in children under the age of 6. The antidote for acute iron intoxication is the parenteral agent deferoxamine (Desferal). This chelating agent binds iron, which is removed by the kidneys, turning the urine a reddish-brown color.

Nursing Responsibilities:

- Obtain a complete health history including allergies, drug history, possible drug reactions, history of PUD, or recent blood loss.
- Obtain baseline levels for RBCs, hematocrit, hemoglobin, and serum ferritin.
- Assess vital signs for signs of cellular hypoxia, such as increased heart rate and respiratory rate.
- Give on an empty stomach if possible because oral iron preparations are best absorbed between meals. If GI adverse effects are prominent, give with or immediately after meals with adequate liquid.
- If the patient experiences difficulty in swallowing tablets or capsules, recommend a liquid formulation or a less corrosive form, such as ferrous gluconate.
- Dilute liquid preparations well and give them through a straw or place them on the back of the tongue with a dropper to prevent staining of teeth and to mask the unpleasant taste.
- Mix Feosol elixir with water as it is not compatible with milk or fruit juice. Fer-In-Sol (drops) may be given in water or in fruit or vegetable juice, according to the manufacturer.
- Monitor laboratory tests for hematocrit and reticulocyte values during therapy. Investigate the absence of satisfactory response after 3 weeks of drug treatment.
- Continue iron therapy for 2 to 3 months after the hemoglobin level has returned to normal (roughly twice the period required to normalize hemoglobin concentration).
- Monitor bowel movements because constipation is a common adverse effect.

Patient and Family Education:

- Do not take tablets or capsules within 1 hour of bedtime.
- Do not crush tablets or empty contents of capsule because this may cause GI distress.
- Take ferrous sulfate with a full glass of water. Rinse mouth with clear water immediately after ingestion.
- Consume citrus fruit or tomato juice with iron preparations (except the elixir form) because ascorbic acid (vitamin C) increases iron absorption.
- Avoid taking drug with milk, eggs, antacids, or caffeine beverages, because these inhibit drug absorption.
- Iron preparations cause dark green or black stools: This is a harmless adverse effect.
- Report constipation or diarrhea to the health care provider. Symptoms may be relieved by adjustments in dosage or diet, or by changing to another iron preparation.

Drugs Similar to Ferrous Sulfate (Feosol, Feostat, Others)

At least eight iron salts are available for administration to patients with iron-deficiency anemia. Iron salts are often classified by their route of administration, either oral (PO) or parenteral.

Oral iron salts: Oral iron salts include ferrous fumarate, ferrous gluconate, polysaccharide-iron complex, and carbonyl iron. The choice of specific agent and dose are based on iron content and degree of GI tolerability. Table 41.4 lists the amount of elemental iron in these drugs.

A large number of brand name iron products and formulations are available, including tablets, drops, elixirs, and suspensions. Nausea, vomiting, constipation, and diarrhea are common adverse effects with all oral iron preparations. Slow-release products, called carbonyl iron (Feosol-caps, Ferronyl), are more expensive, but are less dangerous in children following accidental ingestion because there is a longer period for intervention before toxic effects materialize. Some products have an enteric coating so that the capsule or tablet dissolves in the intestine, thus causing less gastric irritation. Recall, however, that stomach acid is necessary to convert iron to its more absorbable form. In addition, enteric coatings are unreliable in that they may dissolve after the drug has passed the duodenum, which is the primary site for iron absorption. Vitamin C is added to many oral iron supplements because it enhances iron absorption. Some products are formulated as "multivitamins." For example, Niferex PN Forte, which is formulated specifically for pregnant or lactating patients, contains a polysaccharide-iron complex and vitamins A, D, C, folic acid, B complex, calcium, iodine, magnesium, copper, and zinc. Adding extra "enhancers" such as additional vitamins, extended release, or enteric coating increases the cost of the drug but not necessarily its effectiveness. The amount of elemental iron in the product and adverse effects should be the primary factors guiding therapy.

Parenteral iron salts: Iron dextran (Dexferrum, others), iron sucrose (Venofer), and ferric gluconate (Ferrlecit) are parenteral preparations reserved for patients who cannot tolerate oral iron preparations or who have a malabsorption disorder

TABLE 41.4 Iron Content of Oral Iron Formulations

Preparation	Elemental Iron	Dose Needed to Provide 200 mg of Elemental Iron per Day
carbonyl iron	100%	200 mg
ferrous fumarate	33%	600 mg
ferrous gluconate	12%	720 mg
ferrous sulfate: regular	20%	1,000 mg
ferrous sulfate: desiccated	30%	660 mg
polysaccharide iron complex	100%	200 mg

preventing iron absorption from the GI tract. Giving parenteral iron does not lead to a faster recovery for patients with iron-deficiency anemia because the body is limited as to how quickly it can make hemoglobin and new RBCs. These drugs are clearly more toxic than the oral iron products and require careful monitoring during pharmacotherapy.

All three parenteral agents are equally effective at raising iron levels. All are given IV. Iron dextran is also available by the IM route although this is rarely used due to pain at the injection site and unreliable absorption from the muscle. Iron sucrose and iron gluconate have more limited application. They are only approved for patients with iron-deficiency anemia undergoing chronic hemodialysis who are also receiving erythropoietin.

Anaphylaxis has been reported with iron dextran and iron sucrose. Prior to administering an infusion of these agents, the patient must receive a small IV test dose and be observed for 15 to 30 minutes to assess for possible allergic reactions, which may cause respiratory arrest and circulatory collapse. Vital signs should be monitored during the test dose infusion. Some health care providers order test doses conducted prior to every administration of IV iron salts, since anaphylaxis may occur on second and subsequent doses. Ferric gluconate produces a lower incidence of anaphylactic shock; although a test dose is not required, it is good clinical practice to conduct one prior to administration.

Common adverse reactions of iron dextran are hypotension, headache, muscle pain, and joint pain; these are more severe when given IV. Iron dextran appears to increase bone density in the joints, which is the probable cause of the muscle and joint pain. Frequent adverse effects with ferric gluconate include cramping, nausea, vomiting, hypotension, and rash. Iron sucrose is well tolerated, with some patients experiencing leg cramps and hypotension.

CONNECTION *Checkpoint* 41.2

From what you learned in Chapter 10, explain why a patient who is pregnant has a substantially higher iron requirement compared to a nonpregnant woman. (See Answer to Connection Checkpoint 41.2 in Appendix A.)

41.7 Pernicious anemia may be successfully treated with the administration of vitamin B_{12}.

Vitamin B_{12} and folic acid are dietary nutrients essential for rapidly dividing cells. The continuous, high rate of erythropoiesis occurring throughout the life span demands a continuous supply of these vitamins. Without them, the normal production of RBCs is interrupted and large, immature erythrocytes that are unable to carry the same amount of oxygen as normal RBCs are released into the blood, and anemia results.

Vitamin B_{12} is an essential component of two coenzymes required for normal cell growth and DNA replication. Neither plants nor animals synthesize Vitamin B_{12}; only bacteria can make this vitamin. Because the body only requires miniscule amounts of vitamin B_{12} (3 mcg/day), deficiency of this vitamin is usually not due to insufficient dietary intake. Instead, the most common cause of vitamin B_{12} deficiency is absence of **intrinsic factor,** a protein secreted by stomach cells. Intrinsic factor forms a complex with vitamin B_{12}, which is then absorbed into the circulation. Without the formation of this complex, vitamin B_{12} is not absorbed from the intestine. Figure 41.3 illustrates the metabolism of vitamin B_{12}.

Deficiency of intrinsic factor is caused by inflammatory diseases of the stomach or by gastric resection. Inflammatory diseases of the small intestine that affect food and nutrient absorption may also cause vitamin B_{12} deficiency. Because vitamin B_{12} is found primarily in foods of animal origin, strict vegetarians may require a vitamin supplement to avoid deficiency. The center portion of the vitamin B_{12} molecule contains the metal ion cobalt, which is a micromineral essential to human nutrition.

The most profound consequence of vitamin B_{12} deficiency is a megaloblastic anemia called **pernicious anemia,** which affects both the hematologic and nervous systems. In pernicious anemia, the hematopoietic stem cells produce abnormally large erythrocytes that do not fully mature. Although RBCs are most

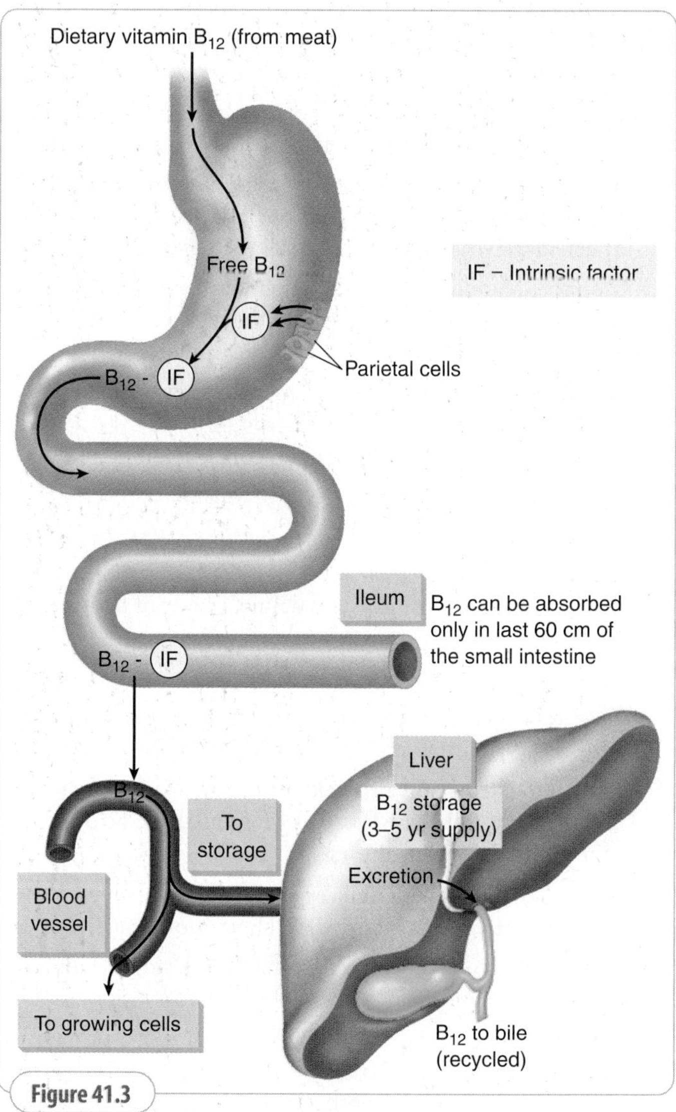

Figure 41.3

Metabolism of vitamin B_{12}.

NURSING PROCESS APPLICATION

Patients Receiving Iron Supplementation

Assessment

Prior to administration:

- Obtain a complete health history including allergies, drug history, possible drug reactions, history of PUD, or recent blood loss.
- Assess the reason for drug administration such as the presence or history of anemia, or prophylaxis during infancy, childhood, and pregnancy.
- Assess CBC, specifically RBCs, hematocrit, hemoglobin levels, and RBC indices to establish baseline values. Assess serum ferritin levels.
- Assess vital signs for signs of cellular hypoxia such as increased heart rate and respiratory rate.

Potential Nursing Diagnoses

- *Risk for Imbalanced Nutrition: Less than Body Requirements,* related to inadequate iron intake
- *Impaired Gas Exchange*, related to low red blood cell count resulting in decreased oxygenation
- *Risk for Injury*, related to weakness, dizziness, and syncope, caused by anemia
- *Deficient Knowledge (Iron Therapy),* related to purpose, precautions, and adverse effects of drug

Planning: Patient Goals and Expected Outcomes

The patient will:

- Exhibit improved serum ferritin level, hematocrit level, and RBC indices.
- Demonstrate improved or diminished symptoms related to anemia such as increased tolerance for activity and decreased fatigability.
- Demonstrate an understanding of the drug's action by accurately describing drug adverse effects and precautions.
- Report significant adverse effects such as GI distress.

Implementation

Interventions and (Rationales)	Patient and Family Education
• Monitor vital signs, especially pulse. (Increased pulse and respiratory rate are indicators of decreased oxygen content in the blood.)	• Instruct the patient to monitor pulse rate and respiratory status. Report irregularities, changes in rhythm, or increased shortness of breath to the health care provider.
• Monitor CBC to evaluate effectiveness of treatment. (Increases in hematocrit and hemoglobin values indicate increased RBC production. RBC indices will show improvement as iron supplementation diminishes anemic state.)	Instruct the patient: • On the need for initial and continuing laboratory blood monitoring. • To keep all laboratory appointments.
• Monitor changes in stool. (May cause constipation, change in stool color, and false positives when stool is tested for occult blood.)	Instruct the patient: • That stool color may change to dark green or black and this is not a cause for alarm. • On measures to relieve constipation, such as including high-fiber vegetables and grains in the diet, and increasing fluid intake and exercise.
• Plan activities and allow for periods of rest to help the patient conserve energy. (Diminished iron levels result in decreased hemoglobin formation leading to weakness and fatigue.)	Instruct the patient to: • Rest when feeling tired and avoid overexertion. • Plan activities to avoid fatigue.
• Administer medication on an empty stomach (if tolerated) at least 1 hour before bedtime. (This maximizes absorption; taking closer to bedtime may increase the chance of GI distress.)	Instruct the patient: • Not to crush or chew sustained-release preparations. • That medication may cause GI upset. • To take medication with food if GI upset becomes a problem. • To take at least 1 hour before bedtime.
• Administer liquid iron preparations through a straw or place on the back of the tongue. (This avoids staining the teeth.)	Instruct the patient to: • Dilute liquid medication before using and to use a straw to take medication. • Rinse the mouth after swallowing to decrease the chance of staining the teeth.
• Administer injectable parenteral iron preparations deep into the muscle using the z-track method. (This ensures absorption and minimizes tissue discolorations.)	• Instruct the patient to report excessive pain at the injection site and to observe for discoloration of the tissue. Report to the health care provider.
• Monitor dietary intake of iron enriched foods. (This ensures adequate intake of foods high in iron.)	• Instruct patient to increase intake of iron-rich foods such as liver, egg yolks, brewer's yeast, wheat germ, and muscle meats.
• Monitor for the potential of child access to medication. (Iron poisoning can be fatal to young children.)	• Advise parents to store iron-containing vitamins out of reach of children and in childproof containers.

Evaluation of Outcome Criteria

Evaluation of the drug's effectiveness occurs by continually assessing and reassign to identify if the patient goals have been met (see "Planning").

affected, lack of maturation of all blood cell types may occur in severe disease. Symptoms of pernicious anemia are often nonspecific and develop slowly, sometimes over several years. Profound nervous system symptoms distinguish this disease from most other anemias and include memory loss, confusion, unsteadiness, tingling or numbness in the limbs, delusions, mood disturbances, and even hallucinations in severe deficiencies. Permanent nervous system impairment may result if the disease remains untreated for 6 to 12 months. Pharmacotherapy includes the administration of cyanocobalamin, a form of vitamin B_{12}. Prior to administration of vitamin B_{12}, the nurse should assess for other causes of anemia including GI bleeding, GI surgery, tapeworm infestation, and gluten enteropathy.

PharmFACT

A deficiency of vitamin B_{12}, folate, or vitamin B_6 may increase the blood level of homocysteine, an amino acid normally found in the blood. An elevated blood level of homocysteine is a risk factor for heart disease and stroke. *Source:* National Institutes of Health Office of Dietary Supplements, 2006.

Folic acid, or **folate**, is B-complex vitamin that is essential for normal DNA and ribonucleic acid (RNA) synthesis. Like B_{12} deficiency, insufficient folic acid levels can manifest as anemia. In fact, the metabolism of vitamin B_{12} and folic acid are intricately linked; a B_{12} deficiency will create a lack of activated folic acid. Folate deficiency is one of the most common types of anemias in the United States.

Folic acid does not require intrinsic factor for intestinal absorption, and the most common cause of deficiency is insufficient dietary intake. This is often observed in patients with chronic alcoholism because their diets are often deficient in this nutrient, and ethanol interferes with folate metabolism in the liver. Fad diets and absorption diseases of the small intestine can also lead to folate-deficiency anemia. Hematopoietic symptoms of folate deficiency are the same as those for B_{12} deficiency; however, no neurologic signs are present. Folate deficiency during pregnancy has been linked to neural birth defects such as spina bifida. Mild deficiency or prophylaxis of folate deficiency is accomplished by increasing the dietary intake of folic acid through fresh green vegetables, dried beans, and wheat products. In cases when adequate dietary intake cannot be achieved, therapy with folate sodium (Folvite) or folic acid is warranted. Folic acid is presented as a drug prototype for water-soluble vitamins in Chapter 62.

PROTOTYPE DRUG Cyanocobalamin (Calomist, Nascobal)

Classification: Therapeutic: Agent for anemia
Pharmacologic: Vitamin supplement

Therapeutic Effects and Uses: Cyanocobalamin is a purified form of vitamin B_{12} that is indicated for patients with vitamin B_{12} deficiency anemia. Treatment of vitamin B_{12} deficiency is most often by weekly, biweekly, or monthly intramuscular (IM) or subcutaneous injections. A typical regimen for pernicious anemia would be 100 mcg IM or subcutaneous once daily for 1 week, followed by 100 mcg on alternate days for 7 doses. Dose reduction continues, with administration every 3 to 4 days for another 2 to 3 weeks, then 100 mcg IM monthly for life. Oral vitamin B_{12} formulations are available primarily as vitamin supplementation, although they are only effective in patients who have sufficient amounts of intrinsic factor and normal absorption in the small intestine. Intranasal spray and gel formulations (Nascobal) are available that provide for once weekly dosage. Because these intranasal formulations exhibit variable absorption and bioavailability, they are used for maintenance therapy after normal vitamin B_{12} levels have been restored by parenteral preparations.

Parenteral administration of cyanocobalamin rapidly reverses most signs and symptoms of B_{12} deficiency, usually within a few days or weeks. If the disease has been prolonged, symptoms may take longer to resolve, and some neurologic damage may be permanent. In most cases, treatment must often be maintained for the remainder of the patient's life. Periodic laboratory blood testing and hemoglobin values are used to gauge the success of pharmacotherapy.

Mechanism of Action: Administration of cyanocobalamin reverses vitamin B_{12} deficiency and results in rapid improvement of anemia symptoms. Normal RBC production resumes, with laboratory evaluation of blood and bone marrow showing continuous improvement over about 7 days. Therapy may extend to several months to restore hepatic stores of the vitamin.

Pharmacokinetics:

Route(s)	PO, IM, deep subcutaneous, intranasal
Absorption	Well absorbed; PO absorption requires intrinsic factor
Distribution	Widely distributed; crosses the placenta; secreted in breast milk
Primary metabolism	Primarily converted in tissues to coenzyme B_{12} and stored in liver; extensive enterohepatic recirculation
Primary excretion	Renal
Onset of action	Peak serum level: 8–12 h (PO), 1–2 h (intranasal), and 1 h (IV)
Duration of action	Half-life: 6 days

Adverse Effects: Adverse effects from cyanocobalamin are uncommon. Because hypokalemia may occur, serum potassium levels are monitored periodically. A small percentage of patients receiving B_{12} exhibit rashes, itching, or other signs of allergy. Anaphylaxis is possible, though rare. Sodium retention occurs in some patients, with possible worsening of HF.

Contraindications/Precautions: Patients with suspected sensitivity to cobalt should receive an intradermal test dose because they may experience allergic reactions or anaphylaxis to the drug. Monotherapy with folic acid will not improve symptoms of vitamin B_{12} deficiency anemia. Cyanocobalamin is contraindicated in patients with severe pulmonary disease and should be used cautiously in patients with heart disease because of the potential for sodium retention caused by the drug.

Drug Interactions: Drug interactions with cyanocobalamin include a decrease in absorption when given concurrently with ethanol, aminosalicylic acid, omeprazole, neomycin, or colchicine. Chloramphenicol may interfere with the therapeutic response to cyanocobalamin. **Herbal/Food:** Unknown.

Pregnancy: Category A (C when used parenterally). Maternal requirements for vitamin B_{12} increase during pregnancy and lactation, although the drug should not be taken in higher than recommended amounts.

Treatment of Overdose: Overdosage is not likely.

Nursing Responsibilities:

- Prior to initiating therapy, monitor laboratory tests such as reticulocyte and erythrocyte counts, hematocrit, hemoglobin, vitamin B_{12}, and serum folate levels. Repeat tests between 5 and 7 days after start of therapy and at regular intervals during therapy. Characteristically, reticulocyte concentration rises in 3 to 4 days, peaks in 5 to 8 days, and then gradually declines as erythrocyte count and hemoglobin rise to normal levels (in 4 to 6 weeks).
- Monitor serum potassium levels during the first 48 hours. Conversion to normal erythropoiesis increases erythrocyte potassium requirement and can result in severe hypokalemia and sudden death.
- Obtain a comprehensive history of hypersensitivities. Sensitization to cyanocobalamin can take as long as 8 years to develop.
- Monitor vital signs in patients with cardiac disease and in those receiving parenteral cyanocobalamin. Be alert to symptoms of pulmonary edema, which frequently occur early in therapy.
- Monitor the effectiveness of pharmacotherapy, as measured by laboratory values and improvement in the symptoms of vitamin B_{12} deficiency. Therapeutic response is often dramatic, occurring within 48 hours.
- Obtain a complete diet and drug history and inquire into alcohol drinking patterns for all patients receiving cyanocobalamin to identify and correct poor dietary habits.

Patient and Family Education:

- Do not discontinue taking this drug without approval of the health care provider. To prevent irreversible neurologic damage, patients with pernicious anemia must continue taking the drug for life.
- Report any disease or infection that occurs during therapy because increased dosage may be required.
- If using the spray form, prime the pump before the first use by pumping the spray a few times until a fine mist appears. If it has been longer than 5 days between uses, prime the pump again. Sniff gently while spraying.
- Eat foods that are rich sources of B_{12} (nonpernicious anemia) such as nutrient-fortified breakfast cereals, vitamin B_{12}-fortified soy milk, organ meats, clams, oysters, egg yolk, crab, salmon, sardines, muscle meat, milk, and dairy products.

Drugs Similar to Cyanocobalamin (Crystamine, Others)

There are no drugs similar to cyanocobalamin.

UNDERSTANDING THE CHAPTER

Key Concepts Summary

41.1 Hematopoiesis is a dynamic process that is responsive to the changing demands of the body.

41.2 Erythropoietin stimulates production of red blood cells and is used to treat anemia.

41.3 Colony-stimulating factors increase the production of leukocytes.

41.4 Platelet production can be increased by administering oprelvekin.

41.5 Anemias may be caused by hemorrhage or a change in red blood cell production or destruction.

41.6 Administration of iron salts can rapidly reverse symptoms of iron-deficiency anemia.

41.7 Pernicious anemia may be successfully treated with the administration of vitamin B_{12}.

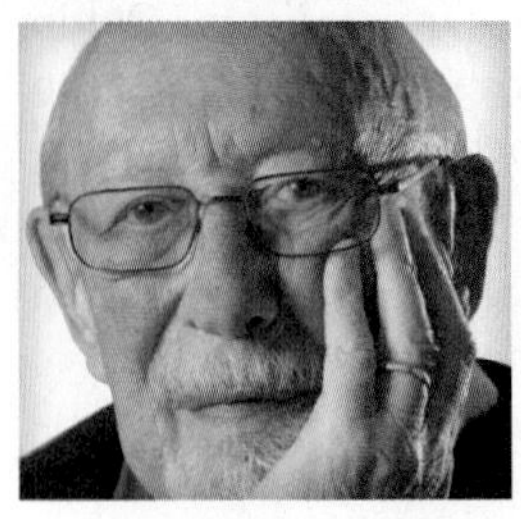

Making the PATIENT Connection

Remember the patient "Carl Guenther" at the beginning of the chapter? Now read the remainder of the case study. Based on the information presented within this chapter, respond to the critical thinking questions that follow.

"A real people person who never met a stranger." That is how family and friends have always described Carl Guenther. His positive and outgoing personality is well known in the community. When Carl was informed about his prostate cancer, he handled the diagnosis well and with his usual optimism. He was confident that the chemotherapy would be successful. His mantra for years had been to "Live every day as if it were your last." However, the treatment for the cancer had presented with adverse effects that he didn't expect and his enthusiasm diminished.

Carl is a 72-year-old retired sales representative for a chain of department stores. His entire career was centered on interacting with all kinds of people. When he retired, his outgoing nature was an asset for the many community agencies that he volunteered to help. He was active in the local Lions Club, with his church's outreach ministry, and as a volunteer at the children's hospital. He had even considered working as a greeter at his neighborhood department store.

As he took chemotherapy, the associated nausea and vomiting were well managed with antiemetic agents. His physical appearance did not change much since Carl had minimal hair loss due to the chemotherapy. Now he faces an exceedingly low white blood cell count and has been advised to avoid potential sources of infection, including people. By far this is the worst adverse effect of the chemotherapy to Carl. He feels socially isolated and depressed. Is this the end he wonders? Am I to die lonely?

Critical Thinking Questions

1. The health care provider orders filgrastim (Neupogen) 10 mcg/kg daily for 4 days. Carl asks you, his nurse, "How does this drug work?" What is your response?
2. List interventions that should be followed during this period of chemotherapy-induced neutropenia to protect Carl from infection.
3. What adverse effects would you monitor in patients receiving Neupogen?

Case Study

When the blood test returned from Betty Arnold's preemployment physical, the results indicated anemia. "No wonder I feel so exhausted all the time," she said. "I thought my fatigue was from taking care of my five children, my home, and my aging parents." When she saw her primary health care provider, she was diagnosed with iron-deficiency anemia and prescribed ferrous sulfate (Feosol) 160 mg sustained release tablets daily.

1. You, as the nurse, will provide teaching for this patient about dietary sources of iron. Create a list of foods high in iron.
2. What adverse effects should Betty watch for while taking Feosol?
3. Is there a best time of the day to take this medication? Why?

NCLEX®-RN Review Questions

1 Which of the following would be included in the care plan for a client receiving epoetin alfa?

1. Avoid fresh fruit and vegetables, or partially cooked meats.
2. Encourage frequent rest periods to minimize fatigue.
3. Limit exposure to direct sunlight and use sunscreen when outdoors.
4. Protect tissues and mucous membranes from traumatic injury.

2 A hematopoietic growth factor is prescribed for each of the following clients. A nurse should question the order for which condition?

1. HIV client receiving zidovudine
2. A client with uncontrolled hypertension
3. A client with chronic renal failure
4. A client with chemotherapy-induced anemia

3 The client is being treated with a filgrastim (Neupogen). Which of the following would the nurse monitor to determine the effectiveness of this drug?

1. White blood cell counts
2. Red blood cell counts
3. Platelet counts
4. Serum potassium level

4 The nurse is teaching the client about oprelvekin (Neumega). Which of the following statements, if made by the client, indicates additional health teaching is needed?

1. "This drug stimulates the production of platelets."
2. "I should weigh myself and watch for fluid retention."
3. "I will report vision changes to my health care provider."
4. "I will add more iron rich foods to my diet."

5 An alcoholic client who is prescribed cyanocobalamin (Crystamine) states, "I don't understand why my health care provider has prescribed B_{12} injections." The nurse's response would be based on which of the following physiologic concepts?

1. Diets of alcohol-dependent clients are often deficient in this nutrient.
2. Ethanol facilitates folate metabolism in the liver.
3. Alcoholic clients are at high risk for pernicious anemia.
4. Liver cirrhosis diminishes natural physiologic deposits of B_{12}.

6 The nurse is teaching the client about ferrous sulfate (Feosol). Which of the following statements should be included in the teaching plan? (Select all that apply.)

1. This drug should be taken on an empty stomach at least 1 hour before or 2 hours after a meal.
2. Getting liquid iron on teeth should be avoided because the drug can cause brown stains.
3. Iron preparation may darken stools and cause constipation.
4. Vitamin E is added to many oral iron supplements because it enhances iron absorption.
5. This drug can be taken with caffeinated beverages.

See Answers to Critical Thinking Questions, Case Study, and NCLEX-RN® Review in Appendix A.

References

Breiterman-White, R. (2007). Hemoglobin variability: Managing the higher end of the target range. *Nephrology Nursing, 34*(2), 201–213.

Coyer, S. M. (2005). Anemia: Diagnosis and management. *Journal of Pediatric Healthcare, 19*(6), 380–385.

Gozzard, D. I. (2006). Diagnosing and treating iron deficiency. *Nursing in Practice: The Journal for Today's Primary Care Nurse, 29*, 57–58, 61.

Holcomb, S. S. (2005). Recognizing and managing anemia. *Nurse Practitioner, 30*(12), 16–18, 23–24, 27–28.

Kaushansky, K., & Kipps, T. J. (2006). Hematopoietic agents: Growth factors, minerals and vitamins. In L. L. Brunton, J. S. Lazo, & K. L. Parker (Eds.), *The pharmacological basis of therapeutics* (11th ed., pp. 1433–1466). New York: McGraw-Hill.

Lichtman, M. A., Williams, W. J., Beutler, E., Kaushansky, K., Kipps, T. J., Seligsohn, U., et al. (Eds.). (2005). *Williams hematology* (7th ed.). New York: McGraw-Hill Professional.

Luggen, A. (2007). Gerontologic nurse practitioner care guidelines: Vitamin B_{12} deficiency in older adults. *Geriatric Nursing, 27*(1), 32–33.

Marcus, R., & Coulston, A. M. (2006). Water-soluble vitamins: The vitamin B complex and ascorbic acid. In L. L. Brunton, J. S. Lazo, & K. L. Parker (Eds.), *The pharmacological basis of therapeutics* (11th ed., pp. 1753–1772). New York: McGraw-Hill.

Marrs, J. (2006). Care of patients with neutropenia. *Clinical Journal of Oncology Nursing, 10*(2), 164–166.

National Institutes of Health Office of Dietary Supplements, 2006. *Dietary supplement fact sheet: Vitamin B_{12}.* Retrieved July 19, 2008, from http://ods.od.nih.gov/factsheets/vitaminb12.asp#h9

Sung, S., Nathan, P. C., Alibhai, S., Tomlinson, G. A., & Beyene, J. (2007). Meta-analysis: Effect of prophylactic hematopoietic colony-stimulating factors on mortality and outcomes of infection. *Annals of Internal Medicine, 147*(6), 400–411.

Yeo, T. P. (2006). Detecting aplastic anemia: A case illustrating the importance of attending to the results of routine test. *American Journal of Nursing, 106*(9), Critical Care Extra: 72AA.

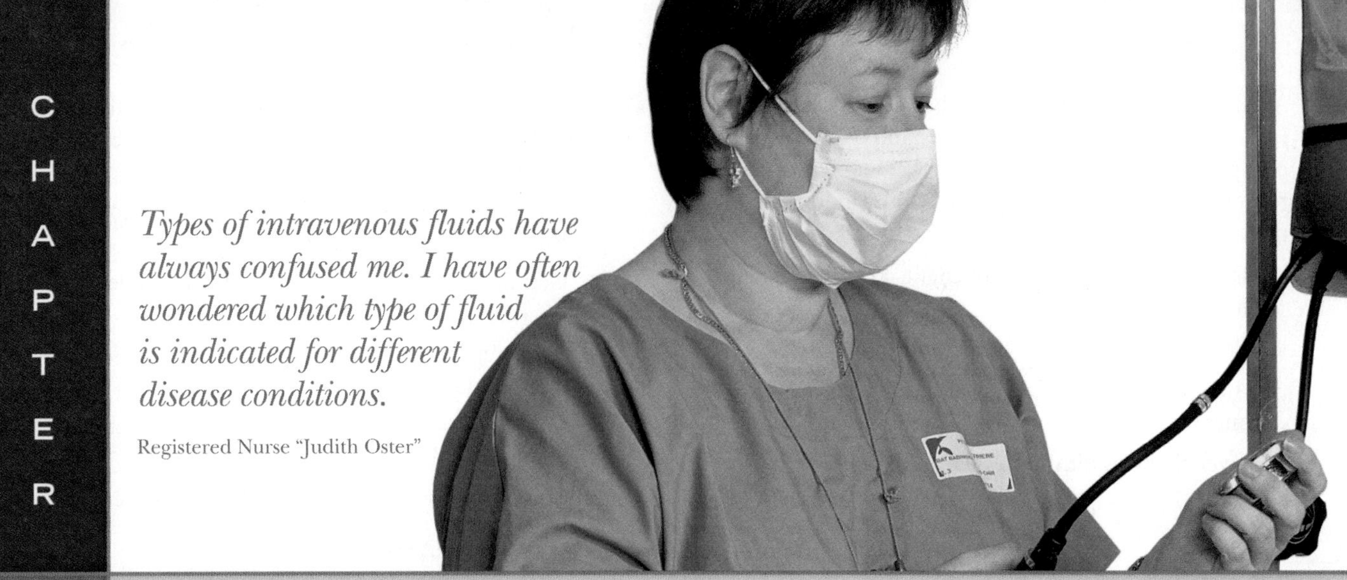

Types of intravenous fluids have always confused me. I have often wondered which type of fluid is indicated for different disease conditions.

Registered Nurse "Judith Oster"

CHAPTER 42

Pharmacotherapy of Fluid Imbalance, Electrolyte, and Acid–Base Disorders

Learning Outcomes

After reading this chapter, the student should be able to:

1. Describe the exchange of fluids that occurs among the different fluid compartments in the body.
2. Identify conditions for which intravenous fluid therapy may be indicated.
3. Explain how changes in the osmolality or tonicity of a fluid can cause water to move to a different compartment.
4. Compare and contrast the use of blood products, crystalloids, and colloids in intravenous therapy.
5. Explain the importance of electrolyte balance in the body.
6. Explain the pharmacotherapy of sodium and potassium imbalances.
7. Discuss medications used to treat acidosis and alkalosis.
8. Describe the nurse's role in the pharmacologic management of fluid imbalance, electrolyte, and acid–base disorders.
9. For each of the classes shown in the chapter outline, identify the prototype and representative drugs and explain the mechanism(s) of drug action, primary indications, contraindications, significant drug interactions, pregnancy category, and important adverse effects.
10. Use the nursing process to care for patients receiving drug therapy for fluid imbalance, electrolyte, and acid–base disorders.

Chapter Outline

Fluid Imbalance

Fluid Replacement Agents

Blood Products

PROTOTYPE **Normal Serum Albumin (Albuminar, Plasbumin, Others)** *p. 690*

Crystalloids

PROTOTYPE **5% Dextrose in Water (D_5W)** *p. 691*

Colloids

PROTOTYPE **Dextran 40 (Gentran 40, Hyskon, 10% LMD, Rheomacrodex)** *p. 692*

Physiology of Electrolytes

Pharmacotherapy of Electrolyte Imbalances

PROTOTYPE **Sodium Chloride (NaCl)** *p. 696*

PROTOTYPE **Potassium Chloride (KCl)** *p. 698*

PROTOTYPE **Magnesium Sulfate ($MgSO_4$)** *p. 700*

Pharmacotherapy of Acid–Base Imbalances

PROTOTYPE **Sodium Bicarbonate** *p. 702*

PROTOTYPE **Ammonium Chloride** *p. 703*

Can too much pure, sparkling water hurt you? As often as people hear "drink plenty of fluids," too much (or too little) can definitely be harmful. The volume and composition of fluids in the body must be maintained within narrow limits. Excess fluid volume can lead to hypertension (HTN), congestive heart failure, or peripheral edema, while depletion results in dehydration.

Body fluids must also contain specific amounts of essential ions or electrolytes, and be maintained at particular pH values. Imbalances in electrolytes or changes in the pH of body fluids may have fatal consequences if left untreated. This chapter will examine drugs used to reverse fluid imbalance, electrolyte, or acid–base disorders.

Key Terms

acidosis, 701
alkalosis, 703
buffers, 701
colloids, 692
crystalloids, 691
electrolyte, 694
extracellular fluid (ECF) compartment, 687
hyperkalemia, 697
hypernatremia, 695
hypokalemia, 697
hyponatremia, 696
intracellular fluid (ICF) compartment, 687
ion trapping, 701
osmolality, 687
osmosis, 688
tonicity, 687

Fluid Imbalance

42.1 Body fluids are exchanged between intracellular and extracellular compartments.

Body fluids travel between compartments separated by semipermeable membranes. Control of water balance in the various compartments is essential to homeostasis. Fluid imbalances are frequent indications for pharmacotherapy.

Not surprisingly, the greatest bulk of body fluid consists of water, which serves as the universal solvent in which electrolytes, minerals, and most nutrients are dissolved. Water alone is responsible for about 60% of the total body weight in a young adult. A newborn may contain 80% water, while an older adult may contain only 40%.

In a simple model, water in the body can be located in one of two places, or compartments. The **intracellular fluid (ICF) compartment,** which contains water that is inside cells, accounts for about two thirds of the total body water. The remaining one third of body fluid resides outside cells in the **extracellular fluid (ECF) compartment.** The ECF compartment is further divided into two parts: fluid in the plasma, or intravascular space, and fluid in the interstitial spaces between cells. The relationship between these fluid compartments is illustrated in Figure 42.1.

Once contained in a compartment, water and minerals do not stay there for very long. There is a continuous exchange, turnover, and mixing of fluids between the various compartments, as the molecules travel across the membranes that separate them. For example, the plasma membranes of cells separate the ICF from the ECF. The capillary membranes separate plasma from the interstitial fluid. Although water travels freely among the compartments, processes of diffusion and active transport govern the movement of large molecules and those with electrical charges. Movement of ions and drugs across membranes is a primary topic of pharmacokinetics (see Chapter 4).

CONNECTION *Checkpoint* 42.1

From what you learned in Chapter 4, what barriers does an oral drug face in moving from the gastrointestinal (GI) tract to the extracellular fluid compartment (plasma)?

See Answer to Connection Checkpoint 42.1 in Appendix A.

42.2 Osmolality or tonicity determines the movement of body fluids.

Osmolality and tonicity are two related terms central to understanding the pharmacotherapy of fluid imbalance disorders. Changes in the osmolality or tonicity of a body fluid can cause significant shifts in water balance between compartments. The nurse will often administer intravenous (IV) fluids to compensate for these changes.

The **osmolality** of a fluid is the number of dissolved particles, or solutes, in 1 kg (1 L) of water. In most body fluids, three solutes determine the osmolality: sodium, glucose, and urea. Sodium is the greatest contributor to osmolality due to its abundance in most body fluids. The normal osmolality of body fluids ranges from 275 to 295 milliosmoles per kilogram (mOsm/kg).

The term **tonicity** is sometimes used interchangeably with osmolality, although they are somewhat different. Tonicity is the ability of a solution to cause a change in water movement across a membrane due to osmotic forces. Whereas osmolality is a laboratory value that can be precisely measured, tonicity is a general term used to describe the relative concentration of IV fluids. The tonicity of normal plasma is considered isotonic and is used as the reference point when administering IV solutions. Solutions that

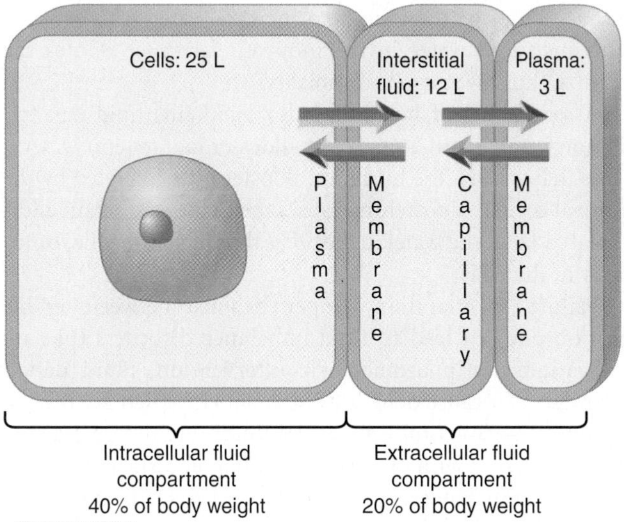

Figure 42.1

Major fluid compartments in the body.

are isotonic have the same concentration of solutes (same osmolality) as plasma. Hypertonic solutions contain a greater concentration of solutes than plasma, whereas hypotonic solutions have a lesser concentration of solutes than plasma.

Through **osmosis,** water moves from areas of low solute concentration (low osmolality), to areas of high solute concentration (high osmolality). If a hypertonic (hyperosmolar) IV solution is administered, the plasma gains more solutes than the interstitial fluid. Water will move, by osmosis, from the interstitial fluid compartment to the plasma compartment. Water will move in the opposite direction, from plasma to interstitial fluid, if a hypotonic solution is administered. Isotonic solutions will produce no net fluid shift. From a pharmacologic perspective, water movement between compartments following an IV infusion can be either a therapeutic effect or an adverse effect depending upon the patient's condition and the expected outcomes of the drug administration.

42.3 Overall fluid balance is regulated primarily by hormones acting upon the kidneys.

The average adult has a water intake of approximately 2,500 mL per day, most of which comes from food and beverages. Water output occurs through the kidneys, lungs, skin, feces, and sweat. To maintain water balance, water intake must equal water output. Net gains or losses of water can be estimated by changes in total body weight.

MyNursingKit | Fluids Animation

The most important physiological mechanism regulating fluid intake is thirst. The sensation of thirst occurs when osmoreceptors in the hypothalamus sense that the ECF has become hypertonic. Saliva secretion diminishes and the mouth dries, driving the individual to ingest fluids. As the ingested water is absorbed, the osmolality of the ECF falls and the thirst center in the hypothalamus is no longer stimulated.

In addition to triggering thirst, the hypothalamus also directs the pituitary gland to release antidiuretic hormone (ADH) when plasma osmolality rises. ADH acts directly on the distal tubules of the kidney to increase water reabsorption. This increased water in the intravascular space dilutes the plasma, thus lowering its osmolality.

A second set of hormones also maintains fluid balance. Through the renin-angiotensin-aldosterone system (RAAS) (see Chapter 34), the hormone aldosterone is secreted by the adrenal cortex. Aldosterone causes the kidneys to retain additional sodium and water in the body, thus increasing the osmolality of the ECF.

Failure to maintain proper balance between intake and output can lead to fluid imbalance disorders that are indications for pharmacologic intervention. Fluid deficit disorders can cause dehydration or shock, which are treated by administering oral (PO) or IV fluids. Fluid excess disorders are treated with diuretics (see Chapter 35). When treating fluid imbalances, the ultimate goal is to diagnose and correct the underlying cause of the disorder, while administering supporting fluids and medications to stabilize the patient.

CONNECTION *Checkpoint* 42.2

From what you learned in Chapter 34, name the two aldosterone antagonists and provide their indications.

See Answer to Connection Checkpoint 42.2 in Appendix A.

Fluid Replacement Agents

42.4 Dehydration may be treated with fluid volume expanders.

When fluid output exceeds fluid intake, volume deficits or contraction may result. Shock, dehydration, or electrolyte loss may occur. Large deficits are fatal, unless treated. The following are some common reasons for fluid depletion:

- Loss of GI fluids due to vomiting, diarrhea, chronic laxative use, or GI suctioning
- Excessive sweating during hot weather, athletic activity, or prolonged fever
- Severe burns
- Hemorrhage
- Excessive diuresis due to diuretic therapy or uncontrolled diabetic ketoacidosis

The immediate goal in treating a volume deficit disorder is to replace the depleted fluid so that blood volume and blood pressure can be maintained. In nonacute circumstances, this may be achieved by drinking more liquids or by administering fluids via a feeding tube. In acute situations, IV fluid therapy is indicated.

Choice of IV fluid therapy depends upon the nature of the volume contraction. Careful attention must be paid to restoring normal levels of blood elements (erythrocytes, leukocytes, and thrombocytes) and electrolytes, as well as fluid volume. If significant blood loss has occurred, blood products may be indicated. Loss of substantial sodium and other salts involves replacement therapy with hypertonic fluids. Excessive sweating can result in water loss that requires hypotonic IV fluids. Treating dehydration with an IV fluid with the incorrect tonicity may worsen the condition. Fluid replacement should always be conducted in a controlled step-wise manner. Rapid infusions can cause fluid overload, pulmonary edema, and cardiovascular stress. Vital signs and plasma electrolytes must be monitored during therapy. Therapy of dehydration is summarized in Table 42.1. The three basic classes of fluid replacement agents are blood products, crystalloids, and colloids.

PharmFACT

Exercise-associated hypernatremia (EAH) is a common condition when an endurance athlete drinks too much water (or electrolyte solutions) during a prolonged exercise. To prevent EAH, marathon runners and others must avoid drinking a larger volume of fluid than their body is losing in sweat and urine. *Source:* Medical News Today, 2008.

TABLE 42.1 Types of Dehydration Disorders and Their Treatment

Type	Isotonic Contraction	Hypotonic Contraction	Hypertonic Contraction
Fluid lost	Water and sodium in equal proportions	Loss of more sodium relative to water	Loss of more water, relative to sodium
Pathophysiology	ECF remains isotonic; no net fluid shift	ECF becomes hypotonic; fluid shifts from ECF to ICF, lowering plasma fluid volume	ECF becomes hypertonic; fluid shifts from ICF to ECF, causing cellular dehydration
Causes	Vomiting, diarrhea, renal disease, diuretics	Diuretics, renal disease	Excessive sweating without replenishment, osmotic diuresis, burns
Treatment	Administer isotonic fluids; e.g., isotonic saline (0.9%)	Administer hypertonic fluids; e.g., isotonic saline (3%)	Administer hypotonic fluids; e.g., hypotonic saline (0.11%) or 5% dextrose

42.5 Transfusions of blood products are used to treat serious conditions that cannot be managed effectively by other means.

About 29 million units of blood products are administered annually in the United States, from about 8 million volunteer donors. Blood products include whole blood, packed red cells, fresh frozen plasma, cryoprecipitate, and platelet infusions. A single unit of whole blood can be separated into its specific constituents (erythrocytes, leukocytes, thrombocytes, plasma proteins, fresh frozen plasma, and globulins), which can be used to treat more than one patient. Indications for the various blood products are shown in Table 42.2.

Blood products may be administered to restore deficient numbers of blood cells or proteins, or to increase fluid volume depending on the clinical situation. Whole blood is indicated for the treatment of acute, massive blood loss (depletion of more than 30% of the total volume) when there is a need to replace plasma volume, as well as supply erythrocytes to increase the blood's oxygen-carrying capacity.

The administration of whole blood has been largely replaced with the use of blood components. There are several reasons

TABLE 42.2 Indications for Blood Products

Product	Description	Indication(s)
Whole blood	Contains all blood components	Rapid, massive blood loss when safer agents are not available
Packed RBCs	One unit of packed RBCs increases hemoglobin by about 1 g/dL and hematocrit by about 3% Washed RBCs are nearly free of plasma, WBCs, and platelets, and are reserved for patients who have severe reactions to plasma components	Product of choice to increase serum hemoglobin level
Fresh frozen plasma (FFP)	An unconcentrated source of all clotting factors, without platelets	Correction of bleeding secondary to factor deficiencies for which specific factor replacements are unavailable, multifactor deficiency states, and rapid warfarin reversal FFP should not be used for simple volume expansion
Cryoprecipitate	A concentrate prepared from FFP Each concentrate contains about 80 units each of factor VIII and von Willebrand factor and about 250 mg of fibrinogen It also contains fibronectin and factor XIII	Originally used for hemophilia and von Willebrand's disease, it is currently used as a source of fibrinogen in acute disseminated intravascular coagulation with bleeding, treatment of uremic bleeding, cardiothoracic surgery, and obstetric emergencies such as abruptio placentae
Immune globulins	Antibody preparations used to provide an immediate boost to the immune system	Rh immune globulin (RhIG) prevents development of maternal Rh antibodies that can result from fetomaternal hemorrhage Other immune globulins are available for postexposure prophylaxis for patients exposed to certain infectious diseases, including cytomegalovirus, hepatitis A and B, measles, rabies, respiratory syncytial virus, rubella, tetanus, smallpox, and varicella
Platelets	One platelet concentrate increases the platelet count by about 10,000/mcL	Used to prevent bleeding in asymptomatic severe thrombocytopenia, for bleeding patients with less severe thrombocytopenia, for bleeding patients with platelet dysfunction due to antiplatelet drugs but with normal platelet count, for patients receiving massive transfusion that causes dilutional thrombocytopenia, and before invasive surgery, particularly if extracorporeal circulation exceeds 2 hours

why whole blood is rarely administered. If the patient only needs one specific component in blood, there is no need to expose the patient to unnecessary components that could potentially trigger an adverse effect. The supply of blood products depends on human donors and may require careful cross matching to ensure compatibility between the donor and the recipient.

The most common complications of whole blood transfusion include febrile nonhemolytic and chill-rigor reactions. The patient experiences symptoms of an allergic reaction that include back pain and low-grade fever and chills. Dizziness, urticaria, and headache may occur during or immediately after the transfusion. Symptoms are generally mild and treated with acetaminophen (Tylenol) and diphenhydramine (Benadryl) as needed.

The most serious adverse effect from administration of whole blood is an acute hemolytic transfusion reaction. This occurs when the patient receiving the transfusion develops antibodies against donor RBC antigens. ABO blood type incompatibility is the most common cause of this rare, though sometimes fatal, disorder. Another uncommon, though serious, adverse effect from whole blood is transfusion-related acute lung injury. This injury occurs when the patient receives donor antibodies that attack normal granulocytes in the lung. Acute respiratory symptoms develop and may be fatal.

Whole blood, despite being carefully screened, also has the potential to transmit serious infections such as hepatitis, cytomegalovirus, malaria, or HIV. In addition, platelet concentrates are stored at room temperature, which may promote the growth of bacteria in the sample. Although disease transmission from donor to recipient is possible, the risk is very low.

PROTOTYPE DRUG Normal serum albumin (Albuminar, Plasbumin, others)

Classification: **Therapeutic:** Fluid replacement agent
Pharmacologic: Blood product, colloid

Therapeutic Effects and Uses: Normal serum albumin is a protein extracted from whole blood, plasma, or placental human plasma that contains 96% albumin and 4% globulins and other proteins. After extraction from blood or plasma, the albumin is sterilized to remove possible contamination by hepatitis viruses or HIV. Albumin naturally comprises 50% to 60% of all blood proteins and the normal serum albumin concentration ranges from 3.5 to 5 g/dL. Plasma protein fraction (Plasmanate) is another albumin product that contains 83% albumin and 17% plasma globulins. Albumin is classified as both a blood product and a colloid.

The functions of endogenous albumin are to maintain plasma osmotic pressure and to bind certain substances traveling through the blood, including fatty acids, hormones, enzymes, and a substantial number of drug molecules. Binding to albumin renders these substances inactive until they become unbound.

Normal serum albumin may be administered to restore plasma volume and maintain cardiac output in patients with hypovolemic shock. It may also be administered to restore the level of blood proteins in patients with hypoproteinemia, which occurs in patients with hepatic cirrhosis. Albumin is occasionally administered to bind and remove toxic bilirubin in hemolytic disease of the newborn. It may also offer protection against kernicterus, a toxic accumulation of bilirubin in infants that causes brain injury. It has an immediate onset of action and is available in concentrations of 5% and 25%.

Mechanism of Action: Administered IV, albumin rapidly increases the osmotic pressure of the blood and causes fluid to move from the tissues to the general circulation.

Pharmacokinetics: Because human albumin is a natural substance, it is not possible to obtain accurate pharmacokinetic values. Endogenous albumin has a half-life of 17 to 19 days.

Adverse Effects: Because albumin is a natural blood product, the patient may have antibodies to the donor albumin and allergic reactions are possible. Because coagulation factors, antibodies, and most other blood proteins have been removed, allergic reactions from albumin are rare. Signs of allergy include fever, chills, urticaria, rash, dyspnea, and possibly hypotension.

Contraindications/Precautions: The drug is contraindicated in patients with severe anemia or cardiac failure in the presence of normal or increased intravascular volume, and in those with known allergy to albumin.

Drug Interactions: There are no clinically significant interactions. **Herbal/Food:** Unknown.

Pregnancy: Category C

Treatment of Overdose: Protein overload may occur if excessive albumin is infused. There is no treatment for overdose.

Nursing Responsibilities:

- Assess vital signs during infusion. Adjust flow rate to prevent too rapid a rise in blood pressure.
- Monitor laboratory tests for dosage of albumin using plasma albumin (normal): 3.5 to 5 g/dL; total serum protein (normal): 6 to 8.4 g/dL; and hemoglobin, hematocrit, and serum electrolytes.
- Assess for signs and symptoms of circulatory overload and pulmonary edema such as dyspnea, shallow breathing, wheezing, or restlessness and slow the infusion rate to keep vein open. Report signs to the prescriber immediately.
- Monitor intake and output ratio and pattern. Report changes in urinary output immediately. Increased colloidal osmotic pressure usually causes diuresis, which may persist from 3 to 20 hours.
- Withhold fluids for 8 hours when albumin is given to a patient with cerebral edema.
- If the patient refuses blood infusions, explain that albumin is a protein found in the blood plasma that will help maintain blood pressure and fluid volume until other conditions can be treated.
- Monitor the infusion site for signs of extravasation or infection.

Patient and Family Education:

- Immediately report chills, nausea, headache, or back pain to the health care provider.
- Report pain or tenderness at the infusion site to the health care provider.

Drugs Similar to Normal Serum Albumin (Albuminar, Plasbumin, Others)

Other blood products are described in Table 42.2 and include whole blood, packed red cells, fresh frozen plasma, cryoprecipitate, and platelet infusions.

42.6 Crystalloids are intravenous solutions that closely resemble the composition of extracellular fluid.

Crystalloids are IV solutions that contain electrolytes and other agents in concentrations that closely mimic the body's extracellular fluid. They are used to replace depleted fluids, and to promote urine output. Crystalloid solutions are capable of quickly diffusing across membranes, leaving the plasma, and entering the interstitial fluid and ICF. Isotonic, hypotonic, and hypertonic solutions are available. Sodium is the most common crystalloid added to solutions, although some crystalloids contain dextrose, a form of glucose. Common crystalloids used in shock include normal saline, lactated Ringer's, Plasmalyte, and hypertonic saline. Selected crystalloids are given in Table 42.3.

Isotonic crystalloids: Infusion of crystalloids will increase the total fluid volume in the body, but the compartment that is most expanded depends on the solute concentration of the fluid administered. Isotonic crystalloids expand the circulating intravascular (plasma) fluid volume, without causing major fluid shifts between compartments. This is because the osmotic pressures of the intravascular and extravascular compartments are equal. Isotonic crystalloids such as normal saline are often used to treat fluid loss due to vomiting, diarrhea, or surgical procedures, especially when blood pressure is low. The isotonic saline solutions may also be used to treat sodium deficiency (hyponatremia) because they contain sodium chloride. Because isotonic crystalloids can rapidly expand circulating blood volume, care must be taken not to cause fluid overload in the patient.

Hypertonic crystalloids: Infusion of hypertonic crystalloids raises the osmolality of the plasma and expands plasma volume by drawing water away from the cells and tissues. These agents may be used to relieve cellular edema, especially cerebral edema. When patients are dehydrated and have hypertonic plasma, hypertonic solutions match the tonicity of the plasma as it is infused, but the dextrose in the IV solution is subsequently metabolized and the solution becomes hypotonic. This hypotonic solution then causes water to shift into the intracellular space, relieving the dehydration within the cells. Overtreatment with hypertonic crystalloids such as 3% normal saline can lead to excessive expansion of the intravascular (plasma) compartment, fluid overload, and HTN.

Hypotonic crystalloids: Hypotonic crystalloid infusions lower the serum osmolality. This causes water to move out of the plasma to the tissues and cells in the intracellular compartment; thus, these solutions are not plasma volume expanders. Hypotonic crystalloids are indicated for patients with hypernatremia and cellular dehydration. Care must be taken not to cause depletion of the intravascular compartment (hypotension) or too much expansion of the intracellular compartment (peripheral edema). Patients who are dehydrated with low blood pressure should be given normal saline; the isotonic saline will expand plasma volume and increase blood pressure while hydrating the patient. Patients who are dehydrated with normal blood pressure should be given a hypotonic solution; this infusion will hydrate cells without expanding plasma volume.

TABLE 42.3 Selected Crystalloid IV Solutions

Drug	Tonicity
normal saline (0.9% NaCl)	Isotonic
hypertonic saline (3% NaCl)	Hypertonic
hypotonic saline (0.45% NaCl)	Hypotonic
lactated Ringer's	Isotonic
plasma-Lyte 148	Isotonic
plasma-Lyte 56	Hypotonic
Dextrose Solutions	
5% dextrose in water (D_5W)	Isotonic*
5% dextrose in normal saline	Hypertonic
5% dextrose in 0.2% saline	Isotonic
5% dextrose in lactated Ringer's	Hypertonic
5% dextrose in plasma-Lyte 56	Hypertonic

*Because dextrose is metabolized quickly, the solution is sometimes considered hypotonic.

PROTOTYPE DRUG 5% Dextrose in water (D_5W)

Classification: Therapeutic: Fluid expander
Pharmacologic: Crystalloid

Therapeutic Effects and Uses: Commonly found in concentrations of 2.5%, 5%, or 10%, dextrose solutions are infused to replace lost water and to enhance renal function. Being a form of glucose, dextrose provides nutritional value: 1 L of 5% dextrose supplies 170 calories. In addition, water is formed during the metabolism of dextrose, adding to the rehydration of the patient. D_5W is also used as a diluent for mixing other medications for IV delivery. Dextrose 50% is indicated for the emergency treatment of insulin hypoglycemia to restore blood glucose levels.

D_5W is isotonic in the container. When infused, however, the dextrose is quickly metabolized in the body, leaving only water, and the solution becomes hypotonic. Water may then move from the plasma to the intracellular spaces, relieving cellular dehydration. Essentially, the infusion of D_5W has the same effect as administration of water. Because this may result in a lower plasma volume, patients needing fluid replacement for hypovolemia should receive lactated Ringer's or normal saline rather than D_5W.

Dextrose is added to other IV solutions, as shown in Table 42.2. It is also available in other concentrations. In all cases, the dextrose is simply added as a source of calories and nutrition.

Mechanism of Action: There are two forms of glucose in nature: L-glucose and D-glucose. Only D-glucose, also called dextrose, can be used by the human body for energy. If insulin is present, glucose (dextrose) enters cells and is converted into adenosine triphosphate (ATP), CO_2, and water.

Pharmacokinetics: Because dextrose and water are natural substances, it is not possible to obtain accurate pharmacokinetic values.

Adverse Effects: Infusion of too much D_5W may cause fluid overload, thus worsening peripheral edema, pulmonary edema, and heart failure. Hyperglycemia is possible, especially in patients with deficient insulin production. Pain may occur at the injection site.

Contraindications/Precautions: Caution must be used when using D_5W in patients with heart failure or who are hyperglycemic. Patients with increased intracranial pressure should not receive hypotonic agents such as D_5W because they may worsen this condition. Dextrose is obtained from corn and patients allergic to this food may be hypersensitive to the drug.

Drug Interactions: There are no significant drug interactions with D_5W. **Herbal/Food:** Unknown.

Pregnancy: Category C.

Treatment of Overdose: Overdose is uncommon, but diuretics may be indicated in cases of fluid overload.

Drugs Similar to 5% Dextrose in Water (D_5W)

Other crystalloids include Ringer's solution and Plasma-Lyte.

Ringer's and Lactated Ringer's: Ringer's solution is named after the pharmacologist Sydney Ringer who created the drug in the mid 1800s. Ringer's solution is an isotonic fluid that contains sodium, chloride, potassium, and calcium ions in concentrations similar to those found in plasma. Lactated Ringer's solution also contains lactate, which serves as a buffer to prevent acidosis. Lactated Ringer's is also available with 5% dextrose. Ringer's solutions are widely administered IV for fluid resuscitation following hemorrhage caused by trauma, surgery, or burns.

Plasma-Lyte: Plasma-Lyte solutions are electrolyte solutions used for fluid resuscitation. Several formulations are available that differ in electrolyte composition and osmolarity. These include Plasma-Lyte-R, Plasma-Lyte-A, Plasma-Lyte-56, and Plasma-Lyte 148.

42.7 Colloids are intravenous solutions containing large molecules that remain in the blood.

Colloids are proteins, starches, or other large molecules that remain in the blood for a long time because they are too large to easily cross the capillary membranes. While circulating, they have the same effect as hypertonic solutions, drawing water molecules from the cells and tissues into the plasma through their ability to increase plasma osmolality and osmotic pressure. These agents are sometimes called plasma volume expanders. Blood product colloids include normal human serum albumin (Section 42.4), plasma protein fraction, and serum globulins. The non-blood product colloids are dextran (40, 70, and high molecular weight) and hetastarch (Hespan). These agents are administered to provide life-sustaining support following massive hemorrhage and to treat shock, as well as for the treatment of burns, acute liver failure, and neonatal hemolytic disease. Selected colloid solutions are given in Table 42.4.

TABLE 42.4 Selected Colloid IV Solutions

Drug	Tonicity
5% albumin	Isotonic
dextran 40 in normal saline	Isotonic
dextran 40 in D_5W	Isotonic
dextran 70 in normal saline	Isotonic
hetastarch 6% in normal saline	Isotonic
plasma protein fraction	Isotonic

PROTOTYPE DRUG Dextran 40 (Gentran 40, Hyskon, 10% LMD, Rheomacrodex)

Classification: **Therapeutic:** Plasma volume expander
Pharmacologic: Colloid

Therapeutic Effects and Uses: Dextran 40 is a synthetic polysaccharide that is too large to pass through capillary walls. It is similar to dextran 70, except dextran 40 has a lower molecular weight. Given as an IV infusion, it has the capability of doubling plasma volume within a few minutes after administration, although its effects last only about 12 hours. Cardiovascular responses include increased blood pressure, increased cardiac output, and improved venous return to the heart. Indications include fluid replacement for patients experiencing hypovolemic shock due to hemorrhage, surgery, or severe burns. When given for acute shock, it is infused as rapidly as possible until blood volume is restored.

Dextran 40 also reduces platelet adhesiveness, and improves blood flow through capillaries by its ability to reduce blood viscosity. These antithrombotic properties have led to its use in preventing deep vein thromboses and postoperative pulmonary emboli. Dextran, however, is less effective than heparin or low molecular weight heparin (LMWH) in preventing thromboembolism (see Chapter 40).

Mechanism of Action: Dextran 40 acts by raising the osmotic pressure of the blood, thereby causing fluid to move from the interstitial spaces of the tissues to the blood. The larger blood volume increases cardiac output, stroke volume, blood pressure, and urinary output. Heart rate and blood viscosity decrease.

Pharmacokinetics:

Route(s)	IV
Absorption	Not absorbed
Distribution	Does not leave the vascular system
Primary metabolism	Unknown
Primary excretion	Renal
Onset of action	Several minutes
Duration of action	12–24 h

Adverse Effects: Vital signs should be monitored continuously during dextran 40 infusions to prevent HTN caused by the plasma volume expansion. Signs of fluid overload include tachycardia, peripheral edema, distended neck veins, dyspnea, or cough. A small percentage of patients are allergic to dextran 40, with urticaria being the most common sign. Anaphylaxis is possible.

Contraindications/Precautions: Dextran 40 is contraindicated in patients with renal failure because fluid overload may result. Adequate fluid intake should be ensured in patients with severe dehydration who receive dextran to prevent renal failure due to high urine viscosity. Other contraindications include severe heart failure and hypervolemic disorders.

Drug Interactions: There are no clinically significant interactions. **Herbal/Food:** Unknown.

Pregnancy: Category C.

Treatment of Overdose: For patients with normal renal function, discontinuing the infusion will reduce adverse effects. Patients with renal impairment may benefit from an osmotic diuretic.

Nursing Considerations:

- Assess the patient's hydration before starting dextran therapy because infusing a severely dehydrated patient can cause renal failure.
- Assess vital signs and observe the patient closely for the first 30 minutes after initiating infusion because this is the period when a hypersensitivity reaction is most likely to occur. Discontinue the infusion if signs of a hypersensitivity reaction occur, such as nausea, epigastric pain, dizziness, swelling of lips and tongue, or hypotension.

NURSING PROCESS APPLICATION

Patients Receiving Fluid Replacement Therapy

Assessment

Prior to administration:

- Obtain a complete health history including allergies, drug history, and possible drug interactions.
- Obtain a complete physical examination.
- Assess for the presence of fluid volume deficit.
- Obtain the following laboratory studies: CBC, serum electrolytes, and renal function (BUN and serum creatinine).

Potential Nursing Diagnoses

- *Risk for Injury*, related to adverse effects of drug therapy
- *Deficient Fluid Volume*
- *Decreased Cardiac Output*, related to low circulatory volume

Planning: Patient Goals and Expected Outcomes

The patient will:

- Immediately report effects such as itching, shortness of breath, flushing, cough, and heart palpitations.
- Exhibit signs of normal fluid volume such as stable blood pressure and adequate urinary output.
- Maintain normal electrolyte levels.
- Demonstrate an understanding of the drug's action by accurately describing drug adverse effects and precautions.

Implementation

Interventions and (Rationales)	Patient and Family Education
• Monitor hemodynamic status every 15 to 60 minutes, including blood pressure, urinary output, and invasive pressure monitoring devices. (Plasma volume expanders cause rapid movement of water into the circulatory system.)	Instruct the patient about: • Reasons for frequently monitoring vital signs and taking other assessments. • Expected outcomes of plasma volume expansion therapy.
• Monitor for hypersensitivity reactions such as urticaria, pruritus, dyspnea, flushing, and anaphylaxis. (These symptoms are used to determine the presence of allergic reactions.)	• Instruct the patient to report itching, shortness of breath, or flushing as symptoms occur.
• Monitor for signs of circulatory overload such as dyspnea, cyanosis, cough, crackles, wheezes, and neck vein distention. (Medication may cause fluid overload quickly.)	• Instruct the patient to report shortness of breath, cough, or heart palpitations as soon as such symptoms occur.
• Monitor for changes in CBC results. (Plasma volume expanders can inhibit coagulation and lower hematocrit and hemoglobin levels. Report reduction of hematocrit below 30% to the prescriber.)	• Instruct the patient to keep appointments for laboratory testing.

Evaluation of Outcome Criteria

Evaluate the effectiveness of drug therapy by confirming that patient goals and expected outcomes have been met (see "Planning").

- Monitor hematocrit before and after infusion initiation because dextran usually lowers hematocrit. Notify the prescriber if hematocrit falls below 30% by volume.
- Monitor central venous pressure (CVP) to estimate status of blood volume and to determine appropriate dosage. Normal CVP is 5 to 10 cm H_2O.
- Observe for signs and symptoms of circulatory overload, such as cough, dyspnea, pulmonary congestion, tachycardia, distended veins in neck, HTN, or headache.
- Before giving dextran, notify the prescriber if the patient is sodium restricted.
- Monitor intake and output including urine specific gravity. If urine specific gravity falls below normal limits, discontinue the therapy and check for dysfunctional renal clearance.
- Assess laboratory tests for possible renal impairment prior to therapy. Report oliguria (scant amount of urine), anuria (no urine output), or lack of improvement in urinary output because dextran usually causes an increase in urinary output. Stop infusion at first sign of renal dysfunction.
- Monitor the infusion site for signs of extravasation or infection.
- High doses are associated with transient prolongation of bleeding time and may interfere with normal blood coagulation; monitor for signs of unusual bleeding.

Patient and Family Education:

- Immediately report signs or symptoms of bleeding, bruising, dark tarry stool, or blood in the urine.
- Immediately report shortness of breath, swelling of feet and ankles, palpitations, or coughing.
- Report pain or tenderness at the infusion site.

Drugs Similar to Dextran 40 (Gentran 40, Hyskon, 10% LMD, Rheomacrodex)

The only solution similar to dextran is hetastarch.

Hetastarch: Hetastarch is a complex mixture of a nonprotein polymer of the starch amylopectin. It is a synthetic colloid with properties similar to 5% albumin, but with an extended duration of action. Hetastarch has a half-life of about 17 days and provides volume expansion for 24 to 36 hours. It is indicated for the treatment and prophylaxis of shock and acute edematous conditions. Hetastarch provides the same physiologic actions as albumin. This drug is pregnancy category C.

Physiology of Electrolytes

42.8 Electrolytes are charged substances that are essential to homeostasis.

Minerals are inorganic substances needed in very small amounts to maintain homeostasis (see Chapter 62). Minerals are held together by ionic bonds and dissociate or ionize when placed in water. The resulting ions have positive or negative charges and are able to conduct electricity, hence the name **electrolyte.** Positively charged electrolytes are called cations; those with a negative charge are anions. Electrolyte levels are measured in units of milliequivalents per liter (mEq/L).

Electrolytes are essential to many body functions, including nerve conduction, membrane permeability, muscle contraction, water balance, and bone growth and remodeling. Levels of electrolytes in body fluids are maintained within very narrow ranges, primarily by the kidneys and GI tract. As electrolytes are lost due to normal excretory functions, they must be replaced by adequate intake, otherwise electrolyte imbalances will result, as shown in Table 42.5. Although imbalances can occur with any ion, sodium,

TABLE 42.5 Electrolyte Imbalances

Ion	Condition	Abnormal Serum Value (mEq/L)	Supportive Treatment*
calcium	Hypercalcemia	Greater than 11	Hypotonic fluid or calcitonin
	Hypocalcemia	Less than 4	Calcium supplements or vitamin D
chloride	Hyperchloremia	Greater than 112	Hypotonic fluid
	Hypochloremia	Less than 95	Hypertonic salt solution
magnesium	Hypermagnesemia	Greater than 4	Hypotonic fluid
	Hypomagnesemia	Less than 0.8	Magnesium supplements
phosphate	Hyperphosphatemia	Greater than 6	Dietary phosphate restriction
	Hypophosphatemia	Less than 1	Phosphate supplements
potassium	Hyperkalemia	Greater than 5	Hypotonic fluid, buffers, or dietary restriction
	Hypokalemia	Less than 3.5	Potassium supplements
sodium	Hypernatremia	Greater than 145	Hypotonic fluid or dietary restriction
	Hyponatremia	Less than 135	Hypertonic salt solution or sodium supplement

*For all electrolyte imbalances, the primary therapeutic goal is to identify and correct the cause of the imbalance.

CONNECTIONS

Lifespan Considerations

Fluid and Electrolytes in the Older Adult

One of the top 10 reasons for hospitalization of Medicare patients is dehydration. These elderly patients may need intravenous (IV) fluids to correct what can be a life-threatening situation. Older adults are more vulnerable to dehydration than the general population for several reasons. As one ages, the thirst mechanism becomes less sensitive. Also, the percentage of water in body weight declines from 70% in younger people to about 60% in seniors. Medications such as diuretics or laxatives can add to fluid and electrolyte depletion. Use of alcohol increases the risk of dehydration as the body uses water to metabolize the alcohol.

Older adults who live alone are considered high risk, especially when they are ill. Dehydration secondary to the flu or stomach virus, with diarrhea and vomiting, can necessitate use of IV fluids. Signs of dehydration, such as confusion and disorientation, can mimic senile dementia or Alzheimer's. Restoration of fluid and electrolyte balance is critical for the older adult.

potassium, and calcium are of greatest importance. The role of calcium in bone homeostasis is presented in Chapter 75.

When an electrolyte imbalance is identified, it is a sign of an underlying medical condition that needs attention. Imbalances are associated with a wide variety of acute and chronic disorders, with renal impairment being the most common cause. In some cases, drug therapy itself can cause the electrolyte imbalance. A classic example is the diuretic furosemide (Lasix), which can cause serious potassium depletion. In all cases, the therapeutic goal is to quickly correct the electrolyte imbalance while the underlying condition is being diagnosed and treated. Treatments for electrolyte imbalances depend upon the severity of the problem and range from simple changes in dietary intake to rapid electrolyte infusions. In acute cases, serum electrolyte levels must be carefully monitored to prevent imbalances in the opposite direction; levels can change rapidly from hypoconcentrations to hyperconcentrations.

Pharmacotherapy of Electrolyte Imbalances

42.9 Sodium balance is closely associated with water balance.

Sodium is the major electrolyte in extracellular fluid. Due to its central roles in neuromuscular physiology, acid–base balance, and overall fluid distribution, sodium imbalances can have serious consequences. Although definite sodium monitors or sensors have yet to be discovered in the body, the regulation of sodium balance is well understood. The normal range of serum sodium is 136 to 145 mEq/L of plasma.

Sodium balance and water balance are intimately connected. As sodium levels increase in a body fluid, solute particles accumulate, and osmolality increases. Water will move toward this area of relatively high osmolality. In simplest terms, water travels toward or with sodium. The physiological consequences of this relationship cannot be overstated: As the sodium and water content of plasma increases, so does blood volume and blood pressure. Thus, sodium movement provides an important link between water retention, blood volume, and blood pressure.

In healthy individuals, sodium intake is equal to sodium output, which is regulated by the kidneys. High levels of aldosterone secreted by the adrenal cortex promote sodium and water retention by the kidneys, as well as potassium excretion. Inhibition of aldosterone promotes sodium and water excretion. When a patient ingests high amounts of sodium, aldosterone secretion decreases, thus sending the excess sodium to the urine. This relationship is illustrated in Figure 42.2.

Hypernatremia: Sodium excess, or **hypernatremia,** occurs when the serum sodium level rises above 145 mEq/L. The most common cause of hypernatremia is decreased sodium excretion due to kidney pathology. Hypernatremia may also be

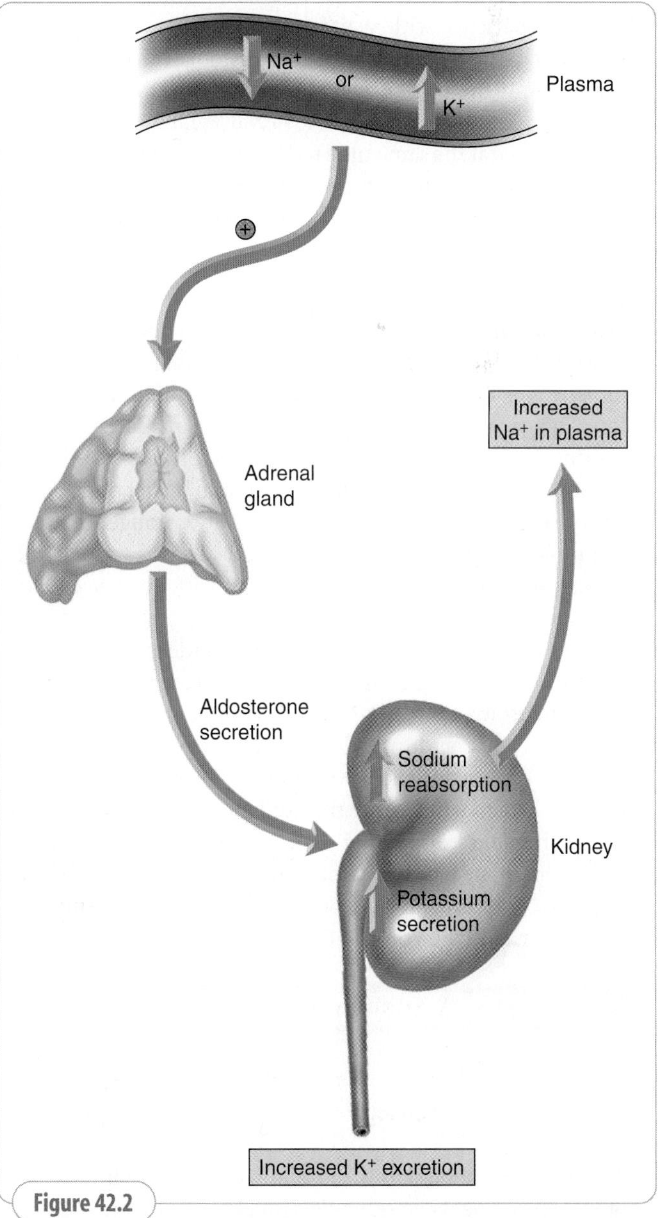

Figure 42.2

Renal regulation of sodium and potassium balance.

caused by excessive intake of sodium, either through dietary consumption or by overtreatment with IV fluids containing sodium chloride or sodium bicarbonate. Overconsumption of table salt (NaCl) or processed foods with high sodium content will quickly exceed the daily amount needed by the body. Patients who drink too little water can develop hypernatremia due to hypertonic plasma. Another cause of hypernatremia is high net water losses, such as that occurring from watery diarrhea, fever, or burns. High doses of glucocorticoids or estrogens also promote sodium retention.

A high serum sodium level increases the osmolality of the plasma, making the intravascular space hypertonic and drawing fluid from interstitial spaces and cells, thus causing cellular dehydration. Ordinarily, a small increase in serum sodium will trigger thirst. Other manifestations of hypernatremia include fatigue, weakness, muscle twitching, convulsions, altered mental status, and a decreased level of consciousness. For minor hypernatremia, a low-salt diet combined with adequate water intake may be effective in returning serum sodium to normal levels. In patients with acute hypernatremia, however, the treatment goal is to rapidly return the osmolality of the plasma to normal. If the patient is hypovolemic, infusing hypotonic fluids such as 5% dextrose or 0.45% NaCl will increase plasma volume, while at the same time reducing osmolality by diluting the plasma. For the patient who is hypervolemic, diuretics may be used to remove sodium and excess water from the body.

Hyponatremia: Hyponatremia is the most common electrolyte abnormality in hospitalized patients and is defined as a serum sodium level less than 135 mEq/L. Hyponatremia may occur through excessive dilution of the plasma caused by administration of hypotonic IV solutions or by high ADH secretion. Hyponatremia may also result from increased sodium loss due to disorders of the skin, GI tract, or kidneys. Significant loss of sodium by the skin may occur in burn patients, and in those experiencing excessive sweating or prolonged fever. GI sodium losses may occur from vomiting, diarrhea, or GI suctioning, and renal sodium loss may occur with diuretic use and in certain advanced kidney disorders.

Early symptoms of hyponatremia include nausea, vomiting, anorexia, and abdominal cramping. Later signs include altered neurologic function such as confusion, lethargy, convulsions, coma, and muscle twitching or tremors. Hyponatremia caused by excessive dilution is treated with loop diuretics, which will remove the fluid overload that caused the hyponatremia (see Chapter 35). Hyponatremia caused by sodium loss may be treated with the administration of oral or parenteral sodium chloride, or with IV fluids containing salt, such as normal saline or lactated Ringer's solution.

PROTOTYPE DRUG Sodium chloride (NaCl)

Classification: **Therapeutic:** Agent for hyponatremia
Pharmacologic: Electrolyte, sodium supplement

Therapeutic Effects and Uses: Sodium chloride is administered for hyponatremia when serum levels fall below 130 mEq/L. The drug is available in several concentrations; the decision on which NaCl concentration to administer is driven by the severity of the sodium deficiency. Normal saline consists of 0.9% NaCl, and is used to treat mild hyponatremia. When serum sodium falls below 115 mEq/L, a highly concentrated 3% NaCl solution may be infused. Other concentrations include 0.45% and 0.22%, and both hypotonic and isotonic solutions are available. For less severe hyponatremia, 1 g tablets are available.

Ophthalmic solutions of NaCl may be used to treat corneal edema, and an OTC nasal spray is available to relieve dry, inflamed nasal membranes. In conjunction with oxytocin, 20% NaCl may be used as an abortifacient late in pregnancy when instilled into the amniotic sac.

Mechanism of Action: Sodium chloride is a replacement solution for lost sodium.

Pharmacokinetics: Because sodium ions form natural electrolytes, it is not possible to obtain accurate pharmacokinetic values. The sodium ions in the drug are widely distributed and excreted by the kidneys in the same manner as endogenous sodium ions.

Adverse Effects: Patients receiving NaCl infusions must be monitored frequently to avoid symptoms of hypernatremia, which include lethargy, confusion, muscle tremor or rigidity, hypotension, and restlessness. Because some of these symptoms are also common to hyponatremia, periodic laboratory assessments must be taken to be certain that sodium values are moving toward the normal range. When infusing 3% NaCl solutions, the nurse should continuously check for signs of pulmonary edema.

Contraindications/Precautions: This drug should not be administered to patients with hypernatremia, congestive heart failure, or impaired renal function.

Drug Interactions: There are no clinically significant drug interactions. **Herbal/Food:** Unknown.

Pregnancy: Category C.

Treatment of Overdose: There is no specific treatment for overdose. If excess fluid accumulation has occurred, diuretics may be administered to remove excess sodium ion and water to reduce pulmonary or peripheral edema.

CONNECTIONS

To the Community

Salt Replacements and Exercise

Athletes are at risk for fluid and electrolyte imbalance when exercising in hot climates. Drinking 400 to 600 mL of fluid 2 hours prior to exertion can lessen the effects of fluid loss. During exercise, the athlete should drink small amounts (150 to 300 mL) every 15 to 20 minutes. If the exercise session is 90 minutes or less, water alone is adequate; if the session exceeds this time, the athlete should consume commercially prepared electrolyte solutions for safety, endurance, and performance. The athlete should eat a balanced diet and may need to add supplemental salt to ensure balance of body sodium.

Drugs Similar to Sodium Chloride (NaCl)

There is no other drug similar to sodium chloride.

42.10 Potassium imbalances must be quickly corrected to prevent serious cardiac consequences.

Potassium is the most abundant intracellular cation; 98% of the potassium present in the body is found inside cells, with the majority found in skeletal muscle. Potassium serves critical roles in muscular contraction and the conduction of nerve impulses.

To prevent imbalances, adequate dietary intake of potassium must be carefully balanced to potassium excretion. Patients with normal diets consume plenty of potassium for bodily functions because the mineral is abundant in fruits, vegetables, and meats.

Insulin is a key hormone for the regulation of potassium homeostasis. The uptake of potassium ion into cells is mediated by insulin. As serum potassium levels rise, the pancreas secretes additional insulin, which causes the ion to move out of the plasma and into cells, thus preventing hyperkalemia. In a typical feedback loop, as serum potassium levels fall, insulin secretion is diminished.

Acid–base imbalances may also affect potassium homeostasis. As the blood becomes acidic, the body attempts to raise plasma pH by pumping hydrogen ions (H^+) into cells. To maintain electrical neutrality, each H^+ entering the cell is exchanged for a K^+ leaving the cell. This can raise the serum potassium level, resulting in hyperkalemia. This is sometimes called a false hyperkalemia because the total body potassium is not actually increased; it has just shifted from intracellular to extracellular spaces.

Potassium ion is freely filtered at the glomerulus, but is entirely reabsorbed as it travels along the kidney tubule. In the distal tubule, however, potassium is secreted back into the renal tubule and exits in the urine. Like sodium, potassium excretion is influenced by the actions of aldosterone on the kidney. In fact, the renal excretion of sodium and potassium ions is closely linked. For every sodium ion that is reabsorbed, one potassium ion is secreted into the renal tubules.

Potassium levels must be maintained within narrow limits. Both hyper- and hypokalemia are associated with fatal dysrhythmias and serious neuromuscular disorders. Because over 98% of potassium is intracellular, serum potassium may not be an accurate reflection of total body potassium. Normal adult values for serum potassium range from 3.5 to 5 mEq/L.

Hyperkalemia: **Hyperkalemia** occurs when the serum potassium level rises above 5 mEq/L. This condition may be caused by excessive consumption of potassium-rich foods or dietary supplements, particularly when patients are taking potassium-sparing diuretics such as spironolactone (see Chapter 35). In fact, overtreatment with potassium supplements is the most common cause of hyperkalemia. Excess potassium may also accumulate when renal excretion is diminished due to kidney pathology. The most serious consequences of hyperkalemia are related to cardiac function: dysrhythmias and heart block. Other symptoms are muscle twitching, fatigue, paresthesias, dyspnea, cramping, and diarrhea. Hyperkalemia is much less common than hypokalemia.

In mild cases of hyperkalemia, potassium levels may be returned to normal by restricting primary dietary sources of potassium such as bananas, citrus and dried fruits, peanut butter, broccoli, and green leafy vegetables. All potassium supplements and the use of salt substitutes containing potassium should be discontinued. If the patient is taking a potassium-sparing diuretic, the dose must be lowered, or a thiazide or loop diuretic substituted.

Several options are available for patients with severe hyperkalemia. Administration of the diuretic furosemide (Lasix) can significantly increase the urinary excretion of potassium within 5 to 15 minutes. Administering glucose or dextrose concurrently with insulin temporarily lowers serum potassium levels by causing potassium to leave the extracellular fluid and enter cells. In all patients who are symptomatic, calcium gluconate or calcium chloride is administered to prevent or treat potassium-induced cardiotoxicity. Sodium bicarbonate is sometimes infused to correct any acidosis that may be concurrent with the hyperkalemia.

Excess potassium may also be eliminated from the body by giving polystyrene sulfonate (Kayexalate) orally or rectally. This agent, which is not absorbed, exchanges sodium ion for potassium ion as it travels through the intestine. The onset of action is 1 hour, and the dose may be repeated every 4 hours as needed. The drug is given concurrently with a laxative such as sorbitol to promote rapid evacuation of the potassium.

Hypokalemia: **Hypokalemia** is one of the most common electrolyte imbalances and occurs when the serum potassium level falls below 3.5 mEq/L. The most frequent cause of hypokalemia is pharmacotherapy with loop and thiazide diuretics. In addition, strenuous muscular activity and severe vomiting or diarrhea can lead to significant potassium loss. Because the body does not have large stores of potassium, adequate daily dietary intake is necessary. Neurons and muscle fibers are most sensitive to potassium loss, and muscle weakness, lethargy, anorexia, dysrhythmias, and cardiac arrest are possible consequences.

Mild hypokalemia is treated by increasing the dietary intake of potassium-rich foods. The foods highest in potassium content include dried fruit, nuts, molasses, avocados, lima beans, and bran cereals. If increasing dietary intake is not possible, a large number of potassium products are available for oral supplementation. The most common supplements are the chloride salts, because these supply both potassium and chloride that are lost during diuretic therapy. Liquid preparations are very effective, although many must be diluted with water or fruit juices prior to administration. Extended release (K-Dur 20, Slow-K, Micro-K) and powders (Klor-Con) are also available.

Severe hypokalemia may require parenteral potassium supplements. Caution must always be used when using IV potassium because rapid administration of the drug can be fatal, especially for patients with significant renal impairment. Cardiac function should be closely monitored during IV potassium therapy.

PROTOTYPE DRUG Potassium chloride (KCl)

Classification: **Therapeutic:** Agent for hypokalemia
Pharmacologic: Electrolyte, potassium supplement

Therapeutic Effects and Uses: Potassium chloride is a drug of choice for preventing or treating hypokalemia because potassium and chloride depletion usually occur concurrently. It is also used to treat mild forms of alkalosis. Oral formulations of potassium chloride include tablets, powders, and liquids, usually heavily flavored due to its unpleasant taste. Because potassium supplements can cause peptic ulcers, the drug should be diluted with plenty of water. When given IV, potassium must be administered slowly, since bolus injections can overload the heart and cause cardiac arrest. Because pharmacotherapy with loop or thiazide diuretics is the most common cause of potassium depletion, patients taking these drugs are usually prescribed PO potassium supplements to prevent hypokalemia.

Mechanism of Action: Potassium chloride is a replacement solution for lost potassium.

Pharmacokinetics: Because potassium chloride is a natural electrolyte, it is not possible to obtain accurate pharmacokinetic values. The potassium ions in the drug are widely distributed and excreted by the kidneys in the same manner as endogenous potassium ions.

Adverse Effects: Nausea, vomiting, diarrhea, and abdominal pain are common, because potassium chloride irritates the GI mucosa. The drug may be taken with meals or antacids to lessen gastric distress. The most serious adverse effects of potassium chloride are related to the possible accumulation of excess potassium. Hyperkalemia may occur if the patient takes potassium supplements concurrently with potassium-sparing diuretics. Because the kidneys perform over 90% of the body's potassium excretion, reduced renal function can rapidly lead to hyperkalemia, particularly in patients taking potassium supplements.

Contraindications/Precautions: Potassium chloride is contraindicated in patients with hyperkalemia, systemic acidosis, severe dehydration, extensive tissue breakdown as in severe burns, or adrenal insufficiency. Oral potassium supplements are contraindicated in any condition for which transit through the GI tract is delayed because prolonged contact may damage the GI mucosa. The drug should be used with extreme caution in patients with chronic or acute renal failure because the drug may accumulate to high levels.

Drug Interactions: Potassium supplements should not be administered to patients who are taking potassium-sparing diuretics because hyperkalemia may result. Angiotensin-converting enzyme (ACE) inhibitors prevent aldosterone secretion and cause potassium retention, thus increasing the risk for hyperkalemia if administered with potassium supplements. Drugs that slow GI transit time, such as anticholinergics, may increase the GI toxicity of potassium supplements. **Herbal/Food:** Unknown.

Pregnancy: Category C.

Treatment of Overdose: Potassium-sparing diuretics and all foods and medications containing potassium should be withheld. Treatment includes IV administration of 10% dextrose solution containing 10 to 20 units of crystalline insulin. Sodium bicarbonate may be infused to correct acidosis. Polystyrene sulfonate may be administered to enhance potassium elimination.

Nursing Considerations:

- Monitor serial serum potassium levels before and during therapy assessing for signs of potassium imbalance and evaluating drug effectiveness.
- Administer oral potassium chloride with the patient sitting upright or standing, because taking this drug in a recumbent position may induce esophagitis.
- Follow directions for diluting various liquid forms of KCl exactly as provided. The usual directions include diluting each 20 mEq potassium in at least 90 mL water or juice and allowing to completely dissolve before administration.
- Dilute liquid forms as directed before administering through a nasogastric tube.
- Never give as an IV push or in concentrated amounts by any route. Infuse at a rate not to exceed 10 mEq/h. Adult patients with severe potassium depletion may be able to tolerate 20 mEq/h. Rapid infusions may cause fatal hyperkalemia.
- Prepare IV potassium chloride by adding desired amount to 100 to 1,000 mL IV solution (compatible with all standard solutions). Usual maximum is 80 mEq/1,000 mL. However, 40 mEq/L is preferred to lessen vein irritation. After adding KCl, invert bag or bottle several times to ensure even distribution. Never add KCl to an existing hanging IV fluid bag.
- Take extreme care to prevent extravasation and infiltration at the IV site. If this occurs, discontinue the infusion immediately, and select another site.
- Assess intake and output ratio and pattern in patients receiving KCl infusions. If oliguria occurs, stop infusion promptly and notify the prescriber.

CONNECTIONS

Patient Safety

Control of Concentrated Electrolyte Solutions

While in the break room, two nurses are discussing problems related to the workflow on a medical surgical unit. Both nurses agree that it would be quicker and faster if the hospital pharmacy would keep a stock of potassium injectable vials on the nursing unit. Then, the nurses could mix their own IV solutions as needed without waiting for the pharmacist. Do you think this is a good idea? Why or why not?

See Answers to Patient Safety Questions in Appendix A.

- Monitor for and report signs of GI ulceration such as epigastric pain, esophageal discomfort, or hematemesis.
- Monitor the patient's heart rate and rhythm with a cardiac monitor while receiving parenteral potassium because irregular rhythm can be an early indication of hyperkalemia.
- Assess for symptoms of hyperkalemia such as diarrhea, nausea, vomiting, dysrhythmias, muscle weakness, and fatigue.
- Understand that the risk of hyperkalemia with potassium supplements increases in older adults with impaired renal function, when dietary intake of potassium suddenly increases, and when kidney function is significantly compromised.
- Teach the patient that the tablet carcass may appear in the stool. The sustained release tablet (e.g., Slow-K) utilizes a wax matrix as a carrier for KCl crystals that passes through the digestive system.
- Administer oral potassium chloride with the patient sitting upright or standing, because taking this drug in a recumbent position may induce esophagitis.

Patient and Family Education:

- Swallow the tablet with a large glass of water or fruit juice (if allowed). Do not crush or chew potassium tablets, although the pills may be large and hard to swallow. Do not suck on the tablet because this could cause ulcerations in the mouth.
- Unless otherwise instructed by the health care provider, avoid foods and drinks high in potassium because this may lead to excessive potassium levels.
- Avoid licorice because large amounts can cause potassium depletion and sodium retention.
- Avoid salt substitutes unless specifically ordered by the health care provider because these contain potassium and other electrolytes.
- Take laxatives only as directed by the health care provider because chronic use can cause diarrhea-induced potassium loss.
- Report persistent vomiting to the health care provider because losses of potassium can occur.
- Report weakness, fatigue, polyuria, or polydipsia to the health care provider because these may indicate potassium deficit.
- Do not unwrap foil containing powders and tablets until ready for use.

Drugs Similar to Potassium Chloride (KCl)

Other potassium salts include acetate, bicarbonate, citrate, and gluconate. Potassium acetate is used as an IV alternative to potassium chloride. Potassium bicarbonate supplies bicarbonate ion, which is alkaline and may be useful in treating acidosis. Potassium citrate makes the urine less acidic and is primarily used to reduce the formation of kidney stones. Potassium gluconate is commonly available in tablet form and dissociates to potassium ion and gluconate ion, a form of glucose.

42.11 Magnesium imbalances significantly affect cardiovascular and neuromuscular function.

Magnesium is the second most abundant intracellular cation and, like potassium, it is essential for proper neuromuscular function. Magnesium also serves a metabolic role in activating certain enzymes in the breakdown of carbohydrates and proteins; it is a cofactor in over 300 biochemical reactions. Patients with disorders of magnesium homeostasis generally present with cardiovascular and neuromuscular symptoms. Because the majority of magnesium is found in bone, serum magnesium levels are not accurate indicators of total body magnesium.

Magnesium levels are primarily controlled by the kidney. The ion is freely filtered and reabsorbed in the loop of Henle and loop diuretics such as furosemide can cause significant magnesium loss. Renal impairment is a major cause of magnesium imbalances. Magnesium is absorbed by the small intestine and small amounts are secreted in intestinal fluid.

Hypomagnesemia: Because it produces few symptoms until serum levels fall below 1 mEq/L, hypomagnesemia is sometimes called the most common undiagnosed electrolyte abnormality. Although the overall incidence for magnesium deficiency is 6% to 12%, the majority of critically ill patients present with this condition. Renal causes of hypomagnesemia include kidney failure and therapy with loop diuretics. GI causes include malabsorption disorders and loss of significant amounts of body fluids due to diarrhea, chronic laxative abuse, or nasogastric suctioning. Hypomagnesemia may also present in alcoholics and in those receiving prolonged parenteral feeding with magnesium-free solutions. Patients may experience general weakness, dysrhythmias, HTN, loss of deep tendon reflexes, and respiratory depression—signs and symptoms that are sometimes mistaken for hypokalemia. Additional signs include muscle twitches, tetany, or seizures.

Magnesium supplements are available by both PO and parenteral routes. Oral formulations are used for minor hypomagnesemia. Because intramuscular (IM) preparations produce significant pain at the injection site, severe cases of hypomagnesemia are normally treated using the IV route. Pharmacotherapy with magnesium sulfate can quickly reverse symptoms of hypomagnesemia. Magnesium sulfate is a central nervous system (CNS) depressant and is sometimes given to prevent or terminate seizures associated with eclampsia.

Hypermagnesemia: Advanced renal failure is the only major cause of hypermagnesemia, although overtreatment with magnesium supplements may also lead to excessive serum magnesium levels. Clinical signs include CNS depression, respiratory depression, hypotension, dysrhythmias, bradycardia, complete heart block, and coma. Infusions of calcium salts will immediately reverse the neuromuscular and cardiovascular signs. If the magnesium elevation is minor, treatment with furosemide to increase urinary excretion may be sufficient to reverse the hypermagnesemia.

PROTOTYPE DRUG Magnesium sulfate ($MgSO_4$)

Classification: **Therapeutic:** Agent for hypomagnesemia
Pharmacologic: Electrolyte, magnesium supplement

Therapeutic Effects and Uses: Severe hypomagnesemia can be rapidly reversed by the administration of IM or IV magnesium sulfate. Parenteral formulations include 4%, 8%, 12.5%, and 50% solutions. After administration, magnesium sulfate is distributed throughout the body, and therapeutic effects are observed within 30 to 60 minutes. Plasma magnesium levels should be monitored frequently during therapy.

Oral forms of magnesium sulfate are used as cathartics, when complete evacuation of the colon is desired. Its action as a CNS depressant has led to its occasional use as an anticonvulsant in patients with preeclampsia or eclampsia.

Mechanism of Action: Magnesium sulfate is a replacement solution for lost magnesium.

MyNursingKit | Understanding Acid–Base Balance

Pharmacokinetics:

Route(s)	PO, IM, IV
Absorption	Not absorbed
Distribution	Widely distributed; crosses the placenta; secreted in breast milk
Primary metabolism	Not metabolized
Primary excretion	Renal
Onset of action	PO: 1–2 h; IM: 1 h
Duration of action	PO: 3–4 h; IV: 30 minutes; half-life: unknown

Adverse Effects: Patients receiving IV infusions of magnesium sulfate require careful observation to prevent toxicity. Early signs of magnesium overdose include flushing of the skin, sedation, confusion, intense thirst, and muscle weakness. Extreme levels cause neuromuscular blockade with resultant respiratory paralysis, heart block, and circulatory collapse. Because of these potentially fatal adverse effects, the use of magnesium sulfate is restricted to patients with severe magnesium deficiency. Mild to moderate hypomagnesemia is treated with oral forms of magnesium such as magnesium gluconate or magnesium hydroxide. Oral magnesium sulfate, also known as Epsom salts, is a saline-type laxative and will cause diarrhea in patients. This may be a dose-limiting adverse effect for some patients.

MyNursingKit | Acid–Base Balance Animation

Contraindications/Precautions: Magnesium is contraindicated in patients with serious cardiac disease. Oral administration is contraindicated in those with undiagnosed abdominal pain, intestinal obstruction, or fecal impaction. The drug should be used cautiously in patients with renal impairment because the drug may rapidly rise to toxic levels.

Drug Interactions: Use with neuromuscular blockers may increase respiratory depression and apnea. Because magnesium sulfate has CNS depression effects, patients receiving other CNS depressants may experience increased sedation. **Herbal/Food:** Magnesium salts may decrease the absorption of certain anti-infectives such as tetracycline.

Pregnancy: Category A.

Treatment of Overdose: Serious respiratory and cardiac suppression may result from overdose. Calcium gluconate or gluceptate may be administered IV as an antidote.

Nursing Responsibilities:

- Assess vital signs every 10 to 15 minutes when the drug is given IV.
- Monitor serum magnesium levels in patients receiving the drug parenterally (normal: 1.8 to 3 mEq/L). Monitor serum calcium and phosphorus levels.
- Assess for early indicators of magnesium toxicity (hypermagnesemia), which include cathartic effect, profound thirst, feeling of warmth, nausea, sedation, confusion, depressed deep tendon reflexes, and muscle weakness. Cardiac arrest may occur at levels in excess of 25 mEq/L.
- Monitor the respiratory rate closely and immediately notify the prescriber if below 12 beats/minute.
- Test the patellar reflex before each repeated parenteral dose. Depression or absence of reflexes can indicate early magnesium intoxication.
- Assess baseline and periodic urinary output, especially in patients with impaired kidney function. Discontinue therapy if urinary output is less than 100 mL during the 4 hours preceding each dose.
- Observe newborns of mothers who received parenteral magnesium sulfate within a few hours of delivery for signs of toxicity such as respiratory and neuromuscular depression.
- Observe patients with hypomagnesemia for signs of improvement such as reduced irritability, tremors, twitching, choreiform movements, tetany, muscle cramps, tachycardia, HTN, or psychotic behavior.
- Keep calcium gluconate readily available in case magnesium sulfate toxicity occurs.

Patient and Family Education:

- Consume plenty of water (1 to 2 L/day) when oral drug is taken to prevent net loss of body water unless otherwise directed by health care provider.
- To prevent future hypomagnesemia, consume rich sources of dietary magnesium such as whole-grain cereals, legumes, nuts, meats, seafood, milk, most green leafy vegetables, and bananas.

Drugs Similar to Magnesium Sulfate ($MgSO_4$)

Several oral magnesium salts may be used for supplementation, but have additional uses. Magnesium citrate (citrate of magnesia) and magnesium hydroxide (milk of magnesia) are classified as laxatives or cathartics. Magnesium oxide (Mag-Ox) is an antacid, and magnesium salicylate (Doan's Pills) is used as an analgesic.

PharmFACT

Although the recommended dietary allowance for magnesium is 420 mg/day in men and 320 mg/day in women, certain patients need higher levels to maintain health. These include those with Crohn's disease, poorly controlled diabetes, pregnant or lactating women, older adults, and alcoholic patients. *Source:* National Institutes of Health Office of Dietary Supplements, n.d.

Pharmacotherapy of Acid–Base Imbalances

42.12 The pH of body fluids must be maintained between very narrow limits.

The degree of acidity or alkalinity of a solution is measured by its pH. A pH of 7.0 is defined as neutral, above 7.0 as basic or alkaline, and below 7.0 as acidic. To maintain homeostasis, the pH of plasma and most body fluids must be kept within the narrow range of 7.35 to 7.45 because nearly all proteins and enzymes in the body function optimally within this range. A few enzymes, most notably those in the digestive tract, require pH values outside the 7.35 to 7.45 range to function properly.

The body generates significant amounts of acids during normal metabolic processes. Without effective means of neutralizing these metabolic acids, the overall pH of body fluids would quickly fall below the normal range. **Buffers** are chemicals that help maintain normal body pH by neutralizing strong acids and bases. The two primary buffers in the body are bicarbonate ions and phosphate ions.

The body uses two mechanisms to remove acid. The acidic carbon dioxide (CO_2) produced during body metabolism is efficiently removed by the lungs during exhalation. The kidneys remove excess acid in the form of hydrogen ion (H^+) by excreting it in the urine. If retained in the body, CO_2 and/or H^+ will lower body pH. Normal acid–base balance is maintained by the lungs and kidneys. Impairment of these organs commonly leads to change in pH.

Acidosis (excess acid) and alkalosis (excess base) are not diseases, but are symptoms of an underlying medical disorder. Acidic drugs and basic drugs are administered to rapidly correct pH imbalances in body fluids, supporting the patient's vital functions while the underlying disease is being treated. The correction of acid–base imbalance is illustrated in Figure 42.3.

42.13 The pharmacotherapy of acidosis includes the administration of alkaline agents.

Acidosis occurs when the pH of the plasma falls below 7.35, which is confirmed by measuring arterial pH, partial pressure of carbon dioxide (P_{CO_2}), and plasma bicarbonate levels. For proper pharmacotherapy, the diagnosis must differentiate between respiratory etiology and metabolic (renal) etiology. Occasionally, the cause has mixed respiratory and metabolic components.

The most profound symptoms of acidosis affect the CNS, and include lethargy, confusion, and CNS depression leading to coma. A deep, rapid respiration rate indicates an attempt by the lungs to rid the body of excess acid. Common causes of acidosis are shown in Table 42.6.

In patients with acidosis, the therapeutic goal is to quickly reverse the adverse effects caused by excess acids in the blood. Mild acidosis may be treated with oral bicarbonate or citrate salts, or other basic substances. For acute acidosis the treatment of choice is to administer infusions of sodium bicarbonate. Bicarbonate ion is a base that can quickly neutralize acids in the blood and other body fluids. The patient must be carefully monitored during infusions because this drug can "overcorrect" the acidosis, causing blood pH to turn alkaline. Sodium citrate, sodium lactate, and sodium acetate are alternative alkaline agents that may be used in place of bicarbonate.

Alkalinizing agents are also used to aid in the renal excretion of toxic substances through a phenomenon called **ion trapping.**

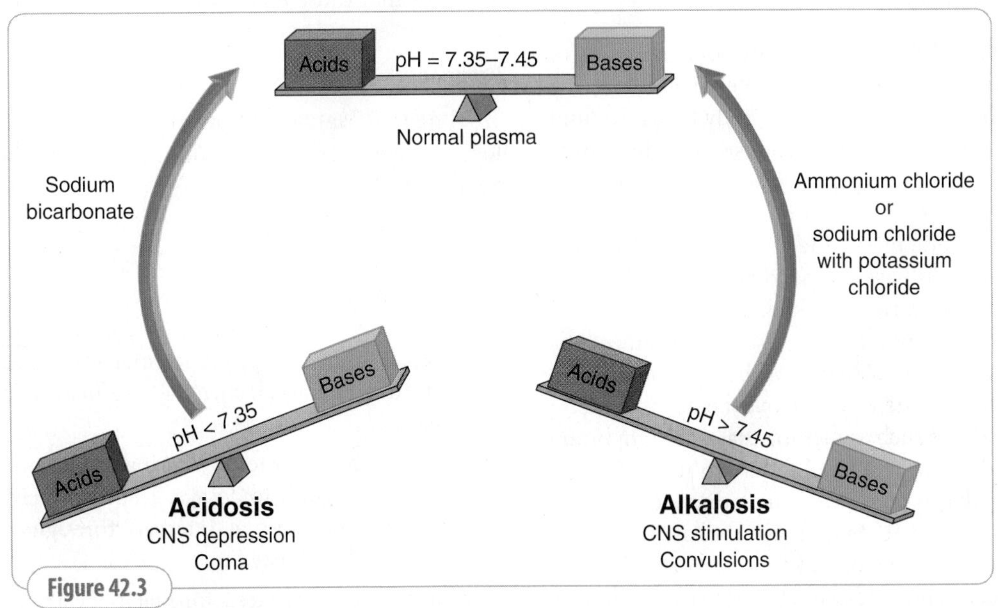

Figure 42.3

Acid–base imbalances.

TABLE 42.6 Causes of Alkalosis and Acidosis

Acidosis	Alkalosis
Respiratory Origins of Acidosis	**Respiratory Origin of Alkalosis**
Hypoventilation or shallow breathing	Hyperventilation due to asthma, anxiety, or high altitude
Airway constriction	
Damage to respiratory center in medulla	
Metabolic Origins of Acidosis	**Metabolic Origins of Alkalosis**
Severe diarrhea	Constipation for prolonged periods
Kidney failure	Ingestion of excess sodium bicarbonate
Diabetes mellitus	Diuretics that cause potassium depletion
Excess alcohol ingestion	Severe vomiting
Starvation	

Whenever a large pH gradient exists across a membrane, drug molecules will accumulate on the side where the opportunity for ionization is greatest. Recall from Chapter 4 that acids ionize in a basic environment; bases ionize in acidic solutions. The infusion of an alkalinizing agent will create an alkaline filtrate in the kidney tubule, a perfect environment for ionization of an acidic drug like aspirin. Rather than being absorbed back into the body, the ionized aspirin remains "trapped" in the filtrate and is excreted in the urine. Thus, through ion trapping, the alkalinizing agent was able to move aspirin from the blood to the urine.

PROTOTYPE DRUG Sodium bicarbonate

Classification: **Therapeutic:** Agent to treat acidosis or bicarbonate deficiency
Pharmacologic: Electrolyte, sodium, and bicarbonate supplement

Therapeutic Effects and Uses: Sodium bicarbonate is a drug of choice for correcting metabolic acidosis. After dissociation, the bicarbonate ion directly raises the pH of body fluids. Sodium bicarbonate may be given PO, if mild acidosis, or IV in cases of acute disease. IV concentrations range from 4.2% to 8.4%. Although sodium bicarbonate also neutralizes gastric acid, it is rarely used to treat peptic ulcers due to its tendency to cause uncomfortable gastric distension. The PO form of sodium bicarbonate is commonly known as baking soda.

Sodium bicarbonate may also be used to alkalinize the urine to speed the excretion of acidic medications such as aspirin and phenobarbital, and as adjunctive therapy for certain chemotherapeutic drugs such as methotrexate. Sodium bicarbonate is also used in chronic renal failure to neutralize the metabolic acidosis that occurs when the kidneys cannot excrete hydrogen ion. When IV sodium bicarbonate is given, it causes the urine to become more alkaline. Less acid is reabsorbed, so more acid and acidic medicine is excreted. This process is known as ion trapping.

Mechanism of Action: The bicarbonate ion in sodium bicarbonate buffers excess acid (H^+) to raise the pH of body fluids.

Pharmacokinetics:

Route(s)	IV, PO
Absorption	Rapidly absorbed
Distribution	Widely distributed in body fluids
Primary metabolism	Not metabolized
Primary excretion	Renal
Onset of action	PO: 15 minutes; IV: immediate
Duration of action	PO: 1–3 h; IV: 8–10 minutes

Adverse Effects: Most of the adverse effects of sodium bicarbonate therapy are the result of metabolic alkalosis created by receiving too much bicarbonate ion. Symptoms may include confusion, irritability, slow respiration rate, and vomiting. Discontinuing the sodium bicarbonate infusion often reverses these symptoms; however, potassium chloride or ammonium chloride may be administered to reverse acute alkalosis. During sodium bicarbonate infusions, serum electrolytes should be carefully monitored because sodium levels may lead to hypernatremia and fluid retention. In addition, high levels of bicarbonate ion passing through the kidney tubules increases potassium secretion that could lead to hypokalemia.

Contraindications/Precautions: Patients who are vomiting, have severe diarrhea, or have continuous GI suctioning will lose acid and chloride and may be in a state of metabolic alkalosis; therefore, they should not receive sodium bicarbonate because it may worsen alkalosis. Due to the sodium content of this drug, it should be used cautiously in patients with cardiac disease, HTN, or renal impairment.

Drug Interactions: Sodium bicarbonate may decrease the absorption of ketoconazole, and may decrease elimination of dextroamphetamine, ephedrine, pseudoephedrine, and quinidine. The elimination of lithium, salicylates, and tetracyclines may be increased. **Herbal/Food:** Chronic use with milk or calcium supplements may cause milk-alkali syndrome, a condition characterized by serious hypercalcemia and possible kidney failure.

Pregnancy: Category C.

Treatment of Overdose: Overdose results in metabolic alkalosis, which is treated by administering acidic agents (see Section 42.10).

Nursing Responsibilities:

- Long-term use of oral sodium bicarbonate with milk or calcium can cause milk-alkali syndrome with symptoms such as nausea, vomiting, anorexia, headache, mental confusion, hypercalcemia, hypophosphatemia, soft tissue calcification, renal and ureteral calculi, renal insufficiency, and metabolic alkalosis.
- Monitor laboratory tests for urinary alkalinization and urinary pH as a guide to dosage. Testing of pH with nitrazine paper may be done at intervals throughout the day so dosage can be adjusted.
- Monitor laboratory tests for metabolic acidosis, and assess for changes in clinical condition and measurements of

acid–base status. Observe for signs of alkalosis such as irritability, muscle twitching, muscle spasms, or muscle weakness or acidosis with signs of rapid breathing, confusion, or lethargy.
- Do not administer this drug to patients with toxemis, because retention of fluids may worsen this condition.
- Administer sodium bicarbonate with caution to patients with HTN because this drug will promote retention of fluids.

Patient and Family Education:
- Do not use sodium bicarbonate as an antacid. Discuss safer alternatives with the health care provider.
- If on a sodium-restricted diet, remember that this drug should be included as part of the total sodium count.
- Avoid taking antacids for longer than 2 weeks except with supervision of the health care provider. Self-treatment with sodium bicarbonate or soda mints may cause sodium retention and alkalosis, especially with impaired renal function.
- Commonly used over-the-counter (OTC) antacid products such as Alka-Seltzer, Bromo-Seltzer, and Gaviscon contain sodium bicarbonate.
- Immediately report any of the following symptoms of too much sodium bicarbonate: confusion, irritability, slow respiration rate, and vomiting.

Drugs Similar to Sodium Bicarbonate
There are no drugs similar to sodium bicarbonate.

42.14 The pharmacotherapy of alkalosis includes the administration of acidic agents.

At plasma pH values above 7.45, **alkalosis** develops. Mortality can reach as high as 80% if the pH rises above 7.65. Like acidosis, alkalosis may have either respiratory or metabolic causes, as shown in Table 42.5. Also like acidosis, the CNS is greatly affected. Symptoms of CNS stimulation occur including nervousness, hyperactive reflexes, and convulsions. In metabolic alkalosis, slow, shallow breathing indicates that the body is attempting to compensate by retaining acid and lowering internal pH. Life-threatening dysrhythmias are the most serious adverse effects of alkalosis.

In mild cases, alkalosis may be corrected by administering sodium chloride combined with potassium chloride. This combination increases the renal excretion of bicarbonate ion, which indirectly increases the acidity of the blood. More severe alkalosis may be treated with infusions of an acidic drug such as ammonium chloride or hydrochloric acid.

PROTOTYPE DRUG Ammonium chloride

Classification: **Therapeutic:** Agent for lowering pH
Pharmacologic: Acidic agent

Therapeutic Effects and Uses: Ammonium chloride is an acidic substance that has been available as a drug for over 80 years. Severe metabolic alkalosis may be reversed by the administration of acidic agents such as ammonium chloride. Ammonium chloride acidifies the urine, which is beneficial in treating certain urinary tract infections. Historically, it has been used as a mild diuretic, though safer and more effective agents have made its use obsolete. By acidifying the urine, ammonium chloride promotes the excretion of alkaline drugs such as amphetamines through ion trapping. Oral and IV forms are available; when given for alkalosis, the IV route is preferred. Because of the potential for causing acidosis, the drug is infused slowly.

Mechanism of Action: During the hepatic conversion of ammonium chloride to urea, Cl^- and H^+ are formed. The H^+ combines with bicarbonate to form the weak acid carbonic acid, which dissociates to water and carbon dioxide. By removing bicarbonate, ammonium chloride decreases the pH of body fluids. The chloride ion also combines with bases to reduce the alkalinity of extracellular fluids.

Pharmacokinetics:

Route(s)	IV, PO
Absorption	Rapidly absorbed
Distribution	Unknown
Primary metabolism	Hepatic
Primary excretion	Renal
Onset of action	Unknown
Duration of action	Unknown

Adverse Effects: Aggressive treatment with ammonium chloride can cause acidosis. Characteristic symptoms of acidosis include CNS depression, drowsiness, confusion, and coma. Periods of CNS excitement may alternate with coma. Oral forms of the drug are irritating to the gastric mucosa and may cause nausea and vomiting.

Contraindications/Precautions: Ammonium chloride should not be administered to patients with serious hepatic or renal impairment because the drug will accumulate to toxic levels. It should not be administered to patients with either metabolic or respiratory acidosis.

Drug Interactions: Ammonium chloride may cause crystalluria when taken with aminosalicylic acid. Antacids should not be administered concurrently because they are alkaline and will antagonize the acidifying effects of ammonium chloride. Ammonium chloride reduces levels of amphetamines, flecainide, mexiletine, methadone, ephedrine, and pseudoephedrine. Urinary excretion of sulfonylureas and salicylates is decreased. Serum magnesium values may decrease. **Herbal/Food:** Unknown.

Pregnancy: Category B.

Treatment of Overdose: Overdose results in metabolic acidosis, which is treated by administering alkaline agents (see Section 42.9).

Nursing Responsibilities:
- Assess IV infusion site for signs of irritation and change site as needed.
- Assess for signs and symptoms of metabolic acidosis such as changes in mental status, confusion, disorientation, and coma or changes in respiratory rate and depth on exertion;

ammonium toxicity has symptoms such as cardiac dysrhythmias and bradycardia, irregular respirations, twitching, or seizures.

- Monitor intake and output ratio and pattern. The diuretic effect of ammonium chloride is compensatory and lasts only 1 to 2 days.
- Monitor laboratory tests for baseline and intermittent determinations of CO_2 combining power, serum electrolytes, and urinary and arterial pH during therapy to avoid serious acidosis.

Patient and Family Education:

- Report pain at the IV injection site to the health care provider.
- Immediately report symptoms of excessive drowsiness or confusion to the health care provider because these are signs of an overdose.

Drugs Similar to Ammonium Chloride

The only similar drug is hydrochloric acid.

Hydrochloric acid: Hydrochloric acid may be administered IV in severe cases of metabolic acidosis. A central venous catheter must be used to administer the drug. Hydrochloric acid is only used when sodium or potassium chloride cannot be administered due to volume overload or advanced renal failure. This drug can cause severe tissue necrosis if it extravasates into the tissues.

UNDERSTANDING THE CHAPTER

Key Concepts Summary

42.1 Body Fluids are exchanged between intracellular and extracellular compartments.

42.2 Osmolality or tonicity determines the movement of body fluids.

42.3 Overall fluid balance is regulated primarily by hormones acting upon the kidneys.

42.4 Dehydration may be treated with fluid volume expanders.

42.5 Transfusions of blood products are used to treat serious conditions that cannot be managed effectively by other means.

42.6 Crystalloids are intravenous solutions that closely resemble the composition of extracellular fluid.

42.7 Colloids are intravenous solutions containing large molecules that remain in the blood.

42.8 Electrolytes are charged substances that are essential to homeostasis.

42.9 Sodium balance is closely associated with water balance.

42.10 Potassium imbalances must be quickly corrected to prevent serious cardiac consequences.

42.11 Magnesium imbalances significantly affect cardiovascular and neuromuscular function.

42.12 The pH of body fluids must be maintained between very narrow limits.

42.13 The pharmacotherapy of acidosis includes the administration of alkaline agents.

42.14 The pharmacotherapy of alkalosis includes the administration of acidic agents.

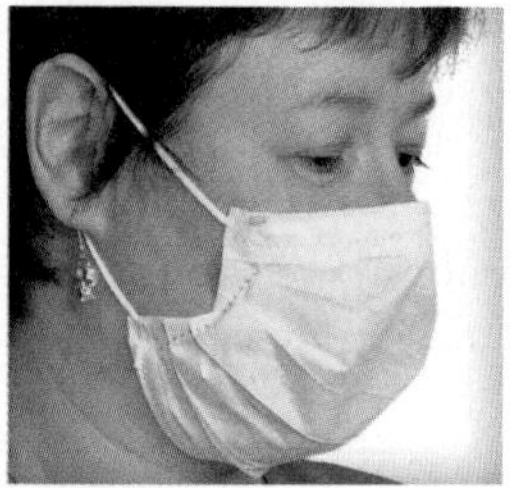

Making the PATIENT *Connection*

Remember "Judith Oster," the nurse at the beginning of the chapter? Now read the remainder of the case study. Based on the information presented within this chapter, respond to the critical thinking questions that follow.

Judith Oster has been a registered nurse for 3 years in a busy emergency department. On a daily basis, Judith cares for older adults, new babies, and everyone in between. She loves her job because she feels that she is learning something new every day. Sometimes it seems that every patient she cares for requires IV fluids. Multiple types of fluids are used, depending on the patient's condition and problem. Although she is proficient in initiating IV lines, she really does not know much about the types of IV fluids. As she drove home after a busy shift, Judith decided that she was going to research the types of IV fluids and their purpose. Her goal is to become the best nurse she can be and learning this was just one part of reaching that goal.

Critical Thinking Questions

1. What are the two major categories of IV solutions?
2. Discuss the indications for each type.
3. Dextrose 5% in water (D_5W) is a common solution. When is it used? What precautions should be taken with this fluid type?
4. What are the indications for the administration of normal serum albumin?
5. When is dextran administered? What are the contraindications for this fluid type?

Case Study

Marvin Fields has been prescribed a loop diuretic, furosemide (Lasix), 40 mg daily, and a potassium supplement 40 mEq tablet daily. As you are preparing to discharge this patient, he states, "I understand why I need the diuretic, but why do I have to take this potassium?"

1. How would you respond to his question?
2. What adverse effect related to potassium supplementation would you advise him to watch for?
3. What advice would you give Marvin about his dietary consumption of potassium-rich foods?

NCLEX-RN® Review

1 The client with a disorder causing acid–base imbalance is being treated with intravenous sodium bicarbonate. The nurse monitors for therapeutic effectiveness by noting which of the following laboratory values?

1. Serum pH
2. Red blood cell count
3. Liver function test
4. Blood urea nitrogen

2 The nurse is teaching the client about a liquid potassium chloride supplement. Which of the following statements, if made by the client, indicates that further teaching is necessary?

1. "I should avoid salt substitutes unless approved by my health care provider."
2. "Liquid preparations should not be diluted with other fluids."
3. "I should report signs of potassium deficit such as weakness and fatigue."
4. "Persistent vomiting will result in significant losses of potassium."

3 The nurse is administering dextran 40 (Gentran 40) to a multiple trauma client post–motor vehicle crash. The nurse knows that one toxic adverse effect of this medication is:

1. Dehydration.
2. Increased urinary output.
3. Hypovolemic shock.
4. Bleeding.

4 The client will be receiving 5% dextrose in water (D_5W) intravenous infusion. Which of the following is correct concerning this therapy? D_5W:

1. Can cause hypoglycemia in the diabetic client.
2. May serve to dilute mixed intravenous drugs.
3. Is considered a colloid solution.
4. Has a sufficient number of calories to supply metabolic needs.

5 The health care provider orders intravenous potassium supplementation for a client with hypokalemia. The nurse should consult with the prescriber about which client assessment finding that may affect the drug therapy?

1. Pupil constriction to direct light
2. Chest congestion and coughing
3. Elevated blood pressure
4. Sudden weight gain and swelling

6 Which of the following nursing actions should be included in the care plan for a client receiving normal serum albumin (Albuminar)? (Select all that apply.)

1. Document past history of blood transfusion reactions.
2. Restrict dietary intake of food high in potassium.
3. Monitor blood pressure and pulse rate.
4. Measure urinary output hourly.
5. Observe for signs related to potassium deficit.

See Answers to Critical Thinking Questions, Case Study, and NCLEX-RN® Review in Appendix A.

References

Ayers, P., & Warrington, L. (2008). Diagnosis and treatment of simple acid-base disorders. *Nutrition in Clinical Practice, 23*(2), 122–127.

Bunn, F., Trivedi, D., & Ashraf, S. (2007). Colloid solutions for fluid resuscitation. *Cochrane Database of Systematic Reviews, 4.* (Art. No.: CD001319, DOI:10.1002/14651858.CD001319.pub2).

Josephson, D. L. (2004). *Intravenous fluid therapy for nurses: Principles and practice* (2nd ed.). Clifton Park, NY: Delmar Publishers.

Joy, M. S., & Hladik, G. A. (2005). Disorders of sodium, water, calcium, and phosphorous homeostasis. In J. T. DiPiro, R. L. Talbert, C. Y. Yee, G. R. Matzke, B. G.Wells, & L. M. Posey (Eds.), *Pharmacotherapy: A pathophysiologic approach* (6th ed., pp. 937–966). New York: McGraw-Hill.

Khanna, A., & Kurtzman, N. A. (2006). Metabolic alkalosis. *Journal of Nephrology, 19*(Suppl 9), S86–S96.

Kraut, J. A., & Kurtz, I. (2005). Metabolic acidosis of CKD: Diagnosis, clinical characteristics, and treatment. *American Journal of Kidney Disease, 45*(6), 978–993.

Mahoney, B. A., Smith W. A. D., Lo, D. S., Tsoi, K., Tonelli, M., & Clase, C. M. (2005). Emergency interventions for hyperkalaemia. *Cochrane Database of Systematic Reviews, 2.* (Art. No.: CD003235, DOI: 10.1002/14651858.CD003235.pub2)

Matzke, G. R., & Palevsky, P. M. (2005). Acid-base disorders. In J. T. DiPiro, R. L. Talbert, C. Y. Yee, G. R. Matzke, B. G. Wells, & L. M. Posey (Eds.), *Pharmacotherapy: A pathophysiologic approach* (6th ed., pp. 51–73). New York: McGraw-Hill.

Medical News Today. (2008). *New statement on exercise-associated hyponatremia issued.* Retrieved July 21, 2008, from http://www.medicalnewstoday.com/articles/27938.php

Mitch, W. E. (2006). Metabolic and clinical consequences of metabolic acidosis. *Journal of Nephrology, 19*(Suppl. 9) S70–S75.

Moritz, M. L., & Ayus, J. C. (2007). *Hospital-acquired hyponatremia—Why Are hypotonic parenteral fluids still being used?* Retrieved July 21, 2008, from http://www.medscape.com/viewarticle/558353

National Institutes of Health Office of Dietary Supplements. (n.d.). *Magnesium.* Retrieved July 21, 2008, from http://ods.od.nih.gov/factsheets/magnesium.asp

UNIT 6

Pharmacology of Body Defenses

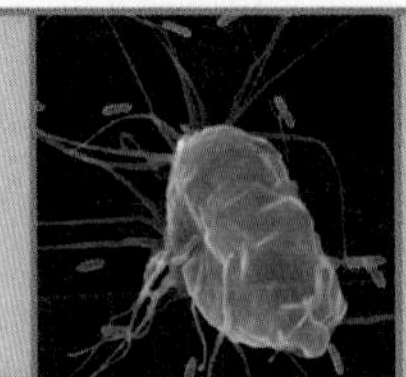
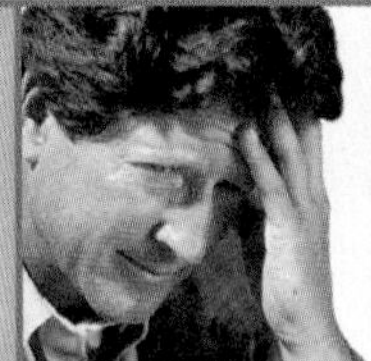
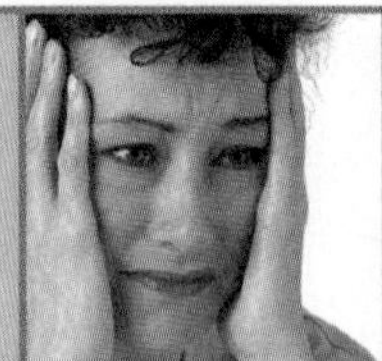
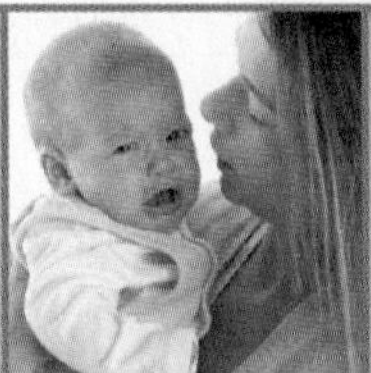

CHAPTER 43 Review of Body Defenses and the Immune System

CHAPTER 44 Pharmacotherapy of Inflammation and Fever

CHAPTER 45 Immunostimulants and Immunosuppressants

CHAPTER 46 Immunizing Agents

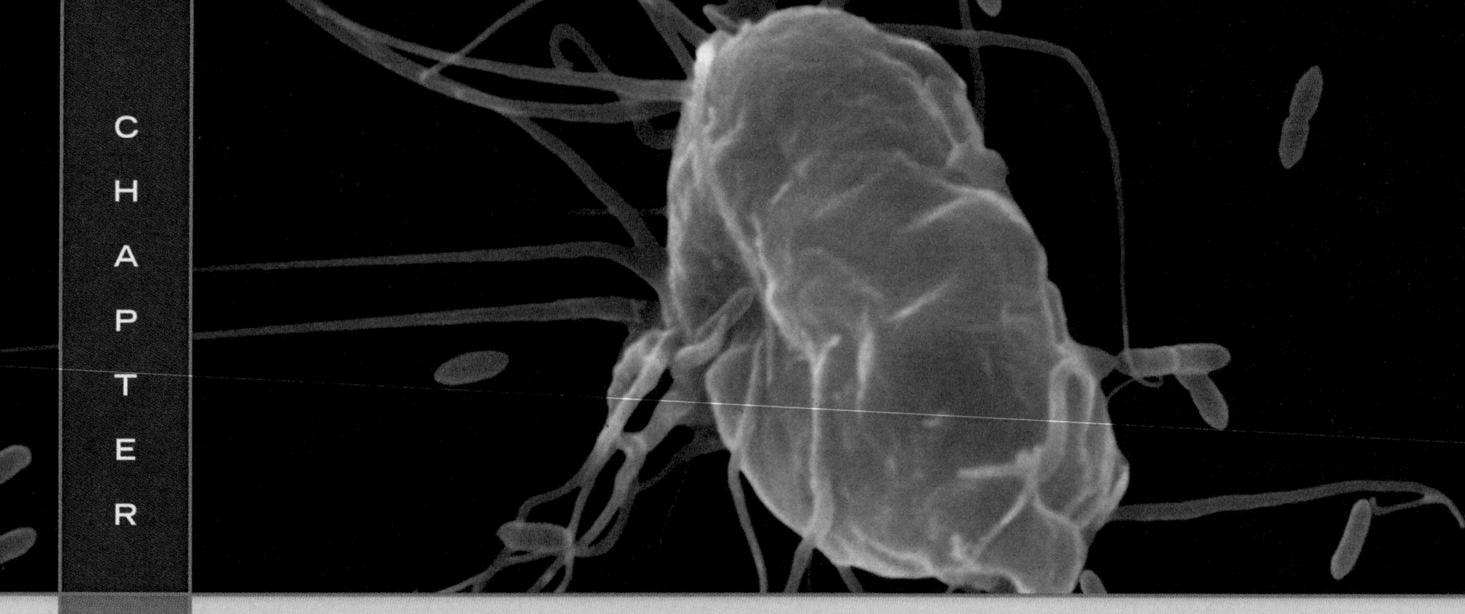

43 Review of Body Defenses and the Immune System

Learning Outcomes

After reading this chapter, the student should be able to:

1. Identify the major components of the lymphatic system.
2. Describe the components of the nonspecific body defense system and their functions.
3. Compare and contrast specific and nonspecific body defenses.
4. Identify the signs and symptoms of inflammation.
5. Outline the basic steps in the acute inflammatory response.
6. Explain the role of histamine and other chemical mediators in the inflammatory response.
7. Compare and contrast the humoral and cell-mediated immune responses.

Chapter Outline

Organization of the Lymphatic System

Nonspecific (Innate) Body Defenses

Inflammation

Specific (Adaptive) Body Defenses

Humoral Immune Response

Cell-Mediated Immune Response

Key Terms

adaptive defenses, 713
antibodies, 713
antigen, 713
B cell, 713
complement system, 711
cytokines, 713
histamine, 711
immunity, 709
inflammation, 711
lymph nodes, 709
lymphatic system, 709
nonspecific body defense system, 709
phagocytes, 710
plasma cell, 713
T cells, 713

The human body is under continuous attack from a host of foreign invaders that include viruses, bacteria, fungi, and even single-celled animals. Some of these pathogens intentionally seek out humans because it is an essential part of their life cycle, whereas others happen to be "at the right place and time" by coincidence when a cut or scrape allows an entrance into the body. Fortunately, the body's extensive defenses are capable of mounting a rapid and effective response against most of these pathogens. Drugs used to modify body defenses, which include anti-inflammatory agents, immunostimulants, immunosuppressants, and vaccines, are presented in Chapters 44 through 46. The purpose of this chapter is to review the fundamental concepts of body defenses that apply to the pharmacotherapy of the immune system and infectious disease. For a more thorough review of this topic, the student should consult an anatomy and physiology textbook.

Organization of the Lymphatic System

43.1 The lymphatic system is the primary organ system that protects the body from invasion by foreign agents.

The components of the lymphatic system provide the body with **immunity,** which is the ability to resist injury and infections. The **lymphatic system** is comprised of a network of cells, vessels, and tissues that provide immune surveillance. This monitoring function begins when fluid leaves the capillaries due to the osmotic forces and high pressure in the capillaries. This fluid, known as lymph, enters blind-ended lymphatic vessels and slowly travels on its journey through the lymphatic system. As much as 3 L of fluid per day travel through the highly branched lymphatic vessel network to eventually return to the cardiovascular circulation.

Lymphatic vessels carry more than escaped fluid. Viruses, bacteria, cellular debris, and even cancer cells can enter these vessels. Should these pathogens or cancer cells be permitted to return to the bloodstream, an infection (or cancer) could quickly spread throughout the body with potentially disastrous consequences. Fortunately, before these pathogens can return to the general circulation, they must pass through dozens of **lymph nodes,** which are the principal lymphoid organs in the body. Lymph nodes are solid, spherical bodies that are packed with macrophages and lymphocytes, which are cells specialized to recognize anything that is "nonself" or foreign to the body. Recognition of these foreign agents activates the immune response, which neutralizes or removes the pathogens before they can reach the general circulation. Each lymph node serves as a minifilter, removing up to 99% of the foreign agents entering the node. Should a pathogen be clever enough to escape surveillance in a lymph node, it is then faced with passing through dozens, and sometimes hundreds, more lymph nodes in the lymphatic system.

In addition to lymph vessels and nodes, lymphoid tissues line connective tissue at every potential portal of entrance into the body, including the gastrointestinal (GI) tract, respiratory tract, and genitourinary tract. Lymphoid tissue contains lymphocytes, which "patrol" the region for potential injury or exposure to microbes. Other large collections of lymphoid tissue include the tonsils, spleen, and thymus. These are considered organs of the lymphatic system.

Although the lymphatic system can be divided into individual structures and components for ease of study, it is best to think of it as an integrated whole. The various components of this system are in continuous communication and work together as a single unit to accomplish effective immune surveillance. A malfunction in any one single component may affect the effectiveness of the entire lymphatic system. An overview of the primary divisions of immunity is shown in Figure 43.1.

PharmFACT

Certain solid tumors secrete growth factors that promote the generation of new lymphatic vessels, or lymphangiogenesis, around the tumor. Scientists are searching for new drugs that might prevent lymphangiogenesis and reduce the risk of tumor metastasis.
Source: Schoppmann, 2005.

Nonspecific (Innate) Body Defenses

43.2 Nonspecific defenses are the body's first line of defense against pathogens.

The first line of protection from pathogens is the **nonspecific body defense system,** which serves as a general barrier to microbes and environmental hazards. The nonspecific defenses are unable to distinguish one type of threat from another; the response is the same regardless of the particular pathogen. The nonspecific portion of the immune system is sometimes referred to as the innate defenses. A summary of nonspecific body defenses is shown in Table 43.1.

The innate defenses provide a comprehensive network of protection for both external and internal body structures. Innate defenses are both physical and cellular. For example, the skin is a formidable mechanical barrier to pathogens as long as it stays intact. The body cavities that are open to the outside environment are lined with a mucosal epithelium that not only provides a physical barrier, but also contains proteins, cilia, lysozymes, and other substances that discourage pathogen growth.

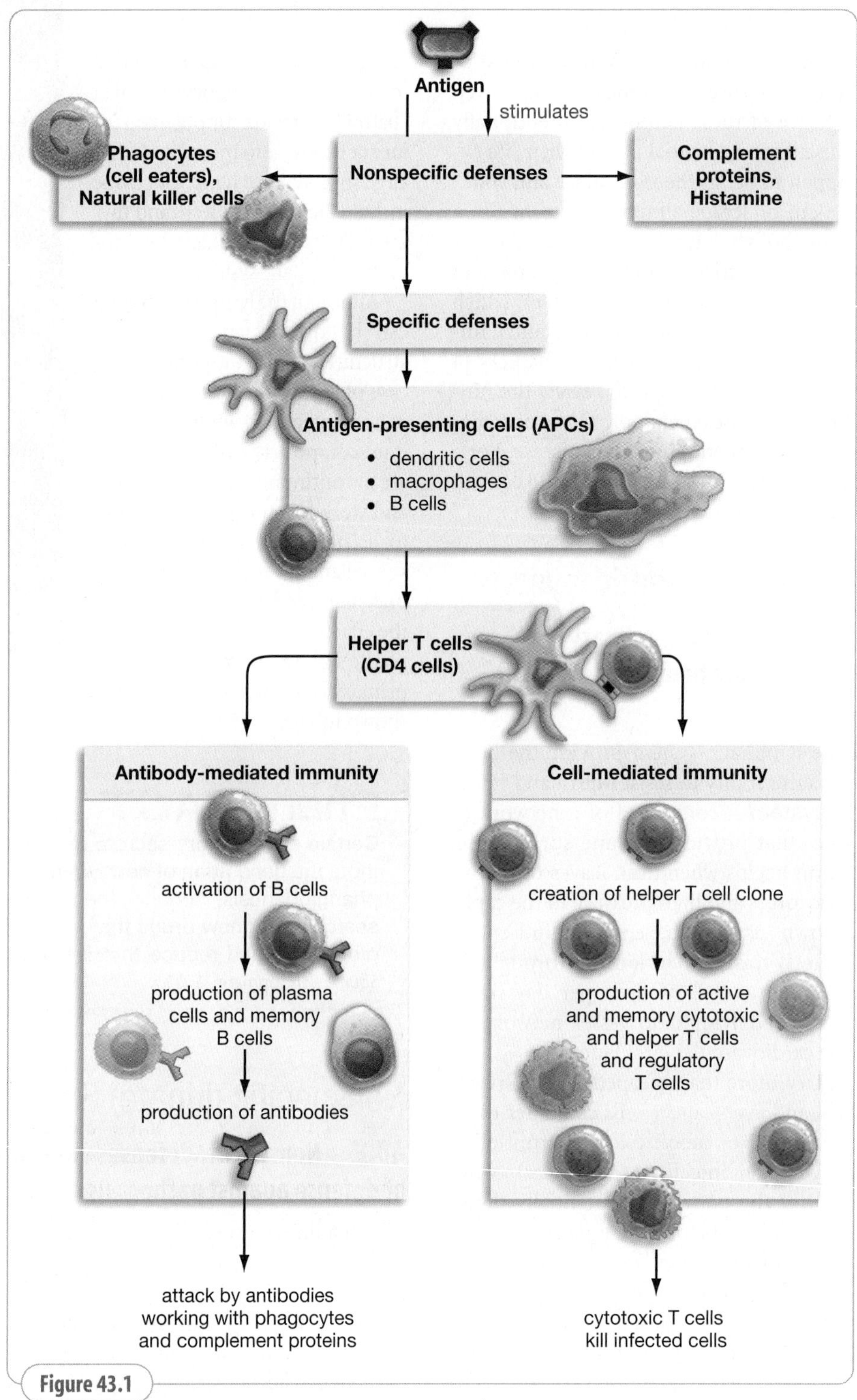

Figure 43.1

Overview of body defenses.
Source: From *Biology: A Guide to the Natural World* (4th ed.), by D. Krogh, 2009, Upper Saddle River, NJ: Prentice Hall.

Pharm*FACT*

The skin surface has a large population of resident bacteria, most of which are associated with sweat glands because these provide warm, humid places to grow. Common residents include *Staphylococcus, Propionibacterium, Acinetobacter*, and *Corynebacterium*.
Source: Madigan & Martinko, 2006.

Internally, the nonspecific defense system consists of proteins, cells, and cellular secretions that are hostile to pathogens that may have penetrated the skin or mucous membrane barriers. These are referred to as the second line of defense. Innate cellular defenses include **phagocytes** and natural killer (NK) cells. The two primary types of phagocytes are neutrophils and macrophages. These phagocytes are either fixed to specific sites (those locations most likely for pathogen entry), or they may

TABLE 43.1 Summary of Nonspecific Body Defenses

Component	Functions
First Line of Defense: Physical Barriers	
Skin	Forms a mechanical barrier to prevent pathogens and other harmful substances from entering the body. Surface contains keratin, which is resistant to water and acid.
Mucous membranes	Line the portals of entry to inhibit the entry of pathogens. Mucus inhibits microbial growth. Cilia in the respiratory tract and saliva in the mouth discourage pathogen entry.
Second Line of Defense	
Phagocytes	Ingest antigens. Specific types include neutrophils, eosinophils, and monocytes, which differentiate into macrophages.
Natural killer (NK) cells	Directly attack virus-infected and cancer cells by releasing substances that are toxic to the antigen.
Interferons	Proteins secreted by cells infected by viruses. They protect uninfected cells and also stimulate the activity of phagocytes and NK cells; used as medications to treat certain types of cancer.
Complement	Promotes inflammation and phagocytosis; lyses microbes.
Fever	Systemic response that increases body temperature to activate body defenses; inhibits the growth of some microbes.
Inflammation	Limits the spread of infection and releases substances that attract phagocytes; initiates repair of the injured area.

migrate throughout the body in search of foreign cells of substances. Natural killer cells are found in most lymphoid organs and are able to kill cancer or virus-infected cells. Although not phagocytic, NK cells release substances that kill the pathogens and that enhance the immune response.

Part of the nonspecific defense system includes the release of antimicrobial proteins. The **complement system** is a cluster of 20 plasma proteins that combine together in a specific sequence and order when an infection occurs. Activation of complement attracts phagocytes to the infection site, attacks and breaks down the cell walls of pathogens, and stimulates the inflammatory process. Interferon is an antimicrobial protein that protects uninfected cells from the pathogen. Interferons have become important drugs in the pharmacotherapy of immune disorders (see Chapter 45) and cancer (see Chapter 58).

Other key processes of the nonspecific defense system are fever and inflammation. Fever accelerates body defenses and associated repair processes by raising the temperature of the body. When excessive, however, fever can harm the body and must be treated with drugs known as antipyretics (see Chapter 44). From a pharmacologic perspective, one of the most important nonspecific defenses is inflammation. Because of its significance, inflammation is presented separately in Sections 43.3 and 43.4.

Inflammation

43.3 Inflammation is a nonspecific defense mechanism that neutralizes or destroys foreign substances and microbes.

Inflammation occurs in response to many different stimuli, including physical injury, exposure to toxic chemicals, extreme heat, invading microorganisms, or death of cells. Inflammation is considered a nonspecific defense mechanism because it proceeds in the same manner regardless of the cause.

The central purposes of inflammation are to contain the injury, destroy the pathogen, and initiate repair of the area. The repair of the injured area can proceed at a faster pace by neutralizing the foreign agent and removing cellular debris and dead cells. Signs of inflammation include swelling, pain, warmth, and redness of the affected area.

Inflammation may be classified as acute or chronic. During acute inflammation, such as that caused by minor physical injury, 8 to 10 days are normally needed for the symptoms to resolve and for repair to begin. If the body cannot neutralize the damaging agent, inflammation may continue for long periods and become chronic. In chronic autoimmune disorders such as lupus and rheumatoid arthritis (RA), inflammation may persist for years, with symptoms becoming progressively worse over time. Other disorders such as seasonal allergy arise at predictable times during each year, and inflammation may produce only minor, annoying symptoms.

43.4 Inflammation proceeds with the release of chemical mediators.

During inflammation, pathogens, chemicals, or physical trauma cause the damaged tissue to release chemical mediators that act as "alarms" to notify the surrounding area of the injury. Chemical mediators of inflammation include histamine, leukotrienes, bradykinin, complement, and prostaglandins. These inflammatory mediators, which are listed in Table 43.2, are sometimes called proinflammatory substances. Some of the inflammatory mediators are important targets for anti-inflammatory drugs. For example, aspirin and ibuprofen are prostaglandin inhibitors that are effective at treating fever, pain, and inflammation.

The rapid release of the chemical mediators of inflammation on a large scale throughout the body is responsible for anaphylaxis, a life-threatening allergic response that may result in shock and death. A number of chemicals, insect stings, foods, and some therapeutic drugs can cause this widespread release of histamine from mast cells if the person has an allergy to these substances.

Histamine is a key chemical mediator of inflammation. It is stored primarily within mast cells located in tissue spaces under epithelial membranes such as the skin, bronchial tree, and digestive tract and along blood vessels. Mast cells detect foreign agents or injury and respond by releasing histamine, which initiates the inflammatory response within seconds. In addition to its role in inflammation, histamine also directly stimulates pain receptors and is a primary agent responsible for the symptoms of seasonal allergies (see Chapter 74).

TABLE 43.2 Chemical Mediators of Inflammation

Mediator	Description
Bradykinin	Protein present in an inactive form in plasma and mast cells; increases vascular permeability and causes pain; effects are similar to those of histamine; broken down by angiotensin-converting enzyme (ACE).
Complement	Series of at least 20 proteins that combine in a cascade fashion to neutralize or destroy an antigen; stimulates histamine release by mast cells; causes cell lysis.
Histamine	Stored and released by mast cells; causes vasodilation, smooth muscle constriction, tissue swelling, and itching.
Leukotrienes	Lipids stored and released by mast cells; effects are similar to those of histamine; synthesized from arachidonic acid; responsible for some symptoms of asthma and allergies.
Prostaglandins	Lipid present in most tissues and stored and released by mast cells; increase capillary permeability, attract white blood cells to the site of inflammation, and cause pain; induce fever; aspirin inhibits their synthesis; some are available as medications.

When released at an injury site, histamine dilates nearby blood vessels, causing the capillaries to become more permeable. Plasma, complement proteins, and phagocytes can then enter the area to neutralize microbes or their toxins. The affected area may become congested with blood, which can lead to significant swelling and pain. Figure 43.2 illustrates the fundamental steps in acute inflammation.

Histamine interacts with two different receptors to elicit an inflammatory response. H_1 receptors are present in the smooth muscle of the vascular system, the bronchial tree, and the digestive tract. Stimulation of these receptors results in itching, pain, edema, vasodilation, bronchoconstriction, and the characteristic symptoms of inflammation and allergy. In contrast, H_2 receptors are present primarily in the stomach, and their stimulation results in the secretion of large amounts of hydrochloric acid.

Drugs that act as specific antagonists for H_1 and H_2 receptors are in widespread therapeutic use. H_1-receptor antagonists, which are used to treat allergies and inflammation, are discussed in Chapter 74. H_2-receptor antagonists are used to treat peptic ulcers and are discussed in Chapter 60.

CONNECTION *Checkpoint* 43.1

In addition to being a mediator of inflammation, bradykinin is responsible for one of the most common adverse effects of ACE inhibitors. From what you learned in Chapter 34, describe this adverse effect.

See Answer to Connection Checkpoint 43.1 in Appendix A.

Specific (Adaptive) Body Defenses

43.5 The specific body defenses include the humoral and cell-mediated immune systems.

The body also has the ability to mount a third line of defense that is specific to certain threats. For example, a specific defense

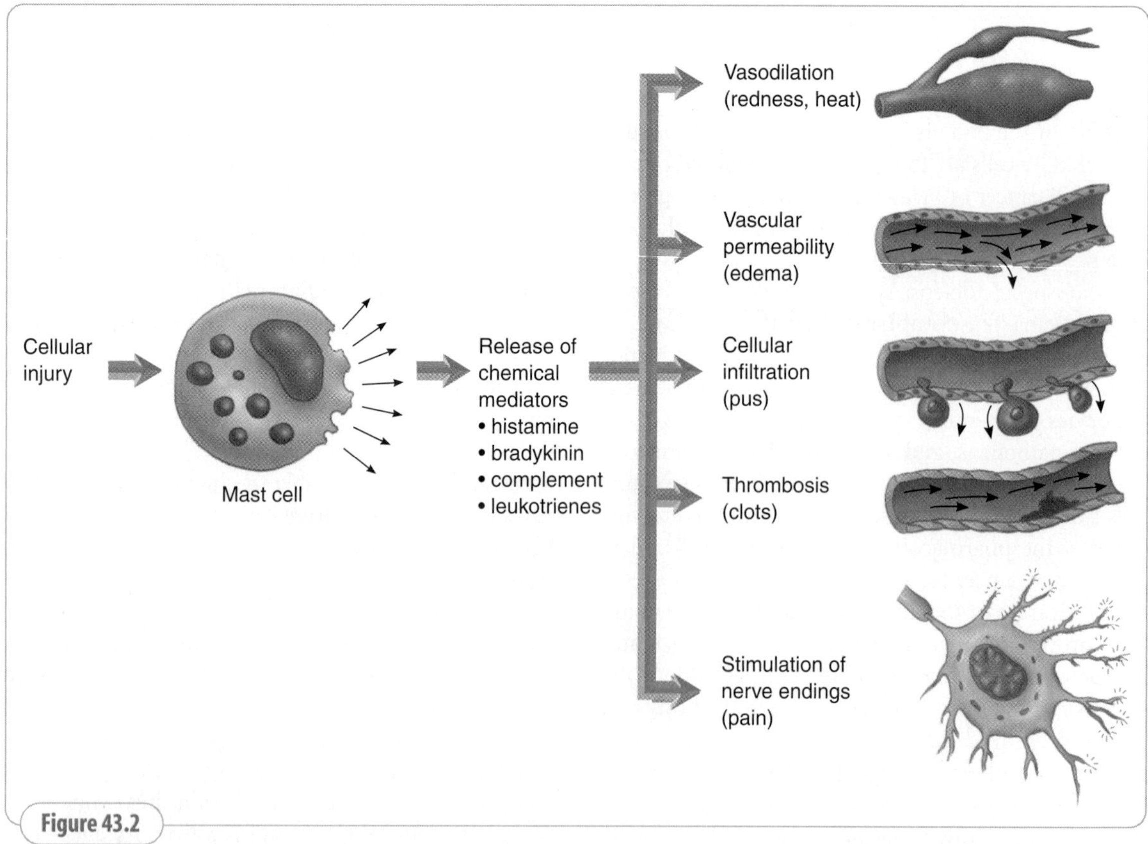

Figure 43.2

Steps in acute inflammation.

may act against only a single species of bacteria and be ineffective against all others. These are known as **adaptive defenses** or, more commonly, the immune response. The primary cell of the immune response is the lymphocyte.

Microbes and foreign substances that elicit an immune response are called **antigens.** Foreign proteins, such as those present on the surfaces of pollen grains, bacteria, nonhuman cells, and viruses, are the strongest antigens. Typically, only a small fragment or piece of a foreign protein is required to activate the immune system. It is estimated that the immune system is able to recognize and react to over a billion different antigens.

The immune response is extremely complex. Following are several important aspects of the immune response.

Specificity: Each aspect of the immune response recognizes only particular pathogens and not others. Recognition of the antigen is dependent on the immune cells interacting with specific foreign proteins. Once an immune response is mounted, it generally only affects the one specific antigen that was recognized.

Systemic: Despite being specific to a particular antigen, the immune response is systemic. Thus antigens that exist beyond the initial site of infection will be neutralized.

Memory: After an interaction with the antigen occurs, the cells of the adaptive immune system remember the immune response. This is different from the components of nonspecific defenses, which have no memory. Upon subsequent exposures to the same antigen, the body is able to mount a stronger and more rapid response.

The basic steps of the immune response involve recognition of the antigen, communication and coordination with other defense cells, and destruction or suppression of the antigen. A large number of chemical messengers and complex interactions are involved in the immune response, many of which have yet to be discovered. The two primary divisions of the immune response are antibody-mediated (humoral) immunity and cell-mediated immunity.

Humoral Immune Response

43.6 The humoral immune response is mediated by B lymphocytes and includes the secretion of antibodies.

The humoral immune response is triggered when an antigen encounters a B lymphocyte, more simply known as a **B cell.** The activated B cell divides to form millions of identical copies of itself in a process known as clonal division. Most cells in this clone are called **plasma cells,** whose primary function is to secrete antibodies specific to the antigen that initiated the challenge. Each plasma cell is capable of manufacturing antibodies at an astounding rate, as many as 2,000 antibodies each second.

Circulating through body fluids are **antibodies,** also known as immunoglobulins (Ig), which physically interact with antigens to neutralize or mark them for destruction by other cells of the immune response. The activation of complement, with subsequent inflammation and enhanced phagocytosis, is a major defense mechanism resulting from the formation of antigen–antibody complexes. Peak production of antibodies occurs about 10 days after an initial antigen challenge. The important functions of antibodies are illustrated in Figure 43.3.

After the antigen challenge, memory B cells are formed that will remember the specific antigen–antibody interaction. Should the body be exposed to the same antigen in the future, the humoral immune system will manufacture even higher levels of antibodies in a shorter period, approximately 2 to 3 days. For some antigens, such as those for measles, mumps, or chickenpox, memory can be retained an entire lifetime. Vaccines are sometimes administered to produce these memory cells in advance of exposure to the antigen, so that when the body is exposed to the actual organism it can mount a fast, effective response (see Chapter 46).

It is important to remember that the body contains millions of different B cells, each programmed to react to a specific antigen. These B cells, in turn, are able to construct millions of different types of antibodies, each specific to a particular antigen. The body is "preprogrammed" with the genetic information to defend against millions of different antigens. Although it is unlikely that an individual will ever be infected during a lifetime with all the different antigens, the body is waiting for the challenge.

Cell-Mediated Immune Response

43.7 The cell-mediated immune response is mediated by T lymphocytes and includes the secretion of cytokines.

A second branch of the immune response involves T lymphocytes, or **T cells.** Two major types of T cells are called helper T cells and cytotoxic T cells. These cells are named after a protein receptor on their plasma membrane. The helper T cells have a CD4 receptor, and the cytotoxic T cells have a CD8 receptor. The helper (CD4) T cells are particularly important because they are responsible for activating most other immune cells, including B cells and other types of T cells. Cytotoxic (CD8) T cells travel throughout the body, directly killing certain bacteria, parasites, virus-infected cells, and cancer cells.

Pharm*FACT*

T cells move quickly throughout the body. In a typical day, a T cell may spend 30 minutes in the blood, 5 to 6 hours in the spleen, and 15 to 20 hours in a lymph node. *Source:* Martini & Nath, 2009.

T cells rapidly form clones after they are activated or sensitized following an encounter with their specific antigen. Unlike B cells, however, T cells do not produce antibodies. Instead, activated T cells produce huge amounts of **cytokines,** which are hormone-like proteins that regulate the intensity and duration of the immune response and mediate cell-to-cell communication. Some cytokines kill foreign organisms directly, whereas others induce inflammation or enhance the killing power of macrophages. Specific cytokines released by activated T cells include interleukins, gamma interferon, tumor necrosis factor (TNF), and perforin. Some cytokines are used therapeutically to stimulate the immune system (see Chapter 45). Small amounts of cytokines are

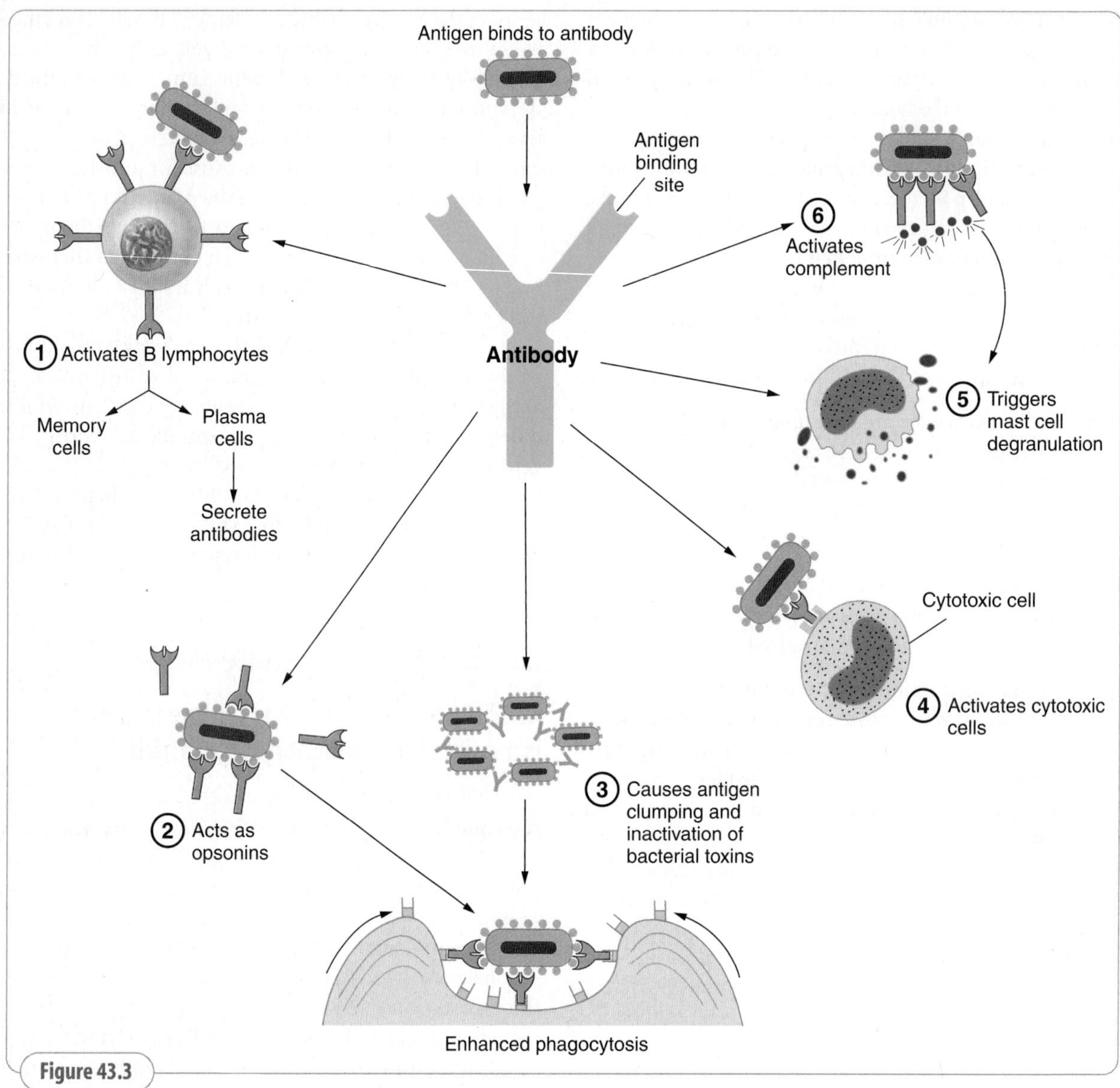

Figure 43.3

Functions of antibodies.

also secreted by certain macrophages, B lymphocytes, mast cells, endothelial cells, and the stromal cells of the spleen, thymus, and bone marrow.

PharmFACT

T cells need help in recognizing intact antigens. Certain macrophages must phagocytize the antigen and present the foreign proteins on their surface to be recognized by T cells. These are called antigen-presenting cells (APCs). *Source:* DiPiro et al., 2005.

Like B cells, some sensitized T cells become memory cells. If the patient encounters the same antigen in the future, the memory T cells assist in mounting a more rapid immune response.

CONNECTION *Checkpoint* 43.2

Proinflammatory cytokines such as interleukin-1 and TNF have been associated with a higher risk of Alzheimer's disease and progression of this disorder. From what you learned in Chapter 25, describe the primary drug classes for treating Alzheimer's disease. See Answer to Connection Checkpoint 43.2 in Appendix A.

UNDERSTANDING THE CHAPTER

Key Concepts Summary

43.1 The lymphatic system is the primary organ system that protects the body from invasion by foreign agents.

43.2 Nonspecific defenses are the body's first line of defense against pathogens.

43.3 Inflammation is a nonspecific defense mechanism that neutralizes or destroys foreign substances and microbes.

43.4 Inflammation proceeds with the release of chemical mediators.

43.5 The specific body defenses include the humoral and cell-mediated immune systems.

43.6 The humoral immune response is mediated by B lymphocytes and includes the secretion of antibodies.

43.7 The cell-mediated immune response is mediated by T lymphocytes and includes the secretion of cytokines.

References

DiPiro, J. T., Talbert, R. L., Yee, G. C., Matzke, G. R., Wells, B. G., & Posey, L. M. (Eds.). (2005). *Pharmacotherapy: A pathophysiologic approach* (6th ed.). New York: McGraw-Hill.

Krogh, D. (2009). *Biology: A guide to the natural world* (4th ed.). Upper Saddle River, NJ: Prentice Hall.

Madigan, M. T., & Martinko, J. M. (2006). *Brock biology of microorganisms* (11th ed.). Upper Saddle River, NJ: Prentice Hall.

Martini, F. H., & Nath, J. L. (2009). *Fundamentals of human anatomy and physiology* (8th ed.). San Francisco: Benjamin Cummings.

Rice, J. (2005). *Medical terminology with human anatomy* (5th ed.). Upper Saddle River, NJ: Prentice Hall.

Schoppmann, S. F. (2005). Lymphangiogenesis, inflammation and metastasis. *Anticancer Research, 25*(6C), 4503–4511.

Silverthorn, D. U. (2006). *Human physiology: An integrated approach* (4th ed.). San Francisco: Benjamin Cummings.

C H A P T E R

My health care provider prescribed ibuprofen for my fever. I thought it was only for inflammation and pain. I don't want to take it. I don't have any pain in my joints.

Patient "Gene Tallo"

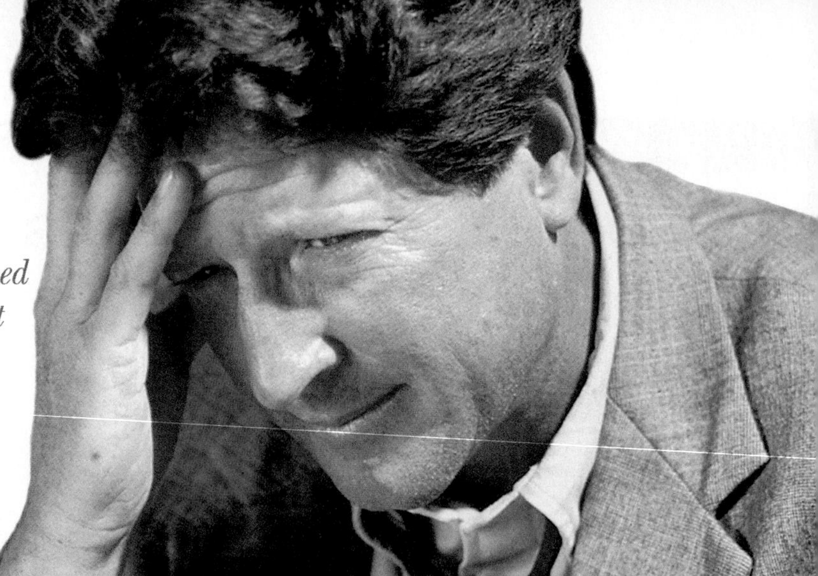

44 Pharmacotherapy of Inflammation and Fever

Learning Outcomes

After reading this chapter, the student should be able to:

1. Explain the pathophysiology of inflammation and fever.
2. Describe the general treatment of inflammation and fever.
3. Explain how aspirin damages the gastrointestinal mucosa.
4. Describe the symptoms and treatment of salicylism.
5. Compare the actions and adverse effects of aspirin to the ibuprofen-like drugs.
6. Compare the actions and adverse effects of the selective cyclooxygenase-2 inhibitors to nonsteroidal anti-inflammatory drugs.
7. Describe the nurse's role in the pharmacologic management of inflammation and fever.
8. For each of the classes shown in the chapter outline, identify the prototype and representative drugs and explain the mechanism(s) of drug action, primary indications, contraindications, significant drug interactions, pregnancy category, and important adverse effects.
9. Use the nursing process to care for patients who are receiving drug therapy for fever or inflammation.

Chapter Outline

Pathophysiology of Inflammation and Fever

Pharmacotherapy of Inflammation

Nonsteroidal Anti-Inflammatory Drugs

Salicylates

PROTOTYPE **Aspirin (Acetylsalicylic Acid)** *p. 721*

Ibuprofen-Like Agents

PROTOTYPE **Ibuprofen (Advil, Motrin, Others)** *p. 725*

Cyclooxygenase-2 Inhibitors

PROTOTYPE **Celecoxib (Celebrex)** *p. 727*

Antipyretic and Analgesic Agent

PROTOTYPE **Acetaminophen (Tylenol)** *p. 729*

Key Terms

anaphylaxis, 717
antipyretics, 718
cyclooxygenase (COX), 719
inflammation, 717
prostaglandins, 718
salicylates, 718
salicylism, 722

Inflammation is a response to injury that destroys agents that could damage human tissue. A large number of conditions can trigger inflammation, including physical trauma, burns, chemical injury, infections, hypersensitivity reactions, or tissue necrosis (death). Inflammation may produce symptoms that range from minor discomfort to severe, disabling pain, fever, and limitation of mobility. This chapter examines drugs used to diminish the inflammatory response and reduce fever.

Pathophysiology of Inflammation and Fever

44.1 Inflammation is a nonspecific body response to antigens and tissue injury.

The basic process of inflammation and the proinflammatory chemical mediators involved are described in Chapter 43. The student should review that chapter before proceeding.

Acute inflammation: Acute inflammation has an immediate onset and lasts 1 to 2 weeks. The inflammatory process is initiated when the body is exposed to a foreign substance, or antigen. The antigen may be anything from ragweed pollen to a microorganism; it may even be a normal cell that has been damaged or changed. Once the inflammation process is initiated, nearby blood vessels become permeable, allowing phagocytic cells to reach and neutralize the antigen. The increased permeability causes edema of the surrounding tissue, which often leads to acute pain and, possibly, joint immobility. The greater the tissue damage from the antigen or the inflammation, the greater will be the edema and the more mobility will be diminished at the site.

Occasionally, acute inflammation is initiated by a rapid, massive release of inflammatory chemical mediators throughout the entire body. This condition, known as **anaphylaxis,** is a life-threatening allergic response that may cause cardiovascular shock and death. A number of chemicals, insect stings, foods, and some therapeutic drugs can cause this widespread release of histamine from mast cells if the person has hypersensitivity to these substances.

The resolution of acute inflammation occurs when damaged tissue begins the process of regeneration and may conclude within a matter of weeks or continue throughout the individual's life with the regeneration of new tissue. Regeneration processes may replace normal cells with scar tissue, especially in nerve, cardiac, and muscle tissues. Replacement with fibrotic tissue can impair the function of the inflamed tissue.

Chronic inflammation: Chronic inflammation has a slow onset and may lack the distinct stages characteristic of acute inflammation. Whereas acute inflammation is the result of an influx of neutrophils, chronic inflammation is caused primarily by lymphocytes and macrophages. The chronic invasion of an area by macrophages and the resultant chemical reaction at the tissue site activates fibroblasts and generates scar tissue, which may limit mobility or narrow vessel lumens. Lymphocytes sometimes surround macrophages, resulting in granulomas. For example, chronic inflammation from *Mycobacterium tuberculosis* in the lung may occur over many years and yield the development of granulomas. The granulomas serve as a means of protection, walling off the agent from the rest of the body. In the event that the host's immune response diminishes, the host is susceptible to the reemergence of inflammation and the possible onset of active infection.

When acute or chronic inflammation is caused by an infection, the patient is prone to the development of a febrile episode, which is characterized by an increase in body temperature due to cytokine-induced changes in the hypothalamus. The systemic manifestations of inflammation associated with an infection are elevated temperature above 39°C (110.4°F), pulse rate greater than 90 beats per minute, respirations greater than 20 per minute, and a white blood cell count greater than 12,000/mm^3.

CONNECTIONS

Complementary and Alternative Therapies Goldenseal

Description: Goldenseal, *Hydrastis canadensis*, is an herb found in North America predominantly in shaded, damp, fertile soil. It is primarily grown in Vermont, Minnesota, Georgia, and Arkansas. The plant produces a fruit, which resembles a raspberry. It is taken internally to improve appetite and decrease dyspepsia.

History and Claims: The goldenseal root was used widely by the North American Indians. The Iroquois used it internally to treat diarrhea, whooping cough, flatulence, bloating, fever, and liver and gallbladder diseases. It is a remedy for inflammation of the mucous membranes. It is also used for gastric inflammation and menstrual pain. The Cherokee used it as a skin wash for local inflammations. The Iroquois used goldenseal internally for fever reduction. Overharvesting and loss of habitat has made goldenseal an endangered species. Goldenseal was declared an official drug in the *United States Pharmacopeia* in 1830. It is one of the top-selling supplements in the United States.

Standardization: The active ingredients of goldenseal include hydrastine and berberine. Goldenseal is standardized by root content. A typical dose is 200 to 500 mg/day of dried root, although some doses are as high as 6 g/day. Some products are standardized by the percentage of hydrastine (usually 5%).

Evidence: Despite its popularity, few controlled research studies have been conducted on goldenseal.

Human clinical studies suggest that it may have some benefit in treating topical infections. There is no direct evidence that goldenseal has any effect on cancer. Goldenseal may be of benefit in treating infections that have a diarrhea component.

Source: From *A Review of Natural Products* (4th ed.), by Facts and Comparisons 4.0, 2005, Philadelphia: Wolters Kluwer Health; and *Herbs at a Glance: Goldenseal*, National Center for Complementary and Alternative Medicine, National Institutes of Health, 2008. Retrieved July 22, 2008, from http://nccam.nih.gov/health/goldenseal/

Pharmacotherapy of Inflammation

44.2 Treatment of inflammation includes nonpharmacologic therapies and the administration of anti-inflammatory drugs.

Because inflammation is a nonspecific process and may be caused by such a variety of physical and infectious etiologies, it may occur in virtually any tissue or organ system. When treating inflammation, the following general principles apply:

- Inflammation is not a disease but a symptom of an underlying disorder. Whenever possible, the cause of the inflammation should be identified and treated.
- Inflammation is a natural process for ridding the body of antigens, and it is usually self-limiting. Nonpharmacologic treatments such as ice packs and rest should be used for mild symptoms whenever applicable.
- Topical drugs should be used when applicable because they cause fewer adverse effects. Inflammation of the skin and mucous membranes of the mouth, nose, rectum, and vagina are best treated with topical drugs. These include creams, ointments, patches, suppositories, and intranasal sprays. Inhalation drugs may be used for pulmonary inflammation.

MyNursingKit | Lupus Foundation

The goal of pharmacotherapy with anti-inflammatory agents is to prevent or decrease the intensity of the inflammatory response and reduce fever, if present. Most anti-inflammatory agents are nonspecific; that is, whether the inflammation is caused by an injury, autoimmune disease, or allergy, the drug will exhibit the same inhibitory actions. Common diseases that benefit from anti-inflammatory agents include allergic rhinitis, anaphylaxis, ankylosing spondylitis, contact dermatitis, Crohn's disease, glomerulonephritis, Hashimoto's thyroiditis, peptic ulcer disease (PUD), rheumatoid arthritis (RA), systemic lupus erythematosus, and ulcerative colitis.

If fever is associated with the inflammation, medications used to reduce body temperature, or **antipyretics,** may be administered. The goal of antipyretic therapy is to lower body temperature while treating the underlying cause of the fever, which is usually an infection. Many of the drugs used for inflammation also reduce fever and relieve mild to moderate pain.

Two major drug classes are used for nonspecific inflammation: nonsteroidal anti-inflammatory drugs (NSAIDs) and the corticosteroids. NSAIDs are the drugs of choice for mild to moderate pain, inflammation, and fever. Should inflammation become severe or disabling, corticosteroid therapy is begun. Due to their serious long-term adverse effects, corticosteroids are usually used for only 1 to 3 weeks to bring inflammation under control. The patient is then switched to NSAIDs. Corticosteroids are used for a large number of conditions, and their pharmacotherapy is presented in Chapter 69.

A few anti-inflammatory drug classes are specific to certain disorders. For example, the 5-aminosalicylic acid drugs such as sulfasalazine (Azulfidine) are specific to treating inflammatory bowel disease (see Chapter 61). Colchicine and allopurinol (Zyloprim) are used for the inflammation specifically caused by gouty arthritis (see Chapter 75). These specific anti-inflammatory agents are more toxic than the NSAIDs.

PharmFACT

In the United States, approximately 70 million NSAID prescriptions are written and 30 billion over-the-counter (OTC) NSAID tablets are sold each year. *Source:* Taha, Angerson, Prasad, McCloskey, & Blatchford, 2007.

Nonsteroidal Anti-Inflammatory Drugs

The NSAIDs consist of three major classes: salicylates, ibuprofen and ibuprofen-like agents, and the selective cyclooxygenase-2 inhibitors. These drug classes are sometimes described as first-generation NSAIDs (salicylates and ibuprofen-like drugs) and second-generation NSAIDs (selective cyclooxygenase-2 inhibitors). This is not a particularly useful means of grouping the drugs because there are over 20 first-generation NSAIDs and only one second-generation NSAID. The ibuprofen-like NSAIDs are described in Section 44.4 and the selective COX-2 inhibitors are presented in Section 44.5.

Salicylates

44.3 Aspirin is an inexpensive, effective, first-generation nonsteroidal anti-inflammatory drug commonly used by adults.

The first of the NSAIDs to be discovered was originally extracted from the bark of the common willow tree. The medical uses of willow bark, especially for pain relief and fever reduction, had been known for centuries but it was not until 1828 that the active ingredient, called salicin, was identified and converted to salicylic acid. Quite toxic in concentrated amounts, salicylic acid was converted into its most useful form, known as aspirin or acetylsalicylic acid, by a scientist at the Bayer Pharmaceutical Company in 1897. The chemical family to which aspirin belongs is known as the **salicylates.** Since its discovery, aspirin has become one of the most highly used therapeutic drugs in the world. Aspirin has the following indications for use:

- Analgesic. The ability to relieve mild to moderate pain.
- Anti-inflammatory. The ability to decrease mild to moderate inflammation.
- Antipyretic. The ability to lower body temperature.
- Anticoagulant. The ability to decrease platelet aggregation.

Understanding the mechanism of action of aspirin is important because it explains both the therapeutic actions of the drug as well as its adverse effects. All NSAIDs act by inhibiting the synthesis of **prostaglandins.** Prostaglandins are local hormones found in virtually every tissue that have many diverse functions depending on their location. Several prostaglandins are available as drugs, including carboprost (Hemabate, prostaglandin F_2 alpha), dinoprostone (Cervidil, prostaglandin E_2), and misoprostol (Cytotec prostaglandin E_1). The physiological properties of prostaglandins include the following:

- Mediation of inflammation. Cause vasodilation, increase capillary permeability, and cause pain.
- GI protection. Increase bicarbonate and mucus production to protect the stomach mucosa from acid.

- **Renal protection.** Help maintain blood flow through the kidneys.
- **Smooth muscle.** Help regulate smooth muscle tone in blood vessels; increase smooth muscle tone in the uterus; may cause bronchodilation or bronchoconstriction.
- **Blood clotting.** Increase platelet aggregation to promote clot formation.

Aspirin blocks the synthesis of prostaglandins by inhibiting the enzyme **cyclooxygenase (COX).** Aspirin and the ibuprofen-like NSAIDs block both forms of the enzyme, known as COX-1 and COX-2, by changing their structures and preventing the formation of prostaglandins. This inhibition of COX is responsible for their therapeutic and adverse effects, depending on the location and function of the prostaglandin that is being blocked. For example, the inhibition of COX in peripheral tissues will reduce the pain and inflammation caused by prostaglandins. The inhibition of COX in the stomach, however, will remove the protective effect of prostaglandins and result in damage to the GI mucosa. The mechanism by which aspirin produces its effects is illustrated in Figure 44.1.

The inhibition of COX in platelets is especially prolonged and may last for the entire 8- to 11-day life span of the platelet. This antithrombotic action inhibits platelet aggregation and reduces the risk of adverse cardiovascular events, including myocardial infarction (MI). The antipyretic effect of aspirin results from a suppression of prostaglandin synthesis in the hypothalamus of the brain. It lowers temperature by indirectly causing centrally medicated peripheral vasodilation and sweating. The principal analgesic effect of aspirin occurs in the peripheral areas of the body and in the central nervous system (CNS). Doses for aspirin and the other salicylates are listed in Table 44.1.

Aspirin is sometimes combined with prescription and over-the-counter (OTC) medications, and its presence is not always obvious unless the label is carefully inspected. This is especially important for patients with aspirin allergy, which is present in about 1% of the population. Patients with asthma or food allergies are most likely to be allergic to aspirin. Aspirin allergy symptoms include rash, urticaria, dyspnea, wheezing, rhinorrhea, and cough. To prevent aspirin allergy the patient should be instructed to read labels carefully and avoid products containing salicylates. This is not always possible because salicylates are naturally found in certain foods and are used as preservatives in others. Patients with aspirin allergies should consult with a dietician regarding which food sources to avoid. Allergists may be able to desensitize patients, if exposure to the drug is unavoidable or if the patient's allergy is severe. Patients who are hypersensitive to aspirin will likely be sensitive to

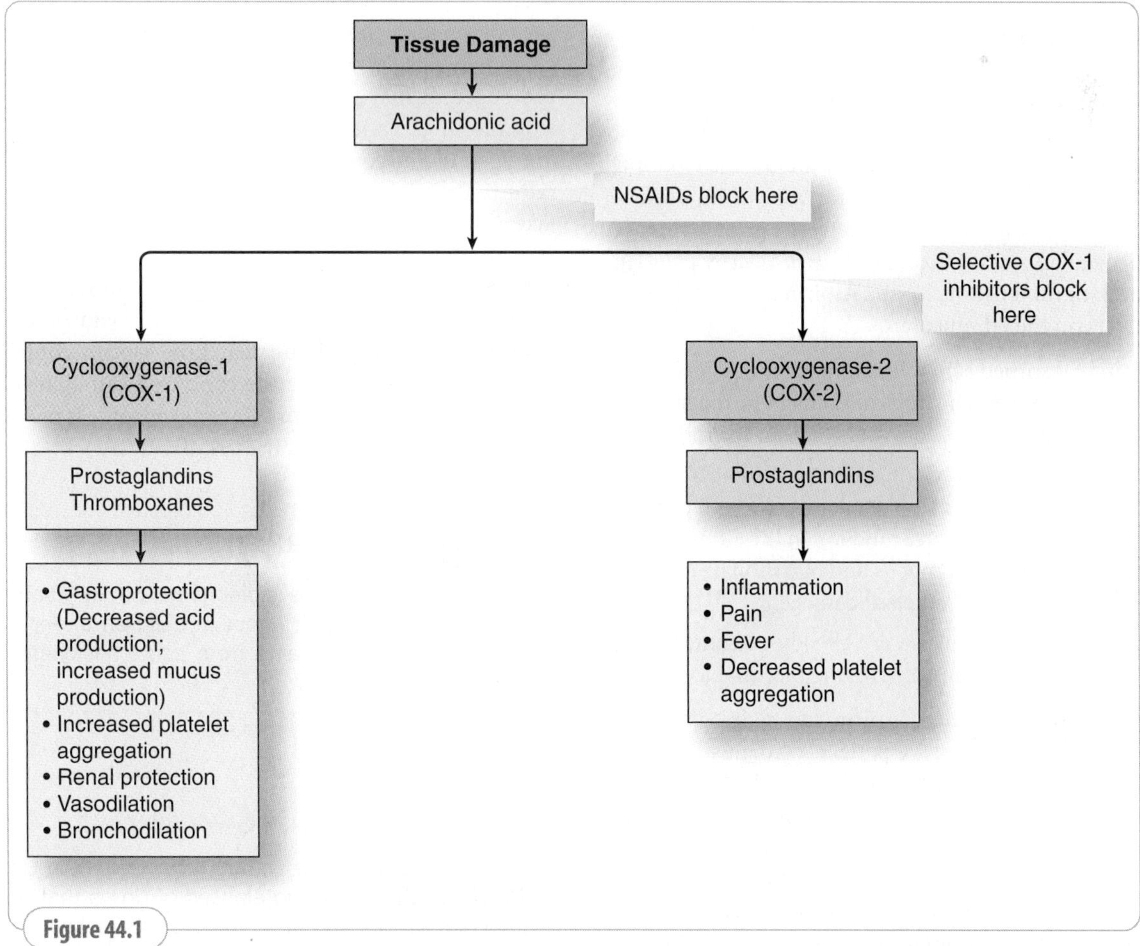

Figure 44.1

Inhibition of cyclooxygenase 1 and 2.

TABLE 44.1 Salicylates

Drug	Route and Adult Dose (maximum dose where indicated)	Adverse Effects
aspirin (Acetylsalicylic Acid)	Mild to moderate pain or fever: PO: 350–650 mg, every 4 h (max: 4 g/day) Arthritic conditions: PO: 3.6–5.4 g/day in four to six divided doses TIA prophylaxis: PO: 5–325 mg/day MI or thromboembolic disorder prophylaxis: PO: 80–325 mg/day	*Tinnitus, deafness, urticaria, nausea, vomiting, confusion, drowsiness, prolonged bleeding time, dyspepsia, stomach pain* Bronchospasm, anaphylactic shock, laryngeal edema, hemolytic anemia, salicylism, angioedema, Reye's syndrome, metabolic acidosis, severe GI bleeding, hepatotoxicity
choline and magnesium trisalicylate (Tricosal, Trilisate)	PO: 1.5–2.5 g/day in one to three divided doses (max: 3 g/day)	
magnesium salicylate (Doan's Pills, Magan, Mobidin)	Analgesic/antipyretic: PO: 650 mg tid or qid Arthritic conditions: PO: 9.6 g/day in divided doses (max: 4.8 g/day)	
salsalate (Amigesic, Salsitab, others)	PO: 325–3,000 mg/day in divided doses (max: 4 g/day)	

Note: *Italics* indicate common adverse effects. Underline indicates serious adverse effects.

other NSAIDs. For pain or fever relief, acetaminophen may be safely used in these patients.

The most significant adverse effect of aspirin and other NSAIDs is GI bleeding, which is shown in Pharmacotherapy Illustrated 44.1. Although the risk is dose related, even low doses of aspirin (75 to 325 mg/day) may double the risk of GI bleeding (Laine, 2006). Risk factors for aspirin-induced GI bleeding include history of peptic ulcers, age greater than 60, use of anticoagulants or corticosteroids, *Helicobacter pylori* infection, smoking, and use of alcohol. Aspirin has the following adverse effects on the GI mucosa:

- As aspirin is absorbed across the stomach mucosa, it causes direct cellular injury. This topical damage to the stomach may be lessened by the use of enteric coated formulations.
- After aspirin is absorbed systemically, it inhibits COX-1 and depletes the GI mucosa of prostaglandins. Prostaglandins normally provide a protective function in the GI mucosa by directing the secretion of mucus and bicarbonate and promoting cellular repair of mucosal damage.
- If GI damage or active ulcers are already present, the antiplatelet effects of aspirin will prolong bleeding.

In addition to GI bleeding, aspirin can cause dyspepsia, nausea, and ulcer perforation. For patients who must take high doses of aspirin, proton pump inhibitors (PPIs), such as omeprazole, may provide some degree of protection against GI damage by reducing acid secretion in the stomach. PPIs are effective and relatively safe drugs (see Chapter 60). An alternative therapy for GI protection is oral misoprostol (Cytotec), which is a prostaglandin. Misoprostol is a pregnancy category X drug, which limits its use in women with childbearing potential.

The antiplatelet effects of aspirin can promote bleeding at sites other than the GI tract. Because it irreversibly inhibits COX-1 in platelets, the antiplatelet action of aspirin can be prolonged. It may take longer for minor cuts and injuries to stop bleeding. Patients undergoing surgical or dental procedures should discontinue aspirin use a week prior to the procedure. Patients with known bleeding disorders should not take aspirin at all.

Children under age 19 should never be administered products that contain aspirin when they have flu symptoms, fever, or chickenpox, due to the risk of Reye's syndrome, a potentially fatal disease. It is unclear how aspirin contributes to Reye's syndrome, because the condition can appear without aspirin use. The incidence of Reye's syndrome is now very rare due to public awareness of the risk associated with aspirin use.

PharmFACT

Over 1,400 salicylate poisonings occur each year, about 4,000 of which occur in children under age 6. Approximately 30 deaths from acute salicylate overdose occur each year. *Source:* Kreplick, 2008.

CONNECTION Checkpoint 44.1

Aspirin is classified as an antiplatelet agent in Chapter 40. Name the other two classes of drugs that are antiplatelet agents and state the prototype drug for each class. See Answer to Connection Checkpoint 44.1 in Appendix A.

PHARMACOTHERAPY ILLUSTRATED 44.1

NSAID-Induced Ulcer Formation

(a)

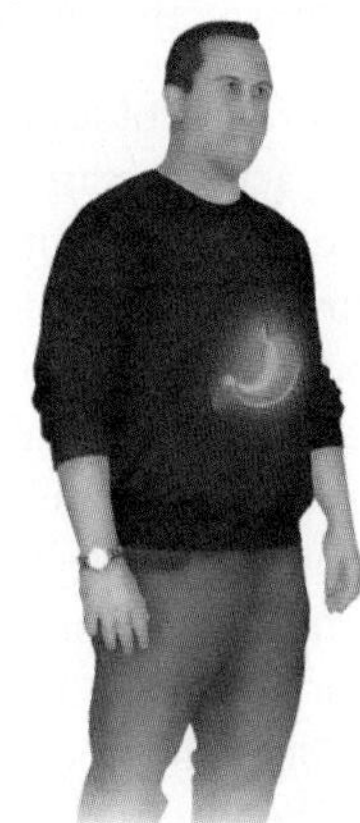

COX converts arachidonic acid to prostaglandins ( ).
- Less acid
- More mucus protection

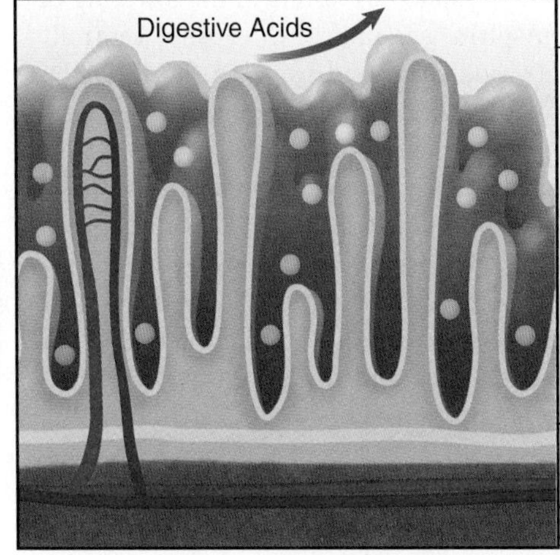

(b)

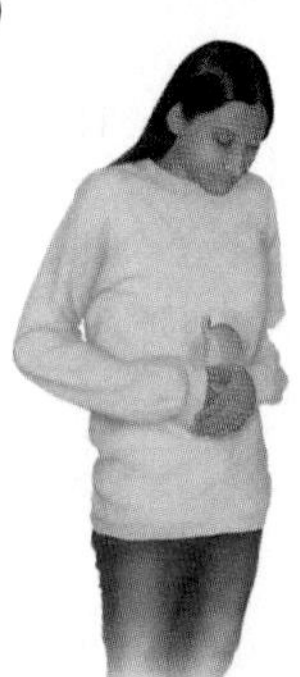

NSAIDs ( ) Inhibit COX and prevent prostaglandin formation.
- More acid/less mucus
- Direct irritation of mucosa

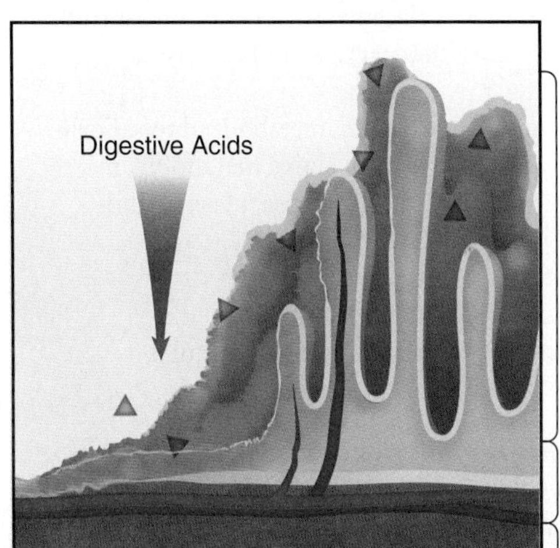

PROTOTYPE DRUG Aspirin (Acetylsalicylic acid)

Classification: **Therapeutic:** Nonnarcotic analgesic, antipyretic, antiplatelet

Pharmacologic: Salicylate, NSAID

Therapeutic Effects and Uses: Approved by the U.S. Food and Drug Administration (FDA) in 1939, aspirin is one of the best known medications. The ability of aspirin to reduce pain, inflammation, and fever makes it an extremely versatile and widely used drug. It is used to reduce pain and inflammation that is mild to moderate in intensity. The doses of aspirin needed to control severe pain or inflammation result in a high incidence of adverse effects.

Aspirin is approved by the FDA for the prevention of thromboembolic events. For example, aspirin is a first-line treatment for stroke prophylaxis in patients with a history of transient ischemic attacks or who have persistent or paroxysmal atrial fibrillation. It is approved for MI prophylaxis in patients who are at risk for a cardiac event and who are not already taking warfarin or an antiplatelet drug, including those with coronary artery disease who have already suffered an MI. To lower the risk of thromboembolic events, emergency medical services professionals administer aspirin to patients with a suspected coronary thrombosis prior to hospital arrival. Patients with a high risk for arterial thromboembolism may receive low-dose aspirin therapy.

An off-label use of aspirin is to prevent colorectal cancer. Regular, long-term aspirin use has been determined to reduce the risk of colorectal cancer. This significant benefit of aspirin is not apparent until more than 10 years of use with doses greater than 14 tablets per week (Chan et al., 2005). It is unclear whether the reduction in the incidence of colorectal cancer from aspirin is worth the increased risk of GI bleeding. The effectiveness of aspirin in preventing cancer is an area of current research.

Mechanism of Action: The anti-inflammatory action of aspirin is caused by the inhibition of COX-1 and COX-2 that leads to reduced prostaglandin synthesis. The analgesic action of aspirin occurs peripherally with limited action in the CNS on the hypothalamus. The suppression of prostaglandin synthesis in or near the hypothalamus results in the lowering of body temperature. Aspirin acts indirectly, causing centrally mediated peripheral vasodilation and sweating. The NSAIDs consist of three major classes: salicylates, ibuprofen and ibuprofen-like agents, and the selective cyclooxygenase-2 inhibitors. These drug classes are sometimes described as first-generation NSAIDs (salicylates and ibuprofen-like drugs) and second-generation NSAIDs (selective cyclooxygenase-2 inhibitors). There are over 20 first-generation NSAIDs and only one second-generation NSAID. The ibuprofen-like NSAIDs are described in Section 44.4 and the selective COX-2 inhibitors are presented in Section 44.5.

Pharmacokinetics:

Route(s)	Oral (PO), rectal
Absorption	80–100% absorbed
Distribution	Widely distributed; crosses the placenta; secreted in breast milk; 80–90% bound to plasma protein
Primary metabolism	Hepatic; metabolized to salicylic acid, an active metabolite, in the GI mucosa, plasma, and erythrocytes
Primary excretion	Renal
Onset of action	Rapid
Duration of action	Half-life: 15–20 minutes

Adverse Effects: A major adverse effect of aspirin is the risk of a serious hypersensitivity reaction, which is noted with symptoms such as bronchospasm, laryngeal edema, and anaphylaxis. It also causes significant stomach irritation, heartburn, nausea, vomiting, diarrhea, and stomach pain in 10% to 30% of patients. The risk of GI bleeding increases with dose. The hematologic adverse effects of aspirin administration include thrombocytopenia, hemolytic anemia, and occult bleeding. Long-term administration of aspirin may produce nephrotoxic effects and hepatotoxicity. Tinnitus and hearing loss are common adverse effects with high doses.

Contraindications/Precautions: Patients who have a hypersensitivity to any salicylate (including that found in foods) should not be administered aspirin or other NSAIDs. Patients who have the "aspirin triad," which includes aspirin allergy, nasal polyps, and asthma, should not be administered aspirin. Aspirin is also contraindicated in chronic rhinitis, acute bronchospasm, agranulocytosis, head trauma, increased intracranial pressure, history of GI bleeding, hypoprothrombinemia, vitamin K deficiency, congestive heart failure (CHF), pregnancy, and lactation. Children and teenagers should not be administered aspirin or products containing aspirin if they have a fever or a flulike illness. Patients over age 60 are especially prone to GI ulceration and bleeding due to aspirin. It should be used cautiously in patients with hypothyroidism, immunosuppression, asthma, and gout. It should also be used cautiously in patients with renal and hepatic impairment, G6PD deficiency, anemia, preoperatively, and in the presence of Hodgkin's disease. Aspirin should not be taken during pregnancy, especially in the third trimester; it may prolong bleeding and inhibit natural contractions caused by prostaglandins in the uterus.

Drug Interactions: Concurrent administration of aspirin with other salicylates such as 5-aminosalicylic acid increases the risk of salicylate toxicity. The combined use of aspirin with acetaminophen may cause additive nephrotoxicity. Ammonium chloride and other acidifying agents decrease the renal elimination of aspirin, resulting in salicylate toxicity. The administration of aspirin with anticoagulants, thrombolytics, or antiplatelet agents increases the patient's risk for bleeding. When oral antidiabetic agents are administered concurrently with high doses of aspirin, hypoglycemic activity increases. Patients who consume three or more alcoholic drinks per day may experience additive GI ulceration. Corticosteroids increase the risk of gastric irritation and result in ulcerogenic effects when administered with aspirin. Methotrexate administered with aspirin results in methotrexate toxicity. Low doses of salicylates may antagonize the uricosuric effects of probenecid and sulfinpyrazone. The antihypertensive effects of beta blockers may decrease if administered concurrently with aspirin. **Herbal/Food:** The administration of dong quai, feverfew, garlic, ginger, horse chestnut, and red clover will increase the patient's risk for bleeding. Taking aspirin with caffeine will increase the rate of aspirin absorption. St. John's wort may increase sedation.

Pregnancy: Categories C (first and second trimester) and D (third trimester).

Treatment of Overdose: Acute or chronic overdose of aspirin is known as **salicylism,** which is defined as a serum salicylate level above 200 mcg/mL. The symptoms depend on the dose but include tinnitus, metabolic acidosis, hyperventilation, respiratory alkalosis (secondary to stimulation of the respiratory center), dehydration, agitation, CNS depression, nausea, and vomiting. Emesis, gastric lavage, and alkalinization of urine are indicated. Hemodialysis is of benefit in severe salicylate poisonings.

Nursing Responsibilities:

- Assess the patient for the effectiveness of the medication, such as reduction in fever, decrease in pain, and decrease in inflammation.
- Prior to administration, obtain a history of salicylate hypersensitivity and GI bleeding or ulcers.
- Assess the prothrombin time (PT) and international normalized ratio (INR) with concurrent anticoagulant use.
- Assess fasting blood glucose in patients with diabetes.
- Assess for aspirin toxicity in the elderly and in patients with asthma, nasal polyps, perennial vasomotor rhinitis, hay fever, or chronic urticaria.

Patient and Family Education:

- Do not administer to children or teenagers who have fever or flulike symptoms.

- Use enteric coated aspirin and take the drug with food if you experience nausea, vomiting, or abdominal pain. Take this drug with a full glass of water and maintain an adequate fluid intake during therapy.
- Do not crush or chew enteric coated or sustained release tablets.
- Discontinue aspirin therapy 7 to 14 days prior to surgery or a dental procedure.
- Discontinue aspirin use and report ringing or buzzing in the ears; impaired hearing; dizziness; unusual bruising or bleeding that is slow to stop; blood in vomit; or black, tarry stools.
- Do not increase the dose of aspirin above label instructions or higher than that recommended by the health care provider.
- Avoid alcohol use because it may irritate the stomach.
- Immediately notify the health care provider of any known or suspected pregnancy.

Drugs Similar to Aspirin (Acetylsalicylic Acid)

Agents that produce similar actions to aspirin include choline and magnesium trisalicylate, magnesium salicylate, and salsalate. Choline salicylate (Arthropan) was discontinued in 1997.

Choline and magnesium trisalicylate (Tricosal, Trilisate): Approved in 1938, this drug combines choline salicylate and magnesium salicylate. It is an oral drug approved for fever and mild to moderate pain and inflammation associated with osteoarthritis, RA, bursitis, and other muscle or joint conditions. This drug causes less GI irritation than aspirin, and it does not have any antiplatelet activity. Choline and magnesium trisalicylate should not be administered to patients with known hypersensitivity to other salicylates. Other contraindications and adverse effects are similar to those of aspirin. This drug is pregnancy category C.

Magnesium salicylate (Doan's Pills, Magan, Mobidin): Approved in 1938, magnesium salicylate is an oral drug approved for fever and mild to moderate pain and inflammation associated with osteoarthritis, RA, bursitis, and other muscle or joint conditions. It inhibits prostaglandin synthesis just as aspirin, but it is less potent and causes less GI irritation. Magnesium salicylate also has less effect on platelet aggregation than aspirin and thus poses less bleeding risk. Magnesium salicylate should not be administered to patients with known hypersensitivity to other salicylates. Other contraindications and adverse effects are similar to those of aspirin. This drug is pregnancy category C.

Salsalate (Amigesic, Salsitab, others): Approved in 1977, salsalate has analgesic properties similar to those of aspirin but it causes less gastric irritation. It is an oral drug approved to treat mild and moderate pain due to osteoarthritis and RA. Like other salicylates, salsalate produces its effects by inhibiting prostaglandin synthesis. It has little antipyretic activity. Salsalate has less effect on platelet aggregation and thus poses less bleeding risk than aspirin does. Salsalate should not be administered to patients with known hypersensitivity to other salicylates. Other contraindications and adverse effects are similar to those of aspirin. This drug is pregnancy category C.

Ibuprofen-Like Agents

44.4 Ibuprofen and similar nonsteroidal anti-inflammatory drugs are the most common drugs for treating mild to moderate pain and inflammation.

In the 1950s researchers began searching for safer alternatives to aspirin or corticosteroids for treating the severe inflammation of RA. An exhaustive search of over 600 potential compounds over a 15-year period resulted in the discovery of ibuprofen, one of the safest and most widely prescribed NSAIDs in the world. The drug was introduced in the United States in 1974, and it became one of the first prescription-only drugs that were changed to OTC status in 1984.

Since the discovery of ibuprofen, over 20 other nonaspirin NSAIDs have been approved by the FDA. Although their chemical structures vary, they are grouped as "ibuprofen-like" because they share the same actions and adverse effects as the original drug. Doses for the NSAIDs are listed in Table 44.2. When used at recommended doses, NSAIDs have the following similarities:

- All have the same mechanism of action: They inhibit both COX-1 and COX-2.
- All have analgesic properties: Most are used to treat mild to moderate pain.
- All have anti-inflammatory properties: Most are specifically approved for osteoarthritis and RA.
- All have antipyretic properties, although not all of them are approved for this indication.
- Most are weak acids that are readily absorbed in the stomach.
- Most are strongly bound to albumin in the blood.
- Most are metabolized in the liver to inactive metabolites, which are excreted by the kidneys.
- All have the ability to cause damage to the GI mucosa, including bleeding and ulcer formation.
- Many pose an increased risk of cardiac events, such as heart failure and MI.
- Many are nephrotoxic at high doses.

From the preceding list, it should be obvious that the various nonaspirin NSAIDs have many similarities. Some of the NSAIDs have slightly different pharmacokinetic profiles. For example, some have longer half-lives or are available in sustained release formulations that permit once-daily dosing. Some are available by the parenteral route, and a few are formulated for children. Some are enteric coated, which may reduce stomach pain but does not appear to be protective against the formation of ulcers. Another consideration that is important to many consumers is cost. A month's supply of generic ibuprofen 200 mg or naproxen 220 mg costs less than $30 and is available OTC (Consumer Reports, 2005). At the opposite extreme are prescription-only celecoxib (Celebrex) 200 mg and flurbiprofen (Ansaid) 100 mg, which cost over $240 for a

TABLE 44.2 Nonaspirin NSAIDs and Acetaminophen

Drug	Route and Adult Dose (maximum dose where indicated)	Adverse Effects
acetaminophen paracetamol (Tylenol, Anacin, others)	PO: 325–650 mg every 4–6 h Rectal: 650 mg every 4–6 h (max: 4 g/day)	*Epigastric pain, abdominal pain* Hepatotoxicity, acute renal failure, GI bleeding
celecoxib (Celebrex)	PO: 100–200 mg bid or 200 mg PO daily (max: 800 mg/day)	*Back pain, peripheral edema, abdominal pain, dyspepsia, flatulence, dizziness, headache, insomnia, HTN* Increased risk of cardiovascular events, acute renal failure
diclofenac (Cataflam, Solaraze, Voltaren, others)	RA and osteoarthritis: PO: 150–200 mg/day in three to four divided doses Ankylosing spondylitis: 25 mg qid and 25 mg PO	*Dyspepsia, dizziness, headache, drowsiness, tinnitus, rash, pruritus, increased liver enzymes, prolonged bleeding time, edema, nausea, vomiting, occult blood loss* Peptic ulcer, GI bleeding, anaphylactic reactions with bronchospasm, blood dyscrasias, renal impairment, MI, CHF, hepatotoxicity
diflunisal (Dolobid)	PO: 1,000 mg followed by 500 mg every 8–12 h (max: 1,500 mg/day)	
etodolac	PO: 600–1,200 mg per day in two to four divided doses (max: 1,200 mg)	
fenoprofen (Nalfon)	PO: 200–600 mg tid or qid (max: 3,200 mg/day)	
flurbiprofen (Ansaid)	PO: 200–300 mg daily in two to four divided doses (max: 300 mg/day and 100 mg/dose)	
ibuprofen (Advil, Motrin, others)	Inflammatory disease: PO: 400–800 mg tid or qid (max: 3,200 mg/day) Pain, fever, dysmenorrhea: PO: 200–400 mg every 4–6 h (max: 1,200 mg/day)	
indomethacin (Indocin)	PO: 25–50 mg bid or tid (max: 200 mg/day and 100 mg/dose)	
ketoprofen	PO: 25–75 mg tid or qid (max: 300 mg/day) PO: 200 mg extended release once daily	
ketorolac (Acular, Toradol)	IM/IV: 30–60 mg loading dose, then 15–30 mg qid (max: 150 mg/day then 120 mg for subsequent days) PO: 10 mg qid prn (max: 40 mg/day) Maximum duration for all routes: 5 days	
meclofenamate	PO: 100–400 mg/day in three to four divided doses (max: 400 mg/day)	
mefenamic acid (Ponstel)	PO: 500 mg loading dose followed by 250 mg maintenance dose qid (max: 1,250 mg/day for no longer than 7 days)	
meloxicam (Mobic)	PO: 7.5–15 mg once daily (max: 15 mg/day)	
nabumetone	PO: 1,000 mg daily as a single dose (max: 2,000 mg/day in one to two divided doses)	
naproxen (Aleve, Anaprox, Naprosyn, others)	PO: 250–500 mg bid (naproxen/naproxen controlled release max: 1,500 mg/day; naproxen sodium max: 1,650/day; nonprescription max: 660 mg/day)	
oxaprozin (Daypro)	PO: 600–1,200 mg daily (max: 1,800 mg/day or 26 mg/kg whichever is lower)	
piroxicam (Feldene)	PO: 20 mg once daily (max: 20 mg/day)	
sulindac (Clinoril)	PO: 150–200 mg bid (max: 400 mg/day)	
tolmetin (Tolectin)	PO: 400 mg tid initially then maintenance dose of 600–1,800 mg/day in three to four divided doses (max: 1,800 mg/day)	

Note: *Italics* indicate common adverse effects. Underline indicates serious adverse effects.

monthly supply. Indications for each of the NSAIDs are shown in Table 44.3.

There are important differences between aspirin and the ibuprofen-like agents in their effects on the blood and heart. Although ibuprofen-like drugs affect blood coagulation, their action is short-lived and they are relatively safe to use with anticoagulants. Because they have less effect on coagulation, the ibuprofen-like agents are not used for the prophylaxis of adverse cardiac events. In fact, some of the nonaspirin NSAIDs such as indomethacin and sulindac significantly increase the risk of cardiovascular events. Caution should be used with all the nonaspirin NSAIDs when they are given for prolonged periods to patients with a history of cardiac disease.

NSAIDs are considered equivalent to aspirin in their effectiveness for treating pain, inflammation, and fever. For the occasional user who takes the medications at recommended doses and who has no risk factors, the drugs are very safe and rarely produce any significant adverse effects. For patients who must take high doses for a chronic illness, ibuprofen appears to cause less GI bleeding than aspirin, although both drugs place patients at high risk for GI damage.

PROTOTYPE DRUG Ibuprofen (Advil, Motrin, others)

Classification: **Therapeutic:** Analgesic, anti-inflammatory drug, antipyretic
Pharmacologic: NSAID

Therapeutic Effects and Uses: Approved in 1974, ibuprofen was the first nonaspirin NSAID marketed in the United States. Like aspirin, it possesses analgesic, anti-inflammatory, and antipyretic properties. It is indicated for the relief of fever and mild to moderate pain associated with chronic symptomatic RA and osteoarthritis, myalgia, headache, dental pain, and dysmenorrhea. Chewable

MyNursingKit Mechanism of Action Animation: Naproxen

TABLE 44.3 Indications for Selected Nonsteroidal Anti-Inflammatory Drugs

NSAID	Arthritis	Mild to Moderate Pain	Fever	Dysmenorrhea	Other Approved Indications
celecoxib (Celebrex)	*A	A		A	Ankylosing spondylitis, familial adenomatous polyposis
diclofenac (Cataflam, Solaraze, Voltaren, others)	A	A		A	Ankylosing spondylitis, actinic keratosis (topical); ocular pain and inflammation (ophthalmic)
diflunisal	A	A			
etodolac	A	A			
fenoprofen (Nalfon)	A	A			
flurbiprofen (Ansaid)	A				Miosis inhibition (ophthalmic)
ibuprofen (Advil, Motrin, others)	A	A	A	A	Acute migraine
indomethacin (Indocin)	A	A			Ankylosing spondylitis; close patent ductus arteriosus (IV)
ketoprofen (Orudis, Oruvail)	A	A	A	A	
ketorolac (Acular, Toradol)		A			Allergic conjunctivitis; reduce ocular pain and inflammation (ophthalmic)
meclofenamate	A	A		A	
mefenamic acid (Ponstel)		A		A	
meloxicam (Mobic)	A				
nabumetone	A				
naproxen (Aleve, Anaprox, Naprosyn, others)	A	A	A	A	Ankylosing spondylitis
oxaprozin (Daypro)	A				
piroxicam (Feldene)	A				
sulindac (Clinoril)	A				Ankylosing spondylitis
tolmetin (Tolectin)	A				

*A = FDA Approved.

tablets, drops, and solutions are available in low doses for administration to children.

Unlike aspirin, ibuprofen is not indicated to treat or prevent any cardiovascular conditions. Ibuprofen inhibits platelet aggregation and prolongs the bleeding time without affecting the PT or whole blood clotting times. Its effects on platelets are reversible within 24 hours after discontinuation of the drug.

Ibuprofen lysine (NeoProfen) is an intravenous (IV) form of the drug that was approved in 2006 to close patent ductus arteriosus in premature infants. The drug has a 75% success rate in infants who are no more than 32 weeks gestational age. Although the mechanism of action is not known, it is believed that prostaglandins delay closing of the ductus. By blocking prostaglandin synthesis with ibuprofen, the ductus closes.

Mechanism of Action: Ibuprofen inhibits COX-1 and COX-2, which block prostaglandin synthesis and modulate T-cell function. Ibuprofen inhibits inflammatory cell chemotaxis, decreases the release of superoxide radicals, and increases the scavenging of these products at the inflammatory sites.

Pharmacokinetics:

Route(s)	PO
Absorption	80% absorbed
Distribution	Crosses the placenta; unknown if secreted in breast milk; highly protein bound
Primary metabolism	Hepatic
Primary excretion	Renal; small amount biliary
Onset of action	1 h
Duration of action	6–8 h

Adverse Effects: In low to moderate doses, ibuprofen is well tolerated and serious adverse effects are uncommon. The most frequent adverse events are GI related and include bleeding, anorexia, heartburn, nausea, vomiting, and constipation or diarrhea. Adverse CNS effects include dizziness, headache, drowsiness, and light-headedness. Other possible adverse effects include hypotension, CHF, peripheral edema, occult blood loss, aplastic anemia, leukopenia, decreased hemoglobin and hematocrit, and increased aspartate transaminase (AST) and alanine transaminase (ALT). Chronic use of ibuprofen may lead to renal impairment, including acute renal failure, polyuria, azotemia, cystitis, hematuria, and increased creatinine and blood urea nitrogen (BUN) levels.

Contraindications/Precautions: Patients who have a known allergy to aspirin or other NSAIDs should not be administered ibuprofen. In addition, patients who have been diagnosed with PUD, bleeding abnormalities, and perioperative pain related to coronary artery bypass graft (CABG) should not receive ibuprofen. The drug should be used cautiously in patients with hypertension (HTN), history of GI bleeding, diabetes mellitus, and impaired renal or hepatic function. It should also be used cautiously in patients who have heart failure, serious HTN, or a history of stroke or MI. Children with asthma may experience diminished respiratory function when administered ibuprofen. Patients with severe hepatic impairment should not receive ibuprofen because the drug can accumulate to toxic levels.

Drug Interactions: Oral anticoagulants taken with ibuprofen may increase the risk of bleeding. Ibuprofen may increase the toxicity of digoxin, lithium, or methotrexate if taken concurrently. Use with other NSAIDs, alcohol, or corticosteroids may cause serious adverse GI events. The antihypertensive action of diuretics, beta blockers, and angiotensin-converting enzyme (ACE) inhibitors may be reduced if taken with ibuprofen. **Herbal/Food:** Ibuprofen combined with feverfew, garlic, ginger, and ginkgo may result in an increased risk of bleeding.

Pregnancy: Categories B (first and second trimesters) and D (third trimester).

Treatment of Overdose: Overdose may lead to acute renal failure, apnea, cyanosis, drowsiness, GI bleeding, nausea, vomiting, and sweating. Treatment is supportive and includes the administration of activated charcoal and nasogastric suction.

Nursing Responsibilities:

- Notify the prescriber before initiating therapy if the patient has a history of PUD, bleeding abnormalities, and perioperative pain related to CABG.
- Assess the patient for the effectiveness of the medication, such as reduction in fever, decrease in pain, or decrease in inflammation.
- Monitor for cardiac responses to the medication and assess for signs and symptoms of fluid retention.
- Monitor BUN and creatinine levels to determine renal toxicity.
- Assess complete blood count (CBC) and liver function studies (AST and ALT), and report abnormal values to the prescriber.

Patient and Family Education:

- Notify the health care provider of blood in vomit, black tarry stools, coffee ground emesis, or GI discomfort.
- Do not take products containing aspirin or other analgesics concurrently with ibuprofen, unless approved by the health care provider.
- Do not drink alcohol because this may cause stomach irritation.
- Refrain from smoking because this may contribute to peptic ulcer formation.
- Take this drug with food or milk to reduce GI discomfort.
- Immediately report unusual bruising to the health care provider.
- Use sun block, wear protective clothing, and avoid prolonged exposure to sunlight.
- Immediately notify the health care provider of any known or suspected pregnancy.
- Immediately report signs of allergic reaction such as difficulty breathing or wheezing, skin rash, hives, itching, or swelling of eyelids, throat, or lips to the health care provider.
- Notify the health care provider if symptoms do not improve within a few days. Do not increase the dose or take the drug more frequently unless approved by the health care provider.

CONNECTIONS

Evidence-Based Practice Nonsteroidal Anti-Inflammatory Drugs

Clinical Question

Can the administration of nonsteroidal anti-inflammatory drugs (NSAIDs) benefit patients with Alzheimer's disease, Parkinson's disease, or Huntington's disease?

Evidence

According to a study that was published in *Current Alzheimer's Research*, inflammation is a characteristic sign of many neurodegenerative diseases such as Alzheimer's disease, Parkinson's disease, and Huntington's disease. Epidemiologic research indicates that anti-inflammatory agents, particularly nonsteroidal anti-inflammatory agents, provide a sparing effect on patients who suffer from these neurodegenerative diseases. The research indicates that the inflammation leads to negative consequences of the diseases. In animal studies classic NSAIDs slowed the progression or delayed the onset of Alzheimer's disease.

Implication

The study suggests that several classes of anti-inflammatory drugs have been identified as beneficial in similar assay systems. It is recommended that a combination therapy of anti-inflammatory agents be studied since they may possess different mechanisms of action which will yield a more beneficial outcome.

Critical Thinking Question

What possible problems could exist if a patient's family member discovers the findings from this study through such venues as the newspaper or television?

Source: From "Nonsteroidal Anti-Inflammatory Drugs (NSAIDs) and Other Anti-Inflammatory Agents in the Treatment of Neurodegenerative Disease," by A. Klegeris and P. L. McGeer, 2005, *Current Alzheimer Research, 2*(3), pp. 355–365.

Drugs Similar to Ibuprofen (Advil, Motrin, Others)

There are a number of subclasses of NSAIDs that are based on the chemical structures of the molecules. These subclasses include the propionic acids (e.g., ibuprofen), phenylacetic acids (e.g., diclofenac), indole acetic acids (e.g., indomethacin), fenamates (e.g., mefenamic acid), ketones (e.g., nabumetone), and oxicams (e.g., piroxicam). From a clinical perspective, the nonaspirin NSAIDs are remarkably similar to ibuprofen. Doses and indications for these drugs differ, as listed in Tables 44.2 and 44.3.

PharmFACT

It is estimated that NSAIDs cause 16,500 deaths annually, largely as a result of GI complications. This is more mortality than is caused from gastric cancer. *Source:* Taha et al., 2007.

CONNECTION *Checkpoint* 44.2

Several NSAIDs are approved to treat mild migraines. From what you learned in Chapter 29, what non-NSAID drug classes are used to terminate severe migraine episodes? See Answer to Connection Checkpoint 44.2 in Appendix A.

Cyclooxygenase-2 Inhibitors

44.5 Celecoxib is an effective second-generation nonsteroidal anti-inflammatory drug, but its use is limited due to an increased risk of myocardial infarction and stroke.

Celecoxib (Celebrex) is a second-generation NSAID that blocks COX-2 without inhibiting COX-1. The selective inhibition of COX-2 produces the analgesic, anti-inflammatory, and antipyretic effects typical of other NSAIDs, but without causing platelet aggregation or GI irritation. The primary advantage of celecoxib is that it causes less GI bleeding and ulcer formation than aspirin or ibuprofen. This medication is the newest and most controversial of the NSAIDs.

The ability to treat arthritis without adverse effects caused excitement throughout the medical field in the 1990s, and the three drugs originally in this class were widely prescribed. This elation quickly ended when postmarketing data revealed that rofecoxib (Vioxx) doubled the risk of MI and strokes in patients taking the drug for extended periods. At that time, more than 84 million people had used rofecoxib since its approval in 1999. Based on the research data, the drug manufacturer voluntarily removed rofecoxib from the market. Shortly afterward a second COX-2 inhibitor, valdecoxib (Bextra), was also voluntarily withdrawn, leaving celecoxib (Celebrex) the sole drug in this class. A large number of lawsuits were subsequently filed, and the marketing of new COX-2 inhibitors has ground to a halt in the United States. Other selective COX-2 inhibitors are still available outside the United States.

PROTOTYPE DRUG Celecoxib (Celebrex)

Classification: **Therapeutic:** Anti-inflammatory
Pharmacologic: COX-2 inhibitor, NSAID

Therapeutic Effects and Uses: Celecoxib is approved to treat mild to moderate pain and inflammation associated with RA, osteoarthritis, dysmenorrhea, dental procedures, headache, and ankylosing spondylitis. It is also an effective antipyretic agent. The effectiveness of celecoxib at reducing pain and inflammation is equivalent to that of other NSAIDs.

In addition to its anti-inflammatory indications, celecoxib also is used for the prohylaxis of adenomas or colorectal polyps in adults with familial adenomatous polyposis (FAP). Patients with this condition have an inherited mutation in a gene that results in hundreds of polyps and an almost 100% risk of colon cancer. Although celecoxib reduces the number of polyps in these patients, it has not been proven to reduce the risk of malignancies.

Mechanism of Action: Celecoxib selectively inhibits the enzyme COX-2. It inhibits prostaglandin synthesis to reduce inflammation. This action relieves pain and inflammation in the joints and smooth muscle tissue.

Pharmacokinetics:

Route(s)	PO
Absorption	Well absorbed
Distribution	Widely distributed; is likely secreted in breast milk; 97% protein bound
Primary metabolism	Hepatic by CYP2C9
Primary excretion	Primarily feces (57%), with some in urine (27%)
Onset of action	Peak: 3 h
Duration of action	Half-life: 11.2 h

Adverse Effects: The selective COX-2 inhibitors have been found to increase the risk of serious cardiovascular events, including fatal MI and stroke. Celecoxib produces the same GI-related adverse effects as other NSAIDs but at a lower rate. GI adverse effects include GI bleeding, ulcers, abdominal pain, diarrhea, dyspepsia, flatulence, and nausea. CNS adverse effects include headache, dizziness, and insomnia. Cardiovascular adverse effects include HTN, MI, and peripheral edema. Adverse effects of the integumentary system are generally rare and include erythema multiforme, exfoliative dermatitis, rash, Stevens-Johnson syndrome, and toxic epidermal necrolysis. Some patients have reported pharyngitis, rhinitis, sinusitis, and upper respiratory infection. The long-term use of celecoxib may cause renal and hepatic impairment.

Contraindications/Precautions: Celecoxib should not be administered to patients with hepatic insufficiency because the primary site of drug metabolism is the liver. It is also contraindicated in patients with advanced renal disease. Celecoxib is contraindicated in patients with anemia or in the postoperative phase of a CABG. Celecoxib is administered cautiously in patients who are CYP2C9 poor metabolizers. This drug is contraindicated in patients with a history of GI bleeding or PUD, and it should be administered with caution to patients receiving anticoagulants. Patients with a history of asthma, bone marrow suppression, cerebrovascular accident (CVA), peripheral vascular disease, elevated liver function tests, heart failure, kidney disease, and fluid retention should be administered celecoxib cautiously.

Drug Interactions: If taken with celecoxib, oral coagulation modifiers such as clopidogrel or warfarin may cause an increased risk of bleeding. Celecoxib may increase the toxicity of lithium if taken concurrently. Use with alcohol, corticosteroids, aspirin, or other NSAIDs may cause serious adverse GI events. The antihypertensive action of diuretics or ACE inhibitors may be reduced if taken with celecoxib. Concurrent use with fluconazole may increase serum celecoxib levels.

Herbal/Food: Feverfew, garlic, ginger, ginkgo, horse chestnut, and red clover may increase the risk of bleeding if used during celecoxib therapy.

Pregnancy: Category C; Category D in the third trimester.

Treatment of Overdose: Overdose may cause acute renal failure, apnea, cyanosis, drowsiness, GI bleeding, nausea, vomiting, and sweating. Treatment is supportive and includes the administration of activated charcoal and nasogastric suction.

Nursing Responsibilities:

- Assess the patient's pain level using a scale of 0 (no pain) to 10 (worst possible pain).
- Notify the prescriber before initiating therapy if the patient has a history of hepatic insufficiency, advanced renal disease, anemia, GI bleeding, or PUD, or if the patient is in the postoperative phase of a CABG.
- Assess the patient for the effectiveness of the medication, such as decreased pain and inflammation.
- Periodically monitor liver enzymes, CBC, and renal function.
- Monitor PT and INR when administered with warfarin.
- Assess for fluid retention and edema in patients with a history of HTN and CHF.
- Monitor for signs of drug-induced heart disease or stroke.

Patient and Family Education:

- Do not drink alcohol because this may cause stomach irritation.
- Promptly report unusual weight gain, fatigue, edema, or rash to the health care provider.
- Report any signs of potential liver toxicity, including jaundice, yellowing of the eyes, clay-colored stools, or dark urine to the health care provider.
- Notify the health care provider of blood in vomit, black tarry stools, coffee ground emesis, or GI discomfort.
- Do not take products containing aspirin or other analgesics concurrently with celecoxib, unless approved by the health care provider.
- Immediately notify the health care provider of any chest pain, slurred speech, or weakness on one side of the body.
- Immediately notify the health care provider of any known or suspected pregnancy.
- Notify the health care provider if symptoms have not improved within a few days. Do not increase the dose or take the drug more frequently unless approved by the health care provider.

Drugs Similar to Celecoxib (Celebrex)

Celecoxib (Celebrex) is the sole medication in this class.

Antipyretic and Analgesic Agent

44.6 Acetaminophen is administered for pain relief and to reduce fever, but it has no anti-inflammatory properties.

Acetaminophen (Tylenol) is administered for pain relief and to reduce fever. Unlike aspirin, ibuprofen, and celecoxib, acet-

CONNECTIONS

Patient Safety

Soundalike Drugs

Mary Clark will be discharged today from the hospital. Earlier this week she slipped on the icy pavement and injured her back. She has been given a prescription for celecoxib (Celebrex). While she is preparing to leave the hospital she mentions to the nurse that the new medication written on the prescription sounded a lot like the medication she routinely takes for depression (Celexa). What should the nurse do?

See Answers to Patient Safety Questions in Appendix A.

aminophen has no anti-inflammatory properties and therefore cannot be classified as an NSAID. Acetaminophen has equal effectiveness to the NSAIDs in reducing pain and fever, and it is often a drug of choice for treating noninflammatory pain. It is the primary alternative to NSAIDs when patients have a contraindication to taking aspirin or ibuprofen. Acetaminophen is frequently combined with other OTC drugs in treating severe flu symptoms. It is often combined with opioid analgesics; adding acetaminophen provides additive pain relief and allows for lower doses of the narcotic (see Chapter 29).

Acetaminophen has no effect on platelet aggregation and does not exhibit cardiotoxicity. Most importantly, it does not cause GI bleeding or ulcers, as do the NSAIDs.

PROTOTYPE DRUG Acetaminophen (Tylenol)

Classification: **Therapeutic:** Nonopioid analgesic, antipyretic
Pharmacologic: Para-aminophenol derivative

Therapeutic Effects and Uses: Approved in 1950, acetaminophen relieves mild to moderate pain but has no effect on

NURSING PROCESS APPLICATION

Patients Receiving NSAID Therapy

Assessment	Potential Nursing Diagnoses
Prior to administration: • Obtain a complete health history (psychosocial and physical), including the origin of fever, recent surgeries, or trauma. • Observe vital signs; assess in context of the patient's baseline values. • Obtain the patient's complete medication history, including nicotine and alcohol consumption and use of herbal supplement and alternative therapies to determine possible drug use of allergies or interactions.	• *Acute Pain,* related to the inflammatory process • *Hyperthermia,* related to the inflammatory process • *Risk for Injury,* related to adverse effects of drug therapy, including occult blood loss, nephrotoxicity, toxic hepatitis, anaphylaxis

Planning: Patient Goals and Expected Outcomes

The patient will:

- Experience decreased pain at the site of injury.
- Experience a reduction in body temperature.
- Experience a decrease in the inflammatory process.
- Demonstrate an understanding of the drug's action by accurately describing the medication's adverse effects, contraindications, precautions, and implications for administration.
- Experience no gastric discomfort and bleeding.

Implementation

Interventions and (Rationales)	Patient and Family Education
	Instruct the patient or family to:
• Monitor current medications for contraindications such as anticoagulants or hypersensitivity to aspirin. (NSAIDs may promote bleeding tendencies)	• Consult with the health care provider prior to taking NSAIDs if concurrently prescribed other medications. • Consult the prescriber for episodes of unexplained bleeding or ecchymosis. Discontinue the use of the NSAID.
• Monitor for gastric irritation and bleeding. (Gastric bleeding is the most significant adverse effect).	• Report gastric pain, chronic indigestion, dyspepsia, or vomiting blood to the prescriber.
• Monitor hepatic and renal function. (Antipyretic agents are metabolized in the liver and excreted in the kidneys)	• Report signs of liver toxicity: nausea, vomiting, anorexia, bleeding, severe upper or lower abdominal pain, heartburn, jaundice, or a change in the color or character of stools to the health care provider.
• Administer with caution to patients with a history of excessive alcohol consumption. (Alcohol increases the risk of liver damage associated with NSAID administration.)	• Abstain from alcohol while taking NSAIDs.

Evaluation of Outcome Criteria

Evaluate the effectiveness of drug therapy by confirming that patient goals and expected outcomes have been met (see "Planning").

MyNursingKit | Mechanism of Action Animation: Acetaminophen

inflammation. Acetaminophen is approved to treat pain associated with osteoarthritis of the hip or knee, dysmenorrhea, dental procedures, headache, and myalgia. It is also an effective antipyretic agent. It is a drug of choice for treating fever. Acetaminophen is administered as a substitute for aspirin when NSAIDs are contraindicated due to age, allergy, or gastric irritation. It is not linked with Reye's syndrome, as is aspirin; thus it is safe to administer to infants, children, and adolescents who have flulike symptoms or chickenpox.

Acetaminophen is available by the oral (suspension, tablets, chewable tablets, extended release tablets, and oral granules) or rectal routes. Childhood and infant preparations are available.

Mechanism of Action: Acetaminophen acts centrally in the CNS by inhibiting COX. It has no effect on COX in peripheral tissues. It also may inhibit the chemical mediators of pain, but its mechanism is unclear. The reduction of fever occurs by its direct action on the heat-regulating center of the hypothalamus to produce peripheral vasodilation, sweating, and dissipation of heat.

Pharmacokinetics:

Route(s)	PO, rectal
Absorption	Rapid and complete absorption
Distribution	Distributed to all body fluids; crosses the placenta; secreted in breast milk; 25% bound to plasma protein
Primary metabolism	Hepatic
Primary excretion	Renal
Onset of action	Peak: 30–60 minutes
Duration of action	1–3 h

Adverse Effects: At recommended doses, acetaminophen is well tolerated and serious adverse effects are rare. The risk for adverse effects is dose related and increases with the long-term use of this drug. Acute acetaminophen poisoning is very serious, and symptoms include anorexia, nausea, vomiting, dizziness, lethargy, diaphoresis, chills, epigastric or abdominal pain, and diarrhea. Excessive acetaminophen use is the number one cause of acute hepatic failure in the United States. The onset of hepatotoxicity is noted with elevated transaminases (ALT, AST) and bilirubin. The patient will also have hypoglycemia, hepatic coma, and acute renal failure. Chronic ingestion of acetaminophen results in neutropenia, pancytopenia, leukopenia, thrombocytopenic purpura, hepatotoxicity in alcoholics, and renal damage.

Contraindications/Precautions: Patients who are allergic to acetaminophen should not be administered this medication. It should be used cautiously in patients with anemia, G6PD deficiency, or hepatic disease. Acetaminophen should be administered cautiously to patients with rheumatoid or osteoarthritis, malnutrition, bone marrow depression, and immunosuppression. Chronic administration of acetaminophen should be avoided in patients with renal impairment because this drug can worsen kidney function.

Drug Interactions: Acetaminophen should not be administered with alcohol or to patients who consume alcohol with regularity because this greatly increases the risk of hepatotoxicity. Alcohol-induced hepatotoxicity can occur at therapeutic doses of acetaminophen. Due to additive hepatotoxic effects, acetaminophen should not be administered with barbiturates, carbamazepine, diphenylhydantoin, isoniazid, rifampin, and sulfinpyrazone. Acetaminophen will decrease lamotrigine levels, if the drugs are administered concurrently. Long-term use of acetaminophen and warfarin will result in increased hypoprothrombinemic effects. Zidovudine administered with acetaminophen may increase the risk of bone marrow suppression. **Herbal/Food:** Caffeine will enhance the analgesic effects of acetaminophen. Hepatotoxicity has been reported with concurrent echinacea use.

Pregnancy: Category B.

Treatment of Overdose: Acetaminophen overdose is treated with oral or IV acetylcysteine (Acetadote). For maximum effectiveness, the antidote should be administered within 8 hours of acetaminophen ingestion. The IV form (Acetadote) is administered by the "three-bag method."

- Loading Dose. Dilute 150 mg/kg in 200 mL of 5% dextrose and administer over 60 minutes.
- Second Dose. Dilute 50 mg/kg in 500 mL of 5% dextrose and administer over 4 hours.
- Third Dose. Dilute 100 mg/kg in 1,000 mL of 5% dextrose and administer over 16 hours.

Nursing Responsibilities:

- Assess the patient's recent drug history. Because many OTC products contain acetaminophen, calculate the total dose accordingly.
- Assess the patient for the effectiveness of the medication, such as reduced fever or decreased pain.
- Perform baseline and periodic liver function tests (AST and ALT) and monitor for signs and symptoms of hepatotoxicity during therapy.
- Assess the patient's level of alcohol use to reveal potential underlying liver disease.

Patient and Family Education:

- Notify the health care provider if symptoms have not improved within a few days. Do not increase the dose or take the drug more frequently unless approved by the health care provider.
- If fever lasts more than 3 days seek immediate medical attention.
- Do not drink alcohol because the combination of alcohol and acetaminophen can cause serious and even fatal liver damage.
- Report any signs of potential liver toxicity, including jaundice, yellowing of eyes, clay-colored stools, or dark urine.
- Keep this drug in a secure location away from small children to prevent accidental overdose, which can be fatal.

Drugs Similar to Acetaminophen (Tylenol)

Acetaminophen is the only medication in this class.

UNDERSTANDING THE CHAPTER

Key Concepts Summary

44.1 Inflammation is a nonspecific body response to antigens and tissue injury.

44.2 Treatment of inflammation includes nonpharmacologic therapies and the administration of anti-inflammatory drugs.

44.3 Aspirin is an inexpensive, effective, first-generation nonsteroidal anti-inflammatory drug commonly used by adults.

44.4 Ibuprofen and similar nonsteroidal anti-inflammatory drugs are the most common drugs for treating mild to moderate pain and inflammation.

44.5 Celecoxib is an effective second-generation nonsteroidal anti-inflammatory drug, but its use is limited due to an increased risk of myocardial infarction and stroke.

44.6 Acetaminophen is administered for pain relief and to reduce fever, but it has no anti-inflammatory properties.

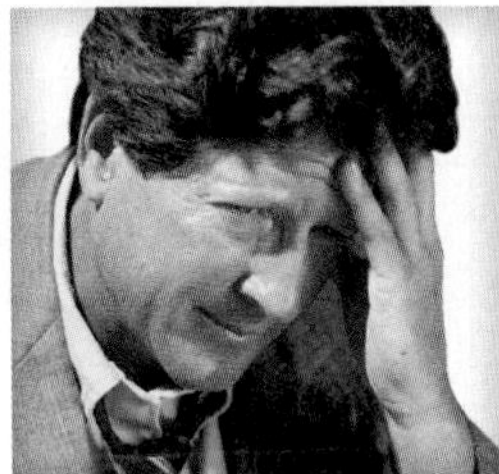

Making the PATIENT *Connection*

Remember the patient "Gene Tallo" at the beginning of the chapter? Now read the remainder of the case study. Based on the information presented within this chapter, respond to the critical thinking questions that follow.

Gene Tallo is a 48-year-old male patient who has developed flulike symptoms, which include muscle aches, sore throat, clear nasal drainage, and cough. His temperature is 39°C (102.4°F); pulse, 88 beats/minute; respiration, 24/minute with scattered wheezes in the upper lobes; and blood pressure of 124/70 mmHg. He developed a temperature today with chills and headache.

The health care provider ordered ibuprofen 400 mg every 4 to 6 hours as needed for muscle aches and fever. The patient is concerned as to why ibuprofen is being given for fever. He understands that ibuprofen is given for inflammation but is concerned about how it will work for fever. As the office nurse you need to provide patient education to the patient.

Critical Thinking Questions

1. Describe the pathophysiology of fever and inflammation.
2. Why is ibuprofen administered for fever?
3. What patient teaching about the administration of ibuprofen and care of flulike symptoms will you provide to Mr. Tallo?

Case Study

Tameeka Jones has a postoperative infection following a vaginal hysterectomy. The infection is noted at the site of the laparoscopic incision of the lower abdomen. She has developed a fever of 38.8°C (102°F). The health care provider has ordered acetaminophen (Tylenol) 650 mg by mouth every 4 to 6 hours as needed for the fever.

1. What is the action of acetaminophen (Tylenol)?
2. What pain medications should be avoided while the patient is receiving acetaminophen (Tylenol) for fever reduction?
3. What patient teaching is important for the patient who has a fever related to infection?

NCLEX-RN® Review

1 A 30-year-old client who suffers from depression has attempted suicide by overdosing on acetaminophen (Tylenol). The nurse in the emergency department will anticipate that the client's treatment will consist of:

1. An intravenous infusion with normal saline to infuse at 1,000 mL per hour.
2. The administration of acetylcysteine (Acetadote) by intravenous infusion.
3. Preparation for cardioversion due to the impending arrhythmia.
4. The assessment of liver enzymes to determine hepatotoxicity.

2 A client suffers from a fever and is allergic to aspirin. Which of the following medications will the nurse anticipate administering to reduce the client's fever?

1. Ibuprofen (Motrin, Advil)
2. Ketorolac tromethamine (Toradol)
3. Acetaminophen (Tylenol)
4. Celecoxib (Celebrex)

3 An anti-inflammatory agent is ordered to be given intravenously to the client for pain. Which of the following anti-inflammatory agents is administered parenterally?

1. Ketorolac (Toradol, Acular)
2. Ketoprofen (Oruvail)
3. Ibuprofen (Motrin, Advil)
4. Celecoxib (Celebrex)

4 An 80-year-old woman, who is scheduled for a total knee replacement next month, currently takes ibuprofen (Motrin, Advil) 600 mg three times per day. Which of the following client teaching interventions is most important?

1. Continue ibuprofen (Motrin, Advil) until surgery.
2. Stop ibuprofen (Motrin, Advil) today.
3. Decrease ibuprofen (Motrin, Advil) to two times per day.
4. Stop ibuprofen (Motrin, Advil) 7 to 14 days before surgery.

5 Acetaminophen (Tylenol) is prescribed for each of the following clients. A nurse should question the order for which client? A client

1. With cirrhosis of the liver.
2. With chronic obstructive pulmonary disease.
3. With breast cancer.
4. Who is taking warfarin (Coumadin).

6 A client takes aspirin (acetylsalicylic acid) daily for pain in the right knee. Which of the following toxic effects may be present with aspirin overdosage? Select all that apply.

1. Tinnitus
2. Hyperventilation
3. Gastrointestinal bleeding
4. Decreased urinary output
5. Peripheral neuropathy

See Answers to Critical Thinking Questions, Case Study, and NCLEX-RN® Review in Appendix A.

References

Ball, J. W., & Bindler, R. C. (2006). *Child health nursing: Partnering with children and families.* Upper Saddle River, NJ: Pearson Education.

Burke, A., Smythe, E. M., & Fitzgerald, G. A. (2006). Analgesic-antipyretic agents: Pharmacotherapy of gout. In L. L. Brunton, J. S. Lazo, & K.L. Parker (Eds.), *The pharmacological basis of therapeutics* (11th ed., pp. 671–716). New York: McGraw-Hill.

Chan, A. T., Giovannucci, E. L., Meyerhardt, J. A., Schernhammer, E. S., Curhan, G. C., & Fuchs, C. S. (2005). Long-term use of aspirin and nonsteroidal anti-inflammatory drugs and risk of colorectal cancer. *Journal of the American Medical Association, 294*(8), 914–923.

Consumer Reports. (2005). *Treating osteoarthritis and pain: The non-steroidal anti-inflammatory drugs: Comparing effectiveness, safety and price.* Retrieved July 22, 2008, from http://www.consumerreports.org/health/resources/pdf/best-buy-drugs/2pager_NSAIDs.pdf

Facts and Comparisons 4.0. (2005). *A review of natural products* (4th ed.). Philadelphia: Wolters Kluwer Health.

Klegeris, A., & McGeer, P. L. (2005). Non-steroidal anti-inflammatory drugs (NSAIDs) and other anti-inflammatory agents in the treatment of neurodegenerative disease. *Current Alzheimer Research, 2,* 355–365.

Kreplick, L. W. (2008). Toxicity, salicylate. *eMedicine.* Retrieved July 28, 2008, from http://www.emedicine.com/emerg/topic514.htm

Laine, L. (2006). Gastrointestinal bleeding with low-dose aspirin: What's the risk? *Alimentary Pharmacology and Therapeutics, 24*(6), 897–908.

National Center for Complementary and Alternative Medicine, National Institutes of Health. (2008). *Herbs at a glance: Goldenseal.* Retrieved July 22, 2008, from http://nccam.nih.gov/health/goldenseal/

Rostom, A., Muir, K., Dube, C., Jolicoeur, E., Boucher, M., Joyce, J., et al. (2007). Gastrointestinal safety of cyclooxygenase-2 inhibitors: A Cochrane collaboration systematic review. *Clinical Gastroenterology and Hepatology, 5*(7), 18–28.

Stillman, M. J., & Stillman, M. T. (2007). Choosing nonselective NSAIDs and selective COX-2 inhibitors in the elderly. A clinical use pathway. *Geriatrics, 62*(2), 26–34.

Taha, A. S., Angerson, W. J., Prasad, R., McCloskey, C., & Blatchford, O. (2007). Upper gastrointestinal bleeding and the changing use of COX-2 non-steroidal anti-inflammatory drugs and low-dose aspirin. *Alimentary Pharmacology and Therapeutics, 26*(8), 471–478. Retrieved July 22, 2008, from http://www.medscape.com/viewarticle/563951

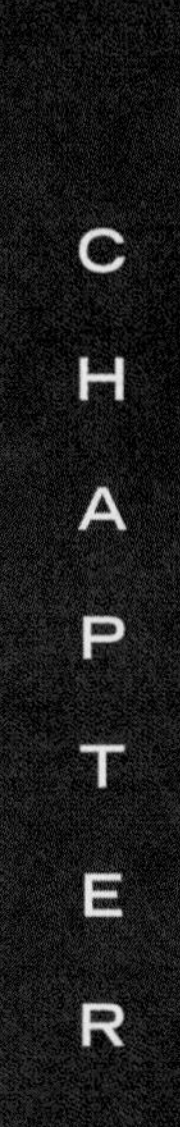

I don't know what's worse—
the symptoms or the treatment.
I feel terrible.

Patient "Carol Banks"

Immunostimulants and Immunosuppressants

45

Chapter Outline

Immunostimulants

Interferons

PROTOTYPE **Interferon Alfa-2b (Intron A)** *p. 735*

Interleukins

PROTOTYPE **Aldesleukin (Proleukin), IL-2** *p. 738*

Other Biologic Response Modifiers

Immunosuppressants

Calcineurin Inhibitors

PROTOTYPE **Cyclosporine (Neoral, Sandimmune)** *p. 743*

Cytotoxic Agents and Antimetabolites

PROTOTYPE **Azathioprine (Azasan, Imuran)** *p. 745*

Antibodies

PROTOTYPE **Muromonab-CD3 (Orthoclone, OKT3)** *p. 747*

Corticosteroids

Learning Outcomes

After reading this chapter, the student should be able to:

1. Describe the two basic types of immunomodulators and their therapeutic applications.
2. Describe the roles of interferons, interleukins, and other cytokines in modulating the immune response.
3. Describe the effects of pegylation on a drug molecule.
4. Explain why therapy with immunosuppressant medications is required following organ transplants.
5. Identify the types of agents used as immunosuppressants.
6. Compare and contrast polyclonal and monoclonal antibodies.
7. For each of the classes shown in the chapter outline, identify the prototype and representative drugs and explain the mechanism(s) of drug action, primary indications, contraindications, significant drug interactions, pregnancy category, and important adverse effects.
8. Use the nursing process to care for patients who are receiving immunostimulants and immunosuppressants.

Key Terms

biologic response modifiers, *734*
calcineurin, *740*
capillary leak syndrome, *738*
cytokines, *734*
cytokine release syndrome, *747*
immunomodulator, *734*
immunostimulant, *734*
immunosuppressant, *734*
interferons (IFNs), *734*
interleukins (ILs), *737*
monoclonal antibodies (MABs), *747*
pegylation, *734*
polyclonal antibodies, *747*
transplant rejection, *740*

The immune system and other body defenses are truly formidable deterrents to invading microorganisms. A healthy defense system can protect the body from life-threatening infections caused by thousands of different species of organisms often over an entire lifetime. In addition, body defenses can protect against "internal" invaders such as cancer cells. There are certain circumstances, however, when drugs may be necessary to modulate body defenses. This chapter examines pharmacotherapy with agents that either stimulate or suppress immune function.

45.1 Immunomodulators are substances that either enhance or suppress the ability of the body to fight infection and disease.

Body defenses are composed of a complex system of cells and tissues designed with a single goal: to protect the body from invasion by foreign substances, or antigens, that may cause harm. Some of these defenses are specific to a single species of microbe, whereas others are nonspecific and provide the same response or protection regardless of the invading pathogen. The student should review the components of body defenses in Chapter 43 before proceeding.

Immunomodulator is a general term referring to any drug or therapy that affects body defenses. There are two basic types of immunomodulators used for pharmacotherapy.

- **Immunostimulants** are drugs that increase the ability of the immune system to fight infection and disease. In most cases, these drugs are used to treat patients with cancer. The use of immunostimulants to treat cancer is called immunotherapy (see Chapter 58). The use of vaccines to boost the immune response is presented in Chapter 46.
- **Immunosuppressants** are drugs that diminish the ability of the immune system to fight infection and disease. Immunosuppressants are used to prevent transplant rejection and to dampen hyperactive immune responses, such as those that may occur during exacerbations of systemic lupus erythematosus (SLE) or rheumatoid arthritis (RA).

Immunostimulants

45.2 Interferons are biologic response modifiers that have antiviral and antineoplastic activity.

When challenged by antigens, certain cells of the immune system secrete **cytokines,** which are substances that help the body mediate and intensify the immune response. Because cytokines have powerful actions on the immune system, the body generally only produces them when challenged by an antigen; their production is rapid though transient. Chronic, high levels of cytokines can contribute to diseases such as psoriasis, Crohn's disease, or RA, and can greatly worsen symptoms of these disorders.

Cytokines exhibit multiple complex actions. A single cytokine can affect multiple target cells, each resulting in a different action. There is also considerable "overlap" or redundancy among the cytokines in that different cytokines can produce the same biologic actions. In addition to affecting their target cells, cytokines interact with each other by turning the synthesis of other cytokines on or off. The physiology of cytokines is complex and is an active research field.

Natural cytokines have been identified and, through recombinant deoxyribonucleic acid (DNA) technology, enough quantity has been made available to treat certain disorders. Also called **biologic response modifiers,** some of these agents have been approved to boost specific functions of the immune system.

Interferons (IFNs) are cytokines secreted by lymphocytes and macrophages that have been infected with a virus. IFNs are unable to protect the infected cell, but they "warn" surrounding cells that a viral infection has occurred. IFNs attach to nearby uninfected cells, inducing the production of protective antiviral proteins. When the virus attempts to attack the protected cell, the pathogen will be inactivated.

IFNs are part of the nonspecific defense system. Their actions slow the spread of viral infections, stimulate the activity of existing leukocytes, increase phagocytosis, and enhance the cytotoxic ability of T cells. Interestingly, IFNs promote apoptosis in infected cells, which is a form of programmed cell death in which the infected cell kills itself to limit the replication and spread of the virus. In addition to their antiviral actions, IFNs also have antineoplastic and anti-inflammatory properties.

Many different cell types produce IFNs. Although their functions are nearly identical, each interferon has a slightly different structure, and some have different receptors. To distinguish among the different IFNs, each type is assigned numbers and a Greek letter. The most common types are IFN alfa-2a, IFN alfa-2b, IFN beta-1a, IFN beta-1b, and IFN gamma-1a. When the drug consists of a mixture of IFNs, the letter "n" is assigned. For example, IFN alfa-n2 contains a mixture of IFN alfa-2a and 2b.

The alfa IFNs, a class of IFNs for which six different formulations are available, have the greatest clinical utility. These include IFN alfa-2a, IFN alfa-2b, IFN alfa-n3, IFN alfa-n1, pegIFN alfa-2a, and pegIFN alfa-2b.

The two "peg" formulations have the molecule polyethylene glycol (PEG) bonded to the IFN. PEG is a polymer with low toxicity that can be found in skin creams, laxatives, lubricants, toothpastes, and many other products. The addition of PEG to another molecule, known as **pegylation,** increases the molecule's solubility and extends its stability. The addition of PEG to an IFN extends the half-life of the drug to allow for once-weekly dosing. Indications for IFN alfa therapy include hairy cell leukemia, acquired immunodeficiency syndrome (AIDS)-related Kaposi's sarcoma, chronic myelogenous leukemia (alfa-2a), and chronic hepatitis B or C (alfa-2b). The use of

TABLE 45.1 Immunostimulants

Drug	Route and Adult Dose (maximum dose where indicated)	Adverse Effects
aldesleukin (Proleukin): interleukin-2	IV: 600,000 units/kg (0.037 mg/kg) every 8 h by a 15-min IV infusion for a total of 14 doses	*Flulike symptoms, rash, anemia, nausea, vomiting, diarrhea, confusion, dyspnea* Cardiac arrest, hypotension, tachycardia, thrombocytopenia, oliguria, anuria, pulmonary edema, capillary leak syndrome
bacillus Calmette-Guérin (BCG) vaccine (Tice, TheraCys)	Interdermal (Tice): 0.1 mL as vaccine Intravesical (TheraCys): bladder instillation for bladder carcinoma	*Flulike symptoms, dysuria, hematuria, anemia, lymphadenopathy* Thrombocytopenia, cystitis, urinary tract infection, disseminated mycobacteria
Interferons		
interferon alfa-2b (Intron-A)	IM/Subcutaneous: hairy cell leukemia: 2 million units/m² 3 times/week Kaposi's sarcoma: 30 million units/m² 3 times/week Hepatitis: 3 million units/m² 3 times/week for 18–24 months	*Flulike symptoms, myalgia, fatigue, headache, anorexia, diarrhea* Myelosuppression, thrombocytopenia, neutropenia, suicide ideation, seizures (IFN beta), MI (IFN gamma), anaphylaxis, hepatotoxicity
interferon alfacon-1 (Infergen)	Subcutaneous: 9 mcg 3 times/week	
interferon alfa-n3 (Alferon N)	Intralesional: 0.05 mL (250,000 international units) per wart twice/week for up to 8 weeks (max: 0.5 mL [2.5 million international units per treatment session])	
interferon beta-1a (Avonex, Rebif)	IM (Avonex): 30 mcg/week Subcutaneous (Rebif): 44 mcg 3 times/week	
interferon beta-1b (Betaseron)	Subcutaneous: 0.25 mg (8 million units) every other day	
interferon gamma-1b (Actimmune)	Subcutaneous: 50 mcg/m², 3 times weekly	
peginterferon alfa-2a (Pegasys)	Subcutaneous: 180 mcg once weekly for 48 weeks	
peginterferon alfa-2b (Peg-Intron)	Subcutaneous: 1.5 mcg/kg/wk	

Note: *Italics* indicate common adverse effects. Underline indicates serious adverse effects.

IFN alfa in the pharmacotherapy of hepatitis is presented in Chapter 55. Doses of the IFNs are listed in Table 45.1.

IFN beta consists of two different formulations, beta-1a and beta-1b, which are primarily reserved for the treatment of severe multiple sclerosis (MS) (see Chapter 25). A third drug in this class, called IFN gamma-1b, has limited clinical application in the treatment of chronic granulomatous disease and severe osteoporosis.

PROTOTYPE DRUG Interferon alfa-2b (Intron A)

Classification: Therapeutic: Immunostimulant
Pharmacologic: Interferon, biologic response modifier

Therapeutic Effects and Uses: Approved in 1986, IFN alfa-2b is a biologic response modifier prepared by recombinant DNA technology that differs from IFN alfa-2a by only one amino acid. Indications include neoplastic conditions such as hairy cell leukemia, malignant melanoma, non-Hodgkin's lymphoma, human papilloma virus, and AIDS-related Kaposi's sarcoma as well as viral infections (chronic hepatitis virus B and C). Off-label indications include chronic myelogenous leukemia, bladder cancer, herpes simplex virus, multiple myeloma, renal cell cancer, human immunodeficiency virus (HIV), varicella-zoster virus (VZV), and West Nile virus. It is available for intravenous (IV), intramuscular (IM), and subcutaneous administration.

Rebetron is a combination drug containing IFN alfa-2b and ribavirin, an antiviral agent. Rebetron is indicated for the pharmacotherapy of hepatitis C infection.

Peginterferon alfa-2b (PegIntron) has a molecule of PEG attached to the IFN molecule, which gives the drug an extended half-life. Peak concentrations can be sustained for 48 to 72 hours, which results in greater antiviral activity. This drug is only approved to treat chronic hepatitis C virus infections, although it may be used off-label to treat chronic hepatitis B infections and neoplastic disease.

Mechanism of Action: IFN alfa-2b has both antiviral and antineoplastic activities. It is a nonspecific inhibitor of viral replication. It affects cancer cells by two mechanisms. First, it enhances the general functions of the immune system: IFNs increase the phagocytic activity of macrophages and monocytes, resulting in enhanced cytotoxicity against tumor cells. Second, this drug suppresses the growth of cancer cells.

Pharmacokinetics:

Route(s)	IV, IM, subcutaneous
Absorption	80% absorbed
Distribution	Unknown if secreted in breast milk
Primary metabolism	Minimal hepatic metabolism
Primary excretion	Renal
Onset of action	Peak: 3–12 h
Duration of action	Half-life: 2 h

Adverse Effects: The most common adverse effect of IFN therapy is a flulike syndrome of fever, chills, dizziness, weight loss, and fatigue that occurs in 50% of patients and which usually diminishes as therapy progresses. Fatigue may be severe at higher doses. Headache, nausea, vomiting, diarrhea, and anorexia are relatively common. Hair loss may occur with prolonged therapy. Depression and suicidal ideation have been reported and may be severe enough to require discontinuation of the drug. The depression may persist after the drug is discontinued. With prolonged therapy, serious adverse effects such as immunosuppression, hepatotoxicity, and neurotoxicity may be observed.

MyNursingKit | Mechanism of Action Animation: Interferon Alpha

Contraindications/Precautions: Contraindications include hypersensitivity to IFNs, autoimmune hepatitis, or hepatic decompensation. Neonates and infants should not receive this drug because it contains benzyl alcohol, which is associated with an increased incidence of neurologic and other serious complications in this age group. If infection occurs during therapy, anti-infectives should be started immediately. Hepatic enzymes may become elevated during IFN therapy and may require discontinuation of the drug. This effect is worse in patients with preexisting hepatic impairment. IFN alfa-2b should be used with caution in patients with cardiac disease, herpes zoster, and recent exposure to chickenpox.

Drug Interactions: IFN alfa-2a may increase theophylline levels. There is additive immunosuppression when IFN alfa-2a is used with antineoplastic drugs. Zidovudine may increase hematologic toxicity and cause immunosuppression. The use of IFN alfa-2a with ethanol may cause excessive drowsiness and dehydration. **Herbal/Food**: Unknown.

Pregnancy: Category C.

Treatment of Overdose: Overdose with IFN may cause lethargy and coma. Treatment is by general supportive measures.

Nursing Responsibilities:

- Obtain baseline laboratory values including a complete blood count (CBC), platelet count, and liver and renal function tests. Monitor laboratory values monthly during treatment.
- Monitor fluid intake and output (I&O) ratio and pattern because adequate hydration is necessary during initial treatment. Encourage increased fluid intake to at least 2,500 mL as tolerated.
- Assess for flulike syndrome such as fever or chills occurring in patients 2 to 6 hours after a dose of IFN. This can be expected so provide supportive care during this phase.
- Monitor body weight daily during therapy. Lack of appetite or anorexia may occur after initial doses with the flulike symptoms but tends to lessen with continued therapy. Loss of body weight and nutrients can be managed with high-calorie, high-protein supplements during an anorexia phase.
- Observe the patient for unexplained bleeding such as ecchymoses and petechiae because this drug can cause thrombocytopenia.
- Provide a safe environment because this drug can cause ataxia, dizziness, and hypotension.
- Monitor for oral superinfection with *Candida albicans.* Alert the prescriber if stomatitis (sore mouth with ulceration), gingivitis, or white patches on the oropharyngeal membrane surfaces are evidenced.
- Monitor blood pressure, vital signs, and cardiac function closely in older adults who are more susceptible to cardiotoxicity.
- Teach patient techniques for self-administration of the medication. Advise the patient to keep the patient information sheet about IFN handy.

Patient and Family Education:

- Do not drive or perform other hazardous activities until the effects of the drug are known because this drug may cause drowsiness or dizziness.
- Avoid exposure to infection. Avoid people who have a sore throat, a cold, the flu, diarrhea, or vomiting, or other kinds of infection. Avoid crowded places such as public transportation.
- Notify the health care provider promptly if symptoms of infection, such as fever, sore throat, vomiting, or diarrhea, occur.
- Keep follow-up appointments with periodic neuropsychiatric monitoring due to possible drug-induced depression. Immediately report any signs of depression, such as lethargy, excessive sleeping, or suicidal ideation.

Drugs Similar to Interferon alfa-2b (Intron A)

Other available IFNs include IFN alfacon-1, IFN alfa-n3, IFN beta-1a, IFN beta-1b, IFN gamma-1b, and peginterferon alfa-2a. IFN alfa-n1 (Wellferon) and IFN alfa-2a are no longer available in the United States.

Interferon alfacon-1 (Infergen): Approved in 1997, IFN alfacon-1 is a drug that contains a mixture of all the IFN alfa subtypes. Given by the subcutaneous route, its only approved indication by the U.S. Food and Drug Administration (FDA) is for the treatment of chronic hepatitis C infection. Contraindications, drug interactions, and adverse effects are the same as those for IFN alfa-2b. Mild flulike symptoms are common adverse effects. Patients should be monitored for depression and suicidal ideation. This drug is pregnancy category C.

Interferon alfa-n3 (Alferon N): Approved in 1989, IFN alfa-n3 is a mixture of IFN alfa subtypes purified from human leukocytes. Indications include genital warts and human papilloma virus. Two injections per week for 8 weeks are usually sufficient to cause warts to disappear. Unlike the other IFNs, this drug is injected directly into lesions (intralesionally). Its off-label indications include treatment of hepatitis C, herpes simplex, and other viral infections by the subcutaneous route. This product may contain egg protein and is contraindicated in patients with egg sensitivity. IFN alfa-n3 exhibits few adverse effects when administered intralesionally. This drug is pregnancy category C.

Interferon beta-1a (Avonex, Rebif): Made through recombinant DNA technology, IFN beta-1a is structurally identical to the natural IFN produced by the body. Approved in 1996, it is one of the few drugs available for treating MS. IFN beta-1a decreases the frequency of clinical exacerbations and slows the progression to physical disability, which is characteristic of MS. The drug acts by inhibiting the release of proinflammatory cytokines that initiate the autoimmune reaction leading to MS. IFN beta-1a also changes the blood–brain barrier and reduces T-lymphocyte migration into the brain, thereby reducing inflammation. It is available by the subcutaneous (Rebif) and IM (Avonex) routes. Adverse effects are similar to those of other IFNs, with flulike symptoms being observed in the majority of patients. Patients should be monitored for depression and suicidal ideation. Decreased peripheral blood counts, including thrombocytopenia and leukopenia, have been reported from postmarketing experience. Rare cases of severe hepatotoxicity, including some cases requiring liver transplantation, have been reported in patients taking IFN beta-1a. Additional details on the pharmacotherapy of MS are presented in Chapter 25. This drug is pregnancy category C.

Interferon beta-1b (Betaseron): Approved in 1993, IFN beta-1b is produced by recombinant DNA technology and is very similar to natural IFN. This drug is available by subcutaneous injection for the treatment of patients with relapsing MS. Its mechanism of action and adverse effects are the same as those of IFN beta-1a. Transient flulike symptoms are frequent adverse effects. Patients should be monitored for depression and suicidal ideation. Injection site inflammation occurs in most patients and may progress to necrosis. This drug is pregnancy category C.

Interferon gamma-1b (Actimmune): Approved in 1999, IFN gamma-1b is produced by recombinant DNA technology and is very similar to natural IFN gamma. IFN gamma-1b has both direct and indirect antiviral activity. This drug activates macrophages to increase the production of interleukin-12 and tumor necrosis factor (TNF), which increases the killing ability of these cells. IFN gamma-1b also promotes the recruitment of leukocytes to the sites of infection or inflammation. IFN gamma-1b is the only IFN indicated for the treatment of chronic granulomatous disease (CGD). CGD is an inherited disorder of phagocytic cells that leads to recurrent life-threatening bacterial and fungal infections. A second characteristic of CGD is the development of nodular granulomas in the skin, gastrointestinal (GI) tract, and genitourinary (GU) tract due to chronic infections at these sites. IFN gamma-1b reduces the frequency and severity of infections in patients with CGD. Off-label indications include infections by *Mycobacterium avium* complex (MAC), pulmonary fibrosis, and ovarian cancer. The most common adverse effects include flulike symptoms, nausea, vomiting, diarrhea, rash, and elevated hepatic enzymes. Because of the potential for neutropenia and thrombocytopenia, periodic CBCs are required. This drug is pregnancy category C.

Peginterferon alfa-2a (Pegasys): Peginterferon alfa-2a is a biologic response modifier that has a molecule of PEG attached to IFN alfa-2a, which is identical to the natural IFN produced by human lymphocytes and macrophages. Approved in 2002, it is prepared through recombinant DNA technology and is available as single-use prefilled syringes and administered by the subcutaneous route. Approved indications for peginterferon alfa-2a include chronic hepatitis B and hepatitis C virus infections that show evidence that the virus is replicating. Off-label uses include renal cell carcinoma and chronic myelogenous leukemia. Patients should be monitored for depression and suicidal ideation. Neutropenia and thrombocytopenia are uncommon but may be severe. Other potential adverse effects include colitis, pancreatitis, hyper- or hypothyroidism, hypertension (HTN), and dysrhythmias. This drug is pregnancy category C.

45.3 Interleukins, vaccines, and colony-stimulating factors are used to boost the immune system.

Interleukins (ILs) are a class of cytokines synthesized by lymphocytes, monocytes, macrophages, and certain other cells in response to antigen exposure. Like IFNs, ILs are signaling molecules that enable cells of the immune system to communicate with each other. The ILs, however, work by different mechanisms than the IFNs. The ILs have widespread effects on immune function that include the following:

- Stimulation of cytotoxic T-cell activity against tumor cells
- Activation and increased production of natural killer (NK) cells
- Increased B-cell and plasma cell production
- Increased neutrophil chemotaxis
- Promotion of inflammation

Over 30 different ILs have been identified, though only a few are available as medications. IL-2, which is derived from helper T cells, promotes the proliferation of both T cells and activated B cells. It is available as aldesleukin (Proleukin), which is approved by the FDA for the treatment of metastatic renal carcinoma. IL-11, which is derived from bone marrow cells, is a growth factor with multiple hematopoietic effects. It is marketed as oprelvekin (Neumega) for its ability to stimulate platelet production in patients with immunosuppression. Oprelvekin is featured as a prototype drug in Chapter 41.

Bacillus Calmette-Guérin (BCG) vaccine (Tice, TheraCys) is a biologic response modifier that is available to enhance the immune system. BCG is an attenuated strain of *Mycobacterium bovis* used for the pharmacotherapy of certain types of bladder cancer.

Vaccines are types of immunostimulants that have the ability to mobilize the body against specific antigens. A small amount of an inactivated antigen is administered and the patient develops an immune reaction. If reexposed to the antigen in future years, memory B or T cells will develop a rapid response, eliminating the antigen before it causes disease. Vaccines are presented in Chapter 46.

CONNECTIONS

To the Community Immunosuppression and Pets

Various restrictions are necessary to maximize the health of those who are prescribed immunosuppressants because these patients are more prone to opportunistic infections. For example, in caring for pets the caregiver may come in contact with bacteria that could cause infections. Because pets can be beneficial to the mental health of the owner or caregiver, taking certain precautions will allow immunosuppressed patients to live successfully with their pets. Following are some guidelines for maintaining a healthy relationship with pets:

- Keep the pet up to date on routine veterinarian checkups and vaccinations. Seek early treatment when the pet becomes ill.
- Feed the pet high-quality food. If cooking for the pet, cook all foods thoroughly, especially eggs and meat.
- Wash hands often, especially when caring for or handling the pet. Wear rubber gloves when cleaning up after a pet, especially when cleaning a birdcage or aquarium.
- If the pet develops diarrhea, have someone other than the immunosuppressed patient clean up for the pet, and take the pet to the veterinarian as soon as possible. A veterinarian can determine if there are bacteria that are harmful to humans.
- Maintain flea control in the pet.
- Do not allow pets to drink from the toilet or go through the garbage.
- Clean the cat litter box daily. If possible have someone other than the immunosuppressed person clean the litter box.
- If possible, keep a cat inside to avoid its natural tendency to hunt and feed on raw meat.
- Avoid adopting stray animals and instead choose a healthy pet from a clean breeding facility, pet store, or animal care facility. Take the new pet to the veterinarian to assess for the presence of disease or harmful bacteria. A pet that is at least 6 months old and free of diarrhea (diarrhea could indicate cryptosporidiosis) is preferred.
- Avoid rough play or teasing that can result in scratches or bites, because bacteria can be passed this way. If a scratch or bite occurs, wash the area immediately with soap and water. Do not allow a cat to lick an open sore or wound on the person with immunosuppression.
- Pets such as turtles, snakes, iguanas, or lizards can transmit the bacteriium salmonella and should be cared for with caution by a person who is immunosuppressed.

The final type of immunostimulants includes the colony-stimulating factors, which are drugs that promote the production of WBCs. For example, filgrastim (Neupogen) stimulates the production of granulocytes, and sargramostim (Leukine) activates multiple types of leukocytes. These agents are used to shorten the length of neutropenia in patients with cancer and in those who have had bone marrow transplant whose bone marrow has been suppressed by drugs. Filgrastim, the prototype, and other colony-stimulating factors are presented in Chapter 41.

CONNECTION *Checkpoint* 45.1

From what you learned in Chapter 41, what is the primary indication of oprelvekin (Neumega) therapy and what is its most important adverse effect? See Answer to Connection Checkpoint 45.1 in Appendix A.

PROTOTYPE DRUG Aldesleukin (Proleukin), IL-2

Classification: **Therapeutic:** Immunostimulant
Pharmacologic: Interleukin, biologic response modifier

Therapeutic Effects and Uses: Approved in 1992, aldesleukin has a structure very similar to natural IL-2, and it has identical actions in the body. It is FDA approved for the pharmacotherapy of metastatic renal cell carcinoma and metastatic malignant melanoma. It has been designated by the FDA as an orphan drug for the chemotherapy of non-Hodgkin's lymphoma and acute myelogenous leukemia. It is used off-label to treat leprosy (see Chapter 52).

Aldesleukin is a very toxic drug that should only be administered by personnel familiar with its use. It must be administered in multiple, brief IV infusions because of its short half-life.

Mechanism of Action: The mechanism of action of aldesleukin is identical to that of endogenous IL-2. It initiates a series of actions that activate IFNs, TNF, and other ILs. The drug promotes proliferation of both B cells and T cells, macrophages, and NK cells, which in turn increase the body's ability to fight cancer cells.

Pharmacokinetics:

Route(s)	IV
Absorption	N/A
Distribution	Widely distributed; unknown if secreted in breast milk
Primary metabolism	Renal
Primary excretion	Renal
Onset of action	Unknown
Duration of action	Half-life: 85 minutes

Adverse Effects: Aldesleukin is a toxic drug that has the potential to cause serious adverse effects in virtually any organ system. Many of the adverse effects are caused by **capillary leak syndrome,** a serious condition in which plasma proteins and other substances leave the blood and enter the interstitial spaces because of porous capillaries. If not monitored carefully, capillary leak syndrome can result in death. Over 70% of patients taking aldesleukin will experience hypotension, which can sometimes be severe enough to cause tissues and organs to receive an insufficient blood supply to function properly. Tachycardia and other dysrhythmias occur in a significant number of patients. Diarrhea, nausea, or vomiting may occur in as many as half the patients taking the drug. Other common adverse effects include confusion, drowsiness, oliguria, stomatitis, anorexia, hyperbilirubinemia, hypothyroidism, elevated hepatic enzymes, weight gain, dyspnea, and pulmonary congestion. Common changes in blood values include thrombocytopenia, anemia, and leucopenia. Flulike symptoms such as fever and malaise occur frequently.

Contraindications/Precautions: There are many contraindications to using aldesleukin, and a thorough baseline assessment of health status is required. Patients with significant cardiac, central nervous system (CNS), pulmonary, renal, or hepatic impairment should not receive this drug. Aldesleukin may cause seizures and should be used with caution in patients with epilepsy. This drug may worsen the condition of patients with autoimmune disease, including those with scleroderma, RA, diabetes mellitus, and thyroiditis.

Drug Interactions: Aldesleukin has the potential to interact with nearly any other drug. Given concurrently with aldesleukin, drugs that affect mental status such as many antianxiety agents, opioids, sedatives, or antipsychotic agents may cause mood disturbances and drowsiness. Concurrent administration with drugs that are hepatotoxic or nephrotoxic may cause additive organ damage. Caution should be used when using agents that modify coagulation such as aspirin, nonsteroidal anti-inflammatory agents (NSAIDs), or platelet inhibitors due to an increased risk of bleeding. Antihypertensive drugs may cause additive hypotension when used with aldesleukin. **Herbal/Food:** None known.

Pregnancy: Category C.

Treatment of Overdose: Dexamethasone may be used to reverse some of the toxicities observed from an overdose of aldesleukin.

Nursing Responsibilities:

- Obtain baseline CBC, electrolytes, renal function, and liver enzymes. Some degree of renal and hepatic impairment is likely during therapy.
- Assess for the presence or history of diseases such as chronic hepatitis, malignant melanoma, hairy cell leukemia, AIDS-related Kaposi's sarcoma, and renal carcinoma to verify the need for this drug.
- Measure vital signs and body weight at the initial assessment and throughout the treatment regimen. Sudden drops in blood pressure 2 to 12 hours after treatment may indicate capillary leak syndrome. If this occurs notify the prescriber immediately.
- Maintain hydration status during therapy to prevent the development of encephalopathy and changes in mental status such as confusion, hallucinations, or agitation. Observe and document any signs and symptoms of depression and suicidal ideation.
- Inspect the oral cavity for sores in the mouth or stomatitis. If present, provide small frequent feedings and mouth care with a non–alcohol-based mouthwash.
- Report any adverse effects such as fever, sore throat, hematuria, petechiae, or tarry stools to the prescriber.
- Assess the electrocardiogram (ECG) for the presence of dysrhythmias.

Patient and Family Education:

- Avoid overscheduling activities and plan specific times for rest. Fatigue is a common adverse effect of this therapy, but energy levels usually return to normal 6 months to a year after treatment.
- Take acetaminophen before injections and every 4 to 6 hours after to manage the common flulike symptoms of fever, headache, chills, and aching muscles and joints.
- Avoid vaccinations while receiving treatment with this drug and for 3 months after completion of treatment.
- Immediately report symptoms of bleeding, infection, or shortness of breath, which can occur due to a temporary drop in the number of blood cells produced by the bone marrow.
- Immediately report hallucinations, agitation, speech or vision changes, palpitations, chest pain, reduced urine output, unusual bruising or bleeding, or yellowing of the eyes to the health care provider.
- Immediately notify the health care provider of any known or suspected pregnancy.
- Do not breast-feed while taking this drug without approval of the health care provider.
- If diarrhea, nausea, or vomiting is present, ask the health care provider for medications that may decrease these symptoms.

Drugs Similar to Aldesleukin (Proleukin), IL-2

The only other IL approved by the FDA is IL-11, a platelet enhancer marketed as oprelvekin (Neumega), which is featured as a prototype in Chapter 41. BCG vaccine is a miscellaneous biologic response modifier. An additional immunostimulant, levamisole (Ergamisol), has been discontinued in the United States.

Bacillus Calmette-Guérin vaccine (Tice, TheraCys): BCG vaccine is a live, attenuated vaccine that is available in two distinct strains with different indications. Both forms are pregnancy category C.

Tice. Tice is used to stimulate immunity against *Mycobacterium tuberculosis*. Vaccination with BCG simulates exposure to tuberculosis and induces an immune response against the organism. This drug is used to prevent tuberculosis and is not given to treat active infections. It is the only FDA-approved treatment for tuberculosis prophylaxis. The drug is not 100% effective and its length of protection is variable. Flulike symptoms often develop 1 to 2 days after administration. Minor skin papules appear at the site of percutaneous puncture.

TheraCys. TheraCys is approved for the prophylaxis and treatment of patients with superficial bladder cancer. This drug is instilled into the urinary bladder for 2 hours, after which the patient voids the medication. The treatment may be repeated at 3-month intervals. TheraCys produces a nonspecific immune reaction in the bladder that attracts lymphocytes, macrophages, and NK cells to the site of the cancer. Adverse effects include local reactions such as bladder irritability, hematuria, dysuria, cystitis, incontinence, and nocturia. A flulike syndrome may occur.

Immunosuppressants

45.4 Immunosuppressants are used to prevent transplant rejection and for the treatment of autoimmune disorders.

Used to inhibit the immune response, immunosuppressants are prescribed for patients who are receiving transplanted tissues or organs and to treat autoimmune disorders. Doses for these agents are listed in Table 45.2.

Transplantation: Transplants may include specific cells, parts of tissues, or complete organs. They may originate from the patient's own body (autografts), genetically identical donors (isografts), or genetically dissimilar donors (allografts). Most transplantation procedures use allografts.

Typing for transplanted tissues includes attempts to match, as closely as possible, donor and recipient human leukocyte antigen (HLA) and ABO blood-type antigens. Despite accurate tissue matching, allografts always contain certain antigens that trigger the patient's immune response. This response, called **transplant rejection,** is often acute; antibodies sometimes destroy the transplanted tissue within 48 hours of the transplant. The cell-mediated branch of the immune system responds more slowly to the transplant, attacking it about 2 weeks following surgery. Chronic rejection of the transplant may occur months or even years after surgery.

MyNursingKit | Xenotransplants

Successful transplantation requires the use of immunosuppressant drugs. One or more immunosuppressants are administered at the time of transplantation and are continued for several months following surgery. In some cases, they are continued indefinitely at low doses. Transplantation would be impossible without the use of effective immunosuppressant drugs. Immunosuppressant therapies have proven very successful at preventing acute transplant rejection but have been mostly unsuccessful at preventing chronic rejection.

Prior to the initiation of immunosuppressant therapy it is critical that the patient be carefully assessed to rule out active infections. This includes screening for viruses such as cytomegalovirus (CMV), hepatitis B and C viruses, Epstein-Barr virus (EBV), VZV, HIV, and herpes simplex virus (HSV). If an active infection is discovered, it should be treated prior to transplantation. In addition, patients should be screened for the presence of cancer prior to surgery because immunosuppressant drugs will allow existing cancers to grow rapidly.

During immunosuppressant therapy the patient will be susceptible to infection from all types of pathogens: viral, bacterial, fungal, or protozoan. Infections in immunosuppressed patients are called opportunistic infections. Opportunistic pulmonary infections are the leading cause of morbidity and mortality in patients receiving a transplant (Duncan & Wiles, 2005). Many patients receive antibiotics for the prophylaxis of opportunistic infections for 4 to 12 months following surgery. Six months following the transplant, 80% of patients will return to their baseline risk of infection, but the remainder will remain at high risk indefinitely.

Long-term survivors of transplants are also at high risk of developing cancers. These include non-Hodgkin's lymphoma, squamous and basal cell skin cancer, cervical cancer, and Kaposi's sarcoma. Regular follow-up monitoring for cancer is required in these patients.

Pharm*FACT*

More than 99,000 patients are waiting for organ transplants. About 75% of these are waiting for a kidney, 16% for a liver, and 2% for a heart. *Source:* United Network for Organ Sharing, 2008.

Autoimmune disorders: Autoimmune disorders are those in which the body creates antibodies against normal tissues. The body attacks its own cells as if they were foreign, resulting in tissue injury. Examples of autoimmune disorders include RA, SLE, myasthenia gravis, and Hashimoto's thyroiditis.

Autoimmune diseases are characterized by symptomatic periods alternating with remissions. Although the remissions may last many months or even years, relapses are often progressive, with worsening symptoms as the disease progresses. During acute relapses, fever and signs of widespread inflammation may be present. Symptoms may affect virtually any tissue or organ, depending on the specific autoimmune disease.

Unlike transplant recipients who may receive immunosuppressants indefinitely, patients with autoimmune disease are usually given these drugs for brief periods in high doses to control relapses. In some cases, however, these patients may receive low doses for longer periods for prophylaxis.

The immunosuppressant class includes drugs that block the immune response by several different mechanisms, as shown in Figure 45.1. These include blocking the receptors and production of IL-2, inhibiting the proliferation of T cells, and using antibodies specific to certain receptors or cells of the immune response. The drugs may be classified into the following categories:

- Calcineurin inhibitors and similar drugs
- Antimetabolites and cytotoxic agents
- Antibodies
- Glucocorticoids

45.5 Calcineurin inhibitors are drugs of choice for the prophylaxis of transplant rejection.

When a T cell encounters an antigen, calcineurin is activated. **Calcineurin** is an enzyme that acts as an intracellular messenger, telling the T cell to begin synthesizing IL-2. As described in Section 45.3, IL-2 is an important chemical mediator in promoting the proliferation of B cells, T cells, macrophages, and NK cells. Blocking IL-2 suppresses the immune response.

Two of the most important drugs in transplant medicine, cyclosporine (Sandimmune, Neoral) and tacrolimus (Prograf), are calcineurin inhibitors. These drugs revolutionized the pharmacotherapy of transplant rejection and have been the mainstay of transplant therapy since the 1980s. Although newer medications have been developed, the calcineurin inhibitors remain critical drugs for transplant recipients. The calcineurin inhibitors allow the doses of corticosteroids to be lowered, thereby reducing the incidence of opportunistic infections following transplants.

TABLE 45.2 Immunosuppressants		
Drug	**Route and Adult Dose (maximum dose where indicated)**	**Adverse Effects**
Antibodies		
basiliximab (Simulect)	IV: 20 mg times two doses (first dose 2 h before surgery; second dose 4 days after transplant)	*Local reactions at the injection site (pain, erythema, myalgia), influenza-like symptoms (malaise, fever, chills), headache, dizziness* Anaphylaxis, HTN, infections (may occur in many different body systems), thrombocytopenia, leukopenia, renal impairment (basiliximab), pulmonary edema (muromonab-CD3 and lymphocyte immune globulin), herpes simplex or cytomegalovirus infections (muromonab-CD3)
daclizumab (Zenapax)	IV: 1 mg/kg; start first dose no more than 24 h prior to transplant, then repeat every 14 days for four more doses	
lymphocyte immune globulin (Antithymocyte Globulin)	IV: 10–30 mg/kg/day	
muromonab-CD3 (Orthoclone OKT3)	IV: 5 mg/day administered in less than 1 min for 10–14 days	
Antimetabolites and Cytotoxic Agents		
anakinra (Kineret)	Subcutaneous: 100 mg (0.67 mL) once daily	*Injection site reactions* Leukopenia, infections, malignancy
azathioprine (Azasan, Imuran)	PO/IV: 3–5 mg/kg/day initially; may be able to reduce to 1–3 mg/kg/day	*Nausea,vomiting, anorexia* Severe nausea and vomiting, bone marrow suppression, thrombocytopenia, infections, malignancy, hepatotoxicity
cyclophosphamide (Cytoxan)	PO: Initial: 1–5 mg/kg/day; maintenance: 1–5 mg/kg every 7–10 days IV: Initial: 40–50 mg/kg in divided doses over 2–5 days up to 100 mg/kg; maintenance: 10–15 mg/kg every 7–10 days or 3–5 mg twice weekly	*Nausea, vomiting, anorexia, neutropenia, alopecia* Anaphylaxis, leukopenia, pulmonary emboli, interstitial pulmonary fibrosis, toxic epidermal necrolysis, Stevens–Johnson syndrome, hemorrhagic cystitis, oligospermia
etanercept (Enbrel)	Subcutaneous: 25 mg twice/week or 0.08 mg/kg or 50 mg once/week	*Injection site reactions (pain, erythema, myalgia), abdominal pain, vomiting, headache* Infections, pancytopenia, leukopenia, anemia, myocardial infarction (MI), heart failure, malignancy
methotrexate (Amethopterin, Folex, Mexate, Rheumatrex, Trexall)	PO/IM/IV: 15–30 mg/day for 5 days; repeat every 12 weeks for three courses	*Headache, glossitis, gingivitis, mild leukopenia, nausea, alopecia* Ulcerative stomatitis, myelosuppression, aplastic anemia, hepatic cirrhosis, nephrotoxicity, sudden death, pulmonary fibrosis, or pneumonia
mycophenolate (CellCept, Myfortic)	PO/IV: 720 mg bid in combination with corticosteroids and cyclosporine; start within 24 h of transplant	*Peripheral edema, diarrhea, headache, tremor, dyspepsia, abdominal pain* Urinary tract infection, leukopenia, anemia, thrombocytopenia, sepsis, HTN
sirolimus (Rapamune)	PO: 6 mg loading dose immediately after the transplant, then 2 mg/day	*Hypercholesterolemia, rash, arthralgia, diarrhea, nausea, vomiting, asthenia, back pain, weight gain, hyperlipidemia* HTN, leukopenia, anemia, thrombocytopenia, sepsis, secondary infections, malignancy
temsirolimus (Torisel)	IV: 25 mg once weekly over 30–60 min	*Rash, asthenia, mucositis, nausea, edema, anorexia, hyperglycemia, hyperlipidemia* Anemia, anaphylaxis, infections, interstitial lung disease or pneumonia, birth defects
thalidomide (Thalomid)	PO: 100–300 mg/day (max: 400 mg/day) for at least 2 weeks	*Rash, mild leukopenia, fever, dizziness, diarrhea, malaise, drowsiness* Toxic epidermal necrolysis, birth defects (pregnancy category X), orthostatic hypotension, neutropenia, peripheral neuropathy
Calcineurin Inhibitors		
cyclosporine (Sandimmune, Neoral)	PO: 250 mg every 12 h for 2 weeks (max: 1 g/day)	*Hirsutism, tremor, nausea, vomiting* HTN, MI, nephrotoxicity, hyperkalemia, seizures, paresthesia, hepatotoxicity
tacrolimus (Prograf)	PO: 0.1–0.15 mg/kg/day in two divided doses every 12 h; start no sooner than 6 h after transplant; give first PO dose 8–12 h after discontinuing IV therapy IV: 0.03–0.05 mg/kg/day as continuous infusion; start no sooner than 6 h after transplant and continue until the patient can take PO therapy	*Oliguria, nausea, constipation, diarrhea, headache, abdominal pain, insomnia, peripheral edema, fever* Infections, HTN, nephrotoxicity, neurotoxicity (tremors, paresthesia, psychosis), hyperkalemia, anemia, hyperglycemia, malignancy, thrombocytopenia, seizures

Note: *Italics* indicate common adverse effects. Underline indicates serious adverse effects.

PHARMACOTHERAPY ILLUSTRATED 45.1

Mechanism of Action of Immunosuppressants

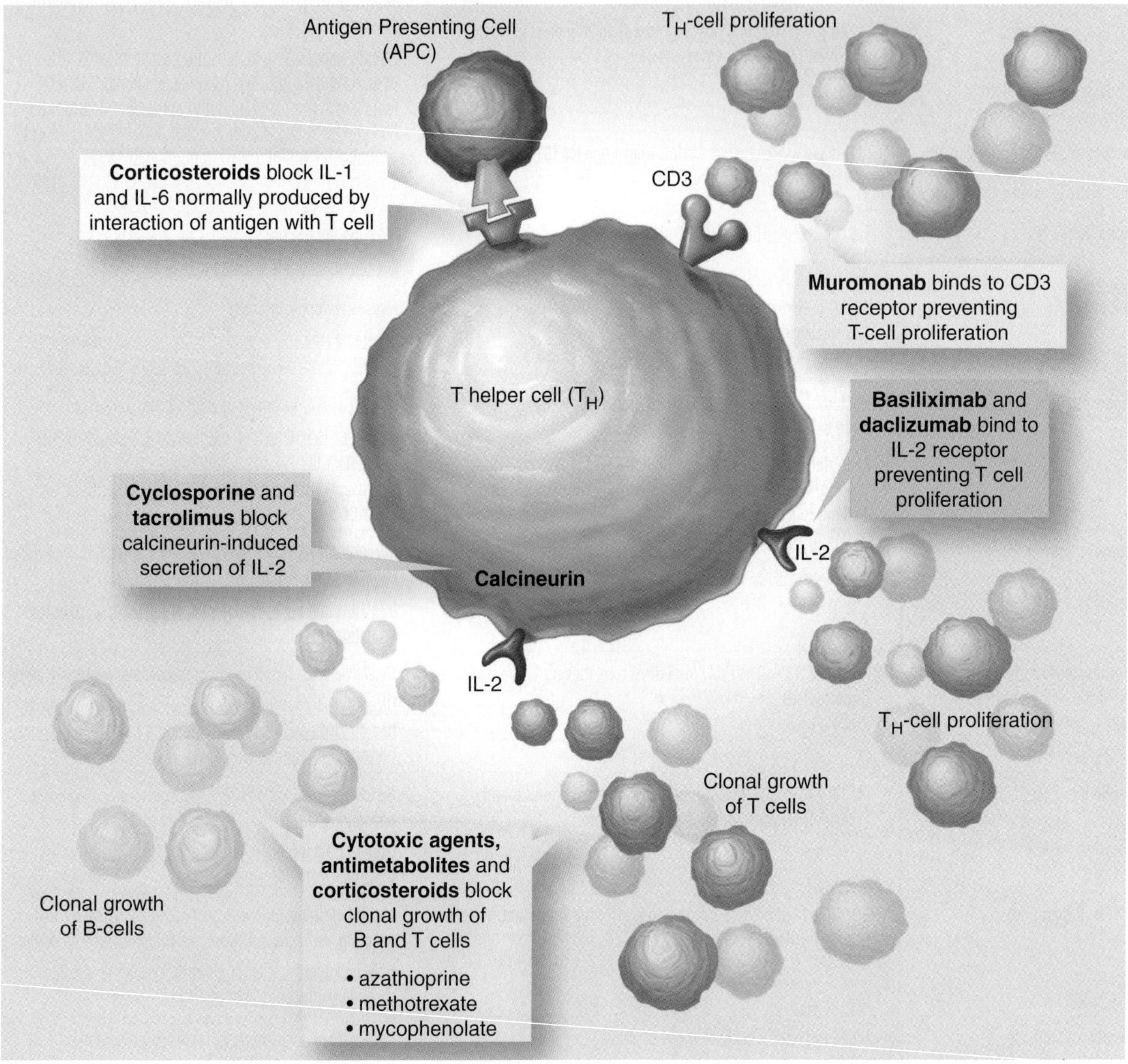

Antigen Presenting Cell (APC)

T_H-cell proliferation

Corticosteroids block IL-1 and IL-6 normally produced by interaction of antigen with T cell

CD3

Muromonab binds to CD3 receptor preventing T-cell proliferation

T helper cell (T_H)

Basiliximab and **daclizumab** bind to IL-2 receptor preventing T cell proliferation

Cyclosporine and **tacrolimus** block calcineurin-induced secretion of IL-2

Calcineurin

IL-2

IL-2

T_H-cell proliferation

Clonal growth of T cells

Clonal growth of B-cells

Cytotoxic agents, antimetabolites and **corticosteroids** block clonal growth of B and T cells

- azathioprine
- methotrexate
- mycophenolate

CONNECTIONS

Treating the Diverse Patient Adherence to Immunosuppressive Medication

Despite the severe consequences, nonadherence to immunosuppressive medication is a problem in elderly African American transplant recipients. Nonadherence rates as high as 35% have been documented in African American kidney transplant recipients as compared with lower rates in non-African Americans. Many factors place older African American recipients at risk for medication nonadherence. These factors may include chronic illness, complex long-term and expensive medications, distressing adverse effects, and social isolation. In a review of the current literature, Russell (2006) examined culturally responsive interventions that enhance immunosuppressive medication adherence in older African American kidney transplant recipients.

The following interventions seem valuable in promoting high adherence behavior in this population:

- Assessing the personal meaning of the illness
- Adapting education materials (appropriate educational level, font size, user friendly)
- Involving health care providers of similar age and ethnicity
- Enhancing access (manageable cost, transportation, and proximity to care)
- Involving family and church members in care

Nonadherence with immunosuppressant therapy can have severe consequences leading to organ rejection, graft loss, and even death.

Source: From "Culturally Responsive Interventions to Enhance Immunosuppressive Medication Adherence in Older African American Kidney Transplant Recipients," by C. L. Russell, 2006, *Progress in Transplantation, 16*(3), pp. 187–196.

Approved in 1983, cyclosporine was the first calcineurin inhibitor and remains the prototype for this class. Tacrolimus appears to be more effective in preventing transplant rejection and reducing the mortality associated with transplants. Recent trends suggest that physicians are shifting from cyclosporine to tacrolimus for transplant maintenance therapy (Basu, Tan, & Shapiro, 2007). The calcineurin inhibitors are also of value in treating the acute inflammation associated with RA and psoriasis, which is an inflammatory disorder of the skin (see Chapter 76).

PROTOTYPE DRUG Cyclosporine (Neoral, Sandimmune)

Classification: **Therapeutic:** Immunosuppressant
Pharmacologic: Calcineurin inhibitor

Therapeutic Effects and Uses: Cyclosporine is a complex chemical obtained from a soil fungus. It is FDA-approved for the prophylaxis of kidney, heart, and liver transplant rejection; psoriasis; and xerophthalmia, an eye condition of diminished tear production caused by ocular inflammation. Off-label indications include a number of autoimmune and inflammatory conditions such as ulcerative colitis, SLE, myasthenia gravis, aplastic anemia, Crohn's disease, psoriatic arthritis, and graft-versus-host disease.

Cyclosporine may be administered as capsules, oral solution, or IV or as an ophthalmic solution (Restasis) for xerophthalmia. Due to the risk of anaphylaxis, the IV route is used only when patients are unable to take oral (PO) medications. Cyclosporine (modified) refers to the capsule, microemulsion dosage formulation of cyclosporine. Cyclosporine (modified) has increased bioavailability as compared to cyclosporine (nonmodified) and cannot be used interchangeably without close monitoring.

Unlike some of the more cytotoxic immunosuppressants, cyclosporine is less harmful to bone marrow cells. When prescribed for transplant recipients, it is often used in combination with a corticosteroid such as prednisone.

Mechanism of Action: Cyclosporine inhibits the function of calcineurin. This diminishes the activity of T cells and B cells and suppresses the immune response.

Pharmacokinetics:

Route(s)	PO, IV, ophthalmic
Absorption	Oral absorption is highly variable
Distribution	Widely distributed; crosses the placenta; secreted in breast milk; 90% bound to lipoproteins
Primary metabolism	Hepatic (CYP3A), extensive first-pass metabolism
Primary excretion	Bile and feces
Onset of action	Peak: 3–4 h
Duration of action	Half-life: 16–27 h

Adverse Effects: The primary adverse effect of cyclosporine is nephrotoxicity, with up to 75% of patients experiencing a reduction in urine flow. Over half the patients taking the drug will experience HTN and tremor. Hirsutism occurs in many patients. Other common adverse effects are elevated hepatic enzymes, headache, and gingival hyperplasia. Infections are common during cyclosporine therapy, including reactivation of latent herpes or varicella infections. Periodic blood counts are necessary to ensure that leukocytes do not fall below 4,000, or platelets below 75,000. Anaphylaxis has been reported with IV administration. Long-term therapy increases the risk of malignancy, especially lymphomas and skin cancers.

Contraindications/Precautions: Patients who are taking cyclosporine should avoid direct exposure to the sun due to an increased risk of skin cancer. Because cyclosporine is nephrotoxic, the drug is either contraindicated or should be used with extreme caution in patients with renal impairment. The drug should not be used during pregnancy or lactation. Because cyclosporine is primarily eliminated via the bile, its dose should be reduced in patients with hepatic or biliary impairment. Patients with active infections should be treated with anti-infectives prior to cyclosporine therapy.

Drug Interactions: Cyclosporine is a major substrate of CYP3A4 and may interact with drugs that inhibit or induce this enzyme. Drugs that may decrease cyclosporine levels include phenytoin, phenobarbital, carbamazepine, and rifampin. Azole antifungal drugs, oral hypoglycemics, and macrolide antibiotics may increase cyclosporine levels. Because cyclosporine increases blood pressure, the doses of antihypertensives will require adjustment. Potassium-sparing diuretics should be avoided because their concurrent use with cyclosporine causes hyperkalemia. Cyclosporine should be given with caution with other nephrotoxic drugs due to the potential for additive kidney damage. Statins should not be used concurrently with cyclosporine due to the potential for myopathy or rhabdomyolysis. **Herbal/Food**: Food decreases the absorption of the drug. Grapefruit juice can raise cyclosporine levels by 50% to 200%. The immune-enhancing effects of astragalus and echinacea may interfere with the action of immunosuppressants.

Pregnancy: Category C.

Treatment of Overdose: An overdose of cyclosporine can result in significant nephrotoxicity and hepatotoxicity. General supportive measures are indicated.

Nursing Responsibilities:

- Establish baseline laboratory values with CBC, platelet count, and liver and renal function tests. Monitor laboratory values monthly during treatment and notify the prescriber of any impending thrombocytopenia or significant changes in renal or hepatic function test values.
- Prior to administering this drug, assess for active infections. Notify the prescriber of any known or suspected infections.
- Observe and continuously assess patients who are receiving parenteral cyclosporine for at least 30 minutes after the start of infusion and at frequent intervals thereafter to detect allergic or other adverse reactions.
- Monitor I&O ratio and pattern because nephrotoxicity occurs in about one third of transplant patients.
- Monitor vital signs periodically during therapy. HTN occurs in over half the patients taking this drug.

- Continually assess for symptoms and signs of local or systemic infection due to fungi, viruses, or bacteria.
- Assess blood or plasma drug concentrations at regular intervals, especially in patients who are receiving this drug PO for prolonged periods, because drug absorption is erratic.

Patient and Family Education:

- Avoid contact with crowds or persons who have infections and immediately report any signs of infection.
- Take this medication at the same time each day to maintain consistent drug blood levels.
- Do not take this drug with grapefruit juice because this can raise cyclosporine levels by 50% to 200%.
- Attend all scheduled follow-up appointments.
- Schedule a dentist appointment prior to starting cyclosporine treatment and practice good oral hygiene because this drug may cause growth of gums. Inspect the mouth daily for white patches, sores, or swollen gums.
- Excessive hair growth is reversible when this drug is discontinued.
- Take this medication with meals to reduce gastric irritation and nausea. The palatability of the oral solution can be improved by mixing it with milk, chocolate milk, or orange juice, preferably at room temperature.
- Take blood pressure frequently. Write down the readings and bring them to each follow-up appointment.
- Avoid direct sunlight and wear protective clothing outdoors because this drug can increase the risk of skin cancer.

Drugs Similar to Cyclosporine (Neoral, Sandimmune)

The only other calcineurin inhibitor is tacrolimus. Although not calcineurin inhibitors, sirolimus and temsirolimus are immunosuppressants similar to tacrolimus and are described next.

Sirolimus (Rapamune): Approved in 1999, sirolimus is a PO drug isolated from a soil bacterium that shares a similar structure and potent immunosuppressant properties with tacrolimus. Sirolimus, however, acts by a unique mechanism; that is, it binds to a protein known as FKBP that prevents T-cell activation and proliferation and the production of antibodies by B cells. Sirolimus does not exhibit the serious organ toxicity characteristic of tacrolimus. This drug appears to be less effective than the calcineurin inhibitors, but it does exert synergistic immunosuppression when used with other immunosuppressive agents. Sirolimus is only approved for use in the prophylaxis of kidney transplant rejection in combination with cyclosporine and corticosteroids for the first year after transplantation. Its safety and effectiveness beyond 1 year have not been established. At 2 to 4 months post-transplantation, the cyclosporine may be gradually withdrawn over a 4- to 8-week period. The serum levels of sirolimus must be adjusted upward when cyclosporine is withdrawn. Adverse effects include hyperlipidemia, hypercholesterolemia, peripheral edema, tremor, azotemia, elevated serum creatinine, HTN, diarrhea, and anemia. As with other immunodepressants, an increase in the incidence of malignancies may occur. This drug is pregnancy category C.

Tacrolimus (Prograf, Protopic): Approved by the FDA in 1994, tacrolimus is available in PO capsule or IV forms for the prophylaxis of heart and liver transplant rejection. It is used off-label for other transplants as well as for graft-versus-host disease, nephritic syndrome, psoriasis, and uveitis. A topical form of tacrolimus (Protopic) is indicated for the short-term treatment of eczema and atopic dermatitis; the topical drug contains a black box warning of possible lymphoma and skin cancer. Tacrolimus is 100 times more potent than cyclosporine and appears to be more effective in some patients at preventing transplant rejection. Nephrotoxicity may occur in half the patients taking this drug. Neurotoxicity symptoms are common and include headache, tremor, paresthesias, insomnia, and dizziness. Hypertension, anemia, hyperglycemia, and GI complaints occur in a significant number of patients who are taking tacrolimus. Like cyclosporine, an increased incidence of infections and malignancies may occur with tacrolimus use. This drug is pregnancy category C.

Temsirolimus (Torisel): One of the newest immunosuppressants approved in 2007, temsirolimus is structurally similar to sirolimus and acts by the same mechanism. In fact, temsirolimus is metabolized in the liver to sirolimus. It is approved to treat patients with advanced renal cell carcinoma that has not responded to other therapies. This drug is administered only by the IV route. Temsirolimus is toxic to the hematologic system; 94% of patients will experience anemia, 53% will experience lymphopenia, and 32% will experience leukopenia. Hyperglycemia occurs in most patients; thus patients with diabetes will require close monitoring. Most patients who are taking the drug will also experience hyperlipidemia that may be serious enough to require pharmacotherapy. Interstitial lung disease is a rare though potentially fatal adverse effect. This drug is pregnancy category D.

Pharm*FACT*

Each day, about 77 people receive organ transplants in the United States, and 19 people die waiting for transplants. *Source:* OrganDonor.Gov, n.d.

45.6 Cytotoxic agents and antimetabolites are used to suppress proliferating B cells and T cells.

Cytotoxic drugs are immunosuppressive agents used to kill B cells and T cells. Antimetabolites do not kill directly, but instead severely restrict the replication of B cells and T cells. Each of these agents acts by a different mechanism. Some of the drugs resemble essential chemical building blocks needed for the biosynthesis of DNA and block replication. Others inhibit protein synthesis. Most of the cytotoxic and antimetabolite immunosuppressants are nonspecific, affecting many different cells of the immune response. They have the same general indications and adverse effects as the calcineurin inhibitors.

CONNECTIONS

Complementary and Alternative Therapies Echinacea

Description: Nine species of echinacea have been identified, and all are native to the midwestern United States and central Canada. *Echinacea purpurea* (purple coneflower) and *Echinacea angustifolia* (narrow-leaf coneflower) are the two most commonly studied species. All portions of the plant contain chemicals that have potential pharmacologic activity.

History and Claims: Echinacea was used by Native Americans to treat various wounds and injuries. Until the widespread manufacture of antibiotics in the late 1940s, echinacea was commonly used as an anti-infective.

Standardization: The flowers, leaves, and stems of this plant are harvested and dried. Preparations include dried powder, tincture, fluid extracts, and teas. No single ingredient seems to be responsible for the herb's activity. A large number of potentially active chemicals have been identified from the extracts. Recommended doses include 300 mg dry powdered extract (standardized to 3.5% echinacoside) or 0.5 to 1 g dried root or tea.

Evidence: There has been wide variation in the quality and doses of echinacea used in research studies, which makes comparisons and conclusions extremely difficult. Echinacea is claimed to boost the immune system by increasing IFN levels, increasing phagocytosis, and inhibiting the bacterial enzyme hyaluronidase. Some substances in echinacea appear to have antiviral activity; thus the herb is sometimes taken to treat the common cold and influenza—an indication for which it has received official approval in Germany. In general, echinacea is used as a supportive treatment for any disease involving inflammation and to enhance the immune system. Adverse effects are rare. However, it may interfere with drugs that have immunosuppressant effects.

Source: From "Echinacea," by B. Kligler, 2003, *American Family Physician, 67*(1), pp. 77–80, 83; "Echinacea for Preventing and Treating the Common Cold," by K. Linde, B. Barrett, R. Bauer, D. Melchart, & K. Woelkart, 2006, *Cochrane Database of Systematic Reviews, 1.* Art. No.: CD000530. DOI: 10.1002/14651858.CD000530.pub2.

PROTOTYPE DRUG Azathioprine (Azasan, Imuran)

Classification: **Therapeutic:** Immunosuppressant
Pharmacologic: Cytotoxic agent

Therapeutic Effects and Uses: An older immunosuppressant approved in 1968, azathioprine is indicated for the prophylaxis of kidney transplant rejection and for the treatment of severe RA. Off-label indications include other inflammatory disorders such as Crohn's disease, autoimmune hepatitis, myasthenia gravis, SLE, and ulcerative colitis. When treating nontransplant conditions, it is generally prescribed only when standard treatments fail.

Azathioprine is usually given PO, but it may be given by the IV route to patients who are unable to take the drug by mouth. When used to prevent transplant rejection, it is usually administered in combination with other immunosuppressants.

Mechanism of Action: Azathioprine inhibits DNA synthesis, resulting in DNA damage and chromosome breakage. The drug is metabolized to mercaptopurine in the liver, an active substance marketed as an antineoplastic drug for leukemia.

Pharmacokinetics:

Route(s)	PO, IV
Absorption	Well absorbed
Distribution	Crosses the placenta; secreted in breast milk; 30% bound to plasma proteins
Primary metabolism	Hepatic; metabolized to mercaptopurine, an active metabolite
Primary excretion	Renal
Onset of action	7–14 days
Duration of action	Half-life: 3 h

Adverse Effects: Azathioprine causes bone marrow suppression that can result in pancytopenia, agranulocytosis, leukopenia, and thrombocytopenia. Serious infections may occur secondary to immunosuppression, and latent herpes or varicella infections may become reactivated during azathioprine therapy. Hepatotoxicity has been reported with this drug. Nausea and vomiting are common, especially during the first few weeks of therapy. Patients who have received a renal transplant and who are being treated with azathioprine have an increased risk of developing skin and lymphoid malignancies. The toxicities of azathioprine are dose related and occur more frequently in patients who have received a renal transplant compared with those who are treated for RA.

Contraindications/Precautions: Azathioprine should be used with extreme caution in patients with preexisting hematologic disease or hepatic impairment. Blood counts and hepatic enzymes must be regularly monitored. Azathioprine is contraindicated during pregnancy and lactation.

Drug Interactions: Additive bone marrow suppression is expected if azathioprine is given concurrently with other immunosuppressants. Concurrent use of allopurinol with azathioprine can result in a large increase in azathioprine activity and hematologic toxicity. The use of angiotensin-converting enzyme (ACE) inhibitors with azathioprine may induce anemia and severe leukopenia. **Herbal/Food**: None known.

Pregnancy: Category D.

Treatment of Overdose: Hemodialysis may be of value in removing some azathioprine from the blood following an overdose. Other treatment measures are supportive.

Nursing Responsibilities:

- Obtain baseline laboratory tests and perform CBCs at least weekly during the first month of therapy, twice monthly during the second and third months, and monthly or more frequently thereafter if needed.
- Regularly assess for adverse effects because this drug has a high potential for toxicity. Report any dramatic or persistent decreases in leukocyte or platelet counts, which may represent irreversible bone marrow depression.

- Continually assess for symptoms and signs of local or systemic infection.
- Monitor kidney function (urine protein, urine electrolytes, creatinine clearance, serum creatinine, blood urea nitrogen [BUN]) and the I&O ratio, noting the color, character, and specific gravity of urine.
- Monitor liver function including alkaline phosphatase, aspartate aminotransferase (AST), alanine aminotransferase (ALT), and serum bilirubin. Repeat at least every 3 months.
- Monitor for abnormal bleeding signs such as easy bruising, bleeding gums, petechiae, purpura, melena, epistaxis, hematuria, hemoptysis, and hematemesis.
- Use protective isolation to reduce infections in the hospitalized patient.
- Avoid invasive procedures such as IM injections if platelet counts are 50,000/mm^3 or less due to the potential for bleeding.

Patient and Family Education:

- Take this drug in divided doses (as prescribed) with meals to reduce gastric irritation and nausea.
- Do not receive any vaccinations during therapy because this could precipitate unusually severe reactions due to the immunosuppressive effects of this drug.
- Avoid contact with crowds or persons who have infections and immediately report any signs of infection.
- Exercise excellent personal hygiene because infection is a constant danger when taking immunosuppressive therapy.
- Use effective birth control during therapy and for 4 months after this drug is discontinued because this drug is associated with birth defects.
- Do not breast-feed while taking this drug without approval of the health care provider.

Drugs Similar to Azathioprine (Azasan, Imuran)

Other cytotoxic and antimetabolite drugs indicated for immunosuppression include anakinra, cyclophosphamide, etanercept, methotrexate, mycophenolate, and thalidomide.

Anakinra (Kineret): Approved in 2001, anakinra is an IL-1 receptor antagonist that prevents the formation of certain inflammatory cytokines. This drug's only indication is for the treatment of RA that has not responded to first-line agents. It is administered only by the subcutaneous route. Injection site reaction is the most frequent adverse effect. Because the drug lowers WBC counts, secondary infections occur in almost 40% of patients taking this drug.

Cyclophosphamide (Cytoxan): Cyclophosphamide is one of the most commonly prescribed drugs for patients with cancer. It acts by forming cross-links in DNA, which prevents cancer cell replication. It is a powerful immunosuppressant, affecting both B cells and T cells. It is used off-label for SLE, graft-versus-host disease, and RA, and for the transplant prophylaxis of solid organs. Hematologic toxicity (pancytopenia, leucopenia, anemia, and thrombocytopenia) is a major dose-limiting adverse effect. Cyclophosphamide is a prototype antineoplastic drug discussed in Chapter 57. This drug is pregnancy category D.

Etanercept (Enbrel): Approved in 1998, etanercept is a protein that mimics the natural receptor for TNF. TNF binds with the drug, rather that its receptors on T cells. This inhibition of TNF activity reduces the levels of damaging cytokines that cause inflammation and joint destruction in patients with RA. The drug is FDA approved to treat RA, psoriatic arthritis, and ankylosing spondylitis. It is administered only by the subcutaneous route. Injection site reactions, headache, infections, nausea, and vomiting are the most frequent adverse effects. This drug is pregnancy category B.

Methotrexate (Amethopterin, Rheumatrex, Trexall): Methotrexate is an older antimetabolite approved in 1953 that acts by inhibiting the enzyme responsible for folic acid metabolism. Like cyclophosphamide, it is indicated for various cancers as well as serious inflammatory disorders such as RA, psoriasis, SLE, and ulcerative colitis. The most frequently reported adverse reactions include nausea, vomiting, stomatitis, esophagitis, oral ulceration, and abdominal distress. Hematologic adverse reactions are common. Methotrexate is a prototype antineoplastic drug discussed in Chapter 57. This drug is pregnancy category X.

Mycophenolate (CellCept, Myfortic): Approved in 1995, mycophenolate is a potent immunosuppressant that acts by inhibiting the DNA synthesis of B cells and T cells. There are two forms of mycophenolate. Mycophenolate mofetil (CellCept) is a prodrug that is converted to its active form, mycophenolic acid, in the body. It is given IV or PO, usually in combination with other immunosuppressants such as cyclosporine and corticosteroids. Mycophenolate sodium (Myfortic) is a delayed release tablet.

Indications for mycophenolate include the prophylaxis of heart, kidney, or liver transplant rejection. Mycophenolate appears to be more effective than azathioprine for the prophylaxis of transplant rejection. This drug was recently given orphan drug status for the treatment of patients with myasthenia gravis and phemigus vulgaris. Off-label indications include SLE, graft-versus-host disease, and atopic dermatitis. GI adverse effects such as nausea, vomiting, constipation, diarrhea, dyspepsia, and abdominal pain are common. Other relatively frequent adverse effects include tachycardia, tremor, back pain, sinusitis, increased urinary frequency, and blood dyscrasias. Weekly CBCs should be obtained and the drug withheld if the absolute neutrophil count (ANC) falls below $1.3 \times (10)^3$ cells/mcL. This is a pregnancy category D drug.

Thalidomide (Thalomid): Thalidomide is an infamous drug that caused serious fetal malformations in patients who were pregnant and took the drug in the late 1950s. At that time the drug was not approved for use in the United States, but it was available in other countries as a sedative. Thalidomide has received orphan drug status for the treatment of a variety of neoplastic and immune-related disorders, including primary brain malignancies, graft-versus-host disease, Crohn's disease, Kaposi's sarcoma, HIV-wasting syndrome, leprosy, stomatitis, *Mycobacterium* infections, and multiple myeloma. Other off-label indications include SLE and renal cell cancer. The drug is highly regulated and is available only through a limited number of pharmacists and physicians. Because the drug is pregnancy category X, a negative pregnancy test is required prior to administration in women with childbearing potential. Adverse effects include teratogenesis, thromboembolic disease, drowsiness, and peripheral neuropathy.

45.7 Antibodies are used to prevent acute transplant rejection, autoimmune disorders, and malignancies.

Recall from Chapter 43 that antibodies are proteins that are produced following an antigen challenge. B cells become plasma cells, which subsequently produce massive amounts of antibodies that help rid the body of the antigen through several mechanisms. Antibodies that are produced by a plasma cell are very specific to the antigen. For example, exposure to *Streptococcus* would result in different antibodies than would *Escherichia coli*. In this example, antibodies boost the immune system. It may seem puzzling then to learn that certain antibodies may be administered to patients to suppress the immune response. How is this possible?

The answer is to somehow create antibodies against human immune cells. A simple method is to inject animals (usually horses, rabbits, or mice) with human T cells, B cells, or thymocytes. The animal creates antibodies against the human immune cells, which can be collected and purified. When injected in humans, the animal's antibodies will attack the T cells (or T-cell receptors). These are called **polyclonal antibodies** because they contain a wide mixture of different antibodies. This polyclonal drug product, called antithymocyte globulin (Atgam, Thymoglobulin), is a potent immunosuppressant and is available for the prophylaxis of kidney transplant rejection and aplastic anemia.

In the 1980s a technique was developed to harvest antibodies produced by a single B cell. Because a single B cell produces a single antibody, it is called a **monoclonal antibody (MAB).** An MAB is very specific, targeting a single type of target cell or receptor. This allows greater effects on the target cell or receptor at lower doses and with fewer adverse effects than using polyclonal antibodies.

The first MABs were derived from mouse cells and had short half-lives. The human immune system quickly recognized them as foreign when they were injected in patients. Through genetic engineering, scientists have been able to replace the mouse portions of the antibody with human sequences, thus allowing it to escape detection by the immune system for longer periods and extending its half-life.

Scientists have created over 20 different MABs to attack a diverse number of targets. The majority of the MABs have been designed to attack specific types of cancer cells (see Chapter 58). Others are used to treat autoimmune or inflammatory disorders by attacking certain cells of the immune system. The FDA-approved MABs are shown in Table 45.3.

Three of the MABs are used as immunosuppressants. Muromonab-CD3 (Orthoclone, OKT3) is administered to prevent the rejection of kidney, heart, and liver transplants and to deplete the bone marrow of T cells prior to marrow transplant. Basiliximab (Simulect) and daclizumab (Zenapax) are given to prevent the acute rejection of kidney transplants.

The MABs are difficult to learn because many have similar names that end in *–mab* (for monoclonal antibody). There is, however, some consistency to the names—they reflect the origin of the antibody.

- MABs of murine (mouse) origin have *–muro* in the name (e.g., muromonab).
- MABs that have 75% human sequences are called chimeric and have *–xi* in the name (e.g., basiliximab).
- MABs that have 90% human sequences are called humanized and have *-zu* in their name (e.g., daclizumab).

PROTOTYPE DRUG Muromonab-CD3 (Orthoclone, OKT3)

Classification: **Therapeutic:** Immunosuppressant
Pharmacologic: Monoclonal antibody

Therapeutic Effects and Uses: Approved by the FDA in 1986, muromonab-CD3 was the first MAB approved for human use. It has been a drug of choice for preventing the acute transplant rejection of solid organs, especially in patients who are resistant to treatment with corticosteroids.

Muromonab-CD3 is administered by the IV route for 10 to 14 days following a diagnosis of acute rejection. The drug immediately causes a reduction in functional T cells. T-cell function returns to baseline levels within 2 to 7 days after discontinuation of this drug.

Mechanism of Action: T lymphocytes have a protein called CD3 on their surface. The normal function of CD3 is to serve as a receptor to bind antigens; the bound antigen then signals the T cell to proliferate and attack the invader. Muromonab specifically binds to the CD3 protein, preventing the T cell from initiating an immune response.

Pharmacokinetics:

Route(s)	IV
Absorption	N/A
Distribution	Widely distributed; unknown if it crosses the placenta or is secreted in breast milk
Primary metabolism	Not fully known; possibly by reticuloendothelial system
Primary excretion	Eliminated by muromonab-CD3 antibodies
Onset of action	Begins within minutes; peak: 2–7 days
Duration of action	7 days

Adverse Effects: Thirty to 60 minutes following the initial IV administration of muromonab, a **cytokine release syndrome** is observed. This occurs because the antibody induces a transient activation of the T cell before blocking it, causing an acute inflammatory response due to massive cytokine release. The most serious symptom of this syndrome is high fever, which

TABLE 45.3 FDA-Approved Monoclonal Antibodies

Drug/Antibody	Approval Date	Target	Approved Treatment(s)
abciximab (ReoPro)	1994	Inhibition of glycoprotein IIb/IIIa	Cardiovascular disease
adalimumab (Humira)	2002	Inhibition of TNF signaling	Inflammatory diseases (mostly autoimmune disorders)
alemtuzumab (Campath)	2001	CD52	Chronic lymphocytic leukemia
basiliximab (Simulect)	1998	IL-2 receptor	Transplant rejection
bevacizumab (Avastin)	2004	Vascular endothelial growth factor	Colorectal cancer, lung cancer
bortezomib (Velcade)	2003	26S proteosome	Multiple myeloma and mantle cell lymphoma
cetuximab (Erbitux)	2004	Epidermal growth factor receptor	Colorectal cancer; head and neck cancer
daclizumab (Zenapax)	1997	IL-2 receptor	Transplant rejection
dasatinib (Sprycel)	2006	Tyrosine kinase enzymes	Chronic myelogenous leukemia; acute lymphoblastic leukemia
eculizumab (Soliris)	2007	Complement system protein C5	Inflammatory diseases, including paroxysmal nocturnal hemoglobinuria
efalizumab (Raptiva)	2002	CD11a	Inflammatory diseases (psoriasis)
gemtuzumab (Ozogamicin, Mylotarg)	2000	CD33	Acute myelogenous leukemia (with calicheamicin)
ibritumomab (Zevalin)	2002	CD20	Non-Hodgkin's lymphoma (with yttrium-90 or indium-111)
infliximab (Remicade)	1998	Inhibition of TNF-a signaling	Inflammatory diseases (mostly autoimmune disorders)
lapatinib (Tykerb)	2007	Epidermal growth factor receptor, human epidermal receptor Type 2 (HER2)	Advanced or metastatic breast cancer
muromonab-CD3 (Orthoclone, OKT3)	1986	T-cell CD3 receptor	Transplant rejection
natalizumab (Tysabri)	2006	T-cell VLA4 receptor	Inflammatory diseases (mainly autoimmune-related MS therapy)
nilotinib (Tasigna)	2007	Kinase enzymes	Chronic myelogenous leukemia
omalizumab (Xolair)	2004	Immunoglobulin E (IgE)	Inflammatory diseases (mainly allergy-related asthma therapy)
palivizumab (Synagis)	1998	An epitope of the F protein of respiratory syncitial virus	Viral infection (especially respiratory syncytial virus [RSV])
panitumumab (Vectibix)	2006	Epidermal growth factor receptor	Colorectal cancer
ranibizumab (Lucentis)	2006	Vascular endothelial growth factor	Macular degeneration
rituximab (Rituxan, Mabthera)	1997	CD20	Non-Hodgkin's lymphoma
sorafenib (Nexavar)	2005	Tyrosine receptor kinases	Advanced renal cell carcinoma
tositumomab (Bexxar)	2003	CD20	Non-Hodgkin's lymphoma
trastuzumab (Herceptin)	1998	ErbB2	Breast cancer

sometimes exceeds 40°C (104°F). Other symptoms of this syndrome include chills, nausea, vomiting, dyspnea, angina, and tremor. Serious pulmonary edema may develop due to fluid overload. Prevention of cytokine release syndrome may be accomplished by administering corticosteroids, antihistamines, and acetaminophen 1 to 4 hours prior to muromonab therapy.

Anaphylaxis has been reported and most commonly occurs within 10 minutes of administration of this drug. Aseptic meningitis syndrome has been reported, with symptoms presenting as headache, fever, meningismus, and photophobia. Patients who have received a transplant and are treated with muromonab have an increased risk of developing infections and secondary malignancies of the skin and lymphoid tissues.

Contraindications/Precautions: Patients with hypervolemia or uncompensated heart failure should not receive muromonab-CD3 due to the risk of severe pulmonary edema. This drug is contraindicated in patients with fever greater than 38°C (100°F). This drug may cause seizures and should be used with caution in those with a prior history of seizure disorders. Muromonab should be used with caution in patients with unstable angina, recent MI, ischemic cardiac disease, coronary artery disease, or pulmonary edema because they are at greater risk of developing serious complications from cytokine release syndrome.

Drug Interactions: The dosage of other immunosuppressant drugs should be reduced during therapy with muromonab.

Cyclosporine therapy should be reduced or withdrawn to prevent nephrotoxicity. **Herbal/Food**: None known.

Pregnancy: Category C.

Treatment of Overdose: Overdose may result in severe symptoms that include hyperthermia, chills, vomiting, diarrhea, pulmonary edema, acute renal failure, and hemolytic anemia. Treatment is supportive.

Nursing Responsibilities:

- Obtain baseline laboratory tests and perform CBCs at least weekly during the first month of therapy, twice monthly during the second and third months, and monthly or more frequently thereafter if needed.
- Regularly assess for adverse effects because this drug has a high potential for toxicity. Report dramatic or persistent decreases in leukocyte or platelet counts, which may represent irreversible bone marrow depression to the prescriber.
- Closely monitor for signs of cytokine release syndrome such as flulike symptoms, dyspnea, chest pain, pulmonary edema, dysrhythmias, and renal impairment. Report any signs of this disorder to the prescriber immediately.
- Continually assess for symptoms and signs of local or systemic infection due to fungi, viruses, or bacteria.
- Assess baseline and periodic fluid status. Monitor kidney function. Report any signs of impending fluid overload to the prescriber immediately.
- Monitor liver function tests including alkaline phosphatase, AST, ALT, and serum bilirubin. Repeat at least every 3 months.
- Monitor for abnormal bleeding signs such as easy bruising, bleeding gums, petechiae, purpura, melena, epistaxis, hematuria, hemoptysis, and hematemesis.
- Prevent infections in the hospitalized patient by using protective isolation.
- Monitor for anaphylaxis for at least 30 minutes following the injection.

Patient and Family Education:

- Avoid contact with crowds or persons who have infections and immediately report any signs of infection to the health care provider.
- Exercise excellent personal hygiene because infection is a constant danger when taking immunosuppressive therapy.
- Immediately report the appearance of rash; hives; shortness of breath; flulike symptoms, including high fever; persistent headache; unusual bruising or bleeding; palpitations; swelling of the feet or ankles; unusual changes in behavior or mood; or seizures.
- Immediately notify the health care provider of any known or suspected pregnancy.

Drugs Similar to Muromonab-CD3 (Orthoclone, OKT3)

Three other antibody drugs are used in transplant medicine: antithymocyte globulin, basiliximab, and daclizumab. The MABs used for RA such as adalimumab (Humira) and infliximab (Remicade) are discussed in Chapter 75.

Antithymocyte globulin (Atgam, Thymoglobulin): Approved in 1981, antithymocyte globulin consists of polyclonal antibodies obtained from the serum of horses (Atgam) or rabbits (Thymoglobulin) exposed to human T cells. Doses of the two are not interchangeable. The drug is a potent immunosuppressant used for the prophylaxis and management of transplant rejection and for the treatment of moderate to severe aplastic anemia in patients who are unable to have bone marrow transplantation. It is used off-label to treat graft-versus-host disease and myelodysplastic syndrome. It is available only by IV infusion and is usually administered once daily for 1 to 2 weeks. A single infusion may lower the lymphocyte count by 85% to 90%. After discontinuation of therapy, T-cell counts take several months to return to baseline levels. The most common adverse effects are fever, chills, malaise, headache, diarrhea, itching, and other flulike symptoms. Corticosteroids, antihistamines, or acetaminophen may be administered 1 hour prior to antithymocyte globulin therapy to prevent cytokine release syndrome. Anaphylaxis has been reported. Like other immunosuppressants, an increased incidence of infections and malignancies is expected. This drug is pregnancy category C.

Basiliximab (Simulect): Basiliximab is a monoclonal antibody against CD25, a receptor on the surface of activated T cells. Under normal conditions, IL-2 binds to the CD25 receptor when antigens are present and the T cell initiates an immune response against the antigen. By binding to CD25, basiliximab stops IL-2 from activating the T cell, and the immune response is prevented. This drug does not lower the total number of circulating T cells; it does, however, lower their ability to respond to an antigen challenge. Administered by IV infusion, the standard regimen is two doses; one is given 2 hours prior to transplantation and the other is given 4 days later. Following the two infusions, the actions of basiliximab may last for 4 to 6 weeks. The only approved indication for basiliximab is for prophylaxis of kidney transplant rejection. It is administered in combination with other immunosuppressants, usually cyclosporine and corticosteroids. Basiliximab causes few adverse effects compared to the calcineurin inhibitors or the cytotoxic immunosuppressants. The most common adverse effects are GI related such as nausea, vomiting, abdominal pain, and diarrhea. Anaphylaxis has been reported. This drug is pregnancy category B.

Daclizumab (Zenapax): Approved in 1997, daclizumab is very similar to basiliximab but has a longer half-life. Like basiliximab, daclizumab is a monoclonal antibody that binds to the CD25 receptor on activated T cells and blocks the effects of IL-2. It is administered IV and acts by the same mechanism of action as basiliximab. The only approved indication for daclizumab is for the prophylaxis of kidney transplant rejection. It is administered in combination with other immunosuppressants, usually cyclosporine and corticosteroids. It has the same adverse effect profile as basiliximab. The standard regimen is five doses, with the first being given just prior to transplantation. The remaining four doses are spaced 2 weeks apart. This drug is pregnancy category C.

CONNECTION Checkpoint 45.2

Patients with hypervolemia should not receive muromonab-CD3 due the risk of severe pulmonary edema. From what you learned in Chapter 35, describe some of the drugs that would likely be used to correct fluid overload prior to muromonab-CD3 therapy. See Answer to Connection Checkpoint 45.2 in Appendix A.

45.8 Corticosteroids are widely used as immunosuppressants but have significant long-term adverse effects.

The corticosteroids, or glucocorticoids, are potent inhibitors of inflammation and are discussed in detail in Chapters 44 and 69. They are often the drugs of choice for the short-term therapy of severe inflammation.

In addition to their anti-inflammatory effects, corticosteroids affect nearly every aspect of the immune response. They intervene at multiple steps in the immune response, including antigen presentation, production of cytokines, and the proliferation of lymphocytes.

- **Lymphocyte effect.** A single dose of corticosteroid reduces circulating lymphocyte counts within a few hours. This inhibits the ability of the body to react to an antigen challenge.
- **Monocyte effect.** Corticosteroids quickly deplete the body of monocytes and macrophages. Macrophages are responsible for presenting antigens to lymphocytes.
- **Neutrophil effect.** Corticosteroids cause neutrophils to move from the bone marrow into the general circulation, resulting in increased numbers of circulating neutrophils. The drug then prevents the neutrophils from migrating out of the circulation to sites of inflammation.

NURSING PROCESS APPLICATION

Patients Receiving Immunomodulators

Assessment	Potential Nursing Diagnoses
Prior to administration: • Obtain a complete health history, including allergies, drug history, and possible drug interactions. • Perform a physical examination, including vital signs, body weight, CBC, liver profile, and serum creatinine levels.	• *Risk for Infection,* related to bone marrow suppression (immunostimulants) or depressed immune response (immunosuppressants) • *Risk for Injury,* related to adverse effects of drug • *Deficient Knowledge (Immunomodulators),* related to purpose, precautions, and adverse effects of drug

Planning: Patient Goals and Expected Outcomes

The patient will:

- Demonstrate therapeutic effect from the drug regimen.
- Demonstrate an understanding of the drug's action by accurately describing the drug's adverse effects and precautions.
- Immediately report significant adverse effects such as shortness of breath, fever, stomatitis, loose stools, cough, bruising, or bleeding.

Implementation

Interventions and (Rationales)	Patient and Family Education
• Monitor vital signs, including body temperature (elevated temperature may indicate the onset of infection or cytokine release syndrome with muromonab-CD3); pulse (immunostimulants may cause dysrhythmias); respiratory rate; and blood pressure (hypotension occurs with capillary leak syndrome).	Instruct the patient to: • Report symptoms associated with infection, including sore throat, myalgia, fever, cough, or dysuria. • Report syncopal or dizziness episodes to the health care provider. • Report palpitations or shortness of breath to the health care provider.
• Monitor laboratory results for leukopenia, neutropenia, thrombocytopenia, anemia, increased liver enzymes, and serum creatinine. (All agents potentially suppress bone marrow function. Patients are at high risk for hepatoxicity and nephrotoxicity.)	Instruct the patient to: • Comply with all ordered laboratory tests. • Immediately report any unusual bleeding or jaundice. • Avoid crowds and people with active infections. • Not receive vaccinations during therapy because they may precipitate unusually severe reactions.
• Monitor the patient's psychological and mental health status. Consult a mental health specialist if necessary. (Interferon may cause depression and suicidal ideation.)	Instruct the patient to: • Report symptoms of mental changes, depression, or suicidal thoughts to the health care provider. • Understand that the depression is related to the medication and will resolve.
• Monitor for non–life-threatening adverse effects such as muscle aches, general malaise, anorexia, and hair changes, and report them to the prescriber at onset. (Simple interventions may minimize non–life-threatening adverse effects. Alopecia may occur with prolonged IFN therapy. Hirsutism is an adverse effect associated with cyclosporine.)	Instruct the patient: • To take acetaminophen for flulike symptoms. • To take the medication at bedtime, if possible, to reduce adverse effects. • To consume small, frequent feedings to maintain nutritional and hydration status. • That changes in body hair are related to the drug therapy.

Evaluation of Outcome Criteria

Evaluate the effectiveness of drug therapy by confirming that patient goals and expected outcomes have been met (see "Planning").

- Other effects. Corticosteroids block the production of prostaglandins and ILs. This results in T cells being unable to react to antigens and proliferate.

Two common drugs in this class, prednisone and methylprednisolone, have been widely used to prevent transplant rejection since the 1960s. When used for a few weeks, the corticosteroids are safe and effective immunosuppressants. The long-term adverse effects of corticosteroids, however, are serious and include osteoporosis, cataract formation, mental status changes, fluid and salt retention, HTN, hyperglycemia, obesity, and adrenal atrophy. Because of their long-term effects, health care providers have begun to look at the possibility of eliminating corticosteroids from the transplant regimen. Some regimens call for the initial use of corticosteroids, with their gradual withdrawal at some point, usually within 3 to 6 months following the transplant. The issue remains unresolved and an area of active research.

UNDERSTANDING THE CHAPTER

Key Concepts Summary

45.1 Immunomodulators are substances that either enhance or suppress the ability of the body to fight infection and disease.

45.2 Interferons are biologic response modifiers that have antiviral and antineoplastic activity.

45.3 Interleukins, vaccines, and colony-stimulating factors are used to boost the immune system.

45.4 Immunosuppressants are used to prevent transplant rejection and for the treatment of autoimmune disorders.

45.5 Calcineurin inhibitors are drugs of choice for the prophylaxis of transplant rejection.

45.6 Cytotoxic agents and antimetabolites are used to suppress proliferating B cells and T cells.

45.7 Antibodies are used to prevent acute transplant rejection, autoimmune disorders, and malignancies.

45.8 Corticosteroids are widely used as immunosuppressants but have significant long-term adverse effects.

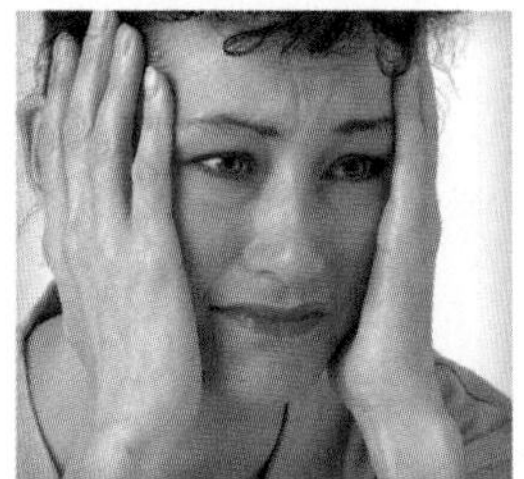

Making the PATIENT Connection

Remember the patient "Carol Banks" at the beginning of the chapter? Now read the remainder of the case study. Based on the information presented within this chapter, respond to the critical thinking questions that follow.

Carol Banks is a 42-year-old woman diagnosed with hepatitis C who was recently seen by her health care provider at an office visit. She complained of right upper quadrant pain, fatigue, anorexia, nausea, and vomiting. She has been feeling progressively worse for the past year but did not seek medical care for her problem. She has lost 12 pounds over the past 6 months.

She was initially hospitalized to receive IV fluids for dehydration and to be further evaluated. Once in the hospital, a full hepatitis panel found that Carol was positive for hepatitis C virus (HCV).

During the initial interview with Carol, she discloses that she was addicted to illegal IV drugs for 15 years and was an alcohol abuser for 20 years. However, Carol claims that she has abstained from substance abuse for the past 5 years. She resides with her husband and three children and is employed as a clerk in a local retail convenience store.

As part of the treatment for Carol's hepatitis she is prescribed interferon alfa-2b (Intron-A). She is taught to self-administer (subcutaneously) the standard dose of IFN, 3 million units given three times weekly.

Critical Thinking Questions

1. Discuss the mechanism of action for interferon alfa-2b (Intron-A) in the treatment of hepatitis C.
2. What are the adverse effects Carol is experiencing with this drug therapy? How can the nurse assist Carol to cope with the related adverse effects?
3. Identify the patient education that Carol will need concerning her drug therapy.

Case Study

Gordon Sharp has been on kidney dialysis since his car accident 2 years ago. He suffered from severe traumatic injuries and subsequently developed renal failure. Gordon's one functioning kidney has been progressively failing, and he is now on the waiting list for a kidney transplant. Preoperatively, Gordon is prescribed prophylactic cyclosporine (Sandimmune).

1. How does cyclosporine work and why is Gordon receiving the drug prior to his surgery?
2. Describe the health teaching that the nurse should present to Gordon concerning this drug therapy.
3. What dietary precautions would be indicated for this patient?

NCLEX-RN® Review

1 The nurse is monitoring the laboratory findings of a client who is taking interferon alfa-2b (Intron-A). Which of the following laboratory findings would indicate that the client is experiencing an expected adverse effect?

1. Increased white blood cell count
2. Decreased hepatic enzymes
3. Increased red blood cell count
4. Declining blood urea nitrogen

2 The client is taking muromonab-CD3 (Orthoclone) and develops a high fever, chills, and dyspnea. The nurse interprets that the client is most likely experiencing:

1. Capillary leak syndrome.
2. Cytokine release syndrome.
3. Restless leg syndrome.
4. Androgen-insensitivity syndrome.

3 The nurse who is caring for a client receiving cyclosporine (Sandimmune) will discontinue the medication immediately and call the prescriber if which of the following occurs?

1. Elevated red blood cell counts
2. Reduced basophil, lymphocyte, and monocyte levels
3. Reduced neutrophils and macrophages
4. Elevated serum creatinine and blood urea nitrogen levels

4 Azathioprine (Imuran) is prescribed to a client who had renal transplant. A nurse reviews the client's medical record and would question the medication order for which of the following clients? The client with:

1. Benign prostatic hyperplasia.
2. Cataract.
3. Cirrhosis.
4. Oliguria.

5 A nurse is instructing a client who is receiving aldesleukin (Proleukin). Which of the following should be included in the teaching plan?

1. Take a "baby" strength aspirin every day.
2. Increase physical activity to avoid weight gain.
3. Record radial pulse rate every morning in a journal.
4. Avoid physical activities such as contact sports.

6 A nurse is particularly cautious in monitoring the client who is prescribed muromonab-CD3 (Orthoclone) if the client has which of the following preexisting conditions? Select all that apply.

1. Pulmonary edema
2. Epilepsy
3. Peptic ulcer disease
4. Coronary artery disease
5. Postoperative renal transplant

See Answers to Critical Thinking Questions, Case Study, and NCLEX-RN® Review in Appendix A.

References

Arbour, R. (2005). Clinical management of the organ donor. *AACN Clinical Issues, 16*(4), 551–580.

Basu, A., Tan, H. P., & Shapiro, R. (2007). Current thinking on calcineurin inhibition in kidney transplantation. *Medscape.* Retrieved August 1, 2008, from http://www.medscape.com/viewprogram/8075

Breslin, S. (2007). Cytokine-release syndrome: Overview and nursing implications. *Clinical Journal of Oncology Nursing, 11*(1), 1092–1095.

Curtis, J. (2006). Corticosteroids and kidney transplantation. *American Journal of Nephrology, 1,* 907–908.

Duncan, M. D., & Wiles, D. S. (2005). Transplant-related immunosuppression: A review of immunosuppression and pulmonary infections. *The Proceedings of the American Thoracic Society, 2,* 449–455.

Flattery, M. P., Salyer, J., Maltby, M. C., Joyner, P. L., & Elswick, R. K. (2006). Lifestyle and health status differ over time in long-term heart transplant patients. *Progress in Transplantation, 16*(3), 232–238.

Hoffman, F. M., Nelson, B. J., Drangstveit, M. B., Flynn, B., Watercott, E. A., & Zirbes, J. M. (2006). Caring for transplant recipients in a nontransplant setting. *Critical Care Nurse, 26*(2), 53–74.

Ingelfinger, J. R., & Schwartz, M. (2005). Immunosuppression—The promise of specificity. *The New England Journal of Medicine, 353*(8), 836–840.

Kligler, B. (2003). Echinacea. *American Family Physician, 67*(1), 77–80, 83.

Krensky, A. M., Strom, T. B., & Bluestone, J. A. (2006). Immunomodulators: Immunosuppressive agents, tolerogens, and immunostimulants. In L. L. Brunton, J. S. Lazo, & K. L. Parker (Eds.), *The pharmacological basis of therapeutics* (11th ed., pp. 1463–1484). New York: McGraw-Hill.

Linde, K., Barrett, B., Bauer, R., Melchart, D., & Woelkart, K. (2006). Echinacea for preventing and treating the common cold. *Cochrane Database of Systematic Reviews, 1.* Art. No.: CD000530. DOI: 10.1002/14651858.CD000530.pub2.

Lloyd, L., & Mizen, J. (2006). A day in the life: Focus on organ transplant nursing. *Australian Nursing Journal, 13*(9), 35.

Moonan, M., Fowler, K., Cook, C., Shermont, H., Powers, D., & O'Sullivan, J. (2007). The gift of life: A nursing grand rounds presentation on organ and tissue donations. *Pediatric Nursing, 33*(5), 458–461.

OrganDonor.Gov. (n.d.). *Be an organ and tissue donor.* Retrieved August 1, 2008, from http://www.organdonor.gov/donor/index.htm

Preet, S., & Tiwari, P. (2007). Therapeutic drug monitoring of immunosuppressants: An overview. *The Indian Journal of Pharmacology, 39*(2), 560–566.

Prescilla, R. P. (2006). Immunosuppression. *Emedicine.* Retrieved August 1, 2008, from http://www.emedicine.com/ped/topic2848.htm

Russell, C. L. (2006). Culturally responsive interventions to enhance immunosuppressive medication adherence in older African American kidney transplant recipients. *Progress in Transplantation, 16*(3), 187–196.

United Network for Organ Sharing. (2008). *About organ allocation.* Retrieved August 1, 2008, from http://transplantliving.org/beforethetransplant/allocation/waitingfororgan.aspx

CHAPTER

I don't think these immunizations are necessary. They made her so sick last time!

Mother of patient "Samantha Abbott"

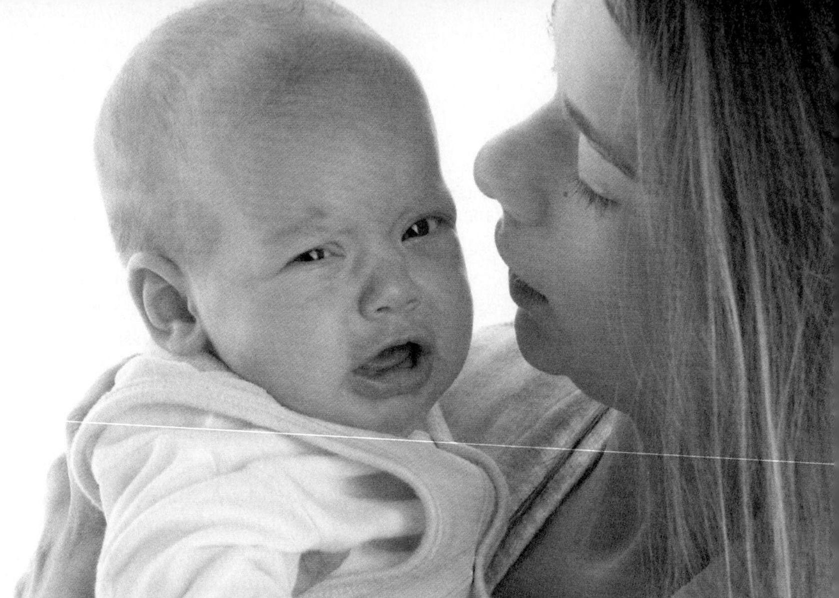

46 Immunizing Agents

Learning Outcomes

After reading this chapter, the student should be able to:

1. Explain why the development of a smallpox vaccine was one of the most significant discoveries of modern medicine.
2. Compare and contrast active and passive immunity.
3. Explain the immune response that leads to the development of active immunity.
4. Prepare a table listing the types of vaccines, their indications, and potential adverse effects.
5. Explain why it is important to administer childhood vaccines at specific ages.
6. Identify contraindications for vaccine administration.
7. Describe the pathogenesis and immunization of bacterial infections, including diphtheria, pertussis, tetanus, pneumococcus, and meningococcus.
8. Describe the pathogenesis and immunization of viral infections, including hepatitis A and B, influenza, rabies, measles, mumps, rubella, polio, varicella zoster, human papillomavirus, and rotavirus.
9. Explain the rationale for administering antibodies to establish passive immunity.
10. For each of the major vaccines and patient age groups, identify the schedule for the recommended dosage sequence established by the Centers for Disease Control and Prevention.
11. Use the nursing process to care for patients receiving immunizing agents.

Chapter Outline

The Discovery of Vaccines

Vaccines and the Immune System

Types of Vaccines

General Principles of Vaccine Administration

Active Immunity: Bacterial Immunizations

Active Immunity: Viral Immunizations

PROTOTYPE **Hepatitis B Vaccine (Engerix-B, Recombivax HB)** *p. 761*

Passive Immunity

PROTOTYPE **Rh_o [D] Immune Globulin (RhoGAM)** *p. 767*

Key Terms

active immunity, 755
antigens, 755
attenuated, 756
boosters, 755
immunization, 755
incubation period, 755
inoculation, 755
interferons, 760
passive immunity, 755
postherpetic neuralgia, 765
shingles, 765
toxoids, 756
vaccination, 755

The earliest attempts at treatments to prevent infection were reported in ancient Indian and Chinese literature when dried, powdered scabs from infected persons were administered to healthy individuals. Vaccinations have since become one of the most important medical interventions for the prevention of serious infectious disease. Routine vaccinations for polio, pertussis, diphtheria, tetanus, and measles is estimated to prevent 3 million deaths annually. This chapter examines the role of vaccines in promoting the health of both children and adults and the potential adverse effects of these drugs.

The Discovery of Vaccines

46.1 The eradication of smallpox was a great triumph in modern medicine.

In the 1790s, Dr. Edward Jenner was experimenting with the use of **inoculation,** the placement of a foreign substance on or in an individual for the purpose of disease prevention. Inoculation uses "live" virus particles obtained from an infected patient. Jenner used the cowpox virus, a benign pathogen in humans, because he predicted that exposure to that virus would provide immunity to smallpox, which was one of the most dreaded human diseases of that era. Case fatality rates of 30% or more were reported with smallpox infections. In the 18th century, the disease was a frequent cause of blindness and death for 400,000 people worldwide annually.

Jenner's inoculation of a single 8-year-old boy ultimately led to one of the greatest triumphs in disease prevention. On May 8, 1980, the World Health Assembly certified that global medical interventions had actually eradicated smallpox infections from the planet (Centers for Disease Control and Prevention [CDC], 2007a). Although this announcement was heralded by the scientific community as proof of the success of routine immunization, it also has presented new challenges. With the last known case of the disease, the need for smallpox immunization ceased and has resulted in a growing, nonimmune population. The widespread release of a modified smallpox organism to an unvaccinated population could be a potential terrorist weapon (see Chapter 78).

Vaccines and the Immune System

46.2 Vaccines are used to activate the immune system for the purpose of disease prevention.

An immune response occurs when an antigen is recognized by the B cells or T cells of the lymphatic system. **Antigens** are foreign substances that include most microbes, non human proteins, and bacterial or plant toxins. Following the first exposure to the antigen, sufficient time is needed for the body to process the antigen and mount an effective response. It is during this time, known as the **incubation period,** that the symptoms of infection and tissue injury develop. During this first antigen exposure, memory B cells or T cells are formed. Should a second or subsequent exposure to the same antigen occur, the memory cells react quickly to produce a more rapid immune response with fewer (or no) symptoms of infection. The student should review Chapter 43 for a summary of the humoral and cell-mediated immune responses before proceeding.

Edward Jenner was the first to use the term *vaccination.* **Vaccination** is the process of introducing foreign proteins or inactive cells (vaccines) into the body to trigger immune activation before the patient is exposed to the real pathogen. As a result of the vaccination, memory B cells or T cells are formed. When later exposed to the real infectious organism, these cells will react quickly by producing large quantities of antibodies and cytokines that help to neutralize or destroy the antigen. Whereas some vaccinations are needed only once, most require follow-up doses, known as **boosters,** to provide prolonged protection. The type of response induced by the real pathogen, or its vaccine, is called **active immunity.** During this response the body produces its own antibodies in response to exposure. The active immunity induced by vaccines closely resembles that caused by natural exposure to the antigen, including the generation of memory cells. The term **immunization** is considered equivalent to the term *vaccination,* and either one may be used to describe this process of disease prevention.

The effectiveness of most vaccines can be assessed by measuring the amount of antibodies produced after the vaccine has been administered, a quantity called titer. If the titer falls below a specified, protective level over time, a booster dose is indicated. Antibodies are a product of the humoral immune system. The cell-mediated immune system is also important in producing immunity, but its cellular responses are less readily measured.

Passive immunity occurs when preformed antibodies are transferred or "donated" from one person to another. For example, maternal antibodies cross the placenta and provide protection for the fetus and newborn. The pharmacotherapy for establishing passive immunity includes the administration of immune globulin following exposure to hepatitis, antivenins for snakebites, and sera to treat botulism, tetanus, and rabies. The drugs for passive immunity are administered when the patient has already been exposed to a virulent pathogen, or when the patient is at very high risk for exposure and there is not sufficient time to develop active immunity. Patients who are immunosuppressed may receive these agents to prevent infections. Because these drugs do not stimulate the patient's immune system, no memory cells are produced and protective effects last only 2 to 3 weeks. Passive immunity is presented in detail in Section 46.6.

Most vaccines are administered with the goal of preventing illness. Common vaccines include those used to prevent patients from acquiring measles, influenza, diphtheria, polio, whooping cough, tetanus, and hepatitis B. Anthrax vaccine has been used to immunize people who are at high risk for exposure to anthrax from a potential bioterrorism incident (see Chapter 78). In the case of infection by the human immunodeficiency virus (HIV), experimental HIV vaccines are given after infection has occurred for the purpose of enhancing the immune response, rather than preventing the disease. Unlike other vaccines, experimental vaccines for HIV have thus far been unable to prevent acquired immune deficiency syndrome (AIDS). The pharmacotherapy of HIV is presented in Chapter 56.

CONNECTION *Checkpoint* 46.1

The humoral and cell-mediated immune responses are components of the specific (adaptive) body defenses. From what you learned in Chapter 43, compare and contrast the humoral and cell-mediated responses to an antigen. See Answer to Connection Checkpoint 46.1 in Appendix A.

Types of Vaccines

46.3 There are four traditional methods of producing vaccines.

The goal of vaccine administration is to induce long-lasting immunity to a pathogen without producing an illness in an otherwise healthy person. Therefore, the microorganisms and other substances used as vaccines must be able to strongly activate the immune system but be modified to pose no significant risk of disease development. The vaccine must be economical to develop and be stable for storage and administration. For disease protection to be long-standing, the vaccine must be able to stimulate the production of memory B cells and T cells. There are four traditional methods of producing safe and effective vaccines, as shown in Table 46.1. All four methods are capable of inducing active immunity.

Attenuated (live) vaccines: Live vaccine products contain microorganisms that are capable of replicating and causing disease. Live vaccines are very effective at inducing immunity but are not used in vaccination because of their risk. However, effective vaccines can be developed from organisms that are **attenuated** or rendered less able to cause disease through the application of heat or chemicals. Attenuated (live) vaccines cause the development of a mild or subclinical case of the disease while still inducing lasting immunity. The type of immune response obtained from the administration of a live or attenuated organism is the same as if the patient had been exposed to the natural, nonattenuated organism. There must, however, be adequate immune functioning for the vaccine to work. The use of attenuated (live) vaccines is dangerous for individuals who are immunosuppressed because the organism may retain some residual ability to replicate and cause disease. In very rare cases, the attenuated virus may mutate to an infectious form in patients who received the vaccine. An example of a live or attenuated vaccine is the measles, mumps, and rubella vaccine (MMR).

Inactivated (killed) vaccines: Inactivated or killed vaccines are of two types: whole agent and subunit. Whole agent vaccines consist of microbes killed by heat or chemicals. Subunit vaccines consist of specific segments of a cell membrane, foreign proteins, or sequences of a chromosome rather than the whole microbe.

Inactivated or killed vaccines are safer than live vaccines because the organism is unable to replicate, mutate, or cause disease. Subsequent booster doses are required to maintain immunity if inactivated or killed vaccines are used. Examples of inactivated or killed vaccines include the influenza and hepatitis A vaccines. Examples of subunit vaccines are the human papillomavirus (HPV) vaccine and the acellular pertussis vaccine.

Toxoid vaccines: Some pathogens secrete toxins, which are responsible for the symptoms of the infection. **Toxoids** are bacterial toxins that have been chemically modified to be incapable of causing disease. When injected as a type of immunization, toxoids induce the formation of antibodies that are capable of neutralizing the real toxins. Toxoids attack the bacterial toxin, not the invading pathogen itself. Examples include the diphtheria and tetanus toxoids.

Recombinant technology vaccines: Modern biologic techniques have allowed the development of vaccines that include partial organisms or proteins that are generated in the laboratory. Perhaps the best example of the use of this form of biotechnology is for the development of the hepatitis B immunization. It was originally obtained from the serum of infected individuals but carried the risk of transmitting HIV when it was administered

TABLE 46.1 Vaccine Types

Type of Vaccine	Immune System Response	Vaccine Examples	Remarks
Attenuated (live) virus	B-cell response; T-cell response	Polio (oral), measles, mumps, rubella, varicella	Risk for disease in persons with reduced immune function
Inactivated (killed) virus	B-cell response	Salk polio, influenza, rabies	Does not confer lifelong immunity
Live attenuated or dead bacteria	B-cell response	Cholera	
Component or subunit vaccine	B-cell response	Tetanus toxoid, diphtheria toxoid	Large quantities of antigen needed
Recombinant technology vaccine	B-cell response	Hepatitis B	Area for current research interest

as a vaccine. Through advances in recombinant deoxyribonucleic acid (DNA) technology, yeast cells have been reengineered to produce protein very similar to those found on the coating of the hepatitis B virus, allowing for the development of safe immune protection from this virus.

General Principles of Vaccine Administration

46.4 Vaccines should be administered by an established schedule with precautions taken for patients who are immunosuppressed or pregnant.

The effective use of vaccines requires that they be delivered according to a specified schedule at the proper dose. Childhood vaccines have a specific age range at which they should be administered. Should the child miss the recommended vaccination, "catch-up" doses can sometimes be administered to provide adequate protection. In addition, comorbid health conditions sometimes cause the delay of vaccinations in certain patients. Although each vaccine has different indications, there are certain general principles that apply to the administration of all or most immunizations.

In the United States, the Centers for Disease Control and Prevention (CDC) is the government agency that establishes immunization schedules. Immunization protocols are reviewed on a regular basis by the CDC's Advisory Committee on Immunization Practices, and revisions are frequently made based on current research. The practicing nurse should refer often to the CDC website for updates.

Dose and timing: The total dose of a vaccine is important for the development of immunity. For some vaccinations, multiple doses are required to achieve immunity. Omitting subsequent doses could result in the lack of full disease protection.

To prevent childhood diseases, certain vaccinations should begin at birth and proceed with booster doses at specific ages according to the schedule recommended by the CDC. The timing established by the CDC allows the vaccine to be given prior to the expected exposure to the pathogen. For example, the pertussis vaccine is begun in the first few months of life because infection by *Bordetella pertussis* often occurs by age 1 or 2. On the other hand, vaccination for HPV is recommended at 11 to 12 years of age because this virus is spread by sexual contact, which often occurs during the teen years. Vaccination outside the guidelines of the vaccination schedule is permitted, but its effectiveness may be reduced.

Route of administration: Vaccines must be administered by the specific route indicated for each product. Failure to follow administration protocol may result in an insufficient immune response. For example, hepatitis B vaccine elicits a satisfactory response when administered into the deltoid muscle but not the gluteus muscle. Injection into the gluteus muscle also risks injury to the sciatic nerve. Attenuated (live) influenza vaccine is administered intranasally, whereas varicella vaccine is given subcutaneously.

Precautions and contraindications: There are few absolute contraindications for the use of vaccines. Caution must be used in immunocompromised patients, such as those with cancer, recent tissue transplant recipients, or those infected with HIV. Patients receiving high-dose, systemic corticosteroid therapy may also have suppressed immune systems. Vaccinations in an immunocompromised patient should be avoided if the patient is having an exacerbation of his or her disorder. In some cases, only inactivated (killed) vaccines are indicated for these patients. Because it is suppressed, the patient's immune system may not be able to develop effective immunity in response to the vaccine, and subsequent laboratory results should be assessed to confirm that immunity has actually occurred.

Although most vaccines are pregnancy category C, vaccinations are often delayed in pregnant patients until after delivery to avoid any potential harm to the fetus. Inactivated (killed) vaccines may be administered to pregnant patients if the benefits of disease prevention outweigh the possible risk to the mother and fetus. For example, exposure to hepatitis B, influenza or tetanus, and diphtheria can have serious or fatal results for the fetus, so immunization of the mother may outweigh the vaccine risks for the fetus. The MMR vaccine should not be administered to pregnant women due to the theoretical risk of transmitting a live virus to the fetus.

Anaphylaxis and allergy: The most common adverse effects of vaccination are pain, swelling, and redness at the injection sites. Allergy or anaphylaxis following vaccination is extremely rare and is estimated at two cases for every 7,644,049 doses (Bohlke et al., 2003). Some preparations may contain preservatives such as gelatin or the mercury compound thimerosal, which could trigger an allergic response. Patients with confirmed vaccine anaphylaxis should not receive subsequent doses of that vaccine.

Adverse event reporting: Health care providers are required to report all vaccine-related adverse events requiring medical attention to the Vaccine Adverse Event Reporting System (VAERS). The VAERS is a postmarketing surveillance program conducted by the CDC and the U.S. Food and Drug Administration (FDA). Voluntary reports may be submitted to the VAERS by patients and parents as well as health care providers. Vaccine manufacturers are required to report any adverse effects of which they are aware.

There are a number of limitations to the VAERS. The VAERS merely collects data and reports incidences of adverse events; it does not attempt to confirm that the reported event was actually caused by the vaccine. Reports are not checked by the FDA or CDC for accuracy or completeness. Despite its limitations, the VAERS serves as an important, central repository of information for identifying potential adverse effects to vaccines.

CONNECTION *Checkpoint* 46.2

Vaccines are sometimes contraindicated if patients are receiving immunosuppressant drugs. From what you learned in Chapter 45, identify the following drugs as being either an immunosuppressant or an immunostimulant: aldesleukin (Proleukin), cyclosporine (Neoral, Sandimmune), muromonab-CD3 (Orthoclone, OKT3), and hydrocortisone. See Answer to Connection Checkpoint 46.2 in Appendix A.

MyNursingKit | Vaccine Updates

Active Immunity: Bacterial Immunizations

46.5 Active immunity can be induced to prevent bacterial infections.

Vaccinations are performed to provide protection against both viral and bacterial pathogens. The role of vaccines is very different for each type of infectious agent. Table 46.2 gives a summary of the epidemiology and immunizations associated with these pathogens. Immunizations against viruses are presented in Section 46.6.

Many bacterial infections cause host cellular injury by releasing toxic substances. Vaccination for bacterial infections, therefore, may be achieved by exposing the immune system to inactive bacterial toxins. When later faced with the actual bacterial infection, the immune system will remember the protein-based toxin and respond rapidly by producing antibodies to neutralize it.

TABLE 46.2 Disease Epidemiology and Immunizations

Disease	Worldwide Incidence	Unites States Incidence	Immunization (age)	Remarks
Cholera	131,943 cases in 52 countries in 2005	35 cases with travel in 1996–2005	Not available in the United States; "boil it, cook it, peel it or forget it"	Route: oral-fecal toxin from bacteria
Diphtheria	Endemic in many developing countries	No reported cases since 1980	2, 4, 6, and 15–18 months; 4–6 years	Mucous membrane bacterial toxin infection
Hepatitis A	Endemic in developing countries	5,683 in 2004	Three-shot series: 0, 1, and 6 months	Route: oral-fecal from carriers; immune globulin available
Hepatitis B	2 billion affected; 350 million chronic carriers worldwide	6,212 in 2004	Three-shot series: 0, 1, and 6 months	Vaccine recommended for all health care providers; immune globulin available
Influenza	Endemic during winter months	More than 36,000 deaths annually (high risk to those older than 65 years of age)	Annual vaccine based on estimated exposure	Vaccine recommended for children, immunocompromised patients, older adults, and health care workers
Measles (Rubeola)	1 million deaths annually in third world countries (mostly children)	Fewer than 150 U.S. cases annually (116 confirmed cases in 2001; 37 in 2002)	MMR: 12–15 months; booster: 4–6 years	Highly contagious; airborne and droplet exposure
Meningococcus	Major outbreaks every 8–12 years	3,000 annual cases; 300 deaths	11–12 years, at high school entry, or college entry	Airborne droplet exposure; antibiotics if known exposure
Mumps	Endemic in many countries; vaccine used in 57% of world	258 cases in 2004	MMR: 12–15 months; booster: 4–6 years	Viral parotitis; respiratory droplet infection
Pertussis	Endemic worldwide	7,580 in 2001; 9,771 in 2002; and 11,647 in 2003	2, 4, 6 and 15–18 months; 4–6 years	Gram-negative bacterial infection, cough; increased incidence in adolescent age group
Poliomyelitis	In 2002–2006, 22 countries previously polio-free reported cases; eight to nine cases VAPP[1] annually	Last case in 1979; five cases in 2005	Inactivated virus: 2, 4, and 12 months; booster: 4–6 years	20% children in Nigeria younger than 5 years are not vaccinated because of fear of AIDS and female infertility
Rabies	Canine rabies epidemic in Africa, Asia, and Central America	Found in all continents	Preexposure vaccine for veterinarians; postexposure immune globulin	Viral infection; transmitted via contaminated saliva; from peripheral nervous system (PNS) to central nervous system (CNS)
Rubella	Common disease worldwide	10 cases in 2004	MMR: 12–15 months; booster: 4–6 years	Mild disease but fetal cataracts, deafness, and cardiac malformations
Smallpox	Global eradication since 1980	Global eradication since 1980	No vaccine in use; concern for bioterrorism use	Live virus vaccine; contagious vesicle
Tetanus	Global health problem; incidence in unvaccinated persons	1995–1997: 124 total cases in the United States; 60% aged 20–59; 35% older than 60 years old	2, 4, 6, and 15–18 months; 4–6 years	Spores in soil; illness follows inadequate or missed immunizations
Varicella (Chickenpox)	Endemic worldwide	90% decline from 1995–2005	One injection between 12 and 18 months old	Highly contagious; airborne spread; latent in nerve ganglia; reoccurs as herpes zoster (shingles)

[1]VAPP: Vaccine-associated paralytic paralysis.

It is common practice to combine several childhood vaccines for a single administration. For example, DTaP combines diphtheria, tetanus, and pertussis into a single injection. Combining vaccines is less traumatic for the child and is more convenient and efficient for the caregiver and the health care provider.

Diphtheria

Pathophysiology: Diphtheria is an infection of the upper respiratory tract caused by the gram-positive bacterium *Corynebacterium diphtheriae.* The bacterium releases a potent toxin that causes a low-grade fever, malaise, and a painful oropharynx. The organism causes the formation of a thick, gray coating across the membranes of the soft palate, tonsillar areas, and uvula. The thickened membranes can partially occlude the airway and cause difficulty swallowing or a feeling of choking. Attempts to remove the membrane result in pain and bleeding. If untreated, the membrane softens and gradually disappears approximately 1 week following its appearance. A majority of deaths associated with diphtheria are related to toxin escape, leading to acute systemic toxicity or myocarditis. Because of effective immunization programs, the disease has almost been entirely eradicated from the United States.

Diphtheria toxoid: Diphtheria toxin is produced by organisms in culture that are rendered inactive by the addition of formalin. The diphtheria toxoid triggers immune memory without producing disease in the upper airways. Currently diphtheria toxin is available as a combination immunization with tetanus toxoid and acellular pertussis (DTaP) as well as in combination with other compatible immunizations. DTaP is part of the recommended routine immunization schedule for infants older than 6 months.

Pertussis (Whooping Cough)

Pathophysiology: Pertussis is a highly contagious infection by the gram-negative bacterium *Bordetella pertussis* that is transmitted via aerosolized droplets from an infected person. Once inhaled, the bacteria attach to the ciliated respiratory epithelial cells and release a toxin. Pertussis begins with a low-grade fever and irritated cough and progresses to spasmodic coughing episodes characterized by an inspiratory "whoop," leading to the common name "whooping cough." The coughing episodes are productive and may be induced by laughing, talking, or activity in children, and lead to gagging or vomiting. The cough will usually resolve at the termination of the infection in approximately 2 to 6 weeks. Exhaustion is common in patients experiencing pertussis, as are secondary respiratory infections. Active pertussis infection is treated with the antibiotic erythromycin, with the best results seen with early and aggressive treatment.

Immunization: Originally the pertussis vaccine was made from inactivated or killed whole cells and was highly effective in providing immunity. The whole cell vaccines, however, were associated with adverse effects that prompted the development of an acellular form (aP). The aP vaccine remains highly effective in producing immunity but has a lower rate of adverse effects than the whole cell vaccine. The acellular form of pertussis vaccine became available in 1996 and has replaced the original form.

Local injection site reactions, drowsiness, persistent crying, and fever occur in 3% to 5% of patients receiving the vaccine. The vaccine is almost always administered concurrently with the diphtheria and tetanus toxoids. The childhood vaccine is called DTaP. The booster vaccine for adults is called Tdap. Children receive five intramuscular (IM) doses of DTaP, one dose at each of the following ages: 2 months, 4 months, 6 months, 15 to 18 months, and 4 to 6 years. Because the severity of pertussis declines with age, vaccination is not recommended for children after age 7 or for adults.

Tetanus

Pathophysiology: *Clostridium tetani* normally lives in soil as a spore but can infect humans when the gram-positive anaerobe enters an open wound. Symptoms of infection may present over a wide range of time, averaging from 3 days to 3 weeks after exposure. *C. tetani* produces a toxin that is one of the most toxic substances known; receiving 2.5 mg (one billionth of a gram) per kilogram of body weight can be lethal. The toxin enters the peripheral nervous system (PNS) and migrates to the central nervous system (CNS). The toxin causes continuous, painful muscular contractions. Symptoms range from local muscle spasm, including the muscles of the jaw ("lockjaw"), to neck stiffness and seizures that are sometimes unresponsive to drug therapy. Treatment includes the administration of antibiotics but is primarily supportive in advanced cases.

Immunization: Tetanus toxoid (TT) is available alone, combined with diphtheria (DT) and combined with both diphtheria and pertussis (DTaP). The initial series of recommended immunizations uses the DTaP and is given in five doses during the first 6 years of the child's life. A contaminated wound in an adult with an appropriate immunization history requires only the booster administration of TT. To retain immunity, the booster for tetanus prevention should be given to adults every 10 years. TT can be injected IM, subcutaneously, or via jet injector. In patients with symptomatic tetanus infection, the TT injection may be coupled with passive immunization of antibodies against the toxin. Effective immunization schedules have nearly eradicated this disease in the United States.

Pneumococcus

Pathophysiology: Infection by *Streptococcus pneumoniae* is the most common cause of bacterial otitis media, meningitis, and pneumonia. Pneumococcal infection begins in the nasopharynx and may spread to the middle ear, sinuses, and lower respiratory tract. It occurs with a higher incidence in the winter months, when air pollution increases, or as a secondary infection following viral disease. The immune health of the patient greatly impacts the progress of *S. pneumoniae* infection and those with decreased immune function are at greater risk for the development of serious infections. Also at risk are patients with diminished cough and gag reflexes who have difficulty clearing secretions from the upper airways, such as those with neuromuscular diseases, or following anesthetic exposure. Smoking is a contributing factor in approximately half of the *S. pneumoniae* infections in nonelderly populations, probably owing to the change in upper airway clearance of secretions in these patients. All strains of *S. pneumoniae* have a common polysaccharide in their cell wall that is used for vaccine development.

Immunization: The immunization for pneumococcal infection has changed over time and currently has two different formulations. The first to be approved by the FDA, called pneumococcal polysaccharide vaccine (PPV), is derived from the cell walls of 23 strains of *S. pneumoniae.* PPV is recommended for those who are age 65 or older and for patients from age 2 to 64 who have a chronic illness or who are living in environments where exposure risk is increased. The vaccine is also recommended in immunocompromised patients (age 2 to 64) who have HIV infection, leukemia, lymphoma, Hodgkin's disease, or multiple myeloma; patients who receive dialysis; patients who are receiving high-dose corticosteroid therapy; and transplant recipients. A booster 5 or more years following the first vaccination is recommended.

Because the administration of PPV to young children with immature immune systems leads to a poor antibody response, this vaccine is not recommended in children under 2 years of age. A second vaccine, called pneumococcal conjugate vaccine (PCV), was specially developed for routine immunization in children under the age of 2. This immunization differs from PPV in that the *S. pneumoniae* polysaccharides are coupled with a protein that leads to improved immune activation in infants with immature immune function. PCV is used in a series of three routine IM injections at 2, 4, and 6 months.

Both PPV and PCV vaccines are well tolerated and only contraindicated in individuals with prior severe reactions to immunizations. The most common symptoms following the administration of either PPV or PCV are local redness, swelling, and pain at the injection site, which lasts from 1 to 3 days.

Meningococcus

Pathophysiology: Meningococcal infection (meningitis) is caused by *Neisseria meningitidis,* a highly virulent gram-negative, toxin-secreting organism. Although meningitis usually occurs sporadically in the United States, it sometimes causes epidemics in other nations. Early meningococcal infection is very difficult to discriminate from other viral or bacterial infections, because it initially presents with nonspecific fever and rash; frequently symptoms appear less than 24 hours before individuals are hospitalized. Neurologic symptoms rapidly develop, including nuchal rigidity, headache, photophobia, and seizures. Infants present with reduced feeding, irritability or lethargy, and bulging fontanels. A rash is seen in most cases, which appears as petechiae or larger purpuric eruptions on the arms, chest, or axilla. Early hospitalization and aggressive treatment with intravenous (IV) penicillin-based antibiotics has reduced the mortality and morbidity of meningococcal infection. About 10% of patients die from the infection and up to 20% suffer some degree of permanent neurologic disability.

Immunization: Routine immunization for meningococcal infection is recommended at age 11. Special populations that should receive vaccination include individuals traveling to regions where meningococcal infection is endemic or those living in crowded conditions, such as college residence halls. Because college freshman living in dormitories are at increased risk for infection, some colleges now require meningococcal vaccination for these students. This practice is required for all college students in the United Kingdom. Once an outbreak (three or more confirmed cases) is documented, immunization is recommended for all potentially exposed individuals, and antibiotic therapy is frequently offered to individuals having close contact with the infected persons.

There are two types of meningococcal vaccine. Meningococcal polysaccharide vaccine (MPSV) is administered by the subcutaneous route and is available for those aged 2 and older. Meningococcal conjugate vaccine (MCV, Menactra) is a newer vaccine that contains *N. meningitidis* polyssacharides conjugated to diphtheria toxoid protein. Given by the IM route, MCV is believed to produce longer lasting immunity than MPSV. Neither vaccine contains live or attenuated organisms. MPSV is recommended for patients aged 2 to 10 and over age 55; MCV is used for ages 11 to 55. Both vaccines are administered as a single dose, with boosters given only if the patient continues at high risk for infection. Neither vaccine protects against meningococcus serogroup B, which is responsible for about one third of all cases of meningitis.

PharmFACT

Approximately 3,000 cases of meningococcal infection are reported annually in the United States. The mortality rate associated with meningococcal infection has declined from 70% to 85% before the availability of antibiotics to 10% to 15% seen today. *Source:* Plotkin & Orenstein, 2004.

Active Immunity: Viral Immunizations

46.6 Effective vaccines that prevent viral infections have been developed.

Vaccinations for viral infections have a different form and function than those for bacterial infections. Viruses are nonliving and only contain strands of nucleic acids (DNA or ribonucleic acid [RNA]), an outer protein coat, and a few viral enzymes. Viruses require a host cell for replication and transmission. The signs and symptoms that follow viral invasion may be caused by either the effects of the viral infection itself or by the host's immune response.

Viral proteins are readily recognized as foreign by the immune system and will normally trigger an immune response. In some cases, immune cells are able to recognize that a virus has entered one of its own cells and has become infected. Recognition of infected cells takes place through the host secretion of special communication proteins called **interferons,** which signal the surrounding noninfected cells of the approaching virus. The infected cells are programmed to undergo cell death, or apoptosis, when they are invaded, thus decreasing the viral spread to adjacent cells. Because viruses undergo rapid mutations that allow them to constantly change structure and evade the host's defense mechanisms, they present enormous challenges for effective vaccine development.

The term "live viral vaccine" is commonly used in clinical practice. The student should understand, however, that viruses are nonliving particles. In vaccine terminology, the term "live" refers to a virus's ability to infect the host and does not indicate that the virus is actually alive.

CONNECTION *Checkpoint* 46.3

From what you learned in Chapter 45, what are the indications for pharmacotherapy with interferons? See Answer to Connection Checkpoint 46.3 in Appendix A.

Hepatitis B

Pathophysiology: Infection with hepatitis B virus (HBV) leads to a range of symptoms, from a self-limiting acute illness to life-threatening liver failure. Patients with HBV infection are at risk for developing a chronic carrier state, which is associated with the development of cirrhosis and hepatic cancer. Of the five viral infections known to cause hepatitis, HBV has the highest incidence worldwide.

Hepatitis B cannot be discriminated from the other forms of viral hepatitis by symptoms alone; serological testing is required for diagnosis. The onset of symptoms ranges between 6 weeks and 6 months postexposure and includes low-grade fever, nausea, vomiting, malaise, fatigue, and anorexia. The patient may present with signs of hepatitis, including jaundice, dark urine, and clay-colored stools that appear 1 to 2 weeks following the onset of symptoms. Approximately 30% of patients are hospitalized during the acute phase of hepatitis infection. End-stage hepatitis includes encephalopathy, confusion and disorientation, and coma, and carries a mortality rate of 60% to 70% without transplantation. Details on the pathophysiology and pharmacotherapy of HBV infections are presented in Chapter 55.

Immunization: The first HBV vaccine became available in 1982 and was derived from the blood of chronic carriers of the disease. Concerns regarding the possibility of transmitting HIV infection with the vaccine resulted in the development of a recombinant form of the vaccine in 1986. Current HBV vaccines contain highly antigenic proteins from the viral coat, which is known as hepatitis B surface antigen (HBsAg). Recombinant hepatitis vaccines contain no blood products and therefore do not represent a risk for HIV infection.

Because of the potential for occupational exposure, health care providers have a 10-fold increased risk of acquiring HBV. Dried HBV can remain infectious on an environmental surface for up to 1 week, and although needlestick injuries have the highest risk of infection (37% to 62%), the virus can gain entry via scratches, rashes, burns, or other disruptions of the mucosal surface. The CDC now recommends preexposure immunization against HBV infection for health care providers. Through the year 2000, approximately 100 million persons have received the HBV vaccine in the United States, and it has been determined to be safe for all age groups.

PROTOTYPE DRUG Hepatitis B vaccine (Engerix-B, Recombivax HB)

Classification: **Therapeutic:** Vaccine
Pharmacologic: Vaccine

Therapeutic Effects and Uses: The HBV vaccine is a noninfectious, highly immunogenic vaccine that provides immunity to HBV in 99% to 100% of patients when given in the recommended three-dose regimen. The effectiveness of the vaccine in producing immunity in adults declines with age. The vaccine is 98% effective in patients aged 20 to 29, 94% in patients aged 30 to 39, and 89% in those age 40 or older. The HBV vaccine may be administered in combination with hepatitis B immunoglobulin for postexposure prophylaxis or to prevent the perinatal transmission of the virus from mother to infant. The vaccine is indicated for immunity against all known subtypes of HBV. Indications for the HBV vaccine include the following:

- Routine infant immunization programs, including those born to hepatitis B infected mothers
- Children born after November 21, 1991, and catch-up immunization of children 11 years old or younger at high risk for infection
- Sexually active adolescents
- Health care workers or caregivers who are at risk for contact with HBV-contaminated blood
- Subpopulations with known high rates of infection, including Alaskan natives, Pacific Islanders, refugees, or persons adopted from areas where HBV infection is endemic
- Persons with high-risk sexual practices, such as heterosexual activity with multiple partners, female prostitutes, homosexual or bisexual practices, or persons who repeatedly contract sexually transmitted infections
- Injecting drug abusers

In adults 19 years or older, the HBV vaccine is administered 10 mcg IM, followed by repeat doses at 1 and 6 months. Travelers to high-risk areas or those who have been recently exposed to the virus may receive 20 mg IM, followed by subsequent doses at 1, 2, and 12 months.

Mechanism of Action: The HBV vaccine consists of HBsAG produced through recombinant DNA technology using yeast cells. Antibodies induced by the HBV vaccine decline over time and may require a booster dose for continued immunization.

Pharmacokinetics:

Route(s)	IM injection in the deltoid or anterolateral thigh in infants and small children
Absorption	Rapid, following IM injection
Distribution	Unknown
Primary metabolism	Unknown
Primary excretion	Unknown
Onset of action	Antibodies to HBV appear within 2 weeks
Duration of action	Immunity lasts 5–7 years

Adverse Effects: The most common adverse effects from HBV vaccination are pain at the injection site and mild to moderate fever. Approximately 15% of patients will experience systemic effects, usually fatigue, dizziness, fever, and headache. Children may experience irritability, fever, diarrhea, fatigue, weakness, diminished appetite, and rhinitis. Anaphylaxis is rare and is usually reported within a few hours after the vaccination. Guillain-Barré syndrome is a very rare potential adverse effect of the HBV vaccine.

Contraindications/Precautions: Known hypersensitivity to yeast or any component of the vaccine is an absolute contraindication. Patients who demonstrated severe hypersensitivity to the first dose should not receive subsequent doses. Although anaphylaxis is rare, proper emergency equipment or facilities should be available. Patients with active infections or unexplained fever should delay the use of the vaccine unless the health of the patient is endangered by withholding the vaccine. Caution should be exercised when administering the vaccine to patients with severe cardiopulmonary impairment. The vaccine should be given to pregnant or lactating women only if clearly needed to protect the health of the mother or child.

Drug Interactions: Hepatitis B immunoglobulin should not be administered in the same syringe or at the same site as the vaccine because it can impair the development of immunity from the vaccine. Patients receiving immunosuppressant drugs may require a higher dose of vaccine. **Herbal/Food:** Unknown.

Pregnancy: Category C.

Treatment of Overdose: Overdose with this drug has not been reported.

Nursing Responsibilities:

- Assess the current health status and previous vaccination history of the patient to determine possible contraindications to the vaccination.
- Record in the patient's permanent record the manufacturer, lot number, date of administration, and the name and address of the person administering the vaccine.
- Use the full recommended dose of the vaccine.
- Because none of the formulas of Recombivax HB contain a preservative, once the single-dose vial has been penetrated, the withdrawn vaccine should be used promptly and the vial must be discarded.
- Shake the vial well before use to maintain the suspension of the vaccine.
- Administer in three dosages; an initial dose is repeated at 1 month and 6 months. A schedule should be given to parents or caregivers to enhance adherence with the dosage schedule.
- Monitor hepatitis B surface antibody levels (anti-HBs) to ensure seroconversion following immunization.

Patient and Family Education:

- Return for all follow-up doses; the vaccination is not effective unless the entire series of doses is completed.
- Immediately report to the health care provider a fever of 39.4C (103°F) or higher, difficulty breathing, confusion, swelling of eyes or face, irritability, or confusion.
- Before receiving this vaccine, inform the health care provider about all the other vaccines you have recently received. Also tell the health care provider if you have received drugs or treatments in the past 2 weeks that can weaken the immune system, including corticosteroid medications; medications to treat psoriasis, rheumatoid arthritis, or other autoimmune disorders; or medicines to treat or prevent organ transplant rejection or cancer.
- Maintain a current and accurate record of all vaccinations received.
- Immediately notify the health care provider of any known or suspected pregnancy before receiving this vaccination.

Drugs Similar to Hepatitis B Vaccine (Engerix-B, Recombivax HB)

There are no other vaccines similar to the HBV vaccine.

Hepatitis A

Pathophysiology: Unlike HBV, which is mostly bloodborne, hepatitis A virus (HAV) is acquired by coming in contact with the stools of an infected person. At highest risk for HAV infection are household contacts or sexual partners of infected persons, and travelers to regions of the world where HAV is endemic (Africa, South America, and most of Asia). Good personal hygiene and proper sanitation can prevent HAV infection. Children are at risk due to generally poor hygiene habits.

Approximately one third of the U.S. population has lifelong immunity to HAV based on a past infection. Symptoms associated with HAV infection are age dependent. In children less than 5 years old, 50% to 90% of infections are asymptomatic, whereas 70% to 95% of adults will exhibit symptoms. Signs and symptoms include elevation in the liver enzyme levels, jaundice, fatigue, anorexia, fever, dull abdominal pain, nausea, and vomiting. Symptoms are often mild, and most patients report the resolution of symptoms in several weeks. The disease is rarely fatal and normally produces no permanent hepatic impairment.

Immunization: When the HAV vaccine became available in 1995, the number of cases of HAV infection in the United States dropped dramatically. Current recommendations for hepatitis A vaccinations include all children at age 12 to 23 months; catch-up vaccination of older children in selected areas; and vaccination of persons at increased risk for hepatitis A, including travelers to endemic areas, illicit drug users, or men who have sex with men (CDC, 2007a).

Given by the IM route, children should receive their initial vaccination at 12 to 23 months of age with a follow-up dose 6 months later. For individuals traveling to endemic regions, three doses may be given with 4 weeks between the three injections. This vaccine is highly immunogenic, with 95% to 100% of vaccinated individuals developing protective antibodies. Antibody coverage persists in both adults and children for 5 to 8 years following vaccination. Adverse effects of the HAV vaccine are mild and include soreness at the injection site, headache, anorexia, and fatigue.

Influenza

Pathophysiology: Influenza, or flu, is a respiratory disease spread by the three forms of the influenza virus: types A, B, and C. Influenza type A is the most dangerous and the primary focus for the annual development of a vaccine for the prevention of epidemic outbreaks. Influenza type A causes seasonal outbreaks during the winter months that are usually self-limiting but may lead to serious health consequences in patients who are debilitated, immunosuppressed, or who have chronic medical conditions. Influenza type A is also harbored in wild aquatic birds and is responsible for outbreaks of "bird flu." Influenza types B and C are less common and generally do not cause epidemics or result in serious symptoms. The influenza viruses mutate at a rapid rate and change their antigenic appearance; almost every time the viral RNA replicates, a new mutant is created. Once an outbreak of influenza occurs, immunization is no longer effective and pharmacotherapy of the active infection may be initiated. Because treatment of influenza infection is minimally effective, the best approach for dealing with this infection is through prevention. The pharmacotherapy of influenza infection is presented in Chapter 55.

Immunization: The first influenza immunization took place in 1945 following a worldwide outbreak during World War II. Throughout the history of influenza immunization, the viral particles used for the inoculation have been incubated in chicken eggs, leading to an increased risk of anaphylaxis in patients with egg allergies. With the development of recombinant human DNA preparations, the risk of allergy has decreased.

The development of the annual influenza vaccine begins with a prediction on the part of scientists as to what strains of the virus are most likely to appear that year. Each year one influenza vaccine is prepared that contains portions of the most likely strains of type A and type B. If their prediction is accurate, the vaccine will prevent 70% to 90% of the flu cases; however, the effectiveness of the vaccine is significantly lower in some years.

Two types of influenza vaccines are available. The trivalent inactivated influenza vaccine (TiIV) is a subcutaneous formulation that is approved for patients older than 6 months, including healthy people, women who anticipate being pregnant during the flu season, and those with chronic medical conditions. The live, attenuated intranasal vaccine (LAIV) is delivered as a nasal spray to healthy people 2 to 49 years of age who are not pregnant. Annual influenza vaccination is recommended for the following groups:

- Everyone over age 50
- Residents of nursing homes or long-term care facilities
- Adults and children who have chronic conditions such as asthma, diabetes, or heart disease
- Anyone whose immune system is compromised due to HIV or AIDS, high-dose corticosteroid therapy, or cancer chemotherapy
- Women who will be pregnant during the influenza season
- Health care providers
- Healthy household contacts (including children) and caregivers of persons at high risk of acquiring influenza

The most common adverse effects of the subcutaneous vaccine are soreness and redness at the injection site. Nasal congestion, headache, and sore throat are common adverse effects of the nasal spray vaccine. About 1% of patients may experience fever, chills, muscle aches, and other symptoms of influenza that last 1 to 2 days. Serious adverse effects are rare. Caution should be used in patients who are allergic to egg or mercury, which is sometimes used as a preservative.

Rabies

Pathophysiology: Rabies is caused by a virus that can invade the nervous system of most mammals. The rabies virus is carried in saliva and is passed to humans through animal bites from infected dogs, coyotes, wolves, foxes, raccoons, skunks, and bats. In unvaccinated individuals, the mortality rate is nearly 100%.

Following the bite of an infected animal, the incubation period for rabies infection is long, from 20 to 60 days. When possible, the biting animal is confined and examined for rabies infection. Because the infection is always fatal if untreated, therapy is immediately implemented while waiting for the results of animal testing.

Pain or paresthesia surrounding the bite is reported by most persons with rabies. Other symptoms include fever, headache, malaise, irritability, anxiety, and insomnia. Short periods of agitation, aggressiveness, hyperactivity, and disorientation are followed by normal behavior. Nuchal rigidity, seizures, bizarre behavior, and hydrophobia indicate a progression of the disease; if untreated, rabies will progress to cardiac or respiratory arrest or paralysis, requiring mechanical ventilation. Death usually occurs within 10 days of the onset of symptoms.

Immunization: pre- and postexposure: Prevention of rabies may be accomplished through vaccination. Although the vaccine is effective, few people are administered preexposure immunization because of the very small risk of coming into contact with a rabid animal during their lifetime. However, this immunization is offered to individuals with potential exposure to rabid animals, such as animal handlers or veterinarians, and to travelers to countries where rabies is prevalent. Cave explorers often receive prophylactic treatment because of their potential exposure to rabid bats. Preexposure immunization includes three inoculations.

Once a potential exposure to rabies is reported, the patient should immediately receive postexposure vaccination. The immune response to dead or attenuated organisms in a rabies vaccine takes approximately 2 weeks to develop, which is well within the incubation period of rabies. Patients receive one dose of rabies immune globulin, which offers immediate protection. Five doses of rabies vaccine are then administered over a 28-day period. If instituted promptly, postexposure vaccination is very successful. If the biting animal is shown not to have rabies, the sequence of vaccinations may be discontinued.

The most common adverse effects of the rabies vaccine are pain and redness at the injection site. Mild, transient flulike symptoms may occur. Pregnant women may receive the vaccine, if exposure to the rabies virus is suspected.

Measles, Mumps, and Rubella

Measles (rubeola) pathophysiology: The measles virus, *Morbillivirus*, is one of the most contagious viral pathogens, being readily transmitted by airborne particles and respiratory secretions. Because humans are the only known reservoir for the virus, routine immunization has eliminated measles as a common childhood disease in the United States. Measles is still widespread in other countries and occasional outbreaks across the United States emphasize the importance of continued MMR immunizations.

Symptoms of measles infection appear 10 to 12 days following airborne exposure and begin with nonspecific cough, malaise, and low-grade fever. The fever can subsequently spike to as high as 40.6°C (105°F). Rash appears first on the oral mucosa but then develops into a reddened, raised rash on the face, hairline, ears, and neck, spreading to the trunk and extremities. The rash lasts approximately 1 week and then fades and disappears. Individuals are considered to be infectious 4 days prior to and after rash appearance. In developing countries, measles infection carries a mortality rate as high as 2% to 15%.

Mumps pathophysiology: Mumps is a viral infection in the parotid salivary glands that is transmitted by exposure to contaminated saliva. Symptoms develop 16 to 18 days after exposure, resulting in mild fever, headache, anorexia, and malaise. The fever usually lasts 1 to 6 days but the swelling in the parotid glands may continue for 10 days or more. The infection is usually self-limiting and mortality is rare. Complications of mumps include orchitis (swelling of the testes) in approximately 37% of infected, postpubescent males and deafness in children.

Rubella or German measles pathophysiology: Rubella, also called German measles, is a viral infection that produces mild symptoms in most people. The rubella virus is transmitted by infected aerosol droplets. Symptoms include enlarged cervical lymph nodes, mild fever, and malaise, followed by a raised rash 14 to 17 days later.

The major concerns with rubella are the consequences of maternal infection during pregnancy. Infection occurring on the first 12 weeks of pregnancy carries the greatest risk of fetal defects. Rubella infection rapidly spreads to all fetal organ systems and may cause a wide variety of consequences. The most frequently described are congenital cataracts and blindness from retinal destruction, heart disease, and deafness in infants. Since the initiation of routine rubella immunization and maternal antibody screening, the incidence of rubella infection of the fetus or newborn has declined to 0.01 per 10,000 pregnancies in the United States. A single, subcutaneous rubella vaccine made from attenuated (live) virus grown in human tissue cultures is available and usually very well tolerated.

Immunization

The MMR vaccine has incorporated live or attenuated viruses since its development in the 1960s, and widespread immunization has led to a 98% decrease in the incidences of these viral infections. Current recommendations include a two-dose subcutaneous immunization, with the first given at 12 to 15 months of age and the second at 4 to 6 years of age. The overall immunity rate for MMR vaccination is 92% to 95%. In 2005, the FDA approved the addition of varicella vaccine to the combination, which is known as MMRV (ProQuad).

A single dose of MMR vaccine is recommended for those individuals born after 1957 without contraindication or past history of measles infection or positive immunity. A second dose of MMR is recommended in the following situations: epidemic outbreak or exposure to measles infection, vaccination with an unknown vaccine between 1963 and 1967 or vaccination with killed organism, health care workers or those traveling internationally, or for nonimmune students in postsecondary educational settings (Tyring, 2005).

Although generally well-tolerated, several groups are usually excluded from vaccination, including:

- Pregnant patients or women planning conception within 3 months of vaccination are contraindicated because the live or attenuated rubella virus poses a hypothetical risk of infection with subsequent congenital malformations.
- Patients who are immunosuppressed are generally contraindicated. However, MMR can be given to individuals living in the same setting with asymptomatic HIV disease and persons with mild immunosuppression.
- Persons reporting an allergy to neomycin or gelatin are contraindicated because the vaccine contains these substances. Persons reporting egg allergy have a very low risk of allergic reaction but it is recommended that these patients be observed for 90 minutes following immunization.

Adverse reactions to MMR vaccination are minimal and include: fever and lymphadenopathy, rare encephalitis (1 occurrence per 1 million vaccinations), and arthralgia in adults. MMR is now available in an aerosolized formulation that has fewer associated adverse effects and an improved immunogenicity as compared to the injected forms.

Polio

Pathophysiology: Poliomyelitis was the leading cause of permanent disability in the era just prior to vaccines. Highly contagious, polio epidemics in the 1800s and early 1900s prompted the search for, and eventual discovery of, vaccines. The virus replicates in the gastrointestinal (GI) tract and is spread by the oral–fecal route via contaminated food and water.

Over 90% of those exposed to the poliovirus are asymptomatic. Rarely (less than 1%), the virus reaches the motor tracts of the spinal cord, where it leads to the development of flaccid muscle paralysis of the infected motor cells. On rare occasions the respiratory muscles are involved, leading to the need for artificial ventilation. Global immunization has made the disease extremely rare and global eradication is possible.

Immunization: There are currently two forms of vaccination for the prevention of poliovirus infection. Developed by Dr. Jonas Salk, the inactivated polio vaccine (IPV) was first marketed in 1955 and later changed to be more potent in 1978. The oral polio vaccine (OPV) was developed in the early 1960s and was used extensively until vaccine-associated paralytic polio (VAPP) was found to be a rare, though devastating, adverse effect. The OPV is still widely used in regions of the world where polio is endemic due to its ease of administration. The OPV also prevents the intestinal spread of the virus, which is of critical importance in areas of the world that have poor sanitation.

Since 2000, the IPV has been exclusively used in the United States for the immunization of infants. Children get four doses of IPV, at 2 months, 4 months, 6 to 18 months, and a booster dose at 4 to 6 years. IPV is available as a single suspension or in combination with DPaT, hepatitis B, or influenza vaccines. Routine IM administration of IPV results in redness, swelling, and tenderness at the administration site. Children receiving the complete IPV regimen are provided 99% to 100% lifelong immunity.

Varicella Zoster

Pathophysiology: Infection by the varicella zoster virus (VZV) leads to the development of two very different diseases. The initial outbreak of VZV, known as chickenpox (varicella), generally occurs during childhood. Following the initial infection, the virus becomes dormant for 30 to 40 years in nerve roots until it reactivates to cause herpes zoster (HZ) or shingles.

The initial VZV infection is transmitted through inhaled droplets or by direct contact with infectious skin lesions. The virus replicates in the local lymph nodes for several days and then becomes bloodborne. By day 10 to 14, a blistered rash appears, with new lesions opening, draining, and crusting within 24 hours. Intense itching may lead to secondary bacterial infections and permanent scarring. General illness is common in individuals for 5 to 7 days with fever, malaise, and anorexia. Adults with chickenpox have more intense symptoms than children and have a seven times greater risk of encephalitis. Furthermore, women who acquire VZV during pregnancy have a small risk of passing the infection to the fetus, resulting in birth defects.

Following the initial infection, the virus migrates to the spinal nerves, where it may remain dormant for the life of the individual. In about 20% of patients, however, the virus becomes reactivated and causes an HZ infection, or **shingles,** usually after age 50; this increases to approximately 50% for individuals over the age of 85. Shingles often begins with a burning or tingling pain, numbness, or itch in one particular location on the surface of the body. After several days or a week, fluid-filled blisters, similar to chickenpox, appear in one area of the body. Shingles lesions can be very painful and may require up to a month for resolution. In immunocompromised individuals the infection may be prolonged, taking 3 to 4 weeks for lesion scabbing and several months for complete resolution. Up to 30% of patients with shingles experience a serious form of the disease called **postherpetic neuralgia** in which the pain lasts for years. In about 15% of patients with shingles, the virus infects the eye and can cause blindness.

Antiviral drugs such as acyclovir (Zovirax) are sometimes administered to reduce the severity and duration of a shingles attack and postherpetic neuralgia. Other treatments for postherpetic neuralgia include corticosteroids and nonsteroidal anti-inflammatory drugs (NSAIDs).

Immunization: An attenuated or live VZV vaccine (Varivax) has been used in the United States since 1995, and it is estimated that widespread vaccination has reduced the incidence of varicella infection by more than 70%. In 2006, new standards were adopted with the following recommendations:

- Implementation of a routine two-dose varicella vaccination schedule for children. The first dose is administered at age 12 to 15 months and the second dose at age 4 to 6 years.
- Routine vaccination of all healthy persons over age 13, without evidence of immunity.
- Prenatal assessment and postpartum vaccination.
- Expanding the use of the varicella vaccine for HIV-infected children.
- Establishing middle school, high school, and college entry vaccination requirements.

There is wide variation in the effectiveness of the vaccine, and 10% to 15% of immunized individuals will still acquire the infection, which is a condition known as breakthrough varicella. Breakthrough varicella infection produces milder symptoms as compared to those in nonimmunized patients.

Also in 2006, an advisory panel of the CDC recommended that all Americans receive the shingles vaccine (Zostavax) at age 60. The shingles vaccine contains a live or attenuated form of the virus and is 60% effective at preventing the reactivation of HZV. The shingles vaccine is essentially a booster of the VZV vaccine administered to prevent chickenpox. It is not effective at treating symptoms of shingles or postherpetic neuralgia once they develop.

Adverse effects associated with HZV vaccine include low-grade fever, tenderness at the injection site, and rash localized to the injection site. The vaccine should be used with caution in persons with a history of allergy to eggs or gelatin. Caution should be exercised with the use of this immunization in pregnant or breast-feeding women. Although there have been no documented problems with receiving the immunization while pregnant, HZV has been linked to the development of birth defects. Finally the administration of this vaccine in immunosuppressed patients may increase the incidence of adverse effects or cause a decrease in the developed immunity.

Pharm*FACT*

Approximately 95% of adults in the United States have antibodies to the varicella-zoster virus, indicating prior exposure to this pathogen. Three out of four patients who experience repeated zoster infections are HIV positive. *Source:* Krause, 2008.

Human Papillomavirus

Pathogenesis: Genital human papillomavirus (HPV), the most common sexually transmitted disease in the United States, is associated with a higher risk of cervical cancer, which is a significant cause of cancer deaths in women. Although there are over 100 different forms of HPV, only 7 are associated with cervical cancer. HPV is associated with a higher risk of other types of cancer, including vaginal, vulvar, and anal. Some types of HPV are responsible for causing genital warts. The virus may infect both males and females, and it may be transmitted from mother to child during vaginal delivery.

Spread through sexual contact, HPV infection may be asymptomatic or lead to the development of a low-grade infection that resolves spontaneously in individuals with a healthy immune system. A high-grade HPV infection may lead to the development of dysplasia, a precancerous change in the cervical cells that is directly related to the viral infection.

Immunization: The HPV vaccine has been created with virus-like particles using recombinant DNA technology. Great caution was necessary in the development of this vaccine because the HPV contains oncogenes, which are modified forms of a gene that are believed to lead to a cancerous transformation. Because of the potential cancer risk, the HPV vaccine is a noninfectious, virus-like particle (VLP) containing only proteins from the coat of the virus, rather than a complete attenuated virus.

The HPV vaccine (Gardasil) is administered through a series of three IM injections. The second and third doses should be given 2 and 6 months after the first dose. The vaccine has close to 100% effectiveness in preventing HPV infection and appears to offer long-lasting protection. The CDC recommends the routine vaccination of females from 11 to 12 years old and for females age 13 to 26 years old who were not vaccinated at an earlier age. Females who have already been infected with a strain of HPV experience less benefit from vaccination. However, it may still prevent infection from additional strains of the virus. It is not licensed for administration to males, although research is being conducted to determine its effectiveness in this population. Mild adverse effects include pain, swelling, and redness of the injection site.

PharmFACT

About 50% of sexually active men and women will acquire the human papillomavirus during their lifetime. Over 6 million new cases of HPV infection occur every year in the United States, with 77% of these occurring between the ages of 15 and 24. *Source:* Centers for Disease Control and Prevention, 2007b.

Rotavirus

Pathophysiology: Approximately 680,000 children die worldwide from rotavirus infection, mostly in developing countries. Although the virus rarely causes death in the United States, it is estimated that nearly every child is infected by age 5 and that most will experience gastroenteritis, resulting in severe diarrhea and dehydration. Viral replication of the rotavirus occurs only in mature red blood cells found in the tips of the intestinal villi, leading to a strictly oral–fecal means of viral transmission.

Immunization: The FDA approved the first rotavirus immunization (RotaShield) in August 1998. In the 10 months following FDA approval, over 1.5 million doses of the vaccine were administered and 15 cases of intussusception (a form of intestinal obstruction from a telescoping of the intestine into itself) were reported. In November 1999, RotaShield was removed from the market due to these safety concerns. A newer live vaccine, RotaTeq, received approval in 2006 as a routine immunization in infants. The CDC recommends rotavirus vaccine in a three-dose oral series in infants 6 to 32 weeks of age for the prevention of gastroenteritis. The vaccine has been shown to reduce the overall incidence of gastroenteritis by 74% and of hospitalization due to the virus by 96%. There are no serious adverse effects associated with immunization with

CONNECTIONS

Lifespan Considerations Vaccine Administration

Pediatric Patients

Young children are at risk for the development of disease because their immune functioning is immature, and although maternal antibodies provide a partial immunity, they rapidly decline in effectiveness in the first 3 months of life. Coupled with reduced immune function are poor communication and hygiene habits, placing infants and young children at significant risk for the development of disease.

Education is extremely important for the parents or caregivers of pediatric patients who are receiving immunizations. Parents and caregivers should be given written material for additional information or reinforcement when at home. Contact information should be provided in case of the development of adverse effect(s). Parents and caregivers should also be instructed not to give children aspirin (acetylsalicylic acid [ASA]) or aspirin-containing products (such as Pepto-Bismol) for the treatment of fever or body aches associated with vaccines. The use of ASA in the event of a viral infection has been associated with the development of Reye's syndrome.

Adolescent Patients

Adolescent patients present specific challenges for the development of infectious disease because they generally are not seen by their health care provider unless they become ill, leading to a potential for lapse in their immunization protection. They require booster immunizations (i.e., tetanus, diphtheria, and MMR booster due 10 years following the initial vaccine series) and rescue immunizations if missed or incorrect series were administered during their childhood. Adolescents who are preparing to leave home to live in college dormitories or residence halls should consider the vaccine for the prevention of meningococcal meningitis. Also important is the vaccine for HPV for the prevention of cervical infection and increased risk for the development of cervical cancer in sexually active female adolescents.

Geriatric Patients

Geriatric patients have an increased incidence of medical illness, predisposing them to a decline in immune functioning and the development of infectious disease. The goal of immunizations in elderly patients is to maintain the immune protection from earlier vaccines and prevent infectious disease. Two forms of vaccines are used in the older population of patients: vaccine boosters, which are designed to reexpose and sensitize the immune system to microorganisms to which they had prior immunity, and the introduction of additional vaccine(s) to prevent disease in at-risk populations.

RotaTeq, but mild cases of diarrhea and vomiting occur in small numbers of patients receiving the drug (Merck, 2008).

Passive Immunity

46.7 Antibodies are administered to provide passive immunity.

Passive immunization is very different from active immunization. Whereas active immunity requires activation of the patient's immune response and leads to the development of memory cells, passive immunity is the administration of preformed antibodies (immunoglobulins): the immune system is not activated and memory cells are not produced.

Passive immunization is typically used to provide immediate protection against a recent infection (or potential infection) or a disease in progress. Several examples serve to illustrate the benefits of passive immunization.

- A person has just been bitten by a potentially rabid dog. It will take several days to determine if the dog is infected with rabies.
- A person has been in a motorcycle accident and suffered serious trauma. He has never had a tetanus vaccination.
- A student nurse has learned that she has been exposed to blood from a patient with confirmed HBV. She has not been vaccinated for HBV.

What do these three scenarios have in common? First, immediate treatment is indicated because the consequences of infection can be serious or fatal. The use of a vaccine requires too much time for the activation of an immune response, and the disease would have the opportunity to create serious illness. In these cases, antibodies against the infection can be administered to provide immediate prevention against rabies, tetanus, or HBV infection. Antibodies are sometimes given concurrently with the vaccine series to provide complete immunity against the disease. For example, following an exposure to rabies the patient is given rabies immunoglobulin (RI) as well as the rabies vaccine.

The preceding scenarios illustrate a second message of importance to the nurse. If the patients had kept their tetanus and HBV vaccinations up to date, they would have developed active immunity to these pathogens and there would be no need to provide passive immunity.

A second indication for the use of passive immunity is for situations where the activation of the immune system and the development of memory are not desirable. In this case, the individual is given the antibodies against the foreign agent and the immune system does not mount a response. The administration of RhoGAM is an example of this type of indication.

Table 46.3 lists selected immune globulin preparations. Pharmacotherapy Illustrated 46.1 shows the development of immunity through vaccines or the administration of antibodies.

PROTOTYPE DRUG Rh_o[D] immune globulin (RhoGAM)

Classification: **Therapeutic:** Immunizing agent (passive)
Pharmacologic: Antibody, immunoglobulin

Therapeutic Effects and Uses: Erythrocytes contain two types of surface antigens that are used to designate the blood type. The first identifier is ABO; the presence or absence of antigen A and antigen B will determine the blood type as A, B, AB, or O. A second identifier on the cell membrane of the red blood cell (RBC) is the Rhesus factor, or Rh antigen. If the antigen is present, the individual is said to be Rh positive (Rh^+) and if it is missing, Rh negative (Rh^-); 85% of individuals living in North America are Rh positive.

Erythroblastosis fetalis (EF), or hemolytic disease of the newborn, is a disorder that was first described in 1940 and that is caused by an Rh incompatibility between the mother and her fetus. This condition can only occur if the mother is Rh negative.

EF does not occur with the first pregnancy because the two types of RBC (Rh^- mother and Rh^+ child) are separated by the placenta and the blood is not physically exchanged. At birth, however, their blood mixes and the mother's immune system reacts by producing antibodies against the foreign Rh^+ antigen. The presence of circulating antibodies against the Rh antigen creates a potential risk for an Rh incompatibility in future pregnancies. If in a subsequent pregnancy the fetus is Rh^+, the mother's antibodies against the Rh^+ antigen will cross the

TABLE 46.3 Immune Globulin Preparations

Drug	Route and Adult Dose (maximum dose where indicated)	Adverse Effects
cytomegalovirus immune globulin (CytoGam)	IV: 150 mg/kg within 72 h of transplantation; then 100 mg/kg for 2, 4, 6, and 8 weeks post-transplant; then 50 mg/kg for 12 and 16 weeks post-transplant	*Local reactions at the injection site (pain, erythema, myalgia), influenza-like symptoms (malaise, fever, chills), headache, joint stiffness* Anaphylaxis
hepatitis B immune globulin (HBIG)	IM: 0.06 mL/kg as soon as possible after exposure, preferably within 24 h, but no later than 7 days; repeat 28–30 days after exposure	
intravenous immune globulin (IVIG, Gammagard, Carimune, Octagam)	IV: 100–200 mg/kg per month IM: 1.2 mL/kg followed by 0.6 mL/kg every 2–4 weeks	
rabies immune globulin (Bayrab, Imogam Rabis-HT, Hyperab)	IM: (gluteal) 20 units/kg as a single dose with rabies vaccine	
Rh_o[D] immune globulin (RhoGAM)	IM/IV: one vial or 300 mcg at approximately 28 weeks; followed by one vial of minidose or 120 mcg within 72 h of delivery if infant is Rh positivete	
tetanus immune globulin (BayTet, HyperTet, HyperTet S/D)	IM: 250 units for prophylaxis	

Note: *Italics* indicate common adverse effects. Underline indicates serious adverse effects.

PHARMACOTHERAPY ILLUSTRATED 46.1

Mechanisms of Active and Passive Immunity

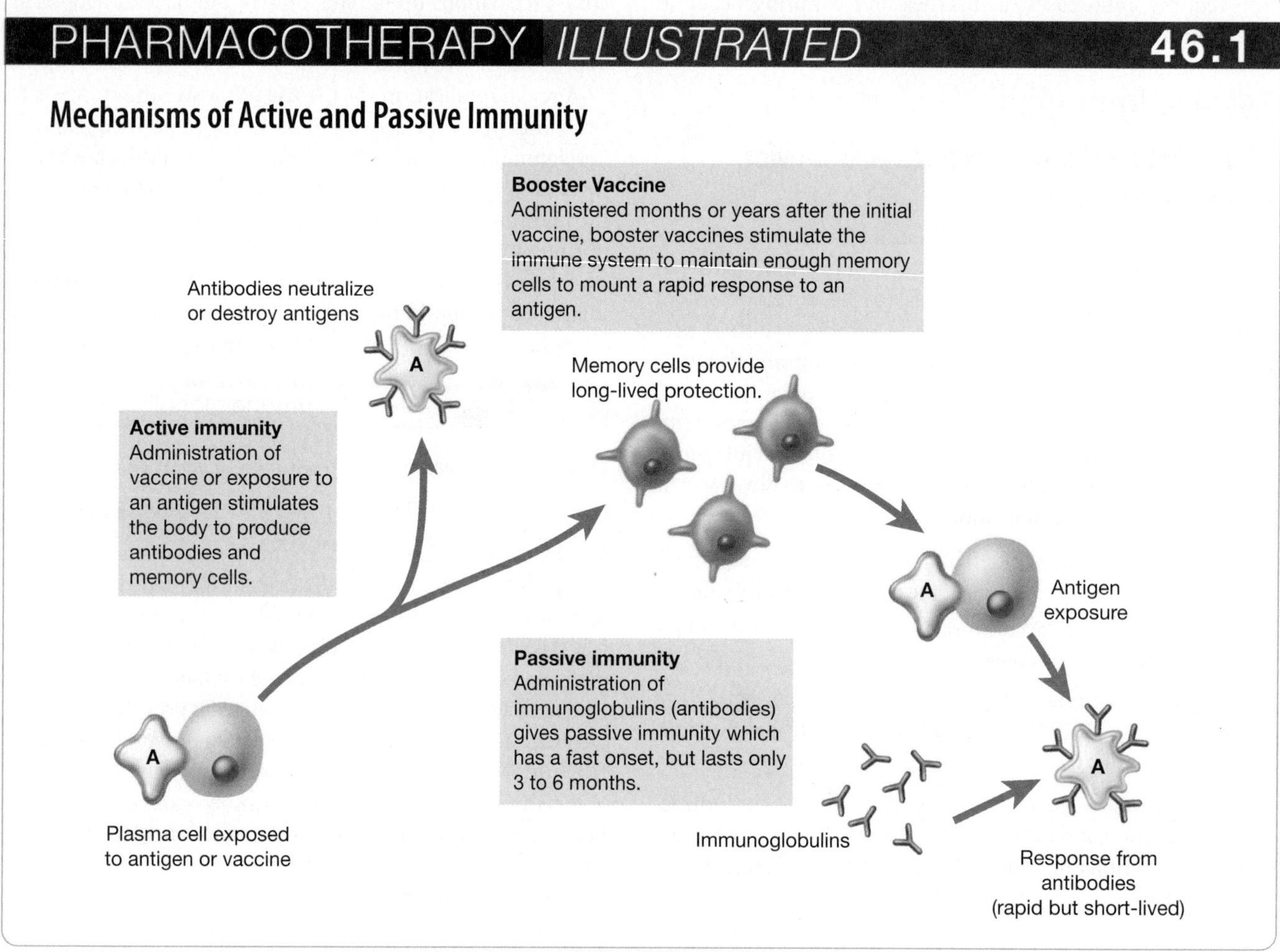

placenta and destroy erythrocytes in the fetus. This may lead to a severe anemia or brain damage in the developing fetus and even fetal death.

Rh_0 immunoglobulins are obtained from filtered human serum for the prevention of Rh incompatibility in Rh^- women. This drug has been used to provide passive immunity since 1968 and has significantly reduced the incidence of EF. Administration of Rh_0 immunoglobulins will prevent the mother from forming Rh antibodies, so that there will be no risk of incompatibility in subsequent pregnancies. Rh_0[D] immune globulin prophylaxis is not indicated if either the father or the fetus is Rh_0[D] negative.

The administration of RhoGAM is recommended:

- At 28 weeks' gestation.
- Within 72 hours postpartum.
- Within 3 hours of spontaneous or induced pregnancy termination.
- Following any event that could lead to transplacental hemorrhage (such as amniocentesis, chorionic villi sampling, or abdominal trauma).

Mechanism of Action: Rh_0[D] antibodies act by suppressing the immune response of Rh^- mothers to Rh^+ fetuses or newborns. Sensitization to Rh_0[D]-positive blood in future pregnancies is therefore less likely to occur.

Pharmacokinetics:

Route(s)	IM, IV
Absorption	Unknown
Distribution	Unknown
Primary metabolism	Unknown
Primary excretion	Unknown
Onset of action	Peak antibody levels: 2 h (IV) or 5–10 days (IM)
Duration of action	Half-life: 24–30 days

Adverse Effects: The most commonly reported adverse reactions include local swelling, redness, and mild pain at the injection site. A small number of patients experience low-grade fever. Hypersensitivity reactions are rare and may include hives, generalized urticaria, tightness of the chest, wheezing, hypotension, and anaphylaxis. Also rarely reported are anemia, anorexia, bruising, disseminated intravascular coagulation (DIC), dyspnea, dysuria, edema, hematuria, hemolysis, hypertension, increased risk of bleeding, lower back pain, malaise, nausea, polydipsia, vomiting, and weight gain.

Contraindications/Precautions: This drug is contraindicated in individuals with a history of hypersensitivity reaction to human immunoglobulin injection. Rh_0[D] antibodies are also contraindicated in patients having immunoglobulin A (IgA) deficiencies or in patients with severe anemia, and should be used with caution in patients who have DIC, hemolysis, renal disease, and splenectomy.

Drug Interactions: No drug interactions have been reported. **Herbal/Food:** Unknown.

Pregnancy: Category C.

Treatment of Overdose: Overdose with this drug has not been reported.

Nursing Responsibilities:

- Monitor patients for at least 20 minutes following the administration of RhoGAM for the potential development of a hypersensitivity reaction.
- Determine the current health status and previous vaccination history of the patient to determine possible contraindications.
- Record in the patient's permanent record the manufacturer, lot number, date of administration, and the name and address of the person administering the vaccine.
- Inspect the prefilled syringe for discoloration or particulate matter prior to administration.

Patient and Family Education:

- Immediately report to the health care provider these serious adverse reactions: fever, difficulty breathing, confusion, swelling of the eyes or face, irritability, or confusion.
- Be aware that mild adverse effects include fever and local injection site swelling, redness, and pain.
- Before receiving this vaccine, inform the health care provider about all other vaccines you have recently received. Also tell the health care provider if you have received drugs or treatments in the past 2 weeks that can weaken the immune system, including corticosteroids; medications to treat psoriasis, rheumatoid arthritis, or other autoimmune disorders; or medicines to treat or prevent organ transplant rejection.
- Notify all health care providers of your Rh status and that you received RhoGAM.

Drugs Similar to Rh_0[D] Immune Globulin (RhoGAM)

Other immunoglobulins include cytomegalovirus immune globulin, hepatitis B immune globulin, and IV immune globulin.

Cytomegalovirus immune globulin (CytoGam): About half of the U.S. adult population has been exposed to cytomegalovirus (CMV). Few people, however, have experienced symptoms because healthy immune systems prevent symptomatic, active infections. When donating organs or tissues, CMV may be inadvertently transferred to a transplant recipient with a suppressed immune system. Cytomegalovirus immune globulin (CMV-IGIV) is recommended for the prevention of CMV infections in at-risk individuals receiving kidney, liver, pancreas, and heart transplants. The drug can lower the incidence of serious CMV-associated disease by 50%. Current dosage recommendations include the IV administration of seven doses, beginning within 72 hours of the receipt of the organ and ending 30 days later. The most common adverse effects are minor and include flushing, chills, muscle cramps, back pain, fever, nausea, vomiting, arthralgia, and wheezing.

Hepatitis B immune globulin (HBIG): The goal of HBIG administration is to prevent the transmission of HBV to those who have been exposed to the virus. The administration of HBIG is recommended for the following instances:

- Nonimmunized individuals who have had acute and significant exposure to hepatitis B–infected blood. This includes accidental needlestick, oral ingestion, or direct mucous membrane contact with infected blood or blood products. One dose is usually given immediately after exposure, and 1 month later. The administration of HBIG is effective in the prevention of clinical hepatitis B infection in approximately 75% of individuals who are treated.
- Infants born to women infected with HBV. These infants should receive HBIG and start the HBV vaccine series within 12 hours of birth. This regimen is 70% to 90% effective in preventing infection in the infant.
- Sexual partners of HBV-infected patients. A single dose of HBIG is 75% effective at preventing HBV infection if the drug is administered within 2 weeks of sexual contact.
- Household exposure of infants less than 12 months of age who are born to a mother or have a primary caregiver who is infected with HBV. These infants should receive HBIG and start the HBV vaccine series before 12 months of age.

The administration of HBIG is effective in the prevention of clinical hepatitis B infection in approximately 75% of individuals who are treated, but this immune protection is temporary, lasting approximately 2 to 3 months. HBIG is usually given concurrently (different IM site) with hepatitis immunization in infants born of hepatitis B–infected mothers. Adverse reactions to HBIG are rare and include local site reactions, such as tenderness, redness, and swelling. Hypersensitivity reactions have also been reported. HBIG is provided in a prefilled, single-dose syringe in either pediatric or adult preparations.

Intravenous immune globulin (IVIG, Gammagard, Carimune, Octagam): Immune globulin contains pooled antibodies obtained from human plasma that is used to provide passive immunity following exposure to an organism for which no active immunization exists, if there is inadequate time to develop active immunity, and as replacement therapy for those with antibody deficiencies. IVIG contains 95% or more immunoglobulin G (IgG). The passive immunity induced by IVIG is capable of attenuating or preventing a wide range of infectious diseases and adverse effects from toxins, mycoplasma, parasites, bacteria, and viruses. IVIG may be thought of as a "generic" treatment for balancing immune systems. It contains components that strengthen immune function as well as substances that can suppress overactive immune systems. Disease protection lasts for 3 weeks or longer. Because this drug contains antibodies to live viruses, active vaccinations should not be given until 3 to 5 months after IVIG has been administered.

NURSING PROCESS APPLICATION

Patient Receiving Immunizations

Assessment	Potential Nursing Diagnoses
Prior to administration: • Determine the current health status, allergies, and previous vaccination history of the vaccine. • Question the patient or caregiver about reactions to previous immunizations. • Follow administration protocol. Immunizations must be administered by the specific route indicated for each product. Failure to follow administration protocol may result in an insufficient immune response. • Record in the patient's permanent record the manufacturer, lot number, date of administration, and the name and address of the person administering the vaccine.	• *Risk for Injury*, related to adverse effects from vaccine administration • *Noncompliance,* related to immunization schedule

Planning: Patient Goals and Expected Outcomes

The patient (or parent or guardian if a minor) will:

- Verbalize an understanding of the rationale for immunizations by describing the purpose of immunizations.
- Verbalize the importance of complying with the immunization schedule by describing the series of immunizations.
- Report any adverse reactions to the health care provider, such as temperature higher than 39.4°C (103°F), convulsions, dyspnea, or alterations in consciousness.

Implementation

Intervention and (Rationales)	Patient and Family Education
• Monitor the patient for expected immune response as evidenced by increased body temperature, general malaise, or redness or soreness at the injection site.	• Inform the patient, parent, or guardian of expected response such as general malaise, slight fever (lower than 39.4°C [103°F]), poor appetite, irritability, and soreness if the immunization is injected.
• Monitor the patient for hypersensitivity reaction symptoms, which include shortness of breath, anxiety, and hypotension.	• Instruct the patient, parent, or guardian to report to the emergency department of the nearest health care facility if the following symptoms develop: temperature higher than 39.4°C (103°F), convulsions, alterations in consciousness, or dyspnea.
• Defer administration of routine immunizing or booster doses in case of acute infection. (Active immunizations require adequate immune response.)	• Explain to the patient that immunizations should not be given when the child has an active infection which requires an unimpeded immune response.
• Provide comfort measures, such as analgesia, warm soaks for the injection site, small meals, and environmental temperature control, to help the patient cope with the discomfort of the injection. (Injectable immunizations are often painful and cause soreness due to the desired immune response.)	• Instruct the patient, parent, or guardian in comfort measures, such as analgesia, warm soaks for the injection site, small meals, and environmental temperature control, to help the patient cope with the discomfort of injection.
• Provide the patient with a written record of immunization and a reminder of when a booster injection is needed. (To ensure optimal immunity some immunizations require boosters, which patients often forget.)	• Inform the patient, parent, or guardian of the benefits and risks associated with the vaccination as well as the importance of completing the immunization series.

Evaluation of Outcome Criteria

Evaluate the effectiveness of drug therapy by confirming that patient goals and expected outcomes have been met (see "Planning").

UNDERSTANDING THE CHAPTER

Key Concepts Summary

46.1 The eradication of smallpox was a great triumph in modern medicine.

46.2 Vaccines are used to activate the immune system for the purpose of disease prevention.

46.3 There are four traditional methods of producing vaccines.

46.4 Vaccines should be administered by an established schedule with precautions taken for patients who are immunosuppressed or pregnant.

46.5 Active immunity can be induced to prevent bacterial infections.

46.6 Effective vaccines that prevent viral infections have been developed.

46.7 Antibodies are administered to provide passive immunity.

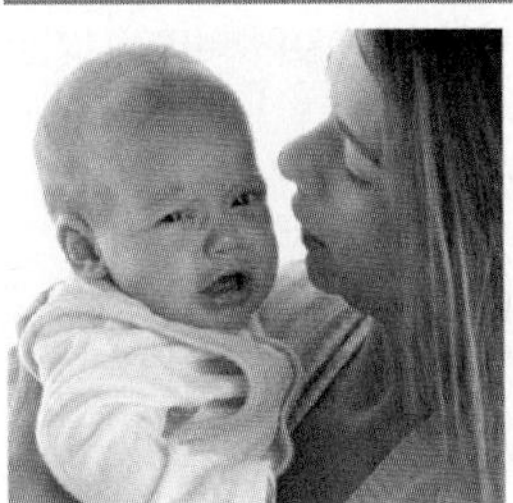

Making the PATIENT Connection

Remember the patient "Samantha Abbott" at the beginning of the chapter? Now read the remainder of the case study. Based on the information presented within this chapter, respond to the critical thinking questions that follow.

Mr. and Mrs. Abbott arrive in the office where you work with their 4-month-old infant, Samantha, for her checkup. She is scheduled to receive the following immunizations today: Rota, DTaP, Hib, PCV, and IPV. Samantha's mother states, "I don't think these immunizations are necessary. Don't these shots usually make children sick?"

As first-time parents, Mr. and Mrs. Abbott are new to the experience of childhood immunizations and require careful teaching. While obtaining her history, you find that 4-month-old Samantha has been doing well and is in the 90th percentile for height and 89th percentile for weight. She has achieved the developmental milestones for her age and is bright and interacts well with her environment.

Critical Thinking Questions

1. What information should be obtained from the Abbotts about Samantha's first response to immunization?
2. Why is it important to discuss the potential adverse effects of vaccines with Samantha's parents?
3. What educational information should be given to the Abbotts?

Case Study

As a nurse working in the intensive care unit, your patient assignment today is to care for a critically ill patient who is known to be HIV positive and hepatitis B and C positive. You are cleaning up after assisting a first-year resident with the insertion of a central line and, as you are putting the disposable drapes into the trash, you feel a sharp pain in your right hand. As you pull your hands away you see a needle protruding through the glove into your hand. You report the incident to your supervisor and report to the emergency department per exposure protocol.

The emergency department physician orders you to have antibody testing for anti-HBsAG, baseline HIV testing, and to receive gamma globulin and antiviral prophylaxis.

1. What is the rationale for the hepatitis B testing?
2. What is the rationale for the HIV testing?
3. Why is gamma globulin ordered?
4. Why is antiviral prophylaxis appropriate?

NCLEX-RN® Review

1 Mary is a 4 month-old infant who is brought to the clinic for her first checkup. Her mother tells the nurse that the child has never been ill. Which of the following factors would the nurse consider most significant in assessing the baby's likelihood of receiving immunizations?

1. Allergies to previously administered medications
2. Mother's preconceptions and reservations relating to vaccines
3. Maternal and paternal allergies or reactions to vaccine administration
4. The nurse's knowledge of the recommended pediatric immunization schedule

2 The nurse is administering RhoGAM to a postpartum client who wants to know how the medication works. The response by the nurse would be based on which of the following physiological concepts? The purpose of RhoGAM administration is:

1. To provide antibodies to destroy foreign fetal red blood cells.
2. To protect the Rh^- fetus during a subsequent pregnancy.
3. To provide antibodies against Rh^+ blood and prevent immune sensitization.
4. To prevent maternal antibodies from crossing the placenta and destroying fetal white blood cells.

3 A 7-year-old girl, who was bitten by a stray dog, is treated in the emergency department. The dog has not been tested to rule out rabies. The nurse will anticipate that this client will receive the following immunizations: (Select all that apply.)

1. Tetanus toxoid
2. DaPT vaccine
3. Rabies immunoglobulin
4. Rabies vaccine
5. Rabies toxoid

4 The nurse determines that the client understands an important principle about toxoids when the client makes which of the following statements? "Toxoids are:

1. Antibodies that have been secreted by a sensitized immune system."
2. Given to counteract the effects of viral interferons."
3. Inactive bacterial toxins used to stimulate antibody production."
4. Rarely used in vaccine development."

5 The occupational health nurse will be administering hepatitis B vaccine to a new employee. Which of the following assessment findings discovered by the nurse would necessitate withholding the injection? The client is:

1. A two-pack per day smoker.
2. Known to have transient hypertension.
3. Allergic to yeast and yeast products.
4. Frightened by needles and injections.

6 A postpartum client received Rh_o immune globulin (RhoGAM) therapy after the delivery of an 8-lb baby boy. The nurse performs what important intervention during the course of this treatment?

1. Monitor the client for 20 minutes following the administration for hypersensitivity reaction.
2. Evaluate the laboratory results for thrombocytopenia, anemia, and increased liver enzymes.
3. Provide the client with the information needed to maintain a low-saturated fat, low-cholesterol diet.
4. Instruct the client to use nonmedicated sugar-free lozenges or hard candies to relieve cough.

See Answers to Critical Thinking Questions, Case Study, and NCLEX-RN® Review in Appendix A.

References

Advisory Committee on Immunization Practices, Centers for Disease Control. Prevention of varicella: Recommendations of the Advisory Committee on Immunization Practices. (2007). *Morbidity and Mortality Weekly Report, 56*(RR-4), 1–40.

Ball, J. W., & Bindler, R. C. (2008). *Pediatric nursing: Caring for children* (4th ed.). Upper Saddle River, NJ: Prentice-Hall.

Bohlke, K., Davis, R. L., Marcy, S. M., Braun, M. M., DeStefano, F., Black, S. B., et al. (2003). Risk of anaphylaxis after vaccination of children and adolescents. *Pediatrics, 112*, 815–820.

Centers for Disease Control and Prevention. (2007a). *Smallpox.* Retrieved July 23, 2008, from http://www.bt.cdc.gov/agent/smallpox/

Centers for Disease Control and Prevention. (2007b). *Vaccines and preventable diseases: HPV vaccination.* Retrieved July 23, 2008, from http://www.cdc.gov/vaccines/vpd-vac/default.htm

Centers for Disease Control and Prevention. (2007c). Update: Prevention of hepatitis A after exposure to hepatitis A virus and in international travelers. Updated recommendations of the Advisory Committee on Immunization Practices (ACIP). *Morbidity and Mortality Weekly Report, 56*(41), 1080–1084.

Centers for Disease Control and Prevention. (2005a). Pertussis—United States, 2001–2003. *Morbidity and Mortality Weekly Report, 54*(50), 1283–1286. Retrieved July 23, 2008, from http://www.cdc.gov/mmwr/preview/mmwrhtml/mm5450a3.htm

Centers for Disease Control and Prevention. (2005b). Prevention and control of meningococcal disease. *Morbidity and Mortality Weekly Report, 54*(RR07), 1–21. Retrieved July 23, 2008, from http://www.cdc.gov/mmwr/preview/mmwrhtml/rr5407a1.htm

Chen, W., & Gluud, C. (2005). Vaccines for preventing hepatitis B in health-care workers. *Cochrane Database of Systematic Reviews, 3.* Art. No.: CD000100. DOI: 10.1002/14651858.CD000100.pub3.

Epocrates online. (2007). *Recombivax HB: Hepatitis B vaccine (recombinant), contraindications and cautions.* Retrieved July 23, 2008, from https://online.epocrates.com/u/1034299/Recombivax+HB/Contraindications+Cautions

Health-Cares.net. (2005). *RH incompatibility: Erythroblastosis fetalis.* Retrieved July 23, 2008, from http://womens-health.health-cares.net/erythroblastosis-fetalis.php

Krause, R. (2008). Herpes zoster. *eMedicine.* Retrieved July 23, 2008, from http://www.emedicine.com/emerg/TOPIC823.HTM

Krensky, A. M., Strom, T. B., & Bluestone, J. A. (2006). Immunomodulators: Immunosuppressive agents, toleragens, and immunostimulants. In L. L. Brunton, J. S. Lazo, and K. L. Parker (Eds.), *The pharmacological basis of therapeutics* (11th ed., pp. 1463–1484). New York: McGraw-Hill.

Medscape. (2008). *BayGam intramuscular: Monograph-immune globulin.* Retrieved July 23, 2008, from http://www.medscape.com/druginfo/monograph?cid=med&drugid=8475&drugname=BayGam+Intramuscular&monotype=monograph&secid=3

Merck. (2008). *RotaTeq (Rotavirus Vaccine, Live, Oral, Pentavalent Oral Solution) prescribing information.* Retrieved July 23, 2008, from http://www.merck.com/product/usa/pi_circulars/r/rotateq/rotateq_pi.pdf

Merck Vaccine Support. (2008). *Gardasil® human papillomavirus quadrivalent (types 6, 11, 16 & 18) vaccine recombinant product monograph.* Retrieved July 23, 2008, from http://www.merckvaccines.com/gardasilProductPage_frmst.html

Ortho-Clinical Diagnostics. (2007). *Rho-GAM ultra filtered PLUS.* Retrieved July 23, 2008, from http://www.rhogam.com/

Plotkin, S. (2003). Vaccines, vaccination and vaccinology. *Journal of Infectious Diseases, 187*, 1349–1359.

Plotkin, S. A., & Orenstein, W. A. (2004). *Vaccines* (4th ed.). Philadelphia: Elsevier.

Tyring, S. K. (2005). *Antiviral agents, vaccines, and immunotherapies.* New York: Marcel Dekker.

UNIT 7

Pharmacology of Infectious and Neoplastic Disease

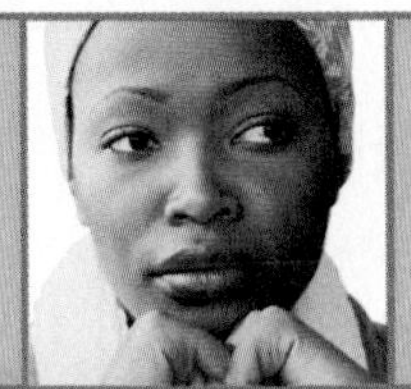
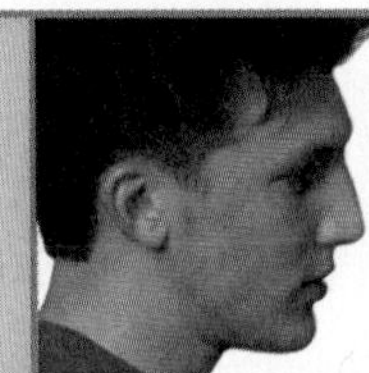
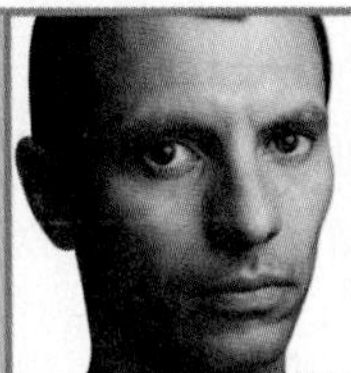
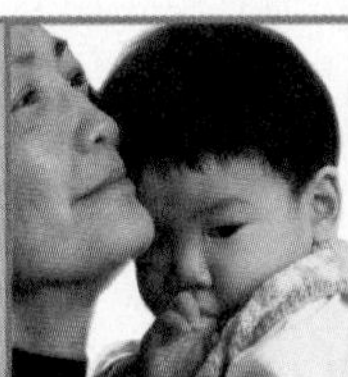

CHAPTER 47	Basic Principles of Anti-Infective Pharmacotherapy
CHAPTER 48	Antibiotics Affecting the Bacterial Cell Wall
CHAPTER 49	Antibiotics Affecting Bacterial Protein Synthesis
CHAPTER 50	Fluoroquinolones and Miscellaneous Antibacterials
CHAPTER 51	Sulfonamides and the Pharmacotherapy of Urinary Tract Infections
CHAPTER 52	Pharmacotherapy of Mycobacterial Infections
CHAPTER 53	Pharmacotherapy of Fungal Infections
CHAPTER 54	Pharmacotherapy of Protozoan and Helminthic Infections
CHAPTER 55	Pharmacotherapy of Non-HIV Viral Infections
CHAPTER 56	Pharmacotherapy of HIV-AIDS
CHAPTER 57	Basic Principles of Antineoplastic Therapy
CHAPTER 58	Pharmacotherapy of Neoplasia

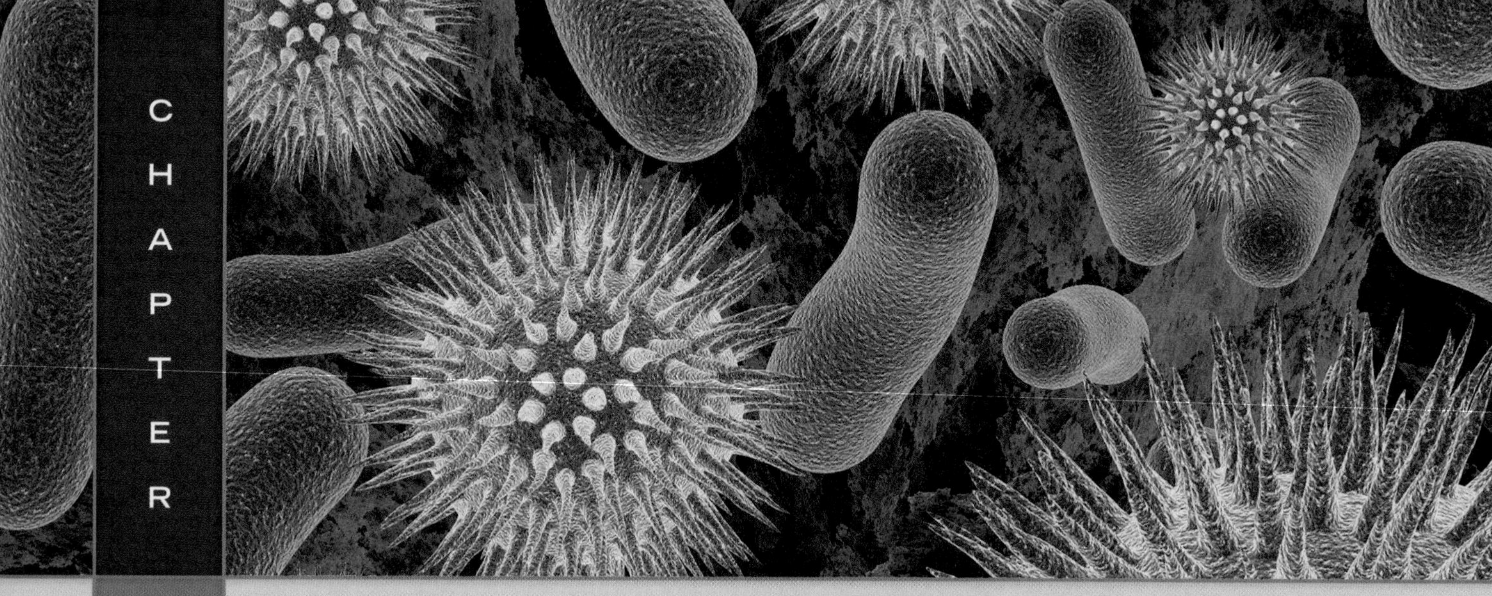

47 Basic Principles of Anti-Infective Pharmacotherapy

Learning Outcomes

After reading this chapter, the student should be able to:

1. Explain the mechanisms by which pathogens infect the body.
2. Derive a method for describing and classifying bacteria.
3. Explain the mechanisms by which anti-infective drugs act to kill pathogens or restrict their growth.
4. Describe the clinical significance of bacterial resistance.
5. Identify steps that the nurse can take to limit the development of resistance.
6. Describe the clinical rationale for selecting specific antibiotics.
7. Identify the role of the nurse in preventing, identifying, and treating adverse effects due to antibiotic therapy.
8. Explain how the patient's immune status, history of allergic reactions, age, pregnancy status, genetics, or local tissue conditions influence anti-infective pharmacotherapy.
9. Explain the clinical importance of selecting the correct antibiotic for the individual patient.
10. Describe the development of superinfections.

Chapter Outline

Pathogenicity and Virulence

Describing and Classifying Bacteria

Classification of Anti-Infectives

Mechanisms of Action of Anti-Infectives

Acquired Resistance

Indications and Selection of Specific Anti-Infectives

Host Factors Affecting Anti-Infective Selection

Superinfections

Key Terms

acquired resistance, 779
aerobic, 776
anaerobic, 776
antibiotic, 776
anti-infective, 776
bacteriocidal, 776
bacteriostatic, 776
broad-spectrum antibiotic, 782
conjugation, 781
culture and sensitivity (C&S) testing, 782
endotoxins, 775
exotoxins, 775
gram negative, 776
gram positive, 776
host flora, 782
invasiveness, 775
microbial antagonism, 784
mutations, 780
narrow-spectrum antibiotic, 782
nosocomial infections, 781
pathogenicity, 775
pathogens, 775
peptidoglycan, 778
superinfections, 784
virulence, 775

The human body has adapted quite well to living in a world teeming with microorganisms (microbes). In the air, water, food, and soil, microbes have been essential components of life on the planet for billions of years. In some cases, these microorganisms coexist in intimate contact with human beings. It is estimated that 10^{14} bacterial cells reside inside or on the surface of the body, which is more than the total number of human cells in an average person. Fortunately, of the millions of species of microbes, only a relative few are harmful to human health. The purpose of this chapter is to present the fundamental principles that apply to the pharmacotherapy of infectious disease in the next nine chapters of this textbook.

PharmFACT

In 1900, 5 of the 10 most frequent causes of death in the United States were infectious diseases. In 2000, only influenza or pneumonia and AIDS are in the top 10 causes of death. *Source:* Madigan, Martinko, Dunlap, & Clark, 2009.

Pathogenicity and Virulence

47.1 Pathogens cause disease due to their ability to invade tissues or secrete toxins.

The first challenge in studying the pharmacotherapy of infectious disease is to understand the terminology that is used to describe the organisms and drugs. Microbes that are capable of causing human disease, or **pathogens,** include viruses, bacteria, fungi, unicellular organisms (protozoans), and multicellular animals (e.g., fleas, mites, and worms).

Some pathogens are extremely infectious and life threatening to humans, whereas others simply cause annoying symptoms or none at all. **Pathogenicity,** the ability of an organism to cause disease, depends on an organism's speed of reproduction and its skill in bypassing or overcoming body defenses. Organisms that usually infect only when the body's immune system is suppressed are called opportunistic pathogens.

Virulence is a quantitative measure of an organism's pathogenicity. A highly virulent microbe is one that can produce disease when present in very small numbers. Virulent pathogens produce their devastating effects through two primary characteristics: invasiveness and toxicity.

Invasiveness is the ability of a pathogen to grow extremely rapidly and cause direct damage to surrounding tissues by their sheer numbers. Because a week or more may be needed to mount an immune response against the organism, this exponential growth can rapidly overwhelm body defenses and disrupt normal cellular function. Some *Streptococci, Staphylococci,* and *Clostridia* secrete hyaluronidase, an enzyme that digests the matrix between human cells, allowing the bacteria to penetrate anatomic barriers more easily. *Staphylococcus aureus* secretes the enzyme coagulase, causing fibrin to be deposited on its cells, thereby protecting it from phagocytes.

The second characteristic of virulence is the production of toxins, or toxicity. **Exotoxins** are proteins released by bacteria into surrounding tissues that have the ability to inactivate or kill host cells. *Clostridium botulinum,* the organism responsible for botulism, produces one of the most potent toxins known that binds to presynaptic motor neurons to prevent the release of acetylcholine. Cholera toxin from *Vibrio cholerae* causes large amounts of fluid to be secreted into the intestinal lumen. Symptoms of exotoxin-producing bacteria are usually caused by the toxin itself, not the bacteria. For example, patients experience food poisoning by ingesting food containing the toxins produced by the organisms; growth of the bacteria in the body is not required. Most exotoxins are water soluble and can readily enter the blood to cause systemic toxemia.

Endotoxins are nonprotein chemicals that are part of the outer layer of the envelope surrounding gram-negative bacteria. After the bacterial cell dies, endotoxins are liberated into the surrounding tissue and induce macrophages to release large amounts of cytokines, causing generalized inflammation, fever, and chills. Rapid decreases in the number of lymphocytes, leukocytes, and platelets may occur. The initial doses of antibiotic therapy may actually worsen symptoms by lysing bacteria and releasing larger amounts of endotoxins. Even very small amounts of some bacterial endotoxins may disrupt normal cellular activity and, in extreme cases, result in death. Examples of organisms producing endotoxins include *Proteus,* a common cause of urinary tract infections (UTIs), and *Neisseria meningitidis,* the agent that causes meningitis.

CONNECTION *Checkpoint* 47.1

From what you learned in Chapter 4, if your patient has a particularly virulent infection, which route of administration would likely be used during antibiotic therapy to most rapidly kill the organisms? See Answer to Connection Checkpoint 47.1 in Appendix A.

Describing and Classifying Bacteria

47.2 Bacteria are described by their staining characteristics, shape, and ability to utilize oxygen.

Because of the enormous number of bacterial species, several descriptive systems have been developed to simplify their study. It is important for nurses to learn these classification schemes, because drugs that are effective against one organism in a class are likely to be effective against other pathogens in the same class. Common bacterial pathogens and their associated diseases are listed in Table 47.1.

One of the simplest methods of classifying microbes is to examine them microscopically after a crystal violet Gram stain has been applied to the microbes. Some bacteria contain a thick cell wall composed of peptidoglycan and retain the violet color after staining. These bacteria are called **gram positive** and include *Staphylococcus, Streptococcus,* and *Enterococcus.* Bacteria that have thinner cell walls will lose the violet stain and are called **gram negative.** Examples of gram-negative bacteria include *Bacteroides, Escherichia, Klebsiella, Pseudomonas,* and *Salmonella.* The distinction between gram-positive and gram-negative bacteria is a profound one that reflects important biochemical and physiological differences between the two groups. Many antibiotics are effective against only one of the two groups. For example, gram-negative bacteria are generally susceptible to the tetracycline class but are resistant to the sulfonamides. This generalization quickly breaks down when resistant strains develop.

Bacteria are often described by their basic shape that can be readily determined microscopically. Those with rod shapes are called bacilli, those that are spherical are called cocci, and those that are spiral are called spirilla. The shape, along with the Gram stain, helps pathologists to identify organisms that are isolated from infectious specimens.

A third factor used to categorize bacteria is their ability to use oxygen. Those that thrive in an oxygen-rich environment are called **aerobic;** those that grow optimally without oxygen are called **anaerobic.** Some organisms have the ability to change their metabolism and survive in either aerobic or anaerobic conditions, depending on their external environment. Antibiotics are often selective for either aerobes or anaerobes.

Classification of Anti-Infectives

47.3 Anti-infective drugs are classified by their susceptible organisms, chemical structures, and mechanisms of action.

Anti-infective is a general term that applies to any medication that is effective against pathogens. In its broadest sense, an anti-infective drug may be used to treat bacterial, fungal, viral, or parasitic infections. To distinguish among the various anti-infectives, these medications are classified as antibacterial, antifungal, antiviral, antiprotozoan, and antihelminthic based on the susceptible organism they treat.

The most frequent term used to describe an antibacterial drug is antibiotic. Technically, **antibiotic** refers to a natural substance produced by a microorganism that can kill other microorganisms. However, many of the newer drugs that are available to treat bacterial infections are now produced synthetically. In clinical practice, the terms antibacterial and antibiotic are used interchangeably to refer to any drug that is effective against bacteria. In this text, antibiotic and antibacterial are used interchangeably.

Classifying drugs only by their susceptible organism, such as an antibacterial, tells us nothing about the properties, actions, or adverse effects of a drug. With over 300 antibacterials available, it is helpful to group these drugs into subclasses that share similar therapeutic properties. Two means of grouping are widely used: chemical classes and pharmacologic classes.

Chemical class names such as aminoglycosides, fluoroquinolones, and sulfonamides refer to the fundamental chemical structure of a group of anti-infectives. Anti-infectives that belong to the same chemical class have close structural similarities and usually share similar antibacterial properties and adverse effects. Although chemical names are often long and difficult to pronounce, placing drugs into chemical classes will assist the student in mentally organizing these drugs into distinct therapeutic groups.

Pharmacologic classes are used to group anti-infectives by their mechanism of action. Like chemical classes, placing an antibiotic into a pharmacologic class allows the nurse to develop a mental framework on which to organize these medications and to predict similar actions and adverse effects. Examples of pharmacologic classes along with their prototype drugs are shown in Table 47.2. It is important that the nurse learn both the chemical class and the pharmacologic class for each antibiotic because this will provide a deeper understanding of the drug's therapeutic action and potential adverse effects.

Mechanisms of Action of Anti-Infectives

47.4 Anti-infective drugs act by selectively targeting a pathogen's metabolism or life cycle.

Although the lymphatic system provides elaborate defenses against microbial invaders, there are times when the immune defenses become overwhelmed by the infection. Furthermore, there are times when acquiring an infection could be a serious health challenge for a patient, and it is best to prevent it. Whether it is used for treating or preventing disease, the primary goal of anti-infective therapy is to assist the body in eliminating a pathogen. Drugs that accomplish this goal by killing bacteria are called **bacteriocidal.** Some drugs do not kill pathogens but instead slow their growth, allowing natural body defenses to eliminate the microorganisms. These growth-slowing drugs are called **bacteriostatic.**

Bacterial cells have distinct anatomic and physiological differences compared to human cells. Bacteria incorporate different chemicals into their membranes and use unique biochemical pathways and enzymes to manage their rapid growth. Even the more complex pathogens such as fungi and protozoans have different cell structures and use certain metabolic pathways not found in human cells. Antibiotics exert selective toxicity by targeting these unique differences between human and bacterial, fungal, and protozoan cells. Through

TABLE 47.1 Common Bacterial Pathogens

Name of Organism	Disease(s)	Description
Gram-Positive Bacilli		
Bacillus anthracis	Anthrax	Aerobe; appears in cutaneous and respiratory forms
Clostridium	Food poisoning, gas gangrene, tetanus	Anaerobe
Corynebacterium	Diphtheria	Aerobe or anaerobe
Gram-Positive Cocci		
Enterococci	Wounds, UTI, endocarditis, bacteremia	Aerobe; part of host flora of the genitourinary and intestinal tracts; common opportunistic pathogen
Staphylococcus aureus	Pneumonia, food poisoning, impetigo, wounds, bacteremia, endocarditis, toxic shock syndrome, osteomyelitis, UTI	Aerobe; some species are part of host flora on the skin and mucous membranes
Streptococci	Pharyngitis, pneumonia, skin infection, septicemia, endocarditis, otitis media, meningitis in children	Aerobe; some species are part of host flora of the respiratory, genital, and intestinal tracts
Gram-Negative Bacilli		
Bacteroides	Peritonitis, abdominal abscess	Anaerobe; part of host flora of the intestinal, respiratory, and genitourinary tracts
Campylobacter	Gastroenteritis, diarrhea	One of the most common causes of diarrheal illness in the United States
Enterobacter	UTI, blood or lung infections	Aerobe or anaerobe
Escherichia coli	Traveler's diarrhea, UTI, meningitis in children, bacteremia	Part of host flora of the intestinal tract
Haemophilus influenzae	Pneumonia, meningitis in children, bacteremia, otitis media, sinusitis	Some species are part of host flora of the upper respiratory tract
Klebsiella pneumoniae	Pneumonia, UTI	Common opportunistic pathogen; often fatal if not treated aggressively
Proteus mirabilis	UTI, skin infection	Part of host flora of the intestinal tract
Pseudomonas aeruginosa	UTI, skin infection, septicemia	Common opportunistic pathogen
Salmonella enteritides	Food poisoning	Acquired from infected animal products: raw eggs, undercooked meat or chicken
Salmonella typhi	Enteric (typhoid) fever	Acquired from contaminated food or water supplies
Serratia	Nosocomial infections of wounds and UTI	Aerobic or anaerobic
Shigella	Dysentery	Aerobic or anaerobic; part of host flora of the gastrointestinal (GI) tract
Vibrio cholerae	Cholera	Gram-negative aerobe; acquired from contaminated food or water
Gram-Negative Cocci		
Neisseria gonorrhoeae	Gonorrhea, urethritis, anorectal infection, pelvic inflammatory disease, neonatal eye infection	Gram-negative aerobe; some species are part of host flora of the upper respiratory tract
Neisseria meningitides	Meningitis, particularly in children	Gram-negative aerobe; may result in death within hours of onset of symptoms
Spirilla/Spirochetes		
Borrelia burgdorferi	Lyme disease	Acquired from tick bites
Treponema	Syphilis	Sexually transmitted infection (STI)
Other Organisms		
Chlamydia trachomatis	Venereal disease, eye infection	Gram-negative; most common cause of sexually transmitted disease in the United States
Mycobacterium leprae	Leprosy	Most cases in the United States occur in immigrants from Africa or Asia
Mycobacterium tuberculosis	Tuberculosis	Very high incidence in patients with human immunodeficiency virus (HIV) or acquired immune disease syndrome (AIDS)
Mycoplasma pneumoniae	Pneumonia	Most common cause of pneumonia in patients age 5–35
Rickettsia rickettsii	Rocky mountain spotted fever	Gram-negative; acquired from tick bites

TABLE 47.2 Classification of Anti-Infective Drugs

Mechanism of Action	Chemical Class	Prototype
Inhibition of cell wall synthesis	Penicillins Cephalosporins Carbapenems	penicillin G cefotaxime (Claforan) imipenem (Primaxin) isoniazid (INH) vancomycin (Vancocin)
Inhibition of protein synthesis	Aminoglycosides Tetracyclines Macrolides Oxazolidinones	gentamicin (Garamycin) tetracycline (Achromycin) erythromycin (E-mycin) linezolid (Zyvox)
Disruption of plasma membrane	Azoles Polyene	amphotericin B (Fungizone) fluconazole (Diflucan) nystatin (Fungizone)
Inhibition of nucleic acid synthesis	Fluoroquinolones	ciprofloxacin (Cipro)
Inhibition of metabolic pathways	Sulfonamides	dapsone (DDS) trimethoprim-sulfamethoxazole (Bactrim, Septra)

this selective action, these pathogens can be killed, or their growth severely hampered, without any major effects on human cells. Of course, there are limits to this selective toxicity, depending on the specific antibiotic and the dose employed. Adverse effects can be expected from all the anti-infectives. There are five major methods by which antibacterials exert their selective toxicity: inhibition of cell wall synthesis, inhibition of protein synthesis, disruption of the plasma cell membrane, inhibition of nucleic acid synthesis, and inhibition of metabolic pathways (antimetabolites).

Inhibition of Cell Wall Synthesis

Unlike human cells, bacteria have rigid cell walls that create a high osmotic pressure within the cells. The cell wall primarily consists of **peptidoglycan,** a substance found only in bacteria that contains sugars bound to peptides. Disruption of this wall causes the cell to absorb water and eventually lyse. The presence of a unique cell wall gives several means by which antibiotics may act. Fungi also have a unique cell wall that contains lipids that are not used in human cells.

The penicillins and cephalosporins bind to specific proteins that are essential to building the bacterial cell wall. Vancomycin acts by preventing the formation of peptide chains that are used in the construction of the cell wall. Several drugs that are effective against *Mycobacterium tuberculosis,* including isoniazid, act by inhibiting the incorporation of mycolic acid, an important component of the cell wall of this mycobacterium. Uses of the cell wall inhibitors are presented in Chapter 48.

Inhibition of Protein Synthesis

Both bacterial and human cells conduct protein synthesis, so this may seem an unlikely target for antibiotics. However, proteins are constructed on the surface of ribosomes, and these organelles have different structures in humans and bacteria. This difference in ribosomal structure accounts for the selective toxicity of certain antibiotics for bacterial cells.

The fact that protein synthesis occurs in several steps affords different mechanisms by which antibiotics may act. For example, the tetracyclines interfere with the transfer of ribonucleic acid (RNA) that carries the amino acids to the ribosome. The aminoglycosides change the shape of the ribosome so that protein synthesis is impeded. Drugs that inhibit protein synthesis are discussed in Chapter 49.

Disruption of the Plasma Cell Membrane

A few antibacterial and antifungal agents act by interfering with the pathogen's plasma membrane. For example, when polymyxin B attaches to the phospholipids in bacterial plasma membranes, the permeability of the membrane changes and substances escape from the cell. The antifungal drug amphotericin B shuts down the synthesis of ergosterol, a lipid essential to the integrity of fungal plasma membranes.

Inhibition of Nucleic Acid Synthesis

Although deoxyribonucleic acid (DNA) and RNA synthesis are complex processes that occur in both human and bacterial cells, the molecular structures of the various enzymes required for these processes differ considerably. The largest group of antibiotics that inhibits DNA synthesis is the fluoroquinolones. These drugs affect bacterial DNA gyrase, an enzyme that uncoils DNA during the replication process. The fluoroquinolones are presented in Chapter 50.

Inhibition of Metabolic Pathways (Antimetabolites)

Because they divide rapidly, bacterial cells need a steady supply of nutrients and metabolites. A few drugs structurally resemble these building blocks and "fool" the bacterial cell into using them for growth. The sulfonamide antibiotics resemble para-amino benzoic acid (PABA), a precursor to folic acid. Folic acid, a B vitamin that is essential to human metabolism, is also essential to bacteria. When the bacteria attempt to use the sulfonamides, bacterial protein synthesis is blocked. The sulfonamides are presented in Chapter 51.

Other Mechanisms of Action

Anti-infectives act by a number of other miscellaneous mechanisms. The antifungal drug griseofulvin inhibits the formation of mitotic microtubules. Antiretrovirals such as zidovudine act by blocking the synthesis of viral DNA by inhibiting the enzyme reverse transcriptase. Mebendazole kills parasitic worms by preventing their absorption of nutrients.

Many other possible mechanisms exist. As the understanding of bacterial physiology increases, it is likely that pharmacologists will develop anti-infectives with entirely new mechanisms of action. The primary mechanisms of action of antibacterial drugs are shown in Pharmacotherapy Illustrated 47.1.

PHARMACOTHERAPY ILLUSTRATED 47.1

Mechanisms of Action of Antimicrobial Drugs

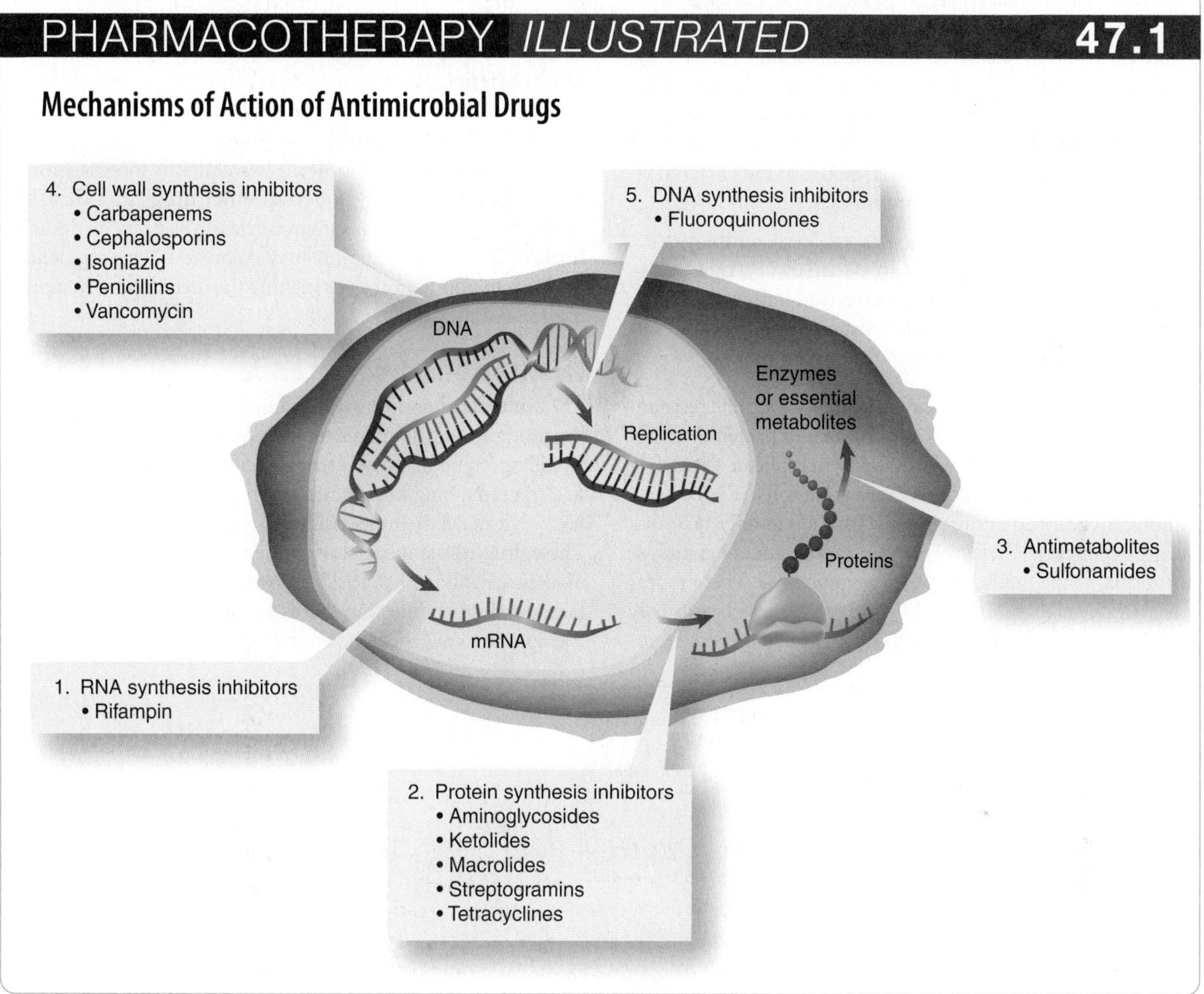

Acquired Resistance

47.5 Acquired resistance is a major clinical problem that is worsened by improper use of anti-infectives.

In the 1950s, health care providers called antibiotics "miracle drugs" and predicted that all infectious disease would one day be eliminated. It did not take long, however, to discover that these miracle drugs were rapidly becoming ineffective. How could a drug that once killed nearly 100% of a species of bacteria soon prove to be ineffective? The answer is acquired resistance.

Acquired resistance is the ability of an organism to become insensitive over time to the effects of an anti-infective. Resistance occurs in antibacterials, antifungals, antivirals, and antiprotozoal drugs. It is a major clinical problem that is growing in importance.

Mechanisms of Resistance

How can an organism become insensitive to a drug that kills other members of its species? Medicine has discovered a number of mechanisms by which pathogens acquire resistance. These include the following:

- **Destruction of the drug.** Organisms can begin producing an enzyme that destroys or deactivates the drug. For example, some bacteria have increased their production of beta lactamase, an enzyme that splits the active portion of the drug molecule. Organisms that produce beta lactamase are resistant to many of the penicillin and cephalosporin antibiotics.
- **Prevention of drug entry into the pathogen.** Some antibiotics must enter the pathogen to cause their action. Some resistant bacteria have developed enzymes that inactivate the drug as it crosses the cell wall. Others have changed the structure of the channels or pores that the antibiotic normally uses to enter the cell. Resistance to penicillins and tetracyclines can occur by these methods.
- **Removal by resistance pumps.** Some bacteria have developed a system that rapidly pumps the antibiotic out of the bacterial cell before it can reach intracellular targets such as ribosomes. Resistant bacteria may actually develop several pumps, each used to remove specific antibiotics.

- **Alteration of the drug's target site.** Most antibiotics have a specific receptor to which they bind that is located on the cell surface or inside the bacteria. In certain resistant bacteria the shape of these receptors has changed, so they no longer bind the drug. This mechanism of resistance is common for the sulfonamides. For the macrolide antibiotics, mutations have resulted in changes to the structure of the bacterial ribosome, which is the receptor for macrolide binding.
- **Development of alternative metabolic pathways.** Some antibiotics act by depleting the pathogen of an essential substance necessary for growth. Some resistant organisms either synthesize larger amounts of the essential substance or find an alternative means of obtaining it from the environment.

How do bacteria change their physiology to become resistant to antibiotics? The answer lies in the nature of bacterial cell division. Microorganisms have the ability to replicate extremely rapidly. Under ideal conditions *Escherichia coli* can produce a million cells every 20 minutes, or 1×10^{21} cells in only 24 hours. During exponential division, bacteria make frequent errors, or **mutations,** while duplicating their genetic code. These mutations, which occur spontaneously and randomly, occasionally result in a change in physiology that gives a bacterial cell a reproductive advantage over its neighbors. For example, the mutated bacterium may be able to survive in harsher conditions, change the shape of its organelles, or perhaps grow faster than other bacterial cells.

One such mutation that is of particular importance to medicine is that which confers drug resistance on a microorganism. Once a resistant strain appears, it permanently loses sensitivity to that specific drug and often to other drugs that share the same pharmacologic and chemical class. Over several decades, these drug-resistant mutants may colonize a large segment of the human population, thus making the medication essentially useless as a first-line antibiotic.

Promotion of Resistance

The widespread and sometimes unwarranted use of antibiotics has promoted the development of drug-resistant bacterial strains. By killing strains of bacteria that are sensitive to the drug, the only bacteria remaining to replicate are those that acquire the mutations that make them insensitive to the effects of the antibiotic. These drug-resistant bacteria are then free to grow, unrestrained by their neighbors that are killed by the antibiotic. Soon the patient develops an infection that is resistant to conventional drug therapy. This concept is shown in Figure 47.1.

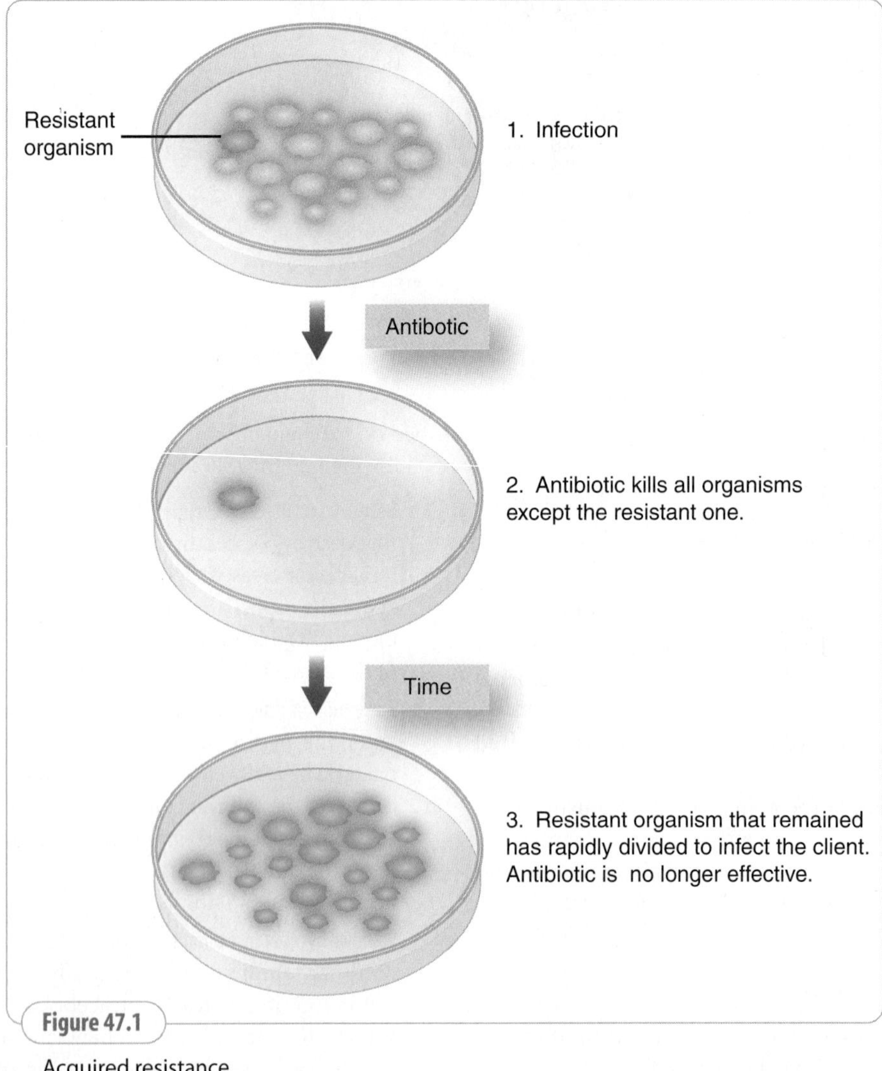

Figure 47.1

Acquired resistance.

After acquiring resistance, the mutated bacterium may pass its resistance gene to other bacteria through **conjugation,** which is the direct transfer of small pieces of circular DNA called plasmids. Through conjugation, it is quite possible for a bacterium that has never been exposed to the antibiotic to become resistant. Furthermore, because conjugation is not species specific, resistance genes may be passed from one species to a totally different species.

It is important to understand that the antibiotic itself does not cause changes in bacterial physiology, nor does the microorganism have a "master plan" to become resistant or to actively "defeat" the drug. The mutation occurs randomly—the result of accident and pure chance. The promotion and growth of the resistant strain, however, is not due to chance. The antibiotic kills the surrounding cells that are susceptible to the drug, leaving the mutated bacterium plenty of room to divide and infect. It should also be understood that it is the bacteria that become resistant, not the patient.

Prevention of Resistant Strains

Patients and their health care providers play important roles in delaying the emergence of resistance to antibiotics. The Centers for Disease Control and Prevention (CDC) has developed a set of guidelines for preventing antimicrobial resistance in the health care setting. These include the following:

- **Prevent infections when possible.** Nurses must always teach their patients that it is always easier to prevent an infection than to treat one. One important aspect of prevention is getting immunizations to protect against diseases such as influenza, tetanus, polio, measles, and hepatitis B (see Chapter 46). Prevention also includes proper care and hygiene of catheters, which are significant sources for microorganisms and provide portals of entry into the body.
- **Diagnose and treat the infection properly.** Infections should be cultured so that the offending organism can be identified and the correct drug chosen, as discussed in Section 47.7.
- **Use antimicrobials wisely.** Antibiotics should only be prescribed when there is a clear rationale for their use. The drugs should be taken for the full length of therapy, and the prescription should not be renewed if the infection has been eliminated or prevented. The more often an antibiotic is prescribed in the population, the larger will be the percentage of resistant strains.
- **Prevent transmission.** Nurses can contain infections and stop the spread of the disease in their work settings by using proper infection control procedures. Additionally, nurses should teach their patients the methods of proper hygiene to prevent the transmission of infectious disease in the home and community settings.

CONNECTION *Checkpoint* 47.2

From what you learned in Chapter 8, explain the difference between resistance and tolerance. See Answer to Connection Checkpoint 47.2 in Appendix A.

47.6 Several specific resistant strains are major clinical challenges due to the lack of therapeutic options.

Infections that are acquired in a health care setting, known as **nosocomial infections,** are often resistant to common antibiotics. Recently, the term *health care associated infection* (HAI) has begun to replace the term *nosocomial.* The most common site of HAIs is the urinary tract, followed by surgical wounds, respiratory tract, and bacteremia. Table 47.3 lists the organisms that are frequently responsible for nosocomial infections.

There are four general sources of HAIs.

- **Patient flora.** Bacteria normally residing on the skin and in the lung or genitourinary tract
- **Invasive devices.** Urinary catheters, vascular catheters, endotracheal tubes, and endoscopes
- **Medical personnel.** Infected health care workers or noninfectious carriers
- **Medical environment.** Contaminated instruments, air, food, or fluids

Many times, patients are at risk for HAIs caused by resistant organisms. Two types of resistant strains are especially important to pharmacotherapy: methicillin-resistant *Staphylococcus aureus* (MRSA) and vancomycin-resistant *Enterococci* (VRE).

Methicillin-Resistant *Staphylococcus aureus* (MRSA): MRSA is a type of bacterium that is resistant to certain antibiotics such as methicillin, amoxicillin, and penicillin. At least 60% of *S. aureus* infections are now resistant to penicillin. The name "methicillin-resistant" is still used for these infections despite the fact that methicillin was removed from the market many years ago.

MRSA infections are most frequently acquired in hospitals and long-term care facilities. These hospital-acquired infections (HA-MRSA) occur primarily in patients with weakened immune systems. MRSA infections that occur in nonhospitalized settings are called community-acquired infections. Community-acquired MRSA (CA-MRSA) infections occur in otherwise healthy people and are usually manifested as skin and soft tissue infections, such as pimples and boils. The strains that

TABLE 47.3 Common Pathogens Associated with Nosocomial Infections

Pathogen	Infection
Acinetobacter species (spp)	Bacteremia
Enterobacter spp	Pneumonia
Enterococci spp	Urinary tract
Escherichia coli	Urinary tract, primary bacteremia, pneumonia
Klebsiella pneumoniae	Pneumonia, urinary tract
Pseudomonas aeruginosa	Pneumonia, urinary tract
Staphylococcus aureus	Surgical wounds, pneumonia, bacteremia
Staphylococci (coagulase negative)	Bacteremia

are responsible for HA-MRSA infections appear to be distinctly different from those that cause CA-MRSA infections; thus the pharmacotherapy of the two infections differs somewhat.

Therapeutic options for patients with serious MRSA infections are limited. In recent years, MRSA strains have developed resistance to most classes of antimicrobials, including fluoroquinolones, macrolides, aminoglycosides, tetracyclines, and clindamycin. In general, the HA-MRSA strains are resistant to more classes than the CA-MRSA infections. Until recently, vancomycin was the only antibiotic effective for treating serious MRSA infections. Unfortunately, MRSA strains that are also resistant to vancomycin have appeared. Several newer antibiotics, including linezolid (Zymox), quinupristin-dalfopristin, and daptomycin are now available to treat multidrug-resistant strains of MRSA.

Vancomycin-Resistant *Enterococci*: *Enterococci* are normal inhabitants of the human GI tract and the female genital tract. *Enterococci* are also frequently found in wounds and pressure ulcers in hospitalized patients or nursing home residents. Patients with compromised immune systems are at greatest risk. Because *Enterococci* are hardy organisms, they can survive for prolonged periods on environmental surfaces, and health care workers using poor infection control techniques can easily spread them. More than 95% of VRE strains in the United States are *E. faecium.*

Like MRSA, VRE infections represent a major therapeutic challenge, and treatment options are limited. Strains that are resistant to the most commonly used classes of antibiotics have been isolated. Virtually all are resistant to high levels of ampicillin, which is the conventional treatment for *Enterococci* infections. In the 1990s, vancomycin became the only antibiotic effective against multidrug-resistant VRE strains. Unfortunately, each year finds more VRE strains becoming resistant to vancomycin, and newer antibiotics must be used for these infections.

PharmFACT

Up to 30% of all *S. pneumoniae* infections in some areas of the United States are resistant to penicillin. Nearly all strains of *S. aureus* in the United States are resistant to penicillin. *Source:* Sherman, 2006.

47.7 Careful selection of the correct antibiotic is essential for effective pharmacotherapy and to limit adverse effects.

It is essential that the health care provider select an antibiotic that will be effective against the specific pathogen that is causing the patient's infection. Selecting an incorrect drug will delay proper treatment, giving the microorganisms more time to invade or secrete toxins. For some infections, treatment delays of just a few hours or days can lead to poorer patient prognosis and even death. Prescribing ineffective antibiotics also promotes the development of resistance and may cause unnecessary adverse effects in the patient.

For the correct antibiotic to be chosen, identification of the causative agent is necessary. Although gathering data on symptoms is important, many infections produce the same signs early in their course; thus more exact laboratory means of diagnosis are necessary.

Infected specimens, such as urine, sputum, blood, or pus, are examined in the laboratory for the purpose of isolating and identifying specific pathogens. After isolation, the microbe is exposed in the laboratory to different antibiotics to determine the most effective ones. This process of isolating the infectious organism and identifying the most effective antibiotic is called **culture and sensitivity (C&S) testing.** Other laboratory techniques include examination of the blood for specific antibodies, direct antigen detection, and DNA probe hybridization.

Ideally, the pathogen should be identified before anti-infective therapy is begun. However, laboratory testing and identification may take several days and, in the case of viruses, several weeks. Indeed, some pathogens cannot be cultured at all. If the infection is severe, therapy is often begun with a **broad-spectrum antibiotic,** which is one that is effective against a wide variety of different microbial species. After C&S testing is completed, the drug may be changed to a **narrow-spectrum antibiotic,** which is one that is effective against a smaller group of microbes or only the isolated species. In general, narrow-spectrum antibiotics have less effect on **host flora,** thus causing fewer adverse effects. Host flora are microorganisms that normally inhabit the human body.

Anti-infectives should not be prescribed for infections such as the common cold or for disorders for which antibiotics serve no therapeutic advantage. Antibiotics do not affect viral diseases such as the common cold, although many patients with this self-limiting disorder believe that these drugs will speed their recovery. Another example of anti-infective misuse is prescribing antibiotics to patients who have a cough due to chronic bronchitis. It should be understood, however, that health care providers may prescribe anti-infectives to prevent a secondary infection from developing. For example, an elderly patient with a severe cold may develop a weakened immune response. Thus the health care provider may order an antibiotic not for the viral infection, but to prevent a secondary bacterial infection from developing.

Indications and Selection of Specific Anti-Infectives

47.8 Depending on the pathogen, anti-infective therapy may be conducted with a single drug or a combination of drugs.

If C&S testing confirms that an infection is caused by a single species of microbe, antibiotic therapy is usually more successful when conducted with one drug. Combining two antibiotics may actually decrease each drug's effectiveness, a phenomenon known as antagonism. For example, giving a drug that slows bacterial growth may interfere with an antibiotic that depends on a high bacterial growth rate to produce its bacteriocidal effect. Use of multiple antibiotics can also promote the emergence of multidrug resistant strains and produce unnecessary adverse effects.

In well-defined circumstances combination therapy with multiple antibiotics is warranted. For example, multiple anti-infective drugs are indicated if several different species of pathogens are causing the infection. Patients may present with a life-threatening infection of unknown etiology and the health care provider may need to prescribe several antibiotics until the specific pathogens can be identified. In some cases, two antibiotics have been shown through clinical research to work synergistically, producing a greater kill than would be achieved by either antibiotic given alone. Examples of situations where multidrug therapy is clearly warranted are for the pharmacotherapy of tuberculosis (see Chapter 52) and HIV-AIDS (see Chapter 56).

CONNECTION *Checkpoint* 47.3

From what you learned in Chapter 6, why would there probably be fewer adverse effects in a patient if two antibiotics are given at lower doses, rather than a single antibiotic given at a higher dose? See Answer to Connection Checkpoint 47.3 in Appendix A.

47.9 Anti-infectives may be administered to prevent infections.

In most cases, anti-infectives are given when there is clear evidence of infection. This is because health care providers have developed clearer rationales for prescribing these drugs due to the widespread use of antibiotics in the population that has promoted the emergence of resistant strains.

Anti-infectives may be administered to prevent infections in certain high-risk patients. In these cases, research has demonstrated that the benefits of infection prophylaxis outweigh the increased risk of adverse effects or the potential for producing resistant strains. Prophylactic anti-infectives are indicated for the following clinical situations:

- Antibiotics for patients with suppressed immune systems, including those with HIV-AIDS or profound neutropenia
- Antibiotics for patients with deep puncture wounds such as from dog bites
- Antibiotics for patients with prosthetic heart valves, prior to receiving medical or dental surgery, to prevent bacterial endocarditis
- Antibiotics for patients who are undergoing specific types of surgery, such as cardiovascular surgery, orthopedic surgery, and surgery of the alimentary canal, where it has been shown that antibiotic use decreases the risk of postoperative infections
- Antimalarial drugs for patients who are entering areas of the world where malaria is endemic
- Antitubercular drugs for close personal contacts of patients who have confirmed or suspected active tuberculosis
- Antiretrovirals to prevent the transmission of HIV to newborns when the mother is HIV positive
- Antiretrovirals for health care workers who have a confirmed exposure to HIV-contaminated body fluids

Prophylactic therapy with anti-infectives is usually conducted using specific protocols that designate the duration of therapy. For example, chloroquine (Aralen) is given 1 week before expected exposure to malaria and continues for 4 weeks following exposure. Zidovudine (AZT) is given to the HIV-positive mother beginning after week 14 of pregnancy until birth, after which the drug is given to the neonate for 6 weeks. Only in rare cases are anti-infectives given prophylactically for indefinite time periods.

Host Factors Affecting Anti-Infective Selection

47.10 Patient factors such as host defenses, local tissue conditions, history of allergic reactions, age, pregnancy status, and genetics influence the choice of anti-infective.

The most important factor in selecting an appropriate antibiotic is to be certain that the microbe is sensitive to the bacteriocidal or bacteriostatic effects of the drug. Once the appropriate drug is chosen the nurse must consider a number of host factors that have the potential to significantly influence the success of anti-infective therapy.

Host Defenses

Remember that the primary goal of antibiotic therapy is to kill enough of the pathogen, or slow their growth, such that natural body defenses can overcome the invading agents. An anti-infective is rarely able to eliminate a pathogen without help from a functioning immune system. Patients with weakened immune defenses often require the administration of prophylactic antibiotics. Should an infection occur, patients with weakened immune defenses would require more aggressive and prolonged anti-infective therapy. Examples of patients who may require this type of antibiotic therapy include those with AIDS and those with neutropenia caused by immunosuppressive or antineoplastic medications.

Local Conditions

Anti-infectives must be able to reach the area of infection in sufficient concentrations to be effective; thus local conditions at the infection site are important to the success of pharmacotherapy. Infections of the central nervous system (CNS) are particularly difficult to treat because many medications have difficulty crossing the blood–brain barrier to reach the brain and its associated tissues. Injury or inflammation at an infection site can cause tissues to become acidic or anaerobic and have poor circulation. Excessive pus formation or large hematomas can impede drugs from reaching their targets. Pathogens such as mycobacteria, salmonella, toxoplasma, and listeria can reside intracellularly and thus be resistant to antibacterial action.

Factors that hinder the drug from reaching microbes will limit therapeutic success, and adjustments in treatment may be necessary. Increasing the dosage or switching to a different route of drug administration may be indicated. Occasionally, it is necessary to switch to a different antibiotic that is more effective for conditions specific to the infection site.

Allergy History

Although not common, serious hypersensitivity reactions to antibiotics may be fatal. The penicillins are the class of antibacterials that have the highest incidence of allergic reactions: Between 0.7% and 4% of all patients who receive these drugs exhibit some degree of hypersensitivity.

Patient assessment must always include a thorough medication history. A previous acute allergic incident with a drug is highly predictive of future hypersensitivity to the same medication. Because the patient may have been exposed to an antibiotic unknowingly, such as through food products or molds, allergic reactions can occur without any apparent previous exposure. If severe allergy to a drug is established, it is best to avoid all drugs in the same chemical class.

Other Host Factors

Age, pregnancy status, and genetics are additional factors that influence anti-infective pharmacotherapy. Infants and elderly patients are less able to metabolize and excrete antibiotics; thus doses are generally decreased. Because of polypharmacy in older patients, this group is more likely to be taking multiple drugs that could interact with antibiotics.

Some antibiotics are readily secreted in breast milk or cross the placenta. For example, tetracyclines taken by the mother can cause teeth discoloration in the newborn, and aminoglycosides can affect hearing. Some anti-infectives are pregnancy category D, such as minocycline, doxycycline, neomycin, and streptomycin. The benefits of antibiotic use in pregnant or lactating women must be carefully weighed against the potential risks to the fetus and neonate.

A genetic absence of certain enzymes can lead to an inability of a patient to metabolize antibiotics to their inactive forms. For example, patients with a deficiency of the enzyme glucose-6-phosphate dehydrogenase should not receive sulfonamides, chloramphenicol, or nalidixic acid due to the possibility of erythrocyte rupture.

CONNECTION *Checkpoint* 47.4

From what you learned in Chapter 45, what classes of drugs are administered to boost immune function so that the patient is less likely to experience an opportunistic infection? See Answer to Connection Checkpoint 47.4 in Appendix A.

Superinfections

47.11 Superinfections can occur when an anti-infective antibiotic kills host flora.

Microorganisms that normally inhabit the human body, or host flora, are present on the surface of the skin, and in the upper respiratory, genitourinary, and intestinal tracts. Some of these microbes serve useful purposes by producing natural antibacterial substances or by breaking down toxic agents. The various host flora are in competition with each other for physical space and nutrients. This **microbial antagonism** helps protect the host from being overrun by pathogenic organisms.

Antibiotics are unable to distinguish between host flora and pathogenic organisms. When an antibiotic kills the host's normal flora, additional nutrients and space are available for pathogenic microorganisms to grow unchecked. These new, secondary infections caused by antibiotic use are called **superinfections,** or suprainfections. The appearance of a new infection while receiving anti-infective therapy is highly suspicious of a superinfection. Signs and symptoms of superinfection commonly include diarrhea, bladder pain, painful urination, or abnormal vaginal discharges.

Broad-spectrum antibiotics are more likely to cause superinfections because they kill many microbial species, which sometimes includes host flora. Organisms that commonly cause superinfections are *Clostridium albicans* in the vagina, *Streptococci* in the oral cavity, and *Clostridium difficile* in the colon.

UNDERSTANDING THE CHAPTER

Key Concepts Summary

47.1 Pathogens cause disease due to their ability to invade tissues or secrete toxins.

47.2 Bacteria are described by their staining characteristics, shape, and ability to utilize oxygen.

47.3 Anti-infective drugs are classified by their susceptible organisms, chemical structures, and mechanisms of action.

47.4 Anti-infective drugs act by selectively targeting a pathogen's metabolism or life cycle.

47.5 Acquired resistance is a major clinical problem that is worsened by improper use of anti-infectives.

47.6 Several specific resistant strains are major clinical challenges due to the lack of therapeutic options.

47.7 Careful selection of the correct antibiotic is essential for effective pharmacotherapy and to limit adverse effects.

47.8 Depending on the pathogen, anti-infective therapy may be conducted with a single drug or a combination of drugs.

47.9 Anti-infectives may be administered to prevent infections.

47.10 Patient factors such as host defenses, local tissue conditions, history of allergic reactions, age, pregnancy status, and genetics influence the choice of anti-infective.

47.11 Superinfections can occur when an anti-infective antibiotic kills host flora.

References

Bartlett, J. G. (2004). *Antimicrobial drug resistance update.* Paper presented at the 44th Interscience Conference on Antimicrobial Agents & Chemotherapy: Antimicrobial Drug Resistance and Emerging Infectious Threats, Washington, DC.

Bauman, R. W. (2009). *Microbiology with diseases by body system* (2nd ed.). San Francisco: Benjamin Cummings.

Chambers, H. F. (2006). General considerations of antimicrobial therapy. In L. L. Brunton, J. S. Lazo, & K. L. Parker (Eds.), *The pharmacological basis of therapeutics* (11th ed., pp. 1095–1110). New York: McGraw-Hill.

Cisneros-Farrar, F., & Parsons, L. (2007). Antimicrobials: Classifications and uses in critical care. *Critical Care Nursing Clinics of North America, 19*(1), 43–51.

Courvalin, P. (2005). Antimicrobial drug resistance: Prediction is very difficult, especially about the future. *Emerging Infectious Diseases, 11*(10), 1503–1506.

Fridkin, S. K., & Gaynes, R. P. (1999). Antimicrobial resistance in intensive care units. *Clinics in Chest Medicine, 20,* 303–316. Retrieved July 24, 2008, from http://www.cdc.gov/ncidod/dhqp/pdf/ar/aricu.pdf

Gilbert, D. N., Moellering, R. C., & Sande, M. A. (2001). *The Sanford guide to antimicrobial therapy 2008* (38th ed.). Sperryville, VA: Antimicrobial Therapy.

Madigan, M. T., Martinko, J. M., Dunlap, P. V., & Clark, D. P. (2009). *Brock biology of microorganisms* (12th ed.). San Francisco: Benjamin Cummings.

Owens, R. C., & Rice, L. (2006). Hospital-based strategies for combating resistance. *Clinical Infectious Diseases, 42*(Suppl. 4), S173–181.

Parsons, L., & Krau, S. (2007). Bacterial infections: Management by acute and critical care nurses. *Critical Care Nursing Clinics of North America, 19*(1), 17–26.

Sherman, M. (2006). An overview of antibiotic resistance. Retrieved July 24, 2008, from http://www.uspharmacist.com/econnect/Default.aspx?tabid=53&page=publish/content/8_1670.htm

Tillotson, G. S., Blondeau, J. M., & Carroll, J. (2007). Hospital-based strategies to reduce antibiotic resistance: Are they valid in the community setting? *Expert Review of Anti-Infective Therapy, 5*(1), 53–59.

Tortora, G. J., Funke, B. R., & Case, C. L. (2007). *Microbiology: An introduction* (9th ed.). San Francisco: Benjamin Cummings.

Woolhouse, M. E. J., & Gowtage-Sequeria, S. (2005). Host range and emerging and reemerging pathogens. *Emerging Infectious Diseases, 11*(12), 1842–1847.

CHAPTER

Last month I underwent surgery for the removal of a skin lesion from my left arm. Unfortunately, I think the wound has become infected. The area is red, swollen, and painful and has a yellowish drainage.

Patient "Katie Dennison"

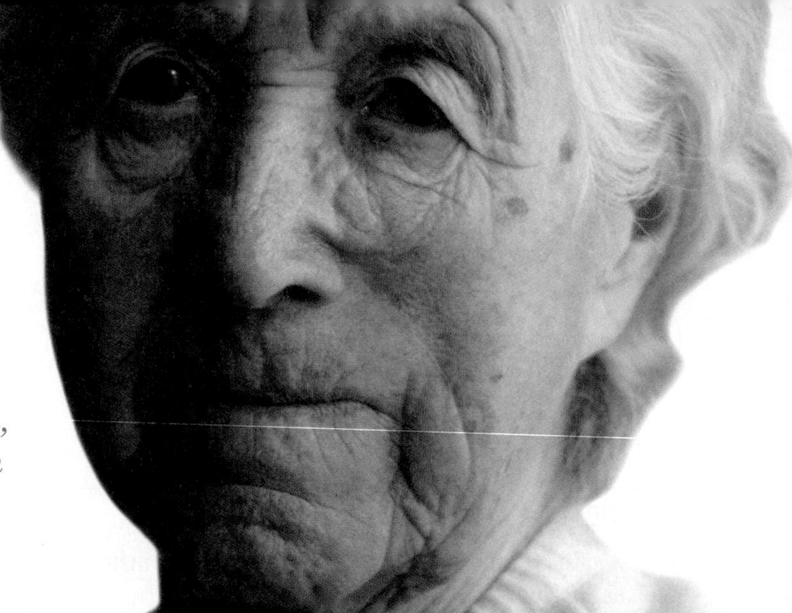

48 Antibiotics Affecting the Bacterial Cell Wall

Learning Outcomes

After reading this chapter, the student should be able to:

1. Explain the structure of a bacterial cell wall and its importance to pharmacotherapy.
2. Identify the classes of antibiotics that act by affecting the synthesis of the bacterial cell wall.
3. Explain the mechanisms by which antibiotics affect the bacterial cell wall.
4. Compare and contrast the four classes of penicillins.
5. Compare and contrast the four generations of cephalosporins.
6. Identify similarities and differences among drugs in the carbapenem class.
7. For each of the classes shown in the chapter outline, identify the prototype and representative drugs and explain the mechanism(s) of drug action, primary indications, contraindications, significant drug interactions, pregnancy category, and important adverse effects.
8. Apply the nursing process to care for patients who are receiving drug therapy with bacterial cell wall inhibitors.

Chapter Outline

Structure of Bacterial Cell Walls

Penicillins

Natural Penicillins

PROTOTYPE **Penicillin G** *p. 791*

Broad-Spectrum Penicillins

PROTOTYPE **Ampicillin (Principen)** *p. 792*

Extended-Spectrum (Antipseudomonal) Penicillins

Penicillinase-Resistant (Antistaphylococcal) Penicillins

Cephalosporins

PROTOTYPE **Cefazolin Sodium (Ancef, Kefzol)** *p. 797*

Carbapenems

PROTOTYPE **Imipenem-Cilastatin (Primaxin)** *p. 800*

Miscellaneous Cell Wall Inhibitors

PROTOTYPE **Vancomycin HCl (Vancocin)** *p. 802*

Key Terms

beta-lactam ring, 788
beta lactamase, 788
penicillinase, 788
penicillin-binding proteins (PBPs), 787
peptidoglycan, 787

The discovery and development of the first anti-infective drugs in the mid-1900s was a milestone in the field of medicine. Humans no longer die in massive numbers from infectious organisms such as *Yersinia pestis*, which killed 25% of the known human population in the 14th century due to the bubonic plague. This chapter examines the penicillins, cephalosporins, and other antibiotic agents that kill bacteria by disrupting their cell walls.

Structure of Bacterial Cell Walls

48.1 Bacterial cell walls consist of layers of carbohydrate and protein chains, which are constructed by enzymes called penicillin-binding proteins.

The cell wall is a structure that sets people apart from the bacterial world. Humans do not have them, but all bacteria do. The osmotic pressure is so high within a bacterial cell that the cell would rupture without the containment of this rigid structure. The cell wall also serves as a barrier to substances that try to enter the cell, including antibiotics. Simply, it protects the bacterial cell from a hostile environment. The cell walls of gram-positive bacteria are very thick, whereas the walls of gram-negative bacteria are thinner. The structure of a bacterial cell wall is illustrated in Figure 48.1.

The primary material in a cell wall is **peptidoglycan,** a strong, repeating network of carbohydrate and protein chains. In gram-negative bacteria, peptidoglycan is laid down in repeated layers that are cross-linked to each other to provide greater stability to the wall. The layers may be compared to a fort that is built to provide protection from invaders. A single wall could be easily destroyed, but five or six repeated walls would provide almost impenetrable protection to those inside.

Because of its critical importance, bacteria spend a lot of time and energy building their cell walls. At least 30 different bacterial enzymes participate in their construction. Some of these enzymes are targets for penicillins and related antibiotics and are called **penicillin-binding proteins (PBPs).** Most penicillins affect transpeptidase, which is the final enzyme in the wall construction process that adds the cross-links to the peptidoglycan layers. Without the cross-linking, the cell wall becomes weakened and bulges due to the high osmotic pressure inside the cell. The bacterial cell eventually lyses (disintegrates). This process is illustrated in Figure 48.2. Because humans do not construct cell walls, they do not have PBPs. Therefore, antibiotics that affect the cell wall have selective toxicity to bacteria.

The PBPs are located on the outside of the plasma membrane of the bacterial cell. This location allows antibiotics to cause their bacteriocidal effect without actually entering the

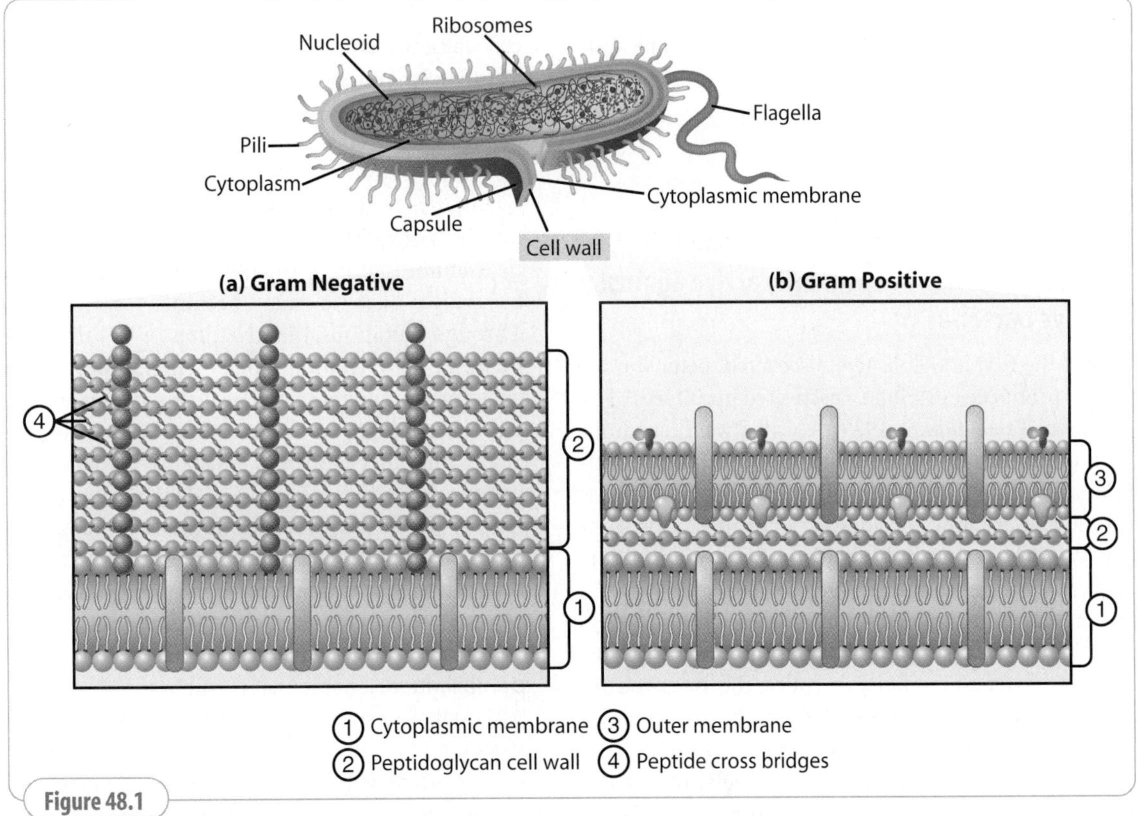

Figure 48.1

The bacterial cell wall: (a) gram-negative bacterium; (b) gram-positive bacterium.

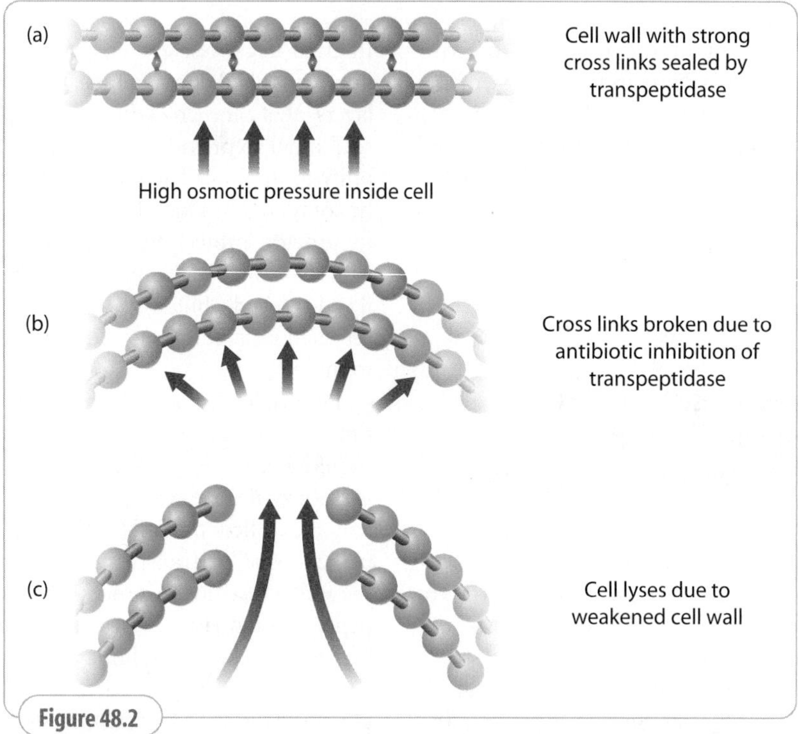

Figure 48.2

Mechanism of penicillin: (a) Bacterial cell wall strengthened by peptide cross-links. (b) Penicillin breaks cross-links. (c) Cell death due to weakened cell walls.

cell. Although all bacteria have a cell wall, the materials and PBPs used in their construction differ among species. Even slight structural changes to a PBP can cause lack of antibiotic binding to the enzyme. This explains why penicillins are not effective against all species of microorganisms. This also provides an explanation as to how an organism develops resistance to the penicillins.

Penicillins

48.2 The penicillins, one of the oldest and safest groups of antibacterials, are primarily active against gram-positive bacteria.

Although not the first anti-infective discovered, penicillin was the first mass-produced antibiotic. Discovered in cultures of the common fungus *Penicillium* in 1929, penicillin was first administered therapeutically in 1941. The medication quickly gathered a reputation as a miracle drug by preventing thousands of deaths from what are now considered minor infections. Penicillins are the most extensively studied of all the antibiotic classes. Doses of the penicillins are listed in Table 48.1.

Penicillins kill bacteria by disrupting their cell walls. The portion of the chemical structure of penicillin that is responsible for its antibacterial activity is called the **beta-lactam ring.** The beta-lactam ring resembles one of the chemical "building blocks" of peptidoglycan. When the PBP enzyme attempts to add the next "link" in the peptidoglycan chain, it binds to the beta-lactam ring, and construction of the cell wall is terminated. Other antibiotic classes that contain a beta-lactam ring include the cephalosporins, monobactams, and carbapenems, as shown in Figure 48.3. These classes are sometimes grouped together and referred to as beta-lactam antibiotics.

Penicillin lyses growing bacterial cells that are building their cell walls; therefore, it is considered bacteriocidal. It has much less toxicity, however, on bacterial cells that have already constructed their cell walls. Like all infections, the body's immune defenses are needed to eliminate stable, slow-growing bacterial cells.

Because of their extensive use over the past 60 years, large numbers of resistant bacterial strains now limit the therapeutic usefulness of the penicillins. There are several mechanisms by which bacteria may become resistant to penicillins. Through mutations, the structures of PBPs have changed such that they no longer bind to penicillin. Indeed, many species of bacteria are inherently insensitive to penicillins because they lack the binding protein target for these antibiotics.

Another mechanism of resistance is that some bacteria secrete enzymes that split the beta-lactam ring, rendering the antibiotic ineffective. **Beta lactamase** is the general term used for any of several enzymes produced by certain bacteria that can split the four-atom beta-lactam ring structure. The action of penicillinase is illustrated in Figure 48.4.

Scientists who first discovered this enzyme named it **penicillinase,** a name that is still frequently used in medicine. Although the terms are sometimes used interchangeably, it should be noted that penicillinase is only one type of beta lactamase—that which splits the ring in penicillin antibiotics. Other forms of beta lactamases exist that can act on cephalosporins, carbapenems, and other antibiotics with this

TABLE 48.1 Penicillins

Drug	Route and Adult Dose (maximum dose where indicated)	Adverse Effects
Natural Penicillins		
penicillin G benzathine (Bicillin)	IM: 1.2 million units as a single dose (max: 2.4 million units/day)	*Rash, pruritus, diarrhea, nausea, fever* Anaphylaxis symptoms, including angioedema, circulatory collapse, and cardiac arrest; nephrotoxicity
penicillin G procaine (Wycillin)	IM: 600,000–1.2 million units daily (max: 4.8 million units/day)	
penicillin G sodium/potassium	IM/IV: 2–24 million units divided every 4–6 h (max: 80 million units/day)	
penicillin V	PO: 125–250 mg qid (max: 7.2 g/day)	
Broad-Spectrum (Aminopenicillins)		
amoxicillin (Amoxil, Trimox)	PO: 250–500 mg tid (max: 1,750 mg/day)	
amoxicillin-clavulanate (Augmentin)	PO: 250- or 500-mg tablet (each with 125 mg clavulanic acid) every 8–12 h	
ampicillin (Principen)	PO/IV/IM: 250–500 mg every 6 h (max: 4 g/day PO or 14 g/day IV/IM)	
ampicillin and sulbactam (Unasyn)	IV/IM: 1.5–3 g every 6 h	
Extended-Spectrum (Antipseudomonal)		
carbenicillin (Geocillin)	PO: 382–764 mg qid	
piperacillin	IM: 2–4 g tid-qid (max: 24 g/day)	
piperacillin-tazobactam (Zosyn)	IV: 3.375 g qid over 30 min	
ticarcillin (Ticar)	IM: 1–2 g qid (max: 24 g/day)	
Penicillinase Resistant (Antistaphylococcal)		
cloxacillin (Cloxapen)	PO: 250–500 mg bid	
dicloxacillin	PO: 125–500 mg qid (max: 4 g/day)	
nafcillin	PO: 250 mg–1 g qid (max: 12 g/day)	
oxacillin	PO: 250 mg–1 g qid (max: 12 g/day)	

Note: *Italics* indicate common adverse effects. Underline indicates serious adverse effects.

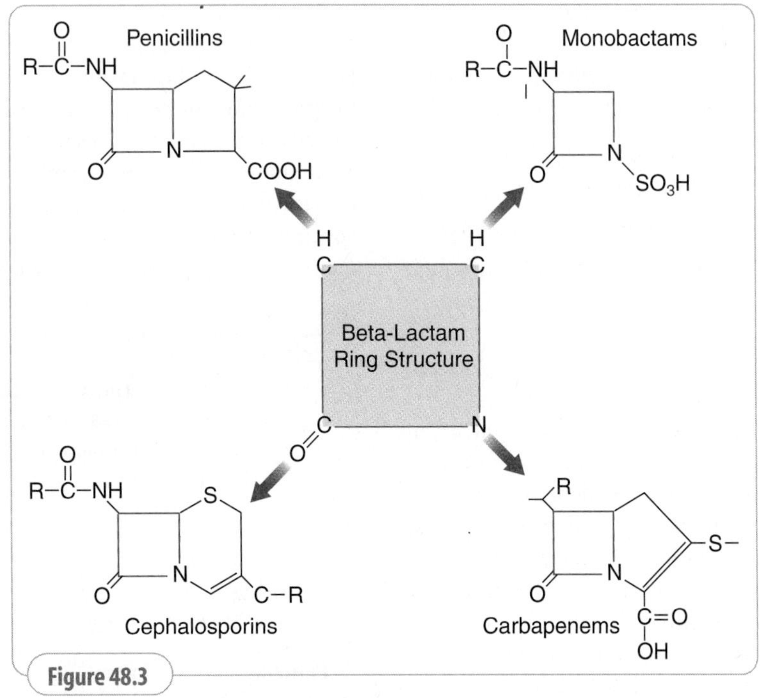

Figure 48.3

Beta-lactam antibiotics: The beta-lactam ring is common to many different classes of antibiotics.

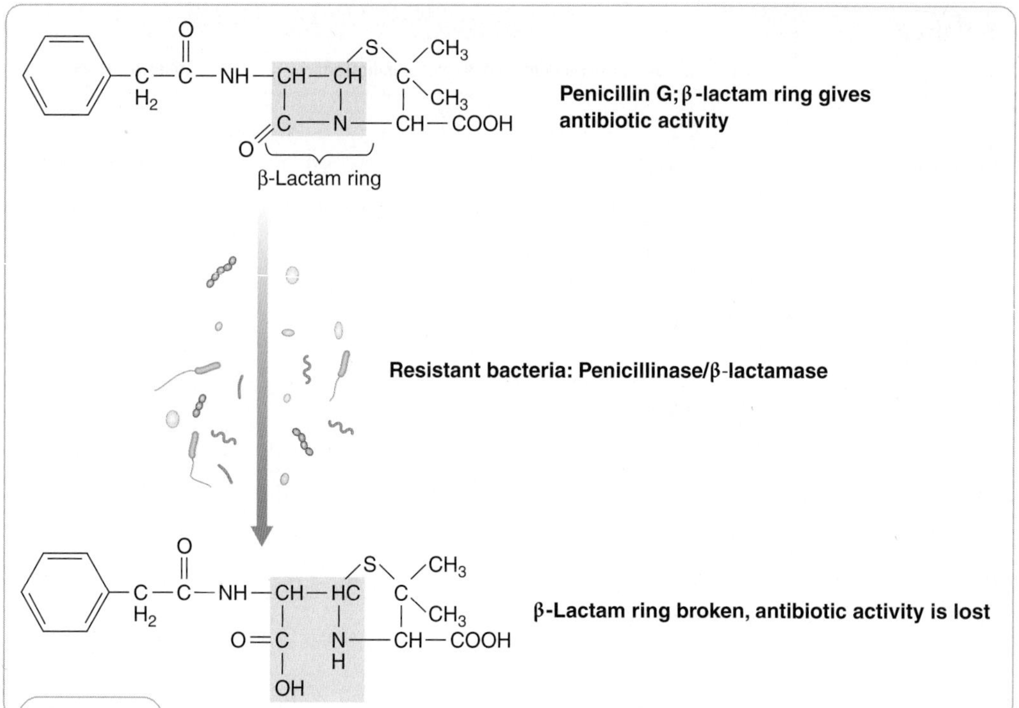

β-Lactam ring

Penicillin G; β-lactam ring gives antibiotic activity

Resistant bacteria: Penicillinase/β-lactamase

β-Lactam ring broken, antibiotic activity is lost

Figure 48.4

Action of penicillinase.

ring structure. In this textbook, the term *penicillinase* is used when referring to this enzyme's action on penicillins, and the term *beta lactamase* is used when referring to other antibiotics. It should be understood, however, that these are two forms of the same enzyme.

To overcome the killing effects of penicillin, some bacteria secrete larger amounts of penicillinase when exposed to antibiotics. In addition, the genes encoding for penicillinase can be transferred to other bacteria through conjugation, thus spreading the development of resistance genes.

Although each drug in this class has certain unique properties, some generalizations may be made about the penicillins.

- Most are more effective against gram-positive bacteria, although a few have activity against gram-negative bacteria.
- Most have a narrow spectrum of antimicrobial activity.
- They are widely distributed to most body tissues, although only small amounts reach the cerebrospinal fluid (CSF).
- Nearly all are rapidly excreted by the kidneys.
- Most have short half-lives.

Allergic reactions are the most common adverse effects of the penicillins and ones that require careful attention by nurses. The overall incidence of penicillin allergy ranges from 1% to 10%. Symptoms range from mild rash and nausea to fever or anaphylaxis. Although the incidence of anaphylaxis is low, ranging from 0.04% to 2%, mortality is high and nurses must take every precaution to identify patients at highest risk. Allergic reactions may occur within minutes after taking the drug, or they may be delayed for several days or weeks.

Prior exposure to penicillin is necessary for an allergic reaction, although this exposure may have occurred inadvertently through exposure to mold or by eating animal products that contain small amounts of penicillin. Allergy to one penicillin increases the risk of allergy to other drugs in this class. There is also a degree of cross-hypersensitivity between penicillins and cephalosporins. The nurse should not give penicillin to a patient who has a medical history of serious penicillin allergy. If penicillin must be given due to a patient's condition, however, there are available skin tests that may be used to assess the probability of the patient experiencing a severe allergic reaction. Giving a small amount of penicillin and waiting to see if anaphylaxis develops is not an acceptable method for assessing the probability of allergy. The size of a dose is not related to the severity of the response, because even very small amounts can elicit anaphylaxis in susceptible patients. Nurses must always be vigilant in observing for signs of allergy following penicillin administration, because there is no infallible method for predicting which patient will experience an allergy to the drug.

CONNECTION *Checkpoint* 48.1

From what you learned in Chapter 6, explain how taking a good medical history can eliminate some allergic reactions to antibiotics. See Answer to Connection Checkpoint 48.1 in Appendix A.

Chemical modifications to the original molecule have produced drugs that offer several advantages over the natural penicillins. These advantages include the following:

- Penicillinase resistance
- Broader antimicrobial spectrum
- Extended spectrum

PharmFACT

The United States Food and Drug Administration (FDA) Nonprescription Drugs Advisory Committee has determined that there is a lack of evidence to support the benefit of using consumer products, including hand washes, body washes, and others, that contain antibacterial additives. *Source:* Centers for Disease Control and Prevention, 2007.

Natural Penicillins

The natural penicillins were the first isolated from the fungus *Penicillium*. They are inexpensive and the drugs of choice for susceptible infections.

PROTOTYPE DRUG Penicillin G

Classification: **Therapeutic:** Antibacterial
Pharmacologic: Cell wall inhibitor, natural penicillin

Therapeutic Effects and Uses: Approved in 1943, penicillin G has a narrow spectrum of activity that includes most gram-positive bacteria. Many gram-negative organisms are resistant to penicillin G. It is a drug of choice for the treatment of infections shown to be susceptible by culture and sensitivity (C&S) testing because it is inexpensive and exhibits few adverse effects. These include susceptible strains of *Staphylococcus, Streptococcus, Neisseria, Actinomyces, Bacillus anthracis, Clostridium, Treponema,* and *Corynebacterium*. Penicillin is given for the prophylaxis of bacterial endocarditis in patients with prosthetic heart valves or congenital heart disease and for those at risk to recurrent bouts of rheumatic fever.

Penicillin G is available as either a potassium or a sodium salt; there is no difference therapeutically between the two salts. Both may be administered intravenously (IV) or intramuscularly (IM). Penicillin G potassium was once available by the oral (PO) route, but the drug had low bioavailability due to destruction by gastric acid. Penicillin V and amoxicillin are more stable in acid and are used when oral penicillin therapy is desired.

Mechanism of Action: This drug inhibits bacterial wall synthesis by binding PBPs. Penicillin G is bacteriocidal and destroyed by penicillinase.

Pharmacokinetics:

Route(s)	IM, IV
Absorption	Rapid absorption (IM)
Distribution	Widely distributed; only small amounts cross the blood–brain barrier; secreted in breast milk; approximately 60% bound to plasma proteins
Primary metabolism	15–30% metabolized, primarily hepatic
Primary excretion	Renal
Onset of action	IM: 15–30 minutes; IV: immediate
Duration of action	4–6 h; half-life: 20–60 minutes

Adverse Effects: Penicillin G is well tolerated by most patients and adverse effects are uncommon. Urticaria and delayed skin reactions occasionally occur. The most serious adverse effect is severe hypersensitivity reaction. The anaphylactic response may include cardiovascular collapse; edema of the mouth, tongue, pharynx, and larynx; confusion; seizures; and hallucinations.

Contraindications/Precautions: Penicillin G is contraindicated in patients who are allergic to any drug in the penicillin class and is used cautiously in those with hypersensitivity to cephalosporins. Because 90% of a dose of penicillin G is excreted unchanged by the kidneys through tubular secretion, patients with significant renal impairment must be carefully monitored. Patients with heart failure should not receive the penicillin sodium salt. Hyperkalemia may result with high doses of the penicillin G potassium salt.

Drug Interactions: Penicillin G may decrease the effectiveness of oral contraceptives. Colestipol will decrease the absorption of penicillin. Probenecid decreases the excretion of penicillin G and can lead to antibiotic toxicity. Potassium-sparing diuretics such as spironolactone may cause hyperkalemia when administered with penicillin G potassium. Because penicillins can antagonize the actions of aminoglycoside antibiotics, drugs from these two classes are not administered concurrently. The bacteriostatic action of tetracyclines may inhibit the bacteriocidal action of penicillin G. **Herbal/Food:** Unknown.

Pregnancy: Category B.

Treatment of Overdose: No specific therapy is available. Patients are treated symptomatically.

Nursing Responsibilities:

- Perform an infection-focused physical examination, including vital signs and a white blood cell (WBC) count. Determine baseline signs and symptoms, indicating the presence of infection.
- Obtain an accurate history from the patient prior to drug administration, including exposure, sensitivity or allergies, and any known reaction to penicillin. Hypersensitivity reactions occur more often with parenteral penicillin than with the oral form of the medication, so monitor the patient closely for 30 minutes after parenteral administration.
- Obtain and assess C&S tests (blood, urine, sputum, wound drainage, other body fluids) before starting therapy.
- Monitor for hypersensitivity reaction, which may be rapid in onset or occur over a period of days or weeks.
- Evaluate renal, hepatic, and hematologic function at regular intervals when a patient is on a high dose of this drug.
- Inject the medication deeply into muscle mass. Rotate injection sites.

Patient and Family Education:

- Immediately report signs of allergy, including rash, difficulty breathing, or swelling of the face, lips, or throat to the health care provider.
- Immediately report severe or persistent diarrhea accompanied by fever to the health care provider. Do not attempt to

MyNursingKit | Mechanism of Action Animation: Penicillin

treat penicillin-related diarrhea with over-the-counter (OTC) products.

- Contact the health care provider if the infection does not begin to improve after a few days of therapy.
- Take this drug exactly as prescribed until the prescription is completed.

Drugs Similar to Penicillin G

Other natural penicillins include penicillin G benzathine, penicillin G procaine, and penicillin V.

Penicillin G benzathine (Bicillin): Approved in 1943, penicillin G benzathine dissociates to form penicillin G; thus they share the same actions, indications, and adverse effects. Penicillin G benzathine is given only by the IM route and is absorbed very slowly, resulting in low peak serum levels with a prolonged duration of action that can last up to 26 days. Neurologic adverse effects have been reported with penicillin G benzathine, including severe agitation, confusion, hallucinations, and seizures. Injections of this drug are painful and injection site reactions may occur. Permanent neurologic damage occurs if this drug is injected near a nerve. This drug is pregnancy category B.

Penicillin G procaine (Wycillin): Approved in 1943, penicillin G procaine is a repository form of penicillin given only by the IM route. Like the benzathine salt, it is absorbed slowly from its injection site and has a prolonged duration of action (15 to 20 hours). It shares the same actions, indications, and adverse effects as penicillin G. The procaine salt is less painful on administration than penicillin G administered by the IM route. Penicillin G procaine can cause neurotoxicity if the drug is accidentally injected near a nerve. Like the benzathine salt, neurologic adverse effects can occur with penicillin G benzathine, including severe agitation, confusion, hallucinations, and seizures. Patients with allergies to the local anesthetic procaine (Novocain) should not receive this drug. This drug is pregnancy category B.

MyNursingKit | Veterinary Antibiotics and Human Health

Penicillin V: Penicillin V is nearly identical to penicillin G, except that it is more acid stable, which allows it to be administered by the PO route. However, it should be taken on an empty stomach to maximize absorption. Approved in 1956, it shares the same actions, indications, and adverse effects as penicillin G. Some patients experience nausea, vomiting, and diarrhea. This drug is pregnancy category B.

Broad-Spectrum Penicillins

A major limitation of the natural penicillins is their lack of activity against gram-negative organisms. The aminopenicillins, amoxicillin and ampicillin, are effective against gram-positive and certain gram-negative bacilli such as *Haemophilus influenzae, Escherichia coli, Salmonella,* and *Shigella.* This distinction is responsible for them being placed into a separate class called broad-spectrum penicillins.

Aminopenicillins are rapidly inactivated by penicillinase, which limits their therapeutic usefulness, particularly against *Staphylococcus aureus* infections. Despite this limitation, the aminopenicillins are some of the most widely prescribed antibiotics for sinus and upper respiratory and genitourinary tract infections. Their widespread use over many decades has resulted in a large number of resistant strains.

Combination drugs have been developed that offer certain advantages over single-drug therapy with aminopenicillins. The fixed-dose combination of Augmentin combines amoxicillin with clavulanate, a beta-lactamase (penicillinase) inhibitor. Another fixed-dose product, Unasyn, contains ampicillin and the beta-lactamase inhibitor sulbactam. By inhibiting penicillinase, these combined agents allow a greater percentage of the aminopenicillin molecules to reach pathogens and affect cell wall synthesis. The beta-lactamase inhibitors are ineffective when used alone and therefore are always used in fixed combination formulations with other drugs.

PROTOTYPE DRUG Ampicillin (Principen)

Classification: **Therapeutic:** Antibacterial
Pharmacologic: Cell wall inhibitor: aminopenicillin

Therapeutic Effects and Uses: Approved in 1963, the actions of ampicillin are similar to those of penicillin G except that ampicillin has a broader spectrum that includes enhanced activity over *Enterococci, E. coli, Proteus mirabilis, Neisseria gonorrhoeae, H. influenzae, Salmonella, Shigella,* and *Bordetella pertussis.* Because a large percentage of resistant strains have developed, ampicillin is no longer the drug of choice for the treatment of gonococcal infections, childhood meningitis, or *Salmonella* or *Shigella* enteritis.

Mechanism of Action: Ampicillin inhibits bacterial wall synthesis by binding PBPs. This drug is bacteriocidal and inactivated by penicillinase.

Pharmacokinetics:

Route(s)	PO, IM, and IV
Absorption	50% absorbed PO
Distribution	Widely distributed; only small amounts cross the blood–brain barrier; secreted in breast milk; plasma protein binding is about 15–20%
Primary metabolism	Largely unmetabolized, 10% hepatic
Primary excretion	Renal
Onset of action	PO: 30–60 minutes; IM: 15–30 minutes
Duration of action	Half-life: 1–2 h

Adverse Effects: Ampicillin is a safe drug that rarely produces serious adverse effects. Rash and diarrhea are the most common adverse effects, and diarrhea occurs more frequently with ampicillin than with the other aminopenicillins. Like all penicillins, anaphylaxis is rare, though potentially fatal. Anaphylactic response may include cardiovascular collapse; edema of the mouth, tongue, pharynx, and larynx; confusion; seizure; and hallucinations. Pseudomembranous colitis is an additional rare, though serious, severe adverse effect. Very high doses may produce confusion and seizures.

Contraindications/Precautions: Ampicillin is contraindicated in patients who are allergic to any drug in the penicillin class and used cautiously in those with hypersensitivity to cephalosporins. Ampicillin is excreted primarily by the kidneys; therefore, drug therapy must be monitored carefully in patients with renal disease.

Drug Interactions: Ampicillin may decrease the effectiveness of oral contraceptives. Probenecid (Benemid) decreases the excretion of ampicillin and can lead to antibiotic toxicity. Penicillins can antagonize the actions of aminoglycoside antibiotics and must be administered at least 2 hours apart. The antibacterial actions of ampicillin are diminished when it is taken concurrently with chloramphenicol, erythromycin, or tetracyclines. **Herbal/Food:** Because food decreases its absorption, ampicillin should be taken on an empty stomach.

Pregnancy: Category B.

Treatment of Overdose: No specific therapy is available. Patients are treated symptomatically.

Nursing Responsibilities:

- Perform an infection-focused physical examination, including vital signs and a WBC count. Determine baseline signs and symptoms, indicating the presence of infection.
- Obtain an accurate history from the patient prior to drug administration, including exposure, sensitivity or allergies, and any known reaction to penicillin. Hypersensitivity reactions occur more often with parenteral penicillin than with the oral form of the medication, so monitor the patient closely for 30 minutes after parenteral administration.
- Obtain and assess C&S (blood, urine, sputum, wound drainage, other body fluids) before starting therapy.
- Monitor for hypersensitivity reaction, which may be rapid in onset or occur over a period of days or weeks.
- Evaluate renal, hepatic, and hematologic function at regular intervals when a patient is on a high dose of this medication.
- Inject the medication deeply into muscle mass. Rotate injection sites.

Patient and Family Education:

- Take this medication with a full 8-oz glass of water on an empty stomach at least 1 hour before or 2 hours after meals for maximum absorption. Food decreases the rate and extent of oral absorption.
- Take this medication around the clock and take all the medication prescribed. This is usually a 10-day course of therapy unless otherwise indicated.
- Immediately report severe or persistent diarrhea accompanied by fever to the health care provider. Do not attempt to treat penicillin-related diarrhea with OTC products.
- Immediately report signs of allergy, including rash, difficulty breathing, or swelling of the face, lips, or throat to the health care provider.
- Contact the health care provider if the infection does not begin to improve after a few days of therapy.

Drugs Similar to Ampicillin (Principen)

The only other aminopenicillin is amoxicillin.

Amoxicillin (Amoxil, Trimox): Approved in 1974, amoxicillin is closely related structurally to ampicillin and has many of the same characteristics. The drug is destroyed by penicillinase-producing organisms. It is more acid stable than ampicillin and offers greater gastrointestinal (GI) absorption with peak serum levels twice as high. It exhibits a lower incidence of diarrhea than ampicillin. Amoxicillin has largely replaced ampicillin, and is one of the most frequently prescribed antibiotics. Amoxicillin should not be administered to patients with hypersensitivity to any penicillin. An extended release form of the drug (Moxatag) was approved in 2008 for treating *Streptococcus pyogenes* infections. This drug is pregnancy category B.

Extended-Spectrum (Antipseudomonal) Penicillins

Carbenicillin, piperacillin, and ticarcillin have broad spectrums of antimicrobial activity similar to those of the aminopenicillins. Their primary advantage is their additional activity against *Pseudomonas aeruginosa*; thus they are called extended-spectrum or antipseudomonal penicillins.

P. aeruginosa is an opportunistic pathogen found in air, soil, and water. It can persist on environmental surfaces such as soap residues and hot tubs and can even survive in some antiseptic solutions. *P. aeruginosa* infections may occur anywhere in the body, primarily causing disease in patients whose health is already compromised in some manner. It is responsible for about 10% of all health care associated infections (HAIs), including serious pneumonia in debilitated patients and a large number of infections in wounds and in patients with extensive burns.

P. aeruginosa has natural resistance to most antibiotics due in part to its ability to rapidly pump out antibiotic molecules that enter its cells. Because pseudomonas infections are often persistent, aggressive combination anti-infective therapy is often indicated. A typical combination includes an aminoglycoside antibiotic with an antipseudomonal penicillin. Because penicillins inactivate aminoglycosides, they must be administered at least 2 hours apart. Other antibiotics such as ceftazidime (Ceptaz, Fortaz, Tazicef), ciprofloxacin (Cipro), or imipenem (Primaxin) may be needed.

As with the other penicillins, drugs in this class inhibit bacterial wall synthesis by binding PBPs. The antipseudomonal penicillins achieve their extended spectrum because they have greater penetration through the outer membrane of gram-negative bacteria and a higher affinity for penicillin-binding proteins. All drugs in this class are similar, and there are few differences on which to distinguish them. Like most penicillins, the antipseudomonal penicillins are widely distributed to tissues and rapidly excreted mostly unchanged in the urine.

Because penicillinase-producing bacteria can inactivate the antipseudomonal penicillins, they are sometimes combined with a beta-lactamase inhibitor. Fixed-dose combinations with beta-lactamase inhibitors include piperacillin and tazobactam (Zosyn) and ticarcillin and clavulanate (Timentin).

Rash and diarrhea are the most common adverse effects of the antipseudomonal penicillins. These drugs prevent the aggregation of platelets, which can prolong bleeding time. Caution must therefore be used when using these drugs concurrently with agents that modify coagulation. Sodium salts of the antipseudomonal penicillins cause sodium overload in patients with heart failure. Carbenicillin exhibits more adverse effects than does ticarcillin or piperacillin. Like all penicillins, anaphylaxis is rare, though potentially fatal. Pseudomembranous colitis is an additional severe adverse effect. Very high doses may produce confusion and seizures. The antipseudomonal penicillins are pregnancy category B.

Carbenicillin indanyl sodium (Geocillin): Approved in 1970, carbenicillin is the only extended-spectrum penicillin available by the PO route. Use of the drug is primarily limited to the treatment of urinary tract infection (UTI) caused by *Pseudomonas* because this drug concentrates in the urine. Serum levels are not high enough for this drug to be clinically useful for systemic infections. The most common adverse effects of carbenicillin are GI related: bad taste, diarrhea, flatulence, nausea, and vomiting. High doses can lead to hypernatremia, platelet dysfunction, and hypokalemia. Electrolytes should be regularly monitored to prevent hypokalemia and hypernatremia. Carbenicillin should not be administered to patients with hypersensitivity to any penicillin. The parenteral form of the drug was discontinued in the United States due to a high incidence of adverse effects.

Piperacillin: Approved in 1981, piperacillin has one of the broadest spectrums of any of the penicillins and is effective against most gram-negative and many gram-positive anaerobic and aerobic microbes. It has been used to treat a variety of serious infections, including those of the skin, blood, sinuses, central nervous system (CNS), respiratory tract, and genitourinary tract. Available by the IM and IV routes, piperacillin is often used in combination with an aminoglycoside antibiotic because together they exert synergistic action on gram-negative microbes. High doses can lead to platelet dysfunction, although piperacillin seems to have less effect than other antipseudomonal penicillins. Electrolytes should be regularly monitored to prevent hypokalemia and hypernatremia. Piperacillin should not be administered to patients with hypersensitivity to any penicillin. Localized injection site reactions include pain, inflammation, phlebitis, and hematomas. Zosyn is a fixed dose combination of piperacillin and tazobactam.

Ticarcillin (Ticar): As with piperacillin, ticarcillin has one of the broadest spectrums of any penicillin. Approved in 1976, it has been used to treat moderate to severe gram-negative infections of the skin, blood, bone and joints, CNS, respiratory tract, and genitourinary tract. Available by either the IM or IV route, high doses can lead to hypernatremia, platelet dysfunction, and hypokalemia. Electrolytes should be regularly monitored to prevent hypokalemia and hypernatremia. Ticarcillin has a high sodium content that could affect patients with preexisting heart disease. Ticarcillin should not be administered to patients with hypersensitivity to any penicillin. Pain and phlebitis with thrombosis may occur at the injection site.

Penicillinase-Resistant (Antistaphylococcal) Penicillins

The final subclass of penicillins includes cloxacillin, dicloxacillin, nafcillin, and oxacillin, which are drugs that are effective against penicillinase-producing bacteria. These agents are less effective than penicillin G against non–penicillinase-producing strains and are ineffective against gram-negative bacteria. This narrow spectrum of activity has largely restricted their use to penicillinase-producing strains of *Staphylococcus*. Because they are often the drugs of first choice for infections by this organism, they are referred to as antistaphylococcal penicillins.

The emergence of many methicillin-resistant *S. aureus* (MRSA) strains has limited the use of this class of drugs. As discussed in Chapter 47, the appearance of MRSA strains that are resistant to all penicillins is an emerging clinical problem. The first drug developed in the penicillinase-resistant class, called methicillin, was removed from the United States market for producing an unacceptable incidence of interstitial nephritis.

Drugs in the penicillinase-resistant class share similar actions and properties with penicillin G. They are only administered by the PO route, where they are readily absorbed, especially on an empty stomach. They are rapidly excreted by the kidneys, having a half-life of 30 to 60 minutes. As with all penicillins, hypersensitivity reactions may occur. Some of these agents are sodium salts, which may cause sodium overload in susceptible patients. Pseudomembranous colitis has been reported in a small number of patients taking these drugs. All are pregnancy category B drugs.

Cloxacillin (Cloxapen): Approved in 1965, cloxacillin is a penicillinase-resistant penicillin available by the PO route. It is used to treat various infections caused by penicillinase-producing *Staphylococcus* but is not effective against MRSA. It has the same indications and adverse effects as other drugs in its class. This drug should not be given to a patient with hypersensitivity to any penicillin.

Dicloxacillin: Approved in 1968, dicloxacillin is a penicillinase-resistant penicillin available by the PO route. As with other drugs in this class, its use is primarily limited to the treatment of susceptible staphylococcal infections. It is not effective against MRSA. It exhibits more reliable GI absorption than nafcillin, but nausea and vomiting are commonly reported adverse effects. It should be taken on an empty stomach to enhance absorption. Dicloxacillin can reach two times the serum blood concentration as cloxacillin. Other adverse effects and contraindications are the same as those of other penicillins. This drug should not be given to a patient with hypersensitivity to any penicillin.

Nafcillin: Approved in 1964, nafcillin is used to treat susceptible infections of the blood, skin, upper and lower respiratory

CONNECTIONS

Lifespan Considerations

Infections in the Older Adult

Infections in older adults are often more severe than those experienced by younger individuals. Scientists believe that one cause of this increased susceptibility is a condition known as immune senescence. Normally, the neutrophil forms the first line of defense against rapidly dividing bacteria. However, as humans age, they become more susceptible to infection due to a decrease of neutrophil function. This produces a reduced response to infectious agents and allows latent infections such as tuberculosis, Epstein-Barr virus, and herpes zoster to become reactivated as one ages. Antibody production also declines with age and may be partially responsible for the high incidence and mortality associated with pneumonia and influenza in older adults.

tract, bone and joints, and urinary tract. It is ineffective against MRSA infections. Unlike most penicillins, nafcillin undergoes enterohepatic circulation and is excreted primarily in the bile: thus dosage adjustments for patients with hepatic disease are necessary. It is available in both oral and parenteral formulations. Because only 10% to 20% of the drug is absorbed when given PO, it should be taken on an empty stomach. The complete blood count (CBC) must be regularly monitored because nafcillin can cause neutropenia and other blood abnormalities in 10% to 20% of the patients taking it. This drug should not be given to a patient with hypersensitivity to any penicillin.

Oxacillin: Approved in 1962, oxacillin is used to treat a variety of staphylococcal infections of the blood, skin, upper and lower respiratory tract, bone and joints, and urinary tract. It is ineffective against MRSA infections. Because oxacillin causes fewer injection-site reactions than nafcillin, it is sometimes the parenteral agent of choice in its class. It is also available by the PO route, but absorption is poor and it should be taken on an empty stomach. Indications and adverse effects are similar to those of other penicillinase-resistant penicillins. This drug should not be given to a patient with hypersensitivity to any penicillin.

Cephalosporins

48.3 The cephalosporins are similar in structure and function to the penicillins and are widely prescribed for gram-negative infections.

Isolated shortly after penicillin, the cephalosporins comprise the largest antibiotic class. Like the penicillins, many cephalosporins contain a beta-lactam ring that is responsible for their antimicrobial activity. In some cephalosporins, the structure of the beta-lactam ring is quite stable and resistant to enzyme destruction. The cephalosporins are bacteriocidal and inhibit cell wall synthesis by binding to PBPs. Growing bacterial cells are unable to build their cell walls properly, and lysis occurs in the same manner as penicillins. The cephalosporins are listed in Table 48.2.

The primary therapeutic use of the cephalosporins is for gram-negative infections and for patients who are allergic to penicillin or who have penicillin-resistant infections. Over 20 cephalosporins are available, all having similar sounding names that can challenge even the best memory. Selection of a specific cephalosporin is first based on the sensitivity of the pathogen, and secondly on possible adverse effects.

The cephalosporins are classified chronologically by their generations, which are loosely based on differences in their spectrums of microbial activity. Table 48.2 shows the four generations of drugs in this class. It is important to note that the placement of a drug in a particular generation is somewhat arbitrary and has little therapeutic usefulness. Drugs within each generation have different chemical structures, routes of administration, and spectrums of activity. Scientists do not always agree on placement. The following generalizations may be made regarding the generations:

- First-generation cephalosporins contain a beta-lactam ring; bacteria-producing beta lactamase are usually resistant to these drugs. They are the most effective cephalosporins against gram-positive bacteria, including *Staphylococci* and *Streptococci* and are sometimes the drugs of choice for these organisms. First-generation cephalosporins have only moderate activity against gram-negative bacteria. First-generation drugs do not cross the blood–brain barrier to any appreciable extent.
- Second-generation cephalosporins exhibit a broader spectrum against gram-negative organisms than do the first-generation agents. They are more potent and less sensitive to beta lactamase than the first-generation drugs. Like the first-generation agents, however, they are unable to enter the CSF in sufficient concentration to treat infections of the CNS. In general, the second-generation agents have largely been replaced by third-generation cephalosporins.
- Third-generation cephalosporins exhibit an even broader spectrum against gram-negative bacteria than the second-generation agents. They generally have a longer duration of action and are resistant to beta lactamase. These cephalosporins are sometimes the drugs of choice against infections by *Pseudomonas, Klebsiella, Neisseria, Salmonella, Proteus,* and *H. influenzae.* Third-generation drugs are able to enter the CSF to treat CNS infections.
- Fourth-generation cephalosporins have a similar antimicrobial spectrum to third-generation agents but are more effective against organisms that have developed resistance to earlier cephalosporins. Fourth-generation drugs are capable of entering the CSF in sufficiently high concentrations to treat CNS infections.

CONNECTION *Checkpoint* 48.2

From what you learned in Chapter 47, what is the primary difference in physiology that distinguishes a gram-positive organism from a gram-negative organism? See Answer to Connection Checkpoint 48.2 in Appendix A.

TABLE 48.2 Cephalosporins

Drug	Route and Adult Dose (maximum dose where indicated)	Adverse Effects
First Generation		
cefadroxil (Duricef)	PO: 500 mg–1 g once or twice a day (max: 2 g/day)	*Diarrhea, abdominal cramping, nausea, fatigue, rash, pruritus, pain at injection sites, oral or vaginal candidiasis* Pseudomembranous colitis, nephrotoxicity, anaphylaxis
cefazolin (Ancef, Kefzol)	IM: 250 mg–2 g tid (max: 12 g/day)	
cephalexin (Keflex)	PO: 250–500 mg qid (max: 4 g/day)	
cephradine (Velosef)	PO: 250–500 mg every 6 h or 500 mg–1 g every 12 h (max: 4 g/day)	
Second Generation		
cefaclor (Ceclor)	PO: 250–500 mg tid (max: 2 g/day)	
cefotetan (Cefotan)	IV/IM: 1–2 g every 12 h (max: 6 g/day)	
cefoxitin (Mefoxin)	IV/IM: 1–2 g every 6–8 h (max: 12 g/day)	
cefprozil (Cefzil)	PO: 250–500 mg 1–2 times/day (max: 1 g/day)	
cefuroxime (Ceftin, Zinacef)	PO: 250–500 mg bid (max: 1 g/day) IM/IV: 750 mg–1.5 g every 8 h (max: 9 g/day)	
Third Generation		
cefdinir (Omnicef)	PO: 300 mg bid (max: 600 mg/day)	
cefditoren (Spectracef)	PO: 400 mg bid for 10 days (max: 800 mg/day)	
cefixime (Suprax)	PO: 400 mg/day or 200 mg bid (max: 800 mg/day)	
cefoperazone (Cefobid)	IV/IM: 1–2 g every 12 h; 16 g/day in two to four divided doses (max: 12 g/day)	
cefotaxime (Claforan)	IM: 1–2 g bid-tid (max: 12 g/day)	
cefpodoxime (Vantin)	PO: 200 mg every 12 h for 10 days (max: 800 mg/day)	
ceftazidime (Fortaz, Tazicef)	IV/IM: 1–2 mg every 8–12 h (max: 6 g/day)	
ceftibuten (Cedax)	PO: 400 mg/day for 10 days (max: 400 mg/day)	
ceftizoxime (Cefizox)	IV/IM: 1–2 g every 8–12 h, up to 2 g every 4 h (max: 12 g/day)	
ceftriaxone (Rocephin)	IV/IM: 1–2 g every 12–24 h (max: 4 g/day)	
Fourth Generation		
cefepime (Maxipime)	IV/IM: 0.5–1 g every 12 h for 7–10 days (max: 6 g/day)	

Note: *Italics* indicate common adverse effects. Underline indicates serious adverse effects.

Over decades of use, many bacterial strains have developed resistance to the cephalosporins. Like the penicillins, the primary mechanism of resistance is the secretion of beta-lactamase enzymes (sometimes called cephalosporinases). Although third-generation agents were initially unaffected by beta lactamase, resistant strains that can inactivate drugs in this generation have been identified. None of the cephalosporins has significant activity against MRSA or penicillin-resistant *Streptococcus pneumoniae.*

In general, the cephalosporins are safe drugs with adverse effects similar to those of the penicillins. Allergic reactions are the most common adverse effect. Although sometimes prescribed for patients who are allergic to penicillin, nurses must be aware that 5% to 10% of the patients who are allergic to penicillin will also exhibit hypersensitivity to cephalosporins. Despite this small incidence of cross-allergy, the cephalosporins offer a reasonable alternative for patients who are unable to take penicillin. Cephalosporins are contraindicated, however, for patients who have experienced anaphylaxis following penicillin exposure.

In addition to allergy, rash, and GI complaints are common adverse effects of cephalosporins. Nurses should continually assess for the presence of superinfections. Because cephalosporins are secreted in small amounts in breast milk, they should be used with caution in nursing mothers.

All cephalosporins, except cefoperazone and ceftriaxone, are eliminated by the kidneys. Earlier-generation cephalosporins exhibited kidney toxicity but this is diminished with the later-generation drugs in this class. Patients with preexisting renal impairment or those who are concurrently receiving nephrotoxic drugs should be monitored carefully during therapy with any cephalosporin. Kidney function tests should be evaluated on a regular basis.

Other adverse effects are specific to particular cephalosporins. For example, cefoperazone and cefotetan interfere with vitamin K metabolism and increase the risk of bleeding due to hypoprothrombinemia. Nurses must carefully monitor prothrombin time (PT) in patients taking these drugs, particularly those who are concurrently taking anticoagulants. Cefoperazone and cefotetan produce a disulfiram-like reaction when taken concurrently with alcohol. Cephalosporins cause pain at IM injection sites, and thrombophlebitis can occur when given IV. Over half of the cephalosporins are only administered parenterally.

PROTOTYPE DRUG Cefazolin sodium (Ancef, Kefzol)

Classification: **Therapeutic:** Antibacterial
Pharmacologic: Cell wall inhibitor: first-generation cephalosporin

Therapeutic Effects and Uses: Approved in 1973, cefazolin is a beta-lactam antibiotic used for the treatment and prophylaxis of bacterial infections, particularly those that are caused by susceptible gram-positive organisms. Its effectiveness extends to nonpencillinase- and penicillinase-producing *S. aureus* and *Streptococci* (except *Enterococci*). Cefazolin is not effective against MRSA. Cefazolin has been used to treat infections of the respiratory tract, urinary tract, skin structures, biliary tract, bones, and joints. It has also been useful in the pharmacotherapy of genital infections, septicemia, and endocarditis. This drug is sometimes used for infection prophylaxis in patients who are undergoing surgical procedures. Cefazolin has a longer half-life than other first-generation cephalosporins, which allows for less frequent dosing. It is one of the most frequently prescribed parenteral antibiotics.

Mechanism of Action: Cefazolin inhibits bacterial wall synthesis by binding to specific PBPs. The drug is bacteriocidal, exhibits a broad spectrum, and is sensitive to beta lactamase.

Pharmacokinetics:

Route(s)	IM and IV
Absorption	Well absorbed when given IM
Distribution	Widely distributed; only small amounts cross the blood–brain barrier; crosses the placenta; secreted in breast milk; about 85% bound to plasma protein
Primary metabolism	Not metabolized
Primary excretion	Renal
Onset of action	Immediate
Duration of action	Half-life: 90–135 minutes

Adverse Effects: Like the penicillins, the cephalosporins are well tolerated by most patients. Rash and diarrhea are the most common adverse effects, and superinfections are likely when the antibiotic is used for prolonged periods. Approximately 1% to 4% of patients will experience some kind of an allergic reaction. Severe hypersensitivity reactions are rare, though potentially fatal. Anaphylactic response may include cardiovascular collapse; edema of the mouth, tongue, pharynx, and larynx; confusion; seizures; and hallucinations. Pain and phlebitis can occur at IM injection sites. However, cefazolin causes less pain than do other cephalosporins. Seizures are a rare, though potentially serious, adverse effect of cephalosporin therapy.

Contraindications/Precautions: Cefazolin is contraindicated in patients who are allergic to any drug in the cephalosporin class and is used cautiously in those with hypersensitivity to penicillins. Because most cefazolin is excreted unchanged by the kidneys, patients with significant renal impairment must be carefully monitored.

Drug Interactions: Probenecid decreases the excretion of cefazolin and can lead to antibiotic toxicity. Concurrent use of cefazolin with nephrotoxic drugs, such as aminoglycosides or vancomycin, increases the risk of nephrotoxicity. Cefazolin may have additive or synergistic antimicrobial action with other antibiotics such as aztreonam, carbapenems, and the penicillins. The anticoagulant effect of warfarin may be increased if given concurrently with cefazolin. **Herbal/Food:** None known.

Pregnancy: Category B.

Treatment of Overdose: No specific therapy is available. Patients are treated symptomatically.

Nursing Responsibilities (includes all generations of cephalosporins):

- Obtain an accurate history from the patient prior to drug administration, including exposure, sensitivity or allergies, and any known reaction to penicillin and cephalosporins.
- Perform an infection-focused physical examination, including vital signs and a WBC count. Determine baseline signs and symptoms, indicating the presence of infection.
- Monitor the patient closely during the first 30 minutes of IV therapy for hypersensitivity and anaphylactoid reaction.
- Obtain and assess C&S testing prior to therapy. Evaluate serum creatinine, creatinine clearance, and blood urea nitrogen (BUN) during and after drug therapy is discontinued. Monitor hepatic and hematologic functions, including PT, international normalized ratio (INR), and partial thromboplastin time (PTT), in prolonged or high-dose therapy.
- Monitor intake and output ratios and patterns and report changes in patients with impaired renal function, chronic UTIs, or when receiving high dosages or an aminoglycoside concomitantly.
- Monitor for any signs or symptoms of superinfections, including vaginal yeast infection or oral fungal infections.
- Report any evidence of bleeding, including ecchymoses, petechiae, bleeding gums, and nosebleeds. Bleeding abnormalities such as thrombocytopenia are more likely to occur in patients with impaired kidney function.
- Assess the IV sites for thrombophlebitis throughout the infusion therapy.

- Inject IM medications deeply into muscle mass and rotate injection sites.
- Report any onset of diarrhea to the prescriber. If diarrhea is mild, discontinuation may be sufficient. If diarrhea is severe, suspect antibiotic-associated pseudomembranous colitis, which is a life-threatening superinfection that may occur in 4 to 9 days or as long as 6 weeks after cephalosporin therapy is discontinued. Most at risk are chronically ill or debilitated older adult patients who are undergoing abdominal surgery, or those in an intensive care unit.

Patient and Family Education:

- Consult the health care provider or pharmacist before drinking alcoholic beverages. For some cephalosporins, this can cause a disulfiram-like reaction with symptoms that include flushing, throbbing in the head and neck, respiratory difficulty, nausea, vomiting, sweating, thirst, chest pain, blurred vision, and confusion.
- Report any signs of a secondary infection (such as vaginal yeast infection or sore mouth) that may occur during therapy to the health care provider.
- Immediately report severe or persistent diarrhea accompanied by fever to the health care provider. Do not attempt to treat penicillin-related diarrhea with OTC products.
- Report any abnormal bleeding or bruising or signs of allergy such as rash or itching to the health care provider.
- Notify the health care provider if the infection does not begin to improve after a few days of therapy.

Drugs Similar to Cefazolin Sodium (Ancef, Kefzol)

First generation: Other first-generation cephalosporins include cefadroxil (Duricef), cephalexin (Keflex), and cephradine (Velosef). All three are administered parenterally and have the same spectrum of microbial activity. All have the same basic indications (primarily gram-positive bacteria) and are eliminated by the kidneys.

Second generation: Second-generation cephalosporins include cefaclor (Ceclor), cefotetan (Cefotan), cefoxitin (Mefoxin), cefprozil (Cefzil), and cefuroxime (Ceftin, Zinacef). All have the same spectrum of microbial activity and there is little difference among the drugs other than the route of administration (see Table 48.2). The kidneys eliminate all second-generation cephalosporins. Cefoxitin and cefotetan are the most active against *Bacteroides fragilis.*

Third generation: Third-generation cephalosporins are the largest group and include cefdinir (Omnicef), cefditoren (Spectracef), cefixime (Suprax), cefoperazone (Cefobid), cefotaxime (Claforan), cefpodoxime (Vantin), ceftazidime (Fortaz, Tazicef), ceftibuten (Cedax), ceftizoxime (Cefizox), and ceftriaxone (Rocephin). The differences among third-generation cephalosporins are minor. Some are available by the PO route, whereas others are given only parenterally (see Table 48.2). Cefixime and ceftriaxone have longer durations that allow for once-daily dosing. Ceftazidime and cefoperazone are the only third-generation drugs with significant activity against *P. aeruginosa.* Cefotaxime (Claforan) is a drug of choice for certain types of meningitis and for infection prophylaxis in patients who are undergoing surgical procedures.

Fourth generation: Cefepime (Maxipime) is the only drug in this generation. It is very similar to the third-generation drugs but appears to have a slightly broader spectrum of activity and is more stable against beta-lactamase-producing organisms. It has been used for the treatment of serious infections in hospitalized patients with gram-positive microorganisms such as *Enterobacteriaceae,* and *Pseudomonas.* It is not effective against MRSA.

Carbapenems

48.4 The carbapenems are resistant to beta lactamase and are broad-spectrum alternatives to penicillin.

Although the penicillins and cephalosporins comprise the largest groups of drugs affecting the bacterial cell wall, several

CONNECTIONS

Complementary and Alternative Therapies Aromatherapy

Description: Aromatherapy is the use of scents to promote healing.

History and Claims: Aromatherapy has existed for 5,000 years and treats various illnesses by administering volatile plant liquids known as essential oils. Proponents of aromatherapy claim that such substances as calendula, geranium, rosemary, tea tree, lavender, eucalyptus, thyme, and bergamot may strengthen the immune system. Many aromas are said to produce a calming effect. A common aroma used to treat upper respiratory congestion is Vicks VapoRub, which is a mixture of camphor, menthol, and eucalyptus oil. In France some essential oils are regulated as prescription drugs, and in many countries they are considered valid treatments.

Standardization: Essential oils are largely unstandardized. Although they may be obtained from an herb or plant, the chemical responsible for the aroma may be manufactured in a laboratory, as are perfumes. Although natural oils are more expensive, it is difficult and often impossible to tell the difference between a natural and a synthetic aroma.

Evidence: Scientific, controlled studies providing evidence for the healing properties of aromatherapy are lacking. At best, evidence is subjective and based on people "liking" the therapy or "feeling better" when using aromatherapy. Some evidence suggests that aromatherapy can have an antianxiety effect. Aromatherapy is harmless so long as patients do not have false beliefs about its healing powers.

Source: From *Complementary and Alternative Therapies for Nursing Practice* (2nd ed., pp. 28–35), by K. L. Fontaine, 2005, Upper Saddle River, NJ: Prentice-Hall Health; *Aromatherapy and Pain,* by L. Vignaroli, 2007, Creighton University School of Medicine. Retrieved July 25, 2008, from http://altmed.creighton.edu/Aromatherapy/

NURSING PROCESS APPLICATION

Patients Receiving Penicillins or Cephalosporins

Assessment	Potential Nursing Diagnoses
Prior to administration: • Obtain a complete health history, including allergies, drug history, and possible drug interactions. • Obtain specimens for C&S testing before initiating therapy. • Perform infection-focused physical examination, including vital signs and WBC count.	• *Risk for Infection* • *Risk for Injury*, related to adverse effects of drug • *Deficient Knowledge (Antibiotic Therapy)*, related to disease process, transmission, and drug therapy • *Noncompliance (Therapeutic Regimen)*, related to complexity

Planning: Patient Goals and Expected Outcomes

The patient will:

- Report reductions in symptoms related to the diagnosed infection and have negative results from laboratory and diagnostic tests for the presenting infection.
- Demonstrate an understanding of the drug's action by accurately describing drug adverse effects and precautions.
- Immediately report significant adverse effects such as shortness of breath, swelling, fever, stomatitis, loose stools, vaginal discharge, or cough.
- Complete the full course of antibiotic therapy and comply with follow-up care.

Implementation

Interventions and (Rationales)	Patient and Family Education
• Monitor vital signs and symptoms of infection to determine antibacterial effectiveness. (Another drug or different dosage may be required.)	• Instruct the patient to notify the health care provider if symptoms persist or worsen.
• Monitor for hypersensitivity reaction. (Immediate hypersensitivity reaction may occur within 2 to 30 minutes, accelerated occurs in 1 to 72 hours; and delayed after 72 hours.)	• Instruct the patient to discontinue the medication and inform the health care provider if symptoms of hypersensitivity reaction develop, such as wheezing; shortness of breath; swelling of face, tongue or hands; and itching or rash.
• Inspect the skin daily for the appearance of rash. Report the presence of rash promptly to the prescriber. (The incidence of ampicillin rash is higher in patients with infectious mononucleosis or other viral infections.)	• Instruct the patient to inspect the skin daily and immediately report the presence of rash to the prescriber.
• Monitor for unexplained bleeding such as epistaxis, purpura, or ecchymoses. Report it to the prescriber. (Some forms of penicillin [mezlocillin] may predispose the patient to thrombocytopenia, particularly if the patient has preexisting renal disease.)	• Instruct the patient to report any unusual bleeding including bleeding from the teeth or gums, or bruising, or unusual bleeding to the prescriber.
• Monitor for severe diarrhea. (This may occur due to superinfection or antibiotic-associated pseudomembranous colitis.)	Instruct the patient to: • Consult the health care provider before taking antidiarrheal drugs because they could cause retention of harmful bacteria. • Consume cultured dairy products with live active cultures, such as kefir, yogurt, or buttermilk, to maintain normal intestinal flora.
• Administer the drug around the clock. (This maintains consistent blood levels of the drug.)	Instruct the patient to: • Take the medication on schedule. • Complete the entire prescription even if he or she is feeling better to prevent the development of resistant bacteria.
• Monitor for superinfection, especially in elderly, debilitated, or immunosuppressed patients. (There is an increased risk for superinfections due to elimination of normal flora.)	• Instruct the patient to report signs and symptoms of superinfection such as fever; black hairy tongue; stomatitis; loose, foul-smelling stools; vaginal discharge; or cough.
• Monitor intake of OTC products such as antacids, calcium supplements, iron products, and laxatives that contain magnesium. (These products interfere with absorption of many antibiotics.)	• Instruct the patient to consult with the health care provider before using OTC medications or herbal products.
• Determine the effect of the prescribed antibiotics on oral contraceptives. (Both penicillins and cephalosporins may reduce the effectiveness of oral contraceptives.)	• Instruct the patient to use an alternate form of birth control while on the antibiotc. Consult the health care provider to determine when to reestablish oral contraceptives.
• Determine the interactions of the prescribed antibiotics with various foods and beverages. (Avoid acidic fruit juices or other acidic beverages within 1 hour of taking penicillin G because this may inactivate the medicine. Some cephalosporins, such as cefamandole, cefoperazone, and cefotetan, cause adverse reactions when taken with alcohol. This disulfiram-like reaction includes flushing, throbbing in the head and neck, respiratory difficulty, nausea, vomiting, sweating, thirst, chest pain, blurred vision, and confusion. This reaction usually begins within 15 to 30 minutes after alcohol is consumed and may last several days after the completion of the antibiotic.)	Instruct the patient to: • Not take penicillins with acidic fruit juices. • Not take alcoholic beverages or alcohol-containing medicine with cephalosporins.
• Monitor the IV site for signs and symptoms of tissue irritation, and extravasation. (Extravasation can cause severe pain.)	• Instruct the patient to report pain or other symptoms of discomfort immediately during IV infusion.
• Implement infection control measures (This prevents cross contamination of infection to other individuals.)	Instruct the patient in infectious control measures: • Avoid sharing contaminated items with others. • Perform frequent hand washing.

(continued)

NURSING PROCESS APPLICATION *(continued)*

• Monitor for adverse effects specific to various antibiotic therapies. (See the specific "adverse effects" for each prototype drug in this chapter.)	• Instruct the patient to report adverse effects specific to the antibiotic therapy prescribed.
• Monitor renal function such as intake and output ratios and urine color and consistency. Monitor laboratory work, including serum creatinine and blood urea nitrogen (BUN). (Penicillins and cephalosporins are eliminated via the renal route.)	• Explain the purpose of required laboratory tests and scheduled follow-up with the health care provider. • Instruct the patient to increase fluid intake to 2,000 to 3,000 mL/day.
• Monitor the patient for adherence with antibiotic therapy. (Stopping therapy early can diminish the success of pharmacotherapy.)	Instruct the patient on the importance of: • Completing the prescription as ordered. • Follow-up care after antibiotic therapy is completed.

Evaluation of Outcome Criteria

Evaluate the effectiveness of drug therapy by confirming that patient goals and expected outcomes have been met (see "Planning").

other antibacterials also act by this mechanism. Doses of these agents are listed in Table 48.3.

Imipenem (Primaxin), ertapenem (Invanz), doripenem (Doribax), and meropenem (Merrem IV) belong to a relatively new class of antibiotics called carbapenems. These drugs are bacteriocidal and have some of the broadest antimicrobial spectrums of any class of antibiotics. They contain a beta-lactam ring and kill bacteria by inhibiting construction of the cell wall. Though similar, the ring in carbapenems has a slightly different structure than other beta-lactam antibiotics that makes it very resistant to destruction by beta lactamase. A disadvantage is that they can only be given parenterally.

All the carbapenems exhibit a low incidence of adverse effects. Diarrhea, nausea, rashes, and thrombophlebitis at injection sites are the most common adverse effects.

PROTOTYPE DRUG Imipenem-cilastatin (Primaxin)

Classification: **Therapeutic:** Antibacterial
Pharmacologic: Cell wall inhibitor, carbapenem

Therapeutic Effects and Uses: Approved in 1985, imipenem is used for the treatment and prophylaxis of susceptible bacterial infections. Of the carbapenems, imipenem has the broadest antimicrobial spectrum and is the most widely used. Because of its broad spectrum and beta-lactamase resistance, it is effective against most gram-positive and gram-negative microbes, including anaerobic bacteria. It is particularly useful for mixed infections containing both aerobic and anaerobic organisms, including those with *S. aureus*. *P. aeruginosa* and strains of MRSA are also susceptible to imipenem.

TABLE 48.3 Carbapenems and Miscellaneous Cell Wall Inhibitors

Drug	Route and Adult Dose (maximum dose where indicated)	Adverse Effects
Carbapenems		
doripenem (Doribax)	IV: 500 mg every 8 h for 5–14 days (max: 500 mg every 8 h)	*Nausea, diarrhea, headache* <u>Anaphylaxis, superinfections, pseudomembranous colitis, confusion, seizures</u>
ertapenem (Invanz)	IV/IM: 1 g/day	
imipenem-cilastatin (Primaxin)	IV: 250–500 mg tid-qid (max: 4 g/day)	
meropenem (Merrem)	IV: 1–2 g tid (max: 2 g tid)	
Miscellaneous Cell Wall Inhibitors		
aztreonam (Azactam)	IM: 0.5–2 g bid-qid (max: 8 g/day)	*Nausea, vomiting, diarrhea, rash, fever, insomnia, injection site reaction* <u>Anaphylaxis, superinfections</u>
fosfomycin (Monurol)	PO: 3 g sachet dissolved in 3–4 oz of water as a single dose	*Nausea, diarrhea, back pain, headache* <u>Anaphylaxis, superinfections</u>
vancomycin (Vancocin)	IV: 500 mg qid; 1 g bid	*Nausea, vomiting* <u>Anaphylaxis, superinfections, nephrotoxicity, ototoxicity, red man syndrome</u>

Note: *Italics* indicate common adverse effects. <u>Underline</u> indicates serious adverse effects.

Although imipenem contains a beta-lactam ring, it is resistant to the actions of beta lactamase. This drug, however, is rapidly destroyed by dipeptidase, an enzyme found in the kidney tubules. Concurrent administration of the drug cilastatin, a renal dipeptidase inhibitor, with imipenem prevents the destruction of imipenem and allows for higher serum levels of the antibiotic. Cilastatin possesses no antimicrobial activity of its own. Imipenem is only marketed with cilastatin in a fixed-dose combination (Primaxin).

Primaxin is sometimes combined with antibiotics from other classes, such as the aminoglycosides or cephalosporins, when treating *P. aeruginosa* infections. Primaxin has a short half-life that requires administration every 6 hours.

Mechanism of Action: Imipenem inhibits bacterial wall synthesis by binding to specific PBPs. Cilastatin blocks renal dipeptidase, which is the enzyme primarily responsible for the excretion of imipenem. The combination of imipenem-cilastatin is bacteriocidal.

Pharmacokinetics:

Route(s)	IM and IV
Absorption	Not absorbed PO
Distribution	Widely distributed, including in the CSF; secreted in breast milk; both imipenem and cilastatin cross the placenta
Primary metabolism	Hepatic
Primary excretion	Renal
Onset of action	IM: rapid; IV: immediate
Duration of action	Half-life: 1 h

Adverse Effects: The most frequent adverse effects of imipenem-cilastatin include nausea, vomiting, diarrhea, rash, and pain and phlebitis at the injection site. Rare, though serious, reactions include confusion, seizures, hallucinations, pseudomembranous colitis, and anaphylaxis. Anaphylactic response may include cardiovascular collapse and edema of the mouth, tongue, pharynx, and larynx.

Contraindications/Precautions: Imipenem-cilastatin is contraindicated in patients who have experienced a severe allergic reaction to this drug, other carbapenems, cephalosporins, or penicillins. Because the kidneys excrete imipenem-cilastatin, patients with significant renal impairment must be carefully monitored and dosages lowered. This drug should be used cautiously in patients with brain lesions, head trauma, or a history of seizures due to an increased risk of seizures.

Drug Interactions: Certain other antibiotics, including penicillins, cephalosporins, and aztreonam antagonize the antimicrobial effects of imipenem-cilastatin; therefore, they should not be given concurrently. Concurrent use with cyclosporine, tramadol, theophylline, or ganciclovir may increase the risk of seizures and other CNS effects. **Herbal/Food:** None known.

Pregnancy: Category C.

Treatment of Overdose: Overdose may result in ataxia and seizures. Patients are treated symptomatically.

Nursing Responsibilities:

- Perform an infection-focused physical examination, including vital signs and a WBC count. Determine baseline signs and symptoms, indicating the presence of infection.
- Assess for previous hypersensitivity to other carbapenems or beta-lactam antibiotics (penicillins and cephalosporins).
- Monitor for signs and symptoms of hypersensitivity. Discontinue this drug and immediately notify the prescriber if symptoms occur.
- Notify the prescriber to adjust the dosage if focal tremors, myoclonus, or seizures occur.
- Assess for any symptoms of superinfections.
- Notify the prescriber promptly of severe diarrhea with fever because this may indicate pseudomembranous colitis (an infection of the colon often caused by the bacterium *Clostridium difficile*).
- Determine the sodium content of this drug when used with patients on sodium restriction.
- Monitor renal, hepatic, and hematologic functions in prolonged or high-dose therapy.
- Do not interchange IM and IV solutions.
- Decrease the rate of IV infusion if nausea is present because this symptom is related to the infusion rate.

Patient and Family Education:

- Immediately report any intense itching, difficulty breathing, or other signs of allergic reaction to the health care provider.
- Report any signs of a secondary infection (such as vaginal yeast infection or sore mouth) that may occur during therapy to the health care provider.
- Report pain or discomfort at the IV infusion site to the health care provider.
- Immediately report severe or persistent diarrhea accompanied by fever to the health care provider. Do not attempt to treat penicillin-related diarrhea with OTC products.
- Immediately report confusion or seizures to the health care provider.
- Immediately notify the health care provider of any known or suspected pregnancy.
- Do not breast-feed while taking this drug without approval of the health care provider.

Drugs Similar to Imipenem-cilastatin (Primaxin)

Other carbapenems include doripenem, ertapenem, and meropenem.

Doripenem (Doribax): Doripenem (Doribax) is a newer drug in this class that was approved in 2007. It is similar to meropenem and has activity against both gram-positive and gram-negative organisms. It is approved to treat complicated intra-abdominal infections and UTIs. It is administered by IV infusion over 60 minutes. Common adverse effects include headache, rash, nausea, vomiting, diarrhea, and phlebitis. Doripenem is contraindicated in patients who have experienced a severe allergic reaction to other carbapenems, cephalosporins, or penicillins. This drug is pregnancy category B.

Ertapenem (Invanz): A newer drug in this class, ertapenem, has a narrower spectrum than the other carbapenems, being active primarily against gram-negative aerobes. Its major advantage is its longer half-life, which allows for once-daily dosing. It is approved for the treatment of serious abdominopelvic and skin infections, community-acquired pneumonia, complicated UTIs, and diabetic foot infections without concomitant osteomyelitis. It is administered by the IV and IM routes. Adverse effects are similar to those of other carbapenems. Ertapenem is contraindicated in patients who have experienced a severe allergic reaction to other carbapenems, cephalosporins, or penicillins. This drug is pregnancy category B.

Meropenem (Merrem): Approved in 1996, meropenem has a similar spectrum of activity to imipenem, although it is only approved for peritonitis and skin and skin structure infections in adults and bacterial meningitis in children. The drug is used off-label for other indications. The antimicrobial spectrum of activity of meropenem is similar to imipenem. Meropenem may be more active against *Enterobacteriaceae, Gonococcus, H. influenzae*, and *P. aeruginosa.* This drug is not destroyed by renal dipeptidase, so it is not administered with cilastatin. Adverse effects are similar to those of imipenem. Meropenem is contraindicated in patients who have experienced a severe allergic reaction to other carbapenems, cephalosporins, or penicillins. It is only available by the IV route. Bolus injections are given IV over 3 to 5 minutes, and infusions over 15 to 30 minutes. This drug is pregnancy category B.

Pharm*FACT*

About 70% of bacteria that cause HAIs are resistant to at least one of the drugs most commonly used to treat infections. Some organisms are resistant to all approved antibiotics and must be treated with experimental and potentially toxic drugs. *Source:* U.S. Food and Drug Administration, n.d.

Miscellaneous Cell Wall Inhibitors

48.5 Several miscellaneous cell wall inhibitors have activity against resistant microbes.

Several other cell wall inhibitors have important roles in the pharmacotherapy of infections. These agents are either new drugs or the only agent in a class.

PROTOTYPE DRUG Vancomycin HCl (Vancocin)

Classification: **Therapeutic:** Antibacterial
Pharmacologic: Cell wall inhibitor

Therapeutic Effects and Uses: Approved in 1964, vancomycin (Vancocin) is used for the treatment and prophylaxis of susceptible bacterial infections. It is effective against most gram-positive organisms, including *Streptococci, Corynebacteria, Clostridia, Listeria,* and *Bacillus* species. Vancomycin is usually administered by slow IV infusion for systemic infections because it is not well absorbed from the GI tract. It has been administered off-label by the intrathecal or intraventricular route to treat meningitis. Oral vancomycin (drinking the IV product) has been used off-label for the treatment of antibiotic-induced pseudomembranous colitis, which is caused by a toxin produced by *C. difficile.*

Current protocols restrict the use of vancomycin to severe infections that have become resistant to safer antibiotics. It is anticipated that this restriction will discourage or delay the appearance of resistant strains. Because vancomycin was used infrequently during the first 30 years following its discovery, the incidence of vancomycin-resistant organisms has been less than with other antibiotics. Vancomycin is the most effective drug for treating MRSA infections. Vancomycin-resistant strains of *S. aureus*, however, have begun to appear in recent years. Vancomycin is often considered the "last chance" antibiotic. Therapeutic options for vancomycin-resistant infections are limited.

Mechanism of Action: Although vancomycin kills bacteria mainly by inhibiting bacterial cell wall synthesis, it also affects the plasma membrane and interferes with ribonucleic acid (RNA) synthesis. The fact that it has multiple mechanisms is probably responsible for the low rate of resistance from the drug. It is bacteriocidal and only effective against gram-positive organisms such as *S. aureus* and *S. pneumoniae.*

Pharmacokinetics:

Route(s)	IV
Absorption	Poorly absorbed PO
Distribution	Widely distributed with small amounts in the CSF; secreted in breast milk; 55% bound to plasma proteins
Primary metabolism	Probably not metabolized
Primary excretion	Renal
Onset of action	IV: immediate
Duration of action	Half-life: 4–8 h

Adverse Effects: Vancomycin may cause a syndrome of flushing, hypotension, tachycardia, and rash on the upper body, a condition called the red man syndrome. This syndrome can be minimized by infusing the drug over at least 60 minutes. Other common adverse effects include nausea, rash, fever, and chills. Serious adverse effects include confusion, seizures, and hallucinations. If extravasation occurs, it may lead to tissue necrosis. Ototoxicity is associated with serum concentrations of vancomycin above 60 to 80 mcg/mL. Tinnitus and high-tone hearing loss precede deafness and may progress even after this drug is discontinued. The most susceptible are older adults and those on high doses. Nephrotoxicity can occur in patients with therapeutic concentrations but is more common if trough serum concentrations are kept above 10 mcg/mL. Anaphylactic response may include cardiovascular collapse or edema of the mouth, tongue, pharynx, and larynx.

Contraindications/Precautions: Vancomycin is contraindicated in patients who have experienced previous hypersensitivity to this drug. The nurse must monitor drug therapy carefully in patients with impaired renal function and those with a history of hearing loss.

Drug Interactions: Vancomycin adds to toxicity of aminoglycosides, amphotericin B, cisplatin, cyclosporine, polymyxin B, and other ototoxic and nephrotoxic medications. Vancomycin may increase the risk of lactic acidosis when administered with metformin, especially in patients with renal impairment. **Herbal/Food:** Unknown.

Pregnancy: Category C.

Treatment of Overdose: Overdose may result in renal impairment. Patients are treated supportively to maintain renal function.

Nursing Responsibilities:

- Perform an infection-focused physical examination, including vital signs and a WBC count. Determine baseline signs and symptoms, indicating the presence of infection.
- Monitor blood pressure and heart rate when administering this drug IV because rapid bolus administration is associated with exaggerated hypotension, including shock and cardiac arrest. Vancomycin should be administered over a period of not less than 60 minutes to avoid rapid infusion-related reactions.
- Monitor for symptoms of the red man syndrome, which include chills or fever; fainting; tachycardia; hives; itching; hypotension; nausea or vomiting; rash; or redness of the face, base of neck, upper body, back, and arms. Notify the prescriber if symptoms develop. Symptoms of the red man syndrome are more common when vancomycin is given by infusion.
- Monitor urinalysis and renal and hepatic functions, and perform hematologic studies.
- Monitor vancomycin blood levels (peak and trough) in patients with borderline kidney function, in infants and neonates, and in patients older than 60 years old. Peak levels are usually collected 1 hour after IV administration. Trough levels are collected 30 minutes before the next dose of the antibiotic.
- Assess baseline and periodic hearing function. This drug may cause damage to the auditory branch of the eighth cranial nerve with consequent deafness, which may be permanent.
- Monitor fluid balance and report changes in intake and output ratio and pattern. Note oliguria or cloudy or pink urine, which is a sign of nephrotoxicity (also manifested by transient elevations in BUN, albumin, and hyaline and granular casts in urine).

Patient and Family Education:

- Immediately report intense itching, difficulty breathing, or other signs of allergic reaction to the health care provider.
- Promptly report ringing in the ears or difficulty hearing to the health care provider.
- Report any signs of a secondary infection (such as vaginal yeast infection or sore mouth) that may occur during therapy to the health care provider.
- Complete the full course of the prescribed drug therapy.
- Notify the health care provider immediately of any known or suspected pregnancy.
- Do not breast-feed while taking this drug without prior approval of the health care provider.
- Maintain adequate fluid intake (2–3 L/day).

Drugs Similar to Vancomycin HCl (Vancocin)

Other miscellaneous cell wall inhibitors include aztreonam and fosfomycin.

Aztreonam (Azactam): Approved in 1986, aztreonam has a beta-lactam ring and belongs to a newer class of antibiotics known as monobactams. Like other cell wall inhibitors, aztreonam binds to specific penicillin-binding proteins to cause a bacteriocidal effect. Although considered narrow-spectrum antibiotics, monobactams are particularly useful against certain gram-negative aerobes, such as *P. aeruginosa.* Other organisms considered susceptible to aztreonam include *Citrobacter, Enterobacter, E. coli, H. influenzae, Neisseria, Proteus, Providencia rettgeri,* and *Shigella.* Monobactams have little or no activity against gram-positive bacteria or anaerobes. Although they have beta-lactam rings, they do not exhibit cross-hypersensitivity with penicillins or cephalosporins. Administered only by the parenteral route, aztreonam exhibits similar adverse effects as those of other cell wall inhibitors including nausea, vomiting, diarrhea, superinfections such as vaginal candidiasis, and local pain or phlebitis at the injection site. Anaphylaxis and pseudomembranous colitis are rare. This drug is pregnancy category B.

Fosfomycin (Monurol): Approved in 1996, fosfomycin is a newer cell wall inhibitor currently approved for the treatment of uncomplicated UTI and bladder infections in women caused by *E. coli* and *Enterococcus faecalis.* It is given as an oral powder, which is mixed with water and taken PO as a single dose. Adverse effects are minor and include asthenia, nausea, vomiting, diarrhea, headache, and vaginitis. This drug is pregnancy category B.

UNDERSTANDING THE CHAPTER

Key Concepts Summary

48.1 Bacterial cell walls consist of layers of carbohydrate and protein chains, which are constructed by enzymes called penicillin-binding proteins.

48.2 The penicillins, one of the oldest and safest groups of antibacterials, are primarily active against gram-positive bacteria.

48.3 The cephalosporins are similar in structure and function to the penicillins and are widely prescribed for gram-negative infections.

48.4 The carbapenems are resistant to beta lactamase and are broad-spectrum alternatives to penicillin.

48.5 Several miscellaneous cell wall inhibitors have activity against resistant microbes.

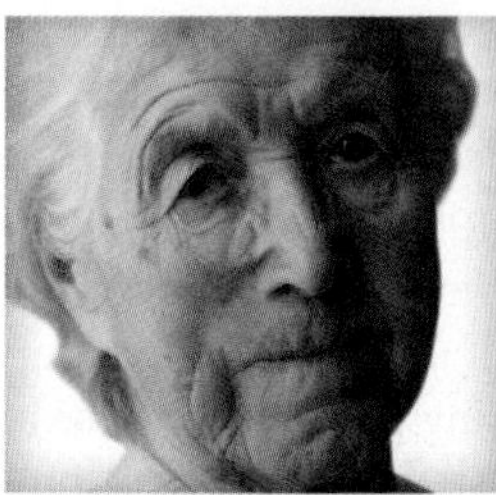

Making the PATIENT *Connection*

Remember the patient "Katie Dennison" at the beginning of the chapter? Now read the remainder of the case study. Based on the information presented within this chapter, respond to the critical thinking questions that follow.

Katie Dennison is an 83-year-old retired school teacher. She was recently seen by her health care provider for removal of a noncancerous skin lesion. Now she suspects that the wound on her arm has become infected. She has attempted to report this condition to her health care provider. However, due to the holidays she has been unable to reach him. Ms. Dennison presents to a local urgent care center for treatment.

The physical examination and diagnostic tests reveal the following findings. Vital signs are: temperature, 38°C (100.9°F); pulse, 110 beats/minute; respiratory rate 20/minute; and blood pressure, 108/68 mmHg. The large dressing on her left arm is saturated with dried yellow-green exudates. She states that it is painful to move her left arm and that the pain has limited her range of motion in the affected extremity. She is pale and has "paper thin" fragile skin.

Katie reports that she accidentally got the dressing wet while taking a shower. She did not change the dressing because she was not told to do so by her health care provider when the skin lesion was removed. A series of laboratory tests were completed. A sterile dressing was applied to the wound. Ms. Dennison was given an injection of cefazolin (Ancef) and a prescription for antibiotics. She was also instructed to follow up with her health care provider within the next 2 to 3 days.

Critical Thinking Questions

1. What factors possibly contributed to the wound infection in this patient?
2. What laboratory tests were probably obtained during this visit to the urgent care center?
3. What information should the nurse provide to the patient concerning the antibiotic?
4. Discuss the mechanism of action for cefazolin.

Case Study

Mrs. Murphy is 80 years old and lives in a retirement community for lower income elderly people. You are the community health nurse visiting with her. As part of your assessment, you ask Mrs. Murphy how she obtains her prescribed medications. The patient explains that most of the time, her neighbor will pick up prescriptions for her. She further explains that in some cases, however, she has "stockpiled" medicines she has been prescribed. When you investigate, you find that the patient has multiple bottles of various types of unused antibiotics. Some of the drugs were prescribed 5 or 6 years ago.

1. Describe how you should respond to this situation.
2. Identify the health teaching needs of this patient regarding "stockpiling" (saving) antibiotics.

NCLEX-RN® Review

1 The nurse should instruct a 21-year-old female client being treated with ampicillin (Principen):

1. To stop taking her oral contraceptives because serious adverse effects could occur.
2. To use oral contraceptives as prescribed because antibiotics do not react with birth control pills.
3. That the antibiotic may decrease the effectiveness of oral contraceptives.
4. That the antibiotic when taken with oral contraceptives causes toxicity.

2 The nurse is caring for a client who is receiving intravenous vancomycin (Vancocin). Which of the following symptoms, if present, may indicate that the client is experiencing drug-induced ototoxicity?

1. Erythema of the earlobes and ear canal
2. Inner ear pruritus after infusion is completed
3. Tinnitus and high-tone hearing loss
4. Ocular pain with purulent drainage

3 The client reports abnormal vaginal discharge after completing a prescription of cefotaxime (Claforan). The nurse recognizes that the client is most likely exhibiting symptoms of:

1. Hypersensitivity reaction.
2. Superinfection.
3. Pseudomembranous colitis.
4. Antibiotic toxicity.

4 The nurse is administering the combination anti-infective amoxicillin with clavulanate (Augmentin). The nurse knows that this combination:

1. Allows a greater amount of the drug to reach pathogens.
2. Prevents the cross contamination of microorganisms.
3. Averts allergic reactions in penicillin-sensitive individuals.
4. Promotes gastric absorption of the drug.

5 The client who is taking imipenem-cilastatin (Primaxin) reports shortness of breath, mouth and tongue swelling, and generalized itching. The nurse initially assesses the client for which of the following?

1. Hypersensitivity reaction
2. Blood dyscrasias
3. Beta-lactamase induction
4. Drug toxicity

6 The nurse is teaching a client who recently was diagnosed with an upper respiratory infection and is prescribed penicillin G (Pentids). The nurse would evaluate the session as being successful if the client states:

1. "I should avoid acidic beverages 1 to 2 hours before taking the medication."
2. "I can expect my tongue to become black and furry."
3. "Once I stop coughing, I should stop taking this medication."
4. "If I miss a dose, I should take two doses together to catch up."

See Answers to Critical Thinking Questions, Case Study, and NCLEX-RN® Review in Appendix A.

References

Centers for Disease Control and Prevention. (2007). *Get smart: Know when antibiotics work. Frequently asked questions.* Retrieved July 25, 2008, from http://www.cdc.gov/drugresistance/community/index.htm

Cleveland Clinic. (2008). *Otitis media.* Retrieved July 25, 2008, from http://www.clevelandclinic.org/health/health-info/docs/1900/1957.asp?index=8613&src=news

Coates, A. R. (2007). Novel approaches to developing new antibiotics for bacterial infections. *British Journal of Pharmacology, 152*(8), 1147–1154.

El-Shaboury, S. R., Saleh, G. A., Mohamed, F. A., & Rageh, A. H. (2007). Analysis of cephalosporin antibiotics. *Journal of Pharmaceutical and Biomedical Analysis, 45*(1), 1–19.

Fontaine, K. L. (2005). *Complementary and alternative therapies for nursing practice* (2nd ed.). Upper Saddle River, NJ: Prentice-Hall Health.

Glasziou P. P., Del Mar, C. B., Sanders, S. L., & Hayem, M. (2003). Antibiotics for acute otitis media in children. *The Cochrane Database of Systematic Reviews, 4.* (Art. No: CD000219.pub2.DOI:10.1002/14651858.CD000219.pub2.)

Goldrick, B. A. (2005). Emerging infections. Infections in older adults: Long term care poses particular risk. *American Journal of Nursing, 105*(6), 31–34.

Hogan, M. A. (2005). *Pharmacology reviews and rationales.* Upper Saddle River, NJ: Prentice-Hall Health.

Larson, E., & Grullon-Figueroa, L. (2004). Availability of antibiotics without prescription in New York City. *Journal of Urban Health: Bulletin of the New York Academy of Medicine, 81*(3), 498.

Nicolau, D. P. (2008). Carbapenems: A potent class of antibiotics. *Expert Opinion on Pharmacotherapy, 9*(1), 23–27.

Schweon, S., & Roman, L. M. (2006). Stamping out surgical site infections, *RN, 69*(8), 36–41.

Tacconelli, E., De Angelis, G., Cataldo, M. A., Pozzi, E., & Cauda, R. (2008). Does antibiotic exposure increase the risk of methicillin-resistant *Staphylococcus aureus* (MRSA) isolation? A systematic review and meta-analysis. *Journal of Antimicrobial Chemotherapy, 61*(1), 26–38.

Turkoski, B. B. (2005). Fighting infection: An ongoing challenge—antibacterials. *Orthopaedic Nursing, 24*(3), 210–223.

U.S. Food and Drug Administration. (n.d.). *Facts about antibiotic resistance.* Retrieved July 25, 2008, from http://www.fda.gov/oc/opacom/hottopics/antiresist_facts.html

Vignaroli, L. (2007). *Aromatherapy and pain.* Creighton University School of Medicine. Retrieved July 25, 2008, from http://altmed.creighton.edu/Aromatherapy/

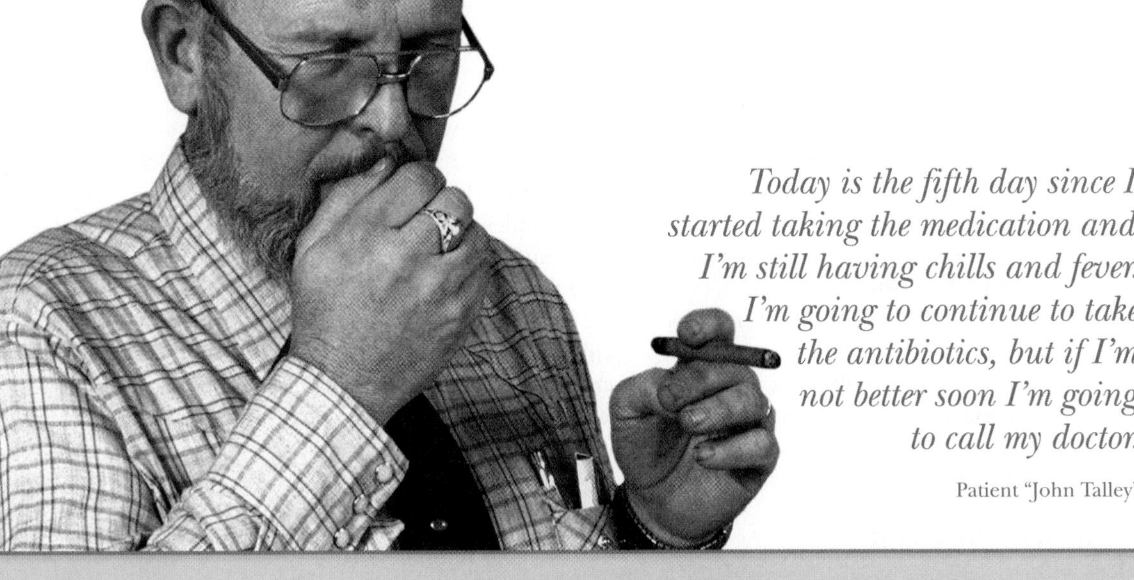

Today is the fifth day since I started taking the medication and I'm still having chills and fever. I'm going to continue to take the antibiotics, but if I'm not better soon I'm going to call my doctor.

Patient "John Talley"

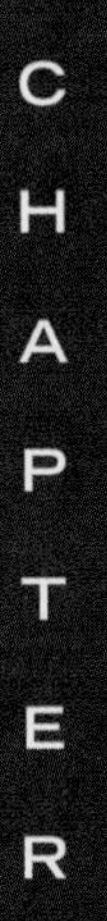

CHAPTER

Antibiotics Affecting Bacterial Protein Synthesis

49

Chapter Outline

Bacterial Protein Synthesis

Mechanisms of Antibiotic Inhibition of Bacterial Protein Synthesis

Tetracyclines

PROTOTYPE **Tetracycline (Sumycin, Others)** *p. 811*

Macrolides

PROTOTYPE **Erythromycin Base (E-Mycin, Others)** *p. 814*

Aminoglycosides

PROTOTYPE **Gentamicin (Garamycin)** *p. 817*

Miscellaneous Inhibitors of Bacterial Protein Synthesis

Learning Outcomes

After reading this chapter, the student should be able to:

1. Explain the steps in the synthesis of bacterial proteins.
2. Identify the classes of antibiotics that act by inhibiting bacterial protein synthesis.
3. Explain mechanisms by which antibiotics inhibit bacterial protein synthesis.
4. Explain how protein synthesis inhibitors exert selective toxicity toward bacterial, rather than human, cells.
5. Describe means by which bacteria become resistant to protein synthesis inhibitors.
6. For each of the classes shown in the chapter outline, identify the prototype and representative drugs and explain the mechanism(s) of drug action, primary indications, contraindications, significant drug interactions, pregnancy category, and important adverse effects.
7. Apply the nursing process to care for patients who are receiving drug therapy with bacterial protein synthesis inhibitors.

Key Terms

cholestatic hepatitis, 814
gray baby syndrome, 821
oxazolidinones, 822
postantibiotic effect, 817
pseudomembranous colitis, 811
streptogramin, 822
Svedberg unit, 809
transcription, 808

To maintain the extreme metabolic rate required for exponential reproduction, bacteria must synthesize huge amounts of protein. Antibacterial drugs that inhibit this high rate of protein metabolism can either kill the bacterial cell or slow its replication rate. Tetracyclines, macrolides, and a few miscellaneous drugs are bacteriostatic inhibitors of protein synthesis. The aminoglycosides are bacteriocidal inhibitors.

Bacterial Protein Synthesis

49.1 Antibiotics inhibit microbial protein synthesis by binding to the bacterial ribosome.

The importance of protein is illustrated by the fact that up to 50% of the dry weight of a bacterial cell consists of protein. Bacterial proteins serve many of the same functions as human proteins. For example, the bacterial enzymes required for all biochemical reactions are proteins. Proteins are studded in the plasma membrane and serve as channels, pores, or transporters, assisting substances as they move into and out of cells. Like human proteins, bacterial proteins are composed of long chains of amino acids.

Several types of proteins, however, are unique to bacteria. Bacterial cells produce protein toxins, which kill other bacteria and can cause serious disease to human cells. The sticky gel-like substance that allows bacterial cells to cling to human epithelial cells on the skin surface, in bronchi, in the gastrointestinal (GI) tract, or in the genitourinary tract is comprised of proteins combined with carbohydrates. The structure of the bacterial cell wall, which is discussed in Chapter 48, consists of peptidoglycan layers of protein and carbohydrates that protect the bacterium from its environment. From these examples, it is easy to understand why proteins are critical to bacterial cells.

An understanding of how proteins are synthesized by bacterial cells is important to understanding how antibiotics act. The basic steps in protein synthesis, or **transcription,** are the same in bacteria as they are in humans. Knowledge of transcription, which is illustrated in Figure 49.1, is necessary to understand the mechanisms of action of antibiotics that inhibit protein synthesis.

Protein synthesis occurs in the cytoplasm and requires the following three components:

- Messenger ribonucleic acid (mRNA)
- Transfer ribonucleic acid (tRNA)
- Ribosomes, which consist of one large and one small subunit

The mRNA carries the encoded message for making a protein from the deoxyribonucleic acid (DNA) to the ribosome, which serves as the site for protein construction. The strand of mRNA squeezes between the two ribosomal subunits and begins to move through the subunits. As it does, a tRNA molecule arrives, carrying the specific amino acid that was encoded in the mRNA strand. As the mRNA proceeds through the ribosome, subsequent amino acids are added one at a time to the growing protein chain. This growing chain is known as a polypeptide. Eventually, a "stop signal" is reached on the mRNA strand, which tells the ribosome that the last amino acid has been added and the protein is ready to be released. The protein may be active immediately, or it may be processed to its active form in the Golgi body. The finished protein may be used within the bacterial cell (enzymes) or be exported outside (toxins).

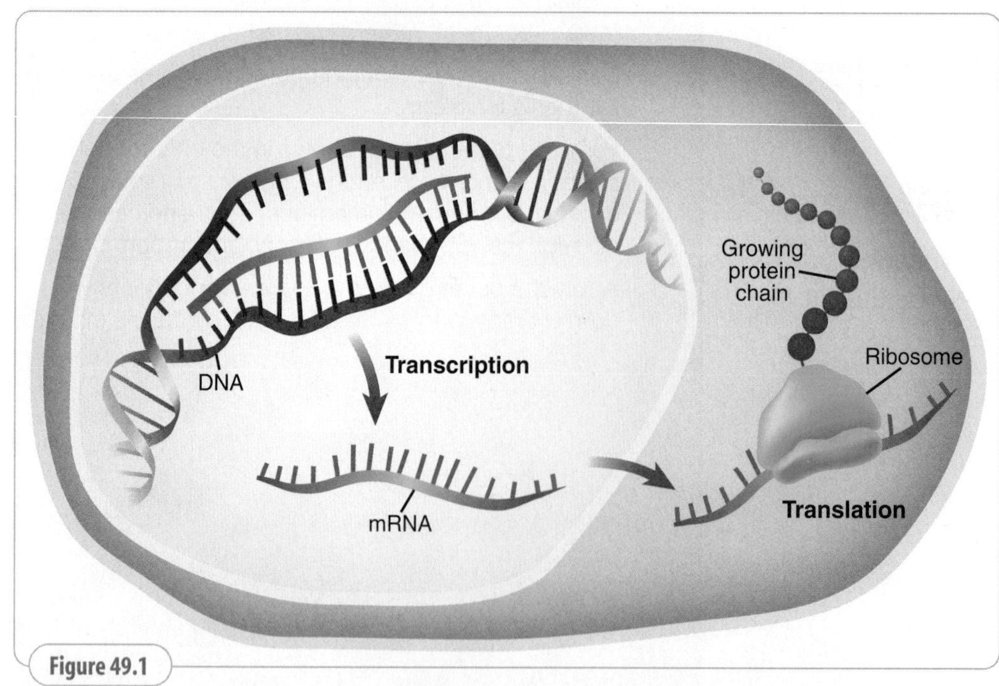

Figure 49.1

Steps in protein synthesis: the DNA is used as a template to make mRNA (transcription); the mRNA is sent to the ribosome to make the protein chain (translation).

All cells, including bacteria, are able to quickly increase protein synthesis to meet their growth demands or to respond to environmental challenges. For example, a bacterium may receive a message that other competitive bacteria are in the vicinity. The gene coding for a toxin or antibiotic may become active, producing large amounts of mRNA and eventually protein toxin, which serves as a defense against the invader.

If both humans and bacteria conduct continuous protein synthesis, why are antibiotics that inhibit protein synthesis not also toxic to human cells? The answer lies in differences in the structures of the bacterial and human ribosomes. Ribosomes are composed of two subunits, one of which is larger and less dense than the other. In bacteria, these ribosomal components are referred to as 30S and 50S subunits. The letter "S" is a unit of measurement, the **Svedberg unit,** which indicates its size or sedimentation rate in a high-speed centrifuge. The entire bacterial ribosome is called a 70S ribosome (Svedberg units are not additive). Antibiotics that inhibit protein synthesis do so by affecting subunits of the bacterial ribosome. Humans have ribosomes that are larger and denser than the 70S bacterial ribosome. The 80S human ribosome is mostly unaffected by antibiotics that bind to the bacterial 70S ribosome, thus providing a degree of "selective toxicity." Interestingly, human mitochondria do contain a 70S ribosome that is affected by several of these antibiotics, thus explaining some of the adverse effects of these drugs.

About 20 drugs that affect the synthesis of bacterial proteins have been discovered. The different steps at which antibiotics inhibit the production of bacterial proteins are shown in Figure 49.2.

Tetracyclines

49.2 Tetracyclines have broad antimicrobial activity against many gram-positive and gram-negative bacteria.

The first tetracyclines were extracted from *Streptomyces* in soil samples in 1948. Unfortunately, their widespread use in the 1950s and 1960s resulted in a large number of resistant strains that now limits the therapeutic usefulness of the drugs in this class.

The five tetracyclines are effective against a large number of aerobic and anaerobic gram-negative and gram-positive organisms: They have one of the broadest antimicrobial spectrums of any class of antibiotics. They are effective against some species that are resistant to penicillins and other cell wall

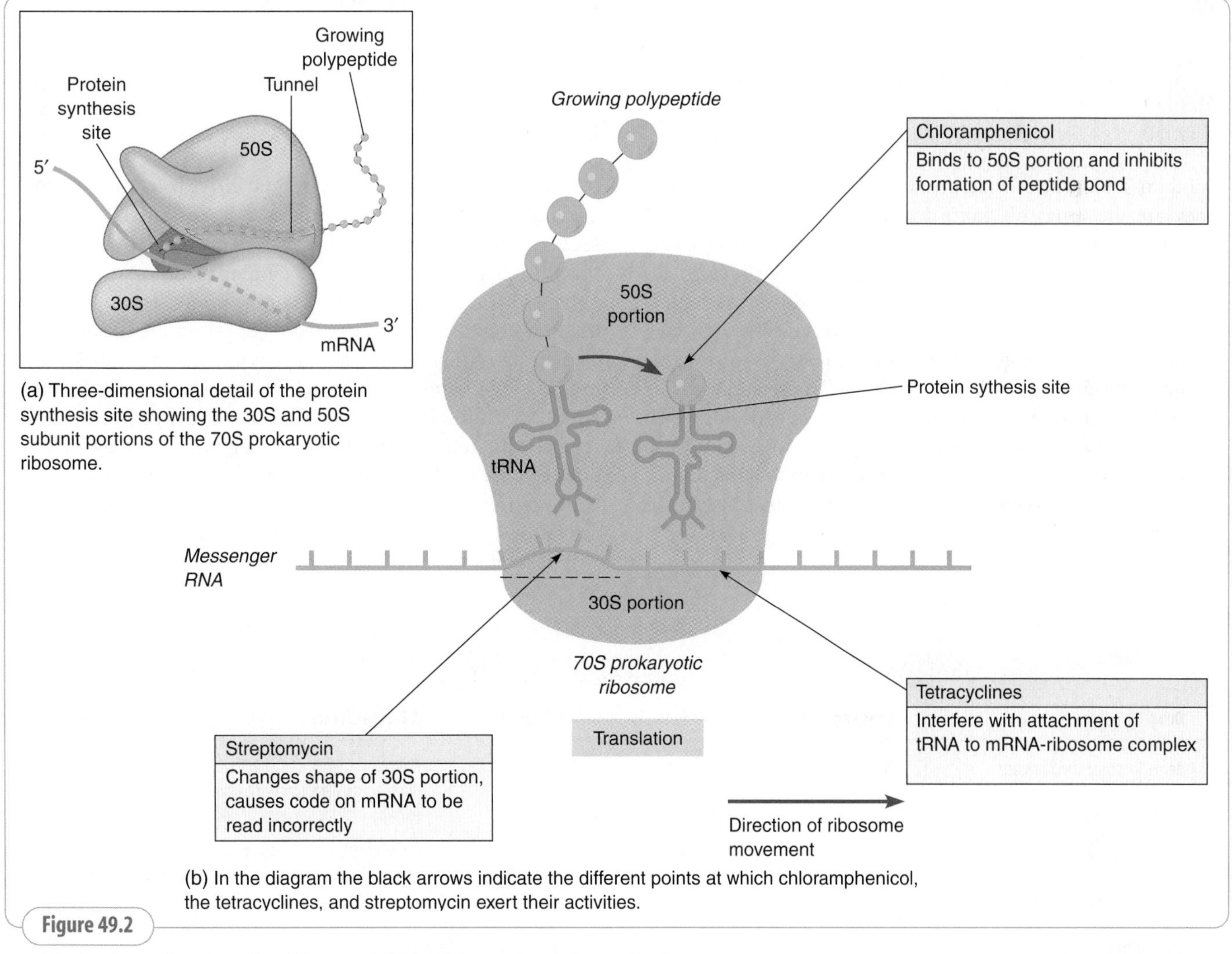

Figure 49.2

Mechanisms of action of antibiotics inhibiting bacterial protein synthesis.
Source: From *Microbiology: An Introduction* (9th ed., p. 563), by G. Tortora, B. Funke, & C. Case, 2007. Reprinted by permission of Pearson Education, Inc., Upper Saddle River, NJ.

CONNECTIONS

Evidence-Based Practice Traveler's Diarrhea

Clinical Question

What are the effects of antibiotics on traveler's diarrhea in relation to duration of illness, severity of illness, and adverse effects of medications?

Traveler's diarrhea frequently attacks people visiting third-world or developing countries, including those located in Africa, the Middle East, and Latin America. Bacteria and the toxins that cause traveler's diarrhea occur in areas with contaminated water supplies, poor sewage systems, or inadequate food handling practices.

Traveler's diarrhea is rarely life threatening for adults. However, antibiotics are sometimes prescribed to reduce the duration and severity of the illness.

Evidence

A review of literature, completed by researchers De Bruyn, Hahn, and Borwick, found that a significant reduction in duration of diarrhea occurred in participants who were treated with antibiotics compared with the placebo. Additionally, a greater number of participants who were taking antibiotics were cured of diarrhea within 72 hours as compared with those treated with the placebo. However, persons taking antibiotics experienced more adverse effects than those taking the placebo.

Implication

More people are traveling to foreign countries than ever before. Nurses can be instrumental in teaching methods to avoid traveler's diarrhea. Clearly, patients can decrease their risk of developing traveler's diarrhea by avoiding drinking tap water and food that may be contaminated. However, other considerations may include not using tap water for brushing teeth, avoiding ice made from tap water, and using only boiled (at least 5 minutes) water for mixing baby formula.

Furthermore, the traveler should be instructed to drink only pasteurized milk and bottled drinks only if the seal has not been broken. Raw fruits and vegetables should be avoided unless peeled. Because raw leafy vegetables (e.g., lettuce, spinach, and cabbage) are hard to clean, they too should not be consumed. Traveler's diarrhea can also be contracted through raw or rare meats and shellfish. Buying food from street vendors increases the risk of contamination because even hot foods left to sit at open air temperatures may become recontaminated.

The patient should be instructed that basic sanitation principles are a key to avoiding contamination. Frequent hand washing is critical to avoid infection. Children should be watched carefully because they may put foreign objects in their mouths or touch contaminated items and then put their hands in their mouths. If possible, keep infants from crawling on dirty floors.

Critical Thinking Question

In what specific patient population is traveler's diarrhea most serious? Why?

See Answers to Critical Thinking Questions in Appendix A.

inhibitors. Because of widespread bacterial resistance, however, they are the drugs of choice for only a few diseases: Rocky Mountain spotted fever, typhus, cholera, Lyme disease, ulcers caused by *Helicobacter pylori*, and chlamydial infections. In addition, *Treponema pallidum* (syphilis) responds well to tetracycline therapy for patients who are allergic to penicillin. Although traditionally used for gonorrhea, most strains of *Neisseria gonorrhoeae* are now resistant to tetracyclines. Drugs in this class are occasionally used for the treatment of acne vulgaris, for which they are given topically or orally (PO) at low doses. Almost all strains of *Pseudomonas aeruginosa* are resistant to tetracyclines. Once resistance develops to one tetracycline, it usually extends to all drugs in this class. Doses for the tetracyclines are listed in Table 49.1.

Tetracyclines exert a bacteriostatic effect by selectively inhibiting bacterial protein synthesis. As illustrated in Figure 49.2, the tetracyclines bind to the 30S bacterial ribosome, thereby preventing the addition of amino acids to the growing polypeptide chain. Resistance to tetracyclines develops when bacteria prevent tetracyclines from concentrating inside their cells, or when their ribosome shape is altered so the antibiotic can no longer bind. In addition to having ribosomes with different structures, human cells lack the active transport system required for tetracyclines to enter their cells. At high doses, however, tetracyclines begin to exert toxicity on human cells.

All tetracyclines have the same spectrum of antimicrobial activity and similar adverse effects. All may be given PO. Several have topical and parenteral formulations. They are sometimes

TABLE 49.1 Tetracyclines

Drug	Route and Adult Dose (maximum dose where indicated)	Adverse Effects
demeclocycline (Declomycin)	PO: 150 mg every 6 h or 300 mg every 12 h (max: 2.4 g/day)	*Nausea, vomiting, abdominal cramping, flatulence, diarrhea, mild phototoxicity, rash, dizziness, stinging or burning with topical applications* <u>Anaphylaxis, superinfections, hepatotoxicity, exfoliative dermatitis, permanent teeth discoloration in children</u>
doxycycline (Vibramycin, others)	PO: 100 mg bid on day 1, then 100 mg daily (max: 200 mg/day)	
minocycline (Minocin, others)	PO: 200 mg as one dose followed by 100 mg bid	
tetracycline (Sumycin, others)	PO: 250–500 mg bid–qid (max: 2 g/day)	
tigecycline (Tygacil)	IV: 100 mg, followed by 50 mg every 12 h	

Note: *Italics* indicate common adverse effects. <u>Underline</u> indicates serious adverse effects.

CONNECTIONS

To the Community Photosensitivity and Antibiotics

Having fun in the sun may be hazardous to some patients. Photosensitivity is a relatively common adverse reaction to some medications, especially antibiotics. Many pharmacologic therapies have photosensitivity as a possible adverse effect. Nurses should provide patients with counseling on the risk of medication-induced photosensitivity and ways to avoid this problem.

Any skin reaction to light is generally defined as photosensitivity. However, this medication-induced adverse effect can present in two categories: phototoxicity and photo allergic reactions. The more common of the two conditions is phototoxicity, which encompasses both sunburn and reactions caused by chemical photosensitizers such as medications. These reactions are typically manifested by delayed redness and edema followed by hyperpigmentation. Phototoxicity may occur after first exposure to a drug.

Photo allergic reactions are less common. These types of reactions are variations of contact dermatitis and are the result of hypersensitivity. In photo allergic reactions, the drug forms an immunogenic complex with cutaneous proteins due to the presence of light energy. Photo allergic reactions tend to become more pronounced with repeat exposures.

Nurses should educate patients about various methods to protect the skin from damage and severe reactions to the sun. Restriction on the amount of time spent in direct sunlight and the proper use of protective clothing and sunscreens are needed to avoid these problems.

described by their duration of action as short acting, intermediate acting, or long acting.

Most PO tetracyclines should be taken on an empty stomach to maximize their absorption. Gastric distress is relatively common with tetracyclines, however, and patients will tend to take tetracyclines with food. Because these drugs bind metal ions such as calcium and iron, tetracyclines should not be taken with milk or iron supplements. Food, milk, or other dairy products can reduce drug absorption by 50% or more. Food does not interfere with absorption of the longer-acting drugs doxycycline and minocycline.

Because most tetracyclines are incompletely absorbed, they remain in the GI tract in high concentrations, often killing normal flora in the colon. Tetracycline-induced diarrhea is common and could indicate toxic effects on normal flora or a bowel superinfection. The presence of diarrhea must be monitored carefully due to the possibility of **pseudomembranous colitis.** Caused by *Clostridium difficile*, this is a rare though potentially severe disorder resulting from therapy with tetracycline and other classes of antibiotics.

When administered parenterally or in high doses, certain tetracyclines can cause hepatotoxicity, especially in patients with preexisting liver disease. Some patients experience photosensitivity during therapy, making their skin especially susceptible to sunburn. Photosensitivity may appear as exaggerated sunburn within minutes to hours of exposure and is often accompanied by a tingling, burning sensation. Because of their broad spectrum, superinfections due to *Candida albicans* are relatively common. Women who are on oral contraceptives may be more susceptible to vaginal candidiasis. Tetracyclines are usually contraindicated in pregnant or lactating women and in children under the age of 8 because these drugs cause yellow-brown teeth discoloration and may slow the overall growth rate in fetuses or children.

PROTOTYPE DRUG Tetracycline (Sumycin, others)

Classification: **Therapeutic:** Antibacterial

Pharmacologic: Protein synthesis inhibitor, tetracycline

Therapeutic Effects and Uses: Approved in 1953, tetracycline is used for the treatment and prophylaxis of susceptible gram-positive and gram-negative bacteria as well as *Chlamydiae, Rickettsiae*, mycoplasmas, and certain protozoa. Tetracycline has one of the broadest spectrums of any antibiotic. Its use has increased over the past decade due to its effectiveness against *H. pylori* in the treatment of peptic ulcer disease. Oral and topical preparations are available for treating inflammatory acne vulgaris.

Mechanism of Action: Tetracycline inhibits bacterial protein synthesis by binding to the 30S ribosomal subunit, interfering with the attachment of the tRNA to the mRNA-ribosome complex. The growing amino acid chain is prematurely terminated and protein synthesis is inhibited. Tetracycline is usually considered bacteriostatic, although it can be bacteriocidal at high concentrations.

Pharmacokinetics:

Route(s)	PO, topical
Absorption	80% is absorbed PO
Distribution	Widely distributed; only small amounts cross the blood–brain barrier; crosses the placenta; secreted in breast milk
Primary metabolism	15–30% metabolized, primarily in the liver
Primary excretion	60% renal, small amounts excreted into bile
Onset of action	1–2 h
Duration of action	Half-life: 6–12 h

Adverse Effects: Being a broad-spectrum antibiotic, tetracycline has a tendency to affect vaginal, oral, and intestinal flora and cause superinfections. Other frequent adverse effects include nausea, vomiting, epigastric burning, diarrhea, discoloration of the teeth, and photosensitivity. Serious adverse reactions include anaphylaxis; fatty degeneration of the liver, producing jaundice; and exfoliative dermatitis. Although not nephrotoxic, tetracycline can worsen kidney impairment in patients with preexisting disease.

Contraindications/Precautions: Tetracycline is contraindicated in patients who are allergic to any drug in the tetracycline class. As a pregnancy category D agent, tetracycline should not be used during pregnancy. Drug therapy must be monitored carefully in patients with impaired hepatic or renal function, because this drug is excreted by these routes.

Drug Interactions: Calcium or iron supplements, magnesium-containing laxatives, and antacids reduce the absorption and serum levels of oral tetracycline. Tetracycline binds with colestipol and cholestyramine, thereby decreasing the antibiotic's absorption. Tetracyclines decrease the effectiveness of oral contraceptives. **Herbal/Food:** Dairy products interfere with tetracycline absorption. Tetracycline eliminates vitamin K producing bacteria in the intestines; patients taking warfarin may experience an increased anticoagulant effect.

Pregnancy: Category D.

Treatment of Overdose: No specific therapy is available. Patients are treated symptomatically.

Nursing Responsibilities:

- Obtain a complete health history, including allergies, drug history, and possible drug interactions.
- Perform an infection-focused physical examination, including vital signs and white blood cell (WBC) count.
- Obtain baseline and intermittent culture and sensitivity (C&S) tests to confirm susceptibility to tetracycline.
- Assess initial and intermittent renal, hepatic, and hematopoietic function test results, especially during high-dose or long-term therapy. Serum tetracycline levels may be indicated for patients at risk for hepatotoxicity, such as with pancreatitis, hepatotoxic drugs, or history of renal or hepatic impairment.
- Administer with a full glass (8 ounces) of water on an empty stomach at least 1 hour before or 2 hours after meals. If the patient experiences nausea, vomiting, or anorexia give this drug with a small amount of food, avoiding foods high in calcium.
- Do not give immediately before sleep because esophagitis and esophageal ulceration are associated with bedtime administration of tetracycline capsules or tablets with insufficient fluid. This is especially true in patients with hiatal hernia or esophageal problems. Report sudden onset of pain or dysphagia to the prescriber.
- Immediately report severe diarrhea to the prescriber. If diarrhea is due to superinfection or pseudomembranous colitis, discontinue tetracycline and begin supportive therapy because this can be life threatening.
- Monitor for evidence of superinfections such as irritation or soreness of the mouth, tongue, throat, vagina, or anus; persistent itching of any area; diarrhea; or foul-smelling excreta or discharge. Inspect the patient's tongue and oral mucous membrane for candidiasis (thrush). Withhold tetracycline and notify the prescriber if superinfection develops.
- Verify eradification of gonococal infection through follow-up cultures from infection sites 3 to 7 days after completion of tetracycline therapy.
- Monitor intake and output (I&O) in patients who are receiving parenteral tetracycline. Report oliguria, any changes in urine appearance, or increase or decrease in I&O.
- Immediately report severe headache or visual disturbances to the prescriber. These possible symptoms of increased intracranial pressure mandate prompt cessation of this drug to prevent irreversible loss of vision.

Patient and Family Education:

- Reduce the incidence of superinfection by using meticulous oral and skin care.
- Before application of the topical drug, clean the affected skin area with soap and water, rinse, and dry well. Protect the eyes, nose, and mouth from topical medication. Topical tetracycline may stain clothing.
- Be aware that maximal results for treating acne may take up to 12 weeks.
- Note that skin color may present as bright yellow to green fluorescence under ultraviolet light and "black light" when treated with the topical drug.
- Report a worsening infection, stinging, or burning sensation with topical applications to the health care provider.
- Do not take antacids, calcium supplements, iron products, and laxatives containing magnesium without approval of the health care provider because this may make tetracycline less effective.
- Avoid unnecessary or prolonged exposure to sunlight and wear protective clothing, sunglasses, and sunscreen.
- Do not breast-feed while taking this drug without approval of the health care provider.
- Immediately notify the health care provider of any known or suspected pregnancy.

Drugs Similar to Tetracycline (Sumycin, Others)

Other tetracyclines include demeclocycline, doxycycline, minocycline, and tigecycline. Oxytetracycline (Terramycin) was discontinued in the United States in 2003.

Demeclocycline (Declomycin): Approved in 1960, demeclocycline has the same spectrum of action and indications as other drugs in this class. It is the only tetracycline that has the ability to stimulate urine flow by blocking the reabsorption of water in the distal renal tubule. Because of this blocking action on antidiuretic hormone (ADH), demeclocycline is used to produce a diuresis in patients with excess ADH secretion. Photosensitivity is more severe with demeclocycline than with any other drug in this class. Demeclocycline undergoes extensive enterohepatic recirculation and is excreted in the bile, thus doses should be reduced for patients with hepatic impairment. This drug is pregnancy category D.

Doxycycline (Vibramycin, others): Approved in 1967, doxycycline is the safest tetracycline for patients with impaired renal function because it is excreted primarily by nonrenal routes. Normally administered PO, an IV form is available for treating severe infections.It is absorbed well, with or without food, and offers the advantage of once- or twice-daily dosing. Doxycycline is included in the *CDC Sexually Transmitted Diseases:*

Treatment Guidelines for treating syphilis, chlamydial infections, and pelvic inflammatory disease. Doxycycline is recommended as an alternative to ciprofloxacin for the prophylactic treatment of *Bacillus anthracis* (anthrax). Adverse effects and contraindications are the same as those of other tetracyclines.

Two doxycycline products are available for the treatment of chronic periodontitis in adults. Atridox is administered as a topical, subgingival controlled release product, and Periostat is given as an oral tablet. Several newer formulations of doxycycline have been approved. In 2005, Doryx, an extended release enteric-coated oral formulation was approved. Approved in 2006, Oracea is a dual-release capsule, containing immediate and delayed release beads for the treatment of inflammatory rosacea. This drug is pregnancy category D.

Minocycline (Minocin, others): Approved in 1971, minocycline offers the advantage of once or twice a day dosing and may be administered without regard to meals or dairy products. It is the only tetracycline that can cause reversible vestibular toxicity, resulting in dizziness, vertigo, and weakness that can limit therapy. Minocycline is active against some strains of bacteria that are resistant to other drugs in the tetracycline class. A microsphere powder formulation, called Arestin, is introduced subgingivally to treat periodontitis. In 2006, Solodyn, an extended release tablet, was approved for the treatment of moderate to severe acne vulgaris. Some research has demonstrated that minocycline is able to reduce symptoms of rheumatoid arthritis. Hepatic function laboratory values should be monitored during therapy to assess for hepatotoxicity. Other adverse effects and contraindications are the same as those of other tetracyclines. This drug is pregnancy category D.

Tigecycline (Tygacil): Tigecycline is the newest tetracycline that was approved in 2005. Available by the intravenous (IV) route, it has more limited indications than other drugs in this class: complicated skin and skin structure infections and complicated intra-abdominal infections. Tigecycline is effective against certain bacterial strains resistant to other antibiotics, including methicillin-resistant *Staphylococcus aureus* (MRSA) and vancomycin-resistant *Enterococci* (VRE). It has not yet shown any cross-resistance with other antibiotics. Nausea and vomiting are the most frequent adverse effects, and these may be severe enough to cause discontinuation of therapy. Other adverse effects and contraindications are the same as those of other tetracyclines. Hepatic function laboratory values should be monitored during therapy to assess for hepatotoxicity. This drug is pregnancy category D.

PharmFACT

The bubonic plague caused by the bacterium *Yersinia pestis* was responsible for killing approximately 50% of the population during the 5th and 6th centuries AD and 40% of the population between the 8th and 14th centuries. If antibiotics had been available back then, most of the estimated 200 million people who died would likely have survived after a 10-day treatment with tetracyclines or aminoglycosides. *Source:* Velendzas & Dufel, 2007.

Macrolides

49.3 The macrolides are safe alternatives to penicillin for many gram-positive infections.

Erythromycin (E-mycin, Erythrocin), the first macrolide antibiotic, was isolated from *Streptomyces* organisms in a soil sample in 1952. The name "macrolide" was chosen for this drug class because they all possess an unusually large 14- to 15-atom ring as part of their chemical structure. Doses for the macrolides are listed in Table 49.2.

Macrolides are considered alternative drugs for patients who are allergic to penicillin. They are widely prescribed although they are the drugs of first choice for relatively few diseases. Most effective against gram-positive bacteria, common indications for macrolides include the treatment of whooping cough, diphtheria, Legionnaire's disease, and infections by streptococci, *Haemophilus influenzae, Mycoplasma pneumoniae,* and chlamydia. Clarithromycin is one of several antibiotics used to treat peptic ulcer disease due to its activity against *H. pylori* (see Chapter 60). The macrolides are the drugs of choice for the prophylaxis of recurring rheumatic fever in patients who are allergic to penicillins.

The macrolides inhibit bacterial protein synthesis by binding to the 50S ribosomal subunit, thus preventing movement of the ribosome along the mRNA. Macrolides do not bind to human ribosomes, thus offering a degree of selective toxicity. These agents are usually bacteriostatic, though they may be bacteriocidal depending on the dose and the target organism.

The newer macrolides have longer half-lives and generally cause less GI irritation than erythromycin, which is the original drug from which macrolides were synthesized. Azithromycin (Zithromax) has an extended half-life such that it can be administered for only 5 days rather than the 10-day therapy required for most antibiotics. A single dose of azithromycin is effective against *N. gonorrhoeae.* The brief duration of therapy is thought to increase patient adherence and to offset the added cost of azithromycin.

Like most of the older antibiotics, macrolide-resistant strains are becoming more common. Many organisms develop

TABLE 49.2 Macrolides

Drug	Route and Adult Dose (maximum dose where indicated)	Adverse Effects
azithromycin (Zithromax, Z-Pak)	PO: 500 mg for one dose, then 250 mg/day for 4 days	*Nausea, vomiting, diarrhea, abdominal cramping, dry skin or burning (topical route)* Anaphylaxis, ototoxicity, pseudomembranous colitis, hepatotoxicity, superinfections, dysrhythmias
clarithromycin (Biaxin)	PO: 250–500 mg bid	
dirithromycin (Dynabac)	PO: 500 mg/day	
erythromycin (E-Mycin, Erythrocin)	PO: 250–500 mg bid or 333 mg tid	

Note: *Italics* indicate common adverse effects. Underline indicates serious adverse effects.

resistance to macrolides by pumping it out of the cell before the antibiotic has a chance to reach an effective concentration. In some cases, bacteria have modified the shape of their 50S ribosomal subunit so that it no longer binds the drug.

The macrolides are well tolerated and considered to be one of the safest antibiotic classes. The most common adverse effects are GI related and include nausea, vomiting, abdominal cramping, and diarrhea. These GI symptoms are observed whether the drug is administered PO or IV. Taking the drug with food can significantly inhibit the absorption of troleandomycin and azithromycin suspension. Thus these drugs should be taken on an empty stomach.

Many macrolides have an enteric coating, which serves two purposes. First, the coating allows the drug to dissolve in the small intestine rather than the stomach, thus causing less gastric irritation. Second, the macrolides are inactivated in gastric acid and the enteric coating allows it to avoid destruction and reach the small intestine where they are readily absorbed in the alkaline environment.

Macrolides are metabolized and concentrated in the liver and excreted into bile. Because macrolides decrease the hepatic metabolism of other drugs, a number of drug–drug interactions are possible. When macrolides prevent the conversion of drugs to their less active form, the serum levels of these other drugs will increase and cause potential toxicity. For example, warfarin (Coumadin) is extensively metabolized to its inactive form in the liver. If given concurrently with erythromycin, the destruction of warfarin is diminished and greater amounts of "active" warfarin remain in the blood for longer periods. Because warfarin increases bleeding time, this could result in unexpected, prolonged bleeding in a patient. In general doses of drugs that are metabolized in the liver should be lowered, or at least carefully monitored, if they are given concurrently with macrolides.

CONNECTION *Checkpoint* 49.1

From what you learned in Chapter 40, what type of laboratory monitoring should be done for a patient who is taking warfarin concurrently with a macrolide? See Answer to Connection Checkpoint 49.1 in Appendix A.

One macrolide, called erythromycin estolate, has been associated with a form of liver damage known as **cholestatic hepatitis.** Cholestatic hepatitis can occur quickly in patients with preexisting liver damage, or it may take 20 or more days before symptoms develop. Laboratory tests for liver injury such as bilirubin and liver transaminases are monitored carefully during therapy with this drug, and signs of hepatic disease such as jaundice or acute pain in the right upper quadrant call for discontinuation of drug therapy. Early identification is important because the liver injury is reversible if the drug is discontinued.

PROTOTYPE DRUG Erythromycin base (E-mycin, others)

Classification: **Therapeutic:** Antibacterial

Pharmacologic: Protein synthesis inhibitor; macrolide

Therapeutic Effects and Uses: Erythromycin base is used for the treatment and prophylaxis of susceptible bacterial infections. The main application for erythromycin is for patients who are allergic to penicillins or who may have a penicillin-resistant infection. It has a spectrum similar to that of the penicillins and is effective against most gram-positive bacteria, including susceptible strains of *Staphylococcus* and *Streptococcus.* Susceptible gram-negative strains include *N. gonorrhea* and *H. influenzae.* It is a drug of choice for infections from *Bordetella pertussis* (whooping cough), *Legionella pneumophila* (Legionnaire's disease), *M. pneumoniae,* and *Corynebacterium diphtheriae.*

Erythromycin is available in a number of salts. All oral forms of erythromycin are considered to have equal effectiveness.

- Erythromycin estolate (Ilosone), erythromycin stearate (Erythrocin), and erythromycin ethylsuccinate (EryPed, Pediamycin) are acid stable and more readily absorbed in the stomach than erythromycin base. These forms are converted to the base form in the liver before they become bacteriostatic. Food interferes with the absorption of erythromycin base, but not the estolate or ethylsuccinate salts.
- Erythromycin gluceptate and erythromycin lactobionate are given IV. They are utilized when the patient is unable to take oral medications, or when the infection is severe enough to warrant a faster onset of action. Topical and ophthalmic formulations are also available.

Mechanism of Action: Erythromycin inhibits bacterial protein synthesis by binding to the 50S ribosomal subunit. Erythromycin is considered bacteriostatic but may be bacteriocidal in high doses.

Pharmacokinetics:

Route(s)	PO, topical, IV (gluceptate and lactobionate salts)
Absorption	Readily absorbed PO; enteric coated
Distribution	Widely distributed; only small amounts cross the blood–brain barrier; secreted in breast milk
Primary metabolism	Hepatic metabolism (CYP3A); concentrates in the liver and bile
Primary excretion	Bile
Onset of action	1 h
Duration of action	Half-life: 1.5–2 h

Adverse Effects: The most common adverse effects from erythromycin are nausea, vomiting, and abdominal cramping, although these are rarely serious enough to cause discontinuation of therapy. Concurrent administration with food reduces these adverse effects. When given by the IV route, phlebitis and intense pain at the injection site are common. One of the most severe adverse effects is cholestatic hepatitis caused by the estolate salt (Ilosone) of this drug. Anaphylaxis is possible. Hearing loss, vertigo, and dizziness may be experienced when using high doses, particularly in older adults and in those with impaired hepatic or renal excretion. High doses of IV erythromycin may be cardiotoxic and pose a risk for torsades de pointes, which is a type of dysrhythmia that is potentially fatal.

Contraindications/Precautions: Erythromycin is contraindicated in patients with hypersensitivity to drugs in the macrolide class and for those who are taking terfenadine, astemizole, or cisapride. Drug therapy must be monitored carefully in patients with impaired hepatic or biliary function, due to the possibility of cholestatic hepatitis.

Drug Interactions: Erythromycin inhibits hepatic CYP450 metabolic enzymes and can interact with many drugs. When used concurrently with erythromycin, the serum levels and toxicities of alfentanil, carbamazepine, cyclosporine, fentanyl, theophylline, and methadone may increase. Because erythromycin may increase the effects of digoxin or warfarin, leading to abnormal bleeding, the doses of these anticoagulants may need to be lowered. Erythromycin competes with clindamycin and chloramphenicol for binding sites on the 50S bacterial ribosomal subunit, causing an antagonistic effect. Thus these antibiotics should not be taken concurrently. The concurrent use of erythromycin with lovastatin or simvastatin is not recommended because it may increase the risk of myopathy and rhabdomyolysis. Because fluconazole also inhibits CYP3A4, especially at high dosages, its concurrent use with erythromycin should be avoided. **Herbal/Food:** Grapefruit juice may increase the bioavailability of erythromycin.

Pregnancy: Category B.

Treatment of Overdose: No specific therapy is available. Patients are treated symptomatically.

Nursing Responsibilities:

- Obtain a complete health history, including allergies, drug history, and possible drug interactions.
- Perform an infection-focused physical examination, including vital signs and WBC count.
- Administer the oral medicine with a full glass (8 ounces) of water on an empty stomach 1 hour before or 3 hours after eating. Avoid administration with, immediately before, or after fruit juices. Give enteric-coated tablets without regard to meals.
- Report nausea, vomiting, and diarrhea to the prescriber. Consult the prescriber to reduce the dosage or administer with a small amount of food.
- Monitor for severe diarrhea because life-threatening pseudomembranous colitis may occur during or after therapy.
- Observe for signs and symptoms of superinfections. Emergence of resistant staphylococcal strains is highly predictable during prolonged therapy.
- Assess intermittent hepatic function tests during prolonged therapy. Monitor for signs and symptoms of hepatotoxicity such as abdominal pain, nausea, vomiting, fever, leukocytosis, and eosinophilia; jaundice may or may not be present. Symptoms may usually occur after 1 to 2 weeks of continuous therapy.
- Report any ototoxic effects such as dizziness, vertigo, nausea, tinnitus, roaring noises, or hearing impairment. These effects occur most frequently in patients who are receiving 4 g/day or more, older adults, female patients, and patients with kidney or liver dysfunction. Ototoxicity is usually reversible with prompt discontinuation of the drug.
- Apply a ribbon of ophthalmic ointment approximately 0.5 to 1 cm long into the lower conjunctival sac of the neonate shortly after birth as a prophylaxis for neonatal eye infection. Use a new tube of erythromycin for each neonate.

Patient and Family Education:

- Immediately report any diarrhea with unexplained fatigue, abdominal pain, or fever to the health care provider because this may indicate pseudomembranous enterocolitis. This may occur even after the drug is discontinued.
- Report any loss of hearing to the health care provider.
- Notify the health care provider if symptoms do not begin to improve in 3 to 4 days.
- Take erythromycin at least 1 hour before or 2 hours after meals. Do not take this medication with, or just after, fruit juices or carbonated drinks. Certain brands of erythromycin may be taken with meals; check with the health care provider or pharmacist.
- Shake liquid and pediatric drops well before each use to mix the medication evenly. Use the bottle dropper to measure the dose of pediatric drops.
- Do not breast-feed while taking this drug without approval of the health care provider.

Drugs Similar to Erythromycin Base (E-Mycin, Others)

Other macrolides include azithromycin, clarithromycin, and dirithromycin.

Azithromycin (Zithromax, Z-pak, Zmax): Approved in 1991, azithromycin has a long duration of action that allows for less frequent dosing. Z-pak allows for 5-day dosing, rather than the conventional 7 to 10 days. For acute otitis media in children, a single dose has been found to be as effective as 3- or 5-day regimens. An IV form for infusions is available for the treatment of pelvic inflammatory disease and community-acquired pneumonia. An ophthalmic solution (AzaSite) was approved in 2007 for treating bacterial conjunctivitis.

Azithromycin causes less nausea than erythromycin and may be taken with or without food. The extended release oral suspension should be administered on an empty stomach. Because azithromycin does not inhibit liver metabolism, it is safer for patients with hepatic impairment and causes fewer drug–drug interactions than erythromycin base. Patients with a known hypersensitivity to any macrolide should not receive azithromycin. This drug is pregnancy category B.

Clarithromycin (Biaxin): Approved in 1991, clarithromycin is similar to erythromycin but causes significantly less nausea, and the regular release tablets may be taken with or without food. The drug is commonly prescribed for infections of the respiratory tract, sexually transmitted infections, *H. pylori*–associated peptic ulcer disease, and otitis media. An extended release (XL) formulation is used to treat sinusitis, chronic bronchitis, and community-acquired pneumonia. The XL form should be administered with food because its absorption is increased. Most adverse effects are GI related and are not serious enough to require discontinuation of therapy. Like erythromycin, a significant number of drug–drug interactions may occur. Patients with a known hypersensitivity to any macrolide should not receive clarithromycin. This drug is pregnancy category C.

- **Dirithromycin (Dynabac):** Approved in 1995, dirithromycin has a longer duration of action and does not inhibit hepatic metabolism. The extended half-life of the drug and its active metabolites allow for once-daily dosing. Indications and adverse effects of dirithromycin are very similar to those for erythromycin. It is available only by the PO route in enteric-coated tablets. Because dirithromycin does not inhibit liver metabolism, it causes fewer drug–drug interactions than erythromycin base. Patients with a known hypersensitivity to any macrolide should not receive dirithromycin. This drug is pregnancy category C.

Aminoglycosides

49.4 The aminoglycosides are effective against aerobic gram-negative organisms but have the potential to cause ototoxicity and nephrotoxicity.

The first aminoglycoside, streptomycin, was named after *Streptomyces griseus*, the soil organism from which it was isolated in 1943. Once widely used, streptomycin is now usually reserved for the treatment of tuberculosis (see Chapter 52) due to the development of safer alternatives and the appearance of a large number of resistant strains. Other aminoglycosides have since been isolated, and several have been produced semisynthetically. All have a chemical structure in common of two or more amino sugars with a glycosidic, or sugar, link. The differences in spelling of some of these drugs, *-mycin* and *-micin*, reflects the different organisms from which the drugs were originally isolated. Doses for the aminoglycosides are shown in Table 49.3.

Aminoglycosides bind irreversibly to the 30S ribosomal subunit of bacteria, changing its shape and preventing the initiation stage of protein synthesis. Some drugs in this class also affect the 50S subunit. In addition, these antibiotics cause mRNA to be read incorrectly, resulting in abnormal proteins that are subsequently inserted into the bacterial plasma membrane, causing it to leak. Whereas most antibiotics that affect protein synthesis are bacteriostatic, aminoglycosides are bacteriocidal.

Although they have the ability to kill many different bacterial species, the aminoglycosides are considered narrow-spectrum drugs because they are normally reserved for serious systemic infections caused by aerobic gram-negative organisms, such as *Pseudomonas* and members of the Enterobacteriaceae family that includes *Escherichia coli, Serratia, Proteus,* and *Klebsiella.* They are ineffective against most gram-positive bacteria. Because oxygen is required for aminoglycoside antibiotics to be transported inside bacterial cells, this class of drugs does not affect anaerobes.

Most aminoglycosides are polar compounds that are poorly absorbed from the GI tract. Because less than 1% of an oral dose is absorbed, they must be administered parenterally to treat systemic infections. Because aminoglycosides travel through the alimentary canal unchanged, they are occasionally given PO to sterilize the bowel prior to intestinal surgery. Neomycin is available for topical infections of the skin, eyes, and ears. Paromomycin (Humatin) is given orally for the treatment of parasitic infections (see Chapter 54).

Due to their polar nature, aminoglycosides cannot enter most human cells. Although distributed to most body fluids, not enough of the drugs enter the cerebrospinal fluid (CSF) for them to treat central nervous system (CNS) infections. Aminoglycosides can, however, cross the placenta. If taken late in pregnancy, streptomycin can cause hearing loss in the child. In addition, aminoglycosides concentrate in renal tissue, which leads to potential nephrotoxicity.

Resistance can occur quickly if aminoglycosides are administered as monotherapy. Resistance occurs when a species acquires an ability to degrade the antibiotic. Once degraded by the bacterial enzymes, these drugs cannot bind to the bacterial ribosome to inhibit protein synthesis. Some resistance also occurs when mutations change the shape of the bacterial ribosome so that it no longer binds the aminoglycoside. The emergence of aminoglycoside-resistant strains of *Enterococcus faecalis* and *Enterococcus faecium* has become a serious clinical problem because there are few therapeutic alternatives to treat

TABLE 49.3 Aminoglycosides

Drug	Route and Adult Dose (maximum dose where indicated)	Adverse Effects
amikacin (Amikin)	IV/IM: 5–7.5 mg/kg as a loading dose, then 7.5 mg/kg bid	*Pain or inflammation at the injection site, rash, fever, nausea, diarrhea, dizziness, tinnitus* Anaphylaxis, nephrotoxicity, irreversible ototoxicity, superinfections
gentamicin (Garamycin, others)	IV/IM: 1.5–2 mg/kg as a loading dose, then 1–2 mg/kg bid-tid	
kanamycin (Kantrex)	IV/IM: 5–7.5 mg/kg bid-tid	
neomycin	PO: 4–12 g/day in divided doses	
paromomycin (Humatin)	PO: 7.5–12.5 mg/kg tid	
streptomycin	IM: 15 mg/kg up to 1 g as a single dose	
tobramycin (Nebcin)	IV/IM: 1 mg/kg tid (max: 5 mg/kg/day)	

Note: *Italics* indicate common adverse effects. Underline indicates serious adverse effects.

these infections. Once resistance develops to an aminoglycoside, the mutant strain is usually resistant to the other drugs in this class. An exception is amikacin, which appears to have some activity against gentamicin-resistant strains.

Several techniques have been used to increase the effectiveness of the aminoglycosides. Administering these drugs in one large dose per day rather than smaller divided doses results in a greater bacteriocidal effect and fewer resistant microbes. A second technique is to administer aminoglycosides and penicillins concurrently (though not mixed in the same IV solution). The penicillin weakens the cell wall, allowing a greater amount of aminoglycoside to enter and reach its ribosomal targets.

Aminoglycosides are excreted almost exclusively by the kidneys. Because certain tissues bind the drugs very tightly, renal excretion may be prolonged up to 20 days after discontinuation of the drug. Although serum drug levels may drop below what is considered a minimally effective concentration, some antimicrobial activity continues during this time. This is known as a **postantibiotic effect.**

The clinical applications of the aminoglycosides are limited by their potential to cause serious adverse effects. The degree and types of potential toxicity is similar for all drugs in this class. For example, all aminoglycosides can impair both hearing and balance. Damage to sensory cells in the cochlea causes hearing loss. Balance is affected by damage to sensory cells in the vestibular apparatus of the inner ear. As high as 25% of patients who are taking aminoglycoside antibiotics may experience some ototoxicity. This effect is more prominent when the medications are used for longer than 10 days, or when the patient has preexisting kidney impairment, causing high serum drug levels. The damage to sensory cells is cumulative; repeated doses of the drug can damage increasing numbers of cells. Because many elderly persons have some degree of preexisting hearing impairment, permanent deafness may occur in this group. Signs of impending inner ear damage include high-pitched tinnitus, headache, nausea, vomiting, and vertigo. Signs of ototoxicity may continue for several weeks after the drugs are discontinued. If hearing and balance functions are not carefully monitored during therapy and proper interventions are not implemented, the ototoxicity may become irreversible.

One of the most serious adverse effects of aminoglycosides is their potential to cause nephrotoxicity. Aminoglycosides directly injure renal tubule cells, and this nephrotoxicity may be severe, affecting up to 26% of patients receiving these antibiotics. As expected, patients who are receiving higher doses for longer periods are most affected. Those with preexisting renal impairment or who are receiving concurrent therapy with other nephrotoxic agents must be monitored carefully: Regular evaluation of urinalysis, blood urea nitrogen (BUN), and serum creatinine results is essential. Serum drug concentrations should be obtained regularly and doses adjusted accordingly to prevent permanent damage. If recognized early, renal damage caused by aminoglycosides is reversible. Impaired kidney function may cause drug serum levels to rise, thus increasing the risk or worsening of ototoxicity.

A less common, though serous adverse effect of aminoglycosides is neuromuscular blockade. Aminoglycosides inhibit the release of acetylcholine at synapses. Giving other drugs that affect acetylcholine release, such as anesthetics or neuromuscular blockers (see Chapter 30) can result in profound apnea and prolonged muscle paralysis. Because they have fewer acetylcholine receptors, patients with myasthenia gravis are especially at risk. To avoid the problem, aminoglycosides may be discontinued prior to surgery. IV calcium salts have been found to reverse aminoglycoside-induced neuromuscular blockade.

CONNECTION *Checkpoint* 49.2

From what you learned in Chapter 18, name the prototype drugs classified as neuromuscular blockers. Is muscle paralysis occurring at a nicotinic or muscarinic synapse? See Answer to Connection Checkpoint 49.2 in Appendix A.

PROTOTYPE DRUG Gentamicin (Garamycin)

Classification: Therapeutic: Antibacterial
Pharmacologic: Protein synthesis inhibitor; aminoglycoside

Therapeutic Effects and Uses: Approved in 1966, gentamicin is used for the treatment and prophylaxis of susceptible bacterial infections. It is prescribed primarily for serious infections caused by aerobic, gram-negative bacilli. Activity includes *Enterobacter, E. coli, Klebsiella, Citrobacter, Pseudomonas,* and *Serratia.* Gentamicin is effective against a few gram-positive bacteria, including some strains of MSRA. It has no activity against anaerobes. This drug is not absorbed by the PO route. A topical formulation (Genoptic) is available for infections of the external eye.

Therapy with gentamicin is generally limited to those cases in which a less toxic alternative is not available. Resistance to gentamicin is increasing, and some patients show cross-resistance to other aminoglycosides such as tobramycin. Gentamicin is sometimes given concurrently with a beta-lactam antibiotic such as a penicillin or cephalosporin to improve bacterial kill and to delay resistance.

Mechanism of Action: Gentamicin inhibits bacterial protein synthesis by binding to the 30S ribosomal subunit. Gentamicin is bacteriocidal by causing premature termination of the growing polypeptide chain.

Pharmacokinetics:

Route(s)	Intramuscular (IM), IV, topical (ophthalmic)
Absorption	Not absorbed PO; readily absorbed IM
Distribution	Distributed to most body tissues and fluids, except the CSF; concentrates in the kidney and inner ear; crosses the placenta; small amounts secreted in breast milk;
Primary metabolism	Not metabolized
Primary excretion	Renal
Onset of action	Rapid
Duration of action	Half-life: 3–4 h

Adverse Effects: Rash, nausea, vomiting, and fatigue are the most common adverse effects. As with other aminoglycosides, some adverse effects from gentamicin may be severe. Ototoxicity can produce a loss of hearing or balance, which may become permanent with continued use. Tinnitus, vertigo, and persistent headaches are early signs of ototoxicity. Aminoglycosides are associated with neuromuscular blockade and may cause severe neuromuscular weakness that lasts for several days. Early signs of neurotoxicity include paresthesias, twitching, and seizures. Signs of reduced kidney function include oliguria, proteinuria, and elevated BUN and creatinine levels. Nephrotoxicity is of particular concern to patients with preexisting kidney disease and may limit pharmacotherapy. Resistance to gentamicin is increasing and some cross-resistance among aminoglycosides has been reported.

Contraindications/Precautions: Gentamicin is contraindicated in patients who are hypersensitive to aminoglycosides. Drug therapy must be monitored carefully in patients with impaired renal function or in those with preexisting hearing loss. Gentamicin should not be used in pregnant or breast-feeding patients.

Drug Interactions: Concurrent use with other nephrotoxic drugs such as acyclovir, amphotericin B, capreomycin, cisplatin, cyclosporine, salicylates, polymyxin B, or vancomycin increases the risk of nephrotoxicity. Other drugs affecting the 8th cranial nerve such as ethacrynic acid and furosemide will increase the risk of ototoxicity if given concurrently with gentamicin. Penicillins can inactivate aminoglycosides if they are mixed together in the same solution. Antiemetics such as dimenhydrinate, meclizine, promethazine, and scopolamine may block the nausea characteristic of vestibular toxicity or motion sickness, thus masking the signs of aminoglycoside-induced ototoxicity. **Herbal/Food:** No significant interactions are known.

Pregnancy: Category D (parenteral).

Treatment of Overdose: Overdose can result in serious kidney damage and ototoxicity. No specific therapy is available. Patients are treated symptomatically.

Nursing Responsibilities:

- Obtain a complete health history, including allergies, drug history, and possible drug interactions.
- Perform an infection-focused physical examination, including vital signs and WBC count.
- Obtain C&S and renal function tests prior to the first dose and intermittently during therapy. Repeat C&S testing if improvement does not occur in 3 to 5 days and reevaluate therapy.
- Determine creatinine clearance and serum drug concentrations at specific intervals, especially for patients with impaired renal function; infants due to immaturity; the elderly; patients receiving high doses or therapy beyond 10 days; and patients with fever or extensive burns, edema, or obesity.
- Draw blood specimens for peak serum gentamicin concentration 30 minutes to 1 hour after IM administration and 30 minutes after completion of a 30- to 60-minute IV infusion. Draw blood specimens for trough levels just before the next IM or IV dose.
- Check vestibular and auditory function before therapy and intermittently. Recheck vestibular and auditory function again 3 to 4 weeks after the drug is discontinued because this is when deafness is most likely to occur. Assess for dizziness, headache, vertigo, nausea and vomiting with motion, ataxia, and nystagmus. Damage to the auditory branch may also occur as tinnitus, fullness in ears, roaring noises, and hearing impairment. Promptly report these to prevent permanent damage.
- Check baseline weight and monitor I&O ratio. Maintain adequate hydration to prevent chemical irritation of the renal tubules. Report oliguria, unusual appearance of urine, change in I&O ratio or pattern, and presence of edema because this drug prolongs elimination time.
- Monitor for signs and symptoms of bacterial overgrowth or opportunistic infections caused by resistant or nonsusceptible organisms.
- Give IM injections deeply into a large muscle.
- Avoid use of topical preparations to large denuded body surfaces due to systemic absorption and toxicity. Wash the affected area with mild soap and water, rinse, and dry thoroughly. Gently apply a small amount of the medication to lesions, then cover with sterile gauze.

Patient and Family Education:

- Avoid direct exposure to sunlight during and for several days after therapy is terminated.
- If exposure to sunlight cannot be avoided, wear protective clothing, sunglasses, and sunscreen.
- Do not breast-feed while taking this drug without prior approval of the health care provider. This drug may affect the teeth of the child.
- Immediately report changes in hearing or low urinary output to the health care provider.
- Notify the health care provider if symptoms do not improve within 3 to 4 days.
- Immediately notify your health care provider of any known or suspected pregnancy.

Drugs Similar to Gentamicin (Garamycin)

Other aminoglycosides include amikacin, kanamycin, neomycin, netilmicin, paromomycin, streptomycin, and tobramycin. All drugs in this class have similar spectrums of activity and adverse effects.

Amikacin (Amikin): Approved in 1976, amikacin has the broadest spectrum and is sometimes effective against organisms that have developed resistance to other aminoglycosides. Amikacin has been used to treat multidrug-resistant tuberculosis (see Chapter 52). It is administered by the IV route. Indications, contraindications, and adverse effects are nearly the same as those for gentamicin. This is a pregnancy category D drug.

Kanamycin (Kantrex): Approved in 1958, kanamycin is the most toxic aminoglycoside, and resistant strains are common. Its use is limited to the adjunctive treatment of hepatic coma and for the short-term treatment of serious infections. Like amikacin, kanamycin may be used to treat multidrug-resistant tuberculosis after first-line agents have failed. Kanamycin can be delivered IV, IM, by inhalation, or by intraperitoneal instillation. Contraindications and adverse effects are the same as for gentamicin. This is a pregnancy category D drug. Concurrent therapy with other nephrotoxic and neurotoxic drugs should be avoided due to the potential for additive adverse effects.

Neomycin: Approved in 1952, neomycin is widely used for topical infections as an over-the-counter (OTC) ointment combined with polymyxin B and bacitracin (Neosporin). It is also combined in OTC creams with hydrocortisone for minor skin irritations and insect bites. Not available in parenteral form due to toxicity, neomycin may be used orally to sterilize the bowel. Oral neomycin can cause headache, lethargy, nausea, and vomiting. This is a pregnancy category C drug.

Paromomycin (Humatin): Approved in 1959, paromomycin is most active against gram-negative aerobic bacteria (with the exception of *Pseudomonas*). The primary use of this drug, however, is for treating intestinal parasitic infections caused by protozoans and tapeworms (see Chapter 54). It is available in both oral and topical formulations. The oral form is not absorbed and is used to sterilize the bowel and remove parasites. This is a pregnancy category C drug.

Streptomycin: The use of streptomycin, the first aminoglycoside approved by the U.S. Food and Drug Administration (FDA) in 1945, was generally discontinued in 1993, but it is still available on a case-by-case basis. It was discontinued due to a large number of resistant strains and its high risk for ototoxicity. It is most often used in combination with other drugs in the pharmacotherapy of multidrug-resistant tuberculosis (see Chapter 52). This is a pregnancy category D drug.

Tobramycin (Nebcin): Approved in 1975, tobramycin has a spectrum of activity similar to that of gentamicin, but it is more effective against *P. aeruginosa* than gentamicin. Most often administered parenterally, tobramycin is also available as an ophthalmic solution and in nebulizer form for patients with cystic fibrosis who have *Pseudomonas* infections. Adverse effects and contraindications are similar to those of gentamicin. This is a pregnancy category D drug.

NURSING PROCESS APPLICATION

Patients Receiving Tetracyclines, Macrolides, and Aminoglycosides

Assessment	Potential Nursing Diagnoses
Prior to administration: • Obtain a complete health history, including allergies, drug history, and possible drug interactions. • Obtain specimens for C&S testing before initiating therapy. • Perform an infection-focused physical examination, including vital signs, WBC count, and sedimentation rate.	• *Risk for Infection* • *Risk for Injury*, related to adverse effects of drug • *Deficient Knowledge (Antibiotic Therapy)*, related to disease process, transmission, purpose, precautions, and adverse effects of drug • *Noncompliance*, related to therapeutic regimen

Planning: Patient Goals and Expected Outcomes

The patient will:

- Report reduction in symptoms related to the diagnosed infection and have negative results for laboratory and diagnostic tests for the presenting infection.
- Demonstrate an understanding of the drug's action by accurately describing drug adverse effects and precautions.
- Immediately report significant adverse effects such as shortness of breath, swelling, fever, stomatitis, loose stools, vaginal discharge, or cough.
- Complete the full course of antibiotic therapy and comply with follow-up care.

Implementation

Interventions and (Rationales)	Patient and Family Education
• Monitor vital signs and symptoms of infection to determine antibacterial effectiveness. (Another drug or a different dosage may be required.)	• Instruct the patient to notify the health care provider if symptoms persist or worsen.
• Monitor for hypersensitivity reaction. (Immediate hypersensitivity reaction may occur within 2 to 30 minutes, accelerated occurs in 1 to 72 hours, and delayed after 72 hours.)	• Instruct the patient to discontinue the medication and inform the health care provider if symptoms of hypersensitivity reaction develop, such as wheezing; shortness of breath; swelling of face, tongue or hands; and itching or rash.
• Monitor for severe diarrhea. (The condition may occur due to superinfection or the possible adverse effect of antibiotic-associated pseudomembranous colitis.)	Instruct the patient to: • Consult the health care provider before taking antidiarrheal drugs, which could cause retention of harmful bacteria. • Consume cultured dairy products with live active cultures, such as kefir, yogurt, or buttermilk, to help maintain normal intestinal flora.
• Administer the drug around the clock. (This is necessary to maintain consistent and effective serum drug levels.)	Instruct the patient to: • Take the medication on schedule. • Complete the entire prescription even if feeling better to prevent the development of resistant bacteria.
• Monitor for superinfection, especially in older adults, debilitated or immunosuppressed patients, and children less than 8 years of age. (There is an increased risk for superinfections due to elimination of normal flora.)	• Instruct the patient to report signs and symptoms of superinfection such as fever; black hairy tongue; stomatitis; loose, foul-smelling stools; vaginal discharge; or cough.

(continued)

NURSING PROCESS APPLICATION *(continued)*

• Monitor intake of OTC products such as antacids, calcium supplements, iron products, and laxatives containing magnesium. (These products interfere with absorption of many antibiotics.)	Instruct the patient: • To consult with the health care provider before using OTC medications or herbal products. • That antacids and calcium supplements specifically block the absorption of tetracyclines.
• Monitor for photosensitivity. (Tetracyclines can increase a patient's sensitivity to ultraviolet light and increase risk of sunburn from 2 weeks to 2 months after taking the medication.)	Encourage the patient to: • Stay out of direct sunlight, especially between the hours of 10:00 A.M. and 3:00 P.M., if possible. • Wear protective clothing, including a hat, and wear sunglasses. • Apply a sun block product that has a skin protection factor (SPF) of at least 15. Some patients may require a product with a higher SPF number, especially if they have a fair complexion. • Apply a sun block lip product that has an SPF of at least 15 to protect lips. • Do not use a sun lamp, tanning bed, or booth.
• Determine the effect of the prescribed antibiotics on oral contraceptives. (Tetracyclines may decrease the effect of oral contraceptives that contain estrogen and increase the chance of unwanted pregnancy.)	• Instruct the patient to use an alternate form of birth control until all the medication is completed.
• Determine the interactions of the prescribed antibiotics with various foods and beverages. (Milk, milk formulas, or other dairy products that are consumed within 1 to 2 hours of administration of tetracyclines, except doxycycline and minocycline, can reduce absorption of these drugs by 50% or more.)	• Instruct the patient regarding foods and beverages that should be avoided with specific antibiotic therapies. • No dairy or calcium products should be consumed with tetracyclines.
• Monitor the IV site for signs and symptoms of tissue irritation, severe pain, and extravasation.	• Instruct the patient to report pain or other symptoms of discomfort immediately during IV infusion.
• Determine the effects of the antibiotic on specific populations. (Tetracyclines may cause permanent discoloration of the teeth and slow down the growth of bones. These medicines should not be given to children 8 years of age or younger or to nursing mothers.)	• Teach the patient that antibiotics act differently in various populations such as pregnant women, breast-feeding mothers, children, and the elderly.
• Monitor renal function such as I&O ratios and urine color and consistency. Monitor laboratory work including serum creatinine and BUN. (Both tetracyclines and aminoglycosides are eliminated via the renal route. Aminoglycosides are particularly nephrotoxic in patients with preexisting renal dysfunction and in older adults.)	• Explain the purpose of required laboratory tests and scheduled follow-up with the health care provider. • Instruct the patient to increase fluid intake to 2,000 to 3,000 mL/day.
• Monitor for hepatic dysfunction with patients who are receiving macrolide therapy. (Macrolides are primarily eliminated via the hepatic route.)	• Instruct the patient to report the onset of nausea, abdominal pain, vomiting, dark urine, pale-colored stool, or jaundice.
• Monitor for symptoms of ototoxicity. (Aminoglycosides may cause vestibular or auditory nerve [8th cranial nerve] damage, resulting in loss of hearing or balance.)	Instruct the patient to report: • Changes in hearing, ringing in the ears, or full feeling in the ears. • Nausea and vomiting with motion, ataxia, nystagmus, or dizziness.
• Monitor the patient for adherence with antibiotic therapy. (Lack of adherence can result in worsening of the infection.)	Instruct the patient in the importance of: • Completing the prescription as ordered. • Follow-up care after antibiotic therapy is completed.

Evaluation of Outcome Criteria

Evaluate the effectiveness of drug therapy by confirming that patient goals and expected outcomes have been met (see "Planning").

Miscellaneous Inhibitors of Bacterial Protein Synthesis

49.5 Several inhibitors of protein synthesis are effective against resistant infections but may have significant adverse effects that limit their use.

Several bacterial protein synthesis inhibitors do not belong to the tetracycline, macrolide, or aminoglycoside classes. These miscel-

PharmFACT

This chapter considered antibiotics selective for bacterial protein synthesis. But bacteria can fight back. *Corynebacterium diphtheriae* produces a toxin that targets human protein synthesis. *Source:* Pilat, Paladino, & Singh, 2006.

TABLE 49.4 Miscellaneous Inhibitors of Protein Synthesis

Drug	Route and Adult Dose (maximum dose where indicated)	Adverse Effects
chloramphenicol	PO: 12.5 mg/kg qid	*Nausea, vomiting, diarrhea* Anaphylaxis, superinfections, pancytopenia, bone marrow depression, aplastic anemia
clindamycin (Cleocin)	PO: 150–450 mg qid IV: 600–1,200 mg/day in divided doses	*Nausea, vomiting, diarrhea, rash, burning, or pruritus (topical forms)* Anaphylaxis, superinfections, cardiac arrest, pseudomembranous colitis, blood dyscrasias
lincomycin (Lincocin)	PO: 500 mg tid-qid (max: 8 g/day) IM: 600 mg every 12–24 h (max: 8 g/day)	*Nausea, vomiting, diarrhea* Anaphylaxis, superinfections, cardiac arrest, pseudomembranous colitis, blood dyscrasias
linezolid (Zyvox)	PO/IV: 600 mg every 12 h (max: 1,200 mg/day)	*Nausea, diarrhea, headache* Anaphylaxis, superinfections, pseudomembranous colitis, blood dyscrasias
quinupristin-dalfopristin (Synercid)	IV: 7.5 mg/kg infused over 60 min every 8 h	*Pain and inflammation at the injection site, myalgia, arthralgia, diarrhea* Superinfections, pseudomembranous colitis
telithromycin (Ketek)	PO: 800 mg once a day	*Nausea, vomiting, diarrhea* Visual disturbances, hepatotoxicity, dysrhythmias

Note: *Italics* indicate common adverse effects. Underline indicates serious adverse effects.

laneous agents, shown in Table 49.4, have varying spectrums of activity and adverse effect profiles and thus must be considered individually. One of the drugs in the miscellaneous class, spectinomycin (Trobicin), has been discontinued in the United States.

Chloramphenicol: Chloramphenicol is an older, broad-spectrum antibiotic that was approved in 1960 and that has been available for nearly 60 years. It binds to the 50S subunit of the bacterial ribosome and may be bacteriostatic or bacteriocidal, depending on species and dose. Chloramphenicol is administered PO or IV as chloramphenicol succinate for serious infections. A topical form is available for ophthalmic and otic infections.

Effective in treating *Salmonella, Rickettsiae, Streptococci,* typhoid fever, and meningitis caused by *H. influenzae*, this agent was widely used before it was found to be associated with bone marrow suppression and a very small, though fatal, incidence of aplastic anemia. Peak and trough serum levels should be monitored regularly during therapy to avoid serious adverse effects. Chloramphenicol is now reserved for meningitis and other infections in which the benefits of the drug clearly outweigh the risks of serious drug toxicity.

Another serious toxicity from chloramphenicol is **gray baby syndrome.** Most often seen in premature or newborn infants, this syndrome occurs when the baby's liver is unable to metabolize or excrete this drug. Symptoms include failure to feed, abdominal distension, cyanosis, and cardiovascular collapse. The syndrome is rapidly fatal and can cause death in a just few hours. If done early, discontinuing chloramphenicol therapy can reverse the syndrome. This is a pregnancy category C drug.

Clindamycin (Cleocin, others): Approved in 1970, clindamycin acts on the 50S bacterial ribosomal subunit in a manner similar to that of the macrolides. It is usually bacteriostatic. A drug of choice for abdominal infections caused by *Bacteroides fragilis*, it is also effective against *Fusobacterium, Actinomyces,* and *Clostridium.*

Three salts of clindamycin are available: clindamycin hydrochloride (PO), clindamycin palmitate (PO), and clindamycin phosphate (parenteral or topical). In 2004, an aerosol topical foam of 1% clindamycin (Evoclin) was approved for the treatment of acne vulgaris, and a single dose suppository vaginal cream (Clindesse) was marketed for bacterial vaginosis.

Once widely prescribed as a penicillin alternative, the use of clindamycin has become limited due to the development of resistant strains, a high incidence of diarrhea, and a potential risk of drug-induced pseudomembranous colitis caused by *C. difficile*, which can be fatal. It is generally only used when safer alternatives are not effective. The nurse must advise patients to report incidences of diarrhea during clindamycin therapy. If pseudomembranous colitis is suspected, clindamycin is discontinued and the patient is placed on a drug that is effective against *C. difficile* such as vancomycin. This is a pregnancy category B drug.

Lincomycin (Lincocin): Approved in 1964, lincomycin is chemically similar to clindamycin. Lincomycin may be used for patients who cannot take penicillins or cephalosporins but it offers no therapeutic advantages over clindamycin. The drug is rarely prescribed due to a relatively high incidence of serious adverse effects, especially pseudomembranous colitis. It is available by both PO and parenteral routes. This is a pregnancy category B drug.

Quinupristin-dalfopristin (Synercid): Approved in 1999, quinupristin-dalfopristin is a fixed-dose bacteriocidal combination used for therapy of life-threatening *E. faecium* infections that are vancomycin resistant and for complicated infections caused by MRSA or *Streptococcus pyogenes.* It is the first in a new class of antibiotics called **streptogramins** that act by binding the 50S bacterial ribosome in a manner similar to that of the macrolides. The combination of the two antibiotics is truly synergistic: The combination has 16 times more antimicrobial activity compared to either drug used alone. Synercid is bacteriocidal and only available by the IV route.

Joint and muscle pain, diarrhea, rash, and pain at the infusion site are common adverse effects. Venous irritation may be severe enough to cause the drug to be discontinued. Synercid inhibits hepatic drug metabolism enzymes, resulting in numerous drug–drug interactions. The nurse should use caution when administering drugs concurrently with Synercid, because those that rely on hepatic metabolism for detoxification may build to toxic levels in the blood. In addition, some cases of pseudomembranous colitis have been reported. Despite its potential for adverse effects, quinupristin-dalfopristin serves an important role in treating multidrug-resistant gram-positive pathogens, which have become a major clinical challenge. Cross-resistance has not yet developed between Synercid and other antibiotic classes. This is a pregnancy category B drug.

Linezolid (Zyvox): Approved in 2000, linezolid is a newer antibiotic that is the first of a new class of antibiotics, the **oxazolidinones** that act by binding to a part of the bacterial 50S ribosome known as the 23S portion. It is unique among antibiotics in that it prevents the first event in protein synthesis, which is the formation of an initiation complex. It is believed to be bacteriocidal. Linezolid is important because it is effective against infections that have become resistant to most other antibiotics, including MRSA and VRE. It is less effective against gram-negative organisms. Although some resistant strains have been identified, this drug does not appear PO. Oral and IV formulations are available.

Adverse effects are usually minor and related to GI distress. Because this drug can cause transient dose-related myelosuppression, laboratory blood counts should be frequently monitored during therapy. Linezolid is a nonselective inhibitor of monoamine oxidase (MAO) and may cause hypertension in some patients. Risk for hypertension and palpitations is increased if the patient is taking sympathomimetics concurrently with linezolid; thus these medications should be avoided. This is a pregnancy category C drug.

Telithromycin: Approved in 2004, telithromycin (Ketek) is a newer, broad-spectrum antibiotic. Structurally similar to the macrolides, telithromycin is the sole member of a new class called ketolides. Ketolides inhibit bacterial protein synthesis by the same mechanism as the macrolides: by binding to the 50S ribosomal subunit. However, telithromycin binds more tightly to the ribosome than other protein synthesis inhibitors and is capable of causing greater bacterial kill. It also exhibits a significant postantibiotic effect in some organisms. Indications for telithromycin are similar to those of the macrolides except it has greater activity against *S. pneumoniae*. Because of this, its primary use is to treat bronchitis, sinusitis, and community-acquired pneumonia. It is effective against many other bacterial strains, including those that show macrolide resistance. This drug is available as oral tablets.

Although most adverse effects are minor and GI related, telithromycin has the potential to cause several serious adverse effects. Hepatotoxicity has occurred in a small number of patients. Those with preexisting hepatic impairment are at greatest risk and should be carefully monitored during therapy. Telithromycin can cause blurred vision, double vision, and difficulty focusing, which can be severe enough to cause discontinuation of therapy. Patients with myasthenia gravis should not take this drug because their symptoms will worsen. As with some of the macrolides, telithromycin may increase the risk for ventricular dysrhythmias such as torsade de pointes and is contraindicated in patients with prolonged QT intervals. This is a pregnancy category C drug.

UNDERSTANDING THE CHAPTER

Key Concepts Summary

49.1 Antibiotics inhibit microbial protein synthesis by binding to the bacterial ribosome.

49.2 Tetracyclines have broad antimicrobial activity against many gram-positive and gram-negative bacteria.

49.3 The macrolides are safe alternatives to penicillin for many gram-positive infections.

49.4 The aminoglycosides are effective against aerobic gram-negative organisms but have the potential to cause ototoxicity and nephrotoxicity.

49.5 Several inhibitors of protein synthesis are effective against resistant infections but may have significant adverse effects that limit their use.

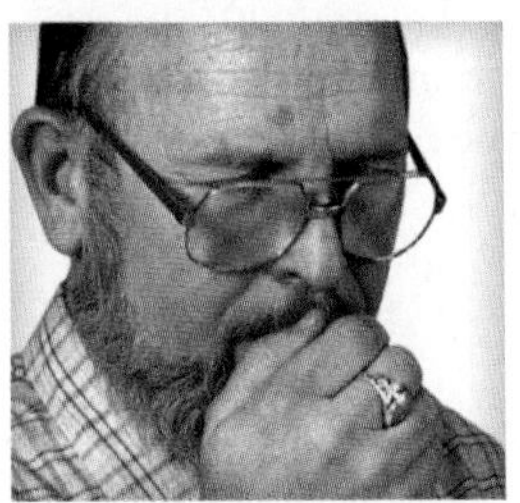

Making the PATIENT Connection

Remember the patient "John Talley" at the beginning of the chapter? Now read the remainder of the case study. Based on the information presented within this chapter, respond to the critical thinking questions that follow.

John Talley, a 51-year-old truck driver, has been suffering from an upper respiratory infection for the last 2 weeks. Although he has seen his health care provider, he does not seem to be improving. He is convinced that if he takes the antibiotic just 1 more day, he will surely improve. However, after 5 days of drug therapy, John continues to experience chills, fever, and a productive cough. His wife insisted that he return to the clinic for further evaluation and treatment.

At the clinic the patient's physical examination and diagnostic tests reveal the following findings: temperature is 39.2°C (102.6°)F, pulse rate is 112 beats/minute, respiratory rate is 30/minute, and blood pressure is 134/88 mmHg. He is visibly short of breath and is experiencing intermittent coughing episodes. On auscultation of his lung fields, bilateral crackles and wheezes are discovered. His WBC count is 14.4 (×10/L). A chest x-ray is taken to confirm a diagnosis of pneumonia and reveals right lower lobe infiltrates (white areas in the lung that indicate infection).

The patient is diagnosed with bacterial pneumonia. He is hospitalized and prescribed IV antibiotic therapy. On the second hospital day you are assigned to care for Mr. Talley. He and his wife have multiple questions about the drug therapy prescribed.

Critical Thinking Questions

1. Why did the first antibiotic prescribed not cure the infection?
2. What is the best way to determine which bacterium is causing the infection?
3. The patient has been told that laboratory personnel will be collecting blood for a peak and trough level this afternoon. What is that?
4. What symptoms would indicate that the patient's condition is worsening?

Case Study

Mr. Klein is an 85-year-old man seen in the outpatient clinic for an acute infection. He has informed the health care provider that he is allergic to a variety of antibiotics and is subsequently prescribed erythromycin estolate. The patient is a recovering alcoholic who has been abstinent for 10 years.

1. What is the significance of Mr. Klein's history of alcoholism?
2. What possible adverse effect should the nurse instruct the patient to watch for?
3. What are the symptoms of this adverse effect?
4. What laboratory diagnostic studies may be indicated in this patient?

NCLEX-RN® Review

1 While teaching the client about taking oral tetracycline, the nurse advises the client to:

1. Consume calcium products to decrease the duration of antibacterial effect.
2. Use a soft toothbrush and floss teeth gently to remove staining on teeth.
3. Weigh each day under standard conditions.
4. Avoid direct exposure to sunlight and apply sun block when outdoors.

2 The nurse determines that the client best understands the use of azithromycin (Zithromax) when the client makes which of the following statements? Azithromycin:

1. Has a longer duration of action that allows for once-daily dosing.
2. Causes more nausea than most other antibiotics in this classification.
3. Must be taken on an empty stomach.
4. Is ineffective if taken with calcium-based foods.

3 The client is receiving amikacin (Amikin) for a bacterial infection. Which of the following adverse effects does the nurse include in the plan of care to monitor the client's status?

1. Weight gain
2. Visual disturbances
3. Mental depression
4. Urinary frequency

4 The health care provider orders gentamicin (Garamycin) for a client with a postoperative wound infection. Which of the following laboratory results should prompt the nurse to consult with the prescriber about possible nephrotoxicity of this drug?

1. Elevated serum creatinine level
2. Decreased blood urea nitrogen (BUN) level
3. Increased white blood cell (WBC) count
4. Elevated serum iron level

5 Which of the following antibiotic therapies would call for the nurse to perform an assessment of baseline hearing and the presence of tinnitus?

1. Tetracyclines
2. Macrolides
3. Aminoglycosides
4. Cephalosporins

6 The client, who has received aminoglycoside for the past 10 days, is experiencing a postantibiotic therapy adverse effect. Due to this development, the nurse should monitor the client for:

1. Neurologic abnormalities.
2. Renal dysfunction.
3. Cardiac complications.
4. Dermatologic problems.

See Answers to Critical Thinking Questions, Case Study, and NCLEX-RN® Review in Appendix A.

References

Centers for Disease Control and Prevention. (2006). *Sexually transmitted diseases: Treatment guidelines 2006.* Retrieved July 25, 2008, from http://www.cdc.gov/std/treatment/default. htm

Hoban, D. J., & Zhanel, G. G. (2006). Clinical implications of macrolide resistance in community-acquired respiratory tract infections. *Expert Review of Anti-Infective Therapy, 4*(6), 973–980.

Kasper, D. L., Braunwald, E., Fauci, A. S., Hauser, S. L., Longo, D. L., & Jameson, J. L. (2005). *Harrison's principles of internal medicine.* New York: McGraw Hill.

McFarland, L., Beneda, H., Clarridge, J., & Raugi, G. (2007). Implications of the changing face of *Clostridium difficile* disease for health care practitioners. *American Journal of Infection Control, 35*(4), 237–253.

Pilat, E., Paladino, L., & Singh, M. K. (2006). Diptheria. eMedicine. Retrieved July 25, 2008, from http://www.emedicine.com/emerg/topic138.htm

Roberts, M. C. (2004). Resistance to macrolide, lincosamide, streptogramin, ketolide, and oxazolidinone antibiotics. *Molecular Biotechnology, 28*(1), 47–62.

Rodriguez, A., Mendia, A., Sirvent, J., Barcenilla, F., de la Torre-Prados, M. V., Sole-Violan, et al. (2007). Combination antibiotic therapy improves survival in patients with community-acquired pneumonia and shock. *Critical Care Medicine, 35*(6), 1493–1498.

Silva, J. G., & Carvalho, I. (2007). New insights into aminoglycoside antibiotics and derivatives. *Current Medicinal Chemistry, 14*(10), 1101–1119.

Velendzas, D. G., & Dufel, S. (2007). CBRNE – Plague. *emedicine.* Retrieved July 25, 2008, from http://www.emedicine.com/emerg/TOPIC428.HTM

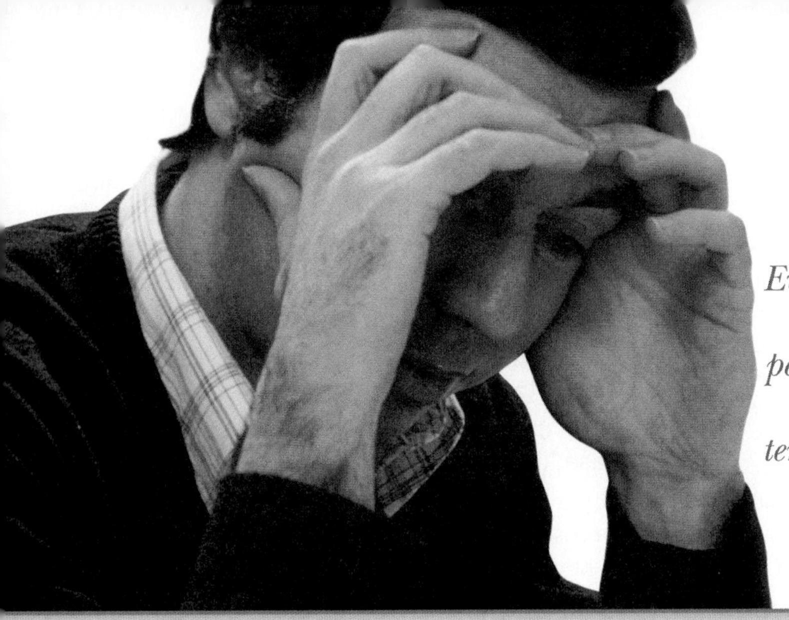

Every morning for the last month I have had terrible headaches with pain directly on my forehead. Then my upper jaw and cheeks became tender to touch and my teeth ached.

Patient "Mike Springs"

CHAPTER 50

Fluoroquinolones and Miscellaneous Antibacterials

Chapter Outline

Bacterial DNA Replication

Inhibition of DNA Replication

Fluoroquinolones

PROTOTYPE DRUG **Ciprofloxacin HCl (Cipro)** *p. 829*

Miscellaneous Antibacterials

Bacitracin

Daptomycin (Cubicin)

Metronidazole (Flagyl)

Polymyxin B

Rifampin (Rifadin)

Telithromycin (Ketek)

Learning Outcomes

After reading this chapter, the student should be able to:

1. Explain the steps in bacterial DNA replication.
2. Identify the classes of drugs that act by affecting bacterial DNA replication.
3. Explain mechanisms by which fluoroquinolones inhibit bacterial DNA replication.
4. Describe means by which bacteria become resistant to fluoroquinolones.
5. For each of the classes shown in the chapter outline, identify the prototype and representative drugs and explain the mechanism(s) of drug action, primary indications, contraindications, significant drug interactions, pregnancy category, and important adverse effects.
6. Explain the nurse's role in the safe administration of fluoroquinolones.
7. Apply the nursing process to care for patients receiving fluoroquinolones and miscellaneous antibacterials.

Key Terms

cyclic lipopeptides, 832
DNA gyrase (topoisomerase II), 826
DNA helicase, 826
DNA polymerase, 826
ketolides, 833
supercoil, 826
topoisomerase IV, 826

With resistance to other antibacterials developing rapidly, drugs in the fluoroquinolone class have become important in the pharmacotherapy of infectious diseases. Fluoroquinolones are bacteriocidal and are effective against many gram-positive and gram-negative microbes. They affect bacterial deoxyribonucleic acid (DNA) synthesis, and are particularly useful in the management of respiratory, genitourinary, and gastrointestinal (GI) infections.

Bacterial DNA Replication

50.1 Bacterial DNA replication requires several different enzymes to uncoil, unwind, and duplicate the DNA.

Under optimal conditions, many pathogenic bacteria can divide every 1 to 3 hours. Under highly favorable conditions, *Escherichia coli* divides every 20 minutes, producing a billion cells in only 10 hours. The most critical step in bacterial reproduction is duplicating the DNA so that each daughter cell contains the same genetic material. Thus, bacteria are in the process of continuously replicating their DNA, as well as constructing cell walls (see Chapter 48) and synthesizing proteins (see Chapter 49).

Like human DNA, bacterial DNA uses the four bases, adenine, guanine, cytosine, and thymidine, and is arranged in a double-helical formation. Most bacteria, however, contain a single circular chromosome as illustrated in Figure 50.1. The helix is then twisted and coiled. This highly twisted arrangement is called a **supercoil.** Immediately prior to replicating its DNA, this supercoil must be relaxed and the two helices unwound so duplication enzymes can reach the bases.

A large number of enzymes are needed for DNA replication, and some of these enzymes are targets for antibiotics. This is a complex process but may be simplified in four steps. The enzymes involved in this four-step process afford different sites at which drugs may act.

1. Relax: Supercoil is "relaxed" by the enzyme **DNA gyrase** (also called **topoisomerase II**).
2. Unwind: After the supercoil is relaxed, the enzyme **DNA helicase** "unwinds" the two strands.
3. Replicate: The enzyme **DNA polymerase** adds the precursor bases to "replicate" the original DNA and form new DNA strands.
4. Migrate: The two newly formed strands are interlocked until the enzyme **topoisomerase IV** frees them to "migrate" to opposite sides of the cell, where they are segregated into the two daughter cells.

Inhibition of DNA Replication

50.2 Drugs have been discovered that inhibit different steps in bacterial DNA replication.

Blocking the DNA replication of a pathogen is a common mechanism used by drugs across several different therapeutic classes. There are three basic ways that drugs can block bacterial DNA replication.

- Drugs can inhibit the synthesis or availability of precursor bases or nucleotides.
- Drugs can interact with or bind to DNA, preventing the uncoiling or relaxation process.
- Drugs can bind to enzymes of DNA replication, halting the formation of new DNA strands.

A number of drugs employed in cancer chemotherapy act by mimicking precursor molecules or by interacting with DNA.

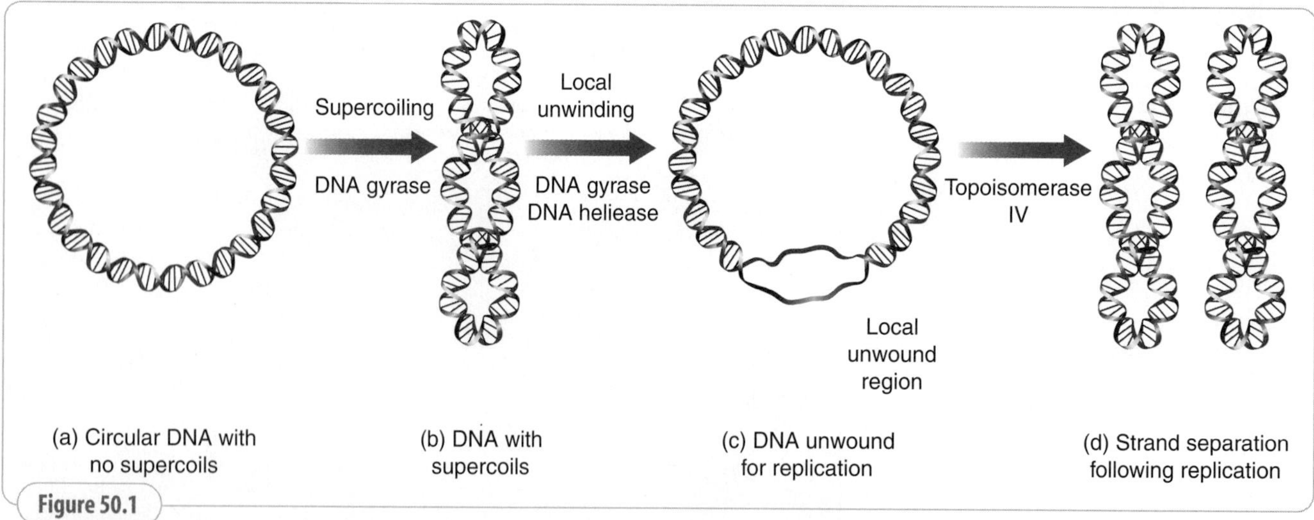

Figure 50.1

Bacterial DNA.

Cytarabine (Cytosar) and fluorouracil (5-FU) resemble nucleotides and are mistakenly incorporated into newly formed DNA strands. Daunorubicin (Cerubidine) and bleomycin are highly toxic antibiotics that interact with DNA to physically block replication. Although classified as antibiotics, these agents are too toxic to be used for infections, but have therapeutic indications in the chemotherapy of specific types of cancer. Antineoplastic drugs are discussed in Chapter 57.

Several drugs act by inhibiting enzymes involved in DNA replication. Acyclovir (Zovirax) inhibits the DNA polymerase of herpesvirus, and is a leading drug for treating this infection (see Chapter 54). Teniposide (Vumon) and etoposide (VePesid) are antineoplastic agents that act by inhibiting topoisomerase I, an enzyme that helps repair DNA damage. By binding in a complex with topoisomerase and DNA, these antineoplastics cause strand breaks that accumulate and permanently damage the DNA.

The fluoroquinolone antibiotics act on two enzymes in the DNA replication process. First, they bind to DNA gyrase, inhibiting its ability to relax the supercoiling of the bacterial DNA. When the replication enzymes reach an area still in a supercoiled state, replication terminates. A second mechanism is binding to topoisomerase IV. When this occurs, the two daughter DNA strands cannot migrate to opposite sides of the cell, and division cannot be completed. It is thought that fluoroquinolones inhibit DNA gyrase in gram-negative organisms, and inhibit topoisomerase IV in gram-positive organisms. However, this is likely an oversimplification of their exact mechanism. These drugs have no effect on human enzymes involved in DNA replication because of significant differences in the chemical structures of the human and bacterial enzymes. These differences account for their selective toxicity on bacteria, and their favorable safety profile.

Fluoroquinolones

50.3 Fluoroquinolones are antibiotics whose therapeutic applications have expanded in recent years to treat many gram-positive and gram-negative infections.

The first drug in this class, nalidixic acid (NegGram), was approved in 1962. Classified as a quinolone, the use of nalidixic acid was restricted to treating urinary tract infections (UTIs) due to its narrow spectrum of activity and a high incidence of bacterial resistance. Nalidixic acid is still used for the pharmacotherapy of UTIs, although it is not a drug of first choice. Nalidixic acid is important because it served as a "building block" for the synthesis of other drugs in this class.

In the late 1980s, the development of quinolones with a fluorine side chain resulted in drugs with wider spectrums of activity, and longer durations of action. The fluoroquinolones, shown in Table 50.1, have become an increasingly important class of antibiotics in the past two decades. Fluoroquinolones are bacteriocidal and affect bacterial DNA synthesis by inhibiting both DNA gyrase and topoisomerase IV.

Four generations of fluoroquinolones are available, based on their antibacterial spectrums. All fluoroquinolones have activity against gram-negative pathogens: The newer drugs are significantly more effective against gram-positive bacteria. The distinctions among the generations are shown in Table 50.2. The newer fluoroquinolones were developed and approved primarily for the treatment of respiratory infections.

Clinical applications of fluoroquinolones include infections of the respiratory, GI, and genitourinary tracts, and some skin and soft tissue infections. Their effectiveness against gram-negative organisms makes them drugs of choice in the

TABLE 50.1 Fluoroquinolones and Quinolones

Drug	Route and Adult Dose (maximum dose where indicated)	Adverse Effects
First Generation		
cinoxacin (Cinobac)	PO: 250–500 mg bid-qid	*Nausea, diarrhea, vomiting, rash, restlessness, pain and inflammation at injection site, local burning, stinging, corneal irritation (ophthalmic)*
nalidixic acid (NegGram)	PO: Acute therapy: 1 g qid PO: Chronic therapy: 500 mg qid	Anaphylaxis, tendon rupture, superinfections, photosensitivity, pseudomembranous colitis, seizure, peripheral neuropathy, hepatotoxicity
Second Generation		
ciprofloxacin (Cipro, Septra)	PO: 250–750 mg bid (max: 1,500 mg/day)	
norfloxacin (Noroxin)	PO: 400 mg bid or 800 mg once daily	
ofloxacin (Floxin)	PO/IV: 200–400 mg bid (max: 800 mg/day)	
Third Generation		
gatifloxacin (Zymar)	Drops (0.3% ophthalmic solution): One drop in each affected eye every 2–4 h	
levofloxacin (Levaquin)	PO/IV: 250–750 mg/day (max: 750 mg/day)	
Fourth Generation		
gemifloxacin (Factive)	PO: 320 mg/day (max: 320 mg/day)	
moxifloxacin (Avelox)	PO/IV: 400 mg/day once daily (max: 400 mg/day)	

Note: *Italics* indicate common adverse effects. Underline indicates serious adverse effects.

TABLE 50.2 Generations of Fluoroquinolones

Generation	Examples	Route of Administration	Spectrum of Activity	Indications
First generation	nalidixic acid, cinoxacin	Oral route	*Enterobacteriaceae*	Uncomplicated UTI
Second generation	ciprofloxacin	Oral and IV routes	*Enterobacteriaceae*, atypical pathogens, *P. aeruginosa*	Complicated UTI, gastroenteritis with severe diarrhea, STDs
Third generation	levofloxacin	Oral and IV routes	*Enterobacteriaceae*, atypical pathogens, some *Streptococci*	Complicated UTI, gastroenteritis with severe diarrhea, STDs, community-acquired pneumonia
Fourth generation	moxifloxacin	Oral routes	*Enterobacteriaceae*, atypical pathogens, some *Streptococci*, MRSA, anaerobes	Bacterial conjunctivitis (ophthalmic drops), acute bacterial sinusitis, exacerbations of chronic bronchitis, community-acquired pneumonia, skin and skin structure infections

treatment of uncomplicated UTIs (see Chapter 48). A newer agent, moxifloxacin (Avelox), is effective against anaerobes, a group of bacteria that are often difficult to treat. Ciprofloxacin (Cipro) is the fluoroquinolone usually selected for infections by *Pseudomonas aeruginosa.* Recent studies have suggested that some fluoroquinolones may be effective against *Mycobacterium tuberculosis*, although the U.S. Food and Drug Administration (FDA) has not approved these drugs for this indication.

Along with doxycycline, streptomycin, and penicillin, several fluoroquinolones are indicated for pathogens that could potentially be used in a bioterrorism incident. Ciprofloxacin (Cipro) is a drug of choice for postexposure prophylaxis to *Bacillus anthracis*, the causative agent of anthrax. Ciprofloxacin is also indicated for postexposure prophylaxis to other potential biologic warfare pathogens such as *Yersinia pestis* (plague), *Francisella tularensis* (tularemia), and *Brucella melitensis* (brucellosis). Details on the pharmacotherapy of bioterrorism agents are presented in Chapter 78.

Fluoroquinolones are well absorbed orally and may be administered either once or twice a day, making them ideal for outpatient therapy. The serum levels of these drugs after oral (PO) administration are nearly equivalent to the levels achieved during IV administration. This allows for a rapid, smooth transition from IV therapy to oral therapy, potentially decreasing the length of the hospital stay. Like aminoglycosides, fluoroquinolones exhibit a postantibiotic effect. Their bacteriocidal actions continue after serum levels fall to below minimum inhibitory concentrations.

Adverse Effects

In the 1990s, fluoroquinolones came into widespread use because they were well tolerated and few serious adverse effects were reported. Over time, several uncommon, although very serious, adverse effects were discovered. Since that time, almost half the fluoroquinolones approved by the FDA have been discontinued in the United States due to safety concerns.

Cartilage toxicity: Animal studies have suggested that fluoroquinolones can affect the extracellular matrix of cartilage during development, and joint toxicity has been reported in children using these drugs. Although these abnormalities ceased upon termination of antibiotic therapy, fluoroquinolones are not approved for patients under 18, and their use in children is restricted to instances where the benefits of pharmacotherapy clearly outweigh the potential risks.

Although rare, tendon abnormalities have also been reported in adults. Tendinitis and rupture of the shoulder, hand, and Achilles tendons have occurred several months after discontinuation of therapy. In 2007, the FDA approved safety labeling revisions that state patients older than 65 years are at increased risk for severe tendon disorders and that this risk is further increased by concurrent use of corticosteroids. Musculoskeletal complaints should be carefully monitored during therapy with fluoroquinolones, and patients should be advised to report unexplained joint pain.

GI toxicity: GI symptoms such as nausea, vomiting, and diarrhea occur in as many as 20% of patients taking fluoroquinolones. Although food does not affect their absorption, certain multivitamins or mineral supplements containing calcium, zinc, iron, aluminum, and magnesium can delay absorption of the antibiotic by as much as 90%. Substances containing these minerals should not be administered at the same time as fluoroquinolones.

In 2007, the FDA approved safety labeling revisions for certain antimicrobials to warn of the risk for *Clostridium difficile*–associated diarrhea. This safety labeling applied to most fluoroquinolones, as well as drugs from several other antibiotic classes.

Hypersensitivity reactions: Certainly not unique to fluoroquinolones, hypersensitivity may occur to any antibiotic. Although the FDA has always required label warnings on quinolones for the risk of hypersensitivity reactions that occur after the first dose, new labels warn of the rare risk for serious, and sometimes fatal, events after multiple doses.

Cardiotoxicity: Some of the most serious adverse effects of drugs in this class are dysrhythmias (gatifloxacin and moxifloxacin). Sparfloxacin and grepafloxacin were removed from the market due to the potential for fatal dysrhythmias. Nearly all fluoroquinolones increase the QT interval.

Central nervous system toxicity: Central nervous system (CNS) effects such as dizziness, headache, and sleep disturbances affect 1% to 8% of patients. Seizures, hallucination, high intracranial pressure, confusion, and toxic psychoses have been reported in patients taking fluoroquinolones. These drugs should be used with caution in patients with preexisting seizure disorders.

Phototoxicity: Moderate to severe phototoxicity may occur in patients exposed to direct or indirect sunlight, or to sunlamps during or following treatment with fluoroquinolones. Recovery may take several weeks.

Hepatotoxicity: Some of the fluoroquinolones elevate hepatic enzymes, which usually return to normal 1 to 2 months following completion of therapy. Trovafloxacin mesylate (Trovan) was discontinued due to an unacceptable incidence of liver damage, including severe hepatic failure.

Resistance: Like other antibiotics, resistance of bacterial species to fluoroquinolones has been increasing and can occur by means of multiple mechanisms. Mutations to DNA gyrase can alter its ability to bind fluoroquinolones, thus rendering the drug less effective. Some bacteria have developed resistance pumps that remove fluoroquinolones from inside their cells, while others have developed a cell wall structure that is less permeable to the drugs. Fluoroquinolones were drugs of choice for treating *Neisseria gonorrhoeae* from 1993–2005. Because of the large number of resistant strains, the CDC no longer recommends fluoroquinolones for the treatment of gonorrhea. Because resistance to one fluoroquinolone sometimes confers resistance to all drugs in this class, resistance is becoming a limiting factor in the clinical utility of these drugs.

PROTOTYPE DRUG Ciprofloxacin HCl (Cipro)

Classification: **Therapeutic:** Antibacterial
Pharmacologic: Bacterial DNA replication inhibitor; fluoroquinolone

Therapeutic Effects and Uses: Ciprofloxacin is a second-generation fluoroquinolone approved in 1987 that is the most widely used drug in this class. It is prescribed for UTI, sinusitis, pneumonia, skin, bone and joint infections, infectious diarrhea, gonorrhea, and certain eye infections. It is a broad-spectrum antibiotic that is more effective against gram-negative organisms. It is active against *Enterobacter, Citrobacter, E. coli, Haemophilus, Klebsiella, Proteus, Staphylococcus, Shigella, Salmonella, Neisseria,* and *Serratia.* It is poorly effective against *Streptococcus pneumoniae* and is inactive against most anaerobic bacteria. Ciprofloxacin is a drug of choice for postexposure prophylaxis of inhalational *B. anthracis* spores.

Several extended release (XR) formulations are available that permit once-daily dosing, usually for treating UTI. Cipro XR contains two different ciprofloxacin salts: ciprofloxacin hydrochloride and ciprofloxacin betaine. Approved in 2005, Proquin XR contains only the hydrochloride salt and has been formulated to cause less nausea, vomiting, and diarrhea than other formulations. Proquin XR is administered for only 3 days and is only approved for uncomplicated UTI (acute cystitis).

Mechanism of Action: By inhibiting bacterial DNA gyrase and topoisomerase, ciprofloxacin affects bacterial replication and DNA repair. Ciprofloxacin is usually considered bacteriocidal and exhibits a prolonged postantibiotic effect.

Pharmacokinetics:

Route(s)	PO, IV, ophthalmic and otic drops
Absorption	60–80% absorbed
Distribution	Widely distributed to all body fluids; crosses the placenta; secreted in breast milk; small amounts in cerebrospinal fluid (CSF); 20–40% bound to plasma proteins
Primary metabolism	Mostly unchanged; small amounts of hepatic metabolism
Primary excretion	Primarily renal; 15% by biliary route
Onset of action	Rapid
Duration of action	Half-life: 1–4 h

Adverse Effects: Ciprofloxacin is well tolerated by most patients, and serious adverse effects are uncommon. GI adverse effects, such as nausea, vomiting, and diarrhea, may occur in as many as 20% of patients taking high doses. Ciprofloxacin may be administered with food to diminish adverse GI effects. The patient should not, however, take this drug with antacids or mineral supplements, since drug absorption will be diminished. Some patients report phototoxicity, headache, and dizziness. Tendonitis and tendon rupture are rare adverse effects with ciprofloxacin. Like most antibiotics, ciprofloxacin can cause serious pseudomembranous colitis. Although rare, seizures and toxic psychosis have been reported in patients receiving fluoroquinolones.

Contraindications/Precautions: Ciprofloxacin is contraindicated in patients who are hypersensitive to fluoroquinolones, and in pregnant patients. Drug therapy must be monitored carefully in patients with suspected CNS disorders, as this drug can be neurotoxic at high doses, and can cause seizures when given by rapid IV infusion. Although prescribed for patients with UTI, the drug should be used with caution in patients with serious renal impairment, as this drug is excreted by this route and may accumulate to toxic levels.

Drug Interactions: Concurrent administration with warfarin may increase anticoagulant effects and result in bleeding due to the decreased metabolism of warfarin. Antacids containing calcium or aluminum, iron or zinc sulfate, and sucralfate decrease the absorption of ciprofloxacin, thus causing decreased effectiveness of the antibiotic. Ciprofloxacin slows the hepatic metabolism of xanthines, including caffeine, theophylline, and theobromine. Theophylline levels may increase 15% to 30%. **Herbal/Food:** Patients ingesting large quantities of caffeinated products may experience excessive nervousness, anxiety, or tachycardia. Calcium-fortified juices may interfere with absorption of the antibiotic.

Pregnancy: Category C.

Treatment of Overdose: No specific therapy is available; patients are treated symptomatically.

MyNursingKit | Mechanism of Action Animation: Ciprofloxacin

Nursing Responsibilities:

- Obtain a complete health history including allergies, drug history, and possible drug interactions.
- Perform an infection-focused physical examination including vital signs and a white blood cell (WBC) count. Determine baseline signs and symptoms that may indicate the presence of infection.
- Assess culture and sensitivity (C&S) tests (blood, urine, sputum, wound drainage, other body fluids) before starting therapy. Treatment may be implemented pending results.
- Monitor intake and output (I&O) ratio and patterns to maintain adequate hydration.
- Assess for GI irritation such as nausea, diarrhea, vomiting, or abdominal discomfort in patients receiving high dosages, and in older adults.
- Monitor coagulation studies closely, including prothrombin times (PTs), and international normalized ratio (INR) in patients receiving warfarin (Coumadin) therapy.
- Assess for signs and symptoms of superinfections such as vaginal itching or discharge, loose or foul-smelling stools, or furry overgrowth on tongue.

Patient and Family Education:

- Immediately report signs of potential allergy such as rash; itching; shortness of breath; swelling of the face, lips, or throat; or palpitations.
- Limit caffeine intake because this may cause insomnia, nervousness, and anxiety.
- Do not take any products containing magnesium or calcium (such as antacids), iron, or aluminum with this drug, or within 2 hours of this drug.
- Avoid sunlight or use sunscreen and protective clothing to prevent burns because this drug can cause photosensitivity.
- Drink 2 to 3 L of fluid per day unless contraindicated by concurrent chronic health problems such as renal disease or heart failure.
- Report sudden, unexplained joint pain.
- Contact the health care provider if the infection does not begin to improve after a few days of therapy.
- Immediately report severe or persistent diarrhea accompanied by fever. Do not attempt to treat antibiotic-related diarrhea with over-the-counter (OTC) products.
- Report nausea, vomiting, or abdominal pain or discomfort.
- Do not drive or perform other hazardous activities until the effects of the drug are known because this drug may cause drowsiness or dizziness.
- Take the drug exactly as prescribed until the prescription is completed.
- Do not breast-feed while taking this drug without approval of the health care provider.

Drugs Similar to Ciprofloxacin HCl (Cipro)

Other fluoroquinolones include gatifloxacin, gemifloxacin, levofloxacin, moxifloxacin, norfloxacin, and ofloxacin. With few exceptions, these drugs have very similar actions and adverse effects to ciprofloxacin. Enoxacin (Penetrex), lomefloxacin (Maxaquin), sparfloxacin (Zagam), and trovafloxacin (Trovan)/alatrofloxacin (Trovan IV) are drugs in this class that have been discontinued in the United States.

Gatifloxacin (Zymar): In 2006, the drug manufacturer discontinued the distribution of the oral and parenteral forms of gatifloxacin. Prior to that time, gatifloxacin was used for UTI, gonorrhea, and respiratory infections caused by organisms resistant to other fluoroquinolones. It is still available as an ophthalmic solution (Zymar) for the treatment of bacterial conjunctivitis. The most frequently reported adverse reactions after ophthalmic administration include increased lacrimation, corneal inflammation, keratitis, papillary conjunctivitis, conjunctival hemorrhage, headache, red eye, and reduced visual acuity. This drug is pregnancy category C.

Gemifloxacin (Factive): Gemifloxacin is a newer drug in this class approved in 2003 for acute bacterial exacerbations of chronic bronchitis and community-acquired pneumonia. It is primarily effective against gram-positive bacteria, most importantly *Streptococcus pneumoniae* and *Staphylococcus aureus*, than many other drugs in this class. It is only available orally. Diarrhea is the most common adverse effect. It is contraindicated in patients with certain dysrhythmias, due to its effects on cardiac conduction. Other contraindications and adverse effects are similar to those of ciprofloxacin. This drug is pregnancy category C.

Levofloxacin (Levaquin): Approved in 1996, levofloxacin is prescribed for UTI, prostatitis, gonorrhea, community-acquired pneumonia, acute sinusitis, acute bacterial exacerbations of chronic bronchitis, skin infections, and bacterial conjunctivitis. It has a long half-life that allows for once-daily dosing. The most common adverse effects are nausea and vomiting. It is available for PO, IV, and ophthalmic (Quixin, Iquix) administration. Adverse effects of ophthalmic levofloxacin include transient blurred vision, foreign body sensation, headache, burning, pharyngitis, and photophobia. Other contraindications and adverse effects are similar to those of ciprofloxacin. This drug is pregnancy category C.

Moxifloxacin (Avelox): Approved in 1999, moxifloxacin is prescribed for skin infections, community-acquired pneumonia, acute sinusitis, and acute bacterial exacerbations of chronic bronchitis. It is available by oral and IV routes, and as an ophthalmic preparation (Vigamox) for bacterial conjunctivitis. The most common adverse effects are dizziness, diarrhea, nausea, and vomiting. Like gemifloxacin, it is contraindicated in patients with certain dysrhythmias, due to its effects on cardiac conduction. This drug is pregnancy category C.

Norfloxacin (Noroxin): Norfloxacin was approved in 1986 and is indicated for UTI and gonorrhea. It has the shortest half-life of all fluoroquinolones and is available only by the PO route. The most common adverse effects are dizziness, nausea, and vomiting. Other contraindications and adverse effects are similar to those of ciprofloxacin. An ophthalmic solution once used for bacterial conjunctivitis is no longer available in the United States. This drug is pregnancy category C.

Ofloxacin (Floxin): Approved in 1990, ofloxacin is indicated for UTI, gonorrhea, lower respiratory tract infections, skin infections, superficial ocular infections (Ocuflox), and otitis media (Floxin Otic). The most common adverse effects are insomnia, nausea, and vomiting. The otic preparation can cause otic pruritus. Other contraindications and adverse effects are similar to those of ciprofloxacin. It is available for the PO, IV, ophthalmic, and otic routes. This drug is pregnancy category C.

NURSING PROCESS APPLICATION

Patients Receiving Fluoroquinolones

Assessment	Potential Nursing Diagnoses
Prior to administration: • Obtain a complete health history including allergies, drug history, and possible drug interactions. • Obtain specimens for C&S before initiating therapy. • Perform infection-focused physical examination including vital signs and WBC count.	• *Risk for Infection* • *Risk for Injury*, related to adverse effects of drug • *Deficient Knowledge (Infection)*, related to disease process, transmission, and drug therapy • *Diarrhea*, related to effects of drug therapy • *Noncompliance (Antimicrobial Therapy)*, related to therapeutic regimen

Planning: Patient Goals and Expected Outcomes

The patient will:

- Report reductions in symptoms related to the diagnosed infection, and have negative results for laboratory and diagnostic tests for the presenting infection.
- Demonstrate an understanding of the drug's action by accurately describing drug adverse effects and precautions.
- Immediately report significant adverse effects such as shortness of breath, swelling, fever, stomatitis, loose stools, vaginal discharge, or cough.
- Complete the full course of antibiotic therapy and comply with follow-up care.

Implementation

Interventions and (Rationales)	Patient and Family Education
• Monitor vital signs and symptoms of infection to determine antibacterial effectiveness. (Another drug or different dosage may be required.)	• Instruct the patient to notify the health care provider if symptoms persist or worsen.
• Monitor for a hypersensitivity reaction. (An immediate hypersensitivity reaction may occur within 2 to 30 minutes; an accelerated reaction may occur in 1 to 72 hours; and a delayed reaction may occur after 72 hours.)	• Instruct the patient to discontinue the medication and inform the health care provider if symptoms of hypersensitivity reaction develop such as wheezing; shortness of breath; swelling of face, tongue, or hands; and itching or rash.
• Monitor for severe diarrhea. (The condition may occur due to superinfection or the possible adverse effect of antibiotic-associated pseudomembranous colitis.)	Instruct the patient to: • Consult the health care provider before taking antidiarrheal drugs, which could cause retention of harmful bacteria. • Consume cultured dairy products with live active cultures, such as kefir, yogurt, or buttermilk, to help maintain normal intestinal flora.
• Administer drug around the clock. (This is necessary to maintain effective blood levels.)	Instruct the patient to: • Take medication on schedule. • Complete the entire prescription even if feeling better, to prevent the development of resistant bacteria.
• Monitor for superinfection, especially in elderly, debilitated, or immunosuppressed patients. (There is an increased risk for superinfections due to elimination of normal flora.)	• Instruct the patient to report signs and symptoms of superinfection such as fever; black hairy tongue; stomatitis; loose, foul-smelling stools; vaginal discharge; or cough.
• Monitor intake of OTC products. (Antacids, dairy products, sucralfate, or vitamin or mineral supplements that contain calcium, iron, or zinc can decrease effects of medication.)	• Advise the patient to consult with the health care provider before using OTC medications or herbal products. • Instruct the patient to administer these substances and medications 2 hours after ciprofloxacin.
• Administer with water and maintain adequate fluid intake. • Monitor I&O. (The drug is excreted by the renal route.)	• Instruct the patient to take each dose with a glass of water and drink several extra glasses of fluid daily.
• Monitor the IV site for signs and symptoms of tissue irritation, severe pain, and extravasation.	• Instruct the patient to immediately report pain or other symptoms of discomfort during intravenous infusion.
• Monitor for adverse effects specific to various antibiotic therapies. (The most serious adverse effects are dysrhythmias [sparfloxacin, gatifloxacin, and moxifloxacin], and liver failure [trovafloxacin].)	• Instruct the patient to report adverse effects specific to the prescribed antibiotic therapy.
• Monitor the patient for adherence to antibiotic therapy. (Patients may stop taking the medication early if feeling better.)	Instruct the patient on the importance of: • Completing the prescription as ordered. • Follow-up care after antibiotic therapy is completed.

Evaluation of Outcome Criteria

Evaluate the effectiveness of drug therapy by confirming that patient goals and expected outcomes have been met (see "Planning").

PharmFACT

In a recent study, *E. coli* culture isolates were examined for resistance to fluoroquinolones. In 2002, 22% of cultures were resistant. In 2005, the percentage of resistant cultures almost doubled to 41%. *Source:* Gerboc, Metro, Ginsberg, & Harkaway, 2008.

Miscellaneous Antibacterials

50.4 A number of miscellaneous antibacterials have specific clinical indications.

Several drugs act by miscellaneous mechanisms, or are the only drugs in their class. Doses for the miscellaneous agents are listed in Table 50.3.

Bacitracin: Bacitracin is an older antibiotic, approved in 1948, that acts by inhibiting cell wall synthesis. It is combined with polymyxin B in OTC first aid products (Neosporin, Polysporin), and is also available as monotherapy in OTC products such as Bacitracin First Aid. It is effective against a variety of gram-positive and a few gram-negative microbes. Although an intramuscular (IM) form is available, bacitracin is almost always used topically due to potential nephrotoxicity. In addition to creams and ointments, bacitracin solutions may be used to soak compresses that can be applied to large areas of the skin. This drug is pregnancy category C.

Daptomycin (Cubicin): Approved in 2003, daptomycin belongs to a new class of antibiotics, the **cyclic lipopeptides.** The spectrum of activity of daptomycin includes a wide variety of gram-positive pathogens. It is indicated for the treatment of complicated skin infections caused by organisms such as *S. aureus*, including methicillin-resistant *S. aureus* (MRSA), *Streptococcus pyogenes*, and *Enterococcus faecalis* (vancomycin-susceptible strains only). Daptomycin is bacteriocidal and its mechanism of action is clearly distinct from any other antibiotic. When binding to bacterial membranes, daptomycin causes a rapid depolarization of membrane potential, leading to inhibition of protein, DNA, and ribonucleic acid (RNA) synthesis. It is given only by IV infusion. Because this drug is new, resistance is not yet a clinical problem. Myopathy has been recorded in a small percentage of patients taking daptomycin. Therefore, the nurse should carefully monitor for muscle pain or weakness. The drug should be withheld if the creatine phosphokinase (CPK) becomes elevated above 1,000 units/L. This drug is pregnancy category B.

Metronidazole (Flagyl): Metronidazole is another older anti-infective, approved in 1963, that is effective against a large number of anaerobes. It acts by interfering with the energy metabolism of pathogens. Metronidazole is one of only a few drugs that have dual activity against both bacteria and multicellular parasites. It is a drug of choice for trichomoniasis, giardiasis, and amebiasis. Unlike most antibiotics, resistance to metronidazole is uncommon. When given orally, adverse effects are generally minor, and include nausea, dry mouth, and headache. High doses can produce neurotoxicity.

As an antibacterial, metronidazole has two indications: serious infections due to anaerobic bacteria, and peptic ulcer disease. Few antibacterials are effective against anaerobes because the organisms reside in sites that have tissue destruction and a poor blood supply. Anaerobic bacteria are common causes of

TABLE 50.3 Miscellaneous Antibacterials

Drug	Route and Adult Dose (maximum dose where indicated)	Adverse Effects
bacitracin	Topical: Apply thin layer of ointment bid or tid or as solution of 250–1,000 units/mL in wet dressing	*Anorexia, nausea, vomiting* <u>Nephrotoxicity, anaphylaxis</u>
daptomycin (Cubicin)	IV: 4–6 mg/kg once every 24 h for 7–14 days	*Nausea, diarrhea, constipation, headache* <u>Anaphylaxis, superinfections, renal failure, myopathy, jaundice, pseudomembranous colitis</u>
metronidazole (Flagyl)	Anaerobic Infections: PO: 7.5 mg/kg every 6 h (max: 4 g/day) IV loading dose: 15 mg/kg IV maintenance dose: 7.5 mg/kg every 6 h (max: 4 g/day)	*Dizziness, headache, anorexia, abdominal pain, metallic taste and nausea, Candida infections* <u>Seizures, peripheral neuropathy, leucopenia</u>
polymyxin B	IV: 15,000–25,000 units/kg/day divided every 12 h IM: 25,000–30,000 units/kg/day divided every 4–6 h	*Urticaria* <u>Nephrotoxicity, neurotoxicity (confusion, blurred vision, paresthesias, paralysis), superinfections</u>
rifampin (Rifadin, Rimactane)	PO/IV: 600 mg/day	*Nausea, vomiting, heartburn, anorexia, diarrhea, orange discoloration of the urine, sweat, and tears* <u>Pseudomembranous colitis, acute renal failure, hepatotoxicity, blood dyscrasias</u>
telithromycin (Ketek)	PO: 800 mg once daily	*Nausea, diarrhea, dizziness, headache* <u>Superinfections, pseudomembranous colitis, hepatotoxicity, dysrhythmias, respiratory failure</u>

Note: *Italics* indicate common adverse effects. <u>Underline</u> indicates serious adverse effects.

abscesses, gangrene, diabetic skin ulcers, and deep wound infections. Serious intra-abdominal infections or septicemia due to *Bacteroides, Clostridium,* and *Streptococci* often respond well to IV infusions of the drug. Metronidazole has found a relatively new use in the treatment of *Helicobacter pylori* infections of the stomach associated with peptic ulcer disease. Metronidazole is featured as a prototype drug in Chapter 54. This drug is pregnancy category B.

Polymyxin B: Approved in 1951, polymyxin B is an older, bacteriocidal drug that acts by disrupting the bacterial cell membrane. The drug is able to penetrate the phospholipid layer, make the membrane leaky, and cause the death of the bacterium. Although parenteral formulations are available, polymyxin B is rarely prescribed by these routes due to potential nephrotoxicity and neurotoxicity. Its primary application is in the treatment of topical infections of the skin, mucous membranes, or eye, caused by gram-negative organisms. It is not effective against gram-positive microbes. It is combined with bacitracin and neomycin in common OTC first aid products such as Neosporin Ointment, Bactine Antibiotic, and Polysporin. Topical application, including to denuded skin, results in negligible systemic absorption. Polymyxin B is combined with neomycin and hydrocortisone in prescription otic preparations. Topical polymyxin B is pregnancy category B.

Rifampin (Rifadin, Rimactane): Approved in 1958, rifampin is administered PO or IV, and is usually associated with the pharmacotherapy of tuberculosis. The drug, however, is effective against a wide range of both gram-positive and gram-negative organisms. As an antibacterial, it is used for prophylaxis in contacts of patients with *Haemophilus influenzae* type B and for the prophylaxis of asymptomatic carriers of meningococcal disease. Occasionally, it is used for Legionnaire's disease, or when therapy with other antibiotics is unsuccessful. The reason its applications are limited is because of the rapid development of resistance, which can appear after only a few days of therapy. A flulike syndrome develops in about half the patients receiving the drug. Rifampin acts by inhibiting bacterial RNA polymerase, the enzyme that makes bacterial RNA. The use of rifampin in the pharmacotherapy of mycobacterial infections is presented in Chapter 52. This drug is pregnancy category C.

Telithromycin (Ketek). In 2004, the FDA approved telithromycin for respiratory infections, the first in a novel class of antibiotics known as the **ketolides.** Telithromycin blocks bacterial protein synthesis by binding to two different sites on the 50S ribosomal subunit. Telithromycin is an oral drug, with the most common adverse effects being diarrhea, nausea, and headache. Originally, its indications included acute bacterial exacerbation of chronic bronchitis due to *S. pneumoniae, H. influenzae,* or *Moraxella catarrhalis*; acute bacterial sinusitis due to *S. pneumoniae, H. influenzae, M. catarrhalis,* or *S. aureus*; and community-acquired pneumonia due to *S. pneumoniae.* Post–market surveillance, however, discovered several cases of hepatic failure in patients receiving this drug. Because of the seriousness of these adverse events, the FDA considered the risks higher than the benefits and withdrew its approval for treating acute bacterial sinusitis and acute bacterial exacerbations of chronic bronchitis. Hepatic function tests must be monitored during therapy. Because of its recent approval, resistance is not yet a clinical problem. This drug is pregnancy category C.

CONNECTION *Checkpoint* 50.1

Some OTC first-aid products contain hydrocortisone. From Chapter 44, what is the expected therapeutic effect of this drug in these OTC products? See Answer to Connection Checkpoint 50.1 in Appendix A.

CONNECTIONS

Patient Safety

Levofloxacin (Levaquin)

Yesterday, Mrs. Rackey received the first dose of IV levofloxacin (Levaquin). While receiving the medication, she reported itching and a slight swelling of the tongue and lips (angioedema). However, later that day she had no discomfort or presence of the previous symptoms. She will receive the second dose of the medication again this morning. What should the nurse do?

See Answers to Patient Safety Questions in Appendix A.

UNDERSTANDING THE CHAPTER

Key Concepts Summary

50.1 Bacterial DNA replication requires several different enzymes to uncoil, unwind, and duplicate the DNA.

50.2 Drugs have been discovered that inhibit different steps in bacterial DNA replication.

50.3 Fluoroquinolones are antibiotics whose therapeutic applications have expanded in recent years to treat many gram-positive and gram-negative infections.

50.4 A number of miscellaneous antibacterials have specific clinical indications.

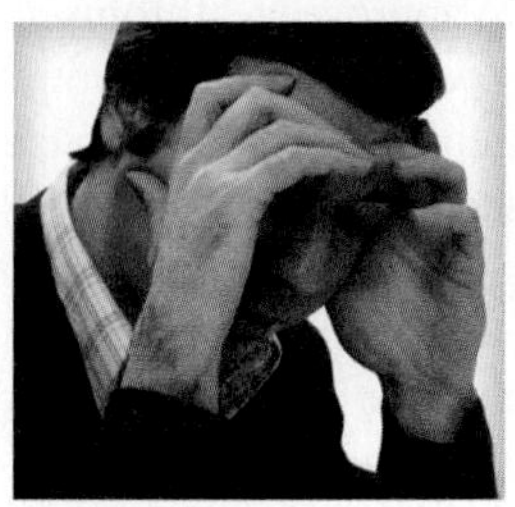

Making the PATIENT *Connection*

Remember the patient "Mike Springs" at the beginning of the chapter? Now read the remainder of the case study. Based on the information presented within this chapter, respond to the critical thinking questions that follow.

Mike Springs presents to the local health clinic. He is a 38-year-old male who has no history of chronic illness. His vital signs are normal with the exception of a slight increase in body temperature, 37.3°C (99.2°F). He denies shortness of breath. However, his nasal passages are congested, causing him to "mouth breathe." Mike is busy with work and family responsibilities. Until this most recent illness, he had started efforts toward a healthier lifestyle and weight reduction. Mike is now jogging for exercise and taking vitamin tablets. He is diagnosed with acute sinusitis and the health care provider orders ciprofloxacin PO 500 mg twice daily for 10 days. Additional medications prescribed include a nasal decongestant and a mild analgesic.

As Mike is leaving the health clinic, he comments that he is responsible for multiple corporate offices and will soon be traveling. He is worried about remembering to take the medication and admits to a history of nonadherence with medication regimens, as he sometimes forgets to take medications.

Critical Thinking Questions

1. Prepare a patient teaching handout for Mike that provides him with information about the antibiotics he is being prescribed.
2. Mike asks you, the nurse, if he should continue jogging and taking vitamins. What would you advise?
3. What tips can you provide someone who forgets to take scheduled medication?

Case Study

Carolyn Ijams is doing her spring cleaning. As she is arranging the content in her medicine cabinet, she notices that there are two tubes of antibiotic ointment. One of the agents is polymyxin B and the other is bacitracin. She read on the Internet that polymyxin can damage the kidney, and because she has had several kidney infections in her life, she is concerned. Approximately half of the content of both tubes has been previously used and Carolyn only has room for one tube.

1. Which antibiotic should she keep? Why?
2. How would you respond to her concerns about polymyxin?

NCLEX-RN® Review

1 The client is prescribed ciprofloxacin (Cipro) and instructed to take each dose of medication on a prescribed time schedule. The nurse recognizes that this instruction is essential because:

1. The medication can cause sleep pattern disturbances.
2. Pathogenic bacteria have extremely rapid growth and reproduction rates.
3. Superinfections may develop if a dose of the medication is missed.
4. Allergic reactions are more likely to occur if a dose is missed.

2 The most important goal of nursing care for a client receiving polymyxin B ointment on a laceration is to:

1. Promote wound healing.
2. Sterilize the skin and mucous membranes.
3. Prevent allergic reaction.
4. Maximize pain relief.

3 A hospitalized patient, who has experienced a sudden onset of diarrhea, is prescribed metronidazole (Flagyl). The nurse knows that the reason this medication is prescribed is because it:

1. Decreases gastric motility and reduces the diarrhea.
2. Has a dual action against both bacteria and multicellular parasites.
3. Reduces diarrhea stool by stimulating the release of peptase.
4. Aids in the fecal elimination of toxic bacteria.

4 A client has been receiving ciprofloxacin (Cipro) for septicemia for 2 weeks and is now ready for discharge. Which discharge instruction would be most appropriate for the nurse to give?

1. Do not take this drug with antacids or any mineral supplements.
2. Report any shortness of breath to your health care provider immediately.
3. Exposure to direct sunlight will help increase absorption of this medication.
4. Limit your fluid intake to less than 1,500 mL per day.

5 Prior to administration, the client asks the nurse how telithromycin (Ketek) works in treating a lower respiratory tract infection. Which nurse response would be correct?

1. "Ketek blocks bacterial protein synthesis by binding to two different sites on the 50S ribosomal subunit."
2. "Ketek alters the DNA of bacteria, rendering the microorganism inactive."
3. "Ketek decreases bacterial folic acid synthesis, stopping the growth of the microorganisms."
4. "Ketek inhibits the protein synthesis of the bacterial cell wall and stops the growth of the microorganism."

6 The client is prescribed fluoroquinolone therapy. The nurse knows that this classification of drugs should be used with caution, or not used at all, in which clients? (Select all that apply.)

1. Clients with serious renal impairment
2. Clients with suspected central nervous system disorders
3. Clients who are pregnant
4. Clients over 65 years old
5. Clients who have anxiety

See Answers to Critical Thinking Questions, Case Study, and NCLEX-RN® Review in Appendix A.

References

Bradbury, B. J., & Pucci, M. J. (2008). Recent advances in bacterial topoisomerase inhibitors. *Current Opinion in Pharmacology, 8*(3), 132–145.

Deshpande, A., Pant, C., Jain, A., Fraser, T. G., & Rolston, D. (2008). Do fluoroquinolones predispose patients to Clostridium difficile associated disease? A review of the evidence. *Current Medical Research and Opinion, 24*(2), 329–333.

Gerboc, J., Metro, M., Ginsberg, P., & Harkaway, R. (2008). *Rapidly developing fluoroquinolone resistance of common uropathogens.* Paper presented at the annual meeting of the American Urological Association, Orlando, FL.

Henderson, D. A., Inglesby, T. V., & O'Toole, T. (2002). *Bioterrorism: Guidelines for medical and public health management.* Chicago: American Medical Association.

Mehlhorn, A. J., & Brown, D. A. (2007). Safety concerns with fluoroquinolones. *The Annals of Pharmacotherapy, 41*(11), 1859–1866.

Owens, R. C., & Ambrose, P. G. (2005). Antimicrobial safety: Focus on fluoroquinolones. *Clinical Infectious Diseases, 41*(2), S144–S157.

Vaughan, D. J., Tillotson, G. S., & Klugman, K. P. (2007). Streptococcus pneumoniae: Review of factors relevant to development and management of fluoroquinolone resistance in a nursing home setting. *Infectious Diseases in Clinical Practice, 15*(2), 92–99.

Yap, R. L., & Schaeffer, A. J. (2004). *Fluoroquinolones: A review and their expanding role in urinary tract infections.* Infectious Disease Infoalert, 19. Tokyo, Japan: Biomedis International LTD.

Zhanel, G., Fontaine, S., Adam, H., Schurek, K., Mayer, M., Noreddin, A., et al. (2006). A review of new fluoroquinolones: Focus on their use in respiratory tract infections. *Treatments in Respiratory Medicine, 5*(6), 437–465.

C H A P T E R

It seems that I have been sick all winter. Yesterday, when I began having a fever, I took some antibiotic tablets that a doctor prescribed when I was sick last month. I'm sure glad I didn't take all of the prescription and had some of the pills left to take.

Patient "Sandra Phillipi"

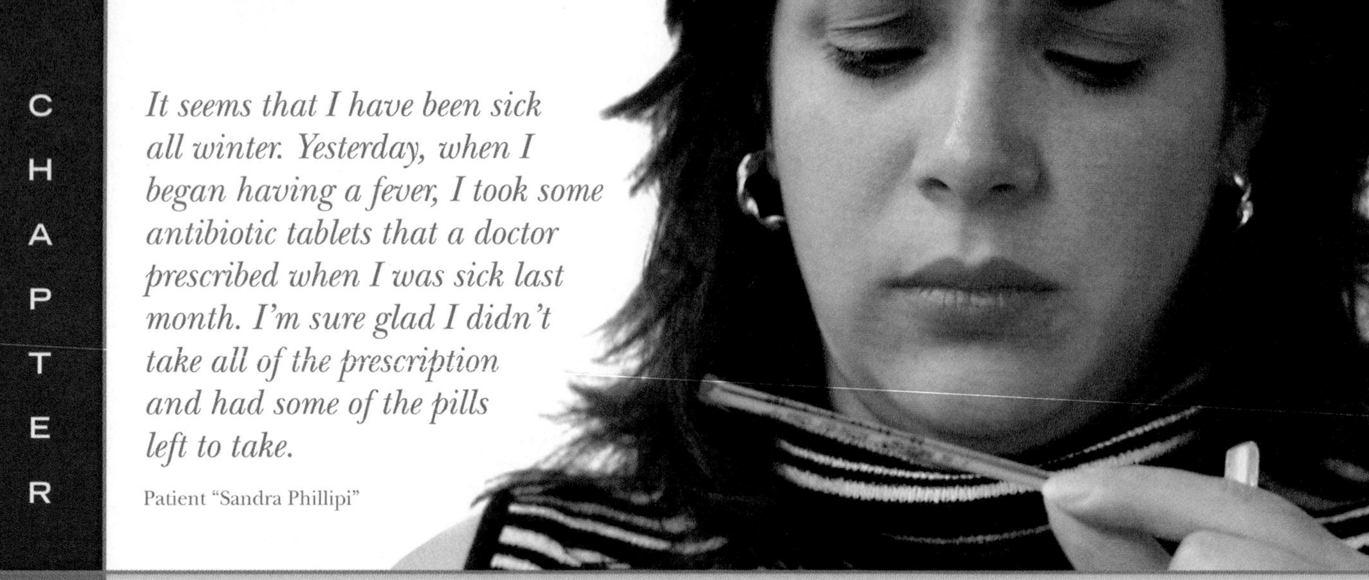

51 Sulfonamides and the Pharmacotherapy of Urinary Tract Infections

Learning Outcomes

After reading this chapter, the student should be able to:

1. Classify types of urinary tract infections based on their anatomic location.
2. Explain the epidemiology and pathogenesis of urinary tract infections.
3. Compare and contrast the pharmacotherapy of complicated versus uncomplicated urinary tract infections.
4. Identify the classes of antibiotics used to treat urinary tract infections.
5. Describe modifications in the pharmacotherapy of urinary tract infections for infants and children, pregnancy, older adults, and those with recurring infections.
6. Explain why folate inhibitors exert selective toxicity toward bacterial cells.
7. For each of the classes shown in the Chapter Outline, identify the prototype and representative drugs and explain the mechanism(s) of drug action, primary indications, contraindications, significant drug interactions, pregnancy category, and important adverse effects.
8. Apply the nursing process to care for patients receiving drugs for urinary tract infections.

Chapter Outline

Pathophysiology of Urinary Tract Infections

Pharmacotherapy of Urinary Tract Infections

Sulfonamides

PROTOTYPE DRUG **Trimethoprim-Sulfamethoxazole (Bactrim, Septra)** *p. 842*

Urinary Antiseptics

PROTOTYPE DRUG **Nitrofurantoin (Furadantin) and Nitrofurantoin Macrocrystals (Macrobid, Macrodantin)** *p. 846*

It is estimated that urinary tract infections (UTIs) account for 8 million office visits and 100,000 hospitalizations per year, making them the most common types of bacterial infections. Although antimicrobial therapy of these infections is often straightforward, UTI is becoming a major clinical challenge in this era of increasing antibiotic resistance. This chapter examines the types of patients most likely to acquire a UTI, and the anti-infective therapy that is most effective against this disease.

Key Terms

- **bacteriuria**, *837*
- **crystalluria**, *842*
- **cystitis**, *837*
- **folic acid**, *841*
- **irritative voiding symptoms**, *837*
- **para-aminobenzoic acid**, *841*
- **prostatitis**, *837*
- **pyelonephritis**, *837*
- **urethritis**, *837*
- **uropathogen**, *837*

> **PharmFACT**
>
> **Fungal urinary infection most commonly occurs in patients who are diabetic, have indwelling urethral catheters, or have received broad-spectrum antimicrobial therapy. *Candida albicans* is the most common isolate.** *Source:* Nicolle, 2005.

Pathophysiology of Urinary Tract Infections

51.1 Infections can occur in any portion of the urinary tract.

The urinary tract consists of the kidneys, ureters, urinary bladder, and urethra. The male and female urinary tracts are identical, with the exception of the urethra, which is shorter in the female and in closer proximity to the anus. This anatomic difference results in the periurethral region of the female being populated by bacteria, normally restricted to the gastrointestinal (GI) tract, that could cause urinary infections. In addition to the male having a longer urethra, the scrotum provides a physical barrier between the urethra and the anus. These anatomic differences result in a higher risk of UTI in females.

The natural, continuous flow of urine from the kidneys, down the ureters, into the bladder, and voiding through the urethra provides a formidable barrier to microorganisms or **uropathogens** attempting to invade the urinary system. Although it is indeed difficult for uropathogens to "go against the flow" and reach beyond the proximal portion of the urethra, this is the means by which the large majority of UTIs are acquired. Infections that travel from the urethra to the bladder or kidney are known as retrograde or ascending infections. The most successful uropathogens are those that secrete "sticky" adhesions, or have structures called fimbriae, that allow them to adhere to the epithelial lining of the urinary tract. Occasionally, pathogens traveling through the blood can infect the kidney. This mode of infection is called the hematogenous route, and is responsible for only 5% of all UTIs.

Any portion of the urinary tract may be infected by uropathogens. Infection of the urethra, or **urethritis,** presents as discomfort during voiding, and occurs in both men and women. It is usually distinguished from a bladder infection, or **cystitis,** because it causes less voiding urgency than cystitis and has a more gradual onset of symptoms. Urethritis is often a sign of a sexually transmitted infection.

A cluster of complaints known as **irritative voiding symptoms** accompanies cystitis. Occurring in both men and women, symptoms include dysuria, and increased voiding urgency and frequency. Despite the increased urgency and frequency, only small volumes of urine are voided during each attempt. During and immediately following voiding, burning or aching may occur. The patient may have suprapubic tenderness upon palpation. Urinalysis usually identifies the presence of an offending uropathogen, or **bacteriuria,** as well as other signs of infection such as pyuria, hematuria, and changes in urine pH, nitrites, or proteins.

In females, symptoms of cystitis are frequently reported following intercourse with a new sexual partner. In males, cystitis is likely to occur following anal intercourse. Cystitis in males may be accompanied by acute **prostatitis.** Normally recognized by palpating the prostate, which will be tender during manual examination, prostatitis may include fever and has the potential to cause urinary obstruction as the prostate swells.

Bacteria that ascend the ureter and reach the kidney can cause **pyelonephritis,** an inflammation of the kidney, pelvis, and other renal cells. Irritative voiding symptoms occur, along with other signs similar to cystitis. More severe symptoms are manifested as nausea, vomiting, fever, chills, and acute costovertebral angle and flank tenderness. Acute pyelonephritis may lead to shock, and may require aggressive anti-infective therapy.

Pharmacotherapy of Urinary Tract Infections

51.2 Choice of pharmacotherapy for acute urinary tract infection depends upon the severity of the infection and the presence of comorbid conditions.

In addition to describing UTIs by their location, these infections may also be classified as complicated or uncomplicated. These

> CONNECTIONS
>
> **To the Community**
>
> **Vaccines to Prevent Urinary Tract Infection**
>
> Scientists have discovered that some women and children lack specific immunoglobulins within the urinary system that fight invading microorganisms. The development of a vaccine to prevent recurrent UTIs has appeared on the "scientific horizon."
>
> Initial studies suggest that these vaccines allow patients to build their own natural defense mechanism. The dead bacteria in the vaccine prompt the body to produce antibodies that can later fight against live organisms. Investigators are piloting both injected and oral vaccines to see which works best. Another route under consideration for this vaccine is a vaginal suppository.

are important distinctions, because the pharmacotherapy for complicated UTI and uncomplicated UTI are quite different.

Acute Uncomplicated Cystitis

Acute uncomplicated cystitis (AUC) occurs in patients who have no serious or chronic health disorders that might impact the spread of the uropathogen or the treatment of the UTI. These infections occur mostly in women of reproductive age, with the highest incidence from 18 to 24 years of age. Adult males rarely have AUC. Common risk factors for AUC include the following:

- Frequent sexual activity
- Use of spermicides for contraception
- Use of a diaphragm for contraception
- Estrogen deficiency

In many cases, a diagnosis of AUC is made by the health care provider based on symptoms and history alone, without additional serologic or urinary testing. Rapid dipstick tests are available to examine for the presence of infection. Women who have experienced a prior AUC are often able to self-diagnose. *Escherichia coli* is the most common causative agent for AUC, responsible for 80% to 90% of UTIs. *Staphylococcus saprophyticus* is isolated in about 10% to 15% of the cases. The most frequent uropathogens are shown in Table 51.1. Follow-up of AUC is usually by routine office visit; no additional testing or cultures are required if the symptoms promptly resolve.

Most patients with AUC begin pharmacotherapy immediately, prior to receiving the results of a urinalysis confirming the specific pathogen. The choice of initial antibiotic and duration of therapy vary widely among practitioners. The choice is often customized to an institution or community, based upon local antibiotic resistance patterns and practitioner experience. Single-dose or short-course therapy is often preferred for patient convenience and to maximize adherence.

Patients often have asymptomatic bacteriuria, discovered on a routine urinalysis: estimates range from 1% to 2% of young adult women to as high as 60% of women over age 60. In general, asymptomatic bacteriuria is not treated. Research has shown that very few of these patients will progress to symptomatic UTI. Widespread therapy would be costly and increase the number of resistant strains in the community. Certain populations of patients, however, are treated when asymptomatic bacteriuria is discovered. These include pregnant patients, those undergoing urologic procedures, and patients who are immunosuppressed or in otherwise poor health.

TABLE 51.1 Most Common Uropathogens

Uncomplicated UTI	Complicated UTI
Escherichia. coli	*E. coli*
Staphylococcus saprophyticus	*Enterobacteriaceae*
Klebsiella	*Klebsiella*
Proteus mirabilis	*Group B streptococci*
Enterobacter	*Enterococcus*
	Pseudomonas
	Proteus mirabilis

The traditional choice for AUC is trimethoprim-sulfamethoxazole (TMP-SMZ), a fixed-dose combination drug that is featured as a prototype in Section 51.4. Given as a 3-day regimen, this agent is effective at eliminating most common uropathogens. The occurrence of many resistant strains, however, has begun to limit its use as a first-line agent.

A second therapy that is equally effective for AUC is a 3-day regimen with a fluoroquinolone such as ciprofloxacin (Cipro). An extended-release form of ciprofloxacin (Cipro XR) that permits once-daily dosing is available. Other fluoroquinolones useful in treating UAC include norfloxacin (Noroxin), ofloxacin (Floxin), and levofloxacin (Levaquin). Fluoroquinolones have become drugs of choice for AUC in many communities because of their safety, and the appearance of sulfonamide-resistant strains. Additional details about the fluoroquinolones are presented in Chapter 50.

An additional choice for AUC therapy in communities where TMP-SMZ resistance is high (over 20%) is urinary antiseptics such as nitrofurantoin, which is featured as a prototype in Section 51.5. If compliance is an issue, a single dose of fosfomycin (Monurol) has proven effective for many patients. Fosfomycin blocks cell wall synthesis, and its only indication is UTI.

CONNECTION *Checkpoint* 51.1

From what you learned in Chapter 50, what is the spectrum of activity of fluoroquinolones? See Answer to Connection Checkpoint 51.1 in Appendix A.

Complicated Urinary Tract Infection

Complicated urinary tract infections (C-UTIs) are defined as infections that occur in a patient who has an underlying comorbid condition that increases the risk of treatment failure. C-UTIs may require aggressive pharmacotherapy, often involving more toxic drugs, higher doses, or prolonged therapy. Comorbid conditions include the following:

- Structural or functional abnormalities in the genitourinary tract such as neurogenic bladder, benign prostatic hyperplasia (BPH), renal tumor, or urinary stones
- Indwelling urinary catheters
- Elderly patients with generally ill health
- Recurring urinary infections
- Identification of resistant uropathogens
- Patients with poor toileting or periurethral hygiene
- All UTIs in men

While nearly all uncomplicated UTIs are caused by *E. coli* and *S. saprophyticus*, C-UTIs are caused by a wider variety of uropathogens (see Table 51.1). Hospital-acquired C-UTIs are sometimes caused by organisms such as *Klebsiella*, *Enterobacter*, *Proteus*, and *Pseudomonas*. When treating C-UTIs, a urine culture should be obtained to identify the specific microbe and the most effective antibiotic based on culture and sensitivity (C&S) testing. Therapy is sometimes begun with a broad-spectrum anti-infective, then adjusted based on C&S results. Patients who have mild or moderate C-UTI can be treated with the same agents used for AUC: fluoroquinolones, TMP-SMZ or nitrofurantoin (Furadantin, Macrobid, Macrodantin). Therapy is often continued for 14 days to be certain all the uropathogens have been eliminated. Severe disease requires hospitalization with parenteral administration of fluoroquinolones, aminoglycosides, cephalosporins, or ampicillin, depending upon the sensitivity of the microbe. Follow-up urine cultures are performed several weeks after completion of therapy to ensure that the uropathogen has been eliminated.

PharmFACT

Urinary tract infections in males usually are caused by an obstruction, such as a urinary stone or enlarged prostate, or from a medical procedure involving a catheter. *Source:* Bowen & Hellstrom, 2007.

51.3 Infants, pregnant patients, older adults, and those with recurring urinary tract infections require modifications to standard pharmacotherapy.

Certain populations require special consideration when selecting and initiating a course of pharmacotherapy to treat UTI. These include infants, children, pregnant women, older adults, and those with recurring infections.

Infants and Children

Although UTIs occur most frequently in sexually active adult women, they are also relatively common in infants and children. Approximately 2.7% of males have a UTI before 12 months of age, a higher percentage than girls of the same age. As many as 3% of all females and 1.2% of males experience a UTI during their school age years. A concern with pediatric patients is that repeated UTIs may cause scarring of the kidneys, resulting in hypertension later in life. With this possibility in mind, health care providers have a goal of preventing recurring infections in kids.

Like adults, *E. coli* causes most pediatric UTIs. Therapeutic options, however, are more limited in children. TMP-SMZ and nitrofurantoin are effective in children. However, fluoroquinolones are contraindicated in children under age 18 because these drugs have been found to affect cartilage development. The safety and efficacy of fosfomycin has not been established in children younger than 12 years old. Recurring UTIs in infants and children may require prolonged, prophylactic antibiotic therapy.

Pregnancy

During pregnancy, the enlarging uterus creates pressure on the urinary bladder, which increases the size of the ureters and promotes urinary stasis and reflux. UTIs in pregnant women are a risk factor for prematurity and newborn low birth weight. In addition, pyelonephritis is one of the most frequent reasons for hospitalization of the pregnant patient.

Urinary screening is routinely performed by the 16th week of pregnancy. Discovery of high levels of bacteria in the urine is an indication for antimicrobial therapy, even if the patient is asymptomatic at the time of testing. A follow-up culture is performed 1 to 2 weeks after therapy is completed. Continued asymptomatic bacteriuria is predictive of symptomatic UTI later in pregnancy. Therapy for asymptomatic bacteriuria is continued until cultures are negative, or until delivery.

During pregnancy, C&S testing is generally conducted to identify the appropriate antibiotic. Pharmacotherapy, however, is limited to drugs that are pregnancy category B, unless the patient is gravely ill. Category B agents include cephalosporins, ampicillin, and nitrofurantoin. Ceftriaxone (Rocephin) is sometimes a drug of choice. Fluoroquinolones are contraindicated during pregnancy due to possible growth inhibition in the fetus, and TMP-SMZ is contraindicated during the first trimester. Asymptomatic patients are often treated for 1 to 3 days, whereas those with clear symptoms of UTI receive a 7-day regimen.

CONNECTION *Checkpoint* 51.2

From what you learned in Chapter 48, if a pregnant patient has a history of serious allergy to ampicillin, should the nurse administer a cephalosporin such as ceftriaxone for UTI? See Answer to Connection Checkpoint 51.2 in Appendix A.

Older Adults

UTIs are common in the geriatric population, especially for those in long-term care (LTC) facilities. Factors that predispose older adults to UTI are BPH, increased postvoid residual urine, and urinary incontinence. Residents of LTC facilities may suffer from chronic diseases and have indwelling catheters or IV lines. The large percentage of patients receiving antibiotics in these facilities promotes the emergence of multidrug-resistant strains, which can be difficult to eliminate in the LTC setting.

Pharmacotherapy in the geriatric population is conducted in the same manner as younger adults, if the geriatric patient is otherwise healthy. Asymptomatic bacteriuria is generally not treated, unless the patient has an underlying comorbid condition. Asymptomatic bacteriuria is present in 30% to 50% of older adults, and such widespread therapy would promote the emergence of resistant strains.

Frail elderly and those with a comorbid condition receive more aggressive pharmacotherapy. These patients may exhibit atypical symptoms, such as altered mental status, sudden incontinence, nausea, or vomiting. If immunosuppressed, an antibiotic may be prescribed for prophylaxis against pneumonia, UTIs, and skin and soft tissue infections, which are the three most common infections in LTC facilities. Because of the prevalence of resistant strains, institutionalized patients with symptomatic UTI should undergo C&S testing to determine the most effective course of therapy. Pharmacotherapy may be prolonged and continue until urine cultures are negative.

By providing a direct route of entry to the bladder for uropathogens, catheter-associated UTI is one of the common hospital-acquired infections. Because the risk of infection increases over time, it is best to remove the catheter as soon as feasible. Patients with catheters should be carefully monitored for signs of UTI. Periodic urinalysis testing should be conducted to check for bacteriuria. Symptomatic UTI with a positive urine culture is an indication for removal of the catheter (if feasible) and initiation of pharmacotherapy.

Recurring Urinary Tract Infections

One in five patients with a UTI will experience a subsequent UTI within 6 months. Recurring UTIs are classified as either relapses or reinfections. A relapse occurs when the patient experiences a second UTI within 2 weeks after completing pharmacotherapy for the original infection. Normally, a relapse is caused by failure of the treatment to totally eliminate the original uropathogen. A reinfection occurs when the patient recovers from the original infection, but acquires another infection weeks or months later. Reinfections may be caused by the original microbe, or by a different uropathogen.

Recurrent UTIs require extended antimicrobial therapy, either with the original antibiotic or with a different agent. It is necessary to identify the pathogen in order to examine for resistant strains.

Women who experience two or more UTIs within 6 months, or three or more UTIs over the course of a year, are candidates for prophylactic therapy. Choices for prophylaxis include administration of antibiotics at low doses either on a daily or three-times-per-week schedule. Another option is to allow the woman to initiate therapy herself. With this type of treatment, the patient is provided with a single dose or 3-day course of therapy, which is initiated by the woman after each act of coitus, or when symptoms first develop. Patients should be advised to see their health care provider if symptoms worsen, or if they do not resolve during prophylactic therapy, because this may be a sign of a more serious infection.

Sulfonamides

51.4 Sulfonamides are the traditional drugs of choice for urinary tract infections, but resistance limits their usefulness.

The discovery of the sulfonamides in the 1930s heralded a new era in the treatment of infectious disease. Effective against both gram-positive and gram-negative bacteria, the sulfonamides significantly reduced mortality from susceptible microbes and earned its discoverer a Nobel Prize in medicine in 1938. Doses for the sulfonamides are listed in Table 51.2.

Sulfonamides are active against a broad spectrum of microorganisms including some staphylococci, many streptococci (except *Enterococcus faecalis*), *Haemophilus influenzae*, *Nocardia*, most *Enterobacteriaceae*, *Neisseria*, and *Chlamydia.* Sulfonamides have also been used to treat mycobacterial infections and some protozoans such as *Toxoplasma gondii.* Agents in this drug class are also given for treatment and prophylaxis of *Pneumocystis carinii* pneumonia and *Shigella* infections of the small bowel. The nurse should keep in mind that although these drugs appear to be effective against many species, the sensitivity of specific strains of these organisms to sulfonamides

TABLE 51.2 Drugs Used for Urinary Tract Infections

Drug	Adult Dose (maximum dose where indicated)	Adverse Effects
Sulfonamides		
sulfadiazine	PO: Loading dose 2–4 g Maintenance dose 2–4 g/day in 4–6 divided doses	*Nausea, vomiting, anorexia, rash, crystalluria* Anaphylaxis, Stevens–Johnson syndrome, blood dyscrasias, fulminant hepatic necrosis, hyperkalemia
sulfadoxine-pyrimethamine (Fansidar)	PO: 1 tablet weekly (500 mg sulfadoxine, 25 mg pyrimethamine)	
sulfisoxazole (Gantrisin)	PO: Loading dose 2–4 g Maintenance dose 1–2 g qid (max: 12 g/day)	
trimethoprim-sulfamethoxazole (TMP-SMZ) (Bactrim, Septra)	PO: 160 mg TMP/800 mg SMZ bid IV: 8–10 mg/kg/day TMP, every 6–12 h infused over 60–90 min	
Urinary Antiseptics and Other Drugs for UTI		
fosfomycin (Monurol)	PO: 3 g sachet dissolved in 3–4 oz of water as a single dose	*Nausea, diarrhea, back pain, headache* Anaphylaxis, superinfections
methenamine hippurate (Hiprex, Urex) or mandelate (Mandelamine)	PO (hippurate): 1 g bid (mandelate): 1 g qid	*Nausea, vomiting, diarrhea, increased urinary urgency* Anaphylaxis, crystalluria
nalidixic acid (NegGram)	PO: Acute infections: 1 g qid Chronic infections: 500 mg qid	*Nausea, vomiting, diarrhea, drowsiness, fatigue, headache, blurred vision* Anaphylaxis, hemolytic anemia
nitrofurantoin (Furadantin, Macrobid, Macrodantin)	PO: 50–100 mg qid (max: 7 mg/kg/day)	*Nausea, vomiting, anorexia, dark urine, rash* Anaphylaxis, superinfections, hepatic necrosis, interstitial pneumonitis, Stevens–Johnson syndrome, hemolytic anemia

Note: *Italics* indicate common adverse effects. Underline indicates serious adverse effects.

in a particular community setting must be confirmed, due to widespread resistance.

Sulfonamides suppress bacterial growth by inhibiting the synthesis of folic acid, or folate. In human physiology, **folic acid** is a water-soluble vitamin that serves a critical role as a coenzyme in the synthesis of ribonucleic acid (RNA) and deoxyribonucleic acid (DNA). But if folic acid is essential to both humans and bacteria, why are the sulfonamides not acutely toxic to humans? The answer lies in differences in the metabolic pathways in humans and bacteria.

Humans must obtain "premade" folic acid by eating foods rich in this vitamin. Humans are unable to synthesize this essential nutrient "from scratch." Bacteria, on the other hand, make their own folic acid using simpler precursor molecules. The steps in this pathway are shown in Figure 51.1. Sulfonamides inhibit the enzyme in Step 1; the drug trimethoprim inhibits the enzyme in Step 3. Note how closely the sulfonamides resemble the precursor molecule, **para-aminobenzoic acid** in Figure 51.2. It is easy to see how an enzyme could confuse the two similar molecules. Once the enzyme binds to the sulfonamide, however, folic acid synthesis stops, and bacterial growth slows. This explains why these agents are bacteriostatic; they slow bacterial growth rather than kill the cells.

The widespread use of sulfonamides for over 60 years has resulted in a substantial number of resistant strains. The mechanism of acquired resistance to sulfonamides is likely a mutation in the enzyme performing Step 1 of folic acid synthesis. Mutant enzymes can still bind PABA, but can no longer bind to sulfonamides. Resistance to one sulfonamide often confers resistance to all members of this class.

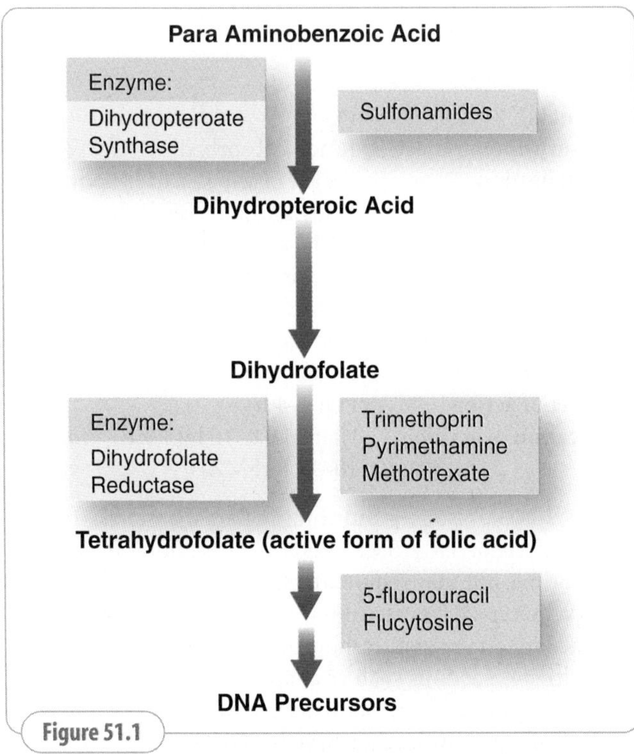

Figure 51.1

Drug inhibition of folic acid metabolism. Drugs inhibit multiple steps in the metabolic pathway leading to folic acid.

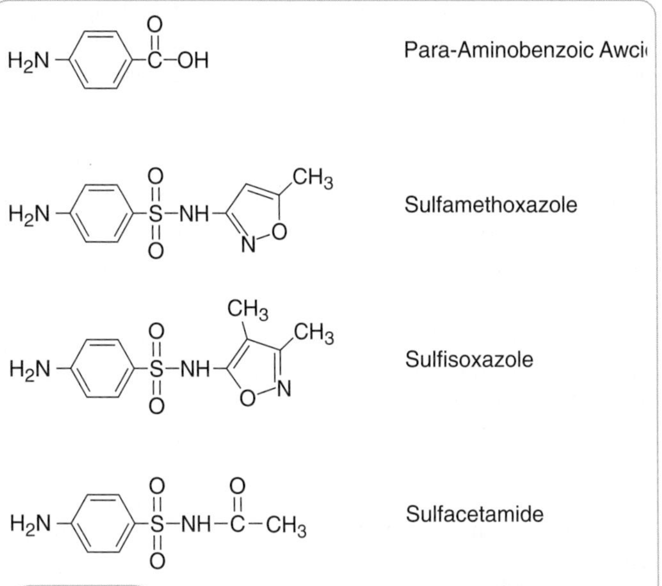

H_2N–C_6H_4–C(=O)–OH — Para-Aminobenzoic Acid

H_2N–C_6H_4–SO_2–NH–(isoxazole, CH_3) — Sulfamethoxazole

H_2N–C_6H_4–SO_2–NH–(isoxazole, CH_3, CH_3) — Sulfisoxazole

H_2N–C_6H_4–SO_2–NH–C(=O)–CH_3 — Sulfacetamide

Figure 51.2

Chemical similarities between para-aminobenzoic acid and sulfonamides.

In addition to resistance, several other factors have led to a significant decline in the use of sulfonamides. The development of the penicillins, cephalosporins, and macrolides gave practitioners larger choices of agents, some of which exhibited an improved safety profile over the sulfonamides. Approval of the combination antibiotic TMP-SMZ marked resurgence in the use of sulfonamides in treating UTIs. Decades of widespread use, however, have now resulted in a large number of strains resistant to TMP-SMZ. In communities with high resistance rates, TMP-SMZ is no longer a drug of first choice, unless C&S testing determines it to be the most effective drug for the specific uropathogen.

Sulfonamides are classified by their absorption and excretion characteristics. These subclasses include:

- Oral (PO) agents that are readily absorbed.
- PO agents that are not absorbed.
- Topical agents.

Agents that are readily absorbed after a PO dose include sulfisoxazole (Gantrisin), sulfadiazine, and TMP-SMZ. These agents are distributed to most tissues in the body, and the amount of plasma protein binding may be significant. Hepatic enzymes convert these drugs to inactive metabolites, and the drugs are excreted rapidly by the kidney. Sulfadoxine is an exception, with an exceptionally long half-life of 7 to 9 days. For malarial prophylaxis, it is combined with pyrimethamine and marketed as Fansidar.

One sulfonamide comprises the second subclass: agents that are given PO but undergo poor, or no, absorption. Sulfasalazine (Azulfidine) remains unabsorbed in the alimentary canal to treat intestinal infections and mild to moderate ulcerative colitis. Some systemic toxicity may be observed with this drug, because one of its metabolic products is absorbed from the intestine and enters the systemic circulation.

The third subclass includes topical sulfonamides. Silver sulfadiazine (Silvadene) is used for the prophylaxis and treatment of topical infections resulting from wounds or burns. Systemic adverse effects may result if the drug is applied to large areas, due to absorption of the antibiotic across the skin. Sulfacetamide (Cetamide, others) is available as a solution to treat ophthalmic infections. Mafenide (Sulfamylon) is applied over burns to prevent infection. Like other topical sulfonamides, the drug may be absorbed across the skin, resulting in significant plasma drug levels.

Adverse Effects

In general, the sulfonamides are safe drugs; however, some adverse effects may be serious. Of most concern are adverse effects on the urinary tract, hypersensitivity reactions, and blood abnormalities. Nausea, vomiting, and anorexia may also occur.

Agents in this class must be used with caution in patients with renal impairment. Sulfonamides have a low solubility, which may cause **crystalluria,** crystals that form in the urine and potentially obstruct the kidneys or ureters. The risk is higher in dehydrated patients and when urine pH is abnormally low. In order to decrease the possibility of crystalluria, fluids in amounts up to 3,000 mL per day should be encouraged to achieve a urinary output of 1,500 mL in 24 hours.

Although not common, sulfonamides can cause potentially fatal blood abnormalities such as aplastic anemia, acute hemolytic anemia, and agranulocytosis. Baseline and periodic blood laboratory values should be assessed to prevent the development of anemia or other hematologic disorders. Patients with preexisting myelosuppression should be monitored carefully during therapy, because this increases the risks associated with drug-induced bone marrow depression.

Hypersensitivity to "sulfa" drugs is well documented. These drugs cause a number of dermal reactions ranging from urticaria to photosensitivity and exfoliative dermatitis. Patients may develop fever and malaise. Cross sensitivity exists with diuretics, such as acetazolamide (Diamox) and the thiazides, and with sulfonylurea antidiabetic agents. These agents should be avoided in patients with a history of hypersensitivity to sulfonamides because this can induce Stevens–Johnson syndrome. At the first signs of rash, the patient should be instructed to stop taking the drug and contact their health care provider.

Most sulfonamides readily cross the placenta, and may reach sufficiently high levels to cause adverse effects in the fetus. Sulfonamides are contraindicated during pregnancy and lactation, because they enter breast milk. They are contraindicated for infants less than 2 months of age and for pregnant patients near term, because sulfonamides displace bilirubin from plasma proteins. The displaced, free bilirubin is toxic to the brain and causes kernicterus, a serious type of jaundice.

CONNECTIONS

Patient Safety

Trimethoprim-Sulfamethoxazole (Bactrim, Septra)

The nurse will administer trimethoprim-sulfamethoxazole (Bactrim, Septra) to a patient with a urinary tract infection. Before giving the medication, the nurse reviews the patient's chart. The nurse notices that the patient is afebrile with a normal pulse, blood pressure, and respiratory rate. The most recent culture indicates a decline in the number of bacteria present in the urine. Other information found in the medical record indicates that the patient routinely takes medication for hypertension and arthritis. The patient has also reported allergies to chocolate and thiazide diuretics. Should the nurse give the medication as prescribed?

PROTOTYPE DRUG Trimethoprim-sulfamethoxazole (Bactrim, Septra)

Classification: **Therapeutic:** Antibacterial

Pharmacologic: Folic acid inhibitor, sulfonamide

Therapeutic Effects and Uses: Approved in 1973, TMP-SMZ is a folic acid inhibitor containing a fixed-dose combination of trimethoprim (TMP) and sulfamethoxazole (SMZ), a sulfonamide. The drug is commonly used for UTI prophylaxis and in the pharmacotherapy of complicated and uncomplicated UTI, depending upon the sensitivity of the specific uropathogen. It is also approved for the treatment and prophylaxis of *P. carinii* pneumonia, *Shigella* infections of the small bowel, and for acute exacerbations of chronic bronchitis. The drug is used off-label for many other indications, depending upon sensitivity of the microbe. PO and IV formulations are available.

Mechanism of Action: Both SMZ and TMP are inhibitors of the bacterial metabolism of folic acid. Each drug inhibits a separate enzyme in the metabolic pathway, creating a synergistic combination: A greater bacterial kill is achieved by the fixed combination than would be achieved with either drug used separately. Because humans obtain folate in their diets, these medications are selective toward bacterial folate metabolism.

Pharmacokinetics:

Route(s)	PO, IV
Absorption	Readily absorbed
Distribution	Widely distributed to all body fluids, including cerebrospinal fluid (CSF); crosses the placenta; secreted in breast milk; protein binding is 70% (SMZ) and 44% (TMP)
Primary metabolism	Hepatic
Primary excretion	Renal
Onset of action	PO: 1–4 h
Duration of action	Half-life: 8–10 h (TMP) and 10–13 h (SMZ)

Adverse Effects: Nausea and vomiting are the most common adverse effects of TMP-SMZ therapy. These normally diminish with time, but may require treatment or cause discontinuation of therapy. Hypersensitivity is relatively common and usually manifests as skin rash, pruritus, and fever. Severe hypersensitivity reactions such as anaphylaxis, Stevens–Johnson syndrome, epidermal necrolysis, agranulocytosis, aplastic anemia, and allergic myocarditis have been recorded. In order to prevent crystalluria and potential damage to tubular cells, it is important to maintain dilute urine during therapy to reduce the concentration of the drugs as they travel through the renal tubule. Due to the potential for photosensitivity, the patient should avoid direct sunlight during therapy.

Contraindications/Precautions: An allergy history should be taken prior to administration because TMP-SMZ is contraindicated in patients with hypersensitivity to sulfites, sulfonamides, or chemically related agents such as thiazide diuretics. TMP-SMZ is contraindicated in patients with folate-deficiency anemia, since a folic acid inhibitor would worsen this condition. This medication is contraindicated in patients with severe renal impairment because this is the primary route of drug excretion and the drug may accumulate to toxic levels in these patients. It should be used with caution in patients with hepatic impairment because the liver metabolizes TMP-SMZ. Trimethoprim decreases potassium excretion and is contraindicated in patients with hyperkalemia.

Drug Interactions: TMP and SMZ may enhance the effects of oral anticoagulants. Since methotrexate also interferes with folate metabolism, concurrent use with TMP-SMZ increases the risk of toxicity. TMP-SMZ exerts a potassium-sparing effect on the nephron and should be used with caution with diuretics such as spironolactone (Aldactone) to prevent hyperkalemia. TMP-SMZ may increase the hypoglycemic response to sulfonylureas due to displacement from protein-binding sites or inhibition of metabolism. **Herbal/Food:** Potassium supplements should not be taken during therapy, unless directed by the health care provider.

Pregnancy: Category C.

Treatment of Overdose: Acidification of the urine will increase the renal elimination of trimethoprim. If signs of bone marrow depression occur during high dose therapy, 5 to 15 mg of leucovorin should be given daily.

Nursing Responsibilities:

- Perform an infection-focused physical examination including vital signs and a white blood cell (WBC) count. Determine baseline signs and symptoms that may indicate the presence of infection.
- Obtain an accurate history from the patient prior to drug administration including exposure, sensitivity, allergies, and any known reaction to sulfites or sulfonamides.
- Give PO doses with a full glass of desired fluid. Maintain adequate fluid intake (at least 2 to 3 L per day) during therapy unless otherwise directed.
- Closely monitor patients with asthma during IV infusion. Intravenous TMP-SMZ contains sodium metabisulfite, which can produce allergic-type reactions in susceptible patients. These reactions include itching and hives, as well as wheezing and anaphylaxis. Adverse effects occur more frequently in asthmatics.
- Monitor baseline and follow-up laboratory test values such as urinalysis, complete blood count (CBC) with differential and platelet count, blood urea nitrogen (BUN), and creatinine clearance, especially during prolonged therapy.
- If the patient is receiving warfarin, monitor laboratory prothrombin time (PT), because TMP-SMZ prolongs PT.
- Monitor intake and output (I&O) for volume and pattern. Report continued symptoms of UTI such as dysuria, frequency, and urgency to the prescriber.
- Monitor older adult patients who are at risk for severe adverse reactions such as those with compromised liver or kidney function or those taking other medications. Frequently observed adverse effects include thrombocytopenia (with concurrent thiazide diuretics), severe drop in platelets with or without purpura, suppression in bone marrow, and severe skin reactions.

Patient and Family Education:

- Immediately report a rash, fever, purpura, sore throat, or jaundice to the health care provider.
- Drink 2 to 3 L (1 liter is approximately equal to 1 quart) of fluids daily, unless otherwise indicated.
- Immediately report severe or persistent diarrhea accompanied by fever to the health care provider. Do not attempt to treat antibiotic-related diarrhea with over-the-counter (OTC) products.
- Notify the health care provider if the infection does not begin to improve after a few days of therapy.
- Do not breast-feed while taking this drug without approval of the health care provider.

Drugs Similar to Trimethoprim-Sulfamethoxazole (Bactrim, Septra)

Other orally absorbed sulfonamides include sulfadiazine, and sulfisoxazole. Sulfadoxine-pyrimethamine (Fansidar) is used exclusively for treating malaria and is discussed in Chapter 54.

Sulfadiazine: Approved in 1941, sulfadiazine is a short-acting, oral sulfonamide that is given every 4 to 6 hours. It has a broad spectrum and is used for diverse infections, including UTI, nocardiosis, meningococcal meningitis, cerebral toxoplasmosis (in combination with pyrimethamine), and resistant malaria. Like other sulfonamides, hypersensitivity may be a major clinical limitation to therapy. Sulfadiazine is poorly soluble in urine and causes more crystalluria than other sulfonamides. Adequate fluid intake and frequent urinary testing is essential to avoid nephrotoxicity. Silver sulfadiazine is a topical medication. This drug is pregnancy category C.

Sulfisoxazole (Gantrisin): Like sulfadiazine, this drug is short acting and must be taken PO every 4 to 6 hours. Approved in 1948, indications include UTI, otitis media due to *H. influenzae*, nocardiosis, and malaria, in combination with other antimalarial agents. It is sometimes preferred over other sulfonamides for UTI because it causes less crystalluria. Hypersensitivity is a common adverse effect. An ophthalmic formulation is available for the treatment of chlamydial conjunctivitis. Pediazole suspension is a combination of sulfisoxazole with erythromycin for the treatment of acute or recurrent otitis media in penicillin-allergic patients. This drug is pregnancy category C.

Trimethoprim (Primsol): In addition to being part of the TMP-SMZ combination, trimethoprim is also available as monotherapy.

Trimethoprim is approved to treat uncomplicated UTI and acute otitis media in children due to *Streptococcus pneumoniae* or *H. influenzae*. It has been used off-label for the treatment of traveler's diarrhea and for *Pneumocystis* pneumonia, in combination with either sulfamethoxazole or dapsone. Rash and pruritus are common adverse effects, and these may appear 1 to 2 weeks after therapy has begun. Some patients experience nausea, vomiting, and diarrhea. Trimethoprim is combined with polymyxin B in an ophthalmic solution for ocular infections. This drug is pregnancy category C.

NURSING PROCESS APPLICATION

Patients Receiving Sulfonamides

Assessment	Potential Nursing Diagnoses
Prior to administration: • Obtain a complete health history including allergies, drug history, and possible drug interactions. • Determine if the patient has ever experienced hypersensitivity reaction to any antibiotics (cross sensitivity is possible with penicillins and cephalosporins). • Obtain specimens for C&S testing before initiating therapy. • Perform infection-focused physical examination including vital signs and WBC count.	• *Risk for Infection* • *Deficient Knowledge (Sulfonamide Therapy)*, related to purpose, precautions, and adverse effects of drug • *Deficient Knowledge (Infection)*, related to disease process and transmission of microorganism • *Noncompliance (Therapeutic Regimen)*, related to completion • *Risk for Impaired Skin Integrity*, related to drug-induced photosensitivity • *Risk for Injury*, related to adverse effects of drug, liver, or kidney dysfunction, or blood dyscrasias

Planning: Patient Goals and Expected Outcomes

The patient will:

- Report a reduction in symptoms related to the diagnosed infection, and have negative results for laboratory and diagnostic tests for the presenting infection.
- Demonstrate an understanding of the drug's action by accurately describing drug adverse effects and precautions.
- Immediately report significant adverse effects such as shortness of breath, swelling, fever, stomatitis, loose stools, vaginal discharge, or cough.
- Complete the full course of antibiotic therapy and adhere to follow-up care.

Implementation

Interventions and (Rationales)	Patient and Family Education
• Monitor vital signs and symptoms of infection to determine antibacterial effectiveness. (Another drug or different dosage may be required.)	• Instruct the patient to notify the health care provider if symptoms persist or worsen.
• Monitor for hypersensitivity reaction. (Immediate hypersensitivity reaction may occur within 2 to 30 minutes, an accelerated reaction may occur in 1 to 72 hours, and a delayed reaction may occur after 72 hours.)	• Instruct the patient to discontinue the medication and inform the health care provider if symptoms of hypersensitivity reaction develop such as wheezing; shortness of breath; swelling of face, tongue, or hands; and itching or rash.
• Encourage fluid intake. (Fluid intake should be 2,000 to 3,000 mL/day to promote urinary output to prevent crystalluria or stone formation.)	• Teach the patient the importance of high intake of fluids. Instruct the patient about alternate forms of fluid intake such as Jell-O, popsicles, and other high-water-content foods.
• Monitor for severe diarrhea. (The condition may occur due to superinfection or the possible adverse effect of antibiotic-associated pseudomembranous colitis.)	Instruct the patient to: • Consult the health care provider before taking antidiarrheal drugs, which could cause retention of harmful bacteria. • Consume cultured dairy products with live active cultures, such as kefir, yogurt, or buttermilk, to help maintain normal intestinal flora.
• Administer the drug around the clock. (This is necessary to maintain effective blood levels.)	Instruct the patient to: • Take the medication on schedule. • Complete the entire prescription even if feeling better, to prevent development of resistant bacteria.
• Monitor for superinfection, especially in elderly, debilitated, or immunosuppressed patients. (There is an increased risk for superinfections due to elimination of normal flora.)	• Instruct the patient to report signs and symptoms of superinfection such as fever; black hairy tongue; stomatitis; loose, foul-smelling stools; vaginal discharge; or cough.
• Monitor for photosensitivity. (Sulfonamides can increase the patient's sensitivity to ultraviolet light and increase the risk of sunburn.)	Encourage the patient to: • Stay out of direct sunlight, especially between the hours of 10:00 A.M. and 3:00 P.M. • Wear protective clothing, including a hat, as well as sunglasses. Apply a sun block product that has a skin protection factor (SPF) of at least 15. Some patients may require a product with a higher SPF number, especially if they have a fair complexion. • Apply a sun block lipstick that has an SPF of at least 15 to protect lips. • Not use a sunlamp, or a tanning bed or booth.

• Determine the effect of sulfonamide on other prescribed medications, if indicated. (Sulfonamides increase bleeding time with oral anticoagulants and decrease blood glucose levels with antidiabetic agents. Iron preparations may interfere with the absorption of the antibiotic.)	• Instruct the patient to report all prescription and OTC medications to the health care provider.
• Determine the interactions of the prescribed antibiotics with food. (Sulfasalazine is best taken after meals to prolong time in the intestines.)	• Instruct the patient when to take the prescribed sulfonamide in relationship to meals.
• Monitor the IV site for signs and symptoms of tissue irritation, severe pain, and extravasation. (Sulfamethoxazole-trimethoprim is the only sulfonamide administered IV.)	• Instruct the patient to report pain or other symptoms of discomfort immediately during IV infusion.
• Monitor for adverse effects specific to various antibiotic therapies. (Nausea and vomiting are the most common adverse effects. Hypersensitivity is also common and usually manifests as skin rash, pruritus, and fever. Severe hypersensitivity reactions such as anaphylaxis, Stevens–Johnson syndrome, epidermal necrolysis, agranulocytosis, aplastic anemia, and allergic myocarditis have been recorded.)	• Instruct the patient to report adverse effects specific to the antibiotic therapy prescribed.
• Monitor renal function such as I&O ratio, urine color, and consistency. Monitor laboratory work including serum creatinine and BUN. (Sulfonamides are eliminated via the kidneys.)	• Explain the purpose of required laboratory tests and scheduled follow-up with the health care provider.
• Monitor the patient for adherence to antibiotic therapy. (Nonadherence to therapy may result in recurrent infections.)	Instruct the patient on the importance of: • Completing the prescription as ordered. • Follow-up care after antibiotic therapy is completed. • Discarding any outdated or unused medication to deter self-medication of drugs with decreased potency.

Evaluation of Outcome Criteria

Evaluate the effectiveness of drug therapy by confirming that patient goals and expected outcomes have been met (see "Planning").

Urinary Antiseptics

51.5 Urinary antiseptics are anti-infective drugs used exclusively for urinary tract infections.

As has been noted throughout this textbook, most medications are totally or partially excreted by the kidney. The majority of drugs and their metabolites travel through the urinary system producing little or no effect on the renal tubular cells or the other parts of the kidney. For the small class of drugs known as the urinary antiseptics, however, the urinary system is their target tissue. Being able to reach the urinary tract in high concentrations is essential to their therapeutic success.

Urinary antiseptics are drugs given by the PO route for their antibacterial action in the urinary tract. While they do not reach high enough levels in the blood to be effective for systemic infections, the kidney concentrates the drugs; thus, their actions are specific to the urinary system. Urinary antiseptics reach therapeutic levels in the kidney tubules, and their anti-infective action continues as they travel to the urinary bladder.

The advantage of the urinary antiseptics is that they are able to treat local infections in the urinary tract without reaching high levels in the blood that might produce systemic toxicity. Although none are usually drugs of first choice for UTI, they serve important roles as secondary medications, especially in patients who present with infections resistant to TMP-SMZ or the fluoroquinolones.

CONNECTIONS

Complementary and Alternative Therapies Cranberry

Description: Cranberry shrubs grow in diverse climates ranging from bogs to forests. The ripe berry is the component used for its potential medicinal effects.

History and Claims: Native Americans used the berries to treat wounds, and to cure anorexia and other digestive complaints. In the early 1900s, it was noted that the acidity of the urine increases after eating cranberries; thus began the belief that cranberry juice is a natural cure for urinary tract infections.

Standardization: The herb is taken as juice or dried extract. Doses generally range from 120 to 4,000 mL of juice or 400 to 500 mg of the extract daily.

Evidence: Cranberry contains a significant amount of vitamin C and other antioxidants that can promote health. Some evidence is available to suggest that cranberry can prevent urinary tract infections. Previously, it was thought that this juice would change the pH of urine to become more acid, discouraging bacteria growth. Although there is some merit to this approach, more recent thought is that chemicals in cranberry juice prevent the bacteria from sticking to the walls of the bladder. This makes it more difficult for the bacteria to colonize and reproduce. The juice should be 100% cranberry and not "cocktail" juice, as that contains sugar which enhances bacteria growth and may be contraindicated in diabetic patients. Some individuals may prefer to take cranberry capsules, which are available at most drug stores.

Source: From "Cranberry Juice and UTI Prevention", by L. Burak, n.d. Retrieved July 28, 2008, from http://altmed.creighton.edu/cranberries/index.html; *Herbs at a Glance: Cranberry,* by National Center for Complementary and Alternative Medicine, 2008. Retrieved July 28, 2008, from http://nccam.nih.gov/health/cranberry/; and "A Systematic Review of the Evidence for Cranberries and Blueberries in UTI Prevention," by R. G. Jepson, and J. C. Craig, 2007, *Molecular Nutrition & Food Research, 51*(6), pp. 738–745.

PROTOTYPE DRUG Nitrofurantoin (Furadantin) and nitrofurantoin macrocrystals (Macrobid, Macrodantin)

Classification: Therapeutic: Antibacterial
Pharmacologic: Urinary tract antiseptic

Therapeutic Effects and Uses: Nitrofurantoin is an older drug that is indicated for the treatment of uncomplicated acute cystitis, most commonly for the prophylaxis of recurrent UTI. Nitrofurantoin is active against the *E. coli, S. saprophyticus,* and many other strains of gram-positive and gram-negative aerobes. It is not effective against the *Pseudomonas, Proteus,* or *Serratia* species. It is not indicated for the treatment of pyelonephritis.

Nitrofurantoin is available in three formulations: a microcrystalline form (Furadantin), a macrocrystalline form (Macrodantin), and a sustained-release macrocrystalline form (Macrobid). The macrocrystalline form is more slowly absorbed than the microcrystalline form and produces fewer GI-related adverse effects.

Despite being approved by the FDA in 1953, development of resistance has not been a significant problem. The broad-based mechanism of action may explain the relative lack of acquired bacterial resistance to nitrofurantoin. Multiple mutations at diverse locations would be necessary for a bacterium to acquire such resistance. Cross resistance with other antibiotics is very rare, if it occurs at all.

Mechanism of Action: Nitrofurantoin acts by several unique mechanisms. When bacteria break down nitrofurantoin, the drug is converted to highly reactive intermediates. These intermediates attack bacterial ribosomal proteins. The drug inhibits bacterial protein synthesis, aerobic energy metabolism, DNA synthesis, RNA synthesis, and formation of the cell wall. Nitrofurantoin is bactericidal in the urine at therapeutic doses.

Pharmacokinetics:

Route(s)	PO
Absorption	Readily absorbed
Distribution	Widely distributed to body fluids; crosses the placenta; secreted in breast milk; 60% bound to plasma proteins
Primary metabolism	Hepatic
Primary excretion	Renal
Onset of action	30 minutes
Duration of action	Half-life: 20 minutes

Adverse Effects: Nitrofurantoin has the potential to produce many adverse effects. Frequent adverse effects include hypersensitivity reactions, anorexia, headache, rash, nausea, and vomiting. Acute and chronic pulmonary toxicity is a serious adverse effect and may include interstitial pneumonitis, persistent cough, and pulmonary fibrosis. Chronic pulmonary toxicity may not appear until months or years after therapy has been completed. Hepatotoxicity is rare, though potentially fatal and may include cholestatic jaundice, hepatic necrosis, or hepatitis.

Contraindications/Precautions: Because nitrofurantoin is excreted by the kidneys, significant renal impairment (creatinine clearance under 60 mL/minute or significant elevated serum creatinine) is a contraindication. Success of treatment depends on achieving high amounts of drug in the urine, which will not occur in patients with oliguria or anuria. Because of the possibility of hemolytic anemia due to immature erythrocyte enzyme systems, the drug is contraindicated in pregnant patients or in neonates less than 1 month of age.

This drug should be used with caution in patients with preexisting pulmonary disease and pulmonary function should be closely monitored throughout therapy. Although rare, reports have cited diffuse interstitial pneumonitis or pulmonary fibrosis as causes of death in patients receiving nitrofurantoin.

Nitrofurantoin should be used with caution in patients with preexisting hepatic disease. The drug should be discontinued immediately if changes are noted in liver function tests.

Drug Interactions: Nitrofurantoin should not be given with antacids containing magnesium because absorption will be decreased. Concurrent administration with nalidixic acid, and possibly fluoroquinolones, may result in antagonism and a decreased drug effect. **Herbal/Food:** Unknown.

Pregnancy: Category B.

Treatment of Overdose: Adequate fluid intake should be provided to ensure renal excretion of the drug. In extreme cases, dialysis may be of value in removing nitrofurantoin.

Nursing Responsibilities:

- Perform an infection-focused physical examination including vital signs and a WBC count. Determine baseline signs and symptoms that may indicate the presence of infection.
- Obtain an accurate history from the patient prior to drug administration including exposure, sensitivity, allergies, and any known hypersensitivity reactions.
- Give drug with food or milk to minimize gastric irritation and discomfort.
- Avoid crushing tablets because of the possibility of tooth staining; rather, dilute oral suspension in milk, water, or fruit juice, and rinse mouth thoroughly after taking drug.
- Monitor results of C&S tests before therapy begins for patients with history of recurrent infections.
- Discontinue the medication if oliguria or anuria occurs and immediately notify the prescriber.
- Assess for signs of urinary tract superinfections such as dysuria, foul-smelling urine, milky colored urine, or perineal irritation.
- Assess for acute pulmonary sensitivity reaction, which usually occurs within the first week of therapy. Symptoms may include mild to severe flulike syndrome and eosinophilia generally developing within a few days. Symptoms usually subside quickly after the medication is discontinued. Pulmonary sensitivity reaction may be more pronounced in older adults.
- Assess for onset of muscle weakness, or numbness and tingling. Note that peripheral neuropathy can be severe and irreversible. Withdraw the medication and immediately notify the prescriber.

Patient and Family Education:

- Report the following symptoms to the health care provider: difficulty breathing, changes in urination (other than brown discoloration), nausea, vomiting, diarrhea, rash, chest pain, cough, fever, vision changes, unusual bleeding, yellowing of skin, or light-colored stools.
- This drug may give a harmless brown color to the urine.
- Consult the health care provider regarding fluid intake. Generally, fluids are not forced; however, intake should be adequate.
- Immediately report severe or persistent diarrhea accompanied by fever. Do not attempt to treat penicillin-related diarrhea with OTC products.
- Contact the health care provider if the infection does not begin to improve after a few days of therapy.
- Do not breast-feed while taking this drug without approval of the health care provider.

Drugs Similar to Nitrofurantoin (Furadantin) and Nitrofurantoin Macrocrystals (Macrobid, Macrodantin)

Other urinary antiseptics include fosfomycin, methenamine, and nalidixic acid.

Fosfomycin (Monurol): Approved in 1996, fosfomycin is approved for the treatment of uncomplicated UTI caused by susceptible organisms. Technically classified as a cell wall inhibitor (see Chapter 48), it reaches high concentrations in the urine and bladder. Thus, it is sometimes called a bladder antiseptic. It is administered as a single PO dose. The most frequent adverse effects are diarrhea, dizziness, dyspepsia, headache, nausea, vomiting, rash, and vaginitis. This drug is pregnancy category B.

Methenamine (Hiprex, Mandelamine, Urex): Methenamine is an older drug approved in 1939 that is available in two salts: hippurate (Hiprex, Urex) and mandelate (Mandelamine). In the very acidic environment of urine, methenamine is metabolized to formaldehyde, a breakdown product toxic to microorganisms. Mandelate and hippurate become acids in the urine, thus providing an even greater environment (lower pH) for the generation of formaldehyde. At therapeutic doses, methenamine is a safe drug, although higher doses can result in dysuria, nausea, vomiting, and hematuria.

The only clinical application of methenamine is for prophylactic treatment of recurrent UTI, especially those with neurogenic bladder. It is effective against most bacteria typically responsible for UTI. Urease-positive bacteria such as *Proteus* are resistant because they produce ammonia in the urine, which prevents the formation of formaldehyde. Concurrent therapy of methenamine with sulfamethoxazole is contraindicated because the combination promotes crystalluria. This drug is pregnancy category C.

Nalidixic acid (NegGram): Approved in 1964, nalidixic acid was the first quinolone anti-infective marketed. Nalidixic acid and newer drugs in this class (fluoroquinolones) act by inhibiting DNA and RNA synthesis (see Chapter 50). While fluoroquinolones are prescribed for many diverse infections, the use of nalidixic acid is limited to UTI. Its spectrum of activity includes most bacteria responsible for UTI. Another first-generation quinolone, cinoxacin (Cinobac), was very similar to nalidixic acid but is no longer marketed in the United States.

Nalidixic acid is readily absorbed in the GI tract and is concentrated in the urine. GI distress is the most common adverse effect. At higher doses, patients may experience drowsiness, fatigue, headaches, and visual disturbances such as blurred vision.

Nalidixic acid is contraindicated in infants less than 3 months of age because it may create intracranial hypertension. The nurse should monitor laboratory blood counts, because nalidixic acid has been reported to cause hemolytic anemia and thrombocytopenia in some patients. This drug displaces warfarin from plasma protein binding sites. Thus, a reduction in dose may be necessary for the anticoagulant. Resistance to nalidixic acid develops rapidly during therapy. This drug is pregnancy category C.

UNDERSTANDING THE CHAPTER

Key Concept Summary

51.1 Infections can occur in any portion of the urinary tract.

51.2 Choice of pharmacotherapy for acute urinary tract infection depends upon the severity of the infection and the presence of comorbid conditions.

51.3 Infants, pregnant patients, older adults, and those with recurring urinary tract infections require modifications to standard pharmacotherapy.

51.4 Sulfonamides are the traditional drugs of choice for urinary tract infections, but resistance has limited their usefulness.

51.5 Urinary antiseptics are anti-infective drugs used exclusively for urinary tract infections.

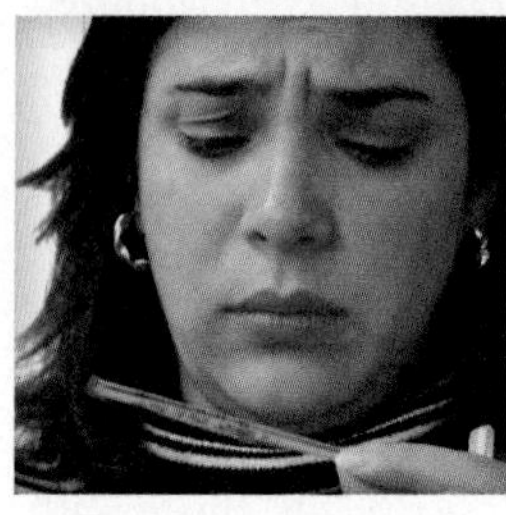

Making the PATIENT Connection

Remember the patient "Sandra Phillipi" at the beginning of the chapter? Now read the remainder of the case study. Based on the information presented within this chapter, respond to the critical thinking questions that follow.

Sandra Phillipi is a 32-year-old woman who has experienced frequent urinary tract infections. She does not have a health care provider, but relies upon the local emergency department for her health care needs. Sandra is married with two children and works in a retail store as a salesperson.

In the emergency department, where you are the nurse, Sandra's physical examination reveals the following findings: temperature 38.4°C (101.2°F), pulse 106 beats/minute, respiratory rate 18/minute, and blood pressure 112/74 mmHg. She complains of dysuria, frequency, urinary urgency, and suprapubic pain. Sandra also reports seeing a small amount of blood in the urine and the sensation of incomplete bladder emptying. She states that recently her urine has become cloudy and smells bad.

As you continue your interview with the patient, she states, "I can't believe I have another urinary tract infection. I had one just last month." The urinalysis reveals microscopic bacteriuria (greater than 10^5/mL). A urine culture is also collected during this visit and the results will be reported within 48 hours.

The patient's preliminary diagnosis is recurrent urinary tract infection, and she receives a prescription for trimethoprim-sulfamethoxazole (TMP-SMZ) (Bactrim, Septra). Sandra is referred to a local health clinic for follow-up care.

Critical Thinking Questions

1. How should you respond to the patient's statements about the recurrent infections?
2. What health teaching regarding antibiotic therapy should you stress to this patient?
3. What information should you give patients about "saving" medications?
4. Why was a urine culture collected prior to initiating the antibiotic therapy?

Case Study

Ms. Dorothy Janes is an 80-year-old female admitted to your unit for hypertension. She is alert and oriented to person, time, and place. Her health care provider ordered Ms. Janes to be restricted to bed rest with bathroom privileges. When the patient's daughter comes to visit, she tells you that sometimes her mother has urinary incontinence due to her slow and unstable ambulation. She wants to know if her mother can have a urinary catheter inserted to prevent "accidents."

1. How would you respond to the daughter's request for her mother to have a urinary catheter inserted?
2. Brainstorm nursing actions that you could implement to avoid urinary incontinence for this patient.

NCLEX-RN® Review

1 An elderly client is prescribed sulfisoxazole (Gantrisin). Knowing that one of the major adverse effects of this drug is crystalluria, the nurse should instruct the client to:

1. Limit intake of foods high in calcium such as milk, cheese, and yogurt.
2. Avoid changing positions (lying down, sitting, or standing) rapidly.
3. Increase fluid intake to 2 to 3 L per day.
4. Avoid consuming alcoholic beverages while taking this medication.

2 The nurse understands that the main purpose of nitrofurantoin (Furadantin) is to:

1. Prevent recurrent urinary tract infections.
2. Relieve the pain associated with urinary tract infections.
3. Promote effective urinary elimination and prevent stasis.
4. Reduce pathogenic microorganisms specific to pyelonephritis.

3 The nurse is collecting health data from a client with a suspected urinary tract infection. Which of the following questions asked by the nurse is least important?

1. "Have you ever had migraine headaches?"
2. "Are you allergic to any sulfa drugs?"
3. "Do you empty your bladder before and after sexual intercourse?"
4. "When was your last menstrual period?"

4 The nurse is providing the client with discharge instructions concerning sulfonamides. Which statement by the client indicates to the nurse that the teaching session was effective?

1. "I can take this medication with an antacid if I experience stomach upset."
2. "This medication will not interact with my anticoagulant."
3. "If nausea continues for more than 24 hours, I will contact my doctor."
4. "I must consume foods high in potassium."

5 The client is to receive trimethoprim-sulfamethoxazole (Bactrim, Septra) for a urinary tract infection. A nurse should question the order for the client with which of the following conditions?

1. Low urinary output renal impairment
2. Elevated blood pressure
3. Expectorating cough and chills
4. Neurologic impairment

6 Trimethoprim-sulfamethoxazole (Bactrim, Septra) is initiated for a client with a urinary tract infection. Which of the following health teachings would be most appropriate for this drug? (Select all that apply.)

1. Stay out of direct sunlight, especially between the hours of 10:00 A.M. and 3:00 P.M.
2. Wear protective clothing, including a hat, as well as sunglasses.
3. Apply a sun block product that has a skin protection factor (SPF) of at least 15.
4. Apply a sun block lipstick that has an SPF of at least 15 to protect lips.
5. Limited use of a sun lamp or tanning bed or booth is acceptable.

See Answers to Critical Thinking Questions, Case Study, and NCLEX-RN® Review in Appendix A.

References

Bowen, A., & Hellstrom, W. J. G. (2007). Urinary tract infections: A primer for clinicians. *Medscape Today.* Retrieved July 28, 2008, from http://www.medscape.com/viewprogram/7049.

Burak, L. (n.d.). *Cranberry juice and UTI prevention.* Retrieved July 28, 2008, from http://altmed.creighton.edu/cranberries/index.html

Gross, P. A., & Patel, B. (2007). Reducing antibiotic overuse: A call for a national performance measure for not treating asymptomatic bacteriuria. *Clinical Infectious Diseases, 45*(7), 1335–1337.

Guay, D. (2008). Contemporary management of uncomplicated urinary tract infections. *Drugs, 68*(9), 1169–1205.

Institute for Clinical Systems Improvement. (2006). *Uncomplicated urinary tract infection in women.* Bloomington, MN: Author. Retrieved July 28, 2008, from http://www.guideline.gov/summary/summary.aspx?ss=15&doc_id=9657

Jepson, R.G., & Craig, J. C. (2007). A systematic review of the evidence for cranberries and blueberries in UTI prevention. *Molecular Nutrition & Food Research, 51*(6), 738–745.

Kimel, H. K. (2005). Managing urinary tract infections: Guide for nursing home practitioners. *Annals of Long Term Care, 13*(9), 25–30.

Lutters, M., & Vogt-Ferrier, N. B. (2008). Antibiotic duration for treating uncomplicated, symptomatic lower urinary tract infections in elderly women. *Cochrane Database of Systematic Reviews,* Issue 3. (Art. No.: CD001535, DOI: 10.1002/14651858.CD001535.pub2).

National Center for Complementary and Alternative Medicine (NCCAM). (2008). *Herbs at a Glance: Cranberry.* Retrieved July 24, 2008, from http://nccam.nih.gov/health/cranberry/

National Center for Complementary and Alternative Medicine (NCCAM). (2004). *Effects of cranberry-containing products in women with recurrent urinary tract infections (UTIs).* Bethesda, MD: National Institutes of Health.

Nicolle, L. E. (2005). Complicated urinary tract infection in adults. *The Canadian Journal of Infectious Diseases & Medical Microbiology, 16*(6), 349–360.

Pohl, A. (2007). Modes of administration of antibiotics for symptomatic severe urinary tract infections. *Cochrane Database of Systematic Reviews,* Issue 4. (Art. No.: CD003237, DOI:10.1002/14651858.CD003237.pub2).

Ribby, K. J. (2006). Decreasing urinary tract infections through staff development, outcomes and nursing process. *Journal of Nursing Care Quality, 21*(3), 272–276.

Skelly, J. (2006). A multifaceted intervention reduced antimicrobial prescriptions for suspected urinary tract infections in nursing home residents. *Evidence-Based Nursing, 9*(2), 59.

CHAPTER

A few years ago I lost my job and was unable to pay my rent. Since then, you could say that I'm homeless. I try to spend my nights at the shelter, but it is sometimes too crowded and I sleep on the street. About a month ago, I started feeling sick with a cough and fever. I'm exhausted and I have no energy.

Patient "Sam Myers"

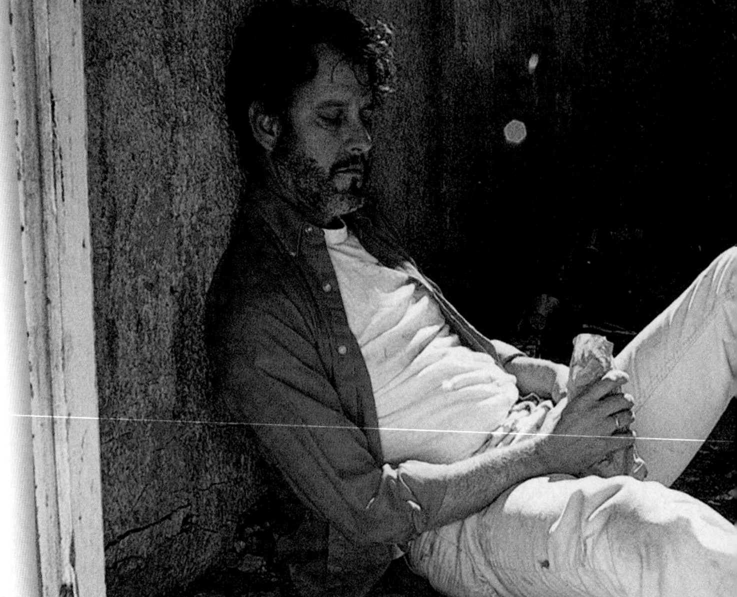

52 Pharmacotherapy of Mycobacterial Infections

Learning Outcomes

After reading this chapter, the student should be able to:

1. Compare and contrast the types of infections caused by mycobacteria.
2. Explain the pathogenesis of tuberculosis.
3. Describe how the pharmacotherapy of tuberculosis differs from that of bacterial infections.
4. Prepare a plan for monitoring the effectiveness of tuberculosis therapy.
5. Identify the most common drug regimens for treating tuberculosis.
6. Describe the pathogenesis and treatment of leprosy.
7. Describe the pathogenesis and treatment of infections caused by *Mycobacterium avium* complex.
8. For each of the classes shown in the chapter outline, identify the prototype and representative drugs and explain the mechanism(s) of drug action, primary indications, contraindications, significant drug interactions, pregnancy category, and important adverse effects.
9. Explain significant patient variables that must be considered for effective pharmacotherapy with antimycobacterial drugs.
10. Apply the nursing process to care for patients receiving drugs for mycobacterial infections.

Chapter Outline

Types of Mycobacterial Infections

Pathogenesis and Diagnosis of Tuberculosis

Pharmacotherapy of Tuberculosis

Antituberculosis Drugs

PROTOTYPE **Isoniazid (INH)** *p. 857*

Drugs for Leprosy

PROTOTYPE **Dapsone (DDS)** *p. 862*

Drugs for *Mycobacterium Avium* Complex (MAC) Infections

Key Terms

acetylation, 857
atypical mycobacterial infections (AMI), 851
directly observed therapy (DOT), 853
leprosy, 862
Mycobacterium avium complex (MAC), 851
mycolic acid, 851
purified protein derivative (PPD), 853
pyridoxine (vitamin B_6), 857
tubercles, 852
tuberculosis (TB), 851

Mycobacterial infections have been responsible for considerable human suffering and death throughout history. Mycobacterial disease was once called *consumption,* because of its ability to cause the body to waste away if left untreated. Although these infections usually respond to modern anti-infectives, therapy is prolonged, and resistant organisms have emerged as major clinical challenges. Despite the effective treatments available for the disease, tuberculosis (TB) still claims about 1.6 million lives each year worldwide. This chapter examines the pharmacotherapy of the three primary infections caused by mycobacteria.

PharmFACT

Over 13,000 Americans have tuberculosis. The TB incidence rate in 2007 was the lowest recorded since national reporting began in 1953. *Source:* Centers for Disease Control and Prevention, 2008.

Types of Mycobacterial Infections

52.1 Several species of mycobacteria are important human pathogens.

The genus *Mycobacterium* consists of about 100 species of aerobic organisms that have in common a unique and complex lipid, **mycolic acid,** which covers their cell surfaces. This waxy coating comprising up to 40% of the cell's weight protects the mycobacterium, making it resistant to many disinfectants, including chlorinated water. About 10 mycobacterial species are potential human pathogens, with *Mycobacterium tuberculosis* being the most common. Robert Koch, a pioneer microbiologist, identified *M. tuberculosis* as the causative agent of TB in 1882.

Nontuberculosis diseases caused by mycobacteria are known as **atypical mycobacterial infections (AMI).** These are considered opportunistic infections because they often appear in people with compromised immune defenses. As the occurrences of human immunodeficiency virus (HIV) infection and acquired immunodeficiency syndrome (AIDS) rose in the 1980s to the 1990s, the once-rare AMIs began to increase in frequency. In addition to HIV-AIDS, AMIs sometimes occurs in patients with leukemia or those who are undergoing antineoplastic or immunosuppressive therapy.

Mycobacterium leprae is an AMI that was identified as the causative agent of leprosy by G. A. Hansen in 1873. Leprosy is still sometimes called Hansen's disease, after its discoverer. The pharmacotherapy of leprosy is presented in Section 52.7.

Unlike *M. tuberculosis* and *M. leprae,* which have been described since antiquity, the characterization of ***Mycobacterium avium* complex (MAC)** infection is relatively recent. MAC usually arises as a secondary infection due to the immunosuppression caused by HIV-AIDS. MAC consists of two predominant species, *Mycobacterium avium* and *Mycobacterium intracellulare.* Whereas *M. avium* is the cause of almost all infections in patients with HIV-AIDS, *M. intracellulare* is more common in immunocompetent patients. The pharmacotherapy of MAC is discussed in Section 52.8.

Several other species can cause AMIs in humans, but their incidence is rare. *Mycobacterium kansasii* is the second most common cause of AMI in patients with HIV-AIDS. *Mycobacterium bovis* is usually acquired from the ingestion of raw, unpasteurized milk. Infections by *M. kansasii* or *M. bovis* cause respiratory symptoms that are almost identical to those of TB.

Mycobacterium scrofulaceum usually affects children 1 to 3 years of age. The target for this pathogen is the lymph nodes, and the infants have mild symptoms, such as low-grade fever. Infections by *Mycobacterium chelonae* and *Mycobacterium abscessus* can cause a variety of clinical syndromes including respiratory disease, local skin disease, osteomyelitis, joint infections, and ocular disease. Surgical site infections due to *M. chelonae* are well documented.

Pathogenesis and Diagnosis of Tuberculosis

52.2 Tuberculosis is a respiratory infection that exhibits both active and latent stages.

Tuberculosis (TB) is a highly contagious infection caused by the organism *M. tuberculosis.* Although tuberculosis has been a major killer throughout human history, its incidence has declined in the United States over most of the 20th century. With the appearance of HIV-AIDS, however, the incidence of TB greatly increased from 1985 to 1992. As many as 20% of all AIDS patients may develop active tuberculosis. High immigration rates from areas of the world where TB is endemic also contributed to increases in this disease in the United States during this period. However, the incidence of TB has declined since 1992.

Patients acquire *M. tuberculosis* by the respiratory route. During its infectious stages, the organism may be transmitted to others via airborne droplets by sneezing, coughing, and even talking. The organism can remain alive in these droplets for several hours outside the body. Unlike most species of mycobacteria, however, *M. tuberculosis* is not an environmental pathogen: It must reside in a living host to survive and reproduce.

TB infections may be classified as primary or post primary. A *primary* TB infection occurs when the patient inhales mycobacteria from a person with an active TB infection. Because they are acquired via inhalation, most primary infections occur in upper lobes of the lungs. The slow-growing mycobacteria activate cells of the immune response, which isolate the microorganisms by creating a wall of macrophages around them. In an attempt to neutralize the mycobacteria, the macrophages ingest them. The pathogens, however, can grow *inside* the macrophages, despite the presence of an ongoing immune response. An acute respiratory infection develops, with symptoms presenting as pneumonia. In those with healthy immune systems, the primary infection lasts a few weeks and then subsides.

Although the macrophages are eventually successful in isolating the pathogen, granulomatous lesions called **tubercles** are formed in the lung. Tissue within the tubercles undergoes necrosis, causing cavities within the lung, which can be identified on chest radiographs. The mycobacteria often become dormant, lying inside the tubercles for an extended time. Indeed, people can retain latent, inactive mycobacteria in tubercles for an entire lifetime.

If the immune system becomes suppressed later in life, the dormant mycobacteria may enter a postprimary or reactivation stage. Once reactivated, *M. tuberculosis* can be disseminated throughout the body via the blood or lymphatic system. Lymph nodes and organs of the genitourinary system are the most common nonrespiratory sites, although infections of the bone marrow and liver are possible. Reactivation frequently occurs in patients with HIV-AIDS, those with poor nutritional status, and those suffering from terminal or debilitating diseases. The pathogenesis of TB is illustrated in Pharmacotherapy Illustrated 52.1.

Some patients with TB remain asymptomatic throughout the infection. In others, the disease progresses so gradually that the individual may not seek medical interventions until the disease becomes advanced. Symptoms are nonspecific and include anorexia, weight loss, night sweats, fatigue, and low-grade fever. Cough becomes progressively worse, producing infectious sputum.

PHARMACOTHERAPY *ILLUSTRATED* 52.1

The Pathogenesis of Tuberculosis

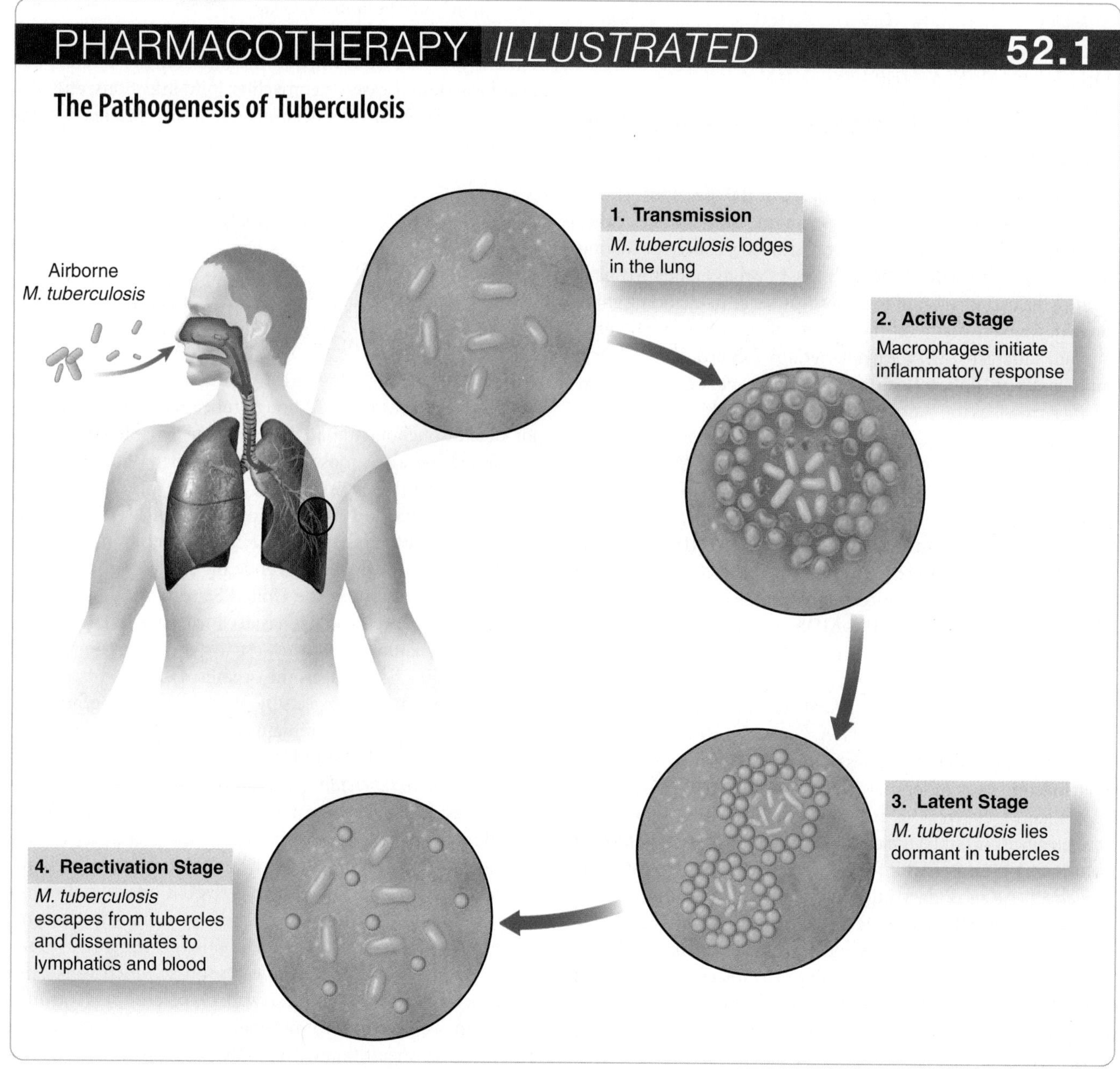

TB is diagnosed by several different means. Each of the following tests has advantages and drawbacks:

- Tuberculin skin test **(purified protein derivative [PPD])**. A positive PPD indicates the presence of memory T cells to *M. tuberculosis*, but cannot determine whether the disease is active or latent. Once a positive PPD occurs, the test will always be positive due to the presence of these memory T cells and the patient should never have subsequent PPDs because skin damage may result.
- Sputum cultures. These are used to culture and identify *M. tuberculosis*. Unfortunately, samples may be negative even when the patient has confirmed TB. Because *M. tuberculosis* grows very slowly on cultured media, results may take several weeks to obtain.
- Chest radiography. Both active and chronic TB infections produce changes in the lung that can be identified on chest radiographs. X-ray evidence is not always specific to TB, however, and other diagnostic evidence is needed to confirm the disease. Annual chest x-rays are used to exclude active TB in patients who exhibit positive PPDs.
- Amplified DNA/RNA tests. Diagnostic laboratory tests such as the Amplicor Diagnostic Mycobacterium Tuberculosis Test can identify the presence of *M. tuberculosis* RNA in a sample. Although these tests are rapid, they are not always used for diagnosis because of their expense.

CONNECTION *Checkpoint* 52.1

From what you learned in Chapter 45, identify immunosuppressant drugs that may cause TB to enter the reactivation stage in a patient who is receiving pharmacotherapy with these agents. See Answer to Connection Checkpoint 52.1 in Appendix A.

Pharm*FACT*

It is estimated that 2 billion people in the world are infected with TB bacilli. This represents almost a third of the world's population. *Source:* World Health Organization, 2008.

Pharmacotherapy of Tuberculosis

52.3 The pharmacotherapy of tuberculosis requires special dosing regimens and schedules.

The primary goal of tuberculosis pharmacotherapy is to eliminate all tubercle mycobacteria, while avoiding the emergence of resistant strains. This involves an initial or induction phase of therapy during which the actively dividing mycobacterial cells are killed, and a continuation phase in which the remaining dormant mycobacteria are eliminated. Special pharmacotherapeutic strategies are required to successfully eradicate this persistent pathogen.

The pharmacotherapy of tuberculosis differs from that of other bacterial infections because the thick mycolic acid layer surrounding the mycobacterium is resistant to penetration by anti-infectives. For the drugs to reach the mycobacteria isolated in tubercles and inside macrophages, therapy must continue for 6 to 12 months. Although the patient is not infectious this entire time and, indeed, may have no symptoms, it is critical that therapy continue the entire period. Patients who develop multidrug-resistant infections may require therapy for as long as 2 years.

A second difference in the therapy of tuberculosis is that a minimum of two—and sometimes as many as seven—antimycobacterial drugs are administered concurrently. During the long treatment period, different combinations of drugs are usually used. Combination drug therapy is necessary because mycobacteria grow slowly and often develop resistance during the course of treatment. The incidence of multidrug-resistant TB is increasing. In some communities, as many as 10% of patients have infections resistant to at least one antituberculosis medication. The use of multiple drugs that kill mycobacteria by different mechanisms lowers the potential for resistance and increases pharmacotherapeutic success. Figure 52.1 illustrates the use of combination therapy during tuberculosis therapy. Doses for the antimycobacterial agents are listed in Table 52.1.

A third difference in therapy is that antimycobacterial drugs are used extensively for preventing the disease, in addition to treating active infections. Because of the acute infectious nature of tuberculosis, prophylactic therapy is indicated for close contacts or family members of recently diagnosed patients. Therapy of infected patients and all close contacts begins immediately after a positive diagnosis has been established. Patients with compromised immune function, such as those with HIV-AIDS or those who are receiving immunosuppressant drugs, may also receive preventative treatment with antimycobacterials. A short-term therapy of 2 months, consisting of combination therapy with isoniazid (INH) and pyrazinamide, is approved for tuberculosis prophylaxis in HIV-positive patients.

A major concern with tuberculosis pharmacotherapy is ensuring that patients fully comply with the prescribed regimen. Nonadherence to pharmacotherapy is the most common cause of treatment failure in tuberculosis patients. In high-risk patients, **directly observed therapy (DOT)** is necessary. DOT requires that a health care provider directly observe the patient swallowing the pills, whether it is in the hospital, office, or home care setting. Nurses serve essential roles in providing education about this disorder to their patients and stressing the importance of adherence.

52.4 The progress of tuberculosis pharmacotherapy must be monitored during the entire treatment period.

Prior to starting TB pharmacotherapy, several baseline assessments should be conducted. Because isoniazid and several other antituberculosis agents are hepatotoxic, the levels of hepatic enzymes and serum bilirubin should be measured. Visual acuity and red-green color vision tests should be obtained because ethambutol may affect these values. Pharmacotherapy with pyrazinamide requires obtaining a baseline serum uric acid level. Audiometry should be performed prior to streptomycin therapy.

During the course of therapy, patients receive monthly follow-up examinations. The nurse should assess for signs of hepatotoxicity, and document any patient symptoms that may

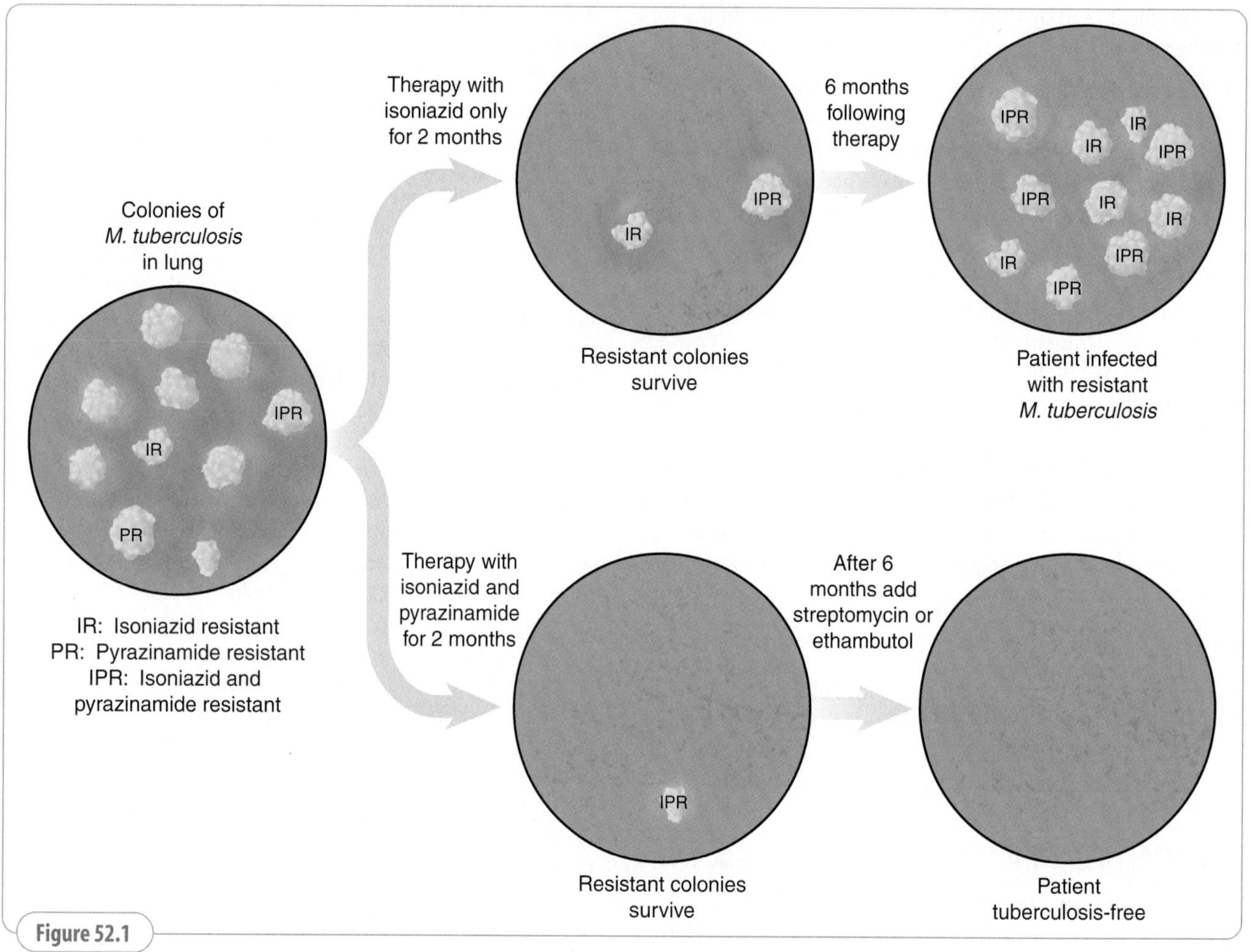

Figure 52.1

Use of combination therapy during tuberculosis therapy to avoid resistance.

suggest adverse drug effects. A complete review of current medications should be conducted to be certain that additional drugs have not been prescribed that could interact with the antimycobacterials. Adherence to the therapeutic regimen must be carefully assessed. For most patients, it is not necessary to perform routine laboratory monitoring for drug toxicity during the treatment period. Patients with known hepatic impairment or who use large amounts of alcohol, however, should receive frequent hepatic enzyme tests.

Sputum smears and cultures are obtained monthly until at least 2 consecutive months of negative values are obtained. Patients with confirmed multidrug-resistant TB should have monthly sputum smears and cultures tests throughout the entire course of pharmacotherapy. At the conclusion of therapy, all patients receive a sputum smear and culture, and a chest radiograph to confirm the absence of active disease. Additional follow-up may be conducted for up to 1 year to exclude the possibility of relapse.

Three months after drug therapy is initiated, approximately 90% of patients will have negative smears and cultures, indicating that the drugs have successfully killed all active mycobacteria. Patients who continue to have positive cultures should be evaluated for the possibility of multidrug-resistant TB. For these patients, drug susceptibility testing is performed and the regimen is adjusted accordingly. The most common cause of treatment failure is poor patient adherence, and the nurse should carefully evaluate any psychosocial factors that may be preventing the patient from taking the medication properly. When multidrug-resistant TB is identified, DOT may be implemented during the remainder of the treatment period to better ensure successful treatment outcomes.

CONNECTION *Checkpoint* 52.2

From what you learned in Chapter 7, identify at least three major factors that might explain why a patient may choose to stop taking antimycobacterials. See Answer to Connection Checkpoint 52.2 in Appendix A.

TABLE 52.1 Antimycobacterial Agents

Drug	Route and Adult Dose (maximum dose where indicated)	Adverse Effects
First-Line Agents		
ethambutol (Myambutol)	Oral (PO): 15–25 mg/kg/day (max: 1,600 mg for daily therapy)	*Nausea, vomiting, headache, dizziness* Anaphylaxis, optic neuritis
isoniazid (INH, Nydrazid)	Latent TB PO: 300 mg/day or 900 mg twice weekly for 6–9 months Active TB PO**:** Daily therapy: 5mg/kg/day or 300 mg/day; if given by DOT: 15 mg/kg or 900 mg twice weekly	*Nausea, vomiting, diarrhea, epigastric pain* Anaphylaxis, peripheral neuropathy, optic neuritis, hepatotoxicity, blood dyscrasias
pyrazinamide (PZA)	PO: 5–15 mg/kg tid-qid (max: 2 g/day)	*Non-gouty polyarthralgia, increase in serum uric acid, rash* Anaphylaxis, hepatotoxicity, fatal hemoptysis, hemolytic anemia
rifabutin (Mycobutin)	TB Prophylaxis PO: 300 mg once daily Active TB 1st phase PO: 5 mg/kg/day 2nd phase PO: 5 mg/kg/day or twice weekly (max: 300 mg/day)	*Nausea, vomiting, heartburn, epigastric pain, anorexia, flatulence, diarrhea, cramping, orange discoloration of the urine, sweat, tears* Pseudomembranous colitis, acute renal failure, hepatotoxicity, hyperuricemia, blood dyscrasias
rifampin (Rifadin, Rimactane)	Latent TB PO: 600 mg/day or 900 mg twice weekly for 4 months Active TB PO: 10 mg/kg/day or 600 mg/day Intravenous (IV) and PO are same dose, but IV needs to be given over 30 min to 3 h and the final concentration should not exceed 6 mg/mL	
rifapentine (Priftin)	PO: 600 mg (four 150-mg tablets) given twice a week for 2 months with an interval of no less than 72 h between doses, then once a week for 4 months	
Second-Line Agents		
aminosalicylic acid (Paser)	PO: 150 mg/kg/day in 3–4 equally divided doses (max: 8g/day)	*GI intolerance, anorexia, diarrhea, fever, leukopenia* Hypersensitivity, inhibition of vitamin B_{12} absorption, hepatotoxicity
amikacin (Amikin)	Intramuscular (IM): 10–15 mg/kg daily for 2 weeks in a large muscle	*Pain or inflammation at injection site, rash, fever, nausea, diarrhea, dizziness, tinnitus* Anaphylaxis, nephrotoxicity, pseudomembranous colitis with prolonged use, irreversible ototoxicity, superinfections
capreomycin (Capastat Sulfate)	IM: 1 g/day (not to exceed 20 mg/kg/day) for 60–120 days, then 1 g 2–3 times/week	*Rash, pain and inflammation at injection site, tinnitus* Blood dyscrasias, nephrotoxicity, ototoxicity, increase in urination, thirst
ciprofloxacin (Cipro)	PO: 250–750 mg bid	*Nausea, diarrhea, vomiting, rash, restlessness, pain and inflammation at injection site, local burning, stinging and corneal irritation (ophthalmic)* Anaphylaxis, tendon rupture, superinfections, photosensitivity, pseudomembranous colitis, seizure, peripheral neuropathy, hepatotoxicity
cycloserine (Seromycin)	PO: 250 mg every 12 h for 2 weeks; may increase to 500 mg every 12 h (max: 1 g/day)	*Drowsiness, headache, lethargy* Convulsions, psychosis, confusion
ethionamide (Trecator-SC)	PO: 750 mg/day (max: 1 gram given in 3–4 divided doses)	*Nausea, vomiting, epigastric pain, diarrhea* Convulsions, hallucinations, mental depression, hepatotoxicity
kanamycin (Kantrex)	IM: 5–7.5 mg/kg bid tid	(see amikacin)
ofloxacin (Floxin)	PO: 200–400 mg bid	(see ciprofloxacin)
streptomycin	IM: 15–30 mg/kg (max: 1–2 g/day) DOT: twice weekly IM: 25–30 mg/kg (max: 1.5 g) DOT: 3 times a week IM: 25–30 mg/kg	*Nausea, vomiting, pain at injection site, drowsiness, headache* Anaphylaxis, ototoxicity, profound CNS depression in infants, respiratory depression, exfoliative dermatitis, nephrotoxicity, teratogenicity

Note: *Italics* indicate common adverse effects. Underline indicates serious adverse effects.

CONNECTIONS

Evidence-Based Practice Direct Observation Therapy Effectiveness

Clinical Question

Some individuals with tuberculosis require drug therapy for at least 6 months. However, many do not complete their course of treatment and may require directly observed therapy (DOT). Does DOT, when compared with self-administration of treatment, affect cure or treatment completion in people receiving treatment for tuberculosis?

Evidence

Investigators Volmink and Garner (2004) examined 11 different research studies to determine the effectiveness of this intervention. Based on the evidence, no statistically significant difference was detected between DOT and self-administration in terms of cure, with similar results for cure plus completion of treatment. When stratified by location, DOT provided at home compared with DOT provided at clinics suggests a possible small advantage for cure with home-based DOT. There was no significant difference detected in clinical outcomes between DOT at a clinic versus DOT provided by a family member or a community health worker (2 trials), or for DOT provided by a family member versus a community health worker.

Implication

Patient adherence to antituberculosis therapy is an issue for the general public since the spread of mycobacterial infections is possible to all those in the community. For this reason, services for people with tuberculosis often use different approaches to encourage people to complete their course of treatment. For many years, health care providers have assumed that DOT by health workers, family members, or community members of people taking their medication showed better cure rates than people having self-administered treatment. However, this intervention is expensive and often difficult to implement and should be closely scrutinized for its effectiveness.

Critical Thinking Question

What criteria would you use determine if the patient needs DOT?

See Answers to Critical Thinking Questions in Appendix A.

Source: From "Directly Observed Therapy for Treating Tuberculosis," by J. Volmink and P. Garner, 2007. Cochrane Database of Systematic Reviews, 3. (Art. No.: CD003343, DOI: 10.1002/14651858.CD003343.pub3)

52.5 First-line or primary antituberculosis drugs are the most efficacious and safest drugs for treating *M. tuberculosis* infections.

MyNursingKit | Tuberculosis Video

Medications for TB are placed into two categories. The safer and more effective agents are called *first-line drugs.* A second group of drugs, which exhibit greater toxicity, are less effective and prescribed when resistance develops to the first-line agents. The *second-line drugs* are discussed in Section 52.6.

The pharmacotherapy regimen for TB depends on drug sensitivity, disease stage, and the patient's immune status. Ideally, results of culture and sensitivity (C&S) testing should be obtained prior to treatment because of the possibility of drug-resistant strains. Definitive C&S results may take several weeks, however, and treatment must begin immediately. Therefore, the initial selection of pharmacotherapy is based on the experience of the prescriber and later adjusted when laboratory results become available.

Standard Regimen

A typical regimen for patients with no complicating factors includes the following:

- Initial phase. 2 months of daily therapy with isoniazid, rifampin (Rifadin, Rimactane), pyrazinamide (PZA), and ethambutol (Myambutol). If C&S results show that the strain is sensitive to the first three drugs, ethambutol is dropped from the regimen.
- Continuation phase. 4 months of therapy with isoniazid and rifampin, 2 to 3 times per week.

The above regimen cures more than 95% of these patients. There are, however, many variations, based on patient variables. In regions where the incidence of isoniazid resistance is 4% or higher, ethambutol (Myambutol) or streptomycin is included as part of the initial therapeutic regimen. Three months of additional therapy may be indicated, depending on whether the sputum cultures have turned negative during therapy. Nine months of therapy is recommended for patients with evidence of nonrespiratory TB. The latest treatment guidelines are published by the Centers for Disease Control and Prevention (CDC).

HIV-Positive Patients

Patients who are HIV positive often respond to the standard regimen. Because nonadherence has been frequently reported, DOT is recommended for HIV-positive patients. In addition, patients taking numerous antiretroviral agents are at greater risk for drug–drug interactions and must be monitored carefully. For example, rifampin and rifabutin can increase the metabolism of some antiretrovirals, thus decreasing their effectiveness against HIV. Certain drug combinations, such as rifampin with single protease inhibitors, should be avoided to the extent possible or dosages adjusted accordingly. Nurses treating HIV-AIDS patients with TB should regularly consult recent pharmacology sources to identify the many drug–drug interactions because serious adverse effects can compromise the success of pharmacotherapy for both TB and HIV.

Pregnant Patients

Pregnant patients with tuberculosis are at risk because drug choices are fewer. The safety of pyrazinamide during pregnancy has not been established; thus, it is usually avoided. Although ethambutol has been used successfully without adverse fetal effects, high doses in laboratory animals produced a low incidence of birth defects; therefore, it is used in pregnancy only if C&S testing shows it to be effective. Streptomycin is contraindicated during pregnancy because it can cause hear-

CONNECTIONS

Treating the Diverse Patient Nursing in Correctional Facilities: High-Risk Populations

Correctional facilities such as prisons and jails present special challenges for tuberculosis (TB) prevention and transmission. Within worldwide prison systems, outbreaks of TB are epidemic. Both case rates and drug resistance rates are increasing, creating an urgent need for more effective TB control.

In correctional facilities, TB infection and active disease occurs in a disproportionate number of inmates dependent on certain exposure factors. Risk factors include overcrowded and inadequately ventilated prison facilities with inmates who are malnourished and infected with HIV or hepatitis B and C viruses. Often, inmates continue substance abuse, which presents an additional risk. A high proportion of inmates are from racial and ethnic minorities and lower socioeconomic populations, which may have inadequate access to or understanding of health care therapies.

The increased transmission of TB in prisons is a health problem for both inmates and the communities into which they return upon release. Inmates infected with *M. tuberculosis* can develop TB disease after their release and infect other persons in the community. Improved health care treatments and monitoring is necessary for both prisoners and the community.

In the late 1970s, nurses became the major providers of health care in correctional facilities. This role includes emergency care, primary care, environmental health care, rehabilitation, health education and promotion, and preventive care. TB surveillance is part of this role as well. Nurses combine knowledge, skills, and experience in the correction field to plan, develop, and manage health care (American Nurses Association [ANA], 1991).

Nurses in correctional facilities identify and manage health care for inmates infected with TB. Professional nurses must assess and promptly report inmates who are diagnosed or suspected of having tuberculosis. Upon confirmation of diagnosis, initiation and completion of safe and effective therapy must be implemented to cure TB, reduce transmission, and prevent the development of drug resistance.

ing impairment in the newborn. Fortunately, these drugs have not been shown to have adverse effects on the breast-feeding neonate; thus, therapy can safely continue during lactation.

Chemoprophylaxis Patients

Treatment of latent or dormant TB reduces the risk that the infection will progress to its active stage, thereby helping to prevent transmission of the disease. Although it would seem prudent to treat everyone suspected of having latent TB, pharmacotherapy is expensive and carries the risk of adverse drug reactions. Patients with a possible latent TB infection are screened and only treated if they fall into a high-risk category. High-risk categories include HIV-positive patients, those receiving immunosuppressive drugs, employees and residents of nursing homes, those living in residential facilities for AIDS patients, prisons, people born in countries where TB is endemic, and those who have been in close contact with patients with active TB. Pharmacotherapy of latent TB normally includes one of the following regimens:

- Nine (9) months of therapy with isoniazid. This is considered the standard treatment. Depending on anticipated patient adherence, the dose may be daily (300 mg) or twice weekly (15 mg/kg).
- Two (2) months of therapy with both rifampin and pyrazinamide. This shorter-duration therapy increases patient adherence, yet it is still effective in eliminating most strains of *M. tuberculosis.*
- Four (4) months of therapy with rifampin. This monotherapy is used for patients who are unable to take isoniazid or pyrazinamide, or who have infections caused by organisms that are resistant to these drugs.

The pharmacotherapy of latent TB is modified for certain patients. Close contacts of HIV-AIDS patients with TB should be treated for at least 12 months. Contacts of patients with confirmed multidrug-resistant TB should receive at least two drugs known to be effective against the resistant *M. tuberculosis* strain. These patients usually require follow-up for 2 years to be certain the resistant strains have been killed. Pregnant patients should receive isoniazid therapy supplemented with **pyridoxine (vitamin B_6),** which has been shown to prevent peripheral neuropathy.

PROTOTYPE DRUG Isoniazid (INH)

Classification: **Therapeutic:** Antituberculosis agent, antimycobacterial

Pharmacologic: Mycolic acid inhibitor

Therapeutic Effects and Uses: Although a patient may take many different drugs during the long treatment period, isoniazid is considered the prototype antituberculosis drug. Approved by the U.S. Food and Drug Administration (FDA) in 1952, it has been a drug of choice for the treatment of *M. tuberculosis* infections because decades of experience have shown it to have a superior safety profile and to be the most effective, single drug for the disease. Isoniazid is used exclusively for the treatment and prophylaxis of mycobacterial infections. Isoniazid may be used alone for chemoprophylaxis, or in combination with other antituberculosis drugs for treating active disease. When used for prophylaxis, therapy may continue for as long as a year. While resistance to isoniazid can develop during therapy, the incidence is only about 10%. Treatment of active disease requires multidrug therapy.

The main route of metabolism of isoniazid is through enzymatic **acetylation** in the liver. Acetylation is a general biochemical process that adds a two-carbon chain to a drug molecule, which usually renders the medication less effective or allows it to be excreted more easily. Not all people are able to acetylate isoniazid at the same rate because of genetic differences in the activity of acetyltransferase, the hepatic enzyme that performs this action. Those of Japanese and Inuit descent often have increased enzyme activity and are known as *fast acetylators.* Those with decreased activity—*slow acetylators*—are most commonly of Scandinavian, North African Caucasian, or Jewish descent. The

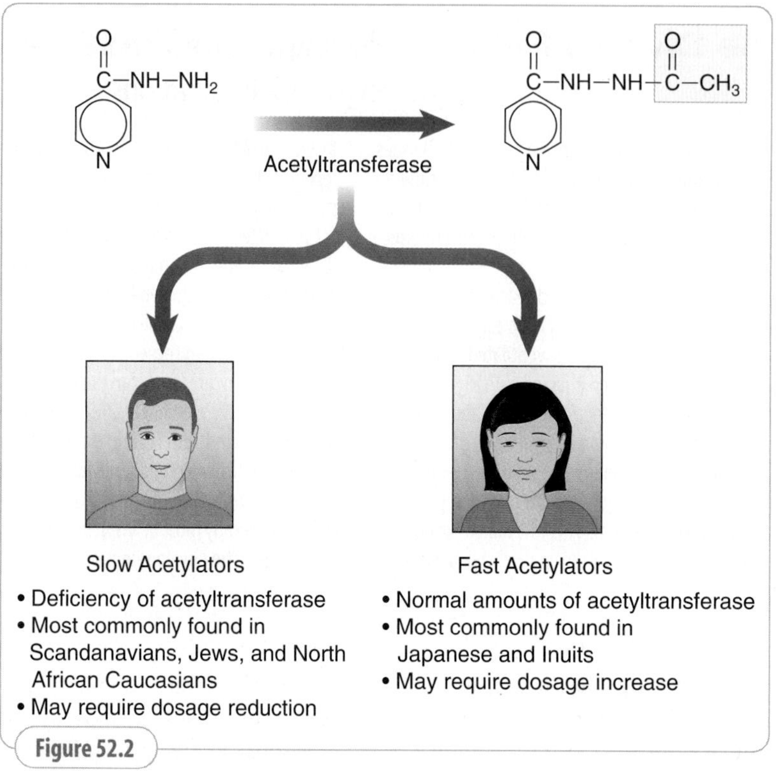

Figure 52.2

Acetylation of isoniazid.

half-life of isoniazid ranges from 70 minutes in fast acetylators to 2 to 5 hours in slow acetylators. Fortunately, isoniazid is safe across a wide range of doses, and these variations do not generally result in toxicity. For optimal therapy, however, doses should be lowered in slow acetylators to avoid adverse effects and increased in fast acetylators to keep plasma levels consistently in the therapeutic range. Dosage reductions should also occur in any patient with significant hepatic impairment because of diminished acetylation. The acetylation of isoniazid is illustrated in Figure 52.2.

Mechanism of Action: Isoniazid acts by inhibiting the synthesis of mycolic acid, an essential cell-wall component of mycobacteria. Because mycolic acids are unique to mycobacteria, isoniazid has no activity for other microbial species. It is bacteriocidal for rapidly dividing organisms but bacteriostatic for dormant mycobacteria.

Pharmacokinetics:

Route(s)	Oral (PO) and intramuscular (IM) (only if PO is unavailable)
Absorption	Readily absorbed
Distribution	Widely distributed (can even enter the necrotic lung tubercles that are characteristic of TB); crosses the placenta, and enters the central nervous system (CNS): secreted in breast milk; about 60% bound to plasma protein.
Primary metabolism	Metabolized by acetylation in the liver
Primary excretion	Renal (75%)
Onset of action	Rapid
Duration of action	Half-life: 1–4 h

Adverse Effects: Isoniazid exhibits few serious adverse effects, which is a major reason why it is a drug of choice for mycobacterial infections. Neurotoxicity is a concern during therapy, and patients may exhibit paresthesia of the feet and hands, convulsions, optic neuritis, dizziness, coma, memory loss, and various psychoses. A major factor responsible for the neurotoxicity of isoniazid is the ability of the drug to cause a deficiency of activated pyridoxine (vitamin B_6), which is required for synthesis of the neurotransmitter gamma-aminobutyric acid (GABA). Many practitioners routinely prescribe pyridoxine during isoniazid therapy to prevent the development of peripheral neuropathy. Pyridoxine is considered the antidote for reversing acute nervous system effects of isoniazid overdose.

Common adverse effects of isoniazid are rash and fever. Although rare, hepatotoxicity is a serious and sometimes fatal adverse effect; thus, the patient should be monitored carefully for jaundice, fatigue, elevated hepatic enzymes, or loss of appetite. Liver enzyme tests are usually performed monthly during therapy to identify early hepatotoxicity. Hepatotoxicity usually appears in the first 1 to 3 months of therapy but may occur at any time during treatment. Older adults appear to be at greater risk to developing hepatotoxicity. Blood dyscrasias such as agranulocytosis and aplastic anemia may occur, although they are uncommon.

Contraindications/Precautions: Isoniazid has no absolute contraindications other than previous allergy to the drug. Pharmacotherapy must be monitored carefully in patients with a history of chronic hepatic disease because the liver metabolizes the drug and fatal hepatitis has been reported. Serum aspartate transaminase (AST) levels should be monitored regularly during therapy in high-risk patients. If AST levels rise to 3 times baseline levels, liver damage is likely and isoniazid should be discontinued. Patients with significant renal impairment usually require lower doses because the kidneys excrete the drug. Patients with seizure disorders should be carefully monitored because isoniazid can increase the incidence of seizures. Patients with a history of seizures often receive pyridoxine supplementation to prevent seizures during isoniazid therapy.

Drug Interactions: Isoniazid is a potent inhibitor of hepatic metabolic enzymes (CYP2C19 and CYP3A4) and is associated with numerous drug–drug interactions. Before adding a new drug to the regimen, the nurse should consult a drug guide for potential interactions. Aluminum-containing antacids should not be administered concurrently because they can decrease the absorption of isoniazid. When disulfiram is taken with isoniazid, lack of coordination or severe psychotic reactions may result. Ethanol use should be avoided because it can increase the risk of hepatotoxicity. Isoniazid inhibits the metabolic breakdown of phenytoin, which may cause the anticonvulsant to build to toxic levels, an effect that occurs more often in slow acetylators. Isoniazid can increase serum levels of carbamazepine and cause carbamazepine toxicity. **Herbal/Food**: Food decreases the absorption of isoniazid.

Pregnancy: Category C.

Treatment of Overdose: Isoniazid overdose may be fatal and treatment is mostly symptomatic. Pyridoxine may be infused in a dose equal to that of the isoniazid overdose to prevent seizures and to correct metabolic acidosis. The dose may be repeated several times until the patient regains consciousness.

Nursing Responsibilities:

- Obtain a complete health history including allergies, drug history, and possible drug interactions. Perform a complete physical examination including vital signs.
- Assess for the presence or history of the following: positive tuberculin skin test, a positive sputum culture or smear, immunosuppressant drug therapy, alcohol abuse, or liver or kidney disease, or close contact with a person recently infected with TB, HIV infection, or AIDS.
- Assess the patient's ability to adhere to long-term therapy.
- Initiate drug therapy after performing appropriate C&S testing to detect possible bacterial resistance.
- Monitor serum drug levels. Remember that inactivation of isoniazid is genetically determined. Be aware that slow inactivation leads to high plasma drug levels and increased risk of toxicity.
- Monitor hepatic function with laboratory tests. Isoniazid hepatitis can be fatal, especially in patients 35 or older and those who ingest alcohol daily. It usually develops during the first 3 to 6 months of treatment but may occur at any time during therapy.
- Administer pyridoxine (vitamin B_6) supplementation (10 to 50 mg). Isoniazid-induced pyridoxine depletion results in neurotoxic effects such as peripheral neuropathy.
- Monitor blood pressure during the period of dosage adjustment to prevent orthostatic hypotension during rapid positional change.
- Monitor serum glucose levels in patients with diabetes. Loss of glycemic control can occur due to drug therapy.
- Monitor for therapeutic effectiveness, which may be observed within the first 2 to 3 weeks of initiating therapy. More than 90% of patients have negative sputum culture reports by the sixth month.

Patient and Family Education:

- Continue therapy until all doses have been taken. The infection may worsen if the instructions for taking the drug are not followed exactly.
- Discontinue the drug and immediately report any allergic reaction, which usually occurs within the 3- to 7-week period after initiating therapy, to the health care provider.
- Discontinue the medication and report dark urine, jaundice, or clay-colored stools, to the health care provider because these symptoms may indicate possible liver toxicity.
- Avoid tyramine-containing foods such as aged cheeses and smoked fish, because these foods may cause flushing, palpitation, and blood pressure elevation.
- Histamine-containing foods such as tuna, sauerkraut in juice, and yeast extracts should be avoided. These foods may result in an exaggerated drug response such as headache, sweating, itching, flushing, hypotension, palpitation, or diarrhea.
- Avoid alcohol while on isoniazid therapy because the risk of liver toxicity is increased.
- Do not breast-feed while taking this drug without approval of the health care provider.
- Keep all appointments for follow-up care because drug resistance and relapse may occur.

Drugs Similar to Isoniazid (INH)

Other first-line antituberculosis drugs include rifampin, rifapentine, rifabutin, pyrazinamide, and ethambutol.

Rifampin (Rifadin, Rimactane): Rifampin is widely used in combination with other drugs in the first-line treatment of TB: It is rarely given as monotherapy for the short-course therapy of latent *M. tuberculosis* infections. Rifampin exerts its bacteriocidal effects by inhibiting RNA synthesis. In addition to treating TB, rifampin is a broad-spectrum antibiotic approved for the short-term treatment of meningococci from the nasopharynx of asymptomatic carriers of *Neisseria meningitidis.* Unlabeled uses include chemoprophylaxis of contacts of patients with *Haemophilus influenza* type B and the treatment of Legionnaire's disease. It is also used to treat leprosy, in combination with dapsone. The drug should only be used when the infectious microbe has been demonstrated to be susceptible to the effects of the medication.

Rifampin is administered by either the PO or intravenous (IV) routes. Hypersensitivity reactions cause flulike symptoms in as many as 50% of the patients taking rifampin. Rash and urticaria are relatively common. Rifampin can be hepatotoxic and caution must be used when administering the drug to patients with preexisting liver disease or who are taking other hepatotoxic antituberculosis drugs such as isoniazid and pyrazinamide.

Rifampin is a potent inducer of cytochrome P450 enzymes. Thus, it has the potential to increase the metabolism of other drugs metabolized by the liver, such as some antiretrovirals for HIV-AIDS, warfarin, and PO contraceptives. Because resistance develops rapidly, rifampin is almost always given in combination with other drugs. This drug is pregnancy category C.

Rifapentine (Priftin) and Rifabutin (Mycobutin): These two drugs are PO agents closely related to rifampin that act by the same mechanism and cause the same adverse effects, including induction of P450 enzymes. There is a high level of cross resistance among rifampin, rifapentine, and rifabutin, which, collectively, are called *rifamycin derivatives.* They are always used in combination with other antituberculosis medications.

Approved in 1998, rifapentine is approved only for the pharmacotherapy of TB and has a longer half-life than rifampin, thus offering the advantage of twice-a-week dosing. Rifabutin was approved in 1992 for the pharmacotherapy of TB and the prophylaxis of MAC in HIV-infected patients. It offers little advantage over rifampin, other than it is thought to have less effect on hepatic enzymes. Rifapentine is pregnancy category C; rifabutin is category B.

Pyrazinamide (PZA): Pyrazinamide is an older drug approved in 1955 that is used for the initial therapy of active or advanced TB in combination with other antimycobacterials. It is usually taken in combination with rifampin, ethambutol, and INH for 8 weeks. If used alone, resistance develops rapidly. Like isoniazid, it acts by inhibiting the synthesis of mycolic acid in *M. tuberculosis.* Given PO, it is distributed to all body fluids and is excreted by the kidneys.

Pyrazinamide causes some degree of dose-related hepatotoxicity in as many as 15% of patients. Great caution should be observed when giving pyrazinamide to patients with preexisting hepatic disease, and frequent laboratory monitoring of liver enzymes must be performed. Frequent use of ethanol increases the risk of hepatotoxicity. Hyperuricemia may be observed in patients because the drug slows the excretion of uric acid. Uric acid levels should be monitored and the nurse should assess for signs of gout or arthralgia, which can occur in up to 40% of the patients taking this drug. This drug is pregnancy category C.

Ethambutol (Myambutol): Approved in 1967, ethambutol is included in multidrug regimens for TB because it is sometimes active against organisms resistant to other first-line agents. It is also effective against atypical mycobacteria such as *M. kansasii.* The mechanism of action of ethambutol is not well understood, although its bacteriostatic effect is thought to be due to the inhibition of cell-wall synthesis and RNA synthesis. It is always given with other antimycobacterials because resistance develops rapidly if the drug is given as monotherapy. It is rapidly absorbed, distributed to most tissues, and excreted by both renal and fecal routes. Ethambutol has a short half-life of 1 to 4 hours; therefore, it must be taken daily.

Ethambutol has a unique adverse effect of optic neuritis that affects visual acuity and the ability to distinguish red from green. This effect is dose related, may be unilateral or bilateral, and is usually reversible when therapy is discontinued. A baseline ophthalmic exam should be conducted prior to therapy. Ethambutol may decrease the excretion of uric acid, causing hyperuricemia; patients with a history of gout should be closely monitored. This drug has few other significant adverse effects. Ethambutol is pregnancy category C.

Combination agents: Rifamate is a capsule that contains both isoniazid and rifampin. Rifater is a tablet containing isoniazid, rifampin, and pyrazinamide. Combining multiple drugs into a single capsule or pill increases their ease of use and promotes patient adherence with therapy.

52.6 Second-line antituberculosis drugs are used when resistance develops to the first-line agents.

If a patient develops multidrug-resistant strains of *M. tuberculosis* during the course of therapy, second-line antibiotics are added to the regimen. These drugs are either more toxic or less effective than the first-line agents. Some of them are occasionally included as part of the initial course of therapy if C&S testing demonstrates their effectiveness. As a rule of therapy, a single antituberculosis agent should never be added to a regimen that fails to control the mycobacterial infection. At least two, and preferably three, new medications to which the organism is likely to be susceptible should be added.

Aminoglycosides: Amikacin (Amikin), kanamycin (Kantrex), and streptomycin are aminoglycosides used as both antibacterials and antituberculosis agents. Like other second-line agents, they are used for multidrug-resistant TB and always in combination with other antimycobacterials. They are administered parenterally because they are not absorbed when given by the PO route.

Approved in 1945, streptomycin has the distinction of being the first clinically effective drug used to treat TB. It was soon noticed, however, that resistance developed quickly when streptomycin was used as monotherapy. Streptomycin use has declined such that it is now a second-line TB drug. This is mostly because of the emergence of numerous streptomycin-resistant strains of *M. tuberculosis* and the need to administer the drug by the IM route. IM injection of the drug is painful and can produce sterile abscesses at the site of injection. Also of serious concern is ototoxicity, which can cause tinnitus, deafness, and vertigo. Streptomycin can accumulate to toxic levels in patients with kidney impairment; thus, renal function tests must be regularly assessed. Other indications for streptomycin include tularemia, plague, brucellosis, and subacute bacterial endocarditis. This drug is pregnancy category D.

Amikacin and kanamycin are closely related structurally and have similar spectrums of activity, actions, and adverse effects. Like other aminoglycosides, these drugs are nephrotoxic, and kidney function must be monitored regularly during therapy. They are also ototoxic and can cause deafness and balance abnormalities. The risk of ototoxicity is higher in patients with impaired renal function. Amikacin appears to be less ototoxic than kanamycin and causes less pain when administered IM. Resistance of mycobacteria to either kanamycin or amikacin sometimes confers resistance to the other.

CONNECTION *Checkpoint* 52.3

From what you learned in Chapter 50, are aminoglycosides bacteriostatic or bacteriocidal? What is the mechanism of action of aminoglycosides? Are they most effective against gram-positive or gram-negative organisms? See Answer to Connection Checkpoint 52.3 in Appendix A.

Aminosalicylic acid (Paser): Aminosalicylic acid (or para-aminosalicylic acid) was widely used to treat TB until more effective and safer drugs were discovered. It is structurally similar to para-aminobenzoic acid, and is thought to have a similar mechanism of action as the sulfonamides. Aminosalicylic acid is given PO, but it has a half-life of only 1 hour. The drug is available as delayed-release granules that are taken several times a day.

The use of aminosalicylic acid is limited to the treatment of multidrug-resistant strains of *M. tuberculosis*. Higher doses can inhibit the acetylation of isoniazid, especially in patients who are rapid acetylators. Concurrent therapy of aminosalicylic acid with isoniazid, however, does not affect the serum level, half-life, or excretion of isoniazid.

Aminosalicylic acid has many adverse effects, the most common of which are gastrointestinal (GI) related and include nausea, vomiting, diarrhea, and abdominal pain. Taking the drug with food can diminish these types of adverse effects. Hypersensitivity is observed in 10% to 15% of patients and may begin with a rapid onset of high fever, lethargy, and joint pain. Aminosalicylic acid reduces the absorption of vitamin B_{12} by as much as 50%; thus, vitamin B_{12} supplements are indicated during long-term therapy. This is a pregnancy category C drug.

CONNECTION *Checkpoint* 52.4

From what you learned in Chapter 52, the synthesis of what essential vitamin is inhibited by the sulfonamides? What is the primary indication for sulfonamide pharmacotherapy? See Answer to Connection Checkpoint 52.4 in Appendix A.

Capreomycin (Capastat): Approved in 1971, the only indication for capreomycin is the pharmacotherapy of multidrug-resistant strains of *M. tuberculosis*. Capreomycin is always given with other antimycobacterials because resistance quickly develops if it is administered alone. It is given only by IM injection. Because it is usually administered daily for the first 120 days of therapy, care must be taken to inject the drug deep into a large muscle mass and to rotate injection sites.

Capreomycin is ototoxic, causing tinnitus and high-frequency hearing loss in up to 9% of patients. Auditory and vestibular function should be assessed prior to starting therapy and retested at least every other month during therapy. Renal toxicity is more common with capreomycin than with streptomycin. Elderly patients are generally more susceptible to the nephrotoxic effects of capreomycin, and the maximal daily dosage should be reduced. Other nephrotoxic drugs such as aminoglycosides should be avoided during capreomycin pharmacotherapy. Renal function tests should be monitored regularly and the drug discontinued if blood urea nitrogen (BUN) levels exceed 30 mg/dL. Because of these adverse effects, capreomycin is sometimes referred to as a "last-line" drug for TB. This is a pregnancy category C drug.

Cycloserine (Seromycin): Approved over 50 years ago, cycloserine is a PO drug used in the pharmacotherapy of multidrug-resistant strains of *M. tuberculosis*. The drug, which resembles the common amino acid D-alanine, acts by blocking mycobacterial cell-wall synthesis. In addition to being an antimycobacterial, cycloserine is also effective against certain gram-negative and gram-positive bacteria and may be used to treat urinary tract infections that are unresponsive to safer antibiotics. It is taken PO, usually twice daily.

Cycloserine use is limited because the difference between a toxic dose and an effective dose is small. Of most concern is neurotoxicity, which can manifest as different symptoms, including headache, lethargy, convulsions, psychotic states with suicidal ideation, depression, confusion, tremor, and paranoid reactions. Concurrent administration of isoniazid and ethionamide can increase the risk of neurotoxicity. The drug is contraindicated in patients with preexisting psychoses or epilepsy because it may worsen these disorders. Because of its toxicity, serum levels of cycloserine are measured frequently during therapy, with normal levels ranging from 25 to 35 mcg/mL. Patients with renal impairment should not receive this drug because the primary route of excretion of this drug is via the kidneys. This is a pregnancy category C drug.

Ethionamide (Trecator-SC): Approved in 1962, ethionamide is a PO drug used as a second-line agent in the pharmacotherapy of multidrug-resistant TB or when patients are unable to tolerate first-line agents. Ethionamide is always used in combination with other agents because resistance develops rapidly if given alone. It is thought to act by inhibiting mycobacterial protein synthesis. The drug has only a 3-hour half-life and therefore must be administered several times daily.

The most common and limiting adverse effects of ethionamide are GI-related and include nausea, vomiting, diarrhea, abdominal pain, excessive salivation, metallic taste, anorexia, and weight loss. GI effects may be diminished by decreasing dosage, by taking the drug with food, or by the concurrent administration of an antiemetic. Concomitant administration of pyridoxine is recommended to decrease the incidence of peripheral neuropathy. Depression and drowsiness are common, and seizures have been reported with ethionamide. Hepatic function should be monitored regularly because hepatitis occurs in about 5% of the patients taking the drug. Alcohol use should be discouraged during ethionamide therapy because of additive harmful effects on the liver. Ethionamide is a pregnancy category C drug.

Fluoroquinolones: Ciprofloxacin (Cipro) and ofloxacin (Floxin) have undergone considerable testing for use as antituberculosis agents. Many multidrug-resistant strains of *M. tuberculosis* are sensitive to the actions of the fluoroquinolones. Because this class of antibiotics is widely used in the pharmacotherapy of bacterial infections, there is concern in the medical community that use of these drugs for TB could produce resistant strains of other pathogens in addition to *M. tuberculosis*. Although they are sometimes given for multidrug-resistant TB, they have not been

CONNECTIONS

To the Community Preventing Transmission of Tuberculosis

Patient education for persons with TB is the responsibility of the professional nurse. To increase patient adherence to the long-term and complicated medication regimen, patients must understand their illness and the measures necessary to cure and decrease further transmission. The nurse should explain the process of transmission through airborne droplets and instruct patients to cover their mouths when coughing or sneezing. The patient and family should be encouraged to open windows and allow proper indoor ventilation when weather allows.

To minimize transmission of TB, nurses should instruct patients with active tuberculosis to refrain from going to work or school and avoid using public transportation until cleared to do so by their health care provider. Also, socialization with friends is important but persons with TB should limit time with visitors. The importance of continuing drug therapy, even if the patient feels better, must be emphasized by the nurse. Nurses must recognize the important role they play in patient education to improve patient health and protect members of the surrounding community. Nurses in ambulatory care settings should reinforce teaching when possible, as well as encourage questions and discussion to ensure that the patients understand the importance of infection control.

approved by the FDA for this indication. They are the safest of the second-line agents available for this infection.

Drugs for Leprosy

52.7 Leprosy is caused by a mycobacterium and is treated by a multidrug regimen.

Leprosy is a chronic infection caused by *M. leprae* that is mentioned in several passages of the Bible. As a historical note, the term *leper* has been used by several cultures to designate someone sinful or unclean, not necessarily someone with the disease we now call leprosy.

Although rare in the United States, it is estimated that 6 million people worldwide have leprosy. Leprosy patients present with macular skin lesions that can become quite large. The organism invades peripheral nervous tissue, causing nerve thickening that results in loss of sensation or paresthesia. If left untreated, the infection causes extreme disfigurement and bone resorption, resulting in loss of digits. The disease is diagnosed through identification of the pathogen from a skin biopsy.

Leprosy may be infectious or noninfectious, depending on the stage of the disease and the progress of pharmacotherapy. Although the mode of transmission is not clear, *M. leprae* is likely spread by the respiratory route. The disease may have a very long incubation period extending from several months to years.

PharmFACT

About 200 to 300 cases of leprosy occur in the United States each year. Nearly all cases are diagnosed in immigrants from countries where leprosy is endemic, such as Southeast Asia, Central Africa, and Central and South America. *Source:* Lewis & Conologue, 2008.

There are two presentations of leprosy, and pharmacotherapy differs for the different types. *Lepromatous* leprosy occurs in patients with defective cell-mediated immunity and is characterized by a slow, progressive development of nodular skin lesions and nerve involvement. Because the patient has an impaired immune system, the mycobacteria may disseminate throughout the body and cause death. *Tuberculoid* leprosy is less progressive and may have long periods of remission followed by reactivation with more severe nerve involvement. These patients have an intact cell-mediated immune response; thus, the disease is more benign and less often fatal.

Like tuberculosis, leprosy is treated with prolonged combination pharmacotherapy because monotherapy causes rapid development of resistant strains. Although improvement in skin lesions may occur within a few months, therapy must continue during the entire treatment period to eliminate all the mycobacteria. A typical regimen includes the following:

- **Lepromatous leprosy.** Initial three-drug regimen that includes dapsone, clofazimine (Lamprene), and rifampin (Rifadin) given for 2 to 5 years.
- **Tuberculoid leprosy.** Initial two-drug regimen with dapsone and rifampin for 6 to 12 months, followed by dapsone alone for 2 to 3 years.

Other drugs may be substituted when the patient cannot tolerate the standard regimen. Ofloxacin (Floxin), clarithromycin (Biaxin), and minocycline (Minocin) are antibacterials that have activity against *M. leprae* and may be used during the long course of leprosy pharmacotherapy.

During the first year of pharmacotherapy, skin lesions may actually worsen because of activation of the cell-mediated immune response. Skin edema may occur and new lesions may appear on normal skin. Most of these reactions occur because immune cells are attacking antigens released by the mycobacteria. If this occurs, corticosteroids such as prednisone are added to the regimen to reduce the severe inflammation.

Leprosy patients are examined monthly throughout the initial course of treatment and less frequently as therapy progresses. Follow-up may continue for several years after the completion of pharmacotherapy. Close contacts of leprosy patients normally do not receive chemoprophylaxis as do those of TB patients, although follow-up examinations are conducted to ensure they have not acquired the infection.

PROTOTYPE DRUG Dapsone (DDS)

Classification: **Therapeutic:** Antileprosy agent, antimycobacterial
Pharmacologic: None

Therapeutic Effects and Uses: Approved in 1955, dapsone is a drug of choice for the treatment of *M. leprae* infections, usually in combination with other antileprosy drugs. It has several off-label uses that include the chemoprophylaxis of malaria in combination with pyrimethamine. In combination with trimethoprim, dapsone is used for the prophylaxis and treatment of *Pneumocystis carinii* pneumonia in patients with AIDS. It may take 3 to 6 months of dapsone therapy before symptoms begin to improve. Pharmacotherapy for the prophylaxis of toxoplasmosis combines dapsone, pyrimethamine, and leucovorin.

Dapsone is the primary therapy for dermatitis herpetiformis, and autoimmune disease characterized by severe blistering skin lesions. Although its name implies herpesvirus as a causative agent, the etiology of the disorder is sensitivity to gluten in the diet. Gluten is a protein found in wheat products.

Mechanism of Action: The mechanism of action of dapsone is incompletely understood, but is thought to be the same as that of the sulfonamides: It inhibits folic acid metabolism.

Pharmacokinetics:

Route(s)	PO
Absorption	Readily absorbed
Distribution	Widely distributed; crosses the placenta; secreted in breast milk
Primary metabolism	Hepatic, through acetylation
Primary excretion	Renal, with small amounts in the feces
Onset of action	4–8 h
Duration of action	Half-life: 20–30 h

Adverse Effects: The most frequent adverse effects of dapsone relate to the hematologic system: dose-related hemolysis and methemoglobinemia with cyanosis. Aplastic anemia and agranulocytosis are rare, though potentially severe, adverse effects. Toxic hepatitis has been reported. The drug concentrates in the skin, causing dermatologic reactions that include photosensitivity and toxic epidermal necrolysis.

Contraindications/Precautions: Contraindications include hypersensitivity to dapsone or related drugs, such as sulfonamides. Because of its adverse effects on the hematologic system, caution should be used in treating patients with preexisting blood disorders. Frequent blood assessments are conducted during therapy to avoid serious adverse effects. Frequent liver enzyme testing should be conducted to monitor for hepatotoxicity, especially in patients with preexisting liver impairment.

Drug Interactions: Some patients receiving pyrimethamine and dapsone concurrently developed agranulocytosis during the second and third month of therapy; therefore, concurrent administration of these drugs must be carefully monitored. Increased dapsone levels have been reported in patients receiving trimethoprim, and patients receiving this combination may be at increased risk for dapsone toxicity. Rifampin may significantly reduce serum levels of dapsone. **Herbal/Food:** Dapsone levels may be decreased by St. John's wort.

Pregnancy: Category C.

Treatment of Overdose: Acute overdose may result in cyanosis, which may be treated by the slow IV administration of 1–2 mg/kg of methylene blue.

Nursing Responsibilities:

- Monitor for serious adverse effects such as GI bleeding, bone and joint pain, or diminished vision. Although reactions are usually reversible, they may require months or years to diminish. Other symptoms include colicky abdominal pain, nausea, and vomiting.
- Monitor periodic laboratory tests including white blood count (WBC) with differential, serum electrolytes, serum albumin, and liver function.
- Assess for any reddish-brown discoloration of skin, cornea, conjunctiva, and body fluids. This adverse effect occurs in 75% to 90% of patients within a few weeks of treatment.
- Assess for tender, erythematous nodules with lymphadenopathy, joint swelling, epistaxis, and iritis, which can suggest a type 2 leprosy reactional state.

Patient and Family Education:

- Maintain strict adherence to the established drug regimen and do not change drug dosage without the approval of the health care provider.
- Do not drive or perform other hazardous activities until the effects of the drug are known because this drug may cause drowsiness or dizziness.
- Minimize the use of soap and rinse thoroughly, especially if the skin is dry.
- Keep all appointments for follow-up care because drug resistance and relapse may occur.
- Immediately report any of the following to the health care provider: changes in vision or hearing, dark urine, unusual fatigue, unusual bruising or bleeding, bluish fingernails, or yellowing of the eyes or skin.

Drugs Similar to Dapsone (DDS)

Other primary antimycobacterial drugs for leprosy include rifampin and clofazimine. Rifampin is also used for TB, and is discussed in Section 52.6.

Clofazimine (Lamprene): Clofazimine is a drug that exhibits selective activity toward mycobacteria. Although its only approved indication is leprosy, clofazimine is sometimes used in the pharmacotherapy of MAC. Given only by the PO route, the drug has a 70-day half-life—one of the longest of any drug. It may take up to 50 days before it exerts a bacteriocidal effect. The drug has anti-inflammatory and immunosuppressive properties. Clofazimine, a bright-red dye, can cause a reddish-brown discoloration of the skin, conjunctiva, and body fluids that may take years to disappear after discontinuing therapy. Therapy of dapsone-resistant infections may require daily administration of clofazimine for several years. This drug is pregnancy category C.

Drugs for *Mycobacterium Avium* Complex (MAC) Infections

52.8 *Mycobacterium avium* complex infections are common in patients with impaired immune function.

MAC is the most common cause of lung disease due to atypical mycobacterial infections. Although rare in healthy people,

NURSING PROCESS APPLICATION

Patients Receiving Antituberculosis Agents

Assessment

Prior to administration:

- Obtain a complete health history including allergies, drug history, and possible drug interactions.
- Perform a complete physical examination including vital signs.
- Assess for the presence or history of the following: positive tuberculin skin test, positive sputum culture or smear, immunosuppressant drug therapy, alcohol abuse, or liver or kidney disease, or close contact with a person recently infected with TB, HIV infection or AIDS.
- Assess cognitive ability to comply with long-term therapy.

Potential Nursing Diagnoses

- *Risk for Infection*
- *Risk for Injury*, related to adverse effects of medication
- *Deficient Knowledge (Antituberculosis Agents)*, related to drug therapy and spread of infection
- *Noncompliance (Therapeutic Regimen)*, related to complexity and long-term nature

Planning: Patient Goals and Expected Outcomes

The patient will:

- Report a reduction in TB symptoms and have negative results for laboratory and diagnostic tests indicating TB infection.
- Demonstrate an understanding of the drug's action by accurately describing drug adverse effects and precautions.
- Immediately report effects such as visual changes, difficulty voiding, changes in hearing, and symptoms of liver or kidney impairment.
- Complete a full course of antituberculosis therapy and comply with follow-up care.

Implementation

<table>
<tr><th>Interventions and (Rationales)</th><th>Patient and Family Education</th></tr>
<tr><td>• Monitor for hepatic adverse effects.
(Antituberculosis agents, such as isoniazid and rifampin, cause hepatic impairment.)</td><td>• Instruct the patient to report yellow eyes and skin, loss of appetite, dark urine, and unusual tiredness.</td></tr>
<tr><td>• Monitor for neurologic adverse effects such as numbness and tingling of the extremities.
(Antituberculosis agents, such as isoniazid, cause peripheral neuropathy and depletion of vitamin B_6.)</td><td>Instruct the patient to:
• Report numbness and tingling of the extremities.
• Take supplemental vitamin B_6 as ordered to reduce risk of adverse effects.</td></tr>
<tr><td>• Collect sputum specimens as directed by the health care provider. (This will determine the effectiveness of the antituberculosis agent.)</td><td>• Instruct the patient in the proper technique needed to collect a quality sputum specimen.</td></tr>
<tr><td>• Monitor for dietary adherence when patient is taking isoniazid. (Foods high in tyramine can interact with the drug and cause palpitations, flushing, and hypertension.)</td><td>• Advise patients taking isoniazid to avoid foods containing tyramine, such as aged cheese, smoked and pickled fish, beer and red wine, bananas, and chocolate.</td></tr>
<tr><td>• Monitor for adverse effects specific to various antituberculosis drugs. (Adverse effects should be reported to the health care provider.)</td><td>Instruct the patient to report adverse effects specific to antituberculosis therapy prescribed:
• Blurred vision or changes in color or vision field (ethambutol)
• Difficulty in voiding (pyrazinamide)
• Fever, yellowing of skin, weakness, and dark urine (isoniazid, rifampin)
• GI system disturbances (rifampin)
• Changes in hearing (streptomycin)
• Numbness and tingling of extremities (isoniazid)
• Red discoloration of body fluids (rifampin)
• Dark concentrated urine, weight gain, edema (streptomycin)</td></tr>
<tr><td>• Establish infection control measures based on the extent of the disease condition and the established protocol. (This will help prevent further spread of infection.)</td><td>• Instruct the patient about infectious control measures, such as frequent hand washing, covering the mouth when coughing or sneezing, and proper disposal of soiled tissues.</td></tr>
<tr><td>• Establish a therapeutic environment to ensure adequate rest, nutrition, hydration, and relaxation. (Symptoms of tuberculosis are manifested when the immune system is suppressed.)</td><td>• Teach the patient to incorporate health-enhancing activities, such as adequate rest and sleep, intake of essential vitamins and nutrients, and intake of 6 to 8 glasses of water per day.</td></tr>
<tr><td>• Monitor the patient's ability and motivation to adhere to the therapeutic regimen. (Treatment must continue for the full length of therapy to eliminate all M. tuberculosis organisms.)</td><td>Explain the importance of adhering with the entire therapeutic plan, including:
• Take all medications as directed by the health care provider.
• Do not discontinue medication until instructed.
• Wear a medical alert bracelet.
• Keep all appointments for follow-up care.</td></tr>
</table>

Evaluation of Outcome Criteria

Evaluate the effectiveness of drug therapy by confirming that patient goals and expected outcomes have been met (see "Planning").

MAC is a frequent cause of infection among those with impaired immune systems and is an expected complication in many patients with AIDS. It is also found in higher incidence in patients with chronic obstructive pulmonary disease (COPD). The infection is caused by *M. avium*, *M. intracellulare*, or a combination of atypical mycobacteria.

Unlike TB, MAC infections are not believed to be contagious or spread by human-to-human contact. The mode of transmission is not understood, although the organisms are widely distributed in soil and water and these may the primary sources of infection. Once inside the body, MAC resides in the lungs like *M. tuberculosis*, and the initial respiratory symptoms are identical. The pathogen may travel through the lymphatics and bloodstream to infect any organ. The frequency of disseminated MAC disease has been markedly reduced in AIDS patients because of successes in the pharmacotherapy of HIV-AIDS.

Treatment of MAC should include at least two drugs (and often three or four) because monotherapy has been shown to promote the emergence of resistant strains. Treatment is prolonged, and relapse rates for treating pulmonary MAC approach 20%. Drugs for this infection include the following:

- **Macrolide antibiotics.** Clarithromycin (Biaxin) and azithromycin (Zithromax) are relatively safe and effective against MAC and are included in most regimens. High doses of clarithromycin (1,000 mg bid) are associated with increased mortality rates.
- **Ethambutol (Myambutol).** Usually used for tuberculosis, this drug may be combined with clarithromycin in the pharmacotherapy of MAC.
- **Rifabutin (Mycobutin).** If a third drug is needed, rifabutin is often effective. Rifabutin, however, can cause many drug interactions, and high doses (600 mg/day) are associated with greater risk of serious uveitis with eye pain. Rifabutin is approved only for the prophylaxis of MAC in HIV-infected patients, although it is also used off-label to treat active infections.

Pharmacotherapy for AIDS patients with MAC infections involves antimicrobial agents with activity against MAC, including clarithromycin, azithromycin, rifabutin, ethambutol, levofloxacin, and amikacin. MAC infections in AIDS patients may be fatal; therefore, chemoprophylaxis is indicated when the CD4 lymphocyte count falls to less than 50 cells/mL. Clarithromycin or azithromycin are drugs of choice for prophylaxis. Rifabutin and ethambutol are alternatives to the macrolides. Many health care providers will discontinue chemoprophylaxis if the HIV-positive patient regains normal immunologic status.

UNDERSTANDING THE CHAPTER

Key Concepts Summary

52.1 Several species of mycobacteria are important human pathogens.

52.2 Tuberculosis is a respiratory infection that exhibits both active and latent stages.

52.3 The pharmacotherapy of tuberculosis requires special dosing regimens and schedules.

52.4 The progress of tuberculosis pharmacotherapy must be monitored during the entire treatment period.

52.5 First-line or primary antituberculosis drugs are the most efficacious and safest drugs for treating *M. tuberculosis* infections.

52.6 Second-line antituberculosis drugs are used when resistance develops to the first-line agents.

52.7 Leprosy is caused by a mycobacterium and is treated by a multidrug regimen.

52.8 *Mycobacterium avium* complex infections are common in patients with impaired immune function.

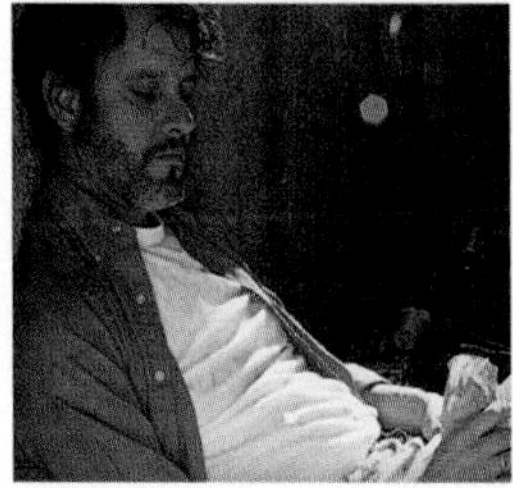

Making the PATIENT *Connection*

Remember the patient "Sam Myers" at the beginning of the chapter? Now read the remainder of the case study. Based on the information presented within this chapter, respond to the critical thinking questions that follow.

Sam Myers is a 58-year-old man who lives on the street. For the past 6 weeks, he has experienced anorexia, weight loss, and low-grade fever. He comes to the local church health center for health problems and now presents with a productive cough that has progressively worsened.

A history and physical examination is completed. Sam is evaluated for TB. The physical examination reveals the following findings: the patient's height is 1.9 meters (6′1″) and his weight is 56.2 kg (124 lb). He is emaciated and obviously malnourished. His vital signs are blood pressure, 112/82 mmHg; heart rate, 102 beats/minute; respiratory rate, 26/minute; and body temperature, 38.2°C (100.9°F). On auscultation, crackles are heard in the upper lung fields. The patient is experiencing moderate dyspnea. Sam's chest x-ray reveals multiple nodular infiltrates in the apical posterior segments of the upper lobes. Sam admits to drinking alcohol almost every day and smoking at least one pack of cigarettes per day. He is admitted to a local acute care hospital for treatment of pulmonary TB.

Critical Thinking Questions

1. Describe the mechanism of transmission for *M. tuberculosis*.
2. Discuss how Sam's living conditions predispose him to pulmonary TB.
3. Why is Sam at high risk for hepatic-related drug adverse effects?

Case Study

When Sam is admitted to the hospital, he is placed in a private room and respiratory isolation procedures are initiated. Additional diagnostic testing is completed that includes a complete blood count (CBC), sputum cultures, and a tuberculin skin test.

M. tuberculosis and positive acid-fast bacilli are reported in the sputum culture. Within 48 hours, Sam's TB skin test is obviously positive (17-mm transverse diameter induration; normal is less than 5 mm). Sam's CBC is within normal limits with the exception of a slight decline in the hemoglobin and hematocrit level. Drug therapy is started immediately. Sam is given isoniazid 5 mg/kg/day, rifampin 600 mg/day, pyrazinamide 25mg/kg/day, ethambutol (Myambutal), and vitamin B_6 supplementation.

1. While Sam is in the hospital, he seems worried and questions the nurse about why he is receiving four different drugs for his tuberculosis. How would you respond?
2. Discuss why Sam is receiving vitamin B_6 supplements.

NCLEX-RN® Review

1 A client who is receiving antituberculosis therapy is complaining of tingling and numbness of the fingers and toes. The nurse knows that these symptoms are most likely due to the drug's ability to:

1. Increase the sensitivity of nerve endings.
2. Decrease the activity of pyridoxine (vitamin B_6).
3. Accelerate the excretion of neurotransmitters.
4. Enhance skin receptors to ascorbic acid (vitamin C).

2 In evaluating the effects of isoniazid (INH), the nurse would monitor the results of which of the following laboratory test(s)?

1. Coagulation studies
2. Sputum cultures
3. Arterial blood gases
4. Pulmonary function test

3 A client's family asks the nurse to explain the most common cause for treatment failure in pulmonary tuberculosis. The nurse knows that treatment failure is most often caused by the client's:

1. Inability to pay for the medication.
2. Poor nutritional intake of complex proteins.
3. Inability or unwillingness to adhere to the therapeutic regimen.
4. Inability to restrict intake of calcium-enriched foods.

4 Which of the following would the nurse expect in the therapeutic management for a client with HIV infection who also has a *Mycobacterium avium* complex infection? (Select all that apply.)

1. Monitoring of the CD4 lymphocyte counts
2. Restricting visitors
3. Using multiple drug therapies
4. Initiating prophylactic treatment of potentially exposed family members.
5. Limiting intake of foods that are high in protein and carbohydrates.

5 The client is diagnosed with *tuberculoid* leprosy and is being treated with dapsone and another antimicrobial drug. Which of the following nursing assessment findings would indicate the client is experiencing adverse effects from this therapy?

1. Discoloration of skin, cornea, and conjunctiva
2. Chronic constipation, chills, and dehydration
3. Hypoglycemia, impaired memory, and impotence
4. Memory loss, nervousness, and pruritus

6 Which of the following clients receiving isoniazid (INH) is most likely to experience hepatotoxicity?

1. A 42-year-old housewife
2. A 22-year-old postpartum female
3. An 82-year-old farmer
4. A 42-year-old marketing executive

See Answers to Critical Thinking Questions, Case Study, and NCLEX-RN® Review in Appendix A.

References

Advisory Council for the Elimination of Tuberculosis. (2006). Prevention and control of tuberculosis in correctional and detention facilities: Recommendations from CDC. *Morbidity Mortality Weekly Report, Recommendations and Reports, 55*(RR09), 1–44.

American Nurses Association (ANA). (1991) *Scope and standards of nursing practice in correctional facilities.* Retrieved July 31, 2008, from http://www.statepen.org/ana.htm

Centers for Disease Control and Prevention (CDC). (2008). Trends in tuberculosis: United States 2007. *Morbidity Mortality Weekly Report, 57*(11), 281–285. Retrieved July 29, 2008, from http://www.cdc.gov/mmwr/preview/mmwrhtml/mm5711a2.htm

Centers for Disease Control and Prevention (CDC). (2005). Trends in tuberculosis. *Morbidity Mortality Weekly Report, 54,* 245–249.

Centers for Disease Control and Prevention (CDC). (2004). Tuberculosis transmission in multiple correctional facilities—Kansas, 2002–2003. *Morbidity Mortality Weekly Report, 52*(32), 734–737.

Centers for Disease Control and Prevention (CDC), Division of Tuberculosis Elimination. (2008). *TB guidelines.* Retrieved July 31, 2008, from http://www.cdc.gov/tb/pubs/mmwr/maj_guide.htm

Klein, G. M., Shack, T. T., & Purcell, B. (2007). Tuberculosis redux: Are you prepared? *Emergency Medicine, 39*(9), 24–26.

Lemone, P., & Burke, K. (2008). *Medical-surgical nursing: Critical thinking in client care* (4th ed.). Upper Saddle River, NJ: Pearson Education, Inc.

Lewis, F. S., & Conologue, D. O. (2008). *Leprosy.* Emedicine. Retrieved July 29, 2008, from http://www.emedicine.com/derm/TOPIC223.HTM

Petri, W. A. (2001). Drugs used in the chemotherapy of tuberculosis, *Mycobacterium avium* complex disease, and leprosy. In J. G. Hardman, L. E. Limbard, & A. G. Goodman (Eds.), *The pharmacological basis of therapeutics* (pp. 1273–1294). New York: McGraw-Hill.

Raviglione, M. C., & O'Brien, R. J. (2005). Tuberculosis. In D. L. Kasper, E. Braunwald, A. Fauci, S. Hauser, D. Longo, & J. L. Jameson (Eds.), *Harrison's principles of internal medicine* (16th ed., Rev., pp. 952–966). New York: McGraw Hill.

Taylor, Z., Nolan, C. M., & Blumberg, H. M. (2005). *Controlling tuberculosis in the United States.* Recommendations from the American Thoracic Society, CDC, and the Infectious Diseases Society of America. *Morbidity Mortality Weekly Report, 54*(RR12), 1–81.

Uthman, M. M. B., Uthman, O. A., & Yahaya, I. (2008). Interventions for the prevention of mycobacterium avium complex in adults and children with HIV (Protocol). *Cochrane Database of Systematic Reviews, 2.* (Art. No.: CD007191, DOI: 10.1002/14651858.CD007191).

Volmink, J., & Garner, P. (2007). Directly observed therapy for treating tuberculosis. *Cochrane Database of Systematic Reviews, 3.* (Art. No.: CD003343, DOI: 10.1002/14651858.CD003343.pub3).

World Health Organization. (2008). *2008 tuberculosis facts.* Retrieved July 29, 2008, from http://www.who.int/tb/publications/2008/factsheet_april08.pdf

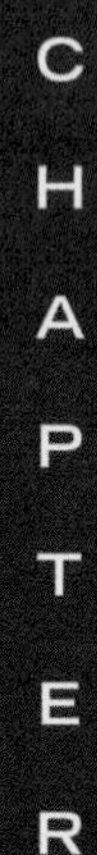

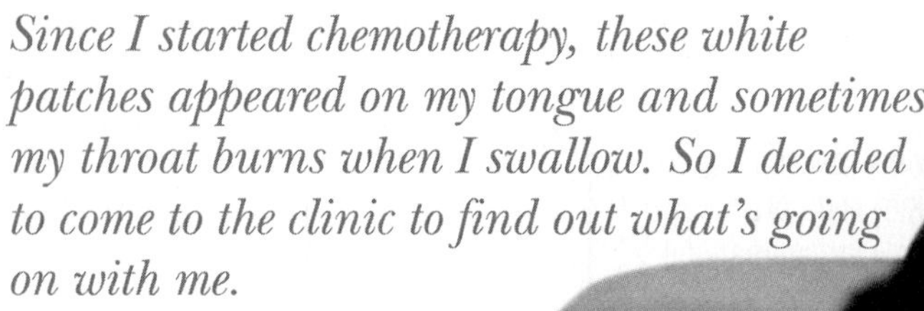

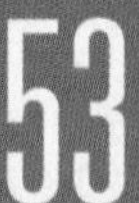

Pharmacotherapy of Fungal Infections

Learning Outcomes

After reading this chapter, the student should be able to:

1. Compare and contrast the pharmacotherapy of fungal and bacterial infections.
2. Classify mycoses based upon the location of the infection and the causative organism.
3. Compare and contrast the pharmacotherapy of superficial and systemic fungal infections.
4. Identify the types of patients at greatest risk of acquiring serious fungal infections.
5. Describe the nurse's role in the pharmacologic management of fungal infections.
6. For each of the classes shown in the chapter outline, identify the prototype and representative drugs and explain the mechanism(s) of drug action, primary indications, contraindications, significant drug interactions, pregnancy category, and important adverse effects.
7. Apply the nursing process to care for patients receiving drug therapy for fungal infections.

Chapter Outline

Characteristics of Fungi and Fungal Infections

Drugs for Systemic Fungal Infections

PROTOTYPE **Amphotericin B Deoxycholate (Fungizone)** *p. 872*

Drugs for Both Systemic and Superficial Fungal Infections

PROTOTYPE **Fluconazole (Diflucan)** *p. 875*

Drugs for Superficial Fungal Infections

PROTOTYPE **Nystatin (Mycostatin, Nystop, Others)** *p. 880*

Key Terms

azole, *875*
β-glucan, *871*
dermatomycoses, *877*
ergosterol, *871*
fungi, *869*
mycoses, *870*
onychomycosis, *877*

The past few decades have seen a dramatic rise in the incidence of fungal infections due to AIDS, aggressive cancer chemotherapy, the widespread use of indwelling intravenous (IV) catheters, and the use of broad-spectrum antibiotics. Fungi are much more complex than bacteria and require a different approach to pharmacotherapy. Because of structural and functional differences, most antibacterial drugs are ineffective against fungi. Although there are fewer drugs to treat fungal infections, the available medications are usually effective.

Characteristics of Fungi and Fungal Infections

53.1 Serious fungal infections are uncommon in people with healthy immune defenses.

Fungi are single-celled or multicellular organisms that serve essential roles on the planet as decomposers of dead plants and animals, returning their elements to the soil for recycling. Fungi include mushrooms, yeasts, and molds. Although 100,000 to 200,000 species of fungi exist in soil, air, and water, only about 50 species are associated with disease in humans. A few species of fungi survive as part of the normal host flora on the skin, mouth, and urogenital tract.

Unlike bacteria, which produce toxins or grow rapidly to overwhelm hosts' defenses, some fungi grow slowly and infections may progress for many months before symptoms develop. With a few exceptions (such as athlete's foot), fungal infections are not easily transmitted through casual contact. In addition to causing infections, fungal antigens may trigger hypersensitivity responses in susceptible patients, resulting in allergies to mold or mildew. A few fungi, such as *Aspergillus flavus,* secrete toxins that can cause illness in humans through ingestion of contaminated grains or other foods.

The human body is remarkably resistant to infection by these organisms and patients with healthy immune defenses experience few serious fungal diseases. However, patients with a suppressed immune system (immunocompromised), especially those infected with HIV, may experience frequent fungal infections and require aggressive pharmacotherapy. A systemic fungal infection in an immunocompromised patient may be rapidly fatal.

The species of pathogenic fungi that attack hosts with healthy immune defenses are often distinct from those that infect immunocompromised patients. Patients with intact immune defenses are afflicted with community-acquired infections such as sporotrichosis, blastomycosis, histoplasmosis, and coccidioidomycosis. Opportunistic fungal infections acquired in a hospital-acquired (nosocomial) setting are more likely to be candidiasis, aspergillosis, cryptococcosis, and mucormycosis. Thus, assessing the immune status of a patient may help in diagnosing the specific infection and in determining the course of pharmacotherapy. Table 53.1 lists the most common fungi that cause disease in humans.

TABLE 53.1 Fungal Pathogens

Name of Fungus	Description
Systemic	
Aspergillus fumigatus and other species	Aspergillosis: Opportunistic; most commonly affects the lungs but can spread to other organs
Blastomyces dermatitides	Blastomycosis: Begins in the lungs and spreads to other organs
Candida albicans and other species	Candidiasis: Most common opportunistic fungal infection; may affect nearly any organ
Coccidioides immitis	Coccidioidomycosis: Begins in the lungs and spreads to other organs
Cryptococcus neoformans	Cryptococcosis: Opportunistic; begins in the lungs but is the most common cause of meningitis in AIDS patients
Histoplasma capsulatum	Histoplasmosis: Begins in the lungs and spreads to other organs
Mucorales species	Mucormycosis: Opportunistic; affects blood vessels, causes sinus infections, stomach ulcers, and others
Pneumocystis carinii	Pneumocystis pneumonia: Opportunistic; primarily pneumonia of the lung but can spread to other organs
Superficial	
Candida albicans and others	Candidiasis: Affects the skin, nails, oral cavity (thrush), vagina
Epidermophyton floccosum	Athletes foot (tinea pedis), jock itch (tinea cruris), and other skin infections
Microsporum species	Ringworm of the scalp (tinea capitis)
Trichophyton species	Affects the scalp, skin, and nails
Cutaneous	
Sporothrix schenckii	Sporotrichosis: Primarily affects the skin and superficial lymph nodes
Mixed Species	Chromoblastomycosis: Chronic skin mycosis

53.2 Mycoses are classified as superficial, subcutaneous, or systemic.

Fungal infections are called **mycoses** (singular, mycosis). A simple and useful method of classifying fungal infections is to consider them as superficial, subcutaneous, or systemic.

Superficial mycoses affect the scalp, skin, nails, and mucous membranes such as the oral cavity and vagina. Only the surface layers of the regions are affected. Mycoses of this type are often treated with topical agents, because these drugs can penetrate into the keratin layer of the skin while producing few systemic adverse effects.

Subcutaneous mycoses are infections that affect deeper skin layers, including the dermis and subcutaneous layers. Often, the organisms that cause subcutaneous infections are different from those that cause superficial infections, as shown in Table 53.1. Because these fungal species often reside in soil, gardeners or people working in occupations involving exposure to soil can acquire these infections through cuts or abrasions on their skin. In addition, these infections occur in greater incidence in regions where the population travels barefoot. Topical antifungal preparations may not penetrate deep enough to reach the pathogen, thus oral (PO) antifungal therapy may be indicated. Some textbooks consider subcutaneous mycoses as subtypes of superficial mycoses.

Systemic mycoses are those that affect internal organs, typically the lungs, brain, and digestive organs. These infections often originate in the lungs, through inhalation of fungal spores. Although less common than superficial or subcutaneous mycoses, systemic fungal infections affect multiple body systems and may be fatal to patients with severely suppressed immune systems. Invasive systemic mycoses require aggressive oral or parenteral medications that produce more adverse effects than the topical agents.

Historically, antifungal drugs used for superficial infections were clearly distinct from those prescribed for systemic infections. In recent years, this distinction has blurred. Some of the newer antifungals may be used for superficial, subcutaneous, or systemic infections. Furthermore, some superficial infections may be treated with parenteral, oral, or topical agents. This therapeutic division between superficial and systemic mycoses is still useful because it separates the pharmacotherapy of relatively benign infections (superficial) from those that may be life threatening (systemic).

PharmFACT

Oropharyngeal candidiasis in the neonate is most commonly acquired from the infected mucosa of the mother during passage of the infant through the birth canal. This condition is 35 times more common in neonates of infected mothers compared to uninfected mothers. *Source:* Scheinfeld, Lambiase, Lehman, & Allan, 2008.

53.3 Antifungal drugs act by disrupting the fungal cell membrane or wall, affecting fungal enzymes or disrupting replication.

Biologically, fungi are classified as eukaryotes: Their cellular organelles and metabolic pathways are more similar to those of humans, than to bacteria. Antibiotics that are efficacious against bacteria are ineffective in treating mycoses due to these

CONNECTIONS

Evidence-Based Practice Reducing Neutropenic Patients' Exposure to Fungal Pathogens

Clinical Question

What factors reduced the neutropenic patient's exposure to fungal pathogens?

Fungal infections are a major factor associated with the mortality and morbidity in cancer patients suffering from neutropenia. Quality of life is severely affected by the symptoms and stress associated with cancer-related fungal invasions. Preventing fungal infection is a priority in the care of both hospitalized and ambulatory patients.

Lessening the exposure to fungal pathogens is one method for decreasing the occurrence of infection in patients both in the hospital and in the community. Nursing professionals must examine environmental factors that may place these patients at risk for infections.

Evidence

Smith and Kagan (2005) explored the empirical literature that examined the clinical question. Their data sources included books, articles, and brochures from 1980 to 2004. Through their comprehensive review of the literature, these two researchers found several factors that reduced the patient's exposure to fungal pathogens. These include:

- Educate health care workers, patients, and visitors about the risk for infection and the procedures to minimize exposure.
- Implement environmental surveillance to eliminate the outbreaks and sources of contamination.
- Use frequent and thorough hand washing techniques.
- Employ meticulous hygiene for the patient's mouth and skin.
- Utilize strict asepsis technique in performing all invasive procedures.
- Modify the environment to minimize airborne contamination.
- Clean the environment daily, including horizontal surfaces and equipment.
- Limit exposure from other living sources such as visitors and pets.
- Eliminate potentially contaminated reservoirs such as soil, damp or moist fabrics, dried or fresh flowers, and standing water.

Critical Thinking Question

What is the role of nurses in minimizing a patient's exposure to fungal pathogens?

See Answers to Critical Thinking Questions in Appendix A.

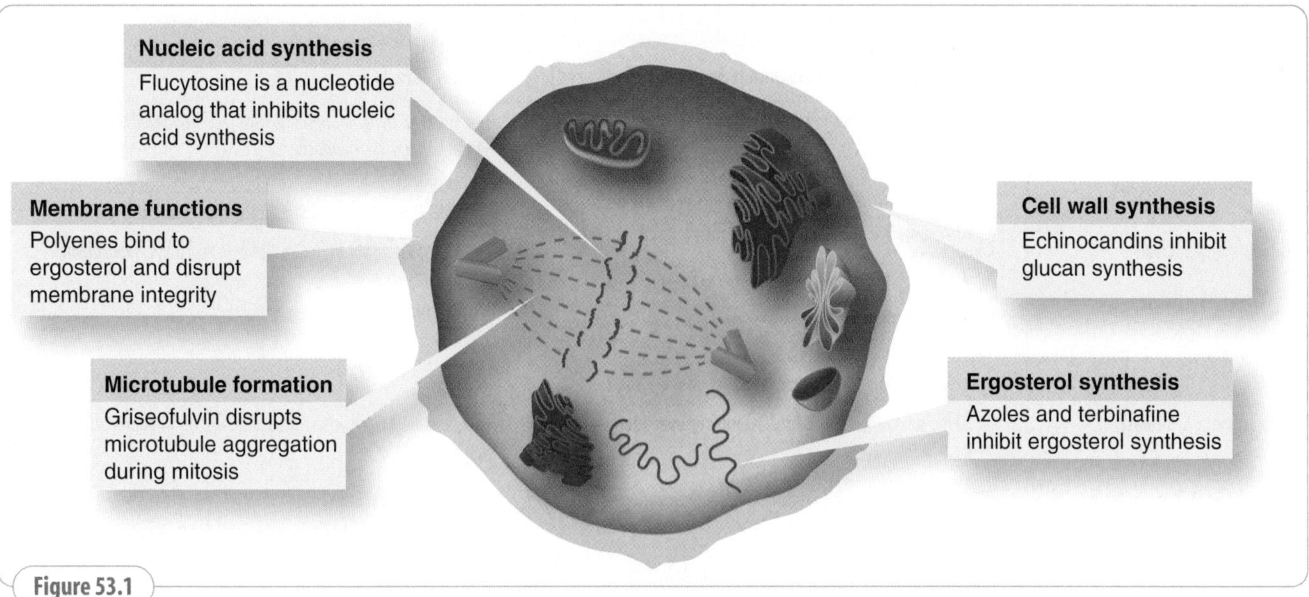

Figure 53.1

Mechanisms of action of antifungal drugs.
Source: From *Broch Biology of Microorganisms* (11th ed., p. 691), by M. Madigan & J. Martinko, 2006. Reprinted by permission of Pearson Education, Inc., Upper Saddle River, NJ.

differences in physiology; thus, an entirely different set of agents is needed to eliminate fungal pathogens.

Like antibacterials, the antifungal drugs may either slow the growth of the organisms (fungistatic) or kill them (fungicidal). The five mechanisms of action of the antifungal drugs are illustrated in Figure 53.1.

One important difference between fungal cells and human cells is the specific steroid used in constructing plasma membranes. While cholesterol is essential for animal cell membranes, **ergosterol** is present in fungi. The largest class of antifungals, the azoles, inhibits ergosterol biosynthesis, causing the fungal plasma membrane to become porous or leaky. Amphotericin B (Fungizone), terbinafine (Lamisil), and nystatin (Mycostatin) also act by this mechanism.

Caspofungin (Cancidas) disrupts fungal cell walls by inhibiting the synthesis of **β-glucan,** an essential component that shapes and strengthens the cell wall. Without sufficient β-glucan, the wall weakens and becomes porous, causing the death of the cell.

Some antifungals act by mechanisms that take advantage of enzymatic differences between fungi and humans. In fungi, flucytosine (Ancobon) is converted to the potent antimetabolite 5-fluorouracil, which inhibits both deoxyribonucleic acid (DNA) and ribonucleic acid (RNA) synthesis. Humans do not have the enzyme necessary for this conversion. 5-Fluorouracil itself is a common antineoplastic medication (see Chapter 58).

A final mechanism is used by the drug griseofulvin. This drug is incorporated into newly formed keratin where it serves a protective effect against fungal invasion. Once entering the fungal cell, it disrupts the mitotic spindle, preventing replication.

CONNECTION *Checkpoint* 53.1

From what you learned in Chapter 48, what major classes of antibacterials act by disrupting cell walls? Why are these agents not effective against fungi? See Answer to Connection Checkpoint 53.1 in Appendix A.

Drugs for Systemic Fungal Infections

53.4 Systemic or invasive fungal disease may require intensive pharmacotherapy for extended periods.

Because human body defenses provide a formidable barrier to fungi, systemic mycoses are rarely encountered in persons with healthy immune systems. The AIDS epidemic, however, resulted in the frequent clinical occurrence of previously rare mycoses, such as cryptococcosis and coccidioidomycosis. The opportunistic disease in AIDS patients spurred the development of several new drugs for systemic fungal infections. In addition to AIDS patients, others who may experience systemic mycoses include patients receiving prolonged therapy with corticosteroids, having extensive burns, receiving antineoplastic agents, having indwelling vascular catheters, or receiving organ transplants. Prophylactic antifungal therapy is sometimes indicated for these high-risk patients.

Pharmacotherapy of systemic mycoses is often continued for many months to fully eliminate the fungus. Unlike the superficial antifungal drugs, systemic agents have the potential to cause serious adverse effects and therapy must be carefully monitored. The systemic antifungal drugs are listed in Table 53.2.

Pharmacologic options for serious systemic mycoses are limited. Amphotericin B (Fungizone) has been the traditional drug of choice for systemic fungal infections since the 1960s. The newer azole drugs such as itraconazole, however, are considerably safer and have become drugs of choice for less severe infections. Although rarely used as a monotherapy, flucytosine (Ancobon) is sometimes used in combination with amphotericin B in the pharmacotherapy of severe *Candida* infections. Caspofungin (Cancidas) is a newer drug that is becoming an important alternative to amphotericin B in the treatment of aspergillosis. Typical protocols for systemic mycoses are shown in Table 53.2.

MyNursingKit Dr. Fungus

TABLE 53.2 Drugs for Systemic Mycoses

Drug	Route and Adult Dose (maximum dose where indicated)	Adverse Effects
amphotericin B (Fungizone, Abelcet, Amphotec, AmBisome)	IV: 0.3–1.5 mg/kg/day, infused over 2–4 h (max: 1.5 mg/kg/day)	*Hypokalemia, hypomagnesemia, rash, fever and chills, nausea, vomiting, anorexia, headache* <u>Nephrotoxicity, liver failure, anaphylaxis, cardiac arrest, thrombocytopenia, leukopenia, agranulocytosis, anemia</u>
anidulafungin (Eraxis)	Candidemia IV: 200 mg on day 1, then 100 mg/day for 14 days Esophageal candidiasis 100 mg on day 1, then 50 mg/day for 7–14 days Infusion rate should not exceed 1.1 mg/min	*Diarrhea, nausea, vomiting, mild allergic reactions, hypokalemia, mild allergic reactions* <u>Neutropenia, dysrhythmias</u>
caspofungin (Cancidas)	IV: 70 mg on day 1, then 50 mg/day infused over 1 h for 14 days	*Fever, headache, infusion-related phlebitis, thrombophlebitis* <u>Anaphylaxis</u>
flucytosine (5-fluorocytosine, Ancobon)	PO: 25 mg/kg every 6 h to reach a peak concentration of 50–100 mcg/mL	*Nausea, vomiting, headache* <u>Blood dyscrasias, cardiac toxicity, renal failure, psychosis</u>
micafungin (Mycamine)	IV: 150 mg/kg/day over 1 h for active *Candida* infection; 50 mg/kg/day over 1 h for *Candida* prophylaxis	*Headache, nausea, rash, phlebitis* <u>Leukopenia, serious allergic reactions, delirium</u>
Azoles		
fluconazole (Diflucan)	PO: 200–400 mg on day 1, then 100–200 mg/day for 2–4 weeks	*Fever, chills, rash, dizziness, drowsiness, nausea, vomiting, diarrhea* <u>Hepatotoxicity, anaphylaxis, blood dyscrasias</u>
itraconazole (Sporanox)	PO: 200 mg/day; may increase to 200 mg bid (max: 400 mg/day)	
ketoconazole (Nizoral)	PO: 200–400 mg/day	
voriconazole (Vfend)	IV: 6 mg/kg on day 1, then 4 mg/kg every 12 h	

Note: *Italics* indicate common adverse effects. <u>Underline</u> indicates serious adverse effects.

PROTOTYPE DRUG Amphotericin B deoxycholate (Fungizone)

Classification: Therapeutic: Antifungal (systemic type)
Pharmacologic: Polyene

Therapeutic Effects and Uses: Approved in 1957, amphotericin B has a broad spectrum of activity that includes most fungi that are pathogenic to humans. It is a drug of choice for treating severe systemic mycoses, and may also be indicated as prophylactic antifungal therapy for patients with severe immunosuppression. Because it is not absorbed from the gastrointestinal (GI) tract, it is normally given by IV infusion. Topical preparations are available for superficial mycoses that have not responded favorably to other antifungals. Several months of pharmacotherapy may be required for a complete cure. Fungal resistance to amphotericin B is not common, but is increasing in incidence.

CONNECTIONS

Lifespan Considerations Oral Candidiasis in Infants

Thrush is commonly seen in infants. It is not considered abnormal in infants unless it lasts longer than a couple of weeks. Oral candidiasis (thrush) is often difficult to distinguish from milk and appears as white adherent patches on the tongue, palate, and inner aspects of the checks. Frequently, the infant with thrush may refuse to suck or feed because of mouth pain.

Thrush appears when the normal flora that resides in the mouth is altered. This can result from antibiotic therapy or poor hand washing by the baby's caregiver. In most cases, thrush is self-limiting and resolves spontaneously. However, it may take as long as 2 months, during which time the fungal infection may spread to the larynx, trachea, bronchi, lungs, and GI tract.

The condition is treated with good hygiene, application of a fungicide, and correction of any underlying disturbance. Since the mother is often the source of the infection, she, too, should be treated to prevent reinfections.

The goals of nursing care include preventing the spread of infection and administering the prescribed topical medication until the infection is resolved.

Antifungal medications should be administered after feeding. Using an applicator or syringe, the medication should be distributed over the entire surface of the oral mucosa and tongue. After swabbing the area, the remainder of the dose is then deposited in the infant's mouth to be swallowed by the infant to treat any GI lesions.

Other measures to control thrush include rinsing the infant's mouth with plain water after each feeding before applying the medication. Instruct caregivers to thoroughly wash reusable nipples and bottles followed by boiling for at least 20 minutes. Pacifiers should also be boiled for at least 20 minutes once daily.

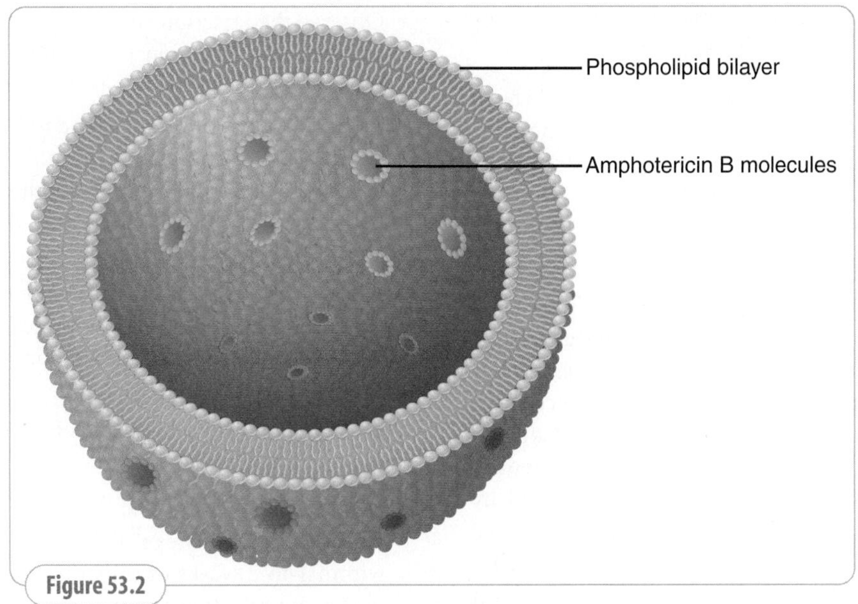

Figure 53.2

Liposomal amphotericin B: Drug molecules are embedded in the lipid bilayer.

To reduce the toxicity of amphotericin B, the original molecule has been formulated with several lipid molecules:

- **Liposomal amphotericin B (AmBisome).** Consists of closed spherical vesicles. Amphotericin B is integrated into the membrane, as illustrated in Figure 53.2.
- **Amphotericin B lipid complex (Abelcet).** Contains amphotericin B complexed with two phospholipids in a 1:1 ratio.
- **Amphotericin B cholesteryl sulfate complex (Amphotec).** Consists of a colloidal suspension of amphotericin B in a 1:1 ratio with the lipid cholesteryl sulfate in microscopic disk-shaped particles.

The principal advantage of the lipid formulations is reduced nephrotoxicity and less infusion-related fever and chills. The reduced toxicity is believed to be due to the decreased plasma levels of the drug. Macrophages ingest the lipid formulations and deliver the medication to its fungal targets before it can accumulate to high serum levels that cause toxicity. Because of their expense, however, the lipid preparations are not considered first-line agents, and are generally used only after therapy with other antifungals has failed. A single treatment with the lipid formulations of amphotericin B can cost several thousand dollars.

Mechanism of Action: Amphotericin B acts by binding to ergosterol in fungal cell membranes, causing them to become permeable.

Pharmacokinetics:

Route(s)	IV, topical
Absorption	Not absorbed topically
Distribution	Widely distributed; very little enters the cerebrospinal fluid (CSF) or amniotic fluid; about 90% bound to plasma protein
Primary metabolism	Hepatic
Primary excretion	Renal
Onset of action	IV: immediate
Duration of action	Half-life: 24–48 h; drug may persist several weeks after therapy is discontinued

Adverse Effects: Amphotericin B can produce frequent and sometimes serious adverse effects. At the onset of therapy, as many as 50% of patients experience acute, infusion-related fever and chills, vomiting, anorexia, and headache. These symptoms usually subside as treatment continues. Pretreatment with corticosteroids, antihistamines, aspirin, or antipyretics may reduce the severity of these distressing symptoms. Although corticosteroids are effective at reducing infusion-related symptoms, care must be taken because drugs in this class may potentiate hypokalemia caused by amphotericin B and predispose a patient to cardiac arrest. Phlebitis is also common during IV therapy, and alternate day dosing is sometimes needed to reduce this adverse effect. Because amphotericin B can cause ototoxicity, the nurse should assess for hearing loss, vertigo, unsteady gait, or tinnitus.

The most limiting effects of amphotericin B are related to its effects on the kidney. Some degree of nephrotoxicity is observed in 80% of the patients taking amphotericin B, thus laboratory tests of kidney function are regularly performed throughout the treatment period. The nurse should monitor for oliguria, changes in intake and output ratios, hematuria, and abnormal renal function tests, and report abnormal values to the health care provider immediately. Ensuring proper fluid and sodium balance during therapy may lessen the nephrotoxic effects of amphotericin B.

Electrolyte imbalance, especially hypokalemia and hypomagnesemia, may develop as a result of renal damage due to amphotericin B. The nurse should monitor for symptoms of low potassium levels, including dysrhythmias. Potassium supplements may be necessary to prevent serious hypokalemia. Because a number of drug–drug interactions are possible during amphotericin B therapy, the nurse should also evaluate all other medication taken by the patient for compatibility with the antifungal agent. Concurrent therapy with other medications that reduce liver or renal function, such as aminoglycosides, is not recommended.

Amphotericin B is occasionally hepatotoxic. Anaphylaxis is possible and cardiac arrest has been reported. Blood abnormalities, including thrombocytopenia, leukopenia, agranulocytosis, and anemia, are potentially serious adverse effects.

Contraindications/Precautions: Amphotericin B should be infused slowly, over 2 to 6 hours, because hypotension, hypokalemia, and shock may result if the medication is administered too rapidly. The drug should be withheld if blood urea nitrogen (BUN) exceeds 40 mg/dL or if serum creatinine rises above 3 mg/dL.

Drug Interactions: Drug interactions with amphotericin B focus on worsening two of its potentially serious adverse effects: nephrotoxicity and hypokalemia. For example, concurrent therapy with aminoglycosides, cyclosporine, vancomycin, carboplatin, and furosemide is not recommended. Corticosteroids, skeletal muscle relaxants, and thiazole may potentiate hypokalemia caused by amphotericin B. Drug-induced hypokalemia will also increase the risk of digoxin toxicity. Because animal studies have indicated an antagonistic effect between amphotericin B and certain azoles (imidazoles), concurrent therapy with this class of antifungals is usually avoided. **Herbal/Food:** Unknown.

Pregnancy: Category B.

Treatment of Overdose: Overdose may result in cardiorespiratory arrest. No specific therapy is available. Patients are treated symptomatically.

Nursing Responsibilities:

- Obtain a complete health history including allergies, drug history, and possible drug interactions.
- Perform infection-focused physical examination including vital signs and white blood cell (WBC) count.
- Premedicate as directed with antipyretics, antihistamines, antiemetics, and corticosteroids to reduce the severity of adverse effects.
- Perform baseline culture and sensitivity (C&S) tests prior to initiating therapy. Other baseline and intermittent laboratory tests include blood urea nitrogen (BUN), serum creatinine, and creatinine clearance; intermittent complete blood counts (CBC); serum electrolytes such as potassium (K^+), magnesium (Mg^{2+}), sodium (Na^+), calcium (Ca^{2+}); and liver function tests.
- Notify the prescriber and reduce or discontinue the drug if BUN exceeds 40 mg/dL or serum creatinine exceeds 3 mg/dL. Monitor for improved renal function before resuming drug therapy.
- Monitor cardiovascular and respiratory status during initial IV therapy. Check vital signs every 30 minutes for at least 4 hours if a test dose is given. Febrile reactions commonly occur within 1 to 2 hours after initiating the infusion. Symptoms usually subside within 4 hours after discontinuing drug and decrease in severity with continued therapy.
- Record intake, output, and weight. Observe and report any change in appearance of urine such as hematuria, presence of sediment, cloudy urine, and any abnormal renal function tests to the prescriber. If the drug is discontinued upon first signs of renal dysfunction, renal damage is usually reversible.
- Observe the injection site for signs and symptoms of local inflammatory reaction or thrombosis, particularly if extravasation occurs.
- Assess for signs of ototoxicity and immediately report any hearing loss or complaints of tinnitus, vertigo, or unsteady gait to the prescriber. Vertigo and hearing loss are more reliable than tinnitus as indicators of ototoxicity in older adults or the very young.
- Assess for the appearance of erythema surrounding topical application to skin lesions. The prescriber may reduce the frequency of topical application to minimize adverse effects.
- Administer IV amphotericin B slowly, over 2 to 6 hours, because hypotension, hypokalemia, and shock may result if the medication is administered too rapidly.

Patient and Family Education:

- Notify the health care provider if symptoms do not improve within 1 to 2 weeks of initiating therapy. Immediately report symptoms that appear worse.
- Do not breast-feed while taking this drug without approval of the health care provider.
- Wash any towels or clothing that contacted the affected lesion area after each treatment.
- Immediately report any of the following symptoms to the health care provider: change in the amount or color of urine, unusual bleeding or bruising, yellowing of eyes or skin, palpitations, or chest pain.
- Report any loss of hearing, dizziness, or ringing in the ears.

Drugs Similar to Amphotericin B Deoxycholate (Fungizone)

Other systemic antifungals include the β-glucan synthesis inhibitors, flucytosine, and certain azole drugs (see Section 53.5).

β-Glucan synthesis inhibitors: Caspofungin (Cancidas), anidulafungin (Eraxis), and micafungin (Mycamine) belong to the newest class of antifungals called echinocandins or β-glucan synthesis inhibitors. Several other drugs in this class are in clinical trials and will likely become available in the near future. Caspofungin is particularly effective against invasive *Candida* and *Aspergillus* species. The drug is not absorbed orally and must be given by the IV route. It is effective against some fungal species that have developed resistance to amphotericin B and the azoles. Micafungin, approved in 2005, is approved to treat *Candida* infections in patients undergoing bone marrow transplants and in those with esophageal candidiasis. Anidulafungin, the newest drug in this class, is approved for candidemia, esophageal candidiasis, and other candida infections. The glucan synthesis inhibitors represent a major development in antifungal drug therapy, although their use is limited by cost. A single treatment can cost as much as $8,000.

The most commonly reported adverse effects with caspofungin are related to histamine release such as fever and rash, and infusion-related reactions including phlebitis, anemia, headache, and nausea. Micafungin creates transient increases in hepatic enzymes, headache, nausea, and vomiting, and some patients have to discontinue therapy due to adverse effects. With anidulafungin, the drug is well tolerated with adverse reactions occurring in 2% or less of patients. These adverse effects are generally not severe; the echinocandins are much better tolerated than amphotericin B and do not exhibit significant nephrotoxicity or hepatotoxicity. All three drugs in this class are pregnancy category C.

Flucytosine (5-fluorocytosine, Ancobon): Unlike amphotericin B and caspofungin, which must be given parenterally, flucytosine is well absorbed from the GI tract. Approved in 1990, flucytosine is structurally similar to cytosine, a nucleotide used in DNA synthesis. When the fungus attempts to use flucytosine to construct its DNA, cell division is inhibited. It is approved to treat septicemia, and pulmonary and urinary tract infections due to *Candida* and *Cryptococcus* species. Unfortunately, resistance to flucytosine is becoming a major clinical problem. The drug is usually used in combination with amphotericin B to reduce the potential for treatment failure due to resistance. Combination therapy also permits the use of lower doses of amphotericin B, thus reducing the risk of nephrotoxicity.

GI adverse effects are common with flucytosine, though symptoms are usually not severe. Flucytosine must be used with extreme caution in patients with renal impairment, as the drug may accumulate to toxic levels in these patients. Hematologic and renal function laboratory tests should be monitored regularly during therapy because the drug can cause bone marrow toxicity, leukopenia, agranulocytosis, and thrombocytopenia. Serum concentrations of flucytosine should be less than 100 g/mL to avoid bone marrow suppression. Flucytosine may cause hepatitis and elevate serum levels of hepatic enzymes. This drug is pregnancy category C.

Drugs for Both Systemic and Superficial Fungal Infections

53.5 Azoles are the drugs of choice for many mycoses due to their efficacy and favorable safety profile.

The **azole** class is the largest and most versatile group of antifungals. These agents have broad spectrums and are used to treat nearly any systemic, subcutaneous, or superficial fungal infection. They have replaced many of the older antifungals because they can be administered PO and have a superior safety profile.

The azoles are sometimes grouped by chemical or therapeutic classes. The azoles form two distinct chemical classes, as follows:

- Imidazoles. Butoconazole, clotrimazole, econazole, ketoconazole, miconazole, oxiconazole, sulconazole, and ticonazole
- Triazoles. Fluconazole, itraconazole, terconazole, and voriconazole

The triazoles are more slowly metabolized and appear to elicit fewer adverse effects than the imidazoles. Most of the newer azoles under development are in the triazole class. In clinical practice, imidazoles and azoles exhibit the same spectrum of activity and act by the same mechanism.

A second method of classifying azoles is by their therapeutic utility as either systemic or topical agents. Fluconazole (Diflucan), itraconazole (Sporanox), ketoconazole (Nizoral), and voriconazole (Vfend) are used for both systemic and topical infections. The remainder of the azoles are prescribed for superficial infections (Section 53.6).

Azoles interfere with the biosynthesis of ergosterol, which is essential for the synthesis of fungal cell membranes. By depleting fungal cells of ergosterol, growth is impaired.

The systemic azoles have a spectrum of activity similar to that of amphotericin B, are considerably less toxic, and have the major advantage that they can be administered PO. Because of these characteristics, azoles have replaced amphotericin B in the pharmacotherapy of less serious systemic fungal infections.

The most common adverse effects of the systemic azoles are nausea and vomiting, which occur in 10% to 20% of patients. Giving the drugs with food or in divided doses may relieve minor GI distress. Severe nausea may require dose reduction or the concurrent administration of an antiemetic. Asymptomatic elevations of serum aminotransferase levels are common. Anaphylaxis and rash have been reported. Fatal drug-induced hepatitis has occurred with ketoconazole, though the incidence is rare and has not been reported with the other systemic azoles. Because of this, itraconazole has largely replaced ketoconazole in the therapy of systemic mycoses. Ketoconazole should not be given to patients with chronic alcoholism due to the possibility of additive liver damage. With all the systemic azoles, liver function tests should be obtained before therapy begins and through the course of treatment. Azoles may affect glycemic control in diabetic patients, so blood glucose should be monitored regularly in these patients.

Various reproductive abnormalities have been reported with systemic azoles, including menstrual irregularities, gynecomastia in males, and drops in plasma testosterone levels. Decreased libido and temporary sterility in males are other potential adverse effects. Fluconazole is teratogenic in laboratory animals and the safety of the azoles during pregnancy has not been established. The risk–benefit ratio should be carefully weighed before initiating azole therapy in a pregnant patient.

PharmFACT

Approximately 75% of all female patients experience vulvovaginal candidiasis at least once during their lifetime. *Source:* Hidalgo & Vazquez, 2008.

PROTOTYPE DRUG Fluconazole (Diflucan)

Classification: **Therapeutic:** Antifungal

Pharmacologic: Inhibitor of fungal cell membrane synthesis, triazole (azole)

Therapeutic Effects and Uses: Approved in 1990, fluconazole is available by tablets, oral suspension, and IV injection. It is particularly effective against *Candida albicans*, and is used to treat oropharyngeal candidiasis, esophageal candidiasis, vulvovaginal candidiasis, and various systemic infections by this species. It is also effective against cryptococcal meningitis and may be used for mycoses that are resistant to other antifungals. Fluconazole is less effective against non-albicans *Candida* species, which account for a significant percentage of opportunistic fungal infections. The drug is approved for prophylaxis of fungal infections in patients with AIDS, those undergoing bone marrow transplants, or those receiving antineoplastic drugs.

Fluconazole offers several advantages over other systemic antifungals. It is rapidly and completely absorbed when given PO. Compared to itraconazole and ketoconazole, it more easily penetrates body membranes to reach infections in the central nervous system (CNS), bone, eye, urinary tract, and respiratory tract.

Mechanism of Action: Like other azoles, fluconazole acts by interfering with the synthesis of ergosterol.

Pharmacokinetics:

Route(s)	IV, PO
Absorption	Readily absorbed PO
Distribution	Widely distributed, including the CSF; secreted in breast milk; 12% bound to plasma protein
Primary metabolism	Hepatic
Primary excretion	Renal
Onset of action	Peak effect: 1–2 h
Duration of action	Half-life: 20–50 h

Adverse Effects: Fluconazole causes few serious adverse effects. Nausea, vomiting, and diarrhea are reported at high doses. Because the kidneys excrete most of the drug, it should be used cautiously in patients with preexisting renal impairment. Unlike ketoconazole, hepatotoxicity with fluconazole is rare. Stevens–Johnson syndrome has been reported in patients with immunosuppression.

Contraindications/Precautions: The only contraindication to fluconazole is hypersensitivity to the drug or another azole. Fluconazole should be used with caution in patients with hepatic impairment because the drug is metabolized in the liver. When given by the IV route, fluconazole is usually prepared without added medications because it is incompatible with a number of drugs. Patients with hypokalemia should be treated with caution because fluconazole may worsen this electrolyte imbalance.

Drug Interactions: Fluconazole is a strong inhibitor of CYP2C9, CYP2C19, and CYP3A4; therefore, it has the potential to interact with several drugs. Use with warfarin (Coumadin) may increase prothrombin time and cause increased risk for bleeding. Hypoglycemia may result if fluconazole is administered concurrently with certain oral hypoglycemics, including glyburide. Fluconazole levels may be decreased with concurrent rifampin or cimetidine use. The effects of fentanyl, alfentanil, benzodiazepines, tricyclic antidepressants, zidovudine, or methadone may be prolonged with concurrent administration of fluconazole. Fluconazole increases the serum level of phenytoin; careful monitoring of phenytoin concentrations is recommended to avoid CNS toxicity. Rifampin increases the metabolism of fluconazole; thus, the dose of fluconazole may need to be increased to maintain therapeutic plasma levels. **Herbal/Food:** Unknown.

Pregnancy: Category C.

MyNursingKit | Mechanism of Action Animation: Fluconazole

Treatment of Overdose: No specific therapy is available; patients are treated symptomatically. Dialysis can be used to lower serum drug level.

Nursing Responsibilities:

- Obtain a complete health history including allergies, drug history, and possible drug interactions.
- Perform an infection-focused physical examination including vital signs and WBC count.
- Monitor BUN, serum creatinine, and liver function laboratory tests. Azoles may elevate laboratory serum values of aspartate aminotransferase (AST), alanine aminotransferase (ALT), alkaline phosphatase, and bilirubin.
- Assess for signs and symptoms of allergic response. Patients who are allergic to one azole may be allergic to others.
- Assess for signs and symptoms of hepatotoxicity.

Patient and Family Education:

- Immediately report signs of liver toxicity, which include right upper quadrant pain, nausea, vomiting, clay-colored stools, yellowing of the skin or eyes, fatigue, or dark orange-colored urine, to the health care provider.
- If diabetic, monitor serum glucose level regularly to ensure proper blood sugar control.
- Disclose all current medications to the health care provider.
- Immediately report signs of drug allergy such as rash, itching, swelling, difficulty breathing, or severe dizziness to the health care provider.
- Immediately notify the health care provider of any known or suspected pregnancy.

Drugs Similar to Fluconazole (Diflucan)

Other systemic azoles include itraconazole, ketoconazole, and voriconazole.

Itraconazole (Sporanox): Approved in 1992, itraconazole is available by PO capsules, PO solution, and IV injection. Its spectrum is similar to other azoles, except it may have greater activity against *Aspergillus.* It is metabolized in the liver to hydoxyitraconazole, which also has antifungal activity. Because the drug may take 2 or more weeks to reach therapeutic levels, a loading dose is infused when treating invasive mycoses. The most common adverse effects of itraconazole are GI related, especially nausea, which occurs in about 10% of patients. Hepatotoxicity is a rare, though potentially serious, adverse effect, which warrants periodic monitoring of liver laboratory tests. The PO capsules should be taken with food to enhance absorption; however, the PO solution should be taken on an empty stomach. Both PO formulations require an acidic stomach environment for absorption and thus should not be taken concurrently with drugs or foods that decrease stomach acidity. Care should be taken when administering itraconazole with other medications, since numerous drug–drug interactions have been reported. Concurrent administration of itraconazole with benzodiazepines or statins is contraindicated. This drug is pregnancy category C.

Ketoconazole (Nizoral): Approved in 1981, ketoconazole is available as tablets for systemic mycoses and as a topical preparation for superficial mycoses. The topical agents are used to treat dandruff and various tinea infections (Section 53.6). As a systemic agent, it is reserved for invasive mycoses, because it is the most hepatotoxic of the azoles. Hepatic function must be monitored regularly during therapy. PO ketoconazole requires an acidic stomach environment for absorption and thus should not be taken concurrently with drugs or foods that decrease stomach acidity. Its most common adverse effects are nausea and vomiting, which can affect over 50% of patients taking high doses of the drug. Like itraconazole, many drug–drug interactions have been reported with ketoconazole. Because the drug inhibits the synthesis of sterols, including testosterone, ketoconazole has been used to treat advanced prostate cancer, although this is not a U.S. Food and Drug Administration (FDA)-approved indication. Ketoconazole may cause a decline in serum testosterone that may lead to male reproductive abnormalities such as gynecomastia and erectile dysfunction. This drug is pregnancy category C.

Voriconazole (Vfend): Approved in 2002, voriconazole is a second-generation triazole synthesized from fluconazole that is approved to treat invasive *Aspergillosis* infections and serious *Candida* infections. It is believed to be safer and more effective than amphotericin B for these indications. It is available by both PO and slow IV infusion routes. Extreme caution should be used when administering voriconazole to patients with severe renal or hepatic impairment, as this can result in toxic accumulation of the drug. The most frequent adverse events affect vision: enhanced brightness, changes in color vision, and blurred vision. Headache, nausea, vomiting, and rash are also common adverse effects. Although visual impairment occurs in 35% to 45% of patients, it is reversible following discontinuation of therapy. Because it participates in many drug interactions, the nurse should seek information from a current drug guide when administering voriconazole concurrently with other medications. This drug causes teratogenicity in laboratory animals and is rated as pregnancy category D.

Drugs for Superficial Fungal Infections

53.6 Drugs for superficial mycoses are safe and effective at eliminating fungi on the skin, nails, or mucous membranes.

Superficial fungal infections of the hair, scalp, nails, and the mucous membranes of the mouth and vagina are rarely medical emergencies. Infections of the nails may be ongoing for months or even years before a patient seeks treatment. Unlike systemic fungal infections, superficial infections may occur in any patient, not just those who have suppressed immune systems. Agents used to treat superficial mycoses are listed in Table 53.3.

Superficial antifungal drugs are much safer than their systemic counterparts because penetration into the deeper layers of the skin is limited, and only small amounts are absorbed into the circulation. Many are available as over-the-counter (OTC) creams, gels, and ointments. If the infection has grown into the deeper skin layers, oral antifungal drugs may be indicated. Extensive superficial or subcutaneous mycoses are sometimes treated with both PO and topical antifungal agents, to ensure that the infection is eliminated from deeper skin layers.

Dermatomycoses: Fungal infections of the skin and hair are called **dermatomycoses.** These infections are named by their Latin terms, beginning with tinea. For example, tinea capitis is an infection of the scalp, and tinea pedis is an infection of the feet.

Fungi that cause dermatomycoses grow in the keratin layer of the skin. Because fungi multiply more rapidly in warm, moist areas, dermatomycoses occur more frequently during the summer months, and in warmer climates. They tend to favor skin creases that stay moist due to sweat or following bathing. Because relapse rates following pharmacotherapy are high, the patient should be taught proper personal hygiene measures to help eliminate the pathogen. These include frequent bathing with thorough drying of the infected area, the use of separate towels for the groin area, and wearing loose clothing.

Tinea corporis is an infection in which the fungus invades relatively hairless skin. The fungus typically appears as a ring pattern, thus resulting in the name ringworm. Transmission may occur through direct contact with infected animals (especially cats and dogs), infected humans, or contaminated furniture or clothing. The most common pathogens are *Trichophyton* and *Microsporum* species. Topical therapies are usually successful in controlling tinea corporis. In cases of inflammatory lesions, oral therapy with griseofulvin (Fulvicin), terbinafine (Lamisil), itraconazole (Sporanox), or fluconazole (Diflucan) is recommended.

Tinea cruris, commonly called jock itch, is a form of tinea corporis that occurs in the groin, perineum, and perianal region. Topical powders and creams are usually sufficient to cure tinea cruris. PO antifungal agents such as griseofulvin (Fulvicin), terbinafine (Lamisil), itraconazole (Sporanox), or fluconazole (Diflucan) may be necessary for severe cases.

Tinea pedis, commonly called athlete's foot, is a type of tinea corporis occurring on the feet, principally occurring between the toes, and on the sole. It is associated with the wearing of shoes and contact with infected bath or pool floors. Tinea pedis is the most common dermatomycosis, affecting about 70% of adults at some time during their life. Topical antifungals are effective for noninflammatory tinea pedis. PO therapy is sometimes used to treat more severe infections and areas such as the soles. Typical therapy includes terbinafine (Lamisil) or itraconazole (Sporanox) for 2 to 4 weeks.

Tinea capitis involves the hair of the head, eyebrows, or eyelashes, and primarily affects children between 4 and 14 years of age. *Trichophyton* is responsible for more than 90% of cases. In contrast with other dermatomycoses, tinea capitis is routinely treated with PO agents. Typical regimens include the following:

- Griseofulvin (Fulvicin). 10 mg/kg/day for 8 to 10 weeks
- Itraconazole (Sporanox). 5 mg/kg/day for 1 to 4 weeks
- Terbinafine (Lamisil). 62.5 to 250 mg/day for 4 weeks

Onychomycoses: **Onychomycosis,** or tinea unguium, is the invasion of the nail plate by a fungus. It is a relatively common

TABLE 53.3 Selected Drugs for Superficial Mycoses

Drug	Route and Adult Dose (maximum dose where indicated)	Adverse Effects
butenafine (Mentax)	Topical: Apply daily for 2–4 weeks for tineas	*Drying of skin, stinging sensation at application site, pruritus, urticaria, contact dermatitis* Granulocytopenia (griseofulvin), cholestatic hepatitis (oral terbinafine), neutropenia (oral terbinafine)
ciclopirox cream, gel, shampoo (Loprox), or nail lacquer (Penlac)	Topical: Apply cream bid for 4 weeks for tineas Topical: Apply lacquer to nail for 48 weeks for onychomycoses	
griseofulvin (Fulvicin)	PO: 500 mg microsize or 330–375 mg ultra microsize daily for tineas and onychomycoses	
naftifine (Naftin)	Topical: Apply cream daily or gel bid for 4 weeks for tineas	
nystatin: topical powder (Mycostatin, Nystop); oral suspension (Nilstat); capsule (Bio-Statin); cream, ointment (Mycostatin, Nystex)	Suspension PO: 400,000–600,000 units 4 times/day Topical: Apply 2–3 times/day to the affected area Capsule: PO: 500,000 to 1 million units every 6 h Vaginal tablets: Insert 1 tablet daily for 2 weeks	
terbinafine (Lamisil)	Topical: Apply once daily or bid for 7 weeks for tineas PO: 250 mg/day for 6–12 weeks for onychomycoses	
tolnaftate (Aftate, Tinactin)	Topical: Apply to the affected area twice daily for 2 weeks for tinea cruris and 4 weeks for tinea pedis or corporis	
undecylenic acid (Fungi-Nail, Gordochom, others)	Topical: Apply once or twice daily for tineas for up to 4 weeks	
Azoles		
butoconazole (Femstat, Gynazole)	Intravaginal: Femstat: 1 applicator for 3 days Gynazole: 1 applicator as a single dose	*Drying of the skin, stinging sensation at application site, pruritus, urticaria, contact dermatitis* No serious adverse effects
clotrimazole: topical cream (Lotrimin AF); intravaginal (Gyne-Lotrimin, Mycelex, others) troche (Mycelex)	Topical: Apply 1% cream bid × 4 weeks Intravaginal: 1 applicator for 7 days; one 100-mg tablet vaginally for 7 days or one 500-mg tablet once Troche: Dissolve one in the mouth over 15–30-min	
econazole (Spectazole)	Topical: Apply 1% cream bid for 4 weeks for tineas or cutaneous candidiasis	
fluconazole (Diflucan)	PO: 150 mg once, for vulvovaginal candidiasis (VVC)	
itraconazole (Sporanox)	PO: 200 mg daily × 1–2 weeks for OPC PO: 200 mg daily for 3 days for VVC PO: 200 mg daily for 3 months for onychomycoses	
ketoconazole (Nizoral)	Topical: Apply 2% cream or shampoo 1–2 times/day to affected area for tineas	
miconazole (Micatin, Monistat)	Topical: Apply 2% cream bid for 2–4 weeks for tineas Intravaginal: 1 suppository daily for 3–7 days	
oxiconazole (Oxistat)	Topical: Apply 1% cream daily for 2 months for tineas and cutaneous candidiasis	
sulconazole (Exelderm)	Topical: Apply 1% cream daily or bid for 2–6 weeks for tineas	
terconazole (Terazol)	Intravaginal: 1 applicator for 3–7 weeks for VVC	
tioconazole (Vagistat-1, Monistat-1)	Intravaginal: 1 applicator as a single dose	

Note: *Italics* indicate common adverse effects. Underline indicates serious adverse effects.

infection, affecting 2% to 3% of Americans. Rates among men are twice that of women, and infections increase with age. The higher incidence in elderly patients is believed to be due to reduced peripheral circulation, general inactivity, increased nail trauma, and difficulty (or inability) in maintaining proper nail hygiene. One in four diabetic patients will acquire an onychomycosis, likely due to reduced circulation to the area.

The most common fungal pathogens responsible for onychomycoses are *Trichophyton* and *Epidermophyton* species. Although any part of the nail may be affected, most commonly the infection begins with invasion of the hyponychium, the place where the nail separates from the nail bed. Toenails are more often affected than fingernails. The nail becomes markedly disfigured and distorted.

Although certainly not a life-threatening infection, onychomycosis is one of the most difficult superficial fungal infections to treat. Nails grow slowly and the nail plate is hard, preventing antifungal agents from penetrating. The traditional drug for onychomycosis has been griseofulvin (Fulvicin), but this drug has a narrow spectrum of activity; in addition, cure rates are low and recurrence is common. In recent years, terbinafine (Lamisil) and itraconazole (Sporanox) have become drugs of choice for onychomycosis. Both of these agents are absorbed into the nail matrix and remain active for several months. Itraconazole can be detected in nail clippings for up to a year after administration and terbinafine for up to 3 months. This long duration is important, as nails may take 9 to 12 months to be totally replaced. Typical therapies have an 80% cure rate and include the following:

- Terbinafine (Fulvicin). 250 mg daily for 3 months
- Itraconazole (Sporanox). 200 mg twice daily for 1 week/month. This cycle is repeated twice for fingernails and three to four times for toenails
- Fluconazole (Diflucan). 150 to 450 mg weekly for 6 to 9 months. This drug is used for patients who are unable to take terbinafine or itraconazole

Until recently, topical therapy alone was not successful for the treatment of onychomycosis because the available drugs could not penetrate deeply enough to eradicate the fungus. Ciclopirox solution (Penlac) is a newer agent applied as a topical nail lacquer for the treatment of mild to moderate onychomycosis. The drug is applied daily, covering the entire nail plate and surrounding skin for 12 months. Ciclopirox has a relatively high relapse rate and does not appear to be as effective as terbinafine or itraconazole.

Pharm*FACT*

Although the overall incidence of onychomycoses is only 2–13% in the United States, this percentage increases to 90% in elderly patients. *Source:* Blumberg, Kantor, & Ratz, 2007.

Superficial Candidiasis: Although there are approximately 10 species of *Candida* that cause disease in humans, *C. albicans* is responsible for nearly 100% of cases of oropharyngeal fungal infections and at least 90% of cases of vulvovaginal candidiasis. A small yeast, *Candida* is often found as part of normal host flora on body surfaces. Candida species are the most common pathogens causing fungal disease in patients with compromised immune defenses.

Oropharyngeal candidiasis (OPC) is an oral mycosis, sometimes called thrush. About 50% of people carry *Candida* in the mouth as part of their host flora. Infection occurs when the patient's defenses are weakened; thus the highest incidence of OPC is seen in AIDS patients, diabetics, cancer patients, and in hospitalized patients. Patients taking inhaled corticosteroids are also at greater risk because these agents cause a local immunosuppression in the oral cavity (see Chapter 73). Although not life threatening, OPC may predispose a patient to esophageal candidiasis, which is a serious, invasive mycosis.

Several options are available for the pharmacotherapy of OPC. Topical therapy is generally preferred and is often successful for milder, uncomplicated infections. Troches and PO suspensions are the most common formulations for topical therapy. Symptoms generally subside in 2 to 3 days but the nurse should encourage the patient to complete the full 1- to 2-week course of therapy. Typical treatments for OPC are as follows:

- Nystatin. Lozenges, 200,000 units or PO suspension, 500,000 units by swish and swallow, four times daily for 7 to 14 days.
- Clotrimazole (Mycelex). 10-mg troche, slowly dissolved in the mouth 5 times a day for 7 to 14 days.
- Fluconazole (Diflucan). 100 to 200 mg/day for 7 to 14 days.
- Itraconazole (Sporanox). Suspension, 200 mg (20 mL) daily by swish and swallow for 7 to 14 days; or capsules, 200 mg/day for 2 to 4 weeks.

Extensive OPC, especially in immunosuppressed patients and in those with esophageal involvement, is treated with systemic therapy. Prolonged therapy with regular follow-up may be required in these patients. Prophylactic therapy of OPC using azole antifungals may be warranted in AIDS patients. Prolonged prophylactic therapy, however, leads to azole-resistant *Candida* species. The practice is generally discouraged, as OPC has a low mortality rate, and empirical treatment of the infection in these patients is generally successful.

Candida species are part of the normal vaginal flora in about 50% of healthy women. Because vulvovaginal candidiasis (VVC) occurs in both healthy and immunosuppressed women, it is not considered an opportunistic infection. The biggest risk factors for VVC are sexual activity, pregnancy, diabetes mellitus, the use of oral contraceptives with high estrogen content, or broad-spectrum antibiotics. *Candida* may be transmitted to male sexual partners. Its highest incidence occurs between the ages of 30 to 40. *C. albicans* is by far the most common species, although *Candida glabrata* is an emerging pathogen for VVC.

Several effective topical agents for VVC are available without a prescription. The various topical regimens have equal efficacy in treating VVC, with response rates of 80% to 90%. Many women prefer PO therapies because of their convenience. Oral therapy has the same efficacy as topical treatment.

Regimens for VVC are classified by their duration of therapy. The most popular therapies are 1-day PO regimens, due to their ease of use. Although 1-day treatments are effective for most women with VVC, there are limitations to this brief therapy. Because 1-day treatments may take up to 48 hours to produce relief, faster-acting topical agents may be more beneficial for patients with severe symptoms. In addition, patients with complicated, persistent, or severe infections require 10 to 14 days of therapy for successful elimination of the pathogen, regardless of the route of administration. Typical therapies for VVC include the following:

- Single topical application. Ticonazole (Vagistat-1, Monistat-1), 6.5% ointment; butoconazole (Gynazole), 2% cream (sustained-released formulation); miconazole, 2% cream
- Single PO dose. Fluconazole, one 150-mg tablet; itraconazole, 200 mg bid for 1 day; clotrimazole, one 500-mg tablet for 1 day
- Multi-day regimens. Butoconazole (Femstat), 2% cream, for 1 to 7 days; clotrimazole (Lotrimin AF), 1% cream or 100-mg tablets for 1 to 7 days; miconazole, 2% cream or 100- to 200-mg suppositories for 1 to 7 days; or nystatin, 100,000-unit vaginal tablet daily for 7 to 14 days

Because recurrent VVC may occur in 5% of patients treated for this infection, cultures may be necessary to identify the specific pathogen. Treatment begins with a 14-day induction phase that uses the same drugs as for nonrecurring infections.

A maintenance phase follows, typically with azole antifungals taken once weekly (fluconazole) or once monthly (itraconazole) for 6 months.

CONNECTION Checkpoint 53.2

From what you learned in Chapter 48, why might broad-spectrum antibacterial therapy cause a *Candida* infection of the vagina? See Answer to Connection Checkpoint 53.2 in Appendix A.

PROTOTYPE DRUG Nystatin (Mycostatin, Nystop, others)

Classification: **Therapeutic:** Antifungal, superficial type
Pharmacologic: Polyene

Therapeutic Effects and Uses: Approved in 1954, nystatin belongs to the same chemical class as amphotericin B, the polyenes. Although they act by the same mechanism, nystatin has very different indications, and is available in a wider variety of formulations, including cream, ointment, powder, tablets, and lozenges. Too toxic for parenteral administration, it is usually used topically to treat *Candida* infections of the vagina, skin, and mouth because it is not absorbed in these areas. Although available as vaginal tablets, the azoles have largely replaced nystatin due to their higher efficacy. PO suspensions are available to treat oropharyngeal candidiasis, using a swish-and-swallow technique. Some formulations, such as Mytrex and Mycolog II cream, combine nystatin with triamcinolone (a corticosteroid) for treating inflamed subcutaneous lesions. It is available as tablets to treat candidiasis of the intestine, since it travels through the GI tract without being absorbed. It is not effective for treating onychomycoses.

Mechanism of Action: Nystatin binds to sterols in the fungal cell membrane allowing leakage of intracellular contents across the weakened membrane.

Pharmacokinetics:

Route(s)	PO suspensions, troches, topical creams, and vaginal tablets; PO tablets for intestinal infections
Absorption	Poorly absorbed
Distribution	Not distributed
Primary metabolism	Not metabolized
Primary excretion	Excreted unchanged in the feces
Onset of action	Rapid
Duration of action	Half-life: 6–12 h

Adverse Effects: When given topically, nystatin produces few adverse effects other than minor skin irritation and burning at the site of application. There is a high incidence of contact dermatitis, related to the preservatives found in some of the formulations. When given PO, it may cause diarrhea, nausea, and vomiting.

Contraindications/Precautions: The only contraindication to nystatin therapy is hypersensitivity to the drug. Although no teratogenic effects have been reported, safety during pregnancy and lactation has not been established.

Drug Interactions: Unknown.

Pregnancy: Category B.

Treatment of Overdose: No specific therapy is available; patients are treated symptomatically.

Nursing Responsibilities:

- Obtain a complete health history including allergies, drug history, and possible drug interactions.
- Perform an infection-focused physical examination.
- Observe for signs of improvement and report persistent infections to the prescriber.
- Avoid any occlusive dressings or ointment applications to moist, dark areas of the body as these conditions may enhance yeast growth.

Patient and Family Education:

- Stop using the drug and report the following symptoms of contact dermatitis to the health care provider: itching, irritation, mild redness, swelling, blistering or scaling of the skin, or temporary thickening of the skin.
- Apply treatments for oral candidiasis (thrush) after meals and at bedtime.
- Dissolve troches in the mouth for about 30 minutes, without chewing or swallowing. Do not take food or drink while dissolving the troche and for 30 minutes after treatment.
- Remove dentures before rinsing with oral suspension as well as dissolving the troche in the mouth. Also remove dentures at night, because oral fungal infections occur more frequently in those wearing dentures 24 hours each day.
- Dust feet, shoes, and stockings with nystatin dusting powder.
- Use cream instead of ointment for use in body folds or areas of skin-to-skin contact. For moist lesions, powder may be most useful. Gently clean infected areas with tepid water before each application.
- Note that treatment of *Candida* skin infections is continued for at least 2 weeks. Therapy can be discontinued after two negative tests for *Candida.*
- Continue medication for vulvovaginal candidiasis during menstruation. Usually therapy lasts about 2 weeks but some cases may require longer therapy.
- Use vaginal tablets up to 6 weeks before the end of the pregnancy term to prevent thrush in the newborn.
- Do not breast-feed while taking this drug without approval of the health care provider.

Drugs Similar to Nystatin (Mycostatin, Nystop, Others)

Other superficial antifungals include terbinafine, topical azoles, and several miscellaneous agents.

Griseofulvin (Grifulvin V, Gris-PEG): Approved in 1959, griseofulvin is an inexpensive antifungal that is indicated for the PO therapy of mycoses of the hair, skin, and nails that have not responded to conventional topical preparations. It is not given topically because the drug is unable to penetrate into the deeper skin layers when given by this route. In an attempt to reduce GI adverse effects and increase its bioavailability, griseofulvin is available as microsize particles (Grifulvin V) and ultramicrosize particles (Gris-PEG). Grifulvin V is 25% to 70% absorbed and Gis-PEG is almost 100% absorbed.

The length of treatment for tinea pedis is 4 to 8 weeks and for tinea unguium, 3 to 6 months. Griseofulvin is deposited in keratin, where it accumulates and inhibits mitosis of the fungal cells. It exhibits few adverse effects, other than headache. Although rare, hepatitis and neutropenia have been reported with prolonged therapy. Griseofulvin has a higher incidence of long-term adverse effects and has a greater relapse rate than some other superficial antifungal agents. This drug is pregnancy category C.

Terbinafine (Lamisil): Approved in 1993, terbinafine may be administered by the PO or topical routes. Terbinafine acts by inhibiting ergosterol biosynthesis. The PO form of the drug is available by prescription to treat onychomycosis. The drug rapidly accumulates in nails, although therapy of persistent onychomycosis may require 6 to 12 weeks. The cure rate for onychomycosis is 50% to 70%, which is higher than that for griseofulvin. Oral preparations are well tolerated, with nausea, vomiting, abdominal pain, and diarrhea being the most common adverse effects. Rare, though serious, adverse effects include Stevens–Johnson syndrome, blood dyscrasias, and hepatic failure.

Nonprescription formulations such as Lamisil AT include topical creams and sprays for treating tinea corporis, tinea pedis, and tinea cruris. Adverse effects are rare with topical terbinafine; irritation or urticaria occurs in less than 1% of patients. The drug is not absorbed when administered topically. Both PO and topical forms of terbinafine are pregnancy category B.

Topical azoles: There are 10 azoles used to treat superficial mycoses. Itraconazole, voriconazole, and fluconazole may be used PO to treat superficial mycoses, whereas the others are topical use only. Among the topical agents, all have equal efficacy and similar adverse effects. Miconazole and clotrimazole are OTC drugs of choice for vulvovaginal candida infections, although there are a number of other azoles available that are equally effective. Transient burning and irritation at the application sites are the most common adverse effects of the topical azoles.

Miscellaneous topical agents: Several agents are less commonly used for superficial fungal infections. These drugs are applied topically, for tineas, or intravaginally, for VVC. The doses and indications for these agents are shown in Table 53.3.

NURSING PROCESS APPLICATION

Patients Receiving Antifungal Therapy

Assessment	Potential Nursing Diagnoses
Prior to administration • Obtain a complete health history including allergies, drug history, and possible drug interactions. • Obtain specimens for C&S before initializing therapy. • Perform infection-focused physical examination including vital signs and WBC count. • Premedicate as directed (antipyretic, antihistamines, antiemetics, and corticosteroids may be given to minimize severity of adverse effects).	• *Risk for Infection* • *Risk for Injury,* related to adverse effects of drug • *Deficient Knowledge (Antifungal Therapy),* related to purpose, precautions, and adverse effects of drug • *Deficient Knowledge (Fungal Infection),* related to disease process and infection transmission • *Noncompliance (Therapeutic Regimen)*

Planning: Patient Goals and Expected Outcomes

The patient will:

- Report a reduction in symptoms related to the fungal infection, and have negative results for laboratory and diagnostic tests for the presenting infection.
- Demonstrate an understanding of the drug's action by accurately describing drug adverse effects and precautions.
- Immediately report significant adverse effects of the specific drug used.
- Complete the full course of antifungal therapy and comply with follow-up care.
- Demonstrate understanding of proper self-administration techniques for topical antifungals.

Implementation: Systemic Antifungals

Interventions and (Rationales)	Patient and Family Education
• Monitor vital signs and symptoms of infection to determine antifungal therapy effectiveness. (Another drug or different dosage may be required.)	• Instruct the patient to notify the health care provider if symptoms persist or worsen.
• Monitor for hypersensitivity reaction. (IV test dose may be given to elicit hypersensitivity response.)	• Instruct the patient to discontinue the medication and inform the health care provider if symptoms of hypersensitivity reaction develop such as wheezing; shortness of breath; swelling of the face, tongue, or hands; and itching or rash.
• Administer IV doses cautiously. (Amphotericin B must be infused slowly, over 2–6 hours, as hypotension, hypokalemia, and shock may result if the medication is administered too rapidly.) • Monitor hydration status before and after drug administration. (Some parenteral antifungal drugs cause nephrotoxicity in the presence of dehydration.)	Instruct the patient to: • Maintain hydration status by increased fluid intake as tolerated. • Report symptoms associated with renal impairment such as sudden weight gain, edema, decreased urinary output, or changes in color or consistency of urine.
• Administer the drug at designated time frames. (This will maintain effective blood levels and "steady state.")	Instruct the patient to: • Take the medication on schedule. • Complete the entire prescription even if feeling better, to prevent the development of resistant bacteria.

(continued)

Implementation: Systemic Antifungals

Interventions and (Rationales)	Patient and Family Education
• Monitor intake of OTC products such as aspirin, nonsteroidal anti-inflammatory drugs (NSAIDs), certain antihistamines, and certain drugs for heartburn and gastroesophageal reflux. (Aspirin and NSAIDs may increase the risk of bleeding; astemizole [Hismanol] and cisapride [Propulsid] may increase the risk of cardiac dysrhythmias.)	• Advise the patient to consult with the health care provider before using OTC, prescribed medications, or herbal products.
• Determine the interactions of the prescribed antifungal therapy with various foods and beverages. (Food intake will affect absorption of antifungal medications.)	Instruct the patient regarding foods and beverages that should be avoided with specific antibiotic therapies: • Itraconazole should be taken with food to enhance absorption. • Ketoconazole may be taken with food to reduce incidence of nausea and vomiting.
• Monitor the IV site for signs and symptoms of tissue irritation, severe pain, and extravasation. (Extravasation of IV antifungal drugs can produce severe tissue damage.)	• Instruct the patient to report pain or other symptoms of discomfort immediately during IV infusion.
• Monitor for adverse effects specific to various antibiotic therapies. (Common adverse effects of a amphotericin B include hypokalemia, hypomagnesemia, rash, fever and chills, nausea, vomiting, anorexia, and headache. Fluconazole causes very few serious adverse effects.)	• Instruct the patient to report adverse effects specific to antibiotic therapy prescribed.
• Monitor renal function such as intake and output ratios, urine color and consistency, serum creatinine and BUN. (Antifungal therapies may be nephrotoxic.)	• Explain the purpose of required laboratory tests and scheduled follow-up with health care provider. • Instruct the patient to increase fluid intake to 2,000 to 3,000 mL/day.
• Monitor hepatic function such as nausea, vomiting, jaundice, dark orange-colored urine, and clay-colored stool. • Monitor laboratory values such as ALT, AST, alkaline phosphatase, and bilirubin. (Some antifungal therapies are hepatotoxic.)	• Instruct the patient to report symptoms that may be associated with hepatic toxicity such as abdominal pain, clay-colored stools, dark concentrated urine, or the presence of jaundice.
• Monitor the patient for adherence to antibiotic therapy. (Because many antifungal agents require long and extensive treatment, some patients may become complacent about therapy.)	Instruct the patient in the importance of: • Completing the prescription as ordered. • Follow-up care after the antibiotic therapy is completed.

Implementation: Topical Agents

Interventions and (Rationales)	Patient and Family Education
• Monitor for possible adverse effects or hypersensitivity. (Minor skin irritation and burning at the site of application may occur.)	• Instruct the patient to discontinue use and notify the health care provider if severe burning, stinging, or eruption occurs.
• Encourage adherence to the proper administration method. (Methods include swish and swallow, suppository insertion, or topical application.) • For application to skin, ALWAYS wear gloves, cleanse area with tepid water, and dry thoroughly prior to application. After removing gloves, wash hands meticulously. (This will avoid cross contamination.)	For oral infections, instruct the patient to: • Swish the oral suspension to coat all mucous membranes, and then swallow medication. • Spit out the medication instead of swallowing, if GI irritation is present. • Allow the troche to dissolve completely, rather than chewing or swallowing it. It may take 30 minutes for it to completely dissolve. • Avoid food or drink for 30 minutes following administration. • Remove dentures prior to using the oral suspension. • Take ketoconazole with water, fruit juice, coffee, or tea to enhance dissolution and absorption. For topical skin application, instruct the patient to: • Avoid wearing tight-fitting undergarments if using ointment in the vaginal or groin area.
• For vulvovaginal application: • Always wear gloves. • Insert one applicator full or one vaginal tablet. • Vaginal medicines are most often administered at bedtime, as the reclined position enhances medication absorption. (Vaginal tissue can be traumatized by the forceful use of applicators or fingernails during medicine administration, so medications should be introduced into the vagina gently.)	• Avoid occlusive dressings because they increase the moisture in these areas and encourage development of additional yeast infections. For vaginal application, instruct the patient: • To relax, as this will decrease resistance to the mode of insertion. • That medicine should not be delivered via the vagina if it is not labeled for vaginal use. • That vaginal medicine should not be taken PO. • That therapy should continue during menstruation. • To refrain from sexual intercourse or have partner wear condom to avoid burning or irritation of the penis or urethra.
• Encourage infection control practices. (This will prevent the spread of infection.)	Instruct the patient to: • Clean the affected area daily. • Apply the medication with a glove. • Wash hands properly before and after application. • Wash clothing and linens that have come in contact with infectious sites after each treatment.

Evaluation of Outcome Criteria

Evaluate the effectiveness of drug therapy by confirming that patient goals and expected outcomes have been met (see "Planning").

UNDERSTANDING THE CHAPTER

Key Concepts Summary

53.1 Serious fungal infections are uncommon in people with healthy immune defenses.

53.2 Mycoses are classified as superficial, subcutaneous, or systemic.

53.3 Antifungal drugs act by disrupting the fungal cell membrane or wall, affecting fungal enzymes or disrupting replication.

53.4 Systemic or invasive fungal disease may require intensive pharmacotherapy for extended periods.

53.5 Azoles are the drugs of choice for many mycoses due to their efficacy and favorable safety profile.

53.6 Drugs for superficial mycoses are safe and effective at eliminating fungi on the skin, nails, or mucous membranes.

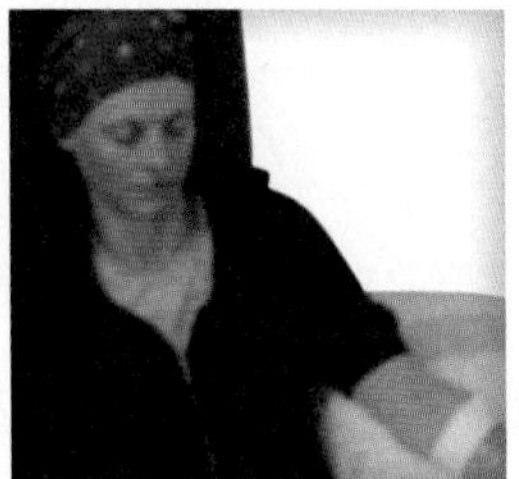

Making the PATIENT Connection

Remember the patient "Sarah Williams" at the beginning of the chapter? Now read the remainder of the case study. Based on the information presented within this chapter, respond to the critical thinking questions that follow.

Sarah Williams is a 58-year-old female with lung cancer who recently finished her second round of chemotherapy. She presents at the clinic with concern about white patches on her tongue and mouth. She states that her mouth is not sore but her throat burns when she swallows. This has made it very difficult for her to eat and drink.

A history and physical exam is completed. The health care provider evaluates Sarah for oropharyngeal candidiasis. She is 5′3″ tall and weighs 52.7 kg (116 lb). Sarah was diagnosed with lung cancer several months prior and is taking chemotherapy and corticosteroids. Upon initial assessment, her vital signs are normal, and she has no complaints except her expressed concerns about her mouth and throat. She has worn dentures for about 5 years.

Critical Thinking Questions

1. Outline the key steps in the initial assessment needed to evaluate Sarah's condition.
2. What are the signs and symptoms you, the nurse, would look for to determine if Sarah is experiencing oropharyngeal candidiasis?
3. Why do you think that Sarah is at risk for this type of infection?

Case Study

The health care provider asks Sarah to remove her dentures to allow a thorough examination of her oral cavity. White patches are apparent on her tongue and throat. The health care provider tells Sarah she has thrush and prescribes the following: 500,000 units nystatin by swish and swallow four times/day for 7 to 14 days, clotrimazole 10 mg troche five times/day for 7 to 14 days, and fluconazole 100 to 200 mg/day for 7 to 14 days.

1. Discuss how Sarah's dentures played a role in her oral infection.
2. What approach does the health care provider take in treating Sarah's thrush?

NCLEX-RN® Review

1 A client is admitted to the acute care hospital for systemic fungal infections. The nurse knows that symptoms most likely develop:

1. Immediately after exposure to fungal spores.
2. Very slowly since fungal infections may progress for many months.
3. 7 to 10 days after exposure to the infecting agent.
4. Any time after exposure to mushrooms, yeast, and molds.

2 The nurse knows that a client's susceptibility to systemic fungal infections is most likely to occur in which of the following client populations?

1. African Americans and Hispanics
2. Clients with cardiovascular disease
3. Immunosuppressed individuals
4. Children and youth

3 In monitoring a client's response to fluconazole (Diflucan), which of the following symptoms would provide the nurse with the earliest indication of drug toxicity?

1. Dark orange-colored urine
2. Tinnitus
3. Tachycardia
4. Difficulty swallowing

4 In caring for a client receiving an intravenous infusion of amphotericin B (Fungizone), the nurse should be alert for which of the following immediate life-threatening complications caused by too-rapid intravenous administration?

1. Myalgia
2. Hypotension
3. Bone marrow suppression
4. Flank pain

5 The nurse knows the reason for pretreatment with corticosteroids, antihistamines, and antipyretics prior to the administration of amphotericin B is to:

1. Enhance the effectiveness of this antifungal agent.
2. Eliminate toxic by-products of this antifungal agent.
3. Reduce the severity of adverse effects associated with this antifungal agent.
4. Increase the half-life of this antifungal agent.

6 Which of the following clients is most likely to develop oral fungal infections? A client taking:

1. Oral diuretics.
2. Inhaled corticosteroids.
3. Sublingual nitrate therapy.
4. Buccal analgesics.

See Answers to Critical Thinking Questions, Case Study, and NCLEX-RN® Review in Appendix A.

References

Bennet, J. E. (2006). Antifungal agents. In L. L. Brunton, J. S. Lazo, & K. L. Parker (Eds.), *The pharmacological basis of therapeutics* (11th ed., pp. 1225–1242). New York: McGraw-Hill.

Blumberg, M., Kantor, G. R., & Ratz, J. (2007). *Onychomycosis.* Emedicine. Retrieved July 30, 2008, from http://www.emedicine.com/derm/topic300.htm

Brown, T., & Chin, T. (2006). Superficial fungal infections. In J. T. De Piro (Ed.), *Pharmacotherapy: A pathophysiologic approach* (6th ed., pp. 2145–2160). New York: McGraw-Hill.

Carver, P. L. (2006). Invasive fungal infections. In J. T. De Piro (Ed.), *Pharmacotherapy: A pathophysiologic approach* (6th ed., pp. 216–219). New York: McGraw-Hill.

Dodds-Ashley, E. (2006). Treatment options for invasive fungal infections. *Pharmacotherapy, 26*(6), 55S–60S.

Enoch, D. A., Ludlam, H. A., & Brown, N. M. (2006). Invasive fungal infections: A review of epidemiology and management options. *Journal of Medical Microbiology, 55*(7), 809–818.

Gupta, A. (2006). Therapies for onychomycosis: A review. *Dermatologic Clinics, 24*(3), 375–379.

Hidalgo, J. A., & Vazquez, J. A. (2008). *Candidiasis.* Emedicine. Retrieved August 4, 2008, from http://www.emedicine.com/med/topic264.htm

Pasqualotto, A. C., & Denning, D. W. (2008). New and emerging treatments for fungal infections. *Journal of Antimicrobial Chemotherapy, 61*(Supplement 1), i19–i30.

Perlroth, J., Choi, B., & Spellberg, B. (2007). Nosocomial fungal infections: Epidemiology, diagnosis, and treatment. *Medical Mycology, 45*(4), 321–346.

Scheinfeld, N. S., Lambiase, M. C., Lehman, D. S., & Allan, J. M. (2008). *Candidiasis, cutaneous.* Emedicine. Retrieved July 29, 2008, from http://www.emedicine.com/derm/topic67.htm

Smith, C. M., & Kagan, S. H. (2005). Prevention of systemic mycoses by reducing exposure to fungal pathogens in hospitalized and ambulatory neutropenic patients. *Oncology Nursing Forum, 32*(3), 565–579.

Wilson, C. (2005). Recurrent vulvovaginitis candidiasis: An overview of traditional and alternative therapies. *Advance for Nurse Practitioners, 13*(5), 24–29.

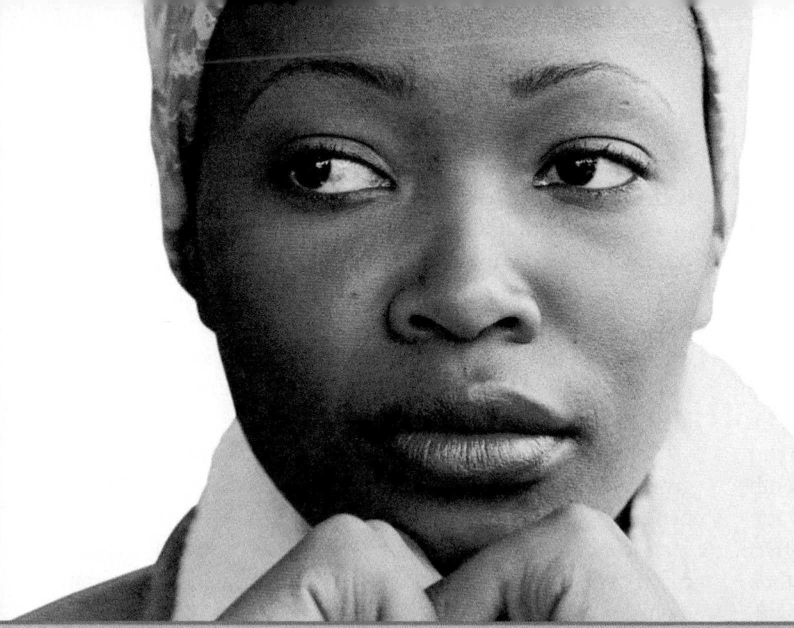

I'm worried about my upcoming trip to the Dominican Republic. I've never been out of the country and don't want to catch anything that will make me sick.

Patient "Harriet Sanchez"

CHAPTER 54

Pharmacotherapy of Protozoan and Helminthic Infections

Chapter Outline

Classification and Pathogenesis of Protozoan Infections

Drugs for Malaria

PROTOTYPE **Chloroquine (Aralen)** *p. 889*

Drugs for Nonmalarial Protozoan Infections

PROTOTYPE **Metronidazole (Flagyl)** *p. 893*

PROTOTYPE **Pyrimethamine and Sulfadiazine (Fansidar)** *p. 897*

Classification and Pathogenesis of Helminthic Infections

Drugs for Helminthic Infections

PROTOTYPE **Mebendazole (Vermox)** *p. 902*

Learning Outcomes

After reading this chapter, the student should be able to:

1. Identify features of protozoa and helminths that distinguish them from bacteria.
2. Identify protozoan and helminthic infections that may benefit from pharmacotherapy.
3. Explain why an understanding of *Plasmodium*'s life cycle is important to the successful pharmacotherapy of malaria.
4. Explain the etiology, pathogenesis, and pharmacotherapy of amebiasis, giardiasis, cryptosporidiosis, toxoplasmosis, trichomoniasis, trypanosomiasis, and leishmaniasis.
5. Explain the etiology, pathogenesis, and pharmacotherapy of ascariasis, enterobiasis, hookworm, and tapeworm infections.
6. Describe the nurse's role in the pharmacologic management of protozoan and helminthic infections.
7. For each of the classes shown in the chapter outline, identify the prototype and representative drugs and explain the mechanism(s) of drug action, primary indications, contraindications, significant drug interactions, pregnancy category, and important adverse effects.
8. Apply the nursing process to care for patients receiving drugs for protozoan and helminthic infections.

Key Terms

cinchonism, *890*
cysts, *886*
erythrocytic stage, *887*
helminths, *898*
malaria, *887*
merozoites, *887*
protozoan, *886*
sporozoite, *887*
trophozoite, *886*
vector, *886*

Protozoa and parasitic worms, or helminths, are more complex than bacteria and cause significant morbidity and mortality worldwide. Pharmacotherapy is complicated by the life cycles of the organisms, during which they may change form and travel to infect distant organs. Some may remain infectious in contaminated soil or water for months or years. With few exceptions, anti-infective drugs used to treat these disorders are different from those for bacterial or fungal infections.

Classification and Pathogenesis of Protozoan Infections

54.1 Protozoa are diverse, single-celled organisms that can cause widespread disease.

A **protozoan** is a single-celled organism that inhabits water, soil, and animal hosts. Although only a few of the more than 20,000 species cause disease in humans, they cause significant morbidity and mortality in Africa, South America, Central America, and Asia. These parasites thrive in conditions where sanitation and personal hygiene are poor and population density is high. The nurse needs to be familiar with these infections because travelers may acquire protozoan diseases overseas and bring them back to the United States and Canada. In addition, some of the protozoan infections frequently occur in patients with immunosuppression, such as those in the advanced stages of acquired immunodeficiency syndrome (AIDS) or who are receiving chemotherapy or immunotherapy. Selected protozoan infections important to human health are listed in Table 54.1.

Protozoa are an extremely diverse group of organisms, with each class having very different physiologies and survival mechanisms. Drugs that are effective against one species of protozoan are often not effective against others.

Some pathogenic protozoa have complex life cycles. The active, growing stage during which the organism feeds, often at the expense of its host, is the **trophozoite** stage. When faced with adverse conditions, some protozoa can form protective capsules called **cysts** that allow the organism to survive in harsh environments in a dormant state for prolonged time periods. Both trophozoite and cyst forms may reside within the human body simultaneously; however, some protozoa enter the cyst stage after they exit from the human body through coughing, sneezing, or fecal excretion. Protozoas remain in the cyst form until the organism is able to reinfect another host. When cysts occur inside the host, the parasite is often resistant to drug therapy.

Several of the major protozoan infections are spread by **vectors,** organisms that harbor the pathogen and carry it from one host to another. Some vectors, such as house flies, simply pick up pathogens on their feet and transport them to human food or water. In other cases, the protozoan lives and multiplies inside the insect, which serves as an intermediate host. The protozoan *Plasmodium*, for example, reproduces in the gut of a mosquito and is transmitted to humans during a mosquito bite, causing malaria. The discovery that mites, ticks, or insects could spread infections was a major advance in medicine because it was then realized that disease outbreaks may be prevented or controlled by eliminating the vectors.

TABLE 54.1 Selected Protozoan Infections

Name of Disease and Protozoan Species	Description	Source of Infection
Amebiasis *Entamoeba histolytica*	Primarily infects the large intestine, causing severe diarrhea; commonly travels to the liver to form liver abscesses; rarely travels to other organs such as the brain, lungs, or kidney	Fecal-contaminated water
Cryptosporidiosis *Cryptosporidium parvum*	Infects the intestines, causing diarrhea; often seen in immunocompromised patients	Fecal-contaminated water; humans and other animals
Giardiasis *Giardia lamblia*	Infects the intestines, causing malabsorption, fatigue, and abdominal pain	Fecal-contaminated water
Leishmaniasis *Leishmania* (various species)	Affects many body systems including the skin, liver, spleen, or blood depending upon the species	Bite of sand fly
Malaria *Plasmodium* (various species)	Infects red blood cells to cause fever, chills, and fatigue; some *Plasmodia* invade the liver and other tissues	Bite of female Anopheles mosquito
Toxoplasmosis *Toxoplasma gondii*	Can invade any organ; causes a fatal encephalitis in immunocompromised patients	Congenital transmission; cat feces
Trichomoniasis *Trichomonas vaginalis*	Common sexually transmitted infection (STI) that causes vaginitis in females and urethritis in males	Transmission through sexual contact with infected fluids
Trypanosomiasis *Trypanosoma cruzi* (American) *Trypanosoma brucei* (African)	The American form (Chagas' disease) invades cardiac tissue and autonomic ganglia; the African form (sleeping sickness) causes fatigue and central nervous system (CNS) depression	Bite of the kissing bug (American) or the tsetse fly (African)

54.2 The female Anopheles mosquito is the carrier of several species of *Plasmodium*, the parasite responsible for malaria.

Although rare in the United States and Canada, 300 to 500 million cases of malaria occur annually worldwide. Approximately 1,300 cases are diagnosed in the United States each year, almost all of which occur in immigrants or travelers returning from regions where the disease is endemic.

> **PharmFACT**
>
> More than 1 million people die of malaria every year. Most of them are infants, young children, and pregnant women, and most of them live in Africa. *Source:* World Health Organization, 2007.

Malaria is caused by four species of the protozoan *Plasmodium*. Each species has a characteristic geographical distribution and pattern of infection, although several species may coexist in the same location. *Plasmodium vivax*, the most common malarial species, occurs predominantly in India, Pakistan, and Central America. *Plasmodium falciparum* occurs with greater incidence in Africa, South America, Haiti, and the Dominican Republic. Although less common, *P. falciparum* causes the most severe symptoms, including a significant number of deaths in endemic areas, and is often more resistant to antimalarial drugs than the other *Plasmodia* species. The fatality rate for *P. falciparum* malaria approaches 10% of the patients infected with the parasite. The other two species, *Plasmodium malariae* and *Plasmodium ovale*, are less common and current medical sources should be consulted for information on these species.

The carrier of the *Plasmodium* protozoan is the female Anopheles mosquito. *Plasmodium* resides in the gut of the female Anopheles mosquito where it matures to its infective form, called a **sporozoite.** When the mosquito bites a human, some of the sporozoites, contained in mosquito saliva, are injected.

Once inside the human host, the blood carries the sporozoites to the liver, where they multiply and transform into millions of progeny called **merozoites.** There is an incubation period of 1 to 6 weeks following the mosquito bite, during which the patient experiences no ill effects.

After the incubation period, merozoites are released into the blood, where they enter red blood cells (RBCs) and multiply. The infected erythrocytes eventually rupture, releasing more merozoites, and causing acute symptoms. This is the **erythrocytic stage** of the infection. Diagnosis is usually confirmed by the identification of *Plasmodium* on a blood smear. The bite of another Anopheles mosquito can pick up the merozoites from infected human blood, and the cycle begins anew. *P. vivax* can remain in body tissues for extended periods to cause relapses months, or even years, after the initial infection. Unlike the human host, which suffers severe illness, the mosquito is unaffected by the presence of *Plasmodium*. The life cycle of *Plasmodium* is shown in Figure 54.1.

Symptoms of *P. vivax* malaria are unusual in that they occur in a predictable, cyclic manner every 48 hours. This is because

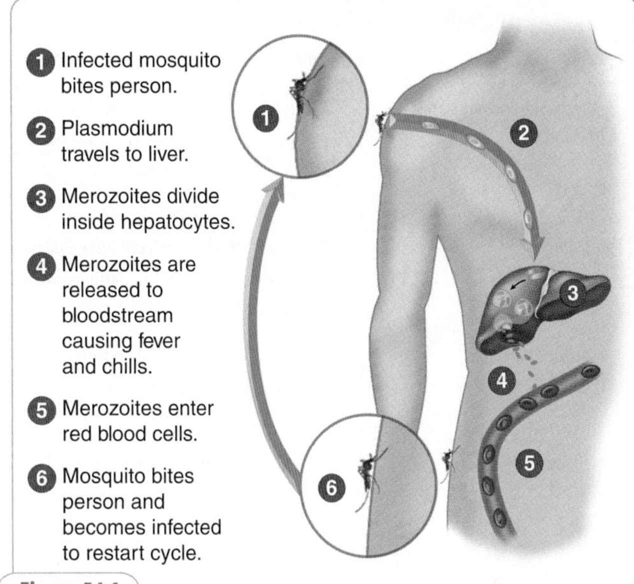

Figure 54.1
Life cycle of *Plasmodium.*

the merozoites grow and rupture erythrocytes on a regular time schedule. The uncomplicated or "classic" malaria attack lasts 6 to 10 hours and occurs in the following stages:

- **Cold stage.** Intense chills and shivering
- **Hot stage.** Fever, headache, vomiting; seizures in young children
- **Sweating stage.** Profuse diaphoresis, followed by return to normal body temperature, and fatigue

Complicated malaria may involve multiple organ failures and can be fatal. Nervous system involvement, called cerebral malaria, leads to abnormal behaviors, impairment of consciousness, seizures, or coma. Loss of large numbers of erythrocytes can cause severe anemia. Pulmonary edema and renal failure can occur. Complicated symptoms are nearly always indicative of infection by *P. falciparum*: The other three species rarely cause severe manifestations or death.

Drugs for Malaria

54.3 The three goals of malaria pharmacotherapy are chemoprophylaxis, treatment of acute attacks, and prevention of relapses.

Pharmacotherapy of malaria attempts to interrupt the complex life cycle of *Plasmodium.* Treatment becomes increasingly difficult as the parasite enters different phases of its life cycle. The goals of antimalarial therapy depend upon the stage of the infection. These goals include chemoprophylaxis, treatment of acute attacks, and prevention of relapse. Drugs for malarial infections are listed in Table 54.2.

Chemoprophylaxis: A rule of thumb to remember about malaria (and many other diseases) is that it is much easier to prevent

TABLE 54.2 Drugs for Malaria

Drug	Route and Adult Dose (maximum dose where indicated)	Adverse Effects
atovaquone and proguanil (Malarone)	For acute infections: PO: 4 tablets as a single daily dose for 3 days For prophylaxis: PO: 1 tablet/day starting 1–2 days before travel and continuing 7 days following return	*Nausea, vomiting, abdominal pain, diarrhea, headache, myalgia* Neutropenia, hypotension
chloroquine hydrochloride (Aralen)	For acute infections: PO: 600 mg initial dose, then 300 mg at 6, 24, and 48 h; IM 200 mg every 6 h prn (max: 800 mg/24 h) For prophylaxis: PO: 300 mg starting 2 weeks before travel and continuing 7–14 days following return	*Nausea, vomiting, diarrhea, visual changes, including blurred vision, photophobia, difficulty focusing* Hemolytic anemia in patients with G6PD deficiency; irreversible retinal damage
hydroxychloroquine (Plaquenil)	For acute infections: PO: 620 mg initial dose, then 310 mg at 6, 18, and 28 h For prophylaxis: PO: 310 mg starting 2 weeks before travel and continuing 4–6 weeks following return	
mefloquine (Lariam)	For acute infections: PO: 1,250 mg as a single dose For prophylaxis: PO: 250 mg once a week for 4 weeks before travel; continuing 250 mg every other week during travel and 2 doses following return	*Vomiting, nausea, diarrhea, myalgia, dizziness, anorexia, abdominal pain* Atrioventricular block, bradycardia, tachycardia, psychosis
primaquine	For acute infection: PO: 15 mg/day for 2 weeks For prophylaxis: PO: 15 mg/day following return for 14 days	*Vomiting, nausea, diarrhea, myalgia, headache, anorexia, abdominal pain* Hemolytic anemia in patients with G6PD deficiency
pyrimethamine (Daraprim)	For prophylaxis: PO: 25 mg once per week for 10 weeks	*Vomiting, nausea, diarrhea, myalgia, abdominal pain* Megaloblastic anemia, leukopenia, thrombocytopenia
quinine (Quinamm)	For acute infections: PO: 650 mg tid for 3 days For prophylaxis: 325 mg bid for 6 weeks	*Vomiting, nausea, diarrhea* Cinchonism (tinnitus, ototoxicity, vertigo, fever, visual impairment), hypothermia, coma, cardiovascular collapse, agranulocytosis

Note: *Italics* indicate common adverse effects. Underline indicates serious adverse effects.

than to treat. The Centers for Disease Control and Prevention (CDC) recommends that travelers to infested areas receive prophylactic antimalarial drugs prior to travel, during their visit, and for at least 1 week after leaving. Chloroquine (Aralen) is the drug of choice, unless travel is to a region known to have a high incidence of chloroquine-resistant strains. Chloroquine therapy begins 1 to 2 weeks before travel, and continues once a week during travel and for 4 weeks after returning.

Several options are available for patients unable to take chloroquine, or who are traveling to areas where chloroquine-resistant species are prevalent. These include the combination drugs atovaquone-proguanil (Malarone), doxycycline, mefloquine (Lariam), or primaquine. Mefloquine is the only medication recommended for prophylaxis during pregnancy.

Treatment of acute attacks: Once a *Plasmodium* infection has occurred, pharmacotherapy of malaria is more successful if it is begun immediately. Treatment is sometimes delayed, however, because the initial symptoms are nonspecific and may resemble the common cold or flu. The patient often does not seek medical attention immediately. Classic malaria symptoms in a patient with a history of recent travel to an endemic region are sufficient evidence to begin antimalarial therapy, without waiting for laboratory confirmation.

Medications are used to interrupt the erythrocytic stage and eliminate the merozoites from red blood cells. Elimination will break the life cycle of the protozoan and stop the acute symptoms. Chloroquine is the traditional antimalarial for treating the acute stage of the disease. It is the drug of first choice for all species of *Plasmodia* causing uncomplicated malarial symptoms.

Several alternatives are available for treating chloroquine-resistant infections. These include primaquine, mefloquine, atovaquone-proguanil, or quinine sulfate. In addition, several antibiotics are effective when used in combination with an antimalarial. Antibiotics used in the pharmacotherapy of malaria include tetracycline, doxycycline, and clindamycin. Tetracycline antibiotics are avoided in pregnant patients because they have the potential to cause birth defects (see Chapter 49).

Patients with complicated malaria are treated aggressively with high doses of parenteral antimalarials. Quinidine gluconate infusions are indicated, along with intravenous (IV) tetracycline, doxycycline, or clindamycin.

Prevention of relapse: Patients who acquire an acute malaria infection will almost always experience subsequent attacks unless drugs are given to eliminate dormant *P. vivax* residing in the liver. Primaquine is one of the few drugs able to eliminate hepatic cysts. To achieve a total cure, primaquine therapy is started near the conclusion of chloroquine therapy. Because *P. falciparum* does not invade the liver, relapses are not a problem with this species; thus, prophylactic drug therapy is unnecessary.

CONNECTION Checkpoint 54.1

From what you learned in Chapter 49, what adverse effects of the tetracyclines cause these drugs to be used with caution during pregnancy? See Answer to Connection Checkpoint 54.1 in Appendix A.

PROTOTYPE DRUG Chloroquine (Aralen)

Classification: Therapeutic: Antimalarial agent
Pharmacologic: Heme complexing agent

Therapeutic Effects and Uses: Developed in response to the high incidence of malaria among American soldiers in the Pacific islands during World War II, chloroquine has been the prototype medication for the prophylaxis and treatment of malaria for over 60 years. Chloroquine is very effective in treating acute symptoms of the erythrocytic stage, but has no activity against dormant *P. vivax* or *P. ovale*. It can reduce the high fever of patients in the acute stage in less than 48 hours. It is also effective for the chemoprophylaxis of malaria caused by *P. malariae* and sensitive strains of *P. falciparum*, when taken 2 weeks before entering an endemic area and continuing 4 to 6 weeks after leaving. Although chloroquine is a drug of choice, many other antimalarials are available because resistance to chloroquine has become a major clinical challenge in certain regions of the world.

Both chloroquine and the closely related drug hydroxychloroquine (Plaquenil) are also used in the treatment of rheumatic and inflammatory disorders, including systemic lupus erythematosus and rheumatoid arthritis. When used for these disorders, doses are higher than those needed for malaria. Because hydroxychloroquine is less toxic at higher doses, this drug is preferred over chloroquine for treating inflammatory diseases. These drugs have also been studied for their effects on HIV, although clinical trials have not yet confirmed their effectiveness.

Mechanism of Action: Chloroquine concentrates in the food vacuoles of *Plasmodia* residing in human red blood cells. Once in the vacuole, the drug likely prevents the destruction of heme and other proteins, which then build to toxic levels within the parasite. The anti-inflammatory effects of chloroquine occur because the drug inhibits the actions of histamine and serotonin, and inhibits prostaglandin synthesis.

Pharmacokinetics:

Route(s)	Oral (PO), intramuscular (IM)
Absorption	Rapid and completely absorbed
Distribution	Widely distributed; crosses the placenta; secreted in breast milk
Primary metabolism	Hepatic; two active metabolites
Primary excretion	Renal
Onset of action	Peak effect: 1–2 h
Duration of action	Half-life: 70–120 h

Adverse Effects: Chloroquine exhibits few serious adverse effects at low to moderate doses. Nausea and diarrhea may occur. At higher doses, central nervous system (CNS) and cardiovascular toxicity may be observed. Symptoms include confusion, delirium, convulsions, reduced reflexes, hypotension, and dysrhythmias. Blood dyscrasias are possible. Chloroquine can cause retinal toxicity, including, blurred vision, photophobia, and difficulty focusing.

Contraindications/Precautions: Patients with preexisting retinal field changes should not receive chloroquine, as the drug concentrates in this tissue and high doses can cause irreversible retinal damage. Baseline and periodic vision screening should be conducted during therapy. Because this drug can affect heme metabolism, it is contraindicated in patients with porphyria. Patients with known glucose-6-phosphate dehydrogenase (G6PD) deficiency should be treated cautiously, if at all, because chloroquine may cause hemolysis in these patients. Because chloroquine is metabolized in the liver, patients with chronic alcoholism or hepatic impairment should be monitored regularly. The drug should be used with caution in patients with eczema or psoriasis, as rare cases of exfoliative dermatitis have been reported. It is also contraindicated in patients with renal impairment and in those with hypersensitivity to the drug. Patients with preexisting hematologic disease should be treated with caution because chloroquine may cause blood dyscrasias.

Drug Interactions: Antacids and laxatives containing aluminum and magnesium can decrease absorption and must not be given within 4 hours of oral chloroquine administration. Cimetidine may also decrease the absorption of chloroquine. Chloroquine may interfere with the antibody response to rabies vaccine. Because chloroquine is associated with an increased risk for QT prolongation and torsades de pointes, it should not be administered concurrently with other drugs known to prolong the QT interval, such as many antidysrhythmics, phenothioazines, and beta-adrenergic agonists. **Herbal/Food:** Unknown.

Pregnancy: Category C.

Treatment of Overdose: Overdose may be fatal. Symptomatic treatment includes anticonvulsants and vasopressors for shock. Ammonium chloride may be used to acidify the urine to hasten excretion of chloroquine.

Nursing Responsibilities:

- Obtain a complete health history including allergies, drug history, and possible drug interactions.
- Obtain baseline vital signs, complete blood count (CBC), and the electrocardiogram (ECG) before initiation of therapy, and then periodically if patient uses this drug long term.
- Monitor for G6PD deficiency and notify the prescriber of this condition prior to administering the drug. G6PD activity testing is used to detect a G6PD deficiency and to determine its potential severity.
- Assess for vision changes and discontinue the drug immediately if these occur. Progressive and irreversible retinopathy can occur even after termination of therapy. Chloroquine can cause retinal toxicity, including blurred vision, photophobia, and difficulty focusing.
- Assess patients on long-term therapy for skeletal muscle weakness and deep tendon reflexes. Discontinue drug if muscle weakness occurs.

Patient and Family Education:

- Notify the health care provider of any of the following conditions: alcohol abuse, blood disorder, dental or eye disease, G6PD deficiency, seizures, psoriasis, liver disease, intestinal disease, or sensitivity to any medicines, foods, dyes, or preservatives.
- Avoid antacids and laxatives containing aluminum and magnesium since these drugs can decrease the absorption of oral chloroquine.
- Do not take any other prescription or nonprescription drugs, dietary supplements, or herbal products without approval of the health care provider.
- Report the following symptoms to the health care provider: visual or hearing problems, loss of balance, muscle weakness, or symptoms of blood dyscrasia such as unusual bruising or bleeding, fever, sore mouth or throat, or unexplained fatigue.
- Wear dark glasses in sunlight or bright light to reduce the discomfort of photophobia and the risk of eye damage.
- Do not drive or perform other potentially hazardous activities until the effects of the drug are known because this drug may cause drowsiness or dizziness.
- Be aware that urine may be colored rusty yellow or brown.
- Immediately notify the health care provider of any known or suspected pregnancy.
- Do not breast-feed while taking this drug without approval of the health care provider.

Drugs Similar to Chloroquine (Aralen)

Other antimalarials include atovaquone, halofantrine, hydroxychloroquine, mefloquine, primaquine, proguanil, pyrimethamine, and quinine. Although halofantrine was approved by the U.S. Food and Drug Administration (FDA) in 1992, it has not been marketed in the United States. It is widely available in other countries. Two combination drugs are available: atovaquone-proguanil (Malarone) and pyrimethamine-sulfadoxine (Fansidar). Fansidar is a prototype drug in Section 54.5. The tetracycline antibiotics are sometimes used for malaria prophylaxis and treatment and are presented in Chapter 49.

Atovaquone-Proguanil (Malarone): The fixed-dose combination drug Malarone was approved in 2000 for the prevention and treatment of malaria. The two drugs have synergistic antimalarial activity and the combination results in less protozoan resistance than when either drug is used as monotherapy. Malarone may be given for prophylaxis or to lessen the severity of acute symptoms. For acute attacks, a 3-day regimen is usually sufficient. For prevention, the drug is begun 1 to 2 days before entering an endemic region, and continued for 7 days after returning. The drug combination is safe and rarely produces serious adverse effects; rash and gastrointestinal (GI) upset are the two most common complaints. Atovaquone (Mepron) is approved as monotherapy to treat *Pneumocystis carinii* pneumonia. This drug is a pregnancy category C.

Hydroxychloroquine (Plaquenil): As its name implies, hydroxychloroquine is closely related to chloroquine, and has essentially the same actions. Approved in 1955, it is indicated for the prevention and treatment of malaria. Like chloroquine, retinal toxicity is a concern. Hydroxychloroquine is also prescribed to treat patients with cutaneous and systemic forms of systemic lupus erythematosus and for rheumatoid arthritis. Hydroxychloroquine is a prototype drug in Chapter 75. It is administered by the oral route. This drug is a pregnancy category C.

Mefloquine (Lariam): Approved in 1989, mefloquine was developed during the Vietnam War to protect American soldiers from multidrug-resistant *P. falciparum* malaria. It is a drug of choice for the prophylaxis of malaria caused by chloroquine-resistant strains of *Plasmodium*. Prophylactic dosing begins 1 week before entering an endemic area and continues for 4 weeks after leaving. Because of the rapid emergence of resistant strains, it is reserved for multidrug-resistant strains of *Plasmodium*. Nausea and vomiting are the most common adverse effects. The primary limitation of mefloquine is nervous system toxicity, including dizziness, nightmares, aggression, and psychoses, which can appear at high doses. Patients with preexisting psychiatric disorders should not take mefloquine. This is a pregnancy category C drug.

Primaquine: Approved in 1951, primaquine is a drug of choice for preventing relapses due to dormant *P. vivax* in the liver. Because it has no activity against the blood forms of *Plasmodium*, it must always be used in combination with other antimalarials. Standard therapy is for 14 days, although 5-day regimens have proven successful. The drug is well tolerated, even at high doses. The most serious adverse effect is hemolytic anemia in patients who are deficient in G6PD. Unlike some of the other drugs in this class, resistance is not a major clinical problem with primaquine. It is also used to treat *P. carinii* pneumonia (PCP) in combination with clindamycin. This is a pregnancy category C drug.

Quinine (Quinamm): First described in the 1600s, quinine is the oldest drug used to treat malaria, and it is still obtained from the bark of the South American cinchona tree. Although safer alternatives have since been discovered, quinine is still occasionally used for chloroquine-resistant *Plasmodia*, in combination with other antimalarials. **Cinchonism,** a syndrome characterized by tinnitus, deafness, headache, vision abnormalities, and diarrhea can occur at therapeutic doses. A major limiting factor is cardiotoxicity, which produces quinidine-like dysrhythmias at high doses. Like primaquine, patients who are deficient in G6PD can experience hemolytic anemia. This drug is pregnancy category X and should never be taken by pregnant patients.

Drugs for Nonmalarial Protozoan Infections

54.4 Amebiasis, giardiasis, and cryptosporidiosis are caused by intestinal parasites and are usually acquired through contaminated water or food.

Although infection by *Plasmodium* is the most significant protozoan disease worldwide, infections caused by other protozoa affect significant numbers of people in endemic areas. Each of the organisms has unique differences in their distribution patterns and in their physiology.

Many areas of the world do not enjoy the high level of sanitation found in the United States and Canada. Drinking water may not be disinfected before consumption and may be contaminated with pathogens from human waste. In regions with poor sanitation, infectious diseases are endemic and contribute significantly to mortality, especially in children who are often more susceptible to the pathogens. Amebiasis, giardiasis, and cryptosporidiosis are protozoan infections of the intestines, spread primarily by poor sanitation.

PharmFACT

It is estimated that 50 million cases of amebiasis occur each year worldwide, resulting in 40,000 to 50,000 deaths annually. Risk factors for severe amebiasis include malnutrition, old age, pregnancy, use of steroids, cancer, alcoholism, and recent travel to a tropical region. *Source:* Medline Plus, 2006.

Amebiasis: Although not endemic to the United States, as much as 10% of the world's population is infected with this protozoan disease. The infection may be carried to the United States by travelers from regions where the disease is endemic, such as Mexico, India, Western and Southern Africa, and portions of Central and South America. The parasite is spread by drinking contaminated water, or by food handlers who transfer the cysts to raw vegetables or other consumables. Less commonly, amebiasis is transmitted through anal sex. Amebiasis also occurs with higher incidence in AIDS patients, due to their inability to mount an effective immune response to the pathogen. The infection is asymptomatic in about 90% of patients.

Amebiasis begins when a person ingests cysts of *Entamoeba histolytica.* The trophozoite form of the protozoan invades the colon mucosa, causing ulcerations and considerable abdominal pain, distention, cramping, and bloody diarrhea. Diagnosis of amebiasis is generally through identification of the trophozoites in the stool; however, serum and stool antigen detection tests specific for *E. histolytica* are available. The life cycle of *E. histolytica* is illustrated in Figure 54.2.

Amebiasis is not restricted to the intestine. The trophozoite may gain access to the general circulation through colon ulcers

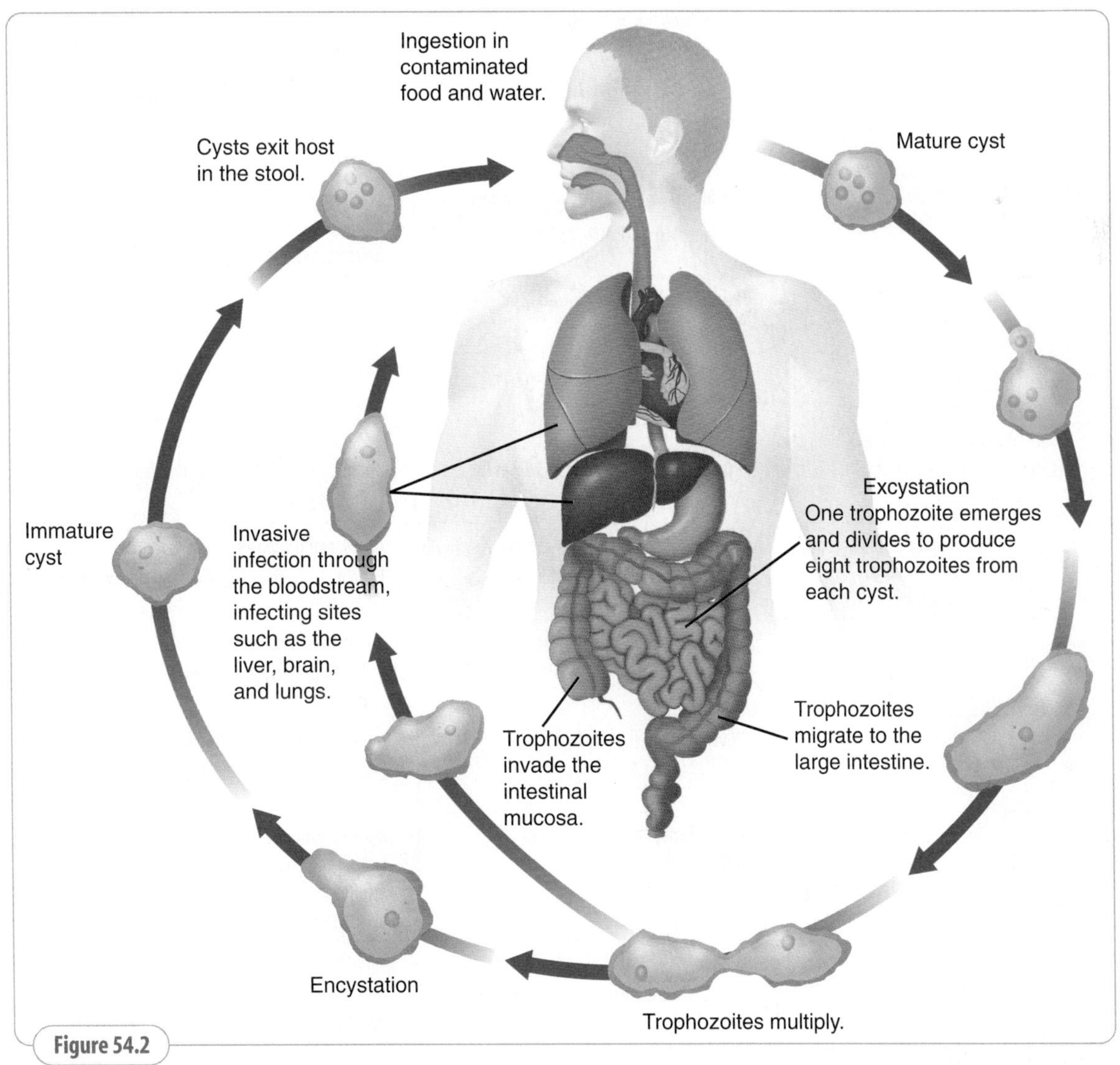

Figure 54.2

Life cycle of *Entamoeba histolytica.*

and travel to other organs, particularly the liver, where it produces hepatic abscesses. Liver involvement causes high fever and right upper quadrant pain. Other possible sites of infection include the brain, genitalia, and lung.

Regimens for amebiasis include combination therapy with two to three agents to eliminate the parasites from their many potential sites. The drug of choice for both intestinal and hepatic amebiasis is metronidazole, due to its safety and efficacy. In cases of acute disease, IV metronidazole may be administered concurrently with an opioid to control severe diarrhea. Second-line therapies such as tetracycline or chloroquine are more toxic and result in higher relapse rates.

If the infection is limited to the intestine, paromomycin (Humatin) and iodoquinol (Yodoxin) are drugs of choice because these agents are able to reach high concentrations in the intestinal lumen without producing significant systemic toxicity. These drugs are sometimes prescribed to eliminate the protozoan in patients who are asymptomatic carriers of the infection.

Pharmacotherapy for amebiasis is continued until multiple negative stool specimens are obtained. Drugs for amebiasis and other nonmalarial protozoan infections are listed in Table 54.3.

Giardiasis: Giardiasis is an infection caused by the protozoan *Giardia lamblia* that has much in common with amebiasis. They are both endemic to regions with poor sanitation, where the water supply is contaminated with human fecal matter. Both affect the intestine, causing acute cramping pain, severe diarrhea, fatigue, and marked weight loss. Both

TABLE 54.3 Drugs for Nonmalarial Protozoan Infections

Drug	Infection	Route and Adult Dose (maximum dose where indicated)	Adverse Effects
eflornithine (Ornidyl)	African trypanosomiasis	IV: 100 mg/kg injected over a period of at least 45 min every 6 h for 14 days	*Nausea, vomiting, diarrhea* Blood dyscrasias, seizures, ototoxicity
iodoquinol (Yodoxin)	Intestinal amebiasis	PO: 650 mg tid for 20 days (max: 2 g/day)	*Nausea, vomiting, headache, dizziness* Loss of vision, agranulocytosis, peripheral neuropathy
melarsoprol (Arsobal)	African trypanosomiasis	IV: 2–3.6 mg/kg for 3 days, then repeated on day 7 and days 10–21	*Fever, albuminuria, transient arthralgias, dermatitis* Encephalopathy, increased mental excitement, twitching, confusion, tremor, seizures
metronidazole (Flagyl)	Trichomoniasis, giardiasis, Gardnerella	For giardiasis: PO: 500 mg bid for 7 days For amebiasis: PO: 500–750 mg tid for 5–10 days	*Dizziness, headache, anorexia, abdominal pain, metallic taste, nausea* Seizures, peripheral neuropathy
nifurtimox (Lampit)	American trypanosomiasis	PO: 8–10 mg/kg 3–4 times/day for 90–120 days	*Rash, dizziness, headache, nausea, vomiting* Seizures, paresthesia with myalgia, pneumonia
nitazoxanide (Alinia)	Diarrhea caused by cryptosporidiosis or giardiasis in children	PO: 100–200 mg every 12 h for 3 days	*Abdominal pain, diarrhea, nausea,vomiting, headache* No serious adverse effects
paromomycin (Humatin)	Intestinal amebiasis	PO: 25–35 mg/kg divided in 3 doses for 5–10 days	*Nausea, vomiting, headache, diarrhea, abdominal cramps* Ototoxicity, nephrotoxicity
pentamidine (NebuPent, Pentam)	Pneumocystis pneumonia, trypanosomiasis, leishmaniasis	IM/IV: 4 mg/kg/day for 14–21 days Inhaled: 300 mg per nebulizer every 3–4 weeks	*Cough, bronchospasm* Hypoglycemia, severe hypotension, kidney failure, pneumothorax
pyrimethamine and sulfadiazine (Fansidar)	Toxoplasmosis	PO: Initial loading dose of pyrimethamine 100–200 mg, then reduced to 25–50 for 4–6 weeks	*Nausea, vomiting, rash* Folic acid deficiency, blood dyscrasias
sodium stibogluconate (Pentostam)	Leishmaniasis	IV or IM: 20 mg/kg/day for 20 days	*Nausea, vomiting, diarrhea, anorexia, cough, substernal pain* ECG changes, pneumonia, blood dyscrasias
suramin (Germanin)	African trypanosomiasis	IV: 1 g on days 1, 3, 7, 14, and 21	*Nausea, vomiting, malaise, fatigue, fever, diarrhea, rash* Loss of consciousness, seizures, nephrotoxicity, adrenal insufficiency, blood dyscrasias, hepatotoxicity, severe hypersensitivity reactions
tinidazole (Tindamax)	Amebiasis Giardiasis Trichomoniasis	For amebiasis: PO: 2 g/day for 3 days For giardiasis or trichomoniasis: PO: 2 g as single dose	*Anorexia, constipation, dyspepsia, dizziness, bitter or metallic taste, nausea, vomiting* Seizures, peripheral neuropathy, angioedema

Note: *Italics* indicate common adverse effects. Underline indicates serious adverse effects.

have a trophozoite and cyst stage, with no intermediate host or vector. Identification of *Giardia* trophozoites or cysts in the stool can help distinguish between the two diseases. Another potential cause of giardiasis in the United States is the unsanitary handling of soiled diapers in day care centers. It is interesting to note that *Giardia* was the very first protozoan discovered, originally identified by the inventor of the microscope, von Leeuwenhoek, in the 1600s.

Giardiasis is more common than amebiasis. It is the most common intestinal parasite responsible for diarrhea symptoms throughout the world. When contaminated food or water is ingested, the acidic environment of the stomach causes the parasite to transform from the cyst to trophozoite stage. The incubation period is 1 to 3 weeks, and symptoms last 2 to 6 weeks. As many as 50% of the patients acquiring *Giardia* are asymptomatic.

Unlike *E. histolytica*, infections of *G. lamblia* remain in the intestine and are often self-limiting. A chronic form of giardiasis, however, can last for months and lead to malabsorption, steatorrhea, weakness, and chronic diarrhea. Although giardiasis is not fatal, it can weaken patients and make them susceptible to infection by opportunistic pathogens. Family members of infected patients, food handlers, and day care workers who are asymptomatic carriers should receive treatment.

Pharmacotherapy of giardiasis includes metronidazole (Flagyl), tinidazole (Tindamax), nitazoxanide (Alinia), or paromomycin (Humatin). Diarrhea generally stops within 48 hours after pharmacotherapy is initiated and a typical regimen continues for 3 to 5 days. Follow-up stool specimens are analyzed to confirm that the pharmacotherapy has been successful.

PharmFACT

According to the Environmental Protection Agency, all surface water in the United States contains Giardia parasites, which means you are at risk if you drink untreated water from shallow wells. *Source:* Mayo Clinic, 2006.

Cryptosporidiosis: Cryptosporidiosis is an infection caused by the protozoan *Cryptosporidium parvum* that causes severe diarrhea. Like *E. histolytica* and *G. lamblia, C. parvum* is primarily an intestinal parasite, acquired through the consumption of fecal-contaminated food or water. It has also been isolated from recreational water. A waterborne outbreak of cryptosporidiosis led to 400,000 cases in Milwaukee, Wisconsin, in 1993, and resulted in at least 100 deaths. This was the largest outbreak of waterborne illness in American history. Cysts of *C. parvum* survive harsh conditions, including chlorination of water: The Milwaukee outbreak occurred despite the fact that the water quality met all existing government standards. Although only about 3,000 cases of cryptosporidiosis are reported in the United States each year, it is responsible for a significant proportion of infectious diarrhea worldwide.

Pharmacotherapy of cryptosporidiosis is targeted at stopping the severe diarrhea through the symptomatic use of antidiarrheal agents. In patients with healthy immune systems, the disease is self-limiting and no antiprotozoan drugs are necessary.

In immunosuppressed patients, cryptosporidiosis has a high mortality rate. Patients with AIDS can develop diarrhea that may cause the loss of as much as 17 L of fluid per day. In addition, the disease can spread to other tissues, especially the gallbladder and biliary tree. Antiprotozoan drug therapy is necessary for these patients, with paromomycin (Humatin) being the drug of choice. Other agents that may be of benefit include azithromycin and nitazoxanide (Alinia). Combination therapy with these drugs may continue for 14 to 28 days, depending upon patient response. Fortunately, the rate of cryptosporidiosis in AIDS patients has declined because antiretroviral therapy has lessened the degree of immunosuppression in many HIV-infected patients.

PROTOTYPE DRUG Metronidazole (Flagyl)

Classification: Therapeutic: Anti-infective, antiprotozoan
Pharmacologic: Nitroimidazole agent

Therapeutic Effects and Uses: Approved in 1963, metronidazole is the prototype medication for amebiasis, being effective against both the intestinal and hepatic phases of the disease. Resistant forms of *E. histolytica* have not yet emerged as a clinical problem with metronidazole. Metronidazole is also a drug of choice for giardiasis (off-label) and trichomoniasis.

In addition to its classification as an antiprotozoan agent, the drug has strong activity against anaerobic bacteria and may be given PO or IV to treat a number of serious respiratory, bone, skin, and CNS infections.

Topical forms of this agent (MetroGel, MetroCream, MetroLotion) are used to treat rosacea, a condition characterized by skin reddening and hyperplasia of the sebaceous glands, particularly around the nose and face. MetroGel-vaginal is approved to treat susceptible vaginal infections. In 1996, the FDA approved Helidac (metronidazole, bismuth, and tetracycline) to eradicate *Helicobacter pylori* infection associated with peptic ulcer disease. Flagyl-ER is an extended duration form of the drug for treating bacterial vaginosis.

Off-label uses of metronidazole include the pharmacotherapy of pseudomembranous colitis, Crohn's disease, and colitis. When used for intestinal pathogens, metronidazole therapy is sometimes followed by administration of iodoquinol, to more effectively eliminate residual parasites harbored in the colon.

Mechanism of Action: Metronidazole enters pathogens and binds to deoxyribonucleic acid (DNA), ribonucleic acid (RNA), and intracellular proteins. Cell death is likely the result of an absence of DNA repair and abnormalities in RNA synthesis.

Pharmacokinetics:

Route(s)	PO, IV, topical
Absorption	Well-absorbed PO (80%)
Distribution	Widely distributed, including the CSF and abscesses; crosses the placenta; secreted in breast milk
Primary metabolism	Hepatic (30–60%)
Primary excretion	Renal (77%), feces (6–15%)
Onset of action	Rapid
Duration of action	Half-life: 6–8 h

Adverse Effects: Although adverse effects are relatively common during metronidazole therapy, most are not serious enough to cause discontinuation of the drug. The most common adverse effects are anorexia, nausea, vomiting, diarrhea, abdominal pain, dizziness, and headache. Dryness of the mouth and an unpleasant metallic taste may be experienced. Seizures and peripheral neuropathy have been reported. Patients receiving the drug by the IV route should be monitored for injection site reactions. Use of the vaginal gel may lead to vaginal candidiasis in over 10% of patients.

Contraindications/Precautions: Although rare, metronidazole can cause bone marrow suppression. Thus, it is contraindicated for patients with blood dyscrasias. CBCs should be monitored during therapy to prevent leukopenia. Metronidazole crosses the blood–brain barrier and is contraindicated in patients with active CNS pathology. Metronidazole should be discontinued if signs of CNS toxicity appear. Liver function tests should be carefully monitored in patients with alcoholism or hepatic impairment, as metronidazole is extensively metabolized in the liver. Doses of metronidazole should be lowered in these patients. The injectable form of metronidazole contains significant amounts of sodium, which can lead to edema in patients with heart failure.

Drug Interactions: Concurrent administration with PO anticoagulants can potentiate hypoprothrombinemia; thus, warfarin doses may require adjustment. Alcohol use may elicit a disulfiram-like reaction. Concurrent use with disulfiram can induce acute psychosis. This includes medications such as cough remedies that contain alcohol. Because metronidazole may elevate lithium levels, doses of lithium may need to be decreased to avoid toxicity. **Herbal/Food**: The extended-release form of the drug should be taken on an empty stomach.

Pregnancy: Category B.

Treatment of Overdose: No specific therapy for overdose is available. Patients are treated symptomatically.

Nursing Responsibilities:

- Obtain a complete health history including allergies, drug history, and possible drug interactions.
- Initiate infection control interventions to prevent the spread of infection, including meticulous hand washing. Monitor other patients on the unit for symptoms of parasitic infection.
- Discontinue therapy immediately and notify the prescriber if CNS symptoms develop such as seizures or peripheral neuropathy, as noted by numbness and paresthesia of the extremities.
- Monitor laboratory tests for total and differential WBC counts before, during, and after therapy. This is especially important if a second course of treatment is necessary.
- Monitor for elevated lithium levels if the patient is on lithium.
- Assess for signs and symptoms of sodium retention, such as weight gain, swelling, or edema, especially in patients with chronic heart failure or who are taking corticosteroid therapy.
- Assess for candidiasis or other mycoses and report infections to the prescriber.
- Obtain repeat fecal examinations for 3 months to determine the effectiveness of the treatment.

Patient and Family Education:

- Follow the therapeutic regimen exactly as prescribed by the health care provider without interruption or changing the dose.
- Refrain from sexual intercourse during therapy for trichomoniasis.
- Report sexual contacts to the health care provider so that they may receive concurrent treatment. Asymptomatic trichomoniasis in the male may cause reinfection of the female.
- Avoid drinking alcohol or using alcohol-containing medications for at least 48 hours after treatment is completed.
- Note that it is normal for urine to become dark or reddish brown during therapy, especially with higher than recommended doses.
- Report symptoms of candidiasis such as vaginitis, milky vaginal discharge, proctitis, furry tongue, glossitis, or stomatitis. Additional treatment with an antifungal agent may be necessary.
- Do not breast-feed while taking this drug without approval of the health care provider.

Drugs Similar to Metronidazole (Flagyl)

Other selected antiprotozoan drugs for amebiasis, giardiasis, or cryptosporidiosis include furazolidone, iodoquinol, nitazoxanide, paromomycin, and tinidazole. Furazolidone (Furoxone) is not available in the United States but is available in other countries.

Iodoquinol (Yodoxin): Approved in 1953, iodoquinol is prescribed for amebiasis to treat the trophozoite and cyst forms of *E. histolytica.* The usual regimen lasts for 20 days. Iodoquinol contains iodine; therefore, it should be used with caution in patients with thyroid disease, and can influence thyroid function tests for as long as 6 months after discontinuation of therapy. Common adverse effects include diarrhea, nausea, vomiting, and stomach pain. Less common, though more serious adverse effects include optic neuritis, loss of vision, anaphylaxis, and agranulocytosis. Iodoquinol also has activity against *Trichomonas vaginalis* and certain bacteria and fungi. This drug is pregnancy category C.

Nitazoxanide (Alinia): Approved in 1996, nitazoxanide is approved for the treatment of infectious diarrhea caused by cryptosporidiosis and giardiasis in adults and pediatric patients, ages 1 through 11. For children, it is formulated as a PO suspension. Off-label uses include diarrhea caused by other agents such as *E. histolytica* and *Clostridium difficile.* Clinical trials are examining its efficacy in AIDS patients with cryptosporidiosis, as this infection can be fatal in immunosuppressed patients. A typical regimen is 500 mg bid for 3 days. The drug is well tolerated, with abdominal pain and GI distress being the most common adverse effects. This drug is pregnancy category B.

Paromomycin (Humatin): Approved in 1959, paromomycin is a broad-spectrum aminoglycoside antibiotic with antiprotozoan activity. The drug has activity against most gram-negative bacteria (except *Pseudomonas aeruginosa*), many gram-positive bacteria, some protozoa, and many parasitic worms. Because it is poorly absorbed from the GI tract, PO dosing is used to kill intestinal bacteria, protozoa, and helminths. It is approved for the treatment of intestinal *E. histolytica* infections, with a typical regimen consisting of 10 to 14 days of therapy. The drug has an orphan drug designation for treating multidrug-resistant tuberculosis and *Mycobacterium avium* complex infections. Although only the oral form is approved for use in the United States, an injectable form of paromomycin is available for the treatment of visceral leishmaniasis in other countries. The most common adverse effects are GI related: nausea, vomiting, cramping, and diarrhea. Like other aminoglycosides, the drug may exhibit ototoxicity and nephrotoxicity. This drug is pregnancy category C.

Tinidazole (Tindamax): Approved in 2004, tinidazole is in the same chemical class as metronidazole, but has a longer half-life that allows for less frequent dosing intervals. Like metronidazole, tinidazole exhibits both antibacterial and antiprotozoan activity. It is highly active against *E. histolytica, T. vaginalis, G. lamblia*, and certain anaerobic bacteria. Typical regimens include single PO doses for giardiasis and trichomoniasis, and 3-day therapy for amebiasis. Tinidazole interacts with anticoagulants to increase the risk of bleeding. When taken concurrently with alcohol, a disulfiram-like reaction occurs. Adverse effects are mild and include bitter or metallic taste and GI distress. Tinidazole is contraindicated during the first trimester of pregnancy (category D) and should be used with caution in the second and third trimesters (category C).

54.5 Other protozoan infections that can cause significant disease include toxoplasmosis, trichomoniasis, trypanosomiasis, and leishmaniasis.

Protozoa can invade nearly any tissue in the body. As has been discussed earlier in this chapter, *Plasmodia* prefer erythrocytes, *Giardia* the colon, and *Entamoeba* travel to the liver. This section presents less common protozoa that invade additional sites. These infections include toxoplasmosis, trichomoniasis, trypanosomiasis, and leishmaniasis.

Toxoplasmosis: Toxoplasmosis is an infection caused by the protozoan *Toxoplasma gondii*. The domestic cat is an intermediate host to the parasite, and serves as a primary means of transmission to humans. The only method of direct human-to-human transmission is from an infected mother to her fetus.

The cycle of *Toxoplasma* infection begins when a cat ingests cysts of *T. gondii*, either through fecal contaminated food or in the flesh of their prey. Once entering the cat, the cysts become trophozoites and invade the small intestine. The cysts are excreted and become infectious after they leave the cat's body. *Toxoplasma* cysts can remain infectious in the environment for up to a year, given ideal conditions such as warm, moist soil.

Toxoplasmosis can occur if humans are exposed to contaminated cat feces, or if they eat raw or undercooked meat containing the cysts. In otherwise healthy persons, toxoplasmosis is usually asymptomatic or presents with mononucleosis-like symptoms such as sore throat, fever, and malaise that rarely require medical intervention. Those who are pregnant or immunosuppressed, however, require pharmacotherapy because the disease can cause significant morbidity in these populations.

Once *T. gondii* enters the body, it can invade nearly any organ. The most common symptom is nonspecific lymphadenopathy. In AIDS patients the brain is sometimes affected, resulting in a variety of CNS symptoms from headache to seizures. The cysts can form necrotic regions in the brain, resulting in focal neurologic abnormalities and changes in mental status. Fatal encephalitis from *Toxoplasma* infection was common in the early years of the AIDS epidemic. Lung infections were also frequent in these patients.

A pregnant patient acquiring *Toxoplasma* during the first two trimesters of pregnancy is at high risk of transmitting the infection to her fetus. The protozoan may cause stillbirth or abortion. Babies may present with ocular toxoplasmosis, a form of the infection that occurs when the cysts are deposited near the retina. Approximately 85% of the newborns who appear normal will develop brain or eye infections from *T. gondii*, sometimes years after birth.

The most effective regimen for acute toxoplasmosis is pyrimethamine with sulfadiazine (Fansidar) for 4 to 5 weeks. Clindamycin may be substituted for sulfadiazine, in patients allergic to sulfonamides. Leucovorin (Folinic acid), a form of folic acid, added to the regimen reduces the potential for pyrimethamine-induced bone marrow suppression.

Patients with AIDS are treated with the same drug combinations as immunocompetent patients, though doses are higher and therapy is more prolonged. Relapse rates for toxoplasmosis in AIDS patients approach 100%. Lifelong prophylaxis with pyrimethamine plus sulfadiazine may be necessary.

Trichomoniasis: Trichomoniasis is a parasitic infection caused by the protozoan *T. vaginalis*. It is a common sexually transmitted infection (STI), affecting approximately 15% of women visiting STI clinics in the United States (2.5 to 3 million women). Coinfection with other STIs is common. The disease is much more common in women: The vagina is a more favorable environment for *T. vaginalis* growth compared to the male reproductive tract.

Because *T. vaginalis* can survive on moist surfaces for several hours, the infection may also be spread by nonsexual means, although this mode of transmission is believed to be uncommon. In addition, there is a small risk of transmission of the infection from mother to baby during childbirth. Thus, trichomoniasis in pregnant patients is considered a treatable condition.

Trichomoniasis most commonly presents with malodorous vaginal discharge, accompanied by vulvar pruritus. Intense scratching may cause erythema and secondary infections in surrounding areas. Dysuria and discomfort during intercourse are common. Fifty percent of *Trichomonas* infections are asymptomatic or subclinical. Most infections in men are asymptomatic, or small amounts of urethral discharge may be noted. Because of the nonspecific nature of the symptoms, diagnosis may be difficult. Culturing of the vaginal discharge is conducted in patients who do not respond to standard therapy and a specific monoclonal antibody test is available, but expense limits its use.

CONNECTIONS

To the Community Sexual Health: Trichomoniasis

Several sexually transmitted infections (STIs) are prevalent in our culture, including trichomoniasis, which is caused by *T. vaginalis*. Trichomoniasis is the most common STI among sexually active young women, with an estimated 7.4 million new cases each year. Women are most frequently affected but men can be as well. Both can transmit this disease to their partners.

Knowing the symptoms of this STI can help both men and women get treatment. Men may not know they are infected because their symptoms may appear vague, with a slight irritation inside the penis, mild discharge, or slight burning after urination or ejaculation. Within 5 to 28 days of exposure, women often experience greenish-yellow frothy, odorous vaginal discharge, painful urination, vaginal irritation and itching, painful sexual intercourse, and sometimes lower abdominal pain.

A laboratory test sample of vaginal fluid in women and urethral fluid in men will provide a diagnosis. Treatment includes the oral antibiotic metronidazole (Flagyl). A woman needs to consult with her health care provider if she is, or suspects she could be, pregnant, as this drug can harm the fetus. All sexual partners must be treated at the same time and avoid sexual contact until treatment is complete and no symptoms exist. Failure to get treatment can result in genital inflammation that increases the risk of being infected with HIV if she comes in contact with someone with HIV. Pregnant women can have adverse outcomes without treatment and need to see a health care provider.

The best way to avoid STIs is to take precautions. These include abstinence, using correctly applied condoms with each sexual contact, and limiting sexual contact to one uninfected partner or limiting the number of partners. Refrain from sex if a sore or any symptoms are present. If infection or exposure to infection is suspected, avoid sex until seen and treated by a health care provider.

With pharmacotherapy, cure rates for trichomoniasis are high. A single PO dose of metronidazole (Flagyl) has been demonstrated to be as effective as prolonged therapy, and more effective than topical agents. The single dose also enhances patient adherence to therapy. However, the higher amount administered as a single dose causes a greater incidence of adverse effects, particularly GI upset. For these patients, 7 days of metronidazole therapy at a lower daily dose is equally effective and produces less GI upset. Therapy should also include the patient's sexual partners, even if they are asymptomatic, to break the cycle of reinfection.

Trypanosomiasis: Trypanosomiasis is actually two distinct parasitic infections: American and African trypanosomiasis. The two infections are caused by different organisms and have different vectors, clinical manifestations, and treatments.

American trypanosomiasis, or Chagas' disease, is caused by *Trypanosoma cruzi*, a parasite found throughout central and northern South America, Central America, and Mexico. The disease is rare in the United States. The vector for Chagas' disease is the "kissing" bug that ingests *T. cruzi* when it feeds on an infected human. The protozoan reproduces in the bug, and is transmitted when the vector defecates on the host's skin at the same time that it feeds. *T. cruzi* usually enters the human host by being rubbed into the vector's bite, an open cut, or the mucous membranes of the eye, nose, or mouth. Other carriers are suspected for *T. cruzi*, including dogs, cats, and rodents. It is estimated that 16 to 18 million people are infected worldwide, and 50,000 die each year from the infection.

Acute Chagas' disease occurs more commonly in children and presents as a granuloma at the entry site, lymphadenography, and hepatomegaly. The acute form is not common, and is often self-limiting. If pharmacotherapy is initiated, the drug of choice is benzimidazole, a medication that is only available in Brazil. Nifurtimox, available from the CDC, has been shown to benefit some patients. Pharmacotherapy for the acute phase is prolonged, at 90 to 100 days.

The chronic stage of Chagas' disease may appear decades after the initial infection and primarily affects the nervous system and heart. Signs and symptoms include cardiomyopathy, and degeneration of autonomic ganglia that can result in megacolon, megaesophagus, and uncoordinated peristalsis. Unfortunately, treating the chronic phase with antiprotozoan agents has not been shown to slow the progression of the disease. The chronic disease is treated symptomatically. Untreated, Chagas' disease is often fatal.

African trypanosomiasis, commonly known as sleeping sickness, is caused by the protozoan *Trypanosoma brucei*. The infection is transmitted to humans by the bite of a tsetse fly carrying *T. brucei*. African trypanosomiasis is restricted to sub-Saharan Africa, and its incidence ranges from 20,000 to 300,000 new infections annually, with about 50,000 deaths a year due to the infection.

Symptoms of *T. brucei* infection include a chancre at the site of the insect bite, extreme malaise (thus the name "sleeping sickness"), intermittent fever, muscle aching, weight loss, and body rash. The parasitic invasion may reach the CNS, causing personality changes, confusion, encephalitis, coma, and possibly death. The infection also affects the liver, heart, and other organs.

Pharmacotherapy of *T. brucei* infection depends on the stage of the disease. Early stages may be treated with suramin (Germanin) or pentamidine (Pentam). These drugs have been available for many decades, and resistance has become a problem. The standard drug for treating the late CNS manifestations is melarsoprol (Arsobal), a medication that has several toxic adverse effects. Eflornithine (Ornidyl), the first new drug for *T. brucei* in over 50 years, also causes serious adverse effects. There is a need for new, effective drugs for this infection.

Leishmaniasis: Most prevalent in Brazil, Peru, Afghanistan, Bolivia, Bangladesh, India, Sudan, Iran, Syria, and Saudi Arabia, leishmaniasis is an infection caused by about 20 different species of the protozoan *Leishmania*. Worldwide, 350 million are believed to be afflicted with the disease. Carriers for *Leishmania* include dogs, foxes, squirrels, and rodents. The disease is transmitted to humans by the bite of the sand fly. Three distinct forms of leishmaniasis have been identified, based on clinical signs and symptoms.

- **Visceral leishmaniasis.** Begins as a skin lesion but progresses to infect the spleen, liver, bone marrow, and lymph nodes. Visceral leishmaniasis is transmitted by contaminated blood or needlesticks, and may occur in patients with advanced AIDS. This infection has a prolonged incubation period of 3 to 8 months. It is usually fatal if untreated. This type most commonly occurs in India, Bangladesh, and Nepal.
- **Cutaneous leishmaniasis.** Characterized by skin lesions that spontaneously heal in 2 to 10 months. Occurs mostly in Mideastern countries such as Afghanistan, Iran, and Saudi Arabia but also is found in Southern Texas, Central America, and South America.
- **Mucocutaneous leishmaniasis.** Characterized by ulcers of the mucous membranes of the nose, pharynx, or oral cavity. Found primarily in South America, these lesions cause severe disfigurement.

The CDC recommends sodium stibogluconate (Pentostam) as the standard treatment for visceral leishmaniasis. This drug, which contains the element antimony, is available only through the CDC. The drug must be administered by the IV or IM routes for 4 to 6 weeks, which makes the treatment of visceral leishmaniasis procedurally difficult in underdeveloped countries where the disease is most prevalent. In addition, resistance to antimony drugs has been a clinical problem, particularly in India, the country with the highest rate of the disease. Relapse may occur as long as 10 years after the initial exposure. Alternative pharmacotherapy for visceral leishmaniasis includes amphotericin B for 20 doses, pentamidine (Pentam) for 15 days, or IM paromomycin (aminosidine) for 30 days.

Cutaneous leishmaniasis heals spontaneously in 5 to 12 months in immunocompetent patients and does not require pharmacotherapy. Mucocutaneous leishmaniasis is a much more serious condition, and secondary bacterial infections are common. Pharmacotherapy of these types of leishmaniasis includes many of the same drugs used for the visceral form. A topical therapy is paromomycin (aminosidine) with methyl benzalkonium chloride that is given for 10 days.

PROTOTYPE DRUG Pyrimethamine and sulfadiazine (Fansidar)

Classification: **Therapeutic:** Antiprotozoan
Pharmacologic: Folic acid antagonist

Therapeutic Effects and Uses: Approved in 1981, Fansidar is a PO, fixed dose combination drug containing two folic acid antagonists: pyrimethamine and sulfadoxine. Fansidar is a drug of choice for treating toxoplasmosis, although this is an off-label indication. Acute toxoplasmosis is treated for 2 to 4 weeks, whereas chronic stages that exhibit organ involvement may require months of therapy. Clinical studies are being conducted to examine its efficacy in the prophylaxis of congenital toxoplasmosis.

Fansidar is approved for the treatment of malaria caused by *P. falciparum* in regions of the world showing high chloroquine resistance. It is considered a second-line antimalarial because adverse effects limit its use and resistance has become a major clinical problem. Because fatalities have occurred due to the development of Stevens–Johnson syndrome, Fansidar is not recommended for malarial prophylaxis.

Because patients may be allergic to sulfadoxine, pyrimethamine (Daraprim) is available as monotherapy for malaria or toxoplasmosis. To boost its efficacy, it is occasionally combined with other anti-infectives such as clindamycin.

Mechanism of Action: Pyrimethamine and sulfadoxine both inhibit the synthesis of folic acid in protozoa. They act synergistically because they block different enzymes in the folic acid pathway, thus inhibiting cell division.

Pharmacokinetics:

Route(s)	PO
Absorption	Pyrimethamine is slowly absorbed; sulfadoxine is rapidly absorbed
Distribution	Both drugs are widely distributed; cross the placenta; secreted in breast milk; about 90% bound to plasma protein
Primary metabolism	Both drugs are metabolized by the liver
Primary excretion	Both drugs are excreted by the renal route
Onset of action	Both drugs have a rapid onset
Duration of action	100 h half-life for pyrimethamine, 200 h half-life for sulfadoxine

Adverse Effects: Common adverse effects of Fansidar include nausea, vomiting, anorexia, abdominal cramping, and rash. Serious adverse effects such folic acid deficiency, megaloblastic anemia, pancytopenia, thrombocytopenia, leucopenia, and Stevens–Johnson syndrome may limit pharmacotherapy with this drug combination.

Contraindications/Precautions: Because pyrimethamine and sulfadoxine are both folic acid inhibitors, they are contraindicated in patients with preexisting megaloblastic anemia caused by folate deficiency. To prevent the development of anemia during therapy, leucovorin (Folinic acid) is administered concurrently. Patients with an allergy to substances containing sulfur should not take Fansidar. Pyrimethamine can stimulate the CNS and cause seizures. Therefore, it is used with caution in patients with seizure disorders. It should be used with caution in patients with significant renal or hepatic impairment, and in those with G6PD deficiency.

Drug Interactions: Few significant drug interactions occur with Fansidar. Other folic acid antagonists such as TMP-SMZ should not be used concurrently with Fansidar, as this will increase the possibility of severe folic acid depletion in the patient. Folic acid supplements should not be given because they will reduce the effectiveness of Fansidar. Fansidar increases the half-life of phenytoin and may cause phenytoin toxicity. **Herbal/Food:** Unknown.

Pregnancy: Category C.

Treatment of Overdose: Overdose can cause seizures and serious blood dyscrasias. Parenteral diazepam may be used to control seizures and leucovorin may be administered to prevent folic acid deficiency.

Nursing Responsibilities:

- Obtain a complete health history including allergies, drug history, and possible drug interactions.
- Initiate infection control interventions to prevent the spread of infection, including meticulous hand washing. Monitor other patients on the unit for symptoms of parasitic infection.
- Discontinue the drug and immediately notify the prescriber if any of the following toxic effects occur: folic acid deficiency, megaloblastic anemia, pancytopenia, thrombocytopenia, leucopenia, and Stevens–Johnson syndrome.
- Monitor laboratory tests such as blood counts, including platelets, twice weekly during therapy.
- Terminate therapy and notify the prescriber if the patient develops hematologic symptoms.

Patient and Family Education:

- Immediately report signs of allergy such as skin rash, itching or hives, or swelling of the face, lips, or tongue to the health care provider.
- Report symptoms of folic acid deficiency such as weakness, anemia with pallor, oral ulcerations, severe or slow-healing infections, diarrhea, poor fat absorption, or fever.
- Do not breast-feed while taking this drug without approval of the health care provider.
- Immediately report any sign of skin rash, redness, or blistering to the helath care provider.
- Avoid direct sunlight and wear protective clothing and sunscreen when going outdoors.

Drugs Similar to Pyrimethamine and Sulfadiazine (Fansidar)

Other selected antiprotozoan drugs for toxoplasmosis, trichomoniasis, trypanosomiasis, or leishmaniasis include eflornithine, melarsoprol, nifurtimox, sodium stibogluconate, and suramin.

Eflornithine (Ornidyl): Eflornithine is prescribed for African trypanosomiasis, especially late-occurring CNS disease. It is less toxic than melarsoprol, but it is more expensive and is thus considered for therapy when melarsoprol fails to provide relief. Given by the IV route, therapy is continued for 7 to 14 days. Close medical supervision is required to monitor for the many serious adverse reactions, such as anemia, diarrhea, seizures, and vomiting. The parenteral form of eflornithine is only available from the World Health Organization. Eflornithine hydrochloride cream (Vaniqa) was approved by the FDA in 2000 as the first topical prescription treatment for women with unwanted facial hair. Adverse effects from the topical formulation are mild and transient. Both IV and topical forms are pregnancy category C.

Melarsoprol (Arsobal): Melarsoprol is an older antiprotozoan, approved in 1949, that is used for the late CNS stages of African trypanosomiasis. It is one of only a few antiprotozoan drugs that can cross the blood–brain barrier to reach the parasite in the CNS. Melarsoprol contains arsenic, an element acutely toxic to life forms. The most common regimen is a series of three IV injections administered with a rest period of 8 to 10 days between each series. Melarsoprol is a toxic drug and severe adverse effects are possible, including fatal encephalopathy convulsions, coma and thrombophlebitis, and necrosis at the injection site, if the drug is extravasated. Significant drug resistance, up to 30% in some regions, has occurred. Melarsoprol is only available from the CDC. This drug is pregnancy category C.

Nifurtimox (Lampit): Nifurtimox is used for the treatment of American trypanosomiasis. It is given PO for 14 to 21 days. Adverse effects include nausea, vomiting, anorexia, and neurologic disturbances. Only 50% to 70% of patients will respond favorably to nifurtimox therapy, indicating a need for additional drugs for this infection. Nifurtimox is only available through the CDC. This drug is pregnancy category D.

Sodium stibogluconate (Pentostam): Sodium stibogluconate is the traditional drug of choice for leishmaniasis; however, decades of use have led to near-total resistance in certain strains of Leishmania. The drug must be given parenterally for 2 to 3 weeks. The most common adverse effects are pain at the injection site, pancreatitis, muscle and joint pain, and decreases in white and red blood cell counts. Treatment failures and relapses are common, indicating a need for more effective drugs for this infection. Sodium stibogluconate is only available through the CDC. This drug is pregnancy category C.

Suramin: Suramin is one of the oldest drugs for African trypanosomiasis, discovered in 1921. It is used exclusively for pharmacotherapy of the initial phase of the infection, since it is unable to cross the blood–brain barrier to treat the CNS symptoms characteristic of late disease. The usual regimen is one IV injection per week for 5 weeks. Nausea and malaise are common during infusions. Renal toxicity is common, though reversible with continued therapy. Suramin is only available through the CDC.

CONNECTION *Checkpoint* 54.2

Sulfonamides have been common antibiotics for many decades. From what you learned in Chapter 51, what are the primary indications for sulfonamide pharmacotherapy? See Answer to Connection Checkpoint 54.2 in Appendix A.

Classification and Pathogenesis of Helminthic Infections

54.6 Helminthic infections cause significant intestinal disease, particularly in areas with poor sanitation.

Helminths consist of various species of parasitic worms. Unlike the single-celled protozoa, helminths have many cells, and thus their anatomy, physiology, and life cycles are more complex. Diseases caused by these pathogens affect more than 2 billion people

NURSING PROCESS APPLICATION

Patients Receiving Pharmacotherapy for a Protozoan Infection

Assessment	Potential Nursing Diagnoses
Prior to administration: • Obtain a complete health history including allergies, drug history, and possible drug interactions. • Obtain a culture and sensitivity test of suspected infection area to determine the need for therapy. • Obtain baseline vital signs, especially pulse and blood pressure. • Obtain a CBC.	• *Risk for Injury*, related to adverse effects of medication • *Deficient Knowledge (Antiprotozoan Therapy)*, related to purpose, precautions, and adverse effects of drug • *Deficient Knowledge (Protozoan Infection)*, related to disease process and infection transmission • *Noncompliance (Therapeutic Regimen)*, related to complexity and cost

Planning: Patient Goals and Expected Outcomes

Patient will:

- Report healing of protozoan infection.
- Demonstrate an understanding of the drug's action by accurately describing drug adverse effects and precautions.
- Immediately report effects such as seizures, numbness in limbs, nausea, vomiting, hives, or itching.

Implementation

Interventions and (Rationales)	Patient and Family Education
• Monitor the CBC periodically. (This drug may cause leucopenia and other blood dyscrasias.)	• Instruct the patient to report fever or other signs of infection.
• Encourage treatment of the sexual partner. (Certain protozoan infections are transmitted through sexual intercourse.)	• Instruct the patient that concurrent treatment of a sexual partner is necessary.
• Monitor the use of alcohol. (The intake of alcohol while taking antiprotozoan medications may produce a disulfiram-like reaction.)	Instruct the patient to: • Abstain from alcohol while taking this medication, including any over-the-counter (OTC) medication that contains alcohol such as liquid cough and cold products. • Report adverse effects such as cramping, vomiting, flushing, and headache, which may result with alcohol use.
• Monitor for CNS toxicity. (Some patients will experience seizures and peripheral neuropathy.)	• Instruct the patient to immediately report seizures, numbness of the limbs, nausea, and vomiting to the health care provider.
• Monitor for hypersensitivity reactions. (Some patients are allergic to these medications.)	• Instruct the patient to immediately report hives and itching, rash, flushing, fever, or joint pain.
• Monitor for GI distress. (The most common adverse effects of many antiprotozoan medications include nausea, vomiting, and abdominal pain.)	Instruct the patient to: • Take this medication with food to decrease GI distress. • Recognize that this medication may cause a metallic taste in the mouth.

Evaluation of Outcome Criteria

Evaluate the effectiveness of drug therapy by confirming that patient goals and expected outcomes have been met (see "Planning").

worldwide, and are quite common in areas of the world lacking high standards of sanitation. Helminth infections in the United States and Canada are neither common nor fatal, although drug therapy may be indicated.

Like protozoa, helminths have stages in their life cycles, which include both immature and a mature forms. Typically, the immature forms enter the body through the skin or the digestive tract. Most attach to the intestinal tract, though some form cysts in skeletal muscle or in organs such as the liver. Helminths are classified as roundworms (nematodes), flukes (trematodes), or tapeworms (cestodes).

Ascariasis: Ascariasis, caused by the roundworm *Ascaris lumbricoides,* is the most common helminth disease worldwide, affecting more than 1.4 billion people. This parasite is endemic to Latin America and Asia and afflicts 4 million Americans, generally in the warm climates of the southeast, and in areas where hygiene and sanitation is poor. This infection occurs most commonly in children between the ages of 3 to 8 years, since this group is most likely to be exposed to contaminated soil without proper hand washing. Although fatalities are rare in the United States, severe infections can lead to complete intestinal obstruction if left untreated. Worldwide, it is estimated that ascariasis causes approximately 60,000 deaths annually, mostly in children.

Transmission of *A. lumbricoides* occurs when a person accidentally ingests eggs from the parasite. Once in the stomach, immature worms hatch from the eggs, and larvae attach to the intestinal wall. The larvae can travel through veins and lymphatics and be carried to the lungs, where they burrow through alveolar walls and migrate up the bronchi. Once reaching the throat, the larvae are swallowed and the cycle begins again.

A. lumbricoides develops into adult worms in the intestines. The female adult worm, which can grow to over 40 cm in length, lays as

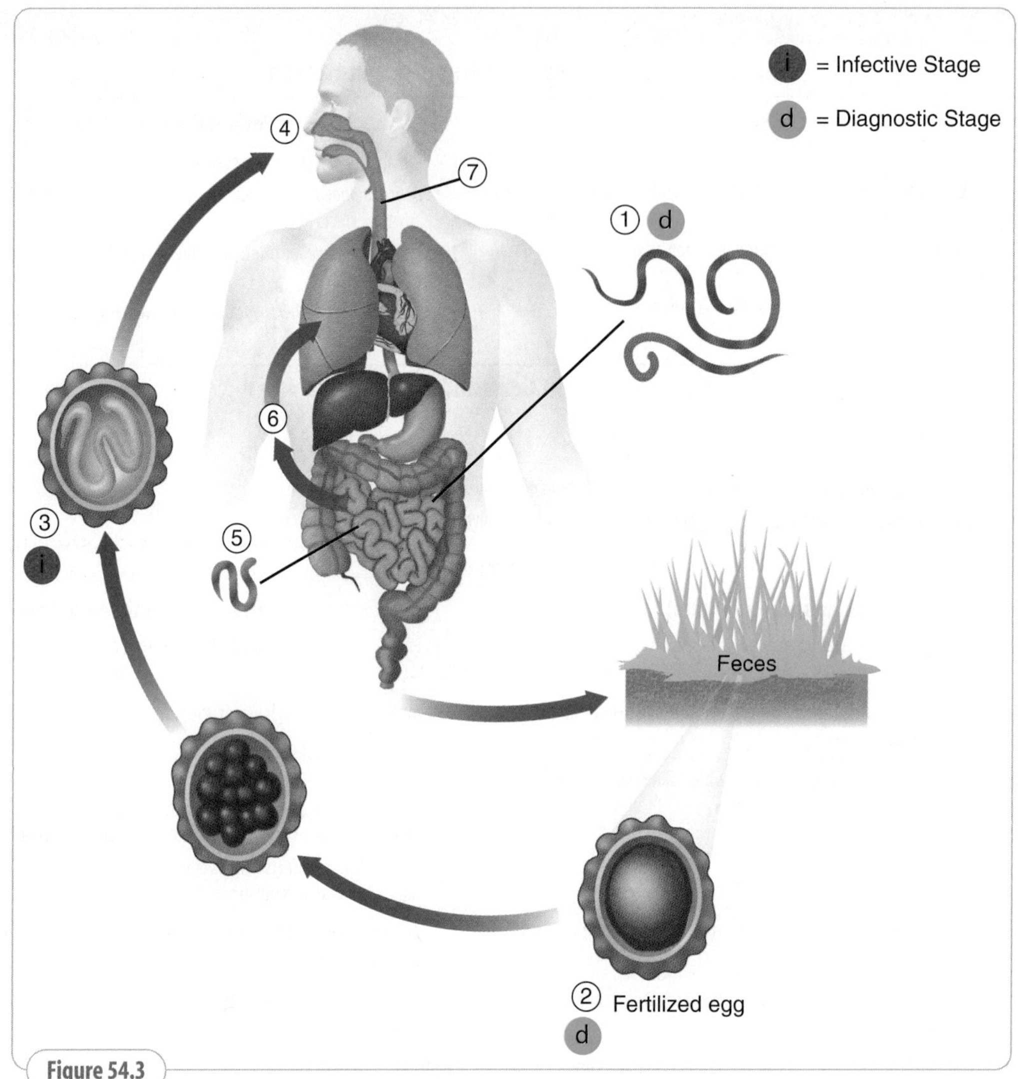

Figure 54.3

Life cycle of *Ascaris*: Adult worms (1) live in the lumen of the small intestine. A female may produce approximately 200,000 eggs per day, which are passed with the feces (2). Fertile eggs become infective after 18 days to several weeks (3), depending on the environmental conditions (optimum: moist, warm, shaded soil). After infective eggs are swallowed (4), the larvae hatch (5), invade the intestinal mucosa, and are carried via circulation to the lungs (6). The larvae mature further in the lungs (10 to 14 days), ascend the bronchial tree to the throat, and are swallowed (7). Upon reaching the small intestine, they develop into adult worms.

many as 240,000 eggs daily, which enter the feces. Under unsanitary conditions, *Ascaris* eggs reach soil where they may remain infective for years. The life cycle of *Ascaris* is shown in Figure 54.3.

Ascariasis presents with both pulmonary and intestinal symptoms. As the larvae reach the lungs, the patient experiences cough, dyspnea, and low-grade fever. The intestinal phase is asymptomatic until large masses of worms are present. Vague upper abdominal pain, distension, and occasional vomiting may be present. Diagnosis is through identification of *Ascaris* eggs or worms in the feces. Occasionally, a worm is observed passing through the anus, mouth, or nose.

Pharmacotherapy for ascariasis is generally successful in eliminating the helminth from the body, without causing significant adverse effects. Oral mebendazole (Vermox) for 3 days is the standard treatment, with albendazole (Albenza) and pyrantel pamoate (Antiminth) as alternative medications. Stools are rechecked 2 weeks after therapy is completed to confirm elimination of the roundworms. When possible, pregnant patients are treated after the first trimester to minimize risks to the fetus.

Enterobiasis: Infection by the pinworm *Enterobius vermicularis* is the most common helminth infection in the United States, afflicting as many as 40 million people, mostly children. The disease causes intense perineal itching due to the presence of deposited *Enterobius* eggs or migrating female worms. The itching is worse at night and may cause restlessness, enuresis, and insomnia. Diagnosis is by identification of eggs on the perianal skin or worms in the stool.

Transmission of *Enterobius* is by diapers, toys, hands, or food contaminated with the eggs. After ingestion, eggs hatch in the duodenum within 6 hours and worms mature in 2 weeks. Only 1 cm in size, adult worms infest the terminal ileum and colon. The female worm is either expelled during defecation or migrates to the perineum where 11,000 eggs per day may be released. After leaving the body, *Enterobius* eggs can remain infectious in the environment for up to 3 weeks. If proper hygiene is not observed, eggs deposited under the fingernails during scratching may be placed in the mouth, renewing the infectious cycle. Like ascariasis, enterobiasis is more common in children, due to the inattention to hand washing. Enterobiasis, however, does not cause mortality.

Pharmacotherapy of enterobiasis includes mebendazole (Vermox), albendazole (Albenza), or pyrantel (Antiminth). A single dose is usually sufficient to eradicate the pinworms, although the dose may be repeated in 2 weeks to maximize therapeutic success. Antipruritic ointments are available for topical application to the perianal region for symptomatic relief of pruritus. Asymptomatic infestation of other household members is frequent; therefore, it is prudent for all close contacts to receive antihelminthic treatment.

Hookworms: Two human hookworms, *Ancylostoma duodenale* and *Necator americanus*, infect 900,000,000 people each year worldwide, usually in warm subtropical and tropical regions. Only about 1 cm in length, the adult hookworms live in the small intestine of the host. The female produces about 10,000 to 25,000 eggs per day, which are passed in the feces. Five days after exiting the body, hookworm eggs hatch, and develop into an infective stage. The parasite is transmitted when an infective larva penetrates the skin, often by a child walking barefoot through contaminated soil. Diagnosis of infestation is confirmed by identification of hookworm eggs in the feces.

The initial symptom of hookworm infection is an itchy "ground rash" at the site of skin penetration. As larvae migrate through the host's blood, they travel to the lung, and up to the throat where they are swallowed and eventually end up in the small intestine. Pulmonary symptoms include cough, blood-tinged sputum, and low-grade fever. Later symptoms include vague abdominal pain, anorexia, and diarrhea.

The mouthparts of hookworms are modified cutting plates that cause hemorrhage when the worms attach to the intestinal mucosa to suck blood from the host. Children are particularly affected by the loss of blood. Although not directly fatal, hookworm infections can weaken the body by causing anemia, and may cause death from infection by opportunistic pathogens.

The larvae of dog and cat hookworms can also infect humans, although they will not mature into adult worms in the human host. Transmitted to humans through contaminated soil or cat litter, these larvae remain in the skin where they migrate for many weeks and cause intense itching. This results in a condition known as *cutaneous larva migrans* or "creeping eruption." Thiabendazole (Mintezol) is a treatment of choice, although therapy with albendazole or ivermectin (Stromectol) may be necessary to eliminate persistent infections.

Mebendazole (Vermox), pyrantel (Antiminth), and albendazole (Albenza) are drugs of choice for hookworm infections. Albendazole and pyrantel are given as a single dose; mebendazole therapy is generally for 3 days. Iron supplements and antianemic drugs may be necessary for patients who have lost an extensive amount of blood.

Tapeworms: Several species of tapeworms infect humans. Beef and pork tapeworms are acquired when raw or undercooked meat is eaten that contains cysts or larvae of the parasites. Similarly, fish tapeworms may be acquired through ingestion of raw or poorly cooked fish containing the parasites. Some of the tapeworms reach enormous lengths; the beef tapeworm, *Taenia saginata*, grows to 25 meters and the pork tapeworm, *Taenia solum*, is 7 meters.

Tapeworm infections may be asymptomatic or produce nonspecific symptoms such as nausea, diarrhea, hunger, fatigue, or abdominal pain. Diagnosis is through identification of perianal eggs or by finding tapeworm eggs in a stool specimen.

The treatment of choice for most tapeworm infections is a single dose of praziquantel (Biltricide). For some infections, a laxative is given 2 hours after treatment, to remove all parts of the worm and its eggs.

Other helminthic infections: Several other helminths cause significant disease worldwide in areas where sanitation is inadequate and food-handling techniques are poor. Drugs used to treat these infections are either the same as those described above, or are only available in other countries. Nurses traveling to these regions should consult medical sources for the most up-to-date pharmacotherapeutic information.

Drugs for Helminthic Infections

54.7 Antihelminthic drugs are usually successful in rapidly eliminating the parasites and have few serious adverse effects.

Drugs used to treat worm infections are called *antihelminthics*. Pharmacotherapy is not indicated for all helminthic infections because some are self-limiting and the adult parasites die without reinfecting the host. When the infestation is severe or if complications occur, however, drug therapy is initiated. Complications caused by extensive infestations may include physical obstruction in the intestine, malabsorption, extensive loss of blood, increased risk for opportunistic bacterial infections, and severe fatigue. Pharmacotherapy is targeted at killing the parasites locally in the intestine, and systemically in the tissues and organs they have invaded. Some antihelminthics have a broad spectrum and are effective against multiple species of worms, while others are indicated for a single species. Resistance is not a clinical problem with antihelminthics. Drugs for helminthic infections are listed in Table 54.4.

Because helminthic infections are often the result of poor sanitation or unhealthy hygiene habits, assessment of the patient's living conditions should be conducted. Often, all family members and close contacts of the patient should be treated in order to prevent reinfestation. Family teaching about ways to prevent reinfestation is essential to break the life cycle of the parasite.

TABLE 54.4 Drugs for Helminthic Infections

Drug	Route and Adult Dose (maximum dose where indicated)	Adverse Effects
albendazole (Albenza)	PO: 400 mg bid with meals (max: 800 mg/day)	*Abnormal liver function tests, abdominal pain, nausea, vomiting* Agranulocytosis, leukopenia
ivermectin (Stromectol)	PO: 150–200 mcg/kg as a single dose	*Fever, pruritus, dizziness, arthralgia, lymphadenopathy* Acute allergic or inflammatory response
mebendazole (Vermox)	PO: 100 mg as a single dose or 100 mg bid for 3 days	*Abdominal pain, diarrhea, rash* Angioedema, convulsions, agranulocytosis
praziquantel (Biltricide)	PO: 5 mg/kg as a single dose or 25 mg/kg tid	*Headache, dizziness, malaise, fever, abdominal pain* cerebrospinal reaction syndrome
pyrantel (Antiminth, Ascarel, Pin-X, Pinworm Caplets)	PO: 11 mg/kg as a single dose (max: 1 g)	*Nausea, tenesmus, anorexia, diarrhea, fever* No serious adverse effects
thiabendazole (Mintezol)	PO: 1.5 g bid for 2 days (max: 3 g/day)	*Dizziness, anorexia, nausea, vomiting* Nephrotoxicity, jaundice, leukopenia

Note: *Italics* indicate common adverse effects. Underline indicates serious adverse effects.

PROTOTYPE DRUG Mebendazole (Vermox)

Classification: **Therapeutic:** Antihelminthic
Pharmacologic: Microtubule inhibitor

Therapeutic Effects and Uses: Mebendazole, albendazole, and thiabendazole belong to the same chemical family, known as the benzimidazoles. Although the three benzimidazoles have similar properties and spectrums of action, mebendazole is the most widely prescribed in the United States.

Approved in 1974, mebendazole is used in the treatment of a wide range of helminthic infections, including those caused by roundworm (Ascariasis), pinworm (Enterobiasis), and hookworm severe species. As a broad-spectrum drug it is particularly valuable in mixed helminthic infections, which are common in areas having poor sanitation. It is effective against both the adult and larval stages of these parasites. For pinworm infections, a single dose is taken, followed by a second dose in 2 weeks. Other helminthic infections require 3 consecutive days of therapy. Although not approved by the FDA for tapeworm infections, it is sometimes prescribed for these parasites.

Mebendazole is poorly absorbed after PO administration, which allows it to maintain high concentrations in the intestine without causing systemic adverse effects.

Mechanism of Action: Mebendazole kills helminths by several biochemical mechanisms, including inhibition of glucose transport and uncoupling energy metabolism in the parasite's mitochondria. The drug binds to β-tubulin and is thought to disrupt the microtubular network in parasitic cells.

Pharmacokinetics:

Route(s)	PO
Absorption	Poorly absorbed
Distribution	Very little reaches the systemic circulation; 95% bound to plasma proteins
Primary metabolism	Hepatic
Primary excretion	Feces
Onset of action	Rapid
Duration of action	Half-life: 3–9 h

Adverse Effects: Because so little of the drug is absorbed, mebendazole does not cause serious systemic adverse effects. As the worms die, some abdominal pain, distension, and diarrhea may be experienced. Rare cases of seizures, agranulocytosis, and angiodema have been reported.

Contraindications/Precautions: Other than hypersensitivity, there are no contraindications for mebendazole. Because it is metabolized by the liver, patients with serious hepatic impairment should be monitored carefully. The drug is a potent teratogen in laboratory animals and should be avoided during pregnancy, especially the first trimester. Use in children under 2 years of age is not advised.

Drug Interactions: Carbamazepine and phenytoin can increase the metabolism of mebendazole, although dosage adjustment is not required because so little of mebendazole is absorbed.

Pregnancy: Category C.

Treatment of Overdose: No specific therapy is available; patients are treated symptomatically.

Nursing Responsibilities:

- Obtain a complete health history including allergies, drug history, and possible drug interactions.
- Initiate infection control interventions to prevent the spread of infection, including meticulous hand washing.
- Monitor other patients on the unit for symptoms of parasitic infection.
- Initiate a second course of treatment if the cure does not occur within 3 weeks.
- Treat all family members simultaneously, because pinworms are readily transmitted from person to person.
- Discontinue the drug if monitoring reveals elevated hepatic enzymes because rare cases of drug-induced hepatitis have been reported.

Patient and Family Education:

- Wash hands thoroughly after touching any item that could be contaminated.
- Maintain good personal hygiene and do not share unwashed clothing, linens, or towels with others.
- Change underclothing, bedclothes, towels, and facecloths daily; bathe frequently, preferably by showering.
- The patient should sleep alone, to limit the spread of the parasites.
- Wash any vegetables or fruits grown in a contaminated area.
- Immediately report unusual fatigue, severe diarrhea, fever, or chills.
- Immediately notify the health care provider, of any known or suspected pregnancy.
- Do not breast-feed while taking this drug without the approval of the health care provider.

Drugs Similar to Mebendazole (Vermox)

Other selected drugs for helminthic infections include albendazole, diethylcarbamazine, ivermectin, praziquantel, pyrantel, and thiabendazole. Bithionol (Bitin) is an antihelminthic available from the CDC for treating *Fasciola hepatica* (a liver fluke). Also available only through the CDC, diethylcarbamazine (Hetrazan) is only used to treat helminthic infections known as lymphatic filariasis, which are caused by various species of threadlike worms found in tropical climates.

Albendazole (Albenza): Approved in 1996, albendazole belongs to the same chemical class as mebendazole. It is incompletely absorbed when given PO, although enough of the drug is distributed to kill parasitic cysts in some tissues. It is a drug of choice for larval forms of the beef tapeworm *T. solium* and for hydatid cysts in the liver that form following infection by the dog tapeworm *Echinococcus granulosus*. Although only approved for these two indications, it is often prescribed off-label for other helminthic infections. Albendazole is well tolerated and exhibits few adverse effects. The most common adverse effect is a transient increase in serum aminotransferase activity caused by its effects on liver function. This is a pregnancy category C drug.

Ivermectin (Stromectol): Approved in 1996, ivermectin has become a mainstay in the pharmacotherapy of several helminthic infections. Its superior safety profile and single-dose efficacy has led to ivermectin replacing thiabendazole and diethylcarbamazine for most helminthic infections. It is a drug of choice in treating onchocerciasis or "river blindness," an especially debilitating filarial infection in Africa, the Middle East, and Latin America. Annual doses have caused a significant reduction of this disease in endemic areas. It is a drug of choice (off-label) for the cutaneous therapy of larva migrans, or "creeping eruption." Because of its wide spectrum of action, it is of great importance in treating mixed helminthic infections, which are so common in third-world countries. Adverse effects are minor and include fever, rash, and pruritus resulting from allergic and inflammatory reactions to the death of the parasites. This is a pregnancy category C drug.

Praziquantel (Biltricide): Approved in 1982, praziquantel is a broad-spectrum antihelminthic drug of choice for schistosomiasis, a helminthic infection caused by blood flukes that affects 200 million people worldwide. People acquire the parasite by bathing or swimming in feces-contaminated water. Although not found in the United States, the parasite is endemic to tropical regions across the globe, causing chronic ill health. Praziquantel is also approved by the FDA for Chinese liver fluke infections, and is prescribed worldwide for other helminthic infections. It is a safe medication, with dizziness, headache, and abdominal pain being the most common adverse effects. This is a pregnancy category B drug.

Pyrantel (Antiminth, Pin-Rid): Approved in 1971, pyrantel is poorly absorbed when given PO; thus, it is only effective against intestinal helminths. As a single dose, it has been a traditional drug of choice for treating enterobiasis, ascariasis, and hookworm infections. It is available over-the-counter (OTC). Adverse effects are usually minor and include nausea, vomiting, headache, dizziness, and rash. Pyrantel is usually considered an alternative to mebendazole. This is a pregnancy category C drug.

Thiabendazole (Mintezol): Like mebendazole and albendazole, this drug belongs to the benzimidazole chemical class. Although it is an effective, broad-spectrum agent, thiabendazole use is limited by a high incidence of adverse effects such as anorexia, nausea, vomiting, and dizziness. Approved in 1967, it is used for various worm infestations, although it has largely been replaced by albendazole and mebendazole for most indications. Topical formulations of thiabendazole cream for "creeping eruption" have been replaced by treatment with PO ivermectin. This is a pregnancy category C drug.

NURSING PROCESS APPLICATION

Patients Receiving Antihelminthic Agents

Assessment	Potential Nursing Diagnoses
Prior to administration: • Obtain a complete health history including allergies, drug history, and possible drug interactions. • Obtain a stool specimen for verification of parasite and determine need for therapy. • Obtain a CBC. • Assess the patient's living situation, including the number of individuals in close contact with the patient.	• *Risk for Injury*, related to adverse effects of medication. • *Deficient Knowledge (Antihelminthic Agents)*, related to purpose, precautions, and adverse effects of drug • *Deficient Knowledge (Helminthic Infection)*, related to disease process and infection transmission • *Acute Pain (Abdominal)*, related to adverse effect of the medication • *Risk for Deficient Fluid Volume*, related to diarrhea, secondary to drug therapy • *Noncompliance (Therapeutic Regimen)*

Planning: Patient Goals and Expected Outcomes

The patient will:

- Report resolution of the parasitic infection.
- Demonstrate an understanding of the drug's action by accurately describing drug adverse effects and precautions.
- Immediately report effects such as itching, hives, diarrhea, and fever.

Implementation

Interventions and (Rationales)	Patient and Family Education
• Monitor the results of stool laboratory diagnostics during treatment. (This will determine the effectiveness of the drug therapy.)	• Instruct the patient to bring a stool sample to the laboratory for testing.
• Monitor for adverse effects. (Antihelminthic drugs are not readily absorbed by the GI system and therefore do not cause serious adverse effects. However, as the worm dies, some patients experience abdominal pain, distention, and diarrhea.)	• Instruct the patient to report transient abdominal pain, diarrhea, and fever.
• Monitor for pregnancy. (Even one dose of this medication during the first trimester may potentially cause fetal damage.)	Instruct the patient to: • Use effective birth control during drug therapy. • Notify the health care provider of any signs of pregnancy.
• Monitor the self-administration of medication. (Some of these medications can cause GI upset.)	• Instruct the patient that tablets can be chewed, swallowed, or crushed, and mixed with food.
• Evaluate health habits. (This will prevent the spread of infestation and prevent future problems.)	Instruct the patient: • That all family members may be treated at the same time to prevent reinfestation. • To wash all fruits and vegetables, and cook meat thoroughly. • To carefully wash hands with soap and water before and after eating and toileting. • To wash toilet seats with disinfectants. • To keep nails clean and out of the mouth. • To not wear tight underwear and change daily. • To sleep alone and wash bedding. • That it is extremely important to complete the entire course of drug therapy.

Evaluation of Outcome Criteria

Evaluate the effectiveness of drug therapy by confirming that patient goals and expected outcomes have been met (see "Planning").

UNDERSTANDING THE CHAPTER

Key Concepts Summary

54.1 Protozoa are diverse, single-celled organisms that can cause widespread disease.

54.2 The female Anopheles mosquito is the carrier of several species of *Plasmodium*, the parasite responsible for malaria.

54.3 The three goals of malaria pharmacotherapy are chemoprophylaxis, treatment of acute attacks, and prevention of relapses.

54.4 Amebiasis, giardiasis, and cryptosporidiosis are caused by intestinal parasites and are usually acquired through contaminated water or food.

54.5 Other protozoan infections that can cause significant disease include toxoplasmosis, trichomoniasis, trypanosomiasis, and leishmaniasis.

54.6 Helminthic infections cause significant intestinal disease, particularly in areas with poor sanitation.

54.7 Antihelminthic drugs are usually successful in rapidly eliminating the parasites and have few serious adverse effects.

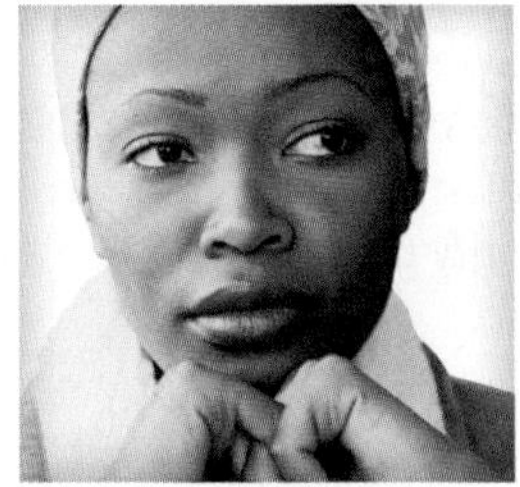

Making the PATIENT Connection

Remember the patient "Harriet Sanchez" at the beginning of the chapter? Now read the remainder of the case study. Based on the information presented within this chapter, respond to the critical thinking questions that follow.

Harriet Sanchez is a 22-year-old nursing student in her second semester. The nursing school is planning an international trip to the Dominican Republic. The students and faculty will be working in rural health clinics providing the community residents with health exams, immunizations, and health teaching. The group will be there for 10 days, and students will reside with various families in the community.

The group's station is a small village called Juan Pablo Duarte. One third of the population in the Dominican Republic lives below the poverty level and this community is no different. The residents are poor and lack many basic services. Most people in this community cannot afford electricity in their homes. Many of the resident families survive by scavenging the local trash dump. Often, both adults and children search through garbage for objects that may be resold for money. Clean water is scarce and most people buy their water from vendors.

Malaria in the Dominican Republic is not uncommon. However, the last reported serious outbreak was in 2004. Health authorities vigilantly monitor the incidence of malaria and try to provide control measures as public finances will allow.

Critical Thinking Questions

1. In your own words, describe the etiology and pathogenesis of malaria.
2. Why is it important to understand the life cycle of *Plasmodium* for pharmacotherapy?
3. Outline the prophylactic treatment for malaria.
4. What adverse effects are associated with chloroquine (Aralen) therapy?

Case Study

Mary Porter is a 19-year-old woman who presents to the local clinic with malodorous vaginal discharge, accompanied by vulvar pruritus. She also complains of dysuria and discomfort during sexual intercourse. Mary is diagnosed with trichomoniasis and started on metronidazole (Flagyl).

1. Why are women clients more likely to contract trichomoniasis?
2. What health teaching would you provide to the patient who is being treated for trichomoniasis?
3. Develop a list of adverse effects this patient may experience while taking metronidazole.

NCLEX-RN® Review

1 The client is taking chloroquine (Aralen) prophylactically before traveling to a third-world country and asks the nurse how long the drug will need to be taken after returning from the trip. Which of the following responses from the nurse would be correct? Chloroquine (Aralen) is:

1. Recommended for 4 weeks after returning from the malaria infested location.
2. Not necessary after leaving the location.
3. Suggested for 3 days after returning from the trip.
4. Optional if the client reports symptoms of malaria.

2 In which of the following community settings would the public health nurse most likely identify potential giardiasis infections?

1. Long-term care facility
2. High school or junior college
3. Child day care centers
4. Meat processing plant

3 A client is being treated with metronidazole (Flagyl) for an intestinal parasitic infection. When instructing the client about this drug, the nurse should caution about the possibility of which adverse reaction?

1. Flatus and intestinal bloating
2. Halitosis
3. Unpleasant metallic taste
4. Alopecia

4 The client is diagnosed with toxoplasmosis and will be treated with pharmacotherapy. Which of the following is a possible source of this infection?

1. Exotic birds
2. Contaminated cat feces
3. Canine dander and fur
4. Bite of the sand fly

5 A nurse would question the order for metronidazole (Flagyl) if prescribed for a client with which of the following conditions? (Select all that apply.)

1. Blood dyscrasias
2. Active central nervous system disease
3. First trimester of pregnancy
4. Pelvic inflammatory disease
5. Trichomoniasis

6 A nurse is monitoring a client receiving metronidazole (Flagyl) for potential adverse effects. Which of the following symptoms, if present, would cause the nurse to discontinue the medication and notify the prescriber?

1. Ataxia and confusion
2. Nausea and diarrhea
3. Anorexia and thirst
4. Weight gain and irritability

See Answers to Critical Thinking Questions, Case Study, and NCLEX-RN® Review in Appendix A.

References

Baird, J. K. (2005). Effectiveness of antimalarial drugs. *New England Journal of Medicine, 352*(15), 1565–1577.

Bethony, J., Brooker, S., Albonico, M., Geiger, S., Loukas, A., Diemert, D., et al. (2007). Soil-transmitted helminthic infections: Ascariasis, trichuriasis, and hookworm. *The Lancet, 67*(9521), 1521–1532.

Davis, A. J., & Kedzierski, L. (2005). Recent advances in antileishmanial drug development. *Current Opinion in Investigational Drugs, 6*(2), 163–169.

Kravetz, J. D., & Federman, D. G. (2005). Toxoplasmosis in pregnancy. *American Journal of Medicine, 118*(3), 212–216.

Legall, D. (2005). Water world. *Gastrointestinal Nursing, 3*(6), 14–17.

Mayo Clinic. (2006). *Giardia infection (giardiasis).* Retrieved August 4, 2008, from http://www.cnn.com/HEALTH/library/DS/00739.html

Medline Plus. (2006). *Amebiasis.* Medline Plus Medical Encyclopedia. Retrieved August 4, 2008, from http://www.nlm.nih.gov/medlineplus/ency/article/000298.htm

Peterson, E. (2007). Prevention and treatment of congenital toxoplasmosis. *Expert Review of Anti-Infective Therapy, 5*(2), 285–293.

Salles, S. M., Salles, M. J., Moraes, L. A., & Silva, M. C. (2007). Invasive amebiasis: An update on diagnosis and management. *Expert Review of Anti-Infective Therapy, 5*(5), 893–901.

Schwebke, J. R., & Burgess, D. (2004). Trichomoniasis. *Clinical Microbiology Reviews, 17*(4), 794–803.

Shapiro, T. A., & Goldberg, D. E. (2006). Chemotherapy of protozoal infections: Malaria. In L. L. Brunton, J. S. Lazo, & K. L. Parker (Eds.). *The pharmacological basis of therapeutics* (11th ed., pp. 869–898). New York: McGraw-Hill.

World Health Organization. (2007). *Malaria.* Retrieved August 4, 2008, from http://www.who.int/mediacentre/factsheets/fs094/en/index.html

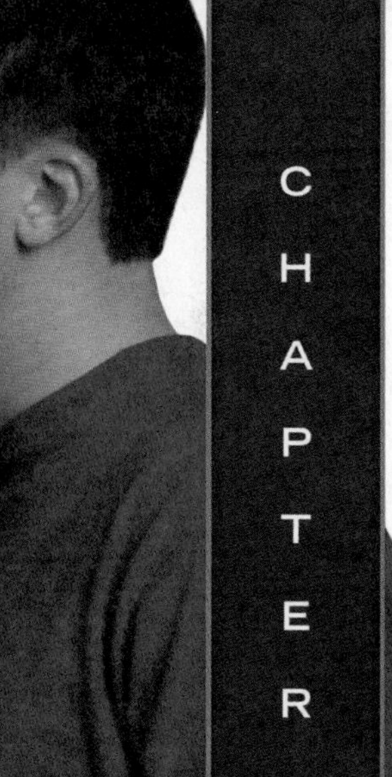

The cold sores are painful and embarrassing. Is there any medication I can take to prevent them from returning?

Patient "Richard Palmer"

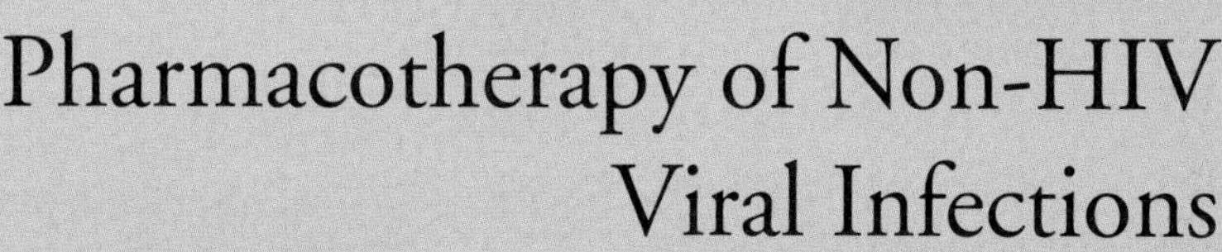

Pharmacotherapy of Non-HIV Viral Infections

55

Chapter Outline

Characteristics of Viruses

Pharmacotherapy of Non-HIV Viral Infections

Agents for Herpesviruses

Antivirals for Herpesviruses

PROTOTYPE **Acyclovir (Zovirax)** *p. 913*

Agents for Influenza Viruses

Antivirals for Influenza Viruses

Neuraminidase Inhibitors

PROTOTYPE **Amantadine (Symmetrel)** *p. 916*

Agents for Hepatitis Viruses

Antivirals for Hepatitis

PROTOTYPE **Lamivudine (Epivir)** *p. 921*

Interferons

Learning Outcomes

After reading this chapter, the student should be able to:

1. Describe the major structural components of viruses.
2. Identify viral infections that benefit from pharmacotherapy.
3. Explain the five principal stages in the pathogenesis of a viral infection.
4. Explain general principles related to the pharmacotherapy of viral infections.
5. Describe the nurse's role in the pharmacologic management of patients receiving medications for herpesviruses, influenza viruses, and hepatitis viruses.
6. For each of the classes shown in the chapter outline, identify the prototype and representative drugs and explain the mechanism(s) of drug action, primary indications, contraindications, significant drug interactions, pregnancy category, and important adverse effects.
7. Apply the nursing process to care for patients receiving drugs for viral infections.

Key Terms

capsid, 908
hemagglutinin, 915
hepatitis, 917
influenza, 915
interferon, 921
intracellular parasites, 908
neuraminidase, 915
provirus, 909
virion, 908
viruses, 908

Viruses are tiny infectious agents capable of causing disease in humans and other organisms. Because they possess only a few simple molecules, viruses use host enzymes and cellular mechanisms to replicate. Although the number of antiviral drugs has increased dramatically in recent years due to research into the AIDS epidemic, antiviral agents remain the least effective of all the anti-infective classes. This chapter will examine the pharmacotherapy of non-HIV viral infections, including herpesviruses, hepatitis viruses, and influenza viruses. Drugs for HIV infection are presented in Chapter 56.

Characteristics of Viruses

55.1 Viruses are infectious agents with simple structures.

Viruses are nonliving agents that contain none of the cellular organelles necessary for self-survival that are present in living organisms. Viruses infect bacteria, plants, and animals by entering a host cell and then using the machinery inside that cell to replicate. Thus, viruses are **intracellular parasites:** They must be inside a host cell to cause infection. A mature infective virus particle is called a **virion.** Figure 55.1 shows the basic structure of a virus.

The structure of viruses is quite primitive, compared to even the simplest bacterial cell. The virus is surrounded by a protein coat or **capsid,** which helps to protect it from the surrounding environment. The structural proteins or glycoproteins that comprise the capsid are arranged in distinct, repeating subunits. These proteins help the virus attach to the cell membrane of its host.

All viruses contain genes, which carry the genetic information needed for viral replication, either in the form of ribonucleic acid (RNA) or deoxyribonucleic acid (DNA). Most possess only a few dozen genes.

Some viruses have an envelope surrounding the capsid and genetic material. The viral envelope consists of phospholipids, glycoprotein, and protein "spikes." The phospholipids actually are derived from the host cell membrane as the virus buds off the host cell. The protein spikes are entirely viral in nature. Recognized as foreign by the host's immune system, viral proteins trigger body defenses that attempt to remove the invader.

Although the host cell supplies most of the machinery needed by the virus, virions contain a few enzymes that serve key roles in the infection process. These enzymes are virus-specific and assist the pathogen in entering the host cell, duplicating its genetic material, inserting its genes into the host's chromosome, or assembling newly formed virions. These unique viral enzymes sometimes serve as important targets for antiviral drug action.

55.2 The replication cycle of a virus occurs in five stages.

Despite their simple structures viruses are diverse, each having a distinct spectrum of infection. While some viruses are lethal, others can coexist with their host and produce no detectable symptoms. Only a handful of viruses cause significant disease in humans. Selected human pathogenic viruses are listed in Table 55.1. Not all viral infections warrant pharmacotherapy. Viruses that may be treated with antiviral medications include herpes simplex, cytomegalovirus, Epstein-Barr, varicella zoster, respiratory syncytial virus, and hepatitis.

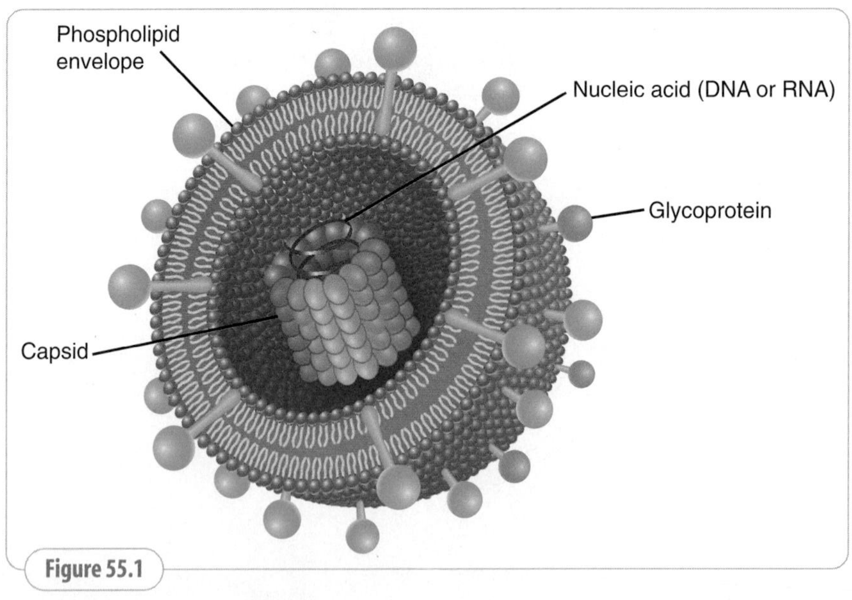

Figure 55.1

General structure of a virus.

TABLE 55.1 Selected Human Viral Diseases

	Virus	Description
DNA viruses	Adenoviruses	More than 40 species that primarily infect the human upper respiratory tract but can also cause conjunctivitis, GI infections, hemorrhagic cystitis, and serious infections in neonates
	Hepadnoviruses	Causes hepatitis B; virus that invades hepatocytes, primarily transmitted by injection of infected blood or by use of contaminated needles
	Herpesviruses	Family of viruses that causes cold sores, genital herpes, infectious mononucleosis, chicken pox, and shingles
	Papovaviruses	Family of viruses that can cause tumors or warts
	Poxvirus	Responsible for smallpox, monkeypox, and molluscum contagiosum (a sexually trasmitted disease)
RNA viruses	Arenaviruses	Family of 15 viruses, one of which causes Lassa fever, a severe form of epidemic hemorrhagic fever that is highly fatal
	Coronaviruses	Family of viruses, some of which cause upper respiratory tract infections with symptoms similar to the common cold
	Myxoviruses and paramyxoviruses	Family of viruses that includes the influenza virus, respiratory syncytial virus, measles virus, and mumps virus
	Orthomyxoviruses	Responsible for human influenza and avian (bird) flu
	Picornaviruses	Large family of viruses that can cause hepatitis A, polio, common cold, meningitis, and myocarditis
	Reoviruses	Large family of viruses that can cause upper respiratory symptoms and gastroenteritis in infants
	Retroviruses	Family includes HIV, the virus responsible for AIDS

Despite their diversity, certain stages are common to most viral infections, as shown in Figure 55.2. The first stage is attachment of the virus to its host cell. In this stage, the proteins on the surface of the virion fuse with protein receptors on the host cell. This attachment is very specific; the "attachment receptor" may be found only in a single species of plant, bacteria, or animal, or even on a single type of cell within an organism. This specificity is why most viruses infect only one species, although a few viruses can mutate and cross species, as is likely the case for HIV.

The second stage of viral infection is penetration of the viral genes and enzymes into the host cell. For some viruses, the entire virion enters the cell, whereas others simply "inject" their genes and enzymes into the host cell.

The third stage is synthesis of viral nucleic acid and proteins by the host cell. Immediately after penetration, a few viral proteins are constructed, which assist in duplication of the viral DNA or RNA. Following duplication of the viral genetic material, two possible events may occur. The virus may immediately begin replicating itself by making viral capsid proteins and viral enzymes, and assembling more virions. In some cases, however, the viral DNA enters the nucleus of the host cell, where it inserts into the chromosome and remains for a period of time ranging from weeks to years before it proceeds to the replication stage. Once the viral DNA integrates into the host chromosome, it is called a **provirus.**

Assembly is the fourth stage of viral infection. All the viral components, structural proteins, enzymes, and nucleic acids, are packaged and made ready for leaving the cell.

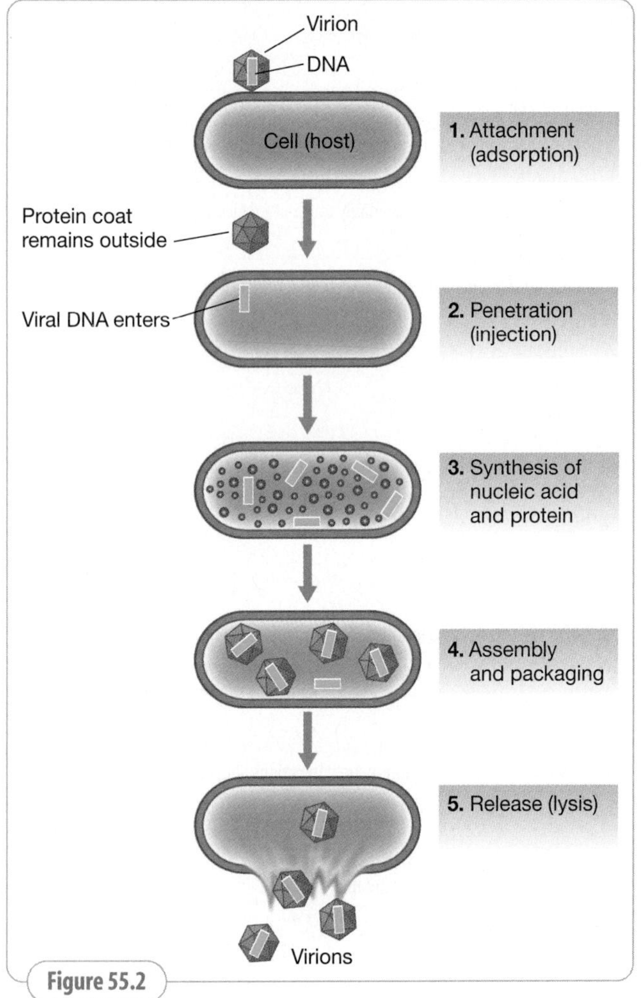

Figure 55.2

The five stages of viral infection.
Source: From *Brock Biology of Microorganisms* (11th ed., p. 238), by M. Madigan & J. Martinko, 2006. Reprinted by permission of Pearson Education, Inc., Upper Saddle River, NJ.

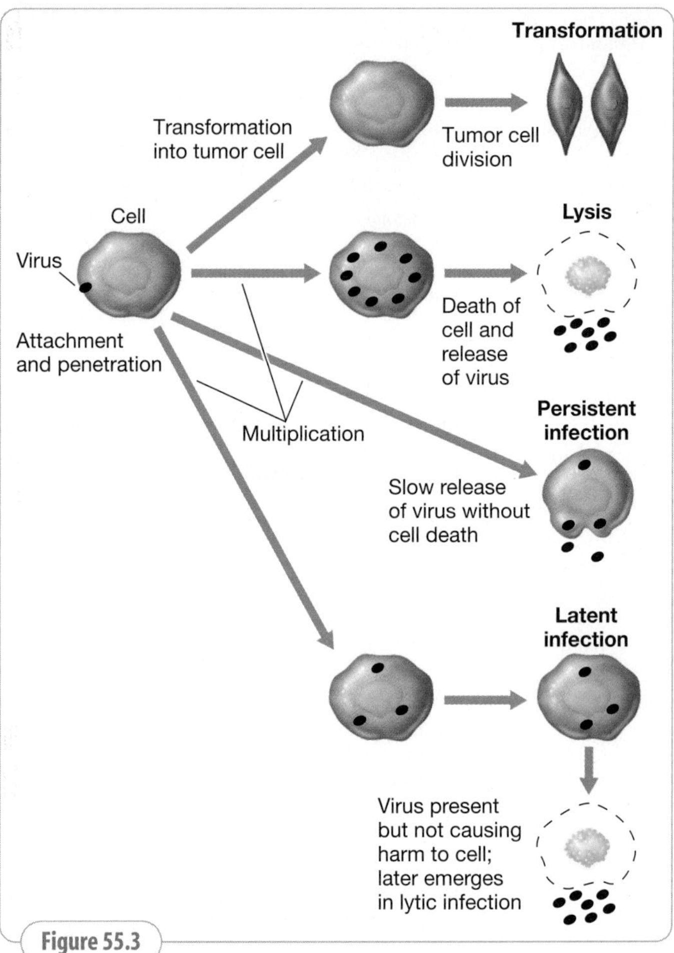

Figure 55.3

Effects of viruses on their host cells.
Source: From *Brock Biology of Microorganisms* (11th ed., p. 251), by M. Madigan & J. Martinko, 2006. Reprinted by permission of Pearson Education, Inc., Upper Saddle River, NJ.

The final stage is the release of virions from the host cell. The number of virions may be so large that the cell bursts, releasing all the infectious particles at one time, killing the cell. In other cases, the virions bud off the host's plasma membrane in a slower, continuous process that does not result in death of the host cell.

Pharmacotherapy of Non-HIV Viral Infections

55.3 Antiviral drugs target a specific viral structure or stage of its replication cycle.

Viruses can have significant effects on their host cells, which are illustrated in Figure 55.3. Some viral infections, such as the common cold, cause acute symptoms but they are self-limiting. While symptoms may be annoying, they resolve in 7 to 10 days and the virus causes no permanent effects, if the patient is otherwise healthy. For these viral infections, drug therapy is not warranted due to the expense and the possibility of producing adverse effects that may be worse than the symptoms of the viral infection itself.

Some viral infections are not self-limiting and drug therapy can be used to prevent the infection or alleviate symptoms. For example, HIV is uniformly fatal if left untreated. Certain hepatitis viruses can result in permanent liver damage and increase a patient's risk of hepatocellular carcinoma. Although not life-threatening in most patients, herpesviruses can cause significant pain and, in the case of ocular herpes, permanent disability.

Antiviral therapy is targeted to a specific structure of the virus or an aspect of its replication cycle. For example, antiviral drugs are available that inhibit specific viral enzymes or change the shape of proteins that can prevent attachment to the host cell. Many of these drugs have only become available recently, due to research prompted by the AIDS epidemic.

Another approach to treating viral infections is to boost the immune system's response to viral antigens. Prevention of some viral infections can be accomplished through vaccines, which prepare body defenses "in advance" of the infection (see Chapter 45). Treatment of acute disease may utilize immunomodulators such as interferons that enhance aspects of the immune response. These are of particular value in treating hepatitis (Section 55.6).

Antiviral pharmacotherapy can be extremely challenging due to the rapid mutation rates of viruses, which can quickly render medications ineffective. Also complicating therapy is the intracellular nature of the virus, which makes it difficult for drugs to find their targets without giving excessively high doses that injure normal cells. Antiviral drugs have narrow spec-

CONNECTIONS

Evidence-Based Practice Human Papilloma Virus Risk Reduction

Clinical Question

Are health education interventions effective in promoting sexual risk reduction behaviors among women to reduce transmission of human papilloma virus (HPV)?

Evidence

Shepherd, Weston, Peersman, and Napuli (1999) examined 30 published research studies to determine the consequence of health education interventions. Studies were included if they evaluated educational interventions targeting women only, and measured the impact on either a behavioral outcome such as condom use for sexual intercourse, partner reduction, or abstinence, or a clinical outcome such as incidence of a sexually transmitted infection (STI). Ten studies showed a statistically significant positive effect on sexual risk reduction, typically with increased use of condoms for vaginal intercourse. This positive effect was generally sustained up to 3 months after the health education interventions.

Implication

The most common cancer affecting women worldwide is cervical cancer. Primary prevention activities include behaviors such as the use of condoms for sexual intercourse (especially among young women), and limiting the number of sexual partners. Health education interventions have been considered one approach to limiting the spread of HPV, a major risk factor for cervical cancer. It is generally assumed that health education is an effective intervention to reduce transmission of HPV, thereby encouraging women to reduce their risk of cancer of the cervix.

According to the *U.S. Cancer Statistics: 2004 Incidence and Mortality* report, 11,892 women in the United States were told that they had cervical cancer in 2004, and 3,850 women died from the disease. It is estimated that more than $2 billion is spent on the treatment of cervical cancer per year in the United States. Educational interventions can encourage at least short-term sexual risk reduction behavior. Health education interventions have the potential to reduce the transmission of HPV, thus possibly reducing the incidence of cervical carcinoma.

Critical Thinking Question

What factors do you think contribute to an individual's inability to sustain health promotion activities that may reduce the transmission of HPV?

See Answers to Critical Thinking Questions in Appendix A.

Source: From "Interventions for Encouraging Sexual Lifestyles and Behaviors Intended to Prevent Cervical Cancer," by J. Shepherd, R. Weston, G. Peersman, and I. Z. Napuli, 1999, *Cochrane Database of Systematic Reviews*, Issue 3. (Art. No.: CD001035, DOI: 10.1002/14651858.CD001035)

trums of activity, usually limited to one specific virus. For most of the viral pathogens, pharmacologic cures are not possible; thus, antivirals remain the least effective of all the anti-infective classes.

Agents for Herpesviruses

55.4 Pharmacotherapy can lessen the severity of acute herpes simplex infections and prolong latency.

Herpes simplex viruses (HSV) are a family of DNA viruses that cause blisterlike lesions on the skin, genitals, and other mucosal surfaces. Herpesviruses are usually acquired through direct physical contact with an infected person, but they can also be transmitted from infected mothers to their newborns, sometimes resulting in severe central nervous system (CNS) disease. Neonatal herpes infection is estimated to have a mortality rate of 50%. The herpesvirus family includes the following:

- HSV-type 1. Primarily infections of the eye, mouth, and lips, although the incidence of genital infections is increasing
- HSV-type 2. Primarily genital infections
- Cytomegalovirus (CMV). Affects multiple body systems in immunosuppressed patients
- Varicella-zoster virus (VZV). Shingles (zoster) and chicken pox (varicella)
- Epstein-Barr virus (EBV). Infectious mononucleosis and a form of cancer known as Burkitt's lymphoma
- Herpesvirus-type 6. Roseola in children and hepatitis or encephalitis in immunosuppressed patients

PharmFACT

About 50 million Americans are infected with genital herpes: 1 out of every 5 of the total adolescent and adult population. Eighty-five percent of adults have serologic evidence of infections by HSV-1. *Source:* Sharma & Brilliant, 2006.

Humans are believed to be the only reservoir for HSV. Following its initial entrance into the human host, HSV may remain in a latent, asymptomatic, nonreplicating state in sensory or autonomic nerve root ganglia for many years. Infection is lifelong. Immunosuppression, physical challenge, or emotional stress can promote active replication of the virus, and the characteristic lesions to reappear. Complications include secondary infections of nongenital tissues.

The pharmacologic goals for the management of herpes infections are twofold: to relieve acute symptoms and to prevent recurrences. It should be noted that the antiviral drugs used to treat herpesviruses do not cure the patient; the virus remains in the patient for the remainder of their life.

Treatment of acute herpesvirus infection: Pharmacotherapy of initial acute HSV-1 and HSV-2 infections is usually accomplished by 5 to 10 days of oral antiviral therapy. Commonly prescribed antivirals for HSV and VZV include acyclovir (Zovirax), famciclovir (Famvir), and valacyclovir (Valtrex). Topical forms of several antivirals are available for local application to herpes lesions, though they are not as effective as the oral medications. In immunocompromised patients, intravenous (IV) agents may be indicated; however, these drugs have a higher risk of serious adverse effects. Antiviral agents for HSV infections are shown in Table 55.2.

TABLE 55.2 Drugs for Herpesvirus Infections

Drug	Route and Adult Dose (maximum dose where indicated)	Adverse Effects
Systemic Agents		
acyclovir (Zovirax)	Initial episode: PO: 200 mg every 4 h while awake for 10 days or 400 tid for 5–10 days Mild HSV labialis (cold sore or fever blister): 400 mg tid for 7 days Mild genital or perirectal HSV: 400 tid for 7 days Severe genital or perirectal HSV: IV 5–10 mg/kg every 8 h for 7–14 days	*Nausea, vomiting, diarrhea, headache, pain, inflammation at injection sites (parenteral agents)* Thrombocytopenic purpura or hemolytic uremic syndrome, nephrotoxicity, seizures (foscarnet), electrolyte imbalances (foscarnet), hematologic toxicity or bone marrow suppression (ganciclovir, valganciclovir)
cidofovir (Vistide)	IV: 5 mg/kg once weekly for 2 weeks	
famciclovir (Famvir)	PO: 500 mg tid for 7 days (max: 1,500 mg/day)	
foscarnet (Foscavir)	IV: 40–60 mg/kg infused over 1–2 h tid (max: 180 mg/kg/day)	
ganciclovir (Cytovene)	IV: 5 mg/kg infused over 1 h bid (max: 6 mg/kg/dose) PO: 1,000 mg TID with food (max: 3,000 mg/day)	
valacyclovir (Valtrex)	PO: 1 g tid (max: 3 g/day)	
valganciclovir (Valcyte)	PO: 900 mg once daily (max: 900 mg/day; 1,800 mg/day during CMV retinitis induction therapy)	
Topical Agents		
docosanol (Abreva)	Topical: 10% cream applied to cold sore up to 5 times/day for 10 days	*Burning, irritation, or stinging at site of application, headache* Photophobia, keratopathy, edema of eyelids (ocular agents)
idoxuridine (Dendrid, Herplex)	Topical: 1 drop in each eye every hour during working hours and 2 hours during the night	
penciclovir (Denavir)	Topical: apply every 2 h while awake for 4 days	
trifluridine (Viroptic)	Topical: 1 drop in each eye every 2 h during waking hours (max: 9 drops/day)	

Note: *Italics* indicate common adverse effects. Underline indicates serious adverse effects.

Recurrent herpes lesions are usually mild and often require no drug treatment. If drug therapy is initiated within 24 hours after symptoms first appear, the length of the acute episode may be shortened, or even prevented.

Herpes of the eye is the most common infectious cause of corneal blindness in the United States. Ocular herpes causes a painful, inflamed lesion on the eyelid or surface of the eye. Prompt treatment with antiviral drugs can stop the herpesvirus from multiplying and destroying epithelial cells. Like genital herpes, once patients acquire ocular herpes they often experience recurrences, which may occur years after the initial symptoms. Use of the antiglaucoma medication latanoprost (Xalatan) (see Chapter 77) has been associated with reactivation of latent ocular HSV.

Pharmacotherapy of ocular herpes is through the local application of drops or ointment. The goal of therapy is to prevent permanent visual disability by limiting corneal involvement of the infection. Trifluridine (Viroptic), vidarabine (Vira-A), and idoxuridine (Herplex) are available in ophthalmic formulations. Oral acyclovir is used in situations where topical drops or ointments are contraindicated. Uncomplicated ocular herpes resolves after 1 to 2 weeks of pharmacotherapy.

Because of the severity of neonatal herpes infections, pregnant patients with the infection are sometimes treated with antivirals. The most extensive clinical experience during pregnancy has been with acyclovir, which has not been associated with teratogenic effects. The safety and effectiveness of these drugs during pregnancy, however, have not been clearly established. The greatest risk for transmission of HSV occurs when the mother acquires the infection late in the pregnancy.

Prophylaxis of herpesvirus infection: Due to the expense and potential adverse effects, antiviral agents are not routinely prescribed for prophylaxis. However, patients who experience particularly severe or frequent recurrences (more than six episodes per year) may benefit from low doses of prophylactic antivirals. Suppressive therapy may also benefit immunocompromised patients, such as those undergoing antineoplastic therapy or those with AIDS.

CONNECTION *Checkpoint* 55.1

From your knowledge of the pharmacokinetics of topical drugs in Chapter 4, why are topical agents not as effective as oral agents in the case of herpes infections? See Answer to Connection Checkpoint 55.1 in Appendix A.

PROTOTYPE DRUG Acyclovir (Zovirax)

Classification: **Therapeutic:** Antiviral for herpesviruses
Pharmacologic: Nucleoside (deoxyguanosine) analog

Therapeutic Effects and Uses: Approved by the U.S. Food and Drug Administration (FDA) in 1982 as one of the first antiviral medications, the activity of acyclovir is limited to the herpesviruses, for which it is a drug of choice. It is most effective against HSV-1 and HSV-2, and effective only at high doses against CMV and varicella-zoster. Acyclovir has no activity against HIV. Resistance has developed to the drug, particularly in patients with HIV-AIDS.

Acyclovir decreases the duration and severity of acute herpes episodes. When given for prophylaxis, it decreases the frequency of herpes recurrences, but it does not cure the patient. It is available in topical form for placing directly on active lesions, in oral (PO) form for prophylaxis, and in an IV form for severe conditions such as herpes simplex encephalitis. Because of its 2.5 to 5 hour half-life, acyclovir is sometimes administered PO up to five times a day. PO formulations include capsule, tablet, and oral suspension. A 5% ointment is available for application to cold sores.

Mechanism of Action: Acyclovir is a nucleoside analog that inhibits viral replication by affecting two viral enzymes. First, it enters the host cell where it is activated by a viral enzyme known as thymidine kinase. The activated drug molecule resembles dGTP, one of the building blocks for DNA. As the virus begins to construct its DNA, it uses acyclovir, rather than dGTP. Once the acyclovir is inserted into the growing DNA chain, viral DNA synthesis is terminated, thus stopping the replication cycle of the virus. Simply stated, acyclovir acts by preventing viral DNA synthesis.

Pharmacokinetics:

Route(s)	PO, IV, topical
Absorption	15–30% is absorbed PO, minimal topical absorption
Distribution	Widely distributed, including the cerebrospinal fluid (CSF); crosses the placenta; secreted in breast milk; 9–33% bound to plasma protein
Primary metabolism	Not metabolized
Primary excretion	Renal exertion, unchanged
Onset of action	Peak effect: 1.5–2 h
Duration of action	Half-life: 2.5–5 h

Adverse Effects: There are few adverse effects to acyclovir when it is administered topically or PO. Nausea, vomiting, anorexia, and elevated hepatic enzymes have been reported. Minor skin irritation, rash, and localized pruritus may occur with the dermatologic formulations.

When given by the IV route, acyclovir is associated with nephrotoxicity, and frequent laboratory tests should be performed to monitor renal function. Ensuring that the infusion is administered slowly and that the patient is properly hydrated can lessen the potential for IV toxicity. Neurotoxicity has also been reported at high doses when acyclovir is given IV, including dizziness, confusion, delirium, and coma.

Contraindications/Precautions: Acyclovir should be used with caution in patients with renal impairment because the antiviral is excreted entirely by the kidneys. Doses should be lowered in these patients and proper hydration should be implemented to prevent crystalluria.

Drug Interactions: Acyclovir interacts with only a few drugs. Probenecid decreases acyclovir elimination and can lead to toxic levels of the antiviral. Zidovudine may increase drowsiness and lethargy. Systemic acyclovir may result in additive nephrotoxicity if used with other drugs affecting renal function such as aminoglycosides. **Herbal/Food**: Unknown.

Pregnancy: Category B.

Treatment of Overdose: Overdose may result in coma, seizures, and renal failure. No specific therapy is available; hemodialysis may be initiated.

Nursing Responsibilities:

- Obtain a complete health history including allergies, drug history, and possible drug interactions.
- For topical administration, wash hands thoroughly before and after treatment of lesions and after disposing of secretions.
- Apply the topical preparation with a finger cot or surgical glove. Apply approximately ½ inch of cream or ointment ribbon for each 4 square inches of surface area. Use sufficient ointment or cream to completely cover lesions.
- Administer the IV infusion for at least 1 hour to prevent renal tubular damage. Monitor the IV flow rate carefully. An infusion pump or microdrip infusion set is preferred.
- When acyclovir is administered IV, monitor intake and output (I&O) ratio and evaluate hydration status. Keep the patient adequately hydrated during the first 2 hours after infusion to maintain sufficient urinary flow and thus prevent precipitation of drug in renal tubules. Encourage PO formulation following IV drug treatment.
- Monitor renal function laboratory tests such as blood urea nitrogen (BUN) and serum creatinine levels. When given by the IV route, acyclovir is associated with nephrotoxicity.
- Monitor for adverse effects and viral resistance with long-term prophylactic use of the PO drug.

Patient and Family Education:

- Start the antiviral therapy as soon as possible after onset of signs and symptoms for best results.
- Do not exceed the recommended dosage, frequency of drug administration, or specified duration of therapy. Contact the health care provider if relief is not obtained or adverse effects appear.
- Cleanse the affected areas with soap and water 3–4 times daily prior to topical application; dry well after application. Following application to the genitals, wear loose-fitting clothes over affected areas.
- Even after herpes simplex infection is controlled, the latent virus can be activated by stress, trauma, fever, exposure to

MyNursingKit | Mechanism of Action Animation: Acyclovir

sunlight, sexual intercourse, menstruation, or treatment with immunosuppressive drugs.

- Refrain from sexual intercourse if either partner has visible lesions or other symptoms of herpes infection; neither the topical nor the systemic drug prevents transmission to other individuals.
- Do not breast-feed while taking this drug without approval of the health care provider.

Drugs Similar to Acyclovir (Zovirax)

Other antivirals effective for treating herpesvirus infections include cidofovir, docosanol, famciclovir, foscarnet, ganciclovir, penciclovir, trifluridine, valacyclovir, and valganciclovir.

Cidofovir (Vistide): Once activated, cidofovir resembles a natural nucleoside (dCTP), and is incorporated into the viral DNA chain, causing premature termination. Approved in 1996, its use is restricted to the prevention or treatment of cytomegalovirus retinitis in patients with AIDS. It has been used off-label to treat HSV, Epstein-Barr, and other viruses. Cidofovir is only available by the IV route. It has an extended intracellular half-life that permits once-weekly dosing, versus foscarnet or ganciclovir, which must be infused daily. The primary dose-limiting adverse effect of cidofovir is nephrotoxicity, which occurs in a large percentage of patients receiving the drug. Because of this, cidofovir should be used with caution in patients with renal impairment, and other drugs that cause nephrotoxicity should be avoided during therapy. Other common adverse effects include rash, headache, alopecia, chills, anorexia, and anemia. This is a pregnancy category C drug.

Docosanol (Abreva): Approved in 2000, docosanol is one of the few nonprescription agents for cold sores and fever blisters. Available as a 10% cream, the drug shortens the healing time and duration of symptoms of the lesions. It acts by blocking the fusion of HSV with its target cells, which is a very different mechanism than other drugs in this class. Docosanol is not absorbed from the skin; thus, no significant adverse effects occur. This is a pregnancy category C drug.

Famciclovir (Famvir): Famciclovir is a nucleoside analog that inhibits viral DNA synthesis in a manner similar to acyclovir, although it has a longer half-life than acyclovir, which permits less frequent dosing. Approved in 1994, it is a prodrug, being activated to penciclovir after gastrointestinal (GI) absorption. When used PO for treating acute genital herpes, it reduces the severity of symptoms and shortens the healing time of the lesions. It is also used for prophylaxis of genital herpes and for treatment of acute herpes zoster (shingles). In herpes zoster management, famciclovir shortens healing time from 7 to 5 days, and reduces pain. It is well tolerated, with headache, nausea, vomiting, and diarrhea being the most common adverse effects. This is a pregnancy category B drug.

Foscarnet (Foscavir): Approved in 1991, foscarnet is an IV medication that is effective against CMV and herpesviruses. It is indicated for CMV retinitis, acyclovir-resistant infections, and HSV infections in AIDS patients. Off-label uses include nonocular CMV infections and VZV infections in AIDS patients. Foscarnet is an expensive drug that exhibits greater toxicity than ganciclovir. Nephrotoxicity is the dose-limiting adverse effect that occurs in about 30% of the patients receiving the drug. Thus, laboratory tests of renal function must be monitored carefully during therapy. Foscarnet is highly ionized in body fluids and may interfere with mineral and electrolyte metabolism, including serum calcium, phosphate, potassium, and magnesium levels. Electrolyte abnormalities with foscarnet use have been associated with seizures and cardiac abnormalities; thus, regular monitoring of serum electrolytes is essential. Headache, nausea, vomiting, and diarrhea are common during therapy. Foscarnet has a short half-life that requires daily infusions throughout the therapy period. This is a pregnancy category C drug.

Ganciclovir (Cytovene): Approved in 1989, ganciclovir is structurally similar to acyclovir and has the same mechanism of action. It is indicated for acute treatment of CMV retinitis and for prophylaxis of CMV infection in immunosuppressed patients. Initial therapy is conducted by IV infusion. Thereafter the patient is switched to PO doses for continued therapy. The principal dose-limiting adverse effect is bone marrow suppression, which can manifest as anemia, neutropenia, thrombocytopenia, or pancytopenia. Laboratory tests must be carefully monitored to assess for leukopenia and thrombocytopenia, as these adverse effects occur in up to 40% of patients taking ganciclovir. Diarrhea, nausea, vomiting, anorexia, abnormal dreams, anxiety, and confusion are frequent adverse effects. Ganciclovir has a short half-life and must be administered daily by slow IV infusion during the treatment period. An intraocular implant containing ganciclovir (Vitrasert) is available that releases the drug slowly over 5 to 8 months. Ganciclovir should be avoided during pregnancy, as the drug is a known teratogen in laboratory animals. This is a pregnancy category C drug.

Penciclovir (Denavir): Approved in 1996, penciclovir is the active metabolite of famciclovir and acts by the same mechanism. Unlike famciclovir, which is taken PO, penciclovir is available only as a 1% cream to apply to recurrent cold sores on the lips or face. It should not be applied to lesions on mucous membranes of the nose or mouth. Penciclovir is not absorbed from the skin; thus, no systemic adverse effects occur. It is a prescription drug, not available OTC. To be effective, it should be applied to lesions every 2 hours while awake. This is a pregnancy category B drug.

Trifluridine (Viroptic): Approved in 1980, trifluridine is a 1% ophthalmic solution indicated for indicated for primary keratoconjunctivitis and recurrent epithelial keratitis due to HSV types 1 and 2. The drug has no systemic adverse effects and causes only minor eye irritation. This is a pregnancy category C drug.

Valacyclovir (Valtrex): Approved in 1995, valacyclovir is a prodrug that is rapidly transformed into acyclovir after oral absorption. It offers the advantage of greater absorption and higher plasma levels than acyclovir. It has the same mechanism of action, indications, and adverse effects as acyclovir. It was originally approved to treat herpes zoster (shingles), but its indications have since been expanded to include initial and recurrent episodes and prophylaxis of herpes genitalis and herpes labialis. This is a pregnancy category B drug.

Valganciclovir (Valcyte): Approved in 2001, valganciclovir is a prodrug that is rapidly converted to ganciclovir after absorption. Given PO, it has the same mechanism of action, indications (cytomegalovirus), and adverse effects as ganciclovir. Patients must be monitored carefully for neutropenia and anemia during therapy. Patients may exhibit cross resistance between the two drugs. This is a pregnancy category C drug.

Agents for Influenza Viruses

55.5 Pharmacotherapy of influenza viruses includes drugs to prevent infection, as well as agents to treat active infections.

Influenza, or flu, is a viral infection characterized by acute symptoms that include sore throat, sneezing, coughing, fever, and chills. The infectious viral particles are easily transmitted via airborne droplets or by hand-to-hand contact. In immunosuppressed patients, an influenza infection may be fatal and flu outbreaks in long-term care facilities can be devastating. In 1919, a worldwide outbreak of influenza killed approximately 20 million people.

Influenza viruses are designated with the letters A, B, or C. Type A is the most common, causes the most severe symptoms, and has been responsible for the serious pandemics throughout history. Due to its rapid mutation rate, there are multiple subtypes of influenza A, and each "flu season" is usually caused by a new subtype. Influenza B is much less common, produces milder symptoms, and has no major subtypes. Type C is even less common and produces symptoms similar to those of the common cold. The influenza viruses should not be confused with *Haemophilus influenza*, a bacterium that causes respiratory symptoms.

PharmFACT

Each year in the United States, 250,000 to 500,000 people get influenza and about 20,000 die from the viral infection. *Source:* Leblebicioglu & Brook, 2007.

The influenza viruses contain single-stranded RNA as their genetic material and have an envelope that contains two types of protein spikes important for pharmacotherapy. One spike contains **hemagglutinin,** an enzyme that facilitates the attachment of the virus to host cells. The other protein spike is composed of an enzyme called **neuraminidase,** which assists the virus in exiting the host cell. Continual mutations to the chemical structures of these spikes creates new influenza strains that are able to evade the immune system. New strains are named by the hemagglutinin (H) and neuraminidase (N) proteins. For example, the Spanish flu subtype is H1N1, whereas the avian (bird) flu subtype is H5N1. Attempts to develop vaccines for influenza strains has been challenging due to these many variants.

The best approach to influenza infection is prevention through annual vaccination. Both inactivated (killed) and live (attenuated) influenza vaccine are available. Those who benefit the most from vaccinations include healthy adults aged 65 or older, residents of long-term care facilities, those with chronic diseases, and women who will be in their second or third trimester during the peak flu season. HIV-AIDS patients are at increased risk of influenza complications and should be immunized using the inactivated vaccine. Influenza vaccination is also recommended for health care workers who deliver direct care to patients at high risk to acquiring influenza, including HIV-infected patients. Adequate immunity is achieved about 2 weeks after vaccination, and lasts for several months up to a year.

CONNECTION *Checkpoint* 55.2

From what you learned in Chapter 46, explain the difference between a live and attenuated vaccine. See Answer to Connection Checkpoint 55.2 in Appendix A.

Only a few antiviral drugs are available to treat influenza. Although these antiviral medications may be useful in preventing influenza or decreasing the severity of influenza symptoms, they should not be considered substitutes for vaccination. The drug amantadine (Symmetrel) has been available to prevent and treat influenza A since 1966. Chemoprophylaxis with amantadine, or the closely related drug rimantadine, is indicated for unvaccinated individuals after a confirmed outbreak of influenza A. Therapy with these antivirals is sometimes begun concurrently with vaccination and continued for 2 weeks. The antiviral offers protection during the period before proper antibody titers are achieved from the vaccine. These drugs are only prescribed for patients who are at greatest risk to the severe complications of influenza due to their expense and the possibility of adverse effects. It is estimated that the antivirals are 70% to 90% effective at preventing influenza A infections. Antivirals for influenza are listed in Table 55.3.

A newer class of drugs, called the *neuraminidase inhibitors*, was introduced in 1999 to treat active influenza infections. Neuroaminidase is a viral enzyme that allows newly-formed, mature virions to bud from infected cells and disperse throughout the respiratory system. Neuraminidase also promotes the penetration of the virus into respiratory epithelial cells and prevents viral inactivation by respiratory mucus. When viral neuraminidase is inhibited, the virions will cling to the surface of the host cell, and be noninfectious.

Given within 48 hours of the onset of symptoms, the two neuraminidase inhibitors, oseltamivir (Tamiflu) and zanamivir (Relenza), will shorten the normal 7-day duration of influenza symptoms to 5 days. Oseltamivir is given PO, whereas zanamivir is inhaled. Oseltamivir is the only antiviral approved to treat both the A and B influenza virus in patients 12 months or older. Cross resistance has been reported between the two drugs in this class. Because these agents are expensive and produce only modest results, prevention through vaccination remains the best alternative.

It is important to remember that these antivirals are not effective against the common cold virus. About 200 different viruses, including rhinoviruses, cause symptoms characteristic of the common cold. Despite considerable attempts to develop a

TABLE 55.3 Drugs for Influenza Infections

Drug	Route and Adult Dose (maximum dose where indicated)	Adverse Effects
Influenza Prophylaxis		
amantadine (Symmetrel)	PO: 100 mg every 12 h continued for at least 10 days after exposure or 2–4 weeks after vaccination (max: 400 mg/day)	*Nausea, dizziness, nervousness, difficulty concentrating, insomnia* Leukopenia, hallucinations, orthostatic hypotension, urinary retention
rimantadine (Flumadine)	PO: 100 mg bid (max: 200 mg/day)	
Influenza Treatment: Neuraminidase Inhibitors		
oseltamivir (Tamiflu)	Treatment: PO: 75 mg every 12 h for 5 days (must be started within 48 hours of symptoms for documented efficacy) Prophylaxis: PO: 75 mg once daily for at least 7 days following close contact, or up to 6 weeks during a community outbreak	*Nausea, vomiting, diarrhea, dizziness* Bronchitis
zanamivir (Relenza)	Treatment: two 5-mg inhalations bid for 5 days (must be administered within 2 days of symptom onset) Prophylaxis: one 5-mg inhalation every 24 h	

Note: *Italics* indicate common adverse effects. Underline indicates serious adverse effects.

vaccine to prevent this annoying infection, success has not yet been achieved. There are drugs, however, that may relieve symptoms of the common cold, and these are presented in Chapter 74.

PROTOTYPE DRUG Amantadine (Symmetrel)

Classification: Therapeutic: Antiviral for influenza
Pharmacologic: Viral replication inhibitor

Therapeutic Effects and Uses: Amantadine has both therapeutic and prophylactic applications for influenza infections. When given during an active infection, amantadine significantly reduces the duration of influenza symptoms. When given for prevention, it is estimated that 70% of the patients taking the drug develop protection against influenza A. Amantadine is sometimes used immediately following influenza vaccination, to give the patient protection during the 2 weeks it takes for protective antibodies to the vaccine to develop.

Use of amantadine is reserved for patients at high risk to influenza exposure. This includes immunocompromised patients, long-term care residents and health care workers, and close personal contacts of high-risk patients. Furthermore, the Centers for Disease Control and Prevention (CDC) has recommended that the distribution of the drug be further restricted due to the large number of influenza strains becoming resistant to amantadine. This drug should not be used as a substitute for influenza virus vaccination (see Chapter 46).

Quite by accident, amantadine was found to have anticholinergic effects that can benefit patients with Parkinson's disease. Its antiparkinson effects are modest, however, and it is not a major drug for this disorder (see Chapter 25).

Mechanism of Action: The precise mechanism of action of amantadine is not known. It is thought to inhibit viral replication by preventing uncoating, although it may also affect assembly of new virions. The antiparkinsonism effects are likely due to the drug's ability to release dopamine and norepinephrine from neuronal storage sites and possibly prevent their reuptake.

Pharmacokinetics:

Route(s)	PO
Absorption	Completely absorbed
Distribution	Widely distributed, including the CSF; crosses the placenta; secreted in breast milk;
Primary metabolism	Not metabolized
Primary excretion	Renal
Onset of action	48 h
Duration of action	Half-life: 20–50 h

Adverse Effects: Up to 33% of patients taking amantadine experience CNS effects that may include insomnia, dizziness, light-headedness, nervousness, loss of concentration, and mental confusion. These symptoms quickly resolve when treatment is stopped. Amantadine can worsen mental problems in patients with a history of psychiatric disorders or substance abuse and cause or increase suicidal ideation. In patients with renal impairment, the drug can build to toxic levels resulting in symptoms such as visual or auditory hallucinations, seizures, coma, or dysrhythmias. Dosage adjustment in these patients is necessary to avoid toxicity. Older adults exhibit a higher incidence of adverse effects and often require reduced dosages.

Contraindications/Precautions: Amantadine should be used cautiously in patients with CNS disease, suicidal ideation, or psychiatric disorders, including seizures or psychoses, as the antiviral may worsen these conditions. Because the drug is excreted almost entirely by the kidneys, patients with preexisting renal disease must be monitored regularly. Although rare, amantadine has caused peripheral edema and congestive heart failure and therefore should be used with caution in patients with preexisting cardiac disease. The drug should not be abruptly withdrawn in patients with Parkinson's disease because symptoms of parkinsonism may dramatically worsen.

Drug Interactions: Patients should avoid alcohol use while taking amantadine, because the combination can lead to increased CNS toxicity, including dizziness, confusion, and orthostatic hypotension. Anticholinergic drugs will exhibit additive effects with amantadine. Dopamine antagonists such as haloperidol will reduce the antiparkinson effects of amantadine. Coadministration with trimethoprim-sulfamethoxazole may impair renal clearance of amantadine, resulting in higher plasma concentrations of the antiviral. **Herbal/Food:** Unknown.

Pregnancy: Category C.

Treatment of Overdose: Overdose of amantadine can result in serious CNS toxicity and death. Physostigmine may be administered by the IV route to control some of the CNS symptoms and anticonvulsants may be necessary. Administration of acidic drugs enhances the renal excretion of the drug. Antidysrhythmics and antihypertensives may be administered to manage cardiovascular toxicity.

Nursing Responsibilities:

- Obtain a complete health history including allergies, drug history, and possible drug interactions.
- Assess for history of suicide attempts or substance abuse because this drug may exacerbate preexisting mental problems. Prescriptions should be written for small quantities.
- For influenza, start drug therapy within 24 hours but no later than 48 hours after the onset of symptoms for effective response, and continue for 24 to 48 hours after symptoms disappear. Contact the prescriber if no improvement is noted within this time.
- Schedule medication administration in the morning or every 12 hours if ordered. The last dose should be scheduled several hours before bedtime to avoid insomnia.
- Assess for CNS effects such as insomnia, hallucinations, light-headedness, nervousness, loss of concentration, and mental confusion. Report unusual CNS effects immediately to the health care provider.

Patient and Family Education:

- Immediately report any of the following to the health care provider: insomnia, hallucinations, light-headedness, loss of concentration, and mental confusion.
- Obtain information from your health care provider regarding the need for annual flu immunization, if appropriate.
- Make position changes slowly when moving from a lying to a sitting position to prevent dizziness and possible fainting.
- Do not drive or perform other hazardous activities until to the effects of the drug are known because this drug may cause drowsiness or dizziness.
- Avoid alcohol intake while taking amantadine, as the combination can lead to increased CNS toxicity.
- Immediately notify the health care provider of any known or suspected pregnancy.

Drugs Similar to Amantadine (Symmetrel)

Other agents for treating influenza include rimantadine, oseltamivir, and zanamivir.

Oseltamivir (Tamiflu): Oseltamivir is a neuraminidase inhibitor available as a PO suspension or capsule that is indicated for the treatment of influenza A or B in patients over 12 months of age. It is also approved for influenza chemoprophylaxis in patients aged 12 months or older. Approved in 1999, the drug must be started within 48 hours of the onset of flu symptoms to be effective. Symptoms in patients infected with influenza resolve 1.3 days (30%) faster if oseltamivir is administered. The drug is well tolerated, with nausea and vomiting being the most common adverse effects. This drug is pregnancy category C.

Rimantadine (Flumadine): Approved in 1993, rimantadine is chemically similar to amantadine, and acts by a similar mechanism. It is approved for the treatment of influenza A infections in adults and for prophylaxis in children. Formulations include tablets, and syrup for pediatric use. Like amantadine, it is not effective against influenza B. Rimantadine is less toxic than amantadine, with GI complaints such as nausea, vomiting and abdominal pain being most commonly reported. Older adults have more adverse effects to rimantadine; thus, doses in this population should be reduced. Like amantadine, the CDC has recommended that use of rimantadine be restricted due to the appearance of resistant viral strains. This drug is pregnancy category C.

Zanamivir (Relenza): Zanamivir is neuraminidase inhibitor available as an inhaled, powdered formulation approved in 1999 for the treatment of active influenza infections in patients aged 7 or older. In 2006, the drug was approved for influenza chemoprophylaxis. Like oseltamivir, the drug must be started within 48 hours of the onset of flu symptoms to be effective. Symptoms in patients infected with influenza resolve 1 to 2 days faster if zanamivir is administered. Zanamivir is well tolerated and devoid of significant adverse effects in most patients. Those with preexisting respiratory disease should use zanamivir with caution, as the drug may initiate bronchospasm in these patients and the use of a bronchodilator may be indicated. This drug is pregnancy category C.

Agents for Hepatitis Viruses

55.6 The most effective therapies for hepatitis infections are antivirals and drugs that boost the immune system to rid the body of the virus.

Hepatitis, or inflammation of the liver, may be caused by drugs, alcohol, autoimmune disorders, metabolic diseases, or infections. Viral hepatitis is a common infection caused by a number of different viruses. Although each virus has its own unique clinical features, they all invade hepatocytes, producing the same symptoms.

Hepatitis may be acute or chronic. Symptoms of acute hepatitis include fever, chills, fatigue, anorexia, nausea, and vomiting. Chronic hepatitis may result in prolonged fatigue, jaundice, liver cirrhosis, and ultimately hepatic failure. Neonates and immunocompromised patients are at higher risk to developing chronic hepatitis. Some patients infected with hepatitis viruses, especially children, are asymptomatic.

The three primary types of viral hepatitis are hepatitis A (HAV), hepatitis B (HAB), and hepatitis C (HAC). The three types are summarized in Table 55.4. Drugs used to manage viral hepatitis infections are listed in Table 55.5.

Hepatitis A: Hepatitis A, an RNA virus, is spread by the oral–fecal route and causes epidemics in regions of the world having poor sanitation. Outbreaks in the United States, however, are most often sporadic events caused by contaminated food.

PharmFACT

The rate of new hepatitis B infections in the United States declined 80% since 1991, due to widespread vaccinations. Still, it is estimated that 46,000 new infections occur annually. *Source:* Centers for Disease Control and Prevention, 2008.

HAV has an incubation period of 4 weeks. During this period, and for 1 to 10 days after symptoms appear, the virus

TABLE 55.4 Summary of Viral Hepatitis Types

Type	Transmission	People at Risk	Prevention	Treatment
Hepatitis A	Primarily through food or water contaminated by feces from an infected person. Rarely, it spreads through contact with infected blood.	International travelers; people living in areas where hepatitis A outbreaks are common; people who live with or have sex with an infected person; and, during outbreaks, day care children and employees, men who have sex with men, and injection drug users	Hepatitis A vaccine; also, avoiding tap water when traveling internationally, and practicing good hygiene and sanitation	Hepatitis A usually resolves on its own over several weeks
Hepatitis B	Through contact with infected blood, through sex with an infected person, and from mother to child during childbirth	People who have sex with an infected person, men who have sex with men, injection drug users, children of immigrants from disease-endemic areas, infants born to infected mothers, people who live with an infected person, health care workers, hemodialysis patients, people who received a transfusion of blood or blood products before July 1992 or clotting factors made before 1987, and international travelers	Hepatitis B vaccine	For chronic hepatitis B: drug treatment with alpha interferon, peginterferon, lamivudine, or adefovir dipivoxil Acute hepatitis B usually resolves on its own; severe cases can be treated with lamivudine
Hepatitis C	Primarily through contact with infected blood; less commonly, through sexual contact and childbirth	Injection drug users, people who have sex with an infected person, people who have multiple sex partners, health care workers, infants born to infected women, hemodialysis patients, and people who received a transfusion of blood or blood products before July 1992 or clotting factors made before 1987	There is no vaccine for hepatitis C; the only way to prevent the disease is to reduce the risk of exposure to the virus. This means avoiding behaviors like sharing drug needles or sharing personal items like toothbrushes, razors, and nail clippers with an infected person.	Chronic hepatitis C: Drug treatment with peginterferon alone or combination treatment with peginterferon and the drug ribavirin Acute hepatitis C: Treatment is recommended if it does not resolve within 2 to 3 months.
Hepatitis D	Through contact with infected blood; this disease occurs only in people who are already infected with hepatitis B	Anyone infected with hepatitis B: Injection drug users who have hepatitis B have the highest risk. People who have hepatitis B are also at risk if they have sex with a person infected with hepatitis D or if they live with an infected person. Also at risk are people who received a transfusion of blood or blood products before July 1992 or clotting factors made before 1987	Immunization against hepatitis B for those not already infected; also, avoiding exposure to infected blood, contaminated needles, and an infected person's personal items	Chronic hepatitis D: Drug treatment with alpha interferon
Hepatitis E	Through food or water contaminated by feces from an infected person; uncommon in the United States	International travelers, people living in areas where hepatitis E outbreaks are common, and people who live or have sex with an infected person	There is no vaccine for hepatitis E; the only way to prevent the disease is to reduce the risk of exposure to the virus. This means avoiding tap water when traveling internationally and practicing good hygiene and sanitation.	Hepatitis E usually resolves on its own over several weeks to months.

TABLE 55.5 Drugs for Viral Hepatitis

Drug	Route and Adult Dose (maximum dose where indicated)	Adverse Effects
Interferons		
interferon alfacon-1 (Infergen)	Subcutaneous: 9 mcg 3 times/week for 24 weeks	*Myalgia, fatigue, headache, anorexia, diarrhea* Myelosuppression, thrombocytopenia, suicide ideation
interferon alfa-n1 (Wellferon)	Subcutaneous/intramuscular (IM): 3 million units 3 times/week for 48 weeks	
interferon alfa-2b (Intron A)	IM/subcutaneous: 2 million units/m^2 3 times/week	
peginterferon alfa-2a (Pegasys)	Subcutaneous: 180 mcg once weekly for 48 weeks	
peginterferon alfa-2b (PEG-Intron)	Subcutaneous: 1 mcg/kg/week for monotherapy; 1.5 mcg/kg/week when given with ribavirin	
Antivirals		
adefovir dipivoxil (Hepsera)	PO: 10 mg once daily	*Headache, nausea, dizziness, fatigue, nasal disturbances (lamivudine)* Nephrotoxicity and lactic acidosis (adefovir, telbivudine), pancreatitis (lamivudine), hepatomegaly with steatorrhea (lamivudine, entecavir), cardiac arrest (ribavirin), hemolytic anemia (ribavirin), apnea (ribavirin), peripheral neuropathy (telbivudine)
entecavir (Baraclude)	PO: 0.5 mg once daily; 1 mg once daily for patients with history of lamivudine resistance	
lamivudine (Epivir HBV)	PO: 150 mg bid	
ribavirin (Copegus, Rebetol, Ribasphere, Virazole)	PO: 3,200-mg capsules in the a.m. and 3,200-mg capsules in the p.m.	
telbivudine (Tyzeka)	PO: 600 mg/day	

Note: *Italics* indicate common adverse effects. Underline indicates serious adverse effects.

is excreted in the stool and the patient is infectious. Clinical presentation includes an abrupt onset of nausea, anorexia, fatigue, and right upper quadrant pain. Hyperbilirubinemia and very high transaminase values are usually observed.

HAV is the most common cause of acute hepatitis in the United States. Although approximately 20% of patients require some hospitalization for symptoms related to the infection, most recover without treatment and develop lifelong immunity to HAV. Fatalities due to chronic disease are rare, with only a small number of patients developing liver failure. Thus, HAV is normally considered an acute disease, having no significant chronic form. This makes HAV very different from hepatitis B or C.

Like all forms of hepatitis, the best approach for HAV is prevention: No antiviral therapy for acute HAV infection is available. Thorough hand washing after toileting is the most effective method for preventing the transmission of HAV. When visiting endemic regions, travelers should drink bottled or boiled water, and not eat raw food.

HAV vaccine (Havrix, VAQTA) has been available since 1995 and consists of inactivated HAV. It is indicated for children living in communities or states with high infection rates, travelers to countries with high endemic HAV infection rates, men who have sex with men, and illegal drug users. When a booster is given 6 to 12 months after the initial dose, close to 100% immunity is obtained. The length of protection has been shown to be 5 to 8 years, although it is predicted that antibody levels may provide protection for 20 years or longer. Adverse effects are mild, and include pain or swelling at the injection site, headache, fatigue, and anorexia. The availability of the HAV vaccine has led to a dramatic drop in the rate of this infection in the United States.

For someone who has been recently exposed to the HAV, hepatitis A immunoglobulin (HAIg), a concentrated solution of antibodies, may provide some degree of passive immunity. HAV immunoglobulin is administered as prophylaxis for patients traveling to endemic areas and to close personal contacts of infected patients to prevent transmission of the virus. A single IM dose of HAIg can provide passive protection and prophylaxis for about 3 months. It is estimated that the immunoglobulins are 85% effective at preventing HAV in patients exposed to the virus. Serious adverse effects to anti-HAV are rare.

CONNECTION *Checkpoint* 55.3

From what you learned in Chapter 46, what is an immunoglobulin? Name some other disease or conditions treated with immunoglobulins. See Answer to Connection Checkpoint 55.3 in Appendix A.

Hepatitis B: Hepatitis B (HBV) is caused by a DNA virus. Although transmission in the United States is primarily through exposure to contaminated blood and body fluids, in endemic regions of the world the infection is widely transmitted by the perinatal route and from child to child.

The incubation period in adults is approximately 4 weeks, while in children the asymptomatic period may last decades. Symptoms of HBV infection are indistinguishable from those of other hepatitis viruses, and include anorexia, nausea, vomiting, fatigue, and abdominal pain. The acute stage can cause severe jaundice. Treatment of acute HBV infection is symptomatic, because no specific antiviral therapy is available. Although infectious, infants are almost always asymptomatic, which is partly responsible for the spread of the virus from child to child. Ninety percent of acute HBV infections in adults resolve with complete recovery and do not progress to chronic disease. Lifelong immunity to HBV is usually acquired following resolution of the infection.

Chronic HBV infection may be asymptomatic, and it may take as long as 10 years before the chronic stage develops. HBV has a much greater incidence of chronic hepatitis and a greater mortality rate, than does HAV. Although adults rarely progress from acute to chronic hepatitis, infants who acquire the infection have a 90% probability of progressing to chronic hepatitis later in life. The final stage of the infection is hepatic cirrhosis. In addition, chronic HBV infections are associated with an increased risk of hepatocellular carcinoma.

Like HAV, the best treatment for HBV infection is prevention through immunization. HBV vaccine (Recombivax HB, Engerix-B) consists of preparations of hepatitis B surface antigen (HBsAg), rather than inactivated virus. Traditionally, the vaccine has been indicated for health care workers and others routinely exposed to blood and body fluids. Because this vaccination protocol failed to address hepatitis B in early childhood, universal vaccination of all children is now recommended and some states require HBV vaccination prior to entry into school. Hepatitis B vaccine is very safe, with mild reactions such as pain at the injection site and low-grade fever being the most frequent adverse effects. Three doses of the vaccine provide up to 90% of the patients with protection against HBV following exposure to the virus. A combination vaccine is available that provides immunity to both HAV and HBV (Twinrix).

For someone who has been recently exposed to the HBV, therapy with hepatitis B immunoglobulins (HBIg) may be initiated. Indications for HBIg therapy include probable exposure to HBV through the perinatal, sexual, or parenteral routes, or known exposure of an infant to a caregiver to HBV. To be effective, HBIg should be administered within 48 hours after parenteral exposure to HBV, within 2 weeks of sexual contact, or to newborns of HBV-positive mothers 12 hours postpartum.

Once chronic hepatitis B becomes symptomatic, pharmacotherapy is indicated with drugs shown in Table 55.2. The two basic strategies to eliminate HBV are to stop viral replication with antivirals, or boost body defenses with immunomodulators. Three different therapies are approved for chronic HBV pharmacotherapy, with no single treatment being clearly superior in all patients.

- Interferon alfa or peginterferon. Thirty to forty percent of patients respond to 4 months of therapy. Five to ten percent of these patients relapse after completing therapy.
- Lamivudine (Epivir). Twenty-five to forty-five percent of the patients respond to therapy, which may last 1 year or longer. Emergence of resistant viral strains is becoming a clinical problem with this drug.
- Adefovir (Hepsera). Approximately 50% of the patients respond to 48 weeks of therapy. The drug is new, and long-term studies are in progress.

Initial therapy of chronic HBV includes either interferon alfa or lamivudine. Interferon has the advantage of being effective against resistant HBV strains, but its use is limited by its cost and numerous adverse effects. Lamivudine has a faster onset and fewer adverse effects but resistant strains may emerge during long-term therapy. Adefovir is relatively new and has not yet been shown to be superior to other therapies. It is prescribed when treatment with interferon or lamivudine fails, or if the established drugs are not well tolerated by the patient. Some health care providers prescribe adefovir in combination with lamivudine to discourage the development of resistant strains. Clinical studies are ongoing to compare the effectiveness of adefovir to lamivudine and interferon; thus, its role in treating HBV infection may change in the future.

In 2005, the FDA approved entecavir (Baraclude), a new drug for chronic HBV. Early data suggests entecavir is as effective, or more effective, than lamivudine. The role of entecavir in treating chronic HBV infection will be established as additional research becomes available.

Because patient symptoms do not reliably indicate the extent of infection, pharmacotherapy is guided by laboratory markers. Hepatic enzymes such as serum alanine transferase (ALT) and aspartate transaminase are used as indicators of liver damage. Hepatitis B DNA, hepatitis B surface antigen (HBsAg), and hepatitis Be antigen (HBeAg) confirm the presence of the virus. Pharmacotherapy is considered successful when hepatic transaminases return to normal values, HBV DNA disappears, and HBeAg is eliminated.

Hepatitis C and other hepatitis viruses: The hepatitis C, D, E, and G viruses are sometimes referred to as non A–non B viruses. Research is continuing to identify additional hepatitis viruses. Of the non A–non B viruses, hepatitis C has the greatest clinical importance.

Transmitted primarily through exposure to infected blood or body fluids, hepatitis C (HCV) is more common than HBV. About 40% to 50% of all HIV-AIDS patients are coinfected with HCV. Perinatal transmission rates are very low.

The incubation period for HAC is 50 days. Like other hepatitis infections, HAC symptoms include nausea, vomiting, anorexia, and jaundice. Although acute HAV infection may be associated with severe symptoms, the majority of patients are asymptomatic. About 70% of patients infected with HCV proceed to chronic hepatitis, and up to 30% may develop end-stage cirrhosis. HCV is the most common cause of chronic hepatitis and is the most frequent indication for liver transplants.

Unlike HAV and HCV, no vaccine is available for hepatitis C due to the very high mutation rate of the virus. In addition, postexposure prophylaxis of HAC with immunoglobulins following exposure to the virus is not recommended because its effectiveness has not been demonstrated.

Current pharmacotherapy for chronic HCV infection includes combination therapy with interferon and the antiviral ribavirin. Combination therapy has been found to produce a more sustained viral suppression than monotherapy with either agent used alone. The sustained success rate for treating hepatitis C is about 50%.

Interferons are immunomodulatory proteins secreted by macrophages, B-lymphocytes, and other body defense cells in response to viral infection. Actions of interferons include suppression of cell division, inhibition of viral replication, and enhancement of macrophage and T lymphocyte activity. Only the alpha family of interferons is used in hepatitis therapy, and each interferon has slightly different applications and indications. Information on interferons used for other indications may be found in Chapters 43 and 46.

PROTOTYPE DRUG Lamivudine (Epivir)

Classification: **Therapeutic:** Antiviral
Pharmacologic: Nucleoside reverse transcriptase inhibitor

Therapeutic Effects and Uses: Originally approved for HIV infection in combination with other antiviral agents in 1995, lamivudine was later approved for chronic hepatitis B infections that have evidence of viral replication and active liver inflammation. For the treatment of chronic HBV infection, lamivudine is given PO, either as monotherapy or in combination with other drugs. In about 14% of patients, the HBV will become resistant to lamivudine after a year of therapy. The dose recommended for treating HBV (100 mg/day) is much less than that recommended for treating HIV (300 mg/day).

When used to treat HIV infection, lamivudine is almost always combined with at least two other agents to delay the development of resistance (see Chapter 56). When used as monotherapy, resistant strains of HBV begin to emerge after about 3 to 6 months of lamivudine therapy. Combivir is a fixed-dose combination tablet containing lamivudine and zidovudine: Trizivir combines lamivudine with abacavir.

Mechanism of Action: Resembling a natural nucleoside, lamivudine inhibits viral DNA synthesis by inhibiting the reverse transcriptase enzyme.

Pharmacokinetics:

Route(s)	PO
Absorption	Rapidly absorbed
Distribution	Distributed to extracellular spaces; enters the CSF in children; crosses the placenta; secreted in breast milk; 36% bound to plasma protein
Primary metabolism	Minimal hepatic metabolism
Primary excretion	Renal
Onset of action	Unknown
Duration of action	Half-life: 2–4 h

Adverse Effects: Lamivudine is a less toxic alternative than interferon therapy, and most patients experience no serious adverse effects. GI adverse effects are relatively common and include nausea, vomiting, abdominal pain, and diarrhea. Ear, nose, and throat infections and fatigue may occur in as many as 25% of the patients taking the drug. Lamivudine can cause an unusual type of liver abnormality called lactic acidosis and hepatomegaly with steatosis. Although rare, this type of hepatotoxicity has resulted in several deaths.

Contraindications/Precautions: Because it is excreted by the kidneys, patients with renal impairment should receive a lower dose and be monitored frequently for changes in urinary laboratory values. Hepatic enzyme values should be monitored regularly during therapy. If any signs of lactic acidosis or hepatotoxicity are noted, the drug should be immediately discontinued. Children with a history of pancreatitis should be carefully monitored, as lamivudine can cause or worsen this condition in pediatric patients. Lactation should be suspended while taking lamivudine therapy. Caution must be used when discontinuing the drug because exacerbations of hepatitis may occur.

Drug Interactions: Lamivudine is frequently used in the multidrug therapy of HIV and HBV. Many complex and unpredictable drug interactions are possible given the nature of these diseases and the multiple drugs administered concurrently during therapy. Nurses who specialize in treating patients infected with HIV or HBV should refer to the most recent drug information provided by the FDA and the drug manufacturer when assessing for potential drug interactions in these patients. In general, any concurrently administered drug that affects the renal excretion or hepatic metabolism of lamivudine has the potential to affect the drug's actions and adverse effects. **Herbal/Food:** May be taken with or without food, although food slows the rate of drug absorption.

Pregnancy: Category C.

Treatment of Overdose: There is no antidote for lamivudine overdose. Patients are treated symptomatically.

Nursing Responsibilities:

- Obtain a complete health history including allergies, drug history, and possible drug interactions.
- Monitor blood counts every 2 to 3 weeks for neutropenia, thrombocytopenia, hemoglobin, and CD4 viral load. If blood counts are low, pharmacotherapy may need to be temporarily discontinued until hematologic function is restored.
- Monitor liver studies such as aspartate aminotransferase (AST), alanine aminotransferase (ALT), bilirubin, and amylase periodically during treatment because the patient is at high risk for hepatotoxicity.

Patient and Family Education:

- Report sore throat, swollen lymph nodes, malaise, fever, and other signs of infection develop to the health care provider. Ear, nose, and throat infections occur in as many as 25% of the patients taking the drug.
- Immediately report the following to the health care provider: yellowing of the skin or eyes, unusual fatigue, or weakness.
- This drug does not cure the disease, but may control the symptoms.

- This drug does not reduce the risk of passing HBV to others.
- Follow-up care is essential. Always comply with appointment schedules.
- Continue taking the drug even if feeling better. Stopping the drug may worsen hepatitis symptoms.
- At least 4 weeks may be needed before any improvement in symptoms are noted.
- Do not breast-feed while taking this drug without approval of the health care provider.
- Immediately notify the health care provider of any known or suspected pregnancy.

Drugs Similar to Lamivudine (Epivir)

Other antivirals for chronic hepatitis include adefovir dipivoxil, lamivudine, ribavirin, and telbivudine. The interferons are discussed separately.

Adefovir Dipivoxil (Hepsera): Approved in 2002, adefovir structurally resembles a natural nucleotide and inhibits viral DNA synthesis of HBV. It is active against several species of viruses, although it is only approved for the oral therapy of chronic HBV infection that shows evidence of active viral replication. Adefovir is an antiviral alternative for patients who have developed resistance to lamivudine. Other than headache and abdominal pain, the drug is well tolerated at the doses used to treat HBV. At high doses and in patients with preexisting renal impairment, urinary laboratory values should be monitored regularly because nephrotoxicity has been reported. Resistance has not been a clinical problem. Severe exacerbation of hepatitis has been reported in patients who have discontinued therapy with adefovir and some other antivirals. This drug is pregnancy category C.

Entecavir (Baraclude): Entecavir is a newer antiviral, approved in 2005 for the treatment of chronic HBV that exhibits evidence of viral replication. Like lamivudine, entecavir is a nucleoside analog that inhibits viral DNA synthesis. Cross resistance has been observed between entecavir and lamivudine. Given PO, the drug is well tolerated and the most common adverse effects include nausea, headache, fatigue, and dizziness. Like lamivudine, a few cases of fatal lactic acidosis and severe hepatomegaly with steatosis have been reported. Exacerbation of hepatitis may occur following discontinuation of therapy with antivirals. This drug is pregnancy category C.

Ribavirin (Copegus, Rebetol): Ribavirin resembles a natural nucleoside and inhibits the viral synthesis of both DNA and RNA. Unlike many antivirals, it has a broad spectrum of activity against both RNA and DNA viruses. Ribavirin is given PO as a tablet (Rebetol) or capsule (Copegus) when treating HCV, always in combination with alfa interferons. The inhalation form (Virazole) was approved in 1985 to treat severe infections from the respiratory syncytial virus. Off-label uses include treatment of influenza, herpes, and other viruses. The most serious adverse effect of ribavirin is hemolytic anemia, and patients must be assessed regularly for changes in laboratory blood values. In addition, the drug can affect the heart and should be used with caution in patients with preexisting cardiac disease. Ribavirin has produced embryotoxicity and fetal defects in every animal studied; it is pregnancy category X. Indeed, pregnant health care workers should not care for patients receiving aerosolized ribavirin due to the risk of incidental exposure. Resistance has not been a clinical problem with ribavirin.

Telbivudine (Tyzeka): Telbivudine is a newer antiviral, approved in 2006, for the treatment of chronic HBV in patients with evidence of active disease. Like lamivudine, it is an oral drug that inhibits viral DNA synthesis by inhibiting the reverse transcriptase enzyme. Viruses may develop cross resistance between lamivudine and telbivudine. The most frequent adverse effects include flulike symptoms, upper respiratory tract infection, fatigue, abdominal pain, and diarrhea. Like lamivudine, a low incidence of lactic acidosis and severe hepatomegaly with steatosis have been reported, including a few fatal cases. This drug is pregnancy category B.

Interferons: Several interferons are commercially available as drugs through recombinant DNA technology. Additional information on these drugs is presented in Chapter 45.

- **Interferon Alfa-2b.** This drug is the only interferon approved for chronic HBV infection. After 4 months of pharmacotherapy, approximately one third of the patients will experience long-term loss of HBV DNA and HBsAg. In the second or third month of therapy, patients may experience an exacerbation of symptoms, probably due to removal of infected hepatocytes by the immune system. Patients most likely to respond to interferon therapy include those with a low viral load (HBV less than 20 copies/mL) and ALT greater than 100. Although the majority of patients respond to interferon monotherapy with normalization of transaminases and a reduction in liver degeneration, relapse rates are high. Permanent resolution of chronic HCV occurs in only about 10% to 25% of patients. Combination therapy with ribavirin increases the therapeutic success rate. Interferon alfa-2b is also used to treat hairy cell leukemia and Kaposi's sarcoma (see Chapter 58).
- **Interferon Alfacon-1 (Infergen).** This drug is approved only for chronic HCV infections. Its antiviral activity is estimated to be 5 times greater than interferon alfa-2a or 2b. Like interferon alfa-2b, it is administered subcutaneously three times per week. Actions and adverse effects are the same as interferon alfa-2b.
- **Interferon Alfa-n1 (Wellferon).** This drug is approved only for chronic HCV infections. Like interferon alfa-2b, it is administered by the subcutaneous route three times per week. Actions and adverse effects are the same as interferon alfa-2b.
- **Peginterferon Alfa-2a (Pegasys) and Peginterferon Alfa-2b (PEG-Intron).** These drugs are pegylated formulations of interferons that produce a more sustained serum drug level over a longer period of time. Pegylation permits the interferon to maintain a consistently high serum level, and to be administered less frequently. Whereas standard interferon formulations must be administered three times per week, pegylated versions require only one dose per week. The PEG molecule is inert and does not influence antiviral activity. Pegasys and PEG-Intron are thought to be equivalent in terms of efficacy. Actions and adverse effects are the same as interferon alfa-2b.

NURSING PROCESS APPLICATION

Patients Receiving Antiviral Agents for Non-HIV Viral Infections

Assessment	Potential Nursing Diagnoses

Prior to drug administration:
• Obtain a complete health history including allergies, drug history, and possible drug interactions.
• Obtain a complete physical examination.
• Obtain the following laboratory studies for systemic antiviral treatment:
  • Liver function
  • Renal function
	• *Risk for Injury,* related to adverse effects of medication.
	• *Deficient Knowledge (Non-HIV Viral Infections Antiviral Agents),* related to purpose, precautions, and adverse effects of drug
	• *Deficient Knowledge (Viral infection)*, related to disease process and infection transmission

Planning: Patient Goals and Expected Outcomes

The patient will:

- Demonstrate knowledge of the disease process, transmission, and treatment.
- Identify adverse effects and report them to the health care provider.
- Complete the full course of therapy and adhere to follow-up care schedule.

Implementation

Interventions and (Rationales)	Patient and Family Education
• Monitor for symptoms of hypersensitivity reactions. (Many antiviral medications can induce a hypersensitivity reaction leading to anaphylaxis.)	• Instruct the patient to discontinue the medication and inform the health care provider if symptoms of hypersensitivity reaction develop such as wheezing, shortness of breath, swelling of face, tongue or hands, itching, or rash.
• Monitor temperature and white blood count and for symptoms of infection. Protect the patient from sources of infection. (Some antiviral drugs may cause agranulocytosis.)	Instruct the patient: • To report symptoms of infections such as fever, chills, sore throat, and cough. • On methods to minimize exposure to infection such as washing hands frequently; avoiding crowds and other people with colds, flu, and other infections; limiting exposure to children and animals; increasing fluid intake; emptying the bladder frequently; and coughing and deep breathing several times per day.
• Monitor I&O ratio and evaluate the patient's hydration status when receiving IV antiviral medications. (Dehydration states will predispose the patient to drug-induced renal damage.)	• Instruct patient on importance of maintaining hydrated state. Encourage intake of oral fluids and food high in water content.
• Determine potential drug–drug and drug–food interactions. (Most antiviral medications have multiple interactions and must be taken exactly as prescribed.)	Instruct the patient: • When to take the specific medication in relationship to food intake (before meals, with meals, or after meals). • About foods or beverages to avoid when taking medication. Some antiviral should not be taken with acidic fruit juice. • To take medication exactly as directed. Do not skip any doses. • To consult with the health care provider before taking any OTC medications or dietary supplements.
• Maintain a safe environment for the patient. (Amantadine may cause dizziness, light-headedness, ataxia, mental confusion, visual and auditory hallucinations, and blurring or loss of vision.)	• Instruct the patient and family members on interventions to avoid potential traumatic injuries: • Avoid driving or operating machinery until the affects of systemic drug are known. • Report symptoms related to neurologic impairment such as confusion, lack of coordination, or visual disturbances.
• Assess the patient's level of understanding regarding use and effect of medication. (Knowledge of the medication's effects is important in reducing the transmission of the virus.)	• Advise the patient to refrain from sexual intercourse if either partner has symptoms of herpes infection; neither topical nor systemic drug prevents transmission to other individuals.

Evaluation of Outcome Criteria

Evaluate the effectiveness of drug therapy by confirming that patient goals and expected outcomes have been met (see "Planning").

UNDERSTANDING THE CHAPTER

Key Concepts Summary

55.1 Viruses are infectious agents with simple structures.

55.2 The replication cycle of a virus occurs in five stages.

55.3 Antiviral drugs target a specific viral structure or stage of its replication cycle.

55.4 Pharmacotherapy can lessen the severity of acute herpes simplex infections and prolong latency.

55.5 Pharmacotherapy of influenza viruses includes drugs to prevent infection, as well as agents to treat active infections.

55.6 The most effective therapies for hepatitis infections are antivirals and drugs that boost the immune system to rid the body of the virus.

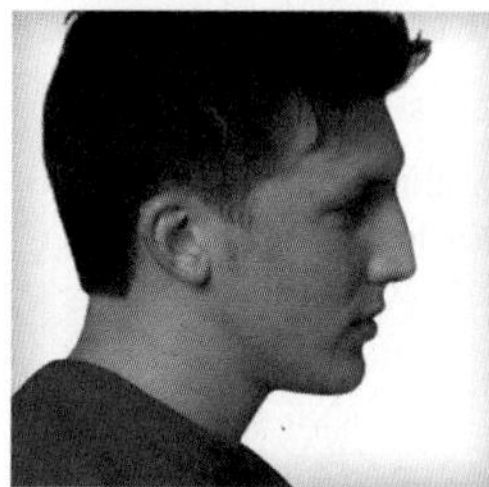

Making the PATIENT *Connection*

Remember the patient "Richard Palmer" at the beginning of the chapter? Now read the remainder of the case study. Based on the information presented within this chapter, respond to the critical thinking questions that follow.

Richard Palmer, a 19-year-old university student, has come to the health clinic. He states that he suffers from cold sores at least 6 to 8 times per year. He informs the nurse that the cold sores usually start with lip pain or tingling, often followed by small, painful, fluid-filled blisters on a raised, red, painful area of his lip. The blisters usually last 2 to 3 days in duration then form yellowish crusts that slough off to reveal pinkish skin.

With his final exams coming up, Richard admits to "feeling the crunch." He also works part time to help meet the expenses of college. Like other college students his age, Richard eats "on the run" and seldom sleeps more than 4 to 5 hours per night. His weekends are even more hectic with the job, school, and keeping up with social activities. Richard requests something to help rid him of the existing cold sore immediately.

Critical Thinking Questions

1. How would you explain the mode of transmission and onset of symptoms for herpes simplex viruses (HSV) to Richard?
2. How would you respond when Richard asked, "Is there any medication that I can take to prevent the cold sores from returning?"
3. Topical acyclovir is prescribed for this patient. What patient education would you provide?

Case Study

Jeanie is a 43-year-old factory worker who has just started a new job. Today, she presents to the employee health services with a fever (temperature: 38.3°C [101.1°F]), headache, myalgia, and cough that developed less than 24 hours ago.

As she is talking to the nurse, she expresses concern that she will lose her job if she is absent from work. "If only I had taken the flu shot, maybe I wouldn't have gotten sick," says Jeanie.

1. Is Jeanie a possible candidate for oseltamivir (Tamiflu)? Why or why not?
2. Paraphrase the mechanism of action for neuraminidase inhibitors.

NCLEX-RN® Review

1 Which of the following women would most likely benefit from annual influenza vaccination? (Select all that apply.)

1. A 69-year-old who lives on a farm in rural Mississippi
2. A 75-year-old who was recently admitted to a long-term care facility
3. A 27-year-old student nurse who currently has influenza symptoms
4. A 28-year-old who is 7 months pregnant and works in a shirt factory
5. A 33-year-old who is HIV positive and uses recreational intravenous drugs

2 The client is receiving an antiviral medication for genital herpes. Which statement, made by the client, would indicate that client teaching for this condition has been successful?

1. "Neither topical nor systemic drug prevents transmission of herpes to other individuals."
2. "I will cleanse the affected areas with soap and water every other day."
3. "I should wear tight-fitting clothes over affected areas to prevent spread of the infection."
4. "I should start the antiviral therapy after the lesion forms a crust."

3 Which of the following laboratory values would be most important for the nurse to monitor in the client receiving intravenous acyclovir (Zovirax)?

1. White blood cell count
2. Serum creatinine
3. Sodium and potassium levels
4. Platelets and coagulation studies

4 The client taking acyclovir (Zovirax) reports sudden onset of herpes lesions. The nurse would initially assess the client for which of the following?

1. Recent stressors such as fever, trauma, or menstruation
2. Increase intake of calcium-based food
3. Exposure to cool moist air
4. Contact with cat or dog dander

5 It is influenza season and an elderly client telephones the clinic asking when it would be appropriate to take oseltamivir (Tamiflu)? Which information provided by the nurse would be correct? Oseltamivir (Tamiflu) is:

1. Given within 48 hours of the onset of symptoms.
2. Administered to prevent influenza.
3. Used to eliminate complications of influenza.
4. Contraindicated for elderly adults.

6 The client is receiving interferon alfacon-1 (Infergen). Which manifestation, if present in the client, would the nurse conclude is an adverse effect of this medication?

1. Neurologic symptoms such as headaches and dizziness
2. Flulike symptoms such as fever and chills
3. Skin disruptions such as acne and ulcerations
4. Gastric discomfort such as dyspepsia and indigestion

See Answers to Critical Thinking Questions, Case Study, and NCLEX-RN® Review in Appendix A.

References

Burkhart, C. G. (2005). Herpes acquisition and transmission. *Journal of Drugs in Dermatology, 3*, 378–383.

Centers for Disease Control and Prevention (CDC). (2008). Prevention and control of influenza: Recommendations of the Advisory Committee on Immunization Practices (ACIP), *Morbidity and Mortality Weekly Report, 57*(Early Release), 1–60.

Centers for Disease Control and Prevention (CDC), Department of Health and Human Services. (2008). *Viral hepatitis: FAQs for health professionals.* Retrieved August 5, 2008, from http://www.cdc.gov/hepatitis/HBV/HBVfaq.htm#overview

Chan, W. F., & Wong, T. (2007). Preparing for pandemic influenza: Revisit the basics. *Journal of Clinical Nursing, 16*(10), 1858–1864.

Chen, X. Y., Wu, T. X., Liu, G. J., Wang, Q., Zheng, J., Wei, J., et al. (2007). Chinese medicinal herbs for influenza. *Cochrane Database of Systematic Reviews, Issue 4.* (Art No.: CD004559, DOI:10.1002/14651858.CD004559.pub3).

Dienstag, J., & McHutchison, J. (2006). American Gastroenterological Association technical review on the management of hepatitis C. *Gastroenterology, 130*(1), 231–264.

Downey, N. H. (2008). Hepatitis C treatment: Special populations. *Gastroenterology Nursing, 31*(2), 162–164.

Ensor, D. (2005). The significance of herpes simplex for school nurses. *The Journal of School Nursing, 21*(1), 10–16.

Hayden, F. G. (2006). Antiviral agents (nonretroviral). In L. L. Brunton, J. S. Lazo, & K. L. Parker (Eds.), *Goodman & Gilman's the pharmacological basis of therapeutics* (11th ed., pp. 1243–1271). New York: McGraw-Hill.

Heathcote, J., & Main, J. (2005). Treatment of hepatitis C. *Journal of Viral Hepatitis, 12*(3), 223–235.

Leblebicioglu, H., & Brook, I. (2007). *Influenza.* eMedicine. Retrieved August 5, 2008, from http://www.emedicine.com/ped/TOPIC3006.HTM

Maltezou, H. C. (2008). Nosocomial influenza: New concepts and practice. *Current Opinion in Infectious Diseases, 21*(4), 337–343.

Sharma, R., & Brilliant, L. C. (2006). *Herpes simplex.* eMedicine. Retrieved August 5, 2008, from http://www.emedicine.com/EMERG/topic246.htm

Shepherd J., Weston, R., Peersman, G., & Napuli, I. Z. (1999). Interventions for encouraging sexual lifestyles and behaviors intended to prevent cervical cancer. *Cochrane Database of Systematic Reviews,* Issue 4. (Art. No.: CD001035,DOI:10.1002/14651858.CD001035).

Wilson, T. R. (2005). The ABCs of hepatitis. *Nurse Practitioner, 30*(6), 12–21.

Wolfe, D. C. (2007). *Hepatitis, viral.* eMedicine. Retrieved August 5, 2008, from http:/www.emedicine.com/med/TOPIC3180.HTM

CHAPTER

Yeah, I admit it. I'm scared and practically out of my mind with worry. I've known several people who have died because of AIDS. What if this happens to me?

Patient "Jim Green"

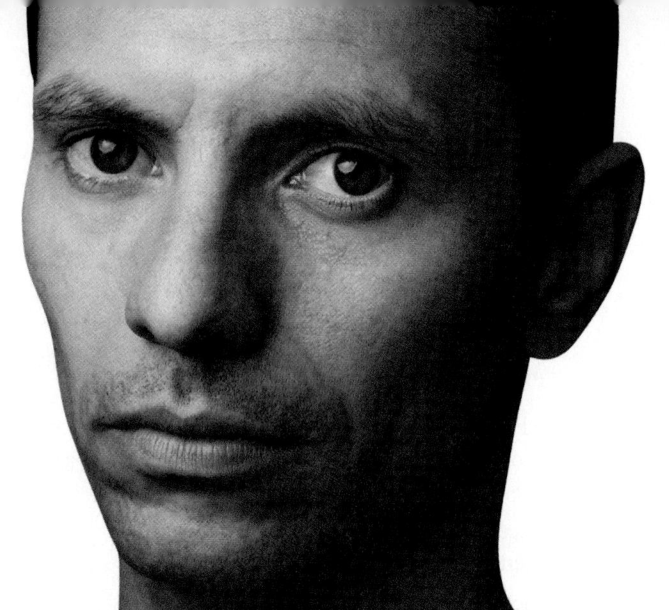

56 Pharmacotherapy of HIV-AIDS

Learning Outcomes

After reading this chapter, the student should be able to:

1. Describe the primary steps in the pathogenesis of HIV infection.
2. Explain reasons for treatment failure during HIV-AIDS pharmacotherapy.
3. Explain the purpose and expected outcomes of HIV-AIDS pharmacotherapy.
4. Describe the advantages of highly active antiretroviral therapy in the pharmacotherapy of HIV infection.
5. Compare and contrast the six classes of antiretroviral medications.
6. Describe the difficulties in developing a vaccine to prevent HIV-AIDS.
7. Explain the protocol and rationale for postexposure prophylaxis following occupational exposure to HIV-infected fluids.
8. Describe the antiretroviral protocol used for reducing the risk of perinatal transmission and for treating pediatric patients with HIV-AIDS.
9. Identify opportunistic infections commonly acquired by AIDS patients and the drugs used to treat them.
10. Describe the nurse's role in the pharmacologic management of patients receiving antiretroviral medications.
11. For each of the classes shown in the chapter outline, identify the prototype and representative drugs and explain the mechanism(s) of drug action, primary indications, contraindications, significant drug interactions, pregnancy category, and important adverse effects.
12. Use the nursing process to care for patients receiving drugs for HIV.

Chapter Outline

Pathogenesis of HIV Infection

General Principles of HIV Pharmacotherapy

Classification of Antiretroviral Drugs

Antiretroviral Drugs

Nucleoside and Nucleotide Reverse Transcriptase Inhibitors

PROTOTYPE **Zidovudine (Retrovir, AZT)** *p. 934*

Nonnucleoside Reverse Transcriptase Inhibitors

PROTOTYPE **Efavirenz (Sustiva)** *p. 936*

Protease Inhibitors

PROTOTYPE **Lopinavir with Ritonavir (Kaletra)** *p. 938*

Fusion Inhibitors, Integrase Inhibitors, and CCR5 Inhibitors

Prophylaxis of HIV Infections

Vaccines

Occupational Exposure to HIV

Perinatal Transmission

Pharmacotherapy of Opportunistic Infections Associated with HIV-AIDS

Key Terms

acquired immunodeficiency syndrome (AIDS), 927
acute retroviral syndrome, 928
antiretroviral, 927
CD4 receptor, 927
highly active antiretroviral therapy (HAART), 932
human immunodeficiency virus (HIV), 927
integrase, 927
lipodystrophy, 934
mitochondrial toxicity, 933
protease, 928
provirus, 927
reverse transcriptase, 927
viral load, 929

Recognized by the medical community as a distinct disease in 1981, the first documented case of **acquired immunodeficiency syndrome (AIDS)** has since been traced back to 1959. The syndrome is characterized by profound immunosuppression, leading to opportunistic infections (OIs) and malignancies not commonly acquired by people with intact immune defenses. The **human immunodeficiency virus (HIV)** was quickly identified as the causative agent for AIDS. HIV-AIDS has resulted in a tragic, worldwide epidemic, causing the deaths of millions of people. The infection continues to be a major public health challenge.

PharmFACT

From 1991 to 2007, the percentage of high school students in the United States who had ever engaged in sexual intercourse decreased by 12%. The percentage who had sexual intercourse with four or more persons during their lifetime decreased by 20%. Among students who were currently sexually active, the prevalence of condom use increased by 33%. *Source:* Morbidity and Mortality Weekly Report, 2008.

Pathogenesis of HIV Infection

56.1 HIV causes a profound loss of immune function.

There are two primary types of HIV: HIV-1 and HIV-2. Because more than 99% of the global AIDS cases are caused by HIV-1, the discussion in this text will apply only to HIV-1. HIV uses the five basic stages of infection described in Chapter 55. There are, however, additional details that are important to understanding the pharmacotherapy of HIV infection.

Transmission: HIV infection occurs by exposure to contaminated body fluids, most commonly blood or semen, since these fluids have the highest concentration of the virus. Transmission may also occur through sexual activity or through contact of infected fluids with broken skin, mucous membranes, or needlesticks. Newborns born to an HIV-infected mother may acquire the virus during birth, or through breast-feeding. Although in industrialized nations the majority of HIV-AIDS patients are men who have sex with other men, heterosexual transmission is significant and is the predominant means of acquiring the infection in developing countries.

PharmFACT

It is estimated that over 509,000 people in the United States are living with HIV-AIDS. Although the largest percentage (43%) is men who acquired the infection through homosexual contacts, a significant percentage (19%) are women who acquired the infection through heterosexual contact. *Source:* Centers for Disease Control and Prevention, 2008.

Replication cycle: Like other viruses, HIV must infect a host cell to duplicate its genetic material and create more virus particles (virions). Knowledge of the replication cycle of HIV is critical to understanding the pharmacotherapy of HIV-AIDS, and is shown in Figure 56.1.

The first stage of HIV pathogenesis is the attachment of the virus to its preferred target: the **CD4 receptor** on the surface of T4 lymphocytes. (Note that the terms CD4 cells, T4 cells, and T4 lymphocytes are used interchangeably in this text.) During this initial stage, structural proteins on the surface of HIV fuse with the CD4 receptor. Because these receptors are also present on monocytes, macrophages, and dendritic cells, multiple cell types become infected. In addition to the CD4 receptor, coreceptors known as CCR5 and CXCR4 have been discovered that assist HIV in binding to the T4 lymphocyte.

The second stage of pathogenesis is the penetration of HIV into the T4 lymphocyte. The virus uncoats and the single stranded ribonucleic acid (RNA) genetic material enters the host cell. HIV converts its RNA strands to double-stranded deoxyribonucleic acid (DNA), using the viral enzyme **reverse transcriptase.** Only a few viruses are able to construct DNA from RNA; no bacteria, plants, or animals are able to perform this unique metabolic function. All living organisms make RNA from DNA. Because of their "backward" or reverse DNA synthesis, these viruses are called *retroviruses* and drugs used to treat HIV infections are called **antiretrovirals.** Although unique, reverse transcriptase is an inefficient enzyme that makes many errors when converting the viral RNA to double stranded DNA. The enzyme has no "proofreading" ability, which allows errors in the viral genetic code to accumulate. This produces a high mutation rate, making it difficult to develop effective vaccines, as discussed in Section 56.9.

The viral DNA eventually enters the nucleus of the T4 lymphocyte where it becomes incorporated into the host's chromosomes. This action is performed by HIV **integrase,** another enzyme unique to HIV. Once incorporated into human chromosomes, the HIV is called a **provirus,** and it remains for the lifetime of the cell. It is impossible to recognize the HIV provirus or remove it. Indeed, despite the fact that the human T4 lymphocyte is infected with a deadly virus, the host's immune system is unable to effectively remove the defective cells.

This *latent phase* of the infection may last only a few weeks, or it may continue for decades. During this phase, patients are asymptomatic and do not realize they are infected. It was once thought that the virus was truly "silent" during the latent phase but research has demonstrated that continuous HIV replication and immune system damage are occurring.

At some point, the latent provirus becomes activated and produces large amounts of viral messenger RNA, with the first

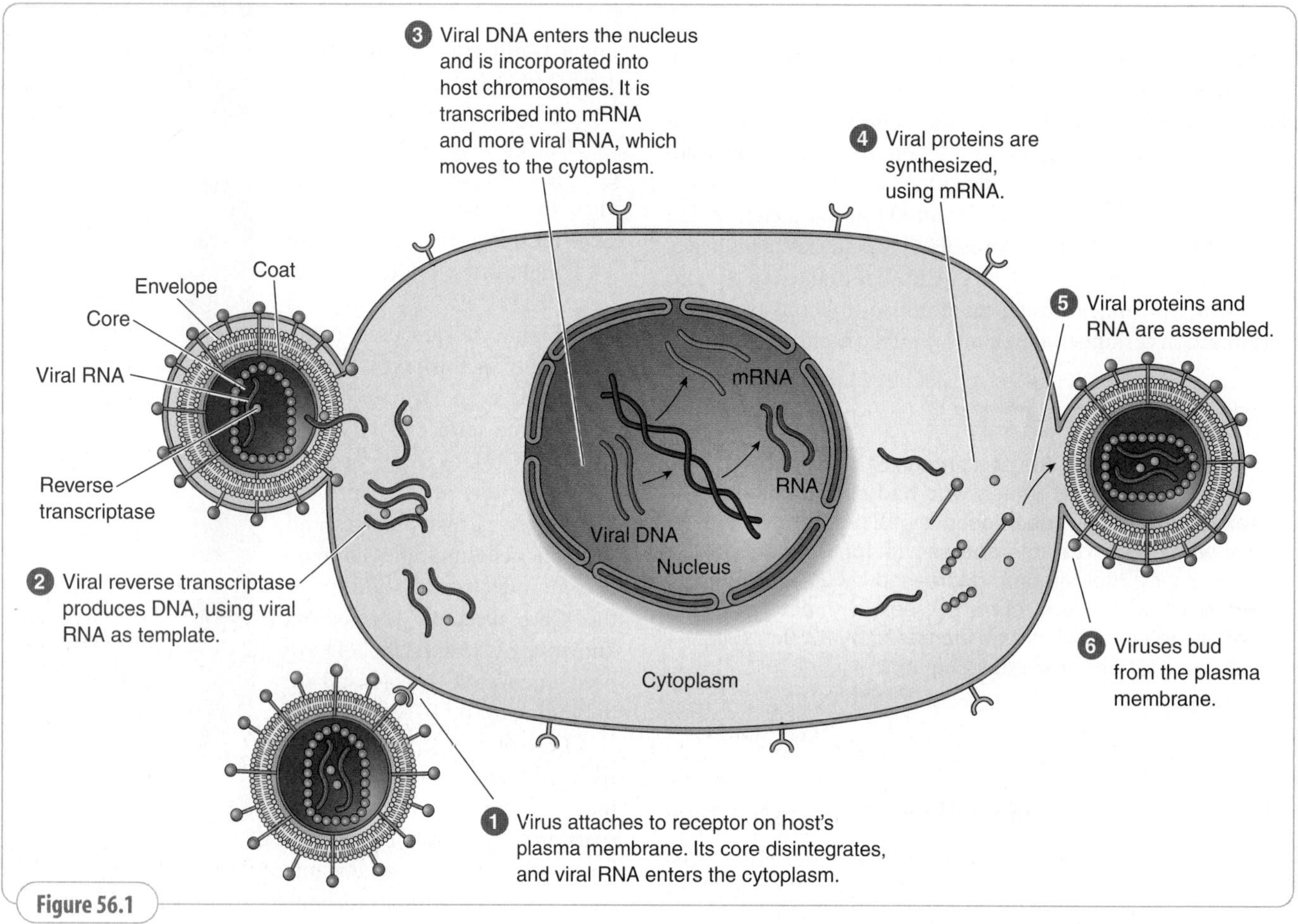

Figure 56.1

Replication of HIV.

strands producing viral proteins that amplify the replication process. All structural components of HIV are subsequently synthesized, and the cell is ready to assemble more virions.

Once synthesized, the individual structural components of HIV migrate to the plasma membrane of the host cell, where they are packaged, and eventually bud from the host cell. The new virions, however, are not yet infectious. As a final step, the viral enzyme **protease** cleaves some of the larger proteins to smaller, functional forms. Once budding occurs, the immune system recognizes that the cell is infected and kills the T4 lymphocyte. Unfortunately, it is too late; it is estimated that an HIV-infected patient may produce as many as 10 billion new virions every day, and the patient's devastated immune system becomes overwhelmed.

Symptoms: Many people incorrectly assume that because the body cannot rid itself of HIV, the immune system does not recognize invasion by the virus. Indeed, the immune system mounts an immediate, massive defense to the entry of HIV, producing an acute inflammatory response that rids the body of many of the infectious virions. It is estimated that a billion HIV virions are destroyed each day during this early stage. Patients experience sore throat, fever, rash, malaise, and weight loss that may last several weeks. However, because patients often mistake these vague symptoms for the common cold or flu, they do not realize HIV infection has occurred and rarely seek medical intervention. Symptoms during this initial phase are known as the **acute retroviral syndrome.** While body defenses may suppress the viral invasion, tragically they are unable to eliminate the virus.

Progression to AIDS is characterized by gradual destruction of the immune system, as measured by the steady decline in the number of CD4 lymphocytes. Unfortunately, the CD4 lymphocyte is the primary cell coordinating the immune response for both the humoral and cell-mediated branches of the immune system (see Chapter 43). When the CD4 cell count falls below a critical level, the patient begins to experience opportunistic bacterial, fungal, and viral diseases, and certain malignancies. Left untreated, the patient eventually is unable to mount any immune defense, and death ensues.

CONNECTION *Checkpoint* 56.1

Patients who are receiving immunosuppressant drugs will have low white cell counts and, like AIDS patients, are at risk to opportunistic infections. From what you learned in Chapter 45, what are the major indications for immunosuppressant therapy? See Answer to Connection Checkpoint 56.1 in Appendix A.

General Principles of HIV Pharmacotherapy

56.2 Treatment of HIV infection is difficult due to the latent nature of the virus and the development of resistant strains.

The widespread appearance of HIV infection in 1981 created enormous challenges for public health and an unprecedented need for the development of new antiviral drugs. HIV-AIDS is unlike any other infectious disease because it is sexually transmitted, uniformly fatal, and demands a continuous supply of new drugs for patient survival. The challenges of HIV-AIDS have resulted in the development of about 20 antiretroviral drugs, with several others in various stages of clinical trials. Unfortunately, the initial hopes of curing HIV-AIDS through antiretroviral therapy or vaccines have not been realized and the disease remains incurable. Although the infection can be managed, stopping antiretroviral therapy always results in a rapid rebound in HIV replication. With HIV mutating extremely rapidly, and resistant strains developing so quickly, the creation of new, novel approaches to antiretroviral drug therapy must remain a high priority in treating HIV infection.

While pharmacotherapy for HIV-AIDS has not produced a cure, it has resulted in a number of therapeutic successes. For example, many patients with HIV infection are able to live symptom-free with their disease for a longer time period due to medications. Furthermore, the transmission of the virus from an HIV-infected mother to her newborn has been reduced dramatically due to intensive drug therapy of the mother prior to delivery, and of the baby immediately following birth. Along with better patient education and prevention, successes in pharmacotherapy have produced a 70% decline in the death rate due to HIV-AIDS in the United States. Unfortunately, this decline has not been observed in African countries, where antiretroviral drugs are not as readily available, largely due to their high cost. A massive global effort will be required to control this infection.

The therapeutic goals for the pharmacotherapy of HIV-AIDS include the following:

- Reduce HIV-related morbidity and prolong survival
- Improve quality of life
- Restore and preserve immunologic function
- Suppress viral load
- Prevent transmission from mother to child in pregnant HIV-infected patients

Initiation of antiretroviral therapy: Should pharmacotherapy of HIV infection start as soon as the disease is diagnosed, or should therapy be postponed until symptoms develop? The optimum time to begin antiretroviral therapy remains controversial, and is a subject of much ongoing debate and research. In current clinical practice, the following serve as guidelines for initiating antiretroviral therapy:

- Antiretroviral therapy should be initiated in patients with a history of an AIDS-defining illness or with a CD4 count below 350 cells/mm^3.
- Antiretroviral therapy should also be initiated in the following groups of infected patients regardless of CD4 count: pregnant women, patients with HIV-associated nephropathy, and patients coinfected with hepatitis B virus (HBV), when HBV treatment is indicated.
- Antiretroviral therapy may be considered in some patients with CD4 T-cell counts above 350 cells/mm^3. These patients include those HIV patients with tuberculosis, Kaposi's sarcoma, non-Hodgkin's lymphoma, and other malignancies.

The primary advantage of initiating therapy during the asymptomatic stage of HIV infection is that the number of replicating virions can be reduced. Early antiretroviral therapy has been shown to delay the onset of acute symptoms and the progression to AIDS. Opportunistic infections (OIs) can be prevented. Early therapy is especially critical for infants under the age of 12 months, since the progression to AIDS can be rapidly fatal for these children.

However, the decision to begin treatment during the asymptomatic stage must be weighed against its negative consequences. Medications for HIV-AIDS are expensive. Treatment with some of the newer agents costs more than $20,000 per year. Antiretrovirals can produce serious adverse effects and may interact with other drugs the patient is taking. Continuous pharmacotherapy over many years promotes viral resistance so that when the acute stage eventually develops, the medications may no longer be effective. These serious consequences must be weighed against the risk of deferring therapy; postponing treatment may cause the disease to reach a critical point where antiretroviral rescue is not possible.

The decision to begin therapy in patients with *symptomatic* HIV disease is a much easier decision, since the severe symptoms of AIDS can rapidly progress to death. Thus, pharmacotherapy nearly always occurs during this phase.

Patients receiving their first treatment for HIV infection are called antiretroviral *naïve*. Therapy for antiretroviral naïve patients is often different from that for antiretroviral experienced patients because drug-resistant strains of HIV develop during therapy.

MyNursingKit | HIV-AIDS Resources at the CDC

Monitoring the progress of antiretroviral therapy: Two laboratory tests used to guide pharmacotherapy are absolute CD4 lymphocyte count and measurement of HIV RNA in the plasma. Figure 56.2 illustrates the value of using these two tests in predicting the prognosis of patients with this infection.

The number of CD4 lymphocytes is an important indicator of immune function that indicates the actual degree of immune system damage caused by the virus. It is a good predictor of the likelihood of the patient acquiring an OI. Normal values range from 500 to 1,600 cells/mcL. HIV-infected patients whose CD4 lymphocyte count falls below 250 cells/mcL are said to have AIDS.

Viral load is determined by measuring the amount of HIV RNA in the blood. The HIV RNA level is an estimate of how rapidly the virus is replicating and is considered a more accurate measure of clinical outcome than CD4 cell counts. Like CD4 lymphocyte counts, HIV RNA levels are determined every 3 to 6 months to monitor progression of the disease and

MyNursingKit | HIV-AIDS Resources at the NIH

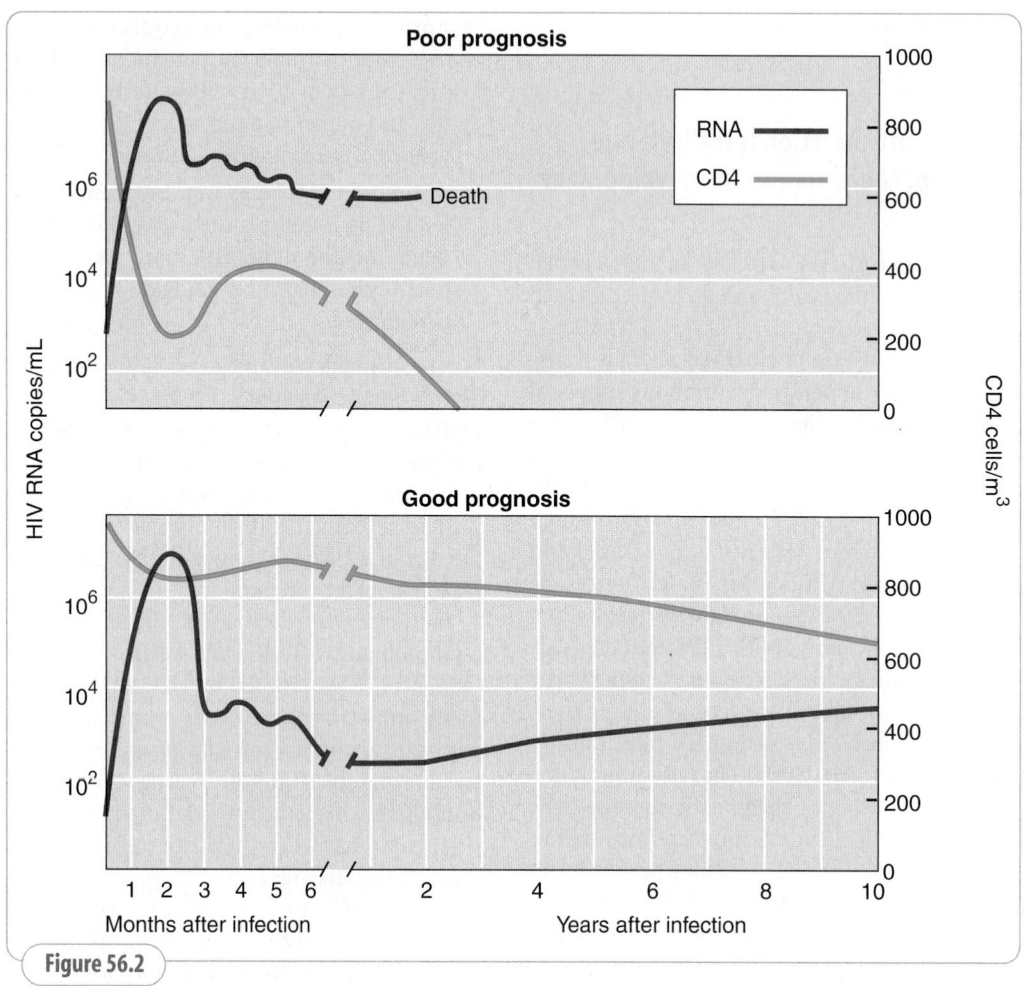

Figure 56.2

Use of CD4 lymphocyte and HIV RNA counts to predict therapeutic outcomes.
Source: From *Broch Biology of Microorganisms* (11th ed., p. 880), by M. Madigan & J. Martinko, 2006. Reprinted by permission of Pearson Education, Inc., Upper Saddle River, NJ.

to assess the degree of success of antiretroviral therapy. The goal of antiretroviral therapy is to reduce HIV RNA in the blood to less than 50 copies/mL.

Treatment failures: Antiretroviral therapy does not totally eliminate HIV from the body and treatment must continue for the remaining lifetime of the patient. Given the high mutation rate of the virus and decades of therapy, it is easy to understand why treatment failures are so common with antiretroviral therapy. Therapeutic failures are extremely challenging for health care providers, nurses, and patients.

Pharmacologic options available for patients with treatment failure are limited. Higher doses are generally not indicated, because they lead to an increased incidence of serious adverse effects. Ideally, the patient is switched to at least two drugs from different chemical classes, which they have not yet received. Because there are only four unique drug classes of antiretroviral agents, this option is not always possible. The primary factors responsible for treatment failure are adverse effects of the medications, lack of adherence to drug therapy, emergence of resistant HIV strains, and the genetic variability among patients.

Antiretroviral drugs cause many adverse effects, including nausea, diarrhea, rash, lipid abnormalities, hepatotoxicity, neuropathy, and increased risk of cardiovascular events. Patients always take at least two of these drugs (and usually more), which often interact with other medications to cause additional adverse effects. Identifying the specific drug interaction causing a toxic effect is challenging for the clinician. Serious adverse effects often require an immediate change in pharmacotherapy. Once the offending drug is identified, it is normally replaced with another drug from the same class. Other times, a simple adjustment such as changing the amount per dose or spacing doses further apart may prevent or eliminate the adverse effect. Adding antinausea drugs or antidiarrheal drugs to the regimen can diminish some of the more common adverse effects.

To be successful, antiretroviral therapy requires strict patient adherence to a complex regimen. Unfortunately, many factors deter patients from complying. Some antiretroviral agents have inconvenient schedules, and must be taken 3 to 4 times per day, or be given parenterally. Some are expensive or simply not available to patients in developing countries. Others make the patient feel quite ill; patients may actually feel much better without taking the drugs. Given these complicating factors, and the prospect of a lifetime of drug therapy, it is easy to understand why adherence to the medication regimen is difficult, even for a motivated patient. The nurse is the key to helping develop a rational daily plan of treatment that best fits the lifestyle of the patient and family.

Drug resistance has become a serious barrier to pharmacotherapeutic success in treating HIV-AIDS. When standard therapies fail, viral resistance must always be considered as a potential source of the failure. Baseline HIV drug resistance testing is now recommended when patients enter care. Follow-up drug resistance testing is performed to determine the future direction of therapy following a failed regimen.

For some drugs such as nevirapine and lamivudine, a single mutation in HIV can produce a strain that will be resistant to all drugs in the same class. Indeed, resistance has been demonstrated after only a single dose of nevirapine. For others, such as the protease inhibitors, several mutations are necessary to confer resistance. Resistant strains may be transmitted between patients through sexual activity or injectable drug abuse. A few cases have been recorded where the HIV strain was resistant to all four classes of antiretrovirals. This situation produces a critical need for the development of new antiretrovirals that act by novel mechanisms. Considerable research is ongoing to determine the optimal therapeutic regimens that delay the emergence of resistant strains. Resistance is always a factor to consider when choosing the optimum regimen in HIV-AIDS patients.

Why do some patients succumb to HIV infections within months after diagnosis, while others survive for decades? Considerable research over three decades has focused on genetic factors that have allowed some individuals to live with HIV for a long time without progressing to AIDS. These patients are known as long-term nonprogressors (LTNPs). Scientists have looked for specific antibodies, cytokines, and protective immune responses in these patients with the hope of developing therapies to help other infected patients. While some progress has been made in this area, researchers are far from understanding the protective genetic make-up of these LTNPs. Until knowledge advances, HIV infection will continue to be potentially fatal in every patient who acquires the infection.

Structured Treatment Interruptions (STIs): Health care providers once recommended the use of structured treatment interruptions: periods of time where all antiretroviral drugs were withdrawn. It was thought that STIs reduced levels of adverse effects, gave patients a welcome drug-free "holiday," and diminished the potential for resistant HIV strains. Research has questioned the effectiveness of STIs; indeed, some studies have suggested that this strategy actually *promotes* drug resistance and hastens disease progression. In all cases, viral load increases when drug therapy is discontinued.

Sexual lifestyle adjustments: Patients with HIV infection often face serious mental health challenges because of their illness. Most are young and sexually active. Knowing that they will likely die prematurely of the infection and that they could kill others through unsafe sexual practices is difficult to accept. Many patients benefit from psychotherapy, and all benefit from compassionate, nonjudgmental, nursing care. Teaching HIV-AIDS patients how to care for themselves and how to protect others from their disease is a major task of the nurse.

Studies have shown that antiretroviral therapy can markedly reduce the amount of HIV RNA in blood and body secretions. This should not be interpreted to mean that the patient is noninfectious. Patients who are asymptomatic, whether they are receiving antiretroviral therapy or not, are still infectious. Patients must observe abstinence or safe sexual practices for the remainder of their lifetimes to protect others from this lethal viral infection.

CONNECTIONS

To the Community Improving Patient Adherence to HIV-AIDS Pharmacotherapy

Highly active antiretroviral therapy (HAART) mandates careful adherence (compliance) to the prescribed drug regimen for optimal positive outcomes. Providing patients with useful tips to help increase adherence can increase the chance of ongoing successful treatment. Desired adherence is at 95% for therapeutic effectiveness.

Patients may miss doses for any number of reasons, such as adverse effects, simple forgetting, a busy life schedule, or not having the medications available. Research studies show that certain factors consistently lead to nonadherence: depression, active use and injection of drugs, or heavy use of alcohol. The patient's social setting can also impact regimen adherence. Living conditions such as unstable housing or a chaotic lifestyle makes adherence to a drug regimen a challenge.

Success is more likely to result when the patient has a supportive and knowledgeable family. Certain strategies can increase HAART therapy adherence. Some of these include the following:

- Start the patient–provider relationship in a positive way and nurture the relationship. Develop a system for easy access to health care providers so that the patient may call and get questions answered at their convenience.
- Assess the patient's readiness for HAART therapy. Investigate the patient's perceptions and beliefs about HAART. Therapy requires commitment and a short delay in starting may be necessary to accommodate individual responses.
- Assess patients for signs and symptoms of depression and treat these before starting HAART therapy.
- Assess the patient for alcohol or drug abuse problems. First, encourage the patient to seek treatment. A possible option is administering medication in a setting where adherence can be monitored.
- Remember that frequent nurse and patient interaction is the key to success, especially during the first month of therapy. This allows time for assessing problems and concerns, as well as strengthening the patient and health care provider relationship.
- Work with social or case worker to assess the patient's support systems and home situation.
- Note the patient's reading skills for appropriate level teaching materials. Know the preferred language for best comprehension.
- Identify a key significant person in the patient's life to support and help with medication adherence. A support group or treatment peer might be useful.
- Help the patient determine the best possible choices for treatment that can easily be incorporated into daily schedules and routines.
- Schedule ongoing individual or group educational sessions to teach the therapeutic effects of HAART as well as how to recognize and manage possible complications associated with pharmacotherapy (Stone, 2001).

Classification of Antiretroviral Drugs

56.3 Six classes of antiretroviral drugs are available to treat HIV infection.

Antiretroviral drugs target specific phases of the HIV replication cycle. The standard pharmacotherapy for HIV-AIDS includes aggressive treatment with multiple drugs concurrently, a regimen called **highly active antiretroviral therapy (HAART)**. The goal of HAART is to reduce the replication of HIV as much as possible, as measured by a reduction in plasma HIV RNA to its lowest possible (or undetectable) level. The simultaneous use of medications from several classes reduces the probability that HIV will become resistant to treatment.

It is important to understand that eliminating the virus from the blood is not a cure because HIV is harbored in locations other than the blood such as lymph nodes. In fact, only a few percent of the total CD4 lymphocytes in the body are circulating in the blood at any given time. Should a patient reach a stage where HIV RNA levels are undetectable, it is important for the nurse to stress that the disease has not been cured and that antiretroviral therapy must be continued for the lifetime of the patient.

Antiretroviral agents, shown in Table 56.1, are classified into the following groups, based upon their mechanism of action:

- Nucleoside/nucleotide reverse transcriptase inhibitors (NRTIs/NtRTIs)
- Nonnucleoside reverse transcriptase inhibitors (NNRTIs)
- Protease inhibitors (PIs)
- Fusion (entry) inhibitors
- Integrase inhibitors
- CCR5 antagonists

Throughout the three decades of the AIDS epidemic, regimens for treating the infection have continuously evolved. While once popular, monotherapy with a single antiretroviral agent, or treatment with three NRTIs are no longer recommended. The development of the protease inhibitor class radically changed the recommended guidelines for antiretroviral therapy. In current clinical practice, the following two regimens have been shown to be the most successful choices for initial therapy:

- One protease inhibitor with two NRTIs; or
- One NNRTI with two NRTIs

To aid in adherence, the FDA has approved several fixed-dose capsules containing two drugs, such as Epzicom (abacavir and lamivudine) and Truvada (tenofovir disoproxil and emtricitabine).

It must be clearly understood that the pharmacotherapy of HIV-AIDS is rapidly evolving. Many of the initial clinical trials for these medications included very small numbers of patients and health care providers are still learning what drug combinations are most effective. The nurse should always review the latest medical literature before treating HIV-AIDS patients.

Pharmacokinetic considerations: Pharmacokinetic variables become very important when treating HIV-AIDS patients and can, in fact, contribute in a major way to the success or failure of pharmacotherapy. The bioavailability of some antiretrovirals is greatly affected by food in the stomach. The absorption of certain antiretrovirals (e.g., indinavir) is decreased in the presence of food. Some (e.g., lopinavir) have a significantly increased absorption with high-fat meals and others (e.g., nevirapine) are not affected by the presence of food.

In addition to changes in absorption, most antiretrovirals are metabolized by the liver. Several can significantly increase or decrease the hepatic metabolism of other drugs, resulting in large numbers of potential drug–drug interactions. These effects differ, even within the same drug class. For example, nevirapine induces the hepatic P450 enzyme system, thus decreasing the levels of other drugs. Delavirdine, an antiretroviral in the same class, inhibits the P450 system, thus increasing the levels of other drugs. Predicting and avoiding complex drug interactions in HIV patients requires truly skilled and dedicated nurses and health care providers who are current on the most recent medical literature.

Antiretroviral Drugs

56.4 Reverse transcriptase inhibitors block the synthesis of viral DNA.

Following penetration into a T4 lymphocyte, the single-stranded viral RNA is used as a template to synthesize double-stranded proviral DNA. HIV virions come "prepackaged" with reverse transcriptase, the enzyme necessary to perform this critical step. Because reverse transcriptase is a viral enzyme not found in human cells, it has been possible to design drugs with the ability to selectively inhibit viral replication.

As proviral DNA is synthesized, biochemical building blocks known as nucleosides and nucleotides are required. Nucleosides/nucleotides form the backbone of the DNA molecule and are composed of the four bases adenine, guanine, thymine, and cytosine. These same nucleosides/nucleotides are used to make human DNA.

Drugs in the nucleoside and nucleotide reverse transcriptase inhibitor classes (NRTIs and NtRTIs) chemically resemble the natural building blocks of DNA. In essence, reverse transcriptase is "fooled" by these drugs, and inserts them into the proviral DNA strand. As the "fake" nucleosides and nucleotides are used to build DNA, however, the proviral DNA chain is prevented from lengthening. Because the growing DNA strand is prematurely terminated, the viral DNA chain is unable to insert into the host chromosome. Reverse transcriptase inhibitors (NRTIs and NtRTIs) have less effect on the progression of the infection if the proviral DNA has already been integrated into the host chromosome.

Although there are differences in pharmacokinetic and toxicity profiles, no single NRTI or NtRTI offers a clear therapeutic advantage over any other. Choice of agent depends upon patient response and the experience of the clinician. With the exception of zidovudine, which is used to prevent perinatal transmission of HIV, the NRTIs and NtRTIs are always used in multidrug combinations in HAART.

The NRTIs are prodrugs. They must first be metabolized to their active, triphosphate form inside their target cells before they become effective. Unlike many other antiretrovirals, the

TABLE 56.1 Antiretroviral Drugs for HIV-AIDS

Drug	Route and Adult Dose (maximum dose where indicated)	Adverse Effects
Nonnucleoside Reverse Transcriptase Inhibitors		
delavirdine (Rescriptor)	PO: 400 mg tid (max: 1,200 mg/day)	*Rash, fever, nausea, diarrhea, headache, stomatitis* Paresthesia, hepatotoxicity (nevirapine), Stevens-Johnson syndrome (SJS), CNS toxicity (efavirenz)
efavirenz (Sustiva)	PO: 600 mg/day (max: 600 mg/day)	
etravirine (Intelence)	PO: 200 mg bid following a meal (max: 400 mg/day)	
nevirapine (Viramune)	PO: 200 mg/day for 14 days, then increase to bid	
Nucleoside and Nucleotide Reverse Transcriptase Inhibitors		
abacavir (Ziagen)	PO: 300 mg bid (max: 600 mg/day)	*Fatigue, generalized weakness, myalgia, nausea, headache, abdominal pain, vomiting, anorexia, rash* Bone marrow suppression, neutropenia, anemia, granulocytopenia, lactic acidosis with steatorrhea, neurotoxicity, peripheral neuropathy (stavudine), pancreatitis (lamivudine)
didanosine (ddI, Videx)	PO: 125–300 mg bid 30 min before a meal	
emtricitabine (Emtriva)	PO: 200 mg once daily (max: 200 mg/day)	
lamivudine (Epivir, 3TC)	PO: 150 mg bid (max: 300 mg/day)	
stavudine (Zerit, D4T)	PO: 40 mg bid (max: 80 mg/day)	
tenofovir (Viread)	PO: 300 mg once daily with a meal	
zidovudine (Retrovir, AZT)	PO: 200 mg every 4 h (1,200 mg/day), after 1 month may reduce to 100 mg every 4 h (600 mg/day) IV: 1–2 mg/kg every 4 h (1,200 mg/day)	
Protease Inhibitors		
atazanavir (Reyataz)	PO: 400 mg daily with food	*Nausea, vomiting, diarrhea, abdominal pain, headache* Anemia, leukopenia, deep vein thrombosis, pancreatitis, lymphadenopathy, hemorrhagic colitis, nephrolithiasis (indinavir), cardiac arrest (atazanavir), thrombocytopenia (saquinavir), pancytopenia (saquinavir)
darunavir (Prezista)	PO: 600 mg taken with 100 mg ritonavir bid with food	
fosamprenavir (Lexiva)	PO: 700–1,400 mg bid in combination with 100–200 mg ritonavir bid (max: 2,800 mg/day)	
indinavir (Crixivan)	PO: 800 mg tid 60 min before a meal	
lopinavir/ritonavir (Kaletra)	PO: 400/100 mg (three capsules or 5 mL of suspension) bid, increase dose to 533/133 mg (four capsules or 6.5 mL) bid, with concurrent efavirenz or nevirapine	
nelfinavir (Viracept)	PO: 750 mg tid with a meal	
ritonavir (Norvir)	PO: 600 mg bid (max: 1,200 mg/day)	
saquinavir (Invirase)	PO: 1,000 mg bid (max: 2,000 mg/day)	
tipranavir (Aptivus)	PO: 500 mg taken with (max 2,000 mg/day) 200 mg ritonavir bid with food	
Miscellaneous Antiretrovirals		
enfuvirtide (Fuzeon)	Subcutaneous: 90 mg bid	*Pain and inflammation at injection site, nausea, diarrhea, fatigue* Hypersensitivity, neutropenia, thrombocytopenia, nephrotoxicity
maraviroc (Selzentry)	PO: 150–600 mg bid (max: 1,200 mg/day)	*Abdominal pain, cough, dizziness, musculoskeletal symptoms, pyrexia, rash, upper respiratory tract infections* Hepatotoxicity, myocardial infarction
raltegravir (Isentress)	PO: 400 mg bid (max: 800 mg/day)	*Headache, diarrhea, nausea* Hypersensitivity reaction

Note: *Italics* indicate common adverse effects. Underline indicates serious adverse effects.

NRTIs do not interact extensively with other drugs undergoing hepatic metabolism. The NtRTIs adefovir and tenofovir are nucleotide inhibitors that are already in their active, triphosphate forms; thus, no metabolic activation is necessary.

Zidovudine was the first antiretroviral used in HIV-AIDS pharmacotherapy. Because zidovudine and some other NRTIs have been used consistently for over 25 years, drug resistance must be considered when selecting the specific agent. There is a high degree of cross resistance among the NRTIs.

As a class, the NRTIs are well tolerated although nausea, vomiting, diarrhea, headache, and fatigue are common during the first few weeks of therapy. Some of the serious adverse effects of NRTIs are caused by **mitochondrial toxicity.** NRTIs inhibit a human enzyme called gamma-polymerase, which is responsible for the replication of DNA in mitochondria. This small, obscure DNA molecule encodes subunits for mitochondrial enzymes in the respiratory chain, which generates ATP. All the NRTIs have been associated with a low incidence of an unusual form of mitochondrial toxicity known as lactic acidosis–severe hepatomegaly with steatosis. This syndrome, which occurs more commonly in women and in those with preexisting hepatic impairment, includes lipid deposits in the liver, elevated transaminase values, and possible hepatic failure. Symptoms are often vague and include nausea, right upper quadrant pain and myalgia. The nurse must carefully monitor liver function tests and assess for hepatic disease, as some fatalities have resulted from this adverse effect.

Another manifestation of mitochondrial toxicity from NRTIs is **lipodystrophy,** a disorder in which fat is redistributed in specific areas in the body. Areas such as the face, arms and legs tend to lose fat, while the abdomen, breasts, and base of the neck (buffalo hump) develop excess fat. The fat redistribution may be associated with hyperlipidemia and hyperglycemia.

Two other serious adverse effects may be associated with mitochondrial toxicity, but the data are inconclusive. Pancreatitis has been reported, particularly with didanosine and stavudine. Peripheral neuropathy, characterized by numbness, pain, or burning in the extremities, sometimes limits therapy with didanosine, zalcitabine, and stavudine.

PROTOTYPE DRUG Zidovudine (Retrovir, AZT)

Classification: **Therapeutic:** Antiretroviral

Pharmacologic: Nucleoside reverse transcriptase inhibitor (NRTI)

Therapeutic Effects and Uses: Zidovudine was first discovered in the 1960s and its antiviral activity was demonstrated prior to the AIDS epidemic. It was approved by the U.S. Food and Drug Administration (FDA) in 1987 for both symptomatic and asymptomatic HIV-infected patients, as well as for postexposure prophylaxis in HIV-exposed health care workers (see Section 56.8). An important indication is to reduce the transmission rate of HIV from an HIV-positive mother to her fetus (see Section 56.9).

Because of its widespread use since the beginning of the AIDS epidemic, HIV strains resistant to zidovudine are common. It is estimated that one third of patients receiving zidovudine will develop resistant HIV strains after 1 year of therapy. Although used as monotherapy during the first decade of the AIDS epidemic, zidovudine is usually prescribed in combination with other antiretrovirals, since this slows the development of resistance and allows HIV to be attacked by several different mechanisms. Most treatment guidelines do not include zidovudine as a drug of first choice due to the potential for resistance. Combination products containing zidovudine include Combivir (zidovudine and lamivudine) and Trizivir (zidovudine, lamivudine, and abacavir).

Mechanism of Action: Structurally, zidovudine resembles thymidine, one of four nucleoside building blocks of DNA. As the reverse transcriptase enzyme begins to synthesize viral DNA, it mistakenly uses zidovudine instead of thymidine, thus terminating the growing chain and creating a defective proviral DNA strand.

Pharmacokinetics:

Route(s)	Intravenous (IV), oral (PO)
Absorption	Readily absorbed
Distribution	Widely distributed, including the cerebrospinal fluid (CSF); secreted in breast milk
Primary metabolism	Hepatic
Primary excretion	Renal
Onset of action	Peak effect: 1–2 h
Duration of action	Half-life: 1 h

Adverse Effects: Zidovudine can cause severe toxicity to bone marrow at high doses; anemia and neutropenia are common and may limit therapy. Many patients experience anorexia, nausea, and diarrhea. Patients may report fatigue, myalgia, and generalized weakness. Headache will occur in the majority of patients taking zidovudine, and more serious central nervous system (CNS) effects have been reported. It is often difficult to determine if adverse effects are due to zidovudine, other drugs the patient is taking concurrently, or the progression of HIV-AIDS illness. Rare cases of fatal lactic acidosis have been reported with zidovudine use.

Contraindications/Precautions: Because zidovudine can suppress bone marrow function after 4 to 6 weeks of therapy, it should be used with caution in patients with preexisting anemia or neutropenia. Blood counts and other laboratory blood tests should be monitored frequently during therapy to prevent hematologic toxicity. Patients with significant renal or hepatic impairment require a reduction in dosage, as zidovudine may accumulate to toxic levels in these patients. Breast-feeding should be suspended because both the virus and the drug may be transmitted through breast milk. Discontinuation of therapy should always be conducted under the guidance of a health care provider.

Drug Interactions: Zidovudine interacts with many drugs. Concurrent administration with other drugs that depress bone marrow function, such as ganciclovir, interferon-alfa, dapsone, flucytosine, or vincristine should be avoided due to cumulative immunosuppression. Stavudine, ribavirin, and doxorubicin compete for intracellular activation sites and will diminish the effects of zidovudine. Probenecid, fluconazole, atovaquone, valproic acid, amphotericin B, and aspirin increase the blood levels of zidovudine and may increase adverse effects from the antiretroviral. Other antiretroviral agents may contribute to the lactic acidosis and hepatomegaly caused by zidovudine. **Herbal/Food:** Zidovudine should be used with caution with herbal supplements such as St. John's wort, which may cause a decrease in antiretroviral activity.

Pregnancy: Category C.

Treatment of Overdose: No specific therapy is available; patients are treated symptomatically.

Nursing Responsibilities:

- Obtain a complete health history including allergies, drug history, and possible drug interactions.
- Perform a complete physical examination and assess for the presence or history of HIV infection.

- Monitor laboratory tests such as complete blood count (CBC), CD4 lymphocyte count, hemoglobin, and granulocyte count to detect potential hematologic toxicity.
- Observe for signs and symptoms of myelosuppression such as anemia and neutropenia, commonly occurring after 4 to 6 weeks of therapy. Note any granulocytopenia within 6 to 8 weeks. Both of these conditions respond to dosage adjustment.
- Monitor for adverse reactions such as nausea, severe headache, insomnia, and myalgia.
- Report anorexia, nausea, and diarrhea to the prescriber. Treat these adverse effects with supportive care.
- Assess for signs and symptoms of OIs, which may indicate treatment failure.

Patient and Family Education:

- Immediately report symptoms of infection such as sore throat, swollen lymph nodes, malaise, or fever to the health care provider.
- Understand that this medication is not a cure for HIV infection, and it does not prevent the spread of HIV to others through sexual contact or blood contamination (e.g., sharing used needles).
- Take HIV-AIDS drugs exactly as ordered and never share prescribed drugs with others.
- Inform the health care provider prior to using any herbal supplements. Herbal supplements such as St. John's wort may decrease the effectiveness of the antiretroviral medication.
- Do not breast-feed while taking this drug without approval of the health care provider.
- Do not discontinue taking this medication without approval of the health care provider.
- Immediately notify the health care provider of any known or suspected pregnancy.

Drugs Similar to Zidovudine (Retrovir, AZT)

Other NRTIs include abacavir, didanosine, emtricitabine, lamivudine, stavudine, and tenofovir. All of the NRTIs are used in combination with other antiretrovirals. Fixed-dose combinations with NRTIs include Combivir (zidovudine and lamivudine), Trizivir (zidovudine, lamivudine, and abacavir), Truvada (tenofovir and emtricitabine), Atripla (emtricitabine, tenofovir, and efavirenz), and Epzicom (abacavir and lamivudine). Zalcitabine (ddC, Hivid) has been discontinued in the United States.

Abacavir (Ziagen): Abacavir chemically resembles the natural nucleoside guanosine, and is indicated for the treatment of HIV infection as part of a multidrug regimen. Approved in 1998, it is given orally once daily and is widely distributed throughout the body, including the CSF. Abacavir is a drug of choice for HIV treatment.

The most common adverse effects are gastrointestinal (GI) related, and include nausea, vomiting, anorexia, and diarrhea. Alcohol use during abacavir therapy should be avoided, as blood levels of the antiretroviral can increase as much as 40%. The most serious concern during abacavir therapy is the development of a unique hypersensitivity syndrome that occurs in 4% to 6% of patients taking the drug. Symptoms, which include fever, rash, dyspnea, cough, or GI distress, occur within the first 6 weeks of treatment. It is essential that these symptoms be monitored and the medication immediately discontinued should allergy be suspected, as deaths have been recorded from this syndrome. Rare cases of fatal lactic acidosis have been reported with abacavir. Cross resistance is common among the NRTIs. This drug is pregnancy category C.

Didanosine (ddI, Videx EC): Approved in 1991, didanosine chemically resembles the naturally occurring nucleoside inosine and is indicated for the treatment of HIV infection as part of a multidrug regimen. An off-label indication is for HIV prophylaxis following suspected occupational exposure to HIV. Given orally once daily, it should be administered on an empty stomach to enhance absorption. The buffered form of didanosine (Videx) was discontinued in 2006. The drug is not widely distributed, and most is excreted unchanged in the urine. Didanosine is not a preferred drug for treating HIV.

Diarrhea and peripheral neuropathy involving numbness and tingling in the hands and feet are common adverse effects occurring in over 20% of patients taking the drug. Of greatest concern is pancreatitis, which is a serious adverse effect that occurs in up to 10% of the patients taking the drug. Patients should be carefully monitored for signs and symptoms that may suggest pancreatitis, such as nausea, vomiting, elevated serum amylase, and increased serum triglycerides because deaths have occurred due to this disorder. Rare cases of fatal lactic acidosis have been reported with didanosine. This drug is pregnancy category B.

Emtricitabine (Emtriva): Approved in 2003, emtricitabine is a cytosine analog, also known as FTC, which is approved for the treatment of HIV infection as part of a multidrug regimen. Although chemically similar to lamivudine, it has the advantages of once-daily dosing and fewer adverse effects. The most frequently reported adverse effects are nausea, headache, skin rash, and skin discoloration on the palms and soles. Of the NRTIs, emtricitabine is believed to have the least mitochondrial toxicity. This drug should not be administered to patients coinfected with HBV because severe exacerbations of hepatitis B symptoms may occur after discontinuation of emtricitabine. Emtricitabine is one of the preferred drugs for initial HIV therapy. This drug is pregnancy category B.

Lamivudine (Epivir): Also known as 3TC, lamivudine is a chemical analog of cytosine, a naturally occurring nucleoside. Approved in 1995, lamivudine is rapidly absorbed orally, and distributed to most body tissues. Better tolerated than most NRTIs, minor adverse effects include transient insomnia and headache. Because significant adverse effects from lamivudine are rare, it is one of the most widely used components of HAART regimens. An off-label indication is for HIV prophylaxis following perinatal or suspected occupational exposure to HIV. Its primary disadvantage is rapid emergence of resistance. As with other drugs in this class, rare cases of fatal lactic acidosis have been reported with lamivudine. This drug is also approved for treatment of hepatitis B (Epivir HBV), and is featured as a prototype drug in Chapter 55. This drug is pregnancy category C.

MyNursingKit | Mechanism of Action Animation: Zidovudine

Stavudine (d4T, Zerit): Approved in 1994, stavudine is a chemical analog of thymidine, a naturally occurring nucleoside that is approved for the treatment of HIV infection as part of a multidrug regimen. An extended release formulation (Zerit XR) was approved in 2002. An off-label indication is for HIV prophylaxis following suspected occupational exposure to HIV. The drug is given orally and is distributed to most compartments, including CSF. Once one of the most frequently prescribed NRTIs, the use of stavudine has declined because the drug exhibits greater mitochondrial toxicity than others in this class. Of special concern is a high degree of lipodystrophy, evidenced by excessive loss of fat tissue, which persists long after the drug is discontinued. Headache and peripheral neuropathy occur in 50% or more of patients taking the drug. Pancreatitis is also possible, but occurs less frequently than with didanosine. This drug is pregnancy category C.

Tenofovir (Viread): Approved in 2001, tenofovir is a nucleotide reverse transcriptase inhibitor (NtRTI), structurally similar to adenosine monophosphate (AMP), which is approved for the treatment of HIV infection as part of a multidrug regimen. Other than having an extra phosphate group, nucleotides are the same as nucleosides, and tenofovir has the same actions on reverse transcriptase as the NRTIs. Tenofovir is administered orally on an empty stomach to increase absorption. Tenofovir is a drug of choice for the initial treatment of HIV.

The most frequently reported adverse effects of tenofovir are nausea, vomiting, and diarrhea. Tenofovir has less effect on mitochondrial enzymes than other drugs in this class; thus, it is better tolerated. Because the drug can lower bone mineral density, patients may be at risk for osteopenia or bone fractures. Due to nephrotoxicity, the use of tenofovir in patients with renal impairment should be carefully monitored, and it should be used cautiously in patients receiving other nephrotoxic drugs. This drug should not be administered to patients coinfected with HBV because severe exacerbations of hepatitis B symptoms may occur after discontinuation of tenofovir. This drug is pregnancy category B.

56.5 The nonnucleoside reverse transcriptase inhibitors inhibit viral DNA replication by binding to reverse transcriptase.

The four nonnucleoside reverse transcriptase inhibitors (NNRTIs) act by a mechanism distinct from the NRTIs. Drugs in this class bind in close proximity to the active site of reverse transcriptase, causing a change in shape of the enzyme molecule. Because of this structural change, reverse transcriptase is unable to add more nucleotides to the proviral DNA chain, resulting in a direct inhibition of enzyme function.

If used as monotherapy, resistance develops rapidly to NNRTIs; thus, they are always used in combination with other antiretrovirals. In fact, a single mutation to an HIV gene can result in resistance to all drugs in this class. However, cross resistance between NNRTIs and drugs from other antiretroviral classes does not occur.

The NNRTIs are generally well tolerated and exhibit few serious adverse effects. The adverse effects are different than the NRTIs. Rash is common with NNRTIs and rare cases of Stevens–Johnson syndrome (SJS) have been reported. Most affect hepatic metabolism, increasing the risk of drug–drug interactions. Liver function should be regularly assessed, especially in patients with preexisting liver disease.

PROTOTYPE DRUG Efavirenz (Sustiva)

Classification: **Therapeutic:** Antiretroviral
Pharmacologic: Nonnucleoside reverse transcriptase inhibitor

Therapeutic Effects and Uses: Approved in 1998, efavirenz is given orally in combination with other antiretrovirals in the treatment of HIV infection. Efavirenz has the advantage of once-daily dosing and penetration into the CSF. Efavirenz is a drug of choice for the initial therapy of HIV infection.

Resistance to NNRTIs can develop rapidly and cross resistance among drugs in this class can occur. High-fat meals increase the absorption by as much as 50% and may cause toxicity. Because of this, efavirenz should be taken on an empty stomach. Atripla is a fixed-dose combination of three antiretroviral drugs: efavirenz, emtricitabine, and tenofovir.

Mechanism of Action: Efavirenz binds directly to reverse transcriptase, disrupting the shape of the enzyme's active site. This inhibition prevents viral DNA from being synthesized from HIV RNA.

Pharmacokinetics:

Route(s)	PO
Absorption	Readily absorbed
Distribution	Widely distributed, including the CSF; unknown if secreted in breast milk; 99% bound to plasma protein
Primary metabolism	Hepatic (CYP3A4 and CYP2B6)
Primary excretion	Renal
Onset of action	Peak effect: 3–5 h
Duration of action	Half-life: 52–76 h

Adverse Effects: CNS adverse effects are observed in at least 50% of the patients when first initiating therapy, including sleep disorders, nightmares, dizziness, reduced ability to concentrate, and delusions. These symptoms gradually diminish after 3 to 4 weeks of therapy. Like other drugs in this class, rash is common and must be monitored carefully. Efavirenz is a known teratogen in laboratory animals and must not be given to pregnant patients.

Contraindications/Precautions: Patients in the childbearing years should be advised to use reliable methods of birth control to avoid pregnancy.

Drug Interactions: Efavirenz induces CYP3A4 and can interact with drugs that are substrates for, or antagonists of, this isozyme. Patients who are receiving antiepileptic medications metabolized by the liver, such as carbamazepine, phenytoin, and phenobarbital, may require periodic monitoring of plasma levels because efavirenz may increase the incidence of seizures. Efavirenz can decrease serum levels of the following: statins, methadone, sertraline, and calcium channel blockers. The CNS adverse effects of efavirenz are worsened if the patient takes psychotropic drugs or consumes alcohol. Levels of warfarin may either increase or decrease. **Herbal/Food:** Efavirenz should be used with caution with herbal supplements, such as St. John's wort, which may cause a decrease in antiretroviral activity.

Pregnancy: Category D.

Treatment of Overdose: No specific therapy is available; patients are treated symptomatically.

Nursing Responsibilities:

- Obtain a complete health history including allergies, drug history, and possible drug interactions.
- Perform a complete physical examination and assess for the presence or history of HIV infection.
- Assess weight, temperature, and respiratory status throughout the drug therapy.
- Monitor for suicidal ideation in patients who are depressed, or who have a history of depression.
- Use bedtime dosing to increase tolerability of CNS adverse effects.
- Monitor GI status and evaluate the patient's ability to maintain a normal diet.
- Obtain periodic liver function and lipid profile tests.
- Assess for signs and symptoms of OIs, which may indicate treatment failure.

Patient and Family Education:

- Immediately report any of the following to the health care provider: skin rash, delusions, inappropriate behavior, or thoughts of suicide.
- Immediately report symptoms of infection such as sore throat, swollen lymph nodes, malaise, or fever to the health care provider.
- Understand that this medication is not a cure for HIV infection, and it does not prevent the spread of HIV to others through sexual contact or blood contamination (e.g., sharing used needles).
- Use barrier contraception if using a hormonal contraceptive.
- Do not discontinue taking this medication without approval of the health care provider because HIV symptoms may worsen.
- Do not drive or perform other hazardous activities until the effects of the drug are known because this drug may cause drowsiness or dizziness.
- Do not breast-feed while taking this drug because both the drug and HIV may be secreted in breast milk.
- Immediately notify the health care provider of any known or suspected pregnancy.

Drugs Similar to Efavirenz (Sustiva)

Other NNRTIs include delavirdine, etravirine, and nevirapine.

Delavirdine (Rescriptor): Approved in 1997, delavirdine is given orally and is very similar to other NNRTIs in actions and adverse effects. It is the least commonly prescribed NNRTI because it must be administered three times per day and does not appear to be as effective as nevirapine or efavirenz. Over 30% of the patients taking this drug develop a skin rash. In most cases, this rash disappears after several weeks of therapy, but it must be monitored carefully, as cases of SJS have been reported in patients receiving this drug. GI distress, headache, and fatigue are also common adverse effects. Because delavirdine can decrease hepatic metabolism, many drug–drug interactions are possible, including those listed for efavirenz. This drug is pregnancy category C.

Etravirine (Intelence): Approved in 2008, etravirine is one of the newest antiretrovirals. Like other NNRTIs, it is used in combination with other oral drugs in the pharmacotherapy of HIV. Because the fasting state can increase absorption of the drug significantly and cause potential toxicity, it should always be taken following a meal. It is excreted primarily in the feces; therefore, no dose adjustment is necessary in patients with renal impairment. Because etravirine can decrease hepatic metabolism, many drug–drug interactions are possible, including those listed for efavirenz. The drug does not exhibit the hepatotoxicity of nevirapine, nor the CNS toxicity of efavirenz. The drug is generally well tolerated, with the most frequently reported adverse effect being rash. This drug is pregnancy category B.

Nevirapine (Viramune): Nevirapine was the first drug in this class, approved in 1996, for the treatment of HIV infection in combination with other antiretroviral agents. Nevirapine is metabolized in the liver by the P450 system. By inducing P450 enzymes, nevirapine increases its own breakdown; thus, dosage may need to be increased after several weeks of therapy to maintain its effectiveness. In addition, because the metabolism of protease inhibitors is decreased, dosage adjustments in these antiretrovirals may be necessary. While efavirenz exhibits a high incidence of CNS effects such as dizziness and fatigue, these symptoms are rare in patients taking nevirapine. Unlike some other antiretrovirals that negatively impact lipid metabolism, nevirapine actually improves the lipid profiles of many patients by increasing HDL. Common adverse effects include nausea, diarrhea, fever, fatigue, and rash, which is occasionally severe enough to require discontinuation of therapy. During the first 18 weeks of therapy, the patient should be carefully monitored for hepatic function because potentially life-threatening hepatotoxicity has occurred with nevirapine. Patients with a history of hepatitis or other liver disease are at greater risk for nevirapine-induced hepatotoxicity. This drug is pregnancy category C.

56.6 Protease inhibitors prevent HIV protease from completing the final step in HIV maturation.

Near the end of its replication cycle, HIV has assembled all the necessary components to create new virions. As the newly formed virions bud from the host cell and are released into the surrounding extracellular fluid, one final step remains before the HIV matures and becomes infectious: A long polypeptide chain must be cleaved to produce the final HIV proteins. The enzyme performing this step is HIV protease.

Drugs in the protease inhibitor (PI) class attach to the active site of HIV protease, thus preventing the final synthesis of HIV proteins. Without this final step in HIV maturation, the virions are noninfectious. When combined with other antiretroviral drug classes in a HAART regimen, the PIs are capable of lowering plasma HIV RNA levels to an undetectable range. When introduced in 1995, the PIs revolutionized the treatment of HIV-AIDS.

PIs are metabolized in the liver and induce hepatic enzymes; thus, they have the potential to interact with numerous medications. In general, they are well tolerated, with GI complaints being the most common adverse effects. Lipodystrophies have been reported, including elevated cholesterol and triglyceride levels, and abdominal obesity. Some of the PIs are associated with hyperglycemia and can cause diabetes or worsen existing diabetes. Blood glucose should be monitored regularly in patients taking PIs.

The available PIs are very similar but there are some noticeable differences in pharmacokinetic properties and adverse effect profiles. Overall, they are very similar. The Panel on Antiretroviral Guidelines for Adults and Adolescents recommends the use of atazanavir, fosamprenavir, or lopinavir (all combined with ritonavir) as drugs of choice for the initial treatment of HIV. Choice of PI therapy is based upon the patient's individual clinical response and the experience of the clinician. Cross resistance among the PIs has been reported.

The initial choice of a primary PI most often includes low doses of ritonavir. Addition of small amounts of ritonavir allows less frequent dosing intervals and increases the plasma concentration of the primary PI. This is known as ritonavir boosting.

PROTOTYPE DRUG Lopinavir with ritonavir (Kaletra)

Classification: Therapeutic: Antiretroviral
Pharmacologic: Protease inhibitor

Therapeutic Effects and Uses: Approved in 2000, Kaletra is a combination drug containing the protease inhibitors lopinavir and ritonavir. Lopinavir is the active component of the combination. Ritonavir inhibits the hepatic breakdown of lopinavir, thus permitting serum levels of lopinavir to increase by more than 100-fold. Kaletra tablets may be taken with or without food, but the oral solution form should be taken with a meal to enhance absorption. It has an extended half-life that allows for once- or twice-daily dosing.

Resistance to lopinavir/ritonavir has been reported in patients treated with other protease inhibitors prior to Kaletra therapy. Kaletra is a drug of choice for the initial therapy of HIV infection.

Mechanism of Action: By effectively inhibiting HIV protease, the final step in the assembly of an infectious HIV virion is prevented.

Pharmacokinetics:

Route(s)	PO
Absorption	Readily absorbed (but quickly destroyed through hepatic first-pass metabolism)
Distribution	Widely distributed; 98% bound to plasma proteins
Primary metabolism	Hepatic (lopinavir is metabolized by CYP3A; ritonavir inhibits CYP3A)
Primary excretion	Renal (10%); feces (83%)
Onset of action	Peak effect: 3–4 h
Duration of action	Half-life: 5–6 h

Adverse Effects: Kaletra is well tolerated by most patients, and the most frequently reported problem is diarrhea. Headache and GI-related effects are common, including nausea, vomiting, dyspepsia, and abdominal pain. Kaletra may cause or worsen symptoms of diabetes mellitus, and hyperglycemia has been reported. Lipodystrophy syndrome occurs in many patients receiving long-term therapy with PIs and large increases in total cholesterol and triglycerides may occur during therapy. This syndrome is associated with hyperglycemia and fat redistribution. Pancreatitis is a rare, though potentially fatal, adverse event.

Contraindications/Precautions: Because of its extensive hepatic metabolism, patients with liver impairment, especially those with preexisting viral hepatitis, should be carefully monitored. Hepatic enzyme levels should be regularly evaluated in these patients to prevent hepatic failure. Patients with diabetes should be monitored regularly because Kaletra may exacerbate this condition. Breast-feeding is contraindicated due to the potential risk of transmitting HIV to the newborn.

Drug Interactions: Lopinavir is extensively metabolized by hepatic enzymes, and drugs that undergo hepatic metabolism may interact with Kaletra. Drugs that increase hepatic P450 enzymes will reduce the effectiveness of the antiretroviral. These include nevirapine, efavirenz, barbiturates, rifampin, rifabutin, phenytoin, and carbamazepine. Conversely, drugs that inhibit the P450 enzymes will increase levels of lopinavir, including aldesleukin, ketoconazole, delavirdine, indinavir, and ritonavir. Statins should not be administered with Kaletra due to an increased risk for myopathy. Concurrent use of rifampin may lower the effectiveness of Kaletra. Potentially life-threatening dysrhythmias may occur if Kaletra is used concurrently with cisapride, pimozide, and certain other antidysrhythmic agents. Kaletra may increase adverse effects associated with selective serotonin reuptake inhibitors (SSRIs), tricyclic antidepressants, and phenothiazines. **Herbal/Food:** St. John's wort should be used with caution, as it may decrease antiretroviral activity.

Pregnancy: Category C.

Treatment of Overdose: No specific therapy is available; patients are treated symptomatically.

Nursing Responsibilities:

- Obtain a complete health history including allergies, drug history, and possible drug interactions.
- Perform a complete physical examination and assess for the presence or history of HIV infection.
- Assess weight, temperature, and respiratory status throughout therapy.
- Administer this drug at evenly spaced intervals because it is most effective when the amount of drug is kept at a constant level.
- Monitor the following: fasting lipid panel at baseline 3 to 6 months after the new regimen starts, then annually or more frequently if baseline levels are abnormal; liver function tests at baseline, then every 3 to 4 months or more frequently if high risk; uric acid at baseline, then periodically; fasting blood glucose 1 to 3 months after new regimen start, then at least every 3 to 6 months thereafter.

- Monitor for the most common adverse reaction, which is diarrhea. Generally, it occurs with mild to moderate severity.
- Monitor blood glucose with diabetic patients because Kaletra may cause or worsen symptoms of diabetes mellitus, and hyperglycemia has been reported.
- Assess for signs and symptoms of OIs, which may indicate treatment failure.

Patient and Family Education:

- Understand that this medication is not a cure for HIV infection, and it does not prevent the spread of HIV to others through sexual contact or blood contamination (e.g., sharing used needles).
- Swallow the tablets whole. Do not crush, break, or chew the tablets.
- Immediately report any of the following to the health care provider: diarrhea, nausea, vomiting, stomach upset, headache, and insomnia.
- Use an additional form of reliable birth control because this medication may decrease the effectiveness of combination-type birth control pills.
- Report changes in body fat while taking this medication (e.g., increased fat in the upper back and stomach areas, decreased fat in the arms and legs) to the health care provider.
- Avoid drinking alcohol while taking this medicine. Lopinavir and ritonavir oral liquid contains a large portion of alcohol.
- Do not take any other prescription or nonprescription medications, dietary supplements, or herbal products without approval of the health care provider.
- Do not discontinue taking this medication without the approval of the health care provider because HIV symptoms may worsen.
- Immediately notify the health care provider of any known or suspected pregnancy.

Drugs Similar to Lopinavir with Ritonavir (Kaletra)

Other PIs include atazanavir, darunavir, fosamprenavir indinavir, nelfinavir, ritonavir, saquinavir, and tipranavir. Amprenavir (Agenerase) has been discontinued in the United States.

Atazanavir (Reyataz): Approved in 2003, atazanavir offers the advantages of once- or twice-daily dosing and fewer adverse effects on lipid levels than other PIs. Along with fosamprenavir and lopinavir, atazanavir is a preferred drug in the initial pharmacotherapy of HIV infection. Pharmacologic boosting of atazanavir with low doses of ritonavir is recommended. Headache and nausea are common adverse effects. Atazanavir increases bilirubin levels in up to 50% of patients taking the drug. Although this does not seem to be associated with liver disease, liver function tests should be regularly monitored during therapy. Atazanavir has been shown to prolong the PR interval of the electrocardiogram (ECG) and produce first-degree atrioventricular block and other conduction abnormalities. Concurrent administration with indinavir can increase the risk of jaundice. Atazanavir may cause hyperglycemia and worsen the symptoms of diabetes. Other adverse effects, contraindications, and drug interactions are similar to those of lopinavir. This drug is pregnancy category B.

Darunavir (Prezista): Approved in 2006, darunavir is a second-generation PI that is indicated for the treatment of HIV infection in treatment-experienced adults, such as those infected with HIV strains resistant to more than one PI. Although cross resistance has been reported, darunavir retains some activity against viral strains resistant to other PIs. Darunavir should be concurrently administered with ritonavir and used as a component of HAART. Because both darunavir and ritonavir decrease hepatic metabolism, numerous drug–drug interactions are possible. Darunavir should be administered with food to increase its absorption. Diarrhea, nausea, headache, and nasopharyngitis are the most common adverse effects. Hepatic enzymes should be monitored to prevent developing hepatotoxicity. Severe rashes are possible, and these often call for discontinuation of therapy. Other adverse effects, contraindications, and drug interactions are similar to those of lopinavir. This drug is pregnancy category B.

Fosamprenavir (Lexiva): Approved in 2003, fosamprenavir is an HIV PI that is almost always administered with low doses of ritonavir as a booster. Fosamprenavir is a preferred drug in the initial pharmacotherapy of HIV infection. Both tablet and oral solution formulations are available and fosamprenavir may be taken with or without food. Like other PIs, fosamprenavir affects the hepatic metabolism of many drugs, making interactions likely. The drug can cause hyperglycemia and thus should be used cautiously in diabetic patients. Other adverse effects, contraindications, and drug interactions are similar to those of lopinavir. This drug is pregnancy category C.

Indinavir (Crixivan): Approved in 1996, indinavir is a PI used to treat HIV infection and for HIV postexposure prophlaxis. It is administered PO, usually with a high-fat meal to increase drug absorption. It has a short half-life that requires three doses per day. Boosting with low doses of ritonavir is recommended. Like other PIs, indinavir should be used cautiously in diabetic patients due to the risk of hyperglycemia. The most serious potential adverse effect is the formation of crystals in the urine, causing nephrolithiasis, which is unique among the protease inhibitors. Renal function should be monitored regularly and the patient should be encouraged to consume adequate amounts of fluid to dilute the urine in order to prevent crystalluria. Because indinavir can decrease the hepatic metabolism of drugs, numerous drug–drug interactions are possible. This drug is pregnancy category C.

Nelfinavir (Viracept): Approved in 1997, nelfinavir was one of the most frequently used PIs for many years. Its use has declined because newer PIs offer a lower pill burden and fewer adverse effects. Nelfinavir is given orally, usually with meals, in order to increase drug absorption. Unlike some other antiretrovirals, nelfinavir is 98% bound to plasma proteins and excreted almost entirely in the feces. Because large amounts of the drug and its metabolites reach the colon, severe diarrhea occurs in about one in four patients. Antidiarrheal medications may be indicated.

Patients taking oral contraceptives should be advised to use other methods of birth control, as nelfinavir decreases plasma levels of ethinyl estradiol. Diabetic patients should be monitored carefully due to the hyperglycemic effect of the antiretroviral. This drug is pregnancy category B.

Ritonavir (Norvir): Approved in 1995, ritonavir is well absorbed orally, and is available in both capsule and solution formulations. Because of low tolerability, the use of ritonavir is now almost entirely limited to boosting the function of other PIs. The drug undergoes extensive hepatic metabolism and is excreted primarily in the feces. Like other PIs, ritonavir inhibits P450 hepatic metabolizing enzymes, which reduces the elimination of many drugs. This is used to advantage in dual PI regimens. Giving low doses of ritonavir as a "boost" to increase serum levels of other PIs permits lower doses of the second PI. Ritonavir increases several other drug metabolizing enzymes in the liver; therefore, drug–drug interactions are common.

Most adverse effects of ritonavir are GI related and may limit therapy. Peripheral and perioral paresthesias are possible. Because ritonavir induces enzymes that increase its own metabolism, its effectiveness will diminish unless doses are increased. This drug is pregnancy category B.

MyNursingKit | Mechanism of Action Animation: Saquinavir

Saquinavir (Invirase): Saquinavir was the original protease inhibitor approved by the FDA in 1995. Recently, an improved formulation of Invirase was developed, allowing for twice-daily dosing. When combined with ritonavir, saquinavir serum levels increase, making the drug more effective. Resistance to saquinavir develops with continued use, and may include cross resistance with other PIs. Saquinavir is well tolerated by most patients, and the most frequently reported problems are GI related, such as nausea, vomiting, dyspepsia, and diarrhea. Other adverse effects are similar to those of lopinavir. Because of its extensive hepatic metabolism, patients with liver impairment should be carefully monitored. This drug is pregnancy category B.

Tipranavir (Aptivus): Approved in 2005, tipranavir shares many characteristics with other drugs in this class. It should always be administered with ritonavir as a booster and it should be taken with food, because high-fat meals will significantly enhance absorption. Tipranavir administered concurrently with enfuvirtide shows activity against HIV strains resistant to other PIs. Because a small number of patients taking this drug have developed liver damage, hepatic function tests should be monitored frequently throughout the duration of treatment. Caution should be used when prescribing tipranavir to patients with elevated transaminases, hepatitis, or other preexisting hepatic impairment. Tipranavir contains sulfur and should be used with caution in patients with allergies to sulfa drugs. Like other PIs, tipranavir may be associated with the development or worsening of diabetes, elevations in cholesterol and triglycerides, and lipodystrophies. Tipranavir has been associated with reports of intracranial hemorrhage. Tipranavir inhibits platelet aggregation and should be used with caution in patients who may be at risk of increased bleeding from trauma, surgery, or other medical conditions, or who are receiving anticoagulants or antiplatelet agents. This drug is pregnancy category C.

56.7 Fusion inhibitors, integrase inhibitors, and CCR5 inhibitors are newer strategies for treating HIV infections.

Because HIV develops resistance to most of the frequently prescribed antiretrovirals, scientists have been looking intensively for unique mechanisms of drug action. In recent years, three such mechanisms have been discovered. Because these drugs are so new, their role in treating HIV infection is evolving.

Fusion inhibitors: In 2003, the FDA approved the first fusion inhibitor. These drugs interfere with the fusion of viral and cellular membranes, thus blocking the entry of HIV into its host cell.

Enfuvirtide (Fuzeon) was welcomed by the medical community as a novel way to attack a key component of the HIV replication cycle. Patients resistant to all other antiretroviral classes are still sensitive to the effects of the fusion inhibitor. Enfuvirtide is given by subcutaneous injection, twice daily. It does not affect hepatic metabolizing enzymes. Its current use is for treating HIV infection in treatment-experienced patients or those with strains that are resistant to other antiretrovirals. Almost every patient taking enfuvirtide will experience an injection site reaction, usually during the first week of therapy. These reactions may involve severe pain, pruritus, erythema, cysts, abscesses, and cellulitis. Nausea, diarrhea, and fatigue are other common adverse effects. Patients should be carefully monitored for lung infections because an increased incidence of pneumonia has been reported in patients taking enfuvirtide. A major advantage is that no significant drug interactions have been found with enfuvirtide. This drug is pregnancy category B.

Integrase inhibitors: In 2007, the FDA approved the first in a new class of antiretroviral drugs called the integrase inhibitors. HIV requires the integrase enzyme to insert its viral DNA into the human chromosome.

Raltegravir (Isentress) PO tablets are indicated for combination therapy with other antiretroviral agents for the treatment of HIV infection in treatment-experienced adult patients who have evidence of viral replication and for strains resistant to multiple antiretroviral agents. Headache and GI-related symptoms such as diarrhea and nausea are the most frequently reported adverse effects. It may be administered with or without food. This drug is pregnancy category C.

CCR5 inhibitors: To enter into human cells, HIV must interact with receptors. CCR5 is the name of one of the coreceptors required for entry. Blocking CCR5 significantly reduces viral load and increases T-cell production.

Maraviroc (Selzentry) PO tablets are indicated for combination therapy with other antiretrovirals in treatment-experienced patients who have evidence of viral replication and strains resistant to multiple antiretroviral agents. The most frequently reported adverse effects are abdominal pain, cough, dizziness, musculoskeletal symptoms, pyrexia, rash, and upper respiratory tract infections. Hepatoxicity has been reported with maraviroc. Caution should be used when administering this drug to patients with preexisting cardiac disease because the drug may increase the risk for myocardial ischemia or infarction. It may be administered with or without food. This drug is pregnancy category B.

NURSING PROCESS APPLICATION

Patients Receiving Antiretroviral Agents

Assessment

Prior to drug administration:

- Obtain a complete health history including allergies, drug history, and possible drug interactions.
- Obtain a complete physical examination.
- Assess for the presence or history of HIV infection.
- Obtain the following laboratory studies: HIV RNA assay / CD4 count, CBC, liver function, renal function, and blood glucose.

Potential Nursing Diagnoses

- *Risk for Infection,* related to compromised immune system
- *Decisional Conflict (Therapeutic Regimen)*
- *Fear,* related to HIV diagnosis
- *Risk for Injury,* related to adverse effects of medications
- *Deficient Knowledge (HIV),* related to disease process, transmission, and treatment
- *Deficient Knowledge (Antiretroviral Agents),* related to purpose, precautions, and adverse effects of drug therapy

Planning: Patient Goals and Expected Outcomes

The patient will:

- Exhibit a decrease in viral load and an increase in CD4 counts.
- Demonstrate knowledge of the disease process, transmission, and treatment.
- Identify adverse effects and report to the health care provider.
- Complete a full course of therapy and adhere to follow-up care.

Implementation

Interventions and (Rationales)	Patient and Family Education
• Monitor for symptoms of hypersensitivity reactions. (Many antiretrovirals may cause anaphylactic reactions.)	• Instruct the patient to discontinue the medication and inform the health care provider if symptoms of hypersensitivity reaction develop such as wheezing, shortness of breath, swelling of face, tongue or hands, itching, or rash.
• Monitor temperature and WBC and for symptoms of infection. Protect the patient from sources of infection. (Some antiretroviral drugs, such as delavirdine, may cause neutropenia.)	Instruct the patient: • To report symptoms of infections such as fever, chills, sore throat, and cough. • On methods to minimize exposure to infection such as washing hands frequently; avoiding crowds and people with colds, flu, and other infections; limiting exposure to children and animals; increasing fluid intake; emptying the bladder frequently; and coughing and deep breathing several times per day.
• Monitor the patient for signs of stomatitis. (Immunosuppression may result in the proliferation of oral bacteria.)	• Advise the patient to recognize and report any mouth ulcers.
• Monitor blood pressure. (Some antiretoviral agents such as abacavir may cause a significant decrease in blood pressure.)	Instruct the patient to: • Rise slowly from a lying or sitting to minimize effects of postural hypotension. • Report changes in blood pressure.
• Monitor HIV RNA assay, CD4 T-cell counts, liver function, kidney function, CBC, blood glucose, and serum amylase and triglyceride levels. (These tests will determine the effectiveness and toxicities of the medication.)	Instruct the patient: • On the purpose of required laboratory tests and schedule follow-up with the health care provider. • To monitor weight and presence of swelling. • To keep appointments for laboratory work.
• Determine the potential drug–drug and drug–food interactions. (Antiretroviral medications produce multiple drug–drug interactions and must be taken exactly as prescribed.) • Saquinavir should be taken with high fat meals or within 2 hours of a full meal. • Ritonavir is unpalatable and can be taken with chocolate milk, nutritional supplement, or food. • Indinavir requires an acidic gastric environment for absorption, and should be taken 1 hour before or 2 hours after a light, low-fat snack.	Instruct the patient: • When to take the specific medication in relationship to food intake (before meals, with meals, or after meals). • About foods or beverages to avoid when taking medication; some antiretrovirals should not be taken with acidic fruit juice. • To take medication exactly as directed. Do not skip any doses. • To consult with the health care provider before taking any OTC medications or dietary supplements.
• Monitor for symptoms of pancreatitis including severe abdominal pain, nausea, vomiting, and abdominal distention. (Some antiretroviral agents such as didanosine may cause pancreatitis.)	• Instruct the patient to immediately report fever, severe abdominal pain, nausea or vomiting, abdominal distention.
• Monitor skin for rash; withhold medication and notify the prescriber at the first sign of rash. (Several antiretroviral medications may cause SJS, which may be fatal).	• Advise the patient to check the skin frequently and notify the health care provider at first sign of any rash.
• Establish a therapeutic environment to ensure adequate rest, nutrition, hydration, and relaxation. (Support of the immune system is essential in HIV patients to minimize opportunistic infections.)	Teach the patient to incorporate health enhancing activities such as: • Adequate rest and sleep. • Proper nutrition that provides essential vitamins and nutrients. • Drinking 6–8 glasses of water per day.

(continued)

NURSING PROCESS APPLICATION *(continued)*

Interventions and (Rationales)	Patient and Family Education
• Monitor blood glucose levels. (Antiretroviral drugs may cause hyperglycemia, especially in patients with type I diabetes.)	• Instruct the patient to report excessive thirst, hunger, and urination to the health care provider. • Instruct diabetic patients to monitor blood glucose levels regularly.
• Monitor for neurologic adverse effects such as numbness and tingling of the extremities. (Some NRTI agents cause peripheral neuropathy.)	Instruct the patient to: • Report numbness and tingling of extremities. • Use caution when in contact with heat and cold due to possible peripheral neuropathy.
• Monitor vision and hearing periodically. (This will assess changes early and detect drug-related adverse effects.)	• Instruct the patient to report any changes in sight or hearing.
• Determine the effect that the prescribed antiretroviral agent has on oral contraceptives. (Many agents reduce the effectiveness of oral contraceptives.)	• Instruct the patient to use an alternate form of birth control to oral contraceptives while taking antiretroviral medications.
• Assess the patient's knowledge level regarding the use and effects of medication. (This is an opportunity to provide additional education.)	Instruct the patient: • That the medication may decrease the level of HIV infection in the blood but will not prevent transmitting the disease. • To use barrier protection during sexual activity. • To avoid sharing needles. • To abstain from donating blood.
• Provide resources for medical and emotional support. (Treatment requires a multidisciplinary approach.)	• Advise the patient about community resources and support groups.

Evaluation of Outcome Criteria

Evaluate the effectiveness of drug therapy by confirming that patient goals and expected outcomes have been met (see "Planning").

Prophylaxis of HIV Infections

56.8 The development of vaccines to prevent HIV has produced disappointing results.

Early in the history of the AIDS epidemic, scientists were optimistic that vaccines could be quickly developed that would prevent the spread of HIV infection. After all, scientists had totally eradicated the smallpox virus as a human threat, and essentially controlled major viral infections such as measles and mumps. Such a vaccine could be given in childhood, offering lifetime protection against the fatal disease.

After decades of research, the FDA has not approved a single vaccine, and scientists are far from developing a vaccine to prevent AIDS. Only a few HIV vaccines are currently in clinical trials, and none are expected to cause a major impact on the HIV epidemic. At best, the HIV vaccines produced thus far only boost the immune response; they are unable to prevent the infection or its fatal consequences. While this may help a patient already infected with the virus to better control the disease, it does not prevent new infections. Why is this the case?

HIV exhibits an extremely rapid replication rate, combined with a high "error" or mutation rate. While creating new viral DNA at a breakneck pace, reverse transcriptase frequently inserts the incorrect nucleotide. It is estimated that, given the size of the HIV genome at 10,000 base pairs, every possible mutation probably occurs at every nucleotide daily in an untreated patient. These errors create huge numbers of genetic variants, or mutant strains, with new and different characteristics from the original. It is not unusual to find dozens of genetic variants of HIV replicating within the same patient. Thus, vaccine development, and indeed antiretroviral therapy, is trying to hit a "moving target" that is changing its genetic makeup literally every minute.

Also challenging is determining the most effective type of vaccine for HIV. The classic type of vaccine uses live, attenuated viruses because this mimics a natural exposure and produces the greatest immunologic response (see Chapter 46). However, given the extreme rate of HIV mutation, scientists are concerned that an attenuated form of HIV could mutate back to a live form and infect the patient. Thus, the approach with HIV has been to take various "pieces" of the virus such as envelope protein subunits and portions of HIV genes, and produce a vaccine "cocktail" to administer to the patient. Unfortunately, these mixes have so far proven ineffective at preventing infection.

An additional challenge is to produce a vaccine-mediated immune response that will reach viruses lying latent inside T cells. HIV-infected cells reside in virtually every compartment in the body and serve as reservoirs for the latent virus, protecting it from the immune response produced by the vaccine. How do scientists coax the immune system to recognize these infected cells and dispose of them? Perhaps a better question is: Can a vaccine be designed to prevent the entry of the virus into cells to begin with? And how can this vaccine be ethically tested, since no animals have the same immune system as humans to serve as an experimental model?

Vaccine research has not been a total failure. Scientists have learned an enormous amount about the immune system's response to HIV infection. This has promoted the development of new drugs and advanced our understanding of how to treat and control the infection. It is likely that a preventative vaccine will become available in the future, but not soon enough for the millions already infected.

CONNECTION *Checkpoint* 56.2

From what you learned in Chapter 46, explain the difference between active immunity and passive immunity. Which type of immunity would an HIV vaccine produce? See Answer to Connection Checkpoint 56.2 in Appendix A.

56.9 Postexposure prophylaxis of HIV infection is designed to prevent transmission to health care workers.

Since the start of the AIDS epidemic, nurses and other health care workers caring for HIV-AIDS patients have been concerned about acquiring the disease from their patients. Fortunately, if proper precautions are observed, the disease is rarely transmitted from patient to health care worker. Accidents have occurred, however, in which the health care worker has acquired the infection by exposure to the blood or body fluids of HIV-infected patients. The risk of transmission through percutaneous exposure (needlestick or sharp cut) to HIV-infected fluid is estimated at 0.3%. Transmission of the virus through contact with a mucous membrane is less, at 0.09%. Approximately 56 cases of seroconversion have been documented in the United States following occupational exposure. Although the risk is small, the question remains, can HIV transmission be prevented following accidental occupational exposure to HIV? The answer is a qualified yes.

The success of postexposure prophylaxis (PEP) for occupational HIV exposure is difficult to assess due to the lack of controlled studies and the small numbers of cases. Enough data has accumulated, however, to demonstrate that PEP is successful in certain circumstances. For prevention to be most successful, PEP should be started within 24 to 36 hours after exposure to a source person who is known to be HIV positive. Although the exact interval remains undefined, longer periods allow the infection to progress to stages where prophylaxis would not be successful. The health care worker should receive a baseline HIV RNA level as soon as possible after exposure.

If the HIV status of the source person is unknown, PEP is decided case by case, based on the type of exposure (percutaneous or mucous membrane) and the likelihood the blood contained HIV. In some cases, PEP is initiated for a few days, until the source person can be tested. PEP should only be initiated if the exposure was sufficiently severe and the source fluid is known, or strongly suspected, to contain HIV. Using PEP outside established guidelines is both expensive and dangerous; the antiretrovirals used for PEP produce adverse effects in over half the recipients.

The selection of drugs for PEP is largely empirical; no established body of evidence exists that clearly demonstrates the success of any specific drug or drug combination. Based on available data, however, current clinical guidelines recommend two classes of PEP: basic and enhanced.

Basic PEP is initiated when the source person is asymptomatic for HIV or is known to have a low viral load (below 1,500 HIV RNA copies/mL). The basic PEP treatment includes one of the following regimens, conducted over a 4-week period:

- Zidovudine and lamivudine, or
- Zidovudine and emtricitabine, or
- Lamivudine and tenofovir, or
- Tenofovir and emtricitabine

If the accidental HIV exposure was particularly severe, and the source is a symptomatic HIV-infected person with a high viral load, a third drug may be added to the regimen. If available, the medical records of the source person should be consulted to determine the possibility of resistance to specific antiretrovirals. The enhanced PEP treatment includes one of the basic regimens listed previously, plus lopinavir/ritonavir. It should be noted that the addition of lopinavir/ritonavir has not been shown to be any more effective than the basic two-drug regimen.

Recently, guidelines have been established for the nonoccupational postexposure prophylaxis (nPEP) of HIV. These guidelines are largely based on animal studies and analysis of the existing data for occupational exposure. Because nPEP is expensive and may result in adverse drug effects, it is only recommended for specific nonoccupational exposures. First, the person must have been exposed to blood or bodily fluids of a person known to be infected with HIV. Second, the nature of the exposure must be such that there is a substantial risk for transmission. Thirdly, the exposure must have occurred no later than 72 hours before antiretroviral therapy is initiated. The sooner nPEP is initiated, the more successful the outcome. The health care provider considers nPEP for exposures outside these guidelines on a case-by-case basis. Recommended therapy is a 28-day regimen of HAART.

56.10 The risk of perinatal transmission of HIV can be markedly reduced by specialized drug protocols.

One of the most tragic aspects of the AIDS epidemic occurs when a mother transmits the virus to her child during pregnancy, delivery, or breast-feeding. Newborns with HIV may succumb to the infection within weeks, or symptoms may be delayed for months or years. The prognosis for these patients is generally poor. The best approach to dealing with HIV infections in neonates is prevention.

In 1994, clinical trials determined that perinatal transmission of HIV could be markedly reduced through pharmacotherapy. This regimen, known as PACTG 076, reduced the perinatal transmission of the virus from 22.6% in the placebo group to 7.6% in the treatment group. This reduction of approximately 70% in transmission was achieved using the following regimen:

- Oral zidovudine administered to the mother, beginning at 14 to 34 weeks of gestation;
- IV zidovudine administered to the mother during labor; and
- PO zidovudine to the newborn for 6 weeks following delivery.

In the years since the PACTG 076 protocol was established, scientists have searched for even more effective means of preventing perinatal transmission. Since monotherapy of HIV has since been abandoned for nonpregnant patients in favor of HAART, should pregnant patients receive drug combinations? Does the administration of antiretrovirals administered to the mother and infant produce congenital or long-term effects on the child? Can changing the PACTG 076 protocol reduce transmission even further?

CONNECTIONS

Lifespan Considerations Children with Human Immunodeficiency Virus

The Joint United Nations Programme on HIV/AIDS (UNAIDS, 2007) reported that in 2007, 2.5 million children 15 years and under were living with HIV-AIDS worldwide. Globally, 17% of all new infections are in this age group. In the United States, new cases of HIV-AIDS in children is quite rare, with only about 38 acquiring this infection in 2006. Clearly, the use of AZT and other antiretroviral therapies by infected women in America has helped decrease the prevalence of HIV-AIDS. However, worldwide numbers are far too high, and the infected children need effective treatment.

HIV can be transmitted in basically two ways. Horizontal transmission occurs through sexual activity or parenteral contact with blood or body fluids. Vertical transmission occurs when an HIV pregnant female passes the HIV to her baby in utero. Over 90% of infected children contract HIV via perinatal transmission. Transmission can also occur by breast-feeding.

Children with HIV require special care from a provider skilled in disease management. Antiretroviral therapy is useful in the treatment of children. Doses may vary based on weight, body surface, height, and weight.

One difficulty is determining when to initiate treatment for children with HIV. Delayed therapy can provide better quality of life and prevent damage to the immune system. However, most HIV babies begin antiretroviral therapy before age 3 months. Children respond differently to anti-HIV therapy with larger increases in CD4 cell counts as well as more diverse CD4 cells. One positive is that children recover more immune response than adults. However, without treatment, about 20% of children will either die or develop AIDS.

Numerous clinical studies worldwide have since examined the three components of the PACTG 076 protocol. To date, there does not appear to be an increased incidence of congenital abnormalities or malignancies among the children born to women receiving the PACTG 076 protocol. However, pediatric patients who were exposed to antiretrovirals in infancy will continue to be monitored into adulthood, because some effects may take decades to appear.

Current clinical practice recommendations for nonpregnant patients are now being applied to pregnant patients. HAART combination therapy is recommended for pregnant patients, as this is the most effective regimen for lowering HIV RNA load, reducing the incidence of viral resistance, and protecting the health of the mother. Due to its success in the PACTG 076 protocol, zidovudine is incorporated into the regimen, unless otherwise contraindicated. The preferred drug to be used in combination with zidovudine is lamivudine. Lamivudine is well tolerated and has been demonstrated as being safe for both mother and fetus in many studies. Should the mother have resistant strains, alternate agents include didanosine, emtricitabine, nevirapine, stavudine, and abacavir. If a PI is necessary, lopinavir/ritonavir has been shown to be safe for the fetus.

A major advantage in treating pregnant patients with antiretrovirals is that when HIV RNA is reduced to less than 1,000 copies/mL, perinatal transmission is very low. However, there is no threshold below which lack of transmission can be guaranteed; thus, perinatal prophylaxis is generally recommended for all patients.

The 6-week zidovudine monotherapy included in the PACTG 076 protocol is still recommended for newborns born to HIV-infected mothers. Therapy should begin immediately after delivery, no later than 6 to 12 hours postpartum. HIV infection is established in infants by age 1 to 2 weeks and beginning antiretroviral therapy more than 48 hours after birth has been shown to be ineffective in preventing the infection. In addition, mothers must be advised not to breast-feed their infants, as this is a possible route of HIV transmission, and many antiretrovirals are secreted in breast milk.

Definitive testing for the presence of HIV can be determined in most infants by age 1 month. If diagnostic testing reveals that the infant is not infected before the 6-week prophylactic treatment period is completed, zidovudine therapy is discontinued. On the other hand, if HIV diagnosis is confirmed during this period, the infant is switched to combination therapy. Both symptomatic and asymptomatic infants under 12 months of age are generally treated with antiretrovirals because HIV infection can rapidly progress to AIDS and death in this age group. Infants receiving early HAART have an improved prognosis over those infants who receive no treatment.

Approximately 12 of the 20 antiretrovirals are approved for pediatric indications. Some of the drugs are too toxic for pediatric use, not available in convenient formulations, or the doses remain to be established. Like adults, the specific regimen is chosen based on the experience of the prescriber and resistance patterns of the HIV strain. The possibility that the child may have inherited a strain already resistant to some of the antiretrovirals must be considered in developing the regimen. Common combinations for infant HIV infections include the following:

- Two NRTIs plus a PI (usually lopinavir with ritonavir)
- Two NRTIs plus an NNRTI (usually efavirenz for children over age 3, or nevirapine for those under age 3 or who are unable to take capsules)

Pharmacotherapy of Opportunistic Infections Associated with HIV-AIDS

56.11 Loss of immune function due to HIV often results in opportunistic infections that require anti-infective therapy.

In the early 1980s, all patients with AIDS acquired serious opportunistic infections (OIs) from pathogenic bacteria, viruses, fungi, and protozoans. Profound loss of immune function allowed dormant pathogens to flourish, as well as lowering the defense barriers for infection by newly acquired organisms. Often, the presentation of an acute OI was the reason the patient first sought medical attention for HIV disease. For example, in the early years of the epidemic, 70% to 80% of all AIDS patients developed *Pneumocystis carinii* pneumonia (PCP), which carried a mortality rate of up to 40% in these patients. Since the advent of HAART, PCP is now rare.

OIs still occur in HIV-AIDS patients; however, they are less common and mortality is diminished. This is because HAART increases the numbers of CD4 lymphocytes, allowing HIV-infected patients to maintain a higher level of immunologic defense. In addition, the anti-infective pharmacotherapy of OIs has evolved due to a better understanding of these diseases. Patients with CD4 counts below 200 cells/mcL are placed on prophylactic antibiotics, because the risk of an OI in these patients is very high. Most other HIV-AIDS patients are monitored carefully for signs of infectious disease, and treated as symptoms indicate.

Drugs used for treating OIs have been presented in previous anti-infective chapters, and the student should refer to those sections for specific drug information. A selected list of preferred drugs for selected OIs is given in Table 56.2.

Concurrent therapy of HIV-AIDS and OIs can create a significant number of drug interactions. In addition, increasing the extensive pill burden of HIV-AIDS patients encourages nonadherence to therapy. For newly diagnosed patients who have not yet received antiretroviral therapy, there is disagreement as to whether the OI therapy should be started before the antiretroviral regimen. In general, the antiretrovirals are begun immediately because, if successful, this will boost the CD4 cell count and allow the immune defenses of the patient to more rapidly eliminate the OI. In some cases, such as cryptosporidiosis, there is no specific anti-infective therapy; therefore, boosting the immune system is imperative. In the case of tuberculosis (TB), which requires prolonged pharmacotherapy with multiple drugs, interactions with antiretrovirals are common, and can be serious. Furthermore, it is often difficult to separate the adverse effects of the antiretroviral from those of the antituberculars. For these reasons, antiretroviral therapy is sometimes postponed 2 to 8 weeks until the antitubercular drug doses have been optimized, and adverse effects have been determined.

CONNECTION *Checkpoint* 56.3

It is common for HIV patients to be treated with antitubercular drugs. From what you learned in Chapter 52, what are the four primary first-line drugs for treating TB? See Answer to Connection Checkpoint 56.3 in Appendix A.

TABLE 56.2 Pharmacotherapy of Selected Opportunistic Infections in HIV-AIDS Patients

Disease	Preferred Drug(s) for Prevention	Comments
Bacterial enteric infections	PO: fluoroquinolone (ciprofloxacin preferred) or TMP-SMX	Most common pathogens are *Salmonella, Campylobacter,* and *Shigella*
Bacterial respiratory infections	Pneumococcal vaccine (PPV); inactivated influenza vaccine	Most common pathogens are *S. pneumoniae* and *H. influenza*
Candidiasis (mucocutaneous)	PO: fluconazole	Topical azoles may be used for vulvovaginal or oropharyngeal disease
Cryptococcosis	No prevention recommended Treatment is with amphotericin B with flucytosine for 2 weeks, followed by fluconazole for 8 weeks	Lifelong prophylaxis with fluconazole is indicated in certain patients
Cryptosporidiosis	No specific anti-infective is indicated; clarithromycin or rifabutin may be effective	Therapy includes symptomatic treatment of diarrhea
Herpes simplex	PO: famciclovir or acyclovir for 7–14 days	IV therapy is indicated in severe infections
Histoplasmosis (disseminated)	PO: itraconazole daily	Lifelong prophylaxis with itraconazole is indicated in certain patients
Mycobacterial infections	PO: Isoniazid plus pyridoxine for 9 months	Serious drug interactions can occur between rifamycin and the NNRTIs and protease inhibitors
Pneumocystis pneumonia (PCP)	PO: TMP-SMX for 21 days	Lifelong prophylaxis is indicated in certain patients; pentamidine may be used for severe cases
Syphilis	IM: benzathine penicillin	
Toxoplasma gondii encephalitis	PO: TMP-SMX	Clindamycin may be used instead of sulfadiazine

UNDERSTANDING THE CHAPTER

Key Concepts Summary

56.1 HIV causes a profound loss of immune function.

56.2 Treatment of HIV infection is difficult due to the latent nature of the virus and the development of resistant strains.

56.3 Six classes of antiretroviral drugs are available to treat HIV infection.

56.4 Reverse transcriptase inhibitors block the synthesis of viral DNA.

56.5 The nonnucleoside reverse transcriptase inhibitors inhibit viral DNA replication by binding to reverse transcriptase.

56.6 Protease inhibitors prevent HIV protease from completing the final step in HIV maturation.

56.7 Fusion inhibitors, integrase inhibitors, and CCR5 inhibitors are newer strategies for treating HIV infections.

56.8 The development of vaccines to prevent HIV has produced disappointing results.

56.9 Postexposure prophylaxis of HIV infection is designed to prevent transmission to health care workers.

56.10 The risk of perinatal transmission of HIV can be markedly reduced by specialized drug protocols.

56.11 Loss of immune function due to HIV often results in opportunistic infections that require anti-infective therapy.

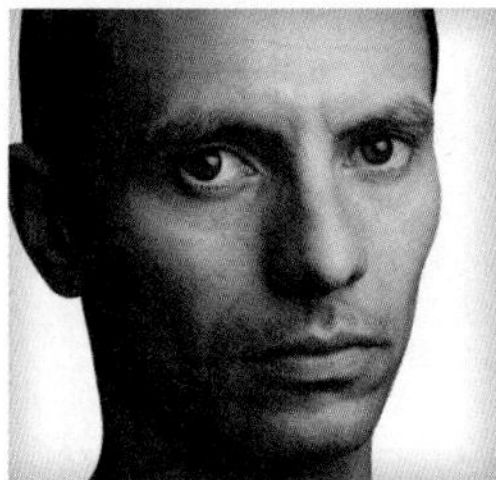

Making the PATIENT Connection

Remember the patient "Jim Green" at the beginning of the chapter? Now read the remainder of the case study. Based on the information presented within this chapter, respond to the critical thinking questions that follow.

Jim Green is a 37-year-old single male who has come to his health care provider because of the recent onset of a chronic sore throat and flulike symptoms, including swollen lymph nodes in the neck and armpits, tiredness, fever, and night sweats. During this office visit, Jim appears extremely anxious and troubled.

When questioned about his apparent nervousness, Jim states, "You don't understand, I'm gay. What if it is discovered that I have AIDS? What will I do? I don't want to die." The health care provider acknowledges the patient's fears and spends additional time allowing the patient to express his concerns. The process of diagnosing HIV is discussed with the patient and initiated.

Jim's medical history reveals he is allergic to penicillin, which results in rash and pruritus. Although Jim does not currently take any prescribed medications, he recently started multivitamin and nutritional supplements due to his recent weight loss. The patient denies any recreational drug use. However, Jim admits he occasionally used IV drugs during his college years. No past history of medical or psychiatric illness exists. He has never had surgery.

Jim does not use tobacco products. He reports drinking alcoholic beverages at least once weekly. Jim explains that he has had numerous sexual (male) partners over the past 10 years with inconsistent use of condoms. Presently he lives alone and works as a sales representative with a local computer firm. A series of laboratory diagnostic tests find the following abnormal results: WBC is decreased with lymphocytes less than 30% of the normal. The lymphocyte screen reveals a reduced $CD4^{-}$/CD8 T-cell ratio, CD4 (helper) lymphocytes decreased, and CD8 lymphocytes increased. Jim is hospitalized with the preliminary diagnosis of sepsis and to rule out HIV.

Critical Thinking Questions

You are the nurse caring for Jim Green in the hospital. On the first evening he is hospitalized, Jim asks if you think his physician will be prescribing antiretroviral therapy.

1. Given this situation, how would you explain the factors that determine when antiretroviral therapy should be initiated?
2. The nursing assistant on the unit states she is afraid to care for this patient for fear of "catching AIDS." In your own words, explain the transmission of HIV.
3. Describe how would you address the nursing assistant's fears.

Case Study

After several days in the hospital, the diagnosis of HIV-AIDS is confirmed. Jim's opportunistic infection has been treated with antibiotic therapy and the patient is discharged from the acute care setting. Jim is referred to the HIV clinic where antiretroviral therapy will be started using a HAART regimen. Although the health care provider has explained the therapy, Jim's anxiety results in his inability to comprehend the entire explanation provided. Jim begins asking you, his nurse, questions about HAART. He states, "I want to learn all I can about my illness and treatment."

1. Using simple language, how would you (the nurse) explain HIV and HAART therapy?
2. Outline the major concepts that Jim will need to understand about his drug treatment.

NCLEX-RN® Review

1 Zidovudine (Retrovir, AZT) is prescribed for a client. Which of the following statements by the client would indicate that further medication-related teaching is needed?

1. "Antiretroviral therapy must be continued for the remainder of my life."
2. "The human immunodeficiency virus vaccine only creates temporary immunity against the disease."
3. "The medication schedule can be adjusted daily depending on my activities."
4. "Many human immunodeficiency virus-infected individuals are able to live symptom-free due to the medication."

2 A client taking a nucleoside reverse transcriptase inhibitor is taught to discontinue the medication and call the health care provider if a redistribution of body fat in the arms, legs, and abdomen are noticed. The nurse knows that these symptoms may be associated with:

1. Renal failure.
2. Lipodystrophy.
3. Hypoaldosteronism.
4. Bone marrow suppression.

3 Because the nurse understands that zidovudine (Retrovir) can cause granulocytopenia, it is essential that the client be taught to:

1. Avoid sources of infection.
2. Schedule frequent rest periods.
3. Arise slowly when moving from a sitting to standing position.
4. Take medication with antacids to enhance absorption.

4 The nurse is aware that myelosuppression may be a problem for some clients receiving antiretroviral therapy. Which of the following findings would indicate that this adverse effect is present?

1. Increase in serum blood urea nitrogen levels
2. Increase in white blood cell count
3. Decrease in platelet counts
4. Decrease in blood pressure

5 The nurse is planning a teaching session with a client who will be receiving antiretroviral drug therapy. Which of the following should be included in the teaching plan? (Select all that apply.)

1. Avoid crowds and other people with colds, flu, and other infections.
2. Notify the health care provider at the first sign of any rash.
3. The medication will prevent transmission of the disease.
4. Cough and deep breathe several times per day.
5. Herbal supplements will not interfere with this therapy.

6 The nurse is collecting the initial health history from the client who will be receiving antiretroviral therapy. The client reports a daily regimen of alternative and complementary health activities. Which of the following may be contraindicated for this client?

1. Yoga and guided imagery
2. St. John's wort
3. Meditation and journaling
4. Weekly visits to a chiropractor

See Answers to Critical Thinking Questions, Case Study, and NCLEX-RN® Review in Appendix A.

References

Ball, S. C. (2004). Postexposure prophylaxis for nonoccupational HIV exposure. *AIDS READ, 14*(11), 587–594.

Bartlett, J. G. (2005). *Antiretroviral therapy: First-line treatment and "switch" strategies.* 12th Conference on Retroviruses and Opportunistic Infections: Treatment and Management of HIV Infection. Retrieved August 19, 2008, from http://www.medscape.com/viewprogram/3952_pnt

Centers for Disease Control and Prevention, Department of Health and Human Services. (2008). *HIV/AIDS Surveillance Report, 2006.* Vol. 18. Retrieved November 1, 2008, from http://cdc.gov/hiv/topics/surveillance/resources/factsheets/prevalence.htm

Hirsch, M. S. (2005). *Highly active antiretroviral therapy in 2005: Recent data for clinical practice.* Retrieved August 19, 2008, from http://www.medscape.com/viewprogram/4116_pnt

Madigan, M. T., Martinko, J. M., Dunlap, P. V., & Clark, D. P. (2006). *Brock biology of microorganisms* (11th ed.). Upper Saddle River, New Jersey: Pearson Education.

Morbidity and Mortality Weekly Report, Centers for Disease Control and Prevention. (2008). *Trends in HIV- and STD-related risk behaviors among high school students: United States 1991–2007, 57*(30), 817–822. Retrieved August 20, 2008, from http://www.cdc.gov/mmwr/preview/mmwrhtml/mm5730a1.htm

Morbidity and Mortality Weekly Report, Centers for Disease Control and Prevention. (2005). *Antiretroviral postexposure prophylaxis after sexual, injection-drug use, or other nonoccupational exposure to HIV in the United States.* Recommendations from the U.S. Department of Health and Human Services, 54(R07), 1–20. Retrieved August 20, 2008, from http://www.cdc.gov/mmwr/preview/mmwrhtml/rr5402a1.htm

Morbidity and Mortality Weekly Report, Centers for Disease Control and Prevention. (2005). *Updated U.S. Public Health Service guidelines for the management of occupational exposures to HIV and recommendations for postexposure prophylaxis, 54*(RR09), 1–17. Retrieved August 20, 2008, from http://www.cdc.gov/mmwr/preview/mmwrhtml/rr5409a1.htm

Morbidity and Mortality Weekly Report, Centers for Disease Control and Prevention. (2004). *Treating opportunistic infections among HIV-infected adults and adolescents.* Recommendations from the CDC, the National Institutes of Health, and the HIV Medicine Association/Infectious Diseases Society of America, 53(RR15), 1–112. Retrieved August 20, 2008, from http://www.cdc.gov/mmwr/preview/mmwrhtml/rr5315a1.htm

National Institutes of Health (NIH), the Centers for Disease Control and Prevention (CDC), and the HIV Medicine Association of the Infectious Diseases Society of America (HIVMA/IDSA). (2008, June 18). *Guidelines for prevention and treatment of opportunistic infections in HIV-infected adults and adolescents.* Retrieved August 20, 2008, from http://aidsinfo.nih.gov/contentfiles/Adult_OI.pdf

Panel on Antiretroviral Guidelines for Adults and Adolescents, Department of Health and Human Services. (2008, January 29). *Guidelines for the use of antiretroviral agents in HIV-1-infected adults and adolescents.* Retrieved August 20, 2008, from http://www.aidsinfo.nih.gov/ContentFiles/AdultandAdolescentGL.pdf

Public Health Service Task Force, Perinatal HIV Guidelines Working Group. (2008, July 8). *Recommendations for use of antiretroviral drugs in pregnant HIV-infected women for maternal health and interventions to reduce perinatal HIV-1 transmission in the United States.* Retrieved August 2, 2008, from http://aidsinfo.nih.gov/contentfiles/PerinatalGL.pdf

Sahloff, E. G. (2005). *Current issues in the development of a vaccine to prevent human immunodeficiency virus, 25*(5), 741–747. Retrieved August 20, 2008, from http://www.medscape.com/viewarticle/504671_print

Stevenson, M., Walker, B. D., & Wainberg, M. A. (2005). *Virus and host factors in HIV-1 pathogenesis.* 12th Conference on Retroviruses and Opportunistic Infections, HIV pathogenesis and immune response, and investigational antiretroviral drugs. Retrieved August 20, 2008, from http://www.medscape.com/viewprogram/3947_pnt

Stone, V. E. (2001). Strategies for optimizing adherence to highly active antiretroviral therapy: Lessons from research and clinical practice. *Clinical Infectious Diseases, 33*(15), 865–872.

UNAIDS. (2007). *AIDS epidemic update: December, 2007.* Retrieved November 1, 2008, from http://data.unaids.org/pub/EPISlides/2007/2007_epiupdate_en.pdf

Working Group on Antiretroviral Therapy and Medical Management of HIV-Infected Children, National Institutes of Health. (2008). *Guidelines on the use of antiretroviral agents in pediatric HIV infection.* Retrieved August 20, 2008, from http://aidsinfo.nih.gov/contentfiles/PediatricGuidelines.pdf

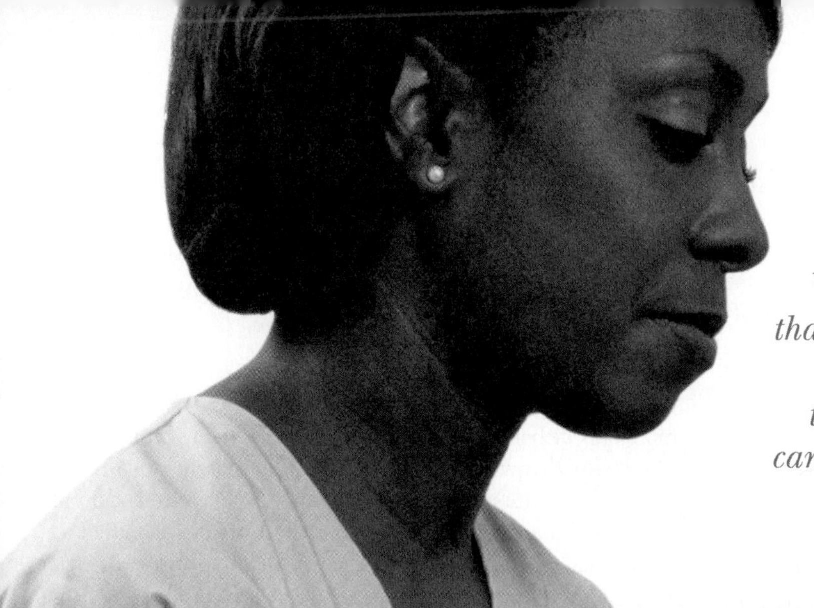

When the doctor first told me that I had cancer, I was scared. Now after hearing all of the things that the chemotherapy can do to my body I'm petrified.

Patient "Cheryl Ogen"

CHAPTER 57

Basic Principles of Antineoplastic Therapy

Chapter Outline

Characteristics of Cancer
Etiology of Cancer
Detection and Prevention of Cancer
Goals of Chemotherapy
Staging and Grading of Cancer
The Cell Cycle and Growth Fraction
Cell Kill Hypothesis
Improving the Success of Chemotherapy
Toxicity of Antineoplastic Agents
Chemotherapeutic Medications and the Nurse
Psychological Issues for the Patient Receiving Chemotherapy

Learning Outcomes

After reading this chapter, the student should be able to:

1. Compare and contrast the differences between normal cells and cancer cells.
2. Identify factors associated with an increased incidence of cancer.
3. Construct a table categorizing the major primary and secondary means of cancer prevention.
4. Compare and contrast the following goals of chemotherapy: cure, control, palliation, prophylaxis, adjuvant, neoadjuvant, and myeloablation.
5. Explain the purposes of staging and grading cancers.
6. Explain the significance of growth fraction and the cell cycle to the success of chemotherapy.
7. Assess the ability of antineoplastic drugs to effect a total cancer cure based on the cell kill hypothesis.
8. Explain how special chemotherapy protocols increase the effectiveness of therapy.
9. Discuss the types of toxicity and adverse effects of chemotherapeutic agents on the various organ systems.
10. Discuss the psychological issues that may impact patients who are receiving chemotherapy in the treatment of cancer.

Key Terms

adjuvant chemotherapy, *953*
alopecia, *960*
angiogenesis, *951*
cachexia, *959*
cancer, *950*
carcinogens, *951*
cell kill hypothesis, *956*
chemotherapy, *952*
emetic potential, *959*
grading, *953*
growth fraction, *955*
metastasis, *951*
mucositis, *959*
myeloablation, *953*
nadir, *958*
neoadjuvant chemotherapy, *953*
neoplasm, *950*
palliation, *952*
peripherally inserted central catheter (PICC) line, *957*
sclerosing, *957*
staging, *953*
telomerase, *951*
telomeres, *951*
tumor, *950*
vesicants, *960*

Cancer is one of the most feared diseases in society for a number of valid reasons. In the United States, cancer accounts for one out of every four deaths. It is often silent, producing no symptoms until it reaches an advanced stage. It sometimes requires painful and disfiguring treatments such as surgery or radiation. Cancer may strike at an early age, even during infancy, to deprive patients of a normal life span. It can affect any system in the body. Perhaps worst of all, the medical treatment of cancer often cannot offer a cure, and progression to death is sometimes slow, painful, and psychologically difficult for patients and their loved ones.

Despite its feared status, many successes have been made in the diagnosis, understanding, and treatment of cancer. Some types of cancer are now curable, and therapies may provide the patient a longer, symptom-free life. This chapter examines the basic principles of cancer therapy. Chapter 58 examines the medications used to treat cancer.

PharmFACT

It is estimated that more than 1,444,920 new cancer cases occur each year in the United States, with more than 559,650 deaths (more than 1,500 people each day). *Source:* American Cancer Society, 2007.

Characteristics of Cancer

57.1 Cancer is characterized by rapid, uncontrolled growth of cells that eventually invade normal tissues and metastasize.

A **tumor** is a swelling, abnormal enlargement, or mass. The word **neoplasm** is often used interchangeably with tumor. Tumors may be benign or malignant. Whereas benign tumors are usually slow growing, remain localized, and rarely cause death, malignant tumors are rapidly growing, invasive, and will kill the host if left untreated. Malignant tumors are classified as carcinomas or sarcomas. Examples of various types of benign and malignant tumors are listed in Table 57.1.

Cancer or carcinoma is a disease characterized by abnormal, uncontrolled cell division. Cell division is a normal process that occurs extensively in most body tissues from conception to late childhood. At some point in time, whether it occurs during fetal life, childhood, or adulthood, the degree of cell division in every tissue must be controlled.

Each cell in the body has the ability to regulate its growth (proliferation) by turning specific genes on and off. For example, growth promoting genes can be turned on when it becomes necessary to replace worn-out cells, as in the case of blood cells, skin cells, and the mucosa of the digestive tract. Growth suppressor genes are responsible for slowing down the duplication rate and can result in a total lack of replication, as in the case of muscle cells and perhaps brain cells. If the suppressor genes become damaged or mutated and do not slow down or stop cell growth, then the cells will undergo abnormal proliferation. Because of the critical importance of cell growth to life, it is likely that each cell has multiple genes that regulate division, all of which are responsive to various chemical signals or messages originating from both inside and outside the cell.

Cancer is thought to result from damage to the genes that control cell growth. Once damaged, the cell is no longer responsive to the chemical signals that normally check its growth. The cancer cells lose their normal functions, dividing rapidly and invading surrounding tissues.

TABLE 57.1 Classification and Naming of Tumors

Name	Description	Examples
Benign tumor	Slow growing; does not metastasize and rarely requires drug treatment	Adenoma, papilloma, lipoma, osteoma, meningioma
Carcinoma	Cancer of epithelial tissue; most common type of malignant neoplasm; grows rapidly and metastasizes	Malignant melanoma, renal cell carcinoma, adenocarcinoma, hepatocellular carcinoma
Glioma	Cancer of glial (interstitial) cells in the brain, spinal cord, and pineal gland	Telangiectatic glioma, brainstem glioma, posterior pituitary gland, or retina
Leukemia	Cancer of the blood-forming cells in bone marrow; may be acute or chronic	Myelocytic leukemia, lymphocytic leukemia
Lymphoma	Cancer of lymphoid tissue	Hodgkin's disease, lymphoblastic lymphoma
Sarcoma	Cancer of connective tissue; grows extremely rapidly and metastasizes early in the progression of the disease	Osteogenic sarcoma, fibrosarcoma, Kaposi's sarcoma, angiosarcoma

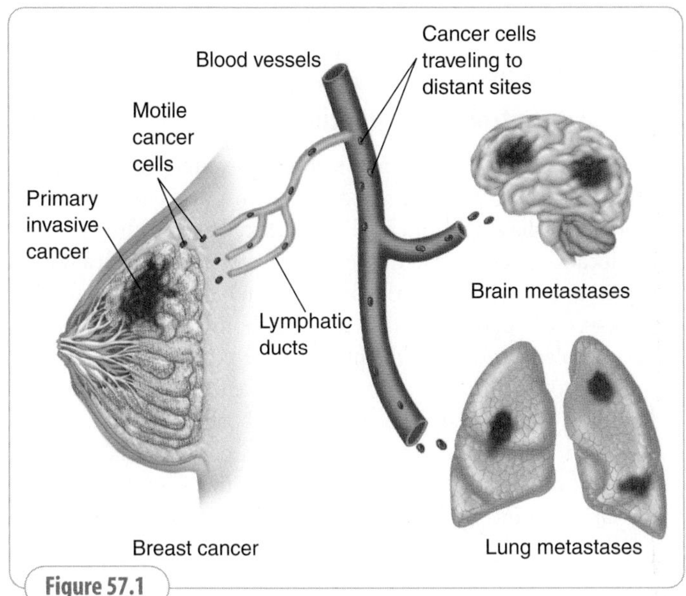

Figure 57.1

Invasion and metastasis by cancer cells.

Unlike most normal cells, cancerous cells are able to move to other places in the body. The abnormal cells often travel to distant sites where they populate new tumors, a process called **metastasis.** Figure 57.1 illustrates some characteristics of cancer cells.

Each time a cell divides it loses small amounts of deoxyribonucleic acid (DNA) from the end of each chromosome. These regions of "extra" repetitive DNA, called **telomeres,** prevent the vital sequences of DNA from being destroyed. Many normal cells are able to undergo mitosis 50 to 60 times before the cell can no longer divide because the telomeres are too short to protect the chromosome from damage. Certain human stem cells contain the enzyme **telomerase,** which can lengthen the DNA chains and allow continued replication. Interestingly, this enzyme is not produced in mature cells, which dooms the cells to eventual death.

Cancer cells are different from normal cells in that they do not die as quickly and can divide and form new cancer cells indefinitely. One explanation for this difference is that most cancer cells produce large amounts of telomerase, which continues to add pieces to the telomeres so that the cell can continue to divide. It is believed that the cancer cell begins to produce telomerase soon after it has mutated and that this may be an important factor in the progression to cancer.

To divide rapidly (and indefinitely) tumor cells need an adequate supply of nutrients. Solid tumors need to create a new capillary network to "feed" themselves. The process of **angiogenesis,** which is the formation of new blood vessels, is controlled by a cascade of events similar to blood coagulation. Some factors that are secreted by cells promote angiogenesis, whereas others inhibit it. Cancer cells appear to have the ability to control angiogenesis and to establish their own blood supply, which not only brings in nutrients, but also provides an "escape route" during metastasis.

Etiology of Cancer

57.2 The etiology of cancer may be chemical, physical, or biologic.

Numerous factors have been found that cause cancer or are associated with a higher risk for acquiring the disease. Agents that cause cancer are known as **carcinogens.**

Many chemical carcinogens have been identified. For example, chemicals in tobacco smoke are probably responsible for about one third of all cancers in the United States. Alcohol ingestion has also been linked to certain cancers, including esophageal, oral, breast, and liver cancers. Chemicals such as asbestos and benzene have been associated with a higher incidence of cancer in the workplace. In some cases, the site of the cancer may be distant from the entry location, as is the case with bladder cancer, which is caused by the inhalation of certain industrial chemicals.

MyNursingKit | CancerNet

A number of physical factors are also associated with cancer. For example, exposure to large amounts of x-rays is associated with a higher risk of leukemia. Ultraviolet (UV) light from the sun is a common cause of skin cancer.

It is estimated that viruses are associated with about 15% of all human cancers. Examples include herpes simplex types I and II, Epstein–Barr, human papillomavirus (HPV), cytomegalovirus, and human T-lymphotrophic viruses. If patients remain free from infection of these viruses, their chances of developing certain types of cancer diminishes greatly. Factors that depress immune function, such as the human immunodeficiency virus (HIV) or immunosuppressant drugs given after transplant surgery, may promote the growth of cancer cells.

Some cancers have a strong genetic component. The fact that close relatives may acquire the same type of cancer suggests that certain genes may predispose close relatives to the condition. These abnormal genes interact with chemical, physical, and biologic agents to promote the formation of cancer. Gender can also be considered a risk factor for certain types of cancer. For instance, breast cancer is more commonly associated with women, whereas bladder cancer is more frequent in men.

Although the development of cancer has a genetic component, it is also greatly influenced by factors in the environment. Maintaining or adopting healthy lifestyle habits may reduce the risk of acquiring cancer. Following proper nutrition, avoiding chemical and physical risks (especially tobacco), and maintaining a regular schedule of health checkups can help prevent cancer from developing into a fatal disease.

Detection and Prevention of Cancer

57.3 The key to successful cancer treatment is prevention and early detection.

If allowed to grow unchecked and untreated, cancer is fatal in nearly 100% of those who acquire it. The key to successful cancer treatment is prevention and early detection. Prevention of cancer falls into two categories: primary prevention and secondary prevention.

Primary prevention of cancer includes interventions that keep cancer from ever developing. Interventions for primary prevention are targeted to avoiding known carcinogens and promoting a healthy lifestyle. Examples of primary prevention include the following:

- Health counseling and education delivered by the nurse
- Elimination of tobacco use to prevent lung, oral, and other cancers
- Receiving the HPV vaccination (Gardasil) to prevent cervical cancer
- Maintaining a healthy diet low in fat and high in fresh vegetables and fruits
- Maintaining weight within recommended levels
- Decreasing excess stress
- Avoiding chronic or prolonged exposure to direct sunlight or wearing protective clothing or sunscreen

Secondary prevention includes interventions leading to the discovery and control of cancerous or precancerous lesions while they are small and localized. Examples of secondary prevention include the following:

- Receiving a Papanicolaou (pap) smear annually, for females older than 18 years or who are sexually active
- Receiving a screening colonoscopy, according to the schedule recommended by the health care provider
- Receiving mammograms, according to the schedule recommended by the health care provider
- Receiving annual prostate exams, for men after age 50
- Performing monthly breast exams, for women of menstruating age and older
- Performing regular skin self-examinations to check for abnormal lesions
- Women between the ages of 9 and 26 years should be vaccinated for human papillomavirus (HPV)

The American Cancer Society recommends using the following acronym to help people remember what to look for when self-assessing for cancer.

Caution

C: change in bowel or bladder habits
A: a sore that does not heal
U: unusual bleeding or discharge
T: thickening or lump in the breast or elsewhere
I: indigestion or difficulty swallowing
O: obvious change in a wart or mole
N: nagging cough or hoarseness

CONNECTION *Checkpoint* 57.1

From what you learned in Chapter 46, describe the immunization schedule for receiving the HPV vaccine.
See Answer to Connection Checkpoint 57.1 in Appendix A.

Goals of Chemotherapy

57.4 The three primary goals of chemotherapy are cure, control, and palliation.

Pharmacotherapy of cancer is sometimes simply referred to as **chemotherapy.** Because drugs are transported through the blood, they have the potential to reach cancer cells in virtually any location. Certain chemotherapeutic drugs are specifically designed to be able to cross the blood–brain barrier to reach brain tumors. Others are instilled directly into body cavities such as the urinary bladder to bring the highest dose possible to the cancer cells without producing systemic adverse effects. Chemotherapy has three general goals: cure, control, and palliation.

When diagnosed with cancer, the primary goal desired by most patients is to achieve a complete cure; that is, permanent removal of all cancer cells from the body. The possibility for cure is much greater if a cancer is identified and treated in its early stages when the tumor is small and localized to a well-defined region. Indeed, the 5-year survival rates for nearly all types of cancers have increased in the past two decades due to improved detection and more effective therapies. Examples in which chemotherapy has been used successfully as curative treatment include Hodgkin's lymphoma, certain leukemias, and choriocarcinoma.

Pharm*FACT*

The highest 5-year survival rates are for cancers of the prostate, testis, and thyroid. The lowest survival rates are for pancreatic and liver cancers. *Source:* American Cancer Society, 2007.

When cancer has progressed and cure is not possible, a second goal of chemotherapy is to control or manage the disease. Although the cancer is not eliminated, preventing the growth and spread of the tumor may extend a patient's life. Essentially, the cancer is managed as a chronic disease, such as hypertension or diabetes.

In its advanced stages, cure or control of the cancer may not be achievable. For these patients, chemotherapy is used as **palliation.** Chemotherapy drugs are administered to reduce the size of the tumor, easing the severity of pain and other tumor symptoms and thus improving the quality of life. Examples of advanced cancers for which palliation is frequently used include osteosarcoma, pancreatic cancer, and Kaposi's sarcoma.

Chemotherapy may be used alone or in combination with other treatment modalities such as surgery or radiation therapy. Surgery is especially useful for removing solid tumors that are localized. Surgery lowers the number of cancer cells in the body so that radiation therapy and pharmacotherapy can be more successful. When only a portion of the tumor is removed it is referred to as debulking. Surgery is not an option for tumors of blood cells or when it would not be expected to extend a patient's life span or improve the quality of life.

Approximately 50% of patients with cancer receive radiation therapy as part of their treatment. Radiation therapy is most successful and produces the fewest adverse effects for cancers that are localized when high doses of ionizing radiation can be aimed directly at the tumor and be confined to a small area. Radiation treatments are frequently prescribed postoperatively to kill cancer cells that may remain following an operation. Radiation is sometimes given as palliation for inoperable cancers to shrink the size of a tumor that may be pressing on vital organs and to relieve pain, difficulty breathing, or difficulty swallowing.

Adjuvant chemotherapy is the administration of antineoplastic drugs after surgery or radiation therapy. The purpose of adjuvant chemotherapy is to rid the body of any cancerous cells that were not removed during the surgery or to treat any micrometastases that may be developing.

Neoadjuvant chemotherapy is the administration of antineoplastic drugs before surgery or radiation therapy with the goal of shrinking a large tumor to a more manageable size. This may also be done if the tumor has invaded vital tissue around it, such as may happen with brain tumors. Shrinking the tumor preoperatively results in less surgical invasion when removing the tumor.

In a few cases, drugs are given as chemoprophylaxis with the goal of preventing cancer from occurring in patients at high risk for developing tumors. For example, patients with a close family history of breast cancer who have had a primary breast cancer removed may receive tamoxifen, even if there is no evidence of metastases. Tamoxifen has been shown to prevent the recurrence of breast cancer in these patients. Chemoprophylaxis of cancer is uncommon because most of these drugs have potentially serious adverse effects.

Certain antineoplastic drugs are highly toxic to bone marrow. The complete destruction of hematopoietic bone marrow cells, known as **myeloablation,** is a very serious adverse effect of these drugs. Myeloablation, however, is often necessary when performing stem cell or bone marrow transplantation. The procedure kills cells in the immune system that could reject the transplant.

CONNECTION *Checkpoint* 57.2

Corticosteroids are administered to most patients who are receiving tissue or organ transplants. From what you learned in Chapter 45, what is the rationale for administering corticosteroids to these patients? See Answer to Connection Checkpoint 57.2 in Appendix A.

Staging and Grading of Cancer

57.5 Cancers are described by their stage and grade.

Staging and grading must be done to determine the extent to which a cancer has invaded the body. These processes are performed on the initial diagnosis of cancer to determine the best course of therapy and predict patient outcomes.

Staging is the process of determining where the cancer is located and the extent of its invasion. Staging helps the health care provider communicate with the patient, caregivers, and other health professionals regarding the involvement of cancer in the patient. It also helps the health care provider determine the best course of treatment.

Once a cancer is staged the level does not change even if the cancer progresses. For instance, if a cancer is staged as level II on diagnosis, the cancer will always be referred to as a stage II even if it spreads to other sites. This is important to understand because patients with cancers that have a lower stage number have a better prognosis than those who are diagnosed with a higher number. For instance if a woman is diagnosed with ovarian cancer and it is staged at a level II, this patient has a better prognosis than another woman who is diagnosed with the same type of cancer at a level IV, even if the level II cancer progresses to a level IV.

During the staging of solid tumors, diagnostic testing determines the size of the tumor, whether the tumor has invaded surrounding tissue, the involvement of lymph nodes, and the presence or absence of metastasis (Table 57.2). Cancer cells may metastasize either via the blood or the lymphatic system. During staging, special lymph nodes called sentinel nodes are biopsied and sent to the laboratory for analysis. If these sentinel nodes are negative for cancer, then it is less likely that the cancer has spread through the lymphatic system. During staging the patient is also assessed for the presence of possible metastases. If no metastases are found, the patient has a better prognosis. Stage 1 is assigned to cancers that are the least invasive. Stage 4 is given for the cancer that is the most aggressive.

Grading is a process that examines potential cancer cells under a microscope and compares their appearance to normal parent cells. Normal cells are highly differentiated: They have

CONNECTIONS

Complementary and Alternative Therapies Selenium

Description: Selenium is an essential trace element that is essential for healthy immune function and is necessary for the metabolism of iodine. It protects cells against breakdown. Selenium can be found in meat and grains, Brazil nuts, brewer's yeast, broccoli, brown rice, dairy products, garlic, molasses, and onions. The amount of selenium in food, however, has a direct correlation to the selenium content of the soil. The soil of much American farmland is low in selenium, resulting in selenium-deficient produce. Low dietary intake of selenium is associated with an increased incidence of several cancers, including lung, colorectal, skin, and prostate.

History and Claims: Selenium is a vital antioxidant, especially when combined with vitamin E. It protects the immune system by preventing the formation of free radicals, which can damage the body.

Standardization: The usual daily dose is 200 mcg of selenium.

Evidence: Selenium supplementation has resulted in increased natural killer cell activity, and studies show its promise as protection against prostate and colorectal cancers, especially among smokers (Lee et al., 2006; Peters et al., 2006; Reid et al., 2006). As an antioxidant, selenium protects the body from the damaging effects of free radicals. Certain breakdown products of selenium are believed to prevent tumor growth by enhancing immune cell activity and suppressing the development of blood vessels to the tumor.

Source: From "An Analysis of Cancer Prevention by Selenium," 2001, by G. F. Combs, L. C. Clark, & B. W. Turnbull, 2001, *BioFactors, 14*(2), pp.153–159; and *Dietary Supplement Fact Sheet: Selenium*, by National Institutes of Health, Office of Dietary Supplements, n.d. Retrieved August 5, 2008, from http://ods.od.nih.gov/factsheets/selenium.asp

TABLE 57.2 Staging of Cancerous Tumors

T Category: describes the original (primary) tumor. Tumor size is usually measured in centimeters. The numbers T1–T4 describe the tumor size and/or level of invasion into nearby structures. The higher the T number, the larger the tumor and/or the further it has grown into nearby structures.

TX	Means the tumor cannot be measured or evaluated
T0	Means there is no evidence of primary tumor (the primary tumor cannot be found)
Tis	Means the cancer is in situ (the tumor has not started growing into the structures around it)

N Category: describes whether or not the cancer has reached nearby lymph nodes. The numbers N1–N3 describe the size, location, and/or number of lymph nodes involved. The higher the N number, the more lymph nodes are involved.

NX	Means the nearby lymph nodes cannot be measured or evaluated
N0	Means nearby lymph nodes do not contain cancer

M Category: tells whether there are distant metastases (spread of cancer to other parts of body).

MX	Means metastasis cannot be measured or evaluated
M0	Means that no distant metastases were found
M1	Means that distant metastases were found (the cancer has spread to distant organs or tissues)

Each type of cancer has its own version of this classification system, so the letters and numbers do not always mean the same thing for every kind of cancer. For example, some cancer classifications may have subcategories, such as T3a and T3b, whereas others may not have an N3 category.

The American Joint Committee on Cancer (AJCC) developed the TNM Classification System as a tool for health care providers to stage different types of cancer based on certain standard criteria. It has replaced many of the older staging systems. In the TNM system, each cancer is assigned a T, an N, and an M category.

Note: From *Making Treatment Decisions: Staging*, by American Cancer Society, 2008. Retrieved December 16, 2008, from http://www.cancer.org/docroot/ETO/content/ETO_1_2X_Staging.asp

TABLE 57.3 Grading of Cancer Cells

The American Joint Committee on Cancer (AJCC) recommends the following cancer grading classifications:

GX	Grade cannot be determined
G1	Well-differentiated (the cancer cells look a lot like normal cells)
G2	Moderately well differentiated (cancer cells look somewhat like normal cells)
G3	Poorly differentiated (the cancer cells do not look much like normal cells)
G4	Undifferentiated (the cancer cells do not look anything like normal cells)

Note: From *Making Treatment Decisions: Staging*, by American Cancer Society, 2008. Retrieved August 5, 2008, from http://www.cancer.org/docroot/ETO/content/ETO_1_2X_Staging.asp

developed, become fully mature, look like the parent cell, and carry on the functions of the parent cell. For example, it is very easy to distinguish a liver cell from a muscle cell or a nerve cell microscopically. When a normal cell becomes cancerous, however, it gradually changes and becomes less differentiated in both structure and function. Once fully undifferentiated, the cancer cell will look very different from the parent cell from which it came and will not carry on the functions of the parent cell.

In the grading process, if the biopsy cells appear differentiated and very similar to the parent cells, the tumor is classified as a Grade 1 (G1) and has the best prognosis. G4 cells are grossly abnormal and clearly different from normal cells. Patients with these malignant and aggressive cells have the worst prognosis. The different grades are described in Table 57.3.

Grading has certain limitations. For instance, solid tumors often contain many different types of cells that vary in appearance from near normal to grossly abnormal. One part of the tumor may have cells consistent with G2, whereas other parts of the same tumor may have cells consistent with G4. Unlike staging, grading may change over time as the tumor evolves.

The Cell Cycle and Growth Fraction

57.6 Many antineoplastic drugs are more effective when given at specific stages of the cell cycle and in tumors with a high growth fraction.

Both normal and cancerous cells go through a sequence of events known as the cell cycle, which is illustrated in Figure 57.2. Knowledge of the cell cycle is important to understanding the effectiveness of anticancer drugs.

In simplest terms, a cell is either performing its daily functions or it is undergoing cell division. There are certain cellular activities that occur in between these two basic functions of the cell that allow its life cycle to be divided into five stages or phases.

Stage G_0: Although sometimes called the resting stage, G_0 is the phase during which cells conduct their everyday activities such as metabolism, impulse conduction, contraction, or secretion. A cell may enter its G_0 phase at any point in the cycle and remain there for extended periods, depending on the specific tissue and surrounding cellular signals. Cells spend most of their lifetime in the G_0 phase.

Stage G_1 (Gap 1): If a cell receives a signal to divide, it leaves the G_0 phase and enters the G_1 phase, during which it synthesizes the ribonucleic acid (RNA), proteins, and other components needed to duplicate its DNA.

Stage S (Synthesis): During the S phase the cell duplicates its DNA.

Stage G_2 (Gap 2): During the G_2 or premitotic phase the cell makes additional proteins and the spindle apparatus that are necessary for cell division or mitosis.

Stage M (Mitosis): The cell undergoes mitosis, which includes prophase, metaphase, anaphase, and telophase. Following mitosis in the M phase, the cell has split into two identical cells that will either start the process over at the G_1 phase or

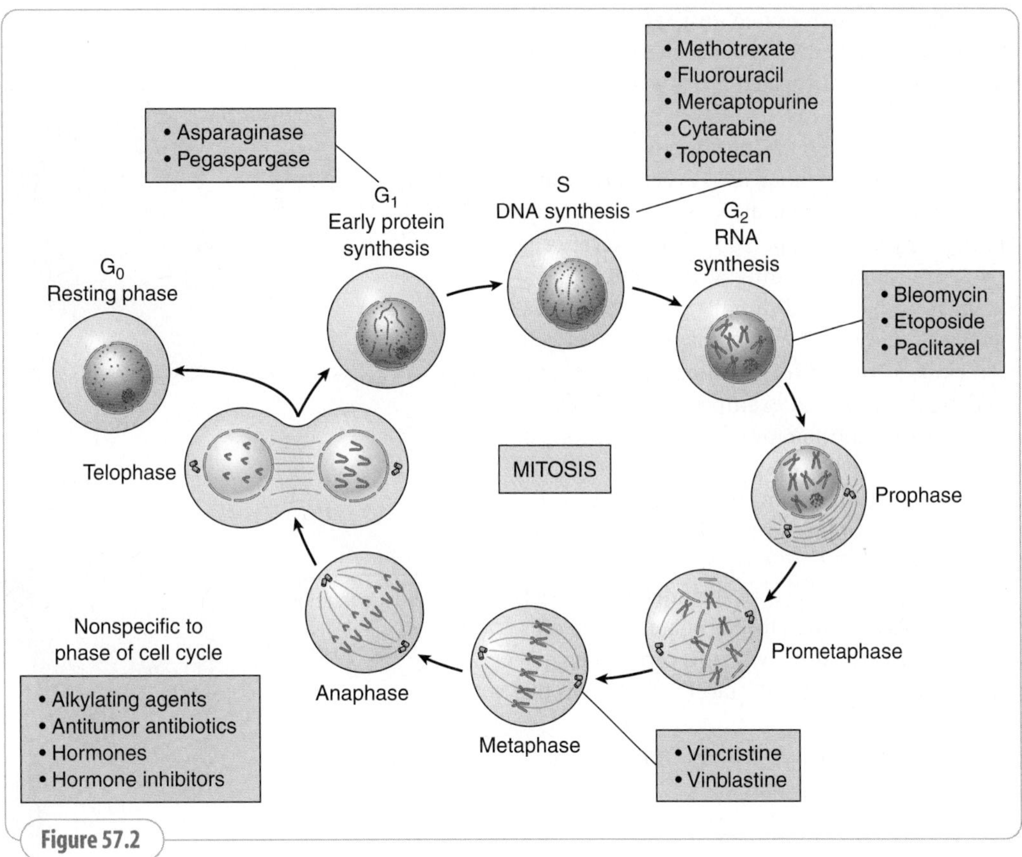

Figure 57.2

Antineoplastic agents and the cell cycle.

enter the G_0 phase depending on the needs of the body. This is the briefest stage of the cell cycle.

The actions of some antineoplastic agents are specific to certain phases of the cell cycle, whereas others are mostly independent of the cell cycle. Cell cycle specific drugs kill the most cancer cells when they are administered in divided but frequent doses. Cell cycle specific drugs are most effective in treating hematologic malignancies and other cancers that have a relatively large proportion of cells proliferating at any given point in time. Examples include mitotic inhibitors such as vincristine (Oncovin), which affect cells in the M phase, and antimetabolites such as fluorouracil (Adrucil), which are most effective against cells during the S phase. In general, cell cycle specific drugs are not effective against tumors that have a large percentage of resting cells.

Cell cycle nonspecific drugs can kill cancer cells in any stage of the cell cycle, including the G_0 resting phase. Often, these drugs are incorporated into resting cancer cells and have no effects until the cells attempt to divide. These drugs act relatively slowly and are given intermittently to give normal cells an opportunity to recover. The effects of alkylating agents such as cyclophosphamide (Cytoxan), antitumor antibiotics, and hormonal therapies are generally independent of the phases of the cell cycle.

The **growth fraction** is a measure of the number of cells undergoing mitosis in a tissue. It is a ratio of the number of replicating cells to the number of resting cells. Antineoplastic drugs are more toxic to tissues and tumors with high growth fractions. For example, certain leukemias and lymphomas have a high growth fraction and therefore have a greater antineoplastic success rate. Solid tumors such as breast and lung cancer generally have a low growth fraction; therefore, they are less sensitive to antineoplastic agents. Because certain normal tissues, such as hair follicles, bone marrow, and the gastrointestinal (GI) epithelium also have high growth fractions, they are sensitive to the effects of the antineoplastics.

With large solid tumors, a high percentage of the cells have entered the G_0 phase, causing the tumor to have a lower growth fraction. Chemotherapeutic drugs are not as effective against cells that are in the G_0 phase. To improve the success of chemotherapeutic drugs, the tumor may be debulked. When a tumor is debulked, a portion is removed surgically, causing the remaining cells to move into the active phases of mitosis. Once the cells enter into mitosis, the chemotherapeutic drugs can more effectively kill the cancer cells.

Cell Kill Hypothesis

57.7 The goal of chemotherapy is to kill as many cancer cells as possible while sparing normal cells.

Measurement of the success of chemotherapy is dependent on the therapeutic goal. If the desirable outcome is a total cure, then success is measured by how long the patient remains cancer-free following treatment. If the goal is palliation, success is measured by the degree to which the patient's quality of life is improved. Because chemotherapy is often prolonged and physically challenging, it is crucial that the patient understand the goals of treatment and how they will be measured. In cases of palliation, the patient must weigh whether the adverse effects associated with treatment are worth the anticipated increase in the quality of life.

Patients who are undergoing chemotherapy usually receive several rounds of treatment spaced over a designated time, usually several weeks or months. This is because each round of chemotherapy kills a set percentage of cancer cells, usually those that are rapidly dividing at the time of treatment. Subsequent rounds kill additional cells. Another reason is that the chemotherapy always damages normal cells and can cause serious adverse effects. Patients need time to recover between treatments. For example, neutrophils are especially sensitive to chemotherapy and the patients' absolute neutrophil count (ANC) will usually plummet after a therapy session. Intervals between treatments allow the body to make more neutrophils so that body defenses are able to fight infections.

The **cell kill hypothesis** is a theoretical model that predicts the ability of antineoplastic drugs to eliminate cancer cells. This hypothesis predicts that a drug will kill a certain percentage, rather than a constant number, of cancer cells. Why is this important?

Theoretically, every single cancer cell in a tumor must be eliminated from the body to cure a patient. Leaving even a single malignant cell could result in regrowth of the tumor. Eliminating every cancer cell, however, is a very difficult task. As an example, consider that a small, 1-cm breast tumor may already contain 1 billion cancer cells before it can be detected during a manual examination. A drug that is able to kill 99% of these cells would be considered a very effective drug indeed. Yet even with this fantastic achievement, 10 million cancer cells would remain, any one of which could potentially cause the tumor to return and kill the patient. The relationship between cell kill and chemotherapy is illustrated in Figure 57.3. It is likely that no antineoplastic drug (or combination of drugs) will kill 100% of the tumor cells. The large burden of cancer cells, however, may be lowered sufficiently to permit the patient's immune system to control or eliminate the remaining cancer cells. Because the immune system is able to eliminate only a relatively small number of cancer cells, it is imperative that as many cancerous cells as possible be eliminated during treatment. This example reinforces the need to diagnose and treat tumors at an early stage when the number of cancer cells is smaller.

Because of their rapid cell division, tumor cells express a high mutation rate, which continually changes their genetic structure, resulting in a more heterogenous mass as the tumor grows. Essentially, the tumor becomes a mass of hundreds of different types of cancer cells with different growth rates and physiological properties. Administration of an antineoplastic drug may kill only a small portion of the tumor, leaving some clones unaffected and able to repopulate the tumor with resistant cells. The appearance of cancer cells that are resistant to antineoplastic drugs complicates the chances for a pharmacologic cure because a therapy that was very successful in reducing the tumor mass at the start of chemotherapy may become less effective over time.

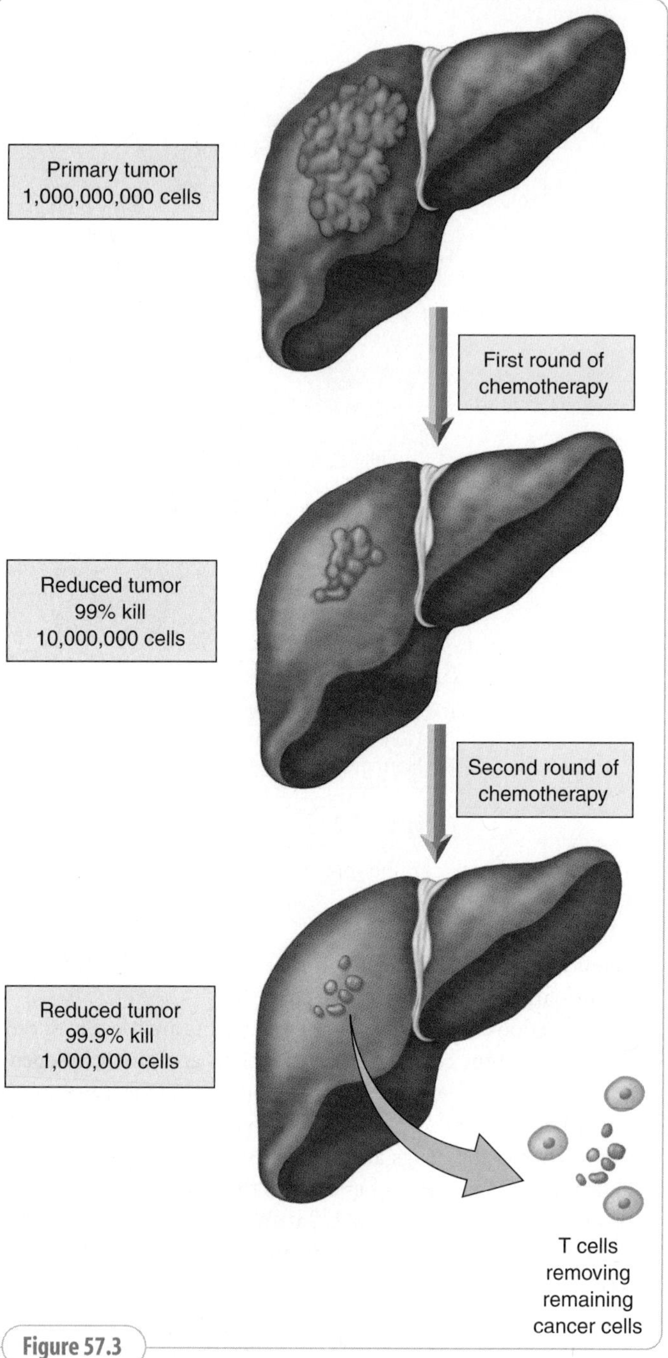

Figure 57.3

Cell kill and chemotherapy.

Improving the Success of Chemotherapy

57.8 Use of multiple drugs and intermittent dosing are strategies that allow for greater success of chemotherapy.

As has been seen throughout this text, the majority of pharmacotherapy is conducted with a single drug given in a constant amount over a specified time period. For most indications, the use of multiple drugs increases the expense of treatment and can cause additional adverse effects. Cancer chemotherapy is an important exception: The concurrent use of multiple drugs, combined with intermittent dosing, results in improved patient outcomes.

Combination Chemotherapy

Chemotherapy is conducted using established protocols that are specific to the type of cancer and its stage. A cancer treatment protocol describes the specific combination of antineoplastic medications that will be given, their doses, and the cycles in which they will be administered. Using multiple drugs affects the different stages of the cancer cell's life cycle and attacks the various clones within the tumor via several mechanisms of action, thus increasing the percentage of cell kill. Combination chemotherapy also allows for lower dosages of each individual agent, thereby reducing toxicity and slowing the development of resistance. Examples of established protocols using combination therapy include cyclophosphamide–methotrexate–fluorouracil (CMF) for breast cancer; cyclophosphamide–doxorubicin–vincristine (CDV) for lung cancer; and daunorubicin-vincristine-prednisone-asparaginase for acute lymphocytic leukemia. Each type of cancer has its own individual protocol, which was established through clinical trials. These protocols are being refined and revised continually based on current research.

> **CONNECTION *Checkpoint* 57.3**
>
> **From what you learned in Chapters 47 through 56, name two infectious diseases that require several years' therapy with anti-infectives, using multiple drugs.** See Answer to Connection Checkpoint 57.3 in Appendix A.

Dosing Schedules

Most chemotherapeutic medications are administered intermittently using specific dosing schedules that have been determined through research to increase the effectiveness of the antineoplastic agents. For example, some of the anticancer drugs are given as a single dose or perhaps several doses over a few days. A few weeks may pass before the next series of doses begins. This gives normal cells time to recover from the adverse effects of the drugs and allows tumor cells that may not have been replicating at the time of the first dose to begin dividing and become more sensitive to the next round of chemotherapy. Sometimes the optimum dosing schedule must be delayed until the patient sufficiently recovers from the drug toxicities, especially bone marrow suppression. Delays or reductions in the planned dosages are likely to affect treatment outcomes. The specific dosing schedule chosen depends on the type of tumor, stage of the disease, and overall condition of the patient.

Route of Administration

Antineoplastic agents are available for administration by virtually any route. Whenever possible, the oral (PO) route is used because it is most acceptable to the patient and eliminates the risk of phlebitis or tissue necrosis due to extravasation that is common with some of the parenteral agents. In addition, antineoplastics may be given locally by topical application to the lesion or through direct instillation into the tumor region. Regional administration causes less systemic toxicity. The most common route for delivering antineoplastics is via the venous system.

Oral: The PO route is the easiest, most convenient, and least expensive route for chemotherapy administration. Patients can self-administer their PO chemotherapy medications at home. It does not necessitate going to a cancer center, health care provider's office, or other location. One problem associated with PO administration is the inconsistency of absorption. Chemotherapeutic agents that are administered PO can and do produce some of the same adverse reactions as the injectable agents, and the patient and caregivers must be aware of these. They must also be taught safe handling and disposal of these drugs. Examples of antineoplastics available as PO preparations include methotrexate, mercaptopurine, cyclophosphamide, and melphalan.

Intravenous: The intravenous (IV) route is the most common route for delivery of chemotherapy agents. One advantage to the IV route is that a constant and consistent serum level of the drug can be obtained by fine adjustments to the infusion rate. A disadvantage is that **sclerosing,** or abnormal tissue hardening of the veins, may occur during prolonged administration. Another disadvantage to the patient is that chemotherapy administration is done in a cancer center, health care provider's office, or some other place away from the patient's home. This may require many miles of commuting, especially in rural areas, and getting there may present a hardship to the patient and family. In addition, traveling out of the home may expose the patient to people with colds and other infections, which can be hazardous to patients with suppressed immune function. In some geographic areas, an oncology nurse will come to the patient's home and administer the chemotherapy, thus enabling the patient to remain at home.

Administration of chemotherapeutic agents can be done through a centrally located access device such as a Groshong catheter, which is inserted by being tunneled under the skin on the chest into a major vein for long-term medication instillation, or through a peripheral vein via a **peripherally inserted central catheter (PICC) line.** A PICC line is a central catheter that is threaded into the vena cava for administration of chemotherapy. The advantage of a central line is that it is less likely to infiltrate and it is inserted in a large vein, which is less likely to become irritated during chemotherapy. A disadvantage of a central line is that it increases the patient's risk of acquiring an infection.

Because IV administration requires a free-flowing IV in a large vein, it is imperative that the nurse constantly assesses the insertion site of the IV for signs of infiltration or phlebitis. Some antineoplastics can cause extreme cellular damage if the solution is allowed to enter surrounding tissues. Because of the potential for tissue damage, most antineoplastics are not administered by the intramuscular (IM) or subcutaneous routes. Examples of IV antineoplastics are carmustine, cisplatin, doxorubicin, and mitomycin.

Intrathecal: Some antineoplastic medications may be delivered intrathecally into the subarachnoid space of the spinal column. In intrathecal administration, the drug bypasses the blood–brain barrier and circulates with the cerebrospinal fluid (CSF) to expose central nervous system (CNS) tumors to high concentrations of the drug. A specially trained individual must conduct the procedure because it requires a lumbar puncture or surgical placement of a reservoir or implanted pump for drug delivery. An advantage to intrathecal administration is that it provides a consistent drug level in the CSF. Potential adverse effects include headaches, confusion, lethargy, seizures, nausea, or vomiting, all of which are signs of increased intracranial pressure.

Intra-arterial: Occasionally the health care provider may choose to administer chemotherapeutic medications through an artery. Intra-arterial administration requires a surgical procedure for catheter placement and, often, special x-ray techniques. In most cases, a catheter is passed via the femoral or brachial artery so that its end lies close to the blood supply of the tumor. Injection creates a very high dose of drug directly to the tumor site. Although the drug subsequently distributes via the circulation to other tissues, the tumor area receives the highest dose.

Intraperitoneal: Intraperitoneal administration via a catheter or port is used to deliver antineoplastic drugs directly to intra-abdominal metastases. The drug is usually slowly absorbed into the systemic circulation. A disadvantage of this method is that it requires the placing of a Tenckhoff catheter, which is a specialized port with one end attached to a catheter that is threaded into a major vein, and the other end under the patient's skin with an access area into which medication is instilled.

Intravesicular: The intravesicular route instills high doses of antineoplastics into the urinary bladder via a Foley catheter to treat tumors of the bladder mucosa. Only small amounts of the drugs are absorbed systemically. The patient retains the drug for a specified period, after which it is voided.

Toxicity of Antineoplastic Agents

57.9 Serious toxicity limits therapy with most antineoplastic agents.

Although cancer cells are clearly abnormal in structure and function, much of their physiology is identical to that of normal cells. Because it is difficult to kill cancer cells selectively without profoundly affecting normal cells, all antineoplastic drugs have the potential to cause serious toxicity. These drugs are often pushed to their maximum dosages to obtain the greatest tumor cell kill. These high dosages always result in adverse effects in the patient, some of which are listed in Table 57.4. Because antineoplastic agents primarily affect cells with a high growth fraction, normal cells that are replicating, such as cells in the hair follicles, GI tract, and hematologic system are most susceptible to adverse effects.

Hematologic System

Erythrocytes, leukocytes, and platelets have relatively short life spans and must be continually replaced by hematopoietic stem cells residing in the bone marrow. These stem cells may be destroyed by antineoplastic agents, resulting in bone marrow suppression (myelosuppression). Myelosuppression is the most common dose-limiting adverse effect of chemotherapy and the one that most often causes discontinuation or delays of chemotherapy. Severe bone marrow suppression is a contraindication to therapy with most antineoplastic drugs.

TABLE 57.4 Examples of Adverse Effects of Anticancer Drugs

Common Expected Adverse Effects	Drug-Specific Adverse Effects	Dose-Limiting Adverse Effects
Nausea, vomiting	Fetal malformations (pemetrexed, methotrexate, mercaptopurine)	Bone-marrow suppression
Stomatitis	Peripheral-sensory neuropathy (cisplatin)	Acute renal failure
Anorexia	Sterility (mechlorethamine)	Pulmonary fibrosis
Alopecia	Cardiotoxicity (doxorubicin, daunorubicin)	Diarrhea
Immunosuppression		
Fatigue		

Chemotherapy causes erythrocyte, leukocyte, and platelet counts to decrease until they reach their lowest value, known as the **nadir.** Patients are most susceptible to the symptoms caused by the myelosuppression, such as anemia, infections, or bleeding, during the nadir. Following the nadir, blood counts begin their recovery back to normal values. The nadir is specific for each chemotherapeutic agent and for each type of blood cell. For example, antimetabolites produce rapid nadirs for neutrophils in 7 to 14 days after the initiation of chemotherapy, with recovery within 7 to 21 days following the nadir. Other agents such as the nitrosoureas produce a delayed nadir for neutrophils at 26 to 63 days, with recovery at 35 to 89 days after the nadir.

Although chemotherapy decreases all types of white blood cells (WBCs), neutrophils are the type most affected. This is primarily because the normal life span of a neutrophil is only 7 to 12 hours, and without continual replacement by stem cells the number of circulating neutrophils quickly falls. A patient is diagnosed with neutropenia when the neutrophil count is less than 1,500 cells/mL. The ANC is calculated by multiplying the WBC count by the percentage of neutrophils. Patients are very susceptible to infections while they are neutropenic. Many times patients who are neutropenic are placed in reverse isolation to protect them from exposure to any infections from family members or health care providers. Even an infection from a mild cold could be fatal to patients with extremely low neutrophil counts. If a patient who is neutropenic and receiving chemotherapy acquires an infection, an increase in WBCs may not be evident. If a patient who is neutropenic does develop a fever, this may be an indication of sepsis, and antibiotics are indicated.

Medications such as colony-stimulating factors (filgrastim [Neupogen] and sargramostim [Leukine]) are sometimes administered to accelerate recovery of suppressed bone marrow and increase the WBC count. The administration of these drugs shortens the time of neutropenia, thus lowering the risk of opportunistic infections and allowing the patient to maintain an optimum dosing schedule for his or her chemotherapeutic medications. Filgrastim is presented as a prototype drug in Chapter 41.

Because the life span of a platelet is only 7 to 8 days, these blood elements require constant replenishment by stem cells in the bone marrow. A patient is diagnosed with thrombocytopenia when the platelet count is less than 100,000 per milliliter of blood. Chemotherapy is often delayed if this occurs. In patients who are receiving chemotherapy, thrombocytopenia usually occurs concurrently with neutropenia. Thrombocytopenia can cause the patient to exhibit abnormal bleeding, with symptoms ranging from bruising to petechiae to serious hemorrhage. Bleeding precautions must be implemented if the platelet count falls below 50,000 per milliliter of blood. To prevent the platelet count from decreasing to a harmful level, platelet infusions may be necessary. Oprelvekin (Neumega) is a thrombopoietic growth factor that may be administered to increase platelet production. This drug is presented as a prototype hematopoietic agent in Chapter 41.

Because erythrocytes have a longer life span (90 to 120 days) than neutrophils or platelets, reductions in red blood cells (RBCs), or anemia, occur later in the course of chemotherapy. A patient is diagnosed with anemia when the RBC count falls to less than 4.2 million/mm^3 for men or 3.6 million/mm^3 for women or when hemoglobin values fall to less than 14 g/dL for men and 12 g/dL for women. Because hemoglobin carries oxygen to all tissues and major organs in the body, anemia may affect every system in the body. An infusion of RBCs may be required to increase a patient's RBC count and hemoglobin value. A medication that the nurse may administer to help increase the number of RBCs is epoetin alfa (Epogen), which is presented as a prototype in Chapter 41. When assessing for anemia, it should be remembered that the etiology may be the result of nonchemotherapy related causes, such as bleeding, iron deficiency, or kidney damage.

Gastrointestinal Tract

The vomiting center in the medulla is triggered by many antineoplastics, resulting in significant nausea and vomiting. Acute nausea and vomiting often begins within minutes of chemotherapy administration and may last for 24 hours. Delayed nausea and vomiting begins 24 hours after chemotherapy and may continue up to 6 days. Anticipatory nausea and vomiting may occur before chemotherapy because the patient may be expecting an unpleasant experience. Antineoplastics are sometimes classified by their **emetic potential.** Before starting therapy with the highest emetic potential agents, patients may be pretreated with antiemetic drugs such as prochlorperazine (Compazine), metoclopramide (Reglan, others), or lorazepam (Ativan). It is not uncommon to administer several different antiemetic medications that have several modes of action. Antiemetic medications are presented in detail in Chapter 61.

The GI tract mucosa is very sensitive to the effects of chemotherapeutic agents. The mucosa commonly becomes inflamed, a condition known as **mucositis.** Consequences of mucositis include painful ulcerations in the mouth and esophagus, difficulty eating or swallowing, GI bleeding, intestinal infections, or severe diarrhea. Some research has shown that eating popsicles during chemotherapy infusions can decrease the severity of mucositis. The nurse may also instruct the patient to eat a bland diet and to use a soft toothbrush for oral care. Some health care providers may order a "medical cocktail," which may include lidocaine viscous, liquid diphenhydramine, and Carafate to decrease the pain associated with the mucositis. The patient should also be instructed to report any signs of thrush, which is an oral yeast infection.

Most patients receiving antineoplastics experience anorexia. This is usually due to a combination of nausea, vomiting, and mucositis. At times the patient's appetite is decreased such that tube feedings or parenteral feedings may be indicated. The body needs sufficient nutrients and calories for normal cells to repopulate and for repair of body tissues. When assessing for anorexia, it should be remembered that this symptom may be the result of direct effects from the tumor itself or from associated psychological changes such as depression or anxiety.

The patient may also experience constipation or diarrhea depending on the specific drugs administered. Some chemotherapeutic medications damage the intestinal lining, thus inhibiting the reabsorption of fluids and producing loose stools. Replacement of fluids and electrolytes as well as treatment with an antidiarrheal drug may be indicated. Some chemotherapeutic medications decrease the motility of the GI tract, resulting in greater reabsorption of fluids that leads to constipation. When assessing for constipation, it should be remembered that other common reasons for this symptom include therapy with opioid analgesics and inadequate water and fiber intake.

Many patients with cancer experience a general wasting of muscle and other tissues referred to as **cachexia.** Cachexia may be caused by toxic effects from the cancer itself or from its treatment. Symptoms from the chemotherapy such as anorexia, mucositis, nausea, and vomiting may contribute to cachexia but there are other non-GI factors that also contribute such as serious chronic pain, depression, and fatigue.

Cardiopulmonary System

Some of the chemotherapeutic medications can be extremely toxic to the heart and lungs. For example, doxorubicin (Adriamycin) is specifically known for its cardiotoxicity and the nurse should monitor the patient for any changes in the electrocardiogram (ECG) and assess for any signs of heart failure. This adverse effect can be serious enough to later cause the patient to need cardiac monitoring or a heart transplant.

Bleomycin (Blenoxane) is specifically known for causing pneumonitis in patients. Nursing care of the patient who is receiving bleomycin should include monitoring the patient's pulse oximeter and respiratory status. Auscultating crackles in the lung fields may be a sign of a developing pneumonitis. Chest x-rays may be necessary two to three times per week to assess for lung changes.

Urinary System

Some of the chemotherapeutic medications can exhibit considerable nephrotoxicity. For example, cisplatin (Platinol) can lead to kidney failure if the dosage limit is exceeded. When administering chemotherapeutic agents that are nephrotoxic, the nurse should closely monitor intake and output. The patient should remain well hydrated during the treatment to help prevent renal damage. Diuretics may be administered to help balance the intake and output of the patient.

Reproductive System

Some antineoplastics, particularly the alkylating agents, affect the gonads and have been associated with infertility in both male and female patients. If a woman is pregnant while receiving treatment, the fetus may be severely damaged due to the high growth fraction of the fetus's cells or may be killed during the treatment. Both male and female patients should be instructed to use reliable contraception if sexually active while receiving chemotherapy and for 3 to 6 months following treatment.

Antineoplastic medications are more likely to cause permanent sterility in men than in women. Some patients choose to have their sperm or eggs harvested prior to treatment in case the chemotherapy does affect their fertility.

Many hospitals have protocols specifying that female nurses and pharmacists not handle chemotherapeutic agents if they are pregnant or are trying to become pregnant due to the toxic effects that the chemotherapy may have on the fetus.

Nervous System

Several chemotherapeutic agents are toxic to the nervous system. For instance vincristine (Oncovin) may cause muscle weakness and peripheral neuritis. It is important for the nurse to assess the patient's neurologic status frequently when administering this medication. Patients should also be made aware of the possible adverse effects so that they may inform the nurse if they begin to notice changes in their strength or any tingling or pain in their extremities.

Cisplatin (Platinol) has been known to cause hearing loss and deafness in some patients. The nurse should assess the patient's hearing throughout the course of treatment and document any changes noted in the patient's ability to hear.

Skin and Soft Tissue

Many antineoplastics are classified as **vesicants,** which are agents that can cause serious tissue injury if they escape from an artery or vein during an infusion or injection. Extravasation or infiltration from an injection site can produce severe tissue and nerve damage, local infection, and even loss of a limb. If a nurse is concerned that a peripheral IV is no longer working properly, the IV should not be used for chemotherapy administration. Although rare, extravasation can still occur with a central line so the nurse should continue to frequently assess the insertion site of a central line while administering chemotherapy. Rapid treatment of extravasation is necessary to limit tissue damage, and certain antineoplastics have specific antidotes. For example, extravasation of carmustine (BiCNU, Gliadel) is treated with injections of equal parts of sodium bicarbonate and normal saline into the extravasation site. Before administering IV antineoplastic agents, the nurse should know the emergency treatment for extravasation. Antineoplastics with the strongest vesicant activity include busulfan, carmustine, dacarbazine, dactinomycin, daunorubicin, idarubicin, mechlorethamine, mitomycin, plicamycin, streptozocin, vinblastine, vincristine, and vinorelbine.

Other Effects

Fatigue is a common complaint during chemotherapy. The precise etiology of the fatigue is often difficult to determine. If the patient has anemia, the lack of hemoglobin to carry oxygen to the tissue can cause the patient to feel fatigued. The patient may be suffering from anxiety or depression due to the diagnosis of cancer, which may lead to sleep deprivation. The process of cellular regeneration after chemotherapy treatments may also cause feelings of fatigue. A nutritional consultation may be helpful in determining if the fatigue has a nutritional origin. Coping strategies for dealing with stress and scheduled periods of rest may benefit the patient.

Hair follicles are damaged by many chemotherapeutic agents, resulting in hair loss or **alopecia.** Hair loss usually begins within 1 to 2 weeks of the first treatment, and regrowth may take 3 to 5 months after the last chemotherapeutic treatment. The potential for alopecia should be discussed with patients before treatment begins so that they may choose to wear a hat, bandana, wig, or other accessory.

One of the ironies of chemotherapy is that the medications that are given to kill the cancer may cause a secondary cancer to develop elsewhere in the patient's body. This is not a common adverse effect but it has been clearly demonstrated in patients. The secondary malignancy usually occurs many years after the initial cancer; thus this adverse effect is of most concern to children being treated with chemotherapy. It is estimated that pediatric cancer survivors have a 10 to 20 times greater risk than other children for developing a secondary malignancy. The most common secondary malignancy is nonlymphocytic leukemia.

Hyperuricemia is most frequently associated after chemotherapy for lymphomas and leukemias due to the rapid cell kill. A patient is diagnosed with hyperuricemia when uric acid levels in the blood are elevated, which can lead to renal failure if the uric crystals deposit in the renal tubules. Signs of hyperuricemia are nausea, vomiting, and oliguria. Keeping the patient well hydrated helps to preserve renal function by "flushing" microscopic crystals out of the kidney before they have a chance to form larger crystals. The nurse who is caring for a patient who is suspected of developing or has been diagnosed with hyperuricemia should monitor the patient's intake and output closely.

Pharm*FACT*

The morbidity and mortality rates for most types of cancer remains higher in the African American population than in Caucasians, with the mortality rates being 38% higher in men and 17% higher in women.
Source: American Cancer Society, 2007.

Chemotherapeutic Medications and the Nurse

57.10 Hospitals, state boards of nursing, and other regulatory agencies have special requirements for nurses who administer chemotherapy.

Most state boards of nursing and hospitals have specific requirements for nurses who administer chemotherapeutic medications. Nurses may be required to take classes in which chemotherapeutic administration and adverse effects of the medications are taught. Other information that may be taught in the chemotherapy class is how to proceed if a vesicant extravasates, what to do if there is a chemotherapy spill or leak, and what precautions to take when administering specific chemotherapies. These classes are generally offered by the institution where the nurse will be administering the chemotherapy.

Many hospitals have specific policies regarding the handling of chemotherapeutic containers and tubing. For instance the nurse may be required to wear gloves and eye shields while administering the chemotherapy. When the chemotherapy is completed, the nurse may be required to return the chemotherapy container and tubing used to administer it to the pharmacy.

Psychological Issues for the Patient Receiving Chemotherapy

57.11 Many patients will experience anxiety, depression, stress, and hopelessness when given the diagnosis of cancer.

Each patient responds to the diagnosis of cancer differently. Many times the initial diagnosis may leave patients feeling shocked and unable to process their feelings. Other times patients may immediately feel depressed or hopeless. Patients may be in a state of denial until chemotherapy begins. The adverse effects of the chemotherapeutic medications will also weigh heavily on the patients' minds. They may question themselves and the nurse as to whether the benefits of the medication outweigh the adverse effects that they experience. They may also be afraid to vocalize the question, "Am I going to die?" even though this question may be at the forefront of their thoughts. If a patient has a poor prognosis, the patient and family may begin to prepare for the end of life. This is a normal process experienced by many patients with cancer.

If a patient is experiencing alopecia or has had to have any surgeries such as a mastectomy or has had a central IV catheter placed, he or she may be experiencing feelings of body image disturbance. Patients may be afraid that family and friends may no longer accept them now that they are physically different. Patients may also have trouble accepting their changed bodies.

Patients may also report feelings of anxiety. This may be due in part to the fear of the unknown. Fears that the patient may have include: Is treatment going to hurt? Am I going to live? Will I have to go through several rounds of cancer treatment and possibly multiple surgeries before I am cured? What will my family do without me? Will the cancer or the treatment be disfiguring? Will my loved ones reject me because of my changed appearance?

Feelings of depression and hopelessness are also common to patients with cancer. If a patient is placed on reverse isolation to protect him or her from other people's germs and those in the environment, the risk for depression is even higher due to the feelings of isolation. The patient may also falsely believe that the rationale behind reverse isolation is that the cancer is contagious or that family and friends believe this so they, therefore, are not visiting as they would if the diagnosis were different.

Chemotherapeutic certified nurses must also be good listeners and have excellent therapeutic communication skills. These nurses must also keep in mind the stress that patients and their family members are feeling during the time of diagnosis and treatment of cancer. It is not uncommon for patients or their families to ask the same questions over and over. It is the nurses' duty to make sure that patients understand the effects that the medication may have on their body as well as the signs and symptoms that they should report to them.

UNDERSTANDING THE CHAPTER

Key Concepts Summary

57.1 Cancer is characterized by rapid, uncontrolled growth of cells that eventually invade normal tissues and metastasize.

57.2 The etiology of cancer may be chemical, physical, or biologic.

57.3 The key to successful cancer treatment is prevention and early detection.

57.4 The three primary goals of chemotherapy are cure, control, and palliation.

57.5 Cancers are described by their stage and grade.

57.6 Many antineoplastic drugs are more effective when given at specific stages of the cell cycle and in tumors with a high growth fraction.

57.7 The goal of chemotherapy is to kill as many cancer cells as possible while sparing normal cells.

57.8 Use of multiple drugs and intermittent dosing are strategies that allow for greater success of chemotherapy.

57.9 Serious toxicity limits therapy with most antineoplastic agents.

57.10 Hospitals, state boards of nursing, and other regulatory agencies have special requirements for nurses who administer chemotherapy.

57.11 Many patients will experience anxiety, depression, stress, and hopelessness when given the diagnosis of cancer.

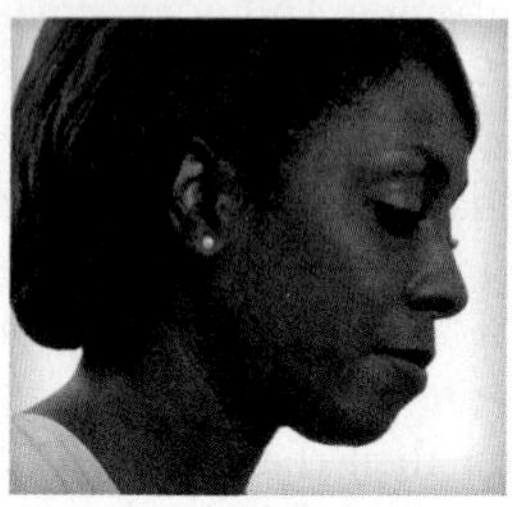

Making the PATIENT Connection

Remember the patient "Cheryl Ogen" at the beginning of the chapter? Now read the rest of the case study. Based on the information presented within this chapter, respond to the critical thinking questions that follow.

Cheryl Ogen is a 39-year-old patient who is employed as a kindergarten teacher. She has been married for 15 years, and has never had any children. Her medical history confirms that both her mother and maternal grandmother died from breast cancer. Now Cheryl has been diagnosed with breast cancer. She is admitted to the hospital for a mastectomy and chemotherapy. Cheryl's breast cancer is Stage T1, N0, M0, and G2. Cheryl has undergone the mastectomy and is now about to begin chemotherapy.

Critical Thinking Questions

1. Cheryl would like to know why she is receiving chemotherapy after the surgeon has removed the cancerous tumor. What would you tell her?
2. Why is it important to understand the staging and grading system used with cancer? How would you interpret the staging and grading of Cheryl's cancer?
3. If you were Cheryl and you were offered the opportunity of participating in a clinical trial for a new chemotherapy medication, would you do it?
4. Identify some of the hematologic changes that Cheryl may experience while receiving chemotherapy.

Case Study

Jonah Cooper is a patient who is newly diagnosed with acute lymphocytic leukemia. He is 28 years old and is the father of two children ages 9 months and 2 years. Jonah is admitted to the hospital for his initial round of chemotherapy.

1. Will Jonah's children be allowed to visit him during his hospital admission?
2. Why is Jonah receiving more than one type of chemotherapy?
3. Why was Jonah's cancer not staged on diagnosis?

NCLEX-RN® Review

1 The health care provider has written in the client's chart that the cancer is at Stage I. The nurse knows that the implications for this staging are that the:

1. Cancer is advanced and the client has a poor prognosis.
2. Cancerous cells are only moderately differentiated from the parent cells.
3. Cancer has been detected at an early stage.
4. Tumor is large and is invading surrounding tissue.

2 The nurse is evaluating the client who is receiving chemotherapy to determine the risk for infection. Which laboratory values would prompt the nurse to implement protective isolation measures for this client?

1. High uric acid level
2. Low neutrophil count
3. High red blood cell count
4. Low platelet count

3 The nurse determines that the client understands an important principle of chemotherapy when the client makes which of the following statements?

1. "The use of multiple chemotherapy drugs affects different stages of the cancer cell's life cycle."
2. "Staging describes the process of determining how responsive the cancer is to the prescribed chemotherapy."
3. "Antineoplastic drugs kill the entire tumor, including the clones, and prevent repopulation."
4. "Combination chemotherapy requires higher dosages of each individual agent and increases toxicity."

4 Chemotherapy is being initiated for a client with prostate cancer who is experiencing mucositis. Which of the following health teaching would be most appropriate for this drug?

1. Use an over-the-counter mouthwash to eliminate bacteria.
2. Increase intake of citrus-containing foods and beverages.
3. Eat a bland diet and use a soft toothbrush for oral care.
4. This adverse effect is expected and will disappear within a few days.

5 The nurse is collaborating with the interdisciplinary team regarding the care of a client with a brain tumor. The nurse knows that the most common reason that subsequent rounds of chemotherapy may be delayed is due to what condition?

1. Myelosuppression
2. Alopecia
3. Mucositis
4. Cachexia

6 A client with cancer is started on a chemotherapeutic agent that is a known vesicant. The nurse performs which priority activity related to this drug? Monitor the client's:

1. Response to antinausea drugs.
2. Intake of calcium-rich foods.
3. Respiratory status for cough.
4. IV site for swelling and pain.

See Answers to Critical Thinking Questions, Case Study, and NCLEX-RN® Review in Appendix A.

References

American Cancer Society. (2008). Making treatment decisions: Staging. Retrieved August 5, 2008, from http://www.cancer.org/docroot/ETO/content/ETO_1_2X_Staging.asp

American Cancer Society. (2007). *Cancer facts & figures for African Americans 2007–2008.* Retrieved August 8, 2008, from http://www.cancer.org/docroot/STT/stt_0.asp

American Cancer Society. (2007). *Cancer facts & figures 2007.* Atlanta: Author. Retrieved August 5, 2008, from http://www.cancer.org/downloads/STT/CAFF2007PWSecured.pdf

ATBC Study Group. (2003). Incidence of cancer and mortality following α-tocopherol & β-carotene supplementation: A postintervention follow-up. *Journal of the American Medical Association, 290*(4), 476–485.

Combs, G. F., Clark, L. C., & Turnbull, B. W. (2001). An analysis of cancer prevention by selenium. *BioFactors, 14*(2), 153–159.

Lee, S., Yeon Chun, J., Nadiminty, N., Trump, D., Ip, C., Dong, Y., et al. (2006). Monomethylated selenium inhibits growth of LNCaP human prostate cancer xenograft accompanied by a decrease in the expression of androgen receptor and prostate-specific antigen (PSA). *The Prostate, 66*(10), 1070–1075.

Lemone, P., & Burke, K. (2008). *Medical-surgical nursing: Critical thinking in client care* (4th ed.). Upper Saddle River, NJ: Pearson Education.

Lutz, C., & Przytulski, K. (2006). *Nutrition and diet therapy. Evidence-based applications* (4th ed.). Philadelphia: F. A. Davis.

National Institutes of Health, Office of Dietary Supplements. (n.d.). *Dietary supplement fact sheet: Selenium.* Retrieved August 5, 2008, from http://ods.od.nih.gov/factsheets/selenium.asp

Pagana, K. D., & Pagana, T. J. (2007). *Mosby's manual of diagnostic and laboratory tests* (3rd ed.). St. Louis: Mosby.

Peters, U., Chatterjee, N., Church, T., Mayo, C., Sturup, S., Foster, C., et al. (2006). High serum selenium and reduced risk of advanced colorectal adenoma in a colorectal cancer early detection program. *Cancer Epidemiology, Biomarkers, and Prevention, 15*(2), 315–320.

Reid, M., Duffield-Lillico, A., Sunga, A., Fakih, M., Alberts, D., & Marshall, J. (2006). Selenium supplementation and colorectal adenomas: An analysis of the nutritional prevention of cancer trial. *International Journal of Cancer, 118*(7), 1777–1781.

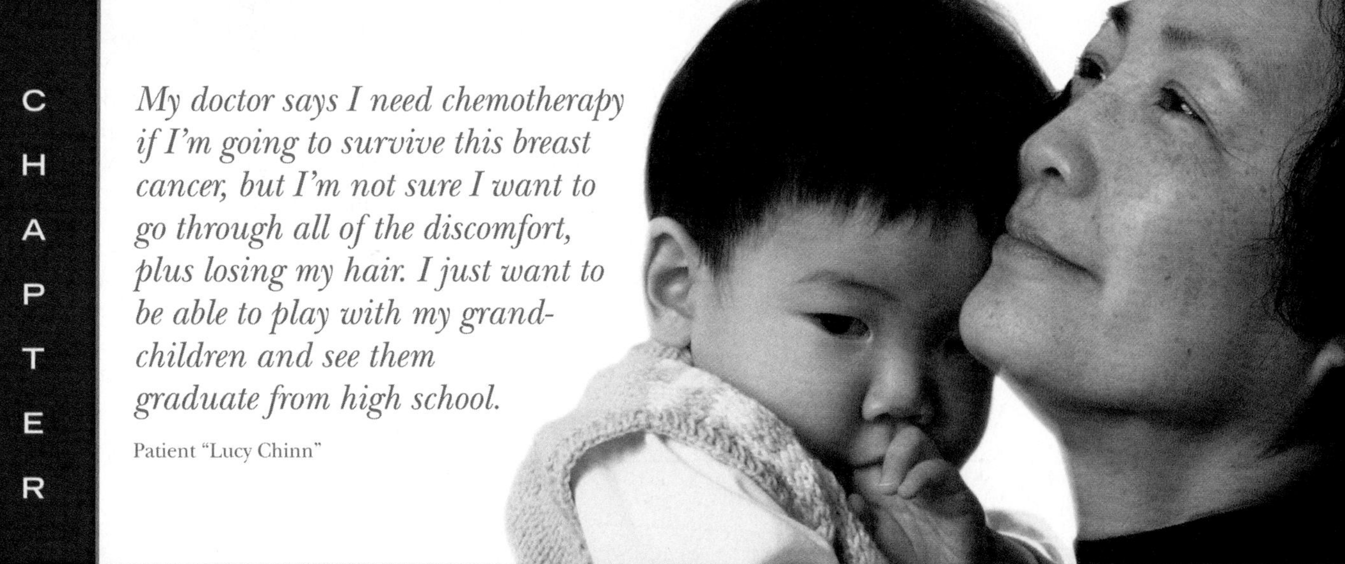

My doctor says I need chemotherapy if I'm going to survive this breast cancer, but I'm not sure I want to go through all of the discomfort, plus losing my hair. I just want to be able to play with my grand-children and see them graduate from high school.

Patient "Lucy Chinn"

58 Pharmacotherapy of Neoplasia

Learning Outcomes

After reading this chapter, the student should be able to:

1. Explain why it is difficult to classify antineoplastic agents.
2. Describe the common and dose-limiting toxicities of antineoplastics.
3. Explain the necessary nursing responsibilities and teaching for the patient who is undergoing chemotherapy.
4. Describe how the process of alkylation can kill rapidly growing cells.
5. Describe how the antimetabolites kill cancer cells.
6. Describe the mechanisms by which antitumor antibiotics kill cancer cells.
7. Explain the mechanisms of action of hormone antagonists.
8. Identify natural products that have the ability to kill tumor cells.
9. Explain the use of biologic response modifiers in cancer chemotherapy.
10. Describe the types of drugs prescribed to reduce or prevent the adverse effects of antineoplastic agents.
11. Discuss ways the nurse can be protected from absorption of the antineoplastics.

Chapter Outline

Classification of Antineoplastic Agents

Nursing Responsibilities for the Patient Undergoing Chemotherapy

Antineoplastic Medications

Alkylating Agents

PROTOTYPE **Cyclophosphamide (Cytoxan)** *p. 967*

Antimetabolites

PROTOTYPE **Methotrexate (MTX, Rheumatrex, Trexall)** *p. 972*

Antitumor Antibiotics

PROTOTYPE **Doxorubicin (Adriamycin)** *p. 977*

Hormones and Hormone Antagonists

PROTOTYPE **Tamoxifen (Nolvadex, Soltamox)** *p. 981*

Natural Products

PROTOTYPE **Vincristine (Oncovin)** *p. 985*

Biologic Response Modifiers and Monoclonal Antibodies

Miscellaneous Antineoplastics

Drugs for Reducing Adverse Effects

Preparing and Administering Antineoplastics

Key Terms

alkylating agents, 966
dose-limiting toxicity, 965
hematopoietic growth factor, 993
leucovorin rescue therapy, 972
molecularly targeted agents, 991
oncology nurse, 993

To begin cancer chemotherapy is a collaborative decision made by the patient, the family, and the health care provider. Chemotherapy is often prolonged and patients will experience adverse effects that can challenge their resolve to complete the regimen. Some of the medications have the potential to produce permanent disability and even death. Nurses must be prepared to assist patients and their families in dealing with the common adverse effects of the antineoplastics, the more serious adverse reactions, and the psychological impact of the decision to continue or discontinue treatment. This chapter examines the types of medications used in cancer chemotherapy and their applications to clinical practice.

Classification of Antineoplastic Agents

58.1 Antineoplastic agents kill or stop the growth of cancer cells and may be classified in multiple ways.

Drugs that are used in cancer chemotherapy come from diverse pharmacologic and chemical classes. Antineoplastics have been extracted from plants and bacteria as well as created entirely in the laboratory. Some of the drug classes attack cellular macromolecules in cancer cells, such as deoxyribonucleic acid (DNA) and proteins, whereas others poison vital metabolic pathways of rapidly growing cells. The common theme among all the antineoplastic agents is their toxicity. They have the ability to kill or stop the growth of cancer cells.

Classification of the antineoplastics is difficult because some of these drugs kill cancer cells by several different mechanisms and have characteristics from more than one class. For example, paclitaxel (Taxol) can be classified as a natural product (it was derived from a plant), a taxane (its chemical structure), a mitotic inhibitor (its mechanism of action), or a cell cycle inhibitor. Furthermore, the mechanisms by which some antineoplastics act are not clearly understood. A simple method of classifying this complex group of drugs includes the following categories:

- Alkylating agents
- Antimetabolites
- Antitumor antibiotics
- Hormones and hormone antagonists
- Natural products
- Biologic response modifiers and monoclonal antibodies
- Miscellaneous antineoplastic drugs

PharmFACT

Prostate cancer is the most common nonskin cancer in America, affecting one in six men. One new case occurs every 2.5 minutes and a man dies from prostate cancer every 19 minutes. *Source:* Prostate Cancer Foundation, 2008.

Nursing Responsibilities for the Patient Undergoing Chemotherapy

58.2 Antineoplastic drugs have serious adverse effects that require skilled nursing assessments and interventions.

Antineoplastic drugs produce the most serious adverse effects of any class of medications. As discussed in Chapter 57, the toxicities of these drugs can affect virtually any body system, organ, or tissue. The student should review Chapter 57 before proceeding.

The majority of antineoplastic agents exhibit bone marrow toxicity that may suppress the numbers of white blood cells (leukopenia, neutropenia), red blood cells (anemia), platelets (thrombocytopenia), or all three types of cells (pancytopenia). Bone marrow suppression may, in turn, lead to opportunistic infections, bleeding, and anemia. In addition, most antineoplastics cause severe nausea, vomiting, stomatitis, diarrhea, constipation, alopecia, and fatigue. A few drugs exhibit neurotoxicity, dermatologic toxicity, nephrotoxicity, and cardiac toxicity.

The fact that most antineoplastic agents are given in combination complicates the ability of the health care provider and nurse to administer care. Toxicities tend to be additive and it is very difficult to determine which specific drug is the one causing the toxicity. Each antineoplastic drug has at least one type of toxicity that could cause discontinuation or temporary delays of therapy. This is called the **dose-limiting toxicity.** In the case of bone marrow suppression, the dose-limiting toxicity is based on laboratory results. When the specific blood cell level falls to a level predetermined by the health care provider, therapy is suspended. In other cases, the dose-limiting toxicity may be based on the patient's subjective symptoms. In all cases, discontinuation or suspension of therapy usually has negative consequences for the patient such that the regimen outcomes will be less effective.

Because the antineoplastics have certain common toxicities, this section lists general nursing responsibilities and patient teaching that should be conducted with most of these drugs. It should be understood, however, that each drug has unique toxicities that require additional monitoring and teaching responsibilities. A current drug guide should always be consulted to obtain current and comprehensive nursing interventions for antineoplastic medications.

Nursing Responsibilities

- Complete a comprehensive baseline assessment, including vital signs, body weight, and general overall health status, and laboratory tests including complete blood count (CBC) with differential, white blood cell (WBC), and platelet counts. If the laboratory tests show that blood counts have dropped below the preestablished standard, hold the drug and notify the prescriber.

- If cardiotoxicity is an anticipated adverse effect, obtain baseline and periodic electrocardiograms (ECGs) during treatment.
- Monitor for ulcerative stomatitis with glossitis and gingivitis. Inspect the mouth daily, and report any patchy necrotic areas, bleeding, discomfort, or overgrowth (black, furry tongue).
- Assess for any signs of infection prior to chemotherapy. Any infections should be treated before starting chemotherapy.
- Assess liver and kidney function because some drugs are contraindicated or their doses may need adjustment if impairment is present.
- Monitor for signs of unusual bleeding during therapy.
- Assess nutritional status and whether nausea or vomiting are present. Recommend treatment with antiemetic drugs as necessary.
- Assess baseline skin integrity frequently during therapy because many antineoplastics cause rash, pruritus, photosensitivity, and discoloration.
- If the patient is receiving a neurotoxic agent such as platinum compounds, assess for baseline auditory and sensory function. If other neurotoxic drugs are used, assess for seizure activity, suicidal ideation, and changes in mental status during therapy.
- Instruct the patient to drink plenty of fluids (2 to 3 L/day) and maintain high urine output (1,500 mL/day). This will dilute the drug metabolites in the bladder and reduce the risk for cystitis.
- When giving intravenous (IV) antineoplastics, assess frequently for extravasation because many of these drugs are vesicants that can cause major tissue damage. When preparing these medications, protective gowns, gloves, and goggles are recommended.

MyNursingKit | Current Indications for Antineoplastics

Patient and Family Education

- Immediately report signs of possible myocardial infarction (MI) to the health care provider. Signs include chest, arm, or back pain, dyspnea, or palpitations, or allergic reaction (facial swelling, tongue thickness, throat tightness, or rash).
- Avoid crowds and persons with known infections and immediately report signs of an infection, such as fever, chills, or sore throat, to the health care provider.
- Perform good oral hygiene, using a soft-bristled toothbrush.
- Eat small, frequent meals of easily digestible foods. Avoid foods high in purine (beans, peas, organ meats) or acid content. Take nutritional supplements if recommended by the health care provider.
- If nausea is present, eat soda crackers and drink ginger ale. Avoid spicy, highly seasoned foods and caffeine.
- Whenever possible, postpone vaccinations during chemotherapy because the body will not be able to mount a sufficient antibody response.
- Suck on ice chips or ice pops if mouth pain is present and also increase fluid intake.
- Know that menstrual irregularities or sterility may occur in premenopausal women and that impotence may occur in men.
- Have routine hearing examinations performed. Immediately report any decreased hearing or other changes, such as ringing, buzzing, or tingling in ears, to the health care provider.
- Know that alopecia may occur and where and when to purchase wigs, if desired.
- If of childbearing age, use effective birth control methods during therapy because many of these drugs can cause birth defects.
- Immediately notify the health care provider of any known or suspected pregnancy.
- Use sunblock and wear protective clothing to avoid direct sun exposure, as recommended by the health care provider.
- Do not breast-feed while undergoing chemotherapy without approval of the health care provider.
- Report significant changes in bowel habits, such as severe diarrhea or chronic constipation, to the health care provider.

CONNECTION *Checkpoint* 58.1

From what you learned in Chapter 46, explain why vaccinations are usually contraindicated in patients who are receiving antineoplastic drugs. See Answer to Connection Checkpoint 58.1 in Appendix A.

Antineoplastic Medications

The antineoplastic medications include alkylating agents, antimetabolites, antitumor antibiotics, hormones and hormone antagonists, natural products, biological response modifiers, monoclonal antibodies, and miscellaneous antineoplastics.

Alkylating Agents

58.3 Alkylating agents change the shape of the deoxyribonucleic acid double helix and prevent cancer cells from dividing normally.

Alkylation, which is the transfer of a carbon group (alkyl group) from one molecule to another, is a common biochemical reaction. In the specific case of chemotherapy, alkylation involves covalent bonding of the antineoplastic drug to the DNA of the cancer cell. The drug may form a "bridge" or cross-link between the two DNA strands and markedly affect the function of the DNA.

The **alkylating agents** kill cancer cells by altering the shape of the DNA double helix and preventing the DNA from duplicating during cell division. Each alkylating agent attaches to DNA in a different manner; however, they all have the effect of inducing cell death or at least slowing the replication of tumor cells. Although the process of alkylation may occur at any time during the cell cycle, the killing action occurs when the affected cell divides because this is when it attempts to duplicate the defective DNA strands. The alkylating agents have a broad spectrum and are used against many types of malignancies, including some lymphomas, myelomas, leukemias, and pancreatic cancers, and some testicular, ovarian, and breast cancers. They are the oldest classification of antineoplastics, having been available since the end of World War II, and are the most widely used antineoplastic drugs. Alkylating agents are sometimes subdivided into chemical classes, which include the nitrogen mustards, nitrosoureas, and platinum compounds. These agents are listed in Table 58.1. Figure 58.1 illustrates the process of alkylation.

Because blood cells are particularly sensitive to the actions of alkylating agents, bone marrow suppression (myelosuppression) is the primary dose-limiting toxicity of these drugs. Within days after administration, the numbers of erythrocytes, leukocytes, and platelets begin to decline, reaching a nadir at 6 to 10 days. These drugs are withheld if red blood cell (RBC), WBC, and platelet counts fall below a predetermined limit during therapy. Epithelial cells lining the gastrointestinal (GI) tract are also damaged with alkylating agents, causing nausea, vomiting, and diarrhea. Alopecia may be expected from most of the alkylating agents. The nitrosoureas and mechlorethamine are also strong vesicants, and great care must be taken to avoid skin contact or extravasation. Secondary malignancies may occur with the alkylating agents. Approximately 5% of the patients treated with alkylating agents develop acute nonlymphocytic leukemia 4 years or more after chemotherapy has been completed.

When alkylating agents are taken for prolonged periods, cancer cells can develop resistance to them. The mechanism of resistance is incompletely understood. However, possible mechanisms include decreased drug uptake by cancer cells, increased cellular inactivation of the drug, and increased production of DNA repair enzymes.

PROTOTYPE DRUG Cyclophosphamide (Cytoxan)

Classification: **Therapeutic:** Antineoplastic

Pharmacologic: Alkylating agent, nitrogen mustard, disease-modifying antirheumatic drug, immunosuppressant

TABLE 58.1 Alkylating Agents

Drug	Route and Adult Dose (maximum dose where indicated)	Adverse Effects
Nitrogen Mustards		
bondamustine (Treanda)	IV: 90–120 mg/m^2 (variable schedule)	*Headache, alopecia, nausea, vomiting, stomatitis, anorexia, rash, fluid retention*
chlorambucil (Leukeran)	PO: 0.1–0.2 mg/kg/day initially; 4–10 mg/day as maintenance	Bone marrow suppression, severe nausea, vomiting, diarrhea, Stevens–Johnson syndrome, hemorrhagic cystitis, neurotoxicity, ototoxicity, pulmonary toxicity, anaphylaxis, and other hypersensitivity reactions
cyclophosphamide (Cytoxan)	PO: 1–5 mg/day initially; 1–5 mg/kg every 7–10 days for maintenance	
estramustine (Emcyt)	PO: 14 mg/kg/day in three to four divided doses	
ifosfamide (Ifex)	IV: 1.2 g/m^2/day for 5 consecutive days	
mechlorethamine (Mustargen)	IV: 6 mg/m^2 on days 1 and 8 of a 28-day cycle	
melphalan (Alkeran)	PO: 6 mg/day for 2–3 weeks	
Nitrosoureas		
carmustine (BiCNU, Gliadel)	IV: 200 mg/m^2 /day	
lomustine (CeeNU, CCNU)	PO: 130 mg/m^2 as a single dose	
streptozocin (Zanosar)	IV: 500 mg/m^2 for 5 consecutive days	
Platinum Compounds		
carboplatin (Paraplatin)	IV: 360 mg/m^2 once every 4 weeks	
cisplatin (Platinol)	IV: 20 mg/m^2/day for 5 days	
oxaliplatin (Eloxatin)	IV: 85 mg/m^2 for 2 h	
Miscellaneous Alkylating Agents		
busulfan (Busulfex, Myleran)	PO: 4–8 mg/day IV: 0.8 mg/kg every 6 hr for 4 days	
dacarbazine (DTIC-Dome)	IV: 2–4.5 mg/kg/day for 10 days, repeated every 4 weeks	
procarbazine (Matulane)	PO: 2–4 mg/kg/day in single or divided dose for 1 week, then 4–6 mg/kg/day until WBCs are less than 4,000/mm^3 or platelets are less than 100,000/mm^3, or when maximum response is obtained	
temozolomide (Temodar)	PO: 150 mg/m^2/day for 5 consecutive days	
thiotepa (Thioplex, TSPA)	IV: 0.3–0.4 mg/kg every 1–4 weeks	

Note: *Italics* indicate common adverse effects. Underline indicates serious adverse effects.

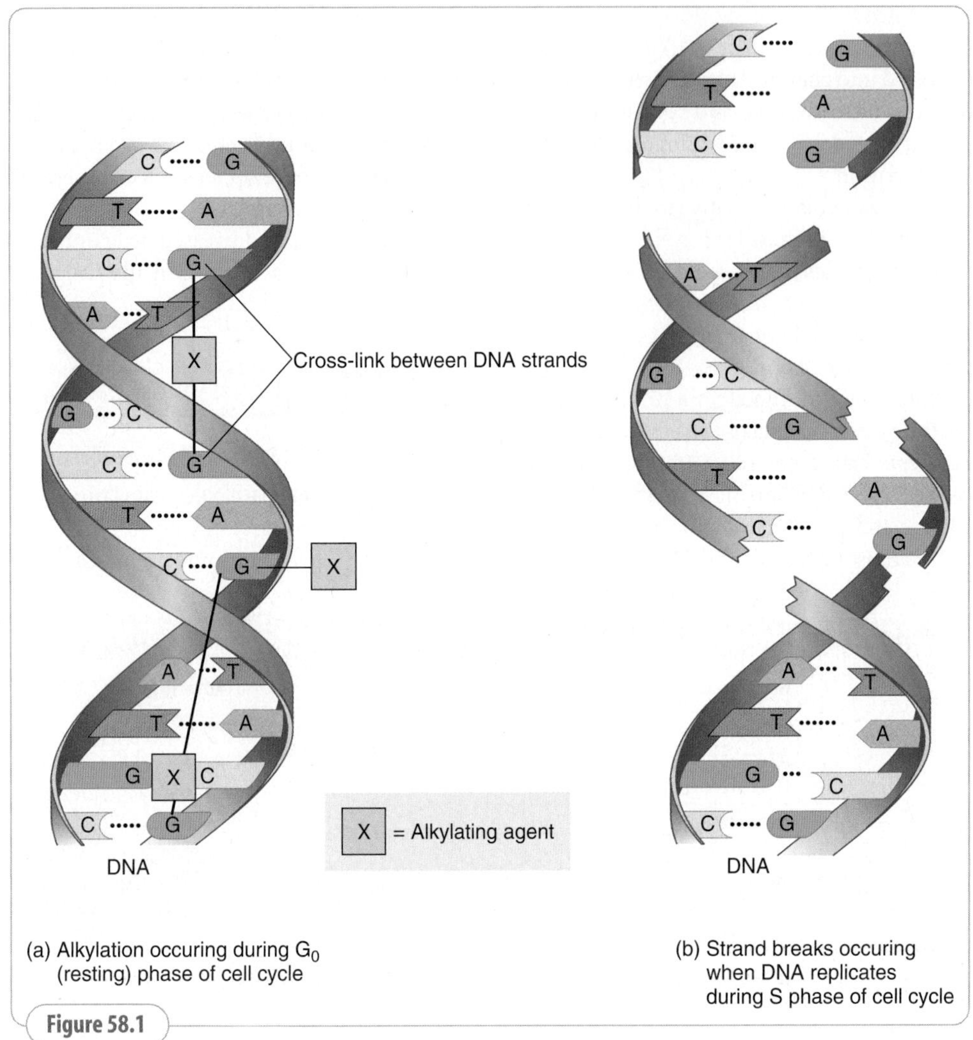

Figure 58.1

Mechanism of action of the alkylating agents.

Therapeutic Effects and Uses: Approved in 1959 by the U.S. Food and Drug Administration (FDA), cyclophosphamide is available as an oral (PO) or injectable preparation. It has a very broad spectrum of action and is approved in combination with other antineoplastics in the chemotherapy of Hodgkin's and non-Hodgkin's lymphoma, acute lymphocytic and myelogenous leukemia, ovarian cancer, breast cancer, multiple myeloma, chronic lymphocytic and myelogenous leukemia, mycosis fungoides, neuroblastoma, sarcomas, and retinoblastoma. It may be used off-label to treat lung cancer, endometrial cancer, Ewing's sarcoma, osteogenic sarcoma, prostate cancer, rhabdomyosarcoma, and other neoplastic conditions. It is used in both children and adults.

Cyclophosphamide is an effective immunosuppressant. Although it is considered an adverse effect during cancer chemotherapy, this drug is used to intentionally cause immunosuppression, often in combination therapy with corticosteroids. Off-label immunosuppressive indications include prophylaxis of organ transplant rejection, nephrotic syndrome, severe progressive rheumatoid arthritis (RA), systemic lupus erythematosus (SLE), and scleroderma.

Mechanism of Action: Cyclophosphamide is a prodrug that is converted to its active form (phosphoramide mustard) in the liver. Cyclophosphamide binds to DNA and forms cross links, which prevent the synthesis of DNA, ribonucleic acid (RNA), and protein. It is a cell cycle nonspecific drug.

Pharmacokinetics:

Route(s)	PO, IV
Absorption	Well absorbed from the GI tract
Distribution	Widely distributed; crosses the placenta; secreted in breast milk; also found in brain tissue
Primary metabolism	Extensive hepatic metabolism by CYP2B6 and other CYP isozymes
Primary excretion	Renal
Onset of action	Peak: 1 h (PO)
Duration of action	Half-life: 3–12 h; metabolites can still be identified in serum after 72 h

Adverse Effects: Adverse effects include those common to other antineoplastic agents, such as anorexia, nausea, vomiting, weight loss, diarrhea, and mouth sores. Alopecia occurs more frequently with cyclophosphamide than with other antineoplastics; 50% of patients will develop total baldness. Other common adverse effects are jaundice, acne, blistered skin, and darkened or thickened skin. Bone marrow suppression is a potentially life-threatening adverse reaction that occurs between days 9 and 14 of therapy; the patient is at dangerous risk for severe infection and sepsis during this period. Bone marrow recovery occurs by days 18 through 25. Other life-threatening adverse effects include secondary cancers, especially of the urinary bladder, cardiotoxicity, and pulmonary fibrosis. Hematuria may signal hemorrhagic cystitis, which can be severe and even fatal. Interference with the ability to reproduce may occur in both males and females, and this may be irreversible. Cyclophosphamide is teratogenic and is associated with increased risk of secondary malignancies that may take several years after completion of chemotherapy to become apparent. The most common secondary malignancies are bladder cancer, lymphoma, and leukemia.

Contraindications/Precautions: The only contraindications to the use of cyclophosphamide are pregnancy, lactation, and severe myelosuppression. The drug must be used cautiously in persons with leukopenia, thrombocytopenia, previous radiation therapy, bone marrow infiltration of tumor cells, impaired renal or hepatic function, recent history of steroid use, or previous therapy that caused cytotoxicity.

Drug Interactions: Many drug interactions are possible with cyclophosphamide due to its extensive hepatic metabolism. This drug has additive immunosuppressive effects if administered with other agents that cause bone marrow toxicity. There may be an increased anticoagulant effect if it is given with anticoagulants. There may be increased cardiotoxicity if it is given with doxorubicin. Insulin may increase hypoglycemia. Lower serum digoxin levels can be expected in the patient who takes digoxin. Phenobarbital use may lead to an increased rate of metabolism of cyclophosphamide, whereas phenytoin use may lead to an increased risk of toxicity. **Herbal/Food:** St. John's wort may increase the toxic effects of cyclophosphamide.

Pregnancy: Category D.

Treatment of Overdose: Overdose can result in severe myelosuppression with the possibility of infection. General supportive measures are administered.

Nursing Responsibilities: (See Section 52.2 for general nursing responsibilities.)

- Monitor laboratory test results. Marked leukopenia is the most serious adverse effect and it can be fatal. Nadir may occur as late as 1 month after a series of daily doses.
- Protect the patient from infection and trauma and from visitors and medical personnel who have colds or other infections during severe leukopenic period.
- Report the onset of unexplained chills, sore throat, and tachycardia to the prescriber. Monitor temperature carefully and report an elevation in temperature immediately. The development of fever in a patient who is neutropenic (granulocyte count less than 1,000) is a medical emergency because sepsis can develop quickly in these patients.
- Monitor intake and output (I&O) ratio and patterns. Increase fluid intake to help prevent renal irritation and hemorrhagic cystitis because this drug is a chemical irritant.
- Promptly report hematuria or dysuria to the prescriber. The drug schedule is usually interrupted and fluids are forced if these conditions occur.
- Record body weight at least twice weekly because this is the basis for dose determination. Alert the prescriber to sudden changes or slow, steady weight gain or loss over a period that appears inconsistent with caloric intake.
- Immediately report diarrhea, which may signal onset of hyperkalemia, particularly if accompanied by colicky pain, nausea, bradycardia, and skeletal muscle weakness, to the prescriber.
- Monitor for hyperuricemia, which occurs commonly during early treatment period in patients with leukemias or lymphoma. Report edema of the lower legs and feet, or joint, flank, or stomach pain to the prescriber.

Patient and Family Education:

- Void frequently, especially after each dose and just before bedtime, to minimize bladder irritation from drug therapy.
- Adhere to the dosage regimen and do not omit, increase, decrease, or delay doses. If for any reason this drug cannot be taken, notify the health care provider.
- Expect hair loss, which occurs in about 33% of patients on cyclophosphamide therapy. Hair loss may be noted 3 weeks after therapy begins; regrowth which often differs in texture and color usually starts 5 to 6 weeks after this drug is withdrawn.
- Use adequate means of contraception during and for at least 4 months after termination of the drug therapy.
- Do not breast-feed during cyclophosphamide therapy without approval of the health care provider.
- Report changes in menstrual cycles to the health care provider. Loss of menstrual periods may last up to 1 year after cessation of therapy in 10% to 30% of women.

MyNursingKit | Mechanism of Action Animation: Cyclophosphamide

Drugs Similar to Cyclophosphamide (Cytoxan)

Alkylating agents include other nitrogen mustards, including chlorambucil, estramustine, ifosfamide, mechlorethamine, and melphalan; the nitrosoureas, including carmustine, lomustine, and streptozocin; and miscellaneous alkylating agents, including busulfan, cisplatin, dacarbazine, procarbazine, temozolomide, and thiotepa.

Busulfan (Busulfex, Myleran): Approved in 1954, busulfan is a potent alkylating agent that is used for palliative treatment of chronic myelogenous leukemia for those patients who are no longer responsive to radiation therapy or other chemotherapeutic agents. It does not appreciably extend survival times. In combination with cyclophosphamide, busulfan is given for bone marrow ablation prior to stem cell transplantation. Busulfan is available as a PO preparation for cancer treatment, and as an IV preparation when used for patients who are undergoing stem cell transplant. Myelosuppression is a serious adverse effect, and blood counts must be closely monitored. Pancytopenia occurs in 100% of patients who are taking high doses of this drug, and this condition may last as long as 2 years. Nausea, vomiting, stomatitis, and anorexia are common adverse effects. Because of the potential for infertility, men and women within child-bearing years should be counseled regarding the drug's reproductive effects. It is a pregnancy category D drug.

Carmustine (BiCNU, Gliadel): Carmustine, a nitrosourea, is an alkylating agent and is one of the few drugs in its class that can penetrate the blood–brain barrier. Thus it used to treat brain tumors such as malignant glioma, astrocytoma, ependymoma, and brain metastases. It is usually administered by the IV route because it is poorly absorbed in the GI tract. A wafer form of the drug (Gliadel) was approved in 1996 for implantation into the cavity created by removal of a brain tumor. The wafer dissolves over 2 to 3 weeks, delivering 1,000 times the amount of carmustine to the tumor site than could be obtained through IV administration. In addition to brain tumors, carmustine is also given for GI tract cancers, lymphomas (including Hodgkin's disease), and melanomas. In combination with other agents, carmustine may be used for bone marrow ablation prior to stem cell transplantation. The most serious rate-limiting toxicity is myelosuppression. Neurologic adverse effects include seizures and encephalopathy. Other adverse effects are those typical of other alkylating agents. This is a pregnancy category D drug.

Chlorambucil (Leukeran): Chlorambucil, a nitrogen mustard alkylating agent, is used to treat chronic lymphocytic leukemia, lymphomas, Hodgkin's disease, giant follicular lymphoma, and cancer of the testes, ovaries, and breast. Because it is an immunosuppressant, chlorambucil is occasionally used off-label to treat nephrotic syndrome, RA, SLE, and other inflammatory disorders. Severe myelosuppression is the major dose-limiting toxicity; blood values usually return to baseline 3 to 4 weeks after administration. In general, chlorambucil produces less toxicity than most other alkylating agents and has a slow onset of action. Approved in 1957, it is available via the PO route. This is a pregnancy category D drug.

Cisplatin (Platinol) and other platinum agents: Cisplatin is a heavy metal complex containing platinum, chloride, and ammonia. It is cell cycle nonspecific and usually used as combination therapy to treat metastatic testicular or ovarian tumors, bladder cancer, osteosarcoma, and soft tissue sarcomas, and as adjuvant therapy in head, neck, esophageal, prostate, lung, and cervical cancers. It is available only as an injectable preparation. Unlike many other alkylating agents, cisplatin does not cause significant myelosuppression. The major dose-limiting toxicity of cisplatin is nephrotoxicity. Acute renal failure may occur within 24 hours after administration, and permanent damage to renal tubular cells may eventually cause chronic renal failure. Extreme caution must be used if cisplatin is to be administered to patients with renal impairment or to those taking other nephrotoxic drugs. Renal function must be closely monitored during therapy. Peripheral neuropathy is another potentially serious adverse effect with symptoms that include numbness that begins in the fingers and toes and proceeds up the limbs toward the trunk. Ototoxicity is common and can result in permanent impairment. The nurse should be prepared for anaphylactic-like reactions that may occur within minutes of cisplatin administration. Cisplatin is a pregnancy category D drug.

Carboplatin (Paraplatin): Approved for the first-line palliative treatment of advanced ovarian cancer, carboplatin is used off-label to treat acute lymphocytic leukemia, acute myelogenous leukemia, bladder cancer, breast cancer, and other tumors. Approved in 1989, carboplatin is administered by the IV route, is structurally similar to cisplatin, and works by the same mechanism but is estimated to be 45 times less toxic. Severe myelosuppression is the dose-limiting toxicity. Neurotoxicity and nephrotoxicity occur less often than with cisplatin. The nurse should be prepared for anaphylactic-like reactions that may occur within minutes of carboplatin administration. This is a pregnancy category D drug.

Oxaliplatin (Eloxatin): Approved in 2002, oxaliplatin is a platinum compound that is approved only to treat advanced colorectal cancer, although it may be used off-label for other solid tumors such as those of the ovary, breast, testes, pancreas, head, or neck. It acts by a different mechanism than cisplatin and thus has very little ototoxicity or nephrotoxicity. It does, however, demonstrate significant levels of peripheral neuropathy, which can be dose limiting. An acute form of peripheral neuropathy begins within days of chemotherapy and resolves in 1 to 2 weeks. A more persistent form has a delayed onset and can cause functional impairment and discontinuation of therapy. Drinking cold beverages or breathing cold air will worsen symptoms of neuropathy. The nurse should be prepared for anaphylactic-like reactions that may occur within minutes of oxaliplatin administration. This is a pregnancy category D drug.

Dacarbazine (DTIC-Dome): Approved in 1998, dacarbazine is an alkylating agent that is available only for IV administration. It has carcinogenic, mutagenic, and teratogenic effects. It is approved to treat metastatic malignant melanoma and refractory Hodgkin's disease, and it may be used off-label for sarcomas and neuroblastomas. Adverse GI effects occur in most patients, but tolerance to these adverse effects may develop over subsequent administrations. Myelosuppression occurs during therapy, although to a lesser extent than many other drugs in this class. Liver function tests should be regularly monitored because dacarbazine has been reported to cause hepatic necrosis. Unlike other alkylating agents, dacarbazine is a pregnancy category C drug although use during the first trimester of pregnancy is contraindicated.

Temozolomide (Temodar): Temozolomide is a prodrug that is metabolized to the same active compound as dacarbazine. Unlike dacarbazine, temozolomide is administered by the PO route. Approved in 1999, it is indicated to treat malignant glioma and astrocytoma and may be used off-label for malignant melanoma. Adverse effects are similar to those of dacarbazine, including myelosuppression and nausea or vomiting. Neurotoxicity, including seizures, hemiparesis, amnesia, and dizziness, occur in a significant number of patients. This is a pregnancy category D drug.

Estramustine (Emcyt): Estramustine is unusual because it is a dual molecule. One portion is a nitrogen mustard alkylating agent and the other is a molecule of estradiol. Thus, the drug may be classified as either an alkylating agent or a hormone. It is administered by the PO route for the palliative therapy of metastatic or advanced prostate cancer and may be used off-label to treat metastatic renal carcinoma. Unlike other alkylating agents, however, myelosuppression is infrequent. Nausea and vomiting are the dose-limiting toxicities. The estrogen component of the drug can cause gynecomastia, mastalgia, thromboembolic disease, and fluid retention. This is a pregnancy category D drug.

Ifosfamide (Ifex): Ifosfamide is one of the newer nitrogen mustard alkylating agents that was approved in 1988 for the treatment of testicular cancer. Off-label indications include breast, lung, pancreatic, bladder and cervical cancers, sarcomas, and non-Hodgkin's lymphoma. Bone marrow suppression is the primary dose-limiting toxicity, with blood count nadirs occurring after 5 days and recovering by 4 weeks. Nephrotoxicity also limits its use and hematuria, hemorrhagic cystitis, and renal insufficiency occur in many patients. Signs of neurotoxicity such as confusion, drowsiness, hallucinations, and depression occur in about 12% of patients who are taking the drug. Cardiac toxicity occurs in as many as 15% of patients and may include dysrhythmias, heart failure, and myocarditis. This is a pregnancy category D drug.

To prevent hemorrhagic cystitis in patients who are taking ifosfamide, the drug mesna (Mesnex) is administered at the time of chemotherapy by the IV route and 2 to 6 hours later by the IV or PO route. Mesna binds the toxic metabolites in the urinary bladder, reducing the incidence of hematuria by 70% to 100%, depending on the dose of ifosfamide. This is the only indication for mesna.

Lomustine (CeeNU, CCNU): Approved in 1976, lomustine is an oral nitrosourea alkylating agent that has actions similar to those of carmustine. Like carmustine, it is able to cross the blood–brain barrier. It is used as palliative therapy in combination with other chemotherapeutic agents or other treatment modalities in primary and metastatic brain tumors and as secondary therapy in Hodgkin's disease. The most serious rate-limiting toxicity is delayed myelosuppression, which may occur up to 6 weeks following administration of the drug. Severe nausea and vomiting occur in most patients and require antiemetic therapy. Taking the drug on an empty stomach can reduce nausea and vomiting symptoms. This is a pregnancy category D drug.

Mechlorethamine (Mustargen): Mechlorethamine is one of the oldest antineoplastics that was approved in 1949. A nitrogen mustard, mechlorethamine produces acute tissue damage with a relatively rapid recovery compared to other antineoplastics. It is available by the IV, intrathecal, or topical routes. It is usually used to provide palliation in patients with Hodgkin's disease (States III and IV), lymphosarcoma, polycythemia vera, bronchogenic carcinoma, and chronic myelocytic or chronic lymphocytic leukemia. It may also be used for palliative treatment of metastatic cancer in intrapleural, intrapericardial, and intraperitoneal spaces when effusion has occurred as a result of the tumor. Nausea and vomiting are acute and require antiemetic therapy. Myelosuppression occurs in 8 to 14 days after drug administration and can be severe. Like cyclophosphamide, infertility is a potential adverse effect. This drug is a vesicant; extravasation requires the administration of sodium thiosulfate to the injection site. This is a pregnancy category D drug.

Melphalan (Alkeran): Melphalan is a nitrogen mustard alkylating agent approved for the palliative treatment of ovarian cancer and multiple myeloma. It may also be used off-label to treat breast or testicular cancer, osteogenic sarcoma, and non-Hodgkin's lymphoma. It is available as both a PO and an IV preparation. Because it has strong immunosuppressive and myelosuppressive effects, it has been used off-label for bone marrow ablation prior to stem cell transplantation in combination with other agents. Hematologic toxicity is the primary dose-limiting toxicity. Blood count nadirs usually occur in 2 to 3 weeks after therapy starts, and recovery is seen 4 to 5 weeks after treatment. Unlike some of the other alkylating agents, melphalan is not highly emetogenic. The nurse should use extra caution to prevent skin exposure (to both nurse and patient) to the drug because it can cause skin necrosis. Because of the potential for infertility, men and women in childbearing years should be counseled regarding the drug's reproductive effects. This is a pregnancy category D drug.

Procarbazine (Matulane): Procarbazine is an oral alkylating agent that was approved in 1969 for the treatment of Hodgkin's disease. However, it may be used off-label for treating non-Hodgkin's lymphomas and central nervous system (CNS) tumors such as medulloblastoma, malignant glioma, and astrocytoma. It is also used as an adjunct in the palliative treatment of Hodgkin's disease. Because it has strong immunosuppressive effects, it may be used off-label for bone marrow ablation prior to stem cell transplantation in combination with other agents. Myelosuppression is the primary dose-limiting toxicity. Blood count nadirs usually occur in week 4 after therapy starts, and recovery is seen 6 weeks after treatment. Nausea and vomiting are also common adverse effects that may be severe. CNS adverse effects are common and may include paresthesias, peripheral neuropathy, seizures, depression, and psychosis. When given by the IV route, neurotoxicity can be dose limiting. This is a pregnancy category D drug.

Streptozocin (Zanosar): Approved in 1982, streptozocin is a nitrosourea alkylating agent that is more toxic and has a lower therapeutic index than many other alkylating agents. It is available as an IV preparation to be used to treat metastatic islet cell cancers of the pancreas either as a single agent or in combination with fluorouracil. It may be used off-label to treat colorectal cancer and other solid tumors. A clinically effective response most likely will be accompanied by some evidence of serious toxicity. The most serious dose-limiting toxicity is nephrotoxicity, which occurs in more than half of the patients taking the drug and can cause permanent impairment and death. Nausea and vomiting are also severe adverse effects of streptozocin. This is a pregnancy category D drug.

Thiotepa: Thiotepa is an alkylating agent that was approved in 1994 to treat bladder, ovarian and breast cancers, and both Hodgkin's and non-Hodgkin's lymphomas. It is administered IV or by the intravesical route for bladder tumors. Myelosuppression is the primary dose-limiting toxicity, although neurotoxicity may also cause delay or discontinuation of therapy. Nausea and vomiting are uncommon. Injections and instillations of thiotepa can cause intense local pain. Intravesical administration causes bladder irritation, dysuria, and increased urgency. It should be noted that the drug may be absorbed during intravesical administration and cause serious myelosuppression. This is a pregnancy category D drug.

Antimetabolites

58.4 Antimetabolites disrupt the critical cellular pathways of cancer cells.

Rapidly growing cancer cells require large quantities of nutrients to construct proteins and nucleic acids. Antimetabolite drugs are structurally similar to these nutrients, but they do not perform the same functions as their natural counterparts. When cancer cells attempt to synthesize proteins, RNA, or DNA using the antimetabolites, metabolic pathways are disrupted and the cancer cells die or their growth is slowed. Some of these structural similarities are illustrated in Figure 58.2.

Some antimetabolites become incorporated into the DNA of cancer cells and interfere with DNA replication and function. Others inhibit the enzymes that synthesize the vital components of the cell. All antimetabolites are cell cycle specific, most affecting the S phase, although some can act during any of the active phases of the cell cycle. The three classes of antimetabolites are the folic acid analogs, the purine analogs, and the pyrimidine analogs. These agents are listed in Table 58.2.

Folic acid analogs: Folic acid, or folate, is vitamin B_9, which is essential for the growth and maintenance of cells. It is especially important during periods of rapid cell growth because this vitamin is needed to replicate DNA. Lack of this vitamin during pregnancy can cause neural tube defects in the fetus. Additional details on folic acid are presented in Chapter 62.

Two folic acid analogs are used as antineoplastic agents. Methotrexate, which was approved in 1953, is the older of the two and is prescribed for several autoimmune disorders in addition to cancer. The second folic acid analog, pemetrexed (Alimta), was approved in 2004 and has very limited therapeutic application. Other folic acid analogs are used as anti-infectives. These include trimethoprim (Primsol), pyrimethamine (Daraprim), and trimetrexate (Neutrexin).

Folic acid analogs are given at very high doses, which can be toxic to normal cells as well as cancer cells. To "rescue" normal cells, the drug leucovorin is administered following chemotherapy with methotrexate. Leucovorin, or folinic acid, is a reduced form of folic acid that is able to enter normal cells but not cancer cells. The normal cells can thus continue replication and development using leucovorin. Available by both the IV and PO routes, **leucovorin rescue therapy** must be initiated at very specific times following the methotrexate dose. Leucovorin is also used to treat overdose or prevent toxicity with other folic acid analogs such as pyrimethamine and trimethoprim. When used with fluorouracil (5-FU) in the treatment of colorectal cancer, leucovorin has been found to enhance cell killing. A new form of leucovorin, levoleucovorin (Fusilev) was approved in 2008. Given by IV infusion, levoleucovorin is an isomer of leucovorin that is reported to have fewer adverse effects.

CONNECTION *Checkpoint* 58.2

Trimethoprim is a folic acid analog that is nearly always combined with another antibiotic medication. From what you learned in Chapter 52, name the antibiotic combination that contains trimethoprim and give its primary indications. See Answer to Connection Checkpoint 58.2 in Appendix A.

PROTOTYPE DRUG Methotrexate (MTX, Rheumatrex, Trexall)

Classification: **Therapeutic:** Antineoplastic

Pharmacologic: Antimetabolite, folic acid analog, immunosuppressant, disease-modifying antirheumatic drug (DMARD)

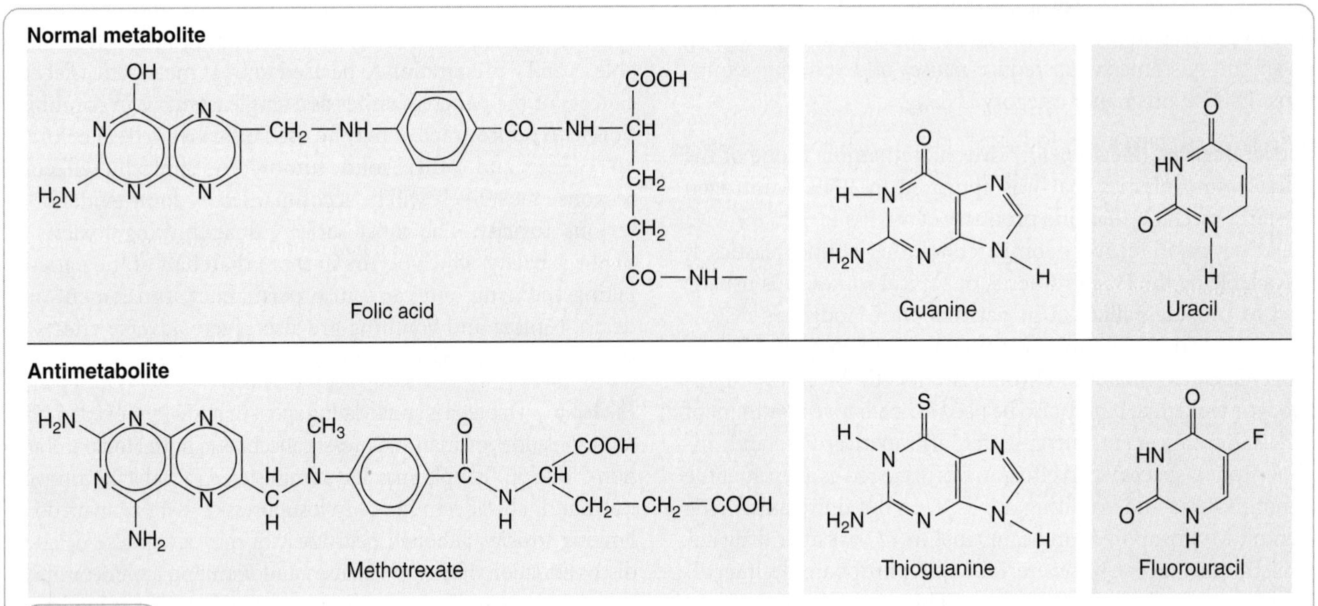

Normal metabolite

Folic acid

Guanine

Uracil

Antimetabolite

Methotrexate

Thioguanine

Fluorouracil

Figure 58.2

Structural similarities between antimetabolites and their natural counterparts.

TABLE 58.2 Antimetabolites

Drug	Route and Adult Dose (maximum dose where indicated)	Adverse Effects
Folic Acid Analogs		
methotrexate (Rheumatrex, Trexall)	PO: 10–30 mg/day for 5 days	*Nausea, vomiting, stomatitis, anorexia, rash, alopecia, headache* Bone marrow suppression, severe nausea, vomiting, diarrhea, mucositis, hepatotoxicity, pulmonary toxicity, neurotoxicity, anaphylaxis, and other hypersensitivity reactions
pemetrexed (Alimta)	IV: 500 mg/m^2 on day 1 of each 21-day cycle	
pralatrexate (Folotyn)	IV: 30 mg over 3 to 5 minutes	
Pyrimidine Analogs		
capecitabine (Xeloda)	PO: 2,500 mg/m^2 /day for 2 weeks	
cytarabine (Cytosar, Cytosine arabinoside, Depot-Cyt)	IV: 200 mg/m^2 as a continuous infusion over 24 h	
floxuridine (FUDR)	Intra-arterial: 0.1–0.6 mg/kg/day as a continuous infusion	
fluorouracil (5-FU, Adrucil, Carac, Efudex)	IV: 12 mg/kg/day for 4 consecutive days	
gemcitabine (Gemzar)	IV: 1,000 mg/m^2 every week for 7 weeks	
Purine Analogs		
cladribine (Leustatin)	IV: 0.09 mg/m^2 /day as a continuous infusion	
clofarabine (Clolar)	IV: 52 mg/m^2/day over 2 h for 5 days	
fludarabine (Fludara)	IV: 25 mg/m^2 /day for 5 consecutive days	
mercaptopurine (6-MP, Purinethol)	PO: 2.5 mg/kg/day	
nelarabine (Arranon)	IV: 1,500 mg/m^2 on days 1, 3, and 5; repeat every 21 days	
pentostatin (Nipent)	IV: 4 mg/m^2 every other week	
thioguanine (6-TG, Tabloid)	PO: 2 mg/kg/day	

Note: *Italics* indicate common adverse effects. Underline indicates serious adverse effects.

Therapeutic Effects and Uses: Approved in 1953, methotrexate is an antimetabolite available by the PO, parenteral, and intrathecal routes. The PO route is preferred for low-dose therapy. It is approved for a large number of neoplastic conditions, including osteosarcoma, acute lymphocytic and lymphoblastic leukemias, and lymphosarcomas in children; certain inoperable head, neck, and pelvic cancers; breast cancers; lung cancers; and advanced stage non-Hodgkin's lymphoma. Its primary use as an antineoplastic agent is in combination therapy to maintain induced remissions in those persons who have had surgical resection or amputation for a primary tumor.

In addition to its role as an antimetabolite, methotrexate is a powerful immunosuppressant. Because of its immunosuppressant properties, methotrexate is used with success in patients with severe RA who have had no response to nonsteroidal anti-inflammatory drugs (NSAIDs) and at least one or more antirheumatic drugs. It also is used to treat severe psoriasis that is unresponsive to other forms of therapy. Off-label uses include other autoimmune disorders such as active Crohn's disease, ulcerative colitis, psoriasis, and SLE. Methotrexate may be used to terminate pregnancy, usually in combination with misoprostol (see Chapter 71).

Mechanism of Action: Methotrexate is specific for the S phase of the cell cycle. It blocks an enzyme that is responsible for converting folic acid to reduced folate, which interferes with DNA synthesis, repair, and cellular replication mainly in actively proliferating tissues. This action is what enables it to be effective in treating psoriasis and arthritis in addition to treating cancer.

Pharmacokinetics:

Route(s)	PO, intramuscular (IM), IV, subcutaneous, intrathecal
Absorption	Variable absorption from the GI tract; well absorbed by the subcutaneous or IM routes
Distribution	Widely distributed; crosses the placenta and blood–brain barrier; secreted in breast milk; 60% bound to plasma protein
Primary metabolism	Hepatic, extensive first pass metabolism
Primary excretion	Renal
Onset of action	Peak: 1–4 h PO, and 0.5–2 h IM, IV
Duration of action	Half-life: 2–4 h

Adverse Effects: Methotrexate has many adverse effects, some of which can be life threatening. These include methotrexate-induced interstitial pneumonitis, sudden death, *Pneumocystis carinii* infection, severe fatal skin reactions, seizures, leukoencephalopathy, hematuria, renal failure, azotemia, uric acid nephropathy, GI hemorrhage, hemorrhagic enteritis, pancreatitis,

MyNursingKit | Mechanism of Action Animation: Methotrexate

pericardial effusion, pulmonary embolism, respiratory fibrosis, respiratory failure, toxic epidermal necrolysis, Stevens–Johnson syndrome, aplastic anemia, abortion, anaphylaxis, tumor lysis syndrome, seizures, or coma (following intrathecal use). The primary dose-limiting toxicities are myelosuppression, GI ulceration, and pulmonary toxicity. Nausea and vomiting are severe at high doses. Low doses will elevate hepatic function enzymes, and high doses can lead to hepatic fibrosis, chronic hepatotoxicity, and possibly cirrhosis.

Contraindications/Precautions: The use of methotrexate as an antineoplastic is contraindicated in thrombocytopenia, anemia, leukopenia, concurrent administration of hepatotoxic drugs and hematopoietic suppressants, alcoholism, or lactation. Precautions must be taken in patients with impaired renal or hepatic function, active infections, ulcerative colitis, and peptic ulcers; in patients with cancer who have preexisting bone marrow impairment; in the very young, elderly, or debilitated; and in those with poor nutritional status. This drug is a confirmed teratogen and precautions must be taken to avoid pregnancy during therapy. Caution should be used in handling this drug because it can cause severe skin reactions.

Drug Interactions: Methotrexate interacts with many drugs. Increased serum methotrexate levels can occur with the penicillins, vancomycin, cyclosporine, and para-amino benzoic acid (PABA). Chloramphenicol may decrease the intestinal absorption of methotrexate. An increased methotrexate effect can occur with probenecid, ibuprofen, aspirin, and tetracyclines. Folic acid may alter the body's response to methotrexate. Methotrexate may cause increased theophylline levels. Sulfonamides can lead to an increased risk of methotrexate-induced immunosuppression. Methotrexate can cause decreased phenytoin effects, leading to increased seizure activity. Methotrexate impairs the immunologic response to smallpox vaccine. Any live vaccine use may lead to a severe reaction that is secondary to the immunosuppressant activity of methotrexate. **Herbal/Food:** Food delays the oral absorption of methotrexate. Echinacea may increase the risk of hepatotoxicity. More than 180 mg per day of caffeine (3 to 4 cups of coffee) may decrease the effectiveness of methotrexate when taken for arthritis.

Pregnancy: Category X.

Treatment of Overdose: Leucovorin or levoleucovorin is given as soon as possible to decrease the toxic effects of methotrexate. Leucovorin can be fatal to the patient if not given in the correct dose at the correct time during methotrexate therapy.

Nursing Responsibilities: (See Section 52.2 for general responsibilities.)

- Prevent exposure to people with infections or colds during periods of leukopenia. Be alert to the onset of agranulocytosis (cough, extreme fatigue, sore throat, chills, fever) and report these symptoms promptly to the prescriber.
- Monitor laboratory tests such as liver and kidney function, CBC with differential, platelet count, and chest x-rays. Frequently monitor blood glucose and periodically monitor the HbA_{1c} of patients with diabetes.
- Inspect the patient's mouth daily; report patchy necrotic areas, bleeding and discomfort, or overgrowth (black, furry tongue) to the prescriber. Monitor for and report ulcerative stomatitis with glossitis and gingivitis, which are often the first signs of toxicity.
- Monitor I&O ratio and pattern. Encourage intake of fluids. Keep the patient well hydrated (about 2,000 mL per 24 hours).
- Be alert for and report symptoms of thrombocytopenia (e.g., ecchymoses, petechiae, epistaxis, melena, hematuria, vaginal bleeding, slow and protracted oozing following trauma) to the prescriber.

Patient and Family Education:

- Avoid alcohol ingestion because this can increase the incidence and severity of methotrexate hepatotoxicity.
- Practice fastidious mouth care to prevent infection, provide comfort, and maintain adequate nutritional status.
- Avoid exposure to sunlight and ultraviolet light. Wear sunglasses and sunscreen.
- Do not self-medicate with vitamins. Some over-the-counter (OTC) compounds may include folic acid (or its derivatives), which alters methotrexate response.
- Avoid taking echinacea because it may increase the risk of hepatotoxicity.
- Limit the intake of caffeine. More than 180 mg per day of caffeine (3 to 4 cups of coffee) may decrease the effectiveness of methotrexate when taken for arthritis.
- Use contraceptive measures during and for at least 8 weeks following therapy.

Drugs Similar to Methotrexate (MTX, Rheumatrex, Trexall)

Pemetrexed is the only other folic acid analog used in cancer chemotherapy. Another analog, trimetrexate (Neutrexin), has been discontinued in the United States. Other antimetabolite medications include the pyrimidine and purine analogs.

Pemetrexed (Alimta): Approved in 2004, pemetrexed is a folic acid analog that is available only as a powder for injection. It is approved to treat malignant pleural mesothelioma that is unresectable or in patients who are not candidates for surgery. It is administered along with cisplatin in these patients. It is also used to treat locally advanced or metastatic non–small cell lung cancer after prior chemotherapy. Off-label indications include solid tumors of the pancreas, kidneys, bladder, breast, colon, stomach, head, and neck. Immunosuppression is the primary dose-limiting toxicity for pemetrexed. GI adverse effects may be serious and include nausea, vomiting, anorexia, diarrhea, constipation, and stomatitis. Patients are usually treated with oral dexamethasone immediately prior to and following pemetrexed therapy in order to prevent serious skin reactions. Caution must be used to ensure adequate kidney function because impairment may cause pemetrexed to accumulate to fatal levels in the blood. This is a pregnancy category D drug.

Pyrimidine analogs: Pyrimidines are bases used in the biosynthesis of DNA and RNA. Because the pyrimidine analogs are structurally similar to naturally occurring pyrimidines, they can act in several ways. They can inhibit the synthesis of pyridine bases, thus limiting the precursors needed for DNA and RNA biosynthesis. Pyrimidine analogs can become incorporated into the structures of DNA and RNA, resulting in a disruption of nucleic acid function.

The pyrimidine analogs include capecitabine (Xeloda), cytarabine (Cytosar, Cytosine arabinoside, Depot-Cyt), floxuridine (FUDR), fluorouracil (5-FU, Adrucil, Carac, Efudex), and gemcitabine (Gemzar). Each of these drugs is a prodrug that is converted to the active form on entering the body.

Capecitabine (Xeloda): Capecitabine is converted into 5-fluorouracil, another antimetabolite by a series of three enzymatic steps. One of these enzymes, thymidine phosphorylase, is found in especially high amounts in cancer cells; thus the drug is converted to a toxic form right in the cancer cell. Capecitabine blocks the synthesis of pyrimidines and can also be incorporated into nucleic acid molecules. It is available as a PO medication used to treat metastatic breast cancer refractory to other treatments, colorectal cancer, or as adjuvant therapy for colon cancer following resection. Capecitabine causes less immunosuppression than many antineoplastic agents. Diarrhea is the dose-limiting toxicity; antidiarrheal therapy with loperamide is often indicated during chemotherapy. Nausea, vomiting, stomatitis, and abdominal pain are common adverse effects. An unusual adverse effect with this drug is palmar-plantar erythrodysesthesia (hand and foot syndrome), which can occur in over half the patients receiving the drug. Hand and foot syndrome is characterized by numbness, tingling, swelling, erythema, blistering, and severe pain. Capecitabine is a pregnancy category D drug.

Cytarabine (Cytosar, Cytosine arabinoside, Depot-Cyt): Approved in 1969, cytarabine is a pyrimidine antimetabolite available for IV, subcutaneous, or intrathecal administration. It is most commonly used to treat hematologic malignancies, including acute myelogenous leukemia, acute lymphatic leukemia, chronic myelogenous leukemia, Hodgkin's and non-Hodgkin's lymphoma, and lymphomatous meningitis. Cytarabine is cell cycle specific in the S phase of the cell cycle. It is converted to its active form, Ara-CTP, and then becomes incorporated into DNA, where it suppresses further DNA synthesis. It has strong myelosuppression activity, with a nadir occurring at week 1 and resolution by week 3 or 4. High-dose therapy can cause severe nausea, vomiting, and other GI toxicities. A cluster of symptoms, called the cytarabine syndrome, can occur within 6 to 12 hours of treatment. Symptoms include bone pain, fever, myalgia, rash, and fatigue. Other serious adverse effects include peripheral neuropathy, respiratory distress, encephalopathy, palmar-plantar erythrodysesthesia, and hepatotoxicity. This is a pregnancy category D drug.

Depot-Cyt, a newer formulation of cytarabine, is a liposomal delivery system that requires less frequent dosing that systemic cytarabine. It is only administered by the intrathecal route for carcinomatous meningitis due to solid tumors. Liposomal cytarabine has been associated with potentially fatal chemical arachnoiditis that occurs within 48 hours of administration. Nervous system symptoms such as confusion, ataxia, dizziness, and impaired cognition are common. When given by the intrathecal route, myelosuppression is minor. This is a pregnancy category D drug.

Floxuridine (FUDR): Floxuridine is a pyrimidine analog antimetabolite that was approved in 1970. Because it is nearly entirely removed by hepatic first pass metabolism, it has very limited applications. Its only approved indication is as a continuous intra-arterial infusion via a hepatic artery catheter for hepatic cancer. Due to its high concentration in the liver, floxuridine can cause elevated liver function enzymes and serious hepatotoxicity. Other adverse effects, such as myelosuppression, nausea, vomiting, anorexia, diarrhea, rash, and alopecia, are common to other antineoplastics. Peptic ulcer disease occurs in about 17% of patients who are taking the drug. This is a pregnancy category D drug.

Fluorouracil (5-FU, Adrucil, Carac, Efudex): Approved in 1962, fluorouracil is an antimetabolite that inhibits DNA and RNA synthesis in the S phase of the cell cycle. It is available as an injection, a topical solution, and a topical cream. It is used singly or in combination to treat solid tumors, including inoperable breast, ovarian, cervical, urinary bladder, liver, colon, rectal, stomach, and pancreatic cancers. As a topical preparation it is used to treat superficial basal cell carcinomas and multiple actinic keratoses. A new formulation of fluorouracil cream using a microsponge delivery system (Carac) was approved in 2000 that allows for once-daily dosing and a sustained release of the drug. Hematologic toxicity may be dose limiting with a nadir at 9 to 14 days and recovery by 30 days. Palmar-plantar erythrodysesthesia occurs in up to 40% of patients receiving a prolonged IV infusion of this drug. Ocular irritation, excessive lacrimation, and conjunctivitis can occur in up to half of the patients taking the drug. Topical applications may cause local photosensitivity, burning, erythema, swelling, and desquamation. Fluorouracil is a pregnancy category D drug.

Gemcitabine (Gemzar): Gemcitabine, available as an injectable preparation, is used to treat locally advanced or metastatic solid tumors of the pancreas, breast, ovary, or lung. It is used in combination with cisplatin or paclitaxel to treat lung cancer. Approved in 1996, the dose-limiting toxicity for gemcitabine is myelosuppression, which occurs in nearly all patients taking the drug. Fever and infection are common adverse effects. Mild to moderate nausea, vomiting, and other GI effects occur in most patients. This is a pregnancy category D drug.

Purine analogs: The last class of antimetabolites is the purine analogs. There are six medications used as antineoplastics in this group: cladribine, fludarabine, mercaptopurine, nelarabine, pentostatin, and thioguanine. Other purine analogs are used for immunosuppression, gout, and antiviral therapy. They are all bases, like the pyrimidines, which are used in the biosynthesis of nucleic acids.

Cladribine (Leustatin): Cladribine is a purine analog that is available as an injectable preparation, which is used as the drug of choice to treat hairy cell leukemia. It is also used off-label to treat chronic lymphocytic leukemia, non-Hodgkin's lymphoma, acute and chronic myelogenous leukemia, and mycosis fungoides. Approved in 1993, cladribine works differently than the other purine analogs in that it is effective against both dividing (S phase) and nondividing cancer cells. Bone marrow suppression is the primary dose-limiting toxicity, with a nadir occurring in 14 days and recovery at 5 weeks. Lymphocyte counts may take up to 34 weeks to a year to return to normal values, resulting in a high number of viral and fungal infections in patients treated with cladribine. Fever and chills, which are often associated with infections, are common. Rash occurs in most patients but is not usually serious. Nausea and vomiting are mild compared to other antineoplastics. Very high doses are neurotoxic and nephrotoxic. This is a pregnancy category D drug.

Clofarabine (Clolar): Clofarabine is a newer purine analog that was approved in 2004 and is administered by IV infusion. It only has one indication: the treatment of relapsed or refractory acute lymphocytic leukemia (ALL) after at least two prior regimens have proven unsuccessful. It is also only approved for patients aged 1 to 21 years. Common adverse events include myelosuppression, opportunistic infections, nausea, vomiting, diarrhea, anorexia, fever, fatigue, abdominal pain, and edema. This is a pregnancy category D drug.

Fludarabine (Fludara): Approved in 1991, fludarabine is a purine analog that is available as an injectable preparation with a similar action to cladribine. It is approved only to treat chronic lymphocytic leukemia (usually with an alkylating agent), but it may be used off-label to treat other leukemias and non-Hodgkin lymphomas. It is believed to be cell cycle specific for the S phase, where it inhibits DNA replication. Severe myelosuppression is the most common dose-limiting toxicity. Like cladribine, lymphocyte levels may take up to a year to return to normal levels. Rare instances of life-threatening autoimmune hemolytic anemia have been reported with this drug. Fever and infections are common, including serious interstitial pneumonitis. Nausea and vomiting are mild compared to other antineoplastics but may be severe at high doses. Edema is a frequent adverse effect. High doses of fludarabine are neurotoxic and can result in blindness, coma, and death. This is a pregnancy category D drug.

Mercaptopurine (6-MP, Purinethol): Mercaptopurine is an older purine analog that was approved in 1953 and is cell cycle specific, being most active in the S phase. It is a prodrug that has very similar actions, indications, and adverse effects to thioguanine. Mercaptopurine is available as a PO preparation and is used mainly to treat acute lymphocytic and myelogenous leukemia in both adults and children. It is less effective in treating adults than children but remains a drug of choice. It can produce a temporary remission in patients with chronic granulocytic leukemia. Due to its powerful immunosuppressant activity, it may be used off-label to produce temporary remissions in patients with ulcerative colitis and Crohn's disease. The most frequent, serious, dose-limiting toxicity of mercaptopurine is myelosuppression, which results in leukopenia, thrombocytopenia, and anemia in nearly every patient. Nausea and vomiting are not severe, but diarrhea may require fluid replacement therapy. This is a pregnancy category D drug.

Nelarabine (Arranon): A newer drug that was approved in 2005, nelarabine is a purine analog given by the IV route to treat T-cell acute lymphoblastic leukemia and T-cell lymphoblastic lymphoma in both adults and children. Its use is limited to patients who have not responded to or have relapsed during treatment with at least two chemotherapy regimens. Neurotoxicity is the major dose-limiting toxicity with nelarabine, and neurologic signs and symptoms may include impaired cognition, severe somnolence, seizures, peripheral neuropathies, ataxia, tremor, dizziness, and cerebral hemorrhage. Myelosuppression occurs in most patients; fatigue, fever, and infection occur frequently. Nausea, vomiting, and other GI complaints are usually not a major cause of discontinuation. Edema is a frequent adverse effect. This is a pregnancy category D drug.

Pentostatin (Nipent): Pentostatin was approved in 1991 to treat hairy cell leukemia that has not responded to interferon alfa, and it may be used off-label to treat other leukemias and lymphomas. It is available as an IV preparation and is cell cycle specific in the S phase. Hematologic toxicity is dose limiting and patients experience a high rate of fever, chills, and infections. Rash and other skin reactions occur in most patients and may be severe. Neurologic toxicity is a serious problem with high doses of pentostatin. Nausea and vomiting are common but can be controlled with antiemetics. This is a pregnancy category D drug.

Thioguanine (6-TG, Tabloid): Approved in 1966, thioguanine is very similar to mercaptopurine in its actions and adverse effects. Like other antimetabolites, it is active in the S phase of the cell cycle. It is available in a PO formulation, and it is used mainly to treat acute nonlymphocytic leukemia. Off-label indications include chronic myelogenous leukemia, psoriasis, refractory ulcerative colitis, and Crohn's disease. Myelosuppression is the most common dose-limiting toxicity. Long-term, continuous use of thioguanine is not recommended due to the risk for serious hepatotoxicity. Adverse GI effects are generally not severe at normal doses. This is a pregnancy category D drug.

Pharm*FACT*

African American women have a higher breast cancer mortality rate at every age and a lower survival rate than Caucasian women. The 5-year survival rate for Caucasian women who were diagnosed with invasive breast cancer is 90%; for African American women the rate is 77%. *Source:* National Breast Cancer Coalition, 2008.

Antitumor Antibiotics

58.5 The antibiotic antineoplastics contain substances obtained from bacteria that have the ability to kill cancer cells.

Antitumor properties have been identified in a number of substances isolated from microorganisms. These chemicals are more cytotoxic than traditional antibiotics, and their use is restricted to treating a few specific types of cancer. For example, the only indication for idarubicin (Idamycin) is acute myelogenous leukemia. Testicular carcinoma is the only indication for plicamycin (Mithramycin). The antitumor antibiotics are listed in Table 58.3.

The antitumor antibiotics bind to DNA and affect its function by a mechanism similar to that of the alkylating agents; therefore, their general actions and adverse effects are similar to those of the

TABLE 58.3 Antitumor Antibiotics

Drug	Route and Adult Dose (maximum dose where indicated)	Adverse Effects
bleomycin (Blenoxane)	IV: 0.25–0.5 unit/kg every 4–7 days	*Nausea, vomiting, stomatitis, anorexia, headache, rash, alopecia* Bone marrow suppression, severe nausea, vomiting, diarrhea, mucositis, pulmonary or cardiac toxicity, anaphylaxis and other hypersensitivity reactions, tissue necrosis (due to extravasation)
dactinomycin (Actinomycin-D, Cosmegen)	IV: 500 mcg/day for a maximum of 5 days	
daunorubicin (Cerubidine)	IV: 30–60 mg/m²/day for 3–5 days	
daunorubicin liposomal (SaunoSome)	IV: 40 mg/m² every 2 weeks	
doxorubicin (Adriamycin, Rubex)	IV: 30–60 mg/m² as a single dose every 21 days, or 30 mg/m² on 3 consecutive days (max: total cumulative dose of 550 mg/m²)	
doxorubicin liposomal (Doxil, Evacet)	IV: 20 mg/m² every 3 weeks	
epirubicin (Ellence)	IV: 100–120 mg/m² as a single dose	
idarubicin (Idamycin)	IV: 8–12 mg/m²/day for 3 days	
mitomycin (Mutamycin)	IV: 2 mg/m² as a single dose	
mitoxantrone (Novantrone)	IV: 12 mg/m² for 3 days	

Note: *Italics* indicate common adverse effects. Underline indicates serious adverse effects.

alkylating agents. Unlike the alkylating agents, however, all the antitumor antibiotics must be administered IV or through direct instillation via a catheter into a body cavity or organ.

As with many other antineoplastics, the major dose-limiting toxicity of drugs in this class is bone marrow suppression. Doxorubicin, daunorubicin, epirubicin, and idarubicin are known as anthracyclines. They are closely related in structure, and cardiac toxicity is a major limiting adverse effect. Cardiotoxicity may occur within minutes of administration, or it may be delayed for months or years after chemotherapy has been completed.

Anthracyclines can cause major damage to the skin, subcutaneous tissue, and nerves should extravasation occur. In 2007, the detoxifying agent dexrazoxane (Totec) was approved to specifically treat anthracycline extravasation. Dexrazoxane is administered by IV infusion as soon as possible after the extravasation occurs.

PROTOTYPE DRUG Doxorubicin (Adriamycin)

Classification: Therapeutic: Antineoplastic
Pharmacologic: Antitumor antibiotic, anthracycline

Therapeutic Effects and Uses: Approved in 1975, doxorubicin is a drug obtained from *Streptomyces* that has a wide spectrum of antitumor activity and is considered one of the most effective single agents against solid tumors. It has strong immunosuppressive activities, is highly toxic to rapidly proliferating cells and slowly developing tumors, and is selectively toxic to cardiac tissue. It is approved to treat neuroblastoma and solid tumors of the bone, bladder, breast, ovary, GI tract, lung, and thyroid. It is also part of many chemotherapy regimens for other tumors, such as acute lymphoblastic and myeloblastic leukemias, Wilm's tumor, soft tissue sarcomas, and multiple myeloma. Given by the IV route, it may be instilled into the bladder for bladder cancer. It is usually used in combination therapy with other antineoplastics, surgery, radiation, and immunotherapy. It is also effective as a preradiation therapy to sensitize superficial tumors.

Doxorubicin liposomal (Doxil, Evacet) is a form of the drug incorporated into a liposomal carrier. The liposomes are closed, spherical molecules that encase the drug. Administered IV the liposomes have a long half-life and produce a more prolonged duration of action. In addition, the liposomes tend to stay in the circulation until they reach tumors which often have leakier capillaries than normal tissues. Once entering the tumor, the drug is released from its carrier. Doxorubicin liposomal is approved for use in patients with Kaposi's sarcoma, refractory ovarian tumors, and relapsed multiple myeloma.

Mechanism of Action: Doxorubicin binds to DNA, causing strand splitting and inhibition of DNA synthesis. It is cell cycle nonspecific.

Pharmacokinetics:

Route(s)	IV
Absorption	N/A
Distribution	Widely distributed, crosses the placenta but does not cross the blood–brain barrier; secreted in breast milk; 75% bound to plasma protein
Primary metabolism	Hepatic
Primary excretion	Bile
Onset of action	Peak: ½–2 h
Duration of action	Triphasic half-life: 12 minutes, 3.3 h, and 30–40 h

Adverse Effects: Doxorubicin has many potentially serious adverse effects. Bone marrow suppression is the major dose-limiting toxicity and may manifest as thrombocytopenia, leukopenia (especially granulocytes), and anemia. The neutropenia nadir occurs at 7 days and recovers by 14 days. Doxorubicin exhibits significant cardiotoxicity, which may be either acute or chronic. Cardiac adverse effects can be life threatening and may include sinus tachycardia, bradycardia, delayed congestive heart failure (CHF), acute left ventricular failure, and myocarditis. Heart failure may occur months or years after the termination of chemotherapy. Other adverse effects include severe nausea, vomiting, mucositis, rash, excessive lacrimation, necrosis at the injection site, severe myelosuppression, hepatotoxicity, anaphylaxis, complete alopecia, and recall phenomenon (a skin reaction due to prior radiation therapy). Doxorubicin turns the urine and tears a red color, which is harmless but anxiety provoking. Secondary malignancies, especially acute myelogenous leukemia, may occur 1 to 3 years following therapy. Temporary decreased fertility is likely in both men and women.

Contraindications/Precautions: Contraindications to the use of doxorubicin include pregnancy, lactation, myelosuppression, thrombocytopenia, preexisting cardiac disease, obstructive jaundice, lactation, or previous treatment with complete cumulative doses of doxorubicin or daunorubicin. Precautions include impaired hepatic or renal function, history of atopic dermatitis, and patients who have received cyclophosphamide or pelvic radiation therapy to areas surrounding the heart. Doxorubicin is a severe vesicant and precautions must be taken to avoid contact with the skin or soft tissue. Skin contact or extravasation should be treated immediately with local ice packs to reduce absorption of the drug.

Drug Interactions: Increased toxicity may occur with other antineoplastics, radiation therapy, or mercaptopurine. Cyclophosphamide may increase the risk of hemorrhagic cystitis or cardiac toxicity. Paclitaxel may decrease the clearance of doxorubicin, leading to more profound neutropenia and stomatitis. Phenobarbital and other barbiturates increase the elimination of doxorubicin. Possible decreased phenytoin levels may occur. Concurrent use with verapamil can raise the serum levels of doxorubicin, thus increasing the risk for cardiotoxicity. Use with paclitaxel will result in an increased incidence of stomatitis, neutropenia, and heart failure. Because doxorubicin causes thrombocytopenia, concurrent use with NSAIDs, anticoagulants, or platelet inhibitors may cause excessive bleeding. **Herbal/Food:** Unknown.

Pregnancy: Category D.

Treatment of Overdose: If myelosuppression occurs, administration of antibiotics, platelets, and granulocytes may be necessary. Symptoms of mucositis and heart failure must be treated symptomatically.

Nursing Responsibilities: (See Section 52.2 for general responsibilities.)

- Prevent the patient from exposure to infections or colds during periods of leukopenia.
- Monitor cardiac function (ECG) prior to the initiation of therapy, at regular intervals, and at the end of therapy. Acute life-threatening dysrhythmias may occur within a few hours of drug administration.
- Monitor baseline and periodic laboratory tests such as hepatic function, renal function, and CBC with differential throughout therapy.
- Report signs of hepatic dysfunction (jaundice, dark urine, pruritus) or kidney dysfunction (altered I&O ratio and pattern, local discomfort with voiding) to the prescriber.
- Stop the infusion, remove the IV needle, and notify the prescriber promptly if the patient complains of stinging or burning sensations at the injection site.
- Promote fastidious oral hygiene, especially before and after meals. Stomatitis, generally maximal in the second week of therapy, frequently begins with a burning sensation accompanied by erythema of oral mucosa that may progress to ulceration and dysphagia in 2 or 3 days.
- Avoid rectal medications and use of a rectal thermometer; rectal trauma is associated with bloody diarrhea resulting from an antiblastic effect on rapidly growing intestinal mucosal cells.

Patient and Family Education:

- Expect complete loss of hair (reversible) as an adverse effect. It may also involve eyelashes and eyebrows, beard and mustache, and pubic and axillary hair. Regrowth of hair usually begins 2 to 3 months after this drug is discontinued.
- Expect urine to become red for 1 to 2 days after administration.

Drugs Similar to Doxorubicin (Adriamycin)

The antineoplastic medications categorized as antitumor antibiotics are divided into two groups: anthracyclines and nonanthracyclines. The nonanthracyclines tend to cause less cardiotoxicity than the anthracyclines. The anthracyclines include doxorubicin, doxorubicin liposomal, daunorubicin, epirubicin, idarubicin, and mitoxantrone. The nonanthracyclines are bleomycin, dactinomycin, and mitomycin. One additional nonanthracycline, valrubicin (Valstar), has been withdrawn by the FDA.

Anthracyclines

Daunorubicin (Cerubidine): Approved in 1979, daunorubicin is an antitumor antibiotic obtained from *Streptomyces* that is available by injection. Daunorubicin binds to DNA, causing strand splitting and inhibition of DNA synthesis. It is cell cycle specific for the S phase. Closely related structurally to doxorubicin, daunorubicin is approved to induce remission in acute myelogenous and lymphocytic leukemia in adults. It is less effective than doxorubicin in treating solid tumors. Bone marrow suppression is the major dose-limiting toxicity. This drug exhibits the same types of cardiotoxicity as doxorubicin although to a lesser extent. Other adverse events, such as nausea, vomiting, alopecia, urine discoloration, and vesicant properties are the same as those of daunorubicin. This drug is pregnancy category D.

Daunorubicin liposomal (SaunoSome) is a formulation of daunorubicin in a liposomal vehicle that was created to increase the amount of the drug delivered to tumor cells while decreasing the amount in normal cells. Administered by the IV route, the only approved use for it is acquired immunodeficiency syndrome (AIDS)-related Kaposi's sarcoma. Off-label indications include acute myelogenous leukemia, breast cancer, multiple myeloma and non-Hodgkin's lymphoma. Adverse effects are the same as those of daunorubicin.

Epirubicin (Ellence): Approved in 1999, epirubicin is closely related to doxorubicin in both structure and function. It is an IV preparation that is highly destructive to rapidly proliferating cells. Epirubicin is approved only for adjuvant therapy for axillary node-positive breast cancer but may be used off-label for bladder, gastric, lung, head, neck, and liver cancers. Epirubicin has the same types of adverse effects as doxorubicin but at a lower incidence. Bone marrow is the major dose-limiting toxicity, with a nadir occurring at 10 to 14 days and recovery at 21 days. The drug exhibits the same types of cardiotoxicity as doxorubicin, such as CHF, although to a lesser extent. Like doxorubicin, moderate to severe nausea, vomiting, and alopecia occur in many patients. Because severe local tissue necrosis can occur, skin contact or extravasation should be treated immediately with local ice packs to reduce absorption of this drug. Secondary acute myelogenous leukemia has been reported in patients treated with epirubicin. This is a pregnancy category D drug.

Idarubicin (Idamycin): Approved in 1990, idarubicin is structurally very similar to daunorubicin. Its only approved indication is for acute myelogenous leukemia in combination with cytarabine, although it may be used off-label to treat refractory acute and chronic myogenous leukemia, advanced metastatic breast cancer, and refractory non-Hodgkin's lymphoma. It is administered by the IV route. Idarubicin is a vesicant, and care must be taken to not allow extravasation or exposure to skin. Like other drugs in this class, bone marrow toxicity is the primary dose limitation, with a nadir by day 15 and recovery by day 25. Other common adverse effects include alopecia, cardiotoxicity, and moderate nausea and vomiting. This is a pregnancy category D drug.

Mitoxantrone (Novantrone): Although not an anthracycline, mitoxantrone is structurally very similar to the anthracyclines and shares some common properties. Approved in 1987, it is approved to treat acute myelogenous leukemia and for the palliation of severe pain associated with advanced prostate cancer. Off-label antineoplastic indications include refractory acute and chronic myelogenous leukemia, breast cancer, metastatic ovarian cancer, liver cancer, and non-Hodgkin's lymphoma. It is one of the few drugs approved to treat secondary, chronic multiple sclerosis. It is usually administered by IV infusion but may be given by the intraperitoneal or intra-arterial routes. The dose-limiting toxicity is myelosuppression, with a nadir at 10 to 14 days and recovery by 2 to 3 weeks. It is considered less cardiotoxic than the anthracyclines, but this is still a significant adverse effect of mitoxantrone. Other adverse effects include stomatitis, moderate nausea, vomiting, alopecia, injection site reactions, and secondary malignancy (leukemia). This is a pregnancy category D drug.

Nonanthracyclines

Bleomycin (Blenoxane): Approved in 1973, bleomycin is an antitumor antibiotic obtained from the *Streptomyces* organism. It is a cell cycle specific drug, being most active in the G_2 phase. Unlike other drugs in this class, bleomycin causes very little bone marrow suppression. Because of this, it is especially useful in combination chemotherapy. Bleomycin is used for palliative therapy for many different cancers, including Hodgkin's and non-Hodgkin's lymphomas, testicular cancer, vulvar cancer, cervical cancer, and squamous cell carcinomas. Bleomycin is available as IM, IV, subcutaneous, and intrapleural preparations. One of its most serious problems is its ability to cause severe and potentially fatal lung injury, with signs such as pulmonary fibrosis, or pleural effusions. Patients who have received radiation treatment to the chest or cumulative doses of bleomycin are at increased risk for lung injury. Serious dermatologic reactions may require lower doses or discontinuation of the drug. Nausea and vomiting are generally mild; however, anorexia and weight loss are common. This is a pregnancy category D drug.

Dactinomycin (Actinomycin-D, Cosmegen): Approved in 1973, dactinomycin is an antitumor antibiotic obtained from the *Streptomyces* organism. Delivered by the IV route, dactinomycin binds to DNA to inhibit RNA synthesis and is cell cycle nonspecific. It is usually used in combination with other antineoplastics. Its primary indication is to treat Wilms' tumor and rhabdomyosarcoma, but it is also approved for choriocarcinoma, Ewing's sarcoma, and testicular carcinoma. Off-label indications include Kaposi's sarcoma, malignant melanoma, and osteogenic sarcoma. Dactinomycin has several dose-limiting toxicities. Myelosuppression can be severe and lead to serious infections with a nadir at 7 to 21 days. Nausea and vomiting are severe and require antiemetic therapy. Other GI effects include severe oral or esophageal ulceration, anorexia, and diarrhea. Hepatotoxicity, including hepatomegaly, ascites, hepatitis, and hyperbilirubinemia, can be severe, especially at high doses. Alopecia and dermatologic skin reactions are common. This drug is extremely irritating to soft tissue if extravasation occurs. This is a pregnancy category D drug.

Mitomycin (Mutamycin): Mitomycin is an antibiotic extracted from *Streptomyces* that was approved in 1974. It is available as an injection and is very effective against both slowly developing and rapidly proliferating cells in solid tumors. It is effective in some tumors that are unresponsive to radiation and other chemotherapeutic agents. It is not recommended for use as a single agent or as a replacement for surgery or radiation. Mitomycin is approved only for gastric and pancreatic cancers but may be used off-label for bladder cancer, colorectal cancer, breast cancer, and squamous cell carcinoma of the head, neck, lung, or cervix. The primary dose-limiting toxicity is bone marrow suppression with a nadir at 3 weeks. Recovery may take 4 to 8 weeks. Severe skin reactions can occur, especially if extravasation occurs. Lung toxicity is rare, but occurrences of interstitial pneumonitis can be fatal. Nausea, vomiting, anorexia, and fatigue may be delayed and persistent during therapy. This is a pregnancy category X drug.

Hormones and Hormone Antagonists

58.6 Hormones and hormone antagonists block the substances necessary for continued growth of tumors.

A number of hormones are used in cancer chemotherapy, including corticosteroids, progestins, estrogens, and androgens. In addition, several hormone antagonists have been found to exhibit antitumor activity. Endocrine, or hormonal therapy, is limited to treating hormone-sensitive tumors of the breast or prostate.

The mechanism of hormone antineoplastic activity is largely unknown. It is likely, however, that these antitumor properties are independent of their normal hormone mechanisms because the doses utilized in cancer chemotherapy are magnitudes larger than the amount normally present in the body. The student should refer to other chapters in this text for a complete discussion of hormone therapy. The antitumor hormones and hormone antagonists are listed in Table 58.4.

In general, the hormones and hormone antagonists act by blocking the substances essential for tumor growth. Because these agents are not cytotoxic, they produce few of the debilitating adverse effects seen with other antineoplastics. They can, however, produce significant adverse effects when given at high doses for prolonged periods. Because they rarely produce cancer cures when used singly, these agents are normally given for palliation. There are four general classes of hormone antagonists.

- Estrogen receptor (ER) blockers
- Aromatase inhibitors
- Gonadotropin-releasing hormone analogs
- Androgen receptor blockers

Estrogen receptor blockers: The hormone estrogen promotes the growth of certain types of breast cancers. The antiestrogens are drugs that block ERs, thus slowing tumor growth. Three of the drugs in this class—raloxifene, tamoxifen, and toremifene—

TABLE 58.4 Hormone and Hormone Antagonists Used for Neoplasia

Drug	Route and Adult Dose (maximum dose where indicated)	Adverse Effects
Hormones		
dexamethasone (Decadron, others)	PO: 0.25 mg bid-qid	*Weight gain, insomnia, abdominal distension, sweating, flushing, diarrhea, nervousness, gynecomastia, hirsutism (testosterone, testolactone)* Thrombophlebitis, muscle wasting (prednisone, dexamethasone), osteoporosis, hepatotoxicity
diethylstilbestrol (DES, Stilbestrol)	PO: for treatment of prostate cancer, 500 mg tid; for palliation, 1–15 mg/day	
ethinyl estradiol (Estinyl, others)	PO: for treatment of breast cancer, 1 mg tid for 2–3 months; for palliation of prostate cancer, 0.15–3 mg/day	
fluoxymesterone (Halotestin)	PO: 10 mg tid	
medroxyprogesterone (Provera, Depo-Provera)	IM: 400–1,000 mg every week	
megestrol (Megace)	PO: 40–160 mg bid-qid	
prednisone (Deltasone, others)	PO: 20–100 mg/m^2/day	
testolactone (Teslac)	PO: 250 mg qid	
testosterone (Andro, Histerone, Testred, Delatest, others)	IM: 200–400 mg every 2–4 weeks	
Hormone Antagonists		
anastrozole (Arimidex)	PO: 1 mg/day	*Hot flashes, insomnia, breast enlargementor pain, headache, diarrhea, asthenia, nausea* Hypersensitivity reactions (including anaphylaxis), thrombophlebitis, CHF (bicalutamide, goserelin), hepatotoxicity (flutamide), sexual dysfunction (goserelin, nilutamide, tamoxifen), ocular toxicity (toremifene)
bicalutamide (Casodex)	PO: 50 mg/day	
degarelix (Firmagon)	Subcutaneous: 240 mg loading dose followed by 80 mg every 28 days	
exemestane (Aromasin)	PO: 25 mg/day after a meal	
flutamide (Eulexin)	PO: 250 mg tid	
fulvestrant (Faslodex)	IM: 250 mg once	
goserelin (Zoladex)	Subcutaneously: 3.6 mg every 28 days	
histrelin (Vantas)	Implant: 1 implant every 12 months (50 mg)	
letrozole (Femara)	PO: 2.5 mg/day	
leuprolide (Eligard, Lupron, Viadur)	Subcutaneously: 1 mg/day	
nilutamide (Nilandron)	PO: 300 mg/day for 30 days; then 150 mg/day	
raloxifene (Evista)	PO: 60 mg once daily (max: 60 mg/day)	
tamoxifen	PO: 10–20 mg 1–2 times/day (morning and evening)	
toremifene (Fareston)	PO: 60 mg/day	
triptorelin (Trelstar)	IM: 3.75 mg once monthly	

Note: *Italics* indicate common adverse effects. Underline indicates serious adverse effects.

CONNECTIONS

Complementary and Alternative Therapies Soy

Description: Soy, or soybean, is a nutritional food that is a major source of protein for many cultures, especially those in China and Japan. In the United States, soy has become increasingly popular and is one of the top 10 most utilized supplements. In addition to its nutritional value, soy contains estrogen-like (phytoestrogen) substances known as isoflavones. Soy milk is made by grinding soybeans into a fine powder, which is then mixed with water. Other products include soy sauce, soy flour, tofu, nutritional snack bars, and soy protein drinks.

History and Claims: Soy has been used as a nutritional source for thousands of years. Claims for soy's benefits include anticancer effects, treatment of osteoarthritis, cholesterol-lowering effects, and reduction of menopausal symptoms. Soy isoflavones have been identified as dietary components that have an important role in reducing the incidence of breast and prostate cancers.

Standarization: Standardization of soy is either to the amount of bean extract or to the amount of isoflavones in the product. The standard dose has not been established.

Evidence: Soy is one of the most studied dietary supplements. For many years soy was believed to provide superlative health benefits, including lowering of low-density lipoprotein (LDL) cholesterol. Both the FDA and the American Heart Association (AHA) gave preliminary approval to soy's benefit in coronary heart disease in the 1990s. However, a 2006 review of 22 studies failed to show any significant benefit in lowering cholesterol with soy protein or isoflavones. Eating soy protein as a replacement for meat and meat products can reduce the risk of heart disease and improve heart health.

Soy isoflavones have antioxidant properties and appear to inhibit angiogenesis and metastasis. Some studies have found a small reduction in prostate cancer and breast cancer risk for those who are taking soy isoflavones. Soy isoflavones may be a promising supplement for cancer chemoprevention or treatment, but more research is needed for definitive conclusions in these areas.

Source: From "Soy Isoflavones and Cancer Prevention," by F. H. Sarkar & Y. Li, 2003, *Cancer Investigation, 21*(5), pp. 744–757; "Meta-Analysis of Soy Intake and Breast Cancer Risk," by B. J. Trock, L. Hilakivi-Clarke, & R. Clarke, 2006, *Journal of the National Cancer Institute, 98*(7), pp. 459–471; "Meta-Analysis of Soy Food and Risk of Prostate Cancer in Men," by L. Yan, & E. L. Spitznagel, 2005, *International Journal of Cancer, 117*(4), pp. 667–669.

are given PO and have both estrogen agonist and estrogen antagonist actions. ERs are activated in some tissues (bone, endometrium) and inhibited in others (breast). Tamoxifen is the most widely prescribed and serves as the prototype.

PROTOTYPE DRUG Tamoxifen (Nolvadex, Soltamox)

Classification: Therapeutic: Antineoplastic
Pharmacologic: Hormonal agent, estrogen receptor blocker

Therapeutic Effects and Uses: Approved in 1985, tamoxifen is an antiestrogen that is available by the PO route. It has an effect on those tumors that have a high ER concentration. It has no effect on ER-negative breast cancers. It is approved for the palliative treatment of advanced, metastatic, ER-positive breast cancer in men and postmenopausal women. Off-label indications include astrocytoma, malignant glioma, malignant melanoma, and ovarian cancer.

A unique feature of tamoxifen is that it is the only antineoplastic that is approved for the prophylaxis of breast cancer for high-risk patients who are at risk of developing the disease. In addition, it is approved as adjunctive therapy in women following a mastectomy to decrease the potential for cancer in the contralateral breast. It is not to be used for prophylaxis in women at low risk to acquiring breast cancer because the risks may outweigh the benefits in this population. Risk factors that may qualify a woman for tamoxifen prophylactic therapy depend on their age but include the following:

- One first-degree relative with a history of breast cancer
- Two or more benign biopsies and a history of a breast biopsy showing atypical hyperplasia
- At least two first-degree relatives with a history of breast cancer and a personal history of at least one breast biopsy
- Lobular carcinoma in situ
- Age at first live birth less than or equal to 25 years of age and age at menarche less than or equal to 11 years
- At least two first-degree relatives with a history of breast cancer and age at first live birth of less than or equal to 19 years
- One first-degree relative with a history of breast cancer and a personal history of a breast biopsy showing atypical hyperplasia

Tamoxifen has several nonneoplastic indications, all of which are off-label. For the treatment of infertility, it may be used to induce ovulation in women who do not ovulate but desire to become pregnant. It may be used to reduce the pain associated with gynecomastia in both women and men. The drug is being examined for its potential use in patients with osteoporosis.

Mechanism of Action: Tamoxifen binds to ERs, producing agonist effects in some tissues (bone) and antagonist effects in other tissues (breast). The binding in breast tissue inhibits DNA replication and affects other growth factors in cancer cells.

Pharmacokinetics:

Route(s)	PO
Absorption	Slowly from the GI tract
Distribution	Widely distributed; crosses the placenta; unknown if secreted in breast milk
Primary metabolism	Hepatic by CYP3A, CYP2C9, and CYP2D6
Primary excretion	Feces
Onset of action	Peak serum concentration: 5 h
Duration of action	Half-life: 5–7 days

Adverse Effects: Tamoxifen has few serious adverse effects other than nausea and vomiting, which occurs in 12% to 25% of patients who are taking the drug. This can be controlled with antiemetics as necessary. Other common adverse effects include hot flashes, vaginal discharge, irregular menses, vaginal bleeding, fluid retention, headaches, light-headedness, and rash. The most serious problem associated with tamoxifen use is the increased risk of endometrial cancer. The benefit far outweighs the risk in women taking tamoxifen to treat breast cancer. The risk versus benefit is not as clear in those women who are taking tamoxifen to prevent breast cancer. There is also an increased but small risk of thromboembolic disease, including cerebrovascular accident (CVA), pulmonary embolism, and deep vein thrombosis (DVT) with the use of tamoxifen. The risk of a thromboembolic event is believed to be about the same as for oral contraceptives.

Contraindications/Precautions: Contraindications to the use of tamoxifen include anticoagulant therapy, preexisting endometrial hyperplasia, history of thromboembolic disease, pregnancy, and lactation. Precautions should be observed in patients with leukopenia, thrombocytopenia, visual disturbances, cataracts, bone marrow suppression, hypercalcemia, and hypercholesterolemia.

Drug Interactions: Tamoxifen is extensively metabolized by hepatic CYP enzymes and may interact with inducers or inhibitors of these enzymes. Use with warfarin increases the risks of bleeding. Cytotoxic antineoplastics may increase the risk of thromboembolism. Bromocriptine may increase tamoxifen levels, whereas aminoglutethimide, medroxyprogesterone, or rifamycin may decrease tamoxifen levels. Selective serotonin reuptake inhibitors (SSRIs) may decrease the effectiveness of tamoxifen. This drug should not be used concurrently with oral contraceptives. **Herbal/Food:** Black cohosh should not be taken unless approved by the health care provider.

Pregnancy: Category D.

Treatment of Overdose: Seizures, neurotoxicity, and QT interval changes may occur with overdose. The patient is treated symptomatically.

Nursing Responsibilities: (See Section 52.2 for general responsibilities.)

- Administer analgesics for pain relief as necessitated by bone and tumor pain or local disease flair. Reassure the patient that this discomfort frequently signals a good tumor response.
- Monitor for local swelling and marked erythema over preexisting lesions or the development of new lesions, which may signal soft tissue disease response to tamoxifen. These symptoms rapidly subside.
- Monitor baseline and periodic laboratory tests. Assess CBC, including platelet counts, periodically. Transient leukopenia and thrombocytopenia (50,000–100,000/mm^3) without hemorrhagic tendency have been reported. Monitor serum calcium periodically.

Patient and Family Education:

- Take the drug exactly as prescribed.
- Immediately report the occurrence of marked weakness, sleepiness, mental confusion, edema, dyspnea, and blurred vision to the health care provider.
- Report drug-induced menstrual irregularities to the health care provider.
- Avoid prolonged sun exposure, especially if the skin is unprotected. Apply sunscreen lotions (SPF 12 or greater) to all exposed skin surfaces.
- Avoid OTC drugs, particularly pain medicines, unless specifically approved by the health care provider.
- Report the onset of tenderness or redness in an extremity.

Drugs Similar to Tamoxifen (Nolvadex, Soltamox)

The drugs in this broad category of antineoplastics are divided into ER blockers, aromatase inhibitors, gonadotropin-releasing hormone analogs, and androgen receptor blockers. The hormone agents such as dexamethasone (Decadron), diethylstilbestrol (DES, Stilbestrol), medroxyprogesterone (Provera, Depo-Provera), prednisone (Deltasone and others), and testosterone (Andro, Histerone, and others) are used for nonneoplastic indications, and information on these drugs may be found in other chapters of this text. Abarelix (Plenaxis) is a hormone antagonist that has been discontinued in the United States.

Estrogen receptor blockers (for tamoxifen, see the prototype feature)

Fulvestrant (Faslodex): Approved in 2002, fulvestrant selectively binds to the ERs of breast cancer cells and inhibits cell division. This drug does not block aromatase and, unlike tamoxifen, fulvestrant has no estrogen agonist activity. It is used to treat advanced breast cancer in ER-positive, postmenopausal women with disease progression following antiestrogen therapy. It appears to be as effective as the aromatase inhibitors. This drug is administered by IM injection once a month. It is generally well tolerated, with the most common adverse effects being nausea, vomiting, constipation, diarrhea, headache, abdominal pain, hot flashes, back pain, and pharyngitis. Temporary injection site pain and inflammation are possible. Fulvestrant is a pregnancy category D drug.

Raloxifene (Evista): Similar to tamoxifen, raloxifene is an oral drug that has agonist and antagonist effects on the ERs in the breast. Unlike tamoxifen, however, it does not have agonist actions on the ERs in the uterus. Originally approved in 1997 for osteoporosis, its indications were expanded in 2007 to include prophylaxis of breast cancer in postmenopausal women who are at high risk for developing the disease. It is used off-label to treat uterine leiomyomata in postmenopausal women. Raloxifene is associated with an increased risk of thromboembolic disorders such as DVT, pulmonary embolism, and retinal thrombosis. Hot flashes and leg cramps are common adverse effects. It is classified as pregnancy category X. A prototype feature for raloxifene is presented in Chapter 75.

Toremifene (Fareston): Approved in 1997, toremifene is a PO medication closely related to tamoxifen that has both agonist and antagonist actions at the ERs. The ERs in the breast are inhibited by this drug, whereas those in the uterus are stimulated. Toremifene is indicated for the treatment of metastatic breast cancer in postmenopausal women with ER-positive or unknown tumors. Common adverse effects include hot flashes, vaginal discharge, diaphoresis, and fluid retention. Serious adverse effects are uncommon but may include CVA, angina, dysrhythmias, and increased intraocular pressure. This is a pregnancy category D drug.

Aromatase inhibitors: Aromatase is the enzyme that catalyzes the last step in the synthesis of estrogen. In premenopausal women, the primary sites of estrogen production are the ovaries. In postmenopausal women estrogen is formed from androgens secreted by the adrenal glands, with only a small amount coming from the ovaries. Aromatase converts androgens (testosterone and androstenedione) to estrogens in the peripheral tissues such as fat and muscle. Aromatase inhibitors dramatically decrease serum estradiol levels, thus starving estrogen-dependent tumors of a major growth stimulus. The American Society of Clinical Oncology recommends adjuvant aromatase inhibitor therapy for all postmenopausal women with ER-positive early breast cancer.

Anastrozole (Arimidex): Anastrozole is a hormone antagonist that is highly specific for the enzyme aromatase. Anastrozole restricts tumor growth by inhibiting the biosynthesis of estrogens, thus depriving the tumor of necessary estrogen. Although first approved in 1995 for the treatment of advanced breast cancer, indications have since been expanded to include the adjuvant treatment of early breast cancer in postmenopausal women with ER-positive disease. An off-label indication of anastrozole is for the treatment of uterine leiomyomata. Serious adverse effects are uncommon during anastrozole therapy. The types of adverse events are similar to those of tamoxifen. Hot flashes occur in 12% to 25% of patients. Nausea, vomiting, and thromboembolic events occur in a small percentage of patients. Osteoporosis during therapy may lead to an increased incidence of spinal fractures. As an antiestrogen, anastrozole will block the effects of oral contraceptives or estrogen replacement therapy. Anastrozole is a pregnancy category D drug.

Exemestane (Aromasin): Exemestane is an oral aromatase inhibitor that reduces serum estradiol concentrations by binding irreversibly and inactivating the aromatase enzyme. Exemestane has greater antiestrogen actions than tamoxifen or anastrozole and is effective when tumors develop resistance to these other agents. First approved in 1999 for the treatment of advanced breast cancer, indications were expanded in 2005 to include the adjuvant treatment of early breast cancer in postmenopausal women with ER-positive disease. It cannot be used in women who are premenopausal or lactating or who have a hypersensitivity to it. Adverse effects are the same as those of other aromatase inhibitors and include hot flashes, nausea, vomiting, and osteoporosis. About 20% of patients with advanced breast cancer will experience lymphopenia. Exemestane is a pregnancy category D drug.

Letrozole (Femara): Letrozole is an oral aromatase inhibitor that prevents the conversion of androgens to estrogens, resulting in reduced serum estrogen levels. First approved in 1997, its indications include the adjuvant treatment of early breast cancer in patients who have received 5 years of adjuvant tamoxifen therapy; first-line treatment of patients with ER-positive or unknown, locally advanced, or metastatic cancer; advanced breast cancer with disease progression following antiestrogen therapy; and the adjuvant treatment of patients with hormone receptor-positive early breast cancer. Treatment is restricted to postmenopausal women. Off-label indications include the treatment of infertility in anovulatory women who wish to become pregnant and to increase the height of boys with idiopathic short stature or delayed puberty. This drug is generally well tolerated, with the most common adverse effects being nausea, vomiting, asthenia, headache, and bone and other musculoskeletal pain. Letrozole is a pregnancy category D drug.

Gonadotropin-releasing hormone analogs: Gonadotropin-releasing hormone (GnRH) analogs closely simulate endogenous GnRH and provide feedback to the pituitary gland. Initially, the effect is to increase the production of interstitial cell-stimulating hormone (ICSH), which increases the production of testosterone by the testes. ICSH is also known as follicle-stimulating hormone (FSH). With continued therapy, the pituitary becomes insensitive to the effects of GnRH, and the production of testosterone falls. In fact, testosterone secretion declines to near zero levels such that treatment with a GnRH analog is considered a type of chemical or pharmacologic castration. The loss of testosterone "starves" prostate cancer cells of the hormone essential for their growth. The GnRH analogs are administered by the subcutaneous or IM routes. All GnRH analogs are pregnancy category X drugs and contraindicated during pregnancy.

Goserelin (Zoladex): Approved in 1993, goserelin is a GnRH antagonist that is administered as a depot implant into the abdominal wall every 1 to 3 months. It reduces testosterone levels in men to castration levels and lowers estrogen levels in women to postmenopausal levels. Approved indications include endometriosis and the palliative treatment of advanced prostate and breast cancer. It may be used off-label to treat uterine leiomyomata or benign prostatic hyperplasia. Hot flashes occur in most patients. Men experience impotence and gynecomastia, whereas women experience amenorrhea. Bone pain and irritation at the injection site are common. Decreased bone density occurs in both men and women. Goserelin is classified as a pregnancy category X drug.

Histrelin (Supprelin, Vantas): Approved in 2004, histrelin is a GnRH analog that is given subcutaneously as an implant, usually in the inner aspect of the upper arm. This drug is slowly released over a period of 12 months, at which time the implant is removed. Its only approved antineoplastic application is for the palliation of advanced prostate cancer. A nonneoplastic indication is for the treatment of central precocious puberty in children. Hot flashes occur in the majority of patients. Men may experience impotence, gynecomastia, and testicular atrophy. Inflammation may occur at the site of implantation. Reduced bone density is an adverse effect in adolescents who are taking the drug. Histrelin is classified as a pregnancy category X drug.

Leuprolide (Eligard, Lupron, Viadur): Leuprolide is a GnRH analog that is an effective androgen antagonist for treating hormone-dependent tumors. It reduces testosterone levels in men to castration levels and lowers estrogen levels in women to postmenopausal levels. It is used as a palliative treatment for advanced prostate cancer as an alternative to orchiectomy or estrogen therapy. It is used off-label to induce ovarian ablation in premenopausal women with ER-positive breast cancer. Nonneoplastic indications include the treatment of benign prostatic hyperplasia, endometriosis, and precocious puberty in children less than 9 years of age. It is occasionally used to treat female infertility by hyperstimulating the ovary (see Chapter 70). This drug is administered by the IM or subcutaneous route. Viadur and Eligard are subcutaneous implants for prostate cancer that release the drug over a period of 1 to 12 months, depending on the formulation. Leuprolide causes nausea, vomiting, hot flashes, and diaphoresis in both men and women. Women develop amenorrhea and men experience testicular atrophy due to reduced testosterone levels. CNS effects such as migraines, depression, insomnia, asthenia, and dizziness may occur. Injection site reactions are frequent. This is a pregnancy category X drug.

Triptorelin (Trelstar): Triptorelin is a GnRH analog that was approved in 2000 for the palliative therapy of advanced prostate cancer. This drug is administered once monthly by the IM route, and most patients achieve the castration levels of androgens in less than a month. Off-label uses include advanced breast cancer, uterine leiomyomata, and precocious puberty. Adverse effects are similar to those of other GnRH analogs. This is a pregnancy category X drug.

Androgen receptor blockers: Growth of prostatic carcinoma is usually androgen dependent. The androgen receptor blockers prevent testosterone and other androgens from reaching their receptors on cancer cells, thus depriving the cells of an important growth promoter. Drugs in this group are all administered PO and are used only to treat prostate cancer. They have an additive or synergistic effect when used in combination with GnRH analogs.

Bicalutamide (Casodex), flutamide (Eulexin), and nilutamide (Nilandron): Bicalutamide, flutamide, and nilutamide are antiandrogen agents that are all closely related in structure and function. All have only one indication: the chemotherapy of metastatic prostate cancer. Bicalutamide and flutamide are used in combination with a GnRH analog such as goserelin or leuprolide. Bicalutamide and flutamide block androgen receptors, whereas the GnRH analog decreases the secretion of testosterone. Nilutamide is given following an orchiectomy. The androgen receptor blockers are administered by the PO route. Adverse effects are mild to moderate and are those expected of blocking androgen secretion such as hot flashes, mastalgia, impotence, decreased libido, and gynecomastia. They are only indicated for prostate cancer and thus should not be administered to women. Bicalutamide and flutamide are pregnancy category X drugs, whereas nilutamide is a pregnancy category C drug.

Natural Products

58.7 Natural products that are derived from plants include the vinca alkaloids, taxanes, and topoisomerase inhibitors.

Agents with antineoplastic activity have been isolated from a number of plants, including the common periwinkle (*Vinca rosea*), Pacific yew (*Taxus baccata*), mandrake (May apple), and the shrub *Campothecus acuminata.* Although structurally very different, medications in this class have the common ability to arrest cell division; thus, some of them are called mitotic inhibitors. The plant extracts, or natural products, are listed in Table 58.5. There are three subdivisions of natural products used as antineoplastics.

- Vinca alkaloids
- Taxanes
- Topoisomerase inhibitors

Vinca alkaloids: The vinca alkaloids vincristine (Oncovin) and vinblastine (Velban) are two older drugs derived from more

CONNECTIONS

Lifespan Considerations Administering Chemotherapy to the Elderly

There is an increased incidence of cancer as a person ages. This may be partially due to the fact that there has been more time for older individuals to be exposed to various carcinogens, and as a person ages, the immune system becomes less and less able to do an adequate job of protecting the body against foreign invasion.

For many years the older person was given a reduced dose of chemotherapy. This was based on the premise that an older body would not be able to tolerate regular doses as well as a younger body and that the nausea and vomiting caused by many of the antineoplastics would be intolerable to the older patient. It has been proven, however, that the older person has no more nausea and vomiting than does a younger person; therefore, the dose of antineoplastics should not be based solely on the patient's age. Doses of antineoplastics should be based on renal, hepatic, and cardiac function. There are a few general things to keep in mind when administering antineoplastics to older patients. A slowed metabolism may have an impact on how quickly the drug is metabolized and excreted. As a person ages, there is an increased chance of major organ function impairments, so a complete assessment must be done before beginning any antineoplastic therapy. The elderly may experience toxicity at a lower dose than a younger person, so the nurse must remain alert to the initial signs of toxicity and intervene as necessary. The nutritional intake of an elderly person may be less than adequate, so the patient and family must be taught about well-balanced diets and ways to substitute healthy foods for other foods. Measures to decrease the chance of developing an infection must be stressed to the elderly patient and family, such as avoiding crowds, avoiding persons with upper respiratory infections, and avoiding sick children.

TABLE 58.5 Natural Products Used as Antineoplastic Therapy

Drug	Route and Adult Dose (maximum dose where indicated)	Adverse Effects
Vinca Alkaloids		
vinblastine sulfate (Velban)	IV: 18.5 mg/m^2 every week	*Nausea, vomiting, stomatitis, anorexia, rash, alopecia, loss of energy and strength*
vincristine (Oncovin)	IV: 1.4 mg/m^2 every week (max: 2 mg/m^2)	Bone marrow suppression, severe nausea, vomiting, diarrhea, mucositis, pulmonary or cardiac toxicity, nephrotoxicity (vincristine), neurotoxicity (vincristine, docetaxel), anaphylaxis or other hypersensitivity reactions, severe fluid retention (docetaxel)
vinorelbine (Navelbine)	IV: 30 mg/m^2 every week	
Taxanes		
docetaxel (Taxotere)	IV: 60–100 mg/m^2 every 3 weeks	
paclitaxel (Taxol)	IV: 135–175 mg/m^2 every 3 weeks	
Topoisomerase Inhibitors		
etoposide (VePesid)	IV: 50/100 mg/m^2/day for 5 days	
irinotecan (Camptosar)	IV: 125 mg/m^2 every week for 4 weeks	
teniposide (Vumon)	IV: 165 mg/m^2 every 3–4 days for 4 weeks	
topotecan (Hycamtin)	IV: 1.5 mg/m^2 /day for 5 days	

Note: *Italics* indicate common adverse effects. Underline indicates serious adverse effects.

than 100 alkaloids isolated from the periwinkle plant. The medicinal properties of this plant were described in folklore in several regions of the world long before their antineoplastic properties were discovered. Despite being derived from the same plant, vincristine, vinblastine, and the semisynthetic vinorelbine (Navelbine) exhibit different effects and toxicity profiles.

PROTOTYPE DRUG Vincristine (Oncovin)

Classification: **Therapeutic:** Antineoplastic
Pharmacologic: Vinca alkaloid, mitotic inhibitor, natural product

Therapeutic Effects and Uses: Vincristine is a cell cycle specific antineoplastic obtained from the periwinkle plant that is active in the M phase of the cell cycle where it inhibits cell division. It is approved to treat acute lymphocytic leukemia, Hodgkin's and non-Hodgkin's lymphomas, lymphosarcoma, malignant glioma, neuroblastoma, rhabdomyosarcoma, soft tissue sarcoma, and Wilms' tumor. It may be used off-label for breast, colorectal, and lung cancers. It is only administered by the IV route.

Mechanism of Action: Vincristine binds to tubulin, which is a protein that makes up the microtubules of the cell that are necessary for cell division. This disrupts the process whereby chromosomes are distributed to the daughter cells during mitosis, resulting in cell death. Paclitaxel and colchicine also produce pharmacologic actions by binding to tubulin, but they bind at a different location than vincristine.

Pharmacokinetics:

Route(s)	IV
Absorption	N/A
Distribution	Widely distributed; does not cross the blood–brain barrier; crosses the placenta; unknown if secreted in breast milk
Primary metabolism	Hepatic
Primary excretion	Bile and feces (80%); renal (20%)
Onset of action	15–20 minutes
Duration of action	Triphasic half-life: 0.85 minute, 7.4 minutes, and 164 minutes

Adverse Effects: Vincristine is a very toxic medication, and even therapeutic doses may result in serious adverse effects. The major dose-limiting toxicity of vincristine is neurotoxicity. This manifests as motor difficulties, peripheral neuropathy, paresthesias (especially of the hands and feet), weakness, cranial nerve palsies (diplopia, hoarseness, deafness, trigeminal neuralgia, vocal cord paralysis), and decreased reflexes. Neurotoxicity may take several months to resolve. CNS effects may include seizures, depression, hallucinations, and coma. GI-related adverse effects include nausea, vomiting, anorexia, stomatitis, severe constipation, and abdominal pain. Other adverse reactions include hepatotoxicity, rash, paralytic ileus (especially in children), and alopecia. Myelosuppression may occur although much less frequently than with other vinca alkaloids. Extravasation can cause intense pain, inflammation, and tissue necrosis. If extravasation occurs, treatment with warm compresses and hyaluronidase is implemented; cold compresses will significantly increase the toxicity of vinca alkaloids.

Contraindications/Precautions: Contraindications to the use of vincristine include obstructive jaundice, men and women of childbearing age, active infection, adynamic ileus, radiation of the liver, infants, pregnancy, and lactation. Cautions must be taken when administering vincristine to patients with leukopenia, preexisting neuromuscular or neurologic disease, hypertension, or hepatic or renal disease; those who are taking drugs with neurotoxic properties; and the elderly. Doses should be reduced in patients with hepatic or biliary disease. Vincristine is a vesicant and caution must be used to avoid exposure of the skin to this drug.

Drug Interactions: Vincristine is a substrate for CYP3A4 and agents that induce CYP3A4 (such as carbamazepine or phenytoin) may increase the metabolism of vincristine and decrease the effects of the drug. Vincristine will increase the action of methotrexate, bleomycin, and anticoagulants. Decreased digoxin and phenytoin levels will occur. Administration of L-asparaginase just prior to vincristine will cause additive neurotoxicity. Concurrent administration with mitomycin may cause acute dyspnea and severe bronchospasm. Neurotoxicity may occur with peripheral nervous system drugs. **Herbal/Food:** Unknown.

Pregnancy: Category D.

Treatment of Overdose: Overdose may cause life-threatening symptoms or death. Symptoms are extensions of the adverse effects of vincristine. There is no antidote and patients are treated symptomatically.

Nursing Responsibilities:

- Prevent exposure to people with infections or colds during periods of leukopenia. Leukocyte count in children usually reaches nadir on the fourth day and begins to rise on the fifth day after drug administration.
- Monitor I&O ratio and pattern, blood pressure, and temperature daily.
- Weigh the patient weekly or more often if ordered. In the presence of edema or ascites, the patient's ideal weight is used to determine dosage. Report a steady gain or sudden weight change to the prescriber.
- Monitor baseline and periodic laboratory tests. Monitor serum electrolytes and CBC with differential. Complete bone marrow remission in leukemia varies widely and may not occur for as long as 100 days after therapy is started.
- Assess for hand muscular weakness, and check deep tendon reflexes (depression of the Achilles reflex is the earliest sign of neuropathy). Also observe for and report mental depression, ptosis, double vision, hoarseness, paresthesias, neuritic pain, and motor difficulties promptly to the prescriber.
- Check the patient's ability to ambulate, and supply support if necessary. Walking may be impaired.
- Take care to distinguish between the depression associated with the realization of neoplastic disease and that which is drug induced.

Patient and Family Education:

- Immediately report stomach, bone, or joint pain and swelling of the lower legs and ankles to the health care provider.
- Start a preventive regimen against constipation that includes adequate fluids, a high-fiber diet, and laxatives at the beginning of treatment, and report to the health care provider changes in bowel habits should they occur.
- Reversible hair loss is reportedly the most common adverse reaction and may persist for the duration of therapy. Regrowth may start before the end of treatment. This is a distressing adverse effect because the scalp hair will drop out in large clumps.

Drugs Similar to Vincristine (Oncovin)

The two additional vinca alkaloids include vinblastine and vinorelbine. Other classes of natural products include the taxames (docetaxel and paclitaxel) and the topoisomerase inhibitors (ironotecan, topotican, etoposide, and teniposide).

Vinblastine (Velban): Vinblastine is obtained from the periwinkle plant and has a chemical structure and mechanism of action very similar to those of vincristine. However, the toxicities and spectrum of actions of the two drugs differ. The use of vinblastine has declined because of the development of newer effective agents, but it has traditionally been used to treat Hodgkin's disease and testicular tumors. Off-label uses include treatment of prostate, bladder, and lung cancers and metastatic malignant melanoma. It is only administered by the IV route. Unlike vincristine, neurotoxicity with vinblastine is infrequent. Instead, myelosuppression is the dose-limiting toxicity (especially neutropenia) with a nadir at 4 to 10 days and recovery between days 7 and 21. An increased risk of infection or bleeding can occur due to the myelosuppressive effects of vinblastine. Nausea and vomiting are generally mild. Extravasation can cause intense pain, inflammation, and tissue necrosis. Other potential adverse effects include hypertension, CVA, dyspnea, and Raynaud's phenomenon. Doses should be reduced in patients with hepatic or biliary disease. This is a pregnancy category D drug.

Vinorelbine (Navelbine): Vinorelbine is a semisynthetic drug derived from vinblastine to which it shares structural and functional similarities. In addition to having the same mechanism of action as the vinca alkaloids, vinorelbine also inhibits RNA synthesis and blocks the cellular use of glutamic acid that is needed for purine synthesis. Its only approved use is to treat non–small cell lung cancer. It may be used off-label to treat metastatic breast cancer, head and neck cancers, ovarian cancer, and Hodgkin's disease. The primary dose-limiting toxicity is myelosuppression (especially neutropenia) with a nadir at 7 to 14 days and recovery between days 14 and 24. The myelosuppressive effects of vinorelbine can increase the risk of infection or bleeding. Like vinblastine neurotoxicity is infrequent. Extravasation can cause intense pain, inflammation, and tissue necrosis. Other adverse effects include mild nausea, vomiting, thromboembolic events, asthenia, fatigue, and pulmonary hypersensitivity. Vinorelbine is a pregnancy category D drug.

Taxanes: The taxanes, which include paclitaxel (Taxol) and docetaxel (Taxotere), were originally isolated from the bark of the Pacific yew, an evergreen found in forests throughout the western United States. More than 19 different taxane alkaloids have been isolated from the tree, and several others are being investigated for potential antineoplastic activity. Although the taxanes are mitotic inhibitors like the vinca alkaloids, they act by a different mechanism. Bone marrow toxicity is usually the dose-limiting factor for the taxanes.

Docetaxel (Taxotere): Approved in 1996, docetaxel is a semisynthetic taxane that is administered only by the IV route. The drug was produced to attain greater antitumor activity and lower toxicity potential than with paclitaxel. Although it affects microtubules and is a mitotic inhibitor, its binding is slightly different than the vinca alkaloids or paclitaxel and thus has a somewhat different action and toxicity. Docetaxel is approved to treat solid tumors, including advanced gastric cancer, head and neck cancers, metastatic breast or prostate cancer, and non–small cell lung cancer that has failed to respond to therapy with platinum antineoplastics. Off-label indications include metastatic malignant melanoma and advanced ovarian cancer. To reduce the incidence and severity of fluid retention and hypersensitivity reactions, all patients who will be receiving docetaxel should be administered dexamethasone for 3 days prior to chemotherapy. Without premedication, a hypersensitivity reaction occurs in about 20% of patients within minutes of the injection. Severe fluid retention occurs in about 7% of patients even with premedication and may include peripheral or generalized edema, dyspnea, pleural effusion, cardiac tamponade, and ascites. The major dose-limiting toxicity is myelosuppression, especially neutropenia, which occurs in nearly all patients. The nadir occurs at 7 days with recovery at 14 days. Skin reactions, primarily erythema, rash, and pruritus on the feet and hands, occur in the majority of patients. Severe skin toxicity occurs in about 5% of patients. Neurologic toxicity such as paresthesias and peripheral neuropathy occur in half the patients taking this drug. Mild to moderate nausea, vomiting, diarrhea, stomatitis, and esophagitis are common. Docetaxel is a pregnancy category D drug.

Paclitaxel (Taxol): Approved in 1992, paclitaxel is a semisynthetic taxane that is administered only by the IV route and approved to treat solid tumors, including metastatic breast cancer, ovarian cancer, Kaposi's sarcoma, and non–small cell lung cancer in combination with cisplatin. Off-label indications include the chemotherapy of bladder, head, and neck cancers. The major dose-limiting toxicity is myelosuppression, especially neutropenia, which occurs in nearly all patients. The nadir occurs at 11 days. This drug is contraindicated in patients with neutrophil counts less than 1,500 cells/mm^3. Anaphylaxis and severe hypersensitivity reaction may occur, usually within an hour after the start of the infusion. To reduce the incidence of severe hypersensitivity reactions, patients should be premedicated with dexamethasone and diphenhydramine prior to paclitaxel administration. Extravasation of paclitaxel can result in an acute and delayed injection site reaction. A local hyaluronidase injection may be beneficial in treating severe extravasation symptoms. Other common adverse events include musculoskeletal pain, asthenia, hypotension, rash, peripheral neuropathy, mild to moderate nausea, vomiting, diarrhea, and stomatitis. Alopecia occurs in nearly every patient. Paclitaxel is a pregnancy category D drug.

Topoisomerase inhibitors: DNA exists in a double stranded supercoiled state. The two strands must be separated if the macromolecule is to replicate or serve as a template for RNA synthesis (see Chapter 57). Topoisomerase is an enzyme that cuts the DNA strand, thus changing it to a more relaxed structure that can be used for DNA and RNA synthesis. The topoisomerase enzyme exists in two closely related forms. Topoisomerase I causes breaks in one strand of the DNA molecule, and topoisomerase II causes breaks in both DNA strands.

Topoisomerase inhibitors bind to the enzyme, preventing it from causing the strand breaks necessary for DNA to perform its functions. The cancer cell is unable to properly uncoil its DNA, and DNA replication terminates prematurely. Topoisomerase inhibitors are natural products, and they are available for IV administration only.

American Indians described uses of the May apple or wild mandrake (*Podophyllum peltatum*) long before pharmacologists isolated podophyllotoxin, which is the primary active ingredient in the plant. As a botanical, podophyllum has been used as an antidote for snakebites, as a cathartic, and as a topical treatment for warts. Teniposide (Vumon) and etoposide (VePesid) are semisynthetic products of podophyllotoxin.

More recently isolated topoisomerase I inhibitors include topotecan (Hycamtin) and irinotecan (Camptosar). These agents are called camptothecins because they were first isolated from *Camptotheca acuminata,* a tree native to China. The camptothecins are administered IV only, and their indications are limited. As with many other cytotoxic natural products, bone marrow suppression is the dose-limiting toxicity for the camptothecins.

Irinotecan (Camptosar): Approved in 1996, irinotecan is a cytotoxic alkaloid obtained from *Camptotheca acuminata.* Like other camptothecin analogs, it acts by inhibiting topoisomerase I, which interferes with DNA replication. It is specific for the S phase of the cell cycle. Irinotecan is approved as the first-line treatment of metastatic colorectal cancer in combination with fluorouracil and for the second-line treatment of colorectal cancer that has progressed despite treatment with fluorouracil. Off-label uses include advanced breast, cervical, ovarian, gastric, and lung cancers. Hematologic toxicity is dose limiting, with anemia, leukopenia, and neutropenia occurring in most patients. Diarrhea is also severe, may be dose limiting, and requires antidiarrheal therapy. The diarrhea may begin immediately after chemotherapy or may be delayed 11 days. Early diarrhea may be accompanied by cholinergic symptoms such as rhinitis, increased salivation, miosis, lacrimation, diaphoresis, and abdominal cramping. These cholinergic symptoms may be prevented by the administration of atropine. Nausea and vomiting are common and severe enough to require pretreatment with antiemetics, which are given on the day of treatment at least 30 minutes before the administration of irinotecan. Other adverse events that occur at a high rate include asthenia, fever, dyspnea, abdominal pain, anorexia, and dizziness. This drug is pregnancy category D.

Topotecan (Hycamtin): Approved in 1996, this drug is an IV camptothecin, topoisomerase I inhibitor very similar to irinotecan, although its indications are different. Topotecan is approved to treat metastatic ovarian cancer after failure of traditional chemotherapy, lung cancer, and inoperable cervical cancer. It may be used off-label to treat rhabdomyosarcoma in children. Like irinotecan, topotecan can cause severe myelosuppression and diarrhea, which are both dose-limiting toxicities. The drug is contraindicated in patients with neutrophil counts less than 1,500 cells/mm^3. Nausea and vomiting are usually mild. Topotecan can cause infertility in both males and females. Other common adverse events include alopecia, fatigue, asthenia, fever, musculoskeletal pain, dyspnea, and headache. This drug is pregnancy category D.

Etoposide (VePesid): Approved in 1983, etoposide is a derivative of podophyllotoxin that inhibits topoisomerase II. It is one of the few antineoplastic natural products that are administered by both PO and IV routes. It is approved for patients with refractory testicular tumors; in patients who have already received surgery, chemotherapy, and radiation without success; and for small cell carcinoma of the lung. Its off-label indications include acute myelogenous and lymphocytic leukemia, Hodgkin's and non-Hodgkin's lymphomas, refractory ovarian cancer, gastric cancer, neuroblastoma, and malignant glioma. Bone marrow toxicity is the dose-limiting toxicity with nadir occurring at day 16 and recovery by days 20 through 22. Nausea, vomiting, and stomatitis are mild. Anaphylaxis has been reported in up to 2% of patients who are receiving this drug. Secondary malignancies, especially acute nonlymphocytic leukemia, may occur in children who are treated with this drug. Etoposide is a pregnancy category D drug.

Teniposide (Vumon): Approved in 1992, teniposide is a derivative of podophyllotoxin that inhibits topoisomerase II. It is only approved to treat refractory childhood acute lymphocytic leukemia but may be used off-label for neuroblastoma, bladder cancer, lung cancer, and non-Hodgkin's lymphoma. Like etoposide, bone marrow toxicity (especially neutropenia) is its most common dose-limiting toxicity. Anaphylaxis has been reported in a significant number of patients, although this may be caused by polyoxyethylated castor oil, which is used as the vehicle for the drug. GI adverse reactions occur in most patients and include severe stomatitis, diarrhea, mild nausea, and vomiting. This drug is pregnancy category D.

NURSING PROCESS APPLICATION

Patients Receiving Cancer Chemotherapy

Assessment

Prior to administration:

- Obtain a complete health history, including allergies.
- Obtain a history of cardiac, hepatic, or renal conditions.
- Obtain laboratory work, especially CBC, platelet count, and hemoglobin and hematocrit counts.
- Assess neurologic status, including mood, affect, and sensory impairment.

Potential Nursing Diagnoses

- *Activity Intolerance,* related to effects of treatment
- *Anxiety,* related to uncertainty of outcome
- *Constipation,* related to adverse effects of medication
- *Ineffective Coping,* related to diagnosis and prognosis
- *Diarrhea,* related to adverse effects of medication
- *Risk for Falls,* related to weakness secondary to effects of treatment
- *Ineffective Health Maintenance,* related to inability to manage adverse reactions of treatment
- *Risk for Infection,* related to myelosuppression
- *Deficient Knowledge (Treatment)*
- *Imbalanced Nutrition: Less than Body Requirements,* related to anorexia, secondary to treatments
- *Impaired Oral Mucous Membrane,* related to adverse effect of medication
- *Self-Care Deficit: Feeding, Bathing/Hygiene,Dressing/Grooming, Toileting,* related to fatigue, secondary to treatment

Planning: Patient Goals and Expected Outcomes

The patient will:

- Experience a reduction in tumor mass or slowed progression of abnormal cell growth.
- Not experience any dose-limiting toxicity or serious adverse effects.
- Explain and demonstrate understanding of the drugs' actions by describing adverse effects, especially those reportable to the health care provider.

Implementation

Interventions and (Rationales)

- Monitor vital signs, especially temperature and laboratory reports. (Antineoplastics may cause immune system suppression and blood dyscrasias.)

Patient and Family Education

Instruct the patient to:

- Take and record vital signs daily (especially temperature).
- Keep the health care provider informed of any changes in vital signs.
- Immediately report any signs of infection, such as sore throat, fever, or increased fatigue.

• Monitor for signs of cardiac or respiratory involvement or ECG changes. (Antineoplastics may cause cardiac or respiratory disorders. Doxorubicin may cause sinus tachycardia, cardiac depression, and delayed-onset CHF. Cyclophosphamide may cause myopericarditis and pulmonary fibrosis.)	Instruct the patient to: • Report immediately any shortness of breath or dyspnea on exertion, cough, or sputum production. • Report tachycardia, edema, or decreased activity tolerance. • Keep all appointments for health care provider follow-up, ECGs, and laboratory work.
• Monitor renal status, character of urine, I&O, daily weight for the patient in the hospital or twice weekly weight for the patient at home, and edema. (Vincristine may cause water retention and concentrated urine. Vincristine and methotrexate may cause increased uric acid levels, renal calculi, or gout. Cyclophosphamide or cisplatin may cause hemorrhagic cystitis.)	Instruct the patient: • To record I&O. • About accurate weight monitoring and recording. • To be alert for and report any changes in urine color, odor, difficulty voiding, or hematuria. • How and where on the body to check for edema. • That doxorubicin will turn urine reddish-brown for 1–2 days after administration.
• Monitor nausea and vomiting. (Most antineoplastics will cause nausea or vomiting, or both.)	• Instruct the patient to report nausea or vomiting, regardless of when in relation to administration of antineoplastics it occurs. • Reassure the patient and family that antiemetics can be administered. • Ensure that the patient has a prescription for prn (as needed) antiemetics for use at home.
• Monitor nutritional status and presence of anorexia. (Anorexia may be present as a result of stomatitis or actual loss of appetite. The patient will eat more if foods that are tolerated are consumed.)	Instruct the patient to: • Keep a food diary to identify which foods are tolerated and which are not. • Ingest easily digested foods and beverages. • Take nutritional supplements, as necessary. • Report any occurrences of nausea, vomiting, diarrhea, or mouth soreness. • Eat small frequent meals, drink cool liquids, and avoid caffeine and spicy or hot foods. • Perform frequent oral hygiene; use only a soft toothbrush; inspect the mouth daily; and avoid using toothpicks.
• Monitor for constipation. (Vincristine, especially when used by elderly patients, may cause severe constipation, fecal impaction, or paralytic ileus.)	Instruct the patient to: • Report changes in bowel patterns. • Increase fiber and fluids in the diet, and increase activity if possible.
• Monitor for conjunctivitis. (Doxorubicin may cause conjunctivitis.)	• Instruct the patient to report any changes in vision and any redness, weepiness, or discomfort.
• Monitor neurologic and sensory status. (Depression and peripheral neuropathy may be caused by antineoplastics. Vincristine may cause ataxia and hand drop or footdrop. Tamoxifen may cause photophobia and decreased vision. These changes may be irreversible.)	• Instruct the patient to report any changes in sensation, numbness, tingling, pain, gait or balance, or mood and affect. • Refer the patient to support groups for those with cancer and encourage attendance. • Instruct the patient to wear sunscreen, long sleeves, and sunglasses, and to limit sun exposure.
• Monitor liver function tests. (Antineoplastics are metabolized by the liver; decreased liver function can lead to toxicity.)	Instruct the patient to: • Monitor for and report any flank pain, jaundice, abdominal pain, bloating, or pale stools. • Keep all appointments for follow-up laboratory tests.
• Monitor for the presence of diabetes mellitus. (Antineoplastics must be administered cautiously to persons with diabetes. Steroid use may lead to hyperglycemia. The combination of insulin and cyclophosphamide may cause hypoglycemia.)	Instruct the patient to: • Recognize signs of hypo- and hyperglycemia and the importance of reporting them. • Monitor and record blood glucose levels daily and report any changes.
• Monitor genitourinary status. (Antineoplastics, especially hormones, may alter the menstrual cycle in women and may lead to impotence in men. Tamoxifen increases the risk of endometrial cancer.)	Instruct the patient and family: • To report changes in menstruation, vaginal discharge, or sexual functioning. • About increased chances of developing endometrial cancer prior to administering tamoxifen.
• Monitor hair and skin status. (Most antineoplastics cause varying degrees of alopecia, which may be a sign of overdose. Methotrexate can cause skin eruptions.)	• Instruct the patient and family to be alert for the appearance of alopecia or skin eruptions. • Refer the patient to the American Cancer Society for assistance in obtaining a wig, if necessary.
• Monitor the use of herbal products. (Herbal products may interact with both antineoplastic and other classifications of medications the patient may be taking.)	• Instruct the patient and family to check with the health care provider before using any herbs or herbal products.

Evaluation of Outcome Criteria

Evaluate the effectiveness of drug therapy by confirming that patient goals and expected outcomes have been met (see "Planning").

Biologic Response Modifiers and Monoclonal Antibodies

58.8 Biologic response modifiers and monoclonal antibodies are agents that use the body's immune system to kill tumor cells.

When body defenses recognize a cancer cell, they react by producing protective substances. These diverse substances, called biologic response modifiers (BRMs), alter the body's defense system to enhance the removal or neutralization of the foreign cell. BRMs include interferons, interleukins, and certain other cytokines. Some of the BRMs are immunostimulants. Although immunostimulants are less toxic than most other classes of antineoplastics, they have limited applications to chemotherapy. When given concurrently with other antineoplastics, however, BRMs help limit the severe myelosuppression caused by other agents. Some of the BRMs are also used for the prophylaxis of transplant rejection to dampen the immune response (see Chapter 45). BRMs, along with some miscellaneous antineoplastics, are listed in Table 58.6. Types of BRMs include the following:

- Interferons are natural proteins produced by T cells in response to viral infection and other antigens. Interferons bind to specific receptors on cancer cell membranes and

TABLE 58.6 Biologic Response Modifiers and Monoclonal Antibodies

Drug	Route and Adult Dose (maximum dose where indicated)	Adverse Effects
Biologic Response Modifiers		
aldesleukin (Proleukin)	IV: 600,000 units/kg (0.037 mg/kg) every 8 h by a 15-min infusion for a maximum of 14 doses	*Flulike symptoms (fever, chills, malaise), rash, anemia, nausea, vomiting, diarrhea, confusion, dyspnea* Cardiac arrest, hypotension, tachycardia, thrombocytopenia, oliguria, anuria, pulmonary edema, capillary leak syndrome
interferon alfa-2 (Roferon-A, Intron A)	Subcutaneous/IM: 2–3 million units/day for leukemia; increase to 36 million units/day for Kaposi's sarcoma	*Flulike symptoms, myalgia, fatigue, headache, anorexia, diarrhea* Myelosuppression, thrombocytopenia, neutropenia, suicide ideation, anaphylaxis, hepatotoxicity
Monoclonal Antibodies and Molecularly Targeted Agents		
alemtuzumab (Campath)	IV: 3–30 mg/day	*Nausea, vomiting, asthenia, stomatitis anorexia, rash, alopecia, tremors (alemtuzumab), fever, chills* Bone marrow suppression (neutropenia, anemia, thrombocytopenia), severe nausea, vomiting, diarrhea, pulmonary toxicity, severe hypersensitivity reactions, pancreatitis (gefitinib,), severe fluid retention (imatinib), CHF (bevacizumab, trastuzumab), dysrhythmias (rituximab), GI perforation (bevacizumab)
bevacizumab (Avastin)	IV: 5 mg/kg every 14 days	
bortezomib (Velcade)	IV: 1.3 mg/m^3 as bolus twice weekly for 2 weeks	
cetuximab (Erbitux)	IV: 400 mg/m^2 over 2 h; then continue with 250 mg/m^2 over 1 h weekly	
dasatanib (Sprycel)	PO: 70 mg bid	
erlotinib (Tarceva)	PO: 150 mg/day	
gefitinib (Iressa)	PO: 250–500 mg/day	
gemtuzumab ozogamicin (Mylotarg)	IV: 9 mg/m^2 for 2 h	
ibritumomab tiuxetan (Zevalin)	IV: 250 mg/m^2 of rituximab is infused followed by 5 mCi of Zevalin in a 10-min IV push	
imatinib (Gleevec)	PO: 400–600 mg/day	
lapatinib (Tykerb)	PO: 1,250 mg (5 tablets) once daily on days 1 to 21 continuously in combination with capecitabine	
nilotinib (Tasigna)	PO: 400 mg bid	
panitumumab (Vectibix)	IV: 6 mg/kg administered over 60 min every 14 days	
rituximab (Rituxan)	IV: 375 mg/m^2/day as a continuous infusion	
scinitinib (Sutent)	PO: 50 mg once daily for 4 weeks followed by 2 weeks off	
sorafenib (Nexavar)	PO: 400 mg bid	
tositumomab (Bexxar)	IV: 450 mg over 60 min	
trastuzumab (Herceptin)	IV: 4 mg/kg as a single dose; then 2 mg/kg every week	

Note: *Italics* indicate common adverse effects. Underline indicates serious adverse effects.

suppress cell division, enhance the phagocytic activity of macrophages, and promote the cytotoxic activity of T lymphocytes. Peginterferon alfa-2a (Pegasys) and interferon alfa-2b (Intron-A) are approved to treat hairy cell leukemia, chronic myelogenous leukemia, Kaposi's sarcoma, and chronic hepatitis B and C. A prototype feature for peginterferon alfa-2b is included in Chapter 45.

- Interleukin-2 activates cytotoxic T lymphocytes and promotes other actions of the immune response. Marketed as aldesleukin (Proleukin), this drug is indicated only for metastatic renal cell carcinoma. A prototype feature for aldesleukin is included in Chapter 45.

Unlike interferons and interleukins, which are immunostimulants, monoclonal antibodies (MABs) suppress immune cells. Several of the MABs are specially engineered to attack the antigens that are present on the surface of specific tumor cells. Because these drugs are very specific, they are sometimes called **molecularly targeted agents.**

Once the MAB binds to its target cell, the cancer cell dies or is marked for destruction by other cells of the immune response. For example, trastuzumab (Herceptin) binds to specific proteins on breast cancer cells (called HER2 proteins) and induces cell death. Alemtuzumab (Campath) binds to a protein known as CD52, which is present on the surface of B and T lymphocytes, monocytes, and other WBCs, and is used to treat chronic lymphocytic leukemia. The key point about MABs is that the tumor cells must posses the specific protein receptor; otherwise, the MAB will be ineffective. Cetuximab (Erbitux) and bevacizumab (Avastin) were both approved in 2006 to treat metastatic colorectal cancer. In the treatment of RA (see Chapter 75) and severe psoriasis (see Chapter 76), MABs are used to dampen overactive inflammatory cells.

Pharm*FACT*

Chemotherapy following surgery increases the 5-year survival rate from Stage I non–small cell lung cancer by 10%. The overall survival rate for the disease, however, remains at only 15% because the cancer is not usually detected until its late stages. *Source:* Erstad, 2006.

CONNECTION *Checkpoint* 58.3

Peginterferon alfa 2a and 2b are used as antineoplastics. From what you learned in Chapter 45, what are the indications for interferon alfacon-1 (Infergen), interferon alfa-n3 (Alferon N), and interferon beta-1a (Avonex, Rebif)? See Answer to Connection Checkpoint 58.3 in Appendix A.

Miscellaneous Antineoplastics

58.9 Several miscellaneous antineoplastics act by unique mechanisms.

Some antineoplastics are classified as miscellaneous because they are structurally dissimilar to any of the previously discussed groups. Because these medications are unique, their adverse reactions vary. Doses for the miscellaneous antineoplastics are listed in Table 58.7.

Angiogenesis inhibitors: Bevacizumab (Avastin), thalidomide (Thalomid) and lenalidomide (Revlimid) are known as angiogenesis inhibitors (antiangiogenic agents) because they prevent the formation of new blood vessels that are vital to the formation of new tumors. These drugs do not kill cancer cells, but they are able to slow tumor growth. Bevacizumab was the first angiogenesis inhibitor approved in 2004 to treat colorectal cancer. It has been approved to treat non-small cell lung cancer and metastatic breast cancer. This drug is a MAB that is targeted to inhibit the function of vascular endothelial growth factor, a natural substance known to promote angiogenesis. Thalidomide is a drug with antiangiogenic properties that acts by multiple mechanisms. Highly teratogenic, thalidomide has limited distribution and is approved to treat multiple myeloma. Lenalidomide is a structural analog of thalidomide that is also indicated for multiple myeloma. It has teratogenic properties and is only available via a limited distribution program.

Altretamine (Hexalen): Altretamine is an oral antineoplastic that is similar to alkylating agents. When metabolized it forms toxic metabolites that bind to cellular macromolecules, resulting in a cytotoxic effect. Its only indication is for refractory ovarian cancer that has not responded well to other therapies. Severe myelosuppression is observed in 15% of patients with a nadir at 3 to 4 weeks and recovery at 6 weeks. The most frequent adverse effects are mild to moderate nausea and vomiting. Altretamine causes mild to moderate neurotoxicity, including peripheral neuropathy, mood disorders, disorders of consciousness, ataxia, dizziness, and vertigo. This is a pregnancy category D drug.

Arsenic trioxide (Trisenox): Approved in 2000, arsenic trioxide is a toxic metal that has only one indication: acute promyelocytic leukemia. Its mechanism of action is incompletely understood but it appears to cause DNA fragmentation that is characteristic of apoptosis. It is administered by IV infusion. Leukocytosis, thrombocytopenia, anemia, nausea, vomiting, abdominal pain, diarrhea, constipation, and anorexia are common adverse effects. Skin reactions include injection site inflammation, dermatitis, and pruritus. Neurotoxicity is relatively common and manifests as headache, insomnia, paresthesias, anxiety, dizziness, and tremors. Because arsenic trioxide can cause QT interval prolongation and complete atrioventricular block, other drugs that prolong the QT interval should be discontinued during therapy. This is a pregnancy category D drug.

Asparaginase (Elspar): Asparaginase is an enzyme that deprives cancer cells of asparagine, an essential amino acid, causing a marked reduction in protein, RNA, and DNA synthesis. It is only approved to treat acute lymphocytic leukemia in combination with other antineoplastics. It is administered by the IM, IV, or subcutaneous routes. Hypersensitivity reactions occur in 40% of patients with symptoms ranging from urticaria to anaphylactic shock. Pretreatment with corticosteroids reduces the incidence of hypersensitivity reactions. This drug is hepatotoxic and may cause hypoalbuminemia and

TABLE 58.7 Miscellaneous Antineoplastics

Drug	Route and Adult Dose (maximum dose where indicated)	Adverse Effects
altretamine (Hexalen)	PO: 65 mg/m² /day	*Hyporeflexia, paresthesias, nausea, vomiting, muscle weakness, peripheral numbness* Leukopenia, thrombocytopenia, parkinson-like tremors
arsenic trioxide (Trisenox)	IV: 0.15 mg/kg/day (max: 60 doses)	*Fever, leukocytosis, nausea, vomiting, diarrhea, abdominal pain, anorexia, rash, pruritus, fatigue, edema, headache, insomnia* Thrombocytopenia, anemia, ecchymosis, epistaxis, bleeding, dysrhythmias
asparaginase (Elspar)	IV, IM: 200 international units/kg/day for 28 days, or 5,000–10,000 units/m²/day every 3 weeks, or 10,000–40,000 units every 2–3 weeks	*Skin rash, urticaria, severe vomiting, nausea, decreased circulating platelets and fibrinogen, reduced clotting factors* Anaphylaxis, fatal hyperthermia, renal failure
bexarotene (Targretin)	PO: 100–400 mg/m²/day; Topical: 1% gel applied to lesion 1–4 times/day	*Hyperlipidemia, leukopenia, rash, pruritus, headache, asthenia, nausea, vomiting* Acute pancreatitis, elevated hepatic enzymes, hypothyroidism
everolimus (Afinitor)	PO: 10 mg once daily	*Stomatitis, infections, asthenia, fatigue, cough, diarrhea* Anemia, respiratory failure, pneumonitis
hydroxyurea (Droxia, Hydrea, Mylocel)	PO: 80 mg/kg every 3 days, or 30 mg/kg/day	*Nausea, vomiting, diarrhea, stomatitis, rash* Myelosuppression
ixabepilone (Ixempra)	IV: 40 mg/m² infused over 3 h every 3 weeks	*Alopecia, diarrhea, fatigue, asthenia, musculoskeletal pain, peripheral sensory neuropathy, stomatitis, mucositis, nausea, and vomiting* anemia, neutropenia, and thrombocytopenia
lenalidomide (Revlimid)	PO: 25 mg/day	*Abdominal pain, nausea, dizziness* Birth defects, neuropathy, neutropenia
mitotane (Lysodren)	PO: 9–10 g/day in divided doses tid or qid	*Anorexia, nausea, vomiting, diarrhea, rash, lethargy, drowsiness* Hemorrhagic cystitis
pegaspargase (Oncaspar)	IV: 2,500 international units/m² every 14 days	Same as asparaginase
thalidomide (Thalomid)	PO: 200–400 mg/day	*Abdominal pain, nausea, dizziness* Birth defects, neuropathy, neutropenia
vorinostat (Zolinza)	PO: 400 mg once daily	*Diarrhea, nausea, vomiting, anorexia, fatigue, chills, taste disorders* Blood dyscrasias, pulmonary embolism
zoledronic acid (Zometa)	IV: 4 mg over at least 15 min	*Flulike symptoms, bone, muscle pain* Dysrhythmias, electrolyte imbalances, osteonecrosis of jaw

Note: *Italics* indicate common adverse effects. Underline indicates serious adverse effects.

decreased synthesis of coagulation factors. Asparaginase may cause fatal pancreatitis. Lethargy, confusion, impaired cognition, and drowsiness are common neurotoxic effects. This is a pregnancy category C drug.

Pegaspargase (Oncaspar) is asparaginase with a molecule of PEG bonded to it. Pegylation increases the half-life of the drug and allows for less frequent dosing: 3 injections of pegaspargase versus 21 injections of asparaginase. The two drugs share the same adverse effects and indications.

Bexarotene (Targretin): Approved in 1999, bexarotene is a retinoid, a group of agents related to vitamin A that are usually used for skin conditions such as psoriasis and acne (see Chapter 76). This drug is approved by the PO and topical routes to treat cutaneous T-cell lymphoma that has not responded to other chemotherapies. Off-label indications include lung cancer, Kaposi's sarcoma, metastatic breast cancer, and severe psoriasis. Adverse effects of the oral formulation include hyperlipidemia, hypothyroidism, acute pancreatitis, leukopenia, headache, asthenia, anemia, anorexia, and photosensitivity. Topical bexarotene can cause rash, erythema, and pruritus. This is a pregnancy category X drug.

Hydroxyurea (Droxia, Hydrea, Mylocel): Hydroxyurea is an oral antineoplastic approved in 1967 for chemotherapy of chronic myelogenous leukemia, head and neck cancers, malignant melanoma, and ovarian cancer. It may be used off-label for acute myelogenous leukemia, astrocytoma, lung cancer, and malignant glioma. Sickle cell anemia is a nonneoplastic indication for the drug. Hydroxyurea causes myelosuppression, especially neutropenia. Nausea, vomiting, stomatitis, and diarrhea are common. Skin ulcers and gangrene have been reported. This is a pregnancy category C drug.

Ixabepilone (Ixempra): A newer drug that was approved in 2007, ixabepilone acts by the same mechanism as the taxanes but it has different pharmacokinetic properties. It is used in combination with capecitabine to treat metastatic or advanced breast cancer resistant to treatment with first-line medications such as the taxanes. At least 20% of patients experience alopecia, diarrhea, fatigue, asthenia, musculoskeletal pain, peripheral sensory neuropathy, stomatitis, mucositis, nausea, and vomiting. More than 40% of patients experience anemia, neutropenia, and thrombocytopenia. This is a pregnancy category D drug.

Mitotane (Lysodren): Mitotane, which is similar to the insecticide DDT, poisons cancer cells by forming links to proteins. Given by the PO route, its only indication is for the chemotherapy of advanced, inoperable adrenocortical cancer. Because the drug is cytotoxic to the adrenal gland, symptoms of acute adrenal insufficiency may emerge. Most patients experience adverse GI effects such as nausea, vomiting, and diarrhea. CNS effects such as lethargy, drowsiness, and vertigo are observed in up to 40% of patients who are taking the drug. Transient skin rashes have been observed in about 15% of the patients. Mitotane is a pregnancy category C drug.

Vorinostat (Zolinza): Approved in 2007, vorinostat arrests the cell cycle and induces apoptosis in cancer cells by inhibiting the activity of the enzyme histone deacetylase. It is only approved for the treatment of cutaneous T-cell lymphoma in patients who have progressive, persistent, or recurrent disease. Fatigue, diarrhea, nausea, altered taste, thrombocytopenia, and anorexia occur in over 20% of patients. Pulmonary embolism is a rare, though serious, adverse effect. Vorinostat may prolong the bleeding time in patients who are taking warfarin. This drug is pregnancy category D.

Zoledronic acid (Reclast, Zometa): Approved in 2001, zoledronic acid is a bisphosphonate, a drug class commonly used to treat osteoporosis. The primary action of the drug is to inhibit bone resorption by osteoclasts. In addition to its use in managing osteoporosis, this drug is approved to treat multiple myeloma in patients with osteolytic metastases, severe hypercalcemia caused by malignancy, and Paget's disease. It is given by IV infusion. Adverse effects include flulike symptoms, fever, fatigue, headache, anemia, anorexia, bone pain, arthralgia, and osteonecrosis of the jaw. Reclast and Zometa are different strengths and may not be used interchangeably. This is a pregnancy category D drug.

Drugs for Reducing Adverse Effects

58.10 Medications are used to relieve the adverse effects of patients undergoing chemotherapy.

Most patients who are undergoing chemotherapy will require drugs to treat the severe adverse effects of antineoplastic medications. In many cases, medications are given to prevent adverse effects from occurring. Some of these are well-established drugs with usefulness that has been proven over the years. Others are drugs that were developed especially to deal with the adverse effects of chemotherapy.

Antiemetics are given to nearly all patients who are undergoing chemotherapy to decrease or prevent nausea and vomiting. Examples include lorazepam (Ativan), dronabinol (Marinol), prochlorperazine (Compazine), and ondansetron (Zofran). The type and dose of the antiemetic is based on the known emetogenic potential of the specific antineoplastic agents employed. Chapter 61 provides complete information on the antiemetics.

Drugs for bowel disorders may be ordered to decrease either constipation or diarrhea. Laxatives or stool softeners may be indicated, such as Milk of Magnesia, psyllium (Metamucil), or docusate (Surfak, Colace). Patients may require a medication such as diphenoxylate with atropine (Lomotil), loperamide (Imodium), or bismuth salts (Pepto Bismol) to stop or decrease diarrhea. The student should refer to Chapter 61 for information on drugs for bowel disorders.

Myelosuppression is a disabling adverse effect of many chemotherapy agents. Three types of drugs are commonly used to prevent serious complications of myelosuppression.

- Epoetin alfa (Epogen, Procrit) is a **hematopoietic growth factor** that stimulates the production of RBCs, which may prevent the development of anemia. A prototype feature for epoetin alfa is included in Chapter 41.
- Colony stimulating factors such as filgrastim (Neupogen) increase neutrophil production in the bone marrow and enhance the phagocytic and cytotoxic functions of existing neutrophils. Administration of filgrastim shortens the length of neutropenia in patients with cancer. A prototype feature for filgrastim is included in Chapter 41.
- Oprelvekin (Neumega) is used to stimulate the production of platelets in patients who are at risk for severe thrombocytopenia caused by chemotherapy. A prototype feature for oprelvekin is included in Chapter 41.

Other medications are ordered as the patient's condition warrants, including analgesics, antibiotics, appetite stimulants, and antidepressants. The pharmacotherapy of neoplasia may include a dozen or more drugs, which makes patient care extremely challenging.

Preparing and Administering Antineoplastics

58.11 Nurses who are preparing and delivering antineoplastics must exercise extreme caution to protect themselves from medication exposure.

Many health care agencies only allow an **oncology nurse** who has received special training to care for patients with cancer and to administer chemotherapy. A large number of antineoplastic medications are absorbed through the skin and mucous membranes, so the person preparing and administering them is at risk for absorbing them. The nurse and other health care professionals engaged in the preparation or administration of antineoplastics must be extremely diligent about always wearing protective clothing, including gloves, whenever handling them. Both the Oncology Nursing Society and the Occupational Safety and Health Administration (OSHA) have established and publicized guidelines for safe handling of antineoplastic medications. The guidelines include information on safe storage and disposal as well as safe handling.

UNDERSTANDING THE CHAPTER

Key Concepts Summary

58.1 Antineoplastic agents kill or stop the growth of cancer cells and may be classified in multiple ways.

58.2 Antineoplastic drugs have serious adverse effects that require skilled nursing assessments and interventions.

58.3 Alkylating agents change the shape of the deoxyribonucleic acid double helix and prevent cancer cells from dividing normally.

58.4 Antimetabolites disrupt the critical cellular pathways of cancer cells.

58.5 The antibiotic antineoplastics contain substances obtained from bacteria that have the ability to kill cancer cells.

58.6 Hormones and hormone antagonists block the substances necessary for continued growth of tumors.

58.7 Natural products that are derived from plants include the vinca alkaloids, taxanes, and topoisomerase inhibitors.

58.8 Biologic response modifiers and monoclonal antibodies are agents that use the body's immune system to kill tumor cells.

58.9 Several miscellaneous antineoplastics act by unique mechanisms.

58.10 Medications are used to relieve the adverse effects of patients undergoing chemotherapy.

58.11 Nurses who are preparing and delivering antineoplastics must exercise extreme caution to protect themselves from medication exposure.

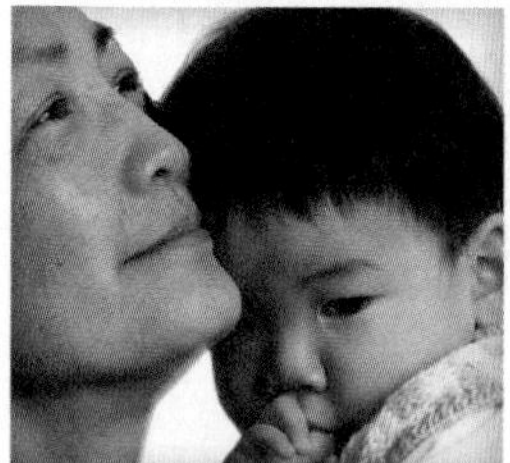

Making the PATIENT *Connection*

Remember the patient "Lucy Chinn" at the beginning of the chapter? Now read the remainder of the case study. Based on the information presented within this chapter, respond to the critical thinking questions that follow.

Lucy is a 55-year-old Asian female in good health presenting with a chief complaint of a small lump in the left breast of approximately 18 months' duration. A mammogram was performed in January 2004 and again in July 2006 and both were normal. At her last check up, Lucy was informed by her health care provider that the lump was fibrocystic and benign. However, the mammogram that was performed 1 week ago was not as optimistic.

Lucy's past medical history indicates that her father died at age 66 from complications associated with diabetes. Her mother and two sisters are alive and healthy. She does not use tobacco or alcohol. Lucy reports that she began her menses at age 13 years. She has been pregnant four times, which resulted in three live births and one miscarriage at 8 weeks' gestation. After seeking a second opinion, Lucy learned that a biopsy revealed Stage IIIa infiltrating lobular carcinoma.

Critical Thinking Questions

1. Lucy's oncologist is deciding which antineoplastic will be best for her. List the antineoplastic agents that are considered effective in treating breast cancer.
2. What do you think are the most important facts that Mrs. Chinn needs to accept at this time in her disease?
3. What long-term medication(s) may be prescribed for Mrs. Chinn, and what is the rationale behind its (their) use?

Case Study

Janet Distretti is a 25-year-old who has recently begun chemotherapy at the local oncology center. She is beginning to feel comfortable with the staff but states: "I never want to look like all of those people who are bald, or nearly bald." She has always been very proud of her long hair, and considers it her most positive feature. She is also experiencing nausea, vomiting, and anorexia with occasional severe diarrhea and constant fatigue. She refuses to speak with any of the other patients who are there at the same time she is, and also refuses to allow anyone in her family to accompany her to the treatments.

1. If you were Janet's nurse, how might you manage her chemotherapy-related nausea?
2. What suggestions might make alopecia easier for her to accept if it occurs?

NCLEX-RN® Review

1 The nurse knows that the most common dose-limiting adverse effect of antineoplastic therapy is:

1. Nausea and vomiting.
2. Myelosuppression.
3. Alopecia.
4. Anorexia.

2 The client is experiencing nausea and vomiting as a result of chemotherapy. Which response, provided by the nurse, would be most appropriate?

1. "Continue taking the chemotherapy. We can help you deal with the nausea and vomiting."
2. "You'll just have to get used to the nausea and vomiting because there is nothing we can do to alleviate it."
3. "Be sure to drink at least a liter of fluid before your chemotherapy treatment; that will help decrease the nausea and vomiting."
4. "Take your chemotherapy on a full stomach."

3 A nurse is caring for a client who is receiving chemotherapy. Which of the following actions should the nurse perform to promote self-protection from the antineoplastic agent?

1. Refuse to handle any antineoplastic medication.
2. Only work with antineoplastics under a specially designed ventilation hood.
3. Always wear protective clothing and gloves, depending on the specific medication.
4. Use universal precautions.

4 A client with pancreatic cancer has started therapy with cisplatin (Platinol). The nurse performs what important intervention during the course of this treatment?

1. Administers a daily laxative
2. Hydrates the client well
3. Administers an antiemetic following chemotherapy
4. Advises the female client to use barrier contraception

5 The client asks the nurse to explain the purpose of leucovorin rescue. Which of the following responses provided by the nurse is correct? Leucovorin rescue:

1. Decreases the amount of time normal cells are exposed to methotrexate.
2. Decreases the incidence of renal failure.
3. Alleviates severe nausea and vomiting.
4. Enhances the client's immune system.

6 The nurse determines that the client understands an important principle of antiestrogen antineoplastic therapy when the client makes which of the following statements? "Antiestrogen antineoplastics therapy:

1. Deprives tumor cells of the growth-promoting influence of estrogen."
2. Prevents breast cancer."
3. Averts the adverse effects of other antineoplastics, including hot flashes and edema."
4. Protects the female from developing osteoporosis."

See Answers to Critical Thinking Questions, Case Study, and NCLEX-RN® Review in Appendix A.

References

American Cancer Society. (2008). *Cancer facts and figures 2008.* Retrieved August 5, 2008, from http://www.cancer.org/docroot/STT/content/STT_1x_Cancer_Facts_and_Figures_2008.asp?from=fast

American Cancer Society News Center. (2006). *A cancer treatment in the spice cabinet? Researchers see promise in turmeric.* Retrieved August 5, 2008, from http://www.cancer.org/docroot/NWS/content/NWS_2_1x_A_Cancer_Treatment_in_the_spice_cabinet.asp

Chabner, B. A., Amrein, P. C., Druker, B., Michaelson, M. D., Mitsiades, C. S., Goss, P. E., et al. (2006). Chemotherapy of neoplastic diseases. In L. L. Brunton, J. S. Lazo, & K. L. Parker (Eds.), *The pharmacological basis of therapeutics* (11th ed., pp. 1315–1403). New York: McGraw-Hill.

Erstad, S. (2006). *Lung cancer survival rates.* Retrieved August 5, 2008, from http://www.revolutionhealth.com/articles/lung-cancer-survival-rates/tw9852

Fitzgerald, M. (2007). Herbal facts, herbal fallacies. *American Nurse Today, 2*(12), 27–33.

Fortenbaugh, C., & Rummel, M. (2004). Chemotherapy safety. *Clinical Journal of Oncological Nursing, 8*(4), 424–425.

Khor, T., Keum, Y., Lin, W., Kim, J., Hu, R., Shen, G., et al. (2006). Combined inhibitory effects of curcurmin and phenethyl isothiocyanate on the growth of human PC-3 prostate xenografts in immunodeficient mice. *Cancer Research, 66,* 613–621.

LeMone, P., & Burke, K. (2008). *Medical-surgical nursing: Critical thinking in client care* (4th ed.). Upper Saddle River, NJ: Pearson Education.

National Breast Cancer Coalition. (2008). *Facts and statistics about breast cancer in the United States: 2008.* Retrieved August 5, 2008, from http://www.stopbreastcancer.org//index.php?option=com_content&task=view&id=493&Itemid=178

National Cancer Institute, U.S. National Institutes of Health. (2008). *Clinical Trials. Pomegranate juice for PSA-only prostate cancer recurrence. Phase III randomized study of pomegranate juice in patients with rising prostate-specific antigen levels after surgery or radiotherapy for localized prostate cancer.* Retrieved August 5, 2008, from http://www.cancer.gov/clinicaltrials/ft-UCLA-0507059-01

Prostate Cancer Foundation. (2008). *FAQs about prostate cancer.* Retrieved August 5, 2008, from http://www.prostatecancerfoundation.org/site/c.itIWK2OSG/b.189965/k.743F/FAQs_About_Prostate_Cancer.htm

Sarkar, F. H., & Li, Y. (2003). Soy isoflavones and cancer prevention. *Cancer Investigation, 21*(5), 744–757.

Szetala, A., & Gibson, D. (2007). How the new oral antineoplastics affect nursing practice. *American Journal of Nursing, 107*(12), 40–49.

Trock, B. J., Hilakivi-Clarke, L., & Clarke, R. (2006). Meta-analysis of soy intake and breast cancer risk. *Journal of the National Cancer Institute, 98*(7), 459–471.

Yan, L., & Spitznagel, E. L. (2005). Meta-analysis of soy food and risk of prostate cancer in men. *International Journal of Cancer, 117*(4), 667–669.

UNIT 8

Pharmacology of the Gastrointestinal System

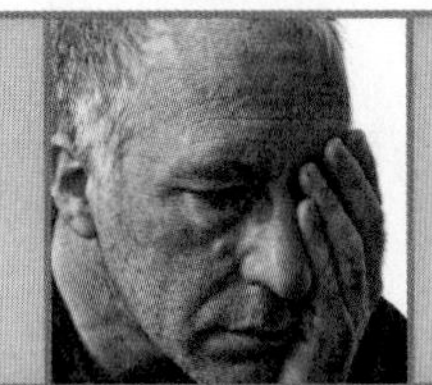 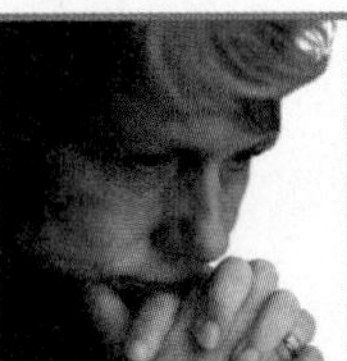 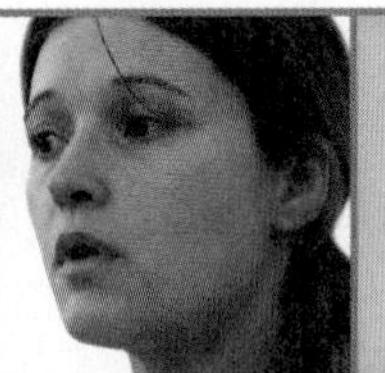 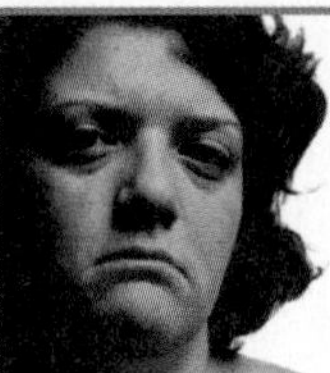

CHAPTER 59	Review of the Gastrointestinal System
CHAPTER 60	Pharmacotherapy of Peptic Ulcer Disease
CHAPTER 61	Pharmacotherapy of Bowel Disorders and Other Gastrointestinal Conditions
CHAPTER 62	Vitamins and Minerals
CHAPTER 63	Enteral and Parenteral Nutrition
CHAPTER 64	Weight Reduction Strategies and the Pharmacotherapy of Obesity

CHAPTER

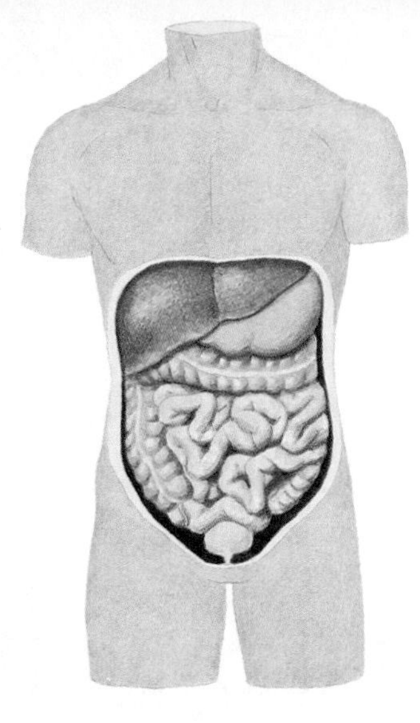

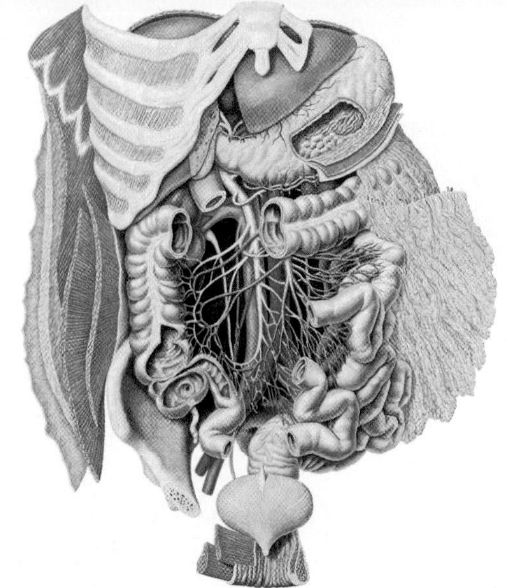

59 Review of the Gastrointestinal System

Learning Outcomes

After reading this chapter, the student should be able to:

1. Describe the major anatomic structures of the digestive system.
2. Outline the steps in the process of digestion.
3. Describe the primary functions of the stomach.
4. Analyze how the anatomical structures of the small intestine promote the absorption of nutrients and drugs.
5. Describe the primary structures and functions of the large intestine.
6. Describe the functions of the liver and their relevance to drug therapy.
7. Explain the hepatic portal system and its importance to drug therapy.
8. Explain the nervous control of digestion.
9. Explain the enzymatic breakdown of nutrients by the digestive system.

Chapter Outline

Overview of the Digestive System

Physiology of the Upper Gastrointestinal Tract

Physiology of the Lower Gastrointestinal Tract

Physiology of the Accessory Organs of Digestion

Regulation of Digestive Processes

Nutrient Categories and Metabolism

Key Terms

absorption, 1000
accessory organs of digestion, 999
alimentary canal, 999
chief cells, 1000
chyme, 1000
defecation, 1000
digestion, 1000
digestive system, 999
enteric nervous system (ENS), 1004
enteroendocrine cells, 1000
enterohepatic recirculation, 1003
first-pass effect, 1003
hepatic portal system, 1003
ingestion, 999
parietal cells, 1000
peristalsis, 1000

Very little of the food we eat is directly available to body cells. Food must be broken down, absorbed, and chemically modified before it is in a form that is useful to cells. The digestive system performs these, and more, functions. This chapter focuses on the aspects of digestion and physiology that are applicable to pharmacotherapy. For a complete review of the digestive system, the student should refer to an anatomy and physiology textbook.

Overview of the Digestive System

59.1 The function of the digestive system is to extract nutrients from food so that they may be used to fuel the metabolic processes in the body.

The **digestive system** consists of two basic anatomic divisions: the alimentary canal and the accessory organs. The **alimentary canal,** or gastrointestinal (GI) tract, is a long, continuous, hollow tube that extends from the mouth to the anus. The **accessory organs of digestion** include the salivary glands, liver, gallbladder, and pancreas. The major structures of the digestive system are illustrated in Figure 59.1.

The overall function of the digestive system is to extract nutrients from food so that they may be used to fuel the metabolic processes in the body. Because food is a complex substance, multiple steps are necessary before cells can use its components. These steps are ingestion, propulsion, digestion, absorption, and defecation.

Ingestion is taking food into the body by mouth. In some

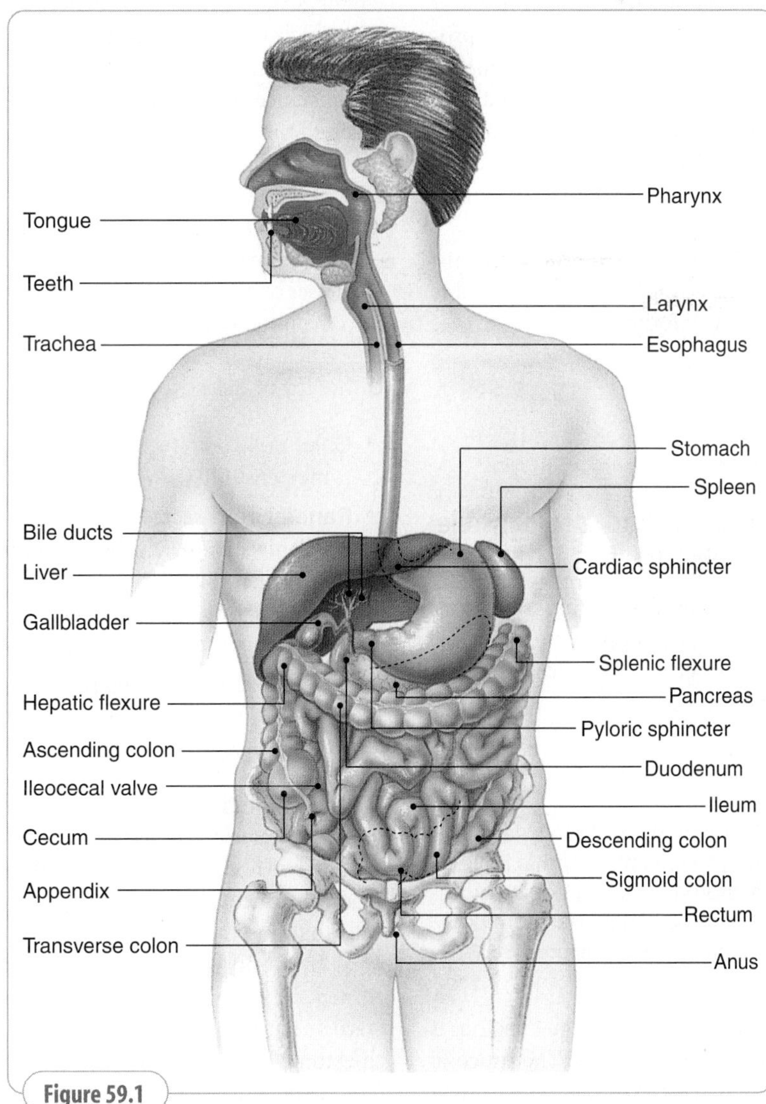

Figure 59.1

The digestive system.
Source: From *Diseases: A Systemic Approach* (6th ed., p. 276), by M. L. Mulvihill, M. Zelman, P. Holdaway, & E. Tompary, 2006. Reprinted by permission of Pearson Education, Inc., Upper Saddle River, NJ.

patients, ingestion bypasses the mouth and delivers nutrients directly into the stomach or small intestine via a feeding tube.

Substances are propelled along the GI tract by **peristalsis,** which is the rhythmic contractions of layers of smooth muscle. The speed at which substances move through the GI tract is critical to the absorption of drugs, nutrients, and water, and for the removal of wastes. If peristalsis is too fast, substances will not have sufficient contact with the GI mucosa to be absorbed. In addition, the large intestine will not have enough time to absorb water, and diarrhea may result. Abnormally slow transit may result in constipation or even obstructions in the small or large intestine.

Digestion is the mechanical and chemical breakdown of food into a form that may be absorbed into the systemic circulation. To chemically break down ingested food, a large number of enzymes and other substances are required. Digestive enzymes are secreted by the salivary glands, stomach, small intestine, and pancreas. The liver makes bile, which is stored in the gallbladder until it is needed for lipid digestion.

Absorption is the movement of nutrients and other substances from the alimentary canal to the circulation. The inner lining of the alimentary canal, called the mucosa layer, provides a surface area for the various acids, bases, and enzymes to break down food. In many parts of the alimentary canal, the mucosa is folded and contains deep grooves and pits. The small intestine is lined with tiny projections called villi and microvilli that provide a huge surface area for the absorption of nutrients and medications.

Not all components of ingested food are useful to the human body or can be digested. The elimination of indigestible substances from the body is called **defecation.**

Physiology of the Upper Gastrointestinal Tract

59.2 The upper gastrointestinal tract is responsible for mechanical and chemical digestion.

The upper GI tract consists of the mouth, pharynx, esophagus, and stomach. From a pharmacologic perspective, the most important regions of the upper GI tract are the buccal and sublingual areas of the mouth, and the stomach.

Pharm*FACT*

Most people believe that obese people have larger stomachs. However, people who are naturally thin have the same size or even larger stomachs than people who have problems with weight control. Weight has nothing to do with the size of the stomach. *Source:* Bouchez, 2008.

The epithelial mucosa of the buccal and sublingual regions is very thin, being only 40 to 50 cells in thickness. The mucosal layer, along with the salivary glands, secretes mucus, which lubricates and moistens the oral cavity. The mucus also serves as a liquid medium for drug administration inside the mouth. The oral mucosa in the sublingual region is relatively permeable, and drugs are rapidly absorbed. The buccal region is less permeable, and drug absorption is slower. The buccal region, however, has less salivary flow and drugs can be retained longer, making it better suited for sustained release delivery systems. For example, Striant is a buccal form of testosterone that is designed to release the drug over an 8- to 12-hour period.

The pharynx and esophagus serve as passageways for ingested food and liquids. Obstruction of these areas, or a loss of the swallowing reflex, precludes the administration of oral drugs. Little absorption occurs across the pharyngeal or esophageal mucosa because drugs travel quickly through these regions of the alimentary canal.

Food passes from the esophagus to the stomach by traveling through the lower esophageal (cardiac) sphincter. This ring of smooth muscle usually prevents the stomach contents from moving backward, a condition known as gastroesophageal reflux. The stomach has both mechanical and chemical functions. The muscular squeezing of the stomach churns and mixes the food, breaking it down mechanically to a semisolid known as **chyme.** Strong peristaltic contractions push the chyme toward the pylorus, where it encounters a second ring of smooth muscle called the pyloric sphincter. Located at the entrance to the small intestine, this sphincter regulates the flow of substances leaving the stomach. Chyme moves in "spurts" through the sphincter into the small intestine. Large pieces of food are refluxed back into the body of the stomach, where they are subjected to more churning to reduce them in size to about 2 mm so that they may pass through the sphincter.

The stomach also secretes substances that promote the processes of chemical digestion. Gastric glands extending deep into the mucosa of the stomach contain several cell types that are critical to digestion and that are important to the pharmacotherapy of digestive disorders.

- **Chief cells** secrete pepsinogen, an inactive form of the enzyme pepsin that chemically breaks down proteins.
- **Parietal cells** secrete 1 to 3 liters of hydrochloric acid each day. This strong acid helps to break down food, activates pepsinogen, and kills microbes that may have been ingested. Parietal cells also secrete intrinsic factor, which is essential for the absorption of vitamin B_{12}.
- **Enteroendocrine cells** secrete hormones that modify the digestive processes. In the stomach, the most important secretion is gastrin, which stimulates acid production.

The combined secretion of the chief and parietal cells, known as gastric juice, is the most acidic fluid in the body, having a pH of 1.5 to 3.5. A number of natural defenses protect the stomach mucosa against this extremely acidic fluid. Certain cells that line the surface of the stomach secrete a thick, mucous layer and bicarbonate ion to neutralize the acid. These form such an effective protective layer that the pH at the mucosal surface is nearly neutral. Once reaching the duodenum, the stomach contents are further neutralized by bicarbonate from pancreatic and biliary secretions.

The pharmacologic importance of the stomach lies in its capacity to absorb drugs. For most oral drugs, the stomach is not the primary site of absorption because the drug does not stay long in the organ. Stomach acidity (pH 1 to 2) can either assist in the absorption process or destroy the drug entirely. Drugs that are weak acids tend to be absorbed in the stomach. Protein drugs are destroyed by pepsin in the stomach before they are absorbed or have a chance to reach the small intestine.

CONNECTION *Checkpoint* 59.1

Nitroglycerin is the most frequently prescribed sublingual medication. From what you learned in Chapter 37, what is the primary indication for nitroglycerin and what is the onset of action time of the drug when it is given by the sublingual route? See Answer to Connection Checkpoint 59.1 in Appendix A.

Physiology of the Lower Gastrointestinal Tract

59.3 The small intestine is the longest portion of the alimentary canal and is the primary organ for absorption.

The lower GI tract consists of the small and large intestines. With its many folds and finger like projections of villi and microvilli, the small intestine is highly specialized for absorption. The lining of each villus is composed of a single layer of epithelial cells and contains blood capillaries, as illustrated in Figure 59.2. Essentially, only a single cell separates a nutrient or drug molecule from the intestinal lumen to the body's circulatory system.

The first 10 inches of the small intestine, known as the duodenum, is the site where chyme mixes with bile from the gallbladder and digestive enzymes from the pancreas. Bile and pancreatic juice enter through an opening in the duodenum known as the duodenal papilla. The duodenum is sometimes considered part of the upper GI tract because of its close proximity to the stomach. The most common disorder of the duodenum, called peptic ulcer, is discussed in Chapter 60.

PharmFACT

A 150-pound person will consume 50 tons of food during his or her lifetime. *Source:* Nexium Research, 2008.

The remainder of the small intestine consists of the jejunum and ileum. Because of its length and enormous absorptive surface, the first 1 to 2 meters of the jejunum is the site of the majority of nutrient and drug absorption. As the jejunum becomes the ileum, the diameter of the intestinal lumen diminishes and the villi become fewer in number. The terminal ileum is a primary site for the absorption of vitamin B_{12}, long chain fatty acids, and fat-soluble vitamins. The ileum empties its contents into the large intestine through the ileocecal valve. Travel time for chyme through the entire small intestine varies from 3 to 6 hours.

The mucosa of the small intestine secretes intestinal juice, which is a mixture of mucus, digestive enzymes, and hormones. The mucus has an alkaline pH, which neutralizes the acidity from the stomach. The small intestine also secretes cholecystokinin, a hormone that promotes pancreatic enzyme secretion and secretin, which stimulates bicarbonate production to make the small intestine more alkaline.

CONNECTION *Checkpoint* 59.2

Many oral drugs have enteric coatings. From what you learned in Chapter 4, what is the purpose of the enteric coating and why are these drugs not to be split or crushed? See Answer to Connection Checkpoint 59.2 in Appendix A.

59.4 The large intestine contains host flora and is a major site of water reabsorption.

The large intestine, or colon, receives chyme from the ileum in a fluid state. The large intestine does not secrete digestive enzymes nor does it have enteroendocrine cells to secrete hormones. With few exceptions, little reabsorption of nutrients occurs during the 12- to 24-hour journey through the colon. The large intestine does secrete a large amount of mucus, which helps lubricate the fecal matter. The major functions of the colon are to reabsorb water and electrolytes from the waste material and excrete the remaining fecal material from the body.

The colon harbors a substantial amount of bacteria and fungi, called the host flora, which serve a useful purpose by synthesizing B-complex vitamins and vitamin K. Disruption of the normal host flora can lead to diarrhea.

From a pharmacologic perspective, the large intestine may be the site of therapeutic or adverse drug effects. A large number of drugs cause either diarrhea or constipation. These effects are usually self-limiting and can be prevented or managed through nursing interventions. When bowel patterns are significantly disrupted, drugs may be given to slow the activity (antidiarrheals) or increase the activity (laxatives) of the large intestine.

Of additional pharmacologic importance are the drugs given by the rectal route. The mucosa of the rectum provides an excellent and rapid absorptive surface for drugs. It is a route of particular importance in children and in patients who are unable to take oral medications due to nausea, vomiting, or other pathology that prevents oral administration. The onset of action is usually slower than the oral route, and drug action is limited by the length of time that the patient can retain the drug without defecation.

Physiology of the Accessory Organs of Digestion

59.5 The liver is the most important accessory digestive organ.

The accessory organs of digestion include the teeth, tongue, salivary glands, pancreas, gallbladder, and liver. Of these, the pancreas and liver have the most pharmacologic importance. The endocrine functions of the pancreas, which include the secretion of insulin and glucagon, are reviewed in Chapter 65.

The liver is one of the most important organs in pharmacology. Along with the kidneys, any drug that reaches the

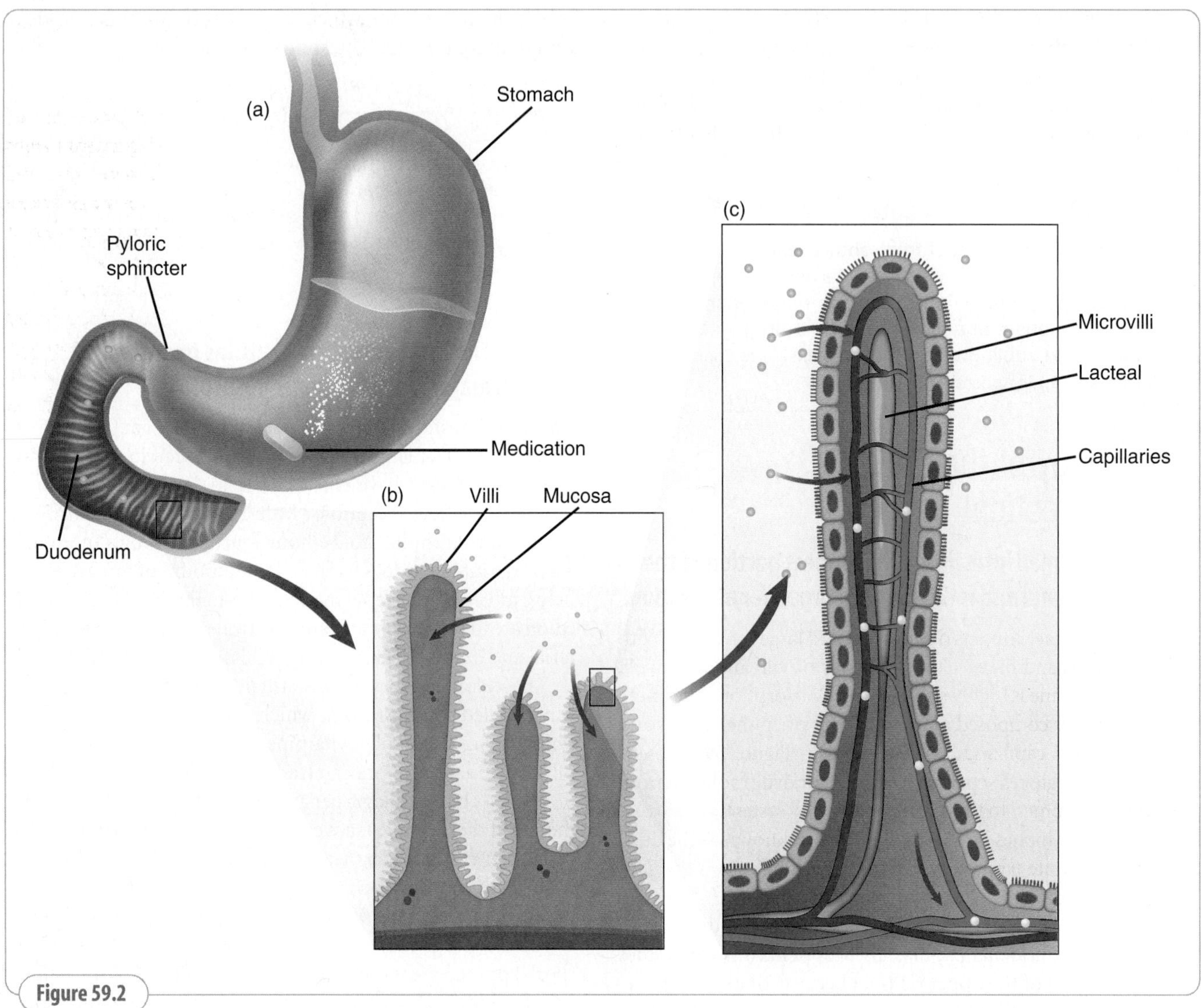

Figure 59.2

Villi and microvilli of the small intestine: (a) Tablet dissolves in the stomach. (b) Medication reaches the villi of the duodenum. (c) Drug molecules are absorbed into the microvilli capillaries.

circulation, regardless of its route of administration, will pass through the liver. The overall function of the liver is to filter and process the nutrients and drugs delivered to it. Substances may be stored, chemically altered, or removed from the blood before they reach the general circulation. The following are some of the primary functions of the liver:

- **Regulation.** Stabilizes the serum levels of glucose, triglycerides, and cholesterol
- **Protection.** Removes toxic substances and waste products such as ammonia
- **Synthesis.** Synthesizes bile, plasma proteins, and certain clotting factors
- **Storage.** Stores iron and fat-soluble vitamins

When most drugs reach the liver, they are metabolized to less toxic substances that are more easily excreted by the kidney. The cytochrome P450 enzyme system in liver cells is especially active at metabolizing drugs; the various isozymes of CYP450 are discussed in Chapter 4. In a few cases, the liver changes the drug to a more active form. It is important to note that the handling of drugs and toxic substances by the liver can damage hepatocytes and impair their functions. This is especially true if the hepatocytes are chronically exposed to harmful substances such as ethanol. Hepatic impairment is a relatively common adverse effect of certain drugs. Whereas drug-induced hepatic impairment is often transient and asymptomatic, some drugs can cause severe, permanent, and even fatal liver damage.

PharmFACT

Acetaminophen (Tylenol) overdose is the leading cause of acute liver failure in the United States. This can occur by taking an overdose of acetaminophen or by taking normal doses in combination with alcohol. *Source:* Lee, 2007.

The hepatic vascular system is different than that in most areas of the body and is important to digestion as well as pharmacology. The liver receives both oxygenated and deoxygenated blood. The **hepatic portal system,** shown in Figure 59.3, is a network of venous vessels that collects blood draining from the stomach, small intestine, and most of the large intestine. This blood is extremely rich in nutrients because it contains substances absorbed during digestion. It is important to know that this blood is delivered to the liver via the hepatic portal vein before it reaches the arterial circulation. The liver then can remove, store, excrete, or perform metabolic functions on these substances before they are sent into the inferior vena cava to reach other organs.

The hepatic portal system serves as an important homeostatic mechanism, allowing a relatively stable composition of blood to circulate through the body. In terms of drug therapy, nearly all oral medications enter the hepatic portal vein for processing by the liver before they reach their target tissue. In some cases, the liver removes a substantial percentage of the drug before it reaches the inferior vena cava, a phenomenon called the **first-pass effect.** Drugs that have a significant first-pass effect may be given by other routes, such as intramuscular, intravenous, subcutaneous, or topical. Although a drug will still eventually reach the liver by these routes, it will have an opportunity to also reach its target tissue. It should be noted that the venous supply of the head and that serving the lower rectum are not parts of the hepatic portal system. Thus, drugs that are given by the buccal, sublingual, or rectal routes bypass the first-pass effect of the liver.

As the liver makes bile it is sent to the gallbladder where it is stored. When lipids enter the small intestine the gallbladder contracts and sends its contents into the duodenum. The bile salts emulsify the lipids, making them easier to digest enzymatically. When bile salts reach the terminal portion of the ileum, 95% are reabsorbed back into the hepatic portal circulation by a process called **enterohepatic recirculation.** This process has direct implications to pharmacotherapy. Certain drugs, including digoxin (Lanoxin), morphine, and estrogens, are eliminated in the bile and are reabsorbed by enterohepatic recirculation. Enterohepatic recirculation recycles the drug multiple times and can significantly extend a drug's half-life. Interactions can occur if one drug interferes with the enterohepatic recycling of another drug. Preventing this recycling can speed the elimination of a drug and reduce its therapeutic effectiveness. An example of such an interaction is when cholestyramine (Questran) interferes with the recycling of lorazepam (Ativan) and increases the clearance of lorazepam from the body.

The pancreas is an essential accessory digestive organ, secreting about a quart of pancreatic fluid into the duodenum each day. This fluid is alkaline (ph 7.5 to 8.8) and contains digestive

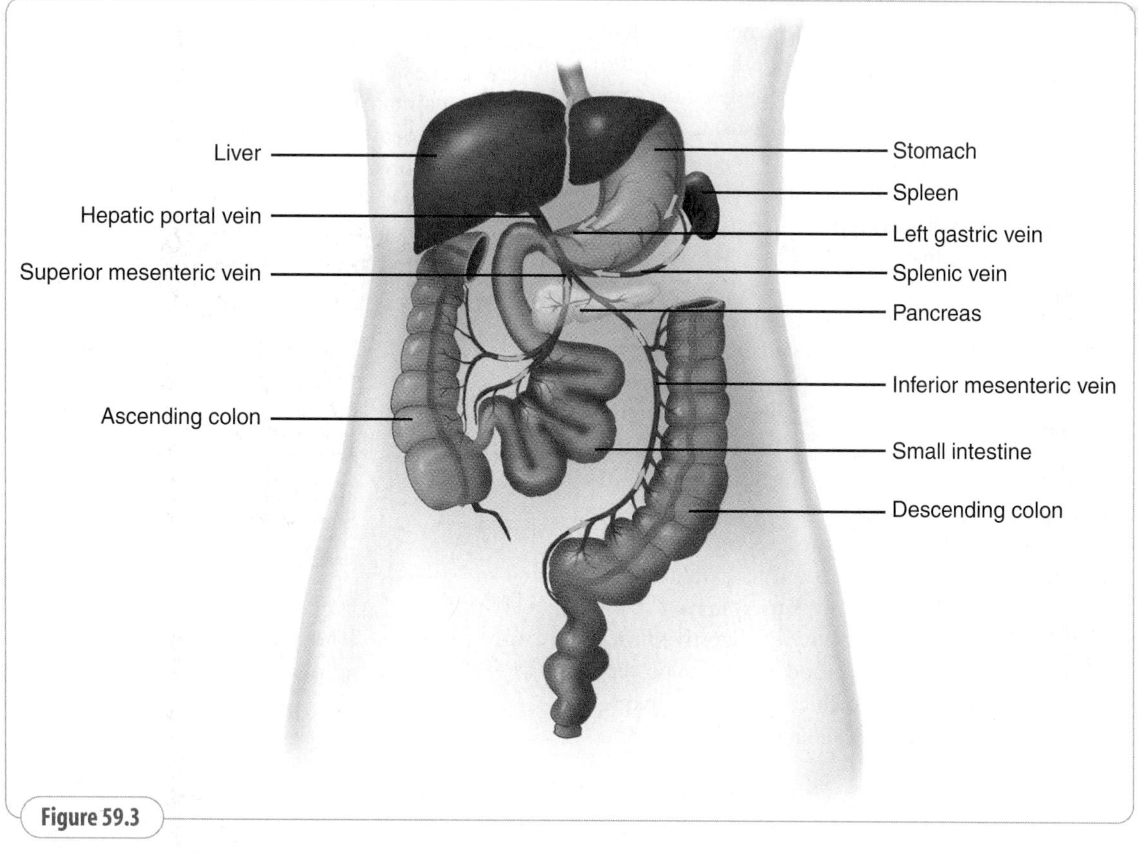

Figure 59.3
Hepatic portal circulation.

enzymes to chemically break down carbohydrates, lipids, proteins, and nucleic acids. From a pharmacologic perspective, the pancreas is relatively protected from drugs and there are only a few therapies for pancreatic digestive disorders.

CONNECTION *Checkpoint* 59.3

The tricyclic antidepressant imipramine is a substrate for the CYP2D6 enzyme, and the selective serotonin reuptake inhibitor (SSRI) fluoxetine is a potent inhibitor of this enzyme. From what you learned in Chapter 6, predict the type of drug interaction that will occur to a patient stabilized on imipramine therapy when fluoxetine is added to the regimen. See Answer to Connection Checkpoint 59.3 in Appendix A.

Regulation of Digestive Processes

59.6 Digestion is regulated by numerous hormonal and nervous factors.

Digestion is controlled through a large number of hormonal and nervous factors that influence the speed of peristalsis and the amount of saliva, mucus, acid, and enzyme secretions. Various negative feedback loops help to regulate these activities so that digestion is a smooth, continuous process. Disruption of normal homeostatic mechanisms can cause cramping, due to excessive peristalsis, or peptic ulcers, due to the overproduction of gastric acid.

The nervous control of digestion is provided at several levels. Chapter 16 discusses the role of the autonomic nervous system (ANS) in controlling the contraction of smooth muscle and glandular secretion. Activation of the parasympathetic nervous system stimulates the digestive processes by increasing peristalsis, salivation, and digestive gland secretion. The sympathetic nervous system has the opposite effects, with beta$_2$-adrenergic receptors in the intestinal wall and alpha$_1$-adrenergic receptors in the salivary glands. Drugs that affect the ANS often affect the digestive processes.

The GI tract is also regulated by local reflexes called the **enteric nervous system (ENS).** This system consists of a vast network of neurons in the submucosa of the alimentary canal that has sensory and motor functions. Chemoreceptors and stretch receptors sense the presence and amount of food in the GI tract and respond accordingly by changing motility without sending signals to the ANS.

The GI tract functions at an automatic level; no conscious thought is required as the system goes about its daily tasks of secretion and digestion. The central nervous system (CNS), however, can greatly influence the activity of digestive functions. For example, merely thinking of food can evoke powerful images. These may be positive, such as perhaps thinking of a steak sizzling on the grill or bread baking in the oven, and increase salivation and peristalsis. Images may also be negative and evoke feelings of nausea and vomiting at the sight of food. Mental health conditions such as depression, anxiety, excessive stress, or bipolar disorder can affect the appetite and digestive processes.

Nutrient Categories and Metabolism

59.7 The chemical breakdown of food is accomplished by digestive enzymes.

The three basic nutrients are carbohydrates, lipids, and proteins. In food these nutrients are large molecules that cannot be absorbed across the mucosa of the alimentary canal. Chemical digestion must break down these complex food molecules into simpler substances so that they can be absorbed and used by the body for metabolic processes.

The breakdown of complex carbohydrates, lipids, and proteins requires digestive enzymes to be delivered when food is present at various parts of the alimentary canal, primarily the stomach and small intestine. These enzymes and their locations are shown in Table 59.1. Secretion of digestive enzymes is regulated by hormones and the nervous system, as described in Section 59.6. Patients who secrete insufficient quantities of digestive enzymes may be administered these substances as drugs.

In addition to the three basic nutrients, the body requires a host of other vitamins and minerals for proper metabolism. Deficiency symptoms will be observed if a patient has insufficient intake of these substances. The pharmacotherapy of vitamins and minerals is presented in Chapter 62.

The intake of various nutrients in sufficient amounts is necessary to maintain good health and to allow the body to heal during periods of illness. The intake of sufficient amounts of proteins, carbohydrates, fats, vitamins, and minerals can often be achieved by eating a well-balanced diet of foods and fluids. When this does not occur, enteral or parenteral therapy may be indicated, as presented in Chapter 63.

TABLE 59.1 Major Digestive Enzymes

Nutrient	Enzyme	Source
Proteins and polypeptides	Pepsin	Gastric glands
	Trypsin, chymotrypsin, carboxypeptidase	Pancreatic juice
	Aminopeptidase	Small intestine
Lipids	Pancreatic lipase	Pancreatic juice
Carbohydrates and starches	Salivary amylase	Saliva
	Pancreatic amylase	Pancreatic juice
	Maltase, sucrose, lactase	Small intestine

UNDERSTANDING THE CHAPTER

Key Concepts Summary

59.1 The function of the digestive system is to extract nutrients from food so that they may be used to fuel the metabolic processes in the body.

59.2 The upper gastrointestinal tract is responsible for mechanical and chemical digestion.

59.3 The small intestine is the longest portion of the alimentary canal and is the primary organ for absorption.

59.4 The large intestine contains host flora and is a major site of water reabsorption.

59.5 The liver is the most important accessory digestive organ.

59.6 Digestion is regulated by numerous hormonal and nervous factors.

59.7 The chemical breakdown of food is accomplished by digestive enzymes.

References

Bouchez, C. (2008). *9 surprising facts about your stomach.* WebMD Digestive Disorders Health Center. Retrieved August 5, 2008, from http://www.webmd.com/digestive-disorders/features/nine-surprising-facts-about-your-stomach

Krogh, D. (2009). *Biology: A guide to the natural world* (4th ed). San Francisco: Pearson/Benjamin Cummings.

Lee, D. (2007). *Acetaminophen (Tylenol) liver damage at a glance.* MedicineNet.com. Retrieved August 5, 2008, from http://www.medicinenet.com/tylenol_liver_damage/page8.htm

Martini, F. H., & Nath, J. L. (2009). *Fundamentals of human anatomy and physiology* (7th ed.). San Francisco: Pearson/Benjamin Cummings.

Nexium Research. (2008). *Digestive system facts.* Retrieved August 5, 2008, from http://www.nexiumresearch.com/digestive_system_facts.html

Rice, J. (2005). *Medical terminology with human anatomy* (5th ed.). Upper Saddle River, NJ: Pearson Education.

Silverthorn, D. U. (2007). *Human physiology: An integrated approach* (4th ed.). San Francisco: Pearson/Benjamin Cummings.

CHAPTER

I was diagnosed with a duodenal ulcer yesterday. Why do I need to take these antibiotics if I don't have an infection?

Patient "Bob Richards"

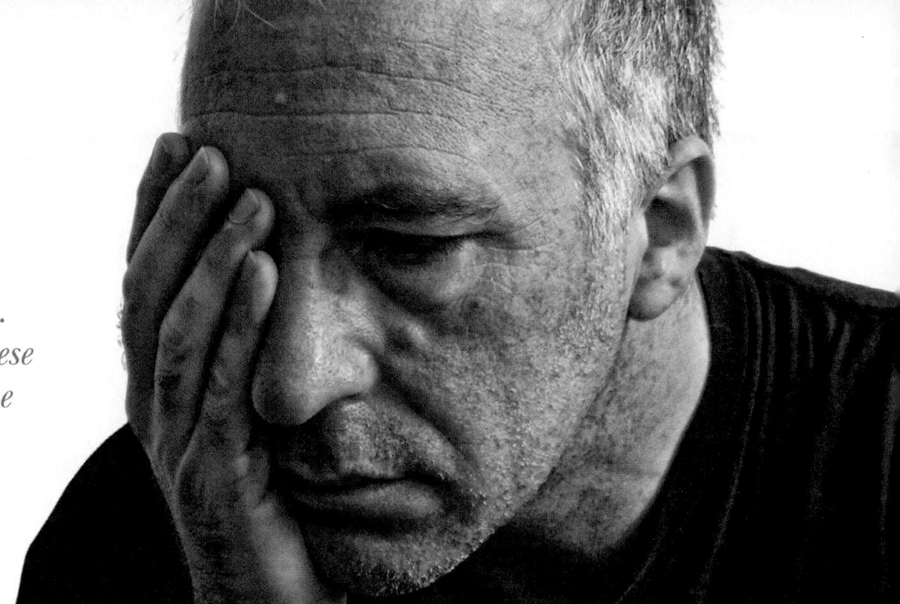

60 Pharmacotherapy of Peptic Ulcer Disease

Learning Outcomes

After reading this chapter, the student should be able to:

1. Explain the physiological regulation of gastric acid secretion.
2. Describe factors that suppress and those that promote the formation of peptic ulcers.
3. Compare and contrast duodenal ulcers and gastric ulcers.
4. Identify the etiology, signs, and symptoms of peptic ulcer disease and gastroesophageal reflux disease.
5. Outline the treatment goals for the pharmacotherapy of peptic ulcer disease and gastroesophageal reflux disease.
6. Identify the classification of drugs used to treat peptic ulcer disease and gastroesophageal reflux disease.
7. Explain the pharmacologic strategies for eradicating *Helicobacter pylori*.
8. Describe the nurse's role in the pharmacologic management of patients with peptic ulcer disease and gastroesophageal reflux disease.
9. For each of the classes shown in the chapter outline, identify the prototype and representative drugs and explain the mechanism(s) of drug action, primary indications, contraindications, significant drug interactions, pregnancy category, and important adverse effects.
10. Use the nursing process to care for patients who are receiving drug therapy for peptic ulcer disease and gastroesophageal reflux disease.

Chapter Outline

Physiology of the Upper Gastrointestinal Tract

Etiology and Pathogenesis of Peptic Ulcer Disease

Etiology and Pathogenesis of Gastroesophageal Reflux Disease

Pharmacotherapy of Peptic Ulcer Disease and Gastroesophageal Reflux Disease

Proton Pump Inhibitors

PROTOTYPE **Omeprazole (Prilosec)** *p. 1014*

H_2-Receptor Antagonists

PROTOTYPE **Ranitidine (Zantac)** *p. 1018*

Antacids

PROTOTYPE **Aluminum Hydroxide (AlternaGEL, Others)** *p. 1021*

Pharmacotherapy of *Helicobacter pylori* Infections

Miscellaneous Drugs Used for Peptic Ulcer Disease and Gastroesophageal Reflux Disease

Key Terms

adhesin, *1023*
antacids, *1019*
antiflatulent, *1021*
Barrett's esophagus, *1010*
gastroesophageal reflux disease (GERD), *1010*
H^+, K^+-ATPase, *1007*
H_2-receptor antagonist, *1016*
milk-alkali syndrome, *1019*
pepsin, *1007*
peptic ulcer, *1007*
prostaglandin E_2, *1007*
proton pump inhibitor (PPI), *1013*
somatostatin, *1007*
Zollinger-Ellison Syndrome (ZES), *1009*

Acid-related diseases of the upper gastrointestinal (GI) tract are some of the most common medical conditions. Drugs for these disorders are available over-the-counter (OTC), and many patients attempt self-treatment before seeking assistance from their health care provider. Signs and symptoms of acid-related conditions of the upper GI tract, however, may indicate more serious disease. This chapter examines the pharmacotherapy of two common disorders of the upper digestive system: peptic ulcer disease (PUD) and gastroesophageal reflux disease (GERD).

Physiology of the Upper Gastrointestinal Tract

60.1 The stomach secretes acid, enzymes, and hormones that are essential to digestive physiology.

The upper GI tract consists of the mouth, pharynx, esophagus, and stomach. The duodenum, the first 10 inches of the small intestine, is sometimes considered part of the upper GI tract because of its close proximity to the stomach. The structures and functions of the upper GI tract are reviewed in Chapter 59.

Gastric glands in the stomach contain several cell types that are critical to digestion and important to the pharmacotherapy of digestive disorders. Chief cells secrete the enzyme pepsinogen, which is then activated to become **pepsin,** which is the digestive enzyme that breaks down proteins from food. Parietal cells secrete gastric (hydrochloric) acid in the stomach, which provides a strongly acidic environment that promotes the conversion of pepsinogen to pepsin, helps to break down food, and kills microbes that may have been ingested. Parietal cells also secrete intrinsic factor, which is essential for the absorption of vitamin B_{12} (see Chapter 62). Parietal cells are targets for the classes of drugs that reduce acid secretion. The cell types present in gastric glands are shown in Figure 60.1.

Parietal cells receive messages from several sources, which tell them to increase or decrease acid production. These cells contain receptors for the hormone gastrin, histamine (H_2), and the neurotransmitter acetylcholine, which are the three principal physiological stimuli that regulate acid secretion from the proton pump, or **H^+, K^+-ATPase,** located on the surface of parietal cells.

Ingestion of food and distension of the stomach stimulate the secretion of the hormone gastrin into the bloodstream. The target cells for gastrin are enteroendocrine cells in the gastric glands. When gastrin binds to their cell surface, the enteroendocrine cells produce and secrete histamine. Histamine then binds to the H_2 receptor on the parietal cell to stimulate acid secretion. In addition to promoting acid secretion, gastrin signals the chief cells to secrete pepsin, promotes the production of pancreatic enzymes, and increases gastric blood flow.

Like most hormones, gastrin is regulated by a negative feedback loop. As the stomach contents reach pH 3 or lower, the hormone **somatostatin** is released by cells in the stomach, small intestine, and pancreas. This hormone suppresses the secretion of gastrin, thus lowering acid secretion. Interestingly, somatostatin is also released by the anterior pituitary gland and is known as growth hormone-inhibiting hormone. However, the nervous system secretion and actions are independent of its digestive actions.

Cells lining the surface of the stomach mucosa secrete a thick mucous layer that provides a continuous, protective physical barrier against acid and pepsin. Bicarbonate ion is also secreted by the epithelial cells in the stomach and serves to neutralize gastric acid on the mucosal surface. The mucus and bicarbonate ion form such an effective protective layer that the pH at the mucosal surface is nearly neutral. Once the stomach contents reach the duodenum, they are further neutralized by the bicarbonate ion from pancreatic and biliary secretions.

Another protective substance is the hormone **prostaglandin E_2.** This hormone stimulates the secretion of mucus and bicarbonate, promotes repair of damaged gastric mucosal cells, and increases blood flow to the mucosa to help maintain optimal mucosal conditions. Several frequently prescribed drugs, including corticosteroids and nonsteroidal anti-inflammatory drugs (NSAIDs), cause peptic ulcers because they are prostaglandin antagonists. The natural defenses of the stomach are shown in Figure 60.2.

Etiology and Pathogenesis of Peptic Ulcer Disease

60.2 Peptic ulcer disease is associated with a number of etiologic risk factors.

A **peptic ulcer** is a lesion or erosion located in either the stomach (gastric) or small intestine (duodenal) mucosa that is usually associated with acute inflammation. PUD was an uncommon condition until the 19th century. Thus it is considered to be a "disease of civilization." Although PUD occurs most often in middle age, it may occur at any time, including infancy and childhood. A significant family history is present in at least half of children with PUD.

PUD occurs when there is an imbalance of protective factors versus aggravating factors: The levels of protective mucus and bicarbonate ion secretions are unable to protect against the aggravating factors of pepsin and gastric acid. Complications of PUD include bleeding, perforation, penetration, and GI obstruction due to scarring. The incidence of PUD is associated with the following risk factors:

- Infection with the bacterium *Helicobacter pylori*
- Close family history of PUD

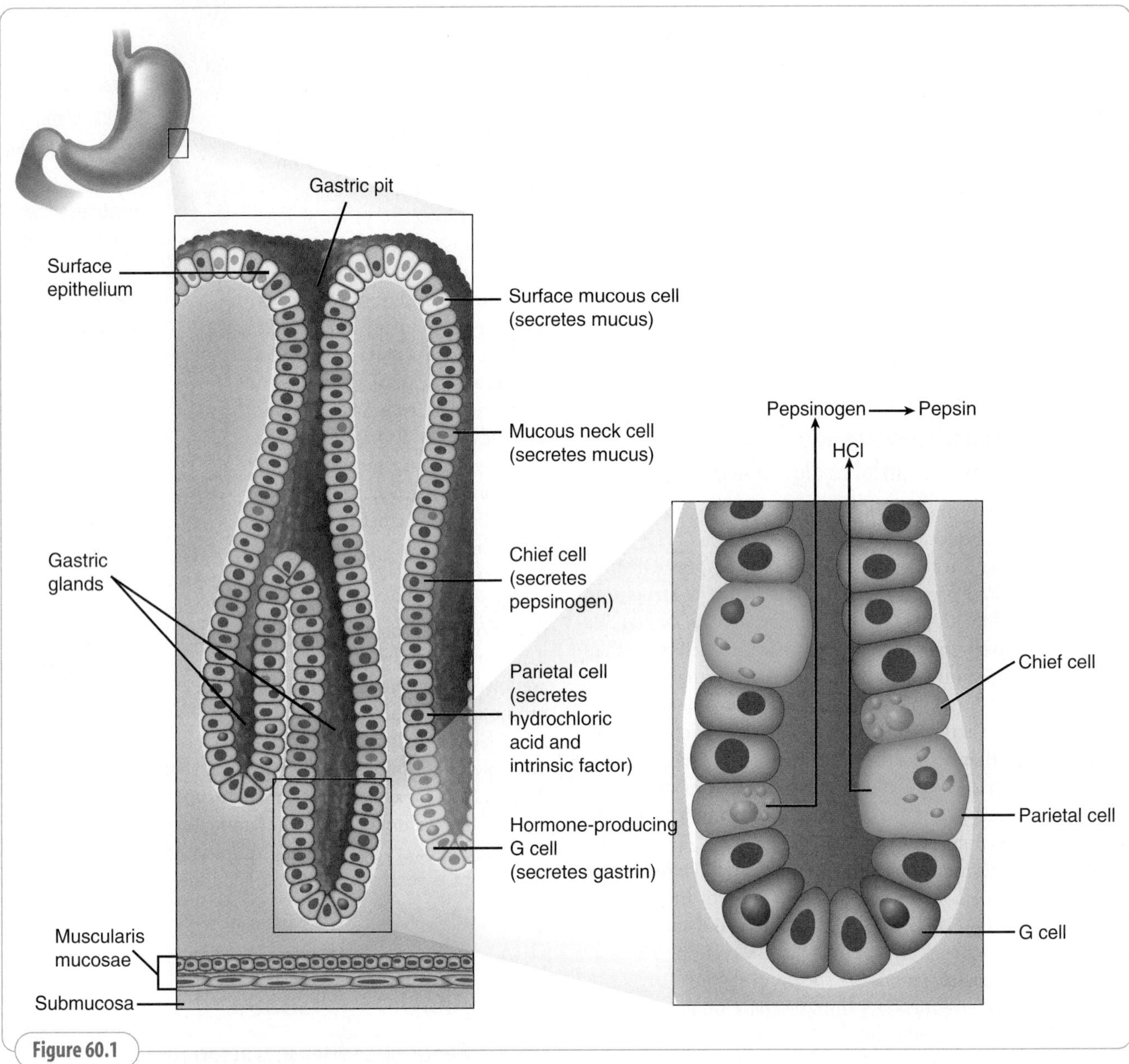

Figure 60.1

The stomach lining: Gastric glands and the secretion of hydrochloric acid.

- Drugs, particularly glucocorticoids, NSAIDs, and platelet inhibitors such as aspirin and clopidogrel
- Blood group O (the antigen may be a target of *H. pylori* attachment)
- Smoking tobacco (increases gastric acid secretion and reduces bicarbonate production)
- Beverages and foods that contain excessive caffeine
- Excessive psychological stress

PharmFACT

Approximately 4.5 million Americans are affected with PUD, and about 10% of Americans will experience an ulcer in their lifetime. *Source: Le & Fantry, 2008.*

For many decades, it was thought that mental and physiological stress, smoking, and spicy foods were the primary causes of PUD. It was theorized that bacteria could not survive the acidic environment of the stomach, thus the hypothesis that an infectious agent could be the cause of PUD was not accepted. In 1982, however, researchers discovered an association between the gram-negative bacterium *Helicobacter pylori* (*H. pylori*) and PUD. Over time, the hypothesis was accepted and treatment of PUD as an infectious disease was aggressively promoted by the Centers for Disease Control and Prevention (CDC). The pharmacotherapy of *H. pylori* is described in Section 60.8.

Many causes of PUD are not related to *H. pylori* infection. For example, drug therapy with NSAIDs is likely responsible for almost half of peptic ulcer cases. Gastric and duodenal ulcers occur in about 20% of patients using NSAIDs on a regular basis, with 4% experiencing serious bleeding.

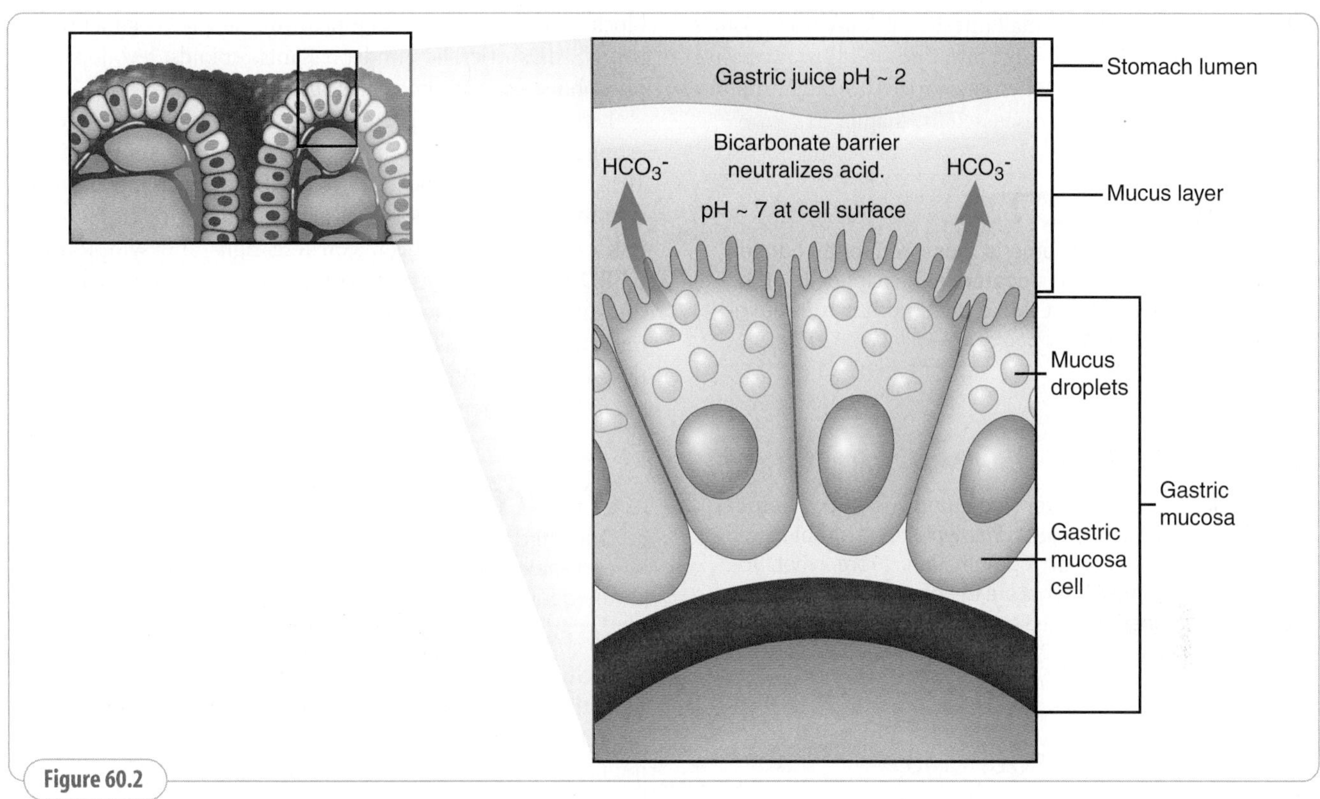

Figure 60.2

Natural defenses against stomach acid.

NSAIDs promote ulcer formation and inflammation both topically and systemically. Topically, NSAIDs cause direct cellular damage to GI mucosal cells. Systemically NSAIDs interfere with prostaglandin synthesis via the enzyme cyclooxygenase (COX) in the stomach, which normally aids in the production of mucus and bicarbonate. NSAIDs decrease gastric blood flow and slow cellular repair. NSAIDs are also weak acids that are nonionized in gastric acid and able to diffuse across the mucous barrier into the gastric epithelial cells, which leads to further cellular damage.

Risk factors for NSAID-induced PUD include long-term use of NSAIDs, advanced age, history of ulcers, concomitant use of corticosteroids, anticoagulants, or alcohol and cigarette smoking. In addition, *H. pylori* infection and NSAIDs act synergistically to promote ulcers. The combination poses a 3.5-fold greater risk of ulcers than either factor alone.

The characteristic symptom of duodenal ulcer is a gnawing or burning, upper abdominal pain that occurs 1 to 3 hours after a meal. The pain is usually worse when the stomach is empty and often disappears with ingestion of food. Night-time pain may awaken the patient. If the erosion progresses deeper into the mucosa, bleeding occurs and may be evident as either bright red blood in vomit or black, tarry stools. Many duodenal ulcers heal spontaneously, although scar tissue remains, predisposing the mucosa to future ulceration, and they frequently recur after months of remission. Perforation and hemorrhage are sometimes the first signs of a duodenal ulcer in infants. Many patients with PUD are asymptomatic.

Gastric ulcers are less common than the duodenal type and have different symptoms. Pain is often relieved with food; however, in some patients the pain is exacerbated with eating. Anorexia, weight loss, and vomiting are more common with gastric ulcers. Remissions may be infrequent or absent. Medical follow-up of gastric ulcers should continue for several years because a small percentage of the erosions become cancerous. The most severe ulcers may penetrate the wall of the stomach and cause death. Whereas duodenal ulcers most frequently occur in males in the 30- to 50-year age group, gastric ulcers are more common in women over age 60. NSAID-related ulcers are more likely to produce gastric ulcers, whereas *H. pylori*–associated ulcers are more likely to be duodenal.

Patients who are experiencing physiological stress resulting from severe trauma, surgery, burns, illness, or shock may experience stress ulcers. Stress ulcers are typically asymptomatic initially, and about 25% of patients present with painless upper GI bleeding. Vasoconstriction secondary to sympathetic nervous system involvement causes decreased blood flow to the small intestine, which may play a role in stress ulcers. Patients who are placed on mechanical ventilation and other seriously ill patients are sometimes administered prophylactic antiulcer drugs to prevent complications due to PUD.

Zollinger-Ellison Syndrome (ZES) is sometimes a hidden cause of PUD. It is caused by a tumor that secretes the hormone gastrin. Because gastrin is the hormonal signal for increasing hydrochloric acid secretion, the huge amounts of acid easily overcome the protective defenses, leading to multiple gastric and duodenal ulcers. Peptic ulcers are persistent, difficult to treat, and slow to heal. Symptoms of ZES are the same as those of PUD. The acid also irritates the GI tract, resulting in diarrhea. Treatment involves aggressive acid suppression with drugs.

MyNursingKit | Peptic Ulcer Disease

MyNursingKit | GERD Video

Ulceration in the distal small intestine is known as Crohn's disease, and erosions in the large intestine are called ulcerative colitis. These diseases, together categorized as inflammatory bowel syndrome (IBS), are discussed in Chapter 61.

PharmFACT

Zollinger-Ellison syndrome is most frequently caused by a tumor (gastrinoma) located in the islet cells of the pancreas. Over 50% of these gastrinomas are malignant and metastasize. *Source: Le & Fantry, 2008.*

CONNECTION *Checkpoint* 60.1

Although surgery is often indicated for ZES, chemotherapy with doxorubicin (Adriamycin) plus streptozocin (Zanosar) is a common combination. From what you learned in Chapter 58, what are the drug classes for these two antineoplastics? See Answer to Connection Checkpoint 60.1 in Appendix A.

Etiology and Pathogenesis of Gastroesophageal Reflux Disease

60.3 Gastroesophageal reflux disease is a chronic condition characterized by persistent heartburn.

Gastroesophageal reflux disease (GERD) results when acidic stomach contents enter the esophagus. Although most often considered a disease of people older than age 40, GERD can also occur in infants. The prevalence of the disease is increasing among both children and adults.

MyNursingKit | GERD in Infants and Children

In adults, the cause of GERD is usually transient weakening or relaxation of the lower esophageal sphincter (LES), a specialized muscle segment at the end of the esophagus. The sphincter may no longer close tightly, allowing movement of gastric contents upward into the esophagus when the stomach contracts. The acidic gastric contents cause an intense burning (heartburn) and, in some cases, injury to the esophagus. In addition, the pathogenesis of GERD involves decreased salivary secretions and diminished esophageal motility. The pathophysiology of GERD is shown in Pharmacotherapy Illustrated 60.1.

Symptoms of GERD include heartburn, dysphagia, dyspepsia, chest pain, nausea, and belching. Symptoms worsen following large meals, exercise, or when in a reclining or recumbent position. There is growing evidence that patients with GERD may also present with symptoms such as chronic cough, wheezing, bronchitis, sore throat, or hoarseness. GERD is a chronic condition with alternating periods of exacerbation and remission.

A large number of substances and conditions can worsen GERD symptoms. These include caffeine, alcohol, citrus fruits, tomato-based products, onions, carbonated beverages, spicy food, chocolate, smoking, pregnancy, and obesity. Certain medications may also contribute to or worsen GERD, including nitrates, benzodiazepines, anticholinergics, beta blockers, alpha blockers, estrogen, progesterone, iron, calcium channel blockers, NSAIDs, tricyclic antidepressants, opioids, levodopa, bisphosphonates, and some chemotherapy agents.

Left untreated, GERD can lead to complications such as esophagitis, esophageal ulcers, or strictures. Approximately 10% of patients diagnosed with GERD will develop **Barrett's esophagus,** a condition that is associated with an increased risk of esophageal cancer. Warning signs and symptoms of GERD that suggest a more complicated disease may include unexplained weight loss, early satiety, anemia, vomiting, initial onset of symptoms after age 50, and prolonged anorexia or dysphagia. Patients who are experiencing these symptoms should notify their health care provider.

PharmFACT

One third of adults in the United States have GERD and males are two to three times more likely to have the condition than females. *Source: Fisichella & Patti, 2008.*

If GERD is associated with obesity, losing weight may eliminate the symptoms. Other lifestyle changes that can improve GERD symptoms include elevating the head of the bed, avoiding fatty or acidic foods, eating smaller meals at least 3 hours before sleep, and eliminating tobacco and alcohol use. Because patients often self-treat this disorder with OTC drugs, a good medication history may give clues to the presence of GERD. Also, patients should be informed that some medications can provoke GERD, so reviewing their medication history may prove helpful. Because drugs provide only symptomatic relief, surgery may become necessary to eliminate the cause of GERD in patients with persistent disease.

An emerging theory suggests that GERD may be a premalignant condition and that chronic acid suppression leads to an increase in esophageal malignancy. This theory is not universally accepted, however, and acid suppression currently remains the mainstay in the treatment of GERD. The presence of GERD does not warrant testing for *H. pylori* infection. Large studies have shown that neither the presence nor absence of *H. pylori* has any influence on the development of GERD.

Pharmacotherapy of Peptic Ulcer Disease and Gastroesophageal Reflux Disease

60.4 Peptic ulcer disease and gastroesophageal reflux disease are best treated with a combination of pharmacotherapy and lifestyle changes.

Before initiating pharmacotherapy, patients are usually advised to change lifestyle factors that may be contributing to the severity of PUD or GERD. For example, eliminating tobacco and alcohol use and reducing stress often allow healing of the ulcer and cause it to go into remission. Avoiding certain foods and beverages can lessen the severity of symptoms. For patients with GERD, losing weight may alleviate symptoms of the disorder.

The goals of PUD pharmacotherapy are to provide immediate relief from symptoms, promote healing of the ulcer, prevent

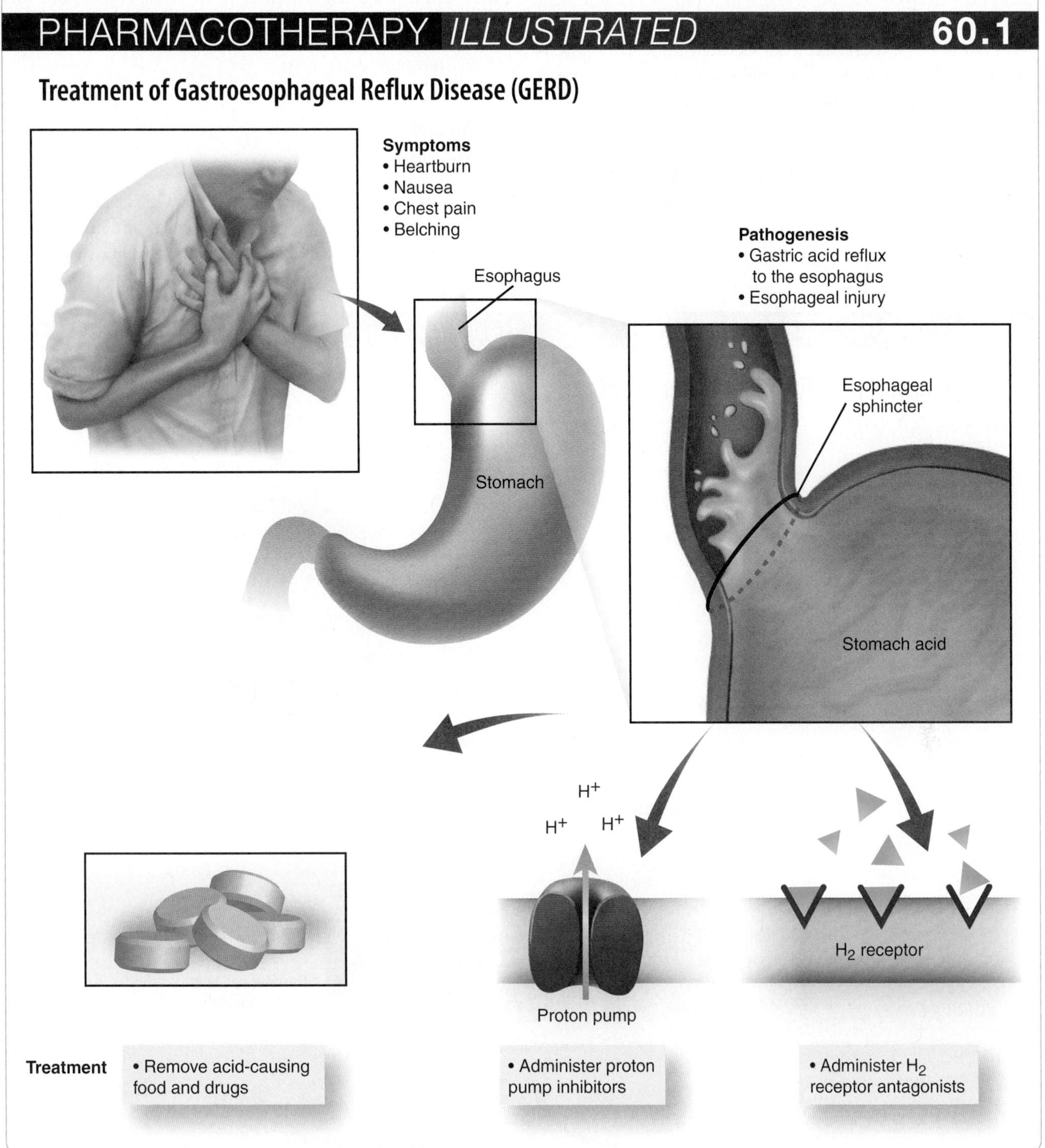

complications, and prevent future recurrence of the disease. Eradication of *H. pylori* and discontinuing NSAIDs or other ulcer-promoting medications when possible are key factors.

For patients who are taking NSAIDs, the initial approach to PUD is to switch to an alternative medication, such as acetaminophen or another analgesic. This is not always possible, however, because NSAIDs are the drugs of choice for treating chronic arthritis and other disorders associated with pain and inflammation. Those with a history of PUD should be advised to avoid NSAIDs in the future to prevent ulcer recurrences. If discontinuation of the NSAID is not possible, concurrent antiulcer drugs are indicated. Platelet inhibitors such as aspirin or clopidogrel should be used cautiously in patients at risk for ulcer complications.

For PUD patients with *H. pylori* infection, elimination of the bacteria using anti-infective therapy is the primary goal of pharmacotherapy (see Section 60.9). If the treatment includes only antiulcer drugs without eradicating *H. pylori*, a very high recurrence rate of PUD is observed. It has also been found that eradicating *H. pylori* infection prophylactically decreases the incidence of peptic ulcers in patients who subsequently take NSAIDs.

Once NSAIDs and *H. pylori* have been addressed, suppressing or neutralizing gastric acid is the aim of the pharmacologic treatment of both PUD and GERD. A wide variety of both prescription and OTC drugs are available to suppress acid secretion. The mechanisms of action of the major drug classes for PUD are shown in Pharmacotherapy Illustrated 60.2. These drugs fall into three primary classes and one miscellaneous group.

- H_2-receptor antagonists
- Proton pump inhibitors
- Antacids
- Miscellaneous drugs

Because medications used in treating GERD and PUD suppress acid, it should be kept in mind that certain nutrients and drugs need an acidic environment for complete absorption.

PHARMACOTHERAPY ILLUSTRATED 60.2

Mechanisms of Action of Antiulcer Drugs

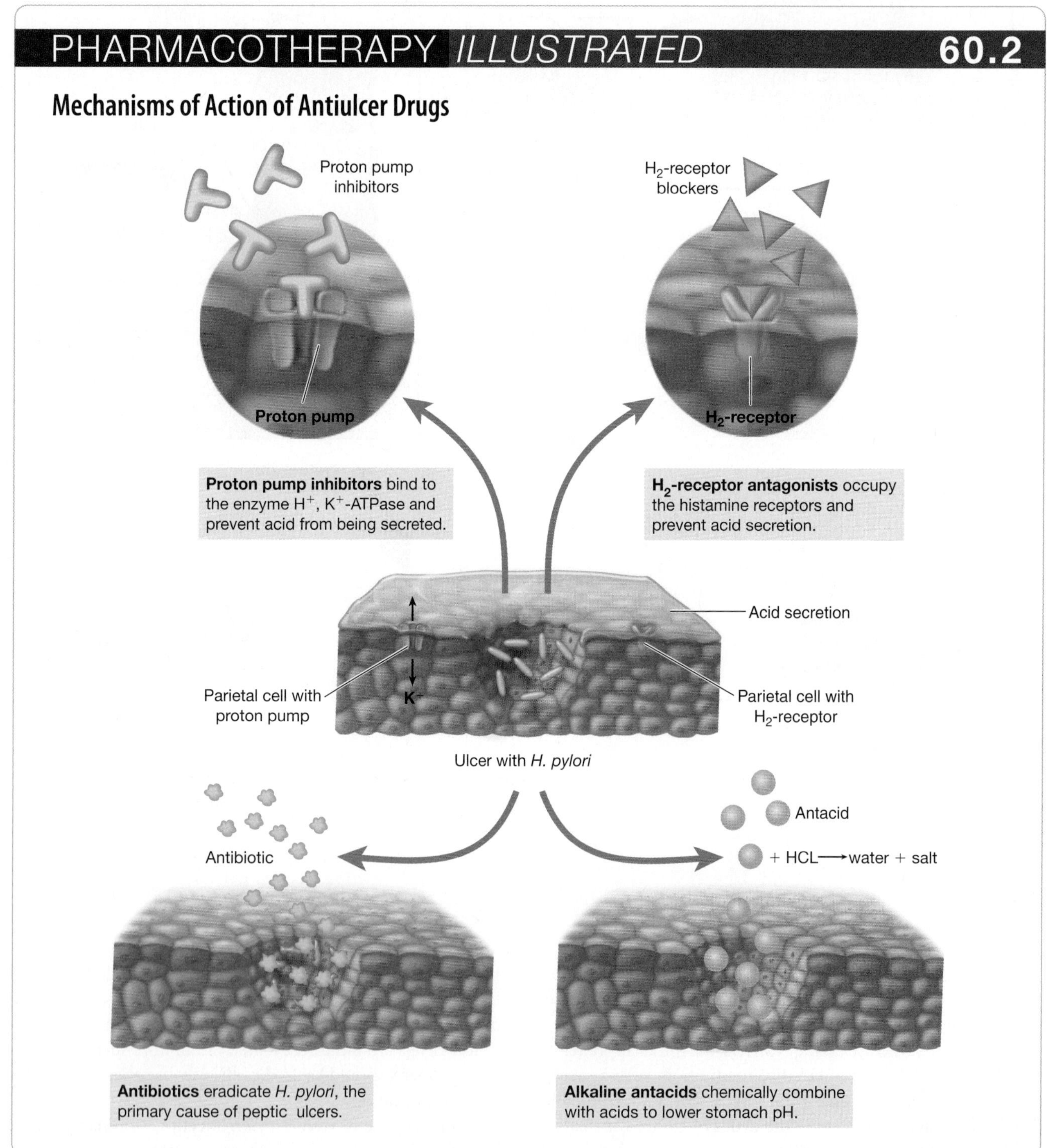

CONNECTIONS

Complementary and Alternative Therapies Ginger's Effect on the Gastrointestinal Tract

Description: Originally from Asia, ginger (*Zingiber officinalis*) is now cultivated in most tropical regions of the world. The active ingredients of ginger, and those that create its spicy flavor and pungent odor, are located in its roots or rhizomes. It has both culinary and medicinal uses.

History and Claims: The use of ginger for medicinal purposes dates to antiquity in India and China, and it is found in many ancient pharmacopeias. Its claimed uses are many and diverse, including antiemetic, antithrombotic, diuretic, anti-inflammatory, to promote gastric secretions, to increase blood glucose, and to stimulate peripheral circulation.

Standardization: Like most herbs, ginger contains multiple substances that may contribute to its pharmacologic activity. It is sometimes standardized according to its active substances, known as gingerols and shogaols. It is sold in pharmacies as dried ginger root powder and is readily available at most grocery stores for home cooking. A typical dose is 250 mg of dried root two to four times per day.

Evidence: Ginger is one of the best studied herbs, and it appears to be useful for a number of digestive-related conditions. Perhaps its widest use is for treating nausea, including that caused by motion sickness, pregnancy morning sickness, and postoperative procedures. It has been shown to stimulate appetite, promote gastric secretions, and increase peristalsis. Newer research has shown that ginger may inhibit the effects of *H. pylori* and may help heal peptic ulcers. Its effects appear to stem from direct action on the GI tract, rather than on the CNS. Ginger has no toxicity when used at recommended doses. Adverse effects include abdominal discomfort and diarrhea. Overdoses may lead to CNS depression, inhibition of platelet aggregation, and cardiotonic effects.

Source: From "The Efficacy of Ginger for the Prevention of Postoperative Nausea and Vomiting: A Meta-Analysis," by N. Chaiyakunapruk, N. Kitikannakon, S. Nathisuwan, K. Leeprakobboon, & C. Leelasettagool, 2006, *American Journal of Obstetrics and Gynecology, 194*(1), pp. 95–99; "Herbal Remedies in Gastroenterology," by K. Comar & D. F. Kirby, 2005, *Journal of Clinical Gastroenterology, 39*(6), pp. 457–468; and "Peptic Ulcer Disease," by R. Podein, 2007, in D. Rakel, *Integrative Medicine* (2nd ed., pp. 279–289), Philadelphia: Elsevier.

For example, long-term acid suppression could lead to a deficiency in folic acid, iron, and vitamin B_{12}. Also, the effects of certain drugs such as fluconazole, tetracyclines, and indomethacin may be decreased because these drugs require an acidic environment for complete absorption.

Pharmacotherapy with Proton Pump Inhibitors

60.5 Proton pump inhibitors block gastric acid secretion and are the drugs of choice in the therapy of peptic ulcer disease and gastroesophageal reflux disease.

The **proton pump inhibitors (PPIs)** act by blocking H^+, K^+-ATPase, the enzyme that is responsible for secreting hydrochloric acid in the stomach. PPIs are indicated for treatment of gastric and duodenal ulcers for 4 to 8 weeks, treatment of GERD, maintenance therapy to prevent recurrence, and treatment of ZES. Omeprazole is available OTC. These agents are listed in Table 60.1.

PPIs reduce acid secretion in the stomach by binding irreversibly to the H^+, K^+-ATPase enzyme at the surface of the parietal cell, thereby blocking the final step in acid production. This enzyme acts as a pump to release acid (also called H^+, or protons) onto the surface of the GI mucosa. The PPIs reduce acid secretion to a greater extent than the H_2-receptor antagonists and have a longer duration of action. About 95% of the acid production is blocked, making the PPIs the most efficient agents available for treating acid-related disease.

Because the proton pump is activated by food intake, the PPI should be taken 20 to 30 minutes before the first major meal of the day. This allows the peak serum drug levels to coincide with the time that the proton pumps are activated. PPIs are formulated in a delayed release formation because the drug would be destroyed in the acidic environment of the stomach.

Although the PPIs have a short serum half-life (about 1.5 hours), they continue to suppress acid for about 24 hours because the inactivation of the proton pump is irreversible. Because not all of the proton pumps are inactivated with the first dose, several days of PPI therapy are needed to achieve maximal acid inhibition. Beneficial effects continue for 3 to 5 days after the drugs have been discontinued. The PPIs are highly protein bound, metabolized in the liver, and excreted in the urine (80%) and feces (20%). Doses do not need to be adjusted for patients with renal insufficiency because there is negligible renal clearance.

All agents in this class have similar effectiveness and adverse effects. The incidence of adverse effects with PPIs is very low,

TABLE 60.1 Proton Pump Inhibitors

Drug	Route and Adult Dose (maximum dose where indicated)	Adverse Effects
esomeprazole (Nexium)	PO: 20–40 mg daily or bid for up to 8 weeks IV: 20–40 mg daily for up to 10 days	*Headache, diarrhea, nausea, rash, dizziness, abdominal pain* <u>Serious adverse effects are rare</u>
lansoprazole (Prevacid)	PO: 15–30 mg daily for 4–8 weeks IV: 30 mg over 30 min daily for up to 7 days	
omeprazole (Prilosec)	PO: 20–60 mg daily or bid	
pantoprazole (Protonix)	PO: 40 mg daily or bid IV: 40 mg IV daily for up to 7 days	
rabeprazole (AcipHex)	PO: 20–60 mg once daily	

Note: *Italics* indicate common adverse effects. <u>Underline</u> indicates serious adverse effects.

CONNECTIONS

Evidence-Based Practice Use of Proton Pump Inhibitors and Gastrointestinal Infection

Clinical Question

The acidic environment of the stomach is known to be a natural barrier to infection from ingested bacteria. The long-term effects of decreasing the acidity of the gastric fluid are uncertain. Because PPIs decrease the acidity, a question to consider would be: Is there an association between PPI use and GI infections?

Evidence

A small increased risk from enteric bacterial infection (such as salmonella) may exist when taking PPIs. There are two situations in which bacterial overgrowth may be of concern: (1) in underdeveloped countries where enteric infections occur more commonly; and (2) in patients who are exposed to PPIs who develop *Clostridium difficile* colitis. Previously, this infection has been associated with prior antibiotic use or immunosuppression. Some reports have shown evidence of an increased risk for the development of *C. difficile* colitis in hospitalized patients who are receiving PPIs.

Implications

The nurse should be alert to the rates of *C. difficile* in patients who are receiving PPIs, especially if these patients have also received antibiotics or are immunosuppressed.

Critical Thinking Question

Considering an association between PPI use and GI infections, what do you think could be the cause?

See Answers to Critical Thinking Questions in Appendix A.

Source: From "Risk of *Clostridium difficile* Among Hospital Inpatients Prescribed Proton Pump Inhibitors: Cohort and Case-Control Studies," by S. Dial, K. Alrascki, C. Manoukian, A. Huang, & D. Manzies, 2004, *Canadian Medical Association Journal, 171*(1), pp. 33–38; and "Use of Gastric Acid-Suppressive Agents and the Risk of Community-Acquired *Clostridium difficile*-Associated Disease," by S. Dial, J. Delaney, A. Barkun, & S. Suissa, 2005, *Journal of the American Medical Association, 294*(23), pp. 2989–2995.

with headache, abdominal pain, diarrhea, nausea, and vomiting being the most commonly reported ones. Rashes and blood dyscrasias are rare. Rebound hypersecretion of acid does not appear to occur after the drugs are discontinued. PPIs can mask an *H. pylori* infection because of the marked reduction in the bacterial load that they initiate.

PPIs heal more than 90% of duodenal ulcers within 4 weeks and about 90% of gastric ulcers in 6 to 8 weeks. GERD may require 8 to 12 weeks of therapy for symptoms to diminish, and long-term maintenance therapy may be needed. PPIs are best suited for the long-term prevention of heartburn rather than the treatment of acute symptoms. In patients with PUD who must take NSAIDs for a chronic pain or inflammatory condition, PPIs taken once daily are effective in reducing the incidence of ulcers.

PROTOTYPE DRUG Omeprazole (Prilosec)

Classification: Therapeutic: Antiulcer drug
Pharmacologic: Proton pump inhibitor

Therapeutic Effects and Uses: Omeprazole was the first PPI to be approved in 1989 for PUD and is available by prescription and OTC. By prescription it is approved for the short-term, 4- to 8-week therapy of active peptic ulcers. OTC, it is indicated for the relief of heartburn. Most patients are symptom-free after 2 weeks of therapy. It is used for longer periods in patients who have ZES. It is combined with antibiotics in regimens for eliminating *H. pylori.* Omeprazole may be prescribed off-label to prevent PUD in patients taking NSAIDs.

Although omeprazole can take 2 hours to reach therapeutic levels, its effects last up to 72 hours. Omeprazole is available only in oral (PO) form in the United States and is approved for pediatric use in children 2 years or older. Zegerid is a combination drug that contains omeprazole and the antacid sodium bicarbonate.

Mechanism of Action: Omeprazole reduces acid secretion in the stomach by binding irreversibly to the enzyme H^+, K^+-ATPase. It inhibits the final pathway involved in acid secretion and effectively inhibits the active proton pumps.

Pharmacokinetics:

Route(s)	PO
Absorption	Rapidly absorbed; food does not influence bioavailability
Distribution	Bioavailability after oral dosing: 50–60%; crosses the placenta; secreted in breast milk; 95% bound to plasma protein
Primary metabolism	Hepatic; significant first-pass effect
Primary excretion	Renal
Onset of action	0.5–3.5 h
Duration of action	3–4 days; half-life: 0.5–1.5 h

Adverse Effects: PPIs are generally well-tolerated drugs. The most common adverse effects are minor and include headache, nausea, diarrhea, rash, and abdominal pain. Although rare, blood disorders may occur, causing unusual fatigue and weakness. Long-term studies have been conducted on the possible effects of omeprazole on cardiovascular events and gastric tumors. None of the studies have shown any significant increase in cardiovascular adverse effects or gastric cancer.

Contraindications/Precautions: The only contraindication is hypersensitivity to the drug. It is not recommended for children under 2 years of age. Patients with hepatic impairment should be treated with caution. The drug should be avoided or used with caution in pregnant or lactating patients.

Drug Interactions: Clinically significant interactions with PPIs are rare. Omeprazole has been shown to both inhibit and induce certain hepatic P450 enzyme systems, although clinically significant interactions are rare. Concurrent use with other drugs using the P450 system, including warfarin, carbamazepine, diazepam, and phenytoin, may inhibit or delay metabolism and cause increased blood levels of these drugs. Thus concurrent use with warfarin may increase the likelihood of bleeding. Coadministration of omeprazole and clarithromycin has been shown to increase plasma levels of both omeprazole and clarithromycin.

PPIs increase gastric pH and have the potential to affect the bioavailability of medications that depend on a lower pH for absorption (e.g., iron salts, digoxin, ampicillin, ketoconazole, atazanavir). Because an acidic environment promotes mineral absorption, mineral deficiencies could occur with long-term PPI use. Decreased vitamin B_{12} absorption may occur because an acid is optimal for vitamin B_{12} absorption. **Herbal/Food:** Ginkgo and St. John's wort may decrease the plasma concentration of omeprazole.

Pregnancy: Category C.

Treatment for Overdose: Overdose is uncommon and is treated symptomatically.

Nursing Responsibilities:

- Obtain a complete medication history, including allergies, drug history, and possible drug interactions.
- Monitor liver function tests during prolonged drug use, as well as serum gastrin, because hypersecretion of gastrin often occurs with constant acid suppression.
- Assess for drug–drug interactions. PPIs increase gastric pH and have the potential to affect the bioavailability of medications that depend on a lower pH for absorption.
- Monitor for vitamin B_{12} and folic acid malabsorption because an acidic environment is necessary for complete absorption of the drug.
- Monitor for adverse effects such as diarrhea, headache, and dizziness.

Patient and Family Education:

- Take this medication 30 minutes before meals, preferably before breakfast.
- Eat foods with beneficial bacteria, such as yogurt, or take *Lactobacillus acidophilus* supplements to replace "friendly" bacteria.
- Sleep with a foam wedge or risers placed under the head of the bed frame or mattress to keep the head elevated 30° if experiencing heartburn.
- Do not crush, break, or chew the tablets or capsules. If taking lansoprazole, the granules from the capsule may be sprinkled into soft foods such as applesauce. Afterward, drink a full glass of water to ensure that all medication is taken.
- Avoid smoking, alcohol use, and foods that cause acid production and gastric discomfort.
- Immediately report GI bleeding, severe diarrhea, abdominal pain, nausea, vomiting, heartburn, pain with urination, or blood in the urine to the health care provider.
- Do not breast-feed while taking this drug without the approval of the health care provider.

Drugs Similar to Omeprazole (Prilosec)

The other PPIs include esomeprazole, lansoprazole, pantoprazole, and rabeprazole.

Esomeprazole (Nexium): Approved in 2001, this drug is very similar in structure, effectiveness, and safety to omeprazole. Its effects may last longer than omeprazole. It is available by the PO and intravenous (IV) routes. Adverse effects include headache, diarrhea, and nausea. Similar to other PPIs, esomeprazole is available as once-a-day dosing for uncomplicated PUD and GERD and twice-daily dosing for complicated conditions such as ZES. It is approved by the U.S. Food and Drug Administration (FDA) for the prophylaxis of ulcers in patients who are taking NSAIDs. Esomeprazole capsules can be opened and the pellets mixed with soft foods and swallowed without chewing. With all PPIs there is a risk of pneumonia due to the elevation in gastric pH. Esomeprazole is pregnancy category B.

Lansoprazole (Prevacid): Approved in 1995, lansoprazole has a similar effectiveness and safety profile to omeprazole and is available by both the PO and IV routes. Its antisecretory effects can last up to 24 hours. Similar to other PPIs, its adverse effects include headache, diarrhea, and nausea. As with other PPIs lansoprazole offers once-a-day dosing for uncomplicated PUD and GERD and twice-daily dosing for ZES. With lansoprazole, as with other PPIs, there is a risk of pneumonia due to the elevation in gastric pH. This drug is eliminated from the body by the biliary system.

For patients who have difficulty swallowing capsules, lansoprazole is available in an oral liquid suspension or the capsule can be easily opened and its contents mixed with soft food and swallowed. Lansoprazole is available as a PO disintegrating tablet (Prevacid SoluTab) that is placed under the tongue and disintegrates within 1 minute. Lansoprazole is pregnancy category B.

Pantoprazole (Protonix): Approved in 2000, pantoprazole has a similar efficacy and safety profile to omeprazole and is available intravenously. Adverse effects include headache, diarrhea, and nausea. Because pantoprazole does not inhibit CYP450 enzymes, it is not likely to affect the metabolism of other drugs.

As with the other PPIs, pantoprazole offers once daily dosing for uncomplicated PUD and GERD and twice daily dosing for ZES. With all PPIs, there is a risk of pneumonia due to the elevation in gastric pH. Omeprazole may be prescribed off-label to prevent ulcers in patients taking NSAIDs. Pantoprazole is pregnancy category B.

Rabeprazole (AcipHex): Although rabeprazole is similar to omeprazole, it causes reversible inhibition of the proton pump; thus its effects are of shorter duration. Approved in 1999, rabeprazole is available by the PO route. The tablets should be swallowed whole and not crushed or chewed. Like other PPIs rabeprazole accentuates the eradication of *H. pylori* when used with appropriate antibiotics. Although rabeprazole is metabolized by the hepatic CYP450 drug metabolizing system, there are no significant clinical drug interactions. Adverse effects are

MyNursingKit | Mechanism of Action Animation: Omeprazole

CONNECTIONS

Evidence-Based Practice Use of Proton Pump Inhibitors and Risk of Bone Fracture

Clinical Question

PPI therapy leads to lower chloride levels, which may lead to decreased calcium absorption. Because decreased calcium absorption is known to be a factor in osteoporosis and bone loss, as a nurse, you may wonder, "Does the use of PPIs increase the risk of bone fracture?"

Evidence

A study from the United Kingdom has linked long-term use (more than 1 year) of PPIs to an increased risk of hip fracture among adults older than 50 years. The risk increased when higher doses were used and when the duration of use was longer. Histamine$_2$- receptor antagonist treatment did not significantly increase hip fracture risk in this study. Further study is needed to replicate and confirm these findings (Yang, Lewis, Epstein, & Metz, 2006).

Implications

PPI therapy leads to lower chloride levels, which may lead to decreased calcium absorption, resulting in increased fracture risk. The nurse should make sure that patients are aware of this and should discuss prevention measures and continued use of PPIs with both the health care provider and the patient.

Critical Thinking Question

Can you think of any long-term safety issues with prolonged PPI use?

See Answers to Critical Thinking Questions in Appendix A.

mild and transient and include headache, diarrhea, nausea, malaise, dizziness, and rash. Rabeprazole is pregnancy category B.

Pharmacotherapy with H$_2$-Receptor Antagonists

60.6 The H$_2$-receptor antagonists suppress gastric acid secretion and are widely prescribed for treating peptic ulcer disease and gastroesophageal reflux disease.

The discovery of the **H$_2$-receptor antagonists,** or H$_2$ blockers, in the 1970s marked a major breakthrough in the treatment of PUD. Since then they have become available OTC and are used extensively in the treatment of mild to moderate hyperacidity disorders of the GI tract. H$_2$-receptor antagonists are indicated for treatment of peptic ulcers and GERD to promote healing and prevent recurrence. Duodenal ulcers usually heal in 6 to 8 weeks, and gastric ulcers may require up to 12 weeks of therapy. All of the H$_2$-receptor antagonists are available OTC for the short-term (2 weeks) treatment of heartburn. These agents are listed in Table 60.2.

Histamine has two types of receptors: H$_1$ and H$_2$. Activation of the H$_1$ receptors produces the classic symptoms of inflammation and allergy, whereas the H$_2$ receptors, which are located on the parietal cells in the stomach, promote gastric acid secretion when activated. The H$_2$-receptor antagonists effectively reduce both fasting and food-stimulated secretion and are also helpful in decreasing nocturnal acid secretion, which is largely dependent on histamine.

Pharmacokinetic properties of drugs in this class include rapid absorption from the small intestine, which is not affected by food, and a 30-minute onset of action. These drugs undergo hepatic metabolism and renal excretion and their half-lives range from 1 to 4 hours. Although there are no known harm-

TABLE 60.2 H$_2$-Receptor Antagonists

Drug	Route and Adult Dose (maximum dose where indicated)	Adverse Effects
cimetidine (Tagamet)	Active ulcers: PO: 300 mg every 6 h or 800 mg at bedtime or 400 mg bid with food; IV: 300 mg every 6 h (over a minimum of 5 min) or 37.5 mg/h by continuous infusion GERD: 400 mg every 6 h or 800 mg bid for 12 weeks	*Diarrhea, constipation, headache, fatigue, nausea, gynecomastia* Rare: hepatitis, blood dyscrasias, anaphylaxis, dysrhythmias, skin reactions, galactorrhea, confusion, or psychoses
famotidine (Pepcid, Mylanta AP)	Active ulcers: PO: 40 mg/day for 4–8 weeks, then 20 mg at bedtime GERD: PO: 20 mg bid for 6 weeks IV: 20 mg every 12 h	*Headache, nausea, dry mouth* Rare: musculoskeletal pain, tachycardia, blood dyscrasia, blurred vision
nizatidine (Axid)	Active ulcers: PO: 150 mg bid or 300 mg at bedtime GERD: PO: 150 mg bid IV: 20 mg every 12 h	
ranitidine (Zantac)	PO: 150 mg bid or 300 mg once daily after the evening meal IV/IM: 50 mg every 6–8 h by intermittent bolus or infusion	

Note: *Italics* indicate common adverse effects. Underline indicates serious adverse effects.

NURSING PROCESS APPLICATION

Patients Receiving Proton Pump Inhibitor Therapy

Assessment	Potential Nursing Diagnoses
Prior to completion of health history: • Obtain a complete history, including allergies, drug history, and possible drug interactions. • Obtain baseline vital signs.	• *Deficient Fluid Volume,* related to GI bleeding • *Acute Pain,* related to disease • *Deficient Knowledge (Peptic Ulcer Disease)*, related to purpose, precautions, and adverse effects of drug therapy

Planning: Patient Goals and Expected Outcomes

The patient will:

- Report episodes of pain or unresolved symptoms.
- Demonstrate an understanding of medication usage, indications, and adverse effects.
- Immediately report adverse effects such as GI bleeding, increased pain, hives, or change in mental status (elderly patients).

Implementation

Interventions and (Rationales)	Patient and Family Education
• Monitor the use of OTC drugs and prescription drugs to assess for drug interactions. (Concurrent use of PPIs with warfarin, carbamazepine, diazepam, or phenytoin can cause increased levels of these drugs. Antacids can decrease the effectiveness of drugs that are given concurrently.)	Instruct the patient: • That some PPIs cause drug interactions and to report all other medications he or she is taking. • To take antacids at least 1 hour after PPIs. • That some drugs (e.g., calcium channel blockers, estrogen, progesterone, beta blockers, anticholinergic drugs, theophylline, and nicotine) aggravate GERD.
• Monitor the use of other supplements and evaluate for symptoms of vitamin B_{12} deficiency. (PPIs can affect mineral absorption. Long-term use of PPIs is associated with slightly decreased levels of vitamin B_{12} and iron.)	Instruct the patient: • To report all vitamins and minerals taken. • About foods high in vitamin B_{12} and iron, including red meats.
• Administer PPIs approximately one half hour before meals because the proton pumps are activated with meals. (PPIs are most effective when proton pumps are most active.)	• Instruct the patient to take medication at the correct time to maximize the drug's effectiveness.
• Monitor smoking and alcohol use. (These can increase gastric acid secretion and aggravate symptoms.)	Instruct the patient: • About the relationship among smoking, alcohol, and acid secretion. • To refrain from smoking and using alcohol.
• Monitor for continued symptoms or exacerbation of symptoms. (Exacerbation of symptoms can suggest a complication such as perforation of an ulcer or esophageal cancer.)	Instruct the patient: • To report continued symptoms and report episodes of blood in the stool, vomiting, or increased abdominal pain immediately. • That GERD is a chronic condition that may require long-term therapy and that an increase or change in symptoms may suggest a complication.
• Monitor the patient for adherence to completing the antibiotic regimen prescribed for *H. pylori* infection. (Incomplete dosing leads to an incomplete cure and the development of antibiotic resistance.)	Instruct patient to: • Complete the antibiotic regimen and to report any adverse effects. • Immediately report itching, hives, shortness of breath, or swelling.
• Advise the patient on healthy lifestyle changes. (Certain lifestyle habits can aggravate symptoms of both PUD and GERD.)	Instruct the patient: • That smoking impairs healing. • To refrain from foods that may aggravate the condition (e.g., spicy foods, peppermint, caffeine, chocolate, fatty foods, tomatoes, and alcohol). • To avoid tight-fitting garments. • To lose weight, if applicable. • To eat small, frequent meals. • To avoid bedtime eating. • To elevate the head of the bed.

Evaluation of Outcome Criteria

Evaluate the effectiveness of drug therapy by confirming that patient goals and expected outcomes have been met (see "Planning").

ful effects on the fetus, these agents cross the placenta and are secreted in breast milk. All drugs in this class have similar safety profiles: Their adverse effects are minor and rarely cause discontinuation of therapy. Patients who are receiving higher doses, those with renal or hepatic disease, or older adults may experience confusion, restlessness, hallucinations, or depression. Antacids should not be taken at the same time as H_2-receptor antagonists because absorption is diminished.

PROTOTYPE DRUG Ranitidine (Zantac)

Classification: Therapeutic: Antiulcer drug
Pharmacologic: H_2-receptor antagonist

MyNursingKit | Mechanism of Action Animation: Ranitidine

Therapeutic Effects and Uses: Approved in 1983, ranitidine has a higher potency than cimetidine, which allows it to be administered once daily, usually at bedtime. Adequate healing of the ulcer takes 4 to 8 weeks, although those at high risk for PUD may continue on drug maintenance for prolonged periods to prevent recurrence. Gastric ulcers heal more slowly than duodenal ulcers and thus require longer therapy. IV and intramuscular (IM) forms are available for the treatment of acute stress-induced bleeding ulcers. Tritec is a combination drug with ranitidine and bismuth citrate. An OTC preparation of ranitidine was approved in 1995.

Ranitidine is indicated for duodenal ulcers, gastric ulcers, hypersecretory conditions, heartburn, and GERD. In some cases, it is used off-label to prevent PUD in those who are taking medications known to cause peptic ulcers. It is not effective as monotherapy for the elimination of *H. pylori.* Ranitidine is available in a dissolving tablet form (EFFERdose) for treating GERD in children and infants older than 1 month of age.

Mechanism of Action: Ranitidine acts by blocking H_2 receptors on the parietal cells in the stomach to decrease acid production. Both daytime and nocturnal basal gastric acids are suppressed.

Pharmacokinetics:

Route(s)	PO, IV, IM (rare)
Absorption	Rapid absorption following PO administration; all three routes achieve comparable blood levels. Food decreases the rate of PO absorption.
Distribution	PO bioavailability is approximately 50%; very little enters the central nervous system; (CNS) crosses the placenta; secreted in breast milk; 15% bound to plasma protein
Primary metabolism	Hepatic
Primary excretion	Renal (mostly unchanged)
Onset of action	30–60 minutes; peak effect: 1–3 h
Duration of action	6–12 h; half-life: 2–3 h

Adverse Effects: Adverse effects are uncommon and transient. Although rare, blood dyscrasias, especially neutropenia and thrombocytopenia, have been reported; thus, periodic blood counts should be performed. Confusion may occur rarely and is usually in the elderly or with IV dosing. High doses may result in gynecomastia, impotence, or loss of libido in men, although these effects are more common with cimetidine.

Contraindications/Precautions: Contraindications include hypersensitivity to H_2-receptor antagonists, acute porphyria, and OTC administration in children less than 12 years of age. The drug should be used with caution in patients with renal impairment; dosages should be reduced.

Drug Interactions: Because ranitidine has much less affinity for CYP450 enzymes, it is less likely to participate in drug–drug interactions than cimetidine. Ranitidine may reduce the absorption of cefpodoxime, ketoconazole, and itraconazole because of the increase in gastric pH induced by H_2-receptor antagonists. Concurrent use can increase the effects of alcohol, sulfonylureas, salicylates, and warfarin. Antacids should not be given within 1 hour of H_2-receptor antagonists because their effectiveness may be decreased due to reduced absorption. Smoking decreases the effectiveness of ranitidine. **Herbal/Food**: Absorption of vitamin B_{12} depends on an acidic environment, so deficiency may occur. Iron is also better absorbed in an acidic environment.

Pregnancy: Category B.

Treatment of Overdose: Overdose is uncommon and is treated symptomatically.

Nursing Responsibilities:

- Obtain a complete history, including allergies, drug history, and possible drug interactions.
- Assess the patient's use of OTC drugs to prevent duplication of treatment. The H_2 blockers are available without prescription.
- Monitor for persistent epigastric pain or heartburn, which may be symptoms of a more serious disease that requires different medical treatment.
- Administer the IV form of this medication slowly over several minutes to prevent bradycardia and hypotension due to the antagonism of histamine receptors located in the heart. IV preparations of H_2-receptor antagonists are utilized for the prevention of stress ulcers seen in an intensive care unit (ICU) setting in critically ill patients.
- Monitor kidney function (blood urea nitrogen [BUN] and serum creatinine) periodically. These drugs are mainly excreted via the kidneys, and patients with diminished kidney function require smaller dosages.
- Assess hepatic function because these medications can cause hepatotoxicity, although rarely.
- Assess elderly patients carefully because they are more prone to adverse effects due to decreased drug clearance.

Patient and Family Education:

- Keep all follow-up appointments and laboratory visits for liver and kidney function tests.
- Unless otherwise directed, take the drug with meals because the buffering effect of food may increase the therapeutic effect.
- Do not take any other prescription or nonprescription drugs, dietary supplements, or herbal products, without approval of the health care provider.

- Do not drink alcohol or smoke while taking this medication because these may worsen the symptoms of PUD.
- Do not breast-feed while taking this drug without approval of the health care provider.
- Immediately notify the health care provider of any known or suspected pregnancy.
- Do not use OTC ranitidine for longer than 2 weeks. Seek medical attention if symptoms persist or recur.
- Immediately report fever, excessive bruising, vomiting of blood, or black-colored stools to the health care provider.

Drugs Similar to Ranitidine (Zantac)

Other H_2-receptor antagonists include cimetidine, famotidine, and nizatidine.

Cimetidine (Tagamet): The first of the H_2 blockers that was approved in 1977, cimetidine is used less frequently than other drugs in this class because (1) it inhibits hepatic drug-metabolizing enzymes and exhibits numerous drug–drug interactions; (2) it has a high incidence of adverse effects; and (3) it must be taken up to four times a day. Because cimetidine interacts with CYP450 enzymes, it may delay the metabolism of other drugs metabolized in the liver, including warfarin, phenytoin, diazepam, and theophylline. Cimetidine also may cause gynecomastia or impotence because it binds to androgen receptors, causing antiandrogenic effects. Cimetidine crosses the blood–brain barrier and therefore is more likely to cause CNS depression and confusion than the other H_2-receptor antagonists. A low-dose OTC preparation is available. Routes of administration include PO, IM, and IV. This drug is pregnancy category B.

Famotidine (Pepcid): Approved by the FDA in 1986, famotidine has indications, actions, and adverse effects that are almost identical to those of ranitidine. Famotidine does not inhibit CYP450 enzymes; therefore, it exhibits fewer drug–drug interactions than cimetidine. Famotidine is the most potent of the H_2-receptor antagonists. It is available OTC and may be given by the PO or IV routes. This drug is pregnancy category B.

Nizatidine (Axid): Although thought to have a similar safety and adverse effect profile to ranitidine and famotidine, nizatidine is not metabolized by the liver CYP450 enzyme system and therefore causes fewer drug interactions. Adverse effects are infrequent and transient. Nizatidine is indicated for up to 8 weeks of PUD therapy (12 weeks for GERD) and is available as PO capsules or a PO solution. Prescription nizatidine was approved in 1988. An OTC preparation was approved in 1995. This drug is pregnancy category B.

CONNECTION *Checkpoint* 60.2

From what you learned in Chapter 4, how is the excretion of drugs affected when they are metabolized through the hepatic CYP450 system? See Answer to Connection Checkpoint 60.2 in Appendix A.

Pharmacotherapy with Antacids

60.7 Antacids are alkaline substances that neutralize stomach acid to treat symptoms of heartburn.

Prior to the development of H_2-receptor antagonists and PPIs, antacids were the mainstay of peptic ulcer and GERD pharmacotherapy. Indeed, many patients still use these inexpensive and readily available OTC drugs. Antacids may provide temporary relief from heartburn or indigestion, but they are no longer recommended as the primary drug class for acid-related disorders. Although antacids relieve symptoms of heartburn, they do not promote ulcer healing or help to eliminate *H. pylori.* These agents are listed in Table 60.3.

Antacids are inorganic compounds that contain aluminum, magnesium, sodium, or calcium that neutralize gastric acid and inactivate pepsin. They are also thought to stimulate prostaglandin production in the mucosa and increase LES tone, which reduces gastroesophageal reflux. These drugs do not protect the stomach by coating the stomach wall. To be considered therapeutic, the dose of antacids should increase the gastric pH to a minimum of 3.5.

Self-medication with antacids is safe when taken in doses as directed on the labels. Although antacids act within 10 to 15 minutes, their duration of action is only 2 hours; thus, they must be taken often during the day. Combinations of aluminum hydroxide and magnesium hydroxide, the most common types, are capable of rapidly neutralizing stomach acid.

All the antacids are equally effective at neutralizing acid and reducing symptoms of heartburn when given in therapeutic doses. Each type has certain disadvantages that may preclude their use.

- **Sodium.** Antacids that contain sodium should not be taken by patients on sodium-restricted diets or by those with hypertension (HTN), heart failure, or renal impairment because they may promote fluid retention.
- **Magnesium.** Absorption of magnesium from high doses of magnesium-containing antacids can cause symptoms of hypermagnesemia (fatigue, hypotension, and dysrhythmias). Magnesium also acts as a laxative when it reaches the large intestine.
- **Calcium.** Antacids that contain calcium can cause constipation and may cause or aggravate kidney stones. When absorbed hypercalcemia is possible and renal failure may occur at very high doses. Administering calcium carbonate antacids with milk or any items with vitamin D can cause **milk-alkali syndrome** to occur. Early symptoms are the same as those of hypercalcemia and include headache, urinary frequency, anorexia, nausea, and fatigue. Milk-alkali syndrome may result in permanent renal damage if the drug is continued at high doses.
- **Aluminum.** Aluminum antacids are not absorbed to any great extent but they can cause constipation. The constipation effect is balanced when aluminum is combined with magnesium salts. Aluminum carbonate and aluminum hydroxide may interfere with dietary phosphate absorption to cause hypophosphatemia.

NURSING PROCESS APPLICATION

Patients Receiving H_2-Receptor Antagonists

Assessment

Prior to administration:

- Obtain a complete health history, including allergies, drug history, possible drug interactions, and family history.
- Assess the patient for signs of GI bleeding.
- Obtain vital signs and the results of CBC, liver, and renal function tests.
- Assess level of consciousness.

Potential Nursing Diagnoses

- *Deficient Knowledge (H_2-Receptor Antagonists)*, related to drug therapy
- *Acute Pain*, related to gastric irritation from ineffective drug therapy
- *Imbalanced Nutrition: Less than Body Requirements*, related to adverse effects of drug
- *Constipation*
- *Diarrhea*, related to drug therapy

Planning: Patient Goals and Expected Outcomes

The patient will:

- Report episodes of drowsiness and dizziness.
- Report episodes of abdominal pain or unresolved symptoms during or after drug therapy.
- Demonstrate an understanding of the drug's actions by accurately describing drug effects, adverse effects, and precautions.
- Adhere to the appropriate course of drug therapy.

Implementation

Interventions and (Rationales)	Patient and Family Education
• Monitor the use of OTC drugs to avoid drug interactions, especially with cimetidine therapy. (The patient should not use any OTC or prescription medications without consulting the health care provider.). Many H_2 receptors are available OTC and may initiate drug interactions (rare except for cimetidine).	• Instruct the patient to consult with the health care provider before taking other medications or herbal products. • Advise the patient that some drugs aggravate GERD, (e.g., calcium channel blockers, estrogen, progesterone, beta blockers, anticholinergic drugs, theophylline, and nicotine).
• Monitor the level of abdominal pain or discomfort to assess the effectiveness of drug therapy. (Abdominal pain or discomfort should decrease with therapy.)	• Advise the patient that pain relief may not occur for several days after beginning therapy. Instruct the patient to report difficulty swallowing, weight loss, increasing pain despite treatment, continuous nausea, vomiting, diarrhea, or black, bloody stools.
• Monitor the patient's use of alcohol. (Alcohol can increase gastric irritation.)	• Instruct the patient to avoid alcohol use.
• Discuss possible drug interactions. (Antacids can decrease the effectiveness of other drugs taken concurrently.)	• Instruct the patient to take H_2-receptor antagonists and other medications at least 1 hour before antacids. Advise the patient not to take an H_2-receptor blocker with a PPI.
• Monitor for continued symptoms or exacerbation in symptoms. (Exacerbation of symptoms can suggest a complication such as perforation of an ulcer or esophageal cancer.) • Observe the patient for signs of GI bleeding. (H_2-receptor antagonists usually do not heal a peptic ulcer. They only decrease acid production; therefore, bleeding may occur from an ulcer.)	Instruct the patient: • To immediately report continued symptoms such as episodes of blood in the stool, vomiting, or increased abdominal pain. • That GERD is often a chronic condition and intermittent or chronic therapy may be needed and that an increase or change in symptoms may suggest a complication.
• Institute effective safety measures regarding falls. (Drugs may cause drowsiness or dizziness.)	• Instruct the patient to avoid driving or performing other hazardous activities until drug effects are known.
• Explain the need for lifestyle changes. (Smoking and certain foods increase gastric acid secretion, and certain factors increase intrathoracic pressure.)	Encourage the patient to: • Stop smoking. Provide information on smoking cessation programs. • Avoid foods that cause stomach irritation or discomfort such as caffeine-containing foods and beverages, citrus and tomato products, and chocolate, if these foods cause discomfort. • Lose weight because obesity may be contributing to symptoms and dietary modifications may be necessary. • Avoid large meals, tight or restrictive clothing, bending and straining, and eating within 4 hours of bedtime. • Sleep with the head of the bed elevated.

Evaluation of Outcome Criteria

Evaluate the effectiveness of drug therapy by confirming that patient goals and expected outcomes have been met (see "Planning").

TABLE 60.3 Antacids

Drug	Route and Adult Dose (maximum dose where indicated)	Adverse Effects
aluminum hydroxide (AlternaGel, others)	PO: 600 mg tid-qid	*Constipation, nausea* Fecal impaction, hypophosphatemia with chronic use
calcium carbonate (Titralac, Tums) calcium carbonate with magnesium hydroxide (Mylanta Gel-caps, Rolaids)	PO: 1–2 g bid-tid PO: 2–4 capsules or tablets prn (max: 12 tablets/day)	*Constipation, flatulence* Fecal impaction, metabolic alkalosis, hypercalcemia, renal calculi
magnesium hydroxide (Milk of Magnesia) magnesium trisilicate and aluminum hydroxide (Gaviscon) magnesium hydroxide and aluminum hydroxide with simethicone (Mylanta, Maalox Plus, others) magaldrate (Riopan)	PO: 5–15 mL or 2–4 tablets as needed up to 4 times daily PO: 2–4 tablets prn (max: 16 tablets/day) PO: 10–20 mL prn (max: 120 mL/day) or 2–4 tablets prn (max: 24 tablets/day) PO: 540–1,080 mg/day (5–10 mL suspension or 1–2 tablets) (max: 20 tablets or 100 mL/day)	*Diarrhea, nausea, vomiting, abdominal cramping* Hypermagnesemia (patients with renal disease), dysrhythmias (when given parenterally)
sodium bicarbonate (Alka-Seltzer, baking soda)	PO: 325 mg–2 g 1 to 4 times/day	*Abdominal distention, belching* Metabolic alkalosis, fluid retention, edema, hypernatremia

Note: *Italics* indicate common adverse effects. Underline indicates serious adverse effects.

- **Bicarbonate.** Being a base, antacids that contain bicarbonate may provoke metabolic alkalosis (e.g., fatigue, mental status changes, muscle twitching, depressed respiratory rate) in patients at risk. Bicarbonate combines with gastric acid to form carbon dioxide, which causes bloating and belching.

Drug interactions with antacids occur by several mechanisms. Because antacids increase stomach pH, they affect the solubility and absorption of many oral drugs. Drugs that are weak acids are nonionized in the acidic environment of the stomach and are thus readily absorbed. If an antacid is given concurrently with a weak acid, the pH of the stomach will rise and result in a more ionized drug that is less readily absorbed. On the other hand, a drug that is a weak base is absorbed in a more alkaline medium. In other words, when taken with antacids, acidic drugs may have less therapeutic effect, and basic drugs may exhibit a greater effect. Examples of acidic drugs include NSAIDs, sulfonylureas, salicylates, warfarin, barbiturates, isoniazid, and digoxin. Basic drugs include morphine sulfate, antihistamines, tricyclic antidepressants, amphetamines, and quinidine.

Enteric-coated or delayed release drugs are designed to dissolve when they reach the alkaline environment in the small intestine. By raising the pH of the stomach, antacids may "fool" enteric-coated tablets into dissolving early and releasing their contents into the stomach. The drug may either irritate the stomach lining, causing nausea or vomiting, or be inactivated.

Drug interactions may also occur if the antacid physically binds to other drugs. For example, certain antacids form chemical complexes with tetracyclines, preventing the antibiotic from being absorbed. Digoxin is another drug whose absorption is affected by binding to antacids.

A third mechanism of drug interaction is due to the effects of antacids on urine pH. Making the urine pH more alkaline increases the excretion of acidic drugs such as aspirin and inhibits the excretion of basic drugs such as amphetamines.

Because antacids are widely used OTC by patients for self-treatment, nurses must emphasize that these drugs be used only as directed on the label due to the potential for adverse effects. To decrease the potential for antacid–drug interactions, nurses should advise that other medications be taken at least 1 hour before or 2 hours after giving an antacid.

Chewable tablets and liquid formulations of antacids are available. A few products combine antacids and H_2-receptor antagonists into a single tablet. For example, Pepcid Complete contains calcium carbonate, magnesium hydroxide, and famotidine. Simethicone is sometimes added to antacid preparations, because it reduces gas bubbles that cause bloating and discomfort. For example, Mylanta contains simethicone, aluminum hydroxide, and magnesium hydroxide. Simethicone is classified as an **antiflatulent** because it reduces gas. It also is available by itself in OTC products such as Gas-X and Mylanta Gas. Some manufacturers advertise their calcium-based antacid products as mineral supplements.

PROTOTYPE DRUG Aluminum hydroxide (AlternaGEL, others)

Classification: Therapeutic: Antiheartburn agent
Pharmacologic: Antacid

Therapeutic Effects and Uses: Aluminum hydroxide is an inorganic agent used alone or in combination with other antacids such as magnesium hydroxide. Combining aluminum compounds with magnesium (Gaviscon, Maalox, Mylanta) increases their effectiveness and reduces the potential for constipation. Unlike calcium-based antacids that can be absorbed and cause systemic effects, aluminum compounds are minimally absorbed. Their primary action is to neutralize stomach acid by raising the pH of the stomach contents. Unlike H_2-receptor antagonists and PPIs, aluminum antacids do

CONNECTIONS

To the Community

Acid Suppression and Vitamin B_{12} in Older Adults

H_2-receptor blockers and PPIs decrease the secretion of hydrochloric acid in the stomach. However, gastric acid is essential for releasing vitamin B_{12} in food, which is bound in a protein matrix. By affecting stomach acidity, these drugs can affect the absorption of this essential vitamin.

These medications are frequently prescribed for elderly patients, who are more likely to have preexisting lower vitamin B_{12} reserves or even deficiencies. With aging the ability to produce adequate amounts of hydrochloric acid, intrinsic factor, and digestive enzymes progressively diminishes. These losses can lead to lower absorption rates, depletion of reserves, and, eventually, vitamin B_{12} deficiency. The nurse must educate older adults who are taking these drugs as to the importance of eating plenty of foods rich in vitamin B_{12} such as red meat, poultry, fish, and eggs. Iron is also best absorbed in an acidic environment. Periodic assessment of the complete blood count (CBC) or serum B_{12} may alert the nurse to vitamin B_{12} deficiency or anemia.

not reduce the volume of acid secretion. They are most effectively used in combination with other antiulcer agents for the symptomatic relief of heartburn due to PUD or GERD. A second aluminum salt, aluminum carbonate (Basaljel), is also available to treat heartburn.

Mechanism of Action: Aluminum hydroxide combines with gastric (hydrochloric) acid to produce aluminum chloride and water. This raises the pH of the stomach contents and inactivates pepsin.

Pharmacokinetics:

Route(s)	PO
Absorption	17–30% absorbed
Distribution	Widely distributed
Primary metabolism	Hepatic
Primary excretion	Renal
Onset of action	20–40 minutes
Duration of action	2 h when taken with food; 3 h when taken 1 h after meals

Adverse Effects: Aluminum antacids frequently cause constipation. At high doses aluminum products bind with phosphate in the GI tract and long-term use can result in phosphate depletion. Those at risk include malnourished people, alcoholics, and those with renal disease. They are often combined with magnesium compounds, which counteract the constipation commonly experienced with aluminum antacids.

Contraindications/Precautions: Prolonged use in patients with low serum phosphate levels should be avoided. This drug should not be used in patients with suspected bowel obstruction.

Drug Interactions: Aluminum compounds should not be taken with other medications because they may interfere with their absorption. Concurrent use decreases the absorption of cimetidine, ciprofloxacin and other fluoroquinolones, digoxin, isoniazid, chloroquine, NSAIDs, iron salts, phenytoin, tetracycline, and thyroxine. Use with sodium polystyrene sulfonate may cause systemic alkalosis. Use of anticholinergic drugs can increase the effects of antacids. **Herbal/Food:** Aluminum antacids may inhibit the absorption of dietary iron.

Pregnancy: Category C.

Treatment of Overdose: There is no specific treatment for overdose

Nursing Responsibilities:

- Obtain a medical history, including the use of OTC and prescription drugs, and assess for signs of renal insufficiency. Magnesium-containing antacids should be used with caution in these patients because the kidneys are unable to excrete excess magnesium.
- Assess for bowel changes. Magnesium-based products may cause diarrhea, and those with calcium and aluminum may cause constipation.
- Monitor the patient for worsening symptoms. Antacids may cause rebound hyperacidity when the stomach responds to the higher pH by producing more gastric acid.
- Monitor laboratory values. Values for serum gastrin and urinary pH may increase. Serum phosphate values may decrease. Report electrolyte changes to the prescriber.
- Hold the drug and notify the prescriber if the patient has symptoms of appendicitis, undiagnosed GI bleeding, or a suspected obstruction, because constipating or laxative effects may exacerbate these conditions.

Patient and Family Education:

- Antacids are for occasional use only. Seek medical attention if symptoms persist or recur. The long-term use of OTC medications can mask the symptoms of more serious disease such as cancer or complicated ulcers.
- Keep all scheduled laboratory visits for phosphorus and calcium levels.
- Do not take antacids with magnesium if you have kidney disease.
- Do not take antacids with sodium if you have heart failure, high blood pressure, or are on a sodium-restricted diet.
- Take antacids at least 2 hours before other PO medications, because drug absorption may be affected. Take antacids 1 hour before meals or at least 2 hours after meals.
- Report any increase in abdominal pain, diarrhea, or constipation.
- This drug may make stools appear white.
- Take this drug with a full glass (8 oz) of water to enhance antacid absorption.
- Shake liquid preparations thoroughly before dispensing and thoroughly chew antacid tablets until wet before swallowing.
- Follow the label instructions carefully and keep within the recommended dosage range.

Drugs Similar to Aluminum Hydroxide (AlternaGEL, Others)

All aluminum salts have similar effects to those of aluminum hydroxide.

Pharmacotherapy of *Helicobacter pylori* Infection

60.8 The gram-negative bacterium *Helicobacter pylori* is associated with approximately 70% of patients with peptic ulcer disease.

It is estimated that 60% to 80% of patients with duodenal ulcers are infected with *H. pylori* and that the majority of patients with gastric ulcers have the bacterium. Research has shown that the eradication of *H. pylori* decreases the recurrence of PUD. Risk factors for *H. pylori* include residing in a developing country, domestic crowding, unclean water, and exposure to the gastric contents of an infected individual. It is the only known microorganism that has been found to survive the hostile conditions in the stomach.

H. pylori has adapted well to the acidic environment in the stomach. It has devised ways to neutralize the high acidity surrounding it and make chemicals called **adhesins** that allow the organism to penetrate the GI mucosa and alter the epithelial cell structure, which initiates inflammation. The inflammatory and immune responses lead to the chronic production of inflammatory cells, including lymphocytes, plasma cells, and macrophages. This response then leads to the formation of immunoglobulin G antibodies and increased production of cytokines, including interleukins and tumor necrosis factor, all of which contribute to the inflammation of the gastric mucosa. Increased gastrin secretion and decreased bicarbonate production also play a role in ulcer formation due to *H. pylori.*

Another mechanism involves ammonia. *H. pylori* produces large amounts of urease, an enzyme that breaks down urea to ammonia and carbon monoxide. Ammonia neutralizes the acid around the bacterium and allows *H. pylori* to survive in the acidic environment of the stomach. Unfortunately, the ammonia is toxic to mucosal cells and erodes the mucous barrier. *H. pylori* then finds its home in the submucosal layer of the stomach, producing damage to the gastric and duodenal mucosae that allows pepsin and gastric acid to further damage the mucosae. There may also be a genetic predisposition that determines one's susceptibility to *H. pylori* infection.

Prior to the identification of the link between *H. pylori* and ulcers, PUD was treated with acid-reducing drugs. Although this therapy was successful at treating symptoms, the majority of patients experienced relapses. This is because the acid-reducing drugs have little effect on *H. pylori,* which can remain active for life if not treated appropriately. Thus for infected patients, elimination of this bacterium is the prime pharmacologic objective. Eradication of the organism allows ulcers to heal more rapidly and remain in remission longer, often permanently.

A combination of antibiotics is used concurrently to eradicate *H. pylori* and help decrease antibiotic resistance. A PPI or bismuth compound is usually included in the regimen. Once eliminated from the stomach, reinfection with *H. pylori* is uncommon. Those with peptic ulcer who are not infected with *H. pylori* should not receive antibiotics because it has been shown that these patients have a worse outcome if they receive *H. pylori* treatment. Thus, patients should be tested for *H. pylori* before initiating treatment for infection. Example regimens used to eradicate *H. pylori* include the following:

- Initial regimen. Omeprazole, clarithromycin (Biaxin), and amoxicillin (Amoxil, others)
- Alternative regimens.
  - Omeprazole (or other PPI), clarithromycin (Biaxin), and metronidazole (Flagyl) or
  - Omeprazole (or other PPI), bismuth subsalicylate (Pepto-Bismol), metronidazole (Flagyl), and tetracycline

Although technically not antibiotics, bismuth compounds inhibit bacterial growth by disrupting their cell wall and preventing *H. pylori* from adhering to the gastric mucosa. The PPI further suppresses *H. pylori,* and the increased pH that results from PPI administration creates a hostile environment for *H. pylori,* thus enhancing the effectiveness of the antibiotics.

H. pylori therapy generally continues for 7 to 14 days. Should resistance occur, rifabutin (Mycobutin) and fluoroquinolones have been and can be used as part of the regimen. Drug regimens continue to evolve as antibiotic resistance patterns change. The American College of Gastroenterology publishes periodic guidelines offering different pharmacologic strategies.

Indiscriminate use of antibiotics can lead to antibiotic resistance; thus treatment should be reserved for patients who would benefit from the regimen. Patient adherence is vital to successful eradication of *H. pylori.* Patients should be instructed on the importance of completing the drug regimen, because discontinuing the anti-infectives too soon may result in reinfection. Interestingly, following treatment for eradicating *H. pylori* infection, certain other conditions such as idiopathic thrombocytopenic purpura (ITP), a blood disorder, have been alleviated.

CONNECTIONS

Lifespan Considerations

Peptic Ulcer Disease and Gastroesophageal Reflux Disease in Children

Antacids, H_2-receptor antagonists, and PPIs are widely used in children in the treatment of GERD. Although rare, PUD does occur in children and these drugs are also used, although in smaller doses than in adults. They are frequently used in critically ill children to prevent GI bleeding. The dosing of PPIs in children is higher per kilogram than for adults (0.7 to 3.3 mg/kg/day). Dietary alterations, including a change in feeding technique, are often included in the treatment. Thickening feedings with cereal has been shown to improve GERD symptoms in infants. A 2-week trial of soy and milk products may be diagnostic and therapeutic in those infants suspected of having intolerance to these foods. Older children are advised to avoid the same aggravating factors as adults, including chocolate, mints, tomatoes, and caffeinated beverages, and to lose weight if applicable.

CONNECTION *Checkpoint* 60.3

From what you learned in Chapter 47, explain why antibiotic resistance has become a major public health problem throughout the world. See Answer to Connection Checkpoint 60.3 in Appendix A.

Miscellaneous Drugs Used for Peptic Ulcer Disease and Gastroesophageal Reflux Disease

60.9 Several miscellaneous drugs, including sucralfate, bismuth subsalicylate, and misoprostol, are beneficial in treating peptic ulcer disease.

There are a few additional drugs used in the pharmacotherapy of PUD and GERD. These agents act by mechanisms other than the ones described for H_2-receptor blockers, PPIs, or antacids.

Sucralfate: Sucralfate (Carafate) is a PO medication that consists of sucrose (a sugar) plus aluminum hydroxide (an antacid). This drug stimulates mucus, bicarbonate, and prostaglandin secretion, all of which enhance mucosal defenses. Sucralfate also acts locally to produce a thick protective barrier that coats and binds to the ulcer, protecting it against further erosion from acid and pepsin to promote healing. It does not affect the secretion of gastric acid. It is intended for short-term therapy (up to 8 weeks). It is sometimes used in critically ill patients to prevent bleeding from stress-related gastritis. Sucralfate is not effective in preventing NSAID-related ulcers.

Other than constipation, the adverse effects of sucralfate are minimal because little of the drug is absorbed from the GI tract. Because sucralfate requires an acid medium to work effectively, concurrent use of antacids, H_2-receptor antagonists, and PPIs will reduce its effectiveness. Sucralfate may bind to other drugs and decrease their absorption, especially digoxin, warfarin, the quinolones and tetracyclines, and phenytoin. Antacids and other medications should be taken 2 hours before or after a dose of sucralfate. A major disadvantage of sucralfate is that it must be taken four times daily.

Bismuth compounds: In the United States the only bismuth compound available is bismuth subsalicylate (Pepto-Bismol), a nonprescription formula containing both bismuth and salicylate. Bismuth subsalicylate stimulates mucosal bicarbonate and prostaglandin production and inhibits *H. pylori* from adhering to the ulcerated tissue. It has been shown to have local antimicrobial actions to *H. pylori* by causing cell wall death to the bacterium. Bismuth is often included as a component of a multidrug regimen containing tetracycline and metronidazole (Pylera, Helidac) to eradicate *H. pylori* infection. As monotherapy, it is approved to treat dyspepsia, heartburn, and diarrhea.

Therapeutic doses of bismuth produce no significant adverse effects. This drug can cause stools to turn black. In stomach acid bismuth subsalicylate is converted to salicylic acid, which is absorbed. Patients who are taking other salicylates, such as aspirin, may experience adverse effects such as tinnitus, headache, nausea, vomiting, or dizziness.

Misoprostol: Misoprostol (Cytotec) is a synthetic form of prostaglandin E_2 that stimulates the production of protective mucus and inhibits gastric acid secretion. Normally, the stomach synthesizes a number of prostaglandins, which suppress acid, promote bicarbonate secretion, and maintain blood flow to the gastric mucosa. The primary use of misoprostol is for the prevention of gastric ulcers in patients who are taking high doses of NSAIDs or corticosteroids. It has a serum half-life of less than 30 minutes and is administered three to four times per day. No reduction is needed in patients with renal insufficiency although the drug is excreted in the urine.

Diarrhea and abdominal cramping are relatively common with misoprostol. Classified as a pregnancy category X drug, misoprostol is absolutely contraindicated during pregnancy. This drug is combined with mifepristone for pregnancy termination (see Chapter 70). The use of misoprostol as an antiulcer agent is not widespread because of the availability of other drugs that are as effective and better tolerated.

Metoclopramide: Approved in 1985, metoclopramide (Reglan) is occasionally used for the short-term (4 to 12 weeks) therapy of symptomatic, documented GERD or PUD in patients who fail to respond to first-line agents. It is more commonly prescribed to treat nausea and vomiting associated with surgery or cancer chemotherapy. Metoclopramide is available by the PO, IM, or IV routes. It causes muscles in the upper intestine to contract, resulting in faster emptying of the stomach. It also decreases esophageal relaxation and blocks food from entering the esophagus, which is of benefit in patients with GERD.

CNS adverse effects such as drowsiness, fatigue, confusion, and insomnia may occur in a significant number of patients. Although uncommon, symptoms of parkinsonism such as bradykinesia, akathisia, and tardive dyskinesia may occur (see Chapter 25). Due to the potential for significant adverse effects and the development of PPIs and H_2-receptor antagonists, metoclopramide is used infrequently. This drug is pregnancy category B.

Anticholinergic drugs: Anticholinergic drugs such as atropine were used to treat peptic ulcers prior to the discovery of safer and more effective drugs. Pirenzepine (Gastrozepine) is a cholinergic blocker (muscarinic) available in Canada that inhibits gastric acid secretion. Although the action of pirenzepine is somewhat selective to the stomach, other anticholinergic effects such as dry mouth and constipation are possible. Anticholinergics are now rarely used for PUD owing to the availability of safer, more effective drugs.

UNDERSTANDING THE CHAPTER

Key Concepts Summary

60.1 The stomach secretes acid, enzymes, and hormones that are essential to digestive physiology.

60.2 Peptic ulcer disease is associated with a number of etiologic risk factors.

60.3 Gastroesophageal reflux disease is a chronic condition characterized by persistent heartburn.

60.4 Peptic ulcer disease and gastroesophageal reflux disease are best treated with a combination of pharmacotherapy and lifestyle changes.

60.5 Proton pump inhibitors block gastric acid secretion and are the drugs of choice in the therapy of peptic ulcer disease and gastroesophageal reflux disease.

60.6 The H_2-receptor antagonists suppress gastric acid secretion and are widely prescribed for treating peptic ulcer disease and gastroesophageal reflux disease.

60.7 Antacids are alkaline substances that neutralize stomach acid to treat symptoms of heartburn.

60.8 The gram-negative bacterium *Helicobacter pylori* is associated with approximately 70% of patients with peptic ulcer disease.

60.9 Several miscellaneous drugs, including sucralfate, bismuth subsalicylate, and misoprostol, are beneficial in treating peptic ulcer disease.

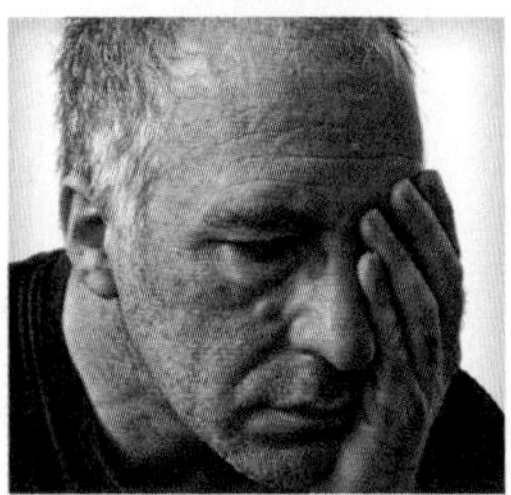

Making the PATIENT *Connection*

Remember the patient "Bob Richards" at the beginning of the chapter? Now read the remainder of the case study. Based on the information presented within this chapter, respond to the critical thinking questions that follow.

Mr. Richards is a 54-year-old man who is employed as a carpenter. He has been taking NSAIDs for a shoulder injury and assumed that this was the cause of his ulcers. He is a 1 pack per day smoker and consumes alcohol. His medical history includes HTN for which he takes a combination diuretic and ACE inhibitor. Because of worsening symptoms, an endoscopy was performed, which confirmed the presence of *H. pylori*. He is worried about using antibiotics because he has been allergic to penicillin in the past.

Critical Thinking Questions

1. Based on the scenario above, what risk factors for PUD does Mr. Richards have?
2. How would you as the nurse describe the recommended treatment for *H. pylori*-induced PUD to him?
3. Why would you be concerned about this patient using NSAIDs with a history of HTN?

Case Study

Sara Gaggi is a 51-year-old overweight white female with HTN who presents for an evaluation of heartburn that has been increasing in both intensity and frequency over the past 18 months. She reports epigastric burning after eating. It is worse after eating spicy foods or drinking red wine. She is occasionally awakened at night with symptoms. OTC antacids and H_2-receptor blockers relieved her symptoms initially, but lately they have provided only minimal relief. Her only routine medication is amlodipine, a calcium channel blocker for her high blood pressure. Because the symptoms are increasing and her current therapy is not relieving her symptoms, an endoscopy was performed, which revealed the presence of GERD.

1. How would you describe the dangers of self-medicating GERD symptoms with OTC medications to Sara?
2. What three risk factors in this case predispose Sara for the development of GERD?
3. What medications will her health care provider likely prescribe?
4. Sara wants to know why symptoms of GERD often increase at night. How would you respond?

NCLEX-RN® Review

1 The client has developed severe diarrhea following 4 days of self-administered antacid preparation. The nurse suspects that the diarrhea may be caused by which type of antacid?

1. Aluminum compounds
2. Magnesium compounds
3. Calcium compounds
4. Sodium compounds

2 Omeprazole (Prilosec) is prescribed for a client with gastroesophageal reflux disease. Which of the following symptoms would the nurse monitor to determine if the drug therapy is effective? A reduction in: (Select all that apply.)

1. Dysphagia.
2. Dyspepsia.
3. Appetite.
4. Nausea.
5. Belching.

3 The nurse is scheduling the client's daily medication. When would be the most appropriate time for the client to receive proton pump inhibitors?

1. At night
2. After fasting at least 2 hours
3. About ½ hour before a meal
4. About 2 to 3 hours after eating

4 A client who has duodenal ulcers is receiving long-term therapy with ranitidine (Zantac). The nurse includes in the care plan that the client should be monitored for which of the following adverse effects?

1. Photophobia and skin irritations
2. Neutropenia and thrombocytopenia
3. Dyspnea and productive coughing
4. Urinary hesitation and fluid retention

5 The prescriber orders sucralfate (Carafate) for a client with peptic ulcer disease. The nurse should question the order if the client is concurrently taking:

1. Proton pump inhibitors.
2. Calcium salt antacids.
3. H_2-receptor antagonists.
4. Aluminum salt antacids.

6 The nurse who is caring for a client with gastroesophageal reflux disease should question the order for which drug?

1. H_2-receptor antagonists
2. Proton pump inhibitors
3. Antibiotics
4. Antacids

See Answers to Critical Thinking Questions, Case Study, and NCLEX-RN® Review in Appendix A.

References

Blair, K., & Beltz, J. (2006, March). Dyspepsia: Is it gastroesophageal reflux disease, or peptic ulcer disease? *The American Journal for Nurse Practitioners*, 157–163.

Chaiyakunapruk, N., Kitikannakon, N., Nathisuwan, S., Leeprakobboon, K., & Leelasettagool, C. (2006). The efficacy of ginger for the prevention of postoperative nausea and vomiting: A meta-analysis. *American Journal of Obstetrics and Gynecology, 194*(1), 95–99.

Chan, F. K. L., Wong, V. W. S., Suen, B. Y., Wu, J. C. Y., Ching, Y. L., Hung, L. C. T., et al. (2007). Combination of a cyclo-oxygenase-2 inhibitor and a proton-pump inhibitor for prevention of recurrent ulcer bleeding in patients at very high risk: A double-blind, randomized trial. *Lancet, 369*(9573), 1621–1626.

Chandrasoma P., & DeMeester, T. (2006). *GERD: Reflux to esophageal adenocarcinoma*. San Diego, CA: Elsevier.

Comar, K., & Kirby, D. F. (2005). Herbal remedies in gastroenterology. *Journal of Clinical Gastroenterology, 39*(6), 457–468.

De Bortoli, N., Leonardi, G., Ciancia, E., Merlo, A., Bellini, M., Costa, F., et al. (2007). *Helicobacter pylori* eradication: A randomized prospective study of triple therapy versus triple therapy plus lactoferrin and probiotics. *American Journal of Gastroenterology, 102*(5), 951–956.

DeVault, K. (2007). Treatment of intermittent reflux symptoms: One size does not fit all. *Journal of Clinical Gastroenterology, 41*(6), 546–547.

Dial, S., Alrascki, K., Manoukian, C., Huang, A., & Manzies, D. (2004). Risk of *Clostridium difficile* among hospital inpatients prescribed proton pump inhibitors: Cohort and case-control studies. *Canadian Medical Association Journal, 171*(1), 33–38.

Dial, S., Delaney, J., Barkun, A., & Suissa, S. (2005). Use of gastric acid-suppressive agents and the risk of community-acquired *Clostridium difficile*-associated disease. *Journal of the American Medical Association, 294*(23), 2989–2995.

Feldman, M., & Le, M. (2007). *Gastroenterology II: Peptic ulcer diseases, May 2007 update.* Philadelphia: APC Medicine.

Fisichella, P. M., & Patti, M. G. (2008). Gastroesophogeal reflux disease. *emedicine.* Retrieved August 5, 2008, from http://www.emedicine.com/med/topic857.htm

Gold, B., Scheiman, J., Sabesin, S., & Vitat, P. (2007). Updates on the management of upper gastrointestinal disorders in the primary care setting: NSAID-related gastropathies and pediatric reflux disease. *Journal of Family Practice, 56*(3), S1–S12.

Goyal, R. (2005). Diseases of the esophagus. In D. L. Kasper, E. Braunwald, A. S. Fauci, S. L. Hauser, D. L. Longo, J. L. Jameson, et al., *Harrison's principles of internal medicine* (16th ed., pp. 217–218). New York: McGraw-Hill.

Gulmez, S., Holm, A., Frederiksen, H., Jensen, T., Pedersen, C., & Hallas, J. (2007). Use of proton pump inhibitors and the risk of community acquired pneumonia: A population based case-control study. *Archives of Internal Medicine, 167*, 950–995.

Kaltenbach, T., Crocket, S., & Gerson, L. B. (2006). Are lifestyle measures effective in patients with gastroesophageal reflux disease? An evidence based approach. *Archives of Internal Medicine, 166*, 965–971.

Le, T. H., & Fantry, G. T. (2008). Peptic ulcer disease. *emedicine.* Retrieved August 5, 2008, from http://www.emedicine.com/med/topic1776.htm

Louw, J. (2006). Peptic ulcer disease. *Current Opinion in Gastroenterology, 22*(6), 607–611.

Lu, H., Hsu, P., Graham, D., & Yamaoka, Y. (2005). Duodenal ulcer promoting gene of *Helicobacter pylori, Gastroenterology, 128*(4), 833.

Podein, R. (2007). Peptic ulcer disease. In D. Rakel, *Integrative medicine* (2nd ed., pp. 279–289). Philadelphia: Elsevier.

Yang, Y., Lewis, J., Epstein, S., & Metz, C. (2006). Long-term proton pump inhibitor therapy and risk of hip fracture. *Journal of the American Medical Association, 296*, 2947–2953.

CHAPTER

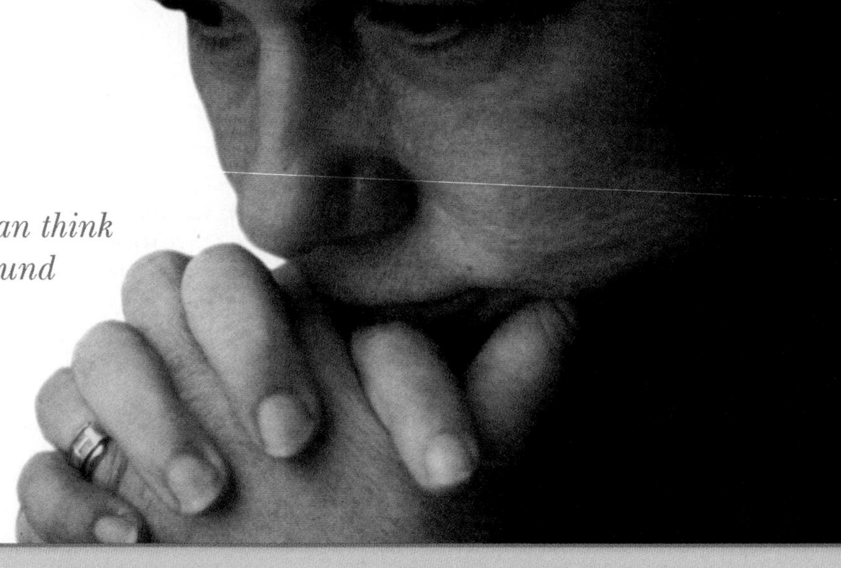

Worried? Lately it's all I can think about. My life revolves around my last bowel movement.

Patient "Marjorie Hatford"

61 Pharmacotherapy of Bowel Disorders and Other Gastrointestinal Conditions

Learning Outcomes

After reading this chapter, the student should be able to:

1. Compare and contrast the definition of constipation used by patients to that used for diagnosis by health care providers.
2. Compare and contrast the different mechanisms of action of laxatives.
3. Explain the pathogenesis of constipation and diarrhea.
4. Compare and contrast the types of drugs used to treat inflammatory bowel disease and irritable bowel syndrome.
5. Explain conditions in which the pharmacotherapy of nausea and vomiting is indicated.
6. Identify drugs that are used to treat acute and chronic pancreatitis.
7. Describe the nurse's role in the pharmacologic management of bowel disorders, nausea and vomiting, and other gastrointestinal conditions.
8. For each of the classes shown in the chapter outline, identify the prototype and representative drugs and explain the mechanism(s) of drug action, primary indications, contraindications, significant drug interactions, pregnancy category, and important adverse effects.
9. Use the nursing process to care for patients who are receiving drug therapy for bowel disorders, nausea and vomiting, and other gastrointestinal conditions.

Chapter Outline

Pathophysiology of Constipation

Pharmacotherapy with Laxatives

Bulk Forming

PROTOTYPE **Psyllium Mucilloid (Metamucil, Others)** *p. 1031*

Stimulant

Stool Softener/Surfactant

Saline/Osmotic

Herbal

Miscellaneous Agents

Pathophysiology of Diarrhea

Pharmacotherapy of Diarrhea

Opioids

PROTOTYPE **Diphenoxylate with Atropine (Lomotil)** *p. 1034*

Miscellaneous Agents

Pharmacotherapy of Inflammatory Bowel Disease

PROTOTYPE **Sulfasalazine (Azulfidine)** *p. 1037*

Pharmacotherapy of Irritable Bowel Syndrome

Pathophysiology of Nausea and Vomiting

Pharmacotherapy of Nausea and Vomiting

PROTOTYPE **Prochlorperazine (Compazine)** *p. 1044*

Pharmacotherapy of Pancreatitis

PROTOTYPE **Pancrelipase (Cotazym, Pancrease, Others)** *p. 1047*

Key Terms

cathartic, 1030
chemoreceptor trigger zone (CTZ), 1041
constipation, 1029
diarrhea, 1032
emetogenic potential, 1041
hyperemesis gravidarum, 1041
inflammatory bowel disease (IBD), 1035
irritable bowel syndrome (IBS), 1039
laxative, 1030
nausea, 1040
pancreatitis, 1045
steatorrhea, 1047
vomiting, 1040
vomiting center, 1041

Bowel disorders, nausea, and vomiting are among the most common complaints for which patients seek medical consultation. Nonspecific symptoms of gastrointestinal (GI) distress may be caused by a large number of infectious, metabolic, inflammatory, neoplastic, or neuropsychological disorders. In addition, nausea, vomiting, constipation, and diarrhea are the most common adverse effects of oral (PO) medications. Although symptoms often resolve without the need for pharmacotherapy, when severe or prolonged, these conditions may lead to serious consequences unless drug therapy is initiated. This chapter examines the pharmacotherapy of these and other conditions associated with the GI tract. The anatomy and physiology of the lower GI tract is reviewed in Chapter 59.

TABLE 61.1 Etiology of Constipation

Condition	Causes
Dietary	Inadequate fluid intake
	Inadequate food intake
	Inadequate fiber intake
	Specific foods: alcoholic beverages, products with a high content of refined white flour, dairy products, and chocolate
Lifestyle	Lack of exercise
GI disorders	Diverticulitis
	Irritable bowel syndrome
	Tumors
	Bowel obstruction
Neurogenic/Central nervous system (CNS) disorders	Diminished peristalsis
	Parkinson's disease
	Cerebrovascular accidents
	Clinical depression
	Head or spinal trauma
Metabolic disorders	Hypothyroidism
	Hypercalcemia or hypocalcemia
	Diabetes
Pregnancy	Diminished exercise, change in diet, pressure of fetus on the colon
Medications	Opioids
	Drugs with anticholinergic action: antihistamines, phenothiazines, tricyclic antidepressants, some antiparkinsonism agents
	Antacids containing bismuth, calcium, or aluminum
	Iron supplements
	Calcium channel blockers
	Nonsteroidal anti-inflammatory agents
	Barium sulfate

Pathophysiology of Constipation

61.1 Constipation is a decrease in the frequency of bowel movements.

Water is reabsorbed as waste material travels through the large intestine. Reabsorption of the proper amount of water results in stools of a normal, soft-formed consistency. If the waste material remains in the colon for an extended period, however, too much water will be reabsorbed, leading to small, hard stools that are difficult to evacuate from the rectum without straining. Abdominal distention, discomfort, and flatulence may occur.

Patients often define **constipation** as a decrease in the frequency of bowel movements. This definition, however, is not entirely satisfactory for diagnosis because the normal frequency of bowel movements varies widely among individuals, from two to three per day to as few as one per week. Constipation occurs more frequently in older adults because fecal transit time through the colon slows with aging. This population also exercises less, has diminished food intake, and uses drugs that cause constipation at a higher rate than in younger adults. All patients should understand that variations in frequency are normal and that a daily bowel movement is not a requirement for good health.

Constipation is not a disease but a symptom of an underlying disorder or condition, some of which are shown in Table 61.1. A diagnosis of chronic constipation includes at least two of the following symptoms without the use of laxatives over the course of a year:

- Two or fewer bowel movements per week
- Lumpy or hard stools at least 25% of the time
- Straining to pass stools at least 25% of the time
- A feeling of incomplete evacuation at least 25% of the time

Occasional constipation is self-limiting and does not require drug therapy. Lifestyle modifications that incorporate increased dietary fiber, fluid intake, and physical activity should be considered before drugs are utilized for constipation. Chronic, infrequent, and painful bowel movements that are accompanied by severe straining may justify initiation of treatment. Excessive straining may lead to anorectal pathology such as anal fissures, hemorrhoids, or rectal prolapse. In its most severe form, constipation can lead to a fecal impaction and complete obstruction of the bowel.

Constipation that is accompanied by acute pain and abdominal distension are signs of a potential bowel obstruction or paralytic ileus. These conditions are medical emergencies, and laxatives, enemas, and other therapies are absolutely contraindicated until the patient receives a full medical evaluation.

Pharmacotherapy with Laxatives

61.2 Laxatives are drugs that increase the frequency and quality of bowel movements.

Laxatives are drugs that promote evacuation of the bowel or defecation and are commonly used to prevent and treat constipation. **Cathartic** is a related term that implies an accelerated, stronger, and more complete bowel emptying. A variety of prescription and over-the-counter (OTC) laxatives, including tablet and liquid formulations, are available. Suppositories are used for infants or patients who are unable to take PO drugs. Laxatives and their doses are listed in Table 61.2.

Laxatives have several important indications. These may be divided into prophylaxis of constipation and treatment of constipation.

- Prophylaxis
  - Prevent straining in patients following a myocardial infarction (MI) or with rectal pathology
  - Patients receiving drug therapies that have constipation as a known adverse effect
  - Patients who are bedridden or otherwise unable to exercise
  - Patients who are pregnant
  - Elderly patients with weak abdominal or perineal muscles
- Treatment
  - Relief of simple, chronic constipation
  - Accelerate the removal of ingested toxic substances following overdose or poisoning
  - Accelerate the removal of dead parasites following antihelminthic drug therapy
  - Cleanse the bowel prior to diagnostic or surgical procedures of the colon or genitourinary tract, including colonoscopy or barium enema

The most common adverse effects of laxatives include abdominal distension and cramping. Diarrhea may result from excessive use. When cleansing the bowel prior to colonoscopy or purging the bowel of toxic substances or parasites, forceful, frequent bowel movements are expected outcomes. Care must be taken to rule out acute abdominal pathology such as bowel obstruction prior to administration because the drugs will increase colon pressure and possibly cause bowel perforation.

TABLE 61.2 Laxatives and Cathartics

Drug	Route and Adult Dose (maximum dose where indicated)	Adverse Effects
Bulk Forming		
calcium polycarbophil (FiberCon, Equalactin, Mitrolan, Konsyl Fiber)	PO: 1 g daily	*Abdominal fullness or cramping, fainting* Esophageal or GI obstruction if taken with insufficient fluid
methylcellulose (Citrucel)	PO: 5–20 mL tid in 8–10 oz liquid	
psyllium mucilloid (Metamucil, Naturacil, others)	PO: 1–2 tablespoons in 8 oz liquid daily prn	
Saline and Osmotic		
magnesium hydroxide (Milk of Magnesia)	PO: 20–60 mL or 6–8 tablets daily prn	*Diarrhea, abdominal cramping* Hypermagnesemia with magnesium hydroxide (dysrhythmias, respiratory failure)
polyethylene glycol (MiraLax)	PO: 17 g/day in 8 oz of liquid daily for 2–4 days	
sodium biphosphate (Fleet Phospho-Soda)	PO: 15–30 mL mixed in liquid daily prn	
Stimulant		
bisacodyl (Correctol, Dulcolax, others)	PO: 10–15 mg daily prn	*Abdominal cramping, nausea, fainting, diarrhea* Fluid and electrolyte loss
castor oil (Emulsoil, Neoloid)	PO: 15–60 mL daily prn	
Stool Softener/Surfactant		
docusate (Colace)	PO: 50–500 mg daily	*Abdominal cramping, diarrhea* No serious adverse effects
Herbal Agents		
castor oil	PO: 15–60 mL daily	*Abdominal cramping, diarrhea* No serious adverse effects
senna	PO: 8.6–17.2 mg daily	
Miscellaneous Agent		
mineral oil	PO: 15–30 mL bid	*Diarrhea, nausea* Nutritional deficiencies, pneumonia (with aspiration)

Note: *Italics* indicate common adverse effects. Underline indicates serious adverse effects.

Laxatives are classified by two primary means: onset of action and mechanism of action. These drugs are often placed into five primary groups and a miscellaneous category. The choice of a particular agent depends on the reason for use (treatment or prophylaxis), the onset of action desired (rapid or slow), and the completeness of evacuation needed (cathartic or laxative).

Bulk-forming laxatives: Bulk-forming agents absorb water, thus adding size to the fecal mass. Because fiber absorbs water and expands to provide "bulk," these agents must be taken with plenty of water. Bulk-forming laxatives are agents of choice for the treatment and prevention of chronic constipation and may be taken on a regular basis without ill effects. Because of their slow onset of action, they are not used when a rapid and complete bowel evacuation is necessary. Bulk-forming laxatives are pregnancy category C, and their onset of action is 24 to 48 hours.

Stimulant laxatives: Stimulant laxatives promote peristalsis by irritating the bowel. They are rapid acting and are more likely to cause diarrhea and cramping than the bulk-forming type of laxatives. They should not be used routinely, because they may cause laxative dependence, abdominal cramping, and depletion of fluid and electrolytes. These products are often used as a "bowel prep" prior to bowel exams or surgeries, sometimes in combination with other laxatives and enemas. Stimulant laxatives are pregnancy category C and their onset of action is 6 to 12 hours (oral) or 1 to 6 hours (rectal).

Surfactant laxatives: Surfactants, commonly called stool softeners, cause more water and fat to be absorbed into the stools. They are ineffective at treating constipation but are most often used to prevent the condition. Stool softeners are generally prescribed for patients who have a condition that puts them at risk for constipation, such as a surgery, an injury, or an MI where straining during defecation should be avoided. Stimulant laxatives are pregnancy category C and their onset of action is 24 to 48 hours.

Saline cathartics: Saline cathartics, also called osmotic laxatives, are poorly absorbed in the intestine. They pull water into the fecal mass to create a more watery stool. These agents can produce a bowel movement very quickly but should not be used on a regular basis due to the possibility of dehydration and fluid and electrolyte depletion. Saline laxatives are highly effective and are an important component of colonoscopy prep and for purging toxins from the body. Most saline cathartics are pregnancy category B. Their onset of action is 1 to 6 hours in high doses.

Herbal laxatives: Herbal agents are natural products that are available OTC and that are widely used for self-treatment of constipation. The most commonly used herbal laxative is senna, a potent herb that stimulates the bowel and increases peristalsis. Other natural laxatives include rhubarb, cascara sagrada, aloe, flaxseed, and dandelion. Patients should be advised to exercise caution when using herbal products because many have not been evaluated through controlled studies for safety or effectiveness. The pregnancy category for natural products has not been determined and their onset of action is variable.

Miscellaneous agents: Mineral oil is a miscellaneous agent that acts by lubricating the stool and the colon mucosa. The use of mineral oil should be discouraged because it may interfere with the absorption of fat-soluble vitamins and can cause other potentially serious adverse effects. Its onset of action is 24 to 48 hours. Approved in 2008, methylnaltrexone (Relistor) is specifically used to treat chronic constipation resulting from the palliative use of opioids. Methylnaltrexone blocks the effects of the opioids in the colon without affecting analgesia. It is administered subcutaneously every other day.

PROTOTYPE DRUG Psyllium mucilloid (Metamucil, others)

Classification: **Therapeutic:** Agent for constipation
Pharmacologic: Bulk-type laxative

Therapeutic Effects and Uses: Psyllium is derived from a natural product—the seeds of the plantain plant. Like other bulk-forming laxatives, psyllium is an insoluble fiber that is indigestible and not absorbed from the GI tract. When taken with a sufficient quantity of water, psyllium swells and increases the size of the fecal mass. The larger the size of the fecal mass, the greater will be the neural stimulus for defecation.

Several doses of psyllium may be needed over 1 to 3 days to produce an optimum therapeutic effect. Several 2.4 g doses may be taken each day. Frequent use of psyllium (7 g/day) may effect a small reduction in blood cholesterol level. This drug is available as granules, powder, and wafers.

Mechanism of Action: Psyllium expands the size of the stool and promotes colon peristalsis that closely resembles a natural bowel movement.

Pharmacokinetics:

Route(s)	PO
Absorption	Not absorbed: remains in the GI tract
Distribution	Not distributed
Primary metabolism	Not metabolized
Primary excretion	Feces
Onset of action	12–24 h
Duration of action	Unknown

Adverse Effects: Psyllium is the safest laxative and rarely produces adverse effects. It generally causes less cramping than the stimulant-type laxatives and results in a more natural bowel movement. If taken with insufficient water, psyllium may swell in the esophagus and cause obstruction.

Contraindications/Precautions: Psyllium should not be administered to patients with undiagnosed abdominal pain, suspected intestinal obstruction, or fecal impaction.

Drug Interactions: Psyllium may decrease the absorption and effects of warfarin, digoxin, nitrofurantoin, antibiotics, and salicylates. **Herbal/Food:** Unknown.

Pregnancy: Category C.

Treatment of Overdose: Overdose from psyllium is unlikely.

Nursing Responsibilities:

- Obtain a complete health history, including allergies, drug history, and possible drug interactions.
- Perform a complete assessment of bowel movements and GI functioning, including constipation frequency, duration, severity, and precipitating factors.
- Mix the powder and granules with at least 8 ounces of a pleasant tasting liquid, such as fruit juice, immediately before use. Insufficient fluid may cause the fiber to swell and cause choking or even rupture of the esophagus. Do not use psyllium if the patient has difficulty swallowing.
- Immediately report complaints of retrosternal pain after taking the drug to the prescriber.
- Monitor therapeutic effectiveness. Laxative effect usually occurs within 12 to 24 hours. Repeat administration for 2 or 3 days may be needed to establish regularity.
- Smaller, more frequent doses spaced throughout the day may be indicated to relieve discomfort of abdominal fullness.
- Monitor warfarin and digoxin levels closely because psyllium may decrease the absorption and effects of these drugs.

Patient and Family Education:

- Drink plenty of fluids, exercise regularly, and eat a high-fiber diet, including whole-grain (e.g., bran) cereals, fruits, and vegetables.
- For new users, start by taking a small amount of the drug and then gradually increase to the recommended dosage to minimize gas and bloating.
- Some preparations contain natural sugars, whereas others contain artificial sweeteners. Note sugar and sodium content of the preparation if on a low-sodium or low-calorie diet.
- Contact the health care provider if constipation persists for more than a week with regular use of a bulk laxative or if rectal bleeding occurs.

Drugs Similar to Psyllium Mucilloid (Metamucil, Others)

Other popular laxatives include bisacodyl, castor oil, docusate, and magnesium salts.

Bisacodyl (Correctol, Dulcolax, others): Bisacodyl is the most frequently used stimulant-type laxative. It acts by irritating the mucosa in the colon and by altering intestinal and electrolyte absorption. Only 15% of the drug is absorbed after oral administration. Onset of action is 8 to 12 hours (PO) if taken at bedtime or 15 to 60 minutes (rectal). Bisacodyl should not be taken with milk or other dairy products because these can dissolve the enteric coating and cause dyspepsia. The enteric-coated tablets should not be crushed or chewed. Minor adverse effects include abdominal pain and cramping. Prolonged use may lead to laxative dependence and fluid and electrolyte loss. Bisacodyl is pregnancy category C.

Castor oil (Emulsoil, Neoloid): Castor oil is one of the oldest and worst-tasting laxatives that was approved by the U.S. Food and Drug Administration (FDA) in 1939. A stimulant-type laxative, castor oil acts on the small intestine and produces a bowel movement in 2 to 6 hours. It causes more adverse effects than other laxatives, including diarrhea, cramping, nausea, vomiting, and dizziness. This drug is pregnancy category X and must not be used during pregnancy.

Docusate (Colace): Docusate is the most frequently prescribed surfactant-type laxative or stool softener. This drug permits additional water and lipids to penetrate the stool, resulting in softer stools. Docusate takes several days to act and therefore is not effective when a rapid and complete bowel evacuation is necessary. Only small amounts are absorbed systemically. Adverse effects are rare. Docusate sodium (Colace) should not be given to patients on sodium restriction. Docusate potassium (Dialose) should not be given to patients with renal impairment. Docusate increases the systemic absorption of mineral oil, so these two medications should not be given concurrently. Docusate should not be taken with certain herbal products such as senna, cascara, rhubarb, or aloe, because it will increase their absorption and the risk of liver toxicity. Docusate is pregnancy category C.

Magnesium hydroxide (Milk of Magnesia, MOM): Magnesium hydroxide has two effects on the GI tract. Taken orally it exerts an antacid effect because this drug neutralizes gastric hydrochloric acid to form magnesium chloride. About 30% of the magnesium chloride is absorbed systemically. The remainder continues along the GI tract and reaches the colon, where it exerts a laxative effect by drawing water and electrolytes to form a larger and softer fecal mass. This drug has a chalky taste and has a small incidence of nausea, vomiting, and abdominal cramping. Patients with impaired renal function should be monitored for hypermagnesemia. Magnesium hydroxide can bind to other drugs, delaying their absorption; thus it should be taken at least 2 hours apart from other medications. Drugs that may result in decreased absorption include H_2-receptor antagonists, iron salts, phenytoin, digoxin, and tetracyclines. Magnesium citrate and magnesium sulfate are other saline-type laxatives with rapid onsets of action, these being 30 minutes to 4 hours.

CONNECTION *Checkpoint* 61.1

From what you learned in Chapter 26, describe the indications for using magnesium to treat seizure disorders.

See Answer to Connection Checkpoint 61.1 in Appendix A.

Pathophysiology of Diarrhea

61.3 Diarrhea is an abnormal increase in the frequency and fluidity of bowel movements.

The small intestine receives about 9 L of fluid, or chyme, daily. Most is reabsorbed, such that only about 1 L reaches the colon. Travel through the colon results in even more reabsorption, and only about 100 mL remains to form stools. Should the small or large intestines fail to reabsorb sufficient fluids, diarrhea may occur. **Diarrhea** is an increase in the frequency and fluidity of bowel movements.

CONNECTIONS

To the Community Laxative Abuse

Laxatives are one of the most frequently abused OTC medication classes. Laxative abuse occurs when patients overuse laxatives in an attempt to have "normal" bowel movements due to a false belief that daily bowel movements are necessary. Laxative abuse is also seen in patients who do not include enough fiber or water in their diets. Patients abuse laxatives to lose weight. Some have eating disorders or are binge eaters who may want to get rid of large meals.

Nurses should monitor for laxative abuse and provide patients with the appropriate education about the use of these drugs. Laxative abuse can have serious effects, such as damage to the muscular function of the bowel and removal of the body's water, vitamins, and minerals. Loss of minerals and salts can cause electrolyte imbalances. Older adults are most vulnerable to these types of changes. Laxatives can also affect the effectiveness of other medications.

The nurse should instruct the elderly individual who expresses concern about overuse of laxatives to see a health care provider to determine the cause of the chronic constipation. Also, the nurse should instruct the patient that tapering off laxative overuse may be better than stopping abruptly. Changing to products containing psyllium may help. Additional alternatives to prevent constipation include the following:

- Drink plenty of water with each meal and throughout the day.
- Eat more fresh fruits, vegetables, and whole grains to increase dietary fiber.
- Go to the bathroom when you feel the urge. (This may occur right after a meal.)
- Exercise regularly to promote bowel movements.

Like constipation occasional diarrhea is a self-limiting disorder that does not warrant drug therapy. Indeed diarrhea in some cases is a type of body defense, rapidly and completely eliminating the body of toxins and pathogens. When prolonged or severe, especially in children, diarrhea can result in a significant loss of body fluids and pharmacotherapy is indicated. In underdeveloped countries, diarrhea is a major cause of illness and death in young children. Prolonged diarrhea may lead to fluid, acid–base, or electrolyte imbalances.

Because diarrhea is a nonspecific symptom of an underlying condition or disease, a primary treatment goal is to identify and treat the underlying condition. Assessing the patient's recent travels, dietary habits, immune system competence, and recent drug history may provide important clues about the etiology. Because such a large number of conditions can cause diarrhea, pinpointing an exact cause may be difficult. Therefore, symptomatic therapy is provided for the diarrhea while identifying its cause. Common etiologies include the following:

- **Infection.** Viral and bacterial infections are the most common cause of diarrhea. Intestinal protozoans and helminths are less common causes. The most frequently encountered diarrhea-producing organisms are *Campylobacter, Salmonella, Cryptosporidium, Giardia, Shigella, Escherichia coli* (traveler's diarrhea), and *Staphylococcus.*
- **Drugs.** Antibiotics often cause diarrhea by killing normal intestinal flora, thereby allowing an overgrowth of opportunistic pathogenic organisms. Laxatives, magnesium antacids, digoxin, orlistat, and nonsteroidal anti-inflammatory drugs (NSAIDs) are also common causes.
- **Inflammation.** Ulcerative colitis, Crohn's disease, and irritable bowel syndrome cause inflammation of the bowel mucosa, leading to periods of intense diarrhea.
- **Foods.** Various foods can cause diarrhea, such as dairy products in lactose intolerant patients, foods with capsaicin (hot pepper), and chronic alcohol ingestion.
- **Malabsorption.** Diseases of the small intestine and pancreas can cause insufficient absorption of foods and fluid.

Pharmacotherapy of Diarrhea

61.4 Opioids are the most effective drugs for controlling severe diarrhea.

Pharmacotherapy related to diarrhea depends on the severity of the condition and any identifiable etiologic factors. If the cause is an infectious disease, then an antibiotic or antiparasitic drug is indicated. Should the etiology be inflammatory, then anti-inflammatory drugs are warranted. When the cause appears to be due to an adverse effect of pharmacotherapy, the health care provider should discontinue the offending medication, lower the dose, or substitute an alternative drug.

The most effective drugs for the symptomatic treatment of diarrhea are the opioids, which can dramatically slow peristalsis in the colon. The most common opioid antidiarrheals are codeine and diphenoxylate with atropine (Lomotil). Diphenoxylate is a Schedule V agent that acts directly on the intestine to slow peristalsis, thereby allowing for more fluid and electrolyte absorption in the large intestine. The opioids cause central nervous system (CNS) depression at high doses and are generally reserved for the short-term therapy of acute diarrhea due to potential adverse effects and the potential for dependence. Details on the indications and adverse effects of opioids are found in Chapter 29.

OTC drugs for diarrhea act by a number of different mechanisms. Loperamide (Imodium) is an analog of meperidine (Demerol), although it has no narcotic effects and is not classified as a controlled substance. Low-dose loperamide is available OTC; higher doses are available by prescription. Other OTC treatments include bismuth subsalicylate (Pepto-Bismol), which acts by binding and absorbing toxins. Psyllium preparations may also slow diarrhea because they absorb large amounts of fluid, which helps to form bulkier stools. Probiotic supplements containing *Lactobacillus,* a normal inhabitant of the human gut and vagina, are sometimes taken to correct the altered GI flora following a serious diarrhea episode. A good source of healthy *Lactobacillus* is yogurt with active cultures, although a freeze-dried form of the bacteria is available in tablets. The antidiarrheals are listed in Table 61.3.

Antidiarrheal medications should never be used to treat diarrhea caused by poisoning or infection by toxin-producing organisms. For these patients, it is important that the toxic substances and organisms be expelled from the body. Use of antidiarrheals will retain these harmful substances. Antidiarrheal use is contraindicated in cases of diarrhea caused by pseudomembranous colitis that is caused by *Clostridium difficile*. This infection can cause fatal toxic megacolon.

PROTOTYPE DRUG Diphenoxylate with atropine (Lomotil)

Classification: Therapeutic: Antidiarrheal
Pharmacologic: Opioid

Therapeutic Effects and Uses: Approved in 1960, diphenoxylate is an oral opioid that is a Schedule IV controlled substance. Like other opioids diphenoxylate slows peristalsis, allowing time for additional water reabsorption from the intestine and the formation of solid stools. It acts within 45 to 60 minutes. It is effective for moderate to severe diarrhea, but it is not recommended for infants. The atropine in Lomotil is not added for its anticholinergic effect but to discourage patients from taking too much of the drug. At recommended doses the effects of atropine are negligible.

Diphenoxylate is discontinued as soon as the diarrhea symptoms resolve. A low-maintenance dose may be continued for up to 10 days if additional diarrhea is anticipated. Lomotil is approved for use in children 2 years and older.

Mechanism of Action: Diphenoxylate acts on the smooth muscle cells of the intestine to slow peristalsis.

Pharmacokinetics:

Route(s)	PO
Absorption	90% absorbed
Distribution	Small amounts are secreted in breast milk
Primary metabolism	Hepatic; metabolized to active metabolite
Primary excretion	Bile and feces
Onset of action	45–60 minutes
Duration of action	3–4 h

Adverse Effects: Unlike most opioids, diphenoxylate has no analgesic properties and has an extremely low potential for abuse. The drug is well tolerated at normal doses. Some patients experience dizziness, lethargy, or drowsiness, and care should be taken not to drive or operate machinery until the effects of the drug are known. At higher doses the anticholinergic effects of atropine, which include drowsiness, flushing, dry mouth, and tachycardia, may be observed.

Contraindications/Precautions: Contraindications to diphenoxylate include hypersensitivity to the drug, severe hepatic impairment, obstructive jaundice, and diarrhea associated with pseudomembranous colitis. Dehydration or electrolyte imbalances should be corrected before diphenoxylate therapy is initiated.

Drug Interactions: Other CNS depressants, including alcohol, will cause additive sedative effects. Opiate antagonists such as naloxone will reduce the effectiveness of diphenoxylate. When taken with monoamine oxidase inhibitors (MAOIs), diphenoxylate may cause hypertensive crisis. **Herbal/Food**: Unknown.

Pregnancy: Category C.

TABLE 61.3 Antidiarrheals

Drug	Route and Adult Dose (maximum dose where indicated)	Adverse Effects
Opioids		
camphorated opium tincture (Paregoric)	PO: 5–10 mL 1–4 times daily	*Drowsiness, light-headedness, nausea, dizziness, dry mouth (from atropine), constipation* Paralytic ileus with toxic megacolon, respiratory depression, CNS depression
difenoxin with atropine (Motofen)	PO: 1–2 mg after each diarrhea episode (max: 8 mg/day)	
diphenoxylate with atropine (Lomotil)	PO: 5 mg 4 times daily (max: 20 mg/day)	
loperamide (Imodium)	PO: 4 mg as a single dose, then 2 mg after each diarrhea episode (max: 16 mg/day)	
Miscellaneous Agents		
bismuth subsalicylate (Kaopectate, Pepto-Bismol)	PO: 2 tablets or 30 mL prn	*Constipation, nausea, tinnitus* Impaction, Reye's syndrome
furazolidone (Furoxone)	PO: 100 mg qid	*Nausea, vomiting* Agranulocytosis, disulfiram-like reaction
octreotide (Sandostatin)	Subcutaneous/intravenous (IV): 100–600 mcg/day in 2–4 divided doses	*Nausea, diarrhea, abdominal pain* Hypo- or hyperglycemia, gallstones, cholestatic hepatitis

Note: *Italics* indicate common adverse effects. Underline indicates serious adverse effects.

Treatment of Overdose: Overdose with Lomotil may be serious. Narcotic antagonists such as naloxone may be administered parenterally to reverse respiratory depression within minutes.

Nursing Responsibilities:

- Obtain a complete health history, including allergies, drug history, and possible drug interactions.
- Perform a complete assessment of bowel movements and GI functioning, including diarrhea frequency, duration, severity, and precipitating factors.
- Assess GI function; report abdominal distention and signs of decreased peristalsis to the prescriber.
- Monitor for signs and symptoms of dehydration such as increased heart rate, increased respiration, decreased sweating, decreased urination, and increased body temperature.
- Monitor young children closely. Dehydration occurs more rapidly in this age group and may influence the variability of response to diphenoxylate and predispose these patients to delayed toxic effects.
- Monitor the frequency and consistency of stools.
- Maintain a safe environment because diphenoxylate with atropine may cause drowsiness or dizziness, resulting in injuries.

Patient and Family Education:

- Do not drive or operate hazardous machinery until the effects of the drug have been determined because diphenoxylate with atropine may cause drowsiness or dizziness.
- Avoid caffeine because it can aggravate diarrhea.
- Avoid alcohol because it may intensify the drowsiness caused by this medicine.
- Do not take this drug if on an antibiotic therapy without approval of the health care provider.
- Report persistent diarrhea to the health care provider or if fever, bloody stools, palpitation, or other adverse reactions occur.
- Take this drug only as prescribed because the long-term use of diphenoxylate with atropine may cause dependency.

Drugs Similar to Diphenoxylate with Atropine (Lomotil)

Other antidiarrheal agents include bismuth subsalicylate difenoxin with atropine, loperamide, octreotide, and paregoric.

Bismuth subsalicylate (Kaopectate, Pepto-Bismol): Bismuth subsalicylate is an oral OTC drug approved for indigestion, heartburn, and diarrhea. Its more recent use is in the treatment of *Helicobacter* infections in patients with peptic ulcer disease (see Chapter 60). Doses may be taken every 30 to 60 minutes (max: 4 doses/day) until the diarrhea resolves. Adverse effects do not occur at recommended doses. Stools may become discolored, although this is not harmful. In stomach acid, bismuth subsalicylate forms salicylic acid, which is absorbed systemically. Thus this drug should be used with caution by patients using aspirin; otherwise salicylate toxicity may result. In addition, this drug should not be used in children with chickenpox of flu symptoms due to the possibility of Reye's syndrome.This drug is pregnancy category C.

Difenoxin with atropine (Motofen): Difenoxin is an opioid that is an active metabolite of diphenoxylate; thus the two drugs have the same actions, contraindications, and adverse effects. Like Lomotil, atropine is added to Motofen to discourage substance abusers from using the drug. It is a Schedule IV controlled substance and is pregnancy category C.

Loperamide (Imodium): Approved in 1976, loperamide is an oral drug that is a drug of choice for the symptomatic treatment of acute diarrhea and the maintenance therapy of chronic diarrhea. Chemically related to the opioids, it shares the antidiarrheal properties of the opioids but has no analgesic action and does not produce dependence. This drug slows peristalsis, increasing the transit time, thus allowing for better formed stools. If diarrhea is not controlled after 48 hours of loperamide therapy, the patient should seek medical attention. Adverse effects are rare. A dose may last up to 24 hours. Safety has been established in children less than 2 years of age. This drug is pregnancy category C.

Octreotide (Sandostatin): Approved in 1988, octreotide is a drug that is closely related to endogenous somatostatin (growth hormone-inhibiting hormone). It is approved to treat acromegaly and severe diarrhea associated with cancer. Octreotide is used off-label to treat a wide variety of other conditions (see Chapter 66), including acquired immunodeficiency syndrome (AIDS)-related diarrhea, ileostomy-related diarrhea, and childhood diarrhea. Octreotide prevents the release of serotonin and other active peptides that promote diarrhea. It also directly inhibits intestinal secretions and enhances absorption. It is only given by the intramuscular (IM) or intravenous (IV) routes. A long-acting depot form (Sandostatin LAR) is available for patients who need to take the drug on a long-term basis. The most frequent adverse effects are GI related, such as nausea, diarrhea, and abdominal pain. During long-term therapy, over half of the patients who are taking octreotide experience gallbladder pathology, including gallstones, or cholestatic hepatitis. This drug is pregnancy category B.

Paregoric (camphorated opium): Paregoric contains opium, which contains morphine and codeine. Although once widely used in the treatment of severe diarrhea, it can cause opioid-related adverse effects and is a Schedule III controlled substance. This drug may also be used to prevent withdrawal symptoms in newborns born to opioid-dependent mothers. Safer agents have replaced paregoric. For short-term use, paregoric is pregnancy category C.

Pharmacotherapy of Inflammatory Bowel Disease

61.5 Inflammatory bowel disease is treated with immunosuppressants and anti-inflammatory drugs.

Inflammatory bowel disease (IBD) is characterized by the presence of ulcers in the distal portion of the small intestine

NURSING PROCESS APPLICATION

Patients Receiving Antidiarrheal Therapy

Assessment	Potential Nursing Diagnoses
Prior to administration: • Obtain a complete health history, including allergies, drug history, and possible drug interactions. • Assess sodium, chloride, and potassium levels. • Evaluate results of a stool culture. • Assess for presence of dehydration. • Obtain vital signs and an electrocardiogram (ECG) as directed.	• *Risk for Deficient Fluid Volume,* related to fluid loss secondary to diarrhea • *Risk for Falls,* related to drowsiness secondary to drug therapy

Planning: Patient Goals and Expected Outcomes

The patient will:

- Report relief of diarrhea.
- Demonstrate an understanding of the drug's action by accurately describing drug adverse effects and precautions.
- Immediately report effects such as persistent diarrhea, constipation, abdominal pain, blood in stool, confusion, dizziness, or fever.

Implementation

Interventions and (Rationales)	Patient and Family Education
• Monitor the frequency, volume, and consistency of stools. (These determine the effectiveness of drug therapy.)	Advise the patient to: • Record the frequency of stools. • Note if any blood is present in stools. • Report any abdominal pain or abdominal distention immediately.
• Minimize the risk of dehydration and electrolyte imbalances by encouraging intake of oral fluids. (These symptoms may occur secondary to diarrhea.)	• Instruct the patient to increase fluid intake and drink electrolyte-enriched fluids.
• Prevent accidental overdosage. (Overdose of opioids in infants may cause serious CNS and respiratory depression.)	• Instruct the patient who is using liquid preparations to use the dropper included to measure the medication dosage and not to use household measurements.
• Monitor for dry mouth. (This is an adverse effect of medications.)	• Instruct the patient to suck on ice or sour candy or to chew gum to relieve the sensation of dry mouth.
• Initiate safety measures to prevent falls. (These medications may cause drowsiness.)	Instruct the patient to: • Refrain from driving or performing other hazardous activities until the effects of the drug are known. • Abstain from using alcohol or other CNS depressants.

Evaluation of Outcome Criteria

Evaluate the effectiveness of drug therapy by confirming that patient goals and expected outcomes have been met (see "Planning").

(Crohn's disease) or mucosal erosions in the large intestine (ulcerative colitis). IBD is treated with medications from several classifications. Over 1 million Americans are estimated to have IBD.

The etiology of IBD remains largely unknown. Several genes involved with immune responses have been identified as being associated with the disorder. It is hypothesized that these defective genes cause hyperactivity of T-cell responses to normal flora in the terminal ileum and colon. These hyperactive responses result in chronic intestinal inflammation.

In addition to genetic susceptibility, it is well established that certain environmental triggers exacerbate symptoms of IBD. The best-studied trigger for Crohn's disease is smoking. Infections, the use of NSAIDs, and a high level of stress are additional environmental factors that have been identified.

Symptoms of IBD range from mild to acute, and the condition is characterized by alternating periods of remission and exacerbation. The most common clinical presentation of ulcerative colitis is abdominal cramping with frequent bowel movements. Severe disease may lead to weight loss, bloody diarrhea, high fever, and dehydration. The patient with Crohn's disease also presents with abdominal pain, cramping, and diarrhea, which may have been present for years before seeking treatment. Symptoms of Crohn's disease are often similar to those of ulcerative colitis.

The expected outcomes for the pharmacotherapy of Crohn's disease are as follows:

- Reduce the acute symptoms of active disease by induction therapy and place the disease in remission.
- Keep the disease in remission with maintenance therapy.
- Change the natural course or progression of the disease.

The mainstays of Crohn's disease induction pharmacotherapy have been the 5-aminosalicylic acid (5-ASA) agents that include sulfasalazine (Azulfidine), olsalazine (Dipentum), balsalazide (Colazal), and mesalamine (Asacol, Canasa, Lialda, others). These agents act rapidly and exhibit a higher safety

TABLE 61.4 Selected Drugs for Inflammatory Bowel Disease and Irritable Bowel Syndrome

Drug	Route and Adult Dose (maximum dose where indicated)	Adverse Effects
Agents for Inflammatory Bowel Disease		
balsalazide (Colazal)	PO: 2.25 g 3 times/day for 8–12 weeks (max: 6.75 g/day)	*Headache, abdominal pain, diarrhea, nausea, vomiting, rash, allergic reactions* Hepatotoxicity, blood dyscrasias salicylate hypersensitivity, crystalluria (sulfasalazine)
mesalamine (Asacol, Canasa, Lialda, others)	PO (delayed release tablets): 800 mg tid for 6 weeks PO (delayed release capsules): 1 g qid for 8 weeks	
olsalazine (Dipentum)	PO: 500 mg bid (max: 3 g/day)	
sulfasalazine (Azulfidine)	PO: 1–2 g/day in four divided doses (max: 8 g/day)	
Agents for Irritable Bowel Syndrome		
alosetron (Lotronex)	PO: Begin with 1 mg daily for 4 weeks; may increase to 1 mg bid (max: 2 mg/day)	*Constipation, abdominal discomfort, nausea, and rash* Ischemic colitis, ileus
dicyclomine (Bentyl)	PO/IM: 20–40 mg qid (max: 160 mg/day PO; 80 mg/day IM)	*Dry mouth, blurred vision, drowsiness, constipation, urinary hesitancy, and tachycardia* Confusion, paralytic ileus
hyoscyamine (Anaspaz, Gastrosed, Levsin)	PO: 0.15–0.3 mg 1–4 times/day	
lubiprostone (Amitiza)	Chronic idiopathic constipation: PO: 24 mcg taken twice daily IBS with constipation: PO: 8 mcg taken twice daily (max: 48 mcg/day)	*Nausea, diarrhea, headache, dyspnea* Allergic reactions

Note: *Italics* indicate common adverse effects. Underline indicates serious adverse effects.

profile than the second-line agents. The 5-ASA agents, however, are not very effective in maintaining remission. Doses for the 5-ASA drugs are listed in Table 61.4.

Once in remission, maintenance therapy of Crohn's disease is started with immunosuppressive agents, which include azathioprine (Imuran), mercaptopurine (Purinethol), or methotrexate (MTX). These drugs are not used for induction therapy because they have a 3-month onset of action. They are, however, effective at extending the time between relapses. For a detailed discussion of immunosuppressant therapy, refer to Chapter 45.

When IBD is especially severe, PO corticosteroids such as prednisone are used as induction therapy. Corticosteroid therapy may also be implemented when patients have not responded well to the 5-ASA drugs. Because of their potentially serious long-term adverse effects, however, they are prescribed for the shortest length of time needed to send the disease into remission. For a detailed discussion of corticosteroid therapy, refer to Chapter 69.

Budesonide (Entocort-EC) is a corticosteroid with interesting properties that allow it to be used as a first-line therapy for IBD. Entocort-EC is encapsulated to avoid significant absorption in the stomach or duodenum. This drug is released slowly and reaches a high concentration in the terminal ileum and proximal colon—the two most frequently affected sites for IBD. Thus budesonide is in direct contact with the GI mucosa and produces a topical anti-inflammatory effect. In addition, when budesonide is absorbed, it is almost entirely removed by first-pass metabolism in the liver. Thus this drug shows few of the adverse effects seen with the long-term use of the other corticosteroids. It is approved for mild to moderate Crohn's disease.

The introduction of biologic therapies in the late 1990s gave clinicians another valuable tool in the pharmacotherapy of IBD. The tumor necrosis factor (TNF) inhibitor infliximab (Remicade) has been shown to effectively reduce the acute symptoms of and provide maintenance therapy for both Crohn's disease and ulcerative colitis. A second anti-TNF drug, adalimumab (Humira), was approved in 2007 for Crohn's disease. Recently a pegylated TNF inhibitor, called certolizumab pegol (Cimzia), was approved that offers dosing at 2- to 4-week intervals. Natalizumab (Tysabri), a monoclonal antibody previously approved for multiple sclerosis, was approved for treating Crohn's disease in 2008. The biologic therapies are expensive and patients experience a much higher rate of serious infections due to their immunosuppressive actions. Natalizumab has other very serious adverse effects that limit its use (see Chapter 25). Biologic therapies are currently recommended only when corticosteroid therapy is unable to control symptoms. Because these drugs cause healing of the GI mucosa, it is possible that early use of these drugs could change the progressive course of IBD. This is an area of active research. For a detailed discussion of biologic therapies and doses of these drugs, refer to Chapter 45.

MyNursingKit | Crohn's and Colitis Foundation

PROTOTYPE DRUG Sulfasalazine (Azulfidine)

Classification: **Therapeutic:** Agent for inflammatory bowel disease
Pharmacologic: 5-aminosalicylate, anti-inflammatory, sulfonamide

Therapeutic Effects and Uses: Approved in 1950, sulfasalazine is a PO drug with anti-inflammatory properties that is approved to treat mild to moderate symptoms of ulcerative colitis for adults and children 6 years and older. Sulfasalazine is used off-label to treat Crohn's disease. It is approved as an alternate drug in the pharmacotherapy of rheumatoid arthritis and is classified as a disease-modifying antirheumatic drug (DMARD) (see Chapter 75).

Colon bacteria metabolize sulfasalazine to two active metabolites: sulfapyridine and 5-ASA (also called mesalamine). These agents are responsible for its anti-inflammatory properties. Mesalamine (Asacol, Canasa, others) is also available as an IBS drug.

Mechanism of Action: Sulfasalazine and its metabolites inhibit the mediators of inflammation in the colon such as prostaglandins and leukotrienes.

Pharmacokinetics:

Route(s)	PO
Absorption	Sulfasalazine is only10–15% absorbed but its metabolites in the colon produce the therapeutic effects
Distribution	Crosses the placenta; secreted in breast milk; 93% bound to plasma protein
Primary metabolism	Hepatic; intestinal metabolism to sulfapyridine and 5-ASA
Primary excretion	Renal; active metabolites in the feces
Onset of action	Peak: 1.5–6 h
Duration of action	Half-life: 5–10 h

Adverse Effects: The most common adverse effects of sulfasalazine are GI related and include nausea, vomiting, diarrhea, dyspepsia, and abdominal pain. Dividing the total daily dose evenly throughout the day and using the enteric-coated tablets may improve adherence. Headache is common. Blood dyscrasias occur infrequently during therapy. Skin rashes are relatively common and may be a sign of a more serious adverse effect such as Stevens–Johnson syndrome. This drug may impair male fertility, which reverses when the drug is discontinued. Sulfasalazine can cause photosensitivity.

Contraindications/Precautions: Sulfasalazine is contraindicated in patients with sulfonamide or salicylate (aspirin or 5-ASA) hypersensitivity. Patients with preexisting anemia, folate, or other hematologic disorders should use this drug with caution because it may worsen blood dyscrasias. Sulfasalazine should be used with caution in patients with hepatic impairment because this drug can cause hepatotoxicity. This drug is contraindicated in patients with urinary obstruction and should be used with caution in dehydrated patients because it may cause crystalluria. Patients with diabetes or hypoglycemia should use sulfasalazine with caution because the drug can increase insulin secretion and worsen hypoglycemia.

Drug Interactions: Sulfasalazine may worsen bone marrow suppression caused by methotrexate and also result in additive hepatotoxicity. Absorption of digoxin may be decreased. Sulfasalazine is a folic acid antagonist and will inhibit absorption of this vitamin. Sulfasalazine can displace warfarin from it protein binding sites, causing increased anticoagulant effects. **Herbal/Food**: Unknown.

Pregnancy: Categories B and D (near term).

Treatment of Overdose: Overdose will cause abdominal pain, anuria, drowsiness, gastric distress, nausea, seizures, and vomiting. Treatment is mostly supportive with gastric lavage, emesis, and alkalinization of urine.

Nursing Responsibilities:

- Obtain a complete health history, including allergies, drug history, and possible drug interactions.
- Perform a complete assessment of GI functioning and symptoms of ulcerative colitis, which include abdominal cramping with frequent bowel movements, weight loss, bloody diarrhea, high fever, and dehydration.
- Monitor for GI distress, including nausea, vomiting, diarrhea, dyspepsia, and abdominal pain. If symptoms persist, the prescriber may withhold the drug for 5 to 7 days and restart it at a lower dosage level.
- Be aware that adverse reactions generally occur within a few days to 12 weeks after the start of therapy. They are most likely to occur in patients who are receiving high doses.
- Monitor laboratory tests for red blood cell counts and folate levels in patients on high doses (more than 2 g/day); a daily supplement may be prescribed. Patients with preexisting anemia, folate, or other hematologic disorders should use the drug with caution because it may worsen blood dyscrasias.
- Response to therapy and duration of treatment are determined by endoscopic examinations.

Patient and Family Education:

- Examine stools and report to the health care provider if enteric-coated tablets have passed intact in feces. If this occurs, a conventional tablet form can be ordered.
- Increase fluid intake to 2 to 3 L/day because this drug may cause crystals in the urine. Be aware that this drug may color urine and skin orange-yellow.
- Attend all follow-up examinations. Relapses occur in about 40% of patients after an initial satisfactory response.
- It is recommended that the interval between doses does not exceed 8 hours (even if administered at night).
- Men may experience a decreased production of sperm and infertility which is reversed with the discontinuation of this drug.
- Avoid driving and performing other hazardous activities until the effects of this drug are known because this drug may cause drowsiness or dizziness.
- Avoid prolonged sun exposure because the skin may be more sensitive. Wear sunscreen, protective clothing, and sunglasses if exposed to direct sunlight.

Drugs Similar to Sulfasalazine (Azulfidine)

Other 5-aminosalicylates include balsalazide, mesalamine, and olsalazine.

Balsalazide (Colazal): Approved in 2000, balsalazide is a PO anti-inflammatory agent approved for the symptomatic treatment of ulcerative colitis in patients age 5 and above. Like sulfasalazine, balsalazide is metabolized in the intestinal mucosa to 5-ASA, which is responsible for its therapeutic effects. Almost 100% of this drug reaches the colon without being absorbed; thus the primary action of the drug is topical rather than systemic. The drug is well tolerated with headache, abdominal pain, diarrhea, nausea, and vomiting being the most common adverse effects. Patients with salicylate hypersensitivity should not take this drug. Rare cases of hepatotoxicity have occurred. This drug is pregnancy category B.

Mesalamine (Asacol, Canasa, Lialda, others): Approved in 1987, mesalamine is sometimes referred to by its chemical name, 5-ASA. It is FDA approved for the treatment of active ulcerative colitis and used off-label for Crohn's disease. A delayed release formulation (Asacol) was developed for maintenance therapy, and a rectal suppository (Canasa) is available to treat ulcerative proctitis. Like other drugs in this class, mesalamine tablets and capsules are designed to release the drug in the terminal ileum and colon to produce its effects topically in the intestinal mucosa. Headache, abdominal pain, diarrhea, nausea, and vomiting are the most common adverse effects. Rectal irritation may be caused by the suppository forms of the drug. Patients with salicylate hypersensitivity should not take this drug. This drug is pregnancy category B.

Olsalazine (Dipentum): Like other drugs in this class, olsalazine is an oral agent that is metabolized in the intestinal mucosa to 5-ASA, which produces a topical anti-inflammatory effect. Nearly 100% of this drug reaches the colon without being absorbed systemically. Approved in 1990, the only indication for this drug is for the maintenance of remission of ulcerative colitis in patients who are unable to tolerate sulfasalazine. The most commonly reported adverse effects are diarrhea, abdominal pain, and rash. Rare cases of hepatotoxicity have occurred. This drug is pregnancy category C.

Pharmacotherapy of Irritable Bowel Syndrome

61.6 Irritable bowel syndrome is treated with dietary management, symptomatic therapy, and drugs that regulate intestinal motility.

Irritable bowel syndrome (IBS), also known as spastic colon or mucous colitis, is a common disorder of the lower GI tract characterized by symptoms that include abdominal pain, visible bloating, excessive gas, and colicky cramping. Bowel habits are altered, with diarrhea alternating with constipation, and there may be mucus in the stool. Pain is usually relieved by defecation, although the patient usually feels as if the evacuation is incomplete. Symptoms of IBS are likely caused by altered GI motility, increased peristalsis, and increased pain sensitivity of the GI tract.

CONNECTIONS

Patient Safety

Infusion Calculations

A nurse is starting an infusion of Remicade on a patient with Crohn's disease. To save time, the nurse prepares the infusion based on the patient's body weight from the last infusion 6 weeks ago.

What error has occurred? How could it have been avoided?

See Answers to Patient Safety Questions in Appendix A.

Pharm*FACT*

Irritable bowel syndrome affects 10% to 20% of adults, and women are twice as likely to have the disorder. *Source:* Olden, 2003.

The diagnosis of IBS is typically one of exclusion, ruling out other diseases such as colon cancer, ulcerative colitis, intestinal infections, Crohn's disease, and diverticulitis. IBS is considered a functional bowel disorder, meaning that the normal operation of the digestive tract is impaired without the presence of detectable organic disease. It is not a precursor of more serious disease. Treatment of IBS is supportive, with drug therapy targeted at symptomatic treatment depending on whether constipation or diarrhea is the predominant symptom. There is no single treatment that is effective for all, or even most, patients.

Lifestyle changes, diet, and aggravating medications: Stress is not a cause of IBS, but it can influence the condition. Attempts should be made to identify stressors and develop positive coping strategies. Psychotherapy, relaxation techniques, and hypnosis may benefit some patients. Food-specific triggers are not always apparent. However, the patient should keep a food diary in an attempt to recognize and avoid foods that appear to worsen the condition. Dietary restriction of caffeine, wheat, or lactose-based products may be attempted. Foods that cause bloating and flatulence such as beans, cabbage, and peas should be avoided.

Part of a medical history for IBS should include drugs that may be contributing to the symptoms of IBS. Common drugs that may cause constipation include NSAIDs, calcium channel blockers, anticholinergics, and opioids. Diarrhea may result from the use of laxatives, magnesium-containing antacids, or antibiotics. Sometimes a change in medication can help reduce IBS symptoms.

Symptom-targeted therapy: Constipation, diarrhea, cramping, painful bowel movements, and rectal urgency occur frequently in patients with IBS. Because constipation and diarrhea often alternate, pharmacotherapy can be challenging. Fiber supplementation with nonprescription bulk laxatives such as psyllium has long been recommended as a treatment for IBS and can help regulate bowel movements to bring relief to some patients. Unfortunately, increased fiber intake will worsen the symptoms in some patients. Loperamide (Imodium), an antidiarrheal, is effective at relieving symptoms of diarrhea in patients with IBS (see Section 61.4).

Antidepressants and antianxiety drugs: For many years the tricyclic antidepressants such as amitriptyline, desipramine (Norpramin), and doxepin (Sinequan) have been used to treat patients with IBS who have pain as a major symptom. Studies on the effectiveness of these drugs in reducing pain and diarrhea in patients with IBS are conflicting, but they may be indicated for those who have depression as a comorbid condition. Selective serotonin reuptake inhibitors (SSRIs) such as paroxetine (Paxil) and the benzodiazepines have also been studied but results suggest that their effectiveness at treating IBS is mild at best. They are not recommended agents.

MyNursingKit | Mechanism of Action Animation: Tegaserod

Antispasmodics and serotonin agents: Antispasmodic drugs are those that relax smooth muscle and slow peristalsis. Dicyclomine (Bentyl) and hyoscyamine (Levsin) are older anticholinergic drugs that are used to reduce bowel spasms in patients with diarrhea-predominant IBS (see Chapter 18). Tegaserod (Zelnorm) is a serotonin (5-HT_4 receptor) agonist and is one of the few drugs approved for the short-term pharmacotherapy of IBS in women presenting with constipation as the primary complaint. It is classified as a serotonin agonist because it acts by binding to serotonin receptors in the GI tract, which stimulates the peristaltic reflex. Alosetron (Lotronex) is a serotonin (5-HT_3) antagonist approved for diarrhea-predominant IBS in women. The two serotonin subreceptors, 5-HT_3 and 5-HT_4, have opposite effects on the colon. Doses for the antispasmodics are listed in Table 61.4.

Drugs that are used to treat IBS do not alter the course of the disease and, in some cases, may worsen patient symptoms. Research has not demonstrated that these drugs are any more effective than nonpharmacologic treatments such as IBS support groups, relaxation therapy, or dietary changes. There is no prototype drug for this condition. Drugs that provide symptomatic relief for some patients include alosetron, dicyclomine, hyoscyamine, and tegaserod.

Alosetron (Lotronex): By inhibiting serotonin (5-HT_3) receptors, alosetron reduces GI-related sensitivity and slows peristalsis in patients with diarrhea-predominant IBS. Alosetron was approved in 2000 but was withdrawn later that same year due to several deaths from ischemic colitis. This drug was allowed to return to the market in 2002 but with severe restrictions on its use. Health care providers who wish to prescribe alosetron must receive special training and testing to learn to appropriately diagnose IBS. Other therapies must have been attempted (and failed) prior to alosetron use. The starting dose was lowered from 1 mg bid to 1 mg daily. No refills are allowed without a follow-up exam by the prescribing health care provider. A risk–benefit statement must be signed by the patient and health care provider that they agree to adhere to therapy plans. Other adverse effects include constipation, abdominal discomfort, nausea, and rash. This drug is pregnancy category B.

Dicyclomine (Bentyl): Dicyclomine is an anticholinergic drug that was approved in 1950 for diarrhea-predominant IBS and other functional disorders of GI motility. Its primary action is antispasmodic, decreasing smooth muscle tone and slowing peristalsis. Dicyclomine may be administered PO or by IM injection. Frequent adverse effects include typical anticholinergic effects such as dry mouth, blurred vision, drowsiness, urinary hesitancy, and tachycardia. Other drugs with anticholinergic activity, such as antihistamines or tricyclic antidepressants, will cause additive adverse effects. This drug is pregnancy category B.

Hyoscyamine (Anaspaz, Gastrosed, Levsin): Available since the FDA was established in 1938, hyoscyamine is an anticholinergic drug that is usually administered PO, but parenteral forms are available. It is approved to treat peptic ulcer disease and diarrhea-predominant IBS because the drug decreases acid secretion of the stomach and slows peristalsis. It has also been used to reverse bradycardia, to relieve symptoms of allergic rhinitis, and to dry respiratory and salivary secretions prior to surgery. Whereas in 1938 hyoscyamine may have been a drug of choice for these conditions, it has been replaced by safer and more effective drugs for nearly every indication. At the doses needed to treat IBS, anticholinergic adverse effects are prominent. This drug is pregnancy category C.

CONNECTION *Checkpoint* 61.2

Anticholinergic drugs can inhibit muscarinic or nicotinic receptors. From what you learned in Chapter 18, which type do dicyclomine and hyoscyamine inhibit? What drug is the prototype for this class? See Answer to Connection Checkpoint 61.2 in Appendix A.

Lubiprostone (Amitiza): Lubiprostone was approved in 2006 for the treatment of chronic idiopathic constipation. In 2008, approval was granted for the use of this drug in treating constipation-predominant IBS in women over age 18. Lubiprostone increases fluid secretion by activating chloride channels in the intestinal luminal cells, thereby altering stool consistency and promoting regular bowel movements. The most common adverse effect is nausea, which can be reduced by taking the drug with food. Lubiprostone should not be administered to patients with diarrhea or suspected GI obstruction. This drug is pregnancy category C.

Tegaserod (Zelnorm): Tegaserod is a serotonin (5-HT_4) agonist that is prescribed for women who have the constipation-dominant form of the disease. This drug decreases abdominal pain and bloating and increases stool formation and the number of bowel movements. It is available in tablet form only. Effectiveness in men is being investigated but has not been established.

Tegaserod was approved in 2002 but postmarketing studies have determined an unacceptable rate of MI, stroke, and unstable angina in patients using this drug. It was withdrawn from the U.S. market in early 2007 due to these safety concerns but returned later that same year with tighter restrictions. Availability is limited to women under age 55 who meet specific guidelines. Patients with a history of cardiovascular disease are excluded from treatment. At this time it is approved for investigational use only for a maximum of 12 weeks of therapy.

Pathophysiology of Nausea and Vomiting

61.7 Nausea and vomiting occur when the vomiting center in the medulla is stimulated.

Nausea is an unpleasant feeling of the need to vomit that is accompanied by weakness, diaphoresis, dizziness, and hyperproduction of saliva. Intense nausea often leads to **vomiting,** or emesis, in which the stomach contents are forced upward into the esophagus and out of the mouth. Vomiting is a defense mechanism used by the body to rid itself of toxic substances.

Vomiting is a reflex primarily controlled by a portion of the medulla of the brain known as the **vomiting center,** which receives sensory signals from the digestive tract, the inner ear, and the **chemoreceptor trigger zone (CTZ)** in the cerebral cortex. Interestingly, the CTZ is not protected by the blood–brain barrier, as is the vast majority of the brain; thus these neurons can directly sense the presence of toxic substances in the blood. Once the vomiting reflex is triggered, wavelike contractions of the stomach quickly propel its contents upward and out of the body.

The treatment outcomes for nausea or vomiting should focus on removal of the cause whenever feasible. Nausea and vomiting are common symptoms associated with a wide variety of conditions. Some conditions originate in the GI tract itself, such as peptic ulcer disease, GI obstruction, gallbladder disease, food poisoning, or ingestion of a toxic substance that irritates the mucosa. The nausea and vomiting may originate from systemic sources such as those caused by cancer, pregnancy, radiation sickness, migraine headache, trauma to the head or abdominal organs, inner ear disorders, extreme pain, diabetes, or systemic drug use. In addition to the CTZ, other parts of the nervous system may promote nausea and vomiting in response to nervousness, emotional imbalances, changes in body position (motion sickness), extreme stress, or when confronted with unpleasant sights, smells, or sounds.

The nausea and vomiting experienced by many women during the first trimester of pregnancy is referred to as morning sickness. The cause of nausea and vomiting during pregnancy is largely unknown but is probably due to hormonal changes, especially in levels of estrogen and human chorionic gonadotropin (HCG). All women of childbearing years who present with nausea or vomiting should receive a pregnancy test because this is such a common explanation for these symptoms. Should this condition become acute, such as continual vomiting, it may lead to **hyperemesis gravidarum,** a situation in which the health and safety of the mother and developing baby can become severely compromised. Complications may include dehydration, electrolyte imbalances, and significant weight loss. Pharmacotherapy with fluid and electrolyte solutions and antiemetics is initiated after other antinausea measures have proven ineffective.

Pharm*FACT*

Although "morning" sickness occurs in 75% to 80% of pregnancies, 83% of the affected women experience the condition throughout the day, not just in the morning. Morning sickness usually ends by week 12. *Source:* Badell, Ramin, & Smith, 2006.

Nausea and vomiting are the most frequently listed adverse effects for oral medications. The nurse should remember that because the vomiting center lies in the brain, nausea and vomiting occur just as frequently with parenteral formulations as with oral drugs. The most extreme example of this occurs with the antineoplastic drugs, most of which cause intense nausea and vomiting regardless of the route they are administered. The capacity of a chemotherapeutic drug to cause vomiting is called its **emetogenic potential.** Nausea and vomiting are common reasons for patient lack of adherence to the therapeutic regimen and for discontinuation of drug therapy.

When large amounts of fluids are vomited, dehydration and significant weight loss may occur. Because the contents lost from the stomach are strongly acidic, vomiting may cause a change in the pH of the blood, resulting in metabolic alkalosis. With excessive loss, severe acid–base disturbances can lead to vascular collapse, resulting in death if medical intervention is not initiated. Dehydration is especially dangerous for infants, small children, and the elderly and is evidenced by dry mouth, sticky saliva, and reduced urine output that is dark yellow-orange to brown in color.

Pharmacotherapy of Nausea and Vomiting

61.8 Antiemetics are prescribed to treat nausea, vomiting, and motion sickness.

Drugs from at least eight different classes are used to prevent or treat nausea and vomiting. Most of these drugs were originally developed for other indications, and their antiemetic characteristics were discovered later. Selection of a particular agent depends on the experience of the health care provider and the cause of the nausea and vomiting.

Patients who are seeking self-treatment can find several options available OTC. For example, simple nausea and vomiting are sometimes relieved by antacids or diphenhydramine (Benadryl). Herbal options include peppermint and ginger, which are the most popular herbal therapies for nausea and vomiting.

Relief of serious nausea or vomiting requires prescription medications. Patients who are receiving antineoplastic drugs may receive three or more antiemetics concurrently to reduce the nausea and vomiting from chemotherapy. In fact, therapy with antineoplastic drugs is one of the most common reasons for prescribing antiemetic drugs. Many antiemetic agents are available through the IM, IV, or suppository routes to prevent loss of the medication due to vomiting. Pharmacotherapy Illustrated 61.1 shows the mechanisms of action of antiemetic medications. Doses for selected antiemetics are listed in Table 61.5.

Anticholinergic agents and antihistamines: These agents are effective for treating simple nausea, with some being available OTC. For example, nausea due to motion sickness is effectively treated with anticholinergics or antihistamines. Motion sickness is a disorder that affects a portion of the inner ear that is associated with significant nausea. The most common drug used for motion sickness is scopolamine (Hyoscine, Transderm), an anticholinergic drug that is usually administered as a transdermal patch. Antihistamines such as dimenhydrinate (Dramamine) and meclizine (Antivert) are also effective but may cause significant drowsiness in some patients. Drugs that are used to treat motion sickness are most effective when taken 20 to 60 minutes before travel is expected.

Antipsychotic agents (antidopaminergics): The primary indication for phenothiazines is the treatment of psychoses (see Chapter 24), but they are also very effective antiemetics. Phenothiazines inhibit dopaminergic receptors in the CTZ, and the severe nausea and vomiting associated with antineoplastic therapy are often treated with these agents. Some of the phenothiazines may cause sedation, and extrapyramidal symptoms (EPS) are a concern with long-term therapy. Promethazine (Phenergan) is an older phenothiazine that is available by the PO, rectal, and parenteral routes that also has significant anticholinergic properties. Nonphenothiazine antipsychotics that have high antiemetic activity include haloperidol (Haldol) and droperidol (Inapsine). Droperidol is only available by the parenteral route.

Benzodiazepines: The primary indication for benzodiazepine is anxiety. Benzodiazepines are ineffective as antiemetics when used as monotherapy. However, they relax the patient and decrease the anxiety associated with chemotherapy and the anticipation of severe nausea and vomiting. Lorazepam (Ativan) is the drug in this class that is most frequently used as an off-label antiemetic adjunct.

PHARMACOTHERAPY *ILLUSTRATED* 61.1

Mechanisms of Action of Antiemetic Medications

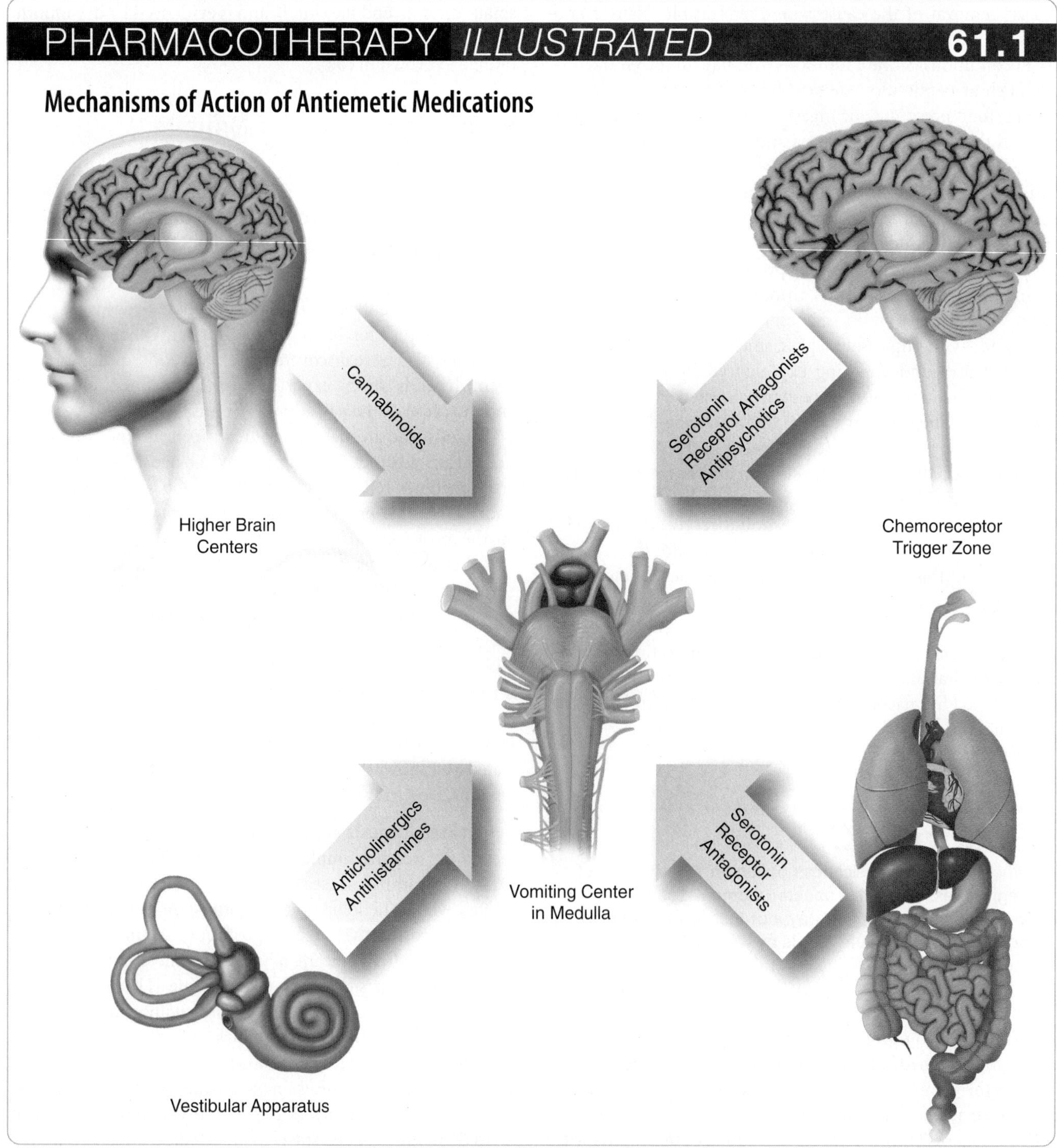

TABLE 61.5 Selected Antiemetics

Drug	Route and Adult Dose (maximum dose where indicated)	Adverse Effects
Anticholinergics-Antihistamines		
cyclizine hydrochloride (Marezine)	PO: 50 mg every 4–6 h (max: 200 mg/day)	*Drowsiness, dry mouth, blurred vision (scopolamine), hypotension (cyclizine)* Hypersensitivity reaction, sedation, tremors, seizures, hallucinations, paradoxical excitation (more common in children), hypotension
dimenhydrinate (Dramamine, others)	PO: 50–100 mg every 4–6 h (max: 400 mg/day)	
diphenhydramine (Benadryl, others)	PO: 25–50 mg tid-qid (max: 300 mg/day)	
hydroxyzine (Atarax, Vistaril)	PO: 25–100 mg tid or qid (max: 400 mg/day)	
meclizine (Antivert, Bonine, others)	PO: 25–50 mg daily, take 1 h before travel (max: 50 mg/day)	
scopolamine (Hyoscine, Transderm-Scop)	Transdermal: 0. 5 mg (patch) every 72 h	
Benzodiazepines		
lorazepam (Ativan)	PO: 0.5–2 mg every 4–6 h (max: 10 mg/day)	*Dizziness, drowsiness, ataxia, fatigue, slurred speech* Paradoxical excitation (more common in children), seizures (if abruptly discontinued), coma
Cannabinoids		
dronabinol (Marinol)	PO: 5 mg/m^2 1–3 h before administration of chemotherapy, then every 2–4 h after chemotherapy for a total of 4–6 doses;	*Dizziness, drowsiness, euphoria, confusion, ataxia, asthenia, increased sensory awareness* Paranoia, decreased motor coordination, hypotension
nabilone (Cesamet)	PO: 1–2 mg bid	
Glucocorticoids		
dexamethasone (Decadron)	PO: 0.25–4 mg bid-qid	*Mood swings, weight gain, acne, facial flushing, nausea, insomnia, sodium and fluid retention, impaired wound healing, menstrual abnormalities, insomnia* Peptic ulcer, hypocalcemia, osteoporosis with possible bone fractures, loss of muscle mass, decreased growth in children, possible masking of infections
methylprednisolone (Medrol, Solu-Medrol, others)	PO: 4–48 mg/day in divided doses	
Neurokinin Receptor Antagonist		
aprepitant (Emend)	PO: 125 mg 1 h prior to chemotherapy	*Fatigue, constipation, diarrhea, anorexia, nausea, hiccups* Dehydration, peripheral neuropathy, blood dyscrasias, pneumonia
Phenothiazine and Phenothiazine-Like		
metoclopramide (Reglan, others)	PO: 1–2 mg/kg 1 h prior to chemotherapy	*Dry eyes, blurred vision, dry mouth, constipation, drowsiness, photosensitivity* EPS, neuroleptic malignant syndrome, agranulocytosis, orthostatic hypotension
perphenazine (Phenazine, Trilafon)	PO: 8–16 mg bid-qid	
prochlorperazine (Compazine, others)	PO: 5–10 mg tid or qid Rectal: 25 mg bid	
promethazine (Phenergan, others)	PO: 12.5–25 mg every 4 hours or qid	
Serotonin (5-HT_3) Receptor Antagonists		
dolasetron (Anzemet)	PO: 100 mg 1 h prior to chemotherapy	*Headache, drowsiness, fatigue, constipation, diarrhea, flulike symptoms* Dysrhythmias, EPS, hepatic failure
granisetron (Kytril, Sancuso)	IV: 10 mcg/kg 30 min prior to chemotherapy PO: 2 mg/day 1 h prior to chemotherapy Transdermal patch: 1 patch 1–2 days prior to chemotherapy	
ondansetron (Zofran)	PO: 4 mg tid prn	
palonosetron (Aloxi)	IV: 0.25 mg 30 min prior to chemotherapy	

Note: *Italics* indicate common adverse effect. Underline indicates serious adverse effects.

Cannabinoids: Cannabinoids are drugs that contain the same active ingredient as marijuana. Dronabinol (Marinol) and nabilone (Cesamet) are given PO to produce antiemetic effects and relaxation with less euphoria compared to marijuana. Cannabinoids are not as effective as other antiemetics.

Corticosteroids: Dexamethasone (Decadron) and methylprednisolone (Solu-Medrol) are used to prevent chemotherapy-induced and postsurgical nausea and vomiting. They are reserved for acute cases due to the possibility of serious adverse effects and are most often used in combination with other antiemetics. Dexamethasone is used for the treatment of delayed nausea and vomiting, which are common problems with certain antineoplastic drugs.

Serotonin (5-HT$_3$) antagonists: The serotonin antagonists include dolasetron (Anzemet), granisetron (Kytril), ondansetron (Zofran), and palonosetron (Aloxi). There are no major differences in effectiveness or toxicity of the serotonin receptor antagonists in treating acute nausea and vomiting. They are available by the PO or parenteral routes. Since the 1990s these drugs have become the most widely prescribed drugs for chemotherapy-induced nausea and vomiting. They exhibit few adverse effects, including headache, constipation or diarrhea, and dizziness.

Other drugs: Aprepitant (Emend) is the first of a new class of antiemetics, known as the neurokinin (NK) receptor antagonists that reduce the level of Substance P, which is involved in the emesis reflex. Aprepitant is FDA approved as part of a 3-day antiemetic regimen for antineoplastic chemotherapy in conjunction with a corticosteroid (dexamethasone) and a 5-HT$_3$ antagonist (odansetron). Aprepitant is pregnancy category B. Tricyclic antidepressants such as amitriptyline (Elavil) have also been used to reduce chronic idiopathic nausea.

On some occasions, it is desirable to stimulate the vomiting reflex with drugs called emetics. Indications for emetics include ingestion of poisons and overdoses of oral drugs. Ipecac syrup, given PO, or apomorphine, given subcutaneously, will induce vomiting in about 15 minutes.

CONNECTION *Checkpoint* 61.3

From what you learned in Chapter 24, define extrapyramidal adverse effects and provide examples of symptoms that a patient with EPS might exhibit. See Answer to Connection Checkpoint 61.3 in Appendix A.

PROTOTYPE DRUG Prochlorperazine (Compazine)

Classification: **Therapeutic:** Antiemetic
Pharmacologic: Phenothiazine

Therapeutic Effects and Uses: Approved in 1982, prochlorperazine is a phenothiazine, which is the largest group of drugs prescribed for severe nausea and vomiting. Prochlorperazine is the most frequently prescribed antiemetic in its class. It is available by the PO (immediate and extended release), IV, IM, and rectal routes. As an antiemetic it is frequently given by rectal suppository. For preoperative nausea prophylaxis, it is administered IV (15 to 30 minutes) or IM (1 to 2 hours) before anesthesia induction. Other FDA-approved indications include anxiety and schizophrenia.

Mechanism of Action: Prochlorperazine acts by blocking dopamine receptors in the brain, which inhibits signals to the vomiting center in the medulla.

Pharmacokinetics:

Route(s)	PO, IM, IV, rectal
Absorption	Rapidly absorbed
Distribution	Widely distributed; crosses the placenta; secreted in breast milk; 91% bound to plasma protein
Primary metabolism	Hepatic
Primary excretion	Renal and biliary
Onset of action	PO: 30–40 minutes; rectal: 60 minutes
Duration of action	PO or rectal: 4–6 h

CONNECTIONS

Complementary and Alternative Therapies *Lactobacillus Acidophilus*

Description: *Lactobacillus acidophilus* is a probiotic bacterium that is normally found in the human alimentary canal and vagina.

History and Claims: *Lactobacillus acidophilus* is considered to be protective flora, inhibiting the growth of potentially pathogenic species such as *E. coli, Candida albicans, H. pylori*, and *Gardnerella vaginalis*. The primary use of *L. acidophilus* is to restore the normal flora of the intestine following diarrhea, particularly from antibiotic therapy.

Standardization: Supplements include capsules, tablets, and granules. Doses are not standardized, and tablet doses range from 50 to 500 mg. *L. acidophilus* may be obtained by drinking acidophilus milk or by eating yogurt or kefir containing live (or active) cultures. Those wishing to obtain *L. acidophilus* from yogurt should read the labels carefully, because not all products contain active cultures. For example, frozen yogurt contains no active cultures.

Evidence: One mechanism used by *L. acidophilus* to limit the growth of other bacterial species is the generation of hydrogen peroxide, which is toxic to most cells. It has also been shown to be effective at shortening episodes of acute infectious diarrhea. These supplements should probably not be used in severely immunosuppressed patients because they may cause infection. Some patients with IBS may benefit from the use of *Lactobacillus* supplements.

Source: From "Lactobacillus: A Review," by C. Slover and L. Danziger, 2007, *Clinical Microbiology Newsletter, 30*(4), 23–27; and "Review Article: Probiotics and Prebiotics in Irritable Bowel Syndrome," by R. Spiller, 2008, *Alimentary Pharmacology and Therapeutics, 28*(4), 385–396.

Adverse Effects: Prochlorperazine produces dose-related anticholinergic adverse effects such as dry mouth, sedation, constipation, blurred vision, orthostatic hypotension, and tachycardia. When used for prolonged periods at higher doses, EPS resembling those of Parkinson's disease are a serious concern. EPS symptoms are more prevalent in older adults. Other dose-related adverse effects include skin hyperpigmentation, agranulocytosis, leukopenia, photosensitivity, neuroleptic malignant syndrome, and retinopathy. In women, the prolonged use of prochlorperazine can alter menstrual patterns and cause breast enlargement with milk production. Men may experience breast enlargement or tenderness, inhibited ejaculation, and priapism (abnormal prolonged erection).

Contraindications/Precautions: This drug should not be used in patients with hypersensitivity to phenothiazines, in comatose patients, or in the presence of profound CNS depression. It is also contraindicated in children under 2 years of age or under 20 pounds. This drug may worsen agranulocytosis, organic brain damage, seizure disorders, or hepatic impairment.

Drug Interactions: Prochlorperazine interacts with alcohol and other CNS depressants to cause additive sedation and respiratory depression. Antacids and antidiarrheals inhibit the absorption of prochlorperazine. When taken with phenobarbital, the metabolism of prochlorperazine is increased. Use with tricyclic antidepressants antihistamines and other agents with anticholinergic activity may produce increased anticholinergic and hypotensive adverse effects. Concurrent use with SSRIs will slow the metabolism of phenothiazine and raise serum concentrations. **Herbal/Food**: Unknown.

Pregnancy: Category C.

Treatment of Overdose: Overdose may result in serious CNS depression and extrapyramidal signs. Patients may be treated symptomatically with anti-Parkinson drugs (for EPS) and possibly a CNS stimulant such as dextroamphetamine.

Nursing Responsibilities:

- Obtain a complete health history, including allergies, drug history, and possible drug interactions.
- Perform a complete assessment, including nausea and vomiting frequency, duration, severity, and precipitating factors.
- Place nauseated patients with altered consciousness in a side-lying position to prevent aspiration of vomitus. Prochlorperazine may depress the cough reflex, thereby placing the patient at greater risk for pulmonary aspiration.
- Withhold foods and fluids until the nausea subsides. Resume food intake gradually with a small amount of clear, cool liquids such as flavored gelatin, carbonated beverages, popsicles, and ice chips.
- Monitor for EPS in older adults, emaciated patients, and children, who are particularly susceptible to these adverse effects. Drug-induced parkinsonism and acute dyskinesia are most frequently seen at the onset of treatment.
- Be aware that the administration of antiemetics may mask other conditions associated with nausea such as intestinal obstruction and increased intracranial pressure.

Patient and Family Education:

- Do not drive or perform other hazardous activities until the effects of the drug are known because this drug may cause drowsiness or dizziness.
- Avoid alcohol while taking this drug because it will cause excessive drowsiness.
- Do not take this drug if tardive dyskinesia, a neurologic disorder with spasms and twitching of the face and arms, has previously occurred when taking other medications.
- Protect the skin from the direct rays of the sun and use a sunscreen lotion (SPF greater than 12) to prevent skin rash or sunburn.
- Immediately report tremor, involuntary twitching, or exaggerated restlessness if they persist more than a few hours to the health care provider. Other reportable symptoms include light-colored stools, changes in vision, sore throat, fever, or rash.

Drugs Similar to Prochlorperazine (Compazine)

The antiemetics have been described earlier in this section.

Pharmacotherapy of Pancreatitis

61.9 Pancreatic enzymes are administered as replacement therapy for patients with chronic pancreatitis.

The pancreas secretes insulin as well as essential digestive enzymes. The enzymatic portion of pancreatic juice contains carboxypeptidase, chymotrypsin, and trypsin, which are converted to their active forms once they enter the small intestine. Three other pancreatic enzymes—lipase, amylase, and nuclease—are secreted in their active form but require the presence of bile for optimum activity. When lack of pancreatic enzyme secretion results in malabsorption disorders, replacement therapy is warranted.

PharmFACT

Drugs are the cause of approximately 1.4% of all cases of pancreatitis. Drugs that are known to be associated with the disorder include corticosteroids, estrogens, sulfonamides, tetracycline, didanosine, furosemide, azathioprine, valproic acid, 5-ASA agents, and pentamidine.

Pancreatitis results when digestive enzymes remain in the pancreas rather than being released into the duodenum. Upon becoming activated and escaping into the surrounding tissue, the enzymes cause inflammation in the pancreas, which can lead to hemorrhage and necrosis. The backed-up enzymes and enteric bacteria may "leak" into the peritoneum, causing a severe systemic reaction and possibly death. Pancreatitis can be either acute or chronic. The two types of pancreatitis have different symptoms, mortality rates, and treatments.

NURSING PROCESS APPLICATION

Patients Receiving Antiemetic Therapy

Assessment	Potential Nursing Diagnoses
Prior to administration: • Obtain a complete health history, including allergies, drug history, and possible drug interactions. • Perform a complete assessment of nausea, including frequency, duration, severity, and precipitating factors, using tools such as self-care journals and visual analog scales. • Assess for the presence of dehydration and electrolyte imbalances. • Obtain vital signs.	• *Risk for Deficient Fluid Volume,* related to fluid loss secondary to vomiting • *Risk for Falls,* related to drowsiness secondary to drug therapy

Planning: Patient Goals and Expected Outcomes

The patient will:

- Report relief of nausea and vomiting.
- Demonstrate an understanding of the drug's action by accurately describing drug adverse effects and precautions.

Implementation

Interventions and (Rationales)	Patient and Family Education
• Monitor frequency, volume, and consistency of vomitus. (This is to determine the effectiveness of drug therapy.)	Instruct the patient to: • Record the frequency of nausea episodes and occurrence of vomiting. • Note if any blood is present in the vomitus. • Report any abdominal pain or abdominal distention immediately.
• Evaluate past experiences with nausea and vomiting such as pregnancy or car sickness. Identify factors that may cause or contribute to nausea such as medications or procedures. (Examining past experiences will aid in determining factors that induce nausea and possible coping strategies.) • Control environmental factors that may evoke nausea such as aversive odors, sounds, and unpleasant visual stimulation. (Health care providers often become immune to such factors and should consider that many factors in the environment may contribute to nausea.)	• Encourage patients to monitor and manage their own nausea. • Identify strategies that have been successful in relieving nausea.
• Monitor intake and output ratio and symptoms associated with dehydration and electrolyte imbalance. (These may occur secondary to vomiting.)	• If vomiting has been prolonged and dehydration is possible, instruct the patient to rise slowly from a recumbent position. • After nausea and vomiting have ceased, gradually increase fluid intake with sips of water or ice chips.
• Initiate safety measures to prevent falls. (Many antiemetics cause drowsiness, which places the patient at risk for injury.)	Instruct the patient to: • Refrain from driving or performing other hazardous activities until the effects of drug are known. • Abstain from using alcohol or other CNS depressants.
• Evaluate the impact of nausea on quality of life factors such as appetite, activity, job performance, role responsibilities, and sleep. (Patients with chronic nausea and vomiting due to various disease conditions or treatments will require individualized therapy to promote optimal outcome.)	• Instruct the patient to report the effectiveness of nausea therapy to the prescriber and its effect on activities of daily living.
• Hold all PO intake of food and beverage until nausea and vomiting have ceased. Incrementally initiate oral intake to prevent recurrence of nausea. (Intake should be withheld until nausea has diminished or vomiting has ceased.)	Instruct the patient to: • Perform frequent oral hygiene to promote comfort unless it stimulates nausea. • Initially resume diet with cold clear liquids and odorless foods. • Eat only small amounts of food that are appealing and that are high-carbohydrate and low-fat.
• Monitor laboratory values. (The loss of fluid associated with vomiting may alter laboratory values.)	Instruct the patient to: • Keep all laboratory appointments. • Report weakness and muscle cramping.

Evaluation of Outcome Criteria

Evaluate the effectiveness of drug therapy by confirming that patient goals and expected outcomes have been met (see "Planning").

Acute pancreatitis: Acute pancreatitis occurs most frequently in middle-aged adults and is often associated with gallstones in women and alcoholism in men. Symptoms of acute pancreatitis present suddenly, often after eating a fatty meal or consuming excessive amounts of alcohol. The most common symptom is a continuous severe pain in the epigastric area often radiating to the back. Fever, tachycardia, abdominal tenderness, and muscular guarding (involuntary spasm of the abdominal muscles when palpated) are common. Although most patients recover from the illness and regain normal pancreatic functions, a small percentage of patients experience recurring attacks and progress to chronic pancreatitis.

Many patients with acute pancreatitis require only bed rest, fasting, and adequate fluid and electrolyte therapy for a few days for the symptoms to subside. For patients with acute pain, an opioid such as hydromorphone (Dilaudid) brings effective relief. To reduce gastric and pancreatic juice secretions, H_2-receptor blockers, such as cimetidine (Tagamet), or proton pump inhibitors, such as omeprazole (Prilosec), may be prescribed. To decrease the amount of pancreatic enzymes secreted, carbonic anhydrase inhibitors, such as acetazolamide (Diamox), or antispasmodics, such as dicyclomine (Bentyl), may be used. In severe cases where enteral nutrition is not tolerated, total parenteral nutrition (TPN) may be necessary.

Cases of pancreatitis accompanied by a high fever and infection have a very high mortality rate. Pharmacotherapy with an antibiotic from the imipenem class is usually begun immediately.

Chronic pancreatitis: Seventy to eighty percent of chronic pancreatitis cases are associated with alcoholism. Other causes include pancreatic cancer and stones. Alcohol is thought to promote the formation of insoluble proteins that occlude the pancreatic duct. Pancreatic juice is prevented from flowing into the duodenum and remains in the pancreas, damaging cells and causing inflammation. Symptoms include chronic epigastric or left upper quadrant pain, anorexia, nausea, vomiting, and weight loss. **Steatorrhea,** the passing of bulky, foul-smelling fatty stools, occurs late in the course of the disease. Chronic pancreatitis causes permanent structural damage to the organ and may cause scarring of the pancreatic duct system. Chronic pancreatitis is a risk factor for the development of pancreatic cancer. The disease eventually leads to pancreatic insufficiency that may necessitate insulin therapy as well as replacement of pancreatic enzymes.

Drugs that are prescribed for the treatment of acute pancreatitis may also be used for patients with chronic pancreatitis. Fasting, IV fluids, and opioid analgesics may be necessary. The chronic, severe pain may lead to high doses of opioids and a possibility of drug dependence. In addition, the patient with chronic pancreatitis may require insulin and antiemetics.

Pancreatic enzyme supplementation is often used in patients with chronic pancreatitis. Supplementation sends a negative feedback message to stop secreting endogenous pancreatic enzymes, which can reduce pain. These supplements are given orally. Pancreatic enzyme supplements such as pancrelipase (Cotazym, Pancrease, others) or pancreatin (Ku-Zyme, Kutrase) help to digest fats and prevent steatorrhea.

PROTOTYPE DRUG Pancrelipase (Cotazym, Pancrease, others)

Classification: **Therapeutic:** Pancreatic enzymes
Pharmacologic: None

Therapeutic Effects and Uses: Pancrelipase contains lipase, protease, and amylase of pork origin and is used as replacement therapy for patients with insufficient pancreatic exocrine secretions, including those with pancreatitis and cystic fibrosis. Given PO the capsule dissolves in the alkaline environment of the duodenum and releases its enzymes. The enzymes act locally in the GI tract and are not absorbed. Pancrelipase is available in powder, tablet, and delayed release capsule formulations.

The different brand names of pancrelipase are not interchangeable because the amounts of pancreatic enzymes in each product are highly variable. Dose is based on the amount of fat in the diet: Approximately 8,000 units of lipase should be given for every 17 g of fat. Doses are taken just prior to meals or with meals.

Mechanism of Action: This agent facilitates the breakdown and conversion of lipids into glycerol and fatty acids, starches into dextrin and sugars, and proteins into peptides.

Pharmacokinetics:

Route(s)	PO
Absorption	Not absorbed
Distribution	Not distributed
Primary metabolism	Metabolized in the small bowel
Primary excretion	Feces
Onset of action	Immediate
Duration of action	Unknown

Adverse Effects: Adverse effects of pancrelipase are uncommon because the enzymes are not absorbed. The most common adverse effects are GI symptoms of nausea, vomiting, and diarrhea. Very high doses are associated with a risk for hyperuricemia.

Contraindications/Precautions: Pancrelipase is contraindicated in patients who are allergic to this drug or to pork products. The delayed release products should not be given to patients with acute pancreatitis.

Drug Interactions: Pancrelipase interacts with iron, which may result in decreased absorption of iron. Calcium and magnesium antacids may diminish the effectiveness of pancrelipase. **Herbal/Food:** Unknown.

Pregnancy: Category C.

Treatment of Overdose: High levels of uric acid may occur with overdose. Patients are treated symptomatically.

Nursing Responsibilities:

- Assess for abdominal pain, noting. Determine the type, intensity, and location of pain.
- Assess the patient for pork allergy because the enzymes in pancrelipase come from pork.

- Monitor intake and output ratio and weight. Note the patient's appetite and quality of stools, weight loss, abdominal bloating, polyuria, thirst, hunger, and itching. Pancreatic insufficiency is frequently associated with steatorrhea, bulky stools, and insulin-dependent diabetes.

Patient and Family Education:

- Take this drug just before, during, or immediately after meals.
- Capsules may be opened and sprinkled over food, but avoid chewing or crushing the microspheres inside the capsules.
- Do not switch to a different brand of pancrelipase without consulting the prescriber.
- Continue to take pancrelipase even if feeling well. Pancrelipase may control symptoms but will not cure the condition.
- Do not take this drug with iron supplements or with calcium or magnesium antacids because they may diminish the effectiveness of this drug.

Drugs Similar to Pancrelipase (Cotazym, Pancrease, Others)

The only other pancreatic enzyme supplement is pancreatin.

Pancreatin (Ku-Zyme, Kutrase): On an equal weight basis, pancrelipase is more potent than pancreatin with 12 times the lipolytic enzyme activity. Pancrelipase also contains at least four times as much trypsin and amylase than does pancreatin. The indications and adverse effects of the two products are the same. This drug is pregnancy category C.

UNDERSTANDING THE CHAPTER

Key Concepts Summary

61.1 Constipation is a decrease in the frequency of bowel movements.

61.2 Laxatives are drugs that increase the frequency and quality of bowel movements.

61.3 Diarrhea is an abnormal increase in the frequency and fluidity of bowel movements.

61.4 Opioids are the most effective drugs for controlling severe diarrhea.

61.5 Inflammatory bowel disease is treated with immunosuppressants and anti-inflammatory drugs.

61.6 Irritable bowel syndrome is treated with dietary management, symptomatic therapy, and drugs that regulate intestinal motility.

61.7 Nausea and vomiting occur when the vomiting center in the medulla is stimulated.

61.8 Antiemetics are prescribed to treat nausea, vomiting, and motion sickness.

61.9 Pancreatic enzymes are administered as replacement therapy for patients with chronic pancreatitis.

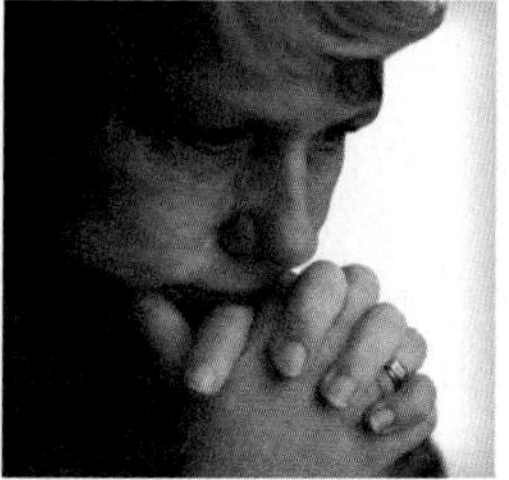

Making the PATIENT *Connection*

Remember the patient "Marjorie Hatford" at the beginning of the chapter? Now read the remainder of the case study. Based on the information presented within this chapter, respond to the critical thinking questions that follow.

Marjorie Hatford, a 71-year-old woman, presented with a history of chronic constipation. She is frustrated with frequent discomfort, abdominal distention, and inability to move her bowels without the use of enemas or digitations. Her bowel frequency is once per week.

Sometimes, Marjorie will take a harsh laxative, which creates uncontrollable liquid bowel movements. Because her bowel movements are often unpredictable, she fears going out in public and has limited her social activities for fear of laxative-induced incontinence. "Why can't I just go to the bathroom every day like I used to?" she asks.

Critical Thinking Questions

1. List the factors related to aging that may contribute to Marjorie's chronic constipation.
2. Create a chart like the one that follows, comparing various types of laxatives.

Laxative Type	How It Works	How Fast It Works	Problems Associated with Use
Bulk forming			
Stimulant			
Surfactant			
Saline			
Herbal			

3. What type of laxative would you suggest for this patient? Why?
4. What lifestyle modification would you recommend to this patient?

Case Study

Scott Mobley is a 57-year-old male with a diagnosis of Crohn's disease. He currently reports having three to five loose bowel movements per day, associated with gas, cramps, and urgency of evacuation. He was diagnosed with Crohn's disease 2 years earlier. Once he is stabilized, he will be placed on sulfasalazine.

1. Scott has asked you, his nurse, how this medication will work. What is your response?
2. What adverse effects of this medication should you share with Scott?
3. What contraindications would you teach Scott about the drug sulfasalazine?

NCLEX-RN® Review

1 The client is taking diphenoxylate with atropine (Lomotil). The nurse monitors for which of the following to determine whether the client is having a therapeutic effect from this medication?

1. Reduction of abdominal cramping
2. Minimal passage of flatus
3. Decrease in loose, watery stools
4. Increased bowel sounds

2 The client who is taking sulfasalazine (Azulfidine) develops a sore throat, bruising, and severe fatigue. The nurse determines that the client is most likely experiencing drug-induced:

1. Stevens–Johnson syndrome.
2. Blood dyscrasias.
3. Idiosyncratic reaction.
4. Hypersensitivity response

3 The nurse teaches the client who is taking prochlorperazine (Compazine) to discontinue the medication immediately and call the prescriber if which of the following occurs?

1. Nausea and vomiting
2. Facial twitching or abnormal involuntary body movements
3. Dry mouth, sedation, and constipation
4. Dizziness, lethargy, and ataxia

4 Zymase (pancrelipase) is prescribed for each of the following clients. A nurse should question the order for which client?

1. The client with allergy to pork products
2. The client with hypertension
3. The client with coronary artery disease
4. The client with hypersensitivity to iodine products

5 A health care provider orders tegaserod (Zelnorm) for a client with irritable bowel syndrome (IBS). The nurse should ask the client about a history of which of the following conditions prior to administration?

1. Multiple sclerosis
2. Femur fracture
3. Anemia
4. Cardiovascular disease

6 A client who has been taking over-the-counter bismuth subsalicylate (Kaopectate, Pepto-Bismol) for diarrhea for several days states that the medication does not seem to be working. Which of the following pharmacologic alternatives would the nurse consider? Select all that apply.

1. Diphenoxylate with atropine (Lomotil)
2. Magnesium hydroxide (Milk of Magnesia)
3. Octreotide (Sandostatin)
4. Metoclopramide (Reglan)
5. Psyllium (Metamucil)

See Answers to Critical Thinking Questions, Case Study, and NCLEX-RN® Review in Appendix A.

References

Badell, M. L., Ramin, S. M., & Smith, J. A. (2006). Treatment options for nausea and vomiting during pregnancy. *Pharmacotherapy, 26*(9), 1273–1287.

Barclay, L. (2007). New guidelines for treatment of irritable bowel syndrome in adults. *Medscape Medical News.* Retrieved August 15, 2008, from http://www.medscape.com/viewarticle/556356

Britt, H., & Fahridin, S. (2007). Presentation of nausea and vomiting. *Australian Family Physician, 36*(9), 682–683.

Feagan, B. G., Dieckgraefe, B. K., & Hanauer, S. B. (2006). *Advances in the treatment of Crohn's disease: From research to clinical practice.* Retrieved August 15, 2008, from http://www.medscape.com/viewprogram/5211

Herrstedt, J. (2008). Antiemetics: An update and the MASCC guidelines applied to clinical practice. *Nature Clinical Practice Oncology, 5*(1), 32–43.

Lehrer, J., & Lichtenstein, G. R. (2007). Irritable bowel syndrome. *Emedicine.* Retrieved August 15, 2008, from http://www.emedicine.com/med/TOPIC1190.HTM#section~Introduction

Liu, J. H., Chen, G. H., Ye, H. Z., Huang, C. K., & Poon, S. K. (1997). Enteric-coated peppermint-oil capsules in the treatment of irritable bowel syndrome: A prospective, randomized trial. *Journal of Gastroenterology, 32,* 765–768.

Metcalf, C. (2007). Chronic diarrhea: Investigation, treatment, and nursing care. *Nursing Standard, 21*(21), 48–56.

Nagel, T., & Roman, L. (2004). Help patients cope with chemo. *RN, 67*(10), 25–31.

Olden, K. W. (2003). *Diagnosis, pathophysiology, and treatment of irritable bowel syndrome.* Retrieved August 15, 2008, from http://www.medscape.com/viewprogram/2749_pnt

Panaccione, R. (2007). Top-down vs step-up therapy in Crohn's disease: What does the evidence say? *Medscape Gastroenterology.* Retrieved January 18, 2008, from http://www.medscape.com/viewarticle/560005_print

Pasricha, P. J. (2006). Treatment of disorders of bowel motility and water flux; antiemetics; agents used in biliary and pancreatic disease. In L. L. Brunton, J. S. Lazo, & K. L. Parker (Eds.), *The pharmacological basis of therapeutics* (11th ed., pp. 983–1008). New York: McGraw-Hill.

Pray, W. S., & Pray, J. J. (2005). Diarrhea: Sweeping changes in the OTC market. *US Pharmacist, 30*(1).

Sanborn, W. J., Feagan, B. G., & Lichtenstein, G. R. (2007). Medical management of mild to moderate Crohn's disease: Evidence-based treatment algorithms for induction and maintenance of remission. *Alimentary Pharmacology and Therapeutics, 26*(7), 987–1003.

Schwartzberg, L. S. (2007). Chemotherapy-induced nausea and vomiting: Which antiemetic for which therapy. *Oncology, 21*(8), 946–953.

Scorza, K., Williams, A., Phillips, J. D., & Shaw, J. (2007). Evaluation of nausea and vomiting. *American Family Physician, 76*(1), 76–84.

Sellin, J. H., & Pasricha, P. J. (2006). Pharmacotherapy of inflammatory bowel disease. In L. L. Brunton, J. S. Lazo, & K. L. Parker (Eds.), *The pharmacological basis of therapeutics* (11th ed., pp. 1009–1020). New York: McGraw-Hill.

Slover, C., & Danziger, L. (2007). Lactobacillus: A review. *Clinical Microbiology Newsletter 30*(4), 23–27.

Spiller, R. (2008). Review article: Probiotics and prebiotics in irritable bowel syndrome. *Alimentary Pharmacology and Therapeutics, 28*(4), 385–396.

Talley, N. J. (2007). Functional nausea and vomiting. *Australian Family Physician, 36*(9), 694–697.

Teitelbaum, J. (2005). Probiotics and the treatment of infectious diarrhea. *The Pediatric Infectious Disease Journal, 24*(3), 267–268.

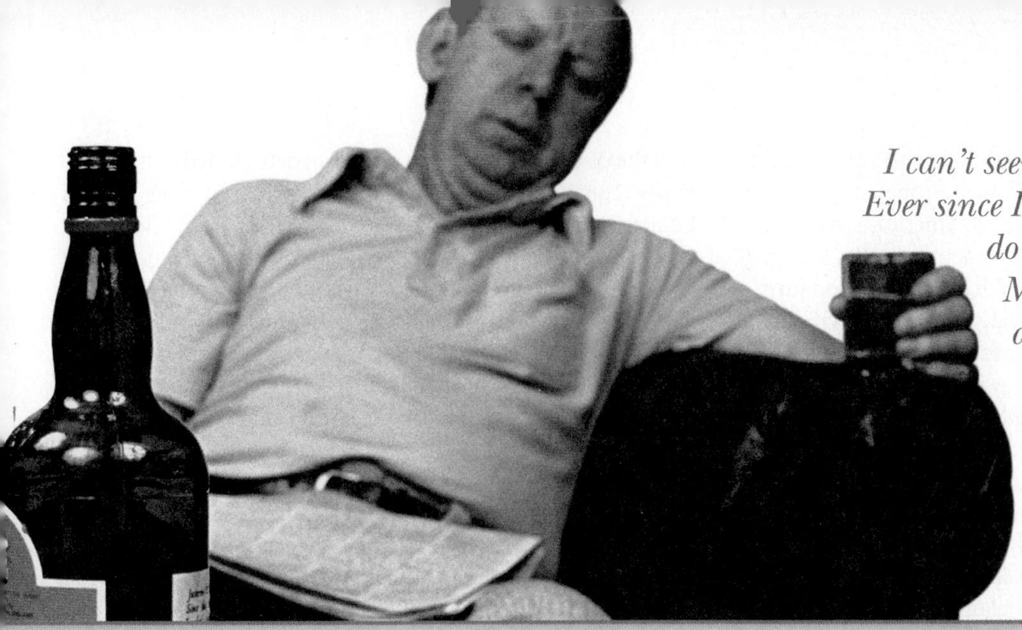

I can't seem to help myself. Ever since I lost my job all I do is drink all day. Most of the time I don't even bother to eat.

Patient "Bill Haywood"

CHAPTER 62

Vitamins and Minerals

Chapter Outline

Role of Vitamins in Health and Disease

Regulation of Vitamins

Recommended Dietary Allowance

Fat-Soluble Vitamins

Water-Soluble Vitamins

Minerals

Macrominerals

Microminerals

Learning Outcomes

After reading this chapter, the student should be able to:

1. Describe the role of vitamins in maintaining wellness.
2. Identify conditions for which vitamin and mineral therapy may be indicated.
3. Explain the importance of vitamins and minerals for optimal health.
4. Discuss the role of the recommended dietary allowance in determining the standardized requirement of various vitamins and minerals.
5. Compare and contrast fat-soluble and water-soluble vitamins.
6. For each of the major vitamins and minerals, identify the mechanism(s) of drug action, primary indications, contraindications, significant drug interactions, pregnancy category, and important adverse effects.
7. Use the nursing process to care for patients who are receiving vitamin and mineral supplements.

Key Terms

Council for Responsible Nutrition (CRN), *1053*
fat-soluble vitamins, *1052*
hypervitaminosis, *1053*
macrominerals, *1062*
microminerals, *1063*
minerals, *1061*
recommended dietary allowance (RDA), *1054*
supplements, *1052*
vitamins, *1052*
water-soluble vitamin, *1052*

The National Institutes of Health (NIH) has estimated that over half of all Americans take vitamin supplements. Recognizing the health benefits of food nutrients, later known as vitamins, dates back 3,500 years ago when the Egyptians discovered that eating certain foods such as liver helped night blindness. Today, this nutrient is known as vitamin A. Through subsequent years the relationship of nutrients in food to disease was largely ignored. Many blamed the occurrence of disease on displeased gods, bad air, or witchcraft. Centuries would pass before a connection was made between vitamins and health. This chapter examines the rationales for vitamin and mineral pharmacotherapy.

Role of Vitamins in Health and Disease

62.1 Although the importance of nutrition has been known for centuries, the specific vitamins were discovered in the 1900s.

When ocean voyages became a preferred way of travel in the Renaissance, extended periods on board a ship often meant limited access to fresh fruits and vegetables. People began to get sick with scurvy, a disease that causes bleeding of the gums, loss of teeth, ulcers on the lower legs, loss of hair, aching joints, fatigue, depression, hallucinations, blindness, and open wounds with decreased ability to heal. In 1774, James Lind, a Scottish surgeon in the Royal Navy, made a major discovery that saved the lives of many sailors. In fact, Lind surmised that more men died from scurvy than from war injuries. Although he knew nothing about vitamins and was not the first person to suspect that citrus fruit had a positive effect on connective tissue, he was the one who performed a systematic clinical experiment to address this illness. He divided the affected sailors into groups and added different substances, such as cider, vinegar, barley water, oranges, or lemons, to their diets. Those who ate citrus fruit recovered from scurvy. He continued to perform experiments using citrus fruit with positive results and published his treatise, recommending lemons and limes in the diet of naval soldiers. Lind was a man before his time because about 40 years passed before authorities accepted the connection between disease and nutrition.

Even in the early 1900s, most people believed that diseases like beriberi and pellagra were infectious processes. Beriberi is now known as a nutritional disease characterized by progressive neuropathy and accompanying dysfunction of the sensory process and an unsteady gait. In the late 1880s, Christian Eijkman studied beriberi in the West Indies and determined the cure for beriberi to be rice. He did not understand that it was a specific substance within the rice that caused the cure. In 1905, Dr. William Fletcher observed inmates who had beriberi at a mental asylum and found that ingesting unpolished rice could prevent the disease. This English physician determined that the rice husks contained some substance (thiamine) that treated beriberi. In 1907, Sir Frederick Gowland, an English biochemist, confirmed the positive relationship of food to health and later joined with Eijkman to win the 1929 Nobel Prize for his work with food nutrients and vitamins. In 1911, a Polish chemist named Casimir Funk coined the term *vitamines,* meaning nutrients vital for life. He discovered that it was the chemical thiamine in the rice husks that cured beriberi.

In the 1920s and 1930s, scientists determined that small amounts of food compounds prevented certain diseases. More than 160 years after Lind's discovery to prevent scurvy, Dr. Albert Szent-Gyorgi, a Hungarian researcher, received the Nobel Prize in medicine by isolating and naming vitamin C. He was interested in the amounts needed as minimum daily doses for disease prevention as compared with *dosis optima quotidiana,* meaning the optimal dose.

62.2 Vitamins are essential for optimal health.

Today **vitamins** are defined as nutrient substances that are required for the health of human body processes. These naturally occurring organic substances are critical for metabolism as well as regulation of cell function and human growth and development. They contain carbon, are found in living organisms such as plants and animals, and function primarily as catalysts that speed up biochemical processes. Vitamins must be taken into the body from the external environment, usually through the diet, and are not manufactured by the body with the exception of vitamin D. Lack of sufficient amounts of vitamins result in symptoms of deficiency. People must consume vitamin supplements when their diet is lacking in these necessary nutrients or when they have health conditions that cause vitamin deficiencies. The vitamins and their functions are summarized in Table 62.1

Vitamins are divided into two basic groups: those that dissolve in water (water soluble) and those that dissolve in lipids (fat soluble). Vitamin C and the B complex vitamins are the primary vitamins that comprise the category of **water-soluble vitamins.** This group of vitamins is stored briefly in the body and then excreted in the urine. A daily intake of water-soluble vitamins is necessary to replenish the necessary supply. One exception is B_{12}, which is stored in the liver. In contrast, **fat-soluble vitamins** are stored in the liver and fatty tissue of the human body and only need intermittent renewal. Because they are stored and not readily excreted, the possibility of toxicity from overdosing is greater with the fat-soluble group, which includes vitamins A, D, E, and K.

For most people there is no need for vitamins if they eat a well-balanced diet. However, many Americans rely on nutrient-poor fast foods and processed edibles as their main diet. Also, vitamins can be destroyed by heat, sunlight, exposure to moisture and air, mold, and oxidation. Although a healthy diet is the best way to increase vitamin and mineral intake, individual vitamin **supplements** are available as an additional way to meet the minimum daily requirements for some people. However, it is important to remember that vitamin and mineral products should supplement a healthy balanced diet; they are not substitutes for good nutrition. Doses for the lipid-soluble vitamin supplements are listed in Table 62.2. The water-soluble vitamin doses are listed in Table 62.3.

TABLE 62.1 Essential Vitamins

Vitamin	Function(s)	Common Cause(s) of Deficiency
A	Visual pigments, epithelial cells	Prolonged dietary deprivation, particularly when rice is the main food source; pancreatic disease; cirrhosis
Cyanocobalamin (B_{12})	Coenzyme in nucleic acid metabolism	Lack of intrinsic factor, inadequate intake of foods with animal origin
Folic acid/Folate (B_9)	Coenzyme in amino acid and nucleic acid metabolism	Pregnancy, alcoholism, cancer, oral contraceptive use
Niacin (B_3)	Coenzyme in oxidation–reduction reactions	Prolonged dietary deprivation, particularly when Indian corn (maize) or millet is the main food source; chronic diarrhea; liver disease; alcoholism
Pyridoxine (B_6)	Coenzyme in amino acid metabolism and red blood cell (RBC) production	Alcoholism, oral contraceptive use, malabsorption diseases
Riboflavin (B_2)	Coenzyme in oxidation–reduction reactions	Inadequate consumption of milk or animal products, chronic diarrhea, liver disease, alcoholism
Thiamine (B_1)	Coenzyme in metabolic reactions, RBC formation	Prolonged dietary deprivation, particularly when rice is the main food source; hyperthyroidism, pregnancy, liver disease, alcoholism
C (ascorbic acid)	Coenzyme and antioxidant	Inadequate intake of fruits and vegetables, pregnancy, chronic inflammatory disease, burns, diarrhea, alcoholism
D	Calcium and phosphate metabolism	Low dietary intake, inadequate exposure to sunlight
E	Antioxidant	Prematurity, malabsorption diseases
K	Cofactor in blood clotting	Newborns, liver disease, long-term parenteral nutrition, certain drugs such as cephalosporins and salicylates

Regulation of Vitamins

62.3 Government regulations and consumer knowledge about vitamins are limited.

A 2007 survey by the **Council for Responsible Nutrition (CRN),** a Washington-based trade association representing ingredient suppliers and manufacturers in the dietary supplement industry, reported that 68% of adults in America take vitamin supplements. Those considered "regular users" increased from 46% in 2006 to 52% in 2007, with 84% believing that these supplements are safe. Most patients are unaware that taking too much of a vitamin or mineral can cause serious adverse effects. **Hypervitaminosis,** or toxic levels of vitamins, has been reported for vitamins A, C, D, E, B_6, niacin, and folic acid. In the United States, it is actually more common to observe syndromes of vitamin excess than of vitamin deficiency.

Consumers may assume that the U.S. Food and Drug Administration (FDA) regulates and approves nutritional supplements,

TABLE 62.2 Fat-Soluble Vitamins for Treating Nutritional Disorders

Drug	Route and Adult Dose (maximum dose where indicated)	Adverse Effects
Vitamin A (Aquasol A)	PO: 500,000 units/day for 3 days, followed by 50,000 units/day for 2 weeks; then 10,000–20,000 units/day for 2 months IM: 100,000 units/day for 3 days followed by 50,000 units/day for 2 weeks	*Uncommon at normal doses* High doses: nausea, vomiting, fatigue, irritability, night sweats, alopecia, dry skin
Vitamin D; calcitriol (Calcijex, Rocaltrol)	PO: 0.25 mcg/day; may be increased by 0.25 mcg/day every 4–8 weeks for patients receiving dialysis or every 2–4 weeks for patients with hypoparathyroid If necessary IV: 0.5 mcg 3 times/week at the end of dialysis; may need up to 3 mcg 3 times/week	*Uncommon at normal doses, metallic taste* High doses: nausea, vomiting, fatigue, headache, polyuria, weight loss, hallucinations, dysrhythmias, muscle, and bone pain
Vitamin E; tocopherol (Aquasol E, vita-Plus E, others)	PO/IM: 60–75 units/day	*Uncommon at normal doses* High doses: nausea, vomiting, fatigue, headache, blurred vision
Vitamin K; phytonadione (AquaMEPHYTON)	PO/IM/subcutaneous: 2.5–10 mg (up to 25 mcg); may be repeated after 6–8 h if needed	*Facial flushing, pain at the injection site* IV route may result in dyspnea, hypotension, shock, cardiac arrest

Note: *Italics* indicate common adverse effects. Underline indicates serious adverse effects.

TABLE 62.3 Water-Soluble Vitamins for Treating Nutritional Disorders

Drug	Route and Adult Dose (maximum dose where indicated)	Adverse Effects
Vitamin B_1: thiamine	IV/IM: 50–100 mg tid PO: 5–30 mg/day	*Pain at the injection site* <u>IV route may result in angioedema, cyanosis, pulmonary edema, GI bleeding, and cardiovascular collapse</u>
Vitamin B_2: riboflavin	PO: 5–10 mg/day	*Adverse effects have not been reported*
Vitamin B_3: niacin (Nicobid, Nicolar, others)	PO: 10–20 mg/day IV/IM/subcutaneous: 25–100 mg 2–5 times/day	*Uncommon at doses used for vitamin therapy* <u>High doses: dysrhythmias</u>
Vitamin B_6: pyridoxine hydrochloride (Besix, Hexa-Betalin, Nestrex)	PO/IM/IV: 2.5–10 mg/day for 3 weeks; then may reduce to 2.5–5 mg/day	*Pain at the injection site* <u>High doses: neuropathy, ataxia, seizures</u>
Vitamin B_9: folic acid (Focalin)	PO/IM/IV/subcutaneous: 0.4–1 mg/day	*Uncommon at normal doses* <u>Parenteral routes: allergic hypersensitivity</u>
Vitamin B_{12}: cyanocobalamin (Betalin 12, Cobex, Cynapin, others)	IM/deep subcutaneous: 30 mcg/day for 5–10 days; then 100–200 mcg/month	*Rash, diarrhea* <u>High doses: thrombosis, hypokalemia, pulmonary edema, heart failure</u>
Vitamin C: ascorbic acid (Ascorbicap, Cebid, Vita-C, others)	PO/IV/IM/subcutaneous: 150–500 mg/day in one to two doses	*Uncommon at normal doses* <u>High doses: deep vein thrombosis (IV route), crystalluria</u>

Note: *Italics* indicate common adverse effects. <u>Underline</u> indicates serious adverse effects.

as it does prescription and over-the-counter (OTC) drugs. However, the legislative regulation of supplements is much more limited as compared to drugs. The FDA regulates herbal, vitamin, and mineral products as "dietary supplements." In 1994, the Dietary Supplement Health and Education Act required labeling of supplements. In 2007, the FDA passed the "current Good Manufacturing Practice" (cGMP) regulations, which mandated manufacturers to evaluate supplements for purity, strength, and composition (see Chapter 15).

The Director of the FDA's Division of Dietary Supplement Programs offers guidelines and tips for consumer safety. The best advice is to be knowledgeable about the purchase and use of supplements. This agency encourages consumers to consult with their health care providers before using supplements and to be leery of false claims. Supplements can be expensive, and choosing foods with needed vitamins and minerals is a more natural way to reach nutritional health goals.

PharmFACT

Vitamins are the seventh most common cause of poisoning in children under the age of 5 in the United States, resulting in about 48,000 cases annually.

Source: Bronstein et al., 2007.

Recommended Dietary Allowance

62.4 The recommended dietary allowance is the dietary intake level that is sufficient to meet the nutrient requirements for most people.

The Food and Nutrition Board of the National Academy of Sciences has established the **recommended dietary allowances (RDAs)** for healthy adults. These values represent the minimum amount of vitamins and minerals needed to prevent disease and are based on scientific nutritional research.

Although a well-balanced diet provides the necessary vitamins and minerals for most people, the amount of vitamins and minerals needed varies based on certain factors. For example, infants, pregnant women, nursing mothers, older adults, those eating a vegan or vegetarian diet, and those with chronic diseases often require larger amounts of vitamins and minerals to maintain optimal health. Men and women can have different vitamin and mineral needs as do persons who participate in vigorous exercise. With normal aging, the absorption of food diminishes and the quantity of ingested food is often reduced, leading to a higher risk of vitamin deficiencies in older adults. Vitamin deficiencies in patients with chronic liver and kidney disease are well documented. In cases where dietary needs are increased, the RDAs will need adjustment and supplements are indicated to achieve optimum wellness.

Certain drugs have the potential to affect vitamin metabolism. Alcohol is known for its ability to inhibit the absorption of thiamine and folic acid: Alcohol abuse is the most common cause of thiamine deficiency in the United States. Folic acid levels may be reduced in patients who are taking phenothiazines, oral contraceptives, phenytoin (Dilantin), or barbiturates. Vitamin D deficiency can be caused by therapy with certain anticonvulsants. Inhibition of vitamin B_{12} absorption has been reported with a number of drugs, including omeprazole (Prilosec) and metformin (Glucophage), alcohol, and oral contraceptives. Nurses must be aware of these drug interactions and recommend vitamin supplements when appropriate.

Vitamin deficiencies follow certain patterns. The following are general characteristics of vitamin deficiency disorders:

- Patients more commonly present with multiple vitamin deficiencies than with a single vitamin deficiency.

CONNECTIONS

Treating the Diverse Patient **Vitamins During Pregnancy**

Pregnancy is a time when vitamin supplements are necessary to provide additional nutritional support. Essentially, the mother is eating for two, because the fetus demands nutritional support as much as the woman's body does. Supplementation with vitamins can support the mother's diet and ensure that both she and her baby get the nutrients they need.

A common practice in prenatal care is for pregnant women to take prenatal vitamin supplements. These vitamins contain numerous nutrients, but calcium, folic acid, and iron are especially important. Each of these substances is necessary for a healthy mother and baby. However, vitamins should be seen as a supplement to a healthy diet during pregnancy.

Folic acid, which is considered part of the B vitamins, is often highlighted as a need in pregnancy because it prevents birth defects such as spina bifida (baby is born without a closed spine), other neural tube problems, and congenital heart conditions. To be certain that the folic acid requirement is met during pregnancy, supplements are recommended. Because birth defects can take place early in pregnancy, taking prenatal vitamins is recommended if a woman is trying to get pregnant.

Calcium is another mineral that is needed during pregnancy. Supplementation can stop the loss of bone density from the mother as the fetus absorbs calcium for bone growth. This is especially important during the second and third trimesters of pregnancy.

Iron is a mineral that is often supplemented in pregnancy because it is the central component in hemoglobin that carries oxygen for both mother and baby. Anemia can occur with insufficient iron intake. Women who experience morning sickness and vomiting are at risk for dietary iron deficiency. Also, women with poor diets or heavy menstrual periods before pregnancy can start their pregnancy with a mineral deficiency. Iron supplements should be taken separately from calcium-rich food and caffeine because these interfere with iron absorption. Vitamin C enhances the absorption of iron so the two can be taken concurrently. Excess iron is poisonous. Therefore, the supplements should be kept away from children to avoid accidental poisoning.

- Symptoms of deficiency are nonspecific and often do not appear until the deficiency has been present for a long period.
- Deficiencies in the United States are most often the result of poverty, fad diets, chronic alcohol or drug abuse, or prolonged parenteral feeding.

Fat-Soluble Vitamins

62.5 Fat-soluble vitamins include vitamins A, D, E, and K.

The fat-soluble vitamins A, D, E, and K are found in fatty foods and oils. Because they are stored in lipid tissue, the body may go several weeks or months with insufficient dietary intake before signs of deficiency are noted. Excessive intake of these vitamins may be harmful.

Vitamin A (Aquasol A, Del-Vi-A)

Therapeutic Effects and Uses: Vitamin A is essential for the normal growth and development of bones and teeth, natural immunity, integrity of epithelial and mucosal surfaces, and vision with the synthesis of visual purple necessary for adaptation to the dark (treats night blindness). Vitamin A replacement therapy is used when metabolic needs are increased such as in pregnancy, during lactation, or with infections. Vitamin A can be used in replacement therapy for conditions affecting the absorption, mobilization, or storage of vitamin A such as steatorrhea, severe biliary obstruction, liver cirrhosis, or total gastrectomy. Some skin conditions such as folliculosis keratosis or psoriasis respond favorably to topical preparations of vitamin A. Vitamin A has antioxidant properties and can be used as a screening test for fat malabsorption.

Mechanism of Action: As a fat-soluble vitamin, vitamin A acts as a cofactor in the synthesis of mucopolysaccharides, synthesis of cholesterol, and the metabolism of steroids. It is easily absorbed through the gastrointestinal (GI) tract with bile salts, pancreatic lipase, and dietary fat, and it is stored in the liver. Small amounts may also be stored in the kidney and body fat. Vitamin A can pass to the newborn through breast milk. Vitamin A is metabolized in the liver and excreted in feces and urine.

Adverse Effects: Adverse effects with vitamin A are rare but the health care provider should be notified of difficulty breathing; hives; swelling of the lips, face, or tongue; or closing of the throat. Overdose may result in hypervitaminosis syndrome symptoms such as fatigue, nausea, vomiting, decreased appetite, headache, gingivitis, dryness or cracking of the lips or skin, irritability, or loss of hair. Rare adverse effects include increased intracranial pressure, jaundice, leukopenia, anemia, and elevated prothrombin time (PT).

Contraindications/Precautions: Contraindications to vitamin A therapy include a history of sensitivity to vitamin A or to any ingredient in the formulation or hypervitaminosis. Oral (PO) administration to patients with malabsorption syndrome is also contraindicated. Its safe use in amounts exceeding 6,000 international units during pregnancy is not established. Vitamin A may falsely increase serum cholesterol determinations or falsely elevate bilirubin determination.

MyNursingKit | QuackWatch

Drug Interactions: The patient should consult with the health care provider if using mineral oil because this can deplete fat-soluble vitamins. Cholestyramine may decrease the absorption of vitamin A. Oral contraceptives can increase the plasma levels of vitamin A.

Pregnancy: Category A (at RDA value).

RDA: 2,500 international units for children, 4,000 international units for women, and 5,000 international units for men.

Nursing Responsibilities:

- Take a patient dietary history that includes normal foods eaten as well as supplements taken. Consider the effective dosage with regard to the patient's dietary intake of foods with vitamin A.
- Women who are taking birth control pills may demonstrate higher plasma vitamin A levels.

- Monitor therapeutic effectiveness. Observe for night blindness, restricted growth and development, susceptibility to infection, renal stones, or unusual dryness of the skin, mouth, and eyes.

Patient and Family Education:

- Consume foods that are rich in vitamin A such as liver, whole milk, cheese, and eggs. Avoid use of mineral oil during vitamin A therapy because it can interfere with the absorption of this vitamin.
- Report adverse symptoms such as nausea, vomiting, anorexia, drying and cracking of the skin or lips, headache, or hair loss.

Vitamin D (Ergocalciferol, Calcitriol)

Therapeutic Effects and Uses: Vitamin D plays a major regulatory role in serum calcium levels. It maintains normal blood calcium and phosphate electrolyte levels by enhancing their intestinal absorption and by promoting mobilization of calcium from bone and the renal reabsorption of phosphate. This fat-soluble vitamin is necessary to develop and maintain strong bones. Vitamin D is used to treat skeletal diseases that weaken the bones such as familial hypophosphatemia (vitamin D-resistant rickets), osteomalacia (adult rickets), osteoporosis, renal osteodystrophy, hypocalcemia associated with hypoparathyroidism, as prophylaxis for and treatment of nutritional rickets, and hypophosphatemia in Fanconi's syndrome. Sometimes vitamin D is helpful in treating psoriasis, rheumatoid arthritis, and lupus vulgaris. A drug prototype feature for calcitriol, the active form of vitamin D, is included in Chapter 75.

Mechanism of Action: Vitamin D is a fat-soluble vitamin that is found in food and that is also made by the body after exposure to ultraviolet (UV) rays from the sun. Sunlight is a significant source of vitamin D because UV rays trigger vitamin D synthesis in the skin. Vitamin D is readily absorbed from the GI tract and distributed in the lymph. The body stores vitamin D in the liver, skin, brain, spleen, and bones. About half of each vitamin D dose is excreted in bile but it may be stored in tissues for months.

Adverse Effects: Adverse effects of vitamin D therapy are rare. Some possible adverse effects include fatigue, weakness, dizziness, ataxia, muscle and joint pain, hypotonia (infants), pruritus, headache, drowsiness, photophobia, or convulsions. GI symptoms include anorexia, nausea, vomiting, diarrhea, metallic taste, dry mouth, constipation, and abdominal cramps. Some patients present with anemia. Musculoskeletal symptoms include calcification of soft tissues in the kidneys, myocardium, lungs, or skin. Nephrotoxicity could occur with symptoms such as polyuria, polydipsia, nocturia, albuminuria, hematuria, and kidney failure. Vitamin D is rarely but possibly implicated in hypertension and some cardiac dysrhythmias. Chronic hypervitaminosis with vitamin D can occur in children, resulting in mental and physical retardation or suppression of linear growth.

Contraindications/Precautions: Precaution should be taken in patients with a known hypersensitivity to vitamin D, hypervitaminosis, hypercalcemia, hyperphosphatemia, renal osteodystrophy with hyperphosphatemia, malabsorption syndrome, or decreased kidney function. Use cautiously in patients with coronary disease, arteriosclerosis (especially in older adults), history of kidney stones, biliary tract disease, or during lactation.

Drug Interactions: Consult with the health care provider if using mineral oil because it can deplete the supply of fat-soluble vitamins in the body. Cholestyramine may decrease the absorption of vitamin D. Vitamin D can cause false increase in serum cholesterol measurements. Prescribers should avoid calcitriol and its analogs because they may increase the incidence of hypercalcemia.

Pregnancy: Category C. The safe use of vitamin D in amounts exceeding 400 international units (10 mcg) daily during pregnancy has not been established.

RDA: Children, men, and women until age 50 need 200 international units of vitamin D per day. For individuals who are age 51 to 70, the minimum dose increases to 400 international units per day. Those who are age 71 and older need 600 international units per day.

Nursing Responsibilities:

- Monitor the patient for common adverse effects of high doses of vitamin D such as anorexia, nausea, vomiting, polydypsia, and polyuria. Discontinue therapy should these symptoms occur.
- Monitor laboratory tests when high therapeutic doses are given with tests of serum calcium, phosphorus, magnesium, alkaline phosphatase, blood urea nitrogen (BUN), and determinations of urine calcium, casts, albumin, and erythrocyte counts every 2 weeks.
- Assess the patient for hypercalcemia, which may occur in patients with osteomalacia. Blood calcium concentration is generally kept between 9 and 10 mg/dL.
- Do not administer vitamin D with magnesium-containing antacids or laxatives in patients with renal impairment because magnesium intoxication may occur.

Patient and Family Education:

- Obtain adequate amounts of sunshine, which is the natural source of vitamin D. Dietary sources include egg yolks, fortified cereals and milk, cod liver oil, and fish such as halibut, mackerel, shrimp, pink salmon, and sardines.
- Do not take vitamin D with magnesium-containing antacids or laxatives.
- Do not take any prescription or nonprescription drugs, dietary supplements, or herbal products without or approval of the health care provider.

PharmFACT

People with dark skin pigmentation may need 20 to 30 times as much exposure to sunlight as fair-skinned people to generate the same amount of vitamin D.
Source: Adams, 2005.

Vitamin E (Tocopherols)

Therapeutic Effects and Uses: Vitamin E has many therapeutic uses. It prevents cell membrane and protein damage, protects against blood clot formation by decreasing platelet aggregation, enhances vitamin A utilization, and promotes the normal growth and development and tone of muscles. As an antioxidant, vitamin E prevents preoxidation, which releases free radicals or highly reactive chemical structures that damage cell membranes and alter nuclear proteins. Free radicals are associated with various conditions such as aging and disease.

Deficiencies of vitamin E often result in hemolytic anemia. Vitamin E therapy can reverse or prevent hemolytic anemia in premature neonates that is caused by vitamin E deficiency. It is also used to prevent retinopathy associated with vitamin E deficiency in neonates, and to treat diseases with secondary erythrocyte membrane abnormalities (e.g., sickle cell anemia and G6PD deficiency), and as a supplement in malabsorption syndromes. Topical vitamin E is used for dry or chapped skin and minor skin disorders.

Some people report improvement in muscular dystrophy symptoms and a number of other conditions although there is no conclusive evidence of its value. Vitamin E is included in most multivitamin formulations and may appear in deodorant preparations as an antioxidant.

Mechanism of Action: When fat absorption is adequate, 20% to 60% of vitamin E is absorbed across the GI tract. It enters blood through the lymph and is stored in adipose (fat) tissue. Vitamin E is metabolized in the liver and is eliminated primarily in bile. Vitamin E crosses the placenta.

Adverse Effects: Adverse reactions to vitamin E are rare. With excessive doses symptoms may include fatigue, headache, skeletal muscle weakness, nausea, diarrhea, intestinal cramps, thrombophlebitis, contact dermatitis, blurred vision, or abnormal bleeding. With toxic levels laboratory tests may reveal increased serum creatine kinase, cholesterol, and triglycerides; decreased serum thyroxine and triiodothyronine; increased urinary estrogens and androgens; and creatinuria.

Contraindications/Precautions: Vitamin E should be used with caution in bleeding disorders and thrombocytopenia or during pregnancy. Vitamin E can prolong the PT by inhibition of vitamin K–dependent carboxylase in someone with abnormally low vitamin K levels. Large doses may worsen iron-deficiency anemia because it may impair the hematologic response to iron.

Drug Interactions: Mineral oil should be avoided because it can deplete fat-soluble vitamins. Cholestyramine may decrease absorption of vitamin E. Vitamin E may enhance the anticoagulant activity of warfarin.

Pregnancy: Category A with doses within the RDA limits.

RDA: Ranges from 4 mg (6 international units) to 11 mg (16.5 international units) in children under 13 years, depending on the age, and 15 mg (22.5 international units) for persons aged 14 through adult. Pregnant women need a minimum of 19 mg (28.5 international units) per day.

Nursing Responsibilities:

- Assess the patient for adverse effects of vitamin E, including muscle weakness, nausea, or diarrhea.
- Encourage the patient to remain under close supervision of the health care provider.
- Monitor for signs of abnormal bleeding, especially if the patient is concurrently taking warfarin.

Patient and Family Education:

- Notify the health care provider if taking iron supplements because the RDA of vitamin E may be increased.
- Consume natural sources of vitamin E such as wheat germ (the richest source) as well as vegetable oils (sunflower, corn, soybean, cottonseed), green leafy vegetables, nuts, dairy products, eggs, cereals, meat, and liver.
- Report for frequent laboratory blood testing if taking vitamin E and warfarin concurrently because PT time may be prolonged.

Vitamin K (Phytonadione)

Therapeutic Effects and Uses: Vitamin K promotes the liver synthesis of clotting factors and is used in the production of red blood cells (RBCs). It helps maintain healthy bones, assists in healing fractures, and minimizes osteoporosis. It is the drug of choice as an antidote for the overdosage of warfarin and indandione PO anticoagulants. Vitamin K reverses hypoprothrombinemia secondary to the administration of PO antibiotics, quinidine, salicylates, sulfonamides, and excessive vitamin A, and secondary to inadequate absorption and synthesis of vitamin K (as in obstructive jaundice, biliary fistula, ulcerative colitis, intestinal resection, or prolonged hyperalimentation). Vitamin K is used as prophylaxis of and therapy for neonatal hemorrhagic disease.

Mechanism of Action: The body makes most of its needed vitamin K through bacteria in the GI tract. Phytonadione is a fat-soluble substance that is chemically identical to and has similar activity as naturally occurring vitamin K. It is absorbed readily in the intestinal lymph if bile is present. Vitamin K is essential for the hepatic biosynthesis of blood-clotting Factors II, VII, IX, and X. Hemorrhage is usually controlled within 3 to 8 hours, with normal PT obtained in 12 to 14 hours after vitamin K administration. Phytonadione is concentrated briefly in the liver after absorption, crosses the placenta, and is secreted in the breast milk of nursing mothers. It is metabolized quickly in the liver and eliminated in the urine and bile.

Adverse Effects: Potential adverse effects include hypersensitivity or anaphylaxis-like reaction, facial flushing, cramp-like pains, convulsive movements, chills, fever, diaphoresis, weakness, dizziness, shock, and cardiac arrest. Other reported effects include headache (after PO dose), brain damage, death, GI upset, paradoxical hypoprothrombinemia (in patients with severe liver disease), severe hemolytic anemia, hyperbilirubinemia, kernicterus, bronchospasm, dyspnea, sensation of chest constriction, and respiratory arrest. Possible pain at the injection site, hematoma and nodule formation, erythematous skin eruptions (with repeated injections), and peculiar taste sensations may occur.

Contraindications/Precautions: Caution should be used in patients with biliary tract disease, obstructive jaundice, or severe liver disease. Patients should be monitored for hypersensitivity to phytonadione, benzyl alcohol, or castor oil. Some interference may occur with diagnostic tests such as falsely elevated urine steroids.

Drug Interactions: Vitamin K can antagonize the anticoagulant effects of warfarin. Patients may have decreased absorption with the use of cholestyramine, colestipol, or mineral oil.

Pregnancy: Category C.

RDA: 80 mcg/day.

Nursing Responsibilities:

- With parenteral use, monitor the patient regularly for severe reactions such as anaphylaxis-like symptoms, because fatalities have occurred during and immediately after intravenous (IV) injection.
- Monitor therapeutic effectiveness, which is indicated by shortened PT, international normalized ratio (INR), bleeding, and clotting times, as well as decreased hemorrhagic tendencies.
- Recognize that patients on large doses may develop temporary resistance to warfarin-type anticoagulants. If a PO anticoagulant is reinstituted, larger doses may be needed or a change to heparin may be indicated.

Patient and Family Education:

- Maintain a well-balanced diet and avoid significant increases in the daily intake of vitamin K–rich foods after the drug regimen is stabilized.
- Dietary sources that are rich in vitamin K include asparagus, broccoli, cabbage, lettuce, turnip greens, pork or beef liver, green tea, spinach, watercress, and tomatoes.

CONNECTION *Checkpoint* 62.1

From what you learned in Chapter 40, describe how vitamin K reverses the therapeutic effects of warfarin (Coumadin). See Answer to Connection Checkpoint 62.1 in Appendix A.

Water-Soluble Vitamins

62.6 Water-soluble vitamins include the B-complex vitamins and vitamin C.

The water-soluble vitamins are found in rich abundance in fresh fruits and vegetables. Unlike the fat-soluble vitamins, vitamin C and most B-complex vitamins are not stored to any great extent, and signs of deficiency may be noted quickly if they are omitted from the diet. Excessive intake of these vitamins is usually not harmful because they are rapidly excreted.

Thiamine (Vitamin B_1 [Thiamine Hydrochloride])

Therapeutic Effects and Uses: Thiamine, also known as vitamin B_1, functions as an essential coenzyme in the metabolism of carbohydrates and has a role in converting tryptophan to nicotinamide. This vitamin is used in the treatment and prophylaxis of beriberi, to correct anorexia due to thiamine deficiency, and in the treatment of neuritis associated with pregnancy, pellagra, and alcoholism. Severe deficiency is characterized by paralysis of the eye muscle (ophthalmoplegia), neuropathy, muscle wasting, edema, serous effusions, and congestive heart failure. Its effectiveness is evidenced by improvement of the clinical manifestations of thiamine deficiency, such as anorexia, gastric distress, depression, irritability, insomnia, palpitations, tachycardia, loss of memory, paresthesias, muscle weakness and pain, elevated blood pyruvic acid level (diagnostic test for thiamine deficiency), and elevated lactic acid level.

Because of its abundance in food, thiamine deficiency in the United States is not common, except in alcoholics and in patients with chronic liver disease. Therapy generally includes other members of the B-complex vitamins because thiamine deficiency rarely occurs alone. Thiamine is sometimes used in combination with other B vitamins to reduce depression and anxiety as well as to prevent motion sickness. Some believe that in certain amounts, this vitamin causes a chemical change on the skin that repels biting insects like mosquitoes.

Mechanism of Action: Thiamine is necessary for the conversion of carbohydrates to energy and is essential in maintaining the proper functioning of the heart, nervous system, and muscles. Thiamine is absorbed from the GI tract and widely distributed, and it is secreted in breast milk. This vitamin is eliminated in the urine.

Adverse Effects: Thiamine has few adverse effects. Excessive doses may cause a feeling of warmth, weakness, sweating, restlessness, tightness of the throat, angioneurotic edema, cyanosis, pulmonary edema, cardiovascular collapse, or hypotension after rapid IV administration. Other adverse effects may include GI hemorrhage, nausea, urticaria, and pruritus.

Contraindications/Precautions: There are no contraindications if the dosage is within the RDA.

Drug Interactions: None known.

Pregnancy: Category A; category C if doses are greater than the RDA.

RDA: 1.5 mg/day.

Nursing Responsibilities:

- Obtain a complete dietary history as an essential part of vitamin replacement therapy.
- Collaborate with the prescriber, dietitian, patient, and responsible family member to develop a dietary teaching plan that can be sustained by the patient.
- Note that the body requirement of thiamine is directly proportional to carbohydrate intake and metabolic rate. The dietary requirement increases when the diet consists predominantly of carbohydrates.
- Assess for signs of thiamine toxicity which may include tachycardia, hypotension, and anaphylaxis-like symptoms.

Patient and Family Education:

- To prevent deficiency, consume dietary sources rich in thiamine such as yeast, pork, beef, liver, wheat and other whole grains, nutrient-added breakfast cereals, and fresh vegetables, especially peas and dried beans.

- Continue taking vitamin supplements exactly as prescribed, even if feeling better.

Riboflavin (Vitamin B_2)

Therapeutic Effects and Uses: Vitamin B_2, or riboflavin, is a component of coenzymes that participate in a number of different oxidation–reduction reactions. As with thiamine, a deficiency of riboflavin is most commonly observed in alcoholics. Clinical symptoms of deficiency include digestive disturbances, headache, burning sensation of the skin (especially "burning" feet), cracking at the corners of the mouth (cheilosis), glossitis, seborrheic dermatitis (and other skin lesions), mental depression, corneal vascularization (with photophobia, burning and itchy eyes, lacrimation, roughness of eyelids), anemia, and neuropathy. Riboflavin therapy is used to prevent riboflavin deficiency and microcytic anemia and to supplement other B vitamins in the treatment of pellagra and beriberi.

Mechanism of Action: As a component of the flavoprotein enzymes, riboflavin works together with a wide variety of proteins to catalyze many cellular respiratory reactions by which the body derives its energy. The vitamin is readily absorbed from the GI tract. Little riboflavin is stored and excess amounts are excreted in urine.

Adverse Effects: Riboflavin is nontoxic. It may discolor urine bright yellow. In large doses, riboflavin may produce yellow-green fluorescence in urine, which can cause false elevations in certain fluorometric determinations of urinary catecholamines.

Contraindications/Precautions: Unknown.

Drug Interactions: Unknown.

Pregnancy: Category A; category C if doses are greater than the RDA.

RDA: 1.7 mg/day.

Nursing Responsibilities:

- Collaborate with the prescriber, dietitian, patient, or caregiver in planning a diet with sufficient riboflavin. A complete dietary history is an essential part of vitamin replacement to identify and correct poor eating habits.
- Note that a deficiency in one B vitamin usually indicates deficiencies in other B vitamins.

Patient and Family Education:

- Large doses may cause an intense yellow discoloration of urine. This is not harmful.
- To prevent deficiency, consume dietary sources rich in riboflavin such as organ meats (liver, kidney, heart), beef, pork, eggs, milk and milk products, yeast, whole-grain cereals and breads, vitamin-enriched breakfast cereals, dark leafy green vegetables, and mushrooms.

Pyridoxine (Vitamin B_6)

Therapeutic Effects and Uses: Pyridoxine deficiency occurs with inadequate dietary intake due to alcoholism, drug-induced deficiency (e.g., isoniazid, oral contraceptives), and inborn errors of metabolism (vitamin B_6–dependent convulsions or anemia). Pyridoxine is used to improve symptoms of vitamin deficiency such as nausea, vomiting, and skin lesions. Other symptoms that resemble those of riboflavin and niacin deficiency include edema, central nervous system (CNS) symptoms, and hypochromic microcytic anemia. Pyridoxine is administered to prevent chloramphenicol-induced optic neuritis. It is used to treat acute toxicity caused by overdosage of cycloserine, hydralazine, or isoniazid (INH); alcoholic polyneuritis; and sideroblastic anemia associated with high serum iron concentration. Pyridoxine has been used to manage many other conditions, including nausea and vomiting in radiation sickness and pregnancy, suppression of postpartum lactation, diabetes, to decrease the symptoms of premenstrual syndrome (PMS), minimize joint pain caused by some types of arthritis, and to treat carpal tunnel syndrome.

Mechanism of Action: Pyridoxine is usually available as part of a water-soluble complex of three closely related compounds with vitamin B_6 activity. Pyridoxine is essential to human nutrition, although a deficiency syndrome is not well defined. It is converted in the body to pyridoxal, a coenzyme that functions in protein, fat, and carbohydrate metabolism and in facilitating the release of glycogen from the liver and muscle. In protein metabolism, pyridoxine participates in many enzymatic transformations of amino acids and in the conversion of tryptophan to niacin and serotonin. It aids in energy transformation in the brain and nerve cells and is thought to stimulate heme production. Pyridoxine is readily absorbed from the GI tract. It is distributed and stored in the liver and crosses the placenta. Metabolism of this vitamin takes place in the liver. Pyridoxine is eliminated in urine.

Adverse Effects: Adverse events are few but the patient could experience paresthesias, slight flushing or feeling of warmth, temporary burning or stinging pain at the injection site, somnolence seizures (particularly following large parenteral doses), low folic acid levels, insomnia, or anxiety.

Contraindications/Precautions: Pyridoxine should be used with caution in patients with renal impairment, neonatal prematurity with renal impairment, or cardiac disease.

Drug Interactions: Use of isoniazid, cycloserine, penicillamine, hydralazine, and oral contraceptives may increase pyridoxine requirements. This vitamin may reverse or antagonize the therapeutic effects of the anti-Parkinson drug levodopa because it reduces the amount of dopamine entering the brain by facilitating the breakdown of levodopa in peripheral circulation.

RDA: 2 mg/day.

Pregnancy: Category C.

Nursing Responsibilities:

- Obtain a complete dietary history to identify and correct poor eating habits.
- Note that a deficiency in one B vitamin usually indicates deficiencies in other B vitamins.
- Monitor neurologic status to determine the therapeutic effect in deficiency states.
- Obtain baseline and periodic laboratory tests for hematocrit, hemoglobin, and serum iron.

Patient and Family Education:

- To prevent deficiency, consume dietary sources rich in vitamin B_6 such as yeast, wheat germ, whole grain cereals, organ meats (especially liver), legumes, leafy green vegetables, and bananas.
- Avoid self-medication with OTC vitamin combinations without first consulting the health care provider.

CONNECTION *Checkpoint* 62.2

From what you learned in Chapter 52, how do antitubercular drugs affect levels of pyridoxine (vitamin B_6)?

See Answer to Connection Checkpoint 62.2 in Appendix A.

Cyanocobalamin (Vitamin B_{12})

Therapeutic Effects and Uses: Cyanocobalamin is used to treat vitamin B_{12} deficiency and anemia due to malabsorption syndrome, such as in pernicious (Addison's) anemia; sprue; GI pathology, dysfunction, or surgery; fish tapeworm infestation; and gluten enteropathy. This drug is also used in vitamin B_{12} deficiency caused by increased physiological requirements or inadequate dietary intake and in vitamin B_{12} absorption (Schilling) test. It may be used to prevent and treat toxicity associated with sodium nitroprusside, to treat asthma, and possibly to aid in healing following surgery. A prototype drug feature for this vitamin is presented in Chapter 41.

Mechanism of Action: Vitamin B_{12} is a cobalt-containing B complex vitamin that is essential for normal growth, cell reproduction, maturation of RBCs, synthesis of nucleoproteins, and maintenance of the nervous system (myelin synthesis). It is believed to be involved in protein and carbohydrate metabolism as well. Vitamin B_{12} deficiency results in megaloblastic anemia, dysfunction of the spinal cord with paralysis, and GI lesions. Intestinal absorption requires the presence of intrinsic factor in the terminal ileum. It is widely distributed and is principally stored in the liver, kidneys, and adrenals. It crosses the placenta and is excreted in breast milk. In metabolism this vitamin is converted in the tissues to active coenzymes and is enterohepatically cycled. Vitamin B_{12} is eliminated in urine in 48 hours.

Adverse Effects: Adverse effects are rare but may include feeling of a swelling body, anaphylactic shock, sudden death, peripheral vascular thrombosis, pulmonary edema, heart failure, mild transient diarrhea, unmasking of polycythemia vera (with correction of vitamin B_{12} deficiency), hypokalemia, itching, rash, flushing, and severe optic nerve atrophy.

Contraindications/Precautions: Contraindications include a history of sensitivity to vitamin B_{12}, other cobalamins, or cobalt; early Leber's disease (hereditary optic nerve atrophy); and indiscriminate use in folic acid deficiency. Caution should be used in patients with heart disease, anemia, or pulmonary disease.

Drug Interactions: Alcohol, aminosalicylic acid, neomycin, and colchicine may decrease the absorption of PO cyanocobalamin. Chloramphenicol may interfere with the therapeutic response to cyanocobalamin.

Pregnancy: Category A; category C (parenteral).

RDA: 2.4 mcg/day for ages 19 and older, 2.6 mcg/day during pregnancy, and 2.8 mcg/day during lactation

Nursing Responsibilities:

- Obtain baseline laboratory values before the initiation of therapy, such as reticulocyte and erythrocyte counts and hemoglobin, hematocrit, vitamin B_{12}, and serum folate levels. Repeat between 5 and 7 days after the start of therapy and at regular intervals during therapy.
- Monitor potassium levels during the first 48 hours. Conversion to normal erythropoiesis increases erythrocyte potassium requirement and can result in severe hypokalemia and sudden death.
- Obtain a careful history of allergies. Sensitization to cyanocobalamin can take as long as 8 years to develop.
- Monitor vital signs in patients with cardiac disease and in those who are receiving parenteral cyanocobalamin. Assess for pulmonary edema, which generally occurs early in therapy.
- The therapeutic response to drug therapy is usually dramatic, occurring within 48 hours. Effectiveness of the therapy is measured by laboratory values and improvement in manifestations of vitamin B_{12} deficiency.
- Obtain a complete diet and drug history and inquire into alcohol drinking patterns for all patients who are receiving cyanocobalamin to identify and correct poor lifestyle habits.

Patient and Family Education:

- Report any new disease or infection because an increase in dosage may be required.
- Continue drug therapy throughout life to prevent irreversible neurologic damage resulting from pernicious anemia.
- To prevent deficiency, consume dietary sources rich in vitamin B_{12} such as nutrient-fortified breakfast cereals, vitamin B_{12}–fortified soy milk, organ meats, clams, oysters, egg yolk, crab, salmon, sardines, muscle meat, milk, and dairy products.

Folic Acid (Vitamin B_9)

Therapeutic Effects and Uses: Folic acid is used to correct folate deficiency, macrocytic anemia, and megaloblastic anemias, which are associated with inadequate dietary intake, alcoholism, primary liver disease, malabsorption syndromes, pregnancy, infancy, and childhood. Studies have shown that up to 80% of neural tube defects in newborns can be prevented with supplementation of folic acid prior to pregnancy.

Mechanism of Action: Vitamin B_9 is essential for the synthesis of nucleoproteins and the maintenance of RBCs, neurons, and proteins. It stimulates production of RBCs, white blood cells (WBCs), and platelets in patients with megaloblastic anemias. Folic acid counters folic acid deficiency, which can result in the production of defective deoxyribonucleic acid (DNA), leading to megaloblast formation and arrest of bone marrow maturation. Folic acid is readily absorbed in the proximal small intestine, is distributed to all body tissues, crosses the placenta in pregnancy, and is secreted in breast milk in lactating women. It is metabolized in the liver and excreted in urine.

Adverse Effects: The patient may feel warmth or flushing with IV doses. Although rare, the possible adverse effects include irritability, depression, loss of appetite, rash, itching, nausea, shortness of breath, or tightness in the chest.

Contraindications/Precautions: Folic acid should not be used in patients with allergic sensitivity to B vitamins. It should be administered with caution if using folic acid alone to correct pernicious anemia or other vitamin B_{12} deficiency states as well as normocytic, refractory, aplastic, or undiagnosed anemia. Caution should be used with neonates. Folic acid can cause false low serum folate levels in patients who are receiving antibiotics such as tetracyclines.

Drug Interactions: Chloramphenicol can antagonize the effects of folate therapy. Folic acid therapy increases the metabolism of phenytoin (Dilantin), possibly causing increased seizure activity.

Pregnancy: Category A.

RDA: 180 to 200 mcg/day.

Nursing Responsibilities:

- Obtain a complete history of dietary intake and any drug or alcohol usage prior to initiating therapy. Recognize that certain drugs such as alcohol, barbiturates, methotrexate, phenytoin, primidone, trimethoprim, and oral contraceptives can cause folate deficiency. Renal dialysis can result in folate deficiency.
- Monitor patients who are taking phenytoin for increased seizure activity.

Patient and Family Education:

- Attend all follow-up appointments while taking folic acid therapy because dosage adjustments may be necessary.
- To prevent deficiency consume dietary sources rich in folic acid such as whole grain cereals and breads, organ meats such as liver and kidney, yeast, fruits, beans, potatoes, and leafy green vegetables.
- Store this vitamin in moderate temperatures and protect it from light and heat, which will make it inactive.

Vitamin C (Ascorbic Acid)

Therapeutic Effects and Uses: Vitamin C is essential for the synthesis and maintenance of collagen and intercellular ground substance of body tissues, blood vessels, cartilage, bones, teeth, skin, and tendons. It helps maintain the functions of the immune system for improved wound healing and increased resistance to infection. Vitamin C is used for both prophylaxis and treatment of scurvy and as a dietary supplement. Off-label uses include acidification of urine, preventing and treating cancer, treating idiopathic methemoglobinemia, and as an adjuvant during deferoxamine therapy for iron toxicity. In megadoses vitamin C may possibly reduce the severity and duration of the common cold. It is used as an antioxidant in formulations of parenteral tetracycline and other drugs.

Mechanism of Action: Vitamin C is readily absorbed and widely distributed to body tissues. It crosses the placenta and is secreted in breast milk. Vitamin C is metabolized in the liver and eliminated rapidly in urine when the plasma level exceeds the renal threshold of 1.4 mg/dL. Unlike most mammals, humans are unable to synthesize ascorbic acid in the body; thus it must be consumed daily.

Adverse Effects: Possible adverse effects from large doses include nausea, vomiting, heartburn, diarrhea or abdominal cramps, acute hemolytic anemia, sickle cell crisis, headache or insomnia, urethritis, dysuria, crystalluria, hyperoxaluria, or hyperuricemia. With rapid IV administration temporary dizziness and soreness at the injection site may occur. Vitamin C may produce false-negative tests for occult blood in stools if taken within 48 to 72 hours of testing.

Contraindications/Precautions: Sodium ascorbate should not be used in patients on sodium restriction; calcium ascorbate is contraindicated in patients who are receiving digoxin (Lanoxin). Excessive doses should be avoided in patients with G6PD deficiency, hemochromatosis, thalassemia, sideroblastic anemia, or sickle cell anemia or in patients prone to gout or renal calculi.

Drug Interactions: Large doses may attenuate the hypoprothrombinemic effects of PO anticoagulants. Aspirin and other salicylates may inhibit ascorbic acid uptake by leukocytes and tissues, and ascorbic acid may decrease elimination of salicylates. Chronic high doses of ascorbic acid may diminish the effects of disulfiram.

Pregnancy: Category C.

RDA: 60 mg/day.

Nursing Responsibilities:

- Obtain baseline and periodic hematocrit and hemoglobin values as well as serum electrolytes.
- Assess for signs and symptoms of acute hemolytic anemia or sickle cell crisis, or both.

Patient and Family Education:

- Do not take vitamin C supplements during pregnancy unless recommended by the health care provider.
- Take large doses of vitamin C in divided amounts because the body only uses what is needed at a particular time and excretes the rest in urine.
- Avoid taking megadoses of vitamin C because this can interfere with the absorption of vitamin B_{12}.
- If taking iron supplements, remember that vitamin C increases the absorption of iron when the two are taken concurrently.
- To prevent deficiency consume dietary sources rich in vitamin C such as citrus fruits, cantaloupe, strawberries, tomatoes, broccoli, cauliflower, and cabbage.

Minerals

Minerals are essential substances that constitute about 4% of the body weight and serve many diverse functions. Some are essential ions or electrolytes in body fluids; others are bound to organic molecules such as hemoglobin, phospholipids, or metabolic enzymes. Those minerals that function as critical electrolytes in the body, most notably sodium and potassium, are covered in more detail in Chapter 42. Sodium chloride, sodium bicarbonate, and potassium chloride are featured as drug prototypes in that chapter.

Because minerals are needed in very small amounts for human metabolism, a balanced diet will supply the necessary quantities for most patients. Like vitamins, excess amounts of minerals can lead to toxicity, and patients should be advised not to exceed the recommended doses. Mineral supplements are, however, indicated for certain disorders. Iron-deficiency anemia is the most common nutritional deficiency in the world and is a common indication for iron supplements. Women at high risk for osteoporosis are advised to consume extra calcium, either in their diet or as a dietary supplement.

62.7 Macrominerals are inorganic substances needed in amounts of at least 100 mg per day for normal body functioning.

Macrominerals are major inorganic substances that must be consumed daily in amounts of 100 mg or higher. Included in this group are calcium, chloride, magnesium, phosphorus, potassium, sodium, and sulfur. Following are brief descriptions of some common macrominerals and their therapeutic uses. Each macromineral is listed in Table 62.4 along with the recommended daily allowance and function.

Calcium: Calcium is primarily stored in the teeth and bones to provide strength. Calcium may also be found in blood, muscle, and in the body fluid between cells. A consistent level of calcium is needed for vital body processes and functions such as bone matrix construction, muscle contraction, hormone and enzymes secretion, hemostasis, and nerve conduction. When a calcium deficiency occurs the patient may become irritable and restless, with muscular cramps, spasms, and cardiac abnormalities. Fractures may result from continued hypocalcemia. Calcium compounds are available for pharmacotherapy in many PO salts such as calcium carbonate, calcium citrate, calcium gluconate, or calcium lactate. IV preparations are administered in severe cases. Calcium gluconate is featured as a prototype drug for hypocalcemia and osteoporosis in Chapter 75.

Chloride: Chloride is a chemical that the human body needs for metabolism and to maintain acid–base balance. In the CNS the inhibitory actions of certain neurotransmitters rely on the entry of chloride into specific neurons. The amount of chloride in the blood is carefully controlled by the kidneys. Isolated imbalances of chloride are due to imbalances in fluid, electrolytes, or acid base. Chloride imbalances are corrected by treating the underlying pathology.

Magnesium: Magnesium is required for more than 300 biochemical reactions in the body. This mineral helps maintain normal muscle and nerve function, keeps cardiac rhythm steady, supports a healthy immune system, and maintains bone strength. The pharmacologic use of magnesium includes multiple pathologic conditions. For example, magnesium citrate is used for bowel evacuation, as is magnesium hydroxide, which can also be used as an antacid. Magnesium salicylate is used for the relief of pain and inflammation in rheumatoid arthritis. Lastly, the mineral can also be used as a CNS depressant because magnesium sulfate is frequently used as an anticonvulsant in labor and delivery. Magnesium sulfate is featured as a drug prototype in Chapter 42.

Most recently, magnesium has been used to help regulate blood sugar levels, promote normal blood pressure, and assist in energy metabolism and protein synthesis. The metabolism of magnesium is important to insulin sensitivity and blood pressure regulation. Magnesium deficiency is common in people with diabetes. Several epidemiologic studies indicate that magnesium may play an important role in regulating blood pressure. Furthermore, magnesium assists in the metabolism of carbohydrates and may influence the release and activity of insulin, which is the hormone that helps control blood glucose (sugar) levels.

Phosphorus: Phosphorus, another essential macromineral, binds to calcium to form calcium phosphate in bones. In addition to playing a role in bone structure, phosphorus is a component of protein, adenosine triphosphate (ATP), and nucleic acids. Dietary sources of phosphorus are widely available; thus hypophosphatemia is most often seen in patients with severe malnutrition, intestinal malabsorption disorders, or kidney impairment that re-

TABLE 62.4 Macrominerals

Mineral	RDA	Function
Calcium	800–1,200 mcg	Forms bony matrix; regulates nerve conduction and muscle contraction
Chloride	750 mcg	Major anion in body fluids; part of gastric acid secretion
Magnesium	Men: 350–400 mg Women: 280–300 mg	Cofactor for many enzymes; necessary for normal nerve conduction and muscle contraction
Phosphorus	700 mg	Forms bone matrix; part of ATP and nucleic acids
Potassium	2 g	Necessary for normal nerve conduction and muscle contraction; principal cation in intracellular fluid; essential for acid–base and electrolyte balance
Sodium	500 mg	Necessary for normal nerve conduction and muscle contraction; principal cation in extracellular fluid; essential for acid–base and electrolyte balance
Sulfur	Not established	Component of proteins, B vitamins, and other critical molecules

sults in excess phosphorus loss in the urine. When serum phosphorus levels fall below 1.5 mEq/L, phosphate supplements are usually administered. Sodium phosphate and potassium phosphate are available for treating phosphorus deficiencies.

62.8 Microminerals are inorganic substances needed in amounts of at least 20 mg per day for normal body functioning.

Commonly called trace minerals, the **microminerals** are required daily in amounts of 20 mg or less. Although they are needed in minute amounts, their functions should not be underestimated. Profound illness may result with deficits of some of the microminerals. Following are brief descriptions of some common microminerals and their therapeutic uses. Each micromineral is listed in Table 62.5 along with the RDA and function.

Iron: Iron is essential to normal human physiology as an integral part of many proteins and enzymes that maintain good health. Iron is an essential component of proteins involved in oxygen transport; a deficiency limits oxygen delivery to cells, resulting in fatigue, poor work performance, and decreased immune function. It is also essential for the regulation of cell growth and differentiation. Dietary sources include meat, shellfish, nuts, and legumes.

Iron can be supplemented using various pharmacologic preparations, which often have ascorbic acid added to improve the absorption of PO iron. Generally, iron supplementation therapy is a PO therapy, and parenteral IV or intramuscular (IM) iron therapy is only given when absorption is seriously compromised by illnesses or when the patient cannot swallow. A prototype drug feature for iron sulfate is presented in Chapter 41.

Iodine: Iodine is a micromineral needed to synthesize thyroid hormone. The most common source of dietary iodine is iodized salt. When dietary intake of iodine is low, hypothyroidism occurs and enlargement of the thyroid gland results. At high concentrations iodine suppresses thyroid function. Lugol's solution, a mixture containing 5% elemental iodine and 10% potassium iodide, is given to hyperthyroid patients prior to thyroidectomy or during a thyrotoxic crisis. Sodium iodide is a drug that acts by rapidly suppressing the secretion of thyroid hormone and is indicated for patients who are having an acute thyroid crisis. Radioactive iodine (I-131) is given to destroy overactive thyroid glands (see Chapter 68). As an expectorant, the iodine ion increases mucus secretion formation in the bronchi and decreases viscosity of the mucus. Iodine salts such as iothalamate and diatrizoate are very dense and serve as diagnostic contrast agents in radiologic procedures of the urinary and cardiovascular systems.

Fluorine: Fluorine, a trace mineral, is best known as the mineral that is helpful for bone and teeth health. Dental professionals may apply concentrated fluoride topically to the teeth to prevent cavities, especially in children. Many cities have added fluoride to the municipal water supply to improve dental health. Because high amounts of fluoride can be quite toxic to children, the use of fluoride-containing products should be closely monitored.

Zinc: Zinc is found in at least 100 enzymes and has a role in regulating nucleic acid synthesis as well as wound healing, bone formation, cell-mediated immunity, and male fertility. Sources of zinc include protein foods, beans, lentils, nuts, seeds, and whole grain cereals. Zinc sulfate, zinc acetate, and zinc gluconate are available to prevent and treat deficiency states at doses of 60 to 120 mg per day. Lozenges that contain zinc can be purchased OTC for treating sore throats and cold symptoms.

TABLE 62.5 Microminerals

Trace Mineral	RDA	Function
Chromium	0.05–2 mg	Potentiates insulin and is necessary for proper glucose metabolism
Cobalt	0.1 mcg	Cofactor for vitamin B_{12} and several oxidative enzymes
Copper	1.5–3 mg	Cofactor for hemoglobin synthesis
Fluorine	1.5–4 mg	Influences tooth structure and possibly affects growth
Iodine	150 mcg	Component of thyroid hormones
Iron	Men: 10–12 mg Women: 10–15 mg	Component of hemoglobin and some enzymes of oxidative phosphorylation
Manganese	2.5 mg	Cofactor in some enzymes of lipid, carbohydrate, and protein metabolism
Molybdenum	75–250 mg	Cofactor for certain enzymes
Selenium	Men: 50–70 mcg Women: 50–55 mcg	Antioxidant cofactor for certain enzymes
Zinc	12–15 mg	Cofactor for certain enzymes, including carbonic anhydrase; needed for proper protein structure, normal growth, and wound healing

NURSING PROCESS APPLICATION

Patients Receiving Vitamin or Mineral Supplementation

Assessment	Potential Nursing Diagnoses
Prior to administration: • Obtain a complete health history, including allergies, drug history, and possible drug interactions. • Obtain a complete physical examination. • Assess for the presence of vitamin and mineral deficits. • Obtain the following laboratory studies: complete blood count (CBC), serum electrolytes, renal function (BUN and serum creatinine).	• *Imbalanced Nutrition, Less than Body Requirements* • *Risk for Injury,* related to adverse effects of vitamin and mineral therapy • *Deficient Knowledge (Vitamin and Mineral Therapy)*

Planning: Patient Goals and Expected Outcomes

The patient will:

- Immediately report symptoms related to hypersensitivity reactions such as itching, shortness of breath, flushing, cough, and heart palpitations.
- Maintain normal vitamin and mineral levels.
- Demonstrate an understanding of the action of the vitamin or mineral by accurately describing adverse effects and precautions.

Implementation

Interventions and (Rationales)	Patient and Family Education
• Monitor for urticaria, pruritus, dyspnea, flushing, and anaphylaxis. (Hypersensitivity reactions may occur with vitamin and mineral supplementation.)	• Instruct the patient to report itching, shortness of breath, or flushing immediately.
• Monitor patient dietary intake, which includes normal foods eaten as well as supplements taken. (This determines preferences and avoidance behavior of specific food groups, which may contribute to deficiency.)	• Instruct the patient to maintain a food log for 3 consecutive days (include one weekend day).
• Encourage natural sources to correct vitamin and mineral deficiencies. (Most vitamins and minerals can be obtained through natural sources, possibly eliminating the need for supplementation.)	Instruct the patient: • On methods to increase dietary intake of needed vitamins or minerals. • To consult the dietitian for alternative forms to increase the dietary intake of the needed nutrient.
• Monitor the therapeutic effectiveness of vitamin and mineral supplementation. (Determine the related symptoms that will resolve once vitamin and mineral levels return to normal state.)	Instruct the patient on: • The symptoms that will resolve once vitamin and mineral levels return to normal. • A timeframe in which to expect improvement.
• Monitor for any adverse effects while administering elevated therapeutic doses of the vitamin or mineral. (Although adverse reactions are rare for most vitamins and minerals, all supplementation has some potential associated adverse effects.)	• Instruct the patient to report adverse effects specific to the vitamin or mineral therapy prescribed.
• Monitor laboratory tests such as serum calcium, phosphorus, magnesium, alkaline phosphatase, and BUN when high therapeutic doses are given. (Toxic states often manifest with abnormal laboratory values.)	• Explain the purpose of required laboratory tests and scheduled follow-up with the health care provider.
• Determine the effect of the vitamin or mineral on other prescribed medications if indicated. (Some vitamin and mineral preparations may interfere with the absorption of medications.)	• Instruct the patient to report all prescription and nonprescription medications to the health care provider.

Evaluation of Outcome Criteria

Evaluate the effectiveness of drug therapy by confirming that patient goals and expected outcomes have been met (see "Planning").

UNDERSTANDING THE CHAPTER

Key Concepts Summary

62.1 Although the importance of nutrition has been known for centuries, the specific vitamins were discovered in the 1900s.

62.2 Vitamins are essential for optimal health.

62.3 Government regulations and consumer knowledge about vitamins are limited.

62.4 The recommended dietary allowance is the dietary intake level that is sufficient to meet the nutrient requirements for most people.

62.5 Fat-soluble vitamins include vitamins A, D, E, and K.

62.6 Water-soluble vitamins include the B complex vitamins and vitamin C.

62.7 Macrominerals are inorganic substances needed in amounts of at least 100 mg per day for normal body functioning.

62.8 Microminerals are inorganic substances needed in amounts of at least 20 mg per day for normal body functioning.

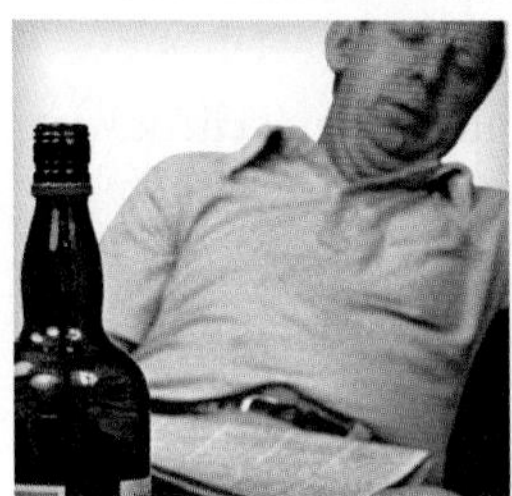

Making the PATIENT *Connection*

Remember the patient "Bill Haywood" at the beginning of the chapter? Now read the remainder of the case study. Based on the information presented within this chapter, respond to the critical thinking questions that follow.

Bill Haywood, a 60-year-old Caucasian male, was brought to the emergency department in an intoxicated state by his family, who found him unconscious in his bathroom. His family states that the patient is a known alcoholic and has been in treatment for alcoholism multiple times. This last drinking binge started 3 weeks ago.

Bill's physical examination reveals the following findings: blood pressure, 104/76 mmHg; pulse 118 beats/minute; respiration 32/minute; temperature 36.1°C (97°F). Although slow to respond to verbal requests, he is intermittently confused and cannot recall recent or past memories. He is pale and frail in appearance. Bill's pupils are reactive to light and present with optic nystagmus. His conjunctiva is markedly jaundiced. His abdomen is slightly distended, indicating possible ascites, and his liver is enlarged and tender. He has 2+ bilateral edema of his legs and feet. Bill is admitted to the intensive care unit with the diagnosis of acute alcohol withdrawal and to rule out Wernicke encephalopathy.

Critical Thinking Questions

1. Upon examination of this patient's laboratory findings, the notable findings are elevated blood pyruvic acid and lactic acid levels. What vitamin deficiency is most likely present given these findings and the patient's previous history?
2. Identify the adverse effects that Bill may experience once vitamin supplement therapy is initiated.
3. Once Bill is stabilized, the nurse will ensure that he receives appropriate referrals to other health care providers. Compile a list of some of the referral sources that would be appropriate in this case.

Case Study

Jerrod is a 16-year-old Hispanic youth with moderate to severe developmental disabilities and mental retardation. He is cared for by his mother in their home. Jerrod has been admitted for possible seizure activity after his mother reported that he began atypical twitching and jerking of the extremities. The mother reports that Jerrod was unresponsive to her commands throughout the episode, which lasted approximately 4 to 5 minutes.

On further questioning, Jerrod's mother discloses that until approximately 6 months ago he attended a day care center for individuals with disabilities. However, due to his increased unpredictable irritability and combative behavior, his mother feared Jerrod venturing outside of the home. Typically, Jerrod spends his days watching television in a dark room or staring endlessly at a fish tank. Additionally, Jerrod is extremely selective about food intake and refuses to consume any dairy products, eggs, fish, or cereals. His daily intake consists mostly of chicken tenders and French fries.

1. One notable laboratory finding is Jerrod's hypocalcemia and hypophosphatemia. What vitamin deficiency is most likely present given these findings and the patient's previous history?
2. What adverse effects should you monitor Jerrod for once the vitamin supplement therapy is initiated?
3. What environmental changes would you recommend to Jerrod's caregivers?

NCLEX-RN® Review

1 A health care provider has ordered oral vitamin A (Aquasol A) supplements for each of the clients with conditions as listed below. A nurse should question the order for which client? The client:

1. With night blindness
2. With malabsorption syndrome
3. Who is lactating
4. With skin conditions

2 Vitamin C (Ascorbic Acid) is being initiated for a postoperative client. What health teaching would be appropriate? Vitamin C:

1. Megadoses can enhance the absorption of vitamin B_{12}.
2. May decrease the incidence of anesthesia-induced complications.
3. Will improve wound healing and increase resistance to infection.
4. Should be taken in large one-time doses.

3 The nurse determines that the client does not understand the important principles of thiamine (vitamin B_1) therapy when the client makes which of the following statements?

1. "I will immediately report tightness of the throat, itching, or swelling of lips."
2. "Sources of thiamine include pork, beef, liver, and other whole grains."
3. "Thiamine may be used with other B vitamins to reduce depression."
4. "Vitamin B_1 maintains normal blood calcium and phosphate levels."

4 A client is receiving vitamin D therapy for nutritional deficiency. The nurse should ask the client about a history of which of the following conditions?

1. Kidney stones
2. Osteomalacia
3. Hypocalcemia
4. Psoriasis

5 A nurse should anticipate the administration of vitamin K (Phytonadione) for which of the following clients? Select all that apply.

1. A newborn infant
2. The client with visual disturbances
3. The client who received an overdosage of certain anticoagulants
4. The client with hypothyroidism
5. A teenager with chronic acne

6 Pyridoxine (vitamin B_6) is being initiated for a client with inadequate dietary intake. What instructions would be inappropriate?

1. Dietary sources of vitamin B_6 include whole grain cereals, liver, and legumes.
2. Record a complete dietary history to identify and correct poor eating habits.
3. Burning or stinging pain at the injection site is a medical emergency.
4. Some medications may increase pyridoxine requirements.

See Answers to Critical Thinking Questions, Case Study, and NCLEX-RN® Review in Appendix A.

References

Adams, M. (2005). *Vitamin D myths, facts and statistics.* Retrieved August 21, 2008, from http://www.naturalnews.com/003069.html

Bronstein, A. C., Spyker, D. A., Cantilena, L. R., Jr., Green, J., Rumack, B. H., & Heard, S.E. (2007). 2006 annual report of the American Association of Poison Control Centers' National Poison Data System (NPDS). *Clinical Toxicology, 45*(6), 815–917.

Jean-Marie, S. (2007). Vitamin supplements: Ensuring a healthy start in life. *Nursing in Practice: The Journal for Today's Primary Care Nurse, 18*(33), 43–44, 46.

More, J. (2007). Who needs vitamin supplements? *Journal of Family Health Care, 17*(2), 57–60.

Prentice, R. L. (2007). Clinical trials and observational studies to assess the chronic disease benefits and risks of multivitamin-multimineral supplements. *American Journal of Clinical Nutrition, 85*(Suppl. 1), 308S–313S.

Rosenberg, I. H. (2007). Challenges and opportunities in the translation of the science of vitamins. *American Journal of Clinical Nutrition, 85*(Suppl. 1), 325S–327S.

Sinatra, S. T. (2007). Cutting edge: Refuel your heart—Four nutritional supplements play critical roles in new approach to heart disease. *Alternative Medicine Magazine, 14*(52), 67–70.

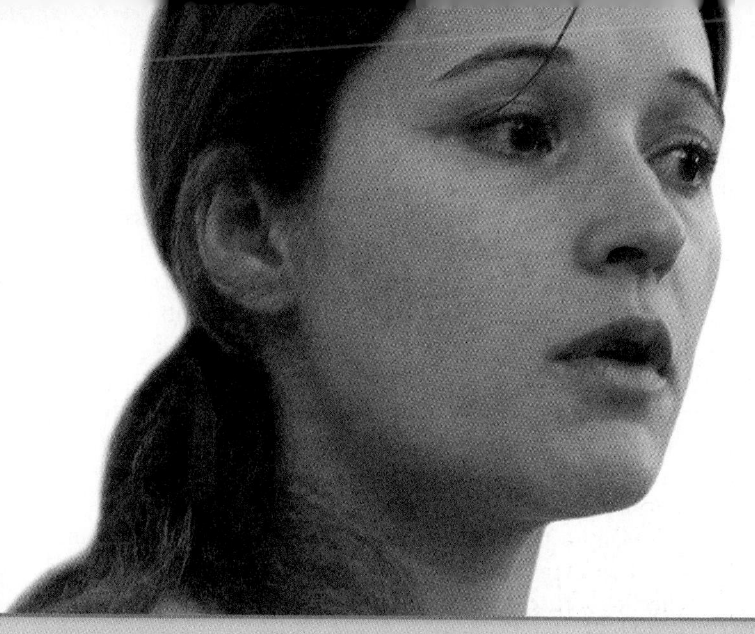

I feel so sick. I can hardly swallow and now I am losing so much weight that I cannot care for my family, let alone myself. My belly is getting big and the cramping keeps me up at night.

Patient "Christine Jones"

CHAPTER 63

Enteral and Parenteral Nutrition

Chapter Outline

Enteral Nutrition

- **Methods of Administration**
- **Enteral Formulations**
- **Elements of Enteral Nutrition**
- **Complications of Enteral Therapy**
- **Drug and Food Interactions**

Parenteral Nutrition

- **Components of Total Parenteral Nutrition Solutions**
- **Monitoring the Patient on Total Parenteral Nutrition**
- **Complications of Parenteral Therapy**
- **Drug and Food Interactions**

Learning Outcomes

After reading this chapter, the student should be able to:

1. Compare and contrast enteral and parenteral methods of nutrition.
2. Distinguish among oligomeric, polymeric, modular, and specialized formulas for enteral nutrition.
3. Identify the possible complications and adverse effects of enteral nutrition administration.
4. Identify and describe the major drug interactions that can occur when enteral nutrition formulas are given.
5. Implement the nursing management for the care of patients receiving enteral feedings.
6. Discuss parenteral protein-sparing nutrition, peripheral vein parenteral nutrition, and central hyperalimentation and the indications for the use of each.
7. Describe the components of total parenteral nutrition solutions and the function of each element in attaining the body's daily requirements.
8. Describe the possible complications of parenteral nutrition therapy.
9. Implement the nursing management for the care of patients receiving total parenteral nutrition.

Key Terms

bolus feedings, *1069*
central vein total parenteral nutrition, *1077*
continuous infusion feedings, *1069*
cyclic feedings, *1069*
dumping syndrome, *1069*
enteral nutrition (EN), *1068*
intermittent feedings, *1069*
modular formulas, *1070*
oligomeric formulas, *1069*
parenteral nutrition, *1068*
partial parenteral nutrition, *1076*
peripheral vein total parenteral nutrition, *1076*
polymeric formulas, *1070*
refeeding syndrome, *1073*
specialized formulas, *1070*
total parenteral nutrition (TPN), *1076*

The intake of various nutrients in predetermined amounts or in combinations is necessary to maintain good health and to allow for the body's healing during periods of illness. The intake of sufficient amounts of amino acids (proteins), carbohydrates, fats, vitamins, and minerals can often be achieved by eating a well-balanced diet of foods and fluids. There are some circumstances, however, where the daily nutritional needs of the body may require supplementation. The purpose of this chapter is to examine the methods and types of products available for providing enteral and parenteral nutrition.

63.1 Nutritional supplementation is required for patients with certain medical conditions.

Ensuring that patients have the necessary nutritional intake for proper health and wellness is a primary responsibility of the nurse. This responsibility extends to all patients, regardless of age, condition, or disease status. Although healthy patients can maintain their required caloric and nutritional requirements by eating a balanced diet, there are certain disease states that may require nutritional intervention. Such conditions include the following:

- Severe infections, such as human immunodeficiency virus-acquired immunodeficiency syndrome (HIV-AIDS)
- States of malnutrition
- Bowel rest for inflammatory bowel disease and disorders of the gastrointestinal (GI) tract
- Coma
- Postsurgical complications
- Major burns and trauma
- Neuromuscular and central nervous system disorders
- Advanced age or prematurity
- Eating disorders
- Cancer-related chemotherapy or radiation therapy

Although mechanical causes such as the inability to chew or swallow properly may limit caloric or nutritional intake, psychological and social reasons also play a role in inadequate nutrition. For example, stress related to a hospitalization may alter a patient's normal eating habits or regimen. Unfamiliar foods and generalized malaise or fear associated with a patient's medical condition may also result in a decreased appetite. Patients may have insufficient funds to purchase adequate amounts or types of foods or may be shunning food as a means of coping with the effects of clinical depression. For the elderly patient, poor fitting dentures or issues with dysphagia may lead to nutritional deficits. Younger patients may be on a fad diet with limited intake of specific nutrients or may be engaging in activities related to bulimia or anorexia.

Clinical nutritional support is utilized in all settings, including hospitals and extended or long-term care facilities, as well as in the individual patient's home. Pediatric patients are now provided various forms of nutritional support at specially trained day care facilities and schools.

Malnutrition in hospitalized persons or residents of nursing homes can result in complications such as delayed wound healing, muscle atrophy, impaired immune function, infection, and death. Secondary complications can include peripheral edema caused by a reduction in plasma proteins and a decreased oncotic pressure (see Chapter 42). Malnourished individuals can also experience dry, flaky skin and hair loss as a result of their poor nutritional state.

63.2 Supplemental nutrition may be provided by the oral or parenteral routes.

There are two basic routes to administer nutritional support: enteral and parenteral. **Enteral nutrition (EN)** is used for patients who have a functioning GI tract but are unable to orally ingest an adequate amount of nutrients to meet their metabolic needs. **Parenteral nutrition** involves the administration of high caloric nutrients via a central vein, such as the subclavian vein.

Before initiating any form of nutritional support therapy, the medical team of health care providers, dietitians, and nurses must thoroughly evaluate the patient and determine which is the best method of treatment. It is also important to examine which route of nutritional support will achieve the desired optimum result. Areas that must be addressed include the amount of weight lost by the individual patient, the percentage of meals consumed, the patient's albumin level, and the patient's overall health and appearance. Other factors to consider when planning nutritional support is the patient's primary diagnosis, the patient's ability to swallow, any anticipated diagnostic testing and treatments (e.g., nothing by mouth [NPO] for more than 3 days), and the patient's overall prognosis. Socioeconomic factors of convenience, feasibility, and cost play a role in the decision-making process as well.

Enteral Nutrition

63.3 There are various methods utilized to administer enteral feedings to the patient.

EN includes products that are administered via the GI tract, either orally or through a feeding tube. When the patient's condition permits, EN is best administered by the oral route. Administering nutrition this way allows the natural digestive process to occur and requires less direct nursing supervision. Oral administration does require patient adherence to the planned feeding regimen and the ability to safely swallow the substance.

If the patient is unable to swallow properly, a feeding tube is passed either through the nose to the GI tract or surgically inserted directly into the stomach or small intestine. A nasogastric (nose to stomach) tube is more commonly used for short-term therapy and is often inserted by the nurse. If the patient displays symptoms of decreased gastric motility, a nasoduodenal or nasojejunal tube is usually inserted by the health care provider. Placement of this tube is confirmed by x-ray, and initiation of its use requires approval from the health care provider. If therapy is expected to last longer than 4 weeks, surgical or percutaneous endoscopic insertion of a gastrostomy or jejunostomy tube by the health care provider may be appropriate. A percutaneous endoscopic gastrostomy (PEG) tube remains the preferred route for long-term therapy and is usually better tolerated than a nasogastric tube.

An advantage of providing nutritional support via a feeding tube is that the amount of enteral solution can be precisely controlled and measured, and calories can be recorded. Contraindications to total enteral nutrition include peritonitis, intestinal obstruction, intractable vomiting, paralytic ileus, intractable diarrhea, and GI ischemia.

Methods of Administration

63.4 Enteral feedings can be delivered by bolus, intermittent drip or infusion, continuous infusion, or cyclic intermittent infusion.

Bolus feedings were the first method introduced and typically deliver 250 to 400 mL of formula every 4 to 6 hours via a syringe or funnel. This method takes about 15 minutes to complete and may not be well tolerated due to the large volume of solution introduced in such a short period. The bolus method can also cause nausea, vomiting, abdominal cramping, and diarrhea, and there is a greater risk of aspiration. It is used with medically stable or ambulatory patients who have adequate absorptive capacity to tolerate the larger volume of fluid.

Intermittent feedings are administered every 3 to 6 hours and take about 30 to 60 minutes to infuse. They can be delivered either by gravity drip or by feeding pump infusion, with 300 to 400 mL of solution administered at each feeding. These feedings commonly use a feeding bag and are considered an inexpensive method of administering EN to the patient.

Continuous infusion feedings are often prescribed for critically ill patients or those with duodenal or jejunal entry feeding tubes. This type of feeding is often delivered by an infusion pump at a slow rate over a 16- to 24-hour period. Studies have shown that continual enteral feeding methods result in the patient meeting his or her nutritional goals much quicker (Rhoney, Parker, Formen, Yap, & Coplin, 2002; Serpa, Kimura, Faintuch & Ceconello, 2003). The continuous method of delivery is more successful because it helps to prevent complications such as the dumping syndrome and avoids the need for frequent irrigation of the tube. **Dumping syndrome** is the result of a sudden influx of feeding into the GI tract and the creation of a high osmotic gradient within the small intestine. This in turn causes a sudden shift of fluid from the vascular compartment to the intestinal lumen. Plasma volume decreases, causing vasomotor responses such as an increased pulse rate, decreased blood pressure, pallor, sweating, weakness, and dizziness. The increased intestinal fluid results in distention and produces a feeling of fullness, abdominal cramping, nausea, vomiting, and diarrhea.

Cyclic feedings are commonly infused over 8 to 16 hours daily (day or night). Infusions during the daytime hours are recommended for patients who are restless during sleep or have a greater risk of aspiration. Night-time infusion allows patients more freedom during the day and is frequently used for ambulatory patients.

Enteral Formulations

63.5 There are several types of liquid nutrition formulas that are commercially available for enteral feedings.

Enteral solutions differ according to the various nutrients, the caloric values, and the osmolality of the solution. There are four basic groups of solutions for EN: oligomeric, polymeric, modular, and specialized. Table 63.1 lists the preparations and commercially produced products on the market.

- **Oligomeric formulas** contain simple or basic forms of free amino acids and peptide combinations that require little or no digestion and are easily absorbed into the body. They are used in patients with digestive disorders such as malabsorption syndrome, partial bowel obstruction, irritable bowel syndrome, short bowel syndrome, bowel fistulas, and antibiotic- or radiation-induced intestinal damage. Because there is little stimulation of digestive secretions, these products are also useful for patients with chronic pancreatitis.

TABLE 63.1 Commercial Enteral Feeding Products

Type	Products	Nursing Responsibilities
Oligomeric	Criticare HN Peptamen Liquid Precision HN, LR Vivonex total enteral nutrition, HN	Formulas are hypertonic and must be started slowly and diluted.
Polymeric	Carnation Instant Breakfast Ensure Ensure HN Ensure Plus	Polymeric formulas can be isotonic or hyperosmolar. Hyperosmolar formulas can cause abdominal cramping and diarrhea. They are started at a slower rate and are administered diluted.
Modular	Casec MCT oil Microlipid Polycose Propac	Most formulas come in powder form, so preparation can be complex and expensive. This product must be stored carefully to prevent contamination.
Specialized	Amin Aid Glucerna Hepatic-Aid II Pulmocare	Formulas may not provide all the necessary nutrients, so careful monitoring of the patient is important.

MyNursingKit | Nursing in Action Video: Patient with a Nasogastric Tube

Oligomeric formulas are more expensive than polymeric preparations, with the main caloric source coming from carbohydrates. They are usually low in fat, which allows for rapid gastric emptying, and many of these preparations are designed for administration directly into the intestines. Flavor packets are available to improve the taste, but they are generally unpalatable and best suited for tube feedings.

- **Polymeric formulas** contain various mixtures of protein, fat, and carbohydrates in high molecular weight form and are considered the most common enteral preparation. These formulas are used in patients who are generally undernourished but have a fully functioning GI tract. Polymeric formulas include blenderized diets and meal replacement formulas. Blenderized diets are generally high-residue, highly viscous products. Meal replacement formulas are either milk based or lactose free. These preparations are nutritionally complete, generally meet the recommended dietary allowance (RDA) for vitamins and minerals (see Chapter 62), and are palatable for oral ingestion.
- **Modular formulas** or supplements contain a single nutrient, protein, carbohydrate, or lipid, and yield a higher caloric density. Although not designed to serve as a sole source of nutrition, they can be added to other products to meet a specific nutrient deficiency. For example, protein modules can be utilized to meet the extra nitrogen needs of patients with burns or severe trauma. Fat modules can be added to the formula of a patient who is ventilator dependent in order to increase the ratio of fat-to-carbohydrate calories and, in turn, decrease the respiratory quotient.
- **Specialized formulas** are designed to fill the specific needs in patients with a particular condition. These conditions include renal failure, hepatic failure, pulmonary disease, or a specific genetic enzyme deficiency.

Elements of Enteral Nutrition

63.6 There are four basic classes of nutrients contained in most enteral nutrition formulas.

There are many different enteral products, each containing various amounts of nutritional substances. The four basic nutrient classes and their functions are as follows.

Carbohydrates: Carbohydrates are the major source of energy in the diet and function to spare body protein, prevent ketosis, and regulate blood glucose levels. Carbohydrate sources in enteral formulas must be soluble, digestible, and have a low osmolality. Commonly used sources of carbohydrates include corn syrup solids, hydrolyzed corn starch, maltodextrin, and other glucose polymers. Some special formulas include various types of fiber, fructose, and fructo-oligosaccharides. Simple sugars, such as sucrose, glucose, dextrose, and lactose, enhance the palatability of the oral preparations but increase the product's osmolality. These simple sugars retain water in the intestinal tract and can therefore promote diarrhea in the patient. The percentage of total calories derived from carbohydrates varies from 30% to 90%, depending on the particular preparation and the specific condition for which it was designed to treat. Most available EN products do not contain lactose and thus should not pose a problem for patients experiencing lactose intolerance.

Proteins: Proteins are essential to the diet because they support cellular growth as well as maintain and repair body tissues. They may be delivered as intact proteins, partially digested (hydrolyzed) protein, or free amino acids. The selection of a particular protein product is based on the patient's medical condition and his or her ability to absorb the protein. Soy protein and caseinates are common sources of intact proteins and are found in polymeric formulas. Oligomeric formulas contain enzymatically hydrolyzed casein or whey. Elemental formulas contain free amino acids. Proteins may make up approximately 4% to 32% of the total calories of enteral formulas, depending on the specific product. Products that are designed for patients with renal impairment may contain no protein, whereas patients who are receiving immune-enhancing formulas may receive as much as 80 g of protein per 1,000 kcal.

Lipids: Lipids provide an isotonic, high caloric source of energy for the body. Soybean and corn oil are commonly used as lipid sources, with canola and safflower oils being recently introduced to the market. Long chain triglycerides provide essential fatty acids, limit the osmolality, and enhance the palatability of the product. The fat content of the enteral product can vary from 1% to 55% of the total calories. Products that are designed for patients with glucose intolerance or pulmonary disease are generally high in fat, whereas products that are designed for patients with intestinal malabsorption contain lower amounts of total fat.

Other nutrients: Most commercially prepared enteral formulas are fortified with vitamins and minerals. When given in adequate volume, they normally provide most of the elements needed for body functioning. However, the volume required to provide the RDA varies greatly among the numerous products available to the consumer. Fiber such as cellulose and pectin is added to enteral formulas to improve stool consistency but can create complications in patients who are fluid restricted or have delayed GI motility. Because most enteral formulas do not provide enough water in solution to maintain adequate hydration, additional free water is needed to meet the minimum fluid requirements.

Complications of Enteral Therapy

63.7 Although considered physiological in nature, total enteral nutrition can predispose the patient to various complications.

Total enteral nutrition therapy poses a risk of mechanical complications such as aspiration, gastroesophageal reflux, diarrhea, metabolic and electrolyte disturbances, and procedural-related problems, such as tube clogging, tube migration, and dislodgment. Localized infections and sepsis are also potential problems during treatment. Table 63.2 summarizes the various complications of EN therapy.

Aspiration: The most serious potential complication for patients who are receiving enteral feedings is tracheobronchial aspiration

TABLE 63.2 Complications of Enteral Nutrition

Complication	Possible Cause	Intervention
Gastrointestinal		
Diarrhea (more than four bowel movements per day or large loose stool)	Medications	• Eliminate antibiotics or antacids if possible.
	Fat intolerance	• Eliminate feedings containing sorbitol. • Change to low-fat formula.
	Bacterial overgrowth	• Culture stool for pathogens. • Administer lactobacillus (acidophilus, Lactinex) if the patient is receiving antibiotics.
	Contaminated formula	• Stop administration of the current formula. • Replace the bag and tubing using aseptic technique. • Adhere to clean standards when changing or manipulating feeding.
	Osmotic overload	• Decrease the concentration of the formula. • Change to an isotonic formula. • Further dilute hypertonic medications.
	Decreased bulk	• Administer medications by an alternate route. • Change to a high-fiber formula. • Administer bulking agents.
	Patient positioning	• Position the patient on the right side to facilitate passage of gastric contents through the pylorus.
	Volume overload	• Decrease the total volume. • Decrease the delivery rate to one previously tolerated. • Advance the delivery rate slowly over 12–24 h. • Stop feeding for 2 hours and check for residuals.
Nausea or vomiting	Delayed gastric emptying	• Change to a low-fat formula. • Administer an agent to stimulate GI tract motility (cisapride, metoclopramide).
	Specific nutrient intolerances	• Change to a lactose-free or low-fat formula.
Constipation (no stool for 3 days)	GI tract obstruction; dehydration and impaction; decreased fiber	• Change to a fiber formula. • Administer a bulking agent. • Stop the feeding. • Provide free water. • Remove impaction.
	GI tract obstruction	• Stop the feeding.
Mechanical		
Pulmonary aspiration	Patient lying flat	• Elevate the head of the bed 30°–45° during continuous feedings or for 30–60 min after bolus feedings.
	Absent or depressed gag reflex	• Infuse feedings into the duodenum or jejunum. • Change to a smaller bore tube.
	Esophageal reflux	• Infuse feedings into the duodenum or jejunum.
	Improper tube placement	• Confirm proper placement of the tube by x-ray after insertion after episodes of severe coughing, vomiting, or a seizure. • Reconfirm placement prior to each feeding by checking for residuals. • Tape the tube in place and mark the tube at the exit point for reference. • Restrain the patient if necessary to prevent the tube from being pulled or dislodged.
Tube obstruction	Acid precipitation of formula	• Flush the tube with water before and after checking for gastric residuals. • Infuse feedings into the duodenum or jejunum. • Do not mix medications with the enteral formula.
	Insufficient tube irrigation	• Flush the tube with warm water before and after each bolus feeding and every 8 hours during continuous feedings or whenever feeding is stopped. • Adequately crush medications and mix powder with water.
	Medications	• Use liquid medications whenever possible. • Flush the tube before and after medication administration with at least 30 mL of warm water.

(continued)

TABLE 63.2 Complications of Enteral Nutrition *(continued)*

Complication	Possible Cause	Intervention
Nasal mucosal damage	Extended use of large-bore tubes	• Avoid administering bulk-forming agents via a small-bore tube. • Alternate nares. • Change to a smaller bore tube. • Change to a permanent gastrostomy or jejunostomy tube for extended enteral support. • Tape the tube in place to minimize rubbing.
Metabolic		
Overhydration	Refeeding syndrome; fluid overload	• Decrease the delivery rate. • Restrict free water. • Change to a concentrated formula. • Administer diuretics. • Change formula.
Dehydration	High osmolality formula; diarrhea; excessive protein intake with inadequate fluid intake; insulin deficiency	• Change formula. • See management of diarrhea. • Change to a decreased protein content formula. • Provide additional water.
Hyperglycemia	Sudden cessation of feedings	• Give insulin via drip. • Change formula to higher fat or lower carbohydrate content. • Taper feedings.
Hypoglycemia	Metabolic acidosis	• Monitor blood sugar if feedings are interrupted. • Reduce potassium intake or use a reduced potassium formula.
Hyperkalemia	Renal insufficiency; anabolic metabolism	• Reduce potassium intake or use a reduced potassium formula. • Administer Kaexalate. • Reduce potassium intake or use a reduced potassium formula.
Hypokalemia	Refeeding syndrome; insulin administration; diuretics; diarrhea	• Monitor serum potassium daily and repeat until the levels stabalize. • Lower dose or discontinue.
Hyperphosphatemia	Renal insufficiency	• Discontinue if possible. • See management above. • Use a reduced phosphate formula. • Administer a phosphate binder.
Hypophosphatemia	Refeeding syndrome, insulin administration	• Monitor serum phosphate daily and repeat until stable.
Hypomagnesemia	Refeeding syndrome, alcoholism	• Monitor serum magnesium daily and repeat until stable.
Hyponatremia	Fluid overload	• Restrict free water. • Use normal saline to flush the tube and provide hydration instead of water. • Reassess medications. • Increase free water.
Elevated BUN	Renal failure, excess protein intake, dehydration, medications (diuretics and steroids)	• Reassess renal function. • Reassess protein needs.
Rapid and excessive weight gain	Excess calories, excess fluid, electrolyte imbalance	• Change the formula. • Evaluate electrolytes.
Insufficient weight gain	Inadequate calories; malabsorption; catabolic state	• Change the formula or increase the delivery rate. • Change to a semielemental formula. • Provide nutrition support for weight maintenance while addressing medical issues.
Depression, withdrawal, nonadherence	Altered body image; loss of oral gratification	• Encourage socialization at mealtimes. • Provide emotional support. • Provide ice chips, sugar-free gum, or hard candy. • Provide oral care during every shift.

of gastric contents. Studies have shown that 70% of aspiration pneumonias occur in patients receiving some form of enteral feeding, whereas more than 40% of nonaspiration pneumonia admissions are patients with a feeding tube (Coutin et al., 2007). Symptoms of aspiration may include dyspnea, tachypnea, wheezing, rales, tachycardia, agitation, and cyanosis. Aspiration of a small amount of enteral formula may not produce immediate symptoms, but a subsequent fever may suggest the development of aspiration pneumonia. The risk for aspiration is increased if the patient is fed while lying flat or if the patient is unconscious. The head of the bed should be elevated at least 30° during the administration of the feeding and should remain elevated for at least 30 minutes after the feeding. The nurse should check for gastric residual volume by gently aspirating the stomach contents before administering the next feeding, or every 4 to 6 hours if the patient is on a continuous infusion. Other risks factors for aspiration include a diminished gag reflex, neurologic injury, gastroesophageal reflux, and the use of large-bore feeding tubes.

Nausea and vomiting: A small percentage of patients who are receiving enteral tube feedings experience nausea and vomiting, which increase the risk of aspiration. The most common cause for this problem is delayed gastric emptying. If this cause is suspected, the following steps should be considered:

- Reduce the doses of opioid or other medications that slow GI motility.
- Switch to a low-fat preparation.
- Administer the feeding at room temperature.
- Reduce the rate of administration.
- Administer a promotility agent such as metoclopramide (Reglan).
- Consider antiemetic medications such as prochlorperazine (Compazine) if gastric residues are low yet nausea persists.

Diarrhea: One of the major problems in tube feeding patients is diarrhea, which is commonly due to the rapid administration of the feeding, high caloric solutions, or bacterial contamination of the feeding formula or equipment. A patient who develops diarrhea while receiving EN should be evaluated for *Clostridium difficile*, which usually results secondary to antibiotic therapy. Drugs that contain magnesium, such as antacids, may contribute to the problem of diarrhea, as well as drugs containing sorbitol, liquid cimetidine (Tagamet), and various multivitamin preparations. Diarrhea frequently coincides with the initiation of the enteral treatments because many of the medications that had been given by the intravenous (IV) route are changed to the PO route when enteral feeding is begun. This frequently causes diarrhea. If diarrhea develops during enteral therapy, the following should be considered:

- Add fiber, such as psyllium (see Chapter 61).
- Consider switching to a formula containing fiber.
- Decrease the rate of infusion.
- Dilute the solution.
- Administer an antidiarrheal agent.

Metabolic complications: **Refeeding syndrome** can occur when nutritional support, including EN therapy, is introduced to severely malnourished patients. This syndrome consists of metabolic complications, such as dehydration, electrolyte imbalances, and hyperglycemia. In severe cases, nervous system complications such as confusion, seizures, and coma may occur.

Careful monitoring can minimize or prevent metabolic complications. To prevent refeeding syndrome, those at high risk should first be identified, including patients with anorexia nervosa, kwashiorkor, chronic alcohol abuse, prolonged fasting, and prolonged IV hydration. Any electrolyte abnormalities should be corrected before starting nutritional support therapy, and vital signs, intake and output (I&O), and laboratory values should all be carefully monitored.

Clogged feeding tube: Tube clogging is more likely to occur with the use of intact protein and high viscous products. Routine flushing of the feeding tube with 20 to 30 mL of warm water every 4 hours during continuous feedings and before and after each intermittent feeding and drug administration can prevent most clogs. Aseptic technique should be utilized in order to minimize formula contamination, and extreme care should be maintained when administering medications via the feeding tube (Table 63.3). Various methods are used to unclog

TABLE 63.3 Drug Administration Guidelines with Enteral Feedings

The following are guidelines for administering medications to patients who are receiving enteral nutrition:

- If the patient is able to take medications by mouth, the PO route is preferred over administration through the tube.
- Alternate routes of administration (IV, intramuscular (IM), rectal, sublingual, or transdermal) should be considered for certain medications that cannot be crushed, are not available in liquid form, or which repeatedly clog or block the tubing.
- Check the compatibility of the medication with the tube feeding formula first before administering it through the tube.
- If a tablet is to be administered through the feeding tube, check with the pharmacist first to make sure that crushing the medication will not alter its effectiveness. Then crush the tablet into a fine powder and mix the powder with warm water before administering the drug.
- For individual doses of most medications, the tube should be flushed with at least 30 mL of water before and after administration. This will serve to clear the tube for the drug delivery, facilitate the transport of the drug to the intestine, and indicate if the tube is patent.
- When several medications are to be administered, all medications should be given separately and the feeding tube flushed with at least 5 mL of water after each medication.
- Most drugs in elixir form are hypertonic. Highly concentrated drug solutions or suspensions should be diluted with at least 60 mL of water before administration in order to decrease gastric mucosal irritation and to prevent osmotic diarrhea.
- Medications should never be added directly to the feeding formula. This may result in a decrease in the potency of the medication as well as a decrease in the stability of the feeding formula.
- For most medications enteral feedings should be stopped for at least 15 min before and after the administration of a drug.

a blocked feeding tube. The first is to instill warm water via a syringe, using slight manual pressure. If this fails, a sodium bicarbonate solution may be instilled in order to break down the clog. Carbonated beverages and cranberry juice have also been known to restore patency to blocked feeding tubes.

Interrupted infusions: In the hospitalized patient, EN may be interrupted for various diagnostic tests and procedures. These may include feedings held due to drug–food incompatibilities, hemodialysis treatment, "NPO after midnight" for surgery or procedures, physical or occupational therapy sessions, transportation from the unit, or GI intolerance (diarrhea, nausea, vomiting). When frequent interruptions are expected, recalculating the goal flow rate on a 22- or 23-hour basis instead of 24 hours may be more practical.

TABLE 63.4 Interaction of Drugs with Enteral Formulas

Interaction with Enteral Formula	Drugs
Physically Incompatible	Dimetapp elixir, Robitussin, thoridazine (Mellaril), iron preparations, KCL liquid, MCT oil, antacids, dicyclomine (Bentyl), cimetidine (Tagamet)
Increased Osmolality	Digoxin (Lanoxin), theophylline, phenytoin (Dilantin), furosemide (Lasix), methyldopa (Aldomet)
Decreased Drug Effect	Warfarin (Coumadin), phenytoin, carbamazepine (Tegretol), ciprofloxacin (Cipro), digoxin, theophylline, lithium, levodopa (L-dopa)

Drug and Food Interactions

63.8 Most medications that are administered orally can also be delivered to the patient via an enteral tube.

Medications that are delivered via an enteral tube must be in a liquid form (elixir or suspension), or finely crushed and dissolved in a liquid vehicle. Drugs that must not be crushed or dissolved are enteric-coated pills, time-release forms, sublingual medications, and bulk-forming laxatives. If a tablet must be administered through the feeding tube, the nurse should check with the pharmacist to make sure that crushing the medication will not alter its effectiveness.

When liquid forms of drugs are mixed with enteral preparations, physical incompatibilities can cause the mixture to thicken and clog the feeding tube. Hyperosmolar liquid medications can also be poorly tolerated by the GI tract, resulting in abdominal distention and cramping, vomiting, and diarrhea. Both of these problems can be avoided by simply flushing the feeding tube with water and by diluting the medication first with warm water before instilling it into the feeding tube.

Enteral feeding products are usually delivered as a constant infusion and contain high concentrations of proteins and certain metals such as calcium, magnesium, and iron. These important nutrients can bind with certain medications, hindering the bioavailability of the drug and, in turn, reducing the total delivered dose of the medication. The fluoroquinalone antibiotics such as ciprofloxacin (Cipro) are a frequently prescribed class of drugs that can interact with these metals. The effectiveness of liquid phenytoin (Dilantin) is often reduced by the drug's ability to bind with proteins in the enteral formula, resulting in subtherapeutic levels of the medication. Likewise, therapeutic levels of warfarin (Coumadin) may also be affected due to protein binding and the presence of vitamin K in the feeding preparation. Holding the enteral feeding for 1 hour before and after an antibiotic dose and 2 hours before and after giving phenytoin or warfarin will help minimize the drug's interaction with the enteral feeding. Table 63.4 lists the various drugs that interact with enteral formulas.

CONNECTION *Checkpoint* 63.1

From what you learned in Chapter 3, explain why drugs that have an enteric coating and those that are extended release should not be crushed and used in enteral feeding. See Answer to Connection Checkpoint 63.1 in Appendix A.

CONNECTIONS

To the Community Enteral Nutrition in the Home Setting

For patients who are receiving home EN therapy via a PEG tube, the impact of this life-altering process may go far beyond the patient to include the family as well. Although the enteral formula can ensure that the patient's nutritional needs are met, the psychological impact can be massive. For some individuals, it may mean never eating another piece of pizza or tasting a spoonful of ice cream ever again. Eating is a comfort, a pleasure, a ritual, and a social occasion. Not being able to orally ingest the food can be devastating to some individuals.

If physically possible, thirst can be eliminated by providing additional water to the tube feeding regimen, rinsing the mouth with water, or by chewing gum or sucking on hard candy. Lubricating the patient's lips with lip balms that now come in various food or fruit flavors can enhance the patient's comfort as well as provide a welcoming taste of food.

It is important for the nurse to stress that the patient needs to keep the teeth, gum, and tongue clean by routine brushing and flossing. Performing oral hygiene at least twice a day will help to decrease bacteria from accumulating in the mouth.

Teach the patient and the family how to administer the feedings and how to care for the enteral tubing. Both the patient and the family need to know what to do if the patient aspirates or if the tube becomes dislodged and how to handle any other complications that may arise. They need to be supplied with emergency contact numbers and be able to recognize which medical situations clearly require emergency treatment.

NURSING PROCESS APPLICATION

Patients Receiving Enteral Nutrition Therapy

Assessment

Prior to administration:

- Obtain a complete health history, including allergies, drug history, and possible drug interactions.
- Obtain a complete physical examination, including height and weight.
- Assess for the presence or history of nutritional deficits, such as inadequate oral intake, GI disease, and increased metabolic need.
- Obtain the following laboratory studies: total protein, albumin levels, serum creatinine, blood urea nitrogen (BUN), complete blood count (CBC), electrolytes, lipid profile, and serum iron.
- Assess that the tube site (once inserted) is secure.
- Assess urine output daily.

Potential Nursing Diagnoses

- *Imbalanced Nutrition: Less than Body Requirements*
- *Deficient Knowledge (Enteral Therapy)*
- *Noncompliance*, related to therapeutic regimen
- *Risk for Injury*, related to tube migration or dislodgment and pulmonary aspiration of enteral feeding solution

Planning: Patient Goals and Expected Outcomes

The patient will:

- Demonstrate improvement or stabilization of nutritional status.
- Demonstrate an understanding of the feeding's action by accurately describing the adverse effects and precautions.
- Immediately report significant adverse effects such as symptoms of hypoglycemia or hyperglycemia, fever, chills, cough, or malaise.
- Maintain laboratory values within the normal limits.

Implementation: Enteral Nutritional Therapy

Interventions and (Rationales)	Patient and Family Education
• Monitor vital signs, observing for signs or infection such as elevated temperature. (Bacterial contamination may occur in high-glucose and high-protein formula.) • Monitor the tube insertion site for signs of redness or skin irritation. (Skin excoriation and infection can occur because the surgical opening penetrates the peritoneum.)	• Instruct the patient to report fever, chills, soreness, drainage at the tube insertion site, cough, or malaise.
• Use aseptic technique with tubing, dressing changes, and feeding solution. (The use of aseptic technique will reduce the incidence of contamination.) • Refrigerate any unused formula and change the feeding bag daily or per institution protocol. (Enteral formulas have a short half-life and the unused formula can sour or spoil if kept uncovered at room temperature. Routinely changing the feeding bag reduces the risk for bacterial contamination.)	Instruct the patient: • That the tube insertion site has a high risk for infection development, hence caution must be taken to keep the area free of irritation or bacteria. • To carefully clean around the tube insertion site and to check that the tube is secure before administering the feeding. • To refrigerate any unused portion of the formula and to monitor the formula for spoilage.
• Monitor weight daily at the same time each day and maintain a record of daily caloric intake. (Weighing the patient at the same time each day will provide a more stable assessment of weight changes and help in assessing the effectiveness of treatment.)	• Instruct the patient to measure weight at home or to keep a record of any oral intake (if permitted).
• Monitor blood glucose levels. Observe for signs of hyperglycemia or hypoglycemia and administer insulin as directed. (Blood glucose levels may be affected by an increase in the rate of formula infusion, if the continuous infusion is stopped, or if the type of formula is changed.)	• Instruct the patient to report symptoms of hyperglycemia (excessive thirst, copious urination, and insatiable hunger) or hypoglycemia (nervousness, irritability, and dizziness).
• Monitor for signs of fluid and electrolyte imbalance by checking electrolyte values. (Electrolytes are indicators of protein nourishment. Electrolyte imbalances may reflect the presence of refeeding syndrome or dumping syndrome, which can occur in patients who receive supplemental nutrition.) • Provide free water to prevent dehydration. (Free water is used by the body to dilute concentrated vascular and cellular spaces, preventing increased serum osmolality.) • Monitor skin turgor and assess the mucous membranes for dryness. (Decreased skin turgor and dry mucous membranes indicate dehydration.)	• Instruct the patient to report any shortness of breath, heart palpitations, and swelling or dryness of mucous membranes, or decreased urine output.
• Monitor renal status. (I&O ratio, daily weight, and laboratory studies, such as serum creatinine and BUN, are used to assess renal function.)	Instruct the patient to: • Weigh self daily. • Monitor I&O. • Report sudden increases in weight or decreased urine output. • Keep all appointments for follow-up care and laboratory testing.

(continued)

NURSING PROCESS APPLICATION *(continued)*

Implementation: Enteral Nutritional Therapy

Interventions and (Rationales)	Patient and Family Education
• Monitor bowel sounds at every shift. (Diarrhea or constipation is a common complication with enteral therapy.) • Record the frequency and consistency of stools. (Patients on enteral therapy can develop *C. difficile* or formula-related diarrhea.) • Monitor the patient's medication regimen for any incompatibilities with the enteral formula. (Many liquid medications contain sorbitol, which can cause diarrhea; other medications may be incompatible with the enteral formula.)	• Instruct the patient to report any abdominal cramping, constipation, nausea, vomiting, or diarrhea.
• Monitor respiratory status at every shift. (Early detection of changes can prevent complications.) Check for signs of respiratory distress, frothy sputum, or abnormal lung sounds. (These may indicate aspiration of the feeding or stomach contents.) • Keep the head of the bed elevated at least 30° for feeding and 1 hour after completion of feeding. (This prevents regurgitation and aspiration.) • Check for proper placement of the tube at every shift by checking for residual volumes. Check prior to each bolus feeding and every 4–6 hours for continuous infusions. (Proper placement helps to reduce the risk of aspiration.) • Hold the feeding if the residual volume is greater than the amount infused in 2 hours of continuous feeding or 50% of the amount of previous bolus feeding. (Increased gastric residual volume may lead to aspiration of the feeding.)	Instruct the patient: • To report any signs of respiratory distress such as shortness of breath, cough, or chest discomfort. • On the proper technique to check for residual volumes, and have the patient or family member demonstrate in return.
• Deliver the enteral feeding according to the method ordered. (Abrupt discontinuation or changes in administration may cause fluctuations in blood glucose levels.) • Flush the tubing accordingly and monitor for occlusion of the tube. (Periodic flushing of the tube with warm water will prevent clogging of the tube with thickened formula.)	Instruct the patient: • About the importance of maintaining the prescribed feeding regimen and rate of infusion. • In techniques to maintain the patency of the feeding tube (flushing the tube with water, properly crushing medications). • In techniques to regain patency if the tube becomes occluded.
• Monitor for signs of depression or withdrawal. (Patients on long-term enteral therapy may experience depression associated with loss of oral gratification from normal ingestion and withdrawal and isolation related to social factors associated with eating.)	• Provide the patient and family with psychological support. • Offer preprinted information and referral to a support group as needed.

Evaluation of Outcome Criteria

Evaluate the effectiveness of drug therapy by confirming that patient goals and expected outcomes have been met (see "Planning").

Parenteral Nutrition

63.9 Parenteral nutrition is used when patients are unable to tolerate enteral feedings.

Parenteral nutrition is often utilized for patients who are unable to eat or tolerate any form of EN. It is frequently given to patients with severe GI disorders such as diseases of the small bowel (Crohn's disease, fistulas, adhesions, postoperative ileus), necrotizing pancreatitis, hyperemesis gravidarum (maternity patients), and pediatric patients with congenital anomalies or prolonged diarrhea. It is also used for patients with demonstrated undernutrition (less than 50% of the metabolic needs met for more than 7 days) as well as patients with AIDs, cancer chemotherapy or radiation-induced enteritis, burns, severe trauma, or anorexia.

Parenteral nutrition is also referred to as **total parenteral nutrition (TPN)** or hyperalimentation and is administered solely by the IV route. It can be delivered via a peripheral line or a central line, depending on the hypertonicity of the solution. TPN can provide all the calories, glucose, protein, fats, minerals, and trace elements needed by the body to sustain growth and to promote weight gain as well as wound healing. **Partial parenteral nutrition** is considered a parenteral solution that lacks an essential element, usually fats or lipids.

Peripheral vein total parenteral nutrition is used when a central venous line cannot be accessed or when it is not appropriate for the patient. These situations may include patients in whom the subclavian vein is inaccessible due to scar tissue from repeated IV line punctures or in patients with extensive trauma, severe burns, or cancer in the region of the upper torso or chest. These patients may be relatively healthy with only a slight nutritional deficit that cannot be met with enteral therapy. Peripheral vein total parenteral nutrition is considered a temporary measure until a central line can be placed, and the solution administered is usually lower in osmolality than the

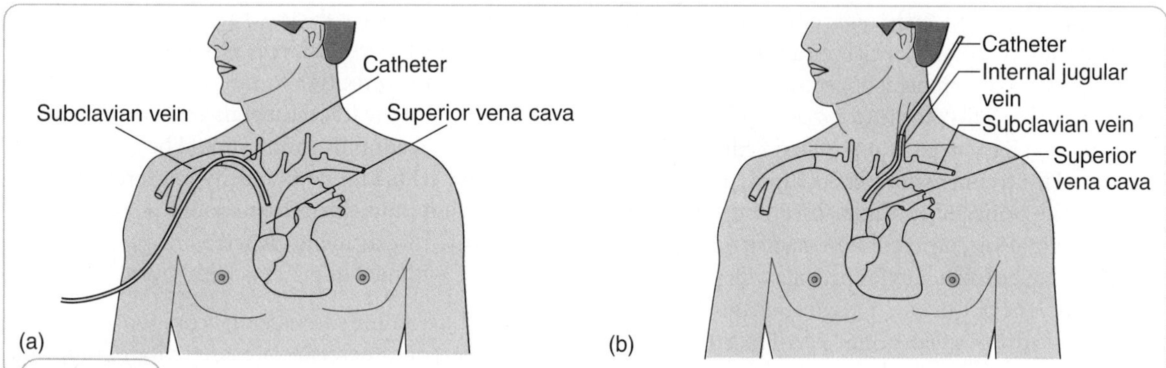

Subclavian vein
Catheter
Superior vena cava
(a)
Catheter
Internal jugular vein
Subclavian vein
Superior vena cava
(b)

Figure 63.1

Central line placement: (a) subclavian vein insertion; (b) left jugular insertion.
Source: From *Kozier & Erb's Fundamentals of Nursing: Concepts, Process, and Practice* (p. 1457), by A. Berman, S. Snyder, B. Kozier, & G. Erb, 2007. Reprinted by permission of Pearson Education, Inc., Upper Saddle River, NJ.

solution delivered through a central line. Peripherally infused parenteral nutrition is advantageous because there are fewer risks associated with the catheter placement, care of the infusion site is simpler, and the complications associated with hyperosmolar solutions can be avoided.

Problems associated with peripheral vein total parenteral nutrition include the need for several large peripheral veins, because the catheter site is routinely rotated to prevent infection. The vein must also be able to accommodate the larger-sized venous catheter. PTPN is associated with a high risk of phlebitis and is therefore reserved for patients with robust veins. Peripherally inserted central catheters (PICC lines) are often inserted in patients for home therapy with peripheral vein total parenteral nutrition.

Central vein total parenteral nutrition is the administration of the solution through a central vein such as the subclavian or the internal jugular vein. Because of the hypertonicity of the parenteral solution, the catheter tip must always be positioned in the superior vena cava so that the solution can be immediately diluted to a more tolerable concentration. The central vein total parenteral nutrition solution usually consists of crystalline amino acids, dextrose, and lipid emulsions with the addition of vitamins, minerals, trace elements, essential electrolytes, and water.

Central vein total parenteral nutrition is used in patients with limited peripheral access or in those patients whose nutritional needs cannot be met by peripheral vein total parenteral nutrition formulas. It is usually considered the access of choice for long-term parenteral therapy and is always administered using an infusion pump in order to precisely monitor the amount of solution given. Figure 63.1 shows the location of a central venous catheter for TPN therapy.

PharmFACT

When assessing undernourished patients for potential enteral therapy, the nurse should consider that the lack of dietary intake may be caused by drugs that cause bleeding gums (anticoagulants), altered taste (captopril), candidiasis (broad-spectrum antibiotics), or nausea and vomiting (antineoplastic drugs and many others). *Source:* Dawodu, Scott, & Chase, 2007.

Components of Total Parenteral Nutrition Solutions

63.10 The basic total parenteral nutrition solution consists of carbohydrates, lipids, amino acids, electrolytes, minerals, and vitamins.

TPN solutions may be modified daily based on the patient's laboratory results, the underlying disorder, the rate of metabolism, and other factors. Like the enteral products, the basic components include carbohydrates, lipids, amino acids, proteins, electrolytes, minerals, and vitamins.

Carbohydrates: Carbohydrates and lipids are the primary sources of calories for the patient on TPN. Dextrose is the most common carbohydrate source because it is inexpensive and readily available from cornstarch, beet, or cane sugar. The RDA of carbohydrates for adult patients ranges from 25 to 35 kcal/kg. When administered through a central line, the concentration of dextrose in the TPN solution usually comprises 25% to 35% of the overall solution.

When dextrose is administered as the primary calorie source (without lipids added), hyperglycemia can occur. Because insulin is required for dextrose utilization, a combination of dextrose and lipids may help reduce the risk of hyperglycemia and the patient's need for supplemental insulin injections. Dextrose increases the metabolic rate and the production of carbon dioxide, which may increase the demands placed on the patient's respiratory system. The addition of lipids will also decrease this risk. Abruptly stopping the TPN solution can result in hypoglycemia due to the continued release of endogenous insulin. This problem can be avoided by substituting a dextrose 10% solution until the new TPN solution bag is available, or by gradually tapering the solution over a 24-hour period when discontinuing parenteral therapy.

CONNECTION *Checkpoint* 63.2

From what you learned in Chapter 42, what are the primary indications for an infusion of dextrose in water (D_5W)? Why should a patient with severe heart failure not receive D_5W? See Answer to Connection Checkpoint 63.2 in Appendix A.

MyNursingKit | American Society for Parenteral and Enteral Nutrition

Lipids: Unlike amino acids and concentrated dextrose solutions, fat emulsions are isotonic, which means that they can be infused through either a peripheral or central line. They are often a requirement for patients who are receiving TPN therapy longer than 5 days. Lipid preparations that are currently available are produced from either safflower oil (Liposyn) or soybean oil (Intralipid). The principal fatty acids used in these preparations are linoleic, linolenic, oleic, palmitic, and stearic acids.

Fat emulsions can be hazardous for patients with liver disease, pulmonary disease, anemia, or blood coagulation disorders, with the most common adverse effect being hyperlipidemia. Fat emboli and death can occur when lipids are administered to premature, preterm, or low-birth-weight infants.

Amino acids: Amino acids are needed by the body to promote the production of proteins, to conserve lean body mass, and to help promote wound healing. The RDA for infants and children ranges from 1.4 to 2.5 g/kg per day, whereas adults require 0.8 to 1 g/kg daily. Essential amino acids cannot be produced by the body, whereas nonessential amino acids can be synthesized from a nitrogen source, such as ammonium salts or urea. Amino acids must be closely monitored in patients with renal failure, because the blood urea nitrogen (BUN) level can become elevated. For the patient with liver failure, the administration of amino acids may result in hepatic coma due to the liver's inability to process nitrogen.

Electrolytes and minerals: Electrolytes, including sodium, potassium, magnesium, calcium, phosphorus, chloride, and acetate, can be added to the TPN formula as salts. Specific electrolyte amounts are ordered daily by the health care provider, based on preexisting deficiencies and the patient's current medical condition. To prevent interactions between specific elements and crystallization of the solution, the pharmacist should add the electrolytes.

Trace mineral mixtures typically contain copper, chromium, manganese, selenium, and zinc and are commercially available to meet the specific nutritional needs of the patient. Trace minerals are metabolic cofactors that are essential for the proper functioning of several enzyme systems.

Although it is routine to monitor serum electrolyte levels, serum levels of the trace minerals are generally not monitored. Trace mineral administration should be decreased or withheld in patients with a limited capacity to excrete them. For example, selenium and chromium should not be used in patients with renal impairment, whereas copper and manganese should be withheld in patients with severe hepatic disease.

Vitamins: Vitamins are essential components of the TPN regimen. Most commercially prepared vitamin formulas can be given on alternate days in order to meet the patient's need for both fat-soluble vitamins as well as the water-soluble vitamins, and they can be added to the existing TPN solution. Vitamin K is usually administered weekly by subcutaneous or intramuscular (IM) injections.

Monitoring the Patient on Total Parenteral Nutrition

63.11 Regular monitoring of the patient on total parenteral nutrition therapy is essential to detect and minimize complications.

Regular monitoring is important during TPN therapy. The patient's individual nutritional requirements should be reviewed regularly, taking into account the patient's current condition, drug therapy, nutritional status, concurrent treatments (e.g., hemodialysis), response to TPN, and supporting laboratory data.

The measurement of daily weights and I&O are essential indices of the patient's response to treatment. Clinical assessment of the patient can reveal physical complications such as ascites, edema, impaired wound healing, or loss of muscle mass that may not be evident if monitoring the patient's weight and laboratory values alone. A suggested schedule for monitoring the patient who is receiving TPN therapy is included on Table 63.5.

TABLE 63.5 Suggested Monitoring Schedule for the Patient on Total Parenteral Nutrition

Assessment Tool	Baseline	Acute Patient	Stable Patient
Electrolytes (sodium [Na], potassium [K]), BUN, creatinine, calcium (Ca), magnesium (Mg), phosphorus	Yes	Daily	1–2 times/week
	Yes	Twice a week	Weekly
Trace elements (zinc, copper, selenium)	Yes	Weekly	Weekly
Triglycerides	Yes	Weekly	Weekly
CBC with differential	Yes	Weekly	Weekly
Prothrombin time (PT), partial thromboplastin time (PTT)	Yes	Weekly	Weekly
Glucose	4 times/day	4 times/day	Daily
Weight	Yes	Daily (same time)	Daily
I&O	Daily	Daily	Daily
Venous access	Yes	Every shift	Every 8 h

Complications of Parenteral Therapy

63.12 As with enteral therapy, patients who are receiving parenteral nutritional therapy can experience various complications.

Despite the vast improvements made in the delivery of parenteral nutrition over the last few years, patients can encounter certain problems during TPN therapy. These may be classified as mechanical, metabolic, or septic in nature.

Mechanical complications: Improper or incorrect placement of the catheter can result in subclavian artery puncture, pneumothorax, hemothorax, carotid artery injury, thromboembolism, catheter malposition, brachial plexus injury, subcutaneous emphysema, endocarditis, cardiac arrhythmias and tamponade, and phrenic nerve paralysis. Venous thrombosis is the most common problem and is associated with significant morbidity rates. Signs of venous thrombosis include distended neck veins as well as swelling of the face and arm on the side of the IV catheter.

Metabolic complications: Metabolic complications of parenteral nutrition therapy fall into two broad categories: early or late complications (Table 63.6). Early complications can usually be anticipated and include fluid volume overload, refeeding syndrome, and various electrolyte and mineral imbalances. Hypertriglyceridemia can lead to pancreatitis and altered pulmonary function if left untreated. The early complications can be prevented by carefully monitoring the patient and adjusting the composition of the TPN formula or the rate of infusion.

Late metabolic complications are less predictable and may be caused by the exacerbation of preexisting conditions, inadequate solution composition, or failure to monitor the patient adequately. Late complications can include fatty acid, mineral, and vitamin deficiencies and metabolic bone disease or bone demineralization, which may develop in patients who receive TPN for periods extending beyond 3 months. Although the exact mechanism is not known, metabolic bone disease can cause severe pain in the lower extremities and the back. The only known treatment is to temporarily or permanently discontinue the TPN infusion. Hepatic steatosis (fatty liver) and gallbladder complications (cholelithiasis and cholecystitis) are also late complications of TPN therapy.

Infectious complications: Parenteral nutrition therapy creates a chronic breach in the patient's physiological line of defense. The IV infusion system from the solution container to the tip of the catheter may serve as a source for the introduction of bacterial or fungal organisms into the patient's bloodstream. The health care provider inserting the venous catheter, the pharmacist mixing the TPN solution, or the nurse hanging the IV bag or changing the central venous catheter dressing may inadvertently contaminate the patient's "lifeline."

Peripheral IV lines are at high risk for infection and infiltration, and the site of the peripheral line should be changed, if possible, every 48 hours in order to eliminate that risk. Unfortunately, severely debilitated patients often have few robust veins available for selection, necessitating the eventual placement of a central line.

Strict asepsis should be maintained when changing the IV tubing and dressings at the IV insertion site. TPN is an excellent medium for the growth of organisms; thus most TPN solutions are prepared by the pharmacist with the use of a laminar airflow

TABLE 63.6 Major Complications of Total Parenteral Nutrition

Complication	Cause	Symptom
Mechanical		
Pneumothorax	Accidental puncture of the pleural cavity by the catheter during insertion.	Sharp chest pain, decreased breath sounds
Hemothorax	Catheter damages a vein with blood entering the chest cavity.	Same as above
Hydrothorax	Catheter perforates a vein, releasing TPN solution into the chest. Clot in the subclavian vein.	Same as above
Venous thrombus	IV tubing is disconnected. Catheter is not clamped. Infusion cap fell off.	Distended neck veins, swelling of the face and arm
Air embolism		Cough, shortness of breath, chest pain, and cyanosis
Metabolic		
Hyperglycemia	Fluid is infused too quickly. Insufficient insulin coverage.	Nausea, headache, weakness, thirst, increased blood glucose level
Hypoglycemia	Fluid stopped abruptly. Too much insulin administered.	Pallor, cold clammy skin, increased pulse, headache, tremors, blurred vision
Fluid overload	Increased IV rate. Fluid shifts from the cellular to the vascular space due to hyperosmolar solution.	Cough, dyspnea, distended neck veins, rales, weight gain
Septic		
Infection	Poor aseptic technique when the catheter is inserted. Contamination of the catheter when changing tubing or when the TPN solution is mixed. Contamination when dressing is changed.	Fever, chills, tachycardia, drainage from the insertion site, lethargy, increased white blood cells (WBCs), positive blood cultures

hood. Whenever possible, the central line should be used exclusively for the infusion of the TPN solution. Other preventive measures to reduce the patient's risk for infection include:

- Changing the dressing routinely (every 48 to 72 hours, per institutional policy) or when it becomes soiled, wet, or loose. The caregiver should wear a mask and gloves while changing the dressing.
- Extending the application of antimicrobial solution (e.g., iodine) at least 1 inch beyond the edges of the final dressing.
- Placing a sterile sponge over the catheter, then covering with an occlusive, waterproof dressing.
- Inspecting the site for signs of tenderness, redness, edema, loose sutures, or any bleeding or drainage.
- Changing the TPN tubing every 24 hours with the first bag of the day. A 0.22 micron inline filter should be used to reduce the introduction of bacteria from the TPN solution.
- Avoiding the use of the TPN catheter for central venous pressure (CVP) monitoring or the administration of IV medications or blood products.

PharmFACT

Catheter-related infections are four to five times higher in patients with diabetes who are receiving TPN compared to those who do not have diabetes and are receiving TPN. *Source:* Davidson, 2000.

Drug and Food Interactions

63.13 Certain drugs are incompatible and should not be added to parenteral nutrition solutions.

The major issue associated with the addition of medications to the parenteral formula is the potential for drug incompatibilities. A significant risk is that of a precipitate forming in the solution but being obscured by the opaque fat emulsion. Therefore, drug additions to the TPN solution should never be undertaken unless sufficient data exist to ensure the stability of the solution. Medications that are routinely added to parenteral preparations and are physiologically stable in solution are the H_2-receptor antagonists, such as ranitidine (Zantac) and insulin.

When there is no other option but to administer a medication through the same access site as the TPN, it is best to use a separate lumen in a multilumen catheter to avoid the potential for incompatibility. The use of a Y site or piggyback drug delivery has helped to decrease the risk of drug compatibility problems. Flushing the IV line prior to and after the medication administration, along with temporarily turning off the TPN infusion during the drug administration for 15 to 30 minutes, will help lower the possibility of interactions.

Drugs with demonstrated physical incompatibilities with TPN include ampicillin, tetracycline, and amphotericin B. For administration of these medications, a second IV line should be sought. Medications that have a decreased therapeutic drug effect when given to patients who are receiving TPN with lipids include kanamycin and warfarin. It is important for the nurse to always check with the pharmacist to confirm compatibility and drug effectiveness when administering TPN with any medication.

CONNECTION *Checkpoint* 63.3

From what you learned in Chapter 60, to what drug class does ranitidine belong? Why would it be added to TPN solutions? See Answer to Connection Checkpoint 63.3 in Appendix A.

CONNECTIONS

To the Community Home Care of Patients on Total Parenteral Nutrition Therapy

The patient and the patient's family should have the opportunity to practice the procedure for delivering TPN therapy at home while they are in the hospital setting under the supervision of the nurse. Review the procedure for the storage of the solution. Instruct the patient to keep the containers refrigerated, but to allow the container to come to room temperature before administering the solution. Instruct the patient not to warm the TPN in the microwave or the oven. Advise the patient to check the expiration date, label of contents, and the appearance of the solution. The patient should not use the solution if the TPN is cloudy, discolored, or has solid pieces floating in it. The solution should not be used if any separation (oil and water) is visible. The patient should check the integrity of the bag by gently squeezing it in order to detect any leakage.

The dressing is to be changed at least every 2 days. Instruct the patient, family, or caregiver to use aseptic technique when changing the dressing. The supplies for the dressing and the infusion should be kept in a clean, dry place when not in use. The IV site should be inspected for any signs of swelling, redness, or drainage, which should be reported to the health care provider immediately. Demonstrate to the family how to irrigate the catheter and how to change the bags and the tubing. Instruct the patient in the various settings of the infusion pump, paying particular attention to reviewing what to do if the alarm goes off during the infusion. Review the local Environmental Protection Agency (EPA) policy regarding the proper disposal of used syringes and IV equipment.

Explain that the patient should be weighed daily, and that the patient's I&O should be closely monitored. Ask the family to observe the patient for signs of edema. Demonstrate to the family how to check the urine glucose level using labsticks. Review the potential complications of TPN, such as chills, fever, dyspnea, chest pain, coughing, reaction to lipid infusion, air embolism, nausea, vomiting, and hypo- or hyperglycemia. Instruct the patient never to stop the TPN infusion without conferring first with the health care provider. Recommend that the family keep the telephone number of the health care provider, the nursing service, and the community emergency services readily available in case an emergency or other need should arise.

NURSING PROCESS APPLICATION

Patients Receiving Total Parenteral Nutrition

Assessment

Prior to administration:

- Obtain a complete health history including allergies, drug history, and possible drug interactions.
- Obtain a complete physical examination including height and weight.
- Assess for the presence or history of nutritional deficits such as inadequate dietary intake, GI disease, and increased metabolic need.
- Obtain the following laboratory studies: total protein, albumin levels, serum creatinine, BUN, CBC, electrolytes, lipid profile, and serum iron levels.

Potential Nursing Diagnoses

- *Risk for Infection,* related to catheter sepsis and high content of protein and glucose solution infusion
- *Risk for Fluid Volume Imbalance,* related to hypertonicity of infusion fluid
- *Deficient Knowledge (Total Parenteral Nutrition)*, related to purpose, precautions, and adverse effects of therapy

Planning: Patient Goals and Expected Outcomes

The patient will:

- Exhibit improvement or stabilization of nutritional status.
- Be free of infection or injury related to TPN.
- Demonstrate an understanding of the parenteral nutrition therapy by accurately describing the care of the catheter, administration of the solution, adverse effects, and precautions.
- Immediately report adverse effects such as symptoms of hypoglycemia or hyperglycemia, fever, chills, cough, or malaise.

Implementation: Total Parenteral Nutrition

Interventions and (Rationales)	Patient and Family Education
• Monitor vital signs, observing for signs of infection such as elevated temperature. (Bacteria may grow in high-glucose and high-protein solutions.)	• Instruct the patient to report fever, chills, soreness, drainage at the infusion site, cough, or malaise.
• Use strict aseptic technique with the IV tubing, dressing changes, and TPN solution, and refrigerate the solution until 30 minutes before using. (Infusion site is at high risk for development of infection.)	• Instruct the patient that the infusion site has high risk for developing an infection; hence, sterile dressings and aseptic technique with the solutions and tubing are needed.
• Monitor blood glucose levels per order. Observe for signs of hyperglycemia or hypoglycemia and administer insulin as directed. (Blood glucose levels may be affected if TPN is turned off, if the rate is reduced, or if excess levels of insulin are added to the TPN solution.)	Instruct the patient to report symptoms of: • Hyperglycemia (excessive thirst, polyuria, and insatiable hunger). • Hypoglycemia (nervousness, irritability, and dizziness).
• Monitor for signs of fluid overload. (TPN is a hypertonic solution and can create intravascular shifting of extracellular fluid.)	• Instruct the patient to report shortness of breath, heart palpitations, swelling, or decreased urine output.
• Monitor renal status. (I&O ratio, daily weight, and laboratory studies such as serum creatinine and BUN are used to assess renal function.)	Instruct the patient to: • Weigh self daily at the same time each day. • Monitor I&O daily. • Report sudden increases in weight or decreased urine output. • Keep all appointments for follow-up care and laboratory testing.
• Monitor respiratory status. Observe for chest pain, cough, shortness of breath, loss of consciousness. (Air embolism can occur when air is siphoned into the catheter when tubing becomes disconnected or with improper priming of the IV line.)	• Instruct the patient in the proper technique for tubing change, use of Luer-lock connections, and priming of the tubing.
• Maintain an accurate infusion rate with the infusion pump; make rate changes gradually, and never discontinue TPN abruptly. (Abrupt discontinuation may cause hypoglycemia, and a sudden change in the flow rate can cause fluctuations in blood glucose levels.)	Instruct the patient: • About the importance of maintaining the prescribed rate of infusion. • Never to stop the TPN solution abruptly unless instructed to do so by the health care provider.

Evaluation of Outcome Criteria

Evaluate the effectiveness of drug therapy by confirming that patient goals and expected outcomes have been met (see "Planning").

UNDERSTANDING THE CHAPTER

Key Concepts Summary

63.1 Nutritional supplementation is required for patients with certain medical conditions.

63.2 Supplemental nutrition may be provided by the oral or parenteral routes.

63.3 There are various methods utilized to administer enteral feedings to the patient.

63.4 Enteral feedings can be delivered by bolus, intermittent drip or infusion, continuous infusion, or cyclic intermittent infusion.

63.5 There are several types of liquid nutrition formulas that are commercially available for enteral feedings.

63.6 There are four basic classes of nutrients contained in most enteral nutrition formulas.

63.7 Although considered physiological in nature, total enteral nutrition can predispose the patient to various complications.

63.8 Most medications that are administered orally can also be delivered to the patient via an enteral tube.

63.9 Parenteral nutrition is used when patients are unable to tolerate enteral feedings.

63.10 The basic total parenteral nutrition solution consists of carbohydrates, lipids, amino acids, electrolytes, minerals, and vitamins.

63.11 Regular monitoring of the patient on total parenteral nutrition therapy is essential to detect and minimize complications.

63.12 As with enteral therapy, patients who are receiving parenteral nutrition therapy can experience various complications.

63.13 Certain drugs are incompatible and should not be added to parenteral nutrition solutions.

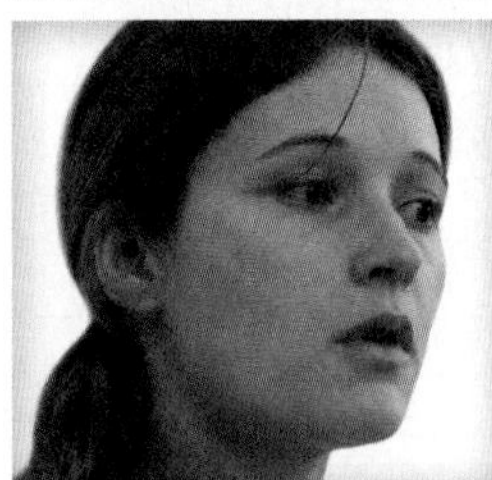

Making the PATIENT *Connection*

Remember the patient "Christine Jones" at the beginning of the chapter? Now read the remainder of the case study. Based on the information presented within this chapter, respond to the critical thinking questions that follow.

Christine Jones, a 32-year-old female, has been admitted to the oncology unit for a course of radiation and chemotherapy, which has been prescribed for her advancing esophageal cancer. Upon admission to the nursing unit, she complained of dysphagia and reported a rapid decrease in her weight over the last 2 weeks. She also noted increasing constipation and abdominal bloating with cramping.

During her 3-week hospitalization, Christine has received a 10-day course of radiation therapy, along with a concurrent course of chemotherapy. Although the cancer has not progressed, she still cannot maintain a proper nutritional state through oral feedings alone. After a lengthy discussion with her health care provider, the option of EN therapy was dismissed due to her high risk for aspiration. A porta-cath, an implantable device placed under the skin of the upper chest into a large vein to provide a pathway for chemotherapy and fluids or to draw laboratory tests, was surgically implanted. Christine was then started on TPN. She is now ready for discharge to home in the care of her husband, Bob, and other family members.

Critical Thinking Questions

1. Christine asks you, the nurse, about storage of the TPN infusion solution. What would you tell her? Give a rationale for your answer.
2. Bob wants to know if there is anything he can do to help while his wife is receiving TPN. What would you tell him?
3. Create a list of potential complications to which Christine and her family should be alerted.

Case Study

Misty Moore is a 36-year-old woman who was admitted to the hospital with a complete bowel obstruction, multiple abdominal adhesions, and a flare-up of Crohn's disease. She stands 5 foot 5 inches and weighs 65 kg. Her usual weight is 75 kg. Her past medical condition includes Crohn's disease since age 16, as well as a 10-year history of type 2 diabetes. Exploratory surgery is scheduled to remove the diseased portion of her small bowel as well as to perform lysis of the adhesions, which occurred as a result of her previous bowel operations. Because of her depleted nutritional state and the 10% drop in her weight, nutritional support is indicated. Her GI tract is not expected to be accessible for at least 10 to 14 days.

1. What type of nutritional support do you think is best for Misty?
2. Considering the patient's condition, what metabolic problem would you suspect she is at risk for developing?
3. How can the risk of developing this problem be reduced?

NCLEX-RN® Review

1 To meet his nutritional goals, the client is placed on enteral feedings via a nasogastric (NG) tube. Which of the following assessments should the nurse perform in order to ensure that the client is maintaining a proper fluid balance?

1. Weigh the client every other day.
2. Maintain a strict record of intake and output, and flush the nasogastric tube once a day.
3. Irrigate the nasogastric tube with water per order, and include this amount on the intake and output record.
4. Assess the skin around the tube insertion site for any drainage or irritation.

2 Before hanging a bag of total parenteral nutrition, the nurse checks the various components of the solution. Which of the following elements would the nurse expect to see on the solution label? Select all that apply.

1. Electrolytes
2. Diuretic
3. Trace minerals
4. Isophane (NPH) insulin
5. Multivitamins

3 The nurse is making rounds at the beginning of the shift and notes that the client's total parenteral nutrition bag is empty. Which of the following solutions should the nurse hang until the total parenteral nutrition solution can be properly prepared and delivered to the nursing unit?

1. 5% dextrose in water (D_5W)
2. 5% dextrose in Ringer's lactate (D_5RL)
3. 5% dextrose in 0.9% sodium chloride (D_5NS)
4. 10% dextrose in water ($D_{10}W$)

4 The client has been discharged home on total parenteral nutrition therapy. When making the home visits, the home care nurse should closely monitor which of the following assessments?

1. Temperature and blood pressure
2. Temperature and weight
3. Pulse and blood pressure
4. Pulse and weight

5 The nurse is preparing to hang a lipid (fat) solution and notes that fat globules are visible at the top of the bag. Which of the following actions should be taken?

1. Roll the solution container gently.
2. Shake the solution container vigorously.
3. Run the solution container under warm water.
4. Obtain a different container of solution.

6 The client who is receiving total parenteral nutrition suddenly spikes a fever of 38.6°C (101.5°F). The nurse notifies the health care provider, who orders that the solution and tubing be changed immediately. The nurse would anticipate that the prescriber may also order that the discontinued unused solution be:

1. Returned to the pharmacy.
2. Sent to the laboratory for culture along with the tubing.
3. Recorded with the lot numbers and the manufacturer's name.
4. Discarded in the client's trash receptacle.

See Answers to Critical Thinking Questions, Case Study, and NCLEX-RN® Review in Appendix A.

References

Berman, A., Snyder, S., Kozier, B., & Erb, G. (2008). *Kozier & Erb's Fundamentals of Nursing: Concepts, Process, and Practice* (8th ed.). Upper Saddle River, NJ: Pearson Education, Inc.

Brotherton, A., & Lyons, C. (2006). The impact of HETF for adults with neurological conditions. *British Journal of Community Nursing, 11*(12), 511–518.

Coutin, I. B., Kejriwal, K., Wilde, V. C., Summers, M., Patel, N., & Apted, P. (2007). Tube feeding and pneumonia: An unhappy couple. *Long-Term Care Interface, 8*(1), 21–25.

Davidson, J. K. (2000). *Clinical diabetes mellitus.* New York: Thieme.

Dawodu, S. T., Scott, D. D., & Chase, M. (2007). Nutritional management in the rehabilitation setting. *Emedicine.* Retrieved August 21, 2008, from http://www.emedicine.com/pmr/TOPIC159.HTM

Huisman-deWaal, G., Schoonhoven, L., Jansen, J., Wanten, G., & vanAchterberg, T. (2007). The impact of home parenteral nutrition on daily life. *Clinical Nutrition, 26*(3), 275–288.

Lauts, N. M. (2005). Management of the patient with refeeding syndrome. *Journal of Infusion Nursing, 28*(5), 337–342.

McCormack, D. (2004). When TPN is indicated. *The World of Irish Nursing, 12*(6), 45–46.

Methany, N. A. (2006). Preventing respiratory complications of tube feedings: Evidence-based practice. *American Journal of Critical Care, 15*(4), 360–369.

Parrish, C. R., & McCray, S. (2003, September). Enteral feeding: Dispelling myths. *Practical Gastroenterology,* 33–50.

Rhoney, D. H., Parker, D., Formen, C., Yap, C., & Coplin, W. (2002, September). Tolerability of bolus versus continuous gastric feeding in brain injured patients. *Neurological Research, 24,* 613–620.

Serpa, L., Kimura, M., Faintuch, J., & Ceconello, I. (2003). Effects of continuous versus bolus infusion of enteral nutrition on critical care patients. *Revista de Hospital das Clinicas, Faculty Med, Sau Paulo, 58*(1), 9–14.

Sudakin, T. (2006). Supporting nutrition with T.E.N or T.P.N. *Nursing 2006, 36*(12), 52–55.

Tharp, R. (2007). *Complications of enteral nutrition.* Retrieved August 21, 2008, from http://www.rxkinetics.com/tpntutorial/2_1.html

The Society of Hospital Pharmacists of Hong Kong. (2006). *Drug-enteral tube feeding interaction.* Retrieved August 21, 2008, from http://www.shphk.org.hk/node/130

University of Washington. (2007). *Clinical nutrition: Enteral nutrition.* Retrieved August 21, 2008, from http://healthlinks.washington.edu/nutrition/section5.html

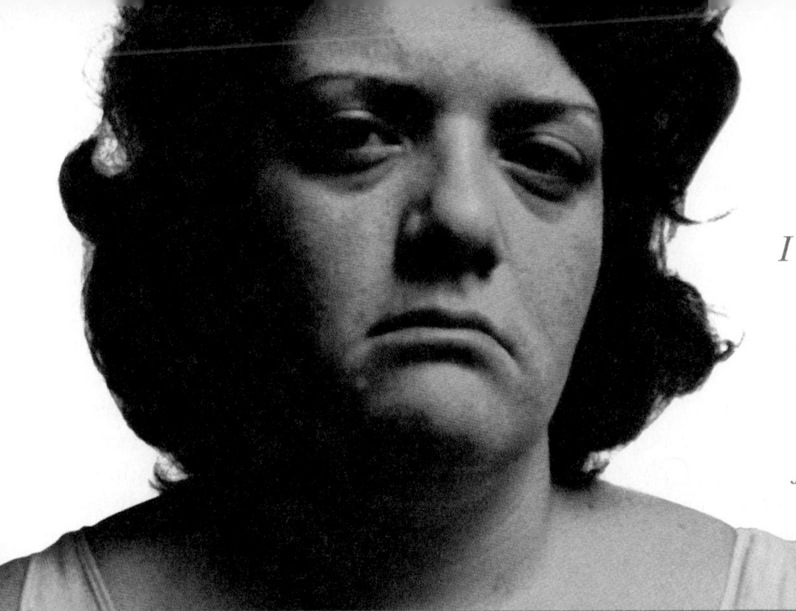

I can't even look at myself in the mirror anymore. Since having my last child, I have gained a tremendous amount of weight. Playing with my kids and finding clothes that fit me have become impossible.

Patient "Rosemary Goodman"

CHAPTER

64 Weight Reduction Strategies and the Pharmacotherapy of Obesity

Chapter Outline

Etiology of Obesity

Pathogenesis of Obesity

Measurement of Obesity

Nonpharmacologic Therapies for Obesity

Pharmacotherapy of Obesity

Anorexiants

PROTOTYPE **Sibutramine (Meridia)** *p. 1090*

Lipase Inhibitors

PROTOTYPE **Orlistat (Alli, Xenical)** *p. 1091*

Adjuncts to Obesity Therapy

Learning Outcomes

After reading this chapter, the student should be able to:

1. Identify genetic and lifestyle factors that contribute to obesity.
2. Explain how energy imbalances can cause weight gain or loss.
3. Describe the role of the hypothalamus in regulating appetite.
4. Explain how leptin and brain neurotransmitters regulate appetite.
5. Describe how obesity is measured.
6. Outline the major components of a successful weight management program.
7. Identify several weight loss agents that were removed from the market due to their adverse effects.
8. Describe the nurse's role in the pharmacologic management of obesity.
9. For each class shown in the chapter outline, identify the prototype and representative drugs and explain the mechanism(s) of drug action, primary indications, contraindications, significant drug interactions, pregnancy category, and important adverse effects.
10. Apply the nursing process to care for patients receiving antiobesity therapy.

Key Terms

adipocytes, *1086*
anorexiants, *1090*
appetite, *1086*
body mass index (BMI), *1087*
cannabinoid receptor (CB1) blockers, *1090*
leptin, *1086*
satiety, *1086*
satiety center, *1086*

Americans spend $30 to $50 billion each year in attempts to lose weight. In the majority of cases, people experience little long-term success in sustaining weight loss. Obesity is closely associated with increased health risks that include premature death, hypertension (HTN), hyperlipidemia, diabetes mellitus, heart disease, sleep apnea, and osteoarthritis. This chapter examines the etiology, pathogenesis, and treatment of obesity.

Etiology of Obesity

64.1 Genetic and lifestyle factors contribute to the etiology of obesity.

Obesity is a growing epidemic in the United States: It is estimated that 95 million adults are overweight or obese. This represents 34% of the adult population over age 20. Along with the increase in adult obesity, infant and childhood obesity has also increased. About 14% of children aged 2 to 5 are now considered obese. All of these percentages have doubled or tripled since the mid-1970s. The trend is expected to continue, as studies have shown that those who were obese as children are more likely to be obese as adults.

Despite considerable research, the specific causes of obesity have not been identified. The etiology is likely a complex combination of genetic, lifestyle, and physiological factors. In a few cases, weight gain can be attributed to medical conditions, the most common being hypothyroidism. Certain rare disorders of the hypothalamus can also cause overeating. Drugs such as corticosteroids are clearly causes of weight gain.

> **Pharm*FACT***
>
> Approximately 30.3% of children (ages 6 to 11) are overweight and 15.3% are obese. For adolescents (ages 12 to 19), 30.4% are overweight and 15.5% are obese. *Source:* National Institute on Media and the Family, 2006.

Studies of family histories and twins support a strong genetic component to obesity. Researchers have identified a few genetic mutations that lead to obesity, although these are rare and do not contribute significantly to the extent of obesity currently observed in the population. While a family history does not cause a person to be obese, it predisposes them to weight gain. The predisposition is best overcome by preventing weight gain. This is particularly important in identifying children at risk of adult obesity and targeting interventions at prevention.

Lifestyle factors play a key role in the development of obesity, the two most obvious factors being diet and physical activity. The fundamental shift in obesity levels in the past three decades has likely been due to high-fat, calorie-dense diets combined with sedentary lifestyles.

There are many theories on the relationship between specific dietary practices and obesity. Often, these are fueled by fad diets rather than research. While it is certainly true that the body metabolizes and stores carbohydrates, lipids, and proteins differently, no specific dietary nutrient limitation has been clearly demonstrated to prevent obesity or to result in more sustainable weight loss.

Despite the ongoing debate on the "best" diet, the fact remains that body weight is determined by energy (calorie) balance. Simply stated, if the number of calories consumed equals the number of calories expended, the person will maintain (balance) body weight at the current level. Changes in weight are due to an energy imbalance. For example, an imbalance of as little as 10 surplus calories per day can lead to a 1 lb weight gain each year. While this seems insignificant, if the imbalance persists over several decades it can lead to obesity in older adults. Of course, this calculation holds true for losing weight, but few are patient enough to wait an entire year to lose a single pound.

Therefore, to lose weight one has to expend more calories than one consumes. In terms of weight loss or gain, the source of the calories, carbohydrates, proteins or lipids, does not matter. Of course, the source is indeed important in terms of overall health and wellness.

The second half of the energy equation is energy expenditure. Physical activity expends calories and can result in either prevention of weight gain or a faster loss of weight. The most successful diet plans always combine a reduction in calories with an increase in physical activity.

Pathogenesis of Obesity

64.2 Appetite is regulated by the satiety center in the hypothalamus and is influenced by various hormones.

Hunger occurs when the hypothalamus recognizes the levels of certain chemicals (glucose) or hormones (insulin) in the blood. Hunger is a normal physiological response that drives people to seek nourishment. Appetite is somewhat different than hunger. **Appetite** is a psychological response that drives food intake based on associations and memory. For example, people often eat, not because they are experiencing hunger, but because it is a particular time of day, or because they find the act of eating pleasurable or social. The psychological feeling of fullness or satisfaction following a meal is called **satiety.** The degree of satiety is directly recognized by a region of the hypothalamus known as the **satiety center.**

> **CONNECTION *Checkpoint* 64.1**
>
> The hypothalamus is part of the limbic system of the brain. From what you learned in Chapter 21, what are the primary functions of the limbic system? See Answer to Connection Checkpoint 64.1 in Appendix A.

Another hormone that regulates hunger and weight balance is **leptin,** a protein secreted by **adipocytes** (fat cells). When a certain amount of fat has been stored, adipocytes increase their secretion of leptin. Receptors for leptin are located in the satiety center in the hypothalamus. Binding of leptin to its receptors signals the hypothalamus that the body has ingested enough food and tells the brain how much adipose tissue is present. Leptin suppresses appetite, and increases body temperature (thermogenic) and energy expenditure. Leptin thus serves as a natural appetite suppressant.

Scientists have intensively searched for a means of reducing appetite by intervening in the leptin pathway. It would seem that administering leptin would be a natural method for suppressing appetite and promoting weight loss. However, obese patients already have high levels of leptin circulating in the blood. Leptin receptors in obese patients appear to have become desensitized and have developed resistance to the satiety effects of leptin. The result is an increase in appetite. At this time, the experimental administration of leptin does not have any effect on obesity.

Binding of the leptin receptors in the hypothalamus creates a signal cascade that leads to the secretion of a number of different hormones. Of primary interest is the action of neuropeptide Y (NPY), a hormone concentrated in the hypothalamus that has been associated with increased appetite and food consumption. If the body has too much adipose tissue, adipocytes will secrete more leptin, which signals the hypothalamus to inhibit NPY release, thus decreasing appetite. Unfortunately, experimental drugs that block NPY receptors have not been found to promote weight loss in obese patients.

Another important finding in the pathogenesis of obesity is the role of neurotransmitters in appetite suppression. Activation of certain subreceptors of the neurotransmitter serotonin (5-HT_{1B} and 5-HT_{2c}) reduces appetite and the consumption of calories at meals. In addition, activation of $alpha_1$- or $beta_2$-adrenergic receptors and the release of norepinephrine seem to decrease appetite. Antiobesity drugs are currently available that promote the release of these neurotransmitters.

Lipids are the most energy-dense nutrients for fueling metabolic processes; more calories can be obtained from lipids than any other molecule. While the body can store only small amounts of protein and carbohydrate, fat stores are nearly unlimited. The ability of adipocytes to increase in size and store a nearly unlimited quantity of fat is likely a consequence of evolutionary adaptation. For most of human history, starvation has been a major cause of death, and hard physical activity was necessary to survive. Those who had more efficient lipid-storage capacity survived the times of famine. Although starvation is still a problem in parts of the world, it is no longer a major cause of death in developed countries. Unfortunately, human metabolic systems are still programmed for low-fat diets, combined with lots of physical exercise. What was once a survival mechanism has become a liability when a person consumes a high-fat diet and chooses a sedentary lifestyle.

Measurement of Obesity

64.3 Obesity is measured by using the body mass index and waist circumference.

Obesity is defined by several different measures. In simple terms, obesity is being more than 20% above the "ideal" weight. The ideal weight fluctuates depending upon the person's gender, height, and general build.

The most commonly accepted measurement of obesity is the **body mass index (BMI).** BMI is determined by dividing body weight (in kilograms) by the square of height (in meters). In adults, a BMI of 25 kg/m^2 indicates the person is overweight. Obesity is defined by a BMI of 30 kg/m^2. Figure 64.1 illustrates a simple graph of BMI for estimating obesity. BMI measurement is not accurate in athletes due to the higher proportion of muscle to fat in these persons.

Another clinical measure of obesity is waist circumference, as measured by a simple tape measure. Waist circumference values of 80 cm (32 in.) for women and 94 cm (37 in.) for men are associated with increased health risk. Waist measurements greater than 88 cm (35 in.) for women and 102 cm (40 in.) for men have the greatest health risks. Waist circumference correlates well with BMI and also provides an estimate of abdominal fat, which is more strongly associated with health risk than fat stored in other regions of the body. Table 64.1 combines the waist circumference and BMI measurements in assessing the health risks for obesity.

PharmFACT

Obesity rates vary considerably by race, ethnic group, and gender. In a 2007 study 53% percent of African American women and 51% of Mexican American women aged 40 to 59 were obese compared with 39% of non-Hispanic white women. *Source:* National Center for Health Statistics, 2007.

Nonpharmacologic Therapies for Obesity

64.4 Nonpharmacologic treatment of obesity should be attempted prior to initiating pharmacotherapy.

Prior to initiation of drug therapy, the health care provider and patient must first attempt to achieve weight management through nonpharmacologic means. This involves making three major lifestyle changes: diet, exercise, and behavior modification. To obtain successful, sustained weight loss, lifestyle changes can be physically and emotionally demanding for an obese patient.

Choosing a sustainable diet is often the biggest hurdle for patients. Although it may have taken decades or longer to become obese, no one wants to take decades to lose weight. Weight loss schemes and fad diets that claim rapid weight loss while making few changes in dietary habits provide strong attractions to obese patients desperate to lose weight. The nurse should assist the patient in setting realistic goals and steer them away from fad diets that may be unhealthy, as well as unsuccessful. Severe restriction of any of the food groups—proteins, carbohydrates, or lipids—is not necessary or recommended by nutritionists. Examining the patient's diet and reducing their normal intake to 1,000 to 1,200 kcal/day for women and 1,200 to 1,600 kcal/day for men is usually sufficient, although small, progressive steps will be needed to achieve these values in patients who are accustomed to consuming 2 to 6 times the recommended daily calorie values. Weight loss of 1 to 2 lb per week is usually a realistic goal and is physically safe.

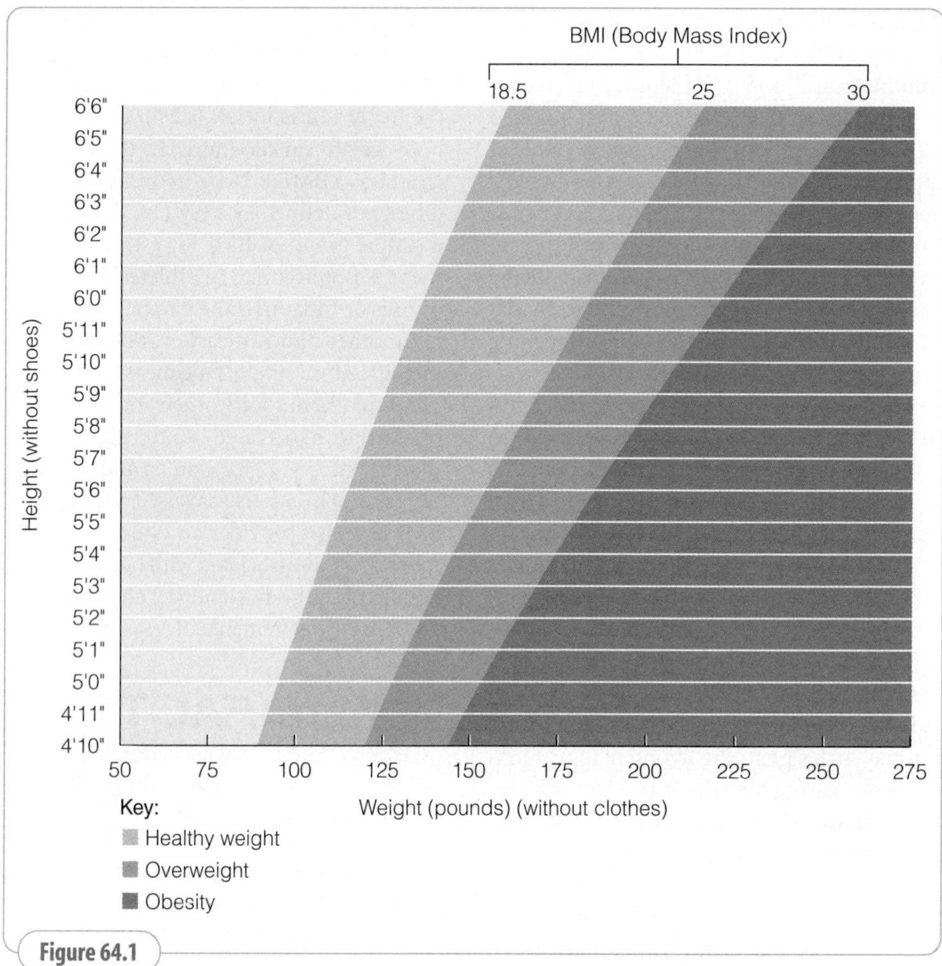

Figure 64.1

Calculation of body mass index. To determine your BMI, find the value for your height on the left and follow this line to the right until it intersects with the value for your weight on the bottom axis. The area in the graph where the two points intersect is your BMI.

Note: From Clinical Guidelines on the Identification, Evaluation, and Treatment of Overweight and Obesity in Adults: The Evidence Report. (1998), by the National Institutes of Health, National Heart, Lung, and Blood Institute, 1998, p. xvii, Washington, DC: U.S. Department of Health & Human Services. Retrieved August 22, 2008, from http://www.nhlbi.nih.gov/guidelines/obesity/ob_gdlns.htm

TABLE 64.1 Classification of Overweight and Obesity by BMI, Waist Circumference, and Associated Disease Risks

			DISEASE RISK* RELATIVE TO NORMAL WEIGHT AND WAIST CIRCUMFERENCE	
	BMI (kg/m²)	**Obesity Class**	**Men 102 cm (40 in.) or less Women 88 cm (35 in.) or less**	**Men > 102 cm (40 in.) Women > 88 cm (35 in.)**
Underweight	< 18.5		—	—
Normal	18.5–24.9		—	—
Overweight	25.0–29.9		Increased	High
Obesity	30.0–34.9	I	High	Very high
	35.0–39.9	II	Very high	Very high
Extreme obesity	40.0 +	III	Extremely high	Extremely high

Note: From *Clinical Guidelines on the Identification, Evaluation, and Treatment of Overweight and Obesity in Adults: The Evidence Report,* by the National Institutes of Health, National Heart, Lung, and Blood Institute, 1998, p. xvii, Washington, DC: Department of Health & Human Services. Retrieved August 22, 2008, from http://www.nhlbi.nih.gov/guidelines/obesity/ob_gdlns.htm

* Disease risk for type 2 diabetes, HTN, and cardiovascular disease.

+ Increased waist circumference can also be a marker for increased risk even in persons of normal weight.

Exercise is an essential component of any weight management program. Many obese patients, however, have other chronic health problems that could impact an exercise program, the most common being diabetes, HTN, and heart disease. The patient should receive a thorough medical work up, to be certain there are no physical contraindications to starting an exercise program. The obese patient should begin with very modest exercise goals and proceed to more challenging physical activity under the guidance of their health care provider. Exercise should be combined with calorie restriction because increased physical activity, by itself, is not an efficient method for losing weight.

Behavior modification is another essential component of successful weight management programs. The patient likely became obese due to poor eating habits and behaviors, which must be changed for the remainder of the person's life. For highly obese patients, the weight loss program will extend a year or longer; therefore, support groups should be encouraged. Breaking learned habits of eating is challenging and relapses always occur. Support groups can provide valuable help in adjusting to new lifestyle patterns.

Surgery is an option for severely obese patients who are at least 80 to 100 lb overweight and who have been unsuccessful in conventional weight loss programs. Surgery involves either restricting the size of the stomach, or bypassing it altogether. Restriction operations remove part of the stomach or place a band around it. This creates a smaller, pouchlike stomach that fills rapidly to give a feeling of fullness. The restriction operations cause weight loss due to less food intake. Bypass operations create a small stomach pouch and attach a portion of the jejunum to the pouch, essentially bypassing most of the stomach and duodenum. Bypass operations lead to weight loss due to less food intake combined with malabsorption. Most patients having obesity surgery experience significant weight loss, 50% to 75% of their excess weight within 1 year. Some do not lose weight, however, and 10% to 20% require additional surgeries. All surgical options carry a risk for complications, some of which may be serious.

Pharmacotherapy of Obesity

64.5 Drugs used for weight management affect appetite or the absorption of fats.

Because of the prevalence of obesity in society and the difficulty most patients experience when following weight reduction plans for extended periods, drug manufacturers have long sought to develop safe drugs that induce and sustain weight loss. The quest for the "magic weight loss pill," however, has been disappointing. In the 1970s, amphetamine and dextroamphetamine (Dexedrine) were widely prescribed to reduce appetite. However, these stimulant drugs are highly addictive and rarely prescribed for weight loss today. In the 1990s, the combination of fenfluramine and phentermine (Fen-Phen) was quite effective at promoting weight loss, but fenfluramine was removed from the market for causing heart valve defects. An over-the-counter (OTC) appetite suppressant, phenylpropanolamine, was removed from the market in 2000 due to an increased incidence of strokes and adverse cardiac events. Until 2004, alternative weight loss products contained ephedra alkaloids, but these have also been removed from the market due to an increased incidence of adverse cardiovascular events. As discussed in Section 64.2, discovery of

CONNECTIONS

To the Community Healthy Weight Reduction Tips

Weight loss is never easy for anyone, but by taking certain health steps, weight loss can become a reality. The nurse must emphasize that weight loss requires lifestyle changes such as healthy eating and exercise. Below are some tips that the nurse can use in teaching the patient who is trying to lose weight:

- Change your lifestyle, which means changing habits. The word *diet* can be considered negative and make you think about deprivation. Everyone has a diet: It is what you eat. The key is to change eating and exercise habits to facilitate weight loss and better health.
- Adopt a positive attitude and seek friendships with positive people. When you feel better, you can more easily embrace dietary and exercise changes.
- Consult your health care provider prior to starting a weight loss and exercise program, especially if you have chronic disease or other health challenges. Your health care provider may also suggest support groups that can help your weight loss success. Online support groups are available for those who do not have time to attend meetings.
- Plan meals in advance. Lack of planning can sabotage any weight loss program. Avoid skipping meals, which can result in hunger and poor choices. Schedule times to exercise in advance and enlist an exercise buddy for added fun. Making diet and exercise social times can improve results.
- Take time to learn about nutrition and try healthy recipes. Eat slowly. Some find that three small meals and two snacks each day stave off hunger and help keep them on track.
- Use natural spices to season foods. Often, these are low in calorie but high in taste.
- Always eat before grocery shopping to minimize impulse buying. Prepare a list of needed items and stick to the list.
- Learn to read labels to know what you are eating and how many calories you are ingesting.
- Understand that a serving size may be less than what you expected and decrease or limit the number of portions you eat. Portion control can make a difference in weight loss success.
- Avoid fad diets or losing weight too quickly. One to two pounds a week is healthy weight loss and is more likely to stay off than fast weight loss.
- Get plenty of sleep. Current research supports the link between sleep deprivation and weight gain. Most people require 7 to 9 hours per night, but this may vary with age.
- Read and research trends in health to stay current but remember that the key to weight loss is healthy lifestyle choices of diet and regular exercise. Weight gain comes to each person over a period of time and weight loss requires time and focus for success. Better health is an added benefit of weight loss in overweight persons.

the hormone leptin led to widespread anticipation that new weight loss products would soon be available, but clinical trials of these agents have not shown any promise.

Current pharmacologic strategies for weight management focus on two sites of action. The appetite suppressants (also called **anorexiants** or anorectics), act centrally by increasing the amounts of norepinephrine, serotonin, and dopamine in regions of the brain that affect appetite. The lipase inhibitors act by reducing the absorption of fats in the small intestine. The approved antiobesity agents produce only modest effects, and pharmacotherapy must be combined with a calorie-restricted diet.

64.6 Anorexiants are drugs used to induce weight loss by suppressing appetite and hunger.

One strategy to reduce weight is to block parts of the nervous system responsible for recognizing and reacting to hunger. Sibutramine (Meridia), a selective serotonin reuptake inhibitor (SSRI), is the most widely prescribed appetite suppressant for the short-term control of obesity. Two other SSRIs, fluoxetine (Prozac) and sertraline (Zoloft), produce a similar loss in weight, although they are not approved by the U.S. Food and Drug Administration (FDA) for this purpose. Phentermine, once part of the now-banned combination of fen-phen is still approved as monotherapy, although it produces only a small, transient weight loss. All of the anorexiants have the potential to produce serious adverse effects, thus their use is limited to short-term therapy. Anorexiants are prescribed for patients with a body mass index (BMI) of at least 30 or greater, or a BMI of 27 or greater, if the patient has other risk factors such as HTN, hyperlipidemia, or diabetes.

Amphetamines were once an accepted therapy for weight loss because they have strong appetite suppressant actions. Their effects on appetite are short-lived, however, due to the development of tolerance. Their continued use leads to higher and higher doses. Amphetamine, methamphetamine, and dextroamphetamine have high abuse potential and the therapy of obesity is no longer an acceptable indication for these drugs. Amphetamine sulfate is featured as a prototype central nervous system (CNS) stimulant in Chapter 28.

CONNECTION *Checkpoint* 64.2

Methylphenidate (Ritalin) is an amphetamine-like drug. From what you learned in Chapter 28, what are the primary indications for amphetamine and methylphenidate? See Answer to Connection Checkpoint 64.2 in Appendix A.

Rimonabant (Acomplia, Zimulti) is the first of a new class of antiobesity agents known as **cannabinoid receptor (CB1) blockers.** The drug is available in over 30 countries but has not yet been approved in the United States. The CB1 receptors are primarily found in the brain, but are also present in some peripheral tissues. Activation of these receptors is responsible for the psychoactive effects of marijuana (see Chapter 8). Overeating activates CB1 receptors in the CNS; blocking them reduces appetite. Tobacco has a similar effect on cannabinoid receptors; thus, rimonabant is also used to promote tobacco cessation. Concerns about adverse effects, especially depression and suicide ideation, have prevented the drug from being marketed in the United States.

PROTOTYPE DRUG Sibutramine (Meridia)

Classification: **Therapeutic:** Antiobesity agent, appetite suppressant
Pharmacologic: Anorexiant, serotonin/norepinephrine reuptake inhibitor

Therapeutic Effects and Uses: Sibutramine is only approved for the adjunctive treatment of obesity when combined with a reduced calorie diet and exercise. The drug is able to produce a 5% to 10% loss of body weight within 6 to 12 months of treatment. Patients who have not lost at least 4 pounds after the first month of therapy require an increase in dose or discontinuation of therapy. Sibutramine therapy is not recommended for longer than 1 year.

Sibutramine is a schedule IV controlled substance, with a very low potential for abuse. It is not approved for use in patients under age 16.

Mechanism of Action: Sibutramine acts by increasing the levels of serotonin and norepinephrine in areas of the brain that regulate hunger. It accomplishes this by inhibiting the reuptake of these neurotransmitters. The level of dopamine is increased to a lesser extent.

Pharmacokinetics:

Route(s)	Oral (PO)
Absorption	Rapidly absorbed
Distribution	Widely distributed; unknown if secreted in breast milk; 97% bound to plasma protein
Primary metabolism	Hepatic (CYP3A4) to active metabolites; extensive first-pass metabolism
Primary excretion	Renal
Onset of action	Peak plasma level: 1.2 h
Duration of action	Half-life: 14–16 h

Adverse Effects: Sibutramine is generally well tolerated and serious adverse effects are uncommon. Headache, constipation, insomnia, and xerostomia are the most common complaints reported during sibutramine therapy. Weight gain may occur after sibutramine is discontinued.

Contraindications/Precautions: Sibutramine is contraindicated in patients with eating disorders (anorexia nervosa or bulimia) because it may worsen these conditions. To prevent a hypertensive crisis, at least 2 weeks should be allowed between discontinuing monoamine oxidase inhibitors (MAOIs) and starting sibutramine. The drug should be used with care in patients with heart disease, dysrhythmias, or stroke, because it may cause tachycardia and raise blood pressure. Because the kidneys excrete the drug, patients with severe renal impairment should be treated with caution. Sibutramine is contraindicated in patients with severe hepatic impairment. Drug therapy should be monitored carefully in patients with a history of drug abuse because it has a potential for dependence.

Drug Interactions: Use with decongestants, cough, and allergy medications may elevate blood pressure. Patients receiving antihypertensive therapy should be monitored for changes in blood pressure during sibutramine therapy. Ketoconazole and erythromycin may inhibit the metabolism of sibutramine. Concurrent use with a MAOI or SSRI may cause serotonin syndrome. Agents such as sibutramine that inhibit serotonin reuptake sometimes affect platelet function; therefore, use with antiplatelet drugs should be monitored carefully. **Herbal/Food:** Unknown.

Pregnancy: Category C.

Treatment of Overdose: Beta-adrenergic blockers may be administered to treat tachycardia and HTN resulting from sibutramine overdose. Patients are treated symptomatically.

Nursing Responsibilities:

- Obtain a complete health history including allergies, drug history, and possible drug interactions.
- Perform a physical assessment including vital signs and apometric measurements such as BMI and body weight.
- Assess laboratory values to determine hepatic and renal function.
- Determine the patient's desire and motivation to reduce weight or body fat.
- Consult a dietitian to prepare and educate the client in the recommended nutritional intake.
- Document weight changes to monitor the therapeutic effect of the drug.
- Monitor blood pressure and heart rate and immediately report any sustained increases to the prescriber.
- Assess and immediately report to the prescriber, any signs or symptoms of serotonin syndrome, a serious and potentially life-threatening drug-related problem characterized by mental confusion and neuromuscular and muscular problems. Serotonin syndrome most often occurs in patients who are taking two or more drugs that can increase CNS levels of serotonin.
- Monitor patients with narrow-angle glaucoma for increasing intraocular pressure.

Patient and Family Education:

- Strictly maintain the diet and exercise program recommended by the health care provider.
- Immediately report to the health care provider, any signs and symptoms of an allergic reaction such as rash or hives, or symptoms of hyperstimulation such as restlessness, shivering, profuse sweating, irritability, and tremor.
- Take the drug in the morning because it may interfere with sleep.
- Check blood pressure and heart rate regularly and report any consistently high readings.
- Avoid taking more medication than prescribed: More is not better.
- Do not take OTC cold, allergy, or cough medications or other OTC weight-loss drugs without the approval of the health care provider.
- Provide the health care provider with a list of all drugs currently taken because adverse effects may be experienced with certain drugs, such as those used to treat depression.
- Keep this medication out of the reach of children.

Drugs Similar to Sibutramine (Meridia)

Other FDA-approved appetite suppressants include diethylpropion and phentermine.

Diethylpropion (Depletite, Durad, others): Diethylpropion is structurally similar to amphetamine and has similar pharmacologic effects. It acts by increasing the levels of norepinephrine in regions of the brain regulating appetite. Given orally, its use is limited to the short-term (up to 12 weeks) therapy of obesity because tolerance develops rapidly to the anorexiant effects of the drug. Nervous system adverse effects include confusion, agitation, nervousness, insomnia, and tremors. Like sibutramine, the drug may worsen HTN or cause dysrhythmias. Although classified as a Schedule IV drug, diethylpropion is not frequently abused because it produces less euphoria than other amphetamine-like drugs. This is a pregnancy category B drug.

Phentermine (Adipex-P, Fastin, Pro-Fast, others): Phentermine is an oral drug approved only for the treatment of obesity. Because tolerance rapidly develops to the appetite suppressant effects, therapy is limited to 8 to 12 weeks. Phentermine is structurally similar to amphetamine, but causes less CNS stimulation and has less potential for abuse. Nervous system adverse effects include nervousness, insomnia, and tremors. Caution should be used in treating patients with HTN or diabetes. Abuse of phentermine causes dependence and psychoses. It is a Schedule IV controlled substance. It is a pregnancy category C drug.

64.7 Lipase inhibitors cause weight loss by interfering with the absorption of fats.

A second strategy to reduce weight is to block the absorption of dietary fats. Lipids are a very dense energy source and most of the accumulated fat in patients is derived from dietary sources.

Chemical digestion of lipids occurs through the enzymatic action of pancreatic lipase, which splits dietary triglycerides into glycerol and free fatty acids. Once absorbed, the fatty acids can be recombined with glycerol and stored in adipocytes. Attempts to produce antiobesity drugs that block lipid absorption have resulted in one approved drug: orlistat (Xenical).

PROTOTYPE DRUG Orlistat (Alli, Xenical)

Classification: **Therapeutic:** Antiobesity agent
Pharmacologic: Lipase inhibitor

Therapeutic Effects and Uses: Approved in 1999, orlistat is indicated for the treatment of obesity, in combination with a reduced calorie diet and exercise. Like the anorexiants, orlistat is indicated for patients with a BMI of 30 or greater, or a BMI of

27 or greater if the patient has other risk factors such as HTN, hyperlipidemia, or diabetes. This drug produces only a modest increase in weight reduction compared to placebos.

The prescription form of orlistat (Xenical) is available at 120 mg, and is given 3 times daily, during or just prior to a meal. In 2007, an OTC dosage form (Alli) was approved at 60 mg. The drug is only effective if taken with meals containing lipids. Orlistat is not approved for children under age 12.

Mechanism of Action: Orlistat inhibits pancreatic lipase and acts by blocking lipid absorption in the gastrointestinal (GI) tract. It primarily lowers the absorption of free fatty acids, but also has an effect on cholesterol absorption. The decreased lipid absorption lowers calories and promotes weight loss. Fat absorption is inhibited by approximately 30% by the drug.

Pharmacokinetics:

Route(s)	PO
Absorption	Minimal absorption
Distribution	Not distributed; remains in the GI tract; does not cross the placenta; is not secreted in breast milk
Primary metabolism	Wall of the GI tract
Primary excretion	Feces
Onset of action	24–48 h
Duration of action	Half-life: 1–2 h

Adverse Effects: Some of the adverse effects of orlistat are directly related to its inhibition of lipid absorption. As more lipids reach the large intestine, flatus with discharge, oily stool, fecal urgency, and abdominal pain are common, especially during the first 4 weeks of therapy. To avoid serious GI adverse effects, patients should restrict their fat intake. Orlistat may also decrease the absorption of other substances, including fat-soluble vitamins and warfarin (Coumadin). Rapid weight loss increases the risk for cholelithiasis. Headache is also a common adverse effect.

Contraindications/Precautions: Orlistat should be used with caution in patients with cholestasis because the drug inhibits gallbladder contractions. Orlistat is contraindicated for patients who have a known cause of obesity, such as hypothyroidism, and in patients with severe malabsorption disorders. The drug is contraindicated in patients with anorexia nervosa or bulimia because it may worsen these disorders.

Drug Interactions: Because orlistat inhibits the absorption of the lipid-soluble vitamins A, D, and E, a supplement containing these vitamins should be taken at least 2 hours before or after a dose of orlistat. Vitamin K levels may decrease in patients taking orlistat, which can affect anticoagulation produced by warfarin. Orlistat decreases the absorption of cyclosporine and the two drugs should not be used concurrently. **Herbal/Food:** Unknown.

Pregnancy: Category B.

Treatment of Overdose: Overdose with orlistat is not a clinical problem because the effects of the drug are rapidly reversible.

Nursing Responsibilities:

- Obtain a complete health history including allergies, drug history, and possible drug interactions.
- Perform a physical assessment including vital signs and apometric measurements such as BMI and body weight.
- Assess laboratory values as indicated to determine hepatic and renal function.
- Determine the patient's desire and motivation to reduce weight.
- Consult a dietitian to prepare and educate the patient on the recommended nutritional intake.
- Administer the drug during or up to 1 hour after a meal containing fat.
- Omit the dose if eating a meal that does not contain fat or if a meal is skipped.
- Monitor weight and BMI; closely monitor diabetics for hypoglycemia.
- Monitor prothrombin time (PT) and international normalized ratio (INR) if the patient is taking warfarin.
- Monitor blood pressure frequently, especially in patients with preexisting HTN.
- Assess for medications that can interact with orlistat such as warfarin, cyclosporine, pravastatin, diabetic drugs, and fat-soluble vitamin supplements such as A, D, E, and K. Vitamin deficiencies can occur, causing changes in eyesight, hair, and skin.

Patient and Family Education:

- Take a daily multivitamin containing fat-soluble vitamins at least 2 hours before or after orlistat.
- GI adverse effects are common but typically resolve after 4 weeks of therapy.
- Avoid high-fat meals to minimize adverse GI adverse effects. Distribute fat calories over three main meals daily. Do not skip meals.
- Monitor weight several times weekly. If diabetic, monitor blood glucose carefully following any weight loss.
- Expect that certain adverse effects can occur such as stomach discomfort, an increased number of stools, loss of control of defecation, gas released with bowel movements, oily stools, or the urgent desire to defecate.
- Increase physical activity as tolerated and approved by the health care provider.
- Provide the health care provider with a list of all drugs and supplements currently taken because orlistat can interact with other drugs and vitamins.
- Immediately notify the health care provider of any known or suspected pregnancy.

Drugs Similar to Orlistat (Alli, Xenical)

Orlistat is the only lipase inhibitor indicated for obesity.

CONNECTION *Checkpoint* 64.3

Orlistat may decrease the absorption of fat-soluble vitamins. From what you learned in Chapter 62, describe the types of effects that could result from deficiencies in the fat-soluble vitamins A and D. See Answer to Connection Checkpoint 64.3 in Appendix A.

Adjuncts to Obesity Therapy

64.8 Artificial sweeteners and fat substitutes are sometimes used as adjuncts to weight management programs.

A primary component of any weight management program is reduction of caloric intake. In an attempt to reduce total calories, many people have turned to artificial sweeteners and fat substitutes.

Artificial sweeteners include saccharin (Sweet'N Low®, SugarTwin®), aspartame (Nutrasweet®, Equal®), acesulfame (ACK, Sweet One®, Sunett®), and sucralose (Splenda®). These agents are 200 to 600 times sweeter than table sugar, or sucrose, and thus less quantity is needed for sweetening food and beverages. Artificial sweeteners are regulated by the FDA because they are classified as food additives. Safety studies suggest that these agents are safe, when used in usual amounts. Consumers should be aware that "sugar-free" foods may contain just as many calories and have a higher fat content than regular foods. Diabetic and pregnant patients should consult with their health care providers before consuming artificial sweeteners.

Stevia is a natural sweetener obtained from an herb in the sunflower family. Three-hundred times sweeter than sucrose, stevia is recognized by the FDA as a dietary supplement, not as a food additive. It has a bitter taste when used in large amounts. Safety concerns have caused it to be banned in several countries.

Fats give food a particular smooth texture, as well as calories. It is not difficult to identify fat-free or low-fat foods because they generally lack the taste and feel of normal fat. Fat substitutes attempt to simulate the feel of normal fat, without the calories or effects of lipid levels in the blood. Olestra is a popular fat substitute that consists of a sucrose molecule surrounded by fatty acids. It has the appeal of fat, but passes through the digestive tract undigested. It offers zero calories and zero fat, but has the unpleasant adverse effects of loose stools and anal leakage. It is primarily restricted to snack foods. Simplesse® is a second fat substitute derived from natural whey protein that is used in baked goods and dairy products. Many other products are under development.

Do artificial sweeteners and fat substitutes actually help obese patients lose weight? The answer depends on the dietary habits of the consumer. Certainly, drinking a liter of a regular soft drink gives one many more calories than the same amount of a diet soft drink. Likewise, 8 ounces of potato chips using olestra gives fewer calories and fat than 8 ounces of regular chips. But patients with serious weight problems should probably make better food choices than soft drinks and chips. A few studies have suggested that the body compensates by craving sucrose and high-fat meals. It should be remembered that the FDA has only evaluated these food additives for safety, not for their effectiveness in maintaining or losing body weight. Just as there are no "miracle pills" for weight loss, there are no "miracle foods" that will promote weight loss. The answer lies in the simple rules of limiting calorie intake, proper nutrition, and exercise.

NURSING PROCESS APPLICATION

Patients Receiving Drugs for Weight Reduction

Assessment	Potential Nursing Diagnoses
Prior to administration: • Obtain a complete health history including allergies, drug history, and possible drug interactions. • Perform a physical assessment including vital signs and apometric measurements such as BMI and body weight. • Assess laboratory values as indicated to determine hepatic and renal function. • Determine the patient's desire and motivation to reduce weight or body fat.	• *Imbalanced Nutrition: More than Body Requirements* • *Deficient Knowledge (Medication)*, related to weight reduction program

Planning: Patient Goals and Expected Outcomes

The patient will:

- State pertinent factors contributing to weight gain.
- Claim ownership for current eating patterns.
- Design dietary modifications to meet individual weight loss goal.
- Adhere to the prescribed medication regimen and report adverse effects to the health care provider.

(continued)

NURSING PROCESS APPLICATION *(continued)*

Implementation

Interventions and (Rationales)	Patient and Family Education
• Focus on lifestyle changes that will have a greater effect on weight reduction in the long term. (Drugs for weight loss have limited effectiveness and some have serious adverse effects.)	• Instruct the patient to: • Set a weekly goal for weight loss. • Weigh weekly—avoid daily weigh in. • Set realistic meal plan to attain goals that include balanced nutritional intake. • Take a daily vitamin supplement with fat-soluble vitamins (orlistat). • Determine current eating habits by keeping a food log for 3 consecutive days. • Establish a gradual exercise plan that incorporates a favored physical activity.
• Encourage participation in weight loss support groups. (Individuals with strong psychosocial support are more likely to adhere to a weight loss regimen.)	• Instruct the patient to: • Investigate weight loss support programs that are available. • Establish a support system (buddy system) to facilitate weight loss. • Set an external reward system for reaching small attainable goals.
• Monitor for adverse effects associated with specific drug therapy. (Weight loss drugs all have associated adverse effects and should be reported to the prescriber.)	• Instruct the patient to: • Report headache, constipation, insomnia, and xerostomia (sibutramine) if unresolved within 1 week of initiating therapy. • Report abdominal pain and uncontrolled diarrhea (orlistat). • Take blood pressure weekly and report consistent changes of 5 mm or more to the health care provider.

Evaluation of Outcome Criteria

Evaluate the effectiveness of drug therapy by confirming that patient goals and expected outcomes have been met (see "Planning").

UNDERSTANDING THE CHAPTER

Key Concepts Summary

64.1 Genetic and lifestyle factors contribute to the etiology of obesity.

64.2 Appetite is regulated by the satiety center in the hypothalamus and is influenced by various hormones.

64.3 Obesity is measured by using the body mass index and waist circumference.

64.4 Nonpharmacologic treatment of obesity should be attempted prior to initiating pharmacotherapy.

64.5 Drugs used for weight management affect appetite or the absorption of fats.

64.6 Anorexiants are drugs used to induce weight loss by suppressing appetite and hunger.

64.7 Lipase inhibitors cause weight loss by interfering with the absorption of fats.

64.8 Artificial sweeteners and fat substitutes are sometimes used as adjuncts to weight management programs.

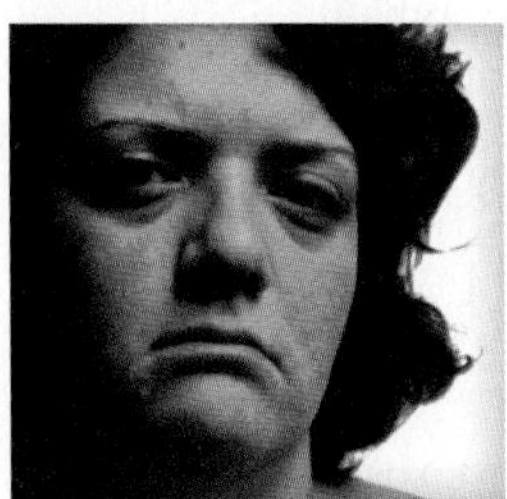

Making the PATIENT *Connection*

Remember the patient "Rosemary Goodman" at the beginning of this chapter? Now read the remainder of the case study. Based on the information presented within this chapter, respond to the critical thinking questions that follow.

Rosemary, a 32-year-old female, has just had her annual physical examination with the advanced practice nurse. The reason for her visit is a complaint of headache and chronic fatigue. Her past medical history reveals "borderline HTN" and "borderline diabetes" but only during her last pregnancy. She is a single mother who works in a fast food restaurant.

Her vital signs are within normal limits with the exception of blood pressure, which is 146/94 mmHg. Her height is 1.6 meters (5 ft 6 in) tall and weighs 119 kg (262 lb). When questioned about her intent to lose weight, Rosemary begins to cry and states she has tried every diet imaginable. "My last diet consisted of eating a lot of grapefruit as my major food source." She further discloses that she has been overweight since childhood. A few years ago, Rosemary used diet pills to lose weight. However, the pill made her feel nervous and irritable. "No matter what I do, the weight always returns, usually more than before!" She further discloses that obesity is common in her family.

Critical Thinking Questions

1. What do you think are the causes of obesity? List the major complications of obesity.
2. Develop a list of drugs commonly used for long-term treatment of obesity. Compare and contrast how these drugs work.
3. What common stereotypes do you think obese individuals face when entering health care facilities? What problem can result from this bias among health care professionals?

Case Study

Kathryn is a 52-year-old woman who has been grossly overweight for more than 15 years. In that time she has tried many diets, exercise regimens, diet clubs, and drug therapies, but all to no avail. She weighs 143 kg (315 lb) and has a BMI of 48. The health care provider has prescribed sibutramine (Meridia). She informs you that she has tried diet pills in the past. She has heard about terrible problems that amphetamines cause other people and is fearful that she will become dependent on the drug, or experience serious complications.

1. Considering this patient's body mass index, do you think she a candidate for sibutramine (Meridia) therapy?
2. Discuss how you can help alleviate Kathryn's concerns about amphetamines and drug dependence.
3. Create a list of adverse effects that are commonly associated with sibutramine (Meridia) that you could give to this patient.

NCLEX-RN® Review

1 The client is receiving sibutramine (Meridia) for the treatment of obesity. The nurse knows that this medication should be:

1. Prescribed in conjunction with a reduced calorie diet and exercise plan.
2. Used only in men and premenopausal women.
3. Recommended only in the absence of adult onset (type 2) diabetes.
4. Increased if the client has not lost 4 pounds in the first week of therapy.

2 The client is taking sibutramine (Meridia). The nurse would monitor for which of the following to determine whether this medication is having a therapeutic effect on the client? A reduction of:

1. 0% to 10% of body weight within 6 to 12 months.
2. 15% to 20% body weight within 3 to 4 months.
3. 12 pounds during the first month of therapy.
4. Adipose tissue surrounding the waist.

3 The client has been started on orlistat (Xenical). The nurse would teach this client to take this medication:

1. Once in the morning.
2. When a feeling of hunger is noticed.
3. Before daily exercise.
4. Just prior to each meal.

4 While taking orlistat (Alli), the nurse would instruct the client to do which of the following?

1. Drink at least 2 to 3 liters of citrus juice (preferably grapefruit juice) per day.
2. Always wear sunscreen when outdoors or when exposed to direct sunlight.
3. Rise slowly from a sitting or supine position.
4. Take a daily vitamin supplement containing fat-soluble vitamins.

5 A nurse is instructing a client taking orlistat (Xenical) about adverse effects to the medication. Which of the following indicates the presence of an expected adverse effect?

1. Flatus with discharge and oily stool
2. Heartburn and dyspepsia
3. Constipation with fecal impaction
4. Nausea with projectile vomiting

6 Which of the following measures is used to assess the presence of obesity? Select all that apply.

1. Body weight
2. Body mass index
3. Waist circumference
4. Treadmill test
5. Buoyancy analysis

See Answers to Critical Thinking Questions, Case Study, and NCLEX-RN® Review in Appendix A.

References

Brown, I. (2007). Management of obesity in primary care: Nurses' practices, beliefs, and attitudes. *Journal of Advanced Nursing, 59*(4), 329–341.

Chaput, J. P., & Tremblay, A. (2006). Current and novel approaches to the drug therapy of obesity. *European Journal of Clinical Pharmacology, 62*(10), 793–803.

Cooke, D. B. (2006). The obesity pipeline: Current strategies in the development of anti-obesity drugs. *Nature Reviews: Drug Discovery, 5*(11), 919.

Fujioka, K., & Lee, M. W. (2007). Pharmacologic treatment options for obesity: Current and potential medications. *Nutrition in Clinical Practice, 22*(1), 50–54.

Halford, J. C. G., Harrold, J. A., Boyland, E. J., Lawton, C. L., & Blundell, J. E. (2007). Serotonergic drugs: Effects on appetite expression and use for the treatment of obesity. *Drugs, 67*(1), 27–55.

Kirkpatrick, P. (2006). Anti-obesity drugs: Fighting fat. *Nature Reviews: Drug Discovery, 5*(8), 634.

Kyrou, I., Valsamakis, G., & Tsigos, C. (2006). The endocannabinoid system as a target for the treatment of visceral obesity and metabolic syndrome. *Annals of the New York Academy of Science, 1083*(1), 270–305.

Lean, M., & Mullan, A. (2007). Review article. Obesity: Which drug and when? *International Journal of Clinical Practice, 61*(9), 1555–1560.

Mackie, K. (2006.) Cannabinoid receptors as therapeutic targets. *Annual Review of Pharmacology and Toxicology, 46*, 101–122.

National Center for Health Statistics. (2007). *New CDC study finds no increase in obesity among adults, but levels still high.* Retrieved August 21, 2008, from http://www.cdc.gov/nchs/pressroom/07newsreleases/obesity.htm

National Institute on Media and the Family. (2006). *Media use and obesity among children.* Retrieved August 23, 2008, from http://www.mediafamily.org/facts/facts_tvandobchild.shtml

Padwal, R., Li, S. K., & Lau, D. C. W. (2004). Long-term pharmacotherapy for obesity and overweight. *Cochrane Database of Systematic Reviews*, (3):CD004094.

Rankin-Box, D. (2007). Nurses have pivotal role in treating morbid obesity. *Nursing Standard, 22*(5), 33.

Schwarz, S., & Freemark, M. (2007). Obesity. Retrieved August 22, 2008, from http://www.emedicine.com/ped/topic1699.htm

Singh, N. (2007). Emergency department equipment for obese patients: Perception of adequacy. *Journal of Advanced Nursing, 59*(2), 140–145.

Snow, T. (2007). Can nurses tackle the obesity crisis? *Nursing Standard 22*(3), 12–13.

Trinko, R., Sears, R. M., Guarnieri, D. J., & Dileone, R. J. (2007). Neural mechanisms underlying obesity and drug addiction. *Physiology & Behavior, 91*(5), 499.

U.S. Department of Health & Human Services, National Heart, Lung, and Blood Institute. (1998). *Clinical guidelines on the identification, evaluation, and treatment of overweight and obesity in adults: The Evidence Report* (p. xvii). Washington, DC: Author. Retrieved August 23, 2008, from http://www.nhlbi.nih.gov/guidelines/obesity/ob_gdlns.htm

Weigle, D. S. (2003). Pharmacological therapy of obesity: Past, present, and future. *Journal of Clinical Endocrinology & Metabolism, 88*, 2462–2469.

UNIT 9

Pharmacology of the Endocrine System

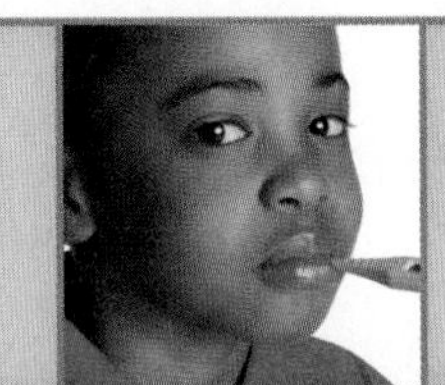
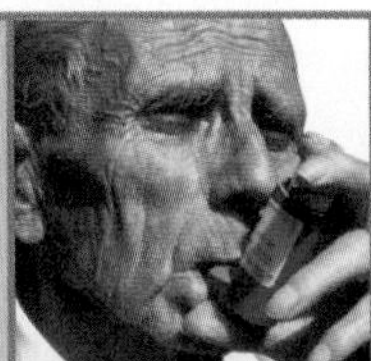
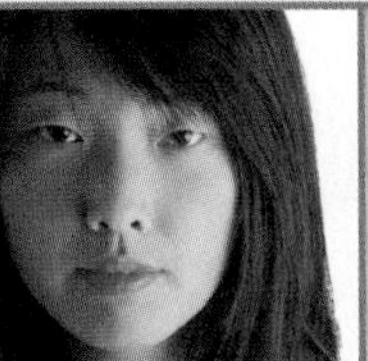
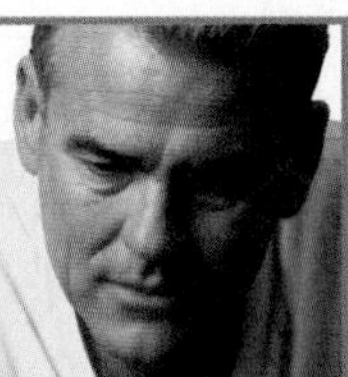

CHAPTER 65 Review of the Endocrine System

CHAPTER 66 Hypothalamic and Pituitary Drugs

CHAPTER 67 Pharmacotherapy of Diabetes Mellitus

CHAPTER 68 Pharmacotherapy of Thyroid Disorders

CHAPTER 69 Corticosteroids and Drugs Affecting the Adrenal Cortex

CHAPTER 70 Estrogens, Progestins, and Drugs Modifying Uterine Function

CHAPTER 71 Drugs for Modifying Conception

CHAPTER 72 Drugs for Disorders and Conditions of the Male Reproductive System

CHAPTER

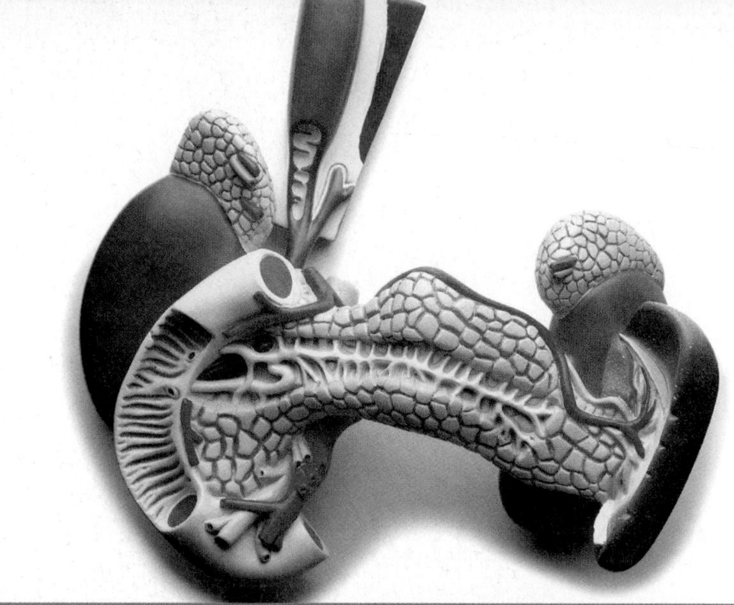

65 Review of the Endocrine System

Learning Outcomes

After reading this chapter, the student should be able to:

1. Describe the general structure and functions of the endocrine system.
2. Compare and contrast the nervous and endocrine systems in the control of homeostasis.
3. Explain circumstances in which hormone receptors may be up-regulated or down-regulated.
4. Through the use of a specific example, explain the concept of negative feedback in the endocrine system.
5. Explain the three primary types of stimuli that regulate hormone secretion.
6. Identify indications for hormone pharmacotherapy.

Chapter Outline

Overview of the Endocrine System
Hormone Receptors
Negative Feedback Mechanisms
Hormone Pharmacotherapy

Key Terms

down-regulation, *1099*
endocrine system, *1099*
hormones, *1099*
negative feedback, *1099*
replacement therapy, *1101*
target cells, *1099*
up-regulation, *1099*

Like the nervous system, the endocrine system is a major controller of homeostasis. Whereas a nerve exerts instantaneous control over a single muscle fiber or gland, a hormone from the endocrine system may affect all body cells and take as long as several days to produce an optimum response. Hormonal balance is kept within a narrow range: Too little or too much of a hormone may produce profound physiological changes. This chapter reviews endocrine anatomy and physiology and its relevance to pharmacotherapy. For a more detailed review of the endocrine system, the student should refer to an anatomy and physiology textbook.

Overview of the Endocrine System

65.1 The endocrine system controls homeostasis through the secretion of hormones.

The **endocrine system** consists of various glands that secrete **hormones,** chemical messengers that the body releases in response to a change in the body's internal environment. The role of hormones is to maintain homeostasis in the body. For example, when the level of glucose in the blood rises above normal, the pancreas secretes insulin to return glucose levels to normal. The various endocrine glands and their hormones are illustrated in Figure 65.1.

After secretion from an endocrine gland, hormones enter the blood and are transported throughout the body. Compared to the nervous system, which reacts to body changes within milliseconds, the endocrine system responds relatively slowly. A few hormones, such as epinephrine, may take a few seconds to cause an effect, while others such as testosterone may take several days or weeks to produce significant changes. Although slower in onset, the effects of hormones have a longer duration than those of the nervous system.

Hormone Receptors

65.2 Hormones must bind to specific receptors to cause physiological changes.

The cells affected by a hormone are called its **target cells.** Target cells have specific protein receptors on their surfaces that bind to the hormone. Once binding occurs, a change is produced in the cell, resulting in an action that is characteristic for the hormone. For example, when epinephrine binds to receptors on smooth muscle cells, they contract. When prolactin binds to secretory cells in the breast, milk production occurs.

It is important to remember that although a hormone travels throughout the body via the circulation, it only affects cells that have receptors for that specific hormone. Epinephrine does not affect breast secretory cells, because these cells have no epinephrine receptors. Prolactin does not cause muscular contraction because smooth muscle cells do not have prolactin receptors.

In some cases, the target cells for a hormone are limited and specific. For example, the only receptors for thyroid-stimulating hormone are in the thyroid gland. However, some hormones, such as insulin and cortisol, have receptors on nearly every cell in the body; thus, these hormones have widespread effects.

The number of protein receptors for a hormone is dynamic, and changes with the needs of the body. Cells can create more receptors on their surface to "capture" hormone molecules as they pass by, a process called **up-regulation.** This may occur if the cell is receiving signals that a hormone action is needed, such as the need for production of more breast milk or additional secretion of thyroid hormone. Once the hormone is up-regulated (secreted in large quantities), the cell no longer needs to "capture" every hormone molecule so it makes fewer receptors on its surface, a process called **down-regulation.** Receptors are very efficient at capturing hormone molecules; although most hormones are secreted only in small amounts, they produce profound changes.

Down-regulation has important implications for pharmacotherapy. When a hormone is administered as pharmacotherapy for long periods, the body recognizes an abundance of the hormone, and cells will down-regulate the number of receptors for that hormone. This causes a desensitization of the target cells; that is, they are less responsive to the effects of the hormone. When therapy is discontinued, the cells will need time, usually several days, to synthesize more protein receptors and adjust to the new hormone level.

It is important to understand that the amount of hormone secreted is only partially responsible for the therapeutic response. Other critical components include the number of receptors and their sensitivity. During pharmacotherapy, raising the doses of hormones will produce little additional pharmacologic effect if the receptors are no longer sensitive to the hormone.

Pharm*FACT*

Growth hormone (GH) is considered a performance-enhancing drug whose use has been banned by major league baseball. Athletes take GH for its supposed ability to aid in the recovery from and prevention of injuries by stimulating the synthesis of collagen, which is necessary for strengthening cartilage, bones, tendons, and ligaments. *Source:* Browning, 2007.

Negative Feedback Mechanisms

65.3 Most hormone action is regulated through negative feedback.

Because hormones can produce profound effects on the body, their secretion and release is regulated by several levels of control. The most important mechanism is **negative feedback,**

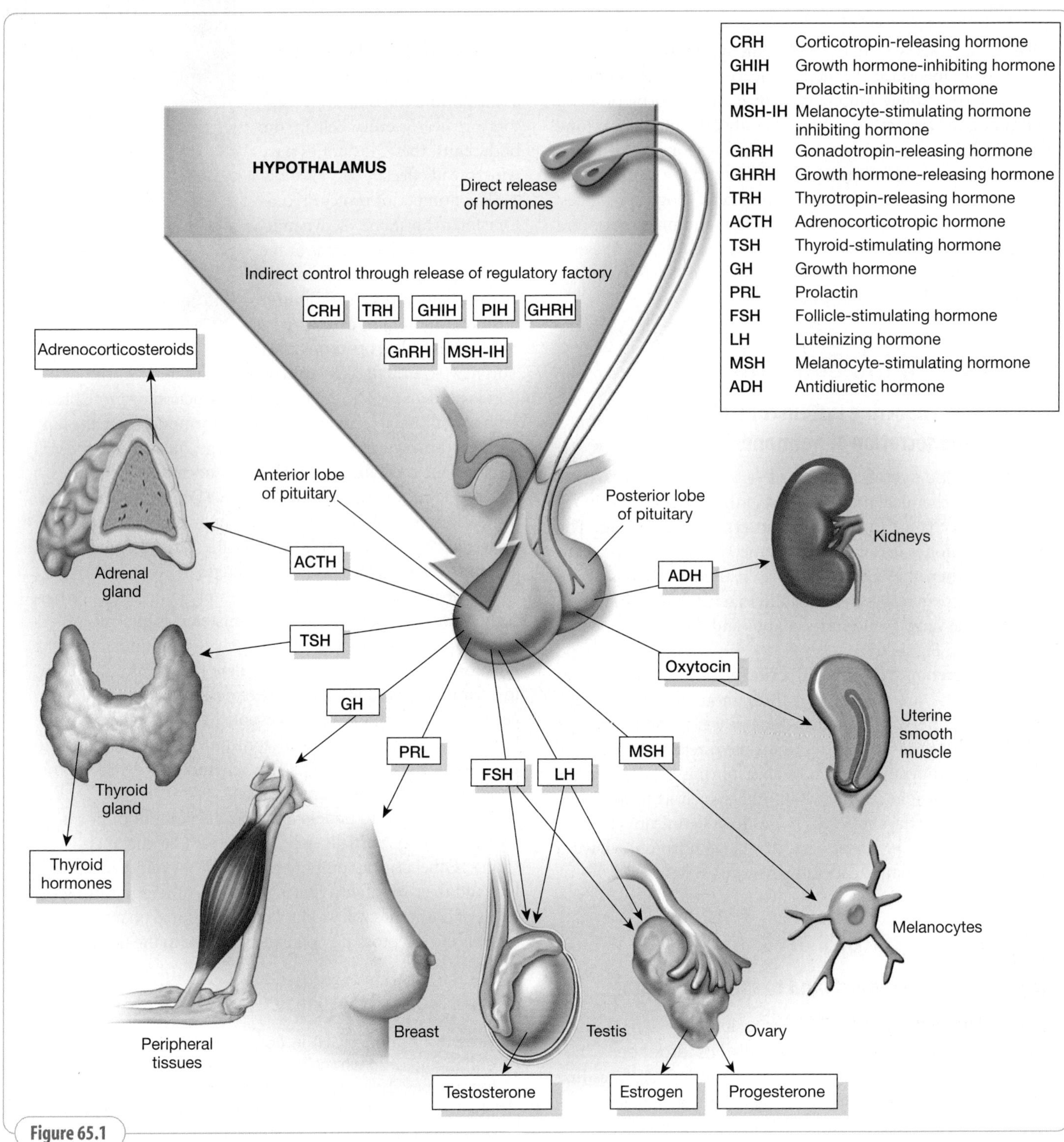

Figure 65.1

Hormones and the endocrine system.

Source: From *Anatomy and Physiology for Health Professions: An Interactive Journey* (p. 233), by B. Colbert, J. Ankney, & K. Lee, 2007. Reprinted by permission of Pearson Education, Inc., Upper Saddle River, NJ.

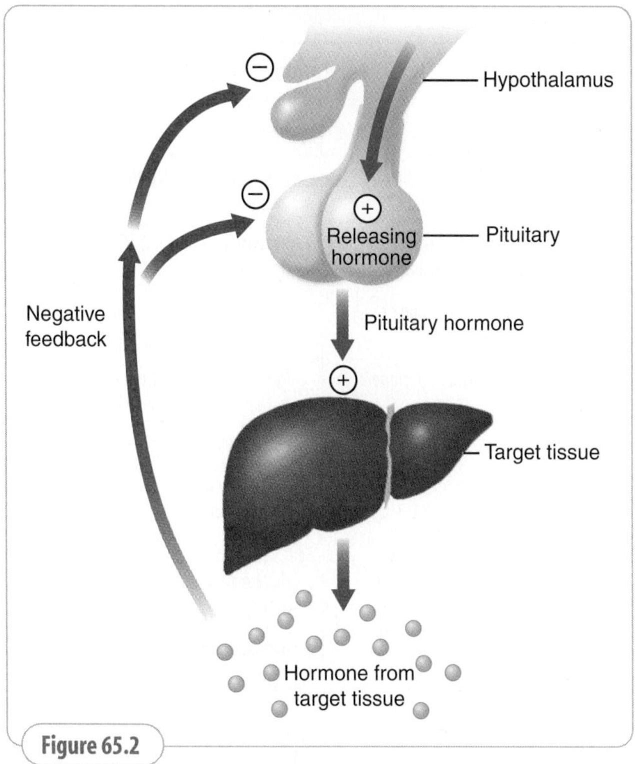

Figure 65.2

Negative feedback mechanism.

which is illustrated in Figure 65.2. When an endocrine tissue receives an appropriate stimulus, a hormone is secreted in larger amounts. The hormone causes an output or action, which is recognized by sensors. The sensors signal the endocrine tissue to stop secreting the hormone; that is, the endocrine tissue provides negative feedback.

Depending on the specific hormone, the negative feedback mechanism may be based on three primary types of stimuli: neuronal, humoral, and hormonal. In some cases, regulation involves multiple stimuli. The various hormones and their regulation are summarized in Table 65.1.

Neuronal stimuli: A few hormones are regulated by nerve impulses. The best example is epinephrine, which is released when a neuronal impulse from the sympathetic nervous system reaches the adrenal medulla. Another example is the release of oxytocin from the pituitary gland.

Humoral stimuli: Some endocrine glands sense the levels of specific substances in the blood and release the hormone when the substance rises above or falls below the normal range. For example, pancreatic islet cells can sense the level of glucose in the blood. If glucose levels become too high, insulin is secreted. Another example is the release of parathyroid hormone when blood calcium levels fall.

Hormonal stimuli: In the endocrine system, it is common for one hormone to control the secretion of another hormone. In some cases, the sequence involves three hormones. For example, thyrotropin-releasing hormone (TRH, from the hypothalamus) stimulates thyroid-stimulating hormone (TSH, from the pituitary), which causes the release of thyroid hormone (TH, from the thyroid gland). In a loop typical of the endocrine system, the last hormone in the pathway (TH) provides negative feedback to shut off secretion of the initial hormone (TRH).

CONNECTION *Checkpoint* 65.1

From what you learned in Chapter 19, identify indications for epinephrine pharmacotherapy. See Answer to Connection Checkpoint 65.1 in Appendix A.

Pharm*FACT*

Recent studies have suggested that working the late shift may increase your risk of cancer. Light at night interferes with melatonin, the "darkness hormone" secreted by the pineal gland at night that inhibits cancers and boosts the immune system. *Source:* Patel, 2006.

Hormone Pharmacotherapy

65.4 Hormone pharmacotherapy is indicated for a diverse variety of conditions.

The goals of hormone pharmacotherapy vary widely. In many cases, a hormone is administered as **replacement therapy** for patients who are unable to secrete sufficient quantities of their own endogenous hormones. Examples of replacement therapy include the administration of thyroid hormone after the thyroid gland has been surgically removed, supplying insulin to patients whose pancreas is not functioning, or administering growth hormone to children with short-stature disorder. The pharmacologic goal of replacement therapy is to supply the same physiological, low-level amounts of the hormone that would normally be present in the body. Selected endocrine disorders and their drug therapy are summarized in Table 65.2.

Some hormones are used in cancer chemotherapy to shrink the size of hormone-sensitive tumors. For example, certain breast cancers are strongly dependent upon estrogen for their growth. Giving the "opposite" hormone, testosterone, will shrink the tumor. In a similar manner, estrogen is used to shrink the size of testicular cancer, which is dependent on testosterone for its growth. Exactly how these hormones produce their antineoplastic action is largely unknown. When hormones are used as antineoplastics, their doses far exceed physiological levels normally present in the body. Hormones are nearly always used in combination with other antineoplastic medications, as discussed in Chapter 58.

TABLE 65.1 Selected Hormones and Their Regulation

Hormone	Target Organ(s) and Action	REGULATION: Stimulation	REGULATION: Inhibition
Adrenocorticotropic hormone (ACTH)	Adrenal cortex; stimulates release of glucocorticoids	Corticotropin-releasing hormone	Negative feedback from glucocorticoids
Aldosterone	Kidneys; promotes reabsorption of sodium and water	Renin-angiotensin pathway, decreased blood volume, hypotension	Increased blood volume or hypertension
Antidiuretic hormone (ADH)	Kidneys; increases water reabsorption	Increased osmolarity of blood or decreased blood volume	Adequate hydration
Follicle-stimulating hormone (FSH)	Ovaries; promotes maturation of ovarian follicles and estrogen production Testes; increases sperm production	Gonadotropin-releasing hormone (GnRH)	Negative feedback from estrogen (females) or testosterone (males)
Glucocorticoids	Most tissues; increases protein breakdown and glucose metabolism, provides resistance to stress, suppresses inflammation and immune response	Adrenocorticotropic hormone (ACTH)	Negative feedback from glucocorticoids
Growth hormone (GH)	Most tissues, including, bone, muscle, liver; stimulates growth and mobilizes lipids	Gonadotropin-releasing hormone (GnRH)	Negative feedback from growth hormone
Insulin	Most tissues; promotes movement of glucose into cells, lowers blood glucose, decreases glycogen synthesis, and increases lipogenesis and protein synthesis	Hyperglycemia	Hypoglycemia
Luteinizing hormone (LH)	Ovaries; stimulates ovulation and production of estrogen Testes; produces testosterone	Gonadotropin-releasing hormone (GnRH)	Negative feedback from estrogen and progesterone (females) or testosterone (males)
Oxytocin	Uterus; stimulates contractions Breasts; ejects milk	Stretching of uterus or infant suckling	Lack of stretching of the uterus or infant suckling
Parathyroid hormone	Kidneys, gastrointestinal tract, bone; increases calcium levels in blood	Hypocalcemia	Hypercalcemia
Prolactin	Breast; promotes lactation	Prolactin-releasing hormone	Prolactin-inhibiting hormone
Thyroid hormone	Most tissues; increases basal metabolic rate and growth	Thyroid-stimulating hormone	Negative feedback from thyroid hormone

TABLE 65.2 Selected Endocrine Disorders and Their Pharmacotherapy

Gland	Hormone(s)	Disorder	Drug Therapy Examples
Adrenal cortex	Corticosteroids	Hypersecretion: Cushing's syndrome	aminoglutethimide (Cytadren) and metyrapone (Metopirone)
		Hyposecretion: Addison's disease	hydrocortisone, prednisone
Gonads	Ovaries: Estrogen	Hyposecretion: Menstrual and metabolic dysfunction	conjugated estrogens and estradiol
	Ovaries: Progesterone	Hyposecretion: Dysfunctional uterine bleeding	medroxyprogesterone (Provera) and norethindrone
	Testes: Testosterone	Hyposecretion: Hypogonadism	testosterone
Pancreatic islets	Insulin	Hyposecretion: Diabetes mellitus	insulin and oral hypoglycemics
Parathyroid	Parathyroid hormone	Hypersecretion: Hyperparathyroidism	surgery (No drug therapy)
		Hyposecretion: Hypoparathyroidism	vitamin D and calcium supplements
Pituitary	Antidiuretic hormone	Hyposecretion: Diabetes insipidus	vasopressin, and desmopressin
	Growth hormone	Hyposecretion: Small stature	somatrem (Protropin) and somatropin (Genotropin)
		Hypersecretion: Acromegaly (adults)	octreotide (Sandostatin)
	Oxytocin	Hyposecretion: Delayed delivery or lack of milk ejection	oxytocin (Pitocin)
Thyroid	Thyroid hormone (T3 and T4)	Hypersecretion: Grave's disease	propylthiouracil (PTU) and I-131
		Hyposecretion: Myxedema (adults)	thyroid hormone and levothyroxine (T4)

Another goal of hormonal pharmacotherapy may be to produce an exaggerated response that is part of the normal action of the hormone. Administering hydrocortisone to suppress inflammation takes advantage of the normal action of the corticosteroids, but at higher amounts than would normally be present in the body. Hydrocortisone is indicated for acute inflammatory disorders such as lupus or rheumatoid arthritis. As another example, supplying estrogen or progesterone at specific times during the menstrual patient can prevent ovulation and pregnancy. In this example, the patient is given natural hormones; however, they are taken at a time when levels in the body are normally low.

Endocrine pharmacotherapy also involves the use of "antihormones." These hormone antagonists block the actions of endogenous hormones. For example, propylthiouracil (PTU) is given to block the effects of an overactive thyroid gland (see Chapter 68). Tamoxifen (Nolvadex) is given to block the actions of estrogen in estrogen-dependent breast cancers (see Chapter 58).

CONNECTION *Checkpoint* 65.2

Glucocorticoids, or corticosteroids, are important drugs in treating inflammation. From what you learned in Chapter 45, explain their role in treating autoimmune disease. See Answer to Connection Checkpoint 65.2 in Appendix A.

UNDERSTANDING THE CHAPTER

Key Concepts Summary

65.1 The endocrine system controls homeostasis through the secretion of hormones.

65.2 Hormones must bind to specific receptors to cause physiological changes.

65.3 Most hormone action is regulated through negative feedback.

65.4 Hormone pharmacotherapy is indicated for a diverse variety of conditions.

References

Browning, K. (2007). *Human growth hormone abuse.* Retrieved August 22, 2008, from http://www.associatedcontent.com/article/139346/human_growth_hormone_abuse.html?cat=5

Colbert, J. B., Ankney, J., & Lee, K. T. (2007). Anatomy and physiology for health professionals: An interactive journey. Upper Saddle River, NJ: Pearson Education.

Greenstein, B., & Wood, D. (2006). *The endocrine system at a glance* (2nd ed.). Malden, MA: Wiley-Blackwell.

Krogh, D. (2009). *Biology: A guide to the natural world* (4th ed.). San Francisco: Benjamin Cummings.

Martini, F. H., & Nath, J. L. (2009). *Fundamentals of human anatomy and physiology* (7th ed.). San Francisco: Benjamin Cummings.

Patel, D. (2006). Shift work, light at night, and risk of breast cancer. *Occupational Medicine 56*(6), 433.

Rice, J. (2005). *Medical terminology with human anatomy* (5th ed.). Upper Saddle River, NJ: Pearson Education, Inc.

Silverthorn, D. U. (2007). *Human physiology: An integrated approach* (4th ed.). San Francisco: Benjamin-Cummings.

CHAPTER

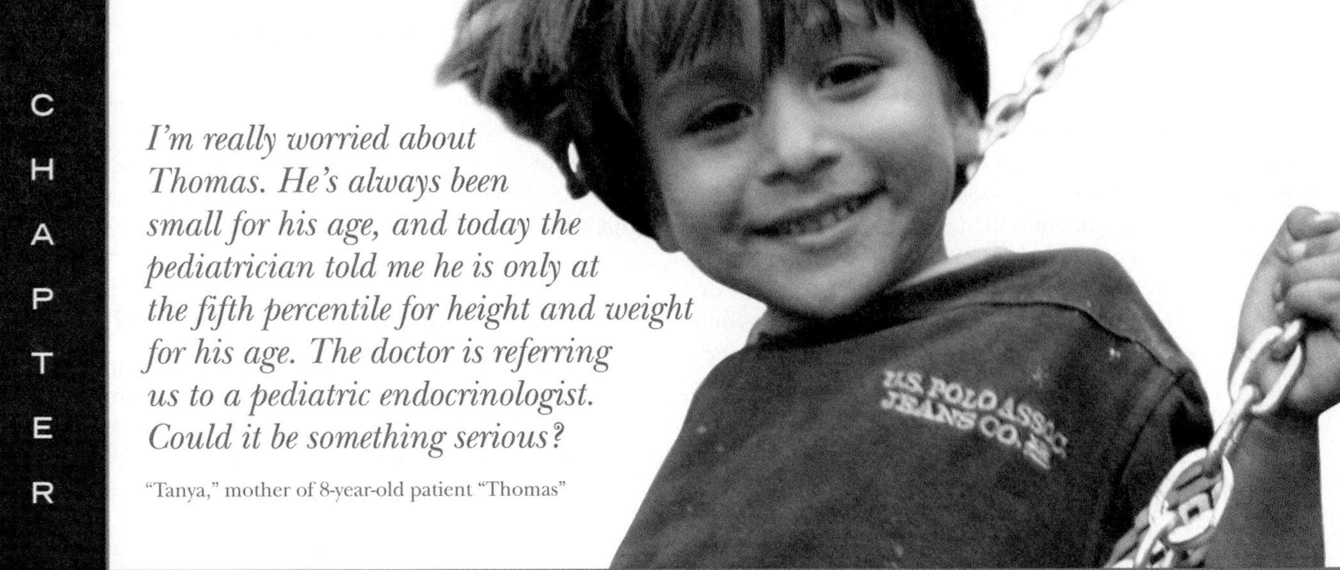

I'm really worried about Thomas. He's always been small for his age, and today the pediatrician told me he is only at the fifth percentile for height and weight for his age. The doctor is referring us to a pediatric endocrinologist. Could it be something serious?

"Tanya," mother of 8-year-old patient "Thomas"

66 Hypothalamic and Pituitary Drugs

Learning Outcomes

After reading this chapter, the student should be able to:

1. Explain the physiology of the hormones secreted by the hypothalamus and pituitary gland.
2. Identify indications for hypothalamic hormones.
3. Explain the pharmacotherapy of growth hormone disorders in children and adults.
4. Explain the pharmacotherapy of antidiuretic hormone disorders.
5. For each of the classes shown in the Chapter Outline, identify the prototype and representative drugs and explain the mechanism(s) of drug action, primary indications, contraindications, significant drug interactions, pregnancy category, and important adverse effects.
6. Use the nursing process to care for patients receiving drug therapy for disorders of the hypothalamus and pituitary gland.

Chapter Outline

Functions of the Hypothalamus

Functions of the Pituitary Gland

Pharmacotherapy of Growth Hormone Disorders

Growth Hormone Analogs

PROTOTYPE **Somatotropin (Accretropin, Genotropin, Humatrope, Norditropin, Nutropin, Saizen, Serostim, Zorbtive)** *p. 1108*

Growth Hormone Antagonists

PROTOTYPE **Octreotide (Sandostatin)** *p. 1111*

Pharmacotherapy of Antidiuretic Hormone Disorders

PROTOTYPE **Desmopressin (DDAVP, Stimate) (Antidiuretic Hormone)** *p. 1114*

Key Terms

acromegaly, *1111*
anterior pituitary gland, *1106*
antidiuretic hormone (ADH), *1112*
diabetes insipidus, *1114*
dwarfism, *1107*
gigantism, *1111*
growth hormone (GH), *1106*
insulin-like growth factor (IGF), *1106*
posterior pituitary gland, *1106*
short stature, *1107*
syndrome of inappropriate antidiuretic hormone (SIADH), *1114*
tropic hormones, *1106*

In the specialty of endocrinology, understanding the complex relationship between the hypothalamus and pituitary gland is important because these organs control so many homeostatic functions. The two collaborate to secrete hormones that control the function of the gonads, adrenal glands, thyroid gland, kidneys, and the milk-producing tissues of the breast. The functioning of these two glands serves as the control center that provides integration between the nervous and endocrine systems. This chapter examines drugs that directly affect the functions of the pituitary and hypothalamus.

Functions of the Hypothalamus

66.1 The hypothalamus controls many diverse body processes and secretes hormones that influence pituitary function.

Roughly the size of an almond, the hypothalamus lies in the center of the diencephalon of the brain, just superior to the brainstem. The overall purpose of the hypothalamus is to maintain balance or homeostasis. To achieve this, the hypothalamus receives input from numerous vital regions of the nervous system, recognizes imbalances, and then makes adjustments to bring the body back to homeostasis. Examples of the multiple and diverse functions of this organ include control of body temperature, thirst, appetite, fatigue, circadian rhythms, anger, and the rate of overall body metabolism. The hypothalamus also controls vital functions of the autonomic nervous system such as heart rate, vasoconstriction, digestion, and sweating. For the purposes of this chapter, only the endocrine functions of the hypothalamus are presented.

As discussed in Chapter 65, every hormone has target cells that possess receptors for that specific hormone. For the hormones secreted by the hypothalamus, there is only one target organ: the pituitary gland. All hypothalamic hormones travel by the blood a short distance to the pituitary, which lies immediately below the hypothalamus. Upon reaching their receptors, the hypothalamic hormones simply increase or decrease the release of hormones by the pituitary gland. Because of this, hormones from the hypothalamus are called releasing hormones or inhibiting hormones. The major hypothalamic hormones and their actions on the pituitary gland are given in Table 66.1

There are very few indications for the administration of hypothalamic hormones: Only one has clinical applications. Rather than give hypothalamic hormones, it is more effective (and less expensive) to administer pituitary hormones, or the secretions of a target endocrine organ such as thyroid hormone, estrogen, testosterone, or corticosteroids.

The hypothalamic hormones that have clinical applications are analogs of gonadotropin-releasing hormone (GnRH): leuprolide (Lupron), goserelin (Zoladex), and nafarelin (Synarel). These drugs are GnRH agonists used to treat endometriosis, a common cause of infertility (see Chapter 70). An additional GnRH analog, histrelin (Supprelin LA) was approved in 2007 to treat central precocious puberty, the premature onset of puberty

TABLE 66.1 Hormones Secreted by the Hypothalamus and Pituitary Gland

Hypothalamic Hormone	Pituitary Hormone	Target Organ	Principle Actions
Corticotropin-releasing hormone (CRH)	Adrenocorticotropic hormone (ACTH)	Adrenal cortex	Stimulates release of corticosteroids
Gonadotropin-releasing hormone (GnRH)	Follicle-stimulating hormone (FSH)	Ovaries, testes	Stimulates release of estrogen and ovarian follicle development in females, and sperm production in males
	Luteinizing hormone (LH)	Ovaries, testes	Triggers ovulation and secretion of estrogen and progesterone in females, increases testosterone secretion in males
None	Melanocyte-stimulating hormone (MSH)	Skin	Stimulates pigmentation
Thyrotropin-releasing hormone (TRH)	Thyroid-stimulating hormone (TSH)	Thyroid gland	Stimulates release of thyroid hormone
Growth hormone–releasing hormone (GHRH) Growth hormone–inhibiting hormone (GHIH)	Growth hormone (GH)	Most body cells	Stimulates growth and development of bones, muscles, cartilage, organs; general body metabolism
Prolactin-releasing hormone (PRH) Prolactin-inhibiting hormone (PIH)	Prolactin	Mammary glands	Promotes lactation

in children. One histrelin implant annually provides negative feedback to shut down the secretion of gonadal hormones, estrogen, and testosterone. Leuprolide, histrelin, and goserelin are also used for the palliative treatment of advanced prostate cancer. Two additional hypothalamic hormone analogs, protirelin (Thyrel), a form of TRH, and sermorelin (Geref), a form of GHRH, were removed from the U.S. market.

CONNECTION *Checkpoint* 66.1

Target tissues can up-regulate or down-regulate the number of receptors for a specific hormone. From what you learned in Chapter 65, which of the two occurs when a hormone is administered as pharmacotherapy for long periods? See Answer to Connection Checkpoint 66.1 in Appendix A.

Functions of the Pituitary Gland

66.2 The pituitary gland secretes hormones that control many diverse body functions.

Although the pituitary gland is often referred to as the "master gland," its function is largely controlled by the releasing or inhibiting hormones from the hypothalamus. The pituitary gland is divided into anterior and posterior lobes, which have very different structures and functions. The anterior lobe comprises the majority of the pituitary gland.

The **anterior pituitary gland** (adenohypophysis) is comprised of glandular tissue that manufactures and secretes hormones that control major body functions and systems. Four of these are called **tropic hormones,** a term that refers to the ability of these hormones to regulate the secretory actions of other endocrine glands. The anterior pituitary hormones are synthesized and stored in the pituitary until they receive a message from the hypothalamus. The hormonal message from the hypothalamus could be to release the hormones (growth hormone-releasing hormone [GHRH], thyrotropin-releasing hormone [TRH], prolactin-releasing hormone [PRH], corticotropin-releasing hormone [CRH], gonadotropin-releasing hormone [GnRH]) or to stop releasing the hormones (growth hormone–inhibiting hormone [GHIH], prolactin-inhibiting hormone [PIH]).

The **posterior pituitary gland** (neurohypophysis), by contrast, consists of nervous tissue and is basically an extension of the hypothalamus. It secretes two hormones: antidiuretic hormone (ADH) and oxytocin. These hormones are manufactured in the hypothalamus and travel down neurons to the posterior pituitary where they are stored, until factors stimulate their release. The primary stimulus causing ADH secretion is an increased serum osmolality, or a high concentration of solutes in the blood. Oxytocin release is stimulated by touch receptors in the nipples of lactating women. Pharmacotherapy with oxytocin is presented in Chapter 70.

Regulation of hormone levels is an essential function because too little or too much of any of these endocrine secretions can cause profound symptoms. Many are controlled by negative feedback loops. As circulating levels of a hormone rise above normal, a message is sent to the hypothalamus, pituitary, or other endocrine gland to shut down the manufacture and secretion of the hormone. This prevents excess hormone levels. When hormones are administered as drug therapy, they can influence this normal negative feedback mechanism. One of the most important examples of this phenomenon is the negative feedback suppression of the adrenal glands caused by administration of corticosteroid medications (see Chapter 69). The student should review the information on negative feedback in Section 65.3 before proceeding.

Because of the widespread effects of the hormones secreted and controlled by the hypothalamus and pituitary glands, disorders of these glands are quite complex. In general, the pathologies of endocrine glands can be categorized as causing hypofunction or hyperfunction of the gland. Pituitary disorders can be the result of tumors, surgery, radiation therapy, infection, injury, infarction (loss of blood supply), or bleeding (hemorrhage) in the area. Congenital defects may also result in absent or impaired function of a hormone, or the lack of an enzyme necessary for hormone production.

Pharmacotherapy of Growth Hormone Disorders

66.3 Growth hormone deficiency in adults and children can be treated by administering recombinant growth hormone.

Growth hormone (GH) is produced and secreted by the anterior pituitary gland. This hormone was once believed to be of importance only during periods of active growth, but it is now recognized that adults produce nearly as much GH as children. Although its major targets are bone and skeletal muscle, GH stimulates many types of body cells to increase in size and replicate. It is considered an anabolic (tissue-building) hormone. The primary effects of GH are as follows:

- Increases length and width of bone.
- Stimulates cartilage growth.
- Stimulates the growth and development of visceral and endocrine organs, skeletal and cardiac muscle, and skin and connective tissue.
- Enhances cellular uptake of amino acids and increased protein synthesis.
- Increases use of fatty acids for fuel with decreased use of glucose; impairs glucose tolerance and insulin resistance in peripheral tissues.

Many of the effects of GH are dependent on **insulin-like growth factors (IGF),** a family of peptides that promote cartilage and bone growth. IGFs are produced in the liver, and released when hepatic cells become activated by growth hormone. Secretion of GH fluctuates during the day, peaking 1 to 4 hours following the onset of sleep. These night-time bursts in GH are greater in children than in adults.

TABLE 66.2 Factors Affecting the Release of Growth Hormone

Factors Increasing Release of GH	Factors Decreasing Release of GH
Amino acids: Leucine, arginine	Beta-adrenergic agonists
Androgens and estrogens	Carbohydrate-rich diet
Clonidine	Cortisol
Elevated body temperature	Free fatty acids
Gamma-hydroxybutyrate	Increased serum glucose level
Growth hormone–releasing hormone (GHRH)	Obesity
Hypoglycemia, fasting, starvation	Somatostatin
L-dopa	
Stress, trauma	
Vigorous exercise	

The overall regulation of serum GH levels resides in the hypothalamus, with the secretion of GHRH and GHIH. There are a large number of secondary factors, such as exercise and sleep, that influence the release of GH, and these are listed in Table 66.2.

In children, GH deficiency results in **dwarfism.** Dwarfism is associated with normal birth length followed by a slowing of the growth rate. These children have normal intelligence, short stature, immature facial features, obesity, and delayed skeletal maturation. In this context, **short stature** is defined as well below the fifth percentile for age and gender, or more than two standard deviations below the mean (average) height for age and gender. Acquired GH deficiency develops later in childhood, and can be caused by a hypothalamic-pituitary tumor, or infection. Children who have been severely neglected or emotionally deprived can develop a psychosocial dwarfism, with poor growth, a potbelly, and poor nutritional habits. GH levels often return to normal once the child is removed from the dysfunctional environment.

PharmFACT

The incidence of short stature associated with childhood GH deficiency is estimated to range between 1 per 4,000 to 1 per 10,000 children. About 20,000 children per year receive growth hormone therapy, and approximately 4,000 new children are diagnosed annually as candidates for GH therapy.

Source: Eledrisi, 2008.

When GH deficiency is the cause of short stature, replacement therapy is the treatment of choice. Until 1985, GH was obtained from the pituitary glands of human cadavers, a practice that was halted following the deaths of several recipients who developed Creutzfeldt-Jakob disease. GH is now obtained using recombinant DNA technology. Doses for the GH analogs are listed in Table 66.3.

Therapy with recombinant GH is expensive, costing approximately $30,000 to $40,000 each year per child. The hormone is administered subcutaneously, several times a week during the period of active growth, and therapy may continue until adulthood. Females with Turner's syndrome and children with chronic renal insufficiency may also be treated with GH. Often, treatment with GH produces only modest gains in final adult height, but these gains are considered beneficial to the psychological well-being of the patient.

Adult GH deficiency is associated with reduced muscle mass, increased cardiovascular mortality, central adiposity and increased visceral fat, insulin resistance, and dyslipidemia. This hormonal deficiency may develop during adulthood, or it may be a continuation of childhood deficiency. Several forms of recombinant human GH formulations (Humatrope and Genotropin) have been approved for use in adults with body-wasting–type disorders. Treatment can result in increased lean body mass, decreased fat mass, increased bone mineral density, and decreased lipid levels.

CONNECTIONS

Evidence-Based Practice Growth Hormone for Age-Appropriate Height

Clinical Question

Is growth hormone effective in helping children born small for gestational age attain age-appropriate height?

Evidence

In a study of long-term responses to growth hormone (GH) therapy among children born small for gestational age, 77 prepubertal children were given daily doses of GH. In a comparison group, 34 similar children were untreated. Significant differences were observed between those treated and those not treated, although height gains were modest. For all children treated, the mean increase in height was 9 cm (3.5 in.) . For children who began treatment more than 2 years prior to puberty, the mean height gain was 12 cm (4.7 in.), while those treated less than 2 years prior to puberty achieved a mean gain of 6 cm (2.3 in.). No adverse effects from the GH were found.

Implication

The younger, shorter, and lighter the child was at the start of GH treatment, the better the response.

Critical Thinking Question

How would you assist the family in determining what would be reasonable goals for height and weight for a child receiving growth hormone therapy?

See Answers to Critical Thinking Questions in Appendix A.

Source: From "Final Height in Short Children Born Small for Gestational Age Treated with Growth Hormone," 2005, by J. Dahlgren, and K.A. Wikland, *Pediatric Research, 57*(2), pp. 216-222.

TABLE 66.3 Hypothalamic and Pituitary Agents

Drug	Route and Adult Dose (maximum dose where indicated)	Adverse Effects
bromocriptine (Parlodel)	PO: 1.25–2.5 mg/day for 3 days, then increase dose every 3–7 days to 30-60 mg/day in divided doses (max: 100 mg/day)	*Orthostatic hypotension, nausea, vomiting, dizziness, headache* Shock, acute MI, cerebral ischemia, confusion, agitation, hallucinations, paranoid delusions
desmopressin (DDAVP, Stimate)	Intranasal: 0.1–0.4 mL (10–40 mcg) in 1–3 divided doses IV/Subcutaneous: 2–4 mcg in 2 divided doses PO: 0.2–0.4 mg/day	*Headache, nasal congestion or irritation, nausea* Water intoxication, coma, thromboembolic disorder, hyponatremia
lanreotide (Somatuline Depot)	Subcutaneous: 60–100 mg every 4 weeks	*Pain at the injection site, nausea, vomiting, diarrhea, itching* Gallstones, bradycardia, hyper- or hypoglycemia
mecasermin (Increlex) mecasermin rinfabate (Iplex)	Subcutaneous: 0.04–0.08 mg/kg twice daily. Must be administered within 20 min of a meal or snack. (max: 0.12 mg/kg given twice daily) Subcutaneous (3 yrs and older): 0.5 mg/kg once daily, up to 1–2 mg/kg/day, given once daily	*Injection site reaction, iron-deficency anemia, goiter, antibody development, headache, hypertrophy of adenoids and tonsils* Hypoglycemia, increased intracranial pressure
octreotide (Sandostatin)	Subcutaneous/IV: 100–600 mcg/day in 2–4 divided doses; after 2 weeks may switch to IM depot, 20 mg every 4 weeks	*Nausea, vomiting, diarrhea, headache, flushing, injection site pain, cholelithiasis* Dysrhythmia, worsening congestive heart failure, sinus bradycardia
pegvisomant (Somavert)	Subcutaneous: 40 mg loading dose, then 10 mg/day (max: 30 mg/day)	*Nausea, diarrhea, injection site pain, flulike symptoms* Liver damage, elevated transaminase levels
somatropin (Accretropin, Genotropin, Humatrope, Norditropin, Nutropin, Serostim, Saizen, Zorbtive)	Humatrope: Subcutaneous: 0.006 mg/kg daily (max: 0.0125 mg/kg/day) Serostim: Subcutaneous: More than 55 kg: 6 mg at bedtime; 45–55 kg: 5 mg at bedtime; 35–45 kg: 4 mg at bedtime; less than 35 kg: 0.1 mg/kg at bedtime Child: Genotropin: Subcutaneous: 0.16–0.24 mg/kg/week in 6–7 doses Norditropin: 0.024–0.034 mg/kg 6–7 times/week	*Pain at injection site, hyperglycemia, arthalgia, myalgia, abdominal pain, otitis media, headache, bronchitis, hypothyroidism, HTN, flulike symptoms* Severe respiratory impairment in severely obese patients with Prader-Willi syndrome, diabetes, pancreatitis, scoliosis of the spine, papilledema, intracranial tumor
vasopressin	IM/subcutaneous: 5–10 units aqueous solution 2–4 times/day IV: 0.2–0.4 units/min up to 1 unit/min	*Tremor, pallor, nausea, vomiting, water retention, intoxication* Angina, acute MI, gangrene, anaphylaxis, cardiac arrest

Note: *Italics* indicate common adverse effects. Underline indicates serious adverse effects.

Human GH has been abused for its anabolic effects. Athletes have used the drug to build muscle, increase strength, and maintain less body fat. It has also been called an "antiaging" drug because it promotes younger-looking skin, improved memory, and reduced wrinkles. The administration of GH for these purposes is illegal, and prolonged use may lead to long-term adverse effects in patients. Despite potential adverse health effects, products advertised as "human growth hormone supplements" are readily marketed without a prescription. These do not contain any GH (which must be administered parenterally) but instead contain a mixture of oral supplements that are claimed to stimulate the pituitary gland. The safety and effectiveness of these products have not been evaluated adequately.

PROTOTYPE DRUG Somatropin (Accretropin, Genotropin, Humatrope, Norditropin, Nutropin, Saizen, Serostim, Zorbtive)

Classification: Therapeutic: Human growth hormone
Pharmacologic: Pituitary hormone

Therapeutic Effects and Uses: Approved in 1987, somatropin is identical to endogenous human GH and is available in several different formulations, which vary by dose and regimen. The preferred route of administration is subcutaneous, although some forms may be given via the intramuscular (IM)

CONNECTIONS

To the Community Inappropriate Adult Use of Growth Hormone to Enhance Athletic Performance and Physical Appearance

GH has been on the list of forbidden substances by international federations and the International Olympics Committee since it became available in its recombinant form in the early 1990s. Although the benefits of GH to enhance athletic performance have not been supported, it is likely used for its anabolic effect on muscle growth. GH is being used in combination with other illegal substances, and that misuse of GH has steadily increased since the late 1980s. Two studies investigated the practice of inappropriate adult use of growth hormone to enhance athletic performance and physical appearance.

Saugy et al. (2006) reviewed the literature regarding the use of GH, its adverse effects, and methods of detection when used for doping. They feel GH is attractive because it is effective in building lean tissue, is hard to detect through testing, and it has no known adverse effects when dosed properly. The authors note that GH is often combined with anabolic steroids when in power sports, and with erythropoietin for endurance sports. Difficulties in detecting GH are due to its pulsatile secretion, and by the recombinant forms being identical to endogenous GH. GH levels vary widely from person to person, and throughout the day. In addition, exercise can cause a five- to ten-fold increase in GH levels. Therefore, with current testing methods it is not possible to say definitely whether a high level is an individual variation or due to exercise, versus due to doping with exogenous forms of the hormone. The only direct evidence of the use of GH as a doping agent comes from it being found by police during doping-related raids. Although immediate adverse effects are not evident, there is concern for the long-term effects of misuse of GH, including an increased risk for cardiovascular disease, diabetes mellitus, edema, and HTN.

In a second study (Parkinson & Evans, 2006), 500 users of anabolic androgenic steroids responded to anonymous questionnaires. The researchers found that the majority of respondents (78.4%) were noncompetitive bodybuilders and nonathletes, who were taking the drugs for cosmetic reasons. In addition to using anabolic steroids, 25% also used GH for its anabolic effects. A total of 13% of those responding reported unsafe injection practices, such as reusing needles. Nearly 100% of the sample reported subjective adverse effects from the steroids, but were nonetheless taking larger doses than had been previously recorded.

route. GH produces growth of long bones in children prior to epiphyseal closure. The gain in growth is very rapid at the initiation of therapy, but slows over time. Treatment may continue until the desired height is achieved, epiphyseal closure occurs, or the patient fails to respond to treatment. If treatment does not result in growth, it is stopped, and the diagnosis is reevaluated. The metabolic effects of the drug include increased protein synthesis, reduced carbohydrate utilization, and increased use of fatty acids for energy.

GH is used in the management of a number of growth-related disorders, including the following:

- Growth failure in children due to GH deficiency or Prader-Willi syndrome (Accretropin and Genotropin)
- Growth failure in children due to chronic renal insufficiency (Nutropin)
- Short stature associated with Turner's syndrome (Accretropin, Genotropin, Humatrope, Norditropin, Nutropin)
- Adult growth hormone deficiency (Genotropin, Humatrope, Norditropin, Nutropin, Saizen)
- AIDS wasting, cachexia, and severe thermal injuries (Serostim)
- Short bowel syndrome in patients receiving specialized nutrition support (Zorbtive)

Although the various brand name products of GH have the same effectiveness, they differ in potency and are not interchangeable. Some are available in prefilled syringes while others are longer acting. The nurse should check the package insert for specific dosing instructions.

Mechanism of Action: Somatropin has the same amino acid sequence as endogenous human growth hormone, and produces the same effects as the naturally occurring form of the hormone. The effects of GH are mediated by IGF.

Pharmacokinetics:

Route(s)	Subcutaneous; IM
Absorption	Well absorbed following injection
Distribution	Distributed to highly perfused organs (liver, kidneys); circulates bound to growth hormone binding protein
Primary metabolism	Hepatic; some metabolism in kidneys
Primary excretion	Renal
Onset of action	Peak action variable: Days to weeks
Duration of action	Half-Life: 3.8–5 h

Adverse Effects: Adverse effects of somatropin include hyperglycemia and insulin resistance, which is made worse in patients with preexisting diabetes mellitus. It can also cause hypothyroidism. Edema of the hands and feet, headache, and hypertension (HTN) often occur initially, but may resolve with continued therapy. Joint pain, muscle aches, and pain at the injection site are common. Carpal tunnel syndrome may occur with use of Serostim. Development of antibodies to growth hormone may rarely occur.

Contraindications/Precautions: Somatropin is contraindicated for use to promote growth in children with epiphyseal closure. It is also contraindicated in patients with severe obesity, respiratory impairment, or sleep apnea due to potentially fatal respiratory impairment. Somatropin is contraindicated in patients with intracranial tumor due to the risk for increased growth, or recurrence of tumor. The drug is contraindicated in patients who are sensitive to glycerin. Somatropin should be used with caution in patients with severe renal or hepatic disease due to reduced clearance, and in patients with diabetes mellitus due to hyperglycemia and insulin resistance. It should be used with caution in pregnant or lactating patients because safety has not been established.

Drug Interactions: Corticosteroids interfere with the bone growth–promoting action of GH; thus, the two should not be given concurrently. Concurrent use with anabolic steroids, androgens, estrogens, or thyroid hormone may increase the rate of epiphyseal closure. **Herbal/Food:** Unknown.

Pregnancy: Category B or C, depending upon the specific formulation.

Treatment of Overdose: Overdose with somatotropin has not been reported.

Nursing Responsibilities:

- Assess baseline height and weight and monitor regularly to determine drug effectiveness. Report lack of growth to the prescriber.
- Reconstitute with the solution provided. Inject the solution carefully, aiming at the side of the vial, and gently swirl to dissolve the drug. Do not shake, as this can break down the drug. Do not use the mixture if it is cloudy or contains particulate matter.
- Monitor laboratory tests for serum protein, serum glucose, and thyroid hormone levels; hypothyroidism may develop during treatment, and would interfere with optimum results.
- Administer the drug in the evening to mimic the body's normal hormone level changes.
- Test for GH antibodies in patients who initially respond to therapy but then fail to respond to the medication.
- Monitor diabetic patients closely because serum glucose levels often increase during therapy and insulin resistance may develop.
- Assess dietary intake because nutritional needs increase with the increased rate of growth. Consult a dietitian or nutritionist as needed.
- Complete a family and caregiver assessment to determine their ability to prepare and administer the medication.
- Determine the family's financial ability to afford medication and consult social services if financial support is necessary.
- Assess for adherence to the drug regimen.

Patient and Family Education:

- Rotate injection sites as directed by the health care provider. The abdomen and thigh are the preferred sites for these subcutaneous injections.
- Immediately report any difficulty walking (limping), or if pain develops in the hip or knee.
- Monitor food intake and report any concerns to the health care provider.
- If diabetic, monitor blood glucose regularly and report significant changes.
- Keep medication refrigerated.

Drugs Similar to Somatropin (Accretropin, Genotropin, Humatrope, Norditropin, Nutropin, Saizen, Serostim, Zorbtive)

Mecasermin is the only other drug that has actions similar to growth hormone.

Mecasermin (Increlex, Iplex): Mecasermin is a newer agent, approved in 2005, that is a solution of insulin-like growth factor (IGF) produced through recombinant DNA technology. This drug is identical to endogenous IGF and therefore has the same actions as growth hormone. Mecasermin is indicated for the long-term treatment of growth failure in children with severe primary IGF deficiency, or for those who have developed

CONNECTIONS

Evidence-Based Practice Long-Term Outcome of Growth Hormone on Pediatric Burn Patients

Clinical Question

Does the use of GH in severely burned pediatric patients improve their long-term outcome?

Evidence

Researchers investigated the beneficial effects of extended GH treatment in severely burned pediatric patients (Przkora et al., 2006). In the study, 44 pediatric patients were randomized into treatment and placebo groups. Those in the treatment group were given GH for 12 months following discharge, then followed for another 12 months after the treatment was discontinued. Effects studied were height, weight, body composition, serum hormone levels, resting energy expenditure, cardiac function, muscle strength, and number of reconstructive procedures performed. The authors found that height, weight, lean body mass, bone mineral content, cardiac function, and muscle strength significantly improved in the treatment group. In addition, the treatment group underwent significantly fewer reconstructive procedures than did the placebo group. The authors found no adverse effects from the GH therapy, and found that the beneficial effects persisted for the 12 months following treatment discontinuation.

Implication

Treatment with GH in severely burned pediatric patients is safe and effective, and facilitates and improves the recovery process.

Critical Thinking Question

Do you think that the child's height and weight at the end of the treatment period are greater than would have been expected without any GH treatment?

See Answers to Critical Thinking Questions in Appendix A.

neutralizing antibodies to GH. It should not be used in adults, after the epiphyses have closed. Increlex is given twice daily by the subcutaneous route, whereas Iplex has a once-daily dosing schedule. Adverse effects include hypoglycemia, headache, dizziness, vomiting, and tonsillar hypertrophy. Rare adverse effects include intracranial HTN and anaphylaxis. This drug is pregnancy category C.

66.4 Overproduction of growth hormone in adults can be treated by administering growth hormone antagonists.

Excessive GH secretion that occurs prior to puberty and the sealing of epiphyseal plates of the long bones results in **gigantism,** or unusual tallness. Gigantism is rare due to early recognition of the cause of the oversecretion: a benign pituitary adenoma. GH excess in children is usually treated with surgery, as soon as the disorder is diagnosed.

Excessive GH secretion in adults causes a condition known as **acromegaly.** Excess levels of GH stimulate the secretion of insulin-like growth factors from the liver, which then produce the clinical manifestations of the disorder. Because the epiphyseal plates are closed in adults, bones become deformed rather than elongated with this disorder. The onset is gradual, with enlargement of the small bones of the hands and feet, face and skull, broad nose, protruding lower jaw, and slanting forehead. The cartilage of the larynx enlarges, deepening the voice. Spinal changes can lead to kyphosis. Arthralgias and degenerative arthritis may occur, and enlargement of organs, including the heart, can result in an early death due to atherosclerosis. Metabolic changes lead to insulin resistance and impaired glucose tolerance. Treatment may consist of a combination of surgery, radiation therapy, and pharmacotherapy to suppress GH secretion and correct metabolic abnormalities. Doses of the GH antagonists are listed in Table 66.3.

PROTOTYPE DRUG Octreotide (Sandostatin)

Classification: **Therapeutic:** Growth hormone antagonist; antidiarrheal

Pharmacologic: Somatostatin

Therapeutic Effects and Uses: Approved in 1988, octreotide, which is commonly called somatostatin, is a long-acting peptide that mimics the actions of the GHIH. Octreotide is effective in both children and adults with GH excess. To treat acromegaly, the drug is initially given three times daily by the subcutaneous route. A long-acting IM form (Sandostatin LAR Depot) is available that reduces dosing to every 4 weeks.

Although GHIH is primarily secreted by the hypothalamus, small amounts are also secreted by the stomach, intestine, and pancreas. Thus, in addition to its effect of blocking GH secretion in the anterior pituitary, octreotide suppresses the release of multiple gastrointestinal (GI) hormones, including gastrin, cholecystokinin (CCK), secretin, vasoactive intestinal peptide, insulin, and glucagon. This has resulted in its use in treating multiple secretory and bleeding conditions of the intestinal tract. Because it stimulates the absorption of fluid and electrolytes from the GI tract and prolongs intestinal transit time, it is approved to treat severe diarrhea and flushing episodes associated with metastatic carcinoid tumors, or vasoactive intestinal peptide tumors. Octreotide inhibits enzymes that cause vasodilation, decreases hepatic and GI blood flow, and reduces hepatic-portal venous pressure. These properties make the drug useful in treating portal HTN and upper GI bleeding caused by esophageal varices. It is also used off-label to reduce the output from pancreatic and other GI fistulas.

Mechanism of Action: Octreotide produces the same effects as the natural hormone somatostatin to suppress secretion of GH. It also suppresses secretion of serotonin, pancreatic peptides, gastrin, vasoactive intestinal peptides, secretin, motilin, insulin, and glucagon.

Pharmacokinetics:

Route(s)	Subcutaneous or IM (depot formulation)
Absorption	Absorbed rapidly following subcutaneous injection
Distribution	May cross the placenta; may be secreted in breast milk
Primary metabolism	Liver
Primary excretion	Renal
Onset of action	15–30 minutes
Duration of action	12 h; half-life: 1.5 h

Adverse Effects: The most common adverse effects of octreotide are related to the GI system: nausea, vomiting, diarrhea, abdominal discomfort, development of gallstones, and elevated liver enzymes. The nausea, vomiting, and abdominal pain diminish with continued therapy. It can also cause headache, fatigue, flushing, and edema. Because hypoglycemia or hyperglycemia can develop with long-term use, an adjustment in insulin doses in diabetic patients may be necessary. It can also cause cardiac dysrhythmias, heart failure, and chest pain. Pain at the injection site is very common.

Contraindications/Precautions: Octreotide is contraindicated in patients who are sensitive to octreotide. It is used with caution in patients with renal impairment or failure, liver disease, cardiac disease, diabetes, and hypothyroidism. Because the drug can cause cholelithiasis, biliary obstruction, or cholecystitis, it should be used cautiously in patients with preexisting gallbladder disease. In addition, it is used with caution in elderly patients due to a significantly longer half-life and delayed clearance; dose adjustments are necessary for these patients.

Drug Interactions: Octreotide may decrease cyclosporine levels, and may alter the absorption of other drugs and nutrients because it slows intestinal motility. Concurrent administration of octreotide with oral antidiabetic agents or insulin can produce hypoglycemia. Additive bradycardia may occur when administered with cardiac agents such as beta-blockers and calcium channel blockers. Concurrent use of octreotide with antidiarrheals and opioids can lead to severe constipation, intestinal obstruction, or paralytic ileus. **Herbal/Food:** Octreotide decreases the absorption of dietary fat and vitamin B_{12}.

Pregnancy: Category B.

Treatment of Overdose: Overdose with octreotide has not been reported.

Nursing Responsibilities:

- Assess baseline height and weight and monitor regularly to determine drug effectiveness.
- Assess baseline and periodic electrocardiograms (ECG) because the drug may cause bradycardia and other dysrhythmias.
- Assess baseline and periodic vitamin B_{12} levels because the drug can reduce the absorption of this vitamin. Recommend supplementation as needed.
- Assess baseline and periodic hepatic and biliary function tests because this drug may cause or aggravate existing gallbladder disease.
- Administer octreotide by subcutaneous injection as the preferred route; the recommended sites are the abdomen, thigh, and buttock. Allow the solution to reach room temperature before administering.
- Monitor serum glucose levels frequently because this drug can cause hypoglycemia and may require adjustments in insulin dose.
- Monitor the patient's cardiac status, thyroid function, and electrolyte balance.

Patient and Family Education:

- Rotate injection sites, and use the preferred sites for injections: the abdomen, thigh, or buttock.
- Administer the drug between meals and at bedtime to minimize adverse GI effects.
- Reconstitute the drug gently, and avoid shaking the vial to prevent damaging the drug. Allow the solution to come to room temperature prior to injecting.
- Immediately report to the health care provider a yellowing of skin or whites of the eyes, sharp right upper abdomen pain, nausea, or vomiting, because these may indicate the development of liver or gallbladder disease.
- Report abdominal pain or changes in bowel habits, either diarrhea or constipation, that is severe or that lasts more than 2 days.
- Be aware that treatment is expensive, and therapy may be prolonged.

Drugs Similar to Octreotide (Sandostatin)

Drugs with similar actions to octreotide include bromocriptine, lanreotide, and pegvisomant.

Bromocriptine (Parlodel): Approved in 1978, bromocriptine is an oral drug that is classified as a dopamine agonist. Dopamine itself is not used for acromegaly due to an unacceptable incidence of adverse effects. Bromocriptine inhibits the secretion of growth hormone as well as prolactin from the pituitary. It is primarily indicated for Parkinson's disease (see Chapter 25) and infertility caused by prolactin excess, but it has been used in combination with octreotide in children with growth hormone excess. The most common dose-limiting adverse effects are psychological reactions including confusion, agitation, hallucinations, paranoid delusions, or nightmares. Other adverse effects include orthostatic hypotension, headache, nausea, vomiting, anorexia, or rash on the face and arms. It is a pregnancy category B drug. Bromocriptine interferes with lactation and should not be used during breast-feeding.

Lanreotide (Somatuline Depot): Approved in 2007, lanreotide is a somatostatin analog indicated for the treatment of patients with acromegaly who have not responded to radiation therapy or who are unable to undergo surgical treatment. The drug lowers levels of growth hormone thus improving symptoms related to acromegaly. Lanreotide is a depot formulation that requires dosing only once per month. It is available in prefilled syringes and is delivered by deep subcutaneous injection. Adverse effects associated with lanreotide include pain at the injection site, nausea and vomiting, diarrhea, gallstones, skin reactions such as itching, bradycardia, and changes in blood glucose levels (either hyper- or hypoglycemia). This drug is pregnancy category C.

Pegvisomant (Somavert): Approved in 1997, pegvisomant is a specific GH receptor antagonist, making it very effective for acromegaly. The drug is structurally very similar to GH, although when it binds to GH receptors, it causes no cellular response. The multiple polyethylene glycol (PEG) molecules attached to the drug prolong its half-life and allow for once-daily dosing. It is administered subcutaneously once daily and is supplied as a powder for reconstitution. Adverse effects include nausea, vomiting, elevated liver enzymes, angina, chest pain and myocardial infarction (MI), HTN, flulike syndrome, and injection site pain. Patients with diabetes should be monitored regularly to avoid hypoglycemia. Therapy for this drug is very expensive, and is continued indefinitely. It is a pregnancy category B drug.

Pharmacotherapy of Antidiuretic Hormone Disorders

66.5 Pharmacotherapy is used to treat deficient or excess secretion of antidiuretic hormone.

It is essential that the concentration of fluids in the body be maintained within narrow limits. Loss of large amounts of water leads to dehydration, a serious condition that can lead to shock and death. Too much body fluid leads to congestion, edema, and water intoxication. **Antidiuretic hormone (ADH)** is one of the most important means the body uses to maintain fluid homeostasis. For a complete discussion of fluid balance and the drugs used as fluid replacement agents, see Chapter 42.

The hypothalamus senses fluid balance by recognizing the osmolarity of the blood. Osmolarity is the number of dissolved particles, or solutes, in a fluid. As water is lost, the osmolality, or concentration of the blood, increases and the hypothalamus directs the posterior pituitary gland to release ADH. This hormone acts on the renal tubules to enhance water reabsorption.

NURSING PROCESS APPLICATION

Patients Receiving Growth Hormone Therapy

Assessment

Prior to administration:

- Obtain a complete health history including allergies, drug history, and possible drug interactions.
- Perform a physical assessment including vital signs. Assess height using a calibrated stadiometer (instrument for measuring height), body weight, and bone age determinations.
- Assess laboratory values as indicated to determine hepatic, renal, and thyroid function.
- Determine serum insulin-like growth factor (IGF-1) and GF binding protein (IGFBP-3).
- Assess for contraindicating factors: GH is contraindicated after epiphyseal closure, in children with Prader-Willi syndrome who are severely obese or have respiratory impairment or sleep apnea, and in patients with intracranial tumor; use cautiously in patients with diabetes mellitus or hypothyroidism.

Potential Nursing Diagnoses

- *Delayed Growth and Development,* related to deficiency of growth hormone
- *Situational Low Self-Esteem,* related to disturbed body image due to decreased height for age

Planning: Patient Goals and Expected Outcomes

The patient will:

- Demonstrate an increase in linear growth.
- Maintain normal metabolic function with adverse effects.
- Verbalize positive self-concept when interacting with others.

Implementation

Interventions and (Rationales)	Patient and Family Education
• Reconstitute drug according to manufacturer's directions; swirl vial to mix, do not shake; discard cloudy solutions or those containing particulate matter. (Proper reconstitution is necessary to have appropriate mixture for injection.)	Instruct the patient: • Not to shake medication vials vigorously. • Not to use cloudy solutions or those with particulate matter.
Follow proper administration techniques: • Inject subcutaneously, using preferred sites: the abdomen and thigh. (The correct injection technique is necessary for proper absorption.) • Administer injections each evening. (This mimics the body's natural release of the hormone.) • Rotate injection sites and record the site used on the medication administration record. (This practice reduces the incidence of local adverse effects.)	Instruct the patient: • On the importance of using sterile technique when administering injections. • On the proper injection procedure. • To report excessive inflammation, pain, or redness at the injection site.

• Obtain measurements of height and weight throughout therapy. (This will help evaluate the progress of therapy.)
  • Plot on growth charts; evaluate for increase in amount and rate of growth; determine goal height.
  • Obtain regular measurements of bone age. (Treatment must be discontinued when the epiphyseal plates closes, as no further effects would occur.)
	Instruct the patient:
	• That treatment is usually discontinued when the epiphyseal plates close.
	• To record the child's height and weight at regular intervals.

• Evaluate the adequacy of nutritional intake. (As growth increases, nutritional needs, especially for protein, increase.)	• Instruct the patient or caregiver on the importance of following a high-protein, nutritionally sound diet.
• Ensure regular testing for serum protein, glucose, and thyroid hormones. Follow patients with diabetes mellitus closely to optimize glycemic control. (HGH therapy can cause hyperglycemia; hypothyroidism can interfere with optimal therapy results.)	Instruct the patient to: • Keep all scheduled laboratory appointments. • Regularly monitor blood glucose levels, if diabetic.
• Monitor for the presence of myalgia, altered gait, or for complaints of pain in the knee or hip. (Avascular necrosis has been known to occur and must be treated as a medical emergency.)	• Inform the patient of adverse effects of the drug, and which to report to the health care provider.

Evaluation of Outcome Criteria

Evaluate the effectiveness of drug therapy by confirming that patient goals and expected outcomes have been met (see "Planning").

TABLE 66.4 Drugs Interacting with Antidiuretic Hormone (ADH)

Drugs Stimulating ADH Secretion	Drugs Inhibiting ADH Secretion
acetaminophen	alcohol
anesthetics	beta-adrenergic agonists
barbiturates	chlorpromazine
carbamazepine	demeclocycline
chlorpropamide	heparin
corticosteroids	lithium
diuretics	norepinephrine
tricyclic antidepressants	opioids
	phenytoin

The increased amount of water in the body reduces serum osmolality to normal levels and ADH secretion stops. Other factors stimulating release of ADH include hypotension, decreased fluid volume, dehydration, pain, nausea, and vomiting. Factors inhibiting ADH release include decreased serum osmolality and increased fluid volume. Many drugs also affect ADH release, as shown in Table 66.4. ADH is also called vasopressin because it has the ability to cause vasoconstriction at high doses.

CONNECTION *Checkpoint* 66.2

In addition to ADH, the renin-angiotensin-aldosterone system (RAAS) is essential for maintaining fluid balance. From what you learned in Chapter 42, how does the RAAS affect sodium and water balance? See Answer to Connection Checkpoint 66.2 in Appendix A.

A deficiency in ADH results in **diabetes insipidus,** a condition characterized by the production of large volumes of very dilute urine, usually accompanied by increased thirst. Diabetes insipidus may be either nephrogenic or neurogenic. Nephrogenic diabetes insipidus is caused by the inability of the kidneys to respond to ADH. Drugs such as lithium (Eskalith), or electrolyte disturbances can cause nephrogenic diabetes insipidus. Because nephrogenic diabetes insipidus results from an inability to respond to ADH, replacement therapy is not effective.

Neurogenic or central diabetes insipidus results from a lack of adequate production or secretion of ADH by the posterior pituitary or the hypothalamus. The etiology of neurogenic diabetes insipidus can be genetic, or acquired following head injury, surgery, tumors, infections, or vascular lesions of the region. Pharmacologic preparations of ADH can be used for replacement therapy for neurogenic diabetes insipidus. The drug of choice for treating chronic neurogenic diabetes insipidus is desmopressin acetate (DDAVP). An oral hypoglycemic agent, chlorpropamide can be used to stimulate ADH release in partial neurogenic diabetes insipidus. Paradoxically, both forms of diabetes insipidus respond in part to thiazide diuretics such as hydrochlorothiazide.

The primary symptoms of diabetes insipidus are polyuria and polydipsia (excessive thirst). Extremely large volumes of fluid (up to 30 L/day) may be ingested and the urine will be very dilute. The intense thirst and frequent urination usually keeps patients awake during the night. Failure to ensure adequate fluid intake will result in hypovolemia and dehydration due to the large renal water loss.

Pharm*FACT*

Diabetes insipidus is uncommon, with a prevalence of 1 case per 25,000 people. The most common form is that which follows trauma or surgery to the pituitary and hypothalamus. *Source:* Cooperman, 2008.

Excess secretion of ADH is the cause of the **syndrome of inappropriate antidiuretic hormone (SIADH),** a condition characterized by marked fluid retention, elevated urine osmolality, low serum osmolality, and sodium loss in the urine. SIADH may occur as a transient or chronic condition. The resulting hyponatremia and water retention cause muscle cramps, weakness, headache, apprehension, nausea, vomiting, and lethargy, progressing to stupor and coma. Treatment involves fluid restriction and diuretics such as mannitol or furosemide (Lasix) to remove excess fluid. Conivaptan (Viprostol) is a vasopressin receptor antagonist that is administered by intravenous (IV) infusion to promote renal water excretion and increase serum sodium levels in patients with SIADH. The antibiotic demeclocycline (Declomycin) is a tetracycline used off-label to treat SIADH due to its ability to cause diuresis through the inhibition of ADH-induced water reabsorption in the tubules and collecting ducts of the kidneys. In severe cases, IV infusion of a hypertonic sodium chloride solution may be necessary to raise serum osmolality. See Chapter 35 for a discussion of diuretic therapy, and Chapter 42 for a discussion of fluid replacement agents.

PROTOTYPE DRUG Desmopressin (DDAVP, Stimate) (Antidiuretic hormone)

Classification: Therapeutic: Antidiuretic hormone replacement
Pharmacologic: Pituitary hormone

Therapeutic Effects and Uses: Approved in 1978, desmopressin is a synthetic analog of human ADH that has a longer duration of action than the natural hormone. It controls the acute symptoms of polyuria and polydipsia in patients with neurogenic diabetes insipidus, but not nephrogenic diabetes insipidus. For DI, the oral (PO) route is preferred, although intranasal, IV, and subcutaneous forms are available.

Desmopressin has vasoconstrictor activity that causes contraction of smooth muscle in the vascular system, uterus, and GI tract. It produces less vasoconstrictive effects than natural vasopressin. Desmopressin also produces an increase in plasma factor VIII and von Willebrand's factor, and is thus indicated for the management of bleeding in patients with hemophilia A and von Willebrand's disease (type I). The use of desmopressin in treating coagulation disorders is presented in Section 40.13. An off-label use for this drug is to control enuresis (bed-wetting) among children.

Mechanism of Action: Desmopressin increases the permeability of renal collecting tubules to water, thereby increasing the reabsorption of water. It produces vasoconstriction of blood vessels at higher doses. The vasoconstriction produced is greatest in portal vessels, and less in cerebral, coronary, pulmonary, and peripheral vessels. Desmopressin enhances GI motility and tone through contraction of smooth muscle in the GI tract.

Pharmacokinetics:

Route(s)	Intranasal, subcutaneous, IV, PO
Absorption	10–20% through nasal mucosa
Distribution	Small amount may cross blood–brain barrier; secreted in breast milk
Primary metabolism	Metabolized rapidly by the liver
Primary excretion	Renal
Onset of action	Intranasal: 10–30 minutes with a peak at 45 minutes PO: 1 h, with a peak at 4–7 h IV: 1 minute with a peak at 30 minutes
Duration of action	Oral, nasal: 8–20 h; IV: 3 h

Adverse Effects: Desmopressin can cause water intoxication. Early signs include drowsiness, headache, and listlessness, progressing to convulsions and coma. Other adverse effects include transient headache, nasal congestion, rhinitis, nausea, mild abdominal pain and cramping, facial flushing, HTN, pain, or swelling at the injection site. A rare adverse effect of desmopressin is a severe allergic reaction or anaphylaxis (IV administration). Tolerance develops to the effects of desmopressin when it is administered more frequently than every 48 hours, or by the IV route.

Contraindications/Precautions: Desmopressin is contraindicated in patients with nephrogenic diabetes insipidus. It is used with caution in patients with coronary artery disease, HTN, and in patients at risk for hyponatremia or thrombi. The drug is contraindicated in patients with moderate or severe renal impairment because the drug can worsen fluid retention and overload. Young children and the elderly should be treated with caution because these patients are more prone to water intoxication and hyponatremia.

Drug Interactions: Increased antidiuretic action can occur with carbamazepine, chlorpropamide, clofibrate, and nonsteroidal anti-inflammatory drugs (NSAIDs). Decreased antidiuretic action can occur with lithium, alcohol, heparin, and epinephrine. **Herbal/Food:** Unknown.

Pregnancy: Category B.

Treatment of Overdose: In case of overdose, or if water intoxication develops, symptomatic treatment with diuretics is recommended.

Nursing Responsibilities:

- Obtain baseline data including blood pressure, weight, and intake and output (I&O) pattern. Continue to monitor blood pressure and weight during the dose regulation period and whenever the drug is administered parenterally.
- Administer desmopressin by direct IV over 30 seconds for diabetes insipidus; administer by IV infusion over 15 to 30 minutes for hemophilia. Do not administer vasopressin tannate (in oil) by the IV route.
- Store parenteral and nasal solutions in the refrigerator; nasal spray may be stored at room temperature. Discard discolored solutions or those containing particulate matter.
- Monitor for early signs of water intoxication; advise patients to decrease fluid intake once treatment begins for diabetes insipidus.
- Monitor electrolytes, particularly sodium levels.
- Weigh the patient daily and assess for edema, auscultate for lung sounds, and monitor blood pressure and heart rate.
- Monitor the serum and urine osmolality; an increased urine osmolality and a decreased serum osmolality indicate treatment effectiveness.
- Assess nasal mucosa for irritation or ulceration during long-term therapy with the nasal spray formulations.

Patient and Family Education:

- Reduce water consumption as directed by the health care provider to prevent symptoms of water intoxication, such as drowsiness, lethargy, or confusion.
- Report nasal congestion or upper respiratory infection to the health care provider.
- Administer the nasal spray high up into the nasal cavity, and not down the throat.
- Maintain a diary of each night's sleep, and record incidents of bed-wetting.
- Do not shake the drug, and avoid temperature extremes to prevent drug breakdown.
- Immediately report rapid increases in weight, heart rate, blood pressure, and shortness of breath to the health care provider because these may indicate water retention.
- Do not take any other prescription or nonprescription drugs, dietary supplements, or herbal products without approval of the health care provider.

Drugs Similar to Desmopressin (DDAVP, Stimate) (Antidiuretic Hormone)

The only drug that is similar to desmopressin is vasopressin.

Vasopressin: A synthetic analog of antidiuretic hormone, vasopressin is given IM or subcutaneously for central or neurogenic diabetes insipidus. Approved in 1941, it has a shorter duration of action than desmopressin and a more pronounced vasoconstrictor action, which can result in serious adverse effects.

NURSING PROCESS APPLICATION

Patients Receiving Antidiuretic Hormone Therapy

Assessment	Potential Nursing Diagnoses
Prior to administration: • Obtain baseline assessments of fluid status: I&O, weight, lung sounds, peripheral edema, thirst, heart rate, and blood pressure. • Obtain baseline measures of serum and urine osmolality or urine specific gravity. • For treatment of enuresis, obtain baseline information on the frequency of bed-wetting episodes, and the amount of sleep obtained each night.	• *Deficient Fluid Volume,* related to water loss and hormonal imbalance • *Excess Fluid Volume,* related to adverse effects of drug therapy • *Impaired Urinary Elimination,* related to enuresis

Planning: Patient Goals and Expected Outcomes

The patient will:

- For treatment of enuresis, have an absence of night-time bed-wetting episodes, and adequate amount of sleep nightly.
- For the treatment of fluid volume deficit, the deficit will be resolved, as evidenced by a decrease in the amount of urine produced to normal levels, serum and urine osmolality in normal ranges, absence of dehydration and excess water retention, and absence of electrolyte imbalances.

Implementation

Interventions and (Rationales)	Patient and Family Education
• Store parenteral and nasal solutions in the refrigerator. Discard solutions that are discolored or contain particulate matter. (Proper storage and handling will maintain the stability of the solution.)	Instruct the patient to: • Not agitate drug. • Avoid temperature extremes to prevent drug breakdown.
• Monitor I&O, daily weight, heart rate, blood pressure, and edema and lung sounds for retained fluids. (Fluid retention can lead to water intoxication and exacerbate cardiac symptoms.)	• Instruct the patient to report sudden increases in weight, edema, heart rate, or blood pressure.
• Monitor for early signs of water intoxication such as drowsiness, listlessness, or headache. (Water intoxication is a severe adverse effect that can usually be prevented through patient teaching.)	Instruct the patient to: • Decrease or limit the amount of fluid intake to prevent water intoxication. • Watch for the early signs of water intoxication. • Immediately report signs to the health care provider.
• Monitor urine specific gravity daily. (A simple method for evaluating the effectiveness of diabetes insipidus treatment is to obtain regular measures of urine specific gravity.)	Instruct the patient: • Regarding symptoms of sodium imbalance. • How to obtain a urine specific gravity measurement. • To keep a log of the urine specific gravity measurements. • When to notify the health care provider regarding measurement.
• For long-term therapy, evaluate nasal mucosa for irritation or ulceration. (Nasal symptoms are a common adverse effect of therapy; nasal symptoms can alter the absorption of the drug and its effectiveness.)	• Instruct the patient to report nasal congestion or upper respiratory infection.
• For patients treated with vasopressin, monitor for excessive vasoconstriction, ischemia, angina, or other signs of tissue anoxia. (The use of vasopressin can precipitate anginal episodes and MI.)	• Instruct the patient to report sudden increases in weight, edema, heart rate, or blood pressure, and any incidents of anginal pain.
• Encourage the patient to take desmopressin as directed. (Using the device as directed will deliver a consistent amount of drug per pump.)	Instruct the patient to: • Administer nasal spray at bedtime for treating enuresis. • Wear a medical alert bracelet specifying therapy. • Correctly administer nasal spray into nasal cavity and not down the throat.

Evaluation of Outcome Criteria

Evaluate the effectiveness of drug therapy by confirming that patient goals and expected outcomes have been met (see "Planning").

Because vasopressin is a potent vasoconstrictor, it is given IV as an alternative to epinephrine for many off-label indications. These include bleeding from esophageal varices or the upper GI tract, cardiac arrest, and the treatment of severe hypotension or shock. Vasopressin may precipitate MI or angina. It may cause water intoxication. When used for its vasopressor effects, possible adverse effects include tissue necrosis and gangrene. Vasopressin is a pregnancy category C drug.

CONNECTION *Checkpoint* 66.3

Desmopressin is used to treat von Willebrand's disease (vWD), the most common inherited coagulation disorder. From what you learned in Chapter 40, what is the function of von Willebrand's factor? See Answer to Connection Checkpoint 66.3 in Appendix A.

UNDERSTANDING THE CHAPTER

Key Concepts Summary

66.1 The hypothalamus controls many diverse body processes and secretes hormones that influence pituitary function.

66.2 The pituitary gland secretes hormones that control many diverse body functions.

66.3 Growth hormone deficiency in adults and children can be treated by administering recombinant growth hormone.

66.4 Overproduction of growth hormone in adults can be treated by administering growth hormone antagonists.

66.5 Pharmacotherapy is used to treat deficient or excess secretion of antidiuretic hormone.

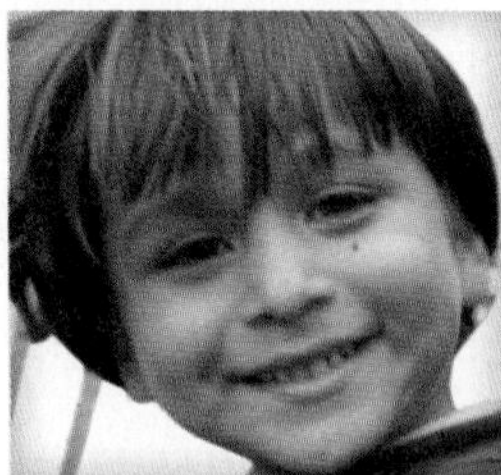

Making the PATIENT Connection

Remember the patient "Thomas" at the beginning of the chapter? Now read the remainder of the case study. Based on the information presented in this chapter, answer the critical thinking questions that follow.

Thomas, an 8-year-old boy, was referred to the pediatric endocrinology clinic with the chief complaint of short stature. He had been healthy and developmentally normal until 3 years ago. Since that time, his growth has been extremely slow and almost imperceptible. On his initial exam, Thomas's weight and height were 17 kg (37.4 lb) and 108 cm (42.5 in.), respectively. His height standard deviation score was -4.0 with a body mass index of 14.6. The remainder of his physical examination was normal.

When the pediatrician reviewed the results of hormonal assay tests with Thomas's parents, everyone was relieved to find out that, although there is a problem, it is not due to a tumor or other life-threatening disorder. Thomas has a congenital deficiency in growth hormone, and the pediatrician begins to discuss replacement therapy with the parents. As the nurse involved in the case, address each of the following questions.

Critical Thinking Questions

1. What teaching will you need to provide to Thomas's parents regarding drug therapy for his disorder?
2. Thomas's father states, "I hope my health insurance will cover this medication." What would you say to this comment?
3. The parents ask about the adverse effects that might occur with this therapy. How would you respond?

Case Study

An 8-year-old boy and his parents visit a pediatrician's office, where you are a nurse. The parents are concerned with the boy's continuing problem with enuresis, or night-time bed-wetting. Increasingly, they see this problem as adversely affecting the boy's self-image, self-esteem, and psychosocial well-being. He is reluctant to take part in sleepovers at friends' houses, or to attend camping trips with his scouting troop.

1. What type of pharmacotherapy do you anticipate for this boy?
2. What information will the boy and parents need as part of patient drug teaching?

NCLEX-RN® Review

1 A teaching plan for a parent whose child is receiving growth hormone would include:

1. Importance of adhering to therapy to prevent mental retardation.
2. The medication cannot be given orally; it can be given only parenterally.
3. If growth hormone is begun in adolescence, it can add up to 6 inches in height.
4. Growth hormone therapy will require frequent blood work.

2 Which of the following findings would the nurse not consider to be effects of growth hormone?

1. Increase in the length and width of long bones
2. Organ, muscle, and connective tissue growth
3. Increased synthesis of proteins
4. Lowering of serum glucose levels

3 The client with neurogenic diabetes insipidus is being started on a nasal spray of desmopressin (DDAVP). Which of the following should the nurse include in the teaching plan?

1. Store the solution in the refrigerator.
2. Use twice the prescribed dose if you have nasal congestion.
3. Obtain weight each morning.
4. If nasal burning occurs, you may use the medicine orally.

4 During the first postoperative day following a craniotomy, a client is noted to have produced 2,400 mL of urine with a specific gravity of 1.001. The nurse suspects that the client has developed:

1. Syndrome of inappropriate antidiuretic hormone.
2. Diabetes insipidus.
3. Excessive urination from fluids given during surgery.
4. Adverse effects of opioids used for pain management.

5 When implementing desmopressin therapy for a client with diabetes insipidus, it is important for the nurse to: (Select all that apply.)

1. Encourage fluids to replace water loss.
2. Restrict fluids to decrease the risk for water intoxication.
3. Monitor serum electrolytes, particularly sodium.
4. Check for hypotension.
5. Suggest increasing the intake of sodium-based foods.

6 Which of the following assessment findings would indicate therapeutic goals have been achieved for a client with diabetes insipidus being treated with vasopressin?

1. Decreasing signs of dehydration
2. Increasing pulse and urine output
3. Decreasing urine specific gravity
4. Decreasing hyperglycemia

See Answers to Critical Thinking Questions, Case Study, and NCLEX-RN® Review in Appendix A.

References

Cooperman, M. (2008). *Diabetes insipidus.* eMedicine. Retrieved August 24, 2008, from http://www.emedicine.com/med/topic543.htm

Corbett, J. V. (2008). *Laboratory tests and diagnostic procedures with nursing diagnoses* (7th ed.). Upper Saddle River, NJ: Prentice-Hall.

Dahlgren, J., & Wikland, K. A. (2005). Final height in short children born small for gestational age treated with growth hormone. *Pediatric Research, 57*(2), 216–222.

Eledrisi, H. S. (2008). *Growth hormone deficiency.* eMedicine. Retrieved August 24, 2008, from http://www.emedicine.com/med/topic930.htm

LeMone, P., & Burke, K. (2008). *Medical-surgical nursing: Critical thinking in client care* (4th ed.). Upper Saddle River NJ: Prentice-Hall.

Liu, H., Bravata, D., Ingram, O., Nayak, S., Roberts, B., Garber, A., et al. (2007). Systematic review: The safety and efficacy of growth hormone in the healthy elderly. *Annals of Internal Medicine, 146*(2), 104–124.

McCance, K. L., & Huether, S. E. (2006). *Pathophysiology: The biologic basis for disease in adults and children* (5th ed.). St. Louis: Mosby.

Nash, K. (2007). HGH: The debate continues. *Dermatology Times, 28*(3), 28–40.

Parkinson, A. B., & Evans, N. A. (2006). Anabolic androgenic steroids: A survey of 500 users. *Medicine & Science in Sports & Exercise, 38(4)*, 644–651.

Porth, C. M. (2005). *Pathophysiology: Concepts of altered health states* (7th ed.). Philadelphia: Lippincott Williams & Wilkins.

Przkora, R., Herndon, D. N., Suman, O. E., Jeschke, M. G., Meyer, W. J., Chinkes, D. L., et al. (2006). Beneficial effects of extended growth hormone treatment after hospital discharge in pediatric burn patients. *Annals of Surgery, 243*(6), 796–803.

Saugy, M., Robinson, N., Saudan, C., Baume, N., Avois, L., & Mangin, P. (2006). Human growth hormone doping in sport. *British Journal of Sports Medicine, 40(Supplement 1)*, i35–i39.

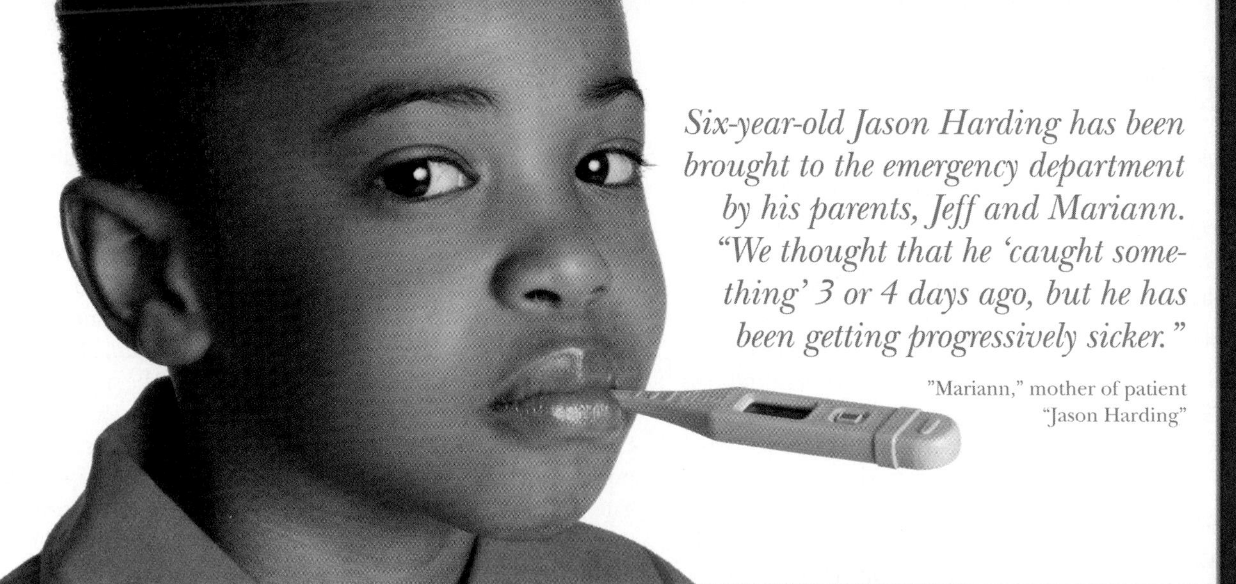

Six-year-old Jason Harding has been brought to the emergency department by his parents, Jeff and Mariann. "We thought that he 'caught something' 3 or 4 days ago, but he has been getting progressively sicker."

"Mariann," mother of patient
"Jason Harding"

CHAPTER 67

Pharmacotherapy of Diabetes Mellitus

Chapter Outline

Physiology of Serum Glucose Control
Pathophysiology of Diabetes Mellitus: Types of Diabetes
Symptoms and Diagnosis of Diabetes
Complications of Diabetes Mellitus
PROTOTYPE **Glucagon (GlucaGen)** *p. 1124*
Drug Therapy for Diabetes: Insulin
PROTOTYPE **Human Regular Insulin (Humulin R, Novolin R)** *p. 1128*
Drug Therapy for Diabetes: Oral Antidiabetic Drugs
Sulfonylureas
PROTOTYPE **Glyburide (DiaBeta, Glynase, Micronase)** *p. 1134*
Biguanides
PROTOTYPE **Metformin (Glucophage, Glucophage XR, Glumetza)** *p. 1135*
Meglitinides
PROTOTYPE **Repaglinide (Prandin)** *p. 1136*
Thiazolidinediones
PROTOTYPE **Rosiglitazone (Avandia)** *p. 1137*
Alpha-Glucosidase Inhibitors
PROTOTYPE **Acarbose (Precose)** *p. 1138*
Oral Combination Products
Drug Therapy for Diabetes: Incretin Therapies
PROTOTYPE **Sitagliptin (Januvia)** *p. 1141*

Learning Outcomes

After reading this chapter, the student should be able to:

1. Explain how blood glucose levels are maintained within narrow limits by insulin and glucagon.
2. Compare and contrast the etiology and pathogenesis of type 1, type 2, and gestational diabetes.
3. Identify the signs and symptoms of diabetes.
4. Describe the acute complications of diabetes.
5. Describe the chronic complications of diabetes.
6. Compare and contrast the pharmacotherapy of the different types of diabetes.
7. For each type of insulin, identify the onset of action, peak action and duration of action, administration routes, when it is given related to meals, compatibility with other insulins, and adverse effects.
8. For each of the classes shown in the Chapter Outline, identify the prototype and representative drugs and explain the mechanism(s) of drug action, primary indications, contraindications, significant drug interactions, pregnancy category, and important adverse effects.
9. Use the Nursing Process to care for patients who are receiving drug therapy for diabetes.

Key Terms

diabetic ketoacidosis (DKA), *1124*
fasting plasma glucose (FPG) test, *1122*
gestational diabetes, *1121*
gluconeogenesis, *1120*
glycogenolysis, *1120*
hemoglobin A1C, *1123*
hyperosmolar hyperglycemic state (HHS), *1124*
incretin enhancer, *1141*
incretin mimetic, *1141*
insulin, *1120*
insulin resistance, *1121*
metabolic syndrome, *1123*
oral glucose tolerance test (OGTT), *1122*
polydipsia, *1122*
polyphagia, *1122*
polyuria, *1122*
prediabetes, *1123*
type 1 diabetes, *1121*
type 2 diabetes, *1121*

It is estimated that nearly 21 million people in the United States have diabetes mellitus, with over 6 million of those being undiagnosed. Diabetes is one of the leading causes of death in the United States. Mortality has been rising in recent years, causing some public health officials to refer to it as an epidemic. Diabetes can lead to serious acute and chronic complications, including heart disease, cerebrovascular accident (CVA), blindness, kidney failure, and amputations. Because nurses frequently care for patients with diabetes, it is imperative that they thoroughly understand the disorder, its treatment, and possible complications. There is an unrelated disorder, diabetes insipidus, which results from a deficiency of antidiuretic hormone (see Chapter 66). When the term *diabetes* is used in this chapter, it is referring to diabetes mellitus.

Physiology of Serum Glucose Control

67.1 Serum glucose is maintained within a narrow range by the hormones insulin and glucagon.

Because diabetes is a disorder of carbohydrate metabolism, it is essential to understand the way the body obtains, metabolizes, and stores glucose. Of all the different molecules available, the body prefers to use glucose as its primary energy source. The brain relies almost exclusively on glucose for its energy needs because it is unable to synthesize glucose and it will exhaust its supply after just a few minutes of activity. Most other tissues can use fatty acids and proteins for energy production, if necessary, but they too prefer to use glucose. The primary role of the liver and pancreas is to regulate the body's fuel supply.

The normal range for serum glucose is considered to be 60 to 100 mg/dL. However, the level is usually tightly regulated by the body to remain between 80 to 90 mg/dL. Although many factors contribute to maintaining a stable serum glucose level, two pancreatic hormones play major roles: **insulin,** which acts to decrease blood glucose levels, and glucagon, which acts to increase blood glucose levels.

Following a meal, glucose is rapidly absorbed from the gastrointestinal (GI) tract and serum levels rise. Some of the glucose is taken up by cells and used for immediate energy needs, but about two thirds is stored in liver and muscle cells as glycogen, the storage form of glucose. When glucose levels fall between meals, glycogen is broken down in a process called **glycogenolysis,** and glucose is released into the bloodstream. Maintaining a stable serum glucose level is simply a matter of storing glucose during times of excess, and returning it to the bloodstream in times of deficiency. The importance of maintaining this delicate balance, however, cannot be overstated. Too much glucose or too little glucose can have lethal consequences.

Following a meal, the pancreas recognizes the rising serum glucose levels and releases insulin. Without insulin, glucose is not able to enter cells of the body. The cells may be surrounded by high amounts of glucose but they are unable to use it until insulin arrives. It may be helpful to visualize insulin as a transporter or "gatekeeper." When present, insulin swings open the gate, transporting glucose inside cells: If there is no insulin, there is no entry. The physiological actions of insulin are summarized as follows:

- Promotes the entry of glucose into cells
- Provides for the storage of glucose, as glycogen
- Inhibits the breakdown of fat and glycogen
- Increases protein synthesis and inhibits **gluconeogenesis,** which is the production of "new" glucose from noncarbohydrate molecules

Insulin is produced in beta cells of the pancreas known as islets of Langerhans, whereas alpha cells in the pancreas secrete glucagon. Glucagon maintains stable blood glucose levels between meals and during periods of fasting and has actions that are opposite to those of insulin. It removes glucose from its storage in the liver and sends it to the blood (glycogenolysis), raising serum glucose within minutes.

The level of glucose in the blood regulates the release of both insulin and glucagon. A hypoglycemic state (low serum glucose) stimulates the release of glucagon and inhibits the release of insulin, whereas a hyperglycemic state (high serum glucose) has the opposite effects and stimulates the release of insulin, and inhibits the release of glucagon. The physiological dynamics of insulin and glucagon release are shown in Figure 67.1.

Additional factors that decrease blood glucose levels are fasting, exercise, and alcohol. Factors that increase blood glucose levels include stress from infection, injury, or surgery, which triggers release of the epinephrine and norepinephrine; large meals or overconsumption of carbohydrates; growth hormone; and corticosteroids.

PharmFACT

The incidence of diabetes mellitus is as follows:

- **1 in every 400–600 children and adolescents has type 1 diabetes.**
- **9.6% of all people 20 years or older has diabetes.**
- **20.9% of all people 60 years or older has diabetes.**
- **The incidence rates for diabetes are higher among non-Hispanic African Americans, Hispanic/Latino Americans, Alaska Natives, Asian Americans, and Pacific Islanders. About 27% of all American Indians in the southern United States have diabetes.** *Source:* Centers for Disease Control and Prevention (CDC), 2005.

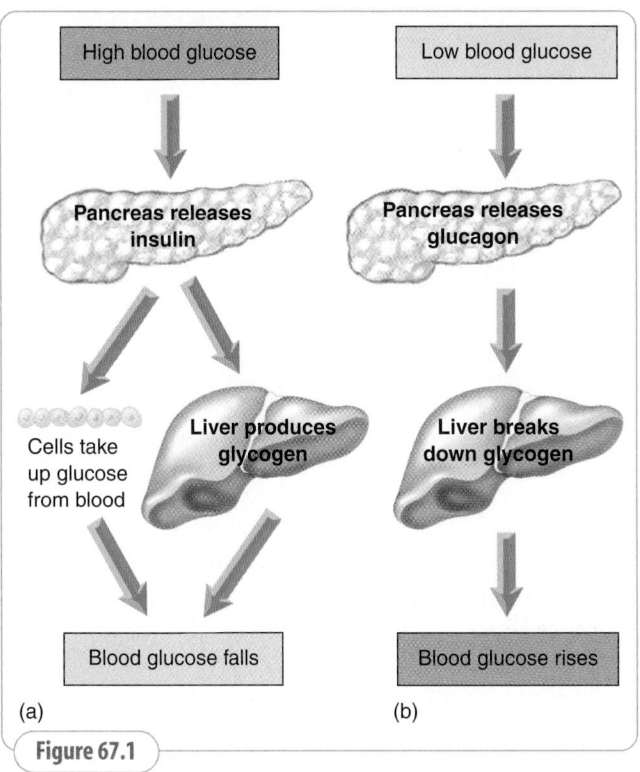

Figure 67.1

Insulin, glucagon, and blood glucose.

Pathophysiology of Diabetes Mellitus: Types of Diabetes

67.2 Type 1 diabetes is characterized by insufficient insulin synthesis by the pancreas, whereas type 2 diabetes is characterized by insulin resistance in the target cells.

The two primary forms of diabetes are called type 1 and type 2. There are significant differences between the two types in terms of pathophysiology and disease management. A third form of the disease occurs during pregnancy and is known as gestational diabetes.

Type 1 diabetes results from the destruction of pancreatic beta cells and their inability to secrete insulin. The destruction of beta cells is believed to result from a combination of autoimmune, genetic, and environmental factors. Type 1 is the less common form of diabetes, accounting for only 5% to 10% of all patients with the disorder. It is seen most frequently among children and young adults, but it may occur at any age.

Because of the lack of sufficient insulin in patients with type 1 diabetes, glucose cannot enter cells and fatty acids are used as a primary energy source. As the body turns to fatty acids for its fuel, acidic, metabolic by-products of lipid metabolism known as ketones will accumulate in the blood. This produces a dangerous and potentially life-threatening condition known as diabetic ketoacidosis (DKA), which is discussed in Section 67.5.

Patients with type 1 diabetes must receive insulin therapy to survive. In the past, type 1 was called juvenile or insulin-dependent diabetes. While these terms are still in use, they do not accurately reflect the nature of the disease.

Type 2 diabetes is the more common form of the disorder, representing 90% to 95% of people with diabetes. The primary physiological characteristic of type 2 diabetes is **insulin resistance,** which is when target cells become unresponsive to insulin due to a defect in insulin receptor function. Essentially, the pancreas is producing sufficient amounts of insulin but target cells do not recognize it.

As cells become more resistant to insulin, blood glucose levels rise and the pancreas responds by secreting even more insulin. Eventually, the hypersecretion of insulin leads to beta cell exhaustion, and ultimately to beta cell death. As type 2 diabetes progresses, it becomes a disorder characterized by insufficient insulin levels as well as insulin resistance. The activity of insulin receptors can be increased by exercise and lowering the level of circulating insulin. In fact, adhering to a healthy diet and regular exercise have been shown to reverse insulin resistance, and to delay or prevent the development of type 2 diabetes.

Eighty percent of persons with type 2 diabetes are overweight, and the degree of obesity directly affects the degree of insulin resistance. In particular, persons with upper body obesity (central obesity) are at increased risk for developing insulin resistance and type 2 diabetes. Although most patients with type 2 diabetes are older, this disease is increasingly being diagnosed in obese adolescents. Risk factors for type 2 diabetes are a family history of diabetes, obesity (body mass index above 27 kg/m^2), and race and ethnicity. African Americans, Native Americans, Hispanic Americans, Asian Americans, and Pacific Islanders are at increased risk for type 2 diabetes (CDC, 2005). Other risk factors are age older than 45 years, a history of elevated fasting serum glucose levels or impaired glucose tolerance, hypertension (HTN), low levels of high-density lipoproteins (HDL below 35 mg/dL), triglycerides above 250 mg/dL, and a history of gestational diabetes, delivery of a baby over 9 pounds, or both. Table 67.1 compares and contrasts type 1 and type 2 diabetes.

Most patients with type 2 diabetes do not require insulin administration, at least initially, but can be managed by oral antidiabetic agents. Type 2 diabetes was formerly called adult-onset diabetes and noninsulin-dependent diabetes but these are not accurate descriptions of the disorder because it occurs in children and may require insulin administration.

Gestational diabetes is a condition resulting from glucose intolerance with an onset, or first recognition, during pregnancy. This is a serious disorder that puts both the woman and fetus at risk for complications, and so requires careful management during pregnancy. In addition, women who develop gestational diabetes are at increased risk for developing diabetes 5 to 10 years after delivery. It occurs most frequently in women with a family history of diabetes, a history of stillbirth or spontaneous abortion, a previous large or heavy-for-date baby, women who are obese or of advanced maternal age, women who have had five or more pregnancies, or women who are members of a high-risk population (Hispanic, Native American, Asian, or African American). If careful nutritional management is unable to normalize serum glucose levels, insulin therapy is initiated. Traditionally, oral antidiabetic drugs have not been used for gestational diabetes due to concerns regarding potential teratogenicity; however, the results of research may change that practice in the future.

TABLE 67.1 Comparison of Type 1 and Type 2 Diabetes Mellitus

Diabetes Mellitus	Type 1	Type 2
Cause	Destruction of beta cells with lack of insulin	Insulin resistance; insulin deficiency may develop
Incidence	5–10%	90–95%
Age at Onset	Children, young adults, usually younger than 35 years	Usually older than 35 years
Symptom Onset	Rapid	Gradual
Body Weight	Usually weight loss	Usually overweight, obese
Symptoms	Polyuria, polydipsia, polyphagia, weight loss	Same (polyuria, polydipsia, polyphagia, weight loss), plus blurred vision, fatigue, recurrent infections
Ketosis	Often present with poor control	Infrequent
Treatment	Insulin replacement, diet, exercise, weight, lipid, and blood pressure control	Oral agents with or without insulin, diet, exercise, weight loss, lipid, and blood pressure control

Symptoms and Diagnosis of Diabetes

67.3 The classic signs and symptoms of diabetes include polyuria, polydipsia, and polyphagia.

The classic triad of signs and symptoms for either type of diabetes is known as the three "polys": **polyuria,** excessive urine production; **polydipsia,** excessive thirst; and **polyphagia,** excessive appetite.

Glucose is one of the body's most valuable molecules, and nondiabetic patients excrete very little. The body normally uses these molecules for energy or stores them for future use. As glucose levels rise in the blood in diabetic patients, however, the kidneys are unable to reabsorb the large amounts passing through the renal tubules, so glucose is eliminated in the urine (glucosuria). Glucose molecules create increased osmotic pressure in body fluids, pulling water along with it; thus, osmotic diuresis (polyuria) occurs. The glucose increases osmotic pressure in the bloodstream, pulling water out of tissue cells, and causing cellular dehydration. This triggers thirst, and increases fluid intake (polydipsia). The excess hunger (polyphagia) occurs primarily with type 1 diabetes, when nutrient stores become too depleted to meet the body's energy needs, and weight is lost. Other signs and symptoms include blurred vision, fatigue, paresthesias, and skin infections. Nocturia, secondary to the polyuria, may occur.

The two primary blood tests for diagnosing diabetes are the **fasting plasma glucose (FPG) test,** and the **oral glucose tolerance test (OGTT).** Testing usually begins with the FPG, obtained following a fast of at least 8 hours. If the FPG results are abnormal (higher than 100 mg/dL), an OGTT is obtained. A loading dose of 75 g glucose is ingested and the plasma glucose level is obtained 2 hours later. In addition, a random glucose level of greater than 200 mg/dL in the presence of symptoms is diagnostic of diabetes, although a FPG or OGTT is usually obtained for verification. Table 67.2 lists the diagnos-

CONNECTIONS

Evidence-Based Practice Oral Hypoglycemic Agents for Gestational Diabetes

Clinical Question

Can oral hypoglycemic agents be used safely and effectively in the treatment of gestational diabetes or in the lactating woman?

Evidence

Traditionally oral hypoglycemic agents have not been widely used during pregnancy for the treatment of gestational diabetes or in women who are lactating due to concerns over teratogenicity. A meta-analysis was done to investigate the effects of an oral hypoglycemic during pregnancy and lactation. The authors note that there is little or no transfer of glyburide or glipizide across the placenta, while metformin and rosiglitazone readily cross. They found that in gestational diabetes, glyburide was safe and effective, although 16% to 19% of women failed to achieve glycemic control. They found no developmental toxicity in infants when metformin was used throughout the pregnancy for women with polycystic ovary syndrome. Information is inadequate to evaluate the risk of glipizide or thiazolidinediones in pregnancy. Finally, they concluded that metformin, glyburide, and glipizide appear to be compatible with breast-feeding, and that neither glyburide nor metformin have been shown to cause developmental toxicity in humans. More trials are necessary to better define the risks and benefits of oral hypoglycemics during pregnancy and lactation.

Implication

These results indicate that treatment of women with type 2 diabetes during pregnancy or the lactation period may be changing in the future as more evidence is gained on the safety of the various drug classes in question (Feig, Briggs, & Koren, 2007).

Critical Thinking Question

How would you respond to the patient with gestational diabetes who asks why she cannot take a pill to control her glucose?

See Answers to Critical Thinking Questions in Appendix A.

TABLE 67.2 Plasma Glucose Levels

	Fasting Plasma Glucose (8-hour fast)	OGTT (2 hours after glucose load)
Diabetes	Equal to or more than 126 mg/dL	Equal to or more than 200 mg/dL
Prediabetes	100–125 mg/dL	140–199 mg/dL
Normal	Less than 100 mg/dL	Less than 140 mg/dL

Note: From *Research in Endocrinology: A Report from the Endocrine Society's 89th Annual Meeting,* by the American Diabetes Association, 2007a, Toronto, Ontario: Author.

tic levels of these tests, based on recommendations of the American Diabetes Association (ADA, 2007a).

Home monitoring of blood glucose is now commonplace, and enables the diabetic patient to maintain tighter control of glucose levels. "Finger-stick" testing involves placing a drop of capillary blood on a test strip, which is then read by a glucose meter. Fasting blood glucose levels, as well as preprandial and postprandial testing, may be employed. Another important laboratory test used in diabetic management is the glycosylated hemoglobin, also called the glycated hemoglobin, or the currently preferred term **hemoglobin A1C.** When glucose levels remain at normal levels, only 4% to 6% of the circulating hemoglobin will have glucose bound to it. Once glucose binds to hemoglobin, it remains bound for the life of the red blood cell (RBC), or roughly 120 days. As serum glucose increases, more glucose becomes bound to hemoglobin. Therefore, the hemoglobin A1C provides a measure of glucose control over the past 8 to 12 weeks. Health care providers recommend that persons with diabetes lower their A1C level to 7% or less. In general, every percentage point drop in A1C levels (e.g., from 8.5% to 7.5%) reduces the risk of vascular complications by 40% (CDC, 2005). Table 67.3 lists the relationship between glucose levels and A1C measures.

Most patients who develop type 2 diabetes go through a period of impaired glucose tolerance referred to as **prediabetes.** In prediabetes, serum glucose levels are elevated but are not high enough to be diagnosed as diabetes. This condition increases the risk for developing diabetes, heart disease, and CVA. Prediabetes may result from impaired fasting glucose, impaired glucose tolerance, or both. Progression from prediabetes to diabetes is not inevitable: Careful management of nutrition, regular exercise, and weight loss (if overweight) may prevent or delay progression to diabetes. Patients with prediabetes should be monitored on an annual basis for the potential development of diabetes and to evaluate the degree of success in managing comorbid conditions such as HTN, hyperlipidemia, and obesity.

TABLE 67.3 Relationship Between Plasma Glucose and Hemoglobin A1C

Mean Plasma Glucose (mg/dL)	Hemoglobin A1C (%)
345	12
310	11
275	10
240	9
205	8
170	7
135	6

CONNECTIONS

Treating the Diverse Patient

Complications of Diabetes in Diverse Populations

The consequences of diabetes can vary by ethnicity. For example, Mexican Americans are almost twice as likely, and non-Hispanic African Americans almost 50% as likely, to develop diabetic retinopathy as non-Hispanic Caucasians. Mexican Americans are 4.5 to 6.6 times more likely, and American Indians are 6 times more likely to suffer from kidney disease than non-Hispanic whites. Mexican Americans, non-Hispanic African Americans, and American Indians are at greater risk for nontraumatic lower limb amputations than are others with diabetes (ADA, n.d.).

A group of abnormalities that tend to occur together has been called insulin resistance syndrome, syndrome X, or the preferred name: **metabolic syndrome.** This syndrome places the patient at increased risk for developing diabetes and vascular complications such as cardiovascular disease, peripheral vascular disease, and CVA. Again, weight loss, exercise, and nutritional management enable people with this syndrome to delay or prevent the progression to type 2 diabetes. The metabolic syndrome is diagnosed by the presence of three or more of the following:

- Central obesity, with waste circumference more than 35 in. for women or more than 40 in. for men
- Serum triglycerides equal to or greater than 150 mg/dL
- High-density lipoprotein (HDL) cholesterol less than 50 mg/dL in women or less than 40 mg/dL in men
- Blood pressure more than 130/85 mm Hg
- Fasting plasma glucose more than 100 mg/dL (Porth, 2005)

Complications of Diabetes Mellitus

67.4 Acute complications of diabetes include hypoglycemia, diabetic ketoacidosis, and hyperosmolar hyperglycemic state.

Uncontrolled diabetes has characteristic complications that occur in most patients. The acute complications of diabetes occur suddenly and require immediate interventions. The diagnosis of diabetes is often made for the first time when a person presents with one of these acute conditions. Hypoglycemia, DKA, and hyperosmolar hyperglycemic state (HHS) are the three primary acute complications. The chronic complications are discussed in Section 67.5.

Hypoglycemia, or abnormally low serum glucose, occurs most often in patients improperly treated with insulin and may occur during therapy with some oral antidiabetic agents. The manifestations of hypoglycemia result from changes in mental status, and by the activation of the sympathetic nervous system. Because the brain relies on a continuous supply of glucose, falling glucose levels may lead to headache, difficulty concentrating, confusion, and behavioral changes, progressing to seizures and coma. The sympathetic nervous system activation results from the body's attempt to increase serum glucose by the release of catecholamines (epinephrine and norepinephrine). These catecholamines cause symptoms that include tachycardia, anxiety, sweating, and the constriction of surface vessels, leading to cool, clammy skin. Acute hypoglycemia is considered a medical emergency, and if prolonged or severe, can lead to brain damage or death.

The symptoms of hypoglycemia may have a very rapid onset. Patients who have had diabetes for an extended time may develop hypoglycemic unawareness, which is the inability to recognize symptoms. Some drugs, such as beta-adrenergic blockers, interfere with the sympathetic symptoms of hypoglycemia, making it more difficult for the patient to recognize the condition and for the body to correct the low glucose levels.

Factors that cause hypoglycemia in diabetic patients include errors in insulin dosage, failure to eat at regular intervals, increased exercise, medication adjustments, or changes in the insulin injection site. Alcohol consumption can lead to hypoglycemia by decreasing gluconeogenesis. The treatment for hypoglycemia is always glucose, given in a concentrated source of 15 to 20 g. This can be repeated as necessary, while taking care not to overtreat the patient and cause hyperglycemia. If the person is unconscious, or unable to swallow safely, a small amount of glucose gel or spray can be administered to the buccal mucosa. Intravenous (IV) glucose is immediately effective in treating hypoglycemia. An alternative therapy is glucagon (see prototype feature later in this section).

Diabetic ketoacidosis (DKA) is an acute condition that occurs primarily in patients with type 1 diabetes. The three major disturbances that occur with DKA are hyperglycemia, metabolic acidosis, and osmotic diuresis. DKA typically develops over several days with symptoms such as polyuria, polydipsia, nausea, vomiting, and severe fatigue, progressing to stupor and eventual coma. The patient may complain of abdominal pain or tenderness, and the breath has a typical fruity smell as the lungs attempt to remove volatile ketoacids. As the acidosis worsens, Kussmaul's respirations may develop, with an increased rate and depth of respirations. Tachycardia and hypotension occur in response to dehydration and fluid depletion.

DKA may be the first presenting symptoms of a person previously undiagnosed with diabetes. The treatment of DKA involves fluid replacement to improve circulating volume and tissue perfusion, normalization of blood glucose levels, correction of electrolyte imbalances and acidosis, and treatment of the underlying cause if needed. Insulin therapy is begun, usually with an IV loading dose, followed by a continuous low dose infusion. Blood glucose levels are lowered gradually because too rapid a drop can cause a fluid shift back into the cells that can lead to cerebral edema. Although DKA is a very serious disorder, the mortality rate for this complication has been reduced to less than 5% with proper treatment (Porth, 2005).

CONNECTION *Checkpoint* 67.1

From what you learned in Chapter 42, what is the clinical definition of acidosis? What is the drug of choice for reversing metabolic acidosis? See Answer to Connection Checkpoint 67.1 in Appendix A.

Hyperosmolar hyperglycemic state (HHS) is another very serious acute complication of diabetes, with a mortality rate of 20% to 40%. HHS is generally seen in persons with type 2 diabetes, and is characterized by extreme hyperglycemia (above 600 mg/dL), hyperosmolarity (above 310 mOsm/L) with dehydration, the absence of ketoacidosis, and central nervous system (CNS) dysfunction. The typical patient is elderly, obese, and has comorbid medical problems, such as heart failure or renal impairment. The elevated serum glucose levels and increased osmolarity produce an osmotic diuresis with marked dehydration, confusion, and lethargy. Other possible neurologic symptoms are seizures, hemiparesis, abnormal reflexes, aphasia, and visual disturbances. Symptoms can progress to stupor and coma. Hemoconcentration increases the risk for clot formation, emboli, and infarction of major organs. Tachycardia and hypotension result from fluid depletion and poor tissue perfusion. Acidosis may develop, but it is caused by an accumulation of lactic acid, and not ketoacids.

The onset of HHS is gradual and insidious and, because of the neurologic manifestations, it may be mistaken for a CVA in elderly patients. Treatment consists of careful fluid replacement while avoiding cerebral and pulmonary edema, correction of electrolyte imbalances, particularly potassium, and insulin to reduce the elevated glucose levels. Low-dose insulin is given by continuous IV infusion to slowly lower glucose levels to 250 to 300 mg/dL. Seizure precautions should be instituted, and hemodynamic monitoring should be used in these critically ill patients. The nurse should closely monitor intake and output, blood pressure, heart rate, lung sounds, weight, peripheral pulses, and neurologic status. Frequent laboratory testing is required. Finally, the underlying cause of the episode should be investigated and treated as needed.

PROTOTYPE DRUG Glucagon (GlucaGen)

Classification: Therapeutic: Hormone: Hypoglycemic agent
Pharmacologic: Pancreatic hormone

Therapeutic Effects and Uses: Glucagon is used for the emergency treatment of severe hypoglycemia in diabetic patients who are unconscious or unable to swallow food or liquids. It is used for radiographic studies to relax the smooth muscle of the GI tract.

Glucagon can be given intramuscularly (IM), subcutaneously, or IV if glucose or dextrose cannot be given IV. Glucagon will raise serum glucose levels, but its onset is 5 to 20 minutes, so recovery is slower than with IV glucose. Because glucagon raises glucose levels by stimulating breakdown of stored glycogen, it is not effective in patients who experience hypoglycemia due to starvation, as their glycogen stores are depleted.

From 1930 to 1950, massive doses of insulin were administered to agitated psychiatric patients with serious mental illnesses to induce seizures and coma, a procedure called insulin shock therapy. Upon administration of glucose or glucagon, the patient awakened in a more sedated state. Although glucagon is still approved for this purpose, this inhumane practice was discontinued when antipsychotic drugs were discovered in the 1950s.

Mechanism of Action: Although glucagon is obtained through recombinant DNA technology, the structure and actions of the drug are identical to those of endogenous glucagon produced by pancreatic alpha cells. Glucagon increases glucose levels by increasing glycogenolysis; therefore, its actions are dependent on the presence of adequate liver glycogen stores. Glucagon stimulates the uptake of amino acids and increases their conversion to glucose (gluconeogenesis), and promotes lipolysis in the liver, with the release of fatty acids and glycerol.

Pharmacokinetics:

Route(s)	IM, subcutaneous, IV
Absorption	Easily absorbed IM or subcutaneous
Distribution	Throughout plasma
Primary metabolism	Liver, plasma, and kidneys
Primary excretion	Renal and through the bile
Onset of action	IV: 5–20 minutes; IM: 30 minutes; subcutaneous: 30–45 minutes
Duration of action	1–1.5 h

Adverse Effects: Glucagon is well tolerated. Adverse effects include nausea, vomiting, hypersensitivity reactions, transient changes in blood pressure (either hypotension or HTN), tachycardia, hyperglycemia, and hypokalemia.

Contraindications/Precautions: Glucagon is contraindicated in patients sensitive to protein compounds, in patients with depleted glycogen stores, or those with insulinoma or pheochromocytoma. It is used with caution in persons with coronary artery disease because it may affect blood pressure or heart rate.

Drug Interactions: Glucagon increases serum glucose and will antagonize the effects of antidiabetic agents. Beta-adrenergic blockers will inhibit the glucose elevating effect of glucagon, and will also increase the risk of blood pressure or heart rate adverse effects associated with glucagon. **Herbal/Food:** None known.

Pregnancy: Category B.

Treatment of Overdose: An overdose can cause hyperglycemia, which may be treated with insulin, IV fluids, and monitoring of electrolytes.

Nursing Responsibilities:

- Assess the patient's blood glucose level before, during, and after glucagon administration.
- Assess the patient's ability to self-administer the drug and monitor blood glucose correctly.
- Assess the patient's adherence to the prescribed dietary and exercise regimen.
- Dilute 1 unit (1 mg) of glucagon with 1 mL of diluent supplied by manufacturer. Administer by direct IV at a rate of 1 unit or fraction thereof over 1 minute. This may be repeated in 20 minutes if the initial dose is ineffective.
- Determine appropriate dosage to be administered. Concentrations greater than 1 mg/mL are not recommended.
- Administer IV glucose solution if patient fails to respond to glucagon.
- Administer supplemental oral carbohydrates once consciousness has been achieved to restore glycogen levels and prevent secondary hypoglycemia.
- Instruct the patient on the proper use of the GlucaGen emergency kit.

Patient and Family Education:

- Immediately report the signs of impending hypoglycemia such as headache, difficulty concentrating, confusion, seizures, palpitations, nervousness, sweating, and cool, clammy skin to the health care provider.
- At the first signs of hypoglycemia, eat sugar or a sweet food product because this may eliminate the need to administer glucagon.
- Do not mix the GlucaGen solution with the powder until it is ready to be used. Discard any unused portion.
- Wear a medical alert bracelet that identifies your medical condition and its treatment.

Drugs Similar to Glucagon (GlucaGen)

There are no drugs similar to Glucagon (GlucaGen).

67.5 Serious, chronic complications of diabetes include neuropathy, nephropathy, retinopathy, and vascular disease.

Most patients with type 2 diabetes experience no symptoms of their illness for many years, perhaps even decades. This is why so many cases of diabetes go undiagnosed. There may be no acute symptoms to motivate the patient to seek medical care. However, while years may pass without symptoms, the effects of uncontrolled blood glucose levels are progressively producing major, irreversible changes on body systems, especially the nervous and circulatory systems.

Teaching patients about the long-term consequences of untreated diabetes can be a major challenge for the nurse. When diagnosed at an asymptomatic stage, it is difficult to convince patients to make radical changes to their lifestyle and to spend money on prescriptions when they do not feel ill. Patients must clearly understand that if they delay treatment until symptoms appear, it will likely be too late to prevent serious, chronic complications. Intensive management of blood glucose levels has been found to dramatically reduce the incidence of long-term complications of diabetes.

Neuropathies are common, affecting an estimated 60% to 70% of persons with diabetes. Diabetic neuropathies affect both the somatic and autonomic nervous systems. Somatic neuropathies include paresthesias, numbness, tingling and pain, motor weakness, and muscle wasting. Autonomic neuropathies include postural hypotension, altered GI functioning including gastroparesis, or gastric atony, diarrhea, altered genitourinary functioning with difficulty voiding or erectile dysfunction, and possible cranial nerve impairment. Intensive management of blood glucose has been shown to reduce the occurrence of neuropathies.

Diabetic nephropathy is the leading cause of end-stage renal disease, which affects patients with both type 1 and type 2 diabetes. Most commonly, the renal glomeruli are damaged, and progressive loss of kidney function leads to eventual renal failure. Comorbid conditions that put the patient at high risk for nephropathy include HTN, poor glucose control, smoking, and hyperlipidemia.

Diabetic retinopathy is the leading cause of acquired blindness in the United States. Twenty years after the onset of diabetes, almost all persons with type 1, and over 60% of those with type 2 diabetes show some degree of retinopathy (Porth, 2005). Regular eye exams are important for all persons with diabetes.

Diabetes is a major risk factor for the development of vascular disease, including premature atherosclerosis, which leads to coronary artery disease, cerebrovascular disease, and peripheral vascular disease. Heart disease and CVA account for about 65% of deaths in persons with diabetes. Preventive measures are directed toward reducing risk factors: control of blood pressure, smoking cessation, lowering lipid levels, and optimal glucose control. In addition, antiplatelet agents are often indicated.

Foot ulcers occur in diabetic patients due to peripheral neuropathies and poor circulation. Neuropathies may impair sensation, so a small area of irritation may go unnoticed. Vascular insufficiency and elevated glucose levels inhibit healing of the ulcer. If the ulcer becomes infected, it is often resistant to treatment, and can ultimately result in the need for amputation. Diabetes is the leading cause of nontraumatic amputations.

Pharm*FACT*

Diabetes is the leading cause of kidney failure and of new cases of blindness in adults 20–74 years of age. Deaths from heart disease and the risk for stroke are two to four times greater for adults with diabetes than for those without diabetes. *Source:* CDC, 2005.

Drug Therapy for Diabetes: Insulin

67.6 Insulin is the cornerstone of therapy for patients with type 1 and gestational diabetes.

Because patients with type 1 diabetes are severely deficient in insulin production, insulin replacement therapy is required to survive. Insulin is also required for those with type 2 diabetes who are unable to manage their blood glucose levels with diet, exercise, and oral antidiabetic agents. Among adults with diabetes in the United States, 16% take only insulin, 12% take insulin with oral agents, 57% take oral agents only, and 15% take neither insulin nor oral medication (CDC, 2005).

The therapeutic goal for patients with type 1 diabetes is to administer insulin as replacement therapy, in normal physiological amounts. Because insulin secretion varies greatly in response to daily activities, pharmacotherapy must be carefully planned in conjunction with proper meal planning and lifestyle habits. The desired outcome of insulin therapy is to prevent the long-term consequences of diabetes by maintaining blood glucose levels strictly within the normal range.

The fundamental principle to remember about insulin therapy is that the right amount of insulin must be available to cells when glucose is present in the blood. Administering insulin when glucose is not available can lead to hypoglycemia and possibly coma. This situation occurs when a patient administers insulin correctly but skips a meal. The insulin is available to cells, but glucose is not. In another example, the patient participates in strenuous exercise. The insulin may have been administered on schedule, and food eaten, but the active muscles quickly use up all the glucose in the blood, and the patient becomes hypoglycemic. Patients with diabetes who engage in competitive sports need to consume food or sports drinks just prior to, and during, the activity to maintain their blood glucose at normal levels. The nurse plays a key role in helping patients plan their meals, activities, and insulin dosages correctly. Figure 67.2 illustrates the management of type 1 diabetes, and correct timing of the insulin dose with meals.

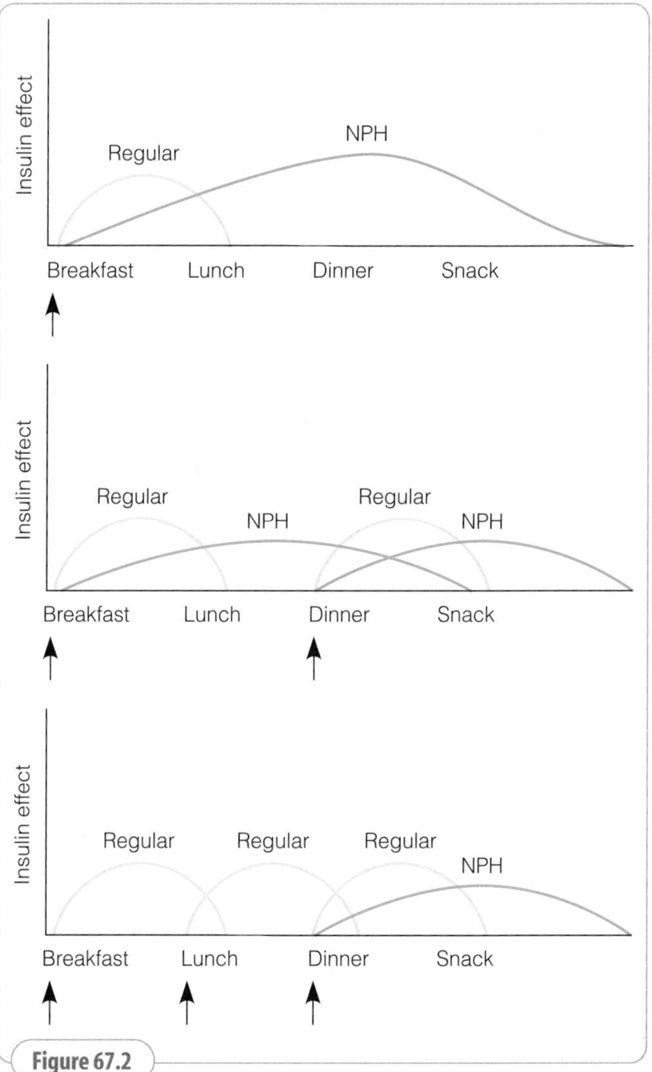

Figure 67.2

Insulin regimens.

Source: From *Medical Surgical Nursing: Critical Thinking in Client Care* (4th ed., p. 577), by P. LeMone & K. Burke, 2008. Reprinted by permission of Pearson Education, Inc., Upper Saddle River, NJ.

TABLE 67.4 Types of Insulin: Actions and Administration

Drug	Action	Onset	Peak	Duration	Administration and Timing	Compatibility
Insulin aspart (NovoLog)	Rapid	10–20 min	1–3 h	3–5 h	Subcutaneous: 5–10 min before meal	Can give with NPH; draw aspart up first, give immediately
Insulin lispro (Humalog)	Rapid	5–15 min	1–1.5 h	3–4 h	Subcutaneous: 5–10 min before meal	Can give with NPH; draw lispro up first, give immediately
Insulin glulisine (Apidra)	Rapid	15–30 min	1 hr	3–4 h	Subcutaneous: 15 min before meal	Can give with NPH; draw glulisine up first, give immediately
Insulin regular (Humulin R, Novolin R)	Short	30–60 min	1–5 h	6–10 h	Subcutaneous: 30–60 min before meal; IV	Can mix with NPH, sterile water, normal saline; do not mix with glargine
Isophane susp (NPH, Humulin N)	Intermediate	1–2 h	6–14 h	16–24 h	Subcutaneous: Mix (cloudy)	Can mix with aspart, lispro, reg; do not mix with glargine
Insulin detemir (Levemir)	Long	Gradual	6–8 h	To 24 h	Subcutaneous: 1/day or 2/day	Do not mix with any other insulin
Insulin glargine (Lantus)	Long	1.1 h	No peak	To 24 h	Subcutaneous: 1/day, same time each day	Do not mix with any other insulin

Many types of insulin are available, differing in their source, time of onset, and peak effect and duration of action. Until the 1980s, the primary source of insulin was beef or pork pancreas. Almost all insulin today, however, is human insulin obtained through recombinant DNA technology because it is more effective, causes fewer allergies, and has a lower incidence of resistance. Pharmacologists have modified human insulin to create certain pharmacokinetic advantages, such as a more rapid onset of action (Humalog) or a more prolonged duration of action (Lantus). These modified forms are called insulin *analogs.* The different types of insulins available are listed in Table 67.4.

Doses of insulin are highly individualized for the precise control of blood glucose levels in each patient. Because the GI tract destroys insulin, it must be given by injection. Some patients require two or more injections daily for proper diabetes management. For ease of administration, two different compatible types of insulin may be mixed, using a standard method, to obtain the desired therapeutic effects. Some of these combinations are marketed in cartridges containing premixed solutions. A long-acting insulin may be taken daily to provide a basal blood level, and supplemented with rapid-acting insulin given shortly before a meal. It is important for nurses and patients to know the time of peak action of any insulin, because that is when the risk for hypoglycemic adverse effects is greatest.

All insulin products used clinically are U-100, meaning 1 mL contains 100 units of insulin, and are administered using U-100 syringes. One type of human regular insulin has been formulated in the U-500 strength, but this is available from the manufacturer only, and is reserved for patients who require very large doses of insulin (more than 200 units/day). Insulin preparations are either clear or cloudy. Those that are cloudy require mixing the solution by rolling the vial prior to drawing out the desired dose. Insulins that are clear do not require mixing. Only regular insulin can be administered by IV injection.

Rapid- or regular-acting insulin can be used in continuous subcutaneous infusion devices, often called insulin pumps. An infusion set, which holds a syringe of the drug, delivers insulin from the pump to a needle anchored in the subcutaneous tissue of the abdomen. The infusion set should be replaced every 3 days, at which time the needle should be moved to a new site, preferably located 1 inch away from the old site. The pump is programmed to release small subcutaneous doses of insulin into the abdomen at predetermined intervals, with larger boluses administered manually at mealtime if necessary. Most pumps contain an alarm that reminds patients to take their insulin. They are generally worn on a belt or tucked into a pocket. Figure 67.3 shows an insulin pump.

The primary adverse effect of insulin therapy is overtreatment; insulin may remove too much glucose from the blood, resulting in hypoglycemia. This may occur when a patient with type 1 DM has more insulin in the blood than is needed to balance the amount of circulating blood glucose. Hypoglycemia may occur when the insulin level peaks, during exercise, when the patient receives too much insulin due to a medication error, or if the patient skips a meal. Some of the symptoms of hypoglycemia are the same as those of DKA. Those that differ and help to determine that a patient is hypoglycemic include pale, cool, and moist skin, with blood glucose less than 50 mg/dL and a sudden onset of symptoms. Left untreated, severe hypoglycemia may result in death.

Other adverse effects of insulin include injection site reactions, generalized urticaria, and swollen lymph glands. Some patients will experience Somogyi phenomenon, a rapid decrease in blood glucose, usually during the night, which stimulates the

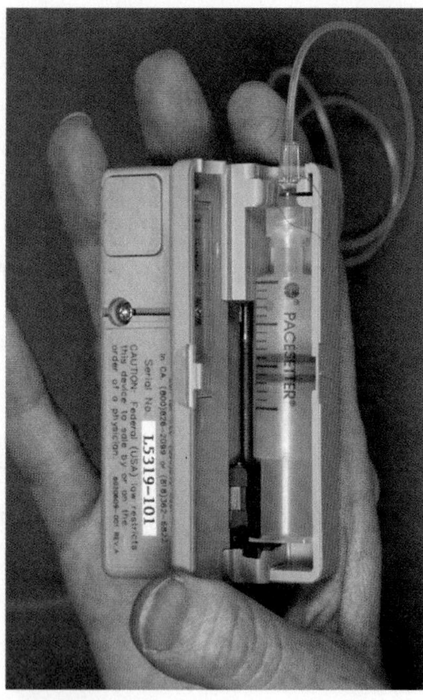

Figure 67.3 Insulin pump.
Source: Pfizer, Inc.

release of hormones that elevate blood glucose (epinephrine, cortisol, and glucagon) resulting in an elevated morning blood glucose level. Administration of insulin above the patient's normal dose may produce a rapid rebound hypoglycemia. The hormone glucagon is administered as a replacement therapy for some diabetic patients when they are in a hypoglycemic state and have impaired glucagon secretion (see Section 67.4).

Patients with diabetes who forget their insulin dose face equally serious consequences. Again, remember the fundamental principle of insulin pharmacotherapy: The right amount of insulin must be available to cells when glucose is present in the blood. Without insulin present, glucose from a meal can build up to high levels in the blood, causing hyperglycemia and possible coma. Proper planning and teaching by the nurse is essential to achieve successful outcomes and maximize patient adherence with therapy.

Insulin Adjunct

Pramlintide (Symlin) is an amylin analog, used along with insulin in persons with type 1 or type 2 diabetes who are not able to achieve glucose control by the use of insulin alone. Amylin is a small peptide released by the beta cells of the pancreas at the same time as insulin. Its natural function is to act synergistically with insulin in glycemic control. The therapeutic actions of pramlintide are to slow gastric emptying time, reduce postprandial glucagon secretion, and increase satiety, thereby leading to reduced calorie intake. Pramlintide is administered subcutaneously immediately prior to each meal, using U-100 insulin syringes. It cannot be mixed with insulin, and must be injected into a different site than insulin. When initiating treatment, rapid- or short-acting insulin doses are usually reduced by 50%. Adverse effects include nausea, vomiting, abdominal pain, headache, dizziness, fatigue, coughing, allergic reaction, or arthralgia. A major adverse effect is hypoglycemia, which is worse in persons with type 1 diabetes, and may be prolonged and severe, occurring within 3 hours following the injection.

PROTOTYPE DRUG Human regular insulin (Humulin R, Novolin R)

Classification: **Therapeutic:** Antidiabetic agent, pancreatic hormone

Pharmacologic: Short-acting hypoglycemic agent

Therapeutic Effects and Uses: Human regular insulin is used to maintain blood glucose levels within normal limits. The primary effects of human regular insulin are: to promote cellular uptake of glucose, amino acids, and potassium; to promote protein synthesis, glycogen formation and storage, and fatty acid storage as triglycerides; and to conserve energy stores by promoting the utilization of glucose for energy needs, and inhibiting gluconeogenesis. Indications for insulin include the following:

- As monotherapy to lower blood glucose levels in patients with type 1 diabetes
- In combination with oral antidiabetic agents in patients with type 2 diabetes
- For the emergency treatment of DKA or hyperosmolar hyperglycemic state
- For gestational diabetes

Because regular insulin is short acting, it is most often used in combination with intermediate or long-acting insulin to achieve 24-hour glucose control. Nondiabetic indications for insulin include stimulation of growth hormone secretion in the evaluation of growth hormone deficiency and the treatment of hyperkalemia to promote a shift of potassium into cells.

Mechanism of Action: Regular insulin is identical to endogenous insulin. Insulin decreases blood glucose levels by increasing cellular uptake of glucose and stimulating storage of glucose as glycogen; it also inhibits the release of glucagon.

Pharmacokinetics:

Route(s)	Subcutaneous; IV (only regular insulin can be given IV); inhalation
Absorption	Rapidly absorbed following subcutaneous injection; absorption time can vary by site of injection
Distribution	Throughout extracellular fluids
Primary metabolism	Hepatic
Primary excretion	Liver and kidneys
Onset of action	Subcutaneous: 30–60 minutes; IV: 15 minutes
Duration of action	6–10 h

Adverse Effects: The most common adverse effect of insulin therapy is hypoglycemia. Rebound hyperglycemia (Somogyi phenomenon) may occur. Irritation at injection sites may occur, including lipohypertrophy, the accumulation of fat in the area of injection. This effect is lessened with rotation of injection sites. Weight gain is a possible adverse effect. Because insulin facilitates the intracellular uptake of potassium, hypokalemia is possible.

Contraindications/Precautions: Beef or pork insulin (which are now rarely used) is contraindicated in persons with hypersensitivity to these animal proteins. Insulin is used with caution in pregnancy, renal impairment or failure, fever, thyroid disease, among the elderly, or in children or infants. Insulin should not be administered to patients with hypoglycemia. Patients with hypokalemia should be monitored carefully because insulin may worsen this condition.

Drug Interactions: Insulin must be used cautiously in conjunction with agents that can produce hypoglycemia, including sulfonylureas, meglitinides, beta-adrenergic blockers, salicylates, anabolic steroids, monamine oxidase inhibitors (MAOIs), and alcohol. Several agents that can antagonize the glucose-lowering effects of insulin include: dextrothyroxine, corticosteroids, epinephrine or norepinephrine, furosemide, and thiazide diuretics. ACE inhibitors increase insulin sensitivity and may enhance the hypoglycemic effects of insulin. Many other drugs can influence blood glucose and the nurse should consult current drug references when treating patients with high insulin doses or who have unstable diabetes. **Herbal/Food:** Garlic, chromium, black cohosh, bitter melon, bilberry, and ginseng may potentiate the hypoglycemic effects of insulin. Cocoa and rosemary may have a hyperglycemic effect.

Pregnancy: Insulin glargine is pregnancy category C; other forms of insulin are category B.

Treatment of Overdose: An overdose of insulin can cause profound hypoglycemia, which is treated with a concentrated source of glucose (dextrose), such as D_5W or glucagon, by the parenteral route.

Nursing Responsibilities:

- Obtain a complete drug history, including the use of herbs and dietary supplements; note any medications that could alter the affects of insulin; assess the patient's alcohol intake because alcohol may increase or decrease insulin's effects.
- Assess the patient's blood glucose level and level of consciousness. Do not administer when blood glucose levels are less than 70 mg/dL or if the patient is exhibiting signs of hypoglycemia.
- Assess the patient's or family members' ability to manage insulin therapy and diabetes.
- Obtain a periodic hemoglobin A1C level to assess serum glucose levels over the past 2 to 3 months.
- Prior to administering rapid-acting insulin, ensure that the patient has consumed, or is capable of consuming, adequate food to prevent a hypoglycemic reaction.
- Prepare the insulin injection using U-100 syringes. Verify the type and dosage with another health care provider to ensure accuracy.
- Rotate the injection sites weekly to prevent lipodystrophy, but bear in mind that insulin absorption can vary by the site used. Use the same locations consistently.
- Assess the patient for knowledge of insulin therapy, diet, and exercise, and how these affect serum glucose levels.
- Administer only regular insulin intravenously.
- Monitor the patient for hypoglycemia, particularly at the time of peak action for the type of insulin used.
- Assess the patient for signs and symptoms of long-term diabetes complications.
- Document the type of insulin, and the amount, using the full term *units,* not the abbreviation *u,* and the site used to administer the drug.
- Teach the patient how to properly prepare an insulin dose.

Patient and Family Education:

- Use low-dose syringes for doses of less than 30 units. Low-dose syringes contain either 30 or 50 units, and make it easier to see and draw up a precise dose.
- Carefully follow the recommended diet and exercise program. Notify the health care provider before beginning any new diet or exercise program because the insulin dose may require adjustment.
- Recognize the signs and symptoms of hypoglycemia and hyperglycemia and report any adverse effects to the health care provider for possible changes in insulin dosing.
- Always carry a supply of readily available sugar or quick-acting carbohydrate for unexpected episodes of hypoglycemia.
- Wear a medical alert bracelet, or carry a medical alert card that explains your condition and treatment.
- Take insulin exactly as prescribed. Do not postpone the dosing time, skip doses, or take a double dose.
- Store insulin as recommended by the health care provider. Unopened vials may be stored in the refrigerator, but do not freeze them. The vial currently being used can be kept at room temperature for up to a month. Avoid exposure to direct sunlight. Discard the vial if the solution becomes cloudy or a precipitate forms.
- Lower the dose of insulin if you are unable to eat, but do not omit the insulin dose because this can result in hyperglycemia. An increased dose may be necessary during periods of high stress or illness.
- Inspect the feet regularly for signs of infection, irritation, and abrasions. Report any slow-healing wounds.

Drugs Similar to Human Regular Insulin (Humulin R, Novolin R)

There are many types of insulin available, which are categorized by their onset of action and duration of action. Table 67.4 compares the different forms of insulin. There are also premixed formulations of insulin available, such as human insulin Humulin 70/30. This type contains 70% NPH and 30% regular insulin, so it can be given before a meal to help control postprandial glucose while also providing longer coverage of insulin needs. Other combination insulins include Humalog 75/25, Humulin 50/50,

TABLE 67.5 Premixed Insulin Combinations

Drug	Description	Route and Adult Dose (maximum dose where indicated)	Onset (min)	Peak (h)	Duration (h)	Adverse Effects
Humulin 70/30	70% NPH insulin/ 30% regular insulin	IM/subcutaneous: individualized doses	30–60	1.5–16	Up to 36	*Pain and swelling at injection site* <u>Hypoglycemia, DKA</u>
Novolin 70/30	70% NPH insulin/ 30% regular insulin	IM/subcutaneous: individualized doses	30–60	2–12	Up to 36	
Humulin 50/50	50% NPH insulin/ 50% regular insulin	IM/subcutaneous: individualized doses	30–60	2–5.5	Up to 24	
NovoLog Mix 70/30	70% insulin aspart protamine/ 30% insulin aspart	IM/subcutaneous: individualized doses	15–60	1–4	Up to 24	
Humalog Mix 75/25	75% insulin lispro protamine/ 25% insulin lispro	IM/subcutaneous: individualized doses	15–60	1–6.5	Up to 24	

Note: *Italics* indicate common adverse effects. <u>Underline</u> indicates serious adverse effects.

Novolin 70/30, and NovoLog 70/30. Selected insulin combinations are listed in Table 67.5.

Insulin aspart (NovoLog): Insulin aspart is a rapid-onset drug, with a structure very similar to endogenous insulin. Insulin aspart has a more rapid onset of action than regular insulin, acting within about 15 minutes when given subcutaneously. Because insulin aspart acts rapidly, injections should be made 5 to 10 minutes before meals. It also has a short duration of action, 3 to 5 hours when compared to regular insulin. Because of its short duration, insulin aspart is usually given in combination with an intermediate or long-acting form of insulin. Insulin aspart is available in 10-mL vials and 3-mL prefilled cartridges.

Insulin detemir (Levemir): Insulin detemir is a long-acting insulin with a slow onset and dose-dependent duration of action. Detemir may be given once or twice a day, depending on the dose; low doses provide shorter durations of action than larger doses, and so dosing is individualized to the patient. At low doses (0.2 units/kg), effects persist about 12 hours. At higher doses (0.4 units/kg), effects last 20 to 24 hours. Because of its slow onset and prolonged duration, insulin detemir is used to provide basal glycemic control. It is not injected before meals to control postprandial hyperglycemia. It cannot be mixed with any other type of insulin and is only given by subcutaneous injection. Insulin detemir is supplied in 10-mL vials, 3-mL cartridges, a 3-mL pen, and a 3-mL InnoLet dosing device. The InnoLet dosing injection device is disposable and has an easy-to-read dial, large push button for injection, and audible clicks that indicate each unit injected.

Insulin glargine (Lantus): Insulin glargine is a newer recombinant insulin analog that exhibits constant, long-duration insulin activity. It has no defined peak effect and provides for the maintenance of steady blood levels; therefore, there is less risk of hypoglycemia with this type of insulin. Insulin glargine allows for once-daily dosing as basal insulin coverage. Although it can be given without regard to meals, it should be given at the same time each day to provide steady blood levels. It cannot be mixed with any other type of insulin and is only given by subcutaneous injection. Research suggests it also helps improve the lipid profiles and A1C levels of type 2 diabetes when added to therapy (Schwartz, 2007). Insulin glargine is supplied in 10-mL vials and in 3-mL cartridges.

Insulin glulisine (Apidra): Insulin glulisine has a rapid onset (10 to 15 minutes) and short duration (3 to 5 hours). Owing to its rapid onset, the drug should be administered no sooner than 15 minutes before eating and no later than 20 minutes after starting a meal. Apidra is only given by subcutaneous injection.

Insulin lispro (Humalog): Insulin lispro is a rapid-acting analog of regular insulin, with effects beginning within 15 to 30 minutes of subcutaneous injection. Insulin lispro acts faster than regular insulin but has a shorter duration of action, 5 hours or less. Because of its rapid onset, insulin lispro should be administered immediately before eating, or even after eating. It is meant to help control the rise in blood glucose brought on by a meal, and is normally given concurrently with an intermediate- or long-acting agent that provides a basal coverage of insulin. It is a clear insulin, and does not require mixing prior to injecting. Lispro cannot be given IV. It is often used with insulin infusion pumps.

Isophane insulin (NPH, Humulin N): Isophane insulin is the only intermediate-acting insulin. It has a slower onset of action (1 to 4 hours) than regular insulin and a duration of action up to 18 to 24 hours. It is used to provide a basal level of insulin coverage for between meals and at night. NPH insulin is normally administered 30 minutes before the first meal of the day, but in some instances a second, smaller dose is taken before the evening meal or at bedtime. Many patients are prescribed insulin that is premixed, such as 70% NPH with 30% regular or rapid acting. If the patient is prescribed a premixed insulin solution, it is important that proper instruction be given, especially if the patient will be using additional regular or rapid-acting insulin on a sliding scale. NPH is a cloudy suspension and requires mixing prior to drawing up a dose. NPH can be given with aspart, lispro, or regular insulin, but cannot be mixed with glargine insulin. When mixed with another type of insulin, NPH should be drawn up after the other insulin, and the mixture should be administered immediately.

CONNECTIONS

Lifespan Considerations Continuous Subcutaneous Insulin Infusion

The ADA has endorsed a consensus statement stating that continuous subcutaneous insulin infusion (CSII) therapy can be appropriate for children and adolescents of all ages proving adequate support personnel are available. This therapy is seen as the most physiologic method of insulin delivery available at this time, providing 24-hour basal delivery of insulin plus postprandial boluses of insulin as needed. A multidisciplinary diabetes team is required to begin CSII, and to supervise the child receiving CSII therapy. Parents and other caregivers require careful education related to diet, exercise, insulin needs, and problems with pump failure, but CSII can be started at any time after the diagnosis. As with any therapy, the benefits must be weighed against potential problems. Benefits of this therapy include a reduction in hemoglobin A1C levels, improved quality of life, decreased variability of glucose levels, and evidence of decreased frequency of severe hypoglycemic episodes. It also seems to be accepted more readily by children with a fear of needles. Indications for use include recurrent severe hypoglycemia, large glucose fluctuations, elevated hemoglobin A1C level, microvascular complications, or risk factors for macrovascular complications, while psychosocial instability or emotional problems in the child may require postponing initiation of pump therapy (Barclay, 2007a).

NURSING PROCESS APPLICATION

Patients Receiving Insulin Therapy

Assessment	Potential Nursing Diagnoses
Prior to administration: • Obtain a complete health history including allergies, drug history, and possible drug interactions. • Assess vital signs. If the patient has a fever or elevated pulse, assess further to determine the cause, because infection can alter the amount of insulin required. • Assess the blood glucose level. • Assess appetite and the presence of symptoms that indicate the patient may not be able to consume or retain the next meal. • Assess subcutaneous areas for potential insulin injection sites. • Assess the patient's knowledge of insulin and ability to self-administer insulin.	• *Risk for Injury,* related to adverse effects of drug therapy • *Deficient Knowledge (Self-Injection)* • *Imbalanced Nutrition: Less than Body Requirements,* related to adverse effects of drug therapy • *Risk for Infection,* related to blood glucose elevations and impaired circulation

Planning: Patient Goals and Expected Outcomes

The patient will:

- Immediately report irritability, dizziness, diaphoresis, hunger, behavior changes, and changes in level of consciousness.
- Demonstrate ability to self-administer insulin.
- Demonstrate an understanding of lifestyle modifications necessary for successful maintenance of drug therapy.
- Demonstrate an understanding of the drug's action by accurately describing drug adverse effects and precautions.

Implementation

Interventions and (Rationales)	Patient and Family Education
• Increase frequency of blood glucose monitoring if the patient is experiencing fever, nausea, vomiting, or diarrhea. (Illness usually requires adjustments in insulin doses.)	• Instruct the patient to increase blood glucose monitoring when experiencing fever, nausea, vomiting, or diarrhea.
• Check urine for ketones if blood glucose is over 300 mg/dL. (Ketones spill into the urine at this glucose level and provide an early sign of DKA.)	Instruct the patient: • To check urine for ketones. • That ketoacidosis normally develops slowly but is a serious problem that needs to be corrected.
• Monitor weight on a routine basis. (Changes in weight alter insulin needs.)	• Instruct the patient to weigh self on a routine basis at the same time each day, and to report significant changes (plus or minus 10 lb).
• Encourage adherence to the prescribed treatment regimen. (Abruptly stopping the medication can precipitate DKA or hyperosmolar hyperglycemic state [HHS].)	• Advise patients to take medication at the same times every day.
• Monitor vital signs. (Increased pulse and blood pressure are early signs of hypoglycemia. Patients with diabetes may have circulatory problems and impaired kidney function that can increase blood pressure.)	• Instruct the patient on how to take blood pressure and pulse, and to report significant changes.
• Monitor potassium level. (Insulin causes potassium to move into the cell and may cause hypokalemia.)	• Instruct the patient to report palpitations or sensations that the heart has skipped a beat.
• Check blood glucose and feed the patient some form of simple sugar at the first sign of hypoglycemia. (Using a simple sugar will raise blood sugar immediately.)	Instruct the patient: • That exercise may increase insulin needs. • To check blood glucose before and after exercise and to keep a simple sugar on hand while exercising. • Before strenuous exercise, to eat some form of simple sugar or complex carbohydrate as a prophylaxis against hypoglycemia.

Evaluation

Evaluate the effectiveness of drug therapy by confirming that patient goals and expected outcomes have been achieved (see "Planning").

CONNECTIONS

Patient Safety

OptiClik Injector Pen

A potential problem that can result in medication errors has been reported by the Institute for Safe Medication Practices (ISMP) involving the use of the OptiClik injector pen for administering insulin glargine or insulin glulisine. Patients who are left handed could administer the wrong dose by using the pen with the dosing window viewed upside down and the needle facing to the right. Because an estimated 20% of people are left handed, there are many opportunities for this error to occur. For example, when the needle is facing to the right (upside down), a dose of 52 units would look like 25 units, 12 units would look like 21 units, and 1 unit will appear to be 10 units (ISMP, 2007). How can the nurse help patients avoid administering the wrong dose?

Drug Therapy for Diabetes: Oral Antidiabetic Agents

67.7 Oral antidiabetic drugs are used to treat type 2 diabetes.

The six primary classes of oral antidiabetic drugs are differentiated by their chemical structures and their mechanisms of action. Oral antidiabetic agents prescribed for patients with type 2 diabetes include sulfonylureas, biguanides, meglitinides, thiazolidinediones (or glitazones), alpha-glucosidase inhibitors, and incretin therapies. Therapy with oral antidiabetic agents is not effective in persons with type 1 diabetes. All oral hypoglycemics have in common the action of lowering blood glucose levels when taken on a regular basis. Many have the potential to cause hypoglycemia; therefore, periodic monitoring of blood glucose levels is necessary. A comparison of the oral antidiabetic drugs is presented in Table 67.6. Doses are listed in Table 67.7.

Therapy of type 2 diabetes is generally initiated with a single agent. If glycemic control is not achieved with monotherapy, then a second agent is added to the therapeutic regimen. Failure to achieve glycemic control with two oral hypoglycemic agents indicates the need for insulin to be added to the regimen, though periodically a third oral agent will be added at the same time as insulin. Doses for selected combination products are listed in Table 67.8.

Sulfonylureas

The first oral hypoglycemics available, sulfonylureas are divided into first- and second-generation categories. Although drugs from both generations are equally effective at lowering blood glucose, the second-generation drugs exhibit fewer drug–drug interactions.

The sulfonylureas act by stimulating the release of insulin from pancreatic islet cells and by increasing the sensitivity of insulin receptors on target cells. The most common adverse effect is hypoglycemia, which is usually caused by taking too

TABLE 67.6 Summary of Oral Hypoglycemic Classes

Drug	Action(s)	Nursing Considerations
Sulfonylureas		
Glyburide (Micronase)	Stimulates insulin release; increases cellular sensitivity to insulin; decreases insulin resistance	Can cause hypoglycemia, GI disturbances, rash; cross sensitivity with sulfa drugs and thiazide diuretics; possible disulfiram response with alcohol
Biguanides		
Metformin (Glucophage)	Decreases hepatic glucose production and release; increases cellular uptake of glucose; lowers lipid levels; promotes weight loss	Common GI adverse effects; risk for lactic acidosis; avoid alcohol; hold 2 days before and after IV contrast; less risk for hypoglycemia
Meglitinides		
Repaglinide (Prandin)	Stimulates insulin release; decreases postprandial glucose and hemoglobin A1C; little effect on fasting glucose	Can cause hypoglycemia, GI effects; well tolerated; administer shortly before meals
Thiazolidinediones		
Rosiglitazone (Avandia)	Decreases hepatic glucose production and secretion; increases cellular sensitivity to insulin	Can cause edema, worsening of heart failure; monitor liver function tests; therapeutic effects take several weeks to develop
Alpha-Glucosidase Inhibitors		
Acarbose (Precose)	Interferes with carbohydrate breakdown and absorption; acts locally in GI tract with little systemic absorption	Common GI effects; hypoglycemia can occur if combined with another oral agent; if this occurs, treat with glucose, not sucrose; take with meals
Incretin Enhancer (Dipeptidyl Peptidase-IV Inhibitor)		
Sitagliptin (Januvia)	Increases synthesis and release of insulin; decreases glucagon production and glucose secretion; increases satiety; supports weight loss	Well tolerated; can cause headache, diarrhea, nasopharyngitis; can cause hypoglycemia if used in combination with another oral agent

much medication or not eating enough food. Hypoglycemia from these agents may be prolonged and require administration of dextrose to return blood glucose to normal levels. Other adverse effects include weight gain, hypersensitivity reactions, GI distress, and hepatotoxicity. When alcohol is taken with sulfonylureas, some patients experience an uncomfortable disulfiram-like reaction, with flushing, palpitations, and nausea.

TABLE 67.7 Oral and Miscellaneous Antidiabetic Agents

Drug	Route and Adult Dose (maximum dose where indicated)	Adverse Effects
Alpha-Glucosidase Inhibitors		
acarbose (Precose)	PO: 25–100 mg tid (max: 300 mg/day)	*Flatulence, diarrhea, abdominal distension* Hypoglycemia (tremors, palpitations, sweating)
miglitol (Glyset)	PO: 25–100 mg tid (max: 300 mg/day)	
Biguanide		
metformin HCL immediate release (Glucophage, Riomet) extended release (Glumetza, Glucophage XR, Fortamet)	PO: 500 mg 2 times/day or 850 mg once daily; increase to 1,000–2,550 mg in 2–3 divided doses/day (max: 2.55 g/day) Glumetza: 1,000–2,000 mg once daily (max: 2 g/day) Glucophage XR: 500 mg once daily (max 2 g/day) Fortamet: 1,000 mg once daily (max: 2.5 g/day)	*Flatulence, diarrhea, nausea, anorexia, abdominal pain, bitter or metallic taste, decreased vitamin B_{12} levels* Lactic acidosis
Meglitinides		
nateglinide (Starlix)	PO: 60–120 mg tid, 1–30 min prior to meals	*Flulike symptoms, upper respiratory infection, back pain* Hypoglycemia (tremors, palpitations, sweating), anaphylaxis, pancreatitis
repaglinide (Prandin)	PO: 0.5–4 mg bid qid, 1–30 min prior to meals (max: 16 mg/day)	
Sulfonylureas, First Generation		
chlorpropamide (Diabinese)	PO: 100–500 mg/day (max: 750 mg/day)	*Nausea, heartburn, dizziness, headache, drowsiness* Hypoglycemia (tremors, palpitations, sweating), cholestatic jaundice, blood dyscrasias
tolazamide (Tolinase)	PO: 100–500 mg 1–2 times/day (max: 1 g/day)	
tolbutamide (Orinase)	PO: 250–1,500 mg 1–2 times/day (max: 3 g/day)	
Sulfonylureas, Second Generation		
glimepiride (Amaryl)	PO: 1–4 mg/day (max: 8 mg/day)	*Nausea, heartburn, dizziness, headache, drowsiness* Hypoglycemia (tremors, palpitations, sweating), cholestatic jaundice, blood dyscrasias
glipizide (Glucotrol)	PO: 2.5–20 mg 1–2 times/day (max: 40 mg/day)	
glyburide (DiaBeta)	PO: 1.25–10 mg 1–2 times/day (max: 20 mg/day)	
glyburide icronized tablets (Micronase)	PO: 0.75–12 mg 1–2 times/day (max: 12 mg/day)	
Thiazolidinediones		
pioglitazone (Actos)	PO: 15–30 mg/day (max: 45 mg/day)	*Upper respiratory infection, myalgia, headache, edema, weight gain* Hypoglycemia (tremors, palpitations, sweating), hepatotoxicity, bone fractures, heart failure, myocardial infarction
rosiglitazone (Avandia)	PO: 4–8 mg 1–2 times/day (max: 8 mg/day)	
Amylinomimetic		
pramlintide (Symlin)	Subcutaneous: Type 1 DM patients: 15–60 mcg prior to meals Type 2 DM patients: 60–120 mcg prior to meals	*Nausea, anorexia, vomiting, dizziness, headache, cough, fatigue* Hypoglycemia (tremors, palpitations, sweating)
Miscellaneous Drugs		
exenatide (Byetta)	Subcutaneous: 5–10 mcg 2 times/day 60 min prior to meal	*Nausea, vomiting, diarrhea, nervousness, decreased vitamin B_{12} levels* Hypoglycemia (tremors, palpitations, sweating)
saxagliptin (Onaluza)	PO: 2.5–5 mg/day	*Headache, upper respiratory infection, nasopharyngitis* Hypoglycemia (tremors, palpitations, sweating), anaphylaxis, angioedema, exfoliative dermatitis, Stevens–Johnson syndrome
sitagliptin (Januvia)	PO: 100 mg once daily	

Note: *Italics* indicate common adverse effects. Underline indicates serious adverse effects.

MyNursingKit | Mechanism of Action Animation: Glipizide

TABLE 67.8 Selected Combination Oral Antidiabetic Agents

Brand Name Drug	Generic Drug Combination	Route and Adult Dose (max dose where indicated)
Actos plus met	pioglitazone/metformin	PO: 15 mg/500–850 mg once or twice daily. Starting dose depends if patient was previously treated with metformin or pioglitazone combination or had an inadequate response with either agent alone (max: 45 mg/2,550 mg daily)
Avandamet	rosiglitazone/metformin	Patients with no prior treatment: PO: 2 mg/ 500 mg once or twice daily. Previously treated patients: PO: 2–4 mg/500–1,000 mg twice daily (max: 8 mg/2,000 mg daily)
Duetact	pioglitazone/glimepride	PO: Start with 30 mg/2 mg once daily (max: 45 mg/8 mg daily)
Glucovance	glyburide/metformin	Patients with no prior treatment: PO:1.25 mg/250 mg once or twice daily. Previously treated patients: PO: 2.5 mg/500 mg to 5 mg/500 mg twice daily (max: 20 mg/2,000 mg daily)
Janumet	sitagliptin/metformin	PO: Starting dose 50 mg/500 mg twice daily with meals. (max: 100 mg/2,000 mg/day)
Metaglip	glipizide/metformin	PO: 2.5 mg/500 mg or 5 mg/500 mg twice daily (max: 20 mg/2,000 mg daily)
Prandimet	repaglinide/metformin	PO: Start with 1 mg/500 mg given twice daily, 15 min. before meals (max: 10 mg/2,500 mg daily)

PROTOTYPE DRUG Glyburide (DiaBeta, Glynase, Micronase)

Classification: Therapeutic: Antidiabetic agent
Pharmacologic: Hypoglycemic agent, sulfonylurea

Therapeutic Effects and Uses: Approved in 1984, glyburide is a second-generation sulfonylurea used to lower blood glucose levels in patients with type 2 diabetes. Glyburide can be used alone or in combination with another oral hypoglycemic agent. It should be used only if diet and exercise have proven ineffective in controlling the elevated blood glucose levels.

Two types of glyburide are available: the conventional form (DiaBeta, Micronase) and a micronized form (Glynase). Glynase allows for lower doses, compared to the conventional forms. Glucovance is a combination product that contains glyburide and metformin.

Mechanism of Action: Glyburide stimulates the release of insulin from pancreatic beta cells, and increases the sensitivity of peripheral tissues to insulin. The stimulation of insulin release relies on some residual beta cell functioning; therefore, the drug is not effective for persons with type 1 diabetes.

Pharmacokinetics:

Route(s)	Oral (PO)
Absorption	Readily absorbed following PO administration
Distribution	Distributed widely to body tissues, with greatest concentrations in liver, kidneys, and intestines; crosses the placenta
Primary metabolism	Extensive hepatic metabolism
Primary excretion	Equal in urine and feces
Onset of action	15–60 minutes
Duration of action	Up to 24 h

Adverse Effects: The primary adverse effect of glyburide is hypoglycemia. Patients at increased risk for hypoglycemia include those with renal or hepatic insufficiency, those consuming an improper diet, and the elderly or malnourished patients. Excessive exercise or alcohol consumption also increases the risk for hypoglycemia. Other adverse effects of therapy include, heartburn, nausea, vomiting, diarrhea, pruritus, erythema, or urticaria, photosensitivity and blurred vision. Rare though serious adverse effects include hepatotoxicity, cholestatic jaundice, aplastic anemia, leucopenia, thrombocytopenia, and agranulocytosis.

Contraindications/Precautions: Glyburide is contraindicated in patients with a known sensitivity to sulfa drugs or thiazide diuretics because sulfonylureas are chemically similar to sulfa drugs. It is contraindicated as the primary treatment for type 1 diabetes, or for diabetic coma or DKA. The drug is used with caution in patients with renal or hepatic disease because the drug may accumulate to toxic levels. If used during pregnancy, glyburide should be discontinued at least 1 month before delivery because newborns exposed to sulfonylureas may develop severe hypoglycemia lasting several days.

Drug Interactions: Using alcohol with glyburide can cause hypoglycemia or hyperglycemia, and has resulted in a disulfiram-type response, with severe nausea, vomiting, flushing, and palpitations. Drugs that can increase hypoglycemia when taken with glyburide are oral anticoagulants, MAOIs, probenecid, sulfonamides, chloramphenicol, oxyphenbutazone, phenylbutazone, salicylates, and clofibrate. Increased risk of hyperglycemia can occur with use of rifampin, and thiazides. **Herbal/Food:** Ginseng, garlic, black cohosh, juniper berries, fenugreek, coriander, or dandelion root can cause hypoglycemia.

Pregnancy: Category C.

Treatment of Overdose: Treatment is the same as for acute hypoglycemia: A concentrated source of glucose is administered.

Drugs Similar to Glyburide (DiaBeta, Glynase, Micronase)

First-generation sulfonylureas are typically less potent, require larger doses, have a shorter duration of action, and require more frequent dosing. Thus, the second-generation agents are more widely prescribed. Acetohexamide (Dymelor), an older first-generation drug, has been discontinued in the United States.

First-generation sulfonylureas:

Chlorpropamide (Diabinese): Approved in 1958, chlorpropamide is the longest acting of the first-generation sulfonylureas, with a duration of action of 24 to 72 hours. In addition to treating type 2 diabetes, an unlabeled use is the treatment of neurogenic diabetes insipidus. Rarely, it can produce an antidiuretic effect, with resulting hyponatremia, water intoxication, and edema. Due to the long half-life of the drug (36 hours), hypoglycemia can be severe and prolonged. It is a pregnancy category C drug.

Tolazamide (Tolinase, Tolamide): Approved in 1965, tolazamide is structurally related to tolbutamide, but is five times more potent. It is taken once daily, with breakfast. It can also be used in patients who fail to respond to other sulfonylureas. It is a pregnancy category C drug.

Tolbutamide (Orinase): Tolbutamide is a short-acting sulfonylurea, with a duration of 6 to 12 hours, given once or twice daily after meals. Approved in 1957, it has been used in patients being treated with insulin who have failed to respond to other sulfonylureas. It is a pregnancy category C drug.

Second-generation sulfonylureas:

Glimepiride (Amaryl): A newer agent approved in 1995, glimepiride can be used alone or in combination with insulin for patients with type 2 diabetes. It is most often given once a day with the first meal of the day. Duetact is a combination oral hypoglycemic approved in 2006 that contains glimepiride and pioglitazone. Avandaryl contains both glimepiride and rosiglitazone.

Glipizide (Glucotrol): Approved in 1984, glipizide is available in a standard tablet form, and an extended release (XL) tablet, which should not be crushed or chewed. In addition to treating patients with type 2 diabetes who do not achieve glucose control with diet alone, it can be used for short-term therapy for those who normally can control their glucose levels by diet. Once-a-day dosing is given 30 minutes before the first meal of the day. Metaglip is a combination product approved in 2002 that contains glipizide and metformin.

CONNECTION *Checkpoint* 67.2

Glyburide combined with alcohol can cause a disulfiram reaction. From what you learned in Chapter 8, what causes the symptoms of the disulfiram reaction?

See Answer to Connection Checkpoint 67.2 in Appendix A.

Biguanides

Metformin (Glucophage), the only drug in this class, acts by decreasing the hepatic production of glucose (gluconeogenesis) and reducing insulin resistance. It does not promote insulin release from the pancreas. Metformin is an oral hypoglycemic agent of choice for managing type 2 diabetes because of its effectiveness and safety.

PROTOTYPE DRUG Metformin (Glucophage, Glucophage XR, Glumetza)

Classification: **Therapeutic:** Antidiabetic agent
Pharmacologic: Hypoglycemic agent; biguanide

Therapeutic Effects and Uses: Approved in 1994, metformin lowers blood glucose levels in patients with type 2 diabetes who are unable to control glucose levels by diet and exercise. It can be used alone or in combination with sulfonylureas, alpha-glucosidase inhibitors, or insulin. It is approved for use in children age 10 or above. Several formulations of metformin are available:

- Regular-release tablets. Administered once or twice daily, absorption is decreased with food, and the peak plasma level is 2.5 hours.
- Solution (Riomet). Administered once or twice daily, absorption is slightly increased with food, and the peak plasma level is 2.3 hours.
- Sustained release (Fortamet, Glucophage XR, and Glumetza). These are extended-duration systems where the drug is slowly released from a semipermeable membrane (Fortamet), gel (Glucophage XR), or gastric-retentive technology (Glumetza). Administered once daily, absorption is significantly increased with food, and the peak plasma level is 6 to 8 hours.

Metformin reduces fasting and postprandial glucose levels. Because it does not promote insulin release, it does not cause hypoglycemia, which is a major advantage of the drug. The drug actions do not depend on stimulating insulin release, so it is able to lower glucose levels in patients who no longer secrete insulin. In addition to lowering blood glucose levels, it lowers triglyceride levels, lowers total and low-density lipoprotein (LDL) cholesterol levels, and promotes weight loss.

Metformin is used off-label to treat women with polycystic ovary syndrome. Women with this syndrome have insulin resistance and high serum insulin levels. Metformin reduces insulin resistance, which in turn lowers insulin and androgen levels, thus restoring normal menstrual cycles and ovulation.

Mechanism of Action: Metformin reduces blood glucose levels by multiple mechanisms. The drug reduces gluconeogenesis, thereby suppressing hepatic production of glucose. In addition, the drug decreases the intestinal reabsorption of glucose and increases the cellular uptake of glucose.

Pharmacokinetics:

Route(s)	PO (regular release tablets, solution, and extended release preparations)
Absorption	Approximately 50–60% of a dose reaches systemic circulation; extended-release forms are absorbed very slowly
Distribution	Distributed to most tissues; crosses the placenta; secreted in breast milk; not protein bound
Primary metabolism	Not metabolized
Primary excretion	Kidneys
Onset of action	Less than 1 h; peak action: 1–3 h
Duration of action	90% excreted within 24 h

Adverse Effects: The most common adverse effects that occur in 30% of patients taking metformin are GI related and include nausea, vomiting, abdominal discomfort, metallic taste, diarrhea, anorexia, and moderate weight loss. It may also cause headache, dizziness, agitation, and fatigue. Unlike the sulfonylureas, metformin rarely causes hypoglycemia or weight gain. The most serious adverse effect is lactic acidosis, which is a rare, though potentially fatal, condition. The risk for lactic acidosis is increased in patients with renal insufficiency, or any condition that puts them at risk for increased lactic acid production, such as liver disease, severe infection, excessive alcohol intake, shock, or hypoxemia. Another drug in this drug class, phenformin, was withdrawn from the market in 1977 due to fatal cases of lactic acidosis.

Contraindications/Precautions: Metformin is contraindicated in patients with impaired renal function, because the drug can rise to toxic levels. It is also contraindicated in patients with heart failure, liver failure, history of lactic acidosis, concurrent serious infection, or with any condition that predisposes the patient to hypoxemia. It is contraindicated for 2 days prior to, and 2 days after, receiving IV radiographic contrast. Metformin is used with caution in patients with anemia, diarrhea, vomiting, dehydration, fever, gastroparesis, or GI obstruction; in older adults; and those with hyperthyroidism, pituitary insufficiency, trauma, or during pregnancy and lactation. Safety in children under age 10 has not been established.

Drug Interactions: Alcohol increases the risk for lactic acidosis, and should be avoided. Captopril, furosemide, and nifedipine may increase the risk for hypoglycemia. Use with IV radiographic contrast may cause lactic acidosis and acute renal failure. The following drugs may decrease renal excretion of metformin: amiloride, cimetidine, digoxin, dofetilide, midodrine, morphine, procainamide, quinidine, ranitidine, triamterene, trimethoprim, and vancomycin. Acarbose may decrease blood levels of metformin. Use with other antidiabetic drugs potentiates hypoglycemic effects. **Herbal/Food:** Metformin decreases the absorption of vitamin B_{12} and folic acid. Garlic and ginseng may increase hypoglycemic effects.

Pregnancy: Category B.

Treatment of Overdose: For overdose or development of lactic acidosis, hemodialysis can be used to correct the acidosis and remove excess metformin.

Drugs Similar to Metformin (Glucophage, Glucophage XR, Glumetza)

Currently, metformin is the only biguanide available.

Meglitinides

The meglitinides are a newer class of oral hypoglycemics that act by stimulating the release of insulin from pancreatic islet cells in a manner similar to that of the sulfonylureas. Both drugs in this class have short durations of action of 2 to 4 hours. Their efficacy is equal to that of the sulfonylureas, and they are well tolerated. Hypoglycemia is the most common adverse effect.

PROTOTYPE DRUG Repaglinide (Prandin)

Classification: **Therapeutic:** Antidiabetic agent
Pharmacologic: Hypoglycemic agent, meglitinide

Therapeutic Effects and Uses: Approved in 1997, repaglinide is used to lower blood glucose levels in patients with type 2 diabetes, as an adjunct to diet and exercise. It may be used alone or in combination with metformin or a thiazolidinedione.

Because repaglinide is rapidly absorbed, it should be taken shortly before each meal. It is effective in lowering postprandial glucose levels, and in reducing hemoglobin A1C levels, but has little effect on fasting glucose levels. It undergoes almost no renal excretion, and so it can be used in patients with renal insufficiency.

Mechanism of Action: Repaglinide lowers glucose levels by stimulating insulin release from pancreatic beta cells. Patients must have some ability to secrete insulin for the drug to be effective.

Pharmacokinetics:

Route(s)	PO
Absorption	Rapidly absorbed following PO administration
Distribution	98% protein bound
Primary metabolism	Hepatic (CYP3A4)
Primary excretion	90% in feces
Onset of action	15–30 minutes; peak: 1 h
Duration of action	4 h

Adverse Effects: Repaglinide is generally well tolerated; the most common adverse effect is hypoglycemia. Other adverse effects include nausea, vomiting, diarrhea, and dyspepsia. Headache, paresthesias, upper respiratory infections, sinusitis, rhinitis, or bronchitis may also occur.

Contraindications/Precautions: Repaglinide is contraindicated in persons with type 1 diabetes or DKA. It should be used with caution in patients with hepatic impairment, during pregnancy or lactation, in elderly patients, or those with systemic infection, surgery, or trauma. Its safety in children has not been established.

Drug Interactions: Drugs that induce hepatic CYP3A4 enzyme such as barbiturates, carbamazepine, rifampin, and pioglitazone may increase repaglinide metabolism and cause hyperglycemia. Drugs that inhibit CYP3A4 such as erythromycin, ketoconazole, and miconazole inhibit repaglinide metabolism and may potentiate hypoglycemia. Gemfibrozil may increase risk for hypoglycemia. Use with isophane insulin may cause myocardial ischemia. **Herbal/Food:** The concurrent intake of grapefruit juice inhibits metabolism and may result in increased repaglinide levels and hypoglycemia. Garlic and ginseng may increase hypoglycemic effects.

Pregnancy: Category C.

Treatment of Overdose: During overdose, provide symptomatic therapy and a concentrated source of glucose for hypoglycemia, preferably by the IV route.

Drugs Similar to Repaglinide (Prandin)

The only other meglitinide is nateglinide.

Nateglinide (Starlix): Approved in 2000, nateglinide has actions and uses similar to repaglinide. It is used alone or in combination with metformin for managing glucose levels in persons with type 2 diabetes who have not achieved glycemic control through diet and exercise. It is not effective for type 1 diabetes. Like repaglinide, it is given 5 to 20 minutes before meals. An important difference between these drugs is that nateglinide is primarily renally excreted, and so should be used with caution in patients with renal impairment. Like repaglinide, nateglinide is well tolerated and hypoglycemia is usually mild. The drug is pregnancy category C.

Thiazolidinediones

The thiazolidinediones (TZDs), or glitazones, reduce blood glucose by decreasing insulin resistance and inhibiting hepatic gluconeogenesis. Optimal lowering of blood glucose may require 3 to 4 months of therapy. The most common adverse effects are fluid retention, headache, and weight gain. Hypoglycemia does not occur with drugs in this class. Liver function should be monitored, because thiazolidinediones may be hepatotoxic; in 2000, troglitazone (Rezulin) was withdrawn from the market because of drug-related deaths due to hepatic failure. Because of their tendency to promote fluid retention, thiazolidinediones are contraindicated in patients with serious heart failure or pulmonary edema.

PROTOTYPE DRUG Rosiglitazone (Avandia)

Classification: **Therapeutic:** Antidiabetic agent
Pharmacologic: Thiazolidinedione

Therapeutic Effects and Uses: Rosiglitazone is used to lower blood glucose levels in persons with type 2 diabetes, as an adjunct to diet and exercise. It can be used as monotherapy or in combination with metformin, a sulfonylurea, or insulin. It is effective in lowering fasting glucose levels and hemoglobin A1C levels. Optimum therapeutic effects take several weeks to occur.

Mechanism of Action: Rosiglitazone lowers blood glucose levels by increasing cellular sensitivity to insulin, thereby reducing insulin resistance. In addition, it decreases gluconeogenesis by the liver.

Pharmacokinetics:

Route(s)	PO
Absorption	Rapidly absorbed
Distribution	Greater than 99% protein bound
Primary metabolism	Hepatic (CYP2C8)
Primary excretion	Primarily renal, with approximately 25% in feces
Onset of action	Within 1 h; peak: 1 h
Duration of action	Greater than 24 h

Adverse Effects: Rosiglitazone is generally well tolerated; the most prominent adverse effect is edema, including macular edema. Anemia, headache, back pain, fatigue, diarrhea, upper respiratory infection, or sinusitis may occur. The drug can also raise serum lipid levels, including HDL cholesterol, triglycerides, and LDL cholesterol. Although no evidence has been found to link this drug to liver damage, it is recommended that baseline liver function tests be obtained prior to initiating treatment, and then assessed every 3 to 6 months while on this drug. Patients should be informed of the signs of liver damage (nausea, fatigue, dark urine, jaundice) as well as the signs of heart failure (dyspnea, weight gain, edema, fatigue) while taking rosiglitazone. Recent research has also raised the concern of increased fracture risk among women taking drugs in this class.

There is current controversy over the cardiovascular effects of rosiglitazone. In 2007, black box warnings for congestive heart failure and for increased risk for myocardial ischemia were added to the rosiglitazone label. Using this drug class in patients with heart failure can increase fluid retention and exacerbate that disorder.

Contraindications/Precautions: Rosiglitazone is contraindicated in persons with severe heart failure, liver disease, or elevated liver enzymes, pregnancy, and lactation. Its safety in children has not been established. Rosiglitazone is contraindicated in persons with type 1 diabetes or DKA.

Drug Interactions: Inducers of hepatic CYP2C8 such as rifampin may decrease the effects of rosiglitazone. Inhibitors of CYP2C8 such as azole antifungal agents, fluvoxamine, gemfibrozil, and trimethoprim may elevate rosiglitazone plasma levels, and increase the risk for adverse reactions. Concurrent use of rosiglitazone with insulin can increase edema and the risk for heart failure and myocardial ischemia. Other antidiabetic agents, angiotensin II receptor antagonists, and gemfibrozil can increase the hypoglycemic effects. Use of rosiglitazone with nitrates is not recommended due to the potential for myocardial ischemia. Thiazide diuretics, phenothiazines, and atypical antipsychotic drugs can decrease the hypoglycemic effects of rosiglitazone by increasing blood glucose levels. **Herbal/Food:** Garlic and ginseng can increase the risk for hypoglycemia if used with rosiglitazone. Cocoa and rosemary may decrease the therapeutic effect and have a hyperglycemic effect.

Pregnancy: Category C.

Treatment of Overdose: Standard treatment for hypoglycemia is initiated during overdose, along with symptomatic treatment of edema or fluid overload.

Drugs Similar to Rosiglitazone (Avandia)

The only other drug in this class is pioglitazone.

Pioglitazone (Actos): Approved in 1999, pioglitazone has actions and uses similar to rosiglitazone. It is rapidly absorbed following PO administration, with peak effects occurring within 7 days of beginning therapy. Pioglitazone has shown more favorable effects on triglyceride and HDL-cholesterol levels than rosiglitazone, with more benefits seen among women than men (ADA, 2007b). Pioglitazone can decrease serum levels of oral contraceptives, and can cause nonovulating premenopausal women to resume ovulation; therefore, a reliable form of contraception is recommended. There is no evidence of liver damage from this drug, but liver function should be assessed for a baseline and periodically thereafter as with rosiglitazone. The cardiovascular safety of the thiazolidinedione drugs has been questioned; black box warnings regarding heart failure and myocardial ischemia were added to labeling in 2007. The drug is pregnancy category C.

Alpha-Glucosidase Inhibitors

The alpha-glucosidase inhibitors act by blocking enzymes in the small intestine responsible for breaking down complex carbohydrates into monosaccharides. Because carbohydrates must be in the monosaccharide form to be absorbed, digestion of glucose is delayed. These agents have minimal adverse effects, with the most common being GI related, such as abdominal cramping, diarrhea, and flatulence. Liver function should be monitored, as a small incidence of liver impairment has been reported. Although alpha-glucosidase inhibitors do not produce hypoglycemia when used alone, hypoglycemia may occur when these agents are combined with insulin or a sulfonylurea.

PROTOTYPE DRUG Acarbose (Precose)

Classification: **Therapeutic:** Antidiabetic
Pharmacologic: Hypoglycemic agent, alpha-glucosidase inhibitor

Therapeutic Effects and Uses: Approved in 1995, acarbose lowers blood glucose levels in persons with type 2 diabetes who cannot adequately manage glucose levels by diet and exercise alone. It may be used alone or in combination with a sulfonylurea, metformin, or insulin. By slowing the breakdown and absorption of carbohydrates, the rise in postprandial glucose level is reduced. Hemoglobin A1C level is lowered as well.

Mechanism of Action: Acarbose lowers glucose levels by interfering with carbohydrate absorption from the GI tract. It acts locally in the GI tract to inhibit the enzyme responsible for carbohydrate breakdown.

Pharmacokinetics:

Route(s)	PO
Absorption	Only 2% absorbed (low absorption is desired because the drug acts locally in the GI tract); some metabolites are absorbed
Distribution	Acts locally in the digestive tract
Primary metabolism	Metabolized in the GI tract by intestinal bacteria and digestive enzymes
Primary excretion	Primarily in feces, 30% in urine
Onset of action	Peak: 1 h
Duration of action	2–4 h

Adverse Effects: The most common adverse effects of acarbose are diarrhea, flatulence, abdominal distention, and borborygmi, anemia (iron deficiency), urticaria, and erythema. The GI-related effects may diminish as therapy progresses; however, they will worsen if the patient does not adhere to the prescribed diabetic diet. Hypoglycemia may occur if acarbose is combined with other hypoglycemic agents. If hypoglycemia does develop, it must be treated with glucose and not sucrose (table sugar), because the drug inhibits the absorption of sucrose. Acarbose may cause elevation of liver enzymes (plasma transaminases), although liver damage has not been reported, and levels return to normal following drug withdrawal.

Contraindications/Precautions: Acarbose is contraindicated in patients with inflammatory bowel disease, bowel obstruction, colon ulcers, or in those predisposed to bowel obstructions. It is used with caution in patients with GI distress, liver disorders, in pregnancy or lactation. Safety in children has not been established.

Drug Interactions: Use with sulfonylureas may increase the risk for hypoglycemia. Drugs that cause hyperglycemia such as thiazide diuretics, corticosteroids, phenothiazines, estrogens, phenytoin, or isoniazid may decrease the effectiveness of acarbose. **Herbal/Food:** Ginseng, garlic, black cohosh, juniper berries, aloe, or dandelion root can cause hypoglycemia. Cocoa and rosemary have a hyperglycemic effect and may decrease the therapeutic effect of acarbose.

Pregnancy: Category B.

Treatment of Overdose: Unlike the sulfonylureas, overdose with acarbose will not cause hypoglycemia. Abdominal pain, flatulence, and diarrhea are treated symptomatically.

Drugs Similar to Acarbose (Precose)

The only other drug in this class is miglitol.

Miglitol (Glyset): Approved in 1996, miglitol is an alpha-glucosidase inhibitor used as monotherapy or in combination with other antidiabetic drugs for the pharmacotherapy of type 2 diabetes. It acts by delaying the conversion of complex carbohydrates to monosaccharides (glucose), thereby lessening the rise in postprandial serum glucose levels. Like acarbose, the drug must be present in the intestine at the same time the carbohydrates are being digested; thus, the drug must be taken with a meal. The adverse effects are similar with the notable exception of not causing increased liver enzymes. Acarbose and miglitol both act locally in the intestine, although miglitol is completely absorbed and has the potential to produce systemic effects. Overdose does not cause hypoglycemia. The drug is pregnancy category B.

Oral Combination Products

Several combination products are available for the treatment of persons with type 2 diabetes. The main advantage of taking a combination drug is that it is more convenient than taking two or more separate drugs, and may improve adherence to the therapeutic regimen.

Glyburide/metformin (Glucovance) can be used for patients who are unable to achieve glucose control by using either product alone. The improvement in glucose control is due to these drugs having different mechanisms of action. Recall that glyburide increases pancreatic insulin secretion, while metformin decreases liver secretion of glucose, and increases cellular uptake of glucose. The adverse effects and contraindications are the same as for each separate drug. Glipizide/metformin (Metaglip) is a similar combination of a sulfonylurea (glipizide) and metformin, with actions similar to Glucovance.

A different type of product combines rosiglitazone and metformin (Avandamet). Rosiglitazone decreases insulin resistance, and metformin decreases hepatic glucose production and increases uptake of glucose. All of these combination products are intended as adjuncts to diet and exercise in blood glucose management. Combination products are not indicated for initial therapy, but are for patients who fail to adequately control glucose levels with the use of a single drug.

Nursing Responsibilities: All Oral Antidiabetic Agents

- Monitor serum glucose levels. Typically, fasting and preprandial glucose levels are obtained, but postprandial levels may also be obtained to evaluate the effectiveness of PO drug therapy.
- Monitor for signs and symptoms of illness or infection, because these may signal that the patient's medication dosage should be adjusted.
- Monitor intake and output, and review laboratory studies for liver function abnormalities.
- Identify patients who are at increased risk for adverse effects of drug therapy:
  - Sulfonylureas are contraindicated during pregnancy or breast-feeding, and are used with caution in persons with renal or liver disease.
  - Metformin is contraindicated in persons who consume excessive alcohol, have renal or liver disease, or any condition that predisposes them to lactic acidosis.
  - Meglitinides are used with caution in persons with liver disease.
  - Glitazones are contraindicated in persons with severe heart failure.
- Administer oral hypoglycemics as directed by the prescriber. Some oral antidiabetic drugs are given 30 minutes before breakfast so that the drug will have reached the plasma when the patient begins to eat.
  - Administer glyburide once or twice a day, 30 minutes before meals.
  - Administer metformin twice a day with the morning and evening meal.
  - Administer meglitinides within 30 minutes before meals.
  - Administer acarbose and miglitol with meals.
- Assess patients for hypoglycemia, hyperglycemia, adverse drug effects, adherence to therapy, and the ability for self-care.

Patient and Family Education:

- Recognize and report the signs and symptoms of hypoglycemia, including rapid heart rate, palpitations, sweating, fatigue, and hunger. Treat these episodes as directed by the health care provider.
- Take sulfonylureas with food if nausea, vomiting, or stomach pain occurs.
- Do not take alcohol with sulfonylureas because uncomfortable symptoms will occur (disulfiram reaction).
- Wear a medical alert bracelet to notify emergency personnel of diabetes. Notify caregivers, coworkers, and others who may be able to provide assistance.
- Recognize and report signs of lactic acidosis with metformin therapy, such as hypoventilation, malaise, body aches, and sleepiness. Do not take alcohol because this increases the risk for lactic acidosis.
- GI upset and diarrhea are common adverse effects of metformin, but these usually subside with continued therapy.
- Take vitamin supplements as directed by the health care provider. Metformin can interfere with the absorption of vitamins B_{12} and folic acid.
- Take medications exactly as prescribed. Do not skip doses or take double doses.
- Immediately report shortness of breath, sudden weight gain, fatigue, or swelling of the hands, feet, or ankles to the helath care provider. Thiazolidinediones can cause edema and weight gain.

NURSING PROCESS APPLICATION

Patient Receiving Oral Antidiabetic Therapy

Assessment

Prior to administration:

- Obtain a complete health history including allergies, drug history, and possible drug interactions.
- Assess blood glucose level.
- Assess knowledge of drug.

Potential Nursing Diagnoses

- *Risk for Injury,* related to adverse effects of drug therapy
- *Deficient Knowledge (Drug Therapy)*
- *Deficient Knowledge (Glucose Testing)*

Planning: Patient Goals and Expected Outcomes

The patient will:

- Immediately report irritability, dizziness, diaphoresis, hunger, behavior changes, and changes in level of consciousness.
- Demonstrate an understanding of lifestyle modifications necessary for successful maintenance of drug therapy.
- Demonstrate an understanding of the drug's action by accurately describing drug adverse effects and precautions.
- Demonstrate an ability to accurately self-monitor blood glucose.
- Maintain blood glucose within a normal range.

Implementation

Interventions and (Rationales)	Patient and Family Education
• Increase the frequency of blood glucose monitoring if the patient is experiencing fever, nausea, vomiting, or diarrhea. (Illness usually requires adjustments in insulin doses.)	• Instruct the patient to increase blood glucose monitoring when experiencing fever, nausea, vomiting, or diarrhea.
• Monitor blood glucose frequently especially at the beginning of therapy, in elderly patients, and in those taking a beta blocker. (Early signs of hypoglycemia may not be apparent.)	• Instruct the patient on symptoms related to hypoglycemia and to report them if they occur.
• Check urine for ketones if blood glucose is over 300 mg/dL. (Ketones spill into the urine at this glucose level and provide an early sign of DKA.)	Instruct the patient: • To check urine for ketones. • That ketoacidosis normally develops slowly but is a serious problem that needs to be corrected.
• Monitor weight, weighing at the same time of day each time. (Changes in weight affect the amount of drug needed to control blood glucose.)	• Instruct the patient to weigh self on a routine basis at the same time each day, and to report significant changes (plus or minus 10 lb).
• Monitor skin for rashes and itching. (These are signs of an allergic reaction to the drug.)	• Instruct the patient on the importance of immediately reporting skin rashes and itching that is unaccounted for by dry skin.
• Monitor activity level. (Dose may require adjustment with change in physical activity.)	Instruct the patient to: • Increase activity level to help lower blood glucose. • Closely monitor blood glucose when involved in vigorous physical activity.
• Encourage adherence with prescribed treatment regimen. (Abruptly stopping the medication can precipitate DKA or HHS. Long-term hyperglycemia can lead to complications of diabetes.)	Instruct the patient: • To take medication at the same times every day. • Not to skip meals. • Follow a diet specified by the health care provider. • Get adequate rest. • Follow healthy routines.
• Monitor vital signs. (Increased pulse and blood pressure are early signs of hypoglycemia. Patients with diabetes may have circulatory problems and impaired kidney function that can increase blood pressure.)	• Instruct the patient how to take blood pressure, temperature, and pulse, and to report significant changes.
• Obtain an accurate history of alcohol use, especially if the patient is receiving a sulfonylurea or biguanide. (These drugs may cause a disulfiram-like reaction.)	• Instruct the patient to abstain from alcohol and to avoid liquid over-the-counter medications that may contain alcohol.
• Check blood glucose and feed patient some form of simple sugar at the first sign of hypoglycemia. (Using a simple sugar will raise blood sugar immediately.)	Teach the patient: • Signs and symptoms of hypoglycemia, such as hunger, irritability, and sweating. • At the first sign of hypoglycemia, to check blood glucose and eat a simple sugar; if symptoms do not improve, call 911. • To monitor blood glucose before breakfast and dinner. • Not to skip meals and to follow a diet specified by the health care provider.

• Review laboratory tests for any abnormalities in liver function. (These drugs are metabolized in the liver and may cause elevations in AST and lactate dehydrogenase [LDH]. Metformin decreases absorption of vitamin B_{12} and folic acid, which may result in deficiencies of these substances.)	• Instruct the patient to report the first sign of yellow skin, pale stools, or dark urine.
• Monitor for signs of lactic acidosis if the patient is receiving a biguanide. (Mitochondrial oxidation of lactic acid is inhibited, and lactic acidosis may result.)	• Instruct the patient to report signs of lactic acidosis such as hyperventilation, muscle pain, fatigue, or increased sleeping.

Evaluation

Evaluate the effectiveness of drug therapy by confirming that patient goals and expected outcomes have been achieved (see "Planning").

- Thiazolidinediones require periodic liver function testing. Immediately report any signs of liver impairment, including fatigue, nausea, vomiting, dark urine, or jaundice.

Drug Therapy for Diabetes: Incretin Therapies

67.8 Incretin therapies offer a new approach to treating type 2 diabetes.

Incretins are hormones released by the mucosa of the small intestine in response to meals. The two incretins, gastric inhibitory peptide (GIP) and glucagon-like peptide (GLP-1), play a major role in regulating blood glucose levels following a meal. Upon secretion the incretins have the following effects:

- Increase the amount of insulin secreted by the pancreas.
- Decrease the amount of glucagon secreted by the pancreas.
- Delay gastric emptying (slow glucose absorption).
- Increase the level of satiety.

Drugs have been developed that augment these natural glucose-lowering hormones. Exenatide (Byetta) is a synthetic drug that acts as an **incretin mimetic.** It has all the actions of natural GLP-1. Sitagliptin (Januvia) is an **incretin enhancer** that prevents the breakdown of incretins, allowing the hormone levels to rise and produce a greater response. Both drugs are effective at lowering blood glucose and have few adverse effects. They work well with other antidiabetic drugs and do not cause hypoglycemia.

PROTOTYPE DRUG Sitagliptin (Januvia)

Classification: **Therapeutic:** Antidiabetic
Pharmacologic: Hypoglycemic agent, DPP-4 inhibitor

Therapeutic Effects and Uses: Approved in 2006, sitagliptin is an incretin enhancer that is used to help lower glucose levels in patients with type 2 diabetes who are unable to achieve normal glucose levels with diet and exercise. The drug is used as adjunct therapy along with diet and exercise, and can be administered as monotherapy or in combination with other oral antidiabetic agents. The drug is given once daily by the PO route.

The actions of sitagliptin are glucose dependent: They occur only in the presence of elevated serum glucose, and so the risk for hypoglycemia is reduced. Sitagliptin has the added benefit of increasing satiety, or the feeling of fullness following a meal, resulting in a lower calorie intake and improved weight control. Sitagliptin lowers both fasting and postprandial glucose levels. Janumet is a fixed-dose combination drug containing sitagliptin and metformin.

Mechanism of Action: Sitagliptin inhibits the enzyme responsible for breaking down incretins: dipeptidyl peptidase-IV (DPP-IV). Inhibition of DPP-IV reduces the destruction of incretins. Levels of incretin hormones increase, thus decreasing blood glucose levels in patients with type 2 diabetes.

Pharmacokinetics:

Route(s)	PO
Absorption	Rapidly absorbed
Distribution	Approximately 38% protein bound
Primary metabolism	20% metabolized in the liver by CYP3A4 and CYP2CB
Primary excretion	Renal
Onset of action	30–60 minutes; peak: 1–4 h
Duration of action	Half-life:12 h

Adverse Effects: Sitagliptin is well tolerated by most patients and adverse effects are generally not serious. Possible adverse effects include headache, diarrhea, nasopharyngitis, and upper respiratory infection. Allergic skin reactions and anaphylaxis have been reported. As monotherapy, sitagliptin does not cause hypoglycemia; however, when used concurrently with a sulfonylurea or insulin hypoglycemia may occur.

Contraindications/Precautions: Sitagliptin is contraindicated in type 1 diabetes and DKA. It is used with caution in persons with renal disorders or renal failure, among older adults, or during pregnancy and lactation. Safety for children under 18 years has not been established.

Drug Interactions: Sitagliptin may increase digoxin levels. **Herbal/Food:** Cocoa and rosemary may decrease the therapeutic effect and have a hyperglycemic effect.

Pregnancy: Category C.

Treatment of Overdose: Overdose is treated symptomatically. If used in combination with other glucose-lowering agents and hypoglycemia occurs, a concentrated source of glucose should be administered by the IV route.

Drugs Similar to Sitagliptin (Januvia)

Saxagliptin (Onglyza) was approved in 2009. Several other incretin enhancers are in the later stages of clinical trials, and may be approved in the near future, including vildagliptin (Galvus), denagliptin (Redona), and aloglipton (Takeda).

Exenatide (Byetta): Exenatide was approved in 2005 for patients with type 2 diabetes who are unable to achieve adequate glycemic control following metformin or sulfonylurea monotherapy. The drug is a synthetic peptide that stimulates the release of insulin from pancreatic beta cells. It mimics the actions of the incretin hormones normally secreted by the intestines, which slow the absorption of glucose. It is effective in lowering fasting and postprandial glucose levels, and causes a consistent, slow weight loss. A major disadvantage of exenatide is that it must be given twice daily by the subcutaneous route, within 60 minutes before the morning and evening meals. It is available as a pen injector. Adverse effects include nausea, vomiting, diarrhea, dyspepsia, anorexia, and gastroesophageal reflux. It can also cause restlessness, a jittery feeling, dizziness, and diaphoresis. Like sitagliptin, it does not cause hypoglycemia. The drug is pregnancy category C.

CONNECTIONS

Complementary and Alternative Therapies Chromium for Hyperglycemia

Description: Chromium is a trace mineral naturally found in various foods, including whole-grain cereals, prunes, nuts, and seafood.

History and Claims: The relationship between chromium intake and glucose metabolism was first reported in the 1950s, when chromium-containing brewer's yeast was reported to prevent diabetes in laboratory animals (Trumbo & Ellwood, 2006). Since that time, the use of chromium supplements among persons with diabetes has become more common practice. Chromium is thought to increase the number of insulin receptors and improve insulin's ability to bind to receptors, therefore lowering blood glucose levels. This, in theory, would lower insulin requirements in persons with type 1 diabetes.

Standardization: The only approved usage for chromium is 4 mcg/mL (chromic chloride injection, USP), which is indicated for use as a supplement to intravenous solutions given for total parenteral nutrition.

Evidence: The evidence for the effects of chromium is inconclusive, with some reporting positive and some negative benefits. Studies in Chinese and Indian populations showed that taking chromium helped people with type 2 diabetes manage their blood glucose levels, while a study of Europeans demonstrated no similar benefit (Kleefstra et al., 2006). VandeLaar, Akkermans, and van Binsbergen (2007) performed a systematic review of studies published outside the United States regarding supplementation and type 2 diabetes. Their analysis showed that many studies have used inappropriate glucose metabolism assessment parameters or have not defined patient populations. In addition, they felt the studies are difficult to compare because they have used different doses (ranging from 200 mcg to 1,000 mcg) and formulations of chromium (such as chromium-rich yeast, chromium chloride, chromium picolinate, and chromium nicotinate), and have been short in duration. Trumbo (2006) summarized the findings of a similar analysis performed by the U.S. Food and Drug Administration (FDA) of studies that originated in the United States. The FDA has concluded that there is no credible evidence to suggest that chromium may reduce the risk of elevated blood glucose levels. More rigorous, blinded, and well-controlled studies are needed to fully assess the efficacy and mechanism of action of chromium supplementation as an adjuvant therapy for type 2 diabetes and impaired glucose tolerance.

UNDERSTANDING THE CHAPTER

Key Concepts Summary

67.1 Serum glucose is maintained within a narrow range by the hormones insulin and glucagon.

67.2 Type 1 diabetes is characterized by insufficient insulin synthesis by the pancreas, whereas type 2 diabetes is characterized by insulin resistance in the target cells.

67.3 The classic signs and symptoms of diabetes include polyuria, polydipsia, and polyphagia.

67.4 Acute complications of diabetes include hypoglycemia, diabetic ketoacidosis (DKA), and hyperosmolar hyperglycemic state.

67.5 Serious, chronic complications of diabetes include neuropathy, nephropathy, retinopathy, and vascular disease.

67.6 Insulin is the cornerstone of therapy for patients with type 1 and gestational diabetes.

67.7 Oral antidiabetic drugs are used to treat type 2 diabetes.

67.8 Incretin therapies offer a new approach to treating type 2 diabetes.

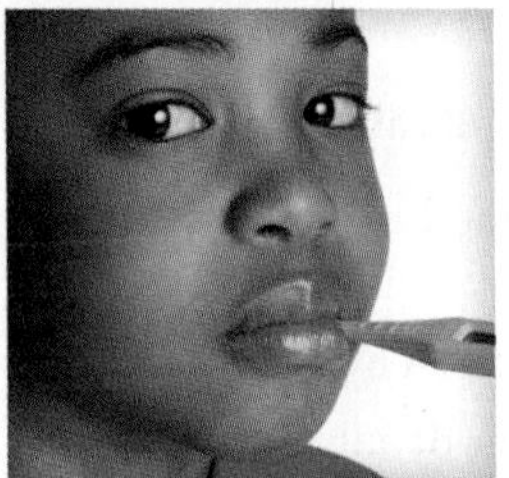

Making the PATIENT Connection

Remember the patient "Jason Harding" at the beginning of the chapter? Now read the remainder of the case study. Based on the information in this chapter, respond to the critical thinking questions that follow.

Jason Harding's parents, Jeff and Mariann, tell the nurse that Jason has been getting progressively sicker over the last 3 to 4 days. They report that he has been having nausea and vomiting, and complaints of vague abdominal pain. The boy appears listless, has dry mucous membranes, and a rapid pulse and respirations. The mother asks the nurse if this could be due to a urinary tract infection, as he has had episodes of bed-wetting in the last week, which is very unusual for him. The health care provider completes a physical examination, and orders laboratory tests.

The nurse gathers and reviews the results of blood and urine tests. The following results are noted: urine, 3+ glucose, 3+ ketones, negative for white blood cells and RBCs; serum glucose 420 mg/dL; serum potassium 6.1 mEq/L; serum bicarbonate 10 mEq/L; pH 7.25.

Critical Thinking Questions

1. How would you, the nurse, explain diabetes mellitus to Jason's parents using simple terminology?
2. What will likely be included in the treatment plan for Jason?
3. What will be the immediate teaching needs of Jason and his parents?

Case Study

A 48-year-old male office manager is seen at a health clinic for his annual physical examination. He is moderately overweight, obtains little or no regular exercise, and eats fast food frequently due to job demands. He has no history of any serious medical conditions, and currently is having no unusual symptoms. He does not smoke or drink alcohol. His blood pressure is 132/86 mmHg; waist circumference 112 cm (44 in.); laboratory results show that his CBC, thyroid, and liver function tests are within normal limits; the lipid profile results are HDL 34 mg/dL, LDL 128 mg/dL, triglycerides 274 mg/dL; fasting glucose 116 mg/dL.

1. What is the most likely cause of this patient's laboratory results?
2. What diabetes classification best describes this patient?
3. What type of treatment is appropriate for this patient? What are his teaching needs?

NCLEX-RN® Review

1 During insulin therapy, nursing interventions to reduce the risk for lipodystrophy include: (Select all that apply.)

1. Monitoring serum glucose levels frequently.
2. Rotating injection sites.
3. Assessing the extremities for normal sensation.
4. Avoiding using any one injection site more often than once a month.
5. Alternating needle sizes weekly.

2 Before administering a morning lispro insulin injection, the nurse should: (Select all that apply.)

1. Obtain a morning urine sample for glucose and ketones.
2. Check that morning's fasting glucose level.
3. Ensure that breakfast trays are present on the unit.
4. Obtain the client's pulse and blood pressure.
5. Assess for symptoms of hypoglycemia.

3 The nurse would attribute which of the following assessment findings as adverse effects to metformin therapy?

1. Hypoglycemia
2. Gastrointestinal distress
3. Lactic acidosis
4. Weight loss

4 A client was started on rosiglitazone for type 2 diabetes. He tells the nurse that he has been taking it for 5 days, but his glucose levels are unchanged. The nurse's best response is:

1. "You should double the dose. It should start helping."
2. "You need to give the drug more time. It can take several weeks before it becomes effective."
3. "You will need to add a second drug since this one has not been effective."
4. "You most likely require insulin now."

5 A young woman calls the clinic and reports that her mother had an insulin reaction, and was found unconscious. The young woman gave her a glucagon injection 20 minutes ago, and her mother woke up, but is still groggy and "does not make sense." The nurse should tell her:

1. "Let her wake up on her own, then give her something to eat."
2. "Place some hard candies in her mouth."
3. "Just let her sleep. People are sleepy after hypoglycemic episodes."
4. "Give her another injection and call the paramedics."

6 The nurse explains to the client that the benefit of using the long-acting insulin glargine over other insulins is that it:

1. Does not need to be administered by injection.
2. Can be given by intramuscular or subcutaneous injection.
3. Does not require blood glucose monitoring.
4. Has no definite peak.

See Answers to Critical Thinking Questions, Case Study, and NCLEX-RN® Review in Appendix A.

References

American Diabetes Association. (2007a). *Research in endocrinology: A report from the Endocrine Society's 89th annual meeting.* Toronto, Ontario: Author.

American Diabetes Association. (2007b). *From insulin to incretins: A report from the 67th Scientific Session of the American Diabetes Association.* Chicago: Author.

American Diabetes Association. (n.d.). *Complications of diabetes in the United States.* Retrieved August 24, 2008, from http://diabetes.org/diabetes-statistics/complications.jsp

Barclay, L. (2007a). Pediatric use of continuous subcutaneous insulin infusion therapy is appropriate. *Medscape Medical News, 2007.* Retrieved August 24, 2008, from http://www.medscape.com/viewarticle/554093

Barclay, L. (2007b). Inhaled human insulin may be safe, effective in adults with type 1 diabetes. *Medscape Medical News.* Retrieved August 23, 2008, from http://www.medscape.com/viewarticle/553399

Buse, J. B., Ginsberg, H. N., Bakris, G. L., Clark, N. G., Costa, F., Eckel, R., et al. (2007). Primary prevention of cardiovascular diseases in people with diabetes mellitus: A scientific statement from the American Heart Association and the American Diabetes Association. *Diabetes Care, 30*(1), 162–172.

Centers for Disease Control and Prevention (CDC). (2005). *National diabetes fact sheet: General information and national estimates on diabetes in the United States.* Atlanta, GA: U.S. Department of Health and Human Services.

Feig, D. S., Briggs, G. G., & Koren, G. (2007). Oral antidiabetic agents in pregnancy and lactation: A paradigm shift? *Annals in Pharmacotherapy, 41*(7), 1174–1180.

The Institute for Safe Medication Practices (ISMP). (2006). *Pharmaceutical industry and medical device companies: Part of the solution?* Retrieved August 24, 2008, from http://www.ismp.org/Newsletters/acutecare/articles/20061116.asp

Kahn, S. (2007). *Increased incidence of fractures in women who receive rosiglitazone in ADOPT.* Presentation at the American Diabetes Association June 2007 Scientific Session, Chicago.

Kleefstra, N., Houweling, S. T., Jansman, F. G., Groenier, K. H., Gans, R. O., Meyboom-de Jong, B., et al. (2006). Chromium treatment has no effect in patients with poorly controlled, insulin-treated type 2 diabetes in an obese Western population: A randomized double-blind, placebo-controlled trial. *Diabetes Care, 29*(3), 521–525.

LeMone, P., & Burke, K. (2008). *Medical-surgical nursing: Critical thinking in client care* (4th ed.). Upper Saddle River, NJ: Prentice-Hall.

National Diabetes Information Clearinghouse (NDIC). (2004). *Complementary and alternative therapy for diabetes.* Retrieved August 24, 2008, from http://diabetes.niddk.nih.gov/dm/pubs/alternativetherapies/

National Institute of Diabetes and Digestive and Kidney Diseases (NIDDK). (2004). *Chromium as adjuvant therapy for type 2 diabetes and impaired glucose tolerance.* Bethesda, MD: Author.

Porth, C. M. (2005). *Pathophysiology: Concepts of altered health states* (7th ed.). Philadelphia: Lippincott Williams & Wilkins.

Schwartz, S. (2007). *Long-acting insulin glargine significantly lowers free fatty acids.* Presentation at the 67th Scientific Sessions of the American Diabetes Association, Chicago.

Trumbo, P., & Ellwood, K. (2006). Chromium picolinate intake and risk of type 2 diabetes: An evidence-based review by the United States Food and Drug Administration. *Nutrition Review 64*(8), 357–363.

VandeLaar, F. A., Akkermans, R. P., & van Binsbergen, J. J. (2007). Limited evidence for effects of diet for type 2 diabetes from systematic reviews. *European Journal of Clinical Nutrition, 61*(8), 929–937.

C H A P T E R

I don't know why I've been so tired lately. Maybe it's just hormones, or my age catching up with me. I've also been gaining weight and it seems like I'm cold all the time. Maybe I should have it checked out.

Patient "Helen Mercado"

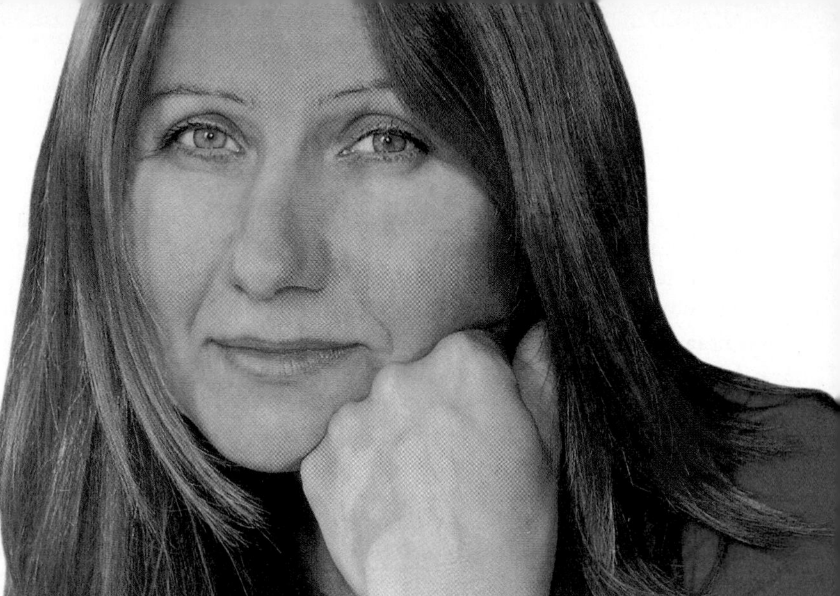

68 Pharmacotherapy of Thyroid Disorders

Learning Outcomes

After reading this chapter, the student should be able to:

1. Explain the functions of thyroid hormone.
2. Explain the negative feedback control of thyroid function.
3. Explain how thyroid disorders are diagnosed.
4. Describe the pathophysiology of hypothyroidism.
5. Describe the pathophysiology of hyperthyroidism.
6. For each of the classes shown in the chapter outline, identify the prototype and representative drugs and explain the mechanism(s) of drug action, primary indications, contraindications, significant drug interactions, pregnancy category, and important adverse effects.
7. Apply the nursing process to care for patients receiving drug therapy for thyroid disorders.

Chapter Outline

Physiology of the Thyroid Gland

Diagnosis of Thyroid Disorders

Hypothyroid Disorders

Pathophysiology

Pharmacotherapy of Hypothyroid Disorders

PROTOTYPE **Levothyroxine (Levothroid, Levoxyl, Synthroid, Thyro-Tabs, Unithroid)** *p. 1151*

Hyperthyroid Disorders

Pathophysiology

Pharmacotherapy of Hyperthyroid Disorders

PROTOTYPE **Propylthiouracil (Propyl-Thyracil, PTU)** *p. 1155*

The thyroid gland affects the function of virtually every organ of the body. It synthesizes and secretes hormones that increase overall body metabolism and protein synthesis. Adequate secretion of these hormones is also necessary for normal growth and development in infants and children, including mental development and attainment of sexual maturity. The thyroid strongly affects cardiovascular and respiratory function, gastrointestinal (GI) function, and neuromuscular function and tone. Thyroid disorders are common, affecting women 5 to 10 times more often than men. This chapter presents the pharmacotherapy for both hypothyroidism and hyperthyroidism.

Physiology of the Thyroid Gland

68.1 Thyroid hormones contain iodine and stimulate the basal metabolic rate of nearly all tissues.

The thyroid gland lies on both sides of the trachea just below the larynx. The gland contains two distinct types of endocrine cell types: follicular cells and parafollicular cells. Follicular cells produce, store, and secrete thyroid hormone. Parafollicular cells produce calcitonin, a hormone totally unrelated to the structure or function of thyroid hormone. Calcitonin regulates calcium metabolism and is used as a drug in the pharmacotherapy of osteoporosis (see Chapter 75).

Thyroid hormone actually consists of two distinct hormones: **tri-iodothyronine (T_3)** and **thyroxine (T_4)**. Both T_3 and T_4 are synthesized from the amino acid tyrosine, and iodine; the subscript numeral refers to the number of iodine molecules each hormone contains. Because the two have very similar actions, they are usually considered a single hormone.

When secreted into the bloodstream, more than 99% of T_3 and T_4 are bound to **thyroxine-binding globulin (TBG)**, a plasma protein produced in the liver. Any condition that causes decreased amounts of plasma proteins, such as protein malnutrition or liver impairment, can lead to a larger percentage of free thyroid hormone, with subsequent symptoms of hyperthyroidism.

Most circulating thyroid hormone is in the form of T_4. To enter target cells, however, T_4 is converted in peripheral tissues to T_3, which is 3 to 5 times more biologically active. This offers an additional level of control (tissue level) of thyroid hormone function.

The two thyroid hormones are metabolized by the liver and excreted by the kidneys, with small amounts excreted in the stool. Iodine is conserved in the process, and returned to the thyroid gland for the production of more hormone molecules. Therefore, only a small intake of iodine is sufficient to meet the demands of the thyroid gland. High amounts of iodine are found in shellfish, but the main dietary source is the use of iodized salt. Thyroid hormones are the only known use for iodine in the body.

Thyroid hormone stimulates the basal metabolic rate of all tissues except the brain, anterior pituitary, spleen, lymph nodes, testes, and lungs. In the presence of large amounts of thyroid hormone, the basal metabolic rate of cells can increase by 60% to 100%. This increases the oxidation of energy sources (glucose, fats, and proteins), which in turn increases oxygen consumption and generates large amounts of heat. Vitamins are used at a faster rate as well, sometimes leading to vitamin deficiencies. Thyroid hormone affects GI function and motility, appetite, and body weight. Thyroid hormone increases the number of $beta_1$- and $beta_2$-adrenergic receptors and enhances their affinity to catecholamines (norepinephrine, epinephrine, and dopamine). The increase in sympathetic activity leads to increased heart rate and force of contraction, cardiac output, and cardiac demands for oxygen. Thyroid hormones also stimulate the secretion of growth hormone (see Chapter 66), and are therefore essential for the normal growth and development of the skeletal and nervous systems, and for the normal functioning of nervous tissue. Thyroid hormone affects reflexes, thought processes, and overall level of consciousness (LOC). Signs and symptoms of thyroid hormone deficiency and excess are presented in Sections 68.3 and 68.5, respectively.

The secretion of thyroid hormone is regulated by the hypothalamus and anterior pituitary gland by way of a negative feedback loop, as shown in Figure 68.1. When blood levels of thyroid hormone are low, the hypothalamus secretes **thyrotropin-releasing hormone (TRH)**. Secretion of TRH stimulates the anterior pituitary to secrete **thyroid-stimulating hormone (TSH)**. TSH then stimulates the thyroid to produce and secrete T_3 and T_4. As blood levels of free, unbound thyroid hormone increase, negative feedback suppresses the secretion of TSH and TRH. High levels of iodine can also cause a temporary decrease in thyroid activity that can last for several weeks. One of the strongest stimuli for increased thyroid hormone production is exposure to cold.

Disorders of the thyroid result from a hypofunction or hyperfunction of the thyroid gland. Abnormal thyroid hormone levels could occur due to disease within the thyroid gland itself, or be caused by abnormalities of the pituitary or

Key Terms

cretinism, *1149*
exophthalmos, *1152*
goiter, *1148*
Graves' disease, *1152*
Hashimoto's thyroiditis, *1149*
iodism, *1156*
myxedema, *1149*
myxedematous coma, *1150*
thyroid crisis, *1154*
thyroid-stimulating hormone (TSH), *1147*
thyroid-stimulating immunoglobulins (TSI), *1154*
thyroid storm, *1154*
thyrotoxicosis, *1154*
thyrotropin-releasing hormone (TRH), *1147*
thyroxine (T_4), *1147*
thyroxine-binding globulin (TBG), *1147*
tri-iodothyronine (T_3), *1147*

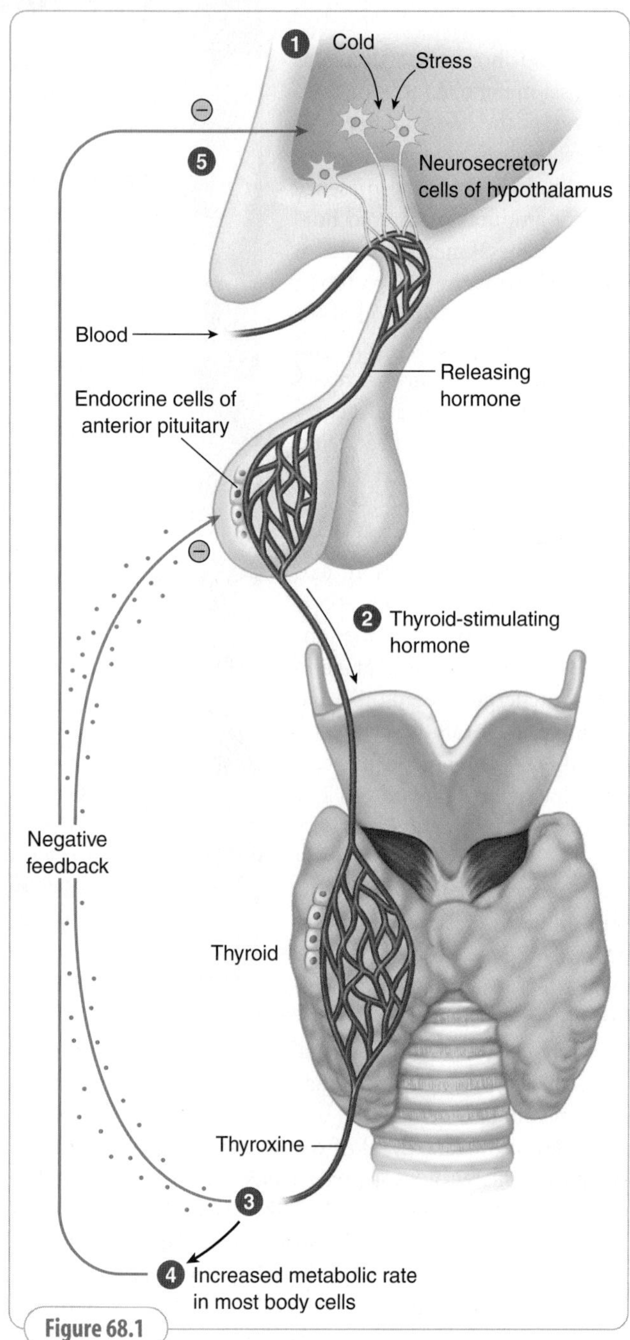

Figure 68.1

Feedback mechanisms of the thyroid gland.

hypothalamus. Table 68.1 compares the signs and symptoms of hyperthyroidism and hypothyroidism.

Thyroid disorders can be due to a congenital defect, or they may develop later in life. They may have an insidious or sudden onset. An increase in the size of the thyroid gland is referred to as a **goiter**. This can occur with normal, high, or low levels of thyroid hormone. Goiters may be diffuse, involving the entire gland, or nodular. When they become considerably enlarged, the goiter can compress the trachea and esophagus, causing difficulty swallowing, a choking sensation, and possibly inspiratory stridor. They may also compress the superior vena cava, causing distention of the neck veins and facial edema.

Diagnosis of Thyroid Disorders

68.2 An accurate diagnosis of thyroid hormone dysfunction is based on the patient's symptoms and the results of diagnostic tests.

Because the thyroid gland is located close to the skin surface, palpation of the thyroid gland is conducted for routine screening of enlargements and nodules. Serum laboratory tests for T_3, T_4, and TSH are commonly used for diagnosis, as shown in Table 68.2. TSH is the preferred laboratory value for diagnosing and monitoring the progression of thyroid disease. Primary hypothyroidism is characterized by a low serum T_4 level and an elevated TSH level.

Abnormal laboratory values must be carefully evaluated because a number of conditions, including stress in critically ill adults, can affect TSH and T_4 levels. In addition, these laboratory values are influenced by abnormalities in serum protein levels because both T_3 and T_4 are heavily protein bound. Any condition that affects protein levels requires careful analysis of these test results. Another laboratory test useful in the diagnosis of thyroid pathology is antithyroid antibody titer. Patients with Hashimoto's thyroiditis, an autoimmune type of thyroid disease, will show abnormal levels of antithyroid antibody titer.

The diagnostic tool of choice for detecting malignancy of a thyroid nodule is the fine needle biopsy. Ultrasonography can be used to assess masses, cysts, and enlargement of the thyroid gland. The radioactive iodine uptake test measures the rate of iodine uptake by the thyroid gland after administration of ^{123}I tracer. This test can detect areas of increased and decreased function. Computed tomography (CT) and magnetic resonance imaging (MRI) scans can be used to determine tracheal compression or pressure on neighboring structures caused by thyroid gland enlargement.

An accurate diagnosis of thyroid hormone dysfunction is essential. Proper treatment of the disorder will depend on whether the abnormality lies within the thyroid gland itself, or is the result of a defect in the negative feedback control by the hypothalamus or pituitary.

PharmFACT

The iodine requirement during pregnancy increases from 150 to 200 mcg/day due to increased renal excretion of potassium iodide. Until week 10 of gestation, the fetus is entirely dependent upon maternal thyroid hormones. *Source:* Weir & Farley, 2006.

Hypothyroid Disorders

68.3 Hypothyroidism, or thyroid deficiency, can occur as a congenital or acquired disorder.

Hypothyroidism may occur as a congenital disorder, or it may be acquired in adulthood. Congenital hypothyroidism is a common, preventable cause of mental retardation. The infant appears normal at birth, due to hormones supplied by the mother while in utero. If untreated, congenital hypothy-

TABLE 68.1 Signs and Symptoms of Thyroid Disorders

Characteristic	Hypothyroidism	Hyperthyroidism
Basal metabolic rate (BMR)	Decreased	Increased
Response to catecholamines	Decreased	Increased
General features	Myxedema, deep voice, impaired growth (child)	Exophthalmos, lid lag, decreased blinking
Blood cholesterol levels	Increased	Decreased
General behavior	Infant: Mental retardation, mentally and physically sluggish, somnolence	Restless, irritable, anxious, hyperkinesis, wakefulness
Cardiovascular function	Decreased cardiac output, bradycardia	Increased cardiac output, tachycardia, palpitations
Gastrointestinal function	Constipation, decreased appetite	Diarrhea, increased appetite
Respiratory function	Hypoventilation	Hyperventilation, dyspnea
Muscle tone and reflexes	Decreased	Increased, muscle tremors
Temperature tolerance	Cold intolerance	Heat intolerance
Skin and hair	Decreased sweating, coarse dry skin and hair	Increased sweating, thin, silky skin and hair
Weight	Increased	Decreased

roidism results in a condition known as **cretinism,** marked by profound mental retardation and impaired growth. Almost half of normal brain development occurs during the first 6 months of life, and thyroid hormone is essential for this to occur. Studies show that if thyroid replacement therapy is begun in the first 6 weeks of life, normal growth and development takes place and cretinism can be prevented. In the United States and Canada, screening for hypothyroidism is conducted for all neonates.

Hypothyroidism in older children and adults results in a general slowing of metabolic processes and **myxedema,** a mucous type of edema caused by an accumulation of hydrophilic substances in connective tissues. Primary hypothyroidism, the most common type in children and adults, results from dysfunction of the thyroid gland. Secondary hypothyroidism is due to pathology of the pituitary gland. Tertiary hypothyroidism is a result of a disorder of the hypothalamus. Causes of hypothyroidism include thyroidectomy or ablation of the thyroid gland with radiation, lithium (used in the treatment of bipolar disorder), or treatment with antithyroid agents. Large amounts of iodine or substances that contain iodine, such as kelp tablets, certain cough syrups, the cardiac drug amiodarone, or iodine-containing radiographic contrast media, can block thyroid hormone production and cause goiter and hypothyroidism. Iodine deficiency is rarely a cause of hypothyroidism in the United States due to the widespread use of iodized salt.

The most common cause of hypothyroidism is an autoimmune disorder known as **Hashimoto's thyroiditis.** This is predominantly a disease of women, striking women 5 to 10 times more often than men. Because hypothyroidism during the first trimester of pregnancy has been shown to cause mental and developmental problems in the fetus, it is recommended that all women receive screening for hypothyroidism early in a pregnancy. By the second trimester when the fetus is able to synthesize thyroid hormone, this threat disappears. Women also experience a high incidence of postpartum thyroiditis, which occurs following approximately 10% of pregnancies.

Hypothyroidism affects nearly all major organ systems, with manifestations arising from two factors: a hypometabolic state and myxedematous changes in body tissues. The hypometabolic state is marked by a gradual onset of weakness and fatigue, a tendency to gain weight despite a decreased appetite, and cold intolerance. Hypotension, bradycardia, hypoventilation, and subnormal temperature may occur. In time, the skin becomes rough and dry, and may have a yellowish cast; the hair becomes course and brittle; and GI motility slows, causing chronic constipation, flatulence, and abdominal distension. Mental dullness, lethargy, slowed reflexes, and memory problems may occur.

TABLE 68.2 Serum Values for Thyroid Function Tests

Thyroid Test	Normal Value	Hypothyroid	Hyperthyroid
Serum T_3	80–200 ng/dL	Decreased	Increased
T_3 uptake	25–35%	No change	Increased
Free T_4	1.0–2.3 ng/dL	Decreased	Increased
Total T_4 (mcg/dL)	4.5–12.5 mcg/dL	Decreased	Increased
TSH (microunits/mL)	2–10 milli international units/mL	Increased	Decreased

CONNECTIONS

Lifespan Considerations Thyroid Disease Among the Elderly

There is a higher prevalence of hypothyroidism among the elderly, with 10% to 15% of older adults having elevated TSH levels. The older adult's signs and symptoms may be similar to those experienced by their younger counterparts: cold intolerance, weight gain, constipation, dry skin, and mental and physical slowing. However, they may be mistaken as normal aging events. Often, the older patient presents with atypical symptoms, such as carpal tunnel syndrome, depression, apathy, dementia, and immobilization.

Hyperthyroidism in the elderly is much less common, but may present with unrecognized, vague symptoms of weight loss, fatigue, palpitations and tachycardia, confusion, and anxiety. These signs and symptoms may be masked by other chronic diseases common to older adults. These symptoms too, are often attributed to normal aging. Older adults may display atypical signs of hyperthyroidism, such as muscle weakness, lethargy, dementia, and osteoporosis. Elevated thyroid levels can cause worsening of heart failure, or unstable angina, and approximately 15% of new cases of atrial fibrillation in the elderly are due to hyperthyroidism.

As fluid accumulates in tissues, the face takes on a puffy look, especially around the eyes; the tongue enlarges; and the voice may be husky. Fluid can accumulate in the pericardial or pleural spaces, causing effusions, cardiac dilatation, and bradycardia. **Myxedematous coma** is a life-threatening end-stage condition of hypothyroidism, characterized by coma, hypothermia, cardiovascular collapse, hypoventilation, hyponatremia, hypoglycemia, and lactic acidosis. This condition occurs most often in elderly women. Even with early detection and treatment the mortality rate is 30% for those who develop myxedematous coma. Treatment consists of supportive measures such as correction of electrolyte and acid–base imbalances, and thyroid replacement therapy. If hypothermia is present, active rewarming is contraindicated, because this may precipitate vasodilation and lead to cardiovascular collapse. Features of thyroid emergencies are described in Table 68.3.

CONNECTION *Checkpoint* 68.1

Patients with hypothyroidism tend to have low rates of angina and myocardial infarction (MI). From what you learned in Chapter 37, explain this link. See Answer to Connection Checkpoint 68.1 in Appendix A.

CONNECTIONS

Lifespan Considerations

Thyroid Hormone Use and Risk of Hip Fracture in Women 65 Years and Older

A case-control study was undertaken to determine if thyroid hormone therapy leads to an increased risk for hip fracture in elderly women. The subjects were 501 women, 65 years of age or older, with 533 age-matched controls who were hospitalized for hip fracture in northern California. No significant difference was found for every use or duration of use of thyroid hormone therapy. Hip fracture was found to correlate with visual impairment, prior use of steroids, and number of falls. These findings are reassuring, given the high number of elderly women on thyroid hormone replacement therapy (Van Den Eeden, Barzilay, Ettinger, & Minkoff, 2003).

TABLE 68.3 Signs and Symptoms of Thyroid Emergencies

Thyroid Storm	Myxedema Coma
Tachycardia	Bradycardia
Hyperthermia	Hypothermia
Tachypnea	Hypoventilation
Hypercalcemia	Hyponatremia
Hyperglycemia	Hypoglycemia
Metabolic acidosis	Respiratory and metabolic acidosis
Cardiovascular collapse: Cardiogenic shock, hypovolemia, arrhythmias	Cardiovascular collapse: Decreased vascular tone
Depressed LOC	Depressed LOC
Emotional lability	Seizures, coma
Psychosis	Hyporeflexia
Tremors, restlessness	

Pharmacotherapy of Hypothyroid Disorders

68.4 Hypothyroidism is treated by replacement therapy with thyroid hormone.

Hypothyroidism is treated by replacement therapy with T_3 or T_4. The standard replacement regimen consists of levothyroxine (T_4), although combined therapy with levothyroxine plus liothyronine (T_3) is an option. Although T_4 is less biologically active than T_3, it is readily converted to T_3 in peripheral tissues. In most cases, replacement therapy must be continued lifelong.

In children with cretinism, therapy should continue for 3 years, after which it should be stopped for 1 month. During this time, thyroid hormone levels are monitored to assess the status of the deficiency and to determine if further treatment is needed.

In adults, serum TSH levels are used to evaluate the progress of therapy. When initiating therapy in elderly patients, the precaution is to "go low and go slow," because there is a risk for inducing acute coronary syndromes in susceptible individuals. Table 68.4 lists the doses of the drugs used to treat hypothyroidism.

TABLE 68.4 Drugs for Hypothyroidism

Drug Name	Dose for Adults (maximum dose where indicated)	Adverse Effects
desiccated thyroid (Armour, Bio-Thyroid, Thyroid USP, others)	PO: 60–180 mg/day	*Weight loss, headache, tremors, nervousness, heat intolerance, irritability, sweating, insomnia, menstrual irregularities*
levothyroxine (Levothroid, Synthroid, Levoxyl, Synthroid, Thyro-Tabs, Unithroid)	PO: 100–400 mcg/day	
liothyronine (Cytomel, Triostat)	PO: 25–75 mcg/day IV: 25–100 mcg/day	Dysrhythmias, hypertension, palpitations, angina
liotrix (Thyrolar)	PO: 12.5–30 mcg/day	

Note: *Italics* indicate common adverse effects. Underline indicates severe adverse effects.

PROTOTYPE DRUG Levothyroxine (Levothroid, Levoxyl, Synthroid, Thyro-Tabs, Unithroid)

Classification: **Therapeutic:** Thyroid hormone
Pharmacologic: Thyroid hormone replacement

Therapeutic Effects and Uses: Levothyroxine is a synthetic form of T_4, with actions identical to endogenous thyroid hormone. It is used for primary or secondary hypothyroidism, congenital hypothyroidism, hypothyroid state resulting from the surgical removal of the thyroid gland, radiation or antithyroid drugs, congenital defect, management of thyroid cancer, or treatment of myxedema coma. The drug is given by the oral (PO) route for routine replacement therapy and intravenously (IV) for myxedematous coma.

To avoid adverse effects, doses of thyroid hormone are highly individualized for each patient. When given by the PO route, 1 to 3 weeks may be required to obtain full therapeutic benefits. Doses for patients with preexisting cardiac disease are usually increased at 4- to 6-week intervals to avoid the possibility of dysrhythmias or angina attacks.

Mechanism of Action: The actions of levothyroxine are identical to endogenous thyroid hormone. The drug increases the metabolic rate, thereby increasing oxygen consumption, respiration, and heart rate; increases the rate of fat, protein, and carbohydrate metabolism; and promotes growth and maturation. Because levothyroxine is converted to T_3, it is not necessary to also give T_3.

Pharmacokinetics:

Route(s)	PO, IV
Absorption	Variable; partial absorption from the GI tract (50% to 80%)
Distribution	Gradually released to peripheral tissues; crosses the placenta; secreted in breast milk; more than 99% bound to protein
Primary metabolism	Hepatic
Primary excretion	Kidneys, with some secreted in bile and excreted in feces
Onset of action	PO: Slow; IV: 6–8 h
Duration of action	1–3 weeks; half-life: 6–7 days

Adverse Effects: At therapeutic doses, adverse effects of levothyroxine therapy are rare. At high doses, treatment may cause central nervous system (CNS) excitability such as tremors, headache, nervousness, or insomnia. Cardiovascular adverse effects include palpitations, tachycardia, angina, and cardiac arrest. Other possible adverse events include allergic skin reactions, diarrhea, nausea, and vomiting. Synthroid 100 mcg and 300 mcg tablets contain tartrazine, which may cause an allergic reaction in some patients, especially those sensitive to aspirin.

Contraindications/Precautions: The use of levothyroxine is contraindicated if the patient is hypersensitive to the drug, is experiencing thyrotoxicosis, or has severe cardiovascular conditions or acute MI. If thyroid hormone is given to patients with adrenal insufficiency, it may cause a serious adrenal crisis; thus, the insufficiency should be corrected prior to administration of levothyroxine. Use of thyroid hormone in the treatment of obesity or weight loss is contraindicated. It should be used with caution in patients with cardiac disease, angina pectoris, cardiac dysrhythmias, hypertension, and impaired kidney function, and in older adults. Symptoms of diabetes mellitus may be worsened with administration of thyroid hormone and doses of antidiabetic drugs may require adjustment.

Drug Interactions: A large number of medications can interact with thyroid hormone and result in either increased or decreased effects. Drugs that decrease the absorption of levothyroxine include cholestyramine, colestipol, calcium- or aluminum-containing antacids, sucralfate, and iron supplements. Several drugs are known to accelerate the metabolism of levothyroxine, including phenytoin, carbamazepine, rifampin, phenobarbital, and sertraline. Levothyroxine increases the effects of warfarin, resulting in an increased risk of bleeding. Digoxin decreases the effectiveness of levothyroxine. Thyroid hormone sensitizes cardiac responsive to catecholamines; therefore, administration of epinephrine or norepinephrine must be carefully monitored in these patients to prevent dysrhythmias. **Herbal/Food:** Soybean flour (infant formula), cottonseed meal, walnuts, and dietary fiber may bind and decrease the absorption of levothyroxine sodium from the GI tract. Calcium or iron supplements should be taken at least 4 hours after taking levothyroxine to prevent interference with drug absorption. The patient should also avoid consuming large amounts of foods that can inhibit thyroid secretion, such as strawberries, peaches, pears, cabbage, turnips, spinach, kale, brussel sprouts, cauliflower, radishes, and peas.

Pregnancy: Category A.

Treatment of Overdose: The treatment of levothyroxine overdose is the same as the treatment of thyroid crisis or thyroid storm, as discussed in Section 68.6. Treatment is directed at reducing the level of circulating thyroid hormone with antithyroid drugs and decreasing sympathetic stimulation with corticosteroids and beta-adrenergic blockers.

Nursing Responsibilities:

- Obtain a complete health history including weight, allergies, drug history, and possible drug interactions.
- Obtain a complete physical examination and vital signs.
- Assess for the presence or history of hypothyroidism symptoms, which include palpitations, excessive nervousness, irritability, insomnia, sweating, diarrhea, and hyperthermia, or intolerance to heat.
- Obtain electrocardiogram (ECG) and laboratory studies including serum T_4, T_3, and TSH levels.
- Monitor the patient's pulse rate before each oral dose during dose adjustment periods; if the heart rate is faster than 100 beats/minute, hold the medication and contact the prescriber.
- Assess periodically for symptoms of hyperthyroidism and hypothyroidism. Levothyroxine has a narrow therapeutic range; dosing that is too high will produce symptoms of hyperthyroidism; doses that are too low produce hypothyroid symptoms.
- Monitor older adults during dose adjustments for angina, dysrhythmias, heart failure, and other cardiac adverse effects.
- Assess vital signs and cardiovascular status if catecholamines (epinephrine, dopamine, and norepinephrine) are used concurrently with thyroid replacement hormones.
- Monitor patients who are taking warfarin for bleeding, and obtain regular laboratory results; the warfarin dose may need to be decreased.
- Assess patients for allergy to aspirin before starting therapy. Synthroid 100 mcg and 300 mcg tablets contain tartrazine, which may cause an allergic reaction in some patients, especially those with sensitivity to aspirin.
- Monitor monthly height and weight, growth and development, and intellectual function in infants treated for thyroid deficiency.
- Monitor blood glucose levels if the patient is diabetic because adjustment of antidiabetic drugs doses may be required.

Patient and Family Education:

- Do not discontinue the medication without consulting the health care provider. Thyroid replacement therapy is lifelong.
- Report chest discomfort, irregular or fast heart rate, pulse rate over 100 beats/minute, excessive nervousness, irritability, insomnia, sweating, diarrhea, and intolerance to heat.
- Take oral levothyroxine once a day, on an empty stomach to maximize absorption, preferably 30 minutes before breakfast.
- Do not change brands of levothyroxine without approval of the health care provider because different brands may not be equivalent. If brands must be changed, the TSH level should be tested after 6 weeks.
- Attend all scheduled follow-up health care provider visits for regular laboratory testing to evaluate thyroid function and the adequacy of the prescribed drug dose.
- Wear a medical alert bracelet to alert emergency medical personnel that this drug is being taken.

Drugs Similar to Levothyroxine (Levothroid, Levoxyl, Synthroid, Thyro-Tabs, Unithroid)

The three other thyroid replacement drugs include desiccated thyroid, liothyronine, and liotrix.

Desiccated thyroid (Armour, Bio-Thyroid, Thyroid USP, others): Desiccated thyroid is an older formulation, approved in 1939, obtained from the dried thyroid glands of pigs. The drug contains T_3 and T_4 in their natural proportions. Desiccated thyroid is less pure and has less reliable content than synthetic formulations, and has largely been replaced by levothyroxine. It is only used for patients who have taken it for years—newly diagnosed cases of hypothyroidism are treated with synthetic thyroid hormone.

Liothyronine (Cytomel, Triostat): Approved in 1954, liothyronine is a synthetic form of T_3 used in replacement therapy for hypothyroidism. Its actions, adverse effects, and contraindications are similar to those for endogenous thyroid hormone. It has a shorter onset, half-life, and duration of action than levothyroxine, and is more expensive. Liothyronine is readily converted to T_3 in the bloodstream. The injectable form of liothyronine is a drug of choice for the treatment of myxedema coma. It is available in oral and IV formulations. This drug is pregnancy category A.

Liotrix (Thyrolar): Liotrix is a synthetic mixture of T_4 and T_3, in a 4:1 ratio, available in PO form only for the treatment of hypothyroidism. Because levothyroxine is readily converted to T_3, there is no apparent advantage in using liotrix over levothyroxine. Its actions, adverse effects, and contraindications are similar to those for endogenous thyroid hormone. This drug is pregnancy category A.

Hyperthyroid Disorders

68.5 Hyperthyroidism, or Graves' disease, is an autoimmune disorder accompanied by ophthalmopathy and goiter.

Symptoms of hyperthyroidism have been recorded in medical documents dating back to the 12th century. The most common cause of hyperthyroidism is **Graves' disease,** named after the Irish doctor Robert Graves who described the disorder in 1835. The condition is characterized by the excessive secretion of thyroid hormone.

The two most visible signs of Graves' disease are goiter and **exophthalmos,** an outward bulging of the eyes. Up to one third of those with Graves' disease develop ophthalmopathy,

NURSING PROCESS APPLICATION

Patients Receiving Thyroid Hormone Replacement Therapy

Assessment

Prior to administration:

- Obtain a complete health history including weight, allergies, drug history, and possible drug interactions.
- Obtain a complete physical examination and vital signs.
- Assess for the presence or history of hypothyroidism symptoms.
- Obtain ECG and laboratory studies including T_4, T_3, and serum TSH levels.

Potential Nursing Diagnoses

- *Activity Intolerance*, related to the disease process
- *Fatigue*, related to impaired metabolic status
- *Deficient Knowledge (Drug Therapy)*
- *Ineffective Health Maintenance*, related to drug adverse effects

Planning: Patient Goals and Expected Outcomes

The patient will:

- Exhibit normal thyroid hormone levels.
- Report a decrease in hypothyroid symptoms.
- Demonstrate an effective knowledge of drug therapy related to drug effects, adverse effects, self-administration, contraindications and precautions, drug interactions, duration of therapy, and follow-up testing needed.

Implementation

Interventions and (Rationales)	Patient and Family Education
• Monitor vital signs; if heart rate is over 100, hold dose and contact the prescriber. (Changes in metabolic rate from therapy are manifested as changes in blood pressure, heart rate, and temperature.) • Monitor for symptoms of hyperthyroidism, including insomnia, tachycardia, heat intolerance, weight loss, chest pain, angina, and diarrhea. (Symptoms of hyperthyroidism may indicate overdosage of thyroid hormone.)	Instruct the patient and family to: • Check heart rate daily prior to taking levothyroxine; if over 100 beats/min, or seems irregular, do not take the drug, and contact the health care provider. • Contact the health care provider should the following occur: chest pain, palpitations, excessive nervousness, inability to sleep, or severe diarrhea. • Remain on the same brand of levothyroxine, as different brands may not be equivalent.
• Monitor for decreased symptoms of hypothyroidism, such as less fatigue, constipation, cold intolerance, depression, and weight gain. (A decrease in symptoms of hypothyroidism would indicate that therapeutic effects of therapy are being attained.)	Instruct the patient and family to: • Notify the health care provider if symptoms persist or worsen. • Not discontinue medication without first consulting with the health care provider, or life-threatening hypothyroidism may result. • Wear a medical alert bracelet to alert emergency medical personnel that this drug is being taken.
• Encourage adherence with prescribed treatment regimen. (Nonadherence with drug therapy may result in myxedema or cretinism.)	Instruct the patient and family to: • Take levothyroxine once a day on an empty stomach to maximize absorption, preferably 30 minutes before breakfast. • Take any calcium or iron supplements at least 4 hours after taking levothyroxine to prevent problems with drug absorption. • Stay on the medication despite not achieving therapeutic effects quickly, as it can take 3 to 4 weeks for levothyroxine to reach a drug plateau, or steady state. • Crush and add medication to food or liquid for pediatric patients. • Avoid foods that can inhibit thyroid secretion, such as strawberries, peaches, pears, cabbage, turnips, spinach, kale, brussels sprouts, cauliflower, radishes, and peas.
• Monitor older patients during dose adjustments for angina, atrial fibrillation or other arrhythmias, heart failure, or other cardiac symptoms. (Reversal of hypothyroidism may cause cardiac symptoms and necessitate an increase in dosages of cardiac medications.)	Instruct the patient and family to: • Check heart rate daily prior to taking levothyroxine; if over 100 beats/min, or seems irregular, do not take the drug, and contact the health care provider. • Check warnings on over-the-counter (OTC) drug labels. Avoid OTC drugs that caution against use by persons with heart or thyroid disease.
• Monitor patients taking anticoagulants such as warfarin for bleeding; obtain prothrombin time (PT) and international normalized ratio (INR) values. (Warfarin dose may need to be decreased when levothyroxine is begun.)	• Instruct the patient and family to report abnormal bruising, nosebleeds, bleeding gums, dark tarry stools, and bright red or "coffee ground" vomiting.
• Monitor the results of thyroid function tests. (TSH levels are used to determine if adequate dosing is being given to maintain therapeutic levels of hormone and achieve desired effects in the patient.)	Instruct the patient and family to: • Obtain regular laboratory testing to evaluate the effectiveness of drug therapy and thyroid function. • If the brands are changed, TSH level should be tested after 6 weeks.
• Monitor infants and children receiving treatment for normal growth and development, bone age, and psychomotor function. (Infants and children receiving replacement therapy should display normal developmental curves.)	• Instruct the family to record the child's weight at weekly intervals.
• If the patient is also being treated for diabetes mellitus, monitor the results of blood glucose levels. (The use of thyroid hormone may decrease the effectiveness of insulin, necessitating a change in hyperglycemic therapy.)	• Instruct the patient and family to report any changes in blood or urine glucose and acetone test results to the health care provider.

Evaluation

Evaluate the effectiveness of drug therapy by confirming the patient goals and expected outcomes have been achieved (see "Planning").

leading to severe eye problems. These include paralysis of the extraocular muscles, damage to the optic nerve with some vision loss, and corneal ulceration due to the inability of the eyelids to close. These eye problems are aggravated by smoking, which should be strongly discouraged in persons with Graves' disease. The ophthalmopathy usually stabilizes with treatment but not all eye changes are reversible with therapy. A rare skin disorder, pretibial myxedema, may also occur, with thickening of the skin, plaques, and nodules over the shins and dorsal surface of the feet. Like the ophthalmic changes, these skin changes may persist despite effective treatment of the hypothyroidism.

Causes of Graves' disease include adenoma and excessive intake of thyroid hormone. The onset is usually between the ages of 20 and 40 years, and it occurs 5 times more often in women than in men. Graves' disease is an autoimmune disorder in which the thyroid gland is stimulated by **thyroid-stimulating immunoglobulins (TSI).** It may occur concurrently with other autoimmune disorders, and there is a familial tendency to the condition.

The manifestations of hyperthyroidism are caused by the hypermetabolic state, and the increase in sympathetic nervous system activity. The symptoms include nervousness, irritability and fatigability, insomnia, weight loss despite a large appetite, tachycardia, palpitations, hypertension, shortness of breath, increased sweating, muscle cramps, hyperthermia, and heat intolerance. A fine muscle tremor may occur. Approximately 15% of elderly patients with new-onset atrial fibrillation, a common cardiac dysrhythmia, have thyrotoxicosis. Table 68.1 summarizes the signs and symptoms of Graves' disease.

Very high levels of circulating thyroid hormone may cause **thyrotoxicosis. Thyroid crisis,** or **thyroid storm** is a rare, life-threatening form of thyrotoxicosis. If untreated, it is associated with mortality rates of 80% to 90%. Even with treatment, mortality from thyroid storm exceeds 20%. It occurs most often in teenage and young adult women with undiagnosed or untreated cases of hyperthyroidism, and can be precipitated by the stress of an acute infection, diabetic ketoacidosis, trauma, or manipulation of the thyroid gland during surgery. Manifestations include high fever, cardiovascular effects (tachycardia, heart failure, angina and MI), and CNS effects (agitation, restlessness, delirium, progressing to coma). It is treated with supportive measures, efforts to reduce body temperature without causing shivering, fluid, glucose and electrolyte replacement, and beta-adrenergic blockers. Aspirin should not be used to lower the body temperature of a person in thyroid storm because it displaces thyroid hormone from its protein binding sites in the serum, increasing the level of free, or active, thyroid hormone, which worsens the condition. Antithyroid drugs may be used to decrease thyroid hormone production.

PharmFACT

Although Graves' disease most commonly occurs in adults, it also occurs in children. About 10% of infants born to women with Graves' disease have hyperthyroidism, but most are asymptomatic. Concordance for Graves' disease is 30% to 50% in identical twins. *Source:* Ferry, 2006.

Pharmacotherapy of Hyperthyroid Disorders

68.6 Hyperthyroidism is treated with surgery or drugs that reduce the production of thyroid hormone.

Treatment of hyperthyroidism often requires surgical removal of all or part of the thyroid gland. In less serious cases of the disorder, pharmacotherapy can be used to diminish the secretion of thyroid hormone.

One strategy to lower thyroid hormone secretion is to destroy part of the gland by administering radioactive iodide (^{131}I). The goal is to use the ionizing radiation from the drug to destroy just enough of the thyroid gland to return the patient to a normal thyroid state.

A second strategy in the treatment of hyperthyroidism is to administer the antithyroid drugs propylthiouracil (PTU) or methimazole (Tapazole), which prevent the incorporation of iodine into the thyroid hormone molecule, and block the conversion of T_4 to T_3 in peripheral tissues. Doses of the antithyroid drugs are listed in Table 68.5.

TABLE 68.5 Antithyroid Agents

Drug Name	Dose for Adults (maximum dose where indicated)	Adverse Effects
methimazole (Tapazole)	PO: 5–15 mg tid (max: 60 mg/day)	*Nausea, rash, pruritus, urticaria, fever, numbness in fingers, peripheral neuropathy, leukopenia, hypothyroidism* Agranulocytosis, bradycardia, hepatotoxicity
potassium iodide and iodine (Lugol's Solution, Pima, SSKI, Thyro-Block)	PO: 250 mg tid	*Diarrhea, nausea, vomiting, stomach pain, fever, weakness, irregular heartbeat, hypothyroidism* Angioneurotic edema, iodine poisoning
propylthiouracil (PTU)	PO: 300–450 mg tid	*Nausea, rash, pruritus, headache, fever, numbness in fingers, diarrhea, myelosuppression, hypothyroidism* Agranulocytosis
radioactive iodide (^{131}I, Iodotope)	PO: 0.8–150 millicurie (a curie is a unit of radioactivity)	*Adverse effects are uncommon* Thyroiditis, hypothyroidism, hypersensitivity

Note: *Italics* indicate common adverse effects. Underline indicates severe adverse effects.

Treatment of thyroid storm is a medical emergency. Propylthiouracil is the preferred drug; however, it can only be given orally. If the oral route is not possible, methimazole can be given rectally. Potassium iodide solution can be given to immediately block the release of thyroid hormone, but should not be given until 1 hour after the administration of antithyroid medications.

Several drugs are used as adjuncts in the therapy of thyroid storm. During hyperthyroid states, beta-adrenergic blocking drugs such as propranolol (Inderal), esmolol (Brevibloc), or metoprolol (Toprol) are given to block the effects of the thyroid hormones on sympathetic receptors in the heart. The actions include a decrease in heart rate and strength of contraction, thereby decreasing myocardial oxygen demands. These effects occur quickly, while the actions of antithyroid drugs take longer to occur. Refer to Chapter 20 for the specific pharmacology of beta-adrenergic blockers.

IV corticosteroids such as hydrocortisone (Solu-Cortef) or dexamethasone (Decadron) may be ordered. Corticosteroids block the conversion of T_4 to T_3 in peripheral tissues. In addition, severe hyperthyroid states create high levels of stress that deplete adrenal corticosteroids in the body and administration of replacement doses is necessary. The pharmacology of the corticosteroids is presented in Chapter 69.

CONNECTION *Checkpoint* 68.2

Patients with Graves' disease have increased hepatic gluconeogenesis, rapid glucose absorption, and increased insulin resistance. From what you learned in Chapter 67, what insulin dosage adjustment is necessary for these patients? See Answer to Connection Checkpoint 68.2 in Appendix A.

PROTOTYPE DRUG Propylthiouracil (Propyl-Thyracil, PTU)

Classification: **Therapeutic:** Antithyroid agent
Pharmacologic: Thyroid hormone inhibitor

Therapeutic Effects and Uses: Approved in 1947, propylthiouracil decreases thyroid hormone levels in hyperthyroid states that are caused by the overproduction of thyroid hormone. It is also used to establish the normal thyroid state prior to surgery or radioactive iodine treatment, and for palliative control of toxic nodular goiter. Propylthiouracil is not effective in treating thyroiditis because this condition is due to over-release, not overproduction, of thyroid hormone.

Mechanism of Action: Propylthiouracil inhibits the first step in the synthesis of thyroid hormone, and suppresses the peripheral conversion of T_4 to T_3. It does not affect thyroid hormone that has already been synthesized, so therapeutic response may be delayed by 3 to 12 weeks, until existing supplies of thyroid hormone have been depleted.

Pharmacokinetics:

Route(s)	PO
Absorption	Rapidly absorbed
Distribution	Concentrated by the thyroid gland; crosses the placenta; secreted in breast milk; 60–80% bound to plasma protein
Primary metabolism	Hepatic
Primary excretion	Kidneys
Onset of action	Absorbed within 30 minutes but therapeutic effects may take several months
Duration of action	Half-life: 1–2 h; peak: 1–1.5 h

Adverse Effects: Approximately 15% to 20% of patients taking this drug will experience leukopenia, which is normally asymptomatic. Serious hypersensitivity reactions are rare, but may be serious and include agranulocytosis, aplastic anemia, thrombocytopenia, rash, urticaria, and glomerulonephritis. The patient may experience liver impairment, including hepatitis and jaundice. Arthralgias and joint swelling occur in 5% of patients. CNS effects include headache, vertigo, neuritis, and paresthesias. Propylthiouracil can also cause hypothyroidism and goiter at high doses.

Contraindications/Precautions: The use of propylthiouracil is contraindicated if the patient has a hypersensitivity to the drug. Although contraindicated during pregnancy, the drug occasionally must be administered to women who experience a thyrotoxic crisis during pregnancy, and it is preferred over methimazole because less of the drug crosses the placenta. It should be used with caution during active infection, during lactation, and bone marrow depression. Because propylthiouracil can cause liver impairment, caution should be used when treating patients with preexisting hepatic disease.

Drug Interactions: Propylthiouracil increases the actions of anticoagulants, which creates an increased risk of bleeding. Iodine-containing agents (amiodarone, potassium iodide, sodium iodide) and thyroid hormones can antagonize the effectiveness of this drug. Altered serum levels of metoprolol, propranolol, and digoxin can occur as the patient moves from a hyperthyroid to a normal thyroid state. Cross hypersensitivity occurs in about 50% of patients who have experienced a hypersensitivity reaction to methimazole, the other major antithyroid medication. **Herbal/Food:** Unknown.

Pregnancy: Category D.

Treatment of Overdose: When propylthiouracil is taken in high doses, it can induce hypothyroidism; the administration of thyroid hormone may be necessary.

Nursing Responsibilities:

- Obtain a complete health history including weight, allergies, drug history, and possible drug interactions.
- Obtain a complete physical examination and vital signs.

- Assess for the presence or history of hypothyroidism symptoms, which include cold intolerance, weight gain, fatigue, bradycardia, constipation, and abdominal distention.
- Obtain ECG and laboratory studies including T_4, T_3, and serum TSH levels, and complete blood count (CBC).
- Monitor patients for response to PTU and other antithyroid drugs: decreased heart rate, weight gain, improved sleep, and reduced serum T_4 levels.
- Monitor for signs of hypothrombinemia such as ecchymoses, purpura, petechiae, or bleeding.

Patient and Family Education:

- Report if pulse rate is greater than 100 beats/minute or less than 60 beats/minute.
- Report significant weight loss, heart rate increases, muscle tremors, and anxiety because these may indicate that the dose needs to be increased.
- Take the medication at the same times every day, at evenly spaced intervals around the clock. Try eating small, frequent meals if nausea is a problem.
- Immediately report severe skin rash or swollen lymph nodes, sore throat, fever; diarrhea, vomiting; irritability; or weakness.
- Avoid using OTC medications without the approval of the health care provider because some products contain iodine, which should be avoided during therapy.
- Do not drive or perform other hazardous activities until the effects of the drug are known because this drug may cause drowsiness or dizziness.
- Do not breast-feed while taking this drug without approval of the health care provider.
- Immediately notify the health care provider of any known or suspected pregnancy.
- Dilute the strong iodine solution with fruit juice or other beverage to make it more palatable.
- Discontinue the drug and contact the health care provider if severe stomach distress develops.

Drugs Similar to Propylthiouracil (Propyl-Thyracil, PTU)

Drugs similar to propylthiouracil (PTU) include Lugol's solution, methimazole, potassium iodide, and radioactive iodide.

Lugol's solution (5% iodine and 10% potassium iodide): This strong iodine solution is given orally to treat hyperthyroidism, as adjunctive therapy 10 to 14 days prior to thyroid surgery, or for the treatment of thyrotoxicosis. Although iodine is necessary for the synthesis of thyroid hormone, high levels inhibit both the synthesis and release of thyroid hormone. The effectiveness of iodine solutions decreases over time, so it is not used for long-term control of hyperthyroidism. Chronic use can result in toxicity known as **iodism,** which is characterized by burning in the mouth and throat, a metallic taste, sore teeth and gums, increased salivation and nasal discharge, swollen eyelids, gastric irritation, and diarrhea. These subside once the drug is discontinued. Potassium iodide is pregnancy category D.

Methimazole (Tapazole): Approved in 1950, methimazole corrects hyperthyroidism by inhibiting the synthesis of thyroid hormone. Like PTU, it does not affect existing stores of thyroid hormone, thus it may take many weeks before a normal thyroid state is achieved. Its uses, contraindications and adverse effects are similar to PTU, except that methimazole does not induce hypothyroidism. Other important differences are that methimazole does not inhibit conversion of T_4 to T_3; therefore, its effects may take longer to occur. Methimazole has a longer half-life, allowing for once-a-day dosing, while PTU must be taken three times a day. This drug is pregnancy category D.

Potassium iodide (Losat, SSKI, Thyro-Block): Potassium iodide is given orally prior to thyroid surgery to reduce the vascularity (to reduce the risk of bleeding), fragility, and size of the thyroid gland. It is also used alone for hyperthyroidism, or in combination with antithyroid drugs and beta-adrenergic blockers in the treatment of thyroid storm. Like other forms of iodide, it suppresses the synthesis and release of thyroid hormone. It is also used to protect the thyroid gland in instances of radiation exposure secondary to a nuclear plant accident. It is taken up by the thyroid gland, thereby blocking the uptake of radiative iodide in the thyroid gland, reducing the risk for developing thyroid cancer. As a protective agent, it must be given immediately prior to, or within 3 hours following, radiation exposure. This drug is pregnancy category D.

Radioactive iodide (^{131}I): Radioactive iodide is an isotope of iodine used for hyperthyroidism. Like all iodine, ^{131}I is taken up by the thyroid gland, where its radioactivity destroys thyroid tissue. The goal is to destroy part of the gland, thereby decreasing the amount of thyroid hormone produced and secreted. In some patients, too much thyroid gland is destroyed and hypothyroidism results, which is then treated with levothyroxine. Approximately two thirds of patients treated with ^{131}I respond to a single treatment, while the rest require two or more treatments. Therapeutic effects develop slowly over 2 to 3 months, and the tissue damage is limited to the thyroid gland, with no surrounding structures affected. While it is contraindicated during pregnancy and breast-feeding, and usually not used in children, ^{131}I has not been known to cause cancer or other serious adverse effects to the thyroid gland or elsewhere in the body. It is used in patients wishing to avoid surgery, or those who do not tolerate antithyroid drugs. It is administered PO, and is also used to treat thyroid cancer (in high doses), and for the diagnosis of thyroid disorders. This drug is pregnancy category X.

NURSING PROCESS APPLICATION

Patients Receiving Antithyroid Therapy

Assessment

Prior to administration:

- Obtain a complete health history including weight, allergies, drug history, and possible drug interactions.
- Obtain a complete physical examination and vital signs.
- Assess for the presence or history of hyperthyroidism symptoms.
- Obtain ECG and laboratory studies including serum T_4, T_3, and TSH levels; and complete blood count (CBC).

Potential Nursing Diagnoses

- *Risk for Infection*, related to drug-induced agranulocytosis
- *Risk for Injury*, related to adverse drug effects
- *Deficient Knowledge (Medication)*
- *Ineffective Health Maintenance*, related to adverse GI drug effects

Planning: Patient Goals and Expected Outcomes

The patient will:

- Exhibit normal thyroid hormone levels.
- Report a decrease in hyperthyroid symptoms.
- Demonstrate an effective knowledge of drug therapy related to drug effects, adverse effects, self-administration, contraindications and precautions, drug interactions, duration of therapy, and follow-up testing needed.

Implementation

Interventions and (Rationales)	Patient and Family Education
• Monitor for decreased symptoms of hyperthyroidism, such as an improvement in insomnia, heat intolerance, anxiety, muscle tremor, tachycardia, diarrhea, and weight loss. (A decline in the symptoms of hyperthyroidism will assist in determining if therapeutic goals are being achieved.) • Monitor for symptoms of hypothyroidism. (Excessive thyroid treatment can result in hypothyroidism and replacement therapy may be indicated.)	Instruct the patient to: • Notify the health care provider if symptoms persist or worsen. • Continue the medication because a prolonged course of treatment (up to 6 to12 months) may be needed to normalize hormone production. • Wear a medical alert bracelet to alert emergency medical personnel that this drug is being taken.
• Monitor vital signs. (Changes in metabolic rate are manifested as changes in blood pressure, pulse, and body temperature.)	Instruct the patient to: • Count the pulse for 1 full minute, and report abnormal rates as directed by the health care provider. • Report any episodes of dizziness, palpitations, and intolerance to temperature changes.
• Monitor thyroid function tests throughout therapy. (Monitoring of TSH, T_3, and T_4 levels will evaluate the effectiveness of therapy.)	Instruct the patient to: • Obtain regular laboratory testing to evaluate the effectiveness of drug therapy and thyroid function. • Continue medication therapy, as a euthyroid state may take 1 month or longer to achieve, depending on the severity of the disease.
• Encourage adherence with prescribed treatment regimen. (Abruptly stopping the medication can precipitate a thyroid crisis.)	• Advise patients to take medication at the same times every day, at regular, evenly spaced times around the clock.
• Monitor for signs of iodine toxicity. (Antithyroid medications may cause iodine toxicity.)	• Instruct the patient to report any burning sensations in the mouth, soreness of the gums and teeth, or brassy taste, as these may indicate iodine toxicity.
• Monitor for drowsiness. (Antithyroid medications may cause drowsiness.)	• Instruct the patient that the medication may cause drowsiness, and to avoid hazardous activities until the effects of the drug are known.
• Monitor for signs of infection, including CBC with white blood cell differential. (Agranulocytosis can result from therapy, increasing the risk of infection.)	• Instruct the patient to monitor for and report severe skin rash, swollen lymph nodes, sore throat, fever, diarrhea, vomiting, or weakness.
• If administering a strong iodine solution, dilute it in fruit juice or other beverage to make it more palatable. Hold the drug if severe stomach distress develops. (Iodine solutions can cause corrosive injury to the GI tract.)	Instruct the patient to: • Eat small, frequent meals if nausea should occur. • Discontinue the drug and notify the health care provider immediately if severe abdominal distress develops.
• Monitor the PT and for the development of any signs of increased bleeding. (If antithyroid therapy is initiated while the patient is receiving warfarin therapy, a dosage reduction of the anticoagulant is often necessary.)	Instruct the patient: • That the dosage of anticoagulants may have to be decreased over the next 1 to 4 weeks. • To report nosebleeds, bleeding gums, dark, tarry stools, and bright red or "coffee ground" vomiting to the health care provider.
• Monitor the patient for pregnancy and lactation. (Antithyroid drugs are contraindicated while pregnant or breast-feeding, as they cross the placenta and enter breast milk, and can affect the thyroid function of the baby.)	• Instruct the patient to immediately report pregnancy or breast-feeding to the health care provider.
• Monitor dietary intake; avoid intake of high iodine foods. (Consuming iodine-rich foods increases the production of thyroid hormones, counteracting the effects of therapy.)	• Instruct the patient to avoid excessive intake of foods high in iodine, including tofu, soy, shellfish, OTC cough medicines, and products containing iodized salt.

Evaluation

Evaluate the effectiveness of drug therapy by confirming the patient goals and expected outcomes have been achieved (see "Planning").

UNDERSTANDING THE CHAPTER

Key Concepts Summary

68.1 Thyroid hormones contain iodine and stimulate the basal metabolic rate of nearly all tissues.

68.2 An accurate diagnosis of thyroid hormone dysfunction is based on the patient's symptoms and the results of diagnostic tests.

68.3 Hypothyroidism, or thyroid deficiency, can occur as a congenital or acquired disorder.

68.4 Hypothyroidism is treated by replacement therapy with thyroid hormone.

68.5 Hyperthyroidism, or Graves' disease, is an autoimmune disorder accompanied by ophthalmopathy and goiter.

68.6 Hyperthyroidism is treated with surgery or drugs that reduce the production of thyroid hormone.

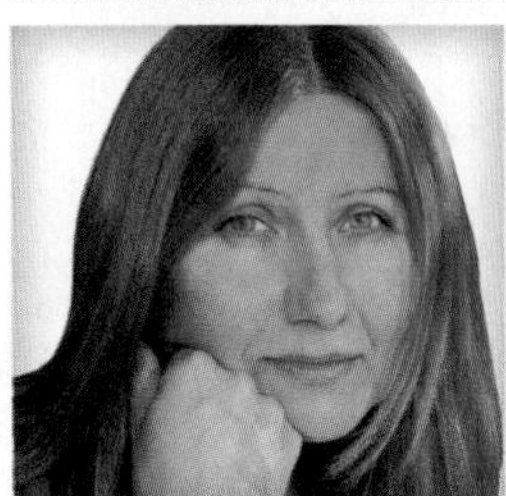

Making the PATIENT *Connection*

Remember the patient "Helen Mercado" at the beginning of the chapter? Now read the remainder of the case study. Based on the information presented within this chapter, respond to the critical thinking questions that follow.

Helen is a 42-year-old mother of three children, who works full time in a department store. She has been feeling tired, gaining weight, and says she feels cold all the time. Acting on her feelings that "something might be wrong," she goes to see her health care provider. Her vital signs at that time are: blood pressure 94/60 mm Hg, heart rate 58, temperature 36.3°C (97.4°F). Her weight has increased 13.6 kg (30 lb) from when she was last seen 6 months ago. She confirms that her appetite has decreased. After completing a physical examination, the health care provider orders some laboratory tests.

Critical Thinking Questions

1. As the nurse, what testing do you anticipate for this patient?
2. Based on the patient's symptoms, what test results would you anticipate?
3. Assuming that you are correct in anticipating the test results, what would be the treatment for this patient?
4. What patient teaching do you believe would be required for this patient?

Case Study

The nurse receives a new patient admission onto a cardiac unit: Mrs. James, a 72-year-old female, with new-onset atrial fibrillation with rapid ventricular response. The nurse connects the patient to a cardiac monitor, then obtains the following vital signs: blood pressure 168/96 mmHg, respirations 28/minute, heart rate 162 beats/minute, temperature 38.7°C (101.6°F). The nurse learns from the patient's daughter that the patient was recently diagnosed with Graves' disease, but that she has not been taking her medications.

1. What diagnostic tests do you expect to see ordered for this patient?
2. What drug therapy do you anticipate for this patient?
3. What long-term therapy do you believe is appropriate for this patient?

NCLEX-RN® Review

1 The client on replacement therapy with levothyroxine (Synthroid) reports feeling nervous and is having palpitations and tremors. The nurse recognizes that the reason for these symptoms is that the client:

1. Is experiencing normal adverse effects of therapy.
2. Now has normal thyroid function and the Synthroid is no longer needed.
3. Has developed a pituitary disorder and needs further evaluation.
4. Is experiencing a hyperthyroid state and the medication dosage needs adjustment.

2 Which of the following assessment findings would the nurse not attribute to the effects of thyroid hormone replacement therapy?

1. Constipation and weight gain
2. Increased heart rate and cardiac output
3. Decreased reports of fatigue
4. Decreased blood cholesterol levels

3 What condition would the nurse suspect in a client being treated with propylthiouracil who also has increased body metabolism, tachycardia, increased body temperature, and anxiety?

1. Graves' disease
2. Myxedema
3. Hashimoto's thyroiditis
4. Cretinism

4 Which of the following assessment findings would cause the nurse to withhold the regularly scheduled dose of levothyroxine?

1. A 2-lb weight gain
2. A blood pressure reading of 100/70 mmHg
3. A heart rate of 110
4. A temperature of 37.9°C (100.2°F)

5 The nurse knows that actions of propylthiouracil include: (Select all that apply.)

1. Inhibition of thyroid hormone synthesis.
2. Suppression of peripheral conversion of T_4 to T_3.
3. Increased breakdown of existing thyroid hormone.
4. Blockage of iodine absorption.
5. Decrease in the actions of anticoagulants.

6 In the administration of a drug such as levothyroxine (Synthroid), the nurse should teach the client:

1. That therapy typically lasts about 6 months.
2. That weekly laboratory tests for T_4 levels will be required.
3. To report weight loss, anxiety, insomnia, and palpitations.
4. That the drug may be taken every other day if diarrhea occurs.

See Answers to Critical Thinking Questions, Case Study, and NCLEX-RN® Review in Appendix A.

References

Corbett, J. V. (2008). *Laboratory tests and diagnostic procedures with nursing diagnoses* (7th ed.). Upper Saddle River, NJ: Prentice-Hall.

Farwell, A. P., & Braverman, L. E. (2006). Thyroid and antithyroid drugs. In L. L. Brunton, J. S. Lazo, & K. L. Parker. (Eds.). *The pharmacological basis of therapeutics* (11th ed., pp. 1511–1540). New York: McGraw-Hill.

Ferry, R. J., & Livitsky, L. L. (2008). *Grave's disease.* eMedicine. Retrieved August 26, 2008, from http://www.emedicine.com/PED/topic899.htm

LeMone, P., & Burke, K. (2008). *Medical-surgical nursing: Critical thinking in client care* (4th ed.). Upper Saddle River, NJ: Pearson Education.

Lenz, S. (2002). Toxicity study of an antidipsotropic Chinese herbal mixture in rats: NPI-028. *Journal of Alternative and Complementary Medicine, 8*(2), 175–183.

Michel, R. H., Neafsey, P. J., & Dzurec, L. C. (2003). Self-medication practices among patients taking levothyroxine. *Internet Journal of Advanced Nursing Practice, 6*(2), 9.

Shah, A. A., & Lettieri, C. J. (2007). *Endocrine emergencies.* Medscape. Retrieved August 26, 2008, from http://www.medscape.com/viewprogram/8373_pnt

Van Den Eeden, S. K., Barzilay, J. I., Ettinger, B., & Minkoff, J. (2003). Thyroid hormone use and the risk of hip fracture in women equal to or greater than 65 years: A case-control study. *Journal of Women's Health, 12*(1), 27–31.

Weir, F. A., & Farley, C. L. (2006). Clinical controversies in screening women for thyroid disorders during pregnancy. *Journal of Midwifery & Women's Health 51*(3), 152–158.

Zimmermann, M. B., Connolly, K., Bozo, M., Bridson, J., Rohner, F., & Grimci, L. (2006). Iodine supplementation improves cognition in iodine-deficient schoolchildren in Albania: A randomized, controlled, double-blind study. *American Journal of Clinical Nutrition, 83*, 108–114.

Zimmermann, M. B., Wegmuller, R., Zeder, C., Torresani, T., & Chaouki, N. (2004). Rapid relapse of thyroid dysfunction and goiter in school-age children after discontinuation of salt iodization. *American Journal of Clinical Nutrition, 79*, 642–645.

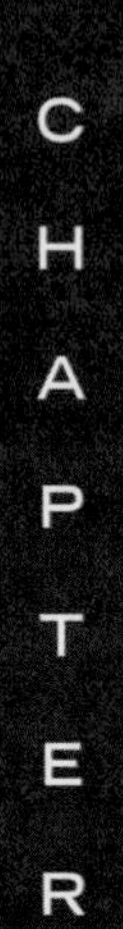

After reading information on the Internet about the adverse effects of my steroid inhaler, I'm really worried. But I can't breathe without it.

Patient "Charlie Harness"

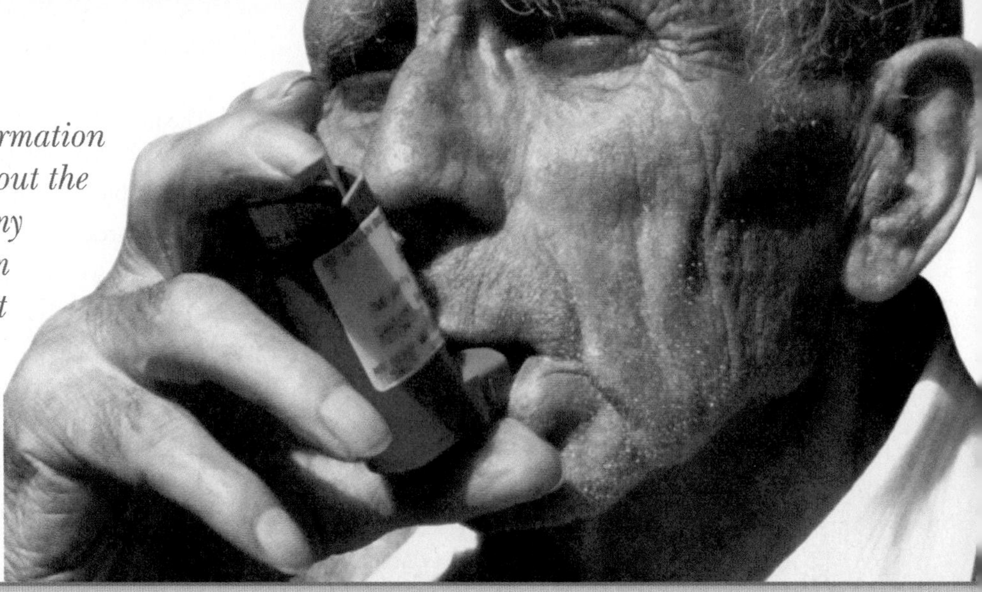

69 Corticosteroids and Drugs Affecting the Adrenal Cortex

Learning Outcomes

After reading this chapter, the student should be able to:

1. Identify the functions of the three major secretions of the adrenal gland.
2. Diagram the negative feedback regulation of corticosteroid secretion.
3. Identify common properties of the corticosteroid medications.
4. Describe the potential adverse effects of long-term corticosteroid therapy.
5. Compare and contrast the pharmacotherapy of acute and chronic adrenocortical insufficiency.
6. Describe how ACTH (cosyntropin) is used to diagnose adrenal disorders.
7. Explain how corticosteroids affect the inflammatory and immune responses.
8. Recognize nonendocrine disorders that respond to corticosteroid therapy.
9. Describe indications for pharmacotherapy with mineralocorticoids.
10. Explain the pharmacotherapy of Cushing's syndrome.
11. Describe the nurse's role in the pharmacologic management of adrenal disorders.
12. For each of the classes shown in the chapter outline, identify the prototype and representative drugs and explain the mechanism(s) of drug action, primary indications, contraindications, significant drug interactions, pregnancy category, and important adverse effects.
13. Use the nursing process to care for patients who are receiving drug therapy with corticosteroids and mineralocorticoids.

Chapter Outline

Physiology of the Adrenal Gland

Overview of Corticosteroid Pharmacotherapy

Adverse Effects of Corticosteroids

Replacement Therapy with Corticosteroids

PROTOTYPE **Hydrocortisone (Aeroseb-HC, Alphaderm, Others)** *p. 1166*

Corticosteroids for Nonendocrine Conditions

Mineralocorticoids

PROTOTYPE **Fludrocortisone (Florinef)** *p. 1170*

Antiadrenal Agents

Key Terms

Addison's disease, *1165*
adrenal atrophy, *1165*
adrenal crisis, *1165*
adrenocortical insufficiency, *1165*
adrenocorticotropic hormone (ACTH), *1162*
Cushing's syndrome, *1171*
glucocorticoids, *1162*
gonadocorticoids, *1162*
hyperaldosteronism, *1170*
hypoaldosteronism, *1170*
mineralocorticoids, *1162*

Though small, the adrenal glands secrete hormones that affect every body tissue. The primary secretions of the adrenal glands, the corticosteroids, are some of the most widely used drugs in medicine. They can be delivered by any route to treat conditions as diverse as dermatitis, lymphoma, ulcerative colitis, allergic rhinitis, and arthritis. This chapter examines the pharmacologic properties of corticosteroids that make them so important to pharmacotherapy.

Physiology of the Adrenal Gland

69.1 The adrenal glands secrete gonadocorticoids, mineralocorticoids, and corticosteroids.

Weighing only two tenths of an ounce, each pyramid-shaped adrenal gland sitting atop each kidney is divided into two major portions: an inner medulla and an outer cortex. The secretions from these two portions have very different functions.

The adrenal medulla secretes 75% to 80% epinephrine, and the remainder of its secretion is norepinephrine. Adrenal release of epinephrine is triggered by activation of the sympathetic division of the autonomic nervous system. Symptoms of the "flight or fright" response resulting from the secretion of these hormones are described in Chapters 16 through 20.

The adrenal cortex secretes three essential classes of steroid hormones: mineralocorticoids, glucocorticoids, and gonadocorticoids. Collectively, the mineralocorticoids and glucocorticoids are called corticosteroids or adrenocortical hormones. Although the terms *corticosteroid* and *glucocorticoid* are sometimes used interchangeably in clinical practice, the term *corticosteroid* technically refers to a hormone or drug that has both glucocorticoid and mineralocorticoid activity. The hormones secreted by the adrenal gland are illustrated in Figure 69.1.

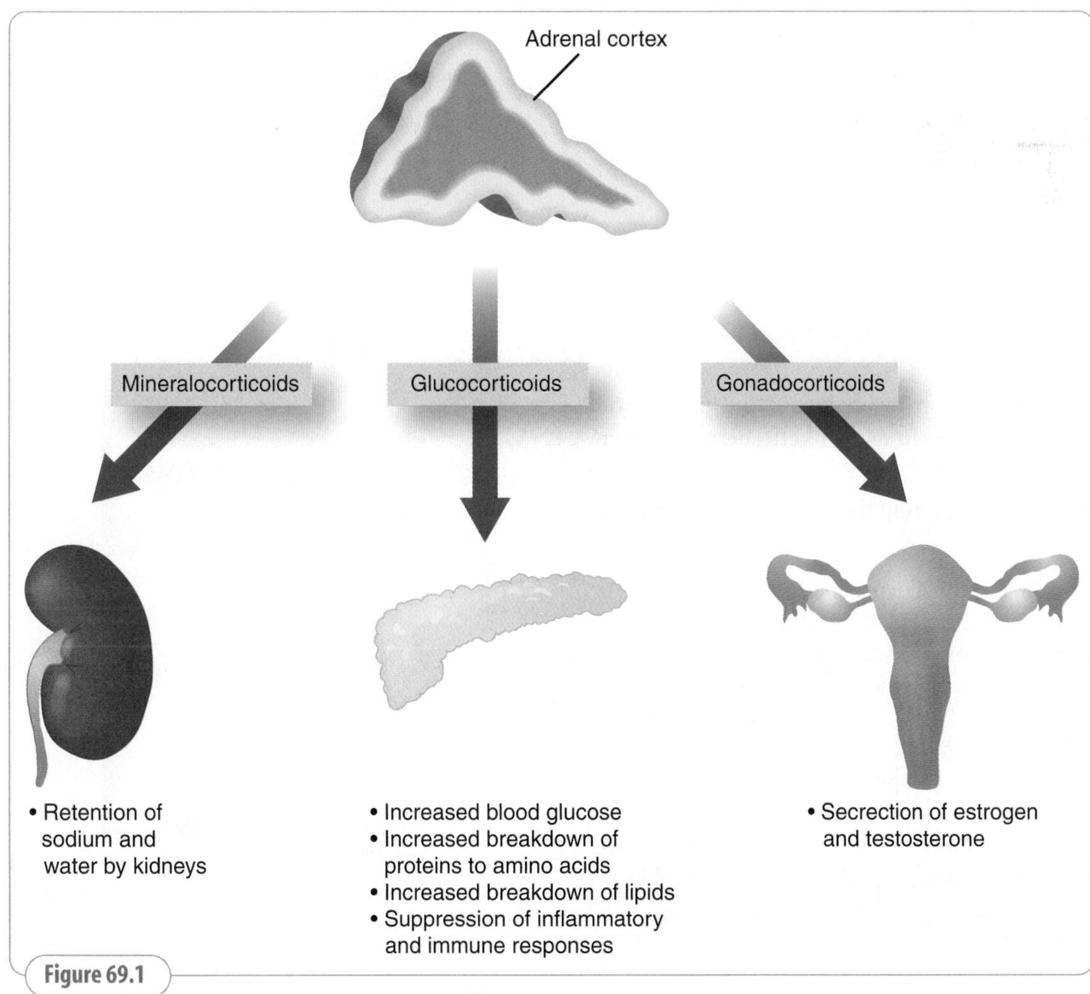

Figure 69.1

Hormonal secretions of the adrenal gland.

Mineralocorticoids: Aldosterone accounts for more than 95% of the **mineralocorticoids** secreted by the adrenal glands. The primary function of aldosterone is to conserve sodium and water and promote the excretion of potassium by the renal tubule, thus regulating plasma volume. Pharmacotherapy with mineralocorticoids is presented in Section 69.6.

Glucocorticoids: More than 30 different **glucocorticoids** are secreted from the adrenal cortex. Cortisol, also called hydrocortisone, is secreted in the highest amount, and is the most important pharmacologically. The liver converts hydrocortisone into cortisone, an active metabolite that is also available as a drug. Corticosterone is an additional steroid secreted by the adrenal cortex.

Glucocorticoids prepare the body for long-term stress and affect the metabolism of nearly every cell. The effects of glucocorticoids are diverse, and include the following:

- Increase the level of blood glucose (hyperglycemic effect) by inhibiting insulin secretion and promoting gluconeogenesis, which is the synthesis of carbohydrates from lipid and protein sources. This decreases glucose utilization by tissues and promotes the storage of glycogen in the liver.
- Increase the breakdown of proteins to amino acids. Amino acids are then converted to glucose and glycogen in the liver, resulting in protein depletion.
- Increase the breakdown of lipids (lipolysis). The fatty acids are then utilized as energy sources.
- Suppress the inflammatory and immune responses.
- Increase the sensitivity of vascular smooth muscle to the actions of norepinephrine and angiotensin II, thus modifying smooth muscle tone.
- Influence the central nervous system (CNS) by affecting mood and maintaining normal nerve excitability.
- Increase the breakdown of bony matrix, resulting in bone demineralization.
- Promote bronchodilation by making bronchial smooth muscle more responsive to sympathetic nervous system activation.
- Stabilize mast cells, inhibiting the release of inflammatory mediators.

As this list confirms, the glucocorticoids are essential hormones for maintaining homeostasis. When given as medications, some of the physiological actions of glucocorticoids in this list are considered therapeutic effects, while others are adverse effects. Unfortunately, it is impossible to totally separate therapeutic effects from adverse effects when drugs with such widespread actions are used in pharmacotherapy.

The physiological levels of glucocorticoids vary based on a circadian rhythm. The lowest serum levels occur during early sleep. Secretion rises during the night, with levels peaking at awakening and declining during the day, depending upon the needs of the body. Stress can cause a rapid increase in glucocorticoid levels; when faced with internal inflammatory or stressful conditions, the synthesis of glucocorticoids can increase to 10 times their baseline level.

Regulation of glucocorticoid levels begins with corticotropin-releasing factor (CRF), secreted by the hypothalamus. CRF travels to the pituitary where it causes the release of **adrenocorticotropic hormone (ACTH).** ACTH then travels via the blood to reach the adrenal cortex, causing it to release glucocorticoids. When the serum level of cortisol rises, it provides negative feedback to the hypothalamus and pituitary to shut off further release of glucocorticoids. This negative feedback mechanism is illustrated in Figure 69.2.

Gonadocorticoids: The **gonadocorticoids** or sex hormones secreted by the adrenal cortex are mostly androgens, though small amounts of estrogens are also produced. The amounts of adrenal sex hormones are far less than the levels secreted by the testes or ovaries during the reproductive years. Though their amount is small, the adrenal gonadocorticoids contribute to the onset of puberty and are the primary source of endogenous estrogen in postmenopausal women (see Chapter 70). Tumors of the adrenal cortex can cause hypersecretion of gonadocorticoids, resulting in hirsutism and masculinization, signs that are more noticeable in women than men. The physiologic effects of androgens are discussed in Chapter 72.

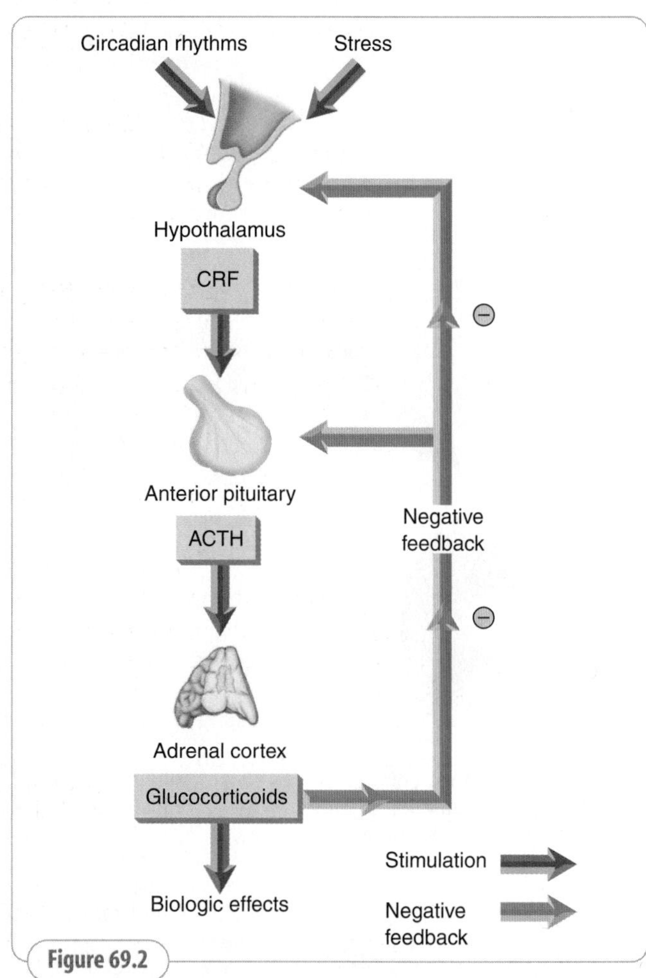

Figure 69.2

Feedback control of the adrenal cortex.

Overview of Corticosteroid Pharmacotherapy

69.2 Corticosteroids are widely used, and all drugs in the class have very similar indications, actions, and adverse effects.

Corticosteroids are some of the most widely prescribed medications because they are useful in treating conditions affecting nearly every body system. Furthermore, some of their indications are for diseases common to all age groups and for diseases that occur frequently in the population. Some are available over-the-counter (OTC) for self-treatment.

There are many ways to classify corticosteroids. One method is based on pathophysiology, such as grouping corticosteroids used for the treatment of inflammation, allergies, or neoplasia. Another method is to group the drugs by body system, such as corticosteroids used for skin conditions, immune disorders, or lung diseases. A third method is to look at corticosteroid use based on their pharmacologic actions, as shown in Table 69.1. In clinical practice, all methods are used.

Regardless of the method of classification, several general statements can be made about the corticosteroid medications:

- All act by the same mechanism.
- Most have the same indications.
- All have the same basic adverse effects, which are dose dependent.
- Indications and adverse effects vary by the dose, length of use, and route of administration.
- They are well absorbed when administered orally or parenterally, and widely distributed to all body tissues. Topical administration (intra-articular, inhalation, skin products, and ocular drops) results in systemic absorption, although at a slow rate.
- Most are highly bound to plasma proteins.
- All are metabolized by the liver and excreted by the kidneys.
- All have the potential to cross the placenta (pregnancy category C) and are secreted in breast milk. Use should be avoided during pregnancy and lactation.

TABLE 69.1 Actions and Indications for Corticosteroids

Pharmacologic Action	Indications
Reduce cell reproduction	Lymphomas and other neoplasms
Reduce joint inflammation	Rheumatoid arthritis, osteoarthritis, bursitis, tendonitis
Reduce lung inflammation	Asthma, chronic obstructive pulmonary disease (COPD)
Reduce skin inflammation	Dermatitis, psoriasis
Supply exogenous corticosteroids	Replacement therapy
Suppress allergic response	Allergic rhinitis; drug reactions
Suppress gastrointestinal (GI) inflammation	Inflammatory bowel disease
Suppress general inflammatory response	Systemic lupus erythematosus
Suppress immune response	Prophylaxis of transplant rejection Autoimmune hemolytic anemia
Suppress ocular inflammation	Conjunctivitis

More than 20 corticosteroids are available as medications, and the choice of a particular agent depends primarily on the pharmacokinetic properties of the drug. The duration of action, which is sometimes used to classify these agents, ranges from short to long acting. Some, such as hydrocortisone, also have mineralocorticoid activity and may cause sodium and fluid retention; others, such as prednisone, have no such effect. Some corticosteroids are available by only one route, such as topical for dermal conditions or intranasal for allergic rhinitis. An overview of the indications for corticosteroid therapy is shown in Table 69.1.

Adverse Effects of Corticosteroids

69.3 Long-term therapy with corticosteroids has the potential to cause serious adverse effects in multiple body systems.

Low-dose or brief-duration regimens of corticosteroids produce few adverse effects. On the other hand, high doses taken for prolonged periods offer a significant risk for serious adverse effects. These adverse effects of corticosteroid therapy are

CONNECTIONS

Complementary and Alternative Therapies Fish Oils for Inflammation

Description: Fish oils, also known as marine oils, are lipids found primarily in coldwater fish. These oils are rich sources of long-chain polyunsaturated fatty acids of the omega-3 type. The two most studied fatty acids found in fish oils are eicosapentaenoic acid (EPA) and docosahexaenoic acid (DHA).

History and Claims: Fish oils are sometimes used for their anti-inflammatory, antithrombotic, antidysrhythmic, and antihyperlipidemic properties.

Standardization: Fish oils are standardized by the amount of omega-3 fatty acids they contain. There is no standard dose; capsules may range from 300 to 2,000 mg.

Evidence: These fatty acids are known for their triglyceride-lowering activity and they also have anti-inflammatory actions (Oh, 2005). Several mechanisms are believed to account for the anti-inflammatory activity of EPA and DHA. The two competitively inhibit the conversion of arachidonic acid to the proinflammatory prostaglandins, thus reducing their synthesis.

Interactions may occur between fish oil supplements and aspirin and other NSAIDs. Although rare, such interactions might be manifested by increased susceptibility to bruising, nosebleeds, hemoptysis, hematuria, and blood in the stool.

well documented and can impact nearly any body system. The following list includes the most significant adverse events from long-term corticosteroid therapy:

- Immune response. Suppression of the immune and inflammatory responses increases patients' susceptibility to infections. Latent infections, such as herpesvirus or tuberculosis, may be reactivated during corticosteroid therapy. In addition, the anti-inflammatory actions of the corticosteroids may mask the signs of an existing infection.
- Peptic ulcers. Prolonged corticosteroid use is associated with the development of peptic ulcers, especially when these agents are combined with nonsteroidal anti-inflammatory drugs (NSAIDs). Both classes of drugs reduce prostaglandin synthesis in the gastric mucosa, which normally provides protection from the high acidity in the stomach. Use of proton pump inhibitors may reduce the incidence of peptic ulcers in these patients (see Chapter 60).
- Osteoporosis. Up to 50% of patients on long-term corticosteroid therapy will suffer a fracture due to osteoporosis. These drugs inhibit calcium absorption, suppress bone formation, and accelerate bone resorption—all actions that weaken the bony matrix. Treatment with a bisphosphonate may reduce the incidence of fractures in these patients (see Chapter 75).
- Behavioral changes. By an unknown mechanism, corticosteroids can induce psychological changes. These may be minor, such as nervousness or moodiness, or may involve hallucinations and increased suicidal tendencies.
- Eye changes. Cataracts and open-angle glaucoma are frequent adverse events of long-term corticosteroid therapy.
- Metabolic changes. Corticosteroids have a hyperglycemic action that raises serum glucose and can cause glucose intolerance, especially in patients with diabetes. Mobilization of lipids may cause hyperlipidemia and abnormal fat deposits. Electrolyte changes include hypocalcemia, hypokalemia, and hypernatremia. Fluid retention, weight gain, hypertension (HTN), and edema are other possible effects.
- Myopathy. Muscle wasting causes weakness and fatigue in many patients. The myopathy may involve ocular or respiratory muscles.

CONNECTIONS

Lifespan Considerations

Corticosteroids in Pediatric Patients

Children taking corticosteroids are of special concern. A child's growth rate may be impaired, ultimately resulting in the delay of puberty. Corticosteroids, such as prednisone, should be used with caution for long-term therapy in children since the drug can cause growth retardation, osteoporosis, avascular necrosis of the femoral heads, glaucoma, or cataracts during prolonged therapy.

Pediatric patients are more likely than adults to absorb topically-applied corticosteroids and experience adrenal suppression. Topical therapy should be conducted only when necessary.

CONNECTION *Checkpoint* 69.1

From what you learned in Chapter 44, what drug class includes drugs of choice for treating mild to moderate inflammation? See Answer to Connection Checkpoint 69.1 in Appendix A.

Corticosteroids interact with many drugs. Their hyperglycemic effects may decrease the effectiveness of antidiabetic agents. Combining glucocorticoids with other ulcerogenic drugs such as aspirin and other NSAIDs markedly increases the risk of peptic ulcer disease. Administration with certain diuretics may lead to hypocalcemia and hypokalemia.

A major goal during long-term corticosteroid therapy is to prevent the development of serious adverse effects. The following strategies are often used to minimize the incidence of serious adverse effects during therapy:

- Doses must be kept to the lowest possible amount that will achieve the therapeutic goal. In some cases, concurrent drug therapy with a noncorticosteroid may be implemented to produce additive therapeutic effects, while keeping the corticosteroid dose low. Careful monitoring of the effectiveness of the drug is necessary.
- Corticosteroids may be administered every other day (alternate-day dosing) to minimize adrenal atrophy (see

CONNECTIONS

To the Community Living with Corticosteroids

Due to chronic illness, many individuals can only manage their disease with the use of corticosteroids. The nurse can be instrumental in teaching the patient how to monitor for adverse effects. In addition, the nurse can aid the patient by providing a few ways to combat or minimize the adverse effects:

- Supplementing a healthy diet with calcium will help to keep bones healthy during a course of corticosteroids and reduce bone density loss.
- Many patients experience weight gain while on corticosteroids. Reducing salt intake can prevent adverse effects associated with fluid retention. Watching fat and calorie intake can help to minimize or prevent weight gain.
- Corticosteroids, when taken early in the day, may reduce adverse effects such as insomnia or night sweats. Corticosteroids may be taken with meals to prevent stomach upset.
- One possible adverse effect of corticosteroids is mood swings and irritability. When family and friends know about this adverse effect, they can provide emotional support when needed.

Section 69.4). This prevents constant, negative feedback on the pituitary and forces the patient's adrenal glands to secrete endogenous corticosteroids every other day.

- For acute conditions, patients are administered large doses of corticosteroids for a few days and then the drug dose is gradually decreased until discontinued. This prevents the severe symptoms of adrenal atrophy from developing.
- Whenever possible, corticosteroids should be administered locally by inhalation, intra-articular injections, or topical applications to the skin, eyes, or ears to diminish the extent of systemic effects. Local administration rarely produces systemic adverse effects.

Replacement Therapy with Corticosteroids

69.4 Adrenocortical insufficiency is treated by administering physiological levels of corticosteroids.

Lack of adequate corticosteroid secretion by the adrenal gland is called **adrenocortical insufficiency.** When pathology of the adrenal glands is the cause of the hyposecretion, it is called primary adrenocortical insufficiency, or **Addison's disease.** The most common etiology of primary adrenocortical insufficiency is the autoimmune destruction of both adrenal glands. Hemorrhage, infections, or metastases in the adrenal glands are other potential causes. Addison's disease is rare and includes a deficiency of both glucocorticoids and mineralocorticoids.

PharmFACT

One of the earliest symptoms of Addison's disease is hyperpigmentation of the sun-exposed areas of the skin, oral mucosa, and vaginal mucosa. This occurs because high ACTH levels stimulate melanocytes to produce excessive amounts of melanin. *Source:* Odeke & Nagelberg, 2006.

Secondary adrenocortical insufficiency occurs due to inadequate secretion of ACTH from the pituitary. If the adrenal gland is not receiving sufficient stimulation from ACTH, hyposecretion of corticosteroids will result. Low serum levels of both ACTH and cortisol are diagnostic of secondary adrenocortical insufficiency because this indicates the adrenal gland is not receiving ACTH stimulation. Secondary adrenocortical insufficiency is much more common than primary and can occur when corticosteroids are suddenly withdrawn during pharmacotherapy. Symptoms of primary and secondary adrenocortical insufficiency are the same because they are both characterized by inadequate corticosteroid secretion.

The onset of chronic adrenocortical insufficiency may take several months or even years before an accurate diagnosis is made. Symptoms include hypoglycemia, fatigue, muscle weakness, hypotension, increased skin pigmentation, and GI disturbances such as anorexia, vomiting, and diarrhea. Replacement therapy with corticosteroids is indicated. The goal of replacement therapy is to achieve the same physiological level of hormones in the blood that would be present if the adrenal glands were functioning properly. Patients requiring replacement therapy usually must take corticosteroids their entire lifetime, and concurrent therapy with a mineralocorticoid such as fludrocortisone (Florinef) is necessary.

Acute adrenocortical insufficiency has a sudden onset and usually occurs when corticosteroids are abruptly withdrawn from a patient who has been on long-term therapy. This is because constant, high amounts of corticosteroid medications provide continuous negative feedback to the hypothalamus and pituitary, shutting down the secretion of ACTH. Without stimulation by ACTH, the adrenal cortex shrinks and stops secreting endogenous corticosteroids, a condition known as **adrenal atrophy.** If the corticosteroid medication is abruptly withdrawn, the shrunken adrenal glands will not be able to secrete sufficient corticosteroids, and symptoms of **adrenal crisis** will appear. Symptoms of this condition include nausea, vomiting, lethargy, confusion, myalgia, arthralgia, fever, asthenia, acute abdominal pain, hypotension, seizures, renal failure, and coma. Immediate administration of IV hydrocortisone is essential because shock may quickly result if symptoms remain untreated. To prevent adrenal crisis, corticosteroids should be discontinued gradually. The mechanism of adrenal atrophy is illustrated in Pharmacotherapy Illustrated 69.1.

The most frequently prescribed corticosteroids for treating adrenal insufficiency are hydrocortisone, prednisone, and dexamethasone. Doses of these drugs are highly individualized to the specific amount of replacement therapy needed by the patient and doses will need to be increased during periods of high stress. Hydrocortisone and dexamethasone are administered by the intramuscular (IM) or intravenous (IV) routes for acute disease, or orally for maintenance doses. Prednisone is administered by the oral (PO) route. Because dexamethasone and prednisone have little or no mineralocorticoid activity, concurrent fludrocortisone therapy is necessary. Hydrocortisone has some intrinsic mineralocorticoid activity; therefore, concurrent administration of fludrocortisone may not be necessary. Doses for common corticosteroids are listed in Table 69.2.

Corticotropin (ACTH) is obtained from the pituitary glands of pigs or other mammals used for food by humans. Another ACTH drug, cosyntropin (Cortrosyn), is more widely used because it more closely resembles human ACTH. The primary use of these agents is to diagnose rather than treat adrenal disorders. Plasma levels of cortisol are measured just prior to, and 60 minutes after, administration of cosyntropin to determine if the adrenal gland responded to the ACTH stimulation. If plasma cortisol levels fail to rise after an injection of cosyntropin, the pathology is at the level of the adrenal gland (primary adrenocortical insufficiency). If the adrenal gland responds by secreting corticosteroids after the cosyntropin injection, the pathology lies at the level of the pituitary or hypothalamus (secondary adrenocortical insufficiency).

CONNECTION *Checkpoint* 69.2

From what you learned in Chapter 46, explain why immunizations are sometimes contraindicated in patients receiving high-dose corticosteroid therapy. See Answer to Connection Checkpoint 69.2 in Appendix A.

PHARMACOTHERAPY *ILLUSTRATED* 69.1

Corticosteroids and Adrenal Atrophy

1. Normal adrenal glands

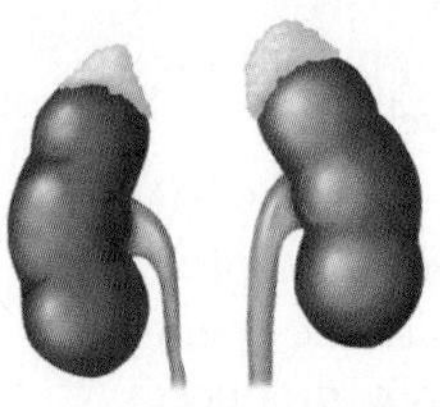

Corticosteroid Therapy

2. Adrenal gland atrophy following corticosteroid therapy

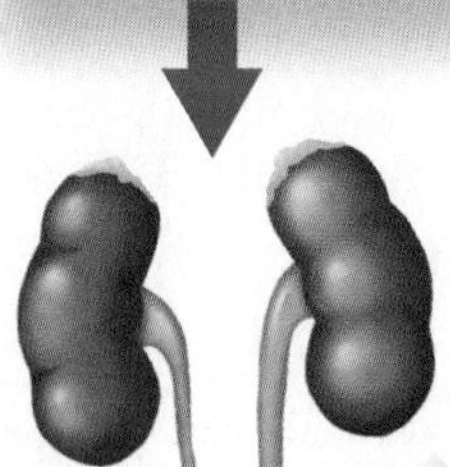

Gradual Discontinuation

Sudden Discontinuation

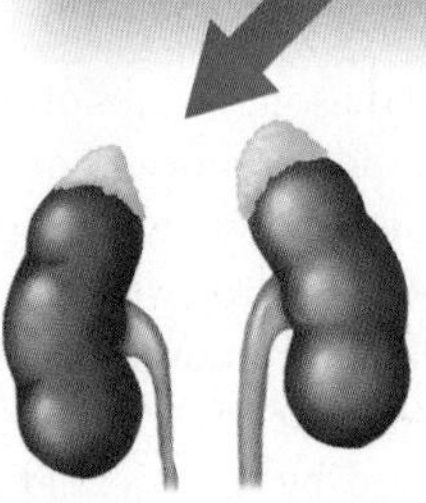

3. Gradual withdrawal of corticosteroids allows adrenal glands to resume normal function

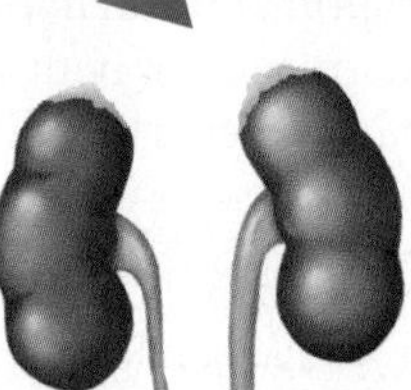

4. Sudden withdraw of corticosteroids leads to acute

- adrenal insufficiency
- hypotension
- lethargy
- renal failure
- asthenia
- nausea/vomiting

PROTOTYPE DRUG Hydrocortisone (Aeroseb-HC, Alphaderm, others)

Classification: Therapeutic: Adrenal hormone

Pharmacologic: Corticosteroid

Therapeutic Effects and Uses: Structurally identical to the natural hormone cortisol, hydrocortisone is a synthetic corticosteroid that is the drug of choice for treating adrenocortical insufficiency. When used for replacement therapy, it is given at physiologic doses. Once proper dosing is achieved, its therapeutic effects should mimic those of endogenous corticosteroids. Hydrocortisone is also available for the treatment of inflammation, allergic disorders, and many other conditions. Intra-articular injections may be given to decrease severe inflammation in affected joints.

Hydrocortisone is available in six different formulations. Hydrocortisone base (Aeroseb-HC, Alphaderm, Cetacort, others), and hydrocortisone acetate (Anusol HC, Cortaid, Cortef Acetate) are available as oral preparations, creams, and ointments. Hydrocortisone cypionate (Cortef Fluid) is an oral suspension. Hydrocortisone sodium succinate (A-Hydrocort, Solu-Cortef) is for parenteral use only. Hydrocortisone valerate (Westcort) is only for topical applications.

TABLE 69.2 Selected Corticosteroids

Drug	Route and Adult Dose (maximum dose where indicated)	Adverse Effects
betamethasone (Celestone, Betacort, others)	PO: 0.6–7.2 mg/day IM: 0.5–9 mg/day	*Mood swings, weight gain, acne, facial flushing, nausea, insomnia, sodium and fluid retention, impaired wound healing, menstrual abnormalities* <u>Peptic ulcer, hypocalcemia, osteoporosis with possible bone fractures, loss of muscle mass, decreased growth in children, possible masking of infections</u>
cortisone (Cortone)	PO: 20–300 mg/day in divided doses	
budesonide (Entocort, Pulmicort, Rhinocort)	Intranasal: 1–2 sprays in each nostril/day (each spray: 32 mcg) PO: 9 mg/day	
dexamethasone (Decadron, others)	PO: 0.25–9 mg/day in divided doses	
hydrocortisone (Cortef, Hydrocortone, others)	PO: 10–320 mg/day in 3–4 divided doses IV/IM: 15–800 mg/day in 3–4 divided doses (max: 2 g/day)	
methylprednisolone (Depo-Medrol, Medrol, others)	PO: 2–60 mg/day in divided doses	
prednisolone (Delta-Cortef, Hydeltrasol, Key-Pred, others)	PO: 5–60 mg 1–4 times/day	
prednisone (Meticorten, others)	PO: 5–60 mg 1–4 times/day	
triamcinolone (Aristocort, Atolone, Kenacort, Kenalog,)	PO: 4–48 mg 1–4 times/day	

Note: *Italics* indicate common adverse effects. <u>Underline</u> indicates serious adverse effects.

Mechanism of Action: The actions of hydrocortisone are complex and the drug is thought to act by multiple mechanisms in different tissues. As a replacement agent, it restores deficient levels of glucocorticoids and, to a lesser extent, mineralocorticoids. As an anti-inflammatory agent, it blocks the actions of various chemical mediators in the inflammatory and allergic responses, including histamine, prostaglandins, and kinins.

Pharmacokinetics:

Route(s)	PO, IV, IM, subcutaneous, rectal, intra-articular, topical
Absorption	Rapid
Distribution	Widely distributed when given PO or parenterally; crosses the placenta; secreted in breast milk; extensively bound to plasma protein
Primary metabolism	Hepatic
Primary excretion	Renal
Onset of action	PO: 1–2 h; IM: 20 minutes
Duration of action	1–1.5 days (PO or IM)

Adverse Effects: When used at low doses for replacement therapy, or by the topical or intranasal routes, adverse effects of hydrocortisone are uncommon. However, signs of Cushing's syndrome can develop with high doses or with prolonged use. Hydrocortisone possesses some mineralocorticoid activity, so sodium and fluid retention may be observed. A wide range of CNS effects have been reported, including insomnia, anxiety, headache, vertigo, confusion, and depression. Cardiovascular effects may include HTN and tachycardia. Long-term therapy may result in peptic ulcer disease, osteoporosis, hyperglycemia, cataracts, HTN, and impaired wound healing.

Contraindications/Precautions: Hydrocortisone is contraindicated in patients who are hypersensitive to the drug or who have known infections, unless the patient is being treated concurrently with anti-infectives. Patients with diabetes, osteoporosis, psychosis, liver disease, or hypothyroidism should be treated with caution. Patients with heart failure (HF) or HTN should be treated with caution due to the possibility of fluid retention with hydrocortisone. If taken for longer than 2 weeks, hydrocortisone should be discontinued gradually. Caution should be used in treating children because the drug may delay normal growth and development. PO corticosteroids must be used with caution in patients with preexisting GI disease such as peptic ulcers or ulcerative colitis because it may worsen these conditions. Use with potassium-wasting drugs such as thiazide or loop diuretics may increase the risk of hypokalemia. Anticholinesterase agents may produce severe weakness. Hydrocortisone may cause a decrease in immune response to vaccines and toxoids. Patients on high doses of hydrocortisone should not receive live vaccines due to the possibility of infection. Because hydrocortisone can cause hyperglycemia, doses of insulin and oral hypoglycemic drugs may require adjustment. Vitamin D supplements are recommended to prevent corticosteroid-induced osteoporosis. **Herbal/Food:** Use with aloe, senna, cascara, or buckthorn may cause potassium deficiency with chronic use.

Pregnancy: Category C.

Treatment of Overdose: Hydrocortisone has no acute toxicity and deaths are rare. No specific therapy is available and patients are treated symptomatically.

Nursing Responsibilities:

- Obtain a complete health history including allergies, drug history, and possible drug interactions.
- Obtain a complete physical examination, focusing on presenting symptoms.
- Obtain serum sodium and potassium levels, hematocrit and hemoglobin levels, blood glucose level, blood urea nitrogen (BUN), and creatinine levels.
- Obtain baselines and continue monitoring blood pressure, weight, fluid and electrolyte balance, and blood glucose.
- Monitor older adults and patients with low serum albumin because these individuals are especially susceptible to adverse effects.
- Recommend ophthalmoscopic examinations every 2 to 3 months, especially if the patient is receiving ophthalmic steroid therapy.
- Monitor for persistent backache or chest pain. Compression and spontaneous fractures of long bones and vertebrae are potential adverse effects.
- Monitor for changes in mood and behavior, emotional instability, or psychomotor activity, especially with long-term therapy.
- Assess for infections prior to initiation of therapy and during therapy. Be alert to the possibility of masked infections and delayed healing due to the immunosuppressive action of the drug.
- Adjust dosage if the patient is subjected to severe stress such as serious infection, surgery, or injury.

Patient and Family Education:

- Expect a slight weight gain with improved appetite. Report any weight gain increase of 2.3 kg (5 lb) per week or greater.
- Avoid alcohol and caffeine because they may contribute to peptic ulcer development during long-term therapy.
- Report symptoms of persistent heartburn or indigestion. Do not self-medicate with antacids or OTC preparations.
- Avoid aspirin or other OTC drugs unless prescribed specifically by the health care provider.
- Eat a high-protein, calcium-, and vitamin D–rich diet to reduce risk of corticosteroid-induced osteoporosis.
- Report slow healing, any vague feeling of being sick, or a return to pretreatment symptoms.
- Do not abruptly discontinue taking the drug. Doses should be gradually reduced to prevent withdrawal symptoms.
- Report any worsening of disease symptoms when the drug is being discontinued.
- Apply topical preparations sparingly in small children because they are more likely to experience adverse effects due to drug absorption.

Drugs Similar to Hydrocortisone (Aeroseb-HC, Alphaderm, Others)

There are many other corticosteroids, all having the same actions. In addition to hydrocortisone, prednisone and dexamethasone are most frequently used for adrenocortical insufficiency.

Dexamethasone (Decadron, Dexacort, others): Dexamethasone is a synthetic corticosteroid that has almost no mineralocorticoid activity. It is 20 to 30 times more potent than hydrocortisone and is available by PO, IV, IM, topical, aerosol, and ophthalmic routes. The parenteral formulations (dexamethasone sodium phosphate) are used for serious disorders such as anaphylaxis, reduction of cerebral edema, or acute adrenocortical insufficiency, or when oral therapy is not possible. Dexamethasone may be injected intra-articularly for the short-term therapy of inflamed joints or intralesionally into acute inflamed lesions associated with discoid lupus, psoriatic plaques, and granulomatous disorders. Systemic forms of the drug are metabolized by the liver to inactive metabolites. Dexamethasone has one of the longest durations of action of any drug in its class. This drug is pregnancy category C.

Prednisone (Deltasone, Sterapred, others): Prednisone is rapidly absorbed and is the most frequently prescribed corticosteroid for oral administration. It is about 4 times more potent than hydrocortisone and has a longer duration of action. It has little mineralocorticoid activity. Prednisone is a synthetic corticosteroid whose actions are the result of being metabolized to an active form, which is also available as the drug prednisolone (Delta-Cortef, others). Although prednisone is only available by the PO route, prednisolone may be administered PO, parenterally, or topically and may be of value in patients with liver impairment because it does not require hepatic activation. When used for inflammation, duration of prednisone therapy is commonly 4 to 10 days. For long-term therapy, alternate-day dosing is used. Prednisone is occasionally used to terminate acute bronchospasm in patients with asthma and as an antineoplastic agent for certain cancers such as Hodgkin's disease, acute childhood leukemias, and lymphomas. Prednisone has the same adverse effects and contraindications as hydrocortisone. This drug is pregnancy category C.

Corticosteroids for Nonendocrine Conditions

69.5 Corticosteroids are frequently used to suppress the inflammatory and immune responses.

One of the most important physiological effects of corticosteroids is their natural ability to dampen the immune response and inhibit the synthesis of inflammatory mediators. When used to treat conditions characterized by hyperactive body defenses, the anti-inflammatory effects of the corticosteroids are therapeutic. When the drugs are administered as replacement therapy, however, suppression of the immune response can result in an increased incidence of infections.

Part of the reason for the effectiveness of the corticosteroids in reducing inflammation and the immune response is that they act by multiple mechanisms. These mechanisms include the following:

- Decreased numbers of circulating lymphocytes, eosinophils, monocytes, and basophils
- Inhibited movement of macrophages and leukocytes to areas of inflammation
- Decreased production of inflammatory cytokines, including histamine, bradykinin, interferons, interleukins, and granulocyte-macrophage colony stimulating factor
- Decreased formation of prostaglandins

It is important to note that the doses necessary to treat inflammatory and other nonendocrine diseases are much higher than those used to treat adrenocortical insufficiency. For example, a daily maintenance dose of prednisone for a patient with Addison's disease is 7.5 mg/day. This amount approximates what would normally be secreted by the adrenal gland. Daily doses of prednisone for nonendocrine disorders range from 5 to 30 mg for transplant prophylaxis; 80 mg for chronic lymphocytic leukemia; 40 to 60 mg for Crohn's disease; and 20 to 300 mg for systemic lupus erythematosus. At these high doses, the adverse effects of corticosteroids will quickly manifest and the adrenal gland will begin to atrophy in only 2 to 4 weeks. It is essential that interventions be planned to prevent adverse effects, as discussed in Section 69.3.

Arthritis: Arthritis is one of the most common diseases affecting older adults. Rheumatoid arthritis (RA) is a chronic autoimmune disease that causes inflammation of joints and is characterized by disfigurement and inflammation of multiple joints. Osteoarthritis (OA) is also a progressive joint disease but it occurs with more advanced age and is characterized by less inflammation than RA. Both types of arthritis are treated with NSAIDs early in the course of the disease. Corticosteroids are administered when inflammation becomes severe, with therapy being limited to 1 to 2 weeks, or until the pain and inflammation subside. If the pain and inflammation is localized to one or two joints, intra-articular injections may be used. Corticosteroids offer only symptomatic treatment and do not alter the course of either type of arthritis. Arthritis pharmacotherapy is presented in Chapter 75.

Inflammatory bowel disease: Inflammatory bowel disease (IBD) is characterized by ulceration in the distal portion of the small intestine (Crohn's disease) or in the large intestine (ulcerative colitis). Various drugs, including the 5-aminosalicylic acid agents, are used to control inflammation, cramping, and diarrhea. Exacerbations are treated with corticosteroids for brief time periods. Budesonide (Entocort-EC) is a corticosteroid that is not absorbed and remains in the intestine to treat the inflammation locally, without causing systemic effects. IBD pharmacotherapy is presented in Chapter 61.

Asthma: Asthma is characterized by chronic inflammation that causes bronchoconstriction in the respiratory passages. Inhaled corticosteroids are drugs of choice for the prevention of asthmatic attacks and the management of chronic asthma. The inhaled agents produce few systemic adverse effects. Oral corticosteroids are used for the short-term management of acute asthma exacerbations. Asthma pharmacotherapy is presented in Chapter 73.

Allergies: Allergic rhinitis is inflammation of the nasal mucosa caused by exposure to allergens. Corticosteroids are applied directly to the nasal mucosa to prevent symptoms of allergic rhinitis. They have largely replaced antihistamines as drugs of choice for this condition. When administered intranasally, the corticosteroids do not exhibit systemic adverse effects. For acute allergies, corticosteroids may be administered parenterally. Because their onset of action is slow, however, they are always administered concurrently with other drugs, such as epinephrine, for this indication. The pharmacotherapy of allergic rhinitis is presented in Chapter 74.

Transplant rejection prophylaxis: Successful tissue transplantation requires the use of immunosuppressant drugs; otherwise, the patient's immune system would reject the transplant. One or more immunosuppressants are administered at the time of transplantation and are continued for several months following surgery. Corticosteroids are part of most therapeutic regimens to prevent transplant rejection. They may be used for several weeks or maintained for 3 to 6 months following surgery. The prophylaxis of transplant rejection is presented in Chapter 45.

Dermatologic conditions: Topical corticosteroids are the most effective therapy for treating the inflammation and itching of dermatitis. These corticosteroids are specially formulated to penetrate deep into the skin layers. Topical corticosteroids such as betamethasone (Diprosone) and hydrocortisone acetate (Cortaid, Caldecort, others) are also the primary, initial treatment for psoriasis. High-potency corticosteroids are used for 1 to 2 weeks, followed by moderate- to low-potency corticosteroids for maintenance therapy. The pharmacotherapy of dermatologic diseases is presented in Chapter 76.

Neoplasms: Corticosteroids such as prednisone (Deltasone, others) and dexamethasone are used as adjuncts in the treatment of certain neoplasms, especially acute childhood leukemias and Hodgkin's disease. They are always used in combination with other antineoplastics. The pharmacotherapy of cancer is presented in Chapter 58.

Edema: Corticosteroids are occasionally used to treat disorders characterized by edema. They have been used for many years to reduce intracranial edema associated with trauma, tumors, and cerebral ischemia. These hormones tend to stabilize capillary membranes. Their effectiveness in treating edema is controversial.

Mineralocorticoids

69.6 Patients with adrenal insufficiency often require replacement therapy with mineralocorticoids.

Aldosterone is the primary hormone regulating sodium and potassium balance in the body. Its actions on the kidney include increased resorption of sodium and water, and increased excretion of potassium. Regulation of aldosterone secretion is through activation of the renin-angiotensin-aldosterone system (RAAS). When plasma volume falls, the kidney secretes renin, which results in the production of angiotensin II. Angiotensin II then promotes aldosterone secretion, which in turn acts on the renal tubules to promote sodium and water retention.

Lack of adequate aldosterone secretion, or **hypoaldosteronism,** may be caused by a number of disorders. The three broad categories of hypoaldosteronism are as follows:

- **Decreased stimulation of the adrenal cortex.** Aldosterone secretion by the adrenal cortex is stimulated by the RAAS (see Chapter 34). Factors that inhibit renin release may cause hypoaldosteronism. Beta blockers, NSAIDs, and calcium channel blockers may reduce renin serum levels and suppress the stimulation of aldosterone secretion. Angiotensin-converting enzyme (ACE) inhibitors block the formation of angiotensin II, which is the normal signal for aldosterone secretion.
- **Hyposecretion of aldosterone.** Low aldosterone secretion may result from primary adrenal insufficiency (Addison's disease), which is usually a deficiency in the secretion of both glucocorticoids and mineralocorticoids. Heparin can also suppress aldosterone synthesis and secretion.
- **Aldosterone resistance.** The renal tubules may become resistant to the actions of aldosterone. Aldosterone resistance occurs during diseases of the renal tubules and may also result from therapy with spironolactone (Aldactone) or progestins.

Whenever possible, the cause of hypoaldosteronism should be identified and treated. In some cases, replacement therapy with fludrocortisone is necessary.

Excessive secretion of aldosterone, or **hyperaldosteronism,** is usually caused by a benign tumor of the adrenal gland. Also known as Conn's syndrome, symptoms include HTN caused by fluid retention, and muscle weakness due to hypokalemia. Surgical excision of the adrenal tumor is the treatment of choice for most patients; however, pharmacotherapy with spironolactone (Aldactone) may be of benefit in patients who are at high surgical risk. Spironolactone is a potassium-sparing diuretic that blocks the actions of aldosterone in the renal tubule. Spironolactone is featured as a drug prototype in Chapter 35.

CONNECTION *Checkpoint* 69.3

From what you learned in Chapter 34, name the two drugs classified as aldosterone antagonists and give their indications. See Answer to Connection Checkpoint 69.3 in Appendix A.

PROTOTYPE DRUG Fludrocortisone (Florinef)

Classification: **Therapeutic:** Agent for hypoaldosteronism
Pharmacologic: Mineralocorticoid

Therapeutic Effects and Uses: Approved in 1954, fludrocortisone is a PO corticosteroid with high mineralocorticoid activity that mimics aldosterone. Although it has some glucocorticoid activity, this action is minimal at therapeutic doses. It is approved for the treatment of adrenocortical insufficiency (Addison's disease) and for salt-losing forms of adrenogenital syndrome, a life-threatening congenital disorder that occurs during the first few weeks of life. It has been used off-label to treat neurogenic orthostatic hypotension.

Mechanism of Action: Fludrocortisone has the same pharmacologic actions as aldosterone. It acts on the distal renal tubule to promote sodium and water reabsorption, and increased urinary potassium excretion.

Pharmacokinetics:

Route(s)	PO
Absorption	Rapidly absorbed
Distribution	Distributed to most tissues; crosses the placenta; secreted in breast milk; highly bound to plasma protein
Primary metabolism	Hepatic to inactive metabolites
Primary excretion	Renal
Onset of action	Peak plasma level: 1.5 h
Duration of action	Half-life: 3.5 h

Adverse Effects: Most adverse effects of fludrocortisone are the result of excessive mineralocorticoid activity: sodium and fluid retention, edema, cardiomegaly, HTN, and HF. Excessive urinary loss of potassium may result in symptoms of hypokalemia: nausea, vomiting, prolongation of the QT interval, muscle cramps, and fatigue.

Contraindications/Precautions: Fludrocortisone must be used with caution if the patient has any disorders in which fluid accumulation could be hazardous, such as HF, HTN, and renal or hepatic impairment. Because the drug has glucocorticoid properties that could lead to immunosuppression, it should not be administered to patients with a known systemic fungal infection.

Drug Interactions: If used with drugs that cause potassium loss, fludrocortisone use will result in additive hypokalemia. Potassium-wasting drugs include thiazide and loop diuretics, and amphotericin B. Fludrocortisone should be used with caution in patients taking digoxin due to the potential for hypokalemia-induced digoxin toxicity. Concurrent use with androgens may cause additive sodium retention and edema. Fludrocortisone may affect glycemic control in diabetic patients; doses of antidiabetic drugs may need to be increased. **Herbal/Food:** Sodium intake should be monitored because high levels may lead to sodium retention.

Pregnancy: Category C.

Treatment of Overdose: Overdosage results in HTN, edema, and hypokalemia. Treatment is symptomatic. Potassium supplements may be beneficial.

Nursing Responsibilities:

- Obtain weight and intake and output ratio to monitor for possible onset of fluid accumulation, especially if the patient is on unrestricted salt intake and not taking a potassium supplement. Report weight gain of 2 kg (5 lb) per week.
- Monitor and record blood pressure daily and report drug-induced HTN to the prescriber.
- Monitor for symptoms of hypokalemia, which include lethargy, fatigue, weakness, discomfort in the legs while sitting still, confusion, and disorientation.
- Monitor for signs of overdosage (hypercorticism) which include psychosis, excess weight gain, edema, congestive HF, ravenous appetite, severe insomnia, and increase in blood pressure.
- Monitor for signs of insufficient dosage (hypocorticism) such as loss of weight and appetite, nausea, vomiting, diarrhea, muscular weakness, increased fatigue, and hypotension.

Patient and Family Education:

- Recognize the signs of potassium depletion associated with high sodium intake: muscle weakness, numbness; and fatigue, anorexia, nausea, and mental depression.
- Eat foods with high potassium content. Reduce sodium intake, if recommended by the health care provider.
- Immediately report swelling or decreased urinary output, which may result from fluid retention edema.
- Weigh self daily under the same conditions and report a steady weight gain of 2 kg (5 lb) per week.
- Report infection, trauma, or unexpected stress of any kind promptly when taking maintenance therapy.

Drugs Similar to Fludrocortisone (Florinef)

Fludrocortisone is the only drug in its class.

Antiadrenal Agents

69.7 Antiadrenal drugs may be administered to lower serum corticosteroid levels in patients with Cushing's syndrome.

Cushing's syndrome occurs when high levels of corticosteroids are present in the body over a prolonged time period. Although hypersecretion of these hormones can occur due to pituitary or adrenal tumors, the most common cause of Cushing's syndrome is long-term therapy with high doses of systemic corticosteroids. Signs and symptoms include adrenal atrophy, osteoporosis, HTN, increased risk of infections, delayed wound healing, acne, peptic ulcers, general obesity, and a redistribution of fat around the face (moon face), shoulders, and neck (buffalo hump). Mood and personality changes are common, and the patient may become psychologically dependent on the drug. Some corticosteroids, including hydrocortisone, also have mineralocorticoid activity and can cause retention of sodium and water. Because of their anti-inflammatory and immunosuppressant properties, corticosteroids may mask signs of infection. It is important to note that corticosteroids do not have anti-infective properties. Even though the patient may not exhibit signs and symptoms of infections, the microorganisms continue duplicating and spreading. This could result in a delay in the initiation of antibiotic therapy.

PharmFACT

Cushing's syndrome caused by adrenal or pituitary tumors has a peak incidence between the ages of 25 to 40 years and afflicts 5 times as many women as men. *Source:* Adler & Dipp, 2008.

Because Cushing's syndrome has a high mortality rate, medical intervention is necessary, with the primary therapeutic goal being to identify and treat the cause of the excess corticosteroid secretion. If the patient is receiving high doses of a corticosteroid medication, gradual discontinuation of the agent is often sufficient to reverse the syndrome. When the cause of the hypersecretion is an adrenal tumor or an ectopic tumor secreting ACTH, surgical removal is indicated.

The antifungal drug ketoconazole (Nizoral) has become a drug of choice for patients with Cushing's syndrome needing long-term therapy. This drug rapidly blocks the synthesis of glucocorticoids, lowering serum levels. Unfortunately, the falling glucocorticoid level signals the pituitary to release more ACTH. Eventually, the very high levels of ACTH may overcome ketoconazole's inhibition of glucocorticoid synthesis. Ketoconazole should not be used during pregnancy because it has been shown to be teratogenic and embryotoxic at high doses in animals. It also causes hepatotoxicity in some patients; liver function should be carefully monitored.

Mifepristone (Mifeprex) is a steroid that has antiadrenal and antiprogesterone activity. It does not affect estrogen or aldosterone synthesis. Mifepristone is a competitive antagonist at glucocorticoid receptors; it does not block the synthesis of glucocorticoids or decrease their amounts. Its primary use in medicine is as an abortifacient: The drug is pregnancy category X and will induce abortion if administered early in pregnancy. Mifepristone has been granted orphan drug status for the treatment of Cushing's syndrome.

Metyrapone (Metopirone) is an antiadrenal drug used for diagnostic purposes. A single dose is administered orally at midnight, and blood samples are taken 8 hours later. Levels of ACTH, glucocorticoids, and their metabolites are measured to see whether the adrenal glands responded to the inhibiting action of metyrapone. The drug inhibits glucocorticoid synthesis and it may be used off-label to treat Cushing's syndrome. Metyrapone is pregnancy category C.

For many years, aminoglutethimide (Cytadren) was used to suppress adrenal function. This antiadrenal drug was removed from the U.S. market early in 2008.

NURSING PROCESS APPLICATION

Patients Receiving Systemic Corticosteroid Therapy

Assessment	Potential Nursing Diagnoses
Prior to administration: • Obtain a complete health history including allergies, drug history, and possible drug interactions. • Obtain a complete physical examination, focusing on presenting symptoms. • Determine the reason the medication is being administered. • Obtain serum sodium and potassium levels, hematocrit and hemoglobin levels, blood glucose level, BUN, and creatinine levels.	• *Risk for Infection*, related to immunosuppression • *Risk for Injury*, related to adverse effects of drug therapy • *Deficient Knowledge (Drug Therapy)*

Planning: Patient Goals and Expected Outcomes

The patient will:

- Exhibit a decrease in the symptoms for which the drug is being given.
- Exhibit no symptoms of infection or adverse effects related to pharmacotherapy.
- Demonstrate an understanding of the drug's action, drug administration, and adverse effects.

Implementation

Interventions and (Rationales)	Patient and Family Education
• Monitor vital signs. (Blood pressure may increase because of increased blood volume and potential vasoconstriction effect.)	• Instruct the patient to report dizziness, palpitations, or headaches.
• Monitor for infection. Protect the patient from potential infections. (Corticosteroids increase susceptibility to infections by suppressing the immune response.)	Instruct the patient to: • Avoid people with colds or other infections. • Report fever, cough, sore throat, joint pain, weakness, and malaise. • Consult with the health care provider before receiving any immunizations.
• Monitor the patient's adherence with the drug regimen. (Sudden discontinuation of these agents can precipitate an adrenal crisis.)	Instruct the patient: • To never suddenly stop taking the medication. • In proper use of self-administering tapering dose pack. • To take oral medications with food.
• Monitor for symptoms of Cushing's syndrome, such as moon face, "buffalo hump," weight gain, muscle wasting, and increased deposits of fat in the trunk. (Symptoms may indicate excessive use of corticosteroids.)	Instruct the patient: • To weigh self daily. • That initial weight gain is expected; provide the patient with weight gain parameters that warrant reporting. • That there are multiple adverse effects to therapy and that changes in health status should be reported.
• Monitor blood glucose levels. (Corticosteroids cause an increase in gluconeogenesis and reduce glucose utilization.)	Instruct the patient to: • Report symptoms of hyperglycemia such as excessive thirst, copious urination, and insatiable appetite. • Adjust insulin dose based on blood glucose level as directed by the health care provider.
• Monitor skin and mucous membranes for lacerations, abrasions, or breaks in integrity. (Corticosteroids impair wound healing.)	Instruct the patient to: • Examine skin daily for cuts and scrapes and to cover any injuries with a sterile bandage. • Watch for symptoms of skin infection such as redness, swelling, and drainage. • Report any nonhealing wound or symptoms of infection.
• Monitor GI status for peptic ulcer development. (Corticosteroids decrease gastric mucus production and predispose the patient to peptic ulcers.)	• Instruct the patient to report GI adverse effects, such as heartburn, abdominal pain, or tarry stools.
• Monitor serum electrolytes. (Corticosteroids cause hypernatremia and hypokalemia.)	Instruct the patient to: • Consume a diet high in protein, calcium, and potassium, but low in fat and concentrated simple carbohydrates. • Keep all laboratory appointments.
• Monitor changes in the musculoskeletal system. (Corticosteroids decrease bone density and strength, and cause muscle atrophy and weakness.)	Instruct the patient: • To participate in exercise or physical activity, to help maintain bone and muscle strength. • That the drug may cause weakness in bones and muscles • To avoid strenuous activity that may cause injury.
• Monitor emotional stability. (Corticosteroids may produce mood and behavior changes such as depression or feeling of invulnerability.)	• Instruct the patient that mood changes may be expected and to report mental status changes to the health care provider.

Evaluation of Outcome Criteria

Evaluate the effectiveness of drug therapy by confirming that patient goals and expected outcomes have been met (see "Planning").

UNDERSTANDING THE CHAPTER

Key Concepts Summary

69.1 The adrenal glands secrete gonadocorticoids, mineralocorticoids, and corticosteroids.

69.2 Corticosteroids are widely used, and all drugs in the class have very similar indications, actions, and adverse effects.

69.3 Long-term therapy with corticosteroids has the potential to cause serious adverse effects in multiple body systems.

69.4 Adrenocortical insufficiency is treated by administering physiological levels of corticosteroids.

69.5 Corticosteroids are frequently used to suppress the inflammatory and immune responses.

69.6 Patients with adrenal insufficiency often require replacement therapy with mineralocorticoids.

69.7 Antiadrenal drugs may be administered to lower serum corticosteroid levels in patients with Cushing's syndrome.

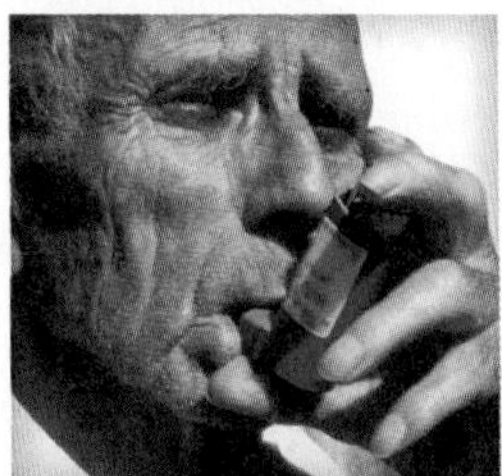

Making the PATIENT Connection

Remember the patient "Charlie Harness" from the beginning of the chapter? Now read the remainder of the story. Based on the information presented in this chapter, answer the critical thinking questions that follow.

Charlie Harness is a 71-year-old man with end-stage COPD. He was admitted to the hospital for severe exacerbation of his lung disease. It was doubtful that Charlie would leave the hospital alive when he was first admitted. His respiratory status was extremely poor. However, Charlie was eventually stabilized and began to improve. A few days before his discharge, the health care provider discussed treatment options with him. In consideration of his pulmonary status, Charlie and his family agreed that home hospice care would be the best alternative. He was subsequently discharged with multiple bronchodilators, analgesics, and corticosteroids. He was also referred to the hospice team.

Previously, Charlie had lived alone, but his daughter has taken a leave of absence from work to care for him in her home. Following 6 weeks of hospice care, you (the nurse) make a home visit. Charlie has done better than expected and is now able to sit up in a chair for short periods. His physical exam reveals that he is experiencing mild to moderate shortness of breath while receiving 2 L of oxygen per minute via binasal cannula. His pulse is 118 beats/minute, respiratory rate 36 breaths/minute, blood pressure 150/80 mmHg, and he is afebrile. The home pulse oximeter reading is 82%. His breath sounds reveal a prolonged expiratory phase and are distant. He denies abdominal distention or tenderness. However, you notice that Charlie has pitting edema in his feet and calves.

Since living with his daughter, Charlie spends much of his time surfing the Internet on a laptop computer. He has recently discovered information about steroids and expresses some concern about the information he has read. He is considering not taking his corticosteroids anymore.

Critical Thinking Questions

1. Create a list of questions you would ask Charlie to determine if he is experiencing any adverse effects from the corticosteroids.
2. What would you tell this patient related to abruptly discontinuing this medication? Why?
3. Charlie's daughter asks you if there are any precautions that should be taken related to corticosteroids. How would you respond?

Case Study

Monica Hamric, a 53-year-old patient, is referred to the endocrinologist for evaluation after being seen by the advanced practice nurse. She presents to the clinic with a history of weight gain, facial hirsutism but thinning of the hair on her head, spontaneous bruising, muscle weakness, and a recent diagnosis of diabetes. She is not taking any medications and has no significant past or family history. The physical examination reveals that Mildred has a "buffalo hump" and red striae in her abdominal and underarm areas. Her blood pressure is also elevated, measuring 162/100 mmHg. The health care provider has diagnosed Monica with Cushing's syndrome and prescribed ketoconazole (Nizoral). Describe the mechanism of action for this drug and what are the signs that indicate that she is experiencing hepatatoxicity?

NCLEX-RN® Review

1 The nurse should advise a client who is receiving parenteral hydrocortisone (Solu-Cortef) about the adverse effects of this medication, which include:

1. Fluid retention.
2. Tinnitus.
3. Urinary retention.
4. Stomatitis.

2 While the client is taking corticosteroids, the nurse will assess for:

1. Irregular heart rate and rhythm.
2. Delayed wound healing.
3. Weight loss of 2 to 3 lb per week.
4. Elevated serum potassium levels.

3 A client with chronic bronchitis is receiving high-dose corticosteroids. The nurse would include in the care plan to monitor which parameter to determine the presence of adverse effects?

1. Breath sounds
2. Blood pressure
3. Bowel sounds
4. Cranial nerve function

4 A client with adrenocortical insufficiency has started therapy with fludrocortisone (Florinef). The nurse performs what important intervention during the course of this treatment?

1. Weigh the client daily.
2. Evaluate the pulse oximetry hourly.
3. Measure the respiratory peak flow.
4. Calculate body surface area.

5 Which of the following assessment findings would indicate that the client taking fludrocortisone (Florinef) for adrenocortical insufficiency (Addison's disease) is experiencing adverse effects?

1. Tingling of the fingers and toes
2. Fluid retention and edema
3. Emotional instability and nervousness
4. Abdominal cramping and diarrhea

6 A client with chronic pulmonary disease is receiving high-dose corticosteroid therapy. The nurse performs what priority intervention during the course of this treatment?

1. Protect the client from sources of potential infection.
2. Teach the client how to self-monitor blood pressure.
3. Encourage ambulation and range-of-motion exercises.
4. Promote dietary intake of sodium-rich foods.

See Answers to Critical Thinking Questions, Case Study, and NCLEX-RN® Review in Appendix A.

References

Adler, G. K., & Dipp, S. L. (2008). *Cushing syndrome.* Retrieved September 1, 2008, from http://www.emedicine.com/med/topic485.htm

Andrioli, M., Giraldi, F. P., De Martin, M., & Cavagnini, F. (2007). Therapies for adrenal insufficiency. *Expert Opinion on Therapeutic Patents, 17*(11), 1323–1329.

Brown, R. L., & Weiss, R. E. (2006). An approach to the evaluation and treatment of Cushing's disease. *Expert Review of Anticancer Therapy,* 6, Supp 1, S37–S46.

Crown, A., & Lightman, S. (2005). Why is the management of glucocorticoid deficiency still controversial: A review of the literature. *Clinical Endocrinology, 63*(5), 483–492.

Diez, J. J., & Iglesias, P. (2007). Pharmacological therapy of Cushing's Syndrome: Drugs and indications. *Mini Reviews in Medicinal Chemistry, 7*(5), 467–480.

Greenspan, F. S., & Gardner, D. G. (Eds.). (2004). *Basic and clinical endocrinology* (6th ed.). New York: McGraw-Hill, pp. 339–401.

Griffiths, H., & Jordan, S. (2002). Corticosteroids: Implications for nursing practice. *Nursing Standards, 17*(12), 43–53.

Jabbour, S. (2006). *Systemic effects of oral glucocorticoids.* ACAAI 2006: Update on corticosteroids. Medscape. Retrieved September 1, 2008, from http://www.medscape.com/viewprogram/6432_pnt

Odeke, S., & Nagelberg, S. B. (2006). *Addison disease.* eMedicine. Retrieved September 1, 2008, from http://www.emedicine.com/med/topic42.htm

Oh, R. (2005). Practical applications of fish oil (omega-3 fatty acids) in primary care. *Journal of the American Board of Family Practice, 18* (1), 28–36.

Turner, M. O. (2008). Inhaled corticosteroids and pneumonia in COPD: An association looking for evidence. *Journal of Respiratory and Critical Care Medicine, 177*(5), 555–556.

CHAPTER

I get fatigued so easily. I'm having mood swings, headaches, bouts of depression, and irritability; but my main concern is that I have absolutely no desire to have sexual intercourse. What's happening to me, and what can I do about it?

Patient "Ileen John"

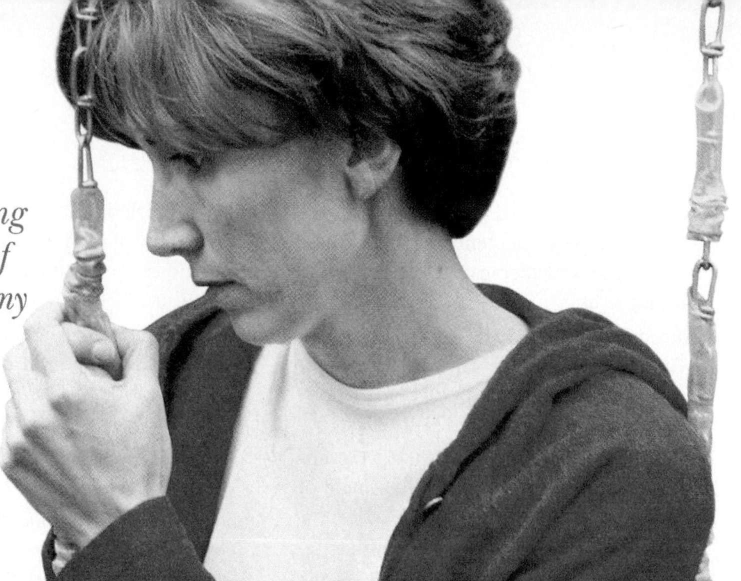

70 Estrogens, Progestins, and Drugs Modifying Uterine Function

Learning Outcomes

After reading this chapter, the student should be able to:

1. Describe the roles of the hypothalamus, pituitary, and ovaries in maintaining female reproductive function.
2. Describe the reproductive and nonreproductive effects of estrogen.
3. Discuss the uses of progestins in the treatment of dysfunctional uterine bleeding.
4. Compare and contrast the advantages and disadvantages of hormone replacement therapy during menopause.
5. Explain the use of uterine stimulants and relaxants in the treatment of antepartum and postpartum women.
6. Explain how drug therapy may be used to treat female infertility.
7. Describe the nurse's role in the pharmacologic management of disorders and conditions of the female reproductive system.
8. For each of the classes shown in the Chapter Outline, identify the prototype and representative drugs and explain the mechanism(s) of drug action, primary indications, contraindications, significant drug interactions, pregnancy category, and important adverse effects.
9. Use the nursing process to care for patients who are receiving drug therapy for disorders and conditions of the female reproductive system.

Chapter Outline

Hormonal Regulation of Female Reproductive Function

Estrogens

PROTOTYPE **Conjugated Estrogens (Cenestin, Enjuvia, Premarin)** *p. 1179*

Progestins

PROTOTYPE **Medroxyprogesterone Acetate (Provera)** *p. 1183*

Hormone Replacement Therapy

Uterine Stimulants: Oxytocics

Ergot Alkaloids

Prostaglandins

PROTOTYPE **Oxytocin (Pitocin)** *p. 1188*

Uterine Relaxants: Tocolytics

Magnesium Sulfate

Calcium Channel Blockers

Beta$_2$-Adrenergic Agonists

Pharmacotherapy of Infertility

PROTOTYPE **Clomiphene Citrate (Clomid, Milophen, Serophene)** *p. 1194*

Key Terms

anovulatory cycles, 1181
climacteric, 1184
corpus luteum, 1177
dysfunctional uterine bleeding, 1181
endometriosis, 1191
hormone replacement therapy (HRT), 1184
infertility, 1191
menopause, 1184
ovarian hyperstimulation syndrome (OHS), 1191
ovulation, 1177
ovulatory dysfunction, 1191
oxytocics, 1186
polycystic ovary syndrome, 1191
preterm labor, 1189
progestin, 1181
tocolytics, 1186

The steroid hormones estrogen and progesterone are responsible for the growth, development, and reproductive health of females throughout the lifespan. Deficiencies or excesses of these hormones can result in profound changes that go beyond the reproductive system. These hormones impact virtually every body system including effects on coagulation, blood vessels, bone, muscles, overall body metabolism, and behavior. Stimulating hormones from the pituitary also affect reproductive function, including fertility, labor, delivery, and the production and ejection of breast milk. This chapter examines hormones and drugs used to treat conditions associated with the female reproductive system.

Hormonal Regulation of Female Reproductive Function

70.1 Regulation of the female reproductive system is achieved by hormones from the hypothalamus, pituitary gland, and ovary.

The two primary hormones of the female reproductive system are estrogen and progesterone. During a woman's childbearing years, nearly all estrogen and progesterone is secreted by the ovaries. Small amounts of estrogen, however, are secreted by other organs, including the adrenal glands, liver, kidney, skeletal muscle, and adipose tissue. In postmenopausal females, nearly all estrogen and progesterone is secreted by nonreproductive tissues. In males, estrogen and progesterone are also secreted in small amounts by the testes.

Unlike males, who secrete steady and continuous levels of testosterone throughout adult life, secretion of the female sex hormones is variable and complex. Knowledge of these complexities is essential to understanding the pharmacotherapy of the female reproductive system. Although this section reviews physiology that is relevant to drug therapy, the student should refer to an anatomy and physiology textbook for more detailed information.

Secretion of female reproductive hormones varies on a 28-day menstrual cycle. The menstrual cycle is described by changes that occur in the ovaries (ovarian cycle) and in the lining of the uterus (uterine cycle). These cycles are controlled by hormones from the hypothalamus and pituitary. The first day of menstruation is considered day 1 of the cycle. The hormonal changes that occur during the ovarian and uterine cycles are illustrated in Figure 70.1.

The hypothalamus secretes gonadotropin-releasing hormone (GnRH), which travels a short distance to the pituitary to stimulate the secretion of the gonadotropins: follicle-stimulating hormone (FSH) and luteinizing hormone (LH). Both of these anterior pituitary hormones act on the ovary and promote the development of immature ovarian follicles. Under the influence of FSH and LH, several ovarian follicles begin the maturation process each month during a woman's reproductive years. As ovarian follicles mature, they secrete increasing amounts of estrogen. On approximately day 14 of the ovarian cycle, a surge of LH (and to a lesser extent FSH) secretion causes one follicle to expel its oocyte (egg), a process called **ovulation.** The LH surge is an absolute requirement for ovulation, and thus conception.

The ruptured follicle, minus its oocyte, remains in the ovary and is transformed into the **corpus luteum,** an endocrine tissue that secretes steadily increasing amounts of progesterone for the next 12 days. The progesterone thickens the uterine mucosa, readying it for implantation and potential pregnancy. The oocyte, on the other hand, begins its journey through the uterine tube and eventually reaches the uterus.

High progesterone and estrogen levels in the final third of the uterine cycle provide negative feedback to shut off GnRH, FSH, and LH secretion, as illustrated in Figure 70.2. Without stimulation from FSH and LH, estrogen and progesterone levels fall sharply, the endometrium is shed, and menstrual bleeding begins a new monthly cycle.

Estrogens

70.2 Estrogens are administered as replacement therapy, to prevent contraception, and for certain neoplasms.

Estrogen is actually a general term for three different steroid hormones: estradiol, estrone, and estriol. The largest amount of estrogen is present as estradiol. Estrogens are responsible for the maturation of the reproductive organs and for the appearance of the secondary sex characteristics of the female during puberty. When women enter menopause at approximately age 50 to 55, the secretion of estrogen by the ovaries diminishes and eventually stops.

Apart from its effects on reproductive functions, estrogen also affects the heart, liver, blood vessels, and bones. Estrogen decreases the levels of low-density lipoprotein (LDL) and increases the amount of high-density lipoprotein (HDL) in the blood. These effects are cardioprotective and help lower the risk of myocardial infarction (MI) in premenopausal women. By blocking resorption of the bony matrix, estrogen causes bones to grow longer and stronger in younger women. The risk of osteoporosis dramatically increases as estrogen levels decrease in postmenopausal women.

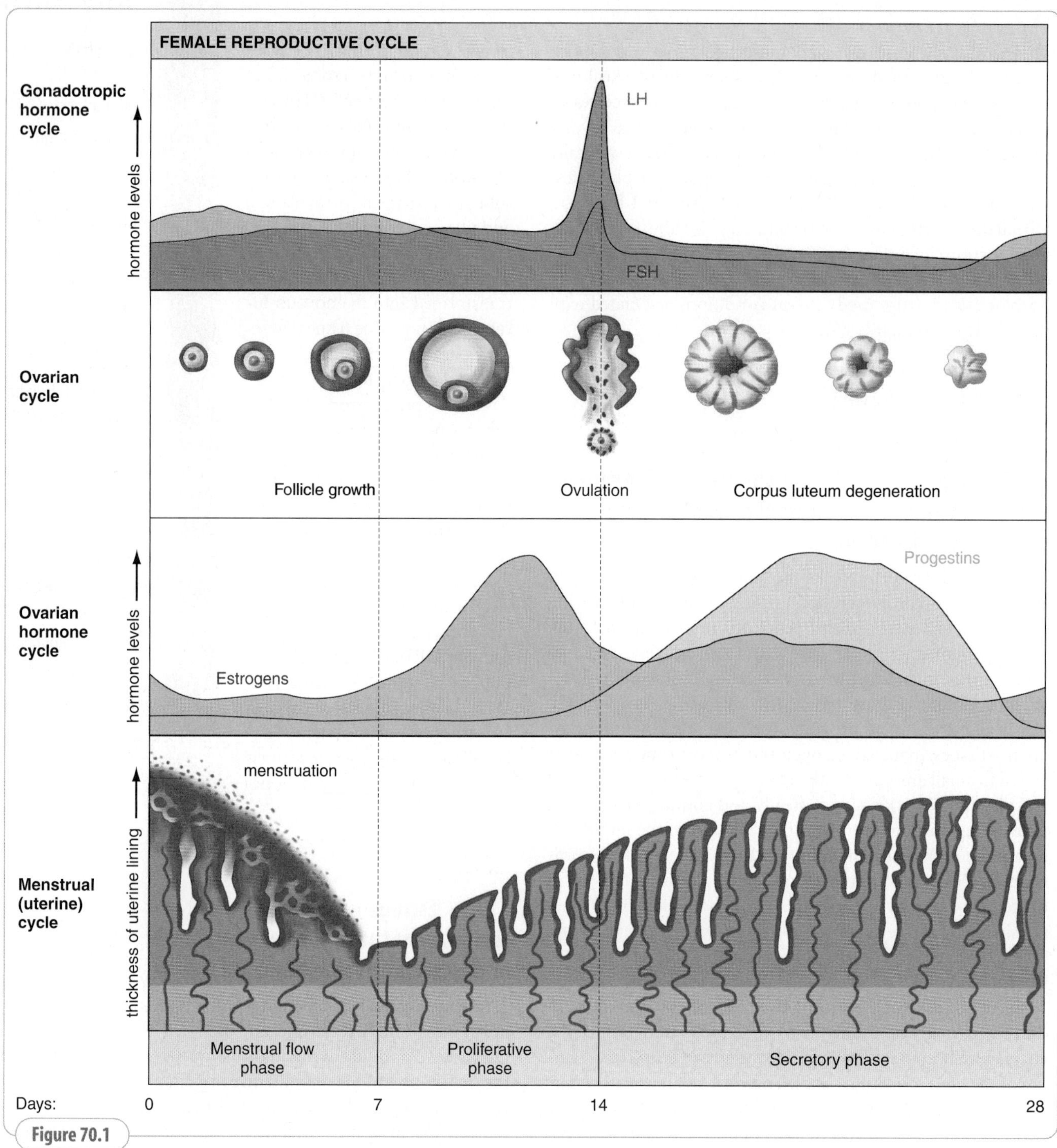

Figure 70.1

Hormonal changes during the ovarian and uterine cycles.

Estrogens are used to treat menopausal symptoms, female hypogonadism, primary ovarian failure, and as contraception. When used as replacement therapy following surgical removal of the ovaries, estrogen is usually combined with a progestin. The purpose of the progestin is to counteract some of the adverse effects of estrogen on the uterus. The use of estrogen in hormone replacement therapy (HRT) is discussed in Section 70.4. The contraceptive uses are presented in Chapter 70. Estrogen drugs are listed in Table 70.1.

High doses of estrogens are sometimes used to treat prostate and breast cancer. Prostate cancer is usually dependent on androgens for growth. Administration of estrogens will suppress androgen secretion. As an antineoplastic hormone, estrogen is rarely used alone. It is one of many agents used in combination for the chemotherapy of cancer.

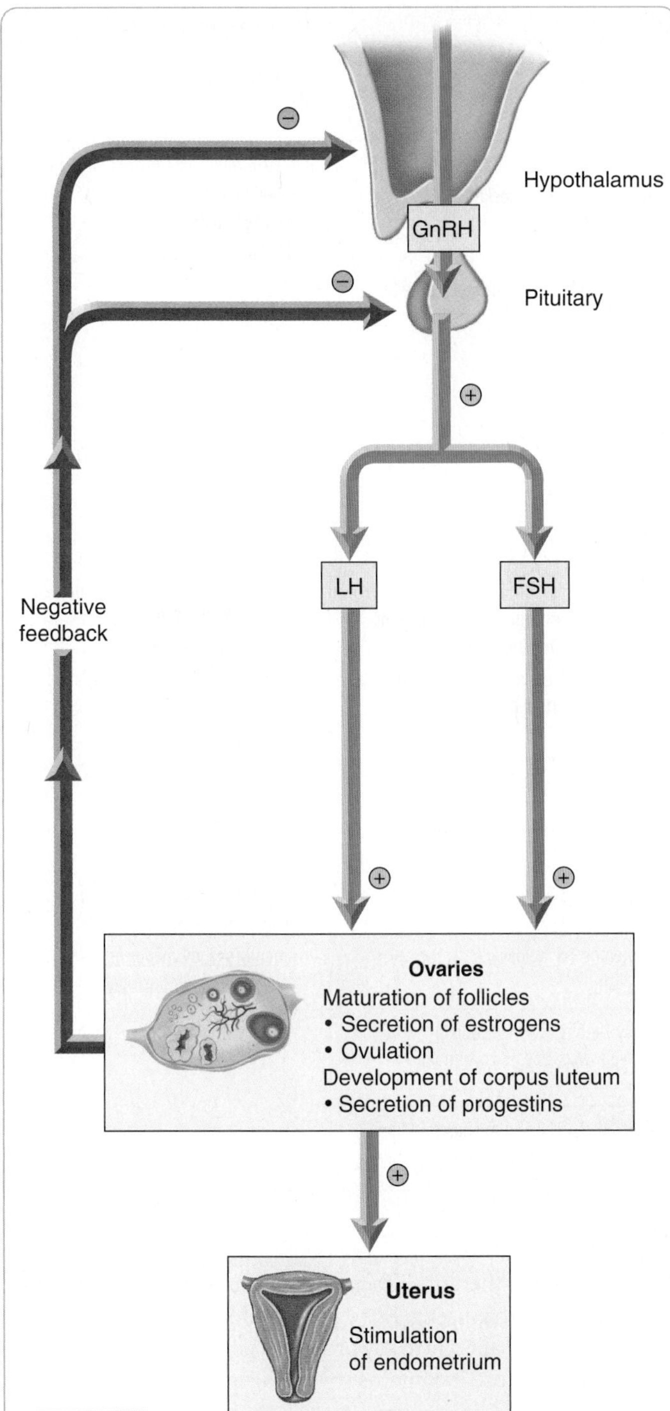

Figure 70.2

Negative feedback control of the female reproductive hormones.

PROTOTYPE DRUG Conjugated estrogens (Cenestin, Enjuvia, Premarin)

Classification: Therapeutic: Hormone

Pharmacologic: Estrogen

Therapeutic Effects and Uses: Conjugated estrogen, equine (Premarin) was approved in 1938 and contains a mixture of different natural estrogens, traditionally obtained from pregnant mares' urine. Conjugated estrogen, A (Cenestin), and conjugated estrogen, B (Enjuvia), contain a mixture of 9 to 10 different synthetic plant estrogens.

The primary indication for conjugated estrogens has been to treat moderate to severe symptoms of menopause caused by diminished estrogen secretion by the ovaries. Other replacement therapies include treatment of female hypogonadism and use after oophorectomy. The drug is approved for the palliative treatment of inoperable prostate cancer. Conjugated estrogens have been used in the past for osteoporosis prophylaxis in postmenopausal women but safer therapies have replaced these drugs for this indication.

Conjugated estrogens are usually administered by the oral (PO) route. For dysfunctional uterine bleeding, they may be administered by the intramuscular (IM) or intravenous (IV) routes. A topical cream is available to treat atrophic vaginitis or vulvar atrophy, which may occur during menopause.

Mechanism of Action: Conjugated estrogens bind to intracellular estrogen receptors that stimulate deoxyribonucleic acid (DNA) and ribonucleic acid (RNA) to synthesize proteins responsible for the biologic effects of estrogens.

Pharmacokinetics:

Route(s)	PO, IM, IV, intravaginal
Absorption	Rapid absorption from the gastrointestinal (GI) tract, readily absorbed through the skin and mucous membranes, slow absorption through IM injections
Distribution	Widely distributed; crosses the placenta; secreted in breast milk; bound primarily to albumin
Primary metabolism	Hepatic metabolism by CYP3A4 to estrone, estradiol, and estriol
Primary excretion	Renal
Onset of action	PO: 30–60 minutes; IM: 15–30 minutes
Duration of action	Half-life: 4–18 h

Adverse Effects: The most frequently reported adverse effects of conjugated estrogens include headache, infections, abdominal cramps and bloating, breast tenderness, and vaginal bleeding. Other less common adverse effects may include thromboembolic events, fluid retention, edema, acute pancreatitis, appetite changes, skin eruptions, mental depression, decreased or increased libido, fatigue, nervousness, and weight gain. The risk of dementia is increased in women older than age 65. Effects are dose dependent.

Estrogens, when used alone, have been associated with a higher risk of endometrial cancer in postmenopausal women (see Section 70.4). Although adding a progestin may exert a protective effect by lowering the risk of uterine cancer, recent studies suggest that progestin may increase the risk of breast cancer following long-term use. The risks of adverse effects increase in patients over age 35.

Contraindications/Precautions: Estrogens should be avoided in patients who have a history of breast cancer, cervical cancer, endometrial cancer, endometrial hyperplasia, prostate cancer, and hepatic diseases or cancer. Additionally, because estrogens

MyNursingKit | Mechanism of Action Animation: Estradiol

TABLE 70.1 Selected Estrogens and Progestins

Drug	Route and Adult Dose (maximum dose where indicated)	Adverse Effects
Estrogens		
estradiol (Climara, Estraderm, Estrace, Vivelle, others)	PO: 0.5–2 mg daily Transdermal patch: 1 patch either once weekly (Climara) or twice weekly (0.025–0.1 mg/day) Topical gel: Approximately 1.25 g/day Intravaginal cream: Insert 2–4 g/day for 2 weeks, then reduce to ½ the initial dose for 2 weeks, then use 1 g 1–3 times/week	*Breakthrough bleeding, spotting, breast tenderness, libido changes* <u>HTN, gallbladder disease, thromboembolic disorders, increased endometrial cancer risk</u>
estradiol valerate (Delestrogen, Duragen-10, Valergen)	IM: 10–20 mg every for 4 weeks	
estrogen, conjugated (Cenestin, Enjuvia, Premarin)	PO: 0.3–1.25 mg daily for 21 days each month	
estropipate (Ogen)	PO: 0.75–6 mg daily for 21 days each month	
Progestins		
medroxyprogesterone (Depot Provera, depo-subQ-Provera, Provera, Cycrin)	PO: 5–10 mg daily on days 1–12 of menstrual cycle IM (Depo-Provera): 150 mg daily for 3 months. Give first dose during the first 5 days of the menstrual period or within the first 5 days postpartum if not breast-feeding. Subcutaneous (depo-subQ-Provera); 104 mg daily for 3 months. Give first dose during the first 5 days of the menstrual period or at the sixth week postpartum if not breastfeeding	*Breakthrough bleeding, spotting, breast tenderness, weight gain* <u>Amenorrhea, dysmenorrhea, depression, thromboembolic disorders</u>
progesterone (Crinone, Endometrin, Prochieve, Prometrium)	Amenorrhea or functional uterine bleeding: IM: 5–10 mg/day Assisted reproductive technology: Intravaginal: 90 mg gel once daily or 100 mg tablets 2–3 times/day	
Estrogen–Progestin Combinations		
conjugated estrogens, equine/medroxyprogesterone (Premphase, Prempro)	PO: Premphase: Estrogen 0.625 mg/daily on days 1–28; add 5 mg medroxyprogesterone daily on days 15–28. PO: Prempro: Estrogen 0.3 mg and medroxyprogesterone 1.5 mg daily Intravaginal Cream: Insert ½ to 2 g daily for 3–6 months	*Breakthrough bleeding, spotting, breast tenderness, weight gain* <u>Amenorrhea, dysmenorrhea, depression, thromboembolic disorders, HTN</u>
estradiol/norgestimate (Prefest)	PO: 1 tablet of 1 mg estradiol for 3 days, followed by 1 tablet of 1 mg estradiol combined with 0.09 mg norgestimate for 3 days. Regimen is repeated continuously without interruption.	
ethinyl estradiol/norethindrone acetate (Activella)	PO: 1 tablet daily, which contains 0.5–0.1 mg of estradiol and 0.5–1 mg norethindrone Transdermal patch: 1 patch, twice weekly	

Note: *Italics* indicate common adverse effects. <u>Underline</u> indicates serious adverse effects.

have been associated with thromboembolic disorders, hypercalcemia and lupus, they should not be prescribed without a thorough investigation of these conditions. Estrogens should be used with caution in patients with lipid disorders because they may increase HDL cholesterol and triglycerides. They are contraindicated in patients with undiagnosed vaginal bleeding. Since estrogens are classified as category X, pregnancy and lactation are contraindications for this drug.

Drug Interactions: Estrogen is metabolized by CYP450 enzymes and may interact with other drugs metabolized in the liver. Interactions include a decreased effect of tamoxifen, enhanced corticosteroid effects, and decreased effects of anticoagulants, especially warfarin. The effects of estrogen may be decreased if taken with barbiturates or rifampin and there is a possible increased effect of tricyclic antidepressants if taken with estrogens. **Herbal/Food:** St. John's wort, red clover, and black cohosh have weak estrogenic effects and may interfere with estrogen therapy. Effects of estrogen may be enhanced if combined with ginseng. Estrogen may decrease the absorption of folic acid. If allergic to soy products, patients should not take Cenestin because it contains soy estrogens.

Pregnancy: Category X.

Treatment of Overdose: Overdose will cause nausea, vomiting, and breakthrough bleeding, which are treated symptomatically.

Nursing Responsibilities:

- Obtain a complete health history including personal or familial history of breast cancer, gallbladder disease, diabetes mellitus, liver, or kidney disease.
- Obtain a drug history to determine possible drug interactions and allergies.
- Assess cardiovascular status including history of hypertension (HTN), MI, cerebrovascular accident (CVA), and thromboembolic disease.

- Determine if the patient is pregnant or lactating prior to drug administration.
- For intravaginal administration, be sure to apply gloves and to wash hands thoroughly before and after application. Use the calibrated dosage applicator dispensed with the cream.
- Advise the prescriber immediately of adverse symptoms such as breakthrough bleeding, excessive fluid retention, leg cramps, vomiting, diarrhea, or bloating.
- Monitor for and report possible signs of thrombophlebitis: redness, pain, and swelling of the calf.
- Inject medication slowly into deep muscle mass. Rotate the injection site.
- Monitor serum phosphatase levels when drug is given for prostate cancer.
- Monitor bone density annually.

Patient and Family Education:

- If depression develops, discontinue the drug and notify the health care provider.
- Take this drug exactly as prescribed. Do not omit, increase, or decrease doses without approval of the health care provider.
- Do not use tampons while using vaginal cream therapy.
- Immediately report any calf pain or redness, dyspnea, and chest pain because these may indicate blood clots.
- Avoid acidic beverages 1 to 2 hours before oral administration because these will destroy the drug.
- Do not breast-feed while taking this drug without the approval of the health care provider.
- Perform a monthly breast self-examination (BSE).
- Do not take any other prescription or nonprescription drugs, dietary supplements, or herbal products without approval of the health care provider.
- Take blood pressure readings periodically and report significant changes to the health care provider.
- Avoid smoking and attend a smoking cessation program if appropriate, because smoking significantly increases the risk for blood clots.

Drugs Similar to Conjugated Estrogens (Cenestin, Enjuvia, Premarin)

Diethylstilbestrol (DES) is a synthetic estrogen used to treat inoperable breast and prostate cancer but it is rarely used.

CONNECTION *Checkpoint* 70.1

The majority of drugs in this chapter are pregnancy category X. From what you learned in Chapter 10, what is the difference between a category D drug and a category X drug? See Answer to Connection Checkpoint 70.1 in Appendix A.

Progestins

70.3 Progestins are administered to treat dysfunctional uterine bleeding, to prevent contraception, and for certain neoplasms.

The general term **progestin** refers to synthetic hormones that have actions identical to natural, endogenous progesterone. In combination with estrogen, progesterone promotes breast development and regulates the monthly changes of the uterine cycle. Under the influence of estrogen and progesterone, the uterine endometrium becomes vascular and thickens in preparation for receiving a fertilized egg. If implantation does not occur, levels of progesterone fall dramatically and menses begins. If pregnancy does occur, the ovary will continue to secrete progesterone, maintaining a healthy endometrium until the placenta develops sufficiently to begin producing the hormone.

Whereas the function of estrogen is to cause proliferation of the endometrium, progesterone limits and stabilizes endometrial growth. Progestins are drugs of choice for treating uterine abnormalities. They are also a component of HRT (see Section 70.4) and may be used as contraceptives (see Chapter 71).

The primary noncontraception indication for progestins is **dysfunctional uterine bleeding,** a condition in which hemorrhage occurs on a noncyclic basis or in abnormal amounts. Dysfunctional uterine bleeding is common in adolescents and menopausal women, and is often associated with **anovulatory cycles.** Anovulatory cycles are those that occur without ovulation.

CONNECTIONS

To the Community Estrogen Use and Psychosocial Issues

Because certain undesirable adverse effects may occur with estrogen use, the nurse should describe them to the patient prior to implementation of drug therapy. The nurse can explore the patient's reaction to these potential risks. The nurse should also assess the patient's emotional support system before initiating drug therapy. Hirsutism, loss of hair, or a deepening of the voice can occur in the female patient. The male patient may develop secondary female characteristics such as a higher voice, lack of body hair, and increased breast size. Impotence may also develop and is typically a concern for many men.

Patients should be taught that these adverse effects are reversible and may subside with adjustment of dosage or discontinuation of estrogen therapy. This knowledge may allow both male and female patients to remain adherent when adverse effects occur. During therapy, patients may need emotional support to assist in dealing with these body image issues. The nurse can encourage this support, discuss these issues with family members, and refer patients for counseling. The nurse can refer the female patient to an aesthetician for hair removal or wig fitting. The male patient and his sexual partner may need a referral to deal with issues surrounding impotence and its effect on their relationship.

NURSING PROCESS APPLICATION

Patients Receiving Estrogen Therapy

Assessment

Prior to administration:

- Obtain a complete health history including personal or familial history of breast cancer, gallbladder disease, diabetes mellitus, liver, or kidney disease.
- Obtain a drug history to determine possible drug interactions and allergies.
- Assess cardiovascular status including HTN, history of MI, CVA, and thromboembolic disease.
- Determine if the patient is pregnant or lactating.

Potential Nursing Diagnoses

- *Excess Fluid Volume*, related to edema secondary to adverse effect of drug
- *Ineffective Tissue Perfusion (Cardiopulmonary, Cerebral)*
- *Ineffective Tissue Perfusion, Peripheral*

Planning: Patient Goals and Expected Outcomes

The patient will:

- Report relief from symptoms of menopause.
- Demonstrate an understanding of the drug's action by accurately describing drug adverse effects and precautions.
- Immediately report such effects as symptoms of thrombophlebitis, difficulty breathing, visual disturbances, severe headache, and seizure activity.

Implementation

Interventions and (Rationales)	Patient and Family Education
• Monitor for thromboembolic disease. (Estrogen increases the risk for thromboembolism.)	• Instruct the patient to report shortness of breath, feeling of heaviness, chest pain, severe headache, warmth, or swelling in the affected part (usually the legs or pelvis).
• Monitor for abnormal uterine bleeding. (If undiagnosed tumor is present, these drugs can increase its size and cause uterine bleeding.)	• Instruct the patient to report excessive uterine bleeding or that which occurs between menstruations.
• Monitor breast health. (Estrogens promote the growth of certain breast cancers.)	• Instruct the patient to have regular breast exams, perform monthly BSE, and obtain routine mammograms, as recommended by the health care provider.
• Monitor for vision changes. (These drugs may worsen myopia or astigmatism and cause intolerance of contact lenses.)	Instruct the patient to: • Obtain regular eye exams during HRT. • Report changes in vision. • Report any difficulty in wearing contact lenses.
• Encourage the patient not to smoke. (Smoking increases risk of cardiovascular disease.)	• Instruct the patient to avoid smoking and participate in smoking cessation programs, if necessary.
• Encourage the patient to avoid caffeine. (Estrogens and caffeine may lead to increased CNS stimulation.)	Instruct the patient to: • Restrict caffeine consumption. • Recognize common foods that contain caffeine: coffee, tea, carbonated beverages, chocolate, and certain over-the-counter (OTC) medications. • Report unusual nervousness, anxiety, and insomnia.
• Monitor glucose levels. (Estrogens may increase blood glucose levels.)	Instruct the patient to: • Monitor blood and urine glucose frequently, if diabetic. • Report any consistent changes in blood glucose.
• Monitor for seizure activity. (Estrogen-induced fluid retention may increase risk of seizures.)	• Instruct the patient to be alert for the possibility of seizures, even at night, and report any seizure-type symptoms.
• Monitor the patient's understanding and proper self-administration. (Improper administration may increase the incidence of adverse effects.)	Instruct the patient to: • Administer proper dose, form, and frequency of medication. • Take with food to decrease GI irritation. • Take daily dose at bedtime to decrease the occurrence of adverse effects. • Document menstruation and any problems that occur.

Evaluation of Outcome Criteria

Evaluate the effectiveness of drug therapy by confirming that patient goals and expected outcomes have been met (see "Planning").

Dysfunctional uterine bleeding is the health problem most frequently reported by women and a common reason for a hysterectomy.

PharmFACT

Dysfunctional uterine bleeding may occur at any time in a woman's reproductive years, but the most severe cases occur in adolescents during the first 18 months after the onset of menstruation. *Source:* Dodds & Sinert, 2007.

Dysfunctional uterine bleeding can have a number of causes, including early abortion, pelvic neoplasms, thyroid disorders, pregnancy, and infection. Types of dysfunctional uterine bleeding include the following:

- **Amenorrhea.** Absence of menstruation
- **Endometriosis.** Abnormal location of endometrial tissues
- **Oligomenorrhea.** Infrequent menstruation
- **Menorrhagia.** Prolonged or excessive menstruation
- **Breakthrough bleeding.** Hemorrhage between menstrual periods
- **Premenstrual syndrome (PMS).** Symptoms developed during the luteal phase
- **Postmenopausal bleeding.** Hemorrhage following menopause
- **Endometrial carcinoma.** Cancer of the endometrium

Dysfunctional uterine bleeding is often due to a hormonal imbalance between estrogen and progesterone. Although estrogen increases the thickness of the endometrium, bleeding occurs sporadically unless it is balanced by adequate progesterone secretion. Administration of a progestin in a regimen starting 5 days after the onset of menses and continuing for the next 20 days can sometimes help to reestablish a normal, monthly cyclic pattern. Oral contraceptives may also be prescribed for this disorder.

The pain, discomfort, and infertility brought on by endometriosis are often treated by danazol, nafarelin, and leuprolide. These drugs suppress the production of estrogen and progesterone resulting in a decrease in growth potential of endometrial tissues (see Section 70.7).

In patients experiencing heavy bleeding, high doses of conjugated estrogens may be administered for 3 weeks prior to adding medroxyprogesterone for the last 10 days of therapy. Treatment with nonsteroidal anti-inflammatory drugs (NSAIDs) helps to ease painful menstrual flow. If aggressive hormonal therapy fails to stop the heavy bleeding, dilation and curettage (D&C) may be necessary.

Progestins are occasionally prescribed for the treatment of metastatic endometrial carcinoma. In these cases, they are used for palliation, in combination with other antineoplastics. Selected progestins and their dosages are shown in Table 70.1.

PROTOTYPE DRUG Medroxyprogesterone acetate (Provera)

Classification: **Therapeutic:** Hormone, agent for dysfunctional uterine bleeding

Pharmacologic: Progestin

Therapeutic Effects and Uses: Approved in 1959, medroxyprogesterone is a synthetic progestin with a prolonged duration of action. Like progesterone, the primary target tissue for medroxyprogesterone is the uterine endometrium. It antagonizes the effects of estrogen on the uterus, thus restoring normal hormonal balance. It also inhibits the midcycle LH surge, which prevents ovulation, and causes a thick cervical mucus that is resistant to the passage of sperm. Approved indications include dysfunctional uterine bleeding, secondary amenorrhea, and contraception.

Medroxyprogesterone may also be given by sustained-release IM (Depo-Provera) or subcutaneous (depo-subQ-Provera) depot injection. This is available in two doses: a lower dose for contraception, and a higher dose for the palliation of inoperable metastatic uterine or renal carcinoma. The use of medroxyprogesterone in contraception is presented in Chapter 71. The drug has been used off-label to treat symptoms of menopause.

Mechanism of Action: This drug is a synthetic derivative of progesterone with prolonged, variable duration of action and androgenic and antiestrogenic activity. The drug inhibits GnRH, thus preventing the LH surge and ovulation.

Pharmacokinetics:

Route(s)	PO, IM, subcutaneous, IV
Absorption	Readily absorbed from the GI tract or IM
Distribution	Crosses the placenta; secreted in breast milk; 90% bound to protein
Primary metabolism	Hepatic
Primary excretion	Feces
Onset of action	PO: 30–60 minutes; IM: 15–30 minutes
Duration of action	Half-life: 30 days (PO) and 50 days (IM)

Adverse Effects: The most common adverse effects of medroxyprogesterone are breast tenderness, and breakthrough bleeding and other menstrual irregularities. Weight gain, depression, HTN, nausea, vomiting, fluid retention, and vaginal candidiasis may also occur. The most serious adverse effect is an increased risk for thromboembolic disease, although the risk is lower than that caused by estrogen.

Contraindications/Precautions: Patients with a history of thromboembolic disorders, or who are pregnant or lactating, should not take progestins. Doses should be reduced in patients with hepatic impairment. Patients with preexisting breast, uterine, or vaginal cancer should not receive medroxyprogesterone unless it is for palliation of advanced cancer. The drug should be used cautiously in patients with a history of psychic depression, and the drug should be discontinued at the first sign of recurring depression. The drug is absolutely contraindicated in patients with known or suspected pregnancy (category X), or in those with undiagnosed vaginal bleeding.

Drug Interactions: Serum levels of medroxyprogesterone are decreased by aminoglutethimide, barbiturates, primidone, rifampin, rifabutin, and topiramate. **Herbal/Food:** St. John's wort may cause intermenstrual bleeding and loss of efficacy.

Pregnancy: Category X.

Treatment of Overdose: Overdose is treated symptomatically.

Nursing Responsibilities:

- Obtain baseline data including blood pressure, weight, and pulse prior to starting therapy. Obtain laboratory tests including complete blood count, liver function, serum glucose, and an electrolyte profile.
- Observe for acute intermittent porphyria during therapy. Symptoms include severe, colicky abdominal pain, vomiting, distention, diarrhea, and constipation.
- Monitor for and report possible signs of thrombophlebitis: redness, pain, and swelling of the calf.
- Administer oral formulation with food to minimize GI distress.
- Inject medication slowly into deep muscle mass. Rotate the injection site.
- Monitor IM injection sites for evidence of sterile abscess. Symptoms include a residual lump and discoloration of tissue at the injection site.

Patient and Family Education:

- Immediately report any calf pain or redness, dyspnea, and chest pain to the health care provider because these may indicate blood clots.
- Immediately notify the health care provider of any known or suspected pregnancy.
- Avoid direct sunlight for extended periods, as progesterone can cause photosensitivity resulting in serious sunburn.
- Report unusual itching, sensitivity to light, acne, rash, and alopecia to the health care provider.
- Immediately report sudden headaches, chest pains, dyspnea, abnormal vaginal bleeding, or depression to the health care provider.
- Perform a monthly breast self-examination (BSE).
- Do not breast-feed while taking this drug without the approval of the health care provider.
- Do not drive or perform other hazardous activities until the effects of the drug are known because this drug may cause drowsiness or dizziness.

Drugs Similar to Medroxyprogesterone Acetate (Provera)

Progestins used in oral contraceptives include norethindrone, norgestrel, desogestrel, and levonorgestrel. These are presented in Chapter 71.

Progesterone (Crinone, Endometrin, Prochieve, Prometrium): Approved in 1978, progesterone is available in a variety of formulations. As a vaginal suppository (Endometrin) or vaginal gel (Crinone, Prochieve), progesterone is used to treat infertile women with progesterone deficiency as part of an assisted reproductive technology system. The vaginal formulations may also be used as progesterone supplements to support embryo implantation and early pregnancy. When used intravaginally, the drug may be absorbed and cause systemic adverse effects such as breast tenderness, bloating, drowsiness, headaches, irritability, and mood swings.

Oral capsules (Prometrium) are approved to treat secondary amenorrhea and may be used off-label to ease symptoms of PMS. Prometrium is also indicated for the prevention of endometrial hyperplasia in postmenopausal women who are receiving conjugated estrogens.

Progesterone IM injections are indicated for amenorrhea and to stop abnormal uterine bleeding. Adverse effects and contraindications are the same as medroxyprogesterone. The PO and IM progesterone formulations are pregnancy category X. The vaginal gel is category B.

Hormone Replacement Therapy

70.4 Hormone replacement therapy provides relief from menopause symptoms but may have serious long-term negative effects.

Menopause is characterized by a progressive decrease in estrogen secretion by the ovaries resulting in the permanent cessation of menses. The **climacteric** is the period of endocrine, somatic, and psychological changes occurring in the transition to menopause. There are over 30 million menopausal women in North America and each decade millions more reach the climacteric. Menopause is neither a disease nor a disorder, but is a natural consequence of aging that is often accompanied by unpleasant symptoms that include hot flashes, night sweats, irregular menstrual cycles, vaginal dryness, and bone mass loss.

> **Pharm*FACT***
>
> **Tobacco smoking is associated with an early onset of menopause (age less than 45 years). Coffee and alcohol consumption do not appear to affect the onset of menopause.** *Source:* Mikkelsen, Graff-Iversen, Sundby, & Bjertness, 2007.

Over the past 40 years, health care providers have commonly prescribed **hormone replacement therapy (HRT)** during menopause. HRT supplies physiological doses of estrogen, sometimes combined with a progestin, to treat unpleasant symptoms of menopause and to prevent the long-term consequences of estrogen loss listed in Table 70.2.

Beginning in the mid-1960s, large numbers of perimenopausal and menopausal women were prescribed estrogens. Estrogens were then promoted as safe and relatively risk free. Conjugated estrogen (Premarin) was the first estrogen product marketed and was widely prescribed, despite lack of research on its effectiveness and long-term effects. The drug's popularity extended several more decades: In 2000, 46 million prescriptions were filled for Premarin, making it the second most frequently prescribed medication in the United States. In that same year, 22.3 million additional prescriptions were written

NURSING PROCESS APPLICATION

Patients Receiving Progestin Therapy

Assessment	Potential Nursing Diagnoses
Prior to administration: • Obtain a complete health history including personal or familial history of breast, endometrial, or renal cancer; liver or kidney disease; dysfunctional uterine bleeding; or endometrial hyperplasia. • Obtain a drug history to determine possible drug interactions and allergies. • Assess cardiovascular status including history of thromboembolic disease.	• *Deficient Knowledge (Drug Therapy)* • *Nausea*, related to adverse effect of drug • *Noncompliance (Drug Regimen)*

Planning: Patient Goals and Expected Outcomes

The patient will:

- Report relief from dysfunctional uterine bleeding or amenorrhea.
- Demonstrate an understanding of the drug's action by accurately describing drug adverse effects and precautions.
- Immediately report effects such as signs of embolism; sudden, severe headache; edema; vision changes; and phototoxicity.

Implementation

Interventions and (Rationales)	Patient and Family Education
• Monitor laboratory tests including liver function, blood glucose, sodium, and chloride levels. (Progestins can affect electrolyte balance and liver function.)	• Instruct the patient to obtain periodic laboratory tests and monitor glucose levels closely if diabetic.
• Monitor for vision changes. (Progestins may cause retinal emboli or cerebrovascular thrombosis.)	• Instruct the patient to report unexplained partial or complete loss of vision, ptosis, or diplopia.
• Monitor for fluid imbalance. (Progestins cause fluid retention and weight gain.)	• Instruct the patient, especially one who has asthma, seizure disorders, cardiac or kidney impairment, or migraines, to monitor for edema or weight gain by weighing self weekly and recording their weight.
• Monitor for integumentary effects of medication. (Progestins have multiple effects on the skin and associated structures.)	Instruct the patient to: • Report itching, photosensitivity, acne, rash, and hair overgrowth or hair loss. • Avoid exposure to UV light and prolonged periods of time in the sun. • Use sunscreen (higher than SPF 12) when outdoors. • Recognize that these changes are temporary and will improve upon discontinuation of this medication.
• Monitor the patient's understanding and proper self-administration. (Improper administration may increase incidence of adverse effects.)	Instruct the patient to: • Administer proper dose, form, and frequency of medication. • Take with food to decrease GI irritation. • Take daily dose at bedtime to decrease occurrence of adverse effects. • Document menstruation and any problems that occur.

Evaluation of Outcome Criteria

Evaluate the effectiveness of drug therapy by confirming that patient goals and expected outcomes have been met (see "Planning").

TABLE 70.2 Potential Consequences of Estrogen Loss Related to Menopause

Stage	Symptoms and Conditions
Early menopause	Mood disturbances, depression, irritability
	Insomnia
	Hot flashes
	Irregular menstrual cycles
	Headaches
Midmenopause	Vaginal atrophy, increased infections, painful intercourse
	Skin atrophy
	Stress urinary incontinence
	Sexual disinterest
Postmenopause	Cardiovascular disease
	Osteoporosis
	Alzheimer's-like dementia
	Colon cancer

for conjugated estrogens combined with medroxyprogesterone (Prempro) (Grady et al., 2002).

In the mid 1970s, studies showed that women who had used estrogen (without progestin) for 7 years or longer were 14% more likely to develop uterine cancer. Progestins were then added to the HRT regimen to lower the risk of endometrial cancer.

Two large, randomized, double-blind, placebo-controlled studies have challenged the safety of using HRT during menopause. The Women's Health Initiative (WHI) and the Heart and Estrogen/Progestin Replacement Study (HERS) helped disprove the benefits of HRT for postmenopausal women. Over 26,000 women were enrolled in these studies, which were discontinued early when it became clear that the potential benefits of long-term HRT were not being realized. The results of the study depended upon whether the HRT consisted of estrogen alone or an estrogen–progestin combination. Researchers reached the following conclusions:

- Women taking an estrogen–progestin-combination HRT experienced a statistically significant increased risk of MI,

CONNECTIONS

Patient Safety

Medication Order

It has been a very busy morning on the nursing unit with multiple patient discharges and several new admissions. One patient is a 35-year-old woman who is being released from the hospital with a discharge order that reads, "Prempro 1 tablet daily at bedtime." Is it necessary for the nurse to clarify this order before the patient leaves the hospital?

See Answers to Patient Safety Questions in Appendix A.

stroke, breast cancer, dementia, and venous thromboembolism. The risks were higher in women older than age 60; women aged 50 to 59 actually experienced a slight decrease in adverse cardiovascular events.

- Women taking estrogen–progestin-combination HRT experienced a decreased risk of hip fractures and colorectal cancer.
- Women taking estrogen alone experienced an increased risk of CVA and thromboembolic disease.
- Women taking estrogen alone did not experience an increased risk for breast cancer or MI.

The adverse effects documented in the WHI study, and others, were significant enough to suggest that the potential benefits of long-term HRT may not outweigh the risks for many women. However, the results of this study remain controversial. HRT does offer relief from the immediate, distressing menopausal symptoms, prevents osteoporosis-related fractures, and may offer some degree of protection from colorectal cancer. These are certainly significant and important benefits from HRT. The risks of HRT include increased incidence of MI, thromboembolic events, breast cancer (estrogen–progestin combinations), ovarian cancer (estrogen alone), and probably dementia, urinary incontinence, and gallbladder disease. Research continues to provide valuable information on the long-term risks of HRT. The data from the WHI study and HERS are still being analyzed and follow-up studies are being conducted to determine which women benefit the most from HRT and which are at greatest risk.

Short-term use of HRT for relieving acute symptoms of menopause may be appropriate for women without a history of cardiovascular disease or cancer. Topical preparations may bring some benefit to women suffering from vulvar and vaginal atrophy. Until research provides more definitive answers, the choice of HRT to treat menopausal symptoms remains a highly individualized one, between the patient and her health care provider.

Uterine Stimulants: Oxytocics

70.5 Oxytocics are drugs used to stimulate the uterus and promote labor and delivery.

Oxytocics are agents that stimulate uterine contractions and promote the induction of labor. **Tocolytics**, discussed in Section 70.6, are agents used to inhibit uterine contractions during premature labor. Doses of these agents are listed in Table 70.3.

The most widely used oxytocic is the natural hormone oxytocin, which is secreted by the posterior pituitary gland. The target organs for oxytocin are the uterus and the breast. Larger and larger amounts of oxytocin are secreted as the uterus is distended by the growing fetus. As blood levels of oxytocin rise, the smooth muscle of the uterus is stimulated to contract, thus promoting labor and the delivery of the baby and the placenta. As pregnancy progresses, the number of oxytocin receptors in the uterus increases, making it even more sensitive to the effects of the hormone.

Oxytocin and other uterine stimulants are only indicated when there are demonstrated risks to the mother or fetus in continuing the pregnancy. Parenteral oxytocin (Pitocin) may be given to induce labor. Doses in an IV infusion are increased gradually, every 15 to 60 minutes, until a normal labor pattern is established. After delivery, IV oxytocin is administered to

CONNECTIONS

Complementary and Alternative Therapies Chaste Berry for Premenstrual Syndrome and Menopause

Description: The chaste tree (*Vitex agnus-castus*) is a shrub common to river banks in the southern Mediterranean region.

History and Claims: The dried berries have been used for thousands of years, with recorded references dating to Hippocrates. The berries are claimed to control vaginal and uterine hemorrhage, and to help expel the placenta following birth. Other claims include reduced pain in women with mastalgia, reduced vaginal dryness, increased amount of breast milk, reduced symptoms of premenstrual syndrome (PMS), and improved libido.

Standardization: Doses are not well standardized. Typical doses may range from 1 to 4 mg of the dried fruit or extracts.

Evidence: Chaste berries contain a number of active substances, some of which are antiadrenogenic and exert effects similar to progesterone. Extracts appear to have a physiological effect on PMS, as well as the unpleasant symptoms of menopause. Women who take the herbal remedy report that PMS symptoms such as bloating, breast fullness, headache, irritability, mood swings, and anger reduce by 50%. There may be better regulation of the menstrual cycle, and less bleeding. When used during menopause, it may help to reverse vaginal changes and diminished libido. Data supporting the claims of increased libido or for increased milk production in lactating women are weak. Adverse effects are minor and include GI upset, rash, and headaches.

Source: From "The Use of Herbs and Dietary Supplements in Gynecology: An Evidence-Based Review," by C. E. Dennehy, 2006, *Journal of Midwifery and Womens Health, 51*(3), pp. 402–409; "Chasteberry," by B. Roemheld-Hamm, 2005, *American Family Physician, 72*(2), pp. 821–824.

TABLE 70.3 Uterine Stimulants and Relaxants

Drug	Route and Adult Dose (maximum dose where indicated)	Adverse Effects
Stimulants (Oxytocics)		
oxytocin (Pitocin)	To control postpartum bleeding: 10–40 units per infusion pump in 1,000 mL of IV fluid at a rate to prevent uterine atony To induce labor: IV: 0.5–2 milliunits/min., gradually increasing the dose no greater than 1–2 milliunits/min. at 30–60-min intervals until contraction pattern is established	*Nausea, vomiting, maternal dysrhythmias* Fetal bradycardia, uterine rupture, fetal intracranial hemorrhage, water intoxication, fetal brain hemorrhage
Ergot Alkaloids		
ergonovine (Ergotrate)	PO: 1 tablet (0.2 mg) tid-qid after childbirth for a maximum of 1 week	*Nausea, vomiting, uterine cramping* Shock, severe HTN, severe dysrhythmias
methylergonovine (Methergine)	PO: 0.2–0.4 mg bid-qid	
Prostaglandins		
carboprost (Hemabate)	IM: Initial: 250 mcg (1 mL) repeated at 1½–3½-h intervals if indicated by uterine response	*Nausea, vomiting, cramping, diarrhea, fever* Uterine laceration, rupture, or hemorrhage
dinoprostone (Cervidil, Prepidil, Prostin E_2)	Intravaginal insert: 10 mg	
misoprostol (Cytotec)	Intravaginal: 25 mcg (1/4 of 100 mcg tablet); may repeat every 3–6 h	
Relaxants (Tocolytics)		
magnesium sulfate	IV: 1–4 g in 5% dextrose by slow infusion (initial max dose: 10–14 g/day, then no more than 30–40 g/day at a max rate of 1–2 g/h)	*Flushing, sweating, muscle weakness* Complete heart block, circulatory collapse, respiratory paralysis
nifedipine (Adalat, Procardia)	PO: Initial dosage of 20 mg, followed by 20 mg after 30 min. If contractions persist, therapy can be continued with 20 mg every 3–8 h for 48–72 h with a maximum dose of 160 mg/day After 72 h, if maintenance is still required, long-acting nifedipine 30–60 mg daily can be used	*Flushing, sweating, muscle weakness* Complete heart block, circulatory collapse, respiratory paralysis
terbutaline sulfate (Brethine)	IV: 2.5–10 mcg/min; increase every 10–20 min; duration of infusion: 12 h (max: 17.5–30 mcg/min) PO: Maintenance dose: 2.5–10 mg every 4–6 h as long as necessary to prevent pregnancy	*Nervousness, tremor, drowsiness* Bronchoconstrictions, dysrhythmias, altered maternal and fetal heart rates

Note: *Italics* indicate common adverse effects. Underline indicates serious adverse effects.

control postpartum uterine bleeding by temporarily restricting blood flow to this organ.

In postpartum women, oxytocin is released in response to suckling, whereby it promotes the ejection (letdown) of milk from the mammary glands. It is important to note that oxytocin does not increase the volume of milk production. This function is provided by the pituitary hormone prolactin, which increases the synthesis of milk. Although rare, deficiencies of prolactin can result in insufficient milk to conduct breast-feeding. The actions of oxytocin during breast-feeding are illustrated in Figure 70.3.

Ergot alkaloids are drugs obtained from a fungus that grows on rye plants that are used as alternatives to oxytocin. They may be used to induce labor or to control postpartum hemorrhage. Although effective at promoting uterine contractions, they are rarely prescribed due to the risk of serious HTN. Available ergot alkaloids include ergonovine (Ergotrate) and methylergonovine (Methergine). Ergot alkaloids are also second-line drugs in the pharmacotherapy of migraines (see Chapter 29).

Several prostaglandins are also used as uterine stimulants. Unlike most hormones that travel through the blood to affect distant tissues, prostaglandins act directly at the site where they are secreted. In the uterus, prostaglandins cause intense smooth muscle contractions. Carboprost (Hemabate) is often used to control postpartum hemorrhage. Dinoprostone (Prepidil, Cervidil) and misoprostol (Cytotec) are prostaglandins used to promote cervical ripening, a softening and dilation of the cervix that must occur prior to vaginal delivery. The prostaglandins may also be used to induce pharmacologic abortion (see Chapter 71).

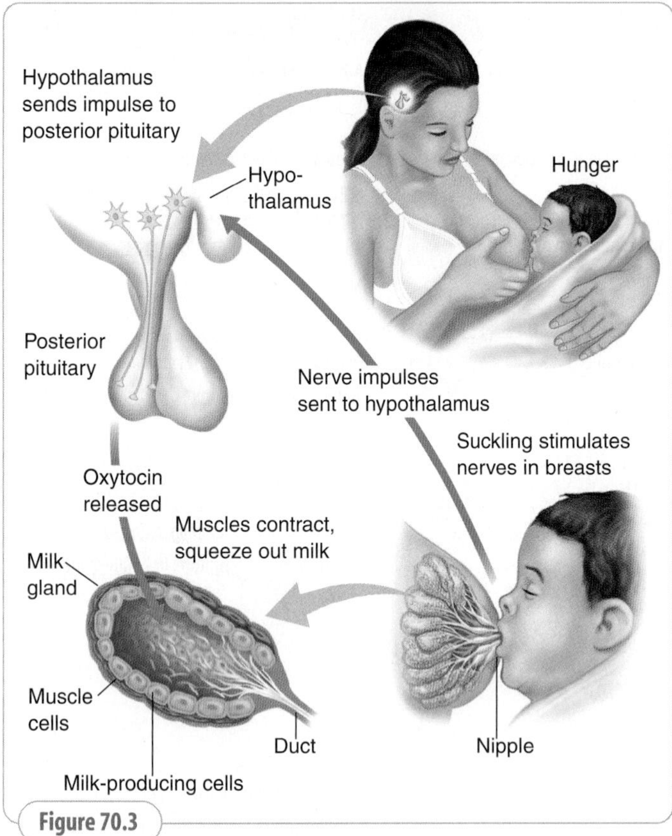

Figure 70.3

Oxytocin and breast-feeding.

PROTOTYPE DRUG Oxytocin (Pitocin)

Classification: **Therapeutic:** Drug to induce labor, uterine stimulant

Pharmacologic: Hormone, oxytocic

Therapeutic Effects and Uses: Oxytocin (Pitocin), identical to the natural hormone secreted by the posterior pituitary gland, is the drug of choice for inducing labor. Given by IV infusion antepartum, oxytocin induces labor almost immediately by increasing the frequency and force of contractions of uterine smooth muscle. It is administered during the final stages of labor, after the cervix is dilated, membranes have ruptured, and presentation of the fetus has occurred. It is also used to induce labor in cases of maternal diabetes, preeclampsia, eclampsia, and erythroblastosis fetalis. It should not be used for elective induction of labor, due to potential adverse effects to the mother or baby.

Oxytocin is also approved to reduce postpartum hemorrhage after expulsion of the placenta, and to aid in returning normal muscular tone to the uterus. This drug is approved at higher doses to induce abortion and for incomplete abortion. Intranasal forms once used to promote milk letdown are no longer available in the United States.

Mechanism of Action: Oxytocin increases the intensity and frequency of uterine smooth muscle contractions. When stimulated by sucking, oxytocin causes smooth muscle in alveolar ducts to contract, thus ejecting milk from the breast.

Pharmacokinetics:

Route(s)	IV or IM
Absorption	Destroyed in the GI tract
Distribution	Widely distributed in the extracellular fluid; small amounts may cross the placenta; secreted in breast milk
Primary metabolism	Rapidly destroyed in the kidney and the liver
Primary excretion	Small amounts via renal
Onset of action	IV: Immediate; IM: 3–5 minutes
Duration of action	Half-life: 3–5 minutes

Adverse Effects: The most common adverse effects of oxytocin are rapid, painful uterine contractions and fetal tachycardia. Uterine rupture or fetal trauma from too-rapid expulsion through the pelvis, seizure, and coma are regarded as the most serious adverse effects. There is an increased risk of uterine rupture in women who have delivered five or more children. When given IV, vital signs of the fetus and mother must be monitored continuously to prevent fetal complications, such as dysrhythmias or intracranial hemorrhage.

Contraindications/Precautions: Oxytocin has an antidiuretic effect and care must be taken to avoid water intoxication. Oxytocin is contraindicated when there is evidence of fetal distress, placenta previa, uterine prolapse, active herpes infection, abnormal fetal position, and cervical cancer. Breast-feeding should be delayed for at least 24 hours after the drug is discontinued.

Drug Interactions: Vasoconstrictors used concurrently with oxytocin may cause severe HTN. Oxytocin may cause adverse cardiovascular effects when administered with fibrinolysin, warfarin, and cyclopropane anesthesia. **Herbal/Food:** Ephedra used with oxytocin may lead to HTN.

Pregnancy: Category X.

Treatment of Overdose: Overdose will cause severe cramping and possible damage to the uterus. Discontinuation of the infusion will result in a rapid resolution of symptoms due to the short half-life of the drug.

Nursing Responsibilities:

- Evaluate the patient for fetal presentation, especially for the presence of cephalopelvic disproportion.
- Monitor and document labor progress. Before and after contractions, record vital signs; input and output (I&O) ratio; weight; strength, duration, and frequency of contractions; and fetal heart tones and rate.
- Monitor vital signs at least every 15 minutes. An increase in the frequency and force of uterine contractions increase the blood pressure and heart rates in the mother, and a decrease in the heart rate of the fetus. If fetal distress is detected, discontinue the infusion in order to prevent fetal anoxia.
- If contractions occur less than 2 minutes apart, stop the infusion, turn the patient on the right side, and notify the prescriber. Administer oxygen as directed.
- Observe for signs of water intoxication due to long-term IV infusion of oxytocin: drowsiness, listlessness, headache, confusion, anuria, and weight gain.

- Check uterine fundus frequently to determine the strength of contractions.
- Note incidence of hypersensitivity or allergic reactions, which are more common when the drug is given by IM or IV injections, rather than through diluted IV solutions.
- Discontinue oxytocin immediately if uterine hyperstimulation is noted. This is characterized by contractions that are less than 2 minutes apart, with greater force than 50 mm Hg, or that last longer than 90 seconds.

Patient and Family Education:

- Notify the health care provider of medical history and all current conditions because oxytocin cannot be used in patients who have had herpes genitalis, invasive cervical cancer, more than five pregnancies, previous traumatic birth, or previous uterine surgery.
- Immediately report unusual swelling, palpitations, or difficulty breathing.

Drugs Similar to Oxytocin (Pitocin)

Uterine stimulants also include prostaglandins (carboprost, dinoprostone, and misoprostol) and the ergot alkaloids (ergonovine and methylergonovine).

Carboprost (Hemabate): Carboprost, equivalent to endogenous prostaglandin F_2 alpha, is approved to induce pharmacologic abortion between weeks 13 and 20 of gestation and for controlling postpartum bleeding that has not responded to oxytocin. For postpartum bleeding, it is administered by the IM route every 15 to 90 minutes until hemorrhage is controlled. Nausea, vomiting, diarrhea, and fever are common adverse effects. This drug is pregnancy category C.

Dinoprostone (Cervidil, Prepidil, Prostin E_2): Dinoprostone, or prostaglandin E_2, is approved to prepare the cervix for labor, or to abort a fetus that has died. To promote cervical ripening, it is administered intravaginally. The gel form is placed into the cervical canal using prefilled syringes that may be repeated every 6 hours, as needed. The vaginal insert releases the drug slowly, over 12 hours. The insert may be quickly and easily removed once labor begins. Both the gel and the insert may stimulate the uterus to begin contracting. Like carboprost, GI effects and fever are very common adverse effects. This drug is pregnancy category C.

Ergonovine (Ergotrate): Ergonovine is an older drug, approved by the U.S. Food and Drug Administration (FDA) in 1960 to treat postpartum bleeding. The drug acts by increasing the frequency and force of uterine contractions to improve uterine tone. Administered by the PO, IV, or IM routes, ergonovine produces uterine contractions within minutes. Parenteral doses may be repeated every 2 to 4 hours and oral doses every 6 to 12 hours until bleeding diminishes. The drug is rarely used off-label to treat variant angina. The drug should not be used to induce labor because it can constrict blood flow through the placenta, and cause fetal harm and possibly uterine rupture. Cramping and GI-related adverse effects are common with ergonovine. This drug is pregnancy category X.

Methylergonovine (Methergine): Approved in 1946, methylergonovine is structurally very similar to ergonovine and acts by the same mechanism. It may be administered by the PO, IM, or IV routes to control postpartum bleeding and restore uterine tone. The IV route is only used in emergency situations because it may produce serious HTN in the mother. Uterine contractions begin in 3 to 5 minutes after an IM dose. The adverse effects are the same as ergonovine. This drug is pregnancy category C.

Misoprostol (Cytotec): Misoprostol is a synthetic analog of prostaglandin E_1 that is approved to treat NSAID-induced peptic ulcers, although it is rarely used for that purpose because safer and more effective drugs are available. Approved in 1988, it is used off-label for pharmacologic abortion, cervical ripening, control of postpartum bleeding, and labor induction. For cervical ripening or labor induction, a 25-mg tablet is placed in the vagina every 3 to 6 hours. For postpartum bleeding, the drug is administered by the PO or rectal route. Misoprostol has a high incidence of uterine hyperstimulation, which can lead to fetal distress and cause uterine damage. Like the other progesterone drugs, GI effects and fever are very common adverse effects. This drug is a pregnancy category X.

Uterine Relaxants: Tocolytics

70.6 Uterine relaxants are used to suppress preterm labor.

Preterm labor is the initiation of labor prior to week 37 of gestation. The most common cause of preterm labor is premature rupturing of membranes or infections of the chorion or uterus. If the organ systems of the fetus are determined to be immature, attempts may be made to delay labor because preterm infants have a high morbidity and mortality rate. Suppressing labor allows additional time for the fetal organs to develop and may permit the pregnancy to reach normal term. Bed rest is mandatory and corticosteroids may be administered to accelerate fetal lung maturity. Antibiotics such as ampicillin or erythromycin are indicated if the preterm labor is due to a uterine or chorionic infection. Preterm labor can be stopped and delivery delayed in about 50% of women, if the membranes have not yet ruptured. The success rate is only 25% in patients with membrane rupture.

Tocolytics are uterine relaxants prescribed to suppress preterm labor contractions. Typically, the mother is given a monitor with a sensor that records uterine contractions and this information is used to determine the doses and timing of tocolytic medications. Tocolytics can generally delay labor by only 24 to 72 hours, but this is often enough time for the fetus to develop normal lung function. The benefits of these drugs must be carefully weighed against their potential adverse effects, which include tachycardia in both the mother and the fetus.

Only a few drugs are available as tocolytics, and none can be realistically considered a prototype. For over 30 years, magnesium sulfate has been the traditional drug of choice for delaying preterm labor, but recent evidence suggests it may be ineffective and poses undue risks to the fetus and mother (Grimes & Nanda, 2006). The only drug that is FDA approved for this indication is ritodrine (Yutopar) but it is no longer being manufactured for

NURSING PROCESS APPLICATION

Patients Receiving Oxytocin (Pitocin)

Assessment	Potential Nursing Diagnoses
Prior to administration: • Obtain a complete health history including past and present gynecologic and obstetric history. • Obtain a drug history to determine possible drug interactions and allergies.	• *Risk for Imbalanced Fluid Volume* • *Risk for Injury,* related to the effects of strong uterine contractions on the fetus

Planning: Patient Goals and Expected Outcomes

The patient will:

- Report an increase in force and frequency of uterine contractions or letdown of milk for breast-feeding.
- Demonstrate an understanding of the drug's action by accurately describing drug adverse effects and precautions.
- Immediately report effects such as listlessness, headache, confusion, anuria, hypotension, nausea, vomiting, and weight gain.

Implementation

Interventions and (Rationales)	Patient and Family Education
• Monitor the fetal heart rate. (Increase in the force and frequency of uterine contractions may cause fetal distress.)	• Instruct the patient about the purpose and importance of fetal monitoring.
• Monitor maternal status including blood pressure, pulse, and frequency; and duration and intensity of contractions.	• Instruct the patient about the importance of monitoring maternal status.
• Monitor fluid balance. (Prolonged IV infusion may cause water intoxication.)	• Instruct the patient to report drowsiness, listlessness, headache, confusion, anuria, and weight gain.
• Monitor for postpartum or postabortion hemorrhage. (Oxytocin can be used to control postpartum bleeding.)	Instruct the patient: • About the importance of being monitored frequently after delivery or after abortion. • To report severe vaginal bleeding or an increase in lochia.
• Monitor lactation status. (Oxytocin causes milk ejection within minutes after administration.)	Instruct the patient: • That oxytocin does not increase milk production. • To monitor for decreased breast pain, redness, or hardness, if taking oxytocin to decrease breast engorgement.

Evaluation of Outcome Criteria

Evaluate the effectiveness of drug therapy by confirming that patient goals and expected outcomes have been met (see "Planning").

use in the United States. Calcium channel blockers and beta-adrenergic agonists appear to be effective but are used off-label for this indication. Doses for these agents are listed in Table 70.3.

Magnesium sulfate: A traditional tocolytic of choice, magnesium sulfate is administered by continuous IV infusion via a controlled pump device until preterm contractions diminish, usually in about 30 minutes. It is used off-label for this indication. During therapy, careful monitoring of deep tendon reflexes, blood pressure, respirations, urinary output, and serum magnesium concentrations are necessary. Early signs of magnesium overdose include flushing of the skin, sedation, confusion, intense thirst, and muscle weakness. Extreme levels cause neuromuscular blockade with resultant respiratory paralysis, heart block, and circulatory collapse. Other indications for magnesium sulfate include treatment of magnesium deficiency and the prevention of seizures in toxemia of pregnancy. This drug is pregnancy category A.

Nifedipine (Adalat, Procardia): Nifedipine is a calcium channel blocker widely prescribed for the treatment of HTN and angina. The drug has been used off-label as a tocolytic as an option to magnesium sulfate. Nifedipine is given either by the PO or sublingual route. A typical regimen includes a loading dose followed by additional PO doses every 15 to 20 minutes until contractions diminish. Nifedipine appears to be as effective as magnesium sulfate and the beta-adrenergic agonists but exhibits fewer adverse effects. Adverse effects include acute pulmonary edema, dysrhythmias, and hypotension. A prototype feature for nifedipine is presented in Chapter 33. This drug is pregnancy category C.

Terbutaline (Brethine): Terbutaline is a beta$_2$-adrenergic agonist that is FDA approved to treat acute bronchospasm due to asthma. It has been used off-label to suppress preterm contractions due to its ability to relax smooth muscle. It is given by the subcutaneous route either by injections every 20 minutes or by using a continuous infusion device and may also be administered orally. Serious adverse reactions may occur. The mother may experience increased heart rate, dysrhythmias, myocardial ischemia, transient hyperglycemia, hypokalemia, and pulmonary edema. The fetus may experience increased heart rate and neonatal hypoglycemia. This drug is pregnancy category B.

CONNECTION *Checkpoint* 70.2

Calcium channel blockers, including nifedipine, are widely used to treat cardiovascular disorders. From Chapter 33, what effects would you expect nifedipine to have on vascular smooth muscle, myocardial oxygen demand, and myocardial conduction? See Answer to Connection Checkpoint 70.2 in Appendix A.

Pharmacotherapy of Infertility

70.7 Female infertility may be treated with drugs that promote oocyte maturation and ovulation.

Infertility is defined as the inability to become pregnant after at least 1 year of frequent, unprotected intercourse. Infertility is a common disorder: 25% of couples experience difficulty in conceiving children at some point during their reproductive lifetimes. It is estimated that female reproductive tract conditions contribute to approximately 60% of the infertility disorders. Agents used to treat infertility are shown in Table 70.4.

PharmFACT

The most important causes of infertility are chlamydia and gonorrhea infections. These infections can cause pelvic inflammatory disease, which can lead to infertility and ectopic pregnancies. *Source:* Centers for Disease Control and Prevention, 2008.

The three primary causes of female infertility are pelvic infections, physical obstruction of the uterine tubes, and lack of ovulation. Extensive testing is often necessary to determine the exact cause, and it is not uncommon to find multiple etiologies for the infertility.

For women whose infertility is due to inadequate ovulation, pharmacotherapy may be of value. **Ovulatory dysfunction** is defined as the presence of abnormal, irregular, or absent ovulation. Signs and symptoms of ovulatory dysfunction include irregular or absent menses, excessive abdominal bloating, and mood lability. Confirmation of the disorder is made by measuring hormone levels.

Ovulatory dysfunction may occur at the level of the hypothalamus, pituitary, or ovary, and pharmacotherapy is targeted to the specific cause of the dysfunction. The most common etiology of ovulatory dysfunction is **polycystic ovary syndrome,** a condition in which the ovaries are filled with follicular cysts and the patient has elevated levels of androgens and estrogen. Hirsutism is commonly observed in these women due to the excessive androgen levels. Another cause of ovulatory dysfunction is hyperprolactinemia, excessive levels of the hormone prolactin, which is most frequently caused by a tumor of the pituitary gland.

Many women with ovulatory dysfunction can be successfully treated with drug therapy; restoring regular, monthly ovulation is an essential goal of fertility management. Ovulation induction protocols are sometimes divided into the following three medication groups, which are shown in Pharmacotherapy Illustrated 70.1:

- Drugs used to promote maturation of ovarian follicles
- Drugs used to trigger ovulation at the end of follicular maturation
- Drugs that promote ovulation to occur on a regular, monthly basis, at the midpoint of the menstrual cycle

Promotion of follicle maturation: Ovulation cannot occur unless the ovarian follicles receive a hormonal signal to mature each month. This signal is normally supplied by LH and FSH during the first few weeks of the menstrual cycle. Clomiphene (Clomid, Milophene, Serophene) is a drug of choice for treating female infertility because it stimulates the release of LH, resulting in the maturation of more ovarian follicles than would normally occur. The rise in LH level induced by clomiphene is sufficient to induce ovulation in about 80% of treated patients. The use of clomiphene assumes that the pituitary gland is able to respond by secreting LH, and that the ovaries are responsive to LH. If either of these assumptions is false, other treatment options should be considered.

If the infertility is a result of endocrine disruption at the pituitary level, therapy with human menopausal gonadotropin (HMG) or GnRH may be indicated. These therapies are generally indicated only after clomiphene has failed to induce ovulation. Also known as menotropins (Pergonal, Humegon), HMG acts on the ovaries to increase follicle maturation, and results in a 25% incidence of multiple pregnancies. Successful therapy with HMG assumes that the ovaries are responsive to LH and FSH. Newer formulations use recombinant DNA technology to synthesize gonadotropins containing nearly pure FSH, rather than extracting the FSH-LH mixture from urine.

Promotion of ovulation: Unless maturing follicles receive the final "burst" of LH, ovulation will not occur. HMG is similar in structure to natural LH and produces the same effect: ovulation.

Restoration of a normal monthly pattern of ovulation: The success of conception will be improved if a regular, monthly pattern of ovulation is established. Premature ovulation, the expulsion of the oocyte from the ovary before it has fully matured, is prevented by the use of two antagonists of GnRH: ganirelix (Antagon) and cetrorelix (Cetrotide).

Stimulation of the ovary by certain fertility drugs causes the ovaries to enlarge. Mild enlargement may cause pelvic pain but is generally benign and disappears when therapy is discontinued. One serious complication of certain fertility drugs is **ovarian hyperstimulation syndrome (OHS).** The onset of OHS is characterized by rapid, massive enlargement of the ovaries accompanied by nausea, vomiting, rapid weight gain, ascites, respiratory difficulties, increased risk of thromboembolism, and progressive kidney impairment. Progressive symptoms call for discontinuation of drug therapy, fluid restriction, bed rest, and symptomatic treatment of nausea, vomiting, and pain. Although OHS can be fatal, most cases resolve in 1 to 2 weeks.

Endometriosis, a cause of infertility, is characterized by the presence of endometrial tissue that has implanted outside the uterus, in locations such as the surface of pelvic organs or the ovaries. Approximately 25% to 50% of infertile women have endometriosis. Being responsive to hormonal stimuli, this abnormal

TABLE 70.4 Agents for Female Infertility

Drug	Route and Adult Dose (maximum dose where indicated)	Adverse Effects
bromocriptine (Parlodel)	PO: 1.25–2.5 mg/daily (max: 2.5 mg 2–3 times/day)	*Nausea, vomiting, cramping, constipation, drowsiness, headache, orthostatic hypotension, anorexia* GI bleeding, psychosis, seizures, syncope
clomiphene (Clomid, Milophene, Serophene)	PO first course: 50 mg/day for 5 days; start on 5th day of cycle following start of spontaneous or induced bleeding (with progestin) Second course if ovulation: Repeat first course until conception or for 3 cycles Second course if no ovulation: 100 mg/day for 5 days as above (max: 100 mg/day)	*Weight gain, symptoms of PMS, hot flashes, dermatitis* Blurred vision, ovarian hyperstimulation, cataracts, thrombosis of temporal arteries
danazol (Danocrine)	PO: 200–400 mg bid for 3–6 months, start during menstruation or if pregnancy test is negative, may extend to 9 months if necessary	*Hirsutism, alopecia, voice deepening, weight gain, vaginal dryness, reduction in breast size, edema, emotional lability, hot flashes* Thromboembolic events, hepatotoxicity, intracranial HTN
FSH- and LH-Enhancing Drugs		
chorionic gonadotropin-HCG (Novarel, Ovidrel, Pregnyl)	IM: 5,000–10,000 units 1 day following last dose of menotropins	Females: *Pelvic pain, depression, fatigue* Ovarian hyperstimulation syndrome Males: *Gynecomastia, acne* Aggressive behavior, depression
follitropin alfa (Gonal-F)	Subcutaneous: 75 international units/day initially, then increased by 37.5 international units at the end of 14 days. Further 37.5-unit dose increases may be made every 7 days if needed (max: 300 international units/day)	*Headache, nausea, abdominal pain, diarrhea, increased infections* Ovarian hyperstimulation syndrome, thromboembolic disorders
follitropin beta (Follistim)	Subcutaneous: 50–75 international units/day initially, then increased by 25–50 international units at the end of 14 days. (max: 300 international units/day)	
menotropins (Humegon, Repronex)	IM: 75 international units of FSH/LH activity given once daily for 7–12 days, followed by HCG 1 day after the last dose of menotropins. The dose may be increased after 2 more cycles to 150 international units	Females: *Ovarian enlargement, pelvic pain* Ovarian hyperstimulation syndrome Males: *Gynecomastia*
		All patients: *Headache, nausea, injection site reaction* Thromboembolic events
urofollitropin (Bravelle)	For ovulatory females: Subcutaneous: 150 international units once daily until sufficient follicular development is attained For anovulatory females: Subcutaneous: 75 international units once daily. The dose should not be increased more than twice in any cycle or by more than 75 international units per adjustment	*Headache, nausea, abdominal pain, diarrhea, increased infections* Ovarian hyperstimulation syndrome, thromboembolic disorders
GnRH Antagonists		
cetrorelix (Cetrotide)	Subcutaneous: 0.25 mg/day during the early to mid follicular phase of the cycle following the initiation of FSH	*Hot flashes, headache, menstrual irregularities* Fetal death, ovarian hyperstimulation syndrome
ganirelix (Antagon)	Subcutaneous: 250 mcg once daily during the early to midfollicular phase of the cycle following the initiation of FSH	
GnRH Analogs/Agonists		
goserelin (Zoladex)	Subcutaneous implant for endometriosis: 3.6 mg every 28 days Subcutaneous implant for advanced carcinoma: 10.8 mg every 3 months	Females: *Headache, depression, sweating, acne, vaginitis, vaginal dryness, menstrual irregularities, bone density loss, emotional lability* Tumor flare (goserelin and leuprolide) Males: *Erectile dysfunction, lethargy, gynecomastia* Heart failure All patients: *Pain at injection site, hot flashes, loss of libido* Bone density loss, fractures
leuprolide (Eligard, Lupron)	IM for endometriosis: 3.75 mg every month or 11.25 mg every 3 months Subcutaneous for infertility: 0.5–1 mg/day. By day 3 of the menstrual cycle, the dosage is typically decreased by 50%	
nafarelin (Synarel)	Intranasal: 2 inhalations/day (200 mcg/inhalation), one in each nostril; begin between days 2 and 4 of menstrual cycle; in patients with persistent regular menstruation after 2 months of therapy, may increase to 800 mcg/day as 2 inhalations (one in each nostril) bid; continue therapy for 6 months	

Note: *Italics* indicate common adverse effects. Underline indicates serious adverse effects.

PATHOPHYSIOLOGY *ILLUSTRATED* 70.1

Mechanisms of Action of Drugs Used to Treat Infertility

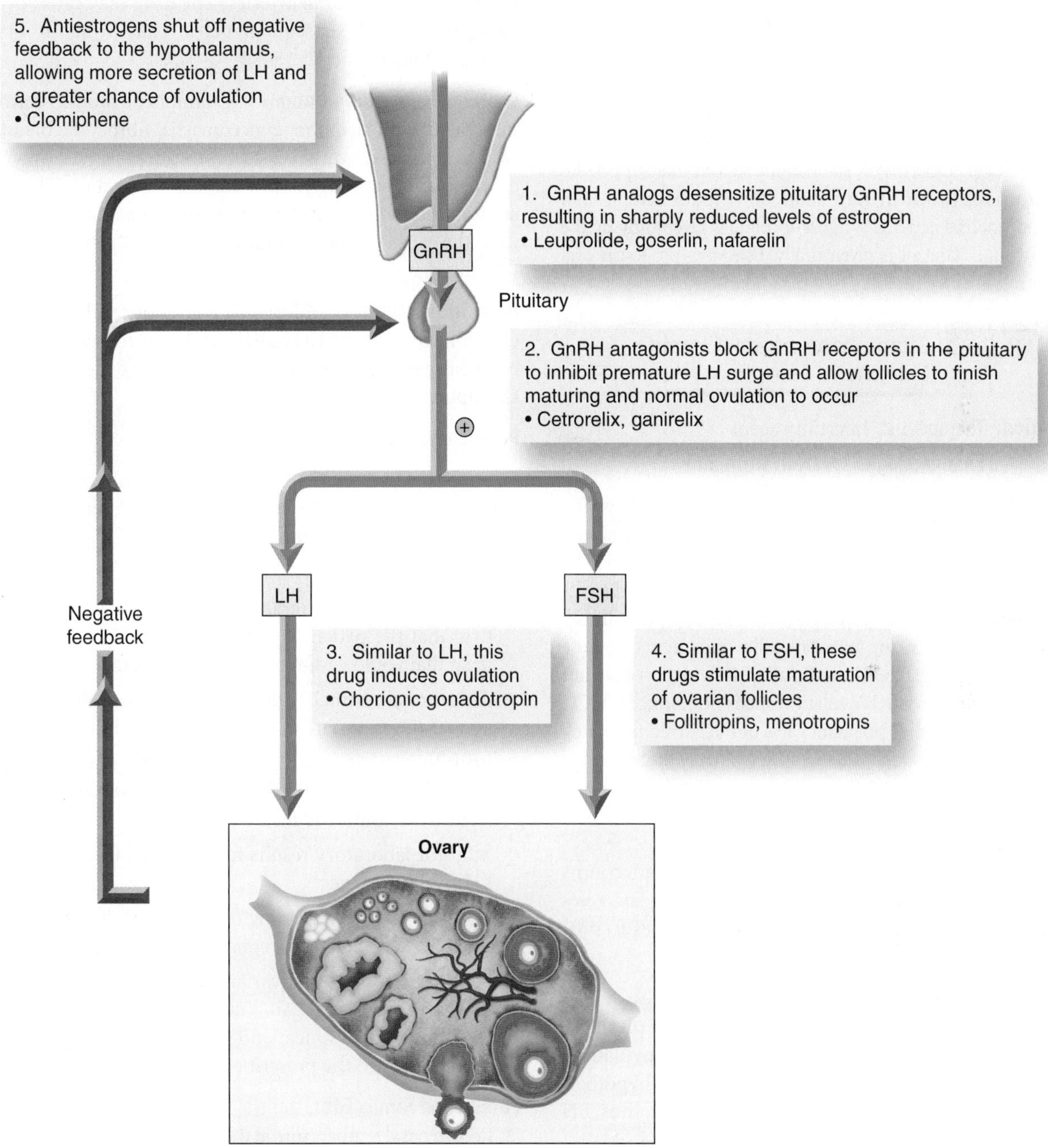

5. Antiestrogens shut off negative feedback to the hypothalamus, allowing more secretion of LH and a greater chance of ovulation
• Clomiphene

1. GnRH analogs desensitize pituitary GnRH receptors, resulting in sharply reduced levels of estrogen
• Leuprolide, goserlin, nafarelin

GnRH

Pituitary

2. GnRH antagonists block GnRH receptors in the pituitary to inhibit premature LH surge and allow follicles to finish maturing and normal ovulation to occur
• Cetrorelix, ganirelix

⊕

LH

FSH

Negative feedback

3. Similar to LH, this drug induces ovulation
• Chorionic gonadotropin

4. Similar to FSH, these drugs stimulate maturation of ovarian follicles
• Follitropins, menotropins

Ovary

tissue can cause pain, dysfunctional uterine bleeding, and dysmenorrhea. Surgical removal, ablation, or laser vaporization of the abnormal endometrial lesions may be necessary. Women who have completed their childbearing, or who are postmenopausal may consider a hysterectomy with oophorectomy.

Leuprolide (Lupron) and nafarelin (Synarel) are GnRH agonists that produce an initial release of LH and FSH, followed by suppression due to the negative feedback effect on the pituitary. Many women experience relief from the symptoms of endometriosis after 3 to 6 months of leuprolide therapy, and the benefits may extend well beyond the treatment period. As an alternative choice, danazol (Danocrine) is an anabolic steroid that suppresses FSH production, which in turn shuts down both ectopic and normal endometrial activity. While leuprolide is given only by the parenteral route, danazol is given orally. Estrogen–progestin oral contraceptives are also useful in treating endometriosis.

PROTOTYPE DRUG Clomiphene citrate (Clomid, Milophene, Serophene)

Classification: **Therapeutic:** Infertility agent
Pharmacologic: Ovarian stimulant

Therapeutic Effects and Uses: Approved in 1967, clomiphene is a drug of choice for female infertility caused by ovulatory dysfunction. It acts by inducing ovulation in anovulatory women. The pregnancy rate of patients taking clomiphene is high, and twins occur in about 3% to 5% of treated patients. Therapy is usually begun with a low dose of 50 mg for 5 days following menses because this is the time of greatest follicle maturation. If ovulation does not occur, the dose is increased. If ovulation still is not induced, HCG is added to the regimen. If pregnancy has not occurred following six cycles of successful ovulation, the drug is usually discontinued and other means of restoring infertility are explored. The use of clomiphene does not permanently restore normal follicle maturation. Its effects diminish once the drug is discontinued.

Clomiphene is used off-label to treat low sperm counts (oligospermia) in men. Just as in females, the drug increases the secretion of LH. In men, LH stimulates the testes to produce testosterone and additional sperm.

Mechanism of Action: Clomiphene acts as an "antiestrogen." Estrogen normally provides negative feedback to the pituitary, shutting off LH secretion, which is required for ovulation. Clomiphene competes for estrogen receptors in the hypothalamus, sending a message that estrogen levels are low; thus, LH is secreted, leading to ovarian stimulation.

Pharmacokinetics:

Route(s)	PO
Absorption	Readily absorbed
Distribution	Crosses the placenta; unknown if secreted in breast milk; 90% bound to protein
Primary metabolism	Hepatic
Primary excretion	Feces; small amounts in urine
Onset of action	30–60 minutes
Duration of action	Half-life: 5–7 days; peak effects: 4–10 days

Adverse Effects: Few serious adverse effects occur during clomiphene therapy. The most common are weight gain, symptoms of PMS, hot flashes, allergic dermatitis, and urticaria. The most serious adverse effects are blurred vision, ovarian hyperstimulation, cataracts and other visual impairments, and thrombosis of temporal arteries. The drug may cause ovarian enlargement with subsequent pelvic pain in about 14% of women taking the drug.

Contraindications/Precautions: Clomiphene should be avoided in patients with lactation, gynecomastia, fibrocystic breast disease, liver disease, ovarian cysts not due to polycystic ovary syndrome, and hepatic, thyroid, or adrenal dysfunction. The drug is contraindicated in patients with dysfunctional uterine bleeding until the cause can be determined. Pregnant patients must not take this drug.

Drug Interactions: Androgens will reduce the success of clomiphene therapy. **Herbal/Food:** Black cohosh and chasteberry have estrogen effects that may reduce the effectiveness of clomiphene.

Pregnancy: Category X.

Treatment of Overdose: Symptoms of overdose include nausea or vomiting, visual blurring, hot flashes, and pelvic pain. The patient is treated symptomatically.

Nursing Responsibilities:

- Prior to beginning therapy, obtain a pregnancy test to confirm that the patient is not pregnant. This is a category X drug that could cause fetal abnormalities.
- Assess for abnormal vaginal bleeding. If present, ensure that neoplastic lesions are not present prior to initiating therapy.
- Prior to initiating therapy, exclude other causes of infertility, such as thyroid disorders, adrenal disorders, hyperprolactinemia, and male factor infertility.
- Monitor laboratory results for increased levels of FSH and LH, and pregnancy.
- Counsel patients regarding the timing of drug therapy and intercourse to achieve pregnancy.
- Monitor for signs of ovarian hyperstimulation syndrome such as rapid weight gain, increased abdominal girth, nausea, vomiting, dyspnea, and chest pain. Report symptoms immediately to the prescriber.

Patient and Family Education:

- Record basal temperature at the same time each day on a graph to determine if ovulation has occurred. Ovulation occurs on days 4 through 10 in women who respond to treatment. There is an increased possibility of a multiple pregnancy.
- Take the medication at the same time each day to maintain consistent drug levels.
- Discontinue the drug and report if pain in the pelvic area or abdominal distention occurs. This may indicate ovarian enlargement or presence of a ruptured ovarian cyst.
- Immediately report blurred vision, spots or flashes in the eyes, severe hot flashes, uterine bleeding, headache, and nausea to the health care provider.

- Do not drive or perform other hazardous activities until the effects of the drug are known because this drug may cause drowsiness or dizziness.
- Report signs of jaundice such as yellowing of the skin or eyes, light-colored stool, and fever.
- Immediately notify the health care provider of any known or suspected pregnancy.

Drugs Similar to Clomiphene Citrate (Clomid, Milophene, Serophene)

Other drugs for female infertility include bromocriptine, cetrorelix, chorionic gonadotropin-HCG, danazol, follitropins, ganirelix, goserelin, leuprolide, menotropins, and nafarelin. Gonadorelin (Lutrepulse) was discontinued in 1997.

Bromocriptine (Parlodel): Approved in 1978, bromocriptine is chemically related to the ergot alkaloids and is indicated for a large number of diverse conditions. The drug is a dopamine agonist, activating dopaminergic receptors in the hypothalamus. For infertility, its primary use is to treat prolactin-secreting tumors of the pituitary, which often cause amenorrhea and female infertility. Normal menses is usually restored after 6 to 8 weeks of therapy. This reduces elevated serum prolactin levels and restores ovulation and ovarian function in amenorrheic women. It is used as a short-term treatment of amenorrhea in the absence of pituitary tumors. It is also FDA approved to treat acromegaly and Parkinson's disease. Off-label indications include mastalgia associated with PMS, alcoholism, cocaine withdrawal, and neuroleptic malignant syndrome. Bromocriptine causes frequent adverse effects that include nausea, vomiting, cramping, constipation, drowsiness, headache, orthostatic hypotension, and anorexia. This drug is pregnancy category C.

Cetrorelix (Cetrotide): Approved in 2000, cetrorelix is a GnRH antagonist given by the subcutaneous route that blocks GnRH receptors in the pituitary. Women undergoing ovarian stimulation with FSH or menotropin therapy experience a sharp rise in estrogen levels due to the maturing follicles, which can trigger an early surge of LH and premature ovulation. Cetrorelix inhibits this premature LH surge in women who are undergoing controlled ovarian stimulation for assisted reproduction, thus allowing follicles to finish maturing and normal ovulation to occur. The only indication for cetrorelix is infertility. Adverse effects are minor and include hot flashes and headache. It is contraindicated for use in primary ovarian failure, renal failure, and pregnancy. This drug is pregnancy category X.

Chorionic Gonadotropin-HCG (Novarel, Ovidrel, Pregnyl): This drug has two forms. HCG is secreted by the placenta and obtained and purified from the urine of pregnant women. Choriogonadotropin alfa (r-HCG, Ovidrel) is a recombinant form with identical actions to HCG. The chorionic gonadotropin drugs have the same actions as LH and can mimic the LH surge that normally causes ovulation. As part of an assisted reproductive program, chorionic gonadotropin is administered at midcycle, after clomiphene or FSH has been used to mature sufficient numbers of ovarian follicles. A single IM dose is sufficient to induce ovulation. The drug has few adverse effects when administered as a single dose in females. This drug is pregnancy category X.

In males, HCG is approved to treat prepubertal cryptorchidism, hypogonadism, and oligospermia. Therapy in males may continue for several months. In males, gynecomastia, acne, and behavioral changes may occur.

Danazol (Danocrine): Danocrine is an oral drug used to treat endometriosis. Approved in 1976, the drug exerts antiestrogenic and weak androgenic properties, which causes ectopic endometrial tissue to atrophy. After 6 weeks of therapy, danazol causes anovulation and amenorrhea, which are its therapeutic effects. When the drug is discontinued, normal ovulation and menstrual cycles return in about 2 to 3 months. Danazol is also FDA approved to treat fibrocystic breast disease and for the prophylaxis of hereditary angioedema. The drug has androgenic actions that may cause permanent masculinization effects such as hirsutism, alopecia, voice deepening, and weight gain. Females may experience effects of estrogen deficiency such as vaginal dryness, reduction in breast size, emotional lability, and hot flashes. Serious adverse effects include thromboembolism, hepatic adenoma, and intracranial HTN. This drug is pregnancy category X.

Follitropins: The follitropins are three different drugs with the same actions. All are versions of human FSH. Urofollitropin (Bravelle) is FSH purified from the urine of postmenopausal females. Follitropin alfa (Gonal-F) and follitropin beta (Follistim) are FSH obtained through recombinant DNA technology. All three FSH products are given by the parenteral route. The function of FSH (and the follitropins) is to stimulate the maturation of ovarian follicles. The drugs are given early in the menstrual cycle, followed by a dose of chorionic gonadotropin, which provides the boost for ovulation. Multiple births, including triplets, quadruplets, and quintuplets, are common during therapy with follitropins. Care must be taken not to "overtreat" with follitropins because this can cause OHS. In males, follitropins are used to stimulate spermatogenesis in patients with hypogonadism and oligospermia. Minor adverse effects include headache, nausea, abdominal pain, diarrhea, and increased infections. The most serious potential adverse effects are OHS and thromboembolism. In addition, serious pulmonary conditions such as acute respiratory distress syndrome and exacerbation of asthma have been reported. The follitropins are pregnancy category X.

Ganirelix (Antagon): Like cetrorelix, ganirelix is a GnRH antagonist given by the subcutaneous route that blocks GnRH receptors in the pituitary. Approved in 1999, its only indication is for female infertility. Ganirelix inhibits the premature LH surge in patients undergoing controlled ovarian stimulation for assisted reproduction. Adverse effects are minor and include hot flashes, menstrual irregularities, and headache. It is contraindicated for use in primary ovarian failure, renal failure, and pregnancy. This drug is pregnancy category X.

Goserelin (Zoladex): Goserelin is a GnRH hormone analog or agonist. It has the same physiological actions as endogenous GnRH; however, the way it is administered causes the opposite effect. Natural GnRH is released by the hypothalamus in an "on–off" pulsatile manner, which stimulates the release of LH and FSH (and eventually estrogen). Like GnRH, goserelin first stimulates LH and FSH secretion. With continuous administration, however, the pituitary receptors become insensitive to the effects of GnRH and the gland stops releasing LH and FSH. Without FSH or LH, the levels of estrogen in females and testosterone in males fall dramatically. This hypoestrogenic state relieves the symptoms of endometriosis. It is also approved for palliative treatment of estrogen-dependent breast cancer and for advanced prostatic cancer, which is dependent upon testosterone. Goserelin is available subcutaneously as a once-monthly implant (for males or females) and a 3-month implant for males with prostate cancer. Females may experience hypoestrogenic effects such as vaginal dryness, depression, menstrual irregularities, bone density loss, emotional lability, and hot flashes. Males may experience erectile dysfunction, gynecomastia, and loss of libido. Pain at the injection site is common. This drug is pregnancy category X.

Leuprolide (Eligard, Lupron): Like goserelin, leuprolide is a GnRH agonist/analog. The two drugs act by the same mechanism: desensitizing pituitary GnRH receptors, resulting in sharply reduced levels of estrogen and testosterone. For relief of endometriosis symptoms, a depot IM injection is given once monthly or once every 3 months, depending upon the dose. Treatment of endometriosis is limited to 6 months. Like goserelin, it is also approved for the palliative treatment of advanced prostatic cancer, and used off-label for breast cancer. Leuprolide is an orphan drug for treating precocious (early) puberty in children less than 9 years old. The drug was once widely used to treat infertility by inhibiting premature LH surges but the GnRH antagonists are now used for this indication. The adverse effects are the same as for goserelin. This drug is pregnancy category X.

Menotropins (Menopur, Repronex): Approved in 1975, menotropins is sometimes referred to as HMG. Menotropins is a product containing a combination of FSH and LH purified from the urine of postmenopausal women. The FSH activity of menotropins is significantly higher than the LH activity. Like the follitropins, menotropins is given by the parenteral route during the first half of the menstrual cycle to promote follicle maturation. At the end of therapy, HCG is often administered to supply the LH surge necessary for ovulation. Menotropins therapy is associated with a 20% to 35% possibility of multiple births. In males, menotropins is FDA approved to stimulate spermatogenesis in patients with hypogonadism and oligospermia. In males, gynecomastia, acne, and behavioral changes may occur. In females, the drug often causes ovarian enlargement and OHS is possible. Serious pulmonary conditions such as acute respiratory distress syndrome and exacerbation of asthma have been reported. This drug is pregnancy category X.

Nafarelin (Synarel): Like goserelin and leuprolide, nafarelin is a GnRH agonist/analog. The three drugs act by the same mechanism: desensitizing pituitary GnRH receptors, resulting in sharply reduced levels of estrogen and testosterone. Unlike the other GnRH analogs, nafarelin is applied topically to the nasal mucosa, where the drug is rapidly absorbed. When used to treat endometriosis, the typical dose is one spray in each nostril daily. It is also approved to treat precocious puberty and used off-label for hirsutism. Nafarelin may be used off-label to prevent premature LH surges in women with infertility; however, ganirelix and cetrorelix are more frequently prescribed for this indication. Adverse effects are the same as the other GnRH agonists goserelin and leuprolide. This drug was approved in 1990 and is pregnancy category X.

UNDERSTANDING THE CHAPTER

Key Concepts Summary

70.1 Regulation of the female reproductive system is achieved by hormones from the hypothalamus, pituitary gland, and ovary.

70.2 Estrogens are administered as replacement therapy, to prevent contraception, and for certain neoplasms.

70.3 Progestins are administered to treat dysfunctional uterine bleeding, to prevent contraception, and for certain neoplasms.

70.4 Hormone replacement therapy provides relief from menopause symptoms but may have serious long-term negative effects.

70.5 Oxytocics are drugs used to stimulate the uterus and promote labor and delivery.

70.6 Uterine relaxants are used to suppress preterm labor.

70.7 Female infertility may be treated with drugs that promote oocyte maturation and ovulation.

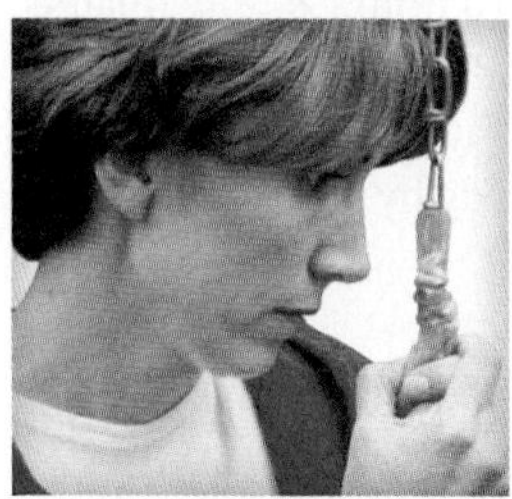

Making the PATIENT Connection

Remember the patient "Ileen John" at the beginning of the chapter? Now read the remainder of the case study. Based on the information presented within this chapter, respond to the critical thinking questions that follow the case study.

Ileen John is 46 years old and exhibiting signs of menopause. She reports a change in her menstrual cycle regularity. For the past year, her periods have occurred between 6 and 8 weeks apart and they lasted only 2 to 3 days. Previously, she experienced her periods approximately every 28 days and they lasted from 4 to 5 days. She reports to the nurse that she is now feeling easily fatigued, has more mood swings, occasional headaches, hot flashes, insomnia, bouts of depression, and irritability. She is concerned about loss of libido. She admits to smoking half a pack of cigarettes a day and drinking several cups of coffee during work hours. She has a family history of HTN, cardiac diseases, and diabetes, but she has never been diagnosed with any of those disorders.

A complete history and physical examination, along with a vaginal examination and a pap smear were performed.

Critical Thinking Questions

1. What do you think is the most likely cause for Ileen's symptoms?
2. Create a list of some treatment options for Ileen.
3. How would you, the nurse, approach caring for Ileen?
4. Ileen asks about the precautions related to suggested treatment options. How would you respond?

Case Study

A 23-year-old woman and her 25-year-old husband attend the infertility clinic for evaluation. Efforts at becoming pregnant naturally for the past 2 years have failed. They inform the nurse that the husband has a 3-year-old son from an earlier relationship. The wife has never conceived. Both denied any sexually transmitted infections. The patient is started on clomiphene citrate (Clomid) 50 mg for 5 days.

1. The young woman asks you, the nurse, "What are some causes for female infertility?" How would you respond?
2. What instructions would you give to the client regarding the administration of this drug?

NCLEX-RN® Review

1 The nurse should include which of the following discharge instructions to the client receiving HRT?

1. Avoid foods that contain caffeine.
2. Take the medication 30 minutes before meals.
3. Discontinue the medication if uterine bleeding begins.
4. Monitor for a sudden increase in low-density lipoprotein cholesterol.

2 The nurse's assessment of the client receiving an intravenous (IV) infusion of oxytocin notes that uterine contractions are 4 minutes apart and 60 seconds in duration. Which of the following nursing interventions is most important based on this assessment?

1. Administer oxygen via face mask.
2. Monitor the client for water intoxication.
3. Position the client on her left side.
4. Discontinue the infusion immediately.

3 The nurse instructs an infertile couple that the drug most commonly used for stimulating ovulation is:

1. Medroxyprogesterone (Provera).
2. Pitocin (Oxytocin).
3. Clomiphene citrate (Clomid).
4. Conjugated estrogens (Premarin).

4 The nurse would identify a patient with which of the following medical conditions as someone who should not be prescribed estradiol/norgestimate (Ortho-Prefest)? (Select all that apply.)

1. Chronic asthma and osteoporosis
2. Diabetes mellitus and hypertension
3. Liver disease and thromboembolic disorders
4. Breast cancer and cervical cancer
5. Scoliosis and kyphosis

5 The client informs the health care provider that she has been trying to become pregnant for more than 2 years and has not used any form of contraception. The health care provider prescribed clomiphene (Clomid) 50 mg/day for 5 days. The nurse should instruct the client to begin taking the drug on the:

1. First day of the menstrual cycle.
2. Fifth day of the menstrual cycle.
3. Fifth day after ovulation.
4. Last day of the menstrual cycle.

6 The client in active labor for over 10 hours is fully dilated but is showing no progress toward delivery. The health care provider orders an oxytocin (Pitocin) injection. The nurse should prepare to give the drug by which route?

1. Intravenously mixed in D_5W
2. Intravenous bolus injection
3. Intramuscularly diluted in saline
4. Nasal spray (both nostrils)

See Answers to Critical Thinking Questions, Case Study, and NCLEX-RN® Review in Appendix A.

References

Bastian, L. A., Smith, C., & Nanda, K. (2003). Is this woman perimenopausal? *Journal of the American Medical Association, 289*(7), 895–902.

Centers for Disease Control and Prevention. (2008). *Infertility and STDs.* Retrieved August 31, 2008, from http://www.cdc.gov/std/infertility/default.htm

Chandiramani, M., & Shennan, A. (2006). Preterm labour: Update on prediction and prevention strategies. *Current Opinion in Obstetrics & Gynecology, 18*(6), 618–624.

Davidson, M. R., London, M. L., & Ladewig, P. L. (2008). *Maternal newborn nursing and women's health across the lifespan* (8th ed.). Upper Saddle River, NJ: Prentice Hall.

Dennehy, C. E. (2006). The use of herbs and dietary supplements in gynecology: An evidence-based review. *Journal of Midwifery and Womens Health, 51*(3), 402–409.

Dodds, N. R., & Sinert, R. (2007). *Dysfunctional uterine bleeding.* eMedicine. Retrieved August 31, 2008, from http://www.emedicine.com/emerg/topic155.htm

Grady, D., Herrington, D., Bittner, V., Blumenthal, R., Davidson, M., Hlatky, M., et al. (2002). Cardiovascular disease outcomes during 6.8 years of hormone therapy: Heart and estrogen/progestin replacement study follow-up (HERS II). *Journal of the American Medical Association, 288*(1), 49–57.

Grimes, D. A., & Nanda, K. (2006). Magnesium sulfate tocolysis: Time to quit. *Obstetrics and Gynecology, 108*(4), 986–989.

Hansen, L. B., & Portman, D. (2006). Hormone therapy update: Current recommendations for menopausal symptoms. *US Pharmacist, 31*(9), 89–96.

Heiss, G., Wallace, R., Anderson, G. L., Aragaki, A., Beresford, S. A. A., Brzyski, R., et al., for the WHI Investigators. (2008). Health risks and benefits 3 years after stopping randomized treatment with estrogen and progestin. *Journal of the American Medical Association, 299*(9), 1036–1045. Retrieved August 31, 2008, from http://www.nhlbi.nih.gov/whi/

Hulley, S., Furberg, C., Barrett-Connor, E., Cauley, J., Grady, D., & Haskell, W. (2002). Noncardiovascular disease outcomes during 6.8 years of hormone therapy: Heart and estrogen/progestin replacement study follow-up (HERS II). *Journal of the American Medical Association, 288*(1), 58–66.

Leeman, L., Fontaine, P., King, V., Klein, M. C., & Ratcliffe, S. (2003). The nature and management of labor pain: Part II. Pharmacologic pain relief. *American Family Physician, 68,* 1115–1120, 1121–1122.

Loose, D. S., & Stancel, G. M. (2006). Estrogens. In L. L. Brunton, J. S. Lazo, & K. L. Parker (Eds.), *The pharmacological basis of therapeutics* (11th ed., pp. 1541–1572). New York: McGraw-Hill.

Ludwig, M., Westergaard, L. G., Diedrich, K., & Andersen, C. Y. (2003). Developments in drugs for ovarian stimulation. *Best Practice & Research, Clinical Obstetrics & Gynaecology, 17*(2), 231–247.

Messina, M. J. (2002). Soy foods and soybean isoflavones and menopausal health. *Nutrition in Clinical Care, 5*(6), 272.

Mikkelsen, T. F., Graff-Iversen, S., Sundby, J., & Bjertness, E. (2007). Early menopause, association with tobacco smoking, coffee consumption, and other lifestyle factors: A cross-sectional study. *BMC Public Health, 7,* 149. Retrieved August 31, 2008, from http://www.biomedcentral.com/1471-2458/7/149/abstract

Roemheld-Hamm, B. (2005). Chasteberry. *American Family Physician, 72*(2), 821–824.

Stearns, V. (2007). Clinical update: New treatments for hot flushes. *The Lancet, 369*(9579), 2062–2064.

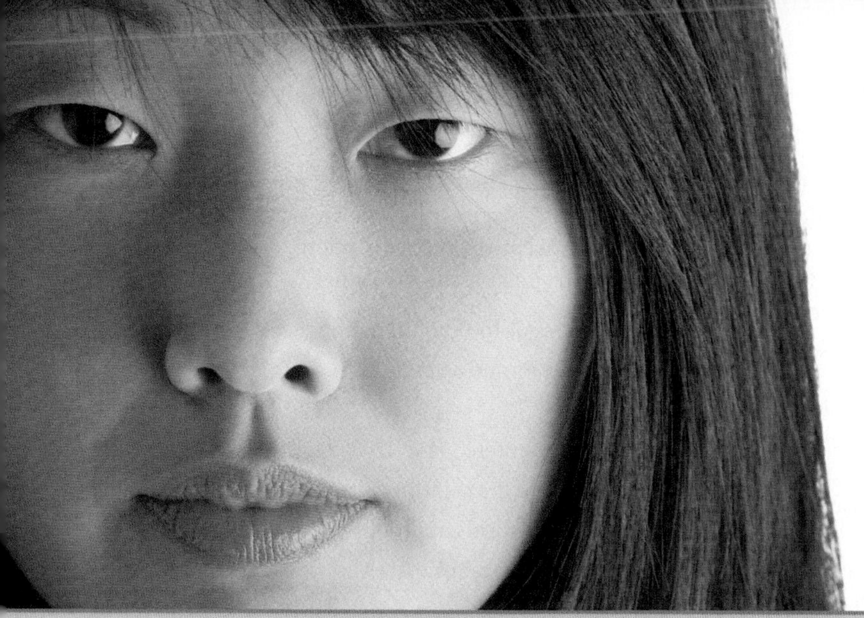

I really don't want to ruin my chances of going to college by becoming pregnant right now in my life. What can I do?

Patient "Lila Bastian," 19 years old

CHAPTER 71

Drugs for Modifying Conception

Chapter Outline

Options and Choices for Birth Control

Combination Oral Contraceptives

Estrogen/Progestin Combinations

PROTOTYPE **Estradiol and Norethindrone (Ortho-Novum)** *p. 1204*

Progestin-Only Oral Contraceptives

Adverse Effects of Combined Oral Contraceptives

Drugs for Long-Term Contraception and Newer Contraceptive Delivery Methods

Spermicides

PROTOTYPE **Nonoxynol-9** *p. 1211*

Emergency Contraception

Drugs for Pharmacologic Abortion

PROTOTYPE **Mifepristone (RU-486)** *p. 1214*

Learning Outcomes

After reading this chapter, the student should be able to:

1. Describe the options and choices available for birth control.
2. Delineate advantages and disadvantages of the different contraceptive modalities.
3. Explain the mechanisms by which estrogens and progestins prevent conception.
4. Discuss the safety and effectiveness of birth control methods.
5. Explain how drugs may be used to provide emergency contraception and to terminate early pregnancy.
6. Describe the nurse's role in the pharmacologic management of patients who are taking oral contraceptives.
7. Compare and contrast the options for long-term contraception.
8. For each of the classes shown in the chapter outline, identify the prototype and representative drugs and explain the mechanism(s) of drug action, primary indications, contraindications, significant drug interactions, pregnancy category, and important adverse effects.
9. Apply the nursing process to care for patients who are receiving drug therapy for contraception.

Key Terms

abortifacients, *1212*
chloasma, *1208*
contraception, *1200*
ectopic pregnancy, *1204*
emergency contraception (EC), *1212*
estrogen, *1200*
progesterone, *1200*
spermicides, *1210*

Currently, approximately 60 million women in the United States are of childbearing age (15 to 44 years). Of these women about 60% practice **contraception,** which is the use of devices, drugs, or surgery to prevent pregnancy. Despite the relatively high percentage of contraceptive use, the rate of unintended pregnancy in the United States remains at approximately 50%. The discovery of the oral contraceptives had a revolutionary impact on society and has given couples a variety of choices for contraception. This chapter discusses the female sex hormones that are used to modify conception, describes other widely used methods of contraception, and identifies the nursing connections to patient and family education.

Pharm*FACT*

In 1989, 20% of all pregnant women smoked during pregnancy. This dropped to 10% in 2004. The smoking rate remains high (24%) for mothers who have less than a high school education. *Source:* National Center for Health Statistics, 2007.

Options and Choices for Birth Control

71.1 Selection of a contraceptive is based on effectiveness, safety, and personal choice.

The decision to engage in sexual activity is one of the most important decisions in life; the choice affects not just the partners, but may impact generations to follow. A couple who is engaging in intercourse on a regular basis without contraceptive protection has a 90% probability of conceiving a child over the course of a year. Thus, the voluntary choice to use contraceptive measures is a critical decision faced by most women in the childbearing years.

Prior to the 1960s, the three primary methods of avoiding pregnancy were total abstinence, abstinence during periods of greatest fertility (rhythm or calender method), and withdrawal prior to ejaculation (coitus interruptus). The discovery of oral contraceptives and the development of novel long-term contraceptives have given couples more effective choices for birth control. Now there are many options that may be considered, each having specific advantages and disadvantages. The primary options are shown in Table 71.1.

Women make personal birth control decisions based on several factors. Regardless of the contraceptive choice, the effectiveness of preventing pregnancy and safety of the medication or device are the highest priorities. Women who engage in intercourse frequently or who are likely to forget to take their medication may prefer the convenience of the long-acting contraceptives. For patients who have a history of thromboembolic disorders, barrier protection or taking progestin-only types of contraceptives are safer options. Factors that influence their decisions include the following:

- Effectiveness of the chosen method
- Adverse effects and safety
- Age
- Frequency of intercourse
- Ease of use and the ability to adhere to the required regimen
- Preexisting medical conditions
- Cultural beliefs and practices

Women who are seeking to prevent conception need to discuss the available options with their health care provider. Final decisions on choosing a contraceptive should be made voluntarily with full knowledge of its advantages and disadvantages, effectiveness, adverse effects, contraindications, and potential long-term risks. When the desire to have children in the future no longer exists, sterilization of either the male or female is the most common and effective option for birth control. Whatever the choice of birth control, personal motivation must be taken into consideration because it is important that the woman be consistent in using the chosen method if pregnancy is to be prevented.

The different contraceptives act in different regions of the female reproductive tract. The student should refer to Pharmacotherapy Illustrated 71.1 on page 1202 often while reading this chapter to obtain an overall perspective on the sites and mechanisms of contraceptive action.

Combination Oral Contraceptives

71.2 The most effective contraceptive agents include combinations of low-dose estrogens and progestins.

The physiology and pharmacologic indications for the female sex hormones estrogen and progesterone are presented in Chapter 70. Because estrogen and progesterone are the two classes of drugs used most frequently for contraception, the student should review that chapter before proceeding.

The most widespread pharmacologic use of estrogen and progesterone is to prevent pregnancy. **Estrogen** is a general term that refers to several female sex hormones. The ones used in oral contraceptives are the synthetic estrogens ethinyl estradiol and, rarely, mestranol. All estrogens have the same pharmacologic actions.

Progestin is a general term that refers to synthetic hormones that have actions identical to natural endogenous progesterone. Although **progesterone** is the natural progestin secreted by the corpus luteum, it is rarely used for contraception. Instead synthetic progestins, including norethindrone, norgestrel, desogestrel, and levonorgestrel, are used. The synthetic progestins have a much longer half-life than progesterone, which allows for the convenience of

TABLE 71.1 Effectiveness of Conception Modifiers

Type	Description	PREGNANCY RATE (%/YEAR)*		Selected Advantages	Selected Disadvantages
		With Perfect Use	With Typical Use		
Hormonal Methods					
Combination oral contraceptives (OCs)	Daily tablets	0.1%	7%	Very effective, decreased risk of ovarian and endometrial cancer	Fluid retention, venous thromboembolism, amenorrhea, nausea, vomiting. irregular bleeding, headache; must be taken daily
Progestin-only oral contraceptives	Daily tablets	0.5%	7%	No estrogen adverse effects; may be used in women with history of thromboembolic disease	Less effective than combination OCs; frequent spotting, amenorrhea, ectopic pregnancy
Progestin injections	Every 3 months	0.3%	3%	Do not have to take daily pills; long-term protection	Amenorrhea, irregular bleeding, headache
Transdermal steroids	Weekly patch	0.3%	8%	Do not have to take daily pills; easy to apply	Similar to OCs; higher risk of thromboembolic disease compared to OCs
Subdermal progestin implants	Every 3 year	0.05%	Not Available	Do not have to take daily pills; long-term protection	Amenorrhea, irregular bleeding, headache
Barrier and Miscellaneous Methods					
Condoms, diaphragms, cervical caps	Coitus based	2–9%	15–18%	Inexpensive; some protection against STIs, no hormonal adverse effects; few significant adverse effects	Less convenient than hormonal methods
Spermicides	Coitus based	5–7% (without condom) 1% (with condom)	18–22% (without condom) 1–2% (with condom)	Inexpensive, no hormonal adverse effects	Ineffective if used without barrier protection; requires reapplication if intercourse lasts longer than 1 hour; inconvenient; vaginal irritation
Contraceptive sponge	Coitus based	9–20%	16–32%	Inexpensive; no hormonal adverse effects; protection lasts 24 hours	Allergic reactions, vaginal dryness or irritation; less convenient
Intrauterine devices/ systems	Mirena, Copper T; every few years	0.5–2%	Not Available	Effective, long-term contraception; decreased menstrual flow and cramping; inexpensive; no hormonal adverse effects (Copper T)	Irregular bleeding, pelvic pain, spontaneous expulsion, uterine perforation
Withdrawal method	Coitus based	4%	27%	Free; no adverse effects	Inconvenient and ineffective
Biological	Calendar/rhythm	1–9%	25%	Free, no adverse effects	Inconvenient and ineffective

*Pregnancy rates from using the various methods listed vary considerably in the scientific literature.

CONNECTIONS

Complementary and Alternative Therapies Black Cohosh

Description: Black cohosh (*Cimicifuga racemosa*) is a perennial that grows in open woods in the eastern United States and parts of Canada. "Black" refers to the color of its roots.

History and Claims: Use of this herb was recorded by Native Americans for more than 100 years. These peoples used the herb for a variety of conditions, including sore throat, kidney ailments, fatigue, menstrual cramps, and to ease the pain of labor. Modern use of this herb has focused on its actions on the female reproductive system.

Standardization: Doses of black cohosh are sometimes standardized by the amount of the chemical 27-deoxyactein, which is an active ingredient. A typical dose of black cohosh ranges from 40 to 80 mg of dried herb per day. (Approximately 1 mg of 27-deoxyactein is present in each 20-mg tablet or in 20 drops of the liquid formulation.)

Evidence: Black cohosh has been shown to be effective in the management of menopausal hot flashes (Osmers et al., 2005). Black cohosh may even help prevent osteoporosis in postmenopausal women. Although black cohosh was once thought to have phytoestrogenic effects, new research questions this fact and further controlled studies are necessary (Borrelli & Ernst, 2008). Its actual mechanism of action is still unknown. Adverse effects include hypotension, uterine stimulation, and gastrointestinal (GI) complaints such as nausea. Black cohosh can increase the action of antihypertensives, so concurrent use should be avoided.

PHARMACOTHERAPY *ILLUSTRATED* 71.1

Mechanisms of Action of Oral Contraceptives

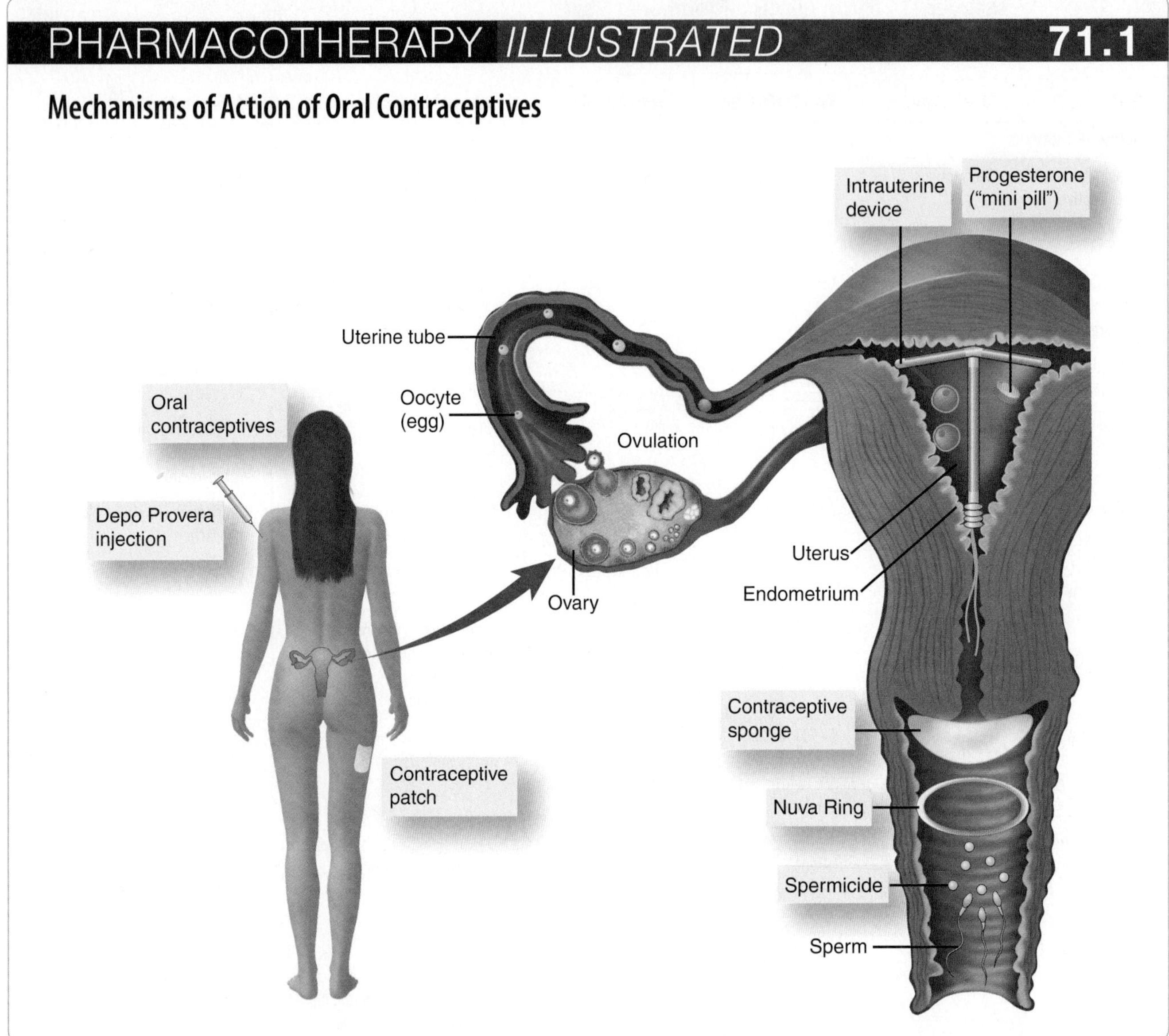

once-daily dosing. All progestins have the same pharmacologic activity.

The majority of oral contraceptives (OCs), known as "the pill," contain combinations of estrogen and progestin. Approximately 30% of the women who choose contraceptive methods select OCs. The drugs are readily available, are inexpensive, and are nearly 100% effective at preventing pregnancy when taken daily. They are excellent methods of contraception for women who are healthy and have no contraindications. One advantage of OCs is that they can be discontinued at any point without long-lasting adverse effects.

A large number of combination OC preparations are available, differing in dose and by type of estrogen and progestin, as illustrated in Table 71.2. Selection of a specific formulation is customized to each patient and determined by which product gives the best contraceptive protection with the fewest adverse effects. Treatment is generally initiated with the lowest dose that effectively provides contraceptive protection. Daily doses of estrogen in OCs have declined from 150 mcg 40 years ago to about 20 mcg in modern formulations. This reduction has resulted in a significant decrease in estrogen-related adverse effects.

Pharm*FACT*

Every year hundreds of millions of women worldwide suffer disability as a result of pregnancy complications, and more than half a million die in pregnancy and childbirth or following unsafe abortion. Almost all of these deaths are preventable. *Source:* Glasier, Gülmezoglu, Schmid, Moreno, & Van Look, 2006.

TABLE 71.2 Selected Oral Contraceptives

Trade Name	Estrogen	Progestin
Monophasic		
Alesse	ethinyl estradiol, 20 mcg	levonorgestrel, 0.1 mg
Desogen	ethinyl estradiol, 30 mcg	desogestrel, 0.15 mg
Loestrin 1.5/30 Fe	ethinyl estradiol, 30 mcg	norethindrone, 1.5 mg
Lo/Ovral	ethinyl estradiol, 30 mcg	norgestrel, 0.3 mg
Ortho-Cyclen	ethinyl estradiol, 35 mcg	norgestimate, 0.25 mg
Yasmin	ethinyl estradiol, 30 mcg	drospirenone, 3 mg
Zovia 1/50E-21 and 28	ethinyl estradiol, 50 mcg	ethynodiol diacetate, 1 mg
Biphasic		
Mircette	ethinyl estradiol, 20 mcg for 21 days; 10 mcg for 5 days	desogestrel, 0.15 mg for 21 days
Ortho-Novum 10/11	ethinyl estradiol, 35 mcg	norethindrone, 0.5 mg (phase 1) and 1 mg (phase 2)
Triphasic		
Ortho-Novum 7/7/7	ethinyl estradiol, 35 mcg	norethindrone, 0.5 mg (phase 1)
	ethinyl estradiol, 35 mcg	norethindrone, 0.75 mg (phase 2)
	ethinyl estradiol, 35 mcg	norethindrone, 1 mg (phase 3)
Ortho Tri-Cyclen	ethinyl estradiol, 35 mcg	norgestimate, 0.18 mg (phase 1)
	ethinyl estradiol, 35 mcg	norgestimate, 0.215 mg (phase 2)
	ethinyl estradiol, 35 mcg	norgestimate, 0.25 mg (phase 3)
Tri-Levlen	ethinyl estradiol, 35 mcg	levonorgestrel, 0.05 mg (phase 1)
	ethinyl estradiol, 40 mcg	levonorgestrel, 0.075 mg (phase 2)
	ethinyl estradiol, 30 mcg	levonorgestrel, 0.125 mg (phase 3)
Triphasil	ethinyl estradiol, 30 mcg	norgestrel, 0.05 mg (phase 1)
	ethinyl estradiol, 40 mcg	norgestrel, 0.075 mg (phase 2)
	ethinyl estradiol, 30 mcg	norgestrel, 1.25 mg (phase 3)
Progestin Only		
Micronor	None	norethindrone, 0.35 mg
Nor-Q.D.	None	norethindrone, 0.35 mg
Ovrette	None	norgestrel, 0.075 mg
Emergency Contraceptive		
Plan B (2 tablets)	None	levonorgestrel, 0.75 mg

Typically, administration of an OC begins on day 5 of the menstrual cycle and continues for 21 days. During the other 7 days of the month, the patient takes a placebo. Although the placebo serves no pharmacologic purpose, it does encourage the patient to take the pills on a daily basis. Some of these placebos contain iron, which replaces iron lost due to menstrual bleeding.

A common problem with OCs, and likely the most frequent reason for treatment failure (pregnancy), is forgetting to take the medication daily. If one dose is missed, two pills taken the following day usually provide for continuous contraception. If two consecutive doses are missed, two tablets should be taken on both the day the missed doses are remembered and the following day. The regular schedule should then be continued, but a second method of contraception should be used for at least 7 days after restarting the pills. If 3 or more consecutive days are missed, the patient should observe other contraceptive precautions until the regimen can be restarted in the next

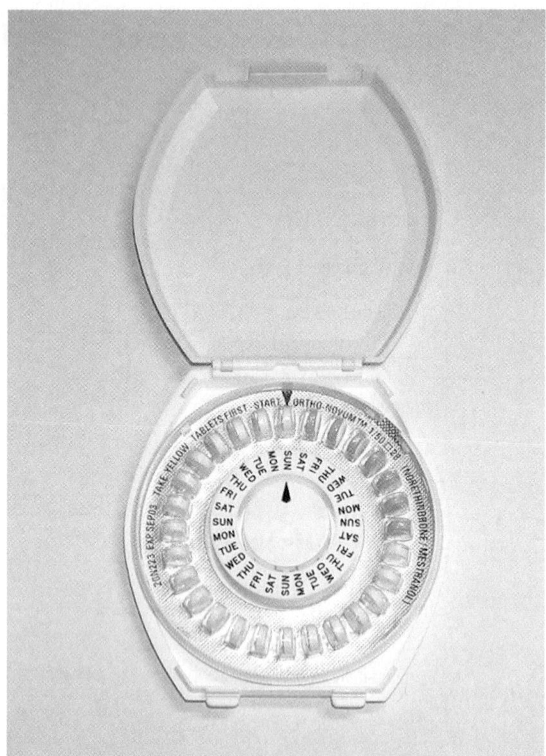

Figure 71.1 An oral contraceptive showing the daily doses and the different formulation taken in the last 7 days of the 28-day cycle.

monthly cycle. Figure 71.1 shows a typical monthly OC packet with the 28 pills.

Estrogen-progestin combination OCs act by preventing ovulation. They accomplish this by providing negative feedback to the pituitary, which suppresses the secretion of leuteinizing hormone (LH) and follicle-stimulating hormone (FSH). Without the influence of LH and FSH, the ovarian follicle cannot mature and ovulation is prevented. The estrogen-progestin agents also make the uterine endometrium less favorable to receive an embryo, thus reducing the likelihood of implantation. In addition the hormones promote the formation of a thick cervical mucus that slows sperm transport and inhibits the process that allows sperm to penetrate the ovum. The student should refer to Figure 70.2 in Chapter 70 for a review of the negative feedback control of female reproductive hormones.

> **CONNECTION *Checkpoint* 71.1**
>
> **Certain drugs that are used to treat infertility block the negative feedback cycle by occupying the estrogen receptors in the hypothalamus. From what you learned in Chapter 70, name this class of drugs and explain how they are used to increase fertility.** See Answer to Connection Checkpoint 71.1 in Appendix A.

There are three types of estrogen-progestin OC formulations: monophasic (e.g., Ortho-Novum 1/35), biphasic (e.g., Ortho-Novum 10/11), and triphasic (e.g., Ortho-Novum 7/7/7). The one most frequently prescribed is the monophasic OC, which delivers a constant dose of estrogen and progestin throughout the 21-day treatment cycle. In biphasic agents, the amount of estrogen in each pill remains constant, but the amount of progestin is increased toward the end of the treatment cycle to better nourish the uterine lining. In triphasic formulations, the amounts of both estrogen and progestin vary in three distinct phases during the treatment cycle.

When discontinuing OCs it may take several months for ovulation to return to normal and for monthly menstrual periods to become regular. Some women can conceive in the first month, whereas others experience a delay for up to a year before fertility is restored. The length of contraceptive use does not appear to affect fertility, except that fertility tapers off in women in their mid to late 30s due to normal aging. The incidence of miscarriage is not increased in women who conceive after having taken OCs.

Although the main purpose for taking combination OCs is to prevent pregnancy, there are several other benefits. Women who are taking OCs report less painful menstruation and may have reduced incidences of the following disorders: **ectopic pregnancy,** which is the development of the fetus elsewhere rather than in the uterus; pelvic inflammatory disease (PID); ovarian and endometrial cancer; colorectal cancer; iron deficiency anemia; and benign breast diseases. Women on OCs also experience a better-regulated menstrual flow and fewer outbreaks of acne.

A newer therapy of "extended regimen" OCs has been developed. Approved in 2003, Seasonale consists of tablets containing levonorgestrel and ethinyl estradiol that are taken for 84 consecutive days, followed by seven placebo tablets (without hormones). This allows for continuous contraceptive protection while extending the time between menses; only four periods are experienced per year. Seasonique is similar, but instead of inert tablets for 7 days, the patient takes low-dose estrogen tablets. Seasonique, which was approved in 2006, is claimed by the manufacturer to have a lower incidence of bloating and breakthrough bleeding.

PROTOTYPE DRUG Estradiol and Norethindrone (Ortho-Novum)

Classification: **Therapeutic:** Combination oral contraceptive
Pharmacologic: Estrogen-progestin

Therapeutic Effects and Uses: Typical of other drugs in this class, the primary use of Ortho-Novum is to prevent pregnancy. It is nearly 100% effective in preventing conception. Ortho-Novum is available in monophasic (1/35), biphasic (10/11), and triphasic (7/7/7) formulations. Off-label indications for the drug include acne vulgaris (in females who have achieved menarche), endometriosis, hypermenorrhea, dysfunctional uterine bleeding, and hirsutism related to hyposecretion of estrogen or oversecretion of androgens. Noncontraceptive benefits of Ortho-Novum include improvement in menstrual cycle regularity and decreased incidence of dysmenorrhea.

CONNECTIONS

Treating the Diverse Patient Cultural Influences in Choosing Contraception

Nurses must assess each woman's cultural beliefs regarding modifying conception. The method of contraception chosen will most likely be influenced by a couple's cultural beliefs and social influences. Because it is not possible for nurses to have knowledge of all cultural practices surrounding contraception, they should listen carefully to what the couples have to say. Here are some general hints that may prove helpful to the nurse during the assessment phase:

- The intrauterine device (IUD) is popularly used by Chinese women.
- African Americans commonly use oral contraceptives.
- Some cultures view contraception as a form of genocide.
- Some cultures use extended breast-feeding as a form of birth control.
- Native Americans are reluctant to control the number of children they have.

Mechanism of Action: Ortho-Novum decreases the chance of pregnancy by inhibiting ovulation. When the right combination of estrogens and progestins is present in the bloodstream, the release of FSH and LH is inhibited, thus preventing ovulation.

Pharmacokinetics:

Route(s)	Oral (PO)
Absorption	83% (norethindrone) and 47–73% (ethinyl estradiol)
Distribution	Widely distributed; secreted in breast milk
Primary metabolism	Hepatic and gastrointestinal (GI) mucosa; extensively metabolized
Primary excretion	Renal and feces
Onset of action	30–60 minutes
Duration of action	Half-life: 3–27 h

Adverse Effects: The most common adverse effects of Ortho-Novum are nausea, breast tenderness, weight gain, and breakthrough bleeding. Less common serious adverse effects include edema, unexplained loss of vision, diplopia, intolerance to contact lenses, gallbladder disease, nausea, abdominal cramps, changes in urinary function, dysmenorrhea, breast fullness, fatigue, skin rash, acne, headache, vaginal candidiasis, photosensitivity, and changes in urinary patterns. Cardiovascular adverse effects, the most serious of all, may include hypertension (HTN) and thromboembolic disorders. The estrogen component of the pill can lead to venous and arterial thrombosis, which results in pulmonary, myocardial, and thrombotic strokes.

Other conditions that are associated with OCs are abnormal uterine bleeding; benign hepatic adenoma; multiple births; elevated plasma glucose; retinal disorder; and melanoderma, a patchy or generalized skin discoloration caused by increased production of melanin. These conditions, though rare, have been reported and tend to disappear immediately after discontinuing the use of OCs.

Contraindications/Precautions: There are many contraindications and precautions regarding the use of OCs. The risk of cancer following long-term OC use has been extensively studied. Because some studies have shown a small increase in the incidence of breast cancer, OCs are contraindicated in patients with known or suspected breast cancer. The incidences of endometrial and ovarian cancers, however, are significantly reduced after long-term OC administration. It is likely that the relationship between the long-term use of these drugs and cancer will continue to be a controversial and frequently researched topic. Obesity is a risk factor for treatment failure and for increased possibilities of thromboembolic events. Smokers have a significantly increased risk of serious thromboembolic events when taking OCs. OCs may significantly worsen symptoms of lupus. Mood disorders, including depression, may be worsened in patients taking OCs. All combination OCs are pregnancy category X and are contraindicated in pregnancy.

Drug Interactions: A number of anticonvulsants (phenobarbital, phenytoin, carbamazepine, and primidone) and antibiotics (tetracyclines, rifampin, and ampicillin) can reduce the effectiveness of OCs, thus increasing a woman's risk of pregnancy. Women who are taking these drugs should be advised to use additional means of birth control or to have their OC dosages revised. Because OCs can reduce the effectiveness of warfarin (Coumadin), insulin, and certain oral hypoglycemic agents, dosage adjustment may be necessary. Tranquilizers are known to cause false-positive pregnancy test results. Patients who are taking theophylline for asthma or imipramine as an antidepressant in conjunction with OCs should be evaluated often because these drugs may accumulate to toxic levels in these individuals. **Herbal/Food:** OCs have been shown to cause breakthrough bleeding when used concurrently with St. John's wort.

Pregnancy: Category X.

Treatment of Overdose: There is no specific treatment for overdose. The patient is treated symptomatically.

Nursing Responsibilities:

- Monitor for adverse effects such as nausea, vomiting, headache, stomach cramping, bloating, dizziness, vaginal discomfort or irritation, increased vaginal fluids, or breast tenderness or enlargement.
- Monitor blood pressure. Increases in blood pressure are more likely in women who have used OCs for many years.

Women with significant HTN should not be started on hormonal contraception.

- Instruct the patient about absolute and relative contraindications to OC use (see Table 71.4).
- Explain the goals of therapy and the reasons for assessing baseline data such as vital signs and the existence of underlying cardiovascular disorders and possible drug adverse effects.
- Discontinue estrogen treatment at least 4 weeks before any surgery that could be associated with a prolonged period of immobilization or vascular complications.
- Monitor blood glucose and glycosylated hemoglobin (HbA1c) laboratory results to determine changes in glycemic control for patients with diabetes.
- Provide information related to tobacco use and refer the patient to a smoking cessation program if appropriate. Cigarette smoking increases the risk of serious cardiovascular adverse effects from OC use. This risk increases with age and with heavy smoking (15 or more cigarettes per day) and is marked in women over 35 years of age.

Patient and Family Education:

- Take OCs exactly as instructed and do not skip doses.
- Report intermittent breakthrough bleeding, spotting, bleeding, or unexplained and sudden abdominal or pelvic pain to the health care provider.
- Weigh one or two times per week and report sudden weight gain or other signs of fluid retention.
- Immediately report signs of positive calf pain on flexing the foot (Homans' sign) and the following symptoms of thromboembolic disorders: tenderness, swelling, and redness in the extremity; sudden, severe headache or chest pain; slurring of speech; change in vision; and tenderness, pain, or sudden shortness of breath.
- Limit caffeine intake because estrogen depresses caffeine metabolism.
- Learn self-examination of breasts and follow a monthly schedule.
- Immediately notify the health care provider of any known or suspected pregnancy.
- Stop smoking and attend a smoking cessation program if appropriate because smoking significantly increases the risk for blood clots.
- Wait at least 3 months after discontinuing the medication before attempting to become pregnant.
- Many antibiotics decrease the effectiveness of OCs. Use a second method of birth control during antibiotic therapy and for at least 7 days after.

Drugs Similar to Estradiol and Norethindrone (Ortho-Novum)

There are dozens of different estrogen-progestin combinations available as OCs. All have the same types of adverse effects. Those with higher doses may be expected to produce more adverse events.

Progestin-Only Oral Contraceptives

71.3 Oral contraceptives that contain only progestin are often used when estrogen is contraindicated.

Although most OCs use a combination of estrogen and progestin, a few products contain only progestin. The progestin-only OCs, sometimes called minipills, are less effective at preventing ovulation. They prevent pregnancy primarily by causing a thick, viscous cervical mucus at the entrance to the uterus that discourages sperm penetration. They also tend to inhibit implantation of a fertilized egg.

Progestin-only oral agents are taken daily throughout the month without the use of placebo tablets. Minipills are somewhat less effective than estrogen-progestin combinations, having a failure rate of 1% to 4%. Their use also results in a higher incidence of irregular menstrual cycles than the combination OCs, including amenorrhea, prolonged bleeding, or breakthrough spotting. Menstrual irregularity is the most frequently reported adverse effect. The risk of ectopic pregnancy is higher with progestin-only products. Progestin-only oral agents are generally reserved for patients who are at high risk for estrogen-related adverse effects. Unlike estrogens, progestins are not associated with a higher risk of thromboembolic events, and they do not have any effect on breast cancer. The progestin-only products are pregnancy category X.

Products that contain norethindrone only include Aygestin, Camila, Errin, Jolivette, Nora-BE, and Ortho Micronor. In addition to contraception, norethindrone therapy is approved to treat amenorrhea, dysfunctional uterine bleeding, and endometriosis (see Chapter 70). The doses used for contraception are only 0.35 mg per day, whereas those for uterine conditions are 2.5 to 10 mg per day. The sole progestin-only product containing norgestrel (Ovrette) was discontinued in 2005. Detailed information on the contraindications, drug interactions, and adverse effects of progestins are included in Chapter 70, along with a prototype feature for medroxyprogesterone (Provera).

Adverse Effects of Combined Oral Contraceptives

71.4 The adverse effects of combined oral contraceptives are uncommon but may be serious in some women.

The adverse effects of combination OCs have been extensively studied, and various risk factors have been identified. These are summarized in Table 71.3. For the large majority of patients, OCs are safe and serious adverse effects are uncommon. A few of the adverse effects, however, may be serious. Because OCs are so widely prescribed, nurses should become familiar with these adverse effects and incorporate them into the teaching component of the treatment plan.

When reading information on the adverse effects of OCs, the nurse should remember that much of the early research was performed on women who were taking high doses of estrogens and

NURSING PROCESS APPLICATION

Patients Receiving Oral Contraceptive Therapy

Assessment	Potential Nursing Diagnoses
Prior to administration: • Obtain a health history, including history of cigarette smoking. • Obtain a drug history to determine possible drug interactions and allergies. • Assess cardiovascular status, including HTN, history of myocardial infarction (MI), cerebrovascular accident (CVA), and thromboembolic disease. • Determine if the patient is pregnant or lactating.	• *Deficient Knowledge (Drug Therapy)* • *Nausea,* related to adverse effects of drug • *Noncompliance (Medication Regimen)*

Planning: Patient Goals and Expected Outcomes

The patient will:

- Report effective birth control by avoidance of pregnancy.
- Demonstrate an understanding of the drug's action by accurately describing drug adverse effects and precautions.
- Take the medication exactly as ordered to prevent pregnancy.
- Immediately report symptoms of thrombophlebitis, difficulty breathing, visual disturbances, and severe headache.

Implementation

Interventions and (Rationales)	Patient and Family Education
• Monitor for the development of breast or other estrogen-dependent tumors. (Estrogen may cause tumor growth or proliferation.)	• Instruct the patient to report if an immediate family relative is diagnosed with any estrogen-dependent tumor. Instruct the patient: • In monthly breast self-examination techniques and to report any unusual lumps. • To know how her breasts look and feel, and to report any changes to the health care provider immediately.
• Monitor for thrombophlebitis or other thromboembolic disease. (Estrogen predisposes to thromboembolic disorders by increasing the levels of clotting factors.)	Instruct the patient to: • Immediately report signs of possible cardiac problems such as chest pain, dyspnea, edema, tachycardia, bradycardia, or palpitations. • Monitor blood pressure regularly. • Report symptoms of HTN such as headache, flushing, fatigue, dizziness, palpitations, tachycardia, or nosebleeds.
• Monitor for cardiac disorders and HTN. (These drugs increase the blood levels of angiotensin and aldosterone, which increase blood pressure.)	Instruct the patient to: • Immediately report signs of possible cardiac problems such as chest pain, dyspnea, edema, tachycardia, bradycardia, or palpitations. • Report symptoms of HTN such as headache, flushing, fatigue, dizziness, palpitations, tachycardia, or nosebleeds.
• Encourage the patient not to smoke. (Smoking increases the risk of thromboembolic disease.)	• Instruct the patient to join a smoking cessation program, because the combination of oral contraceptives and smoking greatly increases the risk of cardiovascular disease, especially MI, particularly if the patient is older than 35 and is smoking 15 or more cigarettes per day.
• Monitor blood and urine glucose levels. (These drugs increase serum glucose levels.)	• Instruct the patient to monitor urine and blood glucose regularly and to contact the health care provider if hyperglycemia or hypoglycemia occurs.
• Monitor the patient's knowledge level of proper administration. (Incorrect use may lead to pregnancy.)	Instruct the patient to: • Discontinue the medication and notify the health care provider if significant bleeding occurs at midcycle. • Take the missed dose as soon as remembered or take two tablets the next day. If three consecutive tablets are missed, begin a new compact of tablets, starting 7 days after the last tablet was taken. • Contact the health care provider if two consecutive periods are missed because pregnancy may have occurred.
• Encourage adherence with follow-up treatment. (Follow-up is necessary to avoid serious adverse effects.)	Instruct the patient to: • Schedule annual Pap smears. • Obtain routine mammograms as recommended by the health care provider.

Evaluation of Outcome Criteria

Evaluate the effectiveness of drug therapy by confirming that patient goals and expected outcomes have been met (see "Planning").

TABLE 71.3 Adverse Effects Associated with Oral Contraceptives

Adverse Effect	Prevention
Breast milk reduction	Some studies suggest that OCs may reduce the quantity of breast milk. They should not be taken until 6 weeks postpartum.
Cancer	Women who test positive for the human papilloma virus have an increased risk of cervical cancer. These patients should have regular checkups. Because estrogens promote the growth of certain types of breast cancer, patients with a history of this cancer should not take OCs.
Glucose elevation	OCs may cause slight increases in blood glucose. Patients with diabetes should monitor their serum glucose carefully during OC therapy.
Hypertension	Risk is increased with age, dose, and length of therapy. Blood pressure should be monitored periodically and antihypertensives prescribed as needed.
Increased appetite, weight gain, fatigue, depression, acne, hirsutism	These are common effects that are often caused by high amounts of progestin. The dose of progestin may need to be lowered.
Lupus exacerbation	Symptoms of systemic lupus erythematosis may worsen in some patients. A progestin-only OC may be an option for these patients.
Menstrual irregularities	Amenorrhea or hypermenorrhea are often caused by low amounts of progestin. The dose of progestin may need to be increased. Breakthrough bleeding and spotting are common with the low-dose OCs. The patient may need a higher dose product.
Migraines	Estrogen may decrease or increase the incidence of migraines. Because migraines are a risk factor for stroke, patients with migraines should seek advice from their health care provider.
Nausea, edema, breast tenderness	These are common effects that are often caused by high amounts of estrogen. The dose of estrogen may need to be lowered.
Teratogenicity	Estrogens are pregnancy category X. Patients should be advised to discontinue OCs if pregnancy is confirmed.
Thromboembolic disorders	Estrogens promote blood clotting. OCs should not be prescribed for patients with a history of thromboembolic disorders, strokes, coronary artery disease, or who are heavy smokers.

progestins. Most, and perhaps all, of the serious adverse effects of OCs are dose dependent. The newer low-dose formulations are likely to result in far less risk than the original OCs. Furthermore, much less research has been conducted on the newer delivery methods for contraception (see Section 71.5), which may have a different spectrum of adverse effects.

According to the World Health Organization absolute contraindications to using OCs exist when the woman has preexisting medical conditions that include breast cancer, cardiac diseases, HTN, hepatitis, and thromboembolic disorders. Relative contraindications exist when there are preexisting disorders such as depression, headaches, epilepsy, and migraine or where the benefits of taking OCs outweigh the risks. Of special concern for OC therapy are women with cardiovascular disorders and women 35 years and older who smoke because of the increased risk of developing thromboembolic events. A summary of the recommendations is listed in Table 71.4. The nurse should discuss nonhormonal contraceptive choices for women who have serious medical conditions for which OCs are contraindicated.

CONNECTION *Checkpoint* 71.2

Thromboembolic events are a serious concern for many patients who are taking OCs. From what you learned in Chapter 40, identify the classes of drugs that may be used to reduce the risk of thromboembolic events in high-risk patients. See Answer to Connection Checkpoint 71.2 in Appendix A.

About 5% of women who are taking OCs will develop HTN because the drugs cause a rise in angiotensin and aldosterone. Angiotensin is a vasopressor agent produced by the kidney, and aldosterone is a hormone secreted by the adrenal cortex of the kidney (see Chapter 34). The action of both substances can result in HTN. The mean elevation from high doses of OCs is about 3 to 6 mmHg systolic and 2 to 5 mmHg diastolic. The current low-dose formulations do not pose a major risk for HTN.

OCs can mimic certain symptoms of pregnancy, including breast tenderness, nausea, bloating, and **chloasma,** which is a darkened pigmentation found on the forehead, temples, cheeks, and upper lips. If a woman suspects pregnancy while taking an OC, the drug should be discontinued immediately because estrogen and progestin can be teratogenic.

Because some types of cancers depend on estrogen and progesterone for their development, the incidence of cancer in women who are taking OCs has been studied for several decades in large numbers of women. Some studies have demonstrated that long-term use may pose a slightly higher risk of breast cancer, whereas others have shown no relationship. Cervical cancer is also slightly increased, and this has been closely associated with human papillomavirus (HPV) infections. However, OCs appear to have a protective effect for ovarian and endometrial cancers that continues for many years after the drugs are discontinued. A protective effect has also been observed for colorectal cancer. Conclusions of these studies are that women who have a personal or very close family history of breast cancer should explore nonhormonal means of contra-

TABLE 71.4 Precautions for the Use of Oral Contraceptives

Absolute Contraindications to Oral Contraceptives	Relative Contraindications to Oral Contraceptives
Acute or chronic liver disorders	Amenorrhea
Breast cancer	Depression
Coronary artery disease	Epilepsy
Diabetes	Interacting drugs (carbamazepine, phenytoin, valproate)
	Migraine headaches
Estrogen-dependent tumors	Oligomenorrhea
Gallbladder disease	Undiagnosed vaginal bleeding
Heavy smoking	
Hemorrhagic disorders	
History of cerebrovascular accident (CVA)	
Hyperlipidemia	
Hypertension (higher than 160/100, or with vascular disease)	
Liver tumors	
Myocardial infarction (MI)	
Pregnancy	
Thromboembolic disorders	
Undiagnosed uterine bleeding	
Women over 35 years who smoke	

ception. All women who are taking OCs should be instructed to perform monthly breast self-examinations and be aware of the importance of routine scheduling of mammograms that are appropriate for their age range.

Other conditions associated with OCs are abnormal uterine bleeding, benign hepatic adenoma, multiple births, retinal disorders, and melanoderma. These conditions, though rare, have been reported and they normally resolve after discontinuing the use of OCs. OCs may accelerate the formation of gallstones in patients who have preexisting gallbladder disease. The drugs may increase glucose levels and suppress insulin responsiveness, although this can be prevented by adjustments in the insulin dose of patients with diabetes.

When discussing the risks and benefits of hormonal contraception with patients, the nurse should place the drug in context with the health risks associated with pregnancy and delivery. Many patients do not understand that pregnancy itself may cause many challenging health conditions for the mother. Maternal morbidity, which is defined as a condition that adversely affects the mother's health beyond what could be expected during childbirth, has been estimated at 43% (Geller, Cox, & Kilpatrick, 2006). Maternal morbidity includes conditions such as hemorrhages, preeclampsia or eclampsia, obstetrical trauma, infections, gestational diabetes, and HTN. Placed in the proper context, the risks of pregnancy for most patients (those without absolute contraindications for OC use) are as great, or greater, than hormonal contraception.

CONNECTIONS

To the Community

Calendar Method of Contraception

Despite several alternative methods of birth control, some women choose the calendar, or rhythm, method as the preferred way to prevent conception. In this method, the woman uses the natural body signals to establish the time in the menstrual cycle when she is most likely to conceive. This information is used to achieve or avoid pregnancy. This type of conception modification is also referred to as the physiological system of contraception. For some religious groups, it is the only acceptable method of contraception.

Drugs for Long-Term Contraception and Newer Contraceptive Delivery Methods

71.5 Long-acting contraceptives and novel delivery methods offer women additional birth control choices.

Long-acting methods that are able to provide effective contraceptive protection for periods lasting from weeks to years have been developed. The long-acting agents and novel delivery systems were developed to offer ease of use and improve adherence. They vary in efficacy, reversibility, and discreteness of use. It is important for nurses and patients to understand that the long-acting methods are not more effective than the daily OCs and that they have the same types of contraindications and adverse effects. These contraceptives are delivered by patches, subdermal implants, injections, and vaginal inserts.

Transdermal delivery method: Transdermal hormonal contraception is a safe, effective, and easy-to-use method of birth control. Approved in 2001, Ortho-Evra is a topical patch worn on the skin of the buttock, arms, or trunk that contains 750 mcg ethinyl estradiol and 6 mg norelgestromin. The patch slowly releases the hormones, which then penetrate the skin, enter the capillaries, and are distributed throughout the body. The patch is changed every 7 days for the first 3 weeks, followed by a patch-free week 4. The patch may be worn during bathing, exercise, and other daily activities. Should the patch fall off, which occurs in about 5% of the applications, it should be replaced as soon as possible. Forgetting to replace or change the patch will result in a rapid loss of contraceptive protection. After the patch is removed, hormone levels return to normal within 3 days.

The serum estrogen levels of patients who use the patch are 60% higher compared to those of patients who take combination OCs. In 2008, the U.S. Food and Drug Administration (FDA) added a warning to the label of Ortho-Evra stating that patients using the patch have an increased risk of venous thromboembolism compared to women taking OCs. The most frequently reported adverse effects of the Ortho-Evra patch include headache, nausea, vomiting, breast discomfort, breakthrough bleeding, and dysmenorrhea. Long-term effects and contraindications are the same as those of OCs. Used patches still contain significant levels of hormones and must be discarded in a waste container away from children. They should not be flushed down the toilet because they can pollute wastewater, lakes, and streams with high levels of estrogen.

Vaginal delivery method: The NuvaRing, illustrated in Figure 3.5 in Chapter 3, is a flexible, soft vaginal ring impregnated with a low-dose, sustained release, combined hormonal contraceptive. It is approximately 2 to 3 inches in diameter and contains 2.7 mg of ethinyl estradiol and 11.7 mg of etonogestrel. The ring is inserted into the vagina once a month to provide 3 weeks of contraceptive protection. The ring slowly releases the hormones, which are absorbed across the vaginal mucosa into the blood and distributed throughout the body. The contraceptive action is systemic in nature and not localized to the vagina. The ring is removed at the end of week 3, and a new ring is inserted a week later during the first week of the next menstrual cycle. If forgotten and left in place for more than 3 weeks, contraceptive action will be lost.

The main adverse effects of NuvaRing are similar to those of combination OCs. Women sometimes discontinue using the vaginal delivery method due to discomfort of the device during intercourse. Women who are suffering from uterine prolapse must monitor the ring frequently because it may fall out. Adverse effects include nausea, bloating, headaches, breast tenderness, and breakthrough bleeding. If the ring is expelled from the vagina, it may be rinsed with water and replaced. Local effects may include vaginal irritation, sensation of a foreign body, and vaginitis. The NuvaRing should be discarded in a waste container away from children and not flushed down the toilet.

Depot injection methods: Intramuscular medroxyprogesterone acetate (DMPA, Depo-Provera) was approved for contraceptive use in the United States in 1992. A single deep intramuscular (IM) injection of 150 mg of Depo-Provera or a subcutaneous injection of 104 mg medroxyprogesterone (depo-subQ Provera) provides 3 months of contraceptive protection. Medroxyprogesterone suppresses ovulation, inhibits sperm from reaching the egg by thickening the cervical mucus, and prevents a fertilized egg from implanting in the uterus. Neither of the depot delivery methods contains estrogen. DMPA is usually given on days 1 through 5 of the menstrual cycle to postpartum women who are not breast-feeding. Breast-feeding women should wait until week 6 postpartum to take the drug. The dose is repeated every 3 months as long as contraception is desired. The depot injection methods are very effective at preventing pregnancy.

Once injected the actions of the drug cannot be reversed. The woman will need to wait at least 3 months, and sometimes up to 12 months, before fertility is restored. Possible adverse effects include menstrual disturbances, abdominal bloating, headache, depression, and decreased libido. Amenorrhea and weight gain are very common. Long-term medroxyprogesterone causes significant bone loss. This drug is pregnancy category X. A prototype feature for medroxyprogesterone may be found in Chapter 70.

Subdermal implant delivery: Marketed from 1996 to 2002, Norplant consisted of six small plastic tubes filled with levonorgestrel that were implanted subcutaneously. Although it provided effective contraception for up to 5 years, the implants were difficult and painful to surgically remove. Implanon is a single rod containing the progestin estanogestrol that is inserted under the skin of the upper arm that provides 3 years of contraceptive protection.

Intrauterine devices: There are three intrauterine devices (IUDs) available. These devices, ParaGard, Progestasert, and Mirena, are all designed in a T shape and have been in use for many years. They are safe, inexpensive, and reliable methods of contraception. They offer a major advantage for women who are likely to forget their daily pill, or who prefer a greater ease of use. The IUD is not felt by the woman or her partner during intercourse. IUDs can be removed at any time. Despite their advantages, only 2% of women who use birth control use IUDs.

The oldest product, ParaGard, also known as Copper T380A, is a plastic device that is partially covered with copper. It is inserted into the vagina, where the copper triggers a spermicidal-like reaction in the body that slows sperm motility and prevents the sperm from reaching the ovum. If fertilization does occur, implantation is not likely to happen because the copper causes endometrial changes to make the lining less favorable. Unlike the hormonal methods, ParaGard has no effect on ovulation. It can be left in place for up to 10 years, and the main adverse effects are bleeding between menses, dysmenorrheal, and expulsion of the device. ParaGard is an important nonhormonal option for patients who have contraindications to using estrogen or progesterone.

Progestasert releases progesterone, which makes the cervical mucus thicker to prevent sperm penetration and changes the endometrium to prevent implantation. This drug often causes less menstrual bleeding and dysmenorrhea. Progestasert is somewhat less effective at preventing contraception than ParaGard or Mirena. Another disadvantage of Progestasert over other IUDs is that it must be replaced annually.

The newer IUD, Mirena, shown in Figure 71.2, is an intrauterine system consisting of a polyethylene reservoir containing levonorgestrel that is slowly released. Contraception results from a thickening of the endometrium and increased cervical mucus that slows down sperm motility. Mirena decreases menstrual pain and lowers blood loss. This drug acts locally to prevent conception over 5 years. The effectiveness of Mirena is similar to that of OCs. This device may be removed at any time, and fertility returns quickly.

Spermicides

71.6 Spermicides are safe but should be combined with barrier protection for maximum effectiveness.

Spermicides are agents that kill sperm. They come in a variety of creams, foams, jellies, and suppositories that immobilize or destroy sperm when inserted into the vagina prior to intercourse. Two spermicides used in contraceptive products are nonoxynol-9 and octoxynol-9. Spermicides are available over-the-counter (OTC).

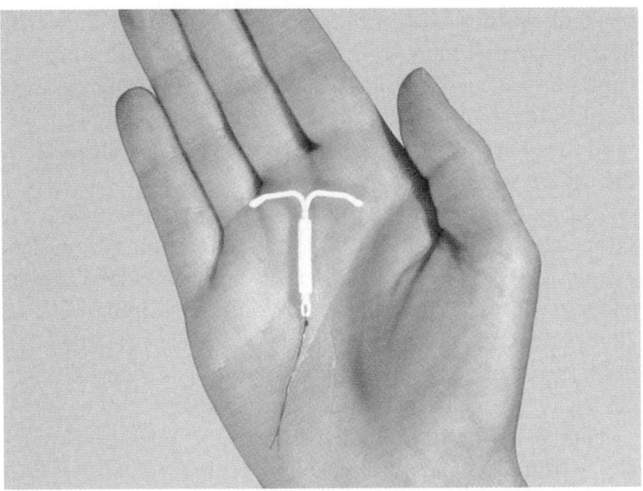

Figure 71.2 The Mirena intrauterine system, which releases levonorgestrel gradually, may be left in place for up to 5 years.
Source: Courtesy of Berlex Laboratories, Wayne, NJ.

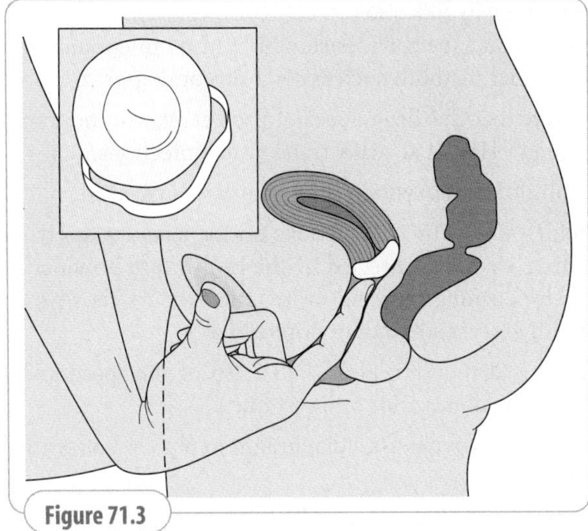

Figure 71.3

The contraceptive sponge is moistened well with water and inserted into the vagina with the concave portion positioned over the cervix.
Source: From *Olds' Maternal-Newborn Nursing & Women's Health Across the Lifespan* (8th ed., p. 97), by M. Davidson, M. London, & P. Ladewig, 2008. Reprinted by permission of Pearson Education, Inc., Upper Saddle River, NJ.

To be effective spermicides must be applied high into the vagina, as close to the cervix as possible, approximately 20 minutes before intercourse. Most spermicides have a duration of action of only 1 hour and must be reapplied if coitus extends beyond this time.

The contraceptive sponge (Today Sponge), which is illustrated in Figure 71.3, is a soft absorbent sponge impregnated with nonoxynol-9. The sponge is moistened with water to activate the spermicides and inserted into the vagina to cover the cervix. The sponge releases the drug slowly and may provide up to 24 hours of contraceptive protection. It is left in place for 6 hours after intercourse but must be removed by 30 hours after insertion. The sponge delivery system has the same effectiveness as spermicidal gels, creams, gels and suppositories. Adverse effects include local irritation and vaginal dryness.

Patients should be informed that spermicides have low levels of effectiveness when used alone and should therefore be used in conjunction with barrier methods such as condoms and diaphragms. Research has also determined that nonoxynol-9 does not offer any protection against chlamydia, gonorrhea, or the human immunodeficiency virus (HIV) as previously thought. In fact, frequent use of spermicides disrupts the vaginal epithelium and may actually increase the risk of HIV transmission from an infected partner. This drug also disrupts the anal mucosa, possibly increasing the risk of HIV transmission and should not be used for anal intercourse. Patients must be instructed to take added precautions to prevent such transmissions.

PROTOTYPE DRUG Nonoxynol-9

Classification: **Therapeutic:** Intravaginal contraceptive
Pharmacologic: Spermicide

Therapeutic Effects and Uses: Originally approved in 1963, nonoxynol-9 is a topical contraceptive agent that acts by inhibiting the ability of sperm to reach the ovum. Most products have a duration of spermicidal action of 60 minutes; the contraceptive sponge provides 24 hours of protection.

Pharmacokinetics: Nonoxynol-9 disrupts the cell membrane of sperm, causing it to lose motility and function. The carrier (foam, sponge, cream, etc.) may also act as a physical barrier to sperm motility.

Route(s)	Apply or insert vaginally
Absorption	Minimal absorption
Distribution	Acts locally, killing the sperm on contact
Primary metabolism	Not metabolized
Primary excretion	Small amounts by the kidneys and in feces
Onset of action	Immediate for creams, foams, gels, and sponge; 5–15 minutes for suppositories
Duration of action	Up to 6 h after intercourse

Adverse Effects: Adverse effects are uncommon. Vaginal irritation and dryness, increase in vaginal infections, irritation of the genitalia of the sexual partner, and toxic shock syndrome have been reported.

Contraindications/Precautions: Persons suffering from cystocele, prolapsed uterus, sensitivity or allergy to nonoxynol-9, vaginitis, or toxic shock syndrome, or those who are pregnant, postabortion, or postpregnancy should avoid this drug.

Drug Interactions: Intravaginal azole antifungals may inactivate the spermicides.

Pregnancy: Category C.

Treatment of Overdose: Overdose is not likely.

Nursing Responsibility:

- Monitor for signs of vaginal infection or irritation.

Patient and Family Education:

- Be aware that spermicides should be used in conjunction with barrier methods such as condoms or diaphragms.
- Be aware that this drug does not protect against the transmission of HIV or sexually transmitted infections.
- Discontinue nonoxynol-9 if pregnancy is suspected.
- Carefully follow the instructions on the label for applying the drug, or use as directed by the health care provider. If excessive burning, stinging, or irritation occurs, try a product with a lower strength of nonoxynol-9.
- If using a diaphragm place 1 to 3 tsp of the spermicidal agent in the dome prior to insertion.
- Leave the spermicide and diaphragm in place 6 hours after intercourse.
- Use the spermicide before the first and every subsequent act of intercourse.
- Report burning; inflammation; intense vaginal and vulvar itching; cheesy, curd-like discharge; painful intercourse; and dysuria to the health care provider.

Drugs Similar to Nonoxynol-9

There are no drugs that are similar to Nonoxynol-9.

Emergency Contraception

71.7 Emergency contraception provides a reproductive option for women who have unprotected sex.

Emergency contraception (EC) is the prevention of implantation following unprotected intercourse. Statistics suggest that almost half the pregnancies in the United States are unplanned. Some of these occur due to the inconsistent use or failure of contraceptive devices. Even OCs have a failure rate of 0.3% to 1%. EC, commonly referred to as the "morning after pill," offers a means of protecting against unwanted pregnancies.

The treatment goal for these patients is to provide effective and immediate contraception. These medications must be taken as soon as possible after unprotected intercourse. They are less effective if taken more than 72 hours after coitus. When used accordingly, these drugs act by preventing ovulation; they do not cause abortion. If implantation of an embryo has already occurred, the drugs used for EC will have no effect on the established pregnancy.

EC can be accomplished pharmacologically by a number of methods. Plan B is the only regimen, however, approved by the FDA that is currently marketed in the United States. A second regimen, the Preven emergency drug kit, was approved in 1998, but marketing was discontinued in the United States in 2004, likely because it caused more adverse effects than Plan B. Table 71.5 lists drugs, routes, and dosages for EC.

In 2006, the FDA approved Plan B for OTC purchase by women 18 years of age or older. Females younger than 18 require a prescription to obtain Plan B. OTC sales are restricted to retail operations with pharmacy services and clinics with health care providers to prevent women who are under 18 from purchasing the drug illegally from convenience stores or retail outlets. Although nonprescription, Plan B is sold "behind the pharmacy counter" so that the pharmacist can verify the patient's age.

The active drug in Plan B is levonorgestrel, which is the same drug used for contraception in the intrauterine system Mirena (see Section 71.5). There is, however, a large difference in doses. Whereas the long-acting Mirena releases 20 mcg per day of levonorgestrel over a 5-year period, Plan B delivers a total of 1,500 mcg levonorgestrel (1.5 mg) in a single day (750 mcg in two doses 12 hours apart).

Plan B is not 100% effective. The normal rate of pregnancy from a single unprotected sex act is 8%; Plan B is estimated to lower this risk to 1% to 2%. Serious adverse effects with Plan B are uncommon. Nausea and vomiting are the most common adverse effects, and abdominal pain, fatigue, headache, irregular (increased or decreased) menstrual bleeding, and dizziness are reported by a number of patients. Plan B is not intended to be a primary method of birth control because the long-term effects of multiple doses have not been established.

Most estrogen-progestin OC agents are also effective for EC if given at sufficient doses and with correct timing. Administration of ethinyl estradiol alone for 5 days is effective, although it causes nausea and vomiting in many patients. Mifepristone (Mifeprex) may be used off-label as EC or to induce abortions (see Section 71.8).

Drugs for Pharmacologic Abortion

71.8 Abortifacients are drugs that are used to terminate pregnancy.

A woman who is in very early pregnancy may decide that she is no longer able to carry the child to term. The nurse should use his or her knowledge of the stages of fetal growth and development to counsel the patient regarding the available options. The risks and benefits of the different options should be provided to the patient. One option for the patient if the pregnancy is 9 weeks or less is a medical abortion. Pharmacologic (medical) abortion is the removal of an embryo by the use of drugs after implantation has occurred. Drugs used to induce abortion are called **abortifacients.**

Once the ovum has been fertilized, several pharmacologic choices are available to terminate the pregnancy, as listed in Table 71.5. A single dose of mifepristone (Mifeprex, RU-486) followed 36 to 48 hours later by a single dose of misoprostol (Cytotec) is a frequently used regimen. Although mifepristone-misoprostol should never be used as a substitute for an effective means of contraception such as abstinence or OCs, these medications do offer women a safer alternative than surgical abortion. The actions of the two drugs are as follows:

- Mifepristone is a synthetic steroid that blocks progesterone receptors in the uterus. If given within 3 days of intercourse, mifepristone alone is almost 100% effective at preventing

TABLE 71.5 Agents for Emergency Contraception and Pharmacologic Abortion

Drug	Route and Adult Dose (maximum dose where indicated)	Adverse Effects
Agents for Emergency Contraception		
levonorgestrel (Plan B)	PO: 2 tablets within 72 h of unprotected intercourse, followed by 2 tablets 12 h later (0.75 mg in each pill)	*Nausea* Serious adverse effects are rare when only two doses are administered.
Agents for Pharmacologic Abortion		
carboprost tromethamine (Hemabate)	IM: Initial: 250 mcg (1 mL) repeated at ½–3½ h intervals if indicated by uterine response. Dosage may be increased to 500 mcg (2 mL) if uterine contractility is inadequate after several doses of 250 mcg (1 mL), not to exceed a total dose of 12 mg or continuous administration for 1 month	*Nausea, vomiting, cramping, diarrhea, fever* Uterine laceration, rupture, or hemorrhage
dinoprostone (Cervidil, Prepidil, Prostin E_2)	Intravaginal: Insert 20-mg suppository high in the vagina; repeat every 2–5 h until abortion occurs or membranes rupture (max: total dose 240 mg)	*Nausea, vomiting, cramping, diarrhea, fever* Uterine laceration, rupture, or hemorrhage
methotrexate with misoprostol	IM methotrexate (50 mg/m^2) followed 5 days later by intravaginal 800 mcg of misoprostol	*Nausea, vomiting, diarrhea* Abdominal pain, headache, uterine hemorrhage, respiratory arrest
mifepristone (Mifeprex) with misoprostol	PO: Day 1: 600 mg of mifepristone; day 3 (if abortion has not occurred): 400 mcg of misoprostol	*Nausea, vomiting, diarrhea* Abdominal pain, headache, uterine hemorrhage

Note: *Italics* indicate common adverse effects. Underline indicates serious adverse effects.

pregnancy. Given up to 9 weeks after conception, mifepristone aborts the implanted embryo.

- Misoprostol is a prostaglandin that causes uterine contractions, thus increasing the effectiveness of the pharmacologic abortion.

Pharmacologic abortion must be conducted under the very close supervision of a health care provider. The patient is required to sign detailed consent forms after it has been determined that the pregnancy is under 49 days. The patient takes mifepristone 600 mg, followed by an assessment by the health care provider 2 days later. If abortion has not occurred, 400 mg of misoprostol is taken. The patient returns to the health care provider in 14 days to confirm that abortion is complete. Occasionally pharmacologic abortion does not occur and the patient is referred for surgical abortion. The primary adverse effect of mifepristone-misoprostol is cramping that occurs soon after taking misoprostol. Nausea is common. The most serious adverse effect is prolonged bleeding, which may continue for 1 to 2 weeks after dosing.

Methotrexate, an antineoplastic agent, is sometimes combined with intravaginal misoprostol (Cytotec). Methotrexate 50 mg/m^2 is given IM, followed in 5 days by 800 mcg of intravaginal misoprostol. If abortion does not occur within 24 hours the misoprostol is repeated. The treatment is 96% effective at causing abortion. Most patients experience adverse effects such as nausea, vomiting, diarrhea, headache, dizziness, abdominal cramping, and hot flashes. Tylenol is often prescribed for pain relief.

Pharm*FACT*

An estimated 19 to 20 million unsafe abortions take place every year; 97% of these are in developing countries. An estimated 68,000 women worldwide die every year from unsafe abortions, and millions more are injured, many permanently. *Source:* Grimes et al., 2006.

Prostaglandins may also be used to induce abortion. Prostaglandins are natural hormones that produce a diverse number of local actions in virtually every body system. In the uterus, the normal function of prostaglandins is to cause contraction of smooth muscle. They have a valuable function in inducing contractions at the beginning of labor and in promoting cervical ripening.

The three approved prostaglandins include dinoprostone (Cervidil, Prepidil, Prostin E_2), carboprost (Hemabate), and misoprostol (Cytotec). All three may be used to induce uterine contractions that can expel an implanted embryo and result in abortion up to the second trimester. Dinoprostone is used early in pregnancy and comes in preparations of vaginal suppositories (Prostin E), vaginal inserts (Cervidil), and gel, which are inserted high into the vaginal canal. Carboprost is administered by deep IM injection and misoprostol by tablet. When used for abortion, misoprostol is administered with either mifepristone or methotrexate. Nausea, vomiting, and diarrhea are common adverse effects of prostaglandins and uterine cramping is expected. Drug-induced fever occurs in

TABLE 71.6 Indications for Prostaglandins

Drug	INDICATIONS				
	Abortifacient	**Control of Postpartum Bleeding**	**Cervical Ripening Induction**	**Labor Induction**	**Other**
carboprost (Hemabate) prostaglandin F_2	A	A	O	O	Hemorrhagic cystitis (O); hydatiform mole (O)
dinoprostone (Cervidil, Prepidil, Prostin E_2) prostaglandin E_2	A	—	A	—	Hydatiform mole (A)
misoprostol (Cytotec) prostaglandin E_1	O	O	O	O	Nonsteroidal anti-inflammatory drug (NSAID)–induced ulcer prophylaxis; (A) kidney transplant rejection prophylaxis (O)

Note: A = FDA-approved indication; O = Off-label indication.

the majority of patients and may last up to 6 hours. Because rare instances of uterine laceration and rupture have been reported, the patient is monitored closely for uterine activity, excessive pain, and vaginal bleeding. Indications for the prostaglandins are shown in Table 71.6.

PROTOTYPE DRUG Mifepristone (RU-486)

Classification: **Therapeutic:** Drug for abortion
Pharmacologic: Abortifacient, progesterone antagonist

Therapeutic Effects and Uses: The only FDA-approved indication for mifepristone is to terminate pregnancies that are less than 49 days' gestation. Due to the controversial nature of this drug, distribution is restricted and tightly controlled. This drug is only available via restricted access to registered prescribers in the United States. The FDA continues to monitor and evaluate reports related to the usage of mifepristone. This drug is not available in pharmacies but is sold directly to approved, registered prescribers. Surgical intervention must be readily available in case of incomplete abortion or severe bleeding or other serious complications. Pharmacotherapy with mifepristone requires three office visits by the patient:

- Day 1: Three 200 mg tablets of mifepristone are taken as a single dose.
- Day 3: If abortion is not confirmed, 400 mg of misoprostol are administered as a single dose. The patient is usually observed for at least 4 hours to determine potential adverse effects. Complete termination usually occurs in 4 to 24 hours.
- Day 14: Confirmation of abortion.

Mifepristone may be used off-label as a means of EC. Given as a single 600-mg dose, it has the same effectiveness and safety profile as Plan B. Other off-label indications include breast cancer, endometriosis, uterine leiomyomata, Cushing's syndrome, and termination of ectopic pregnancy (in combination with methotrexate).

Mechanism of Action: Mifepristone is a strong antagonist of progesterone and corticosteroids. This drug blocks the supportive effects of progesterone on the uterine lining. If given within 72 hours of unprotected intercourse, a fertilized ovum will not be able to implant in the uterus. During early pregnancy, mifepristone acts by increasing the synthesis of prostaglandins and sensitizing the uterus to the effects of prostaglandins. When misoprostol (a prostaglandin) is given on day 3 of treatment, the large amount of prostaglandin promotes increased uterine contractions, which expels the embryo from the uterus.

Pharmacokinetics:

Route(s)	PO
Absorption	Rapidly absorbed
Distribution	Crosses the placenta; it is unknown if secreted in breast milk; 98% bound to plasma protein
Primary metabolism	Hepatic (CYP3A4)
Primary excretion	Mostly feces, small amounts in urine
Onset of action	Rapid
Duration of action	Half-life: 18 h

Adverse Effects: Nearly all patients who take the mifepristone-misoprostol combination experience adverse effects, especially after misoprostol is given on day 3. The most frequent adverse effects of mifepristone are headache, dizziness, nausea, vomiting, fatigue, and abdominal pain or cramping. Vaginal bleeding and spotting will occur for about 16 days. Excessive or continued bleeding may require medical intervention with vasoconstrictor medications or curettage. Rare cases of septic shock have been reported.

Contraindications/Precautions: Because mifepristone is a corticosteroid antagonist, its use in patients who are taking long-term corticosteroid therapy or who have chronic adrenal failure is contraindicated. The mifepristone-misoprostol combination is contraindicated in patients with ectopic pregnancy because the therapy will be ineffective. Those on anticoagulant therapy or who otherwise have an increased risk for bleeding should not receive mifepristone. Patients with an IUD in place should have the device removed before mifepristone is administered. The drug is contraindicated for use in patients who are unable to understand the implications of abortion or who may not comply with the established regimen. Safety in patients under age 18 has not been established. When administered for nonabortion indications, this drug is contraindicated in pregnancy (category X).

Drug Interactions: Because mifepristone is only taken in one or two doses, serious drug interactions are unlikely. This drug does, however, have an extended half-life that may cause interactions after it is discontinued. Mifepristone is metabolized by hepatic CYP450 enzymes and may interact with drugs that induce or inhibit this enzyme system. For example, phenytoin, phenobarbital, and carbamazepine induce CYP3A4, increasing the metabolism of mifepristone and lowering its serum levels. **Herbal/Food**: St. John's wort and grapefruit juice may decrease serum levels of mifepristone.

Pregnancy: Category X.

Treatment of Overdose: Overdose has rarely occurred with mifepristone. Treatment is supportive.

Nursing Responsibilities:

- Conduct a comprehensive health assessment, including the patient's ability to understand the consequences of drug therapy and her ability to comply with the regimen.
- Confirm a positive pregnancy test and that the length of gestation is less than 49 weeks.
- Ensure that the proper emergency medical support is available in case of partial abortion or excessive bleeding.
- Assess for the presence of an IUD, use of anticoagulants, presence of bleeding disorders, or corticosteroid therapy.
- Instruct the patient on the expected adverse effects, especially cramping, and that vaginal bleeding may continue for several weeks to a month.
- Instruct the patient on steps to take in case of emergency, including the phone number and address of the nearest emergency center.

Patient and Family Education:

- Follow the therapeutic regimen exactly as prescribed by the health care provider.
- Attend all follow-up appointments because these are essential for safe and effective drug therapy.
- Immediately report heavy vaginal bleeding (use of more than two thick sanitary pads per hour for 2 consecutive hours), persistent vomiting, severe abdominal cramps, fever of 100.4°F or higher, or weakness to the health care provider.
- Do not take any other prescription or nonprescription drugs, dietary supplements, or herbal products without approval of the health care provider.
- Resume or initiate birth control immediately after the treatment ends or as directed by the health care provider.

Drugs Similar to Mifepristone (RU-486)

There are no drugs that are similar to Mifepristone (RU-486).

UNDERSTANDING THE CHAPTER

Key Concepts Summary

71.1 Selection of a contraceptive is based on effectiveness, safety, and personal choice.

71.2 The most effective contraceptive agents include combinations of low-dose estrogens and progestins.

71.3 Oral contraceptives that contain only progestin are often used when estrogen is contraindicated.

71.4 The adverse effects of combined oral contraceptives are uncommon but may be serious in some women.

71.5 Long-acting contraceptives and novel delivery methods offer women additional birth control choices.

71.6 Spermicides are safe but should be combined with barrier protection for maximum effectiveness.

71.7 Emergency contraception provides a reproductive option for women who have unprotected sex.

71.8 Abortifacients are drugs that are used to terminate pregnancy.

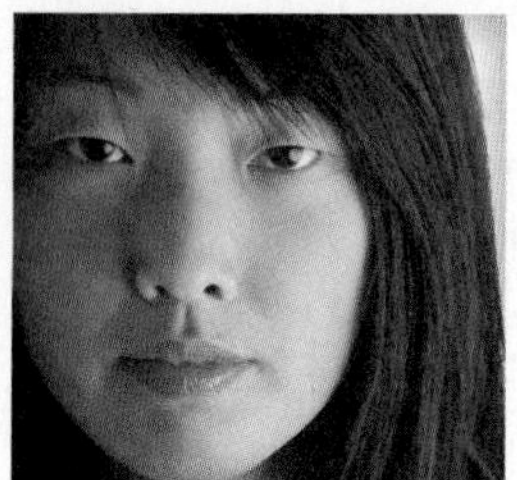

Making the PATIENT Connection

Remember the patient "Lila Bastian" from the beginning of the chapter? Now read the remainder of the case study. Based on the information presented within this chapter, respond to the critical thinking questions that follow.

Lila, a 19-year-old college student, comes to the clinic for renewal of the prescription for her oral contraceptive pills. She finished her last pack of pills (Ortho Novum) 10 days ago. She has been unable to get to the clinic to have her prescription renewed before today. She remembers having unprotected intercourse 2 days ago, and now she is concerned that she will become pregnant. Lila asks the nurse, "How can you help me?"

A complete history and physical finds Lila in very good health. Her vital signs are: temperature, 36.7°C (98°F); pulse, 68 beats/minute; respiratory rate, 18/minute; and blood pressure, 118/71 mmHg. Her weight is 62.6 kg (138 lb) and her height is 1.7 m (5 ft 7 in.). Her skin is dry and warm to the touch, mucous membranes are pink and moist, and there are no outward signs of distress. Her abdomen is soft and not tender, and there are no signs of bloating or distension. She has no vaginal bleeding at this time. Lila emphasizes that she only had sex once, 2 days ago. A urine pregnancy test is negative. A blood specimen was collected for human chorionic gonadotropin (HCG) examination. Lila is prescribed emergency contraceptive pills.

Critical Thinking Questions

1. Lila asks you, the nurse, why both urine and blood samples were collected. How would you respond to her questions?
2. If the prescriber wanted a more sensitive pregnancy laboratory indicator, which test could have been ordered? What is the advantage of this test?
3. What instructions would you give Lila regarding pregnancy and emergency contraception (EC)?

Case Study

Gina Martin, age 22, has been taking combined OCs for the past 2 years. Her health care provider orders antibiotics for a recurrent throat infection. As she is leaving the clinic, she asks you, the nurse, if she should temporarily discontinue her OC.

1. Explain the relationship between antibiotics and oral contraceptives.
2. What advice would you give Gina with regard to continuing the oral contraceptives?

NCLEX-RN® Review

1 Estradiol and norethindrone (Ortho-Novum) is prescribed for each of the following clients. Which clients would the nurse consider at high risk for an adverse response to this therapy? (Select all that apply.)

1. A 38-year-old who is 68.9 kg (152 lb) overweight
2. A 16-year-old athlete with asthma
3. A 22-year-old who smokes two packs of cigarettes per day
4. An 18-year-old with a history of chronic clinical depression
5. A 42-year-old who has delivered four healthy children

2 The client who is taking oral contraceptive therapy informs the nurse that she forgot to take the pill today. Which of the following responses by the nurse would be best when addressing this concern? If one dose is missed:

1. "Two pills taken the following day usually provide adequate contraception."
2. "Take only one pill the next day to prevent overdose of the medication."
3. "Skip another day and then resume the normal medication schedule."
4. "Have a pregnancy test performed as soon as possible."

3 The client who is prescribed progestin-only contraceptives (minipills) asks the nurse how the drug works. Which of the following would be the correct response provided by the nurse? Minipills:

1. "Cause delayed ovulation."
2. "Kill the sperm."
3. "Alter the cervical mucus."
4. "Suppress endometrial development."

4 The nurse has instructed the client to begin taking oral contraceptives on day 5 of her ovarian cycle and to continue for 21 days. During the other 7 days of the month, the client will take a placebo. The nurse knows that the placebo:

1. Contains vitamins and minerals needed for good health.
2. Consists of elements necessary for the other pills to work.
3. Replaces the need for folic acid lost during menstrual bleeding.
4. Encourages the adherence of taking the pill on a daily basis.

5 The nurse is providing health education about contraceptive methods to a group of young adults. Which of the following statements is correct about the use of spermicidal agents? Spermicidal agents:

1. Are extremely effective in preventing pregnancy.
2. Have relatively low levels of effectiveness when used alone.
3. Are the main causes of HIV and pelvic inflammatory disease.
4. Can prevent ectopic pregnancy.

6 Rank the following contraceptive methods in order of effectiveness from most to least effective:

1. Depo Provera
2. Spermicides
3. Calendar rhythm
4. Oral contraceptives
5. Transdermal—Ortho Evra

See Answers to Critical Thinking Questions, Case Study, and NCLEX-RN® Review in Appendix A.

References

Barclay, L. (2007). Oral contraceptive use linked to cancer risk. *Medscape Medical News.* Retrieved September 1, 2008, from http://www.medscape.com/viewarticle/562892

Bensyl, D. M., Iuliano, A. D., Carter, M., Santelli, J., & Gilbert, B. C. (2005). Contraceptive use—United States and territories: Behavioral risk factor surveillance system, 2002. *Morbidity and Mortality Weekly Report, 4*(SS06), 72.

Borrelli, F., & Ernst, E. (2008). Black cohosh (*Cimicifuga racemosa*) for menopausal symptoms: A systematic review of its efficacy. *Pharmacological Research, 57*(7), 502–510.

David, P. S., Boatwright, E. A., Tozer, B. S., Verma, D. P., Blair, J. E., Mayer, A. P., et al. (2006). Hormonal contraception update. *Mayo Clinic Proceedings, 81*(7), 949–955.

Davidson, M. R., London, M. L., & Ladewig, P. L. (2008). *Maternal newborn nursing and women's health across the lifespan.* Upper Saddle River, NJ: Prentice Hall.

Erkkola, R. (2007). Recent advances in hormonal contraception. *Current Opinion in Obstetrics & Gynecology, 19*(6), 547–553.

Geller, S. E., Cox, S. M., & Kilpatrick, S. J. (2006). A descriptive model of preventability in maternal morbidity and mortality. *Journal of Perinatology, 26*(4), 79–84.

Glasier, A., Gülmezoglu, A. M., Schmid, G. P., Moreno, C. G., & Van Look, P. F. (2006). Sexual and reproductive health: A matter of life and death. *Lancet, 368*(9547), 1595–1607.

Grimes, D. A., Benson, J., Singh, S., Romero, M., Ganatra, B., Okonofua, F. E., et al. (2006). Unsafe abortion: The preventable pandemic. *Lancet, 368*(9550), 1908–1919.

Isley, M., & Edelman, M. A. (2007). Contraceptive implants: An overview and update. *Obstetrics and Gynecology Clinics of North America, 34*(1), 73–90.

Kaunitz, A. (2005). Beyond the pill: New data and options in hormonal and intrauterine contraception. *American Journal of Obstetrics and Gynecology, 192*(4), 998–1004.

Kaunitz, A. M. (2006). Contraception 2006: Beyond the pill. *US Pharmacist, 31*(9), 39–48.

National Center for Health Statistics. (2007). *Health, United States, 2007 with chartbook on trends in the health of Americans.* Hyattsville, MD: Author. Retrieved August 30, 2008, from http://www.cdc.gov/nchs/hus.htm

Osmers, R., Friede, M., Liske, E., Schnitker, J., Freudenstein, J., & Henneicke-von Zepelin, H. H. (2005). Efficacy and safety of isopropanolic black cohosh extract for climacteric symptoms. *Obstetrics and Gynecology, 105*(5), 1074–1083.

Prine, L. (2007). Emergency contraception: Myths and facts. *Obstetrics and Gynecology Clinics of North America, 34*(1), 127–136.

World Health Organization. (2004). *Selected practice recommendations for contraceptive use.* Retrieved September 3, 2008, from http://www.who.int/reproductive-health/publications/spr/

CHAPTER

What's wrong with me? Dana excites me so much, but when we get into bed I just can't please her sexually.

Patient "Mike Mayhew"

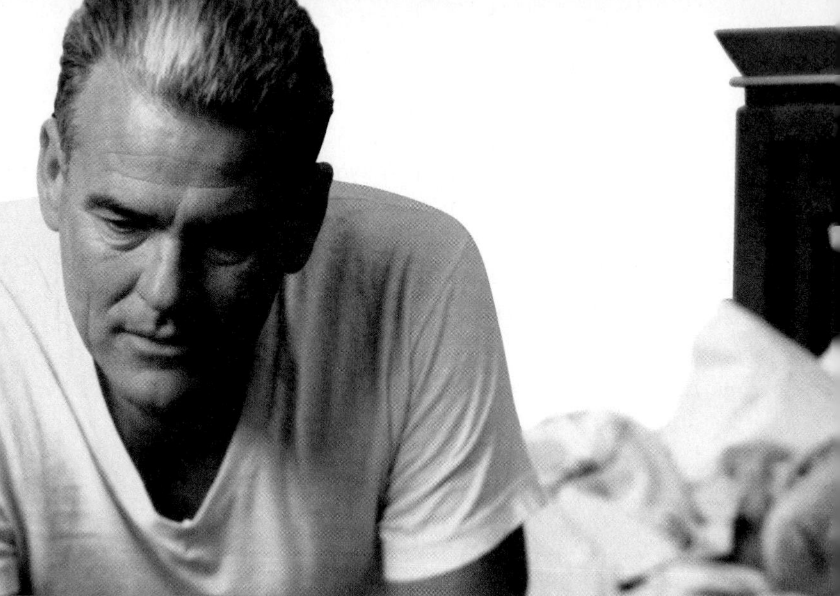

72 Drugs for Disorders and Conditions of the Male Reproductive System

Learning Outcomes

After reading this chapter, the student should be able to:

1. Explain the secretion and physiological effects of androgens.
2. Describe the roles of the hypothalamus, pituitary, and testes in regulating the male reproductive function.
3. Explain the role of androgens in the treatment of male hypogonadism, delayed puberty, and breast cancer.
4. Describe the potential consequences associated with the use of anabolic steroids to enhance athletic performance.
5. Identify the types of male sexual dysfunction and their potential causes.
6. Explain the role of drugs in the therapy of male infertility.
7. Describe the etiology, pathogenesis, and pharmacotherapy of erectile dysfunction.
8. Describe the pathogenesis and pharmacotherapy of benign prostatic hyperplasia.
9. Compare and contrast the nonpharmacologic and pharmacologic management of disorders and conditions of the male reproductive system.
10. For each of the classes shown in the chapter outline, identify the prototype and representative drugs, and explain the mechanism(s) of drug action, primary indications, contraindications, significant drug interactions, pregnancy category, and important adverse effects.
11. Apply the nursing process to care for patients who are receiving drug therapy for disorders and conditions of the male reproductive system.

Chapter Outline

Regulation of Male Reproductive Function

Pharmacotherapy with Androgens

PROTOTYPE **Testosterone** *p. 1221*

Anabolic Steroids

Etiology of Male Sexual Dysfunction

Pharmacotherapy of Male Infertility

Pharmacotherapy of Erectile Dysfunction

PROTOTYPE **Sildenafil (Viagra)** *p. 1228*

Pathophysiology of Benign Prostatic Hyperplasia

Pharmacotherapy of Benign Prostatic Hyperplasia

Alpha$_1$-Adrenergic Blockers

5-Alpha Reductase Inhibitors

PROTOTYPE **Finasteride (Proscar)** *p. 1232*

Key Terms

anabolic effects, *1223*
anabolic steroids, *1223*
androgens, *1219*
azoospermia, *1226*
benign prostatic hyperplasia (BPH), *1229*
corpora cavernosa, *1226*
erectile dysfunction (ED), *1226*
hypogonadism, *1220*
impotence, *1226*
Leydig cells, *1219*
libido, *1220*
oligospermia, *1226*
virilization, *1219*

As in women, reproductive function in men is regulated by a small number of hormones from the hypothalamus, pituitary, and gonads. Because hormonal secretion in men is relatively constant throughout the adult life span, the pharmacologic treatment of reproductive disorders in men is less complex and more limited than in women. This chapter examines the drugs used to treat the disorders and conditions of the male reproductive system.

Regulation of Male Reproductive Function

72.1 Male reproductive function is controlled through the secretion of androgens.

Male reproduction is controlled by hormones secreted by the gonads. **Androgens,** or male sex hormones, are produced primarily by the testes and, to a much lesser extent, the adrenal glands. Testosterone, the primary androgen, is responsible for maturation of the male reproductive system and the secondary sex characteristics of men. Other important androgens include androstenedione and dehydroepiandrosterone (DHEA). The primary cells in the testes that are responsible for androgen secretion are called **Leydig cells.** Androgens are sometimes referred to as anabolic steroids.

Androgens are responsible for the development of the male urogenital system in the fetus. After birth the Leydig cells are quiet until activated by the gonadotropins, which are hormones secreted by the pituitary gland. The resulting increased production of testosterone by the testes begins the cascade of changes that accompany the onset of puberty in the male adolescent. The increased testosterone levels are responsible for the process of **virilization,** or the development of the male sexual characteristics. Over the next several years, the testes, scrotum, and penis enlarge until they reach adult proportions. Pubic and axillary hair grows and other body hair becomes more adult-like in nature. The production of sperm that are capable of fertilizing an ovum begins in the seminiferous tubules of the testes. The cartilage of the larynx grows, causing the deeper toned male voice. Sebaceous gland activity is stimulated, resulting in an increase in the level of acne. The final change is the development of facial hair.

Testosterone has profound metabolic effects in tissues outside the reproductive system. Of particular importance is its ability to enhance skeletal muscle mass and to stimulate the growth of bone, which contributes to the differences in muscle strength and body composition between men and women. Testosterone promotes the synthesis of erythropoietin, resulting in an increased production of red blood cells (RBCs) and accounting for the higher hemoglobin and hematocrit levels found in males.

Androgen secretion is regulated by the same pituitary hormones that control the reproductive function in women. Although the name follicle-stimulating hormone (FSH) applies to its target in the female ovary, this same hormone influences testosterone secretion in men. Leuteinizing hormone (LH), more accurately called interstitial cell–stimulating hormone (ICSH) in the male reproductive system, regulates the production of testosterone by the Leydig cells of the testes. Unlike the 28-day cyclic secretion of estrogen and progesterone in women, testosterone secretion is relatively constant in adult men. Beginning in puberty, testosterone production increases rapidly and continues to maintain a high level of production until later adulthood, after which it slowly declines. Normal plasma concentrations of testosterone are 250 to 1,000 mg/dL. If the level of testosterone in the blood rises above normal, negative feedback to the pituitary shuts off the secretion of LH and FSH. The relationship among the hypothalamus, pituitary, and the male reproductive hormones is illustrated in Figure 72.1.

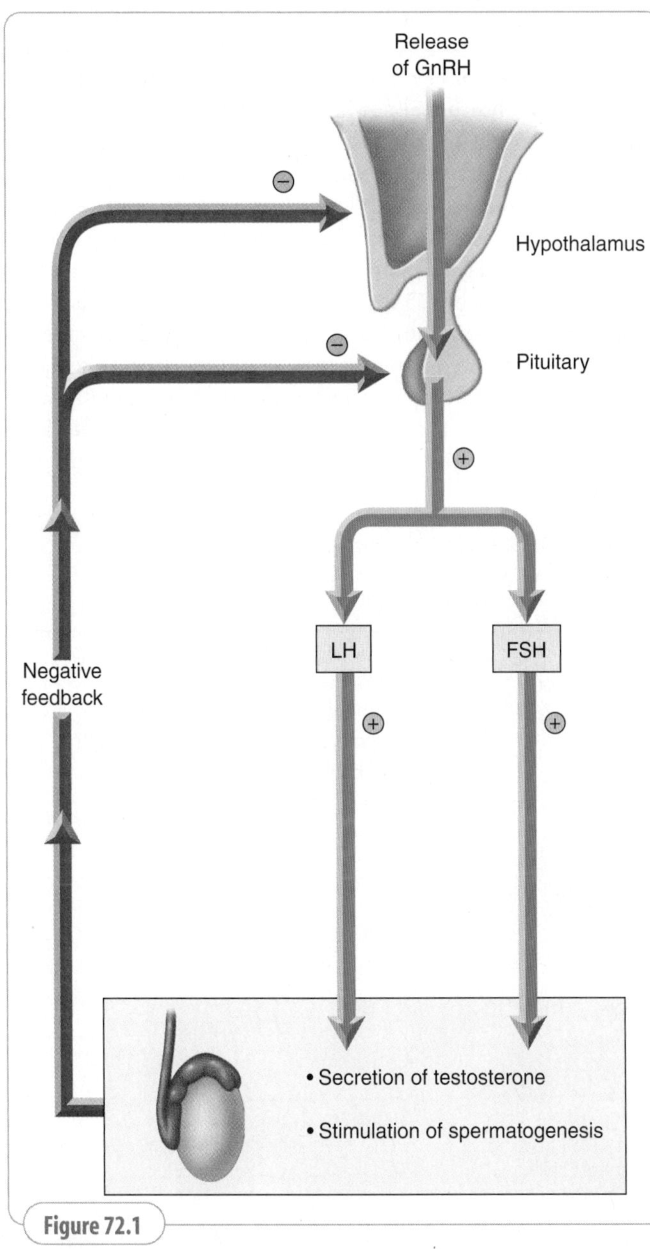

Figure 72.1

Hormonal control of the male reproductive hormones.

Precursor molecules of testosterone (androstenedione and DHEA) are secreted in small amounts by the adrenal glands. Their production in the adrenal gland is controlled by the secretion of adrenocorticotropic hormone (ACTH). These weaker androgens are converted to testosterone once they reach the peripheral tissues. Adrenal androgens have a role in the growth of pubic hair and are thought to influence the skeletal growth spurt in adolescents. In adult males, the adrenal androgens have minimal effects due to the large amount of testosterone produced in the testes.

Pharmacotherapy with Androgens

72.2 Androgens are used to treat hypogonadism and delayed puberty in males and breast cancer in females.

Androgens are used to treat testosterone deficiency in men, delayed puberty, oligospermia, hypogonadism, anemia, muscle-wasting disorders, and certain cancers. These agents are listed in Table 72.1.

Lack of sufficient testosterone secretion by the testes can result in male **hypogonadism.** Hypogonadism may be congenital or acquired later in life. When the condition is caused by a testicular disorder, it is called primary hypogonadism. Examples of disease states that may cause primary testicular failure include mumps, testicular trauma or inflammation, and certain autoimmune disorders.

A deficiency in FSH and LH secretion by the pituitary will result in a lack of stimulus to the testes to produce androgens. Lack of FSH and LH secretion may have a number of causes, including Cushing's syndrome, thyroid disorders, estrogen-secreting tumors, and therapy with gonadotropin-releasing hormone (GnRH) agonists such as leuprolide (Lupron). Hypogonadism that is caused by defects in the pituitary or hypothalamus is known as secondary hypogonadism.

In young men insufficient testosterone secretion may delay the onset of puberty. If total lack of testosterone secretion occurs, puberty will not occur at all. In the adult male the symptoms of hypogonadism include diminished secondary sex characteristics such as sparse axillary, facial, and pubic hair; increased subcutaneous fat; reduced muscle mass; and smaller testicular size. The lack of testosterone can lead to erectile dysfunction (ED); low sperm counts (oligospermia); a decrease in the amount of ejaculate; and decreased **libido,** or a lack of interest in sexual intercourse. Nonspecific complaints may include behavioral and mood changes such as irritability, fatigue, depression, and a general loss of motivation.

Hypogonadism can be easily confirmed by obtaining serum testosterone levels. Testosterone levels are performed early in the day because testosterone is secreted in the morning. Assessment of LH and FSH levels, as well as prolactin, estradiol, and thyroid hormone levels, may be useful in determining causation. Low serum levels of testosterone concurrent with normal or elevated levels of FSH and LH suggest that the testes are unresponsive to hormonal activation, thus the patient has primary hypogonadism. If testosterone, FSH, and LH levels are all low, this would indicate secondary hypogonadism.

Pharmacotherapy of hypogonadism includes replacement therapy with testosterone or other androgens. For young males experiencing delayed puberty, puberty is generally induced when the boy reaches 15 to 17 years of age using a long-acting testosterone preparation. A 6-month period of androgen therapy is given, followed by 6 months without the drug. If further therapy is needed, then testosterone cypionate (Depotest, Andronate) is usually used at a dose of 200 mg every 2 weeks. Therapy can be continued for up to 4 years. Once appropriate

TABLE 72.1 Selected Androgens and Anabolic Steroids

Drug	Route and Adult Dose (maximum dose where indicated)	Adverse Effects
danazol	Oral (PO): 200–400 mg bid for 3–6 months	*Acne, gynecomastia, hirsutism and male sex characteristics (in women), sodium and water retention, emotional lability, amenorrhea, decreased libido, hypercholesterolemia* <u>Anaphylaxis, testicular atrophy and oligospermia at high doses, priapism, peliosis hepatitis, benign intracranial hypertension, thromboembolism</u>
fluoxymesterone (Halotestin)	PO: 5 mg 1–4 times/day	
methyltestosterone capsules (Android, Testred, Virilon); methyltestosterone tablets (Methitest)	PO: 10–50 mg/day Buccal administration: 5–25 mg/day	
nandrolone	IM: 50–200 mg/week	
oxandrolone (Oxandrin)	PO: 2.5–20 mg/day divided 2–4 times/day for 2–4 weeks	
oxymetholone (Androl-50)	PO: 1–5 mg/kg/day	
testosterone (Striant—Buccal Patch) (Testoderm TTS, Androderm, and others—Transdermal Patches) (Androgel, Testim—Topical Gel)	Buccal: 30 mg every 12 h Transdermal: Testoderm TTS patch: Apply 1 daily; Androderm patch: Apply 2.5–7.5 mg patch daily Gel: Apply 5 g daily (max: 10 g)	
testosterone cypionate (Depotest, Andro-Cyp 100 and 200, Depo-Testosterone)	IM: 50–400 mg every 2–4 weeks	
testosterone enanthate (Andro L.A., Delatest, Delatestryl)	IM: 50–400 mg every 2–4 weeks	

Note: *Italics* indicate common adverse effects. <u>Underline</u> indicates serious adverse effects.

physiological hormonal levels are attained, the normal progression of pubertal changes typically occurs.

In the adult patient a variety of testosterone replacement preparations may be administered. Regardless of the type of testosterone chosen, the patient should experience improved libido, increased amount of ejaculate, and correction of ED within days or weeks of initiating therapy. Male sex characteristics become better defined, depression resolves, and muscle strength rapidly improves. Therapy with androgens is targeted to return serum testosterone to normal physiological levels. Above-normal levels serve no therapeutic purpose and increase the risk of adverse effects.

Nonreproductive uses: Because androgens have important physiological effects outside the reproductive system, they have been used to treat certain nonreproductive disorders. Low testosterone levels are a significant risk factor because the hormone promotes the synthesis of erythropoietin, which is essential for RBC production. Administration of testosterone may be used to correct anemia unresponsive to other treatments. These include aplastic anemia and anemias associated with chronic renal disease and chemotherapy. Taking advantage of the anabolic effects of testosterone on bone and skeletal muscle, the drug is sometimes given to debilitated patients who have muscle-wasting disease, such as that seen in patients with acquired immunodeficiency syndrome (AIDS).

High doses of androgens are occasionally used as a palliative measure to treat certain types of breast cancer in combination with other antineoplastic agents. At the high doses required for breast cancer treatment, some virilization will occur in most patients. Androgen therapy is contraindicated in males with breast cancer because it promotes the growth of the cancer. Similarly, because the growth of most prostate carcinomas is testosterone dependent, androgens should not be prescribed for older men unless the possibility of prostate cancer has been ruled out. Patients with prostate carcinoma are sometimes given a GnRH agonist such as leuprolide (Lupron) to reduce circulating testosterone levels.

Testosterone formulations: Testosterone is available in a number of different preparations. All formulations are equally effective and the choice is based on health care provider experience, ease of use, and the personal preference of the patient. Common to all dosage forms is the need for regular follow-up health care visits to ensure that the serum testosterone level is maintained within the designated range.

Intramuscular (IM) testosterone: Testosterone cypionate (Depo-Testosterone) and testosterone enanthate (Delatestryl) are IM forms of testosterone. These drugs tend to be slowly absorbed, are metabolized to free testosterone, and result in blood levels that will vary widely after administration. This variation in serum levels may cause patients to experience fluctuations in their libido and energy and experience mood swings. Patients tend to complain of soreness at the site of injection. IM injections are given deep in the gluteal muscle every 2 to 4 weeks.

Implantable testosterone pellets: Testopel is a long-acting form of testosterone that is implanted subcutaneously, usually on the anterior abdominal wall. Each pellet contains 75 mg of testosterone and one to six are implanted depending on the dose required. Testosterone levels are obtained regularly during therapy and the number of pellets adjusted accordingly. To induce puberty, low doses are used for 4 to 6 months. For adult replacement therapy higher doses are administered, with the effectiveness of the pellets lasting 3 to 4 months.

Transdermal testosterone patch: Androderm is currently the only androgen patch available. Two other patches, Testoderm and Testoderm TTS, have been removed from the market. The Androderm patch is applied to the upper arm, thigh, back, or abdomen, rotating application sites. The patch is not to be applied to the scrotum or to damaged skin. A rash at the site of the application tends to be the only adverse effect noted. Dosages for the patches vary from 2.5 mg to 5 mg over 24 hours depending on the needs of the patient. The patches are applied in the evening and are changed daily. Because the used patches contain some testosterone, they should be disposed of safely, away from children and pets.

Transdermal testosterone gel: AndroGel and Testim are 1% testosterone gels that are applied once daily for treatment of hypogonadism. The alcohol-based gels dry quickly: The testosterone is absorbed in the skin in about 30 minutes and released slowly to the blood. Patients tend to prefer the use of gels because they cause less local irritation, the gel does not fall off like the patches, and there is a more consistent level of testosterone delivered. A major disadvantage is that the gel can be transferred to another person by skin-to-skin contact, causing virilization of female contacts and potential fetal harm. AndroGel is supplied in individual dosed packets, and the drug is applied in the morning to clean and dry skin of the upper arms, shoulders, or abdomen (not the genitals). Testim is supplied in tubes and is applied in the same manner as AndroGel. Showering or swimming should be avoided for several hours after application to avoid washing off this drug. For both of these medications, testosterone levels should be measured after a few weeks of therapy and at various intervals thereafter to ensure that physiological levels have been achieved.

Testosterone buccal tablets: Striant is a form of testosterone that has the ability to produce a continuous supply of testosterone in the blood. Patients are instructed to place a tablet to the gum area just above the incisor, holding it in place for 30 seconds. Usual doses are one tablet (30 mg testosterone) every 12 hours, alternating sides of the cheek. Patients may eat, drink, and chew gum with the buccal tablet in place. There have been only minor adverse effects to this route such as local irritation to the area, bad taste, and altered taste perceptions.

PROTOTYPE DRUG Testosterone

Classification: **Therapeutic:** Male sex hormone
Pharmacologic: Androgen, anabolic steroid, antineoplastic

Therapeutic Effects and Uses: The primary therapeutic use of testosterone is to treat delayed puberty and hypogonadism in males by promoting virilization, including maturation of the sexual organs, growth of facial hair, and a deepening of the voice. In adult males testosterone administration will increase libido and restore masculine characteristics that may be deficient. Testosterone is approved to treat ED when the cause is associated with low androgen levels. The drug is also approved by the U.S. Food and Drug Administration (FDA) for the palliative treatment of inoperable breast cancer in women. Off-label indications for testosterone include treatment of postpubertal cryptorchidism, microphallus, anemia in patients with chronic renal failure, female-to-male gender change, and AIDS-associated wasting syndrome.

Testosterone base is administered by the IM route, although other salts are available for the transdermal, implantable pellets, and buccal routes. Testosterone was classified as a Schedule III controlled substance in 1991 because it was being widely abused by weight lifters and other athletes.

Mechanism of Action: Testosterone binds to specific receptors located in the cell cytoplasm. The hormone-receptor complex then migrates to the cell nucleus where it acts on the deoxyribonucleic acid (DNA) to promote the synthesis of specific messenger ribonucleic acid (RNA) molecules. These form templates for the production of specific proteins that mediate testosterone effects.

Pharmacokinetics:

Route	Buccal, transdermal, IM, implantable pellets
Absorption	Cypionate and enanthate are slowly absorbed from IM sites
Distribution	98% bound to sex hormone-binding globulin; unknown if secreted in breast milk
Primary metabolism	Hepatic
Primary excretion	90% renal, 6% feces
Onset of action	Steady-state levels are reached in 3–4 weeks
Duration of action	2–4 weeks cypionate and enanthate; half-life: 10–100 minutes

Adverse Effects: An obvious adverse effect of testosterone therapy is virilization, which is usually only of concern when the drug is taken by women. Androgens may cause either decreased or increased libido. Salt and water are often retained, causing edema, and a diuretic may be indicated. Liver damage and hepatic cancer are potentially serious adverse effects and are of special concern when high doses are taken for prolonged periods. Acne and skin irritation are common during therapy. Females may experience suppression of ovulation, lactation, or menstruation; hoarseness or deepening of their voice, which is often irreversible; hirsutism; oily skin; clitoral enlargement; regression of breasts; and male-pattern baldness. High doses may suppress spermatogenesis, reduce ejaculatory volume, and cause oligospermia.

Contraindications/Precautions: Testosterone is contraindicated in men with known or suspected breast or prostatic carcinomas because it can promote the growth of these tumors. It is contraindicated in women who are or may become pregnant (category X). The drug may worsen prostatic hyperplasia. Testosterone should be used with caution in patients with preexisting renal or hepatic impairment. Caution must be used if testosterone is administered to patients with diabetes mellitus, history of myocardial infarction (MI), coronary artery disease (CAD), benign prostatic hyperplasia (BPH), and acute intermittent porphyria and in geriatric patients. Monitoring of serum cholesterol, serum electrolytes, as well as liver function tests is needed throughout therapy because testosterone may increase these values.

Drug Interactions: Testosterone may potentiate the effects of oral anticoagulants and increase the risk of severe bleeding. Concurrent use of testosterone with corticosteroids may cause additive edema, which can be a serious concern for those with heart failure. Hepatotoxic drugs should be avoided because their use with testosterone can cause additive liver damage. The 5-alpha reductase agents (finasteride) used to treat prostatic hyperplasia are antiandrogenic and their use with testosterone will inhibit the therapeutic effects of both drugs. **Herbal/Food:** Insulin requirements may decrease, and the risk of hepatotoxicity may increase when used with echinacea. Evaluation of calcium levels is necessary because hypercalcemia may result.

Pregnancy: Category X.

Treatment of Overdose: There is no specific treatment for overdose.

Nursing Responsibilities:

- Obtain a complete health history that includes questions regarding the possibility of impaired sexual functioning and diminished libido.
- Conduct a physical assessment for evidence of decreased hormone production, such as decreased or absent body hair, small testes, or delayed signs of puberty. This assessment should also include the patient's emotional status, because depression and mood swings may be symptoms of decreased hormone secretion.
- Monitor laboratory results, especially liver enzymes, if the patient has a history of anabolic steroid use. Monitor serum cholesterol, especially in patients with a history of MI or angina, because this drug can increase this laboratory value. Monitor testosterone levels to ensure therapeutic levels.
- Evaluate the patient's past medical history for conditions that would contraindicate androgen therapy, including prostatic or male breast cancer, renal disease, cardiac and liver dysfunction, hypercalcemia, BPH, and hypertension (HTN).
- Monitor for adverse effects, including skin reactions such as pruritus or blistering with topical formulations. Adverse reactions that occur in women as a result of androgen use include deepening of the voice, facial hair growth, enlarged clitoris, and irregular menses.

Patient and Family Education:

- Keep all scheduled laboratory visits because testosterone doses may require periodic adjustment based on laboratory results.
- Check weight twice a week and report significant increases of greater than 5 lb per week to the health care provider.
- Immediately report prolonged or painful erection (priapism) that lasts longer than 4 hours to the health care provider.

- If diabetic be alert for signs and symptoms of hypoglycemia (shaking, sweating, hunger, anxiety, and dizziness).
- If taking anticoagulants, immediately report unusual bruising or bleeding to the health care provider.
- Immediately notify the health care provider of any known or suspected pregnancy.
- Use the proper technique in using the medication (transdermal patch, oral [PO] medication, gel, implantable pellets, or injection). Wash hands thoroughly after the application. Allow the medication to dry, and cover the part of the skin on which the medication has been applied. Avoid skin-to-skin contact of that site with other people.
- Apply the buccal tablet to the gum just above the upper incisor tooth, and apply pressure using a finger on the lip to ensure good adhesion.
- Report any changes in libido, growth of facial hair, deepening of voice, or male-pattern baldness.

Drugs Similar to Testosterone

The two other androgens are fluoxymesterone and methyltestosterone.

Fluoxymesterone (Halotestin): Approved in 1983, fluoxymesterone is an oral androgen that is indicated for male hypogonadism and inoperable breast cancer in women. This drug has the same adverse effects, contraindications, and actions as those of testosterone. It is rarely used because it must be taken four times daily and has an increased risk of hepatic damage with long-term use. This drug is pregnancy category X.

Methyltestosterone (Android, Methitest, Testred, Virilon): Methyltestosterone is available as PO tablets, capsules, or buccal tablets. It is indicated for male hypogonadism, delayed male puberty, and inoperable breast cancer in women. This drug has the same adverse effects, contraindications, and actions as those of testosterone. Caution must be used during long-term use because of the potential for hepatotoxicity. This drug is pregnancy category X.

Anabolic Steroids

72.3 Often abused by athletes, anabolic steroids can cause serious adverse effects.

Testosterone has both androgenic and anabolic effects. Its androgenic effects are responsible for creating and maintaining the male sexual characteristics. The hormone's **anabolic effects** relate to its ability to accelerate the growth of RBCs, muscle, bone, and neural tissues.

Anabolic steroids are testosterone-like substances that were originally developed to produce the anabolic effects of androgens while minimizing the androgenic effects. They are rarely prescribed but are often taken inappropriately by athletes who hope to build muscle mass and strength, thereby obtaining a competitive edge. The use of anabolic steroids to improve athletic performance is illegal and strongly discouraged by health care providers. All major athletic organizations prohibit the use of anabolic steroids by their participants.

Interestingly, despite their regulation, many formulations of anabolic steroids can be purchased over-the-counter (OTC) or on Internet websites. They are promoted as natural "steroid alternatives" for building muscle mass. Many anabolic steroid products, including oxymetholone (Anadrol-50) and nandrolone, are potent anabolic steroids that are classified as Schedule III drugs under the Anabolic Steroid Control Act of 2004 because of their abuse potential. The legislation associated with anabolic steroid abuse is presented in Chapter 8.

PharmFACT

Approximately 1 in 35 high school seniors have taken anabolic steroids. The number of high school students trying the drugs peaked in 2000 to 2001 and has been declining since. *Source:* National Institute of Drug Abuse, 2008.

One of the few prescribed anabolic steroids, called oxandrolone (Oxandrin), is used in the treatment of constitutional growth delay, promotion of weight gain in the severely ill, and treatment of delayed puberty in boys. Those who are receiving oxandrolone for growth delay should have bone growth assessed every 6 months. Other steroids are used for the treatment of advanced estrogen-dependent breast cancer and anemia that is unresponsive to other treatment. The anabolic steroids are listed in Table 72.1.

When taken in large doses for prolonged periods, anabolic steroids can produce significant adverse effects, some of which may persist for months after discontinuation of the drugs. When given in higher doses, androgen administration suppresses the release of LH and FSH, resulting in oligospermia, testicular atrophy, and impotence in men. In female athletes menstrual irregularities are likely with an obvious increase in masculine appearance, such as hair growth and reduction in breast size. In teen or preteen males and females, androgens can promote premature epiphyseal plate closure, thereby reducing adult height. Anabolic steroids are hepatotoxic, and permanent liver damage or hepatic carcinoma may result with prolonged use. Accompanying salt and water retention can result in HTN. These agents tend to raise low-density lipoprotein (LDL) and lower high-density lipoprotein (HDL) cholesterol levels, possibly accelerating atherosclerosis. Acne is common. Behavioral changes include an increase in aggressive behavior and psychological dependence. Another unusual adverse effect is peliosis hepatis, which is a condition in which liver and, sometimes splenic, tissue is replaced with blood-filled cysts. These cysts are sometimes asymptomatic and may not be recognized until life-threatening hepatic failure or intra-abdominal hemorrhage occurs. Anabolic steroids are pregnancy category X medications and their use is contraindicated during pregnancy.

NURSING PROCESS APPLICATION

Patients Receiving Androgen Therapy

Assessment	Potential Nursing Diagnoses
Prior to administration: • Obtain a complete health history, including male breast or prostatic cancer; BPH; cardiac, kidney, or liver disease; diabetes; or hypercalcemia. • Obtain laboratory results, including renal function tests, blood urea nitrogen (BUN), creatinine, and prostate-specific antigen (PSA). • Obtain a drug history to determine possible drug interactions and allergies.	• *Disturbed Body Image,* related to effects of decreased or increased hormone function • *Sexual Dysfunction,* related to effects of drug therapy or decreased hormone function • *Deficient Knowledge (Disease Process and Drug Therapy)*

Planning: Patient Goals and Expected Outcomes

The patient will:

- Demonstrate improvement of the underlying condition for which testosterone was ordered.
- Demonstrate an ability to correctly self-administer the prescribed drug.
- Demonstrate an understanding of the drug's action by accurately describing drug adverse effects and precautions.

Implementation

Interventions and (Rationales)	Patient and Family Education
• Monitor serum cholesterol levels. (Elevated cholesterol levels secondary to testosterone administration may increase the patient's risk of cardiovascular disease.)	Instruct the patient to: • Have cholesterol levels measured periodically during therapy. • Modify factors that may lower the risk of hypercholesterolemia, such as decreased fat in the diet, increase exercise, decrease consumption of red meat.
• Monitor calcium levels. (Testosterone can cause hypercalcemia.)	Instruct the patient to: • Be aware of food and over-the-counter (OTC) drugs that contain calcium. • Have calcium levels checked during therapy and be knowledgeable of calcium level results. • Recognize and report symptoms of increased serum calcium, including deep bone and flank pain, anorexia, nausea, vomiting, thirst, constipation, lethargy, and psychoses.
• Monitor bone growth in children and adolescents. (Premature epiphyseal closing may occur, leading to growth retardation.)	• Instruct the pediatric caregiver to have bone-age determinations performed on the child every 6 months.
• Monitor input, output, and patient weight. (Testosterone can cause retention of salt and water, leading to edema.)	• Instruct the patient to check weight twice weekly and report increases, particularly if accompanied by dependent edema.
• Monitor the patient's commitment to the medication regimen. (Maximum therapeutic effects may take several months.)	Instruct the patient to: • Mark the calendar so that the medication can be taken or given at appropriate intervals. • Apply the transdermal patch to dry, clean scrotal skin that has been dry shaved and not to use chemical depilatories. • Notify the female partner of transdermal patch use. There is a chance of absorbing testosterone, resulting in mild virilization. • Avoid showering or swimming for at least 1 hour after gel application.
• Monitor blood glucose, especially in patients with diabetes. (Testosterone therapy may affect glucose tolerance.	Instruct the patient to: • Monitor blood glucose daily and report significant changes. • Recognize that adjustments may need to be made in hypoglycemic medications and diet. • Recognize the importance of routine laboratory studies, so deviations from normal can be corrected immediately.

Evaluation of Outcome Criteria

Evaluate the effectiveness of drug therapy by confirming that patient goals and expected outcomes have been met (see "Planning").

CONNECTION *Checkpoint* 72.1

Anabolic steroids are often taken illegally by "stacking" or "pyramiding." From what you learned in Chapter 8, define the use of these terms in the abuse of these drugs. See Answer to Connection Checkpoint 72.1 in Appendix A.

Etiology of Male Sexual Dysfunction

72.4 Male sexual dysfunction may have both medical and psychological etiologies.

Approximately 50% of males will experience some form of sexual dysfunction during their adult life. The primary types of male dysfunction disorders may be classified as the following:

- Diminished libido: lack of interest in sexual activity
- Erectile Dysfunction (ED): inability to obtain or maintain an erection
- Ejaculation disorder: premature, delayed, or retrograde ejaculation
- Infertility: inability to conceive a child

Certain causes of male sexual dysfunction are treatable, either medically or surgically, or can be improved to the degree that a couple can achieve successful conception or maintain a satisfactory sexual lifestyle. For example, therapy with testosterone can rapidly increase libido in patients who have insufficient serum testosterone levels or hypogonadism. Many men with ED can now be successfully treated with medications.

A large number of drugs that contribute to male sexual dysfunction have been identified and are listed in Table 72.2. In most cases, the dysfunction is dose related and is much less evident when a single drug is taken at low doses. However, taking multiple drugs that have the potential to cause sexual adverse effects may result in additive sexual dysfunction. The two most common drug classes that cause sexual dysfunction are antihypertensives and antidepressants. Because sexual adverse effects are a potential cause of nonadherence, nurses should ask specific questions regarding changes in sexual function when their patients are taking these drugs.

Many comorbid medical conditions are associated with sexual dysfunction. Any condition that results in general debility, such as pain, muscle weakness, shortness of breath, or cerebrovascular accident (CVA), may cause dysfunction. Diabetes and HTN are the two chronic medical conditions most frequently associated with male sexual dysfunction. Patients who present with psychological conditions such as anxiety and depression have a high incidence of sexual dysfunction. Other factors that are associated with ED include obesity and cigarette smoking. Combining multiple risk factors, for example, a patient who has diabetes is obese, takes antihypertensive drugs, and smokes, will result in a high risk for sexual dysfunction.

Nurses play a key role in treating male sexual dysfunction by obtaining a thorough medical history and by recognizing factors that contribute to the disorder. Should patients experience unacceptable sexual adverse effects from their medications, alternative drugs can usually be substituted. Encouraging patients to receive treatment for anxiety, depression, and other comorbid conditions sometimes helps improve the sexual dysfunction. All men at risk should be encouraged to maintain optimum weight, stop smoking, and limit their alcohol use.

TABLE 72.2 Drugs That May Cause or Worsen Male Sexual Dysfunction

Drug/Drug Class	Sexual Adverse Effect(s)
Antihypertensives	
angiotensin-converting enzyme (ACE) inhibitors (e.g., lisinopril)	Erectile dysfunction (ED)
alpha-adrenergic blockers (e.g., prazosin)	Retrograde ejaculation, priapism
beta-adrenergic blockers (e.g., propranolol)	Diminished libido, ED
methyldopa	Diminished libido, ED
spironolactone	Diminished libido, ED
thiazide diuretics	ED
Nervous System Agents	
carbamazepine	ED
haloperidol	Inhibited ejaculation, priapism
lithium carbonate	ED
phenothiazines (e.g., chlorpromazine)	Diminished libido, ED, inhibited ejaculation, priapism
selective serotonin reuptake inhibitors (e.g., fluoxetine)	Anorgasmy, inhibited ejaculation, diminished libido
trazodone	Priapism
tricyclic antidepressants (e.g., imipramine)	Diminished libido, ED, inhibited ejaculation
Other Drugs	
alcohol	ED
anabolic steroids	Infertility
chemotherapy agents (e.g., cyclophosphamide)	Infertility
cimetidine	Diminished libido, ED, gynecomastia
digoxin	ED
finasteride	ED
methotrexate	Infertility

Pharmacotherapy of Male Infertility

72.5 Male infertility is treated with endocrine drugs that boost sperm production.

Infertility affects approximately 6.1 million persons in the United States, or roughly 10% of the reproductive age population. It is estimated that 30% to 40% of infertility among couples is due to difficulties with the male reproductive system.

Like female infertility, male infertility may have a number of complex causes. The most common congenital cause is Klinefelter's syndrome, which is the presence of an extra X chromosome. Acquired infertility may result from testicular trauma; pituitary or hypothalamus disorders; and infections such as mumps, chronic tuberculosis, and sexually transmitted infections. Infertility may occur with or without signs of hypogonadism. Rarely, life-threatening conditions such as testicular cancer and pituitary tumors may be the cause. In addition, the lack of ability to conceive may be caused by factors identified in Section 72.4, such as ED or ejaculation disorders. Identifying the etiology of infertility is important, because not all causes can be successfully treated with pharmacotherapy.

The most obvious etiology of male infertility is lack of sufficient sperm production. **Oligospermia,** is the presence of less than 20 million sperm per milliliter of ejaculate **Azoospermia,** which occurs in 15% of men with infertility, is the complete absence of sperm in an ejaculate. Azoospermia can be caused by severely reduced or absent sperm production or it may indicate an obstruction of the vas deferens or ejaculatory duct that can be corrected surgically. Drug therapy with calcium channel blockers, colchicine, spironolactone, and cimetidine can lower sperm production.

Depending on the cause of the condition, one goal of pharmacotherapy for male infertility may be to increase sperm production. If the cause of the infertility is decreased testosterone secretion due to hypogonadism, administration of this hormone can increase sperm production and cure the condition.

Another method of increasing sperm production is to stimulate the testes with pituitary hormones. Pharmacotherapy often begins with IM injections of human chorionic gonadotropin (HCG) three times per week over 1 year. Although HCG is secreted by the placenta, its effects in men are identical to those of LH: increased testosterone secretion and spermatogenesis. Sperm counts are conducted periodically to assess therapeutic progress. If HCG is unsuccessful, therapy with menotropins (Menopur, Repronex) may be attempted. Menotropins consist of a mixture of purified FSH and LH, which increases testosterone and sperm production.

Once testosterone levels rise, either through the administration of testosterone or HCG, the natural feedback mechanism of the body will signal the pituitary to shut down testosterone secretion in the testes. To boost testosterone levels, antiestrogen drugs such as tamoxifen (Nolvadex) and clomiphene (Clomid) have been used to block the negative feedback of estrogen (from the adrenal glands) to the pituitary and hypothalamus, thus increasing the levels of FSH and LH. Unfortunately, such adverse effects as gynecomastia, decreased libido, and weight gain may be unacceptable to the male patient. Clomiphene is presented as a prototype drug for female infertility in Chapter 70.

Other pharmacologic approaches to treating male infertility have been attempted. Testolactone (Teslac), an aromatase inhibitor, has been administered to block the metabolic conversion of testosterone to estrogen. If retrograde ejaculation has been identified as a probable cause, sympathomimetics may be used to convert to normal, antegrade ejaculation. Various nutritional supplements, such as zinc to improve sperm production, l-carnitine to improve sperm motility and sperm count, and vitamins C and E as antioxidants to reduce reactive intermediates, have been tested. Unfortunately these and other therapies have not conclusively been shown to have any positive effect on male infertility.

Drug therapy of male infertility is not as successful as pharmacotherapy in women because only about 5% of infertile males have an endocrine etiology for their disorder. Many years of therapy may be required. Because of the expense of pharmacotherapy, the large number of injections needed, and the relative lack of success, other means of conception for the infertile man should be explored. There are a wide range of assistive reproduction procedures, including in vitro fertilization or intrauterine insemination that may be pursued.

CONNECTION *Checkpoint* 72.2

Clomiphene is used for both male and female infertility. From what you learned in Chapter 70, how does this drug act to improve female fertility? See Answer to Connection Checkpoint 72.2 in Appendix A.

Pharmacotherapy of Erectile Dysfunction

72.6 Erectile dysfunction is a common disorder that may be successfully treated with inhibitors of the enzyme phosphodiesterase-5.

Erectile dysfunction (ED) is defined as the consistent inability to either attain an erection or to sustain an erection long enough to achieve satisfactory sexual intercourse. **Impotence,** a term often used interchangeably with ED, is the total inability to achieve an erection, an inconsistent ability to achieve an erection, or the ability to have only brief erections. An estimated 15 to 30 million men in the United States have ED. The incidence of ED increases with age, although it may occur in men of any age.

Pharm*FACT*

The landmark study on the prevalence of sexual dysfunction is the Massachusetts Male Aging Study. The study showed that 52% of 1,290 men aged 40 to 70 years had some degree of dysfunction, and almost 10% had total absence of erectile function. Among men in their 70s, the incidence of ED is as high as 70%. *Source:* O'Donnell, Araujo, & McKinlay, 2004.

Penile erection is a complex event that has psychological, neuromuscular, and vascular components. Sexual arousal results in the release of neurotransmitters, primarily nitric oxide and epinephrine, from the hypothalamus. This stimulation along the autonomic nerves results in the release of an enzyme that makes cyclic guanosine monophosphate (cGMP). cGMP causes dilation of the arterioles leading to the major erectile tissues of the penis, called the **corpora cavernosa.** Rigidity of the penis results when the increased local blood flow and pressure fill the vascular spaces within the corpora. This engorgement causes occlusion of the veins that drain blood from the corpora, allowing the penis to remain rigid long enough for successful coitus. When stimulation ends or after ejaculation, cGMP is removed by the enzyme phosphodiesterase-5 (PDE-5). At this point, the pressure in the penis decreases, the veins dilate, blood leaves the corpora, and the penis quickly loses its rigidity. The anatomy of the penis is illustrated in Figure 72.2.

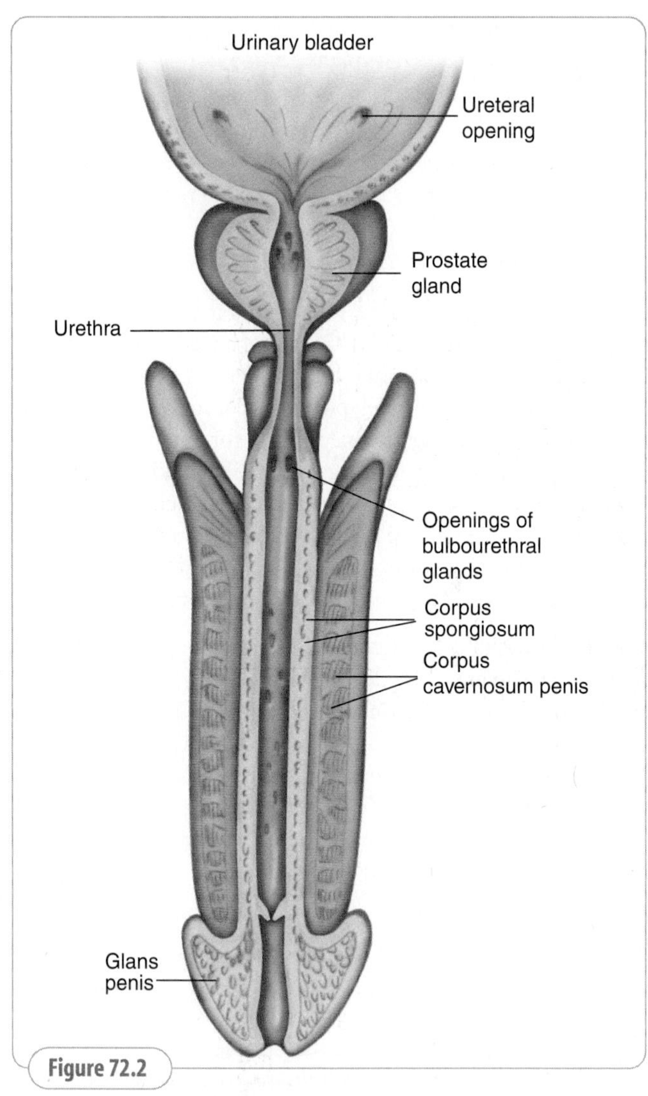

Figure 72.2

Anatomy of the penis.

Source: From *Medical Terminology with Human Anatomy* (5th ed., p. 538), by J. Rice, 2005. Reprinted by permission of Pearson Education, Inc., Upper Saddle River, NJ.

Organic causes of ED may include damage to the nerves serving the penis or a decrease in blood flow though the blood vessels involved in the erection reflex. Many chronic illnesses have the potential to damage the arteries, smooth muscle, and fibrous tissues of the penis, most notably atherosclerosis, diabetes, CVA, kidney disease, and HTN. Psychogenic causes may include depression, fatigue, stress, or fear of sexual failure. In some men, a number of common drugs cause impotence as an adverse effect, including thiazide diuretics, phenothiazines, selective serotonin reuptake inhibitors (SSRIs), tricyclic antidepressants (TCAs), propranolol (Inderal), and diazepam (Valium). Another potential cause of ED is hypogonadism, which can cause an inability to develop an erection, owing to the loss of libido. Nerve innervation and blood flow to the penis may be damaged by surgery, particularly during procedures involving the prostate gland.

A thorough health history of male patients should include questions regarding sexual function. Laboratory tests to check for possible metabolic or hormonal causes of ED include serum testosterone, prostate-specific antigen (PSA), blood chemistries, prolactin, and thyroxin levels. A nocturnal penile tumescence and rigidity (NPTR) test may be ordered. This test monitors the number of erections during sleep and is used to differentiate between the psychological and physiological causes of ED. A penile blood flow test is also used to determine whether there is sufficient arterial and venous flow through the penis. Patients who have diminished or abnormal blood flow may find that the pharmacologic agents to treat ED are not effective. These patients may have more success with penile implants.

The treatment of ED is becoming more prevalent as the population ages because more men are becoming affected by the disorder. If hormones are the cause of the dysfunction, treatment is aimed at correcting the abnormality. In some, testosterone replacement therapy by IM injection or transdermal patches may assist with ED, particularly if associated with hypogonadism or low libido. If the cause is found to be psychological, treatment will usually consist of a combination of psychotherapy and pharmacotherapy.

The development of sildenafil (Viagra), the first PDE-5 inhibitor, revolutionized the treatment of ED. When sildenafil was approved as the first pharmacologic treatment for ED in 1998, it set a record for pharmaceutical sales of any new drug in U.S. history. Two other PDE-5 inhibitors have been approved by the FDA: vardenafil (Levitra) and tadalafil (Cialis). Drugs for ED are listed in Table 72.3.

The PDE-5 inhibitors do not cause an erection. They merely enhance the erection resulting from physical contact or other sexual stimuli by maintaining relaxation of the smooth muscle in the penis and increasing blood flow. These drugs are not as effective in promoting erections in men who do not have ED. Despite considerable research interest, PDE-5 inhibitors have no effects on female sexual function. These drugs are not approved for use by women.

TABLE 72.3 Agents for Erectile Dysfunction

Drug	Route and Adult Dose (maximum dose where indicated)	Adverse Effects
sildenafil (Viagra)	PO: 25–50 mg approximately 30–60 min before intercourse (max: 100 mg once/day)	*Nasal congestion, headache, facial flushing, dizziness, vision abnormalities, myalgia* Hypotension when taken with nitrates, priapism, hearing loss, nonarteritic anterior ischemic optic neuropathy
tadalafil (Cialis)	PO: 10 mg approximately 30 min before intercourse (max: 20 mg/day) Once-daily dosing: 2.5–5 mg daily	
vardenafil (Levitra)	PO: 10 mg approximately 1 h before intercourse (max: 20 mg once/day)	

Note: *Italics* indicate common adverse effects. Underline indicates serious adverse effects.

MyNursingKit | Mechanism of Action Animation: Sildenafil

The three PDE-5 inhibitors are equally effective at promoting erections in 60% to 80% of male patients, and the adverse effects are similar. The most common adverse effects are nasal congestion, headache, facial flushing, and dizziness. These drugs produce a 5- to 10-mm fall in blood pressure, but this drop is usually not clinically important. In patients who are taking nitrates or multiple antihypertensive medications, however, this blood pressure change may produce symptoms of hypotension. Therefore, PDE-5 inhibitors are contraindicated in patients who are taking organic nitrates in any form. Organic nitrates include nitroglycerin and isosorbide mononitrate.

Prior to the discovery of sildenafil, the treatment of ED consisted of rigid or inflatable penile prostheses being implanted into the corpora. As an alternative to prostheses, drugs such as alprostadil (Caverject) or the combination of papaverine plus phentolamine (Pavabid, Genabid, Cerespan) were injected directly into the corpora cavernosa just prior to intercourse. Penile injections cause pain and reduce the spontaneity associated with pleasurable intercourse. Intracavernous injections may cause fibrous tissue within the penis, hypotension, dizziness, pain, and priapism. These alternative therapies are rare today, though they may be used for patients in whom PDE-5 inhibitors are contraindicated.

Alprostadil (Caverject) can be used as a minisuppository that can be administered into the urethra as a medicated urethral system for erection (MUSE) or by direct injection into the cavernosa. As with papaverine, erection results from a relaxation of smooth muscle, increasing blood flow into the corpora. MUSE is available in four dosage strengths: 125, 250, 500, and 1,000 mcg. Alprostadil by either method should not be used more than three times per week and not more than once in 24 hours. Penile pain, burning sensations, and priapism are common adverse effects and, more rarely, penile fibrosis. The effectiveness of alprostadil is less than that of the PDE-5 inhibitors or intracavernosal therapy and the strength of the erection can be improved by using a constriction ring.

PROTOTYPE DRUG Sildenafil (Viagra)

Classification: **Therapeutic:** Agent for treating impotence
Pharmacologic: Phosphodiesterase (PDE)-5 inhibitor

Therapeutic Effects and Uses: Approved in 1998, sildenafil is an PO drug and was the first PDE-5 inhibitor approved for ED. The onset of action is relatively rapid, which is less than 1 hour, and its effects last up to 4 hours.

Sildenafil is also used for the treatment of pulmonary arterial HTN. For this indication, blocking PDE-5 in pulmonary vascular smooth muscle causes vasodilation and reduction in arterial HTN. The drug improves exercise capacity in these patients. Off-label indications include prevention of pulmonary HTN induced by altitude sickness and treatment of Raynaud's phenomena resistant to vasodilator therapy.

Mechanism of Action: Sildenafil inhibits PDE-5 and increases and preserves cGMP levels in the penis. This relaxes smooth muscle in the corpus cavernosum, allowing increased blood flow into the penis and allowing a harder and longer lasting erection in about 70% of men taking the drug.

Pharmacokinetics:

Route	PO
Absorption	Rapid; bioavailability: 40%
Distribution	96% protein bound
Primary metabolism	Hepatic (CYP3A4 and 2C9)
Primary excretion	80% feces, 12% renal
Onset of action	20–60 minutes
Duration of action	24 h; Half-life: 4 h

Adverse Effects: Sildenafil is well tolerated and adverse effects are usually transient and mild. Common adverse effects include headache, dizziness, flushing, rash, and nasal congestion. The most serious adverse effect, hypotension, occurs in patients who are concurrently taking organic nitrates for angina and can result in MI and sudden cardiac death. Sildenafil can produce blurred vision, increased sensitivity to light, or changes in color perception in 10% of the patients. Priapism, a sustained erection lasting longer than 6 hours, has been reported with sildenafil use and may lead to permanent damage of penile tissue.

Contraindications/Precautions: Sildenafil is contraindicated in patients who are taking nitrates and in those with hypersensitivity to this drug. It is contraindicated in patients with severe cardiovascular disease, recent MI, stroke, heart failure, dysrhythmias, and in the presence of anatomic deformities of the penis. This drug should be used with caution in patients with renal or hepatic impairment. Patients with preexisting visual disturbances should not use sildenafil.

Drug Interactions: Cimetidine, erythromycin, and ketoconazole will increase serum levels of sildenafil and necessitate lower drug doses. Concurrent use with nitrates is contraindicated and will result in hypotension and possibly death. Protease inhibitors (ritonavir, amprenavir, others) will cause increased sildenafil levels, which may lead to toxicity. Rifampin may decrease sildenafil levels, leading to decreased effectiveness. Concurrent use of sildenafil with drugs that lower blood pressure, including alpha-adrenergic blockers, should be avoided due to the potential for additive hypotension. **Herbal/Food:** Administration of sildenafil with meals, especially high-fat meals, should be avoided because absorption is decreased. Grapefruit juice increases the plasma concentrations of sildenafil and may cause adverse effects.

Pregnancy: Category B (not approved for females).

Treatment of Overdose: There is no specific treatment for overdose.

Nursing Responsibilities:

- Obtain a complete physical examination, including a history of sexual dysfunction, cardiovascular disease, and presence of emotional disturbances.
- Notify the prescriber if the patient takes nitrates such as nitroglycerin because these drugs may cause a sudden, unsafe drop in blood pressure. Nitrates are also found in recreational drugs, including amyl nitrate or nitrite, commonly called "poppers."
- Administer alpha-adrenergic blockers with caution because coadministration with vardenafil or tadalafil can lead to profound hypotension.

- Assess for any signs or symptoms of cardiovascular distress. Patients with CAD require frequent evaluation to determine if symptoms are due to the CAD or the effects of sildenafil.
- Monitor liver function tests. Patients with cirrhosis or severe decreased liver function should start with lower doses to prevent hepatoxicity.
- Monitor for visual adverse effects such as blurred vision, the inability to differentiate between green and blue, perception of a blue tinge to objects, or photophobia. Observe safety precautions until it is known whether sensory-perceptual alterations occur to prevent falls and other injuries.
- Monitor for presence of headache, dizziness, flushing, rash, and nasal congestion.

Patient and Family Education:

- Keep all laboratory visits to evaluate liver function.
- Take this drug exactly as prescribed. Do not take more than one dose in a 24-hour period.
- Check vital signs routinely and report any significant changes.
- Take this drug 30 to 60 minutes prior to anticipated sexual activity.
- Do not use erectile dysfunction drugs if taking nitrates or alpha blockers.
- Avoid high-fat meals before taking this drug because it may cause a delay in drug action.
- Immediately report chest pain or an erection that lasts longer than 4 hours or is painful to the health care provider.

Drugs Similar to Sildenafil (Viagra)

The two other PDE-5 inhibitors are tadalafil and vardenafil.

Tadalafil (Cialis): Approved in 2003, tadalafil acts by the same mechanism as sildenafil, which is relaxation of penile arterial and trabecular smooth muscle. This drug's absorption is not affected by food. It acts within 30 to 60 minutes and has a longer duration of action than sildenafil: up to 36 hours. The longer duration allows for more spontaneity of sexual activity. Contraindications include patients who take nitrates and dosing can be prescribed every 72 hours. Tadalafil produces less blood pressure decrease than the other drugs in this class, making it safer for patients with congestive heart failure or a history of MI. It also results in a lower incidence of visual disturbances. Other adverse effects are similar to those of sildenafil. A daily dosing of tadalafil was approved in 2008. This drug is pregnancy category B.

Vardenafil (Levitra): Like other drugs in this class, vardenafil allows for relaxation of arterial and trabecular smooth muscle in the penis. Approved in 2003, vardenafil acts within 30 to 60 minutes and its effects continue for 4 to 5 hours. Headache, flushing rhinitis, and dyspepsia are the common adverse effects. Vardenafil may prolong the QT interval and is to be used with caution in patients who are taking nitrates. This drug is pregnancy category B.

CONNECTIONS

Treating the Diverse Patient

Viagra for Women

Many women are asking their health care providers, "Is there a Viagra for me?" The answer right now to that question is no.

It is thought that a greater number of women than men suffer from a degree of sexual dysfunction. In females this dysfunction is characterized by a low libido with a lack of arousal and inability to experience orgasm. The fundamental difference between the sexes though is in the difference in the relationship between arousal and desire. In males simply improving the ability to have an erection will increase their sexual activity. In females, however, the cause of dysfunction is thought to be more psychological in nature, involving complex relationships among mood, self-esteem, and the relationship. So although the enzyme that Viagra affects to increase penile blood flow is found in the pelvic area in women, increasing blood flow to a woman's sexual organs does not cause a woman to feel any more aroused.

Pathophysiology of Benign Prostatic Hyperplasia

72.7 Benign prostatic hyperplasia is an enlargement of the prostate that occurs in older men.

The prostate is a gland the size of a walnut that surrounds the male urethra. Its primary function is to contribute fluids to the ejaculate. The prostate contains two major types of tissues:

- Epithelial tissue. This is the glandular portion of the prostate that secretes fluids for the ejaculate. The growth of prostatic epithelial tissue is controlled by the presence of androgens. Testosterone is converted to its active metabolite, dihydrotestosterone (DHT), in the epithelial cells of the prostate by the enzyme 5-alpha reductase.
- Stomal tissue. This is smooth muscle tissue, which is controlled by alpha$_1$-adrenergic receptors. These receptors cause the smooth muscle to contract around the urethra when activated.

Benign prostatic hyperplasia (BPH), which is an abnormal enlargement of the prostate, is the most common benign neoplasm in men. The exact cause of BPH is unknown, but it exists to some degree in all older men. It is present in 70% of men by age 60 and 90% by age 80. Other than age, the risk factors for BPH include a family history of the disorder, smoking, heavy alcohol consumption, HTN, diabetes, diets high in meats and fats, and African American ancestry. BPH is not considered to be a precursor to prostate carcinoma, though it is well known that many men with BPH eventually experience prostate cancer.

Pharm*FACT*

Screening for BPH and prostate cancer usually begins at age 50. Diagnostic tests include a digital rectal examination and a prostate-specific antigen (PSA) test. Men have a one in six chance of developing prostate cancer in their lifetime. *Source:* Centers for Disease Control and Prevention, 2006.

The characteristic feature of BPH is an enlargement of the prostate gland that decreases the outflow of urine by obstructing the urethra, causing difficult urination. The pathogenesis of BPH involves two components: static and dynamic. The static factors are caused by the physical enlargement of the prostate gland owing to the overgrowth of the epithelial or glandular cells. The gland can double or triple in size with aging, creating a physical block of urine outflow at the neck of the bladder. The dynamic factors are due to excessive numbers of alpha$_1$-adrenergic receptors located in stromal tissue in the neck of the urinary bladder and in the prostate gland. When activated, these receptors compress the urethra and provide resistance to urine outflow from the bladder. The two mechanisms of disease, static and dynamic, have led to two different classes of drugs for treating the symptoms of BPH. BPH is shown in Pharmacotherapy Illustrated 72.1.

Certain frequently used medications worsen symptoms of BPH. Alpha-adrenergic agents, which include decongestants such as pseudoephedrine and phenylephrine, activate alpha$_1$-adrenergic receptors in the bladder neck, causing restriction of urine flow. Drugs with anticholinergic effects such as antihistamines, TCAs, or phenothiazines may worsen the associated urinary retention. Testosterone and other anabolic steroids may increase prostate enlargement which contributes to the physical obstruction of the urethra. Drugs that worsen symptoms of BPH should be avoided in elderly men.

There is not a clear correlation between the symptoms experienced by patients and the size of the prostate. Some men may have minimal enlargement and experience moderate symptoms, whereas others may have extremely enlarged glands and be asymptomatic. This is because the smooth muscle in the urinary bladder has the ability to compensate for the obstruction by contracting with greater force to eject the urine stream. Over time, the bladder is no longer able to compensate and symptoms of BPH manifest, such as increased urinary frequency (usually with small amounts of urine), increased urgency to urinate, postvoid leakage, excessive night-time urination (nocturia), decreased force of the urine stream, and a sensation that the bladder did not completely empty.

Some patients do not seek medical attention until complications caused by the long-standing obstruction at the neck of

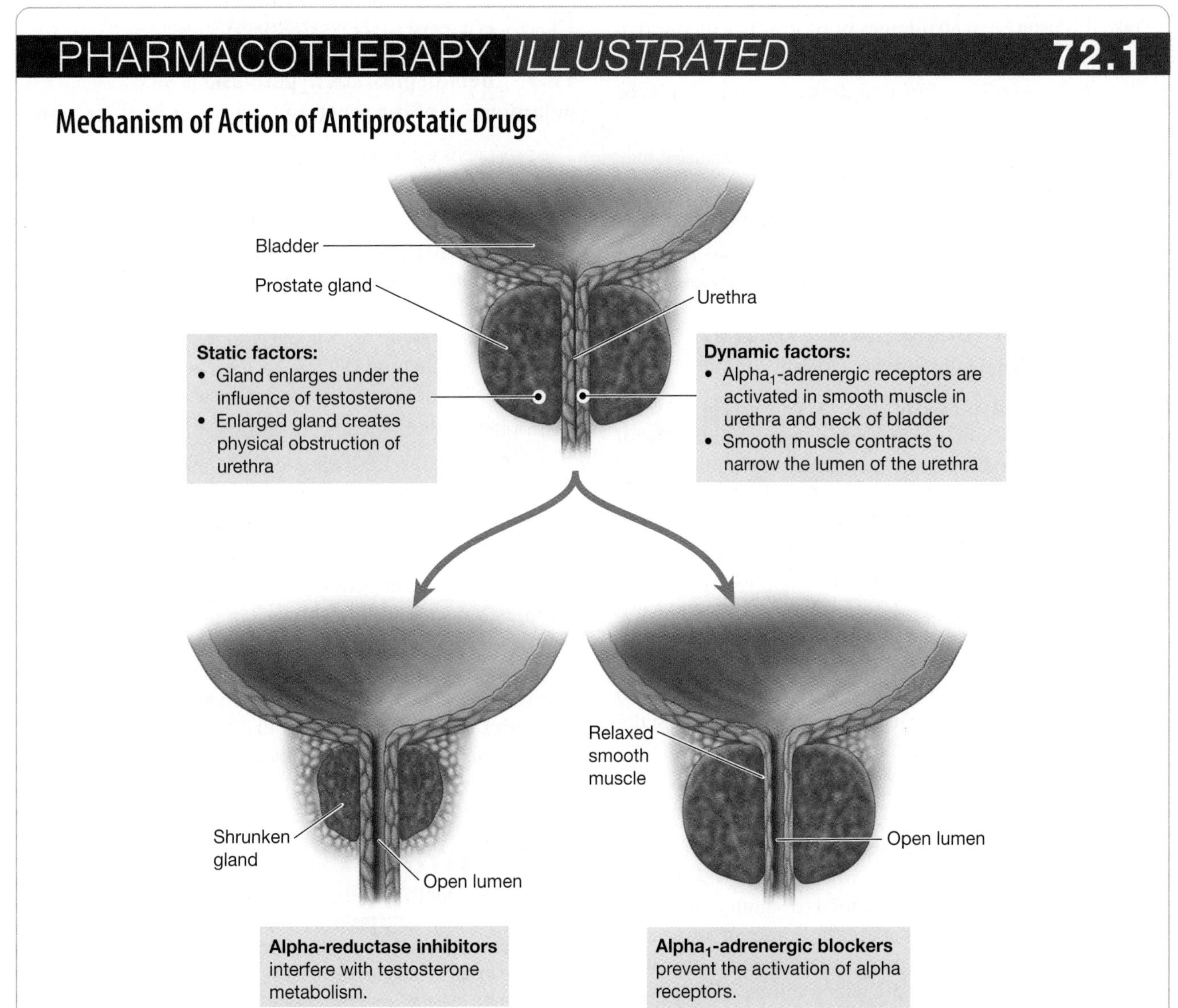

the urinary bladder arise. Serious complications include recurrent urinary infections, incontinence, gross hematuria, bladder stones, and chronic renal failure.

Pharmacotherapy of Benign Prostatic Hyperplasia

72.8 In its early stages, benign prostatic hyperplasia may be treated successfully with drug therapy.

The goal of treatment for patients with BPH focuses on minimizing the urinary obstruction and preventing complications. Drug therapy can only treat symptoms; it cannot reverse or cure BPH. Patients who are asymptomatic or who present with mild symptoms generally do not receive pharmacotherapy. Not all BPH is progressive, and many patients never experience moderate or advanced symptoms. Patient education such as avoiding caffeine or alcohol intake, eliminating drugs that worsen BPH, and restricting fluids close to bedtime may be sufficient to achieve symptomatic improvement. Morning diuretic therapy may be used to lessen night-time diuresis. The patient is reevaluated at 6- to 12-month intervals to assess for worsening symptoms.

When symptoms of BPH worsen, pharmacotherapy is indicated. Only a few drugs are available for the pharmacotherapy of BPH, and these are listed in Table 72.4. Drugs that are used to treat BPH have limited effectiveness and have value only in treating mild to moderate disease as an alternative to surgery. Because pharmacotherapy does not cure the disease, these medications must be taken for the remainder of the patient's life or until surgery is indicated. If the drugs are discontinued, the prostate size increases back to its enlarged state and symptoms of BPH return. In advanced cases, transurethral resection of the prostate or a laser prostatectomy is needed to restore the patency of the urethra.

The two major drug classes for treating BPH are the $alpha_1$-adrenergic blockers and the 5-alpha reductase inhibitors. Research has shown that combination therapy with an $alpha_1$ blocker and a 5-alpha reductase inhibitor is more effective than therapy with either drug alone. This is the treatment of choice for patients with moderate symptoms of BPH.

The $alpha_1$-adrenergic blockers act in the stromal tissue of the prostate to relax smooth muscle in the prostate gland, bladder neck, and urethra, thus easing the urinary obstruction. Doxazosin (Cardura) and terazosin (Hytrin) are of particular value to patients who have both HTN and BPH; these two disorders occur concurrently in about 25% of men older than 60. A third $alpha_1$ blocker, tamsulosin (Flomax), has no effect on blood pressure, and its only indication is BPH. Drugs in this class improve urine flow and reduce other bothersome symptoms of BPH within 1 to 2 weeks of administration. Primary adverse effects include headache, fatigue, and dizziness. Doxazosin and terazosin are not associated with an increased risk of sexual dysfunction, but ejaculatory disorders have been reported with tamsulosin. Reflex tachycardia due to stimulation of baroreceptors is common with $alpha_1$ blockers. Additional information on the $alpha_1$ blockers is presented in Chapter 20.

Some patients are unable to tolerate the cardiovascular adverse effects of the $alpha_1$-adrenergic blockers. For these patients, the 5-alpha reductase inhibitors are used as monotherapy. These agents act by blocking 5-alpha reductase, the enzyme responsible for converting testosterone to DHT, which is its active metabolite. Without DHT the hormonal signal for prostatic epithelial tissue growth is eliminated, thus causing the enlarged prostate to shrink in size. The most commonly prescribed drug in this class is finasteride (Proscar), which is featured as a prototype for BPH. These agents may take several months to shrink the size of the prostate; thus, they are not appropriate for severe disease. The 5-alpha reductase inhibitors produce few adverse effects, although they can cause sexual dysfunction and gynecomastia in some patients. Because they are pregnancy category X, patients who are taking these drugs should not donate blood because of the possibility that the donated blood would be given to a pregnant woman.

CONNECTION *Checkpoint* 72.3

$Alpha_1$-adrenergic blockers are very susceptible to causing the "first-dose phenomenon." From what you learned in Chapter 20, define this phenomenon and describe what should be done to minimize its effects. See Answer to Connection Checkpoint 72.3 in Appendix A.

TABLE 72.4 Agents for Benign Prostatic Hyperplasia

Drug	Route and Adult Dose (maximum dose where indicated)	Adverse Effects
Alpha-Adrenergic Blockers		
alfuzosin (Uroxatral)	PO: 10 mg/day (max: 10 mg/day)	*Orthostatic hypotension, headache, dizziness, decreased libido, decreased ejaculate volume* <u>First-dose phenomenon (severe hypotension and syncope), tachycardia</u>
doxazosin (Cardura)	PO: 1–8 mg/day (max: 8 mg/day)	
doxazosin XL (Cardura XL)	Extended release: 4–8 mg/day (max: 8 mg/day)	
tamsulosin (Flomax)	PO: 0.4 mg 30 min after a meal (max: 0.8 mg/day)	
terazosin (Hytrin)	PO: start with 1 mg at bedtime, then 1–5 mg/day (max: 20 mg/day)	
5-Alpha Reductase Inhibitors		
dutasteride (Avodart)	PO: 0.5 mg/day	*Sexual dysfunction, decreased libido, decreased ejaculate volume, gynecomastia* No serious adverse effects
finasteride (Proscar)	PO: 5 mg/day (max: 5 mg/day)	

Note: *Italics* indicate common adverse effects. <u>Underline</u> indicates serious adverse effects.

CONNECTIONS

Complementary and Alternative Therapies Saw Palmetto

Description: Saw palmetto (*Serona repens*) is a dwarf palm tree that grows in the coastal regions of the southern United States. The portion of the plant that is used in supplements is the berries. More than 2 million men in the United States use saw palmetto each year in the hopes that it will treat their symptoms of benign prostatic hypertrophy (Bent, 2006).

History and Claims: Like finasteride, saw palmetto is thought to help stop a cascade of prostate-damaging enzymes that may create BPH. In theory, it occupies binding sites on the prostate that are typically occupied by DHT, an enzyme that may trigger BPH, inhibiting growth of the prostate gland.

Standardization: Saw palmetto is available in capsule, tablet, and liquid dosage forms. Oral saw palmetto products should be standardized to contain 80% or more of the active ingredients, which are fatty acids.

Evidence: Although several clinical studies have suggested that saw palmetto is as effective as finasteride in treating mild to moderate BPH and produces fewer adverse effects (Fong, Milani, & Djavan, 2005), a landmark study in the *New England Journal of Medicine* indicates that it has no benefit in treating BPH (Bent, 2006). Saw palmetto may cause damage to the liver and pancreas, so it is vital that the nurse obtain a thorough health and supplement use history and advise the patient of its potential adverse effects.

PROTOTYPE DRUG Finasteride (Proscar)

Classification: **Therapeutic:** Drug for BPH
Pharmacologic: Antiandrogen, 5-alpha reductase inhibitor

Therapeutic Effects and Uses: Approved in 1992, finasteride is an PO drug that inhibits the metabolism of testosterone. The drug is sometimes called an antiandrogen. Finasteride promotes shrinkage of enlarged prostates and subsequently helps restore urinary function. It is most effective in patients with larger prostates. This drug is also marketed as Propecia, which is prescribed to promote hair regrowth in patients with male-pattern baldness. Doses of finasteride are five times higher when prescribed for BPH than when prescribed for baldness.

Off-label indications for finasteride take advantage of its antiandrogen effects. The drug has been found to have a slight protective effect when used for prostate cancer prophylaxis. It may be used to treat mild to moderate hirsutism in females.

Mechanism of Action: Finasteride acts by inhibiting 5-alpha reductase, which is the enzyme responsible for converting testosterone to one of its metabolites, 5-alpha dihydrotestosterone. This active metabolite causes proliferation of prostate cells and promotes enlargement of the gland. Finasteride promotes regression of prostate epithelial tissue and decreases mechanical obstruction of the urethra.

Pharmacokinetics:

Route	PO
Absorption	Well absorbed
Distribution	Crosses the blood–brain barrier; found in semen; 90% bound to plasma protein
Primary metabolism	Hepatic (CYP3A4)
Primary excretion	39% renal, 57% feces
Onset of action	Half-life: 5–7 h; maximum effects take 3–6 months
Duration of action	5–7 days

Adverse Effects: Finasteride is well tolerated and adverse effects are generally mild and transient. Finasteride causes various types of sexual dysfunction in up to 16% of patients, including gynecomastia, impotence, diminished libido, and ejaculatory disorders such as decreased volume of ejaculate. The drug reduces sperm production and may impair fertility. The actual incidence of drug-induced sexual dysfunction is difficult to estimate because a large percentage of older males develop these symptoms as a consequence of aging or comorbid conditions. Other minor adverse effects include headache, nausea, rash, dizziness, and asthenia.

Contraindications/Precautions: Contraindications to finasteride include hypersensitivity to the drug, pregnancy (category X), lactation, females, and children. The pregnant nurse or pharmacist should avoid handling crushed medication because it may be absorbed through the skin and cause harm to a male fetus. Caution must be used when administering the drug to patients with hepatic or renal impairment.

Drug Interactions: Use with anticholinergics may decrease the effects of finasteride. Use of finasteride with testosterone will result in a reduction in the effects of both drugs. **Herbal/Food:** Saw palmetto may potentiate the effects of finasteride.

Pregnancy: Category X.

Treatment of Overdose: There is no specific treatment for overdose.

Nursing Responsibilities:

- Obtain a complete physical examination, including a history of cardiovascular disease and sexual dysfunction. The examination should include assessing changes in urinary elimination such as urine retention, nocturia, dribbling, difficulty starting urinary stream, frequency, and urgency.
- Assess vital signs, especially blood pressure and heart rate, if an alpha$_1$-adrenergic antagonist is prescribed. The patient may experience hypotension with the initial doses, and orthostatic hypotension may persist throughout treatment. Syncope can occur.
- Monitor for evidence of orthostatic hypotension, dizziness, and gastrointestinal disturbances. Elderly patients are especially prone to the hypotensive and hypothermic effects related to vasodilation caused by these drugs.
- Monitor patients with asthma or heart failure carefully if alpha$_1$-adrenergic blockers are prescribed concurrently because the drugs may cause bradycardia and bronchoconstriction.

- Assess periodic hepatic function tests because the drugs are metabolized in the liver.
- Monitor the emotional status of patients who are taking alpha blockers because depression is a common adverse effect.
- Monitor for adverse effects, including impotence, decreased volume of ejaculate, or decreased libido.

Patient and Family Education:

- Continue the medication as prescribed. The maximum benefit from the drug is achieved 6 to 12 months of treatment. Improvement will last only as long as the medication is continued.
- Keep all scheduled laboratory visits to evaluate PSA levels.
- Immediately report increased difficulty with urination, impotence, decreased libido, or decreased volume of ejaculate to the health care provider.
- Make position changes slowly when moving from a lying to a standing position to prevent dizziness and possible fainting.
- Women who are pregnant should not handle crushed or broken tablets.
- If sexually active, use a barrier contraceptive to prevent pregnancy.
- Do not take any other prescription or nonprescription drugs, dietary supplements, or herbal products without approval of the health care provider.

Drugs Similar to Finasteride (Proscar)

The only other 5-alpha reductase inhibitor is dutasteride.

Dutasteride (Avodart): Approved in 2001, dutasteride is an PO drug approved only for the treatment of BPH. Compared

NURSING PROCESS APPLICATION

Patients Receiving Therapy with 5-Alpha Reductase Inhibitors

Assessment	Potential Nursing Diagnoses
Prior to administration: • Obtain a complete health history, including liver disease and altered urinary functioning. • Obtain a drug history to determine possible drug interactions and allergies. • Determine whether the patient has a female partner who is pregnant, is planning to become pregnant, or is breast-feeding.	• *Noncompliance (Adverse Effects of Drug Therapy)* • *Deficient Knowledge (Drug Therapy)* • *Sexual Dysfunction,* related to adverse effects of drug therapy

Planning: Patient Goals and Expected Outcomes

The patient will:

- Experience a decreased size of enlarged prostate gland.
- Demonstrate less frequency and urgency and greater force of urine stream.
- Demonstrate an understanding of the drug's action by accurately describing drug adverse effects and precautions.

Implementation

Interventions and (Rationales)	Patient and Family Education
• Monitor prostate and urinary function. (This drug may cause nocturia and changes in urinary frequency and urgency.)	Instruct the patient to: • Schedule prostate and PSA tests periodically during therapy. • Recognize and report symptoms of BPH such as urinary retention, hesitancy, difficulty starting urine stream, decreased diameter of the stream, nocturia, dribbling, and frequency. • Avoid all fluids in the evening, especially those containing caffeine and alcohol, to avoid nocturia. • Drink adequate fluids early in the day to decrease chances of kidney stones and urinary tract infection (UTI).
• Monitor the female partner for pregnancy. (The drugs are teratogenic to the male fetus.)	Instruct the female sexual partner to: • Avoid the semen of the man using the drug. • Avoid touching crushed tablets to prevent transdermal absorption and the transfer of medication through the placenta to the fetus. • Use a reliable barrier contraceptive during therapy.
• Monitor the patient's commitment to the medication regimen. (Maximum therapeutic effects may take several months.)	Instruct the patient to: • Continue the medication even if there is no decrease in symptoms for 6 to 12 months. • Recognize that lifelong therapy may be necessary to control the symptoms of BPH. • Report impotence, decreased volume of ejaculate, or decreased libido.
• Monitor for adverse reactions. (Adverse reactions may require review of the medication by the health care provider.)	Instruct the patient to: • Provide a list of all the medications that the patient is taking, including vitamins and dietary and herbal supplements. • Report any incidents of hypotension, dizziness, or headache.

Evaluation of Outcome Criteria

Evaluate the effectiveness of drug therapy by confirming that patient goals and expected outcomes have been met (see "Planning").

to finasteride, dutasteride causes a greater inhibition of 5-alpha reductase and thus is able to more effectively lower DHT levels. It is estimated that serum DHT levels are lowered 90% to 93% with dutasteride and 70% by finasteride. Dutasteride has a half-life of 5 weeks and it remains in the body for several months after the drug is stopped. Like finasteride, sexual adverse effects such as reduced ejaculate volume, diminished libido, and ED occur in some patients. Dutasteride is taken once a day with or without food. The drug is pregnancy category X. Because it can be absorbed through the skin, pregnant women should not handle the medication without wearing gloves.

UNDERSTANDING THE CHAPTER

Key Concepts Summary

72.1 Male reproductive function is controlled through the secretion of androgens.

72.2 Androgens are used to treat hypogonadism and delayed puberty in males and breast cancer in females.

72.3 Often abused by athletes, anabolic steroids can cause serious adverse effects.

72.4 Male sexual dysfunction may have both medical and psychological etiologies.

72.5 Male infertility is treated with endocrine drugs that boost sperm production.

72.6 Erectile dysfunction is a common disorder that may be successfully treated with inhibitors of the enzyme phosphodiesterase-5.

72.7 Benign prostatic hyperplasia is an enlargement of the prostate that occurs in older men.

72.8 In its early stages, benign prostatic hyperplasia may be treated successfully with drug therapy.

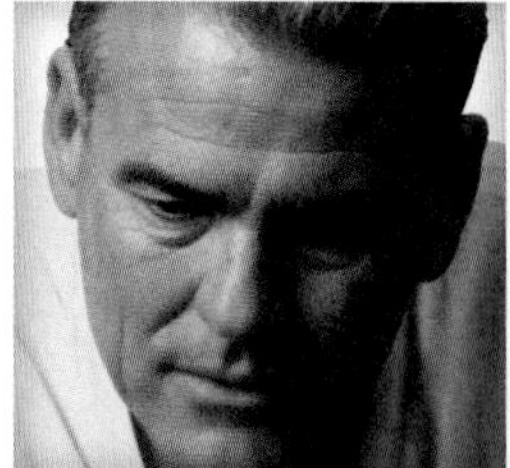

Making the PATIENT *Connection*

Remember the patient "Mike Mayhew" at the beginning of the chapter? Now read the remainder of the case study. Based on the information presented within this chapter, respond to the critical thinking questions that follow.

One year after his divorce, Mike, a 54-year-old white male, began dating and soon met Dana. The couple found that they had a lot in common and enjoyed each other's company. As the relationship grew, the couple became more intimate and sexually involved. However, the emotional scars from his previous marriage were painful and deeply affected him.

After the divorce, Mike suffered from depression and low self-esteem. The condition required short-term hospitalization, and he now follows up on an outpatient basis with a psychiatrist. He has been taking antidepressants and was recently prescribed tadalafil (Cialis) for a diagnosis of ED. Additionally, Mike also has a past history of HTN and is taking nifedipine (Procardia).

Critical Thinking Questions

1. What factors in Mike's life and health history do you think are contributing to the diagnosis of ED?
2. If you were the nurse, what patient education instructions would you provide to Mike regarding administration of tadalafil (Cialis) along with nifedipine (Procardia)?
3. After considering both options, Mike would rather be prescribed sildenafil (Viagra) instead of tadalafil (Cialis). What should the health care provider discuss with Mike about this request?

Case Study

Morrie Jones, a 72-year-old white male, has been having difficulty with urinary frequency and excessive night-time urination. He scheduled an appointment with his health care provider and is diagnosed with benign prostatic hyperplasia (BPH). He is prescribed finasteride (Proscar) and needs to see his health care provider again in 6 months.

1. How would you explain the purpose of finasteride (Proscar) in treating BPH?
2. What education would you provide Mr. Jones that he may find helpful in dealing with BPH?
3. What additional health history and physical assessment findings would be considered in diagnosing this condition?

NCLEX-RN® Review

1 An adult client has been receiving testosterone (Testoderm) for the treatment of primary hypogonadism. Which of the following laboratory tests would the nurse monitor to determine that this drug therapy is effective?

1. Red blood cell count
2. Sperm count
3. FSH
4. LH

2 The client with erectile dysfunction is being evaluated for pharmacotherapy. Which of the following questions should the nurse ask prior to initiating therapy with sildenafil (Viagra)?

1. "Are you currently taking medications for angina?"
2. "Do you have a history of diabetes?"
3. "Have you ever had an allergic reaction to penicillin products?"
4. "Have you ever been treated for gastric ulcers?"

3 The nurse is teaching a class to college men about the dangers of steroid use. Which of the following adverse effects may discourage usage in this particular age group?

1. Liver failure
2. Hypercholesteremia
3. Impotence
4. Heart failure

4 The nurse who is counseling a client about the goal of therapy with sildenafil (Viagra) emphasizes that this drug will:

1. Always result in a penile erection within 10 minutes.
2. Not be effective if dysfunction is psychological in nature.
3. Result in less intense feelings with prolonged use.
4. Heighten sexual response in female partners.

5 The nurse is teaching the client about the use of finasteride (Proscar). What client teaching related to this medication is needed? Select all that apply. Finasteride (Proscar):

1. Promotes shrinkage of an enlarged prostate and helps restore urinary function.
2. Should not be handled by women who may be pregnant.
3. Affects both near and far vision in older adult males.
4. May take 6 to 12 months before the benefit from the drug is achieved.
5. Causes dizziness which can be avoided by making position changes slowly.

6 Which of the following assessment findings would the nurse monitor to determine if a client is achieving a therapeutic effect with finasteride (Proscar)? The client reports:

1. Less hematuria.
2. Decreased flow of urine.
3. Urinating more often.
4. Fewer episodes of nocturia.

See Answers to Critical Thinking Questions, Case Study, and NCLEX-RN® Review in Appendix A.

References

Bent, S. (2006). Saw palmetto for benign prostatic hypertrophy. *New England Journal of Medicine, 354*(6), 557–566.

Centers for Disease Control and Prevention. (2006). *Prostate cancer screening: A decision guide.* Retrieved September 4, 2008, from http://www.cdc.gov/cancer/prostate/publications/decisionguide/

Corbett, J. V. (2008). *Laboratory tests and diagnostic procedures with nursing diagnoses* (7th ed.). Upper Saddle River, NJ: Prentice-Hall.

DiPaola, R. (2006). Proven and unproven therapies for benign prostatic hypertrophy. *New England Journal of Medicine, 354*(6), 632–634.

Ficorelli, C. (2007). Untangling the complexities of male infertility. *Nursing, 2007, 37*(1), 24–26.

Fong, Y. K., Milani, S., & and Djavan, B. (2005). Role of phytotherapy in men with lower urinary tract symptoms: Benign prostatic hyperplasia. *Current Opinion in Urology, 15*(1), 45–48.

Kirby, R. (2004). Selecting long-term medical therapy for BPH. *Contemporary Urology, 16*(1), 12–18.

LeMone, P., & Burke, K. (2008). *Medical-surgical nursing: Critical thinking in client care* (4th ed.). Upper Saddle River, NJ: Prentice-Hall.

McCance, K. L., & Huether, S. E. (2005). *Pathophysiology: The biologic basis for disease in adults and children* (5th ed.). St. Louis: Mosby.

McVary, K. (2007). Erectile dysfunction. *New England Journal of Medicine, 357*(24), 2472– 2481.

National Institute of Drug Abuse. (2008). *NIDA InfoFacts: Steroids (anabolic-androgenic).* Retrieved September 4, 2008, from http://www.drugabuse.gov/infofacts/steroids.html

O'Donnell, A. B., Araujo, A. B., & McKinlay, J. B. (2004). The health of normally aging men: The Massachusetts Male Aging Study (1987–2004). *Experimental Gerontology, 39*(7), 975–984.

Quallich, S. (2006). Examining male infertility. *Urologic Nursing, 26*(4), 277–288.

Spencer, M. (2007, March 30). Management of erectile dysfunction in primary care. *GP: General Practitioner,* 36–37.

UNIT 10

Pharmacology of the Respiratory System and Allergy

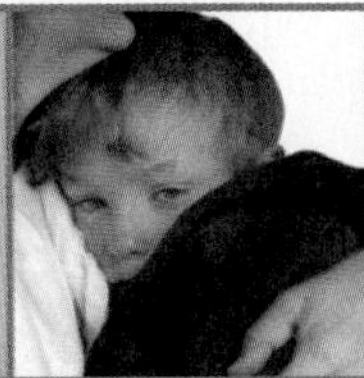

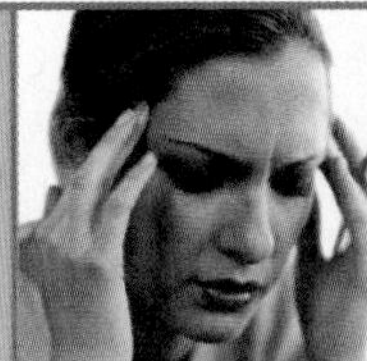

CHAPTER 73 Pharmacotherapy of Asthma and Other Pulmonary Disorders

CHAPTER 74 Pharmacotherapy of Allergic Rhinitis and the Common Cold

CHAPTER

My son can't breathe! Can someone please help me?

Mother of "Jimmy," a 4-year-old with asthma

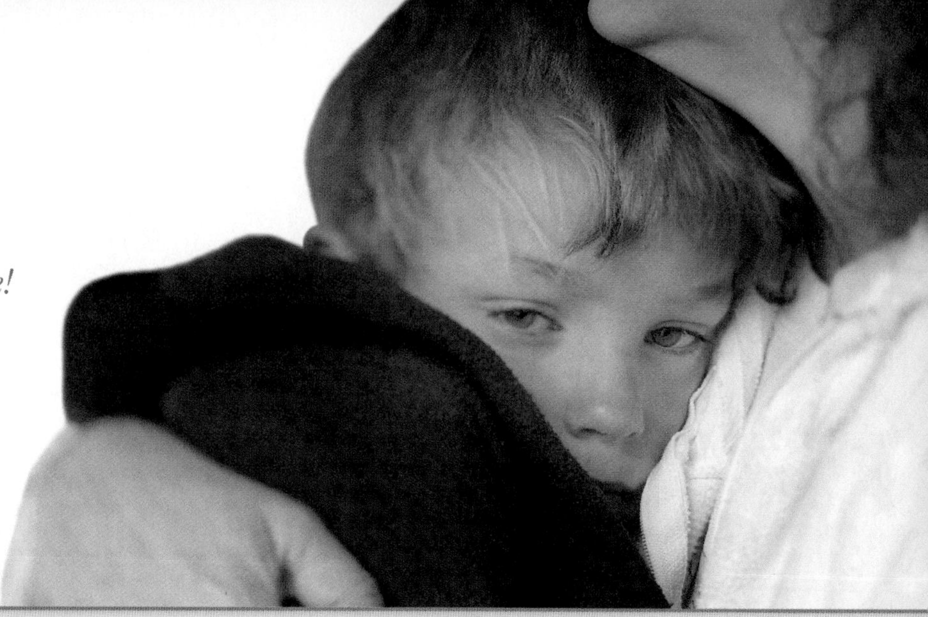

73 Pharmacotherapy of Asthma and Other Pulmonary Disorders

Learning Outcomes

After reading this chapter, the student should be able to:

1. Identify the anatomic structures associated with the lower respiratory tract and their functions.
2. Explain how the autonomic nervous system regulates airway diameter.
3. Explain the role of inflammation and bronchospasm in the pathogenesis of asthma.
4. Compare the advantages and disadvantages of using the inhalation route of drug administration for pulmonary drugs.
5. Describe the types of devices used to deliver aerosol therapies via the inhalation route.
6. Explain the three basic principles of asthma management recommended by the National Asthma Education and Prevention Program.
7. Compare and contrast the indications for pharmacotherapy with the short- versus long-acting beta-adrenergic agonists.
8. Describe the nurse's role in the pharmacologic management of lower respiratory tract disorders.
9. For each of the classes shown in the chapter outline, identify the prototype and representative drugs and explain the mechanism(s) of drug action, primary indications, contraindications, significant drug interactions, pregnancy category, and important adverse effects.
10. Use the nursing process to care for patients who are receiving pharmacotherapy for lower respiratory tract disorders.

Chapter Outline

Physiology of the Lower Respiratory Tract

Pathophysiology of Asthma

Administration of Pulmonary Drugs via Inhalation

Principles of Asthma Pharmacotherapy

Beta$_2$-Adrenergic Agonists

PROTOTYPE **Albuterol (Proventil, Ventolin, VoSpire)** *p. 1246*

Anticholinergics

PROTOTYPE **Ipratropium (Atrovent, Combivent)** *p. 1248*

Corticosteroids

PROTOTYPE **Beclomethasone (Beconase AQ, Qvar)** *p. 1251*

Mast Cell Stabilizers

PROTOTYPE **Cromolyn (Intal) p.** *1252*

Leukotriene Modifiers

PROTOTYPE **Zafirlukast (Accolate)** *p. 1253*

Methylxanthines

PROTOTYPE **Theophylline (Slo-Phyllin, Theochron, Theolair, Uniphyl)** *p. 1255*

Monoclonal Antibodies

Chronic Obstructive Pulmonary Disease

The flow of oxygen, carbon dioxide, and other gases in and out of the human body is dynamic and in constant flux. Minute-by-minute control of the airways is necessary to bring an adequate supply of essential gases to the pulmonary capillaries and to rid the body of some of its most toxic waste products. Any restriction in this dynamic flow, even for brief periods, may result in serious consequences. This chapter examines drugs used in the pharmacotherapy of two primary pulmonary disorders: asthma and chronic obstructive pulmonary disease (COPD).

Physiology of the Lower Respiratory Tract

73.1 The physiology of the respiratory system involves two main processes: perfusion and ventilation.

The primary function of the respiratory system is to bring oxygen into the body and to remove carbon dioxide. The process by which these gases are exchanged is called respiration. The basic structures of the lower respiratory tract are shown in Figure 73.1.

Blood flow through the lung is called pulmonary **perfusion.** The bronchial tree ends in microscopic sacs called alveoli, which have no smooth muscle and inflate like balloons during inspiration. The alveoli are abundantly rich in capillaries. An extremely thin membrane in the alveoli separates the inspired air from the pulmonary capillaries, allowing gases to readily move between the internal environment of the blood and the inspired air. As oxygen crosses this membrane to enter the bloodstream, it is exchanged for carbon dioxide, which is a cellular waste product that leaves the bloodstream to enter the alveoli. The process of gas exchange is illustrated in Figure 73.1.

Ventilation is the process of moving air into and out of the lungs. As the diaphragm contracts and lowers in position, it creates a negative pressure that draws air into the lungs and inspiration occurs. During expiration the diaphragm relaxes and air leaves the lungs passively. Ventilation is a purely mechanical process that occurs approximately 12 to 18 times per minute in adults, which is a rate determined by neurons in the brainstem. This rate may be modified by a number of factors, including emotions, fever, stress, and the pH of the blood.

One of the most important factors that affect ventilation is the size of the thousands of tubes or passageways leading from the outside to the alveoli, collectively known as the airways. The nervous system controls ventilation by changing the diameter of the airways, specifically the very small and abundant bronchioles.

Key Terms

aerosol, *1241*
asthma, *1240*
bronchospasm, *1240*
chronic bronchitis, *1258*
chronic obstructive pulmonary disease (COPD), *1256*
dry powder inhaler (DPI), *1242*
emphysema, *1258*
leukotrienes, *1240*
metered-dose inhaler (MDI), *1242*
methylxanthines, *1255*
mucolytics, *1258*
nebulizer, *1242*
perfusion, *1239*
small volume nebulizer, *1242*
status asthmaticus, *1241*
ventilation, *1239*

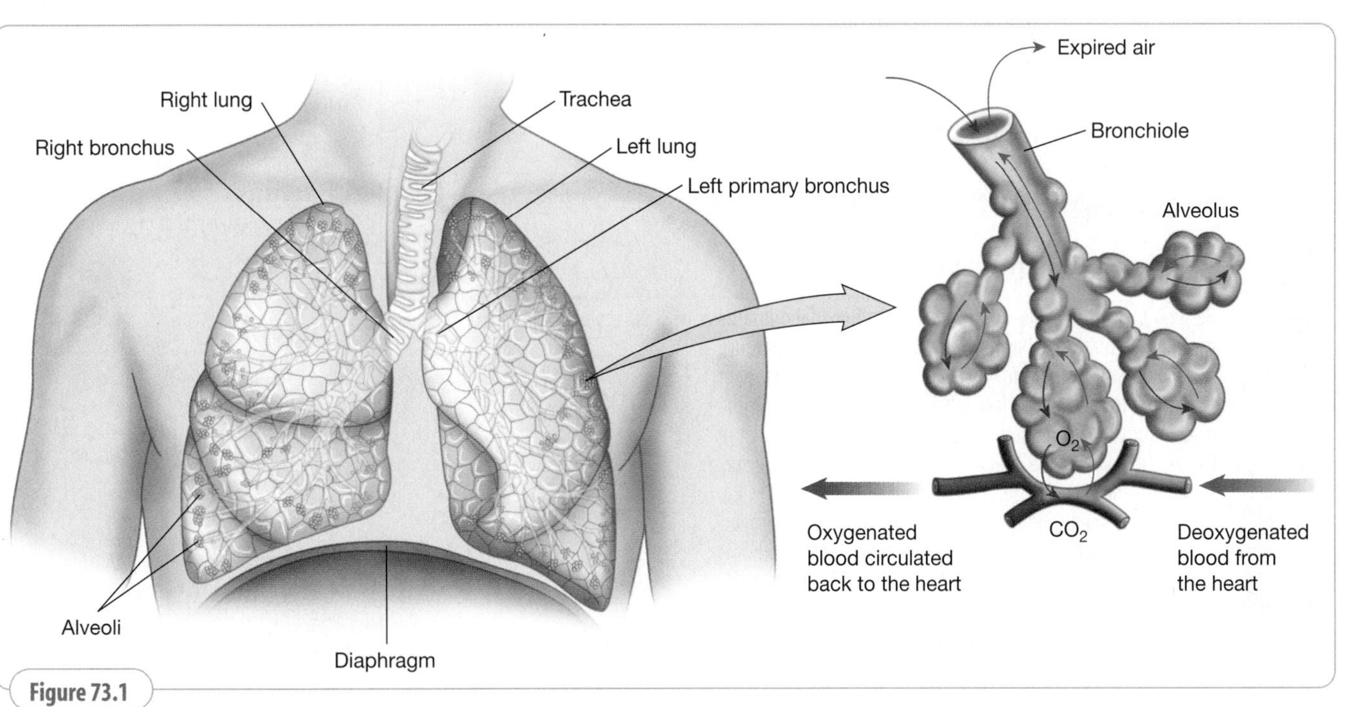

Figure 73.1

The lower respiratory tract and the process of gas exchange.

Bronchioles are muscular, elastic, tubular structures whose diameter, or lumen, varies with the contraction or relaxation of bronchiolar smooth muscle. Bronchodilation allows air to enter the alveoli more freely, thus increasing the supply of oxygen to the body's tissues during periods of exercise. Bronchoconstriction increases airway resistance, resulting in less airflow. Bronchodilation and bronchoconstriction are largely regulated by the two branches of the autonomic nervous system.

- The sympathetic branch activates beta$_2$-adrenergic receptors, which causes bronchiolar smooth muscle to relax, the airway diameter to increase, and bronchodilation to occur.
- The parasympathetic branch causes bronchiolar smooth muscle to contract, the airway diameter to narrow, and bronchoconstriction to occur.

In practical terms, drugs that enhance bronchodilation will cause the patient to breathe easier. On the other hand, drugs that cause bronchoconstriction will cause breathing to become labored and the patient to become short of breath.

Bronchoconstriction is a common indication for the pharmacotherapy of pulmonary disease. Bronchoconstriction may occur through several mechanisms, and the choice of pharmacotherapy will differ depending on the mechanism. An airway may narrow due to **bronchospasm,** which is a sudden contraction of the smooth muscle of the airways that will cause acute dyspnea. Drug treatment for bronchospasm is targeted at immediately relaxing the smooth muscle spasm. A second mechanism of bronchoconstriction is the production of thick, viscous secretions that plug up the airways. Depending on the cause, treatment may involve antibiotics for an infection or drugs that break up viscous secretions (mucolytics). A third mechanism of bronchoconstriction is edema that is caused by engorgement of the pulmonary blood vessels. Treatment may include diuretics and drugs to enhance cardiac function.

CONNECTIONS

Treating the Diverse Patient

Respiratory Distress Syndrome

Respiratory distress syndrome (RDS) is a condition that primarily occurs in premature babies in which the lungs do not produce surfactant. Surfactant forms a thin layer on the inner surface of the alveoli to raise the surface tension, thereby preventing the alveoli from collapsing during expiration. If birth occurs before the pneumocytes in the lung are mature enough to secrete surfactant, the alveoli collapse, and RDS results.

Surfactant medications can be delivered to the newborn, either as prophylactic therapy or as rescue therapy, after symptoms develop. The two natural surfactant agents used for RDS are calfactant (Infasurf) and beractant (Survanta). Calfactant is harvested from calf lungs, and beractant from mature cattle lungs. These drugs are administered intratracheally every 4 to 6 hours until the patient's condition improves.

Pathophysiology of Asthma

73.2 Asthma is a chronic disease that has both inflammatory and bronchospasm components.

Asthma is one of the most common chronic conditions in the United States, and it is increasing at an alarming rate. According to the Centers for Disease Control and Prevention ([CDC], 2006), asthma currently affects more than 20 million Americans. The prevalence of asthma is 74% greater among African Americans compared to European Americans and is 35% higher in females than males. Although often considered a condition of childhood, asthma can occur at any age.

Asthma is characterized by chronic inflammation that occurs when potent mediators of the immune and inflammatory responses are released by mast cells lining the bronchial passageways. These mediators include histamine, **leukotrienes,** prostaglandins, and interleukins. The result of inflammation is an increase in airway edema coupled with increased mucus secretion, which narrows the airways, compromises the process of respiration, and contributes to airway obstruction. This is illustrated in Figure 73.2.

The second component in the pathogenesis of asthma is bronchospasm. The inflammatory conditions in the airway make the smooth muscle hyperresponsive to a variety of stimuli. Stimuli such as breathing smoke, pollutants, or cold air may trigger acute bronchospasm. Specific triggers are listed in Table 73.1. Some patients experience bron-

TABLE 73.1 Common Triggers of Asthma

Cause	Sources
Air pollutants	Tobacco smoke Ozone Nitrous and sulfur oxides Fumes from cleaning fluids or solvents Burning leaves
Allergens	Pollen from trees, grasses, and weeds Animal dander Household dust Mold
Chemicals and food	Drugs, including aspirin, ibuprofen, and beta blockers Sulfite preservatives Food and condiments, including nuts, monosodium glutamate (MSG), shellfish, and dairy products
Respiratory infections	Bacterial, fungal, and viral
Stress	Emotional stress, anxiety, exercise in dry, cold climates

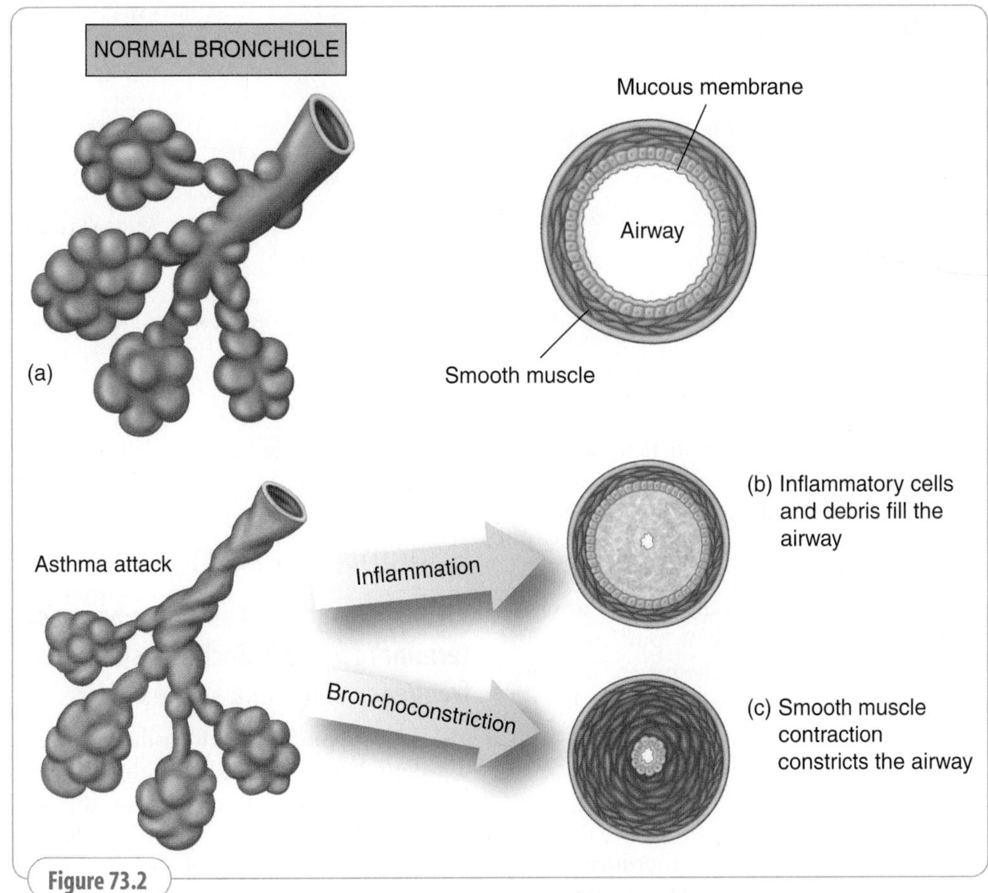

Figure 73.2

Changes in the bronchioles during an asthma attack: (a) Normal bronchiole. (b) The inflammatory component plugs the airway. (c) Bronchoconstriction narrows the airway.

chospasm on exertion, a condition called exercise-induced asthma. Gastroesophageal reflux can trigger an asthma event when acid in the esophagus induces reflex bronchoconstriction.

The patient with asthma may present with a variety of symptoms, including evening cough, shortness of breath, chest tightness, and wheezing. Intervals between symptoms may vary from days to weeks to months. The severity of asthma is often graded by the frequency and intensity of acute episodes, as shown in Table 73.2. **Status asthmaticus,** an emergency situation in which asthma is unresponsive to drug treatment, may lead to respiratory failure. Drugs may be given to prevent asthmatic attacks or to terminate attacks in progress.

PharmFACT

Each day in the United States:

- **40,000 people miss school or work due to asthma.**
- **30,000 people have an asthma attack.**
- **5,000 people visit the emergency department for asthma treatment.**
- **11 people die from asthma.** *Source:* Asthma and Allergy Foundation of America, n.d.

Administration of Pulmonary Drugs via Inhalation

73.3 Inhalation is a common route of administration for pulmonary drugs because it delivers drugs directly to their sites of action.

Many drugs that are used to treat asthma are available for administration by the inhalation route. This route works particularly well because the respiratory system offers a rapid and efficient mechanism for delivering drugs directly to their site of action. The enormous surface area of the bronchioles and alveoli and the rich blood supply to these areas result in an almost instantaneous onset of action for inhaled substances.

Medications are delivered to the respiratory system by aerosol therapy. An **aerosol** is a suspension of minute liquid droplets or fine solid particles suspended in a gas. The major advantage of aerosol therapy is that it delivers the drugs directly to the site of action. Not only does this dramatically decrease the onset of action, but it also allows for much smaller doses of a drug. The small doses of drug given by the inhalation route minimize any systemic effects that might result from absorption across pulmonary capillaries when compared to PO medications. Several devices are used to deliver drugs

TABLE 73.2 Assessment of Asthma

Level	Frequency of Symptoms	Nocturnal Attacks	Activity
Mild intermittent	Less than 2 times/week	Less than 2 times/month	Not limited
Mild persistent	3–6 days/week	More than 2 times/month	Attacks may limit activity
Moderate persistent	Daily	More than 1 time/week	Attacks affect activity
Severe persistent	Continual	Frequent	Attacks limit physical activity

Note: From *Integrated Cardiopulmonary Pharmacology* (2nd ed., p. 263), by B. Colbert and B. L. Kennedy, 2008, Upper Saddle River, NJ: Pearson Education, Inc.

via the inhalation route. The most common are metered-dose inhalers, dry power inhalers, and nebulizers.

The **metered-dose inhaler (MDI),** often simply called an inhaler, is the most common type of aerosol delivery device. It consists of a canister that holds the medicine and a mouthpiece. To use an MDI, the patient presses the canister toward the mouthpiece to deliver a measured dose or "puff" of medication. By inhaling during drug delivery, the patient helps to ensure that the drug reaches the site of action in the lungs. Even when MDIs are used properly, however, the majority of the aerosolized drug never reaches the lungs. There are two primary reasons for this problem. One is that heavier aerosolized particles fall out by gravity and are deposited in the oropharynx. The other reason is that proper coordination of drug delivery with inhalation can be difficult for some patients. To decrease oropharyngeal deposition and to enhance drug delivery to the lungs, many health care providers recommend that patients use a spacer with their MDI. A spacer is a special tube that attaches to the mouthpiece that is designed to hold the cloud of aerosolized medication. This serves two primary purposes. First, the spacer holds drops that fall out of the aerosol so that there is less medication deposited on the oropharynx and in the mouth. Second, because the spacer holds the medication, the patient does not have to precisely coordinate inhalation with activation, so that more drug reaches the site of action.

A **dry powder inhaler (DPI)** delivers the medication as a fine dry powder. Whereas the MDI is activated by pressing the canister, the DPI is automatically activated when the patient inhales through the mouthpiece. Because the timing of drug delivery and inhalation does not have to be coordinated, more medication is delivered to the lung with a DPI. The DPI has no propellants in the canister, which can be harmful to some patients with lung problems.

A **nebulizer** (or **small volume nebulizer**) is a machine that delivers medication as a fine mist. When using a nebulizer, the medication to be delivered is poured into a receptacle. The machine then vaporizes the liquid medication into a mist that is inhaled by using a face mask or other hand-held device. These "breathing treatments" may take up to 30 minutes to administer the drug so it may not work as quickly as a drug taken from an MDI or DPI; however, medication delivered in this fashion is often more effective because it is delivered over many inhalations that occur during the period of medication delivery.

Principles of Asthma Pharmacotherapy

73.4 The goals of asthma pharmacotherapy are to terminate acute bronchospasms and to reduce the frequency of asthma attacks.

The choice of medications for asthma is determined by evidence-based guidelines coupled with the patient's response to therapy and adjusted according to the patient's individual situation. Evidence-based guidelines have been developed by experts in asthma management and are based on research findings. In the United States, the National Asthma Education and Prevention Program (NAEPP) issued guidelines for asthma treatment in 1991, which were updated in 1997, 2002, and 2007. The NAEPP guidelines recommend a stepwise approach to asthma control based on the frequency and severity of symptoms, as shown in Figure 73.3. As patient symptoms worsen, the pharmacotherapy is adjusted accordingly by going to the next "step." This provides for a rational, evidence-based approach to asthma management. The three general strategies for asthma management from the NAEPP are as follows:

- Incorporate four components of care: medications, patient education, environmental control measures, and management of comorbidities.
- Initiate therapy based on asthma severity. For patients not taking long-term control therapy, select the treatment step based on severity. Patients who have persistent asthma require daily long-term control medication.
- Adjust the therapy based on asthma control. Once therapy is initiated, monitor the level of asthma control and adjust the therapy accordingly: step up if necessary and step down if possible to identify the minimum amount of medication required to maintain asthma control.

The goals of asthma pharmacotherapy are twofold: to terminate acute bronchospasms and to prevent or reduce the frequency of asthma attacks. Different medications are

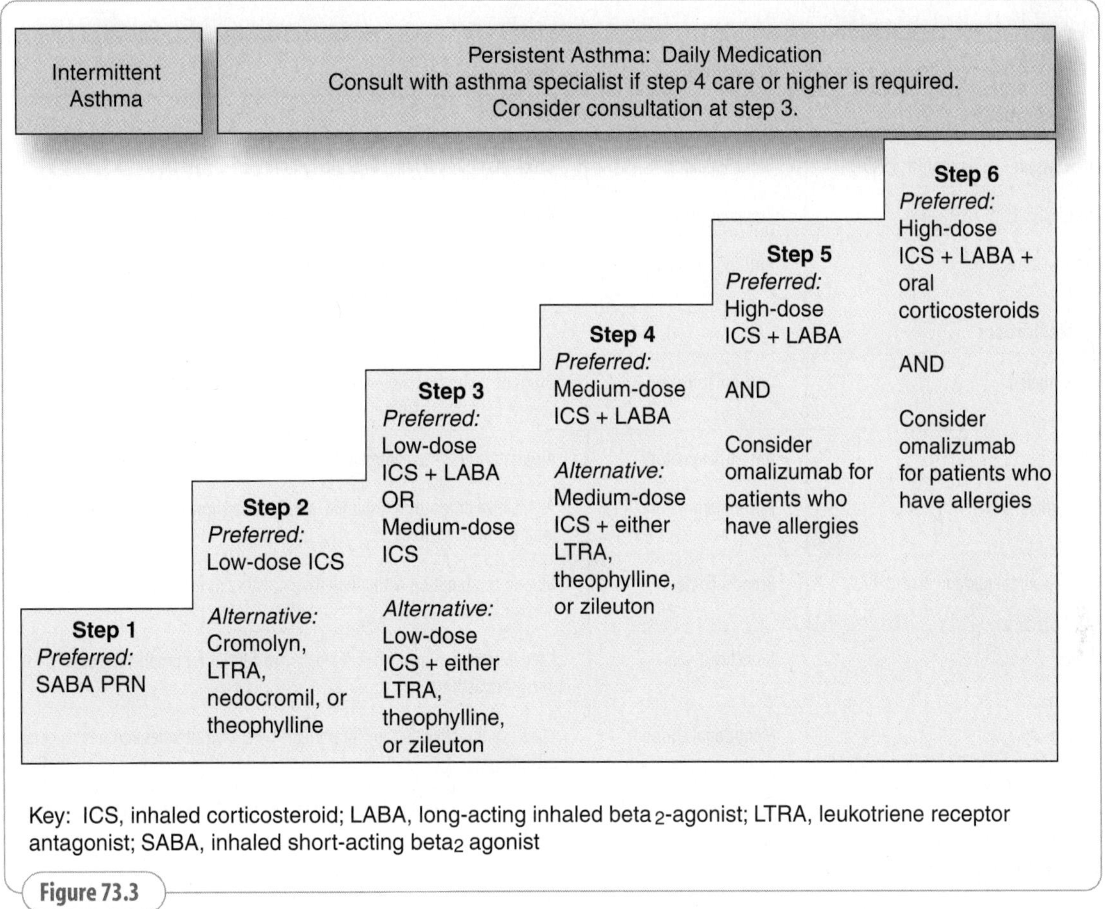

Figure 73.3

Stepwise approach for managing asthma in adults and patients 12 years and older.
Source: From *Expert Panel Report 3 (EPR3): Guidelines for the Diagnosis and Management of Asthma* (p. 343), by the National Asthma Education Prevention Program, coordinated by the National Heart, Lung, and Blood Institute of the National Institutes of Health, 2007. Retrieved September 5, 2008, from http://www.nhlbi.nih.gov/guidelines/asthma/asthgdln.htm

needed to achieve each of these goals. The NAEPP categorizes asthma drugs into two simple classes: quick-relief medications and long-term control medications. A summary of the different classes used for asthma management is shown in Table 73.3.

> **PharmFACT**
>
> **More than 15.7 million adults and 6.8 million children have asthma in the United States. The incidence of childhood asthma doubled from 1980 to the mid-1990s and has remained stable since then.** *Source:* Centers for Disease Control and Prevention, National Center for Health Statistics, 2008.

73.5 Beta$_2$-adrenergic agonists are the most effective drugs for relieving acute bronchospasm.

Beta-adrenergic agonists are some of the most frequently prescribed drugs for treating pulmonary disorders. Beta agonists are drugs that activate the sympathetic nervous system, which relaxes bronchial smooth muscle, resulting in bronchodilation. They are the drugs of choice in the treatment of bronchoconstriction.

Beta agonist medications may act on either beta$_1$ receptors, which are located primarily in the heart, or on beta$_2$ receptors, which are located in smooth muscle of the lung, uterus, and other organs. Beta agonists that activate both beta$_1$ and beta$_2$ receptors are called nonselective bronchodilators. Beta agonists

TABLE 73.3 Overview of Drug Classes for Asthma Management

Class	Mechanism	Use
Quick-Relief Medications		
Short-acting beta$_2$-adrenergic agonists (SABAs)	Bronchodilators	Drugs of choice for relief of acute symptoms.
Anticholinergics	Bronchodilators	Alternate drugs for those who cannot tolerate SABAs.
Corticosteroids: systemic	Anti-inflammatory	Although not rapid acting, these oral agents are used for short periods to reduce the frequency of acute exacerbations.
Long-Acting Medications		
Corticosteroids: inhaled	Anti-inflammatory	Drugs of choice for long-term asthma management. Oral doses may be required for severe, persistent asthma.
Mast cell stabilizers	Anti-inflammatory	Alternative drugs to control mild, persistent asthma or exercise-induced asthma.
Leukotriene modifiers	Anti-inflammatory	Alternative drugs to control mild, persistent asthma or as adjunctive therapy with inhaled corticosteroids.
Long-acting beta$_2$-adrenergic agonists (LABAs)	Bronchodilators	Used in combination with inhaled corticosteroids for prophylaxis of moderate to severe persistent asthma.
Methylxanthines	Bronchodilators	Used in combination with inhaled corticosteroids for prophylaxis of mild to moderate persistent asthma.
Immunomodulators	Monoclonal antibody	Used as adjunctive therapy for patients who have allergies and severe, persistent asthma.

Note: From *Expert Panel Report 3 (EPR3): Guidelines for the Diagnosis and Management of Asthma,* by the National Asthma Education and Prevention Program Coordinating Committee, coordinated by the National Heart, Lung, and Blood Institute of the National Institutes of Health, 2007. Retrieved December 26, 2008, from http://www.nhlbi.nih.gov/guidelines/asthma/asthgdln.htm

CONNECTIONS

Evidence-Based Practice Asthma Management

Clinical Question

What is the standard of asthma management?

Evidence

In 2003, the National Asthma Education and Prevention Program (NAEPP) Expert Panel published the long-awaited document, *Guidelines for the Diagnosis and Management of Asthma–Update on Selected Topics*. This was subsequently updated in 2007. Since its initial publication, although the numbers of asthma diagnoses have increased, asthma morbidity and mortality have been on the decline. The success of the guidelines has been attributed to a reliance on the evidence of hundreds of scientific research findings for guideline development.

The NAEPP guidelines establish some important goals regarding asthma control:

- Minimal or no chronic symptoms day or night
- Minimal or no exacerbations
- No limitations on activities; no school or parent's work missed
- Minimal use of short-acting inhaled beta$_2$ agonist
- Minimal or no adverse effects from medications (NAEPP, 2007)

Implication

Prior to the publication of this document, providers often relied extensively on short-acting beta agonists as rescue therapy when symptoms occurred. To accomplish this new goal of few to no symptoms, the NAEPP designed a stepwise approach to asthma management that worked to prevent rescue therapy from ever being needed in the first place. An important factor in management, however, is that the patient or, if a child, the patient's parents, be able to identify a worsening condition outside of the office visit.

Critical Thinking Question

Use of evidence-based practice guidelines by health care providers has been demonstrated to decrease patient mortality and morbidity. What can the nurse do to promote patient adherence to prescribed management of asthma and self-assessment?

See Answers to Critical Thinking Questions in Appendix A.

- Assess vital signs, particularly the respiratory rate and heart rate prior to administration and 1 to 2 hours following administration.
- Assess the respiratory effort and lung sounds to determine the effectiveness of the drug.
- Assess for cyanosis or pallor, and check oxygen saturation if indicated.
- Assess the patient's peak expiratory flow rate (PEFR) with a peak flowmeter (PFM) and compare this with the patient's personal best recording. Repeat this in 15 to 20 minutes and again in 1 to 2 hours.
- Monitor for conditions that are affected by taking a beta agonist, such as nervousness, tachycardia, or HTN.
- Check the medication record for drugs that interact with beta agonists such as MAOIs and beta blockers.
- Observe for paradoxical bronchospasm, which is an uncommon but dangerous reaction to the drug.
- Evaluate the level of symptom relief at 15 to 20 minutes following administration and again 1 to 2 hours later.

Patient and Family Education:

- Limit intake of caffeine because this substance can increase nervousness and cardiovascular adverse effects.
- Take this medication exactly as prescribed. Acute respiratory distress can be frightening, but taking additional medication can lead to an overdose or serious adverse effects.
- Continue to take this drug even if you are feeling better.
- Immediately report palpitations or shortness of breath that is not relieved by the medication to the health care provider. If the problem is severe, go to the emergency department.
- Rinse the mouth with water and then spit out the water after inhaling the drug to avoid swallowing the medicine that is deposited in the mouth.
- Always consult the health care provider before giving these medicines to children. Albuterol is approved for children aged 2 and older; however, most drugs in this class are limited for children under 6 to12 years of age because insufficient studies have been conducted in this age group.
- Do not breast-feed while taking this drug without approval of the health care provider.
- Immediately notify the health care provider of any known or suspected pregnancy.

Drugs Similar to Albuterol (Proventil, Ventolin, VoSpire)

Other short-acting beta agonists include levalbuterol and pirbuterol. Long-acting beta agonists include arformoterol, formoterol, and salmeterol. Bitolterol mesylate is a drug in this class that has been discontinued in the United States. Adverse effects are the same as those of other beta$_2$ agonists and include tachycardia, nervousness, angina, and headache.

Arformoterol (Brovan): Arformoterol is one of the newer drugs in the class that was approved in 2007 for the treatment of COPD, including chronic bronchitis and emphysema. This drug is an isomer of formoterol and is the first LABA available by inhalation via nebulizer. Formoterol and salmeterol use DPIs. Arformoterol may be administered twice daily. Although it begins to relax bronchi within about 7 minutes, its maximum effects take 1 to 3 hours. Thus this drug is not suitable to terminate acute asthma attacks. Because LABAs have been shown to increase the risk of asthma-related death, the drug should only be prescribed when short- and intermediate-acting drugs are unable to control symptoms. This drug is well tolerated and exhibits few serious adverse effects. This drug is pregnancy category C.

Formoterol (Foradil, Perforomist): Approved in 2001, formoterol is a long-acting, selective beta$_2$ agonist that is administered using a DPI. Because the drug takes 1 to 3 hours for maximum effect, it is not suitable for terminating acute bronchospasm. Due to its long duration of action, formoterol is indicated for asthma prophylaxis, including the prevention of nocturnal symptoms and exercise-induced asthma. It is also approved by the FDA for the relief of bronchospasm due to COPD. Because LABAs have been shown to increase the risk of asthma-related death, this drug should only be prescribed when short- and intermediate-acting drugs are unable to control symptoms. This drug is well tolerated and has the same adverse effect profile as that of other drugs in this class. This drug is pregnancy category C.

Levalbuterol (Xopenex): Approved in 1999, levalbuterol is an isomer of albuterol and has almost identical indications, actions, and adverse effects. This drug is administered via nebulized or aerosolized oral inhalation. It is indicated for the relief of acute bronchospasm symptoms and can be administered three to four times daily. Regular, daily use of levalbuterol is not recommended by the NAEPP as a means to prevent bronchospasm. Like other drugs in this class, levalbuterol has few serious adverse effects, with nervousness and tremor being the most frequently reported. This drug is pregnancy category C.

Pirbuterol (Maxair): Approved in 1986, pirbuterol is a short-acting, selective beta$_2$ agonist that has a structure very similar to albuterol. Its rapid, 5-minute onset of action makes it suitable for the termination of acute bronchospasm symptoms. Doses may be repeated every 4 to 6 hours, as needed. Like the other short-acting beta$_2$ agonists, this drug must not be used on a regular, daily basis to prevent asthmatic attacks. It is also FDA approved for the relief of bronchospasm due to COPD and may be prescribed off-label to prevent exercise-induced bronchospasm. It is available only by the inhalation route. Adverse effects are uncommon and include tachycardia and palpitation. This drug is pregnancy category C.

Salmeterol (Serevent): Approved in 1994, salmeterol is a LABA that is prescribed for asthma prophylaxis and the long-term therapy of bronchospasm associated with COPD. The LABAs salmeterol and formoterol are considered less effective at preventing asthma attacks than the inhaled corticosteroids. Salmeterol has a slow onset of action and should not be used to terminate acute bronchospasm. Because LABAs have been shown to increase the risk of asthma-related death, this drug should only be prescribed when short- and intermediate-acting drugs are unable to control symptoms. The aerosol form of salmeterol has been discontinued in the United States, although the DPI route is still available. Overall, the drug is well tolerated and few serious adverse effects are reported. Pharyngitis and upper respiratory tract infections occur in patients who are taking the drug, and headache is a common adverse effect. This drug is pregnancy category C.

Terbutaline (Brethine): An older drug approved in 1974, terbutaline is indicated for the treatment of bronchospasm. Terbutaline is given by the PO route and may take 30 minutes or longer to act; thus it is too slow to be used for acute conditions. A subcutaneous form of terbutaline can relieve bronchospasm within 15 minutes. PO terbutaline has a shorter duration of action than albuterol or salmeterol and it must be administered three times daily. An inhalation form of the drug (Brethaire) was removed from the U.S. market in 1999. Terbutaline is moderately selective for beta$_2$ receptors but may produce some activation of beta$_1$ receptors in the heart. Adverse effects are similar to those observed with other drugs in this class. Terbutaline is used off-label to delay premature labor contractions due to its effects on beta$_2$ receptors in the uterus that cause smooth muscle relaxation (see Chapter 70). This drug is pregnancy category B.

CONNECTION *Checkpoint* 73.1

The agents for asthma are selective for beta$_2$-adrenergic receptors. From what you learned in Chapter 19, what are the primary indications for the drugs selective for beta$_1$-adrenergic receptors? See Answer to Connection Checkpoint 73.1 in Appendix A.

73.6 The inhaled anticholinergics are used for preventing bronchospasm.

Although short-acting beta agonists are the drugs of choice for treating acute bronchospasm, anticholinergics (cholinergic blockers or antagonists) are alternative bronchodilators. Although anticholinergics such as atropine have been available for many decades, the adverse effect profile of these agents made most anticholinergics poorly suited for the management of asthma. With the delivery of the anticholinergics by inhalation, however, they have become important drugs in the arsenal of asthma pharmacotherapy. There are two inhalation anticholinergic agents available for the treatment of bronchospasm: ipratropium (Atrovent) and tiotropium (Spiriva).

Anticholinergics block the parasympathetic nervous system. Blocking the parasympathetic nervous system results in actions similar to those of stimulating the sympathetic nervous system (see Chapter 16). It is predictable then that anticholinergic drugs would cause bronchodilation and have potential applications in the pharmacotherapy of asthma and COPD. Ipratropium is rapid acting and can be used to relieve acute bronchospasm, whereas tiotropium is better suited for maintenance therapy due to its longer onset.

Anticholinergics have actions that are similar to those of beta-adrenergic agonists and drugs from the two classes may be combined to produce a greater and more prolonged bronchodilation than either drug used separately. This additive effect is particularly useful for patients with persistent bronchospasm for whom either agent alone is inadequate to alleviate bronchoconstriction. Taking advantage of this increased effect, the pharmaceutical companies have developed inhalants that combine both an anticholinergic and a beta agonist into a single canister.

Anticholinergics are available in PO, inhaled, and injection formulations; however, when used for asthma and other respiratory conditions, the inhaled forms are typically prescribed. The inhaled anticholinergics are relatively safe medications. The wide range of anticholinergic adverse effects that is observed when drugs in this class are administered systemically rarely occurs when administered by inhalation.

PROTOTYPE DRUG Ipratropium (Atrovent, Combivent)

Classification: **Therapeutic:** Bronchodilator
Pharmacologic: Anticholinergic

Therapeutic Effects and Uses: Approved by the FDA in 1986, ipratropium is an anticholinergic agent that is delivered by the inhalation and intranasal routes. The inhalation form is approved to relieve and prevent the bronchospasm that is characteristic of asthma and COPD. It is a drug of choice for treating bronchospasms due to COPD, including bronchitis and emphysema. Although it has not received FDA approval for the treatment of asthma, it is nevertheless prescribed off-label for the disorder. NAEPP guidelines state that the role of ipratropium in asthma management is as an alternative to short-acting beta agonists and for patients experiencing severe asthma exacerbations. It is sometimes combined with beta agonists or corticosteroids to provide additive bronchodilation. Ipratropium is much less effective than the beta$_2$ agonists at preventing exercise-induced bronchospasm.

When administered via inhalation, ipratropium can relieve acute bronchospasm within minutes of administration, although peak effects may take 1 to 2 hours. Bronchodilation action may continue for up to 6 hours.

The nasal spray formulation of ipratropium was approved in 1995 for the symptomatic relief of rhinorrhea associated with the common cold and perennial rhinitis. The drug inhibits nasal secretions but does not have decongestant action. Treatment is limited to 3 weeks.

Mechanism of Action: Ipratropium causes bronchodilation by blocking cholinergic receptors in bronchial smooth muscle. Intranasal administration blocks parasympathetic receptors, thus reducing nasal hypersecretion characteristic of the common cold.

Pharmacokinetics:

Route(s)	Inhalation, intranasal
Absorption	Minimal systemic absorption; some of the inhaled drug is swallowed but is not absorbed by the GI tract
Distribution	Small amount is secreted in breast milk; minimally bound to plasma protein
Primary metabolism	Hepatic (CYP450)
Primary excretion	Renal and feces
Onset of action	5–15 minutes; peak effect: 1.5–2 h
Duration of action	3–6 h; half-life: 1.5–2 h

Adverse Effects: Because it is not readily absorbed from the lungs, ipratropium produces few systemic adverse effects. Though rare it can worsen glaucoma with sufficient systemic absorption. Typical anticholinergic adverse effects such as dry mouth, nausea, and gastrointestinal (GI) distress are among the most common adverse effects but occur in less than 3% of patients. Irritation of the upper respiratory tract may result in cough, drying of the nasal mucosa, or hoarseness. Paradoxical acute bronchospasm is a rare adverse effect that may be life threatening. This drug produces a bitter taste that some patients find problematic. Intranasal administration may cause epistaxis and excessive drying of the nasal mucosa.

Contraindications/Precautions: Ipratropium is contraindicated in patients with hypersensitivity to soya lecithin or related food products such as soybean and peanut. Soya lecithin is used as a propellant in the inhaler. Ipratropium is contraindicated in persons who have demonstrated a hypersensitivity to ipratropium. All anticholinergics should be used with caution in patients with closed-angle glaucoma or urinary tract obstruction because they may worsen these conditions.

Drug Interactions: Because it has little systemic absorption, ipratropium interacts with very few drugs. Use with other anticholinergics such as atropine may lead to additive anticholinergic adverse effects. **Herbal/Food:** Unknown.

Pregnancy: Category B.

Treatment of Overdose: Overdose with ipratropium is unlikely because very little of the drug is absorbed.

Nursing Responsibilities:

- Obtain a complete respiratory history and assessment that includes vital signs, particularly respiratory rate and heart rate; respiratory effort; lung sounds; cyanosis or pallor; and oxygen saturation, if indicated.
- Observe for paradoxical bronchospasm, which is an uncommon but dangerous reaction to the drug.
- Assess for the presence or history of glaucoma because this drug is contraindicated for this condition. Assess for visual changes or eye pain.
- Check the medication record for other anticholinergic medications because ipratropium can have additive anticholinergic effects.
- Evaluate adherence to the medication regimen and reinforce the need to take this medicine on a regular basis, if indicated.

Patient and Family Education:

- Do not use this drug to terminate an acute asthma attack.
- Take this drug exactly as prescribed. If respiratory distress continues even though the medications are taken as directed, notify the health care provider because this may indicate a need for medication adjustment.
- Wait 1 or 2 minutes between puffs before inhaling subsequent doses of the medicine.
- After inhaling the medicine, rinse the mouth with water and then spit out the water. This will prevent swallowing of the medication, which could contribute to systemic symptoms, and will help to eliminate any bitter aftertaste.
- Do not give this drug to children without a prescription. Ipratropium is not recommended for children younger than 12 years.
- Do not breast-feed while taking this drug without approval of the health care provider.
- Immediately notify the health care provider of any known or suspected pregnancy.
- Report any new onset of problems or if current problems worsen. Although these drugs are relatively safe, older adults are particularly susceptible to adverse reactions.

Drugs Similar to Ipratropium (Atrovent, Combivent)

The only other anticholinergic currently approved in the United States for inhalation is tiotropium.

Tiotropium (Spiriva): Approved in 2004, tiotropium is closely related to ipratropium and is indicated for the long-term treatment and prophylaxis of bronchospasm in patients with COPD, including chronic bronchitis and emphysema. It is not to be used to terminate acute bronchospasm; short-acting adrenergic agonists are indicated for this condition. An advantage of tiotropium is its long duration of action. Unlike ipratropium, which must be taken four or more times a day, tiotropium only needs to be taken once a day so patients are less likely to miss doses. Another difference between the two agents is that ipratropium is administered by MDI, whereas tiotropium is administered by DPI. For patients with COPD who have difficulty using an MDI device, tiotropium can be a viable alternative. Adverse effects are the same as those of ipratropium. This drug is pregnancy category C.

73.7 Inhaled corticosteroids are the most effective drugs for the long-term control of asthma.

Corticosteroids are the most potent natural anti-inflammatory substances known. Because asthma has a major inflammatory component, it should not be surprising that drugs in this class play a major role in the management of this disorder. Inhaled corticosteroids are the drugs of choice for the prevention of asthmatic attacks and for the management of chronic asthma. Oral corticosteroids are used for the short-term management of acute asthma exacerbations. The therapeutic actions of the corticosteroids have resulted in their widespread use in the pharmacotherapy of allergic rhinitis (see Chapter 74) and other inflammatory disorders (see Chapters 69 and 75). Doses for the inhaled corticosteroids are given in Table 73.5.

Corticosteroids decrease inflammation of the airways by inhibiting the synthesis and release of inflammatory mediators, including histamine, leukotriene, cytokines, and prostaglandins. They also inhibit the number of circulating leukocytes and decrease vascular permeability. This results in diminished mucus production and edema, thus reducing airway obstruction. Although corticosteroids are not bronchodilators, they sensitize the bronchial smooth muscle to be more responsive to beta agonist stimulation. In addition, they reduce the bronchial hyperresponsiveness to allergens, which is responsible for triggering many asthma attacks.

When inhaled on a daily schedule, corticosteroids suppress inflammation without producing major adverse effects. Although symptoms will improve in the first 1 to 2 weeks of therapy, 4 to 8 weeks may be required for maximum benefit. Because of the dangerous adverse effects of long-term therapy, systemic corticosteroids are generally reserved for short-term management of acute asthma exacerbations. For outpatient management in these instances, PO corticosteroids such as prednisone are given for the shortest length of time possible, usually 5 to 7 days. In the hospital setting, intravenous (IV) corticosteroids may be given. Regardless, at the end of the brief treatment period, patients are usually switched to inhaled corticosteroids for long-term management.

When taken long term, both PO and inhaled formulations of corticosteroids have the potential to affect bone physiology in adults and children. Adults who are at risk for osteoporosis should receive periodic bone mineral density tests and possibly pharmacotherapy with bisphosphonates to prevent fractures (see Chapter 75). In children, small decreases in linear bone growth have been documented. Although these effects are usually temporary, growth should be monitored and the prescriber should weigh the risks of growth suppression against the benefits of corticosteroid use. In all cases, effects on bone growth are dose and frequency dependent; thus patients should be administered the lowest doses possible to maintain adequate asthma control.

TABLE 73.5 Anti-Inflammatory Drugs for Asthma

Drug	Route and Adult Dose (maximum dose where indicated)	Adverse Effects
Inhaled Corticosteroids*		
beclomethasone (Beconase AQ, QVAR)	MDI: 1–2 inhalations tid-qid (max: 20 inhalations/day)	*Hoarseness, dry mouth, cough, sore throat* Oropharyngeal candidiasis, hypercorticism, hypersensitivity reactions
budesonide (Pulmicort)	DPI: 1–2 inhalations (200 mcg/inhalation) qid (max: 800 mcg/day)	
flunisolide (Aerobid)	MDI: 2–3 inhalations bid-tid (max: 12 inhalations/day)	
fluticasone (Flovent)	MDI (44 mcg): 2 inhalations bid (max: 10 inhalations/day)	
mometasone (Asmanex)	DPI: 1 inhalation daily (max: 2 inhalations daily)	
triamcinolone (Azmacort)	MDI: 2 inhalations tid-qid (max: 16 inhalations/day)	
Mast Cell Stabilizers		
cromolyn (Intal)	MDI: 1 inhalation qid	*Nausea, sneezing, nasal stinging, throat irritation, unpleasant taste* Anaphylaxis, angioedema, bronchospasm
nedocromil sodium (Tilade)	MDI: 2 inhalations qid	
Leukotriene Modifiers		
montelukast (Singulair)	PO: 10 mg/day in evening	*Headache, nausea, diarrhea* Increased aspartate aminotransferase (AST)
zafirlukast (Accolate)	PO: 20 mg bid 1 h before or 2 h after meals	
5-Lipoxygenase Inhibitor		
zileuton (Zyflo CR)	PO: 1,200 mg bid (max: 2,400 mg/day)	*Headache, nausea, nasal passage irritation, sore throat* Hepatotoxicity

*For doses of systemic corticosteroids, refer to Chapter 69.

Note: *Italics* indicate common adverse effects. Underline indicates serious adverse effects.

PROTOTYPE DRUG Beclomethasone (Beconase AQ, Qvar)

Classification: Therapeutic: Anti-inflammatory
Pharmacologic: Corticosteroid

Therapeutic Effects and Uses: Approved in 1976, beclomethasone is a corticosteroid that is available for administration by aerosol inhalation for asthma (Qvar), or as a nasal spray (Beconase AQ) for allergic rhinitis. Guidelines from the NAEPP place beclomethasone and other drugs in this class as preferred drugs for the long-term management of persistent asthma in both children and adults. Two inhalations, two to three times per day, usually provide adequate prophylaxis, although 3 to 4 weeks of therapy may be necessary before optimum benefits are achieved. In 2000, a double strength formulation (Qvar) was developed with smaller drug particles, which is able to deliver half the usual dose and achieve the same therapeutic effect. Beclomethasone is not a bronchodilator and should not be used to terminate asthma attacks in progress.

The intranasal formulation is effective at reducing the symptoms of allergic rhinitis. Therapeutic effects may take as long as 2 weeks to be fully apparent. Intranasal beclomethasone is also approved to prevent recurrence of nasal polyps following surgical removal. Very little of this drug is absorbed in the systemic circulation when it is administered by this route.

Mechanism of Action: Beclomethasone acts by reducing inflammation and immune responses, thus decreasing the frequency of asthma attacks.

Pharmacokinetics:

Route(s)	Inhalation
Absorption	Minimal systemic absorption
Distribution	Delivered directly to the lungs (site of action); small amountis secreted in breast milk
Primary metabolism	Liver (CYP450: 3A substrate) and lung
Primary excretion	Feces (less than 10% in urine)
Onset of action	Approximately 7 days
Duration of action	Half-life: 15 h

Adverse Effects: Inhaled beclomethasone produces few systemic adverse effects. Because small amounts may be swallowed with each dose, the patient should be observed for signs of corticosteroid toxicity (hypercorticism) when taking this drug for prolonged periods. Local effects may include hoarseness, dry mouth, and changes in taste. Inhaled corticosteroid use has been associated with the development of cataracts in adults. Some studies have shown that long-term intranasal or inhaled corticosteroids may cause growth inhibition in children.

Like all corticosteroids, the anti-inflammatory properties of beclomethasone can mask signs of infections and the drug is contraindicated if active infection is present. A large percentage of patients taking beclomethasone on a long-term basis will develop oropharyngeal candidiasis, a fungal infection in the throat, due to the constant deposits of drug in the oral cavity. Children who have not been vaccinated for varicella should receive the vaccine because of the potential for developing serious disseminated varicella infections during treatment with corticosteroids.

Contraindications/Precautions: The only contraindication to using beclomethasone is hypersensitivity to the drug.

Drug Interactions: Because very little of the drug is absorbed, no clinically significant drug interactions occur. **Herbal/Food:** None known.

Pregnancy: Category C.

Treatment of Overdose: Overdose does not occur when taken by the inhalation route.

Nursing Responsibilities:

- Perform a complete respiratory history and assessment that includes vital signs, particularly respiratory rate and heart rate; respiratory effort; lung sounds; cyanosis or pallor; and oxygen saturation, if indicated.
- Assess for the presence of conditions that could be worsened by taking corticosteroids. These include HTN, heart failure, thromboembolism, peptic ulcers or GI bleeding, and diabetes mellitus.
- Monitor laboratory results for cholesterol and other lipids, complete blood count (CBC), glucose levels, and electrolytes such as potassium. Laboratory analysis for occult blood is needed if the patient develops tarry stools or other evidence of gastric bleeding.
- Monitor the height of children because corticosteroids can slow bone growth.
- Assess bone mineral density test results because corticosteroids can cause osteoporosis. Ensure adequate dietary intake of calcium and vitamin D, or recommend a supplement.
- Monitor for signs and symptoms of infection because corticosteroids decrease the immune response. Assess for oral candidiasis, which is a common oral infection that may occur with inhaled corticosteroids.
- Assess for visual changes in patients who are taking long-term inhaled corticosteroids. Prolonged use of corticosteroids (including inhaled) is known to promote the development of cataracts.

Patient and Family Education:

- Do not take this medication to terminate an acute asthma attack. The maximum benefit of these drugs may not be achieved for 1 to 3 weeks.
- After inhaling, rinse the mouth because the anti-inflammatory properties of the drug may prevent the body from responding to overgrowth of fungi and this may lead to oral fungal infections.
- Watch for signs and symptoms of infections, particularly in the mouth. Report any mouth soreness or white patches in the mouth.
- Take inhaled corticosteroids exactly as prescribed without missing doses.

- Report signs and symptoms such as tarry stools, abdominal pain, or light-headedness or dizziness to the health care provider because these may indicate bleeding.
- Report any lack of improvement or increased incidence of asthma symptoms.
- Schedule an annual visit to the ophthalmologist to determine the presence of cataracts.
- Do not breast-feed while taking this drug without approval of the health care provider.
- Immediately notify the health care provider of any known or suspected pregnancy.

Drugs Similar to Beclomethasone (Beconase AQ, Qvar)

Other corticosteroids for inhalation include budesonide, flunisolide, fluticasone, and triamcinolone.

Budesonide (Pulmicort): Budesonide is a corticosteroid that is available by the intranasal route for allergic rhinitis (Rhinocort), oral inhalation, nebulizer for asthma prophylaxis (Pulmicort), or PO capsules for Crohn's disease (Entocort). The most common adverse effects with the inhaled use of budesonide include respiratory infections, rhinitis, cough, and otitis media. Visual impairment may occur. Growth effects should be monitored in pediatric patients. This drug is pregnancy category B.

Flunisolide (Aerobid): Flunisolide is a corticosteroid that is available by the intranasal route for allergic rhinitis (Nasarel) or by oral inhalation for asthma prophylaxis (Aerobid). The most common adverse effects with inhaled use include upper respiratory infections, dry mouth, hoarseness, nausea, vomiting, and taste changes. Like other drugs in this class, visual impairment may occur and growth effects should be monitored in pediatric patients. This drug is pregnancy category C.

Fluticasone (Flovent): Fluticasone is a corticosteroid that is available by the intranasal route for allergic rhinitis (Flonase); oral inhalation for asthma prophylaxis or COPD (Flovent); or topical cream or ointment for dermatitis, eczema, and other skin conditions (Cutivate). The most common adverse effects with the inhaled use of fluticasone include headache, throat irritation, and upper respiratory tract infections. Visual impairment may occur. Growth effects should be monitored in pediatric patients. Like other inhaled corticoteroids, fluticasone is not indicated for the relief of acute bronchospasm. This drug is pregnancy category C.

Mometasone (Asmanex): Mometasone is an inhaled corticosteroid that is available for the prevention of acute asthmatic attacks. When inhaled it may take an hour or longer to produce its effects; therefore it is not indicated for the relief of acute bronchospasm. Actions and adverse effects are the same as those of other inhaled corticosteroids. An intranasal form is available for allergic rhinitis (Nasonex), and a topical preparation (Elocon) is used to treat various inflammatory skin conditions. This drug is pregnancy category C.

Triamcinolone (Azmacort): Triamcinolone is available in a wide variety of formulations: oral inhalation for asthma (Azmacort), intranasal for allergic rhinitis (Nasacort), ophthalmic for ocular inflammation (Triesence), and various topical formulations for inflammatory skin conditions. Parenteral formulations (Kenalog) are available for a large number of allergic and inflammatory disorders. When inhaled the adverse effects are the same as those of other corticosteroids, such as throat irritation, dry mouth, hoarseness, visual changes, possible growth retardation in children, and upper respiratory tract infections. This drug is pregnancy category C.

CONNECTION *Checkpoint* 73.2

From what you learned in Chapter 69, describe the strategies that are used to limit the incidence of serious adverse effects when corticosteroids must be taken PO for prolonged periods. See Answer to Connection Checkpoint 73.2 in Appendix A.

73.8 Mast cell stabilizers are used for the prophylaxis of asthma and act by preventing the release of histamine.

Mast cell stabilizers serve limited, though important, roles in the prophylaxis of asthma. Mast cells are large cells that contain inflammatory granules, such as histamine, that mediate inflammatory and allergic reactions. When these cells are sensitized, they degranulate and release the inflammatory substances into the body where they initiate an inflammatory response. Mast cell stabilizers are helpful in managing asthma and COPD because they prevent degranulation of the mast cell, preventing the release of histamine and other inflammatory mediators in the airways. There are two currently approved mast cell stabilizers: cromolyn (Intal) and nedocromil (Tilade). Doses of these agents are listed in Table 73.5.

Mast cell stabilizers are administered by inhalation via an MDI or a nebulizer. An intranasal form is available for management of allergic rhinitis.

PROTOTYPE DRUG Cromolyn (Intal)

Classification: Therapeutic: Anti-inflammatory
Pharmacologic: Mast cell stabilizer

Therapeutic Effects and Uses: An older drug that was approved by the FDA in 1973, cromolyn prevents the inflammation that is a characteristic pathophysiologic feature of asthma and COPD. Because it has no effect on previously released inflammatory mediators from mast cell degranulation, the effects will not be noted immediately. The NAEPP guidelines place cromolyn as an alternate drug to be considered for the treatment of mild to moderate asthma when corticosteroids are contraindicated or have not proven effective. This drug should not be used to terminate acute asthma attacks.

For asthma therapy the drug is administered via oral inhalation. An intranasal over-the-counter (OTC) formulation

(Nasalcrom) is available for allergic rhinitis. An ophthalmic solution (Crolom) is used to treat various allergic disorders of the conjunctiva. Gastrocrom is a PO dosage form of cromolyn that is the only FDA approved drug to treat systemic mastocytosis, which is a rare condition in which the patient has excessive numbers of mast cells. Gastrocrom is also used off-label to treat ulcerative colitis and to prevent symptoms associated with food allergies.

Mechanism of Action: By stabilizing mast cells, cromolyn helps to prevent the inflammatory response that occurs when mast cells degranulate.

Pharmacokinetics:

Route(s)	Inhalation
Absorption	Minimal systemic absorption (less than 1%)
Distribution	Delivered directly to the lungs (site of action); small amount crosses the placenta; small amount is secreted in breast milk
Primary metabolism	Hepatic
Primary excretion	Bile (and, subsequently, feces) and renal
Onset of action	Adequate effect may not be noted until 2–4 weeks of use
Duration of action	Unknown

Adverse Effects: Adverse effects are uncommon when the drug is administered by oral inhalation. The most common effects are bronchospasm, cough, and pharyngeal irritation. Intranasal and ophthalmic administration may cause local burning and stinging.

Contraindications/Precautions: As with any drug, persons who have demonstrated a hypersensitivity to this drug should not take it. It should be discontinued if the patient develops pulmonary eosinophilia.

Drug Interactions: No significant interactions are known. **Herbal/Food:** Unknown.

Pregnancy: Category B.

Treatment of Overdose: There are no noted problems associated with overdosage. Toxicity is unlikely.

Nursing Responsibilities:

- Perform a complete respiratory history and assessment that includes vital signs, particularly respiratory rate and heart rate; respiratory effort; lung sounds; cyanosis or pallor; and oxygen saturation, if indicated.
- If a bronchodilator aerosol spray such as albuterol (Proventil) is used in addition to cromolyn, the bronchodilator should be used first, and 5 minutes should elapse before the cromolyn is used.

Patient and Family Education:

- Do not take this drug in an attempt to abort an acute asthma attack. Mast cell stabilizers are ineffective in terminating acute attacks.
- Allow several weeks for the drug to achieve a maximal therapeutic effect. Once this therapeutic level is obtained, take this drug on a regular basis to maintain this benefit.
- Rinse the mouth thoroughly after use or use mints or gum to take away any bitter or unpleasant taste in the mouth. Do not swallow any solution left in the mouth.

Drugs Similar to Cromolyn (Intal)

Nedocromil is the only other mast cell stabilizer.

Nedocromil (Tilade): Approved in 1992, the profile for this agent is similar to that of cromolyn with the exception of a very bitter taste that causes some people to discontinue this drug. This is a particularly important consideration for children who will be less acquiescent to taking distasteful medication. Like cromolyn, nedocromil is to be used only for asthma prophylaxis and not to terminate acute asthma attacks. The drug may require a week of therapy before benefits are obtained and it must be taken on a continuous basis for asthma prophylaxis. An ophthalmic form (Alocril) is available to treat allergic conjunctivitis. This drug is pregnancy category B.

73.9 The leukotriene modifiers, which are primarily used for asthma prophylaxis, act by reducing the inflammatory component of asthma.

Leukotriene modifiers are one of the newest drug classes added to the arsenal of asthma management. They are able to ease bronchoconstriction by reducing inflammation. Because of their delayed onset, leukotriene modifiers are ineffective at terminating acute asthma attacks. The NAEPP guidelines list the leukotriene modifiers as alternative drugs to be considered when inhaled corticosteroids and short-acting beta agonists are unable to control asthma symptoms. Doses for these drugs are listed in Table 73.3.

Leukotrienes are mediators of the immune and inflammatory responses that are involved in allergic and asthmatic reactions. Leukotrienes are synthesized by mast cells as well as neutrophils, basophils, and eosinophils. When released in the airway, they promote edema, inflammation, and bronchoconstriction. Leukotriene modifiers reduce inflammation by either blocking the enzyme that controls leukotriene synthesis or by blocking leukotriene receptors. They are not considered bronchodilators, although they do reduce bronchoconstriction indirectly. The leukotriene modifiers are only available by the PO route.

PROTOTYPE DRUG Zafirlukast (Accolate)

Classification: **Therapeutic:** Agent for asthma prophylaxis, anti-inflammatory

Pharmacologic: Leukotriene modifier

Therapeutic Effects and Uses: Zafirlukast, the first leukotriene modifier that was approved in 1996, is used for the prophylaxis of persistent, chronic asthma. This drug prevents the inflammation that is a characteristic pathophysiologic feature of asthma and COPD. It is less effective than inhaled corticosteroids. Off-label uses include allergic rhinitis and prevention of exercise-induced bronchospasm.

Zafirlukast is given by the PO route. Its relatively long onset of action makes it unsuitable for the termination of acute bronchospasm.

Mechanism of Action: Zafirlukast prevents airway edema and inflammation by blocking leukotriene receptors in the airways.

Pharmacokinetics:

Route(s)	PO
Absorption	Rapidly absorbed, but decreased in presence of food
Distribution	Secreted in breast milk; more than 99% bound to plasma protein
Primary metabolism	Extensive hepatic metabolism (CYP2C9, CYP 3A4)
Primary excretion	Mostly bile; 10% renal
Onset of action	1 week
Duration of action	Unknown; half-life: 10 h

Adverse Effects: Zafirlukast produces few serious adverse effects. Headache is the most common complaint. Rhinitis, nausea, vomiting, and diarrhea are reported by some patients.

Contraindications/Precautions: The only absolute contraindication is hypersensitivity to this drug. Because a few rare cases of fatal hepatic failure have been reported, patients with preexisting hepatic impairment should be treated with caution. This drug should be avoided when breast-feeding.

Drug Interactions: Zafirlukast is metabolized by CYP450 enzymes and has the potential to interact with substrates of the inhibitors of this enzyme. Use with warfarin may significantly increase prothrombin time (PT). Erythromycin and theophylline may decrease the serum levels of zafirlukast. Concurrent use with aspirin can significantly increase zafirlukast levels. **Herbal/Food:** Food can reduce the bioavailability; thus the drug should be taken on an empty stomach.

Pregnancy: Category B.

Treatment of Overdose: Symptoms of overdose include headache, nausea, and vomiting. Treatment is supportive.

Nursing Responsibilities:

- Obtain a complete respiratory history and assessment that includes vital signs, particularly respiratory rate and heart rate; respiratory effort; lung sounds; cyanosis or pallor; and oxygen saturation, if indicated.
- Assess for the presence of hepatic impairment and for a history of alcoholism. This drug is extensively metabolized in the liver.
- Monitor laboratory findings that reflect liver status, including the CBC and periodic hepatic function tests, because this drug may cause hepatitis. Monitor the PT and international normalized ratio (INR) if patients are taking warfarin.
- Check the medication record for medications that interact with leukotriene modifiers such as methylxanthines, warfarin, and beta antagonists.

Patient and Family Education:

- Do not use this drug to terminate an acute asthma attack.
- Immediately report signs and symptoms of liver problems such as jaundice, fatigue, and dark-colored urine to the health care provider.
- Report nausea, itching, or signs and symptoms of infection to the health care provider.
- Take this medication exactly as prescribed, even during symptom-free periods.
- Attend all scheduled appointments with the health care provider and laboratory visits for testing.
- Do not breast-feed while taking this drug without approval of the health care provider.
- Immediately notify the health care provider of any known or suspected pregnancy.
- Watch carefully for signs or symptoms of infection. People older than age 55 may experience an increased frequency of infections when taking these drugs.

Drugs Similar to Zafirlukast (Accolate)

Montelukast and zileuton are other leukotriene modifiers.

Montelukast (Singulair): Given by the PO route, montelukast acts by blocking leukotriene receptors in the airways. Montelukast is the only agent in this category that is approved for very young children, 12 months or older. For pediatric use it is available as chewable tablets and oral granules that may be sprinkled on soft food. The drug is approved for the prophylaxis of persistent, chronic asthma, allergic rhinitis, and exercise-induced bronchospasm. Like other drugs in this class, montelukast should not be used to treat acute asthma attacks. Adverse effects are generally mild. Headache is the most frequently reported adverse effect. This is a pregnancy category B drug.

Zileuton (Zyflo): Approved in 1996, zileuton is an PO drug that acts by inhibiting the lipoxygenase, which is the first enzyme in the pathway of leukotriene synthesis. Like other drugs in this class, zileuton is considered an alternate drug in the prophylaxis of persistent, chronic asthma. In 2007 an extended release formulation (Zyflo CR) was approved that allows for twice-daily dosing. Like other drugs in this class, zileuton should not be used to treat acute asthma attacks. This drug is generally well tolerated, with headache being the most common adverse effect. The most serious concern with zileuton is the potential for liver damage. Zileuton raises liver enzymes (alanine aminotransferase), and cases of jaundice and severe hepatic injury have been reported. This drug is contraindicated in patients with hepatic impairment, and liver function tests should be conducted on a regular basis during therapy. This is a pregnancy category C drug.

73.10 Methylxanthines were once the mainstay of asthma pharmacotherapy but are now rarely prescribed for that disorder.

The **methylxanthines** were considered the drugs of choice for treating asthma 30 years ago. Now they are primarily reserved for the long-term management of persistent asthma that is unresponsive to beta agonists or inhaled corticosteroids. One reason for the lessened use of methylxanthines is that their narrow therapeutic index increases the risk of toxicity, especially with prolonged use. These drugs also have significant interactions with numerous other drugs. Doses for these agents are listed in Table 73.4.

The methylxanthines are modest bronchodilators. They are chemically related to caffeine and share caffeine's stimulant effect. Methylxanthines are available in forms for PO, parenteral, and rectal administration. Because they are not available for inhalation, patients do not benefit from the smaller doses and direct effects that are provided by drugs that can be administered by the inhalation route. Interestingly, theobromine, an ingredient in chocolate, is also a methylxanthine.

PROTOTYPE DRUG Theophylline (Slo-Phyllin, Theochron, Theolair, Uniphyl)

Classification: **Therapeutic:** Bronchodilator
Pharmacologic: Methylxanthine

Therapeutic Effects and Uses: Approved by the FDA in 1940, theophylline is a natural substance found in small amounts in tea. Theophylline relaxes bronchial smooth muscle and may exert some anti-inflammatory action that is beneficial to patients with asthma. It is considered an alternate drug by the NAEPP guidelines, to be considered for asthma prophylaxis when more effective drugs fail to bring symptomatic relief. It may be used in combination with a corticosteroid for persistent asthma. Although FDA-approved for treating acute bronchospasm, theophylline is not recommended by the NAEPP guidelines because the short-acting beta$_2$-adrenergic agonists (SABAs) are more effective.

Theophylline has several off-label indications. As a respiratory stimulant, theophylline and caffeine may be used to treat sleep apnea in neonates and in adults with chronic heart failure. Given IV, theophylline has been found to reduce neurotoxicity resulting from the drug methotrexate.

Mechanism of Action: Theophylline works by two mechanisms. It relaxes bronchial smooth muscle, which promotes bronchodilation, and it suppresses airway responsiveness to stimuli that promote bronchospasm.

Pharmacokinetics:

Route(s)	PO, parenteral, suppository
Absorption	Rapid absorption
Distribution	About 40% protein bound; remainder is distributed well in fluids and less well in body lipids
Primary metabolism	Hepatic (CYP1A2, CYP2E1, CYP3A3)
Primary excretion	Renal
Onset of action	Peak: approximately 60 minutes (highly variable)
Duration of action	Half-life: 6–10 h (highly variable)

Adverse Effects: Theophylline has a very narrow therapeutic index. Therapeutic levels are 10 to 15 mcg/mL and the toxic level is anything above 20 mcg/mL. Serum theophylline levels should be obtained during therapy. Common adverse effects include nausea, vomiting, headache, irritability, and insomnia. More serious reactions include dysrhythmias, hypotension, and seizures.

Contraindications/Precautions: Theophylline should be used with great caution in patients who have seizure disorders, heart failure, or cardiac dysrhythmias. Theophylline has also been shown to increase the production of gastric acid so use in patients with active peptic ulcer disease is not recommended. Because of the extensive hepatic metabolism, theophylline should be closely monitored in patients with a history of liver disease. As with any drug, this drug is contraindicated in persons who have demonstrated a hypersensitivity to it.

Drug Interactions: Because theophylline is highly metabolized by the CYP450 enzyme system, there are numerous drug interactions, including many common antibiotics (ciprofloxacin, clarithromycin, erythromycin), antianxiety agents (diazepam, flurazepam, lorazepam, midazolam), and others. When treating a patient who is receiving multiple drugs concurrently with theophylline, the nurse should consult current sources for potential drug interactions. There are also a number of IV incompatibilities, including emergency medications such as epinephrine, norepinephrine, and isoproterenol. Compatibility of any medication should be checked prior to initiating infusions in the same line.
Herbal/Food: Foods and beverages containing caffeine will cause additive central nervous system (CNS) stimulation. St. John's wort may decrease the effectiveness of theophylline.

Pregnancy: Category C.

Treatment of Overdose: There is no specific antidote to theophylline. Gastric lavage is indicated in the event of an overdose of PO medications. Seizures and other CNS effects may respond to barbiturates or benzodiazepines. Supportive measures need to be provided for hypotension, shock, dysrhythmias, and other toxic effects. Serum levels should be monitored periodically until they are within normal limits.

Nursing Responsibilities:

- Obtain a complete respiratory history and assessment that includes vital signs, particularly respiratory rate and heart rate; respiratory effort; lung sounds; cyanosis or pallor; and oxygen saturation, if indicated.

- Assess for the presence of cardiac impairment, severe renal or liver disorders, and active peptic ulcers.
- Check the medication record for medications that interact with methylxanthines.
- Monitor for common adverse effects such as tachycardia, irritability, restlessness, insomnia, dizziness, headache, palpitations, vomiting, and abdominal pain.
- Monitor serum levels and report inadequate or toxic levels to the prescriber promptly.
- Monitor liver function tests such as bilirubin, alkaline phosphatase (ALP), aspartate aminotransferase (AST), alanine aminotransferase (ALT), and lactate dehydrogenase (LDH).

Patient and Family Education:

- Limit the use of food and beverage products and OTC medications that contain caffeine.
- Report early signs of toxicity such as decreased appetite, nausea, vomiting, dizziness, restlessness, hypotension, or seizures to the health care provider.
- Take this medication at the same time every day exactly as prescribed. Never increase, decrease, omit, or change intervals between doses.
- Limit or eliminate tobacco use because smoking increases the rate of drug clearance from the body, which may diminish the effectiveness of the drug.
- Do not take any other prescription or nonprescription drugs, dietary supplements, or herbal products without approval of the health care provider.
- Attend all scheduled appointments with the health care provider and laboratory visits for testing because they are needed to monitor for safe and effective drug levels.
- Immediately notify the health care provider if breathing problems become worse.
- Do not breast-feed while taking this drug without approval of the health care provider.

Drugs Similar to Theophylline (Slo-Phyllin, Theochron, Theolair, Uniphyl)

Aminophylline and dyphylline are other methylxanthines. Oxtriphylline (Coledyl) is a drug in this class that has been discontinued in the United States.

Aminophylline: Approved in 1975, aminophylline is a theophylline salt that has enhanced water solubility. It is approved to treat symptoms of asthma and COPD. It has the same actions and adverse effects as those of theophylline. Aminophylline is shorter acting than theophylline and is available in PO, rectal, and IV forms. This drug is pregnancy category C.

Dyphylline (Lufyllin): Dyphylline is not a theophylline salt but it has similar actions. It is approved to treat acute bronchospasms associated with asthma and COPD. Approved in 1951, it is available in PO form and has a short half-life of only 2 hours, so it is usually given four times a day. It is 90% less potent than theophylline but exerts fewer adverse effects. The intramuscular (IM) form of the drug has been discontinued in the United States. Indications are the same as those of theophylline. This drug is pregnancy category C.

73.11 Monoclonal antibodies are a newer form of therapy for the prevention of asthma symptoms.

Approved in 2003, omalizumab (Xolair) is the first biologic therapy used to treat asthma, offering a new approach to the management of the disease. This drug is approved for treating allergic rhinitis and moderate to severe, persistent asthma that cannot be controlled satisfactorily with inhaled corticosteroids. To receive omalizumab, the patient must have tested positive for an airborne allergen such as mold, pollen, or animal dander. Although it is only available by the subcutaneous route, injections are scheduled every 2 to 4 weeks, depending on the patient's response to therapy. It is approved for asthma prophylaxis in patients 12 years old or greater.

Omalizumab is a monoclonal antibody. Monoclonal antibodies are designed to attach to a specific receptor on a target cell or molecule. Most monoclonal antibodies are designed to attack cancer cells. However, omalizumab is designed to attach to a receptor on immunoglobulin E (IgE). The normal function of IgE is to react to antigens and cause the release of inflammatory chemical mediators from mast cells and basophils. By binding to IgE, omalizumab prevents inflammation and dampens the body's response to allergens, that sometimes trigger asthma. The student should refer to Chapter 45 for a complete discussion of monoclonal antibodies and a prototype feature for muromonab-CD3 (Orthoclone, OKT3).

Omalizumab is reserved for patients with persistent asthma because of its expense, potential adverse effects, and the need for regular parenteral injections. Although adverse effects are uncommon, they may be serious and include anaphylaxis, bleeding-related events, or severe dysmenorrhea. Less serious adverse effects include rash, headache, and viral infections.

CONNECTION *Checkpoint* 73.3

Most monoclonal antibodies are classified as immunosuppressants. From what you learned in Chapter 45, explain methods by which these drugs can be used to suppress the immune system. See Answer to Connection Checkpoint 73.3 in Appendix A.

Chronic Obstructive Pulmonary Disease

73.12 Chronic obstructive pulmonary disease may be treated with bronchodilators, anti-inflammatory agents, and mucolytics.

Chronic obstructive pulmonary disease (COPD) is a progressive pulmonary disorder characterized by chronic and recurrent obstruction of airflow. The two most common

NURSING PROCESS APPLICATION

Patients Receiving Therapy for Asthma and Chronic Obstructive Pulmonary Disease

Assessment

Prior to administration:

- Obtain a complete health history including allergies, drug history, possible drug reactions, and use of complementary and herbal remedies.
- Assess for symptoms related to respiratory deficiency such as dyspnea, orthopnea, cyanosis, nasal flaring, wheezing, and weakness.
- Obtain vital signs.
- Auscultate bilateral breath sounds for air movement and adventitious sounds such as crackles and wheezes.
- Assess pulmonary function with a pulse oximeter, peak expiratory flowmeter, and arterial blood gases to establish baseline levels.

Potential Nursing Diagnoses

- *Impaired Gas Exchange,* related to bronchial constriction
- *Ineffective Tissue Perfusion (Cardiopulmonary),* related to adverse effects of drugs
- *Deficient Knowledge (Drug Therapy)*
- *Anxiety,* related to difficulty in breathing
- *Sleep Deprivation,* related to adverse effects of drugs
- *Activity Intolerance,* related to ineffective drug therapy

Planning: Patient Goals and Expected Outcomes

The patient will:

- Exhibit adequate oxygenation as evidenced by improved lung sounds and pulmonary function values.
- Report a reduction in subjective symptoms of respiratory deficiency.
- Demonstrate an understanding of the drug's action by accurately describing the drug's adverse effects and precautions.
- Report at least 6 hours of uninterrupted sleep.

Implementation

Interventions and (Rationales)	Patient and Family Education
• Monitor vital signs, including pulse, blood pressure, and respiratory rate. (Baseline data are needed to monitor therapy.)	Instruct the patient to: • Use the medication as directed even if asymptomatic. • Report difficulty with breathing.
• Monitor pulmonary function with a pulse oximeter, peak expiratory flowmeter, or arterial blood gases. (Monitoring is necessary to assess drug effectiveness.)	Instruct the patient to: • Report symptoms of deteriorating respiratory status. • Report increased or unrelieved dyspnea, breathlessness with speech, increased anxiety, or orthopnea.
• Monitor the patient's ability to use an inhaler. (Proper use ensures correct dosage.)	Instruct the patient: • In the proper use of the MDI. • To use the medication strictly as prescribed. Do not "double up" on doses. • To rinse the mouth thoroughly following use.
• Observe for adverse effects specific to the medication used. (Dosage or medication changes may be needed.)	Instruct the patient to report: • Specific drug adverse effects. • Onset of any new symptoms.
• Maintain the environment free of respiratory contaminants such as dust, dry air, flowers, and smoke. (These substances may exacerbate bronchial constriction.)	Instruct the patient to: • Avoid respiratory irritants. • Maintain a "clean air environment." • Stop smoking and avoid secondhand smoke, if applicable.
• Maintain dietary intake that is adequate in essential nutrients and vitamins, and ensure adequate hydration (3–4 L/day). (Dyspnea interferes with proper nutrition. Adequate hydration liquefies pulmonary secretions.)	Instruct the patient to: • Maintain nutrition with foods high in essential nutrients such as protein and carbohydrates. • Consume small frequent meals to prevent fatigue. • Consume 3–4 L of fluid per day if not contraindicated. • Avoid caffeine because this increases CNS irritability.
• Provide emotional and psychosocial support during periods of shortness of breath. (This may decrease anxiety, ease breathing effort, and improve gas exchange.)	Instruct the patient in: • Relaxation techniques. • Controlled breathing techniques.
• Monitor patient adherence to pharmacotherapy. (Maintaining therapeutic drug levels is essential to effective therapy.)	Inform the patient of the importance of: • Ongoing medication adherence. • Regular follow-up with the health care provider.

Evaluation of Outcome Criteria

Evaluate the effectiveness of drug therapy by confirming that patient goals and expected outcomes have been met (see "Planning").

examples of conditions that cause chronic pulmonary obstruction are **chronic bronchitis,** a condition in which excess mucus is produced in the lower respiratory tract, and **emphysema,** a condition in which there is loss of bronchiolar elasticity and destruction of alveolar walls.

The clinical distinction between chronic bronchitis and emphysema is sometimes unclear because patients may exhibit symptoms of both conditions concurrently. Both conditions are strongly associated with smoking tobacco products (cigarette smoking accounts for 85% to 90% of all cases of nonasthmatic COPD) and, secondarily, breathing air pollutants. In chronic bronchitis, excess mucus is produced in the lower respiratory tract due to the inflammation and irritation from cigarette smoke or pollutants. The airway becomes partially obstructed with mucus, thus resulting in the classic signs of dyspnea and coughing. An early sign of bronchitis is often a productive cough that occurs on awakening. Gas exchange may be impaired; thus wheezing and decreased exercise tolerance are additional clinical signs. Microbes thrive in the mucus-rich environment, and pulmonary infections are common.

Because most patients with COPD are lifelong tobacco users, they often have serious comorbid cardiovascular conditions such as heart failure and HTN. Emphysema is most often the result of years of chronic inflammation and is characterized by loss of elasticity of the bronchioles and damage and loss of alveolar wall structures. The loss of elasticity results in partial collapse of the airways on exhalation, leading to air trapping, and the destruction of alveolar walls leads to decreased perfusion and gas exchange at the alveolus. The patient with emphysema may suffer extreme dyspnea from even the slightest physical activity.

Drugs may be used to bring symptomatic relief to patients with COPD, but they do not cure the underlying disorder. The goals of pharmacotherapy of COPD are to relieve symptoms and avoid complications of the condition. Various classes of drugs are used to treat infections, control cough, and relieve bronchospasm. Most patients receive the same bronchodilators and anti-inflammatory agents that are prescribed for asthma. **Mucolytics,** which are agents given to loosen thick viscous bronchial secretions, and expectorants, which are agents given to aid in the removal of mucus, are sometimes prescribed (see Chapter 74). Long-term oxygen therapy is prescribed in later stages and it has been shown to decrease mortality in patients with advanced COPD. Antibiotics may be prescribed for patients who experience multiple bouts of pulmonary infections.

Patients with COPD should not receive drugs that have beta-adrenergic antagonist activity because these agents cause bronchoconstriction. Respiratory depressants such as opioids and barbiturates should also be avoided when possible. An important teaching point for the nurse is to strongly encourage smoking cessation in these patients. Smoking cessation has been shown to slow the progression of COPD and to result in fewer respiratory symptoms; however, it cannot undo damage that has already occurred.

UNDERSTANDING THE CHAPTER

Key Concepts Summary

73.1 The physiology of the respiratory system involves two main processes: perfusion and ventilation.

73.2 Asthma is a chronic disease that has both inflammatory and bronchospasm components.

73.3 Inhalation is a common route of administration for pulmonary drugs because it delivers drugs directly to their sites of action.

73.4 The goals of asthma pharmacotherapy are to terminate acute bronchospasms and to reduce the frequency of asthma attacks.

73.5 Beta$_2$-adrenergic agonists are the most effective drugs for relieving acute bronchospasm.

73.6 The inhaled anticholinergics are used for preventing bronchospasm.

73.7 Inhaled corticosteroids are the most effective drugs for the long-term control of asthma.

73.8 Mast cell stabilizers are used for the prophylaxis of asthma and act by preventing the release of histamine.

73.9 The leukotriene modifiers, which are primarily used for asthma prophylaxis, act by reducing the inflammatory component of asthma.

73.10 Methylxanthines were once the mainstay of asthma pharmacotherapy but are now rarely prescribed for that disorder.

73.11 Monoclonal antibodies are a newer form of therapy for the prevention of asthma symptoms.

73.12 Chronic obstructive pulmonary disease may be treated with bronchodilators, anti-inflammatory agents, and mucolytics.

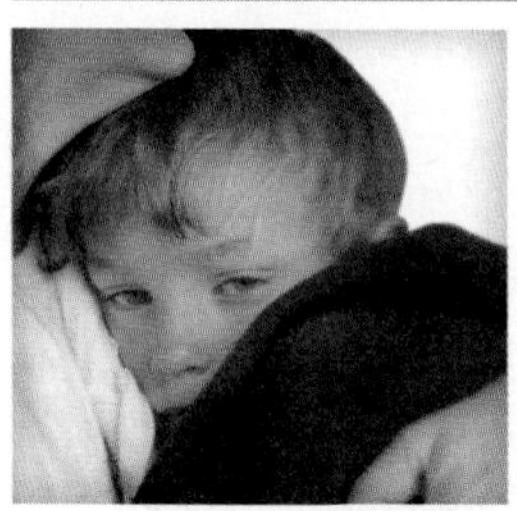

Making the PATIENT *Connection*

Remember the patient "Jimmy" at the beginning of the chapter? Now read the remainder of the case study. Based on the information presented within this chapter, respond to the critical thinking questions that follow.

It is an especially busy night with many very sick children in the emergency department. Then a scream comes from a frantic mother who enters running with a child in her arms. The triage nurse springs into action. The child is in acute respiratory distress with nasal flaring, intercostal retractions, and bilateral wheezing. The nurse asks, "Has this ever happened to your son before?" The mother nods affirmatively, crying, and says, "He has asthma."

Jimmy is a 4-year-old child who was diagnosed with asthma approximately 6 months ago. This is the third asthma attack to occur since his diagnosis. He is awake but visibly gasping for air. His heart rate is 162 beats/minute and his respiratory rate is 48/minute. He is slightly cyanotic around the mouth.

Critical Thinking Questions

1. How would you, the nurse, explain what is causing the symptoms experienced by Jimmy who is in the midst of an acute asthmatic attack?
2. What medications would you anticipate will be prescribed to terminate Jimmy's acute asthmatic attack and why?
3. Jimmy's mother asks you to explain the mechanism of action for the medication of choice in question 2. How would you respond?

Case Study

As the home health nurse, you visit with Mr. Jonas Maxwell weekly to assess his pulmonary status and his adherence to the medication regimen. Mr. Maxwell has end-stage COPD. He was diagnosed with the disease many years ago and his pulmonary status has deteriorated slowly over the past few years. Despite his health care provider's recommendation to change to another medication, Mr. Maxwell insists that theophylline (Theo-Dur) is the only medication that helps him to breathe. He also uses several MDIs with spacer several times per day.

1. What symptoms would you expect to observe in Mr. Maxwell if he is experiencing early signs of toxicity?
2. Create a list of "things to avoid" for an individual who is receiving theophylline therapy.
3. In your own words, how would you describe the function of the spacer used with Mr. Maxwell's MDI?

NCLEX-RN® Review

1 A client with asthma asks which of the prescribed medications should be used in the event of an acute episode of bronchospasm. The nurse will instruct the client to use:

1. Albuterol, a beta agonist bronchodilator, by inhalation.
2. Beclomethasone, a glucocorticoid anti-inflammatory drug, by inhalation.
3. Ipratropium, an anticholinergic bronchodilator, by inhalation.
4. Zafirlukast, a leukotriene modifier, by mouth.

2 A client is prescribed beclomethasone (Beclovent), a glucocorticoid inhaler. Education by the nurse will include:

1. "Check your heart rate because this may cause tachycardia."
2. "Limit your coffee intake while on this drug."
3. "Rinse your mouth out well after each use."
4. "You may feel shaky and nervous after using this drug."

3 The nurse should inform the client who is prescribed a nebulizer treatment with a bronchodilator agent that a common adverse effect is:

1. An increased heart rate with palpitations.
2. Predisposition to infection.
3. Sedation.
4. Temporary dyspnea.

4 The nurse should monitor the client who is taking corticosteroids for evidence of: (Select all that apply.)

1. Infection.
2. Hyperglycemia
3. Urinary retention.
4. Tachycardia.
5. Photophobia.

5 A 4-year-old child with respiratory distress secondary to asthma has an order for a nebulizer treatment. The type of medication most likely to be given for asthma management is a:

1. Beta agonist.
2. Beta antagonist.
3. Corticosteroid.
4. Leukotriene modifier.

6 Despite repeated demonstrations of proper inhaler use by the nurse, the client is unable to return a proper demonstration on the training inhaler. The client is becoming frustrated. The best action for the nurse to take is to:

1. Encourage the client to keep practicing just a little longer.
2. Notify the health care provider that the client is incompetent.
3. Provide a spacer for use with the inhaler.
4. Switch to an oral form of a beta agonist.

See Answers to Critical Thinking Questions, Case Study, and NCLEX-RN® Review in Appendix A.

References

American Lung Association. (2006, July). *Trends in asthma: Morbidity and mortality.* Retrieved September 4, 2008, from http://www.lungusa.org/atf/cf/%7B7A8D42C2-FCCA-4604-8ADE-7F5D5E762256%7D/ASTHMA06FINAL.PDF

American Lung Association. (2006, July). *Trends in chronic bronchitis and emphysema: Morbidity and mortality.* Retrieved September 4, 2008, from http://www.lungusa.org/atf/cf/%7B7A8D42C2-FCCA-4604-8ADE-7F5D5E762256%7D/COPD06.PDF

Asthma and Allergy Foundation of America. (n.d.). *Asthma facts and figures.* Retrieved September 4, 2008, from http://www.aafa.org/display.cfm?id=8&sub=42

Banasiak, N. (2007). Childhood asthma part one: Initial assessment, diagnosis, and education. *Journal of Pediatric Health Care, 21*(1), 44–48.

Centers for Disease Control and Prevention, National Center for Health Statistics. (2008). *Asthma.* Retrieved September 4, 2008, from http://www.cdc.gov/nchs/fastats/asthma.htm

Centers for Disease Control and Prevention, National Center for Health Statistics. (2006). *Asthma prevalence, health care use and mortality, 2003–2005.* Retrieved September 4, 2008, from http://www.cdc.gov/nchs/products/pubs/pubd/hestats/asthma/asthma.htm

Colbert, B., & Kennedy, B. L. (2008). *Integrated cardiopulmonary pharmacology* (2nd ed.). Upper Saddle River, NJ: Pearson Education, Inc.

Dahlin, C. (2006). It takes my breath away end-stage COPD: Part 1: A case study and an overview of COPD. *Home Healthcare Nurse, 24*(3), 148–155.

George, M., Birck, K., Hufford, D. J., Jemmott, L. S., & Weaver, T. E. (2006). Beliefs about asthma and complementary and alternative medicine in low-income inner-city African-American adults. *Journal of General Internal Medicine, 21,* 1317–1325.

Global Initiative for Chronic Obstructive Lung Disease. (2006). *Global strategy for diagnosis, management, and prevention of COPD.* Retrieved September 4, 2008, from http://goldcopd.com/download.asp?intId=379

Joint Task Force on Practice Parameters Representing the American Academy of Allergy, Asthma, and Immunology, the American College of Allergy, Asthma, and Immunology, and the Joint Council of Allergy, Asthma, and Immunology. (2005). Obtaining optimal asthma control: A practice parameter. *Journal of Allergy and Clinical Immunology.* Retrieved September 4, 2008, from http://www.jacionline.org/webfiles/images/journals/YMAI/5412.pdf

Kelly-Shanovich, K., Pulvermacher, A., Sorkness, C., Bhattacharya, A., & Gustafson, B. (2007). The integration of web-based asthma education with nurse case management. *Journal of Allergy and Clinical Immunology, 119*(1), S80.

Lanski, S. L., Greenwalk, M., Perkins, A., & Simon, H. K. (2007). Herbal therapy use in a pediatric emergency department population: Expect the unexpected. *Journal of the American Academy of Child and Adolescent Psychiatry, 42,* 1196.

Markham, A. W., & Wilkinson, J. M. (2004). Complementary and alternative medicines (CAM) in the management of asthma: An examination of the evidence. *Journal of Asthma, 41*(2), 131–174.

National Asthma Education and Prevention Program Coordinating Committee. (2007). *Expert panel report 3 (EPR3): Guidelines for the diagnosis and management of asthma.* Coordinated by the National Heart, Lung, and Blood Institute of the National Institutes of Health. Retrieved September 5, 2008, from http://www.nhlbi.nih.gov/guidelines/asthma/asthgdln.htm

National Heart, Lung, and Blood Institute. (2003). *Expert panel report: Guidelines for the diagnosis and management of asthma* (NIH Publication No. 02-5074). Washington, DC: U.S. Department of Health and Human Services.

O'Hollaren, M. T. (2003). *Middleton's allergy: Principles and practice* (6th ed.). Philadelphia: Mosby.

Sterling, Y. M., & El-Dahr, J. M. (2006). Wheezing and asthma in early childhood: An update. *Pediatric Nursing, 32*(1), 27–31.

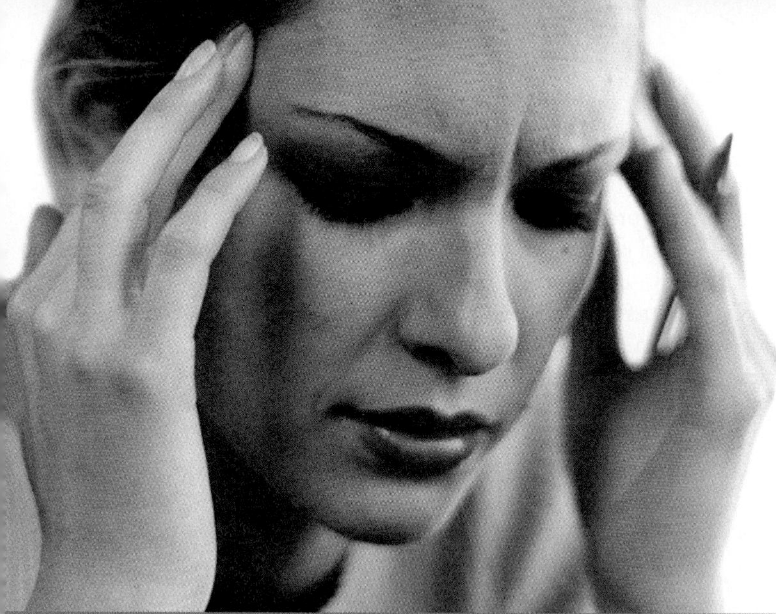

I've been through a lot. But this is starting to get to me. I can't stop coughing, I can't sleep, my head hurts. I thought I had a 'summer cold' but this just drags on. I'm 49 years old and feel like a baby but I need some relief!

Patient "Nancy Williams"

CHAPTER 74

Pharmacotherapy of Allergic Rhinitis and the Common Cold

Chapter Outline

Physiology of the Upper Respiratory Tract

Pathophysiology of Allergic Rhinitis

Pharmacotherapy of Allergic Rhinitis

H_1-Receptor Antagonists (Antihistamines)

PROTOTYPE **Fexofenadine (Allegra)** *p. 1267*

Intranasal Corticosteroids

PROTOTYPE **Fluticasone (Flonase)** *p. 1270*

Mast Cell Stabilizers

Decongestants

PROTOTYPE **Pseudoephedrine (Sudafed)** *p. 1273*

Drugs for the Common Cold

Antitussives

PROTOTYPE **Dextromethorphan (Robitussin, Sucrets, Others)** *p. 1275*

Expectorants and Mucolytics

Learning Outcomes

After reading this chapter, the student should be able to:

1. Identify structures of the upper respiratory tract that serve as body defenses against foreign substances.
2. Describe the common causes and symptoms of allergic rhinitis.
3. Differentiate between H_1 and H_2 histamine receptors.
4. Compare and contrast the first- and second-generation antihistamines.
5. Explain why intranasal corticosteroids are the drugs of choice for the treatment of allergic rhinitis.
6. Compare and contrast the oral and intranasal decongestants.
7. Explain why it is usually better to take individual drugs for the common cold, rather than a multisymptom combination product.
8. Describe the appropriate and inappropriate use of cough suppressants.
9. Describe the use of drugs prescribed to treat thick bronchial secretions.
10. For each of the classes shown in the chapter outline, identify the prototype and representative drugs and explain the mechanism(s) of drug action, primary indications, contraindications, significant drug interactions, pregnancy category, and important adverse effects.
11. Use the nursing process to care for patients who are receiving pharmacotherapy for allergic rhinitis and the common cold.

Key Terms

allergen, 1263
allergic rhinitis, 1263
antitussives, 1275
expectorants, 1277
H_1 receptors, 1264
mast cell stabilizers, 1271
mucolytics, 1277
rebound congestion, 1271

The respiratory system begins at the nose and mouth and ends at the pulmonary capillaries. The pharmacotherapy of asthma and chronic obstructive pulmonary disease (COPD), which are conditions of the lower respiratory tract, are discussed in Chapter 73. This chapter examines the drugs used for two conditions that are primarily associated with the upper respiratory tract: allergic rhinitis and nasal congestion with cough (common cold). Because many of these drugs are readily available over-the-counter (OTC), it is essential for the nurse to provide effective teaching for these agents.

Physiology of the Upper Respiratory Tract

74.1 The upper respiratory tract acts as a defense in preventing systemic infection.

The upper respiratory tract (URT) consists of the nose, nasal cavity, pharynx, and paranasal sinuses. These passageways filter, warm, and humidify air during inhalation. The URT traps particulate matter and many pathogens, preventing them from being carried to the bronchioles and alveoli, where they would have access to the capillaries of the systemic circulation. The mucous membranes of the URT are lined with ciliated epithelium. The cilia projecting from the epithelium are found throughout the nasal passages and help to trap smaller particles. The cilia have a wave-like motion that "sweeps" the pathogens and particulate matter upward toward the oropharynx, where it is swallowed when a person coughs or clears the throat. A sneeze clears the nasal passages. The basic structures of the upper respiratory system are shown in Figure 74.1.

The nasal mucosa is a dynamic structure richly supplied with vascular tissue that is controlled, in part, by the autonomic nervous system. Activation of the sympathetic nervous system constricts the arterioles in the nose, reducing the thickness of the mucosal layer. This serves to widen the airway and allow air to more freely enter the URT. Parasympathetic activation has the opposite effect: The arterioles dilate and more mucus is produced. This difference is important in therapy with drugs affecting the autonomic nervous system. For example, administration of a sympathomimetic will shrink the nasal mucosa, relieving nasal stuffiness associated with the common cold. These agents are classified as decongestants. On the other hand, parasympathetic agents cause increased blood flow to the nose with increased nasal stuffiness and a runny nose as adverse effects.

The oral mucosa serves an important role in body defenses against invasion by microbes. Saliva contains immunoglobulins (IgA) and lysozyme, which break down bacterial cell walls. Swallowed saliva or nasal mucus exposes microorganisms to the hostile environment of the stomach where they contact high gastric acidity and enzymes that kill them.

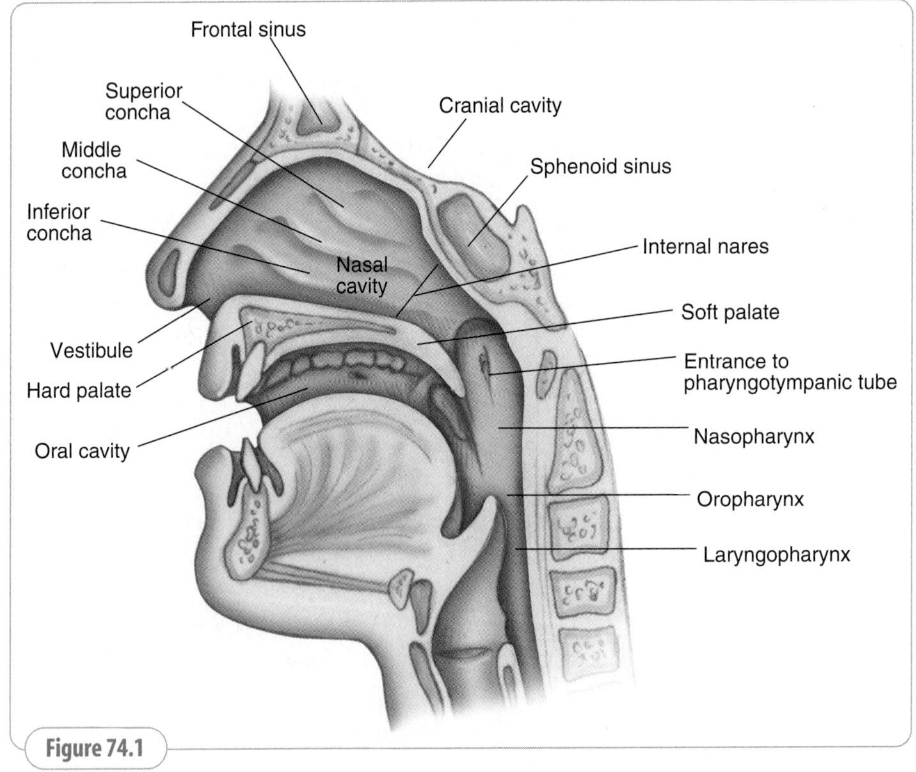

Figure 74.1

The respiratory system.
Source: From *Medical Terminology with Human Anatomy* (5th ed., p. 292), by J. Rice, 2005. Reprinted by permission of Pearson Education, Inc., Upper Saddle River, NJ.

The nasal mucosa is also a first line of immunologic defense, secreting up to a quart of mucus daily. This fluid is rich in immunoglobulins that are able to neutralize airborne pathogens. The nasal mucosa contains numerous nonspecific body defense cells that can activate complement or engulf microbes. Mast cells, which contain histamine, also line the nasal mucosa, and these play a major role in causing the symptoms of allergic rhinitis.

Pathophysiology of Allergic Rhinitis

74.2 Allergic rhinitis is caused by exposure to an environmental allergen, which leads to symptoms that resemble those of the common cold.

Allergic rhinitis is inflammation of the nasal mucosa due to exposure to allergens. Although not life threatening, allergic rhinitis is a condition that affects millions of people and one that is a common indication for pharmacotherapy.

Sometimes called hay fever, the symptoms of allergic rhinitis resemble those of the common cold such as tearing, burning, red, swollen, or itching eyes; sneezing; nasal itching or congestion; postnasal drip; cough; and scratchy throat. In addition to the acute symptoms, complications of allergic rhinitis may include loss of taste or smell, sinusitis, hoarseness, and plugged ears. Some people may not obtain restful sleep and awaken very fatigued. Symptoms can be severe enough to cause poor performance in or absence from school or work. Because of the smaller size of their anatomic structures children are also at increased risk for middle ear infections.

As with other allergies, the cause of allergic rhinitis is exposure to an antigen. An antigen, also called an **allergen,** is anything that is recognized as foreign by the body's defense system. The specific allergen responsible for a patient's allergic rhinitis is often difficult to pinpoint; however, common agents are pollens from weeds, grasses, and trees; mold spores; dust mites; certain foods; and animal dander (skin flakes). Chemical fumes, tobacco smoke, or air pollutants such as ozone are nonallergenic factors that may worsen symptoms. In addition, there is a strong genetic predisposition to allergic rhinitis.

> **Pharm*FACT***
>
> Allergic rhinitis affects 20% of adults and 40% of children. Allergic rhinitis and asthma are the two leading causes of absenteeism due to chronic illness. *Source:* American Academy of Allergy, Asthma, and Immunology, n.d.

Some patients experience symptoms of allergic rhinitis at specific times of the year such as when pollen is at high levels in their environment. These periods are typically in the spring and fall when plants and trees are blooming, thus the name *seasonal* allergic rhinitis. Obviously, the "blooming" season changes with geographic location and with each species of plant. These patients may need symptom relief for only a few months during the year. Others are afflicted with allergic rhinitis symptoms throughout the year because they are continuously exposed to indoor allergens, such as dust mites, animal dander, or mold. This variation is termed *perennial* allergic rhinitis. These patients may require a treatment plan that includes continuous pharmacotherapy.

It is often not clear whether a patient is experiencing seasonal or perennial allergic rhinitis. Patients with seasonal allergies may also be sensitive to some of the perennial allergens. It is also common for one allergen to "sensitize" patients to another allergen. For example, during ragweed season, a patient may become hyperresponsive to other allergens such as mold spores or animal dander. The body's response and the symptoms of allergic rhinitis are the same, however, regardless of the specific allergen(s). Allergy testing can help pinpoint the particular allergens responsible for the symptoms and help direct a treatment plan that includes avoiding allergens that cause the symptoms and treating the symptoms.

The fundamental pathophysiology responsible for allergic rhinitis is inflammation of the mucous membranes in the nose, throat, and airways. The nasal mucosa is rich with mast cells (a type of connective tissue cell) and basophils (a type of leukocyte), both of which synthesize and store histamine. The release of histamine and other compounds such as leukotrienes occurs after a patient has been exposed to specific allergens. The allergen stimulates the production of high amounts of immunoglobulin E (IgE) antibodies. The IgE antibodies then bind to the outer surface of mast cells and basophils, thus sensitizing them. Sometime later when reexposed to the antigen (pollen, etc.) the antigen attaches to the antibody and the antigen–antibody reaction begins. This reaction stimulates a process that begins by mobilizing intracellular calcium and, eventually, the sensitized cells release chemical mediators, including histamine. In certain cases, histamine can be released from mast cells without prior exposure to an antigen (allergen). These nonallergic releases of histamine can occur with cell damage, certain drugs, plasma expanders, or radiographic contrast media.

Patients with allergic rhinitis have greater numbers of mast cells. An immediate (or Type I) hypersensitivity response releases histamine and other chemical mediators such as leukotrienes and prostaglandins from the mast cells and basophils. The body's response to the chemical mediators is to cause vasodilation of arterioles and venules, increase capillary permeability, constrict smooth muscle (bronchioles), increase secretions of glands such as the lacrimals, and act as a neurotransmitter in the central nervous system (CNS). All this, in the case of allergic rhinitis, produces flushing of the skin, sneezing, itching nasal membranes, and watery eyes and can cause drowsiness. A delayed hypersensitivity reaction also occurs 4 to 8 hours after the initial exposure, causing continuous inflammation of the mucosa and adding to the chronic nasal congestion experienced from the allergic response. Because histamine is released during an allergic response, many signs and symptoms of allergy are similar to those of inflammation (see Chapter 44). The mechanism of allergic rhinitis is illustrated in Figure 74.2.

Pharmacotherapy of Allergic Rhinitis

74.3 Drugs for allergic rhinitis include those that prevent the disorder and those that relieve symptoms.

The therapeutic goals of treating allergic rhinitis are to prevent its occurrence and to relieve symptoms. Drugs that are used to

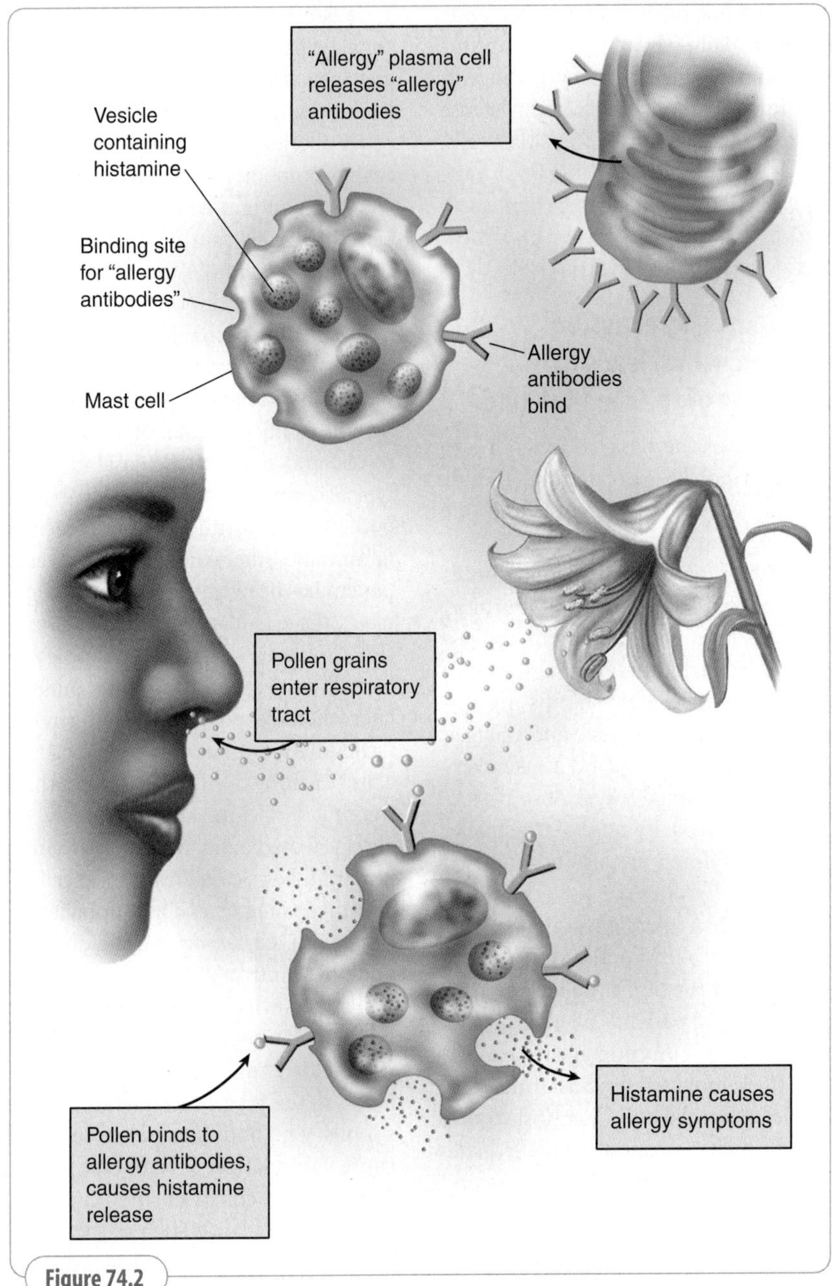

Figure 74.2
Allergic rhinitis.

treat allergic rhinitis may thus be grouped into two simple categories: preventers and relievers.

- Preventers are used for prophylaxis. These include antihistamines, intranasal corticosteroids, and mast cell stabilizers.
- Relievers are used to provide immediate, though temporary, relief for acute allergy symptoms once they have occurred. Relievers include the oral and intranasal decongestants, which usually are drugs from the sympathomimetic class.

In addition to treating allergic rhinitis with drugs, nurses should help patients identify the sources of the allergy and recommend appropriate actions. These may include removing pets from the home environment or limiting their exposure (such as not allowing the pet on furniture); cleaning moldy surfaces; using and routinely cleaning or replacing microfilters on air-conditioning units; and frequent cleaning to remove dust mites from bedding, carpet, or furniture. Although dust mites can never be totally removed from mattresses, regularly decreasing their numbers can help lessen symptoms of allergic rhinitis. It may be interesting to know that dust mites feed primarily on naturally shedding human skin and that it is not the microscopic dust mite itself that a patient inhales and is allergic to, but rather its excrement.

74.4 Antihistamines are widely used to treat allergic rhinitis and other minor allergies.

There are two types of receptors for histamine: H_1 and H_2. The **H_1 receptors** are responsible for producing the typical symptoms of allergy. H_1-receptor antagonists, also called *antihistamines,* are drugs that selectively block histamine from reaching its H_1 receptors, thus alleviating allergic symptoms. Because the term antihistamine is nonspecific and does not indicate which of the two histamine receptors are affected, H_1-receptor antagonist (or blocker) is a more accurate name. In clinical practice, as well as in this text, the two terms are used interchangeably.

Antihistamines that selectively block H_1 receptors are widely used as OTC remedies for the relief of allergy symptoms, motion sickness, and insomnia. Antihistamine agents are listed in Table 74.1.

Drugs that block H_2 receptors such as ranitidine (Zantac) reduce gastric acid secretion and are used to treat peptic ulcer disease and gastroesophageal reflux disease. This histamine receptor activity is not related to allergic responses and is covered in Chapter 60.

The most frequent therapeutic use of antihistamines is for the treatment of allergies. These medications provide symptomatic relief from the characteristic sneezing, runny nose, and itching of the eyes, nose, and throat of allergic rhinitis. Antihistamines are often combined with decongestants and antitussives in OTC cold and sinus medicines. Common OTC antihistamine combinations that are used to treat allergies are listed in Table 74.2.

Antihistamines are most effective when taken prophylactically to prevent allergic symptoms. Their effectiveness in reversing allergic symptoms is limited. This is because antihistamines block the effect of histamine at their receptor sites. They do not prevent the release of histamine from mast cells. Their effectiveness may diminish with long-term use.

In addition to producing antihistamine effects, these drugs also easily cross the blood–brain barrier and block cholinergic receptors to cause typical anticholinergic effects. Anticholinergic effects are responsible for certain beneficial effects of antihistamines, such as drying of mucous membranes, which results in less nasal congestion and tearing.

A large number of H_1-receptor antagonists are available as medications. They all have the same basic mechanism of action and are equally effective in treating allergic rhinitis and other mild allergies. Adverse effects are similar but differ in intensity among the various antihistamines. The older, first-generation antihistamines frequently cause significant drowsiness, which can be a limiting adverse effect in some patients. After a few doses tolerance generally develops to this sedative action. The newer, second-generation antihistamines have less tendency to cause sedation because they do not cross the blood–brain barrier. Alcohol and other CNS depressants should be used with caution when taking antihistamines, because their sedating effects may be additive, even for the second-generation agents. Some patients (especially young children) exhibit CNS stimulation, which can cause insomnia, nervousness, and tremors, or even convulsions. There are other CNS adverse effects such as

TABLE 74.1 H_1-Receptor Antagonists

Drug	Route and Adult Dose (maximum dose where indicated)	Adverse Effects
First-Generation Agents		
azelastine (Astelin, Optivar)	Intranasal: 2 sprays per nostril every 12 h Ocular: 1 drop in each affected eye bid	*Dry mouth, headache, dizziness, urinary retention, thickening of bronchial secretions, nausea, vomiting*
brompheniramine (Dimetapp, others)	PO: 4–8 mg every 4–6 h (max: 40 mg/day)	Paradoxical excitation (usually in children), sedation, hypersensitivity reactions, hypotension, extrapyramidal symptoms (promethazine), agranulocytosis (brompheniramine, promethazine, clemastine)
chlorpheniramine (Chlor-Trimeton, others)	PO: 2–4 mg every 4–6 h (max: 24 mg/day)	
clemastine (Tavist)	PO: 1.34–2.68 mg every 12 h (max: 8.04 mg/day)	
cyproheptadine	PO: 4–20 mg every 6–8 h (max: 0.5 mg/kg/day)	
dexbrompheniramine (Drixoral)	PO: 6 mg bid (max: 12 mg/day)	
dexchlorpheniramine (Dexchlor, Poladex, Polaramine)	PO: 2 mg every 4–6 h (max: 12 mg/day)	
dimenhydrinate (Dramamine)	PO: 50–100 mg every 4 h	
diphenhydramine (Benadryl, others)	PO: 25–50 mg every 6–8 h (max: 300 mg/day)	
promethazine (Phenergan)	PO: 12.5–25 g every 6–24 h (max: 100 mg/day)	
triprolidine (Zymine)	PO: 2.5 mg every 4–6 h (max: 10 mg/day)	
Second-Generation Agents		
cetirizine (Zyrtec)	PO: 5–10 mg/day (max: 10 mg/day)	*Dry mouth, headache, dizziness, nausea, drowsiness (cetirizine), bitter taste (olopatadine)*
desloratadine (Clarinex)	PO: 5 mg/day (max: 5 mg/day)	Paradoxical excitation, hypersensitivity reactions, hypotension
fexofenadine (Allegra)	PO: 60 mg every 12 h or 180 mg once daily	
levocetirizine (Xyzal)	PO: 5 mg (1 tablet or 2 teaspoons) once daily	
loratadine (Claritin)	PO: 10 mg/day (max: 10 mg/day)	
olopatadine (Patanase)	Intranasal: 2 sprays per nostril bid	

Note: *Italics* indicate common adverse effects. Underline indicates serious adverse effects.

MyNursingKit | Mechanism of Action Animation: Diphenhydramine

TABLE 74.2 Selected Over-the-Counter Antihistamine Combinations

Brand Name	Antihistamine	Decongestant	Analgesic
Actifed Cold and Allergy tablets	chlorpheniramine	phenylephrine	—
Actifed Cold and Sinus	chlorpheniramine	pseudoephedrine	acetaminophen
Benadryl Allergy/Cold caplets	diphenhydramine	phenylephrine	acetaminophen
Chlor-Trimeton Allergy/Decongestant tablets	chlorpheniramine	pseudoephedrine	—
Dimetapp Children's Cold and Allergy	brompheniramine	phenylephrine	—
Sudafed PE Sinus and Allergy tablets	chlorpheniramine	phenylephrine	—
Sudafed PE Nighttime Cold	diphenhydramine	phenylephrine	acetaminophen
Tavist Allergy tablets	clemastine	—	—
Triaminic Cold/Allergy	chlorpheniramine	phenylephrine	—
Tylenol Allergy Multi-Symptom Gels	chlorpheniramine	phenylephrine	acetaminophen
Tylenol PM Gelcaps	diphenhydramine	—	acetaminophen

dizziness, confusion, and even fatigue, which more commonly affect the elderly.

The second major adverse effect of antihistamines relates to their anticholinergic effects. Excessive drying of mucous membranes can lead to dry mouth, and urinary hesitancy may be troublesome for patients, especially those with prostatic hyperplasia. Some antihistamines produce more pronounced anticholinergic effects than others. Diphenhydramine and clemastine produce the greatest incidence of anticholinergic adverse effects, whereas the second-generation agents—loratadine, desloratadine, and fexofenadine—produce the least.

Although most antihistamines are given via the oral route (PO), azelastine (Astelin) was the first to be available by the intranasal route. Azelastine is as effective as the PO antihistamines. Although a first-generation agent, azelastine causes less drowsiness than others in its class because it is applied locally to the nasal mucosa, and limited systemic absorption occurs. This may make azelastine slightly safer than PO antihistamines.

Antihistamines are used as adjuncts to the emergency treatment of anaphylaxis, which is the most severe form of allergic reaction. Although massive histamine release causes bronchoconstriction, edema, hypotension, and other symptoms of anaphylaxis, other inflammatory mediators, including leukotrienes and prostaglandins, contribute to the hypersensitivity response. Because antihistamines do not block these other mediators, antihistamines are only effective as adjunctive therapy in anaphylaxis. They are most effective if given as preventive medications before anaphylaxis for patients who are at high risk to an allergic response. The major life-threatening symptoms of anaphylaxis are controlled with epinephrine and other vasoconstrictors.

H_1-receptor antagonists are effective in treating a number of other disorders, including the following:

- **Vertigo and motion sickness.** Nausea resulting from vertigo or motion sickness responds well to antihistamines. These drugs act by suppressing the vomiting center in the medulla and depressing the excitability of the neurons of the vestibular apparatus of the inner ear. To be effective, they must be taken prior to the onset of symptoms. Meclizine (Antivert) and dimenhydrinate (Dramamine) are the two most common antihistamines used for this purpose. Cyclizine (Marezine) is another older antihistamine that is occasionally used to reduce nausea and vertigo. The pharmacotherapy of nausea is discussed in Chapter 61.
- **Parkinson's disease.** Drugs with significant anticholinergic actions are used to treat mild forms of Parkinson's disease. They are also used to treat the tremor and extrapyramidal adverse effects from conventional antipsychotic drugs. Because diphenhydramine exerts great amounts of anticholinergic action, it is sometimes used to treat these conditions.
- **Insomnia.** Many patients become drowsy after taking first-generation antihistamines. OTC sleep aids usually include antihistamines such as diphenhydramine and doxylamine (Unisom Sleep Tabs). After a few days, patients will become tolerant to the drowsiness produced by these drugs; thus they should be used for 2 weeks or less.
- **Urticaria and other skin rashes.** Urticaria or hives is often caused by the release of histamine, and the condition responds well to H_1-receptor blockers. Symptomatic treatment may include any of the first- or second-generation agents, either using PO drugs or topical creams or lotions.

CONNECTION Checkpoint 74.1

Although drugs with anticholinergic action are used to treat Parkinson's disease, they are generally not the drugs of choice. From what you learned in Chapter 25, name the drug most commonly prescribed for Parkinson's disease and the neurotransmitter it replaces. See Answer to Connection Checkpoint 74.1 in Appendix A.

CONNECTIONS

Lifespan Considerations Antihistamines

The elderly generally have a heightened response to antihistamines. This is partly because older adults have decreased cardiac output which causes decreased flow to the liver and kidneys. Elderly patients should be monitored for excessive sedation and altered consciousness because these may contribute to falls or other injuries. Older patients experience a higher incidence of dizziness and confusion when taking these drugs. Use antihistamines with caution in elderly male patients with benign prostatic hyperplasia. They can worsen urinary symptoms by preventing muscles in the prostate and bladder neck from relaxing to allow urine to flow freely.

First-generation antihistamines such as diphenhydramine (Benadryl) remain popular for the treatment of seasonal allergic rhinitis, dermatitis, and urticaria in pediatric patients. However, second generation antihistamines are better for these patients for several reasons. With the less frequent dosing schedule of the second generation agents, administration of the medication is much easier for the parents. Additionally, with less sedation and lower risk of adverse effects, the safety profile of second generation agents appears superior.

PROTOTYPE DRUG Fexofenadine (Allegra)

Classification: **Therapeutic:** Drug for allergic rhinitis and minor allergies

Pharmacologic: H_1-receptor antagonist (second generation), antihistamine

Therapeutic Effects and Uses: Approved in 1996 for the treatment of allergic rhinitis, fexofenadine is a second-generation H_1-receptor antagonist with an effectiveness that is equivalent to that of diphenhydramine. Most effective when taken before symptoms develop, fexofenadine reduces the severity of nasal congestion, sneezing, and tearing of the eyes.

The long half-life of fexofenadine, over 14 hours, allows it to be administered once or twice daily. Fexofenadine is available in PO form as regular tablets, orally disintegrating tablets, and as a suspension. In addition to allergic rhinitis, it is also approved to treat chronic idiopathic urticaria. Allegra-D combines fexofenadine with pseudoephedrine, which is a decongestant.

Mechanism of Action: Fexofenadine acts by competing with histamine for binding to histamine (H_1) receptor sites. It does not prevent the release of histamine.

Pharmacokinetics:

Route(s)	PO (capsules, tablets, and suspension)
Absorption	Rapid
Distribution	Does not cross the blood–brain barrier; unknown if secreted in breast milk; 60–70% bound to plasma protein
Primary metabolism	Hepatic
Primary excretion	80% renal, 11% feces
Onset of action	Usually within 1 h
Duration of action	Half-life: 14.4 h; duration: 12–24 h

Adverse Effects: The major advantage of fexofenadine over first-generation antihistamines is that it does not readily cross the blood–brain barrier, so drowsiness is generally not a major adverse effect. Adverse effects are infrequent and usually minor and include headache, nausea, dyspepsia, and dysmenorrhea. Patients who are taking the drug have an increased incidence of viral infections. Anticholinergic effects such as dry mouth can occur in some patients.

Contraindications/Precautions: The only contraindication to fexofenadine is hypersensitivity to this drug. Patients with advanced renal disease should receive reduced doses.

Drug Interactions: Although considered "nonsedating," fexofenadine can still cause drowsiness in certain patients at high doses and if combined with CNS depressants, including alcohol. Concurrent administration with ketoconazole or erythromycin increases the plasma concentrations of fexofenadine. Prolongation of the QT interval has occurred with other antihistamines but is infrequent with fexofenadine. Antacids that contain aluminum or magnesium may interfere with the absorption of fexofenadine. **Herbal/Food**: Absorption may be decreased when taken with grapefruit, orange, or apple juice, thereby reducing the bioavailability of fexofenadine.

Pregnancy: Category C.

Treatment of Overdose: Overdose may cause CNS depression, dry mouth, and dizziness. There is no specific antidote for overdose, and supportive treatment of symptoms is indicated.

Nursing Responsibilities:

- Prior to initiation of therapy, assess for a history of allergy and the presence of symptoms such as urticaria, angioedema, nausea, vomiting, motion sickness, conjunctivitis, or excess mucus production.
- Prior to the initiation of therapy, obtain a history from the patient, screening for any contraindication or precautionary condition such as renal impairment, pregnancy, or breast-feeding.
- When administering any antihistamine for the first time to patients with a history of heart disease, obtain baseline vital signs and an electrocardiogram (ECG) to detect dysrhythmias. Antihistamines are used with caution in patients with a history of dysrhythmias, heart failure, and hypertension (HTN) because they cause vasodilation due to H_1-receptor stimulation.

Patient and Family Education:

- Do not take other OTC cold, allergy, or sinus medications unless approved by the health care provider.

- Do not drive or perform other hazardous activities until the effects of the drug are known because this drug may cause drowsiness or dizziness.
- Do not consume alcohol while taking antihistamines because of the additive effects that can cause drowsiness.
- Contact the health care provider if symptom improvement does not occur within 2 to 3 weeks.
- Do not breast-feed while taking this drug without approval of the health care provider.
- Immediately notify the health care provider of any known or suspected pregnancy.
- Do not drink grapefruit, apple, or orange juice within 1 hour of taking fexofenadine. Do not eat any of these fruits within 1 hour of taking the medicine.
- Stop taking this drug at least 4 days prior to skin allergy tests; otherwise, false-negative readings may result.

Drugs Similar to Fexofenadine (Allegra)

The second-generation H_1 antagonists include cetirizine, desloratadine, and loratadine. Because the first-generation antihistamines are all very similar, a description of diphenhydramine is included next as an example of this group.

Cetirizine (Zyrtec): Approved in 1995, cetirizine is a second-generation antihistamine that is commonly used for treating allergic rhinitis and itching due to hives. It is used off-label to treat atopic dermatitis and symptoms of allergy-induced asthma. Various PO formulations are available, including tablets to be swallowed, chewable tablets, and syrup. It is well tolerated and approved for children as young as 2 years of age. Adverse effects are uncommon. Cetirizine appears to be somewhat more sedating than other second-generation agents. Xerostomia and fatigue are additional adverse effects. The drug was moved from prescription to OTC status in 2007. Cetirizine is an active metabolite of hydroxyzine (Atarax, Vistaril), a first-generation antihistamine. This drug is pregnancy category B.

In 2007, an isomer of cetirizine was approved by the U.S. Food and Drug Administration (FDA). Levocetirizine (Xyzal) is an PO antihistamine that has the same indications and actions as those of cetirizine but is reported to cause less drowsiness.

Desloratadine (Clarinex): Desloratadine is a nonsedating, second-generation antihistamine that was approved in 2001 for the treatment of allergic rhinitis and itching due to hives. It is the active metabolite of loratadine (Claritin). Desloratadine is administered by the PO route and is approved to treat children 6 months and older. Like other second-generation drugs, sedation is minimal and adverse effects are uncommon. Headache, pharyngitis, and xerostomia are the most frequently reported adverse effects. This drug is pregnancy category C.

Diphenhydramine (Benadryl): Diphenhydramine is a first-generation H_1-receptor antagonist that is commonly used to treat minor symptoms of allergy and the common cold such as sneezing, runny nose, and tearing of the eyes. It exhibits a strong anticholinergic drying action on mucous membranes. OTC diphenhydramine is often combined with an analgesic, decongestant, or expectorant when treating cold symptoms. Diphenhydramine is also used as a topical agent to treat rashes, and intramuscular (IM) and intravenous (IV) forms are available for severe allergic reactions. An elixir and syrup form is available for administration to young children. Other indications for diphenhydramine include Parkinson's disease, motion sickness, and insomnia. Diphenhydramine can cause significant drowsiness, although this usually diminishes with long-term use. Occasionally diphenhydramine is given to produce drowsiness as a treatment for insomnia. This drug may cause paradoxical excitement in some patients, which is an effect most commonly seen in children who are receiving diphenhydramine. This drug may cause anticholinergic adverse effects such as urinary retention, tachycardia, and elevated blood pressure, xerostomia, thickening of bronchial secretions, and blurred vision. This drug is pregnancy category B.

Loratadine (Claritin): Loratadine was the first of the second-generation antihistamines that was approved in 1993 to treat allergic rhinitis and itching due to hives. In 2002, the high safety record of loratadine led to the reclassification of the drug from prescription to OTC. Like other drugs in its class, loratadine causes very little drowsiness, and adverse effects are unusual. It is only available PO and may be administered to children age 2 and older. Drowsiness and headache may occur at higher doses. This drug is pregnancy category C.

74.5 Intranasal corticosteroids are the drugs of choice for allergic rhinitis because of their effectiveness and safety.

Corticosteroids, also known as glucocorticoids, may be applied directly to the nasal mucosa to prevent symptoms of allergic rhinitis. These drugs are listed in Table 74.3.

Although corticosteroids are very effective at reducing allergy symptoms, their oral and parenteral uses are limited by potentially serious adverse effects. Intranasal formulations of these drugs, however, produce virtually no serious adverse effects. Because of their effectiveness and safety, the intranasal corticosteroids have joined antihistamines as first-line drugs in the treatment of allergic rhinitis. They are now considered the most effective drug treatment for allergic and perennial rhinitis. Intranasal corticosteroids are also used for patients undergoing nasal or sinus surgery for their anti-inflammatory action.

When sprayed onto the nasal mucosa, corticosteroids act by multiple mechanisms. They decrease the secretion of inflammatory mediators, reduce tissue edema, and cause a mild vasoconstriction. All agents are administered with a metered-spray device that delivers a consistent dose of drug per spray. All have equal effectiveness. Unlike sympathomimetics, however, the benefits of inhaled corticosteroids are not immediate. To achieve peak response, 1 to 3 weeks (often longer with perennial rhinitis than seasonal rhinitis) may be required. After the patient's symptoms are controlled, the dose of intranasal corticosteroids is reduced to the lowest amount required to control the symptoms. The intranasal corticosteroids must be taken daily to produce maximum benefit.

When administered consistently, the actions of corticosteroids are limited to the nasal passages. The most frequently

NURSING PROCESS APPLICATION

Patients Receiving Antihistamine Therapy

Assessment	Potential Nursing Diagnoses
Prior to administration: • Obtain a complete health history, including information on asthma, cardiac disease, allergies, drug history, and possible drug interactions. • Obtain an ECG and vital signs; assess in the context of the patient's baseline values. • Assess respiratory status, especially breathing pattern. • Assess neurologic status and level of consciousness (LOC).	• *Ineffective Airway Clearance* • *Ineffective Breathing Pattern*

Planning: Patient Goals and Expected Outcomes

The patient will:

- Report a reduction in symptoms related to the allergic rhinitis nasal congestion.
- Accurately describe drug adverse effects and precautions.

Implementation: Antihistamines

Interventions and (Rationales)	Patient and Family Education
• Auscultate breath sounds before administering to rule out lower respiratory problems. Use with extreme caution in patients with asthma or COPD. Keep resuscitative equipment accessible. (Anticholinergic effects of antihistamines may trigger bronchospasm.)	• Instruct the patient to immediately report wheezing or difficulty breathing. • Advise patients with asthma to consult the nurse regarding the use of injectable epinephrine in emergency situations.
• Monitor vital signs (including the ECG in patients with a history of dysrhythmias) before administering. Use with extreme caution in patients with a history of cardiovascular disease. (Anticholinergic effects can increase heart rate and lower blood pressure. Fatal dysrhythmias and cardiovascular collapse have been reported in some patients who are receiving antihistamines.)	Instruct the patient to: • Immediately report dizziness, palpitations; headache; or chest, arm, or back pain, accompanied by nausea, vomiting, or sweating. • Monitor vital signs daily in patients who have cardiac issues, ensuring the proper use of home equipment.
• Monitor thyroid function. Use with caution in patients with a history of hyperthyroidism. (Antihistamines may exacerbate the CNS-stimulating effects of hyperthyroidism and may trigger a thyroid storm.)	• Instruct the patient to immediately report nervousness or restlessness, insomnia, fever, profuse sweating, thirst, or mood changes.
• Monitor for vision changes. Use with caution in patients with narrow-angle glaucoma. (Antihistamines can increase intraocular pressure and cause photosensitivity.)	Instruct the patient to: • Immediately report head or eye pain and visual changes. • Wear dark glasses, use sunscreen, and avoid excessive sun exposure.
• Monitor neurologic status, especially LOC. Use with caution in patients with a history of seizure disorder. (Antihistamines lower the seizure threshold. The elderly are at increased risk of serious sedation and other anticholinergic effects.)	Instruct the patient to: • Immediately report seizure activity, including any changes in character and pattern of seizures. • Avoid driving or performing other hazardous activities until the effects of the drug are known.
• Observe for signs of renal toxicity. Measure intake and output. Use with caution in patients with a history of kidney or urinary tract disease. (Antihistamines promote urine retention.)	• Instruct the patient to immediately report flank pain, difficulty urinating, reduced urine output, or changes in the appearance of urine (cloudy, with sediment or odor).
• Use with caution in patients with diabetes mellitus. Monitor serum glucose levels with increased frequency (e.g., from daily to tid, before meals). (Antihistamines may decrease serum glucose levels.)	Instruct the patient to: • Immediately report symptoms of hypoglycemia. • Consult the health care provider regarding timing of glucose monitoring and reportable results (e.g., "less than 70 mg/dL").
• Monitor for gastrointestinal (GI) adverse effects. Use with caution in patients with a history of GI disorders, especially peptic ulcers or liver disease. (These drugs are metabolized in the liver, increasing the risk of hepatotoxicity.)	Instruct the patient to: • Immediately report nausea, vomiting, anorexia, bleeding, chest or abdominal pain, heartburn, jaundice, or a change in the color or character of stools. • Avoid substances that irritate the stomach such as spicy foods, alcoholic beverages, and nicotine; take the drug with food to avoid stomach upset.
• Monitor for adverse effects such as dry mouth; observe for signs of anticholinergic crisis. (Report adverse effects to the health care provider.)	Instruct the patient to: • Immediately report fever or flushing accompanied by difficulty swallowing ("cotton mouth"), blurred vision, and confusion. • Avoid mixing OTC antihistamines; always consult the health care provider before taking any OTC drugs or herbal supplements. • Suck on sugar-free hard candy to relieve dry mouth, and maintain adequate fluid intake.

Evaluation of Outcome Criteria

Evaluate the effectiveness of drug therapy by confirming that patient goals and expected outcomes have been met (see "Planning").

TABLE 74.3 Intranasal Corticosteroids and Miscellaneous Drugs for Allergic Rhinitis

Drug	Route and Adult Dose (maximum dose where indicated)	Adverse Effects
Intranasal Corticosteroids		
beclomethasone (Beconase AQ, QVAR)	Intranasal: 1 spray bid-qid	*Transient nasal irritation, burning, sneezing, dryness* Hypercorticism (only if large amounts are swallowed)
budesonide (Rhinocort Aqua)	Intranasal: 2 sprays bid	
ciclesonide (Omnaris)	Intranasal: 2 sprays once daily (max: 200 mcg/day)	
flunisolide (Nasalide, Nasarel)	Intranasal: 2 sprays bid; may increase to tid if needed	
fluticasone propionate (Flonase, Veramyst)	Intranasal: 1 spray in each nostril once (Veramyst) or twice (Flonase) daily	
mometasone furoate (Nasonex)	Intranasal: 2 sprays/day	
triamcinolone acetonide (Nasacort AQ)	Intranasal: 2–4 sprays 4 times daily	
Miscellaneous Agents		
cromolyn (NasalCrom)	Intranasal: 1 spray in each nostril tid-qid	*Nasal burning and irritation* Anaphylaxis
montelukast (Singulair)	PO: 10 mg/day	*Headache, nausea, diarrhea* No serious adverse effects

***Note:** Italics* indicate common adverse effects. Underline indicates serious adverse effects.

reported adverse effect is an intense burning sensation in the nose immediately after spraying. Excessive drying of the nasal mucosa may occur, leading to epistaxis (nosebleed).

CONNECTION *Checkpoint* 74.2

Withdrawal of oral or parenteral corticosteroids after long-term use may cause an adrenal crisis. From what you learned in Chapter 69, define *adrenal crisis* and explain its pathogenesis. See Answer to Connection Checkpoint 74.2 in Appendix A.

PROTOTYPE DRUG Fluticasone (Flonase)

Classification: Therapeutic: Agent for allergic rhinitis
Pharmacologic: Intranasal corticosteroid

Therapeutic Effects and Uses: Approved in 1990, fluticasone is an intranasal corticosteroid that is used for the management of nasal symptoms associated with seasonal and perennial rhinitis. Therapy usually begins with two sprays in each nostril, twice daily, and decreases to one dose per day. Prolonged use of corticosteroids can lead to tolerance to the drug's therapeutic effects.

Fluticasone is available in oral inhalation and topical formulations. The oral inhalation product (Flovent) is administered in a metered-dose inhaler (MDI) device for the treatment of asthma and COPD (see Chapter 73). Flovent reduces bronchial inflammation that is characteristic of asthma. Topical ointments and creams are applied to the skin for various inflammatory conditions, including atopic dermatitis, eczema, exfoliative dermatitis, psoriasis, and contact dermatitis (see Chapter 76).

Mechanism of Action: Fluticasone acts to decrease local inflammation in the nasal passages through vasoconstrictor and anti-inflammatory mechanisms. It is thought to inhibit mast cells, macrophages, and inflammatory mediators such as prostaglandins, histamine, kinins, and leukotrienes.

Pharmacokinetics:

Route(s)	Intranasal spray, oral inhalation, topical
Absorption	Intranasal: drug is swallowed, with less than 2% absorbed systemically Oral inhalation: 30% reaches systemic circulation Topical: minimal absorption
Distribution	Widely distributed; 91–99% bound to plasma protein
Primary metabolism	Hepatic, extensive first-pass metabolism by CYP3A4
Primary excretion	Feces
Onset of action	12 h to several days
Duration of action	Several days

Adverse Effects: When administered by the intranasal route, adverse effects of fluticasone are uncommon and include headache, epistaxis, and local burning. Swallowing large amounts increases the potential for systemic corticosteroid adverse effects (see Chapter 69).

Contraindications/Precautions: The only contraindication to fluticasone is prior hypersensitivity to the drug. Because corticosteroids can mask signs of infection, patients with known bacterial, viral, fungal, or parasitic infections (especially of the respiratory tract) should not receive these drugs until the infection has cleared. Safety has not been established in children under 4 years of age.

Drug Interactions: Concurrent use of fluticasone with an intranasal decongestant increases the risk of nasal irritation or bleeding. Use with ritonavir should be avoided, because this drug significantly increases plasma fluticasone levels. **Herbal/Food:** Use with caution with black licorice, which may potentiate the effects of corticosteroids.

Pregnancy: Category C.

Treatment of Overdose: Overdose with intranasal corticosteroids is unlikely. There is no specific treatment.

Nursing Responsibilities:

- Assess the nares for excoriation or bleeding prior to administering the corticosteroid nasal spray. Irritated mucous membranes allow direct access to the bloodstream, increasing the likelihood of systemic adverse effects.
- Do not administer intranasal corticosteroids to patients who have a history of hypersensitivity to any of the ingredients, including preservatives, in the nasal spray.
- Teach the proper technique for priming the drug delivery device as directed by printed instructions that accompany the medication.

Patient and Family Education:

- Carefully follow the directions for use provided by the manufacturer and do not take more than the recommended dose.
- Before the first dose, follow label instructions for priming the device to receive the entire dose of medication.
- Shake inhalers gently before spraying.
- Gently clear (blow) the nose before spraying. Avoid clearing the nose immediately after spraying.
- Avoid swallowing the medication. Spit out the postnasal medication residue and rinse the mouth.
- If a nasal decongestant spray is prescribed with this medication, administer the decongestant spray first to open the nasal passages. This allows the intranasal corticosteroid to be more effective.
- Be aware that it may take 2 to 3 weeks for this drug to reach maximum effectiveness.
- Report nosebleeds, nasal burning, or irritation that lasts more than a few doses to the health care provider.
- Use a humidifier or preservative-free nasal saline spray to ease nasal dryness.

Drugs Similar to Fluticasone (Flonase)

All of the intranasal corticosteroids have the same indications, actions, and adverse effects. Due to individual variation, some patients experience more irritation or burning with one agent over another. All are equally effective when administered at their recommended doses. The other intranasal corticosteroids are listed in Table 74.2.

74.6 Cromolyn and montelukast are alternatives to intranasal corticosteroids in the treatment of allergic rhinitis.

Mast cell stabilizers are drugs that inhibit the release of inflammatory mediators from mast cells. Mast cells contain granules that release histamine and leukotrienes during inflammatory and allergic reactions. Intranasal cromolyn (NasalCrom) is a mast cell stabilizer approved for the treatment of seasonal or perennial allergic rhinitis. Cromolyn is featured as a prototype in Chapter 73.

Most effective when given prior to allergen exposure, cromolyn has few adverse effects and is now designated as an OTC drug for the treatment of allergy and cold symptoms. It is just as effective as antihistamines but less effective than intranasal corticosteroids. This drug is very safe and adverse effects are uncommon. A major disadvantage is that cromolyn must be taken four times daily. If a patient suffers from nasal congestion, a topical decongestant is used prior to administration of cromolyn. When administered by the oral inhalation route cromolyn is approved for the treatment of asthma. A second mast cell stabilizer, called nedocromil (Tilade), is approved only for asthma.

Montelukast (Singulair) is an oral drug that acts by blocking leukotriene receptors. Leukotrienes are associated with inflammation and are responsible for some of the sneezing, nasal itching, and congestion characteristic of allergic rhinitis. Originally approved for the treatment of asthma in 1998, allergic rhinitis was added as an indication in 2003. It is approved for both the seasonal and perennial forms of the disease. Like cromolyn, montelukast is not considered as effective as the intranasal corticosteroids. This drug is well tolerated and produces few serious adverse effects. This drug is pregnancy category B.

CONNECTION *Checkpoint* 74.3

From what you learned in Chapter 73, what is the role of leukotriene antagonists in treating asthma? What drug classes are the drugs of choice for this condition? See Answer to Connection Checkpoint 74.3 in Appendix A.

Decongestants

74.7 Intranasal and oral sympathomimetics are the most effective agents for relieving nasal congestion.

Decongestants are drugs that relieve nasal congestion. They are administered by either the PO or intranasal routes and are often combined with antihistamines in the pharmacotherapy of allergies or the common cold.

Sympathomimetics with alpha-adrenergic activity are effective at relieving the nasal congestion associated with the common cold and allergic rhinitis when given by either the PO or intranasal route. The intranasal preparations such as oxymetazoline (Afrin, others) are available OTC as sprays or drops and produce a noticeable response within minutes. The nasal decongestants are listed in Table 74.4.

Intranasal sympathomimetics produce few systemic effects because only minimal amounts of these drugs are absorbed in the circulation. The most serious, limiting adverse effect of the intranasal preparations is **rebound congestion.** In almost all patients, prolonged use causes hypersecretion of mucus and worsening nasal congestion once the drug effects wear off. This leads to a cycle of increased drug use as the condition worsens to obtain the desired effect from these drugs. Because of this rebound congestion, intranasal sympathomimetics should be used for no longer than 3 to 5 days. Patients who develop dependence

NURSING PROCESS APPLICATION

Patients Receiving Intranasal Corticosteroid Therapy

Assessment	Potential Nursing Diagnoses
Prior to administration: • Obtain a complete health history, including allergies and a drug history. • Monitor the degree of allergic rhinitis symptoms, including nasal congestion, sneezing, and color and amount of nasal discharge.	• *Ineffective Health Maintenance,* related to allergic nasal congestion • *Deficient Knowledge, (Drug Therapy),* related to adverse effects and administration

Planning: Patient Goals and Expected Outcomes

The patient will:

- Report a reduction in symptoms related to the allergic rhinitis nasal congestion.
- Demonstrate the proper method to administer the intranasal drug.
- State the major adverse effects of the drug and what to report to the health care provider.
- State an understanding that the effects of the drug will not be seen for 2 to 3 weeks.
- State an understanding that the drug is for prevention of symptoms.

Implementation: Intranasal Corticosteroids

Interventions and (Rationales)	Patient and Family Education
• Monitor symptoms and anticipate a reduction in 2 to 3 weeks. (Peak response may require 1–3 weeks of therapy)	Instruct the patient to: • Monitor for a reduction in symptoms such as decreased sneezing, watery eyes, and increased ability to breathe nasally. • Report a lack of symptom reduction to the prescriber after consistent use for 3 weeks.
• Follow the drug administration procedure as specified on the drug packaging. (Various intranasal drug administration in devices require specific techniques.)	Follow the package insert for directions on administration, including: • Prime the inhaler prior to first use. • Shake the inhaler prior to each use. • Blow the nose (gently) prior to each use. • Insert the inhaler into the nare away from the septum. • Hold the other nare closed. • Inhale at the same time that the inhaler is depressed. • Repeat the process on the second nare. • If multiple sprays are required for the prescribed dose, alternate nares and wait at least 1–2 minutes between sprays. • The spray may cause nasal irritation. If the irritation continues, report it to the health care provider. • Do not exceed the maximum recommended dose. • Notify the health care provider if signs of infection occur or symptoms do not improve in 1 month. • Rinse the nosepiece in warm water (while holding it upside down to prevent water from entering the container) every day to help prevent bacterial growth. • Use the drug regularly, even if no symptoms are present.

Evaluation of Outcome Criteria

Evaluate the effectiveness of drug therapy by confirming that patient goals and expected outcomes have been met (see "Planning").

should be gradually switched to intranasal corticosteroids because they do not cause rebound congestion. The usual technique for switching to intranasal corticosteroids is by stopping the use of the decongestant in one nostril at a time.

When administered PO, sympathomimetics do not produce rebound congestion. Their onset of action by this route, however, is much slower than when administered intranasally, and they are less effective at relieving severe congestion. The possibility of systemic adverse effects is also greater with the PO drugs. Potential adverse effects include HTN and CNS stimulation that may lead to insomnia and anxiety. Pseudoephedrine and phenylephrine are common sympathomimetics found in oral OTC cold and allergy medicines.

The sympathomimetics relieve only nasal congestion and therefore are often combined with antihistamines to control sneezing and tearing. It is interesting to note that some OTC drugs having the same basic name (Neo-Synephrine, Afrin, and Vicks) may contain different sympathomimetics. For example, Neo-Synephrine decongestants with 12-hour duration contain the drug oxymetazoline; Neo-Synephrine preparations that last 4 to 6 hours contain phenylephrine.

One anticholinergic drug, ipratropium (Atrovent), is indicated for symptoms associated with perennial allergic rhinitis and the common cold. When given by the intranasal route, ipratropium has no serious adverse effects. Its actions are limited to decreasing nasal secretions; it does not stop the sneezing, postnasal drip, or itchy throat or eyes characteristic of allergic rhinitis or the common cold. A more common indication for ipratropium is in the pharmacotherapy of asthma, and a prototype feature for this drug may be found in Chapter 73.

TABLE 74.4 Nasal Decongestants

Drug	Route and Adult Dose (maximum dose where indicated)	Adverse Effects
Sympathomimetics		
ephedrine (Pretz-D)	Intranasal (0.25%): 2–3 sprays/nostril, not more frequently than every 4 h	*Intranasal: transient nasal irritation, burning, sneezing, or dryness, headache* *Oral: CNS stimulation: nervousness, insomnia, headache, dry mouth* Intranasal: rebound congestion Oral: CNS excitation (in people with coronary artery disease or HTN), tremors, dysrhythmias, tachycardia, difficulty in voiding, HTN and peripheral and visceral vasoconstriction
naphazoline (Privine)	Intranasal: 2 drops every 3–6 h	
oxymetazoline (Afrin 12 Hour, Neo-Synephrine 12 Hour, others)	Intranasal (0.05%): 2–3 sprays bid for up to 3 days	
phenylephrine (Afrin 4–6 Hour, Neo-Synephrine 4–6 Hour, others)	Intranasal (0.1%): 1–2 sprays or drop every 4 h, as needed, up to 3 days	
pseudoephedrine (Actifed, Sudafed, others)	PO: 30–60 mg 4–6 h (max: 240 mg/day) Sustained release: 120 mg every 12 h	
Tetrahydrozoline (Tyzine)	Intranasal: 2–4 drops or sprays every 3 h	
xylometazoline (Otrivin)	Intranasal (0.1%): 1–2 sprays bid (max: 3 doses/day)	
Anticholinergic		
ipratropium bromide (Atrovent)	Nasal spray: 2 sprays in each nostril 3–4 times/day up to 4 days	*Transient nasal irritation, burning, sneezing, or dryness, cough, headache* Urinary retention, worsening of narrow-angle glaucoma

Note: *Italics* indicate common adverse effects. Underline indicates serious adverse effects.

PharmFACT

Since legislation restricted the sale of products containing pseudoephedrine, the seizures of illegal methamphetamine laboratories by law enforcement agencies in the United States have decreased 70% from 2003 to 2007. Mexico is the primary source of methamphetamine in the United States. *Source:* Office of National Drug Control Policy, 2008.

PROTOTYPE DRUG Pseudoephedrine (Sudafed)

Classification: Therapeutic: Decongestant

Pharmacologic: Sympathomimetic

Therapeutic Effects and Uses: Approved in 1959, pseudoephedrine is available in tablet and elixir formulations. It is often combined with other medications in OTC preparations used to treat allergic rhinitis, sinus congestion, and the common cold symptoms. Pseudoephedrine promotes sinus drainage and can open obstructed eustachian tubes in adults and children with chronic otic inflammation. It is also used off-label to prevent otitic barotrauma during air travel or diving.

Pseudoephedrine deserves special attention because of its potential for misuse. Pseudoephedrine is the starting chemical for the synthesis of illegal methamphetamine by drug traffickers. As of 2006, pseudoephedrine products must be kept in a locked box behind the pharmacy counter, so that pharmacists can monitor sales and distribution. Although still considered as OTC drugs, pharmacists are required to keep a log of patient names and address, and check the photo identification of the buyer. At least one state has considered making pseudoephedrine a prescription drug. It should be noted that these precautions are not being taken because pseudoephedrine itself is a dangerous drug, but instead to limit the availability of the drug to illicit makers of methamphetamine. Manufacturers have reformulated their OTC cold medicines to contain phenylephrine rather than pseudoephedrine.

Mechanism of Action: Pseudoephedrine activates alpha$_1$-adrenergic receptors, which causes vasoconstriction in the nasal mucosa, resulting in shrinking of mucosal swelling. It also stimulates beta$_2$-adrenergic receptors of the respiratory tract, which may result in some bronchodilation.

Pharmacokinetics:

Route(s)	PO (tablets, elixir)
Absorption	Well absorbed orally
Distribution	Widely distributed, including in cerebrospinal fluid (CSF); crosses the placenta; secreted in breast milk
Primary metabolism	Hepatic
Primary excretion	Renal
Onset of action	30 minutes; extended release: 60 minutes
Duration of action	4–8 h; extended release: 12 h

Adverse Effects: Pseudoephedrine is well tolerated at regular dosage levels. Some patients experience CNS stimulation with symptoms of insomnia, restlessness, anxiety, and dizziness. Excitability is especially a concern in infants and young children.

At high doses, seizures and psychosis may occur. Other sympathomimetic effects include dysrhythmias, HTN, palpitations, tachycardia, dry mouth, and anorexia. Rebound congestion is not usually a concern with PO decongestants. Serious injury and deaths due to overdose have occurred in pediatric patients under 2 years of age who received high doses of cough and cold medicines.

Contraindications/Precautions: Pseudoephedrine should not be used by patients with severe HTN, severe coronary artery disease, hypersensitivity to this drug, or by patients who take monoamine oxidase inhibitor (MAOI) drugs. Alpha-adrenergic agonists should be used with caution in patients with prostatic enlargement, because these drugs increase smooth muscle activity in the prostate gland and may diminish urinary outflow (see Chapter 72). The FDA has issued advisories that nonprescription cough and cold products (including those containing pseudoephedrine) not be used in children under 2 years of age, and that they be used with extreme caution in all children.

Drug Interactions: Pseudoephedrine interacts with MAOIs to cause a hypertensive crisis. Use with other sympathomimetics drugs, including caffeine, can lead to additive cardiovascular and CNS stimulation effects. Beta blockers and pseudoephedrine together can result in HTN or severe bradycardia. Concurrent use with tricyclic antidepressants may result in increased cardiovascular toxicity and severe headaches. Pseudoephedrine can antagonize the effects of antihypertensive drugs. Pseudoephedrine should be avoided in patients who are taking nitrates for angina due to the vasoconstriction caused by the stimulation of alpha-adrenergic receptors on systemic blood vessels. Use with digoxin may cause dysrhythmias. **Herbal/Food:** Bitter orange may increase the risk of HTN.

Pregnancy: Category C.

Treatment of Overdose: Overdose may cause coma, seizures, profuse sweating, and dysrhythmias. No specific treatment exists.

Nursing Responsibilities:

- Assess for the presence or history of nasal or sinus congestion. Also assess the nares for signs of excoriation or bleeding when this medication is used intranasally.
- Before and during pharmacotherapy, assess vital signs, especially pulse and blood pressure, because this drug may cause tachycardia and HTN.
- Assess for benign prostatic hyperplasia (BPH) in men who are older than 40 years old. Drugs in this class can worsen urinary symptoms by preventing muscles in the prostate and bladder neck from relaxing to allow urine to flow freely.
- Assess for cardiovascular disease because oral sympathomimetics are contraindicated in patients with HTN and should be used with caution in patients with coronary artery disease.

Patient and Family Education:

- Limit use of intranasal decongestants to 3 to 5 days.
- Carefully follow the directions for use provided by the manufacturer and do not take more than the recommended dose.
- If taking a prescription decongestant, do not take other OTC cold or allergy preparations (especially those containing antihistamines) without approval of the health care provider because combining these agents may cause excessive drowsiness.
- Immediately report palpitations or chest pain, dizziness or fainting, fever, visual changes, excessively dry mouth, confusion, numbness, or tingling in the face or limbs, severe headache, insomnia, restlessness or nervousness, persistent intranasal pain, nosebleeds, or irritation to the health care provider.
- Do not administer this product to children under the age of 2. For children over age 2, seek advice from the health care provider.

Drugs Similar to Pseudoephedrine (Sudafed)

There are no drugs similar to pseudoephedrine (Sudafed).

Drugs for the Common Cold

74.8 The common cold is caused by a virus and is treated with some of the same drugs as allergic rhinitis.

The common cold is a viral infection of the upper respiratory tract that produces a characteristic array of annoying symptoms. It is fortunate that the disorder is self-limiting, because there is no cure or effective prevention for colds. Therapies used to relieve symptoms include some of the same drugs classes used for allergic rhinitis, including antihistamines and decongestants. A few additional drugs, such as those that suppress cough and loosen bronchial secretions, are used for symptomatic cold treatment.

Many OTC preparations are available to treat cold symptoms. These OTC drugs are often made as combinations containing two or more drugs to treat a variety of symptoms. Some common OTC combination products are listed in Table 74.2. The most common ingredients of combination drugs for the common cold are antihistamines and decongestants; caffeine is sometimes added to combat the adverse effect of drowsiness from first-generation antihistamines. The caffeine is omitted from combination drugs if the medication is to be taken at night, for example, NyQuil. Almost all combination drugs contain some form of analgesic, such as acetaminophen, aspirin, or other nonsteroidal anti-inflammatory agent to help with fever and muscular aches. Many combination products also contain a cough suppressant and an expectorant to help loosen congestion.

The wide variety of combination cold, flu, and sinus products that are available OTC can be confusing for consumers. Multisymptom combination products should only be taken if the patient is experiencing the indicated symptoms. For example, if cough and fever are not present, products that contain cough suppressants, expectorants, or analgesics should not be taken. Consuming combination products without appropriate symptoms can increase the risk of unnecessary adverse effects. It is usually better to take only the drugs needed to treat specific symptoms rather than a combination product.

Drug Interactions: Patients who take MAOIs, triptans, or selective serotonin reuptake inhibitors (SSRIs) should not take dextromethorphan due to the risk of serotonin syndrome (nausea, changes in blood pressure, and confusion). Dextromethorphan has an additive CNS depressant effect with alcohol, antihistamines, antidepressants, and opioids. The analgesic effect of opioids can be almost doubled by giving them with dextromethorphan. **Herbal/Food:** Grapefruit juice can raise serum levels of dextromethorphan and cause toxicity.

Pregnancy: Category C.

Treatment of Overdose: Overdose may result in significant CNS toxicity. Treatment is symptomatic.

Nursing Responsibilities:

- Assess for the presence or history of persistent nonproductive cough, respiratory distress, shortness of breath, and productive cough.
- Monitor for drowsiness because this usually indicates excessive dosage.
- Use extreme caution in administering antitussive drugs to patients with chronic lung conditions because this may result in additive suppression of normal respiratory function.

Patient and Family Education:

- Unless otherwise prescribed by the health care provider, limit use of dextromethorphan to less than a week because cough may be a symptom of other serious pulmonary conditions.
- Do not drive or perform other hazardous activities until the effects of the drug are known because this drug may cause drowsiness or dizziness.
- Avoid alcohol use because this may cause excessive drowsiness.
- Immediately report coughing up green- or yellow-tinged secretions, which may indicate pulmonary infection, difficulty breathing, excessive drowsiness, constipation, and nausea or vomiting.
- Avoid pulmonary irritants, such as smoking or other fumes, because these agents may decrease drug effectiveness.
- If taking a prescription antitussive, do not take OTC cough or cold preparations without approval of the health care provider because these agents may cause excessive drowsiness.
- Carefully follow the directions for use provided by the manufacturer and do not take more than the recommended dose.
- Do not administer this product to children under the age of 2. For children over age 2 seek advice from the health care provider.

Drugs Similar to Dextromethorphan (Robitussin, Sucrets, Others)

The other two nonopioid antitussives are diphenhydramine and benzonatate. Diphenhydramine is discussed in Section 74.4.

Benzonatate (Tessalon): Approved in 1958, benzonatate is an oral, nonopioid antitussive that acts by a unique mechanism. Chemically related to the local anesthetic tetracaine (Pontocaine), benzonatate suppresses the cough reflex by anesthetizing stretch receptors in the lungs. If chewed, this drug can cause numbing of the mouth and pharynx, Adverse effects are uncommon but may include sedation, nausea, headache, and dizziness. This drug should not be used in children under 10 years of age. Like dextromethorphan the effectiveness of benzonatate in treating acute cough has not been clearly established. This drug is pregnancy category C.

Expectorants and Mucolytics

74.10 Expectorants and mucolytics are used to treat thick bronchial secretions.

Several drugs are available to control excess mucus production. **Expectorants** increase bronchial secretions, and **mucolytics** help loosen thick bronchial secretions. These agents are listed in Table 74.6.

Expectorants: Expectorants reduce the thickness or viscosity of bronchial secretions, thus increasing mucus flow that can then be removed more easily by coughing. The only commonly used OTC expectorant is guaifenesin (Mucinex). Like dextromethorphan, guaifenesin produces few adverse effects and is a common ingredient in many combination multisymptom OTC cold and flu preparations. It is most effective in treating dry, nonproductive cough but may also be of benefit for patients with productive cough. Like the antitussives the effectiveness of guaifenesin in reducing acute cold symptoms has been questioned. The dosage range used in cold remedies is usually too low to have much positive benefit for patients. Nonprescription cough and cold products (including those containing guaifenesin) should not be used in children under 2 years of age. High doses can induce nausea, vomiting, and abdominal pain. This drug is pregnancy category C.

Mucolytics: Acetylcysteine (Mucomyst) is one of the few drugs that directly loosen thick, viscous bronchial secretions. Drugs of this type, known as mucolytics, break down the chemical structure of mucus molecules. The mucus becomes thinner and can be removed more easily by coughing. Acetylcysteine is delivered by the PO and inhalation routes and is not available OTC. It is used in patients who have cystic fibrosis, chronic bronchitis, or other diseases that produce large amounts of thick bronchial secretions. Acetylcysteine is also administered by the IV route (Acetadote) to prevent the development of hepatotoxicity in patients who have received an overdose of acetaminophen. Its use in the pharmacotherapy of acetaminophen toxicity is presented in Chapter 44. Adverse effects include bronchospasm, nausea, vomiting, unpleasant odor, and fever. This drug is pregnancy category B.

A second mucolytic, dornase alfa (Pulmozyme), is an enzyme that was approved in 1993 for the management of thick bronchial secretions in patients with cystic fibrosis. Dornase alfa breaks down deoxyribonucleic acid (DNA) molecules in the mucus, causing it to become less viscous. It is administered by the oral inhalation route. Adverse effects include chest pain, conjunctivitis, hoarseness, and pharyngitis. This drug is pregnancy category B.

UNDERSTANDING THE CHAPTER

Key Concepts Summary

74.1 The upper respiratory tract acts as a defense in preventing systemic infection.

74.2 Allergic rhinitis is caused by exposure to an environmental allergen, which leads to symptoms that resemble those of the common cold.

74.3 Drugs for allergic rhinitis include those that prevent the disorder and those that relieve symptoms.

74.4 Antihistamines are widely used to treat allergic rhinitis and other minor allergies.

74.5 Intranasal corticosteroids are the drugs of choice for allergic rhinitis because of their effectiveness and safety.

74.6 Cromolyn and montelukast are alternatives to intranasal corticosteroids in the treatment of allergic rhinitis.

74.7 Intranasal and oral sympathomimetics are the most effective agents for relieving nasal congestion.

74.8 The common cold is caused by a virus and is treated with some of the same drugs as those used to treat allergic rhinitis.

74.9 Antitussives are drugs used to suppress the cough reflex.

74.10 Expectorants and mucolytics are used to treat thick bronchial secretions.

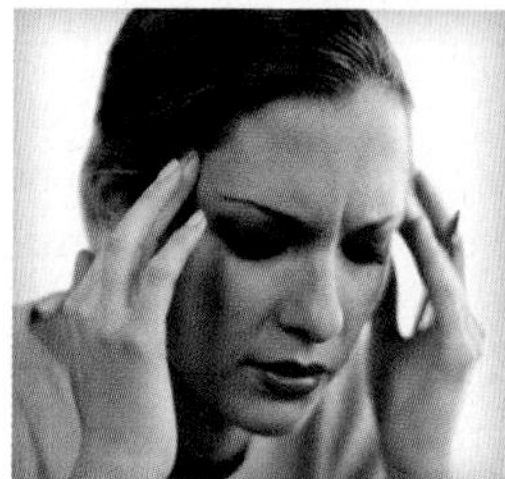

Making the PATIENT *Connection*

Remember the patient "Nancy Williams" at the beginning of the chapter? Now read the remainder of the case study. Based on the information presented within this chapter, respond to the critical thinking questions that follow.

Nancy Williams is a 42-year-old female who is in good health except for her current problem. She has come to the urgent care center because of a stuffy nose; red, itchy eyes; and a slightly sore throat. She takes daily calcium supplements but no other medications. She is 1.68 m (5 ft 6 in.) tall and weighs 67 kg (148 lb).

Ms. Williams is a fourth-grade teacher at a local elementary school and is worried about being able to finish her end of school term activities with the symptoms of a lingering "cold." Ms. William's vital signs are: temperature, 37.4°C (99.4°F); pulse, 102 beats/minute; respirations, 12/minute; blood pressure, 148/88 mmHg; oxygen saturation, 98%.

After taking her vital signs, the nurse learns that Ms. Williams's husband is a medic in the army. Ms. Williams tells the nurse that her mother-in-law bought her a bottle of Neo-Synephrine nasal spray about 10 days ago. It helped, but she tells the nurse that it ran out yesterday and now her nose is even stuffier than before. She had been taking Tylenol but stopped using that, too, because she does not feel like she has a fever and it was not helping much anyway. Ms. Williams says, "I went to the drug store after school and did not stay. I felt so miserable that I couldn't even figure out what medicine does what and I just wanted to get home. I hope the nurse practitioner can help me. I need some rest so I can take care of my girls, do a good job for my students, and get my report cards done." The nurse practitioner observes that Ms. Williams has a cough, runny nose, and inflamed eyes, which she occasionally rubs during the conversation.

Critical Thinking Questions

1. Considering the history and the initial assessment that the nurse practitioner conducted, what further data would you as the nurse want to gather that are not listed in the scenario?
2. If Ms. Williams has no history of heart disease or HTN and takes no medicines to treat those conditions, what do you think might be the cause of her elevated blood pressure and heart rate?
3. Ms. Williams gave her two daughters a golden retriever puppy a few weeks ago. How does this information add to your assessment findings and patient teaching?
4. The nurse practitioner diagnoses Ms. Williams with probable allergic rhinitis and prescribes intranasal Flonase (fluticasone). In addition, the nurse practitioner suggests getting two OTC cough suppressants, one with the main ingredient dextromethorphan and the other one with the main ingredient diphenhydramine. What do you tell Ms. Williams is the reason she is being prescribed each one?

Case Study

A 23-year-old woman arrives with her boyfriend in the emergency department. She is wheezing and short of breath. Her respiratory rate is 23/minute, heart rate is 104 beats/minute, blood pressure is 88/60 mmHg, and she has hives over most of her body. Her boyfriend says she was eating strawberries and suddenly started having trouble breathing. She has eaten strawberries for years and nothing like this has ever happened before. The health care provider prescribes epinephrine for her allergic response.

1. Why did the health care provider not prescribe an antihistamine for this allergic response?
2. A second dose of epinephrine is given and the nurse inserted an IV. With a reduction in her wheezing, the patient's respiratory rate is 18/minute, heart rate is 100 beats/minute, and blood pressure is 98/64 mmHg. The health care provider prescribes Benadryl, 10 mg IV. Describe why the health care provider is now prescribing an antihistamine for the patient.

NCLEX-RN® Review

1 The client has been prescribed fluticasone (Flonase) for allergic rhinitis. Which of the following are appropriate points to include in the teaching plan? Select all that apply.

1. Take with a full glass of water.
2. Prime the inhaler before the first use.
3. Take the drug only when symptoms are present.
4. Take for no more than 5 days to prevent rebound congestion.
5. Effects of the drug may not be noticeable for 2 to 3 weeks.

2 The nurse teaches the client that which type of over-the-counter cough preparations is not effective with coughs associated with the common cold and allergic rhinitis?

1. Dextromethorphan
2. Diphenhydramine
3. Mucolytics
4. Pseudoephedrine

3 An elderly man informs the nurse that he is taking diphenhydramine (Benadryl) to reduce seasonal allergy symptoms. What is the most important topic to include in teaching this client?

1. Do not drive because diphenhydramine is sedating.
2. Obtain an annual eye exam to test for glaucoma.
3. Diphenhydramine may worsen the symptoms of prostatic hyperplasia.
4. Do not stop the drug suddenly because it may cause rebound congestion.

4 The clinic nurse would expect which symptoms to be best treated with intranasal corticosteroids?

1. Acute cough associated with the common cold
2. Nasal stuffiness associated with allergic rhinitis
3. Cough from postnasal drip of allergic rhinitis
4. As a preventive for nasal stuffiness of allergic rhinitis

5 The nurse knows that sympathomimetic decongestants should be avoided by people with which conditions or situations?

1. Hypertension and coronary artery disease
2. Wide-angle glaucoma
3. Breast-feeding women
4. Elderly clients

6 The nurse is teaching the client how to instill intranasal corticosteroids. Which statement would be part of client teaching?

1. "Lie supine for 5 minutes after instillition to absorb all the drug."
2. "Blow your nose after instillition to decrease nasal mucosal irritation."
3. "Expect symptoms to remain for 2 to 3 weeks after beginning the drug."
4. "Prime the instillition device before each use."

See Answers to Critical Thinking Questions, Case Study, and NCLEX-RN® Review in Appendix A.

References

American Academy of Allergy, Asthma, & Immunology. (n.d.). *Allergy statistics.* Retrieved September 4, 2008, from http://www.aaaai.org/media/resources/media_kit/allergy_statistics.stm

Brunton, L. L., Lazo, J. S., & Parker, K. L. (Eds.). (2006). *Goodman & Gillman's The pharmacological basis of therapeutics* (11th ed.). New York: McGraw Hill.

Douglas, R. M, Hemilä, H., D'Souza, R., Chalker, E., & Treacy, B. (2004). Vitamin C for preventing and treating the common cold. *Cochrane Database of Systematic Reviews, 4*: Art. No.: CD000980.pub2.

Eccles, R., Pedersen, A., Regberg, D., Tulento, H., Borum, P., & Stjarne, P. (2007). Efficacy and safety of topical combinations of ipratropium and xylometazoline for the treatment of symptoms of runny nose and nasal congestion associated with acute upper respiratory tract infection. *American Journal of Rhinology, 21* (1), 40–45.

Hayden, M., & Womack, C. (2007). Caring for patients with allergic rhinitis. *Journal of the American Academy of Nurse Practitioners, 19*(6), 290–298.

Hemila, H. (2007, October 15). The role of vitamin C in the treatment of the common cold [Letter to the editor]. *American Family Physician.* Retrieved September 4, 2008, from http://findarticles.com/p/articles/mi_m3225/is_8_76/ai_n27419283

Kim, K. T., Kerwin, E., Landwher, L., Bernstein, J. A., Bruner, D., Harris, D., et al. (2005). Pediatric atrovent nasal spray study group. Use of 0.06% ipratropium bromide nasal spray in children aged 2 to 5 years with rhinorrhea due to a common cold or allergies. *Annals of Allergy, Asthma, and Immunology, 94*(1), 73–79.

Maggini, S., Wintergerst, S., & Hornig, D. H. (2006). Immune-enhancing role of vitamin C and zinc and effect on clinical conditions. *Annals of Nutrition and Metabolism, 50*(2), 85–94.

National Institute of Allergy and Infectious Diseases, National Institutes of Health. (n.d.). *Common Cold.* Retrieved September 4, 2008, from http://www3.niaid.nih.gov/topics/commonCold/overview.htm

Office of National Drug Control Policy. (2008). *Methamphetamine, cocaine, use plummet; new workplace drug testing data show effects of supply crunch.* Retrieved September 4, 2008, from http://www.whitehousedrugpolicy.gov/news/press08/031208.html

Pauling, L. (1970). *Vitamin C, the common cold and the flu.* San Francisco: W. H. Freeman.

Ratner, P. H., Stoloff, S., Metzer, E. O., & Hadley, J. A. (2007). Intranasal corticosteroids in the treatment of allergic rhinitis. *Allergy and Asthma Proceedings, 28*(Suppl. 1), s25–s32.

Smith, S. M., Schroeder, K., & Fahey, T. (2008). Over-the-counter medications for acute cough in children and adults in ambulatory settings. *Cochrane Database of Systematic Reviews 2007, 3.* Art. No.: CD001831. DOI: 10.1002/14651858.CD001831.pub3.

UNIT 11

Miscellaneous Drugs

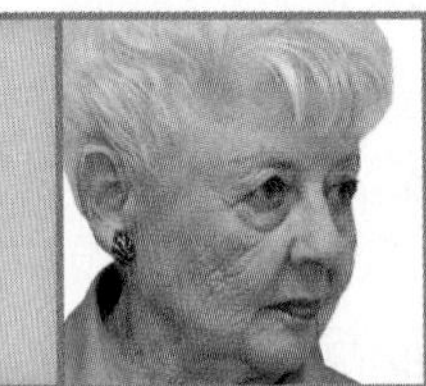
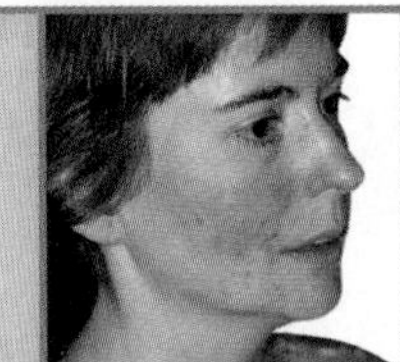
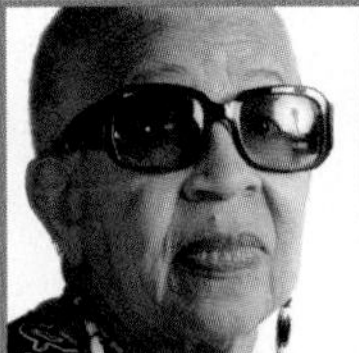
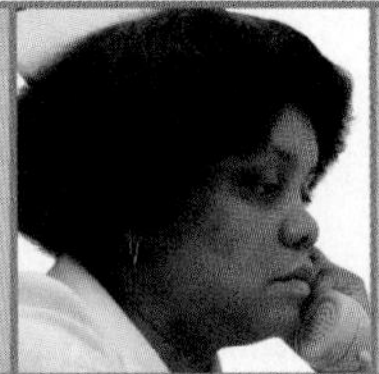

CHAPTER 75 Pharmacotherapy of Bone and Joint Disorders

CHAPTER 76 Pharmacotherapy of Dermatologic Disorders

CHAPTER 77 Pharmacotherapy of Eye and Ear Disorders

CHAPTER 78 Emergency Preparedness: Bioterrorism and Management of Poisoning

CHAPTER

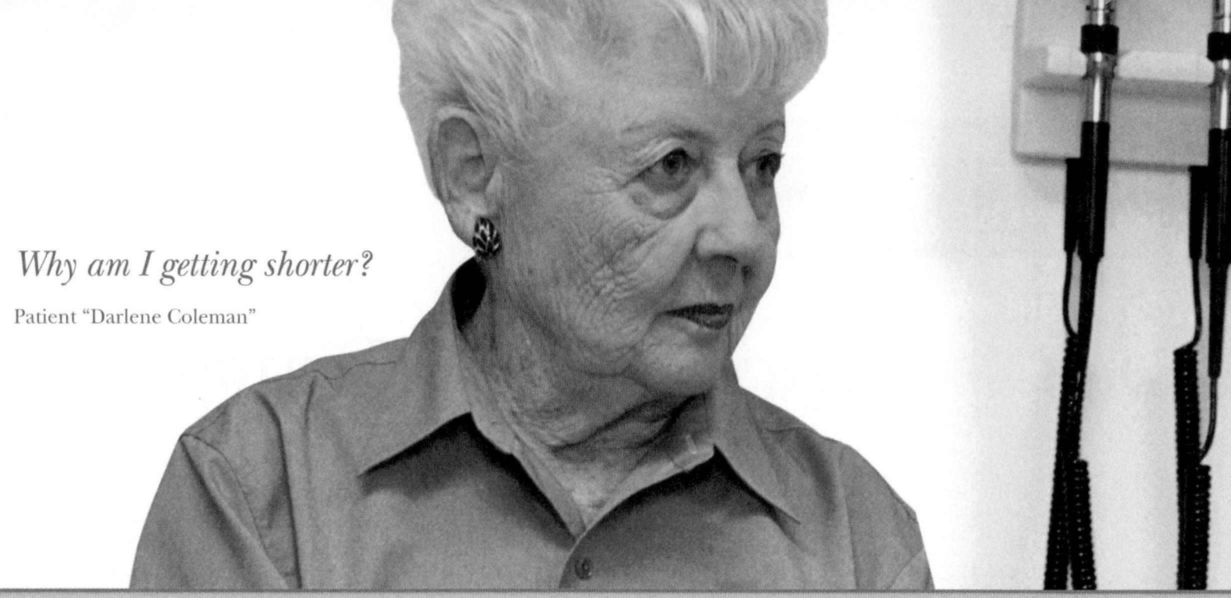

Why am I getting shorter?

Patient "Darlene Coleman"

75 Pharmacotherapy of Bone and Joint Disorders

Learning Outcomes

After reading this chapter, the student should be able to:

1. Describe the role of calcium in maintaining homeostasis in the nervous, muscular, skeletal, and cardiovascular systems.
2. Identify the recommended dietary allowance and the normal serum levels of calcium.
3. Explain the roles of parathyroid hormone, calcitonin, and vitamin D in maintaining calcium balance.
4. Explain the etiology, pathogenesis, and pharmacotherapy for hypocalcemia, osteomalacia, osteoporosis, rickets, osteoarthritis, rheumatoid arthritis, and gout.
5. Describe the nurse's role in the pharmacologic management of bone and joint disorders.
6. For each of the classes shown in the chapter outline, identify the prototype and representative drugs and explain the mechanism(s) of drug action, primary indications, contraindications, significant drug interactions, pregnancy category, and important adverse effects.
7. Apply the nursing process to care for patients who are receiving drug therapy for bone and joint disorders.

Chapter Outline

Role of Calcium in Body Homeostasis

Regulation of Calcium Balance

Pharmacotherapy of Hypocalcemia

Calcium Supplements

PROTOTYPE **Calcium Salts** *p. 1287*

Pathophysiology of Metabolic Bone Disease

Pharmacotherapy of Metabolic Bone Disease

Vitamin D Therapy

PROTOTYPE **Calcitriol (Rocaltrol)** *p. 1292*

Bisphosphonates

PROTOTYPE **Alendronate (Fosamax)** *p. 1296*

Selective Estrogen Receptor Modulators

PROTOTYPE **Raloxifene (Evista)** *p. 1297*

Calcitonin and Miscellaneous Drugs

Pathophysiology and Pharmacotherapy of Joint Disorders

Osteoarthritis

Rheumatoid Arthritis

Disease-Modifying Antirheumatic Drugs (DMARDs)

PROTOTYPE **Hydroxychloroquine (Plaquenil)** *p. 1304*

Pharmacotherapy of Gout

Acute Gouty Arthritis

PROTOTYPE **Colchicine** *p. 1308*

Hyperuricemia

PROTOTYPE **Allopurinol (Zyloprim)** *p. 1309*

Key Terms

acute gouty arthritis, 1307
bisphosphonates, 1294
bone deposition, 1285
bone resorption, 1285
calcitonin, 1285
calcitriol, 1286
cholecalciferol, 1286
disease-modifying antirheumatic drug (DMARD), 1304
gout, 1306
hyperuricemia, 1307
metabolic bone disease (MBD), 1290
osteoarthritis (OA), 1300
osteomalacia, 1291
osteoporosis, 1290
Paget's disease, 1291
rheumatoid arthritis (RA), 1303
selective estrogen receptor modulators (SERMs), 1297
uricosurics, 1309
xanthine oxidase, 1309

The skeletal system and joints are at the core of body movement. Disorders that are associated with bones and joints can lead to immobility and affect a patient's ability to fulfill daily activities. In addition, the skeletal system serves as the primary repository for calcium, which is one of the body's most important minerals.

This chapter focuses on the pharmacotherapy of important skeletal and joint disorders such as osteomalacia, osteoporosis, arthritis, and gout. The importance of calcium balance and the action of vitamin D are stressed because they relate to the proper structure and function of bones.

Role of Calcium in Body Homeostasis

75.1 Adequate levels of calcium in the body are necessary to transmit nerve impulses, to prevent muscle spasms, and for proper bone health.

Calcium balance is critical to the proper functioning of the nervous, muscular, skeletal, and cardiovascular systems. In the nervous system calcium ions influence the release of neurotransmitters and the excitability of all neurons. Contraction is dependent on calcium ion movement in skeletal, smooth, and cardiac muscle cells. Calcium is important for the normal functioning of other body processes such as blood coagulation by converting prothrombin into thrombin and in activating enzymes that catalyze many essential chemical reactions.

Calcium is the major cation for the structure of the bones and teeth. Total body content of calcium is about 1,200 g or approximately 2% of the total body weight. More than 99% of that calcium is in the skeletal system and is bound as a hard matrix known as hydroxyapatite crystals. Only about 1% of the calcium in bone is rapidly exchangeable with blood calcium; the remaining calcium is more stable and slowly exchanged.

Much of the calcium found outside of bone circulates in the blood. Calcium exists in plasma in three forms: ionized, bound, and complexed. About 50% of the serum calcium is in the active, ionized form that participates in intracellular functions, including neuromuscular activity and blood coagulation. This is the only physiologically and clinically significant form of calcium. An adequate amount of free or ionized calcium is required for normal body functions. Most of the remaining 50% of calcium in plasma is bound to plasma proteins, primarily albumin, and other substances and is unavailable for general use by the body.

To maintain homeostasis, the body must obtain sufficient amounts of calcium through proper nutrition and dietary supplements. Unfortunately, only 30% to 50% of dietary calcium is absorbed from the small intestine. The amount absorbed, however, is dynamic and changes with body conditions. Absorption is increased by moderate amounts of fat or high protein intake, high gastric acidity, and the presence of certain hormones that signal low blood calcium. Decreased absorption occurs with vitamin D deficiency, high-fat diet, decreased gastric acidity, certain hormones that signal high blood calcium, and conditions that increase gastrointestinal (GI) motility such as diarrhea. Dietary calcium that remains unabsorbed is excreted in feces. Calcium can also be lost through the nails, hair, sweat, and other bodily fluids. In lactating women, large amounts are lost through breast milk.

The recommended dietary allowance (RDA) of calcium for healthy adults is 800 to 1,200 mg per day. Increased amounts are needed by pregnant and lactating females, growing children, and postmenopausal women, as shown in Table 75.1. The best dietary sources of calcium are dairy products. The calcium found in milk is the most readily available form because milk contains sufficient amounts of vitamin D, which is necessary for calcium absorption. Other rich sources of calcium include seafood, such as salmon, oysters, and clams, and green leafy vegetables, such as kale, broccoli, spinach, and mustard greens. If the body does not obtain enough dietary calcium, it will remove calcium from the bones, resulting in bones that become soft and weakened and that eventually develop osteoporosis. The importance of meeting the daily RDA for calcium is vital to both women and men. Although not as prevalent, men may develop bone conditions such as osteoporosis, and adequate calcium intake should be added to their list of preventive health care interventions.

The normal serum calcium range is 4.5 to 5.5 mEq/L or 8.5 to 10.5 mg/dL. Serum calcium concentrations that exceed 5.5 mEq/L result in hypercalcemia, which causes a decrease in sodium permeability across cell membranes. This is a dangerous state because nerve conduction depends on the proper influx of sodium into cells. When calcium levels in the bloodstream are

TABLE 75.1 Normal Recommended Daily Intakes in Milligrams for Calcium

Persons	United States RDA (mg)
Infants 0–6 months of age	210 mg
Infants 7–12 months of age	270 mg
Infants and children 1–3 years of age	500 mg
Children 4–8 years of age	800 mg
Adolescents 9–18 years of age	1,300 mg
Pregnant and lactating women 14–18 years of age	1,300 mg
Pregnant and lactating women 19–50 years of age	1,000 mg
Adult males and females 19–50 years of age	1,000 mg
Adult males 51+ years of age	1,000 mg
Postmenopausal women	1,500 mg

below 4.5 mEq/L, a state of hypocalcemia develops and the cell membranes become hyperexcitable. If this situation becomes severe, convulsions or muscle spasms may result.

PharmFACT

Approximately one in two women and one in four men over age 50 will have an osteoporosis-related fracture in their remaining lifetime. *Source:* National Osteoporosis Foundation, n.d.

CONNECTION Checkpoint 75.1

Inhibition of calcium transport into cells can have important physiological effects. From what you learned in Chapter 33, what are the primary indications for the pharmacotherapy with calcium channel blockers?
See Answer to Connection Checkpoint 75.1 in Appendix A.

Regulation of Calcium Balance

75.2 Calcium balance is regulated by parathyroid hormone, calcitonin, and vitamin D.

Calcium balance is controlled by parathyroid hormone, calcitonin, and vitamin D. Acting together these three substances regulate the rate of absorption of calcium from the small intestine, the excretion of calcium from the kidney, and the movement of calcium into and out of bone. Calcium balance is illustrated in Figure 75.1.

Parathyroid hormone: Parathyroid hormone (PTH) is secreted from the parathyroid gland, as illustrated in Figure 75.1. The parathyroid glands contain calcium receptors that are able to sense very small changes in serum calcium concentration. When ionized serum calcium levels decrease, the parathyroid glands secrete PTH. PTH directly increases calcium reabsorption in the renal tubule and releases calcium from bone (resorption). PTH indirectly increases serum calcium by

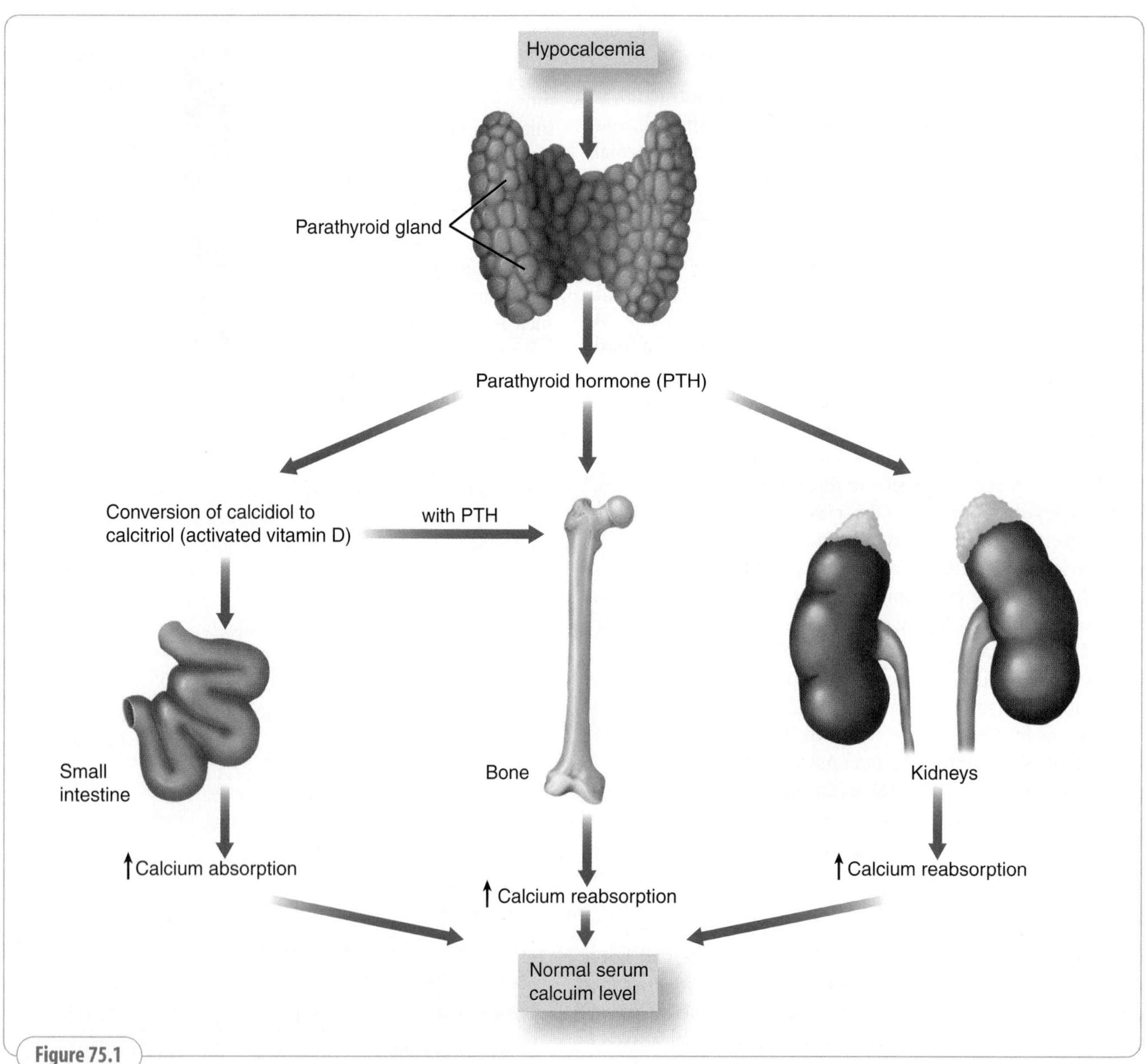

Figure 75.1
Calcium balance.

promoting the formation of activated vitamin D, which then increases calcium absorption from the GI tract. The overall effect of these physiological changes is to rapidly (within minutes) increase serum calcium, returning it to normal levels.

The parathyroid glands are regulated by a typical negative feedback loop. An increase in the ionized serum calcium is recognized by calcium receptors in the parathyroid gland, which suppress PTH secretion. A second piece of the negative feedback loop is that activated vitamin D also shuts down PTH secretion. Without PTH present, the absorption of calcium from the GI tract is diminished, the reabsorption in the kidney tubule decreases, and calcium remains deposited in bone.

The exchange of calcium between the serum and bones is influenced by PTH and calcitonin. PTH stimulates bone cells called osteoclasts. These cells accelerate the process of **bone resorption,** or demineralization, which breaks down bone into its mineral components. Once bone is broken down (resorbed), calcium becomes available to be transported and used elsewhere in the body. The opposite of this process is **bone deposition,** or bone building, which is accomplished by cells called osteoblasts. This process, which removes calcium from the blood to be placed in bone, is stimulated by the hormone calcitonin. It is important to note that maintaining normal serum calcium levels takes precedence over the calcium requirements of the bone. If serum calcium levels are low, bone resorption will occur even if it compromises the structural integrity of the bone matrix.

Calcitonin: When serum calcium levels become elevated, the hormone **calcitonin** is released by the thyroid gland. Calcitonin acts in opposition to PTH and vitamin D to decrease the plasma levels of calcium by inhibiting the resorption of calcium from bone and increasing the excretion of calcium by the kidney, thus decreasing the concentration of serum calcium. It is important to note that calcitonin does not affect the rates of calcium absorption from the small intestine. The actions of calcitonin and PTH are shown in Figure 75.2.

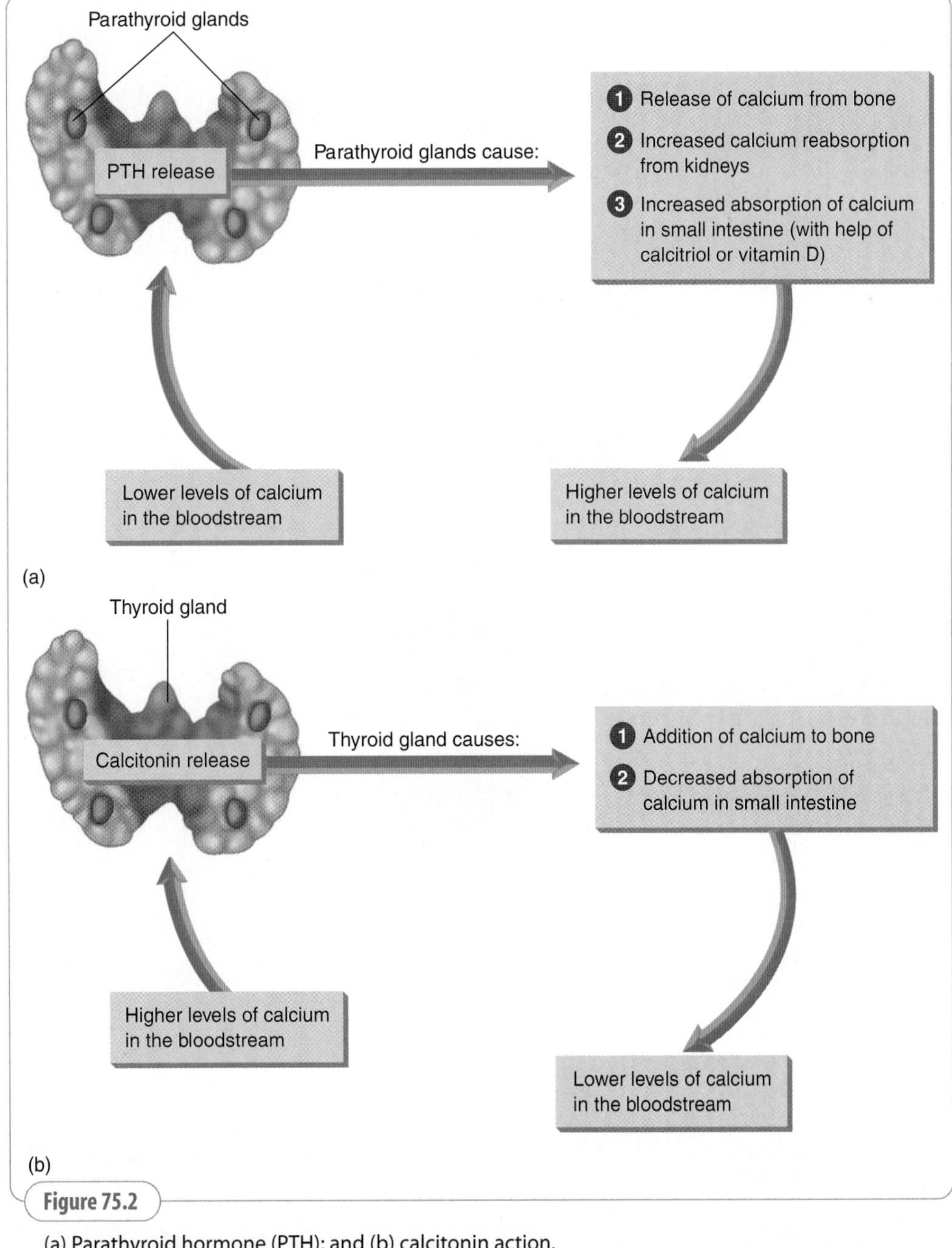

Figure 75.2

(a) Parathyroid hormone (PTH); and (b) calcitonin action.

MyNursingKit | Mechanism of Action Animation: Calcitriol

Calcitonin is available as a medication for the treatment of osteoporosis.

Vitamin D: The regulation of the rate of absorption of calcium from the small intestine is influenced primarily by PTH, but vitamin D is a required component. Vitamin D and calcium metabolism are intimately related: Absorption of calcium is increased in the presence of vitamin D, and absorption is inhibited by vitamin D deficiency. Thus, calcium disorders are often associated with vitamin D disorders.

Vitamin D is unique among vitamins because it is the only vitamin that the body is able to synthesize from precursor molecules. Several steps, however, are required before vitamin D can act on target tissues. Figure 75.3 illustrates the metabolism of vitamin D. In the skin, **cholecalciferol,** the inactive form of vitamin D, is synthesized from cholesterol. Exposure of the skin to sunlight or ultraviolet light increases the level of cholecalciferol in the blood. Cholecalciferol can also be obtained from dietary products such as milk or other foods fortified with vitamin D.

Following its absorption from dietary sources or formation in the skin, cholecalciferol is converted to an intermediate vitamin form called calcifediol. Enzymes in the kidneys then metabolize calcifediol to **calcitriol,** the active form of vitamin D. PTH stimulates the formation of calcitriol at the level of the kidneys. Patients with extensive kidney disease are unable to adequately synthesize calcitriol and thus frequently experience calcium and vitamin D abnormalities. The primary function of calcitriol is to increase calcium absorption from the GI tract. Dietary calcium

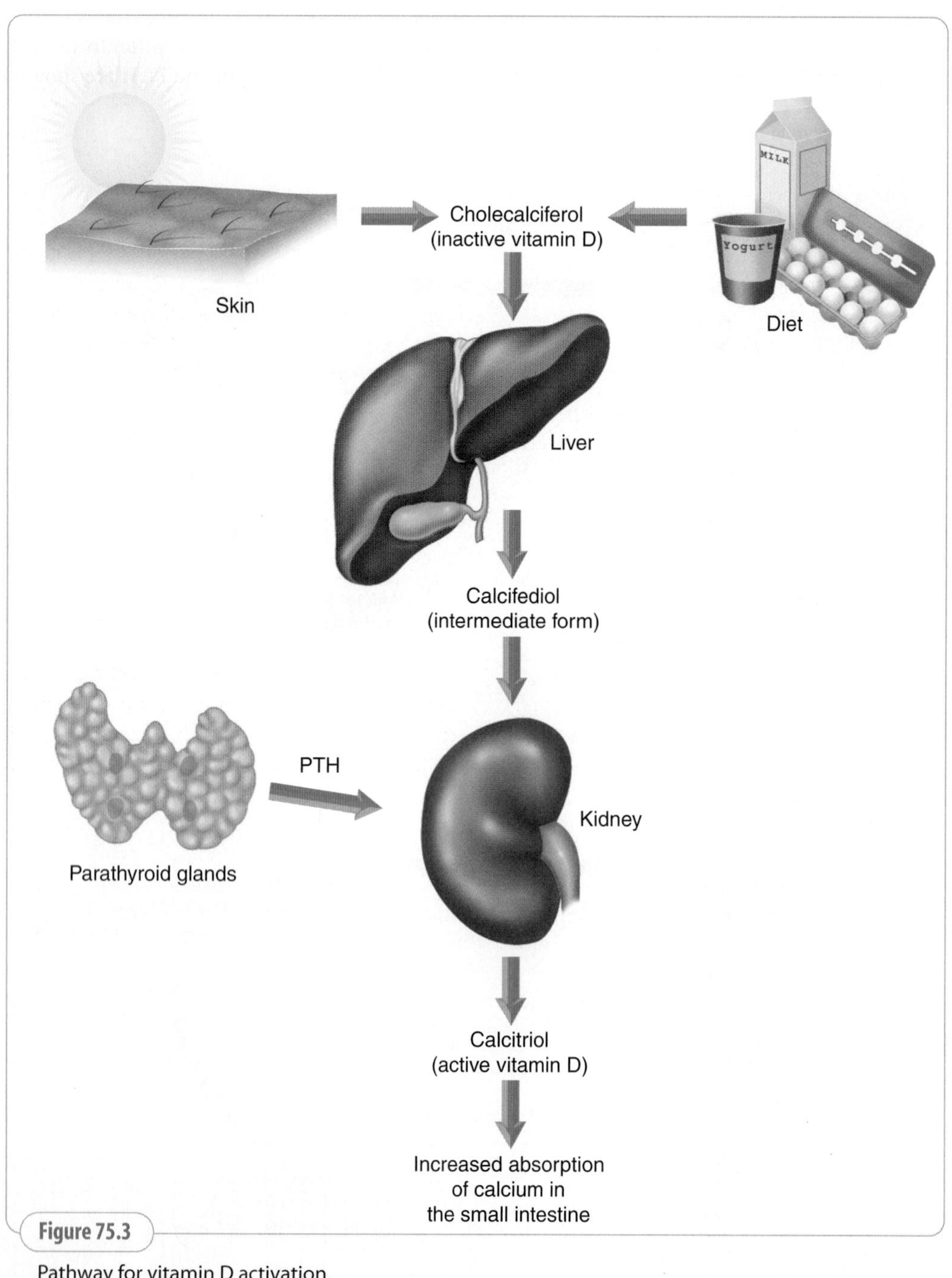

Figure 75.3

Pathway for vitamin D activation.

is absorbed more efficiently in the presence of active vitamin D and PTH, resulting in higher serum levels of calcium, which is then transported to bone, muscle, and other tissues.

Pharmacotherapy of Hypocalcemia

75.3 Hypocalcemia is a condition that requires therapy with calcium supplements, often concurrently with vitamin D.

Hypocalcemia is not a disease but is a sign of underlying pathology. Therefore, diagnosis of the cause of hypocalcemia is essential. Many factors can cause hypocalcemia. Lack of sufficient dietary calcium or vitamin D intake is a common cause and one that can be easily reversed by nutritional adjustments. If hypocalcemia occurs with normal dietary intake, GI causes must be examined, such as excessive vomiting or the presence of malabsorption disorders. Damage to renal tubular cells may cause excessive loss of calcium in the urine. Most patients with chronic kidney disease will require calcium and vitamin D therapy to prevent hypocalcemia.

Another common etiology for hypocalcemia is hypoparathyroidism leading to decreased secretion of PTH, as occurs when the thyroid and parathyroid glands are diseased or surgically removed. A rare cause of hypocalcemia is pseudohypoparathyroidism, which is an uncommon group of genetic disorders characterized not by PTH deficiency but when the target organs for PTH (bone and kidneys) become resistant to the hormone.

Drug therapy is occasionally a cause of hypocalcemia. Blood transfusions and certain anticonvulsants such as phenytoin and phenobarbital can lower serum calcium levels. In addition, overtreatment with drugs that are used to lower serum calcium can result in "overshooting" normal levels. Some of these include furosemide, phosphate therapy, or bisphosphonates. Of special concern is long-term therapy with corticosteroids, which is a very common cause of hypocalcemia and osteoporosis. To help prevent corticosteroid-induced osteoporosis, patients should receive daily supplements of calcium and vitamin D.

Hypocalcemia is frequently asymptomatic. Signs and symptoms of hypocalcemia are those of nerve and muscle excitability. The symptoms include confusion, paresthesias around the mouth and in the digits, carpopedal spasms, and hyperreflexia. Muscle twitching, tremors, or cramping may be evident. Two clinical signs are Chvostek's sign and Trousseau's sign. Chvostek's sign is elicited by tapping on the facial nerve just below the temple. A positive sign is a twitch of the nose or lip. Trousseau's sign is the contraction of the hand and fingers when the arterial blood flow in the arm is occluded for 5 minutes.

Intestinal cramping and hyperactive bowel sounds may be present as the low calcium levels affect the smooth muscle of the GI tract. Severe symptoms include convulsions, laryngeal spasms, and tetany. Tetany is a continuous muscle spasm that can interfere with breathing and even cause death. The characteristic electrocardiogram (ECG) change is a prolonged QT interval, indicating prolonged ventricular depolarization with characteristically weak cardiac muscle contractions.

Unless the hypocalcemia is especially severe or life threatening, adjustments in diet should be attempted prior to initiating therapy with calcium supplements. Increasing the consumption of calcium-rich foods, especially dairy products, fortified orange juice, cereals, and green leafy vegetables, is often sufficient to restore calcium balance.

PROTOTYPE DRUG Calcium salts

Classification: **Therapeutic:** Calcium supplement
Pharmacologic: Drugs for replacement of deficient calcium levels

Therapeutic Effects and Uses: Calcium salts are available in a wide variety of products and formulations. Calcium has two major forms: complexed and elemental. Most calcium supplements are in the form of complexed calcium. These products are often compared on the basis of their ability to release elemental calcium into the bloodstream. The greater the ability of complexed calcium to release elemental calcium, the more potent is the supplement. Table 75.2 lists the doses for selected calcium supplements.

For mild, chronic hypocalcemia, effective and inexpensive calcium supplements are readily available over-the-counter (OTC) in a variety of formulations. Calcium carbonate and calcium citrate are the two most common salts for routine supplementation. Many calcium supplements often contain vitamin D.

The administration of intravenous (IV) calcium salts is required for severe cases of hypocalcemia or if the patient is in tetany. Repeated infusions may be necessary to return serum calcium to normal levels. Constant monitoring of serum calcium is required during IV administration to prevent hypercalcemia.

In addition to preventing or treating hypocalcemia, calcium salts are administered for many other conditions, including osteoporosis, Paget's disease, osteomalacia, chronic hypoparathyroidism, rickets, pregnancy, lactation, and rapid childhood growth. Calcium carbonate is a common antacid used to treat heartburn. It may also be used to bind excessive dietary phosphate in patients with hyperphosphatemia due to end-stage renal disease.

IV calcium gluconate can protect the heart against the hyperexcitability of excessive potassium (hyperkalemia) and help to maintain cardiorespiratory function during magnesium sulfate toxicity (hypermagnesemia). IV calcium salts have been administered during cardiac arrest due to their ability to increase cardiac muscle tone and the force of systolic contraction (positive inotropic effect). However, the use of calcium salts in cardiac resuscitation has declined and is limited to patients with cardiac disease who have hypocalcemia because calcium salts may cause dysrhythmias at high doses.

Mechanism of Action: Calcium salts restore the normal serum levels of calcium, which promotes deposition of the mineral in bone. This helps to restore bone strength and prevent fractures. Calcium also restores normal neuromuscular function and muscular contraction.

Pharmacokinetics: The pharmacokinetics of calcium salts varies by the route of administration and the specific formulation. They are widely distributed and excreted primarily in the feces, with about 20% in the urine. The duration of action of calcium salts is generally only a few hours.

TABLE 75.2 Selected Calcium Salts

Drug	Calcium Content	Route and Adult Dose (maximum dose where indicated)	Adverse Effects
Calcium Supplements (All doses are in terms of elemental calcium.)			
calcium acetate (PhosLo)	25%	Oral (PO): 2–4 tablets with each meal (each tablet contains 169 mg calcium)	*Constipation, nausea, vomiting, metallic taste* <ins>Hypercalcemia (drowsiness, lethargy, headache, anorexia, nausea, vomiting, increased urination, and thirst), dysrhythmias, cardiac arrest, confusion, delirium, stupor, coma</ins>
calcium carbonate (Rolaids, Tums, OsCal, others)	40%	PO: 1–2 g bid-tid	
calcium chloride	27 mg Ca/mL	Intravenous (IV): 0.5–4 g by slow infusion (1 mL/min)	
calcium citrate (Citracal)	21%	PO: 1–2 g bid-tid	
calcium gluconate (Kalcinate)	9% (PO); 9 mg Ca/mL (IV)	PO: 0.5–2 g bid-tid IV: 0.5–4 g by slow infusions (1 g/h)	
calcium lactate (Cal-Lac)	13%	PO: 100–200 mg tid with meals	
calcium phosphate tribasic (Posture)	39%	PO: 1–2 g bid-tid	

Note: *Italics* indicate common adverse effects. <ins>Underline</ins> indicates serious adverse effects.

Adverse Effects: Oral calcium products are safe and produce few adverse effects when used as directed. The most common adverse effect of calcium supplements is hypercalcemia, which is caused by taking too much of this supplement. This can be especially serious in the IV formulations. Symptoms of hypercalcemia include drowsiness, lethargy, weakness, headache, anorexia, constipation, increased gastric acid secretion, nausea, vomiting, a tingling sensation, increased urination, and thirst. IV administration of calcium may cause pain and burning at the IV site, severe venous thrombosis, necrosis, sloughing of the skin (with extravasation) of the skin, hypotension, sensations of heat waves (peripheral vasodilation), fainting, bradycardia, cardiac dysrhythmias, and cardiac arrest. Large doses of supplemental calcium may lead to the formation of symptomatic kidney stones.

Contraindications/Precautions: Calcium salts are contraindicated in patients with ventricular fibrillation, metastatic bone disease, renal calculi, hypercalcemia, predisposition to hypercalcemia, hyperparathyroidism, certain malignancies, and digoxin toxicity. Calcium salts should not be injected into the myocardium or administered by the subcutaneous or intramuscular (IM) routes. Caution must be used with patients who have renal or cardiac insufficiency, dysrhythmias, dehydration, diarrhea, hyperphosphatemia, sarcoidosis, or history of kidney stones. Immobilized patients are at high risk to the development of hypercalcemia.

Drug Interactions: Concurrent use with digoxin increases the risk of dysrhythmias and enhances its inotropic effects. Magnesium may compete for GI absorption. Calcium decreases the absorption of tetracyclines and fluoroquinolones, such as ciprofloxacin. Their use may antagonize the effects of verapamil and possibly other calcium channel blockers. **Herbal/Food:** Zinc-rich foods may decrease the absorption of calcium. Alcohol, caffeine, and carbonated beverages affect the absorption of calcium. Oxalic acid in spinach, rhubarb, Swiss chard, and beets can suppress calcium absorption. Phytic acid, which is present in bran and whole-grain cereals, depresses calcium absorption.

Pregnancy: Category B or C.

Treatment of Overdose: Measures may be taken to treat cardiac abnormalities caused by the resulting hypercalcemia.

Nursing Responsibilities:

- Assess for signs and symptoms of calcium imbalance. For hypercalcemia, assess for drowsiness, lethargy, weakness, headache, anorexia, nausea, vomiting, thirst, and increased urination. Signs and symptoms to assess for hypocalcemia are facial twitching, muscle spasms, paresthesias, and seizures.
- Obtain baseline and periodic vital signs, serum calcium levels, and an ECG to determine the effectiveness of the medication. ECG changes that are associated with hypercalcemia include a decreased QT interval and inverted T waves.
- Obtain a thorough history to determine pregnancy or lactation, past medical history, and current medications, including dietary supplements. Calcium supplements are contraindicated in patients with a history of renal calculi, digoxin toxicity, dysrhythmias, or hypercalcemia.
- Investigate a history of fractures. A fracture experienced by a patient following minimal trauma may be the first indication of osteopenic problems.
- Administer IV calcium salts slowly to avoid hypotension, dysrhythmias, and cardiac arrest. Observe the IV site closely because extravasation may cause tissue irritation and necrosis.
- Monitor electrolyte levels during therapy.

Patient and Family Education:

- Take oral calcium supplements with meals or within 1 hour following meals.
- Report drowsiness, fatigue, lethargy, headache, loss of appetite, nausea, vomiting, increased urination, thirst, facial twitching, weakness of an extremity, muscle spasms, or seizures to the health care provider.
- Immediately report nausea, vomiting, constipation, or difficulty urinating to the health care provider.

- Exercise daily for optimal bone health and to prevent future complications, as recommended by the health care provider.
- Consume adequate amounts of calcium-rich foods such as milk products, dark green vegetables, soybeans, tofu, and canned fish with bones.
- Avoid or limit an excessive intake of zinc-rich foods, because too much zinc may decrease the absorption of calcium. Zinc-enriched foods include nuts, legumes, seeds, and sprouts.
- Avoid or limit alcohol, caffeine, and carbonated beverages, because these affect the absorption of calcium.
- Do not take any other OTC calcium supplements, multivitamins, or antacids without approval of the health care provider.

Drugs Similar to Calcium Salts

A large number of calcium salts are available. A summary of their indications is shown in Table 75.3.

NURSING PROCESS APPLICATION

Patients Receiving Calcium Supplements

Assessment	Potential Nursing Diagnoses
Prior to administration: • Obtain a complete health history, including allergies, drug history, signs of hypercalcemia or hypocalcemia, pregnancy, history of fractures, and possible drug interactions. • Obtain baseline vital signs, especially apical pulse for rate and rhythm, and blood pressure. • Obtain a baseline ECG if parenteral calcium supplement is being administered. • Obtain laboratory tests, including a complete blood count (CBC) and electrolytes, especially calcium and magnesium.	• *Risk for Injury,* related to loss of bone mass and adverse effects of drug • *Deficient Knowledge (Drug Therapy)* • *Deficient Knowledge (Adverse Effects),* related to signs and symptoms to report to health care provider

Planning: Patient Goals and Expected Outcomes

The patient will:

- Have normal serum calcium levels (8.5–11.5 mg/dL).
- Demonstrate an understanding of the drug's action by accurately describing drug adverse effects and precautions.
- Immediately report adverse effects and adverse reactions.

Implementation

Interventions and (Rationales)	Patient and Family Education
• Monitor electrolytes throughout therapy. (Calcium and phosphorus levels tend to vary inversely: Low magnesium levels coexist with low calcium levels.)	• Teach the patient the importance of routine laboratory studies, so deviations from normal can be corrected immediately.
• Monitor for signs and symptoms of hypercalcemia. (Overtreatment may lead to excessive serum calcium levels.)	• Instruct the patient to report signs or symptoms of hypercalcemia such as drowsiness, lethargy, weakness, headache, anorexia, nausea and vomiting, increased urination, and thirst.
• Initiate seizure precautions for patients at risk for hypocalcemia. (Low calcium levels may cause seizures.)	• Instruct the patient to recognize signs of hypocalcemia, such as facial twitching, muscle spasms, seizures, and paresthesias.
• Monitor for musculoskeletal difficulties. (Calcium supplements are used to treat osteoporosis, rickets, and osteomalacia.)	Instruct the patient to: • Take safety precautions to reduce injury and prevent fractures. • Report episodes of sudden pain, joints out of alignment, or inability of the patient to assume normal positioning. • Instruct the patient on the importance of weight-bearing exercises to ensure the bone deposition of calcium.
• Monitor intake and output. Use cautiously in patients with renal insufficiency. (Calcium is excreted by the kidneys.)	Instruct the patient to: • Increase oral fluid intake to 2–3 L/day to prevent the formation of renal stones. • Report any difficulty in urination and measure intake and output.
• Monitor cardiac functioning when the parenteral route is being used. (Possible adverse effects may include short QT wave, heart block, hypotension, dysrhythmias, or cardiac arrest with IV administration.)	• Inform the patient to recognize and report palpitations, light-headedness, dizziness, or shortness of breath.
• Monitor the IV site for infiltration during IV administration. (Extravasation may lead to tissue necrosis.)	• Instruct the patient to report pain or swelling at the IV site.
• Monitor the patient's diet. (Consuming calcium-rich foods may increase the effect of the drug. Consuming foods rich in zinc may decrease calcium absorption.)	• Advise the patient to consume calcium-rich foods and avoid zinc-rich foods.

Evaluation of Outcome Criteria

Evaluate the effectiveness of drug therapy by confirming that patient goals and expected outcomes have been met (see "Planning").

TABLE 75.3 Indications for Selected Calcium Salts

Salt	Antacid	Antihyperkalemic	Antihypermagnesemic	Antihyperphosphatemic	Antihypocalcemic	Cardiotonic	Mineral Supplement	Electrolyte Replenisher
calcium acetate					X			X
calcium carbonate	X			X	X		X	
calcium chloride	X	X	X		X	X		X
calcium citrate				X	X		X	
calcium glubionate					X		X	
calcium gluconate injection		X	X		X	X		X
calcium lactate					X		X	
calcium phosphate, dibasic					X		X	

Pathophysiology of Metabolic Bone Disease

75.4 Metabolic bone disease is characterized by abnormal bone structure.

Metabolic bone disease (MBD) is a general term referring to a cluster of disorders that have in common defects in the structure of bone. MBDs are caused by abnormal amounts of the minerals or hormones responsible for bone homeostasis, such as calcium, phosphate, vitamin D, or PTH. Some MBDs have a genetic etiology, whereas others are iatrogenic and caused by certain drugs and therapies.

Osteoporosis: **Osteoporosis** is an MBD characterized by bone demineralization, decreased bone density, and subsequent fractures. Osteoporosis is the most prevalent MBD in the United States and is responsible for as many as 1.5 million fractures annually. This disorder is usually asymptomatic until the bones become brittle enough to fracture or for vertebrae to collapse.

Normal bone remodeling requires a balance between bone deposition (gain) and bone resorption (loss). The exact pathophysiology of osteoporosis is unknown, but there are two major theories. In the first, osteoporosis may be caused by defective osteoblasts that have an abnormally short life span or work less efficiently, resulting in slow bone deposition. The second and more popular theory suggests that the osteoclasts have increased activity, resorbing bone at an increased rate. The common factor between the two theories is that normal bone turnover is altered, with the rate of resorption greater than bone formation, resulting in a decrease in total bone density and an altered bone structure.

Although the exact cause of osteoporosis is unknown, numerous risk factors have been identified. Women are four times as likely as men to develop osteoporosis, and the most common risk factor associated with the development of osteoporosis is the onset of menopause. When women reach menopause, estrogen secretion declines, and bones become weak and fragile. In women with osteoporosis, fractures often occur in the hips, wrists, forearms, or spine. In some cases, a lack of dietary calcium and vitamin D contributes to bone deterioration. The metabolism of calcium in osteoporosis is illustrated in Figure 75.4.

Major risk factors for osteoporosis include the following:

- Menopause
- Patient age, over 60 years
- Family history of osteoporosis
- White or Asian race
- High alcohol intake
- Estrogen deficiency
- Smoking history
- Androgen deficiency
- Anorexia nervosa
- Low calcium or vitamin D intake
- Physical inactivity
- Thin, lean body build

The World Health Organization has developed a standard for the diagnosis of osteoporosis based on mean bone mineral density (BMD) values of the young adult between the ages of 30 and 35, which is the period of peak bone strength. Through the use of dual-energy x-ray absorptiometry (DEXA), which provides information regarding BMD at the spine and hip, data are analyzed and reported as T scores. DEXA scores are useful in identifying osteopenic and osteoporotic bone and in assessing

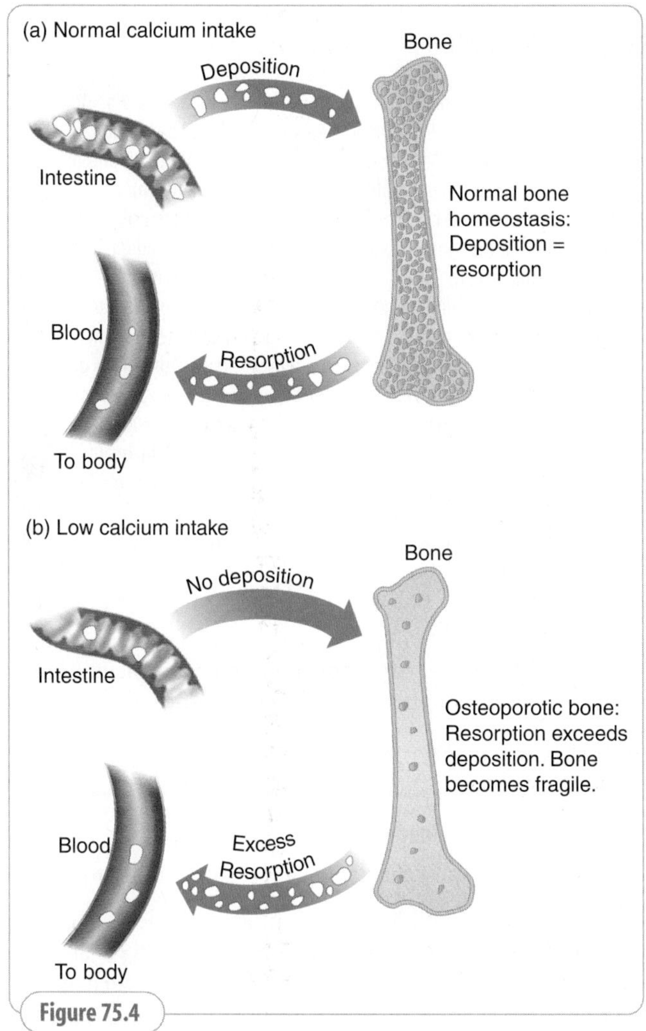

Figure 75.4

Calcium metabolism in osteoporosis.

the response to therapy. Osteopenia, or a low bone mass, is present when the T score is 1 to 2.5 standard deviations below normal. Osteoporosis is defined as a BMD T score of more than 2.5 standard deviations below normal.

Drug therapies for osteoporosis include calcium and vitamin D therapy, estrogen replacement therapy (ERT), estrogen receptor modulators, statins, slow release sodium fluoride, bisphosphonates, and calcitonin. Teriparatide (Forteo) is a new drug for osteoporosis that is a structural analog of PTH produced through recombinant deoxyribonucleic acid (DNA) technology.

Osteomalacia: **Osteomalacia,** referred to as rickets in children, is a disorder characterized by softening of bones without alteration of basic bone structure. Weight-bearing stress on the softened bones causes skeletal deformities. Many factors contribute to the development of osteomalacia and rickets, but the most important is a deficiency of vitamin D and calcium. This risk factor for the disease is extremely rare in the United States, being most prevalent in the elderly, in premature infants, and in individuals on strict vegetarian diets. Other factors that may result in the development of osteomalacia include malabsorption disorders of the small bowel, damage to the renal tubules, adverse effects of anticonvulsant therapy, hepatic impairment, or a limited exposure to sunlight.

Recent research has documented a global resurgence of rickets. The promotion of breast-feeding over vitamin D–fortified formulas is thought to be responsible for part of the increase, particularly in mothers who are vitamin D deficient. In addition, the increased use of sunscreens to prevent skin cancer inhibits the formation of adequate vitamin D by sunlight. The replacement of vitamin D–fortified milk with carbonated beverages by children and teens also contributes to the possibility of rickets. Nurses need to emphasize the importance of including extra dietary vitamin D in children and pregnant women. Drug therapy for children and adults consists of calcium salts and vitamin D.

Symptoms of osteomalacia include hypocalcemia, muscle weakness, muscle spasms, and diffuse bone pain, especially in the hip area. Patients may also experience pain in the arms, legs, and spine. Classic signs of rickets in children include bowlegs and a pigeon breast. Children may also develop a slight fever and become restless at night.

Tests that are performed to verify osteomalacia include bone biopsy; bone radiographs; computed tomography (CT) scan of the vertebral column; and determination of serum calcium, phosphate, and vitamin D levels. Many of these tests are routine for bone disorders and are performed as needed to determine the extent of bone health.

Paget's disease: **Paget's disease,** or osteitis deformans, is a chronic, progressive condition characterized by accelerated remodeling of the bone, producing enlarged and softened bones. With this disorder, the processes of bone resorption and bone formation occur simultaneously but at a very high rate. The rapid turnover causes new bone to be weak and brittle and deformity and fractures may result. Paget's disease can occur in any bone, but it most often affects the vertebrae, skull, sternum, pelvis, femur, and tibia. Paget's disease occurs with equal frequency in men and women over 40 years of age. The cause of Paget's disease is unknown.

Although many patients with Paget's disease are asymptomatic, approximately 10% experience vague, nonspecific complaints for many years. Symptoms include pain of the hips and femurs, joint inflammation, headaches, facial pain, and hearing loss if bones around the ear are affected. Nerves along the spinal column may be pinched because of the abnormal vertebral bone growth.

The evaluation of Paget's disease is based on radiographic and laboratory findings. The enzyme alkaline phosphatase (ALP) is elevated in the blood because of the extensive bone turnover. The disease is usually confirmed by early detection of this enzyme in the blood. Calcium is also liberated because of its close association with phosphate. If diagnosed early enough, symptoms can be treated successfully. If the diagnosis is made late in the progress of the disease, permanent skeletal abnormalities develop and other disorders may appear, including arthritis, kidney stones, and heart disease.

CONNECTIONS

Treating the Diverse Patient Osteoporosis in Men

Osteoporosis is typically thought of as a "woman's disease." However, in recent years, the problem of osteoporosis in men is being recognized as an important public health issue. Osteoporosis poses a significant threat to more than 2 million men in the United States. After age 50, 6% of all men will experience hip fractures and 5% will have vertebral fractures from osteoporosis.

For most persons, bone mass peaks during the third decade of life. At this age, most men generally have a greater bone mass density than women. Men in their 50s do not typically experience the rapid loss of bone mass that women do in the year following menopause. By age 70, however, men and women lose bone mass at the same rates and the absorption of calcium decreases equally for both sexes. In men over the age of 70, age-related bone loss is assumed to be the cause of osteoporosis. The majority of men have at least one other secondary cause that can be attributed to certain lifestyle behaviors, diseases, or medications. The most common causes in men include low levels of testosterone, alcohol use, smoking, GI disease, and long-term exposure to glucocorticoids.

Medications are available to halt bone deterioration. Alendronate (Fosamax) and risedronate (Actonel) have been approved by the United States Food and Drug Administration (FDA) to treat steroid-induced osteoporosis in men. Alendronate is approved for use in men for osteoporosis. None of the other osteoporosis medications that are used with postmenopausal women have been approved for men. If the cause is due to corticosteroid use, the health care provider may try to discontinue the medication when possible or attempt topical administration. If osteoporosis is the result of another condition, such as testosterone deficiency, the health care provider will treat the underlying cause. Other parts of the therapeutic regimen for a male diagnosed with osteoporosis will focus on those measures that maintain bone mass. Interventions would include eating foods high in calcium and vitamin D, regular weight-bearing exercise to maintain proper weight control, and healthy lifestyle guidelines, particularly avoiding smoking and excessive use of alcohol. Evaluation of yearly height and weight measurements need to be included in health care provider assessments.

The pharmacotherapy of patients with Paget's disease includes bisphosphonates and calcitonin. Patients with Paget's disease should consume adequate amounts of calcium and vitamin D on a daily basis.

Pharmacotherapy of Metabolic Bone Disease

75.5 Vitamin D therapy is indicated for treating osteomalacia, hypoparathyroidism, and osteoporosis.

Inactive, intermediate, and active forms of vitamin D are available as medications. Patients' vitamin D needs vary depending on how much sunlight they receive. After age 70, the RDA of vitamin D increases from 400 units per day to 600 units per day. In severe cases of malabsorption disorders, patients may receive 50,000 to 100,000 units per day. Because vitamin D is needed to absorb calcium from the GI tract, many supplements combine vitamin D and calcium into a single tablet.

Several forms of vitamin D are available for therapy. Four of those products—ergocalciferol, cholecalciferol, calcifediol, and calcitriol—are identical to the forms of vitamin D that occur in nature. Each vitamin D product has a slightly different potency and pharmacokinetics. Indications for vitamin D products include the following:

- Hypocalcemia
- Hypophosphatemia
- Osteomalacia or rickets
- Osteoporosis prophylaxis
- Parathyroid dysfunction
- Vitamin D deficiency

Vitamin D is a fat-soluble vitamin that is stored by the body. It is possible to consume too much of this vitamin or to show signs of overdose from prescription medications. Excess vitamin D will cause calcium to leave bones and enter the blood. The signs and symptoms of hypercalcemia, such as anorexia, vomiting, excessive thirst, fatigue, and confusion, may become evident. Kidney stones may occur, and bones may fracture easily.

PROTOTYPE DRUG Calcitriol (Rocaltrol)

Classification: **Therapeutic:** Vitamin D
Pharmacologic: Bone resorption inhibitor

Therapeutic Effects and Uses: Calcitriol is the active form of vitamin D. This medication is used in cases of hypocalcemia and for patients who have hypoparathyroidism. Calcitriol reduces bone resorption and is useful in treating rickets. Patients with chronic kidney disease are unable to synthesize sufficient calcitriol and thus will receive this drug as replacement therapy.

The effectiveness of calcitriol depends on having an adequate amount of calcium; therefore, it is usually prescribed in combination with calcium supplements. It is available for administration via the oral (PO) route in the form of tablets and solutions. An IV solution for injection was approved in 2003.

Mechanism of Action: Calcitriol elevates serum calcium levels, decreases elevated blood levels of phosphate, and decreases bone resorption and demineralization by promoting the intestinal absorption and renal reabsorption of calcium. The rising calcium levels provide negative feedback to the parathyroid glands, reducing the secretion of PTH. Calcitriol itself also provides negative feedback to the parathyroid glands.

Pharmacokinetics:

Route(s)	PO (tablets, capsules, or solution), IV
Absorption	Readily absorbed from the GI tract
Distribution	Widely distributed; crosses the placenta; small amounts are secreted in breast milk; 99% bound to vitamin D-binding protein
Primary metabolism	Hepatic
Primary excretion	Bile/feces
Onset of action	2–6 h
Duration of action	3–5 days

Adverse Effects: The adverse effects of vitamin D therapy include symptoms of hypercalcemia, such as palpitations, anorexia, nausea, vomiting, blurred vision, photophobia, constipation, abdominal cramps, metallic taste, headache, weakness, dry mouth, thirst, increased urination, and muscle or bone pain.

Contraindications/Precautions: This drug should not be given to patients with hypercalcemia or those who have evidence of vitamin D toxicity. Caution must be used in patients with renal failure who are at increased risk for vitamin D-induced hypercalcemia.

Drug Interactions: Thiazide diuretics may enhance the effects of vitamin D, causing hypercalcemia. Too much vitamin D may cause dysrhythmias in patients who are receiving digoxin. Magnesium antacids or supplements should not be given concurrently owing to an increased risk of hypermagnesemia. Orlistat (Xenical) may prevent the absorption of fat-soluble nutrients such as vitamin D. Corticosteroids inhibit the absorption of calcium, which is a major effect of vitamin D. **Herbal/Food:** Unknown.

Pregnancy: Category C.

Treatment of Overdose: Vitamin D overdose results in hypercalcemia, hypercalciuria, and hyperphosphatemia. If the overdosage was recent, emesis should be induced to remove any remaining drug from the stomach. All vitamin D and calcium supplements are discontinued and the patient is placed on a low calcium diet until the hypercalcemia resolves.

Nursing Responsibilities:

- Obtain a thorough history to assess liver function, intake of fat-soluble vitamins, and current medications.
- Assess the sclera, skin pigment, bowel movements, and laboratory test results for evidence of liver dysfunction. Hepatic impairment and an accumulation of fat-soluble vitamins will increase the risk of toxicity from vitamin D supplementation.
- Obtain renal function tests such as serum creatinine and blood urea nitrogen (BUN) and urinalysis to establish baseline data, and regularly monitor these values during the course of treatment. High levels of vitamin D may cause renal impairment.
- Assess for adverse effects of vitamin D therapy, such as hypercalcemia, headache, weakness, dry mouth, thirst, increased urination, and muscular or bone pain.
- Monitor serum calcium, magnesium, alkaline phosphatase, creatinine, and phosphate levels, along with urinary calcium and phosphate levels.
- Monitor for signs of hypercalcemia such as deep bone and flank pain, anorexia, nausea, vomiting, thirst, constipation, muscle hypotonicity, pathologic fracture, bradycardia, lethargy, and psychosis.

Patient and Family Education:

- Consume dietary sources of vitamin D such as fortified milk, eggs, and fish, along with an adequate daily intake of calcium and phosphate.
- Take vitamin D exactly as directed because too much may cause toxic levels.
- Take vitamin D with meals to enhance its absorption.
- Immediately report signs of excess vitamin D, such as fatigue, weakness, nausea, vomiting, and changes in the color or amount of urine, to the health care provider.
- Immediately report yellowing of the skin or eyes, pale bowel movements, and darkened urine to the health care provider.
- Spend at least 20 minutes per day in sunlight to provide enough vitamin D to prevent disease.
- Restrict alcohol consumption while taking vitamin D to avoid liver damage.
- Do not take any other OTC vitamin D supplements or multivitamins without approval of the health care provider.

Drugs Similar to Calcitriol (Rocaltrol)

Other forms of vitamin D for therapy include ergocalciferol, cholecalciferol, calcifediol, dihydrotachysterol, doxercalciferol, and paricalcitol. Doses for the vitamin D preparations are shown in Table 75.4.

Cholecalciferol (Delta-D): Cholecalciferol (vitamin D_3) is the form of vitamin D that is produced in the skin after exposure to ultraviolet (UV) light. It is activated by the liver and kidneys to form calcitriol. Once activated, cholecalciferol produces identical actions and adverse effects as calcitriol. It is an oral dietary supplement for the prophylaxis and treatment of vitamin D deficiency.

Dihydrotachysterol (DHT): Dihydrotachysterol is an oral analog of vitamin D. This drug does not require kidney enzymes for activation and thus is useful in patients with renal impairment. Several weeks of therapy are required for maximum effect. Adverse effects are the same as those of calcitriol. Dihydrotachysterol is excreted primarily in the bile. Its indications include hypocalcemia, hypoparathyroidism, hypophosphatemia, and tetany.

Doxercalciferol (Hectorol): Doxercalciferol is an analog of vitamin D that is given by either the PO or IV route. This drug is activated by the liver alone: No kidney metabolism is necessary. Adverse effects are the same as those of calcitriol. However, caution must be taken to avoid the rapid development of hypercalcemia when this drug is administered by the IV route. Its only approved indication is for the treatment of secondary hyperparathyroidism and resultant bone disease.

Ergocalciferol (Calciferol, Drisdol): Ergocalciferol (vitamin D_2) is a natural vitamin D analog found in plants, fortified milk, eggs, and cereals. Once activated, ergocalciferol produces actions and adverse effects identical to those of calcitriol. Bile is required for its absorption, and the drug requires adequate kidney function to be metabolized to its active form. Indications for therapy with ergocalciferol are the same as those for calcitriol.

Paricalcitol (Zemplar): Paricalcitol is an analog of vitamin D that is given by either the PO or IV route. Adverse effects are the same as those of calcitriol; however, caution must be taken to avoid the rapid development of hypercalcemia when this drug is administered by the IV route. The only indication for paricalcitol is for the treatment of secondary hyperparathyroidism and resultant bone disease.

TABLE 75.4 Vitamin D Preparations

Drug	Route and Adult Dose (maximum dose where indicated)	Adverse Effects
calcitriol (Rocaltrol)	PO: 0.25 mcg/day	*Adverse effects are not observed at normal oral doses.*
cholecalciferol (Delta-D)	PO: 400–1,000 international units daily	Overdose: hypercalcemia, bone pain, lethargy, anorexia, nausea, vomiting, increased urination, hallucinations, dysrhythmias
dihydrotachysterol (DHT, Hytakerol)	PO: 0.75–2.5 mg/day for several days then 0.2–1 mg/day	
doxercalciferol (Hectorol)	PO: 10 mcg, 3 times/week IV: 4 mcg, 3 times/week (max: 60 mcg/week [PO]; 18 mcg/week [IV])	
ergocalciferol (Calciferol, Drisdol)	PO/IM: 25–125 mcg/day for 6–12 weeks	
paricalcitol (Zemplar)	IV: 0.04–0.1 mcg/kg, every other day (max: 24 mcg/kg)	

Note: *Italics* indicate common adverse effects. Underline indicates serious adverse effects.

75.6 Bisphosphonates increase bone density and are used to treat osteoporosis.

The most common drug class for treating osteoporosis is the **bisphosphonates.** These drugs are structural analogs of pyrophosphate, which is a natural substance that inhibits bone resorption. Bisphosphonates bind to hydroxyapatite in bone and suppress osteoclast activity, thus increasing bone mass density and reducing the incidence of fractures by about 50%. Examples include etidronate (Didronel), alendronate (Fosamax), tiludronate (Skelid), zoledronate (Zometa), risedronate (Actonel), and pamidronate (Aredia), which is available as an injectable drug. Etidronate also inhibits bone demineralization that could lead to osteomalacia; the other bisphosphonates do not have this effect. In addition to treating postmenopausal osteoporosis, some of the bisphosphonates are approved to treat corticosteroid-induced osteoporosis. A summary of the indications and their doses for bisphosphonates is shown in Table 75.5 and their doses are listed in Table 75.6.

The beneficial effects of bisphosphonates on bone mass density increase rapidly during the first year of therapy and plateau after 2 to 3 years. Even after discontinuation of therapy, bone density will remain increased for up to a year. For optimum effects, the patient must have adequate dietary consumption of calcium and vitamin D; any deficiencies should be corrected prior to initiating bisphosphonate therapy. Studies suggest that once-weekly dosing with bisphosphonates may give the same bone density benefits as daily dosing because of their extended duration of drug action.

Bisphosphonates are also the drugs of choice for the pharmacotherapy of Paget's disease. For this disorder therapy is usually cyclic, with bisphosphonates administered until serum ALP levels return to normal followed by several months without drugs. When the serum ALP level becomes elevated, therapy is begun again. The pharmacologic goals are to slow the rate of bone reabsorption and encourage the deposition of strong bone.

Several bisphosphonates are used to treat bone metastases and malignant hypercalcemia. Bone metastases are characterized by

TABLE 75.5 Indications of Bisphosphonates

Drug	Osteoporosis in Postmenopausal Women	Osteoporosis in Men	Glucocorticoid-Induced Osteoporosis	Paget's Disease	Hypercalcemia of Malignancy	Breast Cancer/Multiple Myeloma	Multiple Myeloma/Bone Metastases
alendronate (Fosamax)	X	X	X	X			
etidronate (Didronel)					X		
ibandronate (Boniva)	X						
pamidronate (Aredia)				X	X	X	
risedronate (Actonel)	X	X	X	X			
tiludronate (Skelid)				X			
Zoledronate (Reclast, Zometa)	X			X	X		X

TABLE 75.6 Selected Drugs for Osteoporosis and Other Bone Disorders

Drug	Route and Adult Dose (maximum dose where indicated)	Adverse Effects
Hormonal Agents		
calcitonin—salmon (Fortical, Miacalcin)	Hypercalcemia: subcutaneous/IM: salmon, 4 international units/kg bid Osteoporosis: intranasal: 1 spray/day (200 international units) in one nostril, alternating nostrils each day	*Rhinitis, flushing of the face and hands, pain at the injection site* Anaphylaxis
cinacalcet (Sensipar)	PO: start with 30 mg once daily; may increase every 2–4 weeks until target PTH of 150–300 mg/mL (max: 300 mg/day) for secondary hyperparathyroidism	*Dizziness, noncardiac chest pain, hypertension, nausea, anorexia, hypocalcemia, myalgia* Hypocalcemia, seizures
raloxifene (Evista)	PO: 60 mg/day	*Hot flashes, sinusitis, flulike symptoms, nausea* Breast pain, vaginal bleeding, pneumonia, and chest pain, venous thromboembolism, stroke
teriparatide (Forteo)	Subcutaneous: 20 mcg/day	*Dizziness, depression, insomnia, vertigo, rhinitis, increased cough, leg cramps, nausea, arthralgia* Syncope, angina, transient hypercalcemia
Bisphosphonates		
alendronate (Fosamax)	Osteoporosis: PO: 5–10 mg/day Paget's disease: PO: 40 mg/day for 6 months	*Nausea, dyspepsia, diarrhea, bone pain, back pain* Bone fractures, nephrotoxicity, hypocalcemia, hypophosphatemia, gastric ulcer, esophageal perforation, dysrhythmias, anemia, osteonecrosis of the jaw, atrial fibrillation
etidronate (Didronel)	PO: 5–10 mg/kg/day for 6 months or 11–20 mg/kg/day for 3 months	
ibandronate (Boniva)	PO: 2.5 mg/day or one 150-mg tablet per month, taken on the same date each month IV: 3 mg every 3 months	
pamidronate (Aredia)	IV: 15–90 mg in 1,000 mL normal saline or D_5W over 4–24 h	
risedronate (Actonel)	PO: 30 mg/day at least 30 min before the first drink or meal of the day	
tiludronate (Skelid)	PO: 400 mg/day taken with 6–8 oz of water 2 h before or after food for 3 months	
zoledronate (Reclast, Zometa)	IV (Zometa): 4 mg single dose infused over at least 15 min IV (Reclast): 5 mg single dose infused over at least 15 min	

Note: *Italics* indicate common adverse effects. Underline indicates serious adverse effects.

osteoclast hyperactivity, which creates "punched-out," osteolytic lesions that release large amounts of calcium into the blood. Bisphosphonates suppress osteoclast activity, thus slowing the rate of bone resorption and the rate of calcium release. Thus some of these drugs are approved for treating hypercalcemia due to malignancy. It is important to note that bisphosphonates are not antineoplastic agents; they have no effect on tumor cells and are only given as a palliative measure.

The most frequent adverse effects of bisphosphonates include GI symptoms such as nausea, vomiting, abdominal pain, dyspepsia, and esophageal irritation. Because these drugs are poorly absorbed from the intestinal tract, they must be taken on an empty stomach with plain water, at least 30 minutes before any other fluid, food, or medications. To avoid esophageal irritation, the patient should stay in an upright position for at least 30 minutes following the dose. Bisphosphonates are not metabolized and are excreted in the urine.

One unusual adverse effect that may occur during bisphosphonate therapy is osteonecrosis of the jaw. Symptoms include local pain and swelling, loosening of teeth, and infection at the site of the lesion. It is not clear what causes the necrosis. Discontinuing the bisphosphonate does not resolve the lesion because the drugs are incorporated in bone for many months and perhaps years.

CONNECTIONS

Patient Safety

Mistaken Identity

The evening nurse on duty administers medications at 10:15 P.M. When a nurse enters Ms. Brown's room, Ms. Brown is already in bed and falling asleep. The nurse gently shakes her and says, "I have your 10 P.M. medications, Ms. Brown." Although the patient awakens, she is not fully awake. The nurse hands her the medication and a glass of water. Ms. Brown takes the medication and quickly returns to sleeping. In leaving, the nurse notices the room number and realizes that the medication was just given to Ms. Crown, who is in a room down the hall from Ms. Brown.

How could the error have been prevented? What should have been done differently?

PROTOTYPE DRUG Alendronate (Fosamax)

Classification: **Therapeutic:** Drug for osteoporosis
Pharmacologic: Bisphosphonate, bone resorption inhibitor

Therapeutic Actions and Uses: First approved in 1995, alendronate is the best studied drug in this class. Alendronate is approved for the following indications:

- Prevention and treatment of osteoporosis in postmenopausal women
- Treatment of glucocorticoid-induced osteoporosis in both women and men
- Treatment to increase bone mass in men with osteoporosis
- Treatment of symptomatic Paget's disease in both women and men

Alendronate is also used off-label for treating hypercalcemia due to malignancy. Several regimens for alendronate are available: once daily (10 mg), twice weekly (35 mg), or once weekly (70 mg). Although the once weekly is more convenient, higher doses can produce more GI-related adverse effects. All doses must be taken on an empty stomach, preferably in a fasting state 2 hours before breakfast.

Therapeutic effects of alendronate may take 1 to 3 months to appear and may continue for several months after therapy is discontinued. This drug lowers serum alkaline phosphatase, which is the enzyme associated with bone turnover, without major adverse effects.

Mechanism of Action: Alendronate inhibits osteoclast-mediated bone resorption to minimize loss of bone density. Its effects appear to be localized to resorption sites of active bone turnover and it does not interfere with bone mineralization.

Pharmacokinetics:

Route(s)	PO
Absorption	Less than 1% (significantly decreased by food or beverages)
Distribution	Rapid skeletal uptake; unknown if secreted in breast milk; 78% bound to plasma protein
Primary metabolism	Not metabolized
Primary excretion	Up to 50% excreted unchanged in the urine
Onset of action	3–6 weeks
Duration of action	12 weeks or more after discontinuation

Adverse Effects: Adverse effects of alendronate are diarrhea, constipation, flatulence, nausea, vomiting, GI irritation, a metallic or altered taste perception, hypocalcemia, hypophosphatemia, abdominal pain, dyspepsia, arthralgias, myalgias, headache, and rash. Pathologic fractures may occur if the drug is taken longer than 3 months or in cases of chronic overdose. Although rare, this drug may cause serious esophagitis, which is the reason that patients should remain in an upright position at least 30 minutes after receiving a dose.

Contraindications/Precautions: Contraindications include patients with osteomalacia or who have hypersensitivity to this drug. Caution should be used in patients with renal impairment, heart failure, hyperphosphatemia, liver disease, fever or infection, active upper GI problems, and pregnancy. This drug is contraindicated in patients with abnormalities of the esophagus that delay esophageal emptying, such as stricture or achalasia, and in those who are unable to stand or sit upright for at least 30 minutes following administration of the drug.

Drug Interactions: Calcium, iron, antacids containing aluminum or magnesium, and certain mineral supplements interfere with the absorption of alendronate and have the potential to decrease its effectiveness. **Herbal/Food:** The patient's diet must have adequate amounts of vitamin D, calcium, and phosphates. Calcium and food (especially dairy products) reduce alendronate absorption.

Pregnancy: Category C.

Treatment of Overdose: Hypocalcemia is an expected effect of overdose and may be treated with oral or IV calcium compounds.

Nursing Responsibilities:

- Obtain a thorough history to determine risk factors for osteoporosis, history of fractures, GI conditions, and current medications and dietary supplements.
- Administer the medication with a full glass of water (6 to 8 oz) to reduce the potential for esophageal irritation.
- Assess for calcium and vitamin deficiencies. Patients should receive supplemental calcium and vitamin D if dietary intake is inadequate.
- Monitor a complete blood count (CBC), pH, chemistry panel, renal and liver function studies, vital signs, and bone density studies to establish baseline data.

Patient and Family Education:

- Immediately report seizures, muscle spasms, facial twitching, paralysis of extremities, difficulty urinating, decreased urination, darkened urine, nausea, vomiting, diarrhea, or bone pain to the health care provider.
- Take this medication on an empty stomach at least 30 minutes prior to eating—usually in the morning—and sit upright during this time to ensure proper absorption of the medication.
- Do not administer within 2 hours of consuming calcium-containing foods, beverages, or medications. Wait at least 30 minutes after taking an alendronate dose before taking any other drugs.
- Consume calcium-rich foods such as dairy products, dark green vegetables, soybeans, and canned fish with bones such as salmon.
- Report fever, pain, warmth, or inflammation over joints or decreased activity to the health care provider.
- Exercise daily, for optimal bone health and to prevent future complications, as recommended by the health care provider.

Drugs Similar to Alendronate (Fosamax)

Other bisphosphonates include clodronate, etidronate, ibandronate, pamidronate, risedronate, and tiludronate. Clodronate (Bonefos) is a bisphosphonate in the final stages of receiving approval from the FDA. It is available in 67 other countries.

Etidronate disodium (Didronel): Etidronate was the first bisphosphonate approved in the United States in 1977. It is less selective for bone than some of the other drugs in this class and is not a first-choice agent. It is approved for moderate to severe Paget's disease and for hypercalcemia due to malignancy. It is used off-label as an alternative to other bisphosphonates for prevention of postmenopausal and corticosteroid-induced osteoporosis. It is available only PO; the IV preparation was withdrawn from the market in 2005. Like all bisphosphonates, etidronate causes GI mucosa irritation and bone and joint pain. This drug is nephrotoxic and may increase the risk of dysrhythmias. This drug is pregnancy category C.

Ibandronate (Boniva): Ibandronate is one of the newest drugs in this class that was approved in 2003. It is approved for the prevention and treatment of postmenopausal osteoporosis. In addition to its oral formulation, it is the only IV bisphosphonate approved for the prophylaxis of postmenopausal osteoporosis. When administered IV, injections are spaced 3 months apart. Off-label indications include Paget's disease, bone metastases from prostate cancer, and malignant hypercalcemia. Adverse effects are similar to those of other drugs in this class. This drug is pregnancy category C.

Pamidronate (Aredia): Approved in 1991, pamidronate is available by slow IV infusion for hypercalcemia, moderate to severe Paget's disease, and bone metastases due to breast cancer or multiple myeloma. It may be used off-label to treat osteoporosis and osteogenesis imperfecta. Caution must be used when treating patients with renal impairment or who are receiving nephrotoxic drugs because the pamidronate is nephrotoxic. Other common adverse effects are nausea, fever, constipation, and dyspnea. Pamidronate is pregnancy category D.

Risedronate (Actonel): Approved in 1998, risedronate is FDA approved to prevent and treat glucocorticoid-induced and postmenopausal osteoporosis and symptomatic Paget's disease. It may be used off-label to treat osteolytic lesions due to multiple myeloma. Available by the PO route, it is reported to cause less GI distress than other bisphosphonates. Arthralgia, diarrhea, and headache are common adverse effects. This drug is pregnancy category C.

Tiludronate disodium (Skelid): Tiludronate was approved in 1997 to treat symptomatic Paget's disease. It is administered PO and has a similar adverse effect profile to that of other drugs in this class. This drug is pregnancy category C.

Zoledronate (Reclast, Zometa): Zoledronate (also called zoledronic acid) is one of the newer drugs in this class that was originally approved in 2001 for hypercalcemia due to malignancy. Since then indications have been expanded to include multiple myeloma, bone metastases, Paget's disease, and postmenopausal osteoporosis prophylaxis. A major advantage of zoledronate (Reclast) is that its prolonged duration of action results in a once-yearly dose for Paget's disease and osteoporosis prophylaxis. It is only available by IV infusion. Another major advantage is that it can be infused over 15 to 20 minutes compared to 2 to 4 hours for pamidronate. Common adverse effects include a transient flulike syndrome, nausea, constipation, and dyspnea. Zoledronate is nephrotoxic and should be used with caution in patients with renal impairment. Like pamidronate, zoledronate is pregnancy category D and should not be used during pregnancy.

75.7 Selective estrogen receptor modulators increase bone mass density and prevent fractures in postmenopausal women.

Selective estrogen receptor modulators (SERMs), a relatively new class of drugs that bind to estrogen receptors, are used in the prevention and treatment of osteoporosis. When SERMs bind to estrogen receptors, they may activate or inhibit them. Thus, SERMs may be estrogen agonists or antagonists, depending on the specific drug and the tissue involved. For example, raloxifene (Evista) blocks estrogen receptors in the uterus and breast; it has no estrogen-like proliferative effects on these tissues that might promote cancer. Raloxifene does, however, have estrogen-like effects that reduce bone resorption, thus increasing bone density and reducing the likelihood of fractures. It is most effective in preventing vertebral fractures. The dose for raloxifene is shown in Table 75.6. Tamoxifen is a SERM that is used to treat breast cancer (see Chapter 58).

PROTOTYPE DRUG Raloxifene (Evista)

Classification: **Therapeutic:** Agent for osteoporosis prophylaxis
Pharmacologic: Selective estrogen receptor modifier

Therapeutic Effects and Uses: Approved in 1997, raloxifene is primarily used for the prevention or treatment of osteoporosis in postmenopausal women. In 2007, it was approved for the prophylaxis of invasive breast cancer in postmenopausal women at high risk for breast cancer. High risk of breast cancer is defined as at least one breast biopsy showing carcinoma or atypical hyperplasia or having a first-degree relative with breast cancer. Other factors considered are current age, number of breast biopsies, age at menarche, nulliparity, or age of first live birth. It is important for nurses and patients to understand that this drug is for the prevention, not treatment, of breast carcinoma.

Raloxifene increases bone mass density, reducing vertebral fractures. It does not appear to reduce the incidence of fractures at nonvertebral sites. Raloxifene also reduces serum total cholesterol and low-density lipoproteins (LDLs) without lowering high-density lipoproteins (HDLs) or triglycerides. Unlike estrogen, which causes proliferation of uterine and breast tissue causing adverse effects, raloxifene is an estrogen antagonist on these tissues. Raloxifene has been used off-label to treat uterine leiomyomas, for pubertal gynecomastia, and for the prevention of bone loss in men with prostate cancer.

NURSING PROCESS APPLICATION

Patients Receiving Bisphosphonates

Assessment

Prior to administration:

- Obtain a complete health history, including allergies, drug history, and possible drug interactions.
- Assess for the presence or history of pathologic fractures, hypocalcemia, and hypercalcemia.
- Assess nutritional status.
- Obtain laboratory work that includes CBC, pH, electrolytes and renal function studies (BUN, creatinine, uric acid), and serum calcium, phosphorus, and magnesium levels.

Potential Nursing Diagnoses

- *Deficient Knowledge (Drug Therapy)*
- *Risk for Imbalanced Fluid Volume,* related to adverse effects of drug
- *Nausea,* related to adverse effects of drug
- *Acute Pain,* related to adverse drug effects on bone
- *Ineffective Therapeutic Regimen Management,* related to the fact that therapeutic response may take 1–3 months

Planning: Patient Goals and Expected Outcomes

Patient will:

- Demonstrate decreased progression of osteoporosis or Paget's disease and is free of pathologic fractures.
- Demonstrate decreased risk for pathologic fractures.
- Demonstrate an understanding of the drug's action by accurately describing drug adverse effects and precautions.
- Demonstrate an understanding of dietary needs and modifications.
- Maintain adequate fluid volume.

Implementation

Interventions and (Rationales)	Patient and Family Education
• Administer the medication in the morning with at least 8 oz of fluid and 30 minutes before eating or taking other medications (to prevent esophageal irritation and drug–drug interactions). • Keep the head elevated at least 30°. (This prevents esophageal irritation.)	Instruct the patient: • To take bisphosphonates in the morning with a full glass of water at least 30 minutes before eating a meal, drinking a beverage, or taking any other medicine. • To sit or stand (do not lie down) for at least 30 minutes after taking a bisphosphonate. This helps prevent esophageal irritation and ulceration. • Not to take a bisphosphonate late in the day if the patient forgets to take it in the morning.
• Monitor for pathologic fractures and bone pain. (This drug may cause defective mineralization of newly formed bone.)	• Instruct the patient to report any sudden bone or joint pain; difficulty with assuming sitting, standing, or lying positions; or swelling over bone or joints.
• Monitor for GI adverse effects. (There may be problems with absorption if the patient has persistent nausea or diarrhea.)	• Advise patient to immediately report new-onset nausea or diarrhea.
• Monitor calcium laboratory values: Serum calcium levels should be 9–10 mg/dL. (Through inhibition of bone resorption, drug causes blood levels of calcium to fall.)	Advise the patient to: • Keep laboratory appointments for baseline and periodic testing. • Report symptoms of hypocalcemia such as muscle spasms, facial grimacing, convulsions, irritability, depression, and psychoses. • Report symptoms of hypercalcemia such as increased bone pain, anorexia, nausea, vomiting, constipation, thirst, lethargy, fatigue, confusion, and depression.
• Monitor kidney function, especially creatinine level. (Etidronate cannot be used in patients whose creatinine level is greater than 5 mg/dL.)	• Instruct the patient to report any urinary changes, such as decreased urine production or increased urination.
• Monitor BUN, vitamin D, urinalysis, and serum phosphate and magnesium levels. (Bisphosphonates may cause renal dysfunction.) Monitor for toxic vitamin D levels, and assess for decreased serum phosphate and magnesium levels.	• Instruct the patient to report any weakness, persistent headaches, dry mouth, thirst, increased urination, and muscle or bone pain.
• Monitor dietary habits. (Diet must have adequate amounts of vitamin D, calcium, and phosphate.)	• Instruct the patient to include dietary sources of vitamin D, calcium, and phosphate, including dairy products and green leafy vegetables.
• Monitor adherence with the recommended regimen. (Patient may discontinue the drug because of perceived lack of response.)	Advise the patient: • That therapy should continue for 6 months maximum, but full therapeutic response may take 1–3 months. • That effects continue several months after the drug is discontinued. • To avoid vitamins, mineral supplements, antacids, and high calcium products within 2 hours of taking bisphosphonates.

Evaluation of Outcome Criteria

Evaluate the effectiveness of drug therapy by confirming that patient goals and expected outcomes have been met (see "Planning").

Mechanism of Action: As a selective estrogen receptor antagonist or agonist, raloxifene decreases bone resorption while increasing bone mass and density by activating estrogen receptors.

Pharmacokinetics:

Route(s)	PO
Absorption	60% absorbed
Distribution	Crosses the placenta; unknown if secreted in breast milk; 95% bound to plasma protein
Primary metabolism	Hepatic; extensive first-pass metabolism
Primary excretion	Primarily in feces
Onset of action	Unknown
Duration of action	Half-life: 28 h

Adverse Effects: The most common adverse effects of raloxifene therapy are hot flashes, leg cramps, and weight gain. Less common adverse effects include fever, arthralgia, myalgia, arthritis, depression, insomnia, chest pain, peripheral edema, decreased serum cholesterol, nausea, dyspepsia, vomiting, flatulence, GI disorders, gastroenteritis, cystitis, migraine headache, flulike symptoms, endometrial disorder, breast pain, and vaginal bleeding. Raloxifene may cause fetal harm when administered to a pregnant woman.

Contraindications/Precautions: This drug is contraindicated during lactation and pregnancy and in women who may become pregnant. Patients with a history of venous thromboembolism and those who are hypersensitive to raloxifene should not take this drug. Raloxifene should be discontinued 72 hours before prolonged immobilization is anticipated due to risk of thromboembolic events.

Drug Interactions: Concurrent use with warfarin may decrease prothrombin time (PT). Decreased raloxifene absorption will result from concurrent use with ampicillin or cholestyramine. Use of raloxifene with other highly protein-bound drugs (ibuprofen, indomethacin, diazepam, etc.) may interfere with binding sites. Patients should not take cholesterol-lowering drugs or ERT concurrently with this medication. **Herbal/Food:** Black cohosh has estrogenic effects and may interfere with the actions of raloxifene.

Pregnancy: Category X.

Treatment of Overdose: Overdose with raloxifene is uncommon and symptoms are given supportive treatment.

Nursing Responsibilities:

- Obtain a complete history to determine the patient's past medical history, especially uses of hormone replacement therapy, anticoagulants, or cholesterol lowering agents; pregnancy or lactation; or the occurrence of venous thromboembolism.
- Obtain baseline serum lipid and calcium levels, bone density, height, and weight.
- Discontinue this medication at least 72 hours prior or during prolonged immobilization.
- Monitor the patient for signs and symptoms of thromboembolic events, which may include chest pain or shortness of breath. Immediately report these findings to the prescriber.
- Do not give the drug concurrently with cholestyramine (Questran). If unavoidable, space the two drugs as widely apart as possible.
- Monitor laboratory tests periodically to include bone density, liver function, and plasma lipids.
- If the patient is taking oral anticoagulants monitor PT and international normalized ratio (INR).
- Immediately report signs and symptoms of gastric disturbances, headaches, migraines, infection, gynecological abnormalities, chest pain, and rashes to the prescriber.

Patient and Family Education:

- Immediately report unexplained calf pain or leg tenderness to the health care provider. If chest pain or shortness of breath occurs, seek immediate medical attention.
- Avoid restriction of movement during prolonged travel.
- Expect hot flashes during the course of this treatment.
- Do not take this with any other estrogen-containing drug or with any herbal supplement without approval of the health care provider.
- Notify the prescriber if taking any drugs to lower cholesterol.
- Do not breast-feed while taking this drug without approval of the health care provider.
- Immediately notify the health care provider of any known or suspected pregnancy.

Drugs Similar to Raloxifene (Evista)

The only other SERM is tamoxifen, which is a prototype antineoplastic drug in Chapter 58.

CONNECTION *Checkpoint* 75.2

From what you learned in Chapter 58, what are the indications for the pharmacotherapy with tamoxifen (Nolvadex)? See Answer to Connection Checkpoint 75.2 in Appendix A.

75.8 Calcitonin and several miscellaneous drugs are used for osteoporosis and other metabolic bone diseases.

Several miscellaneous drugs are used to treat MBD. Although they act by different mechanisms, they are presented together in this section because each is the only drug in its class.

Calcitonin (Fortical, Miacalcin): Calcitonin is a hormone that is produced and secreted by the thyroid gland in response to elevated serum calcium levels. This hormone directly inhibits osteoclasts. The function of calcitonin is to lower serum calcium levels by decreasing bone resorption and increasing the urinary excretion of calcium. It acts in direct opposition to PTH and vitamin D.

As a drug calcitonin is approved for the treatment of osteoporosis in women who are more than 5 years postmenopause.

Calcitonin increases bone mass density and reduces the risk of vertebral fractures when the diet is adequate for calcium and vitamin D. Because calcitonin is less effective for reducing osteoporosis-related fractures than the bisphosphonates, it is considered a second-line treatment. The dose for calcitonin is shown in Table 75.6.

In addition to treating osteoporosis, calcitonin is indicated for Paget's disease and hypercalcemia. In Paget's disease calcitonin slows the rate of bone turnover and decreases the incidence of bone pain. It is most effective in treating hypercalcemia caused by hyperparathyroidism, prolonged immobility, or that accompanies certain malignancies. Calcitonin is used off-label to reduce neuropathic pain and bone pain associated with metastatic bone cancer and osteoporosis.

Calcitonin-salmon is available by nasal spray or subcutaneous injection. Subcutaneous injections are initially given as a daily dose then decreased to two to three times per week. Calcitonin is also available as an IV injection. Because parenteral forms cause more nausea and vomiting than the intranasal form, they are rarely used except in patients with severe, acute hypercalcemia. When given IV, calcitonin decreases serum calcium levels in approximately 2 hours, with its effects lasting up to 8 hours. Adverse effects of calcitonin-salmon are generally minor; the nasal formulation may irritate the nasal mucosa and cause rhinitis or epistaxis. Generalized flushing of the face and hands may occur and anaphylaxis has been reported. This drug is pregnancy category C.

Cinacalcet (Sensipar): A relatively new drug that was approved in 2004, cinacalcet is a calcium modifier approved to treat hypercalcemia caused by parathyroid gland cancer or for secondary hyperparathyroidism due to chronic kidney disease. Cinacalcet is a calcium mimic; it is recognized as calcium by the parathyroid glands. The parathyroid glands are "tricked" into sensing high levels of calcium and they shut down the production of PTH. With decreased levels of PTH, bone resorption diminishes and serum calcium falls.

Cinacalcet is an oral drug. Its dose is slowly escalated until serum PTH and calcium levels return to normal values. Overtreatment may cause hypocalcemia. Nausea, vomiting, and diarrhea are common during therapy. This drug is a strong inhibitor of CYP450 enzymes and should be used with caution in patients who are receiving other drugs that are CYP450 substrates or inhibitors. This drug is pregnancy category C.

Teriparatide (Forteo): Approved in 2002, teriparatide is a form of human PTH produced by recombinant DNA technology. Its only approved indication is for the treatment of osteoporosis in men and postmenopausal women. This drug is usually reserved for patients with a high risk of bone fractures. Teriparatide is used off-label to treat hypoparathyroidism and corticosteroid-induced osteoporosis.

The actions of teriparatide are identical to those of endogenous PTH. It is the only drug that will increase bone formation. Unlike other medications that simply reduce bone resorption, teriparatide reduces resorption and stimulates the production of new bone. These actions increase bone mass density and reduce the incidence of fractures. A disadvantage of this drug is that it must be given daily by the subcutaneous route. It is available as a prefilled pen injector. Teriparatide is well tolerated, with dizziness and leg cramps being the most frequent adverse effects. This drug should be avoided in patients with an increased risk of bone cancer because it may increase the risks for acquiring osteosarcoma. Because patients with Paget's disease have an increased risk of osteosarcoma, they should not receive teriparatide. Although this drug is rated as pregnancy category C, it has been shown to cause cancer in laboratory animals at 60 times the doses used in patients.

Pathophysiology and Pharmacotherapy of Joint Disorders

75.9 Osteoarthritis is treated with a combination of analgesics and nonpharmacologic therapies.

A simple classification of joint disorders places them into two categories: noninflammatory and inflammatory. The most common of the noninflammatory disorders is osteoarthritis. Common inflammatory joint disorders such as rheumatoid arthritis and gout are covered in Sections 75.10 and 75.11. These joint conditions are frequent indications for pharmacotherapy, with joint pain being common to all disorders. Analgesics and anti-inflammatory drugs are important components of pharmacotherapy. A few additional drugs are specific to the particular joint pathology. Pharmacotherapy Illustrated 75.1 shows the types of joint pathology and their drug therapy.

Osteoarthritis (OA) is a progressive, degenerative joint disease caused by the breakdown of articular cartilage. It is the most common type of arthritis and the second most common cause of disability in the United States, affecting between 20 and 40 million persons. Weight-bearing joints such as the knee, vertebral column, and hip are most commonly affected. The hands are also affected because they are frequently used. OA may be classified as idiopathic or secondary. Idiopathic OA, the most common type, has no known cause but is associated with increasing age. The causes of secondary OA include trauma, mechanical stress, inflammation of the joint structures, neurologic disorders, use of certain medications, and joint instability. Excessive weight contributes to the development of OA, particularly in the knee and hip. Other risk factors associated with OA include decreased estrogen in menopausal women, excessive growth hormone, and increased PTH.

As cartilage thins in the affected joints there is less padding, and, eventually, the underlying bone is exposed. The bone thickens in the exposed areas, forming bone spurs and cysts that narrow the joint space. As these growths enlarge, small pieces may break off, leading to inflammation of the synovial membrane and a loss of lubricating fluid. This leads to further pain, inflammation, and destruction of the synovial membrane lining the joint. The affected joint becomes unstable and more susceptible to injury, with partial joint dislocations and other deformities that are common in advanced disease being seen.

The onset of OA is usually gradual, with pain and stiffness in one or more joints being the first manifestations. The patient with OA typically describes a deep, aching, localized pain, which is usually aggravated by movement and relieved by rest.

PHARMACOTHERAPY ILLUSTRATED 75.1

Joint Disorders

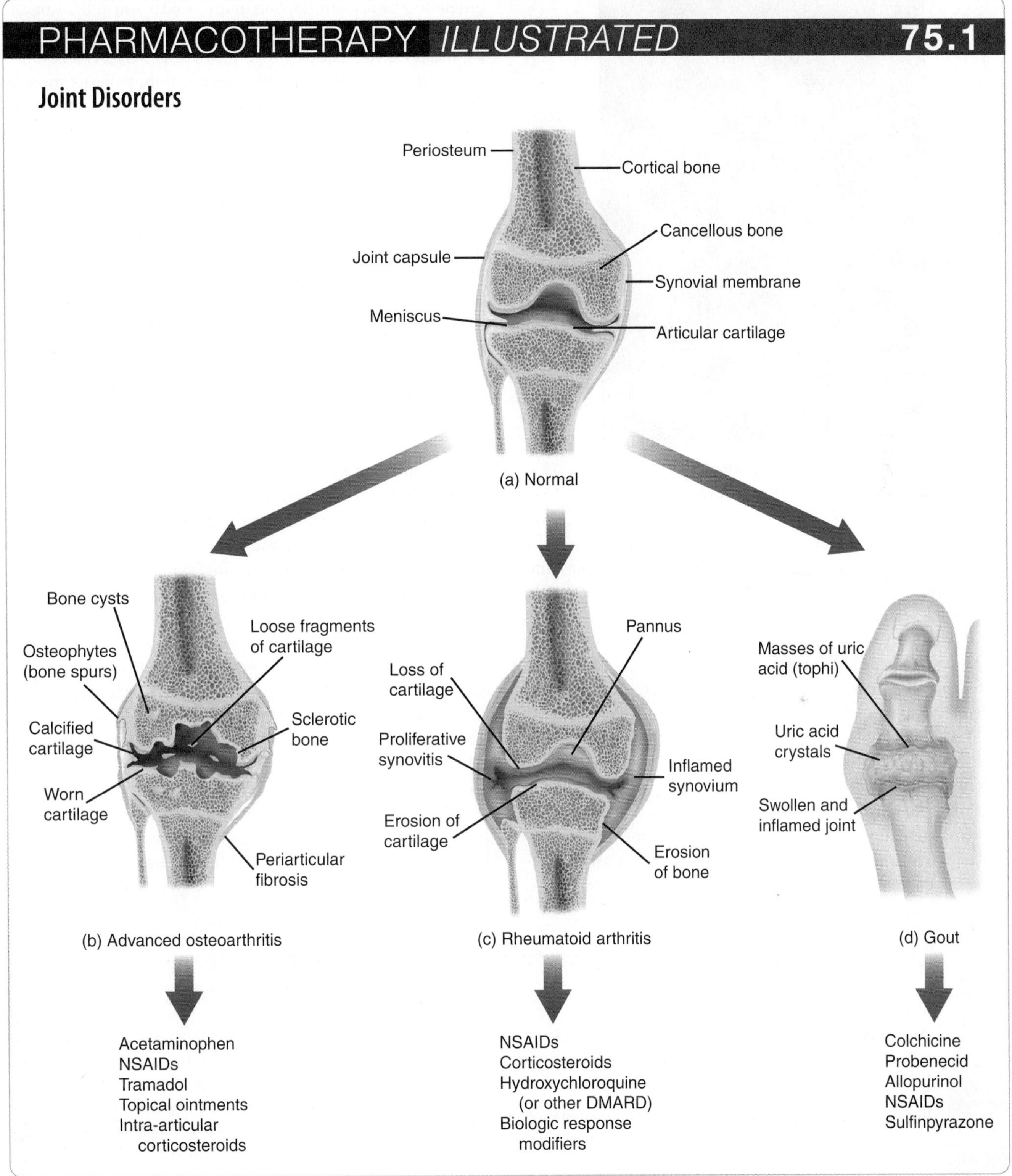

Pain at night may be accompanied by paresthesias. As the disease advances, the range of motion (ROM) of the joint decreases; this is often accompanied by complaints of progressive pain. Bone enlargement can increase joint size; flexion contractures contribute to joint instability. It is important to note that OA is not accompanied by the degree of inflammation associated with other forms of arthritis. The joints of a patient with OA are characteristically hard and cool to palpation. A patient with OA is shown in Figure 75.5. The diagnosis of OA is typically made using a detailed history and physical. Routine x-rays may be useful in determining structural joint changes.

Nonpharmacologic therapies are an essential component of OA management. Walking, nonimpact aerobics, and passive ROM exercises are important to maintain joint flexibility. Improving muscle strength, especially of the quadriceps muscle, will help patients improve their ability to perform activities of

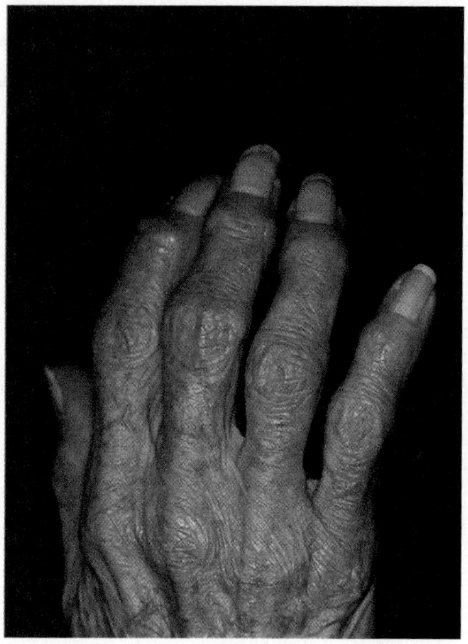

Figure 75.5 Patient with osteoarthritis.
Source: Courtesy of the American College of Rheumatology

daily living. Bracing may help keep joints positioned correctly and relieve pain. Knowledge of proper body mechanics and posture may offer some benefit. Patients who are obese should consider a weight loss program, especially if weight-bearing joints such as the hip and knee are affected. Weight loss has been associated with decreased pain and disability. Surgical procedures such as joint replacement and reconstructive surgery may become necessary when other methods are ineffective.

Drugs should be considered as additions to nonpharmacologic therapies in the overall management of OA. The goals of pharmacotherapy for OA include reducing pain and inflammation and minimizing disability. The initial treatment of choice is acetaminophen. Acetaminophen is inexpensive, participates in few drug–drug interactions, and has fewer serious adverse effects than other analgesics. For patients whose pain is unrelieved by acetaminophen, nonsteroidal anti-inflammatory drugs (NSAIDs), including naproxen and ibuprofen derivatives, are usually given. Because high doses of NSAIDs can result in GI bleeding and affect platelet aggregation, patients must be carefully monitored. Aspirin is no longer recommended because the high doses needed to produce pain relief in patients with OA may cause GI bleeding. Tramadol (Ultram) has become a popular drug for the treatment of moderate to severe pain. Although classified as an opioid, tramadol does not have abuse potential and is not a scheduled drug. Opioids such as codeine may be combined with acetaminophen for severe pain. The student should refer to Chapter 29 for a complete discussion of the actions and adverse effects of analgesics.

In acute cases, intra-articular corticosteroid injections may be used. With intra-articular injections, a long-acting corticosteroid such as triamcinolone is injected directly into the joint space of the affected joint. Pain relief generally lasts 3 months following the injection. Although this procedure relieves pain on a temporary basis, it can speed the destruction of cartilage if it is performed more frequently than every 4 to 6 months.

Many patients use topical medications, including salicylates (Aspercreme and Sportscreme), capsaicin (Capzasin), and counterirritants (Ben-Gay and Icy Hot), which are sold OTC as creams, gels, sprays, patches, or ointments, to relieve OA pain. These therapies are well tolerated and produce few adverse effects. These products should not be used more than four times daily and should be discontinued if irritation occurs.

A newer drug therapy for patients with moderate OA who do not respond adequately to analgesics includes sodium hyaluronate (Hyalgan), a chemical normally found in high amounts within the synovial fluid. Administered by injection directly into the knee joint, this drug replaces or supplements the body's natural hyaluronic acid that deteriorated because of the inflammation of OA. Treatment consists of one injection per week for three to five injections. Hyalgan helps provide a barrier that prevents friction and further inflammation of the joint by coating the articulating cartilage surface. Information

CONNECTIONS

Complementary and Alternative Therapies Glucosamine and Chondroitin for Osteoarthritis

Description: Many patients use OTC herbal medicines to relieve the pain and inflammation associated with OA. Two of the most commonly used agents are glucosamine and chondroitin.

History: Glucosamine is a natural substance that is an important building block of cartilage. With aging, glucosamine is lost with the natural thinning of cartilage. As cartilage wears down, the joints lose their normal cushioning ability, resulting in the pain and inflammation of OA. Chondroitin is another substance that forms part of the matrix between cartilage cells.

Claims: The use of glucosamine is thought to reduce cartilage breakdown and improve cartilage production and repair. Chondroitin is another dietary supplement purported to repair cartilage damaged by inflammation or injury.

Evidence: For the most part the use of these substances is not supported by medical research. Recent research has shown that using these common herbal substances provides minimal or nonexistent benefits. According to the Agency for Healthcare Research and Quality and a Cochrane analysis, these therapies may not benefit patients. The agency examined data from 53 clinical trials of glucosamine, chondroitin, hyaluronan, and arthroscopy and found that there was no evidence that patients with OA got any relief from the dietary supplements (Distler & Anguelouch, 2006; Kuehn, 2007; Reichenbach et al., 2007). However, although there have been some studies that have shown glucosamine to be more effective than a placebo in reducing mild arthritis and joint pain, published research findings for the most part are inconclusive (Clegg et al., 2006; Hampton, 2007). Due to the uncertainty regarding the effectiveness of glucosamine and chondroitin, a common practice among health care providers is that, because the adverse effects associated with the use of these substances are mild, then there is no need to discourage patients from using them if they perceive benefit from their use.

that is given to the patient prior to administration should include adverse effects such as pain or swelling at the injection site and the avoidance of any strenuous activities for approximately 48 hours after injection.

PharmFACT

The rates for rheumatoid arthritis vary from approximately 5% to 6% in Asian and Pacific Islanders to 12% in African Americans and 16% in whites. *Source:* King & Worthington, 2006.

75.10 Pharmacotherapy for rheumatoid arthritis includes analgesics, anti-inflammatory drugs, corticosteroids, and disease-modifying antirheumatic drugs.

Rheumatoid arthritis (RA) is a chronic, progressive autoimmune disease that causes inflammation of the joints. It is characterized by disfigurement and inflammation of multiple joints. RA is less common than OA, with RA affecting about 2.1 million persons in the United States. Typically RA occurs at an earlier age than OA, with the incidence of RA increasing up to age 70. It is important to differentiate between the two types of arthritis because the treatments vary greatly.

In RA, autoantibodies known as rheumatoid factors attack the person's tissues, activating complement and drawing leukocytes into the area, where they attack the cells of the synovial membranes and blood. Inflammation first occurs in the synovial membranes, which line joint cavities, then progresses to the surrounding articular cartilage. The damaged synovial membrane swells and the persistent inflammation spreads and damages the surrounding blood vessels, ligaments, and tendons. The swelling also causes hemorrhage, coagulation, and deposits of fibrin within the joints. This ultimately leads to scar tissue formation that immobilizes the joint.

The exact etiology of RA is not known, but it is likely a combination of environmental and genetic factors. Female reproductive hormones may influence the development of RA because it affects women three to five times more frequently than men. Infectious organisms, such as the Epstein-Barr virus, may play a role in a person developing the autoimmune processes seen with RA.

The course of RA is variable and the rate at which joint deformities develop is not consistent. Disease progression is typically fastest during the first 6 years, slowing thereafter. The onset is typically insidious, though it may be acute if precipitated by a stressor, such as infection. The patient with early RA typically complains of morning joint stiffness, swelling, pain, and generalized fatigue. The joints may be slightly reddened, warm, and tender to palpation. The pattern of joints involved is usually symmetric. The upper extremity joints are often involved, beginning with the hands and wrists, as well as the joints of the toes, ankles, and knees. As the disease worsens, the morning stiffness can extend several hours into the day and occur with any periods of prolonged rest. The persistent inflammation causes deformities of the joints and the supporting ligaments, tendons, and muscles, making activity painful. Muscle weakness and decreased ROM may be apparent. Most or all synovial joints are eventually affected. A patient with RA is shown in Figure 75.6.

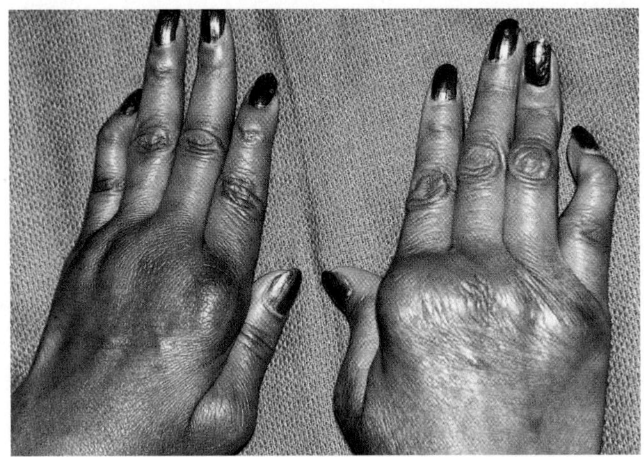

Figure 75.6 Patient with rheumatoid arthritis.
Source: Courtesy of Dr. Jason L. Smith.

Joint manifestations in RA typically precede systemic manifestations, which are associated with advancing disease. Extreme fatigue, anorexia, weight loss, anemia, and low-grade fever are common. Rheumatoid nodules may develop in the subcutaneous tissue of the forearm, toes, and fingers and in the viscera surrounding the heart, lungs, dura, and intestinal tract. Inflammation of the blood vessels can result in vasculitis. Respiratory complications, including pleurisy, pneumonitis, and fibrosis, are common as well as cardiac complications such as pericarditis and myocarditis.

Diagnosis of RA is based on the patient's history and physical and diagnostic tests. Laboratory tests that are helpful in supporting a diagnosis of RA include elevations in the serum rheumatoid factor, erythrocyte sedimentation rate (ESR), antinuclear antibody titers, and serum immunoglobulin levels. Routine x-rays are used to determine the degree of structural joint damage.

Like OA, nonpharmacologic therapies are an essential component of RA management. ROM and joint and muscle strengthening exercises are important if the patient is to continue normal activities of daily living. Psychological counseling may be helpful to help the patient deal with a potentially debilitating disease. Braces, splints, canes, and walkers can assist in ambulation. Loss of excess weight can help take the stress off inflamed joints. Proper rest helps reduce pain.

The primary goals of RA pharmacotherapy are to control inflammation, reduce pain, and maximize physical abilities. Pharmacotherapy for the relief of pain associated with RA includes the same classes of analgesics used for OA. Therapy is begun with NSAIDs, because these agents relieve both pain and inflammation. NSAIDs that are used to treat RA are usually given in doses that are higher than those for the patient with OA. Aspirin is not recommended for long-term therapy due to its adverse effects on the GI system and platelet aggregation. Acetaminophen is effective at relieving pain and fever but has no anti-inflammatory actions. Although the analgesics relieve symptomatic pain, they have little effect on disease progression.

Corticosteroids may be considered for moderate or severe RA. Because of their potent anti-inflammatory action, the goal of therapy with corticosteroids is to relieve the symptoms associated with RA flare-ups. They are not used for long-term therapy because of their adverse effects, including a greater susceptibility to infections, poor wound healing, and osteoporosis. Severe rebound symptoms can occur when these medicines are discontinued. For these reasons, corticosteroids, when used, are given at the lowest daily doses possible.

The progression of tissue damage characteristic of RA can be slowed or modified with a diverse group of drugs called **disease-modifying antirheumatic drugs (DMARDs).** These agents include gold salts, antimalarial agents, D-penicillamine, and drugs that modify immune and inflammatory responses. They have been found to reduce mortality rates, improve symptoms, and enhance the quality of life in patients with RA. Most health care providers begin therapy with a DMARD within 3 months of a confirmed diagnosis of RA. It would not be unusual for a patient to be taking several DMARDs and analgesics. The maximum therapeutic effects from DMARDs often take several months to achieve. All of these drugs can be toxic and close monitoring of patients is required during the course of therapy. Doses of DMARDs are listed in Table 75.7

The choice of a specific DMARD depends on the experiences of the health care provider and the response of the patient to therapy. Therapy often begins with hydroxychloroquine (Plaquenil), methotrexate (Rheumatrex), or sulfasalazine (Azulfidine) because these drugs have the most research-based evidence for reducing mortality. Many rheumatologists consider methotrexate to be the treatment of choice for patients with aggressive RA. Hydroxychloroquine therapy for 3 to 6 months is required to achieve therapeutic effects. Risks of toxicity with this drug are among the lowest associated with DMARDs.

Gold salts, D-penicillamine (Cuprimine), azathioprine (Imuran), cyclosporine (Neoral), and cyclophosphamide (Cytoxan) have been used in the past but are more toxic than many other DMARDs.

Biologic therapies are the newest DMARDs used for the treatment of RA. These biologic agents block steps in the inflammatory response, reduce joint inflammation, and slow the progression of joint damage. Etanercept (Enbrel) and infliximab (Remicade) are both tumor necrosis factor (TNF) antagonists. TNF is a naturally occurring cytokine produced by macrophages and activated T cells that mediates inflammation and modulates cellular immune responses. Elevated levels of TNF are found in the synovial fluid of patients with RA. Adalimumab (Humira) is a biologic response modifier that works to reduce inflammation in patients with polyarthritis. Given as a subcutaneous injection, Humira cannot be administered if the patient has an acute or chronic infection. Patients need to be tested for tuberculosis (TB) prior to initiating therapy. The biologic agents appear to be effective and relatively nontoxic. All of these medications are extremely expensive when compared to first-line therapies.

PROTOTYPE DRUG Hydroxychloroquine (Plaquenil)

Classification: **Therapeutic:** Antirheumatic drug, antimalarial
Pharmacologic: Disease-modifying antirheumatic drug

Therapeutic Effects and Uses: Approved in 1955, hydroxychloroquine is approved for the treatment of RA for which it is a first-line drug. This drug is also used for the prophylaxis and treatment of malaria, but chloroquine (Aralen) is the preferred

TABLE 75.7 Selected Disease-Modifying Antirheumatic Drugs

Drug	Route and Adult Dose (maximum dose where indicated)	Adverse Effects
abatacept (Orencia)	IV: 500–1,000 mg given on 0, 2, and 4 weeks, then every 4 weeks thereafter	*Local reactions at the injection site (pain, erythema, myalgia), headache, nasopharyngitis* <u>Infections: black box warning with adalimumab and TB with infliximab, sepsis, and invasive fungal infections, lupus-like syndrome, positive antinuclear antibodies, tumor lysis syndrome, heart failure exacerbations, Stevens–Johnson syndrome</u>
anakinra (Kineret)	Subcutaneous: 100 mg/day	
etanercept (Enbrel)	Subcutaneous: 25 mg twice weekly; or 0.08 mg/kg or 50 mg once weekly	
infliximab (Remicade)	IV: 3 mg/kg at weeks 0, 2, and 6, then every 8 weeks	
rituximab (Rituxan)	IV: 1,000 mg every 2 weeks for a total of two doses (give a corticosteroid 30 min prior to infusion)	
azathiopurine (Imuran, Azasan)	PO: 1 mg/kg/day once or in divided doses bid for 6–8 weeks (max: 2.5 mg/kg/day); maintenance dose is 1–2.5 mg/kg/day as a single dose or divided	*Chills, fever, malaise, myalgia* <u>Myelosuppression, hepatoxicity, lymphoproliferative disorders</u>
hydroxychloroquine (Plaquenil)	PO: 400–600 mg/day for 4–12 weeks, then 200–400 mg once daily Maintenance dose: 10–20 mg/day	*Anorexia, nausea, vomiting, headache, and personality changes* <u>Retinopathy, agranulocytosis, aplastic anemia, seizures</u>
methotrexate (Rheumatrex, Trexall)	PO: 7.5 mg once/week or 2.5 mg every 12 h for three doses once/week (max: 20 mg/week)	*Headache, glossitis, gingivitis, mild leukopenia, nausea* <u>Ulcerative stomatitis, myelosuppression, aplastic anemia, hepatic cirrhosis, nephrotoxicity, sudden death, pulmonary fibrosis, teratogenicity</u>
sulfasalazine (Azulfidine)	PO: 500–1,000 mg/day (max: 3 g/day)	*Headache, anorexia, nausea, vomiting* <u>Anaphylaxis, Stevens–Johnson syndrome, agranulocytosis, leukopenia, reversible oligospermia</u>

Note: *Italics* indicate common adverse effects. <u>Underline</u> indicates serious adverse effects.

agent for this parasitic infection (see Chapter 54). It may be used to treat systemic lupus erythematosus in patients who have not responded well to other anti-inflammatory drugs. This agent relieves the severe inflammation characteristic of these disorders.

For full effectiveness, hydroxychloroquine is most often prescribed concurrently with salicylates and glucocorticoids. The major advantage of hydroxychloroquine is that it exhibits less bone marrow, renal, and hepatic toxicity than other DMARDs.

Mechanism of Action: The exact mechanism of action of hydroxychloroquine in reducing the symptoms of RA is not known. This drug reduces the migration of neutrophils and eosinophils and likely inhibits the synthesis of histamine and prostaglandins.

Pharmacokinetics:

Route(s)	PO
Absorption	Rapidly and almost completely absorbed
Distribution	Widely distributed; concentrated in the lungs, liver, erythrocytes, eyes, skin, and kidneys; crosses the placenta; secreted in breast milk
Primary metabolism	Partially in the liver to active metabolite
Primary excretion	Renal
Onset of action	Unknown
Duration of action	Unknown

Adverse Effects: The primary adverse effects of hydroxychloroquine are GI-related, such as anorexia, weight loss, nausea, and vomiting. Possible ocular effects include blurred vision, photophobia, diminished ability to read, and blacked-out areas in the visual field. With high doses or prolonged therapy, these retinal changes may be irreversible in some patients. Other adverse effects of hydroxychloroquine include fatigue, anxiety, vertigo, skin rash, itching, bleaching or loss of hair, headache, and mood and mental changes.

Contraindications/Precautions: Patients with known hypersensitivity to this drug or who exhibit retinal or visual field changes associated with quinoline drugs should not receive hydroxychloroquine. Caution should be used in patients with hepatic impairment, alcoholism, impaired renal function, porphyria, metabolic acidosis, and those with a tendency for dermatitis.

Drug Interactions: Antacids that contain aluminum or magnesium may prevent the absorption of hydroxychloroquine. Hydroxychloroquine may increase the risk of liver damage when administered with other hepatotoxic drugs. Alcohol use should be eliminated during therapy. This drug may increase digoxin levels and may interfere with the patient's response to the rabies vaccine. Concurrent administration with cimetidine may increase hydroxychloroquine levels. **Herbal/Food:** None known.

Pregnancy: Category C.

Treatment of Overdose: Overdose may be life threatening, especially in children. Therapy with anticonvulsants, vasopressors, and antidysrhythmics may be necessary.

Nursing Responsibilities:

- Obtain a complete health history, including current medications, vital signs, a complete physical examination, CBC, platelets, liver and renal function tests, uric acid levels, and urinalysis. These test results are obtained as baseline data and performed periodically to assess the effectiveness of the drug.
- Obtain baseline and periodic ophthalmic exams for those requiring long-term therapy.
- Discontinue this drug if the patient develops weakness, visual symptoms, hearing loss, unusual bleeding, or bruising or if skin eruptions occur.

Patient and Family Education:

- Take the medication at the same time every day exactly as directed.
- Administer with milk or food to decrease gastric upset. Do not take OTC antacids unless approved by the health care provider.
- Immediately report any signs of infection to the health care provider.
- Be aware that several months of therapy may be necessary before the maximum benefit is achieved.
- Immediately report changes in vision, muscle weakness, hearing loss, or unusual bleeding to the health care provider.
- Do not drive or perform other hazardous activities until the effects of the drug are known because this drug may cause drowsiness or dizziness.
- Avoid direct sunlight or wear protective clothing outside because this drug may cause photosensitivity.
- Limit or eliminate alcohol consumption to prevent liver damage.

Drugs Similar to Hydroxychloroquine (Plaquenil)

The first- and second-choice DMARDs are described next. Gold salts (Auranofin, Aurothioglucose, and gold sodium thiomalate) and penicillamine (Cuprimine, Depen) are DMARDs that are rarely used and the student should refer to a drug guide for information. Cyclosporine and azathioprine are immunosuppressants that occasionally are used as DMARDs. They are described in Chapter 45.

Adalimumab (Humira): Approved in 2002, adalimumab is a monoclonal antibody that binds to and neutralizes TNF. Approved for adults with RA, adalimumab is administered by the subcutaneous route twice a week. Injection site reactions and adverse effects similar to etanercept are common. There is an increased chance of developing an infection due to its immunosuppressant actions. Reactivation of hepatitis B virus has been reported. Long-term use of adalimumab may lead to a slightly above-normal risk for malignancies, especially lymphoma and melanoma. Adalimumab is pregnancy category B.

Anakinra (Kineret): Approved in 2001, anakinra inhibits interleukin-1 (IL-1), an important chemical mediator of inflammation. It is approved for RA that has not responded to one or more DMARDs. A major disadvantage of this drug is that it must be given daily by the subcutaneous route. Injection site reactions such as pain, swelling, edema, and bruising occur more often than with the other drugs in its class. Ice and hydrocortisone cream are recommended to diminish the pain, along with site rotation. Upper respiratory infections and influenza symptoms occur in many patients. The manufacturer recommends that anakinra not be administered concurrently with TNF inhibitors such as etanercept due to an increased risk of infections. Anakinra is pregnancy category B.

Etanercept (Enbrel): Approved in 1998, etanercept binds specifically to TNF and blocks it from attaching to cell surface TNF receptors. It is approved for the treatment of moderate to severe RA, psoriatic RA in adults, and polyarticular juvenile RA in children with inadequate response to other DMARDs. Etanercept was also approved in 2003 for the treatment of ankylosing spondylitis. Etanercept is administered by the subcutaneous route twice a week. Other than injection site reactions such as pain, swelling, and bruising, adverse effects are uncommon. Adverse effects include serious infection, reactivation of TB, demyelinating disorders, heart failure, and blood dyscrasias. Concurrent use of etanercept with sulfasalazine may result in leukopenia. Etanercept is pregnancy category B.

Infliximab (Remicade): Infliximab is a monoclonal antibody against TNF. It binds to TNF, preventing it from interacting with TNF receptors and causing inflammation. The drug is approved for the treatment of moderate to severe active RA, psoriatic arthritis, spondylitis, ulcerative colitis, and Crohn's disease. For RA infliximab is usually combined with methotrexate and is given as an IV infusion over several hours, followed by subsequent injections in weeks 2 and 6 and every 8 weeks thereafter. Frequent adverse effects are nausea, vomiting, headache, diarrhea, abdominal pain, and infusion-related reactions. Acetaminophen and diphenhydramine (Benadryl) are given prior to infusion to decrease the symptoms of infusion reaction such as chest pain, tachycardia, shortness of breath, and light-headedness. Tuberculosis and other infections commonly occur during therapy. Infliximab is pregnancy category B.

Leflunomide (Arava): Approved in 1998, leflunomide is a DMARD with a unique mechanism of action. It inhibits an enzyme in mitochondria that is responsible for the synthesis of pyrimidines, which are building blocks for DNA and ribonucleic acid (RNA). The result is an inhibition in B-cell and T-cell function. Reduced cytokine and antibody production by these cells reduces inflammation and joint destruction. After a loading dose for 3 days, this drug is given orally once daily. Leflunomide has an exceptionally long half-life, and it can be detected in the blood as long as 2 years after discontinuation. If toxicity occurs, the administration of cholestyramine for 11 days can clear most leflunomide from the body. Common adverse effects include diarrhea, nausea, vomiting, headache, and alopecia. Leflunomide is hepatotoxic and liver function must be regularly monitored during therapy. The possibility of pregnancy should be excluded before therapy is begun because this drug is pregnancy category X.

Methotrexate (Rheumatrex): Methotrexate is a drug used for a number of proliferative and inflammatory diseases, including various carcinomas and leukemias, immunosuppression following kidney transplantation, severe psoriasis, and RA. Methotrexate acts as a folic acid antagonist, and it is a potent immunosuppressant. Gastric irritation and stomatitis are the most frequent adverse effects; these are minimized by the concurrent use of folic acid. Patients, particularly those who are older, obese, or have diabetes or renal disease, need to be monitored for hepatotoxicity, bone marrow suppression, and pneumonitis. The possibility of pregnancy should be excluded before therapy is begun because this drug is pregnancy category X. A prototype feature for methotrexate may be found in Chapter 58.

Sulfasalazine (Azulfidine): Sulfasalazine is a sulfonamide and one of the oldest drugs for RA that was approved in 1950. It is also approved for juvenile RA, Crohn's disease, and ulcerative colitis. It is available as an enteric-coated tablet that must be taken three to four times daily. Its beneficial effects are noted quickly, often after 4 weeks of therapy. GI complaints such as nausea, vomiting, anorexia, diarrhea, and abdominal pain occur in a significant number of patients taking this drug, and these may cause discontinuation of therapy. The GI adverse effects are better tolerated if therapy starts with a low dose that is gradually increased. Headache; blood dyscrasias, especially leukopenia; and skin rashes are also frequent. Regular monitoring of CBCs for bone marrow suppression should be conducted. Patients with allergies to sulfur or other sulfonamides should not receive sulfasalazine. Concurrent administration with iron supplements or antibiotics should be avoided because doing so diminishes the absorption of sulfasalazine. Sulfasalazine is pregnancy category B.

CONNECTION *Checkpoint* 75.3

Chloroquine (Aralen) and hydroxychloroquine (Plaquenil) are very similar, and both may be used to treat malaria. From what you learned in Chapter 54, what organism causes malaria? Describe how these drugs are used for prophylaxis of malaria. See Answer to Connection Checkpoint 75.3 in Appendix A.

Pharmacotherapy of Gout

75.11 Gout is treated with drugs that decrease joint pain and inflammation and lower uric acid levels.

Gout is a form of acute arthritis caused by an accumulation of uric acid (urate) crystals in the joints and other body tissues, causing inflammation. Between 1% and 3% of the U.S. population are affected by gout. Of patients with gout 90% are men, who first manifest symptoms between the ages of 30 and 60; women are affected after menopause.

Gout may be classified as primary or secondary. Primary gout is caused by genetic errors in the metabolism of purines. Uric acid is a waste product created by the metabolic breakdown of the nucleic acids DNA and RNA. The kidneys are responsible for excreting uric acid. High levels of uric acid crystals may result from an increased metabolism of nucleic acids or the reduced excretion of uric acid by the kidneys. Primary gout may therefore be viewed as an imbalance in the uric acid handling by the body. The production of uric acid crystals exceeds the excretion capability of the kidneys. Primary gout is inherited as an X-linked trait; males inherit the disorder through female carriers.

Secondary gout is caused by diseases or drugs that increase the metabolic turnover of nucleic acids or that interfere with the excretion of uric acid. Some examples of drugs that may cause gout include thiazide diuretics, aspirin, cyclosporine, and alcohol, when ingested on a chronic basis. Conditions that can cause secondary gout include diabetic ketoacidosis, hypothyroidism, multiple myeloma, renal impairment, and diseases associated with a rapid cell turnover such as leukemia, hemolytic anemia, and polycythemia.

The primary diagnostic criterion for gout is the serum uric acid level. **Hyperuricemia** is defined as a serum uric acid level of 7 mg/dL. Patients with mild hyperuricemia are asymptomatic. Once the level of uric acid rises to saturation levels in body fluids, urate crystals form and symptoms appear, usually with a sudden onset.

Acute gouty arthritis occurs when needle-shaped uric acid crystals accumulate in joints, resulting in extremely painful, red, and inflamed tissue. Attacks have a sudden onset, often occur at night, and may be triggered by ingestion of alcohol, dehydration, stress, injury to the joint, or fever. Gouty arthritis most often occurs in the big toes, heels, ankles, wrists, fingers, knees, or elbows and may be accompanied by an elevated temperature. With chronic gout, bumps called tophi, or deposits of sodium urate crystals in the subcutaneous tissue, may be present, particularly on the outer ear, arms, and fingers. Deposits of urate crystals in the kidneys may lead to the development of urinary calculi and renal failure. Nephrolithiasis occurs in 10% to 25% of patients with gout and is more likely to occur in patients with low fluid intake and when the urine is acidic.

Gout may be difficult to diagnose because early symptoms may be vague. Although most people with gout have hyperuricemia, the serum levels of uric acid may be normal even during an acute attack. To confirm a diagnosis, a synovial fluid analysis may be performed to evaluate for the presence of uric acid crystals or to rule out synovial fluid infection as the cause of the symptoms.

In its early phases, treatment of gout is very successful. The goals of gout pharmacotherapy are threefold:

- Termination of acute episodes
- Prevention of future attacks
- Avoidance of the formation of gout complications, such as tophi and kidney stones

Combination therapy using uric acid inhibitors such as colchicine and antigout medications such as probenecid (Benemid) and allopurinol (Zyloprim) is the mainstay of gout therapy. Uric acid inhibitors block the accumulation of uric acid in the blood or uric acid crystals within the joints. When uric acid accumulation is blocked, the symptoms associated with gout diminish. These drugs are most effective when taken within the first 12 hours of an acute attack. Oral colchicine may be taken every hour until painful joint symptoms resolve or adverse effects occur. About 80% of the patients using uric acid inhibitors experience GI complaints such as abdominal cramping, nausea, vomiting, and diarrhea. Drugs for gout are listed in Table 75.8.

NSAIDs are the drugs of choice for treating the pain and inflammation of acute episodes of gout. Commonly used NSAIDs include indomethacin (Indocin) and naproxen (Naprosyn), which are taken orally every day. Corticosteroids may be used to treat exacerbations of acute gout, particularly when the symptoms are in a single joint and the medication can be delivered intra-articularly. The most commonly used corticosteroid is prednisone. Most patients report that symptoms improve within a few hours of treatment and the acute episode terminates within a week.

Prophylaxis of gout includes dietary management, avoidance of drugs that worsen the condition, and therapy with antigout medications. Patients should avoid high purine foods such as organ meats, legumes, alcoholic beverages, mushrooms, and oatmeal because these foods form nucleic acids when they are metabolized. Patients should avoid aspirin, niacin, and diuretics because their use can precipitate an acute episode of gout. Renal complications may be avoided by adequate fluid intake and a low protein diet.

TABLE 75.8 Drugs for Gout

Drug	Route and Adult Dose (maximum dose where indicated)	Adverse Effects
allopurinol (Lopurin, Zyloprim)	PO (primary): 100 mg/day; may increase by 100 mg/week (max: 800 mg/day) PO (secondary): 200–800 mg/day	*Drowsiness, skin rash, diarrhea* <u>Severe skin reactions, bone marrow depression, hepatotoxicity, renal failure</u>
colchicine	PO: 0.5–1.2 mg, followed by 0.5–0.6 mg every 1–2 h until pain is relieved (max: 4 mg/attack)	*Nausea, vomiting, diarrhea, GI upset* <u>Bone marrow depression, aplastic anemia, leucopenia, thrombocytopenia, agranulocytosis, severe diarrhea, nephrotoxicity</u>
probenecid (Probalan)	PO: 250 mg bid for 1 week, then 500 mg bid (max: 3 g/day)	*Nausea, vomiting, headache, anorexia, flushed face* <u>Anaphylaxis, severe skin reactions, hepatotoxicity, anemia, aplastic anemia, leukopenia</u>
sulfinpyrazone (Anturane)	PO: 100–200 mg bid for 1 week, then increase to 200–400 mg bid	*GI distress, rash* <u>Blood dyscrasias, nephrolithiasis</u>

Note: *Italics* indicate common adverse effects. <u>Underline</u> indicates serious adverse effects.

PROTOTYPE DRUG Colchicine

Classification: **Therapeutic:** Antigout agent
Pharmacologic: Uric acid inhibitor

Therapeutic Effects and Uses: Colchicine is a natural product obtained from the autumn crocus, which is grown in gardens and found in meadows throughout the United States and Canada. It has been used for centuries as a natural product and was approved by the FDA in 1939. It is the drug of choice for the treatment of acute gouty arthritis. It is much more effective if taken within 24 hours of the onset of symptoms. Colchicine has several off-label indications that include amyloidosis, Paget's disease, hepatic cirrhosis, and Mediterranean fever. This drug is nearly always administered PO. An IV formulation is available but it exhibits considerable toxicity and is rarely used.

Although colchicine has no analgesic properties, patients experience pain relief owing to the reduction in inflammation. Low doses of colchicine may be used as prophylactic therapy for gouty arthritis in patients with normal or slightly elevated serum uric acid levels. Should the patient note the onset of an acute episode, the dose can be increased until symptoms subside. It is important to understand, however, that colchicine does not inhibit uric acid synthesis and does not promote uric acid excretion. Thus, if the patient has escalating serum uric acid levels, allopurinol or sulfinpyrazone is the drug of choice for prophylaxis (see Section 75.12). Patients who are on colchicine prophylaxis therapy may discontinue the drug after they have been symptom free for a year and have normal serum uric acid levels. In some patients, discontinuation may precipitate an acute gout episode.

Mechanism of Action: Colchicine inhibits the migration of neutrophils into the area of inflammation. This drug reduces the inflammation associated with acute gouty arthritis by inhibiting the synthesis of microtubules, which are the subcellular structures responsible for helping white blood cells infiltrate an area.

Pharmacokinetics:

Route(s)	PO
Absorption	Rapidly absorbed
Distribution	Widely distributed, concentrated in leukocytes, kidney, liver, spleen, and intestinal tract
Primary metabolism	Hepatic
Primary excretion	Feces
Onset of action	12 h
Duration of action	Half-life: variable (1.7–20.9 h)

Adverse Effects: The most significant adverse effects of colchicine are GI related and these may occur in up to 80% of patients. These include nausea, vomiting, abdominal pain, anorexia, and diarrhea. This drug may cause bone marrow toxicity, and aplastic anemia, leucopenia, thrombocytopenia, or agranulocytosis may occur. Additional adverse effects include hepatotoxicity, mental confusion, azotemia, proteinuria, hematuria, and oliguria. Severe irritation and tissue damage may occur if the IV formulation leaks around the injection site.

Contraindications/Precautions: This drug is contraindicated in patients with a known hypersensitivity to colchicine, and in those with serious GI, renal, hepatic, pregnancy, or cardiac impairment. Patients with blood dyscrasias should not receive colchicine. Colchicine should be used with caution in older adults and debilitated patients, or in patients with an early manifestation of GI, renal, hepatic, or cardiac disease.

Drug Interactions: Concurrent use with NSAIDs may increase the risk of serious GI symptoms. Colchicine may exhibit additive bone marrow toxicity with cyclosporine, phenylbutazone, and other drugs that adversely affect bone marrow. Erythromycin may increase serum colchicine levels. Loop diuretics may decrease colchicine effects. Alcohol or products that contain alcohol may cause skin rashes and result in additive liver damage. Colchicine may increase a patient's sensitivity to central nervous system (CNS) depressants. Colchicine may also directly interfere with the absorption of vitamin B_{12}. **Herbal/Food:** Alcohol and foods that are rich in purines, including salmon, sardines, and organ meats should be avoided. Foods that cause the urine to become more alkaline, such as milk, fruits, carbonated drinks, most vegetables, molasses, and baking soda, may increase the risk of kidney stones.

Pregnancy: Category C (PO) or D (IV).

Treatment of Overdose: Overdoses (including accidental ingestion of autumn crocus) may cause severe GI distress, shock, paralysis, delirium, respiratory failure, and death. Treatment is symptomatic and may include gastric lavage and hemodialysis.

Nursing Responsibilities:

- Obtain a complete health history, including current medications, vital signs, a complete physical examination, and CBC; platelets; electrolytes; liver and renal function studies; uric acid levels; and urinalysis. These test results are obtained as baseline data and performed periodically to assess the effectiveness of the drug.
- Do not administer parenteral doses to pregnant women (category D).
- Monitor serum uric acid and creatinine throughout therapy.
- Monitor for and report early signs of colchicine toxicity, which include weakness, abdominal discomfort, anorexia, nausea, vomiting, and diarrhea.
- Monitor intake and output and patterns of urination, especially during acute gouty attacks. Increased fluid intake promotes excretion and reduces the risk of urate crystal formation in the kidneys and ureters.

Patient and Family Education:

- Take the medication exactly as ordered. Discontinuing this drug prematurely may result in an acute gout episode.
- Report GI symptoms, rash, headache, loss of appetite, lower back pain, painful urination, or blood in the urine to the health care provider.
- Increase fluid intake to 3 to 4 L per day and report any decrease in urinary output, cloudy urine, unusual color or odor to the urine, pain, or discomfort on urination to the health care provider.

- Avoid alcohol and foods that are rich in purines, including salmon, sardines, legumes, mushrooms, oatmeal, and organ meats.
- Take this drug on an empty stomach when symptoms first appear.
- Limit foods that cause the urine to become more alkaline, which may increase the risk of kidney stones. These foods include milk, fruits, carbonated drinks, most vegetables, molasses, and baking soda.

Drugs Similar to Colchicine

Colchicine is the only drug in this class.

PharmFACT

Pseudogout is a type of arthritis that can cause symptoms similar to gout but involves accumulation of a different type of crystal: calcium pyrophosphate. The patient is treated with analgesics or anti-inflammatory drugs: There is no curative therapy. *Source:* Schumacher, 2006.

75.12 Hyperuricemia is treated with drugs that reduce serum levels of uric acid.

Many patients with increased uric acid levels are asymptomatic. In most cases, pharmacotherapy is not indicated for asymptomatic patients. For patients with repeated acute episodes of chronic gout, however, prophylactic pharmacotherapy should be used to lower serum uric acid levels. Prophylaxis may be obtained by blocking the formation of uric acid or by increasing its excretion.

Allopurinol (Zyloprim) is the drug of choice for the prophylaxis of gout. Allopurinol acts by inhibiting **xanthine oxidase,** which is the enzyme responsible for the formation of uric acid. Blocking the synthesis of uric acid will lower serum uric acid levels, thus preventing gout. It is also used in patients with renal impairment or those who have renal obstruction caused by uric acid stones.

Uricosurics are drugs that increase the rate of excretion of uric acid by blocking its reabsorption in the kidney. These agents are most effective in preventing hyperuricemia and tophi associated with chronic gout and should not be used to treat acute attacks of gouty arthritis. The uricosuric drugs have no analgesic or anti-inflammatory properties. The uricosuric drugs used for gout prophylaxis include probenecid (Benemid) and sulfinpyrazone (Anturane). These drugs may precipitate acute gout during the period of initial therapy because they mobilize the uric acid that has been stored in the body. Concurrent administration of colchicine can help prevent this adverse effect. The mobilization of uric acid may also cause or worsen kidney stones due to the increased amount of uric acid being excreted by the kidneys. To prevent these adverse effects of early therapy, the uricosurics are started at low doses and increased gradually over several weeks. During this initial therapy, the urine may be made more alkaline by the administration of sodium bicarbonate to prevent uric acid crystals from forming. Drugs for hyperuricemia and gout are listed in Table 75.8.

PROTOTYPE DRUG Allopurinol (Zyloprim)

Classification: **Therapeutic:** Antigout agent
Pharmacologic: Xanthine oxidase inhibitor

Therapeutic Effects and Uses: Allopurinol is an older drug that was approved in 1966 for gout and its complications. It is used to control the hyperuricemia that causes severe gout and to reduce the possibility of flare-ups of acute gouty attacks. It is also approved to prevent recurrent nephrolithiasis due to calcium oxalate stones in patients with elevated uric acid levels. It may be used prophylactically to reduce the severity of the hyperuricemia associated with antineoplastic and radiation therapies, both of which increase plasma uric acid levels by promoting nucleic acid degradation. This drug takes 1 to 3 weeks to bring serum uric acid levels to within the normal range.

Allopurinol is available by the PO and IV routes. The IV administration is usually reserved for patients with high uric acid levels resulting from cancer chemotherapy.

Mechanism of Action: Allopurinol reduces uric acid formation by selectively inhibiting the action of xanthine oxidase, which is the enzyme responsible for the formation of uric acid. Lowering the formation of uric acid prevents hyperuricemia. Unlike the uricosuric agents, allopurinol does not increase the renal excretion of uric acid.

Pharmacokinetics:

Route(s)	PO, IV
Absorption	80–90% absorbed in the GI tract
Distribution	Widely distributed; secreted in breast milk
Primary metabolism	Hepatic to the active metabolite oxypurinol
Primary excretion	Renal
Onset of action	24–48 h
Duration of action	18–30 h

Adverse Effects: The most frequent and serious adverse effects are dermatologic. The most common manifestation is a micropapular rash; rare cases of fatal toxic epidermal necrolysis and Stevens–Johnson syndrome have been reported. A rare, sometimes fatal, hypersensitivity syndrome may occur and includes a skin rash, fever, hepatitis, leukocytosis, eosinophilia, and progressive renal failure. Other possible adverse effects include drowsiness, headache, vertigo, nausea, vomiting, abdominal discomfort, malaise, diarrhea, cataracts, retinopathy, and thrombocytopenia.

Contraindication/Precautions: Contraindications include hypersensitivity to allopurinol and idiopathic hemochromatosis. Use cautiously in patients with impaired hepatic or renal function, history of peptic ulcers, lower GI tract disease, bone marrow depression, and pregnancy.

Drug Interactions: Alcohol may inhibit the renal excretion of uric acid. Ampicillin and amoxicillin may increase the risk of skin rashes. An enhanced anticoagulant effect may be seen with the use of warfarin, and toxicity risks increase for azathioprine, mercaptopurine, cyclophosphamide, and cyclosporine. An increased hypoglycemic effect may be seen with chlorpropamide. There is an increased risk of ototoxicity when allopurinol is used with thiazides and ACE inhibitors. Aluminum antacids taken concurrently with allopurinol may decrease its effects. An increased effect may be seen with phenytoin, theophylline, and anticancer drugs, necessitating the need for altered doses of these medications. **Herbal/Food:** Unknown.

Pregnancy: Category C.

Treatment of Overdose: Overdose with allopurinol is rare. There is no specific treatment for an overdose and the patient is treated symptomatically.

Nursing Responsibilities:

- Monitor for therapeutic effectiveness by obtaining serum and urinary uric acid levels 1 to 3 weeks after beginning therapy and by assessing relief of joint pain and increased joint mobility.
- Monitor for signs and symptoms of an acute gouty episode.
- Obtain baseline CBC and liver and kidney function tests before therapy and monthly. Assess the urinary pH at regular intervals to detect the development of renal calculi.
- Discontinue allopurinol at the first sign of a skin rash and immediately notify the prescriber.

Patient and Family Education:

- Increase fluid intake to 3 to 4 L per day and report any decrease in urinary output, cloudy urine, unusual color or odor to the urine, or pain or discomfort on urination to the health care provider.
- Avoid high-purine foods such as alcohol, salmon, sardines, legumes, mushrooms, oatmeal, and organ meats.
- Immediately report itching or rash, diarrhea, stomatitis, flulike symptoms, or a metallic taste in the mouth.
- Do not take large doses of vitamin C because it acidifies the urine and may increase the risk for kidney stones.
- Take this medicine with food or at mealtime to decrease the risk of gastric distress. Tablets may be crushed and taken with fluid or mixed with food.
- Minimize the exposure of the eyes to ultraviolet light or sunlight because it may stimulate the development of cataracts. All patients should have a yearly eye examination.
- Attend all follow-up appointments with the health care provider and for laboratory tests.

Drugs Similar to Allopurinol (Zyloprim)

Additional drugs for gout prophylaxis include probenecid and sulfinpyrazone.

Probenecid (Probalan): Probenecid is an older drug that was approved in 1951. It inhibits the reabsorption of uric acid in the renal tubules, thus increasing its excretion. Given PO, it is effective for prophylaxis but will not terminate acute gout episodes. Probenecid should be taken with meals to decrease gastric irritation. It should be used cautiously when given with other drugs that are highly protein bound. Several combination drugs that contain probenecid and colchicine are available for long-term maintenance therapy. Adverse effects are generally minor and include headache, nausea, vomiting, and anorexia. This drug is pregnancy category C.

Unrelated to its use in treating gout, probenecid blocks the transport of organic acids in the renal tubule. When given concurrently with antibiotics such as penicillins or cephalosporins, the serum levels of antibiotics will be boosted, making them more effective. Because of its effect on renal transport mechanisms, probenecid has the potential to interact with virtually any acidic drug. A drug guide should be consulted when administering probenecid to patients who are taking multiple medications.

Sulfinpyrazone (Anturane): Approved in 1959, sulfinpyrazone is another oral uricosuric agent that is very similar to probenecid. Sulfinpyrazone reduces uric acid levels in patients with chronic gout conditions but is not effective in treating acute episodes. It is more potent than probenecid and its use is generally reserved for patients with symptoms that are resistant to other agents. Although rare, severe blood dyscrasias have been known to occur with its use and should therefore be given with extreme caution to those patients who have a history of hematologic disorders. Sulfinpyrazone also has the potential to cause serious gastric distress, and it should be taken with meals or with antacids to decrease irritation. It is contraindicated in patients with peptic ulcer disease. This drug is pregnancy category C.

NURSING PROCESS APPLICATION

Patients Receiving Antigout Therapy

Assessment	Potential Nursing Diagnoses
Prior to administration: • Obtain a complete health history, including allergies, drug history, and possible drug interactions. • Obtain baseline vital signs. • Obtain laboratory tests that include CBC, platelets, uric acid levels, renal and liver function tests, and urinalysis.	• *Activity Intolerance*, related to joint pain • *Disturbed Body Image*, related to joint swelling • *Deficient Knowledge (Drug Therapy)*

Planning: Patient Goals and Expected Outcomes

The patient will:

- Report a decrease in pain and an increase in function in the affected joints.
- Demonstrate an understanding of the drug's action by accurately describing drug adverse effects and precautions.
- Immediately report adverse effects and adverse reactions.

Implementation

Interventions and (Rationales)	Patient and Family Education
• Monitor laboratory results throughout therapy and perform a Coombs' test for hemolytic anemia. (Agranulocytosis, aplastic anemia, and thrombocytopenia may occur.)	• Instruct the patient about the importance of routine laboratory studies, so that deviations from normal can be corrected immediately.
• Monitor for signs of toxicity. (This will evaluate therapeutic drug regimen and prevent complications.)	• Instruct the patient to report weakness, abdominal pain, nausea, or diarrhea.
• Monitor for signs of renal impairment such as oliguria. Record intake and output. (Monitoring allows prevention of renal complications.)	• Instruct the patient to report a decrease in urine output and to increase fluid intake to 3–4 L/day.
• Monitor dietary habits and intake of high-purine foods. (These foods form nucleic acids when they are metabolized.)	• Instruct the patient to avoid high-purine foods such as organ meats, legumes, alcoholic beverages, mushrooms, and oatmeal.
• Ensure that the medication is administered correctly. (Effectiveness of the drug regimen and prevention of complications depends on adherence.)	• Instruct the patient to take the medication on an empty stomach. Medication should be taken at the first sign of gout attack.
• Monitor for pain and mobility. (This monitoring assesses the effectiveness of the medication.)	• Instruct the patient to report increases or decreases in discomfort and swelling.

Evaluation of Outcome Criteria

Evaluate the effectiveness of drug therapy by confirming that patient goals and expected outcomes have been met (see "Planning").

UNDERSTANDING THE CHAPTER

Key Concepts Summary

75.1 Adequate levels of calcium in the body are necessary to transmit nerve impulses, to prevent muscle spasms, and for proper bone health.

75.2 Calcium balance is regulated by parathyroid hormone, calcitonin, and vitamin D.

75.3 Hypocalcemia is a condition that requires therapy with calcium supplements, often concurrently with vitamin D.

75.4 Metabolic bone disease is characterized by abnormal bone structure.

75.5 Vitamin D therapy is indicated for treating osteomalacia, hypoparathyroidism, and osteoporosis.

75.6 Bisphosphonates increase bone density and are used to treat osteoporosis.

75.7 Selective estrogen receptor modulators increase bone mass density and prevent fractures in postmenopausal women.

75.8 Calcitonin and several miscellaneous drugs are used for osteoporosis and other metabolic bone diseases.

75.9 Osteoarthritis is treated with a combination of analgesics and nonpharmacologic therapies.

75.10 Pharmacotherapy for rheumatoid arthritis includes analgesics, anti-inflammatory drugs, corticosteroids, and disease-modifying antirheumatic drugs.

75.11 Gout is treated with drugs that decrease joint pain and inflammation and lower uric acid levels.

75.12 Hyperuricemia is treated with drugs that reduce the serum levels of uric acid.

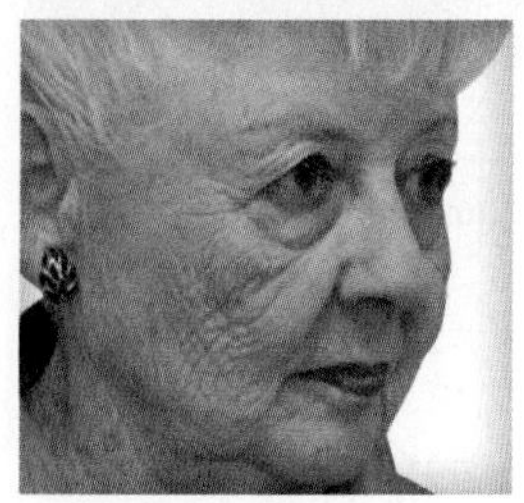

Making the PATIENT Connection

Remember the patient "Darlene Coleman" at the beginning of the chapter? Now read the remainder of the case study. Based on the information presented within this chapter, respond to the critical thinking questions that follow.

Darlene Coleman is a 65-year-old woman who is generally in good health. She has a checkup visit with her gynecologist annually. While assessing Ms. Coleman's vital signs, height, and weight, the nurse notes a significant deviation from the data recorded from last year's visit. Apparently, the patient has lost 1 inch in height during the last year. The nurse then shares this information with Darlene. The patient states, "I have always been short. You should see my mother who is much shorter than I am."

Critical Thinking Questions

1. As the nurse, how would you respond to the patient's statement?
2. As you talk with Ms. Coleman, she asks you, "Is there any way to slow my declining height?" What could you recommend?

Case Study

A young woman calls the triage nurse in her health care provider's office with questions concerning her mother's medication. The mother, age 76, has been taking alendronate (Fosamax) after a bone density test revealed a decrease in bone mass. The daughter is worried that her mother may not be taking the drug correctly and asks for information to minimize the potential for adverse effects.

1. If you were the triage nurse, what information would you include in a teaching plan regarding the PO administration of alendronate?
2. Create a list of adverse effects that the patient's daughter can monitor in her mother.

NCLEX-RN® Review

1 The client who has been prescribed alendronate (Fosamax) demonstrates an understanding of how to correctly take the medication when stating:

1. "I will take my medication prior to eating my lunch or dinner."
2. "I will take my medication immediately before bedtime or at 9 P.M."
3. "I will take my medication with a full glass of water 30 minutes before breakfast."
4. "I should lie flat for at least 30 minutes after I take this medication."

2 Which of the following signs would alert the nurse to the possibility of the development of toxicity to methotrexate (Rheumatrex)?

1. Headache, dizziness, and blurred vision
2. Hematuria, hiccoughs, and jaundice
3. Stomatitis, constipation, and dyspepsia
4. Jaundice, ascites, and edema formation

3 The client asks the nurse to explain how colchicine works. The nurse would base the response on which physiological principle? Colchicine:

1. Increases the deposits of uric acid in the synovial spaces of the joints.
2. Relieves the pain associated with joint inflammation from gouty arthritis.
3. Prevents the accumulation of uric acid crystals in the joints.
4. Increases renal secretion of uric acid crystals.

4 Which of the following laboratory findings would the nurse monitor to determine if pharmacotherapy is helping a client with osteomalacia?

1. Increasing serum calcium and increasing phosphate levels
2. Increasing serum calcium and decreasing phosphate levels
3. Decreasing serum calcium and increasing phosphate levels
4. Decreasing serum calcium and decreasing phosphate levels

5 Which of the following assessment findings in a client who is receiving calcitriol (Calcijex) should the nurse immediately report to the prescriber?

1. Muscle weakness, nausea, and vomiting
2. Diarrhea, abdominal pain, and stomatitis
3. Bone pain, joint stiffness, and fever
4. Photosensitivity, tinnitus, and bone pain

6 Disease-modifying antirheumatic drugs (DMARDs) are prescribed for clients with rheumatoid arthritis. Which of the following statements related to this therapy are correct? (Select all that apply.) The nurse knows that disease-modifying antirheumatic drugs:

1. Include gold salts, antimalarial agents, and drugs that modify the immune response.
2. Enhance the quality of life in clients with rheumatoid arthritis.
3. Often takes several months to achieve maximum therapeutic effects.
4. Are very safe and require very little monitoring during therapy.
5. Are not accepted in modern pharmacotherapy as a viable treatment option.

See Answers to Critical Thinking Questions, Case Study, and NCLEX-RN® Review in Appendix A.

References

Clegg, D. O., Reda, D. J., Harris, C. L., Klein, M. A., O'Dell, J. R., Hooper, M. M., et al. (2006). Glucosamine, chondroitin sulfate, and the two in combination for painful knee osteoarthritis. *New England Journal of Medicine, 354*(8), 795–808.

Corbett, J. V. (2008). *Laboratory tests and diagnostic procedures with nursing diagnoses* (7th ed.). Upper Saddle River, NJ: Prentice-Hall.

Distler, J., & Anguelouch, A. (2006). Evidence-based practice: Review of clinical evidence on the efficacy of glucosamine and chondroitin in the treatment of osteoarthritis. *Journal of the American Academy of Nurse Practitioners, 18*(10), 487–493.

Hampton, T. (2007). Efficacy still uncertain for widely used supplements for arthritis. *Journal of the American Medical Association, 297*(4), 351–352.

Hansberger, J. (2006). Osteoporosis: Review of disease, diagnosis, and treatments for the advanced practice nurse. *The Internet Journal of Advanced Nursing Practice, 8*(1). Retrieved September 7, 2008, from http://www.ispub.com/ostia/index.php?xmlFilePath=journals/ijanp/vol8n1/osteoporosis.xml

King, R. W., & Worthington, R. (2006). Arthritis, rheumatoid. *Emedicine.* Retrieved September 7, 2008, from http://www.emedicine.com/EMERG/topic48.htm

Kuehn, B. (2007). Knee therapies probed. *Journal of the American Medical Association, 298*(20), 2361.

Lemone, P., & Burke, K. (2008). *Medical-surgical nursing: Critical thinking in client care.* Upper Saddle River, NJ: Pearson Education.

Mikuls, T. R. (2007). Quality of care in gout: From measurement to improvement. *Clinical and Experimental Rheumatology, 25*(Suppl. 47), S114–S119.

National Institute of Arthritis and Musculoskeletal and Skin Diseases, the NIH Osteoporosis and Related Bone Diseases National Resource Center. (2006). *Osteoporosis in Men.* Retrieved September 7, 2008, from http://www.niams.nih.gov/Health_Info/Bone/Osteoporosis/men.asp

National Osteoporosis Foundation. (2008). *Osteoporosis: Men.* Washington, DC: Author. Retrieved September 7, 2008, from http://www.nof.org/men/

National Osteoporosis Foundation. (n.d.). *Osteoporosis fast facts.* Retrieved September 7, 2008, from http://www.nof.org/osteoporosis/diseasefacts.htm

Qaseem, A., Snow, V., Shekelle, P., Hopkins Jr., R., Forciea, M. A., & Owens, D. K. (2008). Screening for osteoporosis in men: A clinical practice guideline from the American College of Physicians. *Annals of Internal Medicine, 148*(9), 680–684.

Reichenbach, S., Sterchi, R., Scherer, M., Trelle, S., Bürgi, E., Bürgi, U., et al. (2007). Meta-analysis: Chondroitin for osteoarthritis of the knee or hip. *Annals of Internal Medicine, 146*(8), 580–590.

Schumacher, H. R. (2006). *Pseudogout.* American College of Rheumatology. Retrieved September 7, 2008, from http://www.rheumatology.org/public/factsheets/diseases_and_conditions/pseudogout.asp?aud=pataud=pat

CHAPTER

I hate the way my skin looks. I am always explaining that I have not been in the sun too long.

Patient "Dora McBride"

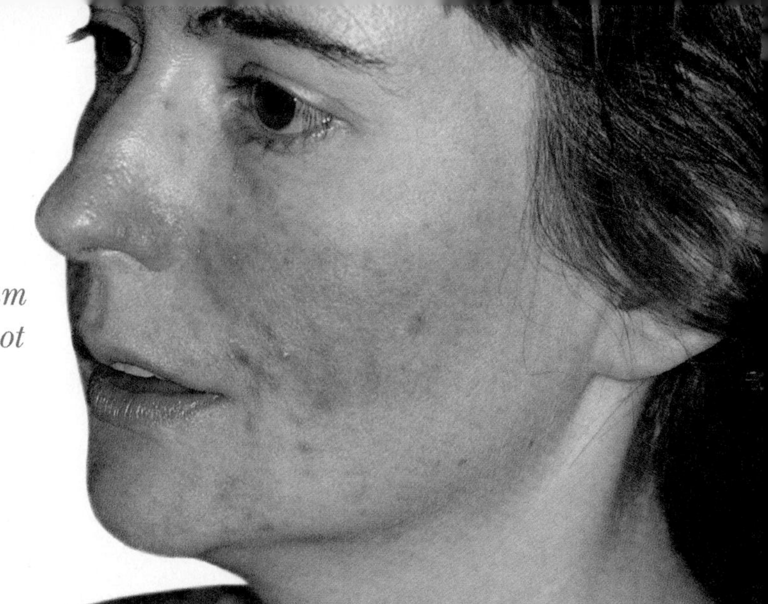

76 Pharmacotherapy of Dermatologic Disorders

Learning Outcomes

After reading this chapter, the student should be able to:

1. Identify the structure and functions of the skin and associated structures.
2. Explain the process by which superficial skin cells are replaced.
3. Explain how skin diseases are classified.
4. Describe the drug therapies for bacterial, fungal, viral, and parasitic infections of the skin.
5. Explain the etiology, pathogenesis, and pharmacotherapy for acne vulgaris, rosacea, dermatitis, and psoriasis.
6. Outline the stepwise approach to treating psoriasis.
7. Describe the prevention and management of minor burns.
8. Describe the nurse's role in the pharmacologic management of skin disorders.
9. For each of the classes shown in the chapter outline, identify the prototype and representative drugs and explain the mechanism(s) of drug action, primary indications, contraindications, significant drug interactions, pregnancy category, and important adverse effects.
10. Use the nursing process to care for patients who are receiving drug therapy for skin disorders.

Chapter Outline

Anatomy of the Integumentary System

Classification of Skin Disorders

Pharmacotherapy of Skin Infections

Scabicides and Pediculicides

PROTOTYPE **Permethrin (Acticin, Elimite, Nix)** *p. 1319*

Pharmacotherapy of Acne and Rosacea

PROTOTYPE **Tretinoin (Avita, Retin-A, Trentin-X)** *p. 1323*

Pharmacotherapy of Dermatitis

Pharmacotherapy of Psoriasis

Pharmacotherapy of Minor Skin Burns

PROTOTYPE **Benzocaine (Americaine, Anbesol, Others)** *p. 1332*

Pharmacotherapy of Alopecia

The integumentary system consists of the skin, hair, nails, sweat glands, and sebaceous glands. The largest and most visible of all organs, healthy skin provides an effective barrier between the outside environment and the body's internal organs, helps to regulate body temperature, and assists in maintaining fluid and electrolyte balance. At times, however, external conditions become too extreme, or conditions within the body change, resulting in unhealthy skin. When this occurs, pharmacotherapy may be utilized to improve the skin's condition. The purpose of this chapter is to examine the broad scope of skin disorders and the drugs used for skin pharmacotherapy.

Anatomy of the Integumentary System

76.1 Three layers of skin, known as the epidermis, dermis, and subcutaneous layers, provide effective barrier defenses for the body.

To understand the actions of dermatologic drugs, it is necessary to have a thorough knowledge of the structure of the skin. The skin comprises three primary layers: the epidermis, dermis, and subcutaneous, as illustrated in Figure 76.1. The epidermis is the visible, outermost layer that constitutes only about 5% of the skin depth. The middle layer is the dermis, which accounts for about 95% of the entire skin thickness. The subcutaneous layer lies beneath the dermis. Some textbooks consider the subcutaneous layer as being separate from the skin and not one of its layers. Each layer of skin is distinct in form and function and provides the basis for how drugs are injected or topically applied.

Epidermis: The epidermis consists of epithelial cells with either four or five sublayers depending on its location. The five layers from the innermost to outermost are the stratum basale (also referred to as the stratum germinativum), stratum spinosum, stratum granulosum, stratum lucidum, and the strongest layer, the stratum corneum. The stratum corneum is referred to as the "horny layer" because of the abundance of the

Key Terms

acne vulgaris, 1320
comedones, 1321
dermatitis, 1325
eczema, 1325
erythema, 1316
excoriation, 1325
keratolytic, 1322
nits, 1318
pediculicides, 1318
plaques, 1328
pruritus, 1316
psoralens, 1331
retinoids, 1322
rhinophyma, 1323
rosacea, 1323
scabicides, 1318
seborrhea, 1320
urticaria, 1316

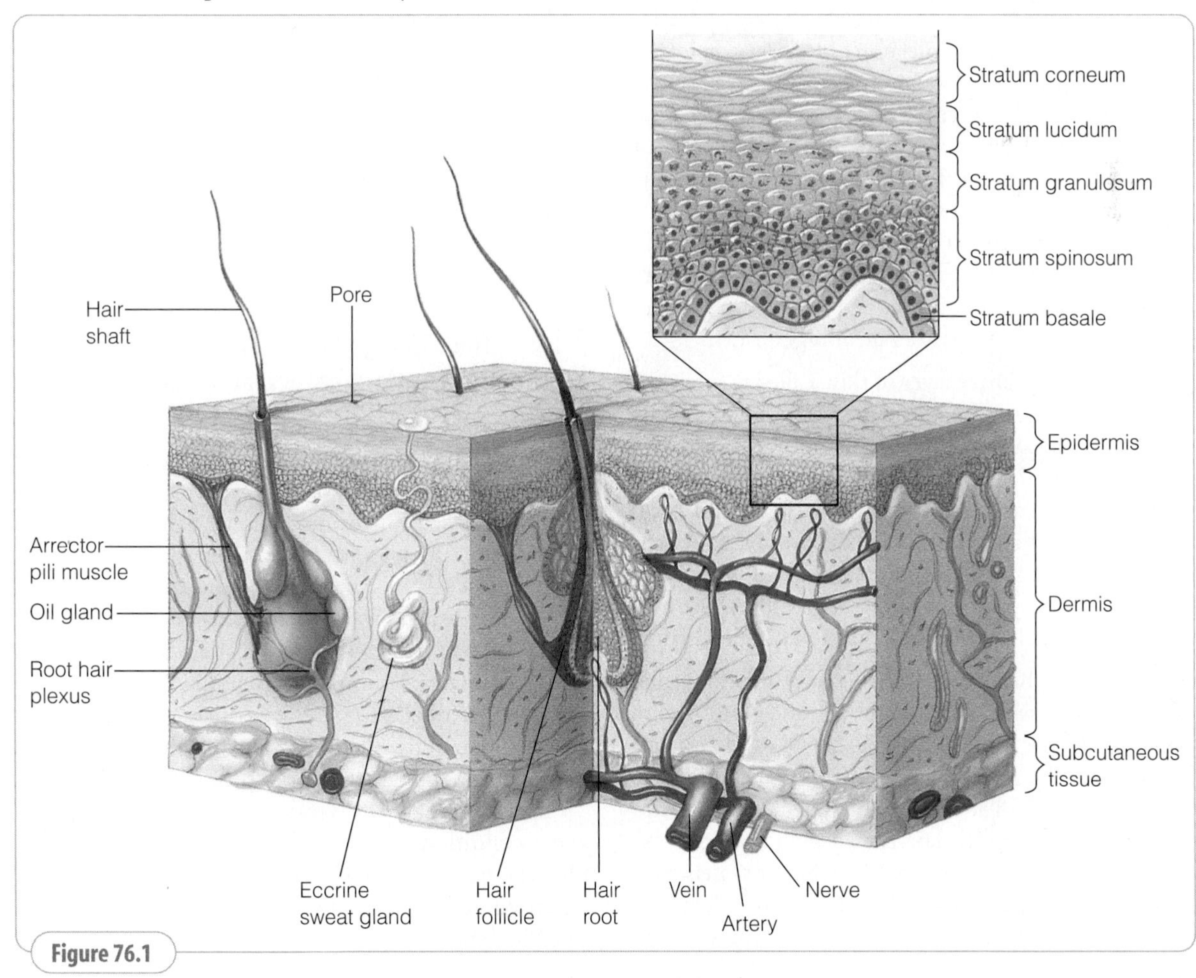

Figure 76.1

Anatomy of the skin.

Source: From *Medical Surgical Nursing* (4th ed., p. 424), by P. LeMone & K. Burke, 2008. Reprinted by permission of Pearson Education, Inc., Upper Saddle River, NJ.

protein keratin, a water-insoluble material secreted by keratinocytes, which is also found in the hair, hooves, and horns of many mammals. Keratin gives the skin its tough, protective seal, forming a barrier that repels bacteria and foreign matter. Most substances cannot penetrate it. The largest amount of keratin is found in those areas subject to mechanical stress, for example, the soles of the feet and the palms of the hands.

The deepest epidermal sublayer, the stratum basale, supplies the epidermis with new cells after older superficial cells have been damaged or lost through normal wear. Over time, these newly created cells migrate from the stratum basale to the outermost layers of the skin. As these cells are pushed to the surface they are flattened and covered with keratin. The outermost skin layer, called the stratum corneum, is composed of these dead cells. On average, it takes a cell about 3 weeks to move from the stratum basale to the body surface.

Specialized cells within the deeper layers of the epidermis, called melanocytes, secrete the dark pigment melanin. Melanin forms a protective shield, which protects the keratinocytes and the nerve endings in the dermis from the sun's ultraviolet (UV) rays. The number and type of melanocytes determine the overall pigment of the skin and determine racial differences in skin tone. Darker skin tones are not caused by an increased number of melanocytes but the size of the pigment melanin that is contained in each cell. The more melanin, the darker the skin color. Freckles, birthmarks, and age spots are caused by the production of melanin. In areas where the melanocytes are destroyed, there are milk-white areas of depigmented skin referred to as vitiligo.

The junction of the epidermis and the dermis is an area of many ridges and furrows called the rete ridges. This area anchors the epidermis to the dermis. The epidermis does not have a separate blood supply. It receives its nutrients by diffusion in the rete ridges from the many blood vessels in the dermis. This surface also provides for the ripples seen on the skin surface, which on the fingertips are called fingerprints.

Dermis: The second primary layer of skin, called the dermis, is a layer of connective tissue that contains no cells. The dermis is composed of collagen fibers and elastic fibers that give the skin both flexibility and strength. It provides a foundation for the epidermis and accessory structures such as hair and nails. Most sensory nerves that transmit the sensations of touch, pressure, temperature, pain, and itch are located within the dermis, as well as the oil glands and sweat glands. A vast network of lymph and capillary vessels is found within the dermis.

Subcutaneous tissue: Beneath the dermis is the subcutaneous tissue, or hypodermis, which lies over muscle and bone. It consists mainly of adipose tissue, which cushions, insulates, and serves as an energy reserve in the event that extra calories are needed to fuel the body. The amount of subcutaneous tissue varies in an individual and is determined by body area, sex, age, nutritional status, and heredity. Many blood vessels pass through the fatty layer and extend into the dermis, forming capillary networks that supply nutrients and remove wastes.

Skin appendages: Hair follicles are located in the dermis. Hair growth varies by race, gender, age, and heredity. Individual hairs vary in both structure and rate of growth, depending on their location. Composed primarily of dead cells, hair consists of a root that begins in the bulb of the hair follicle and grows from the dermis outward. The hair shaft is the portion that projects through the epidermis and exits the skin. Hair growth occurs in cycles; a growth phase is followed by a resting phase during which hair is shed from the body. Stressors can alter the growth cycle and cause temporary hair loss. Permanent baldness is genetic in origin and is seldom influenced by stressors. Hair color is genetically determined by a person's rate of melanin production within the hair shaft.

The sebaceous glands are distributed over the entire skin surface, except for the palms of the hand and the soles of the feet. Most sebaceous glands are directly connected to the hair follicles; the glands of the eyelids, nipple areolae, and genitalia are freestanding. Sebaceous glands produce sebum, which is emptied into the space between the hair follicle and shaft. Sebum lubricates and softens the skin and hair and reduces water loss from the skin surface in low humidity. Sebum also is mildly bacteriostatic. The secretion of sebum is stimulated by hormones, especially androgens.

The skin has two types of sweat glands: apocrine and eccrine. The apocrine glands are directly connected to the hair follicles and are mainly found in the axillary, perineal, nipple areolae, and umbilical areas. The interaction of skin bacteria with the milky secretions of apocrine glands causes distinct body odor. The eccrine glands are found over the entire skin surface. Their ducts open directly onto the skin surface and are not associated with hair follicles. The secretions of the eccrine glands are an important factor in the regulation of body temperature. Sweat is released from the eccrine glands in response to elevated body temperature or ambient temperature and is under control of the sympathetic nervous system.

Classification of Skin Disorders

76.2 The etiology of skin disorders may be classified as infectious, inflammatory, or neoplastic.

Of the many types of skin disorders, some have vague, generalized signs and symptoms, and others have specific and easily identifiable causes. **Urticaria** is a hypersensitivity response that is characterized by hives and is often accompanied by pruritus, or itching. Allergies to foods often manifest as urticaria. **Pruritus** is a general condition that is associated with dry, scaly skin or a parasite infestation. Pruritus may also be a sign of serious systemic pathology, such as cholestatic disease and uremia. A substantial number of drugs have urticaria or pruritus listed as potential adverse effects. Local **erythema** or redness accompanies inflammation and many other skin disorders. Inflammation is a characteristic of burns and trauma to the skin.

Skin disorders are diverse and difficult to classify because some conditions have overlapping components. For example, lesions that are characteristic of acne may be inflamed and become infected. One simple method, which is summarized in Table 76.1, is to group the disorders into the following categories:

- Infectious. Bacterial, fungal, viral, and parasitic infections of the skin and mucous membranes are relatively common

TABLE 76.1 Classification of Skin Disorders

Type	Examples
Infectious	Bacterial infections: boils, impetigo, infected hair follicles
	Fungal infections: ringworm, athlete's foot, jock itch, nail infection
	Parasitic infections: ticks, mites, lice
	Viral infections: cold sores, fever blisters (herpes simplex), chickenpox, warts, shingles (herpes zoster), measles (rubeola), and German measles (rubella)
Inflammatory	Injury and exposure to the sun
	Combination of overactive glands, increased hormone production, and/or infection such as acne and rosacea
	Disorders with itching, cracking, and discomfort such as atopic dermatitis, contact dermatitis, seborrheic dermatitis, stasis dermatitis, and psoriasis
Neoplastic	Skin cancers: squamous cell carcinoma, basal cell carcinoma, and malignant melanoma
	Benign neoplasms include keratosis and keratoacanthoma

and are frequent indications for anti-infective pharmacotherapy. A brief overview of anti-infectives most frequently prescribed for skin conditions is presented in Section 76.3, with further emphasis on parasitic infections in Section 76.4. Greater detail of the individual anti-infective drugs may be found in Chapters 47 through 56.

- **Inflammatory.** Inflammatory disorders encompass a broad range of pathology that includes acne (see Section 76.5), dermatitis (see Section 76.6), burns (see Section 76.7), and psoriasis (see Section 76.8). The pharmacotherapy of inflammatory skin disorders includes many of the agents discussed in Chapter 44, such as corticosteroids.
- **Neoplastic.** Malignant tumors include malignant melanoma and basal cell carcinoma, which are treated with the therapies described in Chapter 58. Warts are a type of benign tumor.

Systemic disease processes that occur in the body may manifest as dermatologic signs and symptoms. Skin abnormalities, including color, sizes, types, and character of surface lesions, and skin turgor and moisture may have systemic causes such as liver or renal impairment, cardiovascular insufficiency, metastatic tumors, recent injury, and poor nutritional status.

Although there are many skin disorders, some warrant only localized or short-term pharmacotherapy. Examples include lice infestation, sunburn with minor irritation, and acne. Eczema, dermatitis, and psoriasis are more serious disorders that require extensive and more prolonged therapy.

Pharmacotherapy of Skin Infections

76.3 When the integrity of the skin is compromised, bacteria, viruses, and fungi can gain entrance and cause infections that require anti-infective therapy.

The skin is normally populated with microorganisms or flora that includes a diverse collection of viruses, fungi, and bacteria. The skin provides an effective barrier against infection from these organisms as long as it remains healthy and intact. The skin is very dry, and keratin is a poor energy source for microbes. Although perspiration provides a wet environment, its high-salt content discourages microbial growth. Furthermore, the outer layer is continually being sloughed off, and the microorganisms leave with the dead skin.

Bacterial skin diseases can occur when the skin is punctured or cut, or when the outer layer is abraded through trauma or removed through severe burns. Some bacteria also infect hair follicles. The most common bacterial infections of the skin are caused by *Staphylococcus* and *Streptococcus,* which are normal skin inhabitants. *Staphylococcus aureus* is responsible for furuncles (boils), carbuncles (abscesses), and other pus-containing lesions of the skin. Both *S. aureus* and *Streptococcus pyogenes* can cause impetigo, which is a superficial skin disorder that commonly occurs in school-age children. Cellulitis is an acute skin and subcutaneous tissue infection caused by *Staphylococcus* and *Streptococcus.* Folliculitis, an infection of hair follicles usually caused by *S. aureus,* is often called a "hot-tub" infection because it is acquired when water in these tubs is not adequately treated with chlorine.

Although many skin bacterial infections are self-limiting, others may be serious enough to require pharmacotherapy. When possible, topical agents are applied directly to the infection site. Topical agents offer the advantage of causing fewer adverse effects, and many are available over-the-counter (OTC) for self-treatment. If the infection is deep within the skin, affects large regions of the body, or has the potential to enter the systemic circulation, oral (PO) or parenteral therapy is indicated. Furthermore, the incidence of methicillin-resistant *S. aureus* (MRSA) skin infections is increasing, which often requires pharmacotherapy with two or more antibiotics. Some of the more common topical antibiotics for skin infections include the following:

- Bacitracin ointment
- Erythromycin ointment (Eryderm, others)
- Gentamicin cream and ointment
- Metronidazole cream and lotion
- Mupirocin (Bactroban)
- Neomycin with polymyxin B (Neosporin), cream and ointment
- Tetracycline

Fungal infections of the skin or nails such as tinea pedis (athlete's foot) and tinea cruris (jock itch) commonly occur in warm, moist areas covered by clothing. Tinea capitis (ringworm of the scalp) and tinea unguium (ringworm of the nails) are also common. These pathogens are responsive to therapy with topical OTC antifungal agents such as undecylenic acid (Cruex, Desenex, others). More serious fungal infections of the skin and mucous membranes, such as *Candida albicans* infections that occur in immunocompromised patients, require systemic antifungals (see Chapter 53). Clotrimazole (Mycelex, Lotrimin, others) and miconazole (Monistat, others) are common antifungals available as creams and lotions that are used for a variety of dermatologic mycoses. Oral fluconazole (Diflucan) is indicated for more serious fungal infections of the skin.

Certain viral infections can manifest with skin lesions. Childhood viral infections that affect the skin include varicella (chickenpox), rubeola (measles), and rubella (German measles). Usually, these infections are self-limiting and nonspecific, so treatment is directed at controlling the extent of skin lesions. Viral infections with skin lesions in adults include herpes zoster (shingles) and herpes simplex (cold sores and genital lesions). Pharmacotherapy of severe or persistent viral skin lesions may include topical or PO antiviral therapy with acyclovir (Zovirax) or other antivirals, as discussed in Chapter 56.

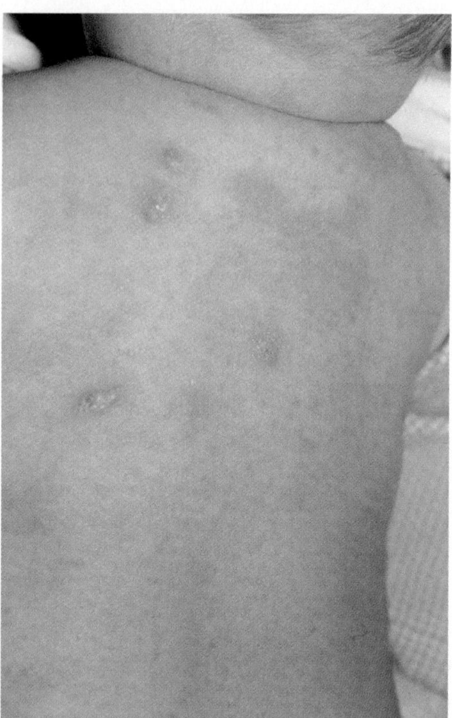

Figure 76.2 Scabies.
Source: Courtesy of Dr. Jason L. Smith

CONNECTION *Checkpoint* 76.1

From what you learned in Chapter 53, what are onychomycoses and what types of drugs are used to treat them? See Answer to Connection Checkpoint 76.1 in Appendix A.

Scabicides and Pediculicides

76.4 Scabicides and pediculicides are used to treat parasitic skin infestations.

Common skin parasites include mites and lice. Scabies is an eruption of the skin caused by the female mite *Sarcoptes scabiei*, which burrows into the skin to lay eggs that hatch after about 5 days. Scabies mites are barely visible without magnification. Scabies lesions most commonly occur between the fingers, on the extremities, in axillary and gluteal folds, around the trunk, and in the genital area, as shown in Figure 76.2. The major symptom is intense pruritus; vigorous scratching may lead to secondary infections. Scabies is easily spread through skin-to-skin contact and from mites living in upholstery, shared bed, and bath linens. Diagnosis is made by visual inspection of the burrows and confirmed by microscopic scrapings of the mite's ova or fecal pellets.

An estimated 3 million new cases of lice infestation or pediculosis are treated each year in the United States. Lice are larger than mites, measuring from 1 to 4 mm in length. They are readily spread by sharing infected hats, hairbrushes, bedding, or clothes or by close personal contact. These parasites require human blood for survival and die within 24 hours without the blood of a human host. Lice (singular: louse) often infest the pubic area or the scalp and lay eggs, referred to as **nits,** which attach to body hairs. Head lice are referred to as *Pediculus humanus capitis* (Figure 76.3), body lice as *Pediculus humanus corporis,* and pubic lice as *Phthirus pubis.* The pubic louse is referred to as a "crab louse," because it looks like a tiny crab when viewed under the microscope. Individuals with pubic lice will sometimes say that they have "crabs." Pubic lice may produce sky-blue macules on the inner thighs or lower abdomen. The bite of the louse and the release of its saliva into the wound both lead to intense pruritus, followed by vigorous scratching. Secondary infections can result from scratching.

The treatment of skin parasites consists of using **scabicides,** which are drugs that kill mites, or **pediculicides,** which are drugs that kill lice. Some drugs are effective against both mites and lice. The choice of drug depends on where the infestation is

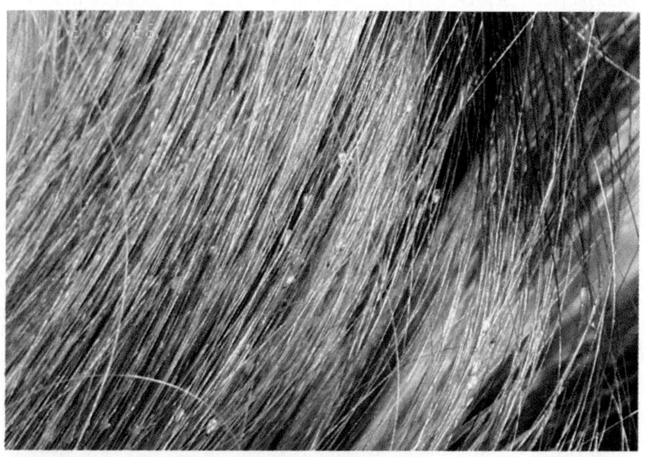

Figure 76.3 Pediculus humanus capitis.
Source: Courtesy of Dr. Jason L. Smith

located as well as other factors such as age, pregnancy, or breast-feeding.

The traditional drug of choice for both mites and lice was lindane. Lindane was also widely used as an agricultural pesticide in the 1950s and 1960s, causing pollution of waterways and prompting restrictions on its use. Because lindane has the potential to cause serious nervous system toxicity, its use is now limited to cases where less toxic drugs have failed to produce an adequate therapeutic response.

The current drug of choice for lice is permethrin, a chemical derived from chrysanthemum flowers and formulated as a 1% liquid (Nix). This drug is considered the safest agent, especially for infants and children. Pyrethrin (RID, others) is a related product that also is obtained from the chrysanthemum plant. Permethrin and pyrethrin, which are also widely used as insecticides on crops and livestock, kill lice and their eggs on contact. These agents are effective in 97% to 99% of patients, although a repeat application may be needed. Adverse effects are generally minor and include stinging, itching, or tingling. If two treatments of pyrethrin-based medications fail to eliminate the infestation, lindane or malathion (Ovide) may be prescribed. Resistant lice are most likely to appear in patients who have received multiple treatments with pyrethrin-based shampoos.

Permethrin is also a preferred agent for scabies. The 5% cream (Elimite) is applied to the entire skin surface and allowed to remain for 8 to 14 hours before bathing. A single application cures 95% of the patients, although itching may continue for several weeks as the dead mites are removed from the skin. Crotamiton (Eurax) is an alternative scabicide that is available by prescription as a 10% cream.

All scabicides and pediculicides must be used strictly as directed, because excessive use can cause serious systemic effects and skin irritation. Drugs for the treatment of lice or mites must not be applied to the mouth, open skin lesions, or eyes, because this will cause severe irritation.

PROTOTYPE DRUG Permethrin (Acticin, Elimite, Nix)

Classification: **Therapeutic:** Antiparasitic
Pharmacologic: Scabicide, pediculicide

Therapeutic Effects and Uses: Nix is marketed as a cream, lotion, or shampoo to kill head and crab lice and mites and to eradicate their ova. A 1% lotion is approved for lice and a 5% lotion for mites. The medication should be allowed to remain on the hair and scalp 10 minutes before removal. Patients should be aware that penetration of the skin with mites causes itching, which lasts up to 2 or 3 weeks even after the parasites have been killed.

Successful elimination of parasitic infections should include removing the nits with a nit comb, washing bedding, and cleaning or removing objects that have been in contact with the head or hair.

Mechanism of Action: Nix affects the nervous system of the parasite, causing paralysis. Because lice are dependent on blood for survival, they die within 24 to 28 hours. It has ectoparasitic and ovicidal activity against *P. humanus capitis*, *P. pubis*, *S. scabiei* (scabies), and against ticks, mites, and fleas.

Pharmacokinetics:

Route(s)	Topical: 5% and 1% formulations
Absorption	Less than 2% is absorbed through intact skin
Distribution	Stored in body fat
Primary metabolism	Hepatic
Primary excretion	Urine
Onset of action	Unknown
Duration of action	3 h

Adverse Effects: Permethrin causes few systemic effects. Local reactions may occur and include pruritus, rash, transient tingling, burning, stinging, erythema, and edema of the affected area.

Contraindications/Precautions: Contraindications include hypersensitivity to pyrethrins, chrysanthemums, sulfites, or other preservatives. Permethrin should be used cautiously on inflamed skin, in those with asthma, or in lactating women.

Drug Interactions: No clinically significant interactions have been documented.

Pregnancy: Category B.

Treatment of Overdose: No specific treatment for overdose with permethrin has been reported. Flush eyes well with water if the medicine accidently gets into the eyes.

Nursing Responsibilities:

- Obtain a thorough history regarding onset of symptoms and possible transmission of the parasite to others. Assess the family members and sexual partners of the affected patients for evidence of lice, nits, or scabies and treat accordingly.
- Obtain a history of pregnancy, lactation, allergies, and use of OTC or other home remedies to treat the current condition.
- Apply gloves before assessing the patient. Assess the hair and skin for evidence of lice, nits, or scabies. Assess the axilla, neckline, hairline, groin, and belt line areas for evidence of lice, such as visualization of nits, erythema, and pruritus.
- If the patient has lesions, assess the skin for abrasions, rashes, and open areas to determine any sites that might be subject to irritation from the topical medication.
- Do not use the liquid formulation on children younger than 2 years; the lotion may not be used on infants younger than 2 months of age.
- Follow application instructions, and wear gloves when applying the medication. Cleanse the lesions and surrounding areas with warm water and soap, and dry thoroughly prior to applying the medication. Cleansing the lesions prior to and between applications of the medication reduces the risk of secondary infections.
- Shake the cream or lotion container well.
- Apply a thin layer of the medication to the affected areas and leave on for the directed amount of time. Then remove the medication by bath or shower.

- Avoid application to the eyes; face; mucous membranes; urethral meatus; open cuts; or raw, weeping surfaces.
- Monitor for local adverse effects, including irritation, pruritus, burning, or stinging.

Patient and Family Education:

- Follow application instructions exactly.
- After treatment for head lice, remove all nits from the hair shaft with a nit comb. Disinfect personal items such as combs and brushes. Remove all nits manually to ensure that the parasite infestation does not recur.
- Notify those who may have been exposed to or have been in close contact with the infected person. For a child in day care, notify the caregivers so that others may be assessed for possible infestation.
- To prevent further infestation or recurrence, wash all bedding in hot water and dry in the dryer on maximum heat. If materials are nonwashable, have them dry cleaned.
- Place stuffed animals or other objects that cannot be washed in plastic bags and ensure that they are sealed completely for 2 weeks.
- Vacuum all carpets and upholstered surfaces. Discard the vacuum bag or empty the container, and place it in the trash container outside the household.
- Keep the environmental temperature at 68° to 72°F and at moderate humidity to reduce itching and drying of the skin.

Drugs Similar to Permethrin (Acticin, Elimite, Nix)

Other drugs for parasitic skin infections include crotamiton, lindane, malathion, and pyrethrin.

Crotamiton (Eurax): Crotamiton is a scabicide and antipruritic that is used to eradicate *S. scabiei* and relieve itching. Available as a 10% cream or lotion, this drug should not be applied to skin that is acutely inflamed, raw, or has weeping surfaces. It should not be instilled into the eyes or mouth. If this drug comes in contact with the eyes, they must be flushed thoroughly with water. Adverse effects may include skin irritation, rash, and erythema. This drug is pregnancy category C.

Lindane: Lindane is a scabicide and pediculicide in a 1% lotion or shampoo form that is applied directly to the skin to be absorbed by parasites and ova (nits), resulting in their death. This drug is commonly used for treatment of head and crab lice and scabies infestations. Although effective, this drug penetrates the skin and may cause significant neurotoxicity; thus its use is limited to cases where safer medications have failed to produce a satisfactory response. Lindane should not be applied to skin that has open cuts, mucous membranes, eyes, or face. It should be used cautiously in infants and patients with a history of seizures, human immunodeficiency virus (HIV) infections, and alcoholism. Disposable or rubber gloves should be worn when applying the medication to reduce exposure to the skin. Adverse effects may include dizziness, tremors, seizures, and death. This drug is pregnancy category C.

Malathion (Ovide): Available as a 0.5% lotion, malathion kills lice and ova by poisoning the nervous system of the parasite. It is contraindicated in children under the age of 6. Care must be taken to keep this drug out of the eyes during treatment because it can cause conjunctivitis. One treatment is all that is needed when using this medication. Because the solution contains alcohol, it is flammable and needs to be kept away from any heat source such as hair dryers or cigarettes. Malathion is very toxic if swallowed. This drug is pregnancy category B.

Pyrethrin (Rid): Pyrethrin is a pediculicide solution or shampoo that poisons the parasite's nervous system, resulting in paralysis and death. Pyrethrin may require a repeat application a week after the first dose. Contraindications include skin infections, abrasions, lactation, and sensitivity to the solution components. Pyrethrin is usually formulated with 4% piperanyl butoxide because this combination results in greater parasite killing. Pyrethrin should be used with caution in ragweed-sensitized patients, infants, and children. This medication is applied to infested areas that are wet, allowing it to stay in place for at least 10 minutes. The areas are then washed and rinsed with warm water. For shampoo applications, the hair is shampooed as usual then a fine-toothed comb is used to remove the lice and eggs from the hair. This drug is pregnancy category C.

Pharmacotherapy of Acne and Rosacea

76.5 The pharmacotherapy of acne includes treatment with benzoyl peroxide, retinoids, and antibiotics; pharmacotherapy for rosacea includes retinoids and metronidazole.

Acne vulgaris and rosacea are two disorders that produce similar appearing lesions on the face. Although the two conditions have some visual similarities and share a few common treatments, the pharmacotherapy of the disorders is very different.

PharmFACT

Acne occurs equally in males and females, but males are likely to have more severe, longer-lasting forms of acne. About 40% of teens seek physician treatment for their acne. *Source:* American Academy of Dermatology, n.d.

Acne vulgaris: **Acne vulgaris,** a disorder of the hair follicles and sebaceous glands, is a common condition that affects 80% of adolescents. Although acne occurs most often in teenagers, it is not unusual to find patients with acne who are older than 30 years, which is a condition referred to as mature acne or acne tardive. Acne vulgaris is more common in men but tends to persist longer in women. Acne affects approximately 17 million persons in the United States, making it one of the most common skin conditions encountered by the nurse.

Although the precise cause of acne is unknown, several factors that are associated with acne vulgaris include abnormal formation of keratin that blocks oil glands and **seborrhea,** the overproduction of sebum by oil glands. The bacterium *Propionibacterium acnes* grows within oil gland openings and changes sebum to an acidic and irritating substance. As a re-

NURSING PROCESS APPLICATION

Patients Receiving Drug Therapy for Lice or Mite Infestation

Assessment	Potential Nursing Diagnoses
Prior to administration: • Obtain a complete history, including age, allergies, drug history, and possible drug interactions. • Obtain a social history of close contacts, including household members and sexual partners. • Assess vital signs. • Assess the skin for the presence of lice or mite infestation, skin lesions, raw or inflamed skin, and open areas. • Assess pregnancy and lactation status.	• *Deficient Knowledge (Drug Therapy)* • *Noncompliance (Drug Therapy)* • *Impaired Skin Integrity,* related to lesions and pruritus

Planning: Patient Goals and Expected Outcomes

The patient will:

- Be free of lice or mites and experience no reinfestation of self or other family members.
- Verbalize an understanding of how lice and mites are spread, proper administration of the drug, necessary household hygiene, and the need to notify household members, sexual partners, and other close contacts such as classmates of the infestation.
- Exhibit skin that is intact and free of secondary infection and irritation.
- Demonstrate an understanding of the drug's action by accurately describing drug adverse effects and precautions.

Implementation

Interventions and (Rationales)	Patient and Family Education

• Monitor for presence of lice or mites. (This determines the effectiveness of drug therapy.)	• Instruct the patient to:
	  • Examine for nits on hair shafts; lice on the skin or clothes, inner thigh areas, seams of clothes that come in contact with the axilla, neckline, or belt line.
	  • Examine for mites between the fingers, on the extremities, in axillary and gluteal folds, around the trunk, and in the pubic area.

• Apply the medication properly. (Proper application is critical to eliminating infestation.)	• Instruct the patient to:
	  • Wear gloves during application.
	  • Remove all skin lotions, creams, and oil-based hair products completely by scrubbing the whole body well with soap and water and drying the skin prior to application.
	  • Apply medication to clean and dry affected body area as directed, using no more than 2 oz per application.
	  • Avoid contact with the product on an infant's skin.
	  • Comb affected hair with a fine-toothed comb, following application of lindane, making sure to remove all nits.
	  • Treat all household members and sexual contacts immediately.
	  • Recheck affected hair or skin daily for 1 week after treatment.

• Inform the patient and caregivers about proper care of clothing and equipment. (Contaminated articles will cause reinfestation.)	• Instruct patient and caregiver to:
	  • Wash all bedding and clothing in hot water, and to dry clean all nonwashable items that came in close contact with the patient.
	  • Clean combs and brushes and rinse thoroughly.

Evaluation of Outcome Criteria

Evaluate the effectiveness of drug therapy by confirming that patient goals and expected outcomes have been met (see "Planning").

sult, small inflamed bumps appear on the surface of the skin. Other factors associated with acne include androgens, which stimulate the sebaceous glands to produce more sebum. This is clearly evident in teenage boys and in patients who are administered testosterone. Studies have indicated that dietary factors do not promote acne. Remissions tend to occur in the summer, perhaps due to more exposure of the skin to the UV rays from sunlight.

The lesions of acne are most frequently distributed on the face, chest, and back. Acne lesions include open and closed **comedones.** Blackheads, or open comedones, occur when sebum has plugged the oil gland, causing it to become black because of the presence of melanin granules. Whiteheads, or closed comedones, develop just beneath the surface of the skin and appear white rather than black. Some closed comedones may rupture, resulting in an inflammatory response. The result is seen as papules, inflammatory pustules, and cysts. Mild papules and cysts drain on their own without treatment. Deeper lesions can cause scarring of the skin. Acne is graded as mild, moderate, or severe, depending on the number and type of lesions present.

The goals of acne therapy are to treat existing lesions and to prevent or lessen the severity of future recurrences. Severe acne can cause permanent scarring of the face. Treatment for acne is directed toward the pathogenesis of the lesion and there is no single effective treatment. The regimen used depends on the extent and severity of the acne. Mechanisms of action of antiacne medications include the following:

- Inhibit sebaceous gland overactivity
- Reduce bacterial colonization
- Prevent follicles from becoming plugged with keratin
- Reduce inflammation of lesions

Many of the mmedications used for acne and related disorders are available OTC. Mild acne is treated by topical therapy with agents such as benzoyl peroxide, topical antibiotics, and salicylic acid. Moderate to severe acne is treated with increasing strengths of tretinoin and the use of systemic antibiotics. Because of their increased toxicity, prescription agents are reserved for more severe, persistent cases. These drugs are listed in Table 76.2.

Benzoyl peroxide (Benzac, Triaz, others) is the most common topical OTC medication for acne. Benzoyl peroxide has a **keratolytic** effect, which helps to treat acne by loosening dry skin and causing an increased shedding of the outer layer of the epidermis. In addition, this drug suppresses sebum production and exhibits antibacterial effects against *P. acnes*. Benzoyl peroxide is available as a topical lotion, cream, or gel in various percent concentrations. Typically the patient applies benzoyl peroxide once daily and, in many instances, this is the only treatment needed. The drug is very safe, with local redness, irritation, and drying being the most common adverse effects. Although the symptoms might worsen during the early weeks of therapy, the skin usually adjusts quickly to its use. Other keratolytic agents that are available by prescription are used for severe acne and include benzoyl peroxide with erythromycin (Benzamycin) and benzoyl peroxide with sulfur (Sulfoxyl).

Retinoids are a class of drug closely related to vitamin A. They are used in the treatment of inflammatory skin conditions, dermatologic malignancies, and acne. The topical formulations are often the drugs of choice for patients with mild to moderate acne, particularly those with the presence of inflammatory cysts. Tretinoin (Retin-A) is an older drug with an irritant action that decreases comedone formation and increases extrusion of comedones from the skin. Tretinoin also has the ability to improve photodamaged skin and is used for wrinkle removal. Other retinoids include isotretinoin (Accutane), an PO vitamin A metabolite medication that aids in reducing the size of sebaceous glands, thereby decreasing oil production and the occurrence of clogged pores. Therapy with retinoids may require 8 to 12 weeks to achieve maximum effectiveness. Common reactions to retinoids include burning, stinging, and sensitivity to sunlight. Adapalene (Differin) is a third-generation retinoid that causes less irritation than the older agents. Additional retinoid-like agents and the related compounds that are used to treat acne are listed in Table 76.2.

Antibiotics are sometimes used in combination with acne medications to lessen the severe redness and inflammation associated with moderate to severe acne, especially when the acne is inflammatory and results in cysts and pustules. Oral doxycycline (Vibramycin, others), minocycline, and tetracycline, which are administered in small doses over a long period, have been the traditional antibiotics used in acne therapy. Erythromycin and clindamycin are frequently used topically and have a low incidence of adverse effects.

Oral contraceptives that contain ethinyl estradiol and norgestimate are also used to help clear the skin of acne by suppressing sebum production and reducing skin oiliness. The agents are reserved for women who are unable to take PO antibiotics or when antibiotic therapy has proved inef-

TABLE 76.2 Drugs for Acne

Drug	Remarks
adapalene (Differin)	Retinoid-like compound used to treat acne formation
azelaic acid (Azelex, Finacea, others)	For mild to moderate inflammatory acne
benzoyl peroxide (Benzalin, Fostex, others)	Keratinolytic available OTC: sometimes combined with erythromycin (Benzamycin) or clindamycin (BenzaClin) for acne caused by *P. acnes*
clindamycin and tretinoin (Ziana)	Combination product with an antibiotic and a retinoid in a gel base; for mild to moderate acne
ethinyl estradiol (Estinyl)	Oral contraceptives are sometimes used for acne; for example, ethinyl estradiol plus norgestimate (Ortho Tri-Cyclen-28)
isotretinoin (Accutane)	For severe acne with cysts, or acne formed in small, rounded masses; pregnancy category X
sulfacetamide sodium (Cetamide, Klaron, others)	For sensitive skin; sometimes combined with sulfur to promote peeling, as in the condition rosacea; also used for conjunctivitis
tazarotene (Tazorac)	A retinoid drug that may also be used for plaque psoriasis; has antiproliferative and anti-inflammatory effects
tetracyclines	Antibiotics; refer to Chapter 49
tretinoin (Retin-A, others)	To prevent clogging of pore follicles; also used for the treatment of acute promyelocytic leukemia and wrinkles

fective. They are most effective for young women when the acne begins somewhat later than usual and tends to flare up at certain times in the menstrual cycle. Estrogen is not administered to male patients because of undesirable adverse effects, such as breast enlargement and decrease in body hair. For the actions and contraindications of oral contraceptives, see Chapter 70.

CONNECTION *Checkpoint* 76.2

Retinoids are derivatives of vitamin A. From what you learned in Chapter 62, what type of vitamin is vitamin A? What are some signs of toxicity due to excess amounts of this vitamin? See Answers to Connection Checkpoint 76.2 in Appendix A.

Rosacea: Rosacea is an inflammatory skin disorder of unknown etiology with lesions affecting mainly the face. Unlike acne, which most commonly affects teenagers, rosacea is a progressive disorder with an onset between 30 and 50 years of age. Rosacea is characterized by small papules or inflammatory bumps without pus that swell, thicken, and become painful, as shown in Figure 76.4. These lesions typically occur in the middle third of the face, including the forehead, nose, cheeks and chin. The face takes on a reddened or flushed appearance with accompanying telangiectasia (dilation of small blood vessels). With time the redness becomes more permanent, and lesions resembling acne appear. The soft tissues of the nose may thicken, giving the nose a reddened, bulbous, irregular swelling called **rhinophyma.** Disorders of the eye frequently accompany rosacea, particularly conjunctivitis, itching, edema, and keratitis.

Rosacea is exacerbated by factors such as sunlight, stress, increased temperature, and agents that dilate facial blood vessels, including alcohol, spicy foods, skin care products, and hot beverages. Rosacea affects more women than men, although men more often develop rhinophyma. Learning and avoiding the environmental triggers that worsen the symptoms of the condition may prevent mild rosacea.

The two most effective treatments for rosacea are topical metronidazole (MetroGel, MetroCream) and azelaic acid (Finacea). Benzoyl peroxide may be applied as needed. Alternative medications include topical clindamycin (Cleocin-T, ClindaMax) and sulfacetamide. Tetracycline antibiotics are of benefit to patients with rosacea who have multiple pustules or ocular involvement. Severe, resistant cases may respond to isotretinoin (Accutane). In addition to medications, some patients receive vascular or carbon dioxide laser surgery to reduce the excessive tissue associated with rhinophyma.

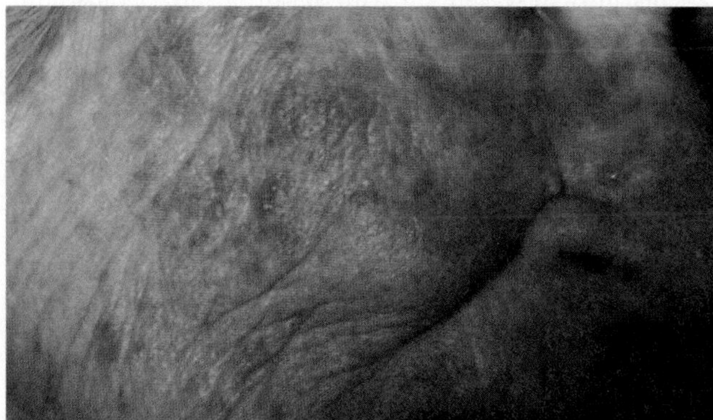

Figure 76.4 Rosacea.
Source: Courtesy of Dr. Jason L. Smith

PROTOTYPE DRUG Tretinoin (Avita, Retin-A, Trentin-X)

Classification: **Therapeutic:** Antiacne agent
Pharmacologic: Retinoid

Therapeutic Effects and Uses: Approved as a topical drug in 1971, tretinoin is a natural derivative of vitamin A. This drug is indicated for the early treatment and control of mild to moderate acne vulgaris. Renova is a topical form of tretinoin that has been approved to treat fine facial wrinkles and hyperpigmentation associated with photodamaged skin. Tretinoin has antineoplastic actions; a PO form (Vesanoid) is approved to treat acute promyelocytic leukemia and may be prescribed off-label for skin malignancies.

Symptoms take 4 to 8 weeks to improve, and maximum therapeutic benefit may take 5 to 6 months. Because of potentially serious adverse effects, this drug is most often reserved for cystic acne or severe keratinization disorders.

Mechanism of Action: The principal action of tretinoin is regulation of skin growth and turnover. As cells from the stratum germinativum grow toward the surface, skin cells are lost from the stratum pore openings, and their replacement is slowed. Tretinoin reverses retention hyperkeratosis and comedone formation, which are the primary events in acne pathology. The drug increases the permeability of the skin and supports conversion of follicular epithelium into a less sturdy and almost fragile condition. Tretinoin also decreases oil production by reducing the size and number of oil glands.

Pharmacokinetics:

Route(s)	Topical, PO
Absorption	Minimally absorbed from intact skin; well absorbed PO
Distribution	Secreted in breast milk; more than 95% bound to plasma protein
Primary metabolism	Hepatic
Primary excretion	Renal
Onset of action	Unknown
Duration of action	Unknown

Adverse Effects: Nearly all patients who use topical tretinoin will experience local effects such as redness, scaling, erythema, crusting, and peeling of the skin with temporary hypopigmentation or hyperpigmentation. Skin irritation can be severe and cause discontinuation of therapy; a lower strength solution may be necessary. Dermatologic adverse effects resolve once therapy is discontinued. Oral therapy can also cause skin adverse effects.

For treatment of acute promyelocytic leukemia, very high PO doses are used and adverse effects are more serious than with topical therapy. The most common effects with PO therapy include bone pain, fever, headache, nausea, vomiting, rash, stomatitis, pruritus, sweating, and ocular disorders. About 25% of patients develop retinoic acid syndrome, which is a serious condition characterized by fever, weakness, fatigue, dyspnea, weight gain, peripheral edema, respiratory insufficiency, and pneumonia. Other adverse effects may include hyperlipidemia, shivering, hemorrhage, pain, dizziness, paresthesias, anxiety, insomnia, depression, cerebral hemorrhage, intracranial hypertension (HTN), hallucinations, dysrhythmias, flushing, hypotension or HTN, heart failure, visual disturbances, abdominal pain, diarrhea, constipation, dyspepsia, GI hemorrhage, renal insufficiency, dysuria, and acute kidney failure.

Contraindications/Precautions: Contraindications for topical administration include eczema, exposure to sunlight or UV rays, sunburn, hypersensitivity to this drug or vitamin A preparation, and children less than 12 years. This drug should be used cautiously in patients who are in an occupation necessitating considerable sun exposure or weather extremes or in patients with hepatic disease. This drug may cause birth defects and is contraindicated during lactation, pregnancy, or suspected pregnancy. Pregnancy testing is advised before starting therapy in female patients of childbearing age. Oral tretinoin is contraindicated in patients who have hepatic disease, leukopenia or neutropenia, or who are hypersensitive to the drug.

Drug Interactions: Topical acne keratinolytics (sulfur, resorcinol, benzoyl peroxide, and salicylic acid) may increase inflammation and peeling; topical products that contain alcohol or menthol may cause stinging. Additive phototoxicity can occur if tretinoin is used concurrently with other phototoxic drugs such as tetracyclines, fluoroquinolone, or sulfonamides. Use of this drug with hypoglycemic agents may lead to a loss of glycemic control and cardiovascular risk, because tretinoin raises serum triglyceride levels. Hepatotoxic drugs may cause additive liver impairment if used concurrently with PO tretinoin. **Herbal/Food:** The PO absorption of tretinoin is increased if taken with a high-fat meal.

Pregnancy: Category C (topical) and D (PO).

Treatment of Overdose: Overuse of the topical drug will lead to excessive skin drying and peeling. Symptoms of PO overdose are nonspecific and resolve with symptomatic treatment.

Nursing Responsibilities:

- Wear gloves when assessing the skin. Assess the facial skin as well as the anterior and posterior thorax because many acne lesions may be found in these areas.
- Obtain a thorough history, including onset of acne, treatments used and their effects, and whether the patient is pregnant. Ask about allergies, past medical history, and current medications.
- Wait for recovery if the patient has been using a desquamative agent before starting any treatment.
- Clean the patient's skin with a mild bland soap and dry the areas thoroughly before applying the medication. It is important to avoid use of any medicated, drying, or abrasive soaps or cleansers.
- Wash hands prior to and after treatment.
- Avoid contact with the eyes, mouth, nose, open wounds, and mucous membranes.
- Dark-skinned individuals may experience unsightly post-inflammatory hyperpigmentation, which is reversible with termination of the drug treatment.
- Response to the therapy should be evident in 2 to 3 weeks but may require 3 to 4 months.

Patient and Family Education:

- Skin redness and drying occur during the first few weeks of treatment. This is a normal response caused by the drug affecting deep, unseen lesions.
- Be aware that scaling and redness will decrease after 8 to 10 weeks of therapy.
- Cleanse the face no more than two to three times a day and prior to each drug application.
- Do not use topical preparations with high concentrations of alcohol, astringents, spices, or lime. Perfumes and shaving lotions should also be avoided during therapy.
- Treatments are not curative and relapses can occur within 3 to 6 weeks after treatment has been discontinued.
- Avoid direct sun exposure during therapy or use a sunscreen with a sun protection factor (SPF) of 15 or higher.
- Do not use other antiacne drugs during therapy due to potential drug interactions, unless approved by the health care provider.

Drugs Similar to Tretinoin (Avita, Retin-A, Trentin-X)

Similar antiacne drugs include adapalene, azelaic acid, isotretinoin, and tazarotene.

Adapalene (Differin): Approved in 1996, adapalene is a topical acne drug that modulates the inflammation, epithelial keratinization, and differentiation of follicular cells. It is very similar to the retinoids but is reported to produce less skin irritation. Optimum results may take up to 12 weeks of therapy. Patients must take caution with sun exposure because this drug can increase the potential for sunburn. Other adverse effects include local burning, pruritus, scaling, and peeling. Only minimal amounts of adapalene are absorbed through the skin. Safety of this drug in patients under age 12 has not been established. This drug is pregnancy category C.

Azelaic acid (Azelex, Finacea, Finevin): Approved in 1995, azelaic acid is a natural product found in wheat, rye, and barley. Azelaic acid is a topical therapy that is effective for the treatment of mild to moderate acne by suppressing the growth of *P. acnes* and decreasing the proliferation of keratinocytes. It is also approved for the topical treatment of inflammatory pustules associated with rosacea. Only 4% is absorbed systemically. Adverse effects are typical of other topical antiacne drugs: local burning, pruritus, scaling, and peeling. Safety of this drug in patients under age 12 has not been established. This drug is pregnancy category B.

Isotretinoin (Accutane): Approved in 1982, isotretinoin is a PO retinoid that is the most effective drug for severe, inflammatory acne. Therapy may require several months for optimum benefit. Off-label uses include rosacia, psoriasis, and the treatment of squamous cell carcinoma of the skin. Because of potentially serious adverse effects, this drug is usually used when other therapies fail to produce satisfactory results. The most serious potential effect is teratogenicity (category X), which can occur after even short courses of isotretinoin therapy. The drug has special requirements for distribution that require patients, physicians, and pharmacists to register and adhere to the iPledge Program, a pregnancy risk management program. Before starting therapy, the patient must submit to two negative pregnancy tests and sign a statement of understanding about the drug's adverse effects. Each subsequent month, the pharmacist must document receipt of a negative pregnancy test and verify that two forms of effective contraception are being utilized by the patient. Males must also register with the iPledge Program because small amounts of isotretinoin are found in semen and could potentially cause birth defects in a pregnant partner. Other common adverse effects include cheilitis, epistaxis, xerostomia, hair loss, eczema, elevated serum lipid levels, myalgia, and arthralgia. Clinical depression, psychosis, and aggression have been reported.

Tazarotene (Avage, Tazorac): Approved in 1997, tazarotene is a topical retinoid derivative of vitamin A that is used for the treatment of acne, fine facial wrinkles, and psoriasis. Patients become sensitive to the sun's UV light and need to wear protective sunscreen and clothing when using this drug. Adverse effects are similar to those of topical tretinoin: local burning, stinging, erythema, and general skin irritation. This drug is metabolized in the skin to an active metabolite; small amounts are absorbed systemically. Safety of this drug in patients under age 12 has not been established. Tazarotene is pregnancy category X.

Pharmacotherapy of Dermatitis

76.6 The most effective treatment for dermatitis is topical corticosteroids, which are classified by their potency.

Dermatitis is a general term that refers to superficial inflammatory disorders of the skin. General symptoms include local redness, pain, and pruritus. Intense scratching may lead to **excoriation,** which are scratches that break the skin surface and fill with blood or serous fluid to form crusty scales. A wide variety of factors can cause dermatitis, with different types of symptoms occurring depending on the causative agent. The three most common types that respond to topical pharmacotherapy are atopic, contact, and seborrheic. Dermatitis may be acute or chronic.

PharmFACT

Allergic dermatitis is the most common skin condition in children younger than 11 years of age. The percentage of children diagnosed with it has tripled in the past two decades. *Source:* American Academy of Allergy, Asthma and Immunology, n.d.

Atopic dermatitis, or **eczema,** is a chronic, inflammatory skin disorder with a genetic predisposition. Patients who present with eczema often have a family history of asthma and hay fever as well as allergies to a variety of irritants such as cosmetics, lotions, soaps, pollens, food, pet dander, and dust. About 75% of patients with atopic dermatitis have had an initial onset before 1 year of age. In those babies predisposed to eczema, breast-feeding seems to offer protection, because it is rare for a breast-fed child to develop eczema before the introduction of other foods. In infants and small children, lesions usually begin on the face and scalp, and then progress to other parts of the body. A frequent and prominent symptom in infants is the appearance of red cheeks.

Contact dermatitis can be caused by a hypersensitivity response, resulting from exposure to specific natural or synthetic allergens such as plants, chemicals, latex, drugs, metals, or foreign proteins. Accompanying the allergic reaction may be various degrees of cracking, bleeding, or small blisters.

Seborrheic dermatitis is a form of eczema that can affect patients at any age. The exact cause of seborrheic dermatitis is unknown, but hormone levels, coexisting fungal infections, nutritional deficiencies, and immunodeficiency states are associated with the disease. Seborrheic dermatitis presents as greasy, not dry, scales that affect the scalp, central face, and anterior chest, often presenting as scalp scaling, or dandruff. Other symptoms may include redness of the nasolabial fold, particularly during times of stress; blepharitis; otitis externa; and acne vulgaris. In infants thick, greasy scales on the vertex of the scalp, commonly known as cradle cap, are seen. These scales can become more widespread, with the central face, forehead, and ears being affected.

Pharmacotherapy of dermatitis is symptomatic and involves lotions and ointments to control itching and skin flaking. Antihistamines may be used to control inflammation and reduce itching, and analgesics or topical anesthetics may be prescribed for pain relief. Atopic dermatitis can be controlled, but not cured, by medications. Part of the management plan must include the identification and elimination of allergic triggers that cause flare-ups.

Topical corticosteroids are the most effective treatment for controlling the inflammation and itching of dermatitis. Creams, lotions, solutions, gels, and pads that contain corticosteroids are specially formulated to penetrate deep into the skin layers. These dermatologic agents are classified by potency, as listed in Table 76.3. The high-potency agents are used to treat acute flare-ups and are limited to 2 to 3 weeks of therapy. The moderate-potency formulations are for more prolonged therapy of chronic dermatitis. The low-potency corticosteroids are prescribed for children.

Long-term corticosteroid use may lead to irritation, redness, hypopigmentation, and thinning of the skin. High-potency

NURSING PROCESS APPLICATION

Patients Receiving Tretinoin (Retin-A) or Isotretinoin (Accutane)

Assessment

Prior to administration:

- Obtain a complete health history, including allergies, drug history, and possible drug interactions.
- Assess for history of psychiatric disorders.
- Assess vital signs to obtain baseline information.

Potential Nursing Diagnoses

- *Disturbed Body Image,* related to presence of acne and possible worsening of symptoms after initiation of treatment
- *Decisional Conflict,* related to desire for pregnancy, and necessity of preventing pregnancy during therapy with tretinoin
- *Noncompliance (Drug Therapy Regimen),* related to time, or failure to use effective contraception
- *Impaired Skin Integrity,* related to inflammation, redness, and scaling, secondary to treatment

Planning: Patient Goals and Expected Outcomes

The patient will:

- Experience decreased acne without adverse effects or adverse reactions.
- Demonstrate acceptance of body image.
- Demonstrate an understanding of the drug's action by accurately describing drug adverse effects and precautions.
- Comply with the treatment regimen by keeping all scheduled appointments and laboratory visits for testing.

Implementation

Interventions and (Rationales)	Patient and Family Education
• Monitor laboratory studies during treatment, including blood glucose. (Monitoring of laboratory values is important in determining complications or serious adverse effects.)	• Instruct the patient to keep laboratory appointments prior to therapy and periodically during therapy, and if the patient has diabetes, he or she must perform home blood glucose monitoring.
• Discuss potential adverse reactions to drug therapy. (Understanding of drug effects is important for adherence.)	• Instruct the patient to avoid using vitamin A products.
• Monitor for cardiovascular problems. (Use tretinoin with caution in patients with heart block, especially if the patient is also taking a beta blocker.)	• Discuss with the patient the importance of complete disclosure regarding the medical history and medications.
• Monitor emotional health. (The patient may become depressed secondary to the acne itself, length of treatment, possibility of worsening symptoms at the beginning of treatment, changed body image, or the drug itself.)	Instruct the patient to: • Report signs of depression immediately and discontinue tretinoin. • Report any feelings of suicide.
• Monitor complete blood count (CBC), blood lipid levels, glucose levels, liver function tests, eye exam, gastrointestinal (GI) status, and urinalysis. (Monitoring of laboratory values is important in assessing for complications or serious adverse effects.)	• Teach the patient the importance of a complete workup prior to starting tretinoin therapy and periodically during the course of treatment.
• Monitor for vision changes. (Corneal opacities or cataracts may develop as a result of drug use. Dryness of the eyes during treatment is common. Night vision may be diminished during treatment.)	Instruct the patient: • To report any decreased vision and to discontinue use of tretinoin. • To avoid driving at night if possible. • That using artificial tears may relieve dry eyes. • That using contact lenses may need to be discontinued during therapy.
• Monitor alcohol use. (Alcohol use leads to increased triglyceride levels.)	Advise the patient to: • Eliminate or greatly reduce alcohol use, including alcohol-containing preparations such as mouthwashes or OTC medications, especially products containing acetaminophen. • Read labels for alcohol content.
• Monitor skin problems. (This will determine the effectiveness of drug therapy.)	Advise the patient: • That acne may worsen during the beginning of treatment. • To monitor the skin for improvement in 4 to 8 weeks; if no improvement is noted, the patient should contact the health care provider.
• Monitor for adverse effects. (Adverse effects may point to potential complications and nonadherence with the drug regimen.)	Instruct the patient to be aware of and to report headache (especially if accompanied by nausea and vomiting), fatigue, depression, lethargy, severe diarrhea, rectal bleeding, abdominal pain, visual changes, dry mouth, hematuria, proteinuria, and liver dysfunction (jaundice, pruritus, dark urine).

Evaluation of Outcome Criteria

Evaluate the effectiveness of drug therapy by confirming that patient goals and expected outcomes have been met (see "Planning").

TABLE 76.3 Selected Topical Corticosteroids for Dermatitis and Related Symptoms

Generic Name	Strength (%)	Trade Names
Very High Potency		
betamethasone dipropionate, augmented, cream	0.05	Diprolene
clobetasol propionate	0.05	Temovate
diflorasone diacetate	0.05	Maxiflor
High Potency		
amcinonide	0.1	Cyclocort
fluocinonide	0.025	Lidex
halcinonide	0.1	Halog
Medium Potency		
betamethasone benzoate	0.025	Uticort
betamethasone valerate	0.1	Valisone
clocortolone pivalate	0.1	Cloderm
desoximetasone, cream	0.025	Topicort
fluocinolone acetonide	0.025	Synalar
flurandrenolide, cream	0.025	Cordran
fluticasone propionate, cream	0.05	Cutivate
hydrocortisone valerate	0.2	Westcort
mometasone furoate	0.1	Elocon
triamcinolone acetonide	0.025–0.1	Aristocort, Kenalog
Low Potency		
alclometasone dipropionate	0.05	Aclovate
desonide	0.05	Desonate, DesOwen, Verdeso
dexamethasone	0.1	Decaspray
hydrocortisone	0.25–1	Cortizone, Hycort

formulations are not advised for the head or neck regions because of potential adverse effects. If absorption occurs, topical corticosteroids may produce undesirable systemic effects, including adrenal insufficiency, mood changes, serum imbalances, and loss of bone mass, as discussed in Chapter 69. To avoid serious adverse effects, careful attention must be given to the amount of corticosteroid applied, the frequency of application, and how long it should be used. For most patients with dermatitis, topical corticosteroids have minimal adverse effects.

Several alternatives to the corticosteroids are available. Patients with persistent atopic dermatitis that does not respond to corticosteroids may benefit from PO immunosuppressive agents, such as cyclosporine. This drug is generally used for the short-term treatment of severe disease. The topical calcineurin inhibitors pimecrolimus 1% (Elidel) and tacrolimus 0.03%, 0.1% (Protopic) are available for patients older than 2 years of age. These medications may be used on all skin surfaces (including the face and neck) because they have fewer adverse effects than the topical corticosteroids. Adverse effects include burning and stinging on broken skin. Pimecrolimus and tacrolimus are not approved for long-term therapy because of a small risk of skin cancer and lymphoma. They are reserved for patients who have not responded to topical corticosteroids. When using these agents occlusive dressings should not be used because this promotes absorption of the drug and can increase the risk of systemic toxicity. The immunosuppressants are presented in Chapter 45.

Topical therapy for seborrheic dermatitis primarily consists of antifungal agents and low-dose topical corticosteroids, depending on the location affected. The first-line therapy for seborrheic dermatitis that affects the scalp should be topical corticosteroids. These may be administered as a shampoo, topical solution, or a lotion applied to the scalp. A typical regimen for an adult would be to use a topical corticosteroid once or twice daily with the use of a medicated shampoo two to three times per week. Shampoos that contain selenium sulfide (Selsun), salicylic acid, zinc pyrithione, or an antifungal azole are most often used. Once-daily antifungal medication with fluconazole (Diflucan), ketoconazole (Nizoral), or ciclopirox (Loprox) combined with 2 weeks of once-daily desonide (DesOwen) is recommended for seborrhoic dermatitis of the face and ears.

CONNECTION *Checkpoint* 76.3

Topical applications of corticosteroids are used for a variety of conditions. What are some indications for corticosteroids given by the following routes of administration: aerosol inhalation (see Chapter 73), intranasal (see Chapter 74), and intra-articular (see Chapter 75)? See Answer to Connection Checkpoint 76.3 in Appendix A.

Pharmacotherapy of Psoriasis

76.7 Psoriasis is a chronic, inflammatory disease that is treated with topical and systemic agents.

Psoriasis is a chronic, inflammatory skin disorder that affects 1% to 2% of the population and appears with greater frequency in people of European ancestry. The onset of psoriasis is generally established by 20 years of age, although it may occur throughout the life span.

Pharm*FACT*

Psoriasis affects more than 4.5 million Americans. About one third of these people have at least one family member with the condition. *Source:* American Academy of Dermatology, n.d.

Although the etiology of psoriasis is incompletely understood, it appears to have both genetic and autoimmune components. About 33% to 50% of the cases have a genetic basis, with a close family member also having the disorder. When one identical twin presents with psoriasis, the other twin has a 70% probability of also acquiring the disease. The immune nature of psoriasis is supported by the discovery that activated T lymphocytes (T cells) migrate to the dermis and release cytokines such as tumor necrosis factor (TNF) that increase the production of skin cells and cause inflammation. Furthermore, suppressing T-cell function through the use of immunosuppressants or biologic therapies improves symptoms of psoriasis.

Specific environmental triggers worsen psoriasis. Factors such as stress, smoking, alcohol, climate changes, and infections can worsen symptoms. In addition, certain drugs, including angiotensin-converting enzyme (ACE) inhibitors, beta-adrenergic blockers, tetracyclines, and nonsteroidal anti-inflammatory drugs (NSAIDs), act as triggers. Persons with psoriasis seem to improve in warmer climates, where there is more exposure to sunlight.

When psoriasis occurs, both the dermis and epidermis become thickened from an extremely fast skin turnover rate, with skin cells reaching the surface in 4 to 7 days instead of the normal 14 days. This rapid proliferation time does not allow for cell maturation and keratinization to occur, giving the skin lesions their characteristic appearance. The typical psoriatic lesions are characterized by red, raised patches of skin covered with flaky, thick, silver scales called **plaques.** Plaques are ultimately shed from the surface while the underlying skin becomes inflamed and irritated. If the scales are scraped away, the dark-red base of the lesion is exposed, producing multiple bleeding points. Lesions vary in size and are usually present on the scalp, elbows, knees, extensor surfaces of the arms and legs, sacrum, and occasionally around the nails. The face is rarely affected. When psoriasis affects the nails, a yellow or brown discoloration may result and the nail itself may separate from the nail bed, thicken, and crumble. The various forms of psoriasis are described in Table 76.4. A patient with the disorder is shown in Figure 76.5.

The goal of psoriasis pharmacotherapy is to reduce erythema, plaques, and scales to improve the cosmetic appearance of the patient, leading to more normal lifestyle activities. This is accomplished by reducing epidermal cell turnover and promoting healing of the psoriatic lesions. The choice of therapy depends on the type and extent of the disease and the history of response to a previous treatment of psoriasis. A number of prescription and OTC drugs are available for the treatment of psoriasis and are listed in Table 76.5. Therapy is often conducted in a stepwise manner. Psoriasis is a lifelong disease and there is no pharmacologic cure.

Topical Drugs

Corticosteroids: Topical corticosteroids are the primary, initial treatment for psoriasis. These drugs are effective, inexpensive, and relatively safe. Examples include betamethasone (Diprosone) and hydrocortisone acetate (Cortaid, Caldecort, others). When they are applied to psoriatic lesions topical corticosteroids suppress cell division, reduce inflammation, re-

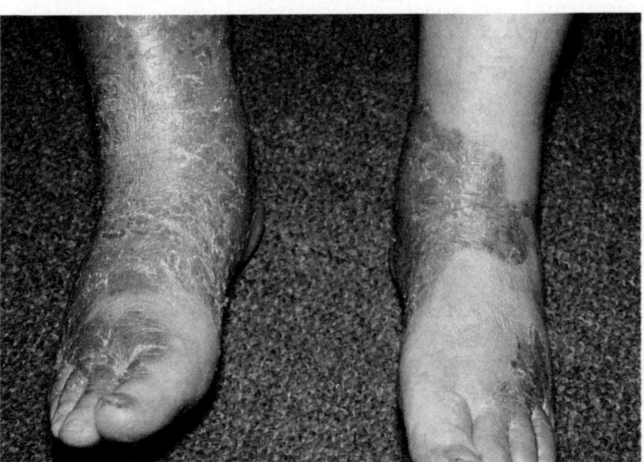

Figure 76.5 Psoriasis.
Source: Courtesy of Dr. Jason L. Smith

TABLE 76.4 Type of Psoriasis

Form of Psoriasis	Description	Most Common Location of Lesions	Comments
Guttate (droplike) or eruptive psoriasis	Lesions smaller than those of psoriasis vulgaris	Upper trunk and extremities	More common in early-onset psoriasis; can appear and resolve spontaneously a few weeks following a streptococcal respiratory infection
Psoriatic arthritis	Resembles rheumatoid arthritis	Fingers and toes at the distal interphalangeal joints; can affect the skin and nails	About 20% of patients with psoriasis also have arthritis
Psoriasis vulgaris	Lesions are papules that form into erythematous plaques with thick, silver or gray plaques that bleed when removed; plaques in dark-skinned individuals often appear purple	Skin over scalp, elbows, and knees; lesions possible anywhere on the body	Most common form; requires long-term specialized management
Psoriatic erythroderma or exfoliative dermatitis	Generalized scaling; erythema without lesions	All body surfaces	Least common form; average
Pustular psoriasis	Eruption of pustules; presence of fever	Trunk and extremities; can appear on the palms, soles, and nail beds	Age of onset is 50 years

lieve pruritus, and delay the movement of keratinocytes that are associated with fast skin turnover. Choosing the correct strength of corticosteroid and the most effective vehicle base are important aspects of treatment because the effectiveness of a topical steroid use depends on its potency and ability to be absorbed into the skin. Initial therapy may begin with a high-potency agent to obtain rapid clearing of the lesions. High-potency agents are also used for acute flare-ups for 2 to 3 weeks. The high-potency formulations are best applied to the areas thickest with plaque, such as the hands or feet, and should not used on the face and genital areas. For chronic maintenance therapy, the patient is switched to moderate- and low-potency corticosteroids because they have a lower potential for adverse effects.

Occlusive dressings may be applied to increase the effectiveness of the corticosteroid. A simple way to enhance drug penetration is to apply the steroid directly to the skin followed by warm, moist dressings and an occlusive outer wrap. Wraps may be large plastic bags, vinyl jogging suits, or rolls of tubular plastic. Care should be taken that the wraps not be left in place longer than 8 hours. The skin should be inspected for atrophy, striae, hypopigmentation, and telangiectasias, which are all adverse effects of topical corticosteroid therapy.

Repeated use of topical corticosteroids will result in tolerance. To delay tolerance, doses of the high-potency drugs are kept as low as possible. Some health care providers discontinue corticosteroids after an adequate response has been obtained and switch to a different therapy such as coal tar for several weeks.

When large areas of the body have psoriatic lesions, topical corticosteroid therapy can be expensive and involve some systemic risk. The larger the area treated, the greater the absorbed doses. The student should refer to Chapter 69 for a discussion of the adverse effects of systemic corticosteroid therapy.

Coal tar and anthralin: Other skin therapies, such as coal tar and anthralin, may be used as monotherapy or in combination with other psoriasis medications. Tar and anthralin inhibit deoxyribonucleic acid (DNA) synthesis and arrest abnormal cell growth as well as reduce inflammation. Coal tar is available as a solution, gel, lotion, and shampoo. Coal tar preparations are messy, staining, and have a foul odor. Therapy with anthralin is similar to that of coal tar. It is applied in a stiff paste to lesions for short periods up to 8 hours. Anthralin is a strong irritant and can cause chemical burns, especially if it comes in contact with uninvolved skin. The use of coal tar and anthralin are considered second-line therapies when the patient develops tolerance to the corticosteroids.

Calcipotriene (Dovonex): Approved in 1993, calcipotriene is a derivative of vitamin D that is available as a cream for use on the body and as a solution for the scalp. The drug binds to vitamin D receptors in the skin, suppresses cellular proliferation, and decreases cellular turnover in the psoriatic plaques. Symptomatic improvement is seen in 2 to 3 weeks. Calcipotriene is an effective alternative to topical corticosteroids. Only about 6% of a topical dose is absorbed systemically. Its most common adverse effect is local irritation. It is not recommended for use by patients over age 65, who have an increased incidence of adverse effects with the drug, or by pregnant and lactating women (category C). Its use may produce hypercalcemia if applied over large areas of the body or if used in higher than recommended doses. Phototherapy of excessive exposure to UV light should be avoided due to the potential for increased tumor incidence. This drug is pregnancy category C.

Tazarotene (Tazorac): Approved in 1997, tazarotene (Tazorac) is a vitamin A retinoid that causes sloughing of the scales covering the psoriatic plaques. For psoriasis this drug is applied once daily in the evening. This drug is also approved for facial wrinkles and acne. This drug is pregnancy category X.

Systemic Drugs

Some patients have severe psoriasis that is resistant to topical therapy. Because these drugs have the potential to cause more serious adverse effects, they are generally only used when topical agents and phototherapy fail to produce an adequate response.

TABLE 76.5 Selected Drugs for Psoriasis and Related Disorders

Drug	Route and Adult Dose (maximum dose where indicated)	Adverse Effects
Topical Medications		
anthralin (Dritho-Scalp, Psoriatec)	Topical: Apply once daily or as directed	*Skin irritation; temporary discoloration of the skin, hair, and fingernails; erythema* No serious adverse effects
calcipotriene (Dovonex)	Topical: Apply a thin layer to the lesions 1–2 times/day up to 8 weeks	*Burning, stinging, folliculitis, itching, dry skin, hyperpigmentation* No serious adverse effects
coal tar (Balnetar, Cutar, others)	Topical: Apply to affected areas once-qid	*Folliculitis, irritation, photosensitivity* No serious adverse effects
salicylic acid (Salax, Neutrogena, others)	Topical: Apply to affected areas tid-qid in concentrations ranging from 2–10%	*Erythema, pruritus, stinging of the skin* No serious adverse effects
tacrolimus (Protopic)	Topical: Apply a thin layer to affected area bid	*Infections, skin burning, pruritus, erythema, headache, fever, hyperesthesia, pain, folliculitis* Skin cancer, lymphoma
tazarotene (Tazorac)	Acne: Apply a thin film to the clean, dry area daily Plaque psoriasis: Apply thin film daily in the evening	*Pruritus, burning, stinging, skin irritation, transient worsening of psoriasis, skin peeling, photosensitivity* Hypertriglyceridemia, teratogenicity
Systemic Medications		
acitretin (Soriatane)	PO: 25–50 mg/day with the main meal	*Dry mouth, alopecia, cheilitis, dry skin, dry mucous membranes* Increased triglycerides and cholesterol, paresthesias, rigors, arthralgia, skin peeling, pseudotumor cerebri, depression, elevated liver function tests, teratogenicity
cyclosporine (Neoral, Gengraf)	PO: 1.25 mg/kg bid (max: 4 mg/kg/day)	*Hirsutism, tremor, vomiting, headache, pruritus, nausea, vomiting, diarrhea* HTN, myocardial infarction (MI), nephrotoxicity, hyperkalemia, gingival enlargement, paresthesias, hepatotoxicity, infection
etanercept (Enbrel)	Subcutaneous: 50 mg twice weekly (given 3–4 days apart) Maintenance dose: 50 mg/week	*Local reactions at the injection site (pain, erythema, myalgia), abdominal pain, vomiting, headache, nasopharyngitis* Infections (tuberculosis, sepsis, and invasive fungal infections), lupus-like syndrome, positive antinuclear antibodies, heart failure exacerbations, pancytopenia
hydroxyurea (Hydrea)	PO: 1,000–1,500 mg/day in single or divided doses	*Chills, edema, fatigue, drowsiness, GI upset* Bone marrow toxicity, leg ulcers, megablastic anemia, hepatotoxicity
methotrexate (Trexall, Rheumatrex)	PO: 2.5–5 mg bid for three doses each week (max: 25–30 mg/week)	*Headache, glossitis, gingivitis, mild leukopenia, nausea* Ulcerative stomatitis, myelosuppression, aplastic anemia, hepatic cirrhosis, nephrotoxicity, sudden death, pulmonary fibrosis, acute renal failure, teratogenicity

Note: *Italics* indicates common adverse effects. Underline indicates serious adverse effects.

In some cases, systemic drugs may be used for a few weeks to produce a rapid improvement in symptoms before beginning topical therapy.

Methotrexate (Rheumatrex, Trexall): The most frequently prescribed systemic drug for severe psoriasis is methotrexate. Methotrexate is an older drug that was approved in 1953 and used in the treatment of a variety of disorders, including carcinomas and rheumatoid arthritis, in addition to being prescribed for psoriasis. For psoriasis, methotrexate inhibits the rapid proliferation of cells in the skin. It is administered either once weekly or bid for 3 days each week. Dosing requires a "rest period" where cells can recover from the cytotoxic effects of the drug. Improvement is noted after several weeks of therapy but maximum effects may take 2 to 3 months. For resistant lesions, methotrexate may be combined with phototherapy or alternated with other systemic drugs. Methotrexate is discussed as a prototype drug in Chapter 58.

Acitretin (Soriatane): Acitretin is a PO retinoid that is approved for severe, resistant psoriasis. Two to three months of therapy may be required for significant symptomatic improvement. Approved in 1997, acitretin acts like other retinoids to inhibit keratin formation and skin inflammation. This drug is very effective at eliminating psoriatic lesions. However, the lesions return soon after therapy is discontinued. The most serious adverse effect is teratogenicity (category X). At least two negative pregnancy tests should be obtained before beginning therapy, and the patient should use effective birth control for 3 years after discontinuing the drug. Many adverse effects occur frequently during therapy, including cheilitis, hair loss, dry skin, pruritus, rash, epistaxis, bleeding gums, and joint pain. The active metabolite of acitretin, etretinate (Tegison), was withdrawn from the market in 1998 due to high toxicity. The patient should refrain from drinking alcohol during acitretin therapy because this converts more of the drug to its toxic metabolite.

Miscellaneous systemic antipsoriatic drugs: Cyclosporine (Sandimmune) is an immunosuppressive agent that is presented as a prototype drug in Chapter 45. It is effective at providing rapid relief from the symptoms of psoriasis and is often combined with other drugs, such as calcipotriene, to provide for a lower dose and reduce toxicity. Hydroxyurea (Hydrea) is a drug that has been approved for various cancers and for sickle cell anemia. It is used off-label to treat psoriasis but bone marrow toxicity limits its use.

Biologic therapies: An understanding of the role of the immune system in the pathogenesis of psoriasis has led to the use of biologic therapies to treat patients with moderate to severe disease. Biologic agents suppress the rate of cell proliferation and have been found to improve the symptoms of psoriasis. Approved biologic agents include alefacept (Amevive), efalizumab (Raptiva), etanercept (Enbrel), and infliximab (Remicade). These agents induce general immunosuppression, and patients are at an increased risk for increased frequency of infection. Etanercept has been shown to be especially useful in treating patients with psoriatic arthritis. A major disadvantage of these drugs is that they are not available in PO formulations. Costs of therapy may exceed $10,000 per year.

Nonpharmacologic therapy: Phototherapy with ultraviolet-A (UVA) and ultraviolet-B (UVB) light is used in cases of severe debilitating psoriasis. Phototherapy with UVA is combined with methoxsalen, a drug from a chemical family known as the **psoralens.** The concurrent use of UVA and the drug is called PUVA therapy. Psoralens are PO or topical agents that produce a photosensitive reaction when exposed to UV light. This reaction reduces the number of psoriatic lesions, but unpleasant adverse effects such as headache, nausea, and skin sensitivity occur that may limit the effectiveness of PUVA therapy. Treatments are limited to two to three times per week and an interim period of 48 hours between treatments is necessary. Because of the strong photosensitizing properties of the psoralens, patients must wear dark glasses during treatment and for the remainder of the day. The use of PUVA has been associated with an increased risk for cataract development.

The second type of phototherapy is with a single UVB light, which is less hazardous than UVA therapy. The wavelength of UVB is similar to sunlight, and it reduces the lesions that cover a large area of the body that normally resist topical treatments. It is usually used in conjunction with topical coal tar. If access to a light treatment unit is not feasible, natural sunlight may be used. The use of commercial tanning beds is not recommended for the patient with psoriasis.

All UV treatments may cause acute sunburn reactions, including generalized redness with edema and tenderness as well as the development of long-term effects of actinic keratosis, premature aging of the skin, and skin cancers. Immunosuppressant drugs such as cyclosporine are not used in conjunction with PUVA therapy, because they increase the risk of skin cancer.

Pharmacotherapy of Minor Skin Burns

76.8 The pharmacotherapy of sunburn includes prevention with sunscreens and treatment with lotions, topical anesthetics, and analgesics.

Sunburn results from overexposure of the skin to UV light and is associated with light skin complexions, prolonged exposure to the sun during the more hazardous hours of the day (10 A.M. until 3 P.M.), and lack of protective clothing when outdoors. Chronic sun exposure can result in serious conditions, including eye injury, cataracts, and skin cancer.

Minor, first-degree burns affect only the outer layers of the epidermis. Excessive exposure to UV light, however, injures the dermis and dilates the capillaries, leading to redness, tenderness, edema, and occasional blister formation. In addition to producing local skin damage, sun overexposure releases toxins that may produce systemic effects. The signs and symptoms of sunburn include erythema, intense pain, nausea, vomiting, chills, edema, and headache. These symptoms usually resolve within a matter of hours or days, depending on the severity of the exposure. Once sunburn has occurred, medications can only alleviate the symptoms; they do not speed recovery time.

The best treatment for sunburn is prevention. Sunscreens are liquids or lotions applied for chemical or physical protection. Chemical sunscreens absorb the spectrum of UV light that is responsible for most sunburns. Chemical sunscreens include those that contain benzophenone for protection against UVA rays; those that work against UVB rays include cinnamates, p-aminobenzoic acid (PABA), and salicylates. Physical sunscreens such as zinc oxide, talc, and titanium dioxide reflect or scatter light to prevent the penetration of both UVA and UVB rays. Parsol is another sunscreen product that is being used more frequently as a key ingredient in lip balm.

The effectiveness of a sunscreen is indicated by its SPF. An SPF of 8 means the product offers eight times more protection than using no sunscreen. Patients with skin that sunburns easily should use products with an SPF of 15 or greater. Waterproof sunscreens are meant to withstand 8 minutes of exposure to water. People tend to apply sunscreen too infrequently and in layers that are too thin. To be effective, sunscreen must be applied generously and often during the exposure period.

Treatment for sunburn consists of addressing symptoms with soothing lotions, rest, prevention of dehydration, and topical anesthetic agents, if needed. Treatment is usually done on an outpatient basis. Topical anesthetics for minor burns include benzocaine (Solarcaine), dibucaine (Nupercainal), lidocaine (Xylocaine), and tetracaine HCl (Pontocaine). Aloe vera is a popular natural therapy for minor skin irritations and burns. Hydrocortisone cream may decrease pain and swelling and assist in the healing of damaged tissue. These same agents may also provide relief from minor pain due to insect bites and pruritus. In more severe cases, PO analgesics and anti-inflammatory agents such as aspirin or ibuprofen may be indicated.

PROTOTYPE DRUG Benzocaine (Americaine, Anbesol, others)

Classification: **Therapeutic:** Topical anesthetic
Pharmacologic: Local anesthetic (ester type), antipruritic

Therapeutic Effects and Uses: Approved in 1938, benzocaine inhibits the conduction of nerve impulses from sensory nerve endings, producing surface anesthesia. It is indicated for the temporary relief of pain and discomfort in patients with pruritic skin problems, minor burns and wounds, and insect bites. It is available in a variety of delivery forms, including sprays, lotions, gels, and lozenges. Several products are available OTC to treat pain due to toothaches, dentures, or canker sores. Because of its short duration of action, it must be applied three to four times a day.

Mechanism of Action: Benzocaine produces surface anesthesia by inhibiting the conduction of nerve endings.

Pharmacokinetics:

Route(s)	Topical
Absorption	Minimally absorbed from intact skin
Distribution	Unknown
Primary metabolism	Hepatic
Primary excretion	Renal
Onset of action	1 minute
Duration of action	15–20 minutes

Adverse Effects: Adverse effects include sensitization in susceptible individuals, allergic reactions, and anaphylaxis. Because it is poorly absorbed, systemic adverse effects are rarely observed.

Contraindications/Precautions: Contraindications include hypersensitivity to benzocaine or other PABA derivatives or to any of the components in the formulation. Caution should be used in patients with a history of drug sensitivity to ester-type anesthetics, denuded skin, or severely traumatized mucosa, and in children under 6 years.

Drug Interactions: Benzocaine may antagonize the antibacterial activity of sulfonamides.

Pregnancy: Category C.

Treatment of Overdose: Overdose with topical benzocaine is unlikely.

Nursing Responsibilities:

- Assess the sunburn, including the location, portion of body surface area, edema, erythema, and blistering.
- Assess for systemic symptoms such as fever, chills, weakness, and shock. These may occur following severe exposure, or when the sunburn affects a large portion of the body surface area.

CONNECTIONS

Complementary and Alternative Therapies Aloe Vera

Description: There are numerous products on the market, including soaps, lotions, creams, and sunscreens that are aimed at the consumer who is seeking the healing properties of aloe vera gel. Health care providers have also prescribed aloe vera gel to treat dermatitis, burns, and a variety of skin disorders.

History and Claims: Aloe vera is derived from the gel inside the leaf of the aloe plant, which is a member of the lily family. Aloe vera contains over 70 active substances, including amino acids, minerals, vitamins, and enzymes. These substances are supposed to kill a variety of microorganisms, decrease pain, and reduce localized inflammation. Aloe vera also has value for its moisturizing and wound healing properties. It has been used medicinally for thousands of years. Early mention is made of aloe's use in ancient Sumaria in 2200 BC, where it was proclaimed a plant of "great healing power" (Goldfaden, 2007).

Standardization: Aloe vera has not been evaluated by the U.S. Food and Drug Administration (FDA) for safety, effectiveness, or purity.

Evidence: There has been minimal standardized clinical research regarding the effectiveness of aloe vera gel. Nurse researchers who have examined the satisfaction level of health care workers who use gloves impregnated with gel note that the use of such gloves tends to result in less contact dermatitis and improved skin integrity (Davis & Harper, 2005; Korniewicz, 2007). A meta-analysis of the management of the skin in patients undergoing radiation therapy found that although aloe vera did not prevent skin burns, there was insufficient evidence regarding the effectiveness it had in the treatment of other skin conditions (McQuestion, 2006). A meta-analysis published in *Burns* (Maenthaisong, Chaiyakunapruk, Niruntraporn, & Kongkaew, 2007) evaluated the effect of aloe vera for burn wound healing. Using duration of wound healing as an outcome measure, there was some evidence to support that aloe vera might be an effective intervention in burn wound healing for first- and second-degree burns. In all cases, further, well-designed trials of aloe vera products are needed to determine their effectiveness.

- Obtain a thorough history, including sunburn and tanning history, the amount of time the patient usually spends in the sun, how easily the patient burns, and what type of sun protection is used. If the patient uses a sunscreen, obtain the SPF rating.
- Obtain an allergy history and use of OTC products or home remedies to treat the sunburn.
- If topical anesthetics or ointments are ordered, assess the skin for secondary infections, in which these medications are contraindicated.
- For patients who are using the medication for the first time, conduct a trial application on a small area of skin to assess for an allergic reaction. If no adverse effects occur within 30 to 60 minutes, the medication may be applied to the entire area of sunburn.

Patient and Family Education:

- Avoid applying the medication to open or infected areas of skin.
- Drink plenty of water to avoid dehydration.
- Report severe, persistent pain.
- Avoid additional sun exposure while receiving treatment.
- Prevent sunburn in the future by wearing protective clothing such as long-sleeved shirts and large-brim hats, and by using sunscreen with an SPF of 15 or greater.
- Follow the directions regarding use and reapplication of sunscreen after swimming or sweating.
- Refrigerate topical lotions so they will provide a soothing, cooling effect when applied.
- Do not apply benzocaine to infants and young children.

Drugs Similar to Benzocaine (Americaine, Anbesol, Others)

Benzocaine is the only drug in its class that is used for minor burns.

Pharmacotherapy of Alopecia

76.9 Several agents are able to stimulate moderate hair regrowth in clients with male- and female-pattern alopecia.

Alopecia is the loss of hair, resulting in baldness. Male-pattern baldness is the most common cause of hair loss in men and is genetically determined. Males affected by this type of alopecia typically experience a loss of hair at the temples, followed by a recession of the hairline and baldness at the crown.

Two drugs are currently available to promote hair regrowth in patients with male-pattern baldness: topical minoxidil (Rogaine) and PO finasteride (Propecia, Proscar). Neither drug was originally developed for baldness. Although the exact mechanism of action is unknown, it is thought that these agents work by stimulating the epithelial cells within the hair follicle. They are most successful in patients with recent onset of symptoms or who are less than 50 years of age. About 40% of patients who are treated two to three times daily for a year will experience moderate regrowth of hair. For both drugs, hair regrowth stops when the drug is discontinued.

Female hair loss differs from hair loss in males and varies by ethnicity. A common type of alopecia in Caucasian women, female-pattern hair loss, typically begins in the early 20s and 30s, with progressive thinning and loss of hair on the top of the scalp but not the back. These females typically do not have a receding hairline. The hair also becomes finer as individual hairs become smaller, resulting in less dense hair. Some females with this pattern of hair loss may have elevated androgen levels or diabetes that requires treatment. Topical minoxidil is currently the only hair regrowth treatment approved for women by the FDA. Applied to the scalp twice daily, it stimulates hairs that are actively growing to have more robust growth.

Women of African descent have a different type of alopecia called central centrifugal alopecia. This type also results in hair loss on the top of the scalp, but it is different from the female-pattern hair loss in that the hair follicles are destroyed. Topical

CONNECTIONS

Lifespan Considerations Stevens–Johnson Syndrome in Children

Stevens–Johnson syndrome (SJS) is a severe form of erythema multiforme that is characterized by an excoriating, blistering skin rash that affects both the skin and the mucous membranes. It often begins with the onset of flulike symptoms, with a rash developing on the upper torso and face that spreads to the rest of the body. Ocular involvement can be one of the adverse effects of SJS. This can range from corneal dryness and conjunctivitis to permanent blindness. The mortality rate is up to 5% due to the risk of accompanying complications, including sepsis and pneumonia (Burfeind, 2007). The exact cause is unknown, but it has often been associated with the use of certain medications, including anticonvulsants, sulfonamide antibiotics, and certain NSAIDs, notably ibuprofen. The time frame from medication administration to the onset of symptoms varies from 12 hours to 15 days.

Four cases of SJS that were directly attributed to ibuprofen therapy from 2001 to 2005 were reported in Canada (World Health Organization, 2005). These cases occurred in individuals between the ages of 13 and 34. Dosages received varied from 200 mg to 1,200 mg daily. In the United States, one research center reported 16 pediatric cases of SJS during an 8-year period. Researchers there identified the most common cause of SJS as being a combination of azithromycin and ibuprofen, followed by ibuprofen alone. Notably, the combination of ibuprofen and another drug was responsible for four additional cases (Dore, 2007). All of the children at this center who experienced complications had received ibuprofen. Although reports of SJS are rare, patients need to be aware of the potential for this reaction to occur and should be instructed to report the development of any rash during the course of treatment.

minoxidil is used in this group to stimulate growth in the unaffected hair follicles, whereas anti-inflammatory medications are used to decrease the destruction of the hair follicles.

Minoxidil (Rogaine): Oral minoxidil (Loniten) was first approved for HTN in 1979. Approval to market the topical solution for hair loss occurred in 1996. The drug is rubbed onto the scalp twice daily. Although the drug is a potent vasodilator, this mechanism is likely not involved in its effectiveness as a hair regrowth agent. The exact mechanism of action is unknown. Only 2% of a topical dose is absorbed systemically; therefore, this route does not affect blood pressure. Various brands of minoxidil include 2% Rogaine for Women, 2% Rogaine for Men Regular Strength, and 5% Rogaine for Men Extra Strength. An off-label use is to treat chemotherapy-induced alopecia. Response rates vary and over half of patients treated do not experience significant regrowth. In patients who are receiving chemotherapy, hair regrowth occurs at a faster rate with minoxidil use. The drug has no significant adverse effects. This drug is pregnancy category C.

Finasteride (Propecia, Proscar): Proscar was approved for benign prostatic hyperplasia (BPH) in 1992. Propecia was later approved to treat male-pattern baldness in 1997. The dose used for treating BPH is five times higher than that used for baldness. Unlike minoxidil, finasteride is a PO medication. This drug is thought to act by reducing the amounts of dihydroxytestosterone (DHT) in hair follicles, thus slowing hair loss. It is less effective than minoxidil at promoting hair regrowth. At the low doses used for hair regrowth, adverse effects are uncommon. It is not approved for use in women. This drug is pregnancy category X. Pregnant women should not touch this drug because it may harm a male fetus if absorbed.

CONNECTION *Checkpoint* 76.4

From what you learned in Chapter 72, describe the mechanism by which finasteride reduces symptoms of BPH. See Answer to Connection Checkpoint 76.4 in Appendix A.

UNDERSTANDING THE CHAPTER

Key Concepts Summary

76.1 Three layers of skin, known as the epidermis, dermis, and subcutaneous layers, provide effective barrier defenses for the body.

76.2 The etiology of skin disorders may be classified as infectious, inflammatory, or neoplastic.

76.3 When the integrity of the skin is compromised, bacteria, viruses, and fungi can gain entrance and cause infections that require anti-infective therapy.

76.4 Scabicides and pediculicides are used to treat parasitic skin infestations.

76.5 The pharmacotherapy of acne includes treatment with benzoyl peroxide, retinoids, and antibiotics; pharmacotherapy for rosacea includes retinoids and metronidazole.

76.6 The most effective treatment for dermatitis is topical corticosteroids, which are classified by their potency.

76.7 Psoriasis is a chronic, inflammatory disease that is treated with topical and systemic agents.

76.8 The pharmacotherapy of sunburn includes prevention with sunscreens and treatment with lotions, topical anesthetics, and analgesics.

76.9 Several agents are able to stimulate moderate hair regrowth in clients with male- and female-pattern alopecia.

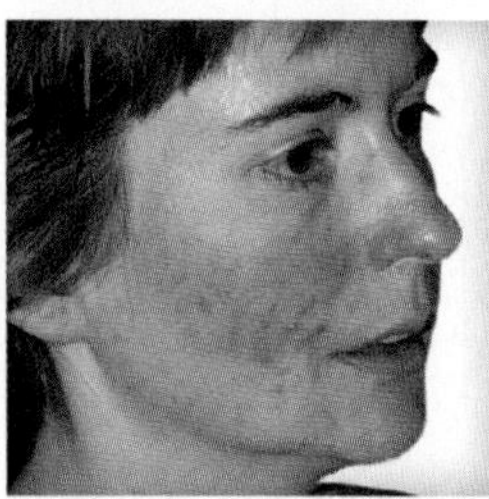

Making the PATIENT Connection

Remember the patient "Dora McBride" at the beginning of the chapter? Now read the remainder of the case study. Based on the information presented within this chapter, respond to the critical thinking questions that follow.

Dora McBride is a 52-year-old woman with a 10-year history of severe redness, flushing, and burning sensations in both ears. She has the condition known as rosacea. As a public relation specialist for a large health care system, she knows that her physical appearance is an important part of her job. Yet, with her skin condition, she appears anything but healthy. She has tried multiple OTC skin preparations to clear her blotchy completion. However, none of them have been successful.

Critical Thinking Questions

1. What would you tell the patient about her condition? Include what rosacea is, who is prone to develop it, and what methods of treatment, both medical and surgical, have been found to be beneficial.
2. What are some reasons why the rosacea exacerbation occurred?

Case Study

During a school nurse screening session on an 8-year-old female, the nurse identifies small groupings of nits in the child's hair and around her ears. The child states, "My head itches all the time." The child presents with long, stringy hair and poor personal hygiene. After further investigation, three other family members who also attend this school have the same presentations.

1. What activities should the nurse include in dealing with this situation?
2. What specific instructions should the parents or caretakers of these children be given in order to disrupt the transmission of the nits in this household?
3. What methods of prevention for further nit infestation would be beneficial for this family to know?

NCLEX-RN® Review

1 An important inclusion in a teaching plan prepared for the client who is taking permethrin (Nix) is:

1. Nix can be applied after body lotion is applied.
2. All body hair, including eyelashes and eyebrows, can be treated with lindane.
3. Lice cannot live outside the body.
4. In addition to hair shafts, examine the inner thigh areas, gluteal folds, and pubic areas for lice.

2 A client is being treated with a course of topical corticosteroid for atopic dermatitis. In planning teaching for this client, the nurse would anticipate which of the following adverse effects?

1. Burning and stinging of the skin in the affected area
2. Development of localized pruritus and hives
3. Hair loss in the application area
4. Worsening of acne vulgaris

3 The client reports using benzoyl peroxide (Benzac) for treatment of acne. The nurse notes that the action of this drug includes all of the following except:

1. Sebum suppression.
2. Antimicrobial effect.
3. Keratolytic effect.
4. Microdermal abrasion.

4 A client has been on tretinoin (Retin-A) for 2 months. What assessment finding would best assist the nurse in determining that treatment with this medication has been effective?

1. Increased hair growth on the scalp
2. Few closed comedones across the nose and forehead
3. Presence of several large sebaceous cysts on the posterior trunk
4. Absence of any new wart growth

5 A priority nursing diagnosis for a 16-year-old client with severe acne is:

1. *Anger,* related to disfigurement.
2. *Disturbed Body Image,* related to facial lesions.
3. *Self-Care Deficit,* related to medication regimen.
4. *Ineffective Health Maintenance,* related to drug therapy.

6 A client with a history of diabetes mellitus is receiving tretinoin (Retin-A) for treatment of acne. Which of the following assessments might indicate an adverse effect of the drug?

1. Dyspnea
2. Blood glucose of 268 mg/dL
3. Blood pressure of 148/88 mm Hg
4. Diarrhea

See Answers to Critical Thinking Questions, Case Study, and NCLEX-RN® Review in Appendix A.

References

American Academy of Allergy, Asthma and Immunology. (n.d.). *Allergy statistics.* Retrieved September 3, 2008, from http://www.aaaai.org/media/resources/media_kit/allergy_statistics.stm

American Academy of Dermatology. (n.d.). *Acne.* Retrieved September 8, 2008, from http://www.skincarephysicians.com/acnenet/acne.html

American Academy of Dermatology. (n.d.). *What is psoriasis?* Retrieved September 8, 2008, from http://www.skincarephysicians.com/psoriasisnet/whatis.html

Bacelieri, R., & Johnson, S. M. (2005). Cutaneous warts: An evidence-based approach to therapy. *American Family Physician, 72*(4), 647–652.

Berman, B., Bienstock, L., Kuritzky, L., Mayaeux, E., & Tyring, S. (2006). Actinic keratoses. *Journal of Family Practice, 55*(5), 1–8.

Burfeind, D. (2007). Severe erythema multiforme: Literature review. *Dermatology Nursing, 19*(2), 188–193.

Canyon, D. V., & Speare, R. (2007). A comparison of botanical and synthetic substances commonly used to prevent head lice. *International Journal of Dermatology, 46*(4), 422– 426.

Davis, D., & Harper, R. (2005). Using gloves coated with a dermal therapy formula to improve skin condition. *AORN Journal, 81*(1), 157–166.

Dore, J. (2007). Morbidity and mortality of mucocutaneous diseases in the pediatric population at a tertiary care center. *Journal of Burn Care & Research, 28*(6), 865–870.

Dorgos, D. (2006). Hair loss in women: More than meets the eye. *Dermatology Nursing, 18*(3), 290–291.

Ebell, M. (2007). Effective topical treatments for nongenital warts. *American Family Physician, 75*(7), 1001–1002.

Goldfaden, G. (2007). Nutrient-rich skin care: Advanced facial masks reverse photoaging, fight blemishes, and rejuvenate skin. *Life Extension, 13*(8), 74–81.

Hall, J. C. (2006). *Sauer's manual of skin diseases* (6th ed.). Philadelphia: Lippincott, Williams & Wilkins.

Jesitus, J. (2007). Rosacea requires multifaceted approach. *Dermatology Times, 28*(1), 50–63.

Korniewicz, D. (2007). Effect of aloe-vera impregnated gloves on hand hygiene attitudes of health care workers. *MEDSURG Nursing, 16*(4), 247–252.

LeMone, P., & Burke, K. (2008). *Medical-surgical nursing: Critical thinking in client care* (4th ed.). Upper Saddle River, NJ: Pearson Education.

Maenthaisong, R., Chaiyakunapruk, N., Niruntraporn, S., & Kongkaew, C. (2007). The efficacy of aloe vera used for burn wound healing: A systematic review. *Burns, 33*(6), 713–718.

McCance, K. L., & Huether, S. E. (2005). *Pathophysiology: The biologic basis for disease in adults and children* (5th ed.). St. Louis: Mosby.

McQuestion, M. (2006). Evidence-based skin care management in radiation therapy. *Seminars in Oncology Nursing, 22*(3), 163–173.

Nash, K. (2007). Options still limited for age-old problem. *Dermatology Times, 28*(6), 40–41.

Schwartz, R. A., Janusz, C. A., & Janniger, C. K. (2006). Seborrheic dermatitis. *American Family Physician, 74*(1), 125–130.

Snow, M. (2007). The truth about scabies. *Nursing, 37*(2), 28–30.

Sunscreen: From buying to applying. (2004). *Mayo Clinic Health Letter, 22*(5), 6.

Torpy, J. M. (2004). Treatment of acne vulgaris. *Journal of the American Medical Association, 292*(6), 726.

World Health Organization. (2005). Ibuprofen: Stevens-Johnson syndrome. *WHO Drug Information, 19*(3), 208–209.

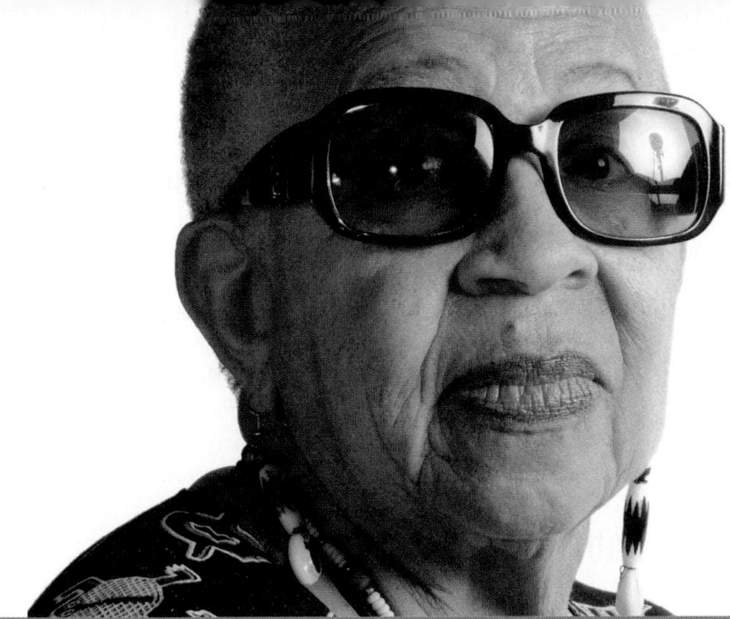

I just cannot see clearly while driving at night-time anymore. All I see are halos around the other cars' headlights.

Patient "Therese Duclos"

CHAPTER 77

Pharmacotherapy of Eye and Ear Disorders

Chapter Outline

Anatomy of the Eye

Pathophysiology of Glaucoma

Pharmacotherapy of Glaucoma

Prostaglandins

PROTOTYPE **Latanoprost (Xalatan)** *p. 1342*

Autonomic Drugs

PROTOTYPE **Timolol (Betimol, Istalol, Timoptic)** *p. 1344*

Miscellaneous Drugs for Glaucoma

Carbonic Anhydrase Inhibitors

Osmotic Diuretics

Pharmacotherapy for Eye Examinations

Anticholinergics

Sympathomimetics

Pharmacotherapy for Other Eye Conditions

Lubricants

Vasoconstrictors

Anatomy of the Ear

Pharmacotherapy with Otic Preparations

Antibiotics

Cerumenolytics

Learning Outcomes

After reading this chapter, the student should be able to:

1. Identify the major anatomical structures of the eye.
2. Identify the major risk factors associated with glaucoma.
3. Compare and contrast open-angle and closed-angle glaucoma.
4. Explain the two major mechanisms by which drugs reduce intraocular pressure.
5. Describe the nurse's role in the nonpharmacologic and pharmacologic management of eye and ear disorders.
6. For each of the classes shown in the chapter outline, identify the prototype and representative drugs and explain the mechanism(s) of drug action, primary indications, contraindications, significant drug interactions, pregnancy category, and important adverse effects.
7. Identify examples of drugs that dilate or constrict pupils, relax ciliary muscles, constrict ocular blood vessels, or moisten eye membranes.
8. Identify the types of ear conditions that could benefit from pharmacotherapy.
9. Apply the nursing process to care for patients who are receiving drug therapy for eye and ear disorders.

Key Terms

aqueous humor, *1338*
cerumenolytics, *1352*
closed-angle glaucoma, *1340*
cycloplegic, *1347*
external otitis, *1350*
glaucoma, *1338*
mastoiditis, *1351*
miosis, *1343*
mydriasis, *1344*
mydriatic, *1347*
open-angle glaucoma, *1340*
otitis interna, *1351*
otitis media, *1351*
tonometry, *1338*

The senses of vision and hearing the primary means for us to communicate with the world around them. Disorders that affect the eye and ear can result in problems with self-care, mobility, safety, and communication. The eye is vulnerable to a variety of conditions, many of which can be prevented, controlled, or reversed with proper pharmacotherapy. The first part of this chapter covers drugs that are used for the treatment of glaucoma and those used routinely by ophthalmic health care providers. The remaining part of this chapter presents drugs that are used for the treatment of common ear disorders, including infections, inflammation, and the buildup of ear wax.

Anatomy of the Eye

77.1 Knowledge of basic eye anatomy is fundamental to understanding eye disorders and their pharmacotherapy.

A firm knowledge of basic ocular anatomy is required to understand eye disorders and their pharmacotherapy. The important structures of the eye are shown in Figures 77.1 and 77.2.

The outermost layer of the eye is composed of the cornea and the sclera. The cornea is the transparent front covering of the eye. It has no blood vessels and receives nutrients from the aqueous humor. The sclera is the thick, white, opaque portion of the eye. In the sclera are the anterior and posterior chambers. The anterior chamber extends from the cornea to the anterior iris; the posterior chamber lies between the posterior iris and the lens. The lens separates these two chambers. In front of the lens is the pigmented iris, which is made up of smooth muscle fibers that change the diameter of the pupil. The pupil is the central opening that allows light to enter. These muscle fibers are under control of the sympathetic nervous system. Pupil constriction is the result of parasympathetic stimulation, and its dilation is a sympathetic response.

The anterior chamber is filled with a fluid called **aqueous humor.** Aqueous humor helps retain the shape of the eye and slowly circulates to bring nutrients to the area and remove wastes. The aqueous humor originates in the posterior chamber from a muscular structure called the ciliary body. From there it flows from the posterior chamber through the pupil and into the anterior chamber. Within the anterior chamber and around the periphery is a network of spongy connective tissue, or trabecular meshwork, that contains an opening called the canal of Schlemm. The aqueous humor drains into the canal of Schlemm and out of the anterior chamber into the venous system, thus completing its circulation. Under normal circumstances, the rate of aqueous humor production is equal to its outflow, maintaining intraocular pressure (IOP) within a normal range. Interference with either the production or outflow of aqueous humor, however, can lead to an increase in IOP.

The posterior chamber is filled with a gel-like substance called vitreous humor that helps the eyeball to maintain its shape and keep the retina in place. The conjunctiva, eyebrows, eyelashes, eyelids, and lacrimal apparatus that produce tears all serve to protect the eye. Infection and inflammatory responses are common conditions in these supporting structures. Redness, edema, and itching are common symptoms.

Pathophysiology of Glaucoma

77.2 The two principal types of glaucoma, closed-angle glaucoma and open-angle glaucoma, are characterized by increased intraocular pressure.

Glaucoma is a condition that is characterized by optic neuropathy with gradual loss of peripheral vision and is usually accompanied by increased IOP. Glaucoma occurs when the IOP becomes high enough to cause optic nerve damage, leading to visual field loss and possibly advancing to blindness. Although the median IOP in the population is 15 to 16 mmHg, this pressure varies greatly with age, daily activities, and even time of day. As a rule, IOPs that are consistently above 21 mmHg are considered abnormal. Many patients, however, tolerate IOPs in the mid to high 20s without damage to the optic nerve. IOPs that are above 30 mmHg require treatment because they are associated with permanent vision changes. Some patients of Asian descent may experience glaucoma at "normal" IOP values, below 21 mmHg.

> **PharmFACT**
>
> The incidence of glaucoma in African Americans is six times higher than in Caucasians. It is the leading cause of blindness in African Americans. *Source:* Glaucoma Research Foundation, n.d.

Glaucoma affects 2.2 million people over the age of 40 in the United States. It is the leading cause of preventable blindness worldwide and the leading cause of blindness in those of Far Eastern ancestry. Primary glaucoma usually occurs without an identifiable cause and is most frequently found in persons older than 60 years of age. In some cases, glaucoma is associated with genetic factors; it can be congenital in infants and children. Glaucoma can also be secondary to eye trauma, infection, diabetes, inflammation, hemorrhage, tumor, or cataracts. Some medications may contribute to the development or progression of glaucoma, including the long-term use of corticosteroids, some antihypertensives, antihistamines, and antidepressants. Other major risk factors associated with glaucoma include hypertension (HTN), migraine headaches, refractive disorders with high degrees of nearsightedness or farsightedness, and normal aging.

Diagnosis of glaucoma can be difficult because it may occur so gradually that patients do not experience symptoms or seek medical attention until late in the disease process. **Tonometry**

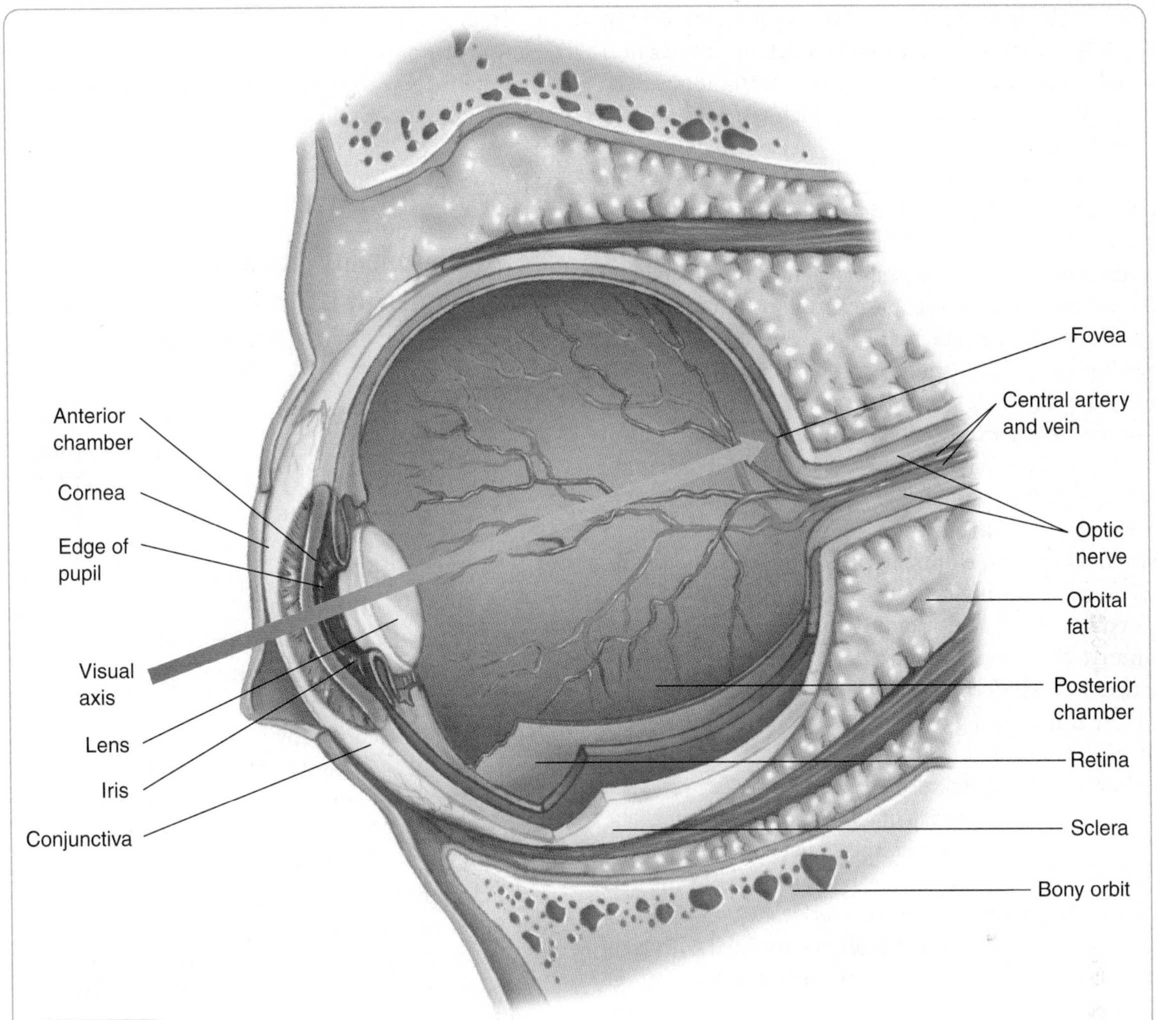

Anterior chamber
Cornea
Edge of pupil
Visual axis
Lens
Iris
Conjunctiva
Fovea
Central artery and vein
Optic nerve
Orbital fat
Posterior chamber
Retina
Sclera
Bony orbit

Figure 77.1

Internal structures of the eye.

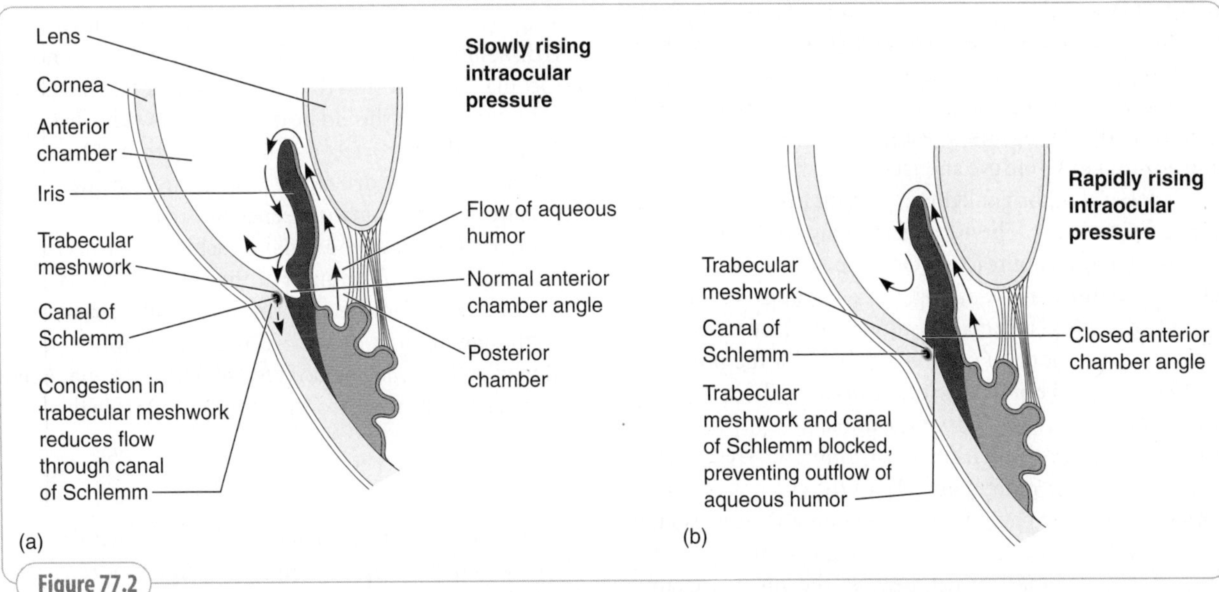

Figure 77.2

Forms of primary adult glaucoma: (a) In chronic open-angle glaucoma, the anterior chamber angle remains open, but drainage of aqueous humor through the canal of Schlemm is impaired. (b) In acute closed-angle glaucoma, the angle of the iris and anterior chamber narrows, obstructing the outflow of aqueous humor.

is a primary ophthalmic technique that tests for glaucoma by measuring IOP. Patients with unusually thick or thin corneas may have false negatives or false positives during tonometry. Patients who have had Lasik surgery, which removes corneal tissue to correct myopia, may appear to have normal IOPs, yet have glaucoma. Gonioscopy uses a gonioscope to measure the depth of the anterior chamber and is useful in distinguishing between open-angle and closed-angle glaucoma. Visual field testing assesses the degree of central visual field narrowing and peripheral vision loss. Funduscopic exams look at retinal field changes that accompany glaucoma.

The two major types of primary glaucoma are closed-angle glaucoma and open-angle glaucoma, as shown in Figure 77.2. Both disorders result from the same problem: a buildup of aqueous humor in the anterior cavity. This buildup is caused either by an excessive production of aqueous humor or by a blockage of its outflow. In either case, IOP increases, leading to progressive damage to the optic nerve. As the optic nerve degenerates, the patient will first notice a loss of visual field, then a loss of central visual acuity, and lastly total blindness. The major differences between closed-angle glaucoma and open-angle glaucoma include how quickly the IOP develops and whether there is narrowing of the anterior chamber angle between the iris and cornea.

Closed-angle glaucoma, also called acute- or narrow-angle glaucoma, accounts for only 5% of all primary glaucoma. The incidence is higher in older adults and in persons of Asian descent. It is typically caused by the normal thickening of the lens and may develop gradually over several years. This type of glaucoma is usually unilateral and is often associated with conditions that result in dilation of the pupil, such as stress, impact injury, or medications. Closed-angle glaucoma occurs when the pressure inside the anterior chamber increases suddenly because the iris is being pushed over the area where the aqueous humor normally drains into the trabecular network and the canal of Schlemm. The displacement of the iris is due in part to the dilation of the pupil or accommodation of the lens, causing the angle between the posterior cornea and the anterior iris to narrow or close.

Signs and symptoms of closed-angle glaucoma are caused by acute obstruction of the outflow of aqueous humor from the eye and include dull to severe eye and facial pain, headaches, seeing colored halos around bright lights, a bulging iris, and a sudden change in visual acuity. The affected eye may appear reddened and the pupil may be nonreactive. Ocular pain may be so severe that it causes nausea and vomiting. Once the outflow is totally closed, closed-angle glaucoma constitutes a medical emergency and laser or conventional surgery is indicated for the preservation of sight. Surgical options include iridectomy, laser trabeculoplasty, trabeculectomy, and drainage implants.

Open-angle glaucoma is the most common type of glaucoma, accounting for more than 90% of the cases. Its cause is not known and many patients are asymptomatic. It is usually bilateral, with the elevated IOP developing over years. Open-angle glaucoma is named as such because the anterior chamber angle is normal; the iris does not completely cover the trabecular meshwork and canal of Schlemm. They remain open with their flow being partially obstructed. This leads to the gradual development of increased IOP with slow degeneration of the optic nerve, resulting in a gradual loss of vision. Most patients with open-angle glaucoma can be successfully treated with medications.

Pharmacotherapy of Glaucoma

77.3 The primary goal of glaucoma pharmacotherapy is to prevent damage to the optic nerve by lowering intraocular pressure.

Intraocular pressure can be controlled and vision preserved if glaucoma is diagnosed and treated with medications early in the course of the disease. Some health care providers initiate pharmacotherapy in all patients with an IOP greater than 21 mmHg. Because of the expense of pharmacotherapy and potential adverse drug effects, other health care providers will instead carefully monitor the patient through regular follow-up exams and wait until the IOP rises to 28 to 30 mmHg before initiating drug therapy. If signs of optic nerve damage or visual field changes are evident, the patient is treated regardless of the IOP.

Once pharmacotherapy is initiated, reevaluation is performed after 2 to 4 months to assess for therapeutic effectiveness. Some of the antiglaucoma drugs take 6 to 8 weeks to reach peak effect. If the therapeutic goals are not achieved with a single agent, it is common to add a second drug from a different class to the regimen to produce an additive decrease in IOP. Some of the agents may continue to have effects on the eye for 2 to 4 weeks after being discontinued.

Maintaining patient adherence with the medication regimen is a key factor in preventing progressive or permanent vision impairment. It is essential that the nurse determine any factors that could decrease adherence, such as insufficient financial resources, lack of knowledge about the disease, lack of dexterity or skill in inserting eyedrops, or difficulty in remembering the dosing schedule. Fear and anxiety about potential blindness and disability may also be evident in the patient diagnosed with glaucoma. Accurate and thorough teaching for the patient and family or caregiver should be directed at how the disease can be managed with the correct use and application of medications.

There are many drugs available to treat glaucoma. These agents work by one of two mechanisms: increasing the outflow of aqueous humor at the canal of Schlemm or decreasing the formation of aqueous humor at the ciliary body. Many agents for glaucoma act by affecting the autonomic nervous system.

Although topical drugs are most commonly prescribed, oral medications may be used for severe glaucoma. Agents for glaucoma, which are listed in Table 77.1, include the following classes:

- Prostaglandins
- Autonomic agents, including beta-adrenergic blockers, nonselective sympathomimetics, $alpha_2$-adrenergic agonists, and cholinergic agonists
- Carbonic anhydrase inhibitors
- Osmotic diuretics

TABLE 77.1 Selected Drugs for Glaucoma

Drug	Route and Adult Dose (maximum dose where indicated)	Adverse Effects
Prostaglandins		
bimatoprost (Lumigan)	1 drop of 0.03% solution daily in the evening	*Increased length and thickness of eyelashes, darkening of the iris, stinging, sensation of foreign body in the eye* Serious adverse effects that may occur with systemic absorption: respiratory infection, flu, angina, muscle or joint pain
latanoprost (Xalatan)	1 drop of 0.005% solution daily in the evening	
travoprost (Travatan)	1 drop of 0.004% solution daily in the evening	
Beta-Adrenergic Blockers		
betaxolol (Betoptic)	1 drop of 0.5% solution bid	*Local burning and stinging, blurred vision, headache* Conjunctival hyperemia; serious adverse effects that may occur with systemic absorption: angina, anxiety, bronchoconstriction, HTN, dysrhythmias
carteolol (Ocupress)	1 drop of 1% solution bid	
levobunolol (Betagan)	1–2 drops of 0.25–0.5% solution 1–2 times/day	
metipranolol (OptiPranolol)	1 drop of 0.3% solution bid	
Timolol (Betimol, Istalol, Timoptic)	1–2 drops of 0.25–0.5% solution 1–2 times/day Gel (salve): apply daily	
Sympathomimetics		
dipivefrin (Propine)	1 drop of 0.1% solution every 12 h	*Local burning and stinging, blurred vision, headache, photosensitivity* Tachycardia, HTN
Cholinergic Agonists		
carbachol (Isoptocarbachol)	1–2 drops of 0.75–3% solution in the lower conjunctival sac up to 3 times/day	*Induced myopia, reduced visual acuity in low light, eye redness, headache* Serious adverse effects that may occur with systemic absorption: salivation, tachycardia, HTN, bronchospasm, sweating, nausea, vomiting, retinal detachment (pilocarpine)
echothiophate iodide (Phospholine Iodide)	1 drop of 0.03–0.25% solution 1–2 times/day	
pilocarpine (Isopto Carpine, Pilopine)	Acute glaucoma: 1 drop of 1–2% solution every 5–10 min for three to six doses Chronic glaucoma: 1 drop of 0.5–4% solution every 4–12 h	
Alpha$_2$-Adrenergic Agonists		
apraclonidine (Iopidine)	1 drop of 0.5% solution bid	*Local itching and burning, blurred vision, dry mouth, headache, eye discharge* Allergic conjunctivitis, conjunctival hyperemia, HTN, bulbar conjunctival follicles
brimonidine tartrate (Alphagan P)	1 drop of 0.1– 0.15% solution in the affected eye tid, 8 h apart	
Carbonic Anhydrase Inhibitors		
acetazolamide (Diamox)	PO: 250 mg 1–4 times/day	*For topical agents: blurred vision, bitter taste, dry eye, blepharitis, local itching, sensation of foreign body in the eye, headache* For oral agents: diuresis, electrolyte imbalances, blood dyscrasias, flaccid paralysis, hepatic impairment
brinzolamide (Azopt)	1 drop of 1% solution tid	
dorzolamide (Trusopt)	1 drop of 2% solution in the affected eye(s) tid	
methazolamide (Neptazane)	PO: 50–100 mg bid-tid	
Osmotic Diuretics		
isosorbide (Ismotic)	PO: 1–3 g/kg 1–2 times/day	*Orthostatic hypotension, facial flushing, headache, palpitations, anxiety, nausea* Severe headache, electrolyte imbalances, edema
mannitol (Osmitrol)	IV: 1.5–2 mg/kg as a 15–25% solution over 30–60 min	

Note: *Italics* indicate common adverse effects. Underline indicates serious adverse effects.

77.4 Prostaglandin analogs are often the drugs of choice for treating high intraocular pressure because of their long durations of action and high safety profiles.

Prostaglandin analogs are a newer and very effective therapy for glaucoma. They are often the drugs of choice for glaucoma because they have long durations of action, allowing for once-daily dosing, and produce fewer adverse effects than the beta-adrenergic blockers. They may be used as monotherapy or combined with drugs from other classes to produce an additive reduction in IOP in patients with resistant glaucoma.

Prostaglandin analogs decrease IOP by enhancing the outflow of aqueous humor. Latanoprost (Xalatan), which is available as a 0.005% eyedrop solution, is one of the most commonly used prostaglandin analogs. Several new ocular prostaglandins have recently been approved, including bimatoprost (Lumigan), and travoprost (Travatan). An occasional adverse effect of these medications is heightened pigmentation, which turns a blue iris to a more brown color. Many patients experience thicker and longer eyelashes. These drugs cause local irritation, stinging of the eyes, and redness during the first month of therapy. Because of these effects, prostaglandins are normally administered just before bedtime.

PROTOTYPE DRUG Latanoprost (Xalatan)

Classification: **Therapeutic:** Drug for glaucoma
Pharmacologic: Prostaglandin analog

Therapeutic Effects and Uses: Approved in 1996, latanoprost is a prostaglandin analog believed to reduce IOP by increasing the outflow of aqueous humor for patients with open-angle glaucoma and ocular HTN. The recommended dose is one drop in the affected eye(s) in the evening. It is used to treat open-angle glaucoma.

Mechanism of Action: Latanoprost reduces elevated IOP in patients with open-angle glaucoma. Latanoprost is a prodrug that is metabolized to its active form in the cornea, reaching its peak effect in about 12 hours.

Pharmacokinetics:

Route	Ophthalmic solution
Absorption	Through the cornea
Distribution	Enters systemic distribution in small amounts
Primary metabolism	Metabolized in the aqueous humor to its active form
Primary excretion	Renal
Onset of action	3–4 h with peak effect at 8–12 h
Duration of action	Unknown

Adverse Effects: Adverse effects include ocular symptoms such as conjunctival edema, tearing, dryness, burning, pain, irritation, itching, sensation of a foreign body in the eye, photophobia, or visual disturbances. The eyelashes on the treated eye may grow thicker or darker. Changes may occur in the pigmentation of the iris of the treated eye and in the periocular skin. Rare, systemic adverse effects include headaches, rashes, flulike symptoms, and abnormal liver function tests.

Contraindications/Precautions: Contraindications include hypersensitivity to the drug or another component in the solution, pregnancy, lactation, intraocular infection, or conjunctivitis. It should not be administered to patients with closed-angle glaucoma. The safety of this drug has not been demonstrated in children.

Drug Interactions: Latanoprost interacts with the preservative thimerosal: If used concurrently with other eyedrops that contain thimerosal, precipitation may occur. **Herbal/Food:** Unknown.

Pregnancy: Category C.

Treatment of Overdose: Overdose with the ophthalmic solution is unlikely.

Nursing Responsibilities:

- Obtain a complete medical history and current medication regimen.
- Remove contact lenses before instilling ophthalmic medications. Do not reinsert the contact lenses for at least 15 minutes.
- Avoid touching the eye or eyelashes with any part of the eyedropper to avoid cross-contamination.
- Apply to only the affected eye(s) or as ordered by the prescriber.
- Wait at least 5 minutes before instilling any other ophthalmic medications.
- Refrigerate and protect the solution from light.

Patient and Family Education:

- This drug may temporarily cause blurred vision. Remove obstacles in the home that may cause falls and other injuries secondary to impaired vision.
- Remove contact lenses before instilling the medication, and wait at least 15 minutes before reinserting them to allow the medication sufficient contact with the eye.
- Do not use any other eye products unless approved by the health care provider.
- Remain immobile after instilling the medication until blurred vision diminishes, approximately 5 minutes.
- Immediately report eye irritation, eye swelling, burning, stinging, redness, blurred vision, pain, irritation, itching, sensation of a foreign body in the eye, photophobia, or visual disturbances.
- Expect increased pigmentation of the iris, eyelid, and additional growth of the eyelashes because these are common adverse effects of the drug.
- Immediately notify the health care provider of any known or suspected pregnancy.

Drugs Similar to Latanoprost (Xalatan)

Bimatoprost and travoprost are other prostaglandin analogs used for glaucoma. A third drug in this class, unoprostone (Rescula), is no longer marketed in the United States.

Bimatoprost (Lumigan): Approved in 2001, bimatoprost is a synthetic prostaglandin analog indicated for the treatment of open-angle glaucoma. It is usually used when the patient has not responded adequately to other antiglaucoma drugs. Use of this drug can cause a gradual increase in the development of brown pigmentation in the iris, which may be irreversible, and includes an increase in pigmentation of the eyelid and growth of the eyelashes. Other adverse effects include blurred vision, eye discomfort, ocular pruritus, conjunctivitis, dry eye, light intolerance, and tearing. It is available as a 0.03% solution applied once daily in the evening. This drug is pregnancy category C.

Travoprost (Travatan): Approved in 2001, travoprost is approved for the treatment of open-angle glaucoma. Travoprost has been found to be more effective in African Americans than in non–African Americans. Like bimatoprost, travoprost is usually used when other drugs have failed to produce a satisfactory response. Use of this drug can cause a gradual increase in the development of brown pigmentation in the iris, which may be irreversible, and includes an increase in pigmentation of the eyelid and growth of the eyelashes. Conjunctival hyperemia has been reported in 35% to 50% of patients treated with travoprost. Some other adverse effects include blurred vision, eye discomfort, ocular pruritus, dry eye, light intolerance, and tearing. It is available as a 0.004% solution, applied once daily in the evening. This drug is pregnancy category C.

CONNECTION *Checkpoint* 77.1

Several prostaglandins are used for their actions on uterine smooth muscle. From what you learned in Chapter 71, what are the primary indications for the prostaglandins carboprost (Hemabate), dinoprostone (Cervidil), and mifepristone (Mifeprex)? See Answer to Connection Checkpoint 77.1 in Appendix A.

77.5 Drugs that affect the autonomic nervous system are sometimes prescribed to treat glaucoma.

Several structures within the eye are activated by the sympathetic and parasympathetic divisions of the autonomic nervous system. As such, a significant number of autonomic agents have been used to treat glaucoma and to aid in ophthalmic examinations of the eyeball.

- Sympathetic activation (or parasympathetic division blockade): Muscles of the iris contract to dilate the pupil; the ciliary muscle relaxes to enhance distance vision.
- Parasympathetic activation (or sympathetic division blockade): Muscles of the iris contract to constrict the pupil; the ciliary muscle contracts to enhance near vision.

The most frequently used autonomic drugs are the beta-adrenergic antagonists or blockers. Alpha$_2$-adrenergic agonists, nonselective sympathomimetics, and cholinergic agonists play minor roles, as discussed next. Prior to reading this section, the student may want to review Chapter 16 to brush up on the terminology and anatomy of the autonomic nervous system.

Beta-adrenergic blockers: Before the discovery of the prostaglandin analogs, beta-adrenergic blockers were the drugs of choice for open-angle glaucoma. These drugs decrease the production of aqueous humor by the ciliary body in the affected eye and can lower IOP by 20% to 30%. There are five beta-adrenergic blockers available as ophthalmic solutions: betaxolol (Betoptic), carteolol (Ocupress), levobunolol (Betagan), metipranolol (OptiPranolol), and timolol (Timoptic, Timoptic XE). These agents generally produce fewer ocular adverse effects than cholinergic agonists or sympathomimetics. In most patients, the topical administration of beta blockers does not result in significant systemic absorption. Should absorption occur, however, systemic adverse effects may include bronchoconstriction, dysrhythmias, and hypotension. Because of the potential for systemic adverse effects, these drugs should be used with caution in patients with asthma, bradycardia, or heart failure. Tolerance will develop with long-term use in about 25% of patients who take these drugs.

Alpha$_2$-adrenergic agonists: Alpha$_2$-adrenergic agonists lower IOP by decreasing the production of aqueous humor and increasing its absorption. Only two alpha$_2$-adrenergic agonists are currently approved for use: apraclonidine and brimonidine. Apraclonidine (Iopidine) is infrequently used but may be prescribed for the prevention or short-term therapy of postoperative increases in IOP. Brimonidine (Alphagan) is more commonly prescribed, either as monotherapy or as an adjunct in combination with a beta-adrenergic blocker, for the long-term treatment of open-angle glaucoma or glaucoma secondary to uveitis, which is an inflammation of the middle layer of the eyeball. Alpha$_2$-adrenergic agonists may be used in combination with other antiglaucoma drugs to cause additive reduction in IOP. In 2007, the U.S. Food and Drug Administration (FDA) approved Combigan, an ophthalmic solution which consists of brimonidine and timolol to treat glaucoma.

Alpha$_2$-adrenergic agonists are contraindicated in closed-angle glaucoma because the pupil dilation that results would worsen the condition. The most significant adverse effect, and one that is a frequent cause for discontinuation of therapy, is an allergic-type reaction that causes sensation of a foreign body, itching, and hyperemia. Other adverse effects include headache, drowsiness, dry mucosal membranes, blurred vision, and irritated eyelids. These drugs produce few cardiovascular or pulmonary adverse effects. Rare systemic adverse effects may occur, including nervousness, anxiety, and muscle tremors. Patients should immediately notify their health care provider if they experience acute eye pain, because this may signal the onset of closed-angle glaucoma.

Cholinergic agonists (miotics): Drugs that directly activate cholinergic receptors in the eye produce **miosis,** or constriction of the pupil, and contraction of the ciliary muscle. These actions physically stretch the trabecular meshwork to allow greater outflow of aqueous humor and a lowering of IOP. Pilocarpine (Isopto Carpine, Pilopine) is the most commonly prescribed antiglaucoma agent in this class. The cholinergic agonists are applied topically to the eye four times daily. Because of their greater toxicity and frequent dosing, these drugs are normally used only in patients with open-angle glaucoma who do not respond to other agents. Local effects include headache, induced myopia, and decreased vision in low light. Systemic absorption can result in hypotension, vomiting, diuresis, bronchoconstriction, diaphoresis, and abdominal pain with diarrhea. Toxic effects include vertigo, bradycardia, tremors, syncope, and cardiac dysrhythmias. Other actions of the cholinergic agonists are presented in Chapter 17.

A second group of cholinergic agonists, the cholinesterase inhibitors, act indirectly to lower IOP. They produce essentially the same actions as the direct-acting agents but exhibit a higher incidence of adverse effects. Cholinesterase inhibitors such as echothiophate cause cataracts in a significant percentage of patients and are only used in those who are resistant to therapy with other agents.

CONNECTION *Checkpoint* 77.2

Cholinergic agonists such as pilocarpine activate muscarinic receptors. From what you learned in Chapter 17, what effect do muscarinic agonists have on lacrimation and how is this used therapeutically? See Answer to Connection Checkpoint 77.2 in Appendix A.

Nonselective sympathomimetics: Nonselective sympathomimetics activate the sympathetic nervous system to produce **mydriasis** (pupil dilation) and increase the outflow of aqueous humor, resulting in a lower IOP. They are not as effective as the beta-adrenergic blockers or the prostaglandin analogs. Agents in this class include epinephrine and dipivefrin, which is converted to epinephrine in the eye. Both are administered topically for open-angle glaucoma and are contraindicated in narrow-angle glaucoma. Epinephrine will increase blood pressure and the heart rate if it reaches the systemic circulation; thus the drug is contraindicated in patients with unstable cardiovascular disease. They also produce a high frequency of ocular adverse effects, including tearing, burning, hyperemia, and stenosis of the nasolacrimal duct. Because of the potential for systemic adverse effects, these agents are third-choice drugs for glaucoma.

PROTOTYPE DRUG Timolol (Betimol, Istalol, Timoptic)

Classification: Therapeutic: Drug for glaucoma
Pharmacologic: Miotic, beta-adrenergic antagonist

Therapeutic Effects and Uses: Approved in 1978, timolol is a nonselective beta-adrenergic blocker available as a 0.25% or 0.5% ophthalmic solution. Its primary indication is chronic open-angle glaucoma. It may also be used for aphakic glaucoma (high IOP in patients with no lens), secondary glaucoma, and ocular HTN. The usual dose is one drop in the affected eye(s) twice a day. Timoptic XE and Istalol allow for once-a-day dosing. Treatment may require 2 to 4 weeks to reach the maximum therapeutic effect. It is also available in tablets (Blocadren), which are prescribed to treat mild HTN.

Mechanism of Action: Timolol topically lowers the elevated and normal IOP by reducing the formation of aqueous humor and possibly increasing outflow. It affects both $beta_1$ and $beta_2$ receptors.

Pharmacokinetics:

Route	Eye solution or gel
Absorption	Small amounts reach the systemic circulation from topical application
Distribution	Secreted in breast milk
Primary metabolism	80% metabolized in the liver to inactive metabolites
Primary excretion	Renal
Onset of action	30 minutes
Duration of action	12–24 h

Adverse Effects: The most common adverse effects from ophthalmic administration are local burning and stinging on instillation. Vision may become temporarily blurred. In most patients there is not significant absorption to cause systemic adverse effects as long as timolol is applied correctly. If absorption occurs, hypotension or dysrhythmias are possible.

Contraindications/Precautions: Although little is absorbed through ocular administration, this drug should be used with caution in certain patients. Timolol is contraindicated in patients with asthma, severe chronic obstructive pulmonary disease (COPD), sinus bradycardia, second- or third-degree atrioventricular block, heart failure, cardiogenic shock, or hypersensitivity to the drug. Safety in children has not been established.

Drug Interactions: Drug interactions may result if significant systemic absorption occurs. Timolol should be used with caution in patients who are taking other beta blockers owing to additive cardiac effects. Concurrent use with anticholinergics, nitrates, reserpine, methyldopa, or verapamil could lead to hypotension and bradycardia. Epinephrine use could lead to HTN followed by severe bradycardia. When given by the ocular route, timolol will produce additive lowering of IOP when given concurrently with other antiglaucoma agents. **Herbal/Food:** There are no known herbal or food interactions with this drug.

Pregnancy: Category C.

Treatment of Overdose: Overdose with ophthalmic solution is unlikely but could result in systemic symptoms such as reduced heart rate and bronchospasm.

Nursing Responsibilities:

- Obtain a complete medical history and current medication regimen.
- Determine if the patient has a history of second- or third-degree heart block, bradycardia, heart failure, or COPD. Antiglaucoma agents that affect the autonomic nervous system may be contraindicated for patients with these conditions because of possible drug absorption into the systemic circulation.
- Establish a baseline blood pressure and pulse prior to starting drug therapy.
- Teach the patient how to check pulse and blood pressure before medication administration. Review the parameters of

the pulse and blood pressure with the patient and family to establish guidelines for notifying the health care provider.

- Remove contact lenses before instilling ophthalmic medications. Do not reinsert contact lenses for at least 15 minutes.

Patient and Family Education:

- Remove obstacles in the home that may cause falls and other injuries secondary to impaired vision. This drug may temporarily cause blurred vision.
- Remove contact lenses before instilling the medication, and wait at least 15 minutes before reinserting them to allow the medication sufficient contact with the eye.
- Remain immobile after instilling the medication until blurred vision diminishes for at least 5 minutes.
- Immediately report eye irritation, eye swelling, burning, stinging, redness, blurred vision, pain, irritation, itching, sensation of foreign body in the eye, photophobia, or visual disturbances to the health care provider.
- Check pulse rate and blood pressure at regular intervals, especially if HTN or severe heart disease are present. This medication can cause a reduction in the resting heart rate and changes in the blood pressure.
- Immediately report any difficulty in breathing to the health care provider.
- Immediately notify the health care provider of any known or suspected pregnancy.

Drugs Similar to Timolol (Betimol, Istalol, Timoptic)

Other beta-adrenergic blockers with ophthalmic indications include betaxolol, carteolol, levobunolol, and metipranolol. Levobetaxolol (Betaxon) is an ophthalmic beta blocker that has been discontinued in the United States.

Betaxolol (Betoptic): Approved in 1985, betaxolol is a selective $beta_1$-adrenergic receptor blocker. This drug reduces IOP by decreasing the production of aqueous humor. Betaxolol is indicated for intraocular HTN and chronic open-angle glaucoma. A tablet form of this drug (Kerlone) is available to treat HTN. Although only small amounts are absorbed from ophthalmic administration, this drug should be used cautiously in patients with heart failure and if used concurrently with a systemic beta-adrenergic blocker. Ocular irritation and tearing are frequent adverse effects. This drug is pregnancy category C.

Carteolol (Ocupress): Carteolol is a nonselective beta-adrenergic blocker that competes for available beta receptor sites and is used for the treatment of chronic open-angle glaucoma. Both $beta_1$ and $beta_2$ receptors are inhibited. Carteolol (Cartrol) was also available as tablets to treat HTN, but it has been discontinued for this indication in the United States. Adverse effects and contraindications are the same as those of other ophthalmic beta blockers. This drug is pregnancy category C.

Levobunolol (Betagan): Approved in 1985, levobunolol is a nonselective beta-adrenergic blocker that is indicated for the treatment of intraocular HTN and chronic open-angle glaucoma. Because small amounts may reach the systemic circulation, caution needs to be practiced when using this drug in patients with asthma, COPD, bradycardia, thyroid conditions, diabetes, and abnormal blood glucose levels. Tolerance can develop with long-term use. Ocular irritation is a frequent, transient adverse effect. This drug is pregnancy category C.

Metipranolol (OptiPranolol): Approved in 1989, this drug is a nonselective beta-adrenergic blocker used for the treatment of elevated IOP and chronic open-angle glaucoma. It is available as a 0.3% solution that is applied to the affected eye(s) twice daily. Small amounts may be absorbed systemically. Contraindications are the same as those of other ophthalmic beta blockers. Ocular irritation is a frequent, transient adverse effect. Although rare, uveitis has been associated with metipranolol use. If this occurs, this drug should be discontinued because uveitis can cause an increase in IOP. This drug is pregnancy category C.

77.6 Carbonic anhydrase inhibitors and osmotic diuretics are occasionally used for treating glaucoma.

Although prostaglandin analogs and beta-adrenergic blockers are the two most frequently prescribed classes for lowering IOP, some patients may experience adverse effects from these agents or have particularly resistant glaucoma. Two additional classes, the carbonic anhydrase inhibitors and the osmotic diuretics, are not routinely prescribed.

Carbonic anhydrase inhibitors: Carbonic anhydrase inhibitors interfere with the synthesis of carbonic acid, which decreases the production of aqueous humor and reduces IOP. They are used as long-term therapy in patients with open-angle glaucoma when prostaglandin inhibitors, beta blockers, and other autonomic agents have not been effective.

Drugs in this class are divided into topical or oral formulations. Dorzolamide (Trusopt) is used topically to treat open-angle glaucoma, either as monotherapy or in combination with other agents. Dorzolamide and other topical carbonic anhydrase inhibitors, including brinzolamide (Azopt), are well tolerated and produce few significant adverse effects other than photosensitivity. PO formulations such as acetazolamide (Diamox) are very effective at lowering IOP in both open-angle and narrow-angle glaucoma but are rarely used because they produce more systemic adverse effects than drugs from other classes. These systemic effects include lethargy, nausea, vomiting, depression, paresthesias, and drowsiness. Patients must be cautioned when taking these medications because they contain sulfur and may cause allergic reactions. Because the oral formulations are diuretics and can reduce IOP quickly, serum electrolytes should be monitored during treatment. A prototype feature for acetazolamide is presented in Chapter 35.

Osmotic diuretics: Osmotic diuretics are occasionally used preoperatively and postoperatively with ocular surgery or as emergency treatment of acute closed-angle glaucoma attacks. Examples include isosorbide (Ismotic), urea, and mannitol (Osmitrol). Because they have the ability to quickly reduce plasma volume (see Chapter 35), these drugs are effective in reducing the formation of aqueous humor, thereby reducing IOP. Adverse

NURSING PROCESS APPLICATION

Patients Receiving Ophthalmic Solutions for Glaucoma

Assessment

Prior to administration:

- Obtain a complete health history, including allergies, drug history, and possible drug interactions.
- Obtain a complete physical examination, focusing on visual acuity and visual field assessments.
- Assess for the presence or history of ocular pain.

Potential Nursing Diagnoses

- *Risk for Injury*, related to visual acuity deficits
- *Self-Care Deficit: Feeding,* related to impaired vision
- *Chronic Pain*, related to disease process
- *Deficient Knowledge (Disease Process)*

Planning: Patient Goals and Expected Outcomes

The patient will:

- Exhibit improvement in visual symptoms.
- Demonstrate an understanding of the disease process.
- Demonstrate an understanding of the drug's action by accurately describing drug adverse effects and precautions.
- Safely function within own environment without injury.
- Report absence of pain.

Implementation

Interventions and (Rationales)	Patient and Family Education
• Monitor visual acuity, blurred vision, pupil reactions, extraocular movements, and ocular pain. (Reporting these signs and symptoms is very important for reducing the chances for serious drug-related interactions.)	• Instruct the patient to report headache and changes in vision.
• Monitor the patient for specific contraindications to the prescribed drug. (Ophthalmic solutions may be contraindicated in many physiological conditions.)	• Instruct the patient to notify the health care provider of all health-related problems and prescribed medications.
• Remove contact lenses before administering ophthalmic solutions. (When contact lenses are in place, the drug is not administered into the eye; therefore, there is no therapeutic effect.)	• Instruct the patient to remove contact lenses prior to administering eyedrops and wait 15 minutes before reinserting them.
• Administer ophthalmic solutions using proper technique. (Improper administration may lead to infection or injury to the eye.)	Instruct the patient to: • Wash hands prior to administering eyedrops. • Avoid touching the tip of the container to the eye because this may contaminate the solution. • Administer the eyedrop in the conjunctival sac. • Apply pressure over the lacrimal sac for 1 minute. • Wait 5 minutes before administering other ophthalmic solutions. • Schedule glaucoma medications around daily routines such as waking, mealtimes, and bedtime to lessen the chance of missed doses.
• Monitor for ocular reaction to the drug such as conjunctivitis and lid reactions. (Reactions may result in further damage to the eye.)	• Instruct the patient to report itching, drainage, ocular pain, or other ocular abnormalities.
• Monitor IOP readings. (These are used to determine the effectiveness of drug therapy.)	• Instruct the patient that IOP readings will be taken before beginning treatment and periodically during treatment.
• Monitor the color of the iris and periorbital tissue of the treated eye. (Evaluation of eye color assists in determining the effectiveness of the drug therapy and potential adverse reactions.)	Instruct the patient that: • More brown color may appear in a lighter-colored iris and in the periorbital tissue of the treated eye only. • Any pigmentation changes develop over months to years. • The eyes may become more bloodshot during the first month of therapy.
• Monitor for the systemic absorption of ophthalmic preparations by taking pulse, blood pressure, and heart rate. (Ophthalmic drugs for glaucoma can cause serious cardiovascular and respiratory complications if the drug is systemically absorbed.)	• Instruct the patient to immediately report palpitations, chest pain, shortness of breath, or irregularities in pulse to the health care provider.
• Monitor and adjust environmental lighting to aid in the patient's comfort. (People who have glaucoma are sensitive to excessive light, especially extreme sunlight.)	Instruct the patient to: • Adjust environmental lighting as needed to enhance vision or reduce ocular pain. • Wear darkened glasses as needed.
• Encourage adherence with the treatment regimen. (Nonadherence with the drug therapy may result in the total loss of vision.)	Instruct the patient to: • Adhere to the medication schedule for eyedrop administration. • About the importance of regular follow-up care with the ophthalmologist or optometrist.

Evaluation of Outcome Criteria

Evaluate the effectiveness of drug therapy by confirming that patient goals and expected outcomes have been met (see "Planning").

CONNECTIONS

Complementary and Alternative Therapies Bilberry for Eye Health

Description: Bilberry (*Vaccinium myrtillus*), a close relative of the blueberry, is a perennial ornamental shrub whose leaves and fruit are used medicinally. It is found throughout central and northern Europe, Asia, and North America.

History and Claims: Bilberry has been used for nearly 1,000 years in traditional European medicine to treat diarrhea, scurvy, and other conditions. Today, the fruit is used in a tea to treat nonspecific diarrhea, menstrual cramps, varicose veins, venous insufficiency and, most importantly, a number of conditions associated with disorders of the eye, including glaucoma, poor night vision, and eye inflammation. A widely circulated story is that bilberry jam was used by pilots in the Royal Air Force during World War II to improve their night vision. Bilberry contains high concentrations of compounds called anthocyanosides, which are thought to assist in the function of the rods in the retina for night vision (Riddle, 2004). Bilberry is believed to have factors that stabilize blood vessels, decreasing blood vessel leakage associated with diabetic retinopathy and macular degeneration. Bilberry has also been used to reduce eye inflammation and to lower the increased IOP associated with glaucoma.

Standardization: Preparations of available bilberry extract are standardized to contain 25% anthocyanidin (Medical Economics, 2007).

Evidence: Bilberry has not been evaluated by the FDA for safety, effectiveness, or purity. It is generally believed to be safe in recommended doses for short periods based on its history as a foodstuff. There are no known reports of serious adverse effects, although when taken in large doses, there is an increased risk of bleeding, upset stomach, or hydroquinone poisoning. To date no clinical studies have shown any association between bilberry intake and a reduction in the incidence of glaucoma or improvements in night vision (Canter, 2004). It has been shown in clinical studies to increase conjunctival capillary resistance in patients with diabetic retinopathy, thereby providing a degree of protection against hemorrhage of the retina (Bell & Gochenaur, 2006).

effects include headache, tremors, dizziness, dry mouth, fluid and electrolyte imbalances, and thrombophlebitis or venous clot formation near the site of intravenous (IV) administration. A prototype feature for mannitol is presented in Chapter 35.

CONNECTION *Checkpoint* 77.3

Mannitol is given by the IV route under controlled conditions. From what you learned in Chapter 35, describe the mechanism of action of osmotic diuretics. See Answer to Connection Checkpoint 77.3 in Appendix A.

Pharmacotherapy for Eye Examinations

77.7 Drugs that are routinely used for eye examinations include mydriatics, cycloplegics, diagnostic dyes, and local anesthetics.

Various drugs are used to enhance diagnostic eye examinations and during ophthalmic surgery. **Mydriatic** drugs cause sympathetic activation that relaxes the ciliary muscle, causing dilation of the pupil and thus allowing for better visualization of retinal structures. **Cycloplegic** drugs not only dilate the pupil but also paralyze the ciliary muscle and prevent the lens from moving during assessment. Mydriatics and cycloplegics are often used in combination to achieve the maximum pupil dilation needed for surgery or during funduscopic exams. Examples of agents used for eye examinations include anticholinergics, such as atropine (Isopto Atropine) and tropicamide (Mydriacyl), and sympathomimetics, such as phenylephrine (Mydfrin). Mydriatic, cycloplegic, and other drugs for eye conditions are listed in Table 77.2.

Mydriatics cause intense photophobia and pain in response to bright light. Mydriatics can worsen glaucoma by impairing aqueous humor outflow and thereby increasing IOP. In addition, strong concentrations of anticholinergics have the potential to have systemic effects on the central nervous system (CNS) and cause confusion, unsteadiness, or drowsiness. Cycloplegics can cause severe blurred vision and loss of near vision. Scopolamine, an anticholinergic often used to prevent motion sickness, can cause blurred vision due to cycloplegia, as well as angle-closure glaucoma attacks. The response to mydriatics and cycloplegics can last 3 hours up to several days. The patient needs to be taught to wear sunglasses and that the ability to drive, read, and perform visual tasks may be affected during treatment.

Diagnostic agents are used to help locate lesions or foreign bodies within the eye and to provide some local anesthesia. Fluorescein sodium is a dye used in assessing the cornea and fitting contact lenses. Scratches may turn bright green; foreign bodies are surrounded by a green halo. Areas where the conjunctiva is damaged show an orange-yellow discoloration. Fluorescein sodium with benoxinate (Fluress) adds local anesthesia, making it useful for the identification and removal of foreign bodies from the cornea.

Local anesthetic agents are used to prevent the pain associated with diagnostic and surgical procedures, suturing and removal of foreign bodies, and ocular injections. The agents used include proparacaine hydrochloride (Alcaine, Ophthaine) and tetracaine hydrochloride (Pontocaine). Application consists of one to two drops applied to the affected eye. Anesthesia typically occurs within 20 seconds and last for 10 to 20 minutes. Adverse effects of their use include local irritation, including conjunctivitis Systemic effects are rarer, but CNS excitation has been known to occur. The nurse must be careful to protect the patient's eye from injury while anesthetized, or corneal damage may occur.

Pharmacotherapy for Other Eye Conditions

77.8 Numerous pharmacologic agents are used to treat minor eye irritation and redness.

Drugs for minor eye irritation and dryness come from a broad range of classes. Some agents lubricate only the eye's surface,

TABLE 77.2 Miscellaneous Agents Used for the Eye

Drug	Route and Adult Dose (maximum dose where indicated)	Adverse Effects
Mydriatics: Sympathomimetics		
phenylephrine HCl (Mydfrin, Neo-Synephrine)	1 drop of 2.5% or 10% solution before eye examination	*Eye pain, photosensitivity, eye irritation, headache* HTN, tremor, dysrhythmias
Cycloplegics: Anticholinergics		
atropine sulfate (Isopto Atropine, others)	Uveitis: 1–2 drops of 1% solution up to 4 times daily; also give 1–2 drops 1 h prior to eye examination	*Eye irritation and redness, dry mouth, local burning or stinging, headache, blurred vision, photosensitivity, eczematoid dermatitis (scopolamine and tropicamide)* Somnolence, tachycardia, convulsions, mental changes, keratitis, increased IOP (homatropine)
cyclopentolate (Cyclogyl, Pentolair)	1 drop of 0.5–2% solution 40–50 min before eye examination	
homatropine (Isopto Homatropine, others)	1–2 drops of 2% or 5% solution before eye examination Uveitis: 1–2 drops of 2–5% solution bid-tid up to every 3–4 h as needed	
scopolamine hydrobromide (Isopto Hyoscine)	1–2 drops of 0.25% solution 1 h before eye examination	
tropicamide (Mydriacyl, Tropicacyl)	1–2 drops of 0.5–1% solution before eye examination	
Anesthetics		
lidocaine (Akten)	2 drops of 3.5% gel before procedure	*Stinging, corneal erosion, headache, slowed healing of corneal abrasions* Anaphylactic reactions
proparacaine (Alcaine, Ophthaine)	1 drop of 0.5% solution in the eye every 5–10 min for 5 to 7 doses	
tetracaine (Altacaine, Pontocaine).	1–2 drops of a 0.5% solution or 1.25–2.5 cm of ointment in the lower conjunctival sac	
Lubricants		
lanolin alcohol (Lacril-lube)	Apply a thin film to the inside of the eyelid	*Temporary burning or stinging, eye itching or redness, headache* No serious adverse effects
polyvinyl alcohol (Liquifilm, others)	1–2 drops tid-qid prn	
Vasoconstrictors		
naphazoline HCl (Albalon Allerest, Clear Eyes, others)	1–3 drops of 0.1% solution every 3–4 h prn	*Temporary burning or stinging, eye itching or redness, headache* No serious adverse effects
oxymetazoline HCl (OcuClear, Visine LR)	1–2 drops of 0.025% solution qid	
phenylephrine (Neo-Synephrine)	1–2 drops of 0.12% solution up to 4 times daily	
tetrahydrozoline HCl (Collyrium, Murine Plus, Visine, others)	1–2 drops of 0.05% solution bid-tid	

Note: *Italics* indicate common adverse effects. Underline indicates serious adverse effects.

whereas others are designed to penetrate and affect a specific area of the eye.

Lubricants are used to lessen the discomfort associated with dryness and maintain the patency of the cornea. They are used as artificial tears in persons who complain of "dry eyes," during anesthesia with acute or chronic nervous system disorders that result in decreased blinking, and as extra moisture for those who have contact lenses or artificial eyes. Artificial tear agents are topical preparations of methyl or vinyl cellulose. These drops can be instilled as often as every hour. A wide variety of over-the-counter (OTC) preparations are available, including eyedrop solutions, ointments, and inserts. There is currently only one prescription drug for dry eye and that is cyclosporine ophthalmic emulsion (Restasis). Restasis is the only agent available that actually stimulates the production of tears. It is most effective when used in combination with artificial tear replacement and is administered as one drop in the affected eye(s) twice daily. Cyclosporine is presented as a prototype immunosuppressant in Chapter 45.

Vasoconstrictors are commonly used to treat minor eye irritation. Common vasoconstrictors include phenylephrine (Neo-Synephrine), naphazoline (Clear Eyes), and tetrahydrozoline (Altazine, Murine Tears Plus, Visine). The adverse effects of the vasoconstrictors are usually minor and include blurred vision, tearing, headache, and rebound vasodilation with redness.

Infection and inflammatory responses are common conditions in the supporting structures of the eye and may result from foreign bodies, bacteria, or viruses. Allergies and irritants such as tobacco smoke are also common sources of inflammation. Redness, edema, and itching are common symptoms. The anti-infectives used to treat eye infections are the same agents used to treat infections in other areas of the body. Applied topically they carry the common adverse effects of conjunctivitis and local skin and eye irritation. Examples of eye infections that are treated with anti-infective medications include:

- Blepharitis. Inflammation of the edges of the eyelids that is commonly seen in older adults and those with dry eyes
- Conjunctivitis. Inflammation or infection of the lining of the eyelids. Bacterial conjunctivitis is often caused by *Staphylococcus aureus*, *Streptococcus pneumoniae*, and *Haemophilus influenzae*. Viral conjunctivitis is highly contagious and treatment is symptomatic
- Chalazion. An infection of the meibomian glands in the eyelids. It is also called an internal stye. Hordeolum, or an external stye, is an infection of the sebaceous glands at the base of the eyelashes. The most common causative agents are seborrhea, streptococcus, and staphylococcal infections
- Keratitis. An inflammation of the cornea that may also be caused by trauma or dryness of the cornea from decreased lubrication. If left untreated, corneal scarring with impaired vision may result

Nonsteroidal anti-inflammatory drugs (NSAIDs), such as ketorolac (Acular), can be used to treat conjunctivitis and other inflammatory conditions. They are also used to reduce inflammation postoperatively and the symptoms associated with seasonal allergies. Topical corticosteroids are also very effective at reducing inflammation in the eye, although they should not be administered if an infection is suspected. The most common adverse effects of topical corticosteroids are cataracts, glaucoma, mydriasis, and ptosis. Cycloplegics can also be used to treat ocular pain caused by almost any inflammatory condition, except glaucoma.

PharmFACT

Steroid-induced glaucoma is usually associated with topical corticosteroid use but it may occur by any route of administration. Elevated IOP (6 mmHg) occurs in 33% of patients with normal eyes after 4 weeks of steroid treatment. *Source:* Rhee & Gedde, 2008.

Several medications, including antihistamines (see Chapter 74), mast cell stabilizers, and combination antihistamine–mast cell stabilizers, are used to decrease the redness and itching associated with allergic conjunctivitis. Systemic antihistamines may be used but they may cause ocular dryness, which could aggravate symptoms. Topical mast cell stabilizers, with or without an antihistamine, are the preferred treatment for allergic conjunctivitis because they do not cause further drying of the eyes. Two new drugs, olopatadine (Patanol) and pemirolast (Alamast), provide for daily dosed treatments for allergic conjunctivitis. Azelastine (Optivar) and epinastine (Elestat) are combination antihistamine–mast cell stabilizers that are indicated for twice-daily dosing. Drugs for the treatment of allergic conjunctivitis are listed in Table 77.3

Anatomy of the Ear

77.9 Knowledge of basic ear anatomy is fundamental to understanding ear disorders and pharmacotherapy.

The ear has two major sensory functions: hearing and maintenance of equilibrium and balance. The three structural areas of the ear—the external, middle, and inner ear—carry out these functions, as shown in Figure 77.3.

The external ear consists of the pinna, which is the visible portion of the ear, and the external auditory canal. The external auditory canal transmits sound waves to the tympanic membrane, or eardrum. This canal is lined with numerous ceruminous glands that protect the canal and help keep the tympanic membrane pliable. The tympanic membrane separates the external ear from the middle ear. The middle ear consists of a bony cavity containing

TABLE 77.3 Drugs for the Treatment of Allergic Conjunctivitis

Drug	Route and Adult Dose	Adverse Effects
Mast Cell Stabilizers		
cromolyn sodium (Crolom)	1–2 drops of 4% solution every 4–6 h	*Dry mouth, headache, nausea, sneezing, nasal symptoms, and transient eye stinging and burning* Bronchospasm, angioedema, anaphylaxis
ketotifen (Alaway, Zaditor)	1 drop bid every 8–12 h	
nedocromil sodium (Alocril)	1–2 drops of 2% solution bid	
pemirolast potassium (Alamast)	1–2 drops of 0.1% solution qid	
Mast Cell Stabilizers and Antihistamines		
azelastine (Astelin, Optivar)	1 drop of 0.05% solution bid	*Fatigue, dizziness, dry mouth, headache, pharyngitis, cough, bitter taste, rhinitis* No serious adverse effects
epinastine (Elestat)	1 drop of 0.05% solution bid	
olopatadine (Patanol)	1 drop of 0.1% solution bid	

Note: *Italics* indicate common adverse effects. Underline indicates serious adverse effects.

CONNECTIONS

To the Community Ophthalmic Drugs in the Home Setting

Older adults who live alone often need to use ophthalmic drugs at home. Assess the ability of the aging individual to safely administer ophthalmic drugs in the home setting. A return demonstration by the patient may be critical to assess the older adult's dexterity and skill in self-administering eye medications. If needed, encourage the patient to seek reasonable alternatives, such as help from a neighbor, family member, or caregiver.

Teaching is critical for positive outcomes in this population. The older adult needs to understand that touching or rubbing the eye can result in infection or damage to the eye. Because vision may already be compromised, the older adult may experience blurred vision that should clear in a reasonable time after using ophthalmic drugs. Caution elderly patients about trying to drive or even ambulate until this unclear vision improves. Additionally, with eye problems, diminished vision puts the older adult at increased risk for falls. Assess the home and make suggestions to improve safety. Care should be taken to label eye medicines to indicate which is for the left eye and which is for the right eye. Scheduling medications around a routine, such as meals, also may help the older adult remember to take the ophthalmic medications as prescribed, increasing adherence, which is necessary for healing.

Pediatric patients are also treated at home for eye disorders. Parents or caregivers in the home are responsible for administering and ensuring the child's adherence with the drug therapy. The same administration instructions apply to both geriatric and pediatric populations. Caution children and family against touching and rubbing the eyes. In the case of infants, toddlers, and very young children, it may be necessary to use elbow splints and guards to prevent them from being able to reach their eyes.

the three ossicles, called the malleus, incus, and stapes, which transmit sound waves to the inner ear. The eustachian tube provides a connection between the middle ear and the oropharynx. It permits equalization of pressure in the middle ear by allowing air to enter or leave the middle ear cavity and for the drainage of secretions. Its mucosa is continuous with the mucosal lining of the throat, providing a means for infectious organisms to enter the middle ear from the nose and throat. The inner ear consists of the semicircular canals, the vestibule, and the cochlea. The cochlea is the main organ of hearing, whereas the semicircular canals and vestibule are responsible for balance and equilibrium.

Pharmacotherapy with Otic Preparations

77.10 Otic preparations treat infections, inflammation, and earwax buildup.

Otitis, or inflammation of the ear, is a common indication for pharmacotherapy. **External otitis,** commonly called swimmer's ear, is an inflammation with or without infection of the outer ear. The acute form is bacterial in origin and most often due to *Pseudomonas aeruginosa* or *S. aureus.* It is associated with water exposure, high humidity, and a history of ear trauma

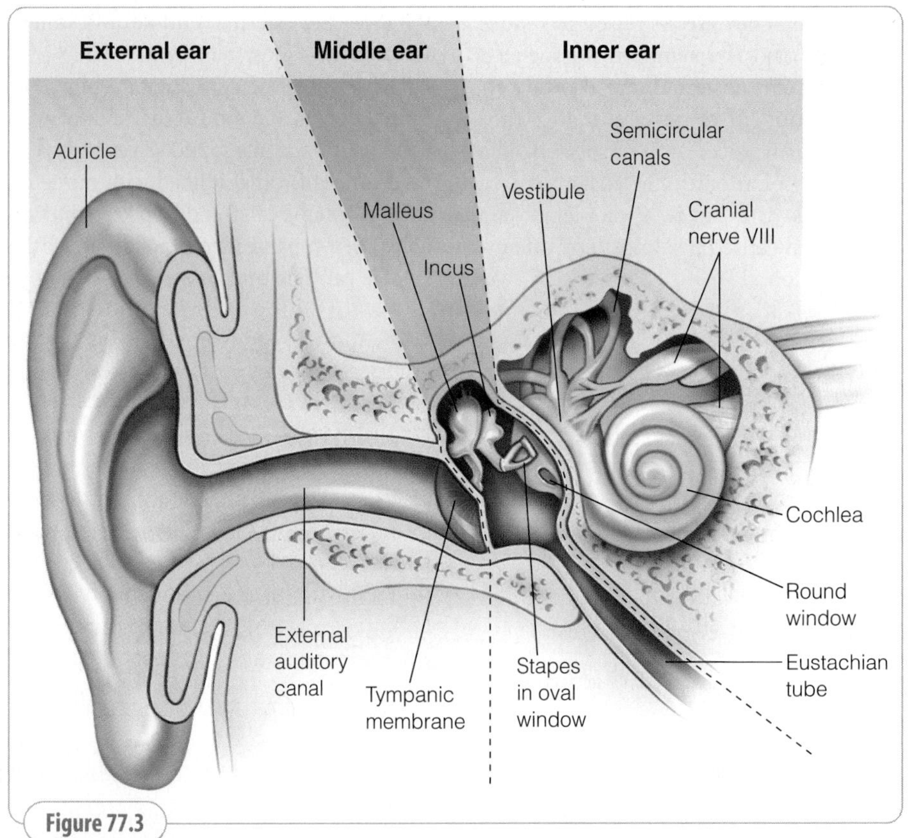

Figure 77.3

Structure of the ear.

Source: From *Health and Physical Assessment in Nursing* (p. 306), by D. D'Amico & C. Barbarito, 2007. Reprinted by permission of Pearson Education, Inc., Upper Saddle River, NJ.

generally from sharp or small objects. Chronic external otitis is most often caused by a fungal infection or an allergic response usually associated with cosmetics, hair products, or devices placed within the ear canal. The typical presentation is that of acute onset ear pain associated with pruritus, swelling, and tenderness to the touch or with movement. A greenish white drainage may accompany symptoms. Hearing impairment may result if the swelling is sufficient to obstruct the auditory canal.

Treatment of external otitis focuses on reducing pain and inflammation, usually with topical corticosteroids, antibiotics, and analgesics, as needed. Neomycin, gentamicin, and ciprofloxacin (Cipro otic) are the most commonly used topical otic antibiotics. Mild fungal infections can be treated with a 90% to 95% alcohol solution; more advanced disease may be treated with topical 1% clotrimazole (Lotrimin) or tolnaftate (Tinactin). If swelling obstructs the external canal, an ear wick may be placed past the blockage and the drops applied to the end. The use of systemic antibiotics may be necessary in cases when outer ear infections are extensive, such as with cellulitis or lymph node involvement.

Otitis media, which is inflammation of the middle ear, is a common disorder that affects infants and young children, although any age may be affected. Among children 75% experience at least one episode of otitis media by their third birthday, and almost half of these children will have three or more ear infections during that time.

There are three common types of otitis media: acute, chronic, and serous. Acute otitis media and chronic otitis media are similar. An infectious agent, most often a viral upper respiratory infection, results in pathogens being introduced into the middle ear through the eustachian tube, leading to swelling and inflammation of the ossicles of the middle ear. Bacterial infection with *S. pneumoniae*, *H. influenzae*, and *Streptococcus pyogenes* cause most cases. Otitis media may also be associated with allergies or eustachian tube dysfunction. Acute otitis has a duration of less than 3 weeks; chronic otitis follows repeated episodes and has a longer duration of symptoms. Sometimes the eardrum ruptures, and pus drains out of the ear. More commonly, the pus and mucus remain in the middle ear due to the swollen and inflamed eustachian tube. This is called middle ear effusion or serous otitis media. After the acute infection has passed, the effusion may remain and become chronic, lasting for weeks, months, or even years.

The chief symptom of otitis media is ear pain with an accompanying sense of fullness in the ear. Headaches are common, along with complaints of malaise and nausea. The patient may complain of tinnitus or "popping" sounds when yawning or swallowing. Otitis media is often difficult to detect because most children affected by this disorder do not yet have sufficient speech and language skills to tell someone what is bothering them. Common signs include the following:

- Unusual irritability
- Difficulty sleeping
- Tugging or pulling at one or both ears
- Fever
- Purulent or bloody drainage from the ear
- Loss of balance
- Unresponsiveness to quiet sounds, or other signs of hearing difficulty such as sitting too close to the television or being inattentive

In 2004, the American Academy of Pediatrics and the American Academy of Family Physicians released guidelines for the treatment of otitis media. The management of pain, especially during the first 24 hours of an episode of acute otitis media, should be part of the plan of care, regardless of the use of antibacterial agents. Whether or not to place a patient on antibiotics or to observe is based on a child's age, diagnostic certainty, and illness severity. The observation option is defined as deferring antibacterial treatment of selected children for 48 to 72 hours and limiting management to symptomatic relief. This option should be limited to otherwise healthy children 6 months to 2 years of age with nonsevere illness at presentation and an uncertain diagnosis and to children 2 years of age and older without severe symptoms at presentation or with an uncertain diagnosis. All children under 6 months of age should receive antibiotic therapy.

Otitis media is treated with a course of systemic rather than topical antibiotics. Amoxicillin, at a dose of 80 to 90mg/kg/day, is prescribed for most children. For patients who have symptoms of a more severe illness and in those for whom additional coverage for β-lactamase-positive *H. influenzae* and *Moraxella catarrhalis* is desired, therapy is initiated with high-dose amoxicillin-clavulanate. For patients with mild penicillin allergy, a cephalosporin may be considered. If the penicillin allergy is more severe, azithromycin or clarithromycin can be used. In the patient who is vomiting or cannot otherwise tolerate oral medication, a single dose of parenteral ceftriaxone has been shown to be effective.

Symptomatic relief for otitis externa and otitis media involves the use of analgesics, such as acetaminophen, or NSAIDs, such as ibuprofen, to relieve pain and reduce fever. Patients with severe pain may require therapy with opioid analgesics such as codeine. A 7-day course of a corticosteroid is often combined with antibiotics when severe inflammation is present. Antihistamines or decongestants may be used to decrease mucus production and fluid levels in the middle ear. Examples of these drugs are listed in Table 77.4.

Labyrinthitis, or **otitis interna,** may occur as the result of chronic otitis media or as part of viral systemic infections, including mononucleosis or an upper respiratory infection. Of all ear infections, otitis interna is the most difficult to treat because the blood-labyrinth barrier makes it difficult for systemic medications to reach the affected areas. **Mastoiditis,** or inflammation of the mastoid sinus, is frequently the result of chronic or inadequately treated bacterial otitis media or inner ear infection. The infection moves into the bone and surrounding structures of the ear. Symptoms of pain, hearing loss, and tenderness typically appear 2 to 3 weeks after an episode of otitis media. Mastoiditis can be a serious problem. If left untreated, it can result in hearing loss.

The treatment of acute mastoiditis involves aggressive antibiotic therapy. IV gentamicin or ticarcillin may be used initially. Therapy may be adjusted once culture and sensitivity results are obtained. Therapy is continued for at least 14 days.

TABLE 77.4 Otic Preparations

Drug	Route and Adult Dose (maximum dose where indicated)	Adverse Effects
acetic acid and hydrocortisone (VoSoL HC)	3–5 drops every 4 h-qid for 24 h, then 5 drops tid-qid	*Ear irritation, local stinging or burning, dizziness* Allergic reactions (antibiotics)
benzocaine and antipyrine (Auralgan)	Fill the ear canal with solution tid for 2–3 days	
carbamide peroxide (Debrox)	1–5 drops of 6.5% solution bid for 4 days	
ciprofloxacin/dexamethasone (CiproDex)	Children to adults: 4 drops in the affected ears bid for 7 days	
ciprofloxacin/hydrocortisone (Cipro)	3 drops of the suspension instilled into the ear bid for 7 days	
polymyxin B, neomycin, and hydrocortisone (Cortisporin)	3 drops in the ear tid-qid	

Note: *Italics* indicate common adverse effects. Underline indicates serious adverse effects.

If the antibiotics are not effective and symptoms persist, surgery such as a mastoidectomy or meatoplasty may be indicated.

Cerumen (earwax) softeners are also used for proper ear health. When cerumen accumulates, it narrows the ear canal and may interfere with hearing. **Cerumenolytics** may be needed to loosen and remove impacted cerumen from the ear canal. Use of these agents usually involves the instillation of an earwax softener and then a gentle lavage of the wax-impacted ear with tepid water using an asepto syringe to gently insert the water. An instrument called an ear loop may be used to help remove earwax but should be used only by health care providers who are skilled in using it. There are three types of cerumen-softening preparations: water based, oil based, and nonwater oil based. Water-based preparations include solutions of triethanolamine, 3% hydrogen peroxide, 10% sodium bicarbonate, and saline or water. The nonwater oil-based preparation available in the United States includes the OTC agent carbamide peroxide (Debrox). Oil-based preparations include household olive, mineral, and almond oils and commercially prepared combinations, such as Cerumol, Earex, and Otocerol. Research has shown that the water-based and nonwater oil agents have equal effectiveness.

CONNECTIONS

Lifespan Considerations

Proper Instillation of Otic Medication

Geriatric and pediatric patients frequently experience ear infections (especially otitis media in children). Proper instruction on the instillation of otic medication is needed. With adults and children older than 3 years, the pinna should be pulled up and back during instillation. With children younger than 3 years of age, the pinna should be gently pulled down and back during instillation. When cerumen accumulates, it narrows the ear canal and may interfere with hearing. This is especially common in older patients and may be part of the changes associated with aging. Health care providers who are working with elderly patients should be trained to take appropriate measures when removing impacted cerumen. Advise patients not to perform earwax removal, especially in children, because of the potential for damage to the eardrum. Eardrops are capable of becoming absorbed by the systemic circulation and being passed on to the fetus or infant in pregnant and lactating women.

Nursing Responsibilities for Otic Medications

- Assess for baseline hearing and auditory status, symptoms, and any current medical conditions before administering otic preparations. The use of otic medications is usually contraindicated in the presence of a perforated eardrum.
- Obtain information regarding hypersensitivity to hydrocortisone, neomycin sulfate, polymyxin B, chloramphenicol, and other medications to be administered.
- Assess for adverse effects that may include burning, redness, rash, swelling, and other signs of topical irritation.
- When instilling cerumenolytics, cleanse the ear thoroughly and remove the cerumen through gentle irrigation. Otic drugs should be warmed to body temperature (but not higher) before instillation.

Patient and Family Education for Otic Medications

- Lie down while instilling eardrops because dizziness may occur.
- Administer eardrops at body temperature by running warm water over the bottle.
- In adults and children older than 3 years, hold the pinna up and back during instillation.
- In children younger than 3 years, gently pull the pinna down and back during instillation.

- Do not touch the ear with the dropper.
- Massage the area around the ear gently after instillation to promote thorough administration to the ear canal.
- Lie on the side opposite the affected ear for 5 minutes after instillation.
- Immediately report any ear pain or discharges from the ear canal.

PharmFACT

Viral labyrinthitis is the most common cause of labyrinthitis, which occurs most frequently in adults aged 30 to 60. The condition usually presents with severe vertigo, nausea, and vomiting. Permanent hearing loss is common in adults and may occur in up to 20% of pediatric cases. *Source:* Boston & Strasnick, 2008.

NURSING PROCESS APPLICATION

Patients Receiving Pharmacotherapy for Otitis Media

Assessment	Potential Nursing Diagnoses
Prior to administration: • Obtain a complete health history, including allergies, drug history, and possible drug interactions. • Obtain a complete physical examination, focusing on evaluation of hearing abilities and deficits. • Assess baseline hearing and auditory status. • Assess for the presence or history of trauma, auditory pain, injury, symptoms, and employment background.	• *Chronic Pain*, related to disease process • *Risk for Injury*, related to impaired hearing abilities • *Deficient Knowledge (Disease Process and Drug Therapy)*

Planning: Patient Goals and Expected Outcomes

The patient will:

- Exhibit no progression of hearing impairment.
- Demonstrate an understanding of the drug's action by accurately describing drug adverse effects and precautions.
- Report the absence of pain.

Implementation

Interventions and (Rationales)	Patient and Family Education
• Monitor hearing abilities and deficits, signs and symptoms such as pain, hearing loss or changes in hearing, tenderness, and drainage. (This helps to establish baseline findings and determine the effectiveness of drug therapy.)	Instruct the patient to report hearing deficits, ear pain, or ear tenderness, to the health care provider.
• Monitor for otic reactions to the drug such as burning, rash, swelling, and other signs of topical irritation. (Some medications are contraindicated in cases of a perforated eardrum.)	Instruct the patient to: • Inform the health care provider of all health-related problems and prescribed medications.
• Remove the hearing aid before administering otic solutions. (With the hearing aid in place, the drug cannot be properly administered into the ear. The hearing aid impedes the medication from reaching its intended target.)	• Instruct the patient to remove the hearing aid(s) related to the affected ear(s) prior to instilling the medications.
• Administer otic solutions using the proper technique. (Improper administration may lead to infection or injury to the ear.)	Instruct the patient to: • Wash the hands prior to handling any medications. • Avoid touching the tip of the dropper to any part of the ear. • Administer eardrops at body temperature by running warm water over the bottle. • In adults and children over the age of 3, pull the pinna up and back during instillation. • In children younger than 3 years, gently pull the pinna down and back during instillation. • Massage the area around the ear gently after instillation to promote thorough administration to the ear canal. • Lie on the side opposite the affected ear for 5 minutes after instillation.
• Assess the patient's complaints of pain. (Otic pain may be treated with nonnarcotic analgesics.)	• Instruct the patient that hearing sensitivity may result due to infection and worsen pain.
• Monitor and adjust the environmental sound to aid in the patient's comfort. (Patients with ear conditions are sensitive to sounds and need to have sound levels adjusted for comfort.)	• Instruct the patient to adjust sound levels of televisions, radios, and the like that may create discomfort to the sensitive ear.
• Encourage adherence to the prescribed treatment regimen. (Nonadherence with drug therapy may result in additional or total loss of hearing.)	• Instruct the patient about regular follow-up care with the health care provider.

Evaluation of Outcome Criteria

Evaluate the effectiveness of drug therapy by confirming that patient goals and expected outcomes have been met (see "Planning").

UNDERSTANDING THE CHAPTER

Key Concepts Summary

77.1 Knowledge of basic eye anatomy is fundamental to understanding eye disorders and their pharmacotherapy.

77.2 The two principal types of glaucoma, closed-angle glaucoma and open-angle glaucoma, are characterized by increased intraocular pressure.

77.3 The primary goal of glaucoma pharmacotherapy is to prevent damage to the optic nerve by lowering intraocular pressure.

77.4 Prostaglandin analogs are often the drugs of choice for treating high intraocular pressure because of their long durations of action and high safety profiles.

77.5 Drugs that affect the autonomic nervous system are sometimes prescribed to treat glaucoma.

77.6 Carbonic anhydrase inhibitors and osmotic diuretics are occasionally used for treating glaucoma.

77.7 Drugs that are routinely used for eye examinations include mydriatics, cycloplegics, diagnostic dyes, and local anesthetics.

77.8 Numerous pharmacologic agents are used to treat minor eye irritation and redness.

77.9 Knowledge of basic ear anatomy is fundamental to understanding ear disorders and pharmacotherapy.

77.10 Otic preparations treat infections, inflammation, and earwax buildup.

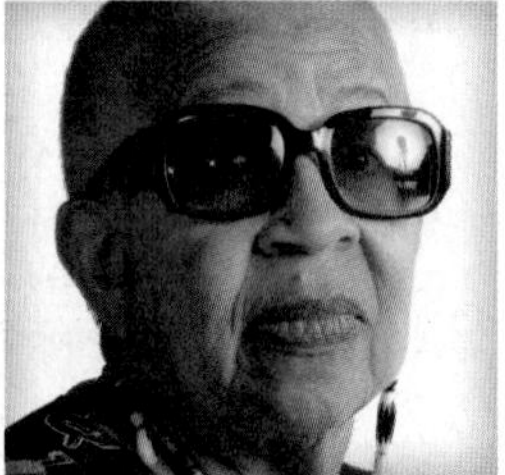

Making the PATIENT *Connection*

Remember the patient "Therese Duclos" from the beginning of the chapter? Now read the remainder of the case study. Based on the information presented within this chapter, respond to the critical thinking questions that follow.

Mrs. Duclos, a 65-year-old African American woman, visits her ophthalmologist with complaints of blurry vision and not being able to see well at night while driving. Her health history includes adult-onset diabetes for the past 10 years and osteoporosis since age 55. Her medical regimen includes diet control for the diabetes and Boniva monthly. She denies any injury to her eyes and last had an eye checkup 1 year ago.

Critical Thinking Questions

1. What factors are presented in Mrs. Duclos's health history that you identify as predisposing conditions for the development of primary open-angle glaucoma?
2. Mrs. Duclos needs to learn the proper administration of eyedrops. What teaching would you provide to ensure that the skill will be performed correctly?
3. Create a list of important facts related to primary open-angle glaucoma that you would discuss with Mrs. Duclos.

Case Study

Zachary, a 4-year-old boy, is complaining of pain in both ears. His mother takes him to his health care provider and he is diagnosed with otitis media. Zachary is prescribed Cortisporin otic drops to be instilled in his right ear four times a day for a week. To ensure that the mother is knowledgeable in this form of administration, the nurse will teach her about the proper technique. Create a patient information sheet for a parent who needs to administer eardrops.

- IM administration is preferred for symptomatic children and recommended for patients with incipient or overt lead-induced encephalopathy.
- Use separate injection sites when dimercaprol (BAL) and calcium EDTA are given concurrently.

Patient and Family Education:

- Immediately report signs of lead toxicity, such as metallic taste in the mouth, seizures, decreased urination, or abdominal cramping to the health care provider.
- Eat foods rich in zinc, calcium, magnesium, iron, and calcium to prevent storage of lead in the body.

PROTOTYPE DRUG Dimercaprol (BAL in Oil)

Classification: **Therapeutic:** Antidote
Pharmacologic: Chelating agent

Therapeutic Effects and Uses: Given by the IM route, dimercaprol is a chelating agent that neutralizes the effects of various heavy metals such as arsenic, gold, and mercury. This drug is also used as an adjunct to edetate calcium disodium (EDTA) in the treatment of lead encephalopathy. Off-label uses include chromium dermatitis and ocular and dermatologic manifestations of arsenic poisoning. Some studies indicate that dimercaprol may be used as an adjunct to penicillamine to increase the rate of copper excretion in Wilson's disease. Wilson's disease is a rare genetic disorder in which copper builds up in the liver and is released into other parts of the body.

Mechanism of Action: Dimercaprol forms ring complexes with some heavy metals, such as arsenic, gold, and mercury, preventing or reversing the binding of metallic cations to body proteins.

Pharmacokinetics:

Route(s)	IM only
Absorption	Well absorbed
Distribution	Distributed mainly in intracellular spaces, including the brain; highest concentration is in the liver and kidneys
Primary metabolism	Unknown
Primary excretion	Urine and feces
Onset of action	Peak: 30–60 minutes
Duration of action	Half-life: unknown

Adverse Effects: About 50% of patients who receive high therapeutic doses have minor reactions, which include nausea, vomiting, fatigue, restlessness, apprehension, headache, burning sensation of the mouth, throat, and eyes, lacrimation, blepharospasm, salivation, tingling of extremities, a feeling of constriction in the chest muscle, diffuse pain and muscle spasm, hypertension (systolic and diastolic), and tachycardia. Most patients report pain at the injection site.

Contraindications/Precautions: Dimercaprol is contraindicated in individuals with hepatic insufficiency (with the exception of postarsenic jaundice); severe renal insufficiency; or poisoning due to cadmium, iron, selenium, or uranium. Because dimercaprol is formulated in peanut oil, patients with a hypersensitivity to peanut products should not receive this drug. This drug should be used cautiously in patients with hypertension, oliguria, G6PD deficiency, and preexisting renal disease.

Drug Interactions: Dimercaprol should not be given when iron, cadmium, selenium, or uranium poisoning is suspected. When this drug is given in the presence of these poisonings, it forms toxic complexes. **Herbal/Food:** Unknown.

Pregnancy: Category C.

Nursing Responsibilities:

- Obtain an allergy history. Hold the drug and notify the prescriber if the patient reports an allergy to peanuts.
- Initiate therapy as soon as possible (within 1 to 2 hours) after ingestion of the poison because irreversible tissue damage may occur, particularly with mercury poisoning.
- Administer dimercaprol by deep IM injection only. Rotate and closley monitor the injection sites because local pain and gluteal abscesses are possible.
- Monitor vital signs. Elevations of systolic and diastolic blood pressure accompanied by tachycardia frequently occur within a few minutes following injection and may remain elevated up to 2 hours.
- Monitor body temperature. Fever occurs in approximately 30% of children receiving treatment and may persist throughout therapy.
- Monitor intake and output ratio because dimercaprol is potentially nephrotoxic. Report oliguria to the prescriber.
- Assess urine daily for albumin, blood, casts, and pH. Blood and urinary levels of the metal serve as guides for dosage adjustments.
- Minor adverse reactions generally reach a maximum 15 to 20 minutes after drug administration and subside in 30 to 90 minutes. Ephedrine or an antihistamine may be administered to prevent symptoms.

Patient and Family Education:

- Drink as much fluid as the health care provider will permit to prevent nephrotoxicity.
- Do not take iron supplements during therapy because this can cause kidney damage.

NURSING PROCESS APPLICATION

Patients Experiencing Poisoning or Overdose

Assessment	Potential Nursing Diagnoses
• Obtain a complete health history, including allergies, drug history, and possible drug interactions. • Assess vital signs, level of consciousness, and cardiopulmonary status.	• *Risk for Poisoning,* related to exposure to toxic hazardous substances • *Risk for Ineffective Breathing Pattern,* related to neurotoxicity • *Risk for Decreased Cardiac Output,* related to cardiotoxicity • *Risk for Peripheral Neurovascular Dysfunction* • *Deficient Knowledge (Health Maintenance),* related to measure to prevent accidental exposure to toxic substances

Planning: Patient Goals and Expected Outcomes

The patient will:

- Maintain stable vital signs and neurologic status.
- Have absorption of drugs minimized and maximal elimination of absorbed drugs.

Implementation

Interventions and (Rationales)	Patient and Family Education
• Maintain airway and provide supplemental oxygen as warranted. (Patients with an overdose or poisoning may be unable to maintain a patent airway, leading to respiratory arrest and death.)	• Instruct the patient to notify the health care provider at the onset of difficulty breathing or swallowing.
• Monitor cardiopulmonary status. (Cardiac dysrhythmias and pulmonary edema may result from overdose of many poisons, including barbiturates, sedatives, hypnotics, and tranquilizers.)	• Explain the reason for frequent monitoring of cardiovascular and pulmonary status.
• Administer IV fluids as ordered. (Crystalloid solutions are used to treat hypovolemia, which may occur because of compromised circulatory status.)	• Instruct the patient and family to report burning, swelling, or discomfort at the IV site.
• Monitor serum glucose levels. Administer concentrated dextrose solution (D_5W) as ordered. (Hypoglycemia may occur due to acute poisoning or overdose with agents such as ethanol and salicylates.)	• Instruct the patient to report symptoms of hypoglycemia such as nervousness, anxiety, hunger, shakiness, perspiration, dizziness, or light-headedness.
• Administer antidotes, if known, once the substance is identified. (Commonly known antidotes include Mucomyst for acetaminophen, flumazenil for benzodiazepines, sodium bicarbonate for cyclic antidepressants, amyl nitrate for cyanide, naloxone for opioids, and osmotic diuretics for methanol and ethylene glycol.)	• Explain the purpose and expected outcome of antidotes administered. • When no antidote exists for the poisonous substance, inform the patient and family what supportive care will be provided.
• Monitor intake and output ratio. (Observe for changes in urine character and color. Myoglobin may be present if rhabdomyolysis occurs as a result of overdose.)	• Inform the patient and family that most poisons are excreted via the kidneys. • Discuss the rationale for close monitoring of urinary output.
• Insert a nasogastric tube, aspirate fluid for analysis, and lavage the stomach. (Lavage removes drugs that may remain in the stomach, preventing further absorption. Aspirate may be sent to the laboratory for analysis of the drugs ingested to provide identification for appropriate treatment.)	• Explain the rationale for gastric lavage and gastric analysis.
• Administer activated charcoal as ordered (Activated charcoal absorbs drugs from gastric content to prevent systemic absorption.)	• Explain the purpose and expected outcome of activated charcoal if administered. • Inform the patient that stools may become temporarily black.
• Prepare the patient for dialysis procedures as ordered. (Hemodialysis or hemoperfusion removes poisons from the system and is used when levels are potentially lethal; otherwise the toxin may be metabolized to a more lethal substance.)	• Explain the rationale for hemodialysis or hemoperfusion.
• Assess for suicidal ideation and refer to a mental health professional as appropriate. (A psychiatric consultation should be ordered for patients who demonstrate suicidal ideations or behaviors.)	• When suicidal ideation is present and poisoning is self-inflicted, explain the reason for referral to a mental health professional. • Explain the importance of follow-up with mental health professionals.
• Assess learning needs and provide education related to poisoning and overdose. (Poisoning may often be prevented by personal and public education efforts.)	• Instruct the patient on the importance of maintaining a safe environment to prevent recurrence of accidental poisonings.

Evaluation of Outcome Criteria

Evaluate the effectiveness of drug therapy by confirming that patient goals and expected outcomes have been met (see "Planning").

UNDERSTANDING THE CHAPTER

Key Concepts Summary

78.1 Emergency preparedness has become an essential competency for all health care professionals.

78.2 Bioterrorism is the intentional release of a virus or microorganism to cause human harm.

78.3 Nurses may have the first opportunity to recognize and initiate a response to bioterrorism.

78.4 The Strategic National Stockpile has large quantities of medicine to protect the public if there is a public health emergency.

78.5 Highly infectious bacteria or viruses could be used as bioterrorist threats.

78.6 There are 13 categories of toxic chemicals that could cause mass casualties if released in the environment.

78.7 Ionizing radiation produces immediate and long-term effects on human tissue.

78.8 The general management of poisoning includes contacting the poison control center or emergency medical services as soon as possible.

78.9 Activated charcoal is effective at adsorbing (binding) most poisons if administered within 60 minutes of ingestion.

78.10 Ion trapping with forced diuresis may be helpful for some poisonings.

78.11 Chelating agents are capable of forming bonds with heavy metals.

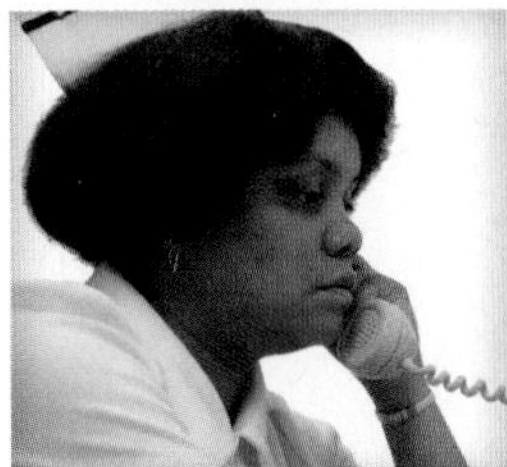

Making the PATIENT *Connection*

Remember the nurse manager "Carol Boler" at the beginning of the chapter? Now read the remainder of the case study. Based on the information presented within this chapter, respond to the critical thinking questions that follow.

As a new nurse manager of a busy urban emergency department, Carol Boler wants her staff to be prepared for mass casualty events and acts of bioterrorism. Although there have been no incidents yet, she knows that with a military base nearby, there is a chance that such an incident could occur. She is planning a series of inservice education meetings with her staff to discuss bioterrorism threats.

Critical Thinking Questions

1. When discussing the bioterrorism threat with a group of staff nurses, which information regarding smallpox should be included?
2. Identify the nursing assessments and interventions that the nurse should initiate when a client is exposed to inhaled anthrax.
3. Discuss the mode of transmission and symptoms associated with *Y. pestis* exposure.

Case Study

As a parish nurse, you have been asked to speak to a group of new mothers about accidental poisonings in young children.

1. Outline the information you need to present to this audience.
2. What recommendations should you give to the group about the use of ipecac syrup?

NCLEX-RN® Review

1 The client is suspected of being exposed to ionizing radiation. Which of the following nursing interventions would have the greatest priority?

1. Provide supportive care for nausea, vomiting, and diarrhea.
2. Limit the client's exposure to ultraviolet light.
3. Avoid contamination of self through limited exposure to the client.
4. Administer antiradiation medications as indicated.

2 The client is exhibiting the symptoms of *Yersinia pestis* exposure. Which of the following pharmacologic therapies would most likely be used in the treatment of this client?

1. Doxycycline
2. Trivalent botulinum antitoxin
3. Ribavirin
4. Atropine sulfate

3 The nurse has received a telephone call from an anxious mother of an 18-month-old child. In a panicked voice, the mother states, "I just discovered that my baby has swallowed an unknown amount of household cleanser." Which of the following would be the appropriate instructions given by the nurse?

1. "Consult the package instructions for information concerning poisoning."
2. "Force your child to vomit using a mixture of warm water and raw eggs."
3. "Take your child immediately to the nearest emergency department or health care agency."
4. "If your child develops seizures or difficulty breathing, call 911."

4 Activated charcoal is ordered for a client who accidently overdosed on prescription medications. For which of the following clients would the nurse question the order for activated charcoal?

1. Acute hepatitis and cirrhosis
2. Impairment of renal function
3. Decreased level of consciousness
4. Anxiety and nervousness

5 The nurse knows that the mechanism of action for chelating therapy is:

1. Removing positively charged metals.
2. Deactivating chemical reaction.
3. Increasing liver metabolism.
4. Decreasing glomerular filtration.

6 Which of the preadministration assessment parameters would the nurse consider before administering edetate calcium disodium (CaEDTA) to a client?

1. Bowel sounds
2. Urinary output
3. Visual acuity
4. Skin turgor

See Answers to Critical Thinking Questions, Case Study, and NCLEX-RN® Review in Appendix A.

References

Bartlett, D. (2005). Tricky toxic presentations at triage. *Journal of Emergency Nursing, 31*(4), 403–404.

Centers for Disease Control and Prevention. (n.d.). *Emergency preparedness & response: Viral hemorrhagic fevers.* Retrieved September 10, 2008, from http://www.bt.cdc.gov/agent/vhf/

Chess, C., & Clark, L. (2007). Weapons of mass destruction: Facilitation of risk communication during the anthrax attacks of 2001. *American Journal of Public Health, 97*(9), 1578–1583.

DePiro, J. T., Talbert, R. L., Yee, G. C., Matzke, G. R., Wells, B. G., & Posey, L. M. (2005). *Pharmacotherapy: A pathophysiologic approach* (6th ed.). New York: McGraw-Hill.

Gracia, R. C., & Snodgrass, W. R. (2007). Lead toxicity and chelation therapy. *American Journal of Health System Pharmacy, 64*(1), 45–53.

Green, S. L., Dargan, P. I., & Jones, A. L.(2005). Acute poisoning: Understanding 90% of cases in a nutshell. *Postgraduate Medicine Journal, 81*, 204–216.

Grey, M., & Spaeth, K. (2006). *The bioterrorism sourcebook.* New York: McGraw-Hill Professional.

Gunnell, D., Ho, D., & Murry, V. (2004). Medical management of deliberate drug overdose: A neglected area for suicide prevention? *Emergency Medicine Journal, 21*(1), 35–38.

Jett, D. A. (2007). Neurological aspects of chemical terrorism. *Annals of Neurology, 61*(1), 9–13.

Mothershead, J. L. (2006). Strategic National Stockpile program: Implications for military medicine. *Military Medicine, 171*(8), 698–702.

Patrick, L. (2006). Lead toxicity: A review of the literature-Part I—Exposure, evaluation, and treatment. *Alternative Medicine Review, 11*(1), 2–22.

Persell, D. J. (2008). Detection and early identification in bioterrorism events. *Family & Community Health, 31*(1), 4–16.

Teshima D., Taniyama T., & Oishi, R. (2001). Usefulness of forced diuresis for acute boric acid poisoning. *Journal of Clinical Pharmacology & Therapeutics, 26*(5), 387–390.

U.S. Army Center for Health Promotion & Preventive Medicine, Office to the Deputy for Technical Services. (1998). *Detailed chemical fact sheets.* Retrieved September 10, 2008, from http://chppm_www.apgea.army.mil/dts/dtchemfs.htm

United States Nuclear Regulatory Commission. (n.d.). *Fact sheet on the Three Mile Island accident.* Retrieved September 11, 2008, from http://www.nrc.gov/reading-rm/doc-collections/ fact-sheets/3mile-isle.html

Vinson, E. (2007). Managing bioterrorism mass casualties in an emergency department: Lessons learned from a rural community hospital disaster drill. *Management & Response, 5*(1), 18–21.

Watson, W. A. (2004). Annual report of the American Association of Poison Control Centers toxic exposure surveillance system. *American Journal of Emergency Medicine, 22*(5), 335–404.

Weiss, M. M., & Weiss, P. D. (2007). Anthrax vaccine and public health policy. *American Journal of Public Health, 97*(11), 1945–1951.

Appendix A

Answers to Critical Thinking Questions, Case Study, and NCLEX-RN® Review

Chapter 1

Answer to Connection Checkpoint 1.1

Colchicine is used for gout. Opium is available as a tincture for diarrhea (Paregoric) but is rarely used therapeutically. Cocaine was once used as an anesthetic but is now considered a major drug of abuse.

Answer to Connection Checkpoint 1.2

Anticoagulant, central nervous system agent, analgesic, and antipyretic describe therapeutic classifications. Salicylate is a pharmacological classification.

Chapter 1 Answers to Critical Thinking Questions

1 The therapeutic classification describes what the drug is treating. These drugs are often identified by the prefix "anti" such as antiseizure, anti-inflammatory, and antihypertensive. The pharmacologic classification describes how the drug acts within the body. A drug's pharmacologic classification is more specific than a therapeutic classification.

2 A barbiturate is the pharmacologic classification for a major sedative. A macrolide is the pharmacologic classification for a major type of antibiotic. Although the words "birth control pills" don't begin with "anti," this classification describes what the drug is being used for (anti-conception). A drug such as ibuprophen (more commonly known as Motrin or Advil) can be classified by its therapeutic use, i.e., anti-inflammatory. Antihypertensives are drugs that lower blood pressure and can also be classified according to their therapeutic use.

3 A prototype is a member of a category that best represents the group as a whole. A prototype is representative of a group, classification, or category. By learning a prototype drug, students can apply their knowledge of the actions and adverse effects of other drugs in the same class.

4 The nurse is a critical member of the health care team and has tremendous responsibility for a patient's drug therapy. The nurse not only administers medication but also closely monitors the patient for the desired outcome and adverse effects. Nurses provide patients with essential drug related education.

Chapter 1 Answers to Case Study Questions

1 Although generic drugs are less expensive than their brand name equivalent, they may vary in their bioavailability. In most cases, this difference does not affect the therapeutic effect of the drug and therefore can be safely substituted. However, in certain critical situations, the onset time of the drug may be extremely important. In such times, such as heart attack, stroke, or shock syndromes, generic forms of a medication may not be recommended.

2 To be safe, you should advise Sarah to talk with her health care provider or nurse practitioner about using generics. Explain to Sarah how important it is to inform her health care providers that her income status is limited. This information will assist the prescriber in determining the best and most cost effective treatment modalities for her.

Chapter 1 Answers to NCLEX-RN® Review

1 Answer: 3 Rationale: The indication is the conditions for which a particular drug is approved. Option 1 is incorrect. A description of how a drug works on its target organs and cells is called the mechanism of action. Option 2 is incorrect. The dosage is the amount of the drug that is given. Option 4 is incorrect. The conditions whereby the drug should be avoided are contraindications. Cognitive Level: Knowledge; Client Need: Safe, Effective Care Management; Nursing Process: Assessment

2 Answer: 3 Rationale: Trade names or proprietary names are designed to help the client remember the name of the drug. There may be multiple trade names for a drug. The chemical name refers to the chemical substances that comprise the drug. These names are often long, complicated, difficult to pronounce, and hard to remember. Most patients do not know the chemical names of their drugs (option 1). A drug's generic name is assigned by the U.S. Adopted Name Council. Drugs only have one generic name. Although generic names are less complicated and easier to remember, these names are often difficult to pronounce. In some cases, different drugs may have very similar generic names such as hydrochlorothiazide, hydromorphone, and hydrocortisone. Most patients will not be familiar with the generic nomenclature (option 2). The naming of drugs does not have a category called "standard" (option 4). Cognitive Level: Application; Client Need: Safe, Effective Care Management; Nursing Process: Assessment

3 Answer: 1 Rationale: Although it would be great if drugs alone could correct human disease and illness, the fact is that drugs are only tools that are part of the overall therapeutic treatment plan. Option 2 is incorrect because drug therapy alone is usually insufficient to correct and cure human illness. Many elements aid in the well-being of clients such as nutrition and sleep. Without the combination of multiple therapeutic interventions, drugs may be less effective. Option 3 is incorrect because nurses play a major role in the drug therapy of clients such as administering, educating, monitoring, and assessing the response to drugs. Option 4 is incorrect because too much reliance on drug therapy can diminish the importance of the nurse-client relationship. Cognitive Level: Application; Client Need: Safe, Effective Care Management; Nursing Process: Assessment

4 Answer: 1, 2, 3, 4 Rationale: Physiological responses to drug therapy are affected by a client's age and gender (option 1). Both race and body mass affect the physiological responses of drug therapies (option 2). A drug's physiological affect is dependent upon a client's health status (option 3). Many diseases such as diabetes have genetic origins. Familial history of disease conditions may reflect potential problems in the client (option 4). Not having medical insurance is not a physiological variable that would affect drug therapy. Cognitive Level: Application; Client Need: Safe, Effective Care Management; Nursing Process: Assessment

5 Answer: 2 Rationale: Bioavailability is the process that promotes drug accessibility to the receptors on body cells. Biotransformation is the chemical alteration of a substance within the body (option 1). Bioengineering is the study of the relationship between living organisms and machinery (option 3). The study of the chemical processes and compounds occurring in living organisms is biochemistry (option 4). Cognitive Level: Application; Client Need: Safe, Effective Care Management; Nursing Process: Assessment

Chapter 2

Answer to Connection Checkpoint 2.1

These are both therapeutic classifications because they describe what the drugs actually do, rather than their mechanisms of action.

Answer to Connection Checkpoint 2.2

The generic name is assigned by the United States Adopted Name Council. The trade, brand, or proprietary name is assigned by the drug manufacturer.

Chapter 2 Answers to Making the Patient Connection

1 Too many people think OTC drugs are harmless. Any drug can have dangerous properties if taken inappropriately, and adverse effects can vary from person to person. OTC drugs may produce toxic results if not used as directed. Also, the use of OTC drugs may prevent individuals from seeking health care when needed. OTC drugs should be used as a temporary measure for minor problems. Individuals who use OTC drugs for recurrent and persistent problems should see a health care provider.

2 Several advantages of OTC medications are: (1) Time—These drugs are available when the patient wants and needs them. They also do not require a visit to a health care provider. (2) Cost—In many cases, OTC drugs are reasonably priced. Many prescription medications are costly and may create financial hardship for individuals with limited resources. (3) Easy administration—Most OTC medications are created so that the administration is fairly simple and does not require any advanced knowledge of human physiology. (4) Readily accessible—OTC medications are sold in a variety of places from grocery stores to vending machines.

The disadvantages of OTC drugs are: (1) Improper use—Some individuals take OTC medications in improper amounts and frequencies. OTC medications should only be used as described in the directions. (2) Self-diagnosis—When patients diagnose themselves, the potential for misdiagnosis of serious and life threatening illnesses occurs. Using OTC medications is not a substitute for physical examination and care by a health care provider when the health problem is persistent. (3) Delay in seeking appropriate health care—When health problems are persistent or intense in nature, individuals should seek medical care. Individuals with conditions such as chest pain, chronic cough, or abdominal pain who prolong seeking medical care by taking OTC medications may increase the risk of disability and mortality.

3 Gertrude can obtain correct information about OTC drugs by talking to a pharmacist or health care provider. Most pharmacists and health care providers will be happy to talk with individuals about possible drug–drug interactions, adverse effects, and contraindications for OTC medications.

Chapter 2 Answers to Case Study

1 The FDA is a federal agency whose function is to protect the public by validating the safety and efficacy of drugs, medical devices, food, and cosmetics. This organization works to provide the public with accurate and scientific-based information related to pharmaceutical products.

2 While the FDA does not necessitate testing of herbal or dietary supplements prior to marketing, it monitors the administration of herbal products, dietary supplements, and cosmetics through the Center for Food Safety and Applied Nutrition (CFSAN).

3 In decades past, the approval of new drugs by the FDA was a long and tedious process. Since the early 1990s, the process has been expedited and now a drug can be approved in approximately 1 year.

Chapter 2 Answers to NCLEX-RN® Review

1 Answer: 2 Rationale: The FDA requires that drug manufacturers demonstrate both safety and efficiency of pharmaceutical products. Option 1 is incorrect because all drugs have potential reactions and adverse effects. Option 3 is incorrect because pharmaceuticals contribute to the overall crisis in health care costs. Government legislation has failed to regulate the cost of drugs. Option 4 is incorrect because most drugs have been tested only with specific populations that do not include women, ethnic groups, children, or the elderly. Cognitive Level: Knowledge; Client Need: Safe, Effective Care Management; Nursing Process: Assessment

2 Answer: 2 Rationale: A placebo is an inactive substance that doesn't produce a physiological reaction. The client should not experience an increase or decrease in symptoms due to taking the placebo (options 1, 3, and 4). Cognitive Level: Application; Client Need: Safe, Effective Care Management; Nursing Process: Evaluation

3 Answer: 2 Rationale: Most drug testing occurs with Caucasian males and therefore limits the generalization of the results to other populations. Drug testing is seldom performed on children, women, or elderly populations (options 1 and 3). Although many drugs are tested using animals, effectiveness in animals does not always verify that the drug will be effective in humans (option 4). Cognitive Level: Knowledge; Client Need: Safe, Effective Care Management; Nursing Process: Assessment

4 Answer: 4 Rationale: Telephone orders are not permissible under federal law for class II controlled substances. Refill prescriptions are usually not any more or less expensive than the original prescription (option 1). The number of listeners is irrelevant (option 2). Prescriptions are not confirmed or verified by the DEA (option 3). Cognitive Level: Application; Client Need: Safe, Effective Care Management; Nursing Process: Assessment

5 Answer: 1 Rationale: The more likely a drug's potential for abuse and dependency, the stricter the regulation to control access to the substance. The cost and production difficulty do not influence the degree of regulation (option 2). Adverse effects and drug or food interactions do not dictate the level of regulatory control (option 3). The length of time taken to confirm that a drug is effective does not affect the degree of regulation (option 4). Cognitive Level: Knowledge; Client Need: Safe, Effective Care Management; Nursing Process: Assessment

Chapter 3

Answer to Connection Checkpoint 3.1

OTC drugs are obtained more easily than prescription drugs. No appointment with a health care provider is required, thus time and money are saved.

Answer to Connection Checkpoint 3.2

Exclusivity prevents other companies from marketing a new drug. The developing pharmaceutical company gains sufficient time to recoup the millions of dollars involved in designing and testing the new drug.

Chapter 3 Answers to Critical Thinking Questions

1 It is important to remember that nonadherence includes not only a failure to take medication as prescribed, but also taking medicine at the wrong time or incorrectly. The most obvious factor that contributes to nonadherence is forgetfulness. Generally, when patients receive multiple medications during various times of the day, the chances of remembering to take the medication decreases.

The nurse should also consider other factors that contribute to nonadherence. The cost of a medication may be a possible reason. Patients may be reluctant to report that their income is limited, and that they cannot afford costly prescriptions. Additionally, the patient may not comprehend the importance of a medication. Some disease conditions may not produce troubling symptoms for a while, allowing the patient to feel well without the medication. Examples of such disease conditions include hypertension and diabetes. Both conditions can be asymptomatic. Some patients will choose to delete a medication due to the distressing adverse effects. Patients should be taught to report adverse effects to the prescriber. In some cases the adverse effects can be diminished by changing the dosage, drug form, or time of day the medication is taken. Many individuals fear dependency on medications and need to be educated about the difference between drug dependence and drug therapy with required medications.

2 One of the most important ways to promote adherence is to determine the reason for nonadherence. Talking with the patient and family members about the medication regimen is critical. In a nonjudgmental manner, the nurse should investigate the reasons for nonadherence and use this information to develop strategies that promote adherence. The nurse can also be instrumental in assisting the patient to adhere to the medication regime. A number of memory joggers can be used to help patients remember such as timers, pill boxes, posted notes, and the assistance of family and friends. If the reason for nonadherence is financial, the nurse can encourage the patient to seek medication assistance with the help of medical social worker, drug-company discount program, or discount pharmacy options. The nurse should also approach the prescriber about alternatives or substitutions when less expensive and just as effective medications may be available.

3 Patients need to learn as much as possible about their medications. They need to understand: the reason for the drug therapy; what the medication is intended to do, how soon the medication is expected to show results, how and when to take the medication, what adverse effects are expected and which ones to report to the prescriber, and what foods or other medications to avoid.

4 Patients vary in what they can and want to understand about their drug therapy. Nurses must assess the patient's ability to manage his/her own medication regimen. Some common factors that should be considered are the patient's age, educational level, and past experiences with medications.

Chapter 3 Answers to Case Study

1 It would be wonderful if we could just take a pill for everything. However, not all medications can be taken orally. In some cases, the route is determined by what will provide the best outcome given the patient's physical condition. Enteral routes require the patient to have fairly healthy gastrointestinal systems. The route may be determined by how rapidly the medication needs to get to the target organs. Lastly, some drug preparations only come in certain forms, thereby mandating the route to be used.

2 The advantages and disadvantages of this patient's medications are: (1) Sublingual medication, placed under the tongue, can be absorbed into the blood vessels and can enter general circulation before passing through the liver. The disadvantage is the patient must be able to cooperate by allowing the medication to dissolve under the tongue without chewing or swallowing it. Oral (PO) medications taken through the mouth, are the most common and convenient way of delivering drugs into the system. Oral drugs do not require special equipment or dispensing apparatus. However, depending on how the drugs interact with the stomach acids and the time needed to pass through the gastrointestinal system, oral drugs may need to be taken with or without food. Also, these drugs are contraindicated for unconscious patients or individuals suffering from nausea and vomiting. (3) A troche is a small, medicated lozenge designed to dissolve in the mouth. The advantages and disadvantages are the same as for sublingual medication. (4) Intravenous (IV) medication is injected into a blood vessel, typically a vein, for direct entry into circulation and can be precisely controlled in the amount given. The disadvantage is that absorption into the blood stream is immediate and can be potentially dangerous. There is also greater risk for infection. (5) Subcutaneous medications are injected in the skin and offer a means of administering drugs to patients who are unable to take medication orally. These drugs avoid digestive enzymes and the hepatic first pass effect. The disadvantage is that only a small amount of medication can be administered via this route and the risk of tissue damage, nerve damage, and infection are greater. (6) Optic solutions are delivered directly into the eye and provide direct medication administration to the target site with minimal systemic absorption. The disadvantage is that individuals with very sensitive eyes may have problems self-administering eye drops. (7) Transdermal patches provide continual and prolonged absorption of the medication. However, in some patients, the patch may cause dermal irritation.

3 Drugs that are enteric-coated and are designated as extended release or sustained release are specifically made to slow the absorption of the medication. For this reason, enteric coated drugs or drugs in extended release form should not be crushed, broken, or manipulated in any way because it will affect the absorption rate of the medication.

Chapter 3 Answers to NCLEX-RN® Review

1 Answer: 4 Rationale: Nonadherence to drug therapy, especially antibiotics, is a major problem. Many people will discontinue the medication when the symptoms disappear. It is critical that the client be instructed to take the medication as prescribed and for the entire specified time. The standards for prescription medications is set by governmental regulation. Consumers and health care providers can trust that medications meet an approved measure of quality (option 1). Toxic adverse effects do not produce the same symptoms of the condition the drug is prescribed for. Most likely when clients experience drug toxicity, an entirely different set of symptoms appear (option 2). Excessive dosage also produces toxicity related adverse effects (option 3). Cognitive Level: Application; Client Need: Safe, Effective Care Management; Nursing Process: Assessment

2 Answer: 2 Rationale: The rule—when in doubt, throw it out—is most often a good one to follow. However, hospital and pharmacies sometimes change brands. Before wasting, a medication it is often wise to consult the pharmacist about any concerns related to the appearance of the medication. The nurse must never administer a medication that has a questionable appearance (option 1). Physicians do not usually administer medications and in some cases are less likely to be capable of identifying what a drug should look like (option 3). Poison control centers are a valuable part of the health care team; however, it is unlikely that these professionals can verify the appearance of a drug (option 4). Cognitive Level: Application; Client Need: Safe, Effective Care Management; Nursing Process: Assessment

3 Answer: 4 Rationale: Vaginal suppositories can be very uncomfortable when the client's bladder is full. Vaginal suppositories dissolve once in place and should not be removed. (option 1). Cleansing the perineal area is not necessarily required before the insertion of a vaginal suppository (option 2). Vaginal suppositories can be used any time during the day and are not restricted to the morning only (option 3). Cognitive Level: Application; Client Need: Safe, Effective Care Management; Nursing Process: Implementation

4 Answer: 4 Rationale: The nurse should contact the prescriber to clarify the order and request another form of the drug be prescribed. The letters SR following Pronestyl indicate that this drug is released over a prolonged time frame. Any drug that has sustained or extended released should never be crushed or tampered with in any way. Altering the form of these medications will radically influence the absorption rate of the drug (option 1). When clients have gastrostomy or any gastric tubes, the nurse should suspect that there is a reason that the oral route cannot be used to administer medication. Prior to administration of this medication, the nurse should first consult the prescriber about giving the medication orally (option 2). Pharmacists are prohibited from changing a drug order without consulting the original prescriber (option 3). Cognitive Level: Application; Client Need: Safe, Effective Care Management; Nursing Process: Assessment

5 Answer: 2 Rationale: Stat is the abbreviation for statim, the Latin word for immediately. Option 1 is incorrect because the order for Lasix has no reference to meal times. Dispensing the medication as the client needs it would most likely be called prn, the abbreviation for pro re nata, which commonly means "as needed" or "as the situation arises" (option 3). Based on the written order, there is no indication that the client should self medicate (option 4). Cognitive Level: Application Client; Need: Safe, Effective Care Management; Nursing Process: Implementation

6 Answer: 1, 2, 5, 6 Rationale: A Drug Enforcement Administration (DEA) number is a series of numbers assigned to a health care provider allowing him or her to write prescriptions for controlled substances such as Lortab (option 1). A prescription must be dated. This prescription does not have a year of issuance (option 2). The prescription fails to state how many tablets the client should take every 6–8 hours (option 5). The number of refills has not been designated (option 6). Options 3 and 4 are incorrect answers. The health care provider has signed the prescription. The drug name and dosage are present. Cognitive Level: Application; Client Need: Safe, Effective Care Management; Nursing Process: Assessment

Chapter 4

Answer to Connection Checkpoint 4.1

Answer: Sustained-release, enteric coated or drugs that are bitter or have damaging effects on the oral mucosa should not be crushed or opened.

Answer to Connection Checkpoint 4.2

Buccal and sublingual are enteral, subcutaneous is parenteral, and intravaginal and rectal are topical.

Chapter 4 Answers to Critical Thinking Questions

1 Mr. Kessler's deteriorating condition will definitely affect drug metabolism. First, the condition of diabetes is an alteration in metabolism and therefore the nurse must always consider that drug therapies given to a diabetic patient may be influenced by this pathology. Additionally, consider Mr. Kessler's heart disease and hepatic function are directly related to cardiovascular function. When perfusion to the liver is less than optimal, it can disturb the hepatic metabolism of drugs and nutrients. Another consideration regarding metabolism involves his lifestyle and ultimately his hepatic function with his habitual use of alcohol. Chronic alcohol abuse is destructive to the liver.

2 The patient has pre-existing kidney disease and requires renal dialysis. Remember that pathological states such as kidney disease can increase the duration and intensity of drug action. The nurse must be particularly vigilant in monitoring the patient for signs of drug toxicity.

3 Both IV and inhalation routes of administration allow the drug to be immediately absorbed and circulated to the target organs. Therapeutic responses to drugs given by these routes are frequently rapid in onset, as are toxic effects. Although, these are the preferred routes of administration for this patient, the nurse must never forget that these techniques can be dangerous.

4 When it is desirable to achieve the target plasma level rapidly a loading dose (also known as bolus dose) is necessary. This large dose of medication is used to load the patient with the drug to achieve the therapeutic range quickly. Since the patient is critically ill, there is no time to wait several days for the desired therapeutic action. He will be given maintenance doses to maintain a steady plasma level of the drug.

Chapter 4 Answers to Case Study

1 There is no way to memorize the half-lives of all drugs. However, this is important information that will guide the nurse in effectively managing the patient's drug therapy. Plasma half-life is the time it takes for half a given amount of a substance, such as a drug, to be removed from the blood plasma. Liver and kidney function may affect the half-life. Drugs with a short half-life leave the body quickly and require more frequent dosing intervals; drugs with long half-lives leave the body more slowly and present a greater risk for medication accumulation and toxicity.

2 The indication for the use of drugs with short half-life is with conditions or procedures that are brief in duration. Patients with chronic illness such as renal and hepatic disease will probably fair better with short half-life drugs in regard to toxicities, but most need the benefits of a long half-life drug.

3 Drugs with long half-lives are particularly useful when it is critical to maintain a constant and consistent level of a drug in the body. Such conditions include hypertension and heart disease.

Chapter 4 Answers to NCLEX-RN® Review

1 Answer: 3 Rationale: This is a false statement. Food decreases the absorption rate of drugs. Options 1, 2, and 4 are incorrect because they are true statements. The liquid form of a drug will be absorbed faster than its tablet form. Greater responses are typically expected with higher doses. Clients should always consult a health care provider should unexpected adverse effects develop. Cognitive Level: Application; Client Need: Safe, Effective Care Management; Nursing Process: Evaluation

2 Answer: 1 Rationale: Infants do not develop a mature microsomal enzyme system until they are a year old and therefore do not metabolize drugs very efficiently. Pregnancy does not affect drug metabolism. The concern with pregnant clients is primarily focused on alterations in distribution due to the fetal-placental barrier (option 2). The presence of kidney stones would not influence drug metabolism (option 3). Hypertension is not a factor that directly results in abnormal metabolism (option 4). Cognitive Level: Application; Client Need: Safe, Effective Care Management; Nursing Process: Assessment

3 Answer: 1 Rationale: Remember that peristalsis is the wavelike muscular contraction that pushes food into the stomach and helps to mix stomach contents. An increase in this activity would decrease the time that drugs would remain in the GI system and therefore decrease absorption. Option 2 is incorrect because excretion for most drugs occurs mostly through the kidneys, lungs, and glands. Peristalsis would not reduce excretions of medications. Option 3 is incorrect because a delay in peristalsis would prolong absorption time. Option 4 is incorrect because peristalsis is not involved in the distribution of drugs to their target sites. Cognitive Level: Application; Client Need: Safe, Effective Care Management; Nursing Process: Assessment

4 Answer: 3 Rationale: Inhaled drugs produce an immediate therapeutic response. Option 1 is incorrect because inhaled medication can be used at any time during the day and are not restricted to the morning. Option 2 is incorrect because doses for inhaled drugs are extremely small compared to orally ingested medications. Option 4 is incorrect. Because these drugs go directly to the lung surface area and are readily absorbed, very little of the substance is lost due to metabolic reaction. Cognitive Level: Application; Client Need: Safe, Effective Care Management; Nursing Process: Evaluation

5 Answer: 4 Rationale: The length of time a drug concentration remains in the therapeutic range is its duration of action. Clients with renal disease are not effectively eliminating metabolized drugs, which increases the duration of action. Option 1 is incorrect because in kidney clients, the duration of action most likely will increase since drug excretion is impaired. Option 2 is incorrect. Although the length of time that the duration of action is extended, the effects of the drug are not improved. Option 3 is incorrect. Renal excretion will increase the duration of action Cognitive Level: Application; Client Need: Safe, Effective Care Management; Nursing Process: Assessment

6 Answer: 1, 2, 4, 5 Rationale: All anatomical structures have increased ability to store drugs in high concentrations. Option 3 is incorrect because blood does not have high affinity characteristics. Cognitive Level: Application; Client Need: Safe, Effective Care Management; Nursing Process: Assessment

Chapter 5

Answer to Connection Checkpoint 5.1

The pharmaceutical company must submit an Investigational New Drug (IND) application that contains all the animal testing data. Approval from the FDA is necessary before the next stage can begin.

Answer to Connection Checkpoint 5.2

By inducing CYP1A2, phenytoin would speed up the metabolism of acetaminophen and inactivate it. Thus phenytoin would be a functional antagonist of acetaminophen.

Chapter 5 Answers to Critical Thinking Questions

1 Potency refers to the amount of drug (usually expressed in milligrams) needed to produce an effect. Efficacy refers to the potential maximum therapeutic response that a drug can produce.

2 In most cases efficacy is more important than potency. However, When judging the relative merits of drugs for a patient, other factors should be considered, such as adverse effects, potential toxicity, duration of effect (which determines the number of doses needed each day), and cost.

3 Comparison of drugs is not always a simple process. Generally, higher doses produce more intense adverse effects. However when two drugs are compared, one cannot assume that the drug with the lower dose produces less adverse effects.

Chapter 5 Answers to Case Study Questions

1 Most drugs work through a mechanism that is similar to a key and lock. Drugs interact with cellular receptors and bind to specific sites to produce actions. When drugs are manufactured, companies attempt to create a drug that is specific to a specific receptor to produce a specific response. However, this is not always possible since receptors are located everywhere in the body. Drugs without a specific receptor site produce more adverse effects than those with specific receptors.

2 Several factors produce variation in drug effects among people. Such factors include an individual's unique metabolism rate, age, weight, sex, and hereditary influences.

3 A drug that is an agonist is a site-specific drug that initiates activity in the cell and triggers activity. A drug classified as an antagonist acts in an opposite way by blocking cellular activity.

Chapter 5 Answers to NCLEX-RN® Review

1 Answer: 1, 2, 3, 5 Rationale: One of the critical determinants of the effectiveness to drug therapy is a physical examination. Nurses will utilize assessment skills to ascertain whether the drug is being effective (option 1). In many cases, a client's vital signs may indicate the effectiveness of a drug such as a decrease in body temperature, a change in blood pressure and pulse or improved respiratory status (option 2). The effects of many drugs are monitored by diagnostic laboratory values such as white blood cell counts, cultures, and various electrolyte values (option 3). Option 4 is incorrect. The dosage time does not directly evaluate the effectiveness of drug therapy. Efficacy is correct because this term describes the ability of a drug to produce the desired therapeutic effect (option 5). Cognitive Level: Application; Client Need: Safe, Effective Care Management; Nursing Process: Implementation

2 Answer: 1 Rationale: Therapeutic index is the ratio between therapeutic dose of a drug and the toxic dose and is used as a measure of the relative safety of the drug. The higher the therapeutic index, the greater the safety of the drug. High therapeutic index doesn't equate to a more dangerous drug (option 2). The higher the therapeutic index, the less risk

of drug toxicity (option 3). A high degree of safety does not signify the degree of effectiveness (option 4). Cognitive Level: Application; Client Need: Safe, Effective Care Management; Nursing Process: Assessment

3 Answer: 1 Rationale: A dose response curve is a graphic representation that shows the relation between the amount of a drug administered and the extent of response it produces. A dose response curve does not illustrate the toxic effects related to a drug or any specific population (option 2). The dose response curve fails to graphically represent duration of action of a drug (option 3). Serum drug levels may be measured using a peak and trough method. However the dose is not decreased and neither parameter is measured with the dose response curve (option 4). Cognitive Level: Knowledge; Client Need: Safe, Effective Care Management; Nursing Process: Assessment

4 Answer: 4 Rationale: The TD_{50} measures the median toxicity dose. This information indicates the dose that will produce a given toxicity in 50% of a group of clients. Effectiveness is not measured using the TD_{50} indicator, which measures toxicity (option 1). A dose response curve measures the relation between the amount of a drug administered and the response it produces (option 2). Receptor subtypes are cellular molecules to which a medication binds to produce its effects and are not directly related to TD_{50} (option 3). Cognitive Level: Application; Client Need: Safe, Effective Care Management; Nursing Process: Assessment

5 Answer: 2 Rationale: Antagonists bind to receptors but do not activate them. Option 1 is incorrect. Antagonists have little or no efficacy. Option 3 is incorrect because antagonists do not activate receptors. Option 4 is incorrect because antagonists have low efficacy. Cognitive Level: Knowledge; Client Need: Safe, Effective Care Management; Nursing Process: Assessment

6 Answer: 1 Rationale: Potency is a reflection of a drugs ability to bind to a receptor. Efficacy and the affinity of drug binding to a receptor are separate variables (option 2). Metabolism is a function of pharmacokinetics not pharmacodynamics (option 3). First-pass effect is a phenomenon that occurs during enteral absorption and would not affect drug affinity (option 4). Cognitive Level: Knowledge; Client Need: Safe, Effective Care Management; Nursing Process: Assessment

Chapter 6

Answer to Connection Checkpoint 6.1

Oral drugs are absorbed into the hepatic-portal circulation which takes them to the liver. The liver can metabolize and inactivate the drug before it ever reaches the general circulation.

Answer to Connection Checkpoint 6.2

Phase 1 is the flat portion of the curve that indicates few target cells have been affected yet by the drug. Phase 2 is the straight-line portion of the curve where there is a linear relationship between the amount of drug administered and the degree of response obtained. In phase 3 a plateau is reached because all the receptors for the drug are occupied.

Chapter 6 Answers to Critical Thinking Questions

1 There are several steps a nurse can take to help Elizabeth minimize adverse drug effects. With the advent of computerized medical records, one can create a list of multiple medical diagnoses and medications. However, many institutions still use paper documents, especially clinics that treat lower socioeconomic patients. The nurses in the clinic may consider proposing a "medical summary page" be added to the medical record that could include medical diagnoses, hospital admissions, and prescribed drug therapies.

Secondly, Elizabeth should be advised to carry a list of her medications with her at all times. When patients are on multiple medications, it is easy to forget one or two when asked about drug therapies. Listing the purpose and dosage for each medication would also be helpful for Elizabeth and the health care provider.

Elizabeth should be instructed to report any symptoms or feelings that "just don't feel right." Furthermore, the nurse should encourage Elizabeth to become more assertive when health care providers suggest a new drug. Assure Elizabeth that it is acceptable to question health care providers when it concerns her health and her drug therapy.

Learning all her drugs and potential adverse effects may be overwhelming for Elizabeth. The nurse can assist her with ongoing education related to her drug therapy at each office visit or with follow-up telephone calls.

2 Several conditions make Elizabeth more susceptible to a drug reaction. The aging process makes the metabolism and excretion of drugs less predictable. Additionally, as the number of drugs a patient takes increases, the greater the risk of adverse drug reactions. Alterations in pharmacokinetics will influence the reactions expected from a given drug. The speed of absorption (specifically enteral drugs) may enhance or reduce the effect of a drug. The distribution of a drug can be altered through modification in protein binding and may produce an unpredicted reaction.

3 As you recall from previous chapters, pharmacokinetics is the movement of drugs from the point of administration to the target cell. Drug reactions can affect each element of pharmacokinetics. Drug–drug reactions that increase or decrease the gastric motility may influence absorption time for enteral drugs. Examples include laxatives and antacids. Additionally, when drugs compete for binding ability to plasma proteins or change the pH of the plasma, drug distribution can be altered. Any drug-generated modification in hepatic enzymes has the ability to cause a drug–drug interaction. Lastly, if a drug changes the rate of renal filtration, a drug interaction may occur.

4 An additive effect occurs when two drugs from a similar therapeutic class generate a combined response. A synergistic effect is the interaction of two or more drugs so that their combined effect is greater than the sum of their individual effects. An antagonistic effect is described as the interaction of two or more drugs that produces a reduced pharmacological response.

Chapter 6 Answers to Case Study

1 Patients are often confused when determining the difference between an adverse effect and a drug allergy. Ask the patient to describe what symptoms occurred related to the medication. Ask how the adverse symptoms were treated because allergic reactions are sometimes treated pharmacologically. It is questionable whether the patient received sufficient drug education or that she understood the possible adverse effects associated with this medication. Adverse effects from codeine almost always include nausea and sleepiness.

2 First, clarify the term drug allergy (known as hypersensitivity reaction). This reaction occurs due to an overactive response from the immune system. In an allergic response, the drug is recognized as the antigen and the body produces antibodies as a defense mechanism. Side effects are a by-product or consequence of a drug. They are usually predictable and characterized by an unwanted effect produced by a medication. An adverse effect is an abnormal, often harmful, undesired, and unintended result of a drug. Adverse effects are not necessarily unexpected. Sometimes, the terms "side effect" and "adverse effect" are used interchangeably.

3 The patient is not experiencing an idiosyncratic reaction. This type of reaction is defined as an unusual or exaggerated reaction to a drug that is not caused by an allergy. Many of these responses are related to the genetic differences between individuals.

Chapter 6 Answers to NCLEX-RN® Review

1 Answer: 1 Rationale: Collecting additional information will guide prescribers with information about other potential adverse effects. Determine which drug produced the adverse reaction as well as the presenting sign and symptoms. The nurse should not notify the prescriber until additional information is collected from the client or family members (option 2). The nurse should be prepared to provide the prescriber with as much information as feasible. Further inquiry is critical. Never administer a medication to a client when allergic sensitivity is suspected (option 3). Although documentation of the event may be in the client's medical record, the reaction may have never been documented. It is best to question the client further about the incident (option 4). Cognitive Level: Application; Client Need: Safe, Effective Care Management; Nursing Process: Assessment

2 Answer: 1 Rationale: When adverse effects are dose related the nurse knows to closely monitor the client for the onset of adverse effects as the dose of the drug is increased. Sometimes adverse effects are noted the first time a drug is administered. However, this is more commonly known as "first-dose effect" (option 2). Specific adverse effects are sometimes more prevalent in various routes of administration. However, this occurrence is more related to the way the drug is given rather than the dose (option 3). The timing of medication is not a factor associated with dose related adverse effects (option 4). Cognitive Level: Application; Client Need: Safe, Effective Care Management; Nursing Process: Assessment

3 Answer: 4 Rationale: Promoting hydration will dramatically reduce the odds of renal damage produced by drug therapies. Avoiding direct sunlight is the information given to clients receiving drugs that cause phototoxicity (option 1). The consumption of potassium-enriched foods will not reduce the chance of drug-induced nephrotoxicity (option 2). Avoiding alcohol consumption will not decrease the likelihood of drug-induced nephrotoxicity (option 3). Cognitive Level: Application; Client Need: Safe, Effective Care Management; Nursing Process: Implementation

4 Answer: 3 Rationale: Urticaria or hives, with raised, itchy areas of skin, is usually a sign of an allergic reaction. Angioedema is a notable swelling around the eyes and lips and sometimes of the hands and feet. The swelling occurs beneath the skin instead of on the surface (option 1). SJS is characterized by a flulike period of fever, sore throat, and headache followed by the sudden development of circular lesions that cover the majority of the skin (option 2). Phototoxicity occurs when a drug renders the skin susceptible to damage by light (option 4). Cognitive Level: Application; Client Need: Safe, Effective Care Management; Nursing Process: Assessment

5 Answer: 2 Rationale: The function of the bone marrow is to produce blood cells. When drugs cause bone marrow toxicity, the condition manifests as a decrease in all blood cell types. Muscle and bone pain are most often associated with muscle toxicity (option 1). Bone marrow toxicity is not related to a decline in an individual's range of motion (option 3). Liver enzymes are not typically affected by bone marrow toxicity (option 4). Cognitive Level: Application; Client Need: Safe, Effective Care Management; Nursing Process: Assessment

6 Answer: 3 Rationale: The presence of right upper quadrant pain and anorexia are the vague symptoms often associated with drug induced liver damage. Option 1 is incorrect because it is a symptom of superinfection which will be discussed with antibiotic therapy in another chapter. Option 2 is incorrect because it describes orthostatic hypotension, which will be discussed with cardiovascular pharmacology. Option 4 is incorrect because it describes symptoms that are characteristic of extrapyramidal symptoms which will be discussed with drugs that affect the neurological system. Cognitive Level: Application; Client Need: Safe, Effective Care Management; Nursing Process: Assessment

Chapter 7

Answer to Connection Checkpoint 7.1

An additive effect occurs when two drugs from a similar therapeutic class produce a combined summation response. A synergistic effect occurs when the response of the two drugs is greater than would be expected from simply adding the two individual drug's responses. Additive or synergistic effects can raise the drug effects to a toxic level.

Answer to Connection Checkpoint 7.2

The USP does not regulate drugs, but it does supply standards for drug purity, strength, and synthesis. Drugs marketed in the U.S. must conform to USP–NF standards to avoid possible charges of adulteration and misbranding.

Chapter 7 Answers to Critical Thinking Questions

1 The nurse is ultimately at fault in this scenario. It is not usual for patients to forget some part of their health history. Although Ross should have notified his health care providers of his suspected cardiac condition, health care professionals must always consider that patient-generated information may not always be totally accurate. The physician certainly should have indicated the route of administration that the drug was to be given. However, a nurse must never take a drug dose or drug route for granted and must clarify before administration. It is critical that nurses have a solid foundation in pharmacology and drug therapies. The administration of drugs must be taken seriously, as it could mean the difference between life and death.

2 Several contributing factors resulted in this fatal error. First, when there is any question, the nurse must be certain that the route of administration is clearly specified. Never assume to know the route or dose of a medication. When unfamiliar with a drug, always take time to look it up in a drug handbook. This would have alerted the nurse of a typical dose, possible adverse reactions to monitor, and the dilution required by the drug. It is virtually impossible to know everything about every drug. To ensure safety, the nurse must rely on quick resources to verify any unknowns. Lastly, not reading a label analytically is inexcusable. Nurses must pay meticulous attention to labels and directions.

3 There are multiple strategies that a nurse can employ to decrease the chances of medication error. The nurse always clarifies a medication order and never assumes dose or route. The nurse also learns to control anxiety. Although not stated in the case study, the nurse may have been anxious about the stat order. Remember that stat means immediately with carefulness and not with recklessness.

4 Health care facilities have taken multiple steps to reduce medication errors. In most hospitals, medications that require pre-mixing or preparation are done within the hospital pharmacy. When this is not the case, the medication is packaged with the solution to be used for dilution. Perhaps if this medication and the diluting solutions had been at least packaged together, the error might not have occurred.

Chapter 7 Answers to Case Study

1 Administering medications to children can be frightening and should never be taken lightly. Problems associated with both pharmacokinetics and pharmacodynamics are influenced by children's complex physiological growth and development. This scenario provides the nurse with an opportunity to develop rapport with the parent. You should discuss the child's health problems and gather other pertinent information that may be needed while the child is at school. Also, you need to determine exactly what this parent's concern is. Is it administration, adverse effects, or something else? As you talk with this parent, be specific in addressing the concerns.

2 Several strategies can help parents safeguard their children and avoid medication errors. Parents should make sure

- the child's health care provider knows the child's weight and has a list of every prescription, OTC medicine, and dietary supplements such as vitamins and herbs the child is taking.
- the child's health care provider knows about any allergies and how the child reacts to medicines.
- they can read the prescriptions written by the health care provider.
- the correct medication is being dispensed by the pharmacist.
- to ask for information about the child's medicines in understandable terms.
- to ask any questions about the directions on the child's medicine labels.
- to ask the pharmacist for the best device to measure the child's liquid medicine.
- to ask for written information about any adverse effects associated with the child's medicine.

3 Parents use many resources to gain information about medication for their children such as the Internet, drug guides, and friends and family. These sources may or may not provide correct information. The best resource a parent can use is the child's health care provider, nurse, or pharmacist who is knowledgeable about the child's health status.

Chapter 7 Answers to NCLEX-RN® Review

1 Answer: 4 Rationale: When medication orders are given via telephone, it is critical that the nurse repeat the order verbatim to the prescriber. Whenever possible it is best for the prescriber to write an order for medication, but this is not always possible (option 1). It is correct that the nurse should attempt to comfort the client using a number of nursing interventions for pain. However, the nurse is required to consult the prescriber when a change in the client's status occurs, regardless of the time (option 2). The nurse is responsible for contacting the prescriber. It is the nurse who can relay clinical findings and assessment (option 3). Cognitive Level: Application; Client Need: Safe, Effective Care Management; Nursing Process: Implementation

2 Answer: 1 Rationale: When in doubt always contact the prescriber, then have the order re-written to prevent future errors. Option 2 is incorrect. What if both nurses conclude on the wrong dosage? Do not take that chance. Contact the prescriber. Option 3 is incorrect. It is possible the pharmacist will also decode the order for the medication incorrectly. Option 4 is incorrect. A drug guide will provide the nurse with the normal dose for most clients. However, it does not consider the client's weight, disease condition, and a multitude of other variables that influence the drug's pharmacokinetic and pharmacodynamic actions. Cognitive Level: Application; Client Need: Safe, Effective Care Management; Nursing Process: Implementation

3 Answer: 2 Rationale: Pharmacies maintain records of medication dispensed to individuals. If a pharmacist can review the client's drug records, he or she can often detect serious potential drug–drug interactions. The insistence on brand names versus generic names does not ensure safe drug administration (option 1). For safety reasons, drugs are dispensed in containers that are sometimes difficult to open. Unless there is a specific reason (such as impaired hand dexterity), medications should be stored in their original safety bottles (option 3). Anyone can post practically anything to the Internet. Information may be incorrect and certainly does not take client specific variables into consideration (option 4). Cognitive Level: Application; Client Need: Safe, Effective Care Management; Nursing Process: Implementation

4 Answer: 3 Rationale: The nurse should always validate a questionable order that a client or a family member verbalizes. Yes, sometimes brands of medications change. However, to be safe, the nurse should withhold the medication and then confirm that the correct drug, dose, and route are being administered (option 1). If a client questions a change in medication or procedure, the nurse should verify the orders (option 2). Giving the drug without validation and advising the patient to talk with the health care provider is after the fact and too late to prevent a drug error (option 4). Cognitive Level: Application; Client Need: Safe, Effective Care Management; Nursing Process: Implementation

5 Answer: 1 Rationale: The nurse's first priority is the always the client. The nurse should determine if any ill effects have occurred. The health care provider should be notified of the medication error. However, this is not the most important action or the nurse's first priority (option 2). All health care agencies have reporting mechanisms for drug errors and the nurse will be responsible for completing this process. However, the assessment of the client must be the first priority for the nurse (option 3). All medication errors should be reported. The reporting mechanism will vary among institutions. Still, this is not the priority action for the nurse when a medication error occurs (option 4). Cognitive Level: Application; Client Need: Safe, Effective Care Management; Nursing Process: Implementation

6 Answer: 3 Rationale: This is the best response because it promotes a collaborative partnership between nurse and client and ensures that the client will receive the medication as ordered. Options 1 and 4 are incorrect. A nurse must ensure that the medication is taken by the client. Both actions are inappropriate and potentially unsafe. The nurse will not know with certainty that the client took the medication. The nurse must be certain that the medication is taken by the person for whom it was prescribed. Option 2 is incorrect. It is not wise, nor professional to place the client in this position. This statement will not foster a positive nurse/client relationship. Cognitive Level: Application; Client Need: Safe, Effective Care Management; Nursing Process: Implementation

Chapter 8

Answer to Connection Checkpoint 8.1

The Harrison Narcotic Act of 1914 was passed to require prescriptions for higher doses of narcotic drugs, and to require pharmacists and physicians to keep narcotic records.

Answer to Connection Checkpoint 8.2

CYP3A is a metabolic enzyme in the liver that alters the structure of many drugs. CYP3A usually detoxifies substances but, in the case of acetaminophen, a toxic substance is produced during metabolism.

Chapter 8 Answers to Critical Thinking Questions

1 J.C.'s substance use is classified as both a physical as well as a psychological dependence. Remember she said that when she is unable to acquire drugs, she feels sick with symptoms of trembling and diaphoresis. This would describe a physiological state that results in a withdrawal syndrome when addictive drug use is stopped. Secondly, her comments about needing drugs just to "get through the night" is characteristic of psychological dependence that is defined as a condition in which a person feels that he or she needs drugs in order to cope with problems.

2 Here are the drugs that J.C. reports using, along with the associated withdrawal symptoms:

Drug Reported	Withdrawal Symptoms
Alcohol	Tremors, anxiety, confusion, seizures
Heroin	Diaphoresis, agitation, dilated pupils (mydriasis), goose bumps (piloerection), and tremors
Crack	Agitation, depression, intense craving for the drug, and extreme fatigue
Valium	Rapid heartbeat, tremor, insomnia, sweating, irritability, anxiety, blurred vision, decreased concentration

It is critical that the nurse realize that patients with substance abuse problems frequently under report drug usage and may not report all substances used or the amount of the drugs consumed.

3 Drug use can trigger serious complications during pregnancy and possibly damage the fetus. Heavy consumption of certain drugs such as alcohol, tobacco, heroin, and tranquilizers taken during pregnancy can lead to premature birth, low birth weight, and increased risk of stillbirth. It is usually advisable for a pregnant woman to stop using drugs during pregnancy. However, this is not always the case when heroin abuse is present. Sudden discontinuation of heroin during pregnancy can be dangerous to the fetus. Some health care professionals believe that it is safer for the mother to continue using the drug until the baby is born.

4 Essential to dealing with a pregnant substance abuser is the development of a non-judgmental attitude. The effect of the substance abuse on the unborn child evokes strong emotions with most people, including nurses. However, little can be accomplished if a patient feels that the health care provider views him or her as evil or unworthy of health care. Obviously, J.C. needs a stabilizing force within her life. The nurse has a tremendous opportunity to assist this patient to seek a healthy lifestyle that will be a positive influence for both mother and baby. A nurse who is open and willing to accept the patient will have a greater chance of referring this patient to critical resources.

5 J.C.'s life has all the variables that trap her in a web of addiction. The drug factor in this case may include the quickness of the substance to relieve her psychological pain. Secondly, the user factors involve her risk-taking behavior (prostitution) and prior history of drug abuse. Lastly, J.C.'s limited opportunities for education and for the development of healthy social norms puts her at risk. Her peer influences were most likely individuals in similar living situations.

Chapter 8 Answers to Case Study

1 Delirium tremens, commonly known as "DTs" is a severe condition that occurs in chronic alcoholism due to sudden withdrawal from alcohol. This condition is complicated by physical and psychological deterioration that can progress from disorientation, hallucinations, and seizures, to death. Characteristic whole body tremors are associated with DTs. Mortality for this condition is reported at 20%. The treatment priority for this condition is prevention of seizure activity. Multiple drug therapies will be initiated to prevent seizure activity including antiseizure medications, sedatives, and vitamin therapy.

2 The key to the level of alcohol intoxication is directly related to the rate of excretion. There are no foods or beverages that will increase the excretion. Therefore, the consumption of coffee, for example, does not produce a sobering effect.

3 Alcohol consumption depresses the CNS. The effects are dose related and produce varying degrees of sedation, relaxation, loss of motor coordination, reduced judgment, and decreased inhibition.

Chapter 8 Answers to NCLEX-RN® Review

1 Answer: 1 Rationale: Addiction is not a problem for the majority of clients who receive narcotic analgesia post operatively. The nurse should administer the dose to treat the pain. It is inappropriate for the nurse to be concerned about addiction in a client who is 3 hours post-op. Reviewing the client's past medical history is an important assessment that should guide nursing practice. However, familiarity with the client's past tendencies toward substance abuse is not critical to the nurse's decision to treat the pain with analgesia (option 2). Pain is best treated in the early stage. If a nurse waits to treat pain until it becomes intolerable, the client will require more (high dose) of the analgesia (option 3). There is no evidence that clients request medication when it is not needed. In fact, some studies reveal that clients will use less pain medication when allowed to self medicate (option 4). Cognitive Level: Application; Client Need: Safe, Effective Care Management; Nursing Process: Assessment

2 Answer: 3 Rationale: Substance abuse users tend to revert back to drug-seeking behavior when they return to the company of other substance abusers. Option 1 is incorrect. A good support system can be extremely beneficial when an individual is attempting to withdraw from physiologically and psychologically addictive substances. Option 2 is incorrect. Clients with substance abuse problems may experience the desire to use drugs long after the drug has physiologically cleared the body. Option 4 is incorrect. Generally speaking, individuals who share a common experience will be perceived as being most helpful to an individual undergoing the same or similar experience. Cognitive Level: Application; Client Need: Safe, Effective Care Management; Nursing Process: Assessment

3 Answer: 4 Rationale: Tachyphylaxis is the rapid decreased response to a drug agent after administration of a few doses. Drug tachyphylaxis is not related to psychological dependence on a substance (option 1). The prompt reversal of a narcotic is accomplished by administering a narcotic antagonist but does not affect tachyphylaxis (option 2). Tachyphylaxis is related to drug tolerance and the physical adaptation of the body to a substance and is not related to psychological dependence (option 3). Cognitive Level: Application; Client Need: Safe, Effective Care Management; Nursing Process: Assessment

4 Answer: 2 Rationale: Sedatives cause a profound suppression of the respiratory system through direct action with the central nervous system. Clients who have overdosed from sedatives are at high risk for respiratory arrest. Sedatives do not typically cause any type of stimulation (option 1). The long-term effects of overdose will most likely manifest through liver and kidney dysfunction. However, this is not the most critical assessment to be done by the nurse (option 3). Level of consciousness is one of the assessments to be made with a client receiving sedatives. However, the nurse should expect a decrease in consciousness with an overdose of sedatives. The most important parameter is to monitor the client's respiratory status (option 4). Cognitive Level: Application; Client Need: Safe, Effective Care Management; Nursing Process: Assessment

5 Answer: 4 Rationale: Typical symptoms of heroin withdrawal include chills, dilated pupils, diarrhea, runny nose, muscle spasms, goose bumps, abdominal pain, sweating, and agitation. Option 1 is incorrect. Heroin is an opiate that depresses the central nervous system. Therefore, the nurse would expect the client to exhibit hyperactive behavior during withdrawal. Option 2 is incorrect. Withdrawal from heroin does not cause these dermatological conditions. Option 3 is incorrect. Paranoia is an over-inflated suspicion and distrust of others not based on fact. Hallucinations are a sensory experience in which a person can see, hear, smell, taste, or feel something that is not there. Delusions are defined as "fixed false beliefs." These symptoms are more typical of hallucinogenic drugs. Cognitive Level: Application; Client Need: Safe, Effective Care Management; Nursing Process: Assessment

6 Answer: 1 Rationale: Disulfiram (Antabuse) is a drug used in the rehabilitation of alcoholism. When clients are taking this drug, even small amounts of alcohol, as found in mouthwash and many over-the-counter medications, can produce flushing, throbbing in the head and neck, respiratory difficulty, nausea, vomiting, sweating, thirst, chest pain, blurred vision, and confusion. There is no reason for a client to avoid dairy products (option 2). Since many alcoholics also have nutritional deficits, it would be beneficial for the client to consume these foods. However, this does not relate to the drug and alcohol interaction that occurs with Antabuse (option 3). There is no reason to limit the client's driving or other activities other than drinking (option 4). Cognitive Level: Application; Client Need: Safe, Effective Care Management; Nursing Process: Assessment

Chapter 9

Answer to Connection Checkpoint 9.1

A medication error is any preventable event that may cause or lead to inappropriate medication use or patient harm while the medication is in the control of the health care professional, patient, or consumer. This example illustrates a preventable medication error.

Answer to Connection Checkpoint 9.2

Excessive cost of medication, forgetting a dose, not understanding instructions from the label or health care provider, not feeling that the therapy is worthwhile.

Chapter 9 Answers to Critical Thinking Questions

1 *Nursing Diagnosis: Fluid Volume Excess* related to compromised regulatory mechanisms.

Goal: By the end of the 12–hour shift, the patient will exhibit improved fluid volume balance AEB (as evidenced by)

Evaluation Criteria: Pitting edema improved to 1+ to 2+; absence of lung crackles; weight decreased by 2–3 pounds; blood pressure decreased to 130–140/80–86; diuresis of 400–600 mL. urine over 2 hours following IV administration of furosemide.

Implementation/Nursing Interventions: note serum potassium level prior to administering furosemide (this drug lowers potassium levels—if the level is abnormally low prior to drug administration, the drug would be held, and the prescriber notified); note the amount of urine output prior to administering the drug; administer the drug, following the 5 rights of drug administration, over the period of time specified in the drug handbook; document medication administration.

Evaluation Criteria: 4 hours after drug administration, the following evaluation data are obtained: 1+ to 2+ dependent pitting edema; lung sounds improved, but fine crackles remain in bilateral bases; blood pressure: 146/88, heart rate: 90; 650 mL urine out since drug administration; weight next morning: 69.4 kg (153 lb) (a decrease of 1.3 kg (3 lb). Evaluation: goal partially met; patient moving toward goal; drug therapy successful in improving problem; continue therapy to completely resolve the problem.

2 *Nursing Diagnosis: Risk for Injury* related to adverse drug effects.

Goal: Absence of injury AEB

Evaluation Criteria: serum potassium remains within normal limits; no change in patient's ability to hear; absence of dehydration: mucous membranes not dry, skin turgor normal, no abnormal thirst; absence of allergic reaction.

Implementation/Nursing Interventions: Prepare drug for administration, follow the 5 rights of drug administration, and identify the patient per institution's policy; review patient allergies; related to IV administration, determine: the need to dilute the drug, compatibility with other substances in the IV line, and the rate of administration (administering this drug too fast increases the risk for ototoxicity and hearing damage).

Evaluation: 4 hours following administration, the following data were gathered: serum potassium = 3.9 mEq/L (normal: 3.5–5.0 mEq/L); no change in hearing; mucous membranes moist, skin turgor normal, patient denies thirst; no signs/symptoms of allergic reaction. Evaluation: goal met; continue interventions for further doses of this drug.

3 *Nursing Diagnosis: Deficient Knowledge (Diuretic Self-Administration)*, related to new medication.

Goal: Knowledge of furosemide adequate to promote safe, effective home self-administration AEB

Evaluation Criteria: By the time of discharge, the patient will be able to state: the drug name, both generic and trade, route, dose, and timing of dose; therapeutic effects of the drug and when to expect them; duration of drug therapy; dietary considerations of drug therapy; main adverse effects, and which ones to report to the health care provider; drug interactions, including OTC drugs, nutritional supplements, or herbal remedies.

Implementation/Nursing Interventions: Provide patient teaching orally and in writing, to include: the drug name and dose; self-administration information: take once a day, by mouth, early in the day to prevent diuresis from disturbing sleep; remain on drug until told to stop; expected effects: increased urine output, ease of heart workload, and ease of breathing; adverse effects: lowered potassium levels; increase intake of potassium-rich foods such as bananas, citrus fruits and juices, potatoes, and tomatoes; dehydration, displayed as dry mouth, excessive thirst; lowered blood pressure (hypotension); monitor blood pressure and notify the prescriber should it lower considerably from normal; ototoxicity, or hearing loss; monitor for, and report to prescriber any changes in ability to hear.

Evaluation Criteria: on completion of patient teaching, gather evaluation data on criteria listed under Goal. Repeat teaching in any area where patient is unable to correctly identify the evaluation criteria.

Chapter 9 Answers to Case Study

1 Related to the drug therapy, the nurse should assess the patient's current medications, past medication use, any drug allergies and the reactions that occurred, and if the patient is pregnant or breast-feeding. Many drugs carry warnings for use during pregnancy or breast-feeding. Related to the disease process, the nurse should assess factors related to the infection including temperature, white blood cell count, the respiratory rate and oxygen saturation level, any shortness of breath, and auscultation of lung sounds.

2 Diagnosis: *Ineffective Airway Clearance* related to excess thick secretions; Goal: effective airway clearance AEB ability to expectorate respiratory secretions, respiratory rate within normal limits, oxygen saturation level 92% or greater on room air, no shortness of breath; Interventions: encourage high fluid intake to help liquefy secretions, encourage deep breathing and coughing, administer, or have patient self-administer antibiotics on a regular schedule to ensure steady serum drug levels.
Diagnosis: *Deficient Knowledge (Antibiotic)*, related to new drug therapy; Goal: adequate drug knowledge for self-administration AEB; able to state, drug name, dose, route, and timing of drug doses, duration of drug therapy, therapeutic effects and when to expect them, major adverse effects and which to report to prescriber, and methods for dealing with minor adverse effects such as nausea. Interventions: develop patient teaching to include the topics above, stress need to remain on antibiotic until prescription is completed, and any follow-up care that is needed.

Chapter 9 Answers to NCLEX-RN® Review

1 Answer: 1 Rationale: Drug allergies, current medications and disease states that could affect drug responses are elements of the baseline data gathered in the assessment phase of the nursing process. Options 2, 3, and 4 are not the appropriate phases of the nursing process for these actions. Cognitive Level: Application; Client Need: Physiological Integrity; Nursing Process: Assessment

2 Answer: Identification of the goal, or outcome, with evaluation criteria, and development of interventions are the two main steps of the planning phase of the nursing process. Cognitive Level: Application; Client Need: Physiological Integrity; Nursing Process: Planning

3 Answer: 3 Rationale: With respect to use with pharmacology, the implementation phase of the nursing process involves administering drugs and providing client drug teaching. Option 1 is incorrect because while performing interventions does belong in the implementation phase, developing interventions is done in the planning phase. Option 2 is incorrect because while providing client teaching is done in the implementation phase, evaluation of that teaching is done in the evaluation phase. Option 4 is incorrect because assessment and evaluation of adverse effects are done in the evaluation phase, rather than in the implementation phase. Cognitive Level: Application; Client Need: Physiological Integrity; Nursing Process: Implementation

4 Answer: 2 Rationale: While each of the answers would be appropriate to evaluate in the evaluation phase of the nursing process, the most important aspect for the nurse to evaluate would be evidence of therapeutic drug effects, since the goal of drug therapy is to cause some beneficial effect. If there is no evidence of therapeutic effects, the drug would likely need to be changed. Cognitive Level: Application; Client Need: Physiological Integrity; Nursing Process: Evaluation

5 Answer: 1, 3, 4 Rationale: Options 1, 3, and 4 are appropriate areas in which to obtain data in the assessment phase. Therapeutic response to a drug (option 2) and prevention of adverse effects (option 5) are determined in the evaluation phase of the nursing process. Cognitive Level: Application; Client Need: Physiological Integrity; Nursing Process: Assessment

6 Answer: 4 Rationale: *Fatigue*, related to sleep deprivation and physical deconditioning, is a properly worded nursing diagnosis. Fatigue is not a disease state, but a response to other causes. It is acceptable to list more than one etiology for a problem, and both the etiologies listed can be addressed by nursing interventions. Option 1 is incorrect because skin integrity related to diabetes gives an etiology (diabetes) that is a medical diagnosis, not something that could be affected by nursing interventions. Option 2 is incorrect because *Risk for Injury* and *Deficient Knowledge*, list two separate diagnoses; these need to be considered by themselves in separate diagnoses. Option 3 is incorrect because pneumonia related to retained secretions uses a medical diagnosis (pneumonia) and not a nursing diagnosis. Cognitive Level: Application; Client Need: Physiological Integrity; Nursing Process: Diagnosis

Chapter 10

Answer to Connection Checkpoint 10.1

Nicotine is a stimulant. The cardiovascular effects of nicotine include an accelerated heart rate and increased blood pressure. Babies born to smoking mothers have lower birth weights and higher risks for respiratory disorders.

Answer to Connection Checkpoint 10.2

Known teratogens may be safely approved for indications in patients who do not have the potential to become pregnant. In most cases these drugs do not affect male reproductive ability, and they are also safe to use in elderly patients.

Answer to Connection Checkpoint 10.3

Each half-life eliminates 50% of the dose. The amount remaining would be 300 mg at 1 half-life (8 h), 150 mg at 2 half-lives (16 h), 75 mg at 3 half-lives (24 h), 37.5 mg at 4 half-lives (32 h) and 18.25 mg at 5 half-lives (40 h).

Chapter 10 Answers to Critical Thinking Questions

1 Once you have established that Ms. David is indeed pregnant, your first concern is to find out whether or not she wishes to continue the pregnancy. If she does, then you must address the issue of her taking the antiseizure medication and the potential harm it may cause to the fetus. In this case it must be determined if the benefits of taking the drug outweigh the risks to the fetus. Studies suggest that pregnant women who take antiepileptic drugs have a higher incidence of bearing children with birth defects such as cleft lip or palate, heart malformations, fetal growth deficiency, and mental deficiency. On the other hand, if the woman discontinues her antiseizure drug, increased seizure activity may occur. The health care provider will provide Ms. David all the pros and cons related to continuing her pregnancy and taking antiseizure medication in order for her to make an informed decision. The decision on whether or not to continue taking the drug is one that Ms. David will make in collaboration with her health care provider and will not be taken lightly.

2 At this early stage of pregnancy the nurse would provide Ms. David with all the standard information regarding caring for herself and her fetus during pregnancy. She should be advised to avoid all medications and herbal supplements unless prescribed by the health care provider and under careful monitoring. You inform Ms. David that smoking, illicit drugs, and alcohol all may have deleterious effect on the fetus and should be avoided. If Ms. David chooses to continue taking her medication, the health care provider will adjust the dose to the lowest effective one and she would be required to have multiple serum checks during the pregnancy. You should advise Ms. David that it is vital that she adhere to the prescribed drug regimen.

3 The FDA has established pregnancy categories A, B, C, D, and X, according to the risk assigned. According to the FDA, category A consists of drugs that have failed to demonstrate a risk to the fetus in the first trimester or subsequent trimesters. Category B means there really is not enough information to determine the risk the drug has on the fetus. Category C means that animal studies have revealed adverse fetal effects but that no controlled studies in women have been done, or that no studies in women or animals are available. With category D drugs there is clear evidence of human fetal risk, but the benefits derived from use in pregnant women may outweigh the risk. Lastly, category X includes drugs which have clearly demonstrated fetal abnormalities, and the risk of using the drug in a pregnant woman clearly outweighs any benefit.

4 Nicotine creates a negative interuterine environment. Smoking nearly doubles a woman's risk of having a low birth-weight baby. Low birth weight can result from poor growth before birth, preterm delivery, or a combination of both. Smoking has long been known to slow fetal growth. Smoking also increases the risk of premature birth. The more a pregnant woman smokes, the greater the risk to her baby.

Chapter 10 Answers to Case Study

1,2 You explain to Irina that using illicit drugs while breast-feeding is an unhealthy behavior that she should avoid. Furthermore, you inform her that the marijuana enters her milk and reaches the baby. It may cause her baby to become sleepy and unable to take in an adequate amount of milk. Insufficient nutrition will ultimately alter his growth and development. Irina may need a referral to other health care professionals such as a mental health counselor to deal with her depression. The nurse should be concerned for both mother and baby since it is typically thought that mothers who use drugs have impaired ability to care for their infants.

Chapter 10 Answers to NCLEX-RN® Review

1 Answer: 2 Rationale: Although many pregnant women find it necessary to take one type of drug or the other during pregnancy and lactation, it is still recommended that all drugs be avoided as much as possible due to the potential effect on the fetus or infant. OTC drugs can be hazardous and may affect the unborn fetus and nursing child (option 1). Drugs used for treating medical conditions such as asthma, hypertension, diabetes and epilepsy should be continued throughout pregnancy for the safety of both mother and infant. There must be close monitoring from the health care provider. In such cases the benefits may outweigh the risks (option 3). The woman should collaborate with her health care provider regarding any drugs taken during pregnancy and lactation (option 4). Cognitive Level: Application; Client Need: Physiological Integrity; Nursing Process: Implementation

2 Answer: 4 Rationale: Drugs within category X are clearly contraindicated because they pose serious risk to the unborn fetus. Category A drugs are safe for the pregnant woman as they demonstrate no risk to injuring the unborn fetus (option 1). Category B consists of drugs that may be given to the mother during pregnancy (option 2). Drugs in category C represent those whereby there is insufficient evidence that the drug is either safe or dangerous to the fetus. Many drugs are in this category simply because the effects on the fetus are unknown (option 3).

3 Answer: 1 Rationale: Although there are multiple factors that impact the transfer of drugs across the placenta, highly lipid soluble drugs will cross the placental barrier more easily than water soluble drugs. Option 2 is an untrue statement. Option 3 is incorrect because small molecules such as alcohol with molecular weights (MW) less than 300 easily cross the placental barrier, while those with higher MW greater than 500 are slower to cross. Option 4 is incorrect because when drugs are highly protein bound, they are too large to cross the placental membrane. Cognitive Level: Application; Client Need: Health Promotion and Maintenance; Nursing Process: Implementation

4 Answer: 1 Rationale: Weeks 1–2 of the first trimester are known as the preimplantation phase. Before implantation, the developing embryo has not yet established a blood supply with the mother. This is sometimes called the "all-or-none" period because exposure to a teratogen either causes death of the embryo or has no effect. Drugs are less likely to cause congenital malformations during this period because the baby's organ systems have not yet begun to form. Options 2, 3, and 4 are incorrect because the embryonic period is 3 to 8 weeks postconception. During the embryonic period there is rapid development of internal structures and maximum sensitivity to teratogens. Teratogenic agents taken during this phase can lead to structural malformation and spontaneous abortion. The specific abnormality depends upon which organ is forming at the time of exposure. Cognitive Level: Analysis; Client Need: Physiological Integrity; Nursing Process: Planning

5 Answer: 4 Rationale: The form of the medication does not affect the passage of drug into the breast milk. The statement in option 1 demonstrates the client knowledge related to the need to use the lowest dose of an OTC drug so it is incorrect. Option 2 is incorrect. It is true that the higher the dose, the more likely the drug will enter the breast milk. Option 3 is incorrect. The client making this statement understands that drugs that work on the nervous system will most likely penetrate the breast milk. Cognitive Level: Application; Client Need: Health Promotion and Maintenance; Nursing Process: Implementation

6 Answer: 3 Rationale: Increased levels of progesterone cause a decrease in gastric tone and intestinal motility resulting in delayed gastric emptying. This leads to extended time for drug absorption. Option 1 is incorrect. Medications may take a longer time to be absorbed and distributed, thus prolonging their onset and durations of action. Option 2 is incorrect. Due to the changes in body fluid volume associated with pregnancy there is greater hemodilution, not hemoconcentration of drugs. Option 4 is incorrect. Of all pharmacokinetic factors, drug metabolism is least affected by pregnancy. Cognitive Level: Knowledge; Client Need: Safe, Effective Care Management; Nursing Process: Implementation

Chapter 11

Answer to Connection Checkpoint 11.1

Food, especially if high in fat, will slow drug absorption. Frequent feedings can slow absorption of drugs given to the baby by the enteral route.

Answer to Connection Checkpoint 11.2

Nursing diagnoses are often stated as a problem, or the risk for a problem, followed by 'related to,' which identifies the etiologies, or those conditions that have caused or contributed to the problem.

Answer to Connection Checkpoint 11.3

This unexpected, unpredictable response is an idiosyncratic effect.

Answer to Critical Thinking Question in Evidence-Based Practice Feature

First the severity of the condition must be verified before any form of treatment is established. Parents must be educated as to the reason for the type of treatment prescribed and be given an option when feasible. Management of symptoms such as earache, fever, and irritability is a priority. There must be access to follow-up care and access to initiation of antibiotic treatment if the condition does not resolve spontaneously. Although only a small percentage of children might suffer increased morbidity if denied antibiotic treatment, the risk of using 'watchful waiting' may result in children developing hearing loss, mastoiditis, meningitis, and recurrent attacks.

Chapter 11 Answers to Critical Thinking Questions

1 The infant's fluid and electrolyte balance is very easily altered when there is vomiting and diarrhea. The infant has a very high (80%) of total body fluid compared to mass. Compared to adults that have a 6% water turnover daily, infants lose and replace up to 25% of their total body water over a period of 24 hours. When an infant stops taking in fluids over a

72-hour period, there is a very high potential for severe dehydration, coupled with the fact that the infant is experiencing diarrhea. Also, the infant has a high metabolic rate that causes increased water loss. Another reason for fluid and electrolyte imbalance is the fact that the infant's immature renal system prevents concentration and retention of fluid.

2 The nurse evaluating a patient experiencing excessive water loss through vomiting and diarrhea will find that the patient has decreased peripheral perfusion. When the body is no longer able to compensate for fluid loss, the total circulating volume is diminished, and peripheral vessels constrict. When assessing the dehydrated infant you will expect to find weak to absent peripheral pulses, slow capillary filling, mottled skin color, tenting of the skin between the thumb and forefinger when picked up, rapid respiration, depressed anterior fontanel, and dry sunken eyes.

3 Acute gastroenteritis is usually attributed mostly to viral infections. The virus alters the balance of fluid and electrolytes in the bowels causing stool and water loss. This patient you may recall was being treated with an oral antibiotic for otitis media, cause undetermined. It is possible that the antibiotic could have caused the diarrhea.

4 Inserting and maintaining an IV line on an infant can be challenging for the nurse. The nurse must accurately calculate the volume of fluid the child needs and set the rate of flow accordingly. The following formula is used to calculate IV fluids. Drops per minute = Total volume ordered × gtt/min/Total infusion time (h). The tiny veins are sometimes hard to find under normal circumstances, and, when the patient is dehydrated it can be twice as difficult. Choosing a site that can be stabilized, easily observed, and does not restrict the infant's movement, is of utmost importance. You would choose superficial veins of the hand, forearm, foot, or ankle. The ultimate goal is to deliver the fluids without complications; thus the right size catheter and tubing must be chosen. In the infant a 22-gauge needle is usually appropriate but the nurse knows to choose the smallest gauge and shortest length catheter that can deliver the prescribed fluid and medication. The IV site must be monitored at least every 15 minutes for redness, swelling, and discoloration. Remove the IV when there is a doubt as to its proper functioning.

5 Acetaminophen was given to correct the fever. It was administered rectally because Timmy has been vomiting and may not tolerate the oral solution.

Chapter 11 Answers to Case Study

1 The first nursing action is to render emergency airway care to insure proper breathing. This includes placing the patient in a sitting position to maintain an open airway and administering oxygen as needed.

2 You would next carry out a full assessment of vital signs including temperature, pulse, respiration, blood pressure, and chest examination for cardiopulmonary status. Vital signs most likely will be elevated with hyperresonance present over the lung fields.

3 You then make sure that epinephrine is on hand. Patients in status asthmaticus can expect to be given epinephrine 1:1000 at a dose of 0.01 mg/kg at a maximum of 0.3 mL subcutaneously along with Terbutaline sulphate treatment 1 mL in 2.5 mL normal saline by nebulizer. A maintenance intravenous drip of D_5W at a rate of 30 mL/h to correct acidosis is also given. Often a dose of steroid such as Solu-Medrol is given to address inflammation.

4 The expected outcome of treatment for status asthmaticus is that the patient will have improved ventilation, correction of dehydration and acidosis, and relief of concurrent infections.

Chapter 11 Answers to NCLEX-RN® Review

1 Answer: 4 Rationale: Delayed gastric emptying causes oral medication to remain longer in the stomach resulting in slowed absorption and more risk for adverse drug reactions. The slow gastric motility will keep the drug longer in the stomach. This will increase the absorption of drugs that are absorbed across the stomach lining, but slow the rate of drug absorption for those that rely upon the intestine for absorption. Options 1–3 are incorrect because increased (not decreased) gastric pH, decreased (not increased) gastric emptying, and low (not high) gastric acid production may enhance the absorption of acid-labile drugs such as ampicillin and slow the absorption of weak acids such as Phenobarbital. Cognitive Level: Application; Client Need: Physiological Integrity; Nursing Process: Assessment

2 Answer: 1 Rationale: The vastus lateralis muscle mass is the most developed in infants and young children and therefore most appropriate for IM injections. The deltoid (option 2), dorsogluteal (option 3), and ventrogluteal (option 4) have very little muscle tissue available for injection and may have erratic blood flow leading to decrease medication absorption. Cognitive Level: Analysis; Client Need: Physiological Integrity; Nursing process: Implementation

3 Answer: 1 Rationale: IM injections in infants are absorbed slowly due to low blood flow to skeletal muscles. Option 2 is incorrect because children experience delayed absorption and distribution of IM drugs. Option 3 is incorrect because IM medications are absorbed slowly and erratically in children. Option 4 is incorrect because children possess very weak muscle contractions that contribute to the delayed absorption and distribution. Cognitive Level: Application; Client Need: Physiological Integrity; Nursing Process: Implementation

4 Answer: 3 Rationale: At 3 years of age the child begins seeking control and independence. Giving the client a choice of liquid with which to combine the medicine will give the client the feeling of control and independence and at the same time encourage cooperation. At age 3 years the child does not yet associate medicine with getting better (option 1). Threatening a child to take medicine is never recommended and may have long-term implications (option 2). 3-year-old clients do not imitate actions unless they want to, and saying that a roommate took their medicine may not result in the client doing the same (option 4). Cognitive Level: Analysis; Client Need: Physiological Integrity; Nursing Process: Implementation.

5 Answer: 3 Rationale: Drugs with extensive protein binding compete for binding sites resulting in increased absorption and high potential for drug interactions. Low potency drugs (option 1), drugs with wide therapeutic index (option 2), and drugs applied to the skin (option 4) are at low risk for drug interactions. Cognitive Level: Application; Client Need: Physiological Integrity; Nursing Process: Implementation

6 Answer: 1 Rationale: Children are most likely to adhere if their medication regimen is simple and inexpensive. Clients are less likely to adhere to the regimen if the medications are costly (option 2), they have to be taken over an extended period of time (option 3), or they have to be taken at varying times during the day (option 4). Cognitive Level: Analysis; Client Need: Physiological Integrity; Nursing Process: Evaluation

Chapter 12

Answer to Connection Checkpoint 12.1

Additive effect: two drugs from a similar therapeutic class produce a summation response. Synergistic effect: effect of the two drugs is greater than would be expected from adding the two drug's responses. Antagonistic effect: effect of the two drugs is less than would be expected from adding the two drugs' responses.

Answer to Connection Checkpoint 12.2

CYP is an enzyme complex named after cytochrome P450, a key component of the hepatic microsomal system. A substrate is a drug that is metabolized by CYP. An inducer is a drug that has the ability to increase metabolic activity in the liver.

Answer to Connection Checkpoint 12.3

This legislation pays 75% of prescription drug spending up to the first $2,250. Those qualifying for the low-income criteria may have their premiums and cost subsidized by the government. Participants are protected against catastrophic costs at $3,600 per year with most beneficiaries paying a co-pay amount of 5%.

Chapter 12 Answers to Critical Thinking Questions

1 Older adults are at increased risk for dehydration because of age-related physiologic changes, including altered thirst perception, reduced total body water, increased proportion of fat to muscle, impaired renal conservation of water, and increased prevalence of multiple chronic diseases. Ms. Smith's risk factors for dehydration are that she is functionally independent, has poor fluid and nutritional intake, is taking four medications, and has a fever. Her depression could be a cause of her inability to fully care for herself and neglect of her fluid intake.

2 The first priority for the nurse is to assess the level of dehydration and begin efforts to rehydrate the patient. Dehydration may present in older adults as confusion, a change in the level of consciousness, and fatigue. Hydration management intervention is determined based on a comprehensive assessment. There are three phases that the nurse uses in caring for this patient. First the nurse must take the patient's vital signs, then perform a head-to-toe assessment, and last, identify risks. Next, laboratory tests are used to predict levels of dehydration. Some laboratory studies may indicate the level of dehydration in this patient. These may include blood urea nitrogen (BUN), urine and serum creatinine levels, and urinalysis. Urinalysis is used to identify or predict impending dehydration. Urine from a dehydrated patient may be concentrated and scant in amount and have a high specific gravity and dark color. The final phase for the nurse is the hydration management. This includes ongoing management of IV and oral fluids. A generally accepted standard for daily fluid intake for adults is 100 mL/kg of weight for the first 10 kg of body weight, 50 mL/kg for the next 10 kg, and 15 mL/kg for the remaining weight.

3 Chronic dehydration manifests as confusion, urinary tract infections, respiratory infections, and constipation. First, complete a full physical assessment including temperature, pulse, and respiration (TPR) and blood pressure (BP). Altered TPR readings can indicate hyperthermia due to dehydration, tachycardia due to hypovolemia, and tachypnea secondary to acidosis. The condition of the skin may reveal tenting secondary to severe dehydration. There may be hypotension secondary both to hypovolemia and response to phenothiazine, an alpha-blocker. Altered mental status or confusion should be assessed because this may be secondary to polypharmacy.

4 The nurse documents expected patient outcomes relevant to hydration management. The outcomes include the patient's ability to maintain body hydration, an improvement in urinary output with urine pH between 4.6 and 8, a urinary specific gravity of 1.005 to 1.025, and urine that is clear and amber in color. The patient should also exhibit decreased acute confusion.

Chapter 12 Answers to Case Study

1 Diphenhydramine has a relatively strong anticholinergic effect. Older people are very susceptible to possible adverse effects of anticholinergic drugs, which can include delirium, memory loss, urinary retention, and constipation. Lorazepam also works on the CNS, and although it may be effective, it can also worsen confusion in older adults.

2 Ms. Brown's underlying dementia is a major risk factor for delirium. Certain medical conditions like pneumonia often cause delirium and worsening confusion. A change in environment (the hospital) can also result in confusion in older adults.

3 The nurse should point out to Ms. Brown that her reaction to the penicillin was due to an allergy. Ms. Brown and her family members should be instructed to always inform her health care provider of this fact and never to take penicillin or its other medicines in the penicillin family. The patient must also be instructed to wear a medic alert bracelet. (See also Chapter 48.)

Chapter 12 Answers to NCLEX-RN® Review

1 Answer: 1 Rationale: Increased gastric pH is a common physiological condition of aging that can affect absorption, distribution, metabolism, and excretion of drugs. Options 2, 3, and 4 are incorrect because blood flow rate, GI motility, and body surface area decrease in the elderly; they do not increase. Cognitive Level: Comprehension; Client Need: Health Promotion and Maintenance; Nursing Process: Implementation

2 Answer: 2 Rationale: A client who is functioning independently in all areas of ADLs should be encouraged to take full responsibility for self-administering medications. This encourages self-efficacy and provides a sense of self-control. Teaching the daughter to administer the insulin should be a choice made by the daughter only (option 1). There is no reason for recommending a home health aide if the client is competent in self-administering (option 3). Since the client's condition calls for insulin there is no need to change to an oral hypoglycemic for the sake of convenience (option 4). Cognitive Level: Application; Client Need: Health Promotion and Maintenance; Nursing Process: Assessment

3 Answer: 3 Rationale: As the person ages lean muscle mass decreases which alters the body's ability to handle drugs. Total body fat increases rather than decreases (option 1). Lean muscle mass decreases rather than increases (option 2). Alteration in serum hemoglobin does not influence the way drugs are prescribed (option 4). Cognitive Level: Application; Client Need: Safe, Effective Care Environment; Nursing Process: Assessment

4 Answer: 1, 2, 3 Rationale: Excessive prescribing, multiple drug therapy, and increased drug sensitivity are all reasons for adverse effects in older adults. As persons age renal function decreases, leading to alteration in pharmacokinetics and pharmacodynamics. Coupled with multiple drug therapy and increased sensitivity, it is not unusual for adverse effects to develop. Body mass decreases as age increases (option 4). Exercise engagement does not influence frequency of adverse effects (option 5). Cognitive Level: Knowledge; Client Need: Health Promotion and Maintenance; Nursing Process: Assessment

5 Answer: 2 Rationale: 36% of clients report that they stop taking their medications once the symptoms go away. Clients should be encouraged to take all medications as prescribed even when they are feeling better. Discontinuing medications prematurely may result in worsening of the client's condition. Options 1, 3, and 4, drugs preventing the client from fully functioning, lack of sufficient funds, and lack of belief of the effectiveness of the drugs have also been cited as reasons for nonadherence, but to a lesser degree. Cognitive Level: Analysis; Client Need: Physiological Integrity; Nursing Process: Implementation

6 Answer: 1 Rationale: Clients will mostly comply with prescribed drug regimens if they believe in the efficacy of the drug, can afford to purchase it, and can see visible improvement in the initial condition. Making the statement, "It doesn't matter if the medication works as long as the doctor prescribed it" should raise a red flag for the nurse as to the level of adherence that may be expected from this client. Options 2, 3, and 4 are positive responses by the client that might indicate potential for adherence. Cognitive Level: Application; Client Need: Health Promotion and Maintenance; Nursing Process: Implementation

Chapter 13

Answer to Connection Checkpoint 13.1

See Figure 5.1 in Chapter 5 on page 56.

Answer to Connection Checkpoint 13.2

Drug A would induce, or increase the activity of CYP enzymes. Because Drug B is inactivated by the same enzymes, more would be removed from the blood and it would exhibit less pharmacological activity.

Chapter 13 Answers to Critical Thinking Questions

1 It is critical that nurses strive to understand the patient's cultural beliefs about health and the attainment of wellness. The nurse must remain non-judgmental about cultural practices that may seem different or unusual to their own. Open communication will establish a rapport with the patient and will allow the nurse to better understand the patient's beliefs and practices. If patients experience prejudicial criticism from health care providers, they are likely to be selective in what they are willing to talk about. When this communication breakdown occurs, an increased risk of potentially harmful drug interactions between conventional and the non-conventional health care practices may occur.

2 Most patients are willing to share cultural beliefs and practices. Often the nurse can engage the patient in casual conversation, which may reveal valuable information. However, this is unlikely to occur if the nurse fails to assess the individual holistically. When health care providers believe in holistic care, the approach to patient care is directed at understanding as much as possible about the individual. Nurses who provide holistic health care believe that understanding all aspects of the patient (physical, spiritual, and psychosocial) is critical to achieving optimal patient outcomes.

3 It is impossible for health care providers to totally understand all cultures. Cultural competence is an ongoing process for all health care providers. Health care providers who support holistic health will clearly understand and respect the cultural differences of their patients.

Chapter 13 Answers to Case Study

1 Caring for her diabetes adequately will be a challenge for this patient. As a patient, Marjorie can benefit from assistance by a knowledgeable and caring nurse. The nurse's role is critical to provide the patient with health information, to connect her to community resources, and to monitor her ability to manage diabetes. Without this support, it is unlikely that she will be capable of managing a chronic disease such as diabetes.

2 Multiple psychosocial factors will influence the patient's ability to care for herself. Being a single mother of three children is a critical factor in this case. Marjorie may be more likely to neglect her own care as she struggles to meet the demands of three small children. Her limited income may also prevent her from purchasing needed supplies and medications that she needs to manage her diabetes. Limited education is also a strong indicator of one's ability to manage chronic disease conditions. Lastly, fear is a psychological factor that will influence the pharmacological treatment of her disease.

3 Self-care of a chronic illness is difficult especially when the patient senses that he/she is dealing with the disease alone. Establishing a therapeutic nurse/patient rapport will be one of the most important components of this patient's care. The nurse can serve a pivotal role in helping the patient understand how to live effectively with diabetes. Secondly, the nurse should ensure that this patient has been referred to other health care providers (such as a dietitian and medical social worker) who can be helpful in securing needed community resources.

Chapter 13 Answers to NCLEX-RN® Review

1 Answer: 2 Rationale: The statement reflects an attempt to understand the client holistically. The nurse understands that multiple contributing factors may contribute to illness. Tylenol should not be recommended initially as it does not address the possible causative factors related to the headaches (option 1). Monitoring the client's pupil response to light, although eventually appropriate, should not be performed initially (option 3). An ophthalmology referral may be inevitable; however, making such a referral should be done after ruling out other sources of the headaches (option 4). Cognitive Level: Application; Client Need: Safe, Effective Care Management; Nursing Process: Assessment

2 Answer: 3 Rationale: Factors associated with a drug's expense and the client's ability to purchase or access needed medication are considered psychosocial variables that may influence adherence to drug therapy. Unpleasant taste may hinder client adherence; however, the problem is physiological rather than psychosocial (option 1). Medications that are difficult to swallow may cause nonadherence; however, difficulty swallowing is a physiological problem (option 2). Liver damage (hepatotoxicity) is a physiological factor (option 4). Cognitive Level: Application; Client Need: Safe, Effective Care Management; Nursing Process: Assessment

3 Answer: 2 Rationale: Cultural beliefs refer to the cumulative ideas of knowledge, experiences, values, attitudes, meanings, and roles acquired by a group of people. Ethnicity is a population of human beings whose members identify with each other either on the basis of common genealogy or ancestry (option 1). Genetic polymorphisms are changes in enzyme structure and function of DNA that occur within a specific subset of the population (option 3). A health-related bias is a prejudice or a sense of preference for one particular point of view and is not specifically culturally related. For example, some clients have a health-related bias toward generic medication and prefer brand name drugs (option 4). Cognitive Level: Application; Client Need: Safe, Effective Care Management; Nursing Process: Assessment

4 Answer: 1 Rationale: Clients who are known as slow acetylators have reduced hepatic metabolism and reduced clearance by the kidney. These clients have a greater potential for drug toxicity. Option 2 is incorrect because acetylation is a metabolic process that does not influence absorption. Option 3 is incorrect because the route or form of administration is not associated with acetylation. Option 4 is incorrect because protein intake does not affect the rate of acetylation. Cognitive Level: Application; Client Need: Safe, Effective Care Management; Nursing Process: Assessment

5 Answer: 1, 2, 3, 4 Rationale: All of these factors: fat-to-muscle ration, cerebral blood flow, limited drug research on women, and health beliefs, may be considered gender factors that influence pharmacotherapy. Option 5, dietary considerations, is more of an ethnic consideration. Cognitive Level: Application; Client Need: Safe, Effective Care Management; Nursing Process: Assessment

Chapter 14

Answer to Connection Checkpoint 14.1

Increased gastric pH, slowed peristalsis, decreased total body water, diminished liver and kidney function, fewer plasma proteins, increased permeability of the blood-brain barrier.

Answer to Connection Checkpoint 14.2

Effects include slurred speech, dizziness, drowsiness, euphoria, and lack of motor coordination. Very high doses can cause brain damage, seizures, cerebrovascular accident, hypothermia, and death.

Chapter 14 Answers to Critical Thinking Questions

1 There are several problems that impact the well-being of this patient. Social isolation is often the most distressing consequence of chronic illness. Frequently involuntary solitude and feelings of detachment place individuals at high risk for social isolation. Depression is one of the most common complications of chronic illness. It is estimated that greater than 30% of individuals with a serious medical condition experience symptoms of depression and loneliness.

Another problem facing this patient is her chronic impaired health status. A chronic illness is one that lasts for a long time and usually must be managed, not cured. Examples of chronic illnesses include diabetes, heart disease, arthritis, kidney disease, HIV/AIDS, lupus, and multiple sclerosis. The management of chronic illness is often difficult and requires a multidisciplinary approach. Myra faces many challenges in managing her illness. She must learn techniques to manage symptoms, avoid complications, and maneuver through a complicated health care system. A complicated medication regimen is yet another challenge that Myra faces. The combination of drugs can cause serious health issues if not managed properly. Lastly, Myra's problem of accessing her needed medications may negatively affect her ability to to adhere to the course of therapy.

2 The parish nurse can help Myra with her medications. However, any assistance must first begin with an assessment of the Myra's ability and willingness to manage the drug therapy. The nurse could assess Myra's understanding and feeling about the insulin therapy. The nurse could also assist by providing Myra with written instructions related to the medication's adverse effects.

The nurse can call the local drugstore and see if they have a delivery service that Myra could access. The nurse could review Myra's health insurance plan and see if bulk delivery of routine medications to her home is available, which will save money.

3 One of the most important functions of the parish nurse is that of ensuring that a parishioner with chronic illness can maintain social contact and use support services within the church. Perhaps the nurse can establish a telephone network with Myra and other church members. Myra may need to be visited regularly by the clergy, the nurse practitioner, and other church members. The church may have a ministry where members pick up medications for persons who no longer drive. Myra might participate in church missions by sending cards or calling shut-ins who belong to her church.

Chapter 14 Answers to Case Study

1 The role of the occupational health nurse is multidimensional. An OHN focuses on promotion and restoration of health, prevention of illness and injury, and protection from work-related and environmental hazards. In this setting, the nurse is a strong advocate for healthy lifestyles which will in turn help to keep employees healthier, thereby reducing health care expenditures.

2 As in any nursing role, assessment is the first step in developing specific interventions to address the population's health needs. One method the nurse could employ is to conduct a health survey with Camden employees. Surveys should be anonymous to protect the employee's privacy. The findings may be very helpful in the development of employee health promotion programs to teach them skills needed to become responsible for their own health.

3 The OHN might consider health programs such as smoking-cessation, exercise and fitness, nutrition, and weight-control. If necessary, the nurse in this setting can educate an employee in the control of chronic illness and can provide information needed to direct them to effective health care resources. Certainly through health promotion activities, there is the potential to reduce the cost of pharmaceuticals. The OHN may also serve as a contact person between the employee and the insurance company. Perhaps the nurse can negotiate with various drug stores or drug companies for a reduced rate on medications for employees.

Chapter 14 Answers to NCLEX-RN® Review

1 Answer: 1 Rationale: The objective of hospice is to provide care or treatment directed toward reducing the severity of symptoms associated with fatal diseases. Nurses in this setting must be knowledgable about ways to to prevent and relieve pain and suffering and to improve quality of life for people facing serious, complex illnesses. Option 2 is incorrect. Although hospice clients may be prescribed drugs for hypertension, the relief of pain and discomfort would be a higher priority in hospice care. Option 3 is incorrect. Diuretic therapy may be used in clients who receive hospice care; however, pain relief is a greater priority for the hospice nurse. Option 4 is incorrect. Hospice nurses do work with clients and families regarding nutritional problems, but pain is considered more critical. Cognitive Level: Application; Client Need: Safe, Effective Care Management; Nursing Process: Assessment

2 Answer: 1, 3, 4 Rationale: The role of the school health nurse is multidimensional. All aspects of health and wellness within this setting are responsibilities of the school health nurse, including teaching students about substance abuse (option 1), assessing the respiratory status of an asthmatic student (option 3), and administering prescribed medication for attention deficit hyperactivity disorder. Option 2 is incorrect. School nurses (except nurse practitioners) do not prescribe medications. Option 5 is incorrect because it is the school nurse's responsibility to check that each medication a student takes is in its own individual container, labeled by the pharmacy. Cognitive Level: Application; Client Need: Safe, Effective Care Management; Nursing Process: Implementation

3 Answer: 1 Rationale: Medications stored in bathrooms are often subjected to changes in temperature and moisture. Although medicine cabinets are frequently found in bathroom areas, it is often the worst place to store medications. Option 2 is incorrect. Many medications are sensitive to light which can cause a loss of potency. Keeping medications in a drawer will protect the medication from exposure to excessive light. Option 3 is incorrect. Many medications come with cotton within the bottle. This small piece of cotton may actually damage the medication due to the moisture wicking action. The client should be instructed to remove the cotton to avoid this from occurring. Option 4 is incorrect. It is best to protect medication from excessive exposure to air. Bottles should be sealed tightly to avoid exposure to air. Cognitive Level: Application; Client Need: Safe, Effective Care Management; Nursing Process: Implementation

4 Answer: 1, 2, 3 Rationale: Smoking, consuming alcohol regularly, and using herbal therapies can all affect drug therapies and should be closely examined. Options 4 and 5 are life style choices and do not affect drug interactions. Cognitive Level: Application; Client Need: Safe, Effective Care Management; Nursing Process: Assessment

5 Answer: 2 Rationale: Clients receiving narcotics in the home setting are at high risk for falls. The hospice nurse will assess the environment for potential fall hazards such as throw rugs and a foot stool and suggest modification in the home to prevent injury. Option 1 is incorrect. Although it is critical that house numbers be easily identifiable, it would not be the priority for a client receiving narcotics in the home setting. Option 3 is incorrect. Vermin infestation is often a problem that many nurses face when making home visits. However, this discovery is not critical to the client receiving narcotic analgesia. Option 4 is incorrect because poor ventilation is not the first priority in this situation, although the nurse will need to address it at some point. Cognitive Level: Application; Client Need: Safe, Effective Care Management; Nursing Process: Assessment

Chapter 15

Answer to Connection Checkpoint 15.1

A pharmacopeia is a medical reference summarizing standards of drug purity, strength, and directions for synthesis. Drugs marketed in the United States must conform to U.S. pharmacopeia (USP) standards to avoid possible charges of adulteration and misbranding.

Answer to Connection Checkpoint 15.2

By inducing CYP enzymes, St. John's wort enhances the metabolic breakdown of antidepressants and benzodiazepines that are substrates for the enzyme. This may reduce their pharmacological activity.

Chapter 15 Answers to Critical Thinking Questions

1 Ginkgo is reported to have some major undesirable effects in individuals taking anticoagulants. This supplement will increase the time required for coagulation and therefore place the patient at risk for bleeding. Although his vital signs do not indicate active bleeding, the bruises on his arms indicate that localized bleeding has occurred in the tissue.

2 Larry should stop taking the Ginkgo immediately. Further doses of this supplement will exacerbate his potential for bleeding. Furthermore, the prescriber may inform the patient to temporarily stop taking the anticoagulant until the risk of hemorrhage subsides. Larry should also be informed not to take any OTC medications that will increase his risk for bleeding. These OTC medications include aspirin and NSAIDs such as ibuprofen (Motrin, Advil).

3 Many complementary and alternative therapies, if used correctly, are considered safe products and are gaining popularity. However, there are some risks involved in taking these preparations. Patients should be told that dietary supplements do not require testing prior to marketing, and additionally, safety does not need to be demonstrated by the manufacturer. Although dietary supplement labels must state that the product is not intended to diagnose, treat, cure, or prevent any disease, it is acceptable for the manufacturer to use statements such as "helps to promote a healthy immune system."

4 Larry's forgetfulness should not be minimized. Several abnormalities can contribute to changes in a patient's mental status including electrolyte disturbances, lack of mental stimulation, diet, and brain pathologies such as a traveling clot from the episode of atrial fibrillation. Larry should receive a diagnostic evaluation to rule out physiologic reasons for his forgetfulness. There are also some psychosocial conditions that can influence a patient's cognitive ability. The nurse should assess the patient for sources of stress or anxiety. In either case, appropriate referral is critical to aid the patient with this problem.

Chapter 15 Answers to Case Study

1 OTC supplements are usually safe if used as directed on the instructions. However, if the patient has pre-existing health problems or is taking other medications, then OTC medications and herbal supplements, can be potentially harmful. Nurses should teach patients to consult a health care professional such as a physician, nurse, or pharmacist before taking these products.

2 When a product is classified as "all natural," it usually implies that the substance is derived from or is made from ingredients found in nature and is not synthetic or man-made. Because a substance comes from a natural product, however, does not make it safe or effective.

3 The role of the nurse is to be sensitive to the patient's need for alternative treatment. Presenting a judgmental attitude about a patient's health practices will reduce open and honest communication. The nurse can provide the patient with information about the advantages and the limitations of complementary and alternative methods. This information allows the patient to make rational and informed decisions about treatment choices.

Chapter 15 Answers to NCLEX-RN® Review

1 Answer: 1 Rationale: Although CAM medications have been used for hundreds of years, many of these drugs lack scientific clinical studies which would verify their effectiveness. Most health care providers are hesitant to recommend a substance that has questionable effectiveness. Option 2 is incorrect because CAM has a rich history. To imply that all alternative therapies are nothing more than fable is incorrect. Many CAM therapies are effective if used correctly. Option 3 is incorrect. There is no evidence that response to CAM therapies is related to the placebo effect. The placebo effect occurs when a client takes an inert substance in conjunction with the suggestion from an authority figure that the pill will aid in healing, and the client's condition actually improves. Option 4 is incorrect. In many cases the CAM therapy may be less expensive than prescription medications. Cognitive Level: Application; Client Need: Safe, Effective Care Management; Nursing Process: Assessment

2 Answer: 3 Rationale: It is best to advise the client to take small amounts of a new supplement to determine any initial intolerance. Doubling dosages can be extremely dangerous and is seldom (if ever) advised. (option 1). There is no indication that fluid intake should be reduced with Echinacea (option 2). Allergic reactions are possible with natural supplements. Clients should be taught to read the label carefully and avoid any supplement that contains any known allergy provoking substances (option 4). Cognitive Level: Application; Client Need: Safe, Effective Care Management; Nursing Process: Implementation

3 Answer: 1 Rationale: Older adults with hepatic disease are at high risk of developing serious drug reactions when taking herbal supplements. The client in option 2 should consult the health care provider before taking any OTC supplements. However, the client is not at a higher risk for developing drug interactions. Option 3 is incorrect. It would not be wise for a client experiencing any acute illness, such as pneumonia, to begin taking supplements until the disease condition is resolved. However, this client is not the most likely to develop drug interactions with the taking of an herbal supplement. Option 4 is incorrect. This client is least likely to experience drug interaction with the use of herbal supplements. However, the client who is taking prescription medication for an acne condition, should consult a health care provider before taking any OTC preparations. Cognitive Level: Application; Client Need: Safe, Effective Care Management; Nursing Process: Assessment

4 Answer: 1, 2, 3, 5 Rationale: Herbal supplements can be found in almost every supermarket, pharmacy, and health food store and are easy to obtain (option 1). Due to aggressive marketing, herbal supplements are extremely popular (option 2). Most herbal supplements are less expensive than prescribed medications and therefore are more appealing to individuals where cost is a critical issue (option 3). Older clients are seeking therapeutic alternatives for chronic health conditions (option 5). Option 4 is incorrect. The myth that natural substances are safer than synthetic products is incorrect. Natural substances can be just as deadly as synthetic substances. Cognitive Level: Application; Client Need: Safe Effective Care Management; Nursing Process: Implementation

5 Answer: 1 Rationale: USP Verified Dietary Supplement Mark is awarded to dietary supplements that pass verification processes. The mark represents that USP has rigorously tested and verified the supplement to ensure that what is on the label is in fact in the bottle and that the supplement does not contain harmful levels of contaminants. Option 2 is incorrect. A DEA number is assigned to a health care provider that allows them to write prescriptions for controlled substances such as a narcotic or antibiotic. Option 3 is incorrect. The FDA does not control herbal supplements and this code is fictitious. Option 4 is incorrect. U.S. Customs is not responsible for ensuring that herbal supplements are pure. Cognitive Level: Application; Client Need: Safe, Effective Care Management; Nursing Process: Assessment

Chapter 16

Answer to Connection Checkpoint 16.1

Nicotine has a direct stimulatory effect on the reticular activating system of the brain, causing symptoms ranging from increased alertness and ability to focus, to feelings of relaxation or light-headedness. The cardiovascular effects of nicotine include an accelerated heart rate and increased blood pressure. Muscular tremors and convulsions may occur. Chronic use leads to emphysema, heart disease, and lung cancer.

Chapter 17

Answer to Connection Checkpoint 17.1

Cholinergic agonists will exert similar actions to those of the adrenergic antagonists.

Answer to Connection Checkpoint 17.2

Efficacy is the greatest maximal response that can be produced by a particular drug. Potency is the amount of a drug needed to produce a response.

Answer to Connection Checkpoint 17.3

Muscarinic receptors are found at postganglionic neurons ending in neuroeffector target tissues in the parasympathetic nervous system. Nicotinic receptors are located at preganglionic neurons ending in ganglia in both the sympathetic and parasympathetic nervous systems. They are also found on skeletal muscle.

Chapter 17 Answers to Critical Thinking Questions

1 The nurse should inform the patient to take the medication 1 hour before or 2 hours after meals to avoid nausea and vomiting. Dizziness, lightheadedness, or fainting may occur with bethanechol, especially when rising from a lying or sitting position. Patients receiving this medication should be instructed not to drive or engage in activities that require alertness until the effects of this drug have been determined. Some minor adverse effects may bethanechol may cause include: belching, stomach rumbling and mild cramps, salivation, diarrhea, and bladder urgency. All are attributable to the stimulation of the parasympathetic system. However, if the patient experiences difficult breathing, chest tightness, or pain, she should immediately contact her health care provider.

2 The nurse can help the patient by providing these tips to help her remember to take her medication. The nurse might suggest the following

- Place your medication next to something you use frequently or in plain sight.
- Post reminder notes on the refrigerator or the bathroom mirror
- Ask a friend or a relative to help remind you to take your medication
- Take the medication the same time every day
- Set an alarm clock or watch to remind you when it is time to take the medication
- Keep a medication diary or checklist so you know when you have taken your pills each day
- Carry your medication in your purse or pocket if you leave your house.
- If you accidentally miss a dose, take the missed dose as soon as you remember it. However, if it is almost time for the next dose, skip the missed dose and continue your regular dosing schedule. Do not take a double dose to make up for a missed one.

3 For this patient, bethanechol is being prescribed to relieve urinary retention. The nurse should monitor the patient's urinary system to determine the effectiveness of this drug therapy. If the therapy is not effective or the dose of the medication is insufficient the patient may complain of a sensation of being unable to empty the bladder even though she feels a strong urge to urinate. Additionally, many people with acute urinary retention also feel pain in the lower abdomen (pelvis) or experience a small amount of urine leaking out of the bladder. If urinary retention is allowed to continue, the patient may demonstrate symptoms of urinary tract infection which include back pain, fever, and painful urination.

Chapter 17 Answers to Case Study

1 Although nicotine replacement therapy will reduce the physical dependence on nicotine, it does not eliminate the psychological dependence. Successful smoking cessation often is dependent on additional assistance such as behavior modification and support groups.

2 Helpful websites include: How to Quit—Quit Tips—sponsored by the Centers for Disease Control and Prevention www.cdc.gov/tobacco/quit_smoking/how_to_quit/quittip.htm Smoking Cessation Support—sponsored by the American Lung Association http://www.lungusa.org/site/c.dvLUK900E/b.4061173/apps/s/content.asp?ct=66740

Chapter 17 Answers to NCLEX-RN® Review

1 Answer: 1 Rationale: Muscarinic agonists may cause reflex tachycardia, which is precipitated by a drop in the client's blood pressure. When this occurs, the baroreceptors recognize the decline in pressure and alert the medulla to increase the heart rate as a compensatory mechanism. Option 2 is incorrect because although the heart rate increases, muscarinic agonists do not directly affect the sinoatrial node. Option 3 is incorrect because hypertension is not a problem with this drug therapy. Option 4 is incorrect because muscarinic agents stimulate bronchial smooth muscles; however this does not impact the heart rate. Cognitive Level: Application; Client Need: Safe, Effective Care Management; Nursing Process: Intervention

2 Answer: 3 Rationale: Pyridostigmine (Mestinon) is used primarily for myasthenia gravis, a neurological disorder characterized by muscle weakness and ptosis. Options 1, 2, and 4 are incorrect because the symptoms listed are not usual problems faced by the client with myasthenia gravis and would therefore be inappropriate outcome statements. Cognitive Level: Application; Client Need: Safe, Effective Care Management; Nursing Process: Planning

3 Answer: 4 Rationale: Bethanechol works on the muscles needed for urination by increasing the ureteral peristalsis and promoting urinary bladder elimination. Option 1 is incorrect because bethanechol (Urecholine) does not diminish the size of structural defects. Options 2 and 3 are incorrect because although bethanechol improves urinary elimination, the mechanism of action occurs at the site of the urinary bladder and ureters rather than the kidney. Cognitive Level: Application; Client Need: Safe, Effective Care Management; Nursing Process: Implementation

4 Answer: 1, 2, 3, 5 Rationale: Common adverse effects of bethanechol include abdominal discomfort, sweating, flushed skin and blurred vision. Option 4 is incorrect because bethanechol increases gastrointestinal peristalsis, and promotes bowel evacuation. Cognitive Level: Application; Client Need: Safe, Effective Care Management; Nursing Process: Assessment

5 Answer: 3 Rationale: Because of the potential for bronchoconstriction, clients with COPD should be treated cautiously with cholinergic agonists. Option 1 is incorrect because neostigmine is used to reduce postoperative abdominal distention. Option 2 is incorrect because urinary retention may be relieved with the administration of neostigmine. Option 4 is incorrect because neostigmine may be used to reverse the effects of nondepolarizing muscle relaxants. Cognitive Level: Application; Client Need: Safe, Effective Care Management; Nursing Process: Assessment

6 Answer: 1 Rationale: If the heart rate falls below 60 beats/min or other established parameter the nurse should consult the prescriber. Atropine will be ordered to restore heart rate. Miosis is constriction of the pupil of the eye and an expected adverse effect of this drug therapy (option 2). Salivation is an expected adverse effect associated with neostigmine (option 3) A respiratory rate of 16 is normal and no need to consult the prescriber (option 4). Cognitive Level: Application; Client Need: Safe, Effective Care Management; Nursing Process: Assessment

Chapter 18

Answer to Connection Checkpoint 18.1

Signs and symptoms of a cholinergic crisis, include miosis, nausea, vomiting, urinary incontinence, increased exocrine secretions, abdominal cramping, tachycardia, hyperglycemia, and progressive muscle weakness. These are all signs of parasympathetic stimulation, which can be reversed with a muscarinic antagonist.

Answer to Connection Checkpoint 18.2

Adrenergic agonists

Answer to Connection Checkpoint 18.3

Pyridostigmine is an inhibitor of acetylcholinesterase used to treat myasthenia gravis. This drug will increase the amount of Ach at nicotinic receptors, which will antagonize the actions of neuromuscular blockers.

Answer to Connection Checkpoint 18.4

A patient with myasthenia gravis has muscular weakness due to a deficiency of Ach at nicotinic receptors. Neuromuscular blockers will further worsen this condition.

Chapter 18 Answers to Critical Thinking Questions

1 Atropine blocks acetylcholine affects on cholinergic receptors in smooth muscle, cardiac muscle, exocrine glands, urinary bladder, and the sinoatrial and atrioventricular nodes of the heart. Due to its diverse and widespread action, atropine has multiple uses that include certain types of bradycardia, spastic disorders of the GI system, and ophthalmic examinations.

2 In Pete's case, the adverse effect of atropine (suppression of exocrine secretions) becomes a therapeutic effect. Atropine is useful in controlling the copious secretions associated with organophosphate poisoning.

3 As the nurse, you would anticipate that Pete will probably experience dry mouth, constipation, urinary retention, increased heart rate, and blurred vision.

Chapter 18 Answers to Case Study

1 Neuromuscular blocking agents are drugs that interfere with the neural transmission between motor neurons and skeletal muscles. These drugs produce paralysis of all muscles, including those used for breathing.

2 Neuromuscular blocking agents such as succinylcholine (Anectine) are sometimes used during short medical surgical procedures. Frequently, when patients are placed on a mechanical ventilator, a neuromuscular agent is given to paralyze the patient during the procedure of inserting the endotracheal tube (a tube or catheter that is inserted into the trachea through the mouth or nose in order to maintain an open air passage or to deliver oxygen).

3 The major problem associated with these drugs is their effect on the respiratory system. Patients will be unable to maintain their own respirations due to the paralysis. The nurse will closely monitor the patient for the absence of respirations and assist the patient mechanically if necessary. Emergency equipment should be in close proximity of any patient is receiving neuromuscular blocking agents. Another associated problem with the administration of neuromuscular blocking agents is that these agents do not produce a decrease in the patient's level of consciousness. Although paralyzed, patients are very aware of their surroundings. An important nursing consideration is communication. Nurses should continue to communicate with the patient by explaining procedures and reassuring the patient while in the paralyzed state.

Chapter 18 Answers to NCLEX-RN® Review

1 Answer: 2 Rationale: Anticholinergic drugs can cause constipation. Therefore, increases in dietary fiber and water intake will help avoid constipation. Option 1 is incorrect because although daily exercise helps in avoiding muscle atrophy, anticholinergic agents are not related to muscle atrophy. Option 3, consuming foods high in iron to increase red blood cell production, is not related to anticholinergic drugs. Option 4 is incorrect because anticholinergic drugs cause tachycardia, not bradycardia. Cognitive Level: Application; Client Need: Safe, Effective Care Management; Nursing Process: Implementation

2 Answer: 1, 2, 3, 4 Rationale: These drugs cause mydriasis and paralysis of the ciliary muscle which is especially useful in ophthalmic examinations (option 1). These agents are extremely therapeutic in correcting cardiac rhythm abnormalities such as bradycardia (option 2). Muscarinic antagonists, most notably ipratropium (Atrovent) and tiotropium (Spiriva), are useful in treating asthma due to their ability to dilate the bronchi (option 3). These drugs are used to reverse the symptoms of overdose of organophosphate insecticides and ingestion of poison mushrooms (option 4). Option 5, urinary retention, is incorrect because this is one of the nontherapeutic adverse effects.) Cognitive Level: Knowledge; Client Need: Safe, Effective Care Management; Nursing Process: Assessments

3 Answer: 2 Rationale: Atropine causes urinary retention to worsen in patients with BPH. Options 1, 3, and 4 are incorrect because these are not contraindications that warrant not using atropine. Cognitive Level: Application; Client Need: Safe, Effective Care Management; Nursing Process: Assessment

4 Answer: 1 Rationale: Muscarinic agents affect the intraocular pressure by causing mydriasis and paralysis of the ciliary muscle. Options 2, 3, and 4 are incorrect because the drug does not promote infections, cause miosis, or affect the retina. Cognitive Level: Knowledge; Client Need: Safe, Effective Care Management; Nursing Process: Assessment

5 Answer: 3 Rationale: Cholinergic antagonists typically cause dry eyes and the client should be encouraged to use lubricating eye drops. Option 1 is incorrect. Clients receiving anticholinergic antagonists frequently complain of extreme dry mouth discomfort. The client should be encouraged to increase the intake of fluids to at least 2 liters per day. Many anticholinergic antagonists may cause drowsiness initially. The client should be instructed to avoid driving or operating heavy machinery until the effects of the drug are known (option 2). Women receiving anticholinergic therapy should be advised to avoid breast-feeding until the medication is discontinued (option 4). Cognitive Level: Application; Client Need: Safe, Effective Care Management; Nursing Process: Implementation

6 Answer: 1 Rationale: The therapeutic effect of succinylcholine is to paralyze skeletal muscles. However this drug does not produce anesthesia or a loss of consciousness. Option 2 is incorrect. Succinylcholine produces no change in the client's sensorium (consciousness). Option 3 is incorrect. The effect of succinylcholine is total muscle paralysis, not muscle relaxation. Furthermore, the client still can experience pain. Option 4 is incorrect. Again, succinylcholine does not affect the mental status of the client. Cognitive Level: Application; Client Need: Safe, Effective Care Management; Nursing Process: Assessment

Chapter 19

Answer to Connection Checkpoint 19.1

Most dopaminergic receptors are in the CNS but some are in the peripheral nervous system. Dopaminergic receptors are important to the action of certain antipsychotic medicines and in the treatment of Parkinson's disease.

Answer to Connection Checkpoint 19.2

Polar drugs are less able to cross nonpolar lipid membranes; thus they are absorbed and enter tissues less efficiently.

Answer to Connection Checkpoint 19.3

Anticholinergic drugs will increase heart rate, thus atropine may counteract reflex bradycardia.

Answer to Connection Checkpoint 19.4

The inhalation route may be used during acute conditions because it has a much faster onset of drug action than the oral or subcutaneous routes.

Chapter 19 Answers to Critical Thinking Questions

1 Albuterol is a sympathomimetic drug that selectively stimulates $beta_2$-adrenergic receptors. The therapeutic responses associated with this drug are bronchodilation and vasodilation. Therefore, it expands constricted bronchial tubes and enhances the passage of airflow into the lungs.

2 Albuterol is used to relieve and prevent bronchospasm in patients with various obstructive diseases such as asthma. The patient is receiving the medication via the inhalation route because it is one of the fastest and most effective routes to administer respiratory medications. Administration of an adrenergic agonist by the parenteral or inhalation routes causes immediate relaxation of bronchial smooth muscle, resulting in bronchodilation.

3 Alexis is demonstrating typical adverse effects associated with the administration of an adrenergic agonist. These adverse effects include CNS stimulation, such as tremor, anxiety, and irritability. Tachycardia is another classic adverse effect related to this classification of medications.

Chapter 19 Answers to Case Study

1 Both epinephrine and pseudoephedrine directly effect alpha receptors, which causes additive vasoconstriction. In Bill's case, the combination of drugs is creating medication-induced HTN.

2 First, you should inform the patient of your suspicions that the combination of drugs is causing his blood pressure to be dangerously high. The patient should be encouraged to stop using the medication immediately and to have his blood pressure rechecked within the next 24 hours. It is essential that you talk with the patient about not using any OTC medications for sinus relief until his health care provider examines him. Lastly, inform the patient that new medications for seasonal allergies are available that are much safer and more effective. Encourage him to ask his health care provider to recommend one.

Chapter 19 Answers to NCLEX-RN® Review

1 Answer: 1 Rationale: This drug activates alpha adrenergic receptors in the peripheral nervous system. Option 2 is incorrect because although phenylephrine has weak beta adrenergic activity, it is not of clinical significance. Options 3 and 4 are incorrect because neither alpha receptors nor beta receptors are found in the CNS, only the peripheral nervous system. Cognitive Level: Knowledge; Client Need: Safe, Effective Care Management; Nursing Process: Implementation

2 Answer: 1, 2, 4 Rationale: Adrenergic agonist nasal sprays should not be shared among individuals due to the risk of spreading any infection. Normally, individuals should be taught the dangers of using adrenergic nasal sprays longer than 3 days. These medications can cause increased blood pressure, increased heart rate, and insomnia. Habitual use of nasal adrenergic agents can also cause necrosis of the nasal mucosa due to the severe vasoconstriction caused by the drug (option 2). Lastly, due to the CNS stimulation, nasal adrenergic agents are not indicated in children and infants (option 4). Option 3 is incorrect because the drug causes CNS stimulation. Lethargy and fatigue are not signs of excessive use. Option 5 is incorrect because when adrenergic agents are used by diabetics, the client's metabolism is increased and hypoglycemia can be problematic. Cognitive Level: Application; Client Need: Safe, Effective Care Management; Nursing Process: Implementation

3 Answer: 4 Rationale: The only rationale for using epinephrine for anaphylaxis is to prevent hypotension and bronchoconstriction. Option 1 is incorrect because the administration of epinephrine for anaphylaxis does not prevent the formation of histamine. Option 2 is incorrect because the administration of epinephrine does not prevent the formation of antibodies in response to an invading antigen. Option 3 is incorrect because in anaphylaxis, white blood cells proliferate as a response to a foreign invader. Epinephrine does not stop this process. Cognitive Level: Knowledge; Client Need: Safe, Effective Care Management; Nursing Process: Assessment

4 Answer: 1 Rationale: When $beta_2$-adrenergic agonists are taken too close to bedtime, the client may experience insomnia. Option 2 is incorrect because all adrenergic agonists act as stimulators. Options 3 and 4 are incorrect because urticaria and tinnitus are not adverse effects associated with this drug therapy. Cognitive Level: Application; Client Need: Safe, Effective Care Management; Nursing Process: Assessment

5 Answer: 2 Rationale: At high dosage, dopamine stimulates alpha 1-adrenergic receptors causing vasodilation and increased blood pressure. Dopamine does not affect the reflexes responsible for pupillary response (option 1). Options 3 and 4 are incorrect because dopamine does not directly affect the client's level of consciousness; nor does it affect the client's gag reflex. Cognitive Level: Knowledge; Client Need: Safe, Effective Care Management; Nursing Process: Assessment

6 Answer: 1, 4 Rationale: The nurse should consult with the prescriber when adrenergic agents are prescribed to individuals with hyperthyroid disease. The medication will further increase an already overactive metabolic system. Also, due to the cardiac excitation induced by these medications, cardiac irregularities such as dysrhythmias will worsen when adrenergic agents are prescribed. Option 2, 3, and 5 are all appropriate reasons to administer adrenergic agonists. Cognitive Level: Knowledge; Client Need: Physiological Integrity; Nursing Process: Assessment

Chapter 20

Answer to Connection Checkpoint 20.1

Indications for cholinergic agonists include open angle glaucoma, Sjögren's syndrome, urinary retention, GI atony, myasthenia gravis, and Alzheimer's disease.

Answer to Connection Checkpoint 20.2

Other catecholamines include norepinephrine, epinephrine, isoproterenol and dobutamine.

Chapter 20 Answers to Critical Thinking Questions

1 Prazosin works decreasing peripheral resistance (relaxing blood vessels) so that blood may flow through the vessels more easily. This effect helps to lower blood pressure. The mechanism of action is based on the drugs ability to block alpha$_1$-adrenergic receptors.

2 Many drugs including antihypertensive medications can induce impotence. The physiological mechanism that creates this situation in male patients is related to the muscle contraction in the vas deferens, which is the main duct through which semen is carried from the epididymis to the ejaculatory duct. When these smooth muscles are inhibited, ejaculation becomes difficult.

3 Many men are reluctant to talk about medication-induced impotence. The nurse must maintain a nonjudgmental attitude if the patient is to develop a trusting relationship with them and the health care provider. The nurse must determine exactly what the patient means by "sexual" adverse effects. Health care providers sometimes must be frank and candid about such matters. The nurse could say "Do you mean problems with erection or problems with ejaculation?" Amos should be informed that just because one medication may have caused sexual dysfunction does not indicate that all antihypertensive medications will do the same. Amos should be assured that his health care providers want to know about such adverse effects and that he needs to report them, especially when a medication creates adverse effects that prompt the patient to discontinue the medication without consulting the health care provider.

Chapter 20 Answers to Case Study

1 There are two reasons why Mr. Perry should not take pseudoephedrine for his allergic symptoms. First, adrenergic agonists such as Sudafed antagonize the antihypertensive action of propranolol, thereby causing the medication to be ineffective. Secondly, adrenergic agonists create vasoconstriction, which will elevate Mr. Perry's blood pressure.

2 A safer medication for this patient would be OTC diphenhydramine (Benadryl). This drug blocks the histamine receptors and reduces allergic symptoms without increasing blood pressure.

Chapter 20 Answers to NCLEX-RN® Review

1 Answer: 1 Rationale: With this drug, the most important action is to monitor the client for adverse effects associated with the cardiovascular system such as changes in pulse and blood pressure. Elevation of the head of bed is not specifically required for this drug regimen (option 2). Inderal can be taken any time regardless of meals (option 3). The therapeutic action of Inderal is not contingent on serum K^+ levels (option 4). Cognitive Level: Application; Client Need: Safe, Effective Care Management; Nursing Process: Assessment

2 Answer: 4 Rationale: Beta-adrenergic antagonists may cause hypoglycemic episodes in diabetic clients. The client should be instructed to monitor blood glucose levels frequently initially, and to notify the prescriber of a decrease. Option 1 is incorrect because insulin dosages are never arbitrarily increased without checking with a health care provider. Diabetic clients should remain on their normal diabetic diets even though they may be taking antihypertensive medications (option 2). Elevation of the extremities is not related to a diabetic taking beta-adrenergic blocker drugs (option 3). Cognitive Level: Application; Client Need: Safe, Effective Care Management; Nursing Process: Implementation

3 Answer: 1 Rationale: Initial therapy of drugs that cause a "first dose phenomenon" are usually prescribed at very low doses and administered at bedtime. The decline in blood pressure due to prazosin is often marked when beginning pharmacotherapy, and when increasing the dose. This "first dose phenomenon" can lead to syncope due to reduced blood flow to the brain. Option 2 is incorrect because doses of antihypertensive medications should never be doubled but should be gradually increased to avoid hypotension. Options 3 and 4 are incorrect because the best time to give prazosin in the initial phases of therapy is at bedtime. Cognitive Level: Application; Client Need: Safe, Effective Care Management; Nursing Process: Implementation

4 Answer: 1 Rationale: The nurse should suspect that the client is describing orthostatic hypotension induced by the medication. Most clients find it helpful to move slowly from a recumbent position to avoid dizziness and syncope. Option 2 is incorrect because although drinking a full glass of water with the medication is a health promotion activity that the nurse might suggest, this action does not eliminate orthostatic hypotension. Option 3 is incorrect because sleeping positions do not influence the presence of orthostatic hypotension. The client should never abruptly stop taking antihypertensive medication. Such action could result in hypertensive crisis, stroke, or heart attack (option 4). Cognitive Level: Application; Client Need: Safe, Effective Care Management; Nursing Process: Implementation

5 Answer: 4 Rationale: One adverse effect of alpha$_1$-adrenergic antagonists is tachycardia. Clients experiencing tachycardia should not receive alpha$_1$ adrenergic antagonists. Alpha$_1$ adrenergic antagonists are often prescribed for benign prostatitic hyperplasia because they relax muscles in the prostate (option 1). A pheochromocytoma is a benign tumor of the adrenal medulla that secretes catecholamines. Alpha$_1$-adrenergic antagonists help to reduce the HTN associated with these tumors (option 2). Alpha$_1$-adrenergic antagonists diminish the vasospasms associated with Raynaud's disease (option 3). Cognitive Level: Knowledge; Client Need: Safe, Effective Care Management; Nursing Process: Assessment

6 Answer: 2, 3, 4 Rationale: Beta adrenergic blockers can have dramatic metabolic effects that produce an increase in serum triglycerides (option 2) and hypoglycemia (option 3). Additionally, these drugs can affect the sexual function of men by producing a decreased libido (option 4). Options 1 (anorexia) and 5 (thrombocytopenia) are not adverse effects associated with beta-adrenergic antagonists. Cognitive Level: Application; Client Need: Safe, Effective Care Management; Nursing Process: Assessment

Chapter 21

Answer to Connection Checkpoint 21.1

The peripheral nervous system has somatic and autonomic divisions. The somatic nervous system provides voluntary control over skeletal muscle. The autonomic nervous system gives involuntary control over functions of the cardiovascular, digestive, respiratory, and genitourinary systems.

Answer to Connection Checkpoint 21.2

Dopamine is used to treat hypovolemic and cardiogenic shock.

Answer to Connection Checkpoint 21.3

Increased brain alertness, increased heart rate and blood pressure, bronchodilation, pupil dilation, increased perspiration.

Chapter 22

Answer to Connection Checkpoint 22.1

Signs and symptoms of amphetamine abuse include increased heart rate, high blood pressure, increased breathing rate, dilated pupils, sweating, and tremors. Long-term use results in feelings of restlessness, anxiety, defensiveness and fits of rage, and a psychosis that closely resembles paranoid schizophrenia.

Answer to Connection Checkpoint 22.2

Sleep difficulties during pregnancy are common due to hormonal changes, emotional stress, and pain or discomfort from the enlarging fetus. Nonpharmacologic means should be attempted to improve sleep. Patients should never take drugs during pregnancy unless approved by their health care provider. The benzodiazepines are pregnancy category D or X.

Answer to Connection Checkpoint 22.3

With these types of names, it is helpful to write both the generic and trade names on the prescription so that the correct drug may be better identified. Typing the name, rather than handwriting it, also helps prevent these types of errors.

Chapter 22 Answers to Critical Thinking Questions

1 Seraphina and Joe have made plans for their retirement, which are probably going to have to be changed, or postponed. They may have financial concerns now. Raising teenagers is costly, and will be difficult if their income is limited to Social Security and pensions. Seraphina feels resentful toward her grandchildren and also feels guilty for being resentful because she recognizes that they did not cause the situation.

2 The health care provider may order antianxiety medications, such as alprazolam (Xanax), buspirone (BuSpar), diazepam (Valium), or lorazepam (Ativan). All of these are administered PO. She may also be prescribed a medication such as zolpidem (Ambien), which is used for short-term treatment of insomnia, while receiving psychotherapy for assistance in resolving her current difficulties.

3 Herbal remedies used by persons of the Latino culture influence the effects of traditional Western medicine. Herbs that are commonly used include kava which promotes muscle relaxation and sleep, and acts as an antidepressant. It may be used in combination with St. John's wort and valerian to promote relaxation. St. John's wort is used for mild depression. It is not effective for moderate to severe depression. If taken with a prescription antidepressant, St. John's wort may increase the risk of suicide. Valerian is a mild sedative, and induces sleep. Its effects are similar to those of the benzodiazepines. Special care must be taken when combining herbs with prescription medications. They can enhance or decrease the actions of the medications. Seraphina must reveal to her health care provider all herbs she is taking so the interactions between them and her ordered medications can be determined, and further patient teaching performed

Chapter 22 Answers to Case Study

1 Adverse effects associated with lorazepam (Ativan) include dizziness, ataxia, drowsiness, blurred vision, vertigo, sedation, and confusion, These effects are dose related and tolerance to them may develop as therapy progresses.

2 Most importantly, instruct the client not to operate machinery or perform potentially hazardous activities that require alert mental status until the effects of the drug are known.

3 The nurse can make several suggestions to Seraphina: Enlist the help of other family members to help with the children, including keeping them for long weekends and part of the summer to reduce some of the burden; help Seraphina to see this situation as something within her control; teach her relaxation techniques; put her in contact with other grandparents who are raising grandchildren, so she can get support from others who are in the same situation; encourage her to continue to call upon her faith

Chapter 22 Answers to NCLEX-RN® Review

1 Answer: 3 Rationale: Ataxia, weakness, restlessness, dizziness, or other motor problems can occur with lorazepam. None of the other options 1, 2, or 4 will occur with lorazepam. Cognitive Level: Application; Client Need: Physiological Integrity; Nursing Process: Assessment

2 Answer: 4 Rationale: Sleeping for 7 hours is the desired effect. The client should not experience periods of sleep lasting only 3 hours (option 1). The client will be taking temazepam to assist with insomnia, not to treat anxiety related to every-day stress (option 2), or to help control panic attacks (option 3). Cognitive Level: Application; Client Need: Physiological Integrity; Nursing Process: Evaluation

3 Answer: 3 Rationale: This medication must be gradually reduced, not abruptly terminated. Abrupt termination may cause withdrawal symptoms (nausea, vomiting, abdominal cramps, diaphoresis, confusion, tremors, seizures). The other options 1, 2, and 4 are correct statements and indicate that the client understands the teaching. Cognitive Level: Application; Client Need: Physiological Integrity; Nursing Process: Evaluation

4 Answer: 2 Rationale: Panic disorder is not an appropriate use for phenobarbital, but the other 3 options are appropriate: treating status epilepticus (option 1), prior to diagnostic testing (option 3), and prior to receiving general anesthesia (option 4). Cognitive Level: Application; Client Need: Safe, Effective Care Environment; Nursing Process: Assessment

5 Answer: 3 Rationale: Client safety is the major issue with sedative-hypnotics, so prevention of falls is the highest priority. The client may experience any of the other 3 options, but none of them is a higher priority than client safety. Cognitive Level: Analysis; Client Need: Safe, Effective Care Environment; Nursing Process: Planning

6 Answer: 1 Rationale: Smoking enhances the metabolism of benzodiazepines, so the medication is broken down and removed from the body more quickly if the client is a smoker. Therefore, a smoker needs a larger dose of a benzodiazepine to get the same effect as that in a nonsmoker. A smaller dose (option 2), or the same dose (option 3) as that given to a nonsmoker would not help relieve the client's symptoms. Cognitive Level: Application; Client Need: Physiological Integrity; Nursing Process: Implementation

Chapter 23

Answer to Connection Checkpoint 23.1

The limbic system is responsible for emotional expression such as anxiety, fear, anger, aggression, depression, sexual drive, and euphoria. Signals routed through the limbic system connect with the hypothalamus and eventually the cerebrum, which allows us to think and reflect on our emotional states such as depression.

Answer to Connection Checkpoint 23.2

Atropine is a prototype anticholinergic drug. The anticholinergic cardiovascular adverse effects can be overcome by the administration of a beta blocker.

Answer to Connection Checkpoint 23.3

Benzodiazepines

Chapter 23 Answers to Critical Thinking Questions

1 The priority is for Jane to receive a complete physical and mental assessment. Any physical cause for the changes in Jane's behavior must be ruled out. After this has been done, a mental status exam must be performed, with emphasis on suicidal ideation.

2 Antidepressants are drugs used to enhance, elevate, or stabilize mood and are often beneficial in treating depression. Most antidepressants act by helping to restore normal neurotransmitter balances of primarily norepinephrine, serotonin, and to a lesser degree, dopamine.

3 To determine if antidepressants are achieving a therapeutic effect the nurse can monitor the client's interest in personal appearance and the performance of normal ADLs. In Jane's case, the clues that clearly demonstrate her depression include lack of interest in her personal appearance, disinterest in her children and their activities, and in day-to-day activities involved in running a home, and her sudden cessation of contact with friends and lack of involvement in former activities.

Chapter 23 Answers to Case Study

1 The nurse must immediately assess Jane for suicidal ideation. If Jane is thinking about suicide, she must be protected. It may be necessary to assign a staff member to be with her 24 hours a day, or it may mean that she must be in sight of a staff member at all times.

2 The SSRIs are the most commonly used antidepressant medications today. Since Jane has no contraindications to any of the SSRIs her health care provider may order sertraline (Zoloft), fluoxetine (Prozac), or one of the other drugs in this category.

3 Patient teaching will include: Maximum therapeutic effects will take 4–5 weeks to occur; weight gain may occur; avoid all other medications and herbal products unless okayed by the prescriber; keep all follow-up health care provider and lab appointments; sexual dysfunction (in women, usually decreased libido and lack of ability to reach orgasm) may occur; sedation may occur (avoid driving or activities requiring alertness until effects of drug are known).

Chapter 23 Answers to NCLEX-RN® Review

1 Answer: 1 Rationale: Imipramine should not be used by patients with seizure disorders because it lowers the seizure threshold. Imipramine is a drug that is effective in treating depression (option 2). Imipramine is one of only two drugs approved for enuresis, or bedwetting in children (option 3). Like other TCAs, imipramine has a number of off-label indications. These include the adjuvant treatment of cancer or neuropathic pain (option 4). Cognitive Level: Knowledge; Client Need: Physiological Integrity; Nursing Process: Assessment

2 Answer: 3 Rationale: Full therapeutic effects of fluoxetine take up to one month. Water and sodium intake are irrelevant (option 1). The patient cannot take an MAOI or a CNS depressant concurrently (option 2). Increased CNS depression may occur, which could lead to deeper depression (option 4). Cognitive Level: Application; Client Need: Physiological Integrity; Nursing Process: Evaluation

3 Answer: 1, 2 Rationale: Persistent GI upset and confusion are signs of lithium levels between 1.5–2.0, which signify early toxicity. Polyuria is not a sign of early toxicity (option 3). Convulsions may occur at levels above 2.5 (option 4). Ataxia is not a sign of early lithium toxicity. (option 5) Cognitive Level: Application; Client Need: Physiological Integrity; Nursing Process: Evaluation

4 Answer: 1 Rationale: The person taking lithium must be conscious of maintaining normal sodium intake. Because lithium is a salt, if sodium intake is low the body will replace the sodium with lithium, leading to lithium toxicity. The other three choices are accurate. The person taking lithium must have regular blood studies (option 2); toxicity is a very real concern, hence the necessity for routine blood studies (option 3); and refrain from breast-feeding (option 4). Cognitive Level: Application; Client Need: Physiological Integrity; Nursing Process: Evaluation.

5 Answer: 3 Rationale: Antidepressants take up to 8 weeks to reach full therapeutic effect, so the patient must continue taking the medication as ordered. It would be detrimental to change to another medication because therapeutic levels would have to start at 0 and take another 8 weeks to build up (option 1). To accuse the patient of not following the recommended regimen (option 2), or to suggest an OTC medication be added (option 4) would be inappropriate. Cognitive Level: Analysis; Client Need: Physiological Integrity; Nursing Process: Implementation.

6 Answer: 3 Rationale: The SSRIs account for over $3 billion in sales every year in the United States, far more than any other classification of antidepressant medications (options 1, 2, and 4). Cognitive Level: Knowledge; Client Need: Physiological Integrity; Nursing Process: Assessment

Chapter 24

Answer to Connection Checkpoint 24.1

Efficacy refers to a drug's ability to produce a therapeutic effect. Potency refers to the dose of drug needed to produce a response. In treating psychoses, the dose is less important than effectiveness.

Answer to Connection Checkpoint 24.2

They usually are used in combination with lithium or valproic acid (Depakene).

Chapter 24 Answers to Critical Thinking Questions

1 Many persons with schizophrenia feel normal when taking their medications as prescribed. These patients may come to believe that they no longer need the medications. George is functioning as any adult does—he goes to work, he coaches his children's sports teams, he provides for his family, and he cares for his wife. Because he views all of these activities as "normal," he convinces himself he no longer has schizophrenia and stops taking his medications.

2 There are many clues, probably subtle at first, then becoming more obvious: George quit coaching his children's sports teams, exhibited a decline in personal hygiene and appearance, and, finally, quit his job without reason.

3 Sheri can be more aware of whether or not George is taking his medications as scheduled (although many psychiatric patients do not want anyone else to manage, or even assist them in managing, their medication regimen). She may need to count his remaining medications, and be sure the appropriate amount of medication remains. She can intervene at the first sign of negative symptoms (decline in personal hygiene, decreased interest in usual activities, etc.) or negative symptoms (delusions, etc.). Other family members can tell Sheri if they notice anything unusual in George's behavior or thought patterns. Sheri is the appropriate person to tell, since George either will not want to admit that he has stopped taking his medication as ordered, or will not recognize that behaviors or thoughts are abnormal.

Chapter 24 Answer to Critical Thinking Question in Evidence-Based Practice Feature

The nurse will be aware of the potential for weight gain, so can teach the patient about proper diet and exercise. The nurse will also be aware of any other health problems the patient has, and can make a comprehensive care plan that takes them into account. The nurse can provide emotional support to the patient who begins to experience weight gain, and assist the patient to explore the advantages and the disadvantages of this particular medication.

Chapter 24 Answer to Critical Thinking Question in Evidence-Based Practice Feature

The patient who discontinues perphenazine in favor of a newer antipsychotic medication will probably have the same potential for discontinuing the new drug. The nurse must remember that different people respond to medications differently; an individual's response is related to the patient's physical and mental state.

Chapter 24 Answers to Case Study

1 Haloperidol (Haldol) is a nonphenothiazine antipsychotic medication that can be used to calm agitation and to decrease psychotic manifestations. Since George is becoming more and more out of control, he would probably refuse to take an oral medication, so an IM preparation is the best choice. Haloperidol will calm him down, slowing his thoughts and his activity so he does not harm himself or anyone else. The onset of the medication is 30–45 minutes, so George must be watched closely during that time. He should be lying down for the entire time (which may be difficult, depending on his level of agitation), and up to 1 hour following administration.

2 Common adverse effects to Haldol are drowsiness and extrapyramidal symptoms, which include involuntary movements, tremors, rigidity, body restlessness, muscle contractions, and changes in breathing and heart rate.

3 George most likely will be hospitalized for less than one week. Psychiatric hospital stays are shorter than ever because most third party payers have decreased the amount of coverage for mental illness. His medication will be restarted, and he will be somewhat stabilized before being discharged. He will also have several chances to speak with a counselor or psychiatric nurse who can try to assist him to gain insight into the reasons behind this current hospitalization. He will be given patient education on his disease, his medication, and the importance of continuing to take his medication even though he feels better.

Chapter 24 Answers to NCLEX-RN® Review

1 Answer: 4 Rationale: "Anti" means against, and "psychotic" means a serious mental disorder; hence, antipsychotic means against the psychosis. Without the medication, the symptoms will return. The other answers are incorrect because they do not speak to the definition of antipsychotic, which is what the question is asking. Cognitive Level: Application; Client Need: Physiological Integrity; Nursing Process: Assessment

2 Answer: 2 Rationale: Acute dystonia, or severe muscle spasms, especially of the back, neck, face, or tongue may appear within hours or days of the first dose of a phenothiazine. Option 1 is incorrect because social withdrawal is a symptom of the disease, and slowed activity may occur as a result of the medication, but the patient's body will become adjusted to it in a short period of time and it will disappear. Option 3 is incorrect because tardive dyskinesia occurs late in therapy, and is more common in the elderly. Option 4 is incorrect because the phenothiazine medications may, and usually do, cause adverse effects even when taken as prescribed. Cognitive Level: Analysis; Client Need: Psychosocial Integrity; Nursing Process: Implementation

3 Answer: 1 Rationale: Benztropine (Cogentin) is classified as an autonomic nervous system agent and an anticholinergic. It suppresses tremor and rigidity by decreasing the excess cholinergic effect associated with dopamine deficiency. Option 2 (Diazepam) and option 4 (Ativan) are antianxiety medications that will not improve the patient's symptoms. Option 3 (Haloperidol) is an antipsychotic medication. Use of it may lead to these symptoms. Cognitive Level: Analysis; Client Need: Physiological Integrity; Nursing Process: Implementation

4 Answer: 2, 4 Rationale: EPS occurs frequently, especially at the beginning of therapy with haloperidol (option 2). A person with Parkinson's disease, seizure disorders, alcoholism, or severe mental depression cannot take haloperidol because they all affect the CNS. If taken with levodopa (the most common medication used to treat Parkinson's disease), the patient may develop dementia. Haloperidol decreases the seizure threshold. Increased CNS depression will occur when mixed with alcohol. The person who is already depressed will become more depressed (option 4). Option 1 is incorrect because it is not necessary to space the administration of haloperidol and antacids. There are no known interactions between these two medications. Option 3 is incorrect because haloperidol must be taken as ordered, on a regular schedule. Taking the drug prn will not reduce symptoms of psychosis because it takes several weeks of regular administration before therapeutic levels are reached. Cognitive Level: Application; Client Need: Health Promotion and Maintenance; Nursing Process: Assessment

5 Answer: 4 Rationale: The patient taking an antipsychotic medication should refrain from consuming alcohol. Concurrent use of alcohol and antipsychotic medication will increase CNS depression. The patient must not substitute alcohol use for medication use; without medications, the symptoms most likely will recur. Option 1, weight gain, option 2, blurred vision, and option 3, hypotension, relate to adverse reactions the patient may experience, and must be monitored and reported if they occur. Cognitive Level: Analysis; Client Need: Health Promotion and Maintenance; Nursing Process: Evaluation

6 Answer: 1 Rationale: Fever, tachycardia, stupor, and incontinence are symptoms of neuroleptic malignant syndrome, a potentially fatal adverse effect of antipsychotics that must be diagnosed and treated immediately. Options 2, 3, and 4 are possible adverse reactions, but are not life threatening, and therefore do not need to be reported with the same urgency as answer 1. Cognitive Level: Analysis; Client Need: Physiological Integrity; Nursing Process: Assessment

Chapter 25

Answer to Connection Checkpoint 25.1

Epinephrine and norepinephrine.

Answer to Connection Checkpoint 25.2

MAOIs were developed to treat hypertension but they have been replaced with safer medications. Tyramine must be strictly avoided.

Answer to Connection Checkpoint 25.3

Neostigmine (Prostigmin) is the prototype cholinesterase inhibitor that acts on nicotinic receptors, and its primary indication is myasthenia gravis. Cholinesterase inhibitors that act on muscarinic receptors may be used to treat open-angle glaucoma.

Chapter 25 Answers to Critical Thinking Questions

1 A complete physical exam is imperative, as well as lab work to determine any electrolyte disturbances, diabetes, or other condition that may be present. A complete personal history, as well as a family history, to determine if any other close family members may have/had AD is necessary. Additionally the assessment should also include cognitive rating scale measurements and assessment of individual and family coping skills.

2 The health care provider will probably recommend that Mary begin taking one of the medications used to treat early Alzheimer's, such as donepezil or tacrine. He will recommend that she not be allowed to drive any longer. He will also recommend that other measures be taken to ensure her safety and the safety of others, including making sure she does not leave home alone, leave pots cooking on the stove, or leave water running in the sink or tub. Things and routines at home must be kept as much the same as possible, including where items are stored and people who come into the home. This will assist Mary in maintaining some semblance of control over her life for as long as possible. As her disease progresses she will not be able to process new information, but she should be able to remember old information for a time.

3 Donepezil may cause some common adverse effects: headache, fatigue, insomnia, nausea, vomiting, diarrhea, anorexia, and abdominal pains. Other adverse effects include vertigo, depression, irritability, syncope, HTN (remember that Mary has mild HTN and takes an antihypertensive), dehydration, incontinence, and blurred vision. Robert will have to be alert for anorexia, and encourage Mary to eat if she loses weight. If she is unable to sleep, she may begin to wander so he may have to install better locks on the doors. She is already depressed at her diagnosis, so if the medication causes increased depression, suicide ideation may appear.

Chapter 25 Answers to Case Study

1 Idiopathic PD, the most common type, has no known cause and is characterized by a progressive loss of neurons from a region of the brain called the substantia nigra. Physiological defects with PD occur in the amounts of neurotransmitters of dopamine and acetylcholine in specific regions of the brain.

2 Drug therapy attempts to restore the functional balance of dopamine and acetylcholine in the striatum of the brain. Levodopa is a precursor in the synthesis of dopamine and helps to restore the imbalance. Levodopa is nearly always combined with carbidopa because the combination increases the effectiveness of levodopa. Carbidopa inhibits the breakdown of levodopa in the intestine and peripheral tissues, which makes more levodopa available to the CNS. Without carbidopa, only 1% of the dose of levodopa reaches the CNS.

3 There are many potential adverse effects of levodopa. Common adverse effects include orthostatic hypotension, nausea, vomiting, anorexia, dry mouth, flatulence, dysphagia, abdominal distress, involuntary movements, hand tremors, fatigue, headache, anxiety, twitching, numbness, confusion, agitation, nightmares, and insomnia. Life-threatening adverse effects include agranulocytosis, leukopenia, and hemolytic anemia.

Chapter 25 Answers to NCLEX-RN® Review

1 Answer: 2 Rationale: Benztropine is frequently used as combination therapy with other antiparkinson drugs leading to decreased tremors. Option 1, amantadine, acts to increase dopamine's release, but only as long as there is dopamine available. Option 3, haloperidol, is a phenothiazine antipsychotic that may lead to pseudo-Parkinson's disease in many persons. Option 4, Donepezil (Aricept) prolongs the time between diagnosis and the institutionalization of the Alzheimer's disease client and is not used for Parkinson's disease. Cognitive Level: Knowledge; Client Need: Physiological Integrity; Nursing Process: Implementation

2 Answer: 3 Rationale: Being independent with ADLs shows an improvement in physical abilities. Option 1, sleep, is a common adverse effect of anti-Parkinson's medications. Option 2 is the opposite of what usually happens; loss of appetite is a common adverse effect. Option 4, itchy skin, is not relevant to PD or to the medications used. Cognitive Level: Application; Client Need: Health Promotion and Maintenance; Nursing Process: Evaluation.

3 Answer: 3 Rationale: It is imperative that the caregivers understand that there is no cure for AD; the best that can happen is that the medication may delay the worsening of symptoms. Option 1 is incorrect because the medication should be given continuously and not only when the symptoms are present. Option 2 is incorrect because the client may become constipated but it is not an emergency. Option 4 is incorrect, because it is not necessary to take the client's vital signs before each dose of medication. Cognitive Level: Application; Client Need: Physiological Integrity; Nursing Process: Evaluation

4 Answer: 1, 4 Rationale: It is difficult to remember to take a medication 4 times a day, and as the client's cognitive functioning declines, it may be increasingly difficult to administer it (option 1). Serious liver damage is a possibility with tacrine (Cognex), which decreases its usefulness (option 4). Options 2 and 3 are incorrect because they are not true. Tacrine may cause weight loss, rather than gain, and does not cause vision difficulties. Option 5 is incorrect because tacrine cannot be purchased over the counter

5 Answer: 1 Rationale: Rivastigmine has no significant drug interactions. This is thought to be true because there is no interaction with enzymes in the liver that metabolize drugs. Options 2, 3, and 4 are incorrect because they do not apply to rivastigmine. Cognitive Level: Knowledge; Client Need: Physiological Integrity; Nursing Process: Planning

6 Answer: 3 Rationale: Depression should never be ignored. Many times a client diagnosed with AD will have enough cognitive functioning to be aware of the ramifications of the diagnosis, and will become depressed. This depression can be decreased with the correct antidepressant. Option 1 is incorrect because depression will not just go away. It is an insensitive remark to say that the client will not remember anything, and it may take several years for the disease to progress to that point (option 2). Estrogen does not reduce the risk of dementia; studies show that it may increase the risk slightly (option 4). Cognitive Level: Application; Client Need: Psychosocial Integrity; Nursing Process: Implementation

Chapter 26

Answer to Connection Checkpoint 26.1

Alcohol withdrawal is severe and may be life-threatening. About 5% to 10% of patients experience delirium tremens, a syndrome of intense agitation, confusion, terrifying hallucinations, uncontrollable tremors, panic attacks, and paranoia.

Answer to Connection Checkpoint 26.2

Benzodiazepines are used primarily for sleep and anxiety. They can be administered as a preoperative sedative, prevention and treatment of delirium tremens in acute withdrawal of alcohol, depression, mania, and psychotic behavior.

Chapter 26 Answers to Critical Thinking Questions

1 Even with multiple medications, Jorge may still continue to experience seizure activity. The patient's family should be told that their primary concern is to protect him from injury. It is important for Jorge's mother to look closely at the home setting for potential hazards. Here are just a few considerations

a. Pad sharp corners
b. Do not leave the patient unattended in a bathtub or swimming pool until the seizures are under control
c. Avoid climbing activities high off the ground (rock or rope climbing)
d. Avoid sleeping in the top bunk
e. Place screen guards around fireplaces
f. Wear a helmet and other protective gear when bicycling

2 Jorge's mother should be instructed on the action, adverse effects, administration guidelines, and nursing implications regarding carbamazepine and phenytoin. It is important that she understand that a dose of medication not be missed, and if it is, to administer it immediately. Instruct her that missing doses of antiepileptic medications could result in status epilepticus. Instruct her to keep using the same brand of phenytoin.

Chapter 26 Answer to Critical Thinking Question in Evidence-Based Practice Feature

Simple partial seizures have an onset that may begin as a small, regional focus, and subsequently progress to a generalized seizure. Patients with simple partial seizures experience a wide array of symptoms depending upon the specific region of brain affected. However, these clients do not lose consciousness. Complex partial seizures (formerly known as psychomotor or temporal lobe seizures) originate from a single focus, usually in the temporal lobe of the brain. Patients exhibit sensory, motor, or autonomic symptoms, with some degree of altered or impaired consciousness.

Chapter 26 Answer to Critical Thinking Question in Evidence-Based Practice Feature

It is critical that the nurse develop a therapeutic rapport with the students. As the school nurse, the students with seizure disorder must feel comfortable and at ease. Otherwise communication will be limited. Spending time and discussing the disorder will allow for open communication and allow the student to explore self esteem issues. The nurse may be providing students with their only opportunity to discuss these sensitive issues.

Chapter 26 Answers to Case Study

1 Valproic acid (Depakene) increases the brain's concentrations of the inhibitory neurotransmitter gamma-aminobutyric acid (GABA), which is a brain chemical that causes sedation.With this drug abnormal electrical impulses in the brain are suppressed, leading to decreased seizure activity.

2 The most common adverse effects are GI-related, such as nausea, vomiting, diarrhea, abdominal pain, and diminished appetite. These effects are usually transient and not severe. An enteric-coated formulation of valproic acid can be used to reduce these uncomfortable effects.

3 One potential adverse effect of valproic acid is increased bleeding tendencies. Matt should inform his dentist that he is taking valproic acid before any dental procedure.

Chapter 26 Answers to NCLEX-RN® Review Questions

1 Answer: 3 Rationale: Staring and transient loss of responsiveness are the most common signs of absence seizures. It is important to implement the diagnostic test of an EEG to rule out absence seizures prior to administering attention deficit disorder medications. The use of the following diagnostic tests: blood glucose analysis (option 1), echocardiogram (option 2), or CT scan (option 4) will not rule out the presence of a seizure disorder. Cognitive Level: Application; Client Need: Physiological Integrity; Nursing Process: Planning

2 Answer: 4 Rationale: Infantile spasms are known as West Syndrome. The drug of choice for West Syndrome is adrenocorticotropic hormone. Valproic acid (Depakote)—option 1, diazepam (Valium)—option 2, and phenytoin (Dilantin)—option 3 are all antiepileptic medications, but are not used in the treatment of West Syndrome. Cognitive Level: Knowledge; Client Need: Physiological Integrity; Nursing Process: Planning

3 Answer: 4 Rationale: Adverse effects of phenobarbital (Luminal) can produce osteomalacia, due to a deficiency in folic acid, calcium, and vitamin D. Hyperkinetic behavior disorder (option 1), sleep apnea (option 2), and cerebrovascular accident (option 3) are not adverse effects of phenobarbital. Cognitive Level: Application; Client Need: Physiological Integrity; Nursing Process: Implementation

4 Answer: 1 Rationale: Long-term use of barbiturates can produce impaired blood coagulation due to a deficiency in vitamin K. The nurse should instruct the patient to consume green leafy vegetables and organ meats to prevent vitamin K deficiency. Cognitive Level: Application; Client Need: Physiological Integrity; Nursing Process: Implementation

5 Answer: 1 Rationale: High doses can cause nystagmus, confusion, ataxia, coma, and seizures and should be reduced. Option 2 is incorrect because increasing the dosage would worsen the symptoms of toxicity. Option 3 is incorrect because maintaining the dose would add to the client's toxicity. Option 4 is incorrect because to discontinue the medication may induce seizure activity.

6 Answer: 2, 3, 4, 5 Rationale: Ethosuximide (Zarontin) is ineffective in treating simple or complex partial seizures, tonic-clonic seizures, and febrile seizures. Option 1 is incorrect because ethosuximide (Zarontin) is used to treat absence seizures.

Chapter 27

Answer to Connection Checkpoint 27.1

Benzodiazepines are indicated for anxiety disorders, insomnia, and certain seizures.

Answer to Connection Checkpoint 27.2

TCAs are approved for depression, and some are approved for social anxiety disorder and panic disorder. Off-label indications include the adjuvant treatment of cancer or neuropathic pain, overactive bladder, attention deficit/hyperactivity disorder, and bulimia.

Answer to Connection Checkpoint 27.3

The most visible symptom is drooping of the eyelids (ptosis) due to muscular weakness. Other symptoms include extreme fatigue, double vision, speech impairment, and difficulty chewing or swallowing. Treatment includes pharmacotherapy with acetylcholinesterase inhibitors, such as pyridostigmine.

Chapter 27 Answers to Critical Thinking Questions

1 The back pain experienced by this patient is a result of excessive use and local injury to the lower back at the lumbosacral region. Other possible causes of muscle spasm include hypocalcemia, debilitating neurological disorders, seizure disorders, and overmedication with antipsychotic agents. Muscle spasms are involuntary contractions of a muscle group or group of muscles. The muscles become tight with a fixed pattern of resistance, which results in diminished function. The disorders associated with movement affect many anatomical systems including the nervous, musculoskeletal, endocrine system, respiratory, and cardiovascular systems.

2 Cyclobenzaprine (Flexeril) is used to relieve muscle spasms associated with acute and painful musculoskeletal disorders. It has been prescribed to relax the muscles of the lumbosacral region. Cyclobenzaprine is similar in action to the TCAs, which produce both sedative and anticholinergic effects. It has the ability to inhibit reflexes and reduce tonic somatic motor activity.

3 Cyclobenzaprine produces muscle relaxation and CNS depression. The patient should be instructed to protect himself from injury and not engage in the operation of machinery while taking the medication; not to consume alcoholic beverages or mood altering drugs. The patient should also be warned against taking OTC medications. The patient should be instructed on all adverse effects and advised to notify the prescriber if adverse effects do not stop in 2–3 weeks. Due to anticholinergic effects the patient should be instructed to void prior to medication administration.

Chapter 27 Answer to Critical Thinking Question in Evidence-Based Practice Feature

Nonpharmacological interventions that might be ordered by the health care provider or physical therapist include the application of heat or cold, hydrotherapy, ultrasound, assisted exercise, massage, traction, and manipulation.

Chapter 27 Answers to Case Study

1 Botulinum toxin, type A is a drug of choice to treat cervical dystonia and is used to improve the severity of abnormal head position. The medication is produced from *Clostridium botulinum* type A. The toxin binds to the motor nerve receptor sites to block neuromuscular conduction, and inhibits the release of acetylcholine. The result of this action is the reduction of muscle activity.

2 Possible adverse effects include injection reactions, headache, dysphagia, muscle weakness, pain, tenderness, bruising, flulike symptoms, dry mouth, upper respiratory infection, and ptosis.

Chapter 27 Answers to NCLEX-RN® Review

1 Answer: 3 Rationale: Malignant hyperthermia is noted in clients with bulky muscles who undergo general anesthesia. Dantrolene is the drug of choice to treat malignant hyperthermia. Although botulinum toxin, type A is a drug of the same class as dantrolene it is not a drug of choice to treat malignant hyperthermia (option 1). Carisoprodol is a centrally-acting skeletal muscle relaxant which is used to treat muscle spasms, not malignant hyperthermia (option 2). Although dantrolene and phenytoin are both hydantoin derivatives, phenytoin is not used to treat malignant hyperthermia (option 4). Cognitive Level: Application; Client Need: Pharmacological and Parenteral Therapies; Nursing Process: Implementation

2 Answer: 1, 3, 4 Rationale: The client should void prior to the administration of cyclobenzaprine due to its anticholinergic effects, which cause urinary retention (option 1). The client should not operate machinery due to the CNS depression effects (option 3). Hard candy reduces dry mouth, which is related to the anticholinergic effects of cyclobenzaprine (option 4). Intake of calcium rich foods is not necessary or indicated with cyclobenzaprine (Flexeril) (option 2). The client should consume a diet high in fiber due to the fact that GI motility is diminished with cyclobenzaprine (option 5). Cognitive Level: Comprehension; Client Need: Physiological Integrity; Nursing Process: Implementation

3 Answer: 2 Rationale: Capsaicin should be applied to the site of pain with a gloved hand. Capsaicin should only be applied to the site of pain not proximal or distal to the pain (option 1). If capsaicin begins to irritate and cause redness it should be discontinued (option 3). Capsaicin should be applied with a gloved hand not a bare hand (option 4). Cognitive Level: Comprehension; Client Need: Physiological Integrity; Nursing Process: Implementation

4 Answer: 1 Rationale: Baclofen (Lioresal) possesses a structure which is similar to the inhibitory neurotransmitter gamma aminobutyric acid. Its off-label use includes treatment of tardive dyskinesia related to long-term treatment with antipsychotic agents. Option 2 is incorrect. Tizanidine (Zanaflex) is a centrally acting alpha$_2$-adrenergic agonist that inhibits motor neurons mainly in the spinal cord. Options 3 and 4 are incorrect. Dantrolene and botulinum toxin, type A are direct acting antispasmodic agents. Cognitive Level: Knowledge; Client Need: Physiological Integrity; Nursing Process: Implementation

5 Answer: 4 Rationale: Physostigmine (Antilirium) may be administered to reverse serious anticholinergic adverse effects. Option 1 is incorrect. Naloxone (Narcan) is often used to decrease the effects of opioids on the CNS, but is not the drug of choice in the treatment of CNS depression with cyclobenzaprine. Meperidine (Demerol) is a CNS depressant and should not be administered with cyclobenzaprine (option 2). Diazepam (Valium) is also a skeletal muscle relaxant and should not be administered with cyclobenzaprine (option 3). Cognitive Level: Application; Client Need: Physiological Integrity; Nursing Process: Implementation

6 Answer: 2 Rationale: Muscle weakness is the most common adverse effect of dantrolene therapy. Muscle tension is not considered a adverse effect of this drug (option 1). If muscle tremors develop, the nurse should investigate other causes. Dantrolene sodium (Dantrium) does not cause tremors (option 3) and is not known to cause muscle pain (option 4). Cognitive Level: Knowledge; Client Need: Physiological Integrity; Nursing Process: Planning

Chapter 28

Answer to Connection Checkpoint 28.1

Club drug refers to substances taken by people at dance clubs, all night parties, and raves. MDMA produces both stimulant and hallucinogenic effects simultaneously. Symptoms include increased wakefulness, increased social and extroversion behaviors and chronic behavioral disorders such as depression, anxiety, sleeplessness, and hostility.

Answer to Connection Checkpoint 28.2

The SSRIs are the drugs of choice for major depressive disorder. Bupropion is an atypical antidepressant.

Answer to Connection Checkpoint 28.3

Most dreaming occurs during the rapid eye movement (REM) stage of sleep.

Chapter 28 Answers to Critical Thinking Questions

1 ADHD is characterized by inattention and hyperactivity. It is four times more common for males to present with inattention and inappropriate behavior than females. A child who is diagnosed with ADHD has difficulty completing tasks, is frequently loud, and interrupts others. Females with ADHD show less aggression but suffer from greater anxiety and mood swings. Jonathon's concerns about entering an evening nursing program are due to the fact that the medications prescribed for ADHD are taken in the morning to assist in the patient's ability to maintain attention throughout the day. By the evening the effect of the medication has declined and the patient may suffer from increased episodes of distraction.

2 The nurse may refer Jonathan to educational counselors or a psychologist for additional testing using an ADHD rating scale. Additional evaluation in the evening may identify the symptoms of ADHD experienced at the time he would be taking classes. It is important that the nurse assess the patient's response to medications administered for ADHD including adverse effects such as CNS depression, effects on the cardiovascular system, particularly the heart rate and blood pressure, and the effect on decreasing the signs and symptoms of ADHD. It is important that the patient be monitored for adverse hepatic effects particularly when administering atomoxetine.

3 The patient should be instructed to contact the prescriber to determine if the dose could be divided so he receives 40 mg in the morning and 40 mg in the evening. This dosing schedule may assist in increasing his attention during the evening class schedule. He should also be instructed to limit caffeine intake. The combination of caffeine and medications for ADHD will increase insomnia. He should be instructed to report any adverse effects to the prescriber. The patient should also have periodic AST/ALT levels tested since this medication is metabolized in the liver.

Chapter 28 Answer to Critical Thinking Question in Evidence-Based Practice Feature

Atomoxetine is administered for the treatment of ADHD in adults and children. The exact mechanism of action is unknown but is thought to be related to selective inhibition of the presynaptic norepinephrine transporter. This action results in the inhibition of norepinephrine reuptake which leads to improved attentiveness and the ability to complete tasks. The patient has decreased episodes of distraction and diminished episodes of hyperactivity. The patient should be educated on the need for long-term use of the medication and for suicidal tendencies and suicidal ideations. The patient should be taught to monitor heart rate and blood pressure with each dosage increase and to not ingest alcohol with this medication due to the risk of liver toxicity. The patient should change positions with caution due to decrease in blood pressure and should not operate machinery when taking this medication.

Chapter 28 Answers to Case Study

1 The action of modafinil is unknown. However, the medication is known to increase extracellular dopamine to enhance alertness. Modafinil increases wakefulness in patients with narcolepsy, excessive sleepiness, and with shift work sleep disorder.

2 The patient should be taught to use a barrier contraceptive if she is of child bearing age. She should not take OTC medications unless approved by her health care provider. She should notify her health care provider if she develops any signs and symptoms of hypersensitivity to the medication. It is important for her to have periodic liver function tests.

3 The patient should be instructed to change positions slowly to reduce the potential for the occurrence of orthostatic hypotension.

Chapter 28 Answers to NCLEX-RN® Review

1 Answer: 4 Rationale: Cerebral stimulants delay growth and the child should have established periods of time without cerebral stimulants. Option 1 is incorrect because the child should be placed in an environment with minimal distractions. Option 2 is incorrect because the use of high calorie snacks is important, as cerebral stimulants will cause weight loss. Option 3 is incorrect because the child should be seated in the front of the classroom. Cognitive Level: Application; Client Need: Health Promotion and Maintenance; Nursing Process: Implementation

2 Answer: 2 Rationale: Atomoxetine should decrease hyperactivity. Option 1 is incorrect—Atomoxetine should increase attention. Options 3 are 4 are incorrect. Adverse effects of atomoxetine include mydriasis and elevated liver enzymes. Cognitive Level: Comprehension; Client Need: Health Promotion and Maintenance; Nursing Process: Evaluation

3 Answer: 1 Rationale: Chlorpromazine is the drug of choice to assist in counteracting amphetamine overdosage. Option 2 is incorrect. Phenytoin is an antiepileptic agent that would only be administered if the client was suffering from status epilepticus. Option 3 is incorrect. Sodium pentothal is an anesthetic agent and would not counteract the effects of amphetamine. Option 4 is incorrect. Dexamethasone (Decadron) is a steroid which would not affect the amphetamine overdosage. Cognitive Level: Application; Client Need: Physiological Integrity; Nursing Process: Implementation

4 Answer: 1 Rationale: Atomoxetine has been linked to suicidal ideations. Options 2, 3, and 4 are incorrect. Amphetamine sulfate, modafinil, and caffeine have not been linked to suicidal ideations. Cognitive Level: Knowledge; Client Need: Psychosocial Integrity; Nursing Process: Evaluation

5 Answer: 2 Rationale: Narcolepsy is noted when the client falls asleep suddenly. The accompanying flaccidity is known as cataplexy. Option 1 is incorrect. Hyperkinetic disorder is noted with periods of inattention not sleep. Option 3 is incorrect. Tonic-clonic seizures are noted with intense muscle contractions followed by alternating contraction and relaxation of muscles. Option 4 is incorrect. TIA has a vascular cause that produces stroke symptoms that resolve in approximately 24 hours. Cognitive Level: Knowledge; Client Need: Physiological Integrity; Nursing Process: Assessment

6 Answer: 4 Rationale: The consumption of caffeinated coffee may interfere with sleep. Option 1 is incorrect. The consumption of alcohol diminishes sleep. Option 2 is incorrect. The consumption of a chocolate bar which contains caffeine diminishes sleep. Option 3 is incorrect. The consumption of a high energy drink which contains caffeine diminishes sleep. Cognitive Level: Application; Client Need: Health Promotion and Maintenance; Nursing Process: Planning

Chapter 29

Answer to Connection Checkpoint 29.1

The abbreviation MS can be confused with magnesium sulfate and result in medication errors.

Answer to Connection Checkpoint 29.2

TCAs are responsible for a high incidence of anticholinergic adverse effects, with symptoms such as dry mouth, blurred vision, constipation, urinary retention and tachycardia. Other adverse effects include orthostatic hypotension cardiac toxicity, sedation, confusion, dizziness, fatigue, sexual dysfunction, and weight gain.

Answer to Connection Checkpoint 29.3

Withdrawal symptoms include dysphoria, diaphoresis, violent yawning, lacrimation, rhinorrhea, pupil dilation, fever, diarrhea, goose bumps, and muscle cramping and tremor. Treatment may include methadone, buprenorphine (Subutex) as monotherapy, or buprenorphine combined with naloxone (Suboxone).

Chapter 29 Answers to Critical Thinking Questions

1 Given the complexity of Mr. Smith's situation, the best solution would be referral to the hospital pain management team (if one exists). In most instances, baseline opioid analgesics would be continued and acute surgical pain management would be superimposed on that baseline. The nurse caring for Mr. Smith after surgery should consider several interventions related to pain management. His age puts him at higher risk for hypotension, respiratory depression, and increased incidence of adverse CNS effects. The nurse would monitor for these problems, and should consider supplemental interventions such as frequent repositioning, relaxation techniques, and distraction.

2 Depending on the type of documentation used in the agency, the nursing plan of care should include *Acute* and *Chronic Pain* as his first nursing diagnoses with a brief note about his chronic pain history. An alert might be placed on the physical chart if electronic medical records are not used. Pain management should be included in all shift reporting, and if possible, the same nurses should be assigned to his care.

3 Hypotension, with unsafe ambulation, and constipation are the most likely adverse effects Mr. Smith will experience. In addition to monitoring vital signs, including respiratory rate and BP, position changes should be made gradually and assisted ambulation would be necessary. A high fiber diet would be started with stool softeners and laxative as needed. He should walk three to four times a day for increasing distances. In addition, nausea from the hydromorphone would need to be assessed and managed if it occurs.

Chapter 29 Answers to Critical Thinking Question in Evidence-Based Practice Feature

1 The nurse should acknowledge that all patients should be routinely assessed for pain, and that assessment should be documented in a standardized manner. Assessment of pain intensity alone is insufficient. Comprehensive pain assessment includes intensity, location, aggravating and alleviating factors, and previous treatments and their effectiveness.

2 When the nurse engages the patient in collaborative care and shared decision making, self-management health outcomes are improved. The nurse should direct attention toward patient and family education that will foster shared management of pain. An emphasis on individualized care and participation of the patient in the treatment plan will produce the best results.

3 Treatment modalities for pain are constantly evolving. For example, pain experts have recently advocated that inappropriate traditional practices such as regular use of IM injections, meperidine, and sole reliance of prn analgesic administration be eliminated. It is critical that nurses stay knowledgeable about pain treatment modalities and the current "best practices" within the literature.

4 One critical role of the nurse, when caring for a patient with pain, is the reassessment and adjustment of the pain management plan. To effectively care for patients with pain, the nurse should respond, not only to pain intensity, but to functional status and adverse effects of the medications.

5 Nurses are called upon to examine their own practices to determine the effectiveness of the nursing care provided to the patient with pain.

Chapter 29 Answers to Case Study

1 Use of IV opioid analgesia with separate anti-emetic therapy would be appropriate. Morphine would most likely be the initial drug of choice.

2 Initially the nurse should assess Rita, including pain and vital signs every 2 hours. An initial dose of morphine IV should be based on her current pain rating, followed by every two hour doses within the ordered range to keep her pain at an acceptable target level. She should be monitored for respiratory depression while keeping pain at alleviated or tolerable levels. The nurse would need to regularly medicate with an IV agent that effectively manages Rita's nausea and vomiting without additional sedation.

3 Adverse effects might include respiratory depression, orthostatic hypotension, nausea, and constipation.

4 Dexamethasone (Decadron), a corticosteroid, is ordered to reduce swelling and pressure on the spinal nerves from the metastases; reducing pressure helps relieve the back pain.

5 The nurse would allow Rita to express her concerns, and then provide teaching to her and her family related to the low incidence of addiction, and the differences between physical dependence and addiction. A conversation about pain control and quality of life would begin the process for a discussion on end-of-life care.

Chapter 29 Answers to NCLEX-RN® Review

1 Answer: 1, 3, 4, 5 Rationale: Common adverse effects of opioids include respiratory depression (option 1), urinary retention (option 3), constipation (option 4), and nausea (option 5). Hypotension, not hypertension is an adverse effect (option 2). Cognitive Level: Knowledge; Client Need: Physiological Integrity; Nursing Process: Evaluation

2 Answer: 4 Rationale: Opioids decrease peristalsis, and bowel surgery produces a temporary cessation of peristalsis (paralytic ileus). Both lead to constipation. Once bowel function has returned enough for the client to start eating, constipation is still likely and needs to be prevented by increased dietary fiber and fluids, as well as taking a stool softener. Respiratory depression (option 1), and urinary retention (option 2), are not likely after several days with decreasing opioid use. Addiction is not a concern in the treatment of acute pain in this scenario (option 3). Cognitive Level: Application; Client Need: Physiological Integrity; Nursing Process: Planning

3 Answer: 3 Rationale: Chest pain is a serious adverse effect of sumatriptan (Imitrex) and needs to be differentiated from angina, which can also be caused by the drug. It needs to be reported to the prescriber immediately (option 2), before using the drug again (option 1). Reclining in a quiet room with cold packs is good advice for migraines, but reporting the adverse effect is more important (option 4). Cognitive level: Application; Client Need: Physiological Integrity; Nursing Process: Implementation

4 Answer: 2 Rationale: The client is describing neuropathic pain which is most likely to respond to the adjuvant analgesic, gabapentin. Nonopioids (ibuprofen) (option 1), or opioids (methadone) (option 4) alone are not appropriate. Naloxone is an opioid antagonist (option 3). Cognitive Level: Application; Client Need: Physiological Integrity; Nursing Process: Planning

5 Answer: 2 Rationale: Ergot alkaloids are one of the two drugs of choice for aborting migraines. Morphine is an opioid agonist and is not effective to abort migraines (option 1). Propranolol is a beta blocker and is used to prevent migraines (option 3). Ibuprofen is a non-opioid analgesic that is used to treat mild to moderate pain (option 4). Cognitive Level: Knowledge Client Need: Physiological Integrity Nursing Process: Planning

6 Answer: 4 Rationale: Elderly clients are at highest risk for hypotension, respiratory depression, and increased incidence of adverse CNS effects such as confusion. Option 1 is incorrect. Most 23-year-old clients can tolerate opioids without adverse effects. Option 2 is incorrect. Individuals who suffer from traumatic injury may receive narcotic analgesia. However, caution should be taken if the individual has also experienced any type of head injury. Option 3 is incorrect. Opioids are often used with individuals who suffer MI. No adverse effects such as hypotension or respiratory depression are usually present if the dose is appropriate for the size of the client. Cognitive Level: Application; Client Need: Physiological Integrity; Nursing Process: Assessment.

Chapter 30

Answer to Connection Checkpoint 30.1

The two classes of analgesics work synergistically to relieve pain, and the dose of opioid can be kept small to avoid dependence and opioid-related adverse effects. Acetaminophen is the nonopioid most frequently used.

Answer to Connection Checkpoint 30.2

Diazepam and lorazepam are utilized in the treatment of status epilepticus.

Answer to Connection Checkpoint 30.3

Atropine blocks receptors in the autonomic nervous system; succinylcholine blocks receptors in the somatic nervous system (skeletal muscle).

Chapter 30 Answers to Critical Thinking Questions

1 Balanced anesthesia is the use of a combination of medications to produce general anesthesia. Balanced anesthetics provide for a rapid and smooth induction. The agents administered include neuromuscular blocking agents, short acting barbiturates, opioids, and nitrous oxide. The purpose of the combination of these medications is to provide muscle relaxation and analgesia along with sedation and loss of sensation. It is important to instruct the patient on balanced and general anesthesia because the administration of a combination of agents rapidly induces unconsciousness and muscle relaxation, and maintains deep anesthesia. The patient is concerned she will awaken during anesthesia, and knowing this information will assist in allaying her fears.

2 The main actions of nitrous oxide are analgesia and reduction in anxiety. Nitrous oxide suppresses the pain mechanism of the CNS. This agent has a low potency and does not produce loss of consciousness or profound skeletal muscle relaxation. Since nitrous oxide does not induce stage 3 surgical anesthesia it is commonly combined with other surgical anesthetic agents.

3 The patient should be educated on the action and effect of balanced anesthesia and the agent to be used to induce and maintain anesthesia. Propofol (Diprivan) is administered to induce and maintain balanced anesthesia. It is important to stress that the patient will continue to receive medication, which will prevent her from awakening during surgery. The patient should also be aware that the medication may cause shivering when she awakens. Inform her that she will be provided with warm blankets to ensure her comfort.

Chapter 30 Answer to Critical Thinking Question in Evidence-Based Practice Feature

Family history of unexplained death following the induction of general anesthetic agents may provide clues that the patient has a genetic disposition for malignant hyperthermia. It is imperative that the patient and family be interviewed prior to surgery to determine if the patient is at risk for the development of malignant hyperthermia. During the surgical procedure and within minutes of the induction of anesthesia the patient should be assessed for tachycardia and hypotension. In the event these symptoms result the anesthesia should be reduced, surgery halted, and the patient's body temperature should be cooled.

Chapter 30 Answers to Case Study

1 Lidocaine blocks the conduction of electrical impulses by reducing the sodium permeability at the cellular level. This prevents pain transmission to the CNS.

2 Lidocaine hydrochloride is a local anesthetic agent with a prompt and intense anesthetic action that lasts longer than procaine. It also exhibits a lower incidence of adverse effects.

Chapter 30 Answers to NCLEX-RN® Review

1 Answer: 2 Rationale: In stage two the client becomes excitable with hyperactivity and irregular heart and respiratory rates. Option 1 is incorrect because in stage one the client loses general sensation, but remains awake. Option 3 is incorrect because in stage three the client's skeletal muscles become relaxed and delirium stabilizes. Option 4 is incorrect because in stage four the client has paralysis of the medulla. Cognitive Level: Knowledge; Client Need: Physiological Integrity; Nursing Process: Assessment

2 Answer: 1 Rationale: Clients who have been diagnosed with a seizure disorder should not receive thiopental sodium due to the risk of status epilepticus. Options 2, 3, and 4 are incorrect because clients with lung cancer, clients who suffer from kidney disease, and clients who suffer from Addison's disease can be administered thiopental sodium cautiously. Cognitive Level: Application; Client Need: Physiological Integrity; Nursing Process: Assessment

3 Answer: 3 Rationale: Succinylcholine is a neuromuscular blocking agent which will provide relaxation of the larynx. Lidocaine is administered as a local anesthetic and will not provide muscle relaxation (option 1). Morphine sulfate is an opioid, which will not provide muscle relaxation (option 2). Atropine will not produce relaxation of the laryngospasm (option 4). Cognitive Level: Knowledge; Client Need: Physiological Integrity; Nursing Process: Implementation

4 Answer: 3 Rationale: Ketamine produces dissociation anesthesia which is a feeling of being separated from the environment. Option 1 is incorrect because anxiety is not the major effect of ketamine. Option 2 is incorrect because ketamine will produce decreased energy. Option 4 is incorrect because dry mouth is not a reaction of ketamine. Cognitive Level: Application; Client Need: Physiological Integrity; Nursing Process: Implementation

5 Answer: 1 Rationale: Epinephrine is administered with lidocaine to decrease bleeding at the site of trauma or surgery. Option 2 is incorrect because epinephrine will cause vasoconstriction, not vasodilation at the site. Option 3 is incorrect because epinephrine will increase blood pressure. Option 4 is incorrect because neither lidocaine nor epinephrine has any antibacterial properties. Cognitive Level: Knowledge; Client Need: Physiological Integrity; Nursing Process: Implementation

6 Answer: 2, 3, 4 Rationale: Alfentanil (Alfenta), is a parenteral opioid agent which promotes general anesthesia. It is an opiate agonist with a rapid onset and short duration of action (option 2). Sufentanil (Sufenta), is an opioid agent that is administered 1–8 micrograms per kilogram (option 3). Regimental (Ultiva), is an opioid agent that is used to induce and maintain general anesthesia (option 4). Option 1 is incorrect because nitrous oxide is not an opioid agent. Option 5 is incorrect because succinylcholine (Anectine) is a neuromuscular blocking agent. Cognitive Level: Knowledge; Client Need: Physiological Integrity; Nursing Process: Assessment

Chapter 31

Answer to Connection Checkpoint 31.1

Plasma proteins, especially albumin, can bind drugs, keeping them in the bloodstream and thus unavailable to reach their target tissues and cause their pharmacotherapeutic effects.

Answer to Connection Checkpoint 31.2

The increased sympathetic stimulation from sympathomimetics and the anticholinergics would speed up heart rate. The increased parasympathetic stimulation from parasympathomimetics and adrenergic antagonists would slow heart rate. The effect of heart rate, however is moderated by compensatory measures such as the baroreceptor reflex.

Answer to Connection Checkpoint 31.3

The beta-adrenergic antagonists (blockers) are the most frequently prescribed autonomic drugs for HTN.

Chapter 32

Answer to Connection Checkpoint 32.1

Prodrugs must be metabolized by the liver to become active. A patient with liver cirrhosis has impairment that will cause lower serum levels of the prodrug. Doses may have to be increased to compensate for hepatic impairment.

Answer to Connection Checkpoint 32.2

The ability of the liver to metabolize drugs diminishes. The doses of prodrugs should be increased, but most other doses should be decreased. Renal function also diminishes with age, causing drugs to remain in the body longer.

Chapter 32 Answers to Critical Thinking Questions

1 The etiology of hyperlipidemia may be inherited or acquired. Certainly, diets high in saturated fats, and lack of exercise contribute greatly to hyperlipidemia and resulting cardiovascular diseases. However, genetics determines one's ability to metabolize lipids, and contributes to high lipid levels in a substantial number of patients. For most patients, dyslipidemias are the result of a combination of genetic and environmental (lifestyle) factors.

2 The patient should be taught the following health concepts related to lowering her LDL level

- Maintain weight at an optimal level.
- Implement a medically supervised exercise plan.
- Reduce dietary saturated fats and cholesterol.
- Increase soluble fiber in the diet.

- Eliminate tobacco use.
- Monitor blood lipid levels regularly, as recommended by the physician.

3 Atorvastatin is an inhibitor of 3-hydroxy-3-methyl-glutaryl coenzyme, a reductase (HMG-CoA), which is essential to hepatic production of cholesterol. Lipitor increases the number of hepatic low-density-lipid (LDL) receptors, thus increasing LDL uptake and catabolism of LDL.

4 Back pain, asthenia, hypersensitivity reaction, myalgia, headache, abdominal pain, constipation, diarrhea, dyspepsia, and flatulence are potential adverse effects.

Chapter 32 Answers to Case Study

1 David needs to understand all the routine concepts related to lowering LDL levels (i.e., weight control, low fat diet, etc). However, for David the problem may not be deficient knowledge. The nurse and the patient need to explore ways in which he can be more consistent with his medication and exercise regimen.

2 Some of the major problems associated with Questran are constipation, fecal impaction, hemorrhoids, abdominal pain and distension, flatulence, bloating sensation, and belching.

3 A lipid profile typically consists of 4–5 different laboratory values. The test usually includes total cholesterol, HDL cholesterol (often called good cholesterol), LDL cholesterol (referred to as bad cholesterol), triglycerides, and HDL/cholesterol ratio. A lipid profile is a group of tests that determine the risks of heart disease.

Chapter 32 Answers to NCLEX-RN® Review

1 Answer: 1 Rationale: Rhabdomyolysis is a serious adverse effect of the statins. During rhabdomyolysis, contents of muscle cells spill into the systemic circulation causing potentially fatal acute renal failure. Early signs of renal failure include decreased urine output, edema, and weight gain. Option 2, rhabdomyoma, is a benign tumor derived from striated muscle. Option 3, rhabdomyosarcoma, is a malignant tumor derived from striated muscle. Option 4, rhinorrhea, is the free discharge of thin nasal mucus. Cognitive Level: Knowledge; Client Need: Physiological Integrity; Nursing Process: Assessment

2 Answer: 2 Rationale: One of the most series adverse effects of this drug is obstruction of the GI tract. Cholestyramine (Questran) does not cause orange urine (option 1). Sore throat and fever are not common adverse effects with cholestyramine (Questran) (option 3). Cholestyramine does not affect capillary refill (option 4). Cognitive Level: Application; Client Need: Physiological Integrity; Nursing Process: Assessment

3 Answer: 1 Rationale: Although there are few contraindications to using bile acid sequestrants, they should be used cautiously in clients with GI disorders such as peptic ulcer disease. Myocardial infarction is not a contraindication for the use of bile acid sequestrants (option 2). Bile acid sequestrant agents do not affect serum sodium levels (option 3). Clients allergic to foods high in tyramine may be prescribed bile acid sequestrants (option 4). Cognitive Level: Application; Client Need: Physiological Integrity; Nursing Process: Implementation

4 Answer: 2 Rationale: Intense flushing and hot flashes occur in almost every client. Option 1, fever and chills, are not an associated adverse effect of nicotinic acid therapy. Option 3, nicotinic acid does not cause tingling of the fingers and toes. Option 4, dry mucous membranes, is not an expected adverse effect with this therapy. Cognitive Level: Application; Client Need: Physiological Integrity; Nursing Process: Assessment

5 Answer: 2 Rationale: Most clients with lipid disorders are asymptomatic. A client should be instructed that maintenance of optimal body weight will help reduce unhealthy lipid levels (option 1). Because cholesterol biosynthesis in the liver is higher at night, statins with short half-lives such as lovastatin should be administered in the evening (option 3). Grapefruit juice inhibits the metabolism of statins, allowing them to reach high serum levels (option 4). Cognitive Level: Application; Client Need: Physiological Integrity; Nursing Process: Evaluation

6 Answer: 2, 3, 4 Rationale: Because bile acid sequestrants are not absorbed into the systemic circulation, adverse effects are limited to the GI tract, causing symptoms such as bloating, abdominal pain, diarrhea, steatorrhea, and constipation (option 2). In addition to binding bile acids, these drugs can bind drugs such as digoxin and warfarin, thus increasing the potential for drug–drug interactions (option 3). Bile acid sequestrants interfere with the absorption of vitamins and minerals, and nutritional deficiencies may occur with extended use (option 4). Option 1 is incorrect. The bile acid sequestrants tend to cause more frequent adverse effects than statins because they are not absorbed into the systemic circulation. Option 5 is incorrect. Medications and vitamins should be taken at least 1 hour before or 4 hours after taking a bile acid sequestrant to avoid drug interactions. Cognitive Level: Knowledge; Client Need: Physiological Integrity; Nursing Process: Assessment

Chapter 33

Answer to Connection Checkpoint 33.1

A CCB has similar cardiovascular actions as anticholinergics thus the two would have additive effects. CCBs have opposite cardiovascular actions to sympathomimetics; thus the two would have antagonistic effects.

Answer to Connection Checkpoint 33.2

Afterload is the pressure that the myocardium must overcome to eject the blood from the ventricles. As afterload increases, cardiac output decreases.

Answer to Connection Checkpoint 33.3

The two drugs would cause additive constipation, orthostatic hypotension and possibly confusion and dizziness. Anticholinergic drugs speed up the heart rate, which could cancel the myocardial depressant actions of verapamil.

Chapter 33 Answers to Critical Thinking Questions

1 Calcium channel blockers slow the rate at which calcium passes into the heart muscle and into the vessel walls. This relaxes the vessels. The relaxed vessels let blood flow more easily through them, thereby lowering blood pressure.

2 HTN is a silent killer. Many people don't experience any symptoms with blood pressure elevations. However, the problem with an elevated blood pressure is that the body's organs fail to work properly under this condition. Complications of HTN include heart attack, heart failure, stroke, kidney failure, aneurysms, and blindness.

3 There is no cure for HTN. However, patients with this chronic disease can live normal lives if lifestyle changes are adopted and adherence to a therapeutic regimen is followed.

4 Adverse effects of CCBs include: hypotension, dizziness, constipation, and dysrhythmias.

Chapter 33 Answers to Case Study

1 The nurse should be empathetic with Mabel's dilemma. After all, she is not having any symptoms. However, you should explain to her that many people have high blood pressure and do not even know it. You should inform Mabel that although high blood pressure usually causes no symptoms, it can cause serious complications.

2 The peripheral vasodilation caused by verapamil (Calan) may trigger flushed skin, headache, dizziness, and light-headedness.

3 Reminders are often helpful when scheduling a patient's medication doses. Some suggestions that the nurse might offer include

- Instruct the patient to time taking medications around daily activities, such as setting an alarm clock, brushing teeth, eating meals, or going to work.
- The patient might consider placing reminder notes in visible places such as the telephone or refrigerator.
- Family members or friends might also offer friendly reminders.
- Some patients find that a medication box that holds an entire day's supply of medicine is helpful.
- Lastly, if the patient continues to have problems remembering, it might be time to have a talk with the prescriber, to see if the medication schedule can be simplified.

4 Certainly, the cost of the medication is a factor that concerns nurses. Many patients will elect not to purchase medication in lieu of other pressing needs. The health care team should be consulted when medication cost becomes an issue. Perhaps there is a less expensive medication that would be just as effective. There may be other community resources available to help with the cost. Medical social workers are often familiar with various strategies to help patients receive medication.

Chapter 33 Answers to NCLEX-RN® Review

1 Answer: 1 Rationale: A major complication associated with the administration of CCBs such as nifedipine is heart failure. Daily weighing will alert the client of signs of fluid retention which may indicate cardiac dysfunction. Nifedipine does not affect the immune system. Clients on this drug should be able to live normal lives. There is no reason to avoid crowds (option 2). There is no relationship between dietary calcium and CCBs (option 3). HTN is asymptomatic. Clients should be instructed to take the medication even when feeling healthy (option 4). Cognitive Level: Application; Client Need: Physiological Integrity; Nursing Process: Implementation

2 Answer: 4 Rationale: Initially, clients may reduce their blood pressure too much, thereby reducing cerebral blood flow. Clients should be instructed to not drive or operate heavy equipment until the affects of the drug are known. Option 1 is incorrect because rash and chills are not associated adverse effects for CCBs. Neither increased urinary output (option 2), nor weight loss (option 3) are associated adverse effects for CCBs. Cognitive Level: Application; Client Need: Physiological Integrity; Nursing Process: Planning

3 Answer: 4 Rationale: An adverse effect of verapamil is heart failure, which will be reflected in the client's intake and output ratio. Verapamil does not affect coagulation (option 1). This drug does not affect thrombocytes (option 2). Verapamil is usually given during hours that the client is awake. However, it can be administered at any time (option 3). Cognitive Level: Application; Client Need: Physiological Integrity; Nursing Process: Implementation

4 Answer: 2 Rationale: Grapefruit juice will enhance the absorption of nifedipine. As a general rule, no medication should be taken with antacids since this will affect the absorption rate of oral medications (option 1). Clients should never double the dose of this drug because life-threatening hypotension could result (option 3). Nifedipine does not affect the efficacy of birth control pills (option 4). Cognitive Level: Knowledge; Client Need: Physiological Integrity; Nursing Process: Implementation

5 Answer: 1, 2, 4 Rationale: Calcium channel blockers reduce the client's blood pressure, which may result in syncope or dizziness. Until the effects of the medication are known the client should avoid driving or other activities requiring mental alertness (option 1). One of the adverse effects associated with CCBs is constipation, which can be reduced by increasing fluid and dietary fiber intake (option 2). CCBs often cause orthostatic hypotension. To ensure safety, clients should be instructed to rise slowly from sitting or lying positions (option 4). Clients should be taught to report a weight gain of .9 kg (2 lb) per day (24-hour time period) (option 3). There are few adverse effects that require immediate discontinuation of the medication by the client but they should be reported to the prescriber. Sudden discontinuation could cause the client to experience hypertensive crisis (option 5). Cognitive Level: Knowledge; Client Need: Physiological Integrity; Nursing Process: Implementation

6 Answer: 3 Rationale: Pulmonary edema calls for discontinuation of the drugs. Therefore the nurse should monitor the client more closely for drug-related problems if the client has a past medical history of pulmonary edema. An appendectomy does not warrant monitoring the client any more than usual (option 1). Renal dialysis clients do warrant close monitoring due to a reduction in renal function. However, these clients are not as high risk as someone with pulmonary edema (option 2). Psychotropic drugs are not known to interact negatively with this drug (option 4). Cognitive Level: Knowledge; Client Need: Physiological Integrity; Nursing Process: Assessment

Chapter 34

Answer to Connection Checkpoint 34.1

Falling blood pressure is sensed by baroreceptors in the aorta and the internal carotid artery. The body responds by increasing heart rate. This accelerated heart rate caused by falling blood pressure is called reflex tachycardia.

Answer to Connection Checkpoint 34.2

$Beta_1$-adrenergic receptors are predominantly located in the heart, and their action will increase heart rate.

Answer to Connection Checkpoint 34.3

The vasopressor action of angiotensin II would increase cardiac output. Increased systemic pressure would cause afterload to increase.

Answer to Connection Checkpoint 34.4

Atropine (a cholinergic blocker) and epinephrine (an adrenergic agonist) would increase sympathetic action and thus antagonize the effects of the ACE inhibitors. Propranolol (a beta-adrenergic blocker) would have additive effects with the ACE inhibitors.

Chapter 34 Answers to Critical Thinking Questions

1 Cozaar works by blocking the action of angiotensin II, which is a chemical produced in the kidneys. Angiotensin II causes the blood vessels to narrow and makes the blood pressure increase. When this chemical is blocked, blood pressure is not elevated.

2 The most common adverse effects associated with losartan (Cozaar) include headache and dizziness. Carlos should be informed that typically these adverse effects disappear after a few days of therapy. However, if these symptoms continue after 1 week, he should notify his health care provider. More severe effects include angioedema and acute renal failure. You should inform Carlos to immediately report edema, decreased urinary output, difficulty breathing, skin rash, and hives to the presriber.

3 Evidence from randomized controlled trials provides overwhelming support for a causal relationship between dietary sodium intake and elevated blood pressure. However, it seems that salt metabolism, and its effects on HTN are extremely complex and are not well understood. The American Heart Association (AHA) strongly supports the reduction of sodium intake for individuals with HTN. Currently the average American adult consumes three times the recommended daily allowance.

Chapter 34 Answers to Case Study

1 Lisinopril binds to and inhibits the action of ACE, thus preventing the conversion of angiotensin I to angiotensin II. Spironolactone acts by blocking aldosterone receptors in the kidney tubules.

2 Spironolactone is used as a diuretic and as an antihypertensive medication. It causes the kidneys to eliminate unneeded water and sodium from the body into the urine but reduces the loss of potassium from the body. The patient should avoid potassium-containing salt substitutes while taking this medication. Ella should also talk with her health care provider about the amount of potassium-rich foods (e.g., bananas, prunes, raisins, and orange juice) that she may eat.

Chapter 34 Answers to NCLEX-RN® Review

1 Answer: 4 Rationale: Lisinopril does not affect serum calcium levels causing an elevated blood pressure. Common adverse effects for lisinopril are cough, headache, dizziness, and orthostatic hypotension. These symptoms should be reported to the prescriber (option 1). Salt substitutes are usually potassium-based products. Individuals taking lisinopril and who are taking potassium supplements are at highest risk for hyperkalemia (option 2). Clients on this medication should be instructed to stay on regular doses of blood pressure medication. If a dose is missed, take it as soon as possible but not too close to the next dose. Never take a double dose (option 3). Cognitive Level: Application; Client Need: Physiological Integrity; Nursing Process: Evaluation

2 Answer: 1 Rationale: Prinivil should be stored in a dry place at room temperature, as heat and moisture may cause drug breakdown. Heat and moisture does not enhance the strength of the drug (option 2). Heat and moisture does not crystallize the medication (option 3). Heat and moisture does not convert the medication to toxic metabolites (option 4). Cognitive Level: Knowledge; Client Need: Physiological Integrity; Nursing Process: Assessment

3 Answer: 3 Rationale: ACE inhibitors also prevent the breakdown of bradykinin. Accumulation of bradykinin in certain tissues such as the lungs can cause adverse effects as manifested by a nonproductive cough. Dry mucous membranes are not adverse effects related to ACE inhibitors (option 1). The expected outcome associated with ACE inhibitors is a decline in blood pressure (option 2). The nurse should expect the blood pressure (both systolic and diastolic) to be reduced (option 4). Cognitive Level: Application; Client Need: Physiological Integrity; Nursing Process: Assessment

4 Answer: 2 Rationale: The most common adverse effects of losartan are headache, dizziness, nasal congestion, and insomnia. Irritability and insomnia are not associated with losartan (option 1). Losartan does not produce sleepiness and slurred speech (option 3). Pruritus and rash are not common adverse effects of this drug (option 4). Cognitive Level: Application; Client Need: Physiological Integrity; Nursing Process: Assessment

5 Answer: 1 Rationale: Clients with severe dehydration may experience hypovolemia and are at high risk of life-threatening hypotension. Losartan may be prescribed for the prevention of diabetic nephropathy (option 2). Losartan is approved for the treatment of HTN (option 3). An off-label use for losartan is heart failure (option 4). Cognitive Level: Application; Client Need: Physiological Integrity; Nursing Process: Assessment

6 Answer: 3 Rationale: Clients receiving Losartan initially should avoid driving or engaging in other potentially hazardous activities until effects of the drug are known. Losartin may cause adverse effects that impair thinking and reaction time. The client or family should be taught methods of home blood pressure measurement and maintenance of a blood pressure log while taking losartan (option 1). OTC medications for colds, sinus or fever, asthma, or appetite control, should be avoided because they may increase blood pressure (option 2). The consumption of alcohol while taking losartan can lower blood pressure which will lead to dizziness and fainting (option 4). Cognitive Level: Application; Client Need: Physiological Integrity; Nursing Process: Evaluation

Chapter 35

Answer to Connection Checkpoint 35.1

When bound to plasma proteins, drugs remain in the blood and are unable to be excreted. Therefore, the half-life of the drug will be prolonged.

Answer to Connection Checkpoint 35.2

Angiotensin II stimulates the adrenal cortex to synthesize and secrete aldosterone. Aldosterone acts on the nephron to increase Na^+ reabsorption and K^+ and H^+ excretion. The increased sodium reabsorption promotes water retention and raises blood pressure.

Answer to Connection Checkpoint 35.3

Lithium is used to treat the acute manic episodes characteristic of bipolar disorder, and in preventing the recurrence of mania or depression. Diuretics can increase the risk of lithium toxicity by promoting sodium loss; the body replaces lost sodium with lithium, which is also a salt.

Answer to Connection Checkpoint 35.4

Hyperkalemia occurs in about 2% to 4% of patients taking ACE inhibitors. Patients with congestive heart failure, renal impairment, or who are taking potassium supplements or potassium-sparing diuretics are at highest risk for hyperkalemia.

Chapter 35 Answers to Critical Thinking Questions

1 Loop diuretics act on the ascending loop of Henle in the kidney. They are primarily used in medicine to treat HTN and edema, often due to CHF or renal insufficiency. Although all electrolytes may be lost due to diuretic therapy, it is potassium that is most severely lost and presents the greatest problem to patients receiving this drug.

Thiazide diuretics are drugs that remove water from the body. These drugs also deplete the body's potassium levels and cause the body to lose magnesium. Thiazides are used to lower blood pressure and are frequently used in combination with other drugs to treat HTN.

Potassium-sparing diuretics do not promote the secretion of potassium into the urine. They are also used as adjunctive therapy in the treatment of HTN and CHF.

Osmotic diuretics work through the diffusion of fluid through semipermeable membranes by creating a shift in fluid from intercellular and interstitial areas to the intravascular space. Initially, due to the increase in the circulating volume, the nurse should monitor the patient for fluid overload.

2 Most diuretics potentially create a deficit of potassium. Hypokalemia predisposes the patient to digoxin toxicity.

3 The patient taking diuretics should be instructed to

- Take the medication exactly as prescribed.
- Watch for electrolyte imbalances and dehydration and steps to prevent such from occurring.
- Weigh weekly and report significant changes to the health care provider such as weight gain of 2 lbs in 2 days.
- Consult prescriber before consuming OTC medications.
- Rise slowly to minimize orthostatic hypotension.

Chapter 35 Answers to Case Study

1 Spironolactone inhibits the action of aldosterone causing the kidneys to excrete sodium and water while retaining potassium. Therefore, spironolactone is classified as a potassium-sparing medication that promotes the output of urine (diuretic).

2 Foods high in potassium include apricots, avocado, banana, cantaloupe, honeydew, kiwi, lima beans, milk, oranges/orange juice, potatoes, prunes, spinach, tomatoes, and vegetable juice.

3 Often hyperkalemia is asymptomatic. Some patients report vague symptoms that include nausea, fatigue, muscle weakness, or tingling. More serious signs include slow heartbeat and weak pulse.

Chapter 35 Answers to NCLEX-RN® Review

1 Answer: 2 Rationale: As a diuretic, Lasix may dramatically reduce the client's circulating blood volume thus producing episodes of orthostatic hypotension. Clients may minimize this effect by rising slowly from sitting or lying positions. The foods listed in option 1 are high in vitamin K but Lasix does not restrict the consumption of these foods. Monitoring pulse rate prior to administration of Lasix is not required (option 3). Lasix is never administered subcutaneously (option 4). Cognitive Level: Application; Client Need: Physiological Integrity; Nursing Process: Implementation

2 Answer: 2 Rationale: Loop diuretics are notorious for producing a significant loss of potassium. Hypokalemia is often the predominant electrolyte imbalance. Hyponatremia is unlikely with the administration of high ceiling diuretics (option 1). Hyperkalemia is inconsistent with the administration of high ceiling diuretics. If elevated potassium levels are present in these clients, other etiologies should be investigated (option 3). Loop diuretics do not cause hypocalcemia (option 4). Cognitive Level: Knowledge; Client Need: Physiological Integrity; Nursing Process: Assessment

3 Answer: 3 Rationale: Muscle cramps and weakness may represent hypokalemia and should be reported to the health care provider. Many clients taking diuretic therapy are instructed to monitor the intake of both sodium and water (option 1). Clients should ingest foods high in potassium, not vitamin K (option 2). It is unlikely that diuretics and antihypertensive drugs will cause sleepiness (option 4). Cognitive Level: Application; Client Need: Physiological Integrity; Nursing Process: Implementation

4 Answer: 1 Rationale: Spironolactone (Aldactone) is a potassium sparing diuretic. This drug does not have a direct effect on magnesium (option 2). This drug saves potassium; it does not excrete it (option 3). This drug does not bind calcium (option 4). Cognitive Level: Knowledge; Client Need: Physiological Integrity; Nursing Process: Assessment

5 Answer: 1, 3, 4 Rationale: These are measures that apply to all clients receiving diuretic therapy. Option 2 is incorrect because spironolactone (Aldactone) is a potassium sparing diuretic and the client is more likely to develop hyperkalemia. Additionally, the client should be taught to avoid foods high in potassium. Option 5 is incorrect because salt substitutes are high in potassium content and should be avoided by a client prescribed spironolactone (Aldactone). Cognitive Level: Knowledge; Client Need: Physiological Integrity; Nursing Process: Planning

6 Answer: 1 Rationale: Clients receiving acetazolamide (Diamox) are at risk for metabolic acidosis due to excess bicarbonate loss. Option 2 is incorrect. Metabolic alkalosis is characterized by a deficit of bicarbonate and is not an adverse effect of acetazolamide (Diamox). Option 3 is incorrect because acetazolamide (Diamox) does not cause respiratory acidosis. Option 4 is incorrect because respiratory alkalosis is not an expected adverse effect of acetazolamide (Diamox). Cognitive Level: Knowledge; Client Need: Physiological Integrity; Nursing Process: Assessment

Chapter 36

Answer to Connection Checkpoint 36.1

Afterload is the systolic pressure in the aorta that must be overcome for blood to be ejected from the left ventricle. As afterload increases, the heart pumps less blood, and stroke volume (and thus CO) decreases.

Answer to Connection Checkpoint 36.2

Thiazide diuretics can deplete the body of potassium. This can cause dysrhythmias in patients taking digoxin.

Answer to Connection Checkpoint 36.3

Verapamil affects both cardiac and vascular smooth muscle. A beta blocker will have additive cardiac suppressant effects. Nifedipine affects vessels but not the heart, thus there will not be additive cardiac effects.

Answer to Connection Checkpoint 36.4

$Beta_1$ blockers are cardioselective and have little effects on bronchial smooth muscle. Nonselective beta blockers may cause bronchoconstriction and worsen asthma.

Answer to Connection Checkpoint 36.5

Pheochromocytoma is a tumor of the adrenal gland that secretes large amounts of epinephrine and norepinephrine. Alpha antagonists block the effects of these catecholamines at the arterioles, thereby reducing blood pressure. Beta blockers do not affect the arterioles.

Chapter 36 Answers to Critical Thinking Questions

1 Elmer is on the right track. Although lifestyle changes aid in high blood pressure reduction, they take time. Plus, even with dietary changes, exercising, and smoking cessation, HTN may still be present. Elmer needs to be informed that it is not unusual that controlling HTN sometimes requires more than one medication, increasing the dosage, or combining various drug therapies.

2 Certainly, Elmer might be depressed about his inability to achieve normal blood pressure. However, there is another factor that should be considered. Some antihypertensive medications such as methyldopa (Aldomet) cause mental depression.

3 HTN is complex and may be caused by a series of physiological factors. It is not unusual for multiple medications to be prescribed before the right type and right dosage brings high blood pressure under control.

4 Elmer should be praised for his efforts. There is a good chance his blood pressure reading would have been much higher had he not initiated the various lifestyle changes. HTN is a chronic disease that can cause some individuals to feel hopeless. Providing the patient with support and encouragement is an important nursing intervention. It may be the determining factor in the patient choosing to adhere to the therapeutic regimen.

Chapter 36 Answers to Case Study

1 Nitroprusadverse acts directly on vascular smooth muscle to produce peripheral vasodilation thereby lowering of arterial blood pressure. It is used for short-term, rapid reduction of blood pressure in hypertensive crises.

2 Nitroprusside is powerful and is only given in critical care or emergency department settings. Adverse effects include profound hypotension, palpitation, bradycardia, and ECG changes.

3 Helen has multiple factors that predispose her to hypertensive crisis: African American, history of HTN, poor adherence to hypertensive management, and obesity.

Chapter 36 Answers to NCLEX-RN® Review

1 Answer: 1 Rationale: Hot baths and showers, prolonged standing in one position, and strenuous exercise may enhance orthostatic hypotension. Methyldopa does not discolor the urine (option 2). Bloating and weight gain are not typical adverse effects of methyldopa (option 3). Methyldopa can be taken without food (option 4). Cognitive Level: Application; Client Need: Physiological Integrity; Nursing Process: Implementation

2 Answer: 4 Rationale: Orthostatic hypotension is a common adverse effect of vasodilators. Vasodilators do not typically cause atelectasis (option 1). Crystalluria is not an adverse effect of vasodilators (option 2). Vasodilators do not cause photosensitivity (option 3). Cognitive Level: Application; Client Need: Physiological Integrity; Nursing Process: Planning

3 Answer: 1 Rationale: Clients who have recently been prescribed apresoline may experience dizziness initially and should be instructed not to engage in activities that may be hazardous. Clients should always consult their health care providers before discontinuing antihypertensive medications (option 2). Clients should report dizziness to the health care provider and should not adjust the dosage until the etiology of the problem is determined (option 3). Clients on this drug have no restriction on air travel (option 4). Cognitive Level: Application; Client Need: Physiological Integrity; Nursing Process: Evaluation

4 Answer: 4 Rationale: The nurse will titrate (adjust) the rate of infusion based on the client's blood pressure. Listening for bowel sounds in the client with hypertensive crisis is not a nursing priority (option 1). Urine specific gravity and glucose levels are not associated with hypertensive crisis or the administration of this drug (option 2). This intervention does not relate to hypertensive crisis or Nipride therapy (option 3). Cognitive Level: Application; Client Need: Physiological Integrity; Nursing Process: Implementation

5 Answer: 2, 3, 4 Rationale: Blood pressure consists of three primary factors that include cardiac output (option 2), peripheral resistance (option 3), and blood volume (option 4). Options 1 and 5 are not factors in blood pressure. Cognitive Level: Knowledge; Client Need: Physiological Integrity; Nursing Process: Assessment

6 Answer: 2 Rationale: Daytime sedation is often a problematic adverse effect for clients taking methyldopa. Taking the dose at night will minimize daytime sedation. Furthermore, some clients reach adequate blood pressure control with a single evening dose. Option 1 is incorrect. Caffeine will increase blood pressure and is not recommended for individuals suffering from hypertension. Option 3 is incorrect. It may not be possible to take a midday nap, especially if the individual works and carries on ADLs. Option 4 is incorrect. Methyldopa is known to cause daytime sedation. However, the client should not discontinue taking the medication since such action can create hypertensive crisis leading to heart attack and stroke. Cognitive Level: Application; Client Need: Physiological Integrity; Nursing Process: Implementation

Chapter 37

Answer to Connection Checkpoint 37.1

A rapid infusion will trigger the atrial reflex. Baroreceptors will recognize stretching of the right atrium and cause the heart rate and cardiac output to increase until the backlog of IV fluid is distributed throughout the body. Patients with angina are at risk for chest pain due to the increased workload on the heart.

Answer to Connection Checkpoint 37.2

The statins are taken to lower LDL-cholesterol levels, which are partially responsible for the lipid deposits on atherosclerotic arteries.

Answer to Connection Checkpoint 37.3

Nonselective beta-adrenergic antagonists block sympathetic receptors on bronchial smooth muscle, which could cause bronchospasm in patients with asthma. Cardioselective $beta_1$ blockers could be used safely.

Chapter 37 Answers to Critical Thinking Questions

1 MI is another name for a heart attack. This occurs when the blood supply to the heart is interrupted, thereby resulting in an oxygen deficit to the heart cells. Heart cells require a steady supply of oxygen. When the supply is decreased or stopped, heart cells begin to die. There are multiple causes for MI. The treatment is aimed at supplying the heart muscle with oxygen enriched blood.

2 Nitroglycerin is a drug which dilates the blood vessels. This dilation allows more blood to reach the oxygen deprived myocardial tissue. Additionally, nitroglycerin causes venous dilation which decreases cardiac preload and oxygen demand of the myocardium.

3 Adverse effects associated with nitroglycerin infusions include hypotension, tachycardia, flushing, and headache.

4 IV nitroglycerin infusions are typically titrated (adjusted) based on the patient's pain and other hemodynamic indicators such as blood pressure and heart rate. Also, IV nitroglycerin must be administered using specialized IV tubing and should always be delivered via infusion pump.

Chapter 37 Answers to Case Study

1 Tolerance is a common problem with nitrates. This condition depends upon the dosage and the frequency of drug administration. Although tolerance develops rapidly, it also disappears rapidly when the drug is withheld. Patients are often instructed to remove the transdermal patch for 6 to 12 hours each day or withhold a night-time dose of the oral medications in order to delay the development of tolerance. Another regimen common to this drug is to instruct the patient to remove the patch at bedtime and cleanse the medication from the skin with soap and water. In the morning, the patient then reapplies a new patch.

2 Headache is a common adverse effect associated with nitrate therapy (approximately 50% of patients). Usually this adverse effect becomes less severe with continued use. Some health care providers may recommend that the patient take acetaminophen or ibuprofen prior to applying the patch to avoid the associated headache.

3 Dizziness upon rising and rapid heart rates are associated with the related drop in systemic blood pressure caused by nitroglycerin. If this adverse effect continues the prescriber should be notified.

Chapter 37 Answers to NCLEX-RN® Review

1 Answer: 3 Rationale: Clients should be taught to remove the old ointment before applying the next dose. Nitroglycerin should be kept at room temperature (option 1). Clients should take the medication before chest pain becomes severe (option 2). Nitroglycerin can be applied to any skin surface. However, there will be a decrease in absorption when applied to hairy areas, soles of feet, and palms (option 4). Cognitive Level: Application; Client Need: Physiological Integrity; Nursing Process: Implementation

2 Answer: 4 Rationale: A decline in blood pressure is an expected adverse effect. The nurse should always assess the blood pressure prior to administering nitroglycerin. Option 1, photosensitivity, is not an expected adverse effect. Option 2 is incorrect because nitroglycerin will cause a decline in blood pressure not an increase. Option 3, vomiting and diarrhea are not expected adverse effects of this medication. Cognitive Level: Application; Client Need: Physiological Integrity; Nursing Process: Assessment

3 Answer: 4 Rationale: Skin irritation due to the nitroglycerin ointment can occur if the same site is used repeatedly. Clients should be instructed to rotate the site of application when using nitroglycerin ointment (option 1). Repeated use of the same application site may actually decrease absorption (option 2). Rebound phenomenon is not an expected occurrence with nitroglycerin (option 3). Cognitive Level: Application; Client Need: Physiological Integrity; Nursing Process: Implementation

4 Answer: 1 Rationale: Clients often complain of a flushing sensation and headache associated with nitroglycerin. This is due to the vasodilation effect of this drug. Tremors and anxiety are not associated adverse effects with this drug (option 2). Although syncope and dizziness may result due to nitroglycerin administration, they are not expected adverse effects (option 3). Nitroglycerin does not cause sleepiness or lethargy (option 4). Cognitive Level: Knowledge; Client Need: Physiological Integrity; Nursing Process: Assessment

5 Answer: 1 Rationale: Atenolol increases blood flow to the myocardium, thereby increasing oxygen supply by reducing the heart rate and decreasing the contractility. Option 2 is incorrect because atenolol is a beta-adrenergic antagonist, which decreases heart rate. This drug does not affect the sodium channels (option 3). Although this drug reduces blood pressure the mechanism of action is not by blocking the $alpha_2$ receptors (option 4). Cognitive Level: Knowledge; Client Need: Physiological Integrity; Nursing Process: Implementation

6 Answer: 1 and 3 Rationale: Atenolol decreases blood pressure and heart rate. The administration of this drug may cause serious cardiac decompensation. Option 2 is incorrect. Atenolol may be used for fast heart rates. Option 4 is incorrect. Tinnitus and hearing loss are not adverse effects associated with atenolol. Option 5 is incorrect. HTN does not warrant holding this medication. Cognitive Level: Application; Client Need: Physiological Integrity; Nursing Process: Assessment

Chapter 38

Answer to Connection Checkpoint 38.1

Propranolol is a nonselective beta-adrenergic antagonist that will block adrenergic receptors on smooth muscle in the lung. This could cause bronchospasms in patients with asthma.

Answer to Connection Checkpoint 38.2

Conn's syndrome, also known as primary hyperaldosteronism will cause the body to retain sodium and water, leading to HTN and increased cardiac workload. Spironolactone (Aldactone) and eplerenone (Inspra) are aldosterone antagonists that could be used to treat this disorder.

Answer to Connection Checkpoint 38.3

The onset of action of nitroglycerin is within minutes. Isosorbide dinitrate should not be used to terminate angina attacks in progress because it takes 20 to 90 minutes to reach therapeutic drug levels.

Answer to Connection Checkpoint 38.4

Cholestyramine binds to other drugs and interferes with their absorption, causing reduced effects. Cholestyramine is used to treat hypercholesterolemia.

Chapter 38 Answers to Critical Thinking Questions

1 Heart failure can be compared to a broken pump as it fails to propel enough blood to meet the metabolic needs of the body. The symptoms presented by this patient represent circulatory congestion due to poor cardiac function. Thelma's irregular labored respirations represent the failure of the heart to adequately pump the fluid thereby causing congestion in the lung which is manifested by crackles. Neck vein distention and pitting edema also represent abnormal accumulation of fluid from an overloaded circulatory system. Typically, the symptoms of HF include dyspnea on exertion, fatigue, pulmonary congestion, and peripheral edema. Lung congestion causes a cough and orthopnea: difficulty breathing in recumbent positions.

2 Digoxin (Lanoxin) is a cardiac glycoadverse that increases the contraction force of the myocardium. It also affects the cardiac conduction system and slows the heart rate. Both actions allow a failing heart to improve its ability to adequately pump blood to the body.

3 Digitalization is a procedure by which doses of digoxin are gradually increased to achieve therapeutic level (saturated tissues), thereby relieving the symptoms of heart failure.

4 The low potassium levels must be corrected, either with PO or IV supplementation, because it may predispose the patient to digoxin toxicity.

Chapter 38 Answers to Case Study

1 The combination of digoxin, furosemide, and potassium supplementation is common. The purpose of the digoxin is to promote effective cardiac pumping and the improvement of the cardiac output. The diuretic (furosemide) eliminates excessive body fluid and reduces the workload of the failing heart. The potassium supplement is prescribed to replace the loss of potassium caused by the diuretic.

2 Serum digoxin levels are blood tests to determine if the correct amount of the drug is in the body. The patient does not need to fast before the test. However, the blood should not be drawn for at least 6 hours after the last dose of digoxin. The patient should write down the time of the last dose.

3 Heart failure patients with normal renal function should be encouraged to consume foods rich in potassium, such as poultry, fish, bananas, cantaloupes, tomatoes, vegetable juice, apple juice, broccoli, and corn.

Chapter 38 Answers to NCLEX-RN® Review

1 Answer: 4 Rationale: A low potassium level, or hypokalemia, can increase the likelihood of toxicity. Hypercalcemia tends to increase the client's sensitivity to digoxin preparations, not hypocalcemia (option 1). Hypomagnesemia, not hypermagnesemia, could potentiate the possibility of digitalis toxicity (option 2). Hyperbilirubinemia does not potentiate the action of digoxin (option 3). Cognitive Level: Comprehension; Client Need: Physiological Integrity; Nursing Process: Assessment

2 Answer: 2 Rationale: The client will be taught to take the pulse daily and to contact the prescriber if the pulse rate is less than 60 or greater than 100 beats per minute. Option 1 is incorrect because the medication should be taken at the same time each day, but preferably after the client has been active for a period of time (midmorning). Typically, the pulse rate will be lower in the morning before the client rises. Option 3 is incorrect because Lanoxin should be withheld if the pulse rate is below 60 beats per minute. Option 4 is incorrect because a high-fiber diet may decrease the absorption of digoxin. Furthermore, foods high in calcium may create hypercalcemia, which will potentiate the possibility of digitalis toxicity. Cognitive Level: Knowledge; Client Need: Physiological Integrity; Nursing Process: Implementation

3 Answer: 1 Rationale: The inotropic effect of digoxin is an increase in the force of the contraction of the heart. Inotropic effects usually increase the volume of the cardiac output (option 2). Inotropic effects do not relax the myocardial muscle (option 3). Although digoxin does affect the cardiac rate and rhythm, this does not define the inotropic effect of the drug (option 4). Cognitive Level: Knowledge; Client Need: Physiological Integrity; Nursing Process: Evaluation

4 Answer: 2 Rationale: A major adverse effect of Primacor is ventricular dysrhythmias which would be manifested by irregularities in the heartbeat. Option 1 is incorrect because typically Primacor does not cause confusion or agitation. Other etiologies such as hypoxia should be investigated. Option 3 is incorrect because Primacor is not known to cause tingling or cramping in the legs. Option 4 is incorrect because brownish discoloration in the skin creases is not an adverse effect related to Primacor therapy. Cognitive Level: Comprehension; Client Need: Safe, Effective Care Environment; Nursing Process: Assessment

5 Answer: 1 Rationale: Research using ACE inhibitors such as captopril (Capoten) and lisinopril (Prinivil) indicate that this classification of drugs used with heart failure clients slows the progression of the disease and reduces mortality. ACE inhibitors do not reduce renal toxicity (option 2). Although treatment for heart failure is aimed at increasing cardiac output this is not accomplished by the impairment of coronary dilation (option 3). Decreasing adrenergic effects is not accomplished with ACE inhibitors (option 4). Cognitive Level: Comprehension; Client Need: Physiological Integrity; Nursing Process: Implementation

6 Answer: 1, 2, 4, and 5 Rationale: These choices are essential pharmacological therapies for heart failure clients. Option 3 is incorrect however, because insulin therapy is not used for the treatment of heart failure. Cognitive Level: Comprehension; Client Need: Safe, Effective Care Environment; Nursing Process: Assessment

Chapter 39

Answer to Connection Checkpoint 39.1

The three channel types are called L, T, and N. The L type is the one blocked by calcium channel antagonists.

Answer to Connection Checkpoint 39.2

There are no $alpha_1$-adrenergic receptors in the heart; therefore $alpha_1$ blockers would be ineffective in treating cardiac dysrhythmias.

Answer to Connection Checkpoint 39.3

The dihydropyridines such as amlodipine (Norvasc), nicardipine (Cardene), and nifedipine (Adalat, Procardia) bind to closed-type calcium channels. These channels are found in greater numbers in vascular smooth muscle than in cardiac muscle; therefore they are primarily used for their vasodilation effect on arterial smooth muscle.

Chapter 39 Answers to Critical Thinking Questions

1 The heart possesses a specialized system to control electrical impulses which are needed for cardiac contraction. Normally the impulse is initiated in a bundle of cells located in the right atrium, called the sinoatrial (SA) node. Once generated, the electrical impulse moves from cell to cell down through the heart until it reaches the atrioventricular (AV) node. This area is located in the middle of the heart, between the atrium and ventricles.

After the AV node, the electrical impulses travel through a bundle of fibers that separate the right and left ventricle. The bundles are known as the Bundle of His. Once the electrical impulse reaches the base of the ventricle (apex), it travels upward and spreads across both ventricles through the Purkinje fibers. SA Node → AV Node → Bundle of His → Purkinje Fibers.

Jada's diagnosis tells what part of the conduction is affected. Atrial fibrillation is a condition that occurs in the upper chambers of the heart. Fibrillation is a rapid uncoordinated twitching movement of the atrium, which impairs cardiac function. This abnormality would be manifested in the P waves of the ECG.

2 Amiodarone when given IV is usually only administered over 2–3 days to achieve a rapid therapeutic blood level. Afterwards, patients are often placed on the oral preparation of this drug. As you explain the mechanism of action to this patient, avoid using difficult medical terms. The patient wants to know how the drug works, not how smart the nurse is. Begin by saying that this drug helps to regulate the electrical condition system of the heart. It slows the rate at which the heart's electrical system recharges and prolongs the electrical phase during which the heart is electrically stimulated. This, in turn, helps to restore the normal heartbeat.

3 Several issues should be discussed with the patient before discharge. The patient should understand that it is important to take amiodarone exactly as directed by the prescriber. If a dose is missed, the patient should take the missed dose as soon as it is remembered; however, never double the doses. For some patients amiodarone causes dizziness, drowsiness, and blurred vision. Until the effects of the drug are fully known, the patient should avoid driving or operating machinery. Additionally, patients should check their pulse daily and report values less than 60 beats/minute to the health care provider. Lastly, some patients receiving amiodarone may suffer from photosensitivity. They should be advised to protect their skin from ultraviolet rays and to wear sunglasses.

4 Jada needs to know that she should avoid grapefruit or grapefruit juice during treatment with amiodarone. Amiodarone can interact with grapefruit and grapefruit juice with dangerous effects.

Chapter 39 Answers to Case Study

1 A prodysrhythmic is a drug, substance, or condition that predisposes an individual to develop cardiac dysrhythmias. HTN, CAD, and MIs are examples of disease conditions that are prodysrhythmic. Practically any drug can become a prodysrhythmic when it reaches toxic levels. Many OTC medications, such as cold remedies or cough and sinus preparations, are capable of stimulating the cardiac electrical system and producing serious heartbeat irregularities.

2 An electrical phenomenon called depolarization is what occurs to produce a cardiac contraction. Each heart cycle consists of two phases: depolarization which represents the myocardial stimulation and repolarization which represents the recovery phase. Drug therapy that treats dysrhythmias effects one or both of these phases (depolarization and repolarization) of the cardiac contraction.

3 Food and beverages that can irritate cardiac cells and cause dysrhythmias include coffee, tea, chocolate, red wine, or simply overeating. Nicotine exposure and any cocaine exposure can cause serious dysrhythmias.

Chapter 39 Answers to NCLEX-RN® Review

1 Answer: 4 Rationale: Procainamide should be avoided in clients suffering from severe heart failure since this drug can worsen the condition. Options 1, 2, and 3 are incorrect because ventricular tachycardia, paroxysmal atrial tachycardia, and atrial fibrillation are sometimes treated with this drug. Therefore the order is not unusual. Cognitive Level: Application; Client Need: Physiological Integrity; Nursing Process: Assessment

2 Answer: 2 Rationale: The client should assume a supine position during IV administration because severe hypotension may occur during the infusion. Additionally, the client should be on continous ECG monitoring while receiving infusion. Option 1 is incorrect. Increased thrombocytes are not related to the administration of procainamide. Option 3 is incorrect. There is no reason to limit the client's intake of calcium when receiving procainamide. Option 4 is incorrect. Although coughing and deep breathing is an effective nursing strategy to maintain pulmonary function, it is not pertinent for the administration of IV procainamide. Cognitive Level: Application; Client Need: Physiological Integrity; Nursing Process: Implementation

3 Answer: 1 Rationale: The therapeutic goal of a potassium channel blocker is not to cause changes in the client's blood pressure. Potassium channel blockers do not increase or decrease the amount of potassium in the serum (option 2). Potassium channel blockers are given to correct dysrhythmias. The nurse will monitor the client's cardiac rhythm to determine the effectiveness of this therapy (option 3). Although renal perfusion may be altered by irregularities in the cardiac rhythm, this drug does not reduce the urinary output (option 4). Cognitive Level: Application; Client Need: Physiological Integrity; Nursing Process: Evaluation

4 Answer: 1 Rationale: The first sign of lidocaine toxicity involves confusion, anxiety, tremors, and paresthesia. If these symptoms are manifested in a client receiving lidocaine, the nurse should withhold the medication and immediately notify the prescriber. Option 2 is incorrect because increasing the infusion rate would increase the serum level of the drug and consequently make the client even more toxic. Calming the client will probably be ineffective, since the anxiety is due to a toxic level of the drug. Option 3 is incorrect because the only way to reduce a toxic serum level of lidocaine is to discontinue the medication and allow the drug to be excreted through physiological mechanisms. There is no antidote. Option 4 is incorrect because simply reducing the infusion rate will be a dangerous action when the client is suffering from toxic drug levels. Cognitive Level: Application; Client Need: Physiological Integrity; Nursing Process: Implementation

5 Answer: 2 Rationale: Beta blockers reduce heart rate and reduce the rate of cardiac conduction. This action decreases the incidence of cardiac dysrhythmias by blocking calcium ion channels in the SA and AV nodes. Option 1 is incorrect because beta-adrenergic antagonist (aka beta-blockers) slow the heart and do not reduce respiratory status. Option 3 is incorrect because phase 4 of the action potential is when the myocardial cell is resting and the exchange of ions (sodium, calcium, and potassium) has not yet started. To eliminate this phase would reduce the resting phase of the heart. Option 4 is incorrect because the assessment findings of a flattened T wave on the ECG complex usually represents ischemia (inadequate blood flow) to the myocardium and is always bad. Cognitive Level: Knowledge; Client Need: Physiological Integrity; Nursing Process: Assessment

6 Answer: 3 Rationale: One problem associated with this drug is photosensitivity. The patient should be instructed to avoid direct sunlight and wear protective clothing and barrier type sunscreen lotions. Option 1 is incorrect. Avoiding crowds is an instruction given to a client who is immune suppressed. Amiodarone is not known to cause this problem. Option 2 is incorrect because amiodarone does not seem to interact with oral contraceptives. Option 4 is incorrect. This is an instruction that a nurse should give the patient when the drug causes bleeding tendencies. This is not a typical adverse effect with amiodarone. Cognitive Level: Application; Client Need: Physiological Integrity; Nursing Process: Implementation

Chapter 40

Answer to Connection Checkpoint 40.1

The extrinsic pathway is activated when blood leaks out of a vessel. The intrinsic pathway is more complex, and is completed within minutes. A common step between the two pathways is the formation of the fibrin clot.

Chapter 40 Answer to Patient Safety Question

Unfortunately, medication errors like this one are common with automated dispensing cabinets. The hospital should avoid pre-made drug preparation on the unit whenever possible and only do it when chances of error have been eliminated. Ultimately, it is the nurse who must be aware that similar packaging can be deceptive and extreme caution is critical, especially when working with infants and children.

Chapter 40 Answers to Critical Thinking Questions

1 It is very common for individuals to think that anticoagulants dissolve blood clots. However, the drug only prevents the thrombus from enlarging or additional thrombi from forming. So what happens to the existing clot? The human body has a natural mechanism called fibrinolysis that occurs on a continual basis. This mechanism will slowly and naturally dissolve any blood clots. However, in the meantime, the heparin will prevent the existing clot from increasing in size.

2 The major emphasis for patients receiving anticoagulation therapy is to prevent injury that may result in internal or external bleeding. It is important to remember that these drugs decrease the patient's ability to form a blood clot, which is essential to prevent exsanguination (bleeding out). Here are a few patient education tips that you will want to share with Ruby.

- Avoid activities that may cause traumatic injury.
- Use soft cloths and mild soap when bathing.
- Avoid wearing clothing that is tight or rubs.
- Avoid blowing or picking the nose.
- Avoid rectal suppositories, tampons, or enemas.
- Watch for bleeding and examine all body fluids for the presence of blood.
- Avoid drugs that contain aspirin or other anticoagulants.

3 An activated partial thromboplastin time (aPTT) is a laboratory test that reports the time required for clot formation in blood plasma after contact activation and the addition of platelet substitutes. This blood test is used to address the intrinsic and common pathways of coagulation. Heparin is titrated according to the aPTT value, which should be between 1.5 to 2 times the patient's baseline when therapeutic anticoagulation is achieved.

4 Long airplane flights can be problematic, especially in patients who have varicose veins (varicosities), irregularly swollen or enlarged veins commonly found in the lower extremities. People who travel on flights that last eight hours or more are four times more likely to develop DVT. Air travel may increase the risk of DVT through one or more of the following mechanisms

- Prolonged sitting and pressure on the calves by the passenger's seat, which can lead to stagnant blood flow in the veins
- Dehydration as a result of low humidity in the cabin and/or the consumption of alcohol and caffeine
- Decreased air pressure and the release of nitric oxide in the plane's cabin
- Aspirin and NSAIDs such as ibuprofen (Motrin/Advil) and naproxen (Aleve) are common OTC medications. Both substances have an anticoagulation effect and can cause bleeding. These drugs should be avoided when the patient is receiving anticoagulation therapy.

Chapter 40 Answers to Case Study

1 Atrial fibrillation is the rapid, uncoordinated firing of electrical impulses from multiple sites in the upper chambers of the heart. This condition causes ineffective cardiac contractions and the heart quivers instead of beating normally. When blood pools in parts of the atrium, subsequent to the poor pumping action, there is an increase in the risk that blood clots will form. Even small blood clots can cause strokes and heart attacks if they leave the heart and are released into the general circulation. Warfarin will prevent the formation of mural thrombi (a thrombus formed on and attached to the endocardium).

2 While taking this medication, Lewis should contact the health care provider immediately if any bleeding or bruising occurs. Lewis should also be told not to take any prescriptions or OTC medications, such as aspirin products, or vitamins and herbal preparations (especially those containing vitamin E or vitamin K), unless ordered by the health care provider. The reason for this is that many of these medications may interact with warfarin. If he forgets to take his medication, warn him not to try to catch up or double up on the dosage. He should contact his health care provider for instructions. Before starting any new medication or having a medical or surgical procedure, Lewis should talk with the health care provider.

3 Liver, broccoli, cabbage, cauliflower, spinach, lentils, chickpeas (garbanzo beans), turnip greens, soybean oil, seaweed, green tea, and herbal teas can all affect Coumadin. He should minimize his intake of these foods.

4 The effects of warfarin are evaluated using blood tests such as prothrombin time (PT) or international normalized ratio (INR). The INR is the ratio of a patient's prothrombin time to a normal (control) sample. Both blood tests measure how long it takes for blood to clot. The warfarin will be adjusted on the time it takes for blood to clot.

Chapter 40 Answers to NCLEX-RN® Review

1 Answer: 1 Rationale: An activated partial thromboplastin time (aPTT) is the appropriate laboratory value that should be monitored with heparin infusions. When the client is receiving this drug, the results should be 1.5 to 2.0 times that client's baseline, or 60–80 seconds. This test is typically performed every 6–8 hours. Option 2 is incorrect. A prothrombin time is used to monitor the effectiveness of warfarin. The normal prothrombin time is 11–15 seconds, although there is some variation depending on the source of the thromboplastin used in the test. For this reason, laboratories report a normal control value along with the client's results. Option 3 is incorrect. Another name for platelets is thrombocytes. They are involved in the cellular mechanism that leads to the formation of a blood clot. However, platelets are not affected by anticoagulants and are therefore not used in the monitoring of these drugs. Option 4 is incorrect. An INR is essentially the same as a prothrombin time (PT) and is used for warfarin monitoring. Cognitive Level: Application; Client Need: Physiological Integrity; Nursing Process: Assessment

2 Answer: 4 Rationale: Dental flossing is prohibited while the client is receiving anticoagulants. The flossing can cause gum irritation and excessive bleeding. Option 1 is incorrect. When heparin is given subcutaneously it is routinely given in the subcutaneous fat found on the abdomen. The reason for this action is twofold. First, the absorption rate is ensured when this location is used. Secondly, most people have sufficient subcutaneous tissue in the abdominal area. Option 2 is incorrect. Clients receiving heparin must be protected from injury. When taking a blood pressure, the cuff pressure must be released as soon as possible to avoid bruising of the upper arm. Option 3 is incorrect. It is critical that the nurse carefully monitor all venipuncture sites for bleeding. When venipuncture is done for laboratory or diagnostic tests, it is important that direct pressure be applied to the site to avoid bleeding into the tissue. Cognitive Level: Application; Client Need: Physiological Integrity; Nursing Process: Planning

3 Answer: 3 Rationale: Many drugs such as aspirin and ibuprofen have strong anticoagulant effects. When the client on Coumadin takes these drugs, essentially more anticoagulant (bleeding) effects can be hazardous. Option 1 is incorrect. Drugs such as aspirin and ibuprofen do not neutralize the effect of an anticoagulant. These drugs enhance the bleeding tendencies of anticoagulants. Option 2 is incorrect. Anticoagulants do not influence the half-life of any drugs. Option 4 is incorrect. The pain associated with arthritis is not worsened by the combination of these drugs. Cognitive Level: Knowledge; Client Need: Physiological Integrity; Nursing Process: Assessment

4 Answer: 2 Rationale: It is critical that the client be told to discontinue the Coumadin prior to dental procedures. Clients should inform health care providers of all medication being taken, especially anticoagulants. Option 1 is incorrect. The INR laboratory test would not be accurate if the client takes any drugs that influence coagulation time. Option 3 is incorrect. Blood pressure and heart rate are not typically affected by anticoagulants. Option 4 is incorrect. A low fat, low carbohydrate diet is not necessary during anticoagulation therapy. Cognitive Level: Application; Client Need: Physiological Integrity; Nursing Process: Implementation

5 Answer: 1 Rationale: Plavix is an antiplatelet drug used to prevent blood clots from forming inside arteries by inhibiting platelet aggregation. Option 2 is incorrect. Heparin is an anticoagulant that blocks the formation of blood clots by activating antithrombin III. Option 3 is incorrect. Coumadin is a vitamin K antagonist used to prevent the blood from clotting. Option 4 is incorrect. The drug alteplase (Activase) is a tissue plasminogen activator that dissolves fibrin clots. Cognitive Level: Knowledge; Client Need: Physiological Integrity; Nursing Process: Assessment

6 Answer: 1, 3, 4, 5 Rationale: Options 1, 3, 4 and 5 are all correct statements. Option 2 is incorrect because vitamin B_{12} does not enhance the response of Refludan. Cognitive Level: Knowledge; Client Need: Physiological Integrity; Nursing Process: Assessment

Chapter 41

Answer to Connection Checkpoint 41.1

The formed elements of the blood are the erythrocytes, leukocytes, and platelets, which comprise about 45% of the composition of blood.

Answer to Connection Checkpoint 41.2

Pregnancy increases the metabolic demands upon the mother, and the mother is making erythrocytes for the growing fetus. Lack of proper iron intake may cause iron-deficiency anemia in the newborn.

Chapter 41 Answer to Patient Safety Questions

In the mid-1980s iron deficiency in children and pregnant women became a health focus. More foods were fortified with iron, and iron supplements were encouraged. Though iron deficiency still exists, the situation has improved. Unfortunately, adults are often unaware that accidental iron poisoning is now the leading cause of deaths by poisoning in children under five years of age. The number of iron poisonings has doubled since the mid-1980s. In 1997 the FDA enforced labeling of all iron-containing drugs to include a warning for young children. To avoid this tragedy, store all iron medicines out of the reach of children. To combat iron deficiency anemia, increase the intake of iron rich foods such as lean red meats, blackstrap molasses, leafy green and yellow vegetables, and selected seafood.

Chapter 41 Answers to Critical Thinking Questions

1 This drug is given when certain white blood cells, called neutrophils, are below normal level. These cells are normally produced in the bone marrow. Filgrastim stimulates the bone marrow to produce these cells, which will reduce the risk of bacterial infections.

2 Neutropenia is an abnormal decrease in the number of neutrophils, which are the most common type of white blood cell. The main function of these cells is to fight infection. Neutropenic patients must take multiple precautions to prevent contact with pathogenic organisms. Some of the precautions include avoiding people with known infections and avoiding uncooked fruits, vegetables, or meats. Vigilant hand washing is essential for neutropenic patients as well as for those caring for them. Patients who experience fever, sore throat, or flulike symptoms should report them immediately to their health care provider.

3 Some common adverse effects of filgrastim include bone pain, nausea, and swelling or redness at the injection site.

Chapter 41 Answers to Case Study

1 Red or organ meats, poultry, and fish have the highest sources of iron. Leafy green vegetables, such as cabbage, broccoli, and turnip greens, are also high in iron content. Dried beans and peas, such as pinto beans and black-eyed peas, and canned baked beans will also add iron to the patient's diet. Enriched white bread, pasta, rice, cereal, and black strap molasses are good sources of iron.

2 The most common adverse effects of PO iron preparations include constipation, darkened or green stools, diarrhea, nausea, and stomach upset. If the GI adverse effects become excessive, the patient should contact the prescriber. Although taking iron with food may reduce the gastric distress, this will also decrease iron absorption.

3 If tolerated, PO iron preparations should be taken on an empty stomach. In most cases, the preparation should be taken 1 hour before a meal or 2 hours after a meal to allow for optimal absorption of the iron. Instruct patients not to take iron within 1 hour of bedtime. For some patients, iron preparations can cause esophageal irritation which can be avoided my not lying flat for at least one hour after taking iron. Lastly, iron supplements should be scheduled 1–2 hours before or after other medications.

Chapter 41 Answers to NCLEX-RN® Review

1 Answer: 2 Rationale: The client who receives epoetin alfa suffers from anemia. This reduction in low red blood cells produces cellular oxygen deficiency, which causes severe fatigue and weakness. Clients receiving this drug therapy should be taught to take scheduled rest periods to avoid over exertion. Option 1 is incorrect. Avoiding fresh fruits and vegetables or uncooked meat would be instructions more appropriate for an individual with neutropenia. Epoetin alfa treats low red blood cell production. Option 3 is incorrect because limiting exposure to direct sunlight and to use sunscreen are the instructions that the nurse should provide if the client is receiving a drug that causes photosensitivity. Epoetin alfa is not associated with this adverse effect. Option 4 is incorrect because when clients are thrombocytopenic, they should be instructed to avoid activities that may cause injury. This would not be appropriate instruction for a client receiving epoetin alfa. Cognitive Level: Application; Client Need: Physiological Integrity; Nursing Process: Implementation

2 Answer: 2 Rationale: This drug should not be given to clients with uncontrolled HTN because hematopoietic growth factors can increase blood pressure. Option 1 is incorrect. The antiretroviral agent, Zidovudine, may cause anemia. HIV clients may receive hematopoietic growth factors such as epoetin alfa. Option 3 is incorrect. With chronic renal failure, clients often suffer from anemia because they are unable to secrete sufficient endogenous erythropoietin. Hematopoietic growth factors are often prescribed for these clients. Option 4 is incorrect. Chemotherapy is notorious for causing anemia. Clients suffering from chemotherapy-induced anemia are often prescribed hematopoietic growth factors. Cognitive Level: Application; Client Need: Physiological Integrity; Nursing Process: Assessment

3 Answer: 1 Rationale: Neupogen increases white blood cell counts. The nurse would monitor for effectiveness by examining this laboratory value. Option 2 is incorrect. Epoetin alfa is the drug that increases red blood cell count. Option 3 is incorrect because platelet counts are not affected by filgrastim. Option 4 is incorrect. Neupogen has no effect on the serum potassium level. Cognitive Level: Application; Client Need: Physiological Integrity; Nursing Process: Evaluation

4 Answer: 4 Rationale: Oprelvekin does not affect iron levels and there would be no reason to instruct the client to increase dietary intake of it. Option 1 is incorrect. Oprelvekin is used to stimulate the production of platelets in clients who are at risk for severe thrombocytopenia. This indicates that health teaching has been effective. Option 2 is incorrect because oprelvekin may cause fluid retention so severe that it may lead to pulmonary edema, pericardial effusion, and ascites. Clients should monitor weight gain and report significant increases to the health care provider. Option 3 is incorrect. Visual impairment, including blurred vision, papilledema, and optic neuropathy may occur with oprelvekin, and vision changes should be reported. Cognitive Level: Application; Client Need: Physiological Integrity; Nursing Process: Evaluation

5 Answer: 1 Rationale: Alcoholics often suffer from a nutritional deficit of vitamin B_{12}, which can manifest as abnormal neurological symptoms. Option 2 is incorrect because ethanol interferes with folate metabolism in the liver. Option 3 is incorrect. Pernicious anemia is caused by a lack of intrinsic factor, a substance needed to absorb vitamin B_{12} from the GI tract. Alcohol-dependent clients do not have a higher incidence of pernicious anemia. Option 4 is incorrect because vitamin B_{12} is a water-soluble vitamin and is not stored in the body. Cognitive Level: Knowledge; Client Need: Physiological Integrity; Nursing Process: Implementation

6 Answer: 1, 2, 3 Rationale: Ferrous preparations bind to many substances including food and other drugs. To ensure complete absorption of the drug, iron supplements should be taken 1 hour before or 2 hours after eating (option 1). Option 2 is correct because liquid iron preparations are most frequently given to children. Such preparations should be given with a straw to prevent contact with the teeth. After swallowing, the client should be instructed to brush the teeth or thoroughly rinse the mouth to prevent staining. Option 3 is correct. The client should be informed that iron preparations can cause dark tarry like stools and may cause constipation. When clients take iron preparations, increased fiber and water intake are measures to take to decrease constipation. Option 4 is incorrect. Vitamin C increases the absorption of iron preparations, not vitamin E. Option 5 is incorrect. Caffeinated beverages inhibit this drug's absorption. Cognitive Level: Application; Client Need: Physiological Integrity; Nursing Process: Implementation

Chapter 42

Answer to Connection Checkpoint 42.1

An oral drug must survive the acid environment of the stomach (and associated enzymes) and then cross the lipid membrane of the GI tract.

Answer to Connection Checkpoint 42.2

Spironolactone (Aldactone) and eplerenone (Inspra) are aldosterone antagonists approved to treat mild to moderate HTN and reduce edema fluid.

Chapter 42 Answers to Patient Safety Questions

Serious patient injury and death can result from concentrated electrolyte solutions such as potassium chloride, now considered a high risk drug. In years past, concentrated electrolyte solutions were kept on the nursing unit. With the removal of these dangerous drugs, fewer accidents from inappropriate use have occurred. Many advocate that these drugs should be treated as controlled substances, removed from nursing units, and kept in the pharmacy. As a precaution for both the patient and nurse, the preparation should be labeled "High Risk," and dosage should be checked by a second nurse prior to administration.

Chapter 42 Answers to Critical Thinking Questions

1 There are two types of IV fluids used in patient care: colloid and crystalloid solutions. The difference lies in the size of the microscopic particles within the solution. Colloid solutions have large particles that do not readily pass through semipermeable membranes. Colloids also increase colloidal osmotic (or oncotic) pressure, pulling water out of the interstitial spaces into the intravascular compartment. Examples of colloid solutions include normal serum albumin, 3% sodium chloride solution, and dextran. The particle sizes within crystalloid solutions are much smaller and cross semipermeable membranes more easily. IV fluids such as D_5W, 0.9% sodium chloride, and lactated Ringer's solution are considered crystalloid solutions.

2 Colloid solutions are useful in situations where the intravascular volume needs to be increased or replaced rapidly. This situation occurs in acute hypovolemic shock, burns, or major multisystem trauma. There are several types of crystalloid solutions used in patient care. A commonly used solution is normal saline (0.9% saline), which contains water and sodium and chloride ions. It is useful for maintaining the daily requirement of salt and water in the body or for replacing GI losses from nasogastric suction or vomiting. Dextrose solution contains water and glucose for energy. This solution is ideal to use in the early postoperative period since it does not cause salt and water overload but provides the patient with some energy. Ringer's lactate solution has an electrolyte profile sim-

ilar to plasma. However, the solution is incapable of transporting oxygen, which is considered a limitation in fluid replacement when red blood cells have been lost and need replenishing.

3 5% dextrose in water (D_5W) is an IV solution given to supply water and calories to the body. It is also used as a mixing solution (diluent) for other IV medications. Dextrose solutions should be used with extreme caution in patients with untreated hyperglycemia.

4 The indications for normal serum albumin administration are

- hypovolemia when the patient is well hydrated,
- malnutrition, burns, major surgery, or conditions leading to hypoalbuminemia,
- pulmonary edema (used in conjunction with a diuretic), or
- binding and removal of toxic bilirubin in hemolytic disease of newborns.

5 A solution that contains dextran is used to replace blood loss in emergency situations when replacement blood is not available. Dextran produces immediate and short-lived expansion of plasma volume by increasing colloidal osmotic pressure and by drawing fluid from interstitial to intravascular space. One problem related to dextran administration is that this solution does not provide electrolytes and can predispose the client to hyponatremia and other electrolyte disturbances. Dextran should not be given to patients suffering from disease conditions that produce hypervolemia, such as renal failure or congestive heart failure.

Chapter 42 Answers to Case Study

1 Loop diuretics are notorious for causing loss of potassium and creating a hypokalemic state. Most of the time, the potassium loss is greater than the patient can consume through daily dietary intake.

2 Patients taking potassium supplementation should be taught the symptoms of hyperkalemia as well as symptoms associated with hypokalemia. Symptoms associated with hyperkalemia include irregular heartbeat, muscle twitching, dyspnea, cramping, and diarrhea. Frequent symptoms of hypokalemia are muscle weakness, lethargy, irregular heartbeat, and anorexia.

3 Because the patient is taking potassium supplements, he should be taught to reduce his intake of potassium-enriched foods. Salt substitutes should be avoided since most contain a high amount of potassium.

Chapter 42 Answers to NCLEX-RN® Review

1 Answer: 1 Rationale: The serum pH is a measure of alkalinity or acidity in the blood. The administration of bicarbonate neutralizes acidic conditions and causes the client's serum to become more alkaline. Option 2 is incorrect because changes in the pH effect the ability of RBCs to release oxygen. However, any changes in pH caused by sodium bicarbonate will not influence the number of RBCs. Option 3 is incorrect because the liver does not metabolize sodium bicarbonate. Liver function tests are not indicators of the drug's effectiveness. Option 4 is incorrect because although sodium bicarbonate excretion occurs in the kidneys, the blood urea nitrogen level will not reveal the effectiveness of this drug Cognitive Level: Application; Client Need: Physiological Integrity; Nursing Process: Evaluation

2 Answer: 2 Rationale: This client needs more teaching. Liquid preparations are very irritating to the gastric mucosa and should always be diluted with juice or water. Option 1 is incorrect because this statement is true. Salt substitutes are high in potassium and should be avoided by clients on potassium supplementation. Option 3 is incorrect because this is a true statement. The client's subjective symptoms may be the first indicators of potassium imbalances. The client should be taught the symptoms of both hyper- and hypokalemia and when to report these symptoms to the health care provider. Option 4 is incorrect because this is a true statement. The GI secretions are rich in potassium. Episodes of persistent vomiting may lead to hypokalemia and should be reported to the health care provider. Cognitive Level: Application; Client Need: Physiological Integrity; Nursing Process: Evaluation

3 Answer: 4 Rationale: Dextran (Gentran 40) interferes with coagulation and reduces blood viscosity. Option 1 is incorrect because Dextran solutions are used to correct low circulating blood volume states. This solution does not cause dehydration. Option 2 is incorrect. Dextran increases the circulating volume and thereby increases urine output, which is a therapeutic effect of the solution. Option 3 is incorrect. Dextran is used for shock (hypovolemia); it does not cause shock. Cognitive Level: Application; Client Need: Physiological Integrity; Nursing Process: Assessment

4 Answer: 2 Rationale: This solution is often used to dilute (reconstitute) powdered forms of drugs that are intended to be given parenterally. Option 1 is incorrect. This solution can cause hyperglycemia in the diabetic client due to the dextrose content. Option 3 is incorrect. D_5W is considered a crystalloid solution. Option 4 is incorrect. One liter of this solution supplies only 170 calories which is not enough to supply the metabolic nutritional needs of adult clients. Cognitive Level: Knowledge; Client Need: Physiological Integrity; Nursing Process: Implementation

5 Answer: 4 Rationale: A sudden increase in body weight and the onset of swelling may indicate renal malfunction. The kidneys are responsible for excretion of excess potassium. Clients will quickly become hyperkalemic if renal insufficiency develops. Option 1 is incorrect because pupillary constriction to light is a normal physiological response, but it is not associated with imbalances of potassium. Option 2 is incorrect because although the nurse should notify the prescriber when the client develops chest congestion and coughing, it is unlikely that these symptoms are associated with potassium supplementation therapy. Option 3 is incorrect because elevated blood pressure is not a symptom associated with potassium imbalance. Cognitive Level: Application; Client Need: Physiological Integrity; Nursing Process: Assessment

6 Answer: 1, 3, 4 Rationale: Normal serum albumin is a product derived from blood. Although rare, transfusion reactions can still occur with normal serum albumin (Option 1). Normal serum albumin causes intercellular and interstitial fluid to move into the intravascular compartment. This movement of fluid will cause an increase in the client's blood pressure and heart rate. The nurse should monitor the client for fluid overload with this solution (Option 3). Urinary output directly relates to the circulating fluid within the vascular system. When fluid volume is low, the kidneys will deliberately conserve fluid and the urinary output will be diminished. As the circulating fluid volume is corrected, the client's urinary output will increase (Option 4). Option 2 is incorrect. Clients receiving normal serum albumin typically do not have any dietary restrictions while receiving this solution.Option 5 is incorrect. Serum albumin (Albuminar) is not administered for potassium imbalances. Cognitive Level: Application; Client Need: Physiological Integrity; Nursing Process: Planning

Chapter 43

Answer to Connection Checkpoint 43.1

ACE inhibitors inhibit the breakdown of bradykinin (also called kinase II), thus preventing bradykinin. The accumulation of bradykinin in certain tissues can cause angioedema and cough, which are adverse effects of ACE inhibitors.

Answer to Connection Checkpoint 43.2

The reversible cholinesterase inhibitors are the most widely prescribed drug class for treating AD. Donepezil (Aricept) is the protype.

Chapter 44

Answer to Connection Checkpoint 44.1

The other antiplatelet drugs include ADP receptor blockers (prototype: clopidogrel bisulfate (Plavix)) and the glycoprotein IIb/IIIa receptor inhibitors (prototype: abciximab (ReoPro)).

Answer to Connection Checkpoint 44.2

Serotonin agonists (triptans) may be indicated for severe migraines. A secondary choice would be a parenteral dopamine agonist, either as monotherapy or in combination with a serotonin agonist. Narcotic analgesics are effective for migraines refractory to other therapies.

Chapter 44 Answers to Critical Thinking Questions

1 During acute inflammation the inflammatory process begins as a response to the invasion of particulate matter, bacteria, or cell damage. Fever results from inflammatory chemical mediators or bacterial toxins.

2 Ibuprofen inhibits COX-I and COX-II, which diminishes inflammation, decreases fever, and reduces pain. It blocks prostaglandin synthesis and modulates T cell function. Ibuprofen inhibits inflammatory cell chemotaxis, decreases the release of superoxide radicals, and increases the scavenging of these products at the inflammatory sites. Ibuprofen is a NSAID, which possesses properties that provide analgesia and fever relief. It inhibits platelet aggregation and prolongs the bleeding time without effecting the prothrombin or whole blood clotting times. It is used for chronic symptomatic rheumatoid arthritis and osteoarthritis. It is administered to relieve mild to moderate pain or menstrual pain.

3 Mr. Tallo should be instructed that ibuprofen has the ability to reduce fever by blocking prostaglandin synthesis, to take the medication with food or milk, and that the maximum dosage is 1200 mg in a 24-hour period. The patient should avoid alcohol and report any signs of dark stools to the health care provider.

Chapter 44 Answer to Critical Thinking Question in Evidence-Based Practice Feature

Alzheimer's disease, Parkinson's disease, and Huntington's disease are progressive chronic illnesses. Although research indicates that NSAIDs can benefit these patients, family members should also be informed that this treatment is not a cure for the disease. Furthermore, family members should be cautioned about medicating with these agents without proper medical supervision since toxic adverse effects can worsen the degenerative diseases. The care of individuals with such chronic and debilitating conditions must be closely supervised by qualified health care providers.

Chapter 44 Answer to Patient Safety Question

It is imperative that the nurse counsel the patient about ways to avoid a self-medication error. Confusing drugs with similar names accounts for about 10 percent of all medication errors according to the FDA, and occurs throughout the medication process, from ordering to administration. One way to avoid error is to instruct the patient to talk with the pharmacist who will be filling the prescription about the "sound-a-like" drugs. The drug may need to be packaged in a distinctly different type of container from the other medication to help prevent confusion. The patient can also label the bottles with large letters using the words ANTIDEPRESSION and PAIN PILLS. Storing the medication in two different locations may also be helpful. While the patient is taking both drugs, it might be best to have someone else double check each dose to ensure that the appropriate medication is being taken.

Chapter 44 Answers to Case Study

1 Acetaminophen reduces fever by direct action on the heat regulating center of the hypothalamus. It promotes peripheral vasodilation, sweating, and heat dissipation.

2 The patient should not be administered any pain medications that contain acetaminophen. The potential for overdosage of acetaminophen is increased when administering pain medication that contains acetaminophen, along with acetaminophen for fever reduction.

3 The patient should be instructed to increase fluid intake, utilize good hand washing and perineal care, and monitor fever before and after the administration of acetaminophen.

Chapter 44 Answers to NCLEX-RN® Review

1 Answer: 2 Rationale: Acetaminophen overdose is treated with PO or IV acetylcysteine (Acetadote). For maximum effectiveness, the antidote should be administered within 8 hours of acetaminophen ingestion. The administration of 1000 mL per hour of normal saline IV would place the client at risk for fluid volume overload (option 1). The client will not be cardioverted to treat acetaminophen poisoning (option 3). The liver enzymes will be assessed on this client but will not provide treatment for acute acetaminophen overdose (option 4). Cognitive Level: Application; Client Need: Physiological Integrit;y Nursing Process: Implementation

2 Answer: 3 Rationale: Acetaminophen is the drug of choice for reduction of fever in the event the client has a hypersensitivity to aspirin. A client who has hypersensitivity to aspirin should not be administered ibuprofen due to the risk of hypersensitivity with the NSAIDs (option 1). Ketorolac tromethamine is not administered for reduction of fever (option 2). Celecoxib reduces fever but will result in the same hypersensitivity as with the administration of aspirin (option 4). Cognitive Level: Comprehension; Client Need: Physiological Integrity; Nursing Process: Planning

3 Answer: 1 Rationale: Ketorolac is administered parenterally for pain. Options 2, 3, and 4 are incorrect because ketoprofen, ibuprofen, and celecoxib are all administered PO. Cognitive Level: Knowledge; Client Need: Physiological Integrity; Nursing Process: Implementation

4 Answer: 4 Rationale: Ibuprofen should be discontinued 7–14 days before surgery. Option 1 is incorrect because ibuprofen should be discontinued 7–14 days prior to surgery to reduce the risk of bleeding. Options 2 and 3 are incorrect because the client should continue her anti-inflammatory agent until 7–14 days before surgery. Cognitive Level: Application; Client Need: Physiological Integrity; Nursing Process: Implementation

5 Answer: 1 Rationale: Acetaminophen is metabolized in the liver. Thus the client with cirrhosis of the liver has impaired liver function and should not receive acetaminophen for pain or fever reduction. A client who has COPD (option 2), a client who has breast cancer (option 3) and a client who is taking warfarin (option 4) can be administered acetaminophen for fever and analgesia. Cognitive Level: Application; Client Need: Physiological Integrity; Nursing Process: Assessment

6 Answer: 1, 2, 3 Rationale: A client who is experiencing toxic effects from aspirin may experience tinnitus (option 1), or hyperventilation (option 2). Aspirin and aspirin-based products are irritants to the GI mucosa and may cause bleeding with frequent use (option 3). Option 4 is incorrect because aspirin does not affect the renal system or cause a reduction in urinary output. Option 5 is incorrect because a client with salicylate toxicity does not experience peripheral neuropathy. Cognitive level: Application; Client Need: Physiological Integrity; Nursing Process: Assessment

Chapter 45

Answer to Connection Checkpoint 45.1

Oprelvekin is used to stimulate the production of platelets in patients who are at risk for severe thrombocytopenia caused by the chemotherapy of nonmyeloid cancers.

Answer to Connection Checkpoint 45.2

Diuretics are most frequently used to remove excess fluid from the body. For severe pulmonary edema, parental loop diuretics such as furosemide (Lasix) are most effective at rapidly resolving edema.

Chapter 45 Answers to Critical Thinking Questions

1 Normally, interferon is produced by body cells to fight infection and tumors. The mechanism of action for these drugs is not fully understood. However, it is thought that interferon boosts the immune system. These substances are secreted by the lymphocytes and macrophages. It is thought that interferon, although unable to protect the infected cell, warns nearby cells of an impending infection. Interferons slow the spread of viral infections, enhance the activity of existing leukocytes, and increase phagocytosis and cytotoxic T cell activity.

2 Common adverse effects of Intron-A include flulike symptoms, increased body temperature, feeling ill, fatigue, headache, muscle pain, convulsion, dizziness, hair thinning, and depression. The nurse can help the patient cope with these symptoms. Analgesics and antipyretics will help the patient feel better. Allowing the patient to express feelings of depression will also be therapeutic. Lastly, the client should be informed that the adverse effects are short term and usually diminish as therapy progresses.

3 Carol will need to learn how to self-administer the injectable interferon. Many patients are fearful of self-administering injectable medication. The nurse will be instrumental in providing the patient with information on injection techniques. Additionally, Carol must be instructed to pace her daily activities to avoid over tiring. The nurse should assist this patient to identify designated rest periods while performing ADLs. The patient must also be encouraged to notify the health care provider promptly if symptoms of infection develop (sore throat, fever, vomiting, and diarrhea.)

Chapter 45 Answers to Case Study

1 Cyclosporine works by targeting the T lymphocytes, thus inhibiting calcineurin, which serves as a chemical mediator involved in the immune response. Cyclosporine suppresses the immune system and prevents actions of certain immune cells.

2 Gordon should be instructed to take this medication with meals to reduce nausea or gastric irritation. Furthermore, he should take medication at the same time each day to maintain therapeutic blood levels. He should avoid sources of infection due to his induced immunosuppression. It is also critical that he keep scheduled follow-up appointments.

3 Because cyclosporine causes immunosuppression, Gordon's food should be well cooked. Any foods that contain harmful microorganisms should be avoided. Secondly, he should be instructed to avoid drinking grapefruit juice since this will increase the serum level of the drug. Lastly, Gordon may be told to limit the amount of foods with potassium in his diet (bananas, prunes, raisins, and orange juice) since this drug may cause hyperkalemia.

Chapter 45 Answers to NCLEX-RN® Review

1 Answer: 1 Rationale: Interferon alpha increases the phagocytic activity of macrophages and monocytes (types of white blood cells), resulting in enhanced cytotoxicity against tumor cells. Option 2 is incorrect because interferon alpha is minimally metabolized by the liver and excreted by the kidneys. However, with prolonged therapy, serious adverse effects such as hepatotoxicity result in elevated hepatic enzymes. Option 3 is incorrect because this drug typically causes anemia, which would manifest as a decrease in red blood cells. Option 4 is incorrect because, although the kidneys excrete this drug, if renal function is affected, it is more likely that the BUN would increase, rather than decrease. Cognitive Level: Application; Client Need: Physiological Integrity; Nursing Process: Assessment

2 Answer: 2 Rationale: A common complication due to anti-T cell antibody infusions is cytokine release syndrome. This syndrome manifests with elevated body temperature (sometimes exceeding 104°F) and can progress to pulmonary edema. Capillary leak syndrome is a condition in which fluid and protein leak out of tiny blood vessels and flow into surrounding tissue. This complication is related to interleukin administration, not muromonab CD3 (option 1). Restless leg syndrome is characterized by leg discomfort during sleep or at night. Muromonab-CD3 is not known to cause this syndrome (option 3). Androgen insensitivity syndrome is a disorder caused by genetic mutation that prevents development of male sexual characteristics in the fetus despite the presence of the Y chromosome. This is not an adverse effect related to Orthoclone (option 4). Cognitive Level: Application; Client Need: Physiological Integrity; Nursing Process: Assessment

3 Answer: 4 Rationale: Elevated serum creatinine and BUN levels indicate renal toxicity. The nurse should immediately contact the prescriber and inform the client to discontinue the drug until further notice. Cyclosporine does not typically affect the erythrocyte count (option 1). Basophils, lymphocytes, and monocytes are types of white blood cells. This drug reduces the white blood cells and it is therefore expected (option 2). Cyclosporine typically creates a neutropenic state in many patients. A reduction in neutrophils and macrophages is most likely expected (option 3). Cognitive Level: Application; Client Need: Physiological Integrity; Nursing Process: Assessment

4 Answer: 3 Rationale: Azathioprine should be used with extreme caution in patients with pre-existing hepatitis impairment such as cirrhosis. Hepatic enzymes must be monitored regularly. Benign prostatic hypertrophy is not a contraindication for this drug therapy (option 1). There is no reason that patients with cataracts should not receive this drug (option 2). Because azathioprine is administered to patients pre- and post renal transplant, it is likely that urinary output may be scant (option 4). Cognitive Level: Application; Client Need: Physiological Integrity; Nursing Process: Assessment

5 Answer: 4 Rationale: Physical activities such as shaving with a blade razor, using dental floss, or participating in contact sports are contraindicated since this drug reduces the patient's ability to form blood clots. Patients receiving aldesleukin may experience thrombocytopenia. Aspirin would increase the patient's risk for hemorrhage (option 1). Many individuals receiving aldesleukin report extreme fatigue. Increasing physical activity during this treatment is not appropriate, and the patient should be taught to conserve energy (option 2). The patient taking aldesleukin is not required to record pulse rates in a journal (option 3). Cognitive Level: Application; Client Need: Physiological Integrity; Nursing Process: Planning

6 Answer: 1, 2, and 4 Rationale: Patients with pulmonary edema are at great risk of developing serious complications due to cytokine-release syndrome (option 1). This drug may cause seizures in patients with a history of seizure disorders (option 2). Cytokine release syndrome has a great risk of developing in patients with coronary artery disease (option 4). Option 3 is incorrect because peptic ulcer disease is not a contraindication for the use of muromonab-CD3. Option 5 is incorrect because renal transplantation is one of the indications for Muromonab-CD3 (Orthoclone). Cognitive Level: Application; Client Need: Physiological Integrity; Nursing Process: Implementation

Chapter 46

Answer to Connection Checkpoint 46.1

Humoral immunity involves the production of antibodies by plasma cells, which neutralize the antigen or mark it for destruction by other defense cells. Cell-mediated immunity involves the activation of specific T cells and the secretion of cytokines such as interferons and interleukins that enhance the immune response and rid the body of the antigen.

Answer to Connection Checkpoint 46.2

Aldesleukin is an immunostimulant. Cyclosporine, muromonab-CD3, and hydrocortisone are immunosuppressants.

Answer to Connection Checkpoint 46.3

Interferon alfas are indicated for malignancies; interferon betas for severe multiple sclerosis; interferon gamma for chronic granulomatous disease and severe osteopetrosis.

Chapter 46 Answers to Critical Thinking Questions

1 It would be important to ask the parents the nature of Samantha's reaction to her first immunization. This should be compared to her office visit record, her immunization schedule, dosage, and the manufacturer information to determine the cause of the reaction.

2 Minor adverse effects are frequently seen with the administration of vaccines and are effectively managed with good education. Clarification of questions will also decrease the fear of the effects of the vaccine and increase adherence. Parental adherence to the recommended pediatric immunization schedule is very important for the health of the child.

3 It would be important to discuss the cause of the symptom(s) and the rationale for the administration of vaccines with the Abbotts. It would also be important to obtain information about their treatment of Samantha's symptoms and to provide them with education regarding the management of symptoms and potential adverse effects in both verbal and written forms.

Chapter 46 Answers to Case Study

1 You received the hepatitis B vaccine upon admission to nursing school four years prior to this exposure. The antibody testing is ordered to check for the presence of anti-hepatitis B antibodies, which would have occurred following your initial vaccination against hepatitis B. As the patient has hepatitis B and you have had a contaminated exposure, you will need antibody protection against hepatitis B to prevent its development.

2 The patient is documented positive for HIV and you will need treatment to prevent your own development of HIV. This serum analysis is ordered to indicate the presence of antibodies against HIV, which would indicate if you have had a prior exposure to HIV and possible infection. There would be no need for antiviral prophylaxis if you are already HIV infected and you would instead need ongoing HIV treatment.

3 Gamma globulins are a major class of immunoglobulins (proteins) found in the blood, that include many of the most common antibodies. When gamma globulin is administered passive immunity occurs. In other words, antibodies are transferred or "donated" from one person to another. Because there is no immunization currently against hepatitis C, you will need to receive a passive immunization against it to prevent its development. This is not a vaccination; instead, it is the use of another person's immunity and antibodies to prevent disease development.

4 Antiviral prophylaxis is necessary because you have had a potentially contaminated exposure to a viral infection. In addition to the administration of passive immunity with gamma globulin, antiviral prophylaxis is recommended and will follow individual institutional protocol for the prevention of viral replication.

Chapter 46 Answers to NCLEX-RN® Review

1 Answer: 2 Rationale: The most important educational priority for this visit is to clarify the caregiver's questions relating to immunization. Option 1 is incorrect because Mary has never been ill and her chance of having a medication allergy is doubtful. Parental reactions to vaccines are unimportant as they are rarely correlated to allergies in offspring (option 3). The printed immunization schedule can be given to parents for their reference, but the nurse's knowledge of the schedule is unimportant to this parent (option 4). Cognitive Level: Comprehension; Client Need: Physiological Integrity; Nursing Process: Assessment

2 Answer: 3 Rationale: Rho-GAM is a passive immunity using another person's antibodies against Rh^+ blood to prevent the sensitization of an Rh^- mother. Option 1 is incorrect. RhoGam does not provide antibodies to destroy red blood cells (RBCs) as the infant has been delivered and the antibodies will have few RBCs to target. Option 2 is incorrect as the problem is not found with Rh^- infants, nor is this even a consideration. Option 4 is incorrect as RBCs carry the Rh antigen and would be targeted by the sensitized maternal immune system and antibodies. Cognitive Level: Comprehension; Client Need: Physiological Integrity; Nursing Process: Implementation

3 Answer: 3, 4 Rationale: This child would need to receive rabies immunoglobulin to provide passive immunity to the potential exposure, as well as a series of 4 rabies vaccines administered on days 3, 7, 14, and 28. Options 1 and 2 are incorrect. Neither tetanus toxoid booster nor DaPT administration is necessary, providing the client is current with her immunization schedule. Option 5 is incorrect. The use of rabies toxoid would be ineffective. Cognitive Level: Application Client Need: Health Promotion and Maintenance Nursing Process: Planning

4 Answer: 3 Rationale: Toxoids are inactive bacterial toxins used to stimulate antibody production. They are not antibodies (option 1), nor are they used to fight the effects of viral interferons (option 2). Toxins are frequently used as a vaccine preparation (option 4). Cognitive Level: Knowledge; Client Need: Physiological Integrity; Nursing Process: Implementation

5 Answer: 3 Rationale: Known hypersensitivity to yeast is an absolute contraindication for Hepatitis B vaccine. If the client is a smoker, he/she should still receive Hepatitis B vaccine (option 1). Hypertension is not a contraindication for Hepatitis B vaccine (option 2). Unfortunately, Hepatitis B vaccine is only available through injection (option 4). Cognitive Level: Knowledge; Client Need: Physiological Integrity; Nursing Process: Assessment

6 Answer: 1 Rationale: Hypersensitivity reactions are likely to occur within the first 20 minutes of administration. The nurse should closely monitor the client's vitals signs during the initial period. Option 2 is incorrect. RhoGAM does not cause thrombocytopenia, anemia, or increase liver enzymes. Option 3 is incorrect. There is no need for a low saturated fat, low cholesterol diet after receiving Rh_0 immune globulin. Option 4 is incorrect. RhoGAM does not cause a cough. Cognitive Level: Knowledge; Client Need: Physiological Integrity; Nursing Process: Implementation

Chapter 47

Answer to Connection Checkpoint 47.1

The IV route usually results in the most rapid onset of action.

Answer to Connection Checkpoint 47.2

Resistance refers to infections, and should not be used interchangeably with tolerance. Microorganisms become resistant, whereas patients become tolerant. Tolerance is a biological condition that occurs when the body adapts to a substance after repeated administration. Over time, larger doses of the drug are required to produce the same initial effect.

Answer to Connection Checkpoint 47.3

For most drugs, the potential for adverse effects increases with the dose. Keeping two drugs below their toxic levels generally results in fewer adverse effects than a single drug that reaches its toxic concentration.

Answer to Connection Checkpoint 47.4

Immunostimulants include interferons, colony-stimulating factors, and interleukins.

Chapter 48

Answer to Connection Checkpoint 48.1

The medical history may reveal previous drug allergies. The nurse may recognize that some of the medications to which the patient is allergic share the same drug class, thus recognizing (and preventing) cross-hypersensitivity.

Answer to Connection Checkpoint 48.2

Gram-positive bacteria contain a thick cell wall that retains a violet color after staining. Gram-negative bacteria have thinner cell walls that lose the violet stain.

Chapter 48 Answers to Critical Thinking Questions

1 Several factors may contribute to the patient's wound infection. First, wet dressings are breeding sites for microorganism since pathogens thrive in warm, moist, dark environments. Patients should be taught to change a wet dressing or return to the health facility for routine dressing changes. Second, elderly patients have an increased risk for infection. Furthermore, proper wound healing is dependent on adequate nutrition. Many elderly adults fail to consume adequate amounts of nutrients needed for wound healing. A diet high in protein, carbohydrates, fats, vitamins, and minerals is critical for proper wound healing.

2 Laboratory studies for this patient might include hematocrit, hemoglobin, and white blood cell counts. Additionally, serum albumin levels may be evaluated. These laboratory values not only indicate the presence or degree of infection, they also may indicate the degree of nutritional impairment that contributes to poor wound healing. Most likely a specimen of the wound drainage will be sent to the laboratory for culture and sensitivity testing to determine the infecting organism, as well as the specific antibiotic therapy that is indicated.

3 Ms. Dennison should be instructed about her prescribed medication including potential adverse effects, when and how to take the medication in relation to meals and food, when to stop taking the prescribed medication, and indicators that would warrant seeking additional health care.

4 Cefazolin (Ancef) inhibits bacterial wall synthesis. It is bactericidal and exhibits a broad spectrum of bacterial coverage.

Chapter 48 Answers to Case Study

1 It is critical that the nurse not overreact to the patient's statements. Open and direct communication will only be facilitated if the patient does not feel judged by the health care provider. The nurse should engage the patient in a dialogue that would clarify the reason for the patient's behavior. The problem of saving outdated antibiotics could be traced to a lack of understanding on the patient's part or to the patient's economic status.

2 The nurse should provide the patient with information about the danger of saving medication in a way that the patient can accept. Additionally, the nurse and patient should explore alternatives that would ensure the patient that she will have access to medication when needed.

Chapter 48 Answers to NCLEX-RN® Review

1 Answer: 3 Rationale: Ampicillin may decrease the effectiveness of oral contraceptives and the client should be instructed to use a barrier method to avoid unwanted pregnancies. The combination of ampicillin and birth control pills will not induce adverse effects (option 1). Oral contraceptive effectiveness may be reduced during ampicillin therapy (option 2). Ampicillin will not create serious toxicity of oral contraceptives (option 4). Cognitive Level: Application; Client Need: Physiological Integrity; Nursing Process: Implementation

2 Answer: 3 Rationale: Ototoxicity is associated with serum concentrations of vancomycin above 60–80 mcg/mL and manifests with tinnitus and high-tone hearing loss. Option 1, redness of the ears, is not indicative of ototoxicity. Option 2, itching of the ears, is not a sign of ototoxicity due to vancomycin administration. Option 4, ocular pain, is associated with the eye, not the ear. Cognitive Level: Knowledge; Client Need: Physiological Integrity; Nursing Process: Assessment

3 Answer: 2 Rationale: Superinfection is a common occurrence in women who have been treated with antibiotic therapy. One symptom may be a vaginal yeast infection with discharge. A hypersensitivity reaction is not usually manifested by vaginal discharge (option 1). The manifestations associated with pseudomembranous colitis are GI related, such as diarrhea (option 3). Vaginal discharge is not a symptom of antibiotic toxicity (option 4). Cognitive Level: Knowledge; Client Need: Physiological Integrity; Nursing Process: Assessment

4 Answer: 1 Rationale: The combination of amoxicillin with clavulanate allows for a greater amount of the drug to reach the pathogenic bacteria. The combination of these two drugs does not prevent cross contamination of microorganisms (option 2). Allergic reactions are not avoided by combining amoxicillin with clavulanate (option 3). The combination of these two substances does not impact the absorption of the drug (option 4) Cognitive Level: Knowledge; Client Need: Physiological Integrity; Nursing Process: Implementation

5 Answer: 1 Rationale: These symptoms are classic signs of hypersensitivity reaction. Option 2 is incorrect because blood dyscrasias includes such problems as thrombocytopenia and neutropenia and the drug does not cause these symptoms. Option 3 is incorrect because beta lactamase is a substance secreted by some bacteria, which renders the antibiotic ineffective. Option 4 is incorrect because drug toxicity implies that the client has received too much of the medication. Hypersensitivity is associated with antigen and antibody reactions. Cognitive Level: Knowledge; Client Need: Physiological Integrity; Nursing Process: Assessment

6 Answer: 1 Rationale: Acidic beverages can destroy the medication. A black and furry tongue is the symptom of an oral superinfection and should be reported (option 2). The client should be taught to take the full prescription even if the symptoms subside (option 3). Clients should never take 2 doses as this will place the client at risk for toxicity (option 4). Cognitive Level: Application; Client Need: Physiological Integrity; Nursing Process: Evaluation

Chapter 49

Answer to Connection Checkpoint 49.1

Prothrombin time (PT) is the standard laboratory test used to monitor the effectiveness of warfarin. The normal PT range is 12–15 seconds. PT is also reported as an international normalized ratio (INR) value. INR values averaging 2.5 are considered therapeutic for most indications.

Answer to Connection Checkpoint 49.2

The two prototype neuromuscular blockers are succinylcholine (Anectine) (depolarizing type) and tubocurarine (nondepolarizing type). Both act on nicotinic receptors in skeletal muscle.

Chapter 49 Answers to Critical Thinking Questions

1 There are multiple reasons that an antibiotic may be ineffective in treating infections. The nurse should investigate any possibilities that could result in unsuccessful antibiotics therapy, such as nutritional status of the patient as well as the timing the patient took the dose in relationship to other medications and foods. Also, the antibiotic prescribed may not have been of sufficient dosage strength to treat the infections, or the pathogen may not be sensitive to the antibiotic. Lastly, the nurse should consider that the patient may not have even taken the antibiotic due to high cost or unpleasant adverse effects.

2 Certainly, the best way to determine the causative pathogen is culture and sensitivity (C & S) testing. A culture determines what kind of organism is causing an illness or infection, whereas sensitivity determines what kind of antibiotic will be most effective in treating the infection. C & S testing is accomplished by collecting a sample of fluid and then applying the sample into a container filled with a specially prepared gelatin (culture). If there are organisms such as bacteria in the sample, they will grow in the culture, usually within 2 days. Viruses usually take longer to grow in a sample. In the meantime, patient treatment will be initiated using a broad-spectrum antibacterial drug known for treating most types of bacterial lung infections.

3 A peak and trough level is comprised of two laboratory tests collectively known as therapeutic drug monitoring (TDM). This type of monitoring is used to confirm a blood drug concentration level that is above or below the therapeutic range. Without drug monitoring, the prescriber cannot be sure if a patient's lack of response to an antibiotic reflects bacterial resistance or is the result of failure to reach the proper therapeutic range of antibiotic concentration in the blood. Blood specimens for drug monitoring can be taken at two different times: during the drug's highest therapeutic concentration (peak level) or its lowest (trough level). Peak levels are usually obtained one to two hours after oral intake, approximately one hour after IM administration, and approximately 30 minutes after IV administration. Trough levels are usually obtained within 15–30 minutes prior to the next scheduled dose.

4 The nurse should monitor the patient for a worsening of his condition. Specific symptoms may include relentless fever, chest pain, increasing shortness of breath, abdominal pain, increase in sputum production, a change in the color and consistency of the sputum, cyanosis of the lips of nail beds, restlessness, confusion, anxiety, hypotension, or tachycardia.

Chapter 49 Answer to Critical Thinking Question in Evidence-Based Practice Feature

Traveler's diarrhea is more serious in children and elders as it can frequently lead to life-threatening dehydration and electrolyte imbalance. Additionally, individuals who are immunosuppressed are at particular high risk for infection due to their inability to ward off invading disease-producing pathogens.

Chapter 49 Answers to Case Study

1 Due to Mr. Klein's past history of alcohol abuse and possible decreased hepatic function, he is at greater risk for the development of cholestatic hepatitis.

2 The most common adverse effects possible for this patient receiving erythromycin may include nausea, abdominal cramping, vomiting, diarrhea, dark urine, pale colored stools, or jaundice.

3 Typical adverse effects of cholestatic hepatitis include loss of appetite, fatigue, mild fever, nausea and vomiting, and abdominal pain. Less common symptoms include dark urine, light-colored stools, jaundice, altered mental state, stupor, or coma.

4 Monitoring the patient's liver function laboratory values will be particularly important. These laboratory values include a series of tests known as a liver panel, liver function tests, or LFT. These tests help to detect liver damage or disease.

Chapter 49 Answers to NCLEX-RN® Review

1 Answer: 4 Rationale: This drug potentially causes photosensitivity. Option 1 is incorrect because calcium products should be avoided with tetracycline therapy. Option 2 is incorrect because brushing will not remove staining. The staining of the teeth due to medication can only be removed by a dental specialist. Option 3 is incorrect because there is no indication for the client taking tetracycline to weigh daily. Cognitive Level: Application; Client Need: Physiological Integrity; Nursing Process: Implementation

2 Answer: 1 Rationale: Longer duration of action is one of the benefits of azithromycin therapy. There is no evidence that azithromycin causes any more nausea than other antibiotics (option 2). Azithromycin is not affected by the gastric content and can be taken any time (option 3). Azithromycin is not affected by calcium-based foods (option 4). Cognitive Level: Application; Client Need: Physiological Integrity; Nursing Process: Evaluation

3 Answer: 1 Rationale: Weight gain will be one of the first signs associated with renal damage secondary to amikacin toxicity. Amikacin toxicity is not manifested by visual disturbances (option 2). Mental depression (option 3) and urinary frequency (option 4) are not expected adverse effects of amikacin therapy. Cognitive Level: Application; Client Need: Physiological Integrity; Nursing Process: Planning

4 Answer: 1 Rationale: Drug-induced nephrotoxicity would cause an elevated serum creatinine level and should be reported to the health care provider. Blood urea nitrogen level would increase in the presence of renal toxicity (option 2). Nephrotoxicity is not typically indicated via the WBC levels (option 3). Serum iron levels are not typically associated with nephrotoxicity (option 4). Cognitive Level: Application; Client Need: Physiological Integrity; Nursing Process: Assessment

5 Answer: 3 Rationale: Aminoglycosides are notorious for causing ototoxicity which manifests as hearing deficit and tinnitus. The nurse should perform baseline assessment of these parameters when this drug therapy is initiated and throughout the course of the treatment. Tetracyclines do not cause ototoxicity (option 1). Macrolides are not associated with these symptoms of toxicity (option 2). Cephalosporins are not known to cause ototoxicity (option 4). Cognitive Level: Application; Client Need: Physiological Integrity; Nursing Process: Assessment

6 Answer: 2 Rationale: Aminoglycosides are toxic to the kidneys. Aminoglycoside therapy does not produce neurological abnormalities (option 1). Cardiac complications are not usual post antibiotic effects with aminoglycosides (option 3). Dermatological problems are not expected post-antibiotic effects of aminoglycosides (option 4). Cognitive Level: Application; Client Need: Physiological Integrity; Nursing Process: Assessment

Chapter 50

Answer to Connection Checkpoint 50.1

Hydrocortisone is a corticosteroid that exhibits strong anti-inflammatory actions. As a topical drug, it can ease the redness and inflammation associated with minor skin cuts and abrasions.

Chapter 50 Answer to Patient Safety Question

It is imperative that the nurse reassesses the patient for drug allergies. Even though patients may initially report their drug allergies to their health care providers, they sometimes forget to mention these during the stressful and hurried admission procedure. Secondly, before the patient receives another dose of this antibiotic, the health care provider should be notified of the reaction, preferably when it occurred, but certainly before the second infusion. Hypersensitivity reactions can worsen with each exposure to an antigen (in this case the antibiotic). The next dose could precipitate an anaphylactic response which is life threatening.

Chapter 50 Answers to Critical Thinking Questions

1 A patient teaching handout should include the following information. This drug can be taken with food or on an empty stomach but should not be taken with dairy products such as milk, yogurt, cheese, or calcium fortified juices. This drug should be taken at about the same time, morning and evening. Take ciprofloxacin for the entire time as prescribed by the health care provider, even after the patient starts to feel better, to be sure the infection is eliminated. If a dose is missed, do not take another or double dose of the medication.

The most common adverse effects of ciprofloxacin are mild and include nausea, diarrhea, vomiting, and abdominal pain or discomfort. Diarrhea that persists with a fever should be reported immediately to the health care provider.

2 You should inform the patient that this medication may cause tendon damage (e.g., tendonitis or tendon rupture). Mike should seek immediate medical attention if he develop joint, muscle, or tendon pain. Also, he should be advised that some OTC medications, multivitamins, and other dietary supplements may contain magnesium, calcium, aluminum, iron, or zinc which can interfere with the absorption of ciprofloxacin and may prevent it from working properly. Advise the patient to read labels to determine if this applies.

3 Remembering to take medication can be problematic especially when the patient begins to feel better. Daily reminders are helpful for scheduling medication doses. One approach is to take medicine around routine activities such as brushing teeth, setting an alarm clock, eating meals, going to work, or performing other daily activities. Other examples include

- Set a timer or watch alarm to go off when it is time to take the medicine.
- Place a reminder card or sticky note in a highly visible place such as on the refrigerator, by the phone, on the medicine cabinet, or even on the bathroom mirror. Change the message frequently, move it to a new spot, or use different colors to get needed attention for adherence.
- Ask a family member or a friend to call and remind the patient of the medication.
- If the patient has a personal computer, free services that send daily email reminders to take medications are available.
- Use a medication box that will hold the entire day's supply of medicine. Load the entire day at one time to decrease the opportunity of a missed or forgotten dose.

Chapter 50 Answers to Case Study

1 If Carolyn is only going to keep one of the medications it would be best to keep the bacitracin. Polymyxin B is not effective against gram-positive microbes, whereas bacitracin is effective against both types of bacteria.

2 Polymyxin can indeed be nephrotoxic, but only if given IM. You can tell Ms. Ijams that polymyxin does not injure the kidneys when used as a topical ointment for minor scrapes and abrasions.

Chapter 50 Answers to NCLEX-RN® Review

1 Answer: 2 Rationale: Because pathogens grow rapidly and are constantly proliferating, all antibiotic therapies should be taken around the clock. This is to ensure a steady serum drug level to fight the bacteria. Ciprofloxacin is not known to cause problems with clients' sleep patterns (option 1). Superinfections occur when an antibiotic eradicates normal flora and an opportunistic organism invades. Although this is a problem associated with antibiotic therapy, it typically is not caused by not adhering to the prescribed schedule (option 3). Allergic reactions are very common with antibiotic therapy. However, the hypersensitivity response occurs due to an antigen or antibody reaction, not from failing to adhere to the medication schedule (option 4). Cognitive Level: Comprehension; Client Need: Physiological Integrity; Nursing Process: Implementation

2 Answer: 1 Rationale: Polymyxin B is a topical antibiotic used to promote wound healing. Skin and mucous membranes cannot be made sterile. Polymyxin B does cause cell death of the invading bacteria. However, it does not sterilize the skin (option 2). Polymyxin B does not prevent allergic reaction (option 3); nor does it provide pain relief to wounds (option 4). Cognitive Level: Comprehension; Client Need: Physiological Integrity; Nursing Process: Planning

3 Answer: 2 Rationale: Metronidazole is one of only a few drugs that have dual activity against both bacteria and multicellular parasites. Often drugs that reduce gastric motility are given for diarrhea. However, metronidazole does not directly affect peristalsis (option 1), it destroys the pathogens causing the diarrhea but not by stimulating the release of peptase (option 3) or aiding in fecal elimination (option 4). Cognitive Level: Comprehension; Client Need: Physiological Integrity; Nursing Process: Implementation

4 Answer: 1 Rationale: When antacids or mineral supplements are taken during ciprofloxacin therapy, drug absorption will be diminished. Dyspnea is a significant finding. However, shortness of breath associated with hypersensitivity reaction most likely would have occurred within the first 2 weeks of the therapy (option 2). Fluoroquinolone therapy may cause photosensitivity in some clients and direct sunlight should therefore be avoided (option 3). The excretion of fluoroquinolones is through the renal system and the client should be encouraged to increase fluid intake to 2–3 liters/day (option 4). Cognitive Level: Comprehension; Client Need: Physiological Integrity; Nursing Process: Implementation

5 Answer: 1 Rationale: Ketek blocks bacterial protein synthesis by binding to two different sites on the 50S ribosomal subunit. Quinolones alter DNA of bacteria and are bactericidal (option 2). Sulfonamides decrease bacterial folic acid synthesis and are bacteriostatic (option 3). Tetracyclines inhibit protein synthesis and cell growth; they are bacteriostatic (option 4). Cognitive Level: Knowledge; Client Need: Physiological Integrity; Nursing Process: Implementation

6 Answer: 1, 2, 3 Rationale: The use of fluoroquinolone should be questioned if any of these conditions is present. Fluoroquinolones are restricted in clients who are less than 18 years of age (option 4). Anxiety is not a contraindication for fluoroquinolone therapy (option 5). Cognitive Level: Knowledge; Client Need: Physiological Integrity; Nursing Process: Assessment

Chapter 51

Answer to Connection Checkpoint 51.1

All fluoroquinolones have activity against gram-negative pathogens: the newer drugs are significantly more effective against gram-positive bacteria.

Answer to Connection Checkpoint 51.2

There is a small incidence of cross-allergy between penicillins and cephalosporins. Ceftriaxone is contraindicated for patients who have experienced anaphylaxis following penicillin exposure.

Chapter 51 Answer to Connections: Patient Safety

Based on the patient's history of allergies to thiazide diuretics, the nurse should withhold the dose of medication. The nurse should withhold the medication and notify the health care provider. TMP-SMZ is contraindicated in patients with hypersensitivity to sulfonamides or chemically related agents such as thiazide diuretics.

Chapter 51 Answers to Critical Thinking Questions

1 You should explain to the patient that urine is sterile. It contains fluids, salts, and waste products, but it is free of bacteria, viruses, and fungi. An infection occurs when microorganisms, usually bacteria from the digestive tract, cling to the opening of the urethra and begin to multiply. Most infections arise from one type of bacteria, *Escherichia coli (E. coli)*, which normally exists in the colon. The urinary system is structured to ward off infection. The ureters and bladder normally prevent urine from backing up toward the kidneys, and the flow of urine from the bladder helps wash bacteria out of the body.

Urinary tract infections (UTIs) are a common complaint in women. Nearly 20% of women will have another UTI after their first occurrence and chances of reoccurrences increase with each infection experienced.

Often, a UTI can be cured with 1–2 days of treatment if the infection is not complicated by other preexisting disease conditions such as urinary obstruction. Still, many health care providers prescribe antibiotics for a week or two to ensure that the infection has been cured.

Women who have had three UTIs are likely to continue having them. Four out of five of these women get another UTI within 18 months of the last one. Additional steps that a woman can take to avoid an infection include: Drink plenty of water (2.5–3L) every day. (1 liter is approximately equal to 1 quart). Urinate when the need is first present; do not resist the urge to urinate. Take showers instead of tub baths. Cleanse the genital area before sexual intercourse. Wipe from front to back to prevent bacteria around the anus from entering the vagina or urethra. Avoid feminine hygiene sprays and scented douches, which may irritate the urethra.

2 Health teaching for the patient receiving Bactrim includes reporting any skin rashes, nausea, vomiting, diarrhea, sore throat, or muscle aches. Teach the patient to avoid direct sunlight due to photosensitivity resulting from the drug. The patient should be taught to drink 2.5–3 liters of water daily, unless otherwise indicated to flush the urinary system. Teach the patient to take the entire prescription of antibiotic and to return to a health care provider for follow up.

3 Teach the patient to use the entire prescription and not save antibiotics for another time for several reasons. Inappropriate use of antibiotics may cause the development of antibiotic-resistant strains of common bacterial diseases. Misuse of antibiotics may result in serious adverse reactions such as diarrhea and abdominal symptoms, rash and allergic reactions, and potentially dangerous interference with other medications. Also, when patients stockpile antibiotics, the drugs may lose potency after expiration dates.

4 A urine culture was collected to determine the pathogen causing the patient's infection. The sensitivity testing was done to determine what antibiotic therapy would be most beneficial.

Chapter 51 Answers to Case Study

1 The nurse should explain to the patient and her daughter that catheter-related bacteruria in the elderly represents the most common nosocomial infection. Approximately 15% to 30% of hospitalized elderly patients with acute conditions undergo urinary catheterization. Indwelling urinary catheterization causes bacteruria to occur at a rate of 3 to 10% of patients per day. A single in-and-out catheterization may cause bacteruria in as many as 20% of patients.

2 The nurse should first assure the patient and family members that several nursing interventions will be implemented to assist the patient with elimination. Relieving the anxiety related to urinary incontinence is an essential part of the nurse's response to the fears of the patient and family. Some of the following interventions may be helpful to address this problem: Establish a time that nursing staff will check with the patient about toileting needs such as every 1–2 hours; provide the patient with a bedside commode or easy access to the toilet; keep the "nurse call" button with the patient for immediate access to help provide the patient with protective garments or incontinence pads; limit the intake of fluids 2–3 hours before sleep time; administer adiuretic-type medication in the daytime hours to prevent nocturia; limit ingestion of bladder irritants such as colas, coffee, and tea.

Chapter 51 Answers to NCLEX-RN® Review

1 Answer: 3 Rationale: Crystalluria is the excretion of crystals in the urine. To prevent this adverse effect, clients are instructed to consume approximately 2–3 liters of fluid per day. This action will flush the crystal from the renal system. Limiting foods high in calcium will not prevent crystalluria (option 1). Positional changes are not related to the adverse effect of crystalluria (option 2). Alcohol should be avoided when taking most medications. However, the effects attributed to alcohol consumption do not include crystalluria (option 4). Cognitive Level: Application; Client Need: Physiological Integrity; Nursing Process: Assessment

2 Answer: 1 Rationale: Nitrofurantoin is prescribed most commonly for the prophylaxis of recurrent UTI. Furadantin has no analgesic effect (option 2). The excretion of urine is not affected by this drug (option 3). Furadantin is not used for pyelonephritis (option 4). Cognitive Level: Knowledge; Client Need: Physiological Integrity; Nursing Process: Assessment

3 Answer: 1 Rationale: The occurrence of migraine headaches is least important since the client has an uncomplicated UTI. Although a common adverse effect of nitrofurantoin is headaches, there is no indication that the client has received this drug. Option 2 is incorrect because it is critical information. Drug therapies for UTIs often include sulfonamides (sulfa drugs). Option 3 is incorrect because UTIs can be prevented if the female client is taught to urinate before and after sexual intercourse. Option 4 is incorrect because determining if the client is possibly pregnant is important. Sulfonamides are contraindicated during pregnancy. Cognitive Level: Application; Client Need: Physiological Integrity; Nursing Process: Assessment

4 Answer: 3 Rationale: Nausea and vomiting are the most common adverse effects of TMP-SMZ therapy. These normally diminish with time, but may require discontinuation of therapy. Antacids will decrease the absorption of the sulfonamide antibiotic (option 1). Sulfonamides increase bleeding time with oral anticoagulants (option 2). Sulfonamides such as TMP-SMZ exert a potassium-sparing effect on the nephron. The client may be at risk for hyperkalemia (option 4). Cognitive Level: Application; Client Need: Physiological Integrity; Nursing Process: Implementation

5 Answer: 1 Rationale: Bactrim is contraindicated in clients with severe renal impairment because this is the primary route of drug excretion, and the drug may accumulate to toxic levels in these clients. A low urinary output would indicate renal impairment. Option 2 is incorrect. HTN is not a contraindication for this medication. Option 3 is incorrect. Cough and chills do not prevent the client from using Bactrim for a urinary tract infection. Option 4 is incorrect. Clients with neurological impairment may be prescribed Bactrim. Cognitive Level: Application; Client Need: Physiological Integrity; Nursing Process: Assessment

6 Answer: 1, 2, 3, 4 Rationale Trimethoprim-Sulfamethoxazole causes photosensitivity. Clients receiving this drug should be given these instructions. Option 5 is incorrect. Individuals taking Trimethoprim-Sulfamethoxazole will not realize the degree of sensitivity experienced with this drug. Sunlamps and tanning beds should be strictly avoided. Cognitive Level: Application; Client Need: Physiological Integrity; Nursing Process: Implementation

Chapter 52

Answer to Connection Checkpoint 52.1

Corticosteroids are the most frequently used immunosuppressants. Other classes include the calcineurin inhibitors (Prototype: cyclosporine) (Neoral, Sandimmune), cytotoxic agents (Prototype: azathioprine) (Azasan, Imuran) and antibodies (Prototype: muromonab-CD3) (Orthoclone, OKT3).

Answer to Connection Checkpoint 52.2

Expense, adverse effects, and inconvenience of taking so many medications for so long.

Answer to Connection Checkpoint 52.3

Aminoglycosides are bacteriocidal drugs that inhibit protein synthesis. They are normally used for serious systemic infections caused by aerobic gram-negative organisms.

Answer to Connection Checkpoint 52.4

Sulfonamides inhibit the bacterial synthesis of folic acid. They are primarily used for urinary tract infections.

Chapter 52 Answers to Critical Thinking Questions

1 *M. tuberculosis* is a communicable disease caused by an aerobic, acid-fast bacillus. The microorganism is acquired by inhalation of small particles. Coughing, talking, laughing, and sneezing transmit infected droplets. Although brief exposure to TB does not usually cause infection, frequent and repeated contact with an infected person increases the risk. High-risk populations include low-income individuals, foreign-born populations, and residents of long-term-care facilities or correctional institutions such as jails or prisons.

2 Sam possibly acquired TB while staying at the homeless shelter. In fact, Sam may have been infected many months before the disease actually developed. In many individuals, the microorganism remains dormant and does not produce symptoms. However, some special circumstances seem to play a role in the progression from dormant TB infection to active disease. These factors include HIV infections, low body weight, advanced age, corticosteroid therapy, and the presence of chronic illness such as diabetes or kidney disease.

3 Sam's tuberculosis is compounded by his chronic use of alcoholic beverages. Many tuberculosis drugs are metabolized in the liver. Liver impairment due to alcohol consumption may affect the drug's metabolism.

Chapter 52 Answer to Critical Thinking Question in Evidence-Based Practice Feature

Based on the research, DOT is not for everyone and should be reserved for individuals who really need the intervention. Typically, when multidrug-resistant TB is identified, DOT may be necessary during the remainder of the treatment period to better ensure successful treatment outcomes. Also, because nonadherence has been frequently reported in this population, DOT is often recommended for HIV-positive patients. Lastly, when patients suffer from psychiatric or mental health problems that prevent them from caring for themselves, then DOT is probably indicated.

Chapter 52 Answers to Case Study

1 It is important to reassure Sam that multiple drugs are given routinely for TBs. The nurse should clarify that combining drug therapies is essential because the bacteria grow slowly and commonly develop resistance to the treatment.

2 One of the most common adverse effects associated with isoniazid therapy is peripheral neuropathy. This drug frequently affects the nervous system and produces tingling and numbness of the hands and feet. Pyridoxine (vitamin B_6) is routinely prescribed by health care providers.

Chapter 52 Answers to NCLEX-RN® Review

1 Answer: 2 Rationale: For some antituberculosis drugs (INH) peripheral neuropathy is problematic. This is due to a decrease in the activity of pyridoxine on the nervous tissue. Often supplemental vitamin B_6 is prescribed to prevent this adverse effect. Antituberculant drugs do not cause an increase in the nerve ending sensitivity (option 1). Antituberculosis therapy does not accelerate the excretion of neurotransmitters (option 3). The drugs used for TB do not affect ascorbic acid (option 4). Cognitive Level: Knowledge; Client Need: Physiological Integrity; Nursing Process: Assessment

2 Answer: 2 Rationale: Once the diagnosis of pulmonary tuberculosis is verified, sputum specimens are routinely collected to determine the effectiveness of the drug therapy. Coagulation studies do not indicate the effectiveness of INH (option 1). Arterial blood gases are used to determine the oxygenation and acid/base status of the client. However, ABGs do not directly indicate the effectiveness of the drug therapy (option 3). Pulmonary function testing is an examination measuring an individual's lung capacity, speed of exhalation, and oxygenation after a period of exertion. This test does not directly evaluate the effectiveness of the antituberculosis therapy (option 4). Cognitive Level: Application; Client Need: Physiological Integrity; Nursing Process: Evaluation

3 Answer: 3 Rationale: For active tuberculosis, treatment is frequently long term and complicated. Clients may tire of the regimen and fail to adhere to the prescribed treatment. Because TB is a national community health problem that potentially affects all citizens, medication is provided to individuals who cannot afford to pay or have no health care insurance (option 1). Although proper nutrition is crucial to support a healthy immune system, it is not considered the cause of treatment failure in clents with TB (option 2). Clients receiving therapy for pulmonary tuberculosis are not limited in the intake of calcium enriched foods (option 4). Cognitive Level: Application; Client Need: Physiological Integrity; Nursing Process: Implementation

4 Answer: 1, 2, 3 Rationale: Monitoring lymphocyte counts in a client with HIV infection is one way to assess the degree of immunosuppression and the risk of developing opportunistic infections (option 1). Due to the immunosuppressed state, visitors may be restricted to protect the client from infections (option 2). Typically, the management for *M. avium* infection in the HIV client requires using multiple drug therapies to eradicate the infection (option 3). Option 4 is incorrect because MAC is not considered a contagious infection. Treating family members to prevent this infection is not necessary. Option 5 is incorrect because limiting the client's intake of foods high in protein and carbohydrates is unnecessary. Cognitive Level: Application; Client Need: Physiological Integrity; Nursing Process: Planning

5 Answer: 1 Rationale: The nurse should observe for any reddish-brown discoloration of skin, cornea, conjunctiva, and body fluids. This adverse effect occurs in 75%–90% of clients within a few weeks of treatment. Even after discontinuation of therapy, skin discoloration may take months or years to fade. The drug does not cause constipation, chills, or dehydration (option 2). Dapsone is not known to cause the adverse effects listed in the question (option 3). Memory loss, nervousness, and pruritus are not adverse effects associated with dapsone (option 4). Cognitive Level: Knowledge; Client Need: Physiological Integrity; Nursing Process: Assessment

6 Answer: 3 Rationale: Elders appear to be at greater risk for developing hepatotoxicity. There is no contraindication to prevent a 42-year-old homemaker from taking this medication (option 1). This drug has not been shown to have adverse effects on the breast-feeding newborn; thus, therapy can safely continue during lactation (option 2). INH is not contraindicated for a 42-year-old marketing executive (option 4). Cognitive Level: Application; Client Need: Physiological Integrity; Nursing Process: Assessment

Chapter 53

Answer to Connection Checkpoint 53.1

The three major classes of cell wall inhibitors are the penicillins, cephalosporins, and carbapenems. These classes inhibit penicillin-binding protein, which is not present in fungi.

Answer to Connection Checkpoint 53.2

Broad spectrum anti-infectives kill many species of organisms, including normal flora. This gives Candida room to grow.

Chapter 53 Answers to Critical Thinking Questions

1 A complete history and a physical exam are necessary to evaluate a patient for an opportunistic infection. Knowing medical diagnoses and medications, along with the current state of the immune system, is key to treating the patient with oropharyngeal candidiasis.

2 *Candida albicans* can reproduce in large numbers in the mouth. Signs and symptoms include red or white colored patches, slightly raised, on mucous membranes, tongue, mouth, and throat. Underneath the patches, the area is raw, may bleed, and can be painful. The throat may be sore and swallowing may be difficult. Taste may diminish.

3 Pathogenic fungi attack hosts with compromised immune systems. Conditions that can weaken the immune system include chemotherapy and corticosteroid use, which both apply to Sarah.

Chapter 53 Answer to Critical Thinking Question in Evidence-Based Practice Feature

Nurses play a pivotal role in preventing the outbreaks of fungal infections. The nurse is responsible for the evaluation of hospitals and home environments for potential sources of pathogens. Secondly, the nurse will provide education to patients on preventive measures that can reduce exposure to fungal pathogens.

Chapter 53 Answers to Case Study

1 Sarah is at higher risk because poor fitting dentures can stress the mucus membranes and result in breaks that allow *Candida* to grow. People with dentures are in the risk group for this fungal infection.

2 Sarah should be told that the first step is to bring the condition causing the thrush under control. In Sarah's case this includes securing better fitting dentures. However, as long as Sarah is taking chemotherapy, her immune system may remain compromised. She will probably need a course of oral treatment using antifungal drugs such as nystatin swish and swallow, clotrimazole troche, and fluconazole. Oral swishes must be held in the mouth before swallowing so the antifungal agent can act locally on the mucous membranes. If the situation cannot be controlled using local measures, systemic treatment may be needed.

Chapter 53 Answers to NCLEX-RN® Review

1 Answer: 2 Rationale: Unlike bacteria, which grow rapidly, fungi grow slowly and infections may progress for many months before symptoms develop. Option 1 is incorrect because fungal infections take time to develop. Clients will not demonstrate symptoms for up to several weeks in most cases. Option 3 is incorrect. It is unlikely that symptoms would be manifested within this time frame after exposure. Option 4 is incorrect. People are exposed to spores, yeast, and molds constantly, and symptoms are most likely to occur in individuals who are immunosuppressed. Cognitive Level: Application; Client Need: Physiological Integrity; Nursing Process: Assessment

2 Answer: 3 Rationale: Clients who have suppressed immune systems, especially those infected with HIV, may experience frequent fungal infections. Option 1 is incorrect. Neither African Americans nor Hispanic individuals have a higher incident rate of fungal infections. Option 2 is incorrect. However, it could be correct if the client has chronic end stage cardiovascular disease with immunosuppression. Option 4 is incorrect. Although children and youth may have immature immune systems, it does not make them more susceptible to systemic fungal infections. Cognitive Level: Application; Client Need: Physiological Integrity; Nursing Process: Assessment

3 Answer: 1 Rationale: Fluconazole (Diflucan) at toxic levels is hepatotoxic. Some symptoms of hepatic toxicity include dark colored orange urine, clay colored stools, right upper quadrant pain, and jaundice. Option 2 is incorrect. Tinnitus is not a typical adverse effect of Diflucan. Option 3 is incorrect. Diflucan is not known to cause tachycardia. Option 4 is incorrect. Dysphagia (difficulty swallowing) is not an expected adverse effect of this drug. Cognitive Level: Application; Client Need: Physiological Integrity; Nursing Process: Assessment

4 Answer: 2 Rationale: Amphotericin B is a very potent antifungal agent. When given intravenously it can precipitate hypotension, hypokalemia, and shock. The drug should be infused slowly over 2–6 hours. Option 1 is incorrect. Amphotericin B can cause a multitude of adverse effects, and myalgia may be one. However this is not a life-threatening complication. Option 3 is incorrect. Amphotericin is a potent antifungal drug and the adverse effects are numerous. However, bone marrow suppression would not be seen immediately due to rapid IV infusion. Option 4 is incorrect. Flank pain is not a life-threatening complication typically seen with intravenous administration of Amphotericin B. Cognitive Level: Application; Client Need: Physiological Integrity; Nursing Process: Assessment

5 Answer: 3 Rationale: Amphotericin B can cause a number of serious adverse effects including fever, chills, and headache. Pretreatment may reduce the severity of these distressing adverse effects. Option 1 is incorrect. Pretreatment with corticosteroids, antihistamines, and antipyretics does not enhance the effectiveness of this antifungal agent. Option 2 is incorrect. The by-products of amphotericin are not affected by the pretreatment of the client. Option 4 is incorrect. Pretreatment does not affect the half-life of the drug. Cognitive Level: Application; Client Need: Physiological Integrity; Nursing Process: Implementation

6 Answer: 2 Rationale: Clients taking inhaled corticosteroid therapy are at greater risk of developing oral fungal infections because these agents cause local immunosuppression in the oral cavity. The nurse should instruct the client to rinse the mouth after using an inhaler that contains corticosteroids. Option 1 is incorrect. Oral diuretics do not increase the client's risk for developing an oral fungal infection. Option 3 is incorrect. The use of sublingual nitrates does not increase the client's susceptibility to oral fungal infections. Option 4 is incorrect. The client's risk for developing an oral fungal infection is not increased with the use of buccal analgesic agents. Cognitive Level: Application; Client Need: Physiological Integrity; Nursing Process: Implementation

Chapter 54

Answer to Connection Checkpoint 54.1

Tetracyclines are pregnancy category D drugs. Tetracyclines have a detrimental effect on the skeletal development of the fetus and should not be used in the second half of pregnancy unless benefits from treatment outweigh the risks to the fetus.

Answer to Connection Checkpoint 54.2

Sulfonamides are indicated for urinary tract infections.

Chapter 54 Answers to Critical Thinking Questions

1 Malaria is caused by the bite of Anopheles mosquitoes infected with the parasite called plasmodium. The four species of the parasite plasmodium include *P. vivax, P. ovale, P. malariae, and P. falciparum.* The female Anopheles mosquito becomes infected by ingesting blood containing the sexual forms of the parasite plasmodium. After the plasmodium reproduces in the mosquito, the mosquito inoculates it into humans.

2 Antimalarial drugs will vary depending upon the different stages of the parasite's life cycle. Through diagnostic evaluation, the health care provider will determine the stage of the infection and prescribe an appropriate treatment plan.

3 Prevention for malaria is based on three factors: 1) evaluating the risk of exposure to infection, 2) preventing mosquito bites by using DEET mosquito repellant, bed nets, and clothing that covers most of the body, and 3) chemoprophylaxis (preventive medications). For travelers, chloroquine therapy is the drug of choice to prevent malaria. This drug is given 1–2 weeks before travel and continues once a week during travel. Once the individual returns from travel, the drug is continued for 4 weeks.

4 Adverse effects of chloroquine include nausea, vomiting, stomach upset, cramps, loss of appetite, diarrhea, tiredness, weakness, and headache.

Chapter 54 Answers to Case Study

1 Trichomoniasis, a common sexually transmitted infection (STI), affects both women and men. The infection is much more common in women because the vagina is a more favorable environment for the pathogen compared to the male reproductive tract.

2 The nurse is in an ideal position to discuss sexual health with clients. The patient should be taught the importance of adherence to the drug therapy and follow-up care. Then a discussion related to sexual practices should follow. Sexual abstinence is the surest method to avoid any STI. The next level of protection includes a long-term mutually monogamous relationship with a partner who is known, through testing, to be uninfected. The use of latex male condoms, when used correctly and consistently can dramatically reduce the transmission of STIs. A person diagnosed with STI should be encouraged to notify all recent sex partners so that they can see a health care provider and be treated. This reduces the risk that the sex partners will develop complications and lessens the risk of reinfection.

3 Common adverse effects of metronidazole include anorexia, nausea, vomiting, diarrhea, abdominal pain, dizziness, headache, dryness of mouth, and metallic taste.

Chapter 54 Answers to NCLEX-RN® Review

1 Answer: 1 Rationale: Chloroquine therapy begins 1–2 weeks before travel, and continues once a week during travel and for 4 weeks after returning. Option 2 is incorrect. Once the prophylaxis is initiated it should be continued for 4 weeks following departure from the site of malaria. Three days is not a sufficient amount of time to ensure the client has adequate protection against malaria infection (option 3). If the client develops symptoms of malaria, prophylaxis is no longer indicated (option 4). Cognitive Level: Application; Client Need: Physiological Integrity; Nursing Process: Implementation

2 Answer: 3 Rationale: A potential cause of giardiasis in the United States is the unsanitary handling of soiled diapers in day care centers. Aggregate living arrangements pose special problems related to infection control. However, giardiasis is not common in long-term care facilities (option 1). Although adolescents and young adults are at high risk for many communicable diseases, giardiasis is not common among this population (option 2). Beef and pork tapeworms are acquired when raw or undercooked meat is eaten that contains cysts or larvae of the parasites (option 4). Cognitive Level: Application; Client Need: Physiological Integrity; Nursing Process: Assessment

3 Answer: 3 Rationale: Many clients complain of an unpleasant metallic taste that can be caused by metronidazole. Flatus and intestinal bloating are not characteristic adverse effects of metronidazole (option 1). Metronidazole does not cause bad breath (halitosis) Other causes of this problem, when chronic, should be explored (option 2). Alopecia (hair loss) is not associated with metronidazole (option 4). Cognitive Level: Application; Client Need: Physiological Integrity; Nursing Process: Assessment

4 Answer: 2 Rationale: Toxoplasmosis can occur if humans are exposed to contaminated cat feces, or eat raw or undercooked meat containing the cysts. Exotic birds can transmit a variety of pathogens; however, toxoplasmosis is not transmitted by birds (option 1). Toxoplasmosis is not transmitted via canine dander and fur (option 3). Leishmaniasis, not toxoplasmosis is transmitted to humans by the bite of the sand fly (option 4). Cognitive Level: Knowledge; Client Need: Physiological Integrity; Nursing Process: Assessment

5 Answer: 1, 2, 3 Rationale: Blood dyscrasia is any abnormal condition of the formed elements of blood or of the constituents required for clotting. Metronidazole can cause bone marrow suppression and is thereby contraindicated for clients with blood dyscrasias (option 1). Metronidazole crosses the blood brain barrier and is contraindicated in clients with active CNS pathology (option 2). Metronidazole may be hazardous to the fetus in the first trimester and should be questioned (option 3). Option 4 is incorrect because pelvic inflammatory disease is an infection (usually sexually transmitted) that spreads from the vagina to the upper parts of a woman's reproductive tract in the pelvic cavity. Metronidazole is often used for this type of infection. Option 5 is incorrect because metronidazole (Flagyl) is used to treat trichomoniasis. Cognitive Level: Knowledge; Client Need: Physiological Integrity; Nursing Process: Assessment

6 Answer: 1 Rationale: An acute onset of any CNS abnormality may manifest as metronidazole toxicity. If ataxia and confusion suddenly develop after the initiation of metronidazole, the nurse should discontinue the medication and contact the health care provider. Adverse effects to metronidazole are rare; however nausea and diarrhea can occur. Should these adverse effects occur, the nurse should notify the prescriber. However, in most cases these adverse effects are transient and do not warrant discontinuation of the medication (option 2). Anorexia and dryness of the mouth are common adverse effects with metronidazole. However, these adverse effect will usually disappear as the therapy continues (option 3). Weight gain and irritability are not typical adverse effects associated with metronidazole (option 4). Cognitive Level: Application; Client Need: Physiological Integrity; Nursing Process: Assessment

Chapter 55

Answer to Connection Checkpoint 55.1

Topical agents are often unable to penetrate to deeper skin layers and may not reach herpesviruses residing in other regions. They also have a slower onset of action.

Answer to Connection Checkpoint 55.2

Live vaccines contain organisms that are rendered less able to infect (attenuated). Inactivated vaccines contain killed organisms that are unable to infect.

Answer to Connection Checkpoint 55.3

Immunoglobulins are antibodies. They may be used to prevent hemolytic disease of the newborn, hepatitis B, or cytomegalovirus.

Chapter 55 Answers to Critical Thinking Questions

1 Herpesviruses are usually acquired through direct physical contact with an infected person. HSV may remain in a latent, asymptomatic, nonreplicating state in sensory or autonomic nerve root ganglia for many years. Infection is lifelong. Immunosuppression, physical challenge, or emotional stress can promote active replication of the virus and reappearance of the characteristic lesions. Antiviral drugs used to treat herpesviruses do not cure the patient.

2 Antiviral agents are not routinely prescribed for prophylaxis due to the cost and potential adverse effects. Patients who experience particularly severe or recurrent episodes may receive low dose antiviral agents.

3 Richard should apply the acyclovir as soon as symptoms of a herpes infection appear. The medication should be applied to all sores every 3 hours (6 times a day) for 7 days, or as directed. Sometimes, this medication may cause burning, stinging, and redness. Cold sores are contagious at all stages and can spread to other people through kissing or sharing things that touch the lips such as towels or utensils. Richard should use disposable gloves when applying the medication to avoid spreading the infection. Lastly, a healthy lifestyle may reduce the recurrence of cold sores. This would include a balanced diet, exercise, restful sleep, and managing emotional stress.

4 There are multiple factors that contribute to preventing individuals from continuing to practice health-promotion activities that reduce the risk for transmission of HPV. Such factors can be categorized into four major areas: (1) personal beliefs about health; (2) lifestyle; (3) cultural norms and values; and (4) social support systems. It is the role of the nurse to examine the barriers that women face when unable to sustain health-promoting activities and to aid the patient in removing obstacles.

Chapter 55 Answers to Case Study

1 The timing and onset of symptoms are critical factors when considering drugs such as oseltamivir. If the drug is given within 48 hours of the onset of symptoms, the drug may shorten the normal 7 day duration of influenza to 5 days. Since Jeanie's symptoms developed 24 hours ago, the health care provider may consider this drug an option for the patient.

2 Neuraminidase is an antigenic enzyme found on the surface of the influenza virus. Neuraminidase aids in the efficiency of virus release from cells. Neuraminidase inhibitors limit the severity and spread of viral infections.

Chapter 55 Answers to NCLEX-RN® Review

1 Answer: 1, 2, 4, 5 Rationale: All adults over the age of 60 should be encouraged to receive an annual influenza vaccine (option 1). The woman in option 2 is nother candidate for influenza vaccination not only due to her age but also because of her living conditions. An outbreak of influenza in a long-term care facility can be lethal for its residents. Due to her pregnant condition, the woman in Option 4 should also be encouraged to receive an annual influenza vaccination. Individuals who are HIV positive should take all precautions to avoid infection such as influenza. Receiving the influenza vaccine would provide the woman in Option 5 with protection against a potentially deadly viral infection. The woman in Option 3 would not benefit from an influenza vaccination because current influenza symptoms are present. Cognitive Level: Application; Client Need: Physiological Integrity; Nursing Process: Assessment

2 Answer: 1 Rationale: Individuals with herpes must understand that transferring the virus remains a possibility even if drug therapies are used. Option 2 is incorrect. Clients with herpes lesions should cleanse affected areas with soap and water 3–4 times daily and dry well prior to application of the topical mediation. Option 3 is incorrect. With application of medication to the genitals, the client should wear loose-fitting clothes over affected areas for comfort. Option 4 is incorrect. For best results, the client should be instructed to start the antiviral therapy as soon as possible after the onset of signs and symptoms. Cognitive Level: Application; Client Need: Physiological Integrity; Nursing Process: Evaluation

3 Answer: 2 Rationale: Acyclovir is associated with nephrotoxicity, and frequent laboratory tests which include serum creatinine levels should be performed to monitor renal function. Option 1 is incorrect. Acyclovir is not known to interfere or affect the white blood cell count. Option 3 is incorrect. Potassium and sodium levels are not affected by acyclovir. Option 4 is incorrect. Acyclovir usually does not affect platelets or coagulation factors. Cognitive Level: Application; Client Need: Physiological Integrity; Nursing Process: Assessment

4 Answer: 1 Rationale: Latent herpesvirus can be activated by stress, trauma, fever, exposure to sunlight, sexual intercourse, and menstruation. Option 2 is incorrect. Calcium-based foods do not precipitate an onset of herpes lesions. Option 3 is incorrect. There is no relationship between the exposure to cool moist air and the onset of herpes lesions. Option 4 is incorrect. Exposure to animal dander is not considered a factor that precipitates the onset of herpes lesions. Cognitive Level: Application; Client Need: Physiological Integrity; Nursing Process: Assessment

5 Answer: 1 Rationale: Most health care providers recommend that Oseltamivir (Tamiflu) be given within the first 48 hours of the onset of the symptoms. Option 2 is incorrect. Tamiflu does not prevent influenza. It minimizes the symptoms and shortens the duration of influenza. Option 3 is incorrect. Complications associated with influenza can be very serious, especially for older adults. Tamiflu does not eliminate the complications of influenza. Option 4 is incorrect. Tamiflu is not contraindicated for older adults. Cognitive Level: Application; Client Need: Physiological Integrity; Nursing Process: Implementation

6 Answer: 2 Rationale: Clients receiving interferon therapy often complain of adverse effects similar to flulike symptoms. Options 1 and 3 are incorrect. Neither neurological symptoms nor skin disruptioare are expected adverse effects related to interferon therapy. Option 4 is incorrect. Interferon does not usually cause gastric discomfort. Cognitive Level: Application; Client Need: Safe, Effective Care; Nursing Process: Evaluation

Chapter 56

Answer to Connection Checkpoint 56.1

Immunosuppressants are used to prevent transplant rejection and to dampen hyperactive immune responses, such as those that may occur during exacerbations of lupus or rheumatoid arthritis.

Answer to Connection Checkpoint 56.2

The type of response induced by the real pathogen, or its vaccine, is called active immunity. Passive immunity occurs when preformed antibodies are transferred from one person to another. A successful HIV vaccine would produce active immunity.

Answer to Connection Checkpoint 56.3

Isoniazid (INH), rifampin (Rifadin, Rimactane), pyrazinamide (PZA), and ethambutol (Myambutol).

Chapter 56 Answers to Critical Thinking Questions

1 The primary concern with this hospitalization is the treatment of the secondary infection. The patient will be more than likely placed on antibiotics and antifungal medication first. Rarely is antiretroviral medication initiated until the presenting infection is treated and under control.

The nurse should realize that the optimal time to start antiretroviral therapy depends on many factors including the presentation of HIV symptoms, CD4 cell counts, and the patient's ability to accept the HIV diagnosis, as well as willingness to comply with the therapy.

2 HIV infections occur when individuals are exposed to contaminated body fluids such as blood or semen. Transmission may occur through sexual activity (oral, anal, or vaginal) or through contact of infected fluids with broken skin, mucous membranes, or needlesticks.

3 The nursing assistant should be taught to use universal standard precautions for all patients no matter the presence or absence of HIV. Below are some preventive measures that all health care providers should take with all patients

- Use appropriate barrier precautions to prevent skin and mucous-membrane exposure when contact with blood or other body fluids of any patient is anticipated. Gloves should be worn for touching blood and body fluids, mucous membranes, or nonintact skin of all patients.
- Gloves should be changed after contact with each patient.
- During procedures that are likely to generate droplets of blood or other body fluids, the nurse should wear a mask and protective eyewear or a face shield to prevent exposure of mucous membranes of the mouth, nose, and eyes.
- Gowns or aprons should be worn during procedures that are likely to generate splashes of blood or other body fluids.
- Hands and other skin surfaces should be washed immediately and thoroughly if contaminated with blood or other body fluids. Hands should be washed immediately after gloves are removed.
- Take precautions to prevent injuries caused by needles, scalpels, and other sharp instruments or devices during procedures, when cleaning used instruments, during disposal of used needles, and when handling sharp instruments after procedures.
- To minimize the need for emergency mouth-to-mouth resuscitation without protection, mouth pieces, resuscitation bags, or other ventilation devices should be available for use in areas where the need for resuscitation is predictable.

Chapter 56 Answers to Case Study

1 Human immunodeficiency virus (HIV) is a microorganism that can kill or damage cells of the body's immune system. HIV progressively destroys the body's ability to fight infections and certain cancers. People diagnosed with HIV may get life-threatening diseases called opportunistic infections, which are caused by microbes such as viruses or bacteria that usually do not make healthy people sick. HIV is the virus that causes AIDS.

HAART is the abbreviation used for highly active antiretroviral therapy. This therapy is indicated in the treatment for HIV infection that employs a combination of several antiretroviral drugs. The drugs inhibit the ability of the virus to multiply in the body and slow down the development of AIDS.

2 Strict adherence to HAART is essential for maintaining treatment benefits and preventing the development of HIV resistance. Safe-sex practices and avoidance of needle-sharing activity is critical, regardless of medication adherence or viral load. Pharmacological treatment only helps prolong life; it does not cure the disease itself.

Chapter 56 Answers to NCLEX-RN® Review

1 Answer: 2 Rationale: This is a false statement. No existing vaccine provides immunity to this disease. Option 1 is incorrect because it is a true statement. Clients should be informed that therapy for HIV will require life long treatment since there is not a cure. Option 3 is incorrect. This is a true statement. Since treatment is often complex and lifelong, whenever possible, the client should be taught how to adjust the daily schedule so as to not interfere with ADLs. Option 4 is incorrect. This is a true statement. With recent advances in pharmacotherapy for HIV infection, many individuals are able to live symptom-free lives. Cognitive Level: Application; Client Need: Safe, Effective Care Management; Nursing Process: Assessment

2 Answer: 2 Rationale: Lipodystrophy is a disorder that is due to mitochondrial toxicity from NRTIs. When this adverse effect occurs, areas such as the face, arms, and legs tend to lose fat, while the abdomen, breasts and base of the neck (buffalo hump) develop excess fat. The fat redistribution may be associated with hyperlipidemia and hyperglycemia. Option 1 is incorrect. A redistribution of body fat is not characteristic of renal failure. Option 3 is incorrect. Hypoaldosteronism refers to decreased levels of the hormone aldosterone. The usual clinical manifestations include hyperkalemia and metabolic acidosis. Option 4 is incorrect. Bone marrow suppression typically manifests by a reduction in blood cell formation. Clients suffer from anemia, thrombocytopenia, and leukopenia. Cognitive Level: Knowledge; Client Need: Physiological Integrity; Nursing Process: Assessment

3 Answer: 1 Rationale: Granulocytopenia is the marked decrease in the number of a type of white blood cell. Granulocytes are part of the nonspecific infection-fighting immune system. When this condition occurs the client is at high risk for infections. Option 2 is incorrect. Granulocytopenia does not produce fatigue. Frequent rest periods are not required due to this adverse effect. Option 3 is incorrect. The adverse effect of granulocytopenia does not affect postural changes or orthostatic hypotension. Rising slowly from a sitting position is not related to the effect of a decline in these blood cells. Option 4 is incorrect. Antacids will diminish absorption. Cognitive Level: Application; Client Need: Physiological Integrity; Nursing Process: Assessment

4 Answer: 3 Rationale: Myelosuppression is the declining ability of the bone marrow to produce blood cells such as platelets, red blood cells and white blood cells. Option 1 is incorrect. Myelosuppression is not reflected in an increase in the serum blood urea nitrogen level (BUN). Option 2 is incorrect. Although the white blood cell count is affected in myelosuppression, this condition causes a decrease in white blood cells rather than an increase. Option 4 is incorrect. A decline in blood pressure is not indicative of myelosuppression. Cognitive Level: Application; Client Need: Physiological Integrity; Nursing Process: Assessment

5 Answer: 1, 2, 4 Rationale: Clients receiving antiretroviral therapy are immunocompromised and should avoid sources of infection such as crowds and individuals who have infections (option 1). The client should be instructed to notify the health care provider at the first sign of a rash. Several antiretroviral medications may cause SJSl, which may be fatal (option 2). Coughing and deep breathing may prevent respiratory infection in the immunosuppressed HIV client (option 4). Option 3 is incorrect. It is imperative that the client understand that HIV may be transmitted to others and that drug therapy does not prevent the transmission. Option 5 is incorrect. Some herbal supplements, such as St. John's wort, interfere with antiretroviral therapy. Cognitive Level: Application; Client Need: Physiological Integrity; Nursing Process: Intervention

6 Answer: 2 Rationale: St. John's wort should be used with caution, because this supplement may decrease the effectiveness of antiviral medications. Option 1 is incorrect. Many clients will turn to alternative therapy when faced with HIV infection. These activities provide the client with a sense of control and comfort and should be supported as long as they are not contraindicated with the prescribed drug therapy. Option 3 is incorrect. Meditation and journaling are not contraindicated. Option 4 is incorrect. If the client wishes to see a chiropractor, there is no reason this should not be allowed. However, the nurse should instruct the client to first consult the health care provider treating the HIV infection. Cognitive Level: Application; Client Need: Physiological Integrity; Nursing Process: Assessment

Chapter 57

Answer to Connection Checkpoint 57.1

HPV immunization (Gardasil) is recommended for three IM doses with the second dose 2 months after the first, and the third dose 6 months after the original. The CDC recommends the routine vaccination of females from 11–12 years old and for females age 13–26 years old who have not been vaccinated at an earlier age.

Answer to Connection Checkpoint 57.2

The corticosteroids are effective immunosuppressants that help prevent transplant rejection.

Answer to Connection Checkpoint 57.3

HIV and tuberculosis.

Chapter 57 Answers to Critical Thinking Questions

1 Even though the surgeon has removed the large part of the tumor, if there is even one cancerous cell left it may repopulate. The goal of chemotherapy is to obtain a total cell kill so that if any cancerous cells were left after the mastectomy the chemotherapy will kill them before the cells have a chance to repopulate the cancer.

2 Staging and grading are important to understand because these systems are used to establish treatment and prognosis for the patient with cancer. T1, N0, M0 tells us that the tumor is relatively small in size and not significantly invading surrounding tissues, no cancerous cells were found in the lymph nodes, and no metastases were found. G_2 tells us that the cells are moderately differentiated and look somewhat like the parent cells. The staging and grading for Cheryl's cancer leads us to believe that she has a good prognosis.

3 A clinical trial is utilized to test new medications or procedures on human subjects. This means that the medication or procedure has been tested on laboratory animals but has not been tested on human subjects. Participants must sign a consent form stating that they have been made aware of all known potential adverse effects and are willingly participating. Participants may withdraw from the study at any time. The decision to participate in clinical trials is a personal choice.

4 Hematological changes that Cheryl may experience during chemotherapy are: thrombocytopenia, neutropenia, and anemia. Thrombocytopenia is defined as a platelet count of less than 100,000 per milliliter of blood. This can cause the patient to exhibit abnormal bleeding. If the platelet count drops to less than 20,000 per milliliter of blood, the patient may begin to bruise easily. They may also exhibit petechiae or purpura. If the platelet count continues to decrease the patient may hemorrhage or die.

A patient is diagnosed with neutropenia when their neutrophil count is less than 1500 cells. The chemotherapy may cause a decrease in all of the patient's white blood cells (leukopenia); however, the neutrophils are usually the type of white blood cells that are affected the most. Cheryl's nadir must be calculated prior to administering any more chemotherapy.

A patient is diagnosed with anemia when their red blood cell count reaches less than 4.2 million/mm^3 for men or 3.6/mm^3 for women, or a hemoglobin count of less than 14 g/dL for men and 12 g/dL for women. Because hemoglobin carries oxygen to all tissues and major organs in the body, anemia may affect every system in the body.

Chapter 57 Answers to Case Study

1 Jonah's children may be allowed to visit him if Jonah does not become neutropenic and the children are free from illness. Some hospitals have policies that children under the age of 13 years are not allowed onto the oncology floors. Because the chemotherapy will decrease his immune system, the risk for Jonah acquiring a bacterial or viral infection is high.

2 The use of multiple drugs affects different stages of the cancer cell's life cycle, and attacks the various clones within the tumor via several mechanisms of action, thus increasing the percentage of cell kill. Combination chemotherapy also allows lower dosages of each individual agent, thus reducing toxicity and slowing the development of resistance.

3 Leukemia is a disseminated cancer not a solid tumor. Only solid tumors may be staged. Leukemias may be graded.

Chapter 57 Answers to NCLEX-RN® Review

1 Answer: 3 Rationale: Stage I suggests that the tumor is relatively small in size, has not invaded the surrounding tissue, and has not been detected in surrounding lymph nodes; thus it has been detected at an early stage. Option 1 is incorrect. Stage I is the earliest staging and has the best prognosis. Option 2 is incorrect. Cell differentiation refers to grading of cancer cells not staging of cancer cells. Option 4 is incorrect. Stage I suggests that the tumor is small and has not begun to invade surrounding tissue. Cognitive Level: Knowledge; Client Need: Physiologic Integrity; Nursing Process: Assessment.

2 Answer: 2 Rationale: A low neutrophil count means that the client has a decreased immune system, thus placing the client at risk for an infection. Protective isolation measures would be initiated to shelter the client from microorganisms. Option 1 is incorrect. A high uric acid level places the client at risk for renal problems. Option 3 is incorrect. A high red blood cell count does not impair the client's immune system. Option 4 is incorrect. A low platelet count places the client at risk for bleeding complications but does not affect the immune system. Cognitive Level: Analysis; Client Need: Physiological Integrity; Nursing Process: Assessment

3 Answer: 1: Rationale: The use of multiple drugs affects different stages of the cancer cell's life cycle, and attacks the various clones within the tumor via several mechanisms of action, thus increasing the percentage of cell kill. Combination chemotherapy also allows lower dosages of each individual agent, thus reducing toxicity and slowing the development of resistance. Option 2 is incorrect. Staging describes the process of determining the extent of cancer in the body and where the cancer is located Option 3 is incorrect. Antineoplastic drugs may kill only a small portion of the tumor, leaving some clones unaffected and able to repopulate the tumor with resistant cells. Option 4 is incorrect. Combination chemotherapy also allows lower dosages of each individual agent, thus reducing toxicity and slowing the development of resistance. Cognitive Level: Comprehension; Client Need: Physiological Integrity; Nursing Process: Evaluation

4 Answer: 3 Rationale: Mucositis is the painful inflammation and ulceration of the mucous membranes lining the digestive tract, that is an adverse effect of chemotherapy and radiotherapy treatment for cancer. Clients experiencing this adverse effect should be instructed to eat a bland diet and to use a soft toothbrush for oral care. Most OTC mouthwashes contain a significant amount of alcohol which will further inflame the oral issue and should be avoided (option 1). Citrus foods and beverages should be avoided since the acidic nature of these foods would cause the client pain (option 2). Mucositis can last the duration of the chemotherapy treatment and should be treated rather than ignored. This condition will prevent intake of adequate nutrition to build new cells (option 4). Cognitive Level: Application; Client Need: Physiological Integrity; Nursing Process: Implementation

5 Answer: 1 Rationale: Myelosuppression is the most common dose-limiting adverse effect of chemotherapy, and the one that most often causes discontinuation or delays of chemotherapy. Although alopecia may be distressing for the client, its presence does not determine when the next round of chemotherapy can be administered (option 2). Mucositis is not a reason that subsequent rounds of chemotherapy should be delayed (option 3). Cachexia is the physical wasting with loss of weight and muscle mass caused by disease. Although it is considered, it is not the most common reason for delaying chemotherapy (option 4). Cognitive Level: Application; Client Need: Physiological Integrity; Nursing Process: Assessment

6 Answer: 4 Rationale: Many antineoplastics are classified as vesicant agents that can cause serious tissue injury if they escape from an artery or vein during an infusion or injection. The nurse should closely monitor the infusion site for swelling and pain. Option 1 is incorrect. Vesicants do not necessarily cause nausea. Option 2 is incorrect. It would be inappropriate for the nurse to monitor the client's intake of calcium-rich foods since this is not related to receiving a chemotherapy classified as a vesicant. Option 3 is incorrect. Respiratory status is not related to the administration of a vesicant type chemotherapy agent. Cognitive Level: Application; Client Need: Physiological Integrity; Nursing Process: Implementation

Chapter 58

Answer to Connection Checkpoint 58.1

Antineoplastic drugs cause immunosuppression; thus there may not be enough B-cells to produce an adequate antibody response. This could cause a lack of immunity. If a live virus is used as a vaccine, it could also result in an active infection.

Answer to Connection Checkpoint 58.2

Trimethoprim-sulfamethoxazole (Bactrim, Septra) is commonly used in the pharmacotherapy of urinary tract infections, Pneumocystis carinii pneumonia, Shigella infections of the small bowel, and acute episodes of chronic bronchitis.

Answer to Connection Checkpoint 58.3

Interferon alfacon-1 is used for chronic hepatitis C infection; interferon alfa-n3 is indicated for genital warts and human papilloma virus; interferon beta-1a is for multiple sclerosis.

Chapter 58 Answers to Critical Thinking Questions

1 Antineoplastics that are proven to have a high rate of cell kill in breast cancer include: cyclophosphamide, doxorubicin, 5-fluorouracil, methotrexate, paclitaxel, or vinorelbine. Most of these antineoplastics are given as part of a combination regimen.

2 Lucy must accept the fact that she has breast cancer, and her best chance of survival lies with a complete course of chemotherapy. Killing as many cancer cells as possible with a complete course of chemotherapy is the only way to decrease or eliminate the chance of the breast cancer metastasizing.

3 Tamoxifen (Nolvadex), an antiestrogen, is used as adjunctive therapy of axillary node-positive or node-negative breast cancer in women following mastectomy, axillary node dissection, or radiation therapy. It is also used to decrease the risk of invasive breast cancer following breast surgery and radiation therapy in women with ductal carcinoma in situ, and to decrease the incidence of breast cancer in high-risk women. The benefits of tamoxifen outweigh the risks in women who have already been diagnosed with breast cancer. Paclitaxel (Taxol) is a miscellaneous antineoplastic that is being used as adjuvant chemotherapy for women whose breast cancer has failed to resolve following combination therapy. At this point in her treatment, we do not know the end result of Mrs. Chinn's chemotherapy regimen, so she may need treatment with paclitaxel after her current chemotherapy series. Another drug available is raloxifene (Evista), classified as an estrogen receptor modulator. Although developed to reduce a postmenopausal woman's risk of developing osteoporosis, or to treat osteoporosis in the same group of women, it is currently an investigational drug being used to reduce the risk of breast cancer in postmenopausal women.

Chapter 58 Answers to Case Study

1 Janet can be told that her health care provider can prescribe medications to decrease the nausea and vomiting. She will be given instructions to take the medication whenever she feels nauseated or begins vomiting. Her eating patterns may have to change, at least temporarily. She should eat more frequent, smaller meals of easily digested foods. She may have to experiment to find those foods that are easiest for her to tolerate. If necessary, she can use prepared food supplements such as Ensure either to supplement what she is able to eat, or to substitute for other foods. She and her family members must be told to make mealtimes more pleasant by removing any unpleasant odors or sights from the area in which Janet is eating her meals. Many antineoplastics cause diarrhea. Occasional diarrhea may not be a problem requiring an intervention, but if it continues she can be given another medication to stop it. She must be taught to increase her fluids as much as she can tolerate without causing more nausea or vomiting, and that IV intake of fluids can be administered if necessary. She must be encouraged to continue the chemotherapy, despite any uncomfortable adverse effects she is experiencing.

2 Janet can be reassured that if alopecia does occur, her hair will regrow in 6–8 weeks after chemotherapy is completed. She can be referred to the American Cancer Society "Look Good, Feel Better" program, for assistance in finding an attractive hairstyle that will minimize the appearance of her hair loss. She can also be referred for wig fitting when she begins to lose her hair. She must be given encouragement that whatever new hairstyle she chooses is attractive and looks good on her. She must also be reminded that different people react to antineoplastics differently. Some people lose all of their hair, some experience thinning, and some lose no or very little hair. She might enjoy talking with another female patient who underwent chemotherapy, suffered with alopecia, and now has a full head of hair. Whatever else is done, she must be encouraged to continue her treatments.

Chapter 58 Answers to NCLEX-RN® Review

1 Answer: 2 Rationale: An antineoplastic cannot be continued if it is reducing the client's ability to protect self against infection. Without this ability, the mildest infectious process may cause the client's death. Options 1, 3, and 4 are incorrect because they are not dose-limiting adverse effects, even though they occur in the majority of persons undergoing chemotherapy. Cognitive Level: Knowledge; Client Need: Physiological Integrity; Nursing Process: Assessment

2 Answer: 1 Rationale: The client must be encouraged to continue with the chemotherapy. Without the full course, the cancer may reactivate and lead to the client's early death. Option 2 is an untrue statement. There are excellent medications available to treat the nausea and vomiting. Options 3 and 4 are incorrect because they are untrue statements. Cognitive Level: Application; Client Need: Physiological Integrity; Nursing Process: Implementation

3 Answer: 3 Rationale: Many antineoplastics can be absorbed through the skin, so the nurse must protect skin surfaces if handling them. Option 1 is incorrect because nurses in general cannot refuse to provide necessary care for their clients, including PO antineoplastic administration. Option 2 is incorrect because nurses do not have access or the need to use a hood; this piece of equipment is used in pharmacies where the antineoplastic medications are prepared. Nurses will not do the preparation of the antineoplastics. Option 4 is incorrect because universal precautions are not applicable to proper handling of medications. Universal precautions are used to prevent the spread of infection from one person to another by proper hand washing, etc., and are appropriate when handling body fluids and bed linens of clients who are receiving chemotherapy. Cognitive Level: Application; Client Need: Physiological Integrity; Nursing Process: Implementation

4 Answer: 2 Rationale: Cisplatin can cause hemorrhagic cystitis. The most effective way to decrease the chances of this occurring is to keep the client well hydrated either with oral or IV fluids for at least 48 hours surrounding the time of administration of cisplatin. Options 1 and 3 may be necessary measures, but neither is a dose-limiting adverse effect. Cisplatin is a pregnancy category D drug so will not be given to the client of child-bearing age unless every other antineoplastic has been tried and failed (option 4). Cognitive Level: Knowledge; Client Need: Physiological Integrity; Nursing Process: Implementation

5 Answer: 1 Rationale: The only use for leucovorin is to reduce the amount of time normal cells are in contact with methotrexate. The other answers are incorrect. Cognitive Level: Knowledge; Client Need: Physiological Integrity; Nursing Process: Implementation

6 Answer: 1 Rationale: Antiestrogen antineoplastics work on ER-positive tumors, or those tumors whose growth depends on a supply of estrogen. If the estrogen is not available to the tumor, it will not survive. They do not prevent breast cancer or the adverse effects of other antineoplastics (options 2 and 3). They do protect the female from developing osteoporosis (option 4). Cognitive Level: Application; Client Need: Physiological Integrity; Nursing Process: Evaluation

Chapter 59

Answer to Connection Checkpoint 59.1

Nitroglycerin is administered to reduce chest pain resulting from angina pectoris. The drug acts within minutes.

Answer to Connection Checkpoint 59.2

An enteric coating is resistant to stomach acid and permits the tablet to reach the small intestine before dissolving. Breaking the tablet will expose the drug to stomach acid, usually resulting in inactivation of the medication.

Answer to Connection Checkpoint 59.3

Fluoxetine will inhibit the metabolism (break down) of imipramine, allowing imipramine to reach higher serum levels and cause possible toxicity.

Chapter 60

Answer to Connection Checkpoint 60.1

Streptozocin is a nitrosourea alkylating agent. Doxorubicin is an anthracycline antitumor antibiotic.

Answer to Connection Checkpoint 60.2

The hepatic CYP450 enzymes metabolize drugs, making them more water soluble and better able to be excreted by the kidneys.

Answer to Connection Checkpoint 60.3

Overuse of antibiotics encourages the emergence of resistant strains. The longer and more often an antibiotic is prescribed, the more likely will be the appearance of resistant bacteria.

Chapter 60 Answers to Critical Thinking Questions

1 Risk factors for the development of PUD include infection with *H. pylori*, use of NSAIDS including aspirin, smoking tobacco, alcohol use, serious illness, and genetic factors.

2 Antibiotics are used to eradicate *H. pylori*. Although he is allergic to penicillin, there are other combinations of drugs available to eradicate *H. pylori*, which may include combinations of the following: clarithromycin, tetracycline, metronidazole, and bismuth compounds. A PPI may also be prescribed which may further decrease bacterial load and suppress acid.

Patient adherence is necessary to eradicate the organism. Patients must understand that they must complete the antibiotic regimen to fully treat the peptic ulcer and combat antibiotic resistance. They should be advised of adverse effects including nausea, diarrhea, and headache.

3 Use of NSAIDs in patients with HTN has been shown to worsen HTN in some patients. The chief mechanism by which NSAIDs contribute to HTN and decrease the effectiveness of antihypertensive drugs appears to be due to the inhibition of prostaglandin synthesis. This inhibition results in an increase in sodium reabsorption and water retention.

Chapter 60 Answer to Critical Thinking Question in Evidence-Based Practice Feature

It is theorized that the increased pH resulting from PPI use allows the organism to survive. Fortunately, although there is evidence of a predisposition to enteric bacterial overgrowth, this is rarely associated with a clinical problem.

Chapter 60 Answer to Critical Thinking Question in Evidence-Based Practice Feature

Long-term safety issues include the effects of prolonged association of gastric atrophy with PPI use, decreased absorption of folate and certain B vitamins, and prolonged elevated gastric pH which may affect the absorption of certain drugs. Finally community acquired pneumonia has been linked to long-term use of PPIs.

Chapter 60 Answers to Case Study

1 OTC medications for GERD are readily available. They are effective for patients with mild and intermittent cases. The danger is that self-medicating may cause a delay in seeking treatment for serious disease. Warning signs and symptoms of GERD that suggest a more complicated disease include unexplained weight loss, early satiety, anemia, vomiting, initial onset of symptoms after age 50, and prolonged anorexia.

2 The cause of GERD is usually transient relaxation of the lower esophageal sphincter (LES), allowing reflux of gastric juices back into the esophagus when the stomach contracts. Since the gastric contents are acidic, they cause injury to the esophagus. Risk factors mentioned in this case study include (1) being overweight, (2) eating spicy foods and red wine, and (3) use of the calcium channel blocker amlodipine. All are known to promote reflux. Other risk factors include tobacco, pregnancy, and other medications including bisphosphonates, nitrates, and theophylline.

3 The PPIs are the most effective medications available for GERD. These are generally safe drugs with few adverse effects. The prototype PPI is omeprazole, which is available by prescription and OTC. H_2 antagonists are also used to treat PUD.

4 Basal acid secretion peaks at night and is minimal in the morning.

Chapter 60 Answer to NCLEX-RN® Review

1 Answer: 2 Rationale: Magnesium compounds, especially in higher doses, often cause diarrhea. Options 1 and 3 are incorrect. Aluminum compounds and calcium compounds may cause constipation. Option 4 is incorrect. Sodium compounds may cause flatulence. Cognitive Level: Application; Client Need: Physiological Integrity; Nursing Process: Assessment

2 Answer: 1, 2, 4, and 5 Rationale: Symptoms of GERD include, dysphagia, dyspepsia, nausea, belching, heartburn, and chest pain. Option 3 is incorrect. The nurse would not expect a decrease in the client's appetite due to this medication. Cognitive Level: Application; Client Need: Physiological Integrity; Nursing Process: Evaluation

3 Answer: 3 Rationale: The proton pump is activated by food intake. Thus, administering it about 20–30 minutes before the first major meal of the day allows peak serum levels to coincide with when the maximum levels of pumps are activated, allowing maximum efficiency of the PPI. The proton pumps are less active at night (option 1), in the fasting state (option 2), or between meals (option 4). Cognitive Level: Application; Client Need: Physiological Integrity; Nursing Process: Planning

4 Answer: 2 Rationale: Blood dyscrasias have been reported, especially neutropenia and thrombocytopenia with long-term use. Periodic blood counts should be performed. Option 1 is incorrect. Ranitidine (Zantac) does not cause photophobia and skin irritations. Option 3 is incorrect. Dyspnea and productive cough are not expected adverse effects for this medication. Option 4 is incorrect. Ranitidine is not known to cause these symptoms. Cognitive Level: Application; Client Need: Physiological Integrity; Nursing Process: Planning

5 Answer: 4 Rationale: Concurrent use of aluminum salts and sucralfate pose a risk for aluminum toxicity. There is no risk of aluminum toxicity with PPIs (option 1), other antacids (option 2), or H_2-receptor antagonists (option 3). Cognitive Level: Knowledge; Client Need: Physiological Integrity; Nursing Process: Implementation

6 Answer: 3 Rationale: Antibiotics have no role in the treatment of GERD. Certain antibiotics are used in treating PUD to eradicate the organism *H. pylori.* H_2-receptor antagonists (option 1) and proton pump inhibitors (option 2) are used routinely to relieve symptoms of GERD. OTC antacids (option 4) provide intermittent relief for mild cases. Cognitive Level: Comprehension; Client Need: Physiological Integrity; Nursing Process: Implementation

Chapter 61

Answer to Connection Checkpoint 61.1

When a pregnant woman is diagnosed with preeclampsia or eclampsia and delivery is not imminent, IV magnesium sulfate may be administered to prevent or terminate seizures. Therapy may continue for 24 hours postpartum, or until hypertension resolves.

Answer to Connection Checkpoint 61.2

These drugs are muscarinic antagonists and atropine is the prototype.

Answer to Connection Checkpoint 61.3

The term extrapyramidal refers to locations in the CNS outside of the cerebrospinal pyramidal tracts of the brain. Extrapyramidal symptoms include acute dystonia, akathisia, parkinsonism, and tardive dyskinesia.

Chapter 61 Answer to Patient Safety Question

This situation places the patient at risk for medication overdose. It is imperative to obtain an accurate assessment of the patient's body weight when a medication dosage is based on that measure. The patient's body weight may fluctuate as in the case of individuals with Crohn's disease. The nurse can never assume that the patient's weight is stable. Also, the nurse should not rely upon the patient's self-reported weight, since this may also be very inaccurate.

Chapter 61 Answers to Critical Thinking Questions

1 Constipation is a common complaint among older persons. Chronic constipation includes at least 2 of the following symptoms: two or fewer bowel movements per week, lumpy or hard stools at least 25% of the time, straining to pass stools at least 25% of the time, and a feeling of incomplete evacuation at least 25% of the time. Constipation occurs more frequently in older adults because fecal transit time through the colon slows with aging. This population also exercises less, has diminished food intake, and often uses drugs that cause constipation at a higher rate than younger adults. All patients should understand that variations in frequency are normal, and that a daily bowel movement is not a requirement for good health. Constipation is more than an annoying problem. Persons with chronic constipation have been shown to have a diminished perception of their quality of life.

Laxative Type	How It Works	How Fast It Works	Problems Associated with Use
Bulk forming	Increases fecal bulk as well as the fluid retained in the bowel lumen	24–48 hours	Increased gas; bloating; bowel obstruction if strictures present; choking if powder forms are not taken with enough liquid
Stimulant	Alters intestinal mucosal permeability Stimulates muscle activity and fluid secretions	6–12 hours	Electrolyte imbalance; abdominal cramping.
Surfactant	Lubricates and softens fecal mass	24–48 hours	Minor effects such as bitter taste and nausea
Saline	Salts lead to retained fluid in the bowel lumen, with a net increase of fluid secretions in the small intestines.	1–6 hours	Electrolyte imbalance; excessive gas; dehydration
Herbal	Stimulates the bowel and increases peristalsis	Unknown	Unknown—depends on the agent.

3 For the immediate problem, perhaps a bulk forming laxative is the drug of choice. Bulk-forming laxatives cause water to be retained in the colon and thereby increase stool bulk. These laxatives have few potential adverse effects and are effective in slowly reversing the symptoms of constipation. In fact, their use is essentially the same as increasing fiber in the diet. Ultimately, Marjorie may need to be given a stool softener on a daily basis. Stool softeners decrease surface tension and therefore allow stool to absorb more water. Stool softeners are generally well tolerated but are ineffective if fluid intake is inadequate.

4 Diet plays a critical role in bowel function, especially in older adults. Evidence has shown that greater intake of dietary fiber is associated with a lesser prevalence of constipation and other GI disorders. To ensure that fiber itself does not become constipating, adequate fluid intake is necessary. The recommended daily requirement for fluids is eight 8-oz glasses, assuming that the patient has no cardiac or renal problems that prohibit intake of this amount. Exercise stimulates defecation and helps strengthen the abdominal muscles that aid defecation.

Chapter 61 Answers to Case Study

1 Sulfasalazine is the combination of two substances: sulfapyridine and an aspirin-like compound. It works to reduce the inflammation in the colon caused by Crohn's disease. The drug tends to be effective in preventing recurrences. However, it does not work as well for relieving severe flare-ups of the disease.

2 The most common adverse effects are nausea and abdominal discomfort, which tend to occur early in the course of treatment. In some cases, sulfasalazine may reduce the number of disease-fighting white blood cells in the body. Other common adverse effects include a skin rash or headache. Sulfasalazine can increase sensitivity to sunlight. Some people taking sulfasalazine develop an orange discoloration of their urine and, occasionally, of their skin. This is usually harmless and should not cause alarm. The discoloration is temporary and goes away after stopping the medication.

3 This drug is contraindicated in the presence of the following conditions: allergies to sulfonamide or aspirin; hematological disorders such as anemia; hepatic impairment; and urinary obstruction.

Chapter 61 Answers to NCLEX-RN® Review

1 Answer: 3 Rationale: Lomotil is given for diarrhea. The client should report a decrease in the number of loose watery stools after administration. Although Lomotil may decrease abdominal cramping, it is not the therapeutic effect desired from this drug (option 1). Because Lomotil slows peristalsis, there may be a decrease in flatus after administration. However, this is not the therapeutic effect desired (option 2). If Lomotil affects the bowel sounds of an individual, it would most likely decrease them by slowing peristalsis (option 4). Cognitive Level: Application; Client Need: Safe, Effective Care Management; Nursing Process: Evaluation

2 Answer: 2 Rationale: One adverse effect of sulfasalazine is blood dyscrasias, which may include anemia, leukopenia, and thrombocytopenia. In Stevens-Johnson Syndrome (SJS) clients suffer from inflammation of the skin and mucous membranes which this client is not experiencing (option 1). Idiosyncratic reactions are aberrant reactions that cannot be explained by the known pharmacologic action of the drug and occur only in a small percent of the population. This client's symptoms are not idiosyncratic but well documented and somewhat expected (option 3). Hypersensitivity responses are due to stimulation of the immune system and are invoked by an antigen or antibody response. The symptoms presented do not reflect hypersensitivity to the drug (option 4). Cognitive Level: Application; Client Need: Safe, Effective Care Management; Nursing Process: Assessment

3 Answer: 2 Rationale: Compazine is a phenothiazine and can cause extrapyramidal symptoms such as facial twitching and involuntary movements. Nausea and vomiting are indications for this drug (option 1). Although troublesome, dry mouth, sedation, and constipation are expected adverse effects of prochlorperazine (option 3). Compazine often can cause dizziness, lethargy, and ataxia due to its effect on the CNS (option 4). Cognitive Level: Application; Client Need: Safe, Effective Care Management; Nursing Process: Assessment

4 Answer: 1 Rationale: The enzymes in pancrelipase come from pork. If the client is allergic to or has religious restrictions on pork, the drug is contraindicated. Zymase is not contraindicated for individuals with HTN (option 2). Typically, clients with coronary artery disease may take pancrelipase if prescribed (option 3). Zymase is not an iodine-based agent. There is no cross sensitivity expected (option 4). Cognitive Level: Application; Client Need: Safe, Effective Care Management; Nursing Process: Assessment

5 Answer: 4 Rationale: In 2007, research conducted by the FDA showed an excess number of serious cardiovascular adverse events, including angina, heart attacks, and stroke in clients taking tegaserod (Zelnorm). Later that year, the FDA approved restricted use of tegaserod (Zelnorm) for clients for whom other treatment options were considered unsafe or ineffective. Its use is now limited by strict criteria to clients without heart disease. Multiple sclerosis is not a contraindication for this medication (option 1). If prescribed, a client with a fracture femur, should not have any problems taking Zelnorm (option 2). Anemia is not a contraindication for this therapy (option 3). Cognitive Level: Application; Client Need: Safe, Effective Care Management; Nursing Process: Assessment

6 Answer: 1, 3 Rationale: Diphenoxylate (an opioid) with atropine is a drug of choice for mild to moderate diarrhea. Octreotide is closely related to endogenous somatostatin, and is approved to treat severe diarrhea. Option 2 is incorrect. Magnesium hydroxide is used to treat constipation and would worsen this client's condition. Option 4 is incorrect. Reglan is used to treat nausea and vomiting, not diarrhea. Option 5 is incorrect. Psyllium (Metamucil) is used for constipation. Cognitive Level: Application; Client Need: Safe, Effective Care Management; Nursing Process: Implementation

Chapter 62

Answer to Connection Checkpoint 62.1

Warfarin acts by creating a functional deficiency of vitamin K, which decreases the amount of certain clotting factors that depend on vitamin K for their synthesis. Adding vitamin K to the diet will reverse the deficiency.

Answer to Connection Checkpoint 62.2

Isoniaxid depletes the body of pyridoxine, which is necessary for the synthesis of the neurotransmitter, gamma-aminobutyric acid. Pyridoxine supplements are necessary to prevent neurotoxicity.

Chapter 62 Answers to Critical Thinking Questions

1 Pyruvic acid and lactic acid play important roles in biochemical processes. Both are involved in the breakdown of glucose. In malnourished individuals, both acids become elevated. In Bill's case, his lack of adequate nutrition, specifically B complex vitamins, is present. Thiamine (Vitamin B_1) is most notably depleted in the alcoholic patient and is often administered IV to prevent and reverse neurological symptoms.

2 When Thiamine (Vitamin B_1) is given IV the nurse should monitor the patient for tightness of throat, angioneurotic edema, anaphylaxis, cyanosis, pulmonary edema, and cardiovascular collapse.

3 Alcoholism is a complex problem with a high rate of recidivism. Health care providers can be instrumental in aiding alcoholic patients. Mental health professionals, dietitians, and spiritual counselors are just a few needed referrals.

Chapter 62 Answers to Case Study

1 Blood calcium and phosphate ion levels are dependent on adequate intake of vitamin D which enhances their intestinal absorption by promoting mobilization of calcium from bone and renal tubular reabsorption of phosphate. Additionally, consider Jerrod's lack of outdoor activities (sunlight) and poor nutritional habits, which increase the potential for Vitamin D deficiency.

2 When patients are prescribed supplemental vitamin D, the nurse should monitor for ataxia, muscle and joint pain, pruritus, headache, and GI upset.

3 Vitamin D is produced photochemically in the epidermal layer of skin, specifically in the stratum basale and stratum spinosum. Therefore, exposing Jerrod to sunlight would increase his levels of Vitamin D.

Chapter 62 Answers to NCLEX-RN® Review

1 Answer: 2 Rationale: Although parenteral vitamin A can be used in replacement therapy for conditions affecting gastric absorption, mobilization, or storage of vitamins, it would be contraindicated if ordered PO. Option 1 is incorrect. In some forms of night blindness there is a deficiency of visual purple, or rhodopsin, which is the pigment in the retina. Rhodopsin maintains photosensitivity only in the presence of vitamin A. Option 3 is incorrect. Vitamin A is not contraindicated for lactating females. Option 4 is incorrect. Some skin conditions, such as folliculosis keratosis or psoriasis, respond favorably to vitamin A. Cognitive Level: Application; Client Need: Safe, Effective Care Management; Nursing Process: Assessment

2 Answer: 3 Rationale: Vitamin C is often prescribed for surgical clients to enhance wound healing. Option 1 is incorrect. Large doses do not increase the absorption of vitamin B_{12}. Option 2 is incorrect. Anesthesia-induced complications are not affected by vitamin C. Option 4 is incorrect. Instruct the patient to take large doses of vitamin C in divided amounts because the body only uses what is needed at a particular time and excretes the rest in urine. Cognitive Level: Application; Client Need: Safe, Effective Care Management; Nursing Process: Implementation

3 Answer: 4 Rationale: Vitamin D is responsible for maintaining normal blood calcium and phosphate levels, not vitamin B_1. Option 1 is incorrect. Symptoms of throat swelling, itching, or swelling of lips are often the first sign of allergic reaction and should be reported. Option 2 is incorrect. Pork, beef, liver, and other whole grains are excellent sources of thiamine. Option 3 is incorrect. Several vitamin and mineral deficiencies, including vitamin B_1, can cause symptoms of depression. Cognitive Level: Application; Client Need: Safe, Effective Care Management; Nursing Process: Assessment

4 Answer: 1 Rationale: Vitamin D should be used cautiously in individuals with a history of kidney stones. Option 2 is incorrect. Osteomalacia is softening of the bones caused by not having enough vitamin D, or by problems with the metabolism of this vitamin. Option 3 is incorrect. A deficiency of vitamin D can lead to hypocalcemia when it is associated with decreased dietary calcium intake. Option 4 is incorrect. Vitamin D has widely been known to help some individuals with psoriasis. Cognitive Level: Application; Client Need: Safe, Effective Care Management; Nursing Process: Assessment

5 Answer: 1, 3 Rationale: Vitamin K is routinely given to newborn infants to prevent bleeding problems related to birth trauma (option 1) . Vitamin K decreases the anticoagulant effects of the drug warfarin (Coumadin) (option 3). Option 2 is incorrect. Vitamin K is not indicated for visual disturbances. Option 4 is incorrect. Vitamin K is not used in the treatment of hypothyroidism. Option 5 is incorrect. Teenagers with chronic acne are not prescribed vitamin K. Cognitive Level: Application; Client Need: Safe, Effective Care Management; Nursing Process: Assessment

6 Answer: 3 Rationale: Injection site discomfort is an expected adverse effect. The nurse should inform the client that it is not uncommon and should disappear in 24–48 hours. Option 1 is incorrect because it is a true statement. Whole grain cereals, liver, and legumes are excellent sources of pyridoxine (vitamin B_6). Option 2 is incorrect because pyridoxine deficiency is often caused by inadequate dietary intake. It would be appropriate to instruct the client to keep a food journal in order to identify nutritional habits. Option 4 is incorrect because isoniazid, cycloserine, penicillamine, hydralazine, and oral contraceptives may increase pyridoxine requirements. Cognitive Level: Application; Client Need: Safe, Effective Care Management; Nursing Process: Implementation

Chapter 63

Answer to Connection Checkpoint 63.1

Enteric coated tablets are designed to dissolve in the small intestine. If they are crushed, their contents will be exposed to stomach acid, which may destroy the drug or cause nausea and vomiting.

Answer to Connection Checkpoint 63.2

Dextrose solutions are infused to replace lost water and to enhance renal function. D5W is also used as a diluent for mixing other medications for IV delivery. Infusion of too much D_5W may cause fluid overload and worsening heart failure.

Answer to Connection Checkpoint 63.3

Ranitidine is an H2-receptor antagonist that reduces both fasting and food-stimulated gastric acid secretion and also decreases nocturnal acid secretion. It is useful in preventing or treating peptic ulcers that arise during TPN therapy.

Chapter 63 Answers to Critical Thinking Questions

1 The family should be taught to store the solution in the refrigerator, removing it one hour before hanging in order to allow it to warm to room temperature. Refrigeration will reduce bacterial growth in the dextrose enriched solution. They should check the expiration date on the bag and not use it if cloudy, discolored, or if precipitates are present. They should be taught to gently squeeze the bag in order to check for any signs of leakage and to wash their hands thoroughly before handling the solution.

2 Explain that the patient should be weighed daily and that I & O needs to be recorded. They should observe Christine for any signs of edema, and instructions should be provided on the use of urine glucose testing strips (lab-sticks).

3 The list should include symptoms such as coughing, chills, fever, chest pain, dyspnea, adverse reactions to lipid infusion, hypo- or hyperglycemia, or air embolism.

Chapter 63 Answers to Case Study

1 Because this patient's GI track is unusable, parenteral nutrition therapy is indicated. Her nutritional needs are too great for PPN; thus a course of TPN is indicated.

2 Because of this patient's poor nutritional state, she is at risk for developing refeeding syndrome once the nutritional therapy is initiated.

3 The deficits in the patient's baseline electrolyte values should be corrected before initiating TPN. They should start the therapy slowly and progress slowly.

Chapter 63 Answers to NCLEX-RN® Review

1 Answer: 3 Rationale: A client receiving enteral feedings can be at risk for dehydration caused by an inadequate intake of free water. It is important to irrigate the tube with water as ordered, or per protocol (before and after an intermittent feeding or medication, or every 4 to 6 hours for continuous feedings), and to include this amount of fluid in the client's I & O record. Option 1 is incorrect, because clients receiving enteral feedings are usually weighed daily. Option 2 is incorrect, because the NG tube is irrigated more than just once a day. Option 4 is incorrect. While assessment of the skin around a PEG tube site is important, it will not indicate the client's fluid balance. This client is receiving the feeding via an NG tube, which is passed through the nose. Cognitive Level: Application; Client Need: Physiological Integrity; Nursing Process: Planning

2 Answer: 1, 3, 5 Rationale: In addition to the base solution, total parenteral nutrition contains electrolytes (sodium, potassium, chloride), trace minerals, and multivitamins. Option 2 is incorrect. If diuretics are needed because of an underlying medical condition, they should be administered separately and not added to the TPN solution. Option 4 is incorrect. Regular insulin may be added to the bag, but not NPH insulin. Cognitive Level: Application; Client Need: Physiological Integrity; Nursing Process: Planning

3 Answer: 4 Rationale: 10% dextrose in water contains the highest concentration of glucose and should be hung until the new TPN bag is available. The solution selected should minimize the risk of hypoglycemia. Options 1, 2, or 3 are incorrect. They will not be effective in preventing hypoglycemia. Cognitive Level: Application; Client Need: Physiological Integrity; Nursing Process: Implementation

4 Answer: 2 Rationale: The client's temperature should be monitored for signs of infection and subsequent sepsis, which are complications of TPN therapy. The weight is monitored to assess the nutritional effectiveness of the TPN and to detect signs of fluid overload. Options 1, 3, and 4 are incorrect. Blood pressure and pulse are important assessments, but do not relate specifically to the effects of TPN. Cognitive Level: Application; Client Need: Physiological Integrity; Nursing Process: Assessment

5 Answer: 4 Rationale: The nurse should not hang the lipids if separation of the emulsion or fat globules is visible in the solution. The solution should be returned to the pharmacy. Options 1, 2, and 3 are inappropriate actions. Cognitive Level: Application; Client Need: Physiological Integrity; Nursing Process: Implementation

6 Answer: 2 Rationale: A catheter-related infection should be suspected if a client receiving TPN spikes a fever during the infusion. Both the unused solution and the tubing should be cultured for infectious organisms. Options 1, 3, and 4 are inappropriate actions. Cognitive Level: Application; Client Need: Physiological Integrity; Nursing Process: Implementation

Chapter 64

Answer to Connection Checkpoint 64.1

The limbic system is responsible for emotional expression, learning, and memory. Emotional states associated with this system include anxiety, fear, anger, aggression, remorse, depression, sexual drive, and euphoria.

Answer to Connection Checkpoint 64.2

Amphetamines and methylphenidate are both used to treat attention deficit/hyperactivity disorder and narcolepsy. Methylphenidate is well tolerated and produces less physical dependence and fewer peripheral adverse effects than amphetamine.

Answer to Connection Checkpoint 64.3

Deficiency of vitamin A can lead to night blindness, diminished natural immunity, and the abnormal growth and development of bones and teeth. Deficiency of vitamin D can cause skeletal diseases that weaken the bones such as rickets, osteomalacia, osteoporosis, renal osteodystrophy, and hypocalcemia.

Chapter 64 Answers to Critical Thinking Questions

1 Although the topic of obesity has been researched extensively, there is not one factor that is considered the underlying etiology. It is most likely due to a combination of factors that are both psychological and physiological. Some pathology can cause obesity such as hypothyroidism. There are also some drug therapies such as corticosteroids, that may induce weight gain. However, there is strong evidence that a sedentary lifestyle and insufficient calorie usage are underlying reasons. Consistently, research indicates that persons who are overweight or obese are at increased risk for hyperlipidemia, hypertension, and cardiovascular disease. Furthermore, obesity is a strong risk factor for the development of Type II diabetes.

2 Currently, there are two drug types that are approved by the FDA for the long-term treatment of obesity. These include sympathomimetic drugs and lipase inhibitors. Sympathomimetic drugs such as sibutramine (Meridia) treat obesity by suppressing one's appetite through restricting the nerve endings' ability to pick up (reuptake) norepinephrine and serotonin. Lipase inhibitors are a class of drugs that prevents the action of enzymes that break down fat (lipase). Orlistat alters the way the body responds to fat intake, allowing the body to excrete fats with absorption.

3 Common weight-related stereotypes are that obese persons are lazy, lack self-discipline, have poor will power, or possess defects of character. In health care facilities, prejudices toward obese patients have been well documented in the literature. Health care providers, including physicians, nurses, psychologists, dietitians, and medical students, are guilty of discrimination. One consequence of bias by health care providers is that obese patients may avoid obtaining medical care because of previous negative experiences.

Chapter 64 Answers to Case Study

1 Body mass index is defined as the individual's body weight divided by the square of their height. Although various tables may differ, it is generally considered that individuals with a BMI of 25 kg/m^2–29.9 kg/m^2 are overweight; 30–34.9 kg/m^2 are in category I obesity, 35–39.9 kg/m^2 are in category II obesity, and greater than 40 kg/m^2 are in category III obesity. With a BMI of 48, Kathryn would be considered a candidate for sibutramine (Meridia) if she is not taking MAOIs, or has a history of heart disease or stroke.

2 Although sibutramine is considered a sympathomimetic, it is not in the same category as amphetamines. The drug has a low potential for dependence and has none of the adverse effects associated with amphetamine-based anorexiants.

3 Common adverse effects related to sibutramine include headache, constipation, insomnia, and abnormal dryness of the mouth (xerostomia).

Chapter 64 Answers to NCLEX-RN® Review

1 Answer: 1 Rationale: Diet and exercise are the mainstays of weight loss. The use of pharmacological regimens are only effective when they are consistently prescribed in conjunction with lifestyle modifications. Option 2 is incorrect because sibutramine can be prescribed for a variety of clients and is not limited to men or premenopausal women. Option 3 is incorrect because although diabetics must be monitored more closely with any type of pharmacologic therapy, type II diabetes is not a contraindication. Option 4 is incorrect because the dosage of this drug most likely will be increased if the client loses less than 1.81 kg (4 lb) the first month, not the first week. However, if the client fails to lose weight, the health care provider should always consider nonadherence with the diet, exercise, and medication plan prescribed before increasing the dose. Cognitive Level: Application; Client Need: Physiological Integrity; Nursing Process: Assessment

2 Answer: 1 Rationale: The suggested weight loss within 6–12 months of initiating sibutramine is approximately 5–10% of the total body weight. Option 2 is incorrect because a weight loss of 15–20% within 3–4 months is not the expected weight loss due to sibutramine. The nurse should consider other reasons. A rapid weight loss could indicate the client is not following the regimen as prescribed, but it can also indicate an underlying pathology. Option 3 is not the best answer, because the nurse is unaware of the client's initial weight. Arbitrarily selecting a number for a weight loss goal can be hazardous to the client's overall health. Option 4 is not as accurate as option 1. Although the client may experience a loss of adipose tissue of the waist, it is not a specific indicator of the therapeutic effects of the drug therapy. Cognitive Level: Knowledge; Client Need: Physiological Integrity; Nursing Process: Evaluation

3 Answer: 4 Rationale: Typically, orlistat is taken just prior to meals so that the drug can inhibit lipase. Option 1 is incorrect because orlistat is taken throughout the day. Frequently the client is instructed to take the orlistat up to 3 times per day. Option 2 is incorrect because this drug does not decrease appetite. It interferes with the absorption of fat in the diet. Option 3 is incorrect because although exercise is a part of the treatment plan for obesity, orlistat does not require administration before exercise. Cognitive Level: Application; Client Need: Physiological Integrity; Nursing Process: Intervention

4 Answer: 4 Rationale: The proper intake of vitamins and nutrients are important in a healthy weight loss program. Since orlistat interferes with lipid absorption, the client should be taught to supplement the diet with a vitamin that contains all the essential fat-soluble vitamins. Option 1 is incorrect. There is a common myth that grapefruit juice magically reduces body weight. The nurse must educate the client about proper nutrition and dispel dietary myths. Option 2 is incorrect. Orlistat does not cause photosensitivity. These instructions would be inappropriate. Option 3 is incorrect. These are instructions the nurse would provide for a client on a drug that causes orthostatic hypotension. Clients on orlistat do not typically experience this adverse effect. Cognitive Level: Application; Client Need: Physiological Integrity; Nursing Process: Assessment

5 Answer: 1 Rationale: Although not serious adverse effects, flatus and oily stools are often troubling to the client. The nurse should inform the client these often occur when taking orlistat. Heartburn and dyspepsia (indigestion) are not adverse effects associated with orlistat (option 2). Many clients initially experience diarrhea with this drug, not constipation (option 3). If the client experiences nausea and vomiting, other causes should be investigated. These are not common adverse effects associated with orlistat (option 4). Cognitive Level: Application; Client Need: Physiological Integrity; Nursing Process: Implementation

6 Answer: 1, 2, 3 Rationale: All are indicators used to assess level of obesity. Option 4 is incorrect because a treadmill test assesses physical fitness, not necessarily obesity. Option 5 is incorrect because buoyancy analysis is not a test used to determine the degree of obesity. Cognitive Level: Knowledge; Client Need: Physiological Integrity; Nursing Process: Assessment

Chapter 65

Answer to Connection Checkpoint 65.1

Epinephrine is a drug of choice in CPR and can quickly reverse many of the symptoms of anaphylaxis. It is sometimes added to cartridges of local anesthetics to cause vasoconstriction of local vessels. Ophthalmic administration of epinephrine may be used to treat glaucoma and intranasal administration can relieve nasal congestion.

Answer to Connection Checkpoint 65.2

Corticosteroids are some of the most effective drugs available for treating inflammation. Because of the potential for long-term, serious adverse effects, their use is limited to short-term therapy.

Chapter 66

Answer to Connection Checkpoint 66.1

When an abundance of hormone is present, such as during hormone pharmacotherapy, a cell down-regulates the number of receptors on its surface.

Answer to Connection Checkpoint 66.2

Through RAAS, the hormone aldosterone is secreted by the adrenal cortex. Aldosterone causes the kidneys to retain additional sodium and water in the body, thus increasing osmolality.

Answer to Connection Checkpoint 66.3

von Willebrand factor is required for platelet adhesion to injured blood vessel endothelium.

Chapter 66 Answers to Critical Thinking Questions

1 Instruct the parents on proper storage, reconstitution, and administration of the drug ordered (somatotropin). Stress that the drug needs to be reconstituted gently, and swirled, not shaken, to prevent the drug from breaking down. Instruct on appropriate injection sites, including the preferred sites (abdomen and thigh), and to rotate sites. Instruct on the time of day to administer the drug: at bedtime to mimic the body's natural release of the hormone. Instruct on the need for follow-up assessments of height, weight, and bone age, and laboratory testing. Provide information on potential adverse effects, especially those that must be reported to the health care provider immediately, such as sudden weight gain, swelling, or severe bone and joint pain.

2 It is important and appropriate to discuss with the parents the ability to afford this medication. Therapy will be expensive, and is not covered by all insurance programs. Therapy is also long-term, usually continuing until closure of the epiphyseal plates and attainment of final adult height. In some cases, you might consider referring the family to a medical social worker who might be able to find other sources of funding if necessary. It is also important to discuss the realistic effects of therapy: that the increases in height are often modest, but still important to the overall well being of the patient.

3 The adverse effects to discuss are hyperglycemia and insulin resistance, with the possibility of developing diabetes mellitus, and hypothyroidism. Routine testing will monitor for these conditions. Other possible adverse effects are edema, headache, and HTN. These usually resolve with continued treatment and dose adjustments. Other adverse effects are joint and bone pain, local pain at the injection site, and the rare possibility of developing antibodies to growth hormone.

Answers to Critical Thinking Question in Evidence-Based Practice Feature

The nurse would review with the family if any of the common risk factors for short stature were present, including a family history of short stature, hypothyroidism, head trauma, or CNS infections, and the presence of growth hormone deficiency. Assess the child's height and weight relative to the sex and age of the child. Compare these to the family history and the child's growth patterns. Some health care providers label patients short for age and sex if they are below a certain percentile on a standard longitudinal height chart. Short stature is a characteristic that must be defined relative to the general population in which people will always be of different heights. Thus, even if GH therapy were available to and effective in all "short" stature children, a population of short children will still exist. They will simply be a few inches taller than those in the former population.

Answers to Critical Thinking Question in Evidence-Based Practice Feature

Delays in growth are commonly observed in children who have sustained a severe burn. The reasons for this growth delay are not completely known, but it is thought that GH levels have been shown to decrease after burn injury. GH, therefore, is thought to maintain growth in severely burned children who would otherwise experience a significant growth delay.

Chapter 66 Answers to Case Study

1 The nurse would anticipate treatment with desmopressin (DDAVP), intranasally, once a day, at bedtime.

2 The boy and his parents will need information on how to store and administer the drug. For intranasal administration, they will need to be instructed on the technique to use to ensure the drug is administered into the nasal cavity, and not down the throat. The drug is supplied with a tube to ensure effective delivery into the nasal cavity. They should also be taught to maintain a diary of night-time trips to the bathroom, or episodes of enuresis to help with dosage adjustments. They need to be informed of adverse effects to monitor for, and which ones need to be reported to the health care provider. Adverse effects include transient headaches, nasal congestion, rhinitis, nausea, abdominal pain, or cramping. The drug could cause fluid retention, with water intoxication a serious adverse effect. Early symptoms of this would be drowsiness, listlessness, and headache. These should be reported immediately to the health care provider.

Chapter 66 Answers to NCLEX-RN® Review

1 Answer: 2 Rationale: Growth hormone cannot be given by a pill; it can only be administered subcutaneously by injections. A lack of growth hormone is not associated with mental retardation (option 1). Children who have had their epiphyseal plates closed are not candidates for growth hormone therapy; therefore most adolescents would see minimal gain in height (option 3). Minimal blood hormone levels are required during therapy (option 4). Cognitive Level: Application; Client Need: Physiological Integrity; Nursing Process: Planning

2 Answer: 4 Rationale: Growth hormone does not result in lowered serum glucose levels. Growth hormone increases the use of fatty acids for fuels, while increasing insulin resistance in peripheral tissues and impaired glucose tolerance, with the overall effect being an increase in serum glucose levels. Growth hormone increases the length and width of long bones (option 1), promotes organ, muscle, and connective tissue growth (option 2), and increases the synthesis of proteins (option 3). Cognitive Level: Application; Client Need: Physiological Integrity; Nursing Process: Evaluation

3 Answer: 3 Rationale: Patients on DDAVP need to obtain a daily weight and monitor for the presence of any pedal edema. Nasal spray does not need to be refrigerated; it may be stored at room temperature (option 1). The patient would not take twice the prescribed dose for nasal congestion (option 2). The patient should always use the medicine in the nasal cavity and not orally (option 4). Cognitive Level: Application; Client Need: Physiological Integrity; Nursing Process: Planning

4 Answer: 2 Rationale: The nurse would suspect diabetes insipidus (DI), which manifests as large amounts of very dilute urine with a specific gravity less than 1.005 due to a lack of antidiuretic hormone. This can occur as an acute problem following surgery or head injury. SIADH occurs as a result of excretion of excess antidiuretic hormone, which results in marked fluid retention (option 1). Excessive use of fluids during surgery would produce an increased amount of urine, but the excess fluids would be eliminated more gradually than 2400 mL and would have a normal specific gravity level (option 3). Opioid analgesics do not cause a large urine output; they are more likely to cause urine retention and difficulty voiding (option 4). Cognitive Level: Analysis; Client Need: Physiological Integrity; Nursing Process: Diagnosis

5 Answer: 2, 3 Rationale: When implementing desmopressin therapy for DI, it is important for the nurse to also restrict fluids to decrease the risk for water intoxication. This serious adverse effect is more likely to occur when excess fluids are taken during desmopressin therapy (option 2). In addition, it is important to monitor electrolytes, particularly sodium levels (option 3). It would be inappropriate to encourage fluids in these patients (option 1). Therapy may cause HTN, not hypotension (option 4). Sodium based foods do not need to be increased in this situation (option 5). Cognitive Level: Application; Client Need: Physiological Integrity; Nursing Process: Planning

6 Answer: 1 Rationale: A client with DI who is responding to therapy with vasopressin would have decreasing signs of dehydration. DI is characterized by large volume urine output with a very low urine specific gravity accompanied by signs of dehydration, including complaints of thirst and an increased pulse rate. Therefore, option 2 is incorrect because the client responding to vasopressin therapy would see a lowered pulse rate related to a decrease in urine output. Vasopressin therapy would cause the urine specific gravity to increase, not decrease (option 3). Blood glucose levels are not affected by vasopressin (option 4). Cognitive Level: Analysis; Client Need: Physiological Integrity; Nursing Process: Evaluation

Chapter 67

Answer to Connection Checkpoint 67.1

Acidosis occurs when the pH of the plasma falls below 7.35. Sodium bicarbonate is the treatment of choice.

Answer to Connection Checkpoint 67.2

A disulfiram reaction occurs when a drug inhibits the enzyme acetaldehyde dehydrogenase, allowing the toxic substance acetaldehyde to build up in the blood.

Chapter 67 Answer to Patient Safety

Nurses should be alert to this problem, and emphasize to patients using this device that when dialing in a dose, they should make sure they are holding the pen so that the "Opticlik" printing on the pen can be read right-side-up (ISMP, 2007).

Chapter 67 Answers to Critical Thinking Questions

1 When describing diabetes mellitus to this patient's parents, it may be helpful to convey the information that will provide them with a mental picture. For example, it may be helpful to visualize insulin as a "gatekeeper." When present, insulin swings open the gate, transporting glucose inside the cell. However, if there is no insulin, there is not entry and the body uses other sources for energy.

2 The nurse anticipates the following treatment: admission to a critical care area; IV placement, and infusion of 0.9% saline to rehydrate the patient; regular insulin, beginning with an IV bolus, followed by a slow, continuous IV infusion until glucose levels are 250 mg/dL or lower; electrolyte and acidosis correction; and frequent laboratory testing of serum glucose and electrolyte levels.

3 The patient and his parents will need extensive teaching on diabetes and its management. Teaching can be organized and directed by a diabetic nurse educator if one is available. The parents will need to understand the disorder, the need for lifelong management, and the possibility of complications, both acute and chronic. They need to understand the relationships between diet, exercise, medications, and glucose levels. They need to understand that glucose levels and insulin needs can vary during times of stress (illness, injury), during growth spurts, and after periods of unusual exercise. They also need medication teaching for insulin. This will include the actions of the drug, and times of onset of action, peak action, and duration of action, how to administer subcutaneous injections and the sites used, and how to store the medication. They will need a registered dietitian to help develop an individualized dietary plan for Jason. They also need to know how to monitor glucose levels using a home glucose meter, and the timing of the insulin injections. They must be taught the signs of hypoglycemia, and the appropriate actions to take should it occur. They should be taught to inform the health care provider of episodes of hypoglycemia so that adjustments in medication can be made. Jason and his parents will need nursing support during this major time of adjustment.

Answer to Critical Thinking Question in Evidence-Based Practice Feature

The nurse would counsel the woman that current practice is for gestational diabetes to be managed with insulin therapy and dietary modifications. This helps to ensure that there are no adverse effects to the developing fetus and that glycemic control is achieved.

Chapter 67 Answers to Case Study

1 These results most likely represent metabolic syndrome.

2 This patient would be classified as having prediabetes.

3 Having prediabetes places the patient at increased risk for developing type 2 diabetes. In addition, the metabolic syndrome places him at increased risk for developing type 2 diabetes, and vascular complications such as cardiovascular disease, peripheral vascular disease, and stroke. He needs to understand these risks, and that he can take actions to delay or prevent the progression to type 2 diabetes. These actions include obtaining regular exercise, maintaining a normal or near-normal weight and blood pressure, and eating a lower fat, lower calorie diet. Patient teaching should include each of these points, and how they can be accomplished by the patient.

Chapter 67 Answers to NCLEX-RN® Review

1 Answer: 2, 4 Rationale: Rotating injection sites and avoiding the use of any one site more often than once a month decrease the risk for lipodystrophy. Monitoring glucose levels (option 1) and assessing sensation (option 3) are both important, but would not alter the risk for lipodystrophy. The client should always use needles specifically designated for insulin use to administer their insulin (option 5). Cognitive Level: Application; Client Need: Physiological Integrity; Nursing Process: Implementation

2 Answer: 2, 3, 5 Rationale: It is always necessary to review the latest glucose level prior to administering any type of insulin (option 2). Because lispro is a rapid-acting insulin, the nurse should ensure that the client will be able to eat a meal shortly after receiving a dose (option 3), and that no signs of hypoglycemia are present (option 5). It is not necessary to check a urine sample for glucose or ketones (option 1). Urine testing does not give exact information, and clients vary on the degree to which glucose and ketones will 'spill' into the urine. It is not necessary to check a pulse or blood pressure prior to giving insulin, as insulin does not directly affect these (option 4). Cognitive Level: Application; Client Need: Physiological Integrity; Nursing Process: Implementation

3 Answer: 3 Rationale: A serious adverse effect of metformin is the risk for developing lactic acidosis. Renal insufficiency and failure, excess alcohol use, and IV contrast agents increase the risk for lactic acidosis, and so are contraindications to its use. The other adverse effects listed, hypoglycemia (option 1), GI distress (option 2), and weight loss (option 4) are adverse effects common among oral hypoglycemic drugs. Cognitive Level: Application; Client Need: Physiological Integrity; Nursing Process: Assessment

4 Answer: 2 Rationale: It can take several weeks for this drug to provide therapeutic effects, so the appropriate response would be to give this drug more time to reach effectiveness. It would not be appropriate for the nurse to change a client's dose (option 1), add a second drug (option 3), or tell the client he will be needing insulin (option 4). Cognitive Level: Application; Client Need: Physiological Integrity; Nursing Process: Implementation

5 Answer: 4 Rationale: Glucagon injections can be repeated if one dose is not effective. Hypoglycemia is a medical emergency, and since this woman has not fully recovered, medical attention is needed. It would not be appropriate to take no action (option 1). It would not be safe to give this client anything by mouth yet, as she is still 'groggy, and not making sense' (option 2). Finally, it would not be normal or expected for a person to remain sleepy following recovery from hypoglycemia (option 3). Cognitive Level: Application; Client Need: Physiological Integrity; Nursing Process: Implementation

6 Answer: 4 Rationale: This insulin has no definite peak, so there is a minimal risk for hypoglycemic reaction. It does have to be given by subcutaneous injection (option 1), cannot be given by IM injection (option 2), and blood glucose monitoring is required for all clients taking any insulin (option 3). Cognitive Level: Knowledge; Client Need: Physiological Integrity; Nursing Process: Implementation

Chapter 68

Answer to Connection Checkpoint 68.1

High metabolic demands of the myocardium are a primary cause of angina. Hypothyroid patients have bradycardia, which places less metabolic demands on the heart.

Answer to Connection Checkpoint 68.2

Hyperthyroidism increases the body's need for glucose as an energy source. Insulin doses would likely have to be increased to prevent hyperglycemia.

Chapter 68 Answers to Critical Thinking Questions

1 Anticipate that this patient will have her T_4 and TSH levels tested for a thyroid dysfunction. Other possible testing could include an ultrasound of her thyroid gland, a radioactive iodine uptake test, or a test for antithyroid antibodies.

2 The patient is displaying symptoms of hypothyroidism, which would likely result in a low level of T_4, and elevated TSH. As thyroid hormone decreases in the serum, the pituitary continues to send out higher and higher levels of TSH, trying to stimulate the production and release of thyroid hormone. The patient may also have an increased titer of antithyroid antibodies, which occurs with Hashimoto's thyroiditis, the most common cause of hypothyroidism.

3 If this patient is diagnosed with hypothyroidism, the treatment consists of thyroid hormone replacement therapy, which continues for life. Most often, patients are given levothyroxine, or T_4 for this replacement therapy, which is evaluated by monitoring levels of TSH. If TSH levels normalize, there is sufficient thyroid hormone in circulation.

4 Patient teaching would include signs and symptoms of hypothyroidism as well as hyperthyroidism, because either can occur related to too high or too low a drug dose. The patient can be taught how to monitor her heart rate, as this is a good indication of hyper vs. hypo metabolic rate. She can also monitor her weight and ability to sleep. She should be informed that pregnancy and breast-feeding require precautions with drug therapy, and to inform her health care provider should these occur. She should also be taught the drugs and substances that interfere with absorption of thyroid hormone, such as calcium, iron, aluminum antacids, and supplements. She should also be informed that levothyroxine has a long half-life and duration of action, and so it will take several weeks of therapy to achieve therapeutic results. Finally, she should be encouraged to use the same brand of levothyroxine, as different brands are not thought to be equivalent. If she does have to change brands, her thyroid testing needs to rechecked, and her dose may need to be adjusted.

Chapter 68 Answers to Case Study

1 The nurse would expect to see the following orders for diagnostic tests: serum T_4, possibly T_3, and TSH levels.

2 Drug therapy for this patient would likely include propylthiouracil to decrease thyroid hormone production and secretion, a beta-adrenergic blocker for blood pressure control and to decrease sympathetic stimulation, and acetaminophen for fever control. Note, aspirin is not given to patients with hyperthyroidism, as the aspirin would displace T_3 and T_4 from their protein binding sites, thereby increasing the amount of free, and thereby, active thyroid hormone, worsening the patient's condition.

3 Long-term therapy for this patient would include antithyroid drugs, suppressive therapy with radioactive iodine, or surgical removal of all or part of the thyroid gland. These therapies may induce hypothyroidism, which is then treated with replacement therapy.

Chapter 68 Answers to NCLEX-RN® Review

1 Answer: 4 Rationale: The administration of too much Synthroid causes hyperthyroidism, characterized by nervousness, palpitations, weight loss, diarrhea, and muscle tremors. These symptoms are not expected effects of therapy (option 1) and care must be taken to avoid overtreatment. The client needs to be taught these symptoms so that dosage adjustments can be made accordingly. Synthroid replacement therapy is life-long; the symptoms would not result from the thyroid gland resuming function (option 2). A pituitary disorder would result in symptoms of hypothyroidism, which the client is not describing, making option 3 incorrect. Cognitive Level: Analysis; Client Need: Physiological Integrity; Nursing Process: Evaluation

2 Answer: 1 Rationale: The effects of thyroid hormone replacement therapy include diarrhea and weight loss, not constipation and weight gain, which are likely to be present due to a deficiency in thyroid hormone (option 1). All the other options: increased heart rate and cardiac output (option 2), decreased reports of fatigue (option 3), and decreased blood cholesterol levels (option 4), are actual effects of thyroid hormone replacement. Cognitive Level: Analysis; Client Need: Physiological Integrity; Nursing Process: Assessment

3 Answer: 1 Rationale: Graves' disease results in hyperthyroidism, which is characterized by an increased body metabolism, increased temperature and pulse rate, and feelings of anxiety. Propylthiouracil is the treatment of choice in clients with Graves' disease. Options 2 (myxedema), 3 (Hashimoto's thyroiditis), and 4 (cretinism), are all hypothyroid disorders. Clients with these conditions would have decreased body metabolism, decreased temperature and pulse, and complaints of lethargy. Treatment with PTU is contraindicated in clients with hypothyroid disorders. Cognitive Level: Analysis; Client Need: Physiological Integrity; Nursing Process: Assessment

4 Answer: 3 Rationale: A heart rate of 110 beats/minute would cause the nurse to hold the scheduled dose of levothyroxine, because it could indicate too high a level of thyroid hormone. A low level of thyroid hormone could cause a weight gain (option 1), or decreased blood pressure (option 2), and so would not cause the nurse to hold the medication. By itself, an elevated temperature, without other signs of hyperthyroidism, would not warrant holding the medication (option 4). Cognitive Level: Analysis; Client Need: Physiological Integrity; Nursing Process: Implementation

5 Answer: 1, 2 Rationale: Propylthiouracil inhibits the synthesis of thyroid hormone (option 1), and suppresses the conversion of T_4 to T_3 (option 2). Propylthiouracil does not cause an increased breakdown of existing thyroid hormone (option 3), or have any effect on the absorption of iodine (option 4). Propylthiouracil increases the actions of anticoagulants, which causes an increased risk of bleeding (option 5) Cognitive Level: Application; Client Need: Physiological Integrity; Nursing Process: Planning

6 Answer: 3 Rationale: The nurse needs to teach the client the symptoms of hyperthyroidism, including weight loss, anxiety, insomnia, and palpitations, because these may indicate over-replacement and require adjustments to therapy. The nurse would also teach the client that therapy will be lifelong, not just for 6 months (option 1), and that periodic monitoring of TSH and T_3 levels will be required, but not on a weekly basis (option 2). Synthroid should be taken on a daily basis, optimally at the same time each day (option 4). Cognitive Level: Application; Client Need: Physiological Integrity; Nursing Process: Implementation

Chapter 69

Answer to Connection Checkpoint 69.1

The NSAIDS are anti-inflammatory drugs of choice because they produce fewer serious adverse effects than the corticosteroids.

Answer to Connection Checkpoint 69.2

Patients receiving systemic corticosteroid therapy may have suppressed immune systems. Immunizations should be avoided because the patient's immune system may not be able to develop effective active immunity in response to the vaccine.

Answer to Connection Checkpoint 69.3

Spironolactone (Aldactone) and eplerenone (Inspra) are aldosterone antagonists used to treat edema and hypertension.

Chapter 69 Answers to Critical Thinking Questions

1 Some questions that the nurse may ask Charlie to determine if any adverse effects are present are: Have you experienced any sore throat, fever, or chills? (immunosuppression); have you noticed any cuts or scrapes that are not healing? (immunosuppression); are you experiencing any abdominal pain? (peptic ulcer formation); have you noticed any changes in your stool color? (bleeding peptic ulcer); are you experiencing any skeletal pain? (skeletal changes); do you seem more irritable or moody? (behavioral changes); have you noticed any changes in your vision? (eye changes); have you notice any swelling or weight gain? (metabolic changes); have you experienced muscle aches? (myopathy).

2 The nurse will inform Charlie that abrupt discontinuation of the medication is very dangerous. Withdrawal from corticosteroids usually causes an exacerbation of disease symptoms. Prednisone mimics the function of the natural hormones produced by the adrenal glands. The adrenal glands stop producing cortisol when someone takes a corticosteroid (like prednisone) at high enough doses for a lengthy period. The nurse could talk with the patient about how to monitor for the adverse effects so that dosage may be reduced if tolerated.

3 Charlie is at high risk for infection, and he should not be exposed to individuals who have active infections such as colds and influenza. Furthermore, Charlie's ability to heal may be impaired so the nurse and daughter could consider potential hazards that would cause skin trauma and avoid this problem. Lastly, reducing salt intake can prevent adverse effects associated with fluid retention.

Chapter 69 Answer to Case Study

Ketoconazol (Nizoral) is an antifungal drug that blocks the synthesis of glucocorticoids. Signs of hepatatoxicity include right upper quadrant abdominal pain, jaundice, clay colored stools, and dark colored urine.

Chapter 69 Answers to NCLEX-RN® Review

1 Answer: 1 Rationale: One of the major adverse effects associated with corticosteroid use, such as hydrocortisone, is weight gain. Corticosteroids cause the body to retain sodium and lose potassium. This combination results in fluid retention, weight gain, and bloating. Measures that can be used to avoid fluid retention are eating a reduced sodium diet, and increasing potassium intake through potassium-rich foods (such as bananas, cantaloupe, grapefruit, and lima beans). Tinnitus is not a typical adverse effect associated with corticosteroid use (option 2). Corticosteroids do not cause urinary retention (option 3). Stomatitis is not associated with the use of corticosteroids (option 4). Cognitive Level: Application; Client Need: Physiologic Integrity; Nursing Process: Implementation

2 Answer: 2 Rationale: Wound healing is dependent on a healthy immune system. Individuals on corticosteroids may experience delayed wound healing because the drug decreases the inflammatory response. Option 1 is incorrect because corticosteroids are not associated with irregularity of the heart rate and rhythm. Option 3 is incorrect because typically, corticosteroids predispose the client to weight gain. Option 4 is incorrect because typically, corticosteroids produce a hypokalemic state. Cognitive Level: Application; Client Need: Physiologic Integrity; Nursing Process: Assessment

3 Answer: 2 Rationale: Clients receiving high dose corticosteroids are at risk of developing hypertension. Therefore, the nurse will monitor the blood pressure. Corticosteroid typically do not alter the client's breath sounds (option 1), or affect the client's bowel function (option 3). The testing of cranial nerves is not indicated if the client is receiving corticosteroids (option 4). Cognitive Level: Application; Client Need: Physiologic Integrity; Nursing Process: Assessment

4 Answer: 1 Rationale: Since fludrocortisone promotes water and sodium retention, the client's body weight should be checked daily. Pulse oximetry is used to measure the oxygen saturation in the blood and would not be indicated in clients receiving Florinef (option 2). Fludrocortisone does not affect the peak flow measure, which evaluates pulmonary function (option 3). The calculation of body surface area is not an intervention associated with this medication (option 4). Cognitive Level: Application; Client Need: Physiologic Integrity; Nursing Process: Implementation

5 Answer: 2 Rationale: Most adverse effects of fludrocortisone are the result of excessive mineralocorticoid activity manifested by fluid retention and edema. Florinef is not known to cause tingling of the digits (option 1). Emotional instability is not associated with fludrocortisones (option 3). Fludrocortisone is not known to cause abdominal cramping or diarrhea (option 4). Cognitive Level: Application; Client Need: Physiologic Integrity; Nursing Process: Assessment

6 Answer: 1 Rationale: Clients receiving high doses of corticosteroids are at high risk for infection. The nurse's priority is to protect the client from sources of infection such as other individuals who are ill, plants, and fresh fruits and vegetables to name a few. Blood pressure instability is usually not a problem for clients receiving corticosteroid therapy and would not be a priority (option1). Ambulation and range of motion exercises are not the priority nursing interventions for this client (Option 3). Option 4 is incorrect because sodium restriction is often necessary to prevent fluid retention for these clients. Cognitive Level: Application; Client Need: Physiological Integrity; Nursing Process: Implementation

Chapter 70

Answer to Connection Checkpoint 70.1

A category D drug has demonstrated a teratogenic risk to the fetus. For a category X drug. Adequate well-controlled or observational studies in animals or pregnant women have demonstrated positive evidence of fetal abnormalities or risks.

Answer to Connection Checkpoint 70.2

Nifedipine reduces blood pressure and myocardial oxygen demand due to the reduced afterload. Nifedipine has no effect on myocardial conduction, except at toxic doses.

Chapter 70 Answer to Patient Safety

Yes, the nurse should clarify the order before the patient leaves. Prempro (conjugated estrogens/medroxyprogesterone acetate) is one of the drugs frequently ordered without specifying the dose. However, the drug is now marketed in two strengths—(0.625 mg/2.5 mg and 0.625 mg/5 mg). With the advent of new drugs and new strengths being developed daily, there is no way to keep current with all the changes. This is why it is imperative to accept only complete orders that specify the strength.

Chapter 70 Answers to Critical Thinking Questions

1 Ms. John is in her mid forties, a time when signs of menopause usually start. It is possible that she is experiencing perimenopause, the period immediately preceding menopause. As women grow older they experience changes in the regularity of menstruation. Menstrual irregularity comes about when there are repeated failures to ovulate. Failure to ovulate is a result of a decrease in the numbers of viable ovarian follicles. Decreased ovulation leads to an increased ratio of estrogen over progesterone. Estrogen excess leads to headache, fluid retention, irritability, and weight gain. Although Ms. John is experiencing signs of perimenopause, there could also be more serious gynecological problems that should not be overlooked. Some of these include uterine tumors or hormone imbalance.

2 Ms. John may be a candidate for HRT. Estrogen, progesterone, and testosterone decrease as a woman approaches menopause. She may also choose to take natural therapies such as black cohosh. Should Ms. John choose to begin medication treatment the aim would be to normalize the ratio between estrogen and progesterone. Testosterone is useful in elevating the woman's mood, sex drive, and energy. The overall goal is to restore balance between the hormones and to diminish the unpleasant symptoms of menopause. Likely drugs are Premarin and Prempro.

3 Perimenopausal symptoms can be annoying and distracting to a woman especially if she does not have a healthy lifestyle or a positive outlook on approaching menopause. First, obtain a complete heath history including family history of breast cancer, gallbladder disease, diabetes mellitus, liver or kidney disease. Obtain a drug history to rule out drug interactions and allergies. Assess cardiovascular status including HTN and history of MI. Determine the patient's pregnancy status. Discuss with the patient her expectations about reaching menopause and what types of adjustments she may need to make. Loss of sex drive, fatigue, memory loss, and irritability are only some of the symptoms Ms. John may experience as she goes from perimenopause to complete menopause.

4 Should this patient choose to begin HRT she will need to adjust her lifestyle. She should discontinue smoking as this increases the risk for cardiovascular disease. She also must reduce or completely discontinue her caffeine intake since estrogens and caffeine may lead to increased CNS stimulation further accentuating her nervousness, anxiety, and insomnia. Since the patient has a strong familial diabetic history, she should be encouraged to monitor her glucose levels because estrogen may increase blood glucose levels. Additionally she should begin a regular exercise program including walking, which retards the chances for osteoporosis.

Chapter 70 Answers to Case Study

1 Female infertility is multifactorial. One of the most common reasons is irregular ovulation. Total absence of ovulation, pelvic inflammatory disease (PID), and obstruction of the uterine tubes may also be reasons. If all the above are ruled out then testing to determine endocrine causes should be carried out. Endocrine causes can be due to conditions in the hypothalamus, pituitary, or ovary.

2 Before administration of clomiphene citrate (Clomid) the nurse would complete a medical history and physical examination. Therapy is usually started with a low dose of 50 mg/day for 5 days. If ovulation does not occur the dose is increased to 100 mg, and then, if still no ovulation, the dose is increased to the maximum of 150 mg/day. If this regimen fails, HCG may be initiated. Inform the couple that the pregnancy rate of persons taking this drug is about 90% and twins occur in about 5% of treated patients. The woman should take the medication at about the same time each day and if a dose is missed it should be taken as soon as remembered. If not remembered until the next day, then take two doses. Report any abnormal bleeding or signs of jaundice such as yellowing of eyes or skin. Discontinue the therapy immediately if pregnancy is suspected.

Chapter 70 Answers to NCLEX-RN® Review

1 Answer: 1 Rationale: The client should avoid caffeine because estrogen and caffeine may lead to increased CNS stimulation and a potential for stroke. Option 2 is incorrect because the medications should be taken with food (option 2). Option 3 is incorrect because the client should report any excessive menstrual bleeding right away (option 3) without discontinuing the medication. HRT causes a lowering, not an increase of LDL (option 4). Cognitive Level: Analysis; Client Need: Physiological Integrity; Nursing Process: Implementation

2 Answer: 2 Rationale: Prolonged use of IV infusion could lead to water intoxication. The client would appear drowsy, listless, and confused. At this stage of therapy the uterine contractions are appropriate in frequency and duration. Hyperstimulation is assessed if the contractions are less than 2 minutes apart and last longer than 90 seconds. Monitoring should be ongoing. Oxygen would be administered via face mask if mother or fetus is in distress (option 1), There is no indication to place the woman on her side (option 3), or to discontinue the infusion at this time (option 4). Cognitive Level: Analysis; Client Need: Physiological Integrity; Nursing Process: Assessment

3 Answer: 3 Rationale: Clomid is an oral nonsteroidal selective estrogen receptor modulator (SERM) that induces ovulation. It is used to treat infertility in women desiring pregnancy whose partners are fertile and potent. Provera is used to correct dysfunctional uterine bleeding and as a contraceptive (option 1). Oxytocin is used to stimulate uterine contractions during labor or to correct post delivery hemorrhage (option 2). Premarin is used to treat atrophic vaginitis and abnormal vaginal bleeding. It is also beneficial in reducing the symptoms of menopause, decreasing the progression of osteoporosis, and treatment of breast and prostate cancer (option 4). Cognitive Level: Knowledge; Client Need: Physiological Integrity; Nursing Process: Assessment

4 Answer: 2, 3, 4 Rationale: HRT should be used cautiously in diabetes and HTN (option 2). It is contraindicated in liver and thromboembolic disorders (option 3), and cancer (option 4). HRT is not contraindicated for the client with chronic asthma and is often prescribed to retard the progression of osteoporosis (option 1). Option 5 is incorrect because clients with scoliosis and kyphosis (abnormal curvatures of the vertebral column) can be prescribed HRT such as estradiol/norgestimate (Ortho-Prefest). Cognitive Level: Analysis; Client Need: Physiological Integrity; Nursing Process: Assessment

5 Answer: 2 Rationale: The standard treatment with Clomid is a low dose of 50 mg for 5 days beginning on the fifth day of the menstrual cycle. If ovulation does not occur, the dose is increased to 100 mg and subsequently to 150 mg. By giving it on the fifth day of the cycle it is hoped that it will be in time to stimulate ovulation. Starting therapy on the first or last day of the cycle would be least effective in stimulating ova because this usually occurs closer to mid cycle (options 1, 4). The woman is anovular, hence the reason for therapy (option 3). Cognitive Level: Application; Client Need: Physiological Integrity; Nursing Process: Implementation

6 Answer: 1 Rationale: A woman in active labor would most likely have an IV infusion going. The standard use of oxytocin during labor is 10 units to 1 L of D_5W or NS to augment contractions. The mixture is delivered at 0.5–1 milliunits/minute to a maximum of 20 milliunits/minute. During labor oxytocin is administered slowly and monitored carefully to avoid overstimulation of the uterus and trauma to mother or fetus. Therefore, any other route would be inappropriate (options 2, 3, and 4). Cognitive Level: Analysis; Client Need: Physiological Integrity; Nursing Process: Implementation

Chapter 71

Answer Connection Checkpoint 71.1

Cetrorelix (Cetrotide) and Ganirelix (Antagon) are antagonists of gonadotropin-releasing hormone (GnRH). They are used in combination with other antifertility drugs to promote a regular ovulatory pattern that is conducive to becoming pregnant.

Answer Connection Checkpoint 71.2

Drugs used to reduce the risk of thromboembolism include aspirin and antiplatelet drugs such as clopidogrel (Plavix). Warfarin may be indicated if the risk for thromboembolism is very high.

Chapter 71 Answers to Critical Thinking Questions

1 Both urine and blood tests were done to detect pregnancy. All pregnancy tests are based on the detection of HCG, which is secreted by the placental trophoblast after the ovum is fertilized. HCG may be detected in the urine and blood of pregnant women as early as 6–8 days after conception. Lila has not taken her birth control pills for more than 10 days. Despite her claims of the last time she had intercourse, it is prudent to carry out these tests before starting any treatment because oral contraceptives can have a teratogenic effect on the embryo.

2 Since Lila is very anxious about not being pregnant, a radioreceptor assay [RRA] serum test for HCG would detect pregnancy within 6–8 days after conception. This test is sensitive and accurate in up to 95% of cases.

3 You are responsible for first discussing with the patient the possibility of her becoming pregnant. You will explain the purpose of the urine and blood tests followed by instructions on how the specimens will be collected. You give the patient a urine container and have her wash her perineal area prior to voiding into the cup. You inform her that even when a test shows negative there still is chance that she may be pregnant if the test is done too early. You will take a careful medication history. If she is taking diuretics or Promethazine the result may be a false negative due to diluted urine. If she is taking antiseizure medicine, hypnotics, or tranquilizers the test may be false positive. Finally, when you prepare to administer the medication you must inform the patient that the adverse effects are nausea and vomiting.

Chapter 71 Answers to Case Study

1 Broad spectrum antibiotics, e.g., tetracyclines and penicillin, destroy bacteria living in the bowel. Bacteria in the intestines are necessary to convert the breakdown products of oral contraceptives (i.e., the products that travel to the bowel following liver metabolism) into a useful form, which are reabsorbed and used. Therefore, the estrogen dose in the circulation will be lower than normal. This increases the risk of pregnancy occurring.

2 You would advise Gina that her oral contraceptives dose would have to be increased. You also advise Gina to use additional precautions during intercourse. Condoms and spermicidal agents are good choices.

Chapter 71 Answers to NCLEX-RN® Review

1 Answer: 1, 3, 4 Rationale: Obesity is a risk factor for treatment failure and for increased possibility of thromboembolic events (option 1). Smokers have a significantly increased risk of serious thromboembolic events when taking OCs (option 3). Mood disorders, including depression, may be worsened in clients taking OCs (option 4). Option 2 and option 5 are incorrect because none of these clients present any causative factors that would influence the likelihood of adverse effects due to OCs. Cognitive Level: Application; Client Need: Physiological Integrity; Nursing Process: Assessment

2 Answer: 1 Rationale: A common problem with OCs, and likely the most frequent reason for treatment failure (pregnancy), is forgetting to take the medication daily. If one dose is missed, two pills taken the following day usually provide adequate contraception. Option 2 is incorrect because taking only one pill the next day will not restore therapeutic levels of the OC. Option 3 is incorrect because omitting another day of therapy would reduce the level of the contraceptive even more. It is highly unlikely that the client will become pregnant (option 4). Cognitive Level: Application; Client Need: Physiological Integrity; Nursing Process: Implementation

3 Answer: 3 Rationale: Minipills consist of progestins only and work by thickening the cervical mucus. The absence of estrogens in these pills reduces the risk of blood clots. The minipills have no effect on ovulations (option 1), do not kill sperm (option 2), and do not suppress endometrial development (option 4). Cognitive Level: Knowledge; Client Need: Physiological Integrity; Nursing Process: Implementation

4 Answer: 4 Rationale: While the placebo serves no pharmacological purpose, it does encourage the client to take the pills on a daily basis. Although some of these placebos contain iron, which replaces iron lost from menstrual bleeding, that is not the most important reason for taking the placebo. OC placebos do not contain vitamins (option 1), or substances that will enhance the function of the other pills (option 2), or folic acid (option 3). Cognitive Level: Application; Client Need: Health Promotion and Maintenance; Nursing Process: Implementation

5 Answer: 2 Rationale: Clients should be informed that spermicidal agents have relatively low levels of efficacy when used alone and should therefore be used only in conjunction with barrier methods such as condoms and diaphragms. Current research suggests that nonoxynol-9 does not offer protection against chlamydia, gonorrhea, or HIV as previously thought. Spermicides are 71–98% effective in preventing pregnancy (option 1). Spermicides do not cause HIV or PID. However, clients should be encouraged to use barrier methods such as a condom to minimize the chances of contracting sexually transmitted infections (STIs) (option 3). Spermicidal agents do not prevent ectopic pregnancy. When used with barrier protection, the chances of contracting infections that cause PIDs are lessened (option 4). Cognitive Level: Application; Client Need: Health Promotion and Maintenance; Nursing Process: Assessment/ Planning

6 Answer: 1, 5, 4, 2, 3

The correct ranking from most effective to least effective is

1. Depo Provera 99% effective
5. Transdermal Ortho 98% effective
4. Oral Contraceptives 96–98% effective
2. Spermicides 71–98% effective
3. Rhythm Method 71–75% effective

Cognitive Level: Knowledge; Client Need: Health Promotion and Maintenance; Nursing Process: Assessment

Chapter 72

Answer to Connection Checkpoint 72.1

Stacking is when the abuser takes two or more different types of steroids concurrently, sometimes by different routes. Pyramiding is when the drugs are taken in a cyclic pattern in which the dose is progressively increased over 6–12 weeks, then is slowly decreased to zero.

Answer to Connection Checkpoint 72.2

Clomiphene acts as an antiestrogen. Estrogen normally provides negative feedback to the pituitary, shutting off LH secretion, which is required for ovulation. Clomiphene blocks the estrogen receptor in the hypothalamus, sending a message to the ovaries that estrogen levels are low. Thus LH is secreted, leading to ovarian stimulation.

Answer to Connection Checkpoint 72.3

Orthostatic hypotension is especially pronounced when beginning pharmacotherapy with alpha$_1$-adrenergic blockers, and when increasing the dose. Because this "first dose phenomenon" can lead to syncope, initial therapy is begun with low doses, usually administered at bedtime.

Chapter 72 Answers to Critical Thinking Questions

1 Common contributing factors to the diagnosis of erectile dysfunction (ED) include recent divorce, a diagnosis of depression, job related stress, use of antidepressants, and a history of HTN.

2 A discussion of the effects of Tadalafil with Mike is needed. The combination of this drug along with antidepressants and nifedipine, which is a nonnitrate vasodilator must be evaluated so as not to develop severe adverse effects. Instruct Mike on the correct administration of the drug and that its effects last up to 36 hours. Encourage continued visits with the psychiatrist.

3 It is important to let Mike know about the differences between these drugs. Sildenafil has an onset of action that is relatively rapid, less than 1 hour, and its effects last up to 4 hours. Tadalafil acts within 30 to 60 minutes and has a longer duration of action than sildenafil: up to 36 hours. The longer duration of tadalafil allows for more spontaneity of sexual activity. Contraindications include patients who take nitrates and dosing can be prescribed every 72 hours. Tadalafil will produce less of a decrease in blood pressure than the other drugs in this class, making it safer for patients like Mike with HTN who are already taking other medications for this condition. Sildenafil is contraindicated in patients who are also taking nitrates.

Chapter 72 Answers to Case Study

1 Finasteride acts in the reproductive tissue to inhibit an enzyme that converts testosterone to dihydrotestosterone, the active form of testosterone in the prostrate. Finasteride allows for a regression of the prostate epithelial tissue, which will decrease any mechanical obstruction in the urethra. This drug is usually well tolerated, but does decrease ejaculate volume and libido in some patients.

2 Avoid caffeine or alcohol intake, eliminate drugs that worsen BPH such as testosterone and other anabolic steroids, and restrict fluids close to bedtime.

3 Complaints of increased urgency to urinate, postvoid leakage, decreased force of the urine stream, and a sensation that the bladder is not completely empty; review of Mr. Jones current medications including herbals, and health history, especially for conditions like HTN; assessment of the patient's liver and pancreas to help prevent adverse effects.

Chapter 72 Answers to NCLEX-RN® Review

1 Answer: 2 Rationale: Primary hypogonadism results in clients with normal pituitary function and testes that are either diseased or unresponsive to FSH and LH. A primary goal of therapy would be increased sperm count with an increase in male masculinization. Testoderm should not affect red blood cell count (option 1). Administering testosterone to the client will not increase FSH (option 3) and LH levels (option 4); decreased levels should result from impact on the feedback loop. Cognitive Level: Knowledge; Client Need: Physiological Integrity; Nursing Process: Evaluation

2 Answer: 1 Rationale: The use of nitrates is contraindicated with Viagra as dangerous hypotension may result. A history of diabetes would not be of concern (option 2). An allergy to penicillin products is not a contraindication for use of sildenafil (option 3). There are no expected adverse reactions with Viagra and the use of antiulcer medication (option 4). Cognitive Level: Application; Client Need: Physiological Integrity; Nursing Process: Assessment

3 Answer: 3 Rationale: While all of the options are potential adverse effects of anabolic steroid use, the possibility of impotence and testicular shrinkage would discourage usage in men of this age group the most, due to their stage of development. Cognitive Level: Application; Client Need: Physiological Integrity; Nursing Process: Implementation

4 Answer: 2 Rationale: For Viagra to be effective, the ED must be physiologic in nature. It is not effective if the dysfunction has solely psychological origins, and therefore does not always cause an erection. Viagra simply enhances rather than causes an erection (option 1). Prolonged use does not result in less intense feelings; some men use Viagra to increase the intensity of the sexual experience (option 3). Research indicates that Viagra has no effect on female sexual function (option 4). Cognitive Level: Application; Client Need: Physiological Integrity; Nursing Process: Implementation

5 Answer: 1, 2, 4, 5 Rationale: Finasteride promotes shrinkage of enlarged prostates and subsequently helps restore urinary function (option 1). Women should avoid handling crushed medication because it may be absorbed through the skin and cause harm to a male fetus (option 2). Maximum benefit may take 6–12 months to be achieved (option 4). Orthostatic hypotension may persist throughout treatment (option 5). Option 3 is incorrect because finasteride (Proscar) does not affect vision. Cognitive Level: Application; Client Need: Physiological Integrity; Nursing Process: Implementation

6 Answer: 4 Rationale: Assessment findings that would indicate that therapeutic benefits have been achieved with therapy would be an easier ability to start the flow of urine, less frequency and hesitancy, increased force of urine, and fewer complaints of nocturia. Hematuria (option 1) is not associated with BPH. Decreased urine flow (option 2), and urinating more frequently (option 3) are not indicative of therapeutic benefits. Cognitive Level: Analysis; Client Need: Physiological Integrity; Nursing Process: Evaluation

Chapter 73

Answer to Connection Checkpoint 73.1

The primary indication for $beta_1$-adrenergic agonists is to stimulate the heart to increase cardiac output for patients in shock.

Answer to Connection Checkpoint 73.2

Corticosteroids are given for the shortest length of time necessary. Oral agents may be taken on alternate days.

Answer to Connection Checkpoint 73.3

Monoclonal antibodies can be designed to neutralize certain components in the inflammatory and immune responses. By neutralizing antibodies, these drugs diminish the extent of immune response by the body.

Chapter 73 Answers to Critical Thinking Questions

1 The respiratory distress that occurs with asthma results from inflammation of the airways coupled with bronchoconstriction. Because children have relatively narrow airways compared to adults, the effects of bronchoconstriction and inflammation are often severe.

2 Short acting inhaled beta-adrenergic agonists are the drugs of choice for terminating asthmatic attacks. The reason they are recommended for this role is because they have a fast onset of action and are effective in reversing the narrowed airways that are creating the respiratory distress.

3 Drugs used in the treatment of asthma are classified as either bronchodilators or anti-inflammatory agents. Beta agonists are in the bronchodilator class. They work by stimulating the sympathetic nervous system, which results in a reversal of bronchoconstriction.

Chapter 73 Answer to Critical Thinking Question in Evidence-Based Practice Feature

Patient teaching plays a critical role in enhancing adherence to the management regimen. In addition to regular patient teaching regarding medications, the patient needs to know the subtle signs and symptoms of a worsening condition. The most important tool for assessing this is the peak flow meter (PFM). It is important to teach on the PFM that the patient will actually use because these instruments vary according to the manufacturer. The patient needs to know how to record findings and when to notify the health care provider. The nurse should require that the patient correctly demonstrate the procedure before discharge. Further, the patient needs to understand the importance of avoiding exposure to communicable respiratory illnesses. Should a communicable illness occur, the provider might need to make a temporary medication adjustment.

Chapter 73 Answers to Case Study

1 Theophylline therapy needs careful monitoring, since patients can easily become toxic to the medication quickly. Early signs of toxicity include such symptoms as decreased appetite, nausea, vomiting, dizziness, and restlessness. Serum drug levels are monitored to ensure that the therapeutic level is maintained.

2 The list of "things to avoid" may include several items. First, many medications interact with methylxanthines. The nurse should check what other medication the patient is taking. Additionally, patients receiving theophylline should limit the use of products that contain caffeine. These include not only food and drink, but also many OTC medications for pain relief. Lastly, smoking increases the rate of drug clearance from the body, which may result in an inadequate level of drug to be therapeutic.

3 The spacer serves two primary purposes. First, the spacer holds drops that fall out of the aerosol so that there is less medication deposited on the oropharynx and in the mouth. Second, because the spacer holds the medication, the patient does not have to precisely coordinate inhalation with activation, so that more drug reaches the site of action.

Chapter 73 Answers to NCLEX-RN® Review

1 Answer: 1 Rationale: There are two important items to consider: (1) the medication and (2) the route. A drug to abort bronchospasm should be given by inhalation in order to ensure rapid action directly at the site. An inhaled beta agonist such as albuterol meets both criteria. Option 2 is incorrect because although inhalants are delivered directly, they do not work quickly and are used for prevention of inflammation. Option 3 is incorrect because this anticholinergic is not approved as rescue therapy for treatment of acute bronchospasm. Option 4 is incorrect because leukotriene modifiers are indicated for prevention of respiratory problems, not for treatment of acute bronchospasm. Furthermore, giving a medication PO would not be appropriate when treating acute bronchospasm. Cognitive Level: Analysis; Client Need: Safe, Effective Care Management; Nursing Process: Implementation

2 Answer: 3 Rationale: Glucocorticoids can decrease the beneficial oral flora that will allow for an overgrowth of fungal infections such as candida. Rinsing the mouth removes any glucocorticoid drug deposited there, and prevents it from being being swallowed. Thus it decreases the likelihood of toxicity through systemic absorption. Option 1 is incorrect because it is the bronchodilators (e.g., adrenergic agonists, anticholinergics, and xanthines) that are likely to cause tachycardia, not glucocorticoids. Option 2 is incorrect because it is the xanthines (e.g., aminophylline and theophylline) that are chemically related to caffeine, not the glucocorticoids. It would not be restricted with a glucocorticoid. Option 4 is incorrect because it is the bronchodilators (e.g., adrenergic agonists, anticholinergics, and xanthines) that are likely to cause the client to feel shaky and nervous. Cognitive Level: Application; Client Need: Safe, Effective Care Management; Nursing Process: Implementation

3 Answer: 1 Rationale: Bronchodilators (e.g., beta agonists, anticholinergics, xanthine derivatives) have an adverse effect on heart rate elevation and palpitations. Option 2 is incorrect because bronchodilators do not decrease the immune response the way certain anti-inflammatory agents do. Option 3 is incorrect because bronchodilator increase alertness. Option 4 is incorrect because bronchodilators relieve dyspnea. While some bronchodilators have been known to cause unexpected problems and paradoxical bronchospasm, this is uncommon and the question asks for a common adverse effect. Cognitive Level: Comprehension; Client Need: Safe, Effective Care Management; Nursing Process: Implementation

4 Answer: 1, 2 Rationale: Because corticosteroids decrease the immune response, the likelihood of infections is increased. Glucocortoids also increase blood glucose thus increasing the likelihood of hyperglycemia. Corticosteroids do not cause urinary retention (option 3) and do not increase the likelihood of tachycardia (option 4). Corticosteroids do not cause photophobia (option 5). Cognitive Level: Application; Client Need: Health Promotion and Maintenance; Nursing Process: Assessment

5 Answer: 1 Rationale: Beta agonists are agents that are used in the management of asthma that may be given to children younger than 5, and are available in formulations suitable for nebulizer treatments. The agents in options 2, 3, and 4 do not meet one or more of the criteria listed above. Cognitive Level: Analysis; Client Need: Health Promotion and Maintenance; Nursing Process: Planning

6 Answer: 3 Rationale: Some clients have difficulty mastering the coordination between inhalation and activation of the medication. In these instances, a spacer will hold the medication cloud so that this is not a concern. The spacer has additional advantages because it results in a more effective delivery of the drug to the site of action and less drug deposition in the mouth and oropharynx. Additional practice may help in the long term, but it is not the priority for an immediate solution to the problem (option 1). The health care provider would not need to be contacted because the client has difficulty learning, provided that a solution is readily available (option 2). Substitution of an oral form of drug is not in the nursing scope of practice and, even if it were, an oral formulation would not be a suitable substitute because the onset of action would be delayed (option 3). Cognitive Level: Analysis; Client Need: Health Promotion and Maintenance; Nursing Process: Planning

Chapter 74

Answer to Connection Checkpoint 74.1

Levodopa is the traditional drug of choice for treating Parkinson's disease. It is used to replenish the neurotransmitter dopamine, which is deficient in these patients.

Answer to Connection Checkpoint 74.2

If the corticosteroid medication is abruptly withdrawn, the shrunken, atrophic adrenal glands will not be able to secrete sufficient corticosteroids, and symptoms of adrenal crisis will appear (nausea, vomiting, lethargy, confusion, myalgia, arthralgia, fever, asthenia, acute abdominal pain, hypotension, seizures, renal failure, and coma).

Answer to Connection Checkpoint 74.3

The leukotriene modifiers are alternative drugs to be considered when intranasal corticosteroids and short-acting beta agonists are unable to control asthma symptoms.

Chapter 74 Answers to Critical Thinking Questions

1 Lung sounds, history of allergies, history of heart disease or HTN, other medicines she is taking, and whether the cough is productive.

2 Many patients who come to health care providers or hospitals have an initially elevated heart rate and blood pressure due to the anxiety of being there. It is called "white coat syndrome." The vital signs will normalize after a few minutes. In Ms. Williams' case she has been taking Neo-Synephrine, an intranasal sympathomimetic (decongestant). The intranasal sympathomimetic does not cause the elevated vital signs as would a PO agent, so she may have anxiety. Taking her vitals again in five to ten minutes may result in a normal set of readings.

3 She may have an allergy to the dog. Because getting rid of the pet may not be an option, suggest that she keep the dog away from her bedroom, or outside, weather permitting. Frequent cleaning of the home and bathing the dog to remove dander may be helpful also.

4 Flonase is a nasal spray that is effective in 90% of patients when they use it to prevent most major symptoms of allergic rhinitis. It may take one to three weeks to see the full effect but an initial effect can bee seen within hours. Ms. Williams' current worsening nasal stuffiness is probably due to the abrupt withdrawal of the Neo-Synephrine. The drug causes rebound congestion if used more than three to five days. Two cough preparations will be taken to help prevent the dry cough. One preparation with dextromethorphan can be used for daytime relief as it does not sedate. The one with diphenhydramine (antihistamine) does have sedating effects and can be used at night to help control the cough and allow the patient to get a better night's sleep.

Chapter 74 Answers to Case Study

1 The patient is having an anaphylactic reaction to strawberries. While this is an allergic reaction, the major cause of the response is not from histamines but from the release of other chemical mediators from mast cells.

2 Once the initial treatment of anaphylaxis (epinephrine) is started, an antihistamine is given as an adjunct to treatment. It will help decrease bronchoconstriction and laryngeal edema that may be caused by small amounts of histamine.

Chapter 74 Answers to NCLEX-RN® Review

1 Answer: 2, 5 Rationale: Priming any inhaler prior to first use ensures that the correct dosage is delivered (option 2). Corticosteroids take about three weeks to become fully effective (option 5). The medication is inhaled so water is not important (option 1). Corticosteroids are used primarily for prophylaxis (option 3). Flonase, like all corticosteroids, is best used as a prophylaxis for symptoms. Unlike inhaled sympathomimetics, corticosteroids do not cause rebound congestion (option 4). Cognitive Level: Application; Client Need: Safe, Effective Care Management; Nursing Process: Implementation

2 Answer: 4 Rationale: Pseudoephedrine is a sympathomimetic and is used only for nasal decongestion. Dextromethorphan and diphenhydramine are both effective for some coughs associated with allergic rhinitis and the common cold (options 1 and 2). Mucolytics are found in some OTC cough preparations used in colds, but are best used to treat chronic productive coughs (option 3). Cognitive Level: Application; Client Need: Physiologic Integrity; Nursing Process: Implementation

3 Answer: 3 Rationale: Diphenhydramine may cause worsening of prostate disease. Driving while taking diphenhydramine may be dangerous; however, there is nothing in the question stem to indicate that the man drives (option 1). Getting an annual eye exam is important, though not the highest priority (option 2). Diphenhydramine is not a sympathomimetic and will not cause rebound congestion on withdrawal (option 4). Cognitive Level: Application; Client Need: Safe, Effective Care Management; Nursing Process: Implementation

4 Answer: 4 Rationale: Intranasal corticosteroids do not treat acute symptoms; rather they are used as a prophylaxis to prevent nasal stuffiness. Intranasal corticosteroids are not used in the treatment of the common cold (option 1). Options 2 and 3 are incorrect because they are acute symptoms for which intranasal corticosteroids are not used. Cognitive Level: Application; Client Need: Physiologic Integrity; Nursing Process: Implementation

5 Answer: 1 Rationale: All sympathomimetics, whether prescription or OTC are CNS stimulants and can increase blood pressure and cause dysrhythmias in people with coronary artery disease. Option 2 is incorrect because wide-angled glaucoma is one contraindication for the use of antihistamines, not decongestants. Option 3 is incorrect because, while some drugs may secrete in breast milk, others may be safe, so taking these should be discussed with the health care provider. Option 4 is incorrect because elderly clients may be more sensitive to any drug, but decongestants are not contraindicated for them. Cognitive Level: Application; Client Need: Physiologic Integrity; Nursing Process: Implementation

6 Answer: 3 Rationale: Intranasal corticosteroids are preventive, so symptoms will not reverse immediately. Lying supine after instillation is unnecessary and takes time (option 1). Blowing the nose after instillation will remove some of the drug and prevent the desired effect (option 2). Priming is done only before the first use of the device; it is wasteful to prime each dose (option 4). Cognitive Level: Application; Client Need: Safe, Effective Care Management; Nursing Process: Implementation

Chapter 75

Answer to Connection Checkpoint 75.1

The calcium channel blockers are used to treat angina and hypertension.

Answer to Connection Checkpoint 75.2

Tamoxifen is approved for the palliative treatment of advanced, metastatic, estrogen receptor-positive breast cancer. Off-label indications include astrocytoma, malignant glioma, malignant melanoma, and ovarian cancer.

Answer to Connection Checkpoint 75.3

Malaria is caused by several species of the protozoan Plasmodium. These drugs are taken 2 weeks before entering an endemic area and continuing 4 to 6 weeks after leaving.

Chapter 75 Answer to Patient Safety Question

The nurse needed to ascertain that the patient receiving the medication was Ms. Brown. Identification needed to be verified by checking the patient's identification band, asking the patient to state her name and date of birth for the nurse, and verifying that these pieces of information matched those listed on the patient's medication administration record.

Chapter 75 Answers to Critical Thinking Questions

1 As the nurse, you are aware that osteoporosis is a condition in which the bone loses minerals and decreases in density, causing a subsequent loss in height. You should explain the details of this condition to the patient. Points to include are

- Risk factors: menopause, age over 60, family history of osteoporosis, Caucasian or Asian race, high alcohol intake, estrogen deficiency, smoking history, androgen deficiency, anorexia nervosa, low calcium or vitamin D intake, physical inactivity, and thin, lean body build.
- Signs and symptoms: fractures seen in the hips, wrists, forearms, or spine, and height loss.
- Diagnosis: height loss, bone fractures, and bone mineral density values.
- Treatments: Many drugs may be helpful. These include calcium and vitamin D therapy, estrogen replacement therapy, estrogen receptor modulators, statins, slow-release sodium fluoride, bisphosphonates, and calcitonin.

2 The nurse should encourage the patient to participate in preventive measures, which include adequate intake of calcium and vitamin D according to age requirements, physical exercise, routine health care follow-up especially in evaluating estrogen needs, use of OTC calcium supplements as recommended by a health care provider, and avoiding alcohol.

Chapter 75 Answers to Case Study

1 As the triage nurse, you should include the following information

- Take the medication in the morning at least 30 minutes before the first food, beverage, or other medication, with an 8 oz glass of plain water.
- Do not take within 2 hours of calcium-containing foods, beverages, or medications, as this will reduce the absorption of the drug.
- Wait at least 30 minutes after alendronate before taking any other drugs, eating, or drinking.
- Sit up or ambulate for 30 minutes after taking the drug. Do not lie down.

2 Adverse effects of alendronate (Fosamax) include diarrhea, constipation, flatulence, gastric irritation, a metallic or altered taste, abdominal pain, muscle aches, headache, and rash.

Chapter 75 Answers to NCLEX-RN® Review

1 Answer: 3 Rationale: Fosamax can cause severe GI adverse effects. To decrease this risk, particularly for esophageal irritation, and to promote the absorption of the medication, Fosamax should be taken with a full glass of water after rising in the morning. The client should not eat or drink anything or lie down for 30 minutes after administration. Option 1 is incorrect. The medication should be taken before breakfast. Options 2 and 4 are incorrect. The client should not lie down after taking Fosamax for at least 30 minutes. Cognitive Level: Application; Client Need: Health Promotion and Maintenance; Nursing Process: Evaluation

2 Answer: 1 Rationale: Headache, dizziness, and blurred vision are all early symptoms of toxicity to methotrexate. Findings of hematuria, jaundice, and ascites (options 2 and 4) would be unrelated to the use of methotrexate. While stomatitis may also occur, constipation would be unrelated to methotrexate (option 3). Cognitive Level: Application; Client Need: Physiological Integrity; Nursing Process: Assessment

3 Answer: 3 Rationale: Colchicine is a uric acid inhibitor, which prevents the accumulation of uric acid in the blood stream or joint cavities, relieving the symptoms of gout and gouty arthritis. Colchicine decreases rather than increases uric acid deposits in the synovial spaces of the joints (option 1). Colchicine does not have any analgesic properties (option 2); clients feel better from decreased inflammation secondary to fewer uric acid crystal deposits. Renal secretion of uric acid is not a mechanism of action of colchicine (option 4). Cognitive Level: Application; Client Need: Physiological Integrity; Nursing Process: Implementation

4 Answer: 1 Rationale: The client with osteomalacia has low serum calcium and low phosphate levels. An indicator that replacement therapy is achieving therapeutic benefits would be increasing serum calcium and phosphate levels. Options 2, 3, and 4 are incorrect because increasing or decreasing actions of the serum calcium and phosphate levels are incorrectly stated. Cognitive Level: Analysis; Client Need: Physiological Integrity; Nursing Process: Evaluation

5 Answer: 1 Rationale: Vitamin D toxicity may occur in the client receiving calcitriol. Symptoms to assess include muscle weakness, fatigue, nausea, vomiting, and changes in the color or amount of urine. Options 2 and 4 are incorrect. Diarrhea, stomatitis, and photosensitivity are not symptoms that would be associated with the effects of Vitamin D therapy. Option 3 is incorrect. Bone pain and fever are symptoms of vitamin D deficiency. Cognitive Level: Analysis; Client Need: Physiological Integrity; Nursing Process: Evaluation

6 Answer: 1, 2, 3 Rationale: DMARDs include gold salts, antimalarial agents, D-penicillamine, and drugs that modify immune and inflammatory responses (option 1). DMARDs have been found to reduce mortality rate, improve symptoms, and enhance the quality of life in clients with rheumatoid arthritis (option 2). Maximum therapeutic effects from DMARDs often take several months to achieve (option 3). Option 4 is incorrect because these drugs can be toxic and close monitoring of clients is required during the course of therapy. Option 5 is incorrect because DMARDs are well-accepted in medical practice because they have been found to reduce mortality rate and improve symptoms of rheumatoid arthritis. Cognitive Level: Knowledge; Client Need: Physiological Integrity; Nursing Process: Implementation

Chapter 76

Answer to Connection Checkpoint 76.1

Onychomycoses are fungal infections of the hair, skin, and nails. Oral antifungal drugs are usually employed over several months of therapy.

Answers to Connection Checkpoint 76.2

Vitamin A is a water-soluble vitamin. Large amounts may cause fatigue, nausea, vomiting, decreased appetite, headache, gingivitis, dryness or cracking of lips or skin, irritability, or loss of hair.

Answer to Connection Checkpoint 76.3

The inhalation route is used for asthma and chronic obstructive pulmonary disease (COPD); the intranasal route is used for allergic rhinitis; the intra-articular route is used for rheumatoid arthritis.

Answer to Connection Checkpoint 76.4

Finasteride inhibits 5-alpha reductase, the enzyme responsible for converting testosterone to 5-alpha dihydrotestosterone. Finasteride promotes regression of prostate epithelial tissue and decreases mechanical obstruction of the urethra.

Chapter 76 Answers to Critical Thinking Questions

1 Explain to the patient that this is an inflammatory skin disorder that primarily affects the face and tends to onset between the ages of 30 and 50. Signs and symptoms of the condition include small papules or inflammatory bumps without pus that swell and become thick and painful. Often the patient's face appears to be sunburned or flushed especially around the forehead, nose, cheeks, and chin. Patients tend to refer to this condition as adult acne. Treatment includes restricting exposure to conditions that would exacerbate the condition along with such medication as Accutane, Finacea, Metronidazole, and systemic antibiotics. Use of laser surgery will assist in reducing the development of excessive tissue that may have developed.

2 Conditions that may exacerbate the rosacea includes sunlight, stress, increased temperatures, alcohol, skin care products, warm beverages, and spicy foods that dilate the facial vessels.

Chapter 76 Answers to Case Study

1 Notify the parents of the situation and assess other members of the family for the presences of nits. Assess the hair especially near the scalp, behind the ears, and at the back of the head; observe for any complaints of pruritus and complaints of dandruff that sticks to the hair or bugs that may be in the hair which could be nits; provide education to the parents, child and other family members about nits and how they are transmitted. Offer empathy to the parents, child, and other family members about this situation. It must be stressed that anyone can get lice.

2 Practice methods of prevention such as not sharing combs, brushes, hats, towels, or bedding among individuals and regularly performing personal hygiene, especially in the hair. Effective treatment involves the use of a pediculicide shampoo (contraindicated in children less than 2 years). Permethrin can be used for children under 2 or pregnant adolescents. Apply shampoo, rub into scalp for 4–5 minutes, rinse, and towel dry. Remove nits with a fine-toothed comb. Repeat the treatment in one week.

3 Do not share brushes, hats, towels, or bedding. Launder bedding and clothing daily, in hot water with detergent and dry with heat. Discard hairbrushes and combs or soak in boiling water for 10–15 minutes. Perform proper hygiene techniques on a regular basis with emphasis on care of the hair.

Chapter 76 Answers to NCLEX-RN® Review

1 Answer: 4 Rationale: Lice and nits can live in areas of the body other than the hair on the client's head. Nix should not be applied after body lotions (option 1). Nix should not be used on eyelashes or eyebrows (option 2). Lice can survive for up to 48 hours on inanimate objects (option 3). Cognitive Level: Application; Client Need: Physiological Integrity; Nursing Process: Implementation

2 Answer: 1 Rationale: Clients taking topical corticosteroids for the treatment of atopic dermatitis may expect to experience a degree of burning and stinging of the skin in the affected area. Localized pruritus and hives (option 2) a loss of hair in the application area (option 3), or a worsening of acne vulgaris (option 4), are not symptoms that would be related specifically to the effects of therapy. Cognitive Level: Application; Client Need: Physiological Integrity; Nursing Process: Assessment

3 Answer: 4
Microdermal abrasion is not a primary action of this drug. Benzoyl peroxide suppresses sebum production (option 1), and has rapid bacteriostatic action against Propionibacterium acnes (option 2). Benzoyl peroxide has a keratolytic effect, which helps to treat the acne by loosening dry skin and causing an increased shedding of the outer layer of the epidermis (option 3). Cognitive Level: Application; Client Need: Physiological Integrity; Nursing Process: Planning

4 Answer: 2 Rationale: A client for whom treatment with tretinoin has been effective would see a decline in the symptoms of acne vulgaris and have fewer open and closed comedones. Tretinoin would not affect the growth of scalp hair (option 1), or decrease the size of warts (option 4).The client would also have a decline in the number of cysts rather than an increase (option 3) . Cognitive Level: Analysis; Client Need: Physiological Integrity; Nursing Process: Evaluation

5 Answer: 2 Rationale: The nurse working with teenagers with acne should establish rapport, as many clients with acne might be embarrassed, or have a *Disturbed Body Image* or low self-esteem because of their acne. Anger (option 1) or a self-care deficit (option 3) are not appropriate diagnoses. *Ineffective Health Maintenance* may be a consideration in some but not all cases (option 4). Cognitive Level: Analysis; Client Need: Physiological Integrity; Nursing Process: Diagnosis

6 Answer: 2 Rationale: Encourage clients to disclose their health history and medications. Concurrent use of tretinoin and hypoglycemic agents could lead to loss of glycemic control, as well as increased triglyceride levels. Dyspnea (option 1), HTN (option 3), and diarrhea (option 4) would not be adverse effects related to tretinoin use. Cognitive Level: Analysis; Client Need: Physiological Integrity; Nursing Process: Assessment

Chapter 77

Answer to Connection Checkpoint 77.1

The prostaglandins stimulate the contraction of uterine smooth muscle. They are used to stimulate labor contractions, or to induce pharmacological abortion.

Answer to Connection Checkpoint 77.2

Muscarinic agonists stimulate lacrimation. They are used to treat xerostomia and Sjögren's syndrome.

Answer to Connection Checkpoint 77.3

Mannitol is filtered by the glomerulus, but is incapable of being reabsorbed from the renal tubule. This creates an osmotic gradient, resulting in decreased water and sodium reabsorption and increased diuresis.

Chapter 77 Answers to Critical Thinking Questions

1 Predisposing factors that Mrs. Duclos presents include the fact that she is an African American, and that she is an elderly adult with a history of diabetes. Other general predisposing factors that may not apply to Mrs. Duclos include Asian descent, genetic factors, congenital defects in infants and children, can be secondary to eye trauma, infection, diabetes, inflammation, hemorrhage, tumors, or cataracts. Long-term use of topical corticosteroids, some antihypertensives, antihistamines, and antidepressants may also contribute to the development or progression of glaucoma. Risk factors associated with glaucoma would include HTN, migraine headaches, and refractive disorders with a high degree of nearsightedness or farsightedness and the normal aging process.

2 Wash hands prior to administering eye drops. Avoid touching the eye or eyelashes with any part of the eyedropper to avoid cross-contamination. Administer the eye drop solution in the conjunctival sac.

Apply pressure over the lacrimal sac for 1 minute. Apply to only the affected eye(s). Ensure that only one drop is instilled. Wait at least 5 minutes before instilling other eye drops. If indicated, refrigerate and protect the solution from light.

3 This condition is caused by excessive production of aqueous humor or by a blockage of the outflow of the aqueous humor. An increase in the intraocular pressure (IOP) is identified by her ophthalmologist by performing tonometry testing. This increase in the IOP will cause damage to the optic nerve resulting in a loss in the visual field, a loss of the central visual acuity and finally total blindness. Treatments for primary open-angle glaucoma consist of drugs that will assist in lowering the IOP. Avoid medications that interfere with glaucoma and its treatment. Proper follow-up with her health care provider needs to be maintained to evaluate the IOP readings and effects of the prescribed medications.

Chapter 77 Answers to Case Study

A patient information sheet could include the following information:

- Wash your hands prior to administering the medication.
- Allow another individual to assist in holding the child in a supine position with the child's head extended.

- Pull the pinna or lower portion of the ear gently down and back to straighten the ear canal for a child younger than 3 years of age, and for the older child, pull the pinna upward and back.
- When the pinna is in the proper position, instill the desired number of drops into the ear.
- Keep the child in the same position for 4–5 minutes to prevent leakage of the medication.
- Gently rub the area just anterior to the ear to facilitate movement of the medication into the ear canal. If desired, a cotton ball may be loosely placed in the ear to promote retention of the medication.

Chapter 77 Answers to NCLEX-RN® Review

1 Answer: 1 Rationale: Cerumenex is used to remove earwax. Ciprofloxacin (Cipro otic) is a topical antibiotic used to treat external otitis (option 2). The best choice of an agent to treat swimmer's ear, not impacted earwax, would be Cortisporin because it combines an antibiotic with an anti-inflammatory agent (option 3). Chloramphenicol is an antibiotic used to treat infections of the external ear canal (option 4). Cognitive Level: Knowledge; Client Need: Physiological Integrity; Nursing Process: Planning

2 Answer: 4 Rationale: Mydriatics cause intense photophobia and pain in response to bright light. Mydriatics can worsen glaucoma by impairing aqueous humor outflow and thereby increasing IOP. Antibiotic drops (option 1), fluorescein sodium (option 2), and proparacaine hydrochloride (option 3), have no effect on IOP. Cognitive Level: Application; Client Need: Physiological Integrity; Nursing Process: Implementation

3 Answer: 1, 2, 4 Rationale: Major risk factors for the development of glaucoma include HTN (option 1), a history of migraine headaches (option 2), and cataracts (option 4). A history of epilepsy (option 3), or Cushing's syndrome (option 5), would not predispose a client to developing glaucoma. Cognitive Level: Knowledge; Client Need: Physiological Integrity; Nursing Process: Assessment

4 Answer: 3 Rationale: Prostaglandin inhibitors, such as Xalatan, decrease intraocular pressure by increasing the outflow of aqueous humor. The actual mechanism by which this occurs is unknown. Beta-blockers and carbonic anhydrase inhibitors, not Xalatan, decrease the production of aqueous humor (option 1). Xalatan does not cause permanent pupil constriction (option 2). Osmotic diuretics are used to quickly reduce the outflow of aqueous humor (option 3), and plasma volume (option 4). Cognitive Level: Application; Client Need: Physiological Integrity; Nursing Process: Implementation

5 Answer: 1 Rationale: Atropine sulfate (Isopto Atropine) is a cycloplegic agent, causing pupil dilation for better visualization of retinal structures and paralyzation of the ciliary muscle. Glycerin anhydrous (Ophthalgan) is an osmotic diuretic used in the treatment of glaucoma (option 2). Proparacaine hydrochloride (Alcaine) is an anesthetic agent (option 3). Acetylcholine causes pupil constriction (option 4). Cognitive Level: Knowledge; Client Need: Physiological Integrity; Nursing Process: Planning

6 Answer: 3 Rationale: Neo-Synephrine causes dilation of the pupil and constriction of the surrounding blood vessels. Neo-Synephrine does not decrease aqueous humor (option 1), and has no lubricating properties (option 2). Cycloplegic agents, not Neo-Synephrine, paralyze the ciliary muscle (option 4). Cognitive Level: Application; Client Need: Physiological Integrity; Nursing Process: Implementation

Chapter 78

Answer to Connection Checkpoint 78.1

Ciprofloxacin is a fluoroquinolone that inhibits the affect of bacterial DNA synthesis by inhibiting both DNA gyrase and topoisomerase IV.

Answer to Connection Checkpoint 78.2

I-131 is used to destroy thyroid cells and shrink the size of an overactive thyroid gland.

Answer to Connection Checkpoint 78.3

Atropine is an antidote used to reverse symptoms of toxicity due to overdose of cholinergic agonists, including organophosphate insecticides and ingestion of mushrooms containing muscarine.

Chapter 78 Answers to Critical Thinking Questions

1 Because smallpox is caused by the variola virus, there is no specific treatment for smallpox disease. The only prevention is vaccination. The virus can be spread from one person to another by direct and prolonged face-to-face contact. Smallpox also can be spread through direct contact with infected bodily fluids or contaminated objects such as bedding or clothing. Exposure to smallpox is followed by an incubation period of 7–17 days during which people do not have any symptoms. Initially, symptoms of smallpox include high fever, malaise, head and body aches, and sometimes vomiting. Often the development of a rash begins in the mouth. However, it quickly spreads to the face and moves to the arms and legs. Supportive care and infection control measures should be instituted for the patient with smallpox.

2 The method of transmission affects the symptoms of anthrax contamination. The most common (cutaneous anthrax) and the most serious (inhalation anthrax) forms of anthrax are transmitted through open skin and inhalation. The nurse should examine the patient's skin for open wounds which may be contaminated. Respiratory assessment and support is imperative for the patient who may have contracted anthrax via respiratory exposure (inhalation).

3 *Yersinia pestis (Y. pestis)* is a gram-negative anaerobic bacterium that causes a life-threatening condition known as pneumonic plague. The isolation of this disease is extremely difficult because it can be spread by aerosol. The person who has the disease would be infectious to everyone with whom they have come in contact within 1–6 days after exposure. If untreated, pneumonic plague will result in respiratory failure with subsequent shock and death.

Chapter 78 Answers to Case Study

1 Poison-proofing a home is the key to preventing childhood poisonings. Always close the container immediately after using it. Properly secure the child-resistant packaging, and put it away immediately in a place where children cannot reach it. Keep pills in their original container. Keep iron-containing tablets and all medications, out of reach, and out of sight of children. Never keep medicines on a countertop or bedside table. Follow medicine label directions carefully to avoid accidental overdoses or incorrect doses that could result in poisoning. Buy the least hazardous products that will serve your purposes and look for products that are safe for children. Never transfer these substances to other containers. The kitchen and bathroom are the most likely unsafe areas. Keep any cabinet containing a potentially poisonous item locked. Remember that child-resistant caps are child-resistant, not childproof. Garages and utility rooms should also be checked for potential poison hazards. Although most houseplants are not poisonous, some are. To be on the safe side, keep houseplants out of the reach of young children. Post your doctor's phone number and the numbers of your regional poison control center (which can be found on the inside cover of the Yellow Pages or in the white pages of your phone directory) by the phone.

2 Never administer Ipecac syrup without first consulting a health care provider.

Chapter 78 Answers to NCLEX-RN® Review

1 Answer: 1 Rationale: No antidote or specific treatment for radiation poisoning. Supportive therapy for the associated symptoms is the only treatment available. Ultraviolet light does not affect individuals who experience radiation poisoning (option 2). An individual with radiation toxicity is incapable of contaminating other individuals (option 3). No anti-radiation medications exist (option 4) Cognitive Level: Application; Client Need: Safe Effective Care Management; Nursing Process: Implementation

2 Answer: 1 Rationale: The drug of choice for *Y. pestis* exposure is doxycycline. Trivalent botulinum antitoxin is one of the two available treatments for botulism. The other antitoxin for botulism is heptavalent botulinum antitoxin (option 2). Ribavirin is an antiviral agent that may be used to treat serious virus infections (option 3). Atropine sulfate is a cholinergic antagonist used for organophosphate poisoning and other health problems (option 4). Cognitive Level: Knowledge; Client Need: Safe, Effective Care Management; Nursing Process: Implementation

3 Answer: 3 Rationale: Time is a critical factor in acute poisonings. The child should be taken to the nearest health care facility immediately. Instructions for poisoning may have changed since the packaging was printed (option 1). Based on the information provided in the question, the nurse does not know what chemicals the child has ingested. Forced vomiting is contraindicated for most poisonings (option 2). Waiting for the child to develop seizures or shortness of breath is too late since the development of these symptoms most likely represents a toxic level of the poison (option 4). Cognitive Level: Application; Client Need: Safe, Effective Care Management; Nursing Process: Implementation

4 Answer: 3 Rationale: Patients with decreased sensorium are at high risk for pulmonary aspiration. Activated charcoal should only be given to these patients if the airway is maintained with an endotracheal tube. Activated charcoal is not absorbed in the GI track and therefore would not be contraindicated in patients with liver pathology (option 1). Activated charcoal is eliminated in the feces and therefore would not be contraindicated in patients with renal impairment (option 2). Anxiety and nervousness are not reasons to withhold the administration of activated charcoal (option 4). Cognitive Level: Application; Client Need: Safe, Effective Care Management; Nursing Process: Assessment

5 Answer: 1 Rationale: Chelating agents capture the toxic metal through a bonding process. The kidneys remove both the chelator and the metal bound to it from the body. Option 2 is incorrect. A chelator binds heavy metals but does not deactivate any chemical reactions. Option 3 is incorrect. Chelation therapy is not involved in metabolism. Option 4 is incorrect. Glomerular filtration is not affected by chelation therapy. Cognitive Level: Knowledge; Client Need: Safe, Effective Care Management; Nursing Process: Assessment

6 Answer: 2 Rationale: Edetate calcium disodium may produce renal damage that may be reduced by ensuring adequate diuresis before therapy begins. Bowel function is not a critical parameter to consider prior to giving this drug (option 1). Edetate calcium disodium administration is not based on visual acuity (option 3). Skin integrity is not a critical parameter to consider prior to giving edetate calcium disodium (option 4). Cognitive Level: Application; Client Need: Safe, Effective Care Management; Nursing Process: Assessment

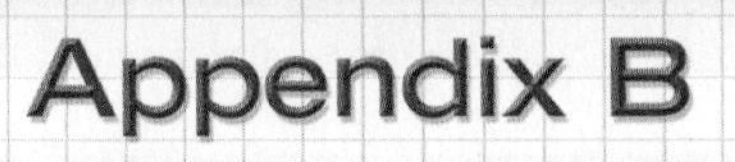

Top 100 Drugs Ranked by Number of Prescriptions

Rank	Top 100 Generic Drugs	Rank	Top 100 Generic Drugs
1.	hydrocodone w/APAP	51.	doxycycline
2.	lisinopril	52.	methylprednisolone tabs
3.	amoxicillin	53.	clonidine
4.	levothyroxine	54.	trimethoprim/sulfa
5.	hydrochlorothiazide	55.	promethazine
6.	azithromycin	56.	isosorbide mononitrate
7.	atenolol	57.	pravastatin
8.	simvastatin	58.	meloxicam
9.	alprazolam	59.	verapamil SR
10.	furosemide	60.	folic acid
11.	metformin	61.	glyburide
12.	sertraline	62.	sulfamethoxazole/trimethoprim
13.	metoprolol tartrate	63.	penicillin VK
14.	ibuprofen	64.	spironolactone
15.	amlodipine	65.	temazepam
16.	oxycodone w/APAP	66.	glimepiride
17.	prednisone	67.	albuterol nebulizer solution
18.	cephalexin	68.	triamcinolone acetonide (topical)
19.	fluoxetine	69.	clindamycin (systemic)
20.	triamterene/HCTZ	70.	metformin HCl ER
21.	propoxyphene N/APAP	71.	glipizide
22.	warfarin	72.	benazepril
23.	lorazepam	73.	metronidazole tabs
24.	omeprazole	74.	amlodipine besylate
25.	clonazepam	75.	metoclopramide
26.	amoxicillin/clavulanate	76.	quinapril
27.	albuterol aerosol	77.	glipizide ER
28.	ciprofloxacin	78.	propranolol
29.	metoprolol succinate	79.	hydroxyzine
30.	cyclobenzaprine	80.	diclofenac
31.	tramadol	81.	estradiol oral
32.	gabapentin	82.	gemfibrozil
33.	fexofenadine	83.	oxycodone ER
34.	lisinopril/HCTZ	84.	doxazosin
35.	citalopram	85.	meclizine
36.	paroxetine	86.	mirtazapine
37.	trazodone	87.	nitrofurantoin
38.	lovastatin	88.	glyburide/metformin
39.	fluticasone	89.	acyclovir
40.	zolpidem	90.	amphetamine salt combination
41.	acetaminophen/codeine	91.	diltiazem
42.	potassium chloride	92.	fentanyl transdermal
43.	amitriptyline	93.	buspirone
44.	diazepam	94.	nabumetone
45.	naproxen	95.	diltiazem CD
46.	enalapril	96.	promethazine/Codeine
47.	ranitidine	97.	methotrexate
48.	fluconazole	98.	bisoprolol/HCTZ
49.	carisoprodol	99.	oxycodone
50.	allopurinol	100.	butalbital/acetaminophen/ caffeine

Rank	Top 100 Brand Name Drugs	Rank	Top 100 Brand Name Drugs
1.	Lipitor	51.	Lamictal
2.	Singulair	52.	Ortho Tri-Cyclen Lo
3.	Lexapro	53.	Xalatan
4.	Nexium	54.	AcipHex
5.	Synthroid	55.	Hyzaar
6.	Plavix	56.	Spiriva
7.	Toprol XL	57.	Wellbutrin XL
8.	Prevacid	58.	Lunesta
9.	Vytorin	59.	Benicar
10.	Advair Diskus	60.	Benicar HCT
11.	Zyrtec	61.	Aricept
12.	Effexor XR	62.	Avapro
13.	Protonix	63.	Detrol LA
14.	Diovan	64.	TriNessa
15.	Fosamax	65.	Cialis
16.	Zetia	66.	Combivent
17.	Crestor	67.	Budeprion XL
18.	Levaquin	68.	Yaz
19.	Diovan HCT	69.	Glycolax
20.	Klor-Con	70.	Imitrex oral
21.	Cymbalta	71.	Evista
22.	Actos	72.	NuvaRing
23.	Premarin-Tabs	73.	Omnicef
24.	Pro-Air HFA	74.	Niaspan
25.	Celebrex	75.	Tri-Sprintec
26.	Flomax	76.	Boniva
27.	Seroquel	77.	Flovent HFA
28.	Norvasc	78.	Avelox
29.	Nasonex	79.	Abilify
30.	Tricor	80.	Avalide
31.	Lantus	81.	Requip
32.	Viagra	82.	Zyrtec Syrup
33.	Altace	83.	Coumadin tabs
34.	Yasmin 28	84.	Zyprexa
35.	Levoxyl	85.	Depakote ER
36.	Adderall XR	86.	Nasacort AQ
37.	Lotrel	87.	Skelaxin
38.	Actonel	88.	Allegra D 12 hr
39.	Ambien CR	89.	Humalog
40.	Cozaar	90.	Vigamox
41.	Coreg	91.	Endocet
42.	Valtrex	92.	Budeprion SR
43.	Lyrica	93.	Depakote
44.	Concerta	94.	Namenda
45.	Ambien	95.	Lidoderm
46.	Risperdal	96.	Strattera
47.	Digitek	97.	Aviane
48.	Topamax	98.	Patanol
49.	Chantix	99.	Proventil HFA
50.	Avandia	100.	Clarinex

Note: From "Top 200 Brand Drugs by Units in 2007." *Drug Topics: The Newsmagazine for Pharmacists,* 2008. Retrieved December 12, 2008, from http://drugtopics.modernmedicine.com/drugtopics/Drugtopics.com+Exclusives/Top-200-Brand-Drugs-By-Units-in-2007/ArticleStandard/Article/detail/491210?searchString=top%20200%20%202007 and "Top 200 Generic Drugs by Units." *Drug Topics: The Newsmagazine for Pharmacists,* 2008. Retrieved December 12, 2008, from http://drugtopics.modernmedicine.com/drugtopics/Drugtopics.com+Exclusives/Top-200-generic-drugs-by-units-in-2007/ArticleStandard/Article/detail/491194?searchString=top%20200%20%202007

Appendix C

Canadian Drugs and Their U.S. Equivalents

U.S. Drug Name	Canadian Drug Name
acebutolol hydrochloride (Sectral)	Monitan, Sectral
acetaminophen (Tylenol)	Abenal, Atasol, Campain, others
acetazolamide (Diamox)	Acetazolam, Apo-Acetazolamide, Diamox
acetohexamide (Dymelor)	Acetohexamide
albuterol (Proventil, Salbutamol)	Salbutamol, Novo-Salmol, and Ventolin
allopurinol (Lopurin, Zyloprim)	Allopurinol, Apo-Alloprin, and Zyloprim
altretamine, hexamethylmelamine (Hexalen)	Hexalen
aminophylline (Truphylline)	Aminophylline
amitriptyline hydrochloride (Elavil)	Apo-Amitripyline, Elavil
amoxicillin (Amoxil, Trimox, Wymox)	Apo-Amoxi, Amoxil
ampicillin (Polycillin, Omnipen)	Novo-Ampicillin, Ampicin, Ampicillin Sodium
asparaginase (Elspar)	Kidrolase
aspirin (ASA, others)	Novasen, Entrophen, others
atenolol (Tenormin)	Apo-Atenolol, Tenormin
atropine sulfate (Isopto Atropine, others)	Atropine Sulfate, Atropine
bacampicillin hydrochloride (Spectrobid)	Penglobe
benztropine mesylate (Cogentin)	Apo-Benztropine, Congentin
betamethasone (Celestone, Betacort, others)	Betaderm, others
bretylium tosylate (Bretylol)	Bretylate
brompheniramine maleate (Codimal-A, Dimetapp)	Dimetane
calcium carbonate (BioCal, Calcite-500, others)	Apo-Cal, Calsan, Caltrate 600
carbamazepine (Tegretol)	Apo-Carbamazepine, Tegretol
cephalexin (Keflex)	Novo-Lexin
cetirizine (Zyrtec)	Reactine
chloral hydrate (Noctec)	Chloral Hydrate
chloramphenicol (Chlorofair, Chloromycetin, Chloroptic, Fenicol)	Pentamycetin
chlordiazepoxide hydrochloride (Librium)	Novo-Poxide
chlorthalidone (Hygroton)	Hygroton
chlorpropamide (Chloronase, Diabinese, Glucamide)	Apo-Chlorpropamide
chlorpheniramine maleate (Chlor-Trimeton, others)	Chlor-Tripolon
chlorpromazine hydrochloride (Thorazine)	Largactil
cimetidine (Tagamet)	Apo-Cimetidine, Novo-Cimetine, Tagamet
cisplatin (Platinol)	Cisplatin Injection
clindamycin hydrochloride (Cleocin)	Dalacin C
clonazepam (Klonopin)	Rivotril
clonidine hydrochloride (Catapres)	Catapres
clorazepate dipotassium (Tranxene)	Novo-Clopate, Tranxene
clotrimazole (Gyne-Lotrimin, Mycelex, Femizole)	Canesten, Clotrimaderm
cloxacillin (Tegopen)	Apo-Cloxi, Novo-Cloxin
codeine	Codeine
colestipol (Colestid)	Colestid, Colestipol HCL
cyclophosphamide (Cytoxan, Neosar)	Procytox
cyproheptadine hydrochloride (Periactin)	Periactin

U.S. Drug Name	Canadian Drug Name
danazol (Danocrine)	Cyclomen
dexamethasone (Decadron, Dexasone, Hexadrol, Maxidex)	Decadron
dextroamphetamine sulfate (Dexedrine)	Dexedrine
diazepam (Valium)	Apo-Diazepam, Diazepam
diethylstilbestrol (DES, Stilbestrol)	Honval
diltiazem (Cardizem, Dilacor, Tiamate, Tiazac)	Apo-Diltiaz, Cardizem
dimenhydrinate (Dramamine)	Apo-Dimenhydrinate, Gravol
diphenhydramine hydrochloride (Benadryl, others)	Benedryl
dipyridamole (Persantine)	Apo-Dipyridamole FC, Persantine
disopyramide phosphate (Norpace, Napamide)	Rythmodan
docusate (Surfak, Dialose, Colace)	Colace
dopamine hydrochloride (Dopastat, Intropin)	Intropin
doxepin hydrochloride (Sinequan)	Sinequin
doxycycline hyclate (Doryx, Doxy, Monodox, Vibramycin)	Apo-Doxy, Doxycin
econazole nitrate (Spectazole)	Ecostatin
epinephrine (Adrenalin, Bronkaid, Primatene)	Adrenalin
ergocalciferol (Deltalin, Calciferol)	Ostoforte
ergotamine tartrate (Ergostat)	Migranal
erythromycin (E-mycin, Erythrocin)	Novo-Rythmo Encap, Erythromid, Erythromycin
estradiol valerate (Delestrogen, Duragen-10, Valergen)	Delestrogen
fluoxymesterone (Halotestin)	Halotestin
flurazepam (Dalmane)	Apo-Flurazepam
furosemide (Lasix)	Lasix
gentamicin sulfate (Garamycin, G-mycin, Jenamicin)	Garamycin
glyburide (DiaBeta, Micronase, Glynase)	Euglucon, Glyburide
griseofulvin (Fulvicin)	Grisovin-FP
haloperidol (Haldol)	Peridol
heparin sodium (Hep-lock)	Hepalean
hydralazine hydrochloride (Apresoline)	Novo-Hylazin, Apresoline
hydrochlorothiazide (HydroDIURIL, HCTZ)	Apo-Hydro
hydrocodone bitartrate (Hycodan)	Robidone
hydrocortisone (Cetacort, Cortaid, Solu-Cortef)	Rectocort, Cortiment
hydroxyzine (Atarax, Vistaril)	Apo-Hydroxyzine
ibuprofen (Advil, Motrin, others)	Amersol, Advil, others
imipramine hydrochloride (Tofranil)	Tofranil
indapamide (Lozol)	Lozide
isoniazid (INH, Laniazid, Nydrazid, Teebaconin)	Isotamine, PMS Isoniazid
isosorbide dinitrate (Isordil, Sorbitrate, Dilatrate-SR)	Isordil
ketoprofen (Actron, Orudis, Oruvail)	Rhodis
lidocaine hydrochloride (Xylocaine)	Xylocard
lithium carbonate (Eskalith)	Carbolith, Duralith
lorazepam (Ativan)	Apo-Lorazepam
loxapine succinate (Loxitane)	Loxapac
meclizine (Antivert, Bonine)	Bonamine
methyldopa (Aldomet)	Apo-Methyldopa, Aldomet
methyltestosterone (Android, Testred)	Metandren
metoclopramide (Reglan)	Maxeran
metoprolol tartrate (Toprol, Lopressor)	Betaloc, Apo-Metoprolol

U.S. Drug Name	Canadian Drug Name
morphine sulfate (Astramorph PF, Duramorph, others)	Epimorph, Statex, and others
naproxen (Naprosyn, Anaprox)	Apo-Naproxen, Naxen, Novo-Naprox
nifedipine (Procardia, Adalat)	Apo-Nifed, Novo-Nifedin
nitrofurantoin (Furadantin, Furalan, Furanite, Macrobid, Macrodantin)	Apo-Nitrofurantoin, Novo-Furantoin
nystatin (Mycostatin, Nilstat, Nystex)	Nyaderm
omeprazole (Prilosec)	Losec
oxazepam (Serax)	Ozazepam
oxymetazoline hydrochloride (Afrin 12 Hour, Neo-Synephrine 12 Hour, others)	New-synephrine
penicillin G sodium/potassium (Pentids)	Penicillin G, Benzathin
penicillin V (Pen-Vee K, Veetids, Betapen-VK)	Apo-Pen-VK, Nadopen-V
pentamidine isoethionate (Pentam 300, Nebupent)	Pentamidine isoethionate
pentobarbital sodium (Nembutal)	Pentobarbitol Sodium IM and IV
phenylephrine hydrochloride (Mydfrin, Neo-Synephrine)	Neo-Synephrine
pilocarpine hydrochloride (Adsorbocarpine, Isopto Carpine, others)	Pilopine HS, Pilocarpine HCL
prednisolone (Delta-Cortef, Key-Pred, Prelone, others)	Pediapred
prednisone (Deltasone, Meticorten)	Apo-Prednisone, Winpred
primidone (Mysoline)	Apo-Primidone
probenecid (Benemid, Probalan)	Benuryl
prochlorperazine (Compazine)	Prorazin, Stemetil
procyclidine hydrochloride (Kemadrin)	Procyclid
promethazine (Pentazine,Phenazine, Phenergan, others)	Phenergen
propoxyphene hydrochloride (Darvon); propoxyphene napsylate (Darvon-N)	Darvon N and Propoxyphene
propranolol hydrochloride (Inderal)	Apo-Propranolol
propylthiouracil (PTU)	Propyl-Thyracil
protriptyline hydrochloride (Vivactil)	Triptil
psyllium hydrophilic mucilloid (Metamucil, Naturcil)	Metamucil
pyrazinamide (PZA)	Tebrazid
quinidine sulfate (Quinidex)	Qunidine Sulfate
ranitidine (Zantac)	Apo-Ranitidine, Zantac
rifampin (Rifadin, Rimactane)	Rofact
scopolamine (Hyoscine, Transderm-Scop)	Transderm-V
secobarbital (Seconal)	Secobarbital
spironolactone (Aldactone)	Novospiroton
sulfasalazine (Azulfidine)	Salazopyrin, Salzopyrin EN-Tabs, others
sulfinpyrazone (Anturan)	Anturane, Anturan, others
tamoxifen citrate (Nolvadex)	Nolvadex-D, Nolvadex, Tamone
testosterone enanthate (Testone LA, Delatest, Delatestryl)	Testosterone Enanthate, Delatestryl
tetracycline hydrochloride (Achromycin, Panmycin, Sumycin)	Novotetra
theophylline (Theo-Dur)	Theo-Dur, Theophylline
thioguanine (TG)	Lanvis
thioridazine hydrochloride (Mellaril)	Mellaril
tolbutamide (Orinase)	Tolbutamide
trifluoperazine hydrochloride (Stelazine)	Stelazine
trihexyphenidyl hydrochloride (Artane)	Apo-Trihex
Tums	Apo-Cal
valproic acid (Depakene)	Epival
verapamil hydrochloride (Calan, Isoptin, Verelan)	Novo-Veramil, Nu-Verap
vinblastine sulfate (Velban)	Velbe
warfarin sodium (Coumadin)	Warfilone

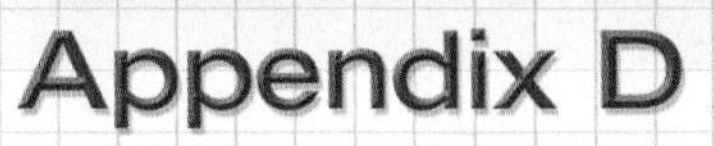

ISMP's List of High-Alert Medications

High-alert medications are drugs that bear a heightened risk of causing significant patient harm when they are used in error. Although mistakes may or may not be more common with these drugs, the consequences of an error are clearly more devastating to patients. We hope you will use this list to determine which medications require special safeguards to reduce the risk of errors. This may include strategies like improving access to information about these drugs; limiting access to high-alert medications; using auxiliary labels and automated alerts; standardizing the ordering, storage, preparation, and administration of these products; and employing redundancies such as automated or independent double-checks when necessary. (Note: manual independent double-checks are not always the optimal error-reduction strategy and may not be practical for all of the medications on the list.)

Classes/Categories of Medications
adrenergic agonists, IV (e.g., epinephrine, phenylephrine, norepinephrine)
adrenergic antagonists, IV (e.g., propranolol, metoprolol, labetalol)
anesthetic agents, general, inhaled and IV (e.g., propofol, ketamine)
antiarrhythmics, IV (e.g., lidocaine, amiodarone)
antithrombotic agents (anticoagulants), including warfarin, low-molecular-weight heparin, IV unfractionated heparin, Factor Xa inhibitors (fondaparinux), direct thrombin inhibitors (e.g., argatroban, lepirudin, bivalirudin), thrombolytics (e.g., alteplase, reteplase, tenecteplase), and glycoprotein IIb/IIIa inhibitors (e.g., eptifibatide)
cardioplegic solutions
chemotherapeutic agents, parenteral and oral
dextrose, hypertonic, 20% or greater
dialysis solutions, peritoneal and hemodialysis
epidural or intrathecal medications
hypoglycemics, oral
inotropic medications, IV (e.g., digoxin, milrinone)
liposomal forms of drugs (e.g., liposomal amphotericin B)
moderate sedation agents, IV (e.g., midazolam)
moderate sedation agents, oral, for children (e.g., chloral hydrate)
narcotics/opiates, IV, transdermal, and oral (including liquid concentrates, immediate and sustained-release formulations)
neuromuscular blocking agents (e.g., succinylcholine, rocuronium, vecuronium)
radiocontrast agents, IV
total parenteral nutrition solutions

Specific Medications
colchicine injection***
epoprostenol (Flolan), IV
insulin, subcutaneous and IV
magnesium sulfate injection
methotrexate, oral, non-oncologic use
opium tincture
oxytocin, IV
nitroprusside sodium for injection
potassium chloride for injection concentrate
potassium phosphates injection
promethazine, IV
sodium chloride for injection, hypertonic (greater than 0.9% concentration)
sterile water for injection, inhalation, and irrigation
(excluding pour bottles) in containers of 100 mL or more

*** Although colchicine injection should no longer be used, it will remain on the list until shipments of unapproved colchicine injection cease in August 2008. For details, please visit: www.fda.gov/bbs/topics/NEWS/2008/NEW01791.html.

Background

Based on error reports submitted to the USP-ISMP Medication Errors Reporting Program, reports of harmful errors in the literature, and input from practitioners and safety experts, ISMP created and periodically updates a list of potential high-alert medications. During February–April 2007, 770 practitioners responded to an ISMP survey designed to identify which medications were most frequently considered high-alert drugs by individuals and organizations. Further, to assure relevance and completeness, the clinical staff at ISMP, members of our advisory board, and safety experts throughout the US were asked to review the potential list. This list of drugs and drug categories reflects the collective thinking of all who provided input.

Glossary

A

Abortifacients drugs used to induce abortion

Absence seizures seizures with a loss or reduction of normal activity, including staring and transient loss of responsiveness

Absorption the process by which drug molecules move from their site of administration to the blood

Accessory organs of digestion include the salivary glands, liver, gallbladder, and pancreas

Acetylation a general biochemical process that adds a two-carbon chain to a drug molecule, which usually renders the drug less effective

Acetylcholine (Ach) primary neurotransmitter of the autonomic nervous system; also present at somatic neuromuscular junctions and at sympathetic preganglionic nerves

Acetylcholinesterase (AchE) enzyme that resides in the synaptic cleft and catalyzes the destruction of Ach

Acetylcholinesterase (AchE) inhibitor indirect-acting cholinergic agonist that is nonselective and affects all Ach synapses

Acidosis condition of having too much acid in the blood; plasma pH below 7.35

Acne vulgaris condition characterized by small inflamed bumps that appear on the surface of the skin

Acquired immunodeficiency syndrome (AIDS) infection caused by the human immunodeficiency virus (HIV)

Acquired resistance when a microbe is no longer affected by a drug following treatment with anti-infectives

Acromegaly excessive growth hormone disorder in which bones become deformed

Action potential electrical change on the surface of a nerve or cardiac muscle cell that allows impulses to be transmitted

Activated partial thromboplastin time (aPTT) blood test used to determine how long it takes clots to form to regulate heparin dosage

Active immunity resistance resulting from a previous exposure to an antigen

Acute dystonia occurs during pharmacotherapy with antipsychotics and involves severe muscle spasms, particularly of the back, neck, tongue, and face

Acute gouty arthritis condition in which uric acid crystals accumulate in the joints of the big toes, ankles, wrists, fingers, knees, or elbows, resulting in red, swollen, or inflamed tissue

Acute retroviral syndrome symptoms during the initial phase of HIV infection

Adaptive defenses defenses that are specific to certain threats; the immune response

Addiction the continued use of a substance despite its negative health and social consequences

Addison's disease hyposecretion of glucocorticoids and aldosterone by the adrenal cortex

Additive effect type of drug interaction in which two agents combine to produce a stronger response or action

Adherence taking medications in the manner prescribed by the health care provider, or in the case of OTC drugs, following the instructions on the label; also called compliance

Adhesin chemicals secreted by certain bacteria that allow *H. pylori* to penetrate the GI mucosa and cause inflammation

Adipocytes fat cells

Adjuvant analgesics drugs that have indications other than pain but are used to enhance analgesia

Adjuvant chemotherapy technique in which antineoplastics are administered *after* surgery or radiation to effect a cure

Adrenal atrophy condition in which the adrenal cortex shrinks and stops secreting endogenous corticosteroids due to lack of stimulation by ACTH

Adrenal crisis condition that occurs when corticosteroid medication is abruptly withdrawn

Adrenergic receptors at the ends of postganglionic sympathetic neurons

Adrenergic agonists agents that activate adrenergic receptors in the sympathetic nervous system, also known as sympathomimetic nervous system

Adrenergic antagonists drugs that block the actions of the sympathetic nervous system

Adrenocortical insufficiency lack of adequate corticosteroid secretion by the adrenal gland

Adrenocorticotropic hormone (ACTH) hormone secreted by the anterior pituitary that stimulates the release of glucocorticoids by the adrenal cortex

Adverse drug effect an undesirable and potentially harmful action caused by the administration of medication

Aerobic pertaining to an oxygen environment

Aerosol suspension of minute liquid droplets or fine solid particles in a gas

Affinity the ability of some tissues to attract, accumulate, and store drugs in high concentrations relative to other tissues

Afterload pressure that must be overcome for the ventricles to eject blood from the heart

Agonist agent that is capable of binding with receptors and producing a response

Agoraphobia an avoidance of closed places where a panic attack might occur such as airplanes, public meetings, or elevators

Akathisia inability to remain still; constantly moving

Alimentary canal a long, continuous, hollow tube that extends from the mouth to the anus; the GI tract

Alkalosis condition of having too many basic substances in the blood; plasma pH above 7.45

Alkylating agents agents that kill cancer cells by altering the shape of the DNA double helix and preventing the DNA from duplicating during cell division

Allergen anything that is recognized as foreign by the body's defense system; also called antigen

Allergic rhinitis inflammation of the nasal mucosa due to exposure to allergens

Allopathy refers to conventional Western medicine that is focused on treating symptoms of the patient without addressing the underlying causes

Alopecia hair loss

Alpha-adrenergic antagonists drugs that block alpha-adrenergic receptors in the sympathetic nervous system

Alzheimer's disease (AD) most common dementia, characterized by loss of memory, delusions, hallucinations, confusion, and loss of judgment

Amide type of chemical linkage found in some local anesthetics involving carbon, nitrogen, and oxygen (–NH–CO–)

Amygdala A key part of the limbic system that generates feelings of anxiety and fear and stimulates several regions of the brain that begin the stress response

Anabolic effects testosterone hormone's ability to accelerate the growth of RBCs, muscle, bone, and neural tissues

Anabolic steroids compounds resembling testosterone with hormonal activity that are commonly abused by athletes

Anaerobic pertaining to an environment without oxygen

Analgesics drugs used to reduce or eliminate pain

Anaphylaxis acute allergic response to an antigen that results in severe hypotension and may lead to life-threatening shock if untreated

Androgens steroid sex hormones that promote the appearance of masculine characteristics

Anemia lack of adequate numbers of red blood cells, or decreased oxygen-carrying capacity of the blood

Angina pectoris acute chest pain on physical or emotional exertion due to inadequate oxygen supply to the myocardium

Angioedema rapid swelling of the throat, face, larynx, and tongue that can lead to airway obstruction and death

Angiogenesis the formation of new blood vessels

Angiotensin I a precursor to the formation of angiotensin II that is produced when angiotensinogen is split by the enzyme renin

Angiotensin II chemical released in response to falling blood pressure that causes vasoconstriction and release of aldosterone

Angiotensin-converting enzyme (ACE) enzyme responsible for converting angiotensin I to angiotensin II

Angiotensinogen protein synthesized by the liver that is continuously circulating in the bloodstream

Anorexiants drugs used to suppress appetite

Anovulatory cycle a menstrual cycle without ovulation

Antacids drugs that neutralize stomach acid

Antagonist agent that blocks the response of another drug

Antagonistic effect type of drug interaction in which adding a second drug results in a diminished pharmacologic response

Anterior pituitary gland comprised of glandular tissue that manufactures and secretes hormones that control major body functions and systems

Anterograde amnesia type of short-term memory loss where the user cannot remember events that occurred while under the influence of a drug

Anthrax an acute infectious disease that results from exposure to the spore-forming bacterium *Bacillus anthracis*

Antibiotic substance produced by a microorganism that inhibits or kills other microorganisms

Antibodies proteins produced by the body in response to an antigen; used interchangeably with the term immunoglobulin

Anticoagulants agents that inhibit the formation of blood clots

Antidepressants drugs that alter levels of two important neurotransmitters in the brain, norepinephrine and serotonin, to reduce depression and anxiety

Antidiuretic hormone (ADH) hormone released by the posterior pituitary gland when blood pressure falls or when the osmotic pressure of the blood increases

Antiflatulent agent that reduces gas bubbles in the stomach and intestines, thereby decreasing bloating and discomfort

Antigens microbes and foreign substances that elicit an immune response

Anti-infective general term for any medication that is effective against pathogens

Antipyretics drugs that lower body temperature

Antiretrovirals drugs that are effective against retroviruses

Antithrombin III (AT-III) protein that prevents abnormal clotting by inhibiting thrombin

Antitussives drugs used to suppress cough

Anxiety state of apprehension and autonomic nervous system activation resulting from exposure to a nonspecific or unknown cause

Anxiolytic drugs that relieve anxiety

Apoprotein protein component of a lipoprotein

Apothecary system of measurement older system on measurement developed in ancient Greece; rarely used in modern medicine

Appetite a psychological response that drives food intake based on associations and memory

Aqueous humor fluid that fills the anterior and posterior chambers of the eye

Assessment appraisal of a patient's condition that involves gathering and interpreting data

Asthma chronic inflammatory disease of the lungs characterized by airway obstruction

Atherosclerosis condition characterized by a buildup of fatty plaque and loss of elasticity of the walls of the arteries

Atonic seizures very short-lasting seizures during which the patient may stumble and fall for no apparent reason

Atrial natriuretic peptide (ANP) hormone secreted by specialized cells in the right atrium when large increases in blood volume produce excessive stretch on the atrial wall

Atrial reflex causes the heart rate and CO to increase until the backlog of venous blood (or IV fluid) is distributed throughout the body

Attention deficit/hyperactivity disorder (ADHD) disorder typically diagnosed in childhood characterized by hyperactivity as well as attention, organization, and behavior control issues

Attenuated organisms that have been rendered less able to cause disease through the application of heat or chemicals from which effective vaccines can be developed

Atypical antidepressant diverse class of drugs that act by mechanisms other than those of the SSRIs, TCAs, and MAOIs

Atypical mycobacterial infections (AMI) nontuberculosis opportunistic diseases caused by mycobacteria

Auras sensory cues such as bright lights, smells, or tastes that precede a migraine

Automaticity ability of certain myocardial cells to spontaneously generate an action potential

Automatisms repetitive arm movements, leg movements, head rolling, chewing, lip-smacking, or swallowing that occur in complex partial seizures

Autonomic nervous system (ANS) portion of the peripheral nervous system that provides involuntary control of vital functions of the cardiovascular, digestive, respiratory, and genitourinary systems

Autonomic tone the background level of autonomic activity that occurs even in the absence of stimuli

Azole term for the major class of drugs used to treat mycoses

Azoospermia complete absence of sperm in an ejaculate

B

B cell lymphocyte responsible for humoral immunity

β-glucan an essential component that shapes and strengthens the cell walls of fungi

Bacteriocidal a substance that kills bacteria

Bacteriostatic substance that inhibits the growth of bacteria

Bacteriuria uropathogens

Balanced anesthesia use of multiple medications to rapidly induce unconsciousness, cause muscle relaxation, and maintain deep anesthesia

Baroreceptors nerves located in the walls of the atria, aortic arch, vena cava, and carotid sinus that sense changes in blood pressure

Barrett's esophagus precancerous condition of the esophagus

Basal ganglia cluster of neurons in the brain that help regulate the initiation and termination of skeletal muscle movement

Basal nuclei area of the brain responsible for starting and stopping synchronized motor activity such as leg and arm motions during walking; also called basal ganglia

Beers criteria list of drugs compiled by physicians that have produced a high incidence of adverse effects in older adults

Belladonna natural source of alkaloids with anticholinergic activity acquired from the deadly nightshade plant, *Atropa belladonna*, which grows throughout the world

Benign prostatic hyperplasia (BPH) nonmalignant enlargement of the prostate gland

Best Pharmaceuticals for Children Act authorizes the FDA to contract for the testing of already approved pediatric drugs, or when the pharmaceutical company declines the option of exclusivity

Beta-adrenergic antagonists also called beta blockers, drugs that block beta-adrenergic receptors; may be nonselective or selective

Beta-lactam ring chemical structure found in most penicillins and some cephalosporins

Beta-lactamase enzyme present in certain bacteria that is able to inactivate many penicillins and some cephalosporins

Bioavailability the rate and extent to which the active ingredient is absorbed from a drug product and becomes available at the site of drug action to produce its effect

Biologic response modifiers natural cytokines that boost specific functions of the immune system

Bioterrorism intentional use of infectious biological agents, chemical substances, or radiation to cause widespread harm or illness

Bipolar disorder syndrome characterized by extreme and opposite moods, such as euphoria and depression

Bisphosphonates class of drugs that block bone resorption by inhibiting osteoclast activity

Blood-brain barrier anatomic structure that inhibits many chemicals and drugs from gaining access to the brain

Body mass index (BMI) measurement of obesity determined by dividing body weight (in kilograms) by the square of height (in meters)

Body surface area (BSA) method method of calculating pediatric dosages using an estimate of the child's BSA

Body weight method method of calculating pediatric dosages which requires a calculation of the number of milligrams of drug, based on the child's weight in kilograms (mg/kg)

Bolus feedings method of enteral feeding that typically delivers 250 to 400 mL of formula every 4 to 6 hours via a syringe or funnel

Bone deposition opposite of bone resorption; the process of depositing mineral components into bone

Bone resorption process of bone demineralization or the breaking down of bone into mineral components

Boosters follow-up doses of vaccines that are required to provide prolonged protection

Botanical plant extract used to treat or prevent illness

Botulism condition caused by *Clostridium botulinum*, an organism that secretes a potent toxin that paralyzes the muscles after a person is poisoned

Bradydysrhythmias disorders characterized by a heart rate of less than 60 beats/minute

Bradykinesia difficulty initiating movement and controlling fine muscle movements

Bradykinin chemical released by cells during inflammation that produces pain and side effects similar to those of histamine

Broad-spectrum antibiotic an anti-infective that is effective against many different gram positive and gram negative organisms

Bronchospasm rapid constriction of the airways

Buffers chemicals that help maintain normal body pH by neutralizing strong acids or bases

C

Cachexia general wasting of muscle and other tissue

Calcineurin intracellular messenger molecule to which immunosuppressants bind

Calcitonin hormone secreted by the thyroid gland that increases the deposition of calcium in bone

Calcitriol substance transformed in the kidneys during the second step of the conversion of vitamin D to its active form

Calcium channel type of voltage-gated channel in cardiac muscle and smooth muscles

Cancer malignant disease characterized by rapidly growing, invasive cells that spread to other regions of the body and eventually kill the host

Cannabinoid receptor (CB1) blockers class of antiobesity agents that block "pleasure" receptors in the brain

Capillary leak syndrome a serious condition in which plasma proteins and other substances leave the blood and enter the interstitial spaces because of porous capillaries

Capsid protein coat that surrounds a virus

Carbonic anhydrase enzyme that forms carbonic acid by combining carbon dioxide and water

Carcinogens agents that cause cancer

Cardiac output (CO) amount of blood pumped by a ventricle in 1 minute

Cardiac remodeling change in the size, shape, and structure of the myocardial cells (myocytes) that occurs over time in heart failure

Cardiotonic drugs agents that increase the force of cardiac contraction; also called inotropic agents

Cardioversion conversion of fibrillation to a normal heart rhythm; also called defibrillation

Cataplexy sudden loss of muscle strength manifested as slurred speech, sagging of the jaw, head nodding, or even complete collapse of the body

Catecholamines class of endogenous hormones involved in neurotransmission that include epinephrine (adrenalin), norepinephrine, and dopamine

Catechol-O-methyltransferase (COMT) enzyme that destroys norepinephrine in kidney and liver cells

Cathartic substance that causes complete evacuation of the bowel

CD4 receptor protein that accepts HIV and allows entry of the virus into the T4 lymphocyte

Cell-kill hypothesis theoretical model that predicts the ability of antineoplastic drugs to eliminate cancer cells

Central nervous system (CNS) stimulants agents that raise the general alertness level of the brain

Central vein total parenteral nutrition the administration of enteral feeding solution through a central vein

Cerumenolytics agent used to loosen and remove impacted cerumen from the ear canal

Chelation therapy use of agents to detoxify poisonous metals such as mercury, arsenic, and lead by converting them to a chemically inert form that can be easily excreted

Chemical name standard nomenclature for a drug assigned by the International Union of Pure and Applied Chemistry (IUPAC)

Chemoreceptors nerves located in the aortic arch and carotid sinus that sense changes in oxygen content, pH, or carbon dioxide levels in the blood

Chemoreceptor trigger zone (CTZ) location in the cerebral cortex which sends sensory signals to the vomiting center

Chemotherapy drug treatment of cancer

Chief cells cells located in the mucosa of the stomach that secrete pepsinogen, an inactive form of the enzyme pepsin that chemically breaks down proteins

Chloasma darkened pigmentation found on the forehead, temples, cheeks, and upper lips

Cholecalciferol vitamin D_3 formed in the skin by exposure to ultraviolet light

Cholestatic hepatitis a form of liver damage associated with the macrolide erythromycin estolate

Cholinergic relating to neurons that release acetylcholine

Cholinergic agonist drugs and chemicals that increase the action of acetylcholine (Ach) at a cholinergic receptor; also called a parasympathomimetic

Cholinergic crisis caused by an overdosage with acetylcholinesterase (AchE) inhibitors or poisoning with organophosphate insecticides or toxic nerve gases; characterized by intense signs of parasympathetic stimulation such as miosis, nausea, vomiting, urinary incontinence, increased exocrine secretions, and abdominal cramping

Cholinesterase inhibitors the most widely prescribed drug class for treating Alzheimer's Disease

Chronic bronchitis recurrent disease of the lungs characterized by excess mucus production, inflammation, and coughing

Chronic obstructive pulmonary disease (COPD) generic term used to describe several pulmonary conditions characterized by cough, mucus production, and impaired gas exchange

Chyme semifluid, partly digested food that is passed from the stomach to the duodenum

Cinchonism syndrome with symptoms such as tinnitus, headache, blurred vision, hearing loss, and dysrhythmias, caused by high doses of quinidine or quinine

Circadian rhythm cyclic basis by which body temperature, blood pressure, hormone levels, and respiration all fluctuate throughout the 24-hour day

Climacteric the period of endocrine, somatic, and psychological changes occurring in the transition to menopause

Clinical phase trials part of clinical investigation, the second stage of drug testing, which involves testing of a new drug in selected patients

Clonic spasms multiple, rapidly repeated muscular contractions

Closed-angle glaucoma acute glaucoma that is caused by decreased outflow of aqueous humor from the anterior chamber

Club drug a diverse group of abused substances taken by people at dance clubs, all-night parties, and raves

Coagulation process of blood clotting

Colloids types of IV fluids consisting of large organic molecules that are unable to cross membranes

Colony-stimulating factors (CSF) hormones that regulate the growth and maturation of specific WBC populations

Combination drug drug product with more than one active generic ingredient

Comedones types of acne lesions that develop just beneath the surface of the skin (whitehead) or as a result of a plugged oil gland (blackhead)

Complement system a cluster of 20 plasma proteins that combine together in a specific sequence and order when an infection occurs

Complementary and alternative medicine (CAM) treatments that consider the health of the whole person and promote disease prevention

Complex partial seizures seizures that originate from a single focus and involve sensory, motor, or autonomic symptoms with some degree of altered or impaired consciousness

COMT inhibitors drugs that prevent the destruction of levodopa in peripheral tissues, thus increasing the amount of levodopa available to enter the brain

Conjugation the direct transfer of small pieces of DNA from one bacterium to another

Constipation infrequent passage of abnormally hard and dry stools

Continuous infusion feeding enteral feedings delivered by an infusion pump at a slow rate over a 16- to 24-hour period

Contraception the use of devices, drugs, or surgery to prevent pregnancy

Contractility the strength with which the myocardial fibers contract

Controlled substance in the United States, a drug whose use is restricted by the Comprehensive Drug Abuse Prevention and Control Act; in Canada, a drug subject to guidelines outlined in the Canadian Narcotic Control Act

Convulsions uncontrolled muscle contractions or spasms that occur in the face, torso, arms, or legs

Coronary artery disease (CAD) a narrowing or occlusion of one or more coronary arteries

Corpora cavernosa tissue in the penis that fills with blood during an erection

Corpus luteum endocrine tissue formed from a ruptured follicle that remains in the ovary after ovulation and secretes progestins

Council for Responsible Nutrition (CRN) trade association that represents suppliers and manufacturers in the dietary supplement industry

Cretinism condition marked by profound mental retardation and impaired growth that results from untreated congenital hypothyroidism

Cross-tolerance situation in which tolerance to one drug makes the patient tolerant to another drug

Crystalloids types of IV fluid resembling blood plasma minus proteins that are capable of crossing membranes

Crystalluria crystals that form in the urine and potentially obstruct the kidneys or ureters

Cultural competence the ability of health care providers to care for people with diverse values, beliefs, and behaviors, including the ability to adapt delivery of care to meet the needs of these patients

Culture set of beliefs, values, religious rituals, language, customs, and behavioral expectations that provide meaning for an individual or group

Culture and sensitivity (C&S) testing a laboratory test used to identify bacteria and to determine which antibiotic is most effective

Curare the first neuromuscular blocker, which was initially extracted from several different plant species native to the rainforests of South America

Cushing's syndrome condition of having an excessive concentration of corticosteroids in the blood; caused by excessive secretion by the adrenal glands or by overdosage with corticosteroid medication

Cyclic feeding enteral feedings that are commonly infused over 8 to 16 hours daily

Cyclic lipopeptides new class of antibiotics that act on gram-positive pathogens

Cyclooxygenase (COX) key enzyme in the prostaglandin metabolic pathway that is blocked by aspirin and other NSAIDs

Cycloplegic drugs that relax or temporarily paralyze ciliary muscles and cause blurred vision

Cystitis bladder infection

Cysts protective capsules formed by some protozoa that allow the organisms to survive in harsh environments in a dormant state for prolonged time periods

Cytokine release syndrome an acute inflammatory response that occurs 30-60 minutes following the initial IV administration of muromonab due to massive cytokine release

Cytokines chemicals produced by white blood cells, such as interleukins, leukotrienes, interferon, and tumor necrosis factor, that guide the immune response

D

Deep vein thrombosis (DVT) thrombosis that occurs in the legs

Defecation evacuation of the colon; bowel movement

Defibrillation conversion of fibrillation to a normal heart rhythm; also called cardioversion

Delirium tremens a syndrome of intense agitation, confusion, terrifying hallucinations, uncontrollable tremors, panic attacks, and paranoia caused by alcohol withdrawal

Delusions false ideas and beliefs not founded in reality

Dementia degenerative disorder characterized by progressive memory loss, confusion, and the inability to think or communicate effectively

Dependence a powerful physiological or psychological need for a substance

Depolarization reversal of the plasma membrane charge such that the inside is made less negative

Depression characterized by a sad or despondent mood that becomes out of proportion to actual life events

Dermatitis inflammatory condition of the skin characterized by itching and scaling

Dermatomycosis fungal infections of the skin and hair

Diabetes insipidus disorder marked by excessive urination due to lack of secretion of antidiuretic hormone

Diabetic ketoacidosis (DKA) a type of metabolic acidosis due to an excess of ketone bodies, most often occurring when diabetes mellitus is uncontrolled

Diarrhea abnormal frequency and liquidity of bowel movements

Dietary supplement nondrug substance regulated by the DSHEA

Dietary Supplement and Nonprescription Drug Consumer Protection Act law that requires companies that market herbal and dietary supplements to include their address and phone number on the product labels so consumers can report adverse events

Dietary Supplement Health and Education Act of 1994 (DSHEA) primary law in the United States regulating herb and dietary supplements

Diffusion the movement of a chemical from an area of higher concentration to an area of lower concentration

Digestion the mechanical and chemical breakdown of food into a form that may be absorbed into the systemic circulation

Digestive system body system consisting of the alimentary canal and the accessory organs

Digitalization procedure in which the dose of cardiac glycoside is gradually increased until tissues become saturated with the drug, and the symptoms of heart failure diminish

Dihydropyridine the largest class of CCBs that bind reversibly to closed-type (inactivated) calcium channels to make them unresponsive to depolarization

Directly observed therapy (DOT) requires that a health care provider directly observe the patient swallowing the pills, whether it is in the hospital, office, or home care setting

Disease-modifying antirheumatic drug (DMARD) drugs that modify the progression of rheumatoid arthritis

Dissociative anesthesia a trance-like feeling of being separated from the environment produced by an anesthetic agent

Distribution the transport of drugs throughout the body after they are absorbed

Diuretic substance that increases urine output

Diuretic resistance phenomenon in some patients who become less responsive as therapy continues with loop diuretics

DNA gyrase (topoisomerase II) in bacterial DNA replication, the enzyme that relaxes the supercoil

DNA helicase in bacterial DNA replication, the enzyme that unwinds the two DNA strands after the supercoil is relaxed

DNA polymerase in bacterial DNA replication, the enzyme that adds the precursor bases to replicate the original DNA and form new DNA strands

Dopamine chemical precursor in the synthesis of norepinephrine; classified as a catecholamine

Dopamine system stabilizer (DSS) drugs that exhibit both antagonist and partial agonist activities on dopamine receptors

Dopamine type 2 (D_2) receptors receptors for dopamine in the basal nuclei of the brain that is associated with schizophrenia and antipsychotic drugs

Dose-limiting toxicity specific types of toxicity that could cause discontinuation or temporary delays of therapy

Dose-response relationship the way a patient responds to varying doses of a drug

Down-regulation the process by which cells make fewer receptors on their surface

Drug any substance that is taken to prevent, cure, or reduce symptoms of a medical condition

Drug allergies a hyperresponse of body defenses to a particular drug that may result in a diverse range of patient symptoms

Drug interaction occurs when a medication interacts with another substance such as another drug, a dietary supplement, an herbal product, or food that is taken concurrently with the medication, and the drug's actions are affected

Drug misuse improper use of drugs that includes overuse, underuse, or, in some cases, erratic use

Drug-protein complex formed when a drug that binds reversibly to a plasma protein, particularly albumin, that makes the drug unavailable for distribution to body tissues

Dry powder inhaler (DPI) device used to convert a solid drug to a fine powder for the purpose of inhalation

Dumping syndrome the result of a sudden influx of enteral feeding into the GI tract and the creation of a high osmotic gradient within the small intestine

Dwarfism a GH deficiency disorder in children associated with normal birth length followed by a slowing of the growth rate

Dysfunctional uterine bleeding hemorrhage that occurs at abnormal times or in excessive quantity during the menstrual cycle

Dyslipidemia abnormal (excess or deficient) level of lipoproteins in the blood

Dysrhythmias abnormality in cardiac rhythm

Dystonia severe muscle spasms, particularly of the back, neck, tongue, and face; characterized by abnormal tension starting in one area of the body and progressing to other areas

E

Eclampsia pregnancy-induced hypertensive disorder

Ectopic foci cardiac tissue outside the normal cardiac conduction pathway that generates action potentials

Ectopic pregnancy the development of the fetus elsewhere rather than in the uterus

Eczema a skin disorder with unexplained symptoms of inflammation, itching, and scaling; also called atopic dermatitis

Efficacy the maximal response that can be produced from a particular drug

Electrocardiogram (ECG) device that records the electrical activity of the heart

Electroconvulsive therapy (ECT) treatment used for serious and life-threatening mood disorders in patients who are unresponsive to pharmacotherapy

Electrolyte charged substance in the blood such as sodium, potassium, calcium, chloride, and phosphate

Emergency contraception (EC) the prevention of implantation following unprotected intercourse

Emergency preparedness the ability to respond quickly and effectively to an unexpected event that may impact human health

Emetic potential usually applied to antineoplastic agents; degree to which an agent is likely to trigger the vomiting center in the medulla, resulting in nausea and vomiting

Emetogenic potential the capacity of a chemotherapeutic drug to cause vomiting

Emphysema terminal lung disease characterized by permanent dilation of the alveoli

Endocrine system body system that consists of various glands that secrete hormones

Endometriosis presence of endometrial tissue in non uterine locations such as the pelvis and ovaries; a common cause of infertility

Endorphins a group of neurotransmitters that function as endogenous opioids or natural pain modifiers in the central nervous system (CNS)

Endotoxins harmful nonproteins that are part of the normal cell wall of gram-negative bacteria

Enteral nutrition (EN) nutrients supplied orally or by feeding tube

Enteral route administration of drugs orally or through nasogastric or gastrostomy tubes

Enteric-coated tablets that have a hard, waxy coating designed to dissolve in the alkaline environment of the small intestine

Enteric nervous system (ENS) network of neurons in the submucosa of the alimentary canal that has sensory and motor functions which regulate the GI tract

Enteroendocrine cells cells that secrete hormones that modify the digestive processes

Enterohepatic recirculation recycling of drugs and other substances by the circulation of bile through the intestine and liver

Enzyme induction process by which a drug increases the activity of the hepatic microsomal enzymes

Ephedra plant species that originally provided the source of the non-catecholamine ephedrine, that activates both alpha and beta receptors

Epilepsy disorder of the CNS characterized by seizures with or without convulsions

Erectile dysfunction (ED) consistent inability to either attain an erection or to sustain an erection long enough to achieve satisfactory sexual intercourse

Ergosterol lipid substance in fungal cell membranes

Erythema redness associated with skin irritation

Erythrocytic stage phase in malaria during which infected red blood cells rupture, releasing more merozoites and causing fever and chills

Erythropoietin hormone secreted by the kidney that regulates the process of red blood cell formation, or erythropoiesis

Esters types of chemical linkage found in some local anesthetics involving carbon and oxygen (–CO–O–)

Estrogen class of steroid sex hormones secreted by the ovary

Ethnicity groups of people with biologic and genetic similarities

Etiologies the part of the nursing diagnosis that identifies those conditions that have caused or contributed to the problem or condition

Euphoria an intense sense of happiness and well-being

Evaluation systematic objective assessment of the effectiveness and impact of interventions

Evaluation criteria specific and measurable achievements that will be used to determine if a particular goal has been met

Evidence-based nursing practice basing nursing practice, especially interventions, on research evidence

Exclusivity after approval of a drug application by the U.S. Food and Drug Administration, a period of time when competing companies are not allowed to market generic versions of a drug

Excoriation scratch that breaks the skin surface and fills with blood or serous fluid to form a crusty scale

Excretion the process of removing substances from the body

Exophthalmos an outward bulging of the eyes

Exotoxin proteins released by bacteria into surrounding tissues that have the ability to inactivate or kill host cells

Expectorants drugs used to increase bronchial secretions

Expiration date approximation of when a drug will begin to lose its effectiveness

Extended release tablets or capsules designed to dissolve very slowly, resulting in a longer duration of action for the medication; also called sustained release

External otitis an inflammation of the outer ear, commonly called *swimmer's ear*

Extracellular fluid (ECF) compartment of body fluid lying outside cells, which includes plasma and interstitial fluid

Extrapyramidal symptoms (EPS) symptoms of acute dystonia, akathisia, parkinsonism, and tardive dyskinesia often caused by antipsychotic drugs

Extrapyramidal system part of the CNS that controls locomotion, complex muscular movements, and posture

Extrinsic pathway activated in response to injury when blood leaks out of a vessel and enters tissue spaces and takes several seconds to complete

F

Fasting plasma glucose (FPG) test a primary blood test for diagnosing diabetes

Fat-soluble vitamins group of vitamins stored in the liver and fatty tissue that include A, D, E, and K

Febrile seizures tonic–clonic motor activity lasting 1 to 2 minutes with rapid return of consciousness that occurs in conjunction with elevated body temperature

Ferritin one of two protein complexes that maintain iron stores inside cells (hemosiderin is the other)

Fetal-placental barrier special anatomic barrier that inhibits many chemicals and drugs from entering the fetus

Fibrin an insoluble protein formed from fibrinogen by the action of thrombin in the blood clotting process

Fibrinogen blood protein that is converted to fibrin by the action of thrombin in the blood coagulation process

Fibrinolysis removal of a blood clot

Fight-or-flight response characteristic set of actions produced when the sympathetic nervous system is activated that prepares the body for heightened activity and for an immediate response to a threat

Filtrate fluid in the nephron that is filtered at Bowman's capsule

First dose phenomenon serious orthostatic hypotension that occurs with the initial doses of $alpha_1$-adrenergic blockers

First-pass effect mechanism whereby drugs are absorbed, enter into the hepatic portal circulation and are inactivated by the liver before they reach the general circulation

Folate B vitamin that is a coenzyme in protein and nucleic acid metabolism

Folic acid B vitamin that is a coenzyme in protein and nucleic acid metabolism

Food and Drug Administration (FDA) U.S. agency responsible for the evaluation and approval of new drugs

Food and Drug Administration (FDA) Modernization Act gave financial incentives for pharmaceutical companies to conduct pediatric research in pharmacology; in exchange for providing pediatric labeling, the legislation gives drug companies the ability to exclusively market the drug for 6 months with no competition

Frequency distribution curve a graphic representation of the actual number of patients responding to a particular drug action at different doses

Formulary list of drug and drug recipes commonly used by pharmacists

Fungi kingdom of organisms that includes mushrooms, yeasts, and molds

G

Gamma aminobutyric acid (GABA) neurotransmitter in the CNS

Ganglia collection of neuron cell bodies located outside the central nervous system

Ganglionic blocker drug that inhibits transmission at the ganglia in the sympathetic and parasympathetic nervous systems

Gastroesophageal reflux disease (GERD) regurgitation of stomach contents into the esophagus

Gate control theory proposes a gating mechanism in the spinal cord that blocks the transmission of pain impulses

General anesthesia medical procedure that produces unconsciousness and loss of sensation throughout the entire body

Generalized anxiety disorder (GAD) difficult-to-control, excessive anxiety that lasts 6 months or more, focuses on a variety of life events, and interferes with normal day-to-day functions

Generalized seizures seizures that travel throughout the entire brain

Generic name name assigned to a drug by the United States Adopted Name Council

Genetic polymorphism changes in enzyme structure and function due to mutation of the encoding gene

Gestational diabetes condition resulting from glucose intolerance with an onset, or first recognition, during pregnancy

Gigantism unusual tallness

Glaucoma condition that is characterized by optic neuropathy with gradual loss of peripheral vision and usually accompanied by increased intraocular pressure

Glomerular filtration rate (GFR) the volume of water filtered through the Bowman's capsules per minute

Glomerulus a specialized capillary in the Bowman's capsule of the kidney that filters the blood during the initial stage of urine formation

Glucocorticoids class of hormones secreted by the adrenal cortex that help the body respond to stress

Gluconeogenesis the production of "new" glucose from noncarbohydrate molecules

Glutamate amino acid that is the most common neurotransmitter in the CNS, found in nearly all regions of the brain

Glycogenolysis the process of glycogen breaking down

Glycoprotein IIb/IIIa enzyme that binds fibrinogen and von Willebrand's factor to begin platelet aggregation and blood coagulation

Goal any object or objective that the patient or nurse seeks to attain or achieve

Goiter refers to an increase in the size of the thyroid gland

Gonadocorticoids sex hormones secreted by the adrenal cortex; also called corticosteroids

Gout metabolic disorder characterized by the accumulation of uric acid in the bloodstream or joint cavities

Grading process that examines potential cancer cells under a microscope and compares their appearance to normal parent cells

Gram negative bacteria that do not retain a purple stain because they have an outer envelope

Gram positive bacteria that stain purple because they have no outer envelope

Graves' disease syndrome caused by hypersecretion of thyroid hormone

Gray baby syndrome serious condition seen most often in premature or newborn infants, that occurs when the baby's liver is unable to metabolize or excrete chloramphenicol

Growth fraction the ratio of the number of replicating cells to resting cells in a tumor

Growth hormone (GH) hormone that is produced and secreted by the anterior pituitary gland

H

H^+, K^+ -ATPase enzyme responsible for pumping acid onto the mucosal surface of the stomach

H_1 receptors sites located on smooth-muscle cells in the bronchial tree and blood vessels that are stimulated by histamine to produce bronchodilation and vasodilation

H_2-receptor antagonist drug that inhibits the effects of histamine at its receptors in the GI tract

Hallucinations seeing, hearing, or feeling things that are not real

Hallucinogens chemicals that have the ability to produce an altered, dreamlike state of consciousness

Hashimoto's thyroiditis an autoimmune disorder that is the most common cause of hypothyroidism

Heart failure (HF) disease in which the heart muscle cannot contract with sufficient force to meet the body's metabolic needs

Helminths type of flat, round, or segmented worms

Hemagglutinin an enzyme that facilitates the attachment of the virus to host cells

Hematopoiesis process of erythrocyte production that begins with primitive stem cells that reside in bone marrow

Hematopoietic growth factor substance that stimulates the production of RBCs, which may prevent the development of anemia

Hemoglobin A1C a laboratory test used in diabetic management; also called glycosylated hemoglobin

Hemophilia hereditary lack of a specific blood clotting factor

Hemopoiesis production and maturation of blood cells which occurs in red bone marrow

Hemosiderin one of two protein complexes that maintain iron stores inside cells (ferritin is the other)

Hemostasis the slowing or stopping of blood flow

Hepatic microsomal enzyme system as it relates to pharmacotherapy, liver enzymes that inactivate drugs and accelerate their excretion; sometimes called the P-450 system

Hepatic portal system a network of venous vessels that collects blood draining from the stomach, small intestine, and most of the large intestine

Hepatitis viral infection of the liver

Herb plant with a soft stem that is used for healing or as a seasoning

High-density lipoprotein (HDL) lipid-carrying particle in the blood that contains high amounts of protein and lower amounts of cholesterol; considered to be "good" cholesterol

Highly active antiretroviral therapy (HAART) drug therapy for HIV infection that includes high doses of multiple medications given concurrently

Histamine chemical released by mast cells in response to an antigen that causes dilation of blood vessels, bronchoconstriction, tissue swelling, and itching

HMG-CoA reductase primary enzyme in the biochemical pathway for the synthesis of cholesterol

Holistic viewing a person as an integrated biologic, psychological, social, cultural, spiritual whole, existing and functioning within the communal environment

Home care nurse monitors the patient's condition, including medication adherence and reporting any adverse effects, and works with the health care provider and pharmacist to achieve optimal therapeutic outcomes

Hormone replacement therapy (HRT) drug therapy, consisting of estrogen and progestin combinations; used to treat symptoms associated with menopause

Hormones chemicals secreted by endocrine glands that act as chemical messengers to affect homeostasis

Hospice nursing the care of terminally ill patients in their homes or in a health care facility and involves effective pain management

Host flora normal microorganisms found in or on a client

Household system of measurement older system of measurement that uses teaspoons, tablespoons, and cups

Human immunodeficiency virus (HIV) the causative agent for AIDS

Hyperaldosteronism excessive secretion of aldosterone

Hypercholesterolemia high levels of cholesterol in the blood

Hyperemesis gravidarum condition of continual vomiting during pregnancy

Hyperkalemia serum potassium level above 5 mEq/L

Hyperkinetic disorder (HKD) refers to the diagnosis of ADHD in Canada

Hyperlipidemia excess amount of lipids in the blood

Hypernatremia high sodium level in the blood

Hyperosmolar hyperglycemic state (HHS) acute complication seen in persons with type 2 diabetes, that is characterized by extreme hyperglycemia, hyperosmolarity with dehydration, the absence of ketoacidosis, and CNS dysfunction

Hypertension (HTN) high blood pressure

Hypertensive emergency (HTN-E) a diastolic pressure of greater than 120 mmHg, with evidence of target-organ system damage; also called hypertensive crisis

Hypertensive urgency severe hypertension, but with no evidence of target-organ damage

Hypertrichosis the elongation, thickening, and increased pigmentation of body hair

Hypertriglyceridemia refers to an increase in triglyceride levels

Hyperuricemia elevated blood level of uric acid, which causes gout

Hypervitaminosis excess intake of vitamins

Hypnagogic hallucinations vivid, dreamlike sensations, sometimes of a frightening nature, that occur with sleep paralysis

Hypoaldosteronism lack of adequate aldosterone secretion

Hypogonadism below-normal secretion of the steroid sex hormones

Hypokalemia serum potassium level below 3.5 mEq/L

Hypomania characterized by the same symptoms as bipolar disorder, but they are less severe and do not cause impaired functioning

Hyponatremia low sodium level in the blood

I

Idiosyncratic response unpredictable and unexplained drug reaction

Immunity ability to resist injury and infections

Immunization process of disease prevention in which the body produces its own antibodies in response to initial exposure to antigens

Immunomodulator general term that refers to drugs that affect body defenses

Immunostimulants drugs that increase the ability of the immune system to fight infection and disease

Immunosuppressants any drug, chemical, or physical agent that lowers the immune defense mechanisms of the body

Implementation when the nurse applies the knowledge, skills, and principles of nursing care to help move the patient toward the desired goal and optimal wellness

Impotence inability to obtain or sustain an erection; also called erectile dysfunction

Incretin enhancer synthetic drug that augments natural glucose-lowering hormones by preventing the breakdown of incretins

Incretin mimetic synthetic drug that augments natural glucose-lowering hormones that has all the actions of the natural drug

Incubation period following the first exposure to the antigen, the time needed for the body to process the antigen and mount an effective response

Indication the medical conditions for which a drug is approved

Infantile spasm also called West syndrome, usually occurs in the first year of life and is characterized by a sudden bending forward, body stiffening, or arching of the torso

Infertility inability to become pregnant after at least 1 year of frequent, unprotected intercourse

Inflammation nonspecific body defense that occurs in response to an injury or antigen

Inflammatory bowel disease (IBD) disease characterized by the presence of ulcers in the distal portion of the small intestine (Crohn's disease) or mucosal erosions in the large intestine (ulcerative colitis)

Influenza a viral infection characterized by acute symptoms that include sore throat, sneezing, coughing, fever, and chills; also called flu

Ingestion the process of taking food into the body by mouth

Inoculation the placement of a foreign substance on or in an individual for the purpose of disease prevention using "live" virus particles obtained from an infected patient

Inotropic agents drugs or chemicals that increase the force of contraction of the heart; also called cardiotonic drugs

Insomnia inability to fall asleep or stay asleep

Insulin pancreatic hormone that acts to decrease blood glucose levels

Insulin resistance occurs in type 2 diabetes mellitus; insulin receptors in target tissues become insensitive to insulin

Insulin-like growth factor (IGF) a family of peptides that promote cartilage and bone growth

Integrase an enzyme unique to HIV which incorporates the viral DNA into the host's chromosomes

Interferons (IFNs) type of cytokine secreted by T cells in response to antigens to protect uninfected cells

Interleukins (ILs) class of cytokines synthesized by lymphocytes, monocytes, macrophages, and certain other cells that enhance the capabilities of the immune system

Intermittent feeding enteral feedings that are administered every 3 to 6 hours

Intervention nursing action that produces an effect or that is intended to alter the course of a disease or condition

Intracellular fluid (ICF) compartment contains water that is inside cells

Intracellular parasite infectious microbe that lives inside host cells

Intrinsic activity the ability of a drug to bind to a receptor and produce a strong action

Intrinsic factor chemical substance secreted by the parietal cells in the stomach that is essential for the absorption of vitamin B_{12}

Intrinsic pathway coagulation pathway activated in response to injury and takes several minutes to complete

Intrinsic sympathomimetic activity (ISA) low level of beta-agonist activity possessed by certain beta adrenergic blockers

Invasiveness is the ability of a pathogen to grow extremely rapidly and cause direct damage to surrounding tissues by their sheer numbers

Investigational new drug (IND) application to the FDA that contains all the animal and cell testing data

Iodism toxicity to Lugol's iodine solution therapy

Ion trapping phenomenon in which alkalinizing agents are used to aid in the renal excretion of toxic substances

Irritable bowel syndrome (IBS) inflammatory disease of the small or large intestine, characterized by intense abdominal cramping and diarrhea

Irritative voiding symptoms syndrome of complaints that accompanies cystitis

Isozyme multiple, similar forms of an enzyme that perform slightly different metabolic functions

J

Juxtaglomerular (JG) cells specialized smooth muscle cells found in the afferent arteriole that sense blood pressure and release rennin

K

Kappa receptors is one of two major endorphin receptors in the CNS where opioids act

Keratolytic action that promotes shedding of old skin

Ketolides class of antibiotics that block bacterial protein synthesis by binding to two different sites on the 50S ribosomal subunit

L

Laxative drug that promotes defecation

Lecithins phospholipids that are an important component of cell membranes

Lennox-Gestaut syndrome mixed seizure that has characteristics of tonic–clonic, atonic, and atypical absence seizures

Leprosy a chronic infection caused by *Mycobacterium leprae*

Leptin hormone that regulates hunger and weight balance

Leucovorin rescue therapy drug therapy administered following chemotherapy with toxic folic acid analogs such as methotrexate to rescue normal cells

Leukotrienes chemical mediators of inflammation stored and released by mast cells; effects are similar to those of histamine

Leydig cells the primary cells in the testes that are responsible for androgen secretion

Libido interest in sexual activity

Limbic system area in the brain responsible for emotion, learning, memory, motivation, and mood

Lipodystrophy a disorder in which fat is redistributed in specific areas in the body

Lipoprotein substance carrying lipids in the bloodstream that is composed of proteins bound to fat

Loading dose relatively large dose given at the beginning of treatment to rapidly obtain therapeutic serum levels of a drug

Local anesthesia loss of sensation to a limited part of the body without loss of consciousness

Locus coeruleus within the brainstem, an area in the pons that has been associated with fear responses and panic attacks

Low-density lipoprotein (LDL) lipoprotein that carries the highest amount of cholesterol

Lymph nodes the principal lymphoid organs in the body

Lymphatic system comprised of a network of cells, vessels, and tissues that provide immune surveillance

M

Macrominerals inorganic compound needed by the body in amounts of 100 mg or more daily

Macula densa specialized cells in the distal convoluted tubule of the nephron that sense the flow rate and osmolality in the filtrate and send a message to the juxtaglomerular cells to release more renin

Maintenance dose amount of drug that keeps the plasma drug concentration in the therapeutic range

Major depressive disorder a depressed mood lasting for a minimum of 2 weeks that is present for most of the day, every day, or almost every day

Malaria tropical disease characterized by severe fever and chills caused by the protozoan *Plasmodium*

Malignant hyperthermia rare condition that is an adverse effect of some general anesthetics characterized by a sudden onset of tachycardia, ventricular dysrhythmia, and hypotension

Mania condition characterized by an expressive, impulsive, excitable, and overreactive nature

Mast cell stabilizers drugs that inhibit the release of inflammatory mediators from mast cells

Mastoiditis inflammation of the mastoid sinus

Median effective dose (ED_{50}) the dose of a drug required to produce a specific therapeutic response in 50% of a group of patients

Median lethal dose (LD_{50}) the dose of a drug that will kill 50% of a group of animals

Median toxicity dose (TD_{50}) dose that will produce a given toxicity in 50% of a group of patients

Medication administration record (MAR) legal documentation of all pharmacotherapies received by the patient

Medication error any preventable event that may cause or lead to inappropriate medication use or patient harm while the medication is in the control of the health care provider, patient, or consumer

Medication error index categorization of medication errors according to the degree of harm an error can cause

Medication reconciliation the process of keeping track of a patient's medications as they proceed from one health care provider to another

Menopause period of time during which females stop secreting estrogen and menstrual cycles cease

Merozoites transformation of sporozoites carried by the blood to the liver inside the human host where they multiply into millions of progeny

Metabolic bone disease (MBD) refers to a cluster of disorders that have in common defects in the structure of bone

Metabolic syndrome a group of abnormalities that tend to occur together that places the patient at increased risk for developing diabetes and vascular complications disease, and CVA

Metabolism the process used by the body to chemically change a drug molecule

Metastasis travel of cancer cells from their original site to a distant tissue

Metered-dose inhaler (MDI) device used to deliver a precise amount of drug to the respiratory system

Methylxanthine chemical class for theophylline and caffeine

Metric system of measurement the most common system of drug measurement that uses liters, milliliters, and grams

Microbial antagonism condition of various host flora in competition with each other for physical space and nutrients that helps protect the host from being overrun by pathogenic organisms

Microminerals inorganic compound needed by the body in amounts of 20 mg or less daily

Migraine severe headache preceded by auras and that may include nausea and vomiting

Milk-alkali syndrome syndrome caused by the administration of calcium carbonate antacids with milk or food containing vitamin D; symptoms include headache, urinary frequency, anorexia, nausea, and fatigue

Mineralocorticoids hormones secreted by the adrenal glands that affect the secretion of sodium and water

Minerals essential substances that constitute about 4% of the body weight and serve many diverse functions

Minimum alveolar concentration describes the potency of inhalation anesthetics

Minimum effective concentration amount of drug required to produce a therapeutic effect

Miosis constriction of the pupil

Mitochondrial toxicity specific type of adverse effects resulting from a drug's toxic actions on mitochondria

Modular formulas enteral feedings that contain a single nutrient, protein, carbohydrate, or lipid, and yield a high caloric density

Molecularly targeted agents refers to certain monoclonal antibodies (MABs) that are engineered to attack the antigens that are present on the surface of specific tumor cells

Monitored anesthesia care (MAC) use of sedatives, analgesics, and other low-dose drugs that allow patients to remain responsive and breathe without assistance

Monoamine oxidase (MAO) enzyme that destroys norepinephrine in the nerve terminal

Monoamine oxidase inhibitor (MAOI) drug inhibiting monoamine oxidase, an enzyme that terminates the actions of neurotransmitters such as dopamine, norepinephrine, epinephrine, and serotonin

Monoclonal antibodies (MABs) antibodies produced by a single B cell that target a single type of cell or receptor

Mood disorder change in behavior such as clinical depression, emotional swings, or manic depression

Mood stabilizer drug that levels mood that is used to treat bipolar disorder and mania

Motor end plate cholinergic synapse on skeletal muscle that allows for communication between the nervous system and skeletal muscle

Mu receptor type of opioid receptor

Mucolytics drugs used to loosen thick mucus

Mucositis inflammation of the epithelial lining of the digestive tract

Muscarinic type of cholinergic receptor found at postganglionic nerve endings in the parasympathetic nervous system that when activated, result in stimulation

Muscarinic agonist drug that is selective for muscarinic receptors

Muscarinic antagonists drugs that block receptors at cholinergic synapses in the parasympathetic nervous system and at a few target organs in the sympathetic nervous system

Muscle rigidity stiffness occurring in Parkinson's Disease that causes difficulty bending over and moving limbs; changes in facial expression, or a lack of facial expression

Muscle spasms involuntary contractions of a muscle or group of muscles, which become tightened, develop a fixed pattern of resistance, and result in a diminished level of functioning

Muscle spasticity condition caused by damage to the CNS in which certain muscle groups remain in a continuous state of contraction

Mutations permanent, inheritable change in the structure of DNA

Myasthenia gravis (MG) muscular disorder caused by a destruction of nicotinic synapses on skeletal muscles and characterized by extreme fatigue, double vision, speech impairment, and difficulty chewing or swallowing

Myasthenic crisis extreme muscular weakness and symptoms similar to those of cholinergic crisis; caused by abrupt discontinuation of medication for myasthenia gravis

***Mycobacterium avium* complex (MAC)** infection that usually arises as a secondary infection due to the immunosuppression caused by HIV-AIDS

Mycolic acid a complex lipid that covers the cell surfaces of the genus *Mycobacterium*, which protects them and makes them resistant to many disinfectants

Mycoses diseases caused by fungi

Mydriasis pupil dilation

Mydriatic agent that causes pupil dilation

Myeloablation complete destruction of hematopoietic bone marrow cells

Myocardial infarction (MI) blood clot blocking a portion of a coronary artery that causes necrosis of cardiac muscle

Myocardial ischemia lack of blood supply to the myocardium due to a constriction or obstruction of a blood vessel

Myocardium the muscular layer of the heart, responsible for its physical pumping action

Myoclonic seizures seizures characterized by brief, sudden contractions of a group of muscles

Myxedema condition caused by insufficient secretion of thyroid hormone

Myxedematous coma a life-threatening end-stage condition of hypothyroidism

N

Nadir lowest values of erythrocyte, leukocyte, and platelet counts caused by chemotherapy

Narcoanalysis a procedure in which the patient is placed in a drug-induced hypnotic state but is able to answer questions or explore painful memories

Narcolepsy sleep disorder that is characterized by severe daytime sleepiness and inability to stay awake

Narcotic natural or synthetic drug related to morphine; may be used as a broader legal term referring to hallucinogens, CNS stimulants, marijuana, and other illegal drugs

Narrow-spectrum antibiotic an anti-infective that is effective against only one or a small number of organisms

Natriuresis sodium excretion in the urine

Natriuretic peptide substances secreted in response to increased pressure in the heart

Nausea uncomfortable wavelike sensation that precedes vomiting

Nebulizer device used to convert liquid drugs into a fine mist for the purpose of inhalation; also called small volume nebulizer

Negative chronotropic effect the property of slowing the speed of electrical conduction across the myocardium

Negative feedback in homeostasis, the shutting off of first hormone in a pathway by the last hormone or product in the pathway

Negative inotropic effect the reduction in the force of myocardial contraction

Negative symptoms in schizophrenia, symptoms that subtract from normal behavior, including a lack of interest, motivation, responsiveness, or pleasure in daily activities

Neoadjuvant chemotherapy the administration of antineoplastic drugs before surgery or radiation therapy with the goal of shrinking a large tumor to a more manageable size

Neoplasm abnormal swelling or mass; same as *tumor*

Nephrons structural and functional units of the kidney

Neuraminidase an enzyme that assists the virus in exiting the host cell

Neurodegenerative disease degenerative diseases of the CNS that include a diverse set of disorders differing in their causes and outcomes

Neuroeffector junction specialized synapse where the postganglionic neuron terminates on smooth muscle, cardiac muscle, or gland

Neurofibrillary tangles bundles of nerve fibers found in the brain of patients with Alzheimer's disease on autopsy

Neurolept analgesia type of general anesthesia that combines fentanyl with droperidol to produce a state in which patients are conscious though insensitive to pain and unconnected with surroundings

Neuroleptic malignant syndrome (NMS) potentially fatal condition caused by certain antipsychotic medications characterized by an extremely high body temperature, drowsiness, changing blood pressure, irregular heartbeat, and muscle rigidity

Neuromuscular blockers drug used to cause total muscle relaxation

Neuron the primary functional cell in all portions of the nervous system; whose purpose is to communicate messages through conduction of an action potential

Neuropathic pain is caused by injury to nerves rather than stimulation of nerves by injury

Neurotransmitter chemicals utilized in the communication of the message from one cell to another, or synaptic transmission

New drug application (NDA) application submitted to the FDA which signals that the pharmaceutical company is ready to sell the new drug

Nicotinic receptor for acetylcholine in the ganglia of both the sympathetic and parasympathetic nervous systems

Nicotinic agonist drug that is selective for nicotinic receptors

Nicotinic antagonists drugs that block receptors at cholinergic synapses in the ganglia or in the somatic nervous system at the neuromuscular junction

Nitric oxide in vascular smooth muscle, an important cell signaling molecule and a potent vasodilator causing relaxation of both arterial and venous smooth muscle

Nits eggs of the louse parasite

Nociceptor pain pain produced by injury to body tissue

Nociceptors receptors connected with nerves that receive and transmit pain signals to the spinal cord and brain

Nomogram a representation by graphs, diagrams, or charts of the relationship between numerical variables; used for drug calculations

Nondepolorizing neuromuscular blockers class of nicotinic antagonists that bind to Ach receptors at motor end plates in skeletal muscle and prevent Ach from reaching its receptors

Nonopioid analgesics have a peripheral site of action, no dependence potential, and provide the baseline pharmacotherapy for pain management; include NSAIDs, acetaminophen, and a few centrally acting agents

Non-rapid eye movement (NREM) sleep phase of sleep during which respirations slow, heart rate and blood pressure decrease, oxygen consumption by muscles decreases, and urine formation decreases

Nonspecific body defense system defense such as inflammation that protects the body from invasion by general hazards

Norepinephrine (NE) primary neurotransmitter in the sympathetic nervous system

Nosocomial infections infections acquired in a health care setting such as a hospital, physician's office, or nursing home

Nursing diagnosis clinically based judgment about the patient and his or her response to health and illness

Nursing process five-part decision-making system that includes assessment, nursing diagnosis, planning, implementation, and evaluation

O

Obsessive–compulsive disorder (OCD) recurrent, intrusive thoughts or repetitive behaviors that interfere with normal activities or relationships

Occupational health nurse (OHN) addresses the health and safety of workers on the job

Oligomeric formulas enteral feeding solutions that contain simple or basic forms of free amino acids and peptide combinations that require little or no digestion and are easily absorbed into the body

Oligospermia presence of less than 20 million sperm in an ejaculate

Oncology nurse nurse who has received special training to care for patients with cancer and to administer chemotherapy

On-off syndrome occurs when a patient with Parkinson's Disease alternates between symptom-free periods (on) and times when the drugs stop working and symptoms abruptly reappear (off)

Onychomycosis the invasion of the nail plate by a fungus; also called tinea unguium

Open-angle glaucoma chronic, simple glaucoma caused by hindered outflow of aqueous humor from the anterior chamber

Opiates substance closely related to morphine that are extracted from the poppy plant

Opioid substance obtained from the unripe seeds of the poppy plant; natural or synthetic morphinelike substance

Opium a milky substance extracted from the unripe seeds of the poppy plant, *Papaver somniferum*, that contains over 20 different chemicals having pharmacologic activity

Oral glucose tolerance test (OGTT) a primary blood test for diagnosing diabetes

Orphan disease serious, though rare, disease that affects less than 200,000 people in the United States

Orthostatic hypotension fall in blood pressure that occurs when changing position from recumbent to upright

Osmolality number of dissolved particles, or solutes, in 1 kg (1 L) of water

Osmosis process by which water moves from areas of low solute concentration (low osmolality) to areas of high solute concentration (high osmolality)

Osmotic pressure force with a vessel caused by differences in the number of large molecules, usually proteins across impermeable membrances

Osteoarthritis (OA) disorder characterized by degeneration of joints; particularly the fingers, spine, hips, and knees

Osteomalacia rickets in children; caused by vitamin D deficiency, characterized by softening of the bones without alteration of basic bone structure

Osteoporosis condition in which bones lose mass and become brittle and susceptible to fracture

Otitis interna condition that may occur as the result of chronic otitis media or as part of viral systemic infections, including mononucleosis or an upper respiratory infection; also called labyrinthitis

Otitis media inflammation of the middle ear

Outcome objective measures of goals

Ovarian hyperstimulation syndrome (OHS) serious complication of certain fertility drugs characterized by rapid, massive enlargement of the ovaries accompanied by physical symptoms

Ovulation release of an egg by the ovary

Ovulatory dysfunction the presence of abnormal, irregular, or absent ovulation

Oxazolidinones class of antibiotics that act by binding to a part of the bacterial 50S ribosome

Oxytocics agents that stimulate uterine contractions and promote the induction of labor

P

Paget's disease disorder of bone formation and resorption characterized by weak, enlarged, and deformed bones

Palliation form of cancer chemotherapy intended to alleviate symptoms rather than cure the disease

Pancreatitis inflammation of the pancreas

Panic disorder anxiety disorder characterized by intense feelings of immediate apprehension, fearfulness, terror, or impending doom, accompanied by increased autonomic nervous system activity

Para-aminobenzoic acid precursor molecule used by bacteria to make their own folic acid

Parasympathetic nervous system portion of the autonomic nervous system that is activated during nonstressful conditions and produces a set of symptoms known as the rest and digest response

Parenteral nutrition the administration of high caloric nutrients via a central vein, such as the subclavian vein

Parietal cells cells in the stomach mucosa that secrete hydrochloric acid

Parish nursing refers to a specialty practice that emphasizes health and healing within a faith community

Parkinsonism having tremor, muscle rigidity, stooped posture, and a shuffling gait

Parkinson's disease (PD) degenerative disorder of the nervous system caused by a deficiency of the brain neurotransmitter dopamine that results in disturbances of muscle movement

Paroxysmal supraventricular tachycardia (PSVT) occurs when episodes of atrial tachycardia alternate with periods of normal rhythm; also called paroxysmal atrial tachycardia (PAT)

Partial agonist medication that produces a weaker, or less efficacious, response than an agonist

Partial fatty-acid oxidation inhibitors a new class of drugs used in the treatment of CAD

Partial (focal) seizures seizures that start on one side of the brain and travel a short distance before stopping

Partial parenteral nutrition a parenteral solution that lacks an essential element, usually fats or lipids

Passive immunity immune defense that lasts 2 to 3 weeks; obtained by administering antibodies

Patent medicines in early America before drug regulation, products that contained an easily identified brand name that claimed to cure just about any symptom or disease

Pathogenicity ability of an organism to cause disease in humans

Pathogens organisms that are capable of causing disease

Pediatric Research Equity Act of 2003 authorizes the FDA to require research of pediatric uses for new drugs

Pediculicides medications that kill lice

Pegylation process that attaches polyethylene glycol (PEG) to a drug molecule to extend its duration of activity

Penicillinase enzyme present in certain bacteria that is able to inactivate many penicillins and some cephalosporins

Penicillin-binding proteins (PBPs) enzymes used by bacteria to build bacterial cell walls that are targets for penicillins and related antibiotics

Pepsin digestive enzyme that breaks down proteins from food

Peptic ulcer erosion of the mucosa in the alimentary canal, most commonly in the stomach and duodenum

Peptidoglycan substance containing sugars bound to peptides which is only found in bacteria

Perfusion blood flow through a tissue or organ

Peripheral resistance amount of friction encountered by blood as it travels through the vessels

Peripheral vein total parenteral nutrition delivery system used when a central venous line cannot be accessed or when it is not appropriate for the patient

Peripherally inserted central catheter (PICC) line a central catheter that is threaded into the vena cava for administration of chemotherapy

Peristalsis involuntary wavelike contraction of smooth muscle lining the alimentary canal

Pernicious anemia type of anemia usually caused by lack of secretion of intrinsic factor

Phagocytes one type of innate cellular defense

Pharmacodynamics study of the mechanisms of drug action and how the body responds to drugs

Pharmacogenetics the study of genetic variations that give rise to differences in the way patients handle medications; branch of pharmacology that examines the role of genetics in drug response

Pharmacokinetics study of how drugs are handled by the body

Pharmacologic classification method of organizing drugs on the basis of their mechanisms of action

Pharmacology the study of medicines; the discipline pertaining to how drugs improve or maintain health

Pharmacopoeia a medical reference summarizing standards of drug purity, strength, and directions for synthesis

Pharmacotherapy the application of drugs for the purpose of disease prevention and treatment of suffering; also called pharmacotherapeutics

Pheochromocytoma a tumor, usually benign, arising from the adrenal medulla that is characterized by excessive secretion of catecholamines

Phobia fearful feeling attached to situations or objects such as snakes, spiders, crowds, or heights

Phosphodiesterase III enzyme in cardiac and smooth muscle; inhibition increases cardiac output due to an increase in myocardial contractility and the decrease in left ventricular afterload

Phospholipid type of lipid that contains two fatty acids, a phosphate group, and a chemical backbone of glycerol

Phototherapy light therapy used for persons suffering from SAD that consists of artificial lighting approximately 5 to 20 times brighter than normal indoor lighting

Physical dependence condition of experiencing unpleasant withdrawal symptoms when a substance is discontinued

Pill rolling common behavior in PD, in which patients rub the thumb and forefinger together in a circular motion, resembling the motion of rolling a tablet between two fingers

Placebo in drug testing, an inert substance that serves as a control "nontreatment" group used to compare the effectiveness of the new drug

Placenta organ that allows for nutrition and gas exchange between the mother and fetus

Planning the linkage of strategies or interventions to established goals and outcomes

Plaque fatty material that builds up in the lining of blood vessels and may lead to hypertension, stroke, myocardial infarction, or angina

Plasma cell cell derived from B lymphocytes that produces antibodies

Plasma half-life ($t_{1/2}$) the length of time required for the plasma concentration of a drug to decrease by one half after administration

Plasminogen protein that prevents fibrin clot formation; precursor of plasmin

Pluripotent stem cell cell that is capable of maturing (differentiating) into any blood cell type

Pneumonic plague life-threatening infectious lung disease that occurs after breathing *Yersinia pestis*, a bacterium found on rodents and their fleas that is responsible for the bubonic plague

Polarized describes a cell that has negative membrane potential

Polyclonal antibodies contain a wide mixture of different antibodies that attack the T cells or T-cell receptors

Polycystic ovary syndrome a condition in which the ovaries are filled with follicular cysts and the patient has elevated levels of androgens and estrogen

Polydipsia excessive thirst

Polymeric formulas solutions that contain various mixtures of protein, fat, and carbohydrates in high molecular weight form and are considered the most common enteral preparation

Polyphagia excessive appetite

Polypharmacy taking multiple drugs concurrently

Polyuria excessive urine production

Positive symptoms in schizophrenia, symptoms that add to normal behavior, including hallucinations, delusions, and a disorganized thought or speech pattern

Postantibiotic effect antimicrobial activity that continues for a time after discontinuation of a drug

Posterior pituitary gland (neurohypophysis), consists of nervous tissue and is an extension of the hypothalamus that secretes antidiuretic hormone (ADH) and oxytocin

Postherpetic neuralgia a serious form of the shingles in which the pain lasts for years

Postictal state period immediately following the seizure

Postmarketing surveillance stage 4 of the drug approval process during which testing is done to survey for harmful drug effects in a larger population

Postpartum onset depression major depression experienced by new mothers following delivery, which is related to hormonal shifts and situational stresses that occur during that period

Post-traumatic stress disorder (PTSD) type of anxiety that develops in response to reexperiencing a previous life event that was psychologically traumatic

Potency the strength of a drug at a specified concentration or dose

Preclinical research first stage of drug development which involves extensive laboratory testing by the pharmaceutical company on human and microbial cells

Prediabetes condition in which serum glucose levels are elevated but are not high enough to be diagnosed as diabetes

Preeclampsia occurs during pregnancy when blood pressure increases to 140/90 mmHg or higher on two separate occasions, and 300 mg of protein is found in the urine over a 24-hour period

Pregnancy categories five classifications developed by the U.S. Food and Drug Administration (FDA) that rate medication risks during pregnancy

Preload degree of stretch of the cardiac muscle fibers just before they contract

Preterm labor the initiation of labor prior to week 37 of gestation

Primary hypertension hypertension having no identifiable cause

Procoagulants agents that promote the formation of blood clots

Prodrug drug that becomes more active after it is metabolized

Prodysrhythmics conditions that promote the formation of cardiac rhythm abnormalities

Progesterone a natural hormone produced by the corpus luteum

Progestin synthetic hormones that have actions identical to endogenous progesterone

Prostaglandin E_2 hormone that stimulates the secretion of mucus and bicarbonate, promotes repair of damaged gastric mucosal cells, and increases blood flow to the mucosa to help maintain optimal mucosal conditions

Prostaglandins class of local hormones that promote local inflammation and pain

Prostatitis bacterial infection of the prostate gland

Protease viral enzyme that is responsible for the final assembly of the HIV virions

Prothrombin blood protein that is converted to thrombin in blood coagulation

Prothrombin time (PT) blood test used to determine the time needed for plasma to clot for the regulation of warfarin dosage

Proton pump inhibitor (PPI) drug that inhibits the enzyme H^+, K^+-ATPase

Prototype drug well-understood model drug to which other drugs in a pharmacological class are compared

Protozoan single-celled animal

Provirus stage of a virus in which the viral DNA integrates into the host chromosome

Pruritus itching associated with dry, scaly skin

Pseudocholinesterase enzyme that rapidly destroys certain drugs in the plasma

Pseudomembranous colitis caused by *Clostridium difficile*, a rare though potentially severe disorder resulting from therapy with tetracyclines and other classes of antibiotics

Psoralens drugs used along with phototherapy for the treatment of psoriasis and other severe skin disorders

Psychological dependence intense craving for a drug that drives people to continue drug abuse

Psychosis general term used in medicine to describe a loss of contact with reality

Psychosocial describes a person's psychological development in the context of one's social environment

Public health nurse has a primary focus on population-level outcomes to promote health and prevent disease for entire population groups

Pulmonary embolism condition that occurs when a venous clot dislodges, migrates to the pulmonary vessels, and blocks arterial circulation to the lungs

Purified protein derivative (PPD) tuberculin skin test

Pyelonephritis an inflammation of the kidney, pelvis, and other renal cells

Pyridoxine (vitamin B_6) B complex vitamin supplement that has been shown to prevent peripheral neuropathy in tuberculosis patients

R

Radiation sickness occurs after exposure to ionizing radiation; symptoms include nausea, vomiting, and diarrhea, weight loss, anorexia, fatigue, and suppression of the bone marrow

Rapid eye movement (REM) sleep stage of sleep characterized by quick, scanning movements of the eyes

Raynaud's disease vasospasms of vessels leading to the fingers and toes can lead to intermittent pain and cyanosis of the digits

Reabsorption movement of filtered substances from the kidney tubule back into the blood

Rebound congestion adverse effect of intranasal decongestants; prolonged use causes hypersecretion of mucus and worsening nasal congestion once the drug effects wear off

Rebound effects symptoms of lethargy and fatigue caused by withdrawal of methamphetamine and other stimulants

Rebound insomnia increased sleeplessness that occurs when long-term antianxiety or hypnotic medication is discontinued

Receptor the structural component of a cell to which a drug binds to produce a response

Recommended dietary allowances (RDAs) amount of vitamins or minerals needed each day to prevent a deficiency in a healthy adult

Rectal route administration of drugs into the rectum for either local or systemic delivery

Refeeding syndrome metabolic complications that can occur when nutritional support, including EN therapy, is introduced to severely malnourished patients

Reflex tachycardia temporary increase in heart rate that occurs when blood pressure falls

Refractory period time during which the myocardial cells rest and are not able to contract

Regional anesthesia similar to local anesthesia except that it encompasses a larger body area, such as an entire limb

Renal failure a condition characterized by a decrease in the kidneys' ability to maintain electrolyte and fluid balance and excrete waste products

Renin an enzyme that is synthesized, stored, and secreted by juxtaglomerular (JG) cells in the kidney

Renin-angiotensin-aldosterone system (RAAS) series of enzymatic steps by which the body raises blood pressure

Replacement therapy hormones administered for patients who are unable to secrete sufficient quantities of their own endogenous hormones

Repolarization return of a negative membrane potential to the cell

Rest-and-digest response signs and symptoms produced when the parasympathetic nervous system is activated

Reticular activating system (RAS) responsible for sleeping and wakefulness and performs an alerting function for the cerebral cortex; includes the reticular formation, hypothalamus, and part of the thalamus

Reticular formation portion of the brain affecting awareness and wakefulness

Retinoids compounds resembling vitamin A used in the treatment of severe acne and psoriasis

Reverse cholesterol transport the process by which cholesterol is transported away from body tissues to the liver

Reverse remodeling occurs after several months of therapy with beta-adrenergic antagonists, when heart size, shape, and function return to normal

Reverse transcriptase viral enzyme that converts RNA to DNA

Rhabdomyolysis breakdown of muscle fibers usually due to muscle trauma or ischemia

Rheumatoid arthritis (RA) systemic autoimmune disorder characterized by inflammation of multiple joints

Rhinophyma reddened, bulbous, irregular swelling of the nose

Risk management system of reducing medication errors by modifying policies and procedures within the institution

Risk-benefit ratio determination of whether the risks or adverse effects from a drug outweigh the potential benefits received by taking the medication

Rosacea chronic skin disorder characterized by clusters of papules on the face

S

Salicylates the chemical family to which aspirin belongs

Salicylism poisoning due to aspirin and aspirin-like drugs

Sarcolemma the muscle membrane

Sarcoplasmic reticula structures within cells that store the calcium that is released by depolarization

Satiety the psychological feeling of fullness or satisfaction following a meal

Satiety center region of the hypothalamus that recognizes satiety

Scabicides drugs that kill scabies mites

Scheduled drug in the United States, a term describing a drug placed into one of five categories based on its potential for misuse or abuse

Schizoaffective disorder psychosis with symptoms of both schizophrenia and mood disorders

Schizophrenia psychosis characterized by abnormal thoughts and thought processes, withdrawal from other people and the outside environment, and apparent preoccupation with one's own mental state

Sclerosing abnormal tissue hardening of the veins

Seasonal affective disorder (SAD) a type of depression experienced during the dark winter months

Seborrhea skin condition characterized by overactivity of oil glands

Second messenger cascade of biochemical events that initiates a drug's action by either stimulating or inhibiting a normal activity of the cell

Secondary hypertension hypertension having a specific identifiable cause

Secretion in the kidney, movement of substances from the blood into the tubule after filtration has occurred

Sedative substance that depresses the CNS and causes drowsiness or sleep

Sedative–hypnotic drug with the ability to produce a calming effect at lower doses and to induce sleep at higher doses

Seizure symptom of epilepsy characterized by abnormal neuronal discharges within the brain

Selective estrogen receptor modulators (SERMs) drug that produces an action similar to estrogen in body tissues; used for the treatment of osteoporosis in postmenopausal women

Serotonin a natural neurotransmitter that is found in high concentrations in the hypothalamus, limbic system, medulla, and spinal cord

Serotonin syndrome (SES) set of signs and symptoms associated with overmedication with antidepressants that includes altered mental status, fever, sweating, and lack of muscular coordination

Shingles herpes zoster (HZ) infection caused by reactivation of the varicella zoster virus (VZV) or chickenpox

Short stature height below the fifth percentile for age and gender, or more than two standard deviations below the mean (average) for age and gender

Side effects types of drug effects that are less serious than adverse effects which are predictable and which may occur even at therapeutic doses

Silent angina myocardial ischemia that occurs in the absence of pain

Simple partial seizures seizures that have an onset that may begin as a small, regional focus, and subsequently progress to a generalized seizure

Sinus rhythm number of beats per minute normally generated by the SA node

Situational anxiety anxiety experienced by people faced with a stressful environment

Sjögren's syndrome chronic autoimmune disorder characterized by excessive dryness of mucous membranes

Sleep attacks sudden bouts of sleep that last 10 to 30 minutes and may occur during the daytime without warning

Sleep paralysis the temporary inability to move after waking up from sleep

Small volume nebulizer device used to convert liquid drugs into a fine mist for the purpose of inhalation; also called nebulizer

Smallpox serious, contagious potentially fatal disease that is caused by the Variola virus

Social anxiety disorders unreasonable and persistent fear of crowds or of being ridiculed or embarrassed in public; also called social phobia

Somatic nervous system nerve division that provides voluntary control over skeletal muscle

Somatostatin synonym for growth hormone inhibiting factor from the hypothalamus

Specialized formulas enteral feeding solution designed to fill the specific needs in patients with a particular condition

Specialty supplements nonherbal dietary product used to enhance a wide variety of body functions

Spermicides agents that kill sperm

Sporozoite mature and infective form of plasmodium that resides in the gut of the female Anopheles mosquito

Stable angina type of angina that occurs in a predictable pattern, usually relieved by rest

Staging the process of determining where the cancer is located and the extent of its invasion

Status asthmaticus condition characterized by repeated seizures or one prolonged seizure attack that continues for at least 30 minutes

Status epilepticus condition characterized by repeated seizures or one prolonged seizure attack that continues for at least 30 minutes

Steatorrhea the passing of bulky, foul-smelling fatty stools

Steroids types of lipids consisting of four rings that is a structural component of certain hormones and drugs

Sterol nucleus ring structure common to all steroids

Strategic National Stockpile (SNS) program designed to ensure the immediate deployment of essential medical materials to a community in the event of a large-scale chemical or biological attack

Streptogramins class of antibiotics that act by binding the 50S bacterial ribosome in a manner similar to that of the macrolides

Striatum location in the brain, where dopamine encounters its receptors and produces multiple actions

Stroke volume amount of blood pumped out by a ventricle in a single beat

Substance abuse self-administration of a drug that does not conform to the medical or social norms within the patient's given culture or society

Substantia nigra location in the brain where dopamine is synthesized that is responsible for regulation of unconscious muscle movement

Substrate drug that is metabolized by a CYP enzyme

Suicide the intentional act of ending one's life

Supercoil the highly twisted arrangement of the helix in bacterial DNA

Superinfection new infection caused by an organism different from the one causing the initial infection; usually an adverse effect of anti-infective therapy

Supplements "extra" vitamins, minerals, or other substances taken by patients to supplement their diets

Surgical anesthesia stage 3 of anesthesia, in which most major surgery occurs

Svedberg unit a unit of measurement represented by the letter "S" which indicates the size or sedimentation rate of the bacterial 70S ribosome

Sympathetic nervous system portion of the autonomic nervous system that is activated under emergency conditions or stress and produces a set of actions called the fight-or-flight response

Sympathomimetic drug that stimulates or mimics the sympathetic nervous system

Symporter a membrane protein that transports two molecules at the same time

Synapse a physical space between two neurons that must be crossed before a message can be transferred from one nerve to another, consisting of a presynaptic nerve, a synaptic cleft, and a postsynaptic nerve

Synaptic cleft space where neurotransmitters enter; which must be crossed for the impulse to reach the postganglionic neuron or effector tissue

Syndrome of inappropriate antidiuretic hormone (SIADH) condition characterized by marked fluid retention, elevated urine osmolality, low serum osmolality, and sodium loss in the urine

Synergistic effect type of drug interaction in which two drugs produce an effect that is much greater than would be expected from simply adding the two individual drugs' responses

T

T cells types of lymphocytes that are essential for the cell-mediated immune response

Tachydysrhythmias disorders exhibiting a heart rate greater than 100 beats/minute

Tachyphylaxis the rapid development of tolerance to any action of a drug, either adverse or therapeutic effects

Tardive dyskinesia (TD) unusual tongue and face movements such as lip smacking and wormlike motions of the tongue that occur during pharmacotherapy with certain antipsychotics

Target cells the cells affected by hormones

Telomerase an enzyme contained in certain human stem cells which can lengthen the DNA chains and allow continued replication

Telomeres regions in chromosomes that prevent the vital sequences of DNA from being destroyed each time a cell divides

Tension headache common type of head pain caused by stress and relieved by nonnarcotic analgesics

Teratogen agent that causes developmental birth defects

Tetrahydrocannabinol (THC) the active chemical in marijuana

Therapeutic classification method of organizing drugs on the basis of what condition is being treated by the drug

Therapeutic index the ratio of a drug's LD_{50} to its ED_{50}

Therapeutic range dosage that produces the desired effects of a drug

Threshold potential an action potential triggered by the membrane potential during myocardial electrical conduction

Thrombin enzyme that causes clotting by catalyzing the conversion of fibrinogen to fibrin

Thrombocytopenia reduction in the number of circulating platelets

Thromboembolic disorder condition in which the body forms undesirable clots

Thrombopoietin hormone produced by the kidneys that controls megakaryocyte activity

Thyroid crisis a rare, life-threatening form of thyrotoxicosis; also called thyroid storm

Thyroid storm a rare, life-threatening form of thyrotoxicosis; also called thyroid crisis

Thyroid-stimulating hormone (TSH) hormone secreted by the anterior pituitary when stimulated by thyrotropin-releasing hormone (TRH)

Thyroid-stimulating immunoglobulins (TSI) stimulates the thyroid gland in Graves' disease

Thyrotoxicosis an acute condition caused by very high levels of circulating thyroid hormone

Thyrotropin-releasing hormone (TRH) hormone secreted by the hypothalamus

Thyroxine (T_4) thyroid hormone that is synthesized from the amino acid tyrosine and 4 atoms of iodine

Thyroxine-binding globulin (TBG) a plasma protein produced in the liver

Tocolytic drug used to inhibit uterine contractions

Tolerance process of adapting to a drug over a period of time and subsequently requiring higher doses to achieve the same effect

Tonic clonic seizures seizures characterized by intense jerking motions and loss of consciousness

Tonic spasm single, prolonged muscular contraction

Tonicity the ability of a solution to cause a change in water movement across a membrane owing to osmotic forces

Tonometry technique for measuring intraocular tension and pressure

Topical route medications applied to the skin or the membranous linings of the eye, ear, nose, respiratory tract, urinary tract, vagina, and rectum

Topoisomerase IV in DNA replication, the enzyme that frees the newly formed interlocked strands, allowing them to migrate into the two daughter cells

Torsades de pointe type of ventricular tachycardia that is characterized by rates between 200 and 250 beats/minute and "twisting of the points" of the QRS complex on the ECG

Total parenteral nutrition (TPN) nutrition provided through a peripheral or central vein

Toxic concentration level of drug that results in serious adverse effects

Toxoids substances that have been chemically modified to remove their harmful nature but are still able to elicit an immune response in the body

Trade name name assigned by the pharmaceutical company marketing a drug; sometimes called the proprietary, product, or brand name

Transcription basic steps in protein synthesis

Transdermal patches topical delivery method that provides for convenient dosing with slow release of the drug

Transferrin protein complex that transports iron to sites in the body where it is needed

Transplant rejection recognition by the immune system of a transplanted tissue as foreign and subsequent attack on the tissue

Tricyclic antidepressant (TCA) class of drugs used in the pharmacotherapy of depression

Triglycerides are types of lipids that contain three fatty acids and a chemical backbone of glycerol

Tri-iodothyronine (T_3) thyroid hormone that is synthesized from the amino acid tyrosine and 3 atoms of iodine

Troche drug formulated to slowly dissolve in the mouth

Trophozoite the active, growing stage during which the protozoan organism feeds, often at the expense of its host

Tropic hormones ability of the anterior pituitary gland hormones to regulate the secretory actions of other endocrine glands

Tubercles cavity-like lesions in the lung characteristic of infection by *Mycobacterium tuberculosis*

Tuberculosis (TB) a highly contagious infection caused by the organism *Mycobacterium tuberculosis*

Tularemia serious infectious disease found in rodents, rabbits, and hares that is caused by the organism *Francisella tularensis*, tularemia

Tumor abnormal swelling or mass

Type 1 diabetes metabolic disease characterized by hyperglycemia caused by a lack of secretion of insulin by the pancreas

Type 2 diabetes chronic metabolic disease caused by insufficient secretion of insulin by the pancreas, and a lack of sensitivity of insulin receptors

Tyramine form of the amino acid tyrosine that is found in foods such as cheese, beer, wine, and yeast products

U

Unstable angina severe angina that occurs frequently and that is not relieved by rest

Up-regulation process by which cells create more receptors on their surface to capture hormone molecules

Urethritis infection of the urethra

Uricosurics drugs that increase the rate of excretion of uric acid by blocking its reabsorption in the kidney

Uropathogen harmful microorganisms that invade the urinary system

Urticaria hypersensitivity response that is characterized by hives and is often accompanied by pruritus, or itching

U.S. Food and Drug Administration (FDA) U.S. agency responsible for the evaluation and approval of new drugs

USP verification program mark on the label of a dietary supplement that indicates to consumers that the product has been manufactured under acceptable standards of purity, has been tested for active ingredients stated on the label, and is free of harmful contaminants

V

Vaccination process of introducing foreign proteins or inactive cells (vaccines) into the body to trigger immune activation before the patient is exposed to the real pathogen

Vaginal route administration of drugs into the vagina to treat local conditions such as infections, pain, and itching

Vasomotor center area of the medulla that controls baseline blood pressure

Vasospastic (Prinzmetal's) angina type of angina in which the decreased myocardial blood flow is caused by spasms of the coronary arteries

Vectors organisms that harbor pathogens and spread several major protozoan infections by carrying them from one host to another

Venous return the volume of blood returning to the heart from the veins

Venous thromboembolism (VTE) occurs when blood flow through a vein is very slow (stasis)

Ventilation process by which air is moved into and out of the lungs

Very low-density lipoprotein (VLDL) lipid-carrying particle that is converted to LDL in the liver

Vesicants agents that can cause serious tissue injury if they escape from an artery or vein during an infusion or injection (extravasation); many antineoplastics are vesicants

Viral load a measurement of HIV RNA levels in the blood which provides an estimate of how rapidly the virus is replicating

Virilization appearance of masculine secondary sex characteristics

Virion particle of a virus capable of causing an infection

Virulence the severity of disease that a pathogen is able to cause

Viruses nonliving particles containing nucleic acid that are able to cause disease

Vitamins organic compounds required by the body in small amounts

Vomiting emesis in which the stomach contents are forced upward into the esophagus and out of the mouth

Vomiting center area in the medulla that controls the vomiting reflex

von Willebrand's disease (vWD) decrease in quantity or quality of von Willebrand factor (vWF)

W

Water-soluble vitamins group of vitamins stored briefly in the body and then excreted in the urine, including the B vitamins and C

Wearing off effect appears gradually near the end of a dosing interval; symptoms become worse because the concentration of the drug has fallen below the therapeutic level

Withdrawal syndrome symptoms that result when a patient discontinues taking a substance on which he or she was dependent

X

Xanthine oxidase enzyme responsible for the formation of uric acid.

Xerostomia dry mouth

Z

Zollinger-Ellison syndrome (ZES) disorder of excess acid secretion in the stomach resulting in peptic ulcer disease

Credits

Chapter Opener Sources

1 Esbin/Anderson/Omni-Photo Communications, Inc.
2 Konstantin Sutyagin/Shutterstock
3 Arni Katz/Phototake NYC
4 Getty Images–Stockbyte, Royalty Free
5 Roy Ramsey/Pearson Education/PH College
6 Michal Heron/Pearson Education/PH College
7 Thinkstock
8 Color Day Production/Getty Images Inc.–Image Bank
9 Samuel Ashfield/Photo Researchers, Inc.
10 © Dorling Kindersley
11 BSIP/Phototake NYC
12 Stevie Grand/Science Photo Library/Photo Researchers, Inc.
13 Daniel Zirinsky/Photo Researchers, Inc.
14 Konstantin Sutyagin/Shutterstock RF
15 TEK Image/Photo Researchers, Inc.
16 Cavallini James/BSIP/Phototake NYC
17 Michal Heron/Pearson Education/PH College
18 DAVID ROCHE/Photolibrary.com
19 Getty Images–Stockbyte, Royalty Free
20 © Dorling Kindersley
21 Studi-Oh Medical Art/Pearson Education/PH College
22 © Roy McMahon/CORBIS All Rights Reserved
23 Michael Newman/PhotoEdit Inc.
24 Robert Harbison
25 Jack Cronkhite/Shutterstock
26 Michael Newman/PhotoEdit Inc.
27 Domenico Gelermo/Shutterstock
28 Patrick White/Merrill Education
29 Juan Silva/Getty Images Inc.–Image Bank
30 © Dorling Kindersley
31 © Marie Schmitt/Image Point FR/CORBIS All Rights Reserved
32 Paul Simcock/Getty Images Inc.–Image Bank
33 Geri Engberg/Geri Engberg Photography
34 Bobby Dea/RealDealPhoto/Shutterstock
35 Crestista/Shutterstock
36 David Young-Wolff/PhotoEdit Inc.
37 Michal Heron/Pearson Education/PH College
38 Michal Heron/Pearson Education/PH College
39 Amos Morgan/Getty Images, Inc.–Photodisc.
40 Shutterstock
41 Shutterstock
42 BSIP/Phototake NYC
43 Dennis Kunkel/Phototake NYC
44 Michael Littlejohn/Pearson Education/PH College
45 © Dorling Kindersley
46 Susanna Price © Dorling Kindersley
47 Tischenko Irena/Shutterstock
48 Ragne Kabanova/Shutterstock
49 Pearson Education/PH College
50 Pearson Education/PH College
51 Eric Fowke/PhotoEdit Inc.
52 Pearson Education/PH College
53 Sam Ogden/Photo Researchers, Inc.
54 Getty Images–Stockbyte, Royalty Free
55 Bill Burlingham/Prentice Hall School Division
56 Rui Vale de Sousa/Shutterstock
57 Keith Brofsky/Getty Images, Inc.–Photodisc.
58 JIM CUMMINS/Getty Images, Inc.–Taxi
59 Giuliano Fornari © Dorling Kindersley
60 Stephen Orsillio/Shutterstock
61 Skjold/Pearson Education/PH College
62 Pearson Education/PH College
63 © Helen King/CORBIS All Rights Reserved
64 Pearson Education/PH College
65 Geoff Brightling © Dorling Kindersley, Courtesy of Denoyer-Geppert Intl.
66 Shawn Talbot/Shutterstock
67 David Mager/Pearson Learning Photo Studio
68 Elena Eliseeva/Shutterstock
69 Garry Watson/Photo Researchers, Inc.
70 Anthony Magnacca/Merrill Education
71 Yuri Arcurs/Shutterstock
72 Getty Images, Inc.
73 Mark Richards/PhotoEdit Inc.
74 Getty Images, Inc.
75 KEN CHERNUS/Getty Images, Inc.–Taxi
76 ISM/Phototake NYC
77 Shutterstock
78 Pearson Education/PH College

Index

Page numbers followed by *f* indicate figures and those followed by *t* indicate tables, boxes, or special features. The titles of special features (e.g., Nursing Process Applications, PharmFacts, Pharmacotherapy Illustrated) are also capitalized.

Prototype drug names appear in color, drug classifications are in SMALL CAPS, and trade names are capitalized and cross-referenced to their generic name.

A

A fibers, 430
abacavir, 935
abatacept, 1304*t*
abbreviations:
  to avoid, 83*t*
  in medication administration, 27*t*
abciximab, 655–56
  adverse effects, 656
  classification, 655
  contraindications/precautions, 656
  drug interactions, 656
  FDA approval, 748*t*
  mechanism of action, 656
  nursing responsibilities, 657
  overdose treatment, 656
  patient and family education, 657
  pharmacokinetics, 656
  pregnancy category, 656
  similar drugs, 657
  for specific conditions
    unstable angina/myocardial infarction, 600
  therapeutic effects and uses, 655–56
Abel, John Jacob, 3
Abelcet. *See* amphotericin B deoxycholate
Abilify. *See* aripiprazole
ABORTIFACIENTS, 1212
  carboprost, 1213, 1213*t*
  dinoprostone, 1213, 1213*t*
  methotrexate with misoprostol, 1213, 1213*t*. *See also* methotrexate
  mifepristone with misoprostol, 1212–13, 1213*t*. *See also* mifepristone
abortion, 1213*t*. *See also* ABORTIFACIENTS
Abreva. *See* docosanol
absence seizures, 372*f*, 374, 376*t*
absorption:
  in digestive process, 1000
  drug, 43
    blood flow at site of administration and, 44
    drug concentration/dose and, 44
    drug interactions and, 45, 71–72, 71*f*
    drug ionization and, 44–45, 44*f*
    in gastrointestinal tract, 44, 1002*f*
    in older adults, 148
    in pediatric patients, 136
    in pregnancy, 123–24
    route of administration and, 43–44
    surface area and, 45
acarbose, 1138–39
  adverse effects, 1133*t*, 1138
  classification, 1138
  contraindications/precautions, 1138
  drug interactions, 1138
  mechanism of action, 1138
  overdose treatment, 1139
  pharmacokinetics, 1138
  pregnancy category, 1138
  route and adult dose, 1133*t*
  therapeutic effects and uses, 1138
accessory organs of digestion, 999. *See also* liver
Accolate. *See* zafirlukast
Accretropin. *See* somatropin
Accupril. *See* quinapril
Accuretic, 572*t*
Accutane, 30*t*. *See also* isotretinoin
ACE (angiotensin-converting enzyme), 530–31
ACE (angiotensin-converting enzyme) inhibitors. *See* ANGIOTENSIN-CONVERTING ENZYME (ACE) INHIBITORS
acebutolol:
  adverse effects, 252*t*, 257
    in breast-feeding infant, 129*t*
  mechanism of action, 257
  route and adult dose, 252*t*
  for specific conditions, 257
    dysrhythmias, 629*t*, 633
Aceon. *See* perindopril
acesulfame, 1093
Acetadote. *See* acetylcysteine
acetaldehyde dehydrogenase, 102
acetaminophen, 729–30
  adverse effects, 724*t*, 730
    in pediatric patients, 142*t*
  classification, 729
  contraindications/precautions, 730
  dosage/routes
    adult, 724*t*
    pediatric, 142*t*
  drug interactions, 101*t*, 730
  mechanism of action, 730
  nursing responsibilities, 730
  overdose treatment, 730, 1364*t*
  patient and family education, 730
  pharmacokinetics, 730
    in older adults, 149
  pregnancy category, 730
  for specific conditions
    osteoarthritis, 1302
  therapeutic effects and uses, 729–30
  toxicity, 46, 1003*t*
acetazolamide, 560–61
  adverse effects, 559*t*, 561, 1341*t*
  classification, 560
  contraindications/precautions, 561
  drug interactions, 561, 842
  mechanism of action, 561
  nursing responsibilities, 561
  overdose treatment, 561
  patient and family education, 561
  pharmacokinetics, 561
  pregnancy category, 561
  route and adult dose, 559*t*, 1341*t*
  for specific conditions
    glaucoma, 1341*t*
  therapeutic effects and uses, 560–61
acetic acid/hydrocortisone, 1352*t*
acetylation, 857–58, 858*f*
acetylcholine (Ach), 188, 266
  actions/effects, 189*t*, 220, 221*f*, 267*t*
  clinical applications, 267*t*
  discovery, 190*t*
  life cycle, 193*f*
  receptors
    muscarinic. *See* muscarinic receptors
    nicotinic. *See* nicotinic receptors
  for specific conditions
    Parkinson's disease, 349
  synthesis and release, 190, 191*f*, 220, 221*f*
  termination of action, 192. *See also* acetylcholinesterase
acetylcholinesterase (AchE), 192, 200
ACETYLCHOLINESTERASE (ACHE) INHIBITORS, 359
  adverse effects, 360
  drugs in class
    ambenonium, 202*t*, 207
    donepezil. *See* donepezil
    echothiophate, 204, 1341*t*, 1344
    edrophonium, 202*t*, 205, 206, 207
    galantamine, 202*t*, 355*t*, 362
    neostigmine. *See* neostigmine
    physostigmine, 202*t*, 204
    pyridostigmine, 202*t*, 204–5, 207
    rivastigmine, 202*t*, 355*t*, 360, 362
    tacrine, 202*t*, 355*t*, 360, 362
  mechanism of action, 201*f*, 359, 361*f*
  Nursing Process Application, 207–8*t*
  for specific conditions
    Alzheimer's disease. *See* Alzheimer's disease, pharmacotherapy
    glaucoma, 204. *See also* glaucoma, pharmacotherapy
    nerve gas poisoning prophylaxis, 204–5
acetylcysteine, 1276*t*, 1277, 1364*t*
acetylsalicylic acid. *See* aspirin
acetyltransferase, 159, 160*t*
Ach. *See* acetylcholine
AchE (acetylcholinesterase), 192, 200
AchE inhibitors. *See* ACETYLCHOLINESTERASE (ACHE) INHIBITORS
acid–base imbalance, 701, 701*f*
  acidosis. *See* acidosis
  alkalosis. *See* alkalosis
acidosis, 701, 701*f*
  causes, 702*t*
  pharmacotherapy, 701–2. *See also* sodium bicarbonate
AcipHex. *See* rabeprazole
acitretin, 1330*t*, 1331
Aclovate. *See* alclometasone dipropionate
acne vulgaris, 1320
  pathophysiology, 1320–21
  pharmacotherapy, 1322–23, 1322*t*
Acomplia. *See* rimonabant
Acova. *See* argatroban
acquired immunodeficiency syndrome (AIDS), 927. *See also* HIV-AIDS
acquired resistance, 779
  incidence, 782*t*, 802*t*
  mechanisms of, 779–80
  medication error, 788
  prevention of, 781
  promotion of, 780–81, 780*f*
acromegaly, 1111

ACTH. *See* adrenocorticotropic hormone
Acticin. *See* permethrin
Actifed. *See* pseudoephedrine
Actifed Cold and Allergy, 1266*t*
Actifed Cold and Sinus, 1266*t*
actigraphy, 279
Actimmune. *See* interferon gamma-1b
Actinomycin-D. *See* dactinomycin
action potentials, 487
Actiq. *See* fentanyl
activated charcoal, 1365
  adverse effects, 1365
  classification, 1365
  contraindications/precautions, 1365
  drug interactions, 1365
  mechanism of action, 1365
  nursing responsibilities, 1365
  patient and family education, 1365
  pharmacokinetics, 1365
  pregnancy category, 1365
  therapeutic effects and uses, 1365
activated partial thromboplastin time (aPTT), 644
active immunity, 755, 758, 760, 768*f*
active transport, 42–43, 43*f*
Activella. *See* ethinyl estradiol; norethindrone
Actonel. *See* risedronate
Actos. *See* pioglitazone
Actos plus met, 1134*t*
Acular. *See* ketorolac
acute dystonia, 331, 331*t*
acute gouty arthritis, 1307. *See also* gout
acute hemolytic transfusion reaction, 690
acute lung injury, transfusion-related, 690
acute myocardial infarction. *See* myocardial infarction
acute otitis media. *See* otitis media
acute pain, 428. *See also* pain
acute retroviral syndrome, 928
acute uncomplicated cystitis (AUC), 838, 838*t*. *See also* urinary tract infections
acute-angle glaucoma, 1340. *See also* glaucoma
acyclovir, 913–14
  adverse effects, 913
  classification, 913
  contraindications/precautions, 913
  drug interactions, 913
  mechanism of action, 827, 913
  nursing responsibilities, 913
  overdose treatment, 913
  patient and family education, 913–14
  pediatric dosage/route, 142*t*
  pharmacokinetics, 913
  pregnancy category, 913
  similar drugs, 914–15
  therapeutic effects and uses, 913
Adalat. *See* nifedipine
Adalat CC, 30*t*. *See also* nifedipine
adalimumab, 748*t*, 1037, 1305
Adamsite-DM, 1362*t*
adapalene, 1322, 1322*t*, 1324
adaptive defenses, 713. *See also* immune response
Adderall. *See* amphetamine sulfate
Adderall XR, 30*t*. *See also* amphetamine sulfate
addiction, 94–95, 429
Addison's disease, 1165
additive effect, 73–74, 73*f*
adefovir dipivoxil, 919*t*, 922
Adenocard. *See* adenosine
Adenoscan. *See* adenosine
adenosine, 629*t*, 637
adenosine diphosphate (ADP) receptor blockers. *See* ANTIPLATELET AGENTS, ADP receptor blockers
adenoviruses, 909*t*
ADH. *See* antidiuretic hormone
ADHD. *See* attention deficit/hyperactivity disorder
adherence, 24, 143, 150
  in older adults, 150–51, 151*t*
  in pediatric patients, 143
adhesins, 1023
Adipex-P. *See* phentermine
adipocytes, 1086
ADJUVANT ANALGESICS, 444, 446
  antidepressants, 446*t*
  antiseizure agents, 446, 446*t*
  benzodiazepines, 447, 446*t*
  bisphosphonates, 446*t*, 447
  clinical applications, 444, 446
  corticosteroids, 446, 446*t*
  indications, 444
  local anesthetics, 446
adjuvant chemotherapy, 953. *See also* ANTINEOPLASTIC AGENTS
adolescents. *See also* pediatric patients
  drug administration in, 139
  obesity rates, 1086*t*
  vaccine administration, 766*t*
ADP (adenosine diphosphate) receptor blockers. *See* ANTIPLATELET AGENTS, ADP receptor blockers
ADR (adverse drug reaction), 151. *See also* adverse drug effects
adrenal atrophy, 1165, 1166*f*
adrenal cortex:
  disorders and pharmacotherapy, 1102*t*
  feedback control, 1162*f*
  hormones secreted by. *See also* CORTICOSTEROIDS
    androgens, 1220
    glucocorticoids, 1161*f*, 1162
    gonadocorticoids, 1161*f*, 1162
    mineralocorticoids, 1161*f*, 1162
adrenal crisis, 1165
adrenal medulla, 195, 1161
Adrenalin. *See* epinephrine
adrenergic, 192
ADRENERGIC AGONISTS, 229
  actions, 229
  classification, 230–31
  mechanism of action, 229–30
  nonselective, 231–33
    amphetamines. *See* AMPHETAMINES
    dopamine, 189*t*, 232*t*, 235
    ephedrine, 232*t*, 235, 1273*t*
    epinephrine. *See* epinephrine
    norepinephrine. *See* norepinephrine
  Nursing Process Application, 241*t*
  selective. *See* ALPHA-ADRENERGIC AGONISTS; BETA-ADRENERGIC AGONISTS
ADRENERGIC ANTAGONISTS, 246
  alpha$_1$-. *See* ALPHA$_1$-ADRENERGIC ANTAGONISTS
  beta-. *See* BETA-ADRENERGIC ANTAGONISTS
  beta$_1$-. *See* BETA$_1$-ADRENERGIC ANTAGONISTS
  mechanism of action, 246, 247*f*
  Nursing Process Application, 258*t*
ADRENERGIC NEURON–BLOCKING AGENTS:
  for hypertension, 574*t*, 578–79
  mechanism of action, 578
adrenergic synapses, 266
adrenergic transmission:
  adrenal medulla in, 195
  alpha-adrenergic receptors, 192. *See also* alpha$_1$-adrenergic receptors; alpha$_2$-adrenergic receptors
  beta-adrenergic receptors, 193–94. *See also* beta$_1$-adrenergic receptors; beta$_2$-adrenergic receptors
  norepinephrine, 192, 194*f*. *See also* norepinephrine
  termination of norepinephrine action, 194–95
adrenocortical insufficiency, 1165
adrenocorticotropic hormone (ACTH), 1162
  regulation, 1102*t*
  target organs and action, 1102*t*, 1105*t*
Adriamycin. *See* doxorubicin
Adrucil. *See* fluorouracil
adverse drug effects, 66
  allergic reactions, 67
  birth defects, 68–69, 69*t*
  drug interactions. *See* drug interactions
  drug-induced cancer, 68, 68*t*
  fetal, 126–27. *See also* teratogens
  hospital admissions due to, 68*t*
  idiosyncratic response, 67–68
  number of drugs taken and, 152*t*
  in older adults, 151–52, 153*t*
  organ-specific toxicity, 69*t*
    bone marrow, 70
    dermatologic, 70
    hepatic, 70
    muscle, 69–70
    neurological, 69
    renal, 69
  in pediatric patients, 140–41, 142*t*, 143
  preventable, 67*t*
  prevention, 66–67
adverse drug reaction (ADR), 151. *See also* adverse drug effects
Advicor. *See* lovastatin; niacin
Advil. *See* ibuprofen
aerobic, 775
AeroBid. *See* flunisolide
aerosols, 1241
affinity, 45
African Americans:
  adherence to immunosuppressive medication, 742*t*
  antihypertensive therapy in, 573
  hypertension in, 567*t*
Afrin. *See* oxymetazoline
Afrin 12 hour. *See* oxymetazoline
Aftate. *See* tolnaftate
afterload, 490, 490*f*
Aggrastat. *See* tirofiban
aging. *See* older adults
agonist, 61, 61*f*
agoraphobia, 275
AIDS (acquired immunodeficiency syndrome), 967. *See also* HIV-AIDS
air embolism, during parenteral nutrition therapy, 1079
akathisia, 331, 331*t*
Akineton. *See* biperiden
Alamast. *See* pemirolast potassium
Alaway. *See* ketotifen

Albalon. *See* naphazoline
albendazole, 902*t*, 903
Albenza. *See* albendazole
Albuminar. *See* normal serum albumin
albuterol, 1246–47
  adverse effects, 232*t*, 1246
  classification, 1246
  contraindications/precautions, 1246
  dosage/routes
    adult, 232*t*
    oral, 239, 240
  drug interactions, 1246
  mechanism of action, 1246
  nursing responsibilities, 1246–47
  overdose treatment, 1246
  patient and family education, 1247
  pharmacokinetics, 1246
  pregnancy category, 1246
  similar drugs, 1247–48
  therapeutic effects and uses, 1246
Alcaine. *See* proparacaine hydrochloride
alclometasone dipropionate, 1327*t*
alcohol:
  adverse effects, 102
  dependence, 101, 102
  drug interactions, 101, 101*t*, 178*t*
  effects, 100–101
  metabolism, 99–100, 100*f*
  in pregnancy, 102
  in schizophrenia, 330
  withdrawal symptoms and treatment, 96*t*, 283*t*
alcohol dehydrogenase, 137
Aldactazide, 549, 572*t*
Aldactone. *See* spironolactone
aldesleukin, 738–39
  adverse effects, 735*t*, 738–39, 990*t*
  classification, 738
  contraindications/precautions, 739
  drug interactions, 739
  mechanism of action, 738
  nursing responsibilities, 739
  overdose treatment, 739
  patient and family education, 739
  pharmacokinetics, 738
  pregnancy category, 739
  route and adult dose, 735*t*, 990*t*
  similar drugs, 739
  therapeutic effects and uses, 738
Aldomet. *See* methyldopa
Aldoril, 572*t*
aldosterone:
  actions/effects, 1169–70
  excessive secretion, 1170
  inadequate secretion, 1170
  regulation, 1102*t*
  release, 532
  target organs and action, 1102*t*
aldosterone antagonists. *See* POTASSIUM-SPARING DIURETICS, aldosterone antagonists
alemtuzumab, 748*t*, 990*t*
alendronate, 1295–96
  adverse effects, 1295*t*, 1296
  classification, 1296
  contraindications/precautions, 1296
  drug interactions, 1296
  mechanism of action, 1296
  nursing responsibilities, 1296
  overdose treatment, 1296
  patient and family education, 1296
  pharmacokinetics, 1296
  pregnancy category, 1296
  route and adult dose, 1295*t*
  similar drugs, 1297
  therapeutic effects and uses, 1294*t*, 1296
Alertec. *See* modafinil
Alesse, 1203*t*
Aleve. *See* naproxen
alfalfa, 129*t*
Alfenta. *See* alfentanil
alfentanil, 460*t*, 462
Alferon N. *See* interferon alfa-n3
alfuzosin, 247, 247*t*, 250
alimentary canal, 999. *See also* gastrointestinal tract
Alimta. *See* pemetrexed
Alinia. *See* nitazoxanide
aliskiren, 532, 575
alkalosis, 701*f*, 703
  causes, 702*t*
  pharmacotherapy, 703. *See also* ammonium chloride
Alka-Seltzer. *See* sodium bicarbonate
Alkeran. *See* melphalan
ALKYLATING AGENTS, 966–67
  adverse effects, 856
  mechanism of action, 968*f*
  miscellaneous
    busulfan, 967*t*, 969–70
    dacarbazine, 967*t*, 970
    procarbazine, 967*t*, 971
    temozolomide, 967*t*, 970
    thiotepa, 967*t*, 971
  nitrogen mustards
    chlorambucil, 967*t*, 970
    cyclophosphamide. *See* cyclophosphamide
    estramustine, 967*t*, 970–71
    ifosfamide, 967*t*, 971
    mechlorethamine, 967*t*, 971
    melphalan, 967*t*, 971
  nitrosoureas
    carmustine, 960, 967*t*, 970
    lomustine, 967*t*, 971
    streptozocin, 967*t*, 971
  platinum compounds
    carboplatin, 967*t*, 970
    cisplatin, 959, 960, 967*t*, 970
    oxaliplatin, 967*t*, 970
Allegra. *See* fexofenadine
Allerest. *See* naphazoline
allergen, 1263
allergic conjunctivitis, 1349, 1349*t*
allergic dermatitis, 1325, 1325*t*
allergic rhinitis, 1263
  incidence, 1263*t*
  pathophysiology, 1263, 1264*f*
  pharmacotherapy, 1263–64
    corticosteroids, 1169, 1268, 1270*t*
      fluticasone. *See* fluticasone
      Nursing Process Application, 1272*t*
    cromolyn. *See* cromolyn
    decongestants, 1271–72, 1273*t*
      pseudoephedrine. *See* pseudoephedrine
    H_1-receptor antagonists, 1264–66, 1265*t*
      fexofenadine. *See* fexofenadine
      Nursing Process Application, 1269*t*
    montelukast, 1270*t*, 1271
allergy, drug, 67
Alli. *See* orlistat
Allium sativum. *See* garlic
allopathy, 157
allopurinol, 1309–10
  adverse effects, 1307*t*, 1309
  classification, 1309
  contraindications/precautions, 1309
  drug interactions, 1309–10
  mechanism of action, 1309
  nursing responsibilities, 1310
  overdose treatment, 1310
  patient and family education, 1310
  pharmacokinetics, 1309
  pregnancy category, 1310
  route and adult dose, 1307*t*
  therapeutic effects and uses, 1309
almotriptan, 450*t*, 452
Alocril. *See* nedocromil sodium
aloe, 177
aloe vera:
  description, 1332*t*
  evidence, 1332*t*
  history and claims, 1332*t*
  standardization, 1332*t*
alopecia, 960, 1333–34
alosetron, 1037*t*, 1040
ALPHA-ADRENERGIC AGONISTS. *See also* ADRENERGIC AGONISTS
  adverse effects, 232*t*, 236, 1230
  clinical applications, 236
  intranasal decongestants. *See* INTRANASAL DECONGESTANTS
  mechanism of action, 236
  midodrine, 232*t*, 238
  ocular decongestants. *See* OCULAR DECONGESTANTS/VASOCONSTRICTORS
  phenylephrine. *See* phenylephrine
  for specific conditions, 231
ALPHA-ADRENERGIC ANTAGONISTS. *See* $ALPHA_1$-ADRENERGIC ANTAGONISTS
$ALPHA_1$-ADRENERGIC ANTAGONISTS, 246, 247*t*
  adverse effects, 248
  drugs in class
    alfuzosin, 246, 247*t*, 250, 1231*t*
    doxazosin, 247*t*, 250, 1220*t*
    phenoxybenzamine, 247*t*, 250
    phentolamine. *See* phentolamine
    prazosin. *See* prazosin
    tamsulosin, 246, 247*t*, 251, 1231*t*
    terazosin, 247*t*, 251, 1231*t*
  mechanism of action, 247*f*
  Nursing Process Application, 258*t*
  for specific conditions
    benign prostatic hyperplasia, 246, 1231, 1231*t*
    hypertension, 246, 574*t*, 576
    hypertensive emergency, 584*t*
    pheochromocytoma, 248
    Raynaud's disease, 248
$alpha_1$-adrenergic receptors:
  locations, 192*t*
  responses, 192, 192*t*
$ALPHA_2$-ADRENERGIC AGONISTS:
  drugs in class
    apraclonidine, 1341*t*, 1343
    brimonidine, 1341*t*, 1343
    clonidine. *See* clonidine
    methyldopa. *See* methyldopa
  for specific conditions
    glaucoma, 1341*t*, 1343
    hypertension, 574*t*, 577

alpha$_2$-adrenergic receptors:
  locations, 192*t*
  responses, 192, 192*t*
alpha-blockers. *See* ALPHA$_1$-ADRENERGIC ANTAGONISTS
ALPHA-GLUCOSIDASE INHIBITORS, 1138
  acarbose. *See* acarbose
  actions, 1132*t*
  mechanism of action, 1138
  miglitol, 1133*t*, 1139
  nursing considerations, 1132*t*
5-alpha reductase inhibitors:
  dutasteride, 1231*t*, 1233–34
  finasteride. *See* finasteride
  mechanism of action, 1230*f*, 1231
  Nursing Process Application, 1233*t*
Alphagan. *See* brimonidine
alprazolam, 101*t*, 282*t*, 283*t*, 285
alprostadil, 1228
Altacaine. *See* tetracaine
Altace. *See* ramipril
alteplase, 658–59
  adverse effects, 659
  classification, 658
  contraindications/precautions, 659
  drug interactions, 659
  mechanism of action, 659
  nursing responsibilities, 659
  overdose treatment, 659
  patient and family education, 659
  pharmacokinetics, 659
  pregnancy category, 659
  similar drugs, 659–60
  therapeutic effects and uses, 659
AlternaGel. *See* aluminum hydroxide
Altoprev. *See* lovastatin
altretamine, 991, 992*t*
aluminum antacids, 1019. *See also* ANTACIDS
aluminum hydroxide, 1021–22
  adverse effects, 1021*t*, 1022
  classification, 1021
  contraindications/precautions, 1022
  drug interactions, 1022
  mechanism of action, 1022
  nursing responsibilities, 1022
  overdose treatment, 1022
  patient and family education, 1022
  pharmacokinetics, 1022
  pregnancy category, 1022
  route and adult dose, 1021*t*
  therapeutic effects and uses, 1021–22
Alzheimer's disease, 358
  anesthesia exposure and risk of, 469*t*
  characteristics, 347*t*
  community issues, 364*t*
  etiology, 358–59
  genetic factors, 359
  pharmacotherapy
    acetylcholinesterase inhibitors, 204
      donepezil. *See* donepezil
      galantamine, 355*t*, 362
      mechanism of action, 359
      rivastigmine, 355*t*, 360, 362
      tacrine, 355*t*, 360, 362–63
    mechanism of action, 361*f*
    memantine, 359*t*, 360
    Nursing Process Application, 363*t*
  symptoms, 358*t*
Amanita muscaria, 203
amantadine, 916–17
  adverse effects, 350*t*, 916, 916*t*
  classification, 916
  contraindications/precautions, 916
  drug interactions, 916–17
  mechanism of action, 916
  nursing responsibilities, 917
  overdose treatment, 917
  patient and family education, 917
  pharmacokinetics, 916
  pregnancy category, 917
  route and adult dose, 350*t*, 916*t*
  similar drugs, 917
  for specific conditions
    influenza, 916*t*
    Parkinson's disease, 350*t*, 354
  therapeutic effects and uses, 916
Amaryl. *See* glimepiride
ambenonium, 202*t*, 207
Ambenyl Cough Syrup, 1276*t*
Ambien. *See* zolpidem
Ambien CR, 30*t*. *See also* zolpidem
AmBisome. *See* amphotericin B deoxycholate
amcinonide, 1327*t*
amebiasis, 886*t*, 891–92, 891*f*, 891*t*, 892*t*
amenorrhea, 1183
Amerge. *See* naratriptan
Americaine. *See* benzocaine
American College of Cardiology/American Heart Association (ACC/AHA), 610*t*
Amethopterin. *See* methotrexate
AMI (acute myocardial infarction). *See* myocardial infarction
AMI (atypical mycobacterial infection), 851
Amicar. *See* aminocaproic acid
amides, 474. *See also* local anesthetics, amide-type
Amigesic. *See* salsalate
amikacin, 818
  adverse effects, 816*t*
  route and adult dose, 816*t*
  for tuberculosis, 855*t*, 860
Amikin. *See* amikacin
amiloride, 556, 556*t*, 558
amino acids:
  as dietary supplement, 179*t*
  in parenteral nutrition, 1078
aminocaproic acid, 661
  adverse effects, 661, 661*t*
  classification, 661
  contraindications/precautions, 661
  drug interactions, 661
  mechanism of action, 661
  nursing responsibilities, 661
  overdose treatment, 661
  patient and family education, 662*t*
  pharmacokinetics, 661
  pregnancy category, 661
  route and adult dose, 661*t*
  similar drugs, 662
  therapeutic effects and uses, 661
aminoglutethimide, 1171
AMINOGLYCOSIDES:
  adverse effects, 816*t*, 817
  drugs in class
    amikacin. *See* amikacin
    gentamicin. *See* gentamicin
    kanamycin, 816*t*, 818–19
    neomycin, 816*t*, 819
    paromomycin, 816*t*, 819
    streptomycin. *See* streptomycin
    tobramycin, 816*t*, 819
  mechanism of action, 816
  Nursing Process Application, 819–20*t*
  resistance to, 816–17
aminopeptidase, 1004*t*
aminophylline, 1245*t*, 1256
aminosalicylic acid, 855*t*, 861
amiodarone, 634–35
  adverse effects, 634
    in breast-feeding infant, 129*t*
  classification, 634
  contraindications/precautions, 634–35
  drug interactions, 178*t*, 635
  mechanism of action, 634
  nursing responsibilities, 635
  overdose treatment, 635
  patient and family education, 635
  pharmacokinetics, 634
  plasma half-life, 50
  pregnancy category, 635
  similar drugs, 635–36
  for specific conditions
    after cardiopulmonary arrest, 602
  therapeutic effects and uses, 634
Amitiza. *See* lubiprostone
amitriptyline:
  drug interactions, 101*t*
  genetic polymorphisms and actions of, 160*t*
  for specific conditions
    anxiety disorders or insomnia, 290*t*, 307
    depression, 304*t*
    migraine prophylaxis, 453
amlodipine:
  adverse effects, 520*t*, 592*t*
  mechanism of action, 521
  potency versus nifedipine, 58
  route and adult dose, 520*t*, 592*t*
  for specific conditions, 519*t*
    angina and myocardial infarction, 592*t*
    hypertension, 521
ammonium chloride, 703–4
  adverse effects, 703
  classification, 703
  contraindications/precautions, 703
  drug interactions, 703
  mechanism of action, 703
  nursing responsibilities, 703–4
  overdose treatment, 703
  patient and family education, 704
  pharmacokinetics, 703
  pregnancy category, 703
  similar drugs, 704
  therapeutic effects and uses, 703
amobarbital, 292, 379, 380*t*
amoxapine, 304*t*, 312
amoxicillin, 793
  adverse effects, 789*t*
    in pediatric patients, 142*t*
  dosage/routes
    adult, 789*t*
    forms not to be crushed or opened, 30*t*
    pediatric, 142*t*
  for specific conditions
    H. pylori infection, 1023
    otitis media, 1351
amoxicillin/clavulanate, 142*t*, 789*t*
Amoxil. *See* amoxicillin

amphetamine sulfate, 415–17
adverse effects, 415, 416*t*, 417
classification, 415
contraindications/precautions, 417
drug interactions, 417
mechanism of action, 415
nursing responsibilities, 417
overdose treatment, 417
patient and family education, 417
pharmacokinetics, 415
pregnancy category, 417
route and adult dose, 416*t*
similar drugs, 417–18
therapeutic effects and uses, 415
AMPHETAMINES:
abuse, 105–6, 415
adverse effects in breast-feeding infant, 129*t*
dosage forms not to be crushed or opened, 30*t*
drugs in class
amphetamine sulfate. *See* amphetamine sulfate
benzphetamine, 416*t*, 417–18
dexmethylphenidate, 416*t*, 418
methylphenidate. *See* methylphenidate
effects in pregnancy, 126
mechanism of action, 415
for specific conditions, 233
attention deficit/hyperactivity disorder, 414
weight loss, 1089, 1090
withdrawal symptoms and treatment, 96*t*
Amphotec. *See* amphotericin B deoxycholate
amphotericin B deoxycholate, 872–74
adverse effects, 872*t*, 873–74
classification, 872
contraindications/precautions, 874
drug interactions, 874
mechanism of action, 873
nursing responsibilities, 874
overdose treatment, 874
patient and family education, 874
pharmacokinetics, 873
pregnancy category, 874
route and adult dose, 872*t*
similar drugs, 874–75
therapeutic effects and uses, 872–73, 873*f*
ampicillin, 792–93
adverse effects, 789*t*, 792–93
in pediatric patients, 142*t*
classification, 792
contraindications/precautions, 793
dosage/routes
adult, 789*t*
pediatric, 142*t*
drug interactions, 793
mechanism of action, 792
nursing responsibilities, 793
overdose treatment, 793
patient and family education, 793
pharmacokinetics, 792
pregnancy category, 793
similar drugs, 793
therapeutic effects and uses, 792
ampicillin/sulbactam, 789*t*
Amrix. *See* cyclobenzaprine
amygdala, 276
amyl nitrite, 592*t*, 594
amyotrophic lateral sclerosis (Lou Gehrig's disease):
characteristics, 347*t*
muscle spasticity in, 403
pharmacotherapy, 366
Amytal. *See* amobarbital
anabolic effects, 1221
ANABOLIC STEROIDS, 1221
abuse, 109, 1221, 1223*t*
adverse effects, 68*t*, 109, 1223
drug interactions, 178*t*
drugs in class
danazol, 1192*t*, 1194, 1195, 1220*t*
nandrolone, 1220*t*, 1223
oxandrolone, 1220*t*, 1223
oxymetholone, 1220*t*, 1223
effects/actions, 108–9
withdrawal symptoms and treatment, 96*t*
Anacin. *See* acetaminophen
Anadrol-50. *See* oxymetholone
anaerobic, 775
Anafranil. *See* clomipramine
anakinra, 741*t*, 746, 1304*t*, 1305–6
analgesics, 429. *See also* pain management
anaphylaxis, 717, 1266
Anaprox. *See* naproxen
Anaspaz. *See* hyoscyamine
anastrozole, 980*t*, 983
Anbesol. *See* benzocaine
Ancef. *See* cefazolin sodium
Ancobon. *See* flucytosine
Ancylostoma duodenale, 901
Andro. *See* testosterone
Androderm, 1221. *See also* testosterone
AndroGel, 1221. *See also* testosterone
ANDROGEN(S), 1219
drugs in class
fluoxymesterone, 980*t*, 1220*t*, 1223
methyltestosterone, 1220*t*, 1223
testosterone. *See* testosterone
testosterone cypionate, 1220, 1220*t*, 1221
testosterone enanthate, 1220*t*, 1221
for hypogonadism, 1220–21
nonreproductive uses, 1221
Nursing Process Application, 1224*t*
regulation, 1219–20
ANDROGEN RECEPTOR BLOCKERS, 984
bicalutamide, 980*t*, 984
flutamide, 980*t*, 984
nilutamide, 980*t*, 984
Android. *See* methyltestosterone
Anectine. *See* succinylcholine chloride
anemia, 675
antineoplastic agents and, 959
assessment, 676
classification, 676, 676*t*
iron deficiency. *See* iron deficiency anemia
in renal failure, 548*t*
Anestacon. *See* lidocaine
anesthesia:
adjunctive agents
neuromuscular blockers, 477
pain management, 477
postoperative medications, 477
preoperative medications, 477
general. *See* general anesthesia
local. *See* local anesthesia
for ocular procedures, 1347, 1348*t*
types, 458
angina pectoris, 589
incidence, 590*t*
pathophysiology, 589–90
pharmacotherapy, 590–91, 591*f*, 592*t*
beta-adrenergic antagonists, 592*t*, 595–98
calcium channel blockers, 519*t*, 592*t*, 598
organic nitrates, 592–95, 592*t*, 595*t*
ranolazine, 591, 592*t*
angioedema, 534, 534*t*
angiogenesis, 951
ANGIOGENESIS INHIBITORS:
bevacizumab, 748*t*, 990*t*, 991
lenalidomide, 991
thalidomide, 14, 741*t*, 746–47, 991
Angiomax. *See* bivalirudin
angiotensin I, 529
angiotensin II:
formation, 529, 531
physiological effects, 531–32
ANGIOTENSIN II RECEPTOR BLOCKERS (ARBs):
versus ACE inhibitors, 539
adverse effects, 575
clinical applications, 538–39
drugs in class
candesartan, 538*t*, 540
eprosartan, 538*t*, 540
irbesartan, 538*t*, 540
losartan. *See* losartan
olmesartan medoxomil, 538*t*, 540
telmisartan, 538*t*, 541
valsartan, 538*t*, 541
mechanism of action, 532, 536, 613
for specific conditions
heart failure, 613
hypertension, 572*t*, 574*t*, 575
angiotensin-converting enzyme (ACE), 530–31
ANGIOTENSIN-CONVERTING ENZYME (ACE) INHIBITORS:
adverse effects, 533*t*, 534, 575, 611, 612*t*, 613
drugs in class
benazepril, 533*t*, 535
captopril, 533*t*, 535, 612*t*
enalapril. *See* enalapril
fosinopril, 533*t*, 536, 612
lisinopril. *See* lisinopril
moexipril, 533*t*, 536
perindopril, 533*t*, 536
quinapril, 533*t*, 536, 612*t*
ramipril, 533*t*, 536, 612*t*
trandolapril, 533*t*, 536
genetic polymorphisms and actions of, 160*t*
mechanism of action, 532–33, 611*f*
Nursing Process Application, 537–38*t*
route and adult dose, 533*t*
for specific conditions
heart failure, 533, 610–11, 611*f*, 612*t*, 613
hypertension, 533, 572*t*, 574*t*, 575
hypertensive emergency, 584*t*
myocardial infarction, 602
angiotensinogen, 160*t*, 529
anidulafungin, 872*t*, 874–75
Anopheles mosquito, 887
anorexia, antineoplastic agents and, 959
ANOREXIANTS, 415, 1090
sibutramine. *See* sibutramine
anovulatory cycles, 1181
ANP (atrial natriuretic peptide), 493, 609
ANS. *See* autonomic nervous system
Ansaid. *See* flurbiprofen
Antabuse. *See* disulfiram

ANTACIDS, 1019
adverse effects, 1019
drug interactions, 1021
drugs in class
aluminum hydroxide. *See* aluminum hydroxide
calcium carbonate, 548*t*, 1021*t*, 1288*t*
magaldrate, 1021*t*
magnesium hydroxide, 1021*t*
magnesium trisilicate, 1021*t*
sodium bicarbonate. *See* sodium bicarbonate
mechanism of action, 1012*f*, 1019
Antagon. *See* ganirelix
antagonist, 61, 61*f*
antagonistic effect, 74, 75*f*
Antara. *See* fenofibrate
anterior pituitary gland, 1106
anterograde amnesia, 98
anthralin, 1329, 1330*t*
anthrax, 828, 1360–61, 1360*t*
antiadrenal drugs, 1171
antibacterials. *See* antibiotics
ANTIBIOTICS, 776
broad-spectrum, 782
cell wall inhibitors
aztreonam, 800*t*, 803
carbapenems. *See* CARBAPENEMS
cephalosporins. *See* CEPHALOSPORINS
fosfomycin. *See* fosfomycin
mechanism of action, 778, 778*t*
penicillins. *See* PENICILLIN(S)
vancomycin. *See* vancomycin HCl
cyclic lipopeptides
daptomycin, 832, 832*t*
DNA synthesis inhibitors
fluoroquinolones. *See* FLUOROQUINOLONES
mechanism of action, 778, 778*t*, 826–27
ketolides
telithromycin, 821*t*, 822, 832*t*, 833
mechanisms of action, 776–77, 778*t*, 779*f*
disruption of plasma membrane, 778, 778*t*
inhibition of metabolic pathways, 778, 778*t*
miscellaneous
bacitracin, 832, 832*t*
metronidazole. *See* metronidazole
polymyxin B, 832*t*, 833
rifampin. *See* rifampin
narrow-spectrum, 782
photosensitivity and, 811*t*
prophylactic use, 783
protein synthesis inhibitors
aminoglycosides. *See* AMINOGLYCOSIDES
chloramphenicol, 821, 821*t*
clindamycin, 821, 821*t*
lincomycin, 821, 821*t*
linezolid, 821*t*, 822
macrolides. *See* MACROLIDES
mechanism of action, 778, 778*t*, 809, 809*f*
quinupristin-dalfopristin, 821–22, 821*t*
tetracyclines. *See* TETRACYCLINES
resistance to. *See* acquired resistance
selection of
host factors affecting, 783–84
pathogen identification and, 782
single versus combination therapy, 782–83
superinfections and, 784
topical, 1317
antibody(ies), 713. *See also* MONOCLONAL ANTIBODIES (MABs)
functions, 714*f*
mechanism of action, 747
anticholinergics. *See* muscarinic antagonists
anticholinesterase agents. *See* ACETYLCHOLINESTERASE (ACHE) INHIBITORS
ANTICOAGULANTS, 642
direct thrombin inhibitors
argatroban, 645*t*, 649
bivalirudin, 645*t*, 649
desirudin, 645*t*, 649
lepirudin. *See* lepirudin
indirect thrombin inhibitors
fondaparinux, 645*t*, 648
heparin. *See* heparin
warfarin. *See* warfarin
low molecular weight heparins
dalteparin, 645*t*, 647
enoxaparin, 645*t*, 647
tinzaparin, 645*t*, 648
mechanism of action, 644*f*
Nursing Process Application, 652*t*
for specific conditions
myocardial infarction, 600–601
anticonvulsants. *See* antiseizure drugs
antidepressants, 303
as adjuvant analgesics, 446, 446*t*
atypical antidepressants. *See* ATYPICAL ANTIDEPRESSANTS
mechanism of action, 303, 305*f*
monoamine oxidase inhibitors. *See* MONOAMINE OXIDASE INHIBITORS (MAOIs)
Nursing Process Application, 315–17*t*
selective serotonin reuptake inhibitors. *See* SELECTIVE SEROTONIN REUPTAKE INHIBITORS (SSRIs)
for specific conditions
anxiety and insomnia, 282*t*, 288–89, 290*t*
attention deficit/hyperactivity disorder, 418
bipolar disorder, 321
cataplexy, 420
depression, 304*t*
irritable bowel syndrome, 1039–40
low-back pain, 398*t*
tricyclic antidepressants. *See* TRICYCLIC ANTIDEPRESSANTS
ANTIDIARRHEALS:
bismuth subsalicylate, 1033, 1034*t*, 1035
furazolidone, 101*t*, 1034*t*
Nursing Process Application, 1036*t*
octreotide. *See* octreotide
opioids, 1033–34
camphorated opium tincture, 1034*t*, 1035
difenoxin with atropine, 1034*t*, 1035
diphenoxylate with atropine. *See* diphenoxylate with atropine
loperamide, 1033, 1034*t*, 1035
antidiuretic hormone (ADH), 493, 493*f*, 1112. *See also* desmopressin; vasopressin
deficiency, 1114
drugs affecting secretion of, 1114*t*
excess, 1114
in fluid balance regulation, 688, 1112
kidney function and, 546
regulation, 1102*t*
target organs and action, 1102*t*
ANTIDYSRHYTHMIC DRUGS:
adenosine, 629*t*, 637
class IA: sodium channel blockers
disopyramide, 629*t*, 632
procainamide. *See* procainamide
quinidine gluconate, 629*t*, 632
quinidine sulfate, 629*t*, 632
class IB: sodium channel blockers
lidocaine, 629*t*, 632. *See also* lidocaine
mexiletine, 629*t*, 632
phenytoin, 629*t*, 632. *See also* phenytoin
class IC: sodium channel blockers
flecainide, 629*t*, 632–33
propafenone, 629*t*, 632
class II: beta-adrenergic antagonists
acebutolol, 629*t*, 633
esmolol, 629*t*, 634
propranolol, 629*t*, 633. *See also* propranolol
class III: potassium channel blockers
amiodarone. *See* amiodarone
dofetilide, 629*t*, 635
ibutilide, 629*t*, 635–36
mechanism of action, 634
sotalol, 629*t*, 636
class IV: calcium channel blockers
diltiazem, 519*t*, 522, 629*t*, 636
mechanism of action, 636
verapamil. *See* verapamil
classification, 627–28, 628*t*
digoxin, 629*t*, 637. *See also* digoxin
mechanism of action, 627–28, 628, 628*t*, 630*f*
Nursing Process Application, 637*t*
ANTIEMETICS, 1041–42
antihistamines/anticholinergics, 1041
cyclizine hydrochloride, 1043*t*
dimenhydrinate, 1043*t*
diphenhydramine. *See* diphenhydramine
hydroxyzine, 1043*t*
meclizine, 1043*t*
scopolamine. *See* scopolamine
benzodiazepines, 1042
lorazepam. *See* lorazepam
cannabinoids, 1044
dronabinol, 1043*t*
nabilone, 1043*t*
corticosteroids, 1044
dexamethasone, 1043*t*
methylprednisolone, 1043*t*
mechanism of action, 1042*f*
neurokinin receptor antagonists
aprepitant, 1043*t*, 1044
Nursing Process Application, 1046*t*
phenothiazines, 333, 1042
metoclopramide, 477, 1043*t*
perphenazine. *See* perphenazine
prochlorperazine. *See* prochlorperazine
promethazine, 477, 1043*t*
selective serotonin receptor inhibitors, 1044
serotonin receptor antagonists, 1044
dolasetron, 1043*t*
granisetron, 1043*t*
ondansetron, 1043*t*
palonosetron, 1043*t*
antiepileptic drugs. *See* ANTISEIZURE DRUGS
antiflatulents, 1021
ANTIFUNGAL DRUGS:
mechanism of action, 870–71, 871*f*
Nursing Process Application, 881–82*t*

for superficial infections
azoles, 878t. *See also* AZOLES
butenafine, 878*t*
ciclopirox, 878*t*, 879
griseofulvin. *See* griseofulvin
naftifine, 878*t*
nystatin. *See* nystatin
terbinafine, 877, 878–79, 878*t*, 881
tolnaftate, 878*t*
undecylenic acid, 878*t*
for systemic and superficial infections
azoles, 872*t*. *See also* AZOLES
for systemic infections, 871, 872*t*
amphotericin B. *See* amphotericin B deoxycholate
anidulafungin, 872*t*, 874–75
caspofungin acetate, 871, 872*t*, 874–75
flucytosine, 871, 872*t*, 875
micafungin, 872*t*, 874–75
antigen, 713, 755
antigen-presenting cells (APCs), 714*t*
antiglaucoma agents. *See* glaucoma, pharmacotherapy
antigout agents:
Nursing Process Application, 1311*t*
uric acid inhibitors
colchicine. *See* colchicine
uricosurics
probenecid, 1307*t*, 1309, 1310
sulfinpyrazone, 1307*t*, 1309, 1310
xanthine oxidase inhibitor
allopurinol. *See* allopurinol
antihelminthic agents. *See* helminthic infections, pharmacotherapy
antihistamines. *See* H_1-RECEPTOR ANTAGONISTS
antihypertensive drugs. *See also* hypertension, pharmacotherapy
combination, 571, 572*t*
mechanism of action, 571*f*
anti-infectives, 776
antibiotics. *See* ANTIBIOTICS
antifungals. *See* ANTIFUNGAL DRUGS
mechanisms of action, 776–77, 778*t*, 779*f*
disruption of plasma membrane, 778, 778*t*
inhibition of cell wall synthesis, 778, 778*t*
inhibition of metabolic pathways, 778, 778*t*
inhibition of nucleic acid synthesis, 778, 778*t*
inhibition of protein synthesis, 778, 778*t*
prophylactic use, 783
resistance to. *See* acquired resistance
selection of
host factors affecting, 783–84
pathogen identification and, 782
single versus combination therapy, 782–83
superinfections and, 784
Antilirium. *See* physostigmine
antimalaria drugs. *See* malaria, pharmacotherapy
ANTIMETABOLITES:
anakinra, 741*t*, 746, 1304*t*, 1305–6
etanercept. *See* etanercept
folic acid analogs, 972, 972*f*
methotrexate. *See* methotrexate
pemetrexed, 973*t*, 974
mechanism of action, 742*f*, 744
purine analogs, 975
cladribine, 973*t*, 975–76
clofarabine, 973*t*, 976
fludarabine, 973*t*, 976
mercaptopurine, 973*t*, 976
nelarabine, 973*t*, 976
pentostatin, 973*t*, 976
thioguanine, 973*t*, 976
pyrimidine analogs, 974–75
capecitabine, 973*t*, 975
cytarabine, 827, 973*t*, 975
floxuridine, 973*t*, 975
fluorouracil, 827, 973*t*, 975
gemcitabine, 973*t*, 975
thalidomide, 14, 741*t*, 746–47, 991
Antiminth. *See* pyrantel
ANTINEOPLASTIC AGENTS:
administration in older adults, 984*t*
adverse effects, 68*t*, 958*t*
alopecia, 960
cardiopulmonary, 959
drugs for reduction of, 992
fatigue, 960
gastrointestinal, 959
hematologic, 958–59
hyperuricemia, 960
nervous system, 960
reproductive system, 960
secondary cancer, 960
skin and soft tissue, 960
urinary system, 959
alkylating agents. *See* ALKYLATING AGENTS
angiogenesis inhibitors. *See* ANGIOGENESIS INHIBITORS
antimetabolites. *See* ANTIMETABOLITES
antitumor antibiotics. *See* ANTITUMOR ANTIBIOTICS
biologic response modifiers, 734, 990
aldesleukin. *See* aldesleukin
interferons. *See* INTERFERON(S) (IFNs)
cell cycle and, 954–55, 955*f*
cell kill hypothesis, 955–56, 956*f*
classification, 965
combination therapy, 957
dosing schedules, 957
hormone antagonists. *See* hormone antagonists, for neoplasia
hormones. *See* HORMONE(S), pharmacotherapy with
miscellaneous
altretamine, 991, 992*t*
arsenic trioxide, 991, 992*t*
asparaginase, 991–92, 992*t*
bevacizumab. *See* bevacizumab
bexarotene, 992, 992*t*
hydroxyurea, 992, 992*t*
mitotane, 992*t*, 993
pegaspargase, 992, 992*t*
zoledronic acid, 992*t*, 993
monoclonal antibodies. *See* MONOCLONAL ANTIBODIES (MABs)
natural products
taxanes. *See* TAXANES
topoisomerase inhibitors. *See* TOPOISOMERASE INHIBITORS
vinca alkaloids. *See* VINCA ALKALOIDS
Nursing Process Application, 988–89*t*
nursing requirements, 960–61
nursing responsibilities, 965–66
patient and family education, 966
preparation and administration, 993
psychological issues for patients, 961
routes of administration, 957–58
ANTIPLATELET AGENTS:
ADP receptor blockers
clopidogrel. *See* clopidogrel
mechanism of action, 653–54
ticlopidine, 653, 653*t*, 655
aspirin. *See* aspirin
dipyridamole, 653*t*, 655
glycoprotein IIb/IIIa receptor inhibitors
abciximab. *See* abciximab
eptifibatide, 653*t*, 657
mechanism of action, 655, 656*f*
tirofiban, 653*t*, 657
mechanism of action, 644*f*, 653
for specific conditions
intermittent claudication, 653*t*
unstable angina/myocardial infarction, 600
antiprostatic drugs. *See* benign prostatic hyperplasia, pharmacotherapy
antipsychotics:
adverse effects, 331–32, 331*t*
in Asian patients, 336*t*
classification, 330
Clinical Antipsychotic Trials of Intervention Effectiveness (CATIE) study, 341*t*
first-generation. *See* FIRST-GENERATION ANTIPSYCHOTICS
genetic polymorphisms and, 160*t*, 336*t*
mechanism of action, 329*f*
Nursing Process Application, 342–43*t*
second-generation (atypical). *See* SECOND-GENERATION (ATYPICAL) ANTIPSYCHOTICS
selection, 330–31
antipyretics, 718
acetaminophen. *See* acetaminophen
nonsteroidal anti-inflammatory drugs. *See* NONSTEROIDAL ANTI-INFLAMMATORY DRUGS (NSAIDs)
salicylates. *See* SALICYLATES
ANTIRETROVIRALS, 927
adverse effects, 930
CCR5 inhibitors
maraviroc, 933*t*, 940
classification, 932
fusion inhibitors
enfuvirtide, 933*t*, 940
integrase inhibitors
raltegravir, 933*t*, 940
nonnucleoside reverse transcriptase inhibitors, 936
delavirdine, 933*t*, 937
efavirenz. *See* efavirenz
etravirine, 933*t*, 937
nevirapine, 933*t*, 937
nucleoside/nucleotide reverse transcriptase inhibitors, 932–34
abacavir, 933*t*, 935
didanosine, 933*t*, 935
emtricitabine, 933*t*, 935
lamivudine. *See* lamivudine
stavudine, 933*t*, 936
tenofovir, 933*t*, 936
zidovudine. *See* zidovudine
Nursing Process Application, 941–42*t*
pharmacokinetics, 932
protease inhibitors, 937–38
atazanavir, 933*t*, 939
darunavir, 933*t*, 939
fosamprenavir, 933*t*, 939

indinavir, 933*t*, 939
lopinavir/ritonavir. *See* lopinavir/ritonavir
nelfinavir, 933*t*, 939–40
ritonavir, 933*t*, 940
saquinavir, 933*t*, 940
tipranavir, 933*t*, 940
resistance to, 931
ANTISEIZURE DRUGS:
as adjuvant analgesics, 446, 446*t*
drug interactions
with herbal products, 178*t*
with oral contraceptives, 372
drugs in class
barbiturates, 379
amobarbital, 379, 380*t*
mephobarbital, 379, 380*t*, 381
phenobarbital. *See* phenobarbital
primidone, 380*t*, 382
benzodiazepines, 283*t*, 382
clonazepam, 380*t*, 383
clorazepate, 380*t*, 383
diazepam. *See* diazepam
lorazepam. *See* lorazepam
midazolam. *See* midazolam
felbamate, 381*t*, 391
gabapentin. *See* gabapentin
hydantoins, 384
fosphenytoin, 380*t*, 385
phenytoin. *See* phenytoin
iminostilbenes, 385
carbamazepine. *See* carbamazepine
oxcarbazepine. *See* oxcarbazepine
lamotrigine. *See* lamotrigine
pregabalin, 381*t*, 391–92
succinimides, 387–88
ethosuximide. *See* ethosuximide
methsuximide, 389
phensuximide, 381*t*
tiagabine, 381*t*, 392
valproic acid. *See* valproic acid
zonisamide, 391*t*, 392
mechanism of action, 377–79, 378*f*
control of electrolyte movement, 377
neurotransmitter balance, 377–79, 379*f*
Nursing Process Application, 393*t*
in older adults, 373–74
selection, 376–77
for specific conditions
bipolar disorder, 319*t*, 320–21
migraine prophylaxis, 453, 453*t*
antithrombin III (AT-III), 645
antithymocyte globulin, 741*t*, 747, 749
ANTITHYROID AGENTS, 1154–55
methimazole, 1154*t*, 1156
Nursing Process Application, 1157*t*
potassium iodide, 1156
potassium iodide and iodine, 1154*t*, 1156
propylthiouracil. *See* propylthiouracil
radioactive iodide, 1154*t*, 1156
antituberculosis drugs. *See* tuberculosis, pharmacotherapy
ANTITUMOR ANTIBIOTICS, 976–77
bleomycin, 827, 959, 977*t*, 978
dactinomycin, 977*t*, 978
daunorubicin, 827, 977*t*, 978
daunorubicin liposomal, 977*t*, 978
doxorubicin. *See* doxorubicin
epirubicin, 977*t*
idarubicin, 977*t*, 978
mitomycin, 977*t*, 978
mitoxantrone. *See* mitoxantrone
ANTITUSSIVES, 1275
nonopioids
benzonatate, 1276*t*, 1277
dextromethorphan. *See* dextromethorphan
opioids
codeine, 1275, 1276*t*
hydrocodone with homatropine, 1275, 1276*t*
Antivert. *See* meclizine
antiviral drugs. *See also* ANTIRETROVIRALS
for non-HIV viral infections
hepatitis. *See* hepatitis, pharmacotherapy
herpes simplex viruses. *See* herpes simplex virus infections, pharmacotherapy
influenza. *See* influenza, pharmacotherapy
mechanism of action, 910–11
Nursing Process Application, 923*t*
Antizol. *See* fomepizole
Anturane. *See* sulfinpyrazone
anxiety, 274. *See also* anxiety disorders
complementary and alternative therapies, 280–81, 281*t*
insomnia and, 280
medications and conditions associated with, 275*t*
model of, 274*f*
pharmacotherapy, 281. *See also specific drugs*
antidepressants, 282*t*, 288–89, 290*t*
barbiturates, 282*t*, 292–93
benzodiazepines, 282*t*, 283–86, 283*t*
nonbenzodiazepine anxiolytics, 282*t*, 288
Nursing Process Application, 293*t*
situational, 275
anxiety disorders:
brain regions responsible for, 276, 277*f*
generalized anxiety disorder, 275
incidence, 275*t*
obsessive–compulsive disorder, 276, 289
panic disorder, 275, 289
pharmacotherapy. *See* anxiety, pharmacotherapy
post-traumatic stress disorder (PTSD), 276, 289
social anxiety disorder, 275, 289
anxiolytic, 281
Anzemet. *See* dolasetron
Apidra. *See* insulin glulisine
apocrine glands, 1316
Apokyn. *See* apomorphine
apomorphine, 350*t*, 354
apoprotein, 496
apothecary system of measurement, 28, 28*t*
appetite, 1086
apraclonidine, 1341*t*, 1343
aprepitant, 1043*t*, 1044
Apresazide, 549, 572*t*
Apresoline. *See* hydralazine
Aptivus. *See* tipranavir
aPTT (activated partial thromboplastin time), 644
Aquasol A. *See* vitamin A
Aquatensen. *See* methyclothiazide
aqueous humor, 1338
Aralen. *See* chloroquine
Aranesp. *See* darbepoetin alfa
Arava. *See* leflunomide
ARBs. *See* ANGIOTENSIN II RECEPTOR BLOCKERS (ARBs)
Aredia. *See* pamidronate
arenaviruses, 909*t*
Arfonad. *See* trimethaphan
arformoterol, 1245*t*, 1247
argatroban, 645*t*, 649
Argesic. *See* salsalate
Aricept. *See* donepezil
Arimidex. *See* anastrozole
aripiprazole, 340–41
adverse effects, 319*t*, 337*t*, 340
classification, 340
contraindications/precautions, 340
drug interactions, 340
mechanism of action, 340
nursing responsibilities, 341
overdose treatment, 341
patient and family education, 341
pregnancy category, 340
route and adult dose, 319*t*, 337*t*
for specific conditions
bipolar disorder, 319*t*
therapeutic effects and uses, 340
Aristocort. *See* triamcinolone
Arixtra. *See* fondaparinux
armodafinil, 421
Armour. *See* desiccated thyroid
Aromasin. *See* exemestane
AROMATASE INHIBITORS, 983
anastrazole, 980*t*, 983
exemestane, 980*t*, 983
letrozole, 980*t*, 983
aromatherapy, 798*t*
Arranon. *See* nelarabine
arsenic trioxide, 991, 992*t*
Arsobal. *See* melarsoprol
Artane. *See* trihexyphenidyl
articaine, 473*t*, 475
artificial sweeteners, 1093
ASA. *See* aspirin
Asacol. *See* mesalamine
ASAP, 27
Ascarel. *See* pyrantel
ascariasis, 899–900, 900*f*
Ascaris lumbricoides, 899–900, 900*f*
ascorbic acid. *See* vitamin C
Asendin. *See* amoxapine
Asian Americans, propranolol sensitivity in, 633*t*
Asian culture, depression treatment in, 300*t*
Asmanex. *See* mometasone
asparaginase, 991–92, 992*t*
aspartame, 1093
Aspercreme, 1302
aspergillosis, 869*t*
Aspergillus fumigatus, 869*t*
aspiration, during enteral nutrition therapy, 1071*t*
aspirin, 722–23
adverse effects, 653*t*, 720, 720*t*, 722
in breast-feeding infant, 129*t*
allergy, 719
classification, 721
contraindications/precautions, 722
dosage forms not to be crushed or opened, 30*t*
drug interactions, 722
with alcohol, 101*t*
with herbal products, 178*t*
enteric coated, 30*t*
mechanism of action, 719, 719*f*, 722
versus nonaspirin NSAIDs, 725
nursing responsibilities, 722
overdose treatment, 722

patient and family education, 722–23
pharmacokinetics, 722
pregnancy category, 722
route and adult dose, 653*t*, 720*t*
similar drugs, 723
for specific conditions
as antiplatelet agent, 653
myocardial infarction, 600
therapeutic effects and uses, 718, 721
assessment, in nursing process, 115
assisted living facilities, 165
Astelin. *See* azelastine
asthma, 1240
incidence, 1240, 1241*t*, 1243*t*
levels, 1242*t*
pathophysiology, 1240–41, 1240*t*, 1241*f*
pharmacotherapy
bronchodilators. *See* BRONCHODILATORS
corticosteroids, 1169, 1244*t*, 1249–50, 1250*t*
beclomethasone. *See* beclomethasone
budesonide. *See* budesonide
flunisolide, 1250*t*, 1252
fluticasone. *See* fluticasone
mometasone, 1250*t*, 1252
triamcinolone, 1167*t*, 1250*t*, 1252
dyphylline, 1256
Evidence-Based Practice, 1244*t*
inhalation route, 1241–42
leukotriene modifiers, 1244*t*, 1250*t*, 1253
montelukast, 1250*t*, 1254
zafirlukast. *See* zafirlukast
zileuton, 1250*t*, 1254–55
mast cell stabilizers, 1244*t*, 1252
cromolyn. *See* cromolyn
nedocromil sodium, 1250*t*, 1253
methylxanthines, 1255
aminophylline, 1245*t*, 1256
theophylline. *See* theophylline
monoclonal antibodies
omalizumab, 748*t*, 1256
Nursing Process Application, 1257*t*
overview of drug classes, 1244*t*
principles, 1242–43
stepwise approach, 1243*f*
Astramorph PF. *See* morphine sulfate
Atabrine. *See* quinacrine
Atacand. *See* candesartan
Atarax. *See* hydroxyzine
atazanavir, 26*t*, 933*t*, 939
atenolol, 597
adverse effects, 252*t*, 257, 597
in breast-feeding infant, 129*t*
classification, 597
contraindications/precautions, 597
drug interactions, 597
mechanism of action, 597
nursing responsibilities, 597
overdose treatment, 597
patient and family education, 597
pharmacokinetics, 597
pregnancy category, 597
route and adult dose, 252*t*
similar drugs, 598
for specific conditions, 257
akathisia, 331, 331*t*
angina, 592*t*
anxiety, 286
therapeutic effects and uses, 597
Atgam. *See* antithymocyte globulin
atherosclerosis, 496, 588, 589*f*
Ativan. *See* lorazepam
Atolone. *See* triamcinolone
atomoxetine, 418–19
adverse effects, 416*t*, 419
classification, 418
contraindications/precautions, 419
drug interactions, 419
mechanism of action, 418
nursing responsibilities, 419
overdose treatment, 419
patient and family education, 419
pharmacokinetics, 418
pregnancy category, 419
route and adult dose, 416*t*
therapeutic effects and uses, 418
atonic seizures, 374–75, 376*t*
atopic dermatitis, 1325
atorvastatin, 504–5
adverse effects, 504*t*, 505
classification, 504
contraindications/precautions, 505
drug interactions, 101*t*, 505
mechanism of action, 504
nursing responsibilities, 505
overdose treatment, 505
patient and family education, 505
pharmacokinetics, 505
pregnancy category, 505
route and adult dose, 504*t*
similar drugs, 505–6
therapeutic effects and uses, 504
atovaquone, 75*t*, 890
atovaquone-proguanil, 75*t*, 888*t*, 890
atracurium, 219*t*, 224, 477
atrial fibrillation, 626. *See also* dysrhythmias
atrial flutter, 626. *See also* dysrhythmias
atrial natriuretic peptide (ANP), 493, 609
atrial reflex, 492
atrial tachycardia, 626. *See also* dysrhythmias
atrioventricular (AV) conduction block, 626. *See also* dysrhythmias
atrioventricular (AV) node, 487
Atromid-S. *See* clofibrate
atropine, 216–17
adverse effects, 214*t*, 216
in pediatric patients, 142*t*
classification, 216
contraindications/precautions, 216
dosage/routes
adult, 214*t*
pediatric, 142*t*
drug interactions, 216–17
history, 215*t*
mechanism of action, 216
nursing responsibilities, 217
overdose treatment, 217
patient and family education, 217
pharmacokinetics, 216
pregnancy category, 217
as preoperative medication, 477
similar drugs, 217–18
for specific conditions
cholinergic crisis, 205
eye examinations, 1347, 1348*t*
therapeutic effects and uses, 216
Atrovent. *See* ipratropium
attention deficit/hyperactivity disorder (ADHD), 106, 413
in adulthood, 414*t*
diagnosis, 413*t*
etiology, 413–14
in girls, 414*t*
pharmacotherapy
amphetamines, 414–18, 416*t*
antidepressants, 418
atomoxetine. *See* atomoxetine
Evidence-Based Practice, 414*t*
Nursing Process Application, 423*t*
symptoms, 413
attenuated, 756
attenuated (live) vaccines, 756, 756*t*
ATYPICAL ANTIDEPRESSANTS, 311
drugs in class
amoxapine, 312
bupropion, 30*t*, 312
duloxetine. *See* duloxetine
mirtazapine, 312
nefazodone, 312–13
reboxetine, 313
trazodone. *See* trazodone
venlafaxine. *See* venlafaxine
mechanism of action, 311
Nursing Process Application, 317*t*
for specific conditions
anxiety, 282*t*, 289
depression, 311
atypical antipsychotics. *See* SECOND-GENERATION (ATYPICAL) ANTIPSYCHOTICS
atypical mycobacterial infection (AMI), 851
AUC (acute uncomplicated cystitis), 838, 838*t*. *See also* urinary tract infections
Augmentin. *See* amoxicillin/clavulanate
Augmentin XR, 30*t*. *See also* amoxicillin/clavulanate
Auralgan. *See* benzocaine/antipyrine
auras, 449
automaticity, 487
automatisms, 375
autonomic drugs, 196, 196*t*. *See also* ADRENERGIC AGONISTS; ADRENERGIC ANTAGONISTS; MUSCARINIC AGONISTS; MUSCARINIC ANTAGONISTS
autonomic nervous system (ANS), 185
activities, 185
drugs affecting. *See* autonomic drugs
parasympathetic division, 186–88
regulation of functions, 195–96, 195*f*
sympathetic division, 185–86
synaptic transmission, 188–90, 188*f*, 189*f*
autonomic tone, 187
AV (atrioventricular) conduction block, 626. *See also* dysrhythmias
AV (atrioventricular) node, 487
Avage. *See* tazarotene
Avalide, 572*t*
Avandamet, 1134*t*
Avapro. *See* irbesartan
Avastin. *See* bevacizumab
Avelox. *See* moxifloxacin
Aventyl. *See* nortriptyline
Avita. *See* tretinoin
Avonex. *See* interferon beta-1a
Axert. *See* almotriptan
Axid. *See* nizatidine
Azactam. *See* aztreonam
Azasan. *See* azathioprine
azathioprine, 745–46
adverse effects, 68*t*, 741*t*, 745, 1304*t*
classification, 745
contraindications/precautions, 745

mechanism of action, 745
nursing responsibilities, 745–46
overdose treatment, 745
patient and family education, 746
pharmacokinetics, 745
pregnancy category, 745
route and adult dose, 741*t*, 1304*t*
similar drugs, 746
for specific conditions
rheumatoid arthritis, 1304*t*
therapeutic effects and uses, 745
azelaic acid, 1322*t*, 1323, 1324–25
azelastine, 1265*t*, 1266, 1349, 1349*t*
Azelex. *See* azelaic acid
azithromycin:
adverse effects, 813*t*, 815
in pediatric patients, 142*t*
dosage/routes
adult, 813*t*
dosage forms, 815
pediatric, 142*t*
drug interactions, 75*t*
indications, 813
for specific conditions
M. avium complex infections, 865
Azmacort. *See* triamcinolone
AZOLES, 875
adverse effects, 875
classification, 875
drugs in class
butoconazole, 878*t*, 879
clotrimazole, 878*t*, 879
econazole, 878*t*
fluconazole. *See* fluconazole
itraconazole. *See* itraconazole
ketoconazole. *See* ketoconazole
miconazole, 878*t*, 879
oxiconazole, 878*t*
sulconazole, 878*t*
terconazole, 878*t*
tioconazole, 878*t*, 879
voriconazole, 872*t*, 877
mechanism of action, 871*f*, 875
for specific conditions
superficial mycoses, 878*t*
systemic mycoses, 872*t*
azoospermia, 1226
Azopt. *See* brinzolamide
Azor, 572*t*
AZT. *See* zidovudine
aztreonam, 800*t*, 803
Azulfidine. *See* sulfasalazine

B

B cell, 713
Bacillus anthracis, 777*t*, 1360. *See also* anthrax
bacillus Calmette-Guérin (BCG) vaccine, 735*t*, 739
bacitracin, 832, 832*t*
baclofen, 400*t*, 401, 402*t*
bacteria:
cell walls, 787–88, 787*f*
classification, 776
DNA replication, 826, 826*f*
gram-negative bacilli, 777*t*
gram-negative cocci, 777*t*
gram-positive bacilli, 777*t*
gram-positive cocci, 777*t*
other, 777*t*
protein synthesis, 808–9, 808*f*
bacteriocidal, 776
bacteriostatic, 776
bacteriuria, 837
Bacteroides, 777*t*
Bactrim. *See* trimethoprim-sulfamethoxazole
baking soda. *See* sodium bicarbonate
BAL in Oil. *See* dimercaprol
balanced anesthesia, 458. *See also* general anesthesia
Balnetar. *See* coal tar
balsalazide, 1037*t*, 1038–39
Banflex. *See* orphenadrine
Baraclude. *See* entecavir
BARBITURATES:
abuse, 98
drug interactions, 178*t*
drugs in class
amobarbital. *See* amobarbital
butabarbital, 282*t*, 292
mephobarbital. *See* mephobarbital
methohexital, 292
pentobarbital, 282*t*, 292
phenobarbital. *See* phenobarbital
secobarbital, 282*t*, 292
thiopental sodium. *See* thiopental sodium
genetic polymorphisms and actions of, 160*t*
mechanism of action, 291
overdose, 98
for specific conditions
anxiety and insomnia, 282*t*, 290*t*, 291–92
general anesthesia, 459–61, 460*t*
seizures, 379, 380*t*, 381–82
tolerance to, 98, 291
withdrawal symptoms and treatment, 96*t*
baroreceptors, 492
Barrett's esophagus, 1010
basal ganglia (nuclei), 270
anatomy, 271*f*
functions, 270
in Parkinson's disease, 348
in schizophrenia, 328
basiliximab, 741*t*, 742*f*, 748*t*, 749
Bayrab. *See* rabies immune globulin
BayTet. *See* tetanus immune globulin
BCG (bacillus Calmette-Guérin) vaccine, 735*t*, 739
beclomethasone, 1251–52
adverse effects, 1250*t*, 1251, 1270*t*
classification, 1251
contraindications/precautions, 1251
drug interactions, 1251
mechanism of action, 1251
nursing responsibilities, 1251
overdose treatment, 1251
patient and family education, 1251–52
pharmacokinetics, 1251
pregnancy category, 1251
route and adult dose, 1250*t*, 1270*t*
similar drugs, 1252
for specific conditions
allergic rhinitis, 1270*t*
therapeutic effects and uses, 1251
Beconase AQ. *See* beclomethasone
Beers criteria, 152
belladonna, 214, 215*t*
Benadryl. *See* diphenhydramine
Benadryl Allergy/Cold caplets, 1266*t*
benazepril, 533*t*, 535
bendroflumethiazide, 554*t*
Benemid. *See* probenecid
Ben-Gay, 1302
Benicar. *See* olmesartan medoxomil
Benicar HCT, 572*t*
benign prostatic hyperplasia (BPH), 1229
pathogenesis, 1229–30
pharmacotherapy
alpha-adrenergic antagonists, 246
alfuzosin, 1231*t*
doxazosin, 1231*t*
doxazosin XL, 1231*t*
tamsulosin, 1231*t*
terazosin, 1231*t*
5-alpha reductase inhibitors
dutasteride, 1231*t*, 1233–34
finasteride. *See* finasteride
mechanism of action, 1230*f*
Nursing Process Application, 1233*t*
screening, 1229*t*
symptoms, 1230
benign tumor, 950*t*
Bentyl. *See* dicyclomine
Benzalin. *See* benzoyl peroxide
Benzamycin. *See* benzoyl peroxide, with erythromycin
benzocaine, 474, 1332–33
adverse effects, 473*t*, 1332
classification, 1332
contraindications/precautions, 1332
drug interactions, 1332
mechanism of action, 1332
nursing responsibilities, 1332–33
overdose treatment, 1332
patient and family education, 1333
pharmacokinetics, 1332
pregnancy category, 1332
route and adult dose, 473*t*
therapeutic effects and uses, 474, 1332
benzocaine/antipyrine, 1352*t*
BENZODIAZEPINES:
abuse, 98
drug interactions
with herbal products, 178*t*
drugs in class
alprazolam, 282*t*, 283*t*, 285
chlordiazepoxide, 282*t*, 283*t*, 285
clonazepam. *See* clonazepam
clorazepate. *See* clorazepate
diazepam. *See* diazepam
estazolam, 282*t*, 283*t*, 286
flurazepam, 282*t*, 283*t*, 286
lorazepam. *See* lorazepam
midazolam. *See* midazolam
oxazepam, 282*t*, 286
quazepam, 282*t*, 286
temazepam, 282*t*, 286
triazolam, 282*t*, 286
in older adults, 152*t*
overdose/poisoning, 284, 1364*t*
for specific conditions, 283*t*
akathisia, 331
in anesthesia, 460*t*, 463–65, 477
anxiety, 282*t*, 283, 285–86
insomnia, 282*t*, 283–84, 286
nausea and vomiting, 1043*t*, 1044
seizures, 380*t*, 382–84
withdrawal symptoms and treatment, 96*t*
benzonatate, 30*t*, 1276*t*, 1277
benzoyl peroxide, 1322, 1322*t*
with erythromycin, 1322
with sulfur, 1322
benzphetamine, 416*t*, 417

benztropine, 355–56
  adverse effects, 214t, 355t, 356
  classification, 355
  contraindications/precautions, 356
  drug interactions, 356
  mechanism of action, 356
  nursing responsibilities, 356
  overdose treatment, 356
  patient and family education, 356
  pharmacokinetics, 356
  pregnancy category, 356
  route and adult dose, 214t, 355t
  similar drugs, 356
  for specific conditions
    acute dystonia, 331t
    Parkinson's disease, 218
  therapeutic effects and uses, 355–56
benzyl alcohol, 137
bepridil, 592t
beractant, 1240t
Best Pharmaceuticals for Children Act, 135
BETA-ADRENERGIC AGONISTS. *See also* ADRENERGIC AGONISTS
  nonselective
    isoproterenol hydrochloride. *See* isoproterenol hydrochloride
  selective. *See* BETA$_1$-ADRENERGIC AGONISTS; BETA$_2$-ADRENERGIC AGONISTS
  for specific conditions, 238
    heart failure, 612t, 618
BETA-ADRENERGIC ANTAGONISTS, 251
  adverse effects, 251–52, 252t, 576, 596, 612t
  discontinuation, 597
  mechanism of action, 247f, 571f, 591f
  nonselective
    betaxolol, 252t, 257, 1341t, 1343, 1345
    carteolol, 252t, 254, 1341t, 1343
    carvedilol. *See* carvedilol
    labetalol. *See* labetalol
    metipranolol, 252t, 255, 1341t, 1343
    nadolol, 252t, 255
    penbutolol, 252t, 255
    pindolol, 251, 252t, 255
    propranolol. *See* propranolol
    sotalol, 252t, 255, 629t, 636
    timolol. *See* timolol
  Nursing Process Application, 258t
  overdose, 252
  selective. *See* BETA$_1$-ADRENERGIC ANTAGONISTS
  for specific conditions, 247f, 251
    akathisia, 331, 331t
    angina, 592t, 595–98
    dysrhythmias, 628t, 629t, 633
    glaucoma, 1341t, 1343
    heart failure, 612t, 613–14
    hypertension, 572t, 574t, 576
    hypertensive emergency, 584t
    migraine prophylaxis, 453, 453t
    myocardial infarction, 592t, 602
    thyroid storm, 1155
BETA$_1$-ADRENERGIC AGONISTS:
  dopamine. *See* dopamine
  epinephrine. *See* epinephrine
  mechanism of action, 238–39
  norepinephrine. *See* norepinephrine
  for specific conditions, 231, 238–39
    heart failure, 612t, 618
BETA$_1$-ADRENERGIC ANTAGONISTS:
  adverse effects, 252t, 255
  clinical applications, 247f, 255
  drugs in class
    acebutolol. *See* acebutolol
    atenolol. *See* atenolol
    betaxolol, 252t, 257
    bisoprolol, 252t, 257
    esmolol. *See* esmolol
    metoprolol. *See* metoprolol
    nebivolol, 252t, 258
  mechanism of action, 247f
  overdose, 255
  for specific conditions
    hypertension, 574t, 576
    hypertensive emergency, 584t
    myocardial infarction, 592t, 602
beta$_1$-adrenergic receptors:
  locations, 192t, 193, 238
  responses, 193, 193t, 238
BETA$_2$-ADRENERGIC AGONISTS:
  adverse effects, 239
  bronchodilators. *See* BRONCHODILATORS
  dobutamine. *See* dobutamine
  genetic polymorphisms and actions of, 160t
  for specific conditions, 231
    asthma, 1243, 1244t, 1245–46, 1245t
    heart failure, 612t, 618
  tocolytics. *See* tocolytics
beta$_2$-adrenergic receptors:
  genetic polymorphisms, 160t
  locations, 192t, 193
  responses, 192t, 193, 1240
beta-blockers. *See* BETA-ADRENERGIC ANTAGONISTS
β-glucan synthesis inhibitors, 874–75
β-glucan, 871
Betacort. *See* betamethasone
Betagan. *See* levobunolol
beta-lactam ring, 788, 789f
beta lactamase, 788
betamethasone, 1167t, 1328
betamethasone benzoate, 1327t
betamethasone dipropionate, 1327t
betamethasone valerate, 1327t
Betapace. *See* sotalol
Betapace AF. *See* sotalol
Betaseron. *See* interferon beta-1b
betaxolol, 252t, 257, 1341t, 1343, 1345
bethanechol chloride, 203–4
  adverse effects, 202t, 203
  classification, 203
  contraindications/precautions, 203
  drug interactions, 203
  mechanism of action, 203
  nursing responsibilities, 203–4
  overdose treatment, 203
  patient and family education, 204
  pharmacokinetics, 203
  pregnancy category, 203
  route and adult dose, 202t
  therapeutic effects and uses, 203
Betimol. *See* timolol
Betoptic. *See* betaxolol
bevacizumab, 748t, 990t, 991
bexarotene, 992, 992t
Bextra. *See* valdecoxib
Bexxar. *See* tositumomab
Biaxin. *See* clarithromycin
bicalutamide, 980t, 984
Bicillin. *See* penicillin G benzathine
BiCNU. *See* carmustine
BIGUANIDES:
  actions, 1132t
  mechanism of action, 1135
  metformin. *See* metformin
  nursing considerations, 1132t
bilberry:
  description, 1347t
  evidence, 1347t
  history and claims, 1347t
  primary uses, 173t
  standardization, 1347t
bile, 49
BILE ACID SEQUESTRANTS (RESINS):
  adverse effects, 504t, 507
  drugs in class
    cholestyramine. *See* cholestyramine
    colesevelam, 504t, 508
    colestipol, 504t, 508
  mechanism of action, 503f, 506–7
  for specific conditions
    dyslipidemias, 504t, 506–8
Biltricide. *See* praziquantel
bimatoprost, 1341t, 1343
bioavailability, 8
BIOLOGIC RESPONSE MODIFIERS, 734, 990
  aldesleukin. *See* aldesleukin
  interferons. *See* INTERFERON(S) (IFNs)
Bio-Statin. *See* nystatin
bioterrorism, 1358. *See also* terrorism
  infectious agents
    anthrax, 1360–61, 1360t
    botulism, 1361
    classification, 1359t
    pneumonic plaque, 1361
    smallpox, 1361
    tularemia, 1361
    viral hemorrhagic fever, 1361
Bio-Thyroid. *See* desiccated thyroid
biotransformation. *See* metabolism, drug
biperiden, 331, 355t
bipolar disorder, 298, 317
  nonadherence to treatment, 318
  pathophysiology, 318
  pharmacotherapy
    antidepressants, 321
    antiseizure drugs, 319t, 320–21
    atypical antipsychotics, 319t, 321
    lithium carbonate. *See* lithium carbonate
    Nursing Process Application, 321t
  symptoms, 317–18
birth control. *See* contraceptive methods
bisacodyl, 30t, 1030t, 1032
bismuth subsalicylate:
  as antidiarrheal agent, 1033, 1034t, 1035
  for *H. pylori* infection, 1023, 1024
  for peptic ulcer disease, 1024
bisoprolol, 252t, 257
BISPHOSPHONATES, 1294
  as adjuvant analgesics, 445, 447, 446t
  adverse effects, 1295
  drugs in class
    alendronate. *See* alendronate
    etidronate, 75t, 1294t, 1295t, 1297
    ibandronate, 1294t, 1295t, 1297
    pamidronate, 1294t, 1295t, 1297
    risedronate, 1294t, 1295t, 1297
    tiludronate, 1294t, 1295t, 1297
    zoledronate (zoledronic acid), 992t, 993, 1294t, 1295t, 1297

Nursing Process Application, 1298*t*
for specific conditions, 1294*t*
osteoporosis, 1294–95, 1295*t*
bitolterol, 240
bivalirudin, 645*t*, 649
black cohosh:
description, 1201*t*
evidence, 1201*t*
history and claims, 1201*t*
labeling, 176*f*
for muscle spasms, 397
primary uses, 173*t*
standardization, 175*t*, 1201*t*
Blastomyces dermatitides, 869*t*
blastomycosis, 869*t*
Blenoxane. *See* bleomycin
bleomycin, 827, 959, 978
blepharitis, 1349
blessed thistle, 129*t*
blister/vesicant agents:
mixture-HL, 1363*t*
mustard-lewisite, 1363*t*
nitrogen mustard-HN-1, HN-2, HN-3, 1363*t*
phosgene oxime, 1363*t*
sulfur mustard agents, 1363*t*
Blocadren. *See* timolol
blood:
functions and properties, 483–85
glucose regulation, 1120, 1121*t*. *See also* diabetes mellitus
blood agents:
cyanogen cyanide, 1362*t*
hydrogen cyanide, 1362*t*
blood–brain barrier, 46, 136, 269, 269*f*
blood pressure, 491. *See also* hypertension
factors affecting, 491, 491*f*
hormones affecting, 493, 493*f*
nervous regulation, 492, 492*f*
self-measurement, 568*t*
variation throughout the life span, 568, 568*t*
BLOOD PRODUCTS:
cryoprecipitate, 689*t*
fresh frozen plasma, 689*t*
immune globulins, 689*t*
normal serum albumin. *See* normal serum albumin
packed RBCs, 689*t*
platelets, 689*t*
principles, 689–90
whole blood, 689*t*, 690
BNP (B-type natriuretic peptide), 609
body mass index (BMI), 1087, 1088*f*
body surface area (BSA) method, dosage calculation, 140
body weight method, dosage calculation, 140
bolus feedings, 1069. *See also* enteral nutrition
bone deposition, 1285
bone marrow, drugs toxic to, 69*t*, 70
bone resorption, 1285
Bonine. *See* meclizine
Boniva. *See* ibandronate
boosters, 755
Bordetella pertussis, 759. *See also* pertussis
Borrelia burgdorferi, 777*t*
bortezomib, 748*t*, 990*t*
botanical, 172
Botox. *See* botulinum toxin type A
botulinum toxin type A, 404*t*, 406, 406*f*
for headache treatment, 453
botulinum toxin type B, 404*t*, 406
botulism, 1361
Bowman's capsule, 545
BPH. *See* benign prostatic hyperplasia
bradydysrhythmias, 625. *See also* dysrhythmias
bradykinesia, 348
bradykinin, 531, 712*t*
brain. *See* central nervous system
brain injury:
ADHD and, 413
muscle spasticity following, 402–3
brainstem, 268*f*, 269
brand name, 7
Bravelle. *See* urofollitropin
breakthrough bleeding, 1183
breast cancer, 976*t*
breast-feeding. *See* lactation
breast milk. *See* lactation
Brethaire. *See* terbutaline
Brethine. *See* terbutaline
Brevibloc. *See* esmolol
Brevital. *See* methohexital
brimonidine, 1341*t*, 1343
brinzolamide, 1341*t*, 1345
broad-spectrum antibiotic, 782
bromocriptine, 354
adverse effects, 350*t*, 354
in breast-feeding infant, 129*t*
route and adult dose, 350*t*
for specific conditions
female infertility, 1192*t*, 1195
growth hormone excess, 1108*t*, 1112
brompheniramine, 1265*t*
bronchioles, 1239*f*, 1240, 1241*f*
BRONCHODILATORS:
anticholinergics
ipratropium. *See* ipratropium
tiotropium bromide, 214*t*, 217, 1245*t*, 1249
beta$_2$-adrenergic agonists
albuterol. *See* albuterol
arformoterol, 1245*t*, 1247
bitolterol, 240
formoterol, 240, 1245*t*, 1247
levalbuterol, 232*t*, 240, 1245*t*, 1247
pirbuterol, 240, 1245*t*, 1247
salmeterol, 240, 1245*t*, 1247–48
terbutaline, 239, 240, 1245*t*, 1248
methylxanthines
aminophylline, 1245*t*, 1256
theophylline. *See* theophylline
bronchospasm, 1240
Brovan. *See* arformoterol
Brucella melitensis, 828
B-type natriuretic peptide (BNP), 609
bubonic plague, 813*t*
buccal route, drug administration, 31, 31*f*
budesonide:
adverse effects, 1167*t*, 1250*t*, 1270*t*
in pediatric patients, 142*t*
dosage/routes
adult, 1167*t*, 1250*t*, 1270*t*
pediatric, 142*t*
pediatric labeling changes, 135*t*
for specific conditions
allergic rhinitis, 1270*t*
asthma, 1250*t*, 1252
inflammatory bowel disease, 1037
buffers, 701
bumetanide, 551*t*, 553, 612*t*
Bumex. *See* bumetanide
bundle of His, 487
bupivacaine, 473*t*, 475–76
Buprenex. *See* buprenorphine
buprenorphine, 99, 436*t*
bupropion:
adverse effects, 304*t*, 312
dosage forms not to be crushed or opened, 30*t*
mechanism of action, 312
route and adult dose, 304*t*
for specific conditions
depression, 304*t*
smoking cessation, 107–8
therapeutic effects and uses, 312
BuSpar. *See* buspirone
buspirone, 282*t*, 287, 288
busulfan, 967*t*, 969–70
butabarbital, 282*t*, 292
butenafine, 878*t*
butoconazole, 878*t*, 879
butorphanol, 436*t*
Byetta. *See* exenatide
Bystolic. *See* nebivolol

C

C fibers, 430
cachexia, 959
CAD. *See* coronary artery disease
Cafergot. *See* caffeine; ergotamine
Cafergot P-B. *See* belladonna; caffeine; ergotamine; pentobarbital
caffeine, 421–22
adverse effects, 416*t*, 422
classification, 421
contraindications/precautions, 422
drug interactions, 422
genetic polymorphisms and actions of, 160*t*
mechanism of action, 107, 422
nursing responsibilities, 422
overdose treatment, 422
patient and family education, 422
pharmacokinetics, 422
pregnancy category, 422
route and adult dose, 416*t*
similar drugs, 422
therapeutic effects and uses, 107, 421–22
withdrawal, 107
Calan. *See* verapamil
Calan SR, 30*t*. *See also* verapamil
Calcidrine Syrup, 1276*t*
Calciferol. *See* ergocalciferol
calcineurin, 740
CALCINEURIN INHIBITORS, 740
cyclosporine. *See* cyclosporine
tacrolimus, 741*t*, 744, 1327, 1330*t*
calcipotriene, 1329, 1330*t*
calcitonin, 1285
for bone pain, 447
in calcium balance regulation, 1285–86, 1285*f*
calcitonin-salmon, 1295*t*, 1299–1300
calcitriol, 1286, 1292–93. *See also* vitamin D
adverse effects, 1293
classification, 1292
contraindications/precautions, 1293
drug interactions, 1293
mechanism of action, 1292
nursing responsibilities, 1293
overdose treatment, 1293
patient and family education, 1293
pharmacokinetics, 1292

pregnancy category, 1293
similar drugs, 1293, 1294*t*
therapeutic effects and uses, 1292
calcium:
balance, regulation of, 1283, 1284*f*, 1285*f*
calcitonin in, 1285–86, 1285*f*
parathyroid hormone in, 1284–85
vitamin D in, 1286–87, 1286*f*
deficiency, 1062
dosage forms, 1062. *See also* calcium salts
functions, 1062, 1062*t*, 1283
imbalances, 694*t*, 1283–84. *See also* hypercalcemia; hypocalcemia
recommended dietary allowance, 1062*t*, 1283*t*
serum ranges, 1283
calcium acetate, 548*t*, 1288*t*, 1290*t*
calcium carbonate, 548*t*, 1019, 1021*t*, 1288*t*, 1290*t*
calcium channel(s), 516
antiseizure drugs and, 377
in muscle contraction, 516, 516*f*
types, 517, 517*f*, 625*t*
CALCIUM CHANNEL BLOCKERS:
actions/effects
on cardiac conduction, 518
on myocardium, 518
on vascular smooth muscle, 518
adverse effects, 520*t*
classification, 518–19
clinical applications, 519*t*
dihydropyridines, 518–19
amlodipine. *See* amlodipine
felodipine. *See* felodipine
isradipine, 519*t*, 520*t*, 521–22
nicardipine. *See* nicardipine
nicardipine SR. *See* nicardipine
nifedipine. *See* nifedipine
nimodipine, 519*t*
nisoldipine, 519*t*, 520*t*, 522
drug interactions, 75*t*
mechanism of action, 591*f*
nondihydropyridines, 519, 519*t*, 522
adverse effects, 522
diltiazem. *See* diltiazem
mechanism of action, 522
verapamil. *See* verapamil
Nursing Process Application, 525*t*
for specific conditions
angina, 519*t*, 592*t*, 598
dysrhythmias, 519*t*, 529*t*
hypertension, 519, 519*t*, 522, 574*t*, 575
hypertensive emergency, 584*t*
migraine prophylaxis, 453, 453*t*
subarachnoid hemorrhage, 519*t*
calcium chloride, 1288*t*, 1290*t*
calcium citrate, 1288*t*, 1290*t*
Calcium EDTA. *See* edetate calcium disodium
calcium glubionate, 1290*t*
calcium gluconate, 1288*t*
calcium lactate, 1288*t*, 1290*t*
calcium phosphate, dibasic, 1290*t*
calcium phosphate tribasic, 1288*t*
calcium polycarbophil, 1030*t*
calcium salts, 1288–89
adverse effects, 1288
classification, 1287
contraindications/precautions, 1288
drug interactions, 1288
examples, 1288*t*
mechanism of action, 1287
Nursing Process Application, 1289*t*
nursing responsibilities, 1288
overdose treatment, 1288
patient and family education, 1288–89
pharmacokinetics, 1287
pregnancy category, 1288
therapeutic effects and uses, 1287, 1290*t*
Caldecort. *See* hydrocortisone acetate
calfactant, 1240*t*
Cal-Lac. *See* calcium lactate
Calphron. *See* calcium acetate
CAM (complementary and alternative medicine), 172. *See also* Complementary and Alternative Therapies
Campath. *See* alemtuzumab
camphorated opium tincture, 1034*t*
Camptosar. *See* irinotecan
Campylobacter, 777*t*
Canada, drug regulations in, 20, 20*t*
Canadian Food and Drugs Act, 20
canal of Schlemm, 1338
Canasa. *See* mesalamine
cancer, 950
characteristics, 950–51, 951*f*
detection and prevention, 951–52
drug-induced, 68, 68*t*
etiology, 951
grading, 953–54, 954*t*
incidence, 950*t*
metastasis, 951, 951*f*
pain management strategies, 429*t*
pharmacotherapy, 952–53. *See also* ANTINEOPLASTIC AGENTS
psychological issues for patients, 961
staging, 953, 954*t*
Cancidas. *See* caspofungin
candesartan, 538*t*, 540
Candida albicans, 811, 869*t*, 879
Candida glabrata, 879
candidiasis, 869*t*. *See also* fungal infections
in HIV-AIDS patients, 945*t*
in infants, 870*t*, 872*t*
micafungin for, 874
oropharyngeal, 870*t*, 872*t*, 879
vulvovaginal, 875*t*, 879–80
cannabinoid receptor (CB1) blockers, 1090
CANNABINOIDS, 1044
dronabinol, 1043*t*
nabilone, 1043*t*
cannabis. *See* marijuana
Cantil. *See* mepenzolate
Capastat Sulfate. *See* capreomycin
capecitabine, 973*t*, 975
capillary leak syndrome, 738
Capoten. *See* captopril
Capozide, 572*t*
capreomycin, 855*t*, 861
capsaicin, 1302
capsid, 908
capsules, 29, 44
captopril, 533*t*, 535, 612*t*
Capzasin, 1302
Carac. *See* fluorouracil
Carafate. *See* sucralfate
carbachol, 202*t*, 204, 1341*t*
carbamazepine, 386–87
adverse effects, 380*t*, 386–87
classification, 386
contraindications/precautions, 387
drug interactions, 387
mechanism of action, 386
nursing responsibilities, 387
overdose treatment, 387
patient and family education, 387
pharmacokinetics, 386
pregnancy category, 387
route and adult dose, 380*t*
similar drugs, 387
for specific conditions
bipolar disorder, 319*t*, 320
seizures, 380*t*, 386
therapeutic effects and uses, 386
carbamide peroxide, 1352, 1352*t*
CARBAPENEMS:
doripenem, 800*t*, 801–2
ertapenem, 800*t*, 802
imipenem-cilastin. *See* imipenem-cilastin
mechanism of action, 800
meropenem, 800*t*, 802
structure, 789*f*
carbenicillin, 789*t*, 794
carbidopa, 30*t*
drug interactions, 178*t*
with levodopa, 349, 350*t*, 351
Carbocaine. *See* mepivacaine
carbohydrates:
in enteral nutrition, 1070
in parenteral nutrition, 1077
carbonic anhydrase, 560
CARBONIC ANHYDRASE INHIBITORS, 549, 559*t*, 560
acetazolamide. *See* acetazolamide
brinzolamide, 1341*t*, 1345
dorzolamide, 1341*t*, 1345
methazolamide, 559*t*, 560, 1341*t*
carboplatin, 967*t*, 970
carboprost:
as abortifacient, 1213, 1213*t*
therapeutic effects and uses, 1214*t*
as uterine stimulant, 1187*t*, 1189
carboxypeptidase, 1004*t*
carcinogens, 951
carcinoma, 950*t*
Cardene. *See* nicardipine
Cardene SR. *See* nicardipine SR
cardiac action potential, 623–25, 624*f*, 630*f*
cardiac conduction system, 487, 489, 489*f*
CARDIAC GLYCOSIDES:
adverse effects, 612*t*, 614
drugs in class
digoxin. *See* digoxin
mechanism of action, 611*f*
Nursing Process Application, 617*t*
for specific conditions
heart failure, 612*t*, 614
cardiac output (CO), 489
cardiac remodeling, 532
cardiotonic drugs, 238
cardiovascular system:
age-related changes, 148, 149*t*
blood, 483–85
blood pressure. *See* blood pressure
cardiac conduction system, 487, 489, 489*f*
cardiac output, 489–90, 490*f*
functions, 483
heart. *See* heart
structure, 484*f*
cardioversion, 627
Cardizem, 30*t*. *See also* diltiazem
Cardizem CD, 30*t*. *See also* diltiazem
Cardizem SR, 30*t*. *See also* diltiazem

Cardura. *See* doxazosin
Carimune. *See* intravenous immune globulin
carisoprodol, 400*t*, 401
carmustine, 960, 967*t*, 970
carnitine (L-carnitine), 616*t*
  description, 616*t*
  evidence, 616*t*
  history and claims, 616*t*
  primary uses, 179*t*
  standardization, 616*t*
carteolol, 252*t*, 254, 1341*t*, 1343, 1345
Cartrol. *See* carteolol
carvedilol:
  adverse effects, 576, 612*t*
  for heart failure, 612*t*
  mechanism of action, 251, 254, 576
  route and adult dose, 612*t*
  for specific conditions, 254
cascara sagrada, 175*t*
Casodex. *See* bicalutamide
caspofungin, 871
caspofungin acetate, 871, 872*t*, 874–75
castor oil, 1030*t*, 1032
Cataflam. *See* diclofenac
cataplexy, 279, 419
Catapres. *See* clonidine
catecholamines, 192, 230–31, 231*f*, 308*f*
catechol-O-methyltransferase (COMT), 194, 231
catechol-O-methyltransferase (COMT) inhibitors, 355
  entacapone, 350*t*, 355
  tolcapone, 350*t*, 355
Category A drugs, 125, 125*t*
Category B drugs, 125, 125*t*
Category C drugs, 125, 125*t*
Category D drugs, 125, 125*t*
Category X drugs, 125, 125*t*
cathartics, 1030, 1031. *See also* LAXATIVES
catheters, urinary tract infection and, 839–40
CATIE (Clinical Antipsychotic Trials of Intervention Effectiveness) study, 341*t*
Caverject. *See* alprostadil
CBER (Center for Biologics Evaluation and Research), 17
CCNU. *See* lomustine
CCR5 INHIBITORS:
  maraviroc, 933*t*, 940
CD4 receptor, 927
CD8 T cells, 713
CDER (Center for Drug Evaluation and Research), 16
Ceclor. *See* cefaclor
Cedax. *See* ceftibuten
CeeNU. *See* lomustine
cefaclor, 796*t*
cefadroxil, 796*t*
cefazolin sodium, 797–98
  adverse effects, 796*t*, 797
  classification, 797
  contraindications/precautions, 797
  drug interactions, 797
  mechanism of action, 797
  nursing responsibilities, 797–98
  overdose treatment, 797
  patient and family education, 798
  pharmacokinetics, 797
  pregnancy category, 797
  route and adult dose, 796*t*
  similar drugs, 798
  therapeutic effects and uses, 797
cefdinir, 796*t*
cefditoren, 796*t*
cefepime, 796*t*, 798
cefixime, 796*t*, 798
Cefizox. *See* ceftizoxime
Cefobid. *See* cefoperazone
cefoperazone, 796*t*, 798
Cefotan. *See* cefotetan
cefotaxime, 796*t*, 798
cefotetan, 796*t*
cefoxitin, 796*t*
cefpodoxime, 796*t*
cefprozil, 796*t*
ceftazidime, 796*t*, 798
ceftibuten, 796*t*
Ceftin. *See* cefuroxime
ceftizoxime, 796*t*
ceftriaxone, 798
  adverse effects
    in pediatric patients, 142*t*
  dosage/routes
    adult, 796*t*
    pediatric, 142*t*
  for urinary tract infection in pregnancy, 839
cefuroxime, 796*t*
Cefzil. *See* cefprozil
Celebrex. *See* celecoxib
celecoxib, 727–28
  adverse effects, 724*t*, 728
  classification, 727
  contraindications/precautions, 728
  cost, 723
  drug interactions, 728
  mechanism of action, 728
  nursing responsibilities, 728
  overdose treatment, 728
  patient and family education, 728
  pharmacokinetics, 728
  pregnancy category, 728
  route and adult dose, 724*t*
  therapeutic effects and uses, 725*t*, 727–28
Celestone. *See* betamethasone
Celexa. *See* citalopram
cell cycle, 954–55, 955*f*
cell kill hypothesis, 955–56, 956*f*
CellCept. *See* mycophenolate
Celontin. *See* methsuximide
Cenestin. *See* conjugated estrogens
Center for Biologics Evaluation and Research (CBER), 17
Center for Drug Evaluation and Research (CDER), 16
Center for Food Safety and Applied Nutrition (CFSAN), 17
central nervous system (CNS), 185, 186*f*
  age-related changes, 148, 149*t*
  damage, muscle spasticity and, 402–3
  degenerative diseases. *See* neurodegenerative diseases
  drug mechanism in, 265
  drugs toxic to, 69, 69*t*
  functional divisions
    basal ganglia, 270, 271*f*
    extrapyramidal system, 270
    limbic system, 270, 270*f*
    reticular activating system, 270, 271*f*
  structure, 268*f*
    blood–brain barrier. *See* blood–brain barrier
    brainstem, 269
    cerebellum, 269
    cerebrum, 267, 269
    hypothalamus, 269
    spinal cord, 269
    thalamus, 269
central nervous system (CNS) depressants:
  abuse
    alcohol. *See* alcohol
    club drugs, 105
    hallucinogens. *See* hallucinogens
    marijuana. *See* marijuana
    opioids, 98–99
    sedatives, 98
  for anxiety and insomnia, 281
    barbiturates. *See* barbiturates
    benzodiazepines. *See* benzodiazepines
  drug interactions, 75*t*, 178*t*
  mechanism of action, 97
central nervous system (CNS) stimulants, 412
  abuse, 105–6
    amphetamines, 105–6
    cocaine. *See* cocaine
    inhalants, 108
    methylphenidate, 106
  amphetamines. *See* AMPHETAMINES
  caffeine. *See* caffeine
  clinical applications, 412
  effects/actions, 412
  modafinil. *See* modafinil
  nicotine, 96*t*, 107
  scheduled drugs, 412*t*
central vein total parenteral nutrition, 1077, 1077*f*. *See also* parenteral nutrition
cephalexin, 142*t*, 796*t*
CEPHALOSPORINS:
  adverse effects, 796–97
  classification, 795
  first-generation, 795, 798
    cefadroxil, 796*t*
    cefazolin. *See* cefazolin sodium
    cephalexin, 142*t*, 796*t*
    cephradine, 796*t*
  fourth-generation, 795
    cefepime, 796*t*, 798
  mechanism of action, 795
  Nursing Process Application, 799–800*t*
  resistance to, 796
  second-generation, 795, 798
    cefaclor, 796*t*
    cefotetan, 796*t*
    cefoxitin, 796*t*
    cefprozil, 796*t*
    cefuroxime, 796*t*
  structure, 789*f*
  third-generation, 795, 798
    cefdinir, 796*t*
    cefditoren, 796*t*
    cefixime, 796*t*, 798
    cefoperazone, 796*t*, 798
    cefotaxime, 796*t*, 798
    cefpodoxime, 796*t*
    ceftazidime, 796*t*, 798
    ceftibuten, 796*t*
    ceftizoxime, 796*t*
    ceftriaxone. *See* ceftriaxone
cephradine, 796*t*
cerebellum, 268*f*, 269
cerebral palsy, 403, 403*t*
cerebrum, 267, 268*f*, 269

Cerebyx. *See* fosphenytoin
Cerespan. *See* papaverine-phentolamine
certolizumab, 1037
Cerubidine. *See* daunorubicin
cerumenolytics, 1352
Cervidil. *See* dinoprostone
Cesamet. *See* nabilone
Cetamide. *See* sulfacetamide
cetirizine, 101*t*, 1265*t*, 1268
cetrorelix, 1192*t*, 1195
Cetrotide. *See* cetrorelix
cetuximab, 748*t*, 990*t*
cevimeline HCl, 202*t*, 204
CFSAN (Center for Food Safety and Applied Nutrition), 17
Chagas' disease (trypanosomiasis), 886*t*, 896
chalazion, 1349
Chantix. *See* varenicline
CharcoAid. *See* activated charcoal
chelation therapy, 1366–67
chemical name, 7
chemoreceptor trigger zone (CTZ), 1041
chemoreceptors, 492
chemotherapy, 952. *See also* ANTINEOPLASTIC AGENTS
chest radiography, in tuberculosis, 853
CHF (congestive heart failure), 607. *See also* heart failure
chickenpox. *See* varicella zoster
chickenpox (varicella zoster), 758*t*, 765, 765*t*
chief cells, 1000
children. *See* pediatric patients
Chlamydia trachomatis, 777*t*
chloasma, 1208
chloral hydrate, 281, 286
chlorambucil, 68*t*, 967*t*, 970
chloramphenicol, 809*f*, 821, 821*t*
chlordiazepoxide, 282*t*, 283*t*, 285
chloride:
  functions, 1062, 1062*t*
  imbalances, 694*t*
  recommended dietary allowance, 1062*t*
chloroprocaine, 473*t*, 474
chloroquine, 889–90
  adverse effects, 889
  classification, 889
  contraindications/precautions, 889
  drug interactions, 889
  mechanism of action, 889
  nursing responsibilities, 889
  overdose treatment, 889
  patient and family education, 890
  pharmacokinetics, 889
  pregnancy category, 889
  prescription ranking, 888
  prophylactic use, 783
  similar drugs, 890
  therapeutic effects and uses, 889
chlorothiazide, 553, 554*t*, 555
chlorpheniramine, 1265*t*
chlorpromazine HCl, 333–34
  adverse effects, 332*t*, 333
  classification, 333
  contraindications/precautions, 333–34
  drug interactions, 101*t*, 334
  mechanism of action, 333
  nursing responsibilities, 334
  overdose treatment, 334
  patient and family education, 334
  pharmacokinetics, 333
  pregnancy category, 334
  route and adult dose, 332*t*
  similar drugs, 334–35
  therapeutic effects and uses, 333
chlorpropamide, 1114, 1133*t*, 1135
chlorthalidone, 553, 554*t*, 555
Chlor-Trimeton. *See* chlorpheniramine
Chlor-Trimeton Allergy/Decongestant tablets, 1266*t*
chlorzoxazone, 400*t*, 401
choking/vomiting agents:
  Adamsite-DM, 1362*t*
  phosgene, 1362*t*
cholecalciferol, 1286, 1293, 1294*t*. *See also* vitamin D
cholera, 758*t*
cholestatic hepatitis, 814
cholesterol, 501, 502*f*. *See also* dyslipidemias
cholesterol absorption inhibitors. *See* ezetimibe
cholestyramine, 507–8
  adverse effects, 507
  classification, 507
  contraindications/precautions, 507–8
  drug interactions, 75*t*, 508
  mechanism of action, 507
  nursing responsibilities, 508
  overdose treatment, 508
  patient and family education, 508
  pharmacokinetics, 507
  pregnancy category, 508
  similar drugs, 509
  therapeutic effects and uses, 507
choline and magnesium trisalicylate, 720*t*, 723
cholinergic, 190
cholinergic agonists, 199. *See also* ACETYLCHOLINESTERASE (ACHE) INHIBITORS; MUSCARINIC AGONISTS; NICOTINIC AGONISTS
  Nursing Process Application, 207–8*t*
cholinergic antagonists. *See also* MUSCARINIC ANTAGONISTS; NICOTINIC ANTAGONISTS
  classification, 213–14
  sites of action, 213*f*
cholinergic crisis, 205, 216
cholinergic receptors. *See* muscarinic receptors; nicotinic receptors
cholinergic synapses, 199, 199*f*, 266
cholinergic transmission:
  acetylcholine. *See* acetylcholine (Ach)
  receptors and neurotransmitters, 190–91, 191*f*, 192*t*. *See also specific receptors*
  termination of acetylcholine action, 192. *See also* acetylcholinesterase
cholinesterase inhibitors, 359. *See also*ACETYLCHOLINESTERASE (ACHE) INHIBITORS
chondroitin, 1302*t*
choriogonadotropin alfa, 1195. *See also* human chorionic gonadotropin (HCG)
Christmas disease, 663
chromium:
  as complementary therapy
    description, 1142*t*
    evidence, 1142*t*
    history and claims, 1142*t*
    primary uses, 179*t*
    standardization, 1142*t*
  functions, 1063*t*
  recommended dietary allowance, 1063*t*
chromoblastomycosis, 869*t*
chronic bronchitis, 1258
chronic obstructive pulmonary disease (COPD), 1256, 1258
  Nursing Process Application, 1257*t*
chronic pain, 428. *See also* pain
chyme, 1000
chymotrypsin, 1004*t*
Cialis. *See* tadalafil
ciclesonide, 1270*t*
ciclopirox, 878*t*, 879, 1328
cidofovir, 912*t*, 914
cilostazol, 653*t*
cimetidine, 45, 152*t*, 1016*t*, 1019
Cimzia. *See* certolizumab
cinacalcet hydrochloride, 1295*t*, 1300
cinchonism, 632, 890
Cinobac. *See* cinoxacin
cinoxacin, 827*t*
Cipro. *See* ciprofloxacin
Cipro XR, 30*t*. *See also* ciprofloxacin
CiproDex. *See* ciprofloxacin-dexamethasone
ciprofloxacin, 829–30
  adverse effects, 827*t*, 829
  classification, 829
  contraindications/precautions, 829
  as CYP1A2 inhibitor, 47
  dosage forms not to be crushed or opened, 30*t*
  drug interactions, 47, 829
  mechanism of action, 829
  nursing responsibilities, 830
  overdose treatment, 829
  patient and family education, 830
  pediatric labeling changes, 135*t*
  pharmacokinetics, 829
  pregnancy category, 829
  route and adult dose, 827*t*
  similar drugs, 830–31
  for specific conditions
    acute uncomplicated cystitis, 838
    anthrax, 1360
    pneumonic plague, 1361
    tuberculosis, 855*t*, 861
  therapeutic effects and uses, 829
ciprofloxacin-dexamethasone, 1352*t*
ciprofloxacin-hydrocortisone, 1352*t*
circadian dysrhythm, 278
circadian rhythm, 278
cisatracurium, 219*t*, 224
cisplatin, 959, 960, 967*t*, 970
citalopram:
  for anxiety disorders, 290*t*
  for depression, 304*t*, 310
Citanest. *See* prilocaine
Citracal. *See* calcium citrate
Citrucel. *See* methylcellulose
cladribine, 973*t*, 975–76
Claforan. *See* cefotaxime
Clarinex. *See* desloratadine
clarithromycin, 815–16
  adverse effects, 813*t*, 816
  dosage/routes
    adult, 813*t*
    pediatric, 142*t*
  for specific conditions
    H. pylori infection, 1023
    leprosy, 862
    M. avium complex infections, 865
Claritin. *See* loratadine
ClearEyes. *See* naphazoline

clemastine, 1265*t*
Cleocin. *See* clindamycin
Cleocin-T. *See* clindamycin/tretinoin
climacteric, 1184
Climara. *See* estradiol
ClindaMax. *See* clindamycin/tretinoin
clindamycin, 821, 821*t*
clindamycin/tretinoin, 1322*t*, 1323
Clinical Antipsychotic Trials of Intervention Effectiveness (CATIE) study, 341*t*
clinical phase trials, 17–18
Clinoril. *See* sulindac
clobetasol dipropionate, 1327*t*
clocortolone pivalate, 1327*t*
Cloderm. *See* clocortolone pivalate
clofarabine, 973*t*, 976
clofazimine, 862, 863
clofibrate, 504*t*, 509
Clolar. *See* clofarabine
Clomid. *See* clomiphene citrate
clomiphene citrate, 1194–95
  adverse effects, 1194
  classification, 1194
  contraindications/precautions, 1194
  drug interactions, 1194
  mechanism of action, 1191, 1194
  nursing responsibilities, 1194
  overdose treatment, 1194
  patient and family education, 1194–95
  pharmacokinetics, 1194
  pregnancy category, 1194
  similar drugs, 1195–96
  for specific conditions
    male infertility, 1226
  therapeutic effects and uses, 1194
clomipramine:
  for anxiety disorders, 289, 290*t*
  for depression, 304*t*, 307
clonazepam:
  adverse effects, 282*t*
  indications, 283*t*
  route and adult dose, 282*t*
  for seizures, 380*t*, 383
clonic spasms, 397
clonidine, 444
  for anxiety, 287
  for hypertension, 578
  for pain, 443*t*, 477
clopidogrel, 654–55
  adverse effects, 653, 654
  classification, 654
  contraindications/precautions, 654
  drug interactions, 654–55
  mechanism of action, 653, 654
  nursing responsibilities, 655
  overdose treatment, 655
  patient and family education, 655
  pharmacokinetics, 654
  pregnancy category, 655
  similar drugs, 655
  therapeutic effects and uses, 654
clorazepate, 285
  adverse effects, 282*t*
  indications, 283*t*
  route and adult dose, 282*t*
  for seizures, 380*t*, 383
closed-angle glaucoma, 1339*f*, 1340. *See also* glaucoma
Clostridium, 777*t*
Clostridium botulinum, 775, 1361
Clostridium difficile, 811, 1014*t*, 1034
Clostridium tetani, 759. *See also* tetanus
clotrimazole, 29, 878*t*, 879, 1318, 1351
clotting factors, for hemophilia, 663
cloxacillin, 789*t*, 794
Cloxapen. *See* cloxacillin
clozapine, 337*t*, 339
Clozaril. *See* clozapine
club drugs, 105
CNP (C-type natriuretic peptide), 609
CNS. *See* central nervous system
CO (cardiac output), 489
coagulation, 485
  disorders, 643–44
  modification of, 644, 644*t*. *See also* ANTICOAGULANTS; ANTIPLATELET AGENTS; HEMOSTATIC AGENTS; THROMBOLYTIC AGENTS
    clotting factors, 663
coagulation cascade, 486, 486*f*
coal tar, 1329, 1330*t*
cobalt, 1063*t*
cocaine:
  abuse, 106–7
  effects/actions, 415
    anesthetic, 472
    in breast-feeding infant, 129*t*
    in pregnancy, 106, 126*t*
  withdrawal symptoms and treatment, 96*t*
coccidioidomycosis, 869*t*
Coccoides immitis, 869*t*
Codamine Syrup, 1276*t*
codeine, 439
  as antitussive, 1275, 1276*t*
  comparison to other opioids, 436*t*
  drug interactions, 101*t*
  genetic polymorphisms and actions of, 159
  metabolism, 46
  route and adult dose, 436*t*
Codiclear DH Syrup, 1276*t*
Codimal DH, 1276*t*
coenzyme Q10:
  description, 507*t*
  evidence, 507*t*
  history and claims, 507*t*
  primary uses, 179*t*
  standardization, 507*t*
Cogentin. *See* benztropine
Cognex. *See* tacrine
cognitive symptoms, schizophrenia, 327, 327*t*
cognitive–behavioral therapy, for depression, 301, 302*t*
Colace. *See* glycerin
Colazal. *See* balsalazide
colchicine, 1308–9
  adverse effects, 1307*t*, 1308
  classification, 1308
  contraindications/precautions, 1308
  drug interactions, 1308
  mechanism of action, 1308
  nursing responsibilities, 1308
  overdose treatment, 1308
  patient and family education, 1308–9
  pharmacokinetics, 1308
  pregnancy category, 1308
  route and adult dose, 1307*t*
  therapeutic effects and uses, 1308
cold therapy, for muscle spasms, 397
colesevelam, 504*t*, 508
Colestid. *See* colestipol
colestipol, 504*t*, 508
COLLOIDS, 692, 692*t*
  dextran 40. *See* dextran 40
  hetastarch, 694
Collyrium. *See* tetrahydrozoline
COLONY-STIMULATING FACTORS (CSFs), 483, 671
  adverse effects, 672–73
  with cancer chemotherapy, 993
  filgrastim. *See* filgrastim
  mechanism of action, 671–72
  pegfilgrastim, 670*t*, 674
  sargramostim, 670*t*, 674
combination drug, 7
combination oral contraceptives. *See* ORAL CONTRACEPTIVES
Combipres, 572*t*
Combivent. *See* ipratropium
comedones, 1321
comfrey, 177
common cold, 1274, 1275*t*
community nurses. *See also* To the Community
  as drug therapy information resource, 167–68
  practice settings
    assisted living facilities, 165
    congregational health, 165
    home care, 164, 164*f*
    hospice, 164–65
    public health, 167
    schools, 165–66, 166*f*, 166*t*
Compazine. *See* prochlorperazine
Compazine Spansule, 30*t*. *See also* prochlorperazine
complement system, 711, 711*t*, 712*t*
complementary and alternative medicine (CAM), 172
Complementary and Alternative Therapies:
  aloe vera, 1332*t*
  aromatherapy, 798*t*
  ascorbic acid, 1275*t*
  bilberry, 1347*t*
  black cohosh, 1228
  carnitine (L-carnitine), 616*t*
  chondroitin, 1302*t*
  chromium, 1142*t*
  coenzyme Q10, 507*t*
  cranberry, 845*t*
  dandelion, 561*t*
  echinacea, 745*t*
  fish oils, 1163*t*
  garlic, 654*t*
  ginger, 1013*t*
  gingko biloba for dementia, 360*t*
  ginseng, 590*t*
  glucosamine, 1302*t*
  goldenseal, 717*t*
  grape seed extract, 569*t*
  hawthorn, 540*t*
  herbal remedies in galactagogues, 129*t*
  kava, 399*t*
  ketogenic diet, 374*t*
  Lactobacillus acidophilus, 1044*t*
  lecithin, 200*t*
  melatonin, 281*t*
  migraine, 453*t*
  saw palmetto, 1232*t*
  selenium, 953*t*
  soy, 981*t*
  St. John's wort for depression, 313*t*

complementary and alternative therapies:
for anxiety and insomnia, 280–81, 280*t*
herbal products/therapy. *See* herbal products/therapy
types, 172, 172*t*
usage statistics, 174
complex partial seizures, 375, 376*t*
compliance. *See* adherence
COMT (catechol-O-methyltransferase), 194, 231
COMT inhibitors. *See* catechol-O-methyltransferase (COMT) inhibitors
Comtan. *See* entacapone
Concerta. *See* methylphenidate
congestive heart failure (CHF), 607. *See also* heart failure
conivaptan, 1114
conjugated estrogens, 1179–81
adverse effects, 1180, 1180*t*
classification, 1179
contraindications/precautions, 1180–81
drug interactions, 1181
mechanism of action, 1179
for menopausal symptoms, 1184
nursing responsibilities, 1181–82
overdose treatment, 1181
patient and family education, 1182
pharmacokinetics, 1180
pregnancy category, 1181
route and adult dose, 1180*t*
therapeutic effects and uses, 1179
conjugated estrogens/medroxyprogesterone, 1180*t*, 1184
conjugation, 781
conjunctivitis, 1349
Conn's syndrome, 1170
constipation, 1029
during enteral nutrition therapy, 1071*t*
etiology, 1029, 1029*t*
opioid therapy and, 436*t*, 437, 437*t*
pharmacotherapy. *See* LAXATIVES
consumption. *See* tuberculosis
contact dermatitis, 1325
continuous infusion feedings, 1069. *See also* enteral nutrition
contraception, 1200
contraceptive methods:
barrier
condoms, diaphragms, cervical caps, 1201*t*
contraceptive sponge, 1201*t*, 1211, 1211*f*
intrauterine devices/systems, 1201*t*, 1210, 1211*f*
spermicides, 1201*t*, 1210–11
nonoxynol-9. *See* nonoxynol-9
biological/calendar, 1201*t*, 1209*t*
emergency. *See* emergency contraception
factors influencing selection, 1200, 1205*t*
hormonal
oral. *See* ORAL CONTRACEPTIVES
progestin injections, 1201*t*, 1210
subdermal progestin implants, 1201*t*, 1210
transdermal steroids, 1201*t*, 1209–10
vaginal delivery, 33, 34*f*, 1210
withdrawal method, 1201*t*
contractility, 490
controlled substances, 20, 94
Controlled Substances Act, 94
convulsions, 371
Copaxone. *See* glatiramer
COPD. *See* chronic obstructive pulmonary disease
Copegus. *See* ribavirin
copper, 1063*t*
Cordarone. *See* amiodarone
Cordran. *See* flurandrenolide
Coreg. *See* carvedilol
Corgard. *See* nadolol
cornea, 1338
coronary arteries, 487, 488*f*
coronary artery disease (CAD), 588, 589*f*. *See also* angina pectoris; myocardial infarction
etiology, 588–89
nonpharmacologic therapy, 590
coronaviruses, 909*t*
corpora cavernosa, 1226
corpus luteum, 1177
correctional facilities, nursing in, 857*t*
Correctol. *See* bisacodyl; phenolphthalein
Cortaid. *See* hydrocortisone acetate
Cortef. *See* hydrocortisone
CORTICOSTEROIDS:
actions, 1163, 1163*t*
as adjuvant analgesics, 446–47, 446*t*
adverse effects, 751, 1163–65, 1164*t*, 1250, 1250*t*
adrenal atrophy/adrenal crisis, 1165, 1166*f*
classification, 1163
drugs in class
beclomethasone. *See* beclomethasone
betamethasone, 1167*t*, 1328
budesonide. *See* budesonide
ciclesonide, 1270*t*
cortisone, 1167*t*
dexamethasone. *See* dexamethasone
flunisolide, 1250*t*, 1252, 1270*t*
fluticasone. *See* fluticasone
hydrocortisone. *See* hydrocortisone
methylprednisolone. *See* methylprednisolone
mometasone, 1250*t*, 1252, 1270*t*
prednisolone, 1167*t*
prednisone. *See* prednisone
triamcinolone, 1167*t*, 1250*t*, 1252, 1270*t*
as immunosuppressants, 742*f*, 750–51
mechanism of action, 742*f*, 750–54, 1168–69
Nursing Process Applications
intranasal administration, 1272*t*
systemic administration, 1172*t*
in pediatric patients, 1164*t*
for specific conditions, 1163*t*
adrenocortical insufficiency, 1165
allergic rhinitis, 1268, 1270*t*
allergies, 1169
arthritis, 1169
asthma, 1169, 1244*t*, 1249–50, 1250*t*
dermatologic conditions, 1169, 1325, 1327*t*
edema, 1169
gout, 1307
inflammatory bowel disease, 1037, 1169
multiple sclerosis, 366
myasthenia gravis, 205–6
nausea and vomiting, 1043*t*, 1044
neoplasia, 1169
ocular conditions, 1349
psoriasis, 1328–29
thyroid storm, 1155
transplant rejection prophylaxis, 1169
topical, 1325, 1327*t*, 1328–29
corticotropin, 1165
corticotropin-releasing hormone (CRH), 1105*t*
cortisone, 1167*t*
Cortisporin. *See* polymyxin B-neomycin-hydrocortisone
Cortizone. *See* hydrocortisone
Cortone. *See* cortisone
Cortrosyn. *See* cosyntropin
Corynebacterium, 777*t*
Corynebacterium diphtheriae, 759. *See also* diphtheria
Corzide, 572*t*
Cosmegen. *See* dactinomycin
cosyntropin, 1165
Cotazym. *See* pancrelipase
Cotazym S, 30*t*. *See also* pancrelipase
Coumadin. *See* warfarin
Council for Responsible Nutrition (CRN), 1053
counterirritants, 1302
Covera-HS, 30*t*. *See also* verapamil
COX (cyclooxygenase), 719, 719*f*
COX-2 (CYCLOOXYGENASE-2) INHIBITORS, 727
celecoxib. *See* celecoxib
Cozaar. *See* losartan
crab louse, 1318
cranberry:
description, 845*t*
evidence, 845*t*
history and claims, 845*t*
primary uses, 173*t*
standardization, 845*t*
Crestor. *See* rosuvastatin
cretinism, 1149
CRH (corticotropin-releasing hormone), 1105*t*
Crinone. *See* progesterone
Crixivan. *See* indinavir
CRN (Council for Responsible Nutrition), 1053
Crohn's disease. *See* inflammatory bowel disease (IBD)
Crolom. *See* cromolyn
cromolyn, 1252–53
adverse effects, 1250*t*, 1253, 1270*t*
classification, 1252
contraindications/precautions, 1253
drug interactions, 1253
mechanism of action, 1253
nursing responsibilities, 1253
overdose treatment, 1253
patient and family education, 1253
pharmacokinetics, 1253
pregnancy category, 1253
route and adult dose, 1250*t*, 1270*t*
similar drugs, 1253
for specific conditions
allergic conjunctivitis, 1349, 1349*t*
allergic rhinitis, 1270*t*, 1271
therapeutic effects and uses, 1252–53
cross-tolerance, 97
crotamiton, 1319, 1320
cryoprecipitate, 689*t*
cryptococcosis, 869*t*, 945*t*
Cryptococcus neoformans, 869*t*
cryptosporidiosis, 886*t*, 892*t*, 893, 945*t*
Cryptosporidium parvum, 886*t*, 893
CRYSTALLOIDS, 691, 691*t*
5% dextrose in water. *See* 5% dextrose in water
hypertonic, 691
hypotonic, 691
isotonic, 691

lactated Ringer's solution, 691*t*, 692
Plasma-Lyte, 691*t*, 692
Ringer's solution, 691*t*, 692
crystalluria, 842
Crystamine. *See* cyanocobalamin
CSFs. *See* COLONY-STIMULATING FACTORS (CSFs)
C-type natriuretic peptide (CNP), 609
CTZ (chemoreceptor trigger zone), 1041
Cubicin. *See* daptomycin
cultural competence, 158, 159*t*
culture, 158
culture and sensitivity (C&S) testing, 782
curare, 223
Cushing's syndrome, 1171, 1171*t*
cutaneous anthrax, 1360*t*
Cutar. *See* coal tar
Cutivate. *See* fluticasone propionate
cyanocobalamin (vitamin B_{12}), 682–83
acid suppression and, 1022*t*
adverse effects, 676*t*, 682, 1054*t*, 1060
classification, 682
contraindications/precautions, 682–83, 1060
deficiency, 680, 682, 682*t*, 1053*t*, 1054. *See also* pernicious anemia
dosage/routes
adult, 676*t*, 1054*t*
intranasal administration, 33
drug interactions, 683, 1060
functions, 1053*t*
mechanism of action, 682, 1060
metabolism, 680, 680*f*
nursing responsibilities, 683, 1060
overdose treatment, 683
patient and family education, 683, 1060
pharmacokinetics, 682
pregnancy category, 683, 1060
recommended dietary allowance, 1060
therapeutic effects and uses, 682, 1060
cyanogen cyanide, 1362*t*
cyclic feedings, 1069. *See also* enteral nutrition
CYCLIC LIPOPEPTIDES, 832
daptomycin, 832, 832*t*
cyclizine hydrochloride, 1043*t*
cyclobenzaprine, 399–401
adverse effects, 399, 400*t*
classification, 399
contraindications/precautions, 399–400
drug interactions, 400
mechanism of action, 399
nursing responsibilities, 400–401
overdose treatment, 400–401
patient and family education, 401
pharmacokinetics, 399
pregnancy category, 400
route and adult dose, 400*t*
similar drugs, 401–2
therapeutic effects and uses, 399
Cyclocort. *See* amcinonide
Cyclogyl. *See* cyclopentolate
cyclooxygenase (COX), 719, 719*f*
CYCLOOXYGENASE-2 (COX-2) INHIBITORS, 727
celecoxib. *See* celecoxib
cyclopentolate, 214*t*, 218, 1348*t*
cyclophosphamide, 746, 967–69
adverse effects, 68*t*, 741*t*, 968–69
classification, 967
contraindications/precautions, 969
drug interactions, 969
mechanism of action, 746, 968
nursing responsibilities, 969
overdose treatment, 969
patient and family education, 969
pharmacokinetics, 968
pregnancy category, 969
route and adult dose, 741*t*
similar drugs, 969–71
therapeutic effects and uses, 746, 968
CYCLOPLEGICS, 1347
atropine, 1348*t*. *See also* atropine
cyclopentolate, 214*t*, 218, 1348*t*
homatropine, 214*t*, 1348*t*
scopolamine hydrobromide, 218, 1347, 1348*t*
tropicamide, 214*t*, 218, 1347, 1347*t*
cycloserine, 855*t*, 861
cyclosporine, 743–44
adverse effects, 68*t*, 741*t*, 743, 1330*t*
classification, 743
contraindications/precautions, 743
drug interactions, 75*t*, 178*t*, 743
mechanism of action, 742*f*, 743
nursing responsibilities, 743–44
overdose treatment, 743
patient and family education, 744
pharmacokinetics, 743
pregnancy category, 743
route and adult dose, 741*t*
similar drugs, 744
for specific conditions
psoriasis, 1330*t*, 1331
therapeutic effects and uses, 743
cyclosporine ophthalmic emulsion, 1348
cyclothymic disorder, 298
Cycrin. *See* medroxyprogesterone acetate
Cyklokapron. *See* tranexamic acid
Cymbalta, 30*t*. *See also* duloxetine
CYP isozymes. *See* cytochrome P450 (CYP) isozymes
CYP1A2, 47*t*
CYP2C9, 47*t*
CYP2C19, 47*t*
CYP2D6, 47*t*
CYP3A4, 47*t*
cyproheptadine, 1265*t*
cystic fibrosis, 1277
cystitis, 837. *See also* urinary tract infections
Cystospaz. *See* hyoscyamine
cysts, 886
Cytadren. *See* aminoglutethimide
cytarabine, 827, 973*t*, 975
cytochrome P450 (CYP) isozymes, 46–47, 47*t*
CytoGam. *See* cytomegalovirus immune globulin
cytokine(s), 713, 734
cytokine release syndrome, 747
cytomegalovirus, 911
cytomegalovirus immune globulin, 767*t*, 769
Cytomel. *See* liothyronine
Cytosar. *See* cytarabine
Cytosine arabinoside. *See* cytarabine
Cytotec. *See* misoprostol
CYTOTOXIC AGENTS:
azathioprine. *See* azathioprine
cyclophosphamide. *See* cyclophosphamide
mechanism of action, 742*f*, 744
mycophenolate, 741*t*, 746
cytotoxic (CD8) T cells, 713
Cytovene. *See* ganciclovir
Cytoxan. *See* cyclophosphamide

D

D4T. *See* stavudine
D_5W. *See* 5% dextrose in water
dacarbazine, 967*t*, 970
daclizumab, 741*t*, 742*f*, 748*t*, 749
dactinomycin, 977*t*, 978
Dalmane. *See* flurazepam
dalteparin, 645*t*, 647
danazol, 1192*t*, 1194, 1195, 1220*t*
dandelion, 561*t*
Danocrine. *See* danazol
Dantrium. *See* dantrolene sodium
dantrolene sodium, 403–6
adverse effects, 404
classification, 403
contraindications/precautions, 404
drug interactions, 404
mechanism of action, 404
nursing responsibilities, 405
overdose treatment, 404
patient and family education, 405–6
pharmacokinetics, 404
pregnancy category, 404
similar drugs, 406
therapeutic effects and uses, 403–4
dapsone, 862–63
adverse effects, 863
classification, 862
contraindications/precautions, 863
drug interactions, 863
mechanism of action, 863
nursing responsibilities, 863
patient and family education, 863
pharmacokinetics, 863
pregnancy category, 863
similar drugs, 863
therapeutic effects and uses, 862–63
daptomycin, 832, 832*t*
Daraprim. *See* pyrimethamine
darbepoetin alfa, 669, 670*t*, 671
darunavir, 933*t*, 939
Darvocet-N. *See* acetaminophen; propoxyphene
Darvon. *See* propoxyphene
Darvon-N. *See* propoxyphene napsylate
dasatinib, 748*t*, 990*t*
daunorubicin, 827, 977*t*, 978
daunorubicin liposomal, 977*t*, 978
Daypro. *See* oxaprozin
Daytrana Transdermal Patch. *See* methylphenidate
DBS (deep brain stimulation), 350*t*
DDAVP. *See* desmopressin
ddl. *See* didanosine
DDS. *See* dapsone
debrisoquin hydroxylase, 160*t*
Debrox. *See* carbamide peroxide
Decadron. *See* dexamethasone
Decaspray. *See* dexamethasone
Declomycin. *See* demeclocycline
DECONGESTANTS:
nasal, 1271–72
ephedrine. *See* ephedrine
ipratropium, 1273*t*. *See also* ipratropium
naphazoline, 1273*t*
oxymetazoline, 1273*t*
phenylephrine. *See* phenylephrine
pseudoephedrine. *See* pseudoephedrine
tetrahydrozoline, 1273*t*
xylometazoline, 1273*t*

ocular, 236
naphazoline, 238, 1273t, 1348t
oxymetazoline, 238, 1348, 1348t
phenylephrine. *See* phenylephrine
tetrahydrozoline, 236, 238, 1348, 1348t
deep brain stimulation (DBS), 350t
deep sedation/analgesia, 458
deep vein thrombosis (DVT), 642, 643t, 648t, 1079t
defecation, 1000
defibrillation, 627
dehydration:
during enteral nutrition therapy, 1072t
etiology, 688
fluid replacement therapy for, 688, 689t. *See also* FLUID REPLACEMENT AGENTS
types, 689t
dehydroepiandrosterone (DHEA), 109, 179t
Delatest. *See* testosterone
delavirdine, 933t, 937
Delestrogen. *See* estradiol valerate
delirium tremens, 102
Delsym. *See* dextromethorphan
Delta-Cortef. *See* prednisolone
Delta-D. *See* cholecalciferol
Deltasone. *See* prednisone
deltoid muscle, for intramuscular injection, 37t
delusions, 326, 327t
Del-Vi-A. *See* vitamin A
Demadex. *See* torsemide
demeclocycline, 810t, 812, 1114
dementia, 358, 360t. *See also* Alzheimer's disease
Demerol. *See* meperidine
Denavir. *See* penciclovir
Depacon. *See* valproic acid
Depade. *See* naltrexone
Depakene, 30t. *See also* valproic acid
Depakote ER, 30t. *See also* valproic acid
dependence, 20, 95–96
Depletite. *See* diethylpropion
depolarization, 624
Depo-Medrol. *See* methylprednisolone
Depo-Provera. *See* medroxyprogesterone acetate
Depo-subQ-Provera. *See* medroxyprogesterone acetate
Depot Provera. *See* medroxyprogesterone acetate
Depot-Cyt. *See* cytarabine
depression, 298
assessment and diagnosis, 300–301
in children and adolescents, 302t
comorbid conditions, 300
Complementary and Alternative Therapies, 313t
cultural influences on treatment, 300t
drug-related, 300
during enteral nutrition therapy, 1072t
genetic factors, 299–300
incidence, 298t, 299t
Lifespan Considerations, 302t
nonpharmacologic therapies, 301–3, 302t
in older adults, 300–301
pathophysiology, 299–300
pharmacotherapy. *See* antidepressants
postpartum onset, 299
suicide and, 301
symptoms, 298, 299t
Treating the Diverse Patient, 300t
dermatitis, 1325
pathophysiology, 1325
pharmacotherapy, 1325, 1327–28, 1327t
dermatologic toxicity, 69t, 70
dermatomycoses, 877
dermis, 1316
DES. *See* diethylstilbestrol
desflurane, 468t, 469
desiccated thyroid, 1151t, 1152
desipramine, 290t, 304t
desirudin, 645t, 649
desloratadine, 1265t, 1268
desmopressin, 662, 1114–15
adverse effects, 1108t, 1115
classification, 1114
contraindications/precautions, 1115
drug interactions, 1115
mechanism of action, 1115
Nursing Process Application, 1116t
nursing responsibilities, 1115
overdose treatment, 1115
patient and family education, 1115
pharmacokinetics, 1115
pregnancy category, 1115
route and adult dose, 1108t
similar drugs, 1115–16
for specific conditions
bleeding in hemophilia, 663
therapeutic effects and uses, 1114–15
Desogen, 1203t
Desonate. *See* desonide
desonide, 1327t, 1328
DesOwen. *See* desonide
desoximetasone, 1327t
Desyrel. *See* trazodone
Detrol. *See* tolterodine
DEXA (dual-energy x-ray absorptiometry), 1290
Dexacort. *See* dexamethasone
dexamethasone:
adverse effects, 1167t
route and adult dose, 1167t
for specific conditions
adrenocortical insufficiency, 1165
dermatitis, 1327t
nausea and vomiting, 1043t, 1044
neoplasia, 980t
therapeutic effects and uses, 1168
dexbrompheniramine, 1265t
Dexchlor. *See* dexchlorpheniramine
dexchlorpheniramine, 1265t
Dexedrine. *See* dextroamphetamine
Dexferrum. *See* iron dextran
dexmethylphenidate, 416t, 418
dextran 40, 692–93
adverse effects, 693
classification, 692
contraindications/precautions, 693
drug interactions, 693
mechanism of action, 692
nursing considerations, 693–94
overdose treatment, 693
patient and family education, 694
pharmacokinetics, 693
pregnancy category, 693
similar drugs, 693
therapeutic effects and uses, 692
dextroamphetamine, 106, 415, 1089
dextromethorphan, 1275–77
abuse, 105, 1275
adverse effects, 1276
classification, 1275
contraindications/precautions, 1276
drug interactions, 1277
mechanism of action, 1276
nursing responsibilities, 1277
overdose treatment, 1277
patient and family education, 1277
pharmacokinetics, 1276
pregnancy category, 1277
similar drugs, 1277
therapeutic effects and uses, 1275
5% dextrose in water, 691–92
adverse effects, 692
classification, 691
contraindications/precautions, 692
drug interactions, 692
mechanism of action, 692
overdose treatment, 692
pharmacokinetics, 692
pregnancy category, 692
similar drugs, 692
therapeutic effects and uses, 691–92
DHE 45. *See* dihydroergotamine
DHEA. *See* dehydroepiandrosterone
DHT. *See* dihydrotachysterol
DiaBeta. *See* glyburide
diabetes insipidus, 1114
diabetes mellitus:
chromium for, 1142t
complications
diabetic ketoacidosis, 1124
in diverse populations, 1123t
hyperosmolar hyperglycemic state, 1124
hypoglycemia, 1123–24
nephropathy, 1126
neuropathy, 1125–26
retinopathy, 1126
vascular disease, 1126
diagnosis, 1122–23, 1123t
gestational, 1121, 1122t
incidence, 1120, 1120t
pathophysiology, 1121
pharmacotherapy
insulin. *See* insulin
oral hypoglycemics. *See* ORAL HYPOGLYCEMICS
symptoms, 1122
type 1, 1121, 1122t
type 2, 286t, 1121, 1122t
diabetic ketoacidosis (DKA), 1124
Diabinese. *See* chlorpropamide
Diamox. *See* acetazolamide
diarrhea, 1032
during enteral nutrition therapy, 1071t, 1073
etiology, 1033
pathophysiology, 1033
pharmacotherapy. *See* ANTIDIARRHEALS
traveler's, 810t
diazepam, 286, 382–83
adverse effects, 380t, 382
classification, 382
contraindications/precautions, 382–83
distribution in older adults, 148–49
drug interactions, 101t, 383
genetic polymorphisms and actions of, 159, 160t
mechanism of action, 382
nursing responsibilities, 383
overdose treatment, 383

parenteral administration, 283
patient and family education, 383
pharmacokinetics, 382
pregnancy category, 383
renal excretion, 49
similar drugs, 383–84
for specific conditions
alcohol withdrawal, 102
in anesthesia, 464
muscle spasms, 398
seizures, 380*t*, 382
therapeutic effects and uses, 283*t*, 382
diazoxide, 580–81, 582, 584*t*
Dibenzyline. *See* phenoxybenzamine
dibucaine, 473*t*, 476
diclofenac, 724*t*, 725*t*
dicloxacillin, 789*t*, 794
dicyclomine, 214*t*, 217, 1037*t*, 1040
didanosine, 933*t*, 935
Didrex. *See* benzphetamine
Didronel. *See* etidronate
Dietary Approaches to Stop Hypertension (DASH) diet, 570*t*
Dietary Supplement and Nonprescription Drug Consumer Protection Act, 176
Dietary Supplement Health and Education Act of 1994 (DSHEA), 14, 175
dietary supplements, 175
regulation, 175–77
specialty, 179, 179*t*
diethylpropion, 1091
diethylstilbestrol (DES), 980*t*, 1181
difenoxin with atropine, 1034*t*, 1035
Differin. *See* adapalene
diffusion, 42, 43*f*
diflorasone diacetate, 1327*t*
Diflucan. *See* fluconazole
diflunisal, 724*t*, 725*t*
digestion, 1000. *See also* gastrointestinal tract
enzymes in, 1004, 1004*t*
in liver, 1003–4, 1003*f*
in lower gastrointestinal tract, 1001
regulation of, 1004
in upper gastrointestinal tract, 1000–1001
digestive system, 999–1000, 999*f*. *See also* gastrointestinal tract
Digibind. *See* digoxin immune fab
digitalization, 614
digitoxin, 614
digoxin, 615–16
adverse effects, 612*t*, 615
biliary excretion, 49
classification, 615
contraindications/precautions, 615
drug interactions, 615
with diuretics, 74
with herbal products, 178*t*
mechanism of action, 615
nursing responsibilities, 616
in older adults, 149, 152*t*
overdose treatment, 615–16, 1364*t*
patient and family education, 616
pharmacokinetics, 615
pregnancy category, 615
route and adult dose, 612*t*
for specific conditions
dysrhythmias, 629*t*, 637
heart failure, 612*t*, 614
therapeutic effects and uses, 615
digoxin immune fab, 1364*t*
dihydroergotamine, 450*t*
dihydropyridines, 518–19. *See also* CALCIUM CHANNEL BLOCKERS
dihydrotachysterol, 1293, 1294*t*
Dilacor. *See* diltiazem
Dilacor XR, 30*t*, 519*t*. *See also* diltiazem
Dilantin. *See* phenytoin
Dilatate. *See* isosorbide dinitrate
Dilatate SR, 30*t*. *See also* isosorbide dinitrate
Dilaudid. *See* hydromorphone
Dilocaine. *See* lidocaine
diltiazem:
adverse effects, 520*t*, 524
dosage forms not to be crushed or opened, 30*t*
mechanism of action, 522, 524
route and adult dose, 520*t*
for specific conditions
angina, 592*t*
dysrhythmias, 519*t*, 629*t*, 636
dimenhydrinate, 1043*t*
dimercaprol, 1367
adverse effects, 1367
classification, 1367
contraindications/precautions, 1367
drug interactions, 1367
mechanism of action, 1367
nursing responsibilities, 1367
patient and family education, 1367
pharmacokinetics, 1367
pregnancy category, 1367
therapeutic effects and uses, 1367
Dimetapp. *See* brompheniramine
Dimetapp Children's Cold and Allergy, 1266*t*
dimethyltryptamine (DMT), 104–5
dinoprostone:
as abortifacient, 1213, 1213*t*
therapeutic effects and uses, 1214*t*
as uterine stimulant, 1187*t*, 1189
Diovan. *See* valsartan
Diovan HCT, 572*t*
Dipentum. *See* olsalazine
DIPEPTIDYL-PEPTIDASE 4 INHIBITOR:
sitagliptin. *See* sitagliptin
diphenhydramine:
adverse effects, 1265*t*, 1268
drug interactions, 101*t*
mechanism of action, 1268
route and adult dose, 1265*t*
for specific conditions
acute dystonia, 331, 331*t*
allergic rhinitis, 1265*t*, 1268
insomnia, 280, 287
nausea and vomiting, 1043*t*
Parkinson's disease, 355*t*
trade names, 7
diphenoxylate, 142*t*
diphenoxylate with atropine, 1034–35
adverse effects, 1034
classification, 1034
contraindications/precautions, 1034
drug interactions, 1034
mechanism of action, 1033, 1034
nursing responsibilities, 1035
overdose treatment, 1035
patient and family education, 1035
pharmacokinetics, 1034
pregnancy category, 1034
similar drugs, 1035
therapeutic effects and uses, 1034
diphtheria:
characteristics, 758*t*
immunization, 758*t*, 759
incidence, 758*t*
pathophysiology, 759
dipivefrin, 1341*t*, 1344
Diprivan. *See* propofol
Diprolene. *See* betamethasone dipropionate
Diprosone. *See* betamethasone
dipyridamole, 653*t*, 655
direct observation of therapy (DOT), 143, 853, 856*t*
direct thrombin inhibitors. *See* ANTICOAGULANTS
dirithromycin, 813*t*, 816
DISEASE-MODIFYING ANTIRHEUMATIC DRUGS (DMARDs), 1304
abatacept, 1304*t*
adalimumab, 748*t*, 1037, 1305
anakinra, 741*t*, 746, 1304*t*, 1305–6
azathioprine. *See* azathioprine
etanercept. *See* etanercept
hydroxychloroquine. *See* hydroxychloroquine
infliximab, 748*t*, 1037, 1304*t*, 1306
leflunomide, 135*t*, 1306
methotrexate. *See* methotrexate
rituximab, 748*t*, 990*t*, 1304*t*
sulfasalazine. *See* sulfasalazine
disopyramide, 629*t*, 632
dissociative anesthesia, 464
distribution, drug, 45
barriers to, 45–46
blood flow to tissues and, 45
drug interactions and, 71*f*, 72
drug solubility and, 45
drug-protein binding and, 45, 46*f*
in older adults, 148–49
in pediatric patients, 136
in pregnancy, 124
tissue storage and, 45
disulfiram, 102
Ditropan. *See* oxybutynin chloride
DIURETIC(S), 548
classification, 549
clinical applications, 548
combination therapy, 550
drug interactions, 178*t*
Lifespan Considerations, 549*t*
mechanism of action, 548–49
Nursing Process Application, 562–63*t*
in older adults, 549*t*
in pediatric patients, 549*t*
sites of action, 550*f*
for specific conditions
heart failure, 612*t*, 613
hypertension, 573, 574*t*
types
carbonic anhydrase inhibitors. *See* CARBONIC ANHYDRASE INHIBITORS
loop (high-ceiling). *See* LOOP (HIGH-CEILING) DIURETICS
osmotic. *See* OSMOTIC DIURETICS
potassium-sparing. *See* POTASSIUM-SPARING DIURETICS
thiazide. *See* THIAZIDE DIURETICS
diuretic resistance, 613
Diuril. *See* chlorothiazide
diversion, of legal drugs, 94
DKA (diabetic ketoacidosis), 1124

DMARDs. *See* DISEASE-MODIFYING ANTIRHEUMATIC DRUGS (DMARDs)
DMT. *See* dimethyltryptamine
DNA gyrase, 826, 826*f*
DNA helicase, 826, 826*f*
DNA polymerase, 826
DNA replication, bacterial, 826, 826*f*
DNA viruses, 909
Doan's Pills. *See* magnesium salicylate
dobutamine:
  adverse effects, 232*t*
  mechanism of action, 240
  route and adult dose, 232*t*
  for specific conditions
    heart failure, 612*t*, 618
    seizures in shock, 240
Dobutrex. *See* dobutamine
docetaxel, 985*t*, 987
docosanol, 912*t*, 914
docusate, 1030*t*, 1032
dofetilide, 629*t*, 635
dolasetron, 1043*t*
Dolobid. *See* diflunisal
Dolophine. *See* methadone
DOM (2,5 dimethoxy-4-methylamphetamine), 105
donepezil, 361–62
  adverse effects, 359*t*, 362
  classification, 361
  contraindications/precautions, 362
  drug interactions, 362
  mechanism of action, 361
  nursing responsibilities, 362
  overdose treatment, 362
  patient and family education, 362
  pharmacokinetics, 362
  pregnancy category, 362
  route and adult dose, 359*t*
  similar drugs, 362–63
  therapeutic effects and uses, 361
dopamine, 266
  actions/effects, 189*t*, 267*t*
  adverse effects, 232*t*, 235, 612*t*
  mechanism of action, 235, 238
  in Parkinson's disease, 348
  route and adult dose, 232*t*, 612*t*
  for specific conditions, 267*t*
    heart failure, 612*t*
    shock, 235
DOPAMINE AGONISTS:
  adverse effects, 353
  drugs in class
    apomorphine, 350*t*, 354
    bromocriptine, 129*t*, 350*t*, 354
    fenoldopam, 584*t*, 724*t*, 725*t*
    pramipexole. *See* pramipexole
    ropinirole, 350*t*, 354
  versus levodopa, 353
  mechanism of action, 349
  for specific conditions
    hypertensive emergency, 584*t*
    Parkinson's disease, 350*t*
  subclasses, 353
dopamine receptors:
  clinical significance, 266
  genetic polymorphisms, 160*t*
DOPAMINE REPLACEMENT AGENTS:
  levodopa. *See* levodopa
  levodopa-carbidopa, 349, 350*t*, 351
  for Parkinson's disease, 350*t*
dopamine system stabilizers, 340. *See also* aripiprazole
dopamine type 2 (D_2) receptors, 328, 329*f*
dopaminergic synapses, 266
Dopastat. *See* dopamine
Doral. *See* quazepam
Doribax. *See* doripenem
Doriglute. *See* glutethimide
doripenem, 800*t*, 801–2
dornase alfa, 1277
dorsogluteal site, intramuscular injection, 37*t*
dorzolamide, 1341*t*, 1345
dose-limiting toxicity, 965
dose–response relationship, 57–58, 58*f*
dosing intervals, 26–27
DOT (direct observation of therapy), 143, 853, 856*t*
Dovonex. *See* calcipotriene
down-regulation, 1099
doxazosin, 247*t*, 250, 1231*t*
doxepin:
  for anxiety disorders, 289, 290*t*
  for depression, 304*t*, 307
doxercalciferol, 1293, 1294*t*
Doxil. *See* doxorubicin liposomal
doxorubicin, 977–78
  adverse effects, 68*t*, 959, 977–78
  classification, 977
  contraindications/precautions, 978
  drug interactions, 978
  mechanism of action, 977
  nursing responsibilities, 978
  overdose treatment, 978
  patient and family education, 978
  pharmacokinetics, 977
  pregnancy category, 978
  similar drugs, 978–79
  therapeutic effects and uses, 977
doxorubicin liposomal, 977*t*
doxycycline, 810*t*, 812–13, 1322, 1361
doxylamine, 283
DPI (dry powder inhaler), 1242
Dramamine. *See* dimenhydrinate
Drisdol. *See* ergocalciferol
Dritho-Scalp. *See* anthralin
Drixoral. *See* dexbrompheniramine
dronabinol, 1043*t*
Droxia. *See* hydroxyurea
drug(s), 4
  of abuse. *See* substance abuse
  administration. *See* drug administration
  approval process
    changes to, 18–19
    limitations, 18
    stages, 17–18, 17*f*
  Canadian regulations, 20, 20*t*
  classification
    pharmacologic, 5–6
    therapeutic, 5–6
  costs of, 5*t*
  definition, 4
  disposal, 26*t*
  do not crush/open list, 30*t*
  as enzyme inducers, 47
  as enzyme inhibitors, 47
  expiration dates, 25
  ideal, characteristics of, 5
  interactions. *See* drug interactions
  legislation, 13–14, 14*t*
  marketing rights, 8
  measurement systems, 27–28, 28*t*
  names
    look-alike/soundalike, 84–85*t*, 729*t*
    medication errors and, 84–86
    types, 7–8, 7*t*
  pharmacokinetics. *See* pharmacokinetics
  prototype, 6–7
  scheduled, 20
  storage, 25, 167
  as substrates, 47
drug administration:
  abbreviations, 27*t*
  in adolescents. *See* pediatric patients
  in children. *See* pediatric patients
  documentation, 28
  dosing intervals, 26–27
  enteral route, 28–31
    absorption and, 44
    buccal, 31, 31*f*
    sublingual, 31, 31*f*
    tablets and capsules, 29
    via gastrostomy tube, 31
    via nasogastric tube, 31
  guidelines, 29*t*
  in infants. *See* pediatric patients
  Lifespan Considerations, 25*t*
  parenteral route, 34–37
    absorption and, 43–44
    intradermal, 35, 35*f*
    intramuscular, 35, 36*f*, 37*t*
    intravenous, 36–37, 37*f*
    subcutaneous, 35, 35*f*
  patient adherence and, 24
  pharmacokinetics. *See* pharmacokinetics
  prescription writing, 25–26, 26*f*
  rights of, 80. *See also* medication error(s)
  by school nurses, 166*t*
  topical route, 31–34
    absorption and, 44
    intranasal, 33, 33*f*
    ophthalmic, 32, 33*f*
    otic, 32, 33*f*
    rectal, 34
    transdermal, 32, 32*f*
    vaginal, 33, 34*f*
drug allergies, 67
drug–drug interactions. *See* drug interactions
drug–food interactions. *See* drug interactions
drug interactions, 70
  with enteral formulas, 1074, 1074*t*
  with food, 45, 74, 75*t*
  with herbal products, 74–75, 75*t*, 177–79, 178*t*
  in hospitalized patients, 74*t*
  mechanisms, 45, 71–72, 71*f*
  in older adults, 153*t*
  patient teaching, 75*t*
  pharmacodynamic, 73–74, 73*f*
drug misuse, 150–51. *See also* substance abuse
drug-protein complexes, 45, 46*f*
dry powder inhaler (DPI), 1242
DTaP. *See* diphtheria, immunization; pertussis, immunization; tetanus, immunization
DTIC-Dome. *See* dacarbazine
dual-energy x-ray absorptiometry (DEXA), 1290
Duetact, 1134*t*
Dulcolax. *See* bisacodyl

duloxetine:
for anxiety or insomnia, 282*t*, 289, 290*t*
for depression, 304*t*, 312
dosage forms not to be crushed or opened, 30*t*
dumping syndrome, 1069
duodenal ulcer, 1009. *See also* peptic ulcer
Duraclon. *See* clonidine
Durad. *See* diethylpropion
Duragen-10. *See* estradiol valerate
Duragesic. *See* fentanyl
Duragesic Transdermal System. *See* fentanyl
Duramorph RF. *See* morphine sulfate
Duricef. *See* cefadroxil
Duvoid. *See* bethanechol chloride
DVT. *See* deep vein thrombosis
dwarfism, 1107. *See also* growth hormone, deficiency
Dyazide, 549, 572*t*
Dynabac. *See* dirithromycin
DynaCirc. *See* isradipine
dyphylline, 1256
Dyrenium. *See* triamterene
dysfunctional uterine bleeding, 1181, 1183
dyslipidemias:
in adolescents, 506*t*
incidence, 496*t*
nonpharmacologic treatment, 500–501, 501*t*
Nursing Process Application, 511*t*
pharmacotherapy, 504*t*
bile acid sequestrants, 504*t*, 506–8
ezetimibe, 504*t*, 510–11
fibric acid agents, 504*t*, 509–10
niacin (nicotinic acid), 504*t*, 509
statins, 501–6, 504*t*
treatment guidelines, 499–500
types, 500*t*
dysrhythmias, 498, 623
acute, 627
asymptomatic, 627
classification, 625–27
diet and, 627*t*
drugs causing, 623*t*
etiology, 623, 623*t*
nonpharmacologic treatment, 627
in pediatric patients, 623*t*
pharmacotherapy, 629*t*. *See also* ANTIDYSRHYTHMIC DRUGS
prophylaxis, 627
dysthymic disorder, 298
dystonia:
acute, 331, 331*t*
chronic, 403, 403*t*

E

ear:
anatomy, 1349–50, 1350*f*
pharmacotherapy
external otitis, 1350–51
Lifespan Considerations, 1352*t*
mastoiditis, 1351–52
nursing responsibilities, 1352
otic preparations. *See* otic preparations
otitis interna, 1351
otitis media, 1351
patient and family education, 1352–53
wax softeners, 1352
EC. *See* emergency contraception
eccrine glands, 1316
ECF (extracellular fluid) compartment, 687, 687*f*
ECG (electrocardiogram), 625, 625*f*, 626*t*
echinacea:
description, 745*t*
drug interactions, 178*t*
evidence, 745*t*
history and claims, 745*t*
primary uses, 173*t*
standardization, 175*t*, 745*t*
Echinacea purpurea. *See* echinacea
echothiophate, 204, 1341*t*, 1344
eclampsia, 373
econazole, 878*t*
Ecotrin, 30*t*. *See also* aspirin
ecstasy. *See* MDMA
ECT (electroconvulsive therapy), 302, 302*t*
ectopic foci, 489
ectopic pregnancy, 1204
eculizumab, 748*t*
eczema, 1325
ED. *See* erectile dysfunction
ED_{50} (median effective dose), 56, 56*f*
Edecrin. *See* ethacrynic acid
edema, corticosteroids for, 1169
edetate calcium disodium, 1366–67
adverse effects, 1366
classification, 1366
contraindications/precautions, 1366
drug interactions, 1366
mechanism of action, 1366
nursing responsibilities, 1366–67
patient and family education, 1367
pharmacokinetics, 1366
pregnancy category, 1366
therapeutic effects and uses, 1366
edrophonium, 202*t*, 205, 206, 207
EEG (electroencephalogram), 372*f*
efalizumab, 748*t*
efavirenz, 936–37
adverse effects, 933*t*, 936
classification, 936
contraindications/precautions, 936
drug interactions, 936–37
with herbal products, 178*t*
mechanism of action, 936
nursing responsibilities, 937
overdose treatment, 937
patient and family education, 937
pharmacokinetics, 936
pregnancy category, 937
route and adult dose, 933*t*
similar drugs, 937
therapeutic effects and uses, 936
Efedron. *See* ephedrine
Effexor. *See* venlafaxine
efficacy, 58–59, 59*f*
eflornithine, 892*t*, 896, 898
Efudex. *See* fluorouracil
Elavil. *See* amitriptyline
Eldepryl. *See* selegiline
elderly patients. *See* older adults
electrocardiogram (ECG), 625, 625*f*, 626*t*
electroconvulsive therapy (ECT), 302, 302*t*
electroencephalogram (EEG), 372*f*
electrolyte(s), 694–95
electrolyte imbalances, 694–95, 694*t*
calcium, 694*t*
hypercalcemia, 694*t*
hypocalcemia. *See* hypocalcemia
chloride, 694*t*
hyperchloremia, 694*t*
hypochloremia, 694*t*
magnesium, 699
hypermagnesemia, 694*t*, 699
hypomagnesemia. *See* hypomagnesemia
phosphate, 694*t*
hyperphosphatemia. *See* hyperphosphatemia
hypophosphatemia, 694*t*, 1072*t*
potassium, 694*t*, 695*f*, 697
hyperkalemia. *See* hyperkalemia
hypokalemia. *See* hypokalemia
sodium, 694*t*, 695, 695*f*
hypernatremia. *See* hypernatremia
hyponatremia. *See* hyponatremia
Elestat. *See* epinastine
eletriptan, 450*t*, 452
Eleutherococcus senticosus. *See* ginseng; goldenseal
Elidel. *See* pimecrolimus
Eligard. *See* leuprolide
Elimite. *See* permethrin
Ellence. *See* epirubicin
Elocon. *See* mometasone furoate
Eloxatin. *See* oxaliplatin
Elspar. *See* asparaginase
Emcyt. *See* estramustine
Emend. *See* aprepitant
emergency contraception (EC), 1212
Plan B, 1203*t*, 1212, 1213*t*
emergency preparedness, 1358
emesis. *See* nausea and vomiting
emetic potential, 959
emetics, 1044
emetogenic potential, 1041
emphysema, 1258
emtricitabine, 933*t*, 935, 943
Emtriva. *See* emtricitabine
Emulsoil. *See* castor oil
E-mycin. *See* erythromycin base
EN. *See* enteral nutrition
enalapril, 535–36
adverse effects, 533*t*, 536
metabolism, 46
route and adult dose, 533*t*
for specific conditions
heart failure, 612*t*
hypertensive emergency, 584*t*
enalaprilat, 536
Enbrel. *See* etanercept
endocrine system, 1099
age-related changes, 149*t*
disorders and pharmacotherapy, 1102*t*
hormone secretion, 1099, 1100*f*
endometrial carcinoma, 1183
Endometrin. *See* progesterone
endometriosis, 1183, 1191
endorphins, 266, 267*t*, 431
endotoxins, 775
Enduron. *See* methyclothiazide
enflurane, 101*t*, 468*t*, 469
enfuvirtide, 933*t*, 940
Engerix-B. *See* hepatitis B vaccine
Enjuvia. *See* conjugated estrogens
enkephalins, 266, 267*t*
enoxaparin, 645*t*, 647
ENS (enteric nervous system), 1004
Ensam. *See* selegiline
entacapone, 350*t*, 355

Entamoeba histolytica, 886*t*, 891, 891f
entecavir, 26*t*, 919*t*, 922
enteral nutrition (EN), 1068
  assessment of need for, 1077*t*
  complications
    aspiration, 1070, 1071*t*, 1073
    constipation, 1071*t*
    diarrhea, 1071*t*, 1073
    interrupted infusions, 1074
    metabolic, 1072*t*, 1073
    nasal mucosal damage, 1072*t*
    nausea and vomiting, 1071*t*, 1073
    tube obstruction, 1071*t*, 1073–74
  drug administration during
    drug interactions, 1074, 1074*t*
    guidelines, 1073*t*
  formulas
    nutrient classes in, 1070
    types, 1069–70, 1069*t*
  in home setting, 1074*t*
  methods, 1068–69
  Nursing Process Application, 1075–76*t*
enteral route, drug administration, 28–29, 44
enteric nervous system (ENS), 1004
enteric-coated, 29
Enterobacter, 777*t*
enterobiasis, 900–901
Enterobius vermicularis, 900–901
Enterococci, 777*t*
  vancomycin-resistant, 782
enteroendocrine cells, 1000
enterohepatic recirculation, 49, 50*f*, 1003
Entocort. *See* budesonide
Entocort-EC. *See* budesonide
enzyme(s), 1004, 1004*t*
enzyme induction, 47
enzyme inhibition, 47
ephedra, 235, 1089
ephedrine, 232*t*, 235, 1273*t*
epidermis, 1315–16, 1315*f*
Epidermophyton, 869*t*, 878
epidural anesthesia, 459*t*, 471, 471*f*
epilepsy, 371, 382*t*. *See also* seizures
epinastine, 1348, 1349*t*
epinephrine, 195
epinephrine, 233–35
  administration precautions, 234*t*
  adverse effects, 232*t*, 233, 612*t*
  classification, 233
  contraindications/precautions, 233
  drug interactions, 233–34
  history, 192*t*
  mechanism of action, 233
  nursing responsibilities, 234
  overdose treatment, 234
  patient and family education, 234–35
  pharmacokinetics, 233
  pregnancy category, 234
  route and adult dose, 232*t*, 612*t*
  similar drugs, 235
  for specific conditions
    heart failure, 612*t*
  therapeutic effects and uses, 233
EpiPen, 235*t*
epirubicin, 977*t*, 978
Epivir. *See* lamivudine
Epivir HBV. *See* lamivudine
eplerenone:
  adverse effects, 538*t*, 541, 556*t*, 558
  mechanism of action, 541, 556, 558
  route and adult dose, 538*t*, 556*t*, 612t
  for specific conditions
    heart failure, 612*t*
epoetin alfa, 669–71
  adverse effects, 670
  classification, 669
  contraindications/precautions, 670
  drug interactions, 670
  mechanism of action, 670
  Nursing Process Application, 672*t*
  nursing responsibilities, 671
  overdose treatment, 671
  patient and family education, 671
  pharmacokinetics, 670
  pregnancy category, 671
  similar drugs, 671
  for specific conditions
    anemia in renal failure, 548*t*
    anemia with cancer chemotherapy, 993
  therapeutic effects and uses, 669–70
Epogen. *See* epoetin alfa
eprosartan, 538*t*, 540
EPS (extrapyramidal symptoms), 331, 331*t*, 349
EPS (extrapyramidal system), 270
Epstein-Barr virus, 911
eptifibatide, 653*t*, 657
Equalactin. *See* calcium polycarbophil
Equanil. *See* meprobamate
Eraxis. *See* anidulafungin
Erbitux. *See* cetuximab
erectile dysfunction (ED), 1226
  pathophysiology, 1227
  pharmacotherapy, 1227–28
    sildenafil. *See* sildenafil
    tadalafil, 1227*t*, 1229
    vardenafil, 1227*t*, 1229
  prevalence, 1226*t*
ergocalciferol, 1293, 1294*t*. *See also* vitamin D
ergonovine, 1187*t*, 1189
Ergostat. *See* ergotamine
ergosterol, 871
ERGOT ALKALOIDS, 451
  contraindications, 451
  dihydroergotamine, 450*t*, 451
  ergonovine, 1187*t*, 1189
  ergotamine, 129*t*, 450*t*, 451
  methylergonovine, 1187*t*, 1189
ergotamine, 129*t*, 450*t*, 451
Ergotrate. *See* ergonovine
erlotinib, 990*t*
ertapenem, 800*t*, 802
Eryc, 30*t*. *See also* erythromycin base
erythema, 1316
Erythrocin. *See* erythromycin base
erythrocytes, 483, 485*t*
erythrocytic stage, malaria, 887
erythromycin base, 814–15
  adverse effects, 814
    in pediatric patients, 142*t*
  classification, 814
  contraindications/precautions, 815
  dosage forms not to be crushed or
      opened, 30*t*
  drug interactions, 815
  mechanism of action, 814
  nursing responsibilities, 815
  overdose treatment, 815
  patient and family education, 815
  pediatric dosage/route, 142*t*
  pharmacokinetics, 814
  pregnancy category, 815
  similar drugs, 815–16
  therapeutic effects and uses, 814
erythropoietin, 483, 668. *See also* epoetin alfa
Escherichia coli:
  replication, 826
  in urinary tract infections, 838, 838*t*
escitalopram:
  for anxiety or insomnia, 282*t*, 289, 290*t*
  for depression, 304*t*, 310
Eskalith. *See* lithium carbonate
Eskalith CR, 30*t*. *See also* lithium carbonate
esmolol:
  adverse effects, 252*t*, 258
  route and adult dose, 252*t*
  for specific conditions, 257–58
    dysrhythmias, 629*t*, 634
    hypertensive emergency, 584*t*
esomeprazole, 30*t*, 1013*t*, 1015
estazolam, 282*t*, 283*t*, 286
esters, 472. *See also* local anesthetics, ester-type
Estinyl. *See* ethinyl estradiol
Estrace. *See* estradiol
Estraderm. *See* estradiol
estradiol, 1180*t*
estradiol/norethindrone, 1204–6
  adverse effects, 1180*t*, 1205
  classification, 1204
  contraindications/precautions, 1205
  drug interactions, 1205
  mechanism of action, 1205
  nursing responsibilities, 1205–6
  overdose treatment, 1205
  patient and family education, 1206
  pharmacokinetics, 1205
  pregnancy category, 1205
  route and adult dose, 1180*t*
  therapeutic effects and uses, 1204
estradiol/norgestimate, 1180*t*
estradiol valerate, 1180*t*
estramustine, 967*t*, 970–71
ESTROGEN(S):
  adverse effects, 68*t*, 1181*t*, 1185–86
  drugs in class
    combinations with progestin
      conjugated estrogens/
        medroxyprogesterone, 1180*t*
      estradiol/norethindrone. *See*
        estradiol/norethindrone
      estradiol/norgestimate, 1180*t*
    conjugated estrogens. *See* conjugated
      estrogens
    estradiol, 1180*t*
    estradiol valerate, 1180*t*
    estropipate, 1180*t*
  loss at menopause, 1184, 1185*t*
  in oral contraceptives, 1200
  replacement therapy
    adverse effects, 68*t*, 1186
    for menopause symptoms, 1184
    Nursing Process Application, 1182*t*
  therapeutic effects and uses, 1177–78
  types, 1177
ESTROGEN RECEPTOR ANTAGONISTS:
  fulvestrant, 980*t*, 982
  raloxifene. *See* raloxifene
  tamoxifen. *See* tamoxifen
  toremifene, 980*t*, 983
estropipate, 1180*t*
eszopiclone, 282*t*, 288

etanercept, 746
adverse effects, 741*t*, 746, 1304*t*, 1306
mechanism of action, 746
route and adult dose, 741*t*, 1304*t*
for specific conditions
psoriasis, 1330*t*, 1331
rheumatoid arthritis, 1304*t*, 1306
therapeutic effects and uses, 746
ethacrynic acid, 551*t*, 553
ethambutol:
for *M. avium* complex infections, 865
for tuberculosis, 855*t*, 858
ethanol. *See* alcohol
ethchlorvynol, 286
ethinyl estradiol:
for acne, 1322*t*
for neoplasia, 980*t*
in oral contraceptives, 1203*t*
ethionamide, 855*t*, 861
Ethmozine. *See* moricizine
ethnic influences, in pharmacotherapy, 158–59
ethnicity, 158
ethosuximide, 388
adverse effects, 388
classification, 388
contraindications/precautions, 388
mechanism of action, 388
nursing responsibilities, 388
overdose treatment, 388
patient and family education, 388
pharmacokinetics, 388
pregnancy category, 388
similar drugs, 388
therapeutic effects and uses, 388
Ethrane. *See* enflurane
ethylene glycol poisoning, 1364*t*
etidronate, 75*t*, 1294*t*, 1295*t*, 1297
etiologies, 115
etodolac, 724*t*, 725*t*
etoposide:
adverse effects, 68*t*, 985*t*, 988
mechanism of action, 827
route and adult dose, 985*t*
therapeutic effects and uses, 988
etravirine, 933*t*, 937
Eulexin. *See* flutamide
euphoria, 412
Eurax. *See* crotamiton
Evacet. *See* doxorubicin liposomal
evaluation criteria, in planning, 117
evaluation, in nursing process, 119–20
evening primrose, 173*t*
evidence-based nursing practice, 117
Evidence-Based Practice:
acute and cancer pain management, 429*t*
acute otitis media, 138*t*
antidepressants for low-back pain, 398*t*
asthma management, 1244*t*
attention deficit/hyperactivity disorder, 414*t*
Clinical Antipsychotic Trials of Intervention Effectiveness (CATIE) study, 341*t*
direct observation therapy effectiveness, 856*t*
growth hormone
for age-appropriate height, 1107*t*
long-term outcome in pediatric burn patients, 1110*t*
human papillomavirus risk reduction, 911*t*
malignant hyperthermia and anesthetic agents, 466*t*
nonsteroidal anti-inflammatory drugs, 727*t*
oral hypoglycemic agents for gestational diabetes, 1122*t*
proton pump inhibitors and bone fracture risk, 1016*t*
proton pump inhibitors and gastrointestinal infection, 1014*t*
reducing neutropenic patients' exposure overdose treatment fungal pathogens, 870*t*
role of school nurses in epilepsy treatment, 386*t*
seizures in older adults, 375*t*
traveler's diarrhea, 810*t*
weight gain with use of atypical antipsychotics, 338*t*
Evista. *See* raloxifene
Evithrom. *See* thrombin
Evoxac. *See* cevimeline HCl
Exanta. *See* ximelagatran
exclusivity, 7
excoriation, 1325
excretion, drug, 48
drug interactions and, 71*f*, 72–73
fecal and biliary, 49, 50*f*
glandular, 49
in older adults, 150
in pediatric patients, 137
in pregnancy, 124
pulmonary, 49
renal, 48–49
Exelderm. *See* oxiconazole
Exelon. *See* rivastigmine
exemestane, 980*t*, 983
exenatide, 1133*t*, 1142
exercise, salt replacements and, 696*t*
exercise-associated hypernatremia, 688*t*
Exforge, 572*t*
Ex-Lax. *See* phenolphthalein
exophthalmos, 1152
exotoxins, 775
EXPECTORANTS, 1277
guaifenesin, 1276*t*, 1277
expiration date, 25
extended release, 29
external otitis, 1350–51
extracellular fluid (ECF) compartment, 687, 687*f*
extrapyramidal symptoms (EPS), 331, 331*t*, 349
extrapyramidal system (EPS), 270
extravasation, of antineoplastic agents, 960
extrinsic pathway, 486, 486*f*
Exubera. *See* insulin human inhaled
eye:
anatomy, 1338, 1339*f*
pharmacotherapy
anesthetic agents, 1347
for examinations, 1347
for glaucoma. *See* glaucoma
in the home setting, 1350*t*
miscellaneous agents, 1347–49, 1348*t*
ezetimibe:
adverse effects, 504*t*, 511
mechanism of action, 503*f*, 510–11
route and adult dose, 504*t*

F

Factive. *See* gemifloxacin
factor IX, 663
factor VIII, 663, 664
factor XI deficiency, 663
famciclovir, 912*t*, 914
familial hypercholesterolemia, 500*t*, 508*t*
famotidine, 477, 1016*t*, 1019
Famvir. *See* famciclovir
Fansidar. *See* pyrimethamine-sulfadiazine
Fareston. *See* toremifene
Faslodex. *See* fulvestrant
Fastin. *See* phentermine
fasting plasma glucose (FPG) test, 1122, 1123*t*
fat substitutes, 1093
fatigue, antineoplastic agents and, 960
fat-soluble vitamins, 1052
vitamin A. *See* vitamin A
vitamin C. *See* vitamin D
vitamin E. *See* vitamin E
vitamin K. *See* vitamin K
FDA. *See* Food and Drug Administration
FDCA (Food, Drug, and Cosmetic Act), 14
febrile seizures, 376, 376*t*
feces, drug excretion in, 49
Feen-a-Mint. *See* phenolphthalein
felbamate, 381*t*, 391
Felbatol. *See* felbamate
Feldene. *See* piroxicam
felodipine:
adverse effects, 520*t*
dosage forms not to be crushed or opened, 30*t*
drug interactions, 74
mechanism of action, 521
route and adult dose, 520*t*
for specific conditions
hypertension, 519*t*
therapeutic effects and uses, 521
female infertility:
causes, 1191, 1191*t*
pharmacotherapy
bromocriptine, 1192*t*, 1195
cetrorelix, 1192*t*, 1195
chorionic gonadotropin-HCG, 1192*t*, 1195
clomiphene citrate. *See* clomiphene citrate
danazol, 1192*t*, 1194, 1195
follitropin alfa, 1192*t*, 1195
follitropin beta, 1192*t*, 1195
ganirelix, 1192*t*, 1195
goserelin, 1192*t*, 1195–96
leuprolide, 1192*t*, 1194, 1196
mechanism of action, 1191, 1193*f*
menotropins, 1191, 1192*t*, 1196
nafarelin, 1192*t*, 1194, 1196
urofollitropin, 1192*t*
female reproductive system:
cycles, 1178*f*
negative feedback control, 1179*f*
regulation, 1177
Femara. *See* letrozole
Femstat. *See* butoconazole
fenfluramine/phentermine, 1089
fenofibrate, 504*t*, 510
fenoldopam, 584*t*
fenoprofen, 724*t*, 725*t*
Fen-Phen. *See* fenfluramine/phentermine
fentanyl, 461–62
adverse effects, 460*t*, 462
classification, 461
contraindications/precautions, 462
disposal, 26*t*
with droperidol, 460*t*
drug interactions, 462

mechanism of action, 462
nursing responsibilities, 462
overdose treatment, 462
patient and family education, 462
pediatric labeling changes, 135*t*
pharmacokinetics, 462
pregnancy category, 462
route and adult dose, 460*t*
similar drugs, 462–63
therapeutic effects and uses, 461
Fentora. *See* fentanyl
fenugreek, 129*t*
Feosol, 30*t*. *See also* ferrous sulfate
Feostat. *See* ferrous fumarate
Fergon. *See* ferrous gluconate
ferric gluconate, 680
ferritin, 677
Ferrlecit. *See* ferric gluconate
ferrous fumarate, 676*t*, 679
ferrous gluconate, 676*t*, 679
ferrous sulfate, 678–79
adverse effects, 676*t*, 678
in pediatric patients, 142*t*
classification, 678
contraindications/precautions, 678
dosage forms not to be crushed or opened, 30*t*
drug interactions, 679
mechanism of action, 678
nursing responsibilities, 679
overdose treatment, 679
patient and family education, 679
pediatric dosage/route, 142*t*
pharmacokinetics, 678
pregnancy category, 679
route and adult dose, 676*t*
similar drugs, 679
therapeutic effects and uses, 678
fetal–placental barrier, 46
fetal tissue transplantation, 350*t*
fetus:
development stage and adverse drug effects, 126–27
drug transfer across placenta to, 124
fever, 711*t*
feverfew, 75*t*, 178*t*
fexofenadine, 1267–68
adverse effects, 1265*t*, 1267
classification, 1267
contraindications/precautions, 1267
drug interactions, 1267
mechanism of action, 1267
nursing responsibilities, 1267
overdose treatment, 1267
patient and family education, 1267–68
pharmacokinetics, 1267
pregnancy category, 1267
route and adult dose, 1265*t*
similar drugs, 1268
therapeutic effects and uses, 1267
FFP (fresh frozen plasma), 689*t*
FiberCon. *See* calcium polycarbophil
FIBRIC ACID AGENTS, 509
adverse effects, 504*t*
drugs in class
clofibrate, 504*t*, 509
fenofibrate, 504*t*, 510
gemfibrozil. *See* gemfibrozil
for dyslipidemias, 504*t*, 509–10
fibrin, 486
fibrinogen, 486
fibrinolysis, 657, 658*f*
fight-or-flight response, 186, 229
filgrastim, 673–74
adverse effects, 673
classification, 673
contraindications/precautions, 673
drug interactions, 673
mechanism of action, 673
nursing responsibilities, 673
overdose treatment, 673
patient and family education, 673–74
pharmacokinetics, 673
pregnancy category, 673
similar drugs, 674
therapeutic effects and uses, 673, 993
filtrate, 545
Finacea. *See* azelaic acid
finasteride, 1232–33
adverse effects, 1231*t*, 1232
classification, 1232
contraindications/precautions, 1232
drug interactions, 1232
mechanism of action, 1232
nursing responsibilities, 1232–33
overdose treatment, 1232
patient and family education, 1233
pharmacokinetics, 1232
pregnancy category, 1232
route and adult dose, 1231*t*
for specific conditions
alopecia, 1333–34
therapeutic effects and uses, 1232
Finevin. *See* azelaic acid
first-dose phenomenon, 248, 576
FIRST-GENERATION ANTIPSYCHOTICS:
in Alzheimer's disease, 360
history, 330
nonphenothiazines
adverse effects, 335
haloperidol. *See* haloperidol
loxapine, 332*t*, 336
molindone, 332*t*, 336
pimozide, 332*t*, 336
therapeutic effects and uses, 335
thiothixene, 332*t*, 336
Nursing Process Application, 342*t*
phenothiazines
chlorpromazine HCl. *See* chlorpromazine HCl
drug interactions, 178*t*
fluphenazine, 332*t*, 334
nonpsychiatric indications, 333
perphenazine, 160*t*, 332*t*, 334
prochlorperazine. *See* prochlorperazine
thioridazine, 332*t*, 335
trifluoperazine, 332*t*, 335
versus second-generation antipsychotics, 330
selection, 332–33
first-pass effect, 48, 48*f*, 1003
fish oil:
description, 1163*t*
evidence, 1163*t*
history and claims, 1163*t*
primary uses, 179*t*
standardization, 1163*t*
Flagyl. *See* metronidazole
flaxseed oil:
drug absorption and, 177
drug interactions, 178*t*
primary uses, 179*t*
flecainide, 629*t*, 632–33
Fleet Phospho-Soda. *See* sodium biphosphate
Flexeril. *See* cyclobenzaprine
Flomax. *See* tamsulosin
Flonase. *See* fluticasone
Flovent. *See* fluticasone
Floxin. *See* ofloxacin
floxuridine, 973*t*, 975
fluconazole, 875–76
adverse effects, 872*t*, 876
in pediatric patients, 142*t*
classification, 875
contraindications/precautions, 876
dosage/routes
adult, 872*t*
pediatric, 142*t*
drug interactions, 876
mechanism of action, 876
nursing responsibilities, 876
overdose treatment, 876
patient and family education, 876
pharmacokinetics, 876
pregnancy category, 876
similar drugs, 876–77
for specific conditions
oropharyngeal candidiasis, 879
seborrheic dermatitis, 1328
superficial mycoses, 877, 878*t*, 879, 1318
systemic mycoses, 872*t*
therapeutic effects and uses, 875–76
flucytosine, 871, 871*f*, 872*t*, 875
Fludara. *See* fludarabine
fludarabine, 973*t*, 976
fludrocortisone, 1170–71
adverse effects, 1170
classification, 1170
contraindications/precautions, 1170
drug interactions, 1170
mechanism of action, 1170
nursing considerations, 1171
overdose treatment, 1170
patient and family education, 1171
pharmacokinetics, 1170
pregnancy category, 1170
therapeutic effects and uses, 1170
fluid compartments, 687, 687*f*
fluid imbalance:
fluid compartments and, 687, 687*f*
fluid movements and, 687–88
physiology, 688
FLUID REPLACEMENT AGENTS:
blood products
cryoprecipitate, 689*t*
fresh frozen plasma, 689*t*
immune globulins, 689*t*
normal serum albumin. *See* normal serum albumin
packed RBCs, 689*t*
platelets, 689*t*
principles, 689–90
whole blood, 689*t*, 690
colloids, 692, 692*t*
dextran 40. *See* dextran 40
hetastarch, 694
crystalloids, 691, 691*t*
5% dextrose in water. *See* 5% dextrose in water
hypertonic, 691

hypotonic, 691
isotonic, 691
lactated Ringer's solution, 691*t*, 692
Plasma-Lyte, 691*t*, 692
Ringer's solution, 691*t*, 692
Nursing Process Application, 693*t*
for specific conditions
dehydration, 688–89, 689*t*
Flumadine. *See* rimantadine
flumazenil, 284, 1364*t*
flunisolide, 1250*t*, 1252, 1270*t*
flunitrazepam, 98
fluocinolone acetonide, 1327*t*
fluocinonide, 1327*t*
fluorescein sodium, 1347
fluorine, 1063, 1063*t*
5-fluorocytosine. *See* flucytosine
FLUOROQUINOLONES:
adverse effects
cardiotoxicity, 828
cartilage toxicity, 828
central nervous system toxicity, 828–29
gastrointestinal toxicity, 828
hepatotoxicity, 829
hypersensitivity reactions, 828
phototoxicity, 829
resistance, 829
clinical applications, 827–28, 828*t*
contraindications, 839
drug interactions, 75*t*
first generation, 828*t*
cinoxacin, 827*t*
nalidixic acid. *See* nalidixic acid
fourth generation, 828*t*
gemifloxacin, 827*t*, 830
moxifloxacin, 827*t*, 830
mechanism of action, 827
Nursing Process Application, 831*t*
resistance to, 832*t*
second generation, 828*t*
ciprofloxacin. *See* ciprofloxacin
norfloxacin, 827*t*, 830, 838
ofloxacin, 827*t*, 831
for specific conditions
tuberculosis, 855*t*, 861–62
third generation, 828*t*
gatifloxacin, 827*t*, 830
levofloxacin, 827*t*, 830, 838
fluorouracil, 827, 973*t*, 975
Fluothane. *See* halothane
fluoxetine, 309–10
adverse effects, 304*t*, 309
in breast-feeding infant, 129*t*
classification, 308
contraindications/precautions, 309
for depression, 304*t*
drug interactions, 309–10
mechanism of action, 309
nursing responsibilities, 310
patient and family education, 310
pediatric labeling changes, 135*t*
pharmacokinetics, 309
pregnancy category, 310
route and adult dose, 282*t*, 304*t*
similar drugs, 310
for specific conditions
anxiety or insomnia, 282*t*, 289, 290*t*
cataplexy, 420
obesity, 1090
therapeutic effects and uses, 308–9
fluoxymesterone, 980*t*, 1220*t*, 1223
fluphenazine, 332*t*, 334
flurandrenolide, 1327*t*
flurazepam, 282*t*, 283*t*, 286
flurbiprofen, 723, 724*t*, 725*t*
flutamide, 980*t*, 984
fluticasone, 1270–71
adverse effects, 1250*t*, 1270, 1270*t*
in pediatric patients, 142*t*
for asthma, 1252
classification, 1270
contraindications/precautions, 1270
drug interactions, 1270–71
mechanism of action, 1270
nursing responsibilities, 1271
overdose treatment, 1271
patient and family education, 1271
pediatric dosage/route, 142*t*
pediatric labeling changes, 135*t*
pharmacokinetics, 1270
pregnancy category, 1271
route and adult dose, 1250*t*, 1270*t*
therapeutic effects and uses, 1270
fluticasone propionate, 1327*t*
fluvastatin, 504*t*, 505–6
fluvoxamine:
for anxiety or insomnia, 282*t*, 289, 290*t*
for depression, 304*t*, 310
focal (partial) seizures, 375. *See also* seizures
Focalin. *See* dexmethylphenidate
Folex. *See* methotrexate
folic acid (folate; vitamin B_9), 841, 1060–61
adverse effects, 676*t*, 1061
contraindications/precautions, 1061
deficiency, 1053*t*, 1054
drug interactions, 1061
functions, 1053*t*
mechanism of action, 1060
metabolism, drug inhibition of, 841, 841*f*
nursing responsibilities, 1061
for nutritional disorders
adverse effects, 1054*t*
route and adult dose, 1054*t*
patient and family education, 1061
for pernicious anemia, 676*t*, 682
pregnancy category, 1061
recommended dietary allowance, 1061
route and adult dose, 676*t*
therapeutic effects and uses, 1060
FOLIC ACID ANALOGS, 972, 972*f*
methotrexate. *See* methotrexate
pemetrexed, 973*t*, 974
folic acid deficiency:
antiseizure drugs and, 373
etiology, 682
homocysteine levels and, 682*t*
management, 682. *See also* folic acid
follicle-stimulating hormone (FSH):
regulation, 1102*t*
target organs and action, 1102*t*, 1105*t*
folliculitis, 1317
Follistim. *See* follitropin beta
follitropin alfa, 1192*t*, 1195
follitropin beta, 1192*t*, 1195
Folvite. *See* folic acid
fomepizole, 1364*t*
fondaparinux, 645*t*, 648
Food and Drug Administration (FDA):
branches and structure, 16–17, 16*f*
drug approval process, 17–18, 17*f*
medication error reporting, 86
pregnancy category ratings, 125–26, 125*t*
Food and Drug Administration (FDA) Modernization Act, 134–35
Food, Drug, and Cosmetic Act (FDCA), 14
food–drug interactions, 45, 74, 75*t*. *See also* drug interactions
Foradil. *See* formoterol
Forane. *See* isoflurane
formoterol, 240, 1245*t*, 1247
formulary, 15
Fortamet. *See* metformin
Fortaz. *See* ceftazidime
Forteo. *See* teriparatide
Fortical. *See* calcitonin-salmon
Fosamax. *See* alendronate
fosamprenavir, 933*t*, 939
foscarnet, 912*t*, 914
fosfomycin:
adverse effects, 800*t*, 840*t*, 847
contraindications, 839
indications, 803, 838, 847
route and adult dose, 800*t*, 840*t*
fosinopril, 533*t*, 536, 612*t*
fosphenytoin, 380*t*, 385
Fosrenol. *See* lanthanum carbonate
Fostex. *See* benzoyl peroxide
FPG (fasting plasma glucose) test, 1122, 1123*t*
Fragmin. *See* dalteparin
Francisella tularensis, 1361
frequency distribution curve, 56, 56*f*
fresh frozen plasma (FFP), 689*t*
Frova. *See* frovatriptan
frovatriptan, 450*t*, 452
5-FU. *See* fluorouracil
FUDR. *See* floxuridine
fulvestrant, 980*t*, 982
Fulvicin. *See* griseofulvin
fungal infections:
candidiasis. *See* candidiasis
characteristics, 869–70
classification, 870
pathogens, 869*t*
pharmacotherapy. *See* antifungal drugs
reducing exposure in neutropenia, 870*t*
subcutaneous, 870
superficial, 870, 877–80
systemic, 870, 871
fungi, 869*t*
Fungi-Nail. *See* undecylenic acid
Fungizone. *See* amphotericin B deoxycholate
Furadantin. *See* nitrofurantoin
furazolidone, 101*t*, 1034*t*
furosemide, 551–52
adverse effects, 551–52, 551*t*, 612*t*
classification, 551
contraindications/precautions, 552
drug interactions, 74, 552
mechanism of action, 551
nursing responsibilities, 552
overdose treatment, 552
patient and family education, 552
pharmacokinetics, 551
pregnancy category, 552
route and adult dose, 551*t*, 612*t*
similar drugs, 553
for specific conditions
heart failure, 612*t*
therapeutic effects and uses, 551
Furoxone. *See* furazolidone

Fusilev. *See* levoleucovorin
FUSION INHIBITORS:
  enfuvirtide, 933*t*, 940
Fuzeon. *See* enfuvirtide

G

G6PD (glucose-6-phosphate dehydrogenase) deficiency, 62*t*
GABA. *See* gamma aminobutyric acid
gabapentin, 389
  adverse effects, 381*t*, 389
  classification, 389
  contraindications/precautions, 389
  drug interactions, 389
  mechanism of action, 389
  nursing responsibilities, 389
  overdose, 389
  patient and family education, 389
  pharmacokinetics, 389
  pregnancy category, 389
  route and adult dose, 381*t*
  therapeutic effects and uses, 389
Gabitril. *See* tiagabine
GAD. *See* generalized anxiety disorder
galactagogues, herbal remedies as, 129*t*
galantamine hydrobromide, 202*t*, 355*t*, 362
gamma aminobutyric acid (GABA), 266–67
  antiseizure drugs and, 377–79, 378*f*, 379*f*
  benzodiazepines and, 283
  clinical applications, 267*t*
  effects, 267*t*
  locations, 189*t*
gamma hydroxybutyrate (GHB), 98. *See also* sodium oxybate
Gammagard. *See* intravenous immune globulin
ganciclovir, 912*t*, 914
ganglia, 188
GANGLIONIC BLOCKERS, 214, 218, 219*t*
  mecamylamine. *See* mecamylamine
ganirelix, 1192*t*, 1195
Gantrisin. *See* sulfisoxazole
Garamycin. *See* gentamicin
Gardasil. *See* human papillomavirus, immunization
garlic:
  description, 654*t*
  drug interactions, 178*t*
  evidence, 654*t*
  history and claims, 654*t*
  primary uses, 173*t*
  standardization, 654*t*
gas exchange, 1239, 1239*f*
GA-Sarin, 1362*t*
GA-Soman, 1362*t*
gastric ulcers, 1009. *See also* peptic ulcer
gastroesophageal reflux disease (GERD), 1010
  complications, 1010
  etiology, 1010
  incidence, 1010*t*
  nonpharmacologic management, 1010
  pathogenesis, 1010, 1011*f*
  in pediatric patients, 1023*t*
  pharmacotherapy, 1011*f*
    bismuth subsalicylate, 1024
    H_2-receptor antagonists. *See* H_2-RECEPTOR ANTAGONISTS
    metoclopramide, 1024
    proton pump inhibitors. *See* PROTON PUMP INHIBITORS (PPIs)
  symptoms, 1010, 1011*f*
gastrointestinal anthrax, 1360*t*
gastrointestinal tract:
  age-related changes, 148, 149*t*
  anatomy, 999, 999*f*
  digestive process. *See* digestion
  drug absorption in, 44, 44*f*, 1000–1001, 1002*f*
  drug excretion in, 49
  ginger's effect on, 1013*t*
  lower, 1001, 1002*f*
  stomach size, 1000*f*
  upper, 1000–1001, 1007, 1008*f*
Gastrosed. *See* hyoscyamine
gastrostomy tube, drug administration via, 31
GA-Tabun, 1362*t*
gate control theory, 430
gatifloxacin, 26*t*, 827*t*, 830
Gaviscon, 1021*t*
gefitinib, 990*t*
gemcitabine, 973*t*, 975
gemfibrozil, 509–10
  adverse effects, 504*t*, 509
  classification, 509
  contraindications/precautions, 510
  drug interactions, 510
  mechanism of action, 509
  nursing responsibilities, 510
  overdose treatment, 510
  patient and family education, 510
  pharmacokinetics, 509
  pregnancy category, 510
  route and adult dose, 504*t*
  similar drugs, 510
  therapeutic effects and uses, 509
gemifloxacin, 827*t*, 830
gemtuzumab, 748*t*, 990*t*
Gemzar. *See* gemcitabine
Genabid. *See* papaverine-phentolamine
gender differences:
  in disease patterns, 160
  in drug response, 160
general anesthesia, 458
  Alzheimer's disease risk following exposure to, 469*t*
  inhalation agents. *See* INHALATION GENERAL ANESTHETIC AGENTS
  intravenous agents. *See* INTRAVENOUS ANESTHETIC AGENTS
  Nursing Process Application, 470*t*
  process, 458–59
  purposes, 458
  stages, 458*t*
generalized anxiety disorder (GAD):
  characteristics, 275
  pharmacotherapy, 283*t*, 289, 290*t*
generalized seizures, 372*f*, 374, 376*t*
generic drugs:
  bioavailability, 8
  versus brand-name drugs, 8
  examples, 7*t*
generic name, 7
genetic polymorphisms, 159–60, 160*t*
Gengraf. *See* cyclosporine
Genotropin. *See* somatropin
gentamicin, 817–18
  adverse effects, 818
    in pediatric patients, 142*t*
  classification, 817
  contraindications/precautions, 818
  drug interactions, 818
  mechanism of action, 817
  nursing responsibilities, 818
  overdose treatment, 818
  patient and family education, 818
  pediatric dosage/route, 142*t*
  pharmacokinetics, 817
  pharmacokinetics in older adults, 148–49
  pregnancy category, 818
  similar drugs, 818–19
  therapeutic effects and uses, 817
Gentran 40. *See* dextran 40
Geocillin. *See* carbenicillin
Geodon. *See* ziprasidone
GERD. *See* gastroesophageal reflux disease
geriatric patients. *See* older adults
German measles. *See* rubella
Germanin. *See* suramin
gestational diabetes, 1121, 1122*t*
gestational epilepsy, 373
GFR (glomerular filtration rate), 547
GH. *See* growth hormone
GH antagonists. *See* growth hormone (GH) antagonists
GHB (gamma hydroxybutyrate), 98. *See also* sodium oxybate
GHIH (growth hormone–inhibiting hormone), 1105*t*
GHRH (growth hormone–releasing hormone), 1105*t*
Giardia lamblia, 886*t*
giardiasis, 886*t*, 892–93, 892*t*, 893*t*
gigantism, 1111
ginger:
  description, 1013*t*
  drug interactions, 177, 178*t*
  evidence, 1013*t*
  history and claims, 1013*t*
  primary uses, 173*t*
  standardization, 175*t*, 1013*t*
ginkgo:
  for dementia, 360*t*
  drug interactions, 75, 177, 178*t*
  primary uses, 173*t*
  standardization, 174, 175*f*, 175*t*
Ginkgo biloba. *See* ginkgo
ginseng:
  description, 590*t*
  evidence, 590*t*
  history and claims, 590*t*
  primary uses, 173*t*
  standardization, 175*t*, 590*t*
glatiramer, 365, 366*t*
glaucoma, 1338
  corticosteroid-induced, 1349*t*
  incidence, 1338, 1338*t*
  pathophysiology, 1338–40, 1339*f*
  pharmacotherapy
    $alpha_2$-adrenergic agonists, 1343
      apraclonidine, 1341*t*, 1343
      brimonidine, 1341*t*, 1343
    beta-adrenergic blockers, 1343
      betaxolol, 252*t*, 257, 1341*t*, 1343, 1345
      carteolol, 252*t*, 254, 1341*t*, 1343, 1345
      levobunolol, 1341*t*, 1343, 1345
      metipranolol, 252*t*, 255, 1341*t*, 1343, 1345
      timolol. *See* timolol
    carbonic anhydrase inhibitors, 1345
      acetazolamide. *See* acetazolamide
      brinzolamide, 1341*t*, 1345
      dorzolamide, 1341*t*, 1345
      methazolamide, 559*t*, 560, 1341*t*

cholinergic agonists
carbachol, 202*t*, 204, 1341*t*
echothiophate, 204, 1341*t*, 1344
pilocarpine, 202*t*, 204, 1341*t*, 1343
isosorbide, 1341*t*
Nursing Process Application, 1346*t*
osmotic diuretics, 1345
isosorbide, 1341*t*
mannitol, 1341*t*. *See also* mannitol
principles, 1340
prostaglandin analogs, 1342
bimatoprost, 1341*t*, 1343
latanoprost. *See* latanoprost
travoprost, 1341*t*, 1343
sympathomimetics, 1344
dipivefrin, 1341*t*, 1344
Gleevec. *See* imatinib
Gliadel. *See* carmustine
glimepiride, 1133*t*, 1135
glioma, 950*t*
glipizide, 1133*t*, 1135
glomerular filtration rate (GFR), 547
glomerulus, 545, 547*f*
GlucaGen. *See* glucagon
glucagon, 1124–25
adverse effects, 1125
classification, 1124
contraindications/precautions, 1125
drug interactions, 1125
mechanism of action, 1125
nursing responsibilities, 1125
overdose treatment, 1125
patient and family education, 1125
pharmacokinetics, 1125
pregnancy category, 1125
therapeutic effects and uses, 1124–25, 1364*t*
glucocorticoids, 1102*t*, 1161*f*, 1162. *See also* CORTICOSTEROIDS
gluconeogenesis, 1120
Glucophage. *See* metformin
Glucophage XR. *See* metformin
glucosamine:
description, 1302*t*
evidence, 1302*t*
history and claims, 1302*t*
primary uses, 179*t*
glucose-6-phosphate dehydrogenase (G6PD) deficiency, 62*t*
Glucotrol. *See* glipizide
Glucotrol XL, 30*t*. *See also* glyburide
Glucovance, 1134*t*
Glumetza. *See* metformin
glutamate:
actions/effects, 267, 267*t*
in Alzheimer's disease, 360
locations, 189*t*
glutamic acid. *See* glutamate
glutethimide, 286
glyburide, 1134–35
adverse effects, 1133*t*, 1134
classification, 1134
contraindications/precautions, 1134
dosage forms not to be crushed or opened, 30*t*
drug interactions, 1134
mechanism of action, 1134
overdose treatment, 1134
pharmacokinetics, 1134
pregnancy category, 1134
route and adult dose, 1133*t*
similar drugs, 1135
therapeutic effects and uses, 1134
glycerin, 559*t*, 560
glycogenolysis, 1120
glycoprotein IIb/IIIa, 600, 655
glycoprotein IIb/IIIa receptor inhibitors. *See* antiplatelet agents
glycopyrrolate, 214*t*, 217
Glynase. *See* glyburide
Glyset. *See* miglitol
GnRH (gonadotropin-releasing hormone), 1105*t*
GnRH analogs/agonists. *See* GONADOTROPIN-RELEASING HORMONE (GNRH) ANALOGS/AGONISTS
GnRH antagonists. *See* GONADOTROPIN-RELEASING HORMONE (GNRH) ANTAGONISTS
goal (outcome), 117
goat's rue, 129*t*
goiter, 1148
goldenseal:
description, 717*t*
drug interactions, 178*t*
evidence, 717*t*
history and claims, 717*t*
standardization, 717*t*
gonadocorticoids, 1161*f*, 1162. *See also* ANDROGEN(S); ESTROGEN(S)
gonadotropic hormone cycle, 1178*f*
gonadotropin-releasing hormone (GnRH), 1105*t*
GONADOTROPIN-RELEASING HORMONE (GNRH) ANALOGS/AGONISTS, 983, 1192*t*
goserelin, 980*t*, 983
histrelin, 980*t*, 983
leuprolide, 980*t*, 983, 1192*t*, 1221
triptorelin, 980*t*, 983
GONADOTROPIN-RELEASING HORMONE (GNRH) ANTAGONISTS, 1191
cetrorelix, 1192*t*, 1195
ganirelix, 1192*t*, 1195
Gonal-F. *See* follitropin alfa
gonioscopy, 1340
Gordochom. *See* undecylenic acid
goserelin, 980*t*, 983, 1192*t*, 1195–96
gout:
diagnosis, 1307
incidence, 1306
pathophysiology, 1301*f*, 1306–7
pharmacotherapy, 1307
allopurinol. *See* allopurinol
colchicine. *See* colchicine
corticosteroids, 1307
nonsteroidal anti-inflammatory drugs, 1307
Nursing Process Application, 1311*t*
probenecid, 1307*t*, 1309, 1310
sulfinpyrazone, 1307*t*, 1309, 1310
grading, cancer, 953–54, 954*t*
gram negative, 776
gram positive, 776
granisetron, 1043*t*
grape seed extract:
description, 569*t*
evidence, 569*t*
history and claims, 569*t*
primary uses, 173*t*
standardization, 569*t*
grapefruit juice, drug interactions with, 74
Graves' disease, 1152. *See also* hyperthyroidism
gray baby syndrome, 821
green tea:
drug interactions, 178*t*
primary uses, 173*t*
Grifulvin V. *See* griseofulvin
griseofulvin:
drug interactions, 101*t*
mechanism of action, 871*f*
for superficial mycoses, 877, 878*t*, 880–81
Gris-PEG. *See* griseofulvin
growth fraction, 955
growth hormone (GH), 1106
deficiency, 1107, 1107*t*
pharmacotherapy
mecasermin, 1108*t*, 1110–11
somatropin. *See* somatropin
Evidence-Based Practice, 1107*t*, 1110*t*
factors affecting release, 1107*t*
Nursing Process Application, 1113*t*
overproduction, 1111
pharmacotherapy
bromocriptine, 1108*t*, 1112
lanreotide, 1108*t*, 1112
octreotide. *See* octreotide
pegvisomant, 1108*t*, 1112
as performance-enhancing drug, 1099*t*, 1108, 1109*t*
regulation, 1102*t*, 1106–7
target organs and action, 1102*t*, 1106
growth hormone (GH) antagonists, 1111
bromocriptine. *See* bromocriptine
lanreotide, 1108*t*, 1112
octreotide. *See* octreotide
pegvisomant, 1108*t*, 1112
growth hormone–inhibiting hormone (GHIH), 1105*t*
growth hormone–releasing hormone (GHRH), 1105*t*
guaifenesin, 1276*t*, 1277
guanadrel, 579
guanethidine, 579
guttate psoriasis, 1329*t*
Gynazole. *See* butoconazole
Gyne-Lotrimin. *See* clotrimazole

H

H+, K+ -ATPase, 1007
H_1-receptor(s), 1265
H_1-RECEPTOR ANTAGONISTS:
adverse effects, 1265–66
first-generation
azelastine, 1265*t*, 1266
brompheniramine, 1265*t*
cetirizine, 1265*t*, 1268
chlorpheniramine, 1265*t*
clemastine, 1265*t*
cyproheptadine, 1265*t*
dexbrompheniramine, 1265*t*
dexchlorpheniramine, 1265*t*
diphenhydramine. *See* diphenhydramine
promethazine. *See* promethazine
triprolidine, 1265*t*
Nursing Process Application, 1269*t*
in older adults, 152*t*, 1267*t*
over-the-counter combinations, 1266*t*
in pediatric patient, 1267*t*
second-generation
desloratadine, 1265*t*, 1268
fexofenadine. *See* fexofenadine
levocetirizine, 1265*t*

loratadine, 1265*t*, 1268
olopatadine, 1265*t*, 1349*t*
for specific conditions
allergic rhinitis, 1264–65
anaphylaxis, 1266
insomnia, 280–81, 1266
Parkinson's disease, 1266
urticaria, 1266
vertigo and motion sickness, 1266
H_2-RECEPTOR ANTAGONISTS, 1016
drugs in class
cimetidine, 45, 152*t*, 1016*t*, 1019
famotidine, 477, 1016*t*, 1019
nizatidine, 1016*t*, 1019
ranitidine. *See* ranitidine
mechanism of action, 1012*f*, 1016
Nursing Process Application, 1020*t*
pharmacokinetics, 1016, 1018
as preoperative medication, 477
HAART (highly active antiretroviral therapy), 932. *See also* ANTIRETROVIRALS
Habitrol. *See* nicotine replacement therapy
Haemophilus influenzae, 777*t*, 833
hair follicles, 1316
halazepam, 283
halcinonide, 1327*t*
Halcion. *See* triazolam
Haldol. *See* haloperidol
Hale's lactation risk categories, 130*t*
half-life. *See* plasma half-life ($t_{1/2}$)
hallucinations, 326, 327*t*
hallucinogens, 103
dimethyltryptamine, 104–5
LSD, 103–4, 104*f*
mescaline, 104, 105*f*
psilocybin, 104, 104*f*
withdrawal symptoms and treatment, 96*t*
Halog. *See* halcinonide
haloperidol, 335–36
adverse effects, 332*t*, 335
in breast-feeding infant, 129*t*
classification, 335
contraindications/precautions, 335
distribution in older adults, 148–49
drug interactions, 335–36
genetic polymorphisms and actions of, 160*t*
mechanism of action, 335
nursing responsibilities, 336
overdose treatment, 336
pharmacokinetics, 335
pregnancy category, 336
route and adult dose, 332*t*
similar drugs, 336
for specific conditions
alcohol withdrawal, 102
therapeutic effects and uses, 335
Halotestin. *See* fluoxymesterone
halothane, 101*t*, 467
Harrison Narcotic Act, 14
hash oil, 102
Hashimoto's thyroiditis, 1149
hashish, 102
Havrix. *See* hepatitis A vaccine
hawthorn, 540*t*
HBIG. *See* hepatitis B immunoglobulin
HCG. *See* human chorionic gonadotropin
HCTZ. *See* hydrochlorothiazide
HDL (high-density lipoprotein), 496, 498*f*, 499*t*
headache, 449, 449*t*. *See also* migraine
Health Canada, 20
health care associated infections. *See* nosocomial infections
health care insurance, ethnic differences in coverage, 159*t*
heart:
coronary arteries, 487, 488*f*. *See also* coronary artery disease
functions, 486–87, 487*t*
structure, 488*f*
heart failure (HF), 607
classification
ACC/AHA stages, 610*t*
NYHA functional classes, 610
drugs that worsen, 609*t*
etiology, 607
in minority populations, 607*t*
nonpharmacologic therapy, 607, 607*t*
pathophysiology, 607–8, 608*f*
natriuretic peptides and neurohumoral factors, 609
plasma volume and preload, 608–9
sympathetic nervous system activation, 608
ventricular hypertrophy, 608
pharmacotherapy, 612*t*
ACE inhibitors, 533, 610–11, 611*f*, 612*t*
beta-adrenergic agonists, 612*t*, 618
beta-adrenergic antagonists, 612*t*, 613–14
cardiac glycosides, 612*t*, 614–16
diuretics, 612*t*, 613
mechanism of action, 611*f*
nesiritide, 619
phosphodiesterase III inhibitors, 612*t*, 618–19
vasodilators, 614
symptoms, 609
in women, 609*t*
heart rate, 490
Hectorol. *See* doxercalciferol
Helicobacter pylori:
in peptic ulcer disease, 1008, 1023
pharmacotherapy, 1023, 1024
helminthic infections:
ascariasis, 899–900
enterobiasis, 900–901
hookworms, 901
pharmacotherapy
albendazole, 902*t*, 903
ivermectin, 902*t*, 903
mebendazole. *See* mebendazole
Nursing Process Application, 904*t*
praziquantel, 902*t*, 903
principles, 901
pyrantel, 902*t*, 903
thiabendazole, 902*t*, 903
tapeworms, 901
helminths, 898
helper (CD4) T cells, 713
Hemabate. *See* carboprost
hemagglutinin, 915
HEMATOPOIETIC GROWTH FACTORS:
with cancer chemotherapy, 993
colony-stimulating factors
filgrastim. *See* filgrastim
mechanism of action, 671–72
pegfilgrastim, 670*t*, 674
sargramostim, 670*t*, 674
erythropoietin
darbepoetin alfa, 670*t*, 671
epoetin alfa. *See* epoetin alfa
Nursing Process Application, 672*t*
mechanism of action, 668–69
platelet enhancer
oprelvekin. *See* oprelvekin
hemoglobin A1C, 1123, 1123*t*
hemophilia, 644
hemophilia A, 662–63
hemophilia B, 663
hemophilia C, 663
hemopoiesis, 484, 668, 669*f*
hemosiderin, 677
hemostasis:
disorders
coagulation, 643–44
thromboembolic, 642–43
normal, 485–86, 485*f*, 642
HEMOSTATIC AGENTS:
adverse effects, 661
aminocaproic acid. *See* aminocaproic acid
desmopressin. *See* desmopressin
mechanism of action, 644*t*, 660–61
thrombin, topical, 661*t*, 662
tranexamic acid, 661*t*, 662
hemothorax, during parenteral nutrition therapy, 1079*t*
heparin, 646–47
adverse effects, 645*t*, 646
classification, 646
contraindications/precautions, 646
drug interactions, 178*t*
mechanism of action, 644–45, 646
monitoring of therapy, 645
nursing responsibilities, 647
overdose treatment, 647
patient and family education, 647
pharmacokinetics, 646
pregnancy category, 647
route and adult dose, 645*t*
similar drugs, 647–48
therapeutic effects and uses, 646
hepatic microsomal enzyme system, 46–48, 47*t*
hepatic portal system, 1003, 1003*f*
hepatitis, 917–18, 918*t*
pharmacotherapy
antivirals
adefovir dipivoxil, 919*t*, 922
entecavir, 26*t*, 919*t*, 922
lamivudine. *See* lamivudine
ribavirin, 919*t*, 922
telbivudine, 919*t*, 922
interferons, 921
interferon alfa-2b. *See* interferon alfa-2b
interferon alfacon-1, 919*t*, 922
interferon alfa-n1, 919*t*, 922
peginterferon alfa-2a, 919*t*, 922
peginterferon alfa-2b, 919*t*
hepatitis A, 909*t*
immunization, 758*t*, 762
incidence, 758*t*
pathophysiology, 762
prevention, 918*t*, 919
risk factors, 918*t*
symptoms, 918–19
transmission, 918, 918*t*
treatment, 918*t*
hepatitis A immunoglobulin (HAIg), 919
hepatitis A vaccine, 919
hepatitis B, 909*t*
immunization, 758*t*, 761, 920. *See also* hepatitis B vaccine
incidence, 758*t*, 918*t*

pathophysiology, 761
pharmacotherapy, 918*t*, 920. *See also* hepatitis, pharmacotherapy
risk factors, 918*t*
symptoms, 920
transmission, 918*t*, 919–20
hepatitis B immunoglobulin (HBIG), 767*t*, 769, 920
hepatitis B vaccine, 761–62
adverse effects, 762
classification, 761
contraindications/precautions, 762
drug interactions, 762
mechanism of action, 761
nursing responsibilities, 762
overdose treatment, 762
patient and family education, 762
pharmacokinetics, 761
pregnancy category, 762
therapeutic effects and uses, 761, 920
hepatitis C:
pharmacotherapy, 918*t*, 921. *See also* hepatitis, pharmacotherapy
prevention, 918*t*
risk factors, 918*t*
symptoms, 920
transmission, 918*t*, 920
hepatotoxicity, 69*t*, 70
Hep-Loc. *See* heparin
Heplock. *See* heparin
Hepsera. *See* adefovir dipivoxil
herb, 172
herbal products/therapy:
best-selling, 173*t*
drug interactions with, 74–75, 75*t*, 177–79, 178*t*
history, 172–74
liquid formulations, 175*t*
in older adults, 177*t*
in pediatric patients, 143*t*
regulation, 175–77
standardization of products, 174–75, 175*t*
Herceptin. *See* trastuzumab
heroin, effects in pregnancy, 126*t*
herpes simplex virus infections:
genital, 911*t*
in HIV-AIDS, 945*t*
ocular, 912
pharmacotherapy
acute infections, 911–12
prophylaxis, 912
systemic agents
acyclovir. *See* acyclovir
cidofovir, 912*t*, 914
famciclovir, 912*t*, 914
foscarnet, 912*t*, 914
ganciclovir, 912*t*, 914
idoxuridine, 912
valacyclovir, 912*t*, 914–15
valganciclovir, 912*t*, 915
topical agents
docosanol, 912*t*, 914
penciclovir, 912*t*, 914
trifluridine, 912, 912*t*, 914
in pregnancy, 912
prophylaxis, 912
herpesviruses, 909*t*
cytomegalovirus, 911
Epstein-Barr virus, 911
herpes simplex viruses. *See* herpes simplex virus infections
herpes zoster. *See* varicella zoster
herpesvirus-type 6, 911
hetastarch, 694
Hexalen. *See* altretamine
HF. *See* heart failure
HHS (hyperosmolar hyperglycemic state), 1124
high-alert medications, 86*t*
high-density lipoprotein (HDL), 496, 498*f*, 499*t*
highly active antiretroviral therapy (HAART), 932. *See also* ANTIRETROVIRALS
hippurate. *See* methenamine hippurate
Hiprex. *See* methenamine hippurate
Hispanic American culture, depression treatment in, 300*t*
histamine, 711–12, 712*t*, 1264
histamine (H_1) receptor antagonists. *See* H_1-RECEPTOR ANTAGONISTS
histamine (H_2) receptor antagonists. *See* H_2-RECEPTOR ANTAGONISTS
Histerone. *See* testosterone
Histoplasma capsulatum, 869*t*
histoplasmosis, 869*t*, 945*t*
histrelin, 980*t*, 983
HIV-AIDS:
in children, 944*t*
incidence, 927*t*
opportunistic infections in
M. avium, 865
pathophysiology, 944–45
pharmacotherapy, 945*t*
tuberculosis, 856
pathogenesis
replication cycle, 927–28, 928*f*
transmission, 927
perinatal transmission, 943–44
pharmacotherapy. *See also* antiretrovirals
improving patient adherence, 931*t*
initiation of therapy, 929
monitoring of progress, 929–30, 930*f*
Nursing Process Application, 941–42*t*
sexual lifestyle adjustments, 931
structured treatment interruptions, 931
therapeutic goals, 929
treatment failures, 930–31
postexposure prophylaxis, 943
symptoms, 928
HKD (hyperkinetic disorder), 413. *See also* attention deficit/hyperactivity disorder
HMG-CoA reductase, 501
holistic, 147
homatropine, 214*t*, 1348*t*
home care nurse, 164, 164*f*
hookworms, 901
HORMONE(S). *See also specific hormones*
endocrine system secretion, 1099, 1100*t*
negative feedback mechanism, 1099–1101, 1101*f*
regulation, 1099, 1102*t*
target organs and actions, 1102*t*
pharmacotherapy with, 1101, 1103
adverse effects, 68*t*
for neoplasia, 979–81, 1101
dexamethasone, 980*t*
diethylstilbestrol, 980*t*
ethinyl estradiol, 980*t*
fluoxymesterone, 980*t*
medroxyprogesterone, 980*t*
megestrol, 980*t*
prednisone, 980*t*
testolactone, 980*t*, 1286
testosterone. *See* testosterone
replacement therapy. *See* hormone replacement therapy
HORMONE ANTAGONISTS:
adverse effects, 68*t*
for neoplasia, 979–81
anastrozole, 980*t*, 983
bicalutamide, 980*t*, 984
exemestane, 980*t*, 983
flutamide, 980*t*, 984
fulvestrant, 980*t*, 982
goserelin, 980*t*, 983
histrelin, 980*t*, 983
letrozole, 980*t*, 983
leuprolide, 980*t*, 984
nilutamide, 980*t*, 984
raloxifene. *See* raloxifene
tamoxifen. *See* tamoxifen
toremifene, 980*t*, 983
triptorelin, 980*t*, 984
hormone receptors, 1099
hormone replacement therapy (HRT), 1101
adverse effects, 1186
for menopause symptoms, 1184
Nursing Process Application, 1182*t*
horny goat weed, 173*t*
horse chestnut, 173*t*
hospice nursing, 165
host flora, 782
household system of measurement, 28, 28*t*
HPV. *See* human papillomavirus
HRT. *See* hormone replacement therapy
HTN. *See* hypertension
HTN-E. *See* hypertensive emergency
Humalog. *See* insulin lispro
Humalog Mix, 1130*t*
human chorionic gonadotropin (HCG):
for female infertility, 1192*t*, 1195
for male infertility, 1226
human immunodeficiency virus (HIV), 927. *See also* HIV-AIDS
perinatal transmission, 943–44
postexposure prophylaxis, 943
replication cycle, 927–28, 928*f*
vaccine development, 942
human integration model, 157, 157*f*
human menopausal gonadotropin, 1191
human papillomavirus (HPV):
immunization, 766
incidence, 766*t*
pathophysiology, 765–66
risk reduction, 911*t*
human regular insulin, 1127*t*, 1128–29
adverse effects, 1128–29
classification, 1128
contraindications/precautions, 1129
drug interactions, 1129
mechanism of action, 1128
nursing responsibilities, 1129
overdose treatment, 1129
patient and family education, 1129
pharmacokinetics, 1128
pregnancy category, 1129
similar drugs, 1129–30
therapeutic effects and uses, 1128
Humatin. *See* paromomycin
Humatrope. *See* somatropin

Humegon. *See* menotropins
Humira. *See* adalimumab
Humulin 50/50, 1130*t*
Humulin 70/30, 1130*t*
Humulin N. *See* isophane insulin
Humulin R. *See* human regular insulin
Huntington's disease, 347*t*
Hyalgan. *See* sodium hyaluronate
Hycamtin. *See* topotecan
Hycodan. *See* hydrocodone
Hycomine Compound, 1276*t*
Hycort. *See* hydrocortisone
Hycotuss Expectorant, 1276*t*
HYDANTOINS, 384
  phenytoin. *See* phenytoin
Hydeltrasol. *See* prednisolone
hydralazine, 579–80
  adverse effects, 580
  classification, 579
  contraindications/precautions, 580
  drug interactions, 580
  genetic polymorphisms and actions of, 160*t*
  mechanism of action, 579
  nursing responsibilities, 580
  patient and family education, 580
  pharmacokinetics, 580
  pregnancy category, 580
  similar drugs, 580–81
  for specific conditions
    heart failure, 614
    hypertensive emergency, 584*t*
  therapeutic effects and uses, 579
Hydrastis canadensis, 178*t*
Hydrea. *See* hydroxyurea
hydrochloric acid, 704
hydrochlorothiazide, 553–55
  adverse effects, 554, 554*t,* 612*t*
  classification, 553
  contraindications/precautions, 554
  drug interactions, 554–55
  mechanism of action, 554
  nursing responsibilities, 555
  overdose treatment, 555
  patient and family education, 555
  pharmacokinetics, 554
  pregnancy category, 555
  route and adult dose, 554*t,* 612*t*
  similar drugs, 555
  for specific conditions
    heart failure, 612*t*
  therapeutic effects and uses, 553–54
hydrocodone, 436*t,* 439, 1275, 1276*t*
hydrocortisone, 1166–68
  adverse effects, 1167, 1167*t*
  classification, 1166
  contraindications/precautions, 1167
  mechanism of action, 1167
  nursing considerations, 1168
  overdose treatment, 1168
  patient and family education, 1168
  pharmacokinetics, 1167
  pregnancy category, 1168
  route and adult dose, 1167*t*
  similar drugs, 1168
  for specific conditions
    adrenocortical insufficiency, 1165
    dermatitis, 1327*t*
  therapeutic effects and uses, 1166
hydrocortisone acetate, 1328
hydrocortisone valerate, 1327*t*
Hydrocortone. *See* hydrocortisone
HydroDIURIL. *See* hydrochlorothiazide
hydrogen cyanide, 1362*t*
hydromorphone, 436*t,* 439
hydrotherapy, for muscle spasms, 397
hydrothorax, during parenteral nutrition therapy, 1079*t*
hydroxychloroquine, 1304–5
  adverse effects, 888*t,* 1305
  classification, 1304
  contraindications/precautions, 1305
  drug interactions, 1305
  mechanism of action, 1305
  nursing responsibilities, 1305
  overdose treatment, 1305
  patient and family education, 1305
  pharmacokinetics, 1305
  pregnancy category, 1305
  route and adult dose, 888*t*
  similar drugs, 1305–6
  for specific conditions
    malaria, 888*t,* 890
  therapeutic effects and uses, 1304–5
hydroxyurea, 992, 992*t,* 1330*t,* 1331
hydroxyzine, 287, 1043*t*
Hygroton. *See* chlorthalidone
Hylorel. *See* guanadrel
Hyoscine. *See* scopolamine
hyoscyamine, 214*t,* 217, 1037*t,* 1040
Hyperab. *See* rabies immune globulin
hyperaldosteronism, 1170
hypercalcemia, 694*t*
hyperchloremia, 694*t*
hypercholesterolemia, 498, 500*t,* 508*t. See also* dyslipidemias
hyperemesis gravidarum, 1041
hyperglycemia. *See also* diabetes mellitus
  during enteral nutrition therapy, 1072*t*
  during parenteral nutrition therapy, 1079
Hypericum perforatum. See St. John's wort
hyperkalemia, 694*t*
  during enteral nutrition therapy, 1072*t*
  etiology, 697
  pharmacotherapy
    polystyrene sulfate, 697
  in renal failure, 548*t*
  supportive treatment, 694*t,* 697
hyperkinetic disorder (HKD), 413. *See also* attention deficit/hyperactivity disorder
hyperlipidemia, 498, 500*t. See also* dyslipidemias
hypermagnesemia, 694*t,* 699
hypernatremia, 694*t*
  exercise-associated, 688*t*
  pathophysiology, 695–96
  supportive treatment, 694*t,* 695
hyperosmolar hyperglycemic state (HHS), 1124
hyperphosphatemia, 694*t*
  during enteral nutrition therapy, 1072*t*
  in renal failure, 548*t*
  supportive treatment, 694*t*
Hyperstat IV. *See* diazoxide
hypertension (HTN), 567
  in African Americans, 567*t,* 573
  body weight and, 533*t*
  cardiovascular effects, 569
  in children, 522*t*
  classification, 567, 567*t*
  consequences, 568–69
  etiology, 568
  nonpharmacologic management, 569–70
    lifestyle modifications, 248*t*
    sodium restrictions, 249*t*
  pharmacotherapy, 574*t*
    ACE inhibitors, 575
    $alpha_2$-adrenergic agonists, 577
    alpha-adrenergic antagonists, 246, 576
    angiotensin II receptor blockers, 575
    beta-adrenergic antagonists, 251, 576
    calcium channel blockers, 575
    choice of medication, 570*t*
    combination medications, 571, 572*t*
    direct-acting vasodilators, 579
    loop diuretics, 573
    mechanism of action, 571*f*
    patient adherence, 572–73
    potassium-sparing diuretics, 573
    thiazide diuretics, 570, 573
  treatment recommendations, 567*t*
  white coat, 518*t*
hypertensive emergency (HTN-E), 581
  mortality from, 582*t*
  Nursing Process Application, 583*t*
  pharmacotherapy, 582, 584*t*
hypertensive urgency, 581
HyperTet. *See* tetanus immune globulin
HyperTet S/D. *See* tetanus immune globulin
hyperthyroidism:
  diagnosis, 1149*t*
  incidence, 1154
  pharmacotherapy, 1154–55
    methimazole, 1154*t,* 1156
    potassium iodide, 1156
    potassium iodide and iodine, 1154*t,* 1156
    propylthiouracil. *See* propylthiouracil
    radioactive iodide, 1154*t,* 1156
  signs and symptoms, 1149*t,* 1152, 1154
hypertrichosis, 581
hypertriglyceridemia, 498, 500*t. See also* dyslipidemias
hyperuricemia, 960, 1307. *See also* gout
hypervitaminosis, 1053
hypervolemia, in renal failure, 548*t*
hypnagogic hallucinations, 279, 420
hypoaldosteronism, 1170
hypocalcemia, 694*t*
  etiology, 1287
  pharmacotherapy
    calcium salts. *See* calcium salts
  in renal failure, 548*t*
  signs and symptoms, 1287
  supportive treatment, 694*t*
hypochloremia, 694*t*
hypoglycemia:
  in diabetes mellitus, 1123–24
  during enteral nutrition therapy, 1072*t*
  during parenteral nutrition therapy, 1079
hypogonadism, 1220–21
hypokalemia, 694*t*
  during enteral nutrition therapy, 1072*t*
  etiology, 697
  pharmacotherapy
    potassium chloride. *See* potassium chloride (KCl)
  supportive treatment, 694*t,* 697
hypomagnesemia, 694*t*
  during enteral nutrition therapy, 1072*t*
  etiology, 699

pharmacotherapy
magnesium sulfate. *See* magnesium sulfate ($MgSO_4$)
signs and symptoms, 699
supportive treatment, 694*t*
hypomania, 298, 318
hyponatremia, 694*t*
during enteral nutrition therapy, 1072*t*
etiology, 696
pharmacotherapy
sodium chloride. *See* sodium chloride (NaCl)
signs and symptoms, 696
supportive treatment, 694*t*
hypoparathyroidism, 1287
hypophosphatemia, 694*t*, 1072*t*
HYPOTHALAMIC AGENTS:
desmopressin. *See* desmopressin
vasopressin, 1108*t*, 1115–16
hypothalamus, 269
anatomy, 268*f*
functions, 276, 1105
hormones secreted by, 1105–6, 1105*t*
hypothyroidism:
congenital, 1148–49
diagnosis, 1149*t*
pathophysiology, 1149
pharmacotherapy
desiccated thyroid, 1151*t*, 1152
levothyroxine. *See* levothyroxine
liothyronine, 1151*t*, 1152
liotrix, 1151*t*, 1152
Nursing Process Application, 1153*t*
regimens, 1150
signs and symptoms, 1149–50, 1149*t*
Hyskon. *See* dextran 40
Hytakerol. *See* dihydrotachysterol
Hytrin. *See* terazosin
Hyzaar, 572*t*

I

^{131}I. *See* radioactive iodide
I-131. *See* radioactive iodide
ibandronate, 1294*t*, 1295*t*, 1297
IBD. *See* inflammatory bowel disease
ibritumomab, 748*t*, 990*t*
IBS. *See* irritable bowel syndrome
ibuprofen, 725–26
adverse effects, 724*t*, 726
in pediatric patients, 142*t*
classification, 725
contraindications/precautions, 726
cost, 723
drug interactions, 726
mechanism of action, 726
nursing responsibilities, 726
overdose treatment, 726
patient and family education, 726
pediatric dosage/route, 142*t*
pharmacokinetics, 726
pregnancy category, 726
route and adult dose, 724*t*
similar drugs, 727*t*
therapeutic effects and uses, 725–26, 725*t*
ibuprofen lysine, 726
IBUPROFEN-LIKE AGENTS:
versus aspirin, 725
costs, 723
diclofenac, 724*t*, 725*t*
diflunisal, 724*t*, 725*t*
etodolac, 724*t*, 725*t*
fenoprofen, 724*t*, 725*t*
flurbiprofen, 724*t*, 725*t*
ibuprofen. *See* ibuprofen
indomethacin, 724*t*, 725*t*
ketoprofen, 724*t*, 725*t*
ketorolac, 724*t*, 725*t*
meclofenamate, 724*t*, 725*t*
mefenamic acid, 724*t*, 725*t*
meloxicam, 724*t*, 725*t*
nabumetone, 724*t*, 725*t*
naproxen, 724*t*, 725*t*
oxaprozin, 724*t*, 725*t*
piroxicam, 724*t*, 725*t*
similarities among, 723
sulindac, 724*t*, 725*t*
tolmetin, 724*t*, 725*t*
ibutilide, 629*t*, 635–36
ICD (implantable cardioverter defibrillator), 627
Icy Hot, 1302
Idamycin. *See* idarubicin
idarubicin, 977*t*, 978
ideal drug, 5
idiosyncratic response, 62, 67–68
idoxuridine, 912
Ifex. *See* ifosfamide
IFNs. *See* INTERFERON(S) (IFNS)
ifosfamide, 967*t*, 971
IGF (insulin-like growth factor), 1106
illusions, 327*t*
ILs. *See* INTERLEUKIN(S) (ILS)
imatinib, 990*t*
imidazoles, 875. *See also* AZOLES
IMINOSTILBENES, 385
carbamazepine. *See* carbamazepine
oxcarbazepine. *See* oxcarbazepine
imipenem-cilastin, 800–801
adverse effects, 800*t*, 801
classification, 800
contraindications/precautions, 801
drug interactions, 801
mechanism of action, 801
nursing responsibilities, 801
overdose treatment, 801
patient and family education, 801
pharmacokinetics, 801
pregnancy category, 801
route and adult dose, 800*t*
similar drugs, 801–2
therapeutic effects and uses, 800–801
imipramine, 306–7
adverse effects, 304*t*, 306
in pediatric patients, 142*t*
classification, 306
contraindications/precautions, 306
dosage/routes
adult, 304*t*
pediatric, 142*t*
drug interactions, 306
genetic polymorphisms and actions of, 160*t*
mechanism of action, 306
nursing responsibilities, 306–7
overdose treatment, 306
patient and family education, 307
pharmacokinetics, 306
pregnancy category, 306
similar drugs, 307
for specific conditions
cataplexy, 420
therapeutic effects and uses, 306
Imitrex. *See* sumatriptan
immune globulins, 689*t*, 767*t*
cytomegalovirus, 767*t*, 769
hepatitis A, 919
hepatitis B, 767*t*, 769, 920
intravenous, 767*t*, 769
rabies, 767*t*
tetanus, 767*t*
immune response:
cell-mediated, 713–14
characteristics, 713
humoral, 713
immunity, 709
active, 755, 758, 760, 768*f*
passive, 755, 767, 768*f*
immunization, 755. *See also* vaccine(s)
immunoglobulin (Ig), 713. *See also* antibody(ies)
IMMUNOMODULATORS, 734
drugs in class
glatiramer, 365, 366*t*
mitoxantrone, 365, 366*t*
immunostimulants. *See* IMMUNOSTIMULANTS
immunosuppressants. *See* IMMUNOSUPPRESSANTS
Nursing Process Application, 750*t*
for specific conditions
asthma, 1244*t*
multiple sclerosis, 365–66, 366*t*
IMMUNOSTIMULANTS, 734
bacillus Calmette-Guérin vaccine, 735*t*, 739
colony-stimulating factors. *See* COLONY-STIMULATING FACTORS (CSFS)
interferons. *See* INTERFERON(S) (IFNS)
interleukins. *See* INTERLEUKIN(S) (ILS)
IMMUNOSUPPRESSANTS, 734
adverse effects, 68*t*
antibodies, 713, 714*f*, 747. *See also* MONOCLONAL ANTIBODIES (MABS)
basiliximab, 741*t*, 742*f*, 748*t*, 749
daclizumab, 741*t*, 742*f*, 748*t*, 749
lymphocyte immune globulin, 741*t*, 747, 749
muromonab-CD3. *See* muromonab-CD3
antimetabolites/cytotoxic agents
anakinra, 741*t*, 746, 1304*t*, 1305–6
azathioprine. *See* azathioprine
cyclophosphamide. *See* cyclophosphamide
etanercept. *See* etanercept
methotrexate. *See* methotrexate
mycophenolate, 741*t*, 746
sirolimus, 741*t*, 744
temsirolimus, 741*t*, 744
thalidomide, 14, 741*t*, 746–47, 991
calcineurin inhibitors, 740
cyclosporine. *See* cyclosporine
tacrolimus, 741*t*, 744, 1328, 1330*t*
corticosteroids, 750–51. *See also* CORTICOSTEROIDS
mechanism of action, 742*f*
in organ transplantation, 740
pet care during therapy with, 738*t*
for specific conditions
autoimmune disorders, 740
inflammatory bowel disease, 1037
Imodium. *See* loperamide
Imogam. *See* rabies immune globulin
implantable cardioverter defibrillator (ICD), 627

implementation, in nursing process, 118–19, 118*f*
impotence, 1226. *See also* erectile dysfunction
Imuran. *See* azathioprine
inactivated (killed) vaccines, 756, 756*t*
inamrinone, 612*t*, 619
Increlex. *See* mecasermin
INCRETIN ENHANCERS, 1141
  actions, 1132*t*
  nursing considerations, 1132*t*
  sitagliptin. *See* sitagliptin
INCRETIN MIMETICS, 1141
  exenatide, 1133*t*, 1142
incubation period, 755
IND (Investigational New Drug), 17
indapamide, 553, 554*t*, 555
Inderal. *See* propranolol
Inderal LA, 30*t*. *See also* propranolol
Inderide, 572*t*
indications, 5
indinavir, 178*t*, 933*t*, 939
indirect thrombin inhibitors. *See* ANTICOAGULANTS
Indocin. *See* indomethacin
Indocin SR, 30*t*. *See also* indomethacin
indomethacin, 30*t*, 724*t*, 725*t*
infantile spasm, 376, 376*t*
infants. *See* pediatric patients
Infasurf. *See* calfactant
Infergen. *See* interferon alfacon-1
infertility, 1191
  female. *See* female infertility
  male, 1225–26
infiltration anesthesia, 471, 471*f*
inflammation, 711, 717
  acute, 717
  chemical mediators, 711–12, 712*t*
  chronic, 717
  classification, 711
  nonpharmacologic management, 718
  pharmacotherapy
    mechanism of action, 915
    nonsteroidal anti-inflammatory drugs. *See* NONSTEROIDAL ANTI-INFLAMMATORY DRUGS (NSAIDS)
  purposes, 711
  steps, 712*f*
inflammatory bowel disease (IBD), 1035
  etiology, 1035
  pharmacotherapy, 1035–36
    balsalazide, 1037*t*, 1038–39
    biologic therapies, 1037
    corticosteroids, 1037, 1169
    maintenance, 1037
    mesalamine, 1037*t*, 1039
    olsalazine, 1037*t*, 1039
    sulfasalazine. *See* sulfasalazine
infliximab, 748*t*, 1037, 1304*t*, 1306
influenza, 915
  immunization, 758*t*, 763
  incidence, 758*t*, 915*t*
  pathophysiology, 763
  pharmacotherapy
    amantadine. *See* amantadine
    oseltamivir, 915, 916*t*, 917
    rimantadine, 915, 916*t*, 917
    zanamivir, 915, 916*t*, 917
  prophylaxis, 915
  vaccine, 915
influenza viruses, 915
ingestion, 999
INH. *See* isoniazid
inhalant abuse, 108, 126*t*
inhalation anthrax, 1360, 1360*t*
INHALATION GENERAL ANESTHETIC AGENTS, 465–66
  gas
    nitrous oxide. *See* nitrous oxide
  volatile liquids, 467
    desflurane, 468*t*, 469
    enflurane, 468*t*, 469
    isoflurane. *See* isoflurane
    sevoflurane, 468*t*, 469
inhalation route, drug administration, 1241–42
Innohep. *See* tinzaparin
InnoPran XL. *See* propranolol
Inocor. *See* inamrinone
inoculation, 755
inotropic agent, 239, 490
insecticide poisoning, 215*t*
insomnia, 279–80, 279*t*
  anxiety and, 280
  causes, 279*t*
  complementary and alternative therapies, 280–81, 280*t*
  pharmacotherapy. *See also specific drugs*
    antidepressants, 282*t*
    barbiturates, 282*t*, 291–92
    benzodiazepines, 282*t*, 283–85, 283*t*, 286
    H_1-receptor antagonists, 1266
    miscellaneous agents, 282*t*, 286–87
    nonbenzodiazepine anxiolytics, 282*t*, 286–88
    nonprescription drugs, 281
    Nursing Process, 293*t*
Inspra. *See* eplerenone
Institute for Safe Medication Practice (ISMP), 86
insulin:
  actions and effects, 1120
  adjunct, 1128
  adverse effects, 1127–28
  doses, 1127
  drug interactions, 178*t*
  Nursing Process Application, 1131*t*
  OptiClik injector pen, 1132*t*
  premixed combinations, 1130*t*
  principles of therapy, 1126, 1126*f*
  regulation, 1102*t*
  subcutaneous infusion, 1127, 1128*f*, 1131*t*
  target organs and action, 1102*t*
  types, 1127, 1127*t*
insulin aspart, 1127*t*, 1130
insulin detemir, 1127*t*, 1130
insulin glargine, 1127*t*, 1130
insulin glulisine, 1127*t*, 1130
insulin human inhaled, 1127*t*
insulin lispro, 1127*t*, 1130
insulin pumps, 1127, 1128*f*
insulin regular. *See* human regular insulin
insulin resistance, 1121. *See also* diabetes mellitus
insulin-like growth factor (IGF), 1106
Intal. *See* cromolyn
integrase, 927
INTEGRASE INHIBITORS:
  raltegravir, 933*t*, 940
Integrilin. *See* eptifibatide
Intelence. *See* etravirine
INTERFERON(S) (IFNs), 711*t*, 734, 760, 921, 990–91
  interferon alfa-2b. *See* interferon alfa-2b
  interferon alfacon-1, 735*t*, 736, 919*t*, 922
  interferon alfa-n1, 919*t*, 922
  interferon alfa-n3, 735*t*, 736–37
  interferon beta-1a, 365, 366*t*, 735*t*, 737
  interferon beta-1b, 365, 366*t*, 735*t*, 737
  interferon gamma-1b, 735*t*, 737
  peginterferon alfa-2a, 735*t*, 737, 919*t*, 922
  peginterferon alfa-2b, 919*t*
  pegylation, 734
interferon alfa-2b, 735–36
  adverse effects, 735*t*, 736, 990*t*
  classification, 735
  contraindications/precautions, 736
  drug interactions, 736
  mechanism of action, 735
  nursing responsibilities, 736
  overdose treatment, 736
  patient and family education, 736
  pharmacokinetics, 736
  pregnancy category, 736
  route and adult dose, 735*t*
  similar drugs, 737–38
  for specific conditions
    hepatitis, 919*t*
    Kaposi's sarcoma, 990*t*
    leukemia, 990*t*
  therapeutic effects and uses, 735
interferon alfacon-1, 735*t*, 736, 919*t*, 922
interferon alfa-n1, 919*t*, 922
interferon alfa-n3, 735*t*, 736–37
interferon beta-1a, 365, 366*t*, 735*t*, 737
interferon beta-1b, 365, 366*t*, 735*t*, 737
interferon gamma-1b, 735*t*, 737
INTERLEUKIN(S) (ILs), 737
  actions/effects, 737
  aldesleukin. *See* aldesleukin
  oprelvekin. *See* oprelvekin
interleukin-2. *See* aldesleukin
interleukin-11. *See* oprelvekin
intermittent feedings, 1069. *See also* enteral nutrition
intermittent infusion, 36
International Union of Pure and Applied Chemistry (IUPAC), 7
interpersonal therapy, for depression, 301, 302*t*
interventions, 116
intra-arterial administration, antineoplastic agents, 958
intracellular fluid (ICF) compartment, 687, 687*f*
intracellular parasites, 908
intradermal administration, 35, 35*f*
intramuscular route, drug administration, 35–36, 36*f*, 37*t*
intranasal administration, 33, 33*f*
INTRANASAL DECONGESTANTS, 236
  oxymetazoline, 238
  pseudoephedrine. *See* pseudoephedrine
  tetrahydrozoline, 238
  xylometazoline, 238
intraperitoneal administration, antineoplastic agents, 958
intrathecal administration:
  antineoplastic agents, 957–58
  baclofen, 402*t*
INTRAVENOUS ANESTHETIC AGENTS:
  barbiturates, 459, 460*t*
    methohexital, 460*t*, 461
    thiopental sodium. *See* thiopental sodium

benzodiazepines, 460*t*
diazepam, 460*t*, 464. *See also* diazepam
midazolam. *See* midazolam
miscellaneous, 460*t*
ketamine. *See* ketamine
propofol, 460*t*, 465
opioids, 460*t*
alfentanil, 460*t*, 462
fentanyl with droperidol, 460*t*. *See also* fentanyl
morphine sulfate, 460*t*. *See also* morphine sulfate
remifentanil, 460*t*, 462–63
sufentanil, 460*t*, 463
intravenous gamma globulin, 366
intravenous immune globulin (IVIG), 767*t*, 769
intravenous route, drug administration, 36–37, 37*f*, 957
intravesicular administration, antineoplastic agents, 958
intrinsic activity, 60
intrinsic factor, 680
intrinsic pathway, 486, 486*f*
intrinsic sympathomimetic activity (ISA), 5
Intron-A. *See* interferon alfa-2b
Intropin. *See* dopamine
Invanz. *See* ertapenem
invasiveness, 775
Invega. *See* paliperidone
Inversine. *See* mecamylamine
Investigational New Drug (IND), 17
Invirase. *See* saquinavir
iodine:
functions, 1063, 1063*t*
recommended dietary allowance, 1063*t*
requirement in pregnancy, 1148*t*
iodism, 1156
iodoquinol, 892, 892*t*, 894
Iodotope. *See* radioactive iodide
ion trapping, 701–2, 1365–66
ionization:
drug absorption and, 44–45, 44*f*
drug transfer across the placenta and, 124
Iopidine. *See* apraclonidine
Iosat. *See* potassium iodide
ipecac syrup, 1044
Iplex. *See* mecasermin rinfabate
ipratropium, 217–18, 1248–49
adverse effects, 1245*t*, 1249
classification, 1248
contraindications/precautions, 1249
drug interactions, 1249
mechanism of action, 1248
nursing responsibilities, 1249
overdose treatment, 1249
patient and family education, 1249
pharmacokinetics, 1249
pregnancy category, 1249
route and adult dose, 214*t*, 1245*t*
similar drugs, 1249
for specific conditions
allergic rhinitis, 1272
therapeutic effects and uses, 1248
Iprivask. *See* desirudin
irbesartan, 538*t*, 540
Iressa. *See* gefitinib
irinotecan, 135*t*, 985*t*, 987
iris, 1338
iron:
deficiency. *See* iron deficiency anemia
metabolism, 677, 677*f*
overdose in children, 678*t*
recommended dietary allowances, 668*t*
iron deficiency anemia:
assessment, 676
etiology, 677–78
pharmacotherapy
iron salts, 676*t*, 677–78, 679*t*
ferrous fumarate, 676*t*, 679
ferrous gluconate, 676*t*, 679
ferrous sulfate. *See* ferrous sulfate
iron dextran, 676*t*, 680
Nursing Process Application, 681*t*
iron dextran, 676*t*, 680
iron poisoning, 1364*t*
iron salts:
oral, 679–80, 679*t*
parenteral, 680
iron sucrose, 680
irritable bowel syndrome (IBS), 1039
incidence, 1039*t*
nonpharmacologic management, 1039
pharmacotherapy
alosetron, 1037*t*, 1040
antidepressants, 1039–40
antispasmodics, 1040
dicyclomine, 1037*t*, 1040
hyoscyamine, 1037*t*, 1040
lubiprostone, 1037*t*, 1040
serotonin agonists, 1040
symptom-targeted, 1039
tegaserod, 1040
irritative voiding symptoms, 837
ISA (intrinsic sympathomimetic activity), 5
Isentress. *See* raltegravir
Ismelin. *See* guanethidine
Ismotic. *See* isosorbide
ISMP (Institute for Safe Medication Practice), 86
Iso-bid. *See* isosorbide dinitrate
Isocaine. *See* mepivacaine
isocarboxazid, 290*t*, 304*t*, 315
isoflurane, 468–69
adverse effects, 468, 468*t*
classification, 468
contraindications/precautions, 468
drug interactions, 468
mechanism of action, 468
nursing responsibilities, 468–69
overdose treatment, 468
patient and family education, 469
pharmacokinetics, 468
pregnancy category, 468
route and adult dose, 468*t*
similar drugs, 469
therapeutic effects and uses, 468
isoniazid, 857–59
acetylation, 857–58, 858*f*
adverse effects, 858
classification, 857
contraindications/precautions, 858–59
drug interactions, 101*t*, 859
genetic polymorphisms and actions of, 159, 160*t*
mechanism of action, 858
nursing responsibilities, 859
overdose treatment, 859, 1364*t*
patient and family education, 859
pharmacokinetics, 858
pregnancy category, 859
similar drugs, 859–60
therapeutic effects and uses, 857–58
isophane insulin, 1127*t*, 1130
isoproterenol hydrochloride, 239–40
adverse effects, 232*t*, 239, 612*t*
classification, 239
contraindications/precautions, 239
drug interactions, 240
mechanism of action, 239
nursing responsibilities, 240
overdose treatment, 240
patient and family education, 240
pharmacokinetics, 239
pregnancy category, 240
route and adult dose, 232*t*, 612*t*
similar drugs, 240
for specific conditions
heart failure, 612*t*
therapeutic effects and uses, 239
Isoptin. *See* verapamil
Isoptin SR, 30*t*. *See also* verapamil
Isopto Atropine. *See* atropine
Isopto Carbachol. *See* carbachol
Isopto-Carpine. *See* pilocarpine
Isopto Hyoscine. *See* scopolamine hydrobromide
Isordil. *See* isosorbide dinitrate
isosorbide, 1341*t*, 1345
isosorbide dinitrate, 594–95
adverse effects, 592*t*
dosage forms not to be crushed or opened, 30*t*
drug interactions, 101*t*
route and adult dose, 592*t*
for specific conditions
angina and myocardial infarction, 592*t*
heart failure, 614
isosorbide mononitrate, 592*t*, 595
isotretinoin, 30*t*, 1322, 1322*t*, 1323, 1325
isozymes, 46–47
isradipine, 519*t*, 520*t*, 521–22
Istalol. *See* timolol
Isuprel. *See* isoproterenol hydrochloride
itraconazole:
adverse effects, 876
mechanism of action, 876
for specific conditions
superficial mycoses, 878–79, 878*t*
systemic mycoses, 872*t*, 876, 877
IV bolus (push) administration, 36, 37*f*
ivermectin, 902*t*, 903
IVIG. *See* intravenous immune globulin
IVIG (intravenous immune globulin), 767*t*, 769
ixabepilone, 992, 992*t*
Ixempra. *See* ixabepilone

J

Jadelle, 1210
Janumet, 1134*t*
Januvia. *See* sitagliptin
Jenner, Edward, 755
Joint Commission on Accreditation of Healthcare Organizations (JCAHO):
emergency preparedness standards, 1359
recommendations for prevention of medication errors, 86, 88
juxtaglomerular (JG) cells, 530, 531*f*

K

Kabikinase. *See* streptokinase
Kalcinate. *See* calcium gluconate
Kaletra. *See* lopinavir/ritonavir
kanamycin, 818–19
  adverse effects, 816*t*
  route and adult dose, 816*t*
  for tuberculosis, 855*t*, 860
Kantrex. *See* kanamycin
Kaon CL, 30*t*. *See also* potassium chloride (KCl)
Kaopectate. *See* bismuth subsalicylate
kappa receptors, 434, 435*t*
kava:
  description, 399*t*
  drug interactions, 177, 178*t*
  evidence, 399*t*
  history and claims, 399*t*
  for specific conditions
    anxiety and insomnia, 280
    muscle spasms, 397
  standardization, 175*t*, 399*t*
Kavatrol. *See* kava
Kayexalate. *See* polystyrene sulfate
KCl. *See* potassium chloride (KCl)
Kefauver-Harris Amendment, 14
Keflex. *See* cephalexin
Kefzol. *See* cefazolin sodium
Kemadrin. *See* procyclidine
Kenacort. *See* triamcinolone
Kenalog. *See* triamcinolone
Keppra. *See* levetiracetam
keratin, 1316
keratitis, 1349
keratolytic, 1322
Kerlone. *See* betaxolol
Ketalar. *See* ketamine
ketamine, 464–65
  abuse, 105, 464
  adverse effects, 460*t*, 464–65
  classification, 464
  contraindications/precautions, 465
  drug interactions, 465
  effects in pregnancy, 126*t*
  mechanism of action, 464
  nursing responsibilities, 465
  overdose treatment, 465
  patient and family education, 465
  pharmacokinetics, 464
  pregnancy category, 465
  route and adult dose, 460*t*
  similar drugs, 465
  therapeutic effects and uses, 464
Ketek. *See* telithromycin
ketoconazole, 877
  adverse effects, 872*t*, 878*t*
  drug interactions, 178*t*
  route and adult dose, 872*t*, 878*t*
  for specific conditions
    Cushing's syndrome, 1171
    seborrheic dermatitis, 1328
    superficial mycoses, 878*t*
ketogenic diet, 373, 374*t*
KETOLIDES, 833
  telithromycin, 821*t*, 822, 832*t*, 833
ketoprofen, 724*t*, 725*t*
ketorolac, 724*t*, 725*t*, 1349
ketotifen, 1349*t*
Key-Pred. *See* prednisolone
kidney(s):
  age-related changes, 148, 149*t*
  in diabetes, 1126, 1126*t*
  drug excretion by, 48–49
  drugs toxic to, 69, 69*t*, 548*t*
  failure. *See* renal failure
  glomerulus, 545, 547*f*
  juxtaglomerular cells, 530, 531*f*
  macula densa, 530, 531*f*
  nephrons, 545, 545*f*
  physiology
    excretion and homeostasis, 545, 546*t*, 547*f*, 688
    reabsorption and secretion, 546, 546*t*, 547*f*
Kineret. *See* anakinra
Klebsiella pneumoniae, 777*t*
Klonopin. *See* clonazepam
Klor-Con, 30*t*. *See also* potassium chloride (KCl)
Klotrix, 30*t*. *See also* potassium chloride (KCl)
Konsyl Fiber. *See* calcium polycarbophil
K-Tab, 30*t*. *See also* potassium chloride (KCl)
Kutrase. *See* pancreatin
Ku-Zyme. *See* pancreatin
Kytril. *See* granisetron

L

labetalol:
  adverse effects, 252*t*, 254
  for hypertensive emergency, 584*t*
  mechanism of action, 254
  route and adult dose, 252*t*
  for specific conditions, 254
labyrinthitis, 1351
Lacril-lube. *See* lanolin alcohol
lactase, 1004*t*
lactated Ringer's solution, 691*t*, 692
lactation:
  antibacterial properties of human milk, 127*t*
  herbal remedies as galactagogues, 129*t*
  oxytocin and, 1188*f*. *See also* oxytocin
  pharmacotherapy during
    with antiseizure drugs, 373
    drug risk categories, 130*t*
    drugs associated with adverse effects in infant, 129, 129*t*
    drugs compatible with, 128*t*
    drugs to avoid, 128*t*
    rationale for, 123
    transfer of drugs from mother to infant in breast milk, 127–28, 128*f*
lactic acidosis, 934
Lactobacillus, 1033
Lactobacillus acidophilus:
  description, 1044*t*
  evidence, 1044*t*
  history and claims, 1044*t*
  primary uses, 179*t*
  standardization, 1044*t*
Lamictal. *See* lamotrigine
Lamisil. *See* terbinafine
lamivudine, 921–22
  adverse effects, 919*t*, 921
  classification, 921
  contraindications/precautions, 921
  drug interactions, 921
  mechanism of action, 921
  nursing responsibilities, 921
  overdose treatment, 921
  patient and family education, 921–22
  pharmacokinetics, 921
  for postexposure prophylaxis of HIV infection, 943
  pregnancy category, 921
  route and adult dose, 919*t*
  similar drugs, 922
  for specific conditions
    hepatitis B, 920
    HIV-AIDS, 933*t*, 935
  therapeutic effects and uses, 921
lamotrigine:
  for bipolar disorder, 319*t*, 320
  for seizures, 381*t*, 391
Lampit. *See* nifurtimox
Lamprene. *See* clofazimine
lanolin alcohol, 1348, 1348*t*
Lanoxin. *See* digoxin
lanreotide, 1108*t*, 1112
lansoprazole, 30*t*, 1013*t*, 1015
lanthanum carbonate, 548*t*
Lantus. *See* insulin glargine
lapatinib, 748*t*, 990*t*
large volume infusion, 36, 37*f*
Lariam. *See* mefloquine
Larodopa. *See* levodopa
Larotid. *See* amoxicillin
Lasix. *See* furosemide
latanoprost, 1342–43
  adverse effects, 1342
  classification, 1342
  contraindications/precautions, 1342
  drug interactions, 1342
  mechanism of action, 1342
  nursing responsibilities, 1342
  ocular herpes infection reactivation and, 912
  overdose treatment, 1342
  patient and family education, 1342
  pharmacokinetics, 1342
  pregnancy category, 1342
  similar drugs, 1342–43
  therapeutic effects and uses, 1342
LAXATIVES, 1030
  abuse, 1032*t*
  adverse effects, 1030
  bulk-forming, 1031
    calcium polycarbophil, 1030*t*
    methylcellulose, 1030*t*
    psyllium mucilloid. *See* psyllium mucilloid
  for constipation, 1030
  herbal agents, 1031
    castor oil, 1030*t*, 1032
    senna, 1030*t*, 1031
  miscellaneous, 1031
    methylnaltrexone, 1031
    mineral oil, 1030*t*, 1031
  prophylactic use, 1030
  saline/osmotic, 1031
    magnesium hydroxide, 1030*t*, 1032
    polyethylene glycol, 1030*t*
    sodium biphosphate, 1030*t*
  stimulant, 1031
    bisacodyl, 1030*t*, 1032
    castor oil, 1030*t*, 1032
    phenolphthalein, 1030*t*
  stool softener/surfactant, 1031
    docusate, 1030*t*, 1032
LD_{50} (median lethal dose), 57
LDL (low-density lipoprotein), 496, 498*f*, 499*t*
L-dopa. *See* levodopa
lecithins, 496
  description, 200*t*, 496
  evidence, 200*t*

history and claims, 200*t*
sources, 496
standardization, 200*t*
uses, 496
leeches, 648
leflunomide, 135*t*, 1306
Leishmania, 886*t*
leishmaniasis, 886*t*, 892*t*, 896–97
lenalidomide, 991
Lennox-Gastaut syndrome, 376, 376*t*
lens, 1338
lepirudin, 648–49
adverse effects, 645*t*, 649
classification, 648
contraindications/precautions, 649
drug interactions, 649
mechanism of action, 648
nursing responsibilities, 649
overdose treatment, 649
patient and family education, 649
pharmacokinetics, 649
pregnancy category, 649
route and adult dose, 645*t*
similar drugs, 649
therapeutic effects and uses, 648
lepromatous leprosy, 862. *See also* leprosy
leprosy, 862
incidence, 862, 862*t*
pharmacotherapy
clofazimine, 862, 863
dapsone. *See* dapsone
regimens, 862
presentations, 862
leptin, 1086
Lescol. *See* fluvastatin
Lescol-XL. *See* fluvastatin
letrozole, 980*t*, 983
leucovorin rescue therapy, 972
leukemia, 950*t*
Leukeran. *See* chlorambucil
Leukine. *See* sargramostim
leukocytes, 483
LEUKOTRIENE MODIFIERS:
for asthma, 1244*t*, 1250*t*, 1253
drugs in class
montelukast, 1250*t*, 1254, 1270*t*, 1271
zafirlukast. *See* zafirlukast
zileuton, 1250*t*, 1254–55
leukotrienes, 712*t*, 1240
leuprolide, 980*t*, 984, 1192*t*, 1194, 1196, 1221
Leustatin. *See* cladribine
levalbuterol, 232*t*, 240, 1245*t*, 1247
Levaquin. *See* levofloxacin
Levarterenol. *See* norepinephrine
Levatol. *See* penbutolol
Levemir. *See* insulin detemir
levetiracetam, 381*t*, 391
Levitra. *See* vardenafil
levoamphetamine, 415. *See also* amphetamine sulfate
levobunolol, 1341*t*, 1343, 1345
levocetirizine, 1265*t*
levodopa, 351–53
adverse effects, 352
with carbidopa, 349, 350*t*, 351
classification, 351
contraindications/precautions, 352
dosage forms not to be crushed or opened, 30*t*
drug interactions, 178*t*, 352
genetic polymorphisms and actions of, 160*t*
mechanism of action, 351*f*, 352
nursing responsibilities, 352
overdose treatment, 352
patient and family education, 353
pharmacokinetics, 352
Pharmacotherapy Illustrated, 351*f*
pregnancy category, 352
similar drugs, 354
therapeutic effects and uses, 351–52
levodopa/carbidopa, 349, 350*t*, 351
Levo-Dromoran. *See* levorphanol
levofloxacin, 827*t*, 830, 833*t*, 838
levoleucovorin, 972
levonorgestrel:
for emergency contraception, 1212, 1213*t*
intrauterine, 43, 1210, 1211*f*
Levophed. *See* norepinephrine
levorphanol, 436*t*, 439
Levothroid. *See* levothyroxine
levothyroxine, 1150–51
adverse effects, 1151, 1151*t*
classification, 1151*t*
contraindications/precautions, 1151
drug interactions, 1151
mechanism of action, 1151
nursing responsibilities, 1151
overdose treatment, 1151
patient and family education, 1151
pharmacokinetics, 1151
pregnancy category, 1151
route and adult dose, 1151*t*
similar drugs, 1152
therapeutic effects and uses, 1151
Levoxyl. *See* levothyroxine
Levsin. *See* hyoscyamine
Lexapro. *See* escitalopram
Lexiva. *See* fosamprenavir
Lexxel, 572*t*
Leydig cells, 1219
LH. *See* luteinizing hormone
Lialda. *See* mesalamine
libido, 1220
Librium. *See* chlordiazepoxide
Lidex. *See* fluocinonide
lidocaine, 474–75
adverse effects, 473*t*, 475, 629*t*
classification, 474
contraindications/precautions, 475
drug interactions, 475
mechanism of action, 475
nursing responsibilities, 475
overdose treatment, 475
patient and family education, 475
pharmacokinetics, 475
pregnancy category, 475
route and adult dose, 473*t*, 629*t*
similar drugs, 475–77
for specific conditions
dysrhythmias, 629*t*, 632
therapeutic effects and uses, 474–75
Lifespan Considerations:
chemotherapy in older adults, 984*t*
children with HIV-AIDS, 944*t*
continuous subcutaneous insulin infusion, 1131*t*
corticosteroids in pediatric patients, 1164*t*
cost of prescription medications, 5*t*, 151*t*
depression in children and adolescents, 302*t*
diuretic therapy in children and geriatric patients, 549*t*
drug monitoring in older adults, 150*t*
fluid and electrolytes in the older adult, 695*t*
H_1-receptor antagonists (antihistamines), 1267*t*
hypertension in children, 522*t*
infections in the older adult, 795*t*
oral candidiasis in infants, 872*t*
otic medication instillation, 1352*t*
pain assessment in the very young, 432*t*
pain expression and management in the elderly, 442*t*
parents' role in preventing medication errors, 82*t*
patient teaching, 118*t*
pediatric medication administration, 25*t*
peptic ulcer disease and gastroesophageal reflux in children, 1023*t*
polyherbacy in older adults, 177*t*
school nurses and medication administration guidelines, 166*t*
sleep–wake patterns, 278*t*
Stevens–Johnson syndrome in children, 1333*t*
thyroid disease in older adults, 1150*t*
thyroid hormone use and hip fracture risk in older women, 1150*t*
vaccine administration, 766*t*
limbic system, 270
anatomy, 270*f*
anxiety disorders and, 276, 277*f*
functions, 270, 276
Lincocin. *See* lincomycin
lincomycin, 821, 821*t*
lindane, 1319, 1320
linezolid, 821*t*, 822
Linum usitatissimum. *See* flaxseed
Lioresal. *See* baclofen
liothyronine, 1151*t*, 1152
liotrix, 1151*t*, 1152
LIPASE INHIBITORS, 1091
orlistat. *See* orlistat
lipid(s). *See also* dyslipidemias
cardiovascular disease and, 496, 498
chemical structure, 497*f*
classification, 496
composition, 498*f*
in enteral nutrition, 1070
in parenteral nutrition, 1078
lipid profile, 499–500, 499*t*
Lipitor. *See* atorvastatin
lipodystrophy, 934
lipoproteins, 496, 498*f*
5-lipoxygenase inhibitor:
zileuton, 1250*t*, 1254–55
Liquifilm. *See* polyvinyl alcohol
lisinopril, 534–35
adverse effects, 533*t*, 534, 612*t*
classification, 534
contraindications/precautions, 534
drug interactions, 534
mechanism of action, 534
nursing responsibilities, 535
overdose treatment, 535
patient and family education, 535
pharmacokinetics, 534
pregnancy category, 534

route and adult dose, 533*t*, 612t
similar drugs, 536
for specific conditions
heart failure, 612*t*
therapeutic effects and uses, 534
lithium carbonate, 318–19
adverse effects, 319, 319*t*
in breast-feeding infant, 129*t*
classification, 318
contraindications/precautions, 319
dosage forms not to be crushed or opened, 30*t*
drug interactions, 319–20
mechanism of action, 318
nursing responsibilities, 320
overdose treatment, 320
patient and family education, 320
pharmacokinetics, 319
pregnancy category, 320
route and adult dose, 319*t*
therapeutic effects and uses, 318
Lithobid. *See* lithium carbonate
liver:
in digestive process, 1003
drug metabolism in, 1002–3
drugs toxic to, 69*t*, 70
failure, acetaminophen and, 1003*t*
functions, 1001–2
hepatic portal circulation, 1003, 1003*f*
10% LMD. *See* dextran 40
LMWHs (low molecular weight heparins), 645–46, 645*t*, 647–48
loading dose, 52
local anesthesia, 458
agents for. *See* local anesthetics
Nursing Process Application, 476*t*
techniques, 471, 471*f*
termination, 471–72
local anesthetics:
as adjuvant analgesics, 447
amide-type, 473*t*, 474
articaine, 473*t*, 475
bupivacaine, 473*t*, 475–76
dibucaine, 473*t*, 476
lidocaine. *See* lidocaine
mepivacaine, 476
prilocaine, 473*t*, 476
ropivacaine, 473*t*, 476
ester-type, 472, 473*t*
benzocaine. *See* benzocaine
chloroprocaine, 473*t*, 474
procaine. *See* procaine
tetracaine, 473*t*, 474
locus coeruleus, 276
Lodine. *See* etodolac
Loestrin 1.5/30 Fe, 1203*t*
Lomotil. *See* diphenoxylate with atropine
lomustine, 967*t*, 971
Loniten. *See* minoxidil
look-alike drug names, 84–85*t*
LOOP (HIGH-CEILING) DIURETICS, 549
adverse effects, 550, 612*t*
clinical applications, 550
drugs in class
bumetanide, 551*t*, 553, 612*t*
ethacrynic acid, 551*t*, 553
furosemide. *See* furosemide
torsemide, 551*t*, 553, 612*t*
route and adult dose, 612*t*
sites of action, 550, 550*f*
for specific conditions
heart failure, 612*t*, 613
hypertension, 573, 574*t*
Lo/Ovral, 1203*t*
loperamide, 1033, 1034*t*, 1035
Lopid. *See* gemfibrozil
lopinavir/ritonavir, 938–39
adverse effects, 933*t*, 938
classification, 938
contraindications/precautions, 938
drug interactions, 938
mechanism of action, 938
nursing responsibilities, 938–39
overdose treatment, 938
patient and family education, 939
pharmacokinetics, 938
pregnancy category, 938
route and adult dose, 933*t*
similar drugs, 939–40
therapeutic effects and uses, 938
Lopressor. *See* metoprolol
Lopressor HCT, 572*t*
Loprox. *See* ciclopirox
Lopurin. *See* allopurinol
Lorabid. *See* loracarbef
loracarbef, 142*t*
loratadine, 101*t*, 1265*t*, 1268
lorazepam, 284–85
adverse effects, 284, 380*t*
classification, 284
contraindications/precautions, 284
drug interactions, 284–85
mechanism of action, 284
nursing responsibilities, 285
parenteral administration, 283
patient and family education, 285
pharmacokinetics, 284
pregnancy category, 285
similar drugs, 285–86
for specific conditions
alcohol withdrawal, 102
initial treatment of psychosis, 328
nausea and vomiting, 1042, 1043*t*
seizures, 380*t*, 383–84
therapeutic effects and uses, 283*t*, 284
Lortab. *See* acetaminophen; hydrocodone
losartan, 539–40
adverse effects, 538*t*, 539
classification, 539
contraindications/precautions, 539
drug interactions, 539
mechanism of action, 539
nursing responsibilities, 539
overdose treatment, 539
patient and family education, 539–40
pharmacokinetics, 539
pregnancy category, 539
route and adult dose, 538*t*
similar drugs, 540–41
therapeutic effects and uses, 539
Lotensin. *See* benazepril
Lotensin HCT, 572*t*
Lotrel, 572*t*
Lotrimin AF. *See* clotrimazole
Lotronex. *See* alosetron
Lou Gehrig's disease. *See* amyotrophic lateral sclerosis
lovastatin, 75*t*, 504*t*, 506
Love-Dromoran. *See* levorphanol
Lovenox. *See* enoxaparin
low molecular weight heparins (LMWHs), 645–46, 645*t*, 647–48
low-back pain. *See also* muscle spasms
antidepressants for, 398*t*
low-density lipoprotein (LDL), 496, 498*f*, 499*t*
loxapine, 332*t*, 336
Loxitane. *See* loxapine
Lozol. *See* indapamide
LSD (lysergic acid diethylamide), 103–4, 104*f*, 126*t*
lubiprostone, 1037*t*, 1040
LUBRICANTS, OCULAR, 1348
lanolin alcohol, 1348, 1348*t*
polyvinyl alcohol, 1348, 1348*t*
Lucentis. *See* ranibizumab
Ludiomil. *See* maprotiline
Lufyllin. *See* dyphylline
Lugol's solution. *See* potassium iodide and iodine
Lumigan. *See* bimatoprost
Luminal. *See* phenobarbital
Lunesta. *See* eszopiclone
lung(s). *See* respiratory system
lung cancer, 991*t*
Lupron. *See* leuprolide
luteinizing hormone (LH):
regulation, 1102*t*
target organs and action, 1102*t*, 1105*t*
Luvox. *See* fluvoxamine
lymph nodes, 709
lymphangiogenesis, 709*t*
lymphatic system, 709
lymphocyte immune globulin, 741*t*, 747, 749
lymphoma, 950*t*
Lyrica. *See* pregabalin
lysergic acid diethylamide (LSD), 103–4, 104*f*, 126*t*
Lysodren. *See* mitotane

M

Maalox Plus, 1021*t*
MABs. *See* MONOCLONAL ANTIBODIES (MABs)
Mabthera. *See* rituximab
MAC (*Mycobacterium avium* complex), 751, 865
Macrobid. *See* nitrofurantoin
Macrodantin. *See* nitrofurantoin
MACROLIDES:
adverse effects, 814
drugs in class
azithromycin. *See* azithromycin
clarithromycin. *See* clarithromycin
dirithromycin, 813*t*, 816
erythromycin. *See* erythromycin base
mechanism of action, 813
metabolism, 814
Nursing Process Application, 819–20*t*
resistance to, 813–14
for specific conditions
M. avium complex infections, 865
therapeutic effects and uses, 813
macrominerals, 1062
calcium. *See* calcium
chloride. *See* chloride
magnesium. *See* magnesium
phosphorus. *See* phosphorus
sodium. *See* sodium
sulfur, 1062*t*
macula densa, 530, 531*f*
mafenide, 842

magaldrate, 1021*t*
Magan. *See* magnesium salicylate
magnesium:
  functions, 699, 1062, 1062*t*
  imbalances, 694*t*, 699
    hypermagnesemia. *See* hypermagnesemia
    hypomagnesemia. *See* hypomagnesemia
  recommended dietary allowance, 701*t*, 1062*t*
magnesium antacids, 1019. *See also* ANTACIDS
magnesium hydroxide, 1021*t*, 1030*t*, 1032
magnesium salicylate, 720*t*, 723
magnesium sulfate ($MgSO_4$), 700
  adverse effects, 700
  classification, 700
  contraindications/precautions, 700
  drug interactions, 700
  mechanism of action, 700
  nursing responsibilities, 700
  overdose treatment, 700
  patient and family education, 700
  pharmacokinetics, 700
  pregnancy category, 700
  similar drugs, 700
  for specific conditions
    hypomagnesemia, 700
    preterm labor, 1190
    seizures in pregnancy, 373
  therapeutic effects and uses, 700
magnesium trisilicate, 1021*t*
maintenance dose, 52
major depressive disorder, 298. *See also* depression
major tranquilizer, 330. *See also* first-generation antipsychotics
malaria, 887
  description, 886*t*
  incidence, 887
  mortality, 887*t*
  pharmacotherapy
    acute attacks, 888
    atovaquone-proguanil, 75*t*, 888*t*, 890
    chemoprophylaxis, 887–88
    chloroquine hydrochloride. *See* chloroquine
    hydroxychloroquine. *See* hydroxychloroquine
    mefloquine, 888, 888*t*, 890
    primaquine, 888*t*, 890
    pyrimethamine, 888*t*
    quinine, 888*t*, 890
    relapse prevention, 888
  stages, 887
Malarone. *See* atovaquone-proguanil
malathion, 1319, 1320
male infertility, 1225–26
male reproductive function, 1219–20, 1219*f*
male sexual dysfunction, 1225, 1225*t*. *See also* erectile dysfunction
malignant hyperthermia, 222, 403–4, 466*t*, 469*t*
malignant tumor, 950*t*. *See also* cancer
maltase, 1004*t*
Mandelamine. *See* mandelate
mandelate, 840*t*, 847
manganese, 1063*t*
mania, 298, 317–18
manic-depression. *See* bipolar disorder
mannitol, 559–60
  adverse effects, 559, 559*t*
  classification, 559
  contraindications/precautions, 559
  drug interactions, 559
  mechanism of action, 559
  nursing responsibilities, 560
  overdose treatment, 559
  patient and family education, 560
  pharmacokinetics, 559
  pregnancy category, 560
  route and adult dose, 559*t*
  similar drugs, 560
  for specific conditions
    glaucoma, 1341*t*
  therapeutic effects and uses, 559
MAO (monoamine oxidase), 194, 231, 308*f*
MAO-B (MONOAMINE OXIDASE-B) INHIBITORS:
  selegiline, 350*t*, 355
MAOIs. *See* MONOAMINE OXIDASE INHIBITORS (MAOIs)
maprotiline, 304*t*, 307
MAR (medication administration record), 28, 87
maraviroc, 933*t*, 940
Marcaine. *See* bupivacaine
Marezine. *See* cyclizine hydrochloride
marijuana:
  effects, 102–3
  medical use, 103
  use in pregnancy, 126*t*
  withdrawal symptoms and treatment, 96*t*
Marinol. *See* dronabinol
Marplan. *See* isocarboxazid
MAST CELL STABILIZERS, 1271
  cromolyn. *See* cromolyn
  ketotifen, 1349*t*
  nedocromil sodium, 1250*t*, 1253, 1349, 1349*t*
  pemirolast potassium, 1349, 1349*t*
  for specific conditions
    allergic conjunctivitis, 1349, 1349*t*
    allergic rhinitis, 1271
    asthma, 1244*t*, 1250*t*, 1252
mastoiditis, 1351
Materia Medica, 3
Matulane. *See* procarbazine
Mavik. *See* trandolapril
Maxair. *See* pirbuterol
Maxalt. *See* rizatriptan
Maxiflor. *See* diflorasone diacetate
Maxipime. *See* cefepime
MBD. *See* metabolic bone disease
MCV (meningococcal conjugate vaccine), 760
MDA (3,4-methylenedioxyamphetamine), 105
MDI. *See* metered-dose inhaler
MDMA (3,4-methylenedioxy-methamphetamine), 105
measles (rubeola):
  characteristics, 758*t*
  immunization, 758*t*, 764
  incidence, 758*t*, 764
  pathophysiology, 764
Mebaral. *See* mephobarbital
mebendazole, 902–3
  adverse effects, 902, 902*t*
  classification, 902
  contraindications/precautions, 902
  drug interactions, 902
  mechanism of action, 902
  nursing responsibilities, 903
  overdose treatment, 902
  patient and family education, 903
  pharmacokinetics, 902
  pregnancy category, 902
  route and adult dose, 902*t*
  similar drugs, 903
  therapeutic effects and uses, 902
mecamylamine, 218–20
  adverse effects, 219, 219*t*
  classification, 218
  contraindications/precautions, 219
  drug interactions, 219
  mechanism of action, 219
  nursing responsibilities, 220
  overdose treatment, 219–20
  patient and family education, 220
  pharmacokinetics, 219
  pregnancy category, 219
  route and adult dose, 219*t*
  therapeutic effects and uses, 218
mecasermin, 1108*t*, 1110–11
mecasermin rinfabate, 1108*t*
mechlorethamine, 967*t*, 971
meclizine, 1043*t*
meclofenamate, 724*t*, 725*t*
median effective dose (ED_{50}), 56, 56*f*
median lethal dose (LD_{50}), 57
median toxicity dose (TD_{50}), 57
Medicare Prescription Drug Improvement and Modernization Act, 14
medication administration record (MAR), 28, 87
medication error(s), 80
  categories, 81*f*, 82*f*
  documentation and reporting, 86–87
  drug names and, 84–85*t*, 84–86
  factors contributing to, 80, 83–84
  impact on health care, 80
  Lifespan Considerations, 82*t*
  packaging and, 648*t*
  prevention
    abbreviations to avoid, 83*t*
    health care policies and procedures, 88
    high-alert drugs, 86*t*
    medical reconciliation, 87
    nursing strategies, 87
    parents' role in, 82*t*
    patient education, 88
  types, 83*t*
medication error index, 80, 81*f*, 82*f*
Medication Error Reporting Program (MERP), 86
medication reconciliation, 88
MEDMARX, 86
Medrol. *See* methylprednisolone
medroxyprogesterone acetate, 1183–84
  adverse effects, 1180*t*, 1183
  classification, 1183
  contraindications/precautions, 1183
  drug interactions, 1183
  mechanism of action, 1183
  nursing responsibilities, 1184
  overdose treatment, 1184
  patient and family education, 1184
  pharmacokinetics, 1183
  pregnancy category, 1184
  route and adult dose, 1180*t*
  similar drugs, 1184
  for specific conditions
    contraception, 1210
    neoplasia, 980*t*
  therapeutic effects and uses, 1183
mefenamic acid, 724*t*, 725*t*

mefloquine, 888, 888*t*, 890
Mefoxin. *See* cefoxitin
Megace. *See* megestrol
megaloblastic anemia. *See* pernicious anemia
megestrol, 980*t*
MEGLITINIDES:
actions, 1132*t*
drugs in class
nateglinide, 1133*t*, 1137
repaglinide. *See* repaglinide
mechanism of action, 1136
nursing considerations, 1132*t*
melarsoprol, 892*t*, 898
melatonin:
cancer risk and, 1101*t*
description, 281*t*
evidence, 281*t*
history and claims, 281*t*
production, 276
standardization, 281*t*
Mellaril. *See* thioridazine
meloxicam, 724*t*, 725*t*
melphalan, 967*t*, 971
memantine, 359*t*, 360
memory B cells, 713
Menactra. *See* meningococcal conjugate vaccine
meningococcal conjugate vaccine (MCV), 760
meningococcal infection:
immunization, 758*t*, 760
incidence, 758*t*, 760*t*
mortality, 760*t*
pathophysiology, 760
prophylaxis, 833
meningococcal polysaccharide vaccine (MPSV), 760
menopause, 1184, 1184*t*, 1185*t*
menorrhagia, 1183
menotropins, 1191, 1192*t*, 1196, 1226
menstrual cycle, 1177, 1178*f*
mental retardation, epilepsy and, 382*t*
Mentax. *See* butenafine
mepenzolate, 214*t*, 217
meperidine, 439–40
comparison to other opioids, 436*t*
disposal, 26*t*
drug interactions, 101*t*
route and adult dose, 436*t*
mephenytoin, 385
mephenytoin hydroxylase, 160*t*
mephobarbital:
adverse effects, 381*t*
route and adult dose, 381*t*
for seizures, 379, 381, 381*t*
therapeutic effects and uses, 292
mepivacaine, 476
meprobamate, 281, 286
Mepron. *See* atovaquone
mercaptopurine, 973*t*, 976
Meridia. *See* sibutramine
meropenem, 800*t*, 802
merozoites, 887
MERP (Medication Error Reporting Program), 86
Merrem. *See* meropenem
mesalamine, 1037*t*, 1039
Mesantoin. *See* mephenytoin
mescaline, 104, 105*f*
Mestinon. *See* pyridostigmine
metabolic acidosis, in renal failure, 548*t*
metabolic bone disease (MBD), 1290
osteomalacia, 1291
osteoporosis. *See* osteoporosis
Paget's disease, 1291–92, 1294
metabolic syndrome, 1123
metabolism, drug, 46
drug interactions and, 71*f*, 72
first-pass effect, 48, 48*f*
hepatic microsomal enzyme system and, 46–48, 47*t*
in older adults, 149–50
patient variation in, 48, 48*t*
in pediatric patients, 136–37
in pregnancy, 124
Metadate. *See* methylphenidate
Metaglip, 1134*t*
Metamucil. *See* psyllium mucilloid
metastasis, 951, 951*f*
metaxalone, 400*t*, 401
metered-dose inhaler (MDI), 1242
metformin, 1135–36
adverse effects, 1133*t*, 1136
classification, 1135
contraindications/precautions, 1136
drug interactions, 1136
mechanism of action, 1135
pharmacokinetics, 1136
route and adult dose, 1133*t*
therapeutic effects and uses, 1135
methadone, 97, 99, 436*t*, 440
methamphetamine:
abuse, 106
addiction, 236*t*
effects in pregnancy, 126
manufacture, 236*t*
methaqualone, 281
methazolamide, 559*t*, 560, 1341*t*
methenamine hippurate, 840*t*, 847
Methergine. *See* methylergonovine
methicillin-resistant *Staphylococcus aureus* (MRSA), 781–82
methimazole, 1154*t*, 1156
Methitest. *See* methyltestosterone
methocarbamol, 400*t*, 401
methohexital, 292, 460*t*, 461
methotrexate, 746, 972–74
adverse effects, 741*t*, 746, 973–74, 1304*t*, 1306
classification, 972
contraindications/precautions, 974
drug interactions, 178*t*, 974
mechanism of action, 973
nursing responsibilities, 974
overdose treatment, 974
patient and family education, 974
pharmacokinetics, 973
pregnancy category, 974
route and adult dose, 741*t*
similar drugs, 974–76
for specific conditions
as abortifacient, with misoprostol, 1213, 1213*t*
psoriasis, 1330, 1330*t*
rheumatoid arthritis, 1304*t*, 1306
therapeutic effects and uses, 973
methscopolamine, 214*t*, 217
methsuximide, 381*t*, 389
methyclothiazide, 554*t*, 555
methyl sulfonyl methane (MSM), 179*t*
methylcellulose, 1030*t*
methyldopa, 577–78
adverse effects, 577
classification, 577
contraindications/precautions, 577
drug interactions, 577
mechanism of action, 577
nursing responsibilities, 578
patient and family education, 578
pharmacokinetics, 577
pregnancy category, 577
similar drugs, 578–79
therapeutic effects and uses, 577
methylene blue, 1364*t*
methylergonovine, 1187*t*, 1189
Methylin. *See* methylphenidate
methylnaltrexone, 1031
methylphenidate:
abuse, 106
for ADHD, 416*t*, 418
administration, 30*t*
adverse effects, 142*t*, 416*t*
disposal, 26*t*
dosage/routes
adult, 416*t*
pediatric, 142*t*
pediatric labeling changes, 135*t*
methylprednisolone:
adverse effects, 1167*t*
for nausea and vomiting, 1043*t*, 1044
route and adult dose, 1167*t*
methyltestosterone, 1220*t*, 1223
METHYLXANTHINES, 421, 1255
aminophylline, 1245*t*, 1256
for asthma, 1244*t*, 1245*t*, 1255
caffeine. *See* caffeine
theobromine, 421
theophylline. *See* theophylline
methysergide, 453
Meticorten. *See* prednisone
metipranolol, 252*t*, 255, 1341*t*, 1343
metoclopramide, 477, 1043*t*
metolazone, 553, 554*t*, 555
Metopirone. *See* metyrapone
metoprolol, 256–57
adverse effects, 252*t*, 256, 612*t*
classification, 256
contraindications/precautions, 256
dosage forms not to be crushed or opened, 30*t*
drug interactions, 256
genetic polymorphisms and actions of, 160*t*
mechanism of action, 256
nursing responsibilities, 256–57
overdose treatment, 256
patient and family education, 257
pharmacokinetics, 256
pregnancy category, 256
route and adult dose, 252*t*, 612*t*
similar drugs, 257–58
for specific conditions
angina, 592*t*
heart failure, 612*t*
therapeutic effects and uses, 256, 286
metric system of measurement, 28, 28*t*
MetroCream. *See* metronidazole
MetroGel. *See* metronidazole
metronidazole, 893–94
adverse effects, 832*t*, 894
classification, 893
contraindications/precautions, 894
drug interactions, 101*t*, 894

mechanism of action, 893
nursing responsibilities, 894
overdose treatment, 894
patient and family education, 894
pharmacokinetics, 893
pregnancy category, 894
route and adult dose, 832*t*
similar drugs, 894–95
for specific conditions
anaerobic infections, 832–33, 832*t*
H. pylori infection, 1023
rosacea, 1323
trichomoniasis, 896
therapeutic effects and uses, 893
metyrapone, 1171
Mevacor. *See* lovastatin
Mexate. *See* methotrexate
mexiletine, 629*t*, 632
Mexitil. *See* mexiletine
$MgSO_4$. *See* magnesium sulfate ($MgSO_4$)
MI. *See* myocardial infarction
Miacalcin. *See* calcitonin-salmon
micafungin, 872*t*, 874–75
Micardis. *See* telmisartan
Micatin. *See* miconazole
miconazole, 878*t*, 879, 1318
microbial antagonism, 784
microminerals:
chromium, 1063*t*
cobalt, 1063*t*
copper, 1063*t*
fluorine, 1063, 1063*t*
iodine. *See* iodine
iron. *See* iron
manganese, 1063*t*
molybdenum, 1063*t*
selenium, 1063*t*
zinc, 1063, 1063*t*
Micronase. *See* glyburide
Microsporum, 869*t*
Midamor. *See* amiloride
midazolam, 463–64
adverse effects, 460*t*, 463
classification, 463
contraindications/precautions, 463
drug interactions, 463
mechanism of action, 463
nursing responsibilities, 464
onset time, 283
overdose treatment, 463–64
patient and family education, 464
pharmacokinetics, 463
pregnancy category, 463
similar drugs, 464
for specific conditions
preoperative medication, 477
for seizures, 380*t*, 384
therapeutic effects and uses, 283*t*, 463
midodrine, 232*t*, 238
Mifeprex. *See* mifepristone
mifepristone, 1214–15
adverse effects, 1214
classification, 1214
contraindications/precautions, 1214–15
drug interactions, 1215
mechanism of action, 1214
nursing responsibilities, 1215
overdose treatment, 1215
patient and family education, 1215
pharmacokinetics, 1214
pregnancy category, 1215
for specific conditions
Cushing's syndrome, 1171
therapeutic effects and uses, 1214
miglitol, 1133*t*, 1139
migraine, 449
characteristics, 449, 449*t*
Complementary and Alternative Therapies, 453*t*
pharmacotherapy, 449–50
ergot alkaloids, 450*t*, 451
triptans, 450*t*, 451–52
prophylaxis, 453, 453*t*
statistics, 449*t*
Migranal. *See* dihydroergotamine
Milk of Magnesia. *See* magnesium hydroxide
milk thistle, 173*t*, 175*t*
milk-alkali syndrome, 1019
Milontin. *See* phensuximide
Milophene. *See* clomiphene citrate
milrinone lactate, 618–19
adverse effects, 612*t*, 618
classification, 618
contraindications/precautions, 618
drug interactions, 618
mechanism of action, 618
nursing responsibilities, 619
overdose treatment, 618
patient and family education, 619
pharmacokinetics, 618
pregnancy category, 618
route and adult dose, 612*t*
similar drugs, 619
for specific conditions
heart failure, 612*t*
therapeutic effects and uses, 618
Miltown. *See* meprobamate
mineral oil, 1030*t*, 1031
MINERALOCORTICOIDS:
adrenal production, 1161*f*, 1162
fludrocortisone. *See* fludrocortisone
for hypoaldosteronism, 1169–70
minerals, 1061–62
macrominerals, 1062–63, 1062*t*
microminerals, 1063, 1063*t*
Nursing Process Application, 1064*t*
in parenteral nutrition, 1078
minimal sedation (anxiolysis), 458
minimum alveolar concentration, 465
minimum effective concentration, 50
Minipress. *See* prazosin
Minizide, 572*t*
Minocin. *See* minocycline
minocycline, 813
adverse effects, 810*t*
for leprosy, 862
pediatric dosage/route, 142*t*
route and adult dose, 810*t*
minoxidil, 581, 1333–34
Mintezol. *See* thiabendazole
miosis, 1343
Miostat. *See* carbachol
MiraLax. *See* polyethylene glycol
Mirapex. *See* pramipexole
Mircette, 1203*t*
Mirena, 43, 1210, 1211*f*
mirtazapine, 304*t*, 312
misoprostol:
as abortifacient, 1212–13, 1213*t*
adverse effects, 1024, 1187*t*
for gastrointestinal protection, 720
for peptic ulcer disease, 1024
route and adult dose, 1187*t*
as uterine stimulant, 1189
mitochondrial toxicity, 933–34
mitomycin, 977*t*, 978
mitotane, 992*t*, 993
mitoxantrone:
adverse effects, 977*t*
for multiple sclerosis, 365, 366*t*
route and adult dose, 977*t*
therapeutic effects and uses, 978
Mitrolan. *See* calcium polycarbophil
Mivacron. *See* mivacurium
mivacurium, 219*t*, 224
mixed opioid agonist-antagonists. *See* OPIOID ANALGESICS
mixture-HL, 1363*t*
MMR vaccine. *See* measles, immunization; mumps, immunization; rubella
Moban. *See* molindone
Mobic. *See* meloxicam
Mobidin. *See* magnesium salicylate
modafinil, 420–21
adverse effects, 416*t*, 420
classification, 420
contraindications/precautions, 420
drug interactions, 420
mechanism of action, 420
nursing responsibilities, 420–21
overdose treatment, 420
patient and family education, 421
pharmacokinetics, 420
pregnancy category, 420
route and adult dose, 416*t*
similar drugs, 421
for specific conditions
narcolepsy, 279
therapeutic effects and uses, 420
moderate (conscious) sedation, 458
modular formulas, for enteral nutrition, 1069*t*, 1070
Moduretic, 572*t*
moexipril, 533*t*, 536
molecularly targeted agents, 991
molindone, 332*t*, 336
molybdenum, 1063*t*
MOM. *See* magnesium hydroxide
mometasone, 1250*t*, 1252, 1270*t*
mometasone furoate, 1327*t*
Monistat. *See* miconazole
Monistat-1. *See* tioconazole
monitored anesthesia care (MAC), 458
monoamine oxidase (MAO), 194, 231, 308*f*
MONOAMINE OXIDASE INHIBITORS (MAOIs), 313
adverse effects, 313–14
for anxiety disorders, 289, 290*t*
drug interactions, 75*t*
with herbal products, 178*t*
with tyramine, 314, 314*t*
drugs in class
isocarboxazid, 290*t*, 304*t*, 315
phenelzine. *See* phenelzine
tranylcypromine sulfate, 290*t*, 304*t*, 315, 317
mechanism of action, 313
Nursing Process Application, 317*t*
MONOAMINE OXIDASE-B (MAO-B) INHIBITORS:
selegiline, 350*t*, 355

MONOCLONAL ANTIBODIES (MABs), 747
drugs in class
abciximab. *See* abciximab
alemtuzumab, 748*t*, 990*t*
basiliximab, 741*t*, 748*t*, 749
bevacizumab, 748*t*, 990*t*
bortezomib, 748*t*, 990*t*
cetuximab, 748*t*, 990*t*
daclizumab, 741*t*, 748*t*, 749
dasatinib, 748*t*, 990*t*
erlotinib, 990*t*
gefitinib, 990*t*
gemtuzumab, 748*t*, 990*t*
ibritumomab, 748*t*, 990*t*
imatinib, 990*t*
lapatinib, 748*t*, 990*t*
muromonab-CD3. *See* muromonab-CD3
natalizumab, 365–66, 366*t*, 748*t*
nilotinib, 748*t*, 990*t*
omalizumab, 748*t*, 1256
panitumumab, 748*t*, 990*t*
rituximab, 748*t*, 990*t*
scinitinib, 990*t*
sorafenib, 748*t*, 990*t*
tositumomab, 748*t*, 990*t*
trastuzumab, 748*t*, 990*t*
FDA-approved, 748*t*
mechanism of action, 742*f*
names, 747
Monoject. *See* heparin
Monopril. *See* fosinopril
montelukast, 1250*t*, 1254, 1270*t*, 1271
Monurol. *See* fosfomycin
mood disorder, 298. *See also* bipolar disorder; depression
MOOD STABILIZERS:
carbamazepine. *See* carbamazepine
lamotrigine, 319*t*, 320
lithium carbonate. *See* lithium carbonate
valproic acid. *See* valproic acid
Morbillivirus, 764. *See also* measles
moricizine, 633
morning sickness, 1041, 1041*t*
morphine sulfate, 437–39
adverse effects, 438
classification, 437
contraindications/precautions, 438
disposal, 26*t*
dosage forms not to be crushed or opened, 30*t*
drug interactions, 101*t*, 438
genetic polymorphisms and actions of, 160*t*
mechanism of action, 438
nursing responsibilities, 438–39
overdose treatment, 438
patient and family education, 439
pharmacokinetics, 438
pregnancy category, 438
similar drugs, 439–40
for specific conditions
intravenous general anesthesia, 460*t*
therapeutic effects and uses, 437–38
motion sickness, 1266
Motofen. *See* difenoxin with atropine
motor end plate, 220, 221*f*
Motrin. *See* ibuprofen
Moxatag. *See* amoxicillin
moxifloxacin, 827*t*, 830
6-MP. *See* mercaptopurine
MPSV (meningococcal polysaccharide vaccine), 760
MRSA (methicillin-resistant *Staphylococcus aureus*), 781–82
MSM (methyl sulfonyl methane), 179*t*
mu receptors, 434, 435*t*
Mucinex. *See* guaifenesin
MUCOLYTICS, 1258, 1277
acetylcysteine, 1276*t*, 1277
for chronic obstructive pulmonary disease, 1258
dornase alfa, 1277
Mucomyst. *See* acetylcysteine
Mucorales, 869*t*
mucormycosis, 869*t*
mucositis, 959
multiple sclerosis (MS):
characteristics, 364
diagnosis, 364
muscle spasticity in, 403
pathophysiology, 364–65, 365*f*
in pediatric patients, 364*t*
mumps:
characteristics, 758*t*
immunization, 758*t*, 764
incidence, 758*t*, 764
pathophysiology, 764
Murine Plus. *See* tetrahydrozoline
muromonab-CD3, 747–49
adverse effects, 741*t*, 747–48
classification, 747
contraindications/precautions, 748
drug interactions, 748–49
mechanism of action, 742*f*, 747
nursing responsibilities, 749
overdose treatment, 749
patient and family education, 749
pharmacokinetics, 747
pregnancy category, 749
route and adult dose, 741*t*
similar drugs, 749
therapeutic effects and uses, 747, 748*t*
muscarinic, 191
MUSCARINIC AGONISTS, 199
clinical applications, 201–3
direct acting
bethanechol chloride. *See* bethanechol chloride
carbachol, 202*t*, 204, 1341*t*
cevimeline HCl, 202*t*, 204
pilocarpine, 202*t*, 204, 1341*t*, 1343
effects/actions, 201–2
indirect acting. *See* ACETYLCHOLINESTERASE (ACHE) INHIBITORS
mechanism of action, 200, 201*f*
Nursing Process Application, 207–8*t*
MUSCARINIC ANTAGONISTS, 200*t*, 213
adverse effects, 214*t*, 215
antisecretory agents, 217
glycopyrrolate, 214*t*, 217
mepenzolate, 214*t*, 217
methscopolamine, 214*t*, 217
propantheline, 214*t*, 217
antispasmodic agents, 217
dicyclomine, 214*t*, 217
hyoscyamine, 214*t*, 217
asthma agents/bronchodilators, 217–18
ipratropium. *See* ipratropium
tiotropium bromide, 214*t*, 217, 1245*t*, 1249
atropine. *See* atropine
centrally acting agents, 218
benztropine. *See* benztropine
trihexyphenidyl. *See* trihexyphenidyl
homatropine hydrobromide, 214*t*
Nursing Process Application, 225*t*
ophthalmic agents, 218
cyclopentolate, 214*t*, 218
tropicamide, 214*t*, 218
overdose, 216*t*, 1364*t*
for Parkinson's disease, 355, 355*t*
routes and adult doses, 214*t*
scopolamine. *See* scopolamine
sites of action, 213, 213*f*
for specific conditions, 214–15
extrapyramidal symptoms, 331, 331*t*
nausea and vomiting, 1043*t*
urge incontinence agents, 218
oxybutynin chloride, 214*t*, 218
tolterodine tartrate. *See* tolterodine tartrate
muscarinic receptors, 191, 191*f*, 203*t*
muscle, drugs toxic to, 69–70, 69*t*
MUSCLE RELAXANTS:
as adjuvant analgesics, 447
adverse effects in older adults, 152*t*
centrally acting skeletal
baclofen, 400*t*, 401, 402*t*
carisoprodol, 400*t*, 401
chlorzoxazone, 400*t*, 401
diazepam. *See* diazepam
metaxalone, 400*t*, 401
methocarbamol, 400*t*, 401
for muscle spasms, 398–99, 400*t*
orphenadrine, 400*t*, 402
tizanidine, 400*t*, 402
direct-acting skeletal
botulinum toxin type A, 404*t*, 406
botulinum toxin type B, 404*t*, 406
dantrolene sodium. *See* dantrolene sodium
mechanism of action, 405*f*
for muscle spasticity, 403–6, 404*t*
Nursing Process Application, 407*t*
in surgery, 406–7
muscle rigidity, 348
muscle spasms, 397
complementary and alternative therapies, 397
nonpharmacologic therapy, 397
Nursing Process Application, 407*t*
pharmacotherapy
centrally acting muscle relaxants, 398–402, 400*t*
nonsteroidal anti-inflammatory drugs, 398
muscle spasticity, 402
direct-acting skeletal muscle relaxants for, 403–6, 404*t*
Nursing Process Application, 407*t*
pathophysiology, 402–3
musculoskeletal system, age-related changes, 149*t*
mushroom poisoning, 203
mustard-lewisite, 1363*t*
Mustargen. *See* mechlorethamine
Mutamycin. *See* mitomycin
mutations, 780
Myambutol. *See* ethambutol

myasthenia gravis:
  characteristics, 347*t*
  nutritional issues, 209*t*
  pharmacotherapy, 205–6
    corticosteroids, 205–6
    neostigmine. *See* neostigmine
  symptoms, 205
myasthenic crisis, 206
Mycamine. *See* micafungin
Mycelex. *See* clotrimazole
Mycelex Troche. *See* clotrimazole
Mycobacterium avium complex (MAC), 751, 865
Mycobacterium bovis, 851
Mycobacterium kansasii, 851
Mycobacterium leprae, 777*t,* 851. *See also* leprosy
Mycobacterium scrofulaceum, 851
Mycobacterium tuberculosis, 777*t,* 851. *See also* tuberculosis
Mycobutin. *See* rifabutin
mycolic acid, 851
mycophenolate, 741*t,* 746
Mycoplasma pneumoniae, 777*t*
mycoses, 870. *See also* fungal infections
Mycostatin. *See* nystatin
Mydfrin. *See* phenylephrine
Mydriacyl. *See* tropicamide
mydriasis, 1344
MYDRIATICS, 1347
  phenylephrine, 1348*t*. *See also* phenylephrine
myeloablation, 953
Myfortic. *See* mycophenolate
Mylanta, 1021*t*
Mylanta AP. *See* famotidine
Mylanta Gel-caps, 1021*t*
Myleran. *See* busulfan
Mylocel. *See* hydroxyurea
Mylotarg. *See* gemtuzumab
Myobloc. *See* botulinum toxin type B
myocardial infarction (MI), 598
  blood test values, 599*t*
  incidence and mortality, 602*t*
  pathophysiology, 598
  pharmacotherapy
    ACE inhibitors, 602
    anticoagulants, 600, 602
    antiplatelet agents, 600
    aspirin, 600
    beta-adrenergic blockers, 602
    glycoprotein IIb/IIIa inhibitors, 600
    goals, 598–99
    nitrates, 602
    pain management, 602
    thrombolytic agents, 599, 601*f*
  sexual activity following, 600*t*
  symptoms, 598
myocardial ischemia, 588
myocardium, 487
myoclonic seizures, 375, 376*t*
Myophen. *See* orphenadrine
Mysoline. *See* primidone
Mytelase. *See* ambenonium
myxedema, 1149
myxedematous coma, 1150, 1150*t*
myxoviruses, 909*t*

N

nabilone, 1043*t*
nabumetone, 724*t,* 725*t*
NaCl. *See* sodium chloride (NaCl)
nadir, 958
nadolol, 252*t,* 255
nafarelin, 1192*t,* 1194, 1196
nafcillin, 789*t,* 794–95
naftifine, 878*t*
Naftin. *See* naftifine
nalbuphine, 436*t*
Nalfon. *See* fenoprofen
nalidixic acid, 827, 827*t,* 840*t,* 847
nalmefene, 447*t,* 448
naloxone, 447–48
  adverse effects, 447*t,* 448
  classification, 447
  contraindications/precautions, 448
  drug interactions, 448
  mechanism of action, 448
  nursing responsibilities, 448
  for opioid dependence, 99
  overdose treatment, 448
  patient and family education, 448
  pharmacokinetics, 448
  pregnancy category, 448
  route and adult dose, 447*t*
  similar drugs, 448
  therapeutic effects and uses, 447, 1364*t*
naltrexone, 102, 448
NANDA (North American Nursing Diagnosis Association), 117
nandrolone, 1220*t,* 1223
NAPAmide. *See* disopyramide
naphazoline, 238, 1273*t,* 1348*t*
Naphcon. *See* naphazoline
Naprosyn. *See* naproxen
naproxen, 101*t,* 723, 724*t,* 725*t*
naratriptan, 450*t,* 452
Narcan. *See* naloxone
narcoanalysis, 459
narcolepsy, 279, 419
  pharmacotherapy, 420
    modafinil. *See* modafinil
    Nursing Process Application, 423*t*
    sodium oxybate, 280, 421
  symptoms, 419–20
narcotic, 434
Nardil. *See* phenelzine
Naropin. *See* ropivacaine
narrow-angle glaucoma, 1340. *See also* glaucoma
narrow-spectrum antibiotic, 782
Nasacort. *See* triamcinolone
Nasacort AQ. *See* triamcinolone
NASAL DECONGESTANTS, 1271–72
  ephedrine. *See* ephedrine
  ipratropium, 1273*t*. *See also* ipratropium
  naphazoline, 1273*t*
  oxymetazoline, 1273*t*
  phenylephrine. *See* phenylephrine
  pseudoephedrine. *See* pseudoephedrine
  tetrahydrozoline, 1273*t*
  xylometazoline, 1273*t*
NasalCrom. *See* cromolyn
Nasalide. *See* flunisolide
Nasarel. *See* flunisolide
nasogastric tube, drug administration via, 31
Nasonex. *See* mometasone
natalizumab, 365–66, 366*t,* 748*t,* 1037
nateglinide, 1133*t,* 1137
National Coordinating Council for Medication Error Reporting and Prevention (NCC MERP), 80, 81*f,* 82*f*
National Formulary (NF), 15–16
National Nurse Emergency Preparedness Initiative, 1358
Native American culture, depression treatment in, 300*t*
Natrecor. *See* nesiritide
natrexone, 447*t*
natriuresis, 549
natriuretic peptides, 609
Naturacil. *See* psyllium mucilloid
nausea, 1040
nausea and vomiting:
  during enteral nutrition therapy, 1071*t,* 1073
  with opioids, 436*t,* 437, 437*t*
  pathophysiology, 1040–41
  pharmacotherapy. *See* ANTIEMETICS
  postanesthesia, 477
  in pregnancy, 1041
Navane. *See* thiothixene
Navelbine. *See* vinorelbine
NCC MERP (National Coordinating Council for Medication Error Reporting and Prevention), 80, 81*f,* 82*f*
NDA (New Drug Application), 18
Nebcin. *See* tobramycin
nebivolol, 252*t,* 258
nebulizer, 1242
NebuPent. *See* pentamidine
Necator americanus, 901
nedocromil sodium, 1250*t,* 1253, 1349*t*
nefazodone, 304*t,* 312–13
negative chronotropic effect, 518
negative feedback, 1099, 1101, 1101*f*
negative inotropic effect, 518
negative symptoms, schizophrenia, 327, 327*t*
NegGram. *See* nalidixic acid
Neisseria gonorrhoeae, 777*t,* 829
Neisseria meningitidis, 760, 777*t*. *See also* meningococcal infection
nelarabine, 973*t,* 976
nelfinavir, 933*t,* 939–40
neoadjuvant chemotherapy, 953. *See also* ANTINEOPLASTIC AGENTS
Neoloid. *See* castor oil
neomycin, 816*t,* 819
neoplasm, 950
NeoProfen. *See* ibuprofen lysine
Neoral. *See* cyclosporine
Neosar. *See* cyclophosphamide
Neosporin, 819
neostigmine, 206–7
  adverse effects, 206
  classification, 206
  contraindications/precautions, 206
  drug interactions, 206
  mechanism of action, 206
  nursing responsibilities, 206–7
  overdose treatment, 206
  patient and family education, 207
  pharmacokinetics, 206
  pregnancy category, 206
  for reversal of nondepolarizing neuromuscular blockers, 223
  similar drugs, 207
  therapeutic effects and uses, 206
Neo-Synephrine. *See* phenylephrine
Neo-Synephrine 4–6 Hour. *See* phenylephrine
nephrons, 545, 545*f*
nephropathy, diabetic, 1126

nephrotoxicity, drugs, 69, 69*t*, 548*t*
Neptazane. *See* methazolamide
nerve agents:
GA-Sarin, 1362*t*
GA-Soman, 1362*t*
GA-Tabun, 1362*t*
prophylaxis, 204–5
VX, 1362*t*
nerve block, 471, 471*f*
nervous system, 185, 186*f*. *See also* central nervous system; peripheral nervous system
Nesacaine. *See* chloroprocaine
nesiritide, 619
Neulasta. *See* pegfilgrastim
Neumega. *See* oprelvekin
Neupogen. *See* filgrastim
neuraminidase, 915
neuraminidase inhibitors:
oseltamivir, 915, 916*t*
zanamivir, 915, 916*t*
neurodegenerative diseases, 347
Alzheimer's disease. *See* Alzheimer's disease
amyotrophic lateral sclerosis. *See* amyotrophic lateral sclerosis
Huntington's disease. *See* Huntington's disease
muscle spasticity in, 402–3
myasthenia gravis. *See* myasthenia gravis
Parkinson's disease. *See* Parkinson's disease
neuroeffector junction, 188
neurofibrillary tangles, 358, 359*f*
neurolept analgesia, 461
neuroleptic, 330. *See also* antipsychotics
neuroleptic malignant syndrome (NMS), 332
NEUROMUSCULAR BLOCKERS, 214, 219*t*
as adjuncts to anesthesia, 477
depolarizing, 220, 221*f*
succinylcholine chloride. *See* succinylcholine chloride
nondepolarizing, 223
atracurium, 219*t*, 224, 477
cisatracurium, 219*t*, 224, 477
mivacurium, 219*t*, 224
pancuronium, 219*t*, 224
rocuronium, 219*t*, 224
tubocurarine. *See* tubocurarine
vecuronium, 219*t*, 224
neurons, 266–67, 270*t*
neuropathic pain, 429, 444, 446
neuropathy, diabetic, 1125–26
neurotoxicity, 69, 69*t*
neurotransmitters, 188. *See also specific neurotransmitters*
actions/effects, 189*t*, 267*t*
in appetite suppression, 1087
clinical applications, 189*t*, 267*t*
in depression, 299
in synaptic transmission, 188, 190, 266–67, 266*f*
Neutrogena. *See* salicylic acid
neutropenia, 672, 674*t*, 959
nevirapine, 933*t*, 937
New Drug Application (NDA), 18
New York Heart Association (NYHA), 610
Nexavar. *See* sorafenib
Nexium, 30*t*. *See also* esomeprazole
NF *(National Formulary)*, 15–16
Niac. *See* niacin
niacin (nicotinic acid; vitamin B_3):
adverse effects, 504*t*, 509
deficiency, 1053*t*
dosage forms not to be crushed or opened, 30*t*
functions, 1053*t*
mechanism of action, 503*f*, 509
for nutritional disorders
adverse effects, 1054*t*
route and adult dose, 1054*t*
route and adult dose, 504*t*
sites of action, 213–14, 213*f*
nicardipine, 522
adverse effects, 520*t*
route and adult dose, 520*t*
for specific conditions
angina, 592*t*
hypertension, 519*t*
hypertensive emergency, 584*t*
nicardipine SR, 519*t*
Nicobid. *See* niacin
Nicoderm. *See* nicotine replacement therapy
Nicorette. *See* nicotine replacement therapy
nicotine:
dependence, 107
effects/actions, 107, 209
toxicity, 209
withdrawal symptoms and treatment, 96*t*
nicotine replacement therapy, 107, 108*f*, 209
nicotinic, 191
nicotinic acid. *See* niacin
NICOTINIC AGONISTS, 199, 209
NICOTINIC ANTAGONISTS, 200*t*, 213, 213*f*
ganglionic blockers, 218, 219*t*
mecamylamine. *See* mecamylamine
neuromuscular blockers. *See* NEUROMUSCULAR BLOCKERS
nicotinic receptors, 191, 191*f*, 192*t*
Nicotrol NS. *See* nicotine replacement therapy
nifedipine, 520–21
adverse effects, 520, 520*t*
classification, 520
contraindications/precautions, 520–21
dosage forms not to be crushed or opened, 30*t*
drug interactions, 521
mechanism of action, 520
nursing responsibilities, 521
overdose treatment, 521
patient and family education, 521
pharmacokinetics, 520
potency versus amlodipine, 58
pregnancy category, 521
route and adult dose, 520*t*
similar drugs, 521–22
for specific conditions, 519*t*
angina, 592*t*
preterm labor, 1187*t*, 1190
therapeutic effects and uses, 520
nifedipine SR, 519*t*. *See also* nifedipine
nifurtimox, 892*t*, 898
Nilandron. *See* nilutamide
nilotinib, 748*t*, 990*t*
Nilstat. *See* nystatin
nilutamide, 980*t*, 984
Nimbex. *See* cisatracurium
nimodipine, 519*t*
Nimotop. *See* nimodipine
Nipent. *See* pentostatin
Nipride. *See* nitroprusside sodium
Nisocor. *See* nisoldipine
nisoldipine, 519*t*, 520*t*, 522
nitazoxanide, 892*t*, 894
nitrates. *See* organic nitrates
nitric oxide, 592
nitrofurantoin, 846–47
adverse effects, 840*t*, 846
classification, 846
contraindications/precautions, 846
drug interactions, 846
mechanism of action, 846
nursing responsibilities, 846
overdose treatment, 846
patient and family education, 847
pharmacokinetics, 846
pregnancy category, 846
route and adult dose, 840*t*
similar drugs, 847
for specific conditions
acute uncomplicated cystitis, 838
therapeutic effects and uses, 846
nitrofurantoin macrocrystals. *See* nitrofurantoin
nitrogen mustard-HN-1, HN-2, HN-3, 1363*t*
NITROGEN MUSTARDS:
chlorambucil, 967*t*, 970
cyclophosphamide. *See* cyclophosphamide
estramustine, 967*t*, 970–71
ifosfamide, 967*t*, 971
mechlorethamine, 967*t*, 971
melphalan, 967*t*, 971
nitroglycerin, 593–94
adverse effects, 592*t*, 593
classification, 593
contraindications/precautions, 593–94
dosage forms not to be crushed or opened, 30*t*
drug interactions, 101*t*, 594
mechanism of action, 593
Nursing Process Application, 596*t*
nursing responsibilities, 594
overdose treatment, 594
patient and family education, 594
pharmacokinetics, 593
pregnancy category, 594
route and adult dose, 592*t*
similar drugs, 594–95
therapeutic effects and uses, 593
Nitropress. *See* nitroprusside sodium
nitroprusside sodium, 582
adverse effects, 582
classification, 582
contraindications/precautions, 582
drug interactions, 582
for hypertensive emergency, 584*t*
mechanism of action, 582
nursing responsibilities, 582
patient and family education, 582
pharmacokinetics, 582
pregnancy category, 582
similar drugs, 582, 584*t*
therapeutic effects and uses, 582
NITROSOUREAS:
adverse effects, 68*t*, 967*t*
carmustine, 960, 967*t*, 970
lomustine, 967*t*, 971
streptozocin, 967*t*, 971
Nitrostat, 30*t*. *See also* nitroglycerin
nitrous oxide, 466–67
adverse effects, 467, 468*t*
classification, 466

contraindications/precautions, 467
drug interactions, 467
effects, 189*t*
mechanism of action, 466–67
nursing responsibilities, 467
overdose treatment, 467
patient and family education, 467
pharmacokinetics, 467
pregnancy category, 467
route and adult dose, 468*t*
therapeutic effects and uses, 466
nits, 1318
Nix. *See* permethrin
nizatidine, 1016*t*, 1019
Nizoral. *See* ketoconazole
NMS (neuroleptic malignant syndrome), 332
nociceptor(s), 428
nociceptor pain, 429
Nolvadex. *See* tamoxifen
nomogram, 140
for body surface area estimation, 140, 141*f*
nonadherence, 24, 24*t*
NONBENZODIAZEPINE ANXIOLYTICS:
for anxiety and insomnia, 282*t*, 285–86
drugs in class
buspirone, 282*t*, 287, 288
eszopiclone, 282*t*, 288
ramelteon, 276, 282*t*, 288
zaleplon, 282*t*, 288
zolpidem. *See* zolpidem
nondepolarizing neuromuscular blocker, 223. *See also* NEUROMUSCULAR BLOCKERS, nondepolarizing
nonmalarial protozoan infections:
amebiasis, 886*t*, 891–92, 891*f*, 891*t*, 892*t*
cryptosporidiosis, 886*t*, 892*t*, 893
giardiasis, 886*t*, 892–93, 892*t*, 893*t*
leishmaniasis, 886*t*, 892*t*, 896–97
Nursing Process Application, 899*t*
pharmacotherapy
eflornithine, 892*t*, 896, 898
iodoquinol, 892, 892*t*, 894
melarsoprol, 892*t*, 898
metronidazole. *See* metronidazole
nifurtimox, 892*t*, 898
nitazoxanide, 892*t*, 894
paromomycin, 892, 892*t*, 894–95
pentamidine, 892*t*
pyrimethamine-sulfadiazine. *See* pyrimethamine-sulfadiazine
sodium stibogluconate, 892*t*, 898
suramin, 892*t*, 898
tinidazole, 892*t*, 895
toxoplasmosis, 886*t*, 892*t*, 895
trichomoniasis, 892*t*, 895–96, 896*t*
trypanosomiasis, 886*t*, 892*t*, 896
NONNUCLEOSIDE REVERSE TRANSCRIPTASE INHIBITORS, 936
delavirdine, 933*t*, 937
efavirenz. *See* efavirenz
etravirine, 933*t*, 937
nevirapine, 933*t*, 937
NONOPIOID ANALGESICS:
acetaminophen. *See* acetaminophen
centrally acting agents
clonidine. *See* clonidine
tramadol. *See* tramadol
ziconotide, 443*t*, 444
nonsteroidal anti-inflammatory drugs. *See* NONSTEROIDAL ANTI-INFLAMMATORY DRUGS (NSAIDs)
Nursing Process Application, 445*t*
nonoxynol-9, 1211–12
adverse effects, 1211
classification, 1211
contraindications/precautions, 1211
drug interactions, 1211
nursing responsibilities, 1211
overdose treatment, 1211
patient and family education, 1212
pharmacokinetics, 1211
therapeutic effects and uses, 1211
nonphenothiazines. *See* FIRST-GENERATION ANTIPSYCHOTICS, nonphenothiazines
non–rapid eye movement (NREM) sleep, 277, 278*t*
nonrestorative sleep, 279
nonspecific body defense system, 709
complements, 711*t*
fever, 711*t*
inflammation. *See* inflammation
interferons, 711*t*. *See also* INTERFERON(S) (IFNs)
mucous membranes, 711*t*
natural killer cells, 711*t*
phagocytes, 711*t*
physical barriers, 709, 711*t*
NONSTEROIDAL ANTI-INFLAMMATORY DRUGS (NSAIDs):
adverse effects, 727*t*
gastrointestinal ulcers, 720, 721*f*, 1009
in older adults, 152*t*
cyclooxygenase-2 (COX-2) inhibitors, 727
celecoxib. *See* celecoxib
drug interactions
with alcohol, 101*t*
with herbal products, 178*t*
Evidence-Based Practice, 727*t*
ibuprofen-like agents
versus aspirin, 725
costs, 723
diclofenac, 724*t*, 725*t*
diflunisal, 724*t*, 725*t*
etodolac, 724*t*, 725*t*
fenoprofen, 724*t*, 725*t*
flurbiprofen, 724*t*, 725*t*
ibuprofen. *See* ibuprofen
indomethacin, 724*t*, 725*t*
ketoprofen, 724*t*, 725*t*
ketorolac, 724*t*, 725*t*
meclofenamate, 724*t*, 725*t*
mefenamic acid, 724*t*, 725*t*
meloxicam, 724*t*, 725*t*
nabumetone, 724*t*, 725*t*
naproxen, 724*t*, 725*t*
oxaprozin, 724*t*, 725*t*
piroxicam, 724*t*, 725*t*
similarities among, 723
sulindac, 724*t*, 725*t*
tolmetin, 724*t*, 725*t*
indications for use, 725*t*
Nursing Process Application, 729*t*
salicylates
aspirin. *See* aspirin
choline and magnesium trisalicylate, 720*t*, 723
magnesium salicylate, 720*t*, 723
poisoning, 720*t*
salsalate, 720*t*, 723
for specific conditions
gout, 1307
muscle spasms, 398
osteoarthritis, 1302
Noradrenaline. *See* norepinephrine
Norco. *See* acetaminophen; hydrocodone
Norcuron. *See* vecuronium
Norditropin. *See* somatropin
norepinephrine (NE), 188, 266
actions/effects, 189*t*, 267*t*
adverse effects, 232*t*, 235, 612*t*
life cycle, 193*f*
receptors, 192, 192*t*
release, 195, 229–30, 230*f*
route and adult dose, 232*t*, 612*t*
for specific conditions, 267*t*
heart failure, 612*t*
shock, 235
termination of action, 194–95
norethindrone, 1206
Norflex. *See* orphenadrine
norfloxacin, 827*t*, 830, 838
normal serum albumin, 690
adverse effects, 690
classification, 690
contraindications/precautions, 690
drug interactions, 690
mechanism of action, 690
nursing responsibilities, 690
overdose treatment, 690
patient and family education, 691
pharmacokinetics, 690
pregnancy, 690
therapeutic effects and uses, 690
Normodyne. *See* labetalol
Noroxin. *See* norfloxacin
Norpace. *See* disopyramide
Norplant, 1210
Norpramin. *See* desipramine
North American Nursing Diagnosis Association (NANDA), 117
nortriptyline:
for anxiety disorders, 290*t*, 307
for depression, 304*t*
Norvasc. *See* amlodipine
Norvir. *See* ritonavir
nosocomial infections, 781–82, 782*t*
Novahistine DH, 1276*t*
Novantrone. *See* mitoxantrone
Novarel. *See* human chorionic gonadotropin (HCG)
Novastan. *See* argatroban
Novocaine. *See* procaine
Novolin 70/30, 1130*t*
Novolin R. *See* human regular insulin
NovoLog. *See* insulin aspart
NovoLog Mix, 1130*t*
NPH. *See* isophane insulin
NSAIDs. *See* NONSTEROIDAL ANTI-INFLAMMATORY DRUGS (NSAIDs)
Nubain. *See* nalbuphine
NUCLEOSIDE/NUCLEOTIDE REVERSE TRANSCRIPTASE INHIBITORS, 932–34
abacavir, 933*t*, 935
didanosine, 933*t*, 935
emtricitabine, 933*t*, 935
lamivudine. *See* lamivudine
stavudine, 933*t*, 936
tenofovir, 933*t*, 936
zidovudine. *See* zidovudine

Nupercainal. *See* dibucaine
nurse(s):
  chemotherapy administration requirements, 960–61
  substance abuse in, 103*t*
nursing diagnosis, 115, 117*t*
nursing process, 115, 116*f*
  assessment, 115
  diagnosis, 115–17
  evaluation, 119–20
  implementation, 118–19, 119*f*
  in medication error prevention, 87
  planning, 117–18
Nursing Process Applications:
  ACE inhibitor therapy, 537–38*t*
  adrenergic agonist therapy, 241*t*
  adrenergic antagonist therapy, 258*t*
  5-alpha reductase inhibitors, 1233*t*
  Alzheimer's disease therapy, 363*t*
  androgen therapy, 1224*t*
  antibiotic therapy
    sulfonamides, 844–45*t*
    tetracyclines, macrolides, and aminoglycosides, 819–20*t*
  anticoagulant therapy, 652*t*
  antidepressant therapy, 315–17*t*
  antidiarrheal therapy, 1036*t*
  antidiuretic hormone therapy, 1116*t*
  antidysrhythmic therapies, 637*t*
  antiemetic therapy, 1046*t*
  antiepileptic medications, 393*t*
  antifungal therapy, 881–82*t*
  antiglaucoma therapy, 1346*t*
  antigout therapy, 1311*t*
  antihelminthic agents, 904*t*
  antipsychotic therapy, 342–43*t*
  antiretroviral therapy, 941–42*t*
  antithyroid therapy, 1157*t*
  antituberculosis therapy, 864*t*
  antiviral drug therapy for non-HIV viral infections, 923*t*
  anxiety or sleep disorders, 293*t*
  asthma, 1257*t*
  attention deficit/hyperactivity disorder therapy, 423*t*
  bipolar disorder therapy, 321*t*
  bisphosphonates, 1298*t*
  calcium channel blocker therapy, 525*t*
  calcium supplements, 1289*t*
  cancer chemotherapy, 988–89*t*
  cardiac glycosides, 617*t*
  cholinergic agonist therapy, 207–8*t*
  chronic obstructive pulmonary disease, 1257*t*
  corticosteroid therapy
    inhaled, 1272*t*
    systemic, 1172*t*
  direct vasodilator therapy, 583*t*
  diuretic therapy, 562–63*t*
  enteral nutrition therapy, 1075–76*t*
  epoetin alfa therapy, 672*t*
  fluid replacement therapy, 693*t*
  fluoroquinolone therapy, 831*t*
  general anesthesia, 470*t*
  growth hormone therapy, 1113*t*
  H_1-receptor antagonists, 1269*t*
  H_2-receptor antagonists, 1020*t*
  hyperlipidemia, 511*t*
  immunizations, 770*t*
  immunomodulators, 750*t*
  insulin therapy, 1131*t*
  iron supplementation, 681*t*
  lice or mite infestation, 1321*t*
  local anesthesia, 476*t*
  muscarinic antagonist (anticholinergic) therapy, 225*t*
  muscle spasms and spasticity therapy, 407*t*
  narcolepsy therapy, 423*t*
  nitroglycerin therapy, 596*t*
  nonopioid analgesic therapy, 445*t*
  nonsteroidal anti-inflammatory drugs, 729*t*
  opioid therapy, 441*t*
  oral contraceptives, 1207*t*
  oral hypoglycemic therapy, 1140–41*t*
  otitis media therapy, 1353*t*
  Parkinson's disease therapy, 357*t*
  penicillin or cephalosporin therapy, 799–800*t*
  progestin therapy, 1185*t*
  proton pump inhibitors, 1017*t*
  protozoan infections, 899*t*
  thrombolytic therapy, 660*t*
  thyroid hormone replacement therapy, 1153*t*
  total parenteral nutrition therapy, 1081*t*
  tretinoin therapy, 1326*t*
  uterine stimulants, 1190*t*
  vitamin or mineral supplementation, 1064*t*
  weight reduction drugs, 1093–94*t*
Nursing Responsibilities:
  abortifacient, 1215
  ACE inhibitors, 535
  acetaminophen, 730
  acetylcholinesterase inhibitors, 362
  activated charcoal, 1365
  adrenergic agonists
    alpha-adrenergic agonists, 237
    $alpha_2$-adrenergic agonists, 578
    beta-adrenergic agonists, 240
    nonselective adrenergic agonists, 234
  adrenergic antagonists
    alpha-adrenergic antagonists, 250
    $beta_1$-adrenergic antagonists, 256–57, 597
    nonselective beta-adrenergic antagonists, 254
  5-alpha reductase inhibitors, 1233–34
  5-aminosalicylates, 1038
  amphetamines, 417
  angiotensin II receptor blockers, 539
  anorexiants, 1091
  antacids, 1022
  antianemic agents
    cyanocobalamin, 683
    ferrous sulfate, 679
  antibiotics
    aminoglycosides, 818
    broad-spectrum penicillins, 793
    carbapenems, 801
    cephalosporins, 797–98
    fluoroquinolones, 830
    macrolides, 815
    natural penicillins, 791
    sulfonamides, 843
    tetracyclines, 812
    urinary tract antiseptics, 846
    vancomycin, 802
  anticoagulants
    oral, 651
    parenteral, 647, 649
  antidepressants
    monoamine oxidase inhibitors, 315
    selective serotonin reuptake inhibitors, 310
    tricyclic antidepressants, 306–7
  antidiarrheals, 1035
  antidiuretic hormone, 1115
  antidysrhythmic drugs
    potassium channel blockers, 635
    sodium channel blockers, 631
  antiemetics, 1045
  antifungal drugs
    amphotericin B, 874
    fluconazole, 876
    nystatin, 880
  antiglaucoma agents, 1342, 1345–46
  antigout agents
    uric acid inhibitors, 1308
    xanthine oxidase inhibitors, 1310
  antihelminthic drugs, 903
  antileprosy drugs, 863
  antimalaria drugs, 889
  antineoplastic agents, 965–66
    alkylating agents, 969
    antimetabolites, 974
    antitumor antibiotics, 978
    hormone antagonists, 982
    vinca alkaloids, 986
  antiplatelet agents
    ADP receptor blockers, 655
    glycoprotein IIb/IIIa receptor inhibitors, 657
  antiprotozoan agents, 894, 898
  antipsychotics
    first-generation, 334
    second-generation (atypical), 338
  antiretrovirals
    nonnucleoside reverse transcriptase inhibitors, 937
    nucleoside/nucleotide reverse transcriptase inhibitors, 934–35
    protease inhibitors, 938–39
  antiseizure drugs
    gabapentin, 389
    hydantoins, 385
    iminostilbenes, 387
    succinimides, 388
    valproic acid, 390–91
  antituberculosis drugs, 859
  antitussives, 1277
  antiviral drugs
    for hepatitis, 921
    for herpesviruses, 913
  barbiturates, 292
  benzodiazepines
    diazepam, 383
    lorazepam, 285
  bile acid sequestrants, 508
  bisphosphonates, 1296
  bronchodilators
    anticholinergics, 1249
    $beta_2$-adrenergic agonists, 1246–47
  calcium channel blockers
    dihydropyridine, 521
    nondihydropyridine, 523–24
  calcium supplements, 1288
  cardiac glycosides, 616
  chelating agents, 1366–67
  cholinergic agonists, 203–4, 207
  CNS stimulants, 417, 420–21, 422
  corticosteroids
    beclomethasone, 1251
    hydrocortisone, 1168
    intranasal, 1271
  direct vasodilators, 580, 582

disease-modifying antirheumatic drugs, 1305
diuretics
carbonic anhydrase inhibitors, 561
loop (high-ceiling), 552
osmotic, 560
potassium-sparing, 557
thiazide, 555
dopamine agonists, 354
dopamine replacement therapy, 352
dopamine system stabilizer, 341
electrolytes
magnesium sulfate, 700
potassium chloride, 698–99
female infertility agents, 1194
fibric acid agents, 510
fluid replacement agents
colloids, 693–94
normal serum albumin, 690
general anesthetics
barbiturate, 461
benzodiazepines, 464
gaseous, 467
intravenous, 465
opioid, 462
volatile liquid, 468–69
glucagon, 1125
H_1-receptor antagonists, 1267
H_2-receptor antagonists, 1018
hematopoietic growth factors
colony-stimulating factors, 673
erythropoietin, 671
platelet enhancers, 675
hemostatic agents, 661
hormones
estrogens, 1180–81
oral contraceptives, 1205–6
testosterone, 1222
immune globulin, 769
immunostimulants
interferons, 736
interleukins, 739
immunosuppressants
antimetabolites/cytotoxic agents, 745–46
calcineurin inhibitors, 743–44
monoclonal antibodies, 749
insulin, 1129
laxatives, 1032
leukotriene modifiers, 1254
lipase inhibitors, 1092
local anesthetics
amides, 475
esters, 474
mast cell stabilizers, 1253
methylxanthines
caffeine, 422
theophylline, 1255–56
mineralocorticoids, 1171
mood stabilizers, 320
muscarinic antagonists
atropine, 217
benztropine, 356
nasal decongestants, 1274
nicotinic antagonists
mecamylamine, 220
succinylcholine, 222
tubocurarine, 224
nonbenzodiazepine anxiolytics, 287
nonopioid centrally acting analgesics, 443–44
nonsteroidal anti-inflammatory drugs
COX-2 inhibitors, 728
ibuprofen-like agents, 726
salicylates, 722
nonstimulant for ADHD, 419
opioid analgesics, 438–39
opioid antagonists, 448
oral hypoglycemics, 1139
organic nitrates, 594
otic medications, 1352
pancreatic enzymes, 1047–48
phosphodiesterase inhibitors, 619
potassium channel blockers, 635
progestins, 1184
proton pump inhibitors, 1015
retinoids, 1324
scabicides/pediculicides, 1319–20
selective estrogen receptor modulators, 1299
skeletal muscle relaxants
centrally acting, 400–401
direct-acting, 405
sodium bicarbonate, 703–4
sodium channel blockers, 631
spermicides, 1211
statins, 505
thrombolytic agents, 659
thyroid replacement agents, 1152
tocolytics, 1188–89
topical anesthetics, 1332–33
triptans, 452
vaccines, 762
vitamins
cyanocobalamin (vitamin B_{12}), 1060
folic acid (vitamin B_9), 1061
pyridoxine (vitamin B_6), 1059
riboflavin (vitamin B_2), 1059
thiamine (vitamin B_1), 1058
vitamin A, 1055–56
vitamin C, 1061
vitamin D, 1056
vitamin E, 1057
vitamin K, 1058
nutritional supplementation, 1068. *See also* enteral nutrition; parenteral nutrition
Nutropin. *See* somatropin
nuts, 501*t*
Nuvagil. *See* armodafinil
NuvaRing, 33, 34*f*, 1210
Nydrazid. *See* isoniazid
NYHA (New York Heart Association), 610
nystatin, 880–81
adverse effects, 880
in pediatric patients, 142*t*
classification, 880
contraindications/precautions, 880
drug interactions, 880
mechanism of action, 880
nursing responsibilities, 880
overdose treatment, 880
patient and family education, 880
pediatric dosage/route, 142*t*
pharmacokinetics, 880
pregnancy category, 880
similar drugs, 880–81
for specific conditions
oropharyngeal candidiasis, 879
therapeutic effects and uses, 880
Nystex. *See* nystatin
Nystop, see nystatin

O

OA. *See* osteoarthritis
oat products, 501*t*
obesity:
in children and adolescents, 1086*t*
classification, 1087*t*
etiology, 1086*t*
incidence, 1086*t*, 1087*t*
measurement of, 1087
medication error, 1087*f*
nonpharmacologic therapy, 1087–89, 1089*t*
pathogenesis, 1086–87
pharmacotherapy, 1089–90
adjuncts
artificial sweeteners, 1093
fat substitutes, 1093
anorexiants. *See* ANOREXIANTS
lipase inhibitors. *See* LIPASE INHIBITORS
Nursing Process Application, 1093–94*t*
OBS (organic brain syndrome), 333
obsessive–compulsive disorder, 276, 289, 290*t*
occupational health nurse (OHN), 166–67
Octagam. *See* intravenous immune globulin
octreotide, 1111–12
adverse effects, 1111
classification, 1111
contraindications/precautions, 1111
drug interactions, 1111
mechanism of action, 1111
nursing responsibilities, 1112
overdose treatment, 1112
patient and family education, 1112
pharmacokinetics, 1111
pregnancy category, 1112
similar drugs, 1112
for specific conditions
diarrhea, 1034*t*, 1035
therapeutic effects and uses, 1111
OcuClear. *See* oxymetazoline
Ocufen. *See* flurbiprofen
OCULAR DECONGESTANTS/VASOCONSTRICTORS, 236
naphazoline, 238, 1273*t*, 1348*t*
oxymetazoline, 238, 1348, 1348*t*
phenylephrine. *See* phenylephrine
tetrahydrozoline, 236, 238, 1348, 1348*t*
OCULAR LUBRICANTS, 1348
lanolin alcohol, 1348, 1348*t*
polyvinyl alcohol, 1348, 1348*t*
Ocupress. *See* carteolol
Ocusert. *See* pilocarpine
ofloxacin, 831
adverse effects, 827*t*, 855*t*
route and adult dose, 827*t*, 855*t*
for specific conditions
leprosy, 862
tuberculosis, 855*t*, 861
Ogen. *See* estropipate
OGTT (oral glucose tolerance test), 1122, 1123*t*
OHN (occupational health nurse), 166–67
olanzapine, 319*t*, 337*t*, 339
older adults:
acid suppression and vitamin B_{12} in, 1022*t*
adherence in, 150–51, 151*t*
adverse drug reactions in, 151–53, 153*t*
chemotherapy administration, 984*t*
definition, 147
demographics, 147*t*
depression in, 300–301
diuretic therapy in, 549*t*
drug interactions in, 153*t*

drug misuse in, 150–51
drug monitoring in, 150*t*
fluid and electrolytes in, 695*t*
H_1-receptor antagonists in, 1267*t*
high-risk drugs, 152*t*
infections in, 795*t*
medication costs and, 151*t*
ophthalmic drug teaching for, 1350*t*
pain expression and management in, 442*t*
pharmacodynamic changes, 150
pharmacokinetic changes
absorption, 148
distribution, 148–49
excretion, 150
metabolism, 149–50
physiologic changes affecting response to drugs, 148, 149*t*, 166*t*
polyherbacy in, 177*t*
polypharmacy in, 147–48, 147*t*
seizures in, 371*t*, 373–74, 375*t*
spending on prescription drugs, 148*t*
teaching tips, 118*t*
thyroid disease in, 1150*t*
thyroid hormone use and hip fracture risk in, 1150*t*
urinary tract infections in, 839–40
vaccine administration, 766*t*
Olestra, 1093
oligomenorrhea, 1183
oligomeric formulas, for enteral nutrition, 1069–70, 1069*t*
oligospermia, 1226
olmesartan medoxomil, 538*t*, 540
olopatadine, 1265*t*, 1349*t*
olsalazine, 1037*t*, 1039
omalizumab, 748*t*, 1256
omega-3 fatty acids, 501*t*
omeprazole, 1014–15
adverse effects, 1014
classification, 1014
contraindications/precautions, 1014
dosage forms not to be crushed or opened, 30*t*
drug interactions, 178*t*, 1014–15
mechanism of action, 1014
nursing responsibilities, 1015
overdose treatment, 1015
patient and family education, 1015
pharmacokinetics, 1014
pregnancy category, 1015
similar drugs, 1015
therapeutic effects and uses, 1014, 1023
Omnaris. *See* ciclesonide
Omnicef. *See* cefdinir
Oncaspar. *See* pegaspargase
oncology nurse, 993
Oncovin. *See* vincristine
ondansetron, 477, 1043*t*
on-off syndrome, 349
onychomycosis, 877–79
open-angle glaucoma, 1339*f*, 1340. *See also* glaucoma
Ophthaine. *See* proparacaine hydrochloride
ophthalmic administration, 32, 33*f*
opiates, 434. *See also* OPIOID ANALGESICS
opioid(s), 98. *See also* OPIOID ANALGESICS; OPIOID ANESTHETICS
abuse, 99
as antidiarrheal agents. *See* ANTIDIARRHEALS, opioids
combination drugs for severe cold symptoms, 1276*t*
dependence, 99
OPIOID ANALGESICS, 434–35
adverse effects, 435, 437, 437*t*
drug interactions, 178*t*
mechanism of action, 435
mixed opioid agonist-antagonists, 434–35, 434*f*
buprenorphine, 436*t*, 440
butorphanol, 436*t*, 440
nalbuphine, 436*t*, 440, 442
pentazocine, 436*t*, 442
Nursing Process Application, 441*t*
opioid agonists, 434, 434*f*
codeine. *See* codeine
fentanyl. *See* fentanyl
hydrocodone, 436*t*, 439
hydromorphone, 436*t*, 439
levorphanol, 436*t*, 439–40
meperidine. *See* meperidine
methadone, 436*t*, 440
morphine sulfate. *See* morphine sulfate
oxycodone. *See* oxycodone
propoxyphene, 436*t*, 440
propoxyphene napsylate, 436*t*
tolerance, 437
withdrawal symptoms and treatment, 96*t*
OPIOID ANESTHETICS, 461
alfentanil, 460*t*, 462
fentanyl. *See* fentanyl
remifentanil, 460*t*, 462–63
sufentanil, 460*t*, 463
OPIOID ANTAGONISTS, 434*f*, 435
indications, 447
nalmefene, 447*t*, 448
naloxone. *See* naloxone
naltrexone, 447*t*, 448
opium, 434
opportunistic infections, in HIV-AIDS:
M. avium, 865
pathophysiology, 944–45
pharmacotherapy, 945*t*
tuberculosis, 856
oprelvekin, 675
adverse effects, 675
classification, 675
contraindications/precautions, 675
drug interactions, 675
mechanism of action, 674, 675
nursing responsibilities, 675
overdose treatment, 675
patient and family education, 675
pharmacokinetics, 675
pregnancy category, 675
therapeutic effects and uses, 675, 993
OptiClik injector pen, 1132*t*
OptiPranolol. *See* metipranolol
Optivar. *See* azelastine
ORAL CONTRACEPTIVES:
for acne vulgaris, 1322–23, 1322*t*
adverse effects, 68*t*, 1206, 1208–9, 1208*t*
combination estrogen-progestin
administration, 1204, 1204*f*
advantages, 1202–4
extended regimen, 1204
failure, 1203
mechanism of action, 1204
preparations, 1203*t*, 1204*f*
return of fertility after, 1204
types, 1204
contraindications, 1209*t*
drug interactions, 178*t*
emergency. *See* emergency contraception
estrogens in, 1200
extended regimen, 1204
mechanism of action, 1202*f*
Nursing Process Application, 1207*t*
progestin-only, 1201*t*, 1203*t*, 1206
progestins in, 1200, 1203*t*
oral glucose tolerance test (OGTT), 1122, 1123*t*
ORAL HYPOGLYCEMICS:
alpha-glucosidase inhibitors, 1138
acarbose. *See* acarbose
actions, 1132*t*
mechanism of action, 1138
miglitol, 1133*t*, 1139
nursing considerations, 1132*t*
biguanides
actions, 1132*t*
mechanism of action, 1135
metformin. *See* metformin
nursing considerations, 1132*t*
combination agents, 1134*t*, 1139
dipeptidyl-peptidase 4 inhibitor
sitagliptin. *See* sitagliptin
drug interactions, 178*t*
for gestational diabetes, 1122*t*
incretin therapies, 1141
actions, 1132*t*
exenatide, 1133*t*, 1142
nursing considerations, 1132*t*
sitagliptin. *See* sitagliptin
meglitinides
actions, 1132*t*
mechanism of action, 1136
nateglinide, 1133*t*, 1137
nursing considerations, 1132*t*
repaglinide. *See* repaglinide
Nursing Process Application, 1140–41*t*
nursing responsibilities, 1139
patient and family education, 1139
principles of therapy, 1132
sulfonylureas. *See* SULFONYLUREAS
thiazolidinediones, 1137
actions, 1132*t*
mechanism of action, 1137
nursing considerations, 1132*t*
rosiglitazone. *See* rosiglitazone
Orap. *See* pimozide
Orencia. *See* abatacept
organ transplantation:
immunosuppressants in, 740, 1169
incidence, 744*t*
waiting lists for, 740*t*
organic brain syndrome (OBS), 333
ORGANIC NITRATES:
administration, 595*t*
drugs in class
amyl nitrite, 592*t*, 594
isosorbide dinitrate. *See* isosorbide dinitrate
isosorbide mononitrate, 592*t*, 595
nitroglycerin. *See* nitroglycerin
mechanism of action, 591*f*, 592–93
Nursing Process Application, 596*t*
for specific conditions
angina, 592–95, 592*t*
myocardial infarction, 602
tolerance to, 593

organophosphate pesticide poisoning, 205
Orinase. *See* tolbutamide
orlistat, 1091–92
  adverse effects, 1092
  classification, 1091
  contraindications/precautions, 1092
  drug interactions, 75*t*, 1092
  mechanism of action, 1092
  nursing considerations, 1092
  overdose treatment, 1092
  patient and family education, 1092
  pharmacokinetics, 1092
  pregnancy category, 1092
  therapeutic effects and uses, 1091–92
Ornidyl. *See* eflornithine
orphan disease, 14
orphenadrine, 400*t*, 402
Ortho Tri-Cyclen, 1203*t*
Orthoclone OKT3. *See* muromonab-CD3
Ortho-Cyclen, 1203*t*
Ortho-Evra, 1209–10
Ortho-Novum 1/35. *See* estradiol/norethindrone
Ortho-Novum 7/7/7, 1203*t*. *See also* estradiol/norethindrone
Ortho-Novum 10/11, 1203*t*. *See also* estradiol/norethindrone
orthostatic hypotension, 248
  with alpha-adrenergic antagonists, 248
  midodrine for, 238
  with opioids, 437, 437*t*
Orudis. *See* ketoprofen
Oruvail. *See* ketoprofen
Os-Cal. *See* calcium carbonate
Os-Cal 500. *See* calcium carbonate
oseltamivir, 915, 916*t*, 917
Osmitrol. *See* mannitol
Osmoglyn. *See* glycerin
osmolality, 687
osmosis, 688
OSMOTIC DIURETICS, 549, 559*t*
  glycerin, 559*t*, 560
  isosorbide, 1341*t*, 1345
  mannitol. *See* mannitol
  sites of action, 550*f*, 558
  toxicity, 558
  urea, 559*t*, 560
osmotic pressure, 558
osteitis deformans, 1291–92
osteoarthritis (OA), 1300
  complementary and alternative therapies, 1302*t*
  nonpharmacologic therapy, 1301
  pathophysiology, 1300, 1301*f*
  pharmacotherapy
    analgesics, 1302
    corticosteroids, 1169, 1302
    sodium hyaluronate, 1302
    topical medications, 1302
  signs and symptoms, 1300–1301, 1302*f*
osteomalacia, 1291
osteopenia, 1291
osteoporosis, 1290
  corticosteroid therapy and, 1164
  diagnosis, 1290–91
  incidence, 1284*t*
  in men, 1292*t*
  pathophysiology, 1290, 1291*f*
  pharmacotherapy, 1291
    bisphosphonates. *See* BISPHOSPHONATES
    hormonal agents
      calcitonin-salmon, 1295*t*, 1299–1300
      cinacalcet hydrochloride, 1295*t*, 1300
      raloxifene. *See* raloxifene
      teriparatide, 1295*t*, 1300
  risk factors, 1290
OTC (over-the-counter) drugs, 19
otic administration, 32, 33*f*
OTIC PREPARATIONS:
  acetic acid/hydrocortisone, 1352*t*
  benzocaine/antipyrine, 1352*t*
  carbamide peroxide, 1352, 1352*t*
  ciprofloxacin/dexamethasone, 1352*t*
  ciprofloxacin/hydrocortisone, 1352*t*
  polymyxin B/neomycin/hydrocortisone, 1352*t*
otitis interna, 1351
otitis media, 1351
  pathophysiology, 1351
  pharmacotherapy, 1351
    Evidence-Based Practice, 138*t*
    guidelines, 1351
    Nursing Process Application, 1353*t*
  signs and symptoms, 1351
Otrivin. *See* xylometazoline
outcome (goal), 117
ovarian cycle, 1177, 1178*f*
ovarian hyperstimulation syndrome, 1191
ovary(ies), disorders and pharmacotherapy, 1102*t*
overhydration:
  during enteral nutrition therapy, 1072*t*
  during parenteral nutrition therapy, 1079*t*
overseas pharmacies, 8
over-the-counter (OTC) drugs, 19
Ovide. *See* malathion
Ovidrel. *See* choriogonadotropin alfa
ovulation, 1177
ovulatory dysfunction, 1191
oxacillin, 789*t*, 794
oxaliplatin, 967*t*, 970
Oxandrin. *See* oxandrolone
oxandrolone, 1220*t*, 1223
oxaprozin, 724*t*, 725*t*
oxazepam, 97, 101*t*, 282*t*, 286
oxazolidinones, 822
oxcarbazepine, 135*t*, 142*t*
oxiconazole, 878*t*
Oxistat. *See* oxiconazole
oxybutynin chloride, 214*t*, 218
oxycodone, 440
  abuse, 99
  administration, 30*t*
  comparison to other opioids, 436*t*
  disposal, 26*t*
  route and adult dose, 436*t*
OxyContin, 30*t*, 99. *See also* oxycodone
oxymetazoline, 238, 1271
oxymetholone, 1220*t*, 1223
oxytocics, 1186. *See also* uterine stimulants
oxytocin, 1188–89
  adverse effects, 1188
  breast-feeding and, 1188*f*
  classification, 1188
  contraindications/precautions, 1188
  drug interactions, 1188
  mechanism of action, 1188
  Nursing Process Application, 1190*t*
  nursing responsibilities, 1188–89
  overdose treatment, 1188
  patient and family education, 1189
  pharmacokinetics, 1188
  pregnancy category, 1188
  regulation, 1102*t*
  similar drugs, 1189
  target organs and action, 1102*t*
  therapeutic effects and uses, 1186–87, 1188
Oxytrol. *See* oxybutynin chloride
Ozogamicin. *See* gemtuzumab

P

P wave, 626*t*
packed RBCs, 689*t*
paclitaxel, 985*t*, 987
Paget's disease, 1291–92, 1294
pain:
  assessment, 431, 432*t*
  classification, 428–29
  Lifespan Considerations, 442*t*
  management. *See* pain management
  physiology, 429–31, 430*f*
    modulation, 431
    perception, 431
    transduction, 430
    transmission, 430
pain management:
  best practices, 429*t*
  equianalgesic dose, 436*t*, 437
  goals and principles, 431–32
  myths, 429
  nonpharmacologic interventions, 431
  pharmacologic therapies, 432–34
    adjuvant analgesics. *See* ADJUVANT ANALGESICS
    nonopioid analgesics. *See* NONOPIOID ANALGESICS
    opioid and nonopioid combinations, 432–34
    opioids. *See* OPIOID ANALGESICS
    patient-controlled analgesia, 432–34
    World Health Organization Analgesic Ladder, 433*f*
  strategies, 428
paliperidone, 337*t*, 339
palivizumab, 748*t*
palliation, 952
palonosetron, 1043*t*
Pamelor. *See* nortriptyline
pamidronate, 1294*t*, 1295*t*, 1297
Pamine. *See* methscopolamine
Panax quinquefolius. *See* ginseng
pancreas, 1003–4
Pancrease, 30*t*. *See also* pancrelipase
pancreatic amylase, 1004*t*
pancreatic islets, disorders and pharmacotherapy, 1102*t*
pancreatic lipase, 1004*t*
pancreatin, 1048
pancreatitis, 1047
  acute, 1047
  chronic, 1047
  pathophysiology, 1045, 1045*t*, 1047
  pharmacotherapy
    pancreatin, 1048
    pancrelipase. *See* pancrelipase
pancrelipase, 1047–48
  adverse effects, 1047
  classification, 1047
  contraindications/precautions, 1047

dosage forms not to be crushed or opened, 30t
drug interactions, 1047
mechanism of action, 1047
nursing responsibilities, 1047–48
overdose treatment, 1047
patient and family education, 1048
pharmacokinetics, 1047
pregnancy category, 1047
therapeutic effects and uses, 1047
pancuronium, 219t, 224
panic disorder:
characteristics, 275
pharmacotherapy, 283t, 289, 290t
panitumumab, 748t, 990t
pantoprazole, 1013t, 1015
papaverine-phentolamine, 1228
papovaviruses, 909t
para-aminobenzoic acid, 841, 841f
Paracetaldehyde. *See* paraldehyde
paracetamol. *See* acetaminophen
Paraflex. *See* chlorzoxazone
Parafon Forte. *See* chlorzoxazone
ParaGard, 1210
paraldehyde, 286
paralysis agitans. *See* Parkinson's disease
paramyxoviruses, 909t
paranoia, 327t
Paraplatin. *See* carboplatin
parasympathetic nervous system, 186–87, 187f
parasympathomimetics. *See* cholinergic agonists
parathyroid gland, disorders and pharmacotherapy, 1102t
parathyroid hormone:
in calcium balance regulation, 1284–85, 1284f, 1285f
target organs and action, 1102t
Paregoric. *See* camphorated opium tincture
parenteral nutrition, 1068
complications
infectious, 1079–80, 1079t
mechanical, 1079, 1079t
metabolic, 1079, 1079t
components of solutions
amino acids, 1078
carbohydrates, 1077
electrolytes and minerals, 1078
lipids, 1078
vitamins, 1078
drug administration during, 1080
home care, 1080t
indications, 1076
Nursing Process Application, 1081t
patient monitoring, 1078, 1078t
types, 1076–77
parenteral route, 34–37
paricalcitol, 1293, 1294t
parietal cells, 1000
parish nursing, 165
parkinsonism, drug-induced, 331, 331t
Parkinson's disease (PD), 348
characteristics, 347t, 348
community issues, 364t
nonpharmacologic treatment, 350t
Nursing Process Application, 357t
on-off syndrome in, 349
pathophysiology, 348–49
pharmacotherapy
amantadine, 350t
COMT inhibitors
entacapone, 350t, 355
tolcapone, 350t, 355
dopamine agonists. *See* dopamine agonists
dopamine replacement agents
levodopa. *See* levodopa
levodopa/carbidopa, 350, 350t
H_1-receptor antagonists, 1266
selegiline, 350t, 355
symptoms, 348
Parlodel. *See* bromocriptine
Parnate. *See* tranylcypromine
paromomycin, 816t, 819, 892, 892t, 894–95
paroxetine:
for anxiety or insomnia, 282t, 289, 290t
for depression, 304t, 310
drug interactions, 101t
paroxysmal supraventricular tachycardia (PSVT), 626
partial agonist, 61, 61f
partial fatty-acid oxidation inhibitors, 591
partial parenteral nutrition, 1076. *See also* parenteral nutrition
partial seizures, 376t
partial (focal) seizures, 375, 376t
Paser. *See* aminosalicylic acid
passive immunity, 755, 767, 768f
passive transport, 42, 43f
Patanase. *See* olopatadine
Patanol. *See* olopatadine
patent medicines, 13, 13f
pathogen(s), 775
pathogenicity, 775
Patient and Family Education:
abortifacient, 1215
ACE inhibitors, 535
acetaminophen, 730
acetylcholinesterase inhibitors, 362
activated charcoal, 1365
adrenergic agonists
alpha-adrenergic agonists, 237–38
$alpha_2$-adrenergic agonists, 578
beta-adrenergic agonists, 240
nonselective adrenergic agonists, 234–35
adrenergic antagonists
alpha-adrenergic antagonists, 250
$beta_1$-adrenergic antagonists, 256–57, 597
nonselective beta-adrenergic antagonists, 254
5-alpha reductase inhibitors, 1233–34
5-aminosalicylates, 1038
amphetamines, 417
angiotensin II receptor blockers, 539–40
anorexiants, 1091
antacids, 1022
antianemic agents
cyanocobalamin, 683
ferrous sulfate, 679
antibiotics
aminoglycosides, 818
broad-spectrum penicillins, 793
carbapenems, 801
cephalosporins, 797–98
fluoroquinolones, 830
macrolides, 815
natural penicillins, 791–92
sulfonamides, 843
tetracyclines, 812
urinary tract antiseptics, 847
vancomycin, 802
anticoagulants
oral, 651–52
parenteral, 647, 649
antidepressants
monoamine oxidase inhibitors, 315
selective serotonin reuptake inhibitors, 310
tricyclic antidepressants, 307
antidiarrheals, 1035
antidiuretic hormone, 1115
antidysrhythmic drugs
potassium channel blockers, 635
sodium channel blockers, 631
antiemetics, 1045
antifungal drugs, 874, 876, 880
antiglaucoma agents, 1342, 1346
antigout agents
uric acid inhibitors, 1308–9
xanthine oxidase inhibitors, 1310
antihelminthic drugs, 903
antileprosy drugs, 863
antimalaria drugs, 890
antineoplastic agents, 965–66
alkylating agents, 969
antimetabolites, 974
antitumor antibiotics, 978
hormone antagonists, 982
vinca alkaloids, 986
antiplatelet agents
ADP receptor blockers, 655
glycoprotein IIb/IIIa receptor inhibitors, 657
antiprotozoan agents, 894, 898
antipsychotic drugs
first-generation, 334
second-generation (atypical), 338–39
antiretrovirals
nonnucleoside reverse transcriptase inhibitors, 937
nucleoside/nucleotide reverse transcriptase inhibitors, 935
protease inhibitors, 939
antiseizure drugs
gabapentin, 389
hydantoins, 385
iminostilbenes, 387
succinimides, 388
valproic acid, 390
antituberculosis drugs, 859
antitussives, 1277
antiviral drugs
for hepatitis, 921–22
for herpesviruses, 913
barbiturates, 292
benzodiazepines
diazepam, 383
lorazepam, 285
bile acid sequestrants, 508
bisphosphonates, 1296
bronchodilators
anticholinergics, 1249
$beta_2$-adrenergic agonists, 1247
calcium channel blockers
dihydropyridine, 521
nondihydropyridine, 524
calcium supplements, 1288–89
cardiac glycosides, 616
chelating agents, 1367
cholinergic agonists, 204, 207
CNS stimulants, 417, 421, 422

    corticosteroids
        beclomethasone, 1251–52
        hydrocortisone, 1168
        intranasal, 1271
    direct vasodilators, 580, 582
    disease-modifying antirheumatic drugs, 1305
    diuretics
        carbonic anhydrase inhibitors, 561
        loop (high-ceiling), 552
        osmotic, 560
        potassium-sparing, 557–58
        thiazide, 555
    dopamine agonists, 354
    dopamine replacement therapy, 353
    dopamine system stabilizer, 341
    electrolytes
        magnesium sulfate, 700
        potassium chloride, 699
    female infertility agents, 1194–95
    fibric acid agents, 510
    fluid replacement agents
        colloids, 694
        normal serum albumin, 690
    general anesthetics
        barbiturate, 461
        benzodiazepines, 464
        gaseous, 467
        intravenous, 465
        opioid, 462
        volatile liquid, 469
    glucagon, 1125
    H_1-receptor antagonists, 1267–68
    H_2-receptor antagonists, 1018–19
    hematopoietic growth factors
        colony-stimulating factors, 673–74
        erythropoietin, 671
        platelet enhancers, 675
    hemostatic agents, 662
    hormones
        estrogens, 1180–81
        oral contraceptives, 1206
        testosterone, 1222–23
    immune globulin, 769
    immunostimulants
        interferons, 736
        interleukins, 739
    immunosuppressants
        antimetabolites/cytotoxic agents, 746
        calcineurin inhibitors, 744
        monoclonal antibodies, 749
    insulin, 1129
    laxatives, 1032
    leukotriene modifiers, 1254
    lipase inhibitors, 1092
    local anesthetics
        amides, 475
        esters, 474
    mast cell stabilizers, 1253
    methylxanthines
        caffeine, 422
        theophylline, 1256
    mineralocorticoids, 1171
    mood stabilizers, 320
    muscarinic antagonists
        atropine, 217
        benztropine, 356
    nasal decongestants, 1274
    nicotinic antagonists
        mecamylamine, 220
        succinylcholine, 222
        tubocurarine, 224
    nonbenzodiazepine anxiolytics, 287–88
    nonopioid centrally acting analgesics, 444
    nonsteroidal anti-inflammatory drugs
        COX-2 inhibitors, 728
        ibuprofen-like agents, 726
        salicylates, 722–23
    nonstimulant for ADHD, 419
    opioid analgesics, 439
    opioid antagonists, 448
    oral hypoglycemics, 1139
    organic nitrates, 594
    otic medications, 1352–53
    pancreatic enzymes, 1048
    phosphodiesterase inhibitors, 619
    potassium channel blockers, 635
    progestins, 1184
    proton pump inhibitors, 1015
    retinoids, 1324
    scabicides/pediculicides, 1320
    selective estrogen receptor modulators, 1299
    skeletal muscle relaxants
        centrally acting, 401
        direct-acting, 405–6
    sodium bicarbonate, 704
    sodium channel blockers, 631
    spermicides, 1212
    statins, 505
    thrombolytic agents, 659
    thyroid replacement agents, 1152
    tocolytics, 1189
    topical anesthetics, 1333
    triptans, 452
    vaccines, 762
    vitamins
        cyanocobalamin (vitamin B_{12}), 1060
        folic acid (vitamin B_9), 1061
        pyridoxine (vitamin B_6), 1060
        riboflavin (vitamin B_2), 1059
        thiamine (vitamin B_1), 1058–59
        vitamin A, 1056
        vitamin C, 1061
        vitamin D, 1056
        vitamin E, 1057
        vitamin K, 1058
Patient Safety:
    control of concentrated electrolyte solutions, 698*t*
    EpiPen use, 235*t*
    infusion, 1039*t*
    iron overdose in children, 678*t*
    levofloxacin, 833*t*
    medication errors due to similar packaging, 648*t*
    medication orders, 1186*t*
    mistaken identity, 1295*t*
    OptiClik injector pen, 1132*t*
    soundalike drugs, 729*t*
    trimethoprim-sulfamethoxazole, 842*t*
patient teaching. *See also* Patient and Family Education
    cultural appropriateness, 119*t*
    implementation, 118–19, 119*f*
    Lifespan Considerations, 118*t*
    planning, 118
    for prevention of medication errors, 88
patient variability, 56, 56*f*
Pavabid. *See* papaverine-phentolamine
Pavulon. *See* pancuronium
Paxil. *See* paroxetine
Paxipam. *See* halazepam
PBPs (penicillin-binding proteins), 787
PCP (phencyclidine), 105, 126*t*
PCV (pneumococcal conjugate vaccine), 760
PD. *See* Parkinson's disease
PDUFA (Prescription Drug User Fee Act), 14, 19
Pedia Care. *See* dextromethorphan
Pediamycin. *See* erythromycin base
pediatric patients:
    acute otitis media in, 138*t*
    adherence issues, 143
    adverse drug effects in, 140–41, 142*t*, 143
    asthma in, 1243*t*
    corticosteroids in, 1164*t*
    depression in, 301, 302*t*
    diuretic therapy in, 549*t*
    dosage calculation, 140, 141*f*
    dosage guidelines for selected drugs, 142*t*
    drug administration in
        adolescents, 139
        infants, 137
        preschoolers, 138
        school-age children, 139
        techniques, 25*t*
        toddlers, 137–38
    drug testing and labeling for, 134–36, 135*t*, 136*t*
    drug utilization patterns, 134*t*
    Evidence-Based Practice, 138*t*
    growth hormone for
        age-appropriate height, 1107*t*
        long-term outcome in burn patients, 1110*t*
    H_1-receptor antagonists in, 1267*t*
    HIV-AIDS in, 944*t*
    hypertension in, 522*t*
    iron overdose in, 678*t*
    medication safety in
        nursing actions and guidelines, 140
        nursing education and communication, 140
    obesity rates, 1086*t*
    ophthalmic drug teaching for, 1350*t*
    oral candidiasis in infants, 872*t*
    oropharyngeal candidiasis in neonates, 870*t*
    pain assessment, 432*t*
    peptic ulcer disease and gastroesophageal reflux in, 1023*t*
    pharmacokinetic responses
        absorption, 136, 136*t*
        distribution, 136
        excretion, 137
        metabolism, 136–37
    seizures in, 373
    SSRIs in, 290*t*
    Stevens–Johnson syndrome in, 1333*t*
    tachycardia in, 623*t*
    teaching tips, 119*t*
    urinary tract infections in, 839
    vaccine administration, 766*t*
Pediatric Research Equity Act of 2003, 136
PEDICULICIDES, 1318
    lindane, 1319
    malathion, 1319, 1320
    Nursing Process Application, 1321*t*
    permethrin. *See* permethrin
    pyrethrin, 1319
Pediculus humanus capitis, 1318*f*
Pediculus humanus corporis, 1318

pegaspargase, 992, 992*t*
Pegasys. *See* peginterferon alfa-2a
pegfilgrastim, 670*t*, 674
peginterferon alfa-2a, 735*t*, 737, 919*t*, 922
peginterferon alfa-2b, 919*t*
PEG-Intron. *See* peginterferon alfa-2b
pegvisomant, 1108*t*, 1112
pegylation, 734
pemetrexed, 973*t*, 974
pemirolast potassium, 1349, 1349*t*
Pen Tsao, 3
Pen Vee K. *See* penicillin VK
penbutolol, 252*t*, 255
penciclovir, 912*t*, 914
PENICILLIN(S):
- adverse effects, 790
- allergy, 790
- broad-spectrum (aminopenicillins)
  - amoxicillin. *See* amoxicillin
  - amoxicillin-clavulanate, 142*t*, 789*t*
  - ampicillin. *See* ampicillin
  - ampicillin/sulbactam, 789*t*
  - characteristics, 792
- characteristics, 790
- combination, 792
- extended-spectrum (antipseudomonal)
  - adverse effects, 794
  - carbenicillin, 789*t*, 794
  - mechanism of action, 793
  - piperacillin, 789*t*, 794
  - piperacillin-tazobactam, 789*t*
  - ticarcillin, 789*t*, 794
- mechanism of action, 788*f*, 789
- natural
  - penicillin G. *See* penicillin G
  - penicillin G benzathine, 789*t*, 792
  - penicillin G procaine, 789*t*, 792
  - penicillin V, 789*t*, 792
- Nursing Process Application, 799–800*t*
- penicillinase-resistant (antistaphylococcal)
  - characteristics, 794
  - cloxacillin, 789*t*, 794
  - dicloxacillin, 789*t*, 794
  - nafcillin, 789*t*, 794–95
  - oxacillin, 789*t*, 794
- resistance to, 788
- structure, 789*f*

penicillin G, 791–92
- adverse effects, 789*t*, 791
- classification, 791
- contraindications/precautions, 791
- drug interactions, 75*t*, 791
- mechanism of action, 791
- nursing responsibilities, 791
- overdose treatment, 791
- patient and family education, 791–92
- pharmacokinetics, 791
- pregnancy category, 791
- route and adult dose, 789*t*
- similar drugs, 792
- therapeutic effects and uses, 791

penicillin G benzathine, 789*t*, 792
penicillin G procaine, 789*t*, 792
penicillin V, 789*t*, 792
penicillin VK, 142*t*
penicillinase, 788
penicillin-binding proteins (PBPs), 787
penis, 1226, 1227*f*
Penlac. *See* ciclopirox
Pentam. *See* pentamidine
pentamidine, 892*t*
pentazocine, 436*t*, 440, 442
pentobarbital, 282*t*, 292
Pentostam. *See* sodium stibogluconate
pentostatin, 973*t*, 976
Pentothal. *See* thiopental sodium
pentoxifylline, 30*t*, 650, 653*t*
Pen-Vee K. *See* penicillin V
PEP (postexposure prophylaxis), HIV, 943
Pepcid. *See* famotidine
pepsin, 1004*t*, 1007
peptic ulcer, 1007
- corticosteroid therapy and, 1164
- etiology, 1008–9
- incidence, 1008*t*
- nonpharmacologic therapy, 1010
- pathogenesis, 1007
- in pediatric patients, 1023*t*
- pharmacotherapy
  - anticholinergics, 1024
  - bismuth subsalicylate, 1024
  - for *H. pylori* infection, 1023, 1024
  - H_2-receptor antagonists. *See* H_2-RECEPTOR ANTAGONISTS
  - mechanism of action, 1012*f*
  - metoclopramide. *See* metoclopramide
  - misoprostol, 1024
  - overview, 1010–13
  - proton pump inhibitors. *See* PROTON PUMP INHIBITORS (PPIs)
  - sucralfate, 1024
- risk factors, 1007–8
- symptoms, 1009

peptidoglycan, 778, 787
Pepto-Bismol. *See* bismuth subsalicylate
Percocet. *See* oxycodone
Percodan. *See* aspirin; oxycodone
Perforomist. *See* formoterol
perfusion, 1239
perindopril, 533*t*, 536
peripheral nervous system, 185, 186*f*. *See also* autonomic nervous system
peripheral resistance, 491
peripheral vein parenteral nutrition, 1076. *See also* parenteral nutrition
peripherally inserted central catheter (PICC) line, 957
peristalsis, 1000
permethrin, 1319–20
- adverse effects, 1319
- classification, 1319
- contraindications/precautions, 1319
- drug interactions, 1319
- mechanism of action, 1319
- nursing responsibilities, 1319–20
- overdose treatment, 1319
- patient and family education, 1320
- pharmacokinetics, 1319
- pregnancy category, 1319
- similar drugs, 1320
- therapeutic effects and uses, 1319

pernicious anemia, 680
- pharmacotherapy
  - cyanocobalamin. *See* cyanocobalamin
  - folic acid. *See* folic acid

perphenazine, 334
- adverse effects, 332*t*
- for nausea and vomiting, 1043*t*
- route and adult dose, 332*t*

Persantine. *See* dipyridamole
Persian Gulf War syndrome, 204–5
pertussis (whooping cough):
- characteristics, 758*t*
- immunization, 758*t*, 759
- incidence, 758*t*
- pathophysiology, 759

Pexeva. *See* paroxetine
pH, drug absorption and, 44, 44*f*
phagocytes, 710
pharmacodynamics, 56
- dose–response relationship, 57–58, 58*f*
- drug interactions and, 73–74, 73*f*
- interpatient variability, 56
- in older adults, 150
- potency and efficacy, 58–59, 59*f*
- receptor theory, 60–61, 60*f*
- therapeutic index, 57, 57*f*

pharmacogenetics, 62, 160
pharmacokinetics, 41, 41*f*
- drug interactions and, 45, 71–73, 71*f*
- in older adults, 148–50, 149*t*
- in pediatric patients
  - absorption, 136–37, 136*t*
  - distribution, 136
  - excretion, 137
  - metabolism, 137
- processes, 42*f*
  - absorption, 43–45, 44*f*
  - distribution, 45–46, 46*f*
  - excretion, 48–49, 50*f*
  - metabolism, 46–48, 47*t*, 48*f*
- time–response relationships
  - plasma concentration, 49–50
  - plasma half-life, 50–51
  - with repeated dosing, 51–52, 52*f*
  - with single-dose administration, 51*f*

pharmacologic classification, 5–6
pharmacology, 4
- clinical nursing practice and, 8–9
- definition, 4
- history, 3

pharmacopeia, 15
pharmacotherapy, 4
- clinical nursing practice and, 7–8
- cultural variables, 158–59, 158*f*
- definition, 4
- ethnic variables, 158–59
- gender influences, 160
- genetic influences, 159–60
- holistic, 157, 157*t*
- nurses as community sources of information, 167–68
- nursing diagnoses in, 117*t*
- in older adults. *See* older adults
- patient adherence in, 24
- in pediatric patients. *See* pediatric patients
- during pregnancy and lactation. *See* lactation; pregnancy
- psychosocial influences, 157–58
- rationale, 4–5, 4*f*

Pharmacotherapy Illustrated:
- acetylcholine life cycle, 193*f*
- active and passive immunity, 768*f*
- alcohol metabolism, 100*f*
- Alzheimer's drugs, 361*f*
- analgesics, 433*t*
- antianginal drugs, 591*f*
- antianxiety medications, 277*f*
- antiemetics, 1042*f*
- antiparkinson drugs, 351*f*

antiprostatic drugs, 1230*f*
antipsychotic drugs, 329*f*
antiseizure drugs, 378*f*
antiulcer drugs, 1012*f*
contraceptives, 1202*f*
corticosteroids and adrenal atrophy, 1166*f*
direct-acting antispasmodics, 405*f*
diuretics, 550*f*
gastroesophageal reflux disease, 1011*f*
heart failure drugs, 611*f*
infertility agents, 1193*f*
joint disorders, 1301*f*
lipid-lowering drugs, 503*f*
norepinephrine life cycle, 193*f*
NSAID-induced ulcer formation, 721*f*
synaptic transmission, 189*f*
thrombolytic therapy, 601*f*
PharmFacts:
abortion, 1213*t*
abuse of OTC drugs, 20*t*
acetaminophen in liver failure, 1003*t*
acetylcholine, 190*t*
acne, 1320*t*
adrenaline/epinephrine, 192*t*
adverse drug reactions, 67*t*, 68*t*, 152*t*
allergic dermatitis, 1325*t*
allergic rhinitis, 1263*t*
Alzheimer's disease, 358*t*
amebiasis, 891*t*
anabolic steroid use, 1223
angina pectoris, 590*t*
angioedema, 534*t*
antibacterial additives, 791*t*
antibacterial properties of breast milk, 127*t*
antibiotic resistance, 782*t*, 802*t*
antidepressant use in pregnancy, 124*t*
antigen-presenting cells, 714*t*
anxiety disorders, 275*t*
assessment for enteral nutrition, 1077*t*
asthma, 1241*t*, 1243*t*
atropine, 215*t*
attention deficit/hyperactivity disorder, 414*t*
belladonna, 215*t*
benign prostatic hyperplasia, 1229*t*
breast cancer mortality, 976*t*
bubonic plague, 813*t*
causes of death, 775*t*
cerebral palsy, 403*t*
common cold, 1275*t*
corticosteroid-induced glaucoma, 1349*t*
Cushing's syndrome, 1171
deep vein thrombosis, 643*t*
depression, 298*t*, 299*t*
diabetes mellitus
complications, 1126*t*
incidence, 1120*t*
dietary supplements, 176*t*
drug approval process, 18*t*, 19*t*
drug costs, 8*t*
drug interactions, 74*t*
drug use in older adults, 150*t*
dysfunctional uterine bleeding, 1183*t*
dyslipidemia, 496*t*, 506*t*
dystonia, 403*t*
elderly population growth, 147*t*
epidural anesthesia, 459*t*
erectile dysfunction, 1226*t*
ethnic differences in insurance coverage, 159*t*
exercise-associated hypernatremia, 688*t*
familial hypercholesterolemia, 508*t*
female infertility, 1191*t*
fluoroquinolones, 832*t*
gastroesophageal reflux disease, 1010*t*
genital herpes, 911*t*
giardiasis, 893*t*
glaucoma, 1338*t*
growth hormone, 1099*t*
growth hormone deficiency, 1107*t*
heart, 487*t*
heart failure, 607*t*
hepatitis B, 918*t*
herbal therapy in pediatric patients, 143*t*
HIV-AIDS, 927*t*
hospice care, 165*t*
human papillomavirus, 766*t*
hypertension, 567*t*
hypertensive crisis, 582*t*
infant death rates, 158*t*
influenza, 915
insomnia, 278*t*
iron, 668*t*
kidney transplants, 545*t*
leprosy, 862*t*
lung cancer, 991*t*
lymphangiogenesis, 709*t*
magnesium, 701*t*
mail order pharmacies, 8*t*
malignant hyperthermia, 469*t*
maternal morbidity and mortality, 1202*t*
medication errors, 80*t*
melatonin, 1101*t*
meningococcal infection, 760*t*
menopause, 1184
mental retardation and epilepsy, 382*t*
migraine statistics, 449*t*
morning sickness, 1041*t*
multiple sclerosis, 364*t*
muscarinic receptors, 203*t*
muscle spasticity, 402*t*
myocardial infarction, 602*t*
neurons, 270*t*
nonadherence, 24*t*
NSAIDs, 718*t*, 727*t*
nurse anesthetists, 461*t*
obesity in children and adolescents, 1086*t*
obesity rates by race and gender, 1087*t*
organ transplantation, 740*t*, 744*t*
oropharyngeal candidiasis in neonates, 870*t*
pain in America, 428*t*
pancreatitis, 1045*t*
Parkinson's disease, 347*t*
pediatric labeling, 136*t*
peptic ulcer disease, 1008*t*
pheochromocytomas, 229*t*
prescription statistics, 26*t*
prescription use, 88*t*
prostate cancer, 965*t*, 1229*t*
pseudoephedrine, 1273*t*
pseudogout, 1309*t*
psoriasis, 1328*t*
Raynaud's disease, 248*t*
renal failure, 546*t*
rheumatoid arthritis, 1303*t*
schizophrenia, 326*t*
seizures in older adults, 371
sexual activity among high school students, 927*t*
sleep duration and type 2 diabetes, 286*t*
Special Considerations, 328*t*
spending on prescription drugs, 148*t*
stomach size, 1000*f*
substance abuse, 94*t*, 95*t*, 98*t*
synapses, 267*t*
T cells, 713*t*
tachycardia in pediatric patients, 623*t*
Three Mile Island nuclear accident, 1363*t*
urinary tract infections in men, 839*t*
varicella zoster, 765*t*
viral hemorrhagic fevers, 1361*t*
vitamin D from sunlight, 1056*t*
vitamin poisoning, 1054*t*
vulvovaginal candidiasis, 875*t*
Zollinger-Ellison syndrome, 1010*t*
Phenazine. *See* perphenazine
phencyclidine (PCP), 105, 126*t*
phenelzine, 314–15
adverse effects, 314
classification, 314
contraindications/precautions, 314
drug interactions, 314–15
mechanism of action, 314
nursing responsibilities, 315
overdose treatment, 315
patient and family education, 315
pharmacokinetics, 314
pregnancy category, 315
similar drugs, 315
for specific conditions
anxiety or insomnia, 290*t*
therapeutic effects and uses, 314
Phenergan. *See* promethazine
Phenergan with Codeine, 1276*t*. *See also* promethazine
phenindione, 129*t*
phenobarbital, 291–92
adverse effects, 291
in breast-feeding infant, 129*t*
classification, 291
contraindications/precautions, 291–92
distribution in older adults, 148–49
drug interactions, 101*t*, 292, 382
as enzyme inducer, 47
mechanism of action, 291
nursing considerations, 292
overdose treatment, 292
patient and family education, 292
pharmacokinetics, 291
pregnancy category, 292
similar drugs, 292
for specific conditions
seizures, 380*t*, 381–82
therapeutic effects and uses, 291
phenolphthalein, 1030*t*
phenothiazines. *See* FIRST-GENERATION ANTIPSYCHOTICS, phenothiazines
phenoxybenzamine, 247*t*, 250
phensuximide, 381*t*
phentermine, 1091
phentolamine, 250–51
adverse effects, 247*t*
for extravasation of dantrolene, 404
for extravasation of dopamine, 235
for hypertensive emergency, 584*t*
mechanism of action, 250
route and adult dose, 247*t*
phenylephrine, 237–38
adverse effects, 232*t*, 237
classification, 236
contraindications/precautions, 237
drug interactions, 237

mechanism of action, 237
nursing responsibilities, 237
overdose treatment, 237
patient and family education, 237–38
pharmacokinetics, 237
pregnancy category, 237
route and adult dose, 232*t*
similar drugs, 238
therapeutic effects and uses, 236–37
eye examinations, 1347
eye irritation, 1348, 1348*t*
phenylpropanolamine, 1089
Phenytek. *See* phenytoin
phenytoin, 384–85
adverse effects, 380*t*, 629*t*
classification, 384
contraindications/precautions, 384–85
drug interactions, 101*t*, 385
mechanism of action, 384
nursing responsibilities, 385
in older adults, 149, 152*t*
overdose treatment, 385
patient and family education, 385
pharmacokinetics, 384
pregnancy category, 385
route and adult dose, 380*t*, 629*t*
similar drugs, 385
for specific conditions
dysrhythmias, 629*t*, 632
therapeutic effects and uses, 384
pheochromocytoma, 229*t*, 248
phobia, 275
phosgene, 1362*t*
phosgene oxime, 1363*t*
PhosLo. *See* calcium acetate
phosphodiesterase III, 618
PHOSPHODIESTERASE III INHIBITORS:
adverse effects, 612*t*, 618
drugs in class
inamrinone, 612*t*, 619
milrinone lactate. *See* milrinone lactate
mechanism of action, 611*f*
for specific conditions
heart failure, 612*t*, 618
PHOSPHODIESTERASE 5 INHIBITORS, 1227–28
sildenafil. *See* sildenafil
tadalafil, 1227*t*, 1229
vardenafil, 1227*t*, 1229
Phospholine Iodide. *See* echothiophate
phospholipids, 496, 497*f*
phosphorus (phosphate):
functions, 1062–63, 1062*t*
imbalances, 694*t*
hyperphosphatemia. *See* hyperphosphatemia
hypophosphatemia, 694*t*, 1072*t*
recommended dietary allowance, 1062*t*
photosensitivity, antibiotics and, 811*t*
phototherapy, 301, 302*t*, 1331
phototoxicity, 70
Phthirus pubis, 1318
physical dependence, 95
physostigmine, 1364*t*
physostigmine salicylate, 202*t*, 204
Phytonadione. *See* vitamin K
picornaviruses, 909*t*
PIH (prolactin-inhibiting hormone), 1105*t*
pill rolling, 348
pilocarpine, 202*t*, 204, 1341*t*, 1343
Pilopine. *See* pilocarpine
Pima. *See* potassium iodide and iodine
pimecrolimus, 1328
pimozide, 332*t*, 336
pindolol, 251, 252*t*, 255
Pin-Rid. *See* pyrantel
Pinworm Caplets. *See* pyrantel
Pin-X. *See* pyrantel
pioglitazone, 1133*t*, 1138
Piper methysticum. See kava
piperacillin, 789*t*, 794
piperacillin-tazobactam, 789*t*
pirbuterol, 240, 1245*t*, 1247
piroxicam, 724*t*, 725*t*
Pitocin. *See* oxytocin
PITUITARY AGENTS:
mecasermin, 1108*t*, 1110–11
oxytocin. *See* oxytocin
somatropin. *See* somatropin
pituitary gland:
disorders and pharmacotherapy, 1102*t*
functions, 1106
hormones secreted by, 1105*t*, 1106
placebo, 18
placenta, 124
Placidyl. *See* ethchlorvynol
Plan B, 1203*t*, 1212, 1213*t*
planning, in nursing process, 117–18
plant sterols, 500–501, 501*t*
plaque, 588–89
Plaquenil. *See* hydroxychloroquine
plaques, in psoriasis, 1328
Plasbumin. *See* normal serum albumin
plasma cell, 713
plasma half-life ($t_{1/2}$), 50
Plasma-Lyte, 691*t*, 692
plasminogen, 657
Plasmodium, 886–87, 886*t*, 887*f*. *See also* malaria
platelets, 689*t*
Platinol. *See* cisplatin
PLATINUM COMPOUNDS:
carboplatin, 967*t*, 970
cisplatin, 959, 960, 967*t*, 970
oxaliplatin, 967*t*, 970
Plavix. *See* clopidogrel
Plendil, 30*t*. *See also* felodipine
pluripotent stem cell, 668
PML (progressive multifocal leukoencephalopathy), 366
PMS (premenstrual syndrome), 1183
pneumococcal conjugate vaccine (PCV), 760
pneumococcal infection:
immunization, 760
pathophysiology, 759–60
pneumococcal polysaccharide vaccine (PPV), 760
Pneumocystis carinii, 869*t*
pneumocystis pneumonia, 869*t*, 945*t*
pneumonic plague, 828, 1361
pneumothorax, during parenteral nutrition therapy, 1079*t*
poisoning:
incidence, 1363
management, 1363–64
activated charcoal. *See* activated charcoal
antidotes, 1364*t*
chelation therapy, 1366
prevention, 215*t*, 1364*t*
Poladex. *See* dexchlorpheniramine
Polaramine. *See* dexchlorpheniramine
polarized, 623
poliomyelitis:
characteristics, 758*t*
immunization, 758*t*, 765
incidence, 758*t*
pathophysiology, 764–65
Polocaine. *See* mepivacaine
POLYCLONAL ANTIBODIES, 747
lymphocyte immune globulin, 741*t*, 747
polycystic ovary syndrome, 1191
polydipsia, 1122
polyethylene glycol, 1030*t*
polymeric formulas, for enteral nutrition, 1069*t*, 1070
polymyxin B, 832*t*, 833
polymyxin B-neomycin-hydrocortisone, 1352*t*
polyphagia, 1122
polypharmacy, 88, 147
in older adults, 147–48, 147*t*
polystyrene sulfate, 548*t*, 697
polyuria, 1122
polyvinyl alcohol, 1348, 1348*t*
Ponstel. *See* mefenamic acid
Pontocaine. *See* tetracaine
positive symptoms, schizophrenia, 327, 327*t*
postantibiotic effect, 817
posterior pituitary gland, 1106
postexposure prophylaxis (PEP), HIV, 943
postherpetic neuralgia, 765
postictal state, 374
postmarketing surveillance, 18
postmenopausal bleeding, 1183
postpartum onset depression, 299
post-traumatic stress disorder (PTSD), 276, 289, 290*t*
Posture. *See* calcium phosphate tribasic
potassium:
functions, 697
imbalances, 694*t*, 697
hyperkalemia. *See* hyperkalemia
hypokalemia. *See* hypokalemia
regulation, 695*f*, 697
POTASSIUM CHANNEL BLOCKERS:
adverse effects, 634
drugs in class
amiodarone. *See* amiodarone
dofetilide, 629*t*, 635
mechanism of action, 634
potassium chloride (KCl), 698–99
adverse effects, 698
classification, 698
contraindications/precautions, 698
dosage forms not to be crushed or opened, 30*t*
drug interactions, 698
mechanism of action, 698
nursing considerations, 698–99
overdose treatment, 698
patient and family education, 699
pharmacokinetics, 698
pregnancy category, 698
similar drugs, 698
therapeutic effects and uses, 698
potassium iodide (KI), 1156, 1363
potassium iodide and iodine, 1154*t*, 1156
POTASSIUM-SPARING DIURETICS, 549, 555–56
adverse effects, 556*t*, 612*t*
aldosterone antagonists, 532, 556
eplerenone. *See* eplerenone
spironolactone. *See* spironolactone
route and adult dose, 556*t*

sites of action, 550*f*
sodium channel inhibitors, 556
amiloride, 556, 556*t*, 558
triamterene, 556, 556*t*, 558
for specific conditions
heart failure, 612*t*, 613
hypertension, 572*t*, 573, 574*t*
potency, 58–59, 59*f*
PPIs. *See* PROTON PUMP INHIBITORS (PPIs)
PPV (pneumococcal polysaccharide vaccine), 760
PQ interval, 626*t*
PQ segment, 626*t*
pralidoxime, 205, 1364*t*
pramipexole, 353–54
adverse effects, 353–54
classification, 353
contraindications/precautions, 353
drug interactions, 353–54
mechanism of action, 353
nursing responsibilities, 354
overdose treatment, 354
patient and family education, 354
pharmacokinetics, 353
pregnancy category, 354
similar drugs, 354
therapeutic effects and uses, 353
pramlintide, 1128, 1133*t*
Prandimet, 1134*t*
Prandin. *See* repaglinide
Pravachol. *See* pravastatin
pravastatin, 504*t*, 506
praziquantel, 901, 902*t*, 903
prazosin, 249–50
adverse effects, 247*t*, 249
classification, 249
contraindications/precautions, 249
drug interactions, 249–50
mechanism of action, 249
nursing responsibilities, 250
overdose treatment, 250
patient and family education, 250
pharmacokinetics, 249
pregnancy category, 250
route and adult dose, 247*t*
similar drugs, 250–51
therapeutic effects and uses, 249
preanesthetic medication, 283*t*
preclinical research, 17
Precose. *See* acarbose
prediabetes, 1123
prednisolone, 1167*t*
prednisone:
adverse effects, 1167*t*
mechanism of action, 1169
route and adult dose, 1167*t*
for specific conditions
adrenocortical insufficiency, 1165
neoplasia, 980*t*
therapeutic effects and uses, 1169
preeclampsia, 373
Prefest. *See* estradiol/norgestimate
pregabalin, 381*t*, 391–92
pregnancy:
alcohol use in, 102
deep venous thrombosis in, 648*t*
drugs of abuse and potential effects in, 126*t*
iodine requirement in, 1148*t*
maternal morbidity and mortality, 1202*t*
nausea and vomiting in, 1041
pharmacotherapy during
drug transfer across placenta, 124
fetal development stage and effect of, 126–27
physiologic changes affecting pharmacokinetics
absorption, 123–24
distribution, 124
excretion, 124
metabolism, 124
pregnancy risk categories, 125–26, 125*t*
rationale for, 123
seizures in, 372–73
tuberculosis infection in, 856–57
urinary tract infections in, 839
vitamins during, 1055*t*
pregnancy categories, 125–26, 125*t*
Pregnyl. *See* human chorionic gonadotropin (HCG)
preload, 490, 490*f*
Premarin. *See* conjugated estrogens
premature infants, respiratory distress syndrome in, 1240*t*
premenstrual syndrome (PMS), 1183
Premphase. *See* conjugated estrogens/medroxyprogesterone
Prempro. *See* conjugated estrogens/medroxyprogesterone
Prepidil. *See* dinoprostone
preschoolers. *See* pediatric patients
prescription(s):
abbreviations on, 27*t*
format, 25–26, 26*f*
statistics, 26*t*
Prescription Drug User Fee Act (PDUFA), 14, 19
preterm labor, 1189
pretibial myxedema, 1154
Prevacid, 30*t*. *See also* lansoprazole
Preven, 1212
Prez-D. *See* ephedrine
Prezista. *See* darunavir
PRH (prolactin-releasing hormone), 1105*t*
Prialt. *See* ziconotide
Priftin. *See* rifapentine
prilocaine, 473*t*, 476
Prilosec, 30*t*. *See also* omeprazole
primaquine, 888*t*, 890
primary hypertension, 568. *See also* hypertension
Primaxin. *See* imipenem-cilastin
primidone:
adverse effects in breast-feeding infant, 129*t*
for seizures, 380*t*, 382
Primsol. *See* trimethoprim
Principen. *See* ampicillin
Prinivil. *See* lisinopril
Prinzmetal's (vasospastic) angina, 589
Privine. *See* naphazoline
prn, 27
ProAmatine. *See* midodrine
Probalan. *See* probenecid
Pro-Banthine. *See* propantheline
probenecid, 1307*t*, 1309, 1310
procainamide, 630–31
adverse effects, 631
classification, 630
contraindications/precautions, 631
dosage forms not to be crushed or opened, 30*t*
drug interactions, 631
genetic polymorphisms and actions of, 160*t*
mechanism of action, 630–31
nursing responsibilities, 631
overdose treatment, 631
patient and family education, 631
pharmacokinetics, 631
pregnancy category, 631
similar drugs, 632–33
therapeutic effects and uses, 630
procaine, 472, 474
adverse effects, 472, 473*t*
classification, 472
contraindications/precautions, 472
drug interactions, 472, 474
mechanism of action, 472
nursing responsibilities, 474
overdose treatment, 474
patient and family education, 474
pharmacokinetics, 472
plasma half-life, 50
pregnancy category, 474
route and adult dose, 473*t*
similar drugs, 474
therapeutic effects and uses, 472
Procan SR. *See* procainamide
Procanbid. *See* procainamide
procarbazine, 967*t*, 971
Procardia. *See* nifedipine
Procardia XL, 30*t*, 519*t*. *See also* nifedipine
Prochieve. *See* progesterone
prochlorperazine, 334–35, 1044–45
adverse effects, 332*t*, 1045
classification, 1044
contraindications/precautions, 1045
dosage forms not to be crushed or opened, 30*t*
drug interactions, 1045
mechanism of action, 1044
nursing responsibilities, 1045
overdose treatment, 1045
patient and family education, 1045
pharmacokinetics, 1044
pregnancy category, 1044
rectal administration, 32
route and adult dose, 332*t*
therapeutic effects and uses, 1044
procoagulants, 642
Procrit. *See* epoetin alfa
procyclidine, 331, 355*t*
prodrugs, 46
product name, 7
prodysrhythmics, 623, 623*t*
Pro-Fast. *See* phentermine
Progestasert, 1210
progesterone, 123–24, 1180*t*, 1184
progestins, 1181
medroxyprogesterone acetate. *See* medroxyprogesterone acetate
Nursing Process Application, 1185*t*
in oral contraceptives, 1200, 1201*t*, 1203*t*, 1206
progesterone, 123–24, 1180*t*, 1184
therapeutic effects and uses, 1181, 1183
Proglycem. *See* diazoxide
Prograf. *See* tacrolimus
progressive multifocal leukoencephalopathy (PML), 366
prolactin, 1102*t*
prolactin-inhibiting hormone (PIH), 1105*t*

prolactin-releasing hormone (PRH), 1105*t*
Proleukin. *See* aldesleukin
promethazine:
  adverse effects, 1265*t*
  for allergic rhinitis, 1265*t*
  for nausea and vomiting, 477, 1042, 1043*t*
Prometrium. *See* progesterone
Pronestyl. *See* procainamide
Pronestyl SR, 30*t*. *See also* procainamide
propafenone, 629*t*, 632
propantheline, 214*t*, 217
proparacaine hydrochloride, 1347, 1348*t*
Propecia. *See* finasteride
Propine. *See* dipivefrin
Propionibacterium acnes, 1320
propofol, 101*t*, 460*t*, 465
propoxyphene, 101*t*, 436*t*, 440
propoxyphene napsylate, 436*t*
propranolol, 253–54
  adverse effects, 253
  Asians' sensitivity to, 633*t*
  classification, 253
  contraindications/precautions, 253
  dosage forms not to be crushed or opened, 30*t*
  drug interactions, 101*t*, 253
  genetic polymorphisms and actions of, 159, 160*t*
  mechanism of action, 253
  nursing responsibilities, 254
  patient and family education, 254
  pharmacokinetics, 253
  pregnancy category, 254
  similar drugs, 254–55
  for specific conditions
    angina, 592*t*
    dysrhythmias, 629*t*, 633
  therapeutic effects and uses, 253, 286
proprietary name, 7
propylthiouracil, 1155–56
  adverse effects, 1154*t*, 1155
  classification, 1155
  contraindications/precautions, 1155
  drug interactions, 1155
  mechanism of action, 1155
  nursing responsibilities, 1155–56
  overdose treatment, 1155
  patient and family education, 1156
  pharmacokinetics, 1155
  pregnancy category, 1155
  route and adult dose, 1154*t*
  similar drugs, 1156
Proscar. *See* finasteride
ProSom. *See* estazolam
prostaglandin(s), 718
  as abortifacients, 1213, 1213*t*
  actions/effects, 712*t*, 718–19
  for glaucoma, 1342
    bimatoprost, 1341*t*, 1343
    latanoprost. *See* latanoprost
    travoprost, 1341*t*, 1343
  indications, 1214
  as uterine stimulants
    carboprost, 1187*t*, 1189
    dinoprostone, 1187*t*, 1189
    misoprostol. *See* misoprostol
prostaglandin E_2, 1007
prostate cancer, 965*t*, 1229*t*
prostate gland, 1229. *See also* benign prostatic hyperplasia
prostatitis, 837
Prostigmin. *See* neostigmine
Prostin E_2. *See* dinoprostone
protease, 928
PROTEASE INHIBITORS, 937–38
  atazanavir, 933*t*, 939
  darunavir, 933*t*, 939
  fosamprenavir, 933*t*, 939
  indinavir, 933*t*, 939
  lopinavir/ritonavir. *See* lopinavir/ritonavir
  nelfinavir, 933*t*, 939–40
  ritonavir, 933*t*, 940
  saquinavir, 933*t*, 940
  tipranavir, 933*t*, 940
protein synthesis, 808–9, 808*f*
proteins, in enteral nutrition, 1070
Proteus mirabilis, 777*t*
prothrombin, 486
prothrombin time (PT), 644
PROTON PUMP INHIBITORS (PPIs):
  adverse effects, 1013–14, 1013*t*, 1014*t*
  bone fracture risk and, 1016*t*
  drugs in class
    esomeprazole, 1013*t*, 1015
    lansoprazole, 1013*t*, 1015
    omeprazole. *See* omeprazole
    pantoprazole, 1013*t*, 1015
    rabeprazole, 1013*t*, 1015–16
  gastrointestinal infection and, 1014*t*
  mechanism of action, 1012*f*, 1013
  Nursing Process Application, 1017*t*
  in pediatric patients, 1023*t*
  for specific conditions
    with aspirin therapy, 720
    peptic ulcer, 1013–14
Protonix. *See* pantoprazole
Protopam. *See* pralidoxime
Protopic. *See* tacrolimus
prototype drug, 6–7
protozoan, 886
protozoan infections, 886*t*
  malaria. *See* malaria
  nonmalarial. *See* nonmalarial protozoan infections
  Nursing Process Application, 899*t*
  pathogenesis, 886
protriptyline, 304*t*, 307
Proventil. *See* albuterol
Proventil Repetabs. *See* albuterol
Provera. *See* medroxyprogesterone acetate
Provigil. *See* modafinil
provirus, 909, 927
Prozac. *See* fluoxetine
pruritus, 1316
pseudocholinesterase, 192, 222
pseudoephedrine, 1273–74
  adverse effects, 1273–74
  classification, 1273
  clinical applications, 238
  contraindications/precautions, 1274
  drug interactions, 1274
  mechanism of action, 1273
  in methamphetamine manufacture, 106, 236*t*
  nursing responsibilities, 1274
  overdose treatment, 1274
  patient and family education, 1274
  pharmacokinetics, 1273
  pregnancy category, 1274
  restrictions on sale, 106, 238, 1273*t*
  therapeutic effects and uses, 1273
pseudogout, 1309*t*
pseudomembranous colitis, 811
Pseudomonas aeruginosa, 777*t*, 793, 828
psilocybin, 104, 104*f*
psoralens, 1331
psoriasis, 1328, 1328*f*
  etiology, 1328
  incidence, 1328*t*
  nonpharmacologic therapy, 1331
  pathophysiology, 1328
  pharmacotherapy
    systemic
      acitretin, 1330*t*, 1331
      cyclosporine. *See* cyclosporine
      etanercept. *See* etanercept
      hydroxyurea, 1330*t*, 1331
      methotrexate, 1330, 1330*t*. *See also* methotrexate
    topical
      anthralin, 1329, 1330*t*
      calcipotriene, 1329, 1330*t*
      coal tar, 1329, 1330*t*
      corticosteroids, 1328–29
      salicylic acid, 1330*t*
      tacrolimus, 1330*t*
      tazarotene, 1329, 1330*t*
  types, 1329*t*
psoriasis vulgaris, 1329*t*
Psoriatec. *See* anthralin
psoriatic arthritis, 1329*t*
psoriatic erythroderma, 1329*t*
PSVT (paroxysmal supraventricular tachycardia), 626
psychodynamic therapy, for depression, 301, 302*t*
psychological dependence, 96
psychosis, 326. *See also* schizophrenia
psychosocial, 157
psyllium mucilloid, 1031–32
  adverse effects, 1031
  classification, 1031
  contraindications/precautions, 1031
  drug absorption and, 177
  drug interactions, 1031
  mechanism of action, 1031
  nursing responsibilities, 1032
  overdose treatment, 1031
  patient and family education, 1032
  pharmacokinetics, 1031
  pregnancy category, 1031
  similar drugs, 1032
  therapeutic effects and uses, 1031
PTSD (post-traumatic stress disorder), 276, 289, 290*t*
PTU. *See* propylthiouracil
pubic lice, 1318
public health nurse, 167
Pulmicort. *See* budesonide
Pulmicort Respules. *See* budesonide
pulmonary embolism, 642
Pulmozyme. *See* dornase alfa
Pure Food and Drug Act (PFDA), 13–14
purified protein derivative (PPD), 853
PURINE ANALOGS, 975
  cladribine, 973*t*, 975–76
  clofarabine, 973*t*, 976
  fludarabine, 973*t*, 976
  mercaptopurine, 973*t*, 976
  nelarabine, 973*t*, 976
  pentostatin, 973*t*, 976
  thioguanine, 973*t*, 976

Purinethol. *See* mercaptopurine
Push Packages, 1359
pyelonephritis, 837
pyrantel, 902*t*, 903
pyrazinamide, 855*t*, 858
pyrethrin, 1319, 1320
pyridostigmine, 202*t*, 204–5, 207
pyridoxine (vitamin B_6):
  adverse effects, 1059
  contraindications/precautions, 1059
  deficiency, 1053*t*
  drug interactions, 1059
  functions, 1053*t*
  mechanism of action, 1059
  nursing responsibilities, 1059
  for nutritional disorders
    adverse effects, 1054*t*
    route and adult dose, 1054*t*
  patient and family education, 1060
  recommended dietary allowance, 1059
  supplement to isoniazid in pregnancy, 857
  therapeutic effects and uses, 1059, 1364*t*
pyrimethamine, 888*t*
pyrimethamine-sulfadiazine, 897–98
  adverse effects, 840*t*, 888*t*, 897
  classification, 897
  contraindications/precautions, 897
  drug interactions, 897
  mechanism of action, 897
  nursing responsibilities, 898
  overdose treatment, 898
  patient and family education, 898
  pharmacokinetics, 897
  pregnancy category, 897
  route and adult dose, 840*t*
  similar drugs, 898
  therapeutic effects and uses, 897
PYRIMIDINE ANALOGS, 974–75
  capecitabine, 973*t*, 975
  cytarabine, 827, 973*t*, 975
  floxuridine, 973*t*, 975
  fluorouracil, 827, 973*t*, 975
  gemcitabine, 973*t*, 975
PZA. *See* pyrazinamide

Q

QRS complex, 626*t*
QT interval, 626*t*
Quaalude. *See* methaqualone
quazepam, 282*t*, 286
Questran. *See* cholestyramine
quetiapine, 319*t*, 337*t*, 339–40
quinacrine, 101*t*
Quinamm. *See* quinine
quinapril, 533*t*, 536, 612*t*
Quinidex. *See* quinidine sulfate
quinidine gluconate, 629*t*, 632
quinidine sulfate, 629*t*, 632
quinine, 888*t*, 890
quinupristin-dalfopristin, 821–22, 821*t*
Qvar. *See* beclomethasone

R

RA. *See* rheumatoid arthritis
RAAS. *See* renin-angiotensin-aldosterone system
rabeprazole, 1013*t*, 1015–16
rabies, 758*t*, 763
rabies immune globulin, 767*t*
Rabis-HT. *See* rabies immune globulin
racemic amphetamine. *See* amphetamine sulfate
radiation sickness, 1363
radiation therapy, 952–53
radioactive iodide, 1154*t*, 1156
raloxifene, 1297–99
  adverse effects, 1295*t*, 1299
  classification, 1297
  contraindications/precautions, 1299
  drug interactions, 1299
  mechanism of action, 1299
  for neoplasia, 980*t*, 982
  nursing responsibilities, 1299
  overdose treatment, 1299
  patient and family education, 1299
  pharmacokinetics, 1299
  pregnancy category, 1299
  route and adult dose, 1295*t*
  therapeutic effects and uses, 1297
raltegravir, 933*t*, 940
ramelteon, 276, 282*t*, 288
ramipril, 533*t*, 536, 612*t*
Ranexa. *See* ranolazine
ranibizumab, 748*t*
ranitidine, 1018–19
  adverse effects, 1016*t*, 1018
    in older adults, 152*t*
  classification, 1018*t*
  contraindications/precautions, 1018
  drug interactions, 1018
  mechanism of action, 1018
  nursing responsibilities, 1018
  overdose treatment, 1018
  patient and family education, 1018–19
  pharmacokinetics, 1018
  pregnancy category, 1018
  for preoperative medication, 477
  route and adult dose, 1016*t*
  similar drugs, 1019
  therapeutic effects and uses, 1018
ranolazine, 591, 592*t*
Rapamune. *See* sirolimus
rapid eye movement (REM) sleep, 278, 278*t*
Raptiva. *See* efalizumab
RAS. *See* reticular activating system
rash, drug-induced, 70
Raynaud's disease, 248, 248*t*
Razadyne. *See* galantamine hydrobromide
RDAs (recommended dietary allowances), 1054
RDS (respiratory distress syndrome), 1240*t*
reabsorption, 546
Rebetol. *See* ribavirin
Rebif. *See* interferon beta-1a
rebound congestion, 1271
rebound effects, 96–97
rebound insomnia, 280
reboxetine, 313
receptor(s), 60, 60*f*
Reclast. *See* zoledronate
recombinant technology vaccines, 756–57, 756*t*
Recombivax HB. *See* hepatitis B vaccine
recommended dietary allowances (RDAs), 1054
Recothrom. *See* thrombin
rectal route, drug administration, 34
red clover, 173*t*
refeeding syndrome, 1073*t*
reflex tachycardia, 202, 492, 579
Refludan. *See* lepirudin
refractory period, 624
regional anesthesia, 458
Reglan. *See* metoclopramide
Relafen. *See* nabumetone
Relenza. *See* zanamivir
Relistor. *See* methylnaltrexone
Relpax. *See* eletriptan
REM (rapid eye movement) sleep, 278, 278*t*
Remeron. *See* mirtazapine
Remicade. *See* infliximab
remifentanil, 460*t*, 462–63
Reminyl. *See* galantamine
Renagel. *See* sevelamer
renal failure, 546
  classification, 547
  diagnosis, 547–48
  drug excretion in, 49
  incidence and causes, 546*t*
  pharmacotherapy, 546–48, 548*t*
renal physiology. *See* kidney(s), physiology
renin, 530, 531*f*
renin inhibitors, 532, 574*t*, 575
renin-angiotensin system, 493, 493*f*
renin-angiotensin-aldosterone system (RAAS), 529
  anatomy, 531*f*
  components, 529–31, 530*f*
  physiological effects, 531–32, 531*f*
  points for drug intervention, 532
Renova. *See* tretinoin
ReoPro. *See* abciximab
reoviruses, 909*t*
repaglinide, 1136–37
  adverse effects, 1133*t*, 1136
  classification, 1136
  contraindications/precautions, 1136
  drug interactions, 1137
  mechanism of action, 1136
  overdose treatment, 1137
  pharmacokinetics, 1136
  pregnancy category, 1137
  route and adult dose, 1133*t*
  similar drugs, 1137
  therapeutic effects and uses, 1136
repetitive transcranial magnetic stimulation (rTMS), for depression, 302*t*, 303
replacement therapy, 1101. *See also* HORMONE(S)
repolarization, 624
Repronex. *See* menotropins
Requip. *See* ropinirole
Rescriptor. *See* delavirdine
reserpine, 578–79
resistance, to antibiotics. *See* acquired resistance
respiratory depression, with opioids, 435, 436*t*, 437, 437*t*
respiratory distress syndrome (RDS), 1240*t*
respiratory system:
  age-related changes, 149*t*
  drug excretion by, 49
  lower, 1239–40, 1239*f*
  upper, 1262–63, 1262*f*
rest-and-digest response, 186
Restasis. *See* cyclosporine ophthalmic emulsion
Restoril. *See* temazepam
Retavase. *See* reteplase
reteplase, 658*t*, 659–60
reticular activating system (RAS), 270
  anatomy, 271*f*
  anxiety disorders and, 276, 277*f*
  functions, 270, 276

reticular formation, 106
Retin-A. *See* tretinoin
RETINOIDS, 1322
  adapalene, 1322, 1322*t*, 1324
  isotretinoin, 30*t*, 1322, 1322*t*, 1323, 1325
  tazarotene, 1322*t*, 1325, 1329, 1330*t*
  tretinoin. *See* tretinoin
retinopathy, diabetic, 1126
Retrovir. *See* zidovudine
retroviruses, 909*t*
reverse cholesterol transport, 498
reverse remodeling, 614
reverse transcriptase, 927
reverse transcriptase inhibitors. *See* NONNUCLEOSIDE REVERSE TRANSCRIPTASE INHIBITORS; NUCLEOSIDE/NUCLEOTIDE REVERSE TRANSCRIPTASE INHIBITORS
Revex. *See* nalmefene
ReVia. *See* naltrexone
Revlimid. *See* lenalidomide
Reyataz. *See* atazanavir
Reye's syndrome, 720
Rezulin. *See* troglitazone
Rh_o [D] immune globulin, 765–69
  adverse effects, 768
  classification, 767
  contraindications/precautions, 768–69
  drug interactions, 769
  nursing responsibilities, 769
  overdose treatment, 769
  patient and family education, 769
  pharmacokinetics, 768
  pregnancy category, 769
  similar drugs, 769
  therapeutic effects and uses, 767–68
rhabdomyolysis, 502
Rheomacrodex. *See* dextran 40
rheumatoid arthritis (RA), 1303
  diagnosis, 1303
  etiology, 1303
  incidence, 1303*t*
  nonpharmacologic therapy, 1303
  pathophysiology, 1301*f*, 1303
  pharmacotherapy
    analgesics, 1303
    corticosteroids, 1169, 1303–4
  signs and symptoms, 1303, 1303*f*
Rheumatrex. *See* methotrexate
Rhinocort. *See* budesonide
Rhinocort Aqua. *See* budesonide
rhinophyma, 1323
RhoGAM. *See* Rh_o [D] immune globulin
Ribasphere. *See* ribavirin
ribavirin, 919*t*, 922
riboflavin (vitamin B_2):
  adverse effects, 1059
  contraindications/precautions, 1059
  deficiency, 1053*t*
  drug interactions, 1059
  functions, 1053*t*
  mechanism of action, 1059
  nursing responsibilities, 1059
  for nutritional disorders
    adverse effects, 1054*t*
    route and adult dose, 1054*t*
  patient and family education, 1059
  pregnancy category, 1059
  recommended dietary allowance, 1059
  therapeutic effects and uses, 1059
Rickettsia rickettsii, 777*t*
RID. *See* pyrethrin
rifabutin:
  drug interactions, 856
  for specific conditions
    H. pylori infection, 1023
    M. avium complex infections, 865
    tuberculosis, 855*t*, 860
Rifadin. *See* rifampin
Rifamate, 860
rifampin:
  clinical applications, 833
  drug interactions, 101*t*, 856, 860
  for specific conditions
    leprosy, 862
    tuberculosis, 855*t*, 859–60
rifapentine, 855*t*, 860
Rifater, 860
Rilutek. *See* riluzole
riluzole, 366
Rimactane. *See* rifampin
rimantadine, 915, 916*t*, 917
rimonabant, 1090
Ringer's solution, 691*t*, 692
ringworm, 869*t*, 877
Riomet. *See* metformin
Riopan. *See* magaldrate
risedronate, 1294*t*, 1295*t*, 1297
risk management, 88
risk-benefit ratio, 68
Risperdal. *See* risperidone
risperidone:
  adverse effects, 319*t*, 337, 337*t*
  classification, 336
  contraindications/precautions, 337
  drug interactions, 337–38
  mechanism of action, 337
  nursing responsibilities, 338
  overdose treatment, 338
  patient and family education, 338–39
  pharmacokinetics, 337
  pregnancy category, 338
  route and adult dose, 319*t*, 337*t*
  for specific conditions
    bipolar disorder, 319*t*
  therapeutic effects and uses, 336–37
Ritalin. *See* methylphenidate
Ritalin SR, 30*t*. *See also* methylphenidate
ritodrine, 240, 1189
ritonavir, 933*t*, 940. *See also* lopinavir/ritonavir
Rituxan. *See* rituximab
rituximab, 748*t*, 990*t*, 1304*t*
rivastigmine, 202*t*, 355*t*, 360, 362
rizatriptan, 450*t*, 452
RNA viruses, 909*t*
Robaxin. *See* methocarbamol
Robinul. *See* glycopyrrolate
Robitussin. *See* dextromethorphan
Robitussin A-C, 1276*t*
Rocaltrol. *See* calcitriol
Rocephin. *See* ceftriaxone
rocuronium, 219*t*, 224
rofecoxib, 727
Rogaine. *See* minoxidil
Rohypnol. *See* flunitrazepam
Rolaids. *See* calcium carbonate
ropinirole, 350*t*, 354
ropivacaine, 473*t*, 476
rosacea, 1323, 1323*f*
rosiglitazone, 1137–38
  adverse effects, 1133*t*, 1137
  classification, 1137
  contraindications/precautions, 1137
  drug interactions, 1137–38
  mechanism of action, 1137
  overdose treatment, 1138
  pharmacokinetics, 1137
  pregnancy category, 1138
  route and adult dose, 1133*t*
  therapeutic effects and uses, 1137
rosuvastatin, 504*t*, 506
RotaShield. *See* rotavirus
rotavirus, 766
Roxanol. *See* morphine sulfate
Rozerem. *See* ramelteon
rTMS (repetitive transcranial magnetic stimulation), for depression, 302*t*, 303
RU-496. *See* mifepristone
rubella (German measles), 758*t*, 764
rubeola. *See* measles
Rubex. *See* doxorubicin
Rythmol. *See* propafenone

S

saccharin, 1093
SAD (seasonal affective disorder), 299
Saizen. *See* somatropin
Salagen. *See* pilocarpine
Salax. *See* salicylic acid
SALICYLATES, 718
  aspirin. *See* aspirin
  choline and magnesium trisalicylate, 720*t*, 723
  magnesium salicylate, 720*t*, 723
  poisoning, 720*t*
  salsalate, 720*t*, 723
  topical, 1302
salicylic acid, 1328, 1330*t*
salicylism, 722
salivary amylase, 1004*t*
salmeterol, 240, 1245*t*, 1247–48
Salmonella enteritides, 777*t*
Salmonella typhi, 777*t*
salsalate, 720*t*, 723
Salsitab. *See* salsalate
salt replacements, exercise and, 696*t*
Sandimmune. *See* cyclosporine
Sandostatin. *See* octreotide
Sansert. *See* methysergide
saquinavir, 178*t*, 933*t*, 940
Sarafem. *See* fluoxetine
sarcolemma, 516
sarcoma, 950*t*
sarcoplasmic reticula, 516
sargramostim, 670*t*, 674
satiety, 1086
satiety center, 1086
SaunoSome. *See* daunorubicin liposomal
saw palmetto:
  description, 1232*t*
  evidence, 1232*t*
  history and claims, 1232*t*
  primary uses, 173*t*
  standardization, 175*t*, 1232*t*
SCABICIDES, 1318
  crotamiton, 1319, 1320
  lindane, 1319, 1320
  Nursing Process Application, 1321*t*

permethrin. *See* permethrin
pyrethrin, 1319, 1320
scabies, 1318, 1318*f*
scheduled drugs, 20, 94, 95*t*, 412*t*
schizoaffective disorder, 327–28
schizophrenia, 326
characteristics, 326
etiology, 328
gender differences, 328*t*
incidence, 326*t*
nonpharmacologic therapy, 330
pharmacotherapy
antipsychotics. *See* antipsychotics
initial treatment, 328
maintenance treatment, 328–29
nonadherence issues, 329–30
prognosis, 330
symptoms, 327–28, 327*t*
school-age children. *See* pediatric patients
school nurses, 165–66, 166*f*, 166*t*, 386*t*
scinitinib, 990*t*
sclera, 1338
sclerosing, 957
scopolamine:
adverse effects, 214*t*, 218, 1043*t*
indications, 218, 1042
route and adult dose, 214*t*, 1043*t*
transdermal administration, 32
scopolamine hydrobromide, 218, 1347, 1348*t*
scurvy, 1052
seasonal affective disorder (SAD), 299
Seasonale, 1204
Seasonique, 1204
sebaceous glands, 1316
seborrhea, 1320
seborrheic dermatitis, 1325, 1327–28
secobarbital, 282*t*, 292
SECOND-GENERATION (ATYPICAL) ANTIPSYCHOTICS:
in Alzheimer's disease, 360
for bipolar disorder, 319*t*, 321
drugs in class
aripiprazole. *See* aripiprazole
clozapine, 337*t*, 339
olanzapine, 319*t*, 337*t*, 339
paliperidone, 337*t*, 339
quetiapine, 319*t*, 337*t*, 339–40
risperidone. *See* risperidone
ziprasidone, 319*t*, 337*t*, 340
mechanism of action, 336
Nursing Process Application, 343*t*
paliperidone, 337*t*, 339
weight gain with use of, 338*t*
second messenger, 60
secondary hypertension, 568. *See also* hypertension
secretion, 546
Sectral. *See* acebutolol
sedative–hypnotic, 281
sedatives, 98
seizures:
classification, 372*f*, 374–76
generalized, 374
partial, 375
pharmacotherapy, 283*t*, 376*t*. *See also* antiseizure drugs
in pregnancy and lactation, 372–73
recurrence rates, 373*t*
school nurses' role in treatment of, 386*t*
SELECTIVE ESTROGEN RECEPTOR MODULATORS (SERMs), 1297
raloxifene. *See* raloxifene
tamoxifen. *See* tamoxifen
SELECTIVE SEROTONIN REUPTAKE INHIBITORS (SSRIs):
as adjuvant analgesics, 446, 446*t*
adverse effects, 308
drug interactions, 75*t*
with herbal products, 178*t*
drugs in class
citalopram, 290*t*, 304*t*, 310
escitalopram, 282*t*, 289, 290*t*, 304*t*, 310
fluoxetine. *See* fluoxetine
fluvoxamine, 282*t*, 289, 290*t*, 304*t*, 310
paroxetine, 282*t*, 289, 290*t*, 304*t*, 310
sertraline, 282*t*, 289, 290*t*, 304*t*, 310–11
mechanism of action, 305*f*
Nursing Process Application, 316*t*
in pregnancy, 124*t*
for specific conditions
anxiety and insomnia, 282*t*, 289, 290*t*
childhood anxiety, 290*t*
nausea and vomiting, 1044
weight loss, 1090
selegiline, 315, 317, 350*t*, 355, 420
selenium, 1063*t*
description, 953*t*
evidence, 953*t*
history and claims, 953*t*
primary uses, 179*t*
standardization, 953*t*
selenium sulfide, 1328
Selzentry. *See* maraviroc
senna, 1030*t*, 1031
Sensipar. *See* cinacalcet hydrochloride
Sensorcaine. *See* bupivacaine
Septocaine. *See* articaine
Septra. *See* trimethoprim-sulfamethoxazole
Serax. *See* oxazepam
Serevent. *See* salmeterol
SERMs. *See* SELECTIVE ESTROGEN RECEPTOR MODULATORS (SERMs)
Seromycin. *See* cycloserine
Serophene. *See* clomiphene citrate
Seroquel. *See* quetiapine
Serostim. *See* somatropin
serotonergic synapses, 267
serotonin (5-HT), 307
actions/effects, 189*t*, 267, 267*t*, 307, 308*f*
clinical applications, 267*t*
in depression, 308. *See also* SELECTIVE SEROTONIN REUPTAKE INHIBITORS (SSRIs)
SEROTONIN (5-HT) AGONISTS:
tegaserod, 1040
SEROTONIN (5-HT) ANTAGONISTS, 1044
alosetron, 1040
dolasetron, 1043*t*
granisetron, 1043*t*
ondansetron, 477, 1043*t*
palonosetron, 1043*t*
serotonin syndrome (SES), 308
Serpalan. *See* reserpine
Serratia, 777*t*
sertraline:
for anxiety or insomnia, 282*t*, 289, 290*t*
for depression, 304*t*, 310–11
drug interactions, 101*t*
for weight loss, 1090
Sertuner, Frederich, 3
serum glucose, 1120, 1121*f*. *See also* diabetes mellitus
SES (serotonin syndrome), 308
sevelamer, 548*t*
sevoflurane, 468*t*, 469
sexual activity:
among high school students, 927*t*
following myocardial infarction, 600*t*
sexual dysfunction:
with alpha-adrenergic antagonists, 248
male, 1225, 1225*t*. *See also* erectile dysfunction
Sherley Amendment, 14
Shigella, 777*t*
shingles (varicella zoster), 674, 758*t*, 765, 765*t*
short stature, 1107, 1107*t*. *See also* growth hormone, deficiency
SIADH (syndrome of inappropriate diuretic hormone), 1114
sibutramine, 1090–91
adverse effects, 1090
classification, 1090
contraindications/precautions, 1090–91
drug interactions, 1091
mechanism of action, 1090
nursing responsibilities, 1091
overdose treatment, 1091
patient and family education, 1091
pharmacokinetics, 1090
pregnancy category, 1091
similar drugs, 1091
therapeutic effects and uses, 1090
sick sinus syndrome, 626. *See also* dysrhythmias
side effects, 66
sildenafil, 1228–29
adverse effects, 1227*t*, 1228
classification, 1228
contraindications/precautions, 1228
drug interactions, 250, 1228
history, 1227
mechanism of action, 1228
nursing responsibilities, 1228–29
overdose treatment, 1228
patient and family education, 1229
pharmacokinetics action, 1228
pregnancy category, 1228
route and adult dose, 1227*t*
similar drugs, 1229
therapeutic effects and uses, 1228
for women, 1229*t*
silent angina, 589. *See also* angina pectoris
Silvadene. *See* silver sulfadiazine
silver sulfadiazine, 842
simethicone, 1021
simple partial seizures, 375, 376*t*
Simplesse, 1093
Simulect. *See* basiliximab
simvastatin, 101*t*, 504*t*, 506
Sinemet. *See* levodopa/carbidopa
Sinemet SR, 30*t*. *See also* levodopa/carbidopa
Sinequan. *See* doxepin
Singulair. *See* montelukast
sinoatrial (SA) node, 487
sinoatrial (SA) node dysfunction, 626. *See also* dysrhythmias
sinus bradycardia, 626. *See also* dysrhythmias
sinus rhythm, 487
sirolimus, 741*t*, 744

sitagliptin, 1141–42
  adverse effects, 1133*t*, 1141
  classification, 1141
  contraindications/precautions, 1141
  drug interactions, 1142
  mechanism of action, 1141
  overdose treatment, 1142
  pharmacokinetics, 1141
  pregnancy category, 1142
  route and adult dose, 1133*t*
  therapeutic effects and uses, 1141
situational anxiety, 275
Sjögren's syndrome, 201
Skelaxin. *See* metaxalone
skeletal muscle relaxants. *See* muscle relaxants
Skelid. *See* tiludronate
skin:
  appendages, 1316
  disorders
    acne vulgaris. *See* acne vulgaris
    classification, 1316–17, 1317*t*
    dermatitis. *See* dermatitis
    infections. *See* skin infections
    psoriasis. *See* psoriasis
    rosacea, 1323, 1323*f*
    sunburn, 1331–33
  drugs toxic to, 69*t*, 70
  layers, 1315–16, 1315*f*
skin infections:
  bacterial, 1317
  fungal, 1318
  parasitic, 1318–20, 1318*f*, 1321*t*
  viral, 1318
sleep:
  amount by population group, 278*t*
  amount required, 277
  function of, 277
  patterns, 278–79, 279*t*
  stages, 277, 278*t*
sleep attacks, 419
sleep disorders:
  evaluation, 279–80
  insomnia. *See* insomnia
  narcolepsy, 279
sleep-maintenance insomnia, 279
sleep-offset insomnia, 279
sleep-onset insomnia, 279
sleep paralysis, 419
sleep–wake patterns, 278–79, 278*t*
Slo-Phyllin. *See* theophylline
Slow-K, 30*t*. *See also* potassium chloride (KCl)
small volume nebulizer, 1242
smallpox, 755, 758*t*, 1361
smoking cessation:
  bupropion for, 107–8
  nicotine replacement therapy for, 107, 108*f*, 209
  varenicline for, 108
SNS (Strategic National Stockpile), 1359
social anxiety disorder, 275, 289, 290*t*
sodium:
  in foods, 249*t*
  functions, 695, 1062*t*
  imbalances
    hypernatremia. *See* hypernatremia
    hyponatremia. *See* hyponatremia
  recommended dietary allowance, 1062*t*
  regulation, 695
sodium antacids, 1019. *See also* ANTACIDS
sodium bicarbonate, 702–3
  adverse effects, 702
  classification, 702
  contraindications/precautions, 702
  drug interactions, 702
  mechanism of action, 702
  nursing responsibilities, 702–3
  overdose treatment, 702
  patient and family education, 703
  pharmacokinetics, 702
  pregnancy category, 702
  therapeutic effects and uses, 702, 1021*t*
sodium biphosphate, 1030*t*
SODIUM CHANNEL BLOCKERS:
  class IA
    disopyramide, 629*t*, 632
    procainamide. *See* procainamide
    quinidine gluconate, 629*t*, 632
    quinidine sulfate, 629*t*, 632
  class IB
    lidocaine. *See* lidocaine
    mexiletine, 629*t*, 632
    phenytoin. *See* phenytoin
  class IC
    flecainide, 629*t*, 632–33
    propafenone, 629*t*, 632
  mechanism of action, 628, 628*t*
sodium channel inhibitors. *See* POTASSIUM-SPARING DIURETICS, sodium channel inhibitors
sodium chloride (NaCl), 696
  adverse effects, 696
  classification, 696
  contraindications/precautions, 696
  drug interactions, 696
  mechanism of action, 696
  overdose treatment, 696
  pharmacokinetics, 696
  pregnancy category, 696
  therapeutic effects and uses, 696
sodium hyaluronate, 1302
sodium nitroprusside. *See* nitroprusside sodium
sodium oxybate:
  for cataplexy/narcoplexy, 22, 280, 421
  disposal, 26*t*
  regulation, 98
sodium stibogluconate, 892*t*, 898
Solaraze. *See* diclofenac
Solarcaine. *See* benzocaine
Soliris. *See* eculizumab
Soltamox. *See* tamoxifen
solubility, drug absorption and, 45
Solu-Medrol. *See* methylprednisolone
Soma. *See* carisoprodol
somatic nervous system, 185
somatostatin, 1007
somatropin, 1108–9
  adverse effects, 1108*t*, 1109
  classification, 1108
  contraindications/precautions, 1109–10
  drug interactions, 1110
  mechanism of action, 1109
  nursing responsibilities, 1110
  overdose treatment, 1110
  patient and family education, 1110
  pharmacokinetics, 1109
  pregnancy category, 1110
  route and adult dose, 1108*t*
  similar drugs, 1110–11
  therapeutic effects and uses, 1108–9
Somatuline Depot. *See* lanreotide
Somavert. *See* pegvisomant
Sonata. *See* zaleplon
sorafenib, 748*t*, 990*t*
Sorbitrate. *See* isosorbide dinitrate
Soriatane. *See* acitretin
Sorine. *See* sotalol
sotalol, 252*t*, 255, 629*t*, 636
soundalike drug names, 84–85*t*
soy:
  description, 981*t*
  drug interactions, 178*t*
  evidence, 981*t*
  history and claims, 981*t*
  primary uses, 173*t*
  products, 501*t*
  standardization, 981*t*
specialized formulas, for enteral nutrition, 1069*t*, 1070
specialty supplements, 179, 179*t*
Spectazole. *See* econazole
Spectracef. *See* cefditoren
SPERMICIDES, 1210–11
  nonoxynol-9. *See* nonoxynol-9
spinal anesthesia, 471, 471*f*
spinal cord, 268*f*, 269
spinal cord injury, 402–3
Spiriva. *See* tiotropium bromide
spironolactone, 556–58
  adverse effects, 541, 556*t*, 557
  classification, 556
  contraindications/precautions, 557
  drug interactions, 557
  mechanism of action, 557
  nursing responsibilities, 557
  overdose treatment, 557
  patient and family education, 557–58
  pharmacokinetics, 557
  pregnancy category, 557
  route and adult dose, 538*t*, 556*t*, 612*t*
  similar drugs, 558
  for specific conditions
    heart failure, 612*t*, 613
    hyperaldosteronism, 1170
  therapeutic effects and uses, 556–57
Sporanox. *See* itraconazole
Sporothrix schenckii, 869*t*
sporotrichosis, 869*t*
sporozoite, 887
Sportscreme, 1302
Sprycel. *See* dasatinib
sputum culture, for tuberculosis, 853
SSKI. *See* potassium iodide
SSRIs. *See* SELECTIVE SEROTONIN REUPTAKE INHIBITORS (SSRIs)
St. John's wort:
  for depression, 313*t*
  drug interactions, 75, 177, 178*t*, 179*t*
  primary uses, 173*t*
  standardization, 175*t*
ST segment, 626*t*
stable angina, 589. *See also* angina pectoris
Stadol. *See* butorphanol
staging, cancer, 953, 954*t*
Staphylococcus aureus, 777*t*
  invasiveness, 775
  methicillin-resistant, 781–82
  in skin infections, 1317
Staphylococcus saprophyticus, 838, 838*t*
Starling's law of the heart, 490

Starlix. *See* nateglinide
STATINS:
  adverse effects, 502–3, 504*t*
  drugs in class
    atorvastatin. *See* atorvastatin
    fluvastatin, 504*t*, 505–6
    lovastatin, 75*t*, 504*t*, 506
    pravastatin, 504*t*, 506
    rosuvastatin, 504*t*, 506
    simvastatin, 504*t*, 506
  mechanism of action, 501–2, 503*f*
  for specific conditions
    in development, 503
    dyslipidemias, 501–6, 504*t*
status asthmaticus, 1241
status epilepticus, 376, 376*t*
stavudine, 26*t*, 933*t*, 936
steatorrhea, 1047
Sterapred. *See* prednisone
stereotactic pallidotomy, 350*t*
steroids, 496, 497*f*
sterol nucleus, 496
Stevens–Johnson syndrome, 1333*t*
stevia, 1093
Stilbestrol. *See* diethylstilbestrol
Stimate. *See* desmopressin
stomach, 1007, 1008*f*
stool softeners, 1030*t*, 1031, 1032
Strategic National Stockpile (SNS), 1359
Strattera. *See* atomoxetine
stratum basale, 1316
stratum corneum, 1315–16
Streptococci, 777*t*
Streptococcus pneumoniae, 759. *See also* pneumococcal infection
Streptococcus pyogenes, 1317, 1351
streptogramins, 822
streptokinase, 658*t*, 660
streptomycin, 819
  adverse effects, 816*t*
  mechanism of action, 809*f*
  route and adult dose, 816*t*
  for specific conditions
    tuberculosis, 855*t*, 860
streptozocin, 967*t*, 971
stress ulcers, 1009. *See also* peptic ulcer
Striant. *See* testosterone
striatum, 348
stroke volume, 489–90
Stromectol. *See* ivermectin
structured treatment interruptions, 931
subcutaneous route, drug administration, 35*f*
subcutaneous tissue, 1316
Sublimaze. *See* fentanyl
sublingual route, drug administration, 31, 31*f*
Suboxone. *See* buprenorphine
substance abuse, 93. *See also specific substances*
  DSM-IV-TR criteria, 93*t*
  effects in pregnancy, 126
  incidence, 94*t*, 95*t*, 98*t*
  legislation of controlled substances, 94
  in nurses, 103*t*
  nurse's role in recognition and treatment, 109
  sedatives and related agents, 98
  types, 93–94
substance P, 189*t*
substantia nigra, 348
substrate, 47
Subutex. *See* buprenorphine
SUCCINIMIDES, 387–88
  ethosuximide. *See* ethosuximide
succinylcholine chloride, 222–23
  as adjunct to anesthesia, 477
  adverse effects, 219*t*, 222
  classification, 222
  contraindications/precautions, 222
  drug interactions, 222
  mechanism of action, 220, 222
  nursing responsibilities, 222
  overdose treatment, 222
  patient and family education, 222–23
  pharmacokinetics, 222
  pregnancy category, 222
  route and adult dose, 219*t*
  similar drugs, 223
  therapeutic effects and uses, 222
sucralfate, 75*t*, 1024
sucralose, 1093
Sucrets. *See* dextromethorphan
sucrose, 1004*t*
Sudafed. *See* pseudoephedrine
Sudafed PE Nighttime Cold, 1266*t*
Sudafed PE Sinus and Allergy tablets, 1266*t*
Sufenta. *See* sufentanil
sufentanil, 460*t*, 463
suicide, 301, 303*t*
Sular. *See* nisoldipine
sulconazole, 878*t*
sulfacetamide, 842, 1322*t*, 1323
sulfadiazine, 840*t*, 841, 842, 843
sulfadiazine-pyrimethamine. *See* pyrimethamine-sulfadiazine
Sulfamylon. *See* mafenide
sulfasalazine, 1037–38
  adverse effects, 1038, 1304*t*, 1306
    in breast-feeding infant, 129*t*
  classification, 1037
  contraindications/precautions, 1038
  drug interactions, 1038
  mechanism of action, 1038
  nursing responsibilities, 1038
  overdose treatment, 1038
  patient and family education, 1038
  pharmacokinetics, 1038
  pregnancy category, 1038
  route and adult dose, 1304*t*
  similar drugs, 1038–39
  for specific conditions
    rheumatoid arthritis, 1304*t*, 1306
  therapeutic effects and uses, 1037–38
sulfinpyrazone, 1307*t*, 1309, 1310
sulfisoxazole, 840*t*, 841, 843
SULFONAMIDES:
  absorption, 841
  adverse effects, 842
  contraindications, 842
  drug interactions, 842
  drugs in class
    mafenide, 842
    sulfacetamide, 842
    sulfadiazine, 840*t*, 841, 842, 843
    sulfadoxine-pyrimethamine, 840*t*, 841
    sulfisoxazole, 840*t*, 841, 843
    trimethoprim, 843–44
    trimethoprim-sulfamethoxazole. *See* trimethoprim-sulfamethoxazole
  excretion, 841
  indications, 840
  mechanism of action, 841, 841*f*
  Nursing Process Application, 844–45t
  resistance to, 841
  structure, 841*f*
  topical, 842
  for urinary tract infections, 840–42, 840*t*
SULFONYLUREAS:
  actions, 1132*t*
  drug interactions, 101*t*, 842
  first generation
    chlorpropamide, 1133*t*, 1135
    tolazamide, 1133*t*, 1135
    tolbutamide, 1133*t*, 1135
  mechanism of action, 1132–33
  nursing considerations, 1132*t*
  second generation
    glimepiride, 1133*t*, 1135
    glipizide, 1133*t*, 1135
    glyburide. *See* glyburide
Sulfoxyl. *See* benzoyl peroxide, with sulfur
sulfur, 1062*t*
sulfur mustard agents, 1363*t*
sulindac, 724*t*, 725*t*
sumatriptan, 451–52
  adverse effects, 450*t*, 451
  classification, 451
  contraindications/precautions, 451
  drug interactions, 452
  mechanism of action, 451
  nursing responsibilities, 452
  overdose treatment, 452
  patient and family education, 452
  pediatric labeling changes, 135*t*
  pharmacokinetics, 451
  pregnancy category, 452
  route and adult dose, 450*t*
  similar drugs, 452
  therapeutic effects and uses, 451
Sumycin. *See* tetracycline
sunburn, 1331–33
sunscreens, 1331
supercoil, 826
superinfections, 784
Supprelin. *See* histrelin
suprachiasmatic nucleus, 276
Suprane. *See* desflurane
Suprax. *See* cefixime
suramin, 892*t*, 898
surface anesthesia, 471*f*
surface area, drug absorption and, 45
surfactants, 1030*t*, 1031, 1032
surgical anesthesia, 459. *See also* general anesthesia
Surmontil. *See* trimipramine
Survanta. *See* beractant
Sustiva. *See* efavirenz
Sutent. *See* scinitinib
Svedberg unit, 809
sweat glands, 1316
Symlin. *See* pramlintide
Symmetrel. *See* amantadine
sympathetic nervous system, 186–87, 187*f*
  adrenal medulla, 195
  in heart failure, 608
sympathomimetics, 229. *See also* adrenergic agonists
symporter, 549, 551*f*
Synagis. *See* palivizumab
Synalar. *See* fluocinolone acetonide
synapses, 188, 266–67, 266*f*
synaptic cleft, 188

synaptic transmission, 188–90, 188*f*, 189f
Synarel. *See* nafarelin
syndrome, 267*t*
syndrome of inappropriate diuretic hormone (SIADH), 1114
Synercid. *See* quinupristin-dalfopristin
synergistic effect, 73*f*, 74, 84*t*
Synthroid. *See* levothyroxine
syphilis, in HIV-AIDS, 945*t*

T

T cells, 713, 713*t*
T wave, 626*t*
T_3 (tri-iodothyronine), 1147
T_4 (thyroxine), 1147
tablets, 29, 44
Tabloid. *See* thioguanine
tachydysrhythmias, 626–27. *See also* dysrhythmias
tachyphylaxis, 97
tacrine, 202*t*, 355*t*, 360, 362–63
tacrolimus, 741*t*, 742*f*, 744, 1327, 1330*t*
tadalafil, 1227*t*, 1229
Taenia saginata, 901
Taenia solum, 901
Tagamet. *See* cimetidine
Talwin. *See* pentazocine
Tambocor. *See* flecainide
Tamiflu. *See* oseltamivir
tamoxifen, 981–82
  adverse effects, 68*t*, 982
  classification, 981
  contraindications/precautions, 982
  drug interactions, 982
  mechanism of action, 981
  nursing responsibilities, 982
  overdose treatment, 982
  patient and family education, 982
  pharmacokinetics, 981
  pregnancy category, 982
  similar drugs, 982–84
  therapeutic effects and uses, 981
    for male infertility, 1226
tamsulosin, 246, 247*t*, 251
Tanacetum parthenium. See feverfew
Tapazole. *See* methimazole
tapeworms, 901
Tarceva. *See* erlotinib
tardive dyskinesia (TD), 331, 331*t*
target cells, 1099
Targretin. *See* bexarotene
Tarka, 572*t*
Tasigna. *See* nilotinib
Tasmar. *See* tolcapone
Tavist. *See* clemastine
Tavist Allergy tablets, 1266*t*
TAXANES, 986–87
  docetaxel, 985*t*, 987
  paclitaxel, 985*t*, 987
Taxol. *See* paclitaxel
Taxotere. *See* docetaxel
tazarotene, 1322*t*, 1325, 1329, 1330*t*
Tazicef. *See* ceftazidime
Tazorac. *See* tazarotene
TBG (thyroxine-binding globulin), 1147
3TC. *See* lamivudine
TD (tardive dyskinesia), 331, 331*t*
TD_{50} (median toxicity dose), 57
Tdap. *See* pertussis, immunization
tegaserod, 1040
Tega-Tussine Syrup, 1276*t*
Tekturna. *See* aliskiren
Tekturna HCT, 572*t*
telbivudine, 919*t*, 922
telithromycin, 821*t*, 822, 832*t*, 833
telmisartan, 538*t*, 541
telomerase, 951
telomeres, 951
temazepam, 282*t*, 286
Temodar. *See* temozolomide
Temovate. *See* clobetasol dipropionate
temozolomide, 135*t*, 967*t*, 970
temsirolimus, 741*t*, 744
Tenckhoff catheter, 958
tenecteplase, 658*t*, 660
teniposide, 68*t*, 827, 985*t*, 988
tenofovir, 933*t*, 936, 943
Tenoretic, 572*t*
Tenormin. *See* atenolol
Tensilon. *See* edrophonium
tension headache, 449
Tequin. *See* gatifloxacin
teratogens, 68–69, 69*t*, 126–27
Terazol. *See* terconazole
terazosin, 247*t*, 251
terbinafine, 877, 878–79, 878*t*, 881
terbutaline, 239, 240
  as bronchodilator, 1245*t*, 1248
  as tocolytic, 1187*t*, 1190
terconazole, 878*t*
teriparatide, 1295*t*, 1300
terrorism:
  chemical agents, 1362, 1362*t*
    blister/vesicant agents. *See* blister/vesicant agents
    blood agents. *See* blood agents
    choking/vomiting agents. *See* choking/vomiting agents
    nerve agents. *See* nerve agents
  infectious agents, 1359*t*, 1360–61, 1360*t*
  ionizing radiation, 1363
Teslac. *See* testolactone
Tessalon. *See* benzonatate
Tessalon Perles, 30*t*. *See also* benzonatate
testes, disorders and pharmacotherapy, 1102*t*
Testim, 1221. *See also* testosterone
testolactone, 980*t*, 1226
Testopel, 1221. *See also* testosterone
testosterone, 1221–23
  actions/effects, 1219
  adverse effects, 1222
  buccal administration, 32, 1221
  classification, 1221
  contraindications/precautions, 1222
  drug interactions, 1222
  formulations, 1221
  mechanism of action, 1222
  nursing responsibilities, 1222
  overdose treatment, 1222
  patient and family education, 1222–23
  pharmacokinetics, 1222
  pregnancy category, 1222
  similar drugs, 1223
  therapeutic effects and uses, 1221–22
    for neoplasia, 980*t*
testosterone cypionate, 1220, 1220*t*, 1221
testosterone enanthate, 1220*t*, 1221
Testred. *See* testosterone
tetanus:
  characteristics, 758*t*, 759
  immunization, 758*t*, 759
  pathophysiology, 759
tetanus immune globulin, 767*t*
tetanus toxoid, 759
tetracaine, 473*t*, 474, 1347, 1348*t*
tetracycline, 811–12
  adverse effects, 810*t*, 811
  classification, 811
  contraindications/precautions, 811–12
  drug interactions, 812
  mechanism of action, 811
  nursing responsibilities, 812
  overdose treatment, 812
  patient and family education, 812
  pharmacokinetics, 811
  pregnancy category, 812
  route and adult dose, 810*t*
  similar drugs, 812–13
  therapeutic effects and uses, 811
    acne vulgaris, 1322*t*
TETRACYCLINES:
  adverse effects, 811
  drug interactions, 45, 75*t*
  drugs in class
    demeclocycline, 810*t*, 812
    doxycycline, 810*t*, 812–13
    minocycline. *See* minocycline
    tetracycline. *See* tetracycline
    tigecycline, 810*t*, 813
  indications, 810
  mechanism of action, 809–10, 809*f*
  Nursing Process Application, 819–20*t*
tetrahydrocannabinol (THC), 102. *See also* marijuana
tetrahydrozoline, 236, 238, 1348, 1348*t*
Teveten. *See* eprosartan
Teveten HCT, 572*t*
6-TG. *See* thioguanine
thalamotomy, 350*t*
thalamus, 268*f*, 269
thalidomide, 14, 741*t*, 746–47, 991
Thalomid. *See* thalidomide
Theochron. *See* theophylline
Theolair. *See* theophylline
theophylline, 421, 422, 1255–56
  adverse effects, 1245*t*, 1255
  classification, 1255
  contraindications/precautions, 1255
  drug interactions, 1255
  mechanism of action, 1255
  nursing responsibilities, 1255–56
  overdose treatment, 1255
  patient and family education, 1256
  pharmacokinetics, 1255
  pregnancy category, 1255
  route and adult dose, 1245*t*
  similar drugs, 1256
  therapeutic effects and uses, 1255
TheraCys. *See* bacillus Calmette-Guérin (BCG) vaccine
therapeutic classification, 5–6
therapeutic index, 57, 57*f*
Therapeutic Products Directorate (TPD), 20
therapeutic range, 50, 51*f*
thiabendazole, 902*t*, 903
thiamine (vitamin B_1):
  adverse effects, 1058
  contraindications/precautions, 1058
  deficiency, 1053*t*, 1054
  drug interactions, 1058

functions, 1053*t*
mechanism of action, 1058
nursing responsibilities, 1058
for nutritional disorders
adverse effects, 1054*t*
route and adult dose, 1054*t*
patient and family education, 1058–59
pregnancy category, 1058
recommended dietary allowance, 1058
therapeutic effects and uses, 1058
THIAZIDE DIURETICS, 549
adverse effects, 553, 554*t*, 612*t*
clinical applications, 553
drug interactions, 842
drugs in class
bendroflumethiazide, 554*t*
chlorothiazide, 553, 554*t*, 555
chlorthalidone, 553, 554*t*, 555
hydrochlorothiazide. *See* hydrochlorothiazide
indapamide, 553, 554*t*, 555
methyclothiazide, 554*t*, 555
metolazone, 553, 554*t*, 555
route and adult dose, 554*t*
sites of action, 550*f*, 553
for specific conditions
heart failure, 612*t*, 613
hypertension, 570, 572*t*, 573, 574*t*
THIAZOLIDINEDIONES, 1137
actions, 1132*t*
mechanism of action, 1137
nursing considerations, 1132*t*
rosiglitazone. *See* rosiglitazone
thioguanine, 973*t*, 976
thiopental sodium, 459–61
adverse effects, 460, 460*t*
classification, 459
contraindications/precautions, 460
drug interactions, 460
mechanism of action, 459
nursing responsibilities, 461
patient and family education, 461
pharmacokinetics, 459
pregnancy category, 461
route and adult dose, 460*t*
similar drugs, 461
for specific conditions, 292
therapeutic effects and uses, 459
Thioplex. *See* thiotepa
thioridazine, 332*t*, 335
thiotepa, 967*t*, 971
thiothixene, 332*t*, 336
threshold potential, 624
thrombin, 486, 661*t*, 662
Thrombinar. *See* thrombin
thrombocytopenia, 643, 643*t*, 959
thromboembolic disorder, 642
THROMBOLYTIC AGENTS:
drugs in class
alteplase. *See* alteplase
reteplase, 658*t*, 659–60
streptokinase, 658*t*, 660
tenecteplase, 658*t*, 660
mechanism of action, 601*f*, 644*t*, 657–58
for myocardial infarction, 599, 601*f*
Nursing Process Application, 660*t*
thrombopoietin, 484, 674
thrush. *See* candidiasis
Thymoglobulin. *See* antithymocyte globulin
Thyro-Block. *See* potassium iodide
thyroid crisis (thyroid storm), 1150, 1150*t*, 1154, 1155
thyroid function tests, 1149*t*
thyroid gland:
disorders, 1102*t*
diagnosis, 1148, 1149*t*
emergency, 1150, 1150*t*, 1154, 1155
hyperthyroidism. *See* hyperthyroidism
hypothyroidism. *See* hypothyroidism
in older adults, 1150*t*
physiology, 1147–48, 1148*f*
thyroid hormone, 1102*t*
thyroid-stimulating immunoglobulins (TSI), 1154
thyroid storm. *See* thyroid crisis
Thyroid USP. *See* desiccated thyroid
Thyrolar. *See* liotrix
Thyro-Tabs. *See* levothyroxine
thyrotoxicosis, 1154
thyrotropin-releasing hormone (TRH), 1105*t*, 1147
thyrotropin-stimulating hormone (TSH), 1147
thyroxine (T_4), 1147
thyroxine-binding globulin (TBG), 1147
tiagabine, 381*t*, 392
Tiazac. *See* diltiazem
Ticar. *See* ticarcillin
ticarcillin, 789*t*, 794
Tice. *See* bacillus Calmette-Guérin (BCG) vaccine
Ticlid. *See* ticlopidine
ticlopidine, 653, 653*t*, 655
tigecycline, 810*t*, 813
Tilade. *See* nedocromil sodium
tiludronate, 1294*t*, 1295*t*, 1297
Timolide, 572*t*
timolol, 1344–45
adverse effects, 252*t*, 255, 1344
classification, 1344
contraindications/precautions, 1344
drug interactions, 1344
mechanism of action, 1344
nursing responsibilities, 1344–45
overdose treatment, 1344
patient and family education, 1345
pharmacokinetics, 1344
pregnancy category, 1344
route and adult dose, 252*t*
similar drugs, 1345
for specific conditions, 255
angina, 592*t*
therapeutic effects and uses, 1344
topical, 255
Timoptic. *See* timolol
Timoptic XE. *See* timolol
Tinactin. *See* tolnaftate
Tindamax. *See* tinidazole
tinea capitis, 869*t*, 877, 1318
tinea corporis, 877
tinea cruris, 869*t*, 877, 1318
tinea pedis, 869*t*, 877, 1318
tinea unguium, 1318
tinidazole, 892*t*, 895
tinzaparin, 645*t*, 648
tioconazole, 878*t*, 879
tiotropium bromide, 214*t*, 217, 1245*t*, 1249
tipranavir, 933*t*, 940
tirofiban, 653*t*, 657
Titralac. *See* calcium carbonate
tizanidine, 400*t*, 402
TMP-SMZ. *See* trimethoprim-sulfamethoxazole
TNKase. *See* tenecteplase
To the Community:
accidental insecticide poisoning, 215*t*
acid suppression and vitamin B_{12} in older adults, 1022*t*
adherence to antiretroviral therapy, 931*t*
antidepressants for childhood anxiety, 290*t*
blood pressure self-measurement, 568*t*
body weight and hypertension, 533*t*
calendar method of contraception, 1209*t*
DASH diet, 570*t*
dietary measures to lower cholesterol, 501*t*
dysrhythmia and diet, 627*t*
enteral nutrition in the home setting, 1074*t*
estrogen use and psychosocial issues, 1181*t*
food–drug interactions, 75*t*
growth hormone, inappropriate use of, 1109*t*
home care of patients during total parenteral nutrition therapy, 1080*t*
immunosuppression and pets, 738*t*
intrathecal baclofen pump, 402*t*
laxative abuse, 1033*t*
lifestyle modifications for hypertension, 248*t*
lipid profiles, 499*t*
living with Alzheimer's or Parkinson's disease, 364*t*
long-term corticosteroid therapy, 1164*t*
methamphetamine, 236*t*
myasthenia gravis, 209*t*
ophthalmic drugs in the home setting, 1350*t*
photosensitivity and antibiotics, 811*t*
poisoning prevention, 1364*t*
polypharmacy in older adults, 147*t*
prevention of tuberculosis transmission, 862*t*
public health challenges and community programs, 570*t*
salt replacements and exercise, 696*t*
sexual activity following myocardial infarction, 600*t*
sodium restrictions, 249*t*
teaching patients about dietary sodium, hypertension, and food labels, 529*t*
teaching patients with neutropenia, 674*t*
trichomoniasis, 896*t*
vaccines for prevention of urinary tract infections, 837*t*
weight reduction tis, 1089*t*
white coat hypertension, 518*t*
tobramycin, 816*t*, 819
TOCOLYTICS, 239, 1186, 1189–90
magnesium sulfate. *See* magnesium sulfate
nifedipine, 1187*t*, 1190. *See also* nifedipine
ritodrine, 240, 1189
terbutaline, 240, 1187*t*, 1190
tocopherols. *See* vitamin E
toddlers. *See* pediatric patients
Tofranil. *See* imipramine
Tolamide. *See* tolazamide
tolazamide, 1133*t*, 1135
tolbutamide, 1133*t*, 1135
tolcapone, 350*t*, 355
Tolectin. *See* tolmetin
tolerance, 97, 437
Tolinase. *See* tolazamide

tolmetin, 724*t*, 725*t*
tolnaftate, 878*t*, 1351
tolterodine tartrate, 135*t*, 214*t*, 218
tonic spasm, 397
tonic–clonic seizures, 372*f*, 374, 376*t*
tonicity, 687
tonometry, 1338
topical anesthesia, 471, 471*f*
topical route, drug administration, 31–32, 44
Topicort. *See* desoximetasone
TOPOISOMERASE INHIBITORS, 987
- etoposide. *See* etoposide
- irinotecan, 135*t*, 985*t*, 987
- teniposide, 68*t*, 827, 985*t*, 988
- topotecan, 985*t*, 987–88

topoisomerase IV, 826, 826*f*
topotecan, 985*t*, 987–88
Toprol. *See* metoprolol
Toprol XL, 30*t*. *See also* metoprolol
Toradol. *See* ketorolac
toremifene, 980*t*, 983
Torisel. *See* temsirolimus
Tornalate. *See* bitolterol
torsades de pointes, 627
torsemide, 551*t*, 553, 612*t*
tositumomab, 748*t*, 990*t*
total parenteral nutrition (TPN), 1076. *See also* parenteral nutrition
Tourette's syndrome, 333
Tovalt. *See* zolpidem
toxic concentration, 50
toxoid vaccines, 756, 756*t*
toxoids, 756
Toxoplasma gondii, 886*t*, 895
toxoplasmosis, 886*t*, 892*t*, 895, 945*t*
TPD (Therapeutic Products Directorate), 20
Tracrium. *See* atracurium
traction, for muscle spasms, 397
trade name, 7
tramadol, 442–44
- adverse effects, 443, 443*t*
- classification, 442
- contraindications/precautions, 443
- drug interactions, 443
- mechanism of action, 442–43
- nursing responsibilities, 443–44
- overdose treatment, 443
- patient and family education, 444
- pharmacokinetics, 443
- pregnancy category, 443
- route and adult dose, 443, 443*t*
- similar drugs, 444
- for specific conditions
  - osteoarthritis, 1302
- therapeutic effects and uses, 442

Trandate. *See* labetalol
trandolapril, 533*t*, 536
tranexamic acid, 661*t*, 662
transcription, 808, 808*f*
transdermal patches, 32, 32*f*
Transderm-Scop. *See* scopolamine
transferrin, 677
transfusions:
- blood. *See* BLOOD PRODUCTS
- fluid. *See* FLUID REPLACEMENT AGENTS

transplant rejection, 740, 1169
Tranxene. *See* clorazepate
tranylcypromine, 290*t*, 304*t*, 317
trastuzumab, 748*t*, 990*t*
Travatan. *See* travoprost
traveler's diarrhea, 810*t*
travoprost, 1341*t*, 1343
trazodone:
- for anxiety disorders, 290*t*
- for depression, 304*t*, 313
- drug interactions, 178*t*

Treating the Diverse Patient:
- anesthesia exposure and risk of Alzheimer's disease, 469*t*
- antipsychotics in Asian patients, 336*t*
- attention deficit/hyperactivity disorder in girls, 414*t*
- cultural influences and depression treatment, 300*t*
- cultural influences in contraceptive selection, 1205*t*
- culturally appropriate treatment, 119*t*
- culturally competent care, 159*t*
- diabetes complications, 1123*t*
- enzyme deficiencies, 62*t*
- heart failure in women, 609*t*
- high-risk populations in correctional facilities, 857*t*
- immunosuppressive medication in older African Americans, 742*t*
- nurses and substance abuse, 103*t*
- osteoporosis in men, 1292
- pregnancy and deep venous thrombosis, 648*t*
- propranolol sensitivity in Asians, 633*t*
- respiratory distress syndrome, 1240*t*
- sildenafil for women, 1229*t*
- variations in drug metabolism, 48*t*

Trecator-SC. *See* ethionamide
Trelstar. *See* triptorelin
Trental, 30*t*. *See also* pentoxifylline
Trentin-X. *See* tretinoin
Treponema, 777*t*
tretinoin, 1323–24
- adverse effects, 1323–24
- classification, 1323
- contraindications/precautions, 1324
- drug interactions, 1324
- mechanism of action, 1323
- Nursing Process Application, 1326*t*
- nursing responsibilities, 1324
- overdose treatment, 1324
- patient and family education, 1324
- pharmacokinetics, 1323
- pregnancy category, 1324
- similar drugs, 1324–25
- therapeutic effects and uses, 1322, 1322*t*, 1323

Trexall. *See* methotrexate
TRH (thyrotropin-releasing hormone), 1105*t*, 1147
triamcinolone, 1167*t*, 1250*t*, 1252, 1270*t*
triamcinolone acetonide, 1327*t*
Triaminic Cold/Allergy, 1266*t*
Triaminic Expectorant DH, 1276*t*
triamterene, 556, 556*t*, 558
triazolam, 282*t*, 286
triazoles, 875. *See also* AZOLES
Trichomonas vaginalis, 886*t*, 895
trichomoniasis, 892*t*, 895–96, 896*t*
Trichophyton, 869*t*, 878
TriCor. *See* fenofibrate
Tricosal. *See* choline and magnesium trisalicylate
TRICYCLIC ANTIDEPRESSANTS, 303
- as adjuvant analgesics, 446, 446*t*
- advantages, 305
- adverse effects, 305, 447
  - in older adults, 152*t*
- drug interactions, 178*t*
- drugs in class
  - amitriptyline. *See* amitriptyline
  - clomipramine, 289, 290*t*, 304*t*, 307
  - desipramine, 290*t*, 304*t*
  - doxepin, 289, 290*t*, 304*t*, 307
  - imipramine. *See* imipramine
  - maprotiline, 304*t*, 307
  - nortriptyline, 290*t*, 304*t*
  - protriptyline, 304*t*, 307
  - trimipramine, 304*t*, 307
- mechanism of action, 305, 305*f*
- Nursing Process Application, 316*t*
- overdose/poisoning, 1364*t*
- for specific conditions
  - anxiety disorders, 289, 290*t*
  - attention deficit/hyperactivity disorder, 418
  - depression, 304*t*
  - migraine prophylaxis, 453, 453*t*

Triescence. *See* triamcinolone
trifluoperazine, 332*t*, 335
trifluridine, 912, 912*t*, 914
triglycerides, 496, 497*f*, 499*t*
trihexyphenidyl:
- adverse effects, 214*t*
- for Parkinson's disease, 218, 355*t*, 356
- route and adult dose, 214*t*

tri-iodothyronine (T_3), 1147
Trilafon. *See* perphenazine
Trileptal. *See* oxcarbazepine
Tri-Levlen, 1203*t*
Trilisate. *See* choline and magnesium trisalicylate
trimethaphan, 218
trimethoprim, 843–44
trimethoprim-sulfamethoxazole, 842–43
- adverse effects, 840*t*, 842–43
  - in pediatric patients, 142*t*
- classification, 842
- contraindications/precautions, 843
- drug interactions, 843
- mechanism of action, 842
- nursing responsibilities, 843
- overdose treatment, 843
- patient and family education, 843
- Patient Safety, 842*t*
- pediatric dosage/route, 142*t*
- pharmacokinetics, 842
- pregnancy category, 843
- route and adult dose, 840*t*
- similar drugs, 843–44
- for specific conditions
  - acute uncomplicated cystitis, 838
- therapeutic effects and uses, 842

trimipramine, 304*t*, 307
Trimox. *See* amoxicillin
Triostat. *See* liothyronine
Triphasil, 1203*t*
triprolidine, 1265*t*
TRIPTANS:
- almotriptan, 450*t*, 452
- eletriptan, 450*t*, 452
- frovatriptan, 450*t*, 452
- naratriptan, 450*t*, 452
- rizatriptan, 450*t*, 452
- sumatriptan. *See* sumatriptan
- zolmitriptan, 450*t*, 452

triptorelin, 980*t*, 984
Trisenox. *See* arsenic trioxide
troches, 29
troglitazone, 1137
trophozoite, 886
tropic hormones, 1106
Tropicacyl. *See* tropicamide
tropicamide, 214*t*, 218, 1347, 1348*t*
Truphylline. *See* aminophylline
Trusopt. *See* dorzolamide
Trypanosoma brucei, 886*t*, 896
Trypanosoma cruzi, 886*t*, 896
trypanosomiasis, 886*t*, 892*t*, 896
trypsin, 1004*t*
TSH (thyrotropin-stimulating hormone), 1147
TSI (thyroid-stimulating immunoglobulins), 1154
TSPA. *See* thiotepa
tubercles, 852
tuberculin skin test, 853
tuberculoid leprosy, 862. *See also* leprosy
tuberculosis (TB), 851
  diagnosis, 853
  incidence, 851, 853*t*
  pathogenesis, 852, 852*f*
  pharmacotherapy
    combination, 853, 854*f*, 860
    dosing regimens and schedules, 853
    first-line agents
      ethambutol, 855*t*, 858
      in HIV-positive patients, 856, 945*t*
      isoniazid. *See* isoniazid
      in pregnancy, 856–57
      pyrazinamide, 855*t*, 858
      rifabutin, 855*t*, 860
      rifampin. *See* rifampin
      rifapentine, 855*t*, 860
      standard regimen, 856
    monitoring, 853–54
    Nursing Process Application, 864*t*
    second-line agents
      amikacin. *See* amikacin
      aminosalicylic acid, 855*t*, 861
      capreomycin, 855*t*, 861
      ciprofloxacin. *See* ciprofloxacin
      cycloserine, 855*t*, 861
      ethionamide, 855*t*, 861
      kanamycin. *See* kanamycin
      ofloxacin. *See* ofloxacin
      streptomycin. *See* streptomycin
  postprimary, 852
  primary, 851–52
  prophylactic therapy, 853, 857
  transmission, 851, 862*t*
tubocurarine, 223–24
  adverse effects, 224
  classification, 223
  contraindications/precautions, 224
  drug interactions, 224
  mechanism of action, 223
  nursing responsibilities, 224
  overdose treatment, 224
  patient and family education, 224
  pharmacokinetics, 224
  pregnancy category, 224
  similar drugs, 224
  therapeutic effects and uses, 223
tularemia, 1361
tumor, 950, 950*t*
Tums. *See* calcium carbonate
Tussionex, 1276*t*
Tygacil. *See* tigecycline
Tykerb. *See* lapatinib
Tylenol. *See* acetaminophen
Tylenol Allergy Multi-Symptom Gels, 1266*t*
Tylenol PM Gelcaps, 1266*t*
type 1 diabetes, 1121, 1122*t*. *See also* diabetes mellitus
type 2 diabetes, 286*t*, 1121, 1122*t*. *See also* diabetes mellitus
tyramine, 314, 314*t*
Tysabri. *See* natalizumab
Tyzeka. *See* telbivudine
Tyzine. *See* tetrahydrozoline

U

Ultane. *See* sevoflurane
Ultiva. *See* remifentanil
Ultram. *See* tramadol
ultrasound, for muscle spasms, 397
ultraviolet-A (UVA) therapy, 1331
ultraviolet-B (UVB) therapy, 1331
Unasyn. *See* ampicillin/sulbactam
undecylenic acid, 878*t*, 1318
Uniphyl. *See* theophylline
Uniretic, 572*t*
United States Pharmacopeia (USP), 15, 16*f*
  Verification Program, 176, 176*f*
United States Pharmacopeia-National Formulary (USP-NF), 16
Unithroid. *See* levothyroxine
Univasc. *See* moexipril
unstable angina, 589. *See also* angina pectoris
up-regulation, 1099
urea, 559*t*, 560
Ureaphil. *See* urea
Urecholine. *See* bethanechol chloride
urethritis, 837. *See also* urinary tract infections
Urex. *See* methenamine hippurate
URIC ACID INHIBITORS, 1307
  colchicine. *See* colchicine
URICOSURICS, 1309
  probenecid, 1307*t*, 1309, 1310
  sulfinpyrazone, 1307*t*, 1309, 1310
urinalysis, 547
URINARY ANTISEPTICS, 845
  fosfomycin. *See* fosfomycin
  mandelate, 840*t*
  methenamine hippurate, 840*t*, 847
  nalidixic acid. *See* nalidixic acid
  nitrofurantoin. *See* nitrofurantoin
urinary retention, with opioids, 437, 437*t*
urinary system, age-related changes, 149*t*
urinary tract infections (UTIs):
  incidence, 837
  in men, 839*t*
  pathophysiology, 837
  pharmacotherapy, 840*t*
    acute uncomplicated cystitis, 838
    complicated, 838–39
    in older adults, 839–40
    in pediatric patients, 839
    in pregnancy, 839
    recurrence, 840
    sulfonamides. *See* SULFONAMIDES
    urinary antiseptics. *See* URINARY ANTISEPTICS
  symptoms, 837
  vaccines for prevention of, 837*t*
urofollitropin, 1192*t*
uropathogens, 837, 838*t*
Uroxatral. *See* alfuzosin
urticaria, 1316
  drug-induced, 70
  pharmacotherapy, 1266
USP. *See United States Pharmacopeia*
USP Verification Program, 176, 176*f*
USP-NF *(United States Pharmacopeia-National Formulary)*, 16
uterine relaxants. *See* TOCOLYTICS
uterine stimulants:
  ergot alkaloids
    ergonovine, 1187*t*, 1189
    methylergonovine, 1187*t*, 1189
  oxytocin. *See* oxytocin
  prostaglandins
    carboprost, 1187*t*, 1189
    dinoprostone, 1187*t*, 1189
    misoprostol. *See* misoprostol
Uticort. *See* betamethasone benzoate

V

vaccination, 755
vaccine(s):
  administration principles
    in adolescents, 766*t*
    adverse event reporting, 757
    anaphylaxis and allergy, 757
    dose and timing, 757
    in older adults, 766*t*
    in pediatric patients, 766*t*
    precautions and contraindications, 757
    route, 757
  bacillus Calmette-Guérin, 735*t*, 739
  diphtheria, 758*t*, 759
  hepatitis A, 758*t*, 919
  hepatitis B. *See* hepatitis B vaccine
  in HIV-AIDS patients, 945*t*
  human immunodeficiency virus, 942
  human papillomavirus, 766
  immune system and, 755
  influenza, 758*t*, 763, 915
  measles, 758*t*
  meningococcal, 758*t*, 760
  mumps, 758*t*, 764
  Nursing Process Application, 770*t*
  pertussis, 758*t*, 759
  pneumococcal, 758*t*, 760
  poliomyelitis, 764–65
  rabies, 793
  rubella, 758*t*, 764
  tetanus, 758*t*, 759
  types, 756–57, 756*t*
  for urinary tract infection, 837*t*
  varicella zoster, 758*t*, 765
Vaccine Adverse Event Reporting System (VAERS), 757
vaginal route, drug administration, 33, 34*f*
Vagistat-1. *See* tioconazole
vagus nerve stimulation (VNS), for depression, 302*t*, 303
valacyclovir, 912*t*, 914–15
Valcyte. *See* valganciclovir
valdecoxib, 727
Valergen. *See* estradiol valerate
valerian:
  for anxiety and insomnia, 280
  drug interactions, 177, 178*t*
  primary uses, 173*t*
Valeriana officinalis. *See* valerian

valganciclovir, 912*t*, 915
Valisone. *See* betamethasone valerate
Valium. *See* diazepam
valproate. *See* valproic acid
valproic acid, 390–91
  adverse effects
    in pediatric patients, 142*t*
  classification, 390
  contraindications/precautions, 390
  dosage forms not to be crushed or opened, 30*t*
  drug interactions, 390
  mechanism of action, 390
  nursing responsibilities, 390–91
  overdose treatment, 390
  patient and family education, 391
  pediatric dosage/route, 142*t*
  pharmacokinetics, 390
  pregnancy category, 390
  for specific conditions
    anxiety, 286
    bipolar disorder, 319*t*, 320
    seizures, 380*t*, 390
  therapeutic effects and uses, 390
valsartan, 538*t*, 541
Valtrex. *See* valacyclovir
Vancocin. *See* vancomycin HCl
vancomycin HCl, 802–3
  adverse effects, 800*t*, 802
  classification, 802
  contraindications/precautions, 803
  drug interactions, 803
  mechanism of action, 802
  nursing responsibilities, 803
  overdose treatment, 803
  patient and family education, 803
  pharmacokinetics, 802
  pregnancy category, 803
  route and adult dose, 800*t*
  similar drugs, 803
  therapeutic effects and uses, 802
vancomycin-resistant *Enterococci* (VRE), 782
Vantas. *See* histrelin
Vantin. *See* cefpodoxime
VAQTA. *See* hepatitis A vaccine
vardenafil, 1227*t*, 1229
varenicline, 108
varicella zoster (chickenpox/shingles):
  characteristics, 758*t*
  immunization, 758*t*, 765
  incidence, 758*t*, 765*t*
  pathophysiology, 765
variola virus, 1361
Varivax. *See* varicella zoster, immunization
Vascor. *See* bepridil
Vaseretic, 572*t*
vasoconstrictors, ocular. *See* OCULAR DECONGESTANTS/VASOCONSTRICTORS
VASODILATORS, DIRECT-ACTING:
  drugs in class
    diazoxide, 580–81, 584*t*
    hydralazine. *See* hydralazine
    minoxidil, 581
    nitroprusside sodium. *See* nitroprusside sodium
  mechanism of action, 611*f*
  Nursing Process Application, 583*t*
  for specific conditions
    heart failure, 612*t*, 614
    hypertension, 574*t*, 579
vasomotor center, 492
vasopressin, 602, 1108*t*, 1115–16
vasospastic (Prinzmetal's) angina, 589
Vasotec. *See* enalapril
Vasotec IV. *See* enalaprilat
vastus lateralis muscle, intramuscular injection, 37*t*
Vaughan Williams classification, 627
V-Cillin K. *See* penicillin VK
Vectibix. *See* panitumumab
vectors, 886
vecuronium, 219*t*, 224
Vee-Cillin-K. *See* penicillin V
Veetids. *See* penicillin V
Velban. *See* vinblastine sulfate
Velcade. *See* bortezomib
Velosef. *See* cephradine
venlafaxine, 311–12
  adverse effects, 304*t*, 311
  classification, 311
  contraindications/precautions, 311
  drug interactions, 311–12
  mechanism of action, 311
  nursing responsibilities, 312
  overdose treatment, 312
  patient and family education, 312
  pediatric labeling changes, 135*t*
  pharmacokinetics, 311
  pregnancy category, 312
  route and adult dose, 304*t*
  similar drugs, 310–11
  for specific conditions
    anxiety or insomnia, 282*t*, 289, 290
  therapeutic effects and uses, 311
Venofer. *See* iron sucrose
venous return, 490
venous thromboembolism (VTE), 642
ventilation, 1239
Ventolin. *See* albuterol
ventricular fibrillation, 627. *See also* dysrhythmias
ventricular tachycardia, 626–27. *See also* dysrhythmias
ventrogluteal site, intramuscular injection, 37*t*
VePesid. *See* etoposide
Veramyst. *See* fluticasone
verapamil, 523–24
  adverse effects, 520*t*, 523
  classification, 523
  contraindications/precautions, 523
  dosage forms not to be crushed or opened, 30*t*
  drug interactions, 523
  injection, 519*t*
  mechanism of action, 523
  nursing responsibilities, 523–24
  overdose treatment, 523
  patient and family education, 524
  pharmacokinetics, 523
  pregnancy category, 523
  route and adult dose, 520*t*
  similar drugs, 524
  for specific conditions
    angina, 592*t*
    dysrhythmias, 629*t*, 636
  therapeutic effects and uses, 523
Verdeso. *See* desonide
Verelan. *See* verapamil
Vermox. *See* mebendazole
Versed. *See* midazolam
vertigo, 1266
very low-density lipoprotein (VLDL), 496, 498*f*
Vesanoid. *See* tretinoin
vesicant, 960
Vestra. *See* reboxetine
Vfend. *See* voriconazole
Viadur. *See* leuprolide
Viagra. *See* sildenafil
Vibramycin. *See* doxycycline
Vibrio cholerae, 775, 777*t*
Vicodin. *See* acetaminophen; hydrocodone
Vicodin ES. *See* acetaminophen; hydrocodone
Videx. *See* didanosine
vinblastine sulfate, 985*t*, 986
VINCA ALKALOIDS:
  vinblastine sulfate, 985*t*, 986
  vincristine. *See* vincristine
  vinorelbine, 985*t*, 986
vincristine, 985–86
  adverse effects, 94, 985–86
  classification, 985
  contraindications/precautions, 986
  drug interactions, 986
  mechanism of action, 985
  nursing responsibilities, 986
  overdose treatment, 986
  patient and family education, 986
  pharmacokinetics, 985
  pregnancy category, 986
  similar drugs, 986
  therapeutic effects and uses, 985
vinorelbine, 985*t*, 986
Vioxx. *See* rofecoxib
Viprostol. *See* conivaptan
Viracept. *See* nelfinavir
viral hemorrhagic fevers, 1361, 1361*t*
viral infections:
  hepatitis. *See under* hepatitis
  herpesvirus. *See* herpesviruses
  influenza. *See* influenza
  pharmacotherapy principles, 910–11, 910*f*
viral labyrinthitis, 1353*t*
viral load, 929
Viramune. *See* nevirapine
Viread. *See* tenofovir
virilization, 1219
Virilon. *See* methyltestosterone
virion, 908
Viroptic. *See* trifluridine
virulence, 775
virus(es), 908. *See also specific viruses and infections*
  DNA, 909*t*
  effects on host cells, 910, 910*f*
  replication, 908–10, 910*f*
  RNA, 909*t*
  structure, 908, 908*f*
Visine. *See* tetrahydrozoline
Visine LR. *See* oxymetazoline
Visken. *See* pindolol
Vistaril. *See* hydroxyzine
Vistide. *See* cidofovir
vitamin(s), 1052
  deficiencies, 1054–55
  discovery, 1052
  fat-soluble, 1052
    vitamin A. *See* vitamin A
    vitamin C. *See* vitamin D
    vitamin E. *See* vitamin E
    vitamin K. *See* vitamin K

government regulations, 1053–54
in parenteral nutrition, 1078
poisoning, 1054*t*
during pregnancy, 1055*t*
recommended dietary allowances, 1054
supplements, 1052–64
water-soluble, 1052
vitamin B_1. *See* thiamine
vitamin B_2. *See* thiamine
vitamin B_3. *See* niacin
vitamin B_6. *See* pyridoxine
vitamin B_9. *See* folic acid
vitamin B_{12}. *See* cyanocobalamin
vitamin C. *See* vitamin C
vitamin A:
adverse effects, 1055
contraindications/precautions, 1055
deficiency, 1053*t*
drug interactions, 1055
functions, 1053*t*
mechanism of action, 1055
nursing responsibilities, 1055–56
for nutritional disorders
adverse effects, 1053*t*
route and adult dose, 1053*t*
patient and family education, 1056
pregnancy category, 1055
recommended dietary allowance, 1055
therapeutic effects and uses, 1055
vitamin B_1. *See* thiamine
vitamin B_2. *See* riboflavin
vitamin B_3. *See* niacin
vitamin B_6. *See* pyridoxine
vitamin B_9. *See* folic acid
vitamin B_{12}. *See* cyanocobalamin
vitamin C (ascorbic acid):
adverse effects, 1061
contraindications/precautions, 1061
deficiency, 1053*t*
as dietary supplement, 179*t*, 1275*t*
drug interactions, 1061
evidence, 1275*t*
functions, 1053*t*
history and claims, 1275*t*
mechanism of action, 1061
nursing responsibilities, 1061
for nutritional disorders
adverse effects, 1054*t*
route and adult dose, 1054*t*
patient and family education, 1061
pregnancy category, 1061
recommended dietary allowance, 1061
standardization, 1275*t*
therapeutic effects and uses, 1061, 1366
vitamin D. *See also* calcitriol
adverse effects, 1056
in calcium balance regulation, 1286–87, 1286*f*
contraindications/precautions, 1056
deficiency, 1053*t*, 1054
drug interactions, 1056
functions, 1053*t*
mechanism of action, 1056
nursing responsibilities, 1056
for nutritional disorders
adverse effects, 1053*t*
route and adult dose, 1053*t*
patient and family education, 1056
pregnancy category, 1056
recommended dietary allowance, 1056
sun exposure and, 1056*t*
therapeutic effects and uses, 1056, 1292
vitamin E:
adverse effects, 1057
contraindications/precautions, 1057
deficiency, 1053*t*
drug interactions, 1057
functions, 1053*t*
mechanism of action, 1057
nursing responsibilities, 1057
for nutritional disorders
adverse effects, 1053*t*
route and adult dose, 1053*t*
patient and family education, 1057
pregnancy category, 1057
recommended dietary allowance, 1057
therapeutic effects and uses, 1057
vitamin K:
adverse effects, 1057
contraindications/precautions, 1058
deficiency, 1053*t*
drug interactions, 1058
with warfarin, 74
functions, 1053*t*
mechanism of action, 1057
nursing responsibilities, 1058
for nutritional disorders
adverse effects, 1053*t*
route and adult dose, 1053*t*
patient and family education, 1058
pregnancy category, 1058
recommended dietary allowance, 1058
therapeutic effects and uses, 1057
vitiligo, 1316
Vitrasert. *See* ganciclovir
Vivactil. *See* protriptyline
Vivelle. *See* estradiol
Vivitrol. *See* naltrexone
VLDL (very low-density lipoprotein), 496, 498*f*
VNS (vagus nerve stimulation), for depression, 302*t*
Voltaren. *See* diclofenac
vomiting, 1040. *See also* nausea and vomiting
vomiting center, 1041
von Willebrand's disease (vWD), 664
voriconazole, 872*t*, 877
vorinostat, 992*t*, 993
VoSol HC. *See* acetic acid/hydrocortisone
VoSpire. *See* albuterol
VoSpire ER. *See* albuterol
VRE (vancomycin-resistant *Enterococci*), 782
VTE (venous thromboembolism), 642
Vumon. *See* teniposide
VX, 1362*t*
Vytorin. *See* ezetimibe; simvastatin

W

waist circumference, 1087, 1088*t*
warfarin, 650–52
adverse effects, 645*t*, 650
in older adults, 149
classification, 650
contraindications/precautions, 650
drug interactions, 650, 650*t*
with alcohol, 101*t*
with cimetidine, 45
with ciprofloxacin, 47
with erythromycin, 814
food and herbal, 75*t*
with herbal products, 178*t*
with vitamin K, 74
genetic polymorphisms and actions of, 159, 160*t*
mechanism of action, 650
monitoring therapy, 650
nursing responsibilities, 650
overdose treatment, 650
patient and family education, 650–51
pharmacokinetics, 650
pregnancy category, 650
route and adult dose, 645*t*
therapeutic effects and uses, 650
water-soluble vitamins, 1052
vitamin B_1. *See* thiamine
vitamin B_2. *See* thiamine
vitamin B_3. *See* niacin
vitamin B_6. *See* pyridoxine
vitamin B_9. *See* folic acid
vitamin B_{12}. *See* cyanocobalamin
vitamin C. *See* vitamin C
wearing off effect, 349
WelChol. *See* colesevelam
Wellbutrin. *See* bupropion
Wellbutrin SR, 30*t*. *See also* bupropion
Wellbutrin XL, 30*t*. *See also* bupropion
Wellferon. *See* interferon alfa-n1
West nomogram, 141*f*
Westcort. *See* hydrocortisone valerate
white coat hypertension, 518*t*
whole blood, 689*t*, 690
whooping cough (pertussis), 758*t*, 759
withdrawal syndrome, 96–97, 96*t*
World Health Organization Analgesic Ladder, 433*f*
Wycillin. *See* penicillin G procaine

X

Xalatan. *See* latanoprost
Xanax. *See* alprazolam
xanthine oxidase, 1309
xanthine oxidase inhibitors. *See* allopurinol
Xeloda. *See* capecitabine
Xenical. *See* orlistat
xerostomia, 201
ximelagatran, 650
Xolair. *See* omalizumab
Xopenex. *See* levalbuterol
Xylocaine. *See* lidocaine
xylometazoline, 238
Xyrem. *See* sodium oxybate
Xyzal. *See* levocetirizine

Y

Yasmin, 1203*t*
Yersinia pestis, 828, 1361
Yodoxin. *See* iodoquinol
yohimbe, 173*t*, 248–49
Yutopar. *See* ritodrine

Z

Zaditor. *See* ketotifen
zafirlukast, 1253–54
adverse effects, 1250*t*, 1253–54, 1254
classification, 1253
contraindications/precautions, 1254
drug interactions, 1254
mechanism of action, 1254
nursing responsibilities, 1254
overdose treatment, 1254

patient and family education, 1254
pharmacokinetics, 1254
pregnancy category, 1254
route and adult dose, 1250*t*
similar drugs, 1254–55
therapeutic effects and uses, 1253–54
zaleplon, 282*t*, 288
Zanaflex. *See* tizanidine
zanamivir, 915, 916*t*, 917
Zanosar. *See* streptozocin
Zantac. *See* ranitidine
Zarontin. *See* ethosuximide
Zaroxolyn. *See* metolazone
Zebeta. *See* bisoprolol
Zelapar. *See* selegiline
Zelnorm. *See* tegaserod
Zemplar. *See* paricalcitol
Zemuron. *See* rocuronium
Zenapax. *See* daclizumab
Zerit. *See* stavudine
ZES (Zollinger-Ellison syndrome), 1009–10, 1010*t*
Zestoretic, 572*t*
Zestril. *See* lisinopril
Zetia. *See* ezetimibe
Zevalin. *See* ibritumomab
Ziac, 572*t*
Ziagen. *See* abacavir
Ziana. *See* clindamycin/tretinoin
ziconotide, 443*t*
zidovudine, 934–35
adverse effects, 933*t*, 934
classification, 934
contraindications/precautions, 934
drug interactions, 75*t*, 934
mechanism of action, 934
nursing responsibilities, 934–35
overdose treatment, 934
patient and family education, 935
pharmacokinetics, 934
for postexposure prophylaxis of HIV infection, 943
pregnancy category, 934
for prevention of perinatal transmission of HIV, 943–44
prophylactic use, 783
route and adult dose, 933*t*
similar drugs, 935–36
therapeutic effects and uses, 934
zileuton, 1250*t*, 1254–55
Zimulti. *See* rimonabant
Zinacef. *See* cefuroxime
zinc, 1063, 1063*t*
zinc pyrithione, 1328
Zingiber officinale. See ginger
ziprasidone, 319*t*, 337*t*, 340
Zithromax. *See* azithromycin
Zmax. *See* azithromycin
Zocor. *See* simvastatin
Zofran. *See* ondansetron
Zoladex. *See* goserelin
zoledronate (zoledronic acid), 992*t*, 993, 1294*t*, 1295*t*, 1297
Zolinza. *See* vorinostat
Zollinger-Ellison syndrome (ZES), 1009–10, 1010*t*
zolmitriptan, 450*t*, 452
Zoloft. *See* sertraline
zolpidem, 287–88
adverse effects, 287
classification, 287
contraindications/precautions, 287
dosage forms not to be crushed or opened, 30*t*
drug interactions, 287
mechanism of action, 287
nursing responsibilities, 287
overdose treatment, 287
patient and family education, 287–88
pharmacokinetics, 287
pregnancy category, 287
similar drugs, 288
therapeutic effects and uses, 287
Zometa. *See* zoledronate
Zomig. *See* zolmitriptan
Zonegran. *See* zonisamide
zonisamide, 391*t*, 392
Zorbtive. *See* somatropin
Zorcaine. *See* articaine
Zostavax. *See* varicella zoster, immunization
Zosyn. *See* piperacillin-tazobactam
Zovia 1/50E-21 and 28, 1203*t*
Zovirax. *See* acyclovir
Z-pak. *See* azithromycin
Zyban. *See* bupropion
Zyflo. *See* zileuton
Zyloprim. *See* allopurinol
Zymar. *See* gatifloxacin
Zymine. *See* triprolidine
Zyprexa. *See* olanzapine
Zyrtec. *See* cetirizine
Zyvox. *See* linezolid

Special Features

Connections: Complementary and Alternative Therapy
Aloe Vera 1332
Aromatherapy 798
Ascorbic Acid (Vitamin C) 1275
Bilberry for Eye Health 1347
Black Cohosh 1201
Carnitine (L-Carnitine) 616
Chaste Berry for Premenstrual Syndrome and Menopause 1186
Chromium for Hyperglycemia 1142
Coenzyme Q10 507
Cranberry 845
Dandelion 561
Echinacea 745
Fish Oils for Inflammation 1163
Garlic 654
Ginger's Effect on the Gastrointestinal Tract 1013
Ginkgo Biloba for Treatment of Dementia 361
Ginseng 590
Glucosamine and Chondroitin for Osteoarthritis 1302
Goldenseal 717
Grape Seed Extract 569
Hawthorn 540
Herbal Remedies as Galactogogues 129
Kava 399
Lactobacillus acidophilus 1044
Lecithin 200
Melatonin 281
Natural Therapies for Migraines 453
Saw Palmetto 1232
Selenium 953
Soy 981
St. John's Wort for Depression 313
The Ketogenic Diet 374

Connections: Evidence-Based Practice
Acute Otitis Media 138
Asthma Management 1244
Best Practices in Acute and Cancer Pain Management 429
Controlling Symptoms of Attention Deficit/Hyperactivity Disorder 414
Direct Observation Therapy Effectiveness 856
Growth Hormone for Age-Appropriate Height 1107
Human Papilloma Virus Risk Reduction 911
Long-Term Outcome of Growth Hormone on Pediatric Burn Patients 1110
Low-Back Pain and Antidepressants 398
Seizures in the Older Adult 375
Malignant Hyperthermia and Anesthetic Agents 466
Nonsteroidal Anti-Inflammatory Drugs 727
Oral Hypoglycemic Agents for Gestational Diabetes 1122
Reducing Neutropenic Patients' Exposure to Fungal Pathogens 870
Role of the School Nurse in Treating Epilepsy 386
The Clinical Antipsychotic Trials of Intervention Effectiveness (CATIE) Study 341
Traveler's Diarrhea 810
Use of Proton Pump Inhibitors and Gastrointestinal Infection 1014
Use of Proton Pump Inhibitors and Risk of Bone Fracture 1016
Weight Gain with Use of Atypical Antipsychotics 338

Connections: Lifespan Considerations
Administering Chemotherapy to the Elderly 984
Antihistamines 1267
Corticosteroids in Pediatric Patients 1164
Challenges of Pediatric Medication Administration 25
Children with Human Immunodeficiency Virus 944
Continuous Subcutaneous Insulin Infusion 1131
Cost of Prescription Medications 5
Depression in Children and Adolescents 302
Diuretic Therapy 549
Drug Monitoring in the Older Adult 150
Fluid and Electrolytes in the Older Adult 695
High Blood Pressure in Children 522
Infections
Infections in the Older Adult 795
Influence of Age on Pain Expression and Perception 442
Older Adults at Risk for Polyherbacy 177
Oral Candidiasis in Infants 872
Pain Assessment in the Very Young 432
Parents' Role in Preventing Medication Errors: Ask Before You Act 82
Peptic Ulcer Disease and Gastroesophageal Reflux Disease in Children 1023
Proper Instillation of Otic Medication 1352
Reducing the Cost of Medications for Older Adults 151
School Nurses and Medication Administration Guidelines 166
Sleep–Wake Patterns 278
Stevens–Johnson Syndrome in Children 1333
Teaching Throughout the Life Span 118
Thyroid Disease Among the Elderly 1150
Thyroid Hormone Use and Risk of Hip Fracture in Women 65 Years and Older 1150
Vaccine Administration 766

Connections: Patient Safety
Be Aware of Similar Packaging 648
Control of Concentrated Electrolyte Solutions 698
Fat Emulsions and Infants
Infusion Calculations 1039
Iron Overdose in Children 678
Levofloxacin (Levaquin) 833
Medication Order 1186
Mistaken Identity 1295
OptiClik Injector Pen 1132
Proper Use of the EpiPen® 235
Soundalike Drugs 729
Trimethoprim-Sulfamethoxazole (Bactrim, Septra) 842

Connections: To the Community
Acid Suppression and Vitamin B12 in Older Adults 1022
Avoiding Accidental Insecticide Poisoning 215
Avoiding Accidental Poisonings 1364
Blood Pressure Self-Measurement 568
Body Weight and Hypertension 533
Calendar Method of Contraception 1209
Dysrhythmias and Diet 627
Enteral Nutrition in the Home Setting 1074
Estrogen Use and Psychosocial Issues 1181
Food–Drug Interactions 75
Healthy Weight Reduction Tips 1089
Home Care of Patients on Total Parenteral Nutrition Therapy 1080
Improving Patient Adherence to HIV-AIDS Pharmacotherapy 931
Immunosuppression and Pets 738
Inappropriate Adult Use of Growth Hormone to Enhance Athletic Performance and Physical Appearance 1109
Laxative Abuse 1033
Lifestyle Modifications for Hypertension 248
Lifestyle Modifications to Control Heart Failure 607
Living with Alzheimer's or Parkinson's Disease 364
Living with Corticosteroids 1164
Methamphetamine: When a Good Drug Goes Bad 236
Myasthenia Gravis?Medications and Nutrition 209
Patients with Multiple Sclerosis
Ophthalmic Drugs in the Home Setting 1350
Photosensitivity and Antibiotics 811
Reducing Medication Errors in Older Adults 147
Preventing Transmission of Tuberculosis 862
Public Health Challenges and Community Programs 570
Salt Replacements and Exercise 696
Sexual Activity: Just Another Form of Exercise 600
Sexual Health: Trichomoniasis 896
Sodium Restrictions: How Much Is Too Much? 249
Teaching Patients About Dietary Measures to Lower Cholesterol 501
Teaching Patients About Dietary Sodium, Hypertension, and Food Labels 529
Teaching Patients About a Lipid Profile 499
Teaching Patients with Neutropenia 674
The DASH Diet 570
The Intrathecal Baclofen Pump 402
Treating Childhood Anxiety with Antidepressants 290
Vaccines to Prevent Urinary Tract Infection 837
White Coat Hypertension 518

Connections: Treating the Diverse Patient
Adherence to Immunosuppressive Medication 742
Asian Patients' Sensitivity to Propranolol 633
Attention Deficit/Hyperactivity Deficit Increase in Girls 414
Complications of Diabetes in Diverse Populations 1123
Cultural Influences and the Treatment of Depression 300
Cultural Influences in Choosing Contraception 1205
Enzyme Deficiencies in Ethnic Populations 62
Exposure to Anesthesia and the Risk of Alzheimer's Disease 469
Genetic Lack of Enzyme 336
One Size Does Not Fit All 48
Osteoporosis in Men 1292
Nurses and Substance Abuse 103
Nursing in Correctional Facilities: High-Risk Populations 857
Pregnancy and Deep Vein Thrombosis 648
Providing Culturally Appropriate Teaching119
Providing Culturally Competent Care 159
Respiratory Distress Syndrome 1240
Viagra for Women 1229
Vitamins During Pregnancy 1055
Women and Heart Failure 609

Prototype Drugs
abciximab (ReoPro) 655
acarbose (Precose) 1138
acetaminophen (Tylenol) 729
acetazolamide (Diamox) 560
activated charcoal (CharcoAid) 1365
acyclovir (Zovirax) 913
albuterol (Proventil, Ventolin, VoSpire) 1246
aldesleukin (Proleukin), IL-2 738
alendronate (Fosamax) 1296
allopurinol (Zyloprim) 1309
alteplase (Activase) 658
aluminum hydroxide (AlternaGEL, others) 1021